*Enzinger and Weiss's*

# Soft Tissue Tumors

*Enzinger and Weiss's*

# Soft Tissue Tumors

**Fourth edition**


**Sharon W. Weiss, M.D.**
Professor and Vice Chair
Director of Anatomic Pathology
Department of Pathology and
Laboratory Medicine
Emory University
School of Medicine
Atlanta, Georgia

**John R. Goldblum, M.D.**
Staff Pathologist
Department of Anatomic Pathology
The Cleveland Clinic Foundation
Cleveland, Ohio



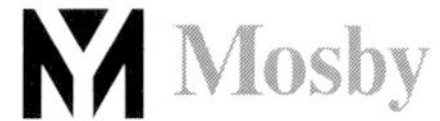


*A Harcourt Health Sciences Company*

St. Louis London Philadelphia Sydney Toronto

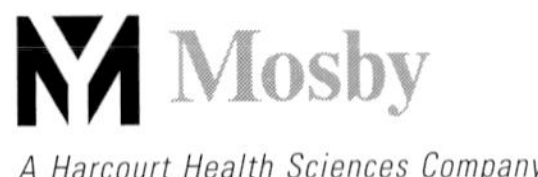
A Harcourt Health Sciences Company

*Editor:* Marc Strauss
*Developmental Editor:* Lynne Gery

FOURTH EDITION


Mosby, Inc.
*A Harcourt Health Sciences Company*
11830 Westline Industrial Drive
St. Louis, Missouri 63146

Printed in the United States of America

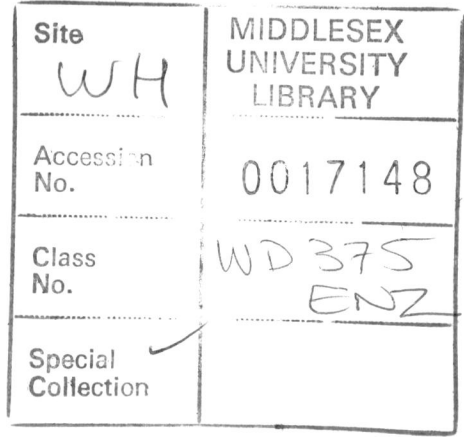


**Library of Congress Cataloging-in-Publication Data**

Weiss, Sharon W.
Enzinger and Weiss's soft tissue tumors / Sharon W. Weiss, John R. Goldblum—4th ed.
p.; cm
Rev. ed. of Soft tissue tumors / Franz M. Enzinger, Sharon W. Weiss, 3rd. ed. © 1995.
Includes bibliographical references and index.
ISBN 0-323-01200-0
1. Soft tissue tumors. I. Title: Soft tissue tumors. II. Goldblum, John R. III. Enzinger, Franz M. Soft tissue tumors. IV. Title.
[DNLM: 1. Soft Tissue Neoplasms. WD 375 W432e 2001]
RC280.S66 E56 2001
616.99′2—dc21 2001030975

Last digit is the print number: 9 8 7 6 5 4 3 2

# DEDICATION

*To the loving memory of our fathers*

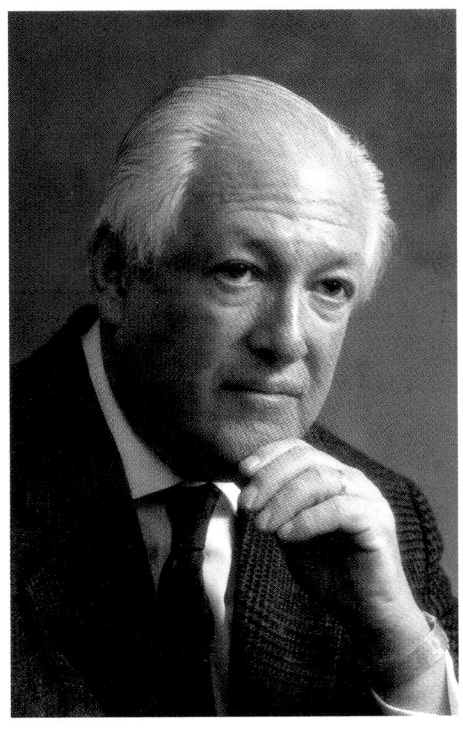

Raymond Walter Goldblum, M.D.
1924–1998

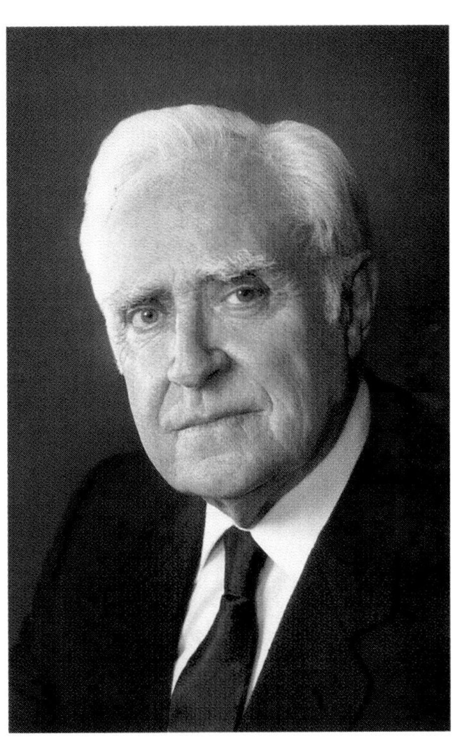

Thomas Joseph Whelan Jr., M.D.
1921–1999

# CONTRIBUTORS


FADI W. ABDUL-KARIM, M.D.
Professor of Pathology,
Case Western Reserve University Institute of Pathology;
Director of Anatomic Pathology,
University Hospitals of Cleveland,
Cleveland, Ohio
*Fine Needle Aspiration Biopsies of Soft Tissue Tumors*

ALFRED E. CHANG, M.D.
Professor of Surgery,
University of Michigan Medical School,
Ann Arbor, Michigan
*Clinical Evaluation and Treatment of Soft Tissue Tumors*

JONATHAN A. FLETCHER, M.D.
Associate Professor of Pathology and Pediatrics,
Harvard Medical School;
Associate Pathologist,
Brigham and Women's Hospital,
Boston, Massachusetts
*Cytogenetic Analysis of Soft Tissue Tumors*

ANDREW L. FOLPE, M.D.
Assistant Professor,
Department of Pathology and Laboratory Medicine,
Emory University,
Atlanta, Georgia
*Immunohistochemistry for Analysis of Soft Tissue Tumors*

KIM R. GEISINGER, M.D.
Professor of Pathology,
Wake Forest University School of Medicine;
Director, Surgical Pathology and Cytopathology,
North Carolina Baptist Hospital,
Winston-Salem, North Carolina
*Fine Needle Aspiration Biopsies of Soft Tissue Tumors*

ALLEN M. GOWN, M.D.
Clinical Professor,
Department of Pathology,
University of British Columbia,
Vancouver, British Columbia, Canada;
Medical Director and Chief Pathologist,
PhenoPath Laboratories,
Seattle, Washington
*Immunohistochemistry for Analysis of Soft Tissue Tumors*

PAUL S. MELTZER, M.D., Ph.D.
Head,
Section of Molecular Genetics,
Cancer Genetics Branch,
National Human Genome Research Institute,
National Institutes of Health,
Bethesda, Maryland
*Molecular Genetics of Soft Tissue Tumors*

RICHARD P. MOSER, JR., M.D.
Professor of Radiology and Orthopaedic Surgery,
Penn State University College of Medicine;
Acting Chair,
Department of Radiology,
The Milton S. Hershey Medical Center,
Hershey, Pennsylvania
*Radiologic Evaluation of Soft Tissue Tumors*

WILLIAM M. PARRISH, M.D.
Assistant Professor of Orthopaedic Surgery,
Penn State University College of Medicine;
The Milton S. Hershey Medical Center,
Hershey, Pennsylvania
*Radiologic Evaluation of Soft Tissue Tumors*

VERNON K. SONDAK, M.D.
Professor of Surgery,
University of Michigan Medical School,
Ann Arbor, Michigan
*Clinical Evaluation and Treatment of Soft Tissue Tumors*

# PREFACE
## to the Fourth Edition

Each new edition of a textbook bears its unmistakable marks. Ours, appearing at the dawn of a new millennium, is no exception. The familiar cover, with its adaptation of a Vesalius drawing, suggests a comforting continuity with the past, a reassurance that questions posed will still be answered, that illustrations will again serve to guide one to a particular diagnosis, and that novel ideas will be presented in a manner understandable by the practicing physicians for whom this book has always been intended. Yet there is a significant difference. The authorship has for the first time in nearly 20 years changed, and I would like to take this opportunity to acknowledge the extraordinary influence that Franz Enzinger, the senior author of previous editions, has had on this book and in soft tissue pathology in general. Franz represents one of the generation of great diagnostic pathologists, the likes of which we may never again see. Their generation was one that never fully knew the advantages of immunohistochemistry, cytogenetics, and molecular biology, and as a result their raw diagnostic skills reached heights that our trainees today can only imagine. Franz's descriptions of new lesions, epitomized by his classic paper on epithelioid sarcoma, serve as models for the power of observation and the nuances of detail. His seminal paper on liposarcoma, published with Dr. Winslow, presented a classification that today stands largely intact, firmly validated by cytogenetic and molecular findings.

The first edition of this book in many areas represented a distillate of this great man's personal observations, buttressed by the enormous treasure trove of cases accessioned at the Armed Forces Institute of Pathology. In preparing this fourth edition, we have strived to build on that extraordinary foundation, while embracing new ideas and technologies. Although I have missed Franz's wisdom and counsel in preparing this edition, I have found great personal satisfaction in working with a new colleague and former resident, Dr. John Goldblum, whose ebullience and energy have served as a mainstay in assuring the timely completion of this edition.

In addition to the change in authorship, our readers will note that this edition has been converted almost entirely to color, and a substantial number of new illustrations have been added. We are indebted to Dr. Irving Dardick, who is responsible for the outstanding color renditions in this book. New chapters have been written on the topics of "Fine Needle Aspiration Biopsies of Soft Tissue Tumors" by Drs. Geisinger and Fadi-Karim and "Immunohistochemistry for Analysis of Soft Tissue Tumors" by Drs. Folpe and Gown. Drs. Jonathan Fletcher and Paul Meltzer have again provided superlative updates in the fast-moving fields of cytogenetics and molecular biology of soft tissue tumors, while Drs. Sondak and Chang and Moser and Parrish have expanded their respective clinical and radiologic chapters. All of our authors are preeminent authorities who have graciously taken time from their busy lives to share their expertise. We thank them very much.

We are indebted to our publisher and their outstanding staff who have facilitated our work on this edition. These include Marc Strauss, Lynne Gery, Joan Sinclair, and Berta Steiner. We deeply appreciate the help of our secretaries, Susan Raven, Kathleen Ranney, and Sandy Swanson, and the residents and fellows who performed the proofreading: Drs. Steve Billings, Edward Garcia, Jessica Leiden, and Jessica Sigel. Finally, without the love and support of our families—Bernie, Francine, Asmita, Andrew, Ryan, Janavi, and Raedan, we doubt any of this would have been possible. We could tell them this book is also theirs, but we suspect in their hearts they know this already.

*Sharon W. Weiss, M.D.*
*Atlanta, 2001*

# PREFACE
## to the First Edition

Since the publication of the *AFIP Fascicle on Soft Tissue Tumors* by A.P. Stout in 1957 and the revised edition by A.P. Stout and R. Lattes in 1967, there have been numerous advances and changes both in the diagnosis and treatment of soft tissue tumors. This book combines traditional views, which have stood the test of time, and newer concepts and observations accrued over the past 20 years. Because a precise diagnosis is essential for planning of treatment and assessment of prognosis, emphasis has been placed throughout the book on clear and concise descriptions and differential diagnoses of the tumors discussed. Each chapter has been freely illustrated, and comprehensive references have been added with emphasis on recent publications.

The WHO Classification of Soft Tissue Tumors provided the basis for the classification in this book. However, since its publication in 1969 several modifications have become necessary. Fibrohistiocytic and extraskeletal cartilaginous and osseous tumors have been included as separate groups, and a number of changes have been made, especially in the classification of fibrous, vascular, and neural tumors. The role of histochemistry, electron microscopy, and immunohistochemistry has been noted when applicable. Relatively less emphasis, however, has been placed on the specifics of therapy because of the rapidly changing nature of this discipline. It is our hope that this blending of old and new will make this book valuable not only as a reference book for those specifically interested in soft tissue tumors but also as a diagnostic aid for the practicing general pathologist.

In many areas the contents of this book reflect our personal experience derived from approximately 5000 cases reviewed annually in the Department of Soft Tissue Pathology of the Armed Forces Institute of Pathology. The large number of cases has afforded us a unique opportunity for which we are extremely grateful.

We also wish to express our appreciation and gratitude to the many contributing pathologists who not only shared their interesting and problematic cases with us but also provided additional teaching material in the form of photographs, roentgenograms, and electron micrographs. We also owe thanks to our professional colleagues for their advice and support in this endeavor, to the photographic staff of the Institute, especially Mr. C. Edwards and Mr. B. Allen, for their skill and assistance in preparing the photographs, and to Mrs. P. Diaz and Mrs. J. Kozlay for typing the manuscript. We are also greatly indebted to our publishers for their cooperation and help throughout the production of this book. We are particularly indebted to our families for their patience and tolerance.

*Franz M. Enzinger*
*Sharon W. Weiss*

# CONTENTS

# CHAPTER 1

# GENERAL CONSIDERATIONS

Soft tissue can be defined as nonepithelial extraskeletal tissue of the body exclusive of the reticuloendothelial system, glia, and supporting tissue of various parenchymal organs. It is represented by the voluntary muscles, fat, and fibrous tissue, along with the vessels serving these tissues. By convention it also includes the peripheral nervous system because tumors arising from nerves present as soft tissue masses and pose similar problems in differential diagnosis and therapy. Embryologically, soft tissue is derived principally from mesoderm, with some contribution from neuroectoderm.

Soft tissue tumors are a highly heterogeneous group of tumors that are classified on a histogenetic basis according to the adult tissue they resemble. Lipomas and liposarcomas, for example, are tumors that recapitulate to a varying degree normal fatty tissue; and hemangiomas and angiosarcomas contain cells resembling vascular endothelium. Within the various histogenetic categories, soft tissue tumors are usually divided into benign and malignant forms.

*Benign tumors,* which more closely resemble normal tissue, have a limited capacity for autonomous growth. They exhibit little tendency to invade locally and are attended by a low rate of local recurrence following conservative therapy.

*Malignant tumors,* or *sarcomas,* in contrast, are locally aggressive and are capable of invasive or destructive growth, recurrence, and distant metastasis. Radical surgery is required to ensure total removal of these tumors. Unfortunately, the term sarcoma does not indicate the likelihood or rapidity of metastasis. Some sarcomas, such as dermatofibrosarcoma protuberans, rarely metastasize, whereas others, such as malignant fibrous histiocytoma, do so with alacrity. For these reasons it is important to qualify the term sarcoma with a statement concerning the degree of differentiation or the histologic grade. "Well differentiated" and "poorly differentiated" are qualitative, and hence subjective, terms used to indicate the relative maturity of the tumor with respect to normal adult tissue. Histologic grade is a means of quantitating the degree of differentiation by applying a set of histologic criteria. Usually well differentiated sarcomas are low grade lesions, whereas poorly differentiated sarcomas are high grade neoplasms. There are also borderline lesions for which it is difficult to determine the malignant potential, and there are benign neoplastic and nonneoplastic lesions that morphologically appear to be malignant but follow a benign clinical course (*pseudosarcomas*).

## INCIDENCE

The incidence of soft tissue tumors, especially the frequency of benign tumors relative to malignant ones, is nearly impossible to determine accurately. Benign soft tissue tumors outnumber malignant tumors by a margin of about 100:1 in a hospital population, and their annual incidence is approximately 300 per 100,000 population.[100,101] The fact that many benign tumors, such as lipomas and hemangiomas, do not undergo biopsy makes direct application of data from most hospital series invalid for the general population, however.

Malignant soft tissue tumors, on the other hand, ultimately come to medical attention. Soft tissue sarcomas, compared with carcinomas and other neoplasms, are relatively rare and constitute fewer than 1% of all cancers.[86] Based on data from the American Cancer Society, it was estimated that 8100 new soft tissue sarcomas would develop during 2000 in the United States (Table 1–1). The incidence varies among age groups; it also depends on the definition

**TABLE 1–1 ESTIMATED NEW CASES OF CANCER BY SITE (UNITED STATES, 2000)**

| Site | No. of Cases |
|---|---|
| Lung | 164,000 |
| Colon and rectum | 130,200 |
| Breast | 184,200 |
| Central nervous system | 16,500 |
| Soft tissue | 8,100 |
| Bone | 2,500 |

Data from Cancer Statistics, 2000. CA Cancer J Clin 50:12, 2000.

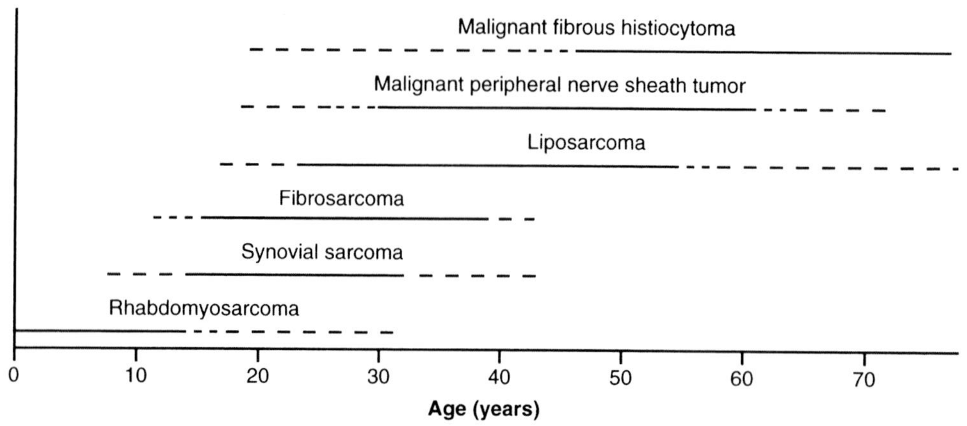


**FIGURE 1–1.** Approximate relation of age to incidence of various types of sarcoma. Continuous line indicates peak incidence of tumor. Dotted line indicates reduced incidence of tumor.

of soft tissue sarcomas and the types of neoplasm included among these tumors. For example, in one study of sarcomas of the locomotor system,[101] the overall annual incidence rate was 1.4 per 100,000, whereas the age-specific incidence for patients 80 years or older was 8.0 per 100,000. Moreover, in the National Cancer Survey,[21] retroperitoneal, mesenteric, and omental sarcomas are counted among the neoplasms of the digestive system, and pleural sarcomas (malignant mesotheliomas) are included among the tumors of the respiratory tract.

There seems to be an upward trend in the incidence of soft tissue sarcomas, but it is not clear whether this represents a true increase or reflects better diagnostic capabilities and greater interest in this type of tumor. According to Ross et al.,[97] with data from the National Cancer Institute's Surveillance, Epidemiology, and End Results Program (SEER), there was a marked increase in the age-adjusted incidence of soft tissue sarcomas between 1981 to 1987. However, when patients with Kaposi's sarcoma were eliminated from this analysis, the rates remained relatively unchanged throughout that time period. Judging from the available data, the incidence and distribution of soft tissue sarcomas seem to be similar in different regions of the world. Soft tissue sarcomas may occur anywhere in the body, but most arise from the large muscles of the extremities, the chest wall, the mediastinum, and the retroperitoneum. They occur at any age and, like carcinomas, are more common in older patients; about 15% affect persons younger than 15 years, and about 40% affect persons 55 years or older.

Soft tissue sarcomas occur more commonly in males, but gender and age-related incidences vary among the histologic types (Fig. 1–1). For instance, embryonal rhabdomyosarcoma occurs almost exclusively in young individuals, whereas malignant fibrous histiocytoma is predominantly a tumor of old age and is rare in children younger than 10 years. There is also no proven racial variation, even though the annual age-adjusted incidence rates have been reported to be higher for Blacks than Whites in the United States.[90]

## PATHOGENESIS

As with other malignant neoplasms, the pathogenesis of most soft tissue tumors is still unknown. Recognized causes include various physical and chemical factors, exposure to ionizing radiation, and inherited or acquired immunologic defects. Evaluation of the exact cause is often difficult because of the long latent period between the time of exposure and the development of sarcoma, as well as the possible effect of multiple environmental and hereditary factors during the induction period. Origin of sarcomas from benign soft tissue tumors is rare, except for malignant peripheral nerve sheath tumors arising in neurofibromas, which are nearly always in patients with the manifestations of type 1 neurofibromatosis (von Recklinghausen's disease).

### Environmental Factors

*Trauma* or *past injury* is frequently implicated in the development of sarcomas. Many of these reports are anecdotal, however, and the integrity of the injured part was not clearly established before injury. Consequently, trauma often seems to be an event that merely calls attention to the underlying neoplasm. Occasionally there is reasonable evidence to suggest a causal relation. Rare soft tissue sarcomas have been reported as arising in scar tissue following surgical procedures or thermal or acid burns, at fracture sites, and in the vicinity of plastic or metal implants, usually after a latent period of several years.[13,84] We reviewed material from a patient who developed flexion contractures and extensive heterotopic ossification after electrical injury to the arm followed 9 years later by an osteosarcoma.[1] The temporal sequence provided strong circumstantial evidence that the sarcoma had arisen at a preexisting site of severe tissue injury. More recently, Kirkpatrick et al.[54] studied the histologic features in capsules surrounding the implantation site of a variety of biomaterials. Interestingly, these authors noted a spectrum of change, from focal proliferative lesions through preneoplastic proliferations to incipient sarcomas and suggested a model of multistage tumorigenesis akin to the adenoma–carcinoma sequence.

*Environmental carcinogens* have been related to the development of sarcomas, but their role is largely unexplored, and only a few substances have been identified as playing a role in the induction of sarcomas in humans. A variety of animal models exist to induce sarcomas, including the subcutaneous implantation of methylcholanthrene-induced sarcoma in Fischer rats[129] and the induction of angiosarcomas in mice using dimethylhydrazine.[66]

*Asbestos,* a hydrated silicate, is the most important known environmental carcinogen. Exposure to this substance, principally in the form of crocidolite or chrysotile, occurs in asbestos miners and industrial workers who process, install, or repair electrical and thermal insulation, brake linings, cement tiles, or pipes. Inhaled as a microscopic particle, asbestos ultimately reaches the pulmonary parenchyma and pleural surface, where after many years it may be associated with the development of pleural and peritoneal mesotheliomas or pulmonary carcinomas. Important risk factors are the intensity and duration of asbestos exposure, the type of asbestos, and the submicroscopic fiber diameter.[72] The risk is greatest with crocidolite, the blue asbestos mined in South Africa; the risk is much less with chrysotile, the white asbestos chiefly found in Canada and Russia, which amounts to more than 95% of the asbestos used commercially[6,57] (see Chapter 29).

Phenoxyacetic acid herbicides, chlorophenols, and their contaminants such as 2,3,7,8-tetrachlorodibenzo-para-dioxin (dioxin) have been linked to sarcoma genesis.[11,34,36,109] A series of case–control studies from Sweden from 1979 to 1990 reported an up to a sixfold increased risk of soft tissue sarcoma associated with exposure to phenoxyacetic acids or chlorophenols in individuals exposed to these herbicides in agricultural or forestry work.[30,31,39,40,128] Similar reports of an increased risk of sarcoma associated with these herbicides were reported from Italy,[103,122] Great Britian,[7] and New Zealand.[104] Although a study by Leiss and Savitz[62] linked use of phenoxyacetic acid lawn pesticides with soft tissue sarcomas in children, several other studies with more detailed exposure histories did not show this to be the case.[131] These inconsistencies may be due in part to the predominant phenoxyacetic herbicide used in different locations. In the United States 2,4-dichlorophenoxyacetic acid is the primary phenoxyacetic herbicide used, whereas in Sweden the main herbicides contain 2,4,5-trichlorophenoxyacetic acid and 2-methyl-4-chlorophenoxyacetic acid, both of which are more likely contaminated with dioxin.[131] High levels of dioxin exposure due to accidental environmental contamination near Seveso from an explosion at a chemical factory was followed by a threefold increased risk of soft tissue sarcomas reported among individuals living near this factory.[10,19] In addition, the possibility of an increased incidence of sarcomas was claimed for some of the 2 million soldiers stationed in Vietnam between 1965 and 1970 who were exposed to Agent Orange, a defoliant that contained dioxin as a contaminant.[55,102] However, in several case–control and proportional mortality studies, no excess risk of soft tissue sarcoma was reported among those Vietnam veterans who were directly involved with the spraying of Agent Orange.[43,131]

*Vinyl chloride* exposure is clearly associated with the development hepatic angiosarcoma.[25,32] There are also rare reports of extrahepatic angiosarcoma associated with this agent.[94]

*Radiation* exposure has been related to the development of sarcomas; but considering the frequency of radiotherapy, radiation-induced soft tissue sarcomas are uncommon, and there is no doubt that the benefit of radiation for treatment of malignant neoplasms outweighs the risk of developing a sarcoma. The incidence of postradiation sarcoma is difficult to estimate, but reports generally range from 0.03% to 0.80%.[3,69] Much of the data regarding the incidence of postradiation sarcomas are derived from large cohorts of breast cancer patients treated with postoperative radiation therapy. For example, Taghian et al.[111] found 11 postradiation sarcomas among 7620 patients with breast carcinoma treated with postoperative irradiation, for a cumulative incidence of 0.2% at 10 years. Similarly, Pierce et al.[89] reported three cases of postradiation sarcoma in 1624 women undergoing lumpectomy and postoperative irradiation at the Joint Center for Radiation Therapy between 1968 and 1985, for a 10-year actuarial risk of 0.8%. Similar data have been reported from the Swedish Cancer Registry.[48,49]

To qualify as a postradiation sarcoma, the criteria proposed by Cahan et al.[14] and later modified by Arlen et al.[4] must be met. They include documentation that the sarcoma developed in the irradiated field, histologic confirmation of the diagnosis, a period of latency of at least 3 years between irradiation and the appearance of tumor, and documentation that the region bearing the tumor was normal prior to administration of the radiation. Nearly all postradiation sarcomas occur in adults, and women develop them more frequently, an observation that reflects the common use of radiation for treatment of breast and gynecologic malignancies. In our experience, the most common disease for which patients receive radiation are lymphomas and breast, ovarian, and endometrial carcinomas.

Although it was anticipated that the use of megavoltage radiation would reduce the incidence of postradiation sarcomas, this has not proved to be true. Both orthovoltage and megavoltage radiation may be associated with the subsequent development of sarcomas, and there do not appear to be differences in the type of sarcoma or survival rates between the two groups, although the average dosages associated with orthovoltage radiation are lower and the latency periods longer.[69,119,127]

Postradiation sarcomas do not display the wide range of appearances associated with sporadic nonradiation-induced tumors. The most common postradiation soft tissue sarcoma is malignant fibrous histiocytoma, which accounts for nearly 70% of cases, followed by osteosarcoma, fibrosarcoma, malignant peripheral nerve sheath tumor, chondrosarcoma, and angiosarcoma. Unfortunately, most postradiation sarcomas are high grade lesions and are detected at a relatively higher stage than their sporadic counterparts. Thus the survival rate associated with these lesions has been poor, as most studies report overall 5-year survival rates of 10–30%.[42,58,78,95]

The prognosis is most closely related to the site of the postradiation sarcoma, which in turn probably reflects resectability.[87] Patients with radiation-induced sarcomas of the extremities have the best survival (approximately 30% at 5 years), whereas those with lesions arising in the vertebral column, pelvis, and shoulder girdle generally have survival rates of less than 5% at 5 years.[69,87,123]

The total dose of radiation seems to influence the incidence of postradiation sarcoma, as most of these tumors are reported to occur at doses of 5000 cGy or more.[69,87] Mutations of the *p53* gene have been implicated in the pathogenesis of these tumors.[83] Extravasated Thorotrast (thorium dioxide), although no longer used for diagnostic or therapeutic purposes, has induced soft tissue sarcomas, particularly angiosarcomas, at the site of injection.[91,92]

## Oncogenic Viruses

The role of oncogenic viruses in the evolution of soft tissue sarcomas is still poorly understood, although there is strong evidence that the human herpesvirus 8 (HHV8) is the causative agent of Kaposi's sarcoma[15,16,23,46,65] (see Chapter 25). In addition, there is a large body of literature supporting the role of the Epstein-Barr virus in the pathogenesis of smooth muscle tumors in patients with immunodeficiency syndromes or following therapeutic immunosuppression in the transplant setting.[53,60,61,71,105,112,120] Aside from these settings, there is no conclusive evidence that human-transmissible viral agents constitute a major risk factor in the development of soft tissue sarcomas, although electron microscopy has revealed virus particles repeatedly in a variety of soft tissue tumors.

## Immunologic Factors

As mentioned above, immunodeficiency and therapeutic immunosuppression are also associated with the development of soft tissue sarcomas, particularly leiomyosarcomas. In addition, acquired regional immunodeficiency, or loss of regional immune surveillance, may also be the underlying mechanism in the development of the relatively rare angiosarcomas that arise in the setting of chronic lymphedema, secondary to radical mastectomy (Stewart-Treves syndrome),[74,81,107] or congenital or infectious conditions.[24,75,77]

## Genetic Factors

A number of genetic diseases are associated with the development of soft tissue tumors, and the list will undoubtedly lengthen as we begin to understand the molecular underpinnings of mesenchymal neoplasia. Neurofibromatosis 1 and neurofibromatosis 2, previously referred to as the peripheral and central forms of the disease, respectively, are classic examples of genetic disease associated with soft tissue tumors.

Neurofibromatosis 1, which commences early in life with the onset of café au lait spots, is later characterized by numerous neurofibromas. Inherited as an autosomal dominant trait, the disease is primarily a neuroectodermal dysplasia, although nonneural tumors may occur as well. In 1–5% of cases, malignant peripheral nerve sheath tumors develop as a result of malignant degeneration of neurofibromas (see Chapter 31). The gene for neurofibromatosis 1 was localized to the pericentromeric region of chromosome 17 and was subsequently cloned. Its gene product is ubiquitously distributed in normal tissues and appears to have tumor suppressor activity.[68]

Neurofibromatosis 2, though lumped with neurofibromatosis 1 in early clinical descriptions, is a clinically and genetically distinct disease. Characterized by bilateral acoustic neuromas, its gene has been localized to chromosome 22[115] (see Chapter 4).

Familial adenomatous polyposis and Gardner syndrome are associated with mutations in the adenomatosis polyposis coli (*APC*) gene on chromosome 5q.[33,82] These syndromes, which are inherited as an autosomal dominant trait, may be associated with mesenteric fibromatosis, and mutations of the *APC* gene have also been detected in these tumors.[76] Studies suggest that mutations of this gene result in a

**TABLE 1–2 SOFT TISSUE TUMORS OCCURRING ON AN INHERITED BASIS OR FOLLOWING A FAMILIAL DISTRIBUTION**

| Tumor Type | Comments |
|---|---|
| Fibrous tumors | |
| Palmar, plantar, and penile fibromatosis | Occasionally in several generations of one family and in twins |
| Deep fibromatosis (desmoid tumor) | Rare familial cases |
| Mesenteric fibromatosis | Frequently associated with familial polyposis coli and Gardner syndrome |
| Fibromatosis colli | Occasionally in twins |
| Myofibromatosis | Rarely in siblings or increased familial incidence |
| Hyaline fibromatosis | Frequently in siblings |
| Fatty tumors | |
| Lipoma | About 5% familial |
| Multiple lipomas | Increased familial incidence |
| Angiolipoma | About 5% familial |
| Angiomyolipoma | Manifestations of tuberous sclerosis complex in about one-third of patients |
| Fibrohistiocytic tumors | |
| Xanthoma tuberosum | Occurs in familial hyperlipidemia |
| Tendinous xanthoma | Occurs in familial hyperlipidemia and in cerebrotendinous xanthomatosis; autosomal recessive mode of inheritance |
| Muscular tumors | |
| Cutaneous leiomyoma | Occasional familial cases with pattern suggesting autosomal dominant mode of inheritance |
| Familial gastrointestinal stromal tumor | Germlike mutation of c-*kit* |
| Vascular tumors | |
| Glomus | Occasional familial cases following an autosomal dominant mode of inheritance |
| Osler-Weber-Rendu disease (hereditary hemorrhagic telangiectasia) | Autosomal dominant mode of inheritance |
| Blue rubber bleb nevus syndrome (cavernous hemangiomas of the skin and gastrointestinal tract) | Autosomal dominant mode of inheritance in some cases |
| Neural tumors | |
| Neurofibromatosis 1 | Autosomal dominant mode of inheritance; *NF1* gene localized to chromosome 17 |
| Neurofibromatosis 2 | Autosomal dominant mode of inheritance; *NF2* gene localized to chromosome 22 |
| Bilateral (inherited) retinoblastoma | Germline deletion of *Rb1* locus on chromosome 13; associated with secondary sarcomas |
| Neuroblastoma | Rare familial cases |
| Paraganglioma | Occasional familial cases suggesting autosomal dominant mode of inheritance |
| Osseous tumors | |
| Fibrodysplasia ossificans progressiva | Occasionally increased familial incidence, including in homozygotic twins; autosomal dominant mode of inheritance |
| Miscellaneous tumors | |
| Tumoral calcinosis | Increased familial incidence; about 40% in siblings |
| Li-Fraumeni syndrome | Germline deletion of *p53* locus resulting in familial rhabdomyosarcoma, early onset of breast carcinoma, and other neoplasms |

protein product that loses the ability to degrade β-catenin, resulting in an elevated β-catenin protein level, which promotes fibroblastic proliferation.[2,63] Soft tissue sarcomas may also be a component of a variety of neoplastic disorders that may affect multiple relatives in a single family (so-called cancer family syndromes). Mutations of the *p53* tumor suppressor gene are critical to sarcoma genesis in patients with Li-Fraumeni syndrome.[64,67,106,113] The inherited, or bilateral, form of retinoblastoma is associated with the development of sarcomas, usually osteosarcomas. In this disease a germline mutation of the *Rb1* locus occurs. When a "second hit" develops in the other allelic site in somatic cells (i.e., retinoblasts), tumors develop. A number of other soft tissue tumors are known to occur in families, but the rarity of these reports indicates that collectively they do not account for a significant proportion of cases. These lesions, which are enumerated in Table 1–2, include various fibromatoses, lipomas, xanthomas, leiomyomas, neurofibromas, neuroblastomas, gastrointestinal stromal tumors, and paragangliomas. An excellent review of familial cancer syndromes was reported by Tsao.[117]

## CLASSIFICATION OF SOFT TISSUE TUMORS

Development of a useful, comprehensive histologic classification of soft tissue tumors has been a relatively slow process. Earlier classifications have been largely descriptive and have been based more on the nuclear configuration than the type of tumor cells. Terms such as "round cell sarcoma," "spindle cell sarcoma," and "pleomorphic sarcoma" may be diagnostically convenient but should be discouraged because they are meaningless and convey little information as to the nature and potential behavior of a given tumor. Moreover, purely descriptive classifications do not clearly distinguish between tumors and tumor-like reactive processes. More recent classifications have been based principally on the line of differentiation of the tumor, that is, the type of tissue formed by the tumor rather than the type of tissue from which the tumor arose.

Over the past two to three decades there have been several attempts to devise a useful, comprehensive classification of soft tissue tumors. They include the Armed Forces Institute of Pathology (AFIP) classifications published in the *Atlas of Tumor Pathology* in 1957,[108] 1967, and 1983[59] and the World Health Organization (WHO) classification published first in 1969[29] and revised in 1994.[126] The classification used herein is similar but not identical to the 1994 WHO classification, a collective effort by pathologists in nine countries.

Each of the histologic categories is divided into a benign group and a malignant group. The various tumors are named according to the tissue they most closely resemble. Rhabdomyosarcomas, for example, show rhabdomyoblastic differentiation rather than that of tumors that arise from voluntary or striated muscle tissue. Most tumors retain the same pattern of differentiation in the primary and recurrent lesions, but occasionally they change their pattern of differentiation or may even differentiate along several cellular lines.

Malignant fibrous histiocytoma and liposarcoma are the most common soft tissue sarcomas of adults; together they account for 35–45% of all sarcomas. The incidence of the different types, however, varies in different series. For example, among 1116 soft tissue sarcomas reviewed by Hashimoto et al.,[41] malignant fibrous histiocytoma (25.1%) and liposarcoma (11.6%) were the most common, followed by rhabdomyosarcoma (9.7%), leiomyosarcoma (9.1%), synovial sarcoma (6.5%), malignant peripheral nerve sheath tumor (5.9%), and fibrosarcoma (5.2%). In the series by Markhede et al.[70] the three most common sarcomas were malignant fibrous histiocytoma (28%), fibrosarcoma (14%), and liposarcoma (9%). Rhabdomyosarcoma, neuroblastoma, and the extraskeletal Ewing's sarcoma/primitive neuroectodermal tumor (PNET) family are the most frequent soft tissue sarcomas of childhood. A histologic classification of soft tissue tumors is presented in Table 1–3.

## STAGING AND GRADING SOFT TISSUE SARCOMAS

The histologic type of sarcoma does not always provide sufficient information for predicting the clinical course, and grading and staging soft tissue sarcomas are essential for an accurate prognosis for planning and evaluating therapy, and for comparing and exchanging data. *Grading* determines the degree of malignancy and is based on an evaluation of several histologic parameters. *Staging* provides shorthand information regarding the state or extent of the disease at a designated time, preferably at the time of the initial histologic diagnosis. Grading and staging are complicated by numerous, often interrelated variables that are likely to affect clinical behavior. In fact, a grading or staging system that is comprehensive and gives full consideration to all factors that might affect the course of the disease and the results of therapy is too complex for practical purposes. On the other hand, a more limited, more practical system may suffer from the hazards of oversimplification and may result in data that are neither meaningful nor reliable, thereby defeating the purpose for which the system was designed.

The accuracy of grading and staging obviously depends on the input of adequate, precise clinical and pathologic data; staging is best accomplished following biopsy and histologic diagnosis of the primary tumor. Grading and staging of recurrent tumors are of much less significance because they are influenced by the preceding therapy. In fact, grading may not be reliable in some cases following therapy. Moreover, the type of tumor, rather than its grade, provides information as to the likelihood of lymph node metastasis. For instance, lymph node metastasis is common with rhabdomyosarcomas and epithelioid sarcomas but is rare with liposarcomas and malignant peripheral nerve sheath tumors. As with all grading and staging systems, the data are recorded in a standard checklist or protocol.[5]

## GRADING

Traditionally, as outlined by Broders et al.[12] in 1939, the grade of a malignancy is determined by a combined assessment of several histologic features: (1) degree of cellularity; (2) cellular pleomorphism or anaplasia; (3) mitotic activity (frequency and abnormality of mitotic figures); (4) degree of necrosis; and (5) expansive or infiltrative and invasive growth. Additional factors include the amount of matrix formation and the presence or absence of hemorrhage, calcification, and inflammatory infiltrate. The amount of matrix formation, such as collagen or mucoid material, is

## TABLE 1–3 HISTOLOGIC CLASSIFICATION OF SOFT TISSUE TUMORS

- Fibrous tumors
  - Benign
    - Nodular fasciitis (including intravascular and cranial types)
    - Proliferative fasciitis and myositis
    - Organ-associated pseudosarcomatous myofibroblastic proliferations
    - Ischemic fasciitis (atypical decubital fibroplasia)
    - Fibroma (dermal, tendon sheath, nuchal types)
    - Elastofibroma
    - Nasopharyngeal angiofibroma
    - Giant cell angiofibroma
    - Keloid
    - Desmoplastic fibroblastoma (collagenous fibroma)
    - Fibrous hamartoma of infancy
    - Infantile digital fibromatosis
    - Myofibroma and myofibromatosis
    - Hyalin fibromatosis
    - Gingival fibromatosis
    - Fibromatosis colli
    - Calcifying aponeurotic fibroma
    - Calcifying fibrous pseudotumor
    - Infantile-type fibromatosis
  - Intermediate
    - Adult-type fibromatosis
      - Superficial (including palmar, plantar, penile fibromatosis, knuckle pads)
      - Deep (including extraabominal, abdominal, intraabdominal, mesenteric, pelvic fibromatosis)
    - Inflammatory myofibroblastic tumor (inflammatory fibrosarcoma)
    - Infantile fibrosarcoma
  - Malignant
    - Adult-type fibrosarcoma
      - Usual type
      - Myxoid type (myxofibrosarcoma, low grade myxoid malignant fibrous histiocytoma)
      - Low grade fibromyxoid type with or without rosettes (low grade fibromyxoid sarcoma)
      - Sclerosing epithelioid type
- Fibrohistiocytic tumors
  - Benign
    - Fibrous histiocytoma (cutaneous and deep)
      - Cellular
      - Epithelioid
    - Juvenile xanthogranuloma
    - Reticulohistiocytoma
    - Xanthoma
    - Extranodal (soft tissue) Rosai-Dorfman disease
  - Intermediate
    - Atypical fibroxanthoma
    - Dermatofibrosarcoma protuberans (including pigmented forms)
    - Giant cell fibroblastoma
    - Angiomatoid fibrous histiocytoma
    - Plexiform fibrohistiocytic tumor
    - Soft tissue giant cell tumor of low malignant potential
  - Malignant
    - Malignant fibrous histiocytoma
      - Storiform-pleomorphic type
      - Myxoid type
      - Giant cell type (malignant giant cell tumor of soft parts)
      - Inflammatory type
- Lipomatous tumors
  - Benign
    - Lipoma [solitary, multiple, cutaneous, deep (including intramuscular and perineural)]
    - Angiolipoma
    - Myolipoma
    - Chondroid lipoma
    - Spindle cell/pleomorphic lipoma
    - Angiomyolipoma
    - Myelolipoma
    - Hibernoma
    - Lipoblastoma or lipoblastomatosis
    - Lipomatosis
      - Diffuse lipomatosis
      - Cervical symmetric lipomatosis (Madelung's disease)
      - Pelvic lipomatosis
  - Intermediate
    - Atypical lipoma (well differentiated liposarcoma of superficial soft tissue, atypical lipomatous tumor)
  - Malignant
    - Well differentiated liposarcoma
      - Lipoma-like
      - Sclerosing
      - Inflammatory
      - Spindle cell
    - Myxoid-round cell liposarcoma
    - Pleomorphic liposarcoma
    - Dedifferentiated liposarcoma
- Smooth muscle tumors and related lesions
  - Benign
    - Leiomyoma
    - Angiomyoma
    - Angiomyofibroblastoma
    - Palisaded myofibroblastoma of lymph node
    - Intravenous leiomyomatosis
    - Leiomyomatosis peritonealis disseminata
  - Malignant
    - Leiomyosarcoma
- Extragastrointestinal (soft tissue) stromal tumors
  - Benign
    - Benign extragastrointestinal stromal tumor
    - Benign extragastrointestinal autonomic tumor
  - Malignant
    - Malignant extragastrointestinal stromal tumor
    - Malignant extragastrointestinal autonomic nerve tumor
- Skeletal muscle tumors
  - Benign
    - Cardiac rhabdomyoma
    - Adult rhabdomyoma
    - Fetal rhabdomyoma
      - Myxoid (classic)
      - Intermediate (cellular, juvenile)
  - Malignant
    - Embryonal rhabdomyosarcoma
      - Usual type
      - Botryoid type
      - Spindle cell type
    - Alveolar rhabdomyosarcoma
    - Pleomorphic rhabdomyosarcoma
    - Rhabdomyosarcoma with ganglion cells (ectomesenchymoma)
- Tumors of blood and lymph vessels
  - Benign
    - Papillary endothelial hyperplasia
    - Hemangioma
      - Capillary hemangioma (including juvenile)
      - Cavernous hemangioma (including sinusoidal)
      - Venous hemangioma
      - Epithelioid hemangioma (angiolymphoid hyperplasia)
      - Pyogenic granuloma
      - Acquired tufted hemangioma
      - Hobnail hemangioma
      - Spindle cell hemangioma
    - Lymphangioma
    - Lymphangiomyoma and lymphangiomyomatosis

*Table continued on following page*

**TABLE 1–3** HISTOLOGIC CLASSIFICATION OF SOFT TISSUE TUMORS *Continued*

    - Angiomatosis
    - Lymphangiomatosis
  - Intermediate
    - Epithelioid hemangioendothelioma
    - Hobnail hemangioendothelioma
      - Retiform type (retiform hemangioendothelioma)
      - Dabska type (endovascular papillary angioendothelioma)
    - Kaposiform hemangioendothelioma
  - Malignant
    - Angiosarcoma
    - Kaposi's sarcoma
- Perivascular tumors
  - Benign
    - Glomus tumor
      - Usual type
      - Glomangioma
      - Glomangiomyoma
      - Glomangiomatosis
    - Benign hemangiopericytoma/solitary fibrous tumor
    - Myopericytoma
  - Malignant
    - Malignant glomus tumor
    - Malignant hemangiopericytoma/malignant solitary fibrous tumor
- Synovial tumors
  - Benign
    - Tenosynovial giant cell tumor
      - Localized type
      - Diffuse type
  - Malignant
    - Malignant tenosynovial giant cell tumor
- Mesothelial tumors
  - Benign
    - Adenomatoid tumor
  - Intermediate
    - Multicystic mesothelioma
    - Well differentiated papillary mesothelioma
  - Malignant
    - Diffuse mesothelioma
      - Epithelial type
      - Sarcomatoid type
      - Biphasic type
- Peripheral nerve sheath tumors and related lesions
  - Benign
    - Traumatic neuroma
    - Glial heterotopia
    - Mucosal neuroma
    - Pacinian neuroma
    - Palisaded encapsulated neuroma
    - Morton's interdigital neuroma
    - Nerve sheath ganglion
    - Neuromuscular hamartoma
    - Neurofibroma and neurofibromatosis
      - Usual type (localized)
      - Diffuse
      - Plexiform
      - Epithelioid
    - Schwannoma and schwannomatosis
      - Usual type
      - Cellular schwannoma
      - Plexiform schwannoma
      - Degenerated (ancient) schwannoma
      - Epithelioid schwannoma
      - Neuroblastoma-like schwannoma
    - Melanotic schwannoma
    - Perineurioma
      - Intraneural perineurioma (localized hypertrophic neuropathy)
      - Extraneural (soft tissue) perineurioma
    - Granular cell tumor
    - Neurothekeoma
    - Ectopic meningioma
  - Malignant
    - Malignant peripheral nerve sheath tumor (MPNST)
      - Usual type
      - MPNST with rhabdomyoblastic differentiation (malignant Triton tumor)
      - Glandular malignant schwannoma
      - Epithelioid MPNST
      - MPNST arising in a schwannoma
      - MPNST arising in a ganglioneuroma
    - Malignant granular cell tumor
    - Clear cell sarcoma of the tendon and aponeurosis
    - Malignant melanocytic schwannoma
    - Ectopic ependymoma
- Primitive neuroectodermal tumors and related lesions
  - Benign
    - Ganglioneuroma
    - Pigmented neuroectodermal tumor of infancy (retinal anlage tumor)
  - Malignant
    - Neuroblastoma
    - Ganglioneuroblastoma
    - Ewing's sarcoma/primitive neuroectodermal tumor
    - Malignant pigmented neuroectodermal tumor of infancy (retinal anlage tumor)
- Paraganglionic tumors
  - Benign
    - Paraganglioma
  - Malignant
    - Malignant paraganglioma
- Extraskeletal osseous and cartilaginous tumors
  - Benign
    - Panniculitis ossificans and myositis ossificans
    - Fibroosseous pseudotumor of the digits
    - Fibrodysplasia ossificans progressiva
    - Extraskeletal chondroma or osteochondroma
    - Extraskeletal osteoma
  - Malignant
    - Extraskeletal chondrosarcoma
      - Well differentiated chondrosarcoma
      - Myxoid chondrosarcoma
      - Mesenchymal chondrosarcoma
    - Extraskeletal osteosarcoma
- Miscellaneous tumors
  - Benign
    - Congenital granular cell tumor
    - Tumoral calcinosis
    - Myxoma
      - Cutaneous
      - Intramuscular
    - Juxtaarticular myxoma
    - Aggressive angiomyxoma
    - Parachordoma
    - Amyloid tumor
    - Pleomorphic hyalinizing angiectatic tumor of soft parts
  - Intermediate
    - Ossifying fibromyxoid tumor of soft parts
    - Inflammatory myxohyaline tumor
  - Malignant
    - Synovial sarcoma
    - Alveolar soft part sarcoma
    - Epithelioid sarcoma
    - Desmoplastic small round cell tumor
    - Malignant extrarenal rhabdoid tumor

**TABLE 1–4 GRADING SYSTEMS: HISTOLOGIC PARAMETERS USED IN VARIOUS GRADING SYSTEMS**

| Parameter | Markhede | Myhre Jensen | Costa | Coindre |
|---|---|---|---|---|
| Cellularity | + | + | + | − |
| Differentiation | − | − | − | + |
| Pleomorphism | + | + | + | − |
| Mitotic rate | + | + | + | + |
| Necrosis | − | − | + | + |

usually inversely proportional to the cellularity and degree of differentiation. The depth of the tumor is another important prognostic factor.

Because the various parameters are closely interrelated, almost any combination provides useful information as to the grade of the tumor. The two most important parameters for grading soft tissue sarcomas seem to be the number of mitotic figures and the extent of necrosis[17,20,116] (Table 1–4).

The number of grades varies among staging systems: two, three, and four grades have been distinguished. Three-grade systems seem best suited for predicting patterns for survival and likely response to therapy.[47] Four-grade systems usually show little difference between the two lowermost grades; two-grade systems, which distinguish only between low grade and high grade sarcomas, are more readily related to the two surgical therapies but make it difficult to grade tumors of intermediate malignancy accurately, such as well differentiated fibrosarcomas.

The histologic type and subtype may be used as a shortcut to establish the tumor grade.[5,20,79] For example, alveolar rhabdomyosarcoma, neuroblastoma, and the extraskeletal Ewing's sarcoma/PNET family are high grade sarcomas. In contrast, well differentiated liposarcomas, infantile fibrosarcoma, and dermatofibrosarcoma protuberans are low grade sarcomas.

Ancillary procedures such as immunohistochemical, ultrastructural, and molecular genetic studies are useful for establishing the type of tumor. The extent to which molecular alterations are important in determining malignancy is still in its evolutionary stages. It is well established that N-*myc* amplification provides additional prognostic information among tumors of comparable stage. In other tumors, however, genetic alterations may parallel other findings, such as the mitotic index, so it is difficult to know the value of these studies when determining grade or therapy. More recent data suggest that identification of specific fusion transcripts secondary to translocations may be of prognostic significance for certain tumors, such as alveolar rhabdomyosarcoma,[51] synovial sarcoma,[50] and the Ewing's sarcoma/PNET family.[22] The extent to which some of these findings can provide incremental or independent prognostic information, apart from factors such as grade, is not fully defined.

## LIMITATIONS AND PITFALLS OF GRADING

The significance and predictive value of the various histologic parameters differ for various sarcomas. Mitotic activity, for example, is important when grading leiomyosarcomas but is of much less significance when grading the various subtypes of malignant fibrous histiocytoma. Malignant granular cell tumor and alveolar soft part sarcoma behave more aggressively than is implied by their moderate degree of cellular pleomorphism and paucity of mitotic figures. Likewise, mitotic figures are rare in many diffuse and highly malignant mesotheliomas. Infantile fibrosarcoma, on the other hand, is a tumor of relatively low grade malignancy despite its cellularity and prominent mitotic activity.

Occasional problems may also be caused by morphologic variations in different portions of the same tumor. At times well differentiated and poorly differentiated portions are encountered in leiomyosarcomas, malignant peripheral nerve sheath tumors, and liposarcomas (dedifferentiated liposarcomas). In these cases the grade should be determined on the basis of the least differentiated area, but the extent of the less differentiated portion of the neoplasm must also be taken into consideration. For instance, a small focus of round cell liposarcoma in the center of a myxoid liposarcoma does not necessarily indicate a poor prognosis. In a small percentage of cases, a higher degree of malignancy may be present in the recurrent or the metastatic growth. These changes may be spontaneous or may be the effect of treatment, particularly radiotherapy. On the other hand, there are also occasional rhabdomyosarcomas in which the recurrent lesion after therapy shows a higher degree of differentiation than the primary tumor.

Grading is not a substitute for a histologic diagnosis and does not permit distinguishing benign and malignant lesions; in fact, it may be misleading with tumors and tumor-like lesions. Nodular and proliferative fasciitis and early stages of myositis ossificans are typical of these reactive, sarcoma-like lesions, which are marked by a high degree of cellularity, markedly increased mitotic activity, and even, infrequently, areas of necrosis. Caution in this regard is particularly indicated because by no means have all of these benign mesenchymal lesions that occur in the guise of sarcomas been defined or recognized.

Grading, like diagnosing soft tissue sarcomas, requires representative, well fixed, well stained histologic material. Thick sections may be misleading as to the degree of cellularity and mitotic activity, and heavily stained sections may suggest less cellular differentiation than is actually present. Selection of the tissue sample and the length of fixation may also influence artificially the degree of necrosis and the mitotic index. Necrosis may also be more prominent in ulcerated tumors or those previously operated on.

## GRADING SYSTEMS

Grading and staging systems should be based on soft tissue tumors of one specific type, as the predictive significance of the various grading and staging parameters varies among sarcomas. However, in many systems assessment of the results and the prognostic significance of grading and staging soft tissue sarcomas is based on soft tissue tumors as a general group rather than on a specific tumor entity because of the relative rarity of these tumors and the difficulty of assembling a large number of sarcomas of any specific type. Therefore with many staging systems the predictive value of the histologic type is incorporated into the histologic grade of the tumor.

In 1982 Markhede et al.[70] suggested a grading system that used four grades of malignancy based on cellularity, cellular pleomorphism, and mitotic activity. In their study the grade correlated well with survival rates. Patients with grade 1 and 2 tumors had similar clinical courses, and no patients died from these tumors. The 5- and 10-year survival rates with grade 3 tumors were 68% and 55%, respectively, and with grade 4 tumors they were 47% and 26%, respectively.

In 1983, Myhre Jensen et al.[80] graded 261 soft tissue sarcomas from the Aarhus Musculoskeletal Tumour Centre. They employed three grades, with 5-year survival rates of 97% for grade 1 tumors, 67% for grade 2 tumors, and 38% for grade 3 tumors. The respective 10-year survival rates were 93%, 57%, and 23%. The authors concluded that mitotic activity was the main discriminating criterion but warned that delay in fixation, especially in the center of large tumors, may artificially reduce mitotic counts (Fig. 1–2).

Costa et al.[20] described a grading system based on a review of 163 sarcomas from the National Cancer Institute (NCI). They used a combination of histologic diagnosis (Table 1–5), cellularity, cellular pleomorphism, and mitotic rate as criteria for grading; but they also included necrosis as an important determinant for predicting recurrence and survival rates. They employed a three-grade system and stressed that grade 2 and 3 tumors that exhibited moderate or marked necrosis (> 15%) had a significantly poorer prognosis; thus necrosis emerged as a major discriminating variable. The respective 5-year survival rates of patients with the three grades were 100%, 73%, and 46%.

In 1984 Trojani et al.[116] presented a grading system known as the FNCLCC (Fédération Nationale des Centres de Lutte Contre le Cancer) system, developed by the French Federation of Cancer Centers Sarcoma Group based on an analysis of 155 adult patients with soft tissue sarcomas. On the basis of a multivariate analysis of the various histologic features, they selected a combination of cellular differentiation, mitotic rate, and tumor necrosis as parameters for their grading system. The authors assigned a score to each of these parameters and added the scores together for a combined grade (Table 1–6). They concluded that

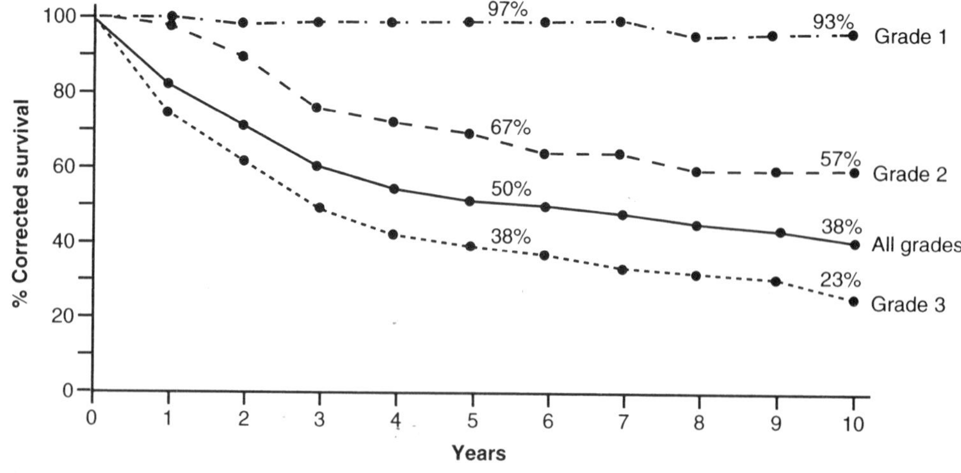


**FIGURE 1–2.** Grading system for soft tissue sarcomas based on three grades of malignancy. (From Myhre Jensen O, Kaae S, Madsen EH, et al. Histopathological grading in soft-tissue tumours: relation to survival in 261 surgically treated patients. Acta Pathol Microbiol Immunol Scand 91A:145, 1983.)

**TABLE 1–5 ASSIGNED HISTOLOGIC GRADE ACCORDING TO HISTOLOGIC TYPE IN THE NCI SYSTEM**

| Histologic Type | Grade 1 | Grade 2 | Grade 3 |
|---|---|---|---|
| Well differentiated liposarcoma | + | | |
| Myxoid liposarcoma | + | | |
| Round cell liposarcoma | | + | + |
| Pleomorphic liposarcoma | | | + |
| Fibrosarcoma | | + | + |
| MFH, pleomorphic type | | + | + |
| MFH, inflammatory type | | + | + |
| MFH, myxoid type | | + | |
| DFSP | + | | |
| Malignant granular cell tumor | | + | + |
| Leiomyosarcoma | + | + | + |
| Malignant hemangiopericytoma | + | + | + |
| Rhabdomyosarcoma (all types) | | | + |
| Chondrosarcoma | + | + | + |
| Myxoid chondrosarcoma | + | + | |
| Mesenchymal chondrosarcoma | | | + |
| Osteosarcoma | | | + |
| Extraskeletal Ewing's sarcoma | | | + |
| Synovial sarcoma | | | + |
| Epithelioid sarcoma | | + | + |
| Clear cell sarcoma | | + | + |
| Superficial MPNST | | + | |
| Epithelioid MPNST | | + | + |
| Malignant Triton tumor | | | + |
| Angiosarcoma | | + | + |
| Alveolar soft part sarcoma | | | + |
| Kaposi's sarcoma | | + | + |

Modified from Costa J, Wesley RA, Glatstein E, et al. The grading of soft tissue sarcomas: results of a clinicopathologic correlation in a series of 163 cases. Cancer 53:530, 1984.
NCI, National Cancer Institute; MFH, malignant fibrous histiocytoma; DFSP, dermatofibrosarcoma protuberans; MPNST, malignant peripheral nerve sheath tumor.

**TABLE 1–6 DEFINITIONS OF GRADING PARAMETERS FOR THE FNCLCC SYSTEM**

| Parameter | Criterion |
|---|---|
| Tumor differentiation | |
| Score 1 | Sarcoma closely resembling normal adult mesenchymal tissue (e.g., well differentiated liposarcoma) |
| Score 2 | Sarcoma for which the histologic typing is certain (e.g., alveolar soft part sarcoma) |
| Score 3 | Embryonal and undifferentiated sarcomas; sarcoma of uncertain type |
| Mitosis count | |
| Score 1 | 0–9/10 HPF |
| Score 2 | 10–19/10 HPF |
| Score 3 | ≥20/10 HPF |
| Tumor necrosis (microscopic) | |
| Score 0 | No necrosis |
| Score 1 | ≤50% Tumor necrosis |
| Score 2 | >50% Tumor necrosis |
| Histologic grade | |
| Grade 1 | Total score 2, 3 |
| Grade 2 | Total score 4, 5 |
| Grade 3 | Total score 6, 7, 8 |

Modified from Coindre JM, Trojani M, Contesso G, et al. Reproducibility of a histopathologic grading system for adult soft tissue sarcomas. Cancer 58:306, 1986.
FNCLCC, Fédération Nationale de Centres de Lutte Contre le Cancer; HPF, high-power fields.

the histologic grade was the single most important factor for predicting survival rates; tumor depth (superficial versus deep) was another important prognostic parameter. The reproducibility of this system was tested by 15 pathologists[18]; an agreement was reached in 81% of the cases for tumor necrosis, 74% for tumor differentiation, 73% for mitotic rate, and 75% for overall tumor grade, although the agreement as to histologic type was only 61%.

In 1997, Guillou et al.[37] performed a comparative study of the NCI and FNCLCC systems in 410 adult patients with nonmetastatic soft tissue sarcomas. By univariate analysis, both systems were of prognostic value for predicting metastasis and overall survival. By multivariate analysis, a tumor size of 10 cm or more, a deep location, and a high tumor grade, irrespective of the system used, were found to be independent prognostic factors for the advent of metastases. Interestingly, there were grade discrepancies using these two grading systems in 34.6% of the cases. Use of the FNCLCC system resulted in an increased number of grade 3 tumors, a reduced number of grade 2 tumors, and a better correlation with overall and metastasis-free survival when compared with the NCI system.

Although the FNCLCC system is perhaps the best documented and tested system thus far, there are nonetheless certain inherent problems in its usage. Perhaps the most problematic is the way in which one derives the "differentiation score." It is defined as the extent to which a tumor resembles adult mesenchymal tissue (score 1), the extent to which the histologic type is known (score 2), or the observation that the tumor is undifferentiated. Although a listing of the differentiation scores for the common tumors has been reported (Table 1–7), the rationale for some of

**TABLE 1–7 TUMOR DIFFERENTIATION SCORE ACCORDING TO HISTOLOGIC TYPE IN THE UPDATED VERSION OF THE FNCLCC SYSTEM**

| Histologic Type | Tumor Differentiation Score |
|---|---|
| Well differentiated liposarcoma | 1 |
| Myxoid liposarcoma | 2 |
| Round cell liposarcoma | 3 |
| Pleomorphic liposarcoma | 3 |
| Dedifferentiated liposarcoma | 3 |
| Well differentiated fibrosarcoma | 1 |
| Conventional fibrosarcoma | 2 |
| Poorly differentiated fibrosarcoma | 3 |
| Well differentiated MPNST | 1 |
| Conventional MPNST | 2 |
| Poorly differentiated MPNST | 3 |
| Epithelioid MPNST | 3 |
| Malignant triton tumor | 3 |
| Well differentiated malignant hemangiopericytoma | 2 |
| Conventional malignant hemangiopericytoma | 3 |
| Myxoid MFH | 2 |
| Typical storiform/pleomorphic MFH | 2 |
| Giant-cell and inflammatory MFH | 3 |
| Well differentiated leiomyosarcoma | 1 |
| Conventional leiomyosarcoma | 2 |
| Poorly differentiated/pleomorphic/epithelioid leiomyosarcoma | 3 |
| Biphasic/monophasic synovial sarcoma | 3 |
| Embryonal/alveolar/pleomorphic rhabdomyosarcoma | 3 |
| Well differentiated chondrosarcoma | 1 |
| Myxoid chondrosarcoma | 2 |
| Mesenchymal chondrosarcoma | 3 |
| Conventional angiosarcoma | 2 |
| Poorly differentiated/epithelioid angiosarcoma | 3 |
| Extraskeletal osteosarcoma | 3 |
| Ewing's sarcoma/PNET | 3 |
| Alveolar soft part sarcoma | 3 |
| Epithelioid sarcoma | 3 |
| Malignant rhabdoid tumor | 3 |
| Clear cell sarcoma | 3 |
| Undifferentiated sarcoma | 3 |

Modified from Guillou L, Coindre J-M, Bonichon F, et al. Comparative study of the National Cancer Institute and French Federation of Cancer Centers Sarcoma Group grading systems in a population of 410 adult patients with soft tissue sarcoma. J Clin Oncol 15:350, 1997.

PNET, primitive neuroectodermal tumor; see Tables 1–5 and 1–6 for other abbreviations.

these scores is not clear. For example, malignant fibrous histiocytoma is accorded a score of 2, whereas the inflammatory variant, an essentially identical lesion but having inflammatory cells as its sole difference, is given a score of 3. Differentiation scores of 1, 2, or 3 may be given to fibrosarcoma, but the criteria for these distinctions is elusive. It must also be remembered that this system has been derived from resected specimens unmodified by treatment, a situation that is not analogous to our current practices, which are heavily weighted toward grading on biopsies or on resection specimens following irradiation or chemotherapy.

Numerous additional studies have confirmed the utility of histologic grading of soft tissue sarcomas.[85,96,118] In a study by Hashimoto et al. of 1116 patients with soft tissue sarcomas,[41] histologic grade significantly correlated with survival in certain tumor types (malignant fibrous histiocytoma, leiomyosarcoma, liposarcoma) but not in others (rhabdomyosarcoma, synovial sarcoma, malignant peripheral nerve sheath tumor). The authors concluded, "it seems to be difficult to choose a single prognostic factor that is valid for all types of soft tissue sarcomas, and therefore we believe that the predictive significance of the various histologic parameters should be based on each specific sarcoma." An extension of this view has found its way into several recent publications on synovial sarcomas,[9] extraskeletal myxoid chondrosarcomas,[73] and extragastrointestinal stromal tumors[93] that define low or high risk lesions depending on a number of variables including histologic and clinical parameters. Figure 1–3 provides putative guidelines for grading soft tissue sarcomas; it gives the estimated range of malignancy for each type of sarcoma, which in turn serves as baseline for determining the histologic grade by using standard cytologic criteria such as cellularity, mitotic activity, and necrosis. The historical aspects of the various proposed grading systems have been excellently reviewed by Kilpatrick.[52] More recently, Ki-67 reactivity,[44,45,110,121] the argyrophilic stain for nucleolar organizer regions (AgNOR counts),[56,114,130] and mast cell counts[114] have been investigated as potential histologic markers for assessing the proliferative activity of soft tissue sarcomas.

In conclusion, despite all of the problems inherent in grading sarcomas, it still remains one of the most powerful tools in assessing prognosis, and a grade should be given in addition to histopathologic type whenever possible. Admittedly, needle biopsies repre-

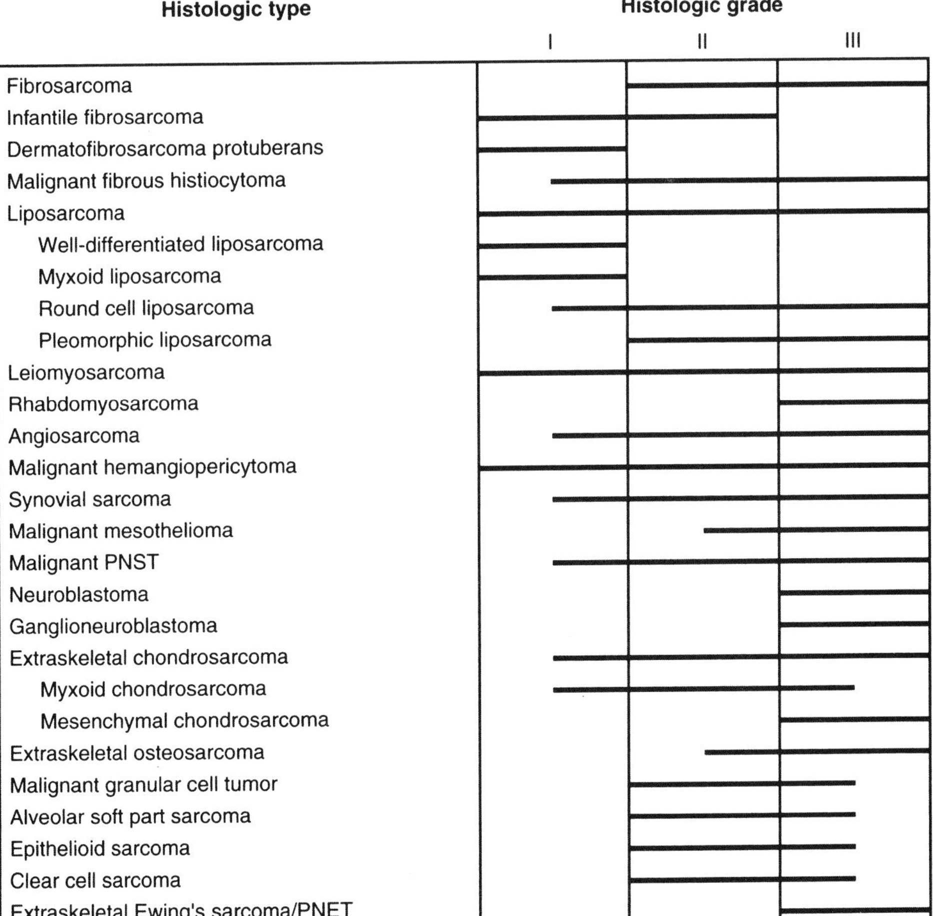


**FIGURE 1–3.** Soft tissue sarcomas. Estimated range of degree of malignancy based on histologic type and grade. Grade within the overall range depends on specific histologic features such as cellularity, cellular pleomorphism, mitotic activity, amount of stroma, infiltrative or expansive growth, and necrosis.

sent a distinct challenge and in these circumstances grade may be viewed as a "minimum" grade. Since each grading system which has been used in recent years has been validated and has proven efficacy, the choice of which to use may be one of personal or institutional choice. To derive a modified "grading" or "risk assessment" system for each type of sarcoma, as discussed above, has some appeal, but as an overall initiative would result in so many systems with different parameters that its sheer complexity might defeat its purpose. Thus, it is our belief that general grading systems supplemented where necessary by specific "risk assessment" systems for unusual sarcomas (e.g. epithelioid sarcoma, clear cell sarcoma, angiosarcoma) may be the most reasonable compromise.

## STAGING SYSTEMS

Several staging systems have been developed for soft tissue sarcomas in an attempt to predict prognosis and to evaluate the effect of therapeutic intervention by stratifying similar tumors according to prognostic factors such as histologic grade, tumor size, compartmentalization of the tumor, and the presence or absence of metastasis.[88] The two major staging systems used at present for adult soft tissue sarcomas were developed by The American Joint Committee on Cancer (AJCC)[8,35,98,99] and the Musculoskeletal Tumor Society as described by Enneking et al.[26–28] Each of these systems has advantages and disadvantages, as described below.

### AJCC Staging System

The original AJCC staging system was based on data obtained from a retrospective study of 702 sarcomas collected from 13 institutions. The study included only tumors that were diagnosed during the 15-year period 1954–1969, were histologically confirmed, had adequate follow-up information, and underwent primary treatment in the institution that contributed the specimen. Because the sample was too small to gain sufficient data on all well defined soft tissue sarcomas, the staging system was limited to the eight most common types.[98,99] This system is based on the TNM staging system used for staging carcinomas, with the addition of histologic grade as a prognostic variable. Thus the AJCC system, published in 1992,[8] is based on the size of the primary tumor (T), the involvement of lymph nodes (N), the presence of metastasis (M), and the type and grade of sarcoma (G). In 1997 several important modifications were made to the AJCC staging system.[35] Tumor depth, first shown to have prognostic significance in a large series of malignant

**TABLE 1–8 DEFINITIONS AND STAGING SYSTEM OF THE AMERICAN JOINT COMMITTEE ON CANCER**

Primary Tumor (T)
- TX Primary tumor cannot be assessed
- T0 No evidence of primary tumor
- T1 Tumor 5 cm or less in greatest dimension
  - T1a superficial tumor
  - T1b deep tumor

Regional Lymph Nodes (N)
- NX Regional lymph nodes cannot be assessed
- N0 No regional lymph node metastasis
- N1 Regional lymph node metastasis

Distant Metastasis (M)
- MX Distant metastasis cannot be assessed
- M0 No distant metastasis
- M1 Distant metastasis

HISTOPATHOLOGIC GRADE
- GX Grade cannot be assessed
- G1 Well differentiated
- G2 Moderately differentiated
- G3 Poorly differentiated
- G4 Undifferentiated

| Stage | Grade | Primary Tumor | Regional Lymph Nodes | Distant Metastasis |
|---|---|---|---|---|
| IA | G1 or G2 | T1a or T1b | N0 | M0 |
| IB | G1 or G2 | T2a | N0 | M0 |
| IIA | G1 or G2 | T2b | N0 | M0 |
| IIB | G3 or G4 | T1a or T1b | N0 | M0 |
| IIC | G3 or G4 | T2a | N0 | M0 |
| III | G3 or G4 | T2b | N0 | M0 |
| IV | Any G | Any T | N1 | M0 |
| | Any G | Any T | Any N | M1 |

From AJCC Cancer Staging Handbook, 5th ed. Lippincott-Raven, Philadelphia, 1998; and Peabody TD, Gibbs CP, Simon MA. Evaluation and staging of musculoskeletal neoplasms. J Bone Joint Surg [Am] 86:1207, 1998.

* Superficial tumor is located exclusively above the superficial fascia without invasion of the fascia; deep tumor is located either exclusively beneath the superficial fascia, or superficial to the fascia with invasion of or through the fascia, or superficial and beneath the fascia. Retroperitoneal, mediastinal, and pelvic sarcomas are classified as deep tumors.

**TABLE 1–9 DEFINITIONS OF ANATOMIC EXTENT IN THE MUSCULOSKELETAL TUMOR SOCIETY STAGING SYSTEM**

| Intracompartmental (T1) | | Extracompartmental (T2) |
|---|---|---|
| Intraarticular | → | Soft tissue extension |
| Superficial to deep fascia | → | Deep fascial extension |
| Paraosseous | → | Intraosseous or extrafascial extension |
| Intrafascial compartment | → | Extrafascial compartment |

Modified from Enneking WF, Spanier SS, Goodman MA. A system for the surgical staging of musculoskeletal sarcoma. Clin Orthop 153:106, 1980 and Peabody TD, Gibbs CP, Simon MA. Evaluation and staging of musculoskeletal neoplasms. J Bone Joint Surg [Am] 80:1204, 1998.

fibrous histiocytomas by Weiss and Enzinger[124,125] and endorsed in an early soft tissue tumor textbook,[38] was subsequently incorporated into this staging system. In addition, grades 1 and 2 were grouped as low grade and grades 3 and 4 as high grade. In a four-tiered system this grouping works well. It is less clear-cut whether a grade 2 lesion in a three-tiered staging system is better classified as "low grade" or "high grade." The AJCC staging system is summarized in Table 1–8.

### Musculoskeletal Tumor Society Staging System

The Enneking system, designed for sarcomas of both soft tissue and bone, distinguishes two anatomic settings: T1, intracompartmental tumors confined within the boundaries of well defined anatomic structures, such as a functional muscle group, joint, and subcutis; and T2, extracompartmental neoplasms that arise within or involve secondarily extrafascial spaces or planes that have no natural anatomic barriers to extension. There are two grades (G1 and G2) and three stages. In this system, two grades are favored because they can be better related to the two surgical procedures (wide and radical excision) and because of the reported lack of any difference in the metastatic rate between intermediate and high grade tumors. This staging system is summarized in Tables 1–9 and 1–10.

### Advantages and Disadvantages of Staging Systems

These two staging systems serve as a valuable guide to therapy and provide useful prognostic information. Although the AJCC system is applicable to soft tissue sarcomas at any site, the development of this system was based on studies that included lesions from a variety of anatomic locations, including the extremities, retroperitoneum, and head and neck. It is difficult to compare data from patients with tumors at these sites given the differences in the ability to eradicate tumors surgically in these anatomic locations. The AJCC system also uses 5 cm as an important dimension for determining prognosis, although the designation is somewhat arbitrary. The Musculoskeletal Tumor Society (Enneking) system, with its emphasis on compartmentalization, is best suited for well documented sarcomas arising in the extremities. It does not include the type, size, or depth of the tumor as separate parameters; and its two-tiered grading system is probably too narrow for the wide biologic range of soft tissue sarcomas. Because of the need for adequately defining compartmentalization, the system does not lend itself to retrospective staging. Further-

**TABLE 1–10 MUSCULOSKELETAL TUMOR SOCIETY STAGING SYSTEM**

| Stage | Grade | Site | Metastasis |
|---|---|---|---|
| IA | G1 | T1 | M0 |
| IB | G1 | T2 | M0 |
| IIA | G2 | T1 | M0 |
| IIB | G2 | T2 | M0 |
| III | G1 or G2 | T1 or T2 | M1 |

Modified from Enneking WF, Spanier SS, Goodman MA. A system for the surgical staging of musculoskeletal sarcoma. Clin Orthop 153:106, 1980 and Peabody TD, Gibbs CP, Simon MA. Evaluation and staging of musculoskeletal neoplasms. J Bone Joint Surg [Am] 80:1204, 1998.

more, this system was devised before the routine use of advanced imaging techniques such as magnetic resonance imaging and before the widespread use of adjuvant therapy.[88]

Obviously, staging soft tissue sarcomas requires a multidisciplinary approach with close cooperation among clinician, oncologist, and pathologist. In view of the relative rarity of these tumors, staging and grading are ideally carried out in large medical centers with special interest and experience in the diagnosis and management of soft tissue sarcomas. Moreover, prospective rather than retrospective studies are necessary to test the value of the various staging systems.

## REFERENCES

1. Aboulafia AJ, Brooks F, Piratzky J, et al. Osteosarcoma arising from heterotopic ossification after an electrical burn. J Bone Joint Surg Am 81:564, 1999.
2. Alman BA, Li C, Pajerski ME, et al. Increased $\beta$-catenin protein and somatic APC mutations in sporadic aggressive fibromatoses (desmoid tumors). Am J Pathol 151:329, 1997.
3. Amendola BE, Amendola MA, McClatchey KD, et al. Radiation-associated sarcoma: a review of 23 patients with postradiation sarcoma over a 50 year period. Am J Clin Oncol 12: 411, 1989.
4. Arlen M, Higinbotham NL, Huvos AG, et al. Radiation-induced sarcoma of bone. Cancer 28:1087, 1971.
5. Association of Directors of Anatomic and Surgical Pathology. Recommendations for the Reporting of Soft Tissue Sarcomas. Hum Pathol 30:3, 1999.
6. Attanoos RL, Gibbs AR. Pathology of malignant mesothelioma. Histopathology 30:403, 1997.
7. Balarajan R, Acheson ED. Soft tissue sarcomas in agricultural and forestry workers. J Epidemiol Community Health 38:113, 1984.
8. Beahrs OH, Henson DE, Hutter RVP, et al. Manual for Staging of Cancer, 3rd ed. Lippincott, Philadelphia, 1992.
9. Bergh P, Meis-Kindblom JM, Gherlinzoni F, et al. Synovial sarcoma: identification of low and high risk groups. Cancer 85:2596, 1996.
10. Bertazzi P, Pesatori A, Consonni D, et al. Cancer incidence in a population accidentally exposed to 2,3,7,8-tetrachlorodibenzo-para-dioxin. Epidemiology 4:398, 1993.
11. Breslin P, Kang HK, Lee Y, et al. Proportionate mortality study of US Army and US Marine Corps veterans of the Vietnam war. J Occup Med 30:412, 1988.
12. Broders AC, Hargrave R, Meyerding HW. Pathological features of soft tissue fibrosarcoma with special reference to the grading of its malignancy. Surg Gynecol Obstet 69:267, 1939.
13. Burns WA, Kanhauwand S, Tillman L, et al. Fibrosarcoma occurring at the site of a plastic vascular graft. Cancer 29:66, 1972.
14. Cahan WG, Woodard HQ, Higinbotham NL, et al. Sarcoma arising in irradiated bone. Cancer 1:3, 1948.
15. Cathomas G, Stalder A, McGandy CE, et al. Distribution of human herpes virus 8 DNA in tumorous and nontumorous tissue of patients with acquired immunodeficiency syndrome with and without Kaposi's sarcoma. Mod Pathol 11:415, 1998.
16. Chang Y, Cesarman E, Pessin MS, et al. Identification of herpesvirus-like DNA sequences in AIDS-associated Kaposi's sarcoma. Science 266:1865, 1994.
17. Coindre J-M, Terrier P, Bui MB, et al. Prognostic factors in adult patients with locally controlled soft tissue sarcoma: a study of 546 patients from the French Federation of Cancer Centers Sarcoma Group. J Clin Oncol 14:869, 1996.
18. Coindre JM, Trojani M, Contesso G, et al. Reproducibility of a histopathologic grading system for adult soft tissue sarcoma. Cancer 58:306, 1986.
19. Collins JJ, Strauss ME, Levinskas GJ, et al. The mortality experience of workers exposed to 2,3,7,8-tetrachlorodibenzo-p-dioxin in a tricholophenol process accident. Epidemiology 4:7, 1993.
20. Costa J, Wesley RA, Glatstein E, et al. The grading of soft tissue sarcomas: results of a clinicohistopathologic correlation in a series of 163 cases. Cancer 53:530, 1984.
21. Cutler SJ, Young IL. Third National Cancer Survey: incidence data. Natl Cancer Inst Monogr 41:1, 1975.
22. De Alava E, Kawai A, Healey JH, et al. EWS-FLI 1 fusion transcript structure is an independent determinant of prognosis in Ewing's sarcoma. J Clin Oncol 16:1248, 1998.
23. Dictor M, Rambech E, Way D, et al. Human herpes virus 8 (Kaposi's sarcoma-associated herpes virus) DNA in Kaposi's sarcoma lesions, AIDS Kaposi's sarcoma cell lines, endothelial Kaposi's sarcoma simulators, and the skin of immunosuppressed patients. Am J Pathol 148:2009, 1996.
24. Dubin HU, Creehan EP, Headington JT. Lymphangiosarcoma and congenital lymphedema of the extremity. Arch Dermatol 110:608, 1974.
25. Elliot P, Kleinschmidt I. Angiosarcoma of the liver in Great Britain in proximity to vinyl chloride sites. Occup Environ Med 54:14, 1997.
26. Enneking WF. Musculoskeletal Tumor Surgery. Churchill Livingstone, New York, 1983.
27. Enneking WF, Spanier SS, Goodman MA. A system for the surgical staging of musculoskeletal sarcoma. Clin Orthop 153: 106, 1980.
28. Enneking WF, Spanier SS, Malawar MM. The effect of the anatomic setting on the results of surgical procedures for soft part sarcoma of the thigh. Cancer 47:1005, 1981.
29. Enzinger FM, Lattes R, Torloni R. Histological typing of soft tissue tumours. In: International Histological Classification of Tumours, No. 3. World Health Organization, Geneva, 1969.
30. Eriksson M, Hardell L, Adami H-O. Exposure to dioxins as a risk factor for soft tissue sarcoma: a population-based case-control study. J Natl Cancer Inst 82:486, 1990.
31. Eriksson M, Hardell L, Berg NO, et al. Soft-tissue sarcomas and exposure to chemical substances: a case-referent study. Br J Ind Med 38:27, 1981.
32. Evans DM, Williams WJ, Jung IT. Angiosarcoma and hepatocellular carcinoma in vinyl chloride workers. Histopathology 7:377, 1983.
33. Fearon ER, Vogelstein B. A genetic model for colorectal tumorigenesis. Cell 61:759, 1990.
34. Fingerhut MA, Halperin WE, Marlow DA. Cancer mortality in workers exposed to 2,3,7,8-tetrachlorodibenzo-p-dioxin. N Engl J Med 324:212, 1991.
35. Fleming ID, Cooper JS, Henson GE, et al. AJCC Cancer Staging Manual, 5th ed. Lippincott-Raven, Philadelphia, 1997.
36. Greenwald P, Kovasznay B, Collins DN, et al. Sarcomas of soft tissues after Vietnam service. J Natl Cancer Inst 73:1107, 1984.
37. Guillou L, Coindre J-M, Bonichon F, et al. Comparative study of the National Cancer Institute and French Federation of Cancer Centers Sarcoma Group grading systems in a population of 410 adult patients with soft tissue sarcoma. J Clin Oncol 15: 350, 1997.
38. Hajdu SI. Pathology of Soft Tissue Tumors. Lea & Febiger, Philadelphia, 1979.
39. Hardell L, Axelson O. Soft-tissue sarcoma, malignant lym-

phoma, and exposure to phenoxy acids or chlorophenols. Lancet 1:1408, 1982.
40. Hardell L, Sandstrom A. Case-control study: soft-tissue sarcomas and exposure to phenoxyacetic acids or chlorophenols. Br J Cancer 39:711, 1979.
41. Hashimoto H, Daimaru Y, Takeshita S, et al. Prognostic significance of histologic parameters of soft tissue sarcomas. Cancer 70:2816, 1992.
42. Huvos A, Woodard H, Cahan W, et al. Postradiation osteogenic sarcoma of bone and soft tissues: a clinicopathologic study of 66 patients. Cancer 55:1244, 1985.
43. Institute of Medicine: Veterans and Agent Orange: Health Effects of Herbicides Used in Viet Nam. National Academy of Sciences, National Academy Press, Washington, DC, 1994.
44. Jensen V, Hoyer M, Sorensen FB, et al. MIB- 1 expression and iododeoxyuridine labelling in soft tissue sarcomas: an immunohistochemical study including correlations with p53, bcl-2 and histological characteristics. Histopathology 28:437, 1996.
45. Jensen V, Sorensen FP, Bentzen SM, et al. Proliferative activity (MIB-1 index) is an independent prognostic parameter in patients with high-grade soft tissue sarcomas of subtypes other than malignant fibrous histiocytoma: a retrospective immunohistological study including 216 soft tissue sarcomas. Histopathology 32:536, 1998.
46. Jin YT, Tsai ST, Yan JJ, et al. Detection of Kaposi's sarcoma-associated herpes virus-like DNA sequence in vascular lesions: a reliable diagnostic marker for Kaposi's sarcoma. Am J Clin Pathol 105:360, 1996.
47. Kandel RA, Bell RS, Wunder JS, et al. Comparison between a 2- and 3-grade system in predicting metastatic-free survival in extremity soft-tissue sarcoma. J Surg Oncol 72:77, 1999.
48. Karlsson P, Holberg E, Johansson KA, et al. Soft tissue sarcoma after treatment for breast caancer. Radiother Oncol 38: 25, 1996.
49. Karlsson P, Holmberg E, Samuelsson A, et al. Soft tissue sarcoma after treatment for breast cancer: a Swedish population-based study. Eur J Cancer 34:2068, 1998.
50. Kawai A, Woodruff J, Healey JH, et al. SYT-SSX gene fusion as a determinant of morphology and prognosis in synovial sarcoma. N Engl J Med 338:153, 1998.
51. Kelly KM, Womer RV, Sorensen PHB, et al. Common and variant gene fusions predict distinct clinical phenotypes in rhabdomyosarcoma. J Clin Oncol 15:1831, 1997.
52. Kilpatrick SE. Histologic prognostication in soft tissue sarcomas: grading versus subtyping or both? A comprehensive review of the literature with proposed practical guidelines. Ann Diagn Pathol 3:48, 1999.
53. Kingma DW, Shad A, Tsokos M, et al. Epstein-Barr virus (EBV)-associated smooth muscle tumor arising in a post-transplant patient treated successfully for two PT-EBV-associated large cell lymphomas. Am J Surg Pathol 20:1511, 1996.
54. Kirkpatrick CJ, Alves A, Kohler H, et al. Biomaterial-induced sarcoma: a novel model to study preneoplastic change. Am J Pathol 156:1455, 2000.
55. Kogan MD, Clapp RW. Soft tissue sarcoma mortality among Viet Nam veterans in Massachusetts, 1972 to 1983. Int J Epidemiol 17:39, 1988.
56. Kuratsu S, Myoui A, Tomita Y, et al. Usefulness of argyrophilic nucleolar organizer staining for histologic grading of soft tissue sarcomas. J Surg Oncol 54:139, 1993.
57. Landrigan PJ. Asbestos: still a carcinogen. N Engl J Med 338: 1618, 1998.
58. Laskin WB, Silverman TA, Enzinger FM. Postradiation soft tissue sarcomas: an analysis of 53 cases. Cancer 62:2330, 1988.
59. Lattes R. Tumors of the soft tissue. In: Atlas of Tumor Pathology, Second Series, Fascicle 1, Revised. Armed Forces Institute of Pathology, Washington, DC, 1983.
60. Le Bail B, Morel D, Merel P, et al. Cystic smooth-muscle tumor of the liver and spleen associated with Epstein-Barr virus after renal transplantation. Am J Surg Pathol 20:1418, 1996.
61. Lee ES, Locker J, Nalesnik M, et al. The association of Epstein-Barr virus with smooth muscle tumors occurring after organ transplantation. N Engl J Med 332:19, 1995.
62. Leiss JK, Savitz DA. Home pesticide use and childhood cancer: a case control study. Am J Public Health 85:249, 1995.
63. Li C, Bapat B, Alman BA. Adenomatous polyposis coli gene mutation alters proliferation through its $\beta$-catenin-regulatory function in aggressive fibromatosis (desmoid tumor). Am J Phathol 153:709, 1998.
64. Li FP, Fraumeni JF. Soft tissue sarcomas, breast cancer, and other neoplasms: a familial syndrome? Ann Intern Med 71:747, 1969.
65. Li JJ, Huang YQ, Cockerell CJ, et al. Localization of human herpes-like virus type 8 in vascular endothelial cells and perivascular spindle shaped cells of Kaposi's sarcoma lesions by in situ hybridization. Am J Pathol 148:1741, 1996.
66. Madarnas P, Dube M, Rola-Pleszozynski M, et al. An animal model of Kaposi's sarcoma: pathogenesis of dimethyl hydrazine induced angiosarcoma and colorectal cancer in three mouse strains. Anticancer Res 12:113, 1992.
67. Malkin D, Li F, Strong LC, et al. Germ line p53 mutations in a familial syndrome of breast cancer, sarcomas, and other neoplasms. Science 250:1233, 1990.
68. Marchuk DA, Saulino AM, Tavakkol R, et al. cDNA cloning of the type 1 neurofibromatosis gene: complete sequence of the NF1 gene product. Genomics 11:931, 1991.
69. Mark RJ, Poen J, Tran LM, et al. Postirradiation sarcomas: a single institution study and review of the literature. Cancer 73: 2653, 1994.
70. Markhede G, Angervall L, Stener B. A multivariate analysis of the prognosis after surgical treatment of malignant soft tissue tumors. Cancer 49:1721, 1982.
71. McClain KL, Leach CT, Jenson HB, et al. Association of Epstein-Barr virus with leiomyosarcomas in young people with AIDS. N Engl J Med 332:12, 1995.
72. McDonald JC, Armstong B, Case B, et al. Mesothelioma and asbestos fiber type. Cancer 63:1544, 1989.
73. Meis-Kindblom JM, Bergh P, Gunterberg B, et al. Extraskeletal myxoid chondrosarcoma: a reappraisal of its morphologic spectrum and prognostic factors based on 117 cases. Am J Surg Pathol 23:636, 1999.
74. Meis-Kindblom JM, Kindblom L-G. Angiosarcoma of soft tissue: a study of 80 cases. Am J Surg Pathol 22:683, 1998.
75. Merrick T, Erlandson RA, Hajdu SI. Lymphangiosarcoma of a congenitally lymphedematous extremity. Arch Pathol 91:365, 1971.
76. Miyaki M, Konishi M, Kikuchi-Yanoshita R, et al. Coexistence of somatic and germ-line mutations of APC gene and desmoid tumors from patients with familial adenomatous polyposis. Cancer Res 53:5079, 1993.
77. Muller R, Hajdu SI, Brennan MF. Lymphangiosarcoma associated with chronic filarial lymphedema. Cancer 59:174, 1987.
78. Murray EM, Werner D, Greef EA. Postradiation sarcomas: 20 cases and a literature review. Int J Radiat Oncol Biol Phys 45: 951, 1999.
79. Myhre Jensen O, Hgh J, Stgaard SE, et al. Histopathological grading of soft tissue tumours: prognostic significance in a prospective study of 278 consecutive cases. J Pathol 163:19, 1991.
80. Myhre Jensen O, Kaae S, Madsen EH, et al. Histopathological grading in soft-tissue tumours: relation to survival in 261 surgically treated patients. Acta Pathol Microbiol Immunol Scand 91A:145, 1983.

81. Naka N, Ohsawa M, Tomita Y, et al. Angiosarcoma in Japan: a review of 99 cases. Cancer 75:989, 1995.
82. Nakamura Y, Nishisho I, Kinzler KW, et al. Mutations of the adenomatous polyposis coli gene in familial polyposis coli patients and sporadic colorectal tumors. Princess Takamatsu Symp 22:285, 1991.
83. Nakanishi H, Tomita Y, Myoui A, et al. Mutation of the p53 gene in postradiation sarcoma. Lab Invest 78:727, 1998.
84. Ozyazghan I, Kontas O. Burn scar sarcoma. Burns 25:455, 1999.
85. Parham DM, Webber BL, Jenkins JJ, et al. Non-rhabdomyosarcomatous soft tissue sarcomas of childhood: formulation of a simplied system for grading. Mod Pathol 8:705 1995.
86. Parker SL, Tong T, Bolder W, et al. Cancer statistics, 1996. CA Cancer J Clin 46:5, 1996.
87. Patel SG, See ACH, Williamson PA, et al. Radiation induced sarcoma of the head and neck. Head Neck 21:346, 1999.
88. Peabody TD, Gibbs CP, Simon MA. Evaluation and staging of musculoskeletal neoplasms. J Bone Joint Surg [Am] 80:1204, 1998.
89. Pierce SM, Recht A, Lingos TI, et al. Long-term radiation complications following conservative surgery and radiation therapy in patients with early stage breast cancer. Int Radiat Oncol Biol Phys 23:915, 1992.
90. Polednak AP. Incidence of soft-tissue cancers in blacks and whites in New York State. Int J Cancer 38:21, 1986.
91. Przygodzki RM, Finkelstein SD, Keohavong P, et al. Sporadic and Thorotrast-induced angiosarcomas of the liver manifest frequent and multiple point mutations in K-ras 2 Lab Invest 76:153, 1997.
92. Rademaker J, Widjaja A, Galanski M. Hepatic hemangiosarcoma: imaging findings and differential diagnosis. Eur Radiol 10:129, 2000.
93. Reith JD, Goldblum JR, Lyles RH, et al. Extragastrointestinal (soft tissue) stromal tumors: an analysis of 48 cases with emphasis on histologic predictors of outcome Mod Pathol 13:577, 2000.
94. Rhomberg W. Exposure to polymeric materials in vascular soft-tissue sarcomas. Int Arch Occup Environ Health 71:343, 1998.
95. Robinson E, Neugut AI, Wylie P. Clinical aspects of postirradiation sarcomas. J Natl Cancer Inst 80:233, 1988.
96. Rooser B, Attewell R, Berg MO, et al. Prognostication in soft tissue sarcoma: a model with four risk factors. Cancer 61:817, 1988.
97. Ross JA, Severson RK, Davis S, et al. Trends and the incidence of soft tissue sarcomas in the United States from 1973 through 1987. Cancer 72:486, 1993.
98. Russell WO, Cohen J, Cutler S, et al. Staging system for soft tissue sarcoma. In: American Joint Committee for Cancer Staging and End Results Reporting. Task Force on Soft Tissue Sarcoma. American College of Surgeons, Chicago, 1980.
99. Russell WO, Cohen J, Enzinger FM, et al. A clinical and pathological staging system for soft tissue sarcomas. Cancer 40: 1562, 1977.
100. Rydholm A. Management of patients with soft tissue tumors: strategy developed at a regional oncology center. Acta Orthop Scand Suppl 203:13, 1983.
101. Rydholm A, Berg NO, Gullberg B, et al. Epidemiology of soft tissue sarcoma in the locomotor system: a retrospective population-based study of the interrelationships between clinical and morphological variables. Acta Pathol Microbiol Immunol Scand 92A:363, 1984.
102. Sarma PR, Jacobs J. Thoracic soft-tissue sarcoma in Viet Nam veterans exposed to Agent Orange. N Engl J Med 306:1109, 1992.
103. Serraino D, Franceschi S, La Vecchia C, et al. Occupation and soft-tissue sarcoma in northeastern Italy. Cancer Causes Control 3:25, 1992.
104. Smith AH, Pearce NE, Fisher DO, et al. Soft tissue sarcoma and exposure to phenoxyherbicides and chlorophenols in New Zealand. J Natl Cancer Inst 73:1111, 1984.
105. Somers GR, Tesoriero AA, Hartland E, et al. Multiple leiomyosarcomas of both donor and recipient origin arising in a heart-lung transplant patient. Am J Surg Pathol 22:1423, 1998.
106. Srivastava S, Zou Z, Pirollo K, et al. Germ-line transmission of a mutated p53 gene in a cancer-prone family with Li-Fraumeni syndrome. Nature 348:747, 1990.
107. Stewart FW, Treves M. Lymphangiosarcoma in postmastectomy lymphedema. Cancer 1:64, 1949.
108. Stout AP. Tumors of soft tissue. In: AFIP Atlas of Tumor Pathology, Fascicle 1, First Series. Armed Forces Institute of Pathology, Washington, DC, 1957.
109. Suruda AJ, Ward EM, Fingerhut MA. Identification of soft tissue sarcoma deaths in cohorts exposed to dioxin and to chlorinated naphthalenes. Epidemiology 4:14, 1993.
110. Swanson SA, Brooks JJ. Proliferation markers Ki-67 and p105 in soft tissue lesions: correlation with DNA flow cytometric characteristics. Am J Pathol 137:1491, 1990.
111. Taghian A, De Vathaire F, Terrier P, et al. Long-term risk of sarcoma following radiation therapy for breast cancer. Int J Radiat Oncol Biol Phys 21:361, 1991.
112. Timmons CF, Dawson DB, Richards CS, et al. Epstein-Barr virus associated leiomyosarcomas in liver transplantation recipients: origin from either donor or recipient tissue. Cancer 76:1481, 1995.
113. Toguchida J, Yamaguchi T, Dayton SH, et al. Prevalence and spectrum of germline mutations of the p53 gene among patients with sarcoma. N Engl J Med 326:1301, 1992.
114. Tomita Y, Aozasa K, Myoui A, et al. Histologic grading in soft-tissue sarcomas: an analysis of 194 cases including AgNOR count and mast-cell count. Int J Cancer 54:194, 1993.
115. Trofatter JA, MacCollin MM, Rutter JL, et al. A novel moesin-, ezrin-, radixin-like gene is a candidate for the neurofibromatosis 2 tumor suppressor. Cell 72:791, 1993.
116. Trojani M, Contesso G, Coindre JM, et al. Soft tissue sarcomas of adults: study of pathological and prognostic variables and definition of a histological grading system. Int J Cancer 33:37, 1984.
117. Tsao H. Update of familial cancer syndromes and the skin. J Am Acad Dermatol 42:939, 2000.
118. Tsujimoto M, Aozasa K, Ueda T, et al. Multivariate analysis for histologic prognostic factors in soft tissue sarcomas. Cancer 62:994, 1988.
119. Tucker M, D'Angio G, Boice JD, et al. Bone sarcomas linked to radiotherapy and chemotherapy in children. N Engl J Med 317:588, 1987.
120. Tulbah A, Al-Dayel F, Fawaz I, et al. Epstein-Barr virus-associated leiomyosarcoma of the thyroid in a child with congenital immunodeficiency: a case report. Am J Surg Pathol 23:473, 1999.
121. Ueda T, Aozasa K, Tsujimoto M, et al. Prognostic significance of Ki-67 reactivity in soft tissue sarcomas. Cancer 63:1607, 1989.
122. Vineis P, Terracini B, Ciccone G, et al. Phenoxy herbicides and soft-tissue sarcomas in female rice weeders: a population-based case-referent study. Scand J Work Environ Health 13:9, 1987.
123. Weatherby RP, Dahlin DC, Ivins JC. Postradiation sarcoma of bone: review of 78 Mayo Clinic cases. Mayo Clin Proc 56:294, 1981.
124. Weiss SW, Enzinger FM. Malignant fibrous histiocytoma: an analysis of 200 cases. Cancer 41:2250, 1978.

125. Weiss SW, Enzinger FM. Myxoid variant of malignant fibrous histiocytoma. Cancer 39:1672, 1977.
126. Weiss SW, Sobin L. Histological typing of soft tissue tumours. In: World Health Organization International Histological Classification of Tumours, 2nd ed. Springer-Verlag, Berlin, 1994.
127. Wiklund TA, Blomqvist CP, Raty J, et al. Postirradiation sarcoma: analysis of a nationwide cancer registry material. Cancer 68:524, 1991.
128. Wingren G, Fredrikson M, Brage HN, et al. Soft tissue sarcoma and occupational exposures. Cancer 66:806, 1990.
129. Wolf RF, Ng B, Wekeler B, et al. Effect of growth hormone on tumor and host in an animal model. Ann Surg Oncol 1:314, 1994.
130. Wrba F, Augustin I, Fertl H. Nucleolar organizer regions in soft tissue sarcomas. Oncology 48:166, 1991.
131. Zahm SH, Fraumeni JF. The epidemiology of soft tissue sarcoma. Semin Oncol 24:504, 1997.

# CHAPTER 2

# CLINICAL EVALUATION AND TREATMENT OF SOFT TISSUE TUMORS

VERNON K. SONDAK AND ALFRED E. CHANG

Soft tissue sarcomas are a heterogeneous group of malignant neoplasms that can arise from mesenchymal elements anywhere in the body. Despite the fact that soft tissues and bone comprise almost two-thirds of the mass of the human body, sarcomas are uncommon tumors. Benign neoplasms of the soft tissues, in contrast, are commonplace and rarely consequential. These facts explain a number of clinical observations about the management of soft tissue sarcomas. Because of the relative rarity of sarcomas compared to benign soft tissue tumors, both patients and clinicians frequently fail to appreciate the significance of an enlarging soft tissue mass, and a tissue diagnosis is commonly obtained only after a significant delay. Few pathologists accumulate extensive experience with these rare tumors; hence, once biopsied, pathologic classification may be incomplete or inaccurate. After the diagnosis is made, many oncologists lack sufficient knowledge of the behavior of specific soft tissue sarcomas to provide appropriate therapy. The goal of this chapter is to review the clinical evaluation and treatment of soft tissue tumors in hopes of facilitating the prompt diagnosis and proper multimodality management of these challenging lesions. This chapter reflects current approaches to the treatment of adult soft tissue sarcomas.

Beginning with the initial biopsy, information provided by the pathologist assumes a critical role in the management algorithm of soft tissue sarcomas. Once the diagnosis of sarcoma has been established, the most important consideration when determining treatment strategy is the histologic grade of the tumor.[19,55] Sarcomas are usually assigned a grade from 1 to 3, with 1 being the lowest. Low grade sarcomas rarely metastasize, although they can be locally aggressive. Higher grade sarcomas (grade 2 or 3) pose a significant threat of metastasizing and present problems of local control. Assigning a pathologic grade to an individual tumor can be a difficult, subjective task; the specific details of the criteria used to grade soft tissue sarcomas are discussed elsewhere in this book. The clinical importance of the tumor grade cannot be overstressed, and an ideal biopsy allows a confident grade assignment.

Next in clinical significance is the location of the primary tumor. The location of a soft tissue sarcoma influences the treatment options; for instance, retroperitoneal tumors require an approach different from that for extremity tumors. The sites of soft tissue sarcomas from five reported series are presented in Table 2–1. In virtually all series of adult soft tissue sarcomas the extremities represent the predominant site of origin. Approximately 45% of soft tissue sarcomas occur in the lower extremity, 15% in the upper extremity, 15% in the retroperitoneum, 10% in the head and neck region, and nearly all the rest in the abdominal and chest walls. Visceral sarcomas, which arise from the connective tissue stroma found in all organs, account for a small number of cases. Although their overall behavior may be similar to that of sarcomas found elsewhere, treatment of a visceral sarcoma is highly dependent on the organ in which it is located.

## BIOPSY AND PREOPERATIVE EVALUATION

Both benign and malignant soft tissue tumors commonly present as a painless mass. There are no reliable findings on physical examination to indicate

**TABLE 2–1** ANATOMIC SITES OF SOFT TISSUE SARCOMAS, BASED ON LARGE SERIES

| Study | No., By Site | | | | | |
|---|---|---|---|---|---|---|
| | *Lower Extremity* | *Upper Extremity* | *Head and Neck* | *Trunk* | *Retroperitoneum* | *Total* |
| Abbas et al.[1] | 81 | 42 | 24 | 66 | 38 | 251 |
| Potter et al.[59] | 152 | 59 | 12 | 48 | 36 | 307 |
| Torosian et al.[88] | 208 | 81 | 21 | 92 | 90 | 492 |
| Lawrence et al.[42] | 2110 | 594 | 406 | 872 | 568 | 4550 |
| *Total* | 2551 (46%) | 776 (14%) | 463 (8%) | 1078 (19%) | 732 (13%) | 5600 (100%) |

whether a soft tissue mass is benign or malignant. Benign soft tissue tumors far outnumber their malignant counterparts. By virtue of these facts, prolonged delays before definitive treatment are common in patients with sarcoma. A survey of more than 5800 sarcoma patients revealed that about half waited at least 4 months before seeing a physician, and 20% experienced delays of 6 months or more *after* seeking treatment before a correct diagnosis was made.[42] Often sarcoma patients are diagnosed clinically as having a "chronic hematoma" or "pulled muscle" and undergo prolonged observation or treatment for these conditions. In fact, nonathletic adults rarely develop persistent soft tissue masses from either of these causes in the absence of a history of unusually strenuous activity or significant trauma unless they are on chronic anticoagulant therapy. These diagnoses should be entertained only in the setting of clear-cut local trauma or in the anticoagulated patient. When a soft tissue mass arises in a patient with no history of trauma or persists more than 6 weeks after local trauma, further evaluation or biopsy (or both) is usually indicated.

Virtually all soft tissue masses more than 5 cm in diameter and any new, enlarging or symptomatic lesions, should be biopsied. Only small subcutaneous lesions that have persisted unchanged for many years should be considered for observation rather than biopsy. The best way to avoid undue diagnostic delay during evaluation of a soft tissue mass is for the physician always to remain cognizant of the possibility of malignancy.

## Biopsy Techniques

Properly performed, a timely biopsy is the critical first step in a multimodality treatment approach. Improperly done, it can complicate patient care and sometimes even eliminate treatment options. Several biopsy techniques are available to the clinician: fine-needle aspiration, core-needle biopsy, incisional biopsy, and excisional biopsy. The choice of biopsy is dictated by the size and location of the mass and the experience of the pathologist. Excisional biopsy should be reserved for small (<3–5 cm in greatest diameter) and superficial soft tissue masses where the chance of malignancy is low and where complete excision would not jeopardize subsequent treatment in the event a sarcoma is found (Fig. 2–1).

*Fine-needle aspiration* (FNA) involves use of a fine-gauge needle (usually 21–23 gauge) to aspirate individual tumor cells from a mass. FNA cytology has a role to play in the diagnosis of some soft tissue lesions, but its use should be limited because even experienced cytopathologists are often unable to discern the grade and histologic type of a sarcoma from the small cellular sample of an aspirate.[8] The advantage of FNA is that it is relatively atraumatic and hence can be used to sample deep-seated tumors (e.g., retroperitoneal masses) under computed tomography (CT) guidance. FNA minimizes the potential for tumor spillage in the peritoneal cavity that can accompany open surgical biopsy of a retroperitoneal sarcoma. CT-guided FNA has proven helpful for diagnosing intraabdominal and retroperitoneal tumors but is rarely needed for extremity sarcomas. FNA biopsy is also acceptable for documenting local or distant recurrence in patients with a previously diagnosed sarcoma, where the cytology findings can be directly compared with the prior histology specimens.

*Core-needle biopsy* results in the retrieval of a thin sliver of tissue (approximately 1 × 10 mm). Here again, the small sample size may make it difficult for a pathologist to diagnose the tumor accurately, or the tissue obtained may not be representative of the entire tumor, leading to an underestimate of the grade. Tissue necessary for special stains or electron microscopy may not be available with this technique. Previously expressed fears that core-needle biopsy of extremity sarcomas would result in a significant number of hematomas—and hence the dissemination of tumor cells beyond the confines of the primary lesion—appear groundless. Several series have compared core-needle and open biopsies of soft tissue tumors and documented that both the histologic type and grade of a sarcoma could be correctly determined by core-needle biopsy in about 90% of cases.[5,6,34] Moreover, the core-needle biopsy approach is more

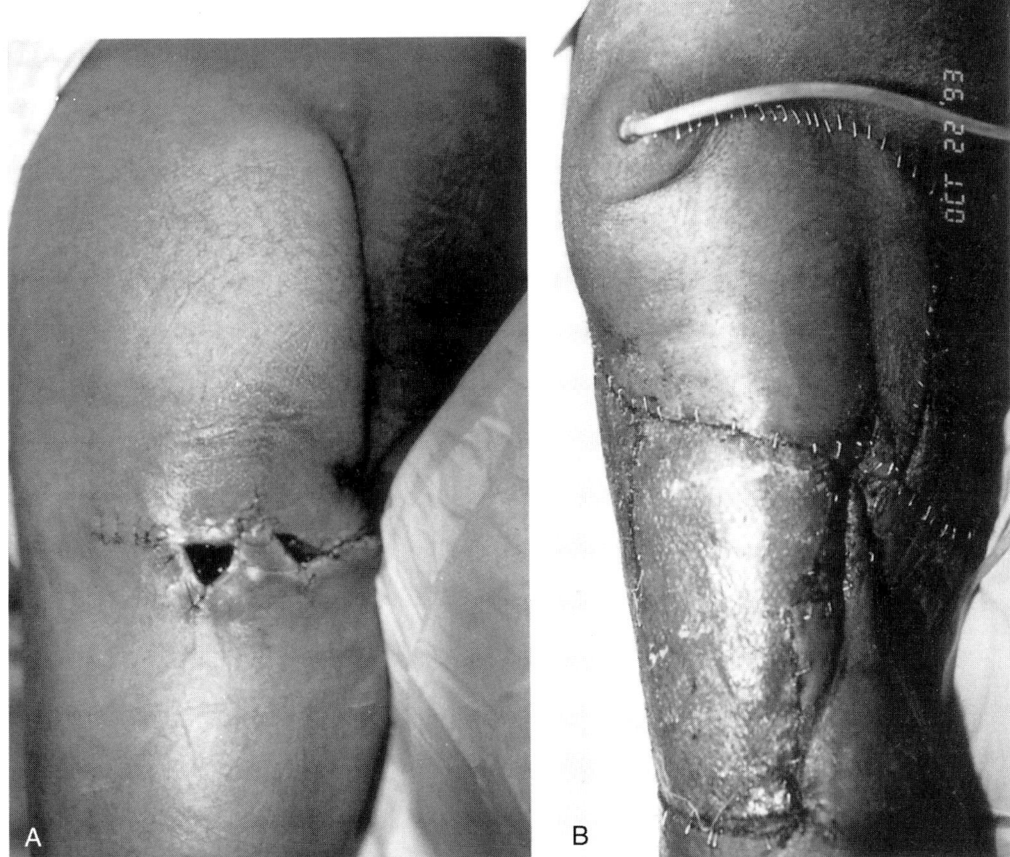


**FIGURE 2–1.** (**A**) Excisional biopsy was carried out on a large mass in the posterior compartment of the upper thigh using a transverse incision. The biopsy site subsequently became infected, leading to wound breakdown. The combination of the transverse orientation of the incision, the excisional biopsy with positive margins, and the postbiopsy wound complication significantly compromised the ability to carry out a definitive resection. (**B**) Ultimately, wide excision of the biopsy site, tumor bed, and surrounding normal tissue required reconstruction with a tensor fascia lata myocutaneous flap and split-thickness skin grafts.

cost-effective.[75] These results have encouraged wider use of this technique, including core-needle biopsies using CT guidance.[80]

*Excisional biopsy* refers to removal of the entire grossly evident lesion, usually without a significant margin of normal tissue. Many sarcomas appear to be encapsulated at the time of open biopsy. In actuality, these tumors have a "pseudocapsule" (Fig. 2–2), and removing the tumor through its pseudocapsule leaves gross or microscopic cancer behind in many cases.[31,50] "Shellout," or excisional biopsy, should be reserved for lesions less than 3–5 cm in diameter or for extremely superficial tumors. Excisional biopsies of large or deep sarcomas are undesirable as they can contaminate surrounding tissue planes, which may compromise the subsequent definitive surgical procedure (Fig. 2–1).

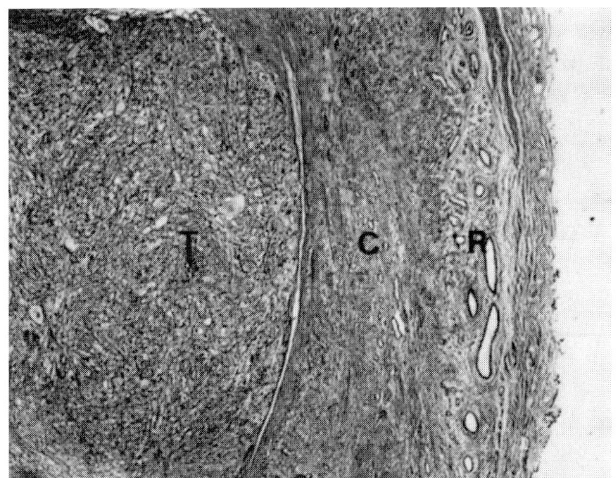


**FIGURE 2–2.** High-grade sarcoma tumor (T) surrounded by a pseudocapsule composed of a compression zone (C) and a reactive zone (R). (× 15)

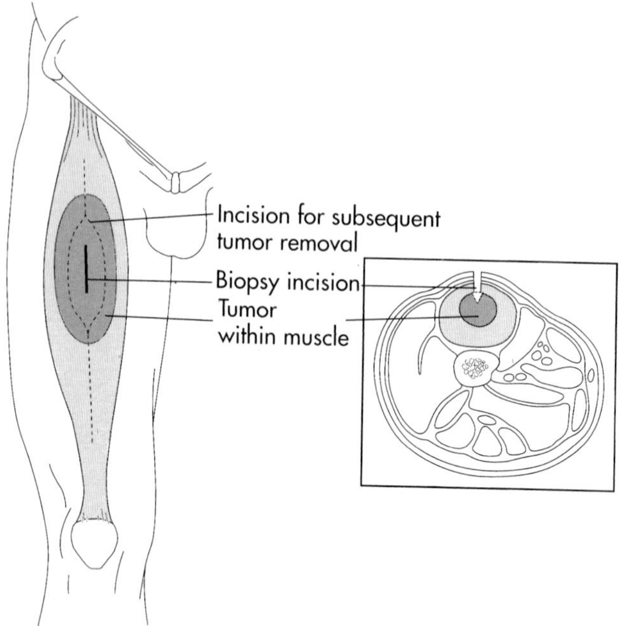


**FIGURE 2–3.** Technique for biopsy of an extremity soft tissue mass suspected of being a sarcoma. The mass should not be enucleated within the pseudocapsule; rather an incisional biopsy leaving the bulk of the lesion undisturbed should be carried out. (From Sondak VK. Sarcomas of bone and soft tissue. In Greenfield LJ, et al. (eds) Surgery: Scientific Principles and Practices. Lippincott, Philadelphia, 1993.)

*Incisional biopsy* involves removal of a generous wedge of tissue that is minimally manipulated at the time of surgery. There are several important technical factors when performing an incisional biopsy.[4,80] For extremity lesions, the incision is oriented along the long axis of the extremity. For truncal or retroperitoneal lesions, the biopsy incision is situated so it can be readily excised along with the tumor if a sarcoma is diagnosed. The biopsy site should be directly over the tumor, at the point where the lesion is closest to the surface, and there should be no raising of flaps or disturbance of tissue planes superficial to the tumor (Fig. 2–3). Prior to wound closure, careful attention is paid to hemostasis to minimize the likelihood of a hematoma, which could disseminate tumor cells through normal tissue planes. Drains are not used routinely; in the uncommon case where a drain is required, it should exit either through or near the biopsy incision. If malignancy is diagnosed, the drain tract must be excised in continuity with the tumor mass.

A *frozen section* examination at the time of biopsy can be useful for determining whether the specimen contains viable lesional tissue for examination, in contrast to nonviable tumor or nonlesional reactive tissue surrounding the tumor. Because of the subtle criteria necessary to distinguish benign from malignant soft tissue tumors and the importance of proper grade assignment, treatment planning (including definitive resection) is almost always deferred until a definitive report based on permanent sections is available.

## Staging and Preoperative Evaluation

### *GTNM Staging System*

Because of the prognostic importance of the histologic grade, the staging of soft tissue sarcomas is based on both clinical and histologic information. The familiar TNM classification is modified to a GTNM system (Table 2–2). This system was modified extensively and now incorporates the depth of the tumor relative to the investing muscular fascia as a criterion. Size $\leq$ 5 cm, superficial location, and low histologic grade are considered "favorable" factors. The T stage is assigned based on size (T1 $\leq$ 5; T2 $>$ 5 cm) and depth relative to the fascia (a, entirely above the fascia; b, invasion of or entirely below the fascia). Thus a 6 cm sarcoma located entirely in the subcutaneous tissue above the muscular fascia would be categorized as T2a, whereas the same tumor involving the fascia would be T2b. All intraabdominal and intrathoracic sarcomas are by definition "b" lesions. For the pur-

**TABLE 2–2 AMERICAN JOINT COMMISSION ON CANCER GTNM CLASSIFICATION AND STAGE GROUPING OF SOFT TISSUE SARCOMAS**

| | |
|---|---|
| **Tumor grade** | |
| G1 | Well differentiated |
| G2 | Moderately differentiated |
| G3 | Poorly differentiated |
| G4 | Undifferentiated |
| **Primary tumor** | |
| T1 | Tumor ≤ 5 cm in greatest diameter |
| T1a | Superficial tumor |
| T1b | Deep tumor |
| T2 | Tumor > 5 cm in greatest diameter |
| T2a | Superficial tumor |
| T2b | Deep tumor |
| **Regional lymph node involvement** | |
| N0 | No known metastases to lymph nodes |
| N1 | Verified metastases to lymph nodes |
| **Distant metastasis** | |
| M0 | No known distant metastasis |
| M1 | Known distant metastasis |
| **Stage grouping** | |
| Stage IA | Low grade, small (G1–2, T1a or b,N0,M0) |
| Stage IB | Low grade, large, superficial (G1–2, T2a,N0,M0) |
| Stage IIA | Low grade, large, deep (G1–2, T2b,N0,M0) |
| Stage IIB | High grade, small (G3–4, T1b,N0,M0) |
| Stage IIC | High grade, large, superficial G3–4, T2a,N0,M0 |
| Stage III | High grade, large, deep G3–4, T2b,N0,M0 |
| Stage IV | Nodal or distant metastases Any G, any T,N1,M0 or any G, any T, any N,M1 |

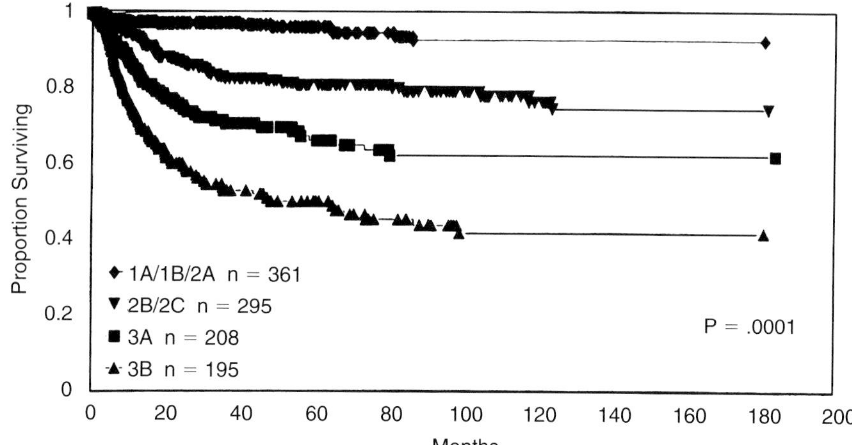


**FIGURE 2-4.** Overall survival for soft tissue sarcoma patients based on tumor grade, size, and depth at the time of presentation. Stage 3 tumors are further subdivided by size 5-10 cm (3A) or >10 cm (3B). (From Brennan MF. Staging of soft tissue sarcomas. Ann Surg Oncol 6:8, 1999.)

pose of staging, well differentiated and moderately differentiated tumors (grade 1 and grade 2, respectively) are considered together as "low grade," and poorly differentiated and undifferentiated tumors (grade 3 and grade 4, respectively) are considered together as "high grade." All small low grade tumors (regardless of depth) and all superficial low grade tumors (regardless of size) are classified as stage I. Stage II sarcomas are either low grade, large, and deep (stage IIA); high grade and small (stage IIB); or high grade, large, and superficial (stage IIC). All high grade, large, and deep sarcomas are stage III tumors. Any tumor with regional or distant metastatic disease, regardless of the grade of the primary tumor, is classified as stage IV. This staging system is clinically useful, as it distinguishes patients into groups with clearly differing prognoses (Fig. 2–4).

Some limitations of the current TNM system are apparent. The revised TNM system no longer recognizes any difference between well and moderately differentiated tumors, although there are significant data to suggest that grade 2 tumors fare worse than grade 1 lesions.[49] Regarding size, it is clear that the larger the primary sarcoma, the greater is the risk of metastasis and death.[55,62] Size is also a significant predictive factor with respect to the ability to achieve local control by surgery alone or with irradiation.[18,60,84] In the TNM system, tumors ≤ 5 cm in greatest diameter are classified as T1, and tumors > 5 cm are classified as T2. Although the GTNM size cutoff is 5 cm, tumors > 10 cm have an even worse prognosis.[11,62] Table 2–3 documents the correlation between tumor size and 5-year disease-free survival rates in patients with intermediate and high grade sarcomas that were locally controlled by surgery and irradiation. (It is of note that in the same series from which Table 2–3 was taken none of 38 grade 1 tumors that were successfully controlled locally developed distant metastases within 5 years.[84]) Future versions of the staging system could incorporate more than two T categories to reflect the variations in prognosis more accurately with increasing size. Also, the current TNM system appropriately recognizes that superficially located tumors (i.e., those situated entirely

**TABLE 2–3** FIVE-YEAR DISEASE-FREE SURVIVAL RATES BY TUMOR SIZE FOR PATIENTS WITH INTERMEDIATE AND HIGH GRADE SARCOMAS TREATED WITH SURGERY AND IRRADIATION

| Tumor Size (cm) | No. of Patients* | % Disease-free at 5 Years |
|---|---|---|
| <2.5 | 17 | 94 |
| 2.6–4.9 | 48 | 77 |
| 5.0–10.0 | 55 | 62 |
| 10.1–15.0 | 24 | 51 |
| 15.1–20.0 | 9 | 42 |
| >20.0 | 6 | 17 |
| *Total* | 159 | 65 |

From Suit HD, Mankin HJ, Wood WC, et al. Treatment of the patient with stage M0 soft tissue sarcoma. J Clin Oncol 6:854, 1988.

*Only patients in whom local control was achieved were included.

above the deep or muscular fascia of the body) have a more favorable prognosis. One recent series of 215 patients with superficial extremity sarcomas documented a 10-year survival rate of 85% despite the fact that 53% of tumors were high grade and 25% were ≥5 cm.[12] The relation between size, grade, depth, and prognosis has not been fully defined. Specifically, confirmation that a small, superficial high grade sarcoma (stage IIB) truly has a prognosis similar to that of a large, deep, low grade tumor (stage IIA) or a large, superficial high grade sarcoma (stage IIC) is needed.

Regional lymph node involvement is uncommon in soft tissue sarcomas, with fewer than 4% of cases having nodal metastases at presentation. When node involvement occurs, it conveys essentially the same prognosis as distant metastatic disease and is therefore classified as stage IV (Fig. 2–5). In a review of more than 2500 patients in the world literature, the incidence of lymph node metastases from each of the major histologic types of soft tissue sarcomas was analyzed.[90] Only 5% of patients with soft tissue sarcomas developed nodal metastases at any point in the course of their disease. The incidence of lymph node metastases was slightly higher in epithelioid sarcomas, rhabdomyosarcomas, and clear cell sarcomas than in other histologic types. Similar findings were noted in a review of a large, prospective sarcoma database containing 1772 patients.[29] Forty-six patients (2.6%) developed lymph node metastases at some time during their lives. All but 1 of the 46 patients had a high grade primary tumor, with epithelioid sarcomas, embryonal rhabdomyosarcomas, and angiosarcomas being the histologic types most often associated with nodal involvement (13–17%). Because of the rarity of lymphatic involvement by sarcoma at the time of presentation, the differential diagnosis of spindle cell tumors presenting with lymph node metastases should always include carcinoma and melanoma.

### *Preoperative Evaluation*

Once a diagnosis of sarcoma is established, the extent of the primary tumor must be assessed and a search for the presence of metastatic disease conducted. Physical examination is important when determining the size of the tumor, any fixation to adjacent structures, the relation of the tumor to the biopsy site, the functional status of the involved part, lymph node involvement, and any confounding conditions that could compromise optimal surgical or radiation treatment. Distant metastatic disease is found in a significant number of patients with soft tissue tumors at the time of presentation. Two large-scale surveys, together comprising about 13,500 patients with soft tissue sarcomas, found that 20–23% of patients had evidence of metastases at the time of presentation.[42,58] By far the most frequent site of metastases is the lungs. In extremity sarcoma patients who ever develop metastases, the lungs are involved more than 75% of the time. About half of all sarcoma patients who die of metastatic disease have lung metastases as their only site of distant spread. Liver involvement is rare except in intraabdominal and retroperitoneal sarcomas. In one series, 61 of 65 patients (94%) with hepatic metastases from sarcoma had intraabdominal primary tumors, mostly leiomyosarcoma.[36] Occasional patients develop bone or central nervous system metastases; these sites are uncommon in patients who do not already have lung metastases.[59]

For patients with a newly diagnosed soft tissue sarcoma, a chest radiograph and chest CT scan are appropriate to search for pulmonary metastases. For intraabdominal or retroperitoneal tumors, a CT scan that includes the liver should be added. Other studies

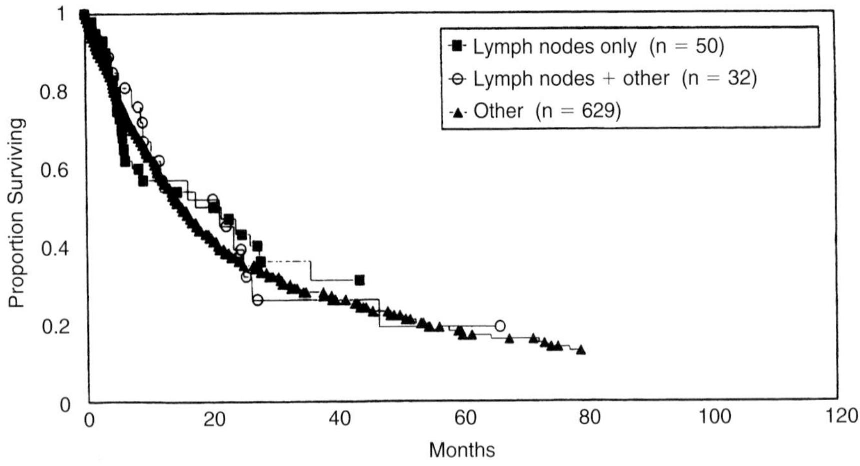


**FIGURE 2–5.** Disease-specific survival for 711 patients with soft tissue sarcoma metastatic to lymph nodes alone, lymph nodes and other distant sites, or non-lymph-node distant sites only. (From Brennan MF. Staging of soft tissue sarcomas. Ann Surg Oncol 6:8, 1999.)

aimed at detecting metastases, such as radionuclide bone scans, CT scans, and magnetic resonance imaging (MRI) of the head, are not indicated in the absence of symptoms suggestive of metastatic involvement.

In addition to assessing prognosis, the initial evaluation provides information about the extent of the primary tumor. Bone films can indicate cortical bone destruction or that the mass is a primary bone tumor rather than a soft tissue tumor.[40] Tumors adjacent to bone may result in a periosteal reaction, which can be detected by a bone scan.[25] In most cases, because soft tissue sarcomas rarely invade bone, neither plain radiographs of the bone nor bone scans prove helpful. CT scans and MRI are the most important radiologic studies for assessing the extent and resectability of soft tissue sarcomas, regardless of the site of origin. These studies permit definition of the primary tumor in relation to bone, muscle, neurovascular structures, and adjacent organs—critical information when planning treatment. Both CT scans and MRI can provide this information, and in most cases either study alone is sufficient. The choice between them is based primarily on availability, cost, and the experience of the radiologist. The advantages and disadvantages of each modality should be considered on a case-by-case basis.

Computed tomography is widely available, and both the primary site and the lungs (the major site of metastasis) can be imaged during the same session. Most radiologists have more experience reading CT scans than magnetic resonance (MR) images. Tumor involvement of bone is generally more clearly discernible on CT scan, whereas bone marrow invasion can be better defined by MRI. Disadvantages of CT scanning include the ionizing radiation and the need for iodinated contrast administration.

Magnetic resonance imaging has several advantages when evaluating a primary sarcoma. The plane of imaging is not limited to the transverse (axial) plane of CT scanning. Coronal, sagittal and even oblique planes may be imaged. Comparative studies have also suggested that MR scans may better define the relation between tumor and muscle.[10,16] Because of the strong magnetic fields required, MRI may not be feasible for patients with implanted metallic objects, such as pacemakers, artificial joints, or some vena caval filters. Although the information obtained from CT scans and MRI of the primary tumor is occasionally complementary, for most patients either study alone suffices.

Sarcomas have a characteristic arteriographic appearance, with prominent neovascularity and displacement of normal vessels. Angiography is rarely necessary for extremity lesions, although it may be useful for some retroperitoneal tumors. Increasingly, information on the proximity of a tumor to major vessels, once provided by angiography, is now being obtained from specially sequenced MRI (*magnetic resonance angiography*) (Fig. 2–6).[40]

Recently, a consortium of sarcoma experts undertook to establish guidelines for the preoperative and postoperative (follow-up) evaluation of patients with soft tissue sarcomas.[20] Although beyond the scope of this chapter, the reader is referred to these guidelines as a resource for cost-effective patient management.

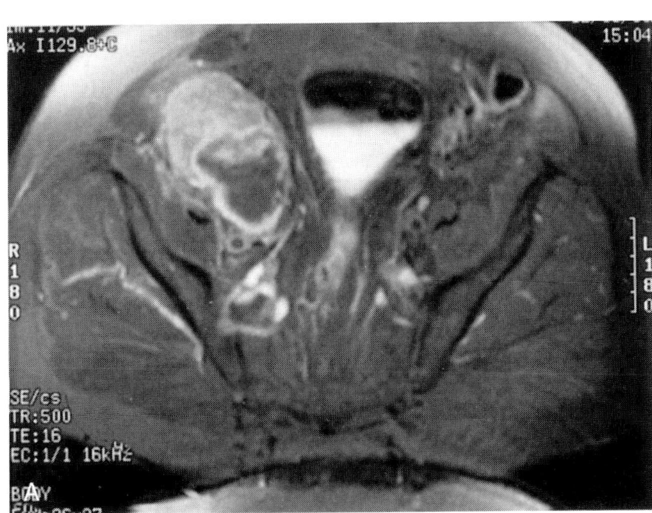


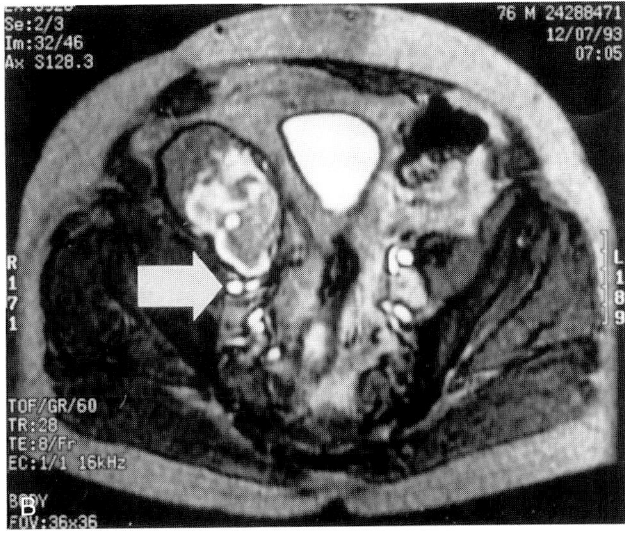


**FIGURE 2–6.** (**A**) Standard magnetic resonance scan of a recurrent soft tissue sarcoma in the pelvic retroperitoneum. (**B**) Magnetic resonance angiography was performed to determine the relation of the tumor to the iliac vessels (*arrow*) more precisely.

## NATURAL HISTORY

### Local Recurrence

One of the major clinical problems when treating soft tissue sarcomas is the propensity of the primary tumor to recur locally. Soft tissue sarcomas enlarge in a centrifugal fashion and compress normal tissue, giving the appearance of encapsulation. This pseudocapsule is actually composed of an inner compressed rim of normal tissue (compression zone) and an outer rim of edema and small newly formed vessels (reactive zone) (Fig. 2–2). Fingers of tumor can extend into and through this pseudocapsule and give rise to satellite lesions. Although the pseudocapsule provides surgeons with a tempting plane for dissection and invites a shellout procedure, such an excision leaves microscopic and often gross tumor in the wound.[31,50] Excision of any sarcoma in the pseudocapsule is inadequate therapy and results in the development of local recurrences in up to 90% of patients.

The site of a soft tissue sarcoma can certainly influence the technical ease with which resectability can be accomplished; hence it affects the potential for local control. For instance, lesions of the head and neck regions, where abutment to vital structures is often the case, are less likely to be controlled than lesions in the extremities.[89] In the extremity, the site of the tumor may also have prognostic implications. Local control may be more difficult to achieve for proximal tumors than those more distally located, possibly because they achieve a larger size before detection. Simon and Enneking[72] reported local recurrences following surgery alone in the buttock, groin, thigh, and areas below the knee to be 38%, 14%, 15%, and 0%, respectively. Potter et al.[60] reported that among 115 patients with thigh sarcomas disease-free and overall survival was significantly worse for patients with tumor spread into the upper half of the thigh than for those with involvement limited to the distal thigh. In contrast, Yang et al.[93] found that patients undergoing multimodality treatment for sarcomas in the popliteal, axillary, or antecubital fossae had local control and overall survival rates similar to those for patients with purely intracompartmental extremity tumors. Hence, the significance of location in the extremity may be less with multimodality therapy than with surgery alone.

The time to local recurrence following surgery follows a predictable pattern. In one series of patients treated with surgery alone, approximately 80% of all lesions that were destined to recur locally did so within 2 years (Fig. 2–7).[13] Simon and Enneking[72] reported that all of the local recurrences seen in 54 patients they treated surgically occurred within 30 months of resection. The impact of adjuvant therapy on local recurrence is discussed later in the chapter.

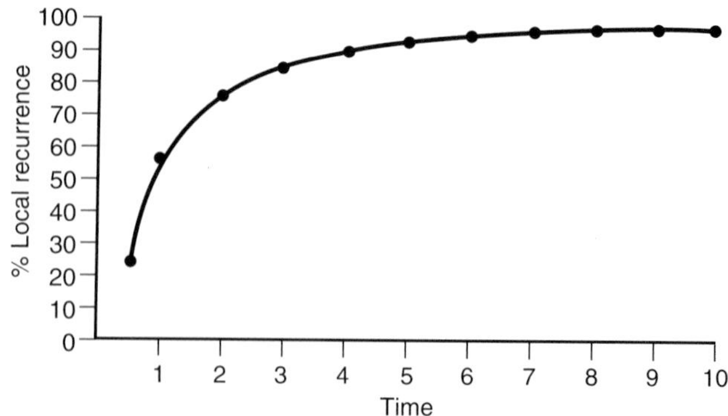


**FIGURE 2–7.** Percentage of local recurrences versus time from definitive surgery for soft tissue sarcomas. (Adapted from Cantin J, McNeer GP, Chu FC, Booher RJ. The problem of local recurrence after treatment of soft tissue sarcoma. Ann Surg 168:47, 1968.)

Isolated local recurrences of soft tissue sarcomas, regardless of site, should be considered for further resection. A thorough evaluation for the presence of disseminated disease should be performed before contemplating resection of a local recurrence. In one series of patients, 20 of 21 (96%) isolated local recurrences were surgically resectable.[59] Figure 2–8**A** shows the actuarial continuous disease-free survival rate for the 20 patients who underwent resection of isolated local recurrences: 7 patients developed subsequent tumor recurrences. The median disease-free interval had not been reached. Figure 2–8**B** shows a 69% actuarial 3-year survival rate for these 20 patients. This encouraging long-term survival rate after resection of isolated local recurrence has been documented by other investigators as well.[35,48] Moreover, limb-sparing resection of locally recurrent extremity sarcomas is often feasible. In a series of 52 patients with locally recurrent extremity sarcomas, 75% underwent successful resection without amputation.[48]

### Distant Metastasis

Despite adequate local control of the primary lesion, many patients with high grade and a few patients with low grade soft tissue sarcomas succumb to metastatic disease. Although most patients with soft tissue sarcomas present without obvious metastases, many harbor occult micrometastases that eventually become clinically evident. These patients represent a population who could benefit from adjuvant systemic chemotherapy along with removal of the primary tumor (this topic is presented in more detail later).

As with local recurrence, the incidence and pattern of distant metastasis depends on the site of the primary sarcoma. Potter et al.[59] analyzed 307 patients who underwent complete resection of high-grade sarcomas followed by irradiation and chemotherapy. A

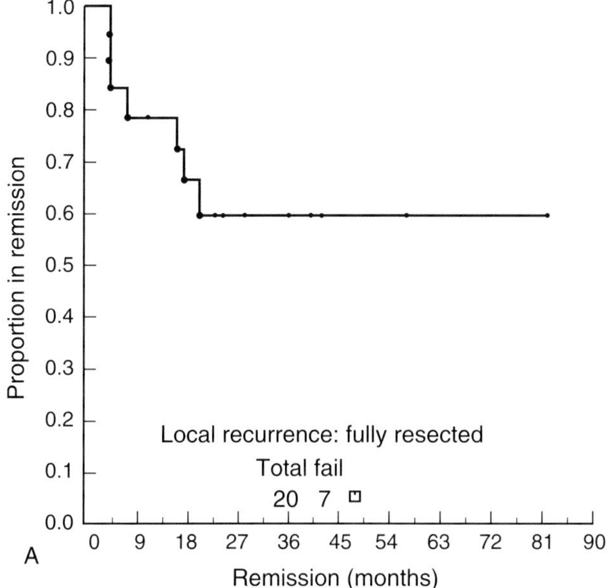


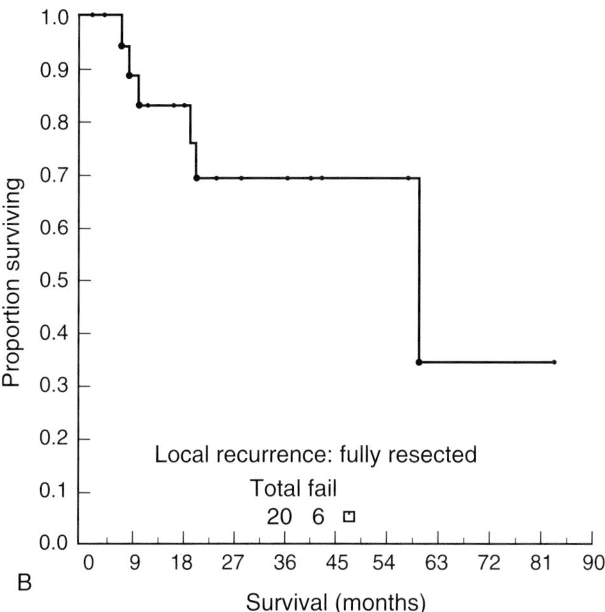


**FIGURE 2–8.** Disease-free survival (**A**) and overall survival (**B**) in patients rendered free of disease after resection of isolated locally recurrent sarcoma. (From Potter DA, Glenn J, Kinsella T, et al. Patterns of recurrence in patients with high-grade soft-tissue sarcomas. J Clin Oncol 3:353, 1985.)

total of 107 patients (35%) developed local recurrence or distant metastases; they are listed in Table 2–4 according to the site of the primary tumor. The predominant site of first recurrence was in the lung, seen in 52% of patients who developed local or distant disease (70% of patients with extremity primaries). Patients with retroperitoneal sarcomas had a greater tendency for local recurrence and disseminated disease throughout the abdomen. Patients with head and neck and truncal sarcomas had a higher local recurrence rate than those with extremity sarcomas. Treatment options for patients with metastatic disease include surgical resection if the tumor is localized to one organ system or systemic cytotoxic chemotherapy if it is not. These treatment options are discussed in detail later in this chapter.

## TREATMENT OF LOCALIZED TUMORS

Benign soft tissue tumors require only complete local excision for adequate treatment. By contrast, a variety of treatment approaches to localized primary and recurrent sarcomas have been reported, including surgery alone or in combination with irradiation or chemotherapy.

### Extremity Sarcomas

#### *Surgical Therapy*

Surgery is the mainstay of any treatment approach for a clinically localized primary or recurrent soft tissue sarcoma. As has been described, however, removal of the gross tumor mass from within its pseudocapsule is associated with a prohibitively high likelihood of local recurrence. With the appreciation of the infiltrative nature of these tumors, radical procedures such as amputation came to be accepted as the standard for surgical therapy. Enneking classified surgical procedures for extremity sarcomas according to the margins achieved.[24] He described four types of excision.

1. *Intracapsular excisions* are performed inside the pseudocapsule and are often piecemeal in nature. An amputation that passes within the pseudocapsule is called an *intracapsular amputation.* The likelihood of local recurrence with intracapsular procedures is virtually 100%.
2. *Marginal excisions* are en bloc resections performed through the reactive zone (pseudocapsule) surrounding the tumor. Excisional biopsies and "shellout" procedures fall into this category. An amputation performed through this marginal zone is called a *marginal amputation.* Local recurrences are expected 60–80% of the time.
3. *Wide excisions* are en bloc resections done through normal tissue beyond the reactive zone but within the muscular compartment of origin, leaving in place some portion of that compartment. The pseudocapsule is removed en bloc, and the tumor is never visualized during the procedure. The reported local recurrence rate following wide excision alone varies depending on

**TABLE 2–4 PATTERNS OF LOCAL RECURRENCE AND METASTASIS IN PATIENTS WITH HIGH GRADE SOFT TISSUE SARCOMAS BY SITE OF PRIMARY TUMOR**

| | Site of Primary Tumor | | | | | |
|---|---|---|---|---|---|---|
| **Site of Initial Failure** | ***Extremity*** | ***Breast*** | ***Head and Neck*** | ***Trunk*** | ***Retroperitoneum*** | ***Total*** |
| Isolated local recurrence | 7 (10%) | 0 | 2 (50%) | 7 (41%) | 5 (30%) | 21 (20%) |
| Isolated lung metastases | 43 (70%) | 3 (75%) | 2 (50%) | 5 (29%) | 3 (17%) | 56 (52%) |
| Isolated other metastases | 11 (15%) | 1 (25%) | 0 | 2 (12%) | 1 (6%) | 15 (14%) |
| Multiple sites | 4 (5%) | 0 | 0 | 3 (18%) | 8 (47%) | 15 (14%) |
| *Total* | 65 | 4 | 4 | 17 | 17 | 107 (100%) |

From Potter DA, Glenn J, Kinsella T, et al. Patterns of recurrence in patients with high grade soft-tissue sarcomas. J Clin Oncol 3:353, 1985.

selection criteria and the adequacy of the margin as assessed histologically, but overall it is approximately 30%. An amputation can be considered a *wide amputation* if it is performed through normal tissue proximal to the reactive zone but remains within the compartment of involvement.

4. *Radical excisions* are en bloc resections of the tumor and the entire compartment of origin, leaving no remnant of the compartment intact. A *radical amputation* usually requires disarticulation of the joint proximal to the involved compartment and results in removal of the entire compartment at risk. Local recurrence rates are the lowest with these procedures and are discussed below.

The following surgical procedures are commonly employed when radical excision is chosen, generally as the sole modality of treatment for extremity soft tissue sarcomas.

## COMPARTMENT EXCISIONS

For tumors that arise entirely within an anatomically defined muscular compartment, excision of the muscles comprising that compartment from origin to insertion is often successful in achieving local control. The thigh, which is the site of more than 50% of all extremity sarcomas, has three major compartments bound by the fascia lata and its extensions. The anterior compartment includes primarily the quadriceps and sartorius muscles, which can be removed along with the femoral nerve. An anterior compartment excision results in knee weakness and instability, which can be improved with the use of the transplanted gracilis and short head of the biceps. Even without such reconstruction, patients can ambulate after an anterior compartment excision by using the hip flexors to throw the leg forward; gait is improved with the use of a locking knee brace. The medial thigh compartment consists of the gracilis, adductors (minimus, brevis, longus, and magnus), and pectineus muscles. Medial compartment excision is generally well tolerated, with only limited functional deficit. Posterior compartment excision removes the hamstring muscles (semimembranosus and semitendinosus and biceps femoris), as well as the posterior portion of the adductor magnus muscle. Ambulation is surprisingly well maintained after this surgery, with knee flexion brought about by the action of the gracilis and soleus muscles on the distal femur. Buttockectomy entails removal of the entire gluteus maximus muscle for tumors localized entirely within this muscle.

## RADICAL AMPUTATIONS

Below-knee amputation is performed through the tibia and fibula and allows a stump to be used for fitting a prosthetic device. Rehabilitation from this procedure is usually satisfactory. Below-knee amputation is the radical resection for any soft tissue sarcoma of the foot. Above-knee amputation can be performed at any level distal to the lesser trochanter to allow enough stump for a prosthesis. This amputation does not constitute a radical excision for tumors above the knee, as the entire compartment is not removed. Hip disarticulation entails complete removal of the femur at the hip joint. Most muscles attached to the lower extremity are removed in their entirety. This procedure constitutes one option for radical excision for patients with lesions of the middle and lower thigh. Hemipelvectomy involves removal of the entire lower extremity and hemipelvis, with disarticulation of the sacroiliac joint and pubic symphysis. This procedure is a radical amputation for patients with proximal thigh and buttock tumors. The standard hemipelvectomy utilizes a posterior flap of skin and subcutaneous tissue overlying the buttock. For buttock and posterior thigh lesions, it is possible to construct an anterior myocutaneous flap based on the quadriceps muscles and superficial femoral artery to cover the surgical defect. Modified hemipelvectomy preserves the iliac wing, which allows improved patient rehabilitation. It is similar to the standard hemipelvectomy except the sacroiliac joint is preserved and the iliac bone is divided below the level of the

**TABLE 2–5** LOCAL CONTROL AND AMPUTATION RATES IN PATIENTS WITH SOFT TISSUE SARCOMAS OF THE EXTREMITY TREATED WITH RADICAL SURGERY AS THE SOLE MODALITY OF THERAPY

| Parameter | Simon and Enneking[72] | Shiu et al.[71] |
|---|---|---|
| Total no. of patients | 54 | 297 |
| Radical compartment excision | 25 (46%) | 158 (53%) |
| Radical amputation | 29 (54%) | 139 (47%) |
| Patients with local control | | |
| Radical compartment excision | 88% | 72% |
| Radical amputation | 79% | 93% |
| Overall | 83% | 82% |

sciatic notch. Because this involves transection of muscles in the buttock, it is not suitable for lesions in this area. Internal hemipelvectomy is not generally employed for soft tissue tumors; it involves removal of the hemipelvis without amputation of the extremity and can be useful for management of bony tumors of the hemipelvis.[3]

For tumors of the hand and wrist requiring radical amputation, below-elbow amputation is used. Above-elbow amputation is used for tumors of the forearm. Shoulder disarticulation is reserved for distal arm and elbow lesions. Forequarter amputation (interscapulothoracic amputation) is applied to the treatment of lesions of the axilla, shoulder girdle, or proximal arm. This procedure includes removal of the entire upper extremity along with the scapula and clavicle. Detailed descriptions of all these procedures are provided in atlases devoted to soft tissue tumor surgery.[9,21,83]

The means required to achieve a radical excision depend in part on the anatomic location of the tumor and its size. Many tumors of the extremities are not located in distinct anatomic compartments, and hence a radical excision cannot be achieved except by amputation. Similarly, large tumors localized to one compartment but that abut bone or major neurovascular structures cannot be radically excised without amputation. A radical excision, as defined by Enneking, is ***not*** required for all sarcomas. With the use of adjuvant radiation therapy, local control rates with less radical resections have improved and match those achievable with radical surgery. Currently, wide excision is the procedure of choice for low grade sarcomas or higher grade tumors that are to be treated with multimodality therapy. Marginal excision is frequently all that can be achieved for treatment of retroperitoneal and head and neck sarcomas; intracapsular excision is not generally performed except for the occasional low grade tumor for which any other type of excision would cause an unacceptable loss of function. Adjuvant irradiation should almost always be considered when tumors must be treated with marginal or intracapsular excisions.

The experiences of Shiu et al.[71] and Simon and Enneking[72] using radical surgical procedures as single modality therapy are summarized in Table 2–5. Overall local control was obtained in approximately 80% of patients undergoing radical resection, regardless of whether amputation was performed. Unfortunately, even a "radical" excision is not always associated with an adequate margin when the resected specimen is examined histologically. When histologic evaluation verified that adequate margins were obtained with the radical procedure, the local failure rate was 5% (Table 2–6). If microscopic tumor was found at or within 1 mm of the surgical margin, the

**TABLE 2–6** LOCAL FAILURE RATES AFTER RADICAL EXCISION WITH HISTOLOGICALLY NEGATIVE VERSUS POSITIVE MARGINS

| | No. of Local Failures/Total No. of Patients | |
|---|---|---|
| **Study** | ***Negative Margins*** | ***Positive Margins*** |
| Simon and Enneking[72] | 1/46 | 8/8 |
| Markhede et al.[45] | 5/76 | 16/19 |
| *Total* | 6/122 (5%) | 24/27 (89%) |

local failure rate rose to 89%. Inadequate margins were most commonly associated with large proximal thigh and groin tumors. More distal extremity tumors rarely had tumor at or close to the surgical margin after appropriate radical excision, and the local control rate can be expected to approach 100% after radical amputation of distal extremity sarcomas.[52]

Although radical excisions that achieve a histologically negative margin are associated with high rates of local tumor control, the functional, psychological, and cosmetic costs can be high.[77] For this reason, radical surgery as single modality therapy has gradually been replaced by more conservative resection performed as part of multidisciplinary, multimodality treatment approaches. Nowhere is this trend more evident than during treatment of extremity soft tissue sarcomas with multimodality, limb-sparing therapy.

### LIMB-SPARING PROCEDURES

Rosenberg et al. compared radical amputation to wide local excision plus postoperative irradiation in a prospective, randomized trial. Patients who underwent limb-sparing surgery had a survival rate identical to those undergoing amputation, despite a slightly higher local recurrence rate (19% vs. 6%, a difference that was not statistically significant).[66] This study demonstrated the merit of limb-sparing approaches to extremity sarcomas. Radical amputation is currently reserved for patients who are not suitable candidates for limb-sparing approaches, usually because of abutment to bone or major neurovascular structures or an extremely large tumor size. It is of note that the location of the tumor distally in the extremity (hand or foot) is not necessarily an indication for amputation. Local control with acceptable function can be achieved with limb-sparing approaches in most of these cases.[37,70]

Most current limb-salvage protocols include wide excision as the definitive surgical procedure. Wide excision involves gross total removal of the tumor with a wide margin of normal tissue, but no attempt is made to resect an entire muscle compartment. Rather, a margin of 3–5 cm of normal tissue is obtained proximally and distally. It includes excision of some overlying skin to encompass all previous scars or biopsy sites. Tumor should not be visualized during the excision so tumor cells are not spilled into the surgical bed. On the lateral and deep margins, at least one grossly uninvolved fascial plane is resected en bloc with the tumor. For large or deep-seated tumors, resection of uninvolved periosteum or adventitia may represent the deep margin. Removal of periosteum should be limited to areas directly abutting tumor to minimize the likelihood of postirradiation pathologic fracture.[44] If necessary, major vascular structures may be resected and reconstructed with graft material. On occasion, major nerves (e.g., sciatic nerve) are sacrificed to preserve a functional albeit neurologically compromised extremity. Because of their less aggressive nature, when low grade lesions are resected major vessels or nerves are not taken along with the tumor. Placement of titanium clips outlining the limits of the excision is essential as a guide to the radiation therapist for constructing the radiation treatment portal. Suction catheters are placed at the end of the dissection to allow evacuation of any blood and serous fluid from the operative bed and to promote the adherence of skin flaps.

The use of multimodality therapy (particularly preoperatively) is associated with a high incidence of wound complications.[51] These complications can be disastrous in an irradiated wound or if major vessels, nerves or bone become exposed. To minimize the likelihood of wound breakdown, consideration should always be given to reconstructing the surgical defect with free or pedicled myocutaneous flaps. Barwick et al.[7] articulated the criteria for primary closure of a wide excision wound in patients undergoing multimodality therapy: The skin edges should be approximated without tension, and the resection site must not have exposed bone, nerve, blood vessel, or tendon present. If the skin edges cannot be approximately without tension but the base of the resection is entirely muscle, a split-thickness skin graft should be applied; otherwise, a flap reconstruction is performed. Irradiated wounds in the trunk and retroperitoneum may present a formidable technical challenge to the reconstructive surgeon.[41]

## *Radiation Therapy*

For patients with small, superficial or low-grade tumors, wide local excision alone is associated with a low rate of local recurrence.[68] Most other patients undergoing surgical excision receive additional therapy to improve the chances for local control. In most cases this additional therapy includes irradiation. Irradiation has been shown to be effective as sole therapy for extremity sarcomas in patients who refused or could not tolerate surgery. Of 26 patients treated with radiation alone (dose 65 Gy; 100 rad = 1 Gy), a local control rate of 61% was achieved at 4 years.[86] Although treatment with radiation alone was not as successful as treatment with radical surgery, the success rate was high enough to argue strongly for including radiation therapy in multimodality treatment approaches.

### POSTOPERATIVE RADIATION THERAPY

Postoperative radiation therapy after wide excision provides excellent local control for primary extremity sarcomas up to 10 cm in size. The randomized trial of amputation versus wide local excision previously cited validated the concept of limb-sparing surgery combined with postoperative irradiation.[66] Generally, a total of 60 Gy or more is required to ensure local control. At these dose levels the entire circumference of the extremity must not be irradiated, in order to avoid massive lymphedema. In practice, a strip of skin and subcutaneous tissue away from the tumor is excluded from the treatment field to prevent this complication.

Radiation can also be delivered to the tumor bed postoperatively by means of implanted radioactive sources, a technique referred to as *brachytherapy*. This approach has the advantage of a much shorter time to initiation and completion of therapy (usually begun within a week of operation and completed in 4–5 days, compared with 6–7 weeks of external beam radiation beginning a month or more postoperatively). On the other hand, brachytherapy is technically complex and requires the presence of an experienced radiation oncologist in the operating room. A randomized trial demonstrated a significant decrease in local recurrences for high grade sarcomas after combined surgery and postoperative brachytherapy compared with surgery alone.[54] Patients with low grade sarcomas did not benefit from adjuvant brachytherapy, although a recent randomized trial showed that external beam radiation effectively decreased local recurrence of these tumors.[91] Otherwise, brachytherapy and external beam radiation appear to be equivalent when properly administered. The data from these two randomized trials provide strong support for the routine inclusion of radiation therapy (by some technique) in all patients with high grade, and many if not most patients with low grade, extremity sarcomas undergoing limb-sparing surgery.

#### PREOPERATIVE RADIATION THERAPY

Preoperative irradiation followed by conservative surgery offers several theoretic advantages. The treatment volume is restricted to the known or probable extension of tumor. This means that a smaller volume can be treated than is the case with postoperative irradiation, as the latter must cover all tissues manipulated or handled during the surgical procedure. The resection may be of a lesser magnitude if tumor regression is obtained with preoperative irradiation. Seeding the surgical bed with viable tumor cells may be reduced. Several centers have used this approach; local control rates for large tumors appear to be improved with preoperative treatment (Table 2–7), and in some cases tumors initially considered unresectable without amputation shrank sufficiently to permit limb-sparing resection.[57,84]

Enneking and McAuliffe[26] have reported their experience utilizing preoperative irradiation followed by wide or marginal resection of low and high grade extremity sarcomas. They compared their results with comparably staged, matched controls who underwent either a limb-sparing procedure or amputation without preoperative irradiation (Table 2–8). Local recurrence rates were highest in the group undergoing limb-sparing surgery alone (37%) and were significantly higher than in those undergoing preoperative irradiation plus surgery (5%). In the same series, patients undergoing limb-sparing procedures reported substantially better postoperative function than those with amputation. The use of preoperative treatment for large extremity sarcomas has increased the number of patients who can be considered for limb-sparing surgery.

### Adjuvant Chemotherapy

Although multimodality treatments achieve local control without amputation in a large percentage of patients with intermediate and high grade soft tissue sarcomas, metastatic disease ultimately develops and

**TABLE 2–7** LOCAL CONTROL RATES 5 YEARS AFTER WIDE EXCISION WITH POSTOPERATIVE VERSUS PREOPERATIVE EXTERNAL BEAM IRRADIATION

| | Postoperative Irradiation | | Preoperative Irradiation | |
|---|---|---|---|---|
| Tumor Size (cm) | *No. of Patients* | *% Locally Controlled* | *No. of Patients* | *% Locally Controlled* |
| <2.5 | 14 | 82 | 5 | 100 |
| 2.6–4.9 | 45 | 85 | 9 | 89 |
| 5.0–10.0 | 29 | 84 | 32 | 91 |
| 10.1–15.0 | 8 | 83 | 17 | 100 |
| 15.1–20.0 | 5 | 0 | 9 | 73 |
| >20.0 | 1 | 0 | 6 | 100 |
| *Total* | 102 | 80 | 78 | 92 |

From Suit HD, Mankin HJ, Wood WC, et al. Treatment of the patient with stage M0 soft tissue sarcoma. J Clin Oncol 6: 854, 1988.
Note: Allocation to therapy was by physician choice, not randomization.

**TABLE 2–8 OUTCOMES FOR EXTREMITY SARCOMA PATIENTS AFTER PREOPERATIVE IRRADIATION/ WIDE OR MARGINAL EXCISION COMPARED TO STAGE-MATCHED PATIENTS WITH AMPUTATION OR WIDE OR MARGINAL EXCISION WITHOUT IRRADIATION**

| Type of Treatment | No. of Patients | Local Recurrence | Disease-free Survival | Satisfactory Function |
|---|---|---|---|---|
| Amputation/no irradiation | 16 | 2 (13%) | 11 (69%) | 2 (13%) |
| Wide or marginal excision/no irradiation | 19 | 7 (37%)* | 7 (37%) | 13 (68%) |
| Excision/preoperative irradiation | 19 | 1 (5%) | 11 (58%) | 12 (63%) |

From Enneking WF, McAuliffe JA. Adjunctive preoperative radiation therapy in treatment of soft tissue sarcomas: a preliminary report. Cancer Treat Symp 3:37, 1985.
* $p < 0.05$ compared with preoperative irradiation plus excision; not significantly different from amputation group.

results in the death of about 50% of patients in most reported series (Fig. 2–9). This figure is even higher if only stage III (large, high grade, deep) tumors are considered. For this reason, the use of effective systemic adjuvant chemotherapy would be desirable following definitive treatment of local disease. Indeed, adjuvant chemotherapy is now the standard for patients with localized extremity osteosarcomas and has been repeatedly shown to increase overall survival. To date, however, conclusive evidence that administration of adjuvant chemotherapy to patients with localized extremity sarcomas can increase overall survival is lacking. Several prospective, randomized, controlled trials and numerous retrospective studies examining the role of adjuvant chemotherapy in sarcoma patients have been reported. A variety of factors limit the extent to which definitive conclusions can be drawn from these studies, including (1) the relatively small number of patients in each study and hence the low statistical power to detect a clinically meaningful benefit; (2) the variety of eligibility criteria used, particularly in regard to tumor size, grade, and primary site; (3) the differing and often relatively ineffectual chemotherapeutic regimens employed; and (4) variations among study pathologists in the histopathologic grading of the tumors.[94]

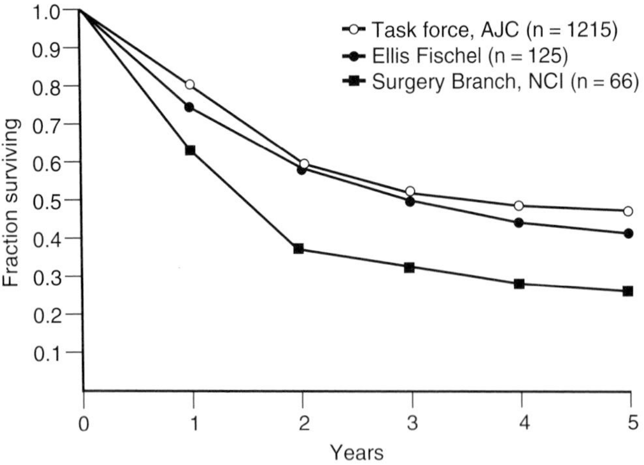


**FIGURE 2–9.** Five-year survival rate of patients with extremity soft tissue sarcomas from three reported series. (From Rosenberg SA, Suit HD, Baker LH. Sarcomas of soft tissues. In DeVita VT, et al. (eds) Cancer: Principles and Practice of Oncology, 2nd ed. Lippincott, Philadelphia, 1985.)

Retrospective reviews employing historical controls are difficult to interpret because of the selection bias inherent in such studies; this has been amply demonstrated in adjuvant studies of osteosarcoma patients.[85] Although some authors have cited a benefit from adjuvant chemotherapy in retrospective reviews of soft tissue sarcoma patients, many have not. On occasion, subsequent updates of patients from the same institution where initially favorable results were reported have shown a lack of effect. In any case, virtually all these retrospective series are sufficiently flawed that only prospective, randomized, controlled trials can be looked on to provide information regarding the effectiveness of adjuvant chemotherapy. To date, all the randomized trials for soft tissue sarcomas have utilized postoperative chemotherapy, administered after the performance of and successful recovery from amputation or wide excision (generally along with irradiation).

Doxorubicin is the most commonly used cytotoxic drug for management of metastatic sarcoma. Consequently, this agent has undergone extensive evaluation as single-agent adjuvant chemotherapy for resected soft tissue sarcomas. Randomized trials, however, have demonstrated that adjuvant doxorubicin does not improve overall survival compared with surgery alone.[23] A randomized, controlled trial of multiagent chemotherapy (doxorubicin, cyclophosphamide, and methotrexate) after surgery showed improved disease-free survival for patients with high grade extremity sarcomas but not for those of the trunk or retroperitoneum.[65] Toxicity with this regimen proved substantial. Symptomatic cardiac toxicity developed in 14% of patients, and many asymptomatic patients demonstrated decreased cardiac function on noninvasive testing. A subsequent study comparing this regimen to one with a lower doxorubicin dose (to limit cardiotoxicity) suggested that the less toxic program was equivalent to the higher-dose regimen.[15] More recently, a randomized trial evaluating adjuvant therapy with doxorubicin and ifosfamide (the two most active agents in metastatic soft tissue sarcoma) showed significant disease-free and overall survival benefits for adjuvant chemotherapy.[30] The magnitude of the benefit was sufficiently great that the trial was terminated early, after only 104 patients of a planned 200 had been enrolled.

Despite the favorable findings from these trials, other studies of adjuvant multidrug chemotherapy for soft tissue sarcomas have failed to demonstrate improvement in overall survival rates. A meta-analysis of existing randomized trials pooled the available data to minimize the limitations imposed by sample size in any one study. This analysis showed that the likelihood of disease recurrence was decreased 10% at 10 years in patients who received adjuvant chemotherapy. Overall survival increased by 4% at 10 years.[87] In this meta-analysis, the best evidence for a beneficial effect of adjuvant chemotherapy was seen in patients with extremity sarcomas. Whether the magnitude of this benefit is sufficient to justify the significant toxicity of adjuvant chemotherapy must be determined on an individual basis.

Increasingly, preoperative chemotherapy regimens are being employed in patients with extremity sarcomas.[22] This approach has become the treatment of choice for most patients with osteosarcomas of the extremity[47] but has yet to be established as superior to conventional therapy for soft tissue tumors. The use of preoperative chemotherapy has been termed *neoadjuvant chemotherapy;* it has been used alone or with preoperative irradiation. One of the main theoretic advantages of neoadjuvant chemotherapy is that the effectiveness of the drug regimen can be directly assessed by monitoring the clinical response and evaluating the degree of necrosis of the primary tumor at the time of resection.[14,56] As yet, however, there is no proof that patients whose primary tumor responds to the preoperative regimen are protected from developing metastases, or that patients whose tumors fail to respond benefit from switching to alternate therapy postoperatively. Given the numerous remaining questions regarding preoperative and postoperative adjuvant chemotherapy, patients with stage III (large, high-grade, deep) extremity sarcomas should be enrolled in an established clinical trial whenever possible.

#### *Isolation Limb Perfusion*

Several investigators have treated extremity sarcomas with a technique known as isolation limb perfusion.[43,92] Isolation perfusion is performed by cannulating the artery and vein to an extremity (e.g., iliac artery and vein) and directing all the blood flow for that extremity through a cardiopulmonary bypass pump. The temperature of the perfusate can be regulated, and generally hyperthermic perfusion is employed. Initially, limb perfusion was carried out using standard cytotoxic agents such as melphalan. More recently, the addition of tumor necrosis factor-$\alpha$ (TNF$\alpha$) and interferon-$\gamma$ (IFN$\gamma$) to melphalan has been reported to increase response rates dramatically. In most cases responses to perfusion have been of short duration, but in at least some cases resection of lesions initially thought to be unresectable without amputation has been achieved after perfusion.

### Treatment of Nonextremity Sarcomas

Unlike sarcomas of the extremity, lesions that arise in the head and neck, thoracic or abdominal wall, mediastinum, or retroperitoneum are rarely amenable to true "radical" resection. Furthermore, many of these tumors are situated in areas where nearby normal tissues impose limitations on the amount of radiation that may be delivered to the tumor or tumor bed. Because of these factors, multimodality therapy approaches have in general been less successful for sarcomas in these sites than for extremity sarcomas. Local recurrences are more common and, particularly for retroperitoneal tumors, often lead to the demise of the patient before disseminated metastases become evident. Given the current state of the art, improvements in techniques for achieving local control of nonextremity tumors offers promise for greater increases in patient survival rates than is the case with primary sarcomas of the extremities.

General principles of evaluation and management of nonextremity sarcomas parallel those for extremity tumors. Long delays before diagnosis and initiation of therapy can be avoided only by maintaining a high index of suspicion and promptly performing a biopsy for any new, persistent, or enlarging soft tissue mass. Fine-needle and core-needle biopsies play a major role, especially for relatively inaccessible sites such as the retroperitoneum. There is no situation in which definitive surgical therapy should be performed without a tissue diagnosis, and frozen section examination is rarely relied on to provide a definitive diagnosis. The possibility that the tumor is actually a primary bone sarcoma, lymphoma, or a metastasis from a carcinoma located elsewhere should always be kept in mind; this practice avoids the pitfall of applying radical surgical resection to lesions best treated in another fashion. Characteristic features of soft tissue sarcomas at various nonextremity sites are noted in the following sections.

### Sarcomas of the Head and Neck

Approximately 8–10% of all soft tissue sarcomas are located in the head and neck region (Table 2–1). For soft tissue sarcomas of the neck it is sometimes possible to obtain wide or radical margins with procedures similar to those employed for neck dissection; resecting sarcomas arising in the region of the mandible, maxilla, and base of the skull may prove challenging (Fig. 2–10). Farr reported on 285 patients with soft tissue sarcomas of the head and neck with an absolute 5-year survival rate of 32%.[28] This experience represented a diverse group of patients who were subjected to different forms of therapy over an extended period of time. A more recent review from the same institution focused on 176 adult patients treated between 1950 and 1985 and who were followed a minimum of 2 years.[27] In this cohort, the 5-year survival rate was 55%, with 40% of patients alive at 10 years. Patients with high grade tumors, however, had a 10-year survival rate of only 20%. Univariate analysis of prognostic factors identified a tumor size of ≥ 5 cm, positive margins, bone involvement, and high histologic grade to be significantly associated with low survival rates. In the absence of multivariate analysis, it is impossible to know to what extent these adverse features are independent prognostic factors (e.g., large size, positive margins, and bone involvement were all far more common in high grade tumors than low grade tumors in this series). More recently, a registry of head and neck sarcomas comprising 214 patients from a number of institutions was reported. The resectability rate was 84%, and the 5-year survival rate was 70%, with 56% of patients disease-free after 5 years.[89]

### Sarcomas of the Body Wall

Sarcomas of the thoracic or abdominal wall constitute approximately 15% of all soft tissue sarcomas. These lesions can usually be adequately encompassed by a wide, full-thickness excision to achieve negative margins. Abdominal wall defects can be reconstructed in straightforward fashion with the use of a nonabsorbable mesh prosthesis. Significant portions of the bony thorax can be resected without compromising respiratory function, even though nonrigid prosthetic materials are utilized. Extensive defects of the thoracic cage require a rigid reconstruction, generally employing a shaped prosthesis formed of methylmethacrylate cement between two pieces of polypropylene mesh.[53] Reconstruction of the chest wall and large abdominal wall defects also frequently requires coverage with myocutaneous flaps, which have a better blood supply than standard skin flaps or split-thickness skin grafts. The use of myocutaneous flaps is associated with decreased wound complications if postoperative radiotherapy is required.

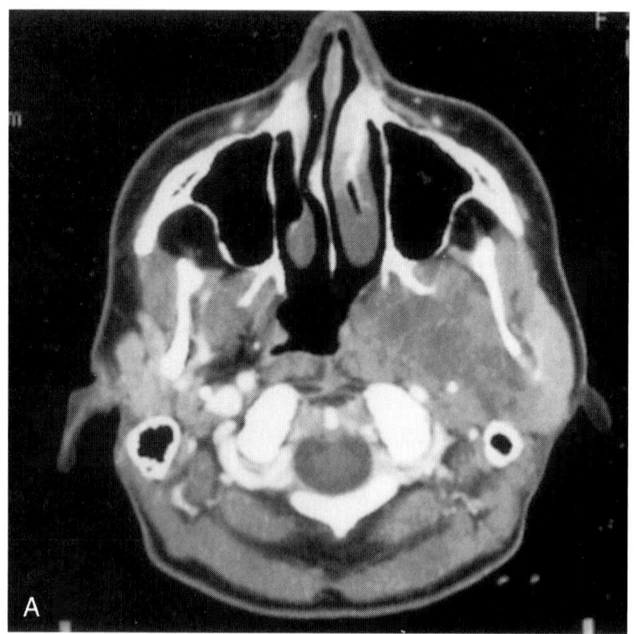


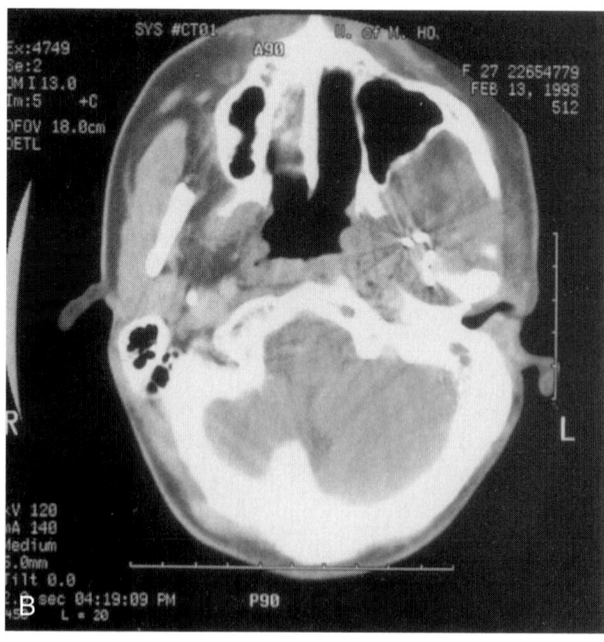


**FIGURE 2–10.** (**A**) Computed tomography (CT) scan demonstrating a large, high grade fibrosarcoma involving the left mandible, infratemporal fossa, and masticator space. To facilitate resection, the patient was treated with preoperative external beam radiation along with the radiation sensitizer iododeoxyuridine. (**B**) Appearance after resection and reconstruction with bone grafts.

### *Sarcomas of the Retroperitoneum*

Retroperitoneal sarcomas are perhaps the most difficult sarcomas to manage.[76,82] These tumors do not come to the attention of the patient until they are large; retroperitoneal sarcomas less than 5 cm are rarely seen.[81] Even massive tumors may present with only minimal symptoms (Fig. 2–11). Most retroperitoneal sarcomas are liposarcomas, leiomyosarcomas, or malignant fibrous histiocytomas,[38,82] and they may weigh several kilograms at the time of excision. Clinical evaluation of these tumors should include a CT scan of the chest and abdomen; MRI is helpful for defining the extent of vascular involvement and has largely replaced the need for arteriography and vena cavography (Fig. 2–6).

The surgical approach to retroperitoneal tumors requires exploration through a transperitoneal approach using either a midline or bilateral subcostal incision. Experience has shown that retroperitoneal approaches via the flank, as are often used for nephrectomy, do not allow adequate visualization for safe resection.[81] The approach to resecting retroperitoneal sarcomas has been well outlined by Storm and Mahvi[82] and is shown in Figure 2–12. The initial maneuver is to establish a plane of dissection of the tumor from major intraabdominal vascular structures. Subsequently, a retroperitoneal plane is established to allow complete tumor removal. When resecting a retroperitoneal sarcoma, it is nearly impossible to achieve the type of wide or radical margins that would be considered standard when excising an extremity tumor. Nonetheless, gross total resection of all visible tumor should be the goal of any surgical procedure, even if it involves resecting other intraabdominal organs or vessels.[69] Incomplete resection or "debulking" of a retroperitoneal tumor is not associated with improved long-term survival rates compared with biopsy and subsequent nonsurgical treatment.[46,82] With aggressive surgical approaches and a willingness to resect adjacent organs, most retroperitoneal sarcomas are now amenable to gross total excision.[38] After complete tumor resection, the major determinant of overall sur-

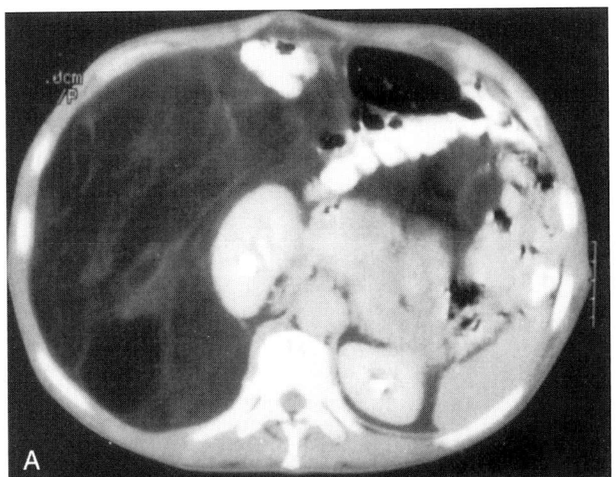


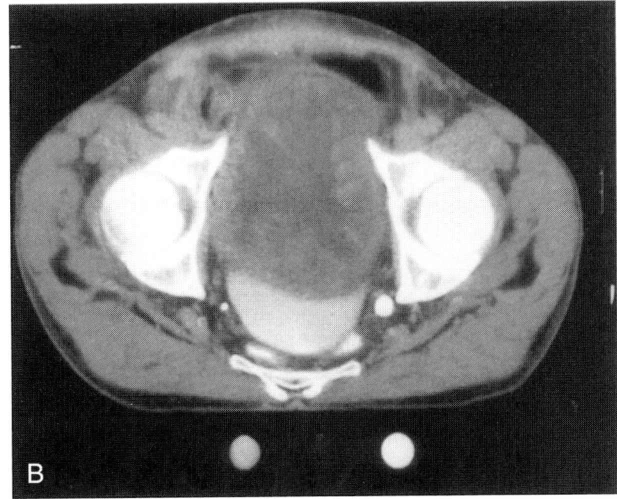


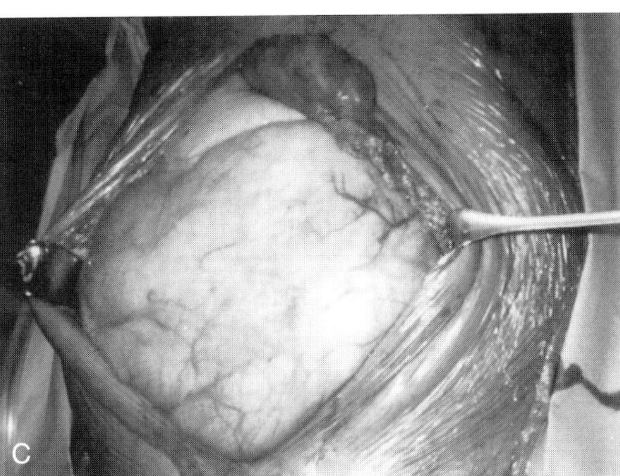


**FIGURE 2–11.** (**A, B**) CT scans demonstrating massive retroperitoneal liposarcoma, which presented as an otherwise asymptomatic increase in abdominal girth. The tumor consisted predominantly of low grade elements (**A**), but a 20 cm region of high grade dedifferentiated liposarcoma was also present (**B**). (**C**) Appearance of the abdomen at laparotomy for tumor resection, showing the fatty tumor virtually filling the abdomen. Fifteen years previously the patient had undergone a cholecystectomy and was told that he had "excessive fat" in his right retroperitoneum; no biopsy was obtained at that time.

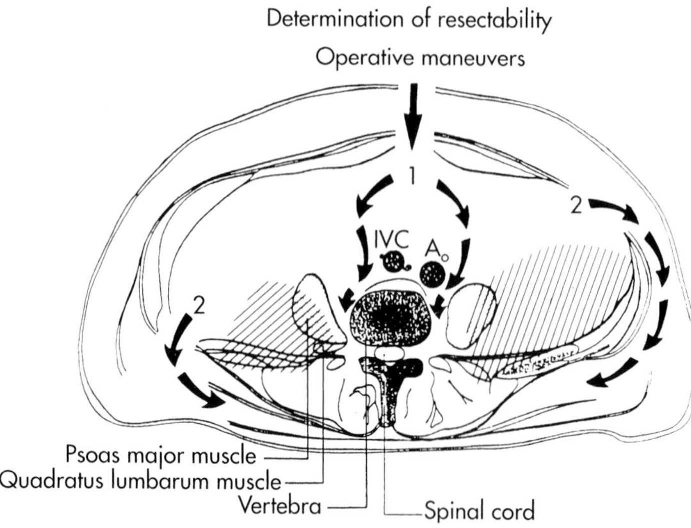


**FIGURE 2–12.** Initial intraoperative maneuvers to assess resectability of retroperitoneal sarcomas (represented by cross-hatched regions). (1) A plane of dissection between the tumor and the major vascular structures is established. (2) A retroperitoneal plane is established to evaluate areas adjacent to the spinal foramina and allow resection of the tumor. (From Storm FK, Mahvi DM. Diagnosis and management of retroperitoneal soft-tissue sarcoma. Ann Surg 214:2, 1991.)

vival is the histologic grade of the tumor (Fig. 2–13).[82] Unlike low grade extremity sarcomas, where tumor-related mortality is rare, only 42% of patients with completely resected low grade retroperitoneal sarcomas were alive at 10 years. For patients with high grade tumors, the prognosis is far worse: 24% were alive at 5 years and only 11% at 10 years despite complete tumor resection.

Local recurrence, with or without distant disease, is common after surgical therapy of retroperitoneal sarcomas (Table 2–4). A randomized study was performed to investigate the efficacy of intraoperative radiotherapy in decreasing local recurrence rates. Thirty-five patients were randomly assigned to either postoperative external beam radiotherapy (50–55 Gy) or intraoperative radiotherapy (20 Gy in a single dose delivered immediately after removal of the tumor) plus lower-dose postoperative external beam radiotherapy (35–40 Gy). All patients had large intermediate or high grade tumors and were treated after exploration revealed no evidence of metastases and determined that the tumor was resectable. Overall survival rates were virtually identical for the two groups (median survival 52 months for external beam radiation only versus 45 months for intraoperative radiotherapy; a nonsignificant difference). After a median follow-up of 8 years, 26 of 35 patients had experienced disease recurrence: 16 of 20 patients in the external beam radiation group (all with local recurrence) and 10 of 15 patients in the intraoperative radiotherapy group. Only 6 of the 15 patients who received intraoperative radiotherapy had local failure, indicating that the intensive radiotherapy sterilized residual tumor cells in the treatment field in some cases.[73] The logistic difficulties, expense, and toxicity of intraoperative radiotherapy are clearly not justified given the minimal overall benefit. This trial illustrates the unsatisfactory results that are currently achieved with aggressive surgical resection and intraoperative or postoperative irradiation in patients with retroperitoneal sarcomas.

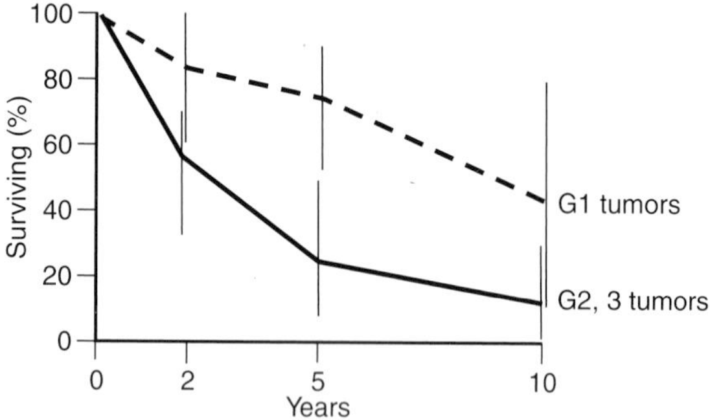


**FIGURE 2–13.** Overall survival by tumor grade for completely resected retroperitoneal sarcomas based on cumulative data from published series. In all, 49 low-grade (G1) and 80 intermediate or high grade (G2,3) sarcomas were included in this analysis. The range of values reported in the individual series from which these data were derived is indicated by the vertical bars. (Modified from Storm FK, Mahvi DM. Diagnosis and management of retroperitoneal soft-tissue sarcoma. Ann Surg 214:2, 1991.)

Glenn et al. explored the use of multimodality therapy with irradiation and chemotherapy for retroperitoneal sarcomas.[33] A group of 37 patients with completely resected high grade retroperitoneal tumors went on to receive postoperative adjuvant therapy. All 37 patients underwent postoperative radiotherapy; 21 also received chemotherapy, but the other 16 did not. The actuarial 3-year survival rate was 43%, and it did not appear to be affected by chemotherapy. Irradiation and chemotherapy were both poorly tolerated and were associated with significant long-term toxicity in these patients, who were treated while still recovering from major operative procedures.

Attention has turned to preoperative multimodality approaches for treatment of retroperitoneal sarcomas. Cytotoxic chemotherapy[17] and radiation sensitizers[63,78] have been successfully administered along with external beam radiation prior to resection. Preoperative therapy is advantageous because it is administered when the patient is most able to withstand the rigors of therapy, potentially minimizing the magnitude of the resection or allowing initially unresectable tumors to be completely excised (Fig. 2–14). Also under active investigation is the use of intraperitoneal chemotherapy administered during the early postoperative period after complete or partial tumor resection.[39] At present, however, none of these alternatives can be considered standard of care.

### *Adjuvant Therapy for Nonextremity Sarcomas*

Because nonextremity sarcomas are rarely amenable to resection with the wide or radical margins achievable in the extremity, radiation is employed after surgery in most cases. As with extremity tumors, there are clearly some cases in which postoperative irradiation is not mandatory: Low grade tumors that are completely excised with histologically negative margins may be observed without adjuvant treatment, provided that any subsequent recurrence would again be amenable to excision. Most authorities advocate irradiation after resection of nonextremity low grade sarcomas with close or positive margins and after resection of any intermediate or high grade tumors. The efficacy of adjuvant chemotherapy for patients with nonextremity sarcomas has not been established to date. Only one randomized trial examined the efficacy of adjuvant chemotherapy in patients with soft tissue sarcomas of the head and neck, breast, and trunk, all of whom also received postoperative radiotherapy.[32] Adjuvant chemotherapy consisted of doxorubicin, cyclophosphamide, and methotrexate, a regimen no longer commonly used for sarcoma treatment. The 3-year actuarial disease-free survival rate in the chemotherapy group was 72% compared with 60% in the group without chemotherapy; the 3-year overall survival rates were 71% and 60%, respectively (Fig. 2–15). These differences were not statistically significant ($p$ values of 0.27 and 0.92, respectively). Virtually all other randomized trials of adjuvant chemotherapy that involved patients with nonextremity sarcomas lumped them together with extremity tumors. A meta-analysis of all these clinical trials, previously cited, suggested a small benefit for adjuvant chemotherapy in terms of improved survival rates. The evidence for benefit of adjuvant chemotherapy was strongest with extremity tumors.[87] So long as local recurrence rates for nonextremity sarcomas remain high, the benefits of adjuvant chemotherapy on survival are likely to be limited. Conversely, improvements in local therapy highlight the need for improved systemic therapy, as more patients die from distant disease who might otherwise have succumbed to local recurrence.[78]

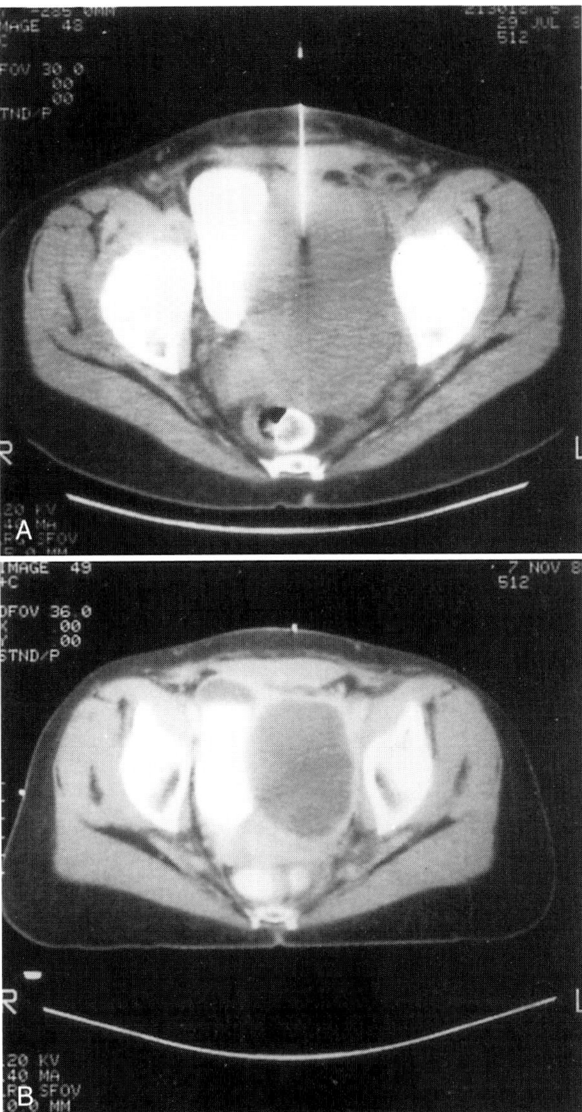


**FIGURE 2–14.** (**A**) CT scan demonstrating a large high grade pelvic malignant fibrous histiocytoma considered unresectable because of involvement of the pelvic side wall. (**B**) CT scan of the same patient after preoperative treatment with 62.5 Gy external beam radiation along with iododeoxyuridine. The tumor is significantly smaller, is more homogeneous, and has regressed away from the pelvic side wall sufficiently to permit resection. The resected specimen was composed entirely of nonviable tumor tissue (100% necrosis after preoperative treatment). (From Sondak VK, Economou JS, Eilber FR. Soft tissue sarcomas of the extremity and retroperitoneum. Adv Surg 24:333, 1991.)

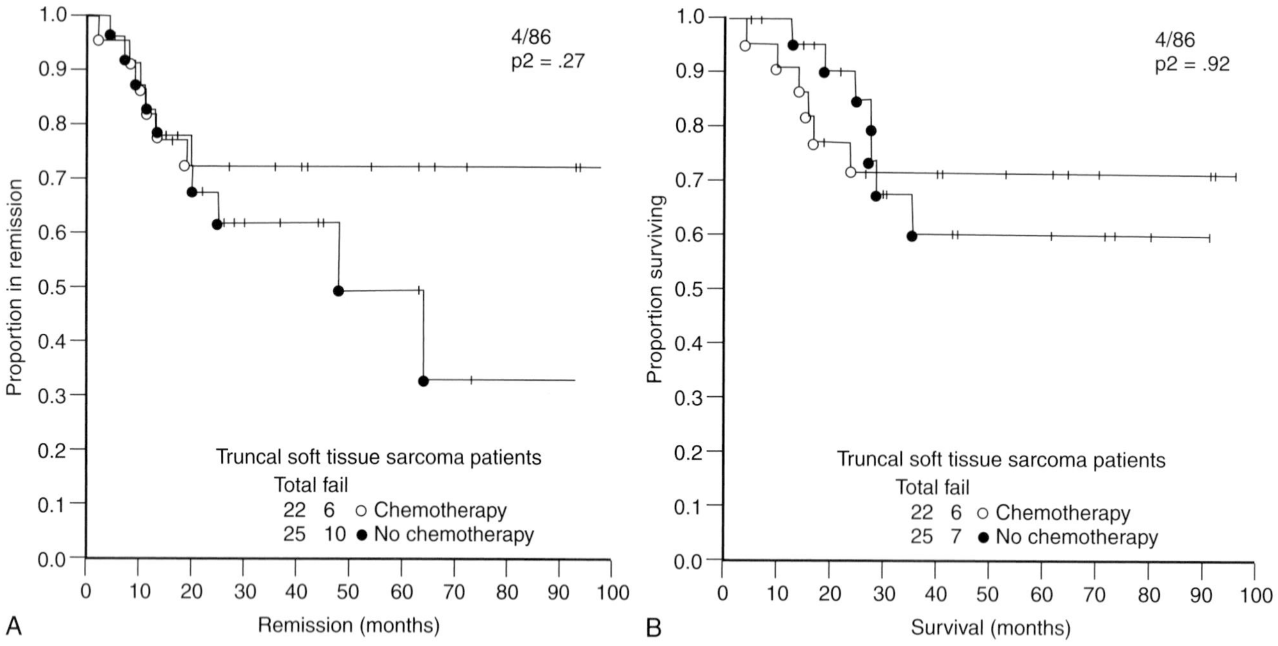


**FIGURE 2–15.** Disease-free survival rates (**A**) and overall survival rates (**B**) in patients entered onto a randomized trial of adjuvant chemotherapy versus observation after resection of high grade truncal, breast, or head and neck sarcomas. After a median follow-up of 5 years, there are no significant differences between the two groups. (From Glenn J, Kinsella T, Glatstein E, et al. A randomized prospective trial of adjuvant chemotherapy in adults with soft tissue sarcomas of the head and neck, breast, and trunk. Cancer 55:1206, 1985.)

## TREATMENT OF METASTATIC DISEASE

### Surgery

The sites of initial tumor recurrence in 307 patients after primary treatment of a soft tissue sarcoma were reviewed.[59] Primary therapy in these patients consisted of complete surgical resection, often in combination with postoperative chemotherapy and radiation therapy. A total of 107 patients (35%) developed local recurrence or distant metastases at the sites identified in Table 2–4; the lung was the predominant site of disease in 52% of patients. Isolated local recurrences were the second most common, seen 20% of the time. As indicated earlier, the pattern of recurrence was dependent on the site of the primary sarcoma. Patients with sarcomas of the head and neck, retroperitoneum, and chest or abdominal wall had a higher local recurrence rate than those with tumors of the extremities. Approximately 80% of all local recurrences and disseminated metastases became evident within 5 years.

Removal of clinically normal lymph nodes generally has no role in the treatment of soft tissue sarcomas; dissection of tumor-containing lymph node basins, documented by fine-needle or excisional biopsy, should be performed if no other metastatic disease is evident. Radical lymphadenectomy for patients with nodal involvement in the absence of metastasis elsewhere was associated with a 34% five-year survival, fully justifying an aggressive surgical approach in these patients.[29]

As is the case for patients with isolated local or regional recurrence, aggressive surgical treatment of pulmonary metastases should be attempted when technically feasible. Patients who are found to have pulmonary metastases by plain radiography or CT of the chest should have a thorough evaluation for extrapulmonary tumor, particularly in the primary site. For sarcomas of the extremities or trunk, this can be accomplished by physical examination and CT scan or MRI of the primary site. For patients with intraabdominal or retroperitoneal sarcomas, a CT scan of the liver should be performed to exclude metastases there. Patients with extrapulmonary tumor are not considered candidates for curative resection of pulmonary metastases. The patient's pulmonary function should also be evaluated to ensure that the patient can tolerate a thoracotomy and will have adequate ventilatory reserve after resection. In one representative series, 40 of 56 patients (72%) with isolated pulmonary metastases were rendered disease-free with surgery, with an actuarial 3-year survival rate of 38%.[59] Several studies evaluating factors that might be significant in predicting outcome from pulmonary metastasectomy have been reported.[61] Univariate analyses have generally identified a small number of metastatic nodules seen on preoperative CT scans (fewer than three or four), a long disease-free interval prior to appearance of the lung nodules, and a long tumor doubling time (> 40 days) as being correlated with a longer median postoperative survival. It should be noted that no single criterion is sufficiently accurate to exclude any patient from resection; even patients with several unfavorable factors occasionally are long-term survivors. Overall, the 5-year survival ranges from 10% to 35% in most reported series. With osteosarcoma metastatic to the lung, adjuvant systemic chemotherapy before or after pulmonary resection appears to convey additional benefit[74]; whether this will hold true for soft tissue sarcomas remains to be determined.

## Chemotherapy

Systemic cytotoxic chemotherapy is generally not considered curative for patients with metastatic soft tissue sarcomas. Osteogenic sarcomas, Ewing's sarcomas, and childhood rhabdomyosarcomas are associated with much higher response rates to chemotherapy. Nonetheless, for adult soft tissue sarcoma patients without a curative surgical option, chemotherapy represents the best currently available palliative treatment. Objective tumor regression and relief of symptoms can be achieved in a significant fraction of patients, with acceptable toxicity. Cytotoxic drugs that are or have been commonly employed in the treatment of metastatic sarcomas include doxorubicin, cyclophosphamide, ifosfamide, methotrexate, vincristine, cisplatin, dactinomycin and dacarbazine. Of these agents, doxorubicin and ifosfamide appear to have the highest degree of activity when administered as single agents. Most often, combination regimens are employed; the combination of doxorubicin and ifosfamide, with or without dacarbazine, appears to be particularly active (Fig. 2–16).

A multiinstitutional cooperative group study of 340 patients with metastatic soft tissue sarcoma compared response rates and survival times following treatment with doxorubicin and dacarbazine alone or combined with ifosfamide and mesna (a uroprotective agent utilized to minimize the incidence of ifosfamide-induced hemorrhagic cystitis). The addition of ifosfamide increased the response rate significantly (32% for all three drugs versus 17% for doxorubicin plus dacarbazine). Toxicity was also greater, and overall survival did not differ significantly based on treatment.[2] The authors suggested that ifosfamide be included in the initial therapy for patients receiving preoperative chemotherapy and for younger patients better able to tolerate the toxicity. For older patients and those whose original tumor was of low or intermediate histologic grade, they recommended the use of doxorubicin and dacarbazine initially, followed if necessary by ifosfamide upon progression.

Patients who achieve a partial response to chemotherapy but are left with one or several potentially

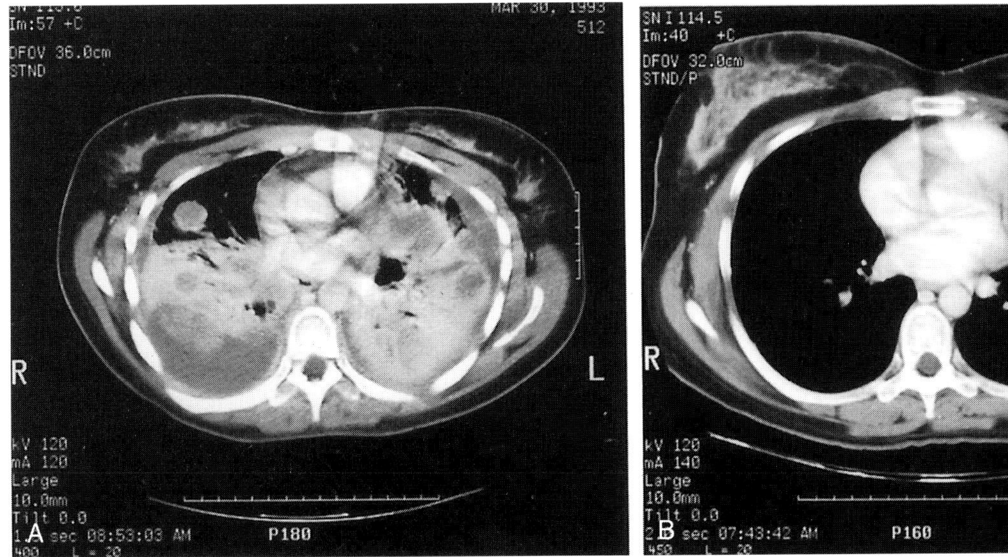


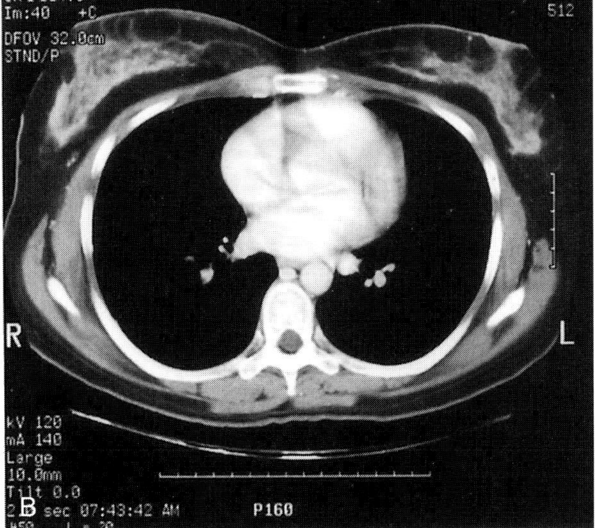


**FIGURE 2–16.** (**A**) Pretreatment chest CT scan demonstrating metastatic high grade sarcoma with associated malignant pleural effusion. (**B**) CT scan obtained after 6 months of treatment with doxorubicin and ifosfamide shows complete resolution of the effusion and virtually complete disappearance of the pulmonary nodules. The response lasted 9 months and was associated with excellent palliation of the patient's shortness of breath. (Courtesy of Dean Brenner, MD, Section of Hematology/Oncology, University of Michigan.)

resectable metastases should be considered for surgical excision. Conversion of a chemotherapy-induced partial response to a complete response can enhance the duration of response and is associated with a survival time equivalent to that obtained with complete response to chemotherapy alone. Similarly, the occasional patient with one or several metastatic lesions not amenable to resection can be treated effectively with localized irradiation to consolidate the response to chemotherapy.

To date, immunotherapeutic approaches including monoclonal antibodies, cytokines, and adoptive cellular therapies have found only a limited role in the management of metastatic sarcoma. Rosenberg et al.[64] reported that none of six sarcoma patients treated with high dose interleukin-2 responded, and enthusiasm for immunotherapy of sarcomas waned. Evidence has mounted that sarcomas do indeed express tumor antigens that are potentially recognizable by the human immune system.[79] Such evidence, combined with the successful use of TNF$\alpha$ during isolation limb perfusion, has led to an increase in the number of research protocols investigating the use of immunotherapy (including gene transfer therapy) for advanced sarcomas.

The clinical evaluation and treatment of patients with soft tissue sarcomas remains a challenge. Since the early 1980s, aggressive treatment approaches by experienced multidisciplinary oncology teams have improved the outlook for these patients. The feasibility and appropriateness of limb-sparing therapies for patients with high grade extremity sarcomas, many of whom would have been treated by amputation in the past, are now firmly established. The multidisciplinary team should include surgeons, radiation oncologists, medical oncologists, pathologists, radiologists, rehabilitation therapists, oncology nurses and social workers. The contribution of the pathologist and the need for a thorough, detailed enumeration of the histologic features of the tumor relevant to therapy cannot be overstressed. Because of the relatively low incidence of these tumors, patients with soft tissue sarcomas should generally be referred to medical centers with experience in sarcoma management.[67] Nonetheless, it remains for every practicing physician to be aware of soft tissue sarcomas and their behavior, so patients with soft tissue masses can be promptly and appropriately evaluated, a diagnosis made, and optimal therapy initiated.

## REFERENCES


1. Abbas JS, Holyoke ED, Moore R, Karakousis CP. The surgical treatment and outcome of soft-tissue sarcoma. Arch Surg 116: 765, 1981.
2. Antman K, Crowley J, Balcerzak SP, et al. An intergroup phase III randomized study of doxorubicin and dacarbazine with or without ifosfamide and mesna in advanced soft tissue and bone sarcomas. J Clin Oncol 11:1276, 1993.
3. Apffelstaedt JP, Zhang PJ, Driscoll DL, Karakousis CP. Various types of hemipelvectomy for soft tissue sarcomas: complications, survival and prognostic factors. Surg Oncol 4:217, 1995.
4. Arca MJ, Sondak VK, Chang AE. Diagnostic procedures and pre-treatment evaluation of soft tissue sarcomas. Semin Surg Oncol 10:323, 1994.
5. Ball AB, Fisher C, Pittam M, et al. Diagnosis of soft tissue tumours by Tru-cut biopsy. Br J Surg 77:756, 1990.
6. Barth RJ Jr, Merino MJ, Solomon D, et al. A prospective study of the value of core needle biopsy and fine needle aspiration in the diagnosis of soft tissue masses. Surgery 112:536, 1992.
7. Barwick WJ, Goldberg JA, Scully SP, Harrelson JM. Vascularized tissue transfer for closure of irradiated wounds after soft tissue sarcoma resection. Ann Surg 216:591, 1992.
8. Bennert KW, Abdul-Karim FW. Fine needle aspiration cytology vs. needle core biopsy of soft tissue tumors: a comparison. Acta Cytol 38:381, 1994.
9. Bland KI, Karakousis CP, Copeland EM III (eds). Atlas of Surgical Oncology. WB Saunders, Philadelphia, 1995.
10. Bland KI, McCoy DM, Kinard RE, Copeland EM III. Application of magnetic resonance imaging and computed tomography as an adjunct to the surgical management of soft tissue sarcomas. Ann Surg 205:473, 1987.
11. Brennan MF. Staging of soft tissue sarcomas. Ann Surg Oncol 6:8, 1999.
12. Brooks AD, Heslin MJ, Leung DH, et al. Superficial extremity soft tissue sarcoma: an analysis of prognostic factors. Ann Surg Oncol 5:41, 1998.
13. Cantin J, McNeer GP, Chu FC, Booher RJ. The problem of local recurrence after treatment of soft tissue sarcoma. Ann Surg 168: 47, 1968.
14. Casper ES, Gaynor JJ, Harrison LB, et al. Preoperative and postoperative adjuvant chemotherapy for adults with high grade soft tissue sarcoma. Cancer 73:1644, 1994.
15. Chang AE, Kinsella T, Glatstein E, et al. Adjuvant chemotherapy for patients with high-grade soft-tissue sarcomas of the extremity. J Clin Oncol 6:1491, 1988.
16. Chang AE, Matory YL, Dwyer AJ, et al. Magnetic resonance imaging versus computed tomography in the evaluation of soft tissue tumors of the extremities. Ann Surg 205:340, 1987.
17. Chawla SP, Rosen G, Eilber F, et al. Cisplatin and Adriamycin as neoadjuvant and adjuvant chemotherapy in the management of soft tissue sarcomas. In: Salmon SE (ed) Adjuvant Therapy of Cancer VI. WB Saunders, Philadelphia, 1990.
18. Collin CF, Friedrich C, Godbold J, et al. Prognostic factors for local recurrence and survival in patients with localized extremity soft-tissue sarcoma. Semin Surg Oncol 4:30, 1988.
19. Costa J, Wesley RA, Glatstein E, Rosenberg SA. The grading of soft tissue sarcomas. Cancer 53:530, 1984.
20. Demetri GD, Pollock R, Baker L, et al. NCCN sarcoma practice guidelines. Oncology 12:183, 1998.
21. Economou SG, Economou TS. Atlas of Surgical Techniques. WB Saunders, Philadelphia, 1996.
22. Eilber FR, Eckardt JJ, Rosen G, et al. Preoperative chemotherapy for soft tissue sarcoma. Hematol Oncol Clin North Am 9: 817, 1995.
23. Elias AD, Antman KH. Adjuvant chemotherapy for soft-tissue sarcoma: a critical appraisal. Semin Surg Oncol 4:59, 1988.
24. Enneking WF. Staging of musculoskeletal neoplasms. In: Current Concepts of Diagnosis and Treatment of Bone and Soft Tissue Tumors. Springer-Verlag, Heidelberg, 1984.

25. Enneking WF, Chew FS, Springfield DS, et al. The role of radionuclide bone-scanning in determining the resectability of soft-tissue sarcomas. J Bone Joint Surg Am 63:249, 1981.
26. Enneking WF, McAuliffe JA. Adjunctive preoperative radiation therapy in treatment of soft tissue sarcomas: a preliminary report. Cancer Treat Symp 3:37, 1985.
27. Farhood AI, Hajdu SI, Shiu MH, Strong EW. Soft tissue sarcomas of the head and neck in adults. Am J Surg 160:365, 1990.
28. Farr HW. Soft part sarcomas of the head and neck. Semin Oncol 8:185, 1981.
29. Fong Y, Coit DG, Woodruff JM, Brennan MF. Lymph node metastasis from soft tissue sarcoma in adults: analysis of data from a prospective database of 1772 sarcoma patients. Ann Surg 217:72, 1993.
30. Frustaci S, Gherlinzoni F, De Paoli A, et al. Preliminary results of an adjuvant randomized trial on high risk extremity soft tissue sarcomas (STS): the interim analysis. Proc Am Soc Clin Oncol 16:496a, 1997.
31. Giuliano AE, Eilber FR. The rationale for planned reoperation after unplanned total excision of soft-tissue sarcomas. J Clin Oncol 3:1344, 1985.
32. Glenn J, Kinsella T, Glatstein E, et al. A randomized prospective trial of adjuvant chemotherapy in adults with soft tissue sarcomas of the head and neck, breast, and trunk. Cancer 55: 1206, 1985.
33. Glenn J, Sindelar WF, Kinsella T, et al. Results of multimodality therapy of resectable soft tissue sarcomas of the retroperitoneum. Surgery 97:316, 1985.
34. Heslin MJ, Lewis JJ, Woodruff JM, Brennan MF. Core needle biopsy for diagnosis of extremity soft tissue sarcoma. Ann Surg Oncol 4:425, 1997.
35. Huth J, Eilber FR. Patterns of metastatic spread following resection of extremity soft-tissue sarcomas and strategies for treatment. Semin Surg Oncol 4:20, 1988.
36. Jaques DP, Coit DG, Casper ES, Brennan MF. Hepatic metastases from soft-tissue sarcoma. Ann Surg 221:392, 1995.
37. Johnstone PA, Wexler LH, Venzon DJ, et al. Sarcomas of the hand and foot: analysis of local control and functional result with combined modality therapy in extremity preservation. Int J Radiat Oncol Biolo Physics 29:735, 1994.
38. Karakousis CP, Gerstenbluth R, Kontzoglou K, Driscoll DI. Retroperitoneal sarcomas and their management. Arch Surg 130: 1104, 1995.
39. Karakousis CP, Kontzoglou K, Driscoll DL. Intraperitoneal chemotherapy in disseminated abdominal sarcoma. Ann Surg Oncol 4:496, 1997.
40. Kransdorf MJ, Murphey MD. Imaging of Soft Tissue Tumors. Saunders, Philadelphia, 1997.
41. Ladin D, Rees R, Wilkins E, et al. The use of omental transposition in the treatment of recurrent sarcoma of the back. Ann Plast Surg 31:556, 1993.
42. Lawrence W Jr, Donegan WL, Natarajan N, et al. Adult soft tissue sarcomas: a pattern of care survey of the American College of Surgeons. Ann Surg 205:349, 1987.
43. Lienard D, Ewalenko, P, Delmotte J-J, et al. High-dose recombinant tumor necrosis factor alpha in combination with interferon gamma and melphalan in isolation perfusion of the limbs for melanoma and sarcoma. J Clin Oncol 10:52, 1992.
44. Lin PP, Schupak KD, Boland PJ, et al. Pathologic femoral fracture after periosteal excision and radiation for the treatment of soft tissue sarcoma. Cancer 82:2356, 1998.
45. Markhede G, Angervall L, Stener B. A multivariate analysis of the prognosis after surgical treatment of malignant soft-tissue tumors. Cancer 49:1721, 1982.
46. McGrath PC, Neifeld JP, Lawrence W Jr, et al. Improved survival following complete excision of retroperitoneal sarcomas. Ann Surg 200:200, 1984.
47. Meyers PA, Heller G, Healey J, et al. Chemotherapy for nonmetastatic osteogenic sarcoma: the Memorial Sloan-Kettering experience. J Clin Oncol 10:5, 1992.
48. Midis GP, Pollock RE, Chen NP, et al. Locally recurrent soft tissue sarcoma of the extremities. Surgery 126:666, 1998.
49. Myhre Jensen O, Kaae S, Madsen EH, Sneppen O. Histopathological grading in soft-tissue tumors: relation to survival in 261 surgically treated patients. Acta Pathol Microbiol Immunol Scand 91A:145, 1983.
50. Noria S, Davis A, Kandel R, et al. Residual disease following unplanned excsion of a soft-tissue sarcoma of an extremity. J Bone Joint Surg Am 78:650, 1996.
51. O'Sullivan B, Davis A, Bell R, et al. Phase III randomized trial of pre-operative versus post-operative radiotherapy in the curative management of extremity soft tissue sarcoma: a Canadian Sarcoma Group and NCI Canada Clinical Trials Group study. Proc Am Soc Clin Oncol 18:535a, 1999.
52. Owens JC, Shiu MH, Smith R, Hajdu SI. Soft tissue sarcomas of the hand and foot. Cancer 55:2010, 1985.
53. Perry RR, Venzon D, Roth JA, Pass HI. Survival after surgical resection for high-grade chest wall sarcomas. Ann Thorac Surg 49:363, 1990.
54. Pisters PW, Harrison LB, Leung DH, et al. Long-term results of a prospective randomized trial of adjuvant brachytherapy in soft tissue sarcoma. J Clin Oncol 14:859, 1996.
55. Pisters PW, Leung DH, Woodruff J, et al. Analysis of prognostic factors in 1,041 patients with localized soft tissue sarcomas of the extremities. J Clin Oncol 14:1679, 1996.
56. Pisters PW, Patel SR, Varma DG, et al. Preoperative chemotherapy for stage IIIB extremity soft tissue sarcoma: long-term results from a single institution. J Clin Oncol 15:3481, 1997.
57. Pollack A, Zagars GK, Goswitz MS, et al. Preoperative vs. postoperative radiotherapy in the treatment of soft tissue sarcomas: a matter of presentation. Int J Radiat Oncol Biol Physics 42:563, 1998.
58. Pollock RE, Karnell LH, Menck HR, Winchester DP. The National Cancer Data Base report on soft tissue sarcoma. Cancer 78:2247, 1996.
59. Potter DA, Glenn J, Kinsella T, et al. Patterns of recurrence in patients with high grade soft-tissue sarcomas. J Clin Oncol 3: 353, 1985.
60. Potter DA, Kinsella T, Glatstein E, et al. High-grade soft tissue sarcomas of the extremities. Cancer 58:190, 1986.
61. Putnam JB Jr, Roth JA. Resection of sarcomatous pulmonary metastases. Surg Oncol Clin North Am 2:673, 1993.
62. Ramathan RC, A'Hern R, Fisher C, Thomas JM. Modified staging system for extremity soft tissue sarcomas. Ann Surg Oncol 6:57, 1999.
63. Robertson JM, Sondak VK, Weiss SA, et al. Preoperative radiation therapy and iododeoxyuridine for large retroperitoneal sarcomas. Int J Radiat Oncol Biol Phys 31:87, 1995.
64. Rosenberg SA, Lotze MT, Muul LM, et al. A progress report on the treatment of 157 patients with advanced cancer using lymphokine-activated killer cells and interleukin-2 or high dose interleukin-2 alone. N Engl J Med 316:889, 1987.
65. Rosenberg SA, Tepper J, Glatstein E, et al. Prospective randomized evaluation of adjuvant chemotherapy in adults with soft tissue sarcomas of the extremities. Cancer 52:424, 1983.
66. Rosenberg SA, Tepper J, Glatstein E, et al. The treatment of soft-tissue sarcomas of the extremites: prospective randomized evaluations of (1) limb-sparing surgery plus radiation therapy compared with amputation and (2) the role of adjuvant chemotherapy. Ann Surg 196:305, 1982.

67. Rydholm A. Improving the management of soft tissue sarcoma; diagnosis and treatment should be given in specialist centres. BMJ 317:93, 1998.
68. Rydholm A, Gustafson P, Rööser B, et al. Limb-sparing surgery without radiotherapy based on the anatomic location of soft tissue sarcoma. J Clin Oncol 9:1757, 1991.
69. Sarkar R, Eilber FR, Gelabert HA, Quinones-Baldrich WJ. Prosthetic replacement of the inferior vena cava for malignancy. J Vasc Surg 28:75, 1998.
70. Selch MT, Kopald KH, Ferreiro GA, et al. Limb salvage therapy for soft tissue sarcomas of the foot. Int J Radiat Oncol Biol Physics 19:41, 1990.
71. Shiu MH, Castro EB, Hajdu SI, Fortner JG. Surgical treatment of 297 soft tissue sarcomas of the lower extremity. Ann Surg 182:597, 1975.
72. Simon MA, Enneking WF. The management of soft-tissue sarcomas of the extremities. J Bone Joint Surg Am 58:317, 1976.
73. Sindelar WF, Kinsella TJ, Chen PW, et al. Intraoperative radiotherapy in retroperitoneal sarcomas: final results of a prospective, randomized, clinical trial. Arch Surg 128:402, 1993.
74. Skinner KA, Eilber FR, Holmes EC, et al. Surgical treatment and chemotherapy for pulmonary metastases from osteosarcoma. Arch Surg 127:1065, 1992.
75. Skrzynski MC, Biermann JS, Montag A, Simon MA. Diagnostic accuracy and charge-savings of outpatient core needle biopsy compared with open biopsy of musculoskeletal tumors. J Bone Joint Surg Am 78:644, 1996.
76. Sondak VK, Economou JS, Eilber FR. Soft tissue sarcomas of the extremity and retroperitoneum: advances in management. Adv Surg 24:333, 1991.
77. Sondak VK, Leonard JA Jr, Robertson JM, et al. Limb-sparing surgery for extremity soft tissue sarcomas: functional and rehabilitation considerations. Surg Oncol Clin North Am 2:657, 1993.
78. Sondak VK, Robertson JM, Sussman JJ, et al. Preoperative idoxuridine and radiation for large soft tissue sarcomas: clinical results with five-year follow-up. Ann Surg Oncol 5:106, 1998.
79. Song S, Stastny JJ, Chen H, Das Gupta TD. Expression of sarcoma-associated antigens p102 and p200 in human sarcoma cell lines. Anticancer Res 16:1171, 1996.
80. Springfield DS, Rosenberg A. Biopsy: complicated and risky. J Bone Joint Surg Am 78:639, 1996.
81. Storm FK, Eilber FR, Mirra J, Morton DL. Retroperitoneal sarcomas: a reappraisal of treatment. J Surg Oncol 17:1, 1981.
82. Storm FK, Mahvi DM. Diagnosis and management of retroperitoneal soft-tissue sarcoma. Ann Surg 214:2, 1991.
83. Sugarbaker PH, Nicholson TH. Atlas of Extremity Sarcoma Surgery. Lippincott, Philadelphia, 1984.
84. Suit HD, Mankin HJ, Wood WC, et al. Treatment of the patient with stage M0 soft tissue sarcoma. J Clin Oncol 6:854, 1988.
85. Taylor WF, Ivins JC, Pritchard DJ, et al. Trends and variability in survival among patients with osteosarcoma: a 7-year update. Mayo Clin Proc 60:91, 1985.
86. Tepper JE, Suit HD. Radiation therapy of soft tissue sarcomas. Cancer 55:2273, 1985.
87. Tierney JF, Stewart LA, Parmar MKB, et al. Adjuvant chemotherapy for localised resectable soft-tissue sarcoma of adults: meta-analysis of individual data: Sarcoma Meta-analysis Collaboration. Lancet 350:1647, 1997.
88. Torosian MH, Friedrich C, Godbold J, et al. Soft-tissue sarcoma: initial characteristics and prognostic factors in patients with and without metastatic disease. Semin Surg Oncol 4:13, 1988.
89. Wanebo HJ, Koness RJ, MacFarlane JK, et al. Head and neck sarcoma: report of the Head and Neck Sarcoma Registry: Society of Head and Neck Surgeons Committee on Research. Head Neck 14:1, 1992.
90. Weingrad DN, Rosenberg SA. Early lymphatic spread of osteogenic and soft-tissue sarcomas. Surgery 84:231, 1978.
91. Yang JC, Chang AE, Baker AR, et al. Randomized prospective study of the benefit of adjuvant radiation therapy in the treatment of soft tissue sarcomas of the extremity. J Clin Oncol 16:197, 1998.
92. Yang JC, Fraker DL, Thorn AK, et al. Isolation perfusion with tumor necrosis factor-alpha, interferon-gamma, and hyperthermia in the treatment of localized and metastatic cancer. Recent Results Cancer Res 138:161, 1995.
93. Yang RS, Lane JM, Eilber FR, et al. High grade soft tissue sarcoma of the flexor fossae: size rather than compartmental status determine prognosis. Cancer 76:1398, 1995.
94. Zalupski MM, Baker LH. Systemic adjuvant chemotherapy for soft tissue sarcomas. Hematol Oncol Clin North Am 9:787, 1995.

# CHAPTER 3

# RADIOLOGIC EVALUATION OF SOFT TISSUE TUMORS

RICHARD P. MOSER JR. AND WILLIAM M. PARRISH

Beginning with the second edition, this textbook included a chapter entitled the "Radiologic Evaluation of Soft Tissue Tumors." The first word was carefully selected because *radiologic* refers to all imaging modalities, including magnetic resonance imaging, computed tomography, angiography, ultrasonography, and scintigraphy, in addition to plain x-ray films, or radiographs, whereas *radiographic* refers only to "plain films," "plain x-ray films," or merely "x-ray films." Although all of these diverse modalities, on occasion, are useful and important when evaluating a suspected soft tissue tumor, the most indispensable technique is unmistakably magnetic resonance imaging.

When the second edition of this textbook appeared in 1988, clinical magnetic resonance imaging (commonly abbreviated in the literature as MR or MRI) was still in its relative infancy in the United States and elsewhere. Since then, there have been numerous marvelous, even spectacular, advances (technologic and otherwise).[32,37,68,134] Perhaps the single most important change has been the sheer proliferation in the overall number of MR scanners throughout the United States, notwithstanding the relentless penetration nationwide of managed care organizations and initiatives, whose common efforts and near-total focus are medical cost containment. It is difficult if not impossible to put the "technologic genie back into the bottle." As the twenty-first century begins, most hospitals in the United States have at least one clinical MR scanner, with many providing continuous daily, year-round service and immediate access especially for patients with intracranial or spinal cord-related medical emergencies.

The use of MR has dramatically increased for diverse reasons beyond the mere introduction of increasingly sophisticated body coils and innovative new pulse sequences. Most important, perhaps, has been the decremental cost of the equipment, which coincided with substantial technologic advances in both computer hardware and software design. The latter typically results in MR scanners with better spatial resolution and faster scanning times. In turn, the faster scanning times result in quicker patient "through-put" and less degradation in image quality due to patient motion. There have been important, concurrent advances in magnet shielding and configuration as well, including widening the bore of the magnet. The wider bore diameter substantially decreases problems related to "claustrophobia," a major problem with most early magnets that prevented many patients (particularly the obese) from being scanned. In fact, a successful "niche" market has recently developed based solely on low field strength: "open" (i.e., nonclaustrophobic) MR scanners. These stunning advances have contributed to the proliferation of magnets throughout the United States, so much so that, for example, there are currently more MR scanners in the Washington, DC metropolitan area alone than there are in most other countries of the world.

With many of these MR instruments scanning 3000–6000 patients per year (or even more), many more soft tissue tumors are scanned than ever before, and our experience with these lesions has substantially increased. Consequently, the medical literature detailing the strengths and weaknesses of MR for making preoperative diagnoses (which must be confirmed pathologically) and facilitating management has grown enormously. In fact, an entire book has been devoted to expanding the principles we presented in an earlier version of this chapter.[99] It was based on case material from the Armed Forces Institute of Pathology (AFIP). This updated chapter refines the basic principles we previously presented and augments them with extensive new experience, illustrated by many new figures.

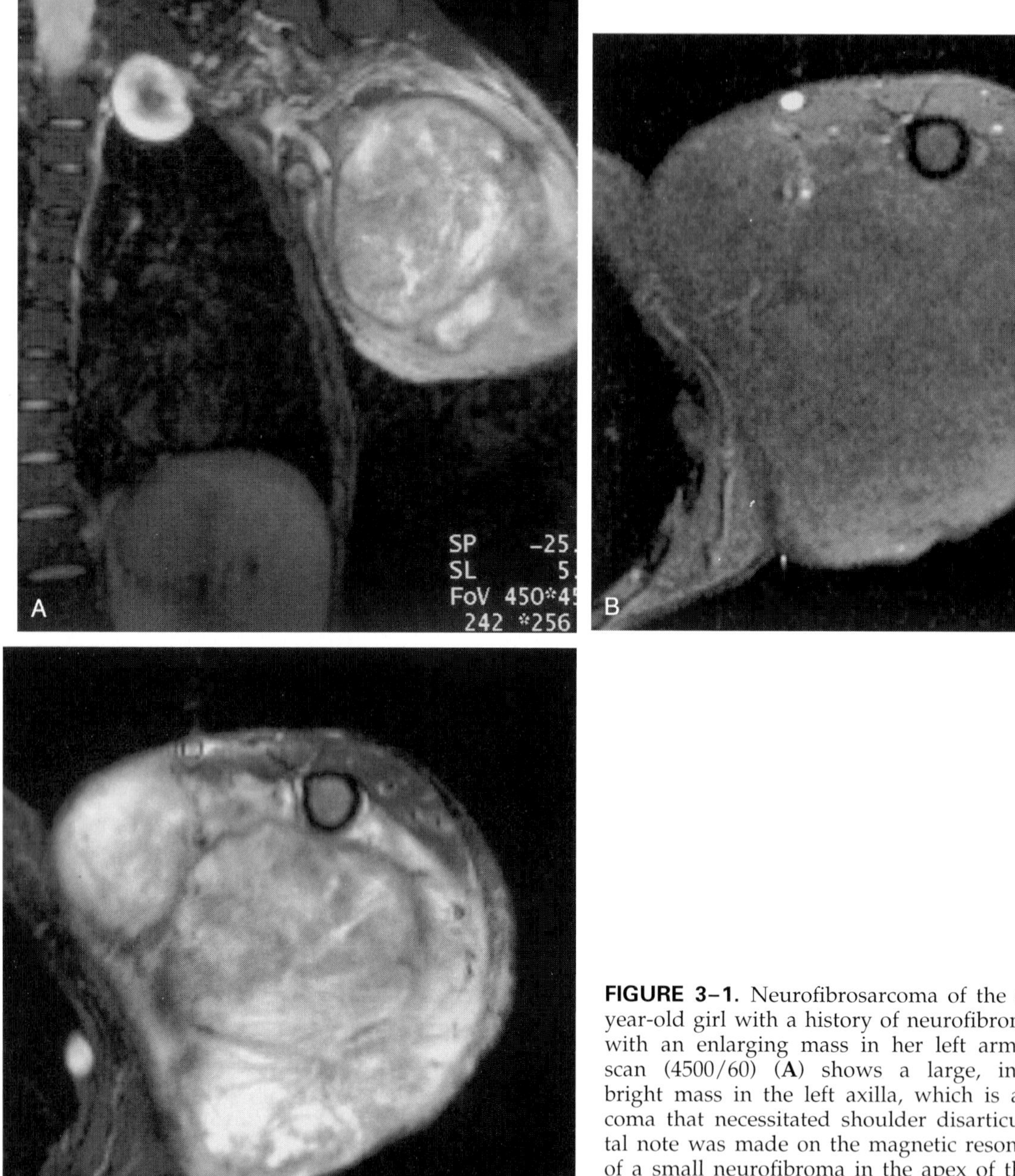


**FIGURE 3–1.** Neurofibrosarcoma of the shoulder. A 19-year-old girl with a history of neurofibromatosis presents with an enlarging mass in her left arm. Coronal STIR scan (4500/60) (**A**) shows a large, inhomogeneously bright mass in the left axilla, which is a neurofibrosarcoma that necessitated shoulder disarticulation. Incidental note was made on the magnetic resonance (MR) scan of a small neurofibroma in the apex of the left hemithorax. The complex nature of the neurofibrosaroma, which nearly surrounds the humerus and encompasses the neurovascular bundle, is shown to good advantage on axial 2D Flash (31/10) (**B**) and STIR (4000/60) (**C**) MR scans.

## OVERVIEW

Soft tissue tumors constitute a large, heterogeneous group of benign and malignant entities. In most cases the clinical findings associated with the tumors are disappointingly nonspecific. The typical clinical presentation is of a patient with a soft tissue mass of variable duration. Coexistent pain is an inconstant finding. Infrequently, the clinical findings themselves are highly suggestive of the specific nature of the tumor, as when an infant with a large arteriovenous malformation in the arm or leg presents with congestive heart failure, or a patient with hyperpigmented cutaneous lesions presents with subcutaneous or deep-seated neurofibromas (or both) or rarely a malignant peripheral nerve sheath tumor (Fig. 3–1).

In a predictably parallel fashion, the radiologic patterns exhibited by soft tissue tumors are also diverse and frequently nonspecific. Exceptions are infrequent but include fatty soft tissue tumors (Figs. 3–2, 3–3)* and soft tissue hemangiomas (Figs. 3–4, 3–5).† Imaging studies most commonly utilized to assess soft tissue tumors are (1) conventional radiographs, (2) MR imaging, and (3) computed tomography (CT). Since the previous editions of this book, MR has clearly emerged as the best method for cross-sectional imaging of soft tissue tumors, so much so that CT is necessary as a supplemental imaging modality in only a few cases. Sonography and angiography are utilized even less commonly. These various imaging modalities play a major role in detecting, localizing, characterizing, and determining the extent of the tumor. The last three, because they substantially affect the patient's management, represent the primary function of radiologic imaging of soft tissue masses.

Soft tissue tumors are usually round or oval. Far less commonly, they are elliptical (Fig. 3–6) or even exhibit a dumbbell shape (Figs. 3–2, 3–3) (in at least one plane—axial, coronal, sagittal—of the MR scan). These tumors vary widely in size and may arise in the skin, subcutaneous tissues, muscle, or other deep soft tissues. Superficial lesions of the skin are best assessed by clinical inspection and palpation. Masses arising in the subcutaneous and deeper soft tissues should be evaluated by radiologic studies, which can detect calcification, ossification, or radiolucency in the lesion. Cross-sectional imaging can determine the homogeneity (or lack thereof) of the lesion, the extent of the mass (including involvement of adjacent bones, joints, neurovascular structures, or other soft tissues), and the epicenter of the lesion. The challenges to the radiologist are to (1) suggest an appropriate sequencing of radiologic studies that permits timely, accurate evaluation of the tumor while simultaneously minimizing expense and discomfort to the patient; (2) determine the extent of the lesion and its impact on adjacent structures; and (3) suggest an appropriate differential diagnosis. Whereas MR plays a vital role in all three of these areas, under no circumstances should the MR scan be interpreted without correlation with the radiographs, which should always be obtained first.

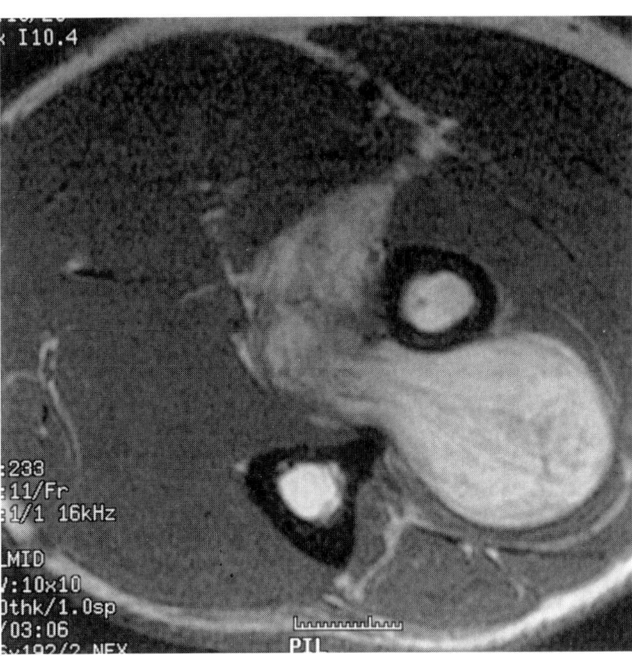


**FIGURE 3–2.** Intramuscular lipoma of the forearm. A 46-year-old man presented with an enlarging forearm mass and limited supination. Axial SE T1 MR scan (233/11) shows a large "dumbbell-shaped" mass insinuating itself between the radius and ulna. The lesion is predominantly bright, similar in signal intensity to subcutaneous fat, but contains streaks of linear fibrous septa. The latter are frequently encountered in soft tissue lipomas.

Unfortunately, in most cases radiologic features cannot reliably distinguish between benign and malignant soft tissue tumors. This important caveat cannot be overemphasized. Radiologic studies are invaluable tools for assessing the "macroscopic" but not the "microscopic" features of a soft tissue tumor or tumor-like process. Note that MR plays a vitally important role in the evaluation of patients afflicted with bone tumors too, but there is an interesting difference. The differential diagnosis of a bone lesion is almost always based on the radiograph, whereas the differential diagnosis of a soft tissue mass or tumor is almost always based on the MR scan [except for le-

*References 3, 5, 12, 21, 35, 36, 62, 87, 92, 97, 99, 100, 104, 115, 117, 122, 123, 126, 143, 174.

†References 19, 20, 26, 27, 40, 51, 60, 83, 89, 90, 112, 116, 128, 129, 133, 143, 147, 156, 157, 197.

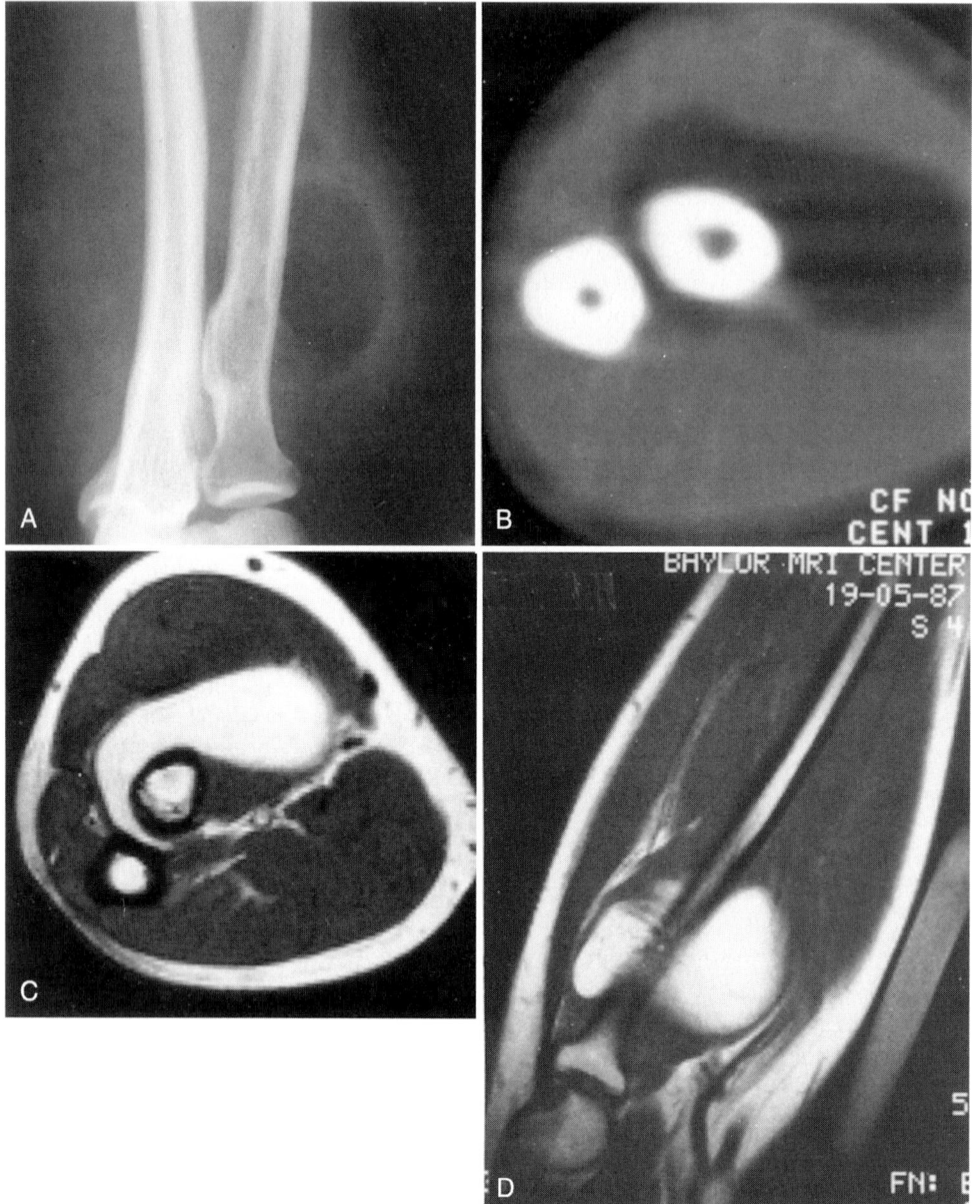


**FIGURE 3–3.** Lipoma of the proximal forearm. (**A**) Plain radiograph demonstrates the fatty nature (radiolucency) and sharp margins of the lipoma, adjacent to the proximal radius. (**B**) The fatty nature of the tumor is also readily apparent on the computed tomography (CT) scan as a region of decreased attenuation (i.e., attenuation of the lipoma is less than that of adjacent muscle) that partly envelops the radius. On the CT scan, the exact extent of the tumor remains uncertain. (**C**) Axial MR scan (534/34) at the same level as the CT scan (**B**) shows the excellent soft tissue contrast of MR and extension of the lipoma around the radius, with insinuation of the "tail" of the lesion between the radius and ulna in a "dumbbell" configuration. The bright or high-signal intensity signal of the lipoma on this T1-weighted image is typical of fatty tissue. (**D**) Coronal T1-weighted MR scan (534/34) reveals to better advantage the three-dimensional nature of the lipoma, its sharp margins, and its substantial encirclement of the radius. The radial cortex, which is black (due to an absence of signal, or "signal void," in the calcified bony cortex) on the MR scan, is intact and easily identified because of the contrasting high signal from the marrow fat in the bone and the high, fatty signal in the adjacent soft tissue lipoma.

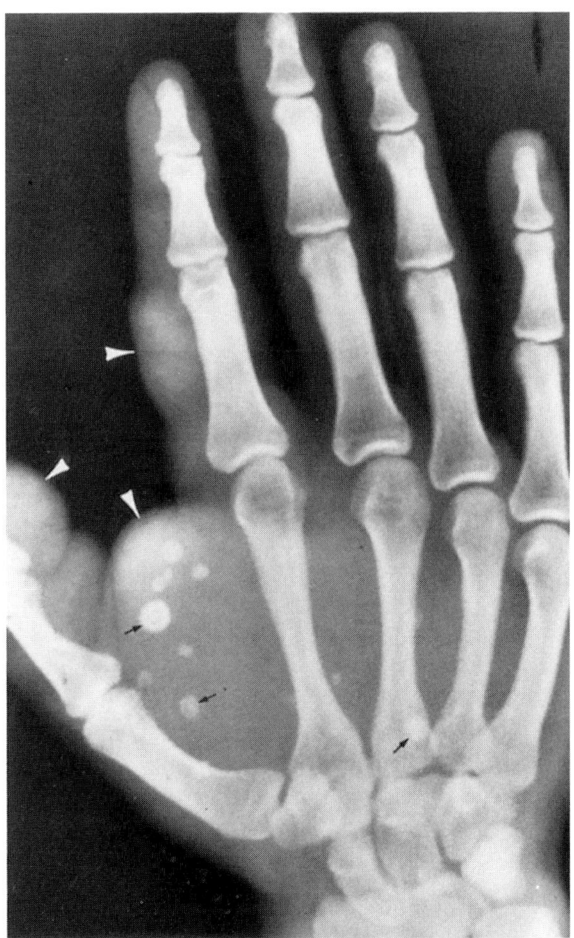

**FIGURE 3–4.** Hemangioma of the hand with calcified phleboliths. The hemangioma causes extensive soft tissue swelling (arrowheads) with increased density involving the thumb, index finger, and thenar region. Multiple small calcified phleboliths (small arrows) are seen in a typical configuration of spherical rings.

sions such as hemangiomas, which demonstrate calcification that is better assessed by radiography (Figs. 3–4, 3–5) or CT scans].

## SOFT TISSUE VERSUS BONY ORIGIN OF THE SOFT TISSUE MASS

In most instances, modern imaging modalities can reliably determine whether the mass arises from bone (i.e., cortex or marrow space) or from adjacent soft tissues (Fig. 3–7). The relation between a soft tissue tumor and adjacent structures may assume one of three patterns (Fig. 3–8): (1) The soft tissue mass may be completely distinct from the adjacent bone, separated by an uninvolved soft tissue plane. This situation is most common. The margin of any soft tissue mass, best assessed on MR, may be characterized as "sharp" or "ill-defined." (2) Occasionally, the soft tissue mass barely touches or contacts the outer cortical surface of an adjacent bone (Fig. 3–8), thereby creating acute angles between the mass and the bone (Fig. 3–9). (3) The mass directly affects the bone, a situation that may take many forms, varying from extrinsic bony erosion, with or without an associated periosteal reaction, to frank invasion of the marrow space of the affected bone.

Depending on the location of the soft tissue tumor, one or more bones can be affected. The area of extrinsic erosion of bone by the soft tissue mass may exhibit sharp, well defined margins that are round or scalloped in contour (Fig. 3–10) and that occasionally exhibit bony sclerosis in their margins (Fig. 3–10). Conversely, there may be an ill-defined interface between the soft tissue mass and the adjacent, affected bone (Fig. 3–8), sometimes with associated ill-defined bony erosion or even complete cortical destruction with extension of the tumor into the bone marrow (Fig. 3–11). In the latter case, it is occasionally difficult to predict confidently whether the lesion arose in the soft tissues and secondarily invaded the adjacent bone or vice versa.

A soft tissue origin of the lesion should immediately be suspected when multiple bones are eroded (Fig. 3–8). These bones are typically adjacent to each other, with the tumor surrounding or insinuated between them (Figs. 3–12, 3–13). Predictably, this situation is encountered most frequently in the carpals, metacarpals, tarsals, and metatarsals and less frequently in the bones of the forearm (radius and ulna) or lower leg (tibia and fibula). This situation occurs least frequently in adjacent ribs or vertebrae. An analogous situation exists when a soft tissue mass arises in or adjacent to a joint and secondarily erodes or invades the bony structures that constitute that joint.

The bone adjacent to a soft tissue mass may demonstrate periosteal new bone formation with or without direct tumor invasion. Indolent lesions produce solid cortical thickening and more aggressive ones an interrupted periosteal reaction (Figs. 3–8, 3–14, 3–15). Periosteal reactions are most commonly encountered in association with hypervascular soft tissue neoplasms. Benign and malignant vascular soft tissue tumors may produce such periosteal reactions. The solid periosteal reaction reflects slower, or more indolent, biologic activity and therefore is more typical of benign tumors, particularly hemangiomas. The interrupted periosteal reaction, on the other hand, reflects more aggressive biologic activity and, accordingly, is more commonly encountered in association with malignant soft tissue tumors.

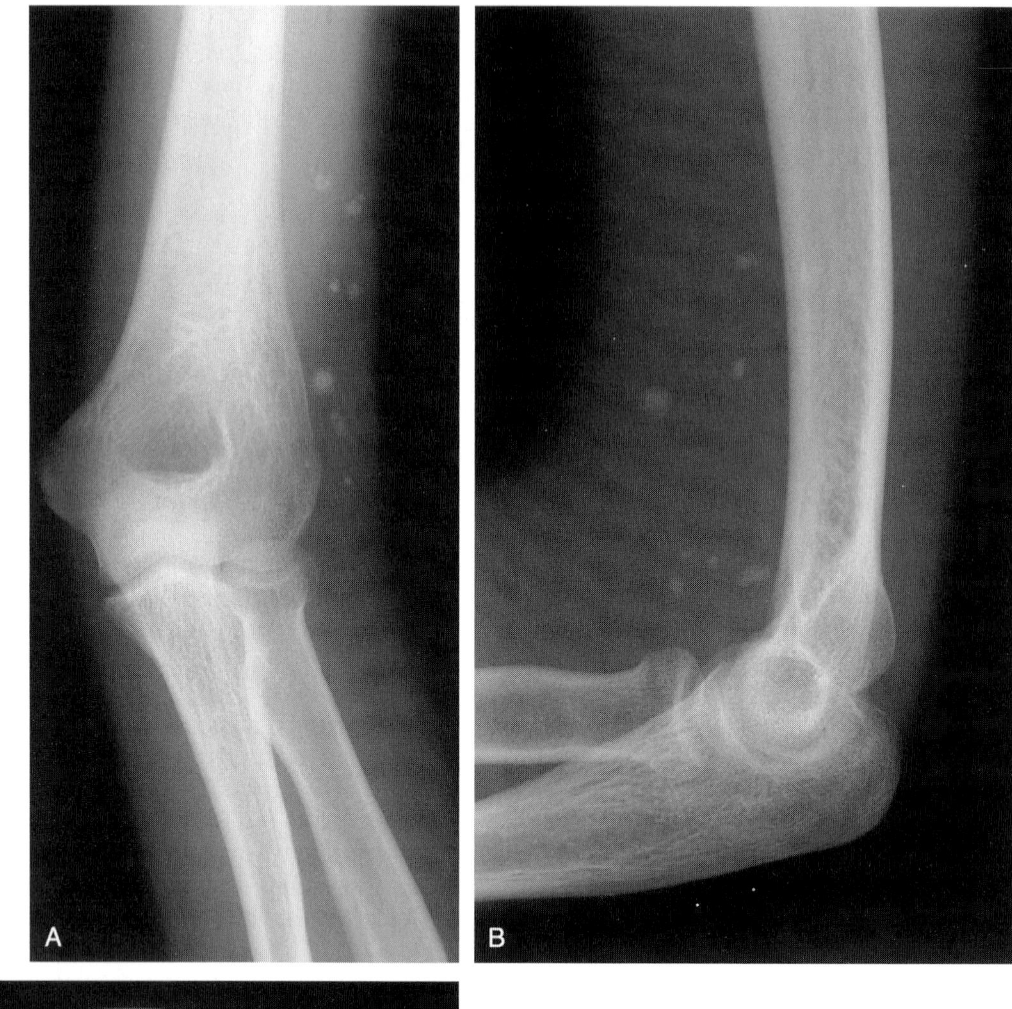

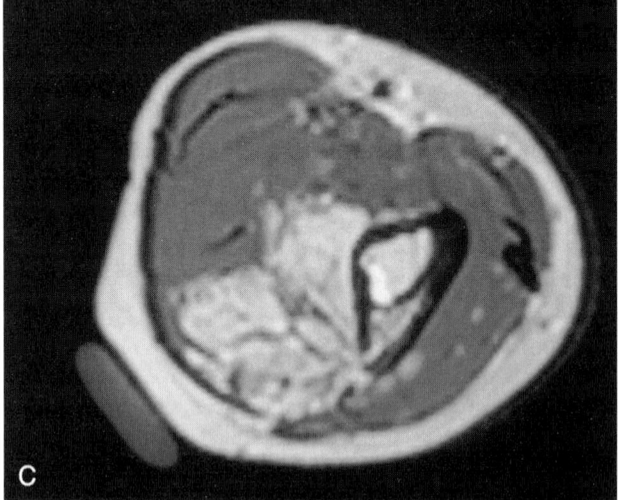

**FIGURE 3–5.** Hemangioma of the upper extremity. A 15-year-old girl presents with painful swelling near the left elbow. The pain and swelling worsened following physical activity. Anteroposterior (AP) (**A**) and lateral (**B**) radiographs of the elbow demonstrate multiple calcified phleboliths. The T2 axial MR scan (2500/30) (**C**), and coronal T1 (500/15)

*Illustration continued on opposite page*

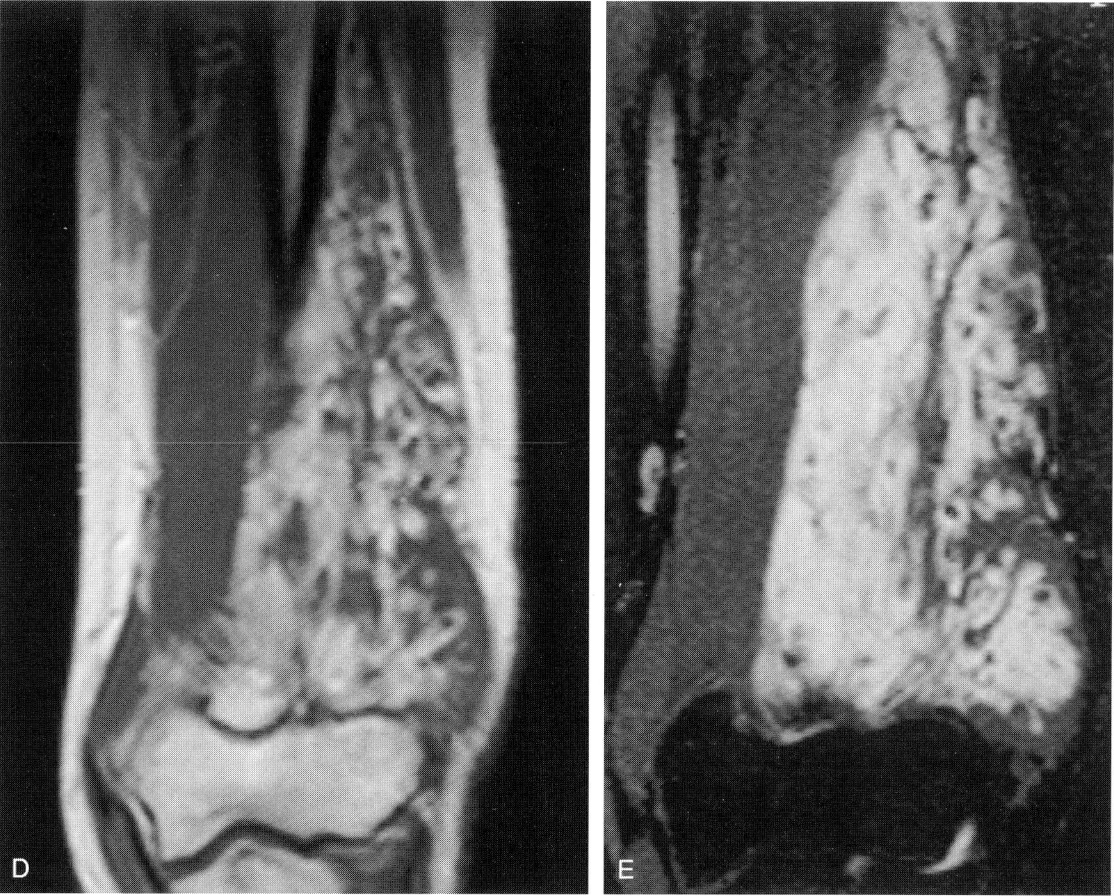


**FIGURE 3–5** *(Continued).* (**D**) and inversion recovery (2000/30) (**E**) MR images well demonstrate abundant fat and numerous vessels in the lesion. This contellation of findings is characteristic of a large intramuscular hemangioma.

The spectrum of patterns (Fig. 3–8) described above are typical manifestations of soft tissue tumors restricted to soft tissue or secondarily affecting adjacent bone. When determining whether a lesion is "primary" in soft tissue or "primary" in bone, it is usually correct that the site of the most extensive abnormality represents the origin, or "epicenter," of the process. Comparison of plain radiographs with cross-sectional imaging studies such as MR or CT scans can usually determine the epicenter of the lesion, thereby localizing the origin of the lesion primarily to soft tissue or bone and resolving the dilemma of "inside out" or "outside in." The "reference" frame used here is from the perspective of the skeleton. Therefore "inside out" refers to the situation in which the tumor arises in the bone and secondarily invades the adjacent soft tissues. Conversely, "outside in" refers to the situation in which the tumor arises in soft tissues and secondarily invades adjacent bone.

Bone tumors may be completely or partially contained in the affected bone. The first radiologic indication of bone destruction may be endosteal cortical erosion, which can progress to complete cortical destruction with periosteal elevation and reaction and eventually frank invasion of the adjacent soft tissues. The soft tissue mass associated with a primary skeletal neoplasm ("inside out") has its epicenter in the affected bone, just the opposite of the situation that exists for a primary soft tissue tumor that subsequently affects the adjacent bone ("outside in"). In the latter situation (soft tissue tumor or mass secondarily invading the adjacent bone), the epicenter of the soft tissue mass is outside the bone. Also the outer, cortical bony surface (rather than the inner or endosteal surface) is eroded first by tumors of soft tissue origin. On rare occasions aggressive neoplasms such as Ewing's sarcoma, poorly differentiated chondrosarcoma, and leukemia have such extremely high biologic activity they infiltrate the microscopic haversian canals of cortical bone into the adjacent periosteal structures and present as a lesion of suspected soft tissue origin

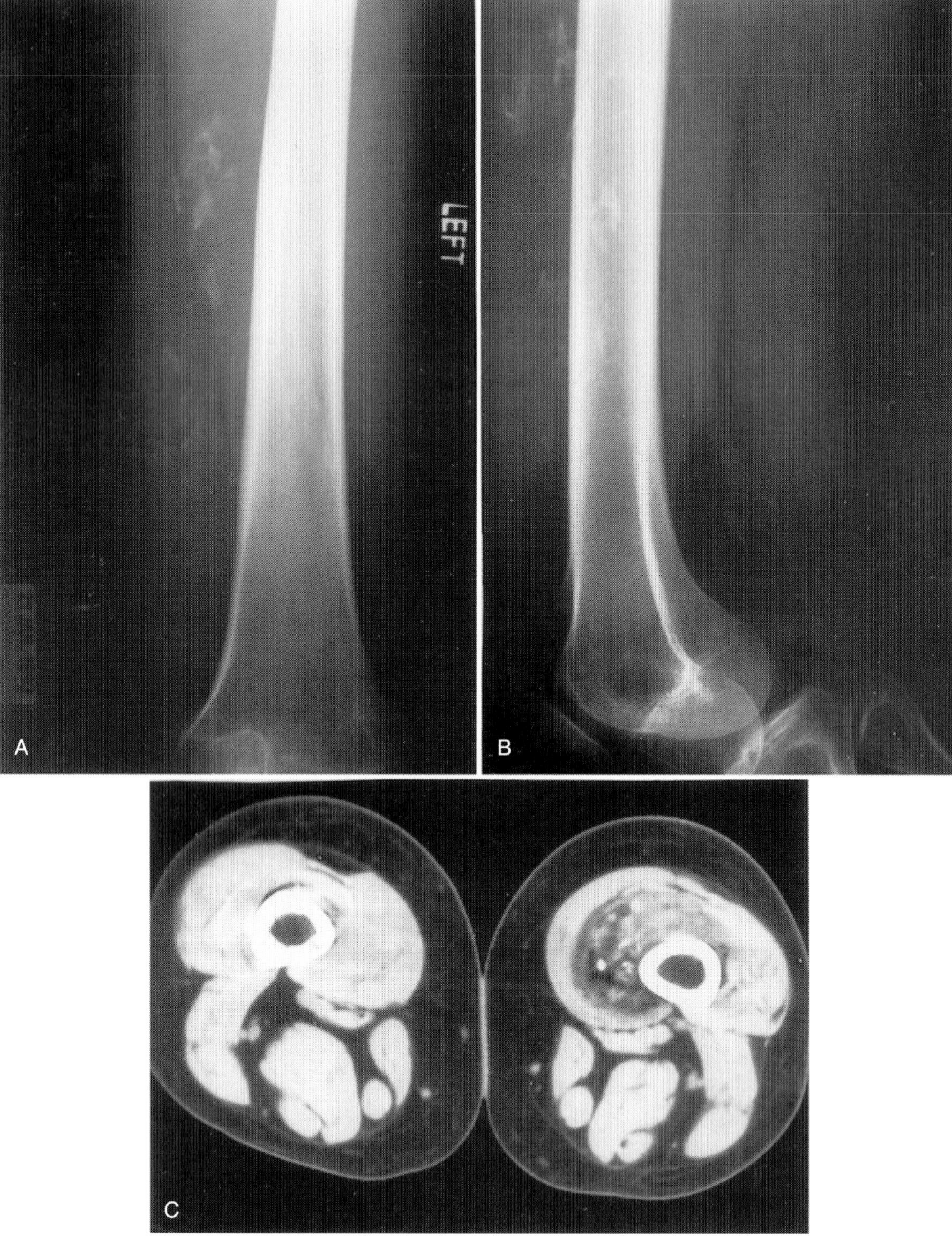


**FIGURE 3–6.** Hemangioma of the thigh. AP (**A**) and lateral (**B**) radiographs show peculiar, discrete "chicken-wire" calcifications in the soft tissues of the anteromedial thigh. Axial CT scans, with soft tissue (**C**) and bone.

*Illustration continued on opposite page*

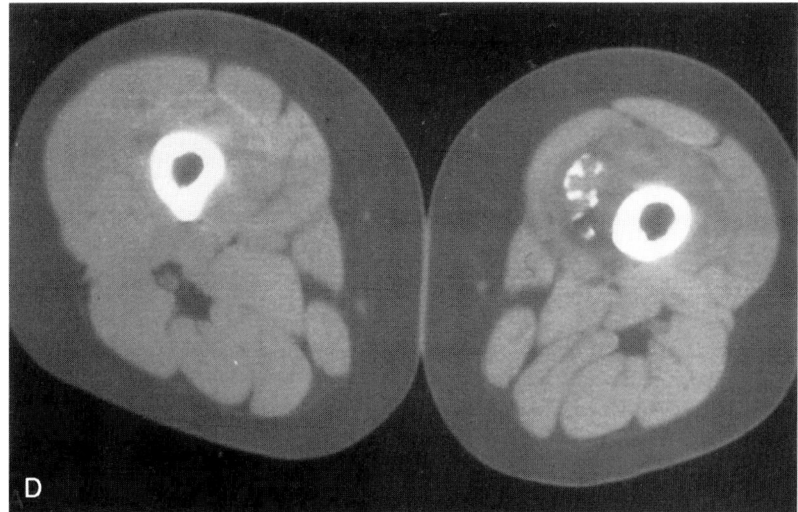


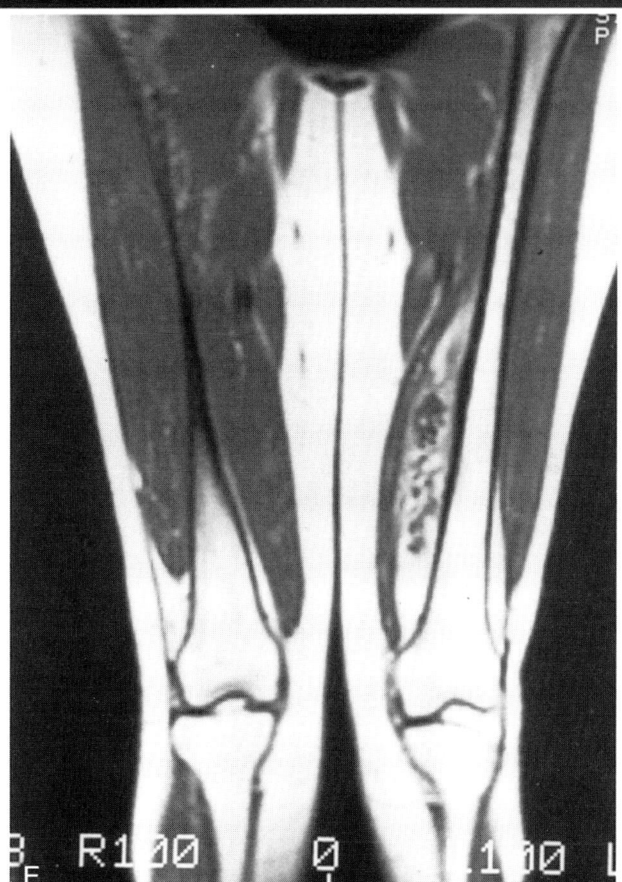


**FIGURE 3–6** *(Continued)*. (**D**) Windows, show a large inhomogeneous soft tissue mass encircling the medial aspect of the femur. The margins of the mass are ill-defined, particularly anteriorly. The configuration of some of the soft tissue calcifications is best appreciated on the bone windows (**D**). Coronal T1-weighted (350/10) MR scan (**E**) shows an interesting "elliptical" configuration to the inhomogeneous hemangioma. Note how the lesion abuts the medial femoral cortex.

*Illustration continued on following page*

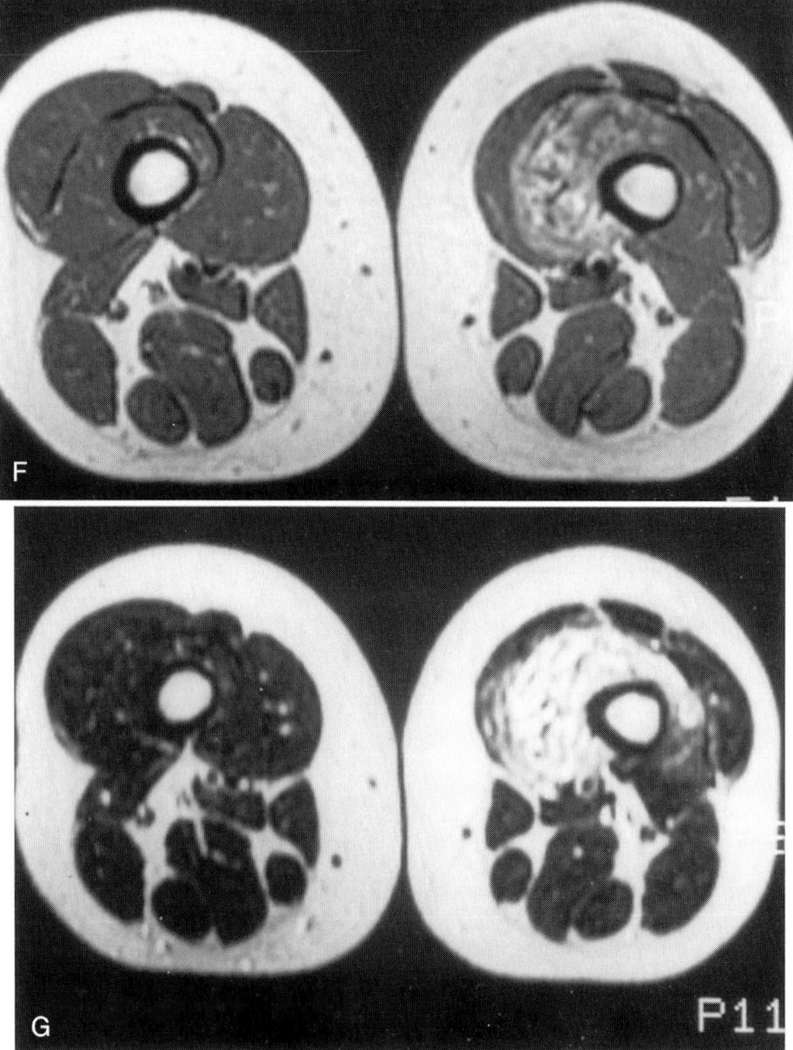


**FIGURE 3–6** *(Continued).* Axial T1-weighted (700/16) (**F**) and T2-weighted (300/85) (**G**) MR scans also show the inhomogeneous nature of the soft tissue hemangioma and its relation to the femoral cortex. The MR images well demonstrate abundant fat and numerous vessels in the lesion, typical features of a soft tissue hemangioma.

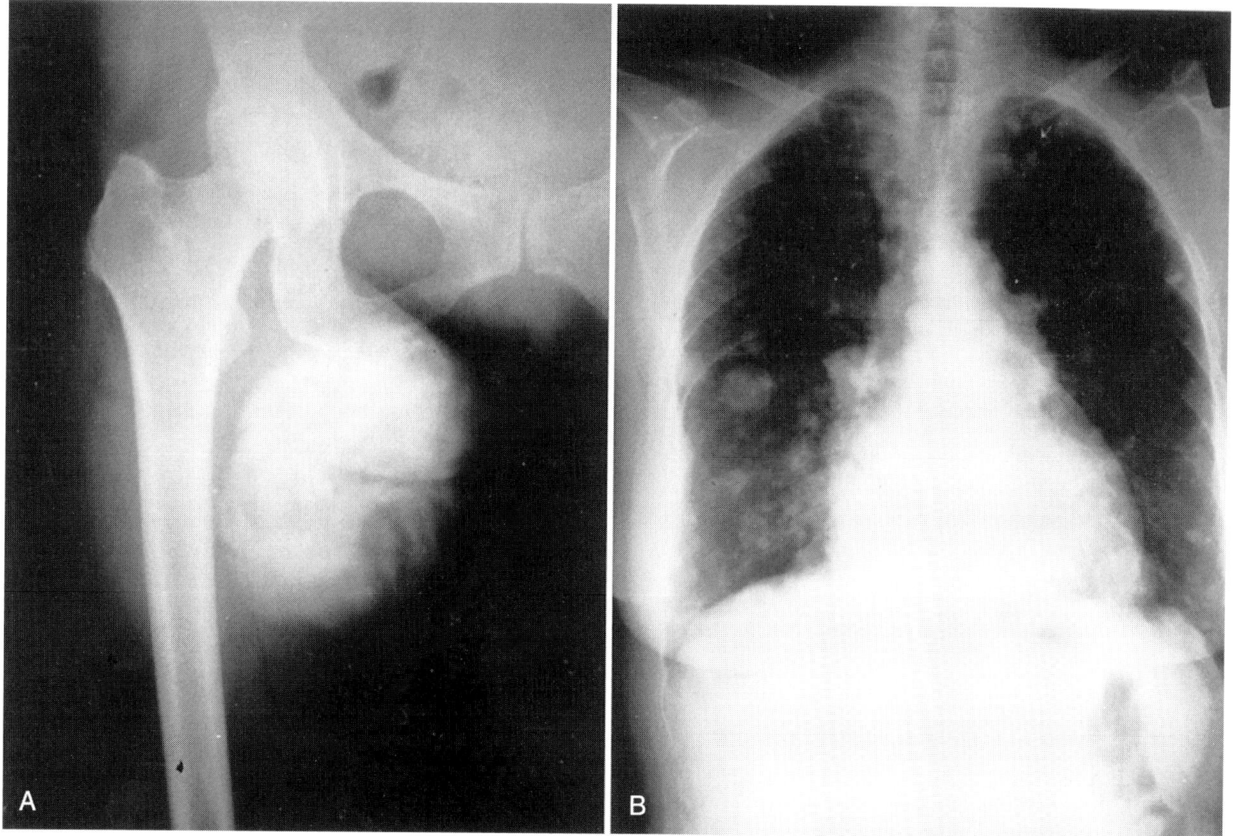


**FIGURE 3–7.** Extraskeletal osteosarcoma of the thigh with several suspected skeletal metastases and extensive metastases to the chest. (**A**) Frontal radiograph of the thigh shows a large, densely calcified mass (diameter 13 cm) in the medial soft tissues of the right thigh. (**B**) Posteroanterior (PA) chest radiograph demonstrates diffuse, bilateral pulmonary metastases of varying size. For unknown reasons these metastases are disproportionately located adjacent to the heart.

*Illustration continued on following page*

due to the absence of radiographically demonstrable cortical destruction. Because of the exquisite sensitivity of MR for detecting bone marrow involvement, however, the surgeon should rarely be mistaken as to the epicenter of the disease process.

## RADIOLOGIC CRITERIA FOR DISTINGUISHING BENIGN AND MALIGNANT SOFT TISSUE TUMORS

Imaging features useful for distinguishing benign from malignant soft tissue tumors have been discussed extensively in the medical literature.* There are numerous ways to characterize a soft tissue tumor radiologically, including size, shape, or configuration, rate of growth, location, number of tumors, radiodensity, homogeneity, evidence of osseous involvement, and interface with adjacent soft tissues. Unfortunately, none of these features is reliably pathognomonic for distinguishing between benign and malignant tumors. It is possible, however, to characterize the features of a "classic" benign soft tissue tumor and the "typical" malignant soft tissue lesion. This characterization is helpful during preoperative staging and for alerting the treating physician to the fact that the tumor has predominantly benign or predominantly malignant radiologic features. Understandably, this judgment also affects management of the neoplasm.

The margin or interface of the tumor with the uninvolved adjacent soft tissues may be sharply demarcated or ill-defined. Benign tumors are usually sharply circumscribed, whereas malignant tumors

*References 1, 2, 4, 11, 23, 28, 29, 45, 46, 56, 58, 64, 65, 73, 76, 77, 79, 81, 86, 88, 94, 95, 103, 110, 119, 132, 140, 142, 153, 155, 162, 164, 172, 173, 180, 188, 189, 204.

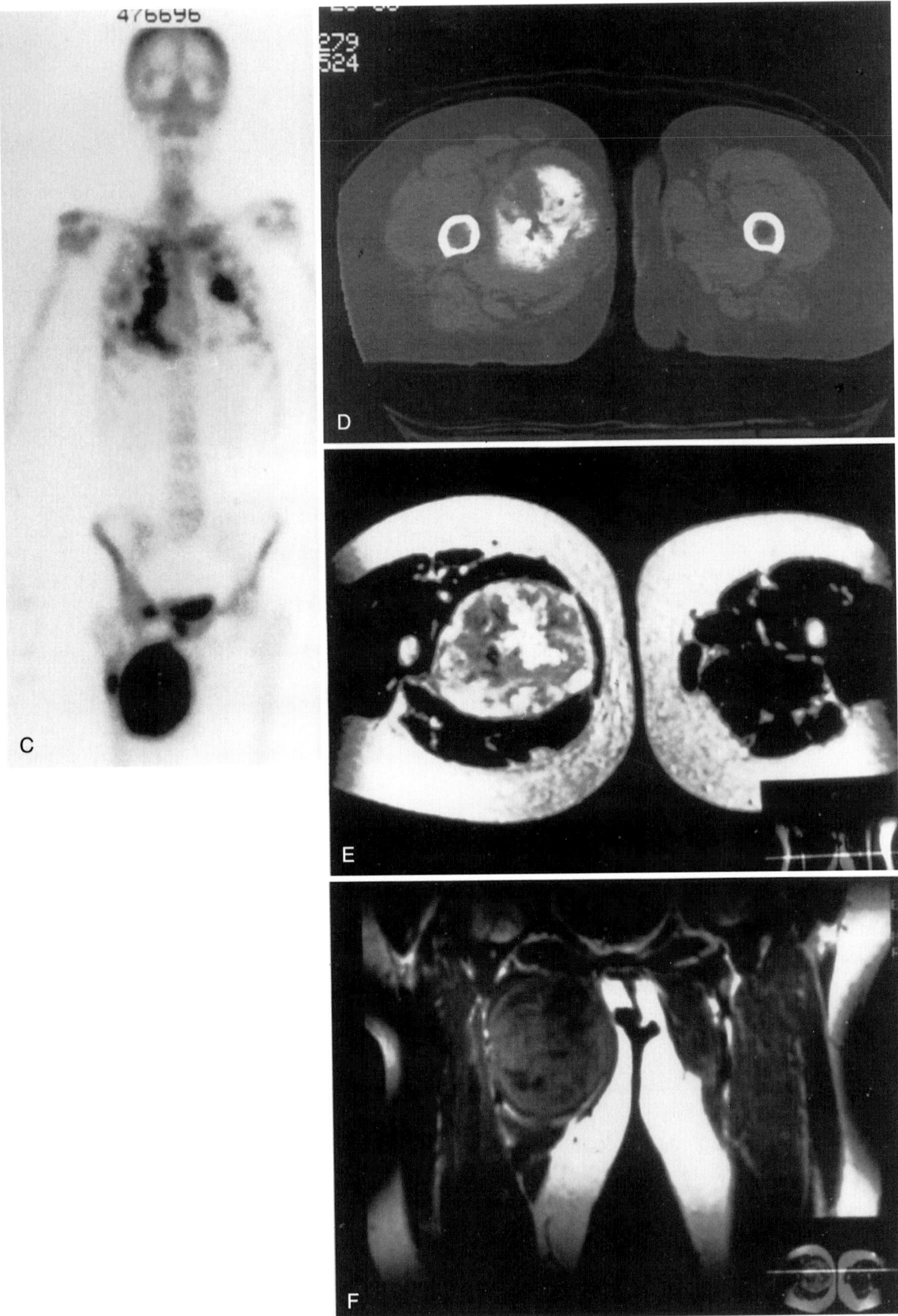


**FIGURE 3–7** *(Continued). See legend on opposite page*

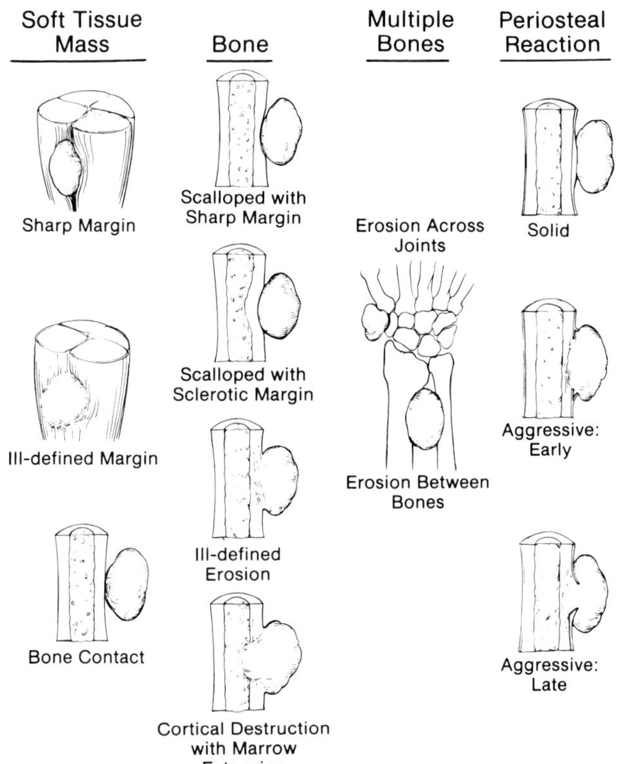


**FIGURE 3–8.** Spectrum of radiologic patterns of soft tissue tumors.

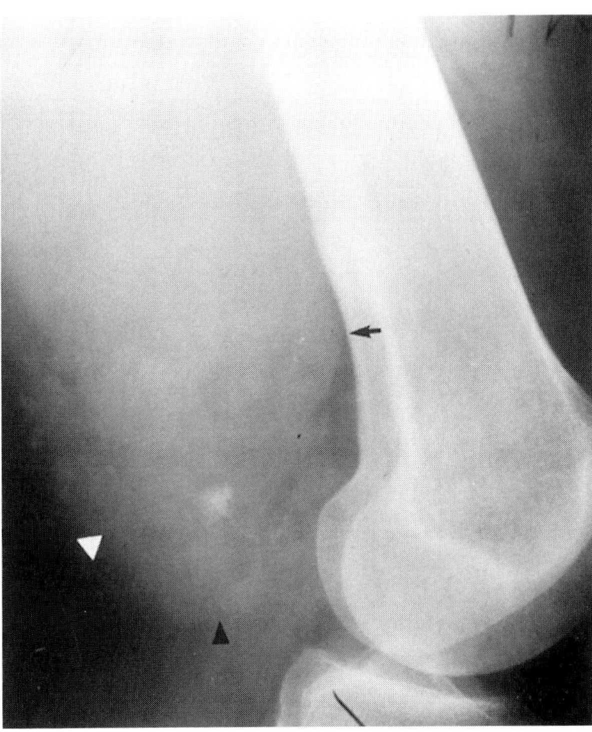

**FIGURE 3–9.** Synovial sarcoma of the distal thigh. The mass in the posterior soft tissues contacts the adjacent, posterior femur. Contact point demonstrates an acute angle (arrow) between the tumor and the femur. Also of note is that the mass has an ill-defined distal margin (arrowheads) and contains several small calcifications.

**FIGURE 3–7** *(Continued).* (**C**) Methylene diphosphonate (MDP) scintigram demonstrates marked radionuclide accumulation in the soft tissue lesion in the thigh and diffuse uptake in the chest. Based exclusively on the scintigram, it is impossible to localize precisely the sites of the lesions in the chest (e.g., pulmonary parenchymal, pericardial, or osseous or in mediastinal lymph nodes). Also noted are several foci of increased radionuclide uptake in the proximal right femur adjacent to the soft tissue mass and in the right hemipelvis. (**D**) Axial CT scan with bone windows demonstrates a large, sharply demarcated, densely, but inhomogeneously calcified mass in the medial soft tissues of the right thigh. On all CT cuts, although the medial border of the mass is in close anatomic proximity to the adjacent femoral cortex, there was a distinct separation between the mineralized soft tissue mass and the femur. Overall, there was more extensive mineralization toward the center of the soft tissue mass. (**E**) Axial MR scan (2500/30) demonstrates a large, sharply demarcated, inhomogeneous soft tissue mass in the medial thigh. An interesting nodular pattern is noted in the lesion. (**F**) Coronal MR scan (600/30) also demonstrates an inhomogeneous signal throughout the sharply demarcated lesion in the medial soft tissues of the right thigh. This case clearly demonstrates that highly malignant soft tissue masses can exhibit sharply demarcated margins on MR scans. The importance of this point cannot be overemphasized. The MR scan shows "macroscopic," not "microscopic," boundaries of the soft tissue mass.

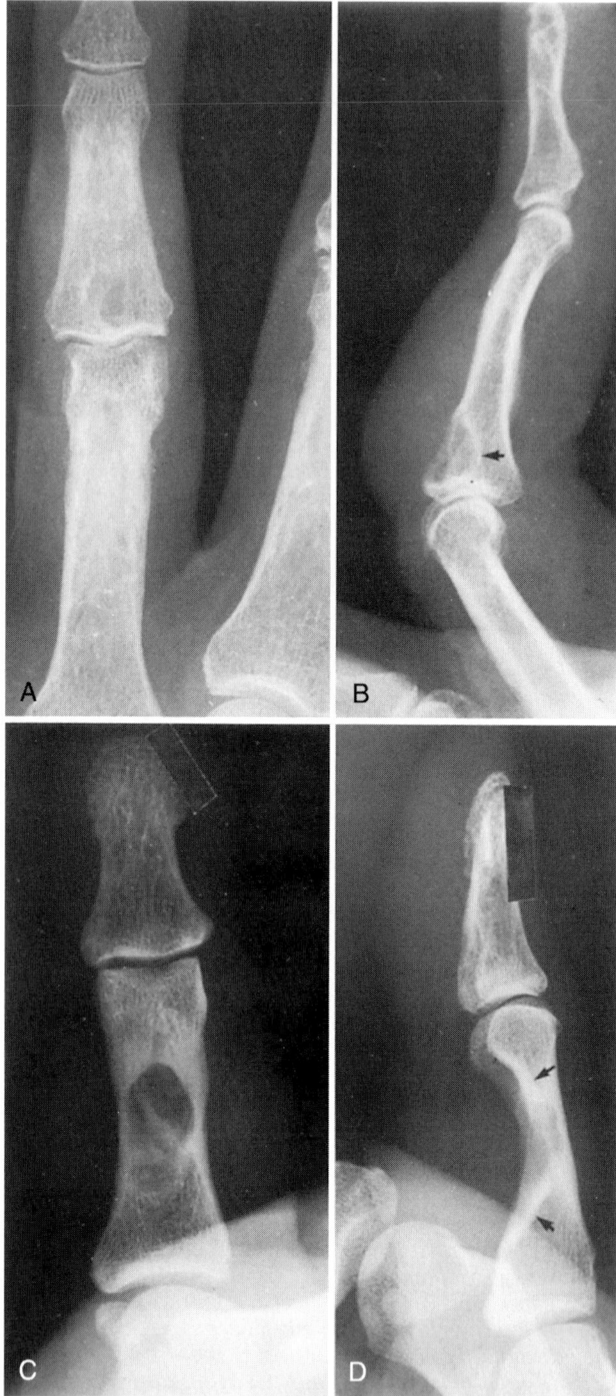


**FIGURE 3–10.** Scalloped bony margins in two patients. Case 1: Synovial chondromatosis of the finger. AP (**A**) and lateral (**B**) radiographs show a soft tissue mass adjacent to the middle phalanx, producing a scalloped, sclerotic margin (arrow). Scalloping of the phalanx is due to the extrinsic erosion by the soft tissue mass into the adjacent bone and is seen best on the lateral view. Case 2: Giant cell tumor of the tendon sheath involving the thumb. The lesion could be easily mistaken for an intraosseous lesion in the proximal phalanx based on the frontal radiograph (**C**), but the extrinsic nature and scalloped sclerotic margins (arrows) are seen in excellent detail on the lateral radiograph (**D**).

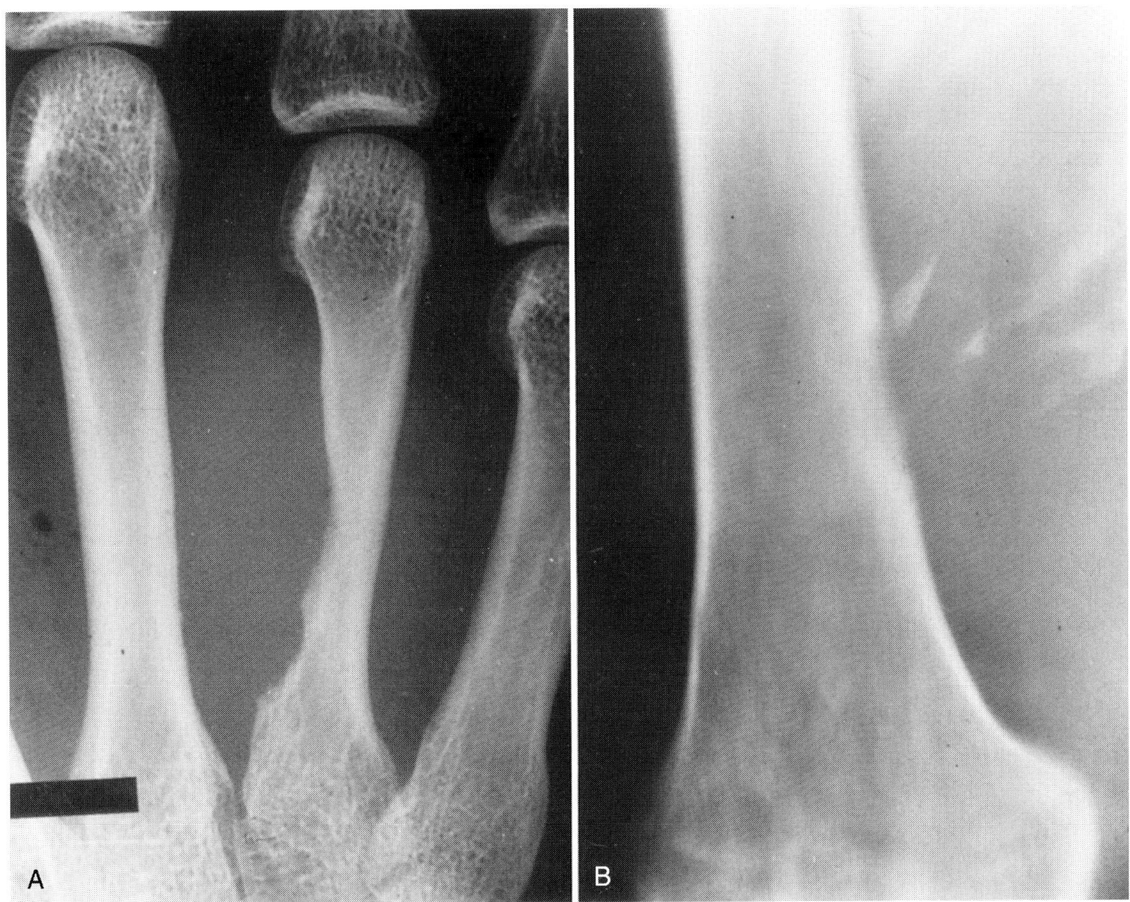


**FIGURE 3–11.** Cortical destruction with marrow extension. (**A, B**) Two different patients with synovial sarcoma show cortical destruction and marrow extension. The latter is indicated by destruction of endosteal cortex, although the marrow involvement can be imaged more convincingly on magnetic resonance scans. Both patients presented with a soft tissue mass. Coexistent calcification was noted in the synovial sarcoma of the thigh, where the tomogram (**B**) clearly demonstrates both the endosteal destruction and the areas of calcification.

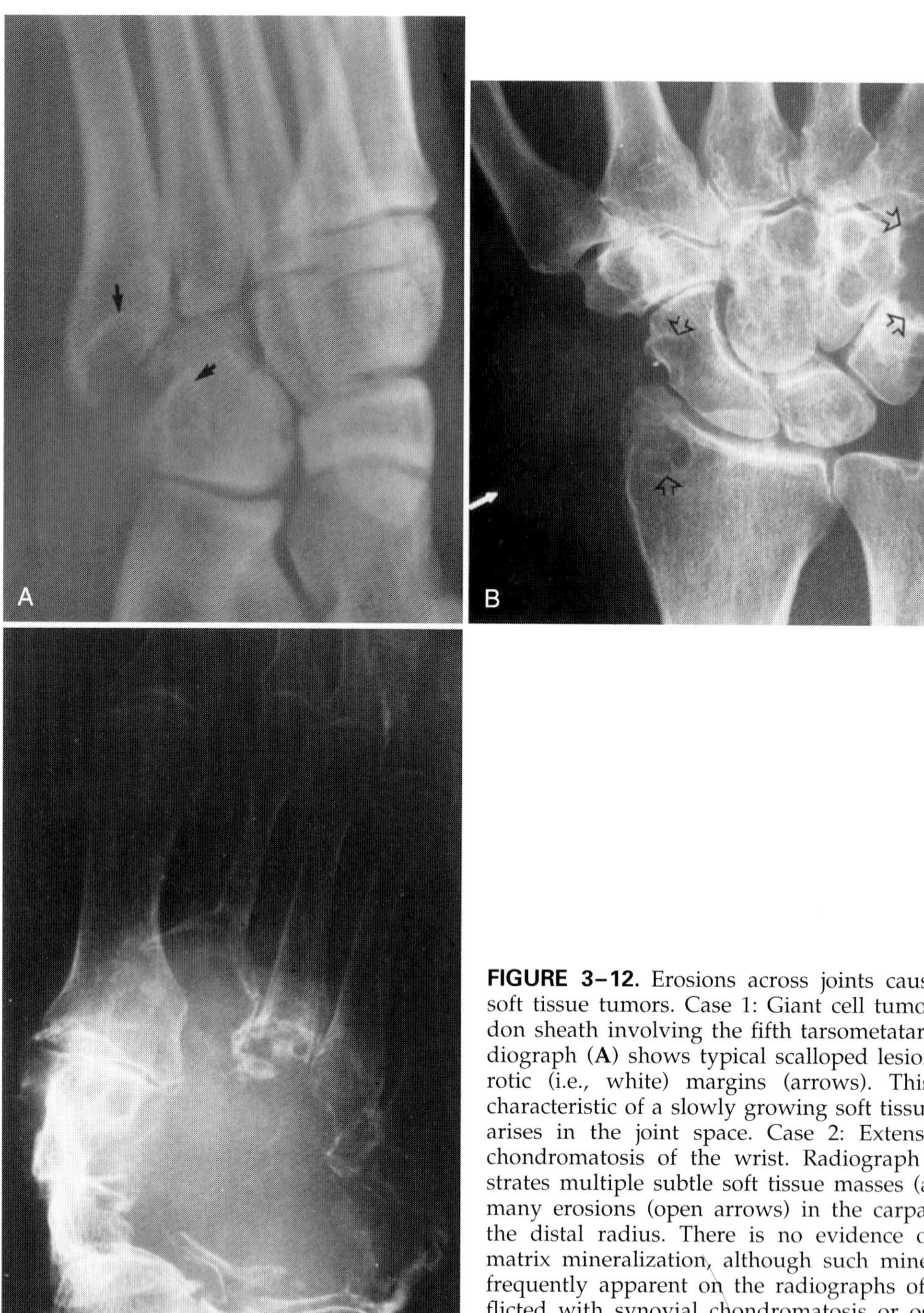


**FIGURE 3–12.** Erosions across joints caused by three soft tissue tumors. Case 1: Giant cell tumor of the tendon sheath involving the fifth tarsometatarsal joint. Radiograph (**A**) shows typical scalloped lesions with sclerotic (i.e., white) margins (arrows). This pattern is characteristic of a slowly growing soft tissue tumor that arises in the joint space. Case 2: Extensive synovial chondromatosis of the wrist. Radiograph (**B**) demonstrates multiple subtle soft tissue masses (arrows) with many erosions (open arrows) in the carpal bones and the distal radius. There is no evidence of chondroid matrix mineralization, although such mineralization is frequently apparent on the radiographs of patients afflicted with synovial chondromatosis or osteochondromatosis. Case 3: Neurilemoma of the soft tissues of the mid-foot. The radiograph (**C**) shows extensive destruction of both tarsal and metatarsal bones. The osseous margins are smooth and predominantly sclerotic.

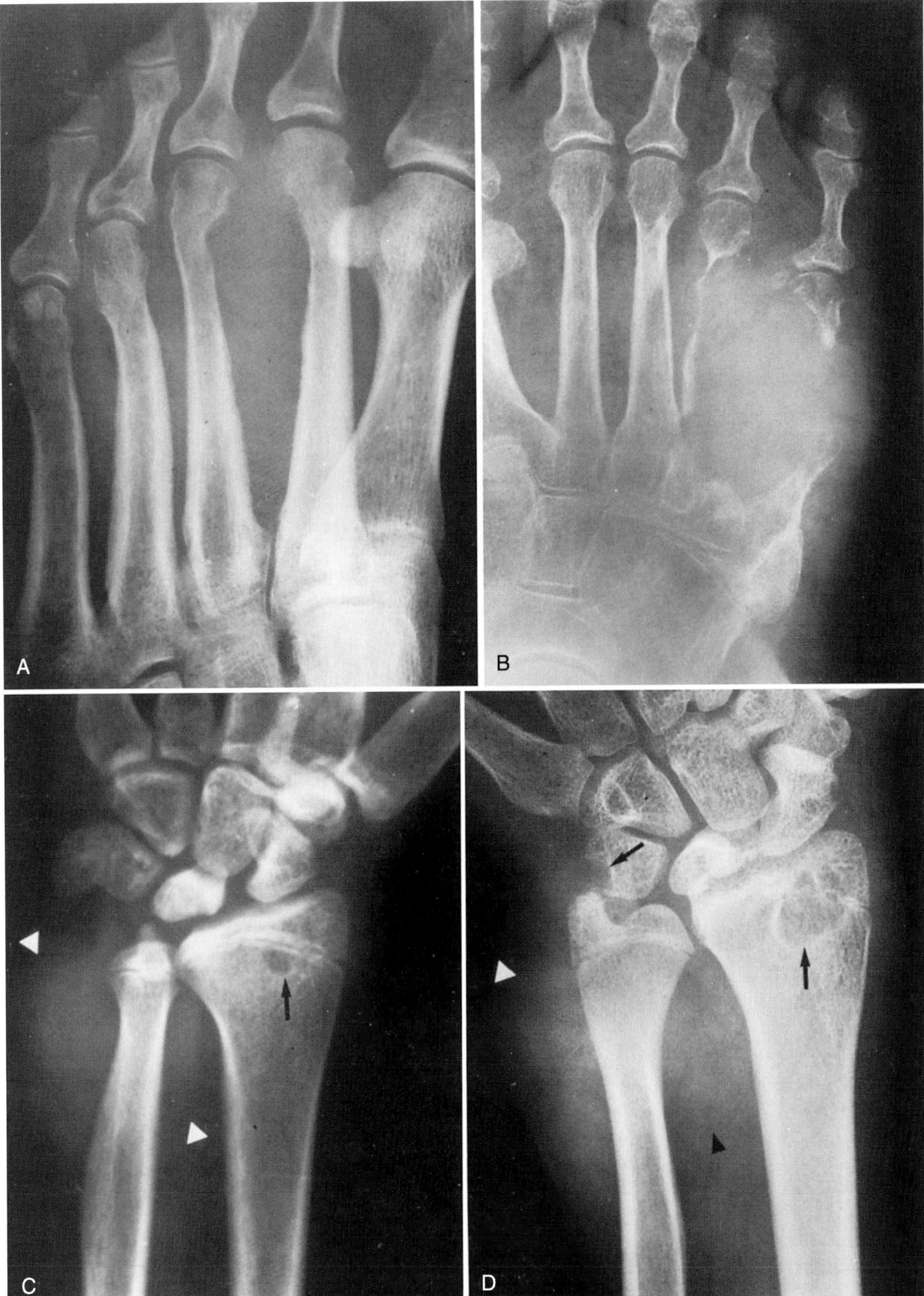


**FIGURE 3–13.** Erosions between bones caused by three soft tissue masses. Case 1: Malignant schwannoma involving the soft tissues and bones of the foot. Radiograph (**A**) shows a soft tissue mass that separates and erodes the adjacent second and third metatarsals, with subtle ill-defined cortical destruction of the affected bones. Case 2: Chondrosarcoma of soft tissue of the foot. Coned-down radiograph (**B**) shows aggressive and near-total destruction of the fourth and fifth metatarsal bones by a large soft tissue mass. There are ill-defined bony erosions in the affected metatarsals. Case 3: Pigmented villonodular synovitis of the wrist. Radiographs (**C, D**) show slowly progressive bony destruction with smooth sclerotic margins (arrows) and enlargement of the sort tissue mass (arrowheads) between the initial radiograph (**C**) and the radiograph obtained 3 years later (**D**).

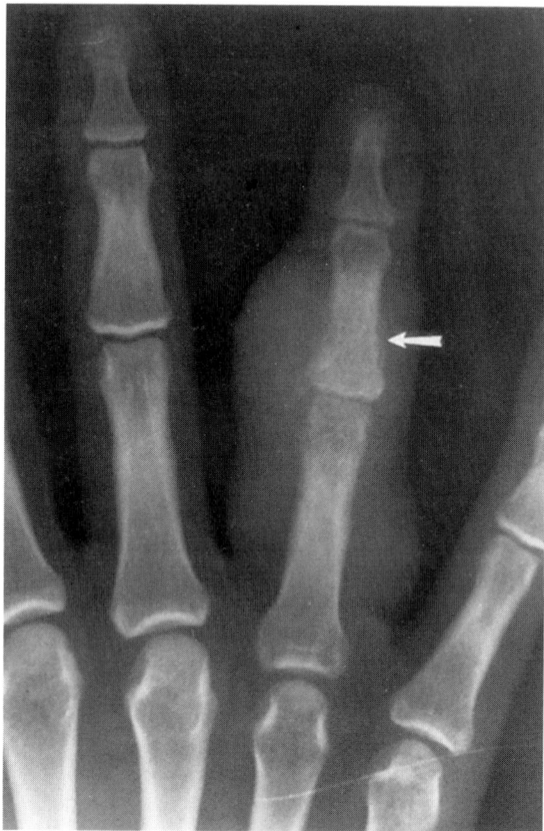

**FIGURE 3–14.** Chondrosarcoma of the synovium of the finger causing an aggressive periosteal reaction. Anterior view of the fourth finger shows a large soft tissue mass that extends from the base of the finger to the distal interphalangeal joint. It contains several small, subtle calcifications. Proximal interphalangeal joint is narrowed, and there is aggressive cortical destruction and a periosteal reaction (arrow) involving the middle phalanx and, to a lesser extent, the distal aspect of the proximal phalanx.

generally have an ill-defined interface, in at least a portion of their peripheral margin. An important caveat must be added, however. Both benign and malignant tumors on occasion exhibit sharp or ill-defined margins. Therefore analysis of the margin of the soft tissue tumor is not absolute for determining the benign versus malignant nature of the tumor. In fact, a sharp margin is not uncommon in malignant soft tissue tumors, and the inexperienced surgeon may merely "shell out" such a tumor when more extensive surgery is required. Understandably, "shelling out" the tumor is inadequate surgery for malignant disease, as this procedure leaves residual tumor, increasing the likelihood of local recurrence and eventually distant metastases. Inflammatory and posttraumatic conditions in the soft tissues can also produce sharp or ill-defined demarcation and occasionally are confused with soft tissue tumors.[1]

The size of these tumors can vary dramatically and is usually of minimal help when distinguishing benign from malignant soft tissue tumors. Generally speaking, of course, "big is bad." Ironically, however, some of the largest tumors recorded in the earlier literature were benign fatty tumors weighing as much as, or even more than, the patient weighed otherwise. The shape of the mass also has minimal prognostic value for distinguishing benign from malignant soft tissue tumors. Because benign tumors generally remain stable or grow slowly and malignant tumors grow rapidly (Fig. 3–15), monitoring the pattern or rate of growth clinically and radiologically provides useful information (Fig. 3–15). Unfortunately, rapid growth is not completely specific for malignant tumors. For example, benign tumors, with or without associated hemorrhage or infection, occasionally demonstrate rapid enlargement.

The location of the soft tissue tumor sometimes helps with the differential diagnosis. For instance, nodular synovitis (giant cell tumor of the tendon sheath)[4,79,162,164,188] (Figs. 3–10C, D, 3–12A) and superficial fibromatoses predominate in the soft tissues of the hands and feet. Xanthomatosis usually affects the tendons about the elbows, hands, and feet; whereas synovial sarcomas frequently involve the soft tissues of the thigh and lower extremities near the knee (Fig. 3–9) but usually do not involve the joint. Synovial chondromatosis[64,153] and synovial osteochondromatosis most frequently occur in the knee, hip, and shoulder, although almost any joint can be affected (Figs. 3–10A, B, 3–12B). The radiologic appearance of synovial osteochondromatosis is quite characteristic, however.

Nonneoplastic soft tissue masses (which might be confused with soft tissue tumors) occur in predictable locations. For example, popliteal cysts (Baker's cysts)[67,105,106,146] are characteristically located in the posterior aspect of the knee joint and exhibit a typical appearance on MR scan and sonography. Ganglion cysts[189] are most common near the wrist; but because they are typically small and readily palpable, MR is rarely indicated for their assessment. Overall there is such wide variation in the location of soft tissue tumors that location, by itself, is of limited use for distinguishing benign from malignant tumors. The trite saying "it must be taken out to be spelled out" remains applicable in most cases.

Benign and malignant soft tissue tumors are most commonly solitary, although both are occasionally multiple. Multiple benign lesions are more common and include multiple fibromas, lipomas, hemangiomas, glomus tumors, xanthomas, myxomas, and neurofibromas. Multiple malignant lesions are less frequent and include multiple soft tissue metastases such as occur in epithelioid sarcomas, Kaposi's sarcomas, and angiosarcomas. Detection of multiple lesions

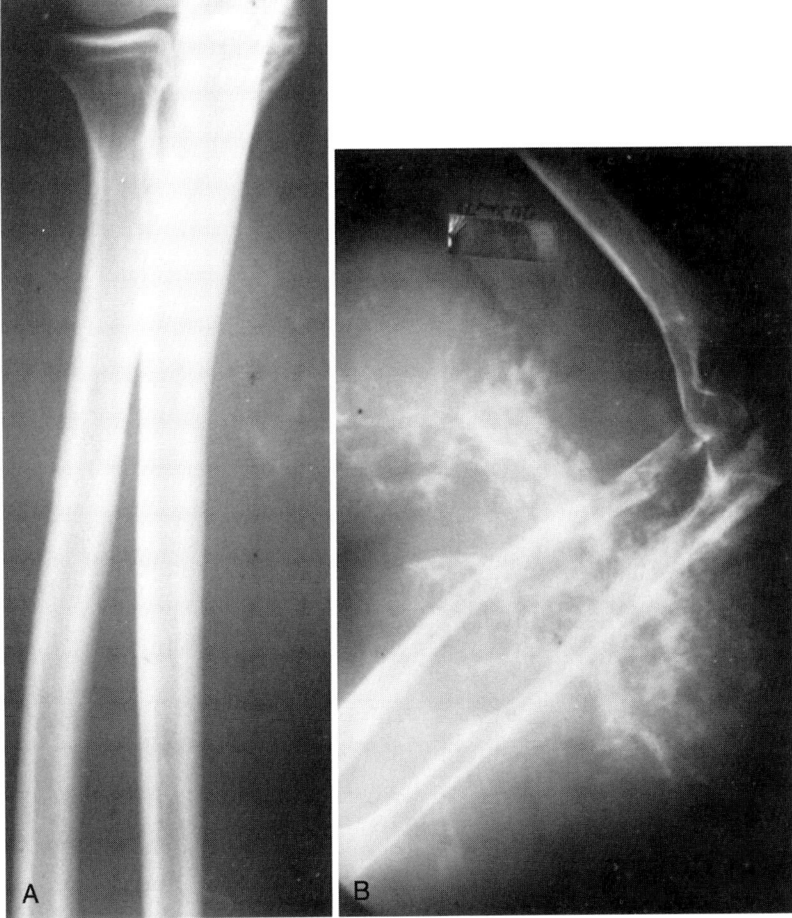


**FIGURE 3–15.** Synovial sarcoma of the forearm causing an aggressive periosteal reaction, a bizarre pattern of calcification in the soft tissue mass, and dramatic growth. (**A**) At clinical presentation the AP radiograph of the proximal forearm shows only subtle calcification in the soft tissue mass. (**B**) Follow-up oblique radiograph obtained approximately 1 year later reveals an extensive, rapidly growing tumor containing abundant, bizarre calcification and evoking an aggressive periosteal reaction in the radius and ulna. Portions of the radial and ulnar cortices are destroyed, and marrow invasion is suspected. From an imaging perspective, the marrow invasion and overall configuration and extent of the soft tissue mass would be best demonstrated on MR scans.

is helpful for staging the tumor preoperatively as it is important for the surgeon planning the type of operation to appreciate the extent of the disease. Unfortunately, multiplicity per se does not indicate whether the soft tissue lesion is benign or malignant.

The radiodensity of a soft tissue mass provides important clues for the preoperative diagnosis. The spectrum of radiodensity ranges from radiolucency to water (unit) density to radiopacity. Radiolucency is consistent with fatty tissue (Figs. 3–2, 3–3, 3–16, 3–17, 3–18)* and sometimes myxomatous tissue.[95] Rarely, air is seen in the soft tissues, allowing a specific diagnosis of abscess (Fig. 3–19) (in the absence of a history of recent penetrating trauma). Water or unit density is nonspecific and typical of most soft tissue tumors. Radiopacity may be due to calcification, chondrification, or ossification in the soft tissue tumor, depending on the specific radiologic pattern. These patterns of radiopacity, best demonstrated on plain radiographs, are important as they may allow a specific preoperative diagnosis. An example is the formation of phleboliths (Figs. 3–4, 3–5), a structure that is quite specific and is detected in some hemangiomas, particularly those with cavernous features (Figs. 3–4, 3–5, 3–6, 3–20). Mature cartilage appears on radiographs as radiodense "rings" or curvilinear "arcs" (Fig. 3–21). This finding, which signifies that at least a portion of the soft tissue tumor has cartilaginous differentiation, indicates either a cartilaginous tumor or a tumor with secondary cartilaginous metaplasia. Unfortunately, the presence of radiodense arcs and rings does not indicate whether it is a benign or a malignant cartilaginous lesion. Osteoid may be produced by soft tissue tumors in a radiologic pattern of homogeneous "cloud-like" densities (Fig. 3–7) or mature trabecular bone formation (Fig. 3–22). The presence of mature trabecular or lamellar bone is reassuring because it suggests a slowly growing (and hence benign) lesion, such as an ossifying lipoma, chondroma, hemangioma, or rarely a well differentiated liposarcoma.

*Text continued on page 67*

*References 3, 5, 12, 35, 36, 38, 74, 80, 87, 92, 97–100, 104, 115, 117, 122, 123, 143, 174.

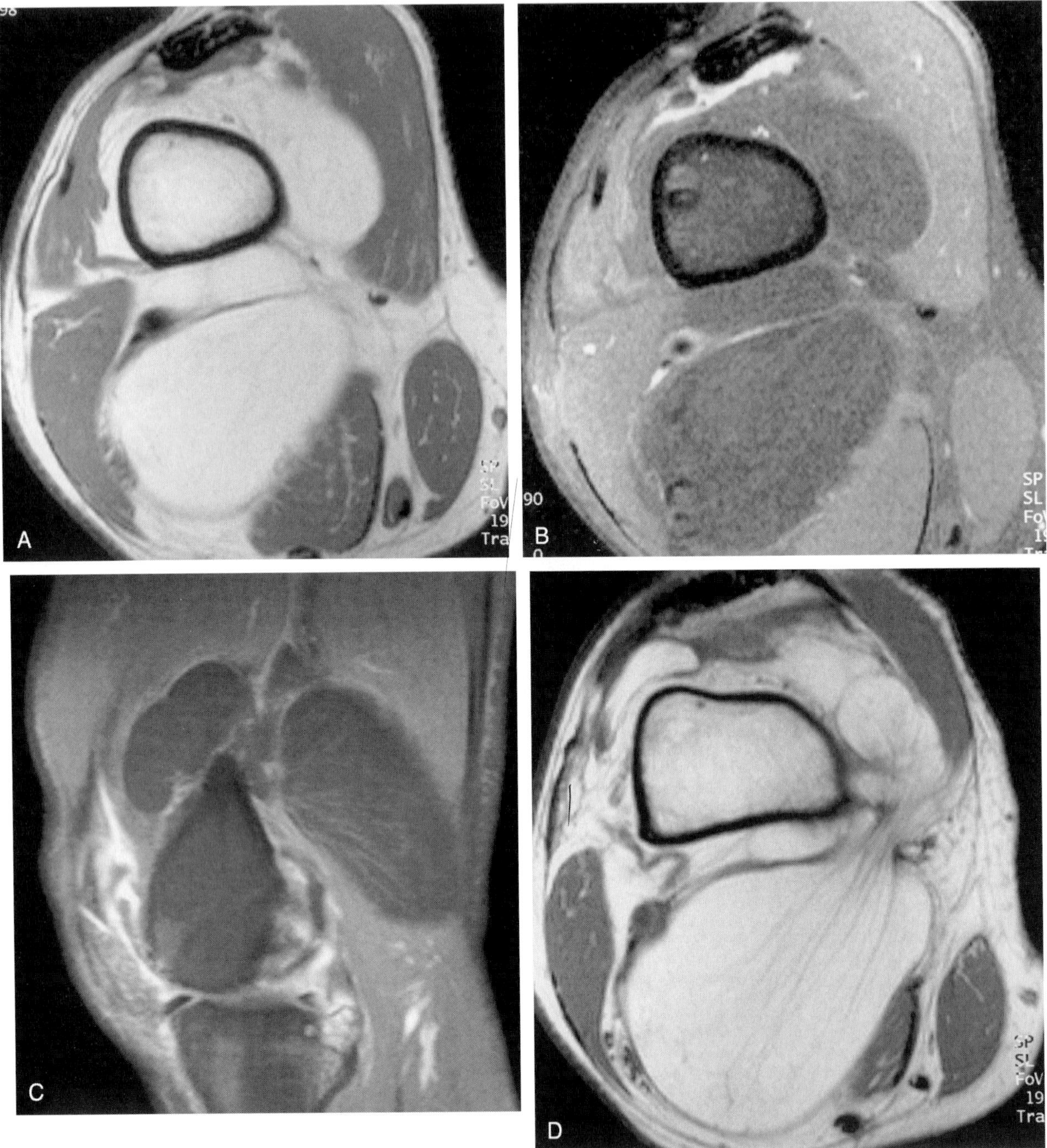

**FIGURE 3–16.** Lipoma of the thigh. A 62-year-old man presented with a long history of a gradually enlarging thigh mass. (**A**) Axial T1 (748/12) MR image shows that the large lipoma involves the posterior and anterior compartments of the distal thigh. It is insinuating itself around the neurovascular bundle. (**B**) These findings are also clearly demonstrated on the gadolinium-enhanced axial T1 (782/12) MR image. (**C**) Simultaneous anterior and posterior compartment involvement is clearly demonstrated on the gadolinium-enhanced, fat-suppressed sagittal T1 (782/12) MR scan. (**D**) On some of the cuts the MR scans demonstrated interesting linear, fibrous striae crossing the lipoma, which is particularly apparent on the axial T1 (748/12) MR scan. The lipoma was marginally resected through a single popliteal approach, at which time the neurovascular structures were carefully dissected from the neoplasm.

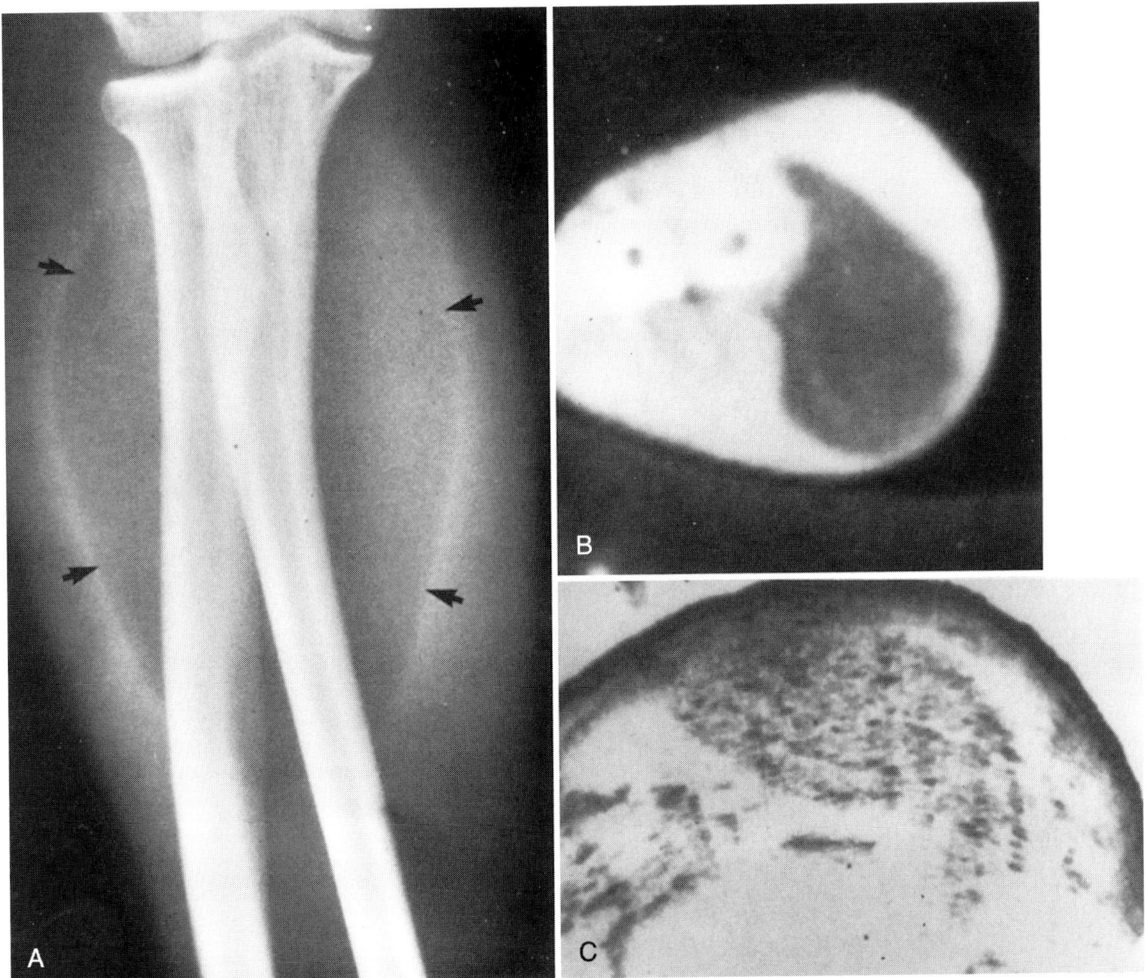


**FIGURE 3–17.** Lipoma of the proximal foream. (**A**) AP radiograph demonstrates the sharply marginated radiolucent mass (arrows) with uniform fatty density. This radiographic appearance is classic for a soft tissue fatty tumor. (**B**) The fatty nature, sharp margins, and typical homogeneous fatty density of the lesion are confirmed on the CT scan. Note that the fatty tissue is dark (decreased attenuation) on the CT scan, whereas on MR it is more commonly bright or white (high signal intensity unless a "fat suppression" pulse sequence has been employed). (**C**) Sonography demonstrates the well defined mass with uniform echogenicity throughout the lesion.

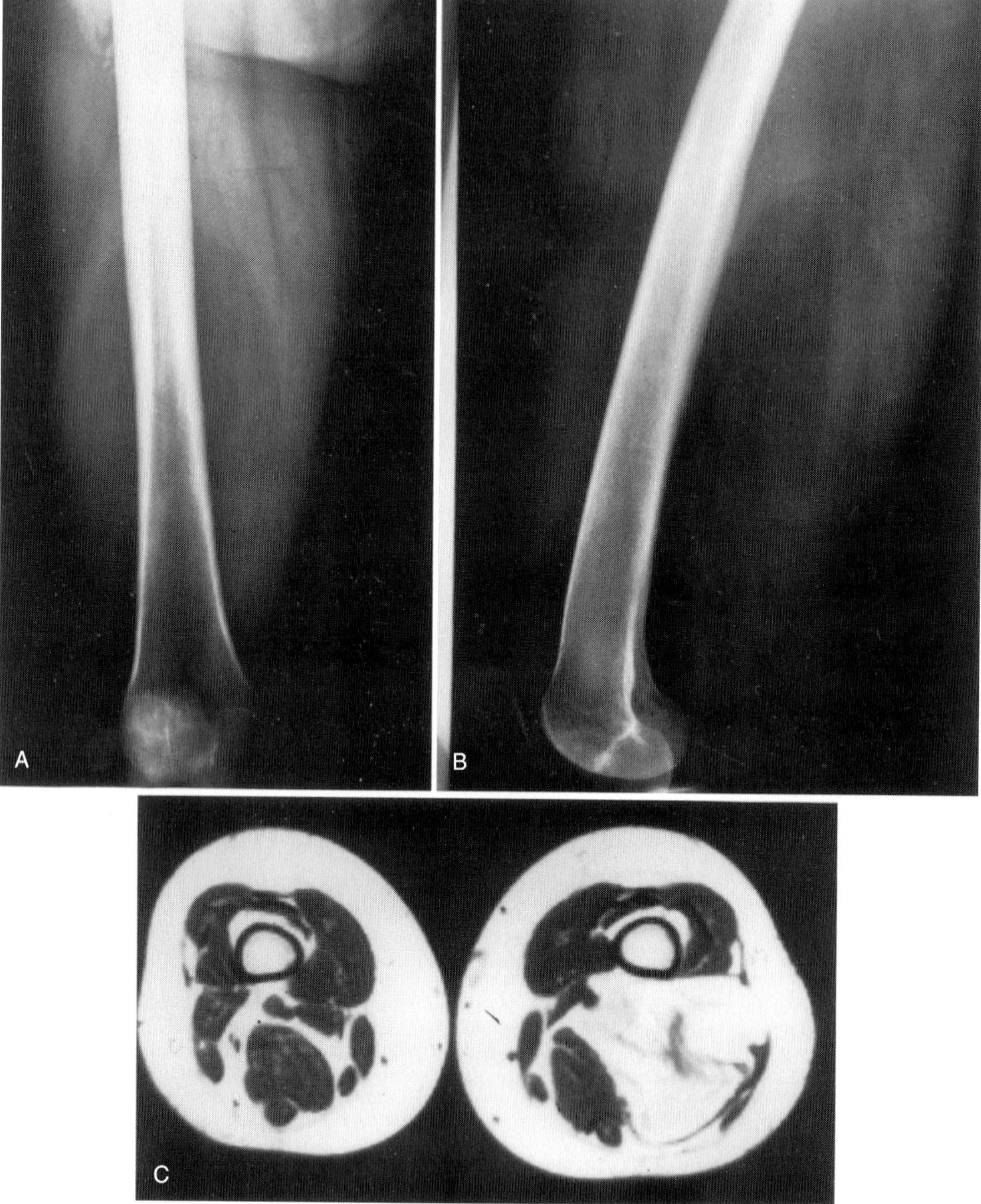


**FIGURE 3–18.** Well differentiated soft tissue liposarcoma of the thigh. AP (**A**) and lateral (**B**) radiographs demonstrate an oval, fatty soft tissue mass in the posterior aspect of the distal thigh. The lesion is inhomogeneous, and its posterior and distal margins are indistinct, best appreciated on the lateral radiograph (**B**). Axial T1-weighted (600/15) (**C**) and T2-weighted (2500/90).

*Illustration continued on opposite page*

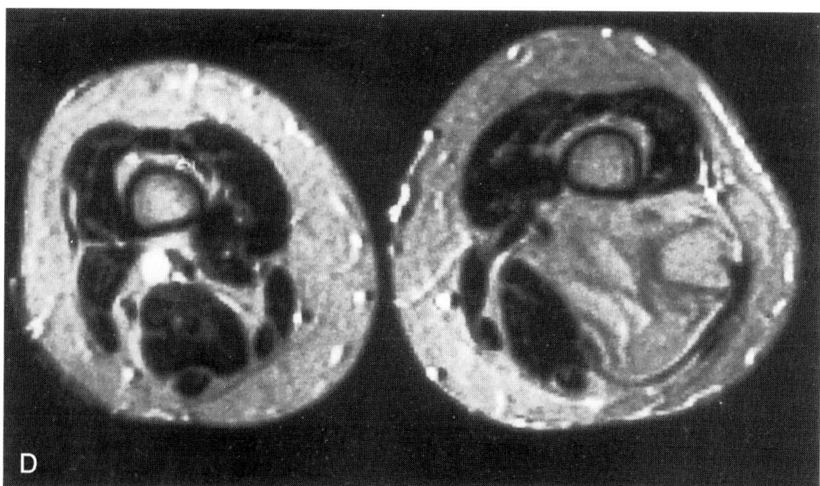

**FIGURE 3–18** *(Continued).* (**D**) MR scans define the borders of the liposarcoma to better advantage. Although the tumor is inhomogeneous, in most areas of the lesion the signal characteristics are identical to those in subcutaneous fat. Note how the liposarcoma abuts the adjacent posterior femoral cortex. (Courtesy of Mark J. Kransdorf, MD.)

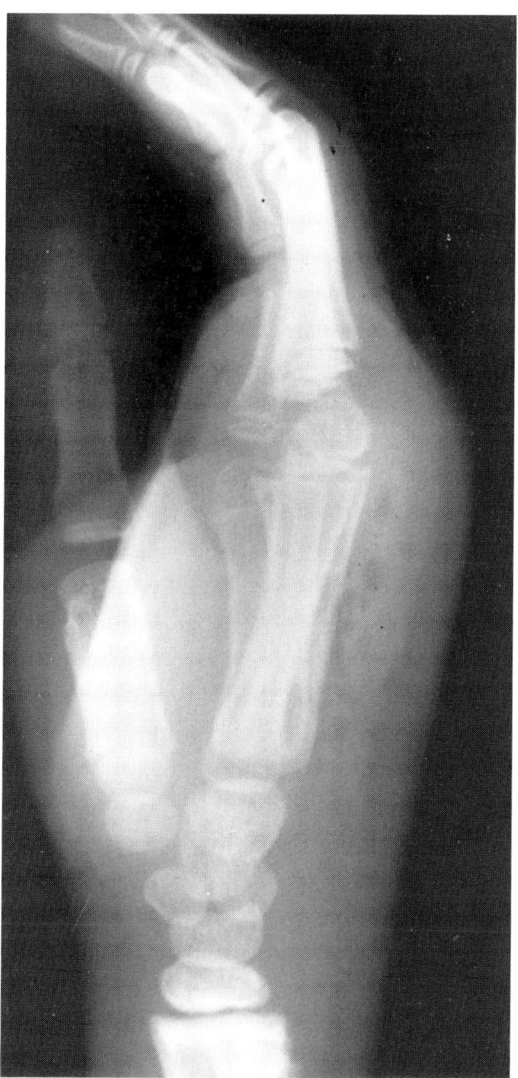

**FIGURE 3–19.** Osteomyelitis of the hand with a secondary soft tissue abscess. Lateral radiograph of the hand reveals soft tissue swelling with gas collection in the soft tissues surrounding the metacarpals of digits 2 through 5. (Courtesy of Dr. Ruppert David.)

Calcification may occur in both benign and malignant soft tissue lesions (Fig. 3–23).* Nodular (pseudosarcomatous) fasciitis and myositis ossificans are only two of the benign conditions associated with soft tissue calcification. Without a recognized structure (i.e., amorphous configuration), calcification is nonspecific and is merely another general feature of the tumor. However, amorphous calcifications are frequently present in up to 30% of patients with synovial sarcomas (Figs. 3–9, 3–15),† so this entity should always be considered in the differential diagnosis of a soft tissue mass with amorphous calcification. Occasionally, peripheral maturation and calcification are seen during the end-stage of myositis ossificans (Figs. 3–24, 3–25).

Tumoral calcinosis with homogeneous, extremely dense, lobulated calcific masses about the joint has a typical radiographic appearance (Fig. 3–26). This rare condition consists of calcium salt deposition in extracapsular soft tissues about the joints, most commonly the shoulders, hips, and elbows. Although usually idiopathic, tumoral calcinosis has been associated with metabolic disorders (e.g., hyperparathyroidism), collagen vascular disease, and prior trauma. The deposits tend to enlarge gradually and may recur after surgery.

Bony involvement adjacent to a soft tissue tumor can be extremely informative. Smooth scalloping with an intact sclerotic bony margin separating the cortex from the adjacent soft tissue mass indicates slow growth (i.e., low biologic activity) and is typically encountered in benign soft tissue tumors. However, this pattern is rarely seen in slowly growing malig-

*References 17, 18, 39, 44, 49, 57, 61, 91, 93, 101, 136, 145, 170, 193, 197, 202.

†References 9, 10, 13, 22, 31, 33, 70, 75, 82, 131, 137, 139, 144, 175, 187, 200.

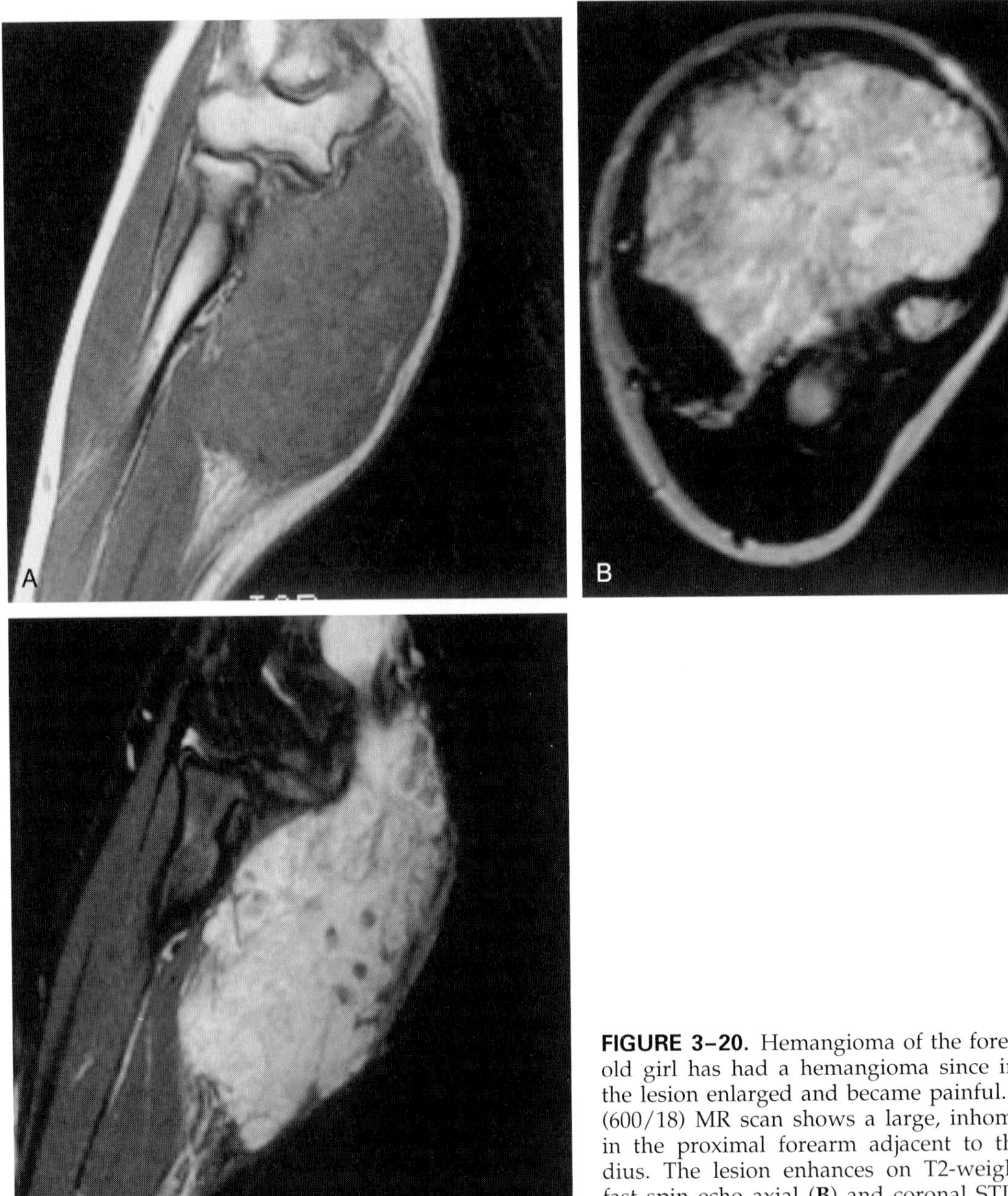


**FIGURE 3–20.** Hemangioma of the forearm. A 15-year-old girl has had a hemangioma since infancy; recently the lesion enlarged and became painful. (**A**) Coronal T1 (600/18) MR scan shows a large, inhomogeneous mass in the proximal forearm adjacent to the proximal radius. The lesion enhances on T2-weighted (6500/144) fast spin echo axial (**B**) and coronal STIR (3000/38) (**C**) MR images. Numerous vessels are noted in the lesion on the STIR coronal image (**C**).

nant neoplasms such as synovial sarcoma. Thus when present it implies a slowly developing interface between the soft tissue mass and the adjacent bone and is usually encountered in benign tumors. Irregular or ill-defined cortical destruction, whether limited to the cortex or associated with frank marrow invasion, is indicative of a rapidly growing lesion (i.e., high biologic activity), suggesting a malignant soft tissue tumor. Other rapidly progressive disorders (e.g., acute infection) arising in bone or soft tissue with secondary invasion of adjacent bone may simulate this pattern; however, the clinical presentation of the affected patient differs markedly from that of a patient with a soft tissue tumor. Occasionally, bone adjacent to the soft tissue mass is not eroded but exhibits only a periosteal reaction. Single-layered, multilayered, interrupted, or otherwise complex periosteal reaction (Fig. 3–15) patterns indicate high biologic activity and usually a malignant process. Conversely, a solid periosteal reaction and cortical hyperostosis suggest slow biologic activity and usually a benign process. Frequently, this hyperostotic pattern occurs in associa-

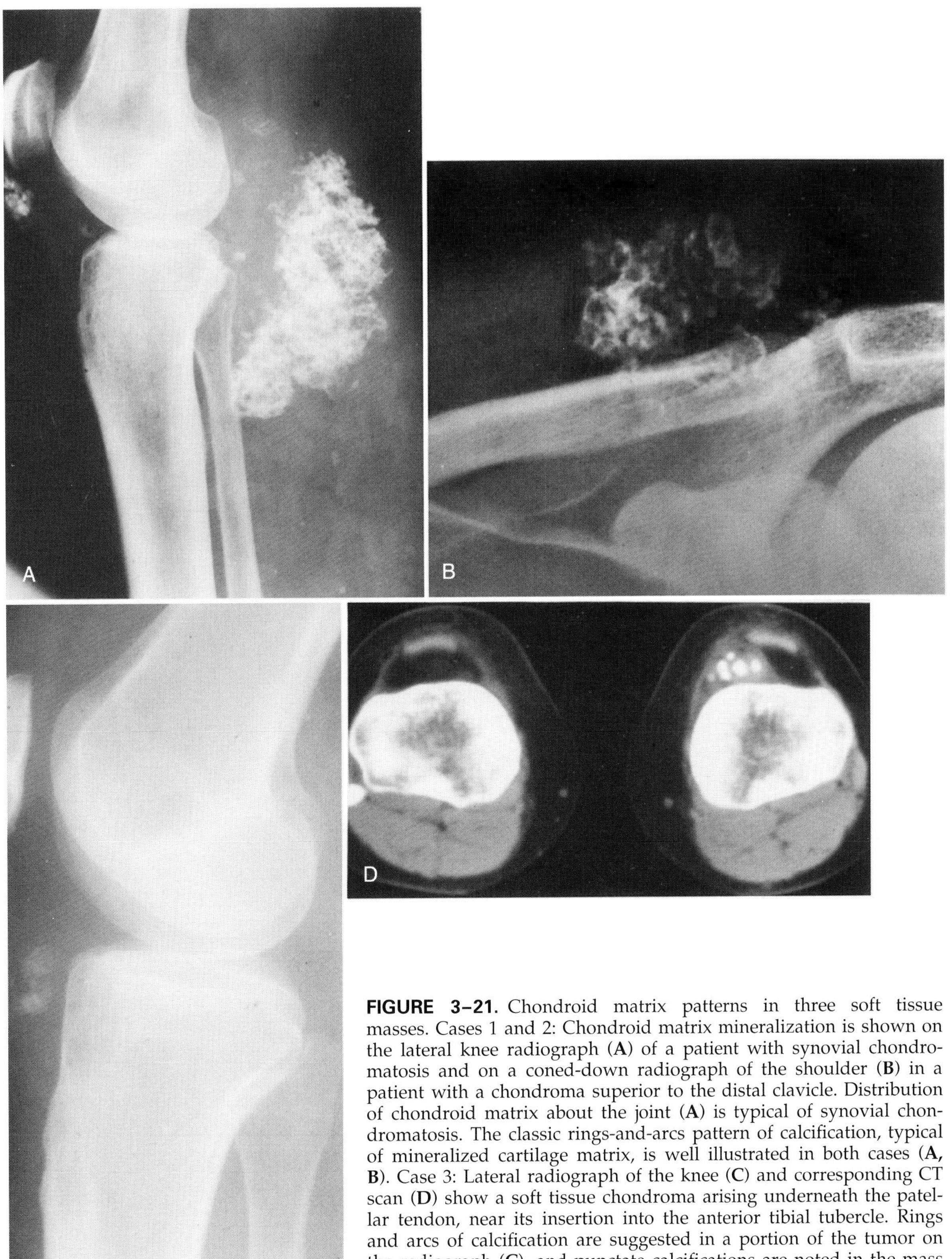


**FIGURE 3–21.** Chondroid matrix patterns in three soft tissue masses. Cases 1 and 2: Chondroid matrix mineralization is shown on the lateral knee radiograph (**A**) of a patient with synovial chondromatosis and on a coned-down radiograph of the shoulder (**B**) in a patient with a chondroma superior to the distal clavicle. Distribution of chondroid matrix about the joint (**A**) is typical of synovial chondromatosis. The classic rings-and-arcs pattern of calcification, typical of mineralized cartilage matrix, is well illustrated in both cases (**A, B**). Case 3: Lateral radiograph of the knee (**C**) and corresponding CT scan (**D**) show a soft tissue chondroma arising underneath the patellar tendon, near its insertion into the anterior tibial tubercle. Rings and arcs of calcification are suggested in a portion of the tumor on the radiograph (**C**), and punctate calcifications are noted in the mass on the CT scan (**D**).

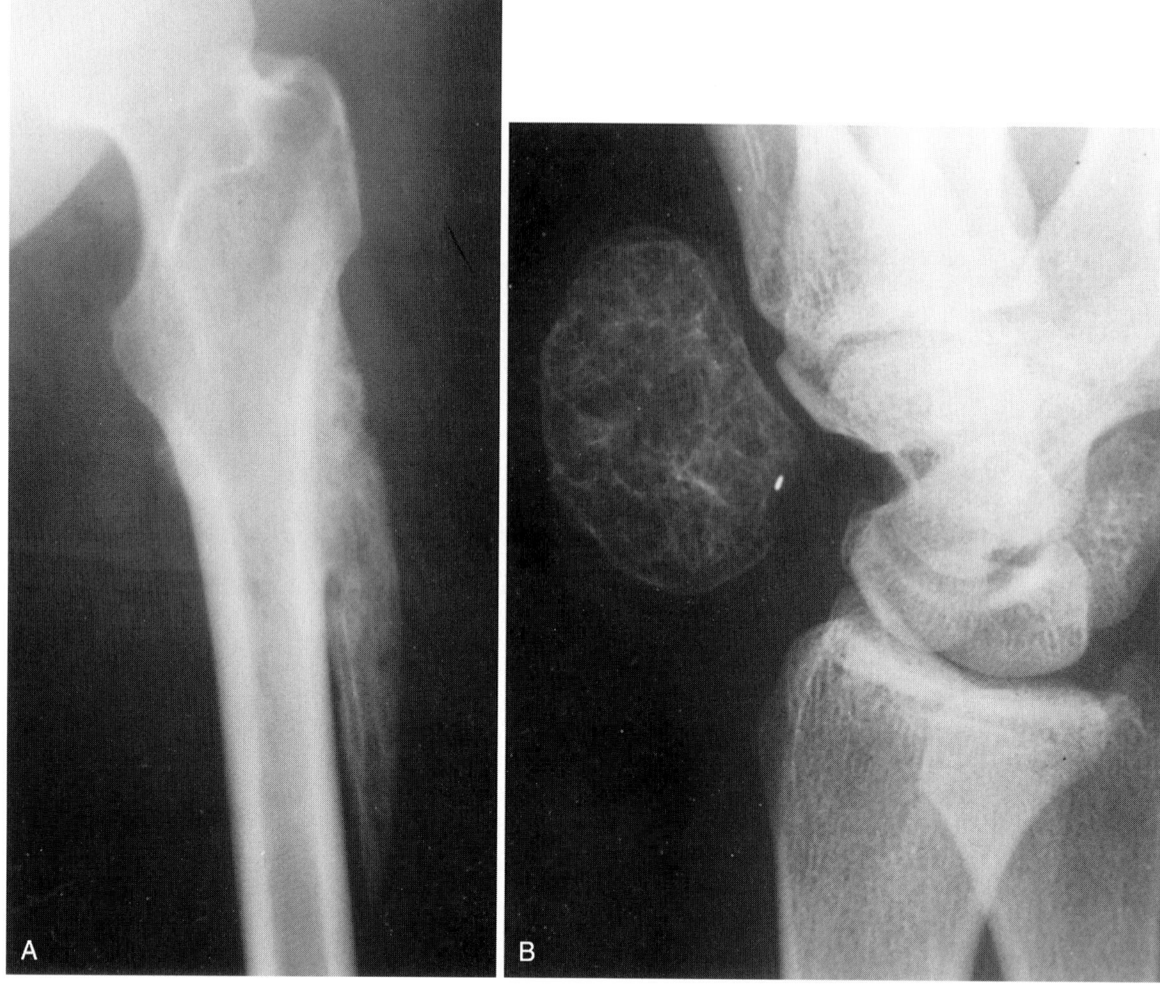


**FIGURE 3–22.** Trabecular bone formation in two patients. Case 1: Well formed heterotopic bone formation with a trabecular pattern is noted on the AP radiograph of the hip (**A**) along the muscle planes of the lateral thigh in this paraplegic patient. The proximal extent of the heterotopic bony mass is attached to the femur, and its margins are well defined. Case 2: Lateral radiograph (**B**) of the wrist shows a chondroma of the soft tissue of the dorsum of the wrist with a well developed trabecular pattern and a smooth peripheral shell. This is due to mature enchondral bone formation.

tion with vascular soft tissue tumors, especially hemangiomas.

## IMAGING MODALITIES EMPLOYED TO EVALUATE SOFT TISSUE TUMORS

Multiple imaging modalities are useful for evaluating soft tissue masses.* These studies are invaluable for detecting the lesion, localizing its anatomic extent, and determining its effect on adjacent structures. Such findings are accurately predicted by radiologic imaging and are extremely helpful when staging the tumor and planning surgical or medical management. A specific diagnosis, based exclusively on radiologic criteria, is usually not possible. As mentioned previously, however, radiologic findings indicating the presence of phleboliths (Figs. 3–4, 3–5), fat (Figs. 3–2, 3–3, 3–16, 3–17, 3–18), trabecular bone formation (Figs. 3–23A, 3–24, 3–25), or cartilage mineralization (Figs. 3–21, 3–23B) are important clues for identifying the lesion.

*References 6–8, 14–16, 24, 25, 30, 34, 41–43, 47, 48, 50, 52–55, 59, 63, 66, 69, 71, 72, 78, 84, 85, 96, 102, 107–109, 111, 113, 114, 118, 120, 121, 124, 125, 127, 130, 135, 138, 149–152, 154, 158–161, 163, 165–169, 171, 176–179, 181–186, 190–192, 194–196, 198, 199, 201, 203.

### Conventional Radiographic Studies

The plain film radiograph obtained with low kilovoltage technique (below 50 kvp) enhances the difference

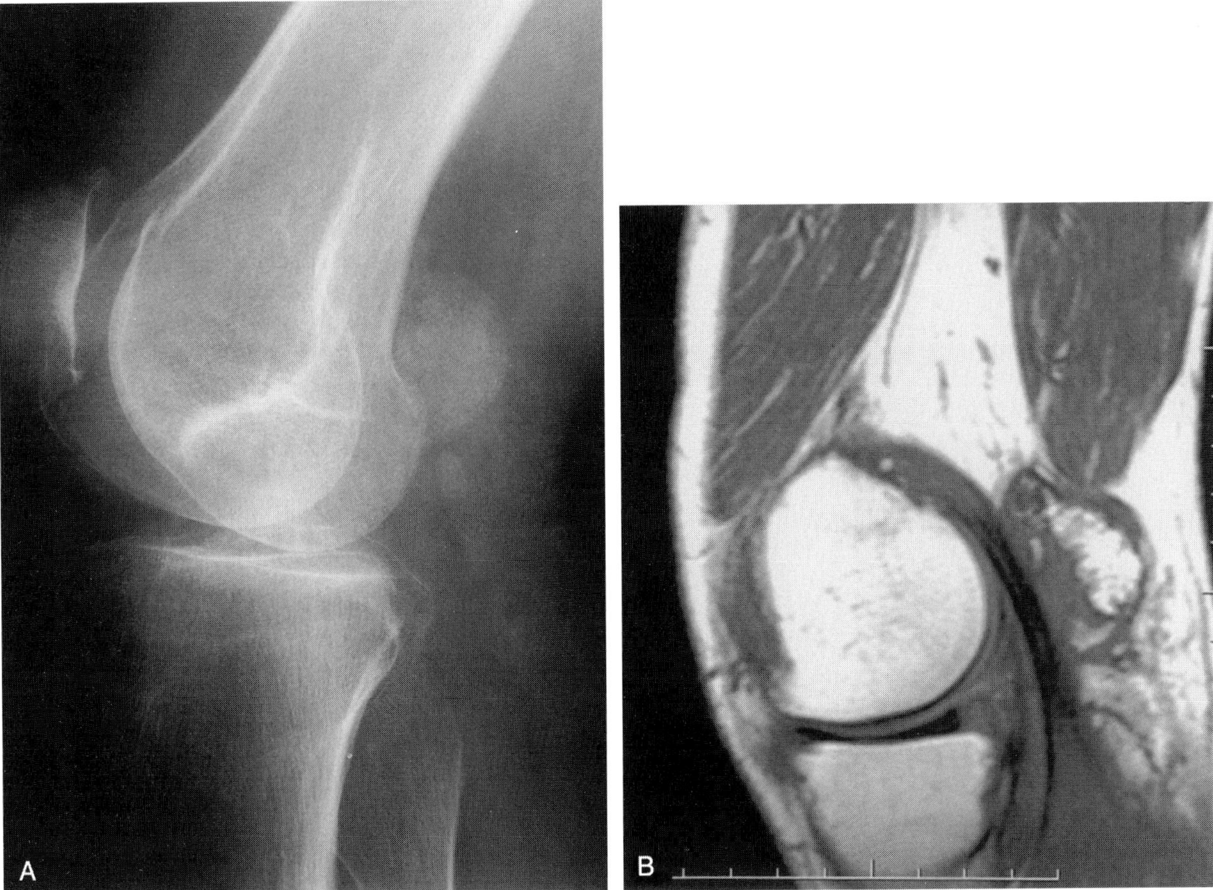


**FIGURE 3–23.** Synovial chondromatosis or osteochondromatosis of the knee. A 33-year-old man presents with knee pain. (**A**) Lateral radiograph of the knee demonstrates several varying-sized calcifications behind the knee. (**B**) Sagittal T1 MR scan (500/14) clearly delineates the mass, part of which demonstrates a signal consistent with bone marrow in the osteochondroma.

in radiographic density between fat and muscle and accentuates the soft tissue detail. Routine (Fig. 3–26) or overpenetrated radiographs best demonstrate involvement of adjacent bone. Plain tomography is of particular value for assessing calcifications in soft tissue masses and for delineating soft tissue abnormalities adjacent to complex bony structures (pelvis, spine, chest wall, shoulder). Plain tomography augments, but does not replace, the plain radiograph. The plain film is still invaluable for predicting the presence and nature of bony involvement. Although the plain radiograph remains the best imaging modality for bone tumors, MR imaging is the best technique for formulating the differential diagnosis of a soft tissue mass because of its ability to discriminate fat from muscle and to clearly demarcate muscle groups, neurovascular structures, and other soft tissue structures. When adjacent bone is involved by a slowly growing soft tissue mass, local pressure by the mass results in a scalloped pattern with a well defined sclerotic margin (Figs. 3–10, 3–12, 3–13), which is most frequently encountered in benign processes. Irregular cortical destruction is usually associated with fast-growing, frequently malignant lesions (Figs. 3–11, 3–13A, B, 3–14, 3–15). Obliteration or displacement of normal fascial planes due to soft tissue infiltration is common in both benign and malignant tumors. Occasionally this interface is lobulated and smooth, suggesting the presence of a confining capsule. Few soft tissue tumors have a true capsule, and what resembles a capsule is simply a compressed rim of normal structures. Thus a smooth margin can be deceptive (Fig. 3–7) if it is automatically equated with benignancy.

## Arthrographic Studies

Overall, arthrography plays a limited role in assessing soft tissue masses but may be utilized to demonstrate synovial lesions and secondary involvement of the synovium by adjacent soft tissue or bony tumors. It may also be helpful for demonstrating synovial

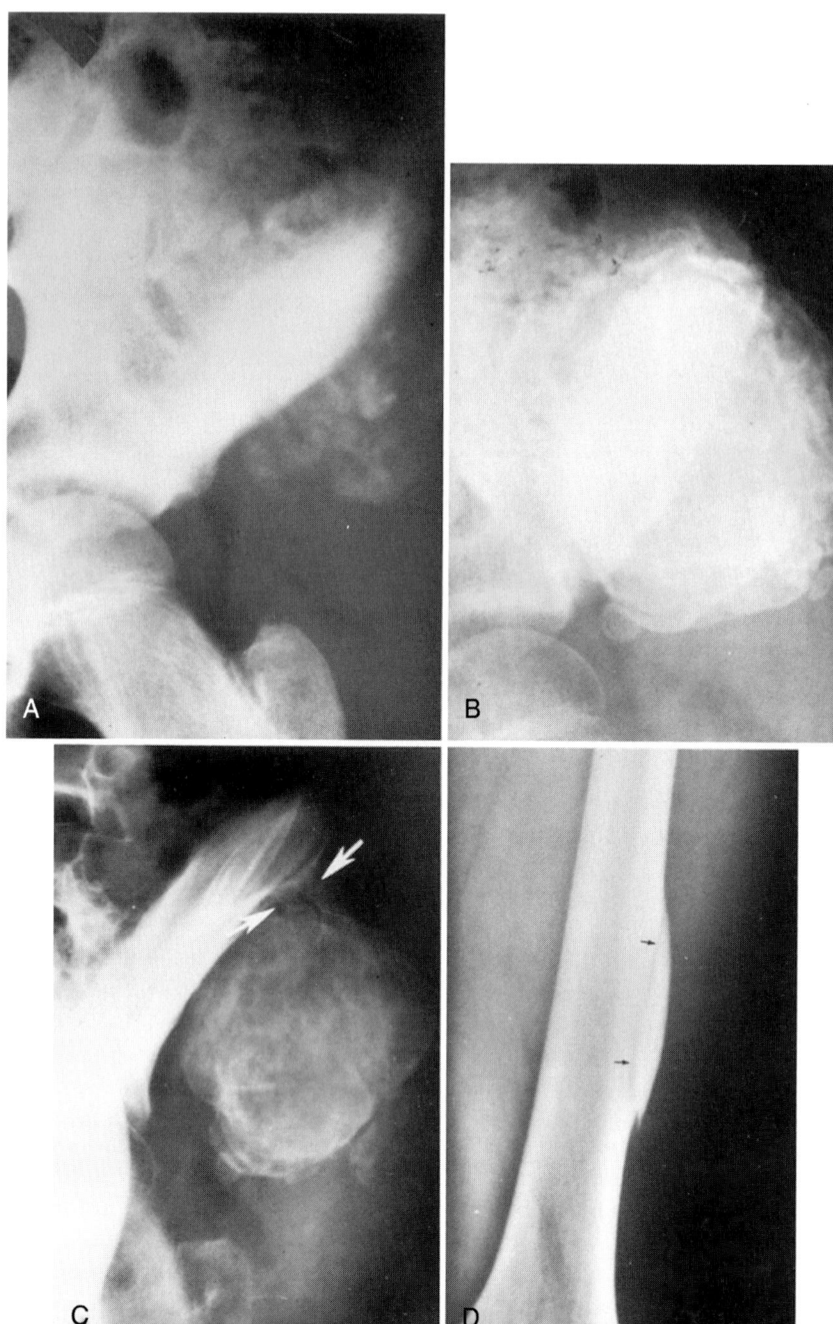


**FIGURE 3–24.** Myositis ossificans in the healing stage in two patients. Case 1: Coned-down serial radiographs of myositis ossificans of the buttocks show progressive healing (over 8 weeks) with typical peripheral maturation and calcification. Initial radiograph (**A**) of the hip reveals a pattern of nonspecific, amorphous calcification in the buttocks. A mature shell and adjacent small "satellites" are noted on the follow-up coned-down radiograph (**B**). The oblique film (**C**), obtained at the same time as the radiograph shown in (**B**), demonstrates attachment (arrows) of the myositis ossificans to the superior ilium. Case 2: Radiograph of the thigh (**D**) shows mature dense myositis ossificans involving the deep soft tissue of the thigh attached to the adjacent femoral cortex. The radiolucent line at its base (arrows) is a nonmineralized soft tissue band at the edge of the lesion.

herniations or cysts that present as soft tissue masses. Most of this information, however, is readily apparent on the MR scan.

## Scintigraphic Studies

Radionuclide scanning with phosphate and other radiopharmaceutical agents demonstrates uptake in soft tissue tumors (Fig. 3–7C; see also Figs. 3–31A and 3–35C, below).[18,34,84,124,158,159,185] However, detection is inconsistent; and if isotopic uptake occurs, the margins and local extent of the lesion may be poorly defined, and false-negative scans can occur. Although invasion of the adjacent bone is detectable by bone scanning, the bony involvement is usually already apparent on plain radiographs. Dynamic scintigraphy clearly identifies vascular soft tissue lesions (see Fig. 3–31A, below). Positive scans can occur in many diverse diseases such as soft tissue neoplasm or infection or in association with local or widespread soft tissue min-

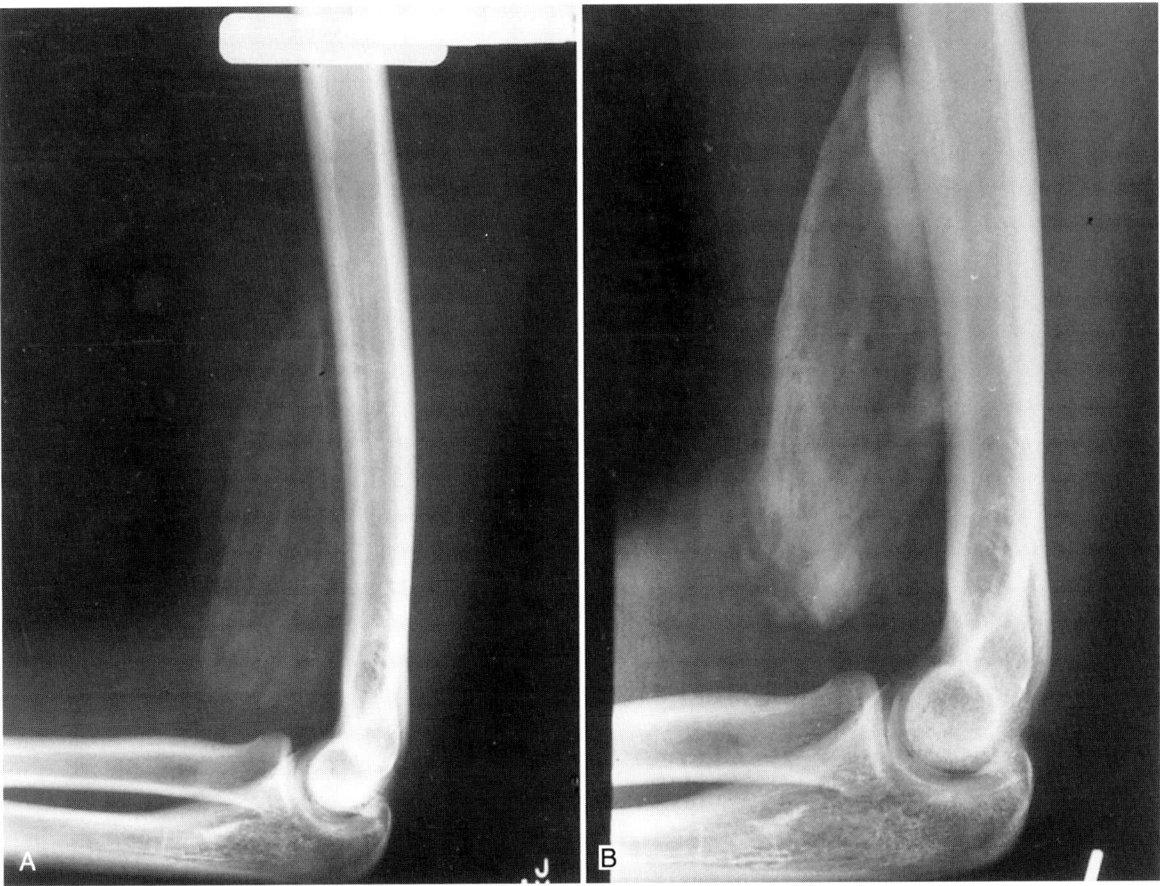


**FIGURE 3–25.** Myositis ossificans of the arm. (**A**) Lateral radiograph shows subtle triangular calcification in the anterior soft tissues of the arm. (**B**) Follow-up lateral radiograph 6 months later shows progressive "maturation" of the calcification in the soft tissue mass and attachment of the lesion to the anterior humeral cortex.

eralization (Fig. 3–26B). Scintigraphy is most helpful for identifying additional noncontiguous skeletal or soft tissue lesions that may not be suspected clinically or detected on conventional radiographs. Such findings are significant for patient management, as they may alter the choice of therapeutic procedure.

## Sonographic Studies

Sonography provides an accurate method for detecting and determining the size (Fig. 3–17C) of the soft tissue mass in the extremities due to differential patterns of echoes detected in the mass compared to those in normal muscle and fascia This modality is far less reliable than CT or MR when the mass occurs in complex anatomic locations such as the pelvis, is located in deep soft tissues adjacent to bone, or occurs in the thorax surrounded by the lung. When the soft tissue mass occurs in other locations, particularly in the abdomen or extremities, sonography precisely establishes anatomic relations and tumor margins but generally provides considerably lesser anatomic detail than is available on CT or MR. Most soft tissue tumors have an echogenicity distinct from the adjacent soft tissues, which provides an interface between the tumor and surrounding soft tissues. The size and configuration of the mass can be accurately determined by sonography because the lesion can be visualized in both the transverse (axial) and longitudinal (sagittal) planes. Therefore sonography may be useful for following the size of the soft tissue mass on serial studies or the response of the lesion to treatment by nonsurgical means such as chemotherapy or radiation therapy. The echo pattern of solid masses is nonspecific, but a fluid-filled mass such as a synovial cyst (popliteal cyst) can be easily differentiated from a solid mass by sonography. Perhaps the best utility for sonography is an ultrasound-guided biopsy of a relatively superficial soft tissue mass.

## Angiographic Studies

Angiography is most helpful for evaluating the vascular supply of a soft tissue mass and the impact of

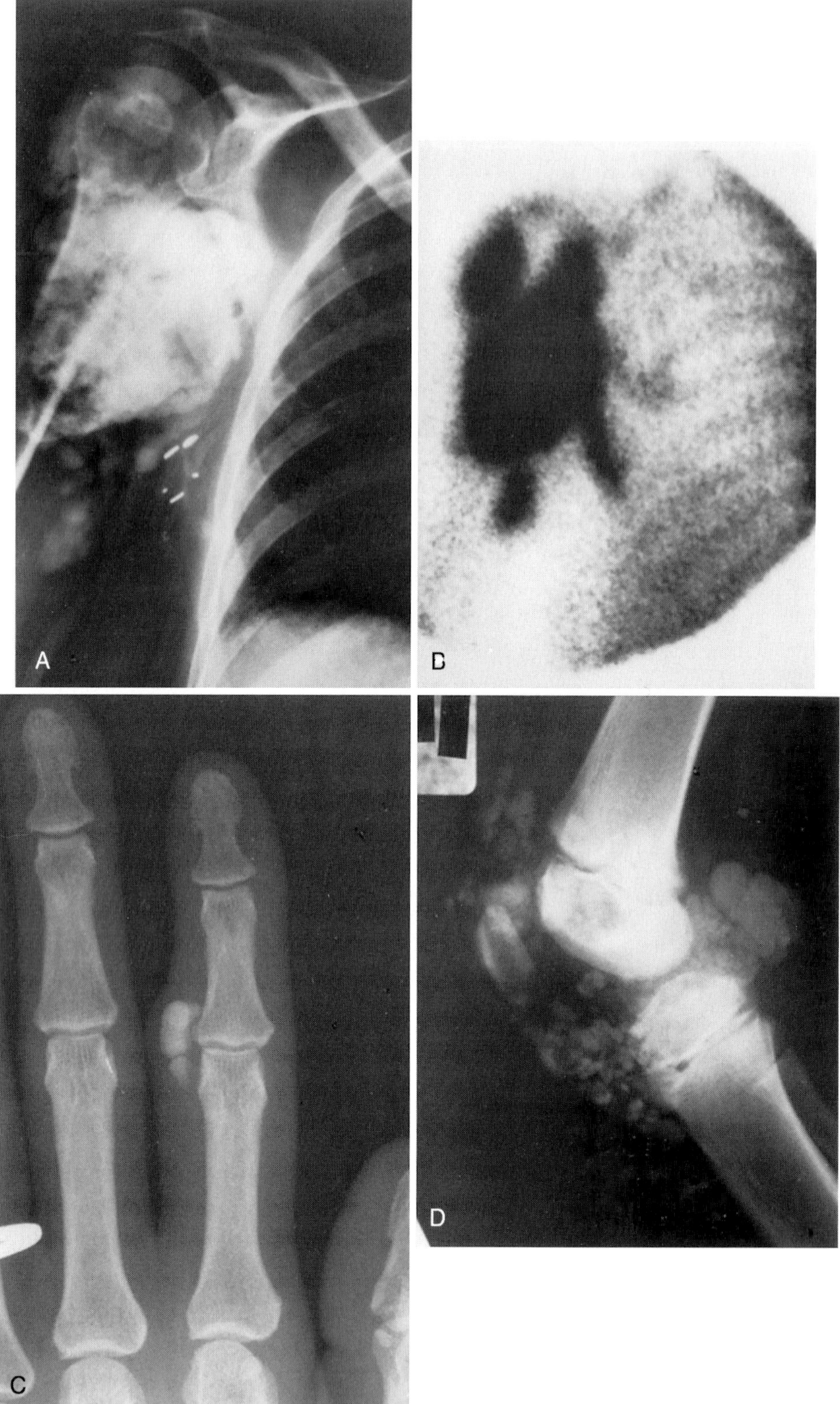


**FIGURE 3–26.** Tumoral calcinosis in three patients. Case 1: Patient with renal osteodystrophy demonstrates tumoral calcinosis on the oblique radiograph (**A**) with extensive, relatively homogenous calcification about the right shoulder. Bone scintigram (**B**) of the same patient reveals increased radionuclide uptake in the mass. Cases 2 and 3: AP radiograph of the fingers (**C**) and lateral radiograph of the knee (**D**) of two patients with idiopathic tumoral calcinosis show the typical multiple lobules of relatively homogeneous calcification about the joint. They are actually located outside the joint capsule, however.

the mass on adjacent structures (Fig. 3–27).* The angiogram, typically performed with the digital subtraction technique (digital subtraction angiography, or DSA), provides information about the anatomic extent of the tumor, including its effect on adjacent structures, the arterial supply, and venous drainage (Fig. 3–28). Because these features influence the choice of operative procedures, angiography is a valuable adjunct to patient management.[141] Much of this anatomic information can also be obtained in a noninvasive fashion via magnetic resonance angiography (MRA). Because the patient with a soft tissue tumor is likely to undergo MR scanning anyway, the referring physician should discuss with the radiologist the appropriateness of performing MRA as a supplement to the routine MR pulse sequences. Interventional angiographic procedures are sometimes necessary, occasionally to embolize a highly hypervascular soft tissue mass preoperatively or, rarely, to embolize a persistent arterial bleeder following surgical resection of the lesion.

Malignant soft tissue tumors have angiographic patterns that range from hypervascular (Figs. 3–29, 3–30, 3–31) to hypovascular. The angiographic features of neovascularity, puddling, and tumor blush are typical of malignant tumors, although benign tumors also occasionally demonstrate neovascularity. Malignant soft tissue tumors are frequently heterogeneous and contain less-vascular areas, corresponding to areas of hemorrhage and necrosis along with hypervascular areas that correspond to viable tumor. Unsuspected satellite tumors adjacent to a primary mass may also be discovered by angiography.

Certain angiographic patterns are suggestive of specific histologic diagnoses such as hemangiomas and vascular malformations. Hemangiopericytoma is another tumor that may exhibit a unique and striking hypervascular pattern.[2,58,76,140,172,204] A frequent angiographic feature of hemangiopericytoma is that early during the arterial phase the main arteries are displaced around the periphery of the tumor. Later, the feeding arteries spread in a meshwork pattern before penetrating the lesion. This peripheral vascular distribution noted at angiography correlates well with the plexiform meshwork of vessels covering the tumor seen on inspection of the gross specimen. This angiographic pattern is highly suggestive of hemangiopericytoma. In most soft tissue masses, however, a specific pathologic diagnosis cannot be predicted reliably by angiography.

*References 25, 51, 69, 72, 102, 103, 107, 108, 120, 129, 169, 184, 204.

## CT Scanning

Computed tomography has proved helpful for detecting soft tissue tumors and monitoring the patient for local recurrence and distant metastases (Figs. 3–3, 3–6, 3–7, 3–17, 3–31, 3–32). Therefore if a patient is to undergo CT scanning or MR imaging, it is imperative that it be done prior to any biopsy or surgical intervention. If this principle is ignored, the value of the combined imaging studies is dramatically diminished because it becomes difficult, or even impossible, to assess how much of the soft tissue abnormality is due to the lesion versus surgically induced changes such as edema and hemorrhage. CT scanning is most useful for defining the extent of the soft tissue mass and its relation to adjacent structures, especially in complex anatomic sites such as the pelvis. This exquisite anatomic detail enables the surgeon to perform more complete resection of the tumor and the radiotherapist to define a more precise radiation therapy field. Occasionally, CT scanning can help establish a diagnosis, especially with regard to detection of adipose tissue in tumors whose fatty component may not be appreciated on plain radiographs. Contrast enhancement is valuable for assessing the vascularity of the soft tissue mass and distinguishing the mass from adjacent structures, especially the vascular bundle. Soft tissue tumors can also be isodense with normal muscle on precontrast CT scans and become evident only following contrast infusion. CT scanning is superior to MR imaging for detecting and characterizing calcification in the soft tissue mass and detecting subtle cortical erosion and periosteal reaction in the bone adjacent to the mass. The ability of CT scanning to detect calcification in the soft tissue mass can prove invaluable for suggesting a specific diagnosis. For example, phleboliths suggest hemangiomas; calcified rings and arcs suggest a cartilaginous lesion; amorphous calcification in a large soft tissue mass suggests a soft tissue osteosarcoma or synovial sarcoma; and peripheral calcification surrounding a soft tissue mass suggests myositis ossificans, whereas calcification throughout the lesion favors tumoral calcinosis.

## Magnetic Resonance Imaging

Magnetic resonance imaging is arguably the most important technologic innovation in medicine during the last 15 years. Both CT and MR are expensive and depend on sophisticated computers that rapidly analyze millions of complex differential equations. There are significant differences between the two methods. CT provides cross-sectional images primarily confined to the axial plane. Rarely, when imaging the face, coronal imaging can be accomplished directly with

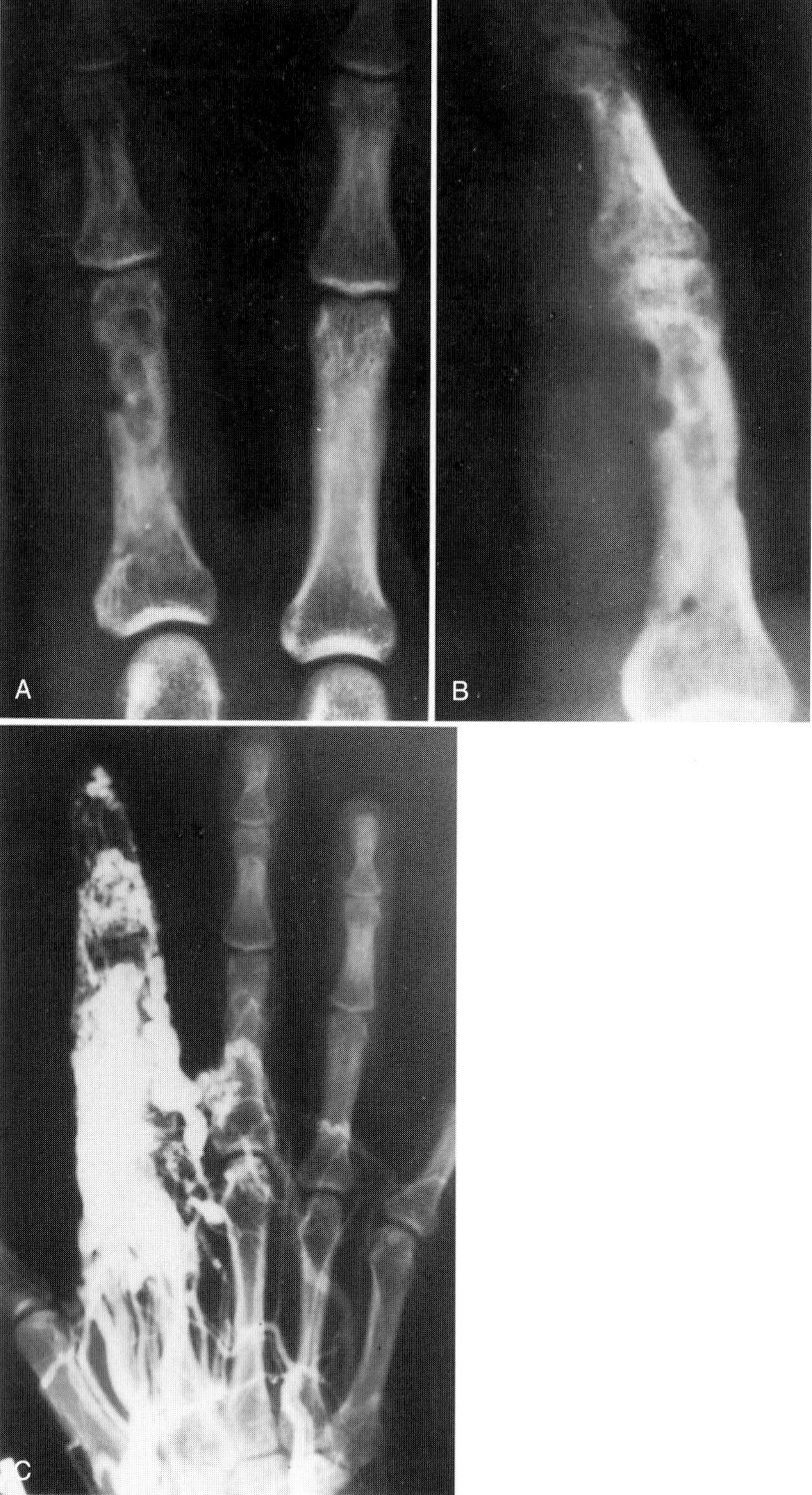


**FIGURE 3–27.** Hemangioma (arteriovenous malformation type) of the soft tissue of the finger with bony involvement. AP (**A**) and oblique (**B**) radiographs show soft tissue swelling along the radial aspect of the proximal phalanx of the index finger with extensive, tortuous scalloped bony erosions on the periosteal and endosteal cortical surfaces. (**C**) Angiogram demonstrates that the bony erosions are caused by dilated blood vessels. Enlarged arteries and early draining veins are noted. The process extends from the palm of the hand to the distal phalanx of the index finger, with definite but less, involvement of the third digit.

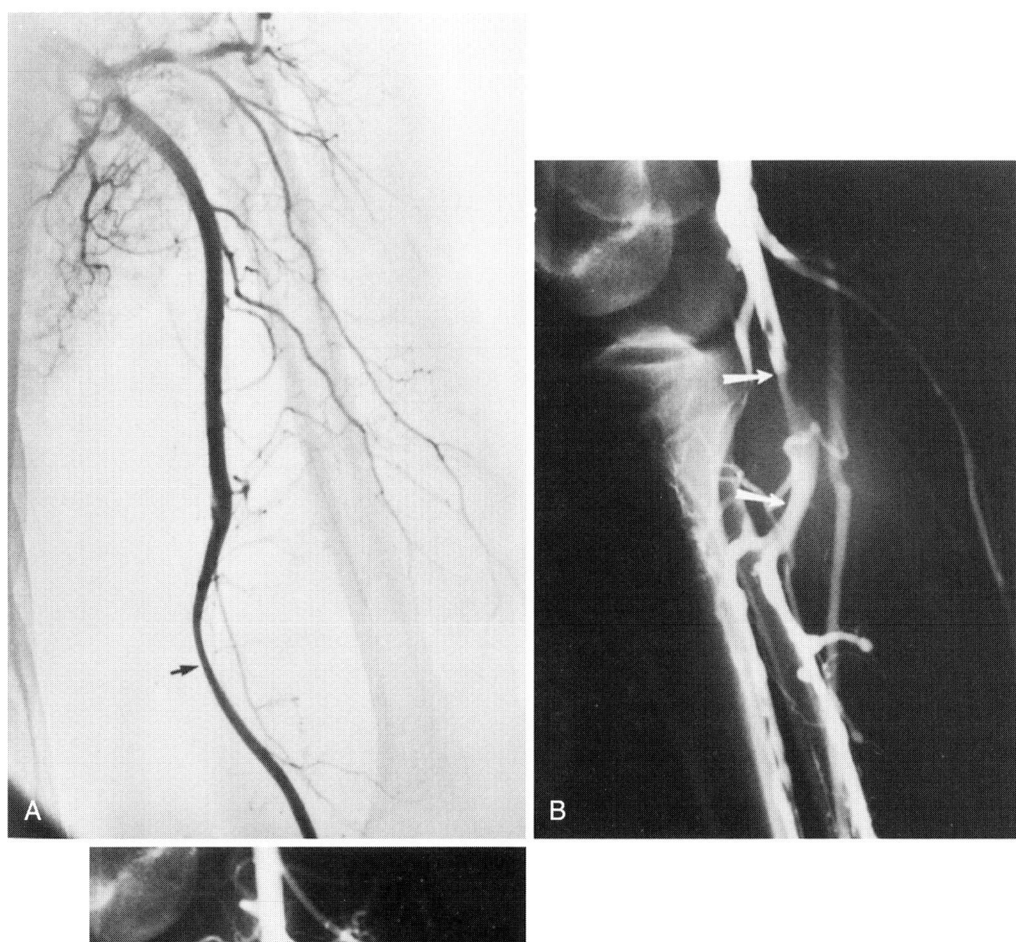


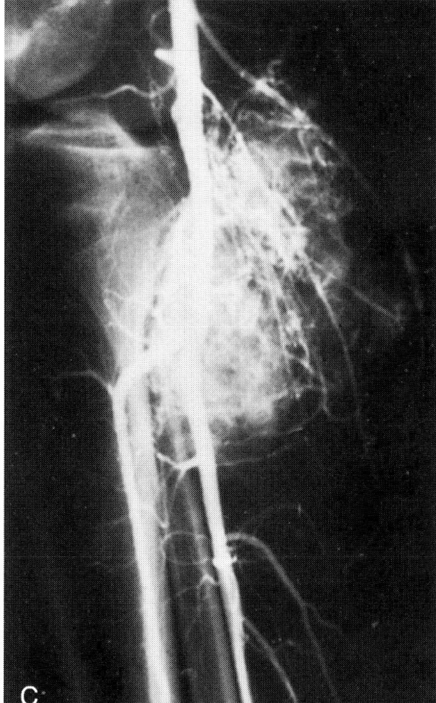


**FIGURE 3–28.** Vascular bundle involvement by two tumors. Case 1: Malignant schwannoma arises in the soft tissues of the arm, just above the elbow. Angiogram (**A**) demonstrates narrowing and displacement of the brachial artery (arrow) as it drapes around the tumor. Case 2: Fibrosarcoma of the soft tissues of the upper calf has grown with displacement of and extension into the popliteal vein (arrows), as demonstrated on the venogram (**B**). Angiogram (**C**) of this same patient reveals the hypervascular nature of the tumor, with tumor blush and multiple feeding arteries, mostly from the popliteal artery.

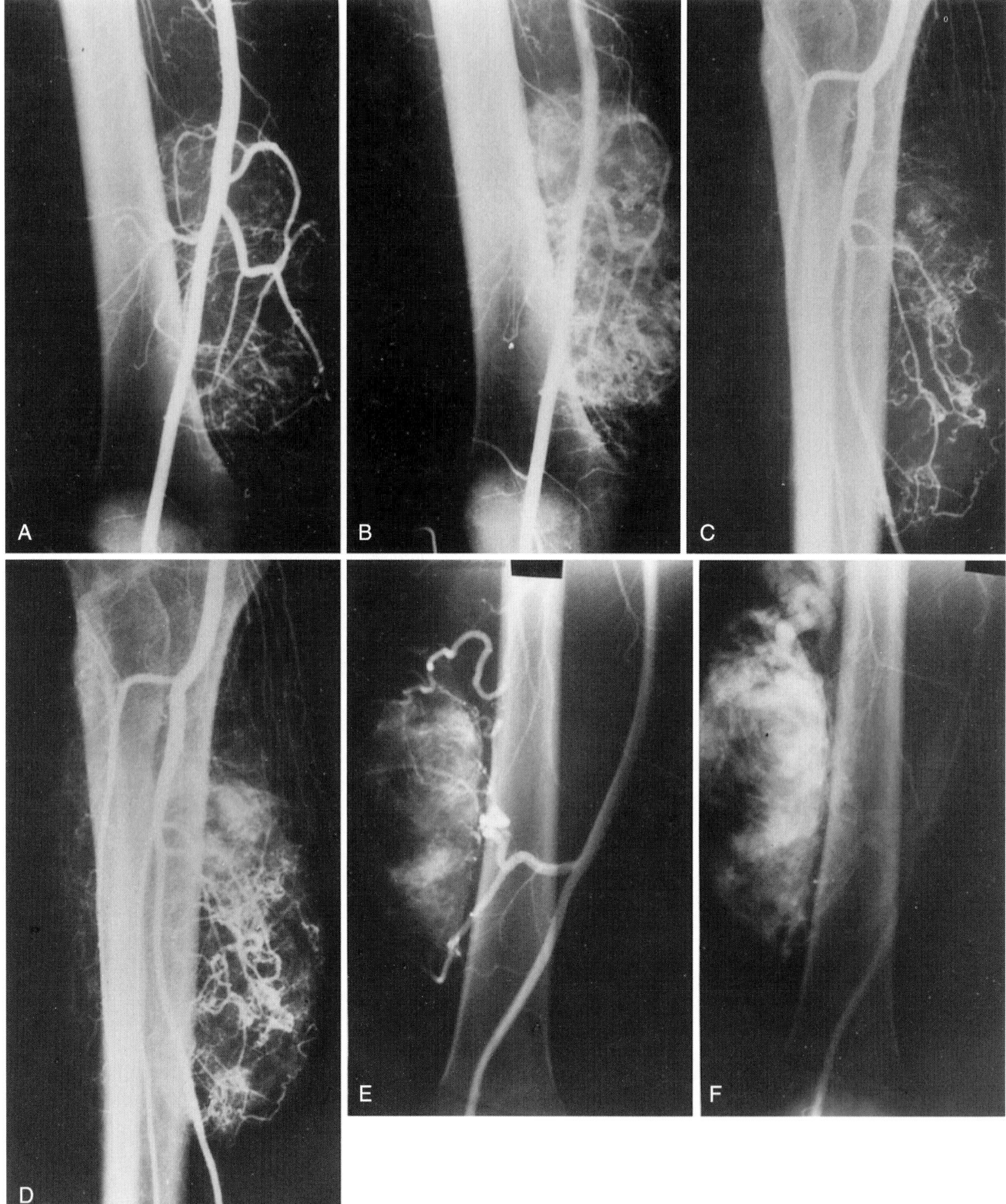


**FIGURE 3–29.** Hypervascular pattern of three malignant soft tissue tumors. Angiography demonstrates the hypervascularity, neovascularity, vascular displacement, and tumor blush most frequently seen in malignant tumors. Case 1: Malignant fibrous histiocytoma (**A, B**) of the thigh. Case 2: Leiomyosarcoma (**C, D**) of the calf. Case 3: Synovial sarcoma (**E, F**) of the thigh. A large draining vein is also noted near the superior aspect of the synovial sarcoma (**F**). The vascular pattern is similar in all three disease entities and is not unique for any specific diagnosis.

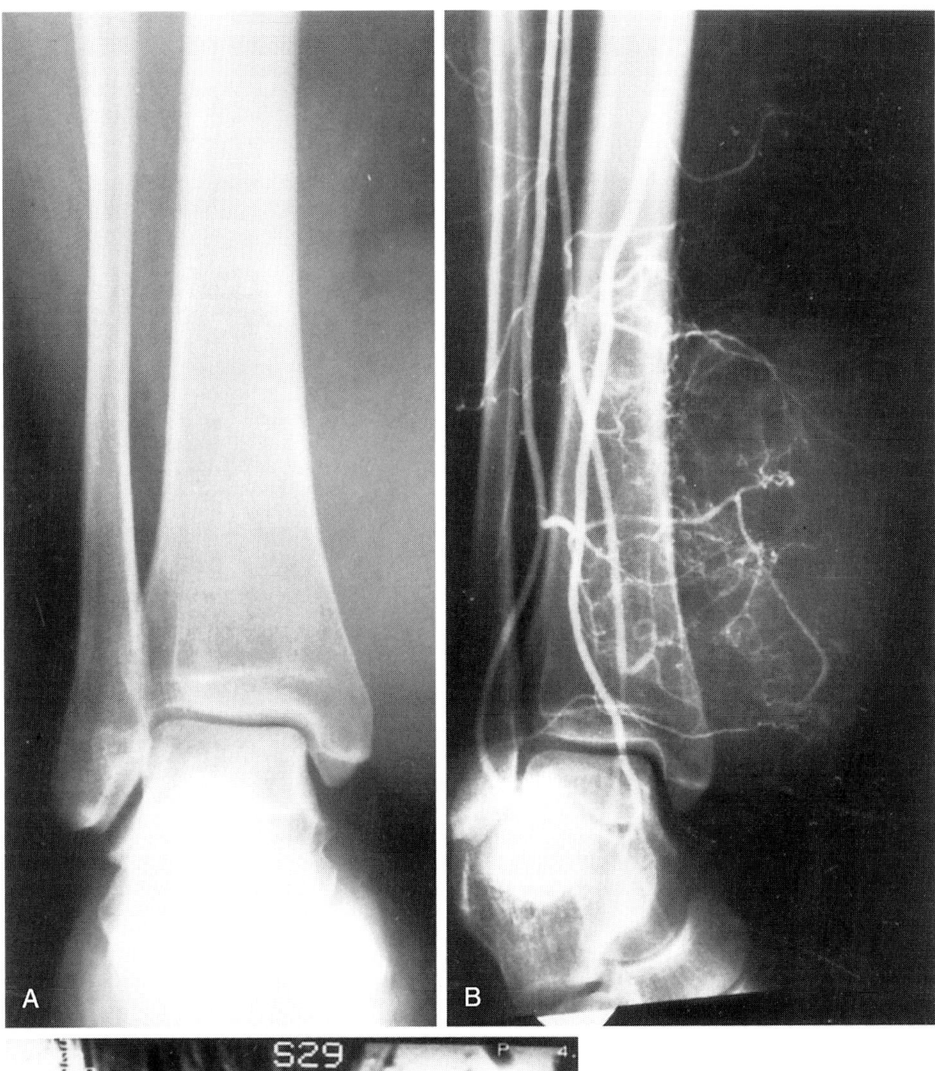


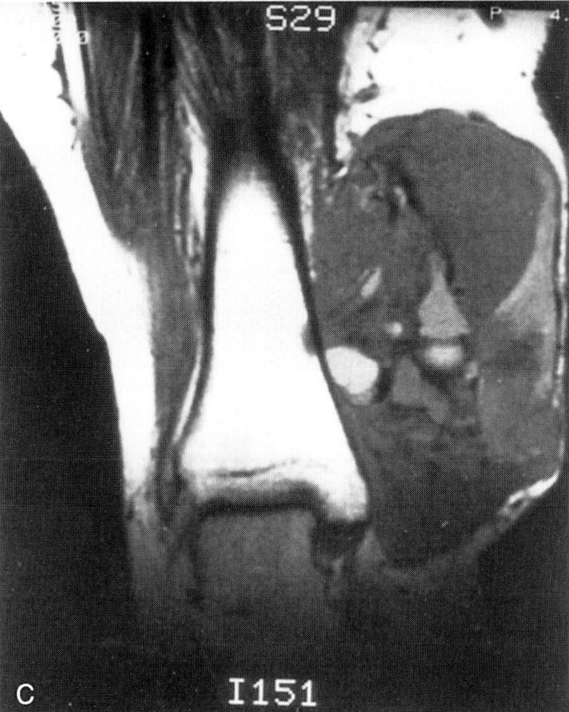


**FIGURE 3–30.** Synovial sarcoma of the medial soft tissues near the ankle. (**A**) AP radiograph reveals a large, nondescript soft tissue mass in the medial soft tissues just above the ankle. (**B**) AP angiogram shows hypervascularity and neovascularity in the lesion. (**C**) Coronal T1-weighted (600/20) MR scan shows a large, heterogeneous soft tissue mass corresponding to the abnormalities noted on the radiograph and angiogram. This scan also shows one small focus of adjacent tibial invasion that was not apparent on the radiograph. (Courtesy of Mark J. Kransdorf, MD.)

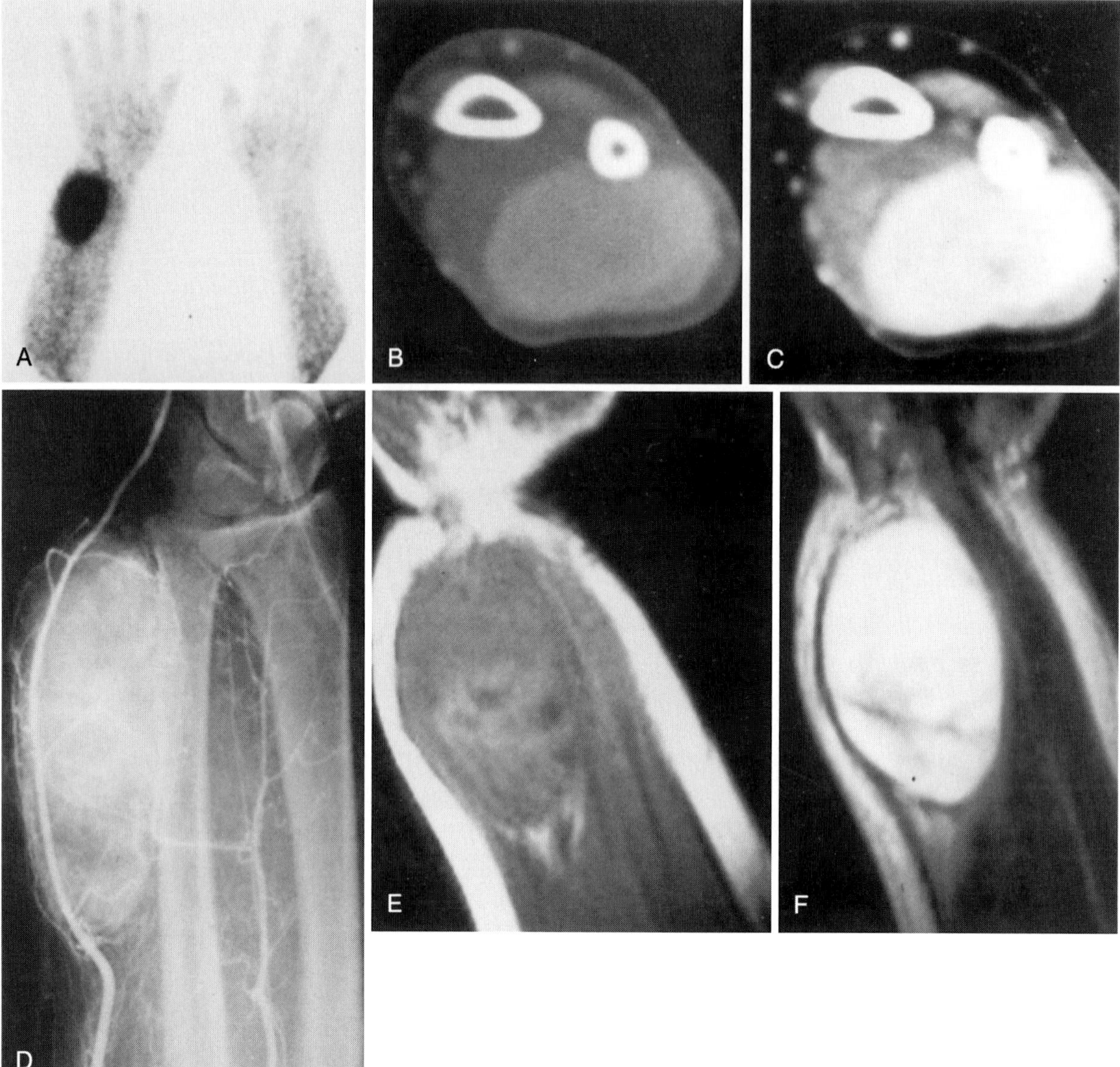


**FIGURE 3–31.** Malignant fibrous histiocytoma involving the soft tissues of the forearm. Plain radiographs (not shown) demonstrated a sharply marginated soft tissue mass without bony erosion. (**A**) Blood pool scintigram shows focal increased tracer uptake in the tumor, consistent with its increased vascularity. (**B**) Unenhanced CT scan reveals muscle displacement by the mass, which is in contact with the adjacent ulna. (**C**) Contrast-enhanced CT scan shows a sharply marginated, enhancing tumor. (**D**) Oblique angiogram demonstrates displaced vessels, neovascularity, and tumor blush. (**E**) On the T1-weighted MR scan study the signal intensity of the tumor is similar to that of adjacent muscles, with little contrast differentiation. (**F**) On the T2-weighted MR scan there is excellent contrast differentiation, and the increased signal of the tumor contrasts markedly with that of the surrounding soft tissues. This case clearly demonstrates that a malignant soft tissue tumor can exhibit sharp or well defined margins on cross-sectional imaging modalities (CT and MR scans).

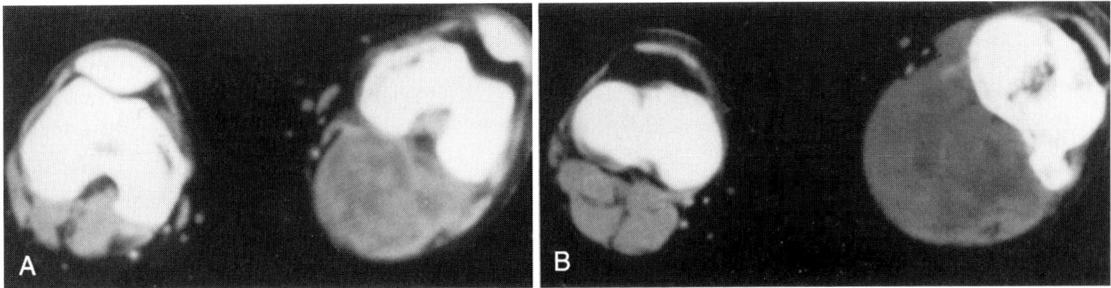


**FIGURE 3–32.** Synovial sarcoma arising in the posterior soft tissues of the left knee. Axial CT scans are obtained through the femoral condyles (**A**) and upper calf (**B**). The scans show the extent of the tumor, which has a heterogeneous consistency, typically due to necrosis or hemorrhage in the tumor. There is extension into the area of the popliteal artery, tibial nerve, and adjacent muscles, although these features could be better illustrated on MR scans.

CT scanning. When other anatomic sites are scanned, computer-derived reconstructed images can be obtained in the coronal or sagittal plane, although these images are typically inferior in quality to those obtained via MR. A major advantage of MR imaging is its ability to image the region of anatomic interest directly in orthogonal planes (i.e., axial, coronal, and sagittal planes). This capability and the excellent soft tissue contrast of the image are invaluable when assessing the extent of a soft tissue mass.

Another major difference between CT and MR is the underlying physics principle responsible for the images. CT scans, like radiographs, employ ionizing radiation, which is attenuated by the physical characteristics of normal or diseased tissues. MR imaging is different and more complicated. MR utilizes magnets weighing as much as several tons and with magnetic field strengths typically between 0.3 and 1.5 T. In addition to the magnets, there are transmitting and receiving antennas. The strong magnetic field causes the atomic nuclei (usually hydrogen nuclei) to line up and undergo precession; that is, the magnet causes the nucleus to wobble at a specific frequency rate. If the nuclei are exposed to pulses of radio waves they absorb energy, and the excess energy in the nuclei is then released in the form of radio waves, which serve as the MR signal.

Multiple factors affect the signal: T1, the longitudinal or spin-lattice relaxation rate; T2, the spin-spin relaxation rate; TR, the pulse repetition time; and TE, the echo time. In general, short TR and TE times accentuate T1 differences between tissues; and long TR and TE times accentuate T2 differences. The parameters are selected by the radiologist, who then monitors the images. Since clinical MR scanning was introduced in the United States during the early and mid-1980s, countless articles have addressed an evolution of innovative techniques (e.g., STIR, proton density, fat suppression) to delineate the soft tissue masses.[32,37,68,134] Understandably, therefore, there is no one best MR technique for evaluating soft tissue tumors.

Most soft tissue tumors exhibit a low signal intensity (i.e., they appear dark) or intermediate signal intensity on T1-weighted scans; and they exhibit a high signal intensity (i.e., they are bright or white) on T2-weighted scans (Figs. 3–33 to 3–44). Therefore MR provides little diagnostic specificity for most soft tissue tumors, as explained earlier in the chapter. However, one group of tumors typically have a high signal on T1-weighted scans, including hematomas, lipomas, liposarcomas, hemangiomas, and lesions complicated by hemorrhage into a preexisting tumor. The histologic picture of these lesions varies, but all contain blood or fat. In contrast, flowing blood, unlike the stagnant blood in a hematoma, has a low signal intensity, permitting assessment of vessel patency. Lesions that are predominantly fibrous[28,73,81,83,103,119,142,155] exhibit low signal intensity on both T1- and T2-weighted images. A detailed discussion of the wide assortment of available MR pulse sequences is beyond the scope of this chapter but is readily available in numerous focused publications.[99]

Most soft tissue masses have a nonspecific appearance on MR imaging; but even so, this technique is the imaging modality of choice for determining (in three orthogonal planes) the extent of the lesion. If the plain radiograph obtained from the patient with a palpable soft tissue mass fails to demonstrate bony involvement or calcification in the soft tissue lesion, only MR imaging (not CT scanning) need be performed.

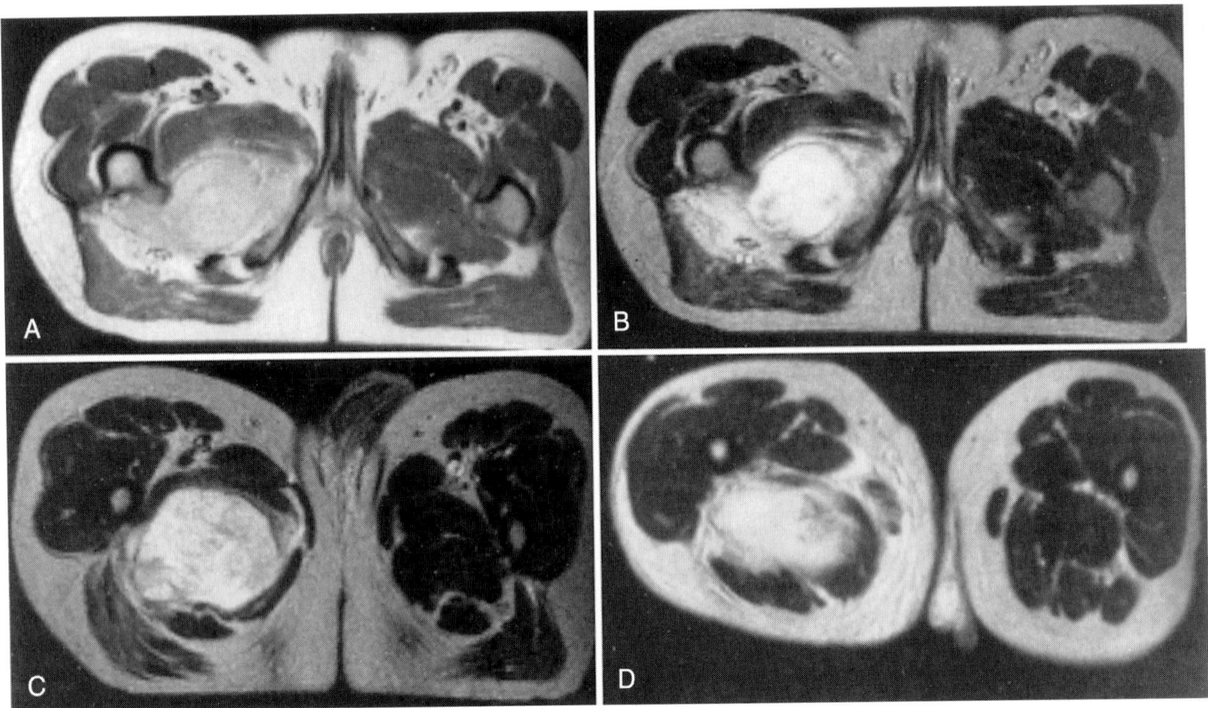


**FIGURE 3–33.** Myxoid liposarcoma of the thigh. The lesion involves the soft tissues of the upper medial right thigh. (**A**) T1-weighted, spin density mixed MR scan indicates involvement of the posterior aspect of the proximal femur. (**B**) T2-weighted MR scan demonstrates increased contrast resolution and the high signal intensity of the tumor. (**C, D**) More distal T2-weighted MR scans show that although the femoral artery and vein are separate from the tumor the mass is infiltrating adjacent muscle and soft tissue planes. Understandably, ill-defined margins on cross-sectional imaging (CT or MR scans) raise the concern that a soft tissue tumor is malignant.

Several investigators initially proposed that if MR scanning showed a mass with a sharply defined margin it was likely to be benign; unfortunately, there are many exceptions to that "rule," as mentioned earlier in the chapter. As a final caveat, during a cost-conscious era that has witnessed a proliferation of freestanding imaging centers, it is imperative that a final interpretation of CT scanning or MR studies of musculoskeletal tumors must never be rendered until the radiologist correlates the cross-sectional imaging study with the plain radiograph. Failure to adhere to this principle results in serious mistakes in patient management.

## CONCLUSIONS

Several factors influence the choice and results of the operative procedure during surgical management of soft tissue tumors: histologic diagnosis, anatomic extent of the tumor, and a desire to prevent contamination of uninvolved tissues during surgical manipulation. Information concerning the last two factors is best obtained by multiple diagnostic imaging, which includes plain radiographs, MR imaging, and possibly CT scanning. To a lesser extent, sonography, angiography, and scintigraphy also are useful.

It is important to understand that even though all these modalities assist in obtaining significant morphologic information about the soft tissue mass a final diagnosis almost invariably depends on a tissue diagnosis. If necessary, percutaneous biopsy can be performed successfully by the interventional radiologist under guidance with sonographic studies or CT scanning. Under no circumstances, however, should the soft tissue mass be needled or biopsied before an MR scan is performed unless the mass is on the skin surface.

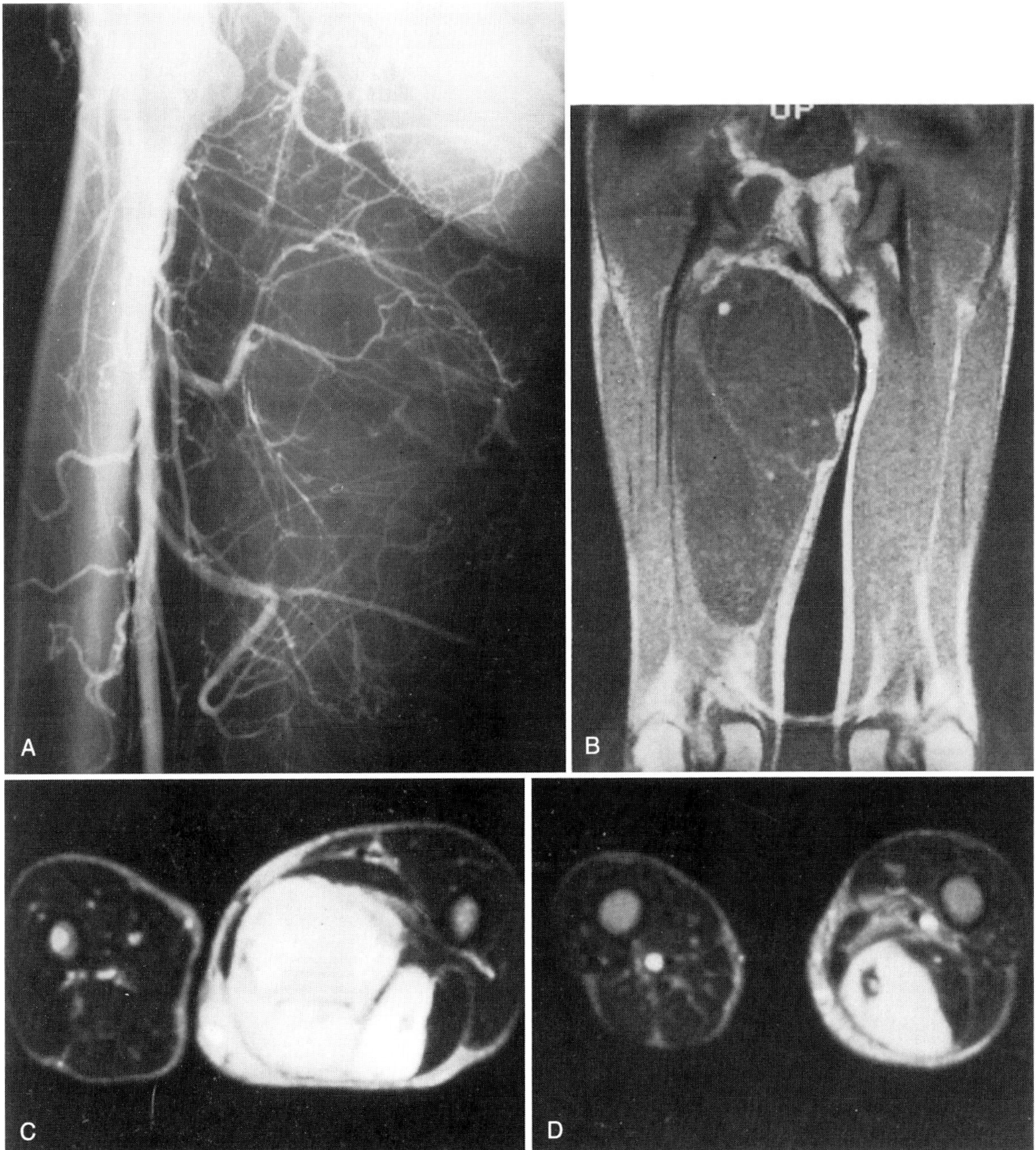


**FIGURE 3–34.** Malignant fibrous histiocytoma of the medial thigh. (**A**) Angiogram demonstrates the hypervascularity of the lesion. (**B**) Coronal T1-weighted MR scan clearly demonstrates the extent of the tumor and its interface with adjacent structures. (**C, D**) Two axial T2-weighted MR scans reveal increased signal in the tumor as well as extensive edema and swelling of the subcutaneous tissues and fascial planes.

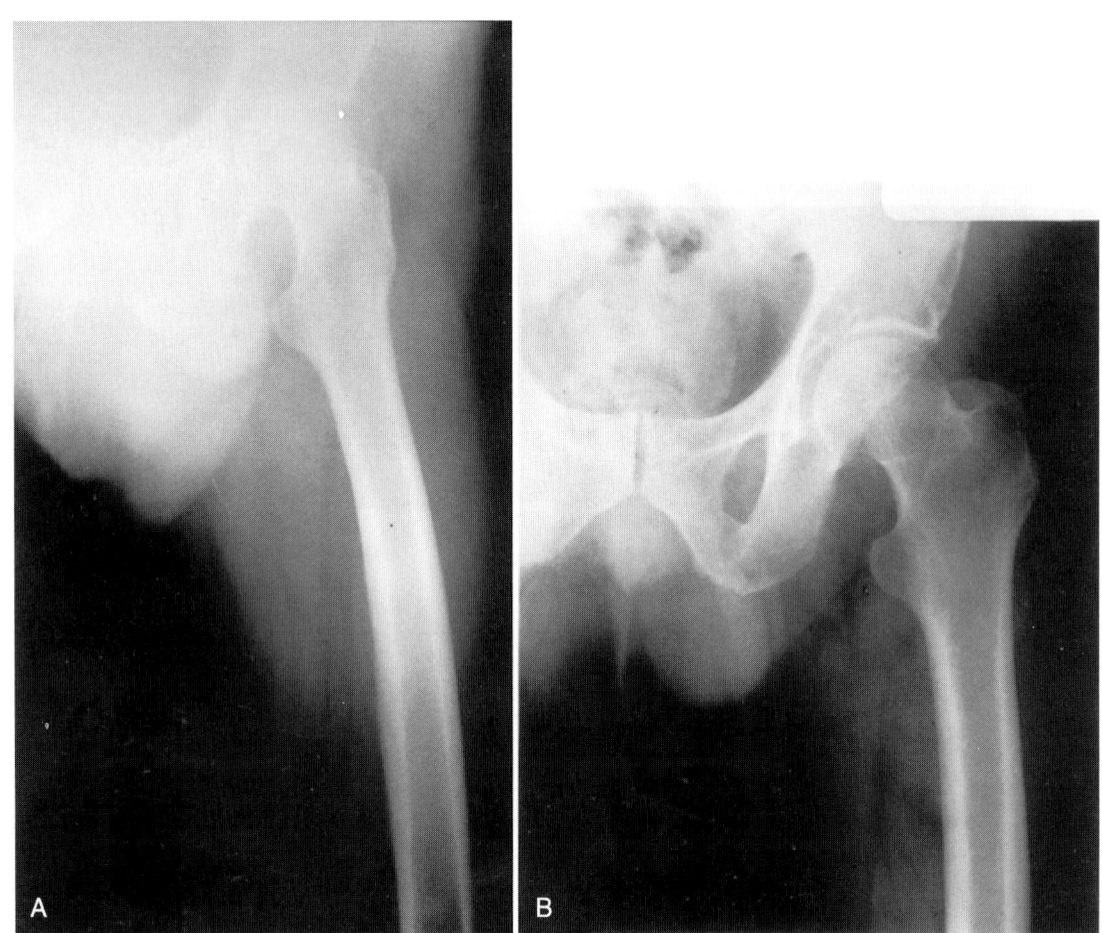


**FIGURE 3–35.** Hibernoma of the thigh. (**A, B**) AP radiographs of the thigh demonstrate bizarre linear lucencies in the medial soft tissues of the left thigh.

*Illustration continued on opposite page*

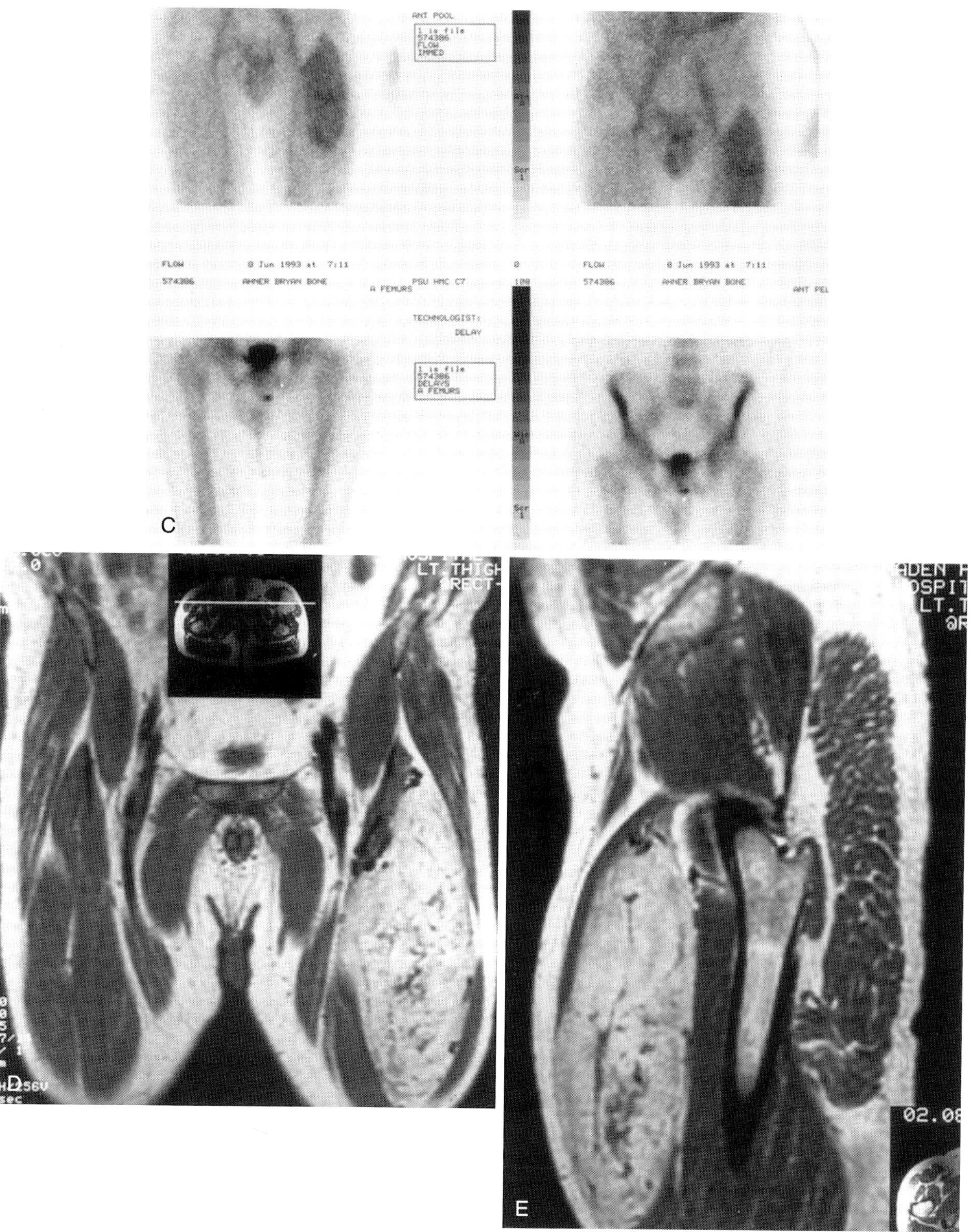


**FIGURE 3–35** *(Continued).* (**C**) Scintigram demonstrates a large hypervascular soft tissue mass in the proximal thigh. The mass is readily apparent on the flow portion of the study but is subtle on the delayed images. T1-weighted (600/25) coronal (**D**) and sagittal (**E**) MR scans demonstrate a large soft tissue mass in the proximal left thigh. The predominant signal in the inhomogeneous lesion approximates that of fat. The sagittal image clearly demonstrates a soft tissue muscle plane separating the mass from the underlining femoral cortex.

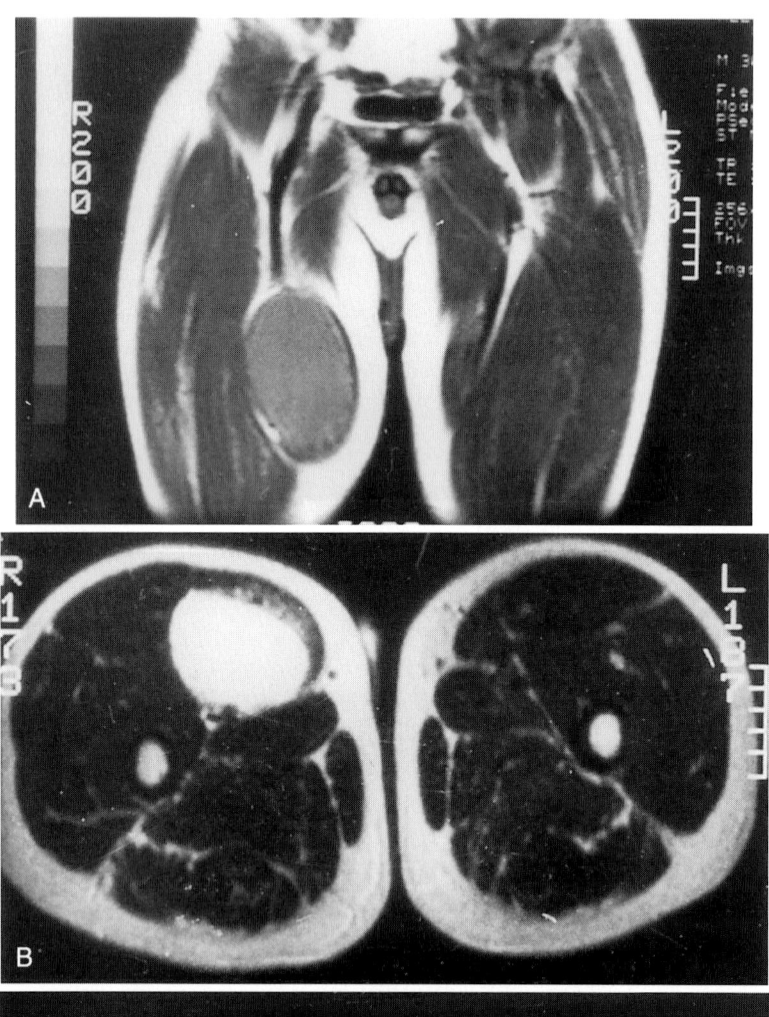


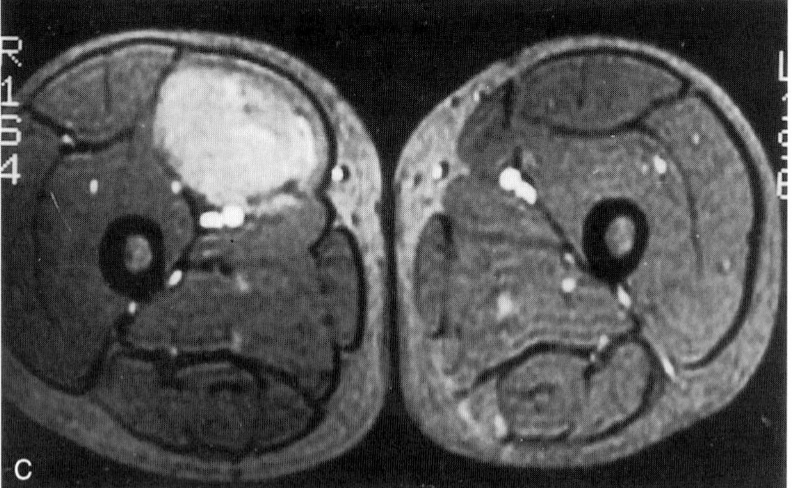


**FIGURE 3–36.** Synovial sarcoma of the thigh. (**A**) Coronal T1-weighted (600/20) MR scan demonstrates a sharply marginated, oval soft tissue mass in the medial right thigh. At this pulse sequence, the signal of the mass is intermediate between that of subcutaneous fat and muscle. Axial T2-weighted MR scan (2000/80) (**B**) and GRE MR scan (33/13, with a 60-degree flip angle) (**C**) clearly demarcate the lesion, which is surrounded by a small amount of edema. There is evidence of muscle separating the mass from the femur. This case illustrates a malignant soft tissue tumor that exhibits sharp or well defined margins on cross-sectional imaging (in this case on MR scans). (Courtesy of Mark J. Kransdorf, MD.)

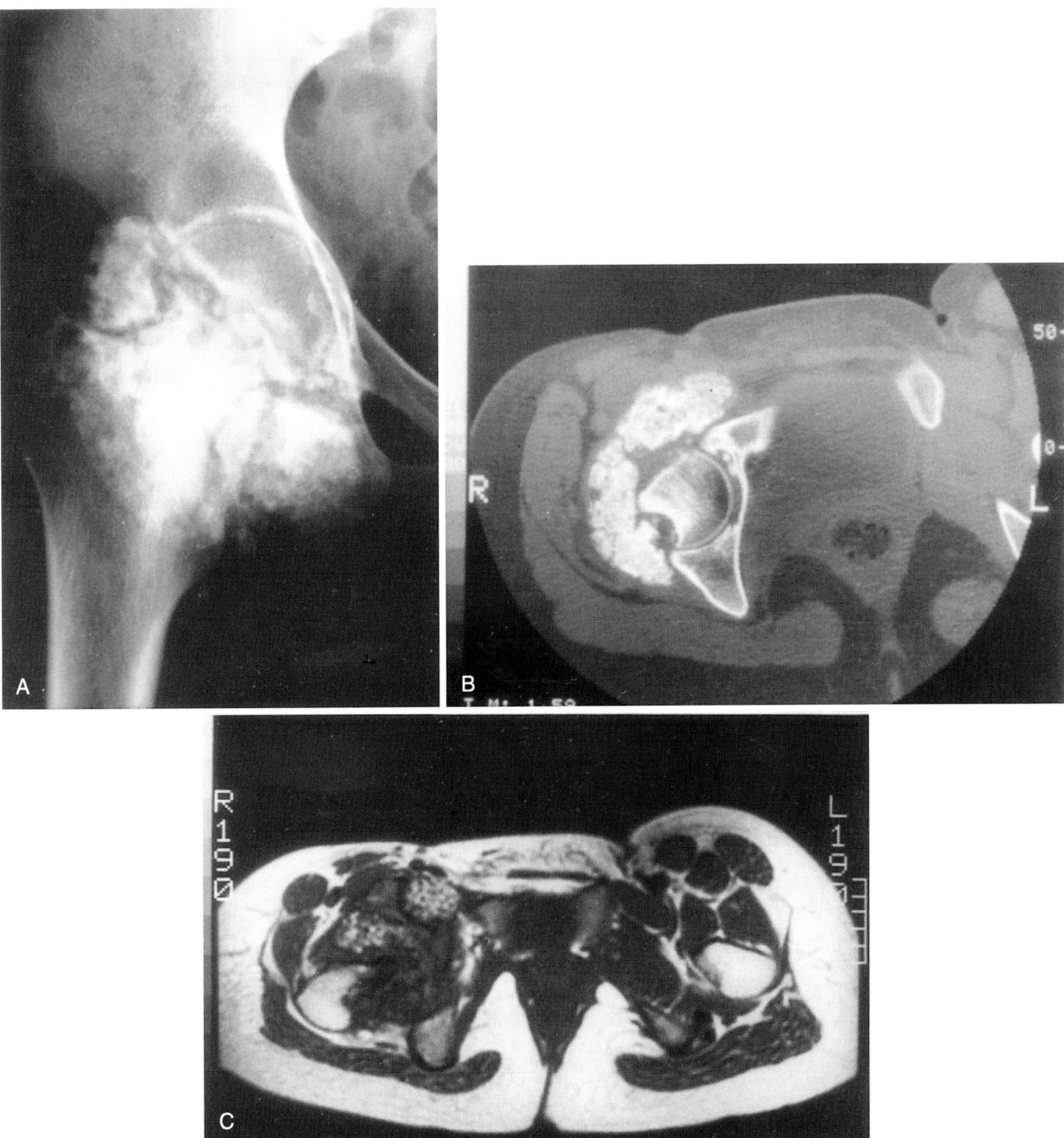


**FIGURE 3–37.** Synovial chondromatosis of the hip. (**A**) AP radiograph demonstrates extensive soft tissue calcification overlying the right hip. (**B**) Axial CT scan imaged at bone windows demonstrates that the calcification is in the hip joint and causes some remodeling of the posterior aspect of the right femoral head. The appearance of the mineralization on both the radiograph and CT scan is strongly suggestive of a cartilaginous lesion. (**C**) Axial T1-weighted (300/15) MR scan demonstrates cartilaginous masses anterior to the right femoral neck. As is readily apparent, the CT scan (**B**) is more suitable for characterizing the calcification in the lesion. (Courtesy of Mark J. Kransdorf, MD.)

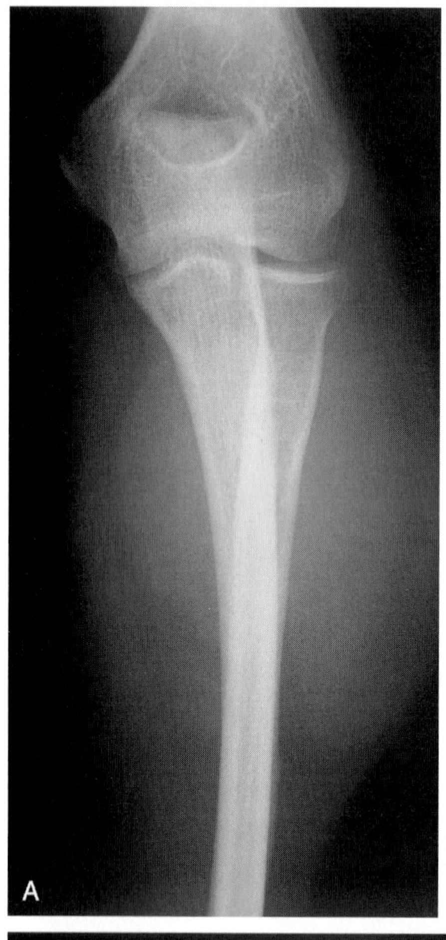


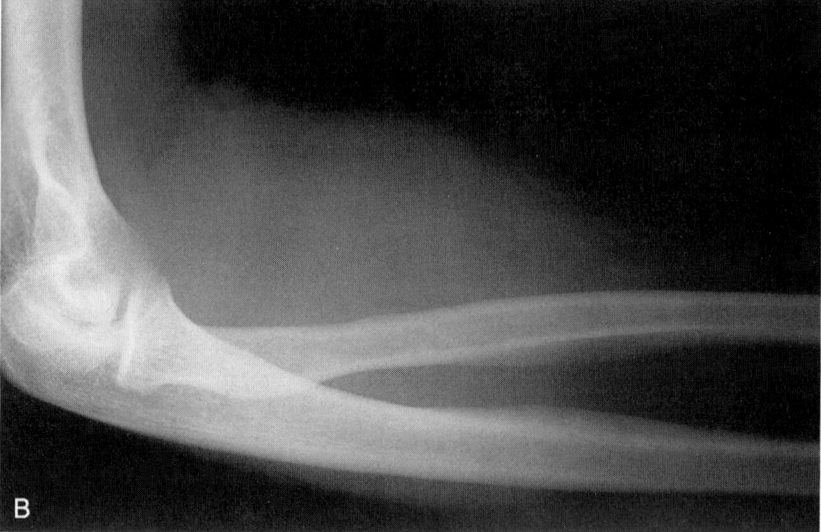


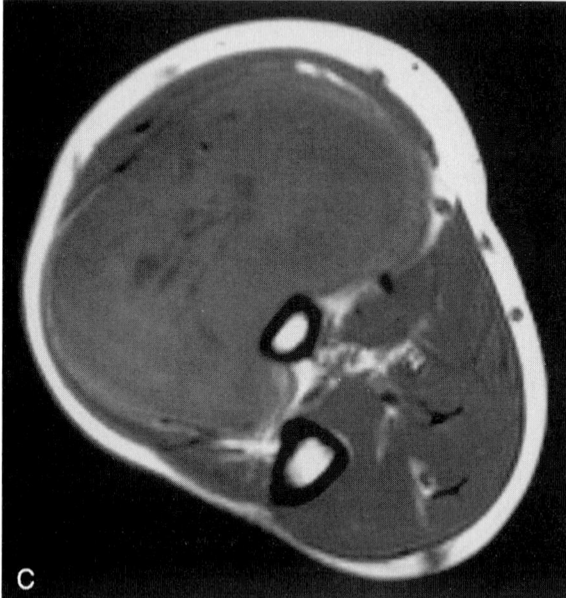


**FIGURE 3–38.** Neurofibroma of the proximal forearm in a 32-year-old man with known neurofibromatosis. Because the patient presented with a rapidly enlarging mass of the forearm, there was grave concern that the lesion was malignant. Frontal (**A**) and lateral (**B**) radiographs demonstrate a large soft tissue mass in the proximal forearm. The extent of the lesion cannot be accurately determined from the radiographs. (**C**) Unenhanced axial T1 (600/15) MR scan demonstrates a large, inhomogeneous soft tissue mass replacing most of the anterior soft tissues with marked compression and displacement of the adjacent muscle. There was a substantial inhomogeneous increase in signal on T2-weighted MR images (not shown).

*Illustration continued on opposite page*

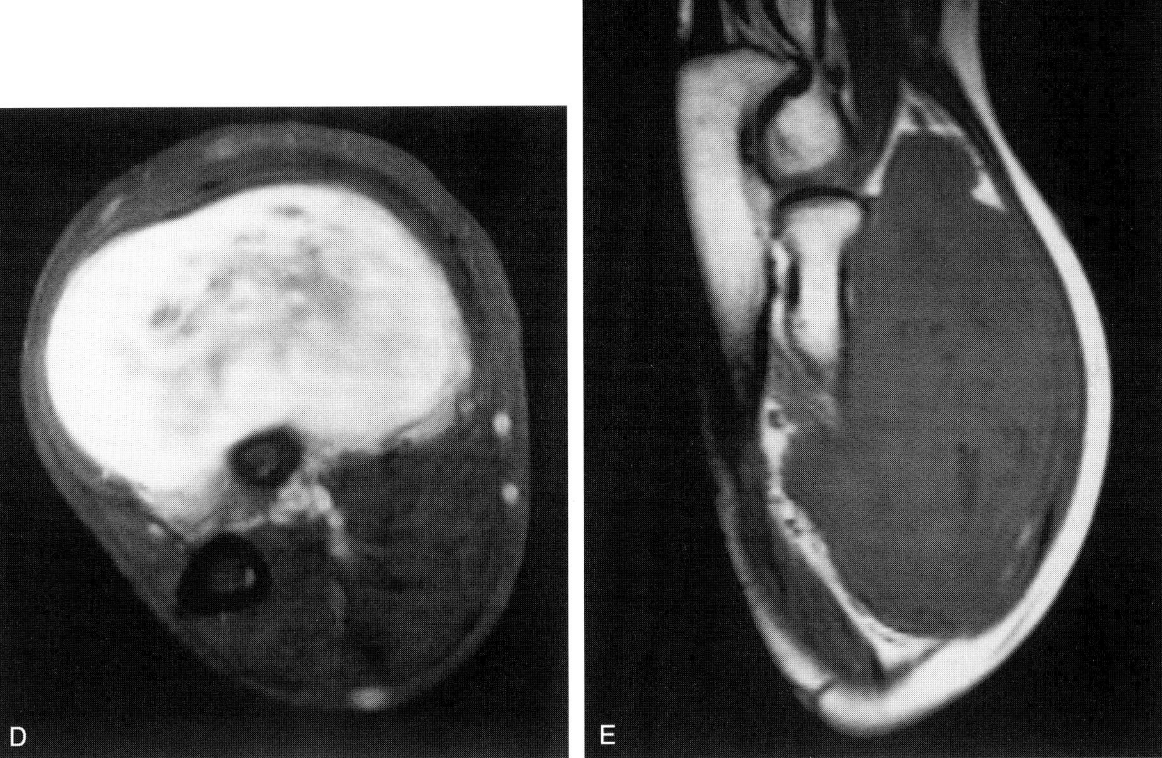


**FIGURE 3-38** *(Continued).* (**D**) Enhanced axial T1-weighted (650/15) MR scan confirms the size and location of the large soft tissue neurofibroma, which is inhomogeneous but sharply marginated. (**E**) Size of the lesion is also well demonstrated on the unenhanced T1 sagittal/coronal image (E-600/15), where the mass and radial head are easily seen. The MR scans were performed prior to resection, which revealed a large neurofibroma.

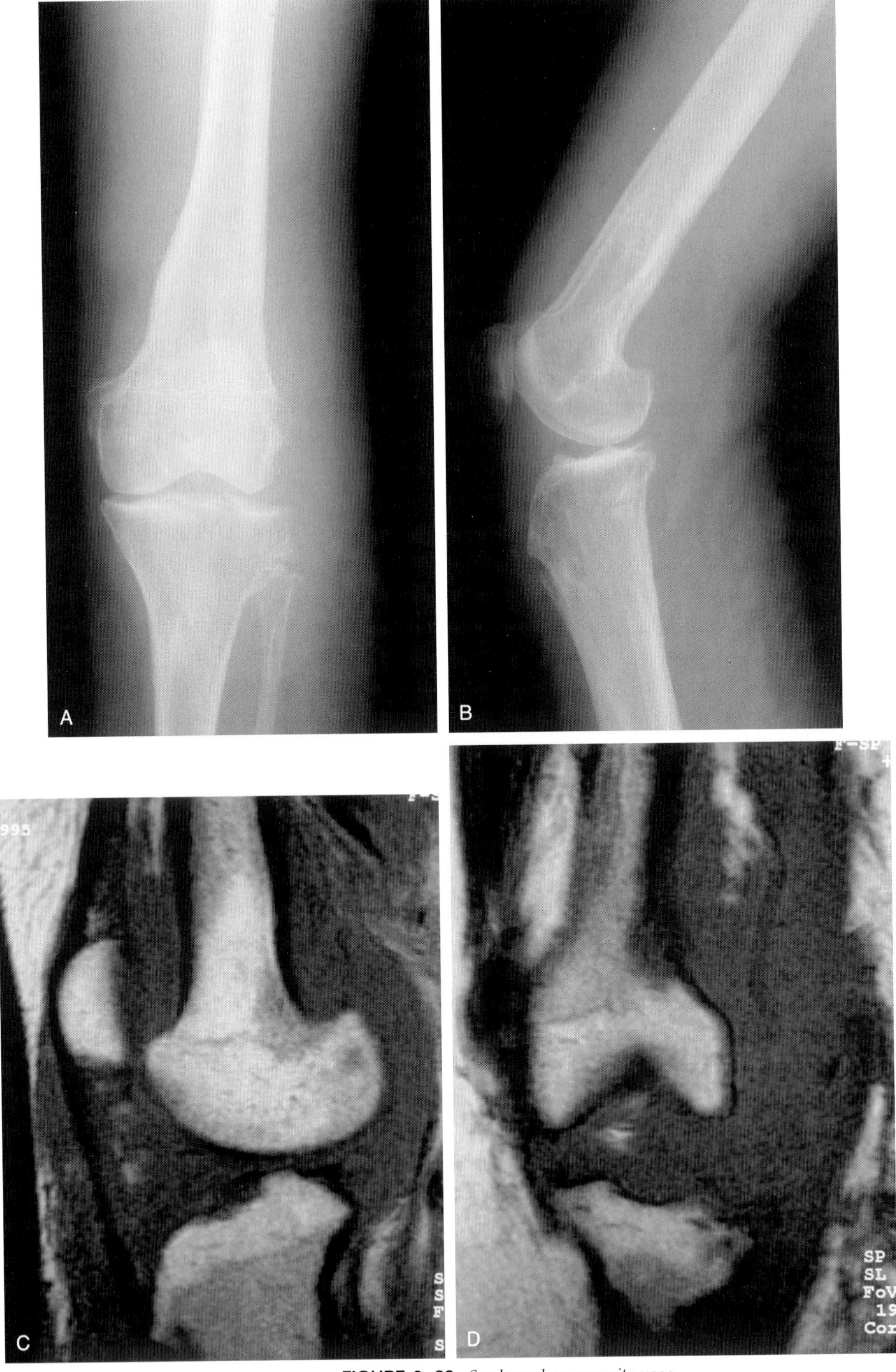

**FIGURE 3–39.** *See legend on opposite page*

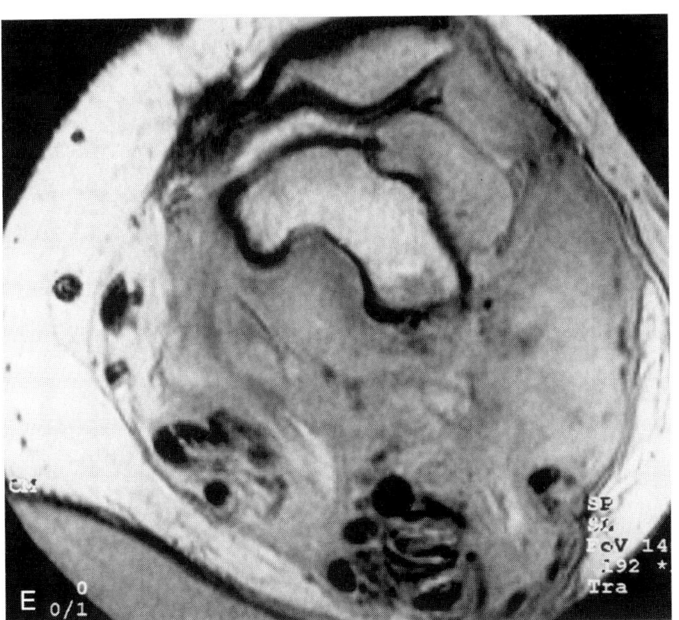


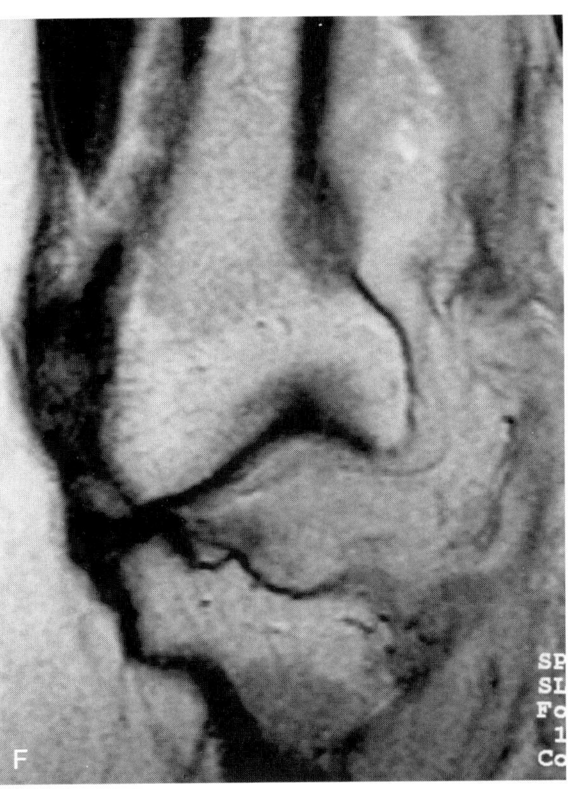


**FIGURE 3–39** *(Continued).* Neurofibroma of the knee. This 47-year-old woman with a long history of neurofibromatosis presented with an unstable knee joint due to disruption of the collateral and cruciate ligaments. AP (**A**) and lateral (**B**) radiographs demonstrate a large soft tissue mass about the knee. On the AP view there is mild scalloping of the medial distal femur due to the adjacent soft tissue mass but no evidence of frank invasion of the bone. Sagittal (**C**) and coronal (**D**) unenhanced T1 (700/15) MR images clearly demonstrate the large soft tissue mass, which is insinuating itself into the knee joint. Definite intraarticular extension of the neurofibroma is readily appreciated on the axial (**E**) and coronal (**F**) gadolinium-enhanced T1 (700/15) MR images. On the axial image the plexiform neurofibroma is insinuated between the distal femur and patella and is nearly encircling the distal femur. A stabilizing total knee arthroplasty was performed; the patient developed a Charcot joint, and the prosthesis subsequently loosened.

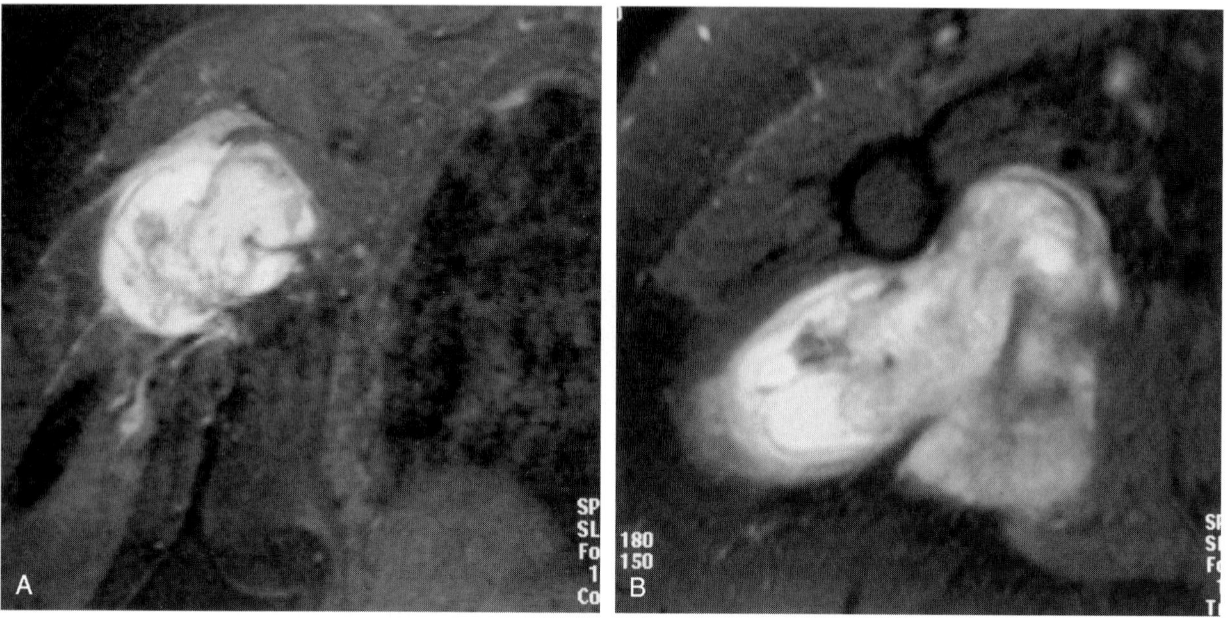


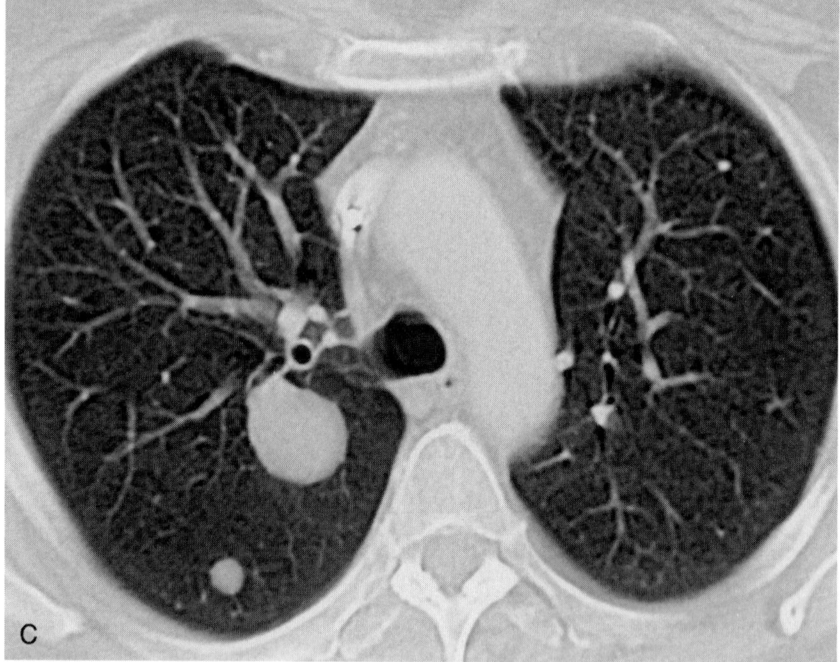


**FIGURE 3–40.** Metastatic angiosarcoma of the arm. This 65-year-old woman presented with a painful, enlarging arm mass. Biopsy had been performed several months earlier at another institution. Coronal (**A**) and axial (**B**) STIR (4800/30) MR scans demonstrate a large, lobulated, inhomogeneous soft tissue mass in the right axilla. The mass displaces adjacent neurovascular structures. Despite four-quarter amputation and chemotherapy, the patient developed chest metastases approximately 18 months after presentation. The chest metastases are easily identified on the axial CT scan (**C**) of the chest.

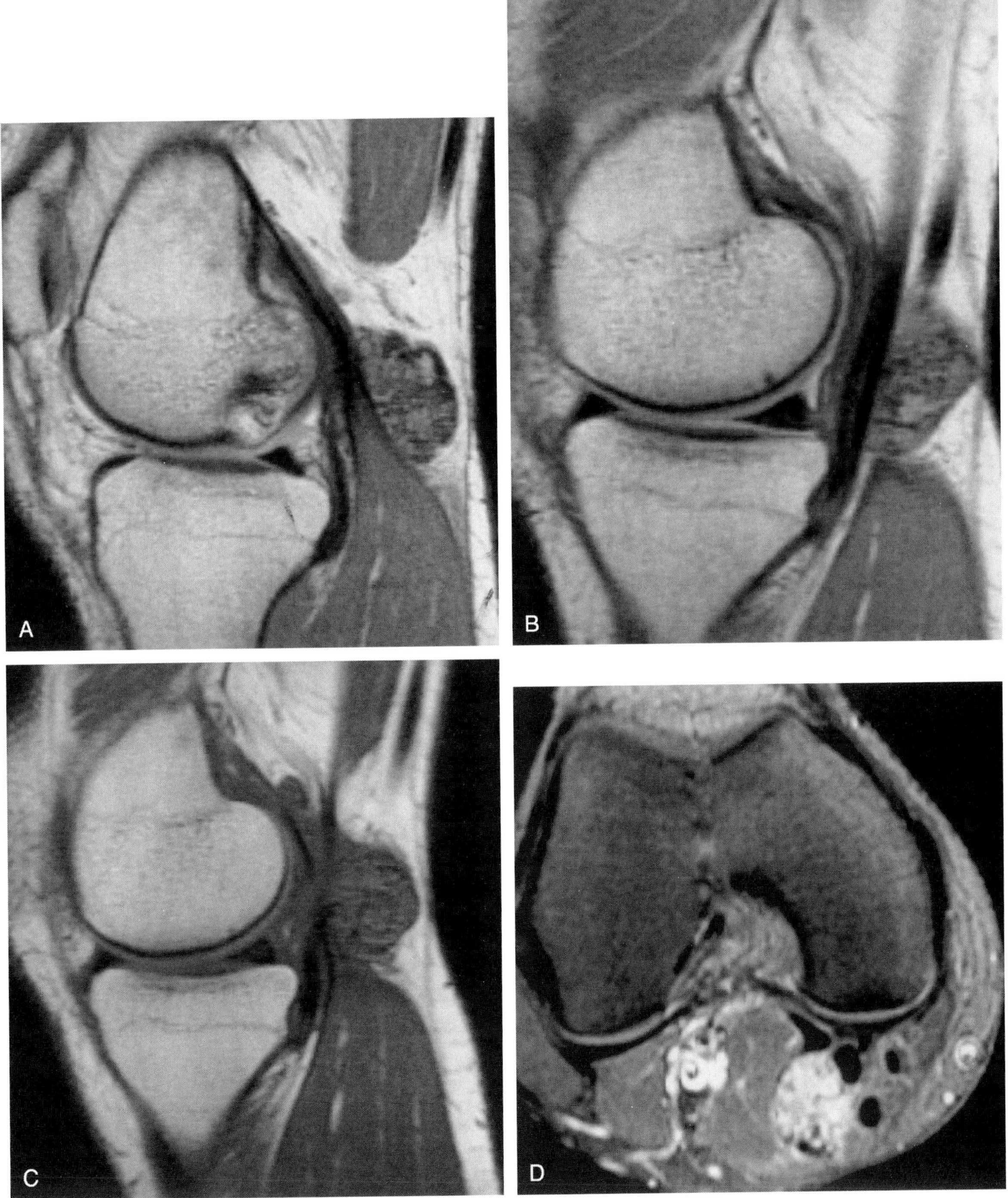


**FIGURE 3–41.** Giant cell tumor of the tendon sheath. A 32-year-old woman presented with chronic, atraumatic knee pain with a stable, palpable mass behind the right knee. Sagittal proton density, fast spin echo MR images (**A, B**) show the mass in the posterior soft tissues of the distal thigh. Lesion is somewhat lobulated in configuration and inhomogeneous in appearance, and it abuts the hamstring tendon. (**C**) Similar findings are noted on the sagittal T1 (433/12) MR scan. (**D**) Axial T1 (500/13) gadolinium-enhanced, fat-suppressed MR scan shows the gastrocnemius muscle belly located between the popliteal neurovascular bundle and the lesion. The patient underwent resection with tenosynovectomy.

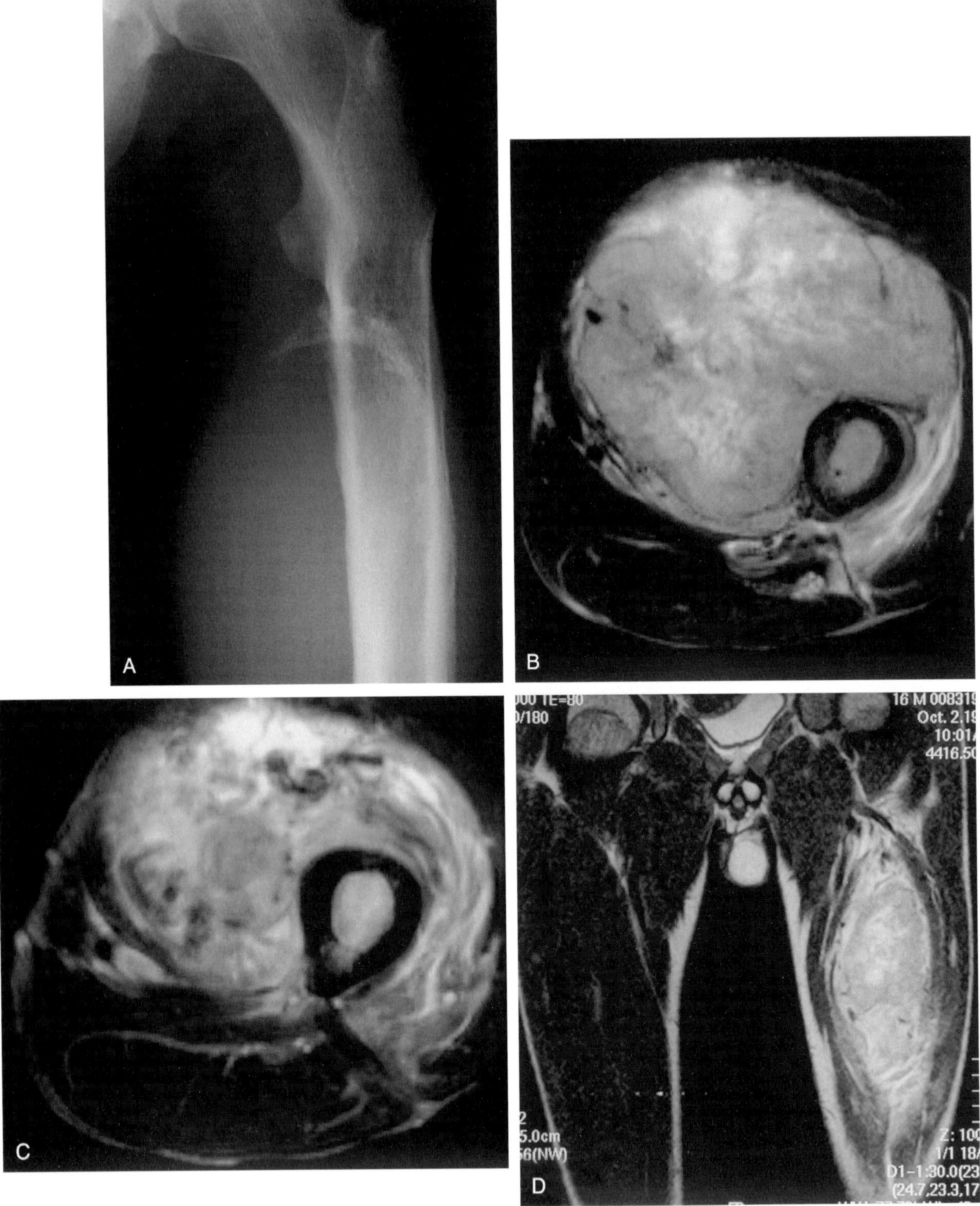


**FIGURE 3–42.** Alveolar soft-part sarcoma of the thigh. A 16-year-old boy presented with a painful, enlarging soft tissue mass in the left thigh. (**A**) AP radiograph of the left thigh shows a large medial soft tissue mass with a bizarre periosteal reaction and infratrochanteric bony lysis consistent with intraosseous extension of the soft tissue mass. (**B, C**) The large, inhomogeneous soft tissue mass, with the epicenter in the proximal, medial soft tissues, is clearly seen on axial T2 (5000/96) MR images. The mass extends up to the anterior skin surface; and in many areas the margins of the tumor are poorly defined. The extent of the lesion is better appreciated on coronal fast spin echo T2 (4000/80) (**D**) and sagittal

*Illustration continued on opposite page*

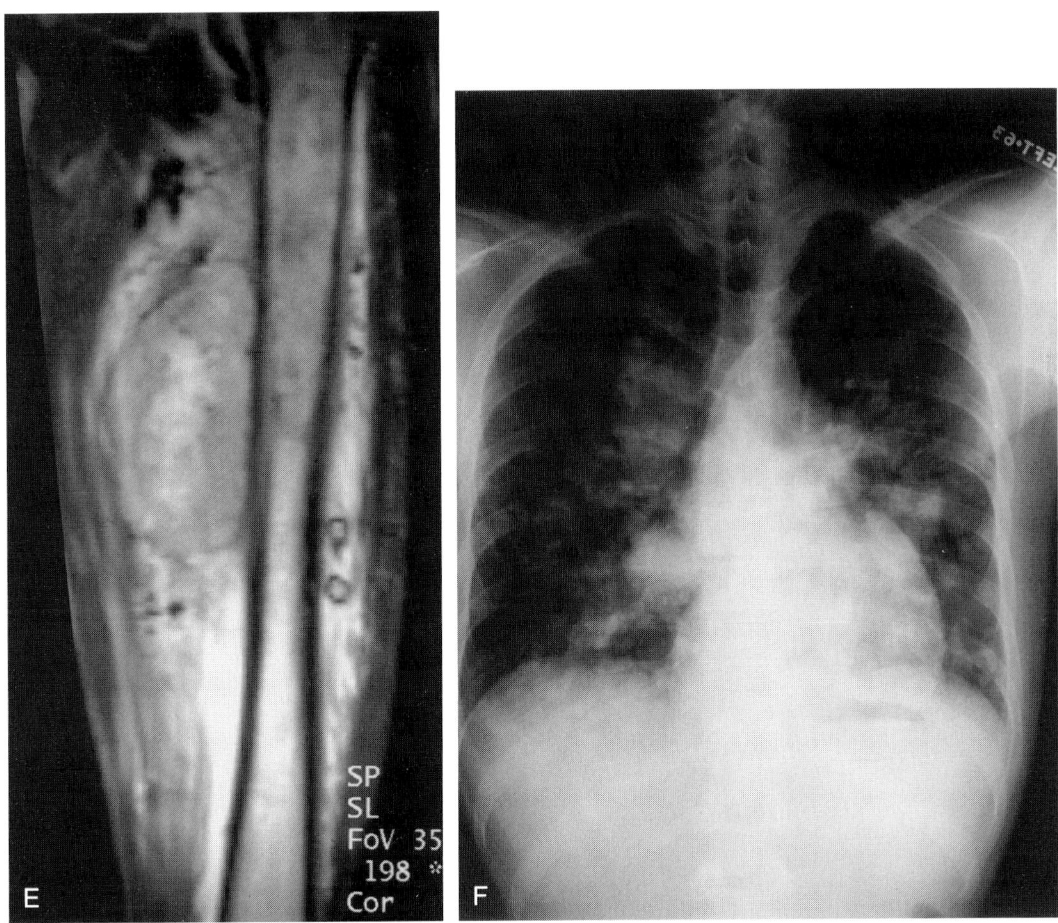


**FIGURE 3–42** *(Continued).* (**E**) STIR (5000/60) MR images. The image in **E** clearly demonstrates involvement of the femoral bone marrow. (**F**) Chest radiograph shows pulmonary metastases that are too numerous to count.

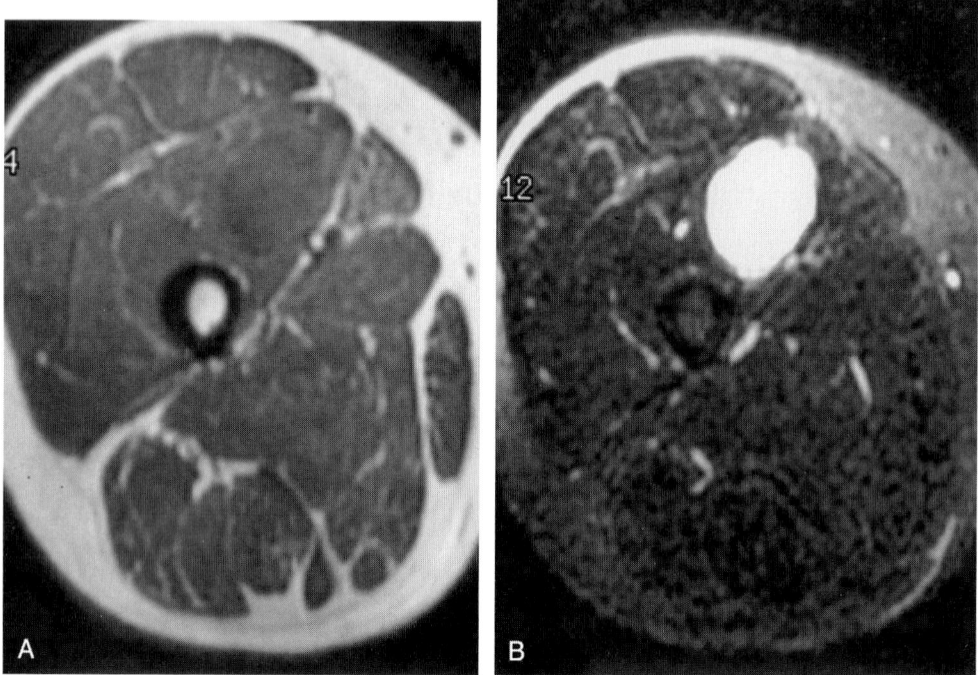


**FIGURE 3–43.** Intramuscular myxoma of the thigh. A 38-year-old man presented with a slowly enlarging mass in the anterior left thigh. Radiographs (not shown) were unremarkable. The mass was near-isointense with muscle on the T1-weighted (733/17) axial MR scan (**A**) but is conspicuous on the T2-weighted (5000/96) axial MR scan (**B**). It was an intramuscular myxoma that was marginally resected.

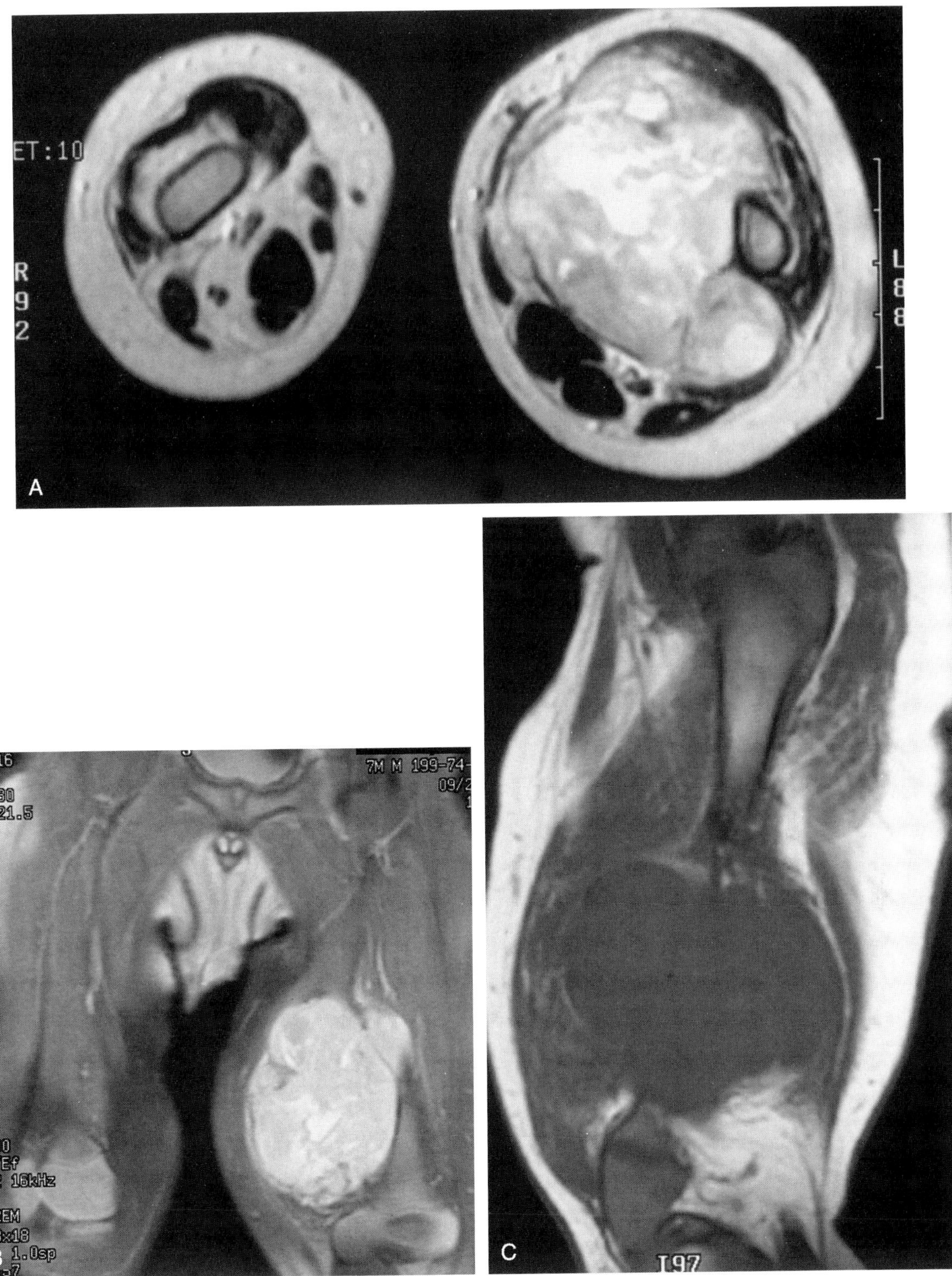


**FIGURE 3–44.** Rhabdomyosarcoma of the thigh. A 7-month-old male infant presented with a rapidly enlarging left thigh mass. Axial T2 (4100/100) (**A**), coronal proton density (5300/21) (**B**), and sagittal T1 (500/16) (**C**) MR scans all reveal a large, inhomogeneous medial left thigh mass. Open biopsy revealed rhabdomyosarcoma. Despite hip disarticulation, the lesion metastasized rapidly, resulting in death within 6 months of surgery.

## REFERENCES


1. Adams EM, Chow CK, Premkumar A, et al. The idiopathic inflammatory myopathies: spectrum of MR imaging findings. Radiographics 15:563, 1995.
2. Alpern MB, Thorsen MK, Kellman GM, et al. CT appearance of hemangiopericytoma. J Comput Assist Tomogr 10:264, 1986.
3. Alvine G, Rosenthal H, Murphey M, et al. Hibernoma. Skeletal Radiol 25:493, 1996.
4. Balsara ZN, Stainken BF, Martinez AJ. MR image of localized giant cell tumor of the tendon sheath involving the knee. J Comput Assist Tomogr 13:159, 1989.
5. Bartis JR. Massive lipoma of the foot: a case report. J Am Podiatr Assoc 64:874, 1974.
6. Benedikt RA, Jelinek JS, Kransdorf MJ, et al. MR imaging of soft-tissue masses: role of gadopentetate dimeglumine. J Magn Reson Imaging 4:485, 1994.
7. Berger PE, Kuhn JP. Computed tomography of tumors of the musculoskeletal system in children. Radiology 127:171, 1978.
8. Bernardino ME, Jing BS, Thomas JL, et al. The extremity soft tissue lesion: a comparative study of ultrasound, computed tomography, and xeroradiography. Radiology 139:53, 1981.
9. Bernreuter WK, Sartoris DJ, Resnick D. Magnetic resonance imaging of synovial sarcoma. J Foot Surg 29:94, 1990.
10. Berquist TH, Ehman RL, King BF, et al. Value of MR imaging in differentiating benign from malignant soft-tissue masses: study of 95 lesions. AJR 155:1251, 1990.
11. Binkovitz LA, Berquist TH, McLeod RA. Masses of the hand and wrist: detection and characterization with MR imaging. AJR 154:323, 1990.
12. Blacksin M, Barnes FJ, Lyons MM. MR diagnosis of macrodystrophia lipomatosa. AJR 158:1295, 1992.
13. Blatt CJ, Hayt DB, Desai M, et al. Soft tissue sarcomas imaged with technetium-99m pyrophosphate. NY State J Med 77:2118, 1977.
14. Bohndorf K, Reiser M, Lochner B, et al. Magnetic resonance imaging of primary tumours and tumour-like lesions of bone. Skeletal Radiol 15:511, 1986.
15. Bradley WG, Waluch V, Lai KS, et al. The appearance of rapidly flowing blood on magnetic resonance images. AJR 143: 1167, 1984.
16. Braunstein EM, Silver TM, Martel W, et al. Ultrasonic diagnosis of extremity masses. Skeletal Radiol 6:157, 1981.
17. Broder MS, Leonidas JC, Mitty HA. Pseudosarcomatous fasciitis: an unusual cause of soft tissue calcification. Radiology 107: 173, 1973.
18. Brown M, Thrall J, Cooper R, et al. Radiography and scintigraphy in tumoral calcinosis. Radiology 124:757, 1977.
19. Buetow PC, Kransdorf MJ, Moser RP Jr, et al. Radiologic appearance of intramuscular hemangioma with emphasis on MR. AJR 154:563, 1990.
20. Burrows PE, Mulliken JB, Fellows KE, et al. Childhood hemangiomas and vascular malformations: angiographic differentiation. AJR 141:483, 1983.
21. Bush CH, Spanier SS, Gillespy T. Imaging of atypical lipomas of the extremities: a report of three cases. Skeletal Radiol 17: 472, 1988.
22. Cadman NL, Soule EH, Kelly PJ. Synovial sarcoma: an analysis of 134 tumors. Cancer 18:613, 1965.
23. Cerofolini E, Landi A, DeSantis G, et al. MR of benign peripheral nerve sheath tumors. J Comput Assist Tomogr 15:593, 1991.
24. Chang AE, Matory YL, Dwyer AJ, et al. Magnetic resonance imaging versus computed tomography in the evaluation of soft tissue tumors of the extremities. Ann Surg 205:240, 1987.
25. Cockshott WP, Evans KT. The place of soft tissue arteriography. Br J Radiol 37:367, 1964.
26. Cohen E, Kressel HY, Perosio T, et al. MR imaging of soft tissue hemangiomas: correlation with pathologic findings. AJR 150:1079, 1988.
27. Cohen JM, Weinreb JC, Redman HC. Arteriovenous malformations of the extremities: MR imaging. Radiology 158:475, 1986.
28. Cotten A, Flipo RM, Chastanet P, et al. Pigmented villonodular synovitis of the hip: review of radiographic features in 58 patients. Skeletal Radiol 24:1, 1995.
29. Crim JR, Seegar LL, Yao L, et al. Diagnosis of soft tissue masses with MR imaging: can benign masses be differentiated from malignant ones? Radiology 185:581, 1992.
30. Dalinka MK, Zlatkin MB, Chao P, et al. Use of magnetic resonance imaging in the evaluation of bone and soft-tissue tumors. Radiol Clin North Am 28:461, 1990.
31. Davis B, Sundaram M, Kransdorf MJ. Synovial sarcoma: imaging findings in 34 patients. AJR 161:827, 1993.
32. Delfaut EM, Beltran J, Johnson G, et al. Fat suppression in MR imaging: techniques and pitfalls. Radiographics 19:373, 1999.
33. Demas BE, Heelan RT, Lane J, et al. Soft tissue sarcomas of the extremities: comparison of MR and CT in determining the extent of disease. AJR 150:615, 1988.
34. Desai A, Eymontt M, Alavi A, et al. 99mTc-MDP uptake in nonosseous lesions. Radiology 135:181, 1980.
35. DeSantos LA, Goldstein HM, Murray JA, et al. Computed tomography in the evaluation of musculoskeletal neoplasms. Radiology 128:89, 1978.
36. Deseran MW, Seeger LL, Doberneck SA, et al. Case report 840: hibernoma of the right gracilis muscle. Skeletal Radiol 23:301, 1994.
37. Disler DG, McCauley TR, Ratner LM, et al. In-phase and out-of-phase imaging of bone marrow: prediction of neoplasia based on the detection of coexistant fat and water. AJR 169: 1439, 1997.
38. Dooms GC, Hricak H, Sotlitto RA, et al. Lipomatous tumors with fatty component: MR imaging potential and comparison of MR and CT results. Radiology 157:479, 1985.
39. Doud TM, Moser RP, Giudici MAI, et al. Case report 704: extraskeletal osteosarcoma of the thigh with several suspected skeletal metastases and extensive metastases to the chest. Skeletal Radiol 20:628, 1991.
40. Drape JL, Idy-Peretti I, Goettmann S, et al. Subungual glomus tumors: evaluation with MR imaging. Radiology 195:507, 1995.
41. Edelman RR. MR angiography: present and future. AJR 161:1, 1993.
42. Edelman RR, Mattle HP, Atkinson DH, et al. MR angiography. AJR 154:937, 1990.
43. Egund N, Ekelund L, Sako M, et al. CT of soft-tissue tumors. AJR 137:725, 1981.
44. Engelsted BL, Gilula LA, Kyriakos M. Ossified skeletal muscle hemangioma: radiologic and pathologic features. Skeletal Radiol 5:35, 1980.
45. Enneking WE. Staging of musculoskeletal neoplasms, from the Musculoskeletal Tumor Society. Skeletal Radiol 13:183, 1985.
46. Enneking WF, Spanier SS, Malawar MM. The effect of the anatomic setting on the results of surgical procedures for soft part sarcoma of the thigh. Cancer 47:1005, 1981.
47. Erlemann R, Reiser MF, Peters PE, et al. Musculoskeletal neoplasms: static and dynamic Gd-DTPA-enhanced MR imaging. Radiology 171:767, 1989.
48. Erlemann R, Vassalio P, Bongartz G, et al. Musculoskeletal neoplasms: fast low-angle shot MR imaging with and without Gd-DTPA. Radiology 176:489, 1990.
49. Eugenidis N, Locher J. Tumoral calcinosis imaged by bone scanning: case report. J Nucl Med 18:34, 1977.
50. Feldman F, Singson RD, Staron RB. Magnetic resonance imaging of paraarticular and ectopic ganglia. Skeletal Radiol 18:353, 1989.

51. Finck EJ, Moore TM. Angiography for mass lesions of bone, joint, and soft tissue. Orthop Clin North Am 8:999, 1977.
52. Fletcher BD, Reddick WE, Taylor JS. Dynamic MR imaging of musculoskeletal neoplasms. Radiology 200: 869, 1995.
53. Fornage BD, Rifkin MD. Ultrasound examination of the hand and foot. Radiol Clin North Am 26:109, 1988.
54. Frantzell A. Soft tissue radiography: technical aspects and clinical applications in the examination of limbs. Acta Radiol Suppl 85:1, 1951.
55. Fujimoto H, Murakami K, Ichikawa T, et al. MRI of soft-tissue lesions: opposed-phase T2*-weighted gradient-echo images. J Comput Assist Tomogr 17:418, 1993.
56. Galant J, Marti-Bonmati, L, Soler R, et al. Grading of subcutaneous soft tissue tumors by means of their relationship with the superficial fascia on MR imaging. Skeletal Radiol 27:657, 1998.
57. Goldman AB. Myositis ossifcans circumscripta: a benign lesion with malignant differential diagnosis. AJR 126:32, 1976.
58. Grant EG, Gronvall S, Sarosi TE, et al. Sonographic findings in four cases of hemangiopericytoma. Radiology 142:447, 1982.
59. Greenfield GB, Arrington JA, Kudryk BT. MRI of soft tissue tumors. Skeletal Radiol 22:7, 1993.
60. Greenspan A, Azouz EM, Matthews J, et al. Synovial hemangioma: imaging features in eight histologically proven cases, review of the literature, and differential diagnosis. Skeletal Radiol 24:583, 1995.
61. Harkness J, Peters H. Tumoral calcinosis: a report of six cases. J Bone Joint Surg Am 49:721, 1967.
62. Heelan RT, Watson RC, Smith J. Computed tomography of lower extremity tumors. AJR 132:933, 1979.
63. Heiken JP, Lee JKT, Smathers RL, et al. CT of benign soft-tissue masses of the extremities. AJR 142:575, 1984.
64. Hermann G, Abdelwahab IF, Klein M, et al. Synovial chondromatosis. Skeletal Radiol 24:298, 1995.
65. Hermann G, Abdelwahab IF, Miller TT, et al. Tumour and tumour-like conditions of the soft tissue: magnetic resonance imaging features differentiating benign from malignant masses. Br J Radiol 65:14, 1992.
66. Hermann G, Rose JS. Computed tomography in bone and soft tissue pathology of the extremities. J Comput Assist Tomogr 3: 58, 1979.
67. Hermann G, Yeh HC, Lehr-James C, et al. Diagnosis of popliteal cysts: double-contrast arthrography and sonography. AJR 137:369, 1981.
68. Hernandez RJ, Keim DR, Chenevert TL, et al. Fat suppressed magnetic resonance imaging of myositis. Radiology 182:217, 1992.
69. Herzberg DL, Schreiber MH. Angiography in mass lesions of the extremities. AJR 111:541, 1971.
70. Horowitz AL, Resnick D, Watson RC. The roentgen features of synovial sarcomas. Clin Radiol 24:481, 1973.
71. Hudson TM, Hamlin DJ, Enneking WF, et al. Magnetic resonance imaging of bone and soft tissue tumors: early experience in 31 patients compared with computed tomography. Skeletal Radiol 13:134, 1985.
72. Hudson TM, Hass G, Enneking WF, et al. Angiography in the management of musculoskeletal tumors. Surg Gynecol Obstet 141:11, 1975.
73. Hughes TH, Sartoris DJ, Schweitzer ME, et al. Pigmented villonodular synovitis: MRI characteristics. Skeletal Radiol 24:7, 1995.
74. Hunter JC, Johnston WH, Genant HK. Computed tomography evaluation of fatty tumors of the somatic soft tissues: clinical utility and radiologic-pathologic correlation. Skeletal Radiol 4: 79, 1979.
75. Israels SJ, Chan HS, Daneman A, et al. Synovial sarcoma in childhood. AJR 142:803, 1984.
76. Jaffe N. Hemangiopericytoma: angiographic findings. Br J Radiol 33:614, 1960.
77. Janzen L, Logan PM, O'Connell JX, et al. Intramedullary chondroid tumors of bone: correlation of abnormal peritumoral marrow and soft-tissue MRI signal with tumor type. Skeletal Radiol 26:100, 1997.
78. Jelinek J, Kransdorf MJ. MR imaging of soft tissue masses: mass-like lesions that simulate neoplasms. Magn Reson Imaging Clin N Am 3:727, 1995.
79. Jelinek JS, Kransdorf MJ, Shmookler BM, et al. Giant cell tumor of the tendon sheath: MR findings in nine cases. AJR 162: 919, 1994.
80. Jelinek JS, Kransdorf MJ, Shmookler BM, et al. Liposarcoma of the extremities: MR and CT findings of the histologic subtypes. Radiology 186:445, 1993.
81. Jelinek JS, Kransdorf MJ, Utz JA, et al. Imaging of pigmented villonodular synovitis with emphasis on magnetic resonance imaging. AJR 152:337, 1989.
82. Jones BC, Sundaram M, Kransdorf MJ. Synovial sarcoma: MR imaging findings in 34 patients. AJR 161:827, 1993.
83. Kaplan PA, Williams SM. Mucocutaneous and peripheral soft-tissue hemangiomas: MR imaging. Radiology 163:163, 1987.
84. Kaufman JH, Cedermark BJ, Parthasarathy KL, et al. The values of $^{67}$Ga scintigraphy in soft-tissue sarcoma and chondrosarcoma. Radiology 123:131, 1977.
85. Kilcoyne RF, Richardson ML, Porter BA, et al. Magnetic resonance imaging of soft tissue masses. Clin Orthop 228:13, 1988.
86. Kim YS, Yeh LR, Trudell D, et al. MR imaging of the major nerves about the elbow: cadaveric study examining the effect of flexion and extension of the elbow and pronation and supination of the forearm. Skeletal Radiol 27:419, 1998.
87. Kransdorf MJ. Benign soft-tissue tumors in a large referral population: distribution of diagnoses by age, sex, and location. AJR 164:395, 1995.
88. Kransdorf MJ, Jelinek JS, Moser RP Jr, et al. Magnetic resonance appearance of fibromatosis: a report of 14 cases and review of the literature. Skeletal Radiol 19:495, 1990.
89. Kransdorf MJ, Jelinek JS, Moser RP Jr, et al. Soft tissue masses: diagnosis using MR imaging. AJR 153:541, 1989.
90. Kransdorf MJ, McFarland DR, Moser RP Jr, et al. Case report 649: arteriovenous malformation of the distal thigh with bone involvement. Skeletal Radiol 20:63, 1991.
91. Kransdorf MJ, Meis JM. Extraskeletal osseous and cartilaginous tumors of the extremities. Radiographics 13:853, 1993.
92. Kransdorf MJ, Meis JM, Jelinek JS. Dedifferentiated liposarcoma of the extremities: imaging findings in four patients. AJR 161:127, 1993.
93. Kransdorf MJ, Meis JM, Jelinek JS. Myositis ossificans: MR appearance with radiologic-pathologic correlation. AJR 157: 1243, 1991.
94. Kransdorf MJ, Meis JM, Montgomery E. Elastofibroma: MR and CT appearance with radiologic-pathologic correlation. AJR 159:575, 1992.
95. Kransdorf MJ, Moser RP Jr, Jelinek JS, et al. Intramuscular myxoma: MR features. J Comput Assist Tomogr 13:836, 1989.
96. Kransdorf MJ, Moser RP Jr, Jelinek JS, et al. Soft tissue masses: diagnosis using MR imaging. AJR 153:541, 1989.
97. Kransdorf MJ, Moser RP Jr, Madewell JE. Imaging techniques. In: Bogumill GP, Fleegler EJ, McFarland GB (eds) Tumors of the Hand and Upper Limb. Churchill Livingstone, New York, 1993.
98. Kransdorf MJ, Moser RP Jr, Meis JM, et al. Fat containing soft tissue masses of the extremities. Radiographics 11:81, 1991.
99. Kransdorf MJ, Murphey MD. Imaging of Soft Tissue Tumors. Saunders, Philadelphia, 1997.
100. Krinsky G, Rofsky NM, Weinreb JC. Nonspecificity of short inversion time inversion recovery (STIR) as a technique of fat

suppression: pitfalls in image interpretation. AJR 166:523, 1996.
101. Lafferty F, Reynolds E, Pearson O. Tumoral calcinosis: a metabolic disease of obscure etiology. Am J Med 38:105, 1965.
102. Lagergren C, Lindbom A. Angiography of peripheral tumors. Radiology 79:371, 1962.
103. Lagergren C, Lindbom A, Soderberg G. Vascularization of fibromatous and fibrosarcomatous tumors: histopathologic, microangiographic, and angiographic studies. Acta Radiol 53:1, 1960.
104. Lateur L, Van Ongeval C, Samson I, et al. Case report 842: benign hibernoma. Skeletal Radiol 23:306, 1994.
105. Lawson TL, Mittler S. Ultrasonic evaluation of extremity soft-tissue lesions with arthrographic correlation. J Can Assoc Radiol 29:58, 1978.
106. Lec KR, Cox GG, Neff JR, et al. Cystic masses of the knee: arthrographic and CT evaluation. AJR 148:329, 1987.
107. Levin DC, Gordon DH, McSweeney J. Arteriography of peripheral hemangiomas. Radiology 121:625, 1976.
108. Levin DC, Watson RC, Baltaxe HA. Arteriography in the diagnosis and management of acquired peripheral soft-tissue masses. Radiology 104:53, 1972.
109. Levin DN, Herrmann A, Spraggins T, et al. Improved visualization of musculoskeletal tumors using linear combinations of conventional MR images. In: Book of Abstracts: Society of Magnetic Resonance in Medicine, vol 5. SMRM, Berkeley, CA, 1986.
110. Levine E, Huntrakoon M, Wetzel LH. Malignant nerve-sheath neoplasms in neurofibromatosis: distinction from benign tumors by using imaging techniques. AJR 149:1059, 1987.
111. Levine E, Lee KR, Neff JR, et al. Comparison of computed tomography and other imaging modalities in the evaluation of musculoskeletal tumors. Radiology 131:431, 1979.
112. Levine E, Wetzel LH, Neff JR. MR imaging and CT of extrahepatic cavernous hemangiomas. AJR 147:1299, 1986.
113. Levinsohn EM, Bryan PJ. Computed tomography in unilateral extremity swelling of unusual cause. J Comput Assist Tomogr 3:67, 1979.
114. Levitt RG, Sagel SS, Stanley RJ, et al. Computed tomography of the pelvis. Semin Roentgenol 13:193, 1978.
115. Lewandowski PJ, Weiner SD. Hibernoma of the medial thigh: case report and literature review. Clin Orthop 330:198, 1996.
116. Llauger J, Monill JM, Palmer J, et al. Synovial hemangioma of the knee: MRI imaging findings in two cases. Skeletal Radiol 24:578, 1995.
117. London J, Kim EE, Wallace S, et al. MR imaging of liposarcomas: correlation of MR features and histology. J Comput Assist Tomogr 18:832, 1989.
118. Ma LD, Frassica FJ, McCarthy EF, et al. Benign and malignant musculoskeletal masses: MR imaging differentiation with rim-to-center differential enhancement ratios. Radiology 202:739, 1997.
119. Mahajan H, Kim EE, Wallace S, et al. Magnetic resonance imaging of malignant fibrous histiocytoma. Magn Reson Imaging 7:283, 1989.
120. Margulis AR, Murphy TO. Arteriography in neoplasms of extremities. AJR 80:330, 1958.
121. Martel W, Abell MR. Radiologic evaluation of soft tissue tumors. Cancer 32:352, 1973.
122. Martin DS, Sharafuddin M, Boozan J, et al. Multiple symmetric lipomatosis (Madelung's disease). Skeletal Radiol 24:72, 1995.
123. Math KR, Pavlov H, DiCarlo E, et al. Spindle cell lipoma of the foot: a case report and literature review. Foot Ankle Int 16: 220, 1995.
124. Matsui K, Yamada H, Chiba K, et al. Visualization of soft tissue malignancies by using $^{99m}$Tc polyphosphate, pyrophosphate, and diphosphonate ($^{99m}$TcP). J Nucl Med 14:632, 1973.
125. May DA, Good RB, Smith DK, et al. MR imaging of musculoskeletal tumors and tumor mimickers with intravenous gadolinium: experience with 242 patients. Skeletal Radiol 26:1, 1997.
126. McEachern A, Janzen DL, O'Connell JX. Shoulder girdle lipomatosis. Skeletal Radiol 24:471, 1995.
127. McLeod RA, Gisvold JJ, Stephens DH, et al. Computed tomography of soft tissues and breast. Semin Roentgenol 13:267, 1978.
128. McMaster MJ, Soule EH, Ivins JC. Hemangiopericytoma: a clinicopathologic study and long-term follow-up of 60 patients. Cancer 36:2232, 1975.
129. McNeill TW, Chan GE, Capek V, et al. The value of angiography in the surgical management of deep hemangiomas. Clin Orthop 101:176, 1984.
130. Melson GL, Staple TW, Evens RG. Soft tissue radiographic technique. Semin Roentgenol 8:19, 1973.
131. Meyer CA, Kransdorf MJ, Jelinek JS, et al. Case report 716: soft tissue metastasis in synovial sarcoma. Skeletal Radiol 21: 128, 1992.
132. Meyer CA, Kransdorf MJ, Jelinek JS, et al. Radiologic appearance of nodular fasciitis with emphasis on MR and CT. J Comput Assist Tomogr 15:276, 1991.
133. Meyer JS, Hoffer FA, Barnes PD, et al. Biological classification of soft-tissue vascular anomalies: MR correlation. AJR 157:559, 1991.
134. Mirowitz SA. Fast scanning and fat-suppression MR imaging of musculoskeletal disorders. AJR 161:1147, 1993.
135. Mirowitz SA, Totty WG, Lee JK. Characterization of musculoskeletal masses using dynamic GD-DTPA enhanced spin-echo MRI. J Comput Assist Tomogr 16:120, 1992.
136. Mitnick P, Goldfarb S, Slatopalsky E, et al. Calcium and phosphate metabolism in tumoral calcinosis. Ann Intern Med 92: 482, 1980.
137. Mizutani H, Yanagi T, Suzuki H, et al. Synovial sarcoma in the prevertebral space of the neck: CT and MR findings. Radiat Med. 15:121, 1997.
138. Moon KL, Genant HK, Helms CA, et al. Musculoskeletal applications of nuclear magnetic resonance. Radiology 147:161, 1983.
139. Morton MJ, Berquist TH, McLeod RA, et al. MR imaging of synovial sarcoma. AJR 156:337, 1991.
140. Mujahed Z, Vasilas A, Evans JA. Hemangiopericytoma: a report of four cases with a review of the literature. AJR 82:658, 1959.
141. Murphy MD, Fairbairn KJ, Parman LM, et al. Musculoskeletal angiomatous lesions: radiologic-pathologic correlation. Radiographics 15:893, 1995.
142. Murphy MD, Gross TM, Rosenthal HG. Musculoskeletal malignant fibrous histiocytoma: radiologic-pathologic correlation. Radiographics 14:807, 1994.
143. Murphy WD, Hurst GC, Duerk JL, et al. Atypical appearance of lipomatous tumors on MR images: high signal intensity with fat-suppression STIR sequences. J Magn Reson Imaging 1: 477, 1991.
144. Murray JA. Synovial sarcoma. Orthop Clin North Am 8:963, 1977.
145. Norman A, Dorfman HD. Juxtacortical circumscribed myositis ossificans: evolution and radiographic features. Radiology 96: 301, 1970.
146. Pathria MN, Zlatkin M, Sartoris DJ, et al. Ultrasonography of the popliteal fossa and lower extremities. Radiol Clin North Am 26;77, 1988.
147. Pearce WH, Rutherford RB, Whitehill TA, et al. Nuclear magnetic resonance imaging: its diagnostic value in patients with

congenital vascular malformations of the limbs. J Vasc Surg 8: 64, 1988.
148. Peh WCG, Trouong NP, Totty WG, et al. Pictorial review: magnetic resonance imaging of benign soft tissue masses of the hand and wrist. Clin Radiol 50:519, 1995.
149. Petasnick JP, Turner DA, Charters JR, et al. Soft-tissue masses of the locomotor system: comparison of MR imaging with CT. Radiology 160:125, 1986.
150. Petterson H, Gillespy T, Hamlin DJ, et al. Primary musculoskeletal tumors: examination with MR imaging compared with conventional modalities. Radiology 164:237, 1987.
151. Petterson H, Hamlin DJ, Mancuso A, et al. Magnetic resonance imaging of the musculoskeletal system. Acta Radiol (Diagn) (Stockh) 26:225, 1985.
152. Pirkey EL, Hurt J. Roentgen evaluation of the soft tissues in orthopedics. AJR 82:271, 1959.
153. Pope TL, Keats TE, deLange EE, et al. Idiopathic synovial chondromatosis in two unusual sites: inferior radioulnar joint and ischial bursa. Skeletal Radiol 16:205, 1987.
154. Preidler KW, Brossmann J, Daenen B, et al. Measurements of cortical thickness in experimentally created endosteal bone lesions: a comparison of radiography, CT, MR imaging, and anatomic sections. AJR 168 1501, 1997.
155. Quinn SF, Erickson SJ, Dee PM, et al. MR imaging in fibromatosis: results in 26 patients with pathologic correlation. AJR 156:539, 1991.
156. Rak KM, Yakes WF, Ray RL, et al. MR imaging of symptomatic peripheral vascular malformations. AJR 159:107, 1992.
157. Rauch RF, Silverman PM, Korobkin M, et al. Computed tomography of benign angiomatous lesions of the extremities. J Comput Assist Tomogr 8:1143, 1984.
158. Richman LS, Gumerman LW, Levine G, et al. Localization of Tc99m polyphosphate in soft tissue malignancies. AJR 124:577, 1975.
159. Rosenthal L. $^{99m}$Tc-Methylene diphosphonate concentration in soft tissue malignant fibrous histiocytoma. Clin Nucl Med 3: 58, 1978.
160. Rubin DA, Kneeland JB. MR imaging of the musculoskeletal system: technical considerations for enhancing image quality and diagnostic yield. AJR 163:1155, 1994.
161. Russell WO, Cohen J, Cutler S, et al. Staging system for soft tissue sarcoma. American Joint Committee for Cancer Staging and End Results Reporting: Task Force on Soft Tissue Sarcoma. American College of Surgeons, Chicago, 1980.
162. Savage RC, Mustafa EB. Giant cell tumors of tendon sheath (localized nodular tenosynovitis). Ann Plastic Surg 13:205, 1984.
163. Schumacher IM, Genant HK, Korobkin M, et al. Computed tomography: its use in space-occupying lesions of the musculoskeletal system. J Bone Joint Surg Am 60:600, 1978.
164. Sherry CS, Harms SE. MR evaluation of giant cell tumors of tendon sheath. J Magn Reson Imaging 7:195, 1989.
165. Shuman WP, Pattern RM, Baron RI, et al. Comparison of STIR and spin-echo MR imaging at 1.5T in 45 suspected extremity tumors: lesion conspicuity and extent. Radiology 179:247, 1991.
166. Sonin AH, Tutton SM, Fitzgerald SW, et al. MR imaging of the adult elbow. Radiographics 16:1323, 1996.
167. Sostman HD, Prescott DM, Dewhirst MW, et al. MR imaging and spectroscopy for prognostic evaluation in soft-tissue sarcomas. Radiology 190:269, 1994.
168. Soye I, Levine E, DeSmet AA, et al. Computed tomography in the preoperative evaluation of masses arising in or near the joints of the extremities. Radiology 143:727, 1982.
169. Stanley P, Miller JA. Angiography of extxemity masses in children. AJR 130:1119, 1978.
170. Steinbach LS, Johnston JO, Teper EF, et al. Tumoral calcinosis: radiologic-pathologic correlation. Skeletal Radiol 24:573, 1995.
171. Stess RM, Ariza J, Goodling GA. Preoperative imaging for soft tissue tumors of the foot. J Foot Ankle Surg 33:295, 1994.
172. Stout AP, Murray MR. Hemangiopericytoma: vascular tumor featuring Zimmerman's pericytes. Ann Surg 116:26, 1942.
173. Stull MA, Moser RP, Kransdorf MJ, et al. Magnetic resonance appearance of peripheral nerve sheath tumors. Skeletal Radiol 20:9, 1991.
174. Sundaram M, Baran G, Merenda G, et al. Myxoid liposarcoma: magnetic resonance imaging appearances with clinical and histologic correlation. Skeletal Radiol 19:359, 1990.
175. Sundaram M, McGuire MH, Fletcher J, et al. Magnetic resonance imaging of lesions of synovial origin. Skeletal Radiol 15: 110, 1986.
176. Sundaram M, McGuire MH, Herbold DR, et al. High signal intensity soft tissue masses on T1-weighted pulsing sequences. Skeletal Radiol 16:30, 1987.
177. Sundaram M, McGuire MH, Herbold DR. Magnetic resonance imaging of soft tissue masses: an evaluation of fifty-three histologically proven tumors. Magn Res Imaging 6:237, 1988.
178. Sundaram M, McGuire MH, Schajowicz F. Soft tissue masses: histologic basis for decreased signal (short T2) on T2-weighted MR images. AJR 148:1247, 1987.
179. Sundaram M, McLeod RA. MR imaging of tumor and tumor-like lesions of bone and soft tissue. AJR 155:817, 1990.
180. Suzuki Y, Ehara S, Shiraishi H, et al. Embryonal rhabdomyosarcoma of foot with expansive growth between metatarsals. Skeletal Radiol 26:128, 1997.
181. Swan JS, Grist TM, Sproat IA, et al. Musculoskeletal neoplasms: preoperative evaluation with MR angiography. Radiology 194:519, 1995.
182. Swensen SJ, Keller PL, Berquist TH, et al. Magnetic resonance imaging of hemorrhage. AJR 145:921, 1985.
183. Tehranzadeh J, Mnaymneh W, Ghavam C, et al. Comparison of CT and MR imaging in musculoskeletal neoplasms. J Comput Assist Tomogr 13:466, 1989.
184. Templeton AW, Stevens E, Jansen C. Arteriographic evaluation of soft tissue masses. South Med J 59:1255, 1966.
185. Thrall JH, Ghaed N, Geslien GE, et al. Pitfalls in $Tc^{99}m$ polyphosphate skeletal imaging. AJR 121:739, 1974.
186. Totterman S, Weis SL, Szumouski J, et al. MR fat suppression technique in the evaluation of normal structures of the knee. J Comput Assist Tomogr 13:473, 1989.
187. Totty WG, Murphy WA, Lee JKT. Soft-tissue tumors: MR imaging. Radiology 160:135, 1986.
188. Ushijma M, Hashimoto H, Tsuneyoshi M, et al. Giant cell tumor of the tendon sheath. Cancer 57:875, 1986.
189. Valls R, Melloni P, Darnell A, et al. Diagnostic imaging of tibial periosteal ganglion. Eur Radiol 7:70, 1997.
190. Vande Berg BC, Malghem J, Lecouvet FE, et al. Magnetic resonance imaging of the normal bone marrow. Skeletal Radiol 27: 471, 1998.
191. Van der Woude HJ, Verstraete KL, Hogendoorn PCW, et al. Musculoskeletal tumors: does fast dynamic contrast-enhanced subtraction MR imaging contribute to the characterization? Radiology 208:821, 1998.
192. Vanel D, Shapeero LG, De Baere T, et al. MR imaging in the follow-up of malignant and aggressive soft-tissue tumors: results of 511 examinations. Radiology 190:263, 1994.
193. Varma DG, Ayala AG, Guo SQ, et al. MRI of extraskeletal osteosarcoma. J Comput Assist Tomogr 17:414, 1993.
194. Verstraete KL, De Deene Y, Roels H, et al. Benign and malignant musculoskeletal lesions: dynamic contrast-enhanced MR imaging: parametric "first pass" images depict tissue vascularization and perfusion. Radiology 192:835, 1994.
195. Verstraete KL, van der Woude HJ, Hogendoorn PCW, et al. Dynamic contrast-enhanced MRI in the musculoskeletal system. J Magn Reson Imaging 6:311, 1996.

196. Viamonte M Jr, Roen S, LePage J. Nonspecificity of abnormal vascularity in the angiographic diagnosis of malignant neoplasms. Radiology 106:59, 1973.
197. Wang YC, Jeng CM, Wu DY, et al. Giant ossified cavernous hemangioma of an extremity associated with an equinovarus deformity. Skeletal Radiol 27:522, 1998.
198. Weekes RG, Berquist TH, McLeod RA, et al. Magnetic resonance imaging of soft tissue tumors: comparison with computed tomography. Magn Res Imag 3:45, 1985.
199. Weekes RG, McLeod RA, Reiman HM, et al. CT of soft-tissue neoplasms. AJR 144:355, 1985.
200. Weinberger G, Levinsohn EM. Computed tomography in the evaluation of sarcomatous tumors of the thigh. AJR 130:115, 1978.
201. Wetzel LH, Levine E, Meuphy MD. A comparison of MR imaging and CT in the evaluation of musculoskeletal masses. Radiographics 7:851, 1987.
202. Wilbur J, Slatopalsky E. Hyperphosphatemia and tumoral calcinosis. Ann Intern Med 68:1044, 1980.
203. Wilson JS, Korobkin M, Genant HK, et al. Computed tomography of musculoskeletal disorders. AJR 131:55, 1978.
204. Yaghmai I. Angiographic manifestations of soft tissue and osseous hemangiopericytomas. Radiology 126:653, 1978.

# CHAPTER 4

# MOLECULAR GENETICS OF SOFT TISSUE TUMORS

PAUL S. MELTZER

The pathogenesis of cancer is one of the most difficult and complex problems in biology. Many aspects of the process by which a normal cell becomes transformed into a cancer cell remain elusive, although modern cell and molecular biology has had a profound impact on the understanding of carcinogenesis. This chapter focuses on the molecular genetics of soft tissue tumors, an aspect of tumor biology that has become central to the entire discipline. For definitions of terms used in this chapter, see the glossary in Table 4–1.

It has been suspected for decades that tumors arise by a multistep process involving sequential genetic alterations in normal progenitor cells. In this model elaborated by Nowell, each step confers a selective advantage leading to clonal expansion and phenotypic transformation until ultimately a fully malignant tumor develops.[170] It is now possible to assign specific genes to some of the steps involved in tumorigenesis, and technology is available that enables the elucidation of those that remain.[243] Certain difficulties persist, however. For example, there is no unitary pathway that accounts for all forms of cancer; rather, multiple genetic targets are altered in a combinatorial fashion characteristic of each tumor category. The requirement for multiple genetic alterations before a cell becomes malignant explains the tendency for most human cancers to occur in the elderly. Despite impressive technical advances, limitations exist in the ability of tumor biologists to study alterations in rare tumors or those that are difficult to cultivate in the laboratory. Considering the current pace of progress, however, there is justifiable cause for optimism. The explosion of knowledge in cancer genetics has already contributed to and will continue to add to diagnostic refinements, prognostic markers, and novel therapeutic targets.

Many of the specific molecular events associated with human malignancy have been elucidated in the hematopoietic neoplasms. Solid tumors have been less tractable, although in recent years significant progress has been made in the molecular analysis of solid tumors. Despite their rarity relative to the intensively studied common solid tumors (e.g., colorectal carcinoma), important progress has been made in elucidating the molecular alterations present in soft tissue tumors. In part, this has been due to the unanticipated relevance to soft tissue tumors of genes that were first recognized in other cancers or in hereditary cancer predisposition syndromes. In other instances, highly tumor-specific molecular genetic anomalies have been identified in individual soft tissue tumors.

## TARGETS OF GENETIC ALTERATION IN HUMAN CANCERS

The development of recombinant DNA technology has facilitated analysis of the molecular events that occur during tumorigenesis. An understanding of the fundamental principles of molecular biology has become essential for readers of the current literature in oncology. The techniques used to characterize genes and gene expression in tumor cells depend on the principle of basepair complementarity in the DNA double helix. DNA rendered single-stranded (denatured) readily returns to the double-stranded configuration in which guanine is paired with cytosine and thymine is paired with adenine (Fig. 4–1). Even though the human genome consists of more than a billion basepairs, a segment of DNA corresponding to a specific gene, under appropriate laboratory conditions, finds the correct target sequence in single-stranded genomic DNA and forms a double-stranded hybrid. If this segment of DNA is labeled so it can be

**TABLE 4-1 GLOSSARY**

**Codon**—the fundamental unit of the genetic code, which specifies a single amino acid; composed of three "letters" selected from the four-letter "alphabet" that makes up a DNA sequence: G (guanine), A (adenine), T (thymine), and C (cytosine).
**Differential oligonucleotide hybridization**—a technique for identifying mutations in polymerase chain reaction (PCR)-amplified DNA using small synthetic DNA probes (oligonucleotides) of known DNA sequence.
**Denaturing gradient gel electrophoresis**—a technique for screening PCR products for mutations by exploiting the subtle effects of sequence changes on the stability of the double-stranded DNA.
**Loss of heterozygosity (LOH)**—use of genetic markers to determine loss of chromosomal segments in tumor cells, which may be associated with loss of a functional tumor suppressor gene during tumor progression.
**Mismatch error repair**—DNA normally contains two perfectly complementary strands in which G-C and A-T basepairs are matched at all positions. Errors may occur during DNA replication and later may be corrected by a "proofreading" system that scans the newly replicated DNA for mismatches in the normal pattern of basepairing.
**Missense**—a mutation that results in substitution of an incorrect amino acid in a protein.
**Nonsense**—a mutation that results in premature termination of a polypeptide.
**Positional cloning**—isolation of a gene based on genetic information that determines its position on a given chromosome.
**Positive regulatory element**—a DNA sequence in proximity to a given gene that provides recognition sites for the transcription factors that control that gene's expression.
**Single-stranded conformation polymorphism assay**—a technique for screening PCR products for mutations by exploiting the abnormal migration of mutant DNA strands.
**Transcription factor**—a protein that binds to DNA at a specific site and promotes the expression of genes located in that region. Many distinct families of transcription factors have been identified, and aberrations of their function appear to be important events in solid tumors and leukemias. Transcription factors are multifunctional proteins that may be composed of several regions (domains) that interact with DNA or other components of the transcription apparatus. Among the several DNA binding domains that have been identified is the ETS domain named after the prototypic gene in this family. Structural alterations of genes of the *ETS* family have been identified in solid tumors. The bZIP (basic zipper) structural motif characterizes a family of transcription factors that function as dimers (either heterodimers or homodimers) with dimerization depending on the "zipper" sequence.
**Transfection**—the transfer of exogenous DNA into cells in tissue culture. Genes encoded in the transferred DNA may be expressed, altering the phenotype of the recipient cells.
**Transgenic mouse**—animal in which a genetic alteration has been engineered by introducing a foreign gene or inactivating an endogenous gene ("knockout"). This technology has proven to be a powerful tool for studying gene function.
**Transition**—a mutation in which one pyrimidine (T or C) or one purine (A or G) is substituted for the other.
**Transversion**—a mutation in which a purine (A or G) is substituted for a pyrimidine (T or C) or vice versa.

detected in the laboratory, it becomes a probe for the gene in question.

A DNA probe may be synthetic, or it may be a small segment of human DNA that has been propagated as a recombinant DNA clone in a microbial host. A cloned human DNA fragment can be of genomic origin or can be prepared from messenger RNA (mRNA), in which case it is designated a complementary DNA (cDNA). There is currently an international effort to sequence the entire human genome that has resulted in a rough draft" consisting of a nearly complete sequence, with completion anticipated by 2002. The impact of this complete catalog of

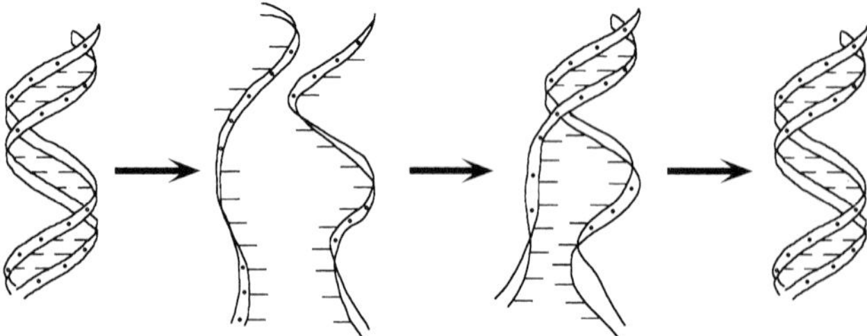

**FIGURE 4-1.** DNA double helix. Denaturating conditions dissociate the two strands, which can then reanneal to each other or to a complementary DNA probe.

human genes on all aspects of medical science is difficult to overstate and will be felt in cancer research as an acceleration of cancer gene discovery. This information will also encourage the development of diagnostic tools applicable to clinical specimens and ultimately lead to a refined characterization of individual tumors that can be used to establish prognosis and guide therapy.

Procedures based on the principle of DNA hybridization are exquisitely sensitive and can easily detect target molecules in the picogram range. Frequently these experiments are conducted using target nucleic acids (e.g., DNA or RNA extracted from tumor specimens) that have been immobilized to a solid support such as a nylon membrane. Detection of DNA digested by a restriction endonuclease (an enzyme that cleaves DNA at a specific sequence) and size fractionated by gel electrophoresis prior to transfer to a solid support is referred to as Southern blot hybridization[223] (Fig. 4-2). The mRNA transcribed from a given gene can be similarly detected following electrophoresis and transfer to a membrane in a Northern blot procedure.

The polymerase chain reaction (PCR) has become an important technique of DNA analysis.[196] PCR uses

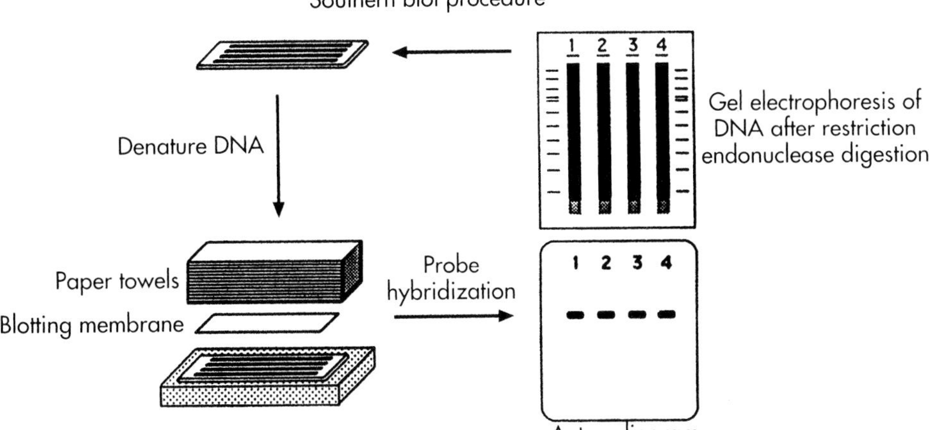


**FIGURE 4–2.** Southern blot procedure can be used to detect gross alterations in gene structure, such as chromosome translocations and gene amplification. DNA fragments generated by restriction endonuclease cleavage are size-fractionated by gel electrophoresis, transferred to a solid support, and detected by DNA hybridization.

specific synthetic oligonucleotides to amplify a section of a given gene in vitro. With automated equipment, it is possible to carry out this procedure in a few hours starting with the DNA from a few cells (Fig. 4–3). This technology enables the analysis of genetic changes in the DNA from tumor biopsies including paraffin-embedded material. PCR products can be analyzed for the presence of mutations by a variety of electrophoretic or hybridization techniques as well as DNA sequence analysis. With an additional step (reverse transcription) PCR can be carried out on RNA (RT-PCR). This is particularly useful for analysis of the abnormal mRNAs that occur in some tumors. The implementation of these and related techniques has led to the identification of many of the genes critical for growth of human cancers.

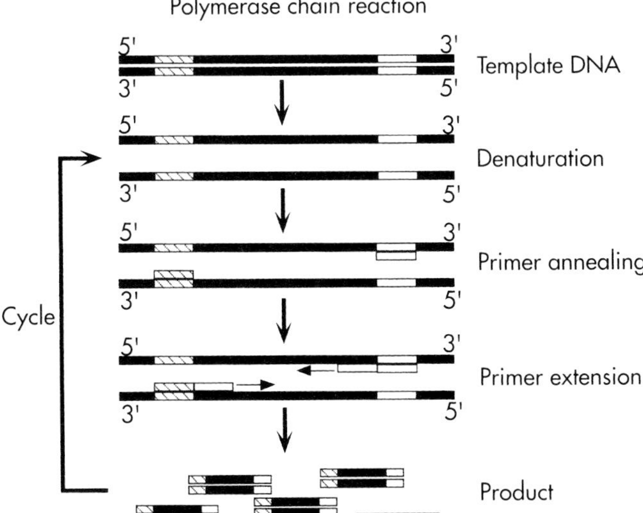


**FIGURE 4–3.** Polymerase chain reaction (PCR) forms the basis of techniques used to analyze genes in minute specimens. PCR can generate microgram quantities of DNA starting from a few template molecules by successive cycles of denaturation, primer annealing, and primer extension. Expressed genes can be studied by first converting mRNA to cDNA and then amplifying the product by PCR.

Genes that contribute to tumorigenesis fall into several broad categories: those with functions that drive cells toward proliferation (oncogenes), those that normally function to restrain cell proliferation (tumor suppressor genes),[115] and those that protect the integrity of the genome. The study of tumorigenic retroviruses in animal systems has led to the identification of numerous oncogenes.[27] Some retroviruses have acquired and subverted the function of host genes that, when normally regulated, function in growth and development but can cause neoplasia when aberrantly expressed or mutated. Other retroviruses inappropriately activate growth-promoting host genes upon integration into the host genome. With a few important exceptions, most of the several dozen oncogenes identified in this fashion are not now known to be targets of genetic alteration in human cancers. Although viral infection does not appear to be a common cause of human soft tissue tumors, Kaposi's sarcoma, which is strongly associated with a specific herpes virus infection (human herpes virus 8, or HHV8), is an important exception.[7,197] Nonetheless the study of animal retroviruses has contributed significantly to the elucidation of the complex regulatory networks that control the process of cell proliferation.

## Mechanisms of Oncogene Activation in Human Cancers

Direct analysis of human tumors has led to the identification of a number of oncogenes of importance in human tumorigenesis. Two approaches have been particularly productive: DNA transfection and positional cloning. DNA transfection exploits the propensity of nontumorigenic immortalized cells (classically NIH 3T3 cells) to take up exogenous tumor DNA and become transformed when they express a transferred oncogene.[178,231] This type of experiment has led to the identification of several human oncogenes, including the *ras* family of guanosine triphosphate (GTP)-binding proteins, which normally function in the transmission of mitogenic signals. Three members of the *ras* gene family, H-*ras*, K-*ras*, and N-*ras*, are now recognized in the human genome.[30] Remarkably, H-*ras* and K-*ras* had also been identified as retroviral oncogenes. DNA sequence analysis of the transforming *ras* genes demonstrated that they had undergone point mutations. These mutations are not random but cluster in codons 12, 13, and 61, where they lead to amino acid substitutions, which confer transforming activity by degregulating *ras* guanosine triphosphatase (GTPase) activity. Analysis of *ras* mutations, which are now known to occur with varying frequency in a large variety of cancers, provided decisive proof of the somatic mutation theory of cancer. These mutations are considered to be among the early steps of transformation in colorectal and pancreatic carcinomas.

Although many human oncogenes fall outside the spectrum of sensitivity of the NIH 3T3 assay, alternative approaches have been productive. It would be a daunting prospect to search the billions of nucleotides in the human genome for oncogenic mutations. Fortunately, in many cases markers have been provided in the form of tumor-specific chromosome translocations. Although most of these translocations have been described in the hematopoietic neoplasms,[143] several have been described in solid tumors (see Chapter 5). The presence of a specific translocation facilitates the positional cloning of the gene(s) at the breakpoint. In this fashion, numerous translocation breakpoints have been analyzed in leukemias and lymphomas.[44,143] Two general categories of events have been described. One type of event leads to overexpression of an oncogene that has been translocated into a chromosomal region associated with the immunoglobulin genes or T cell receptor genes. Because these gene clusters have been studied intensively, it is relatively straightforward to characterize translocations in these regions. Positive regulatory elements derived from the lymphoid-specific genes presumably act on the translocated oncogene, leading to inappropriately high levels of oncogene expression. An example of this category is t(8:14), which occurs in Burkitt's lymphoma, in which the *myc* oncogene is translocated into the immunoglobulin heavy chain locus. The second category of translocation involves the juxtaposition of two genes, one from each translocation partner, resulting in the formation of a fusion gene product, an abnormal protein that is never seen in normal cells and is highly characteristic of the malignant disorder in which it is found. This is the underlying molecular event in the t(9:22) chromosome in chronic myelogenous leukemia that fuses the *bcr* and *abl* genes.[53,83] As discussed below, a number of soft tissue tumor-specific translocations have been characterized at the molecular level, and all result in the formation of fusion proteins.

Gene amplification can be defined as the accumulation of additional copies of a gene out of proportion to the modal chromosome number of the cell.[109] This phenomenon was originally studied in tissue culture cells that had acquired resistance to methotrexate through exposure to an incrementally increasing drug concentration in the medium. Although a number of mechanisms may contribute to this phenomenon, resistance is frequently associated with accumulation of extra copies of the gene encoding dihydrofolate reductase (*DHFR*), the target of methotrexate action. Increased transcription from the increased copies of the *DHFR* gene leads to increased production of the dhfr protein. Cytologically, the increased copies of the *DHFR* gene can be localized either extrachromosomally as small paired chromatin bodies called double minutes (DMIN) or intrachromosomally as homogeneously staining regions (*HSRs*). Although originally described in the methotrexate/*DHFR* system, a similar phenomenon has been described with multiple additional selective agents.

Gene amplification can be viewed as a mechanism by which cells can acquire increased expression of genes that confer a selective advantage. The propensity to undergo gene amplification is clearly enhanced in malignant cells. Although the mechanisms that underlie this phenomenon are incompletely understood, gene amplification is part of the genetic instability of cancer cells that in some experimental systems is related to specific abnormalities such as alterations in the *TP53* gene.[142] In view of these considerations, it is not surprising that gene amplification has been described in tumor specimens. However, in contrast to laboratory systems designed to study drug resistance, the targets of spontaneous amplification in tumor cells are oncogenes rather than drug resistance genes. In this situation oncogene amplification can be viewed as a genetic alteration that contributes a proliferative advantage to a clone of tumor cells, which then comes to predominate in the tumor population. Amplification of a given gene can be readily determined in tumor specimens by Southern blot, PCR, or fluorescence in situ hybridization analysis.

Oncogene amplification has been described in a wide variety of cancers including soft tissue tumors.[4] Cytogenetic studies frequently provide evidence for the occurrence of gene amplification through the identification of HSR and DMINs. When amplified DNA is identified in tumor cells, the problem remains to identify the target gene encoded in the amplified sequences that drives the amplification process. When a well known oncogene is mapped to the amplified region, as in the case of *MYCN* amplification in neuroblastoma, it may be straightforward, but, not all instances are as easily analyzed. Because the DNA contained in the form of DMINs or HSRs may be megabases in size, several genes may be contained in the amplified region. Characterization of these genes and their pattern of amplification and expression in many tumors is necessary to define the actual target gene.

## Tumor Suppressor Genes

If normal cells are induced to fuse with tumor cells, the hybrid cell frequently loses its ability to form tumors in experimental animals.[225] This effect can be demonstrated to depend on the introduction of specific normal chromosomes, suggesting that normal genes may suppress the ability of a cancer cell to form tumors. This is the operational definition of the term tumor suppressor gene. Tumor suppressor genes may be inactivated by somatic mutation via changes at the DNA sequence level or by gross rearrangement. In the latter case, loss of an allele in tumor cells may be defined with polymorphic DNA markers. Such loss of heterozygosity (LOH) studies comprise an important tool for mapping regions of chromosomal loss in tumors. Ideally, this lengthy process concludes with the identification of a gene that undergoes somatic mutation in tumors and suppresses tumorigenicity when reintroduced into tumor cells.

Tumor suppressor genes have been identified by two routes, the genetic analysis of tumors, and genetic mapping studies in families with hereditary predisposition to cancer. Although most familial cancer predisposition syndromes do not increase the risk for sarcomas, there are some important exceptions, such as Li-Fraumeni syndrome and hereditary retinoblastoma. With each newly identified gene comes an opportunity to scrutinize affected kindreds for less common manifestations, which may include soft tissue tumors. Two important tumor suppressor genes, *TP53* and *RB1*, are of particular relevance to soft tissue tumors. *RB1*, the hereditary retinoblastoma gene, is the prototypic tumor suppressor gene. Knudson's observations of the rate of onset of sporadic versus hereditary retinoblastoma led him to the "two hit" hypothesis, which correctly predicted that two mutations were necessary for the initiation of retinoblastoma.[116,117] In hereditary cases, one of these mutations has already occurred in the germline, accounting for early onset and high tumor probability (multifocality and bilaterality). In sporadic cases the coincidence of two mutational events in a single cell is much less frequent, resulting in unilateral disease of later onset. The *RB1* gene was identified by positional cloning relative to markers associated with hereditary retinoblastoma.[68,69,131] It encodes a nuclear phosphoprotein that appears to have a central role in cell cycle regulation.[86,141] It has binding affinity for other cell cycle proteins, and this affinity is modulated by cyclic phosphorylation during the cell cycle by cyclin-dependent kinases. It is not clear why germline mutations in *RB1* have such a strongly tissue-specific oncogenic effect resulting in early-onset retinoblastoma. Most likely it is related to the existence of parallel regulatory pathways in most cell lines. It should be noted that in patients with hereditary retinoblastoma the oncogenic propensity conferred by the *RB1* mutation is not strictly limited to retinoblastoma. In fact, these patients carry a high risk of second malignancies, particularly sarcomas.[2,163,164] Although some occur within prior orbital radiation fields, many originate out of field and must be related to the underlying genetic lesion. It is therefore not surprising, as discussed below, to find that some sporadic sarcomas also acquire defects in the *RB1* gene.

The effects of *RB1* on the cell cycle introduce an important theme in the molecular biology of sarcomas that provides a useful conceptual framework for considering a number of the genes important in the development of these tumors. Several of the genes altered in sarcomas can be related to the cell cycle, and these apparently disparate genes are related functionally (Fig. 4–4). Disturbance of the orderly process of regulating the replication of DNA and cell division is a central theme in the development of sarcomas. Loss of function of genes that can arrest the cell cycle (e.g., *TP53*, *RB1*, *CDKN2A*) or gain of function of genes that promote cell cycle progression (*MDM2*, *CDK4*) are frequent events in sarcomas. In fact, whereas changes in individual genes may be present in only a small proportion of cases of a given histologic type, alterations in at least one of the genes affecting cell cycle progression are present in a larger proportion of cases.

The most intensively studied tumor suppressor gene is *TP53* (commonly referred to as *p53*), originally identified as a tumor antigen in SV40-infected cells.[133,242] Because of its increased expression in tumor cells, it was initially misclassified as an oncogene. Loss of heterozygosity analysis of colorectal cancer suggested the importance of a gene on chromosome 17p in the region where *TP53* had been previously mapped. When the DNA sequence of the remaining *TP53* allele was determined, inactivating mutations were identified.[13] The normal *TP53* gene functions to restrain cell growth, and mutations in this gene promote unregulated cell growth. Activated

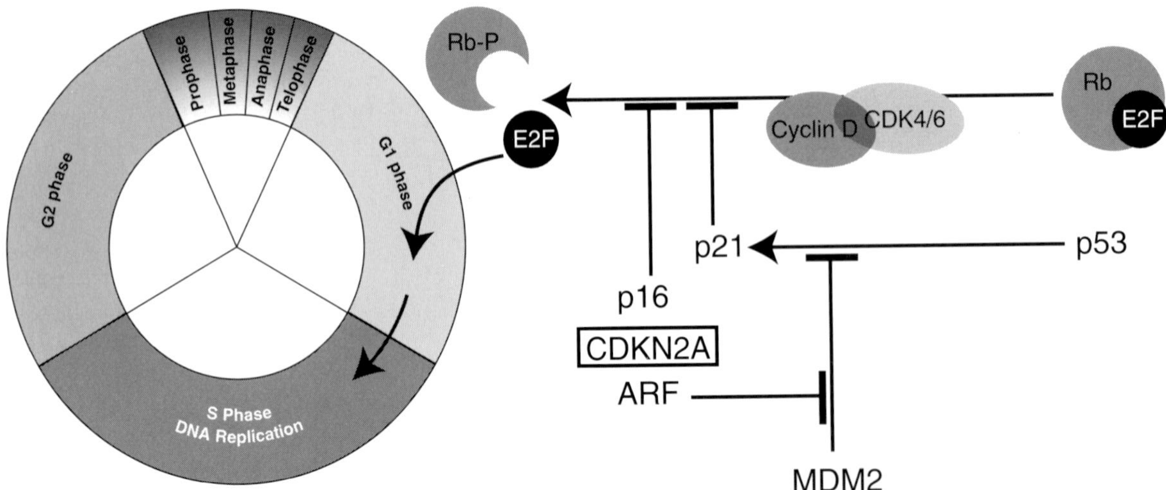


**FIGURE 4–4.** Cell cycle illustrating key regulators of the $G_1$-to-S phase transition of the cell cycle mediated by phosphorylation of Rb and subsequent release of the transcription factor E2F. Genes in this pathway are frequent targets of genetic alteration in cancer, either by loss of function (as is the case for *RB1, TP53,* and *CDKN2A*) or by gain of function (exemplified by *CDK4* and *MDM2*). *CDKN2A* encodes two distinct cell cycle regulators, *p16* and *ARF,* through the use of alternative reading frames.

by DNA damage, *TP53* is a key regulator of the cell cycle through its function as a tetrameric transcription factor regulating the expression of other genes.[156] Thus *TP53* has been termed "guardian of the genome."

Hundreds of *TP53* mutations have been identified in a wide variety of human cancers.[88] The mutations are not distributed at random but cluster at certain highly conserved locations in the *TP53* gene. Mutations of most tumor suppressor genes are null mutations that eliminate the protein product from the cell. In contrast, although total loss of *p53* is occasionally observed, most *p53* mutations are true missense mutations that interfere with the activity of the protein as a transcription factor. Tumors with such mutations accumulate the mutant protein. Although the mechanisms favoring this mutation are not completely understood, it appears that by interacting with residual normal p53 protein, mutant *p53* can act to inactivate *p53* in tumors that retain a normal *TP53* allele.[110] An important gene induced by *TP53* in response to genotoxic stress has been identified as *CDKN1A* (*p21*).[61] *CDKN1A* exerts an inhibitory effect on the cyclin kinase/cyclin pathway and provides a direct biochemical connection between *TP53* and the cell cycle. Although somatic alterations of *p21* do not appear to be important in tumors, mutations in a similar negative regulator of the cyclin-dependent kinase function, *CDKN2A* (*p16*), have been identified in families with a predisposition to melanoma.[91] Although mutations of this gene seem to be infrequent in soft tissue tumors, loss of function through deletions has been observed in aggressive tumors.[174]

Transgenic mouse technology has become an important tool tor studying gene function.[3] It is possible to insert exogenous genes and delete normal genes from the mouse germline. Mice lacking a functional *TP53* gene are viable but highly tumor-prone.[58,80] Heterozygous mice, carrying only one functional *TP53* allele, developed osteosarcomas (32%), lymphomas (32%), angiosarcomas (10%), rhabdomyosarcomas (5%), undifferentiated sarcomas (3%), malignant peripheral nerve sheath tumors (3%), and a variety of less common tumors. Mice carrying homozygous defective *TP53* genes developed tumors more rapidly than heterozygotes, with a preponderance of lymphomas (59%), angiosarcomas (18%), testicular tumors (7%), and undifferentiated sarcomas (5%). The mouse model can be compared to the phenotype observed kindreds with the Li-Fraumeni cancer syndrome who carry germline mutations in the *TP53* gene.[148–150] Li-Fraumeni syndrome patients are predisposed to a characteristic constellation of tumors.[228] Bone and soft tissue sarcomas, brain tumors, breast cancer, adrenal cortical carcinoma, and leukemia account for most of the tumors. As with all hereditary cancer syndromes, onset is early, with the cancer risk nearly 50% by age 35. Fortunately, new germline mutations in *TP53* appear to be rare and therefore account for only a few of the sporadic tumors that fall within the Li-Fraumeni spectrum. The presence of a heritable *TP53* mutation should be suspected in patients with a family history consistent with Li-Fraumeni syndrome, in individuals who develop two independent primary tumors of certain histologic types, and in children who develop rhabdomyosarcoma at an age of less than 3 years.[57,134,149] Not all Li-Fraumeni syndrome families carry *TP53* mutations. Recently, mutations in another cell cycle gene, *hCHK2*, were found in patients with Li-Fraumeni syndrome.[21]

### Genes that Protect the Integrity of the Genome

Genes that protect the integrity of the genome are the most recently recognized category of genetic alteration in human cancers. Initial observations using PCR to amplify polymorphic dinucleotide repeat sequences in tumor specimens (a procedure used to identify LOH) unexpectedly revealed sequences of altered repeat length in the tumor DNA that were not present in the patient's normal DNA.[1,95,233] They must have arisen as a result of somatic mutation during DNA replication. This phenotype of somatic dinucleotide repeat instability has been associated with the hereditary nonpolyposis colon cancer syndrome (HNPCC). The genes *hMSH2* and *hMLH1* are mutated in HNPCC kindreds linked to chromosomes 2 and 3, respectively.[127,177] These genes are part of the DNA mismatch error repair system, and cells from HNPCC patients are highly defective in DNA repair.[180] It is likely that this defect contributes to the evolution of cancer in these families through an increased rate of somatic mutation at other sites. Of importance, the DNA replication error phenotype is not confined to HNPCC families or to the tumors associated with this syndrome (colorectal, endometrial, and ovarian carcinomas) but also occurs in sporadic colorectal tumors and non-HNPCC tumors including sarcomas, where it presumably indicates loss of function in one or more components of the mismatch repair pathway. Data on the frequency of this phenomenon in sarcomas is inconclusive, and mutations in mismatch repair genes have not been reported in sarcomas.[20,155,200,230,240]

Additional genes related at least in part to the cellular response to DNA damage include *TP53* (Li-Fraumeni syndrome), *ATM* (ataxia telangiectasia), and *BRCA1* and *BRCA2* (hereditary breast and ovarian cancers). In each case, germline mutations confer a predisposition to cancer, but sarcomas are a clear part of only the Li-Fraumeni syndrome. Recently attention has turned to genes involved in the orderly distribution of chromosomes to daughter cells during mitosis. Somatic mutations have been identified in one such gene, *BUB1*, in colorectal carcinoma.[35] It is likely that important mutational targets of genetic instability in sarcomas remain to be identified.

## SPECIFIC GENETIC ALTERATIONS IN SOFT TISSUE TUMORS

### Analysis of Tumor Specimens

As the genetic targets of tumorigenesis are uncovered, their role in the full spectrum of human tumors is gradually being defined. A significant difficulty with clinical studies of germ mutations in cancer is that mutations in patients are typically scattered throughout the gene in question. This poses a significantly more complex analytic problem than, for example, typing a series of known allelic variants as is done routinely for the HLA locus. Because DNA is stable in banked frozen tissues, it is feasible to perform retrospective analyses. A few milligrams of tumor tissue provides enough DNA for several Southern blots. The PCR-based methods[196] require only a few cells for analysis and can be applied to paraffin-embedded material. Although PCR is capable of amplifying a given gene from minute specimens, PCR products typically span only small segments of DNA, requiring the use of multiple reactions to fully characterize a given gene. Techniques for screening PCR products for mutation include differential oligonucleotide hybridization and gel electrophoresis techniques such as the single-stranded conformation polymorphism assay (SSCP) or denaturing gradient gel electrophoresis (DGGE).[81,90,147] Chromatographic techniques are promising alternatives to gel-based methods.[140] These methods are screening techniques, and their validation and precise characterization of mutations depends on DNA sequence analysis. All current techniques favor the analysis of small genes or those where mutations tend to cluster (e.g., *TP53*). Large genes (e.g., *RB1*) pose more difficulties for screening. In general, unless the entire gene in question is sequenced, the data obtained by screening tests tend to underestimate the true frequency of mutation.[82] The development of automated fluorescent DNA sequencing instruments has considerably facilitated the documentation of specific mutations. The use of dense arrays of synthetic oligonucleotides attached to a solid matrix (DNA microarrays) holds some promise for mutation detection in large genes, but technical and cost concerns have limited the development of this technology for diagnostic purposes.[78] Because of the importance of mutation testing for genetic diseases, it is anticipated that technologies for mutation screening will be optimized for clinical application.

In contrast to mutational analysis, assays for tumor-specific chromosome translocations are more straightforward and can be readily accomplished by RT-PCR.[221] In principle, a PCR product can be obtained only if the fusion gene is present in the specimen.

However, even this analysis is complicated by the occurrence of variant translocations, which requires confirmation of the PCR product by hybridization with an internal sequence or by DNA sequencing.

### Tumor Suppressor Genes in Soft Tissue Tumors

Although all of the currently recognized tumor suppressor genes were originally discovered in other cancers, several of these genes have considerable relevance to soft tissue tumors. Observations of *TP53* mutations in the Li-Fraumeni syndrome, the occurrence of sarcomas in survivors of hereditary retinoblastoma, and the rare association of sarcomas with some familial cancer syndromes have motivated the study of these genes in soft tissue tumors.

Because most inactivating mutations of *TP53* are concentrated in a relatively small region, the application of PCR-based techniques to *TP53* is particularly straightforward.[29] Additionally, immunohistochemical studies have frequently been used as surrogates for DNA analysis of *TP53*.[23] Immunohistochemistry, which is less definitive than DNA sequencing, exploits the tendency of mutant forms of *TP53* to accumulate to much higher levels than are observed for the wild-type protein. A number of series of various size have been reported but are difficult to compare because of variations in technique (immunostaining versus mutation screen; complete versus partial gene analysis), limiting the precision with which the incidence of *TP53* mutation can be estimated in each diagnostic category. Nonetheless, there are sufficient data to establish a role for *TP53* mutation in the evolution of certain soft tissue tumors. Overall, it can be concluded that *TP53* mutations are found in most categories of soft tissue tumor with an incidence usually less than 20%.[8,36,64,139,187,198,199,220,235,257,260] In contrast, *TP53* mutations do not appear to be important in neuroblastoma.[46,89,92,118,151,241] There is a significant incidence of *TP53* mutation in osteosarcoma[8,37,186,201–203,217,235,245], and Ewing's sarcoma.[79,118,119,245] In some instances, the precise pattern of *TP53* alteration may be relevant to mechanisms of damage by carcinogens. For example, in a study of angiosarcomas of the liver in vinyl chloride-exposed patients, two of four patients carried A to T missense transversions in *TP53*.[87] Molecular epidemiologic studies of this type may open new possibilities for cancer prevention.[219]

The retinoblastoma gene is significantly larger than *TP53* and is proportionately more difficult to study; only limited data at the DNA level are available. Some investigators have examined tumors for loss of the RBI protein by immunohistochemistry as a surrogate marker for gene inactivation. In sarcomas, total of partial gene deletions appear to be important mechanisms of *RB1* inactivation. This type of event is clearly important in osteosarcoma,[160,190,244] but less information is available for soft tissue sarcomas. In a study of the *RB1* gene at the gross structural level in DNA and RNA from a series of soft tissue sarcomas, *RB1* deletions were found in two of five malignant fibrous histiocytomas, two of four liposarcomas, the one extraosseous osteosarcoma and the one mesenchymoma; they were absent from the few studied, leiomyosarcomas, hemangiopericytomas, and extraosseous chondrosarcomas[254] Additional examples of deletion and rearrangement of *RB1* have been reported in single cases of spindle cell sarcoma, leiomyosarcoma, and fibrosarcoma.[227] Rearrangement was accompanied by loss of the normal allele. In contrast, genetic alterations and reduced expression *RB1* were not found in 18 rhabdomyosarcoma specimens.[51] Studies of *RB1* protein expression by immunhistochemistry have identified frequent loss of expression in soft tissue sarcomas.[40,102] Given the spectrum of second malignancies observed in survivors of bilateral retinoblastoma, it is likely that as improved technologies for scanning large genes become available a significant role for *RB1* alterations will become apparent in some soft tissue tumors.

Neurofibromatosis type 1 (von Recklinghausen's disease) is due to defects in the *NF1* gene on chromosome 17.[153] At the biochemical level, *NF1* functions as a GTPase-associated protein (GAP) with a negative regulatory influence on *ras*.[77] It therefore can be considered a candidate tumor suppressor gene. Indeed, loss of the normal *NF1* allele is observed in neurofibromas occurring in *NF1* patients.[208] Similarly, malignant tumors arising in *NF1* patients have shown loss of chromosome 17 alleles consistent with the second hit predicted by Knudson's hypothesis.[75,132,136,144,259] In addition, a few sporadic somatic mutations of *NF1* have been identified in various cancers including neuroblastoma (two cell lines), individual anaplastic astrocytomas, myelodysplastic syndrome, and colorectal carcinoma.[98,136,232] Another study failed to find *NF1* mutations by PCR-SSCP analysis of 50 neuroblastoma specimens.[92] *NF-1* mutations do not seem to be frequent in sporadic tumors. Interestingly, although the cyclin-dependent kinase inhibitor *CDKN2A* does not appear to be a frequent mutational target in soft tissue sarcomas, mutations are observed in osteosarcomas and in the progression of neurofibromas to neurofibrosarcoma.[94,146,159,161,166,167,179] The related syndrome neurofibromatosis type II is caused by mutations in the *NF-2* gene. Alterations in this gene conforming to the two-hit hypothesis are found in tumors developing in *NF-2* patients and in sporadic tumors, notably mesothelioma.[25,26,206,236]

Both familial adenomatous polyposis and Gardner syndrome (GS) are associated with mutations in the

*APC* (adenomatosis polyposis coli) gene on chromosome 5q.[63,165] The *APC* gene acts though its interaction with $\beta$-catenin.[229] *APC* mutations appear to be one of the earliest events in the progression of adenomas to sporadic colorectal carcinoma. Desmoid tumors are the principal soft tumor associated with GS. For sporadic desmoid tumors, *APC* mutations have been detected in a subset of patients.[5,73] It is of interest that mutations in the *APC* target $\beta$-catenin appear to be more frequent and occur in other soft tissue tumors as well.[96,162]

Survivors of a malignant rhabdoid tumor may develop a second rhabdoid tumor, suggesting that these individuals carry a predisposing mutation. This suspicion has been confirmed with the discovery that malignant rhabdoid tumors carry mutations in the *hSNF5/INI1* gene.[193,210,239] This gene encodes a transcription factor that is part of a complex of proteins with ATP-dependent helicase activity. It is of interest that mutations in this gene have also been identified in sporadic medulloblastomas, choroid plexus carcinomas, and rhabdomyosarcoma.[52,209]

No significant data are available that implicate any of the other known tumor suppressor genes in soft tissue tumors, and it is likely that many of the relevant genetic targets have yet to be identified. A number of approaches are being used to search for novel tumor suppressor genes in various cancers.[43,195,250] Polymorphic DNA markers can be used to compare normal and tumor tissues from the same individual, thereby detecting loss of chromosomal segments in a given tumor. A molecular cytogenetic technique, comparative genome hybridization, can be used to screen the entire genome of a tumor cell for chromosomal gains and losses.[100] Comparisons between tumor and normal DNA using representational difference analysis (RDA) have been productive.[135] Gene expression-based techniques such as differential display and cDNA microarray analysis have been applied to look for genes with reduced expression in tumor tissue relative to their normal progenitor.[56,137] Using these and other approaches, several chromosome regions that may be relevant to soft tissue tumors are currently being characterized. Of course, the role of the astute clinician in identifying familial cancer clusters remains important. Although identification of genes inactivated in tumors remains a complex and challenging process, careful comparison of normal and tumor tissues can be expected to define additional specific targets of genetic loss in sarcomas.

## Activation of *ras*

Mutations of *ras* are known to occur in soft tissue sarcomas, but studies to date are limited. In one study, H-*ras* mutations were found in codon 12 in two of six malignant fibrous histiocytomas and one of three embryonal rhabdomyosarcomas; they were absent from one case each of alveolar rhabdomyosarocma, pleomorphic rhabdomyosarcoma, and leiomyosarcoma.[251] In contrast, a series of 35 malignant fibrous histiocytomas failed to show any H-*ras* mutations.[191] There may well be epidemiologic differences that account for the variation in the frequency of *ras* mutations. It has been noted that H-*ras* mutations were common in Korean patients relative to a group of U.S. patients analyzed in the same laboratory.[261,262] K-*ras* mutations were identified in codon 13 of five of six angiosarcomas from vinyl chloride-exposed workers.[154] Thorotrast-induced and spontaneous angiosarcomas have been shown to carry a high frequency of K-*ras* mutations.[184] These studies of *ras* and *TP53* illustrate the potential of molecular epidemiology to provide insights into the mechanism of carcinogenesis in response to particular mutagenic agents.[87]

## Tumor-specific Translocations

Several soft tissue tumor-specific translocations have now been characterized in detail. To date, all translocations cloned from soft tissue tumors lead to the creation of unique tumor-specific fusion proteins. The biochemical mechanisms by which these proteins contribute to tumor growth remain to be fully elucidated. However, their consistent presence in tumors of a given histologic type and the nature of the genes involved provide a strong basis for concluding that these fusion proteins must be central to the pathogenesis of the tumors in which they occur. Identification of their molecular basis provides insights into the fundamental processes regulating the growth and differentiation of connective tissue cells and provides a framework for the categorization of tumors based on their molecular pathology. Many of the translocation-encoded fusion genes are transcription factors. This observation suggests that disturbance of the orderly program of gene expression associated with cell growth and differentiation is a central mechanism in the development of soft tissue tumors. Ewing's sarcoma was the first tumor in which the rearranged gene was identified, and the ramifications of this discovery are significant.

## Ewing's Sarcoma

A characteristic recurrent t(11;22) occurs in Ewing's sarcoma (both osseous and extraosseous) and peripheral neuroepithelioma. This is now the best-studied example of a solid tumor chromosome translocation. This rearrangement leads to juxtaposition of a gene, designated *EWSR1* (also called *EWS*), on chromosome 22 with the *FLI1* gene on chromosome 11 (Fig. 4–5).[55]

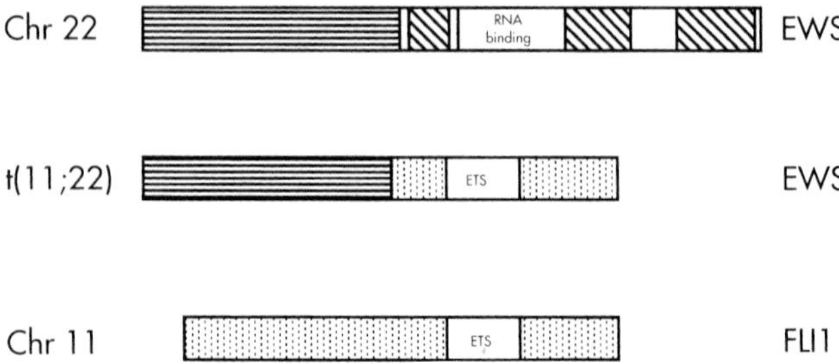


**FIGURE 4–5.** In the Ewing's sarcoma fusion protein, the *ETS* DNA binding protein provides sequences that replace the *EWSRI* RNA binding domain.

The normal function of *EWSR1* is unknown, although it contains an RNA-binding domain in its C-terminal portion and a region with transcriptional activating properties in its N-terminal half. *FLI1* is a member of the ETS family of transcription factors and is known to contain a DNA-binding domain.[189,264] The EWSR1-FLI1 fusion protein replaces the RNA binding domain with sequences from FLI1. In the initial cases studied, the entire DNA binding domain and C-terminus of FLI1 were contributed to the fusion protein. This suggests that an abnormal protein is formed that retains the effector portion of EWSR1, with its usual RNA binding function replaced by the DNA binding activity of FLI1. Biochemical studies have demonstrated that the fusion protein is a potent transcriptional activator.[157] In a series of 89 Ewing's sarcomas and peripheral neuroepitheliomas, the breakpoints in the *EWSR1* and *FLI1* genes were identified in 80 and 66 cases, respectively. *EWSR1* always contributed at least its first 7 exons, including the transcriptional activating domain, to the fusion protein, with the breaks tending to fall in a hinge region that joins this region to the RNA binding domain.[267] The contribution of *FLI1* was considerably more variable. In 13 cases *EWSR1* was joined not to *FLI1* but to a closely related gene, *ERG,* normally found on chromosome 21. Although occasional aberrations of chromosome 21 had been previously described, a balanced t(21;22) has not been described. The EWSR1-ERG fusion proteins have a structure and range of breakpoints within ERG similar to those of the EWSR1-FLI fusion proteins. Although *FLI1* and *ERG* account for most of the EWSR1 fusions in Ewing's sarcoma, additional rare variants have been described that fuse EWSR1 to the ETS proteins ETV1, EIAF, and FEV.[97,181,238] In all cases, a fusion gene of similar structure is formed. Evidence is beginning to accumulate that variations in the structure of the fusion gene may have clinical correlations. Although cases with *FLI1* and *ERG* fusions behave similarity,[74] the precise breakpoint *FLI1* appears to affect the activity of the resultant transcription factor. The most common form (type 1), which includes exons 6–9 of *FLI1,* exhibits reduced activity relative to the type 2 variant, which includes exons 5–9.[138] Additionally, evidence has been presented that the type I translocation has a favorable impact on prognosis.[49,50]

The ability to verify the presence of *EWSR1* rearrangements by molecular techniques means that it is possible to place unambiguously a small round blue cell tumor in the group of disorders characterized by *EWSR1-ETS* gene rearrangements.[226] However, the variability of the breakpoints places significant demands on the laboratory performing the analysis. Determining the presence of a fusion gene by RT-PCR is rapid, but the existence of multiple partners for *EWSR1* means that multiple primer pairs must be used to be sure of finding the fusion transcript.[125,221] Additionally, because the size of the RT-PCR product depends on the precise breakpoint, confirmatory hybridization with an oligonucleotide probe is essential for diagnostic certainty. Also, samples must be obtained with a technique that ensures the recovery of adequate numbers of viable tumor cells and then processed in the operating room with appropriate techniques to allow preservation of RNA. These conditions are most easily met by open biopsy rather than fine-needle aspiration, which may provide insufficient quantities of RNA for RT-PCR.

## Myxoid Liposarcoma

Myxoid liposarcoma is characterized by the presence of t(12;16). Through a candidate gene approach, a transcription factor designated DDIT3 (also called CHOP and GADD153) was mapped to the breakpoint.[6] DDIT3 is a member of the C/EBP family of transcription factors, which is not expressed in proliferating cells but is induced by growth arrest or DNA damage and probably exerts an antiproliferative effect.[192] It contains a dimerization domain through which it can interact with other proteins, its principal partner being the C/EBP$\beta$ transcription factor. Probes for *DDIT3* recognize altered restriction fragments on Southern blots of myxoid liposarcoma DNA (Fig. 4–6). The rearranged *DDIT3* gene is joined to the gene encoding a previously unknown protein FUS (also

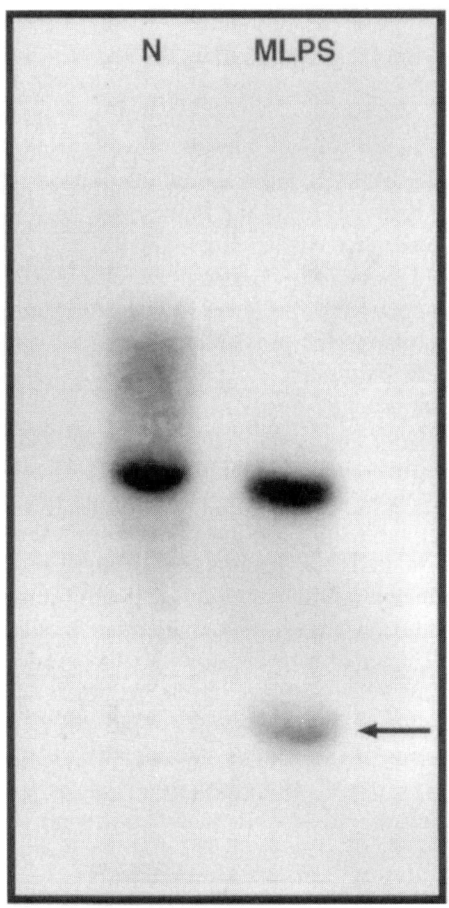


**FIGURE 4–6.** Southern blot illustrating rearrangement of the *DDIT3* gene in myxoid liposarcoma. Tumor DNA (right lane) contains an extra band derived from the t(12;16), which is not present in normal DNA (left lane).

called TLS) (Fig. 4–7)[45,185] Structural analysis of this protein reveals 55.6% identity with the *EWSR1* gene, target of the Ewing's sarcoma translocation (discussed below). The normal function of FUS is unknown. It is a nuclear protein, and its C-terminal portion, like that of EWSR1, contains an RNA binding domain. In myxoid liposarcoma, a fusion transcript is expressed from t(12;16) in which the RNA binding domain of TLS/FUS is replaced by *DDIT3* sequences including the bZIP dimerization domain. Remarkably, myxoid liposarcomas have been described that carry fusions of EWSR1 with DDIT3, further emphasizing the close functional similarity of EWSR1, and FUS.[175]

## Additional *EWSR1* Fusions

*EWSR1* fusions, always with a transcription factor, have been described in several other rare sarcomas. Clear cell sarcoma (also referred to as malignant melanoma of the soft parts) contains a t(12;22) translocation involving the *EWSR1* gene.[266] As in Ewing's sarcoma, in clear cell sarcoma the RNA binding domain of the *EWSR1* gene is replaced by sequences from a transcription factor *ATF1*. Another fusion gene has been described in desmoplastic small round cell tumor linking *EWSR1* to the Wilms' tumor suppressor gene *WT1*.[22,124] *WT1* is itself a transcription factor, but fusion of this tumor suppressor gene with *EWSR1* converts it to an oncogene. Of interest *EWSR1-WT1* appears to induce expression of the platelet-derived growth factor $\alpha$ chain, which may account for the desmoplastic character of this tumor.[129] In myxoid chondrosarcoma, *EWSR1* is fused with an orphan nuclear receptor, *TEC*.[34,121,122] An interesting variant has been observed in this disease in which a more distant relative of *EWSR1*, *TAF2N* (also called *RBP56*), is utilized with the same partner gene.[176,215] The mechanism by which the FUS/EWSR1 fusion proteins promote the proliferation of sarcoma cells has not been determined in detail but is certainly a consequence of disturbances in gene expression caused by the presence of the abnormal transcription factor. The recurring theme of *EWSR1* and *FUS* translocations in various sarcomas suggests that mechanisms linked to the function of these genes are of critical importance in the growth of soft tissue tumors.

## Alveolar Rhabdomyosarcoma

Most alveolar rhabdomyosarcoma cells exhibit t(2;13). The genetic consequences of this rearrangement have been determined[15,70,211] (Fig. 4–8). As in the case of myxoid liposarcoma, a candidate gene approach was successful in defining the translocation breakpoint, which involves the paired box developmental transcription factor *PAX3*. Interestingly, mutations in *PAX3* give rise to Waardenburg syndrome (characterized by partial albinism and deafness). Studies of the mouse orthologus of *PAX3* demonstrated that it is a key developmental regulator of limb myogenesis.[152] A subset of tumors carry a variant t(1;13), which involves the close *PAX3* relative *PAX7*.[48] Sequence analysis of the fusion partner utilized in both translocations identifies it as a member of the fork head (so

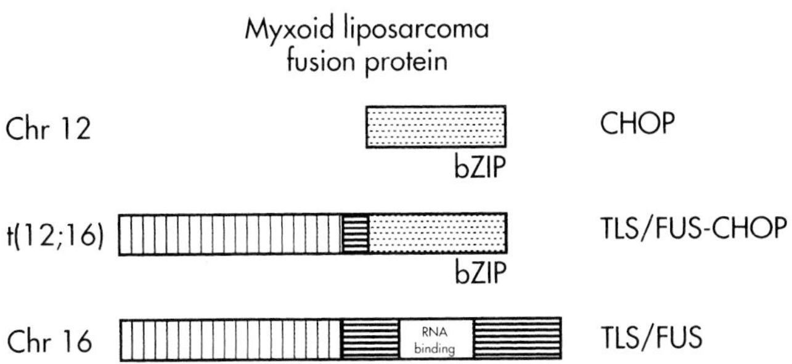


**FIGURE 4–7.** In the myxoid liposarcoma fusion protein, the *DDIT3* transcription factor provides sequences that replace the RNA binding domain in TLS/FUS protein.

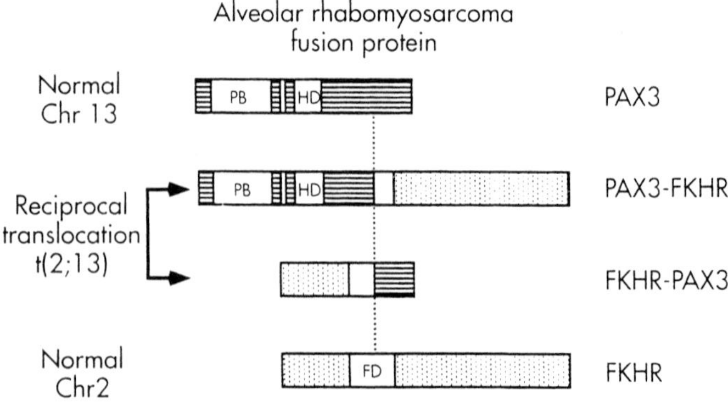


**FIGURE 4–8.** In alveolar rhabdomyosarcoma, fusion protein sequences from *PAX3* are joined to sequences from *FKHR*, generating a chimeric transcription factor. Two chimeric proteins are potentially formed by the reciprocal translocation; but based on the pattern of expression, the PAX3-FKHR protein is the oncogenic product. PB, HD, and FD indicate paired box, homeodomain, and forkhead domains, respectively.

named because of the phenotype caused by mutations in the *Drosophila* homologue) domain family of transcription factors designated *FOXO1A* (also called *FKHR*). The predicted fusion transcripts are detectable in and highly specific for alveolar rhabdomyosarcoma[60,70] (Fig. 4–9). Interestingly, amplification of the *PAX7-FKHR* variant fusion gene has been reported as a mechanism underlying its overexpression.[16,47,248] As in the translocations discussed above, the mechanism underlying the oncogenic impact of the *PAX3-FOXO1A* fusion product is related to the dysregulation of gene expression in the tumor progenitor cell. The myogenic character of the *PAX3-FOXO1A* gene is readily detected on cDNA microarrays when this gene is introduced into NIH 3T3 cells.[111]

## Synovial Sarcoma

Synovial sarcoma is characterized by t(X;18), which leads to the formation of a fusion gene between the *SSXT*(also called *SYT*) on chromosome 18 and one of two adjacent genes on the X chromosome, *SSX1* or *SSX2*.[39,42,54] A rare variant involving *SSX4* also has been reported.[216] This fusion gene produces a nuclear protein with a probable effect on gene expression, but in this instance the fusion protein appears to lack a DNA-binding domain.[31] Using RT-PCR, it is possible to detect the *SYT-SXX* fusion transcript and to distinguish the variants.[10,65,169,237,252] Of interest, there appears to be a correlation between histologic type and translocation type, with biphasic and monophasic histologies being more characteristic of the *SSXT-SSX1* and *SSXT-SSX2* fusions, respectively.[9,103] Comparison of tumors containing these variant translocations also suggests that the *SSXT-SSX1* fusion is associated with high proliferative activity and an adverse prognosis.[93,168]

## Congenital Fibrosarcoma

In congenital fibrosarcoma of infancy, a recurrent t(12;15)(p13;q25) has been shown to result in a fusion gene between *ETV6* and *NTRK3*.[114] The dimerization domain of *ETV6* (also known as *TEL*) is fused with the tyrosine kinase domain of *NTRK3*, a neurotrophin receptor. This change probably disturbs signaling through this *NTRK3*. Remarkably, the same gene fusion is found in congenital mesoblastic nephroma, a histologically similar neoplasm and suggests a unified pathogenetic mechanism underlying these neoplasms.[113]

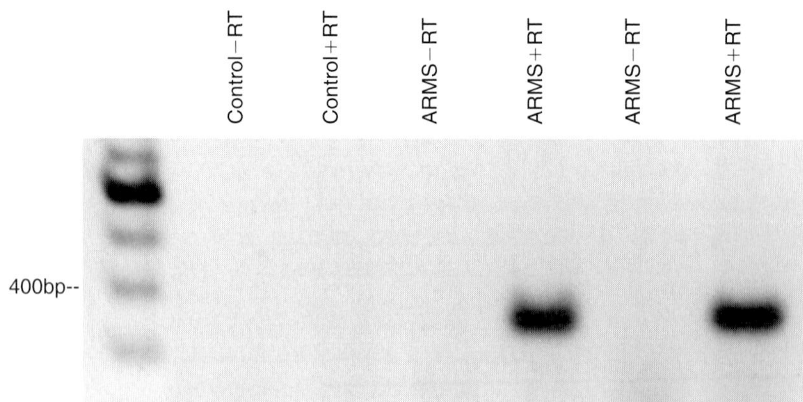


**FIGURE 4–9.** Detection of the *PAX3-FKHR* fusion gene by reverse transcriptase-polymerase chain reaction (RT-PCR). A specific product is found only in alveolar rhabdomyosarcoma (ARMS) samples that contain this rearrangement and not in negative controls. The product is formed only after reverse transcriptase (RT) treatment, indicating that it is derived from mRNA and not from a DNA contaminant.

### Dermatofibrosarcoma Protuberans

Dermatofibrosarcoma protuberans frequently exhibits rearrangements of chromosome 17 and 22, as translocations or as supernumerary ring chromosomes. These cytogenetic aberrations result in generation of a fusion gene between the platelet-derived growth factor B chain (*PDGFRB*) and collagen type I alpha 1 (*COL1A1*).[214] A number of variants have been described.[171] The oncogenic mechanism is presumably related to abnormal growth factor activity, as the fusion removes elements that normally negatively regulate *PDGFRB*. The fusion gene can be detected by RT-PCR.[246]

### Benign Tumors

Remarkably, tumor-specific gene fusions also occur in benign tumors, notably lipoma and leiomyoma. These rearrangements involve the *HMGIC* gene on 12q15.[12,105] Diverse partner chromosomes have been observed linked to 12q14–q15 in various tumors. In addition to lipoma and leiomyoma, rearrangements of *HMGIC* have been observed in pulmonary chondroid hamartoma, pleomorphic adenomas of the salivary gland, endometrial polyps, and a variety of benign tumors of mesenchymal origin.[28,71,72,84,85,107,108,224,234,247] *HMGIC* is the human orthologue of the murine pygmy gene and is a member of the HMGI family of small nuclear proteins including *HMGIC* and *HMGIY*, which are characterized by the presence of a DNA binding domain called the AT hook, which binds to the minor groove of AT-rich DNA and induces DNA bending.[265] The HMGIC protein consists of only 109 amino acids encoded by 5 exons, with the three AT hook domains being encoded by the first three exons.[11,38] The third intron is large (140 kb) and is the site of the translocations that fuse sequences from almost every chromosome to the AT hook domains of *HMGIC*. The precise biochemical effects of the fusion proteins have not been established, and the multiple partner genes have not yet been fully characterized. In one instance [a lipoma with t(3:12)], the partner gene contains two tandem LIM motifs, sequences known to function as protein interaction domains.[12,182] Variant translocations in benign tumors may involve a second gene in the *HMGI* family, *HMGIY*, located on chromosome 6p21 rather than *HMGIC*.[104,106,222,253,258]

Tumors carrying rearrangements of the *HMGI* genes are remarkable for their benign behavior. Despite the presence of this genetic abnormality, benign lipomas and leiomyomas do not appear to evolve into malignant tumors. It is remarkable that cells that have acquired *HMGIC* translocations appear to have increased proliferative capacity without the tendency to accumulate the further genetic alterations that would lead to malignant progression.

### Sarcomas that Lack Specific Fusion Genes

Despite the growing catalog of fusion genes associated with soft tissue tumors, it should be noted that not all sarcomas carry these characteristic abnormalities. Notable exceptions include leiomyosarcoma, embryonal rhabdomyosarcoma, malignant fibrous histiocytoma, osteosarcoma, and well differentiated liposarcoma. Although additional specific fusion proteins will undoubtedly be described, it appears that the foregoing sarcomas, like most carcinomas, arise as the consequence of loss of tumor suppressor gene function, oncogene activation, and disruption of the mechanisms protecting genomic integrity rather than as a consequence of fusion gene formation.

### Gene Amplification in Soft Tissue Tumors

Gene amplification is an important mechanism of oncogene activation in soft tissue tumors. The most intensively studied amplification is that of the *MYCN* oncogene in neuroblastoma. It might be expected that oncogene amplification would be associated with more aggressive clinical behavior. Initially recognized by virtue of its similarity to the c-*myc* oncogene, *MYCN* belongs to the helix-loop-helix family of transcription factors.[204] Amplified *MYCN* sequences in tumors are usually carried extrachromosomally as DMINs, which can integrate and form HSRs on culture.[205] A particularly striking feature of *MYCN* amplification is the high level of amplification, often several hundredfold, in some neuroblastomas. Remarkably, the level of amplification tends to be consistent in a given patient, not changing on serial biopsies.[33] *MYCN* amplification is associated with high levels of MYCN protein expression, presumably leading to deregulated gene expression and a proliferative advantage to the tumor.[206] *MYCN* amplification is found in about half of patients with advanced-stage poor-prognosis disease.[206] It is a prognostic variable that is sufficiently strong that its status should be determined in every neuroblastoma.[32] *MYCN* is also amplified in some rhabdomyosarcomas,[59] and the related gene *MYC* is also an amplification target in sarcomas.[17–19]

In contrast to neuroblastoma, in which a single target gene was readily identified in the *MYCN* amplification unit, a more complex problem has been posed by the identification of amplified sequences from chromosome 12q in soft tissue tumors where the amplification encompasses a highly gene-dense chromosomal segment (Fig. 4–10). A wide variety of tumors have been affected at varying frequency, including malignant fibrous histiocytoma, liposarcoma, rhabdomyosarcoma, osteosarcoma, and Ewing's sarcoma.[66,67,101,123,126,158,183,188,218,249,255] The region amplified

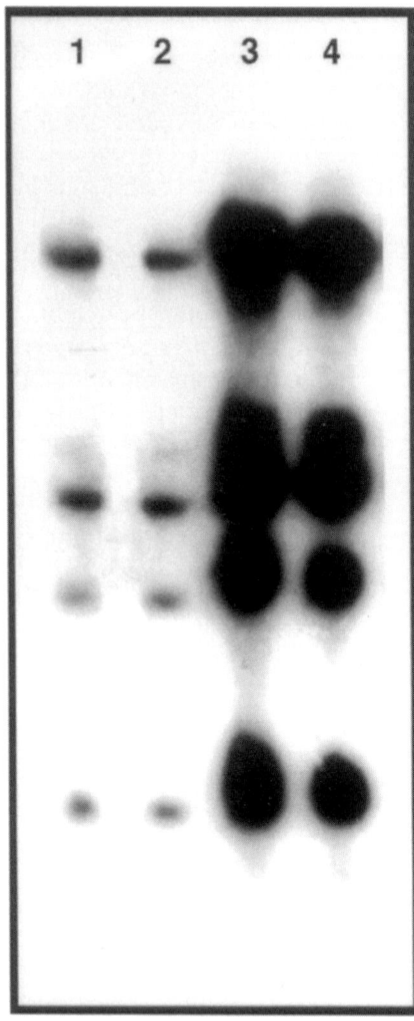


**FIGURE 4–10.** Southern blot analysis illustrating amplification of *MDM2* sequences in malignant fibrous histiocytoma. Note the increased intensity of hybridization in lanes 2 and 4 compared to lanes 1 (normal DNA) and 2 (malignant fibrous histiocytoma without amplification).

varies in size from tumor to tumor but may be quite large, encompassing several genes, each of which potentially has an effect on tumor growth. Mapping studies have shown that 12q amplification involves two distinct regions, each containing an important cell cycle-related gene. In a given tumor, these segments of 12q may be amplified individually or together. The region closer to the centromere includes the cyclin-dependent kinase *CDK4* and more distally carries the negative regulator of *TP53*, *MDM2*.[24,62,112]

*MDM2* (murine double minute 2), originally described in a murine DMIN-bearing cell line, also falls within the chromosome 12q amplification unit.[172] *MDM2* has transforming activity in vitro, and its function has been studied in some detail, as it has been recognized as a modulator of the tumor suppressor gene *TP53*.[173] The MDM2 protein interacts directly with the TP53 protein and exerts a negative effect on the transcriptional activation activity of TP53. There is also evidence of transcriptional induction of MDM2 by normal TP53, suggesting that there is a regulatory feedback loop involving these two proteins.[14] These observations have led to the hypothesis that MDM2 overexpression may be an alternative pathway to TP53 inactivation. Supporting this concept, in a small series of MFH and liposarcoma specimens, *TP53* mutation and *MDM2* amplification always occurred independently.[128] Antibodies are available for the MDM2 protein and have been applied in an immunhistochemical study of 211 adult sarcomas also analyzed for *TP53* expression.[41] Altogether, 37% overexpressed *MDM2*, and 26% expressed *TP53*. These groups were not mutually exclusive, with approximately 10% of tumors expressing both antigens. It is of some interest that not all tumors carrying apparent *MDM2* amplification exhibited high levels of immunohistochemically detectable MDM2 expression. In this patient cohort both TP53 and MDM2 positivity were independent predictors of survival. A synergistic interaction between MDM2 and p53 immunohistochemical staining was found in another study of extremity sarcomas.[256]

## Clinical Implications of Molecular Genetics

The rapid progress in molecular characterization of human cancers leads to consideration of how this information might be applied in the diagnostic laboratory.[194] At present, it is clear that molecular genetics is of most importance to investigators studying the fundamental biology of cancer. Nonetheless, DNA-based markers or their immunochemical surrogates clearly have valuable diagnostic and prognostic correlations in specific situations. Perhaps the most well established example in a solid tumor is *MYCN* amplification in neuroblastoma. As usual in oncology, the importance of potential prognostic markers depends on the availability of effective therapeutic interventions for aggressive tumors. In this regard, the availability of bone marrow transplantation for neuroblastoma has provided impetus for identifying patients with clinically low stage tumors who actually are at high risk because their tumors carry *MYCN* amplification. For many soft tissue tumors, their relative rarity and pathologic complexity renders meaningful clinical correlative studies more difficult. Additionally, several factors limit the clinical implementation of molecular genetics. At present, the technical expertise necessary for analysis of tumor DNA and RNA is usually available only at tertiary care centers, and the use of immunohistochemical techniques, although useful, does not directly address the question of genetic mutation. In the future, improved cost-effective molecular diagnostic technologies are likely to be widely disseminated. Much of the impetus for such technology development is related to the rapid progress in identifying human genes that may predispose to a wide variety of diseases including but not limited to cancer.

Despite these considerations, several of the molecular alterations now recognized in soft tissue tumors are candidates for transfer to the clinical laboratory. Of particular importance are the fusion proteins derived from chromosome translocations. Because the anomalous mRNAs for these proteins can be amplified by RT-PCR, they are detectable in tissue samples of minimal size. In addition, PCR-based technology does not suffer from the requirement of cytogenetic analysis for living cells and should facilitate the diagnosis of these translocations in a larger number of specimens than presently possible. An additional application of PCR is the detection of minimal residual disease in the bone marrow or harvested peripheral blood stem cells in the transplantation setting. Pioneered in leukemias, this approach may prove valuable for some solid tumors such as Ewing's sarcoma. Fluorescence in situ hybridization is an alternative technology that can detect specific translocations and gene amplifications in small tissue specimens. It has proven valuable in leukemia, and its use has been extended to solid tumors.[76,99,120,130,145,212,213,263] Another potential implication of tumor-specific fusion proteins is that, in theory, they may give rise to unique epitopes, which could be used to develop monoclonal antibodies. The latter would allow diagnosis of these translocations on tissue sections.

Although many of these applications await further clinical correlative studies and technologic development, the importance of molecular diagnostics will continue to increase. For example, most clinical correlative studies in soft tissue tumors have utilized only one or two molecular markers, but a more complete genotypic analysis is clearly necessary to explore the relation between clinical variables and tumor molecular genetics. It must be recognized that only parts of the puzzle posed by the molecular genetics of soft tissue tumors are in hand. As the remaining pieces of the puzzle are identified, the overall picture of molecular aberrations in cancer will inevitably become more apparent.

## REFERENCES


1. Aaltonen LA, Peltomaki P, Leach FS, et al. Clues to the pathogenesis of familial colorectal cancer. Science 260:812, 1993.
2. Abranson DH. Second nonocular cancers in retinoblastoma: a unified hypothesis: the Franceschetti lecture. Ophthalmic Genet 20:193, 1999.
3. Adams JM, Cory S. Transgenic models of tumor development. Science 254:1161, 1991.
4. Alitalo K, Schwab M. Oncogene amplification in tumor cells. Adv Cancer Res 47:235, 1986.
5. Alman BA, Li C, Pajerski ME, et al. Increased beta-catenin protein and somatic APC mutations in sporadic aggressive fibromatoses (desmoid tumors). Am J Pathol 151:329, 1997.
6. Aman P, Ron D, Mandahl N, et al. Rearrangement of the transcription factor gene CHOP in myxoid liposarcomas with t(12;16)(q131). Genes Chromosomes Cancer 5:278, 1992.
7. Ambroziak JA, Blackbourn DJ, Herndier BG, et al. Herpes-like sequences in HIV-infected and uninfected Kaposi's sarcoma patients. Science 268:582, 1995.
8. Andreassen A, Oyjord T, Hovig E, et al. p53 abnormalities in different subtypes of human sarcomas. Cancer Res 53:468, 1993.
9. Antonescu CR, Kawai A, Leung DH, et al. Strong association of SYT-SSX fusion type and morphologic epithelial differentiation in synovial sarcoma. Diagn Mol Pathol 9:1, 2000.
10. Argani P, Zakowski MF, Klimstra DS, et al. Detection of the SYT-SSX chimeric RNA of synovial sarcoma in paraffin-embedded tissue and its application in problematic cases. Mod Pathol 11:65, 1998.
11. Ashar HR, Cherath L, Przbysz KM, Chada K. Genomic characterization of human HMGIC, a member of the accessory transcription factor family found at translocation breakpoints in lipomas. Genomics 31:207, 1996.
12. Ashar HR, Fejzo MS, Tkachenko A, et al. Disruption of the architectural factor HMGI-C: DNA-binding AT hook motifs fused in lipomas to distinct transcriptional regulatory domains. Cell 82:57, 1995.
13. Baker SJ, Fearon ER, Nigro JM, et al. Chromosome 17 deletions and p53 mutations in colorectal carcinomas. Science 244: 217, 1989.
14. Barak Y, Juven T, Haffner R, et al. mdm2 expression is induced by wild type p53 activity. Embo J 12:461, 1993.
15. Barr FG, Galili N, Holick J, et al. Rearrangement of the PAX3 paired box gene in the paediatric solid tumour alveolar rhabdomyosarcoma. Nat Genet 3:113, 1993.
16. Barr FG, Nauta LE, Davis RJ, et al. In vivo amplification of the PAX3-FKHR and PAX7-FKHR fusion genes in alveolar rhabdomyosarcoma. Hum Mol Genet 5:15, 1996.
17. Barrios C, Castresana JS, Kreicbergs A. Clinicopathologic correlations and short-term prognosis in musculoskeletal sarcoma with c-myc oncogene amplification. Am J Clin Oncol 17:273, 1994.
18. Barrios C, Castresana JS, Ruiz J, et al. Amplification of c-myc oncogene and absence of c-Ha-ras point mutation in human bone sarcoma, J Orthop Res 11:556, 1993.
19. Barrios C, Castresana JS, Ruiz J, et al. Amplification of the c-myc proto-oncogene in soft tissue sarcomas. Oncology 51:13, 1994.
20. Belchis DA, Meece CA, Benko FA, et al. Loss of heterozygosity and microsatellite instability at the retinoblastoma locus in osteosarcomas. Diagn Mol Pathol 5:214, 1996.
21. Bell DW, Varley JM, Szydlo TE, et al. Heterozygous germ line hCHK2 mutations in Li-Fraumeni syndrome. Science 286:2528, 1999.
22. Benjamin LE, Fredericks WJ, Barr FG, et al. Fusion of the EWS1 and WT1 genes as a result of the t(11;22)(p13;q12) tranlocation in deoplastic small round cell tumors. Med Pediatr Oncol 27:434, 1996.
23. Bennett WP, Hollstein MC, Hsu IC, et al. Mutational spectra and immunohistochemical analyses of p53 in human cancers. Chest 101:19S, 1992.

24. Berner JM, Forus A, Elkahloun A, et al. Separate amplified regions encompassing CDK4 and MDM2 in human sarcomas. Genes Chromosomes Cancer 17:254, 1996.
25. Bianchi AB, Hara T, Ramesh V, et al. Mutations in transcript isoforms of the neurofibromatosis 2 gene in multiple human tumour types. Nat Genet 6:185, 1994.
26. Bianchi AB, Mitsunaga SI, Cheng JQ, et al. High frequency of inactivating mutations. in the neurofibromatosis type 2 gene (NF2) in primary malignant mesotheliomas. Proc Natl Acad Sci USA 92:10854, 1995.
27. Bishop JM. Viral oncogenes. Cell 42:23, 1985.
28. Bol S, Wanschura S, Thode B, et al. An endometrial polyp with a rearrangement of HMGI-C underlying a complex cytogenetic rearrangement involving chromosomes 2 and 12. Cancer Genet Cytogenet 90:88, 1996.
29. Borresen AL, Hovig E, Smith SB, et al. Constant denaturant gel electrophoresis as a rapid screening technique for p53 mutations. Proc Natl Acad Sci USA 88:8405, 1991.
30. Bos JL. The ras family and human carcinogenesis. Mutat Res 195:255, 1988.
31. Brett D, Whitehouse S, Antonson P, et al. The SYT protein involved in the t(X;18) synovial sarcoma translocation is a transcriptional activator localised in nuclear bodies. Hum Mol Genet 6:1559, 1997.
32. Brodeur GM, Azar C, Brother M, et al. Neuroblastoma: effect of genetic factors on prognosis and treatment. Cancer 70(Suppl):1685, 1992.
33. Brodeur GM, Hayes FA, Green AA, et al. Consistent N-myc copy number in simultaneous or consecutive neuroblastoma samples from sixty individual patients. Cancer Res 47:4248, 1987.
34. Brody RI, Ueda T, Hamelin A, et al. Molecular analysis of the fusion of EWS to an orphan nuclear receptor gene in extraskeletal myxoid chondrosarcoma. Am J Pathol 150:1049, 1997.
35. Cahill DP, Lengauer C, Yu J, et al. Mutations of mitotic checkpoint genes in human cancers. Nature 392:300, 1998.
36. Castresana JS, Rubio MP, Gomez L, et al. Detection of TP53 gene mutations in human sarcomas. Eur J Cancer 31A:735, 1995.
37. Chandar N, Billig B, McMaster J, et al. Inactivation of p53 gene in human and murine osteosarcoma cells. Br J Cancer 65: 208, 1992.
38. Chau KY, Patel UA, Lee KL, et al. The gene for the human architectural transcription factor HMGI-C consists of five exons each coding for a distinct functional element. Nucleic Acids Res 23:4262, 1995.
39. Clark J, Rocques PJ, Crew AJ, et al. Identification of novel genes, SYT and SSX, involved in the t(X;18)(p11.2;q11.2) translocation found in human synovial sarcoma. Nat Genet 7:502, 1994.
40. Cohen JA, Geradts J. Loss of RB and MTS1/CDKN2 (p16) expression in human sarcomas. Hum Pathol 28:893, 1997.
41. Cordon-Cardo C, Latres E, Drobnjak M, et al. Molecular abnormalities of mdm2 and p53 genes in adult soft tissue sarcomas. Cancer Res 54:794, 1994.
42. Crew AJ, Clark J, Fisher C, et al. Fusion of SYT to two genes, SSX1 and SSX2, encoding proteins with homology to the Kruppel-associated box in human synovial sarcoma. Embo J 14:2333, 1995.
43. Croce CM. Genetic approaches to the study of the molecular basis of human cancer. Cancer Res 51:5015S, 1991.
44. Croce CM, Tsujimoto Y, Erikson J, et al. Chromosome translocations and B cell neoplasia. Lab Invest 51:258, 1984.
45. Crozat A, Aman P, Mandahl N, et al. Fusion of CHOP to a novel RNA-binding protein in human myxoid liposarcoma. Nature 363:640, 1993.
46. Davidoff AM, Pence JC, Shorter NA, et al. Expression of p53 in human neuroblastoma- and neuroepithelioma-derived cell lines. Oncogene 7:127, 1992.
47. Davis RJ, Barr FG. Fusion genes resulting from alternative chromosomal translocations are overexpressed by gene-specific mechanisms in alveolar rhabdomyosarcoma. Proc Natl Acad Sci USA 94:8047, 1997.
48. Davis RJ, Bennicelli JL, Macina RA, et al. Structural characterization of the FKHR gene and its rearrangement in alveolar rhabdomyosarcoma. Hum Mol Genet 4:2355, 1995.
49. De Alava E, Kawai A, Healey JH, et al. EWS-FLI1 fusion transcript structure is an independent determinant of prognosis in Ewing's sarcoma. J Clin Oncol 16:1248, 1998.
50. De Alava E, Panizo A, Antonescu CR, et al. Association of EWS-FLI1 type 1 fusion with lower proliferative rate in Ewing's sarcoma. Am J Pathol 156:849, 2000.
51. De Chiara A, T'Ang A, Triche TJ. Expression of the retinoblastoma susceptibility gene in childhood rhabdomyosarcomas. J Natl Cancer Inst 85:152, 1993.
52. DeCristofaro MF, Betz BL, Wang W, et al. Alteration of hSNF5/INI1/BAF47 detected in rhabdoid cell lines and primary rhabdomyosarcomas but not Wilms' tumors. Oncogene 18:7559, 1999.
53. De Klein A, van Kessel AG, Grosveld G, et al. A cellular oncogene is translocated to the Philadelphia chromosome in chronic myelocytic leukaemia. Nature 300:765, 1982.
54. De Leeuw B, Balemans M, Olde Weghuis D, et al. Identification of two alternative fusion genes, SYT-SSX1 and SYT-SSX2, in t(X;18)(p11.2;q11.2)-positive synovial sarcomas. Hum Mol Genet 4:1097, 1995.
55. Delattre O, Zucman J, Plougastel B, et al. Gene fusion with an ETS DNA-binding domain caused by chromosome translocation in human tumours. Nature 359:162, 1992.
56. DeRisi J, Penland L, Brown PO, et al. Use of a cDNA microarray to analyse gene expression patterns in human cancer. Nat Genet 14:457, 1996.
57. Diller L, Sexsmith E, Gottlieb A, et al. Germline p53 mutations are frequently detected in young children with rhabdomyosarcoma. J Clin Invest 95:1606, 1995.
58. Donehower LA, Harvey M, Slagle BL, et al. Mice deficient for p53 are developmentally normal but susceptible to spontaneous tumours. Nature 356:215, 1992.
59. Driman D, Thorner PS, Greenberg ML, et al. MYCN gene amplification in rhabdomyosarcoma. Cancer 73:2231, 1994.
60. Edwards RH, Chatten J, Xiong QB, et al. Detection of gene fusions in rhabdomyosarcoma by reverse transcriptase-polymerase chain reaction assay of archival samples. Diagn Mol Pathol 6:91, 1997.
61. El Deiry WS, Tokino T, Velculescu VE, et al. WAF1, a potential mediator of p53 tumor suppression. Cell 75:817, 1993.
62. Elkahloun AG, Bittner M, Hoskins K, et al. Molecular cytogenetic characterization and physical mapping of 12q13-15 amplification in human cancers. Genes Chromosomes Cancer 17: 205, 1996.
63. Fearon ER, Vogelstein B. A genetic model for colorectal tumorigenesis. Cell 61:759, 1990.
64. Felix CA, Kappel CC, Mitsudomi T, et al. Frequency end diversity of p53 mutations in childhood rhabdomyosarcoma. Cancer Res 52:2243, 1992.
65. Fligman I, Lonardo F, Jhanwar SC, et al. Molecular diagnosis of synovial sarcoma and characterization of a variant SYT-SSX2 fusion transcript. Am J Pathol 147:1592, 1995.
66. Florenes VA, Maelandsmo GM, Forus A, et al. MDM2 gene amplification and transcript levels in human sarcomas: relationship to TP53 gene status. J Natl Cancer Inst 86:1297, 1994.
67. Forus A, Florenes VA, Maelandsmo GM, et al. Amplification and expression of genes in the q13-14 region of chromosome 12 in human sarcomas. Cell Growth Differ 4:1065, 1993.

68. Friend SH, Bernards R, Rogelj S, et al. A human DNA segment with properties of the gene that predisposes to retinoblastoma and osteosarcoma. Nature 323:643, 1986.
69. Friend SH, Horowitz JM, Gerber MR, et al. Deletions of a DNA sequence in retinoblastomas and mesenchymal tumors: organization of the sequence and its encoded protein. Proc Natl Acad Sci USA 84:9059, 1987.
70. Galili N, Davis RJ, Fredericks WJ, et al. Fusion of a fork head domain gene to PAX3 in the solid tumor alveolar rhabdomyosarcoma. Nat Genet 5:230, 1993.
71. Geurts JM, Schoenmakers EF, Roijer E, et al. Expression of reciprocal hybrid transcripts of HMGIC and FHIT in a pleomorphic adenoma of the parotid gland. Cancer Res 57:13, 1997.
72. Geurts JM, Schoenmakers EF, Roijer E, et al. Identification of NFIB as recurrent translocation partner gene of HMGIC in pleomorphic adenomas. Oncogene 16:865, 1998.
73. Giarola M, Wells D, Mondini P, et al. Mutations of adenomatous polyposis coli (APC) gene are uncommon in sporadic desmoid tumours. Br J Cancer 78:582, 1998.
74. Ginsberg JP, de Alava E, Ladanyi M, et al. EWS-FLI1 and EWS-ERG gene fusions are associated with similar clinical phenotypes in Ewing's sarcoma. J Clin Oncol 17:1809, 1999.
75. Glover TW, Stein CK, Legius E, et al. Molecular and cytogenetic analysis of tumors in von Recklinghausen neurofibromatosis. Genes Chromosomes Cancer 3:62, 1991.
76. Gray JW, Pinkel D. Molecular cytogenetics in human cancer diagnosis. Cancer 69(Suppl):1536, 1992.
77. Gutmann DH, Wood DL, Collins FS. Identification of the neurofibromatosis type 1 gene product. Proc Natl Acad Sci USA 88:9658, 1991.
78. Hacia JG. Resequencing and mutational analysis using oligonucleotide microarrays. Nat Genet 21:42, 1999.
79. Hamelin R, Zucman J, Melot T, et al. p53 mutations in human tumors with chimeric EWS/FLI-1 genes. Int J Cancer 57:336, 1994.
80. Harvey M, McArthur MJ, Montgomery CJ, et al. Spontaneous and carcinogen-induced tumorigenesis in p53-deficient mice. Nat Genet 5:225, 1993.
81. Hayashi K. PCR-SSCP: a method for detection of mutations. Genet Anal Tech Appl 9:73, 1992.
82. Hayashi K, Yandell DW. How sensitive is PCR-SSCP? Hum Mutat 2:338, 1993.
83. Heisterkamp N, Stephenson JR, Groffen J, et al. Localization of the c-abl oncogene adjacent to a translocation break point in chronic myelocytic leukaemia. Nature 306:239, 1983.
84. Hennig Y, Rogalla P, Wanschura S, et al. HMGIC expressed in a uterine leiomyoma with a deletion of the long arm of chromosome 7 along with a 12q14-15 rearrangement but not in tumors showing del(7) as the sole cytogenetic abnormality. Cancer Genet Cytogenet 96:129, 1997.
85. Hennig Y, Wanschura S, Deichert U, et al. Rearrangements of the high mobility group protein family genes and the molecular genetic origin of uterine leiomyomas and endometrial polyps. Mol Hum Reprod 2:277, 1996.
86. Hollingsworth RJ, Hensey CE, Lee WH. Retinoblastoma protein and the cell cycle. Curr Opin Genet Dev 3:55, 1993.
87. Hollstein M, Marion MJ, Lehman T, et al. p53 mutations at A: T base pairs in angiosarcomas of vinyl chloride-exposed factory workers. Carcinogenesis 15:1, 1994.
88. Hollstein M, Sidransky D, Vogelstein B, et al. p53 mutations in human cancers. Science 253:49, 1991.
89. Hosoi G, Hara J, Okamura T, et al. Low frequency of the p53 gene mutations in neuroblastoma. Cancer 73:3087, 1994.
90. Hovig E, Smith SB, Brogger A, et al. Constant denaturant gel electrophoresis, a modification of denaturing gradient gel electrophoresis, in mutation detection. Mutat Res 262:63, 1991.
91. Hussussian CJ, Struewing JP, Goldstein AM, et al. Germline p16 mutations in familial melanoma. Nat Genet 8:15, 1994.
92. Imamura I, Bartram CR, Berthold F, et al. Mutation of the p53 gene in neuroblastoma and its relationship with N-myc amplification. Cancer Res 53:4053, 1993.
93. Inagaki H, Nagasaka T, Otsuka T, et al. Association of SYT-SSX fusion types with proliferative activity and prognosis in synovial sarcoma. Mod Pathol 13:482, 2000.
94. Iolascon A, Faienza MF, Coppola B, et al. Analysis of cyclin-dependent kinase inhibitor genes (CDKN2A, CDKN2B, and CDKN2C) in childhood rhabdomyosarcoma. Genes Chromosomes Cancer 15:217, 1996.
95. Ionov Y, Peinado MA, Malkhosyan S, et al. Ubiquitous somatic mutations in simple repeated sequences reveal a new mechanism for colonic carcinogenesis. Nature 363:558, 1993.
96. Iwao K, Miyoshi Y, Nawa G, et al. Frequent beta-catenin abnormalities in bone and soft-tissue tumors. Jpn J Cancer Res 90:205, 1999.
97. Jeon IS, Davis JN, Braun BS, et al. A variant Ewing's sarcoma translocation (7;22) fuses the EWS gene to the ETS gene ETV1. Oncogene 10:1229, 1995.
98. Johnson MR, Look AT, DeClue JE, et al. Inactivation of the NF1 gene in human melanoma and neuroblastoma cell lines without impaired regulation of GTP.Ras. Proc Natl Acad Sci USA 90:5539, 1993.
99. Kallioniemi OP, Kallioniemi A, Kurisu W, et al. ERBB2 amplification in breast cancer analyzed by fluorescence in situ hybridization. Proc Natl Acad Sci USA 89:5321, 1992.
100. Kallioniemi OP, Kallioniemi A, Sudar D, et al. Comparative genomic hybridization: a rapid new method for detecting and mapping DNA amplification in tumors. Semin Cancer Biol 4:41, 1993.
101. Kanoe H, Nakayama T, Murakami H, et al. Amplification of the CDK4 gene in sarcomas: tumor specificity and relationship with the RB gene mutation. Anticancer Res 18:2317, 1998.
102. Karpeh MS, Brennan MF, Cance WG, et al. Altered patterns of retinoblastoma gene product expression in adult soft-tissue sarcomas. Br J Cancer 72:986, 1995.
103. Kawai A, Woodruff J, Healey JH, et al. SYT-SSX gene fusion as a determinant of morphology and prognosis in synovial sarcoma. N Engl J Med 338:153, 1998.
104. Kazmierczak B, Dal Cin P, Wanschura S, et al. HMGIY is the target of 6p21.3 rearrangements in various benign mesenchymal tumors. Genes Chromosomes Cancer 23:279, 1998.
105. Kazmierczak B, Hennig Y, Wanschura S, et al. Description of a novel fusion transcript between HMGI-C, a gene encoding for a member of the high mobility group proteins, and the mitochondrial aldehyde dehydrogenase gene. Cancer Res 55:6038, 1995.
106. Kazmierczak B, Meyer-Bolte K, Tran KH, et al. A high frequency of tumors with rearrangements of genes of the HMGI(Y) family in a series of 191 pulmonary chondroid hamartomas. Genes Chromosomes Cancer 26:125, 1999.
107. Kazmierczak B, Pohnke Y, Bullerdiek J. Fusion transcripts between the HMGIC gene and RTVL-H-related sequences in mesenchymal tumors without cytogenetic aberrations. Genomics 38:223, 1996.
108. Kazmierczak B, Rosigkeit J, Wanschura S, et al. HMGI-C rearrangements as the molecular basis for the majority of pulmonary chondroid hamartomas: a survey of 30 tumors. Oncogene 12:515, 1996.
109. Kellems RE. Gene Amplification in Mammalian Cells: A Comprehensive Guide. Marcel Dekker, New York, 1993.
110. Kern SE, Pietenpol JA, Thiagalingam S, et al. Oncogenic forms of p53 inhibit p53-regulated gene expression. Science 256:827, 1992.
111. Khan J, Bittner ML, Saal LH, et al. cDNA microarrays detect activation of a myogenic transcription program by the PAX3-

FKHR fusion oncogene. Proc Natl Acad Sci USA 96:13264, 1999.
112. Khatib ZA, Matsushime H, Valentine M, et al. Coamplification of the CDK4 gene with MDM2 and GLI in human sarcomas. Cancer Res 53:5535, 1993.
113. Knezevich SR, Garnett MJ, Pysher TJ, et al. ETV6-NTRK3 gene fusions and trisomy 11 establish a histogenetic link between mesoblastic nephroma and congenital fibrosarcoma. Cancer Res 58:5046, 1998.
114. Knezevich SR, McFadden DE, Tao W, et al. A novel ETV6-NTRK3 gene fusion in congenital fibrosarcoma. Nat Genet 18: 184, 1998.
115. Knudson AG. Antioncogenes and human cancer. Proc Natl Acad Sci USA 90:10914, 1993.
116. Knudson AJ. Mutation and cancer: statistical study of retinoblastoma. Proc Natl Acad Sci USA 68:820, 1971.
117. Knudson AJ, Hethcote HW, Brown BW. Mutation and childhood cancer: a probabilistic model for the incidence of retinoblastoma. Proc Natl Acad Sci USA 72:5116, 1975.
118. Komuro H, Hayashi Y, Kawamura M, et al. Mutations of the p53 gene are involved in Ewing's sarcomas but not in neuroblastomas. Cancer Res 53:5284, 1993.
119. Kovar H, Auinger A, Jug G, et al. Narrow spectrum of infrequent p53 mutations and absence of MDM2 amplification in Ewing tumours. Oncogene 8:2683, 1993.
120. Kumar S, Pack S, Kumar D, et al. Detection of EWS-FLI-1 fusion in Ewing's sarcoma/peripheral primitive neuroectodermal tumor by fluorescence in situ hybridization using formalin-fixed paraffin-embedded tissue. Hum Pathol 30:324, 1999.
121. Labelle Y, Bussieres J, Courjal F, et al. The EWS/TEC fusion protein encoded by the t(9;22) chromosomal translocation in human chondrosarcomas is a highly potent transcriptional activator. Oncogene 18:3303, 1999.
122. Labelle Y, Zucman J, Stenman G, et al. Oncogenic conversion of a novel orphan nuclear receptor by chromosome translocation. Hum Mol Genet 4:2219, 1995.
123. Ladanyi M, Cha C, Lewis R, et al. MDM2 gene amplification in metastatic osteosarcoma. Cancer Res 53:16, 1993.
124. Ladanyi M, Gerald W. Fusion of the EWS and WT1 genes in the desmoplastic small round cell tumor. Cancer Res 54:2837, 1994.
125. Ladanyi M, Lewis R, Garin-Chesa P, et al. EWS rearrangement in Ewing's sarcoma and peripheral neuroectodermal tumor: molecular detection and correlation with cytogenetic analysis and MIC2 expression. Diagn Mol Pathol 2:141, 1993.
126. Ladanyi M, Lewis R, Jhanwar SC, et al. MDM2 and CDK4 gene amplification in Ewing's sarcoma. J Pathol 175:211, 1995.
127. Leach FS, Nicolaides NC, Papadopoulos N, et al. Mutations of a MutS homolog in hereditary nonpolyposis colorectal cancer. Cell 75:1215, 1993.
128. Leach FS, Tokino T, Meltzer P, et al. p53 mutation and MDM2 amplification in human soft tissue sarcomas. Cancer Res 53(Suppl):2231, 1993.
129. Lee SB, Kolquist KA, Nichols K, et al. The EWS-WT1 translocation product induces PDGFA in desmoplastic small round-cell tumour. Nat Genet 17:309, 1997.
130. Lee W, Han K, Harris CP, et al. Use of FISH to detect chromosomal translocations and deletions: analysis of chromosome rearrangement in synovial sarcoma cells from paraffin-embedded specimens. Am J Pathol 143:15, 1993.
131. Lee WH, Bookstein R, Hong F, et al. Human retinoblastoma susceptibility gene: cloning, identification, and sequence. Science 235:1394, 1987.
132. Legius E, Marchuk DA, Collins FS, et al. Somatic deletion of the neurofibromatosis type 1 gene in a neurofibrosarcoma supports a tumour suppressor gene hypothesis. Nat Genet 3:122, 1993.
133. Levine AJ. The p53 tumor-suppressor gene [editorial]. N Engl J Med 326:1350, 1992.
134. Li FP, Garber JE, Friend SH, et al. Recommendations on predictive testing for germ line p53 mutations among cancer-prone individuals. J Natl Cancer Inst 84:1156, 1992.
135. Li J, Yen C, Liaw D, et al. PTEN, a putative protein tyrosine phosphatase gene mutated in human brain, breast, and prostate cancer. Science 275:1943, 1997.
136. Li Y, Bollag G, Clark R, et al. Somatic mutations in the neurofibromatosis 1 gene in human tumors. Cell 69:275, 1992.
137. Liang P, Pardee AB. Differential display of eukaryotic messenger RNA by means of the polymerase chain reaction. Science 257:967, 1992.
138. Lin PP, Brody RI, Hamelin AC, et al. Differential transactivation by alternative EWS-FLI1 fusion proteins correlates with clinical heterogeneity in Ewing's sarcoma. Cancer Res 59:1428, 1999.
139. Liu FS, Kohler MF, Marks JR, et al. Mutation and overexpression of the p53 tumor suppressor gene frequently occurs in uterine and ovarian sarcomas. Obstet Gynecol 83:118, 1994.
140. Liu W, Smith DI, Rechtzigel KJ, et al. Denaturing high performance liquid chromatography (DHPLC) used in the detection of germline and somatic mutations. Nucleic Acids Res 26: 1396, 1998.
141. Livingston DM, Kaelin W, Chittenden T, et al. Structural and functional contributions to the $G_1$ blocking action of the retinoblastoma protein. (the 1992 Gordon Hamilton Fairley memorial lecture). Br J Cancer 68:264, 1993.
142. Livingstone LR, White A, Sprouse J, et al. Altered cell cycle arrest and gene amplification potential accompany loss of wild-type p53. Cell 70:923, 1992.
143. Look AT. Oncogenic transcription factors in the human acute leukemias. Science 278:1059, 1997.
144. Lothe RA, Saeter G, Danielsen HE, et al. Genetic alterations in a malignant schwannoma from a patient with neurofibromatosis (NF1). Pathol Res Pract 189:465, 1993.
145. Lu YJ, Birdsall S, Summersgill B, et al. Dual colour fluorescence in situ hybridization to paraffin-embedded samples to deduce the presence of the der(X)t(X;18)(p11.2;q11.2) and involvement of either the SSX1 or SSX2 gene: a diagnostic and prognostic aid for synovial sarcoma. J Pathol 187:490, 1999.
146. Maelandsmo GM, Berner JM, Florenes VA, et al. Homozygous deletion frequency and expression levels of the CDKN2 gene in human sarcomas—relationship to amplification and mRNA levels of CDK4 and CCND1. Br J Cancer 72:393, 1995.
147. Makino R, Yazyu H, Kishimoto Y, et al. F-SSCP: fluorescence-based polymerase chain reaction-single-strand conformation polymorphism (PCR-SSCP) analysis. PCR Methods Appl 2:10, 1992.
148. Malkin D, Friend SH. The role of tumour suppressor genes in familial cancer. Semin Cancer Biol 3:121, 1992.
149. Malkin D, Jolly KW, Barbier N, et al. Germline mutations of the p53 tumor-suppressor gene in children and young adults with second malignant neoplasms. N Engl J Med 326:1309, 1992.
150. Malkin D, Li FP, Strong LC, et al. Germ line p53 mutations in a familial syndrome of breast cancer, sarcomas, and other neoplasms. Science 250:1233, 1990.
151. Manhani R, Cristofani LM, Odone Filho V, et al. Concomitant p53 mutation and MYCN amplification in neuroblastoma Med Pediatr Oncol 29:206, 1997.
152. Mansouri A. The role of Pax3 and Pax7 in development and cancer. Crit Rev Oncog 9:141, 1998.
153. Marchuk DA, Saulino AM, Tavakkol R, et al. cDNA cloning of the type 1 neurofibromatosis gene: complete sequence of the NF1 gene product. Genomics 11:931, 1991.
154. Marion MJ, Froment O, Trepo C. Activation of Ki-ras gene by

point mutation in human liver angiosarcoma associated with vinyl chloride exposure. Mol Carcinog 4:450, 1991.

155. Martin SS, Hurt WG, Hedges LK, et al. Microsatellite instability in sarcomas. Ann Surg Oncol 5:356, 1998.
156. May P, May E. Twenty years of p53 research: structural and functional aspects of the p53 protein. Oncogene 18:7621, 1999.
157. May WA, Lessnick SL, Braun BS, et al. The Ewing's sarcoma EWS/FLI-1 fusion gene encodes a more potent transcriptional activator and is a more powerful transforming gene than FLI-1. Mol Cell Biol 13:7393, 1993.
158. Meddeb M, Valent A, Danglot G, et al. MDM2 amplification in a primary alveolar rhabdomyosarcoma displaying a t(2;13)(q35;q14). Cytogenet Cell Genet 73:325, 1996.
159. Meye A, Wurl P, Hinze R, et al. No p16INK4A/CDKN2/MTS1 mutations independent of p53 status in soft tissue sarcomas. J Pathol 184:14, 1998.
160. Miller CW, Aslo A, Won A, et al. Alterations of the p53, Rb and MDM2 genes in osteosarcoma. J Cancer Res Clin Oncol 122:559, 1996.
161. Miller CW, Yeon C, Aslo A, et al. The p19INK4D cyclin dependent kinase inhibitor gene is altered in osteosarcoma. Oncogene 15:231, 1997.
162. Miyoshi Y, Iwao K, Nawa G, et al. Frequent mutations in the beta-catenin gene in desmoid tumors from patients without familial adenomatous polyposis. Oncol Res 10:591, 1998.
163. Mohney BG, Robertson DM, Schomberg PJ, et al. Second nonocular tumors in survivors of heritable retinoblastoma and prior radiation therapy. Am J Ophthalmol 126:269, 1998.
164. Moll AC, Imhof SM, Bouter LM, et al. Second primary tumors in patients with retinoblastoma: a review of the literature. Ophthalmic Genet 18:27, 1997.
165. Nakamura Y, Nishisho I, Kinzler KW, et al. Mutations of the adenomatous polyposis coli gene in familial polyposis coli patients and sporadic colorectal tumors. Princess Takamatsu Symp 22:285, 1991.
166. Nielsen GP, Burns KL, Rosenberg AE, et al. CDKN2A gene deletions and loss of p16 expression occur in osteosarcomas that lack RB alterations. Am J Pathol 153:159, 1998.
167. Nielsen GP, Stemmer-Rachamimov AO, Ino Y, et al. Malignant transformation of neurofibromas in neurofibromatosis 1 is associated with CDKN2A/p16 inactivation. Am J Pathol 155:1879, 1999.
168. Nilsson G, Skytting B, Xie Y, et al. The SYT-SSX1 variant of synovial sarcoma is associated with a high rate of tumor cell proliferation and poor clinical outcome. Cancer Res 59:3180, 1999.
169. Nilsson G, Wang M, Wejde J, et al. Reverse transcriptase polymerase chain reaction on fine needle aspirates for rapid detection of translocations in synovial sarcoma. Acta Cytol 42:1317, 1998.
170. Nowell PC. The clonal evolution of tumor cell populations. Science 194:23, 1976.
171. O'Brien KP, Seroussi E, Dal Cin P, et al. Various regions within the alpha-helical domain of the COL1A1 gene are fused to the second exon of the PDGFB gene in dermatofibrosarcomas and giant-cell fibroblastomas. Genes Chromosomes Cancer 23:187, 1998.
172. Oliner JD, Kinzler KW, Meltzer PS, et al. Amplification of a gene encoding a p53-associated protein in human sarcomas. Nature 358:80, 1992.
173. Oliner JD, Pietenpol JA, Thiagalingam S, et al. Oncoprotein MDM2 conceals the activation domain of tumour suppressor p53. Nature 362:857, 1993.
174. Orlow I, Drobnjak M, Zhang ZF, et al. Alterations of INK4A and INK4B genes in adult soft tissue sarcomas: effect on survival. J Natl Cancer Inst 91:73, 1999.
175. Panagopoulos I, Hoglund M, Mertens F, et al. Fusion of the EWS and CHOP genes in myxoid liposarcoma. Oncogene 12:489, 1996.
176. Panagopoulos I, Mencinger M, Dietrich CU, et al. Fusion of the RBP56 and CHN genes in extraskelatal myxoid chondrosarcomas with translocation t(9;17)(q22;q11). Oncogene 18:7594, 1999.
177. Papadopoulos N, Nicolaides NC, Wei Y-F, et al. Mutation of a mutL homolog in hereditary colon cancer. Science 263:1625, 1994.
178. Parada LF, Tabin CJ, Shih C, et al. Human EJ bladder carcinoma oncogene is homologue of Harvey sarcoma virus ras gene. Nature 297:474, 1982.
179. Park YK, Chi SG, Kim YW, et al. Mutational alteration of the p16CDKN2a tumor suppressor gene is infrequent in Ewing's sarcoma. Oncol Rep 6:1261, 1999.
180. Parsons R, Li GM, Longley MJ, et al. Hypermutability and mismatch repair deficiency in RER+ tumor cells. Cell 75:1227, 1993.
181. Peter M, Couturier J, Pacquement H, et al. A new member of the ETS family fused to EWS in Ewing tumors. Oncogene 14:1159, 1997.
182. Petit MMR, Mols R, Schoenmakers EF, et al. LPP, the preferred fusion partner gene of HMGIC in lipomas, is a novel member of the LIM protein gene family. Genomics 36:118, 1996.
183. Pilotti S, Della Torre G, Lavarino C, et al. Molecular abnormalities in liposarcoma: role of MDM2 and CDK4-containing amplicons at 12q13-22. J Pathol 185:188, 1998.
184. Przygodzki RM, Finkelstein SD, Keohavong P, et al. Sporadic and Thorotrast-induced angiosarcomas of the liver manifest frequent and multiple point mutations in K-ras-2. Lab Invest 76:153, 1997.
185. Rabbitts TH, Forster A, Larson R, et al. Fusion of the dominant negative transcription regulator CHOP with a novel gene FUS by translocation t(12;16) in malignant liposarcoma. Nat Genet 4:175, 1993.
186. Radig K, Schneider-Stock R, Haeckel C, et al. p53 gene mutations in osteosarcomas of low-grade malignancy. Hum Pathol 29:1310, 1998.
187. Radig K, Schneider-Stock R, Oda Y, et al. Mutation spectrum of p53 gene in highly malignant human osteosarcomas. Gen Diagn Pathol 142:25, 1996.
188. Ragazzini P, Gamberi G, Benassi MS, et al. Analysis of SAS gene and CDK4 and MDM2 proteins in low-grade osteosarcoma. Cancer Detect Prev 23:129, 1999.
189. Rao VN, Ohno T, Prasad DD, et al. Analysis of the DNA-binding and transcriptional activation functions of human Fli-1 protein. Oncogene 8:2167, 1993.
190. Reissmann PT, Simon MA, Lee W-H, et al. Studies of the retinoblastoma gene in human sarcomas. Oncogene 4:839, 1989.
191. Rieske P, Bartkowiak J, Szadowska A, et al. Malignant fibrous histiocytomas and H-ras-1 oncogene point mutations. Mol Pathol 52:64, 1999.
192. Ron D, Habener JF. CHOP, a novel developmentally regulated nuclear protein that dimerizes with transcription factors C/EBP and LAP and functions as a dominant-negative inhibitor of gene transcription. Genes Dev 6:439, 1992.
193. Rousseau-Merck MF, Versteege I, Legrand I, et al. hSNF5/INI1 inactivation is mainly associated with homozygous deletions and mitotic recombinations in rhabdoid tumors. Cancer Res 59:3152, 1999.
194. Rowley JD, Aster JC, Sklar J. The impact of new DNA diagnostic technology on the management of cancer patients: survey of diagnostic techniques. Arch Pathol Lab Med 117:1104, 1993.

195. Sager R. Tumor suppressor genes in the cell cycle. Curr Opin Cell Biol 4:155, 1992.
196. Saiki RK, Gelfand DH, Stoffel S, et al. Primer-directed enzymatic amplification of DNA with a thermostable DNA polymerase. Science 239:487, 1988.
197. Schalling M, Ekman M, Kaaya EE, et al. A role for a new herpes virus (KSHV) in different forms of Kaposi's sarcoma. Nat Med 1:707, 1995.
198. Schneider-Stock R, Onnasch D, Haeckel C, et al. Prognostic significance of p53 gene mutations and p53 protein expression in synovial sarcomas. Virchows Arch 435:407, 1999.
199. Schneider-Stock R, Radig K, Oda Y, et al. p53 gene mutations in soft-tissue sarcomas—correlations with p53 immunohistochemistry and DNA ploidy. J Cancer Res Clin Oncol 123:211, 1997.
200. Schneider-Stock R, Szibor R, Walter H, et al. No microsatellite instability, but frequent LOH in liposarcomas. Int J Oncol 14: 721, 1999.
201. Scholz RB, Kabisch H, Weber B, et al. Studies of the RB1 gene and the p53 gene in human osteosarcomas. Pediatr Hematol Oncol 9:125, 1992.
202. Schreck RR. Tumor suppressor gene (Rb and p53) mutations in osteosarcoma. Pediatr Hematol Oncol 9:ix 1992.
203. Schwab M, Alitalo K, Klempnauer KH, et al. Amplified DNA with limited homology to myc cellular oncogene is shared by human neuroblastoma cell lines and a neuroblastoma tumour. Nature 305:245, 1983.
204. Schwab M, Varmus HE, Bishop JM, et al. Chromosome localization in normal human cells and neuroblastomas of a gene related to c-myc. Nature 308:288, 1984.
205. Seeger RC, Wada R, Brodeur GM, et al. Expression of N-myc by neuroblastomas with one or multiple copies of the oncogene. Prog Clin Biol Res 271:41, 1988.
206. Sekido Y, Pass HI, Bader S, et al. Neurofibromatosis type 2 (NF2) gene is somatically mutated in mesothelioma but not in lung cancer. Cancer Res 55:1227, 1995.
207. Sekine K, Tsuchiya T, Hinohara S, et al. Analysis of the p161NK4, P14ARF, p15, TP53, and MDM3 genes and their prognostic implications in osteosarcoma and Ewing's sarcoma. Cancer Genet Cytogenet 120:91, 2000.
208. Serra E, Puig S, Otero D, et al. Confirmation of a double-hit model for the NF1 gene in benign neurofibromas. Am J Hum Genet 61:512, 1997.
209. Sevenet N, Lellouch-Tubiana A, Schofield D, et al. Spectrum of hSNF5/INI1 somatic mutations in human cancer and genotype-phenotype correlations. Hum Mol Genet 8:2359, 1999.
210. Sevenet N, Sheridan E, Amram D, et al. Constitutional mutations of the hSNF5/INI1 gene predispose to a variety of cancers. Am J Hum Genet 65:1342, 1999.
211. Shapiro DN, Sublett JE, Li B, et al. Fusion of PAX3 to a member of the forkhead family of transcription factors in human alveolar rhabdomyosarcoma. Cancer Res 53:5108, 1993.
212. Shipley J, Crew J, Birdsall S, et al. Interphase fluorescence in situ hybridization and reverse transcription polymerase chain reaction as a diagnostic aid for synovial sarcoma. Am J Pathol 148:559, 1996.
213. Shipley JM, Jones TA, Patel K, et al. Ordering of probes surrounding the Ewing's sarcoma breakpoint on chromosome 22 using fluorescent in situ hybridization to interphase nuclei. Cytogenet Cell Genet 64:233, 1993.
214. Simon MP, Pedeutour F, Sirvent N, et al. Deregulation of the platelet-derived growth factor B-chain gene via fusion with collagen gene COL1A1 in dermatofibrosarcoma protuberans and giant-cell fibroblastoma. Nat Genet 15:95, 1997.
215. Sjogren H, Meis-Kindblom J, Kindblom LG, et al. Fusion of the EWS-related gene TAF2N to TEC in extraskeletal myxoid chondrosarcoma. Cancer Res 59:5064, 1999.
216. Skytting B, Nilsson G, Brodin B, et al. A novel fusion gene, SYT-SSX4, in synovial sarcoma. J Natl Cancer Inst 91:974, 1999.
217. Smith SB, Gebhardt MC, Kloen P, et al. Screening for TP53 mutations in osteosarcomas using constant denaturant gel electrophoresis (CDGE). Hum Mutat 2:274, 1993.
218. Smith SH, Weiss SW, Jankowski SA, et al. SAS amplification in soft tissue sarcomas. Cancer Res 52:3746, 1992.
219. Smith SJ, Li Y, Whitley R, et al. Molecular epidemiology of p53 protein mutations in workers exposed to vinyl chloride. Am J Epidemiol 147:302, 1998.
220. Soini Y, Vahakangas K, Nuorva K, et al. p53 immunohistochemistry in malignant fibrous histiocytomas and other mesenchymal tumours. J Pathol 168:29, 1992.
221. Sorensen PH, Liu XF, Delattre O, et al. Reverse transcriptase PCR amplification of EWS/FLI-1 fusion transcripts as a diagnostic test for peripheral primitive neuroectodermal tumors of childhood. Diagn Mol Pathol 2:147, 1993.
222. Sornberger KS, Weremowicz S, Williams AJ, et al. Expression of HMGIY in three uterine leiomyomata with complex rearrangements of chromosome 6. Cancer Genet Cytogenet 114:9, 1999.
223. Southern E. Detection of specific sequences among DNA fragments separated by gel electrophoresis. J Mol Biol 98:503, 1975.
224. Staats B, Bonk U, Wanschura S, et al. A fibroadenoma with a t(4;12) (q27;q15) affecting the HMGI-C gene, a member of the high mobility group protein gene family. Breast Cancer Res Treat 38:299, 1996.
225. Stanbridge EJ. Functional evidence for human tumour suppressor genes: chromosome and molecular genetic studies. Cancer Surv 12:5, 1992.
226. Stephenson CF, Bridge JA, Sandberg AA. Cytogenetic and pathologic aspects of Ewing's sarcoma and neuroectodermal tumors. Hum Pathol 23:1270, 1992.
227. Stratton MR, Moss S, Warren W, et al. Mutation of the p53 gene in human soft tissue sarcomas: association with abnormalities of the RB1 gene. Oncogene 5:1297, 1990.
228. Strong LC, Williams WR, Tainsky MA. The Li-Fraumeni syndrome: from clinical epidemiology to molecular genetics. Am J Epidemiol 135:190, 1992.
229. Su LK, Vogelstein B, Kinzler KW. Association of the APC tumor suppressor protein with catenins. Science 262:1734, 1993.
230. Suwa K, Ohmori M, Miki H. Microsatellite alterations in various sarcomas in Japanese patients. J Orthop Sci 4:223, 1999.
231. Tabin CJ, Bradley SM, Bargmann CI, et al. Mechanism of activation of a human oncogene. Nature 300:143, 1982.
232. The I, Murthy AE, Hannigan GE, et al. Neurofibromatosis type 1 gene mutations in neuroblastoma. Nat Genet 3:62, 1993.
233. Thibodeau SN, Bren G, Schaid D. Microsatellite instability in cancer of the proximal colon. Science 260:816, 1993.
234. Tkachenko A, Ashar HR, Meloni AM, et al. Misexpression of disrupted HMGI architectural factors activates alternative pathways of tumorigenesis. Cancer Res 57:2276, 1997.
235. Toguchida J, Yamaguchi T, Ritchie B, et al. Mutation spectrum of the p53 gene in bone and soft tissue sarcomas. Cancer Res 52:6194, 1992.
236. Trofatter JA, MacCollin MM, Rutter JL, et al. A novel moesin-, ezrin-, radixin-like gene is a candidate for the neurofibromatosis 2 tumor suppressor. Cell 72:791, 1993.
237. Tsuji S, Hisaoka M, Morimitsu Y, et al. Detection of SYT-SSX fusion transcripts in synovial sarcoma by reverse transcription-polymerase chain reaction using archival paraffin-embedded tissues. Am J Pathol 153:1807, 1998.
238. Urano F, Umezawa A, Yabe H, et al. Molecular analysis of Ewing's sarcoma: another fusion gene, EWS-E1AF, available for diagnosis. Jpn J Cancer Res 89:703, 1998.

239. Versteege I, Sevenet N, Lange J, et al. Truncating mutations of hSNF5/INI1 in aggressive paediatric cancer. Nature 394:203, 1998.
240. Visser M, Bras J, Sijmons C, et al. Microsatellite instability in childhood rhabdomyosarcoma is locus specific and correlates with fractional allelic loss. Proc Natl Acad Sci USA 93:9172, 1996.
241. Vogan K, Bernstein M, Leclerc JM, et al. Absence of p53 gene mutations in primary neuroblastomas. Cancer Res 53:5269, 1993.
242. Vogelstein B, Kinzler KW. p53 function and dysfunction. Cell 70:523, 1992.
243. Vogelstein B, Kinzler KW. The multistep nature of cancer. Trends Genet 9:138, 1993.
244. Wadayama B, Toguchida J, Shimizu T, et al. Mutation spectrum of the retinoblastoma gene in osteosarcomas. Cancer Res 54:3042, 1994.
245. Wadayama B, Toguchida J, Yamaguchi T, et al. p53 expression and its relationship to DNA alterations in bone and soft tissue sarcomas. Br J Cancer 68:1134, 1993.
246. Wang J, Hisaoka M, Shimajiri S, et al. Detection of COL1A1-PDGFB fusion transcripts in dermatofibrosarcoma protuberans by reverse transcription-polymerase chain reaction using archival formalin-fixed, paraffin-embedded tissues. Diagn Mol Pathol 8:113, 1999.
247. Wanschura S, Kazmierczak B, Pohnke Y, et al. Transcriptional activation of HMGI-C in three pulmonary hamartomas each with a der(14)t(12;14) as the sole cytogenetic abnormality. Cancer Lett 102:17, 1996.
248. Weber-Hall S, McManus A, Anderson J, et al. Novel formation and amplification of the PAX7-FKHR fusion gene in a case of alveolar rhabdomyosarcoma. Genes Chromosomes Cancer 17: 7, 1996.
249. Wei G, Lonardo F, Ueda T, et al. CDK4 gene amplification in osteosarcoma: reciprocal relationship with INK4A gene alterations and mapping of 12q13 amplicons. Int J Cancer 80:199, 1999.
250. Weinberg RA. Tumor suppressor genes. Science 254:1138, 1991.
251. Wilke W, Maillet M, Robinson R. H-ras-1 point mutations in soft tissue sarcomas. Mod Pathol 6:129, 1993.
252. Willeke F, Mechtersheimer G, Schwarzbach M, et al. Detection of SYT-SSX1/2 fusion transcripts by reverse transcriptase-polymerase chain reaction (RT-PCR) is a valuable diagnostic tool in synovial sarcoma. Eur J Cancer 34:2087, 1998.
253. Williams AJ, Powell WL, Collins T, et al. HMGI(Y) expression in human uterine leiomyomata: involvement of another high-mobility group architectural factor in a benign neoplasm. Am J Pathol 150:911, 1997.
254. Wunder JS, Czitrom AA, Kandel R, et al. Analysis of alterations in the retinoblastoma gene and tumor grade in bone and soft-tissue sarcomas. J Natl Cancer Inst 83:194, 1991.
255. Wunder JS, Eppert K, Burrow SR, et al. Co-amplification and overexpression of CDK4, SAS and MDM2 occurs frequently in human parosteal osteosarcomas. Oncogene 18:783, 1999.
256. Wurl P, Meye A, Schmidt H, et al. High prognostic significance of Mdm2/p53 co-overexpression in soft tissue sarcomas of the extremities. Oncogene 16:1183, 1998.
257. Wurl P, Taubert H, Bache M, et al. Frequent occurrence of p53 mutations in rhabdomyosarcoma and leiomyosarcoma, but not in fibrosarcoma and malignant neural tumors. Int J Cancer 69: 317, 1996.
258. Xiao S, Lux ML, Reeves R, et al. HMGI(Y) activation by chromosome 6p21 rearrangements in multilineage mesenchymal cells from pulmonary hamartoma. Am J Pathol 150:901, 1997.
259. Xu W, Mulligan LM, Ponder MA, et al. Loss of NF1 alleles in phaeochromocytomas from patients with type I neurofibromatosis. Genes Chromosomes Cancer 4:337, 1992.
260. Yoo J, Lee HK, Kang CS, et al. p53 gene mutations and p53 protein expression in human soft tissue sarcomas. Arch Pathol Lab Med 121:395, 1997.
261. Yoo J, Robinson RA. H-ras and K-ras mutations in soft tissue sarcoma: comparative studies of sarcomas from Korean and American patients. Cancer 86:58, 1999.
262. Yoo J, Robinson RA, Lee JY. H-ras and K-ras gene mutations in primary human soft tissue sarcoma: concomitant mutations of the ras genes. Mod Pathol 12:775, 1999.
263. Zhang J, Meltzer P, Jenkins R, et al. Application of chromosome microdissection probes for elucidation of BCR-ABL fusion and variant Philadelphia chromosome translocations in chronic myelogenous leukemia. Blood 81:3365, 1993.
264. Zhang L, Lemarchandel V, Romeo PH, et al. The Fli-1 proto-oncogene, involved in erythroleukemia and Ewing's sarcoma, encodes a transcriptional activator with DNA-binding specificities distinct from other Ets family members. Oncogene 8:1621, 1993.
265. Zhou X, Benson KF, Ashar HR, et al. Mutation responsible for the mouse pygmy phenotype in the developmentally regulated factor HMGI-C. Nature 376:771, 1995.
266. Zucman J, Delattre O, Desmaze C, et al. EWS and ATF-1 gene fusion induced by t(12;22) translocation in malignant melanoma of soft parts. Nat Genet 4:341, 1993.
267. Zucman J, Melot T, Desmaze C, et al. Combinatorial generation of variable fusion proteins in the Ewing family of tumours. Embo J 12:4481, 1993.

# CHAPTER 5

# CYTOGENETIC ANALYSIS OF SOFT TISSUE TUMORS

JONATHAN A. FLETCHER

Most malignant soft tissue tumors contain clonal chromosome aberrations, many of which are diagnostic for particular tumor types.[50,67,145,146,174] Demonstration of characteristic chromosome abnormalities can be especially useful for diagnosing undifferentiated small round-cell or spindle cell soft tissue tumors.[50] The characteristic chromosome aberrations in these tumors appear to be critical for maintaining neoplastic transformation, and they are retained as a given tumor becomes progressively less differentiated. Hence evaluation of specific chromosome abnormalities is often informative in tumors that have lost diagnostic immunohistochemical or ultrastructural features (or both). Notably, the presence of any clonal chromosome aberration was once regarded as strong evidence of malignancy. Such views changed during the 1980s when characteristic cytogenetic aberrations were described in various benign mesenchymal tumors. The evidence to support a clonal origin of benign entities such as leiomyoma and lipoma is now overwhelming.[102,126,137]

Although most soft tissue tumors contain clonal cytogenetic aberrations, the traditional detection methods—in which karyotypes are assembled after chromosome banding—have many limitations. Classic cytogenetic banding methods are labor-intensive, and successful analyses are predicated on the ability of the cytogeneticist to culture the tumor cells in question. Several alternate methods (e.g., fluorescence in situ hybridization) permit evaluation of chromosomal aberrations in archival soft tissue tumor specimens.

## METHODOLOGIC CONSIDERATIONS

Normal human somatic cells contain two sex chromosomes and 22 pairs of autosomal chromosomes. Each chromosome has a short arm (designated *p*) and a long arm (designated *q*), with a centromere separating the two arms. Before 1970 it was exceedingly difficult to assess cytogenetic aberrations because the various human chromosomes could be distinguished based only on the gross morphologic features of overall chromosome size and centromere location. It was subsequently discovered that both fluorescent and nonfluorescent stains bind selectively and reproducibly to certain chromosome regions. This selective staining yields patterns of alternating light and dark bands in each chromosome arm, and knowledge of the characteristic normal banding patterns has facilitated studies of chromosomal alterations in neoplastic proliferations. Cytogenetic laboratories employ a number of stains that highlight different chromosome regions, the most widely used being quinacrine staining for fluorescence studies[26] and Giemsa staining for nonfluorescent banding.[157]

Soft tissue tumors have been karyotyped extensively since the mid-1980s, and virtually all malignant soft tissue tumors contain clonal chromosome aberrations (Table 5–1).[50] Although the presence of clonal chromosome aberrations was once assumed to be de facto evidence of cancer, it is now clear that such aberrations are found in many benign soft tissue tumors (Table 5–2). Cytogenetic aberrations are only one subset of all the genetic mutations found in malignant and benign soft tissue tumors. It is likely that all neoplastic soft tissue tumors contain multiple clonal genetic mutations, which are responsible collectively for deregulated cell growth. Many mutations are cytogenetically evident (e.g., chromosome translocations or deletions of large chromosomal regions), whereas others (e.g., deletions or substitutions of individual DNA nucleotides) cannot be detected at the cytogenetic level of resolution. Point mutations are evaluated using molecular methods.

**TABLE 5–1 CHARACTERISTIC CYTOGENETIC ABERRATIONS IN MALIGNANT SOFT TISSUE TUMORS**

| Histologic Finding | Characteristic Cytogenetic Events | Molecular Events | Frequency (%) | Diagnostic Utility? |
|---|---|---|---|---|
| Chondrosarcoma, extraskeletal myxoid | t(9;22)(q31;q12) | *EWS-CHN* fusion | >75 | Yes |
| Clear cell sarcoma | t(12;22)(q13;q12) | *EWS-ATF1* fusion | >75 | Yes |
| Desmoplastic small round cell tumor | t(11;22)(p13;q12) | *EWS-WT1* fusion | >75 | Yes |
| Dermatofibrosarcoma protuberans | Ring form of chromosomes 17 and 22 | *COL1A1-PDGFB* fusion | >75 | Yes |
| | t(17;22)(q21;q13) | *COL1A1-PDGFB* fusion | 10 | Yes |
| Ewing's sarcoma | t(11;22)(q24;q12) | *EWS-FLI1* fusion | >80 | Yes |
| | t(21;22)(q12;q12) | *EWS-ERG* fusion | 5–10 | Yes |
| | t(2;22)(q33;q12) | *EWS-FEV* fusion | <5 | Yes |
| | t(7;22)(p22;q12) | *EWS-ETV1* fusion | <5 | Yes |
| | t(17;22)(q12;q12) | *EWS-E1AF* fusion | <5 | Yes |
| Fibrosarcoma, infantile | t(12;15)(p13;q26) | *ETV6-NTRK3* fusion | >75 | Yes |
| | Trisomies 8, 11, 17, and 20 | | >75 | Yes |
| Gastrointestinal stromal tumor | Monosomies 14 and 22 | | >75 | Yes |
| | Deletion of 1p | | >25 | No |
| | | *KIT* mutation | >90 | Yes |
| Leiomyosarcoma | Deletion of 1p | | >50 | No |
| Liposarcoma | | | | |
| Well differentiated | Ring form of chromosome 12 | | >75 | |
| Myxoid/round cell | t(12;16)(q13;p11) | *TLS-CHOP* fusion | >75 | Yes |
| | t(12;22)(q13;q12) | *EWS-CHOP* fusion | >5 | Yes |
| Pleomorphic | Complex* | | 90 | No |
| Malignant fibrous histiocytoma | | | | |
| Myxoid | Ring form of chromosome 12 | | ? | ? |
| High grade | Complex* | | >90 | No |
| Myxofibrosarcoma | See Malignant fibrous histiocytoma | | | |
| Malignant peripheral nerve sheath tumor | | | | |
| Low grade | None | | >90 | No |
| High grade | Complex* | | | |
| Mesothelioma | Deletion of 1p | | >50 | Yes |
| | Deletion of 9p | p15, p16, and p19 inactivation | >75 | Yes |
| | Deletion of 22q | *NF2* inactivation | >50 | Yes |
| | Deletions of 3p and 6q | | >50 | Yes |
| Neuroblastoma | | | | |
| Good prognosis | Hyperdiploid, no 1p deletion | | 90 | Yes |
| Poor prognosis | 1p deletion | | 90 | Yes |
| | Double minute chromosomes | N-*myc* amplification | >25 | Yes |
| Primitive neuroectodermal tumor | (see Ewing's sarcoma) | | | |
| Rhabdoid tumor | Deletion of 22q | *INI1* inactivation | >90 | Yes |
| Rhabdomyosarcoma | | | | |
| Alveolar | t(2;13)(q35;q14) | *PAX3-FKHR* fusion | >75 | Yes |
| | t(1;13)(p36;q14), double minutes | *PAX7-FKHR* fusion | 10–20 | Yes |
| Embryonal | Trisomies 2q, 8 and 20 | | >75 | Yes |
| | | Loss of heterozygosity at 11p15 | >75 | Yes |
| Synovial sarcoma | | | | |
| Monophasic | t(X;18)(p11;q11) | *SYT-SSX1* or *SYT-SSX2* fusion | >90 | Yes |
| Biphasic | t(X;18)(p13;q11) | *SYT-SSX1* fusion | >90 | Yes |

*Consistent finding of extremely complex karyotypes containing multiple numerical and structural chromosomal aberrations.

**TABLE 5–2 CONSISTENT CYTOGENETIC ABERRATIONS IN BENIGN SOFT TISSUE TUMORS**

| Histologic Findings | Characteristic Cytogenetic Events | Molecular Events | Frequency (%) | Diagnostic Utility |
|---|---|---|---|---|
| Desmoid tumor | Trisomies 8 and/or 20 | | 25 | No |
| | Deletion of 5q | *APC* deletion | 10 | ? |
| Hibernoma | Translocation at 11q13 | | >50 | Yes |
| Leiomyoma, uterine | t(12;14)(q15;q24) | *HMGIC* and *RAD51* translocation | 20 | Yes |
| | Deletion of 7q | | 20 | ? |
| | Trisomy 12 | | 10 | ? |
| Lipoblastoma | Rearrangement of 8q12 | *PLAG1* fusions | >50 | Yes |
| Lipoma | | | | |
| Solitary | Rearrangement of 12q15 | *HMGIC* fusions | 75 | Yes |
| Multiple | None | | | |
| Neurofibroma | None | | | |
| Schwannoma, benign | Deletion of 22q | *NF2* inactivation | >75 | Yes |

The cytogenetic approach requires fresh, viable, tumor specimens that should be processed rapidly and transported to the cytogenetics laboratory in sterile tissue culture medium or in a physiologic buffer such as Hanks buffered salt solution. It is important that the cytogenetic sample be removed from the overall tumor specimen with sterile scalpel blades or scissors. Otherwise, bacterial or fungal contamination may lead to microbial overgrowth in the subsequent tissue cultures. Because viable tumor cells are essential for establishing the tissue cultures, it is also important that the specimen be selected carefully so it contains a minimum of necrotic tissue. Finally, it is crucial to minimize nonneoplastic components, particularly fibroblasts, lest these cells overwhelm the tumor cell population after the cultures are established. The success of the cytogenetic analysis depends largely on the quality of the tumor specimen, whereas the amount of tumor is less important; thus percutaneous needle biopsies of small round-cell tumors and other cellular sarcomas can be karyotyped routinely.[1,50,70,86,143] At least 80% of all soft tissue tumors can be cultured successfully if the specimens are carefully selected to minimize necrotic and nonneoplastic components.

Chromosome banding is most successful during metaphase when the chromosomes are maximally contracted. To obtain metaphase cells, tumor specimens are first disaggregated mechanically or enzymatically into single cells and small cell clusters.[92] Metaphase cells can often be extracted directly from disaggregated high-grade tumors if less than 1 hour has passed from the time of biopsy.[50] Lower-grade tumors must be placed in tissue culture for several days to improve the tumor cells' mitotic index. It is imperative that the cytogeneticist be acquainted with the characteristic tissue culture morphologic characteristics of the various tumor and nonneoplastic cell types. Daily inspection of the tissue cultures by inverted microscopy reveals when the tumor population is growing rapidly, and a mitotic spindle inhibitor (e.g., Colcemid) can then be added to arrest the growth of proliferating cells during metaphase. The time frame within which cytogenetic findings can be determined varies widely depending on the type and grade of the tumor. Metaphase preparations from high-grade tumors can often be obtained by direct harvesting or after 1–4 days in culture. Low-grade tumors, by contrast, often must be cultured for up to 1 week before metaphase preparations can be obtained. Longer culture periods (e.g., 2–3 weeks) should be avoided because genetic artifacts often develop in long-term cultures. The most frequent artifact is loss of the neoplastic clone due to overgrowth by fibroblasts or other nonneoplastic cells; such overgrowth results in a spurious diploid karyotype.

## CYTOGENETIC TERMINOLOGY

Karyotypes are described by means of an intricate shorthand system (Table 5–3)[111] that details both chromosome number and the location and mechanism of chromosome rearrangements. Numeric abnormalities are indicated by a plus or minus sign before a specific chromosome number (e.g., −22 indicates loss of one copy of chromosome 22). Chromosome rearrangements are indicated by abbreviations signifying the mechanism of the rearrangements. These rearrangement abbreviations are followed by one or more sets of parentheses, which describe the chromosome bands affected by the rearrangements. An example of this shorthand is 47,XX,+8,t(12;16)(q13;p11), in which 47 indicates the total chromosome number, XX indicates a female cell, and +8 indicates an extra copy, or trisomy, of chromosome 8. The t indicates a translocation (i.e., a reciprocal exchange of material

**TABLE 5-3 CYTOGENETIC ABBREVIATIONS**

| Abbreviation | Meaning |
|---|---|
| cen | Centromere |
| del | Deletion |
| dmin | Double minute chromosome |
| hsr | Homogeneously staining region |
| ins | Insertion |
| inv | Inversion |
| mar | Marker chromosome (aberrant chromosome whose origin cannot be ascertained) |
| p | Chromosome short arm |
| q | Chromosome long arm |
| r | Ring chromosome |
| t | Translocation |
| tel | Telomere |

between two different chromosome arms) and the first set of parentheses indicates that chromosomes 12 and 16 are involved in the translocation. The second set of parentheses indicates that the translocation breakpoint on chromosome 12 is on the long arm (q) at band 13, whereas the translocation breakpoint on chromosome 16 is on the short arm (p) at band 11. The translocation (12;16) is a characteristic rearrangement in myxoid liposarcoma (Table 5–1), and trisomy 8 is a frequent secondary aberration in these tumors.[173,188] A useful guide to chromosome nomenclature, the International System for Human Cytogenetic Nomenclature, was most recently updated in 1995.[111]

## IN SITU HYBRIDIZATION

Whereas conventional cytogenetic analyses are performed using various staining techniques that highlight chromosome bands, the newer discipline of "molecular cytogenetics" involves evaluation of particular chromosome regions using DNA probes.[49,91,134,138] Most molecular cytogenetic methods are based on in situ hybridization (ISH). That is, the DNA probes are hybridized and evaluated in the cellular (in situ) context. ISH assays are generally referred to as fluorescence in situ hybridization (FISH) when the hybridization reaction is detected by fluorescence microscopy. ISH reactions are also evaluable by brightfield microscopy using peroxidase or alkaline phosphatase detection strategies.[71,168] Fluorescence detection is generally the most sensitive, whereas peroxidase or alkaline phosphatase reaction products are more stable and, for most pathologists, more conveniently analyzed. FISH can be carried out using DNA probes that have been directly labeled with fluors such as fluorescein isothiocyanate (FITC) and rhodamine. The sensitivity of FISH can often be enhanced by indirect detection (e.g., hybridization with a biotinylated probe followed by detection with avidin-FITC). The FITC signals, with this indirect detection approach, can then be amplified further by successive incubations with biotinylated anti-avidin and avidin-FITC.

In situ hybridization to paraffin tissue sections is useful for demonstrating chromosome aberrations among particular cell populations,[80,116] but a drawback of this approach is that nuclei are often incomplete owing to the necessary thinness (typically 4–6 μm) of the sections.[80,116] ISH can also be carried out against intact nuclei that have been disaggregated from thick (50–60 μm) paraffin sections[152,153] or frozen tumor specimens, avoiding the problem of nuclear slicing artifacts (Fig. 5–1).[196] These hybridizations have been carried out successfully using tumor nuclei disaggregated from paraffin blocks that were more than 20 years old.[152] The DNA probes used for ISH can be directed against whole chromosomes or localized chromosome regions. "Cocktails" of probes that target an entire chromosome are referred to as chromosome "paints"; they are especially useful for confirming chromosome translocations in metaphase preparations.[134] DNA probes that target specific chromosome regions are employed to demonstrate chromosome deviations in both metaphase and interphase cells. These localized probes are particularly useful for demonstrating chromosome translocations,[13] chromosome deletions,[178] and gene amplifications[110,160] in archival pathology specimens (Fig. 5–2).

The ISH methods will likely play an increasing role as diagnostic adjuncts in soft tissue tumor pathology.

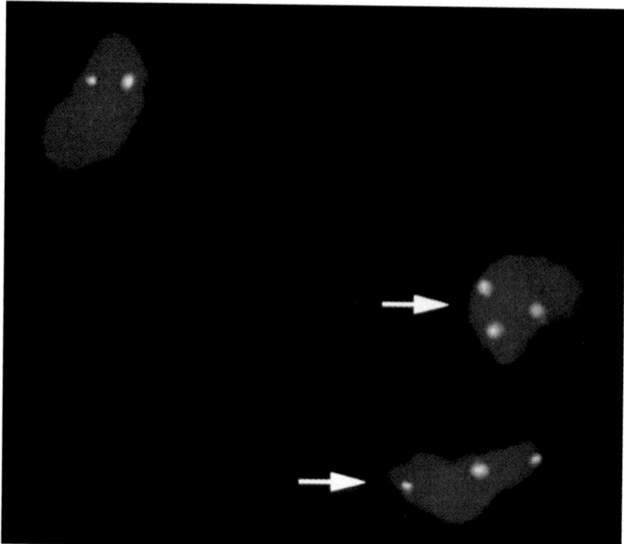

**FIGURE 5–1.** Fluorescence in situ hybridization (FISH) demonstration of trisomy 8 in nuclei disaggregated from a frozen desmoid specimen. In situ hybridization was carried out using a biotinylated chromosome 8 centromere probe and probe detection was with avidin-FITC. Two nuclei (arrows) have triple hybridization signals.

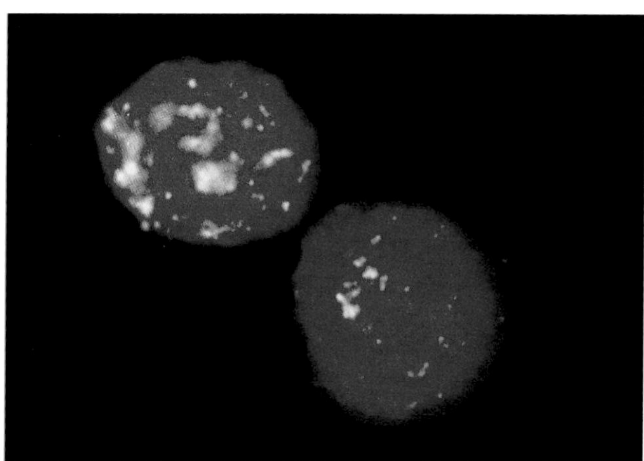

**FIGURE 5–2.** Fluorescence in situ hybridization demonstration of N-*myc* amplification in neuroblastoma nuclei. In situ hybridization was carried out using a biotinylated N-*myc* probe, and probe detection was with avidin-FITC. Both nuclei have marked amplification of N-*myc*.

Certain ISH probe sets can be used to address many diagnostic possibilities, particularly if the ISH assay is performed as a "special stain" in relation to the overall histologic evaluation. For example, ISH probes flanking the Ewing's sarcoma gene (*EWS*) can reveal diagnostic chromosome rearrangements in several soft tissue tumors (Table 5–1). Akin to Southern blotting, this approach demonstrates *EWS* region rearrangement but does not specify the *EWS* translocation partner (fusion) gene (Fig. 5–3). Identification of the partner gene, if desired, can be obtained subsequently by the reverse transcriptase polymerase chain reaction (RT-PCR) or by using additional ISH probes.

Several molecular cytogenetic methods have greatly expanded the capabilities of ISH. Examples include comparative genomic hybridization[76] and spectral karyotyping,[155] both of which permit genome-wide evaluation of chromosomal aberrations.

*Comparative genomic hybridization* is performed by extracting total genomic DNAs from a tumor of interest and from a nonneoplastic control cell population. These DNAs are differentially labeled (e.g., tumor DNA with fluorescein and control DNA with rhodamine) and then co-hybridized against normal metaphase cells. Chromosomal regions overrepresented (amplified) or underrepresented (deleted) in the tumor DNA manifest as color shifts of the corresponding chromosome regions in the normal metaphase target cells. An advantage of comparative genomic hybridization compared to conventional karyotyping is that tumor DNA can be isolated from archival specimens. There is no need for cell culture. Comparative genomic hybridization does not, however, detect balanced chromosomal rearrangements (e.g., balanced translocations), which are diagnostic markers in many soft tissue tumors.

*Spectral karyotyping* is a new method in which a complex panel of DNA probes is co-hybridized against tumor chromosome preparations. Whereas most ISH techniques involve hybridization of one or two fluorescence-tagged probes, spectral karyotyping probe panels generally include probes for each chromosome or chromosome arm (24 or more probes). Each probe is detected using different ratios of fluorescence markers, such as fluorescein and rhodamine. By varying the ratio of each fluor, chromosomes can be given a unique color. Thus spectral karyotyping enables a comprehensive ISH screen of the entire tumor cell karyotype.

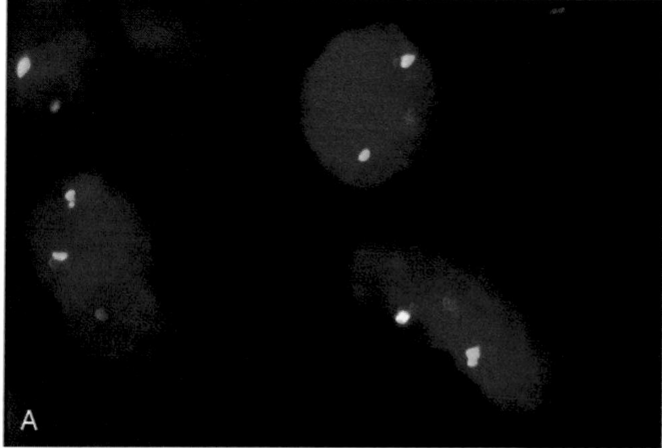


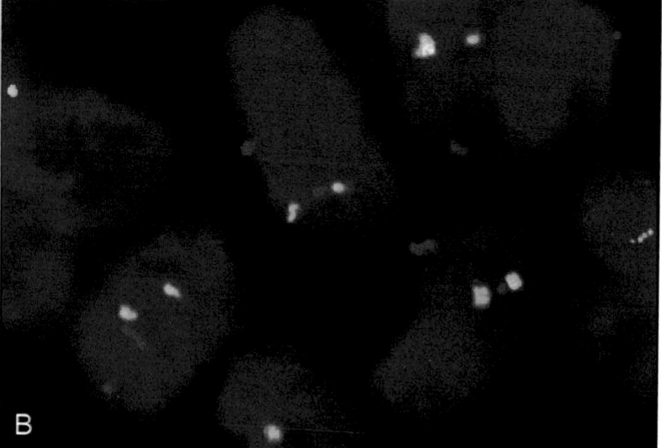


**FIGURE 5–3.** Fluorescence in situ hybridization demonstration of probes on the centromeric and telomeric sides of the chromosome 22 *EWS* gene. Hybridizations were performed using 4-$\mu$m paraffin sections of (**A**) Ewing's sarcoma and (**B**) clear cell sarcoma. The centromeric and telomeric probes are detected with FITC (green) and Texas red, respectively. One pair of green-red probe signals is split apart, in each case, due to rearrangement of the *EWS* region. (From Davison JM, Morgan TW, Hsi B-L et al. Subtracted, unique-sequence, in situ hybridization: experimental and diagnostic applications. Am J Pathol 153:1401, 1998. Copyright © American Society for Investigative Pathology.)

Comparative genomic hybridization and spectral karyotyping are powerful research tools, but they have not been adopted widely for routine clinical applications. They require specialized microscopy and image analysis capabilities and are relatively time-consuming in their present form.

## CYTOGENETIC MECHANISMS

The recurring soft tissue tumor chromosome rearrangements, particularly those that serve as diagnostic or prognostic markers, are often critical events in tumorigenesis. The nature of each chromosome rearrangement (whether translocation, deletion, or amplification) often suggests the mechanism by which specific genes participate in tumorigenesis. Certain soft tissue tumor translocation breakpoints interrupt genes directly, resulting in novel "fusion" oncogenes. Other translocation breakpoints are adjacent to a particular gene and result in deregulated expression (typically overexpression) of the gene. Deletions (whether involving whole chromosomes or chromosomal regions) generally signify loss of one or more tumor-suppressor genes. Amplification events, whether extrachromosomal (double minute chromosomes) or intrachromosomal (homogeneously staining regions), generally signify increased copies (and associated overexpression) of one or more oncogenes. Ring chromosomes generally form when a given chromosome loses one or both of its telomeres. Telomeres ordinarily serve to stabilize the chromosome ends. Once telomeres have been lost, the chromosome ends become "sticky" and tend to fuse, often in a circular ring form, with some other chromosomal region.

## CYTOGENETIC ANALYSIS OF SPECIFIC TUMORS

### Adipose Tumors

Most adipose tumors, whether benign or malignant, contain distinctive chromosome aberrations (Tables 5–1, 5–2). Useful diagnostic markers include the 12q rearrangement in lipomas, ring chromosomes in atypical lipomas (well-differentiated liposarcoma), t(12;16) translocations in myxoid/round-cell liposarcomas, and cytogenetic complexity in pleomorphic liposarcomas. Each of these associations is discussed below.

Solitary lipomas can be assigned to one of three general cytogenetic categories: (1) those with rearrangements of the mid-portion of the chromosome 12 long arm (band 12q15); (2) those with clonal aberrations not involving 12q15; and (3) those with normal karyotypes.[46,98,175] Chromosome 12q15 rearrangements target the *HMGIC* (high mobility group IC) gene, giving rise to *HMGIC* fusion oncogenes that most likely encode constitutively active transcriptional regulators.[5,151] The chromosome 12q15 rearrangements are generally accomplished by translocations with a variety of partner chromosomes, the most frequent translocation partner being the long arm of chromosome 3.[98] Lipomas with 12q15 rearrangements are no different, histologically or clinically, from those that lack such aberrations. Other nonrandom aberrations in lipomas include rearrangement of the chromosome 6 short arm and deletion of the chromosome 13 long arm, which are each seen in fewer than 10% of cases.[98] Another is deletion of the chromosome 16 long arm, which is associated with spindle cell and pleomorphic histology.[46,99] Given the high frequency of cytogenetic aberrations in solitary lipomas, it is notable that multiple lipomas from the same patient invariably have normal karyotypes. Patients with multiple lipomas likely have an underlying genetic predisposition (e.g., a DNA point mutation) that is not evident by cytogenetic analysis.

Characteristic cytogenetic aberrations are found in several other benign adipose tumors. Most lipoblastomas have rearrangements of the chromosome 8 long arm,[35,52] whereas hibernomas generally have rearrangements of the chromosome 11 long arm.[36,107,114]

The most diagnostically useful aberration in malignant adipose tumors is a translocation of chromosomes 12 and 16: t(12;16)(q13;p11). This translocation is found in most myxoid liposarcomas[46,173,188] and is retained in those cases that acquire round cell features.[69,87] The t(12;16) translocation results in fusion of the *CHOP* gene on chromosome 12 with the *TLS* gene on chromosome 16[2,32] and the resultant fusion oncoprotein is an activated transcription factor. The t(12;16) translocation appears to be diagnostic for myxoid liposarcoma and has not been found in other liposarcoma subtypes or in other myxoid soft tissue tumors.[96,187] Detection can be accomplished by cytogenetics or RT-PCR.

Well-differentiated liposarcomas (atypical lipomas) contain large unidentifiable "giant marker" chromosomes or ring chromosomes composed of chromosome 12 material (Fig. 5–4).[46,129] The biologic significance of these ring and "giant marker" chromosomes remains to be determined. Well-differentiated liposarcoma karyotypes are generally noncomplex, often containing the ring or giant marker chromosomes (or both) as isolated aberrations. Pleomorphic liposarcomas, by contrast, have exceedingly complex karyotypes with multiple clonal chromosome aberrations.[50,173] The karyotypic complexity in pleomorphic liposarcomas has hampered attempts to define consistent chromosome aberrations that might be of diagnostic use.

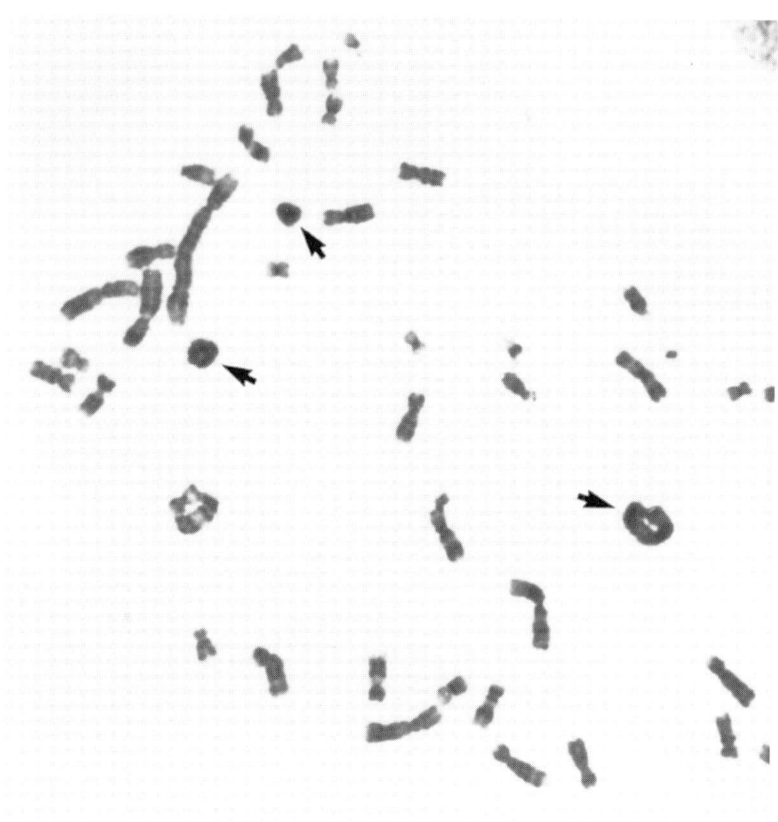

**FIGURE 5-4.** Partial metaphase from a well-differentiated liposarcoma showing three ring chromosomes (arrows) of varying size.

## Clear Cell Sarcoma (Malignant Melanoma of Soft Parts)

Clear cell sarcomas of soft tissues, also referred to as melanomas of the soft parts, share many phenotypic features with cutaneous malignant melanomas. Hence it may be difficult to distinguish between clear cell sarcoma and cutaneous melanoma diagnostically. Despite the histologic similarities between clear cell sarcoma and cutaneous melanoma, these two tumors are clinically different. Clear cell sarcomas usually present as isolated masses located in deep soft tissues without apparent origin from skin. It is notable, therefore, that more than 75% of clear cell sarcomas contain the chromosome translocation t(12;22)(q13;q12) (Fig. 5-5), which has never been reported in cutaneous melanoma.[20,47,133,170,176,182] The t(12;22) translocation fuses the *ATF1* gene on chromosome 12 with the *EWS* gene on chromosome 22.[24,200] *ATF1* encodes a transcription factor, and the biologic implications of the translocation are probably similar to those of Ewing's sarcoma translocations (discussed below). The clear cell sarcoma t(12;22) translocation can be detected by karyotyping or in situ hybridization (Fig. 5-3B), whereas the associated *EWS-ATF1* fusion can be detected conveniently by RT-PCR.

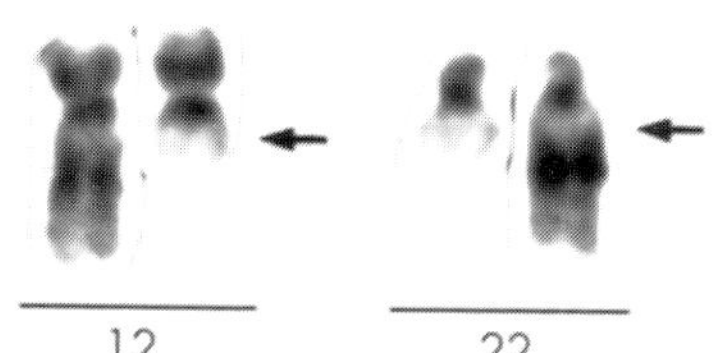


**FIGURE 5-5.** Partial karyotype of a clear cell sarcoma showing translocation of chromosomes 12 and 22. Arrows indicate translocation breakpoints on the rearranged chromosomes.

## Desmoplastic Small Round-Cell Tumor

Desmoplastic small round-cell tumors are composed of undifferentiated malignant small round-cells within a florid desmoplastic reaction.[61] Most desmoplastic small round-cell tumors contain a unique translocation of chromosomes 11 and 22: t(11;22)(p13;q11-12).[12,139] The desmoplastic small round-cell tumor translocation fuses the Ewing's sarcoma gene (chromosome 22) with the Wilms' tumor 1 gene (*WT1*) on the chromosome 11 short arm.[60,88] This translocation is cytogenetically distinct from the classic Ewing's sarcoma translocation, t(11;22), which involves the chromosome 11 long arm. The chromosome 11 breakpoint in intraabdominal desmoplastic small round-cell tumors is on a different arm from that of the classic breakpoint in Ewing's sarcoma and primitive neuroectodermal tumors.

## Ewing's Sarcoma and Primitive Neuroectodermal Tumors

Most Ewing's sarcomas and peripheral primitive neuroectodermal tumors contain chromosome translocations involving the Ewing's sarcoma gene, *EWS*. Although Ewing's sarcomas and peripheral primitive neuroectodermal tumors were once believed to be unrelated neoplasms, they are now viewed as a single neoplastic entity with a spectrum of differentiation. For simplicity, both Ewing's sarcomas and peripheral primitive neuroectodermal tumors are referred to as *Ewing tumors* in this chapter.

More than 80% of Ewing tumors contain a cytogenetic translocation in which material is exchanged between the long arms of chromosomes 11 and 22 (Fig. 5–6).[185] The cytogenetic shorthand description of this translocation is t(11;22)(q24;q12), and the translocation results in fusion of the chromosome 11 *FLI1* gene with the chromosome 22 *EWS* gene.[41,42,185,190] *FLI1* encodes a transcription factor (a protein that regulates expression of other genes); and the oncogenic *EWS–FLI1* fusion gene encodes an activated version of this transcription factor. A smaller subset of Ewing tumors, perhaps 5–15% of the total, have variant translocations in which the Ewing's sarcoma gene is fused with other transcription factor genes that are structurally related, by virtue of encoding ETS domains, to *FLI1* (Table 5–1).[72,74,78,132,166] The Ewing's sarcoma gene translocations are considered to be "primary" genetic aberrations in Ewing tumors because they are found in virtually all cases and are assumed to be the critical genetic aberration in these tumors. However, several other nonrandom cytogenetic abnormalities are found in subsets of Ewing tumors, including trisomy 8, trisomy 12, and translocation of chromosomes 1 and 16.[50,115] Each of these aberrations is found in fewer than 40% of Ewing tumors. Although presumably associated with "neoplastic progression," their prognostic relevance is uncertain.[4,103]

Several investigators have pointed out that the shared cytogenetic translocation in Ewing's sarcoma and primitive neuroectodermal tumors provides additional evidence of a close relation between these tumors.[27,89,94] Indeed, specific chromosome translocations in human cancers are generally observed in closely related cell types. Such translocations are presumably nononcogenic in more distantly related cells. Thus it is possible that Ewing's sarcoma and primitive neuroectodermal tumors result from transformation of closely related cells that differ only in their degree of neuroectodermal differentiation. It is also notable that an identical t(11;22)(q24;q12) translocation has been detected occasionally in other small round-cell tumors, including some cases of olfactory neuroblastoma (esthesioneuroblastoma),[194] small-cell osteosarcoma,[122] and mesenchymal chondrosarcoma.[144] The t(11;22) translocation in olfactory neuroblastomas is perhaps not a surprising finding because one subgroup of these tumors resembles primitive neuroectodermal tumor morphologically.[109] Notably, the Ewing's translocation, t(11;22), was detected frequently in one series of olfactory neuroblastomas,[167] whereas it was not detected at all in another.[3] Therefore it is unlikely that the t(11;22) translocation characterizes a major subgroup of olfactory neuroblastomas. Likewise, the description of chondroid differentiation in an experimental primitive neuroectodermal tumor model[63] suggests the possibility that mesenchymal chondrosarcomas with t(11;22)(q24;q12) translocation are simply Ewing's sarcomas with chondroid differentiation. The collective experimental evidence indicates that non-Ewing tumors with the t(11; 22) translocation are simply Ewing's sarcomas with atypical histology.

The t(11;22)(q24;q12) translocation is detected readily by conventional cytogenetic methods because Ewing's sarcoma and primitive neuroectodermal tumor cells grow well in tissue culture. In fact, the translocation can generally be detected in needle biopsy specimens.[1,50,70] It can also be detected by FISH, using probes to the *EWS* and *FLI1* regions,[43] and by RT-PCR.[6] One advantage of FISH is that "screening" approaches can be used to detect both the classic t(11; 22) translocation and the occasional chromosome 22 variant translocations (Table 5–1; Fig. 5–3A).[74,78,132,166] Advantages of PCR include superior sensitivity and identification of breakpoint locations within the translocated genes. Several studies have indicated that *EWS–FLI1* breakpoint locations might be prognostic in the family of Ewing tumors.[39,48,199]

## Fibromatoses, Fibrosarcomas, and Related Tumors

### *Dermatofibrosarcoma Protuberans*

The most consistent cytogenetic abnormality in dermatofibrosarcoma protuberans is a ring chromosome that is often superimposed on an otherwise normal karyotype (Fig. 5–7).[21,117,123,128] The ring chromosomes in dermatofibrosarcoma protuberans are invariably composed of intermixed sequences from chromosomes 17 and 22 (Fig. 5–8).[117,130] Rings composed of chromosomes 17 and 22 material have not been described in other types of sarcoma, and this cytogenetic finding is a useful diagnostic marker. The oncogenic mechanism in dermatofibrosarcoma protuberans ring chromosomes involves multiple copies of a fusion gene, *COL1A1–PDGFB*, in which *COL1A1* (a collagen gene) is contributed by chromosome 17 and *PDGFB* (platelet-derived growth factor-$\beta$ gene) by

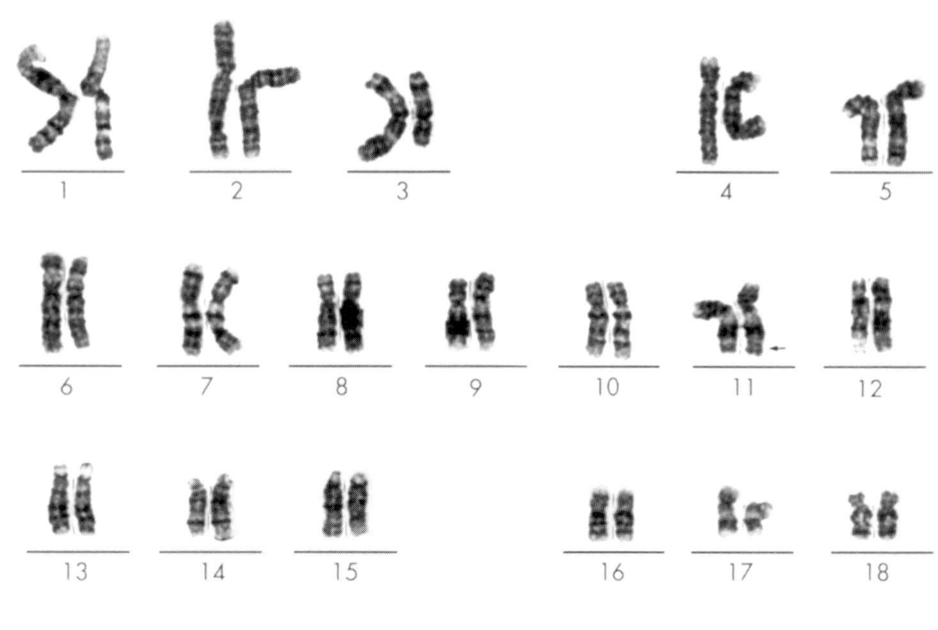


**FIGURE 5–6.** Karyotype of a Ewing's tumor showing translocation of chromosomes 11 and 22. Arrows indicate translocation breakpoints on the rearranged chromosomes. Chromosome 3 on the right is shorter than its partner because of a deletion; this was another clonal mutation in the tumor.

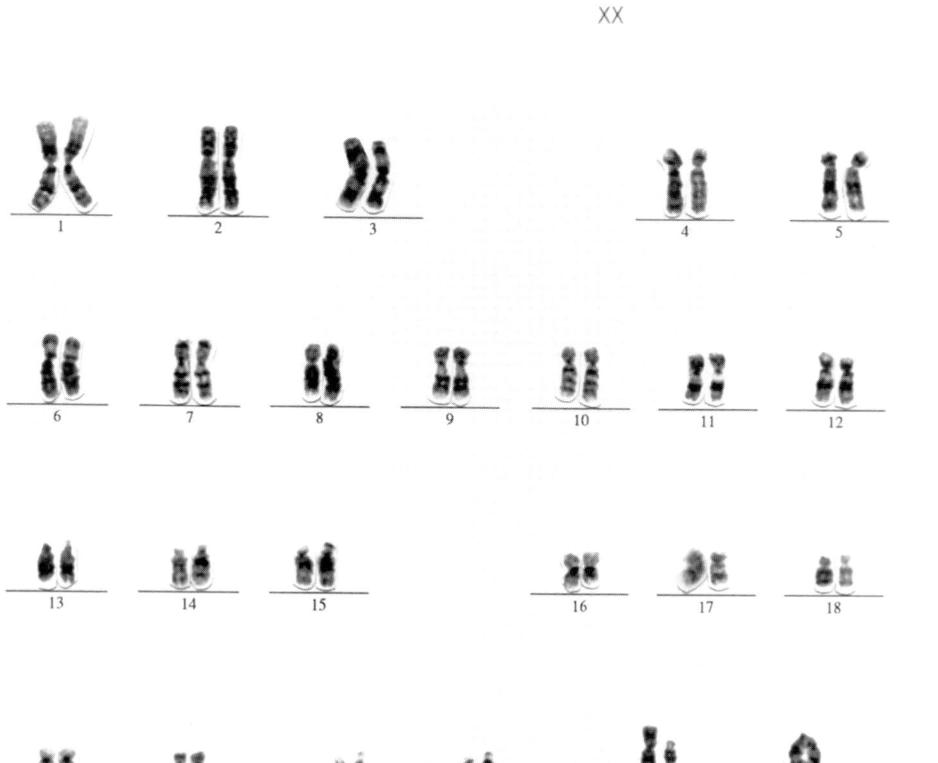


**FIGURE 5–7.** Karyotype of a dermatofibrosarcoma protuberans in which the only cytogenetic aberration is a supernumerary ring chromosome.

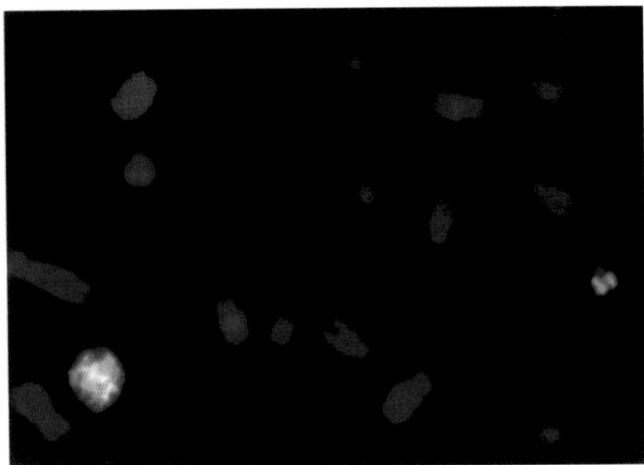

**FIGURE 5–8.** Fluorescence in situ hybridization analysis of a dermatofibrosarcoma protuberans ring chromosome (lower left). The ring is composed of alternating chromosome 17 (red) and chromosome 22 (green) sequences. (From Naeem R, Lux ML, Huang SF, et al. Ring chromosomes in dermatofibrosarcoma protuberans are composed of interspersed sequences from chromosomes 17 and 22. Am J Pathol 147:1553, 1995. Copyright © American Society for Investigative Pathology.)

chromosome 22.[123,164] The diagnostic *COL1A1–PDGFB* oncogene fusion can be demonstrated by FISH or RT-PCR. Additional cytogenetic abnormalities are seen in association with the ring chromosomes in some dermatofibrosarcoma protuberans tumors, the most frequent being trisomy for chromosome 8.[21,117,123,128] However, it is not known whether trisomy 8, or any other abnormality, is a marker of recurrence or fibrosarcomatous transformation. Occasional dermatofibrosarcoma protuberans tumors have balanced t(17;22) translocations (associated with the *COL1A1–PDGFB* fusion gene) rather than the usual ring chromosomes. Notably, such translocations are also characteristic of giant cell fibroblastomas.[123,164] This shared cytogenetic feature supports the notion that giant cell fibroblastoma is a pediatric form of dermatofibrosarcoma protuberans.[163]

#### Desmoid Tumors

Deep fibromatoses (desmoid tumors) often appear normal on cytogenetic studies, but trisomies for chromosomes 8 or 20 have been reported in approximately 20% of these tumors (Fig. 5–1).[34,54,108] The chromosomal trisomies are typically found in only a small number of the desmoid tumor cells (10–30%) and may be secondary mutations rather than primary tumorigenic events.[34,54,108] Preliminary data suggest that desmoid tumors with trisomy 8 are at increased risk of subsequent local recurrence.[54,85] A less common aberration in desmoid tumors is deletion of the chromosome 5 long arm, which is found in fewer than 10% of cases overall; it is more common in desmoid tumors from familial adenomatous polyposis (Gardner syndrome) patients.[22,37,198] The chromosome 5 deletions result in loss of the adenomatous polyposis coli (*APC*) tumor-suppressor gene; the remaining *APC* allele in such cases is typically inactivated by a point mutation.[113,158]

#### Fibrosarcoma (Infantile/Congenital) and Mesoblastic Nephroma

Trisomies of chromosomes 8, 11, 17, and 20 are characteristic aberrations in infantile fibrosarcomas.[153] It is interesting that one or more of this same group of trisomies are also found in the cellular variant of mesoblastic nephroma, which is an infantile renal tumor having substantial histologic overlap with infantile fibrosarcoma.[154] In addition, most infantile fibrosarcomas and cellular mesoblastic nephromas contain the same diagnostic chromosome translocation, t(12;15)(p13;q26) (Fig. 5–9).[82,83,142] This translocation results in fusion of the chromosome 12 *ETV6* (also known as *TEL*) gene with the chromosome 15 *NTRK3* (also known as *TRKC*) gene. The t(12;15) translocation is difficult to detect by conventional cytogenetic banding approaches, so it was rarely mentioned in descriptions of congenital fibrosarcoma or mesoblastic nephroma karyotypes prior to 1998. The t(12;15) translocation can be demonstrated readily by FISH (Fig. 5–9) or RT-PCR.[82,83,142] From a clinical standpoint, infantile fibrosarcomas and cellular mesoblastic nephromas are undifferentiated, mitotically active tumors that nonetheless have an excellent prognosis after excisional biopsy.[19,28] These tumors appear to be closely related at the pathogenetic, morphologic, and clinical levels. It is likely that they represent a single neoplastic entity, arising in either renal or soft tissue locations.

#### Inflammatory Myofibroblastic Tumor

Inflammatory myofibroblastic tumor (also known as inflammatory pseudotumor) is composed of fascicles of bland myofibroblastic cells admixed with a prominent inflammatory infiltrate. The myofibroblastic cells, which can be distinguished from the inflammatory component in tissue culture, often contain clonal chromosome aberrations.[165,179,183] No diagnostic cytogenetic aberration has been identified in these tumors. The cytogenetic clonality confirms a neoplastic myofibroblastic pathogenesis.

### Gastrointestinal Stromal Tumors

Gastrointestinal stromal tumors have distinctive karyotypes that generally include deletion of chromosomes 14 and 22.[45,101,147] Less often, gastrointestinal

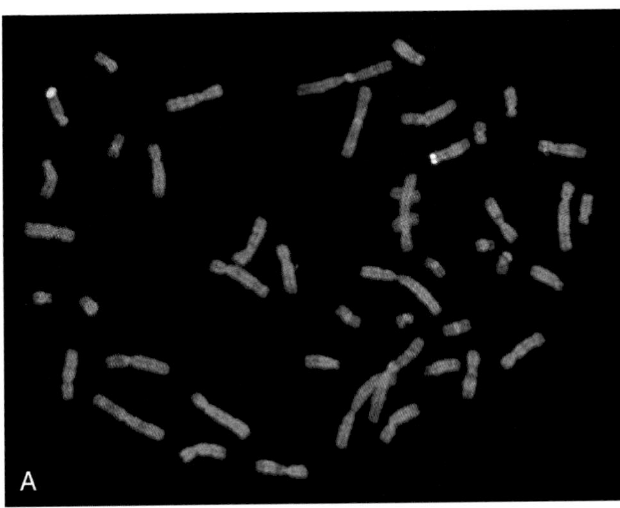


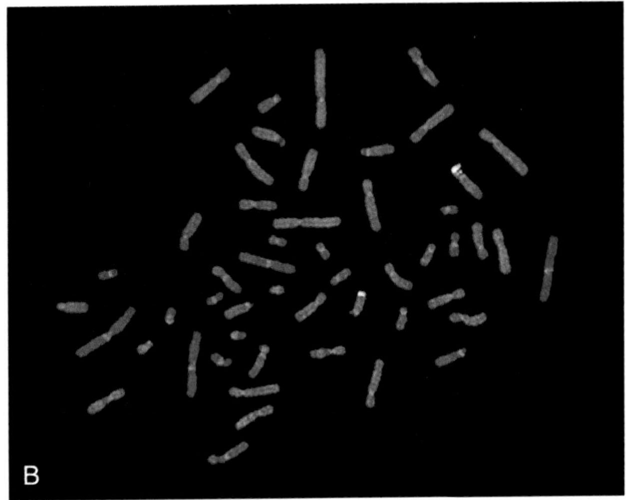


**FIGURE 5-9.** Fluorescence in situ hybridization analysis of the *ETV6 (TEL)* region in metaphase cells from congenital mesoblastic nephroma (**A**) and infantile fibrosarcoma (**B**). The centromeric and telomeric probes are detected with Texas red and FITC (green), respectively; and normal, unrearranged *ETV6* loci are evidenced by yellow fusion signals. One pair of green-red probe signals is split apart, in both tumors, owing to rearrangement of the *ETV6* region. (From Rubin BP, Chen CJ, Morgan TW, et al. Congenital mesoblastic nephroma t(12;15) is associated with ETV6-NTRK3 gene fusion: cytogenetic and molecular relationship to congenital (infantile) fibrosarcoma. Am J Pathol 153:1451, 1998. Copyright © American Society for Investigative Pathology.)

stromal tumors contain deletions of the chromosome 1 short arm (Table 5-1). Virtually all gastrointestinal stromal tumors display strong immunostaining for the KIT receptor tyrosine kinase protein, and most cases also contain activating mutations of the *KIT* oncogene.[68,118] In addition, germline (inherited) *KIT* mutations are responsible for a rare syndrome of familial, multifocal, gastrointestinal stromal tumors.[121] Both germline and somatic *KIT* aberrations are point mutations that are not evident at the cytogenetic level of resolution. However, the gastrointestinal stromal tumor cytogenetic profile—particularly the concomitant loss of chromosomes 14 and 22—is different from that in potential histologic mimics, including smooth muscle and peripheral nerve sheath tumors (Table 5-1).[45,147]

## Hemangiopericytoma

The most consistent cytogenetic abnormality in hemangiopericytoma is rearrangement of the chromosome 12 long arm, which is found in approximately 30-50% of cases.[100,131,171] The chromosome 12 rearrangements are not diagnostic, however, because similar aberrations are found occasionally in other spindle cell sarcomas.[112]

## Malignant Fibrous Histiocytoma

Most high-grade malignant fibrous histiocytomas have complex karyotypes[96,97,106] containing numerous clonal chromosome abnormalities. Superimposed on the clonal aberrations are many nonclonal aberrations that are unique to individual metaphase cells. The cytogenetic complexity in these tumors suggests that specific factors are continually promoting chromosome disarray. This "genetic instability" might account for the pleomorphism and immunohistochemical heterogeneity of high-grade malignant fibrous histiocytomas. Most myxoid malignant fibrous histiocytomas, by contrast, are lower-grade tumors that lack the karyotypic complexity of high-grade malignant fibrous histiocytomas. Ring chromosomes are found in more than 50% of myxoid malignant fibrous histiocytomas,[96,124] whereas no diagnostically useful chromosome rearrangements have been defined in high-grade malignant fibrous histiocytomas.

## Mesothelioma

Virtually all mesotheliomas contain clonal cytogenetic aberrations, the most characteristic being a group of deletions involving chromosomes 1, 3, 6, 9, and 22 (Table 5-1; Fig. 5-10).[65,135,180,181] These chromosome deletions are found in mesotheliomas irrespective of primary location (pleural versus peritoneal) or histologic type (epithelial versus sarcomatoid versus mixed). None of the deletions is specific for mesothelioma; in fact, the same chromosome deletions are found in non-small-cell lung carcinomas. Accordingly, cytogenetic demonstration of chromosome deletions is unlikely to be of value for distinguishing epithelial mesothelioma from bronchogenic adenocarcinoma. Cytogenetic analyses are useful for confirming a neoplastic proliferation, however, because the characteris-

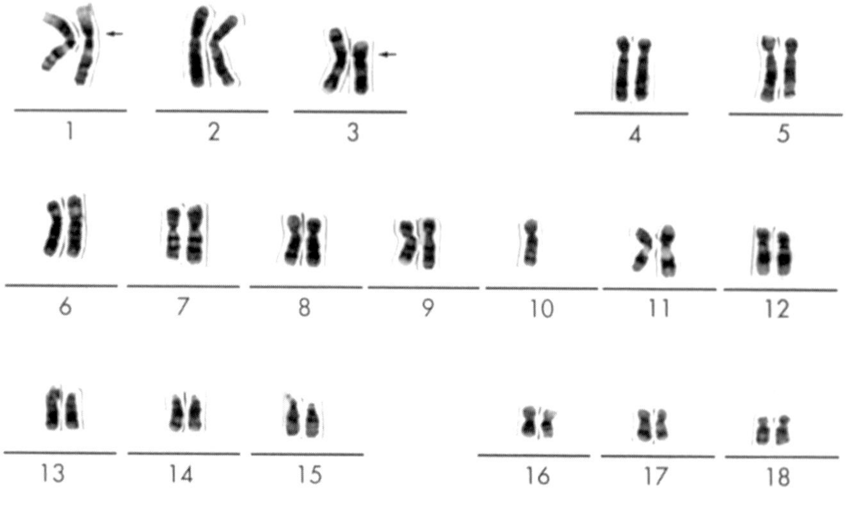


**FIGURE 5–10.** Karyotype of a pleural mesothelioma in which arrows indicate rearrangements resulting in loss of material from the chromosome 1 short arm, chromosome 3 short arm, and chromosome 22 long arm.

tic chromosome deletions of mesothelioma have not been found in reactive mesothelial hyperplasias.[64]

## Neuroblastoma

Most neuroblastomas can be assigned to one of two genetic categories. The first category includes neuroblastomas that are responsive to nonintensive therapy and that sometimes undergo spontaneous regression. These favorable-prognosis neuroblastomas typically have near-triploid DNA content, lack cytogenetically evident chromosome 1 short arm deletions, and lack N-*myc* amplification.[23,66,77] The second neuroblastoma category includes tumors with unfavorable prognostic markers: near-diploid or near-tetraploid DNA content, deletion of the chromosome 1 short arm, and in many cases amplification of the N-*myc* oncogene (Figs. 5–2, 5–11).[23,25,77] N-*myc* amplification, typically manifesting as double minute chromosomes, is arguably the most ominous of the adverse prognostic

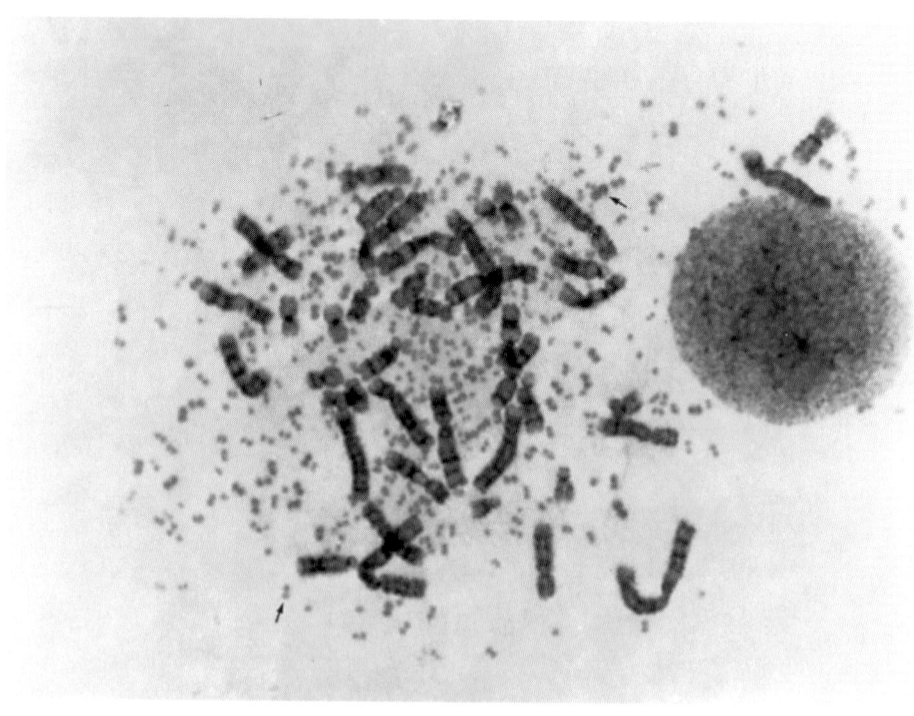

**FIGURE 5–11.** Neuroblastoma metaphase cell with numerous double minute chromosomes of varying size (arrows).

markers. N-*myc*-amplified neuroblastomas in children are rarely curable, although complete remissions are sometimes obtained using intensive myeloablative chemotherapy. Therefore genetic parameters can be useful for determining the appropriate intensity of therapy for children whose prognoses cannot be established using clinical parameters.[23] Cytogenetic analyses of neuroblastoma have been difficult, however, because the tumor cells from most favorable-prognosis neuroblastomas fail to divide in culture.[23] It is notable, therefore, that both N-*myc* amplification and chromosome 1 deletions can be demonstrated in interphase cells by in situ hybridization.[84,160,178]

## Peripheral Nerve Sheath Tumors

Benign and malignant peripheral nerve sheath tumors are seen with high frequency in patients with the hereditary neurofibromatosis syndromes. Neurofibromas and malignant peripheral nerve sheath tumors are common in individuals with neurofibromatosis type 1 (von Recklinghausen neurofibromatosis), whereas benign schwannomas are associated with neurofibromatosis type 2 (central neurofibromatosis).

Characterization of the neurofibromatosis syndrome genes has shed substantial light on the pathogenesis of peripheral nerve sheath tumors. The neurofibromatosis type 1 and type 2 genes are located on chromosomes 17 and 22, respectively; and both of these genes encode tumor-suppressor proteins that normally constrain cell proliferation.[8,40,90,95,141,184,191] Both sporadic malignant peripheral nerve sheath tumors and cases associated with hereditary neurofibromatosis commonly have deletions of the neurofibromatosis type 1 gene. However, those deletions are difficult to prove cytogenetically, as the karyotypes in most malignant peripheral nerve sheath tumors are complex (Fig. 5–12).[62,75,136] Neurofibromatosis type 1 gene mutations are also found in some neurofibromas.[30,149] Notably, the mutations in neurofibromas are found only in the Schwann cell component.[81] This observation supports the view that neurofibromas are clonal schwannian neoplasms, whereas the other admixed cell lineages, including fibroblasts, mast cells, and perineural cells, are reactive. Neurofibroma mutations can be demonstrated by molecular methods, whereas karyotyping studies are invariably normal. The normal cytogenetic patterns likely reflect tissue culture overgrowth of the neoplastic Schwann cells by reactive fibroblasts. Most benign schwannomas, whether sporadic or syndromic, feature noncomplex karyotypes with deletions of the neurofibromatosis type 2 gene region on chromosome 22. Generally, an entire

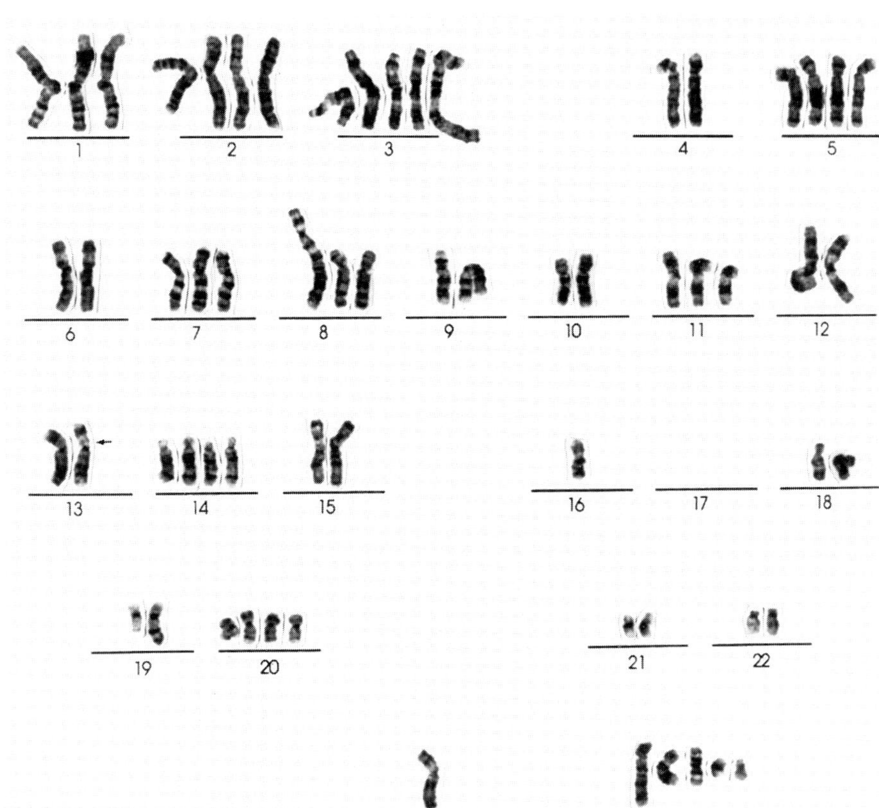


**FIGURE 5–12.** Complex karyotype of a malignant peripheral nerve sheath tumor. The karyotype is aneuploid with numerous chromosome gains, losses, and rearrangements.

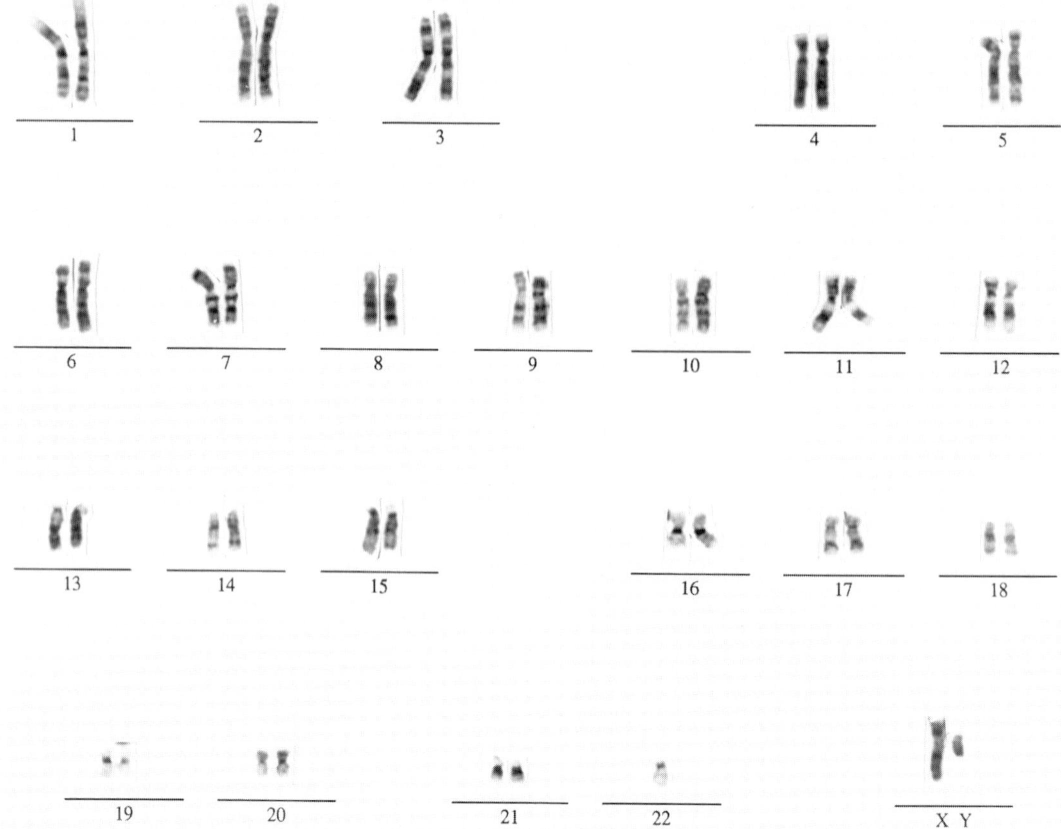


**FIGURE 5–13.** Noncomplex karyotype of a benign schwannoma with loss (monosomy) of chromosome 22 as an isolated chromosomal abnormality.

copy of chromosome 22 is lost (Fig. 5–13).[9,16,31] These deletions are typically associated with mutational inactivation of the remaining allele of the neurofibromatosis type 2 gene.[17,104,105]

### Rhabdoid Tumor

Most malignant rhabdoid tumors, whether arising in soft tissues, kidney, or the central nervous system, are characterized by deletions of the chromosome 22 long arm.[11,14,140,161] The chromosome 22 deletions target a tumor-suppressor gene, *INI1,* which encodes a protein involved in chromatin remodeling.[15,192] The rhabdoid tumor karyotypic profile is characteristic inasmuch as the chromosome 22 deletion is often the only detectable cytogenetic aberration. Chromosome 22 deletions are encountered occasionally in other (nonrhabdoid) high-grade soft tissue tumors. However, nonrhabdoid high-grade sarcomas almost never have karyotypes in which chromosome 22 deletion is the only clonal aberration.

### Rhabdomyosarcoma

Cytogenetic analyses have been useful for reaffirming the distinct nature of embryonal and alveolar forms of rhabdomyosarcoma. Alveolar rhabdomyosarcomas are characterized by reciprocal chromosome translocations involving the *FKHR* (Forkhead transcription factor) gene on chromosome 13. In most alveolar rhabdomyosarcomas the *FKHR* gene is fused with the *PAX3* gene on chromosome 2,[7,59,159] but a few cases contain fusions of *FKHR* with the *PAX7* gene on chromosome 1.[38] *FKHR, PAX3,* and *PAX7* encode transcription factors; and the *PAX3/FKHR* and *PAX7/FKHR* fusion oncogenes encode activated forms of those transcription factors.[10,58] The alveolar rhabdomyosarcoma chromosome translocations—and the associated fusion oncogenes—can be demonstrated by karyotyping, FISH, or RT-PCR.[6,13,44,127,189,193,195] Some alveolar rhabdomyosarcomas grow poorly in tissue culture; hence FISH and RT-PCR are more reliable than karyotyping.

Embryonal rhabdomyosarcomas lack *FKHR* translocations. In fact, no diagnostic translocations of any type have been described in embryonal rhabdomyosarcoma, although embryonal-type cases often contain extra copies of chromosomes 8 and 20 and the chromosome 2 long arm.[193] These aberrations are typically accompanied by deletions of the chromosome 11 short arm.[51,156] The chromosome 11 losses are read-

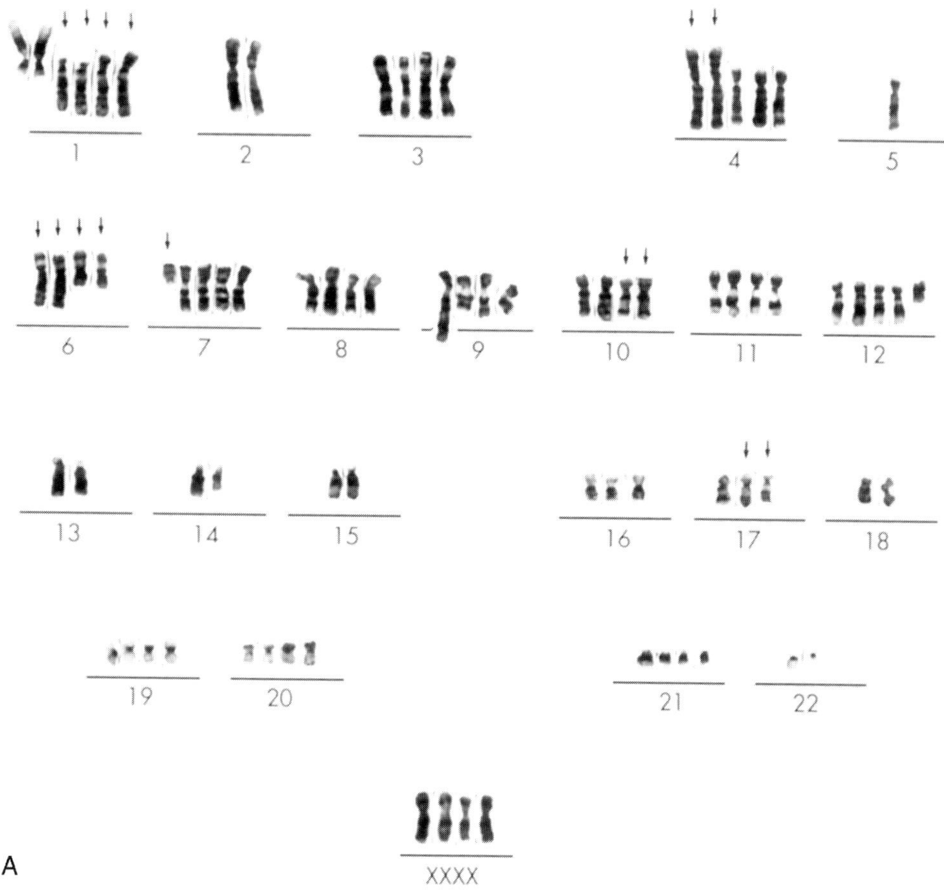


**FIGURE 5-14.** Karyotypes of two cells from a well-differentiated pelvic leiomyosarcoma. Arrows indicate clonal chromosome rearrangements that were found in all cells analyzed from this tumor. "Mar" = marker, which indicates an abnormal chromosome of uncertain origin. The karyotypes in **A** and **B** share numerous clonal abnormalities but differ in total chromosome number (80 versus 156 chromosomes). Chromosome rearrangements not designated by arrows (e.g., the bizarre chromosome 7 rearrangements at lower left in **B**) were not present consistently and reflect the genetic heterogeneity in this tumor. (From Fletcher JA, Morton CC, Pavelka K, Lage JM. Chromosome aberrations in uterine smooth muscle tumors: potential diagnostic relevance of cytogenetic instability. Cancer Res 50:4092, 1990.)

*Illustration continued on following page*

ily demonstrated by molecular methods[51,156] but are usually not obvious by cytogenetic studies.

## Smooth Muscle Tumors

Leiomyosarcomas contain heterogeneous chromosome aberrations,[112,172] but the most consistent finding has been deletion of the chromosome 1 short arm (Table 5-1). These deletions are probably not useful diagnostically because similar deletions are found occasionally in malignant fibrous histiocytomas, rhabdomyosarcomas, malignant peripheral nerve sheath tumors, and gastrointestinal stromal tumors.[112] The cytogenetic literature for leiomyosarcomas is misleading in that many of the reported karyotypes are likely those of gastrointestinal stromal tumors. Hence a unique leiomyosarcoma cytogenetic category characterized by deletion of the chromosome 1 short arm, monosomy 14, and monosomy 22 has been reported in several papers.[18,33,148,172] These cases, invariably abdominal in location, are presumably gastrointestinal stromal tumors. The only consistent finding with true leiomyosarcomas is that the karyotypes are generally complex. Most leiomyosarcomas contain numerous clonal and nonclonal chromosome aberrations, and this complexity can be striking even in low-grade specimens (Fig. 5-14).[53]

Many leiomyomas contain clonal chromosome aberrations, and the evidence for a clonal origin in most benign smooth muscle tumors is compelling.[119,126,137] Leiomyomas lacking clonal chromosome aberrations probably contain oncogenic DNA point mutations that cannot be visualized at the cytogenetic level of resolution.[102] Most leiomyoma karyotypes are far simpler than those seen in leiomyosarcomas.[119,126,137] Uterine leiomyomas, in particular, are known to have several recurrent chromosome aberrations. Deletion of the chromosome 7 long arm is found in 15–25% of

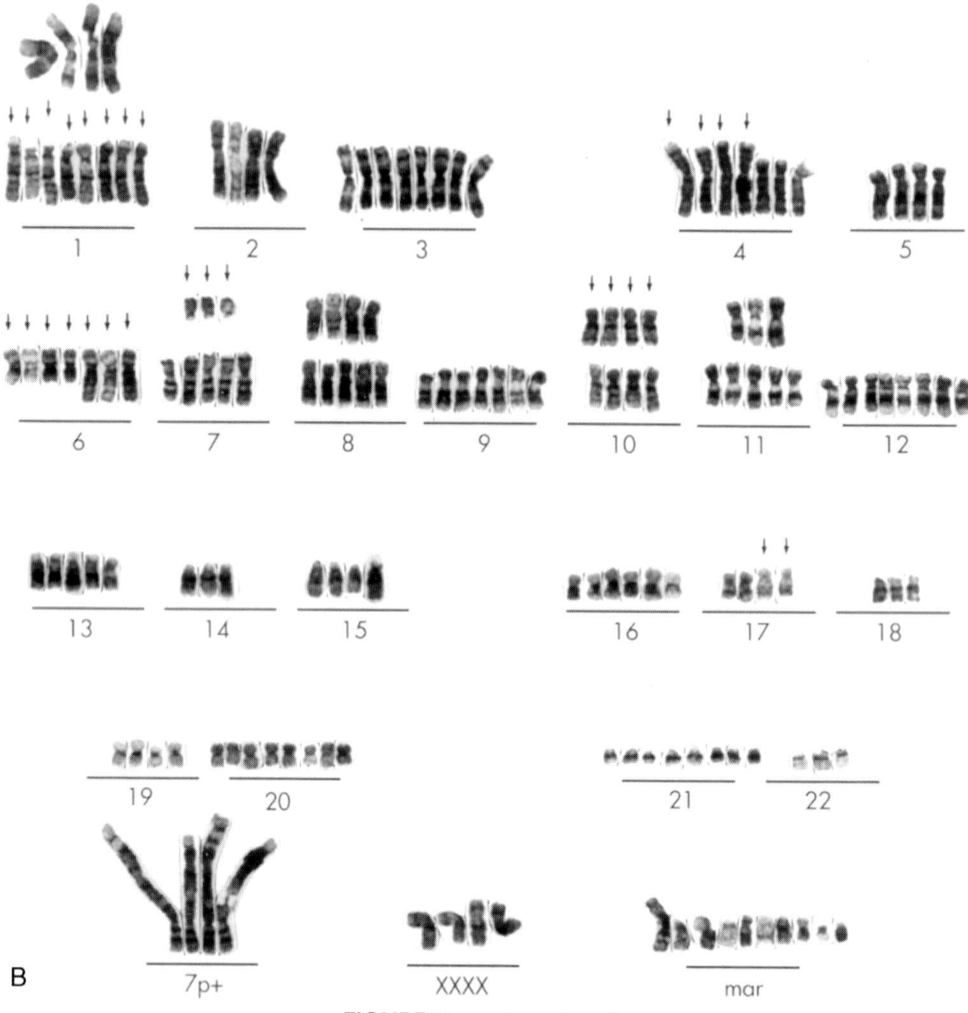


**FIGURE 5–14** *(Continued).*

cases, whereas trisomy 12 and rearrangements of the chromosome 6 short arm are each found in approximately 10–15% of cases.[119,120,126,137,197] The most distinctive leiomyoma cytogenetic abnormality is a translocation of chromosomes 12 and 14, which is found in approximately 20% of cases. This translocation results in overexpression of the chromosome 12 *HMGIC* gene by virtue of juxtaposition with the chromosome 14 *RAD51* (recombinational repair) gene.[150] The various leiomyoma cytogenetic aberrations are not characteristic of leiomyosarcomas, and cytogenetic aberrations in leiomyomas do not appear to be associated with increased risk of tumor progression (malignant transformation).

## Synovial Sarcoma

Both biphasic and monophasic synovial sarcomas are characterized by a reciprocal translocation of chromosomes X and 18: t(X;18)(p11;q11).[93,186] The t(X;18) translocation is found in more than 90% of synovial sarcomas but is not found in potential histologic mimics such as hemangiopericytoma, mesothelioma, leiomyosarcoma, or malignant peripheral nerve sheath tumor. The molecular underpinnings of the t(X;18) translocation are somewhat complex in that the oncogene on chromosome 18 (*SYT*) can be fused with either of two nearly identical genes (*SSX1* or *SSX2*) on chromosome X.[29] The *SSX1* and *SSX2* genes are adjacent to each other in the same Xp11 chromosome band, and one gene presumably arose from the other, evolutionarily, via a duplication event. Given their close proximity, it is impossible to distinguish *SYT–SSX1* from *SYT–SSX2* translocations using conventional chromosomal banding methods. However, the alternate *SSX* fusions can be demonstrated readily using FISH or RT-PCR.[73,162] The specific *SSX* fusion type might be relevant clinically. Kawai et al. demonstrated *SYT–SSX1* fusions in each of 12 biphasic synovial sarcomas, whereas monophasic synovial sarcomas had either *SYT–SSX1* or *SYT–SSX2* fusion oncogenes.[79] Patients with *SYT–SSX2* fusions appeared to have a better metastasis-free survival than those with *SYT–SSX1* fusions.[79]

### Benign Mesenchymal-Epithelial Tumors

Breast fibroadenomas, pulmonary chondroid hamartomas, and endometrial polyps are benign tumors composed of mesenchymal and epithelial cells. Some of these tumors have been considered historically as nonneoplastic hamartomas or hyperplasias, but recent cytogenetic studies have demonstrated clonal chromosome aberrations indicating a neoplastic origin for each of these entities.[55–57,125,169,177] Immunohistochemical analyses of the clonal aberrant metaphase cells demonstrates that these cells are mesenchymal. By contrast, the epithelial components lack clonal aberrations and are presumably reactive.[55–57] The cytogenetic and molecular aberrations in these tumors are related to those in other benign mesenchymal neoplasms, particularly mature lipomas and uterine leiomyomas. Most pulmonary hamartomas and endometrial polyps and some breast fibroadenomas have rearrangements of the chromosome 6 short arm or chromosome 12 long arm. As discussed above for lipomas and leiomyomas, these cytogenetic abnormalities invariably affect the *HMGIY* and *HMGIC* genes.

## RECENT DEVELOPMENTS

Several new cytogenetic correlations were reported after this chapter went to press. First, *alveolar soft part sarcomas* were found to have a recurrent translocation, t(X;17)(p11;q25), resulting in fusion of the *ASPL* and *TFE3* genes.[1] Second, a subset of *endometrial stromal sarcomas* were found to have a translocation, t(7;17), resulting in fusion of the *JAXF1* and *JJAZ1* genes.[2] Third, a subset of *inflammatory myofibroblastic tumors* were found to have chromosome 2p23 rearrangements, resulting in oncogenic fusions of the *ALK* (anaplastic lymphoma kinase) gene.[3–5] Fourth, chromosome 8q12 rearrangements, in *lipoblastoma,* were found to target the *PLAG1* transcription factor gene.[6]

### REFERENCES


1. Akerman M, Dreinhofer K, Rydholm A, et al. Cytogenetic studies on fine-needle aspiration samples from osteosarcoma and Ewing's sarcoma. Diagn Cytopathol 15:17, 1996.
2. Aman P, Ron D, Mandahl N, et al. Rearrangement of the transcription factor gene CHOP in myxoid liposarcomas with t(12;16)(q13;p11). Genes Chromosomes Cancer 5:278, 1992.
3. Argani P, Perez-Ordonez B, Xiao H, et al. Olfactory neuroblastoma is not related to the Ewing family of tumors: absence of EWS/FLI1 gene fusion and MIC2 expression. Am J Surg Pathol 22:391, 1998.
4. Armengol G, Tarkkanen M, Virolainen M, et al. Recurrent gains of 1q, 8 and 12 in the Ewing family of tumours by comparative genomic hybridization. Br J Cancer 75:1403, 1997.
5. Ashar HR, Fejzo MS, Tkachenko A, et al. Disruption of the architectural factor HMGI-C: DNA-binding A-T hook motifs fused in lipomas to distinct transcriptional regulatory domains. Cell 82:57, 1995.
6. Barr FG, Chatten J, D'Cruz CM, et al. Molecular assays for chromosomal translocations in the diagnosis of pediatric soft tissue sarcomas. JAMA 273:553, 1995.
7. Barr FG, Galili N, Holick J, et al. Rearrangement of the PAX3 paired box gene in the paediatric solid tumour alveolar rhabdomyosarcoma. Nat Genet 3:113, 1993.
8. Basu TN, Gutmann DH, Fletcher JA, et al. Aberrant regulation of ras proteins in malignant tumour cells from type 1 neurofibromatosis patients. Nature 356:713, 1992.
9. Bello MJ, de Campos JM, Kusak ME, et al. Clonal chromosome aberrations in neurinomas. Genes Chromosomes Cancer 6:206, 1993.
10. Bennicelli JL, Fredericks WJ, Wilson RB, et al. Wild type PAX3 protein and the PAX3-FKHR fusion protein of alveolar rhabdomyosarcoma contain potent, structurally distinct transcriptional activation domains. Oncogene 11:119, 1995.
11. Besnard-Guerin C, Cavenee W, Newsham I. The t(11;22)(p15.5;q11.23) in a retroperitoneal rhabdoid tumor also includes a regional deletion distal to CRYBB2 on 22q. Genes Chromosomes Cancer 13:145, 1995.
12. Biegel JA, Conard K, Brooks JJ. Translocation (11;22)(p13;q12): primary change in intra-abdominal desmoplastic small round cell tumor. Genes Chromosomes Cancer 7:119, 1993.
13. Biegel JA, Nycum LM, Valentine V, et al. Detection of the t(2;13)(q35;q14) and PAX3-FKHR fusion in alveolar rhabdomyosarcoma by fluorescence in situ hybridization. Genes Chromosomes Cancer 12:186, 1995.
14. Biegel JA, Rorke LB, Packer RJ, Emanuel BS. Monosomy 22 in rhabdoid or atypical tumors of the brain. J Neurosurg 73:710, 1990.
15. Biegel JA, Zhou JY, Rorke LB, et al. Germ-line and acquired mutations of INI1 in atypical teratoid and rhabdoid tumors. Cancer Res 59:74, 1999.
16. Bijlsma EK, Brouwer-Mladin R, Bosch DA, et al. Molecular characterization of chromosome 22 deletions in schwannomas. Genes Chromosomes Cancer 5:201, 1992.
17. Bijlsma EK, Merel P, Bosch DA, et al. Analysis of mutations in the SCH gene in schwannomas. Genes Chromosomes Cancer 11:7, 1994.
18. Boghosian L, Dal Cin P, Turc-Carel C, et al. Three possible cytogenetic subgroups of leiomyosarcoma. Cancer Genet Cytogenet 43:39, 1989.
19. Bolande RP. Congenital mesoblastic nephroma of infancy. Perspect Pediatr Pathol 1:227, 1973.
20. Bridge JA, Borek DA, Neff JR, Huntrakoon M. Chromosomal abnormalities in clear cell sarcoma: implications for histogenesis. Am J Clin Pathol 93:26, 1990.
21. Bridge JA, Neff JR, Sandberg AA. Cytogenetic analysis of dermatofibrosarcoma protuberans. Cancer Genet Cytogenet 49:199, 1990.
22. Bridge JA, Sreekantaiah C, Mouron B, et al. Clonal chromosomal abnormalities in desmoid tumors: implications for histopathogenesis. Cancer 69:430, 1992.
23. Brodeur GM, Azar C, Brother M, et al. Neuroblastoma: effect of genetic factors on prognosis and treatment. Cancer 70:1685, 1992.
24. Brown AD, Lopez-Terrada D, Denny C, Lee KA. Promoters containing ATF-binding sites are de-regulated in cells that express the EWS/ATF1 oncogene. Oncogene 10:1749, 1995.
25. Caron H, van Sluis P, de Kraker J, et al. Allelic loss of chro-

mosome 1p as a predictor of unfavorable outcome in patients with neuroblastoma. N Engl J Med 334:225, 1996.
26. Caspersson T, Zech L, Johansson C. Differential binding of alkylating fluorochromes in human chromosomes. Exp Cell Res 60:315, 1970.
27. Cavazzana AO, Miser JS, Jefferson J, Triche TJ. Experimental evidence for a neural origin of Ewing's sarcoma of bone. Am J Pathol 127:507, 1987.
28. Chung EB, Enzinger FM. Infantile fibrosarcoma. Cancer 38:729, 1976.
29. Clark J, Rocques PJ, Crew AJ, et al. Identification of novel genes, SYT and SSX, involved in the t(X;18)(p11.2;q11.2) translocation found in human synovial sarcoma. Nat Genet 7:502, 1994.
30. Colman SD, Williams CA, Wallace MR. Benign neurofibromas in type 1 neurofibromatosis (NF1) show somatic deletions of the NF1 gene. Nat Genet 11:90, 1995.
31. Couturier J, Delattre O, Kujas M, et al. Assessment of chromosome 22 anomalies in neurinomas by combined karyotype and RFLP analyses. Cancer Genet Cytogenet 45:55, 1990.
32. Crozat A, Aman P, Mandahl N, Ron D. Fusion of CHOP to a novel RNA-binding protein in human myxoid liposarcoma. Nature 363:640, 1993.
33. Dal Cin P, Boghosian L, Sandberg AA. Cytogenetic findings in leiomyosarcoma of the small bowel. Cancer Genet Cytogenet 30:285, 1998.
34. Dal Cin P, Sciot R, Aly MS, et al. Some desmoid tumors are characterized by trisomy 8. Genes Chromosomes Cancer 10: 131, 1994.
35. Dal Cin P, Sciot R, De Wever I, et al. New discriminative chromosomal marker in adipose tissue tumors: the chromosome 8q11-q13 region in lipoblastoma. Cancer Genet Cytogenet 78:232, 1994.
36. Dal Cin P, Van Damme B, Hoogmartens M, Van Den Berghe H. Chromosome changes in a case of hibernoma. Genes Chromosomes Cancer 5:178, 1992.
37. Dangel A, Meloni AM, Lynch HT, Sandberg AA. Deletion (5q) in a desmoid tumor of a patient with Gardner's syndrome. Cancer Genet Cytogenet 78:94, 1994.
38. Davis RJ, D'Cruz CM, Lovell MA, et al. Fusion of PAX7 to FKHR by the variant t(1;13)(p36;q14) translocation in alveolar rhabdomyosarcoma. Cancer Res 54:2869, 1994.
39. De Alava E, Kawai A, Healey JH, et al. EWS-FLI1 fusion transcript structure is an independent determinant of prognosis in Ewing's sarcoma. J Clin Oncol 16:1248, 1998.
40. DeClue JE, Papageorge AG, Fletcher JA, et al. Abnormal regulation of mammalian p21ras contributes to malignant tumor growth in von Recklinghausen (type 1) neurofibromatosis. Cell 69:265, 1992.
41. Delattre O, Zucman J, Melot T, et al. The Ewing family of tumors—a subgroup of small-round-cell tumors defined by specific chimeric transcripts. N Engl J Med 331:294, 1994.
42. Delattre O, Zucman J, Plougastel B, et al. Gene fusion with an ETS DNA-binding domain caused by chromosome translocation in human tumours. Nature 359:162, 1992.
43. Desmaze C, Zucman J, Delattre O, et al. Interphase molecular cytogenetics of Ewing's sarcoma and peripheral neuroepithelioma t(11;22) with flanking and overlapping cosmid probes. Cancer Genet Cytogenet 74:13, 1994.
44. Downing JR, Khandekar A, Shurtleff SA, et al. Multiplex RT-PCR assay for the differential diagnosis of alveolar rhabdomyosarcoma and Ewing's sarcoma. Am J Pathol 146:626, 1995.
45. El-Rifai W, Sarlomo-Rikala M, Miettinen M, et al. DNA copy number losses in chromosome 14: an early change in gastrointestinal stromal tumors. Cancer Res 56:3230, 1996.
46. Fletcher CD, Akerman M, Dal Cin P, et al. Correlation between clinicopathological features and karyotype in lipomatous tumors: a report of 178 cases from the Chromosomes and Morphology (CHAMP) Collaborative Study Group. Am J Pathol 148:623, 1996.
47. Fletcher JA. Translocation (12;22)(q13-14;q12) is a nonrandom aberration in soft-tissue clear-cell sarcoma. Genes Chromosomes Cancer S:184, 1992.
48. Fletcher JA. Ewing's sarcoma oncogene structure: a novel prognostic marker? J Clin Oncol 16:1241, 1998.
49. Fletcher JA. DNA in situ hybridization as an adjunct in tumor diagnosis. Am J Clin Pathol 112 (Suppl 1):511, 1999.
50. Fletcher JA, Kozakewich HP, Hoffer FA, et al. Diagnostic relevance of clonal cytogenetic aberrations in malignant soft-tissue tumors. N Engl J Med 324:436, 1991.
51. Fletcher JA, Kozakewich HP, Pavelka K, et al. Consistent cytogenetic aberrations in hepatoblastoma: a common pathway of genetic alterations in embryonal liver and skeletal muscle malignancies? Genes Chromosomes Cancer 3:37, 1991.
52. Fletcher JA, Kozakewich HP, Schoenberg ML, Morton CC. Cytogenetic findings in pediatric adipose tumors: consistent rearrangement of chromosome 8 in lipoblastoma. Genes Chromosomes Cancer 6:24, 1993.
53. Fletcher JA, Morton CC, Pavelka K, Lage JM. Chromosome aberrations in uterine smooth muscle tumors: potential diagnostic relevance of cytogenetic instability. Cancer Res 50:4092, 1990.
54. Fletcher JA, Naeem R, Xiao S, Corson JM. Chromosome aberrations in desmoid tumors: trisomy 8 may be a predictor of recurrence. Cancer Genet Cytogenet 79:139, 1995.
55. Fletcher JA, Pinkus GS, Donovan K, et al. Clonal rearrangement of chromosome band 6p21 in the mesenchymal component of pulmonary chondroid hamartoma. Cancer Res 52:6224, 1992.
56. Fletcher JA, Pinkus GS, Weidner N, Morton CC. Lineage-restricted clonality in biphasic solid tumors. Am J Pathol 138: 1199, 1991.
57. Fletcher JA, Pinkus JL, Lage JM, et al. Clonal 6p21 rearrangement is restricted to the mesenchymal component of an endometrial polyp. Genes Chromosomes Cancer 5:260, 1992.
58. Fredericks WJ, Galili N, Mukhopadhyay S, et al. The PAX3-FKHR fusion protein created by the t(2;13) translocation in alveolar rhabdomyosarcomas is a more potent transcriptional activator than PAX3. Mol Cell Biol 15:1522, 1995.
59. Galili N, Davis RJ, Fredericks WJ, et al. Fusion of a fork head domain gene to PAX3 in the solid tumour alveolar rhabdomyosarcoma. Nat Genet 5:230, 1993.
60. Gerald WL, Ladanyi M, de Alava E, et al. Clinical, pathologic, and molecular spectrum of tumors associated with t(11; 22)(p13;q12): desmoplastic small round-cell tumor and its variants. J Clin Oncol 16:3028, 1998.
61. Gerald WL, Miller HK, Battifora H, et al. Intra-abdominal desmoplastic small round-cell tumor: report of 19 cases of a distinctive type of high-grade polyphenotypic malignancy affecting young individuals. Am J Surg Pathol 15:499, 1991.
62. Glover TW, Stein CK, Legius E, et al. Molecular and cytogenetic analysis of tumors in von Recklinghausen neurofibromatosis. Genes Chromosomes Cancer 3:62, 1991.
63. Goji J, Sano K, Nakamura H, Ito H. Chondrocytic differentiation of peripheral neuroectodermal tumor cell line in nude mouse xenograft. Cancer Res 52:4214, 1992.
64. Granados R, Cibas ES, Fletcher JA. Cytogenetic analysis of effusions from malignant mesothelioma: a diagnostic adjunct to cytology. Acta Cytol 38:711, 1994.
65. Hagemeijer A, Versnel MA, Van Drunen E, et al. Cytogenetic analysis of malignant mesothelioma. Cancer Genet Cytogenet 47:1, 1990.
66. Hayashi Y, Inaba T, Hanada R, Yamamoto K. Chromosome

findings and prognosis in 15 patients with neuroblastoma found by VMA mass screening. J Pediatr 112:567, 1988.
67. Heim S, Mitelman F. Cancer Cytogenetics. Wiley-Liss, New York, 1995.
68. Hirota S, Isozaki K, Moriyama Y, et al. Gain-of-function mutations of c-kit in human gastrointestinal stromal tumors. Science 279:577, 1998.
69. Hisaoka M, Tsuji S, Morimitsu Y, et al. Detection of TLS/FUS-CHOP fusion transcripts in myxoid and round cell liposarcomas by nested reverse transcription-polymerase chain reaction using archival paraffin-embedded tissues. Diagn Mol Pathol 7:96, 1998.
70. Hoffer FA, Gianturco LE, Fletcher JA, Grief HE. Percutaneous biopsy of peripheral primitive neuroectodermal tumors and Ewing's sarcomas for cytogenetic analysis. AJR 162:1141, 1994.
71. Hopman AH, Claessen S, Speel EJ. Multi-colour brightfield in situ hybridisation on tissue sections. Histochem Cell Biol 108: 291, 1997.
72. Ishida S, Yoshida K, Kaneko Y, et al. The genomic breakpoint and chimeric transcripts in the EWSR1-ETV4/E1AF gene fusion in Ewing sarcoma. Cytogenet Cell Genet 82:278, 1998.
73. Janz M, de Leeuw B, Weghuis DO, et al. Interphase cytogenetic analysis of distinct X-chromosomal translocation breakpoints in synovial sarcoma. J Pathol 175:391, 1995.
74. Jeon IS, Davis JN, Braun BS, et al. A variant Ewing's sarcoma translocation (7;22) fuses the EWS gene to the ETS gene ETV1. Oncogene 10:1229, 1995.
75. Jhanwar SC, Chen Q, Li FP, et al. Cytogenetic analysis of soft tissue sarcomas: recurrent chromosome abnormalities in malignant peripheral nerve sheath tumors (MPNST). Cancer Genet Cytogenet 78:138, 1994.
76. Kallioniemi A, Kallioniemi OP, Sudar D, et al. Comparative genomic hybridization for molecular cytogenetic analysis of solid tumors. Science 258:818, 1992.
77. Kaneko Y, Kanda N, Maseki N, et al. Different karyotypic patterns in early and advanced stage neuroblastomas. Cancer Res 47:311, 1987.
78. Kaneko Y, Yoshida K, Handa M, et al. Fusion of an ETS-family gene, EIAF, to EWS by t(17;22)(q12;q12) chromosome translocation in an undifferentiated sarcoma of infancy. Genes Chromosomes Cancer 15:115, 1996.
79. Kawai A, Woodruff J, Healey JH, et al. SYT-SSX gene fusion as a determinant of morphology and prognosis in synovial sarcoma. N Engl J Med 338:153, 1998.
80. Kim SY, Lee JS, Ro JY, et al. Interphase cytogenetics in paraffin sections of lung tumors by non-isotopic in situ hybridization: mapping genotype/phenotype heterogeneity. Am J Pathol 142:307, 1993.
81. Kluwe L, Friedrich R, Mautner V. Loss of NF1 allele in Schwann cells but not in fibroblasts dervied from an NF1-associated neurofibroma. Genes Chromosomes Cancer 24:283, 1999.
82. Knezevich SR, Garnett MJ, Pysher TJ, et al. ETV6-NTRK3 gene fusions and trisomy 11 establish a histogenetic link between mesoblastic nephroma and congenital fibrosarcoma. Cancer Res 58:5046, 1998.
83. Knezevich SR, McFadden DE, Tao W, et al. A novel ETV6-NTRK3 gene fusion in congenital fibrosarcoma. Nat Genet 18: 184, 1998.
84. Komuro H, Valentine MB, Rowe ST, et al. Fluorescence in situ hybridization analysis of chromosome 1p36 deletions in human MYCN amplified neuroblastoma. J Pediatr Surg 33:1695, 1998.
85. Kouho H, Aoki T, Hisaoka M, Hashimoto H. Clinicopathological and interphase cytogenetic analysis of desmoid tumours. Histopathology 31:336, 1997.
86. Kullendorff CM, Donner M, Mertens F, Mandahl N. Chromosomal aberrations in a consecutive series of childhood rhabdomyosarcoma. Med Pediatr Oncol 30:156, 1998.
87. Kuroda M, Ishida T, Horiuchi H, et al. Chimeric TLS/FUS-CHOP gene expression and the heterogeneity of its junction in human myxoid and round cell liposarcoma. Am J Pathol 147: 1221, 1995.
88. Ladanyi M, Gerald W. Fusion of the EWS and WT1 genes in the desmoplastic small round cell tumor. Cancer Res 54:2837, 1994.
89. Ladanyi M, Heinemann FS, Huvos AG, et al. Neural differentiation in small round cell tumors of bone and soft tissue with the translocation t(11;22)(q24;q12): an immunohistochemical study of 11 cases. Hum Pathol 21:1245, 1990.
90. Legius E, Marchuk DA, Collins FS, Glover TW. Somatic deletion of the neurofibromatosis type 1 gene in a neurofibrosarcoma supports a tumour suppressor gene hypothesis. Nat Genet 3:122, 1993.
91. Lichter P, Tang CJ, Call K, et al. High-resolution mapping of human chromosome 11 by in situ hybridization with cosmid clones. Science 247:64, 1990.
92. Limon J, Dal Cin P, Sandberg AA. Application of long-term collagenase disaggregation for the cytogenetic analysis of human solid tumors. Cancer Genet Cytogenet 23:305, 1986.
93. Limon J, Mrozek K, Mandahl N, et al. Cytogenetics of synovial sarcoma: presentation of ten new cases and review of the literature. Genes Chromosomes Cancer 3:338, 1991.
94. Llombart-Bosch A, Carda C, Peydro-Olaya A, et al. Soft tissue Ewing's sarcoma: characterization in established cultures and xenografts with evidence of a neuroectodermic phenotype. Cancer 66:2589, 1990.
95. Lutchman M, Rouleau GA. The neurofibromatosis type 2 gene product, schwannomin, suppresses growth of NIH 3T3 cells. Cancer Res 55:2270, 1995.
96. Mandahl N, Heim S, Arheden K, et al. Rings, dicentrics, and telomeric association in histiocytomas. Cancer Genet Cytogenet 30:23, 1988.
97. Mandahl N, Heim S, Willen H, et al. Characteristic karyotypic anomalies identify subtypes of malignant fibrous histiocytoma. Genes Chromosomes Cancer 1:9, 1989.
98. Mandahl N, Hoglund M, Mertens F, et al. Cytogenetic aberrations in 188 benign and borderline adipose tissue tumors. Genes Chromosomes Cancer 9:207, 1994.
99. Mandahl N, Mertens F, Willen H, et al. A new cytogenetic subgroup in lipomas: loss of chromosome 16 material in spindle cell and pleomorphic lipomas. J Cancer Res Clin Oncol 120:707, 1994.
100. Mandahl N, Orndal C, Heim S, et al. Aberrations of chromosome segment 12q13–15 characterize a subgroup of hemangiopericytomas. Cancer 71:3009, 1993.
101. Marci V, Casorzo L, Sarotto I, et al. Gastrointestinal stromal tumor, uncommitted type, with monosomies 14 and 22 as the only chromosomal abnormalities. Cancer Genet Cytogenet 102: 135, 1998.
102. Mashal RD, Fejzo ML, Friedman AJ, et al. Analysis of androgen receptor DNA reveals the independent clonal origins of uterine leiomyomata and the secondary nature of cytogenetic aberrations in the development of leiomyomata. Genes Chromosomes Cancer 11:1, 1994.
103. Maurici D, Perez-Atayde A, Grier HE, et al. Frequency and implications of chromosome 8 and 12 gains in Ewing sarcoma. Cancer Genet Cytogenet 100:106, 1998.
104. Merel P, Hoang-Xuan K, Sanson M, et al. Predominant occurrence of somatic mutations of the NF2 gene in meningiomas and schwannomas. Genes Chromosomes Cancer 13:211, 1995.
105. Merel P, Khe HX, Sanson M, et al. Screening for germ-line mutations in the NF2 gene. Genes Chromosomes Cancer 12: 117, 1995.

106. Mertens F, Fletcher CD, Dal Cin P, et al. Cytogenetic analysis of 46 pleomorphic soft tissue sarcomas and correlation with morphologic and clinical features: a report of the CHAMP Study Group: chromosomes and morphology. Genes Chromosomes Cancer 22:16, 1998.
107. Mertens F, Rydholm A, Brosjo O, et al. Hibernomas are characterized by rearrangements of chromosome bands 11q13-21. Int J Cancer 58:503, 1994.
108. Mertens F, Willen H, Rydholm A, et al. Trisomy 20 is a primary chromosome aberration in desmoid tumors. Int J Cancer 63:527, 1995.
109. Mills SE, Frierson HF Jr. Olfactory neuroblastoma: a clinicopathologic study of 21 cases. Am J Surg Pathol 9:317, 1985.
110. Misra DN, Dickman PS, Yunis EJ. Fluorescence in situ hybridization (FISH) detection of MYCN oncogene amplification in neuroblastoma using paraffin-embedded tissues. Diagn Mol Pathol 4:128, 1995.
111. Mitelman F. ISCN (1995): An International System for Human Cytogenetic Nomenclature. Karger, Basel, 1995.
112. Mitelman F. Catalog of Chromosome Aberrations in Cancer '98. Wiley-Liss, New York, 1998.
113. Miyaki M, Konishi M, Kikuchi-Yanoshita R, et al. Coexistence of somatic and germ-line mutations of APC gene in desmoid tumors from patients with familial adenomatous polyposis. Cancer Res 53:5079, 1993.
114. Mrozek K, Karakousis CP, Bloomfield CD. Band 11q13 is nonrandomly rearranged in hibernomas. Genes Chromosomes Cancer 9:145, 1994.
115. Mugneret F, Lizard S, Aurias A, Turc-Carel C. Chromosomes in Ewing's sarcoma. II. Nonrandom additional changes, trisomy 8 and der(16)t(1;16). Cancer Genet Cytogenet 32:239, 1988.
116. Mydlo JH, Shore N, Reuter V, Herr HW. Perirenal lipoma versus renal cell carcinoma. Urology 38:67, 1991.
117. Naeem R, Lux ML, Huang SF, et al. Ring chromosomes in dermatofibrosarcoma protuberans are composed of interspersed sequences from chromosomes 17 and 22. Am J Pathol 147:1553, 1995.
118. Nakahara M, Isozaki K, Hirota S, et al. A novel gain-of-function mutation of c-kit gene in gastrointestinal stromal tumors. Gastroenterology 115:1090, 1998.
119. Nilbert M, Heim S. Uterine leiomyoma cytogenetics. Genes Chromosomes Cancer 2:3, 1990.
120. Nilbert M, Heim S, Mandahl N, et al. Trisomy 12 in uterine leiomyomas: a new cytogenetic subgroup. Cancer Genet Cytogenet 45:63, 1990.
121. Nishida T, Hirota S, Taniguchi M, et al. Familial gastrointestinal stromal tumours with germline mutation of the kit gene. Nat Genet 19:323, 1998.
122. Noguera R, Navarro S, Triche TJ. Translocation (11;22) in small cell osteosarcoma. Cancer Genet Cytogenet 45:121, 1990.
123. O'Brien KP, Seroussi E, Dal Cin P, et al. Various regions within the alpha-helical domain of the COL1A1 gene are fused to the second exon of the PDGFB gene in dermatofibrosarcomas and giant-cell fibroblastomas. Genes Chromosomes Cancer 23:187, 1998.
124. Orndal C, Mandahl N, Rydholm A, et al. Supernumerary ring chromosomes in five bone and soft tissue tumors of low or borderline malignancy. Cancer Genet Cytogenet 60:170, 1992.
125. Ozisik YY, Meloni AM, Stephenson CF, et al. Chromosome abnormalities in breast fibroadenomas. Cancer Genet Cytogenet 77:125, 1994.
126. Pandis N, Heim S, Bardi G, et al. Chromosome analysis of 96 uterine leiomyomas. Cancer Genet Cytogenet 55:11, 1991.
127. Parham DM, Shapiro DN, Downing JR, et al. Solid alveolar rhabdomyosarcomas with the t(2;13): report of two cases with diagnostic implications. Am J Surg Pathol 18:474, 1994.
128. Pedeutour F, Coindre JM, Nicolo G, et al. Ring chromosomes in dermatofibrosarcoma protuberans contain chromosome 17 sequences: fluorescence in situ hybridization. Cancer Genet Cytogenet 67:149, 1993.
129. Pedeutour F, Forus A, Coindre JM, et al. Structure of the supernumerary ring and giant rod chromosomes in adipose tissue tumors. Genes Chromosomes Cancer 24:30, 1999.
130. Pedeutour F, Simon MP, Minoletti F, et al. Ring 22 chromosomes in dermatofibrosarcoma protuberans are low-level amplifiers of chromosome 17 and 22 sequences. Cancer Res 55: 2400, 1995.
131. Perez-Atayde AR, Kozakewich HP, McGill T, Fletcher JA. Hemangiopericytoma of the tongue in a 12-year-old child: ultrastructural and cytogenetic observations. Hum Pathol 25:425, 1994.
132. Peter M, Couturier J, Pacquement H, et al. A new member of the ETS family fused to EWS in Ewing tumors. Oncogene 14: 1159, 1997.
133. Peulve P, Michot C, Vannier JP, et al. Clear cell sarcoma with t(12;22) (q13-14;q12). Genes Chromosomes Cancer 3:400, 1991.
134. Pinkel D, Landegent J, Collins C, et al. Fluorescence in situ hybridization with human chromosome-specific libraries: detection of trisomy 21 and translocations of chromosome 4. Proc Natl Acad Sci USA 85:9138, 1988.
135. Popescu NC, Chahinian AP, DiPaolo JP. Nonrandom chromosome alterations in human malignant mesothelioma. Cancer Res 48:142, 1988.
136. Rao UN, Surti U, Hoffner L, Yaw K. Cytogenetic and histologic correlation of peripheral nerve sheath tumors of soft tissue. Cancer Genet Cytogenet 88:17, 1996.
137. Rein MS, Friedman AJ, Barbieri RL, et al. Cytogenetic abnormalities in uterine leiomyomata. Obstet Gynecol 77:923, 1991.
138. Ried T. Interphase cytogenetics and its role in molecular diagnostics of solid tumors. Am J Pathol 152:325, 1998.
139. Rodriguez E, Sreekantaiah C, Gerald W, et al. A recurring translocation, t(11;22)(p13;q11.2), characterizes intra-abdominal desmoplastic small round-cell tumors. Cancer Genet Cytogenet 69:17, 1993.
140. Rosty C, Peter M, Zucman J, et al. Cytogenetic and molecular analysis of a t(1;22)(p36;q11.2) in a rhabdoid tumor with a putative homozygous deletion of chromosome 22. Genes Chromosomes Cancer 21:82, 1998.
141. Rouleau GA, Merel P, Lutchman M, et al. Alteration in a new gene encoding a putative membrane-organizing protein causes neuro-fibromatosis type 2. Nature 363:515, 1993.
142. Rubin BP, Chen CJ, Morgan TW, et al. Congenital mesoblastic nephroma t(12;15) is associated with ETV6-NTRK3 gene fusion: cytogenetic and molecular relationship to congenital (infantile) fibrosarcoma. Am J Pathol 153:1451, 1998.
143. Saboorian MH, Ashfaq R, Vandersteenhoven JJ, Schneider NR. Cytogenetics as an adjunct in establishing a definitive diagnosis of synovial sarcoma by fine-needle aspiration. Cancer 81: 187, 1997.
144. Sainati L, Scapinello A, Montaldi A, et al. A mesenchymal chondrosarcoma of a child with the reciprocal translocation (11;22)(q24;q12). Cancer Genet Cytogenet 71:144, 1993.
145. Sandberg AA, Bridge JA. The Cytogenetics of Bone and Soft Tissue Tumors. R.G. Landes, Austin, TX, 1995.
146. Sandberg AA, Turc-Carel C, Gemmill RM. Chromosomes in solid tumors and beyond. Cancer Res 48:1049, 1988.
147. Sarlomo-Rikala M, el-Rifai W, Lahtinen T, et al. Different patterns of DNA copy number changes in gastrointestinal stromal tumors, leiomyomas, and schwannomas. Hum Pathol 29:476, 1998.

148. Saunders AL, Meloni AM, Chen Z, et al. Two cases of low-grade gastric leiomyosarcoma with monosomy 14 as the only change. Cancer Genet Cytogenet 90:184, 1996.
149. Sawada S, Florell S, Purandare SM, et al. Identification of NF1 mutations in both alleles of a dermal neurofibroma. Nat Genet 14:110, 1996.
150. Schoenmakers EF, Huysmans C, van de Ven WJ. Allelic knockout of novel splice variants of human recombination repair gene RAD51B in t(12;14) uterine leiomyomas. Cancer Res 59:19, 1999.
151. Schoenmakers EF, Wanschura S, Mols R, et al. Recurrent rearrangements in the high mobility group protein gene, HMGI-C, in benign mesenchymal tumours. Nat Genet 10:436, 1995.
152. Schofield DE, Fletcher JA. Trisomy 12 in pediatric granulosa-stromal cell tumors: demonstration by a modified method of fluorescence in situ hybridization on paraffin-embedded material. Am J Pathol 141:1265, 1992.
153. Schofield DE, Fletcher JA, Grier HE, Yunis EJ. Fibrosarcoma in infants and children: application of new techniques. Am J Surg Pathol 18:14, 1994.
154. Schofield DE, Yunis EJ, Fletcher JA. Chromosome aberrations in mesoblastic nephroma. Am J Pathol 143:714, 1993.
155. Schrock E, du Manoir S, Veldman T, et al. Multicolor spectral karyotyping of human chromosomes. Science 273:494, 1996.
156. Scrable H, Witte D, Shimada H, et al. Molecular differential pathology of rhabdomyosarcoma. Genes Chromosomes Cancer 1:23, 1989.
157. Seabright M. A rapid banding technique for human chromosomes. Lancet 2:971, 1971.
158. Sen-Gupta S, Van der Luijt RB, Bowles LV, et al. Somatic mutation of APC gene in desmoid tumour in familial adenomatous polyposis. Lancet 342:552, 1993.
159. Shapiro DN, Sublett JE, Li B, et al. Fusion of PAX3 to a member of the forkhead family of transcription factors in human alveolar rhabdomyosarcoma. Cancer Res 53:5108, 1993.
160. Shapiro DN, Valentine MB, Rowe ST, et al. Detection of N-myc gene amplification by fluorescence in situ hybridization: diagnostic utility for neuroblastoma. Am J Pathol 142:1339, 1993.
161. Shashi V, Lovell MA, von Kap-Herr C, et al. Malignant rhabdoid tumor of the kidney: involvement of chromosome 22. Genes Chromosomes Cancer 10:49, 1994.
162. Shipley JM, Clark J, Crew AJ, et al. The t(X;18)(p11.2;q11.2) translocation found in human synovial sarcomas involves two distinct loci on the X chromosome. Oncogene 9:1447, 1994.
163. Shmookler BM, Enzinger FM, Weiss SW. Giant cell fibroblastoma: a juvenile form of dermatofibrosarcoma protuberans. Cancer 64:2154, 1989.
164. Simon MP, Pedeutour F, Sirvent N, et al. Deregulation of the platelet-derived growth factor B-chain gene via fusion with collagen gene COL1A1 in dermatofibrosarcoma protuberans and giant-cell fibroblastoma. Nat Genet 15:95, 1997.
165. Snyder CS, Dell'Aquila M, Haghighi P, et al. Clonal changes in inflammatory pseudotumor of the lung: a case report. Cancer 76:1545, 1995.
166. Sorensen PH, Lessnick SL, Lopez-Terrada D, et al. A second Ewing's sarcoma translocation, t(21;22), fuses the EWS gene to another ETS-family transcription factor, ERG. Nat Genet 6:146, 1994.
167. Sorensen PH, Wu JK, Berean KW, et al. Olfactory neuroblastoma is a peripheral primitive neuroectodermal tumor related to Ewing sarcoma. Proc Natl Acad Sci USA 93:1038, 1996.
168. Speel EJ, Ramaekers FC, Hopman AH. Cytochemical detection systems for in situ hybridization, and the combination with immunocytochemistry, "who is still afraid of red, green and blue?" Histochem J 27:833, 1995.
169. Speleman F, Cin PD, Van Roy N, et al. Is t(6;20)(p21;q13) a characteristic chromosome change in endometrial polyps? Genes Chromosomes Cancer 3:318, 1991.
170. Speleman F, Colpaert C, Goovaerts G, et al. Malignant melanoma of soft parts: further cytogenetic characterization. Cancer Genet Cytogenet 60:176, 1992.
171. Sreekantaiah C, Bridge JA, Rao UN, et al. Clonal chromosomal abnormalities in hemangiopericytoma. Cancer Genet Cytogenet 54:173, 1991.
172. Sreekantaiah C, Davis JR, Sandberg AA. Chromosomal abnormalities in leiomyosarcomas. Am J Pathol 142:293, 1993.
173. Sreekantaiah C, Karakousis CP, Leong SP, Sandberg AA. Cytogenetic findings in liposarcoma correlate with histopathologic subtypes. Cancer 69:2484, 1992.
174. Sreekantaiah C, Ladanyi M, Rodriguez E, Chaganti RS. Chromosomal aberrations in soft tissue tumors: relevance to diagnosis, classification, and molecular mechanisms. Am J Pathol 144:1121, 1994.
175. Sreekantaiah C, Leong SP, Karakousis CP, et al. Cytogenetic profile of 109 lipomas. Cancer Res 51:422, 1991.
176. Stenman G, Kindblom LG, Angervall L. Reciprocal translocation t(12;22)(q13;q13) in clear-cell sarcoma of tendons and aponeuroses. Genes Chromosomes Cancer 4:122, 1992.
177. Stephenson CF, Davis RI, Moore GE, Sandberg AA. Cytogenetic and fluorescence in situ hybridization analysis of breast fibroadenomas. Cancer Genet Cytogenet 63:32, 1992.
178. Stock C, Ambros IM, Mann G, et al. Detection of Ip36 deletions in paraffin sections of neuroblastoma tissues. Genes Chromosomes Cancer 6:1, 1993.
179. Su LD, Atayde-Perez A, Sheldon S, et al. Inflammatory myofibroblastic tumor: cytogenetic evidence supporting clonal origin. Mod Pathol 11:364, 1998.
180. Taguchi T, Jhanwar SC, Siegfried JM, et al. Recurrent deletions of specific chromosomal sites in 1p, 3p, 6q, and 9p in human malignant mesothelioma. Cancer Res 53:4349, 1993.
181. Tiainen M, Tammilehto L, Mattson K, Knuutila S. Nonrandom chromosomal abnormalities in malignant pleural mesothelioma. Cancer Genet Cytogenet 33:251, 1998.
182. Travis JA, Bridge JA. Significance of both numerical and structural chromosomal abnormalities in clear cell sarcoma. Cancer Genet Cytogenet 64:104, 1992.
183. Treissman SP, Gillis DA, Lee CL, et al. Omental-mesenteric inflammatory pseudotumor: cytogenetic demonstration of genetic changes and monoclonality in one tumor. Cancer 73:1433, 1994.
184. Trofatter JA, MacCollin MM, Rutter JL, et al. A novel moesin-, ezrin-, radixin-like gene is a candidate for the neurofibromatosis 2 tumor suppressor. Cell 72:791, 1993.
185. Turc-Carel C, Aurias A, Mugneret F, et al. Chromosomes in Ewing's sarcoma. I. An evaluation of 85 cases of remarkable consistency of t(11;22)(q24;q12). Cancer Genet Cytogenet 32:229, 1988.
186. Turc-Carel C, Dal Cin P, Limon J, et al. Involvement of chromosome X in primary cytogenetic change in human neoplasia: nonrandom translocation in synovial sarcoma. Proc Natl Acad Sci USA 84:1981, 1987.
187. Turc-Carel C, Dal Cin P, Rao U, et al. Recurrent breakpoints at 9q31 and 22q12.2 in extraskeletal myxoid chondrosarcoma. Cancer Genet Cytogenet 30:145, 1988.
188. Turc-Carel C, Limon J, Dal Cin P, et al. Cytogenetic studies of adipose tissue tumors. II. Recurrent reciprocal translocation t(12;16)(q13;p11) in myxoid liposarcomas. Cancer Genet Cytogenet 23:291, 1986.
189. Turc-Carel C, Lizard-Nacol S, Justrabo E, et al. Consistent chromosomal translocation in alveolar rhabdomyosarcoma. Cancer Genet Cytogenet 19:361, 1986.

190. Turc-Carel C, Philip I, Berger MP, et al. Chromosome study of Ewing's sarcoma (ES) cell lines: consistency of a reciprocal translocation t(11;22)(q24;q12). Cancer Genet Cytogenet 12:1, 1984.
191. Twist EC, Ruttledge MH, Rousseau M, et al. The neurofibromatosis type 2 gene is inactivated in schwannomas. Hum Mol Genet 3:147, 1994.
192. Versteege I, Sevenet N, Lange J, et al. Truncating mutations of hSNF5/INI1 in aggressive paediatric cancer. Nature 394:203, 1998.
193. Wang-Wuu S, Soukup S, Ballard E, et al. Chromosomal analysis of sixteen human rhabdomyosarcomas. Cancer Res 48:983, 1988.
194. Whang-Peng J, Freter CE, Knutsen T, et al. Translocation t(11;22) in esthesioneuroblastoma. Cancer Genet Cytogenet 29:155, 1987.
195. Whang-Peng J, Knutsen T, Theil K, et al. Cytogenetic studies in subgroups of rhabdomyosarcoma. Genes Chromosomes Cancer 5:299, 1992.
196. Xiao S, Renshaw AA, Cibas ES, et al. Novel fluorescence in situ hybridization approaches in solid tumors: characterization of frozen specimens, touch preparations, and cytologic preparations. Am J Pathol 147:896, 1995.
197. Xing YP, Powell WL, Morton CC. The del(7q) subgroup in uterine leiomyomata: genetic and biologic characteristics; further evidence for the secondary nature of cytogenetic abnormalities in the pathobiology of uterine leiomyomata. Cancer Genet Cytogenet 98:69, 1997.
198. Yoshida MA, Ikeuchi T, Iwama T, et al. Chromosome changes in desmoid tumors developed in patients with familial adenomatous polyposis. Jpn J Cancer Res 82:916, 1991.
199. Zoubek A, Dockhorn-Dworniczak B, Delattre O, et al. Does expression of different EWS chimeric transcripts define clinically distinct risk groups of Ewing tumor patients? J Clin Oncol 14:1245, 1996.
200. Zucman J, Delattre O, Desmaze C, et al. EWS and ATF-1 gene fusion induced by t(12;22) translocation in malignant melanoma of soft parts. Nat Genet 4:341, 1993.

## Recent Developments

1. Ladanyi M, Lui MY, Antonescu CR, et al. The der(17)t(X;17)(p11;q25) of human alveolar soft part sarcoma fuses the *TFE3* transcription factor gene to *ASPL,* a novel gene at 17q25. Oncogene, in press.
2. Koontz J, Soreng AL, Nucci M, et al. Frequent fusion of two previously unknown genes, *JAXF1* and *JJAZ1,* in endometrial stromal tumors. Submitted for publication, 2000.
3. Griffin CA, Hawkins AL, Dvorak C, et al. Recurrent involvement of 2p23 in inflammatory myofibroblastic tumors. Cancer Res 59:2776, 1999.
4. Lawrence B, Perez-Atayde A, Hibbard MK, et al. TPM3-ALK and TPM4-ALK oncogenes in inflammatory myofibroblastic tumors. Am J Pathol 157:377, 2000.
5. Ladanyi M. Aberrant ALK tyrosine kinase signaling. Different cellular lineages, common oncogenic mechanisms. Am J Pathol 157:341, 2000.
6. Hibbard MK, Kozakewich HP, Dal Cin P, et al. PLAG1 fusion oncogenes in lipoblastoma. Cancer Res 60:4869, 2000.

CHAPTER 6

# FINE NEEDLE ASPIRATION BIOPSIES OF SOFT TISSUE TUMORS

KIM R. GEISINGER AND FADI W. ABDUL-KARIM

Fine needle aspiration biopsies (FNABs) have become an established tool in the diagnostic armamentarium of many clinical practices. The initial diagnosis of many mass lesions in both superficial (e.g., breast and thyroid) and deep (e.g., lung and pancreas) body sites can often be readily and safely assessed by FNAB. One of the few remaining frontiers for FNAB is evaluation of primary soft tissue tumors.[1,7,8,17,18,22,26,27,33,38,41,49,51–53,60,65,82,92,109]

## GENERAL CONSIDERATIONS

Several important challenges are inherent to the FNAB evaluation of soft tissue neoplasms. First, many of these lesions, especially the sarcomas, are rare. Accordingly, most practicing pathologists do not encounter them on a routine basis and may not be familiar with their morphologic, clinical, and radiographic features. Another reason pathologists may be reluctant to evaluate soft tissue tumors is that they have overlapping histopathologic and cytomorphologic attributes that are further compounded by the morphologic heterogeneity present in some of these mass lesions. The increasing recognition of borderline tumors or neoplasms of intermediate malignancy make the interpretation of FNAB of soft tissue masses even more problematic. For these reasons, some pathologists and surgeons, particularly those from Scandinavia, have advocated that the diagnosis and treatment of many soft tissue lesions, especially sarcomas, take place in centralized medical facilities.[7,8,85]

The FNAB has a number of distinct, well recognized advantages that require consideration for its application to orthopedic neoplasms.[1,8,49] Aspiration biopsy, compared to other techniques, is a rapid outpatient procedure that can provide an immediate diagnosis. It permits the orthopedic surgeon to discuss potential additional diagnostic procedures and therapy with the patient during the initial visit. It also facilitates further processing or triaging of the patient by the surgeon. Patients suffer relatively little pain or discomfort from the aspiration procedure, and in most circumstances local anesthesia is not necessary. The needle for administering the local anesthetic has a larger caliber (and therefore more potential for pain) than the diameter of the aspiration needle. A major advantage of FNAB over core-needle biopsies is the much greater sampling of a mass lesion. By altering the direction of the needle during a single puncture, multiple portions of the mass can be aspirated. If necessary, multiple separate needle punctures can be performed during a single patient visit. Cellular material may be obtained during the same biopsy setting for cell blocks. Cell blocks are preferred to direct smears for immunocytochemical studies that assist in determining the histogenesis of a neoplasm. Material may also be obtained by FNAB for electron microscopy, cytogenetics, and molecular biologic analysis.

The FNAB has a low rate of significant clinical complications, and most patients there are none. Others may suffer bleeding, edema, or tenderness at the biopsy site. The procedure does not disrupt tissue planes or contaminate the subsequent surgical site. Thus "no bridges are burned," and if not diagnostic the FNAB can be followed by another biopsy procedure. There has not been any documented instance of needle tracking of sarcomatous tumor cells by a fine needle. Finally, compared to all other biopsy techniques, FNAB is relatively inexpensive and viewed as cost-effective in our current medical economic milieu.

Unfortunately, however, FNAB has several disadvantages, some of which are relatively specific for orthopedic lesions.[1,8,39,49,67,76] FNAB always results in relatively small samples of a tumor. There is dispersion of individual cells inherent in the aspiration technique and at least partial loss of recognizable diagnostic tissue patterns. These limitations inevitably can result in less-specific diagnoses with regard to histologic type and subtype of tumors. Thus, even if the neoplasm can be identified as sarcomatous, the cytopathologist may not be able to define more specifically the exact type of malignant mesenchymal tumor. It may also be difficult to distinguish among benign cellular lesions, borderline tumors, and low grade sarcomas. As discussed later in this chapter, accurate grading of many sarcomas is impossible when utilizing current histopathologic classification schemes. As with other types of tumors, in densely collagenized or sclerotic masses or highly vascular lesions FNAB may provide only sparse cellularity on the smear, making a benign versus malignant distinction impossible.

It is important to emphasize that diagnosis of a soft tissue tumor by aspiration biopsy always requires the intimate cooperation and interaction of orthopedic surgeons, radiologists, and pathologists. This is absolutely necessary to optimize the integration of all clinically relevant information to achieve the best cytologic diagnosis. Whenever possible, an on-site evaluation of the aspirate by the pathologist is preferred. It provides the opportunity for the pathologist to provide an on-site evaluation of adequacy and to review important imaging studies, discuss the mass lesion with the surgeon, and possibly examine the patient.[8,49]

## ACCURACY

Several factors must be considered prior to determining the diagnostic accuracy of FNAB of musculoskeletal masses. Only a few series with large numbers of patients have been published.[7,8,18,22,27,51,53,60,65,69,109] In addition, there appears to be a lack of standardization or uniformity among these reports. Some studies have included patients with both benign and malignant neoplasms,[7,8,18,22,53,60,109] whereas others addressed only sarcomas.[27,51] A number of series are dedicated to the primary diagnosis of a mass, whereas others include many patients with recurrent sarcomas. Several studies have included aspiration biopsies of bone and soft tissue lesions.[27,60] The manner in which the data are analyzed varies from series to series as well. Some authors have provided only the number of cases, whereas others have reported levels of diagnostic sensitivity and specificity, rates of false-negative and false-positive diagnoses, or both. Several excellent studies have details of cytomorphologic features of aspirates of soft tissue lesions but provide little or no numeric data regarding accuracy.[26,50,94]

Akerman and Willén from Sweden have described the largest series of FNAB of soft tissue lesions.[8] Over a 20-year period these investigators evaluated 517 patients with an aspirate for a primary diagnosis of a soft tissue neoplasm; of these lesions, 315 were benign and 202 were sarcomas. These authors were able to distinguish benign from malignant in 94% of the patients as proven by clinical follow-up, resection or both.[8] Their errors were equally divided between 14 false-negative interpretations and 14 false-positive diagnoses (Table 6–1). Among the latter, two patients underwent excessive surgical therapy. In their experience, and we agree, the area of greatest difficulty for morphologic interpretation is the spindle cell neoplasms followed by lipomatous tumors.[8]

From Sweden, Brosjö et al. evaluated 342 patients with a relatively equal distribution between benign and malignant soft tissue tumors.[22] The FNAB diagnosis was conclusive in 300 of these patients (88%). There was a 5% false-negative rate among the 153 benign cytologic diagnoses, and a 2% false-positive rate resulted among the 147 malignant cytologic diag-

**TABLE 6–1 DIAGNOSTIC ACCURACY OF FNAB OF SOFT TISSUE TUMORS**

| Study | Benign Tumors (no.) | Sarcomas (no.) | False-positive Rate (%) | False-negative Rate (%) |
|---|---|---|---|---|
| Akerman and Willén[8] | 315 | 202 | 4 | 7 |
| Brosjö et al.[22] | 149 | 151 | 2 | 5 |
| Oland et al.[69] | 17 | 25 | 0 | 6 |
| Miralles et al.[65] | 34 | 60 | 4 | 0 |
| Layfield et al.[53] | 63 | 51 | 2 | 4 |
| Bennert and Abdul-Karim[18] | 16 | 37 | 0 | 0 |
| Costa et al.[27] | * | 41 | 8 | 7 |
| Kilpatrick et al.[51] | ** | 68 | ** | 3 |

* Not clear from published data.
** Only examined sarcomas.

noses. Accordingly, a correct diagnosis was rendered in 97% of this population.

From Israel, Oland and colleagues reported their experience with 196 patients, including children, who underwent FNAB of a soft tissue mass.[69] Altogether,[132] patients had a benign cytologic diagnosis (tumor or inflammation) and were followed medically. Another 16 patients were diagnosed with metastatic carcinoma, without subsequent surgery. A total of 48 patients underwent histologic examination of their masses following the FNAB, and all 25 FNAB diagnoses of frank sarcoma were confirmed; thus there were no false-positive interpretations. Of the 17 benign soft tissue tumors diagnosed by cytology, one was a false-negative interpretation: A diagnosis of fibroma was rendered in an individual who was proven to have a fibrosarcoma. The final six patients had an FNAB diagnosis that did not commit between benign and malignant; their subsequent histologic evaluations all proved to be benign.[69]

Miralles et al. reported a series of 117 soft tissue FNABs from Spain,[65] with the lesions relatively evenly divided between benign and malignant tumors. Unlike the above cited studies in which FNAB was used for primary evaluation of a soft tissue mass, many specimens studied by Miralles et al. were clinically suspected recurrences or metastases of previously documented sarcomas.[65] These investigators had no false-negative interpretations, but they did report a 4% false-positive diagnosis rate. One of the two patients with a false-positive result actually had fat necrosis that was diagnosed in the smears as a liposarcoma; excessive surgery was the unfortunate result. Importantly, their paper contained a statement that makes us ponder whether the statistics were completely accurate. The authors stated in their discussion of pseudosarcomatous mass lesions that "we encountered difficulties in the correct diagnosis of these lesions and thus recommend an open biopsy for their exact diagnosis." None of the benign specimens in their series, however, were considered among the traditional pseudosarcomatous lesions. If the latter had been included, we suspect that their false-positive rate might have been higher.

In the United States, Layfield et al.[53] and Bennert and Abdul-Karim[18] reported series of similar size. Layfield et al.'s series included 114 sufficient aspirates from patients with benign and malignant soft tissue lesions, including 51 individuals with histologically documented soft tissue sarcomas.[53] These authors had false-positive and false-negative rates of 2% and 4%, respectively. Two patients in whom lipomas were aspirated had a cytologic diagnosis of liposarcoma. The authors did not inform the reader if there were any adverse clinical outcomes for these two patients. The study by Bennert and Abdul-Karim specifically compared the results of FNAB and subsequent tissue core needle biopsies.[18] Among the 117 soft tissue lesions, 38% of the aspirates were considered unsatisfactory for evaluation (insufficient cellularity), and 17% were inflammatory. The remaining 53 aspirates (45%) were considered diagnostic of a soft tissue tumor. All 16 benign aspiration interpretations were correct, as were the 37 aspiration diagnoses of sarcoma. Although the core needle biopsies provided more specific typing of the sarcoma than did the FNAB in 19% of the malignant diagnoses, the overall clinical management of the patients was not improved by the use of the tissue core biopsies. In their cases with histologic confirmation, the levels of diagnostic sensitivity and specificity were both 100% for the cytologic interpretations.

A series by Costa et al. included 52 FNABs of 46 soft tissue and 6 bone neoplasms.[27] Among the biopsies, 43 were for a primary diagnosis, and 9 were for clinically suspected recurrence. Costa et al. reported a 7% false-negative rate and an 8% false-positive diagnostic rate; most of the latter occurred during evaluation of potential recurrent tumors. This suggests to us that some pathologists may be more comfortable rendering a malignant interpretation in patients with a previous histologic diagnosis of sarcoma.[27] In our opinion, the same strict cytomorphologic criteria for recurrent sarcoma should be applied as when making a primary diagnosis of the same neoplasm.

Liu et al. systematically examined a series of 89 aspirates that included samples derived from 20 benign and 69 malignant masses including 11 metastatic malignant melanomas.[60] Among the aspirates,[69] were from soft tissue lesions. Each FNAB was independently evaluated by four pathologists who differed in their years of experience in performing and interpreting aspiration biopsies. Each pathologist evaluated these specimens in two settings: without and then later with the clinical history. In each of the two scenarios, each pathologist provided a precise cytopathologic diagnosis for the aspiration smears and classified the smears into one of four categories: benign, probably benign, probably malignant, or definitely malignant. These data were then utilized to create receiver operator characteristic (ROC) curves. Without benefit of the clinical history, the proportion of precise correct diagnoses ranged from 0.19 to 0.44. With addition of the clinical history, the proportions of precise interpretations improved to a range of 0.48–0.66. The proportion of correct diagnoses improved for all four cytopathologists. These results strongly support our contention that one must integrate relevant clinical data and radiographic interpretations whenever evaluating aspiration biopsies of soft tissue lesions.[60] Without addition of the clinical history, the proportion of correct classifications (as measured by the area under the ROC curve) ranged from 0.81 to 0.90. The range of correct classification improved to 0.89–0.90 with addition of the clinical history. Difficulty was especially noted for benign spindle cell tumors, including hemangiomas and nerve sheath neoplasms. Integration of the clinical history with the cytomorphology proved to be most useful for evaluating lipomatous neoplasms and particularly for diagnosing liposarcomas as definitely malignant. Interestingly, the clinical information was, in some cases, misleading in that the proportion of correct classifications declined for both hemangiomas and myositis ossificans. In the diagnostic exercises, the more experienced cytopathologists fared better when designating a precise diagnosis and determining the correct benign/malignant ratio. Overall, knowledge of the clinical history provided greater assistance for the less experienced pathologists. This reiterates the crucial premise that FNAB of soft tissue lesions should be interpreted in conjunction with the clinical and radiographic information pertaining to that specific mass.

Although the exact role to be played by FNAB in the clinical evaluation of soft tissue mass lesions remains controversial, we believe that the bulk of the reported data and our own practices strongly support its ability to distinguish accurately between benign and malignant soft tissue tumors (Table 6–1). The levels of diagnostic specificity and sensitivity are approximately 95% for establishing a frank diagnosis of sarcoma.[8,49] In addition, FNAB can accurately differentiate sarcomas from other forms of malignancy extending to or metastatic to soft tissues.

We are also of the opinion that FNAB can accurately subclassify soft tissue tumors (especially sarcomas) into general, clinically relevant categories (see below) that permit initiation of therapy in many patients. Specific subtyping is usually not necessary for this step, with the obvious exception of the round cell sarcomas. We believe that many pathologists are remiss when interpreting a proportion of soft tissue tumors in histologic preparations as to specific subtypes without the aid of ancillary diagnostic procedures such as immunohistochemistry and cytogenetic studies. With few exceptions, these same procedures can be readily applied to aspirated material; thus specific subtyping may be provided in a large proportion of nonpleomorphic sarcomas with the combination of cytomorphology and ancillary testing. A major limitation, however, may be retrieval of sufficient material to perform extensive testing. As discussed later, preoperative grading of sarcomas by FNAB may be problematic in a significant proportion of patients, but it does not prevent the oncologist from treating many patients appropriately. With more experience by a larger number of practicing pathologists, we are confident that FNAB will become a well accepted practice for initial evaluation of superficial and deep soft tissue lesions.

In a number of clinical investigations, the histologic grade of a sarcoma has been demonstrated to be an important, (perhaps the most crucial) single prognostic factor when predicting the risk of metastasis. Many histologic grading classifications have several microscopic features in common, including tumor cellularity. In general, cellularity is inversely related to the amount of extracellular matrix material. Other microscopic attributes include mitotic figure counts, the amount of tumor necrosis, nuclear pleomorphism, and the degree of tumor differentiation or histogenetic type of neoplasm.

Little attention has been paid to grading sarcomas in aspiration smears.[49,51,108] Willén et al. briefly discussed grouping sarcomatous aspirates into low and high grade neoplasms.[109] Within certain restrictions, we believe that many soft tissue sarcomas can be accurately graded by FNAB in a clinically relevant manner. To discuss this further, we introduce our classification of soft tissue sarcomas based on direct aspiration smears.

## GENERAL SARCOMA CLASSIFICATION

Soft tissue sarcomas can be classified into six general categories on the basis of the predominant appearance of the specimen in aspiration smears: myxoid, spindle cell, pleomorphic, polygonal cell, round cell, and miscellaneous.[49] The round cell and pleomorphic sarcomas are, by definition, high grade sarcomas, whereas most myxoid sarcomas fall into the low grade category. Accurate grading of the spindle cell and polygonal cell sarcomas is more challenging. The miscellaneous category includes diverse entities that may be difficult to distinguish from benign mesenchymal proliferations, the best example of which is well differentiated liposarcoma.

## MYXOID SARCOMAS

The myxoid sarcomas include myxoid liposarcoma, myxoid malignant fibrous histiocytoma (myxofibrosarcoma), and extraskeletal myxoid chondrosarcoma.[39,49,103] At low magnification the most apparent feature of the aspirate smears of these sarcomas is voluminous extracellular matrix material. Often this material presents as irregularly shaped, moderately sized fragments with or without embedded tumor cells (Figs. 6–1, 6–2). With the Romanowsky stains, the matrix appears as a reddish purple substance and varies from fibrillar to structureless and homogeneous

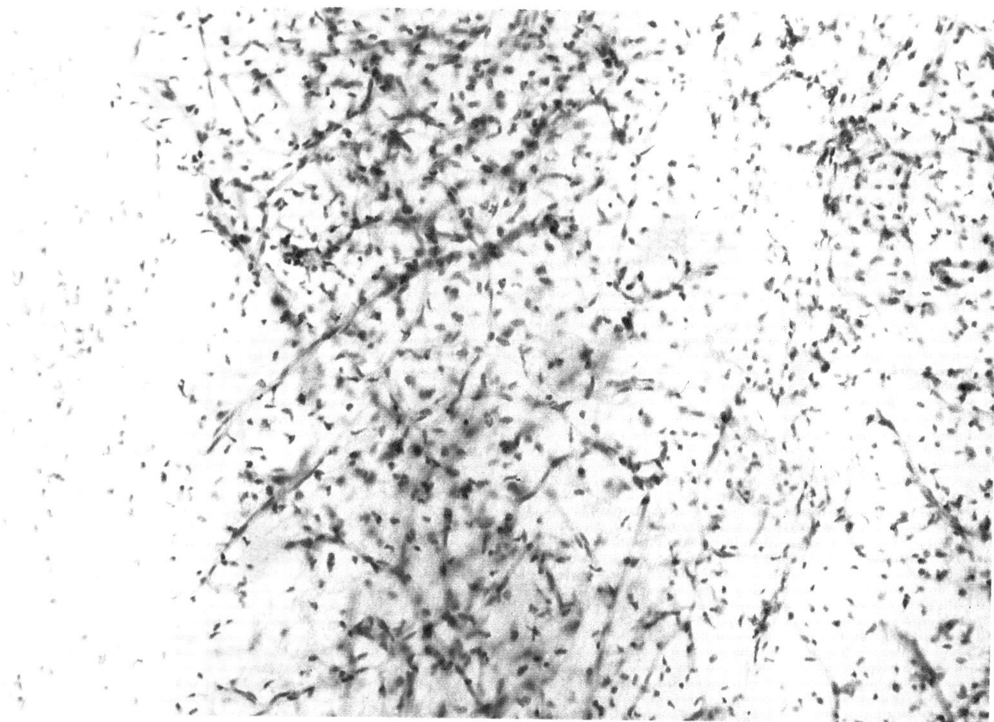

**FIGURE 6–1.** Myxoid liposarcoma. A moderate number of small, uniform neoplastic cells with solitary hyperchromatic nuclei are set in an abundant cyanophilic matrix, which also contains an obvious network of branched capillaries. Similar-appearing malignant cells are scattered adjacent to the fragment of matrix. (Papanicolaou stain, ×40)

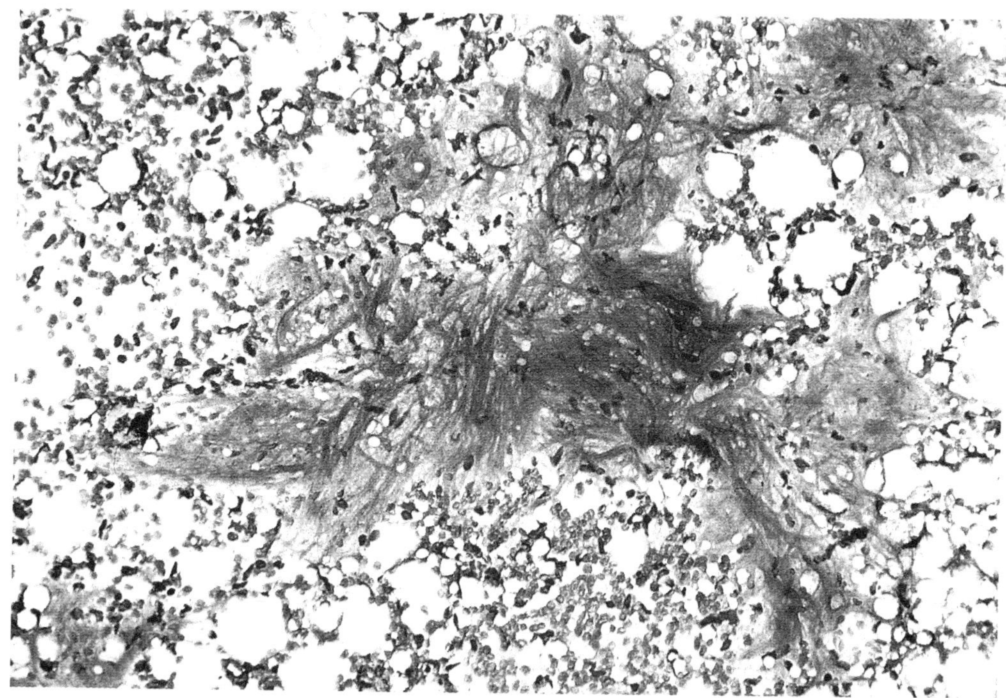

**FIGURE 6–2.** Myxoid liposarcoma. Fibrillar matrix contains a small number of small homogeneous malignant cells. Some of the neoplastic cells have one or more lipid vacuoles. (Diff-Quik stain, ×40)

in appearance (Figs. 6–2, 6–3). The matrix may appear metachromatic, especially in extraskeletal chondrosarcomas. The matrix is cyanophilic, and with the Papanicolaou stain it typically appears as a relatively watery pale green substance (Fig. 6–1). The edges of the fragments of matrix material may be sharply defined or blend irregularly with the background as delicate spicules extending from the body of the fragment. In the smear the sarcomatous cells are present as individually dispersed elements and in small aggregates, both embedded in the matrix material and free in the smear background. Typically, the malignant cells are relatively small and have stellate, spindled, or rounded contours. Their precise shapes are more apparent when they are unencumbered by the matrix. Most cells have a small to moderately sized, often densely hyperchromatic solitary nucleus. Nucleoli are generally small and inconspicuous. A few multinucleated giant tumor cells may also be randomly distributed in the smears.[64,70]

Gonzalez-Campora et al. reported an FNAB series of 16 myxoid soft tissue tumors, 5 of which were benign and 11 malignant.[39] We concur with their opinion that the only cells of diagnostic value in smears of lipomatous tumors are lipoblasts (Fig. 6–4). In our experience, lipoblasts may be sparse, requiring a careful search. Lipoblasts are characterized by rounded contours and scant to moderate volumes of cytoplasm that is occupied by one or more sharply defined lipid vacuoles. These vacuoles may be uniform in size or vary in diameter, but they characteristically displace the solitary nucleus to an eccentric cellular position and indent its membrane with a resultant scalloped contour.[103] Their nuclei show mild to moderate variability in size and are generally hyperchromatic. Another highly distinctive feature in smears of myxoid liposarcomas is the presence of branched delicate capillaries in the matrix material, a feature apparent at low magnification[8,66,98,103] (Figs. 6–1, 6–3). The smears also contain unspecialized small mesenchymal cells with high nuclear/cytoplasmic ratios and spindled or stellate contours; they are indistinguishable from many tumor cells in myxoid malignant fibrous histiocytomas. Poorly differentiated myxoid liposarcomas present in smears as large, round tumor cells with high nuclear/cytoplasmic ratios and occasional lipid vacuoles (Fig. 6–5). Finding a low grade component mixed with the obviously malignant round cells in the same aspirate is a helpful clue to correct classification of the latter. Only rarely has the aspiration appearance of lipoblastoma been described.[75] It may be indistinguishable from myxoid liposarcoma, making it essential that one is apprised of the age of the patient, as lipoblastoma occurs virtually only in children, and myxoid liposarcoma virtually never arises in patients less than 10 years of age.

Aspirates from myxoid malignant fibrous histiocy-

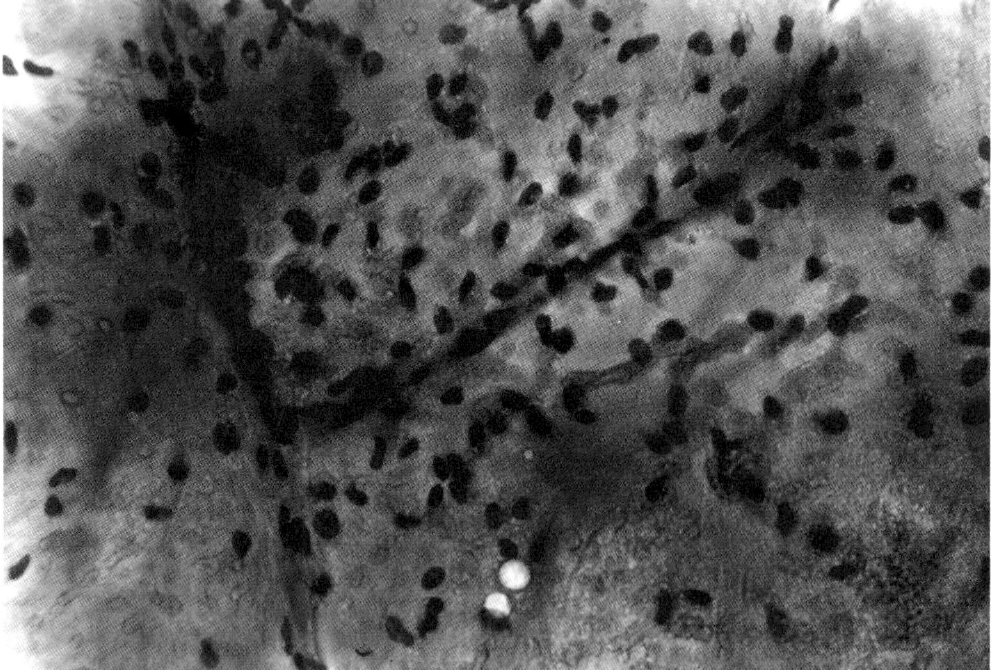

**FIGURE 6–3.** Myxoid liposarcoma. The small malignant cells are characterized by solitary darkly stained nuclei and high nuclear/cytoplasmic ratios. They appear to be fairly evenly scattered in the metachromatic matrix, which also contains a branched capillary. (Diff-Quik stain, ×400)

**FIGURE 6–4.** Myxoid liposarcoma. Small mononucleated neoplastic cells have one or more lipid vacuoles in the cytoplasm. In some cells multiple vacuoles indent the hyperchromatic nucleus. (Diff-Quik stain, ×400)

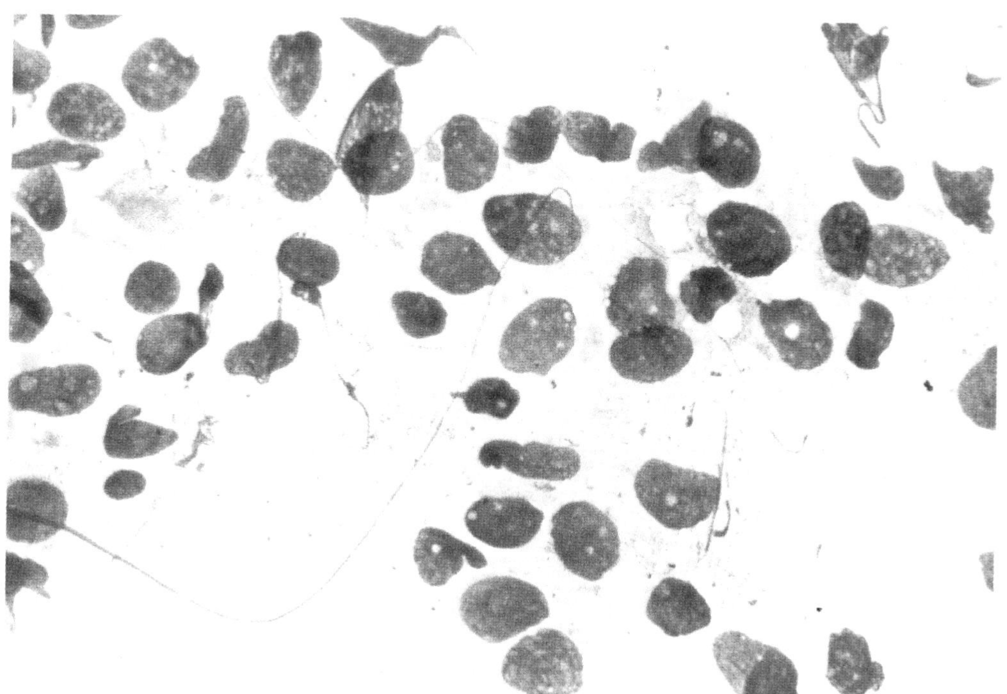

**FIGURE 6–5.** Round cell liposarcoma. The poorly differentiated variant of myxoid liposarcoma is composed of relatively small, uniform malignant cells characterized by large round nuclei, scanty cytoplasm, and occasionally prominent nucleoli. Cytoplasmic lipid vacuoles are seen in some of the neoplastic cells. (Diff-Quik stain, ×400)

tomas have abundant matrix material in the smears with three morphologic cell types: small spindle-shaped fibroblast-like cells, histiocytic cells, and multinucleated tumor giant cells[64] (Figs. 6–6, 6–7). In our experiences, it is the last cell type that distinguishes this tumor from other myxoid sarcomas. Aspirate smears from intramuscular myxomas are poorly cellular; they are characterized by voluminous matrix material with scattered spindled and stellate cells manifesting no atypia and fragments of atrophic muscle fibers.[39] Gonzalez-Campora et al. warned of two potential diagnostic pitfalls in this setting: misidentification of macrophages as lipoblasts and misinterpretation of atrophic muscle fibers as multinucleated tumor giant cells.[39] In the former situation, the histiocytic nucleus has a smooth, round or ovoid shape not indented by cytoplasmic vacuoles. The latter structures are not as sharply defined in histiocytes, conferring a foamy to granular quality to the cytoplasm. Atrophic muscle fibers have uniform round nuclei that do not manifest atypia or nucleoli.

Wakely and colleagues reported a series of 33 aspirates of myxoid lesions of soft tissue origin[103]; 22 were sarcomas, and 11 were benign. The amount of stroma in the smears, the degree of cellularity, and the density or opaqueness of the matrix material were semiquantified. For inclusion in the study, at least one slide from each case had to have three or more intermediate-power fields occupied by matrix material. The matrix had a relatively watery or translucent appearance on the smears from many of the specimens derived from both benign and malignant lesions. The fragments of matrix had relatively poorly defined outlines that conferred an amorphous appearance. However, most of the sarcomas also included matrix material with a different quality; specifically, it appeared much denser with sharply defined smooth edges. The latter was most evident in extraskeletal myxoid chondrosarcomas (Fig. 6–8).

For Gonzalez-Campora et al. the most distinctive feature of their solitary extraskeletal myxoid chondrosarcoma was the extreme metachromatic nature of the matrix material.[39] After Romanowsky staining, it varied from brilliant red to pink to intensely blue-red; and with the Papanicolaou preparation it appeared violet to red. Such dense stromal matrix was only infrequently seen by us in aspirates of benign preparations.[103] In this analysis, moderate to high levels of cellularity were found in 95% of the sarcomas but in only 18% of the benign tumors.[103] Similarly, moderate to marked nuclear atypia was found in 59% of the malignant lesions and 9% of the benign samples. The sole benign specimen with marked nuclear atypia was a pleomorphic lipoma. Malignant tumor giant cells, often multinucleated, were most characteristic of the myxoid malignant fibrous histiocytomas (Fig. 6–

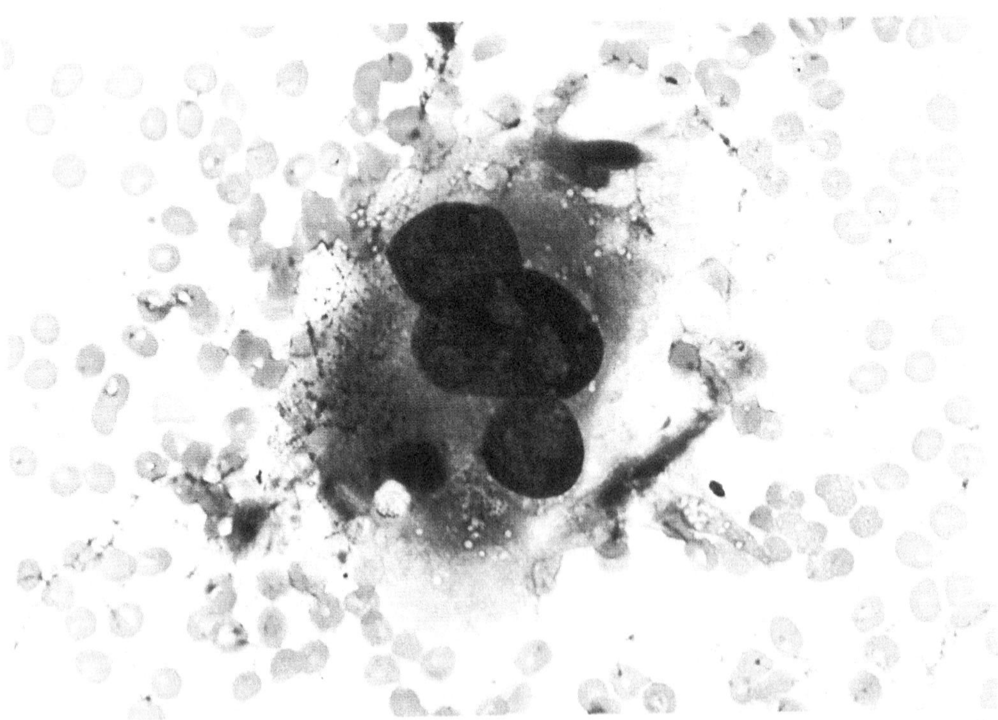

**FIGURE 6–6.** Myxoid malignant fibrous histiocytoma (MFH). Scattered bizarre-appearing tumor giant cells are characteristically present in small numbers in aspirates of many of these neoplasms. This one is characterized by multiple variably sized nuclei with prominent nucleoli and abundant cytoplasm. The latter has indistinct edges that appear to blend into the smear background. (Diff-Quik stain, ×400)

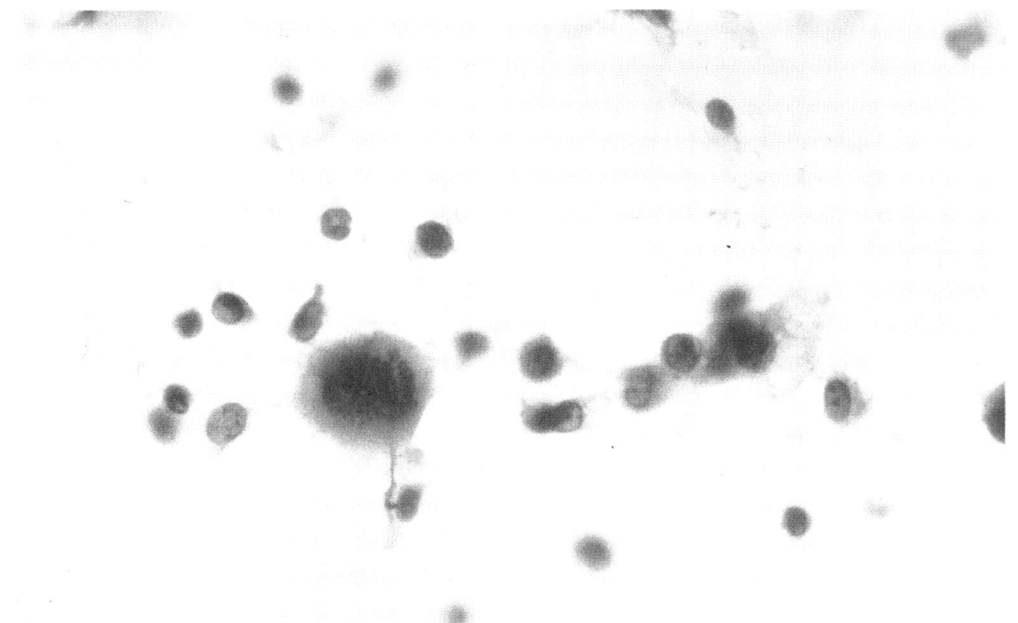

**FIGURE 6–7.** Myxoid MFH. An obviously malignant tumor giant cell is seen among individually dispersed tumor cells. The latter are much more typical of this neoplasm, being characterized by solitary small dark nuclei, minute nucleoli, and high nuclear/cytoplasmic ratios. (Papanicolaou stain, ×100)

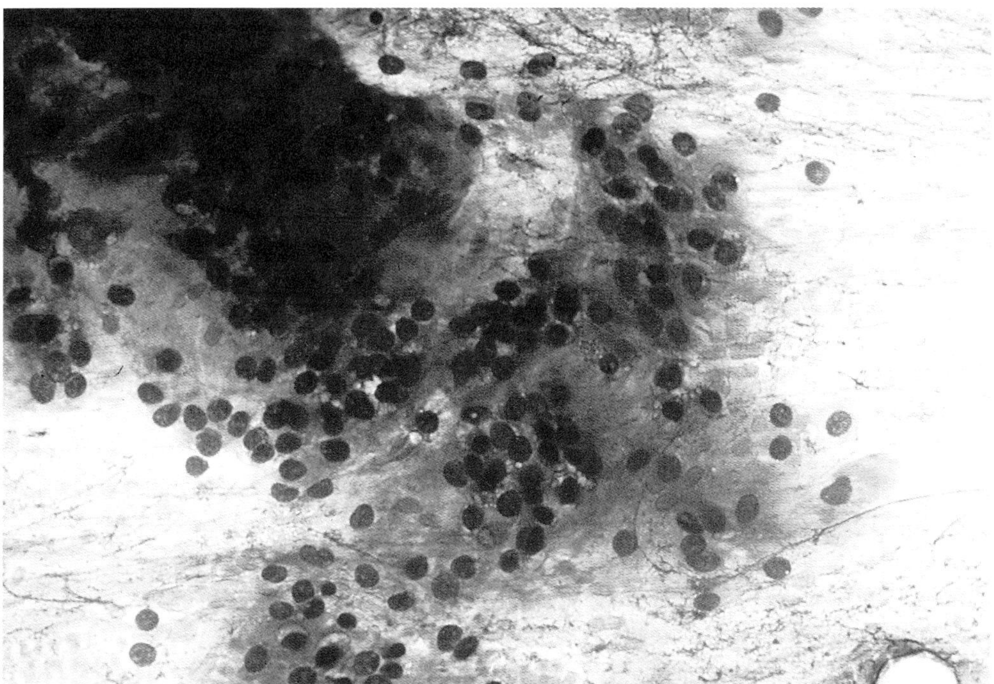

**FIGURE 6–8.** Myxoid chondrosarcoma. Abundant dense homogeneous metachromatic stroma is occupied by numerous small homogeneous neoplastic cells. The latter have solitary round nuclei and apparently high nuclear/cytoplasmic ratios. Rare tumor cells are present in lacunae. (Diff-Quik stain, ×100)

6). Five of the six myxoid chondrosarcomas contained neoplastic cells in lacunae-like spaces in the matrix (Fig. 6–8). For the most part, the benign specimens reported by Wakely et al. were characterized by a combination of low cellularity or the smear and a lack of nuclear atypia.[103] Furthermore, the matrix had an amorphous, semitransparent appearance that seemed not to be fragments but a thin, diffuse film.

The differential diagnoses of the myxoid sarcomas include benign myxoid soft tissue lesions and several other nonsarcomatous malignancies. Ganglion cysts may yield moderate amounts of viscous fluid on aspiration that may be difficult to smear on the slide. The smears are extremely hypocellular and are dominated by a granular-appearing myxoid substance. The few cells present have a histiocytic appearance and are clearly benign. The combination of clinical and microscopic features allows recognition of this lesion and distinguishes it from myxoid sarcomas. As stated earlier, aspirates of soft tissue myxomas are also characterized by low cellularity on the smear.[5,25,39] The cells are round to elongated with solitary small nuclei containing bland chromatin. The abundant pale matrix material may appear granular or fibrillary. The aspirates of ganglion cysts and true myxomas are thus morphologically indistinguishable, as they are closely related. Although mitotic figures are sparse in aspirates of myxoid sarcomas, they would not be expected in aspirates of these benign entities. Furthermore, multinucleated tumor giant cells are not observed. Other benign soft tissue lesions that may have a myxoid background include nodular fasciitis and myxoid neurofibroma.[15,28,96] These lesions are better considered under the spindle cell category.

Once a myxoid neoplasm is identified as sarcoma, it is not always possible to subtype it histologically, although some specimens do provide histogenetic clues. Specimens that contain clearly identifiable lipoblasts and a well defined branched capillary network in the matrix indicate a myxoid liposarcoma[6,66,98,103] (Figs. 6–3, 6–4). Although other sarcomas have tumor cells with cytoplasmic vacuoles, they should not be confused with those of a lipoblast. In the other myxoid sarcomas the vacuoles are generally quite small and do not affect the nuclear contour or position. In myxoid malignant fibrous histiocytomas it may be relatively easy to find isolated, obviously malignant, even bizarre-appearing tumor giant cells[64,103] (Figs. 6–6, 6–7). The latter may have one or more huge nuclei with coarsely granulated chromatin and prominent nucleoli. Their nuclear/cytoplasmic ratios may not be high, as the cells may have voluminous cytoplasm with indistinct borders that tend to blend imperceptibly into the smear background. In addition, large curvilinear blood vessels may be present at the periphery of matrix fragments in myxoid malignant fibrous histiocytomas. Myxoid chondrosarcomas may have cells in a dense, highly metachromatic matrix material.[103] Only rarely has low grade fibromyxoid sarcoma been reported in aspirates dominated by myxoid material and not by spindle-shaped tumor cells; we do not believe the changes are diagnostically specific.[57]

Chordomas must be included in the differential diagnosis of myxoid sarcomas in the pelvis and retroperitoneum. Based purely on cytomorphologic attributes, chordomas may be difficult or even impossible to distinguish from myxoid sarcomas. These smears are characterized by moderate cellularity and abundant extracellular matrix material. Several potential microscopic clues suggest the correct diagnosis. In chordomas the neoplastic cells tend to be larger, have more abundant cytoplasm, and have a relatively "epithelial" appearance. Although their nuclei may be larger than those expected in most tumor cells from myxoid sarcomas, their nuclear/cytoplasmic ratios are relatively low. Furthermore, more distinct separation of tumor cells and matrix may be seen in chordomas. Immunocytochemistry can be definitive; chordoma tumor cells are strongly and diffusely positive for cytokeratin, unlike the myxoid sarcomas.

## SPINDLE CELL SARCOMAS

The spindle cell sarcomas include fibrosarcoma, leiomyosarcoma, synovial sarcoma, malignant peripheral nerve sheath tumor, Kaposi's sarcoma, and some forms of malignant fibrous histiocytoma and angiosarcoma.[32,49,58,59,75,108] This group of malignancies poses the greatest diagnostic difficulties for the FNAB and has the greatest potential for both false-positive and false-negative diagnoses due to the difficulty of distinguishing benign and low grade tumors. In our experience, the two major attributes that allow an aspirate to be designated a sarcoma are moderate to high smear cellularity and hyperchromatic nuclei in almost all sampled cells[49] (Figs. 6–9, 6–10, 6–11). Based purely on cytomorphology, however, it may be difficult to distinguish among the various spindle cell sarcomas and to grade the neoplasm accurately. It is our notion that neither nuclear configurations nor cytoplasmic features are of value in distinguishing among the spindle cell sarcomas, especially those of high grade.

In general, aspiration biopsies yield moderately to highly cellular smears.[49] The main feature of these smears is a predominance of cells with elongated or spindled nuclei, paralleling the shape of the cell. The degree of intercellular cohesion may vary markedly from patient to patient and among the various spindle cell sarcomas. Some specimens are dominated by individually dispersed neoplastic cells and small,

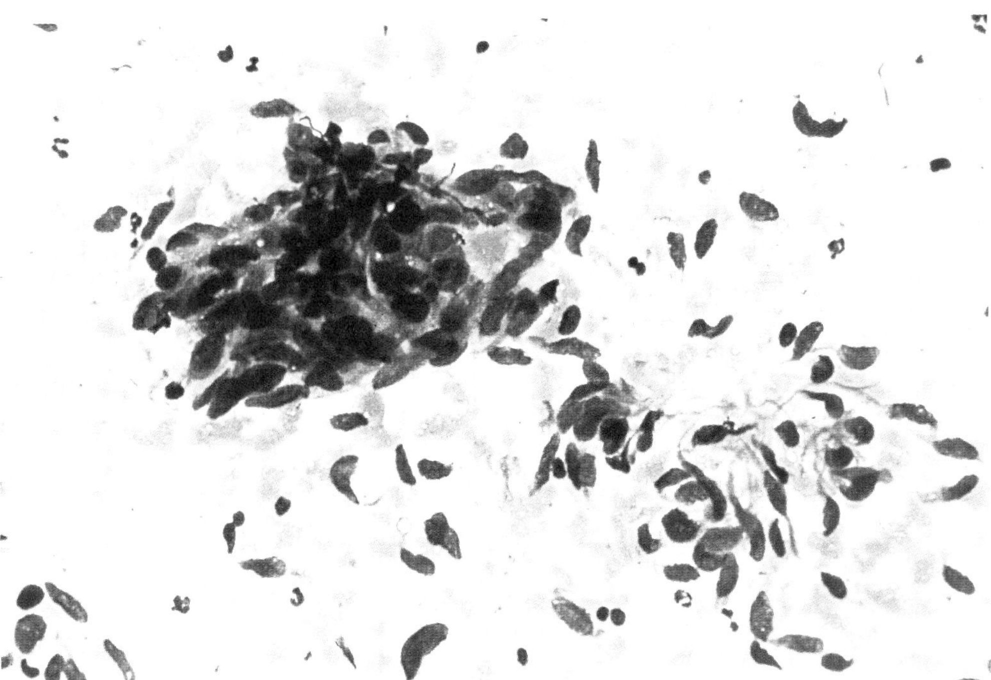

**FIGURE 6–9.** Synovial sarcoma. This highly cellular aspirate smear contains individual tumor cells, loose clusters, and a three-dimensional cohesive tumor fragment. The malignant cells are uniform, each with a single elongated nucleus and high nuclear/cytoplasmic ratio. Nuclear contours vary from plump and ovoid to markedly elongated to comma-shaped. Little matrix material is evident in this sample. (Diff-Quik stain, ×250)

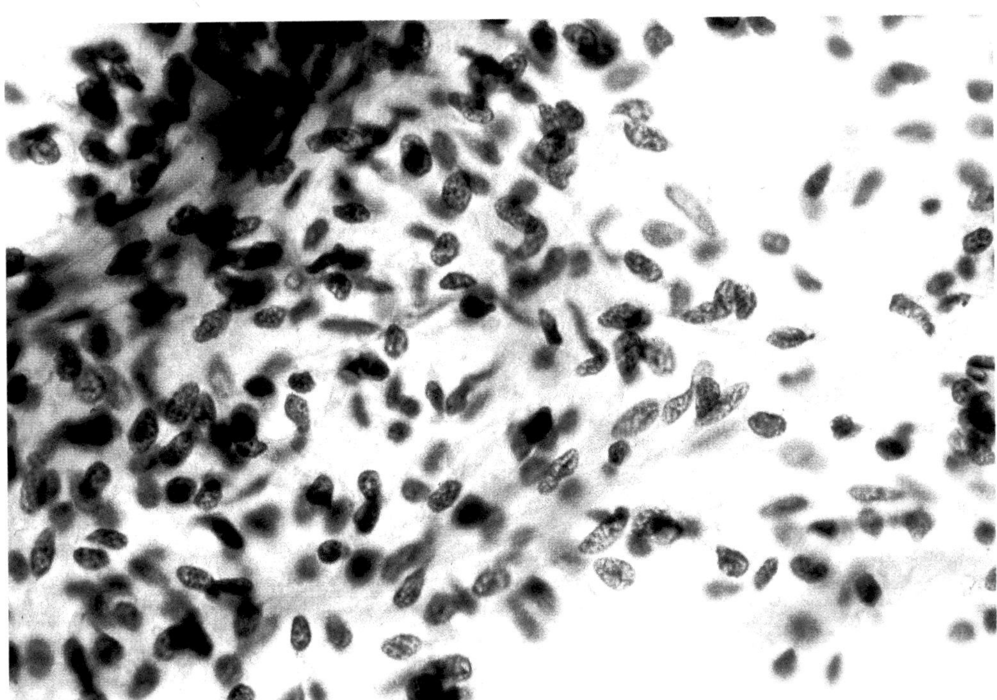

**FIGURE 6–10.** Fibrosarcoma. This aspirate smear is characterized by numerous homogeneous malignant cells, each with a solitary elongated nucleus with hyperchromatic chromatin. The neoplastic cells appear to be arranged haphazardly in delicate matrix material. Pleomorphism is minimal. (Papanicolaou stain, ×250)

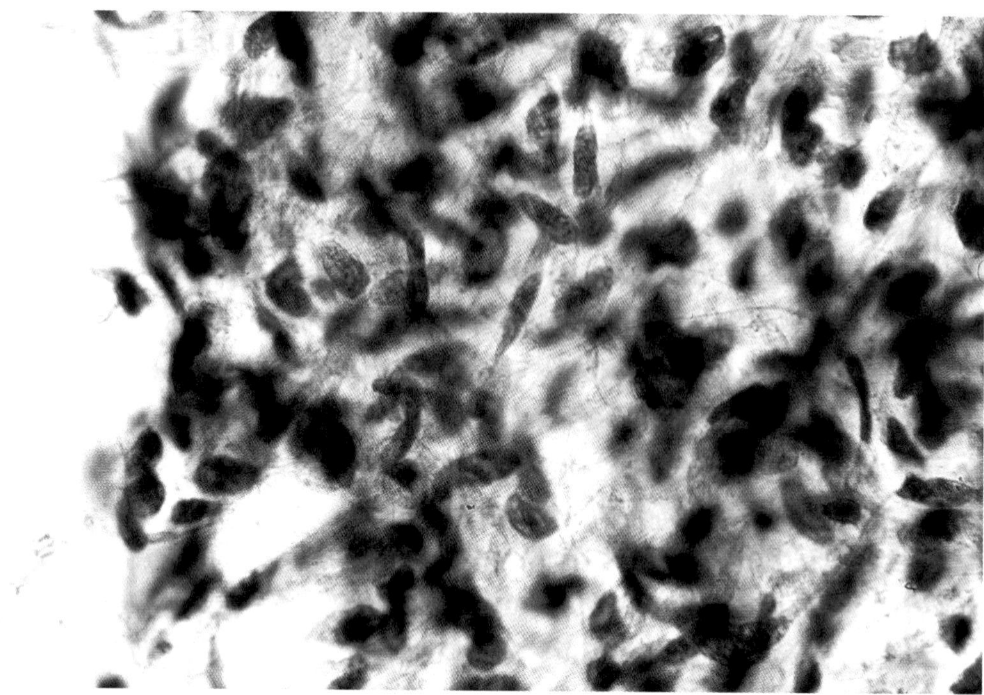

**FIGURE 6–11.** Fibrosarcoma. Coarsely granular, darkly stained chromatin and generally inconspicuous nucleoli are the major features of the spindle-shaped nuclei of this sarcoma. Cellularity is high, and there is no apparent arrangement of the malignant cells. (Papanicolaou stain, ×400)

loose aggregates, whereas in smears from other tumors large tissue fragments predominate. In our experience, the latter situation is most characteristic of leiomyosarcomas. The edges of the neoplastic fragments are often indistinct, as the peripheral-most cells appear to be "exfoliating" from the surface of the fragment (Fig. 6–9). This is in contrast to the sharply defined edges of cellular aggregates in aspirates of carcinomas. The neoplastic cells are usually mononuclear, although multinucleated tumor giant cells are seen in some of the more poorly differentiated sarcomas. Their chromatin is finely to coarsely granular and may be either evenly or irregularly distributed (Figs. 6–10, 6–11). Although nucleoli may be present, in general they are neither large nor prominent. The volume of cytoplasm varies from scant to moderate; and in some neoplasms the tumor cells have long, tapering cytoplasmic tails. Although spindle cell sarcomas may be difficult to subclassify based purely on their cytomorphology, ancillary diagnostic procedures such as immunocytochemistry, cytogenetics, and molecular assays help pinpoint a specific histologic interpretation.

The more frequently aspirated benign spindle cell soft tissue tumors are nerve sheath neoplasms and nodular fasciitis (Figs. 6–12 to 6–17). Cellularity on the smears of most benign nerve sheath tumors is generally low to moderate.[30,31,43,44,80,84,111] The most consistent feature of these specimens is that most of the aspirated neoplastic cells are present in cohesive fragments with irregular contours and consisting of interlacing fascicles (Fig. 6–12). Most of the neoplastic cells have a solitary elongated nucleus with sharply pointed tips. Furthermore, some of the nuclei have a wavy or buckled contour (Figs. 6–13, 6–14). Their chromatin is usually finely granular and uniformly distributed. In some specimens the chromatin is darkly stained. For the most part, nucleoli are not recognized. On the other hand, intranuclear vacuoles are present with some frequency. In the fragments the neoplastic cells are embedded in collagenous matrix material that stains reddish pink with Diff-Quik and green with the Papanicolaou stain. The matrix material may have a fibrillar or granular appearance. The cytoplasm is generally inconspicuous, as it appears to blend imperceptibly with the surrounding collagen. In most tumors only a small number of individually scattered neoplastic cells are present. Many of these cells are not intact but, rather, consist of "stripped" nuclei with no visible attached cytoplasm. In some aspirates rows of parallel nuclei form palisades, and rarely Verocay bodies are recognized (Fig. 6–14). In neurofibromas the neoplastic nuclei do not exhibit any such orientation but, rather, appear to be scattered haphazardly in the aspirated fragments of collagen. Mitotic figures are not usually present in benign

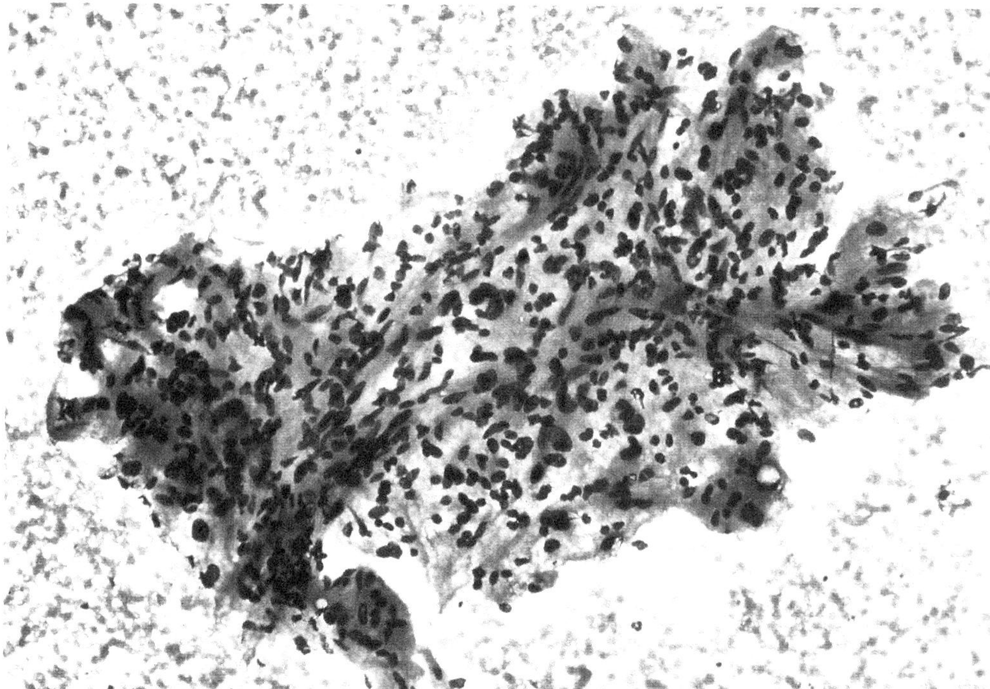

**FIGURE 6–12.** Schwannoma. This aspirate smear is characterized by a large cohesive fragment of tumor. Moderate numbers of neoplastic cells are situated in an abundant matrix. Pink-staining material represents both cytoplasm and collagen. Note the complete absence of individually dispersed tumor cells. (Diff-Quik stain, ×40)

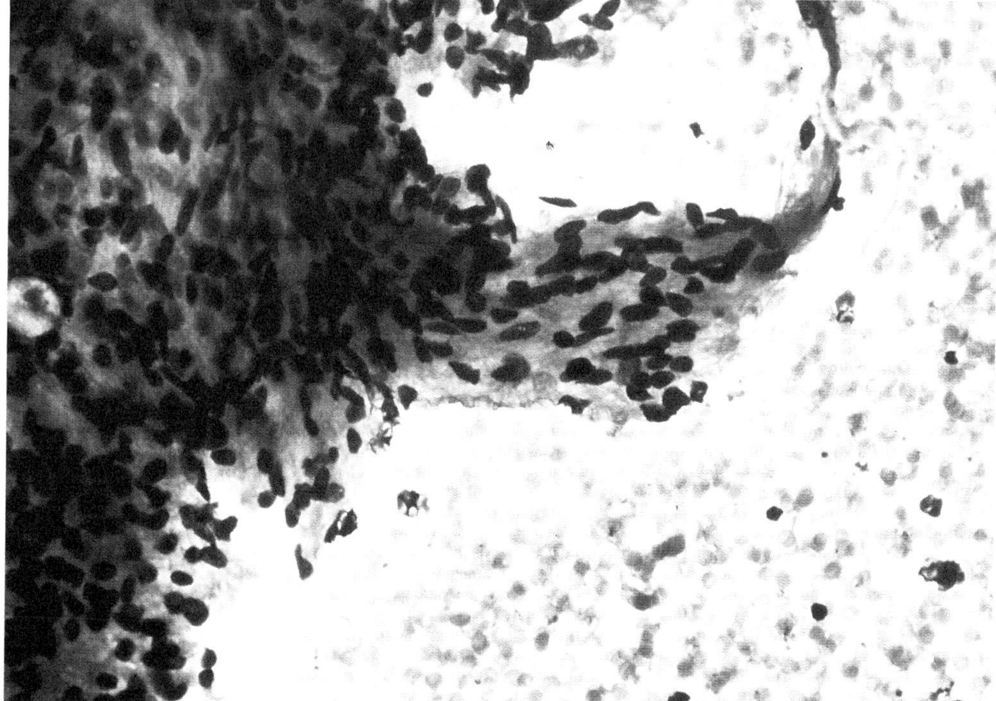

**FIGURE 6–13.** Schwannoma. In this cohesive tumor fragment it is evident that the neoplastic cells have elongated darkly stained nuclei and scant to moderate volumes of cytoplasm. Some of the tumor cells appear to be arranged in parallel bundles. Some of the nuclei are straight and smooth, whereas others have a serpentine configuration. (Diff-Quik stain, ×100)

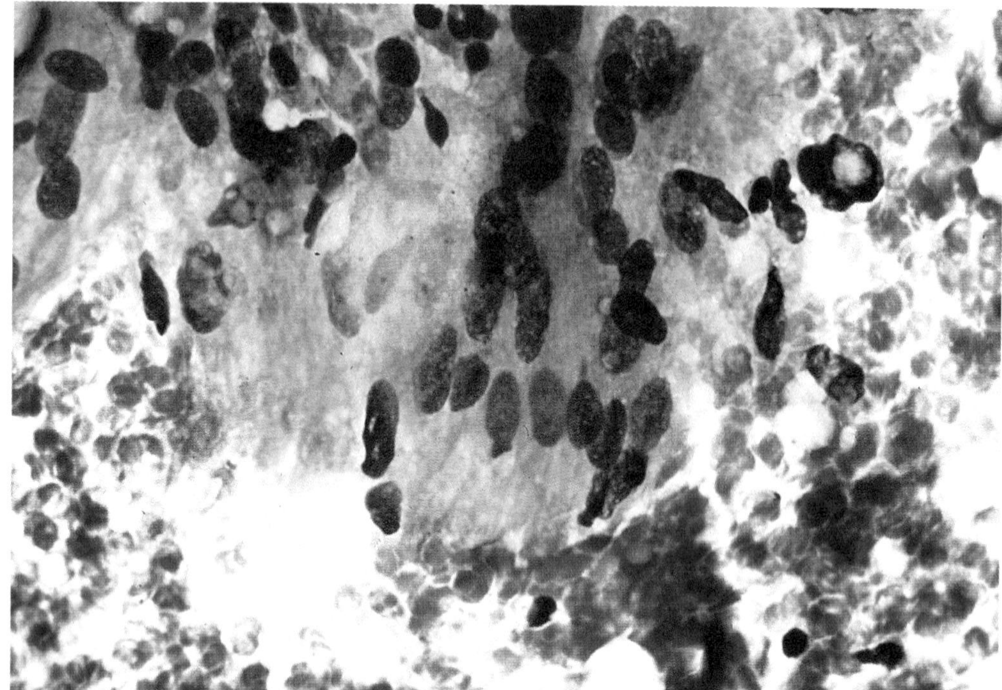

**FIGURE 6–14.** Schwannoma. The elongated neoplastic nuclei appear to be lined up in a single row, or palisade, possibly in an attempt to form a Verocay body. Their cytoplasm blends imperceptibly into the adjacent collagen. Again, there are no isolated neoplastic cells. (Diff-Quik stain, ×400)

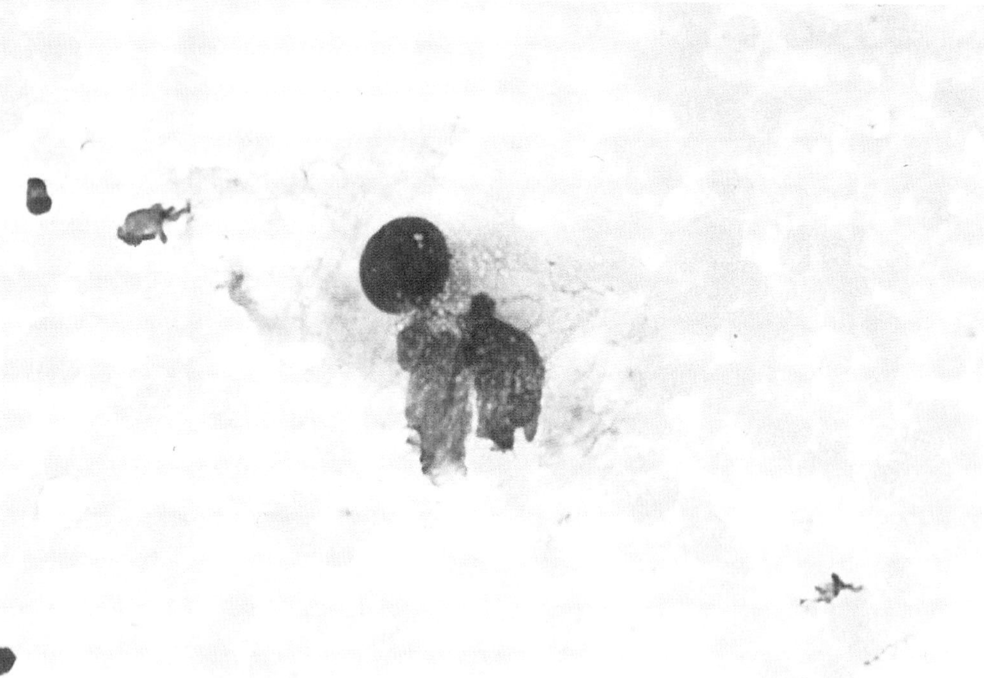

**FIGURE 6–15.** Ancient schwannoma. This huge multinucleated tumor giant cell was present in an aspirate that otherwise completely resembled a conventional schwannoma. Although somewhat difficult to appreciate, the chromatin is rather amorphous. Such cells tend to be isolated and rare in aspirates of this neoplasm. (Diff-Quik stain, ×400)

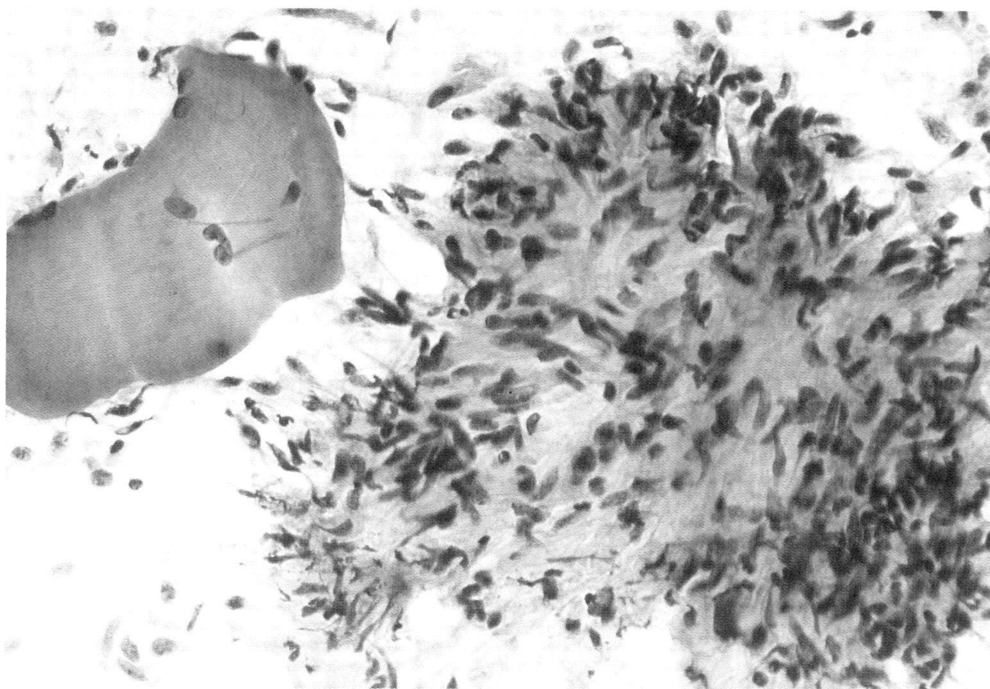

**FIGURE 6–16.** Nodular fasciitis. The classic loosely textured "tissue culture" appearance of nodular fasciitis is evident. Haphazardly positioned proliferating myofibroblasts are present in a pale-stained, fibrillated myxoid matrix that also contains scattered lymphocytes. Although some of the nuclei of the proliferating cells are darkly stained, most are euchromatic. Adjacent to this fragment are individual myofibroblasts and skeletal muscle fibers. (Papanicolaou stain, ×40)

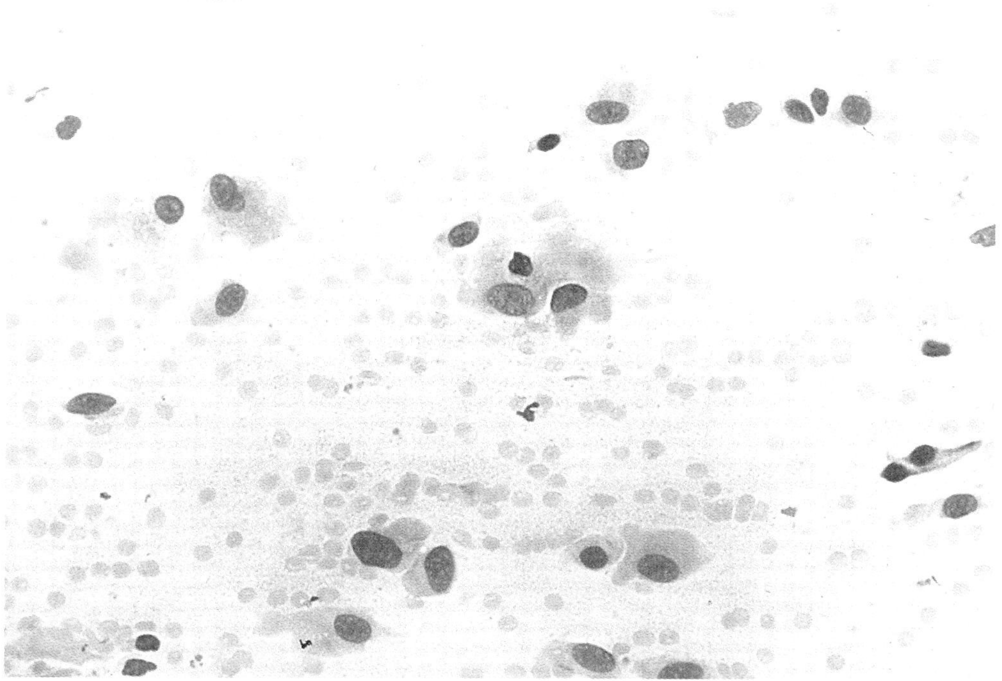

**FIGURE 6–17.** Nodular fasciitis. Scattered myofibroblasts are characterized by solitary nuclei with smooth, delicate membranes; fine, even chromatin; and small but distinct nucleoli. The cells have moderate volumes of cytoplasm and are polygonal to elongated. (Diff-Quik stain, ×100)

nerve sheath tumors. In the series of 29 benign nerve sheath neoplasms reported by Resnick et al., 55% of the specimens were considered nondiagnostic.[80] The remaining 45% manifested attributes of a benign nerve sheath tumor, and four were specifically interpreted as neurilemomas. An important clinical clue is intense pain radiating distally during aspiration.

A potential diagnostic pitfall for FNAB of benign nerve sheath tumors may be observed in the aspirates of ancient schwannomas.[31,84] Aspirated cells may be large with one or more huge hyperchromatic, irregularly contoured nuclei (Fig. 6–15). Careful attention to the chromatin structure is important, as it appears completely homogeneous and smudged or pyknotic-like. These cells may be individually dispersed in the smears that otherwise resemble a typical schwannoma. These huge cellular elements should not be mistaken for malignancies. Helpful clues include a sparsity of such tumor giant cells, a degenerative chromatin pattern, lack of mitotic activity, and overall preservation of cohesion. The cellular schwannoma represents another potential diagnostic problem. In our limited experience, a major clue to recognizing the benign nature is the retention of almost all of the neoplastic cells in the cohesive tumor fragments. The presence of diffuse and intense immunoreactivity for S-100 protein is also useful, as malignant peripheral nerve sheath tumors rarely retain this antigen to this degree. Henke et al. reported a patient in whom the preoperative aspiration biopsy was misinterpreted as sarcoma on the basis of high smear cellularity, mitotic activity, and focal necrosis.[43]

The differential diagnosis must include malignant peripheral nerve sheath tumors.[44,47,63,100] Generally, smears of these tumors have a somewhat higher degree of cellularity than do those of their benign counterparts (Figs. 6–18, 6–19). We believe that the single most important attribute for distinguishing benign from malignant is the presence of a much greater proportion of individually dispersed neoplastic cells in the sarcomas (Fig. 6–18). In the more well differentiated tumors, most neoplastic cells have solitary uniform elongated nuclei, sometimes with a serpentine configuration (Fig. 6–19). In less well differentiated nerve sheath tumors, a larger proportion of the cells are pleomorphic and may include multinucleated malignant tumor giant cells. As the histologic grade of these neoplasms increases, the amount of extracellular matrix material in the smears declines. Mitotic figures are usually readily recognizable. Our experience is thus mirrored by that of Jiménez-Heffernan et al., who described aspiration biopsies from 10 malignant peripheral nerve sheath tumors.[47] Four of these lesions were histologically relatively well differentiated;

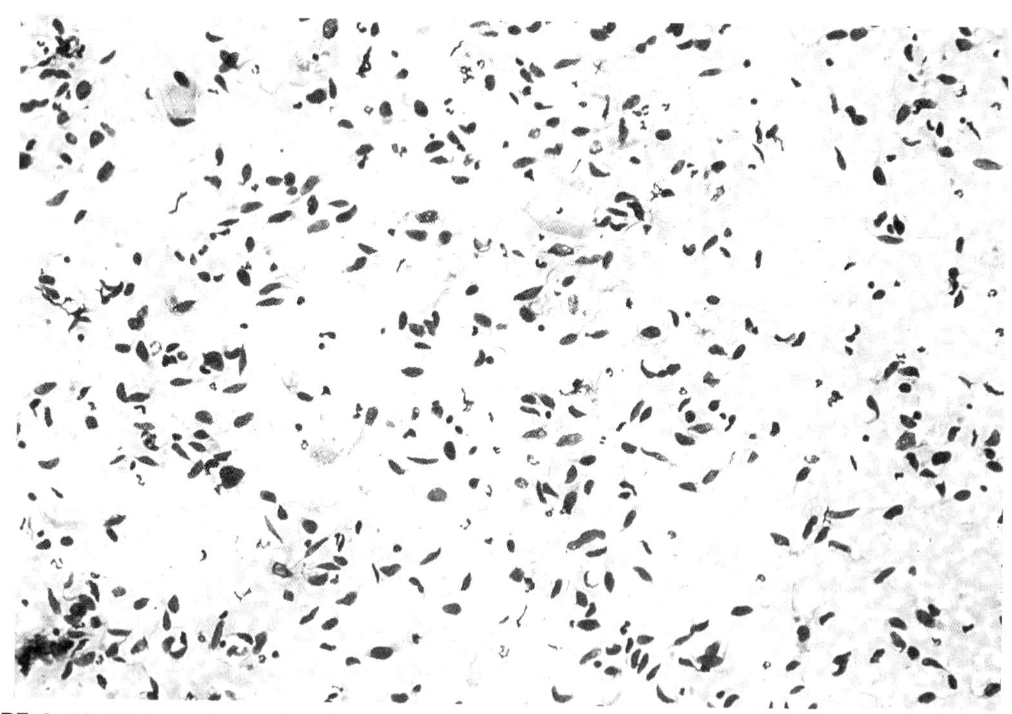

**FIGURE 6–18.** Malignant peripheral nerve sheath tumor. This extremely cellular aspirate is dominated by mildly pleomorphic and dissociated malignant spindle-shaped neoplastic cells. There is almost no evidence of intercellular cohesion. The nuclear/cytoplasmic ratios appear high, although some of the cells have elongated cytoplasmic tails. Spindle-shaped nuclei vary from smooth to buckled to wavy. (Diff-Quik stain, ×40)

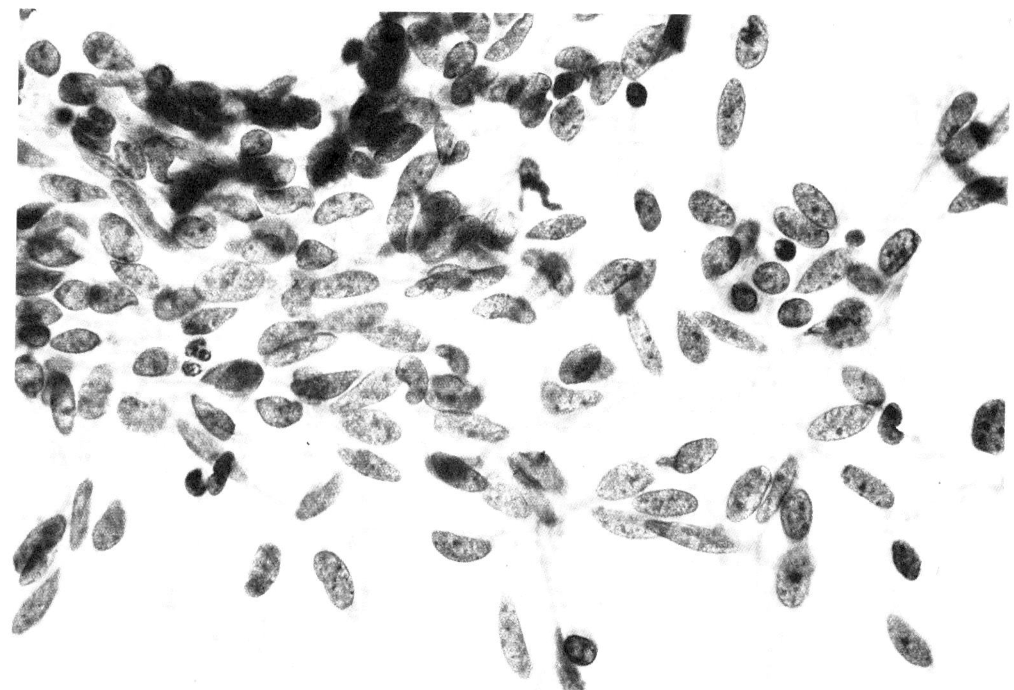

**FIGURE 6–19.** Malignant peripheral nerve sheath tumor. This highly cellular aspirate contains a loose aggregate of malignant cells. The edges of the aggregate appear irregular, resulting from individual cells falling away from its surface. Each cell has a solitary elongated nucleus with finely granulated, evenly distributed hyperchromatic chromatin and an occasional minute nucleolus. No evidence of specific differentiation is seen in this specimen. (Papanicolaou stain, ×400)

these smears could be recognized as malignant and derived from peripheral nerve sheath. Four others were high grade spindle cell neoplasms that could be easily recognized as sarcomatous but did not manifest histogenetic clues. The remaining two cases had a more epithelioid appearance. In contrast to schwannomas, aspirated cellular material from malignant peripheral nerve sheath tumors is either negative or only focally and weakly positive for S-100 protein immunocytochemically.

Aspiration biopsies of synovial sarcomas yield moderately and, more frequently, highly cellular smears.[4,9,45,50,83,101] Each cell has a solitary ovoid nucleus with finely granular, evenly dispersed, hyperchromatic chromatin with inconspicuous nucleoli (Figs. 6–9, 6–20). Most neoplastic elements have scanty cytoplasm, resulting in high nuclear/cytoplasmic ratios. A small number of neoplastic cells in many cases have more abundant cytoplasm, which characteristically appears as bipolar tapered cytoplasmic tails. Some of these malignant cells are individually scattered, a manifestation of reduced intercellular cohesion, as is the frayed edges of many of neoplastic aggregates. The shapes of the individual neoplastic nuclei vary from blunt and ovoid to much more elongated. The number of mitotic figures in a given specimen is variable. Aspirates from histologically documented biphasic synovial sarcomas are dominated by these spindled neoplastic cells (Fig. 6–21). However, in some tumors neoplastic elements exhibit distinct epithelial differentiation, evidenced by polygonal contours and solitary round hyperchromatic nuclei (Fig. 6–21).[49,83,101] The nuclei are either centrally or eccentrically positioned in the cytoplasm, which may appear finely vacuolated. Mononucleated and multinucleated tumor giant cells are not usually seen, as pleomorphism is minimal.

The specific FNAB diagnosis of synovial sarcoma is markedly enhanced by the use of ancillary diagnostic procedures. Immunocytochemically, positive reactivity for epithelial markers (e.g., the various cytokeratins) assists in the differential diagnosis with other spindle cell sarcomas.[9,49] Aspirated cellular material provides an excellent specimen for cytogenetic analysis, specifically to demonstrate the characteristic reciprocal translocation.[9,49] Using the reverse transcription-polymerase chain reaction (RT-PCR), Inagaki et al. were able to identify the specific SYT-SSX fusion products of synovial sarcomas in aspiration specimens.[45]

Similar to peripheral nerve sheath neoplasms, benign and malignant smooth muscle tumors can gener-

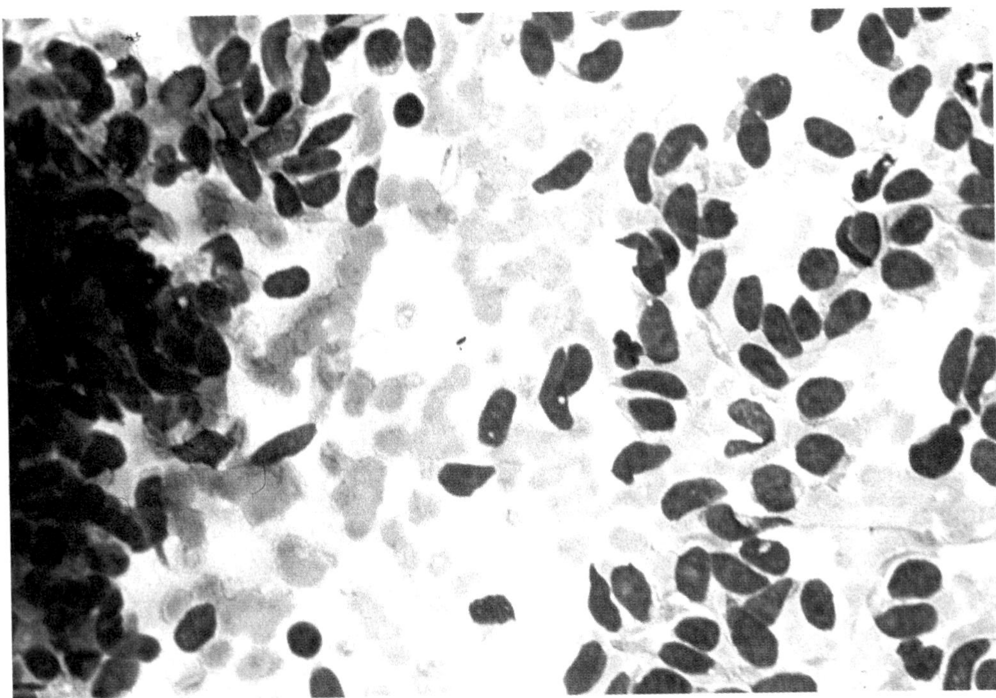

**FIGURE 6–20.** Synovial sarcoma. Both individual neoplastic cells and a cohesive tumor fragment are present in this field. Note the striking uniformity of the malignant cells. Each has a single ovoid nucleus with fine, even chromatin and a high nuclear/cytoplasmic ratio. (Diff-Quik stain, ×400)

ally be distinguished from each other on the basis of their cellularity or smears and the presence or absence of well developed intercellular cohesion.[16,29,94,99] Cellularity is much higher with the sarcomas. Generally, in aspiration biopsy specimens of leiomyomas most of the neoplastic cells are present in cohesive tissue fragments, whereas a larger proportion of the tumor cells from leiomyosarcomas are individually dispersed or in loosely cohesive clusters without intervening matrix (Figs. 6–22 to 6–25). The elongated nuclei may have a "cigar" shape in benign and malignant neoplasms, whereas in other cells the nuclei have a nonspecific spindled contour. The cells have eosinophilic cytoplasm that appears to blend with the collagen matrix. Mitotic figures are not recognized in aspiration smears of these benign neoplasms.

Vascular and perivascular neoplasms also must be considered in the differential diagnosis of spindle cell sarcomas,[21,37,42,68,71] especially Kaposi's sarcoma and hemangiopericytoma. In general, samples contain a prominent background of blood, so cellularity on the smear may not be as high as would be expected for many other sarcomas.

Kaposi's sarcoma generally yields moderately cellular samples dominated by large tissue fragments composed of homogeneous spindle-shaped cells.[42] Although matrix material may be seen in some of the fragments (especially in air-dried preparations), they are usually densely cellular with characteristically overlapping elongated neoplastic cells. Smears of the aspirates also contain small aggregates of loosely cohesive neoplastic cells. Individually scattered tumor cells and stripped elongated nuclei are present as well. The cells are characterized by ovoid to more elongated nuclei with finely granular, evenly dispersed chromatin and inconspicuous nucleoli. A characteristic attribute is nuclear fragility, which manifests as streaks of chromatin material in the aggregates.[42] The neoplastic cells have scanty, weakly basophilic cytoplasm with poorly defined cell borders. Pleomorphism is minimal. Although the cytomorphologic findings are not specific, in the proper clinical setting and in particular in a patient known to have acquired immunodeficiency syndrome (AIDS), this picture is consistent with the diagnosis of Kaposi's sarcoma. Demonstration of vascular differentiation markers such as CD31 and CD34 by immunocytochemistry is useful for supporting the diagnosis. Using PCR, Alkan et al. demonstrated the presence of human herpes virus-8 in all aspiration biopsy specimens of Kaposi's sarcoma; aspirates of all other spindle cell proliferations were negative for this agent.[12]

Similarly, hemangiopericytomas do not produce a specific diagnostic cytomorphologic picture on smears.[37,68] The specimens, however, may have a typical appearance. Smears are moderately to highly cel-

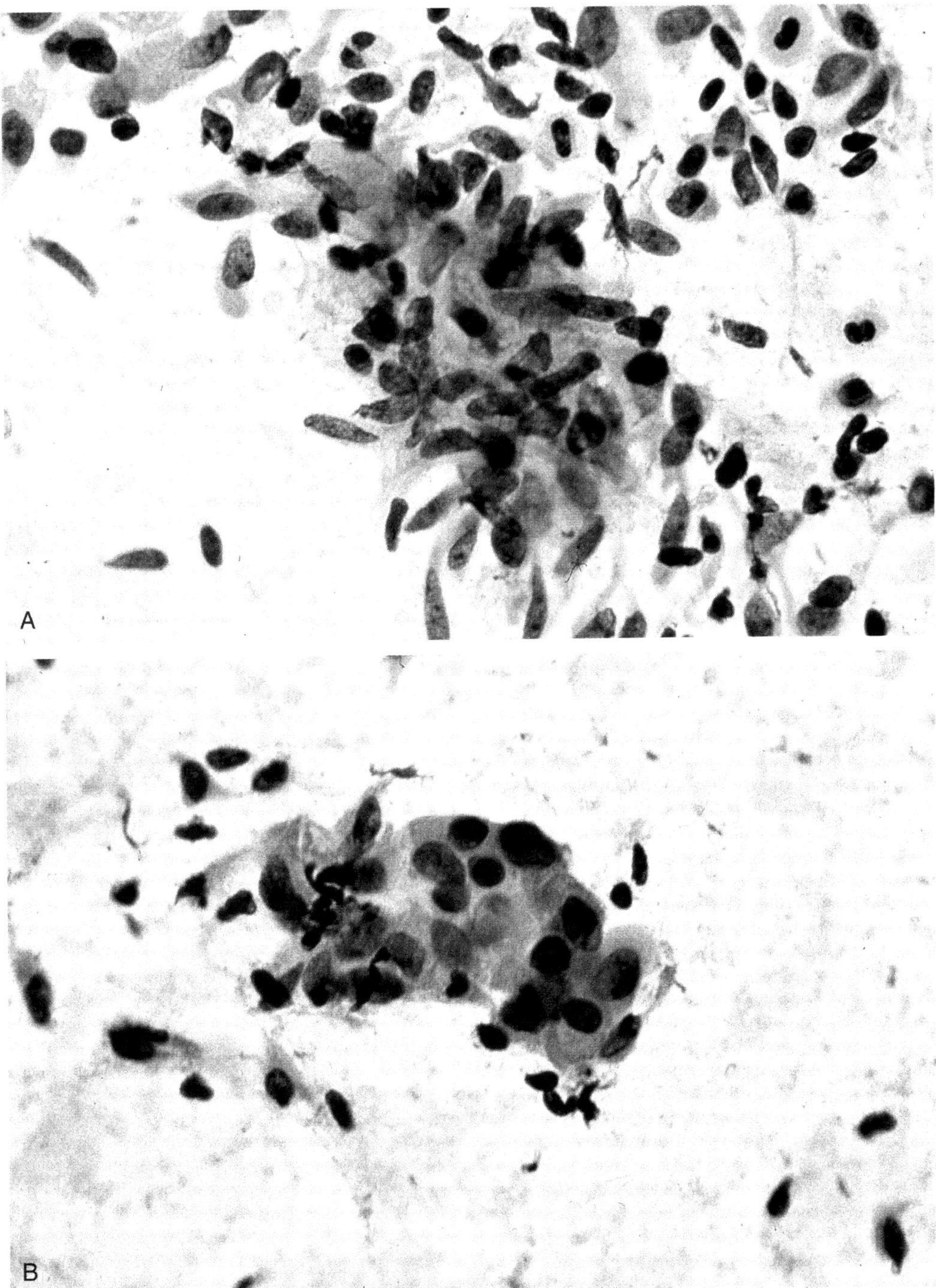


**FIGURE 6–21.** (**A**) Biphasic synovial sarcoma. Most of the malignant cells in this field have solitary elongated hyperchromatic nuclei and spindled cellular contours. A few of the neoplastic cells have more polygonal shapes and obvious cytoplasm. (Papanicolaou stain, ×400) (**B**) Biphasic synovial sarcoma. This cluster of malignant cells has an epithelial appearance in that the cells have round to polygonal configurations with more-or-less central round to ovoid nuclei. The latter have darkly stained chromatin. A few scattered spindle-shaped neoplastic cells are also apparent. (Papanicolaou stain, ×400)

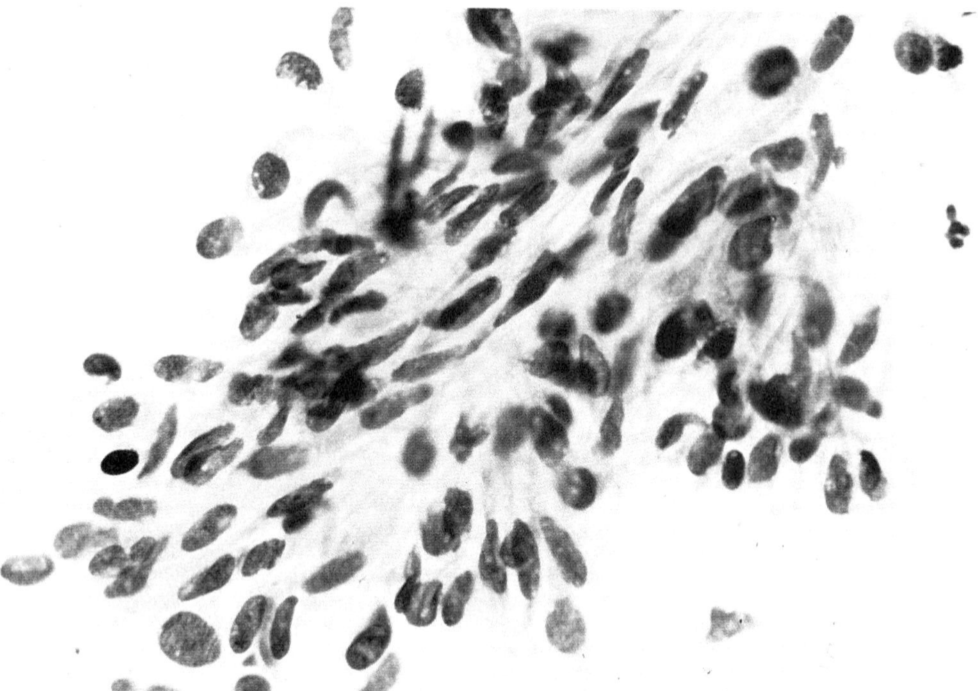

**FIGURE 6–22.** Leiomyoma. This cohesive fragment of spindled to ovoid neoplastic cells is characteristic of this neoplasm in aspirate smears. Although their shapes are somewhat variable, the nuclei have relatively uniform sizes and appearances with fine, even, almost structureless euchromatic chromatin. The cells seem to have moderate volumes of pale cytoplasm. (Papanicolaou stain, ×400)

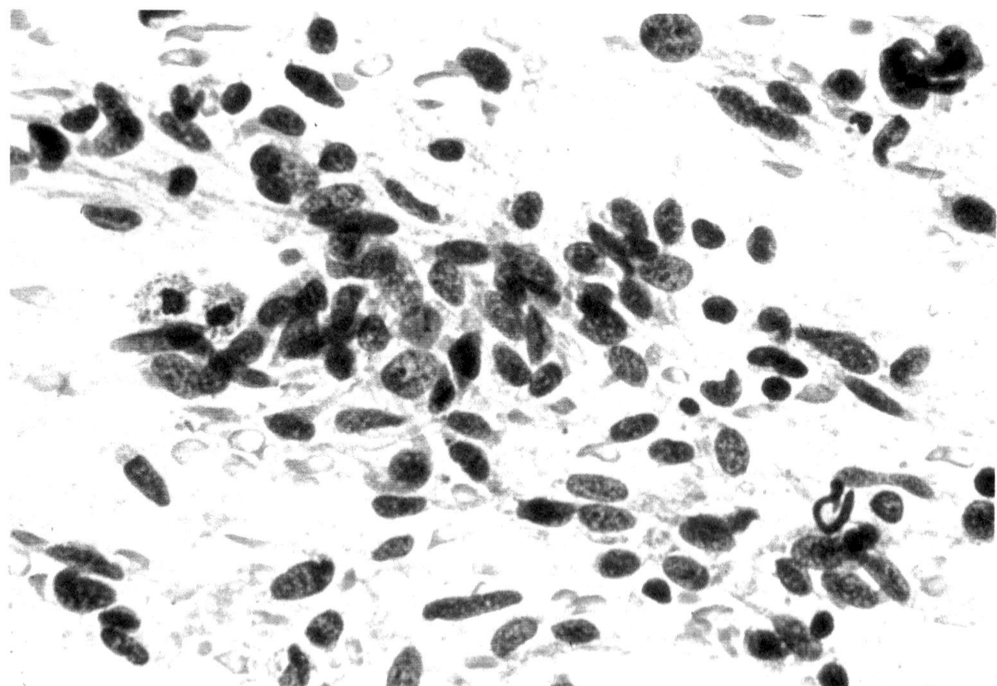

**FIGURE 6–23.** Leiomyosarcoma. Compared to the leiomyoma in Figure 6–22, intercellular cohesion is markedly reduced, manifested by small, loose clusters and individual neoplastic cells. The malignant cells have elongated nuclei with coarse, dark chromatin and inconspicuous cytoplasm. (Papanicolaou stain, ×400)

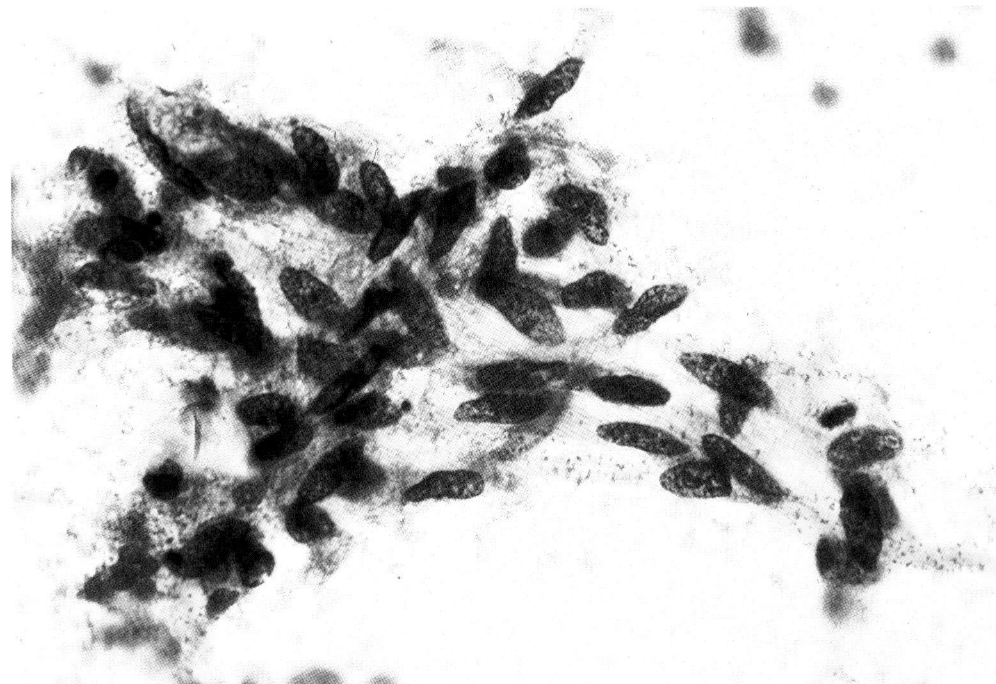

**FIGURE 6–24.** Leiomyosarcoma. Compared to Figure 6–22, the sarcomatous nuclei are larger and hyperchromatic. Although the cells have obvious dense cytoplasm, the cells appear crowded owing to a high nuclear/cytoplasmic ratio. (Papanicolaou stain, ×400)

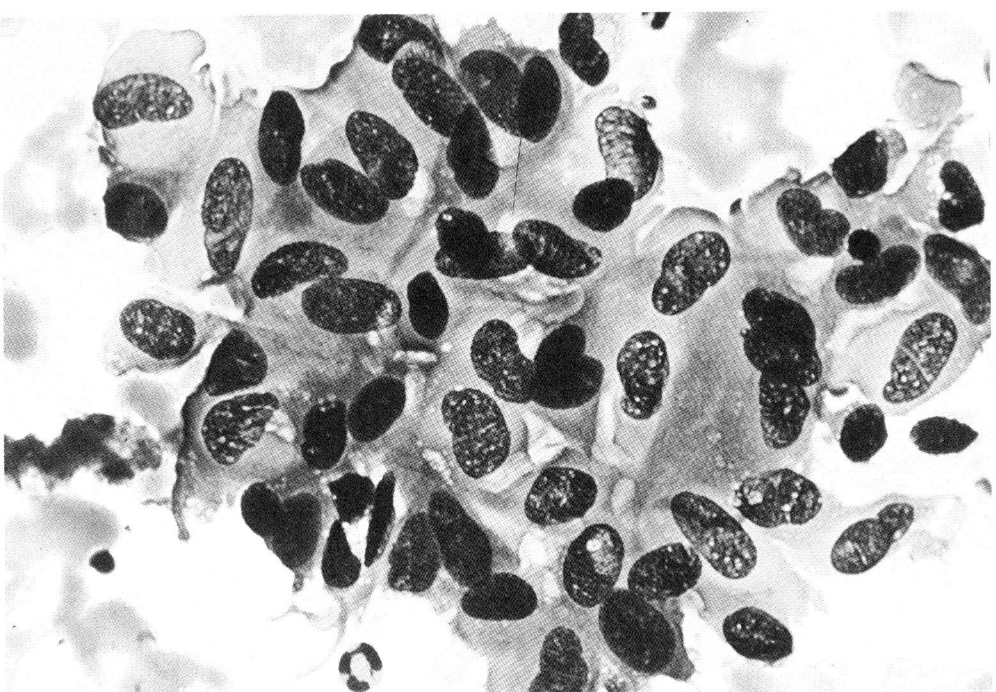

**FIGURE 6–25.** Leiomyosarcoma. Although some of the malignant cells and their nuclei here have elongated contours, others have a more polygonal or rounded contour, corresponding to a more epithelioid histologic appearance in portions of the resected neoplasm. Note that the cells have moderate volumes of cytoplasm but still have rather high nuclear/cytoplasmic ratios. (Diff-Quik stain, ×400)

lular with a bloody background. Similar to Kaposi's sarcoma, they are often predominated by cellular cohesive tissue fragments. A characteristic feature of some of the aspirated fragments is that they are traversed by endothelial cell-lined capillaries. The neoplastic cells are larger and have plumper nuclei than the benign endothelial cells. This is in contrast to Kaposi's sarcoma in which capillaries do not course through the tumor fragments. According to some, "staghorn" vessels are not recognized in the neoplastic fragments.[37,68] In addition, the smears contain small, loosely cohesive monolayers of tumor cells and individually dispersed neoplastic cellular elements. Pleomorphism is mild to moderate, and most of the neoplastic cells have solitary ovoid or somewhat elongated nuclei with scanty, ill-defined cytoplasm. Their chromatin is finely granular, uniformly dispersed, and variably stained. In most cases at least some of the nuclei appear hyperchromatic.

Aspiration biopsies of angiosarcomas present a more diverse cytomorphologic array.[2,21,94] Some tumors are dominated by distinctly spindle-shaped neoplastic cells, whereas in others the malignant elements have rounded or polygonal contours. In addition, tumor fragments are less pervasive than in either Kaposi's sarcoma or hemangiopericytoma. Rather, a much larger proportion of the cells are isolated or present in small, loosely cohesive clusters. Distinct vasoformative channels are recognized in some samples. Individual cells typically have a solitary elongated or round nucleus with definite hyperchromasia and variably clumped chromatin granules. In general, prominent nucleoli are not evident, but we have seen some tumors with large macronucleoli. Pleomorphism may be more extensive than that seen in either Kaposi's sarcoma or hemangiopericytoma. Although some suggest that cytoplasmic hemosiderin is characteristic of angiosarcomas in aspiration biopsy specimens, others have not found this to be helpful.[21,60] Immunocytochemistry to identify endothelial differentiation markers may be useful for confirming the diagnosis of angiosarcoma.

Aspiration biopsies of benign vascular tumors generally are uncommon.[71] These smears are dominated by blood and in many cases do not demonstrate any other cell types. An occasional aggregate of bland-appearing spindle-shaped endothelial cells and fibroblasts set in scanty collagenous matrix material may be randomly scattered in the specimen. Fragments of degenerating skeletal muscle fibers may also be recognized in the aspirates from intramuscular hemangiomas.[1]

The final group of soft tissue lesions to be considered on an aspiration smear dominated by spindle-shaped cells are the fibrous and fibrohistiocytic proliferations. The prototype, fibrosarcoma, has only rarely been described in cytologic samples.[1] The cellularity and the degree of pleomorphism on the smear depend largely on the histologic grade of the fibrosarcoma; in general, high cellularity and prominent anisonucleosis are associated with poorly differentiated minors. On smears, the cells are present both singly and in generally loose clusters. With more differentiated neoplasms, the tumor cells are rather homogeneous in size and appearance. Most cells have a solitary ovoid to elongated nucleus with evenly dispersed, finely granulated chromatin with small nucleoli. The neoplastic cells have variable amounts of cytoplasm, ranging from scanty to moderate. Many have a distinctly spindled contour with unipolar or bipolar tails. Although it would be unusual to find multinucleated giant cells in aspirates of poorly differentiated fibrosarcomas, these neoplasms may yield moderate variability in nuclear size and contour. Mitotic figures are usually evident on the smears. Fragments of collagenized stroma may be present.

Based purely on cytomorphologic features, aspirates of well differentiated fibrosarcomas may be difficult or impossible to distinguish from the fibromatoses, dermatofibrosarcoma protuberans, synovial sarcomas, and well differentiated peripheral sheath tumors.[1] The poorly differentiated fibrosarcomas must be distinguished from malignant fibrous histiocytomas and high grade leiomyosarcomas. Nonneoplastic proliferative lesions such as nodular fasciitis must also be considered in the differential diagnosis of fibrosarcoma.

The fibromatoses are characterized in smears by a variable cellularity that tends to be low to moderate and therefore is less than that seen in frank sarcomas.[78,105] The proliferating fibroblasts present with solitary uniform, elongated nuclei with delicate membranes, fine even chromatin, and inconspicuous nucleoli. Similar to fibrosarcoma, the predominant cellular contour is spindled, and the volume of cytoplasm is variable. Characteristically, one may find bipolar, tapering, long cytoplasmic tails. Importantly, mitotic figures should not be identified. The cells occur both singly and in small, loose aggregates; at times they are situated in collagenized stromal tissue. A similar cytomorphologic picture may be seen with idiopathic retroperitoneal fibrosis.[97]

On aspiration smears, dermatofibrosarcoma protuberans may be considered a bridge between the fibrous and fibrohistiocytic neoplasms.[77] Smears are moderately to highly cellular and contain both individually dispersed and loosely aggregated spindled cells (Fig. 6–26). The smears also usually contain neoplastic cells in fragments of stroma. The individual cells have solitary ovoid nuclei with delicate chromatin that may stain darkly. Nucleoli are small and inconspicuous. Typically, the cells have moderate vol-

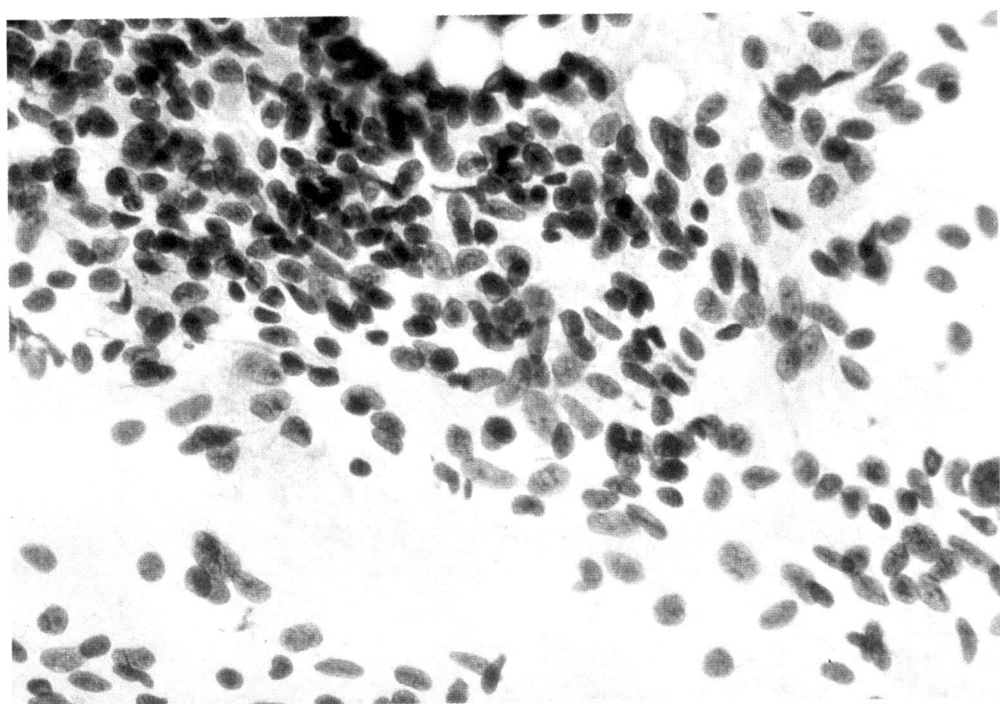

**FIGURE 6–26.** Dermatofibrosarcoma protuberans. This highly cellular aspirate is dominated by haphazardly patterned cells with spindled to ovoid configurations. Their cytoplasm is scanty and inconspicuous. At one edge, the neoplastic cells appear to infiltrate around adipocytes. (Papanicolaou stain, ×100) (Courtesy of Dr. Celeste Powers.)

umes of pale basophilic cytoplasm that may present as long bipolar tails. The presence at low magnification of a whorled or storiform arrangement of the cells and infiltration of fatty tissue by the proliferating spindle cells is useful for rendering a specific diagnosis.[77] The cytomorphologic features of malignant fibrous histiocytoma is presented in the discussion of the pleomorphic sarcomas below.

Although not pathognomonic, the distinctive cytomorphology of nodular fasciitis, in conjunction with the appropriate clinical presentation, allows a confident diagnosis of this lesion.[15,28,96] The smears are moderately to frequently highly cellular and are composed of singly dispersed cells, loose aggregates, and tissue fragments all set in a highly characteristic metachromatic myxoid background (Fig. 6–16). The latter is better appreciated with the Romanowsky stain, with which it appears red to violet. With the Papanicolaou stain it appears pale green. In the fragments, the proliferating cells appear loosely and haphazardly arranged, creating the characteristic tissue culture pattern. Although cellular contours are variable, most of the lesional cells are spindle-shaped with moderate volumes of faintly basophilic cytoplasm and one or two blunt-to-long cytoplasmic tags. A few of the proliferating cells have ovoid or polygonal contours with similar-appearing cytoplasm (Fig. 6–17). Most of the cells have a solitary nucleus, although binucleation also occurs. Characteristically, the nuclei are perfectly round with distinct thin membranes, generally vesicular chromatin, and distinct small to large nucleoli. The latter vary in shape from smooth and round to angulated. Nucleolar prominence results from their large size and the pale-stained chromatin. Mitotic figures may be evident in the smears and in some tumors are numerous. Thus the fibroblastic cells have a reparative look.[46] The cytologic picture is rounded out with an admixture of predominantly mononuclear inflammatory cells in the background.

Nonsarcomatous malignancies must also be considered in the differential diagnosis of spindle cell sarcomas. Sarcomatoid carcinomas and mesotheliomas may present on smears as predominantly elongated neoplastic cells with obviously malignant nuclear attributes. In a few malignant melanomas, most of the sampled cells have distinctly spindled contours and may closely simulate a sarcoma. Appropriate immunocytochemical stains can often clarify this issue. The patient's previous medical history may also be helpful. A proportion of non-Hodgkin's lymphomas may present, at least focally, on smears as a spindle cell proliferation. This typically occurs in mediastinal and retroperitoneal lymphomas associated with dense sclerosis. The collagenous material compresses some of the lymphoma cells, creating elongated contours that may persist in aspiration smears. However, the characteristic features of an aspirated non-Hodgkin's lymphoma can be seen elsewhere in the sample, allowing the correct diagnosis. Again, the use of immunocytochemistry is helpful.

## PLEOMORPHIC SARCOMAS

On aspiration smears the pleomorphic sarcomas are almost always readily recognized as malignant and often as sarcomatous at low magnification.[49] The direct smears are usually highly cellular with little tendency for the malignant cells to aggregate (Fig. 6–27). An admixture of small round cells with high nuclear/cytoplasmic ratios, large polygonal or spindled cells with scant to moderate volumes of cytoplasm, and numerous bizarre tumor giant cells may be observed in a single field (Figs. 6–28, 6–29, 6–30). The latter are characterized by one or more large hyperchromatic nuclei, some with huge nucleoli. Some of the nuclei appear highly contorted or have many lobes. These cells typically have moderate to abundant cytoplasm with cell borders that appear to blend imperceptibly into the background. The latter frequently contains necrotic debris. Pleomorphic malignant fibrous histiocytomas and liposarcomas account for almost all of the neoplasms on aspiration smears from this category. In many instances, it is not possible to distinguish between these two tumors on the basis of aspiration cytomorphology, but this situation does not appear to be highly relevant clinically.[6,36,66,107] However, if lipoblasts (cells with cytoplasmic lipid vacuoles that indent the nucleus) are identified, a specific diagnosis may be offered.[6,107]

In smears of malignant fibrous histiocytoma, the cells are dispersed singly and are present in loose clusters.[19,106] Personally, we find the combination of high cellularity, mostly single malignant cells, and marked pleomorphism characteristic of this neoplasm. Similar to our own experiences, Liu et al. identified the combination of fibroblastic cells, multinucleated cells, and abundant myxoid matrix material as features supporting the interpretation of malignant fibrous histiocytoma.[59] On the other hand, Berardo et al. did not find a single cytomorphologic feature that allowed them to distinguish reliably malignant fibrous histiocytoma from other cytologically high grade pleomorphic neoplasms.[19]

Although most of the entities included in the differential diagnosis of pleomorphic sarcomas are other malignant neoplasms, a few benign proliferations also must be considered, including pleomorphic lipoma, giant cell tumors, ancient schwannoma, and proliferative fasciitis/myositis. The aspiration cytomorphology

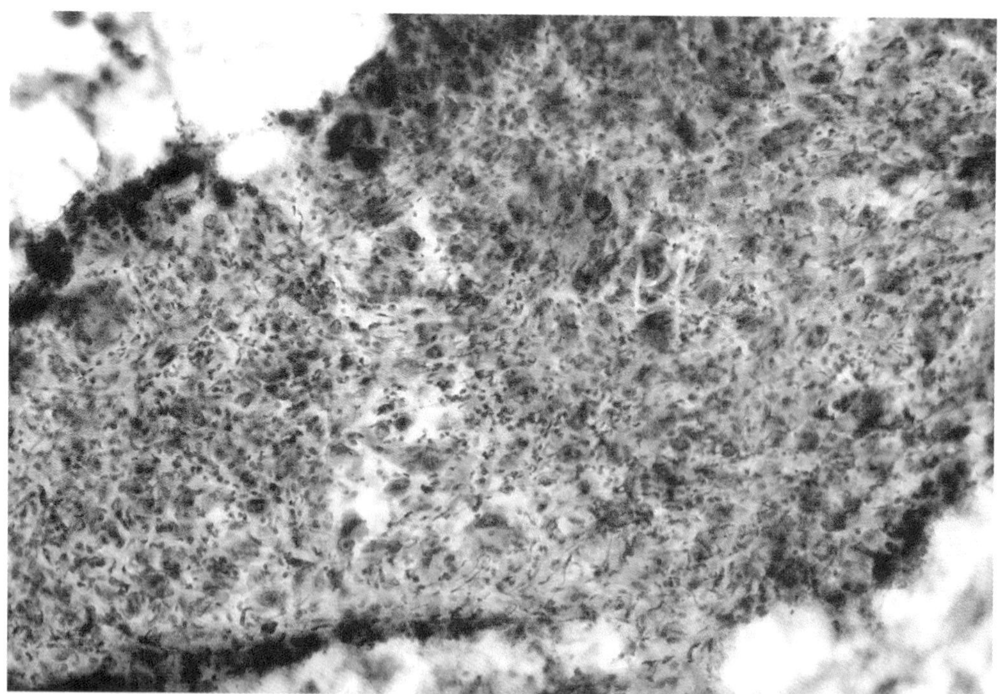

**FIGURE 6–27.** Pleomorphic MFH. This aspirate smear demonstrates the characteristic feature of pleomorphic sarcomas: extremely high smear cellularity, striking variability in size and shapes of the malignant cells, and lack of cohesion. (Hematoxylin and eosin, ×40)

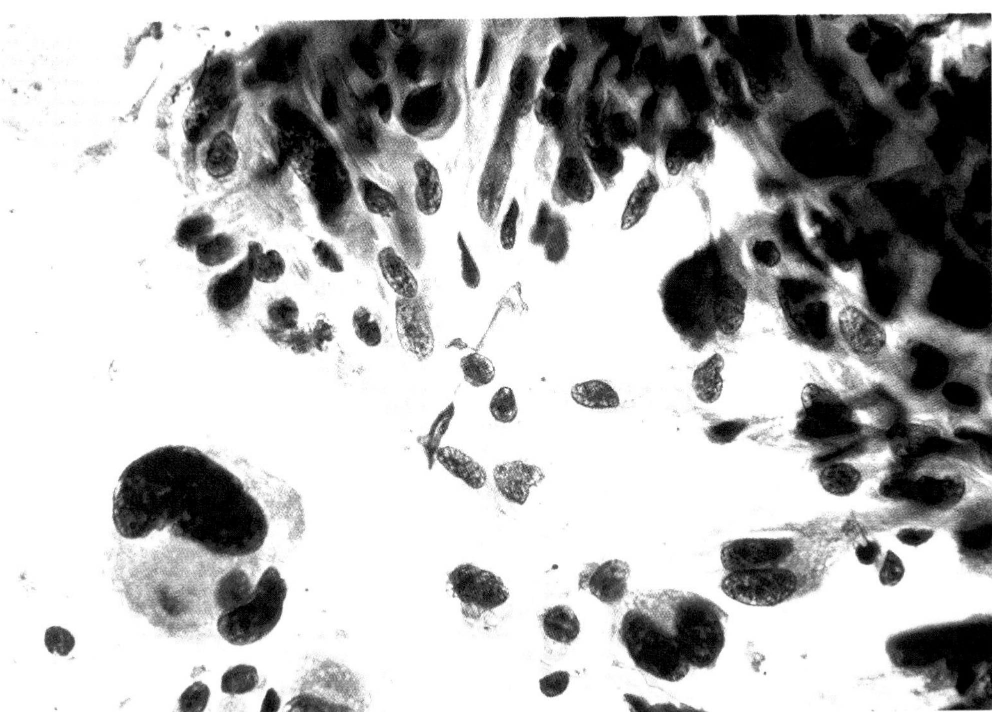

**FIGURE 6–28.** Pleomorphic MFH. Marked variability in the size and appearance of the malignant cells is apparent. Some of the tumor cells are relatively small with solitary hyperchromatic nuclei and inapparent cytoplasm. Others are large with more polygonal or spindled shapes. Also present are several multinucleated tumor giant cells. The latter have two or more darkly stained nuclei and moderate to voluminous cytoplasm. Note that in several of the tumor giant cells the nuclei form a characteristic acute angle with each other. (Papanicolaou stain, ×400)

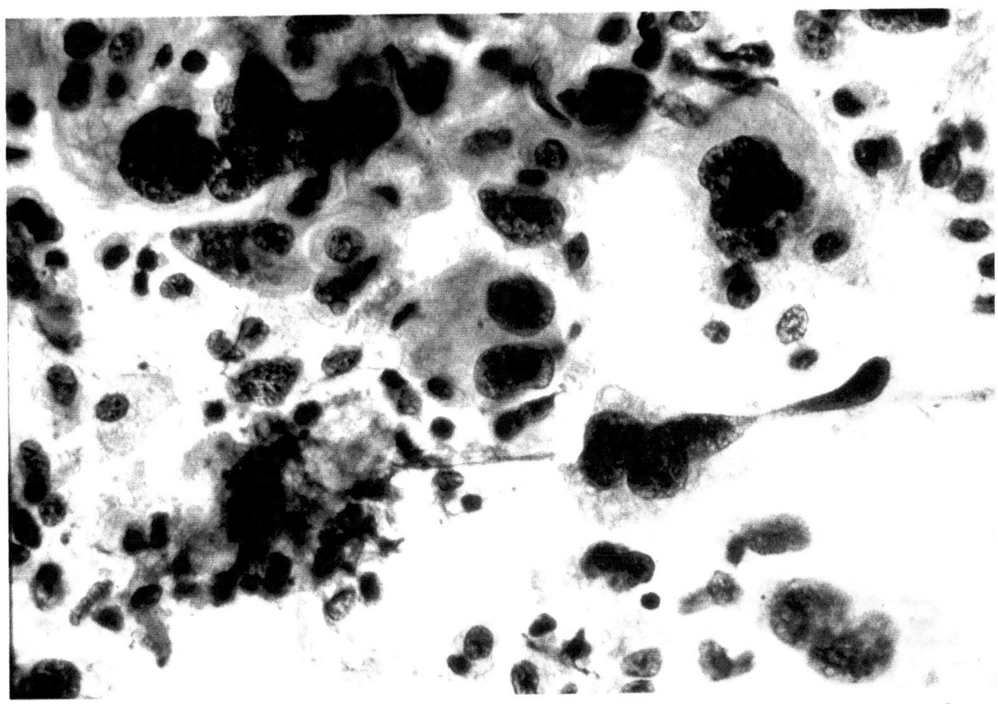

**FIGURE 6–29.** Pleomorphic MFH. Striking hyperchromasia and pleomorphism characterize the neoplastic nuclei and cells in this smear. Multinucleated tumor giant cells, some with bizarre appearances, are evident in association with malignant cells having a more histiocytoid appearance. (Papanicolaou stain, ×400)

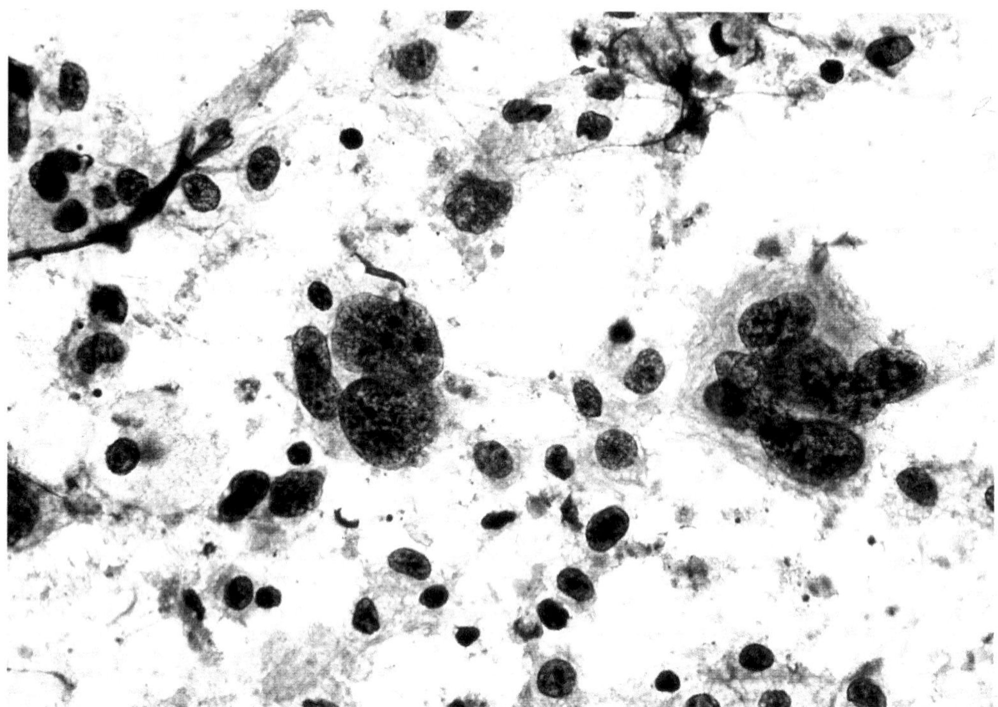

**FIGURE 6–30.** Pleomorphic MFH. Dispersed monstrous tumor giant cells are present containing multiple irregularly shaped and sized nuclei in their cytoplasm. The chromatin is coarsely granular and darkly stained; nucleoli are evident in some of the cells. Also note that the small malignant cells have round to ovoid to spindled contours. (Papanicolaou stain, ×400)

of pleomorphic lipoma has been described only rarely.[6,81,103] According to Akerman and Rydholm, the smears consist largely of tissue fragments and aggregates, indicating that intercellular cohesion is relatively well preserved.[6] The smears contain an admixture of bland to reactive fibroblast-like spindled cells, unremarkable adipocytes, multinucleated tumor giant cells, and lipoblasts (Fig. 6–31). The lipoblasts typically have a centrally or eccentrically located solitary hyperchromatic nucleus, the contours of which are deformed by lipid vacuoles impinging on it. Although these pleomorphic cells may simulate those of a sarcoma, strikingly bizarre and obviously malignant tumor giant cells are absent, the cellularity is relatively low on the smear, and intercellular cohesion is preserved. The giant cells in aspirates of tenosynovial giant cell tumors also should not be mistaken for the anaplastic giant cells of sarcomas (Fig. 6–32).[55,102,110] We have examined (courtesy of Dr. M.W. Stanley) a striking example of proliferative myositis. Admixed with reactive fibroblasts and muscle fragments were dispersed giant cells, some of which clearly resembled ganglion cells whereas others had large, irregular, dark nuclei. Their homogeneous smudged chromatin was diagnostically helpful, as was recognition of the benign and mixed nature of most of the aspirated cells.

The most common entities in the differential diagnosis are pleomorphic carcinomas of diverse sites.[90] Notable examples are giant cell or sarcomatoid carcinomas of the lung, thyroid, kidney, and pancreas. Some aspirates are completely indistinguishable from those of sarcomas on the basis of cytomorphology alone. In addition to the clinical history, the smears should be carefully searched for the presence of residual epithelial differentiation in the form of cohesive aggregates of carcinoma cells with polygonal to columnar configurations. In general, expression of epithelial markers such as cytokeratin is more striking in carcinomas than sarcomas.

Rarely, sarcomatoid mesotheliomas in FNABs completely simulate a pleomorphic soft tissue sarcoma. Positive immunostaining for cytokeratin and calretinin are the only pathologic clues to the appropriate diagnosis. Melanomas may simulate not only spindle cell sarcomas but also the pleomorphic variants. Cytoplasmic melanin pigment is not usually recognized; and again the clinical history of a prior melanoma or immunostaining for melanoma-related antigens (especially HMB-45) allows one to render the correct diagnosis. Anaplastic lymphomas, especially those positive for Ki-1, may simulate pleomorphic sarcomas in aspiration smears. These specimens are generally highly cellular with a strikingly dissociative pattern

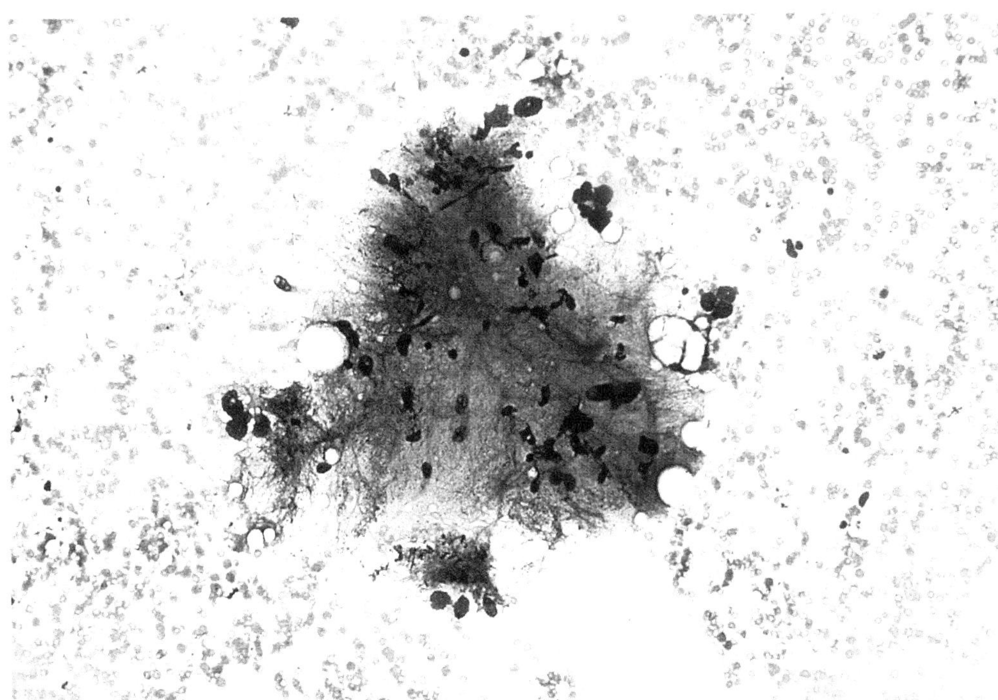

**FIGURE 6–31.** Pleomorphic lipoma. Scant cellularity characterizes this aspirate. Although most of the cells are small with solitary nuclei and apparently high nuclear/cytoplasmic ratios, others are larger. They vary from spindled to multinucleated tumor giant cells. A few neoplastic cells have prominent cytoplasmic lipid vacuoles. (Diff-Quik stain, ×40)

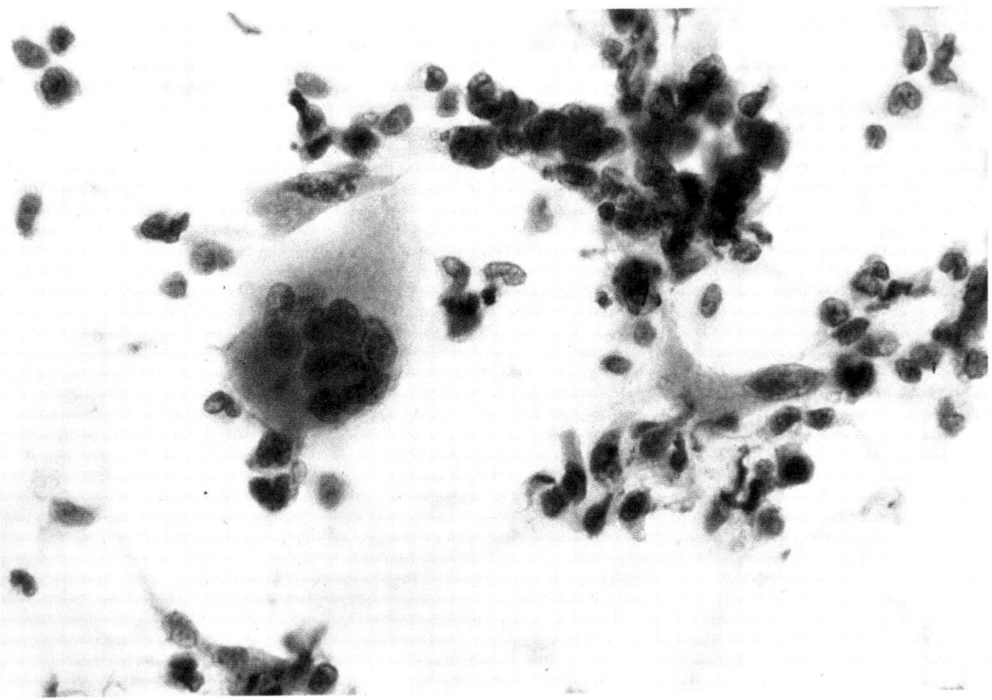

**FIGURE 6–32.** Giant cell tumor of tendon sheath. In contrast to the pleomorphic sarcomas, the nuclei in the giant cells are much smaller and more homogeneous. They have fine, even chromatin and small but distinct nucleoli. These giant cells have much more abundant cytoplasm and hence lower nuclear/cytoplasmic ratios. In the proper clinical setting this tumor should never be confused with a pleomorphic sarcoma. (Papanicolaou stain, ×100)

and marked variability in size and shape of the cells, including multinucleated tumor giant cells. Characteristic wreath cells and the presence of lymphoglandular bodies suggest the correct neoplasm. In contrast to most lymphomas, however, the latter bodies may not be easily found in smears. Rarely, granulocytic sarcomas, especially those of the $M_7$ type, resemble a pleomorphic sarcoma.[61,92] Finding small malignant cells with the characteristics of myeloblasts may facilitate the proper interpretation.

## POLYGONAL CELL SARCOMAS

The least frequent of the FNAB categories of soft tissue sarcomas is the polygonal or epithelial-like group,[49] which includes epithelioid sarcoma, alveolar soft part sarcoma, clear-cell sarcoma, and the predominantly epithelioid types of sarcoma. Although cellularity on the smear is variable, it is usually moderate to high, often with a largely dissociative pattern (Fig. 6–33). These smears contain, therefore, numerous individually dispersed malignant cells and small, generally flat aggregates. The malignant cells have round or polygonal shapes, well defined cellular borders, and at least moderate volumes of cytoplasm (Figs. 6–34, 6–35). Typically, they have a solitary, often eccentrically positioned round nucleus with a thick distinct membrane, vesicular chromatin, and one or more large nucleoli. In any of the polygonal cell sarcomas, some neoplastic cells are binucleated or even multinucleated. A few of the neoplastic cells have a spindled shape (Fig. 6–36).

The aspiration cytomorphologic attributes of epithelioid sarcoma, alveolar soft part sarcoma, and clear-cell sarcoma overlap,[3,13,24,47,48,68,74,89] although certain features point to a specific lesion. Optically clear cytoplasm and well developed intranuclear cytoplasmic pseudoinclusions indicate a clear-cell sarcoma.[13,24] In alveolar soft part sarcoma, some of the neoplastic cells have filamentous structures or distinct vacuoles in their abundant, finely granulated cytoplasm.[47,68,89] Benign and malignant granular cell tumors may also be considered in this category, as the neoplastic cells have voluminous, distinctly granular cytoplasm[34,35] (Fig. 6–37). A panel of antibodies may allow distinction of these neoplasms immunocytochemically.

The differential diagnosis of polygonal cell sarcomas in aspiration biopsies is relatively limited. A diagnosis of polygonal cell sarcoma can be rendered in the appropriate clinical scenario: A soft tissue mass presents in an extremity of a relatively young adult patient. Although unlikely, one must exclude a metastatic carcinoma or melanoma mimicking a primary soft tissue sarcoma. In general, a greater degree of intercellular cohesion and three-dimensional aggregates favor metastatic carcinoma. Clinical data includ-

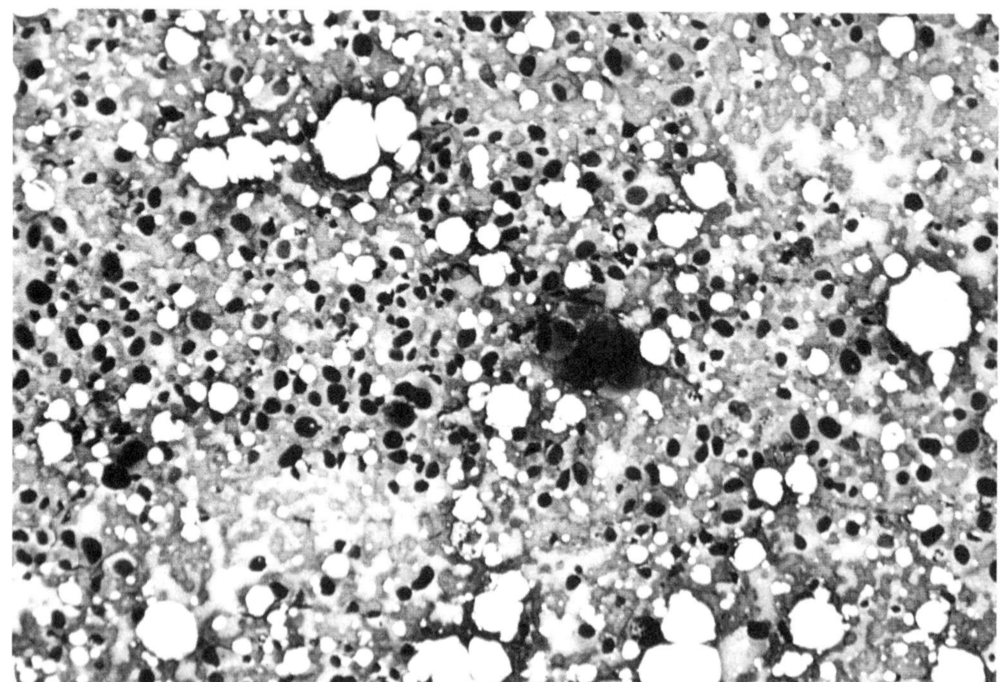

**FIGURE 6–33.** Clear-cell sarcoma. High cellularity and a lack of cohesion characterize this aspirate. Most of the cells have large single nuclei with prominent nucleoli and scanty cytoplasm. A few large, multinucleated neoplastic cells are also evident. (Diff-Quik stain, ×40)

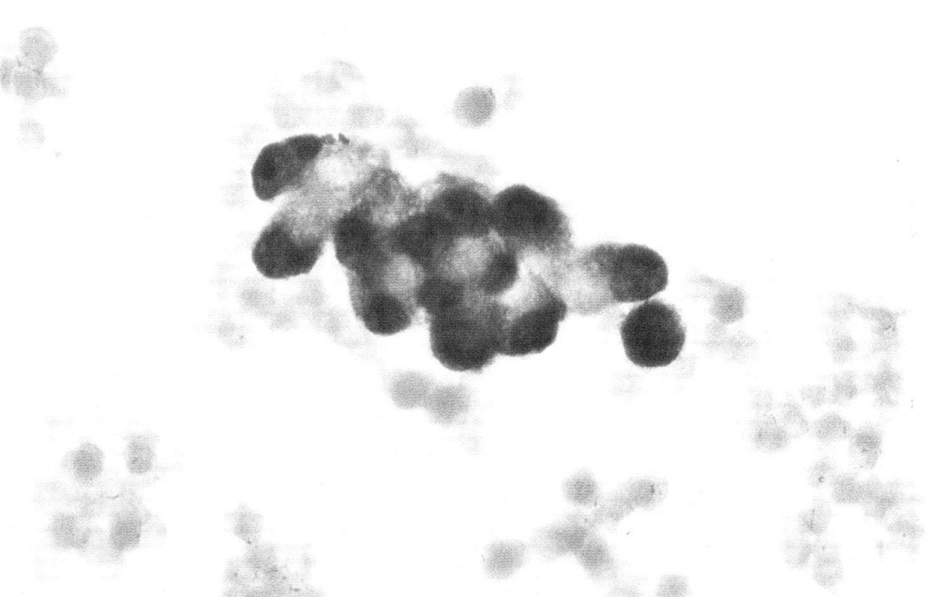

**FIGURE 6–34.** Clear-cell sarcoma. The neoplastic cells in this cohesive cluster have a distinct epithelioid appearance that is related to their polygonal contours, moderate volumes of cytoplasm, and eccentrically located round nuclei. The latter have prominent nucleoli. The cytoplasm is vacuolated, and in some cells it occurs to the extent that the cytoplasm appears clear. (Diff-Quik stain, ×250)

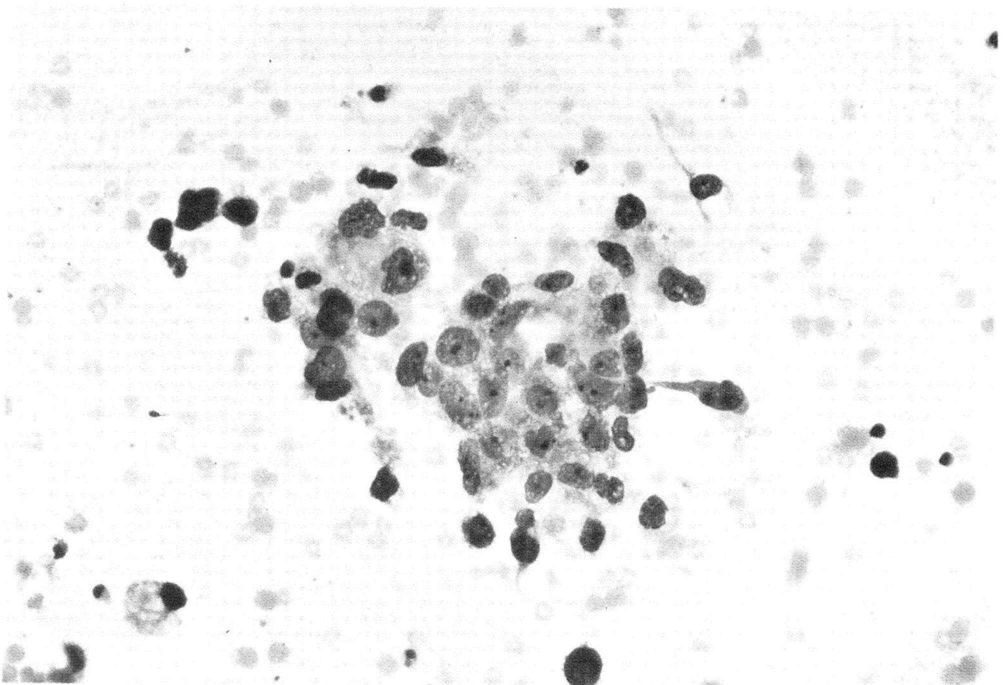

**FIGURE 6–35.** Epithelioid sarcoma. This cohesive aggregate has a distinct epithelioid appearance with maintenance of cohesion, polygonal contours, and peripherally situated round nuclei. Nucleoli are also strikingly prominent. (Diff-Quik stain, ×250)

**FIGURE 6–36.** Epithelioid sarcoma. Cohesion is reduced in this neoplasm compared to that in Figure 6–35. Cellular contours vary from round to polygonal to spindled. The nuclei have coarse, dark chromatin and distinct nucleoli. Overall, the nuclear/cytoplasmic ratios are not particularly high. (Papanicolaou stain, ×250)

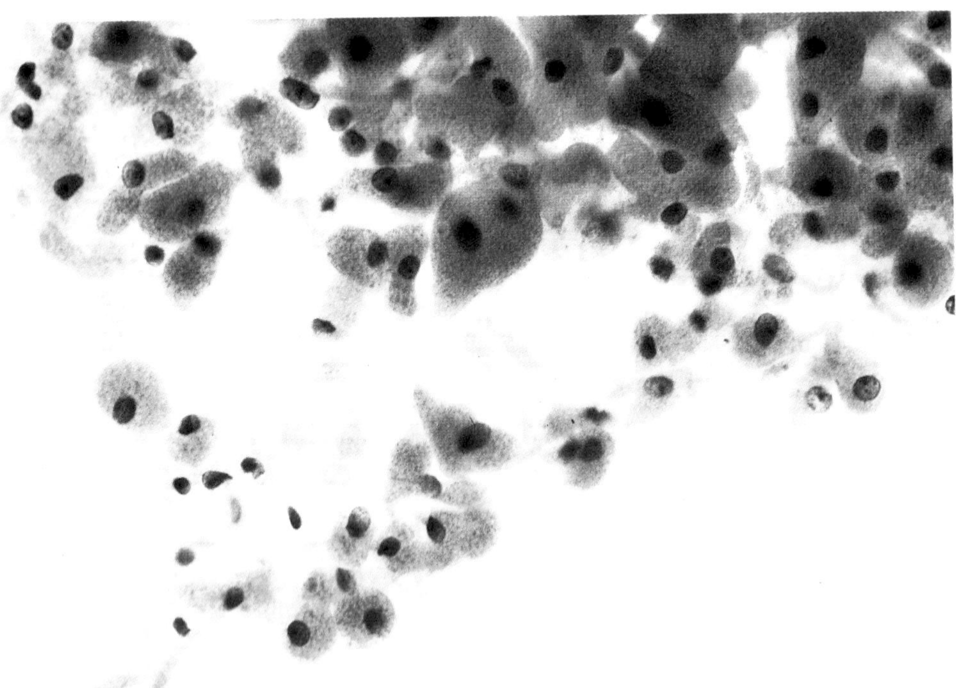

**FIGURE 6–37.** Granular cell tumor. This moderately cellular sample is characterized by uniform-appearing cells. Each cell has a round to polygonal shape, abundant distinctly granulated cytoplasm, and relatively small round nuclei. The latter, for the most part, are hyperchromatic and structureless, although nucleoli are evident in some. Obviously, the nuclear/cytoplasmic ratios are low. (Papanicolaou stain, ×250)

ing the medical history and imaging studies should assist in this differential diagnosis. Based solely on the findings in a single aspiration biopsy, it may be impossible to distinguish a clear-cell sarcoma from a metastatic melanoma. Renal and extrarenal rhabdoid tumors should also be considered in the differential diagnosis of some of these neoplasms.[104]

## ROUND CELL SARCOMAS

Although most soft tissue sarcomas occur predominantly in adult patients, the round cell sarcomas largely affect the pediatric population.[49] The most common is rhabdomyosarcoma. Other entries in this category include extraskeletal Ewing's sarcoma (ES)/primitive neuroectodermal tumor (PNET) and intra-abdominal desmoplastic small round-cell tumor. Aspiration biopsies of round cell sarcomas typically yield highly cellular smears composed of relatively small, homogeneous malignant cells.[11,49,54,93] These neoplastic elements typically have a solitary nucleus with high nuclear/cytoplasmic ratios. The major exception is the embryonal rhabdomyosarcoma in which a proportion of the neoplastic cells have abundant cytoplasm and multiple nuclei. Nuclear chromatin is generally hyperchromatic, and nucleoli may or may not be prominent.

Aspiration biopsies of rhabdomyosarcoma yield moderately to highly cellular samples.[10,14,72,86–88] The appearance depends partly on the histologic subtype. A large proportion of the cells are individually dispersed with no evidence of intercellular cohesion. With alveolar rhabdomyosarcoma, it is more likely that a proportion of the neoplastic cells are present in large, loosely cohesive aggregates (Fig. 6–38). Although some have suggested that these aggregates manifest a pseudoalveolar arrangement, we believe this pattern is difficult to recognize.[87] A large proportion of the neoplastic cells appear quite primitive in that they have a solitary round nucleus and a high nuclear/cytoplasmic ratio with no evidence of specific differentiation (Figs. 6–39, 6–40, 6–41). The chromatin is finely granular, evenly dispersed, and darkly stained. Nucleoli tend to be small and inconspicuous but may be large. In a study of 15 aspirated rhabdomyosarcomas, Akhtar and colleagues grouped the aspirated tumor cells into three categories: early, intermediate, and late rhabdomyoblasts.[10] They stated that in alveolar rhabdomyosarcomas most of the neoplastic cells were early rhabdomyoblasts, resembling

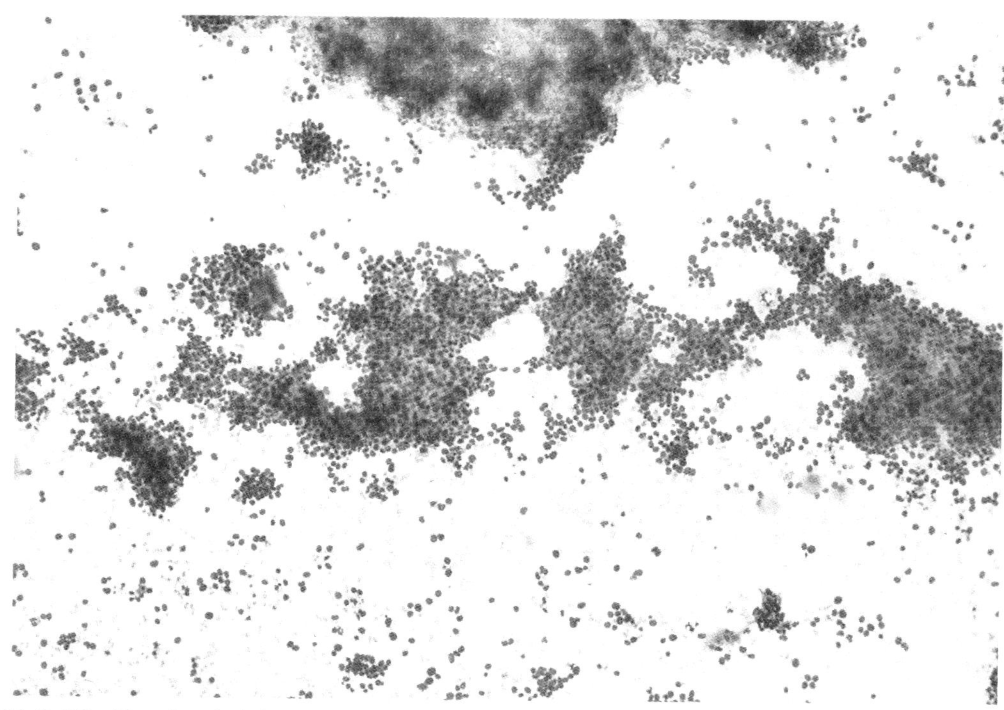

**FIGURE 6–38.** Alveolar rhabdomyosarcoma. In this scanning lens view, high smear cellularity is apparent, with many of the tumor cells present in loosely cohesive fragments. It almost suggests a pseudoalveolar arrangement. In addition, individually dispersed neoplastic cells are evident. Even at this low magnification, the striking uniformity of the cells is evident. Each cell has a solitary round nucleus surrounded by only a scanty rim of cytoplasm. (Diff-Quik stain, ×20)

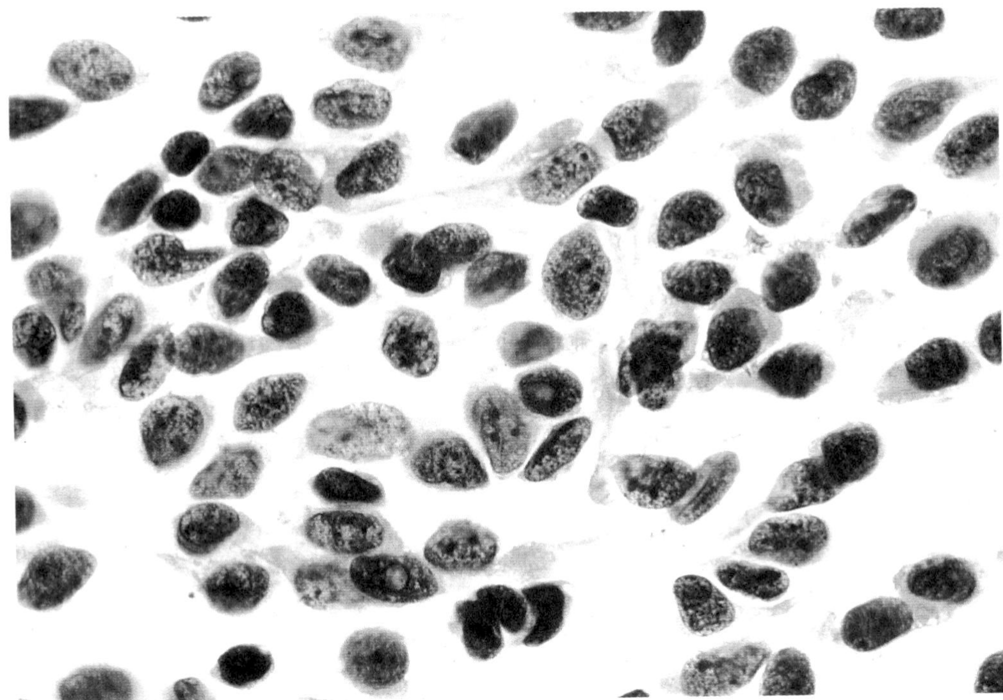

**FIGURE 6–39.** Embryonal rhabdomyosarcoma. The neoplastic cells are quite homogeneous in appearance. Each has a single ovoid nucleus with fine, even hyperchromatic chromatin and minute nucleoli. Most cells have scant cytoplasm in which the nucleus appears to be eccentrically positioned. A few tumor cells have long, tapering cytoplasmic tails. Cellularity is high, and cohesion is poorly preserved. (Hematoxylin and eosin, ×400)

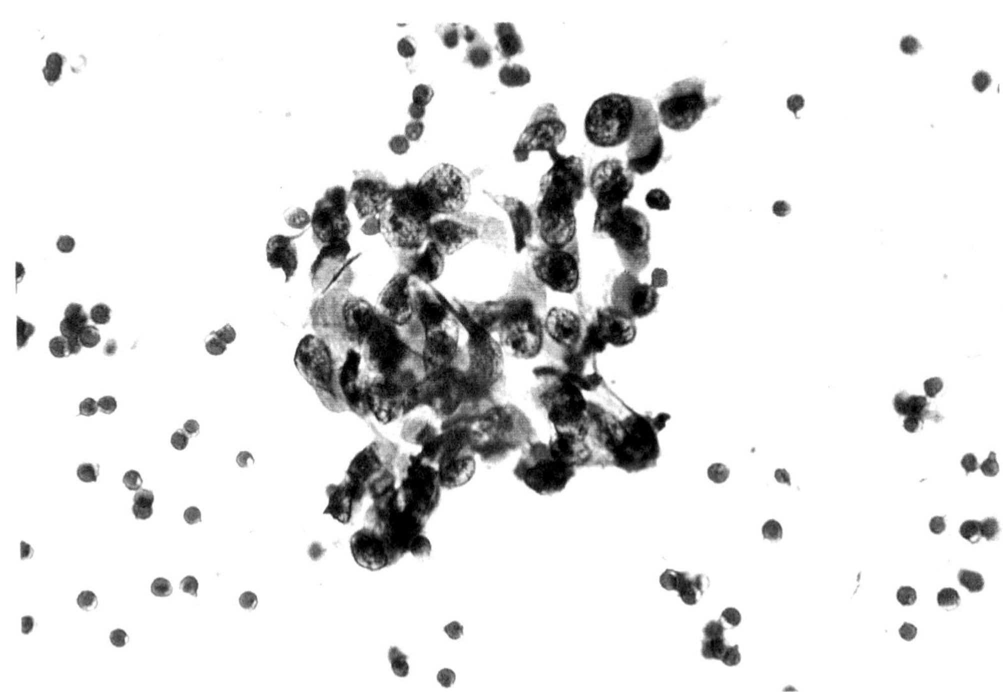

**FIGURE 6–40.** Embryonal rhabdomyosarcoma. The neoplastic cells in this example have more round or polygonal configurations. Despite the darkly stained chromatin, nucleoli are prominent. (Papanicolaou stain, ×250)

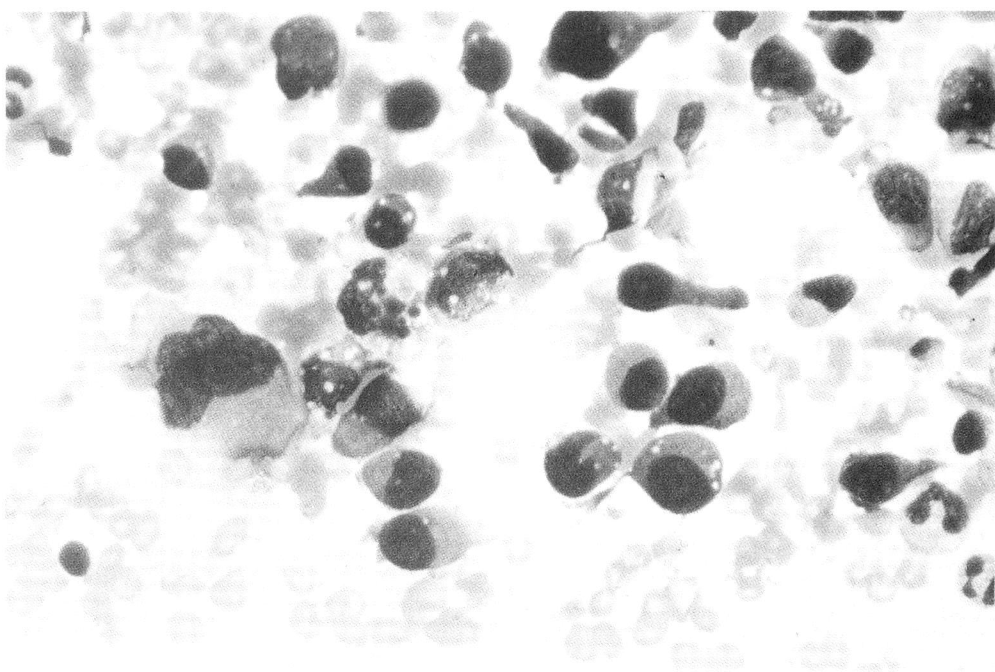

**FIGURE 6–41.** Embryonal rhabdomyosarcoma. A spectrum of cellular appearances is apparent. Most of the cells have solitary small round nuclei and rather high nuclear/cytoplasmic ratios. A tadpole cell is evident in the center of the field. Note also the presence of a large multinucleated tumor giant cell and the absence of intercellular cohesion. (Diff-Quik stain, ×400)

the undifferentiated cells described above. The intermediate rhabdomyoblasts had more abundant cytoplasm that tended to be palely stained and at times vacuolated. Voluminous, relatively opaque cytoplasm characterized the late rhabdomyoblasts. Cell contours varied from round to highly elongated or strap-like.

With the Romanowsky stain, some of the neoplastic elements have dense inclusion-like foci in the cytoplasm that correspond ultrastructurally to concentrated aggregates of sarcomeres. A proportion of these cells are multinucleated and sometimes include highly pleomorphic nuclei with prominent nucleoli. Embryonal rhabdomyosarcoma contains varying admixtures of rhabdomyoblasts at the three levels of differentiation. Needless to say, these categories are artificial, with no distinct lines of separation, so in an individual patient the distinction is difficult. Clinical data and karyotypic analysis are more useful. More importantly, it is the presence of the relatively large cells with abundant dense cytoplasm and multinucleation that allows the pathologist to distinguish rhabdomyosarcomas from other small round-cell tumors by FNAB (Fig. 6–41). This suggestion is supported by the recent logistic regression analysis of Layfield et al., in which the presence of strap, or "tadpole"-shaped, cells correlated well with the interpretation of rhabdomyosarcomas among small round-cell tumors.[54]

Aspirates of ES/PNET present a much more homogeneous cytomorphologic picture (Figs. 6–42, 6–43, 6–44). Aspiration biopsy specimens consistently yield high cellularity with numerous solitary mononucleated neoplastic cells.[20,79] The nuclei appear perfectly round with uniformly dispersed fine chromatin and inconspicuous nucleoli. For the most part, the nuclear/cytoplasmic ratios are extremely high. Occasionally, cytoplasmic blebs or sharply "punched-out" glycogen vacuoles are seen (Figs. 6–43, 6–44). Pseudorosettes may be evident in cohesive monolayers of neoplastic cells. The smear background does not demonstrate matrix material or lymphoglandular bodies. Although not totally specific, the diagnosis of ES/PNET can be supported by a positive immunocytochemical reaction for CD99. Furthermore, aspirated material may be submitted for karyotypic analysis; it would demonstrate an 11;22 reciprocal translocation.

The desmoplastic small round-cell tumor is another consideration in this category. This high grade, generally fatal cancer typically affects male adolescents; it presents as a primary mass involving the peritoneum or omentum. Infrequently, these neoplasms arise in extraabdominal locations. Aspiration biopsies yield

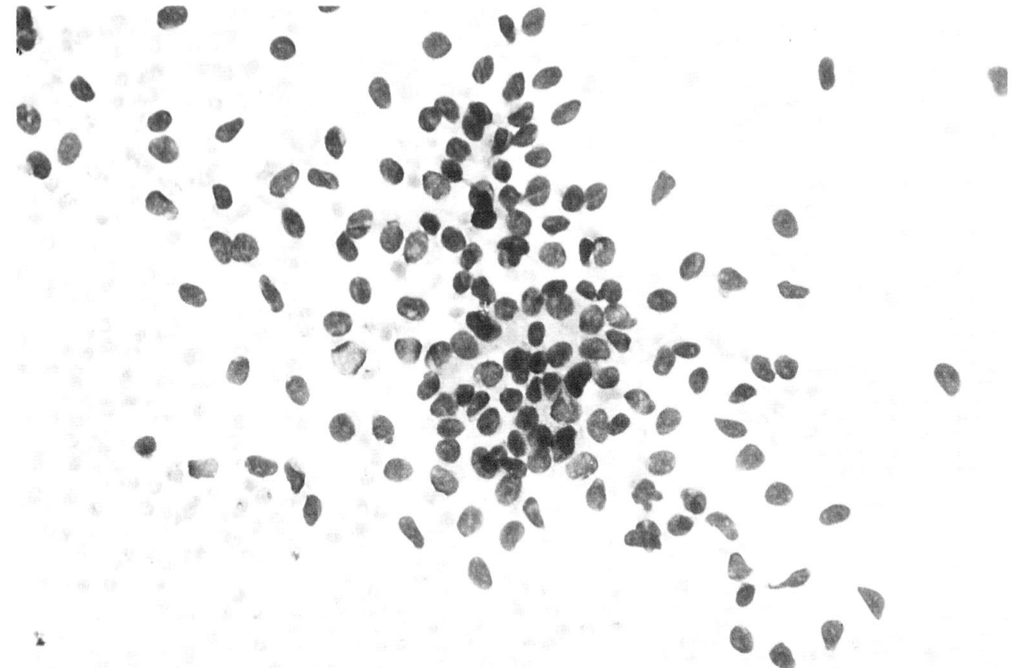

**FIGURE 6–42.** Primitive neuroectodermal tumor (PNET). Although the malignant cells are loosely arrayed, a suggestion of pseudorosette formation is evident in the central aggregate. The neoplastic cells are strikingly homogeneous, each with a solitary round nucleus and an extremely high nuclear/cytoplasmic ratio. The chromatin is finely reticulated, and nucleoli are not evident. (Diff-Quik stain, ×100)

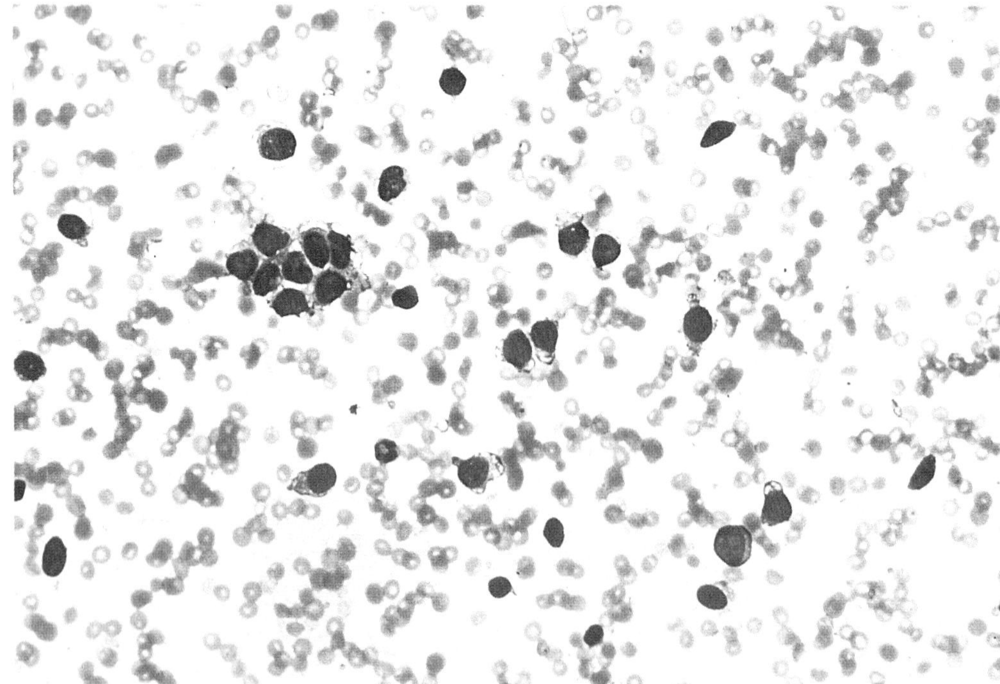

**FIGURE 6–43.** PNET. The cytoplasm of some of the malignant cells contain one or more glycogen vacuoles. As in the tumor in Figure 6–42, the tumor cells are strikingly uniform. (Diff-Quik stain, ×100)

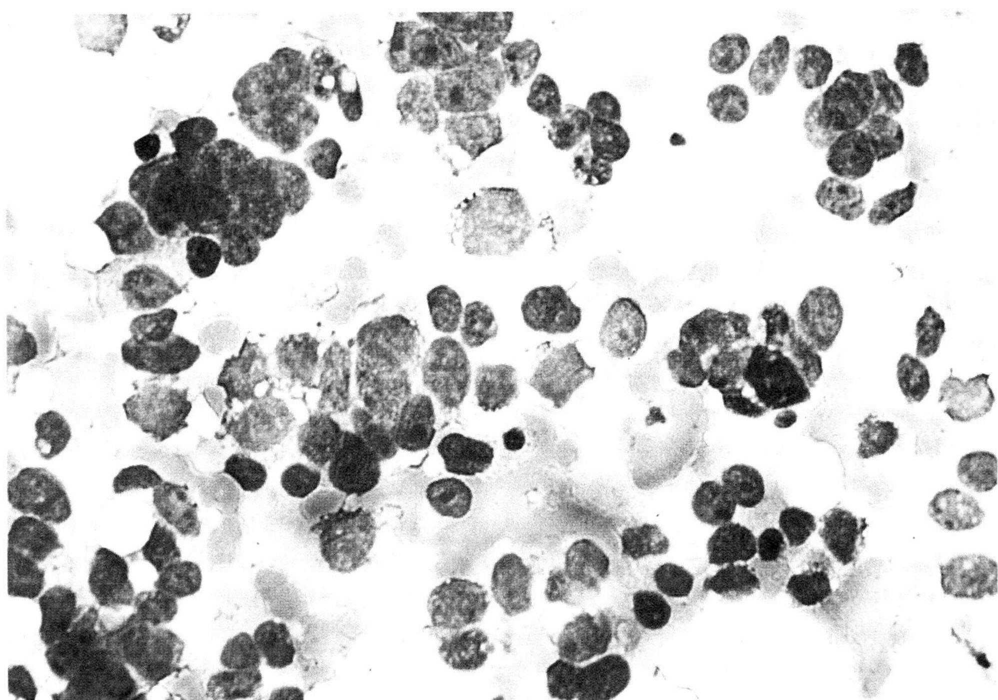

**FIGURE 6–44.** PNET. Each malignant cell has a single round nucleus with finely reticulated, evenly dispersed chromatin. For the most part, nucleoli are inconspicuous. In many cells the cytoplasm is barely visible, whereas others have small to large glycogen vacuoles. The presence of cohesion and the lack of lymphoglandular bodies helps distinguish this lesion from lymphoma. (Diff-Quik stain, ×400)

variably cellular smears, which presumably is a reflection of the prominent desmoplastic stroma in the tumor.[23,62] The smears reveal uniform, small, round malignant cells present as individual cells and in aggregates (Fig. 6–45). Each neoplastic cell has single round nucleus with hyperchromatic and chromatin inconspicuous nucleoli. Generally, the cytoplasm is scanty. Thus on smears the cells resemble those of Ewing's sarcoma. The smears may also show fragments of cellular collagen. If this diagnosis is considered, the results of immunocytochemistry on aspirated material may be supportive. These neoplastic cells exhibit multidirectional differentiation, typically being positive for cytokeratin, desmin, and neuron-specific enolase. Material obtained by FNAB may demonstrate an 11;22 reciprocal translation by cytogenetics, which differs from that found in ES/PNET, or a specific gene fusion product seen by the PCR.

In intraabdominal aspiration biopsy specimens, two other entities must be entertained in the differential diagnosis: neuroblastoma and Burkitt's lymphoma. Aspirates of neuroblastoma yield moderately to highly cellular samples dominated by small primitive malignant cells characterized by solitary nuclei and extremely high nuclear/cytoplasmic ratios.[54,91] Each nucleus has a round, ovoid, or slightly irregular contour with even, fine chromatin that stains darkly. Nucleoli are either absent or small and inconspicuous. Although many of the neoplastic cells show no specific differentiation, the smears may provide important diagnostic clues. One is the presence of pseudorosettes,[54,91] which consist of one or more layers of nuclei surrounding central fibrillar material. True lumens are not evident. Similar filamentous material corresponding to the neuropil may be present in the background; and a large proportion of the cells appear embedded in this material. With the Diff-Quik stain it appears pink to gray, and with the Papanicolaou stain it is green. Another potentially helpful diagnostic clue is the presence of neoplastic ganglion cells. These elements are characterized by a large size, polygonal contours, moderate to voluminous basophilic cytoplasm, and one or more nuclei. The latter often appear perfectly round and have distinct membranes, vesicular chromatin, macronucleoli, and eccentric locations. Smaller cells may represent partially differentiated neuroblasts.

Burkitt's lymphoma presents a characteristic picture in the FNAB aspirate. The smears are highly cellular and composed of discohesive, homogeneous, round blasts. These cells have diameters approximately three times that of a small mature lymphocyte. Each neoplastic cell has a solitary, often perfectly round-appearing nucleus with moderately clumped chromatin

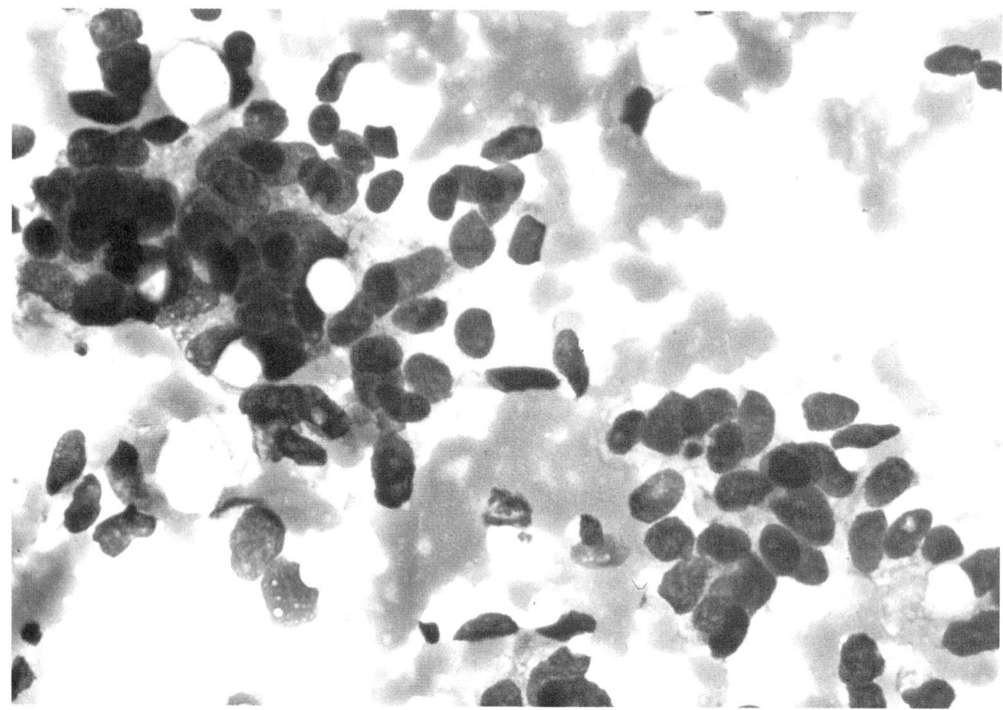

**FIGURE 6–45.** Intraabdominal desmoplastic small round-cell tumor. The malignant cells demonstrate no evidence of specific differentiation. The cohesive clusters are occupied by cells with solitary round nuclei, finely reticulated chromatin, small nucleoli, and scanty cytoplasm. (Diff-Quik stain, ×400)

and one or more distinct nucleoli. In general, multiple small nucleoli are evident. The volume of cytoplasm varies from scanty to moderate; it is distinctly basophilic and may contain round lipid vacuoles. With alcohol fixation both the cytoplasmic basophilia and the vacuoles are lost; on the other hand, the tumor cells appear even more homogeneous. The background contains numerous lymphoglandular bodies. Cytogenetic analysis of aspirated cellular material shows an 8;14 reciprocal translocation.

## MISCELLANEOUS SARCOMAS

A neoplasm that does not fit neatly into any of the above categories is the well differentiated liposarcoma (Figs. 6–46, 6–47). The aspiration cytomorphology of this tumor has only rarely been detailed.[6,66,107] Smears are only moderately cellular at best, and the sample may be mistaken for benign adipose tissue owing to the presence of mostly (or exclusively) mature-appearing fat cells, often in fragments. The latter are huge univacuolated cells with small, dark, round peripheral nuclei. The diagnosis of liposarcoma requires finding unequivocal lipoblasts with cytoplasmic lipid vacuoles that compress and distort the hyperchromatic nucleus. Although some have described complex arrays of branching capillaries in well differentiated liposarcomas, this has not been our experience and we would not expect them to be prominent.[108]

As implied, the FNAB diagnosis of well differentiated liposarcoma is difficult. As with other neoplasms, additional studies are needed when doubt exists. With well differentiated liposarcoma, we recommend a tissue examination. If the mass is in the retroperitoneum and sampling is guided radiologically, a needle core biopsy may suffice; otherwise, an open biopsy is performed.

The major entity in this differential diagnosis is benign fat, either normal tissue or a lipoma. These two entities are morphologically indistinguishable in aspirates. To diagnose a lipoma, a distinct mass must be detected clinically. Smears contain variable numbers of flat to three-dimensional aggregates of benign adipocytes (Fig. 6–48).[6,66] On smears, elastofibromas may closely simulate lipomas, as they contain clusters of mature adipocytes plus small fragments of fibrous connective tissue. The characteristic thick elastic fibers are not evident with conventional stains. In the scenario where an elastofibroma is suspected clinically, smears may be destained and then restained for elastic fibers. This maneuver permits an accurate diagnosis.[73]

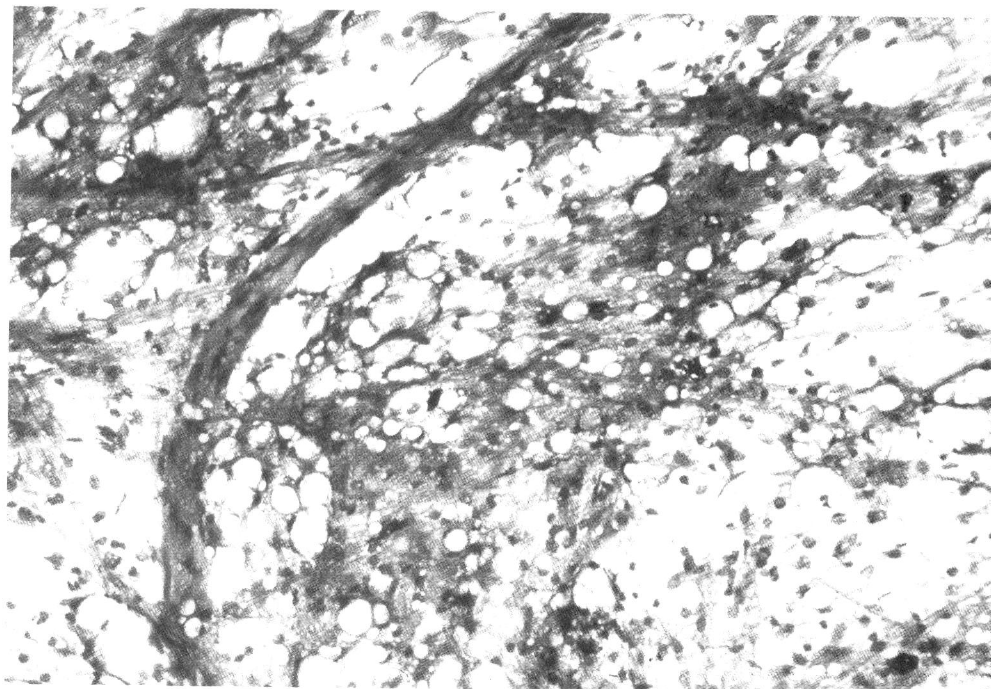

**FIGURE 6–46.** Well differentiated liposarcoma. Unremarkable-appearing adipocytes appear to be embedded in fibrous connective tissue. In addition, however, scattered cells have large nuclei, some of which appear to have cytoplasmic lipid vacuoles. In the proper clinical setting, this picture is diagnostic of liposarcoma. Vascularity is prominent. (Diff-Quik stain, ×40)

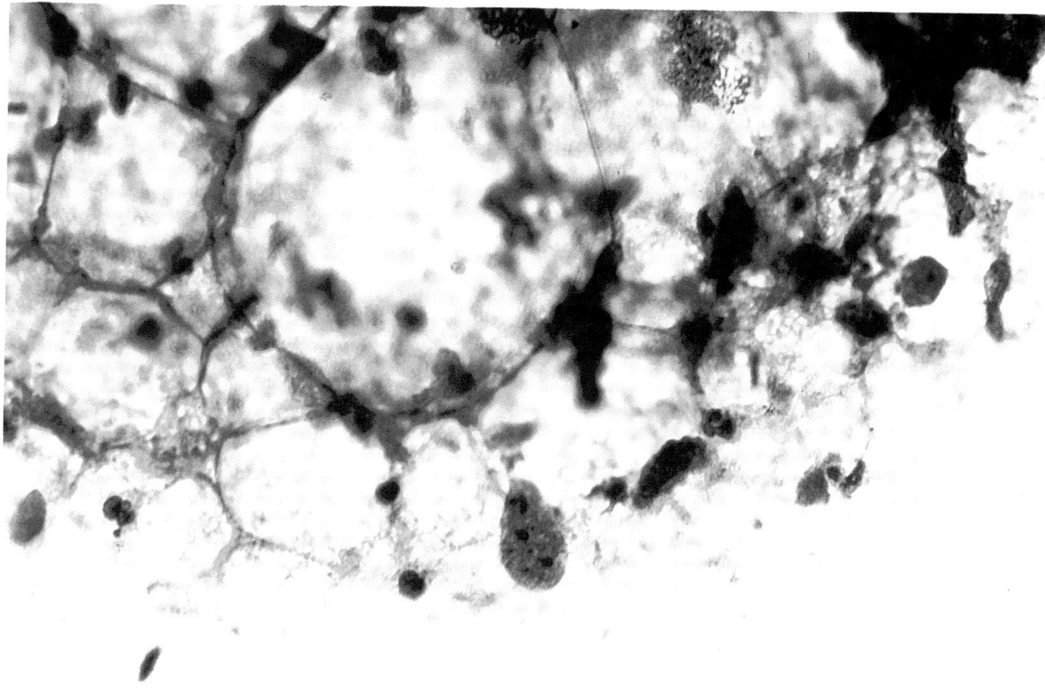

**FIGURE 6–47.** Well differentiated liposarcoma. Although most of the adipocytes in this field appear unremarkable, one has a large, irregularly shaped nucleus with darkly stained and variably granular chromatin. (Papanicolaou stain, ×400)

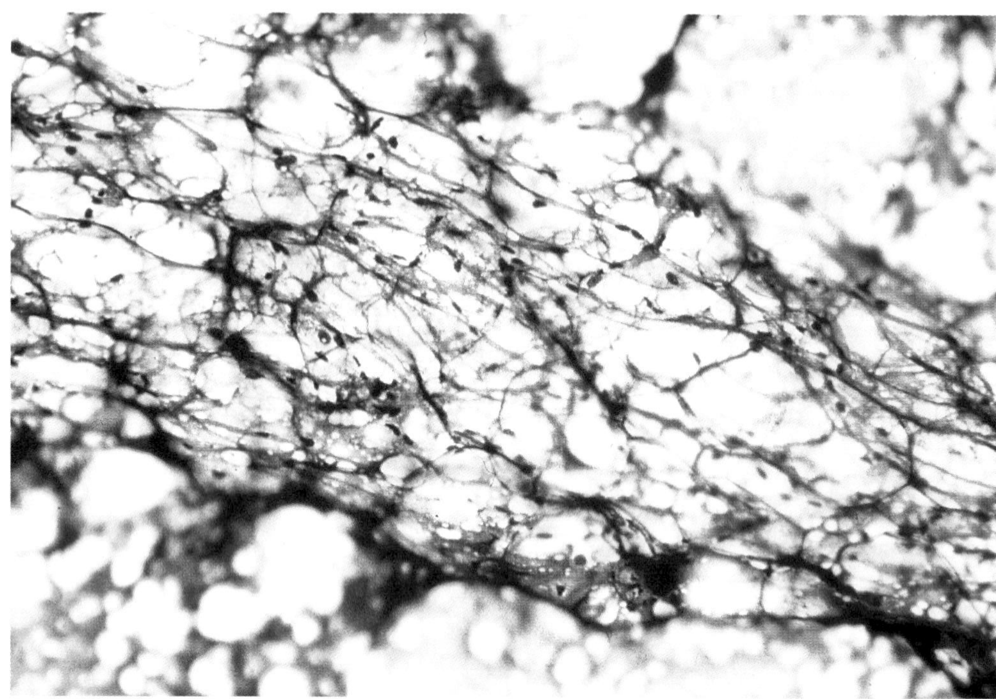

**FIGURE 6–48.** Lipoma. This large cohesive fragment of benign adipose tissue is composed of large unremarkable fat cells. Cell borders are distinct, cytoplasm is clear, and nuclei are extremely small and peripherally located. Occasional capillaries are seen coursing throughout the fragment. (Diff-Quik stain, ×40)

## GRADING SARCOMAS

Among the prognostic factors in patients with soft tissue sarcomas, histologic grade is consistently one of the most significant.[40,56] Accordingly, it is important to consider the possibility of accurately grading soft tissue sarcomas by FNAB. Although several grading schemes exist for these neoplasms, most of them consistently incorporate several microscopic attributes: mitotic activity, amount of necrosis, and degree of differentiation or histologic subtype. Guillou and Coindre stated, "The risk of underestimating necrosis or mitotic activity is directly related to the low quantity of material provided. Grading sarcomas on fine needle or core biopsy should be discouraged. The risk of error is too high, and diagnosis of a histologic type of sarcoma is uncertain if not impossible."[40] According to these experts, grading sarcomas on aspiration smears should not and cannot be accomplished reliably and accurately. As stated subsequently, we do not totally agree. One can certainly make general predictions, although currently final grading is usually based on the findings of incisional biopsies or definitive excisions.

There are several reasons for these authors to have made this statement. First, counting mitotic figures in aspiration biopsies of any tumor type is not a standardized practice, to say the least. Although mitotic figures can certainly be seen on direct smears, we are unaware of anyone who consistently and routinely uses mitotic figure counts on smears of any type of neoplasm. If for no other reason, the variability in cellularity from field to field would be prohibitive. Similarly, the proportion of the tumor that is necrotic prior to chemotherapy or radiotherapy cannot be predicted on the basis of aspiration biopsy results. Thus the cytologist can state only that necrotic debris is absent or present in scant or large amounts on the smears. A third feature, the degree of differentiation or histologic subtype, is somewhat different. With FNAB a specific cell type can be identified in a large proportion of soft tissue sarcomas. This is especially true if one utilizes ancillary diagnostic procedures such as immunocytochemistry and cytogenetics directly on aspirated cellular material.

With all of this in mind, many soft tissue sarcomas can be graded in a clinically relevant manner on the basis of aspiration biopsies.[51] Specifically, round cell sarcomas are almost always high grade neoplasms. Furthermore, with the use of ancillary diagnostic testing, specific diagnoses can be rendered in a large proportion of these cases. Although the specific cell type of a pleomorphic sarcoma cannot always be determined on smears, these neoplasms can almost always be recognized as high grade. Conversely, if they can be identified accurately, well differentiated liposarcomas are consistently low grade. Most of the myxoid sarcomas are low grade neoplasms. It is the polygonal cell and especially the spindle cell categories that pose the greatest difficulty.[51,108] In our limited experience, we do not believe that the polygonal cell sarcomas can be stratified accurately into grades on the basis of aspiration biopsy results.

## CONCLUSIONS

Without a doubt, FNAB of soft tissue neoplasms has important limitations that must be recognized. Samples of the neoplasm may be limited in cellularity to the point of being insufficient for diagnosis. As a generalization, soft tissue neoplasms have several attributes that may lead to poor cellularity on the smear. As with other tumor types, the pathologist should never feel compelled to "force" a diagnosis on limited samples. There are certain neoplasms for which a benign versus malignant designation cannot be made with certainty from aspiration smears. In addition, it may be impossible to predict the grade to some extent on the basis of smear preparations. Based purely on cellular morphology, the exact cell type of many soft tissue neoplasms cannot be stated accurately. However, many of these problems are obviated with the use of ancillary diagnostic procedures. Obviously, there is the need for a cytopathologist with interest and knowledge in soft tissue pathology. Furthermore, the diagnostician must be willing to state in some cases that the diagnosis is uncertain.

The FNAB procedure does have a number of advantages that overall outweight the disadvantages. Aspiration biopsy provides a rapid, relatively nontraumatic procedure for sampling both superficial and deep-seated mass lesions. With experience, soft tissue neoplasms can be recognized and accurately diagnosed in many instances. Another advantage is that multiple samples can be obtained during a single clinic visit, which is especially relevant when on-site evaluation of the smear is available at the time of the biopsy. FNAB is easily performed on orthopedic neoplasms in the outpatient setting. Finally, compared to other diagnostic procedures, FNAB is relatively inexpensive. Thus in many patients a tumor can be accurately typed and graded with high levels of diagnostic sensitivity and specificity. At the very least, FNAB permits rapid triage of the patient for diagnosis by more traditional methods.

### REFERENCES

1. Abdul-Karim FW, Rader AE. Fine needle aspiration of soft-tissue lesions. Clin Lab Med 18:507, 1998.
2. Abele J, Miller T. Cytology of well differentiated and poorly differentiated hemangiosarcoma in fine needle aspirates. Acta Cytol 26:341, 1992.
3. Ahmen MN, Feldman M, Seemayer TA. Cytology of epithelioid sarcoma. Acta Cytol 18:459, 1974.
4. Aisner SC, Seidman JD, Burke KC, Young JWR. Aspiration cytology of biphasic and monophasic synovial sarcoma. Acta Cytol 37:413, 1993.
5. Akerman M, Rydholm A. Aspiration cytology of intramuscular myxoma: a comparative clinical, cytologic, and histologic study of ten cases. Acta Cytol 27:505, 1983.
6. Akerman M, Rydholm A. Aspiration cytology of lipomatous tumors: a 10 year experience at an orthopedic oncology center. Diagn Cytopathol 3:295, 1987.
7. Akerman M, Rydholm A, Persson BM. Aspiration cytology of soft tissue tumors; the 10 year experience at an orthopaedic oncology center. Acta Orthop Scand 56:407, 1985.
8. Akerman M, Willén H. Critical review of the role of fine needle aspiration in soft tissue tumors. Pathol Case Rev 3: 111, 1998.
9. Akerman M, Willén H, Carlén B, et al. Fine needle aspiration (FNA) of synovial sarcoma: a comparative histological-cytological study of 15 cases including immunohistochemical, electron microscopic and cytogenetic examination and DNA-ploidy analysis. Cytopathology 7:187, 1996.
10. Akhtar M, Ali MA, Bakry M, et al. Fine needle aspiration biopsy of childhood rhabdomyosarcoma: cytologic, histologic, and ultrastructural correlations. Diagn Cytopathol 8:465, 1992.
11. Akhtar M, Ashraf AM, Sabbah R, et al. Small round cell tumor with divergent differentiation: cytologic, histologic and ultrastructural findings. Diagn Cytopathol 11:159, 1994.
12. Alkan S, Eltoum IA, Tabbara S, et al. Usefulness of molecular detection of human herpesvirus-8 in the diagnosis of Kaposi sarcoma by fine-needle aspiration. Am J Clin Pathol 111:91, 1999.
13. Almeida MM, Nunes AM, Frable WJ. Malignant melanoma of soft tissue: a report of three cases with diagnosis by fine needle aspiration cytology. Acta Cytol 38:241, 1994.
14. Almeida M, Stastny JF, Wakely PE Jr, Frable WJ. Fine needle aspiration biopsy of childhood rhabdomyosarcoma: re-evaluation of the cytologic criteria for diagnosis. Diagn Cytopathol 11:231, 1994.
15. Azua J, Arraiza A, Delgado B, Romeo C. Nodular fasciitis initially diagnosed by aspiration cytology. Acta Cytol 29:562, 1985.
16. Barbazza R, Chiarelli S, Quintarelli GF, Manconi R. Role of fine-needle aspiration cytology in the preoperative evolution of smooth muscle tumors. Diagn Cytopathol 16:326, 1997.
17. Barth RJ, Merino MJ, Solomon D, et al. A prospective study of the value of core needle biopsy and fine needle aspiration in the diagnosis of soft tissue masses. Surgery 112:536, 1992.
18. Bennert KW, Abdul-Karim FW. Fine needle aspiration cytology vs. needle core biopsy of soft tissue tumors: a comparison. Acta Cytol 38:381, 1994.
19. Berardo MD, Powers CN, Wakely P Jr, et al. Fine-needle aspiration cytopathology of malignant fibrous histiocytoma. Cancer Cytopathol 81:228, 1997.
20. Berhant LE, Anderson LH, Taylor DA. Extraskeletal Ewing's sarcoma: diagnosis of a case by fine needle aspiration cytology. Acta Cytol 30:683, 1986.
21. Boucher LD, Swanson PE, Stanley MW, et al. Cytology of angiosarcoma: findings in fourteen fine-needle aspiration biopsies and one pleural fluid. Am J Clin Pathol 114:210, 2000.
22. Brosjö O, Bauer HCF, Kreisbergers A, et al. Fine needle aspiration biopsy of soft tissue tumors. Act Orthop Scand 65(Suppl 256):108, 1994.
23. Caraway NP, Fanning CV, Amato RJ, et al. Fine-needle aspi-

ration of ultra-abdominal desmoplastic small round cell tumor. Diagn Cytopathol 9:465, 1993.
24. Caraway NP, Fanning CV, Wojeik EM, et al. Cytology of malignant melanoma of soft parts: fine needle aspirates and exfoliative specimens. Diagn Cytopathol 9:632, 1993.
25. Caraway NP, Staerkel GA, Fanning CV, et al. Diagnosing intramuscular myxoma by fine needle aspiration: a multidisciplinary approach. Diagn Cytopathol 11:255, 1994.
26. Cohen MB, Layfield LJ. Fine needle aspiration biopsy of soft tissue tumors. In: Schmidt WA, Miller TR (eds) Cytopathology Annual 1994. ASCP Press, Chicago, 1994, pp 101–132.
27. Costa MJ, Campman SC, Davis RL, Howell LP. Fine-needle aspiration cytology of sarcoma: retrospective review of diagnostic utility and specificity. Diagn Cytopathol 15:23, 1996.
28. Dahl I, Akerman M. Nodular fasciitis: a correlative cytologic and histologic study of 13 cases. Acta Cytol 25:215, 1981.
29. Dahl I, Hagmar B, Angervall L. Leiomyosarcoma of the soft tissue: a correlative cytological and histological study of 11 cases. Acta Pathol Microbiol Scand 89:285, 1981.
30. Dahl I, Hagmar B, Idvall I. Benign solitary neurilemoma (schwannoma): a correlative cytological and histological study of 28 cases. Acta Pathol Microbiol Immunol Scand 92: 91, 1984.
31. Dodd LG, Marom EM, Dash RC, et al. Fine-needle aspiration cytology of "ancient" schwannoma. Diagn Cytopathol 20:307, 1999.
32. Ferretti M, Gusella PM, Mancini AM, et al. Progressive approach to the cytologic diagnosis of retroperitoneal spindle cell tumors. Acta Cytol 41:450, 1997.
33. Finley JL, Silverman JF, Cappellari JO, Geisinger KR. Fine needle aspiration cytology of gynecologic sarcomas and mixed tumors. In: Schmidt WA, Miller TR (eds) Cytopathology Annual, ASCP Press, Chicago, 1996, pp 267–287.
34. Franzen S, Stenkvist B. Diagnosis of granular cell myoblastoma by fine needle aspiration biopsy. Acta Pathol Microbiol Scand 72:391, 1968.
35. Geisinger KR, Kawamoto EH, Marshall RB, et al. Aspiration and exfoliative cytology, including ultrastructure, of a malignant granular cell tumor. Acta Cytol 29:593, 1985.
36. Geisinger KR, Naylor B, Beals TF, Novak PM. Cytopathology, including transmission and scanning electron microscopy of pleomorphic liposarcomas in pleural fluids. Acta Cytol 24: 435, 1980.
37. Geisinger KR, Silverman JF, Cappellari JO, Dabbs DJ. Fine-needle aspiration cytology of malignant hemangiopericytomas with ultrastructural and flow cytometric analyses. Arch Pathol Lab Med 114:705, 1990.
38. Gonzalez-Campora R, Munoz-Arias G, Otal-Salaverri C, et al. Fine needle aspiration cytology of primary soft tissue tumors: morphologic analysis of the most frequent types. Acta Cytol 36:905, 1992.
39. Gonzalez-Campora R, Otal-Salaverri C, Helvia-Vazquez A, et al. Fine needle aspiration in myxoid tumors of the soft tissues. Acta Cytol 34:179, 1990.
40. Guillou L, Coindre J-M. How should we grade soft tissue sarcomas and what are the limitations? Pathol Case Rev 3: 105, 1998.
41. Hajdu SI. Diagnosis of soft tissue sarcomas on aspiration smears. Acta Cytol 40:604, 1996.
42. Hales M, Bottles K, Muller T, et al. Diagnosis of Kaposi's sarcoma by fine-needle aspiration biopsy. Am J Clin Pathol 88:20, 1987.
43. Henke AC, Salomão DR, Hughes JH. Cellular schwannoma mimics a sarcoma: an example of a potential pitfall in aspiration cytodiagnosis. Diagn Cytopathol 20:312, 1999.
44. Hood IC, Qizilbash AH, Young JEM, Archibald SD. Needle aspiration cytology of a benign and a malignant schwannoma. Acta Cytol 28:157, 1984.
45. Inagaki H, Murase T, Otsuka T, Eimoto T. Detection of SYT-SSX fusion transcript in synovial sarcoma using archival cytologic specimens. Am J Clin Pathol 111:528, 1999.
46. James LP. Cytopathology of mesenchymal repair. Diagn Cytopathol 1:91, 1985.
47. Jiménez-Heffernan JA, López-Ferrer P, Vicandi B, et al. Cytologic features of malignant peripheral nerve sheath tumor. Acta Cytol 43:175, 1999.
48. Kapila K, Chopra P, Verma K. Fine needle aspiration cytology of alveolar soft-part sarcoma. Acta Cytol 29:559, 1985.
49. Kilpatrick SE, Geisinger KR. Soft tissue sarcomas: the utility and limitations of fine needle aspiration biopsy. Am J Clin Pathol 110:50, 1998.
50. Kilpatrick SE, Teot LA, Stanley MW, et al. Fine needle aspiration biopsy of synovial sarcoma. Am J Clin Pathol 106:769, 1996.
51. Kilpatrick SE, Ward WG, Cappellari JO, Bos GD. Fine-needle aspiration biopsy of soft tissue sarcomas: a cytomorphologic analysis with emphasis on histologic subtyping, grading, and therapeutic significance. Am J Clin Pathol 112:179, 1999.
52. Kindblom L-G, Walaas L, Widelin S. Ultrastructural studies in the preoperative cytologic diagnosis of soft tissue tumors. Semin Diagn Pathol 3:317, 1986.
53. Layfield LJ, Anders KH, Glasgow BJ, Mirra JM. Fine needle aspiration of primary soft tissue lesions. Arch Pathol Lab Med 110:420, 1986.
54. Layfield LJ, Liu K, Dodge RK. Logistic regression analysis of small round cell neoplasms: a cytologic study. Diagn Cytopathol 20:271, 1999.
55. Layfield LJ, Moffatt EJ, Dodd LG, et al. Cytologic findings in tenosynovial giant cell tumors investigated by fine-needle aspiration cytology. Diagn Cytopathol 16:317, 1997.
56. Levine EA. Prognostic factors in soft tissue sarcoma. Semin Surg Oncol 17:23, 1999.
57. Lindberg GM, Maitra A, Gokaslan ST, et al. Low grade fibromyxoid sarcoma: fine-needle aspiration cytology with histologic, cytogenetic, immunohistochemical, and ultrastructural correlation. Cancer Cytopathol 87:75, 1999.
58. Liu K, Dodge RK, Dodd LG, Layfield LJ. Logistic regression analysis of low grade spindle cell lesions: a cytologic study. Acta Cytol 43:143, 1999.
59. Liu K, Dodge RK, Layfield LJ. Logistic regression analysis of high grade spindle cell neoplasms: a fine needle aspiration cytologic study. Acta Cytol 43:593, 1999.
60. Liu K, Layfield LJ, Coogan AC, et al. Diagnostic accuracy in fine-needle aspiration of soft tissue and bone lesions: influence of clinical history and experience. Am J Clin Pathol 111: 632, 1999.
61. Liu K, Mann KP, Garst JL, et al. Diagnosis of posttransplant granulocytic sarcoma of fine-needle aspiration cytology and flow cytometry. Diagn Cytopathol 20:85, 1999.
62. Logrono R, Kurtycz DF, Sproat IA, et al. Diagnosis of recurrent desmoplastic small round cell tumor by fine needle aspiration: a case report. Acta Cytol 41:1402, 1997.
63. McGee RS Jr, Ward WG, Kilpatrick SE. Malignant peripheral nerve sheath tumor: a fine needle aspiration biopsy study. Diagn Cytopathol 17:298, 1997.
64. Merck C, Hagmar B. Myxofibrosarcoma: a correlative cytologic and histologic study of 13 cases examined by fine needle aspiration cytology. Acta Cytol 24:137, 1980.
65. Miralles TG, Gosalbez F, Menéndez P, et al. Fine needle

aspiration cytology of soft-tissue lesions. Acta Cytol 30:671, 1986.

66. Nemanqani D, Mourad WA. Cytomorphologic features of fine-needle aspiration of liposarcoma. Diagn Cytopathol 20: 67, 1999.
67. Nguyen GK. What is the value of fine needle aspiration biopsy in the cytodiagnosis of soft tissue tumors? Diagn Cytopathol 4:352, 1988.
68. Nickols J, Koivuniemi A. Cytology of malignant hemangiopericytoma. Acta Cytol 23:119, 1979.
69. Oland J, Rosen A, Reif R, et al. Cytodiagnosis of soft tissue tumors. J Surg Oncol 37:168, 1986.
70. Ordóñez NG, Hickey RC, Brooks TE. Alveolar soft-part sarcoma: a cytologic and immunohistochemical study. Cancer 61:525, 1988.
71. Pérez-Guillermo M, Pérez JS, Rojo B, Gil AH. FNA cytology of cutaneous vascular tumors. Cytopathology 3:231, 1992.
72. Pettinato G, Swanson PE, Insabato L, et al. Undifferentiated small round-cell tumors of childhood: the immunocytochemical demonstration of myogenic differentiation in fine needle aspirates. Diagn Cytopathol 5:194, 1989.
73. Pisharodi LR, Cary D, Bernacki EG Jr. Elastofibroma dorsi: diagnostic problems and pitfalls. Diagn Cytopathol 10:242, 1994.
74. Pohar-Marinsek Z, Zidar A. Epithelioid sarcoma in FNAB smears. Diagn Cytopathol 11:367, 1994.
75. Pollono DG, Tomarchio S, Drut R, et al. Retroperitoneal and deep-seated lipoblastoma: diagnosis by CT scan and fine-needle aspiration biopsy. Diagn Cytopathol 20:295, 1999.
76. Powers CN, Berardo MD, Frable WJ. Fine needle aspiration biopsy: pitfalls in the diagnosis of spindle-cell lesions. Diagn Cytopathol 10:232, 1994.
77. Powers CN, Hurt MA, Frable JW. Fine needle aspiration biopsy: dermatofibrosarcoma protuberans. Diagn Cytopathol 9: 145, 1993.
78. Raab SS, Silverman JF, McLeod DL, et al. Free needle aspiration biopsy of fibromatoses. Acta Cytol 37:323, 1993.
79. Renshaw AA, Pérez-Atayde AR, Fletcher JA, Granter SR. Cytology of typical and atypical Ewing's sarcoma/PNET. Am J Clin Pathol 106:620, 1996.
80. Resnick JM, Fanning CV, Caraway NP, et al. Percutaneous needle biopsy diagnosis of benign neurogenic neoplasms. Diagn Cytopathol 16:17, 1997.
81. Rigby HS, Wilson V, Cawthorn S, Ibrahim N. Fine needle aspiration of pleomorphic lipoma: a potential pitfall of cytodiagnosis. Cytopathology 4:55, 1993.
82. Ryan M. Cytology and mesenchymal pathology: how far will we go? Am Clin Pathol 106:561, 1996.
83. Ryan MR, Stastny JF, Wakely PE Jr. The cytopathology of synovial sarcoma: a study of six cases, with emphasis on architecture and histopathologic correlation. Cancer Cytopathol 84:42, 1998.
84. Ryd W, Mugal S, Ayyash K. Ancient neurilemoma: a pitfall in the cytologic diagnosis of soft tissue tumors. Diagn Cytopathol 2:244, 1986.
85. Rydholm A. Centralization of soft tissue sarcoma: the southern Sweden experience. Acta Orthop Scand 68(Suppl 273):4, 1997.
86. Salomão DR, Sigman JD, Greenebaum E, Cohen MB. Rhabdomyosarcoma presenting as a parotid gland mass in pediatric patients: fine-needle aspiration biopsy findings. Cancer Cytopathol 84:425, 1998.
87. Seidal T, Mark J, Hagmar B, Angervall L. Alveolar rhabdomyosarcoma: a cytometric and correlated cytological and histological study. Acta Pathol Microbiol Scand (A) 90:345, 1982.
88. Seidal T, Walaas L, Kindblom LG, Angervall L. Cytology of embryonal rhabdomyosarcoma: a cytologic, light microscopic, electron microscopic, and immunohistochemical study of seven cases. Diagn Cytopathol 4:292, 1988.
89. Shabb N, Sneige N, Fanning CV, Dekmezian R. Fine needle aspiration cytology of alveolar soft-part sarcoma. Diagn Cytopathol 7:293, 1991.
90. Silverman JF, Dabbs DJ, Finley JL, Geisinger KR. Fine-needle aspiration biopsy of pleomorphic (giant cell) carcinoma of the pancreas: cytologic, immunocytochemical, and ultrastructural findings. Am J Clin Pathol 89:714, 1988.
91. Silverman JF, Dabbs DJ, Ganick DJ, et al. Fine needle aspiration cytology of neuroblastoma, including peripheral neuroectodermal tumor, with immunocytochemical and ultrastructural confirmation. Acta Cytol 32:367, 1988.
92. Silverman JF. Geisinger KR, Park HK, et al. Fine-needle aspiration cytology of granulocytic sarcoma and myeloid metaplasia. Diagn Cytopathol 6:106, 1990.
93. Silverman JF, Joshi VV. FNA biopsy of small round cell tumors of childhood: cytomorphological features and the role of ancillary studies. Diagn Cytopathol 10:245, 1994.
94. Silverman JF, Lannin DL, Larkin EW, et al. Fine needle aspiration cytology of post-irradiation sarcomas, including angiosarcoma, with immunocytochemical confirmation. Diagn Cytopathol 5:275, 1989.
95. Smith MB, Silverman JF, Raab SS, et al. Fine-needle aspiration cytology of hepatic leiyomyosarcoma. Diagn Cytopathol 11:321, 1994.
96. Stanley MW, Skoog L, Tani EM, Horwitz CA. Spontaneous resolution of nodular fasciitis following diagnosis by fine needle aspiration. Acta Cytol 35:616, 1991.
97. Stein AL, Bardawil RG, Silverman SG, Cibas ES. Fine needle aspiration biopsy of idiopathic retroperitoneal fibrosis. Acta Cytol 41:461, 1997.
98. Szadowska A, Lasota J. Fine needle aspiration cytology of myxoid liposarcoma: a study of 18 tumors. Cytopathology 4: 99, 1993.
99. Tao LC, Davidson DD. Aspiration biopsy cytology of smooth muscle tumors: a cytologic approach to the differentiation between leiomyosarcoma and leiomyoma. Acta Cytol 37:300, 1993.
100. Vendraminelli R, Cavazzana AO, Poletti A, et al. Fine needle aspiration cytology of malignant nerve sheath tumors. Diagn Cytopathol 8:559, 1992.
101. Viguer JM, Jiménez-Heffernan JA, Vicandi B, et al. Cytologic features of synovial sarcoma with emphasis on the monophasic fibrous variant: a morphologic and immunocytological analysis of bcl-2 protein expression. Cancer Cytopathol 84:50, 1998.
102. Wakely PE Jr, Frable WJ. Fine needle aspiration biopsy cytology of giant cell tumor of tendon sheath. Am J Clin Pathol 102:87, 1994.
103. Wakely PE Jr, Geisinger KR, Cappellari JO, et al. Fine-needle aspiration cytopathology of soft tissue: chromyxoid and myoid lesions. Diagn Cytopathol 12:101, 1995.
104. Wakely PE Jr, Giacomantonio M. Fine needle aspiration cytology of metastatic malignant rhabdoid tumor. Acta Cytol 30:533, 1986.
105. Wakely PE Jr, Price WG, Frable WJ. Sternomastoid tumor of infancy (fibromatosis colli): diagnosis by aspiration cytology. Mod Pathol 2:378, 1989.
106. Walaas L, Angervall L, Hagmar B, Save-Soderberg J. A correlative cytologic and histologic study of malignant fibrous histiocytoma: an analysis of 40 cases examined by fine needle aspiration cytology. Diagn Cytopathol 2:46, 1986.
107. Walaas L, Kindblom LG. Lipomatous tumors: a correlative

cytologic and histologic study of 27 tumors examined by fine needle aspiration cytology. Hum Pathol 16:6, 1985
108. Weir MM, Rosenberg AE, Bell DA. Grading of spindle cell sarcomas in fine-needle aspiration biopsy specimens. Am J Clin Pathol 112:784, 1999.
109. Willén H, Akerman M, Carlén B. Fine needle aspiration (FNA) in the diagnosis of soft tissue tumours; a review of 22 years experience. Cytopathology 6:236, 1995.
110. Yu GH, Staerkel GA, Kershnisnik MM, Varma DGK. Fine needle aspiration of pigmented villonodular synovitis of the temporomandibular joint masquerading as a primary parotid gland lesion. Diagn Cytopathol 16:47, 1997.
111. Zbieranowski I, Bedard YC. Fine needle aspiration of schwannomas: value of electron microscopy and immunocytochemistry in the preoperative diagnosis. Acta Cytol 33:381, 1989.

CHAPTER 7

# APPROACH TO THE DIAGNOSIS OF SOFT TISSUE TUMORS

## CLINICAL INFORMATION

The diagnosis of a soft tissue lesion, as with other tumors, presupposes that the pathologist has a modicum of clinical information and adequate, well processed tissue. At a minimum, the pathologist should be apprised of the age of the patient, the location of the tumor, and its growth characteristics. In some cases the results of radiographic studies, particularly computed tomography (CT) scans, enhance one's understanding of the clinical extent of the lesion (see Chapter 3).

Although age rarely, if ever, suggests a particular diagnosis, the importance of this information is knowing if the patient is a child. In general, there is little overlap between soft tissue tumors occurring in children and those seen in adults. Therefore this critical piece of information essentially presents the patholgist with two groups of tumors from which a differential diagnosis can be constructed. For example, malignant fibrous histiocytoma is essentially unheard of during childhood, so one should consider other diagnoses for a pleomorphic tumor in a child. On the other hand, neuroblastoma and angiomatoid fibrous histiocytoma rarely occur after childhood, and such diagnoses should always be made cautiously in adults.

Location, too, provides ancillary help in the differential diagnosis. Sarcomas, for the most part, develop as deeply located masses and infrequently present as superficial lesions. Exceptions do occur, however, and include lesions such as dermatofibrosarcoma protuberans, epithelioid sarcoma, and angiosarcoma (Table 7–1). It is also useful to recall that when carcinomas or melanomas metastasize to soft tissue, it is usually as small, superficial nodules rather than as large, deeply situated masses. In our experience the most common carcinomas that present as soft tissue metastases are pulmonary and renal carcinomas, the former usually appearing as a subcutaneous mass on the chest wall and the latter as a soft tissue mass in nearly any location.

Unfortunately, there is a great deal of overlap between the manner of presentation of benign and malignant soft tissue masses, so this information may be least helpful to the pathologist. Most soft tissue sarcomas of the extremities are detected by the patient as a slowly growing mass that has been present for about 6 months at the time of diagnosis. The duration of benign lesions may be similar, although such lesions are generally described as static or slowly growing. An exception to the foregoing observation is the rapid development of some cases of nodular fasciitis. These superficial, reactive lesions may develop rapidly over a period of 1–3 weeks, and we have even encountered some that evolved in a few days, a pattern of growth that seldom if ever is encountered with a sarcoma. Thus an astute general surgeon can sometimes suggest the diagnosis of fasciitis for a rapidly evolving superficial lesion of the extremity.

## DIAGNOSTIC MATERIAL

Material for diagnosis can be obtained by needle biopsy or excisional or incisional biopsy, the choice largely depending on the size and location of the lesion (see Chapter 2). From a pathologist's perspective, the latter two specimens are preferable, as they yield a higher volume of tissue; but excisional biopsy of large, deep tumors in undesirable because it may interfere with further surgical procedures and may lead to complications such as a massive hematoma and disturbed wound healing. The biopsy procedure should always be planned in such a manner that the biopsy tract can be excised together with the tumor during the definitive surgical procedure.

**TABLE 7–1 SUPERFICIAL SOFT TISSUE SARCOMAS**

Dermatofibrosarcoma protuberans
Epithelioid sarcoma
Angiomatoid fibrous histiocytoma
Plexiform fibrohistiocytic tumor
Myxoid malignant fibrous histiocytoma (myxofibrosarcoma)
Angiosarcoma
Kaposi's sarcoma
Atypical fibroxanthoma

Needle biopsy may be adequate for documenting recurrent or metastatic disease in a patient with a known diagnosis of sarcoma; but it should be used with caution when major surgical procedures depend on the diagnosis. In the past, frozen sections examinations were performed commonly with the expectation that definitive surgery would be accomplished during the same intraoperative procedure; but this trend is changing. Frozen sections are now obtained primarily to assure the surgeon that she or he has obtained representative, viable tissue that is adequate for a permanent section diagnosis. This may be accomplished by freezing a portion of the biopsy material or sometimes, as in the case of a needle biopsy, performing a touch preparation. The presence of malignant cells in a nonnecrotic background on a touch preparation ensures that the specimen is adequate. A background of reactive or necrotic cells suggests that a pseudocapsule has been biopsied or that the specimens is largely necrotic, requiring additional material depending on the clinical impression.

Because there is a growing tendency to perform limb-sparing surgery for sarcomas of all types, the number of major amputation specimens received in the surgical pathology laboratory has markedly decreased compared to one to two decades ago. Most extremity sarcomas are removed with a wide local excision, usually combined with preoperative or postoperative radiotherapy. As with many other surgical specimens, the margins should be marked with permanent ink and blotted dry prior to the dissection of the specimen. Once incised, the gross characteristics of the tumor should be noted. If malignancy is suspected, careful assessment of the tumor as to its surroundings is mandatory. This includes the location of the lesion (subcutis, muscle) its size, its relation to vital structures (e.g., bone, neurovascular bundle), and the relative amount of necrosis present if it can be judged grossly. Size is important for providing an accurate T descriptor for the surgeon if the lesion is a sarcoma. Lesions less than 5 cm are classified as T1, whereas those larger than 5 cm are classified as T2. Assessment of the degree of necrosis is important for untreated sarcomas, as this parameter is used in some grading systems. The extent of necrosis in lesions treated with preoperative irradiation or chemotherapy is also important, as it helps the clinical staff assess the efficacy of preoperative irradiation or chemotherapy, although it does not carry the same implication as necrosis in an untreated lesion. Often the gross appearance of the tumor is deceptive. Sarcomas may appear to be well circumscribed, for example, whereas some benign tumors suggest an infiltrative or invasive growth pattern. Also, the term *encapsulation* is often misleading and may invite inadequate excision by shelling out or enucleation of the tumor.

There are no standard guidelines for sampling soft tissue tumors; to some extent, sampling is dictated by the specific case. In the case of a known benign lesion, a few representative sections suffice (or the entire lesion if it is small). With a sarcoma, the questions to be answered are different. For example, it may be less important to submit numerous sections for a high grade sarcoma than for a low grade lesion in which the sampling is being driven by the need to document the presence of high grade areas. We have generally obtained one section for each centimeter of tumor diameter, with no more than about 10 sections if the lesion appeared more or less uniform. Representative sections of the margins or sections designed to show impingement of vital structures are also obtained. We select blocks for margins judiciously, depending on the gross appearance of the lesion. Lesions several centimeters away from a margin seldom have positive margins microscopically, so extensive margin sampling in these situations is less critical than with excisions containing grossly close margins. One exception is epithelioid sarcoma, a lesion that may be deceptive in its clinical extent grossly. Polaroid prints or Xerox impression of a specimen can be useful for providing visual data as to the orientation of the specimen and sampling sites.

Most specimens are handled adequately as described above. However, in cases in which diagnostic difficulty is anticipated, it is useful to have frozen (and less often glutaraldehyde-fixed) tissue in reserve in the event ancillary studies are important. It should be emphasized that there are certain tumors in which ancillary studies are essential. Notably, frozen tissue should be reserved for N-*myc* amplification studies of childhood neuroblastoma, and frozen tissue is highly recommended for use in national protocol studies for childhood rhabdomyosarcoma. Although we often perform cytogenetic studies on a wide variety of soft tissue lesions, for the most part they do not contribute directly to the diagnosis or therapy; an exception is the differential diagnosis of round cell sarcoma in which the question of an extraskeletal Ewing's sarcoma has been raised but for which the histologic features do not permit an unequivocal diagnosis.

## MICROSCOPIC EXAMINATION

The first and most important step in reaching a correct diagnosis is careful scrutiny of conventionally stained sections with light microscopy under low-power magnification. Useful microscopic features that can be identified at this point include the size and depth of the lesion, its relation to overlying skin and underlying fascia, and the nature of the borders (pushing, infiltrative).

Perhaps the most important question at this juncture is whether the lesion under study is a reactive process or a neoplasm. Reactive lesions may occur in superficial or deep soft tissue but tend to be more frequent in the former location. (Table 7–2). A number of histologic features are suggestive of a reactive process. First, some reactive lesions display a distinct zonal quality. For example, in the case of fascial forms of nodular fasciitis and ischemic fasciitis one encounters a cuff of proliferating fibroblasts that surround a central hypocellular zone of fibrinoid change. Myositis ossificans too displays a zonation that consists of centrifugal maturation of fibroblastic to osteoblastic mesenchyme. Cells comprising reactive lesions often have the apppearance of tissue culture fibroblasts with large vesicular nuclei, prominent nucleoli, and striking cytoplasmic basophilia, reflecting the presence of abundant rough endoplasmic reticulum. Although mitotic figures may be numerous, important negative observations include no atypical mitotic figures or nuclear atypia, as one would expect in a sarcoma.

Once satisfied that a reactive lesion can be excluded, the pathologist is justified in proceeding with analysis of the neoplasm. At low power, one is usually struck with the architectural pattern, the appearance of the cells, and the characteristics of the stroma. These characteristics can lend themselves to the development of a number of differential diagnostic categories.

1. *Fasciculated spindle cell tumors.* These lesions comprise a large group of tumors (e.g., fibrosarcoma and synovial sarcoma) characterized by long fascicles (Table 7–3). Cellular schwannoma and fibromatosis must be distinguished from the others because they are nonmetastasizing tumors. Unlike the others, fibromatosis is typically a lesion of low cellularity and nuclear grade. Cellular schwannoma, unlike the others, is characterized by diffuse, intense S-100 protein immunoreactivity.

2. *Myxoid lesions* (Table 7–4). Although nearly any soft tissue tumor may appear myxoid from time to time, a number of lesions display myxoid features consistently. In adults the differential diagnosis of myxoid tumors includes myxoma, myxoid malignant fibrous histiocytoma (myxofibrosarcoma), myxoid liposarcoma, and myxoid chondrosarcoma. Analysis of the vascular pattern, degree of nuclear atypia, and occasionally the staining characteristics of the matrix aid in this distinction. For example, an intricate vasculature is a feature of both myxoid liposarcoma and myxoid malignant fibrous histiocytoma, but it is not a feature of myxoid chondrosarcoma or myxoma.

3. *Epithelioid tumors* (Table 7–5). For the differential diagnosis of epithelioid tumors, it is important to rule out metastatic carcinoma, melanoma, and even large-cell lymphomas before assuming that one is dealing with an epithelioid soft tissue tumor. Immunohistochemistry plays a decidedly pivotal role in this regard (discussed in greater detail in Chapter 8).

**TABLE 7–2 REACTIVE LESIONS SIMULATING A SARCOMA**

Nodular fasciitis
Intravascular and cranial fasciitis
Ischemic fasciitis (atypical decubital fibroplasia)
Organ-based fibromyxoid pseudotumors/postoperative spindle cell nodules
Proliferative fasciitis and myositis
Intravascular papillary endothelial hyperplasia
Myositis and panniculitis ossificans
Fibrodysplasia ossificans progressiva
Fibroosseous pseudotumor of the digits

**TABLE 7–3 FASCICULATED SPINDLE CELL TUMORS**

Fibromatosis (desmoid tumor)
Cellular schwannoma
Fibrosarcoma
Leiomyosarcoma
Spindle cell rhabdomyosarcoma
Synovial sarcoma
Malignant peripheral nerve sheath tumor

**TABLE 7–4 MYXOID SOFT TISSUE LESIONS**

Myxoma, cutaneous, intramuscular*
Aggressive angiomyxoma
Myxoid neurofibroma
Neurothekeoma
Myxoid chondroma
Myxoid lipoma (including myxoid spindle cell lipoma)
Lipoblastoma
Ossifying fibromyxoid tumor of soft parts
Myxoid liposarcoma*
Myxoid chondrosarcoma*
Myxoid dermatofibrosarcoma protuberans
Myxoid malignant fibrous histiocytoma (myxofibrosarcoma)*
Botryoid embryonal rhabdomyosarcoma
Myxoid leiomyosarcoma

* Most commonly encountered myxoid tumors.

| TABLE 7–5 EPITHELIOID SOFT TISSUE TUMORS |
|---|
| Alveolar soft part sarcoma |
| Epithelioid sarcoma |
| Epithelioid angiosarcoma |
| Epithelioid hemangioendothelioma |
| Epithelioid hemangioma |
| Extragastrointestinal stromal tumor (epithelioid leiomyoma/leiomyosarcoma) |
| Epithelioid variant of malignant peripheral nerve sheath tumor |
| Epithelioid schwannoma |
| Malignant rhabdoid tumor |
| Malignant mesothelioma |
| Synovial sarcoma (biphasic and predominantly monophasic epithelial) |

4. *Round cell tumors* (Table 7–6). Like epithelioid lesions, the differential diagnosis of round cell lesions can be broad; it presupposes excluding non-soft-tissue lesions that may mimic a round cell sarcoma (e.g., lymphoma, carcinoma) and is greatly facilitated by the use of immunohistochemistry. It should also be borne in mind that the round cell tumor is not synonymous with round cell sarcoma, as benign lesions (e.g., glomus tumor, giant-cell-poor forms of tenosynovial giant cell tumor) also enter the differential diagnosis. In general, the age of the patient helps narrow the possibilities. In children these lesions include neuroblastoma, rhabdomyosarcoma, Ewing's sarcoma/primitive neuroectodermal tumor (ES/PNET), and the rare desmoplastic small round cell tumor. Most of these diagnoses would not be considered in adults.

5. *Pleomorphic tumors* (Table 7–7). The differential diagnosis of pleomorphic sarcomas relies heavily on tumor sampling to identify areas of specific differentiation, sometimes in conjunction with immunohistochemistry. Malignant fibrous histiocytoma is by far the most common pleomorphic sarcoma, but it should not be diagnosed in unusual situations unless carcinoma, melanoma, and lymphoma have been excluded.

| TABLE 7–6 ROUND CELL SOFT TISSUE TUMORS |
|---|
| Alveolar rhabdomyosarcoma |
| Desmoplastic small cell round cell tumor of childhood |
| Embryonal rhabdomyosarcoma |
| Extraskeletal Ewing's sarcoma/primitive neuroectodermal tumor (PNET) |
| Round cell liposarcoma |
| Cellular forms of extraskeletal myxoid chondrosarcoma |
| Mesenchymal chondrosarcoma |
| Small-cell osteosarcoma |
| Malignant hemangiopericytoma |
| Glomus tumor |
| Tenosynovial giant cell tumor |

| TABLE 7–7 PLEOMORPHIC SARCOMAS |
|---|
| Malignant fibrous histiocytoma |
| Pleomorphic liposarcoma |
| Pleomorphic rhabdomyosarcoma |
| Pleomorphic malignant peripheral nerve sheath tumor |
| Pleomorphic leiomyosarcoma |

6. *Hemorrhagic and vascular lesions* (Table 7–8). Although sarcomas are generally highly vascularized, the number of soft tissue lesions that present as a hemorrhagic mass is limited and, interestingly, includes many nonvascular (i.e., nonendothelial) tumors. Conversely, many vascular tumors, such as intramuscular hemangiomas, do not have a hemorrhagic appearance. When evaluating vascular lesions, a good starting point is to ascertain whether the lesion is predominantly intravascular or extravascular[18] (Table 7–9). Intravascular lesions are nearly always benign and include primarily organizing thrombus/hematoma followed by the occasional angiocentric vascular tumor (Table 7–10). Extravascular lesions may be benign or malignant; features that favor benignancy include sharp circumscription, lobular arrangement of vessels, and the presence of both large (thick-walled) and small vessels. Angiosarcomas, on the other hand, have irregular margins, lack a lobular arrangement of vessels, and are composed of naked endothelial cells that dissect randomly through tissue planes. They usually occur in adults in the superficial soft tissues.

Further study of the sections can provide important information about the growth pattern, degree of cellularity, and amount and type of matrix formation. Growth patterns vary considerably, ranging from a fascicular, herringbone, or storiform (cartwheel, spiral nebula) pattern in fibroblastic, myofibroblastic, and fibrohistiocytic tumors to plexiform or endocrine patterns, palisading, and Homer-Wright and Flexner-Wintersteiner rosettes in various benign and malignant neural tumors. Biphasic cellular patterns with epithelial and spindle cell areas are characteristic of synovial sarcoma and mesothelioma. Although not all growth patterns permit a definitive diagnosis, they are of great help in narrowing the various differential diagnostic possibilities. Table 7–11 lists some of the

| TABLE 7–8 HEMORRHAGIC LESIONS OF SOFT TISSUE |
|---|
| Organizing hemorrhage/hematoma |
| Aneurysmal fibrous histiocytoma |
| Angiomatoid fibrous histiocytoma |
| Angiosarcoma |
| High grade sarcomas of various type (occasional) |

**TABLE 7–9 EVALUATION OF VASCULAR LESIONS**

| Parameter | Benign Vascular Lesion | Angiosarcoma |
|---|---|---|
| Age | All | Adults |
| Anatomic site | All | Superficial soft tissues usually |
| Predisposing factors | | Lymphedema, radiation |
| Intravascular vs. extravascular | Either | Virtually always extravascular |
| Lobular growth | Often, particularly capillary hemangioma | No |
| Circumscription | Variable | No |
| Thick-walled vessels | Yes, particularly intramuscular hemangioma, angiomatosis | No |

most common architectural patterns in soft tissue pathology and relates them to the type of tumor in which they are found most frequently.

Other features, such as the amount and type of extracellular matrix, can be helpful in the differential diagnosis. Abundant myxoid material is produced by a variety of benign and malignant soft tissue tumors, ranging from myxoma and myxoid neurofibroma to myxoid liposarcoma and myxoid chondrosarcoma. It is usually an indication of a relatively slow-growing tumor, and it has been shown that the degree of myxoid change in some malignant tumors is inversely related to the metastatic rate (e.g., myxoid malignant fibrous histiocytoma, myxoid liposarcoma). Abundant collagen formation is also found more often in slowly growing tumors than in rapidly growing ones. However, this finding is not always significant and also may be a prominent feature of some highly malignant sarcomas, such as synovial sarcoma, malignant fibrous histiocytoma, and postirradiation sarcomas. Examination may also provide information as to the presence of calcification and metaplastic changes, especially metaplastic cartilage and bone formation. Table 7–12 summarizes these changes in a variety of soft tissue tumors.

The degree and type of cellular differentiation is best obtained under high-power examination. Lipoblasts, for example, are characterized by the presence of sharply defined intracellular droplets of lipid and one or more centrally or peripherally placed round or scalloped nuclei. Round and spindle-shaped rhabdomyoblasts can be usually identified in conventionally stained hematoxylin-eosin sections by their deeply eosinophilic cytoplasm with whorls of eosinophilic fibrillary material near the nucleus and cytoplasmic cross-striations. When interpreting these cells, however, caution is indicated because occasionally entrapped normal or atrophic fat or muscle tissue may closely resemble lipoblasts or rhabdomyoblasts, respectively. Differentiated smooth muscle cells are characterized by their elongated shape, eosinophilic longitudinal fibrils, and long slender (cigar-shaped) nuclei, often with terminal juxtanuclear vacuoles. Other spindle cells are even more difficult to identify. Distinguishing fibroblasts, myofibroblasts, Schwann cells, and the spindle cells of synovial sarcoma and mesothelioma is more often based on the location and growth pattern than on cytologic characteristics; positive identification of these cells frequently requires immunohistochemical studies or electron microscopic analysis. Cellular inclusions are rare in soft tissue pathology; alveolar soft part sarcoma can be identified by the characteristic intracellular periodic acid-schiff (PAS)-positive crystalline material, and digital fibromatosis can be identified by eosinophilic inclusions consisting of actin-like microfilaments.

High-power examination is also essential for mitotic counts [e.g., the number of mitotic figures per 10 high power fields (HPF)]. Atypical mitotic figures are rare in benign soft tissue tumors and almost always indicate malignancy. Mitotic counts are useful for diagnosing benign and malignant nerve sheath tumors and tumors of smooth muscle tissue, but they are of little importance for the diagnosis of nodular fasciitis, localized and diffuse giant cell tumors, or malignant fibrous histiocytoma. Although nuclear atypia is more often associated with malignancy, it may occur as a degenerative feature in benign lesions (Table 7–13).

**TABLE 7–10 INTRAVASCULAR TUMORS AND PSEUDOTUMORS**

Organizing thrombi and papillary endothelial hyperplasia
Intravascular fasciitis
Spindle cell hemangioma
Epithelioid hemangioendothelioma
Epithelioid hemangioma
Intimal sarcoma

## HISTOCHEMISTRY AND IMMUNOHISTOCHEMISTRY

Hematoxylin-eosin-stained sections represent the mainstay of diagnosis but occasionally must be supported by ancillary techniques. Formerly, histochemistry was commonly used for the diagnosis, but a burgeoning number of antibodies and refinement of the techniques have made immunohistochemistry the an-

**TABLE 7–11 CORRELATION OF GROWTH PATTERN AND TUMOR TYPE**

| Growth Pattern | Tumor Type |
|---|---|
| Alveolar | Alveolar soft part sarcoma; alveolar rhabdomyosarcoma |
| Acinar | Synovial sarcoma; mesothelioma |
| Biphasic | Synovial sarcoma; mesothelioma |
| Cording | Epithelioid hemangioendothelioma; myxoid chondrosarcoma; malignant peripheral nerve sheath tumor, epithelioid type; round cell liposarcoma (rare) |
| Fascicular | Fibromatosis (desmoid tumor); cellular schwannoma; fibrosarcoma; malignant peripheral nerve sheath tumor; synovial sarcoma |
| Endocrinoid (zellballen) | Paraganglioma; alveolar soft part sarcoma |
| Lobular, nodular nest-like | Lipoblastoma; liposarcoma; epithelioid sarcoma; clear-cell sarcoma; fibrous hamartoma of infancy |
| Palisading | Schwannoma; malignant peripheral nerve sheath tumor; leiomyosarcoma; extragastrointestinal stromal tumor; synovial sarcoma (rare) |
| Plexiform | Neurofibroma; schwannoma (neurilemoma); plexiform fibrohistiocytic tumor |
| Plexiform capillary | Myxoid liposarcoma; myxoid malignant fibrous histiocytoma |
| Pericytoma | Hemangiopericytoma; solitary fibrous tumor; synovial sarcoma; mesenchymal chondrosarcoma; malignant peripheral nerve sheath tumor; myofibromatosis; juxtaglomerular tumor; liposarcoma (rare) |
| Rosettes, pseudorosettes | Neuroblastoma; neuroepithelioma; malignant peripheral nerve sheath tumor (rare) |
| Storiform (cartwheel) | Dermatofibrosarcoma protuberans; fibrous histiocytoma; malignant fibrous histiocytoma; neurofibroma; perineurioma |
| Tubulopapillary | Mesothelioma |

cillary modality of choice for most diagnostic situations. Still, there are a few specific situations in which histochemistry provides information not easily obtained by immunohistochemistry. For example, identification of PAS-positive/diastase-resistant crystals represents the cornerstone for the diagnosis of alveolar soft part sarcoma; distinguishing epithelial mucin from mesenchymal mucin is best done by histochemistry. Although immunohistochemistry has improved the accuracy of diagnosis, one must be aware of the potential problems and limitations when interpreting these stains. Not only is it important to know the specificity of the antibody, one must also be aware of the artifacts that can occur in these preparations, such as nonspecific staining of the edge of the tissue section (edge artifact) or necrotic zones, diffusion or uptake of antigen into adjacent tissues or cells (e.g., myoglobin diffusion from necrotic muscle tissue into

**TABLE 7–12 CALCIFICATION, CHONDROID, AND OSSEOUS METAPLASIA IN SOFT TISSUE TUMORS**

| Lesion | Calcification | Chondroid | Osteoid |
|---|---|---|---|
| Calcifying aponeurotic fibroma | + | + | − |
| Fibrodysplasia ossificans progressiva | + | + | + |
| Giant cell tumor | + | − | + |
| Hemangioma | + | − | + |
| Lipoma | + | + | + |
| Leiomyoma | + | − | − |
| Malignant fibrous histiocytoma | − | − | + |
| Melanocytic schwannoma | + | − | − |
| Mesenchymal chondrosarcoma | − | + | + |
| Mesothelioma | − | + | − |
| Myofibromatosis | + | − | − |
| Myositis ossificans | − | + | + |
| Myxoid liposarcoma | − | + | − |
| Malignant mesenchymoma | − | + | + |
| Malignant peripheral nerve sheath tumor | − | + | − |
| Myxoid chondrosarcoma | − | + | − |
| Ossifying fibromyxoid tumor | − | + | + |
| Osteosarcoma | + | + | + |
| Panniculitis ossificans | − | − | + |
| Synovial sarcoma | + | + | + |
| Tumoral calcinosis | + | − | − |

+, present (variable); −, usually absent.

**TABLE 7–13 BENIGN SOFT TISSUE TUMORS WITH NUCLEAR ATYPIA**

Pleomorphic fibroma of the skin
Fibrous histiocytoma with bizarre cells
Pleomorphic lipoma
Pleomorphic leiomyoma
Ancient schwannoma
Symplastic glomus tumor

histiocytes), and the cross-reactivity of some antibodies (a phenomenon encountered more often with monoclonal than polyclonal antibodies).

To use immunostains in the most effective and cost-efficient way, it is useful to have an algorithmic approach in mind and to use these reagents in panels (see Chapter 8). For example, a panel of antibodies to differentiate carcinomas, melanomas, sarcomas, and lymphomas from one another would be selected before a series of B and T cell markers. In our experience, immunohistochemistry is an important if not obligate part of the workup of certain soft tissue lesions, such as round cell sarcomas, epithelioid tumors, and pleomorphic tumors particularly in the skin.

## ELECTRON MICROSCOPY

Electron microscopy plays a far less prominent role in the diagnosis of soft tissue lesions than previously. This change is explained not only by the growing popularity of immunohistochemistry but also by the high cost and labor-intensive nature of electron microscopy, the relative inexperience of most pathologists in interpreting these studies, and the sampling inherent in this technique. Moreover, only a few ultrastructural markers lead to a specific histologic diagnosis, such as melanosomes in clear-cell sarcoma and malignant melanoma and Weibel-Palade bodies in vascular tumors. In most instances the pathologist is called on to evaluate a constellation of less specific features and to decide, based on their frequency or prominence, the probability of a certain diagnosis, recognizing that a loss of differentiation by light microscopy is usually paralleled by a similar loss ultrastructurally.

Traditionally, electron microscopy has been most useful in the diagnosis of round cell sarcoma, but it should be pointed out that this is also the area in which immunohistochemistry and cytogenetics has made important strides. It is now rare that a diagnosis hinges on the results of electron microscopic analysis alone. Still, electron microscopy has yielded interesting information regarding the participation of myofibroblasts in most benign and malignant soft tissue lesions.

## DIAGNOSTIC NOMENCLATURE

Even with complete sampling and ancillary studies, it may not be possible to classify all sarcomas accurately. In our consultation practice approximately 10% of all sarcomas do not lend themselves to a definitive classification. Nonetheless, it is often possible for the pathologist to provide the clinician with sufficient information so therapy can proceed unencumbered. For example, when evaluating moderately differentiated spindle cell sarcomas, one cannot always distinguish a malignant peripheral nerve sheath tumor from a fibrosarcoma. Yet this distinction is not clinically important if the pathologist can assure the clinician that the lesion is malignant and can provide a histologic grade. Likewise, it is not worthwhile to labor exhaustively over classifying a pleomorphic sarcoma when the therapy does not differ. Thus in these ambiguous diagnostic situations, there is no substitute for a constructive dialogue among the surgeon, pathologist, and oncologist to define the therapeutically relevant

**TABLE 7–14 MANAGERIAL DISEASE CATEGORIES**

| Clinical Status | Behavior | Usual Therapy | Examples |
|---|---|---|---|
| Benign | Local excision usually curative; rare recurrence but not destructive; no metastasis | Local excision | Histologically benign tumors and pseudotumors |
| Borderline or intermediate | Local recurrence common and often destructive; metastases vary from none to few | Extended local to wide excision depending on circumstances | Fibromatosis (nonmetastasizing); dermatofibrosarcoma protuberans (rare metastasis) |
| Malignant | Local recurrence common; metastasis common; systemic disease sometimes present at onset | Wide excision; possible adjuvant therapy | Malignant fibrous histiocytoma |

Modified from Kempson RL, Hendrickson MR. In: Weiss SW, Brooks JSJ (eds) An Approach to the Diagnosis of Soft Tissue Tumors in Soft Tissue Tumors. Williams & Wilkins, Baltimore, 1996, with permission.

**TABLE 7–15 EMORY UNIVERSITY HOSPITAL TEMPLATE REPORTING OF SARCOMAS**

Histologic type:
Grade: I, II, III
Size: greatest diameter (in centimeters)
Location: subcutis, muscle, body cavity
Margins: positive/negative (if <1.5 cm, give measurement)
Nodes: positive/negative
Necrosis: absent/present (microscopic)/present (macroscopic—approximate %)
Ancillary studies: state if tissue was sent for cytogenetics, molecular diagnostics, flow cytometry, or tissue banking
TNM code:

pathologic information. This has led to a managerial classification of soft tissue lesions[10] (Table 7–14). Such a system emphasizes the expected behavior rather than the histologic type. When the pathologist cannot be certain of the exact diagnosis, a managerial system can bridge the gap. For example, a low grade myxoid sarcoma that does not seem to fall clearly into a specific diagnostic category could be labeled "low grade myxoid sarcoma" with a comment that local recurrence rather than metastasis would be the expected behavior. The diagnosis "myxoid tumor with locally recurring potential" expresses the same information.

## STANDARDIZED REPORTING OF SOFT TISSUE SARCOMAS

To convey the pathologic findings to clinicians unambiguously, we have found it useful to standardize our reports (Table 7–15) using guidelines recently proposed by the Association of Directors of Anatomic and Surgical Pathology.[2] The three most important pieces of information the pathologist supplies in a surgical pathology report, apart from the diagnosis of "sarcoma," are the grade, size, and depth of the lesion; each is an independent prognostic variable that figures prominently in the clinical stage (see Chapter 1).[1]

- *Grading system.* The choice of a grading system is largely one of institutional, regional, or national preference, as all reported grading systems can be correlated with outcome (see Chapter 1).[4,6] The report should make clear the number of tiers in the grading system; for example, it is important to know whether a lesion is grade 2 of a four-tiered system or a three-tiered system. Alternatively, some prefer the simple labels "low grade" or "high grade."
- *Tumor.* The maximum dimensions of a tumor is given in metric units and in three dimensions if possible.
- *Location and depth.* These tumor parameters are addressed by indicating whether it is superficial (above the fascia), deep (below the fascia or in muscle), or in a body cavity. For purposes of staging, deep lesions are defined as those in muscle, a body cavity, or the head and neck.[1]
- *Margins.* It is believed that sarcomas excised with a less than 1.5–2.0-cm margin are prone to local recurrence[13] unless they are bordered by unbreached fascia or periosteum.[15] For this reason we comment on all positive margins (ink on the tumor) and the distance and location of all margins less than 1.5 cm. Positive margins imply a greater chance for distant metastasis with high risk extremity sarcomas.[9]
- *Necrosis.* Because necrosis is an integral part of some grading systems, it is useful to indicate whether necrosis is absent, microscopically present, or macroscopically present. If macroscopically present, we attempt to give some estimate of the amount. It should be kept in mind, however, that grading systems that rely on assessment of necrosis imply examination of surgical specimens that have not been altered by preoperative irradiation or chemotherapy. Once therapy is given, it is difficult to know to what extent necrosis is spontaneous versus therapy-induced. Nonetheless, if preoperative irradiation or chemotherapy has been undertaken, clinicians usually find that a statement as to the amount of viable tumor that remains is helpful.
- *Ancillary studies.* It is useful if the report indicates what tissue has been archived for future use (tissue bank) or referred to other laboratories for additional tests or consultation.
- *Optional information.* There are several other features on which pathologists may comment, including the mitotic rate, vascular invasion, nature of the margin (circumscribed, infiltrating), presence of an inflammatory infiltrate, and a preexisting benign lesion (e.g., sarcoma arising in a neurofibroma). None translates directly into patient management, and therefore they are considered optional in the report. In most instances, however, mitotic activity is assessed prior to arriving at a histologic grade.

## REFERENCES

1. AJCC Cancer Staging Handbook, 5th ed. Lippincott Williams & Wilkins, Philadelphia, 1998, pp. 139–146.
2. Association of Directors of Anatomic and Surgical Pathology. Recommendations for the reporting of soft tissue sarcomas. Mod Pathol 11:1257, 1998.
3. Brooks AD, Meslin MJ, Leung DHY, et al. Superficial extremity soft tissue sarcoma: an analysis of prognostic factors. Ann Surg Oncol 5:41, 1998.
4. Coindre J-M, Terrier P, Bui NB, et al. Prognostic factors in adult patients with locally controlled soft tissue sarcomas: a

study on 546 patients from the French Federation of Cancer Centers Sarcoma Group. J Clin Oncol 14:869, 1996.
5. Erlandson RA, Woodruff JM. Role of electron microscopy in the evaluation of soft tissue neoplasms with emphasis on spindle cell and pleomorphic tumors. Hum Pathol 29:1372, 1998.
6. Guillou L, Coindre J-M, Bonichon F, et al. Comparative study of the National Cancer Institute and French Federation of Cancer Centers Sarcoma Group grading systems in a population of 410 adult patients with soft tissue sarcomas. J Clin Oncol 15: 350, 1997.
7. Heslin MJ, Lewis JJ, Nadler E, et al. Prognostic factors associated with long term survival for retroperitoneal sarcoma: implications for management. J Clin Oncol 15:2832, 1997.
8. Heslin MJ, Lewis JJ, Woodruff JM, Brennan MF. Core needle biopsy for diagnosis of extremity soft tissue sarcoma. Ann Surg Oncol 44:425, 1997.
9. Heslin MJ, Woodruff JM, Brennan MF. Prognostic significance of a positive microscopic margin in high risk extremity soft tissue sarcoma: implications for management. J Clin Oncol 14: 473, 1996.
10. Kempson RL, Hendrickson MR. In: Weiss SW, Brooks JSJ (eds) An Approach to the Diagnosis of Soft Tissue Tumors in Soft Tissue Tumors. Williams & Wilkins, Baltimore, 1996.
11. Mackay B, Osborne BM. The contribution of electron microscopy to the diagnosis of tumors. Pathol Annu 8:359, 1978.
12. Markhede G, Angervall L, Stener B. A multivariate analysis of the prognosis after surgical treatment of malignant soft tissue tumors. Cancer 49:1721, 1982.
13. Pisters PWT, Leung DHY, Woodruff J, et al. Analysis of prognostic factors in 1,041 patients with localized soft tissue sarcomas of the extremeties. J Clin Oncol 14:1679, 1996.
14. Rydholm A. Management of patients with soft tissue tumors: strategy developed at a regional oncology center. Acta Orthop Scand Suppl 203:13, 1983.
15. Rydholm A, Rooser B. Surgical margins for soft tissue sarcoma. J Bone Joint Surg Am 69:1074, 1987.
16. Singer S, Corson JM, Gonin R, et al. Prognostic factors predictive of survival and local recurrence for extremity soft tissue sarcoma. Ann Surg 219:165, 1994.
17. Taxy JB, Battifora H. The electron microscope in the study and diagnosis of soft tissue tumors. In: Trump BF, Jones TT (eds) Diagnostic Electron Microscopy. Wiley, New York, 1980.
18. Weiss SW. The Vincent McGovern Memorial Lecture: Vascular tumors: a deductive approach to diagnosis. Surg Pathol 2:185, 1989.
19. Weiss SW, Sobin LH. Histological typing of soft tissue tumors. In: World Health Organization International Histological Classification of Tumors, 2nd ed. Springer-Verlag, Berlin, 1994.

# CHAPTER 8

# IMMUNOHISTOCHEMISTRY FOR ANALYSIS OF SOFT TISSUE TUMORS

ANDREW L. FOLPE AND ALLEN M. GOWN

Immunohistochemistry is the use of antibody-based reagents for localization of specific epitopes in tissue sections. In recent years, immunohistochemistry has become a powerful tool to assist the surgical pathologist in many clinically critical settings. It is important to recognize that immunohistochemistry has two components, each with its own strengths and weaknesses. These components may be thought of as the "hardware" (i.e., antibodies, detection systems) and the "software" (i.e., analytic processes). No matter how selective are the antibodies or how powerful the detection system, the method fails if the analytic tools are inadequate. The reader is referred to several books for updates on the methodologic component of the hardware of immunohistochemistry[60,216]; this chapter focuses on the antibody component of the hardware and the ways in which immunohistochemistry assists in the diagnosis of soft tissue neoplasms.

It is critical to recognize that immunohistochemistry is an adjunctive technique that does not supercede or replace the traditional morphologic diagnosis. Indeed, the interpretation of immunohistochemical results ex vacuo is perhaps the surest route to an incorrect diagnosis in soft tissue pathology. Second, as powerful as the technique of immunohistochemistry may be for identifying tumors or cell types, there are some cases in which no specific diagnosis can be reached despite intensive histologic and immunohistochemical study. In these cases, electron microscopic, cytogenetic, and molecular genetic studies may be informative.

The expression of certain antigens, or clusters of antigens, is characteristic of some tumors. Whereas there are thousands of monoclonal and polyclonal antibodies available to assist in tumor diagnosis, only a small subset has proved to be of practical value in the diagnosis of soft tissue neoplasms. Tables 8–1 and 8–2 present an overview of the markers discussed in the sections below. The question-marks highlight the gaps in our understanding of the cellular biology of many soft tissue tumors.

## INTERMEDIATE FILAMENTS

The intermediate filaments comprise the major component of the cytoskeleton and consist of five major subgroups [vimentin, cytokeratins, desmin, neurofilaments, glial fibrillary acidic protein (GFAP)] and a small number of minor subgroups (e.g., nestin, peripherin).[41,48,177] Ultrastructurally, the intermediate filaments appear as wavy unbranched filaments that often occupy a perinuclear location in the cell. Whereas it was originally thought that intermediate filament expression was restricted to specific cell types (e.g., cytokeratins in carcinomas, vimentin in sarcomas), this is not the case. The following sections on intermediate filaments concentrate not only on the normal pattern of expression of these proteins but also on the situations in which intermediate filaments show "anomalous expression."

### Vimentin

Vimentin, a 57-kDa intermediate filament protein, is expressed in all mesenchymal cells. Vimentin is ubiquitously expressed in all cells during early embryogenesis and is gradually replaced in many cells by type-specific intermediate filaments.[40,41] In some mesenchymal tissues vimentin is typically co-expressed along with the type-specific intermediate filaments

**TABLE 8–1 COMMON IMMUNOHISTOCHEMICAL MARKERS**

| Antibodies To | Expressed By |
|---|---|
| Cytokeratins | Carcinomas, epithelioid sarcoma, synovial sarcoma, some angiosarcomas and leiomyosarcomas, mesothelioma, extrarenal rhabdoid tumor |
| Vimentin | Sarcomas, melanoma, some carcinomas and lymphomas |
| Desmin | Benign and malignant smooth and skeletal muscle tumors |
| Glial fibrillary acidic protein | Gliomas, some schwannomas |
| Neurofilaments | Neuroblastic tumors |
| Pan-muscle actin | Benign and malignant smooth and skeletal muscle tumors, myofibroblastic tumors and pseudotumors |
| Smooth muscle actin | Benign and malignant smooth muscle tumors, myofibroblastic tumors and pseudotumors |
| Myogenic nuclear regulatory proteins (myogenin, MyoD1) | Rhabdomyosarcoma |
| S-100 protein | Melanoma, benign and malignant peripheral nerve sheath tumors, cartilaginous tumors, normal adipose tissue, Langerhans cells |
| Epithelial membrane antigen | Carcinomas, epithelioid sarcoma, synovial sarcoma, some nerve sheath tumors (perineurioma), meningiomas, anaplastic large-cell lymphoma |
| CD31 | Benign and malignant vascular tumors |
| Von Willebrand factor (factor VIII-related protein) | Benign and malignant vascular tumors |
| CD34 | Benign and malignant vascular tumors, solitary fibrous tumor, hemangiopericytoma, epithelioid sarcoma, dermatofibrosarcoma protuberans |
| CD99 (*MIC2* gene product) | Ewing's sarcoma/primitive neuroectodermal tumor, some rhabdomyosarcomas, some synovial sarcomas, lymphoblastic lymphoma, mesenchymal chondrosarcoma, small-cell osteosarcoma |
| CD45 (leukocyte common antigen) | Lymphoma |
| CD30 (Ki-1) | Anaplastic large-cell lymphoma |
| CD68 | Macrophages, fibrohistiocytic tumors, granular cell tumors, various sarcomas, melanomas, carcinomas |
| Melanosome-specific antigens (HMB-45, Melan-A, tyrosinase, microphthalmia transcription factor) | Melanoma, angiomyolipoma, clear-cell sarcoma, melanotic schwannoma |

**TABLE 8–2 SPECIFIC TUMOR TYPES, NORMAL COUNTERPARTS, AND USEFUL MARKERS**

| Tumor Type | Normal Cell Counterpart | Useful Marker(s) |
|---|---|---|
| Angiosarcoma | Endothelium | Type IV collagen, von Willebrand factor, ulex lectin, CD34, CD31 |
| Leiomyosarcoma | Smooth muscle | Type IV collagen, muscle (smooth) actins, desmin |
| Rhabdomyosarcoma | Skeletal muscle | MyoD1, myogenin; muscle (sarcomeric) actins; desmin |
| Ewing's sarcoma | ? | CD99 (*p30/32-MIC2*) |
| Synovial sarcoma | ? | Cytokeratin, EMA |
| Epithelioid sarcoma | ? | Cytokeratin, CD34 |
| Malignant nerve sheath tumor | Nerve sheath (e.g., Schwann cell, perineurial cell) | S-100, CD57, NGF receptor, type IV collagen, EMA |
| Liposarcoma | Adipocyte | ?, Type IV collagen, S-100 protein |
| Chondrosarcoma | Chondrocyte | ?, Type IV collagen, S-100 protein |
| Osteogenic sarcoma | Osteocyte | ?, Osteocalcin |
| Kaposi's sarcoma | ? | Ulex lectin, CD34, VEGFR-3, podoplanin |
| Malignant fibrous histiocytoma | ? | ? |
| Myofibroblast lesions (e.g., nodular fasciitis) | Myofibroblast | Smooth muscle actins |
| Gastrointestinal stromal tumor | Cells of Cajal | Muscle actins, CD34, CD117a (c-*kit*) |
| Hemangiopericytoma, solitary fibrous tumor | ? | CD34 |

(e.g., desmin and vimentin co-expression in muscle cells, vimentin and GFAP in some Schwann cells). Reversion to a pattern of vimentin expression is typically seen in cultured cells of many lineages.[37,234] Vimentin is also commonly expressed by sarcomatoid carcinomas at any site, an unfortunate fact that greatly limits its utility in the immunohistochemical distinction of carcinomas from sarcomas.[2,58,139,145,206] As a diagnostic reagent, antibodies to vimentin are of greatest utility in the diagnosis of carcinomas of uncertain primary site, where strong co-expression may be a clue to renal, endometrial, and thyroid carcinomas.[8] Vimentin immunoreactivity has been touted as a good marker of tissue preservation. However, vimentin expression, similar to that of all the intermediate filaments, is rather hardy and may remain present in tissues in which all other immunoreactivity has been lost.[108]

## Cytokeratins

Cytokeratins, the most complex members of the intermediate filament protein family, are a collection of more than 20 proteins. The cytokeratins may be grouped by their molecular weights (40–67 kDa) into acidic and basic subfamilies, or by their usual pattern of expression in simple or complex epithelium (Fig. 8–1). In practice, the cytokeratins are most commonly thought of in terms of low-molecular-weight cytokeratins (generally cytokeratins 8, 18, and 19) and high-molecular-weight cytokeratins (generally cytokeratins 1, 5, 10, and 14). Cytokeratins are highly sensitive markers for identifying carcinomas and are generally employed as markers distinguishing epithelial from nonepithelial tumors (i.e., lymphomas, sarcomas, melanomas) (Fig. 8–2). Recently it has been demonstrated that cytokeratin expression is not restricted to carcinomas.

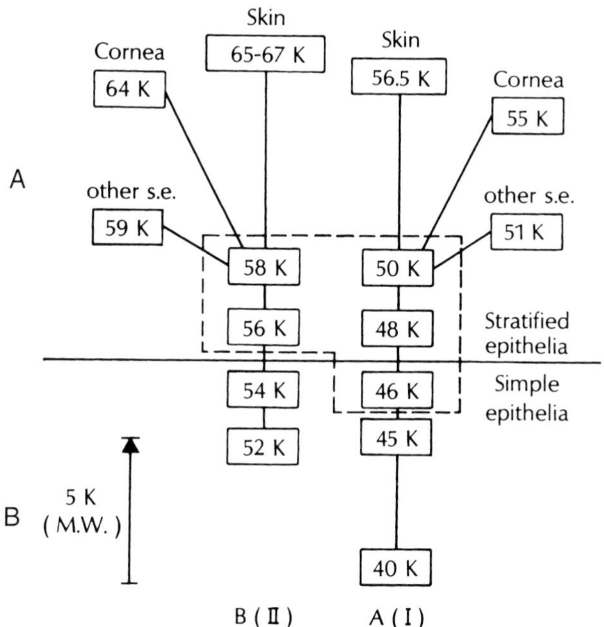


**FIGURE 8–1.** Subcategorization of acidic (**A**) and basic (**B**) cytokeratin subgroups within various tissues. (Modified from Cooper D, Schermer A, Sun TT. Classification of human epithelium and their neoplasms using monoclonal antibodies to keratins: strategies, applications, and limitations. Lab Invest 52:243, 1985, with permission.)

### *Sarcomas with "True" Epithelial Differentiation: Epithelioid Sarcoma and Synovial Sarcoma*

Among the sarcomas there are two classes of cytokeratin expression. A small subset of sarcomas display true epithelial differentiation as defined by usual expression of cytokeratin and other epithelial proteins such as the desmoplakins (e.g., synovial sarcomas and epithelioid sarcomas).[149] Additionally, there is a larger group of tumors that occasionally display "anomalous" cytokeratin (i.e., cytokeratin expression by cells and tumors without true epithelial differentiation). Synovial sarcomas and epithelioid sarcomas are the best, if not the only, examples of sarcomas manifesting true epithelial differentiation (Fig. 8–3). (Indeed, some have questioned the validity of the nomenclature of these tumors based on this observation.[158]) In contrast, anomalous cytokeratin expression is characterized by immunostaining (even under optimal technical conditions) in a subset of the target cell population. In those cells cytokeratin is present in only a portion of the cytoplasm, often yielding a "perinuclear" or "dot-like" pattern of immunostaining. This dot-like pattern is not always an indication of anomalous cytokeratin, however, as it is typically seen in some neuroendocrine carcinomas, including small-cell carcinomas and Merkel cell tumors, and in extrarenal rhabdoid tumors[64,101,154] (Fig. 8–4). In addition, it is rare to find cytokeratins other than those corresponding to the Moll catalog 8 and 18 (corresponding to positivity with antibodies CAM5.2 or 35BH11) in tumors manifesting anomalous cytokeratin expression.[149]

Contrary to some earlier suggestions, anomalous cytokeratin expression is not a universal feature of sarcomas. It is, instead, a feature of a limited subset of nonepithelial tumors, particularly smooth muscle tumors, melanomas, and endothelial cell tumors; as such, it may serve as a clue to the diagnosis of these tumors. Interestingly, the normal cell counterparts of some of these tumors (i.e., smooth muscle cells and

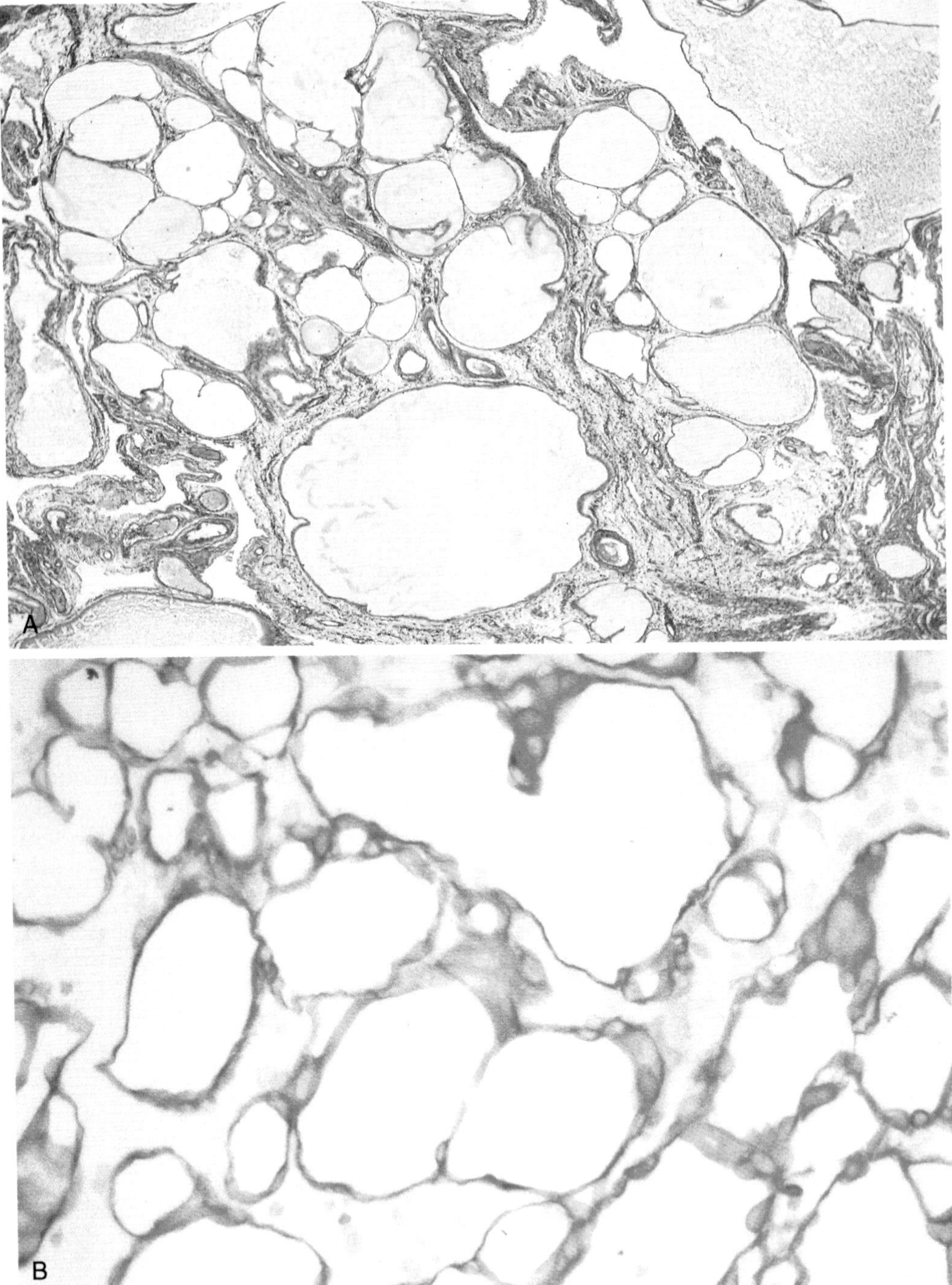


**FIGURE 8–2.** Cystic mesothelioma (**A**) immunostained for cytokeratin (**B**). Demonstration of strong cytokeratin expression is useful for distinguishing this entity from cystic lymphangioma.

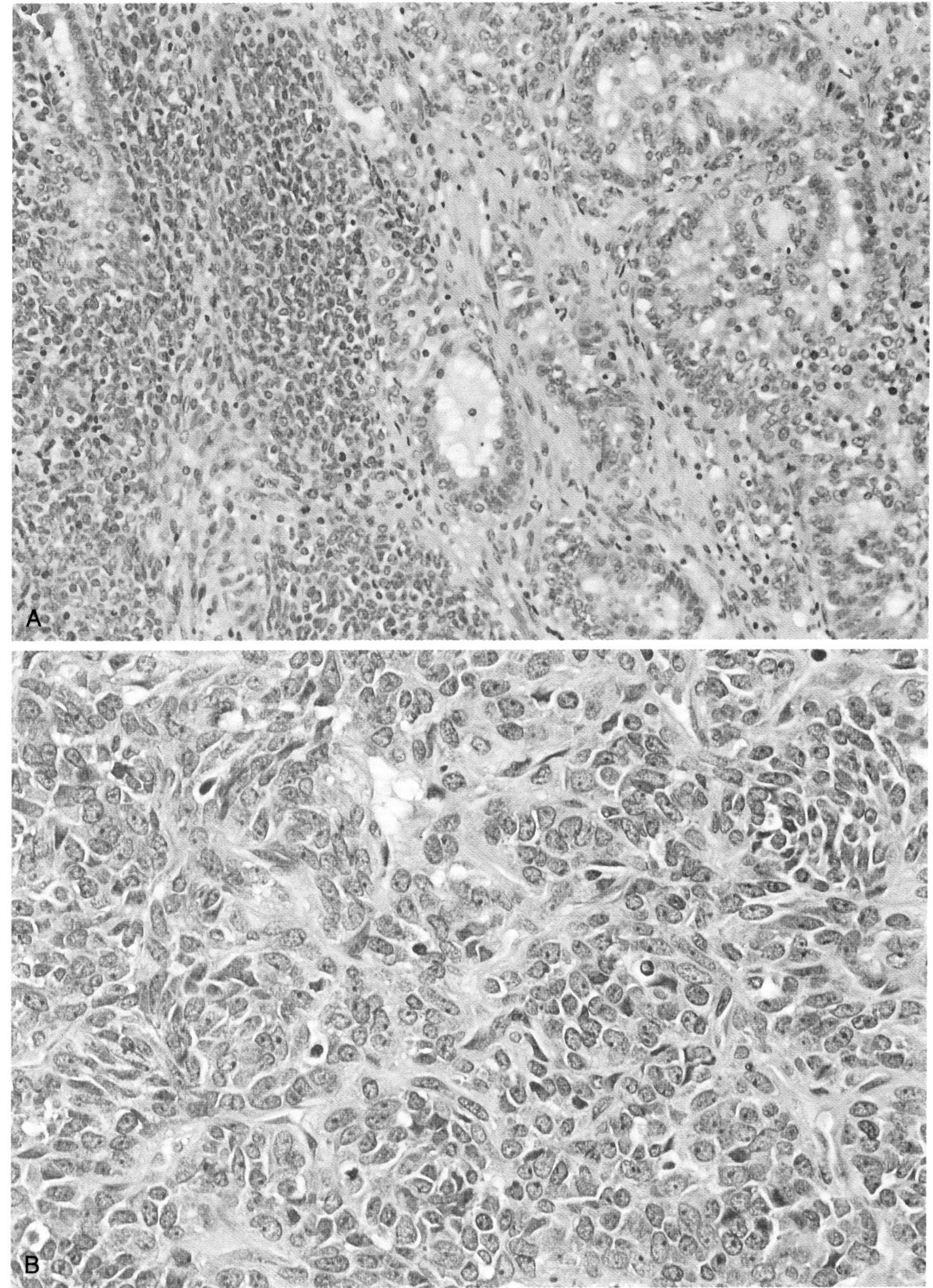


**FIGURE 8–3.** Biphasic synovial sarcoma with an evolving poorly differentiated cell population (**A**). Poorly differentiated synovial sarcoma (**B**) demonstrating focal expression of high-molecular-weight cytokeratins

*Illustration continued on following page*

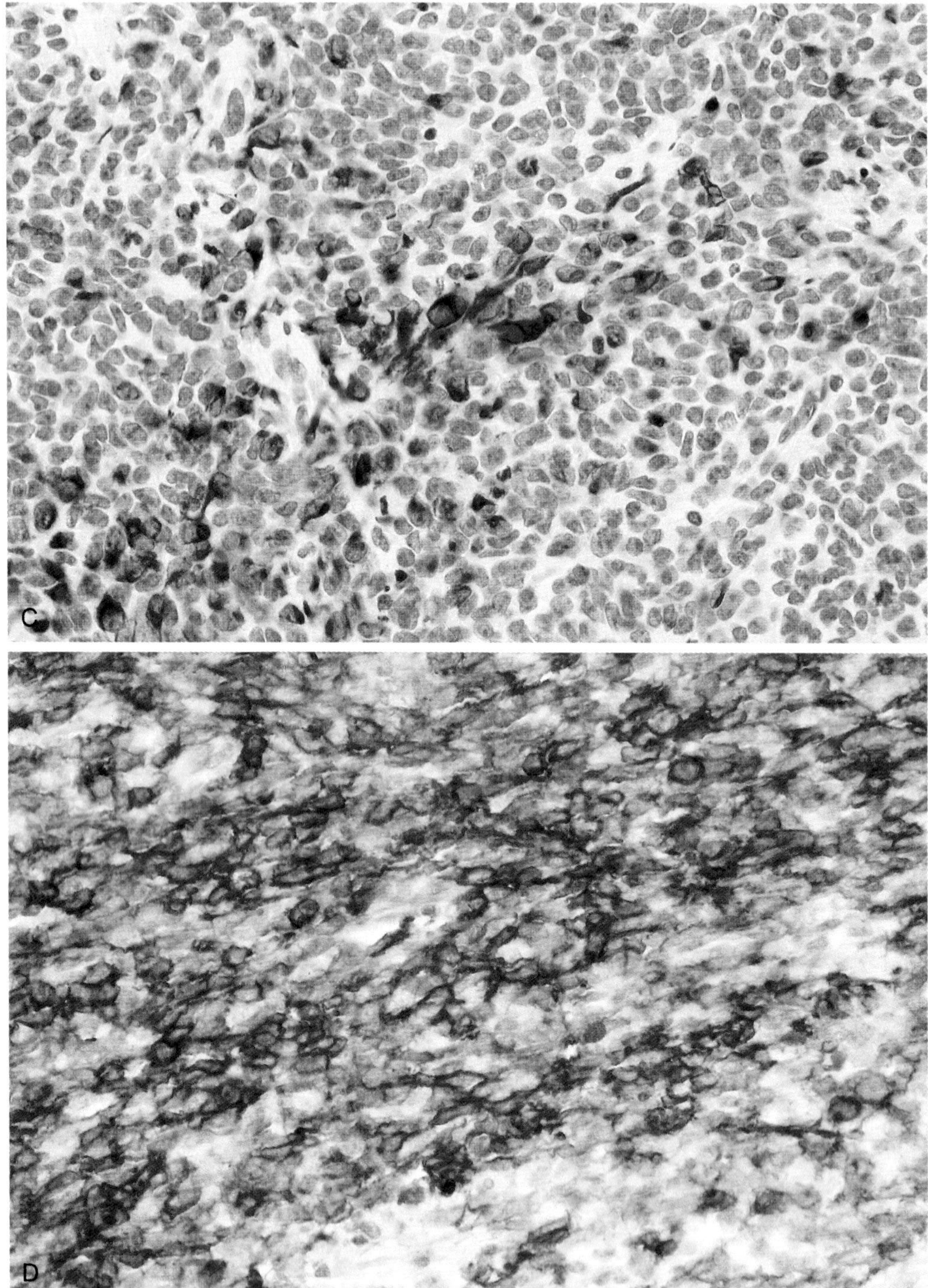

**FIGURE 8–3** (*Continued*). (**C**). Expression of cytokeratin in synovial sarcomas may be focal, and some express only high-molecular-weight isoforms. Many poorly differentiated synovial sarcomas also express CD99 (**D**), and it is important not to mistake them for primitive neuroectodermal tumors.

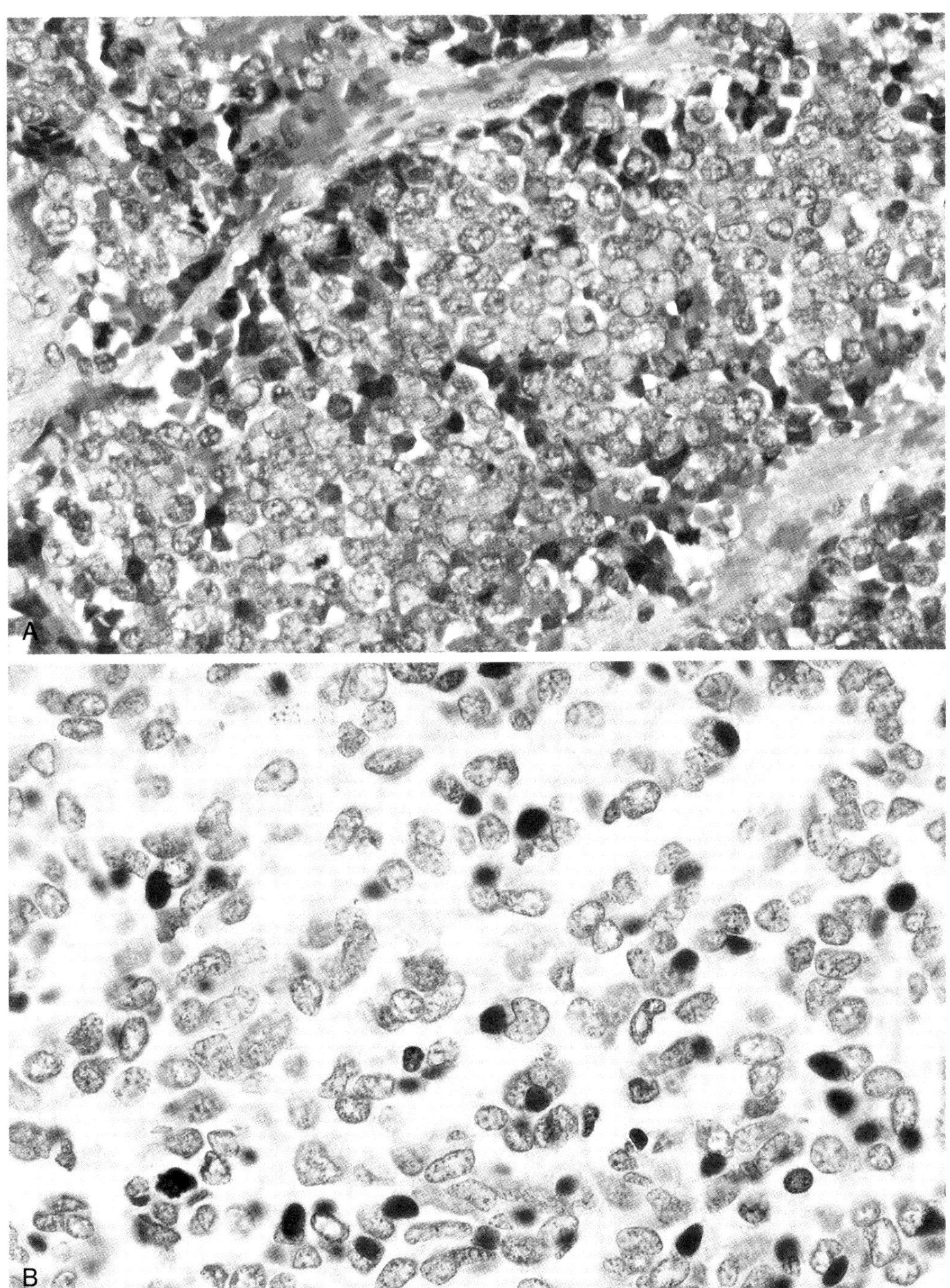

**FIGURE 8–4.** Merkel cell carcinoma (**A**) demonstrating characteristic expression of cytokeratin in a dot-like pattern (**B**). Dot-like expression of cytokeratin and other intermediate filaments is not specific for neuroendocrine carcinomas and may be seen in any "small, blue round cell." Dot-like expression may also be a clue to anomalous intermediate filament expression.

endothelial cells) have been found to express cytokeratins in nonmammalian species.[105]

### Smooth Muscle Cells and Smooth Muscle Tumors

Frozen sections of the smooth muscle cell-rich myometrium of the uterus (along with myocardial cells) were first reported to "react with" various anti-cytokeratin antibodies. Brown et al.[22] and Norton et al.[164] verified these findings using slightly different techniques, although Norton et al. failed to find corroborative biochemical evidence of cytokeratin expression by these smooth muscle cells. Biochemical documentation of true "anomalous" cytokeratin expression of cytokeratins 8 and 18 was first presented by Gown and colleagues,[87] in which immunostaining was corroborated by Western blots; it was further documented by two-color immunofluorescence studies of myometrial smooth muscle cells grown in vitro. Subsequent studies have shown that at least 30% of leiomyosarcomas manifest cytokeratin,[148,186,215] and this percentage may increase in the post-heat-induced epitope retrieval era.

### Melanomas

Despite the fact that many studies completed during the mid-1980s concluded that melanomas were vimentin-positive, cytokeratin-negative tumors,[88,251] Zarbo et al. first confirmed the cytokeratin positivity of many melanomas and demonstrated the positive immunostaining as a function of tissue preparation and fixation (with 21% of cases positive in frozen sections but far fewer in formalin-fixed, paraffin-embedded sections).[251] Zarbo et al. also performed one- and two-dimensional gel electrophoresis with immunoblotting, confirming that cytokeratin 8 was expressed by the tumor cell population.[251] Anomalous cytokeratin expression is generally a feature of metastatic, but not primary, melanomas.[15]

### Angiosarcomas

Early reports suggested that vascular tumors manifesting epithelioid histologic features (e.g., epithelioid hemangioendothelioma and epithelioid angiosarcoma) express cytokeratin in most cases[14,91,166,231,242] (Fig. 8–5). It has been recognized, however, that angiosarcomas other than those with epithelioid features express cytokeratin in about one-third of cases.[146]

### Small Blue Round Cell Tumors

A surprising number of tumors in the category of "small, blue round cell tumors" of childhood, typically co-express cytokeratin in a pattern much like that of anomalous cytokeratin expression. These tumors include Ewing's sarcoma/primitive neuroectodermal tumor,[92,159] rhabdomyosarcoma,[36,156] Wilms' tumor,[56,246] and desmoplastic small round-cell tumor of childhood.[169,181]

### Cytokeratin Expression in Other Sarcomas

The literature is replete with reports of cytokeratin expression in other sarcomas, including malignant fibrous histiocytoma,[137,157,191,239] chondrosarcoma,[1,95] osteosarcoma,[42] and malignant peripheral nerve sheath tumors.[69,99,149] Nonetheless, in our experience cytokeratin expression in these tumors is rare.

It is important to remember that immunoreactivity and true antigen expression are not necessarily synonymous[12] (Fig. 8–6). Several factors can theoretically account for positive cytokeratin immunostaining in tumors without true cytokeratin expression. This include the use of antibodies at inappropriately high concentrations,[212] potentially altered specificities following the use of heat-induced epitope retrieval techniques ("antigen retrieval"),[213] and the cross-reactivity of anti-cytokeratin antibodies with other proteins.[11] As with any antibody, it is also critical to distinguish reactive cytokeratin-positive cells, such as submesothelial fibroblasts, from the neoplastic cell population (Fig. 8–7). By employing an approach to immunohistochemistry that includes use of a panel of antibodies, the pathologist can generally avoid misinterpretation that might result from "misbehavior" of one antibody.

## EPITHELIAL MEMBRANE ANTIGEN

Epithelial membrane antigen (EMA) is an incompletely characterized antigen that is present in a group of carbohydrate-rich, protein-poor, high-molecular-weight molecules present on the surface of many normal types of epithelium, including that in the pancreas, stomach, intestine, salivary gland, respiratory tract, urinary tract, and breast.[98,184] Among normal mesenchymal cells, EMA expression is limited to perineurial cells[61,217,219] and meningeal cells.[197,218] There are a limited number of uses for EMA in sarcoma diagnosis. EMA expression is a more sensitive, but less specific, marker of poorly differentiated synovial sarcomas; it may be helpful in cases with only focal (or absent) cytokeratin expression.[75] Perineuriomas and malignant peripheral nerve sheath tumors with perineurial differentiation are characterized by a sometimes subtle expression of EMA along cell processes, as well as by type IV collagen expression[61,100,217,219,250]

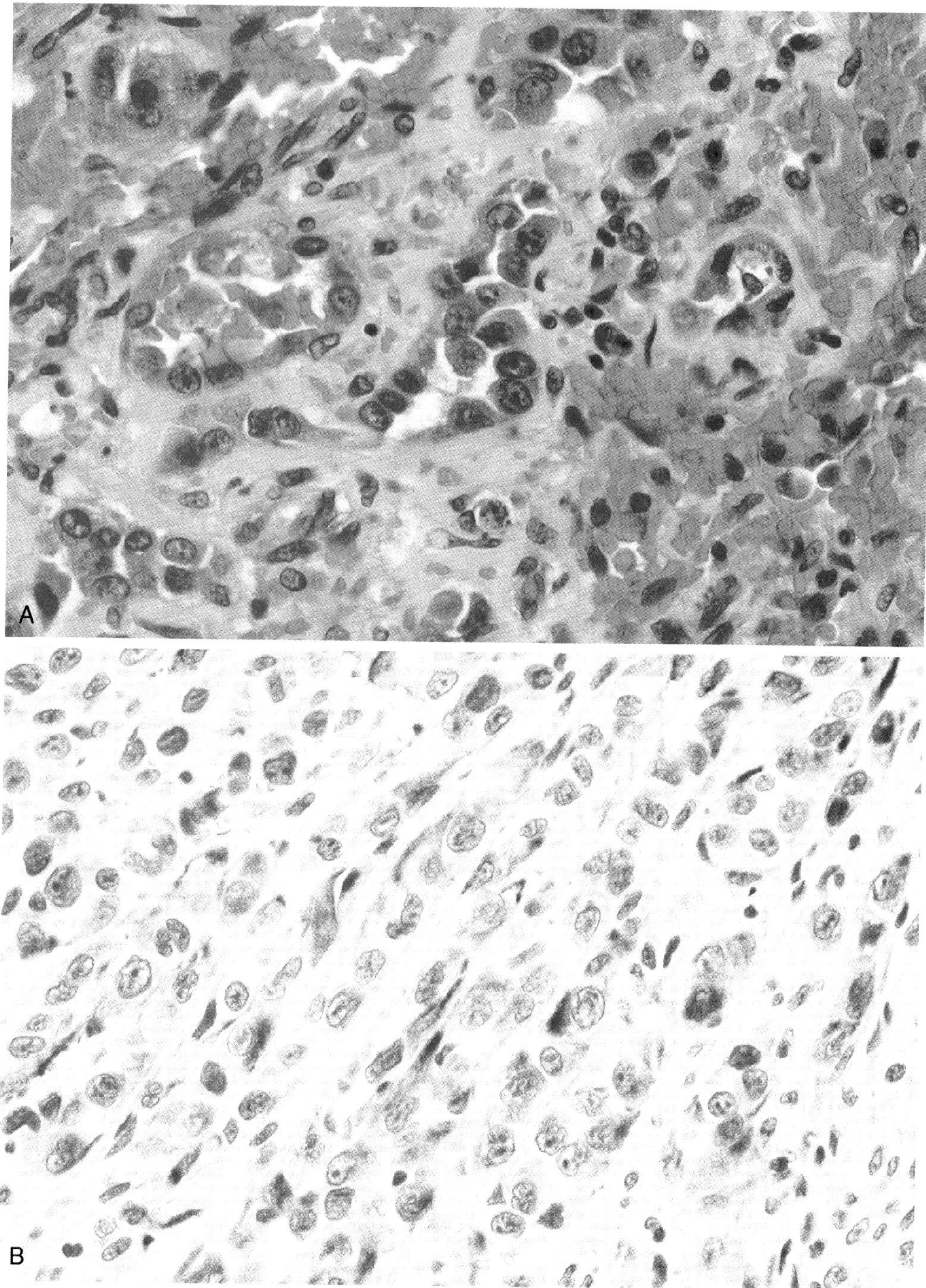


**FIGURE 8–5.** Epithelioid angiosarcoma (**A**) with strong expression of low-molecular-weight cytokeratin (**B**). Vascular tumors, particularly epithelioid ones, commonly express low-molecular-weight cytokeratins and may be mistaken for carcinoma.

*Illustration continued on following page*

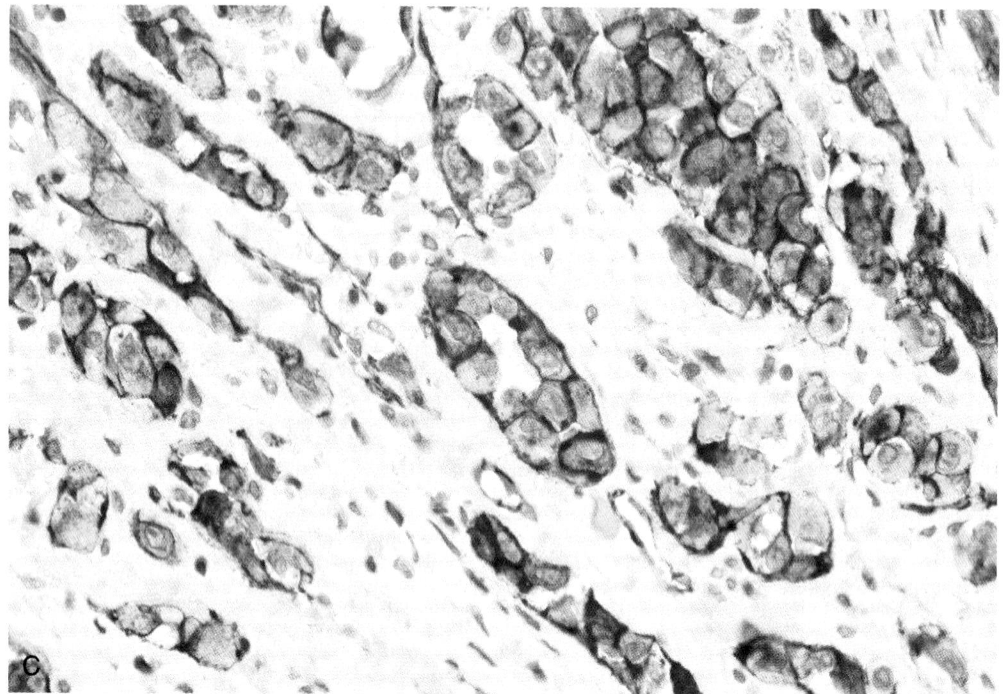


**FIGURE 8–5** (*Continued*). Expression of CD31 (**C**), a highly specific marker of endothelium, serves to distinguish keratin-positive angiosarcoma from carcinoma or epithelioid sarcoma.

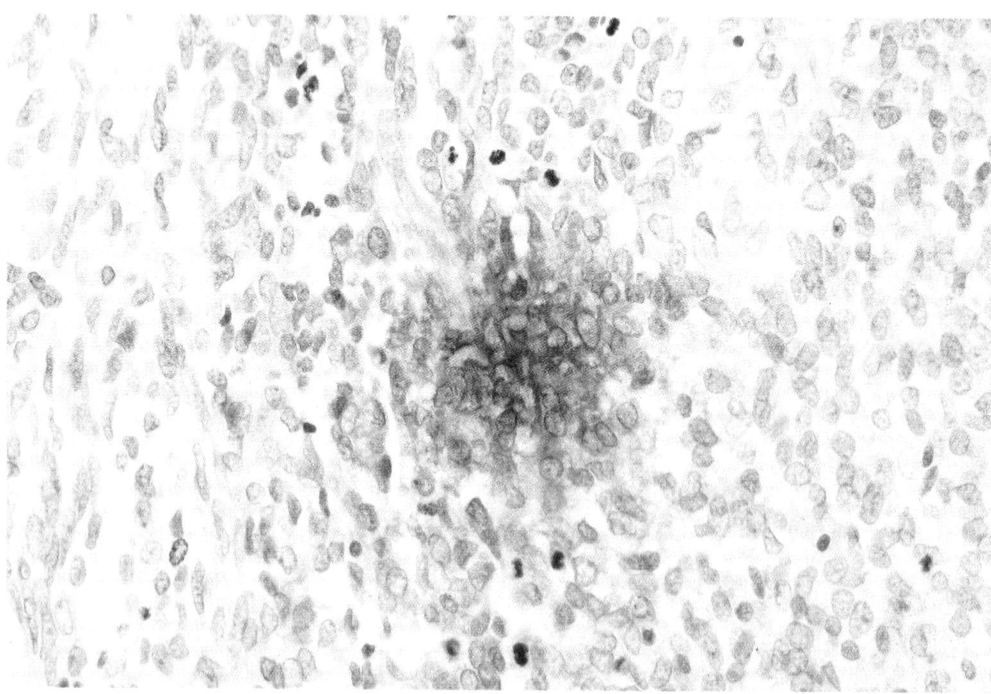

**FIGURE 8–6.** Overlay of dandruff on a slide, creating apparent focal cytokeratin expression.

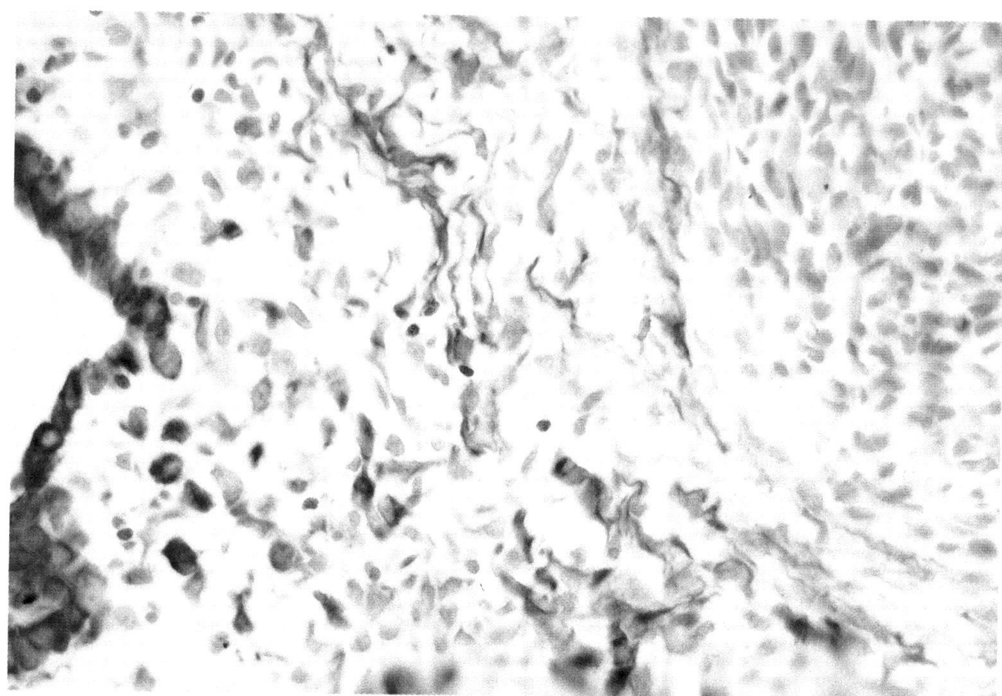

**FIGURE 8–7.** Low-molecular-weight cytokeratin expression in mesothelium (top) and in spindled submesothelial fibroblasts (middle). Expression of cytokeratin in these reactive submesothelial fibroblasts should be distinguished from cytokeratin expression in the adjacent infiltrating sarcoma (bottom).

(Fig. 8–8). Ectopic meningiomas, like their meningeal counterparts, are characterized by EMA and vimentin expression in the absence of cytokeratin expression.[197,218]

## MARKERS OF MUSCLE DIFFERENTIATION

There are three types of muscle differentiation. The first is skeletal muscle differentiation, as recapitulated in rhabdomyoma and rhabdomyosarcoma. The second is "true" smooth muscle differentiation, reflected in leiomyoma and leiomyosarcoma. The third is "partial" smooth muscle differentiation, as seen in the myofibroblasts that constitute a significant population of cells in healing wounds and the stromal reaction to tumors. There is a also subset of soft tissue tumors (e.g., nodular fasciitis and myofibroblastoma), the phenotype of which bears great resemblance to myofibroblasts rather than true smooth muscle cells. The principal markers of muscle differentiation are the intermediate filament desmin, the various actin isoforms, and the myogenic regulatory proteins.

### Desmin

Desmin is the intermediate filament protein associated with both smooth and skeletal muscle differentiation; it is rarely expressed by myofibroblasts and their corresponding tumors. In skeletal muscle desmin is localized to the Z-zone between the myofibrils, where it presumably serves as binding material for the contractile apparatus.[120] In smooth muscle it is associated with cytoplasmic dense bodies and subplasmalemmal dense plaques. Desmin may also be expressed by nonmuscle cells, including the fibroblastic reticulum cell of the lymph node,[6,33] the submesothelial fibroblast,[232] and endometrial stromal cells.[79] It is among the earliest muscle structural genes expressed in the myotome of embryos and has been regarded by some as the best single marker for the diagnosis of poorly differentiated rhabdomyosarcoma.[4,223] Although the early literature on desmin questioned its sensitivity in formalin-fixed, deparaffinized tissue sections,[9,132,180] more recent studies have borne out its excellent sensitivity. In our experience, with the use of heat-induced epitope retrieval techniques and modern antibodies such as D33, desmin is the most sensitive marker of skeletal and smooth muscle differentiation in terms of both the fraction of tumors so identified and the fraction of tumor cells in given tumors that are positive. We have detected desmin expression in nearly 100% of rhabdomyosarcomas, including poorly differentiated ones[73,238] (Fig. 8–9).

Desmin expression is apparently not as specific for muscle tumors as was originally thought, as it has also been described in primitive neuroectodermal tu-

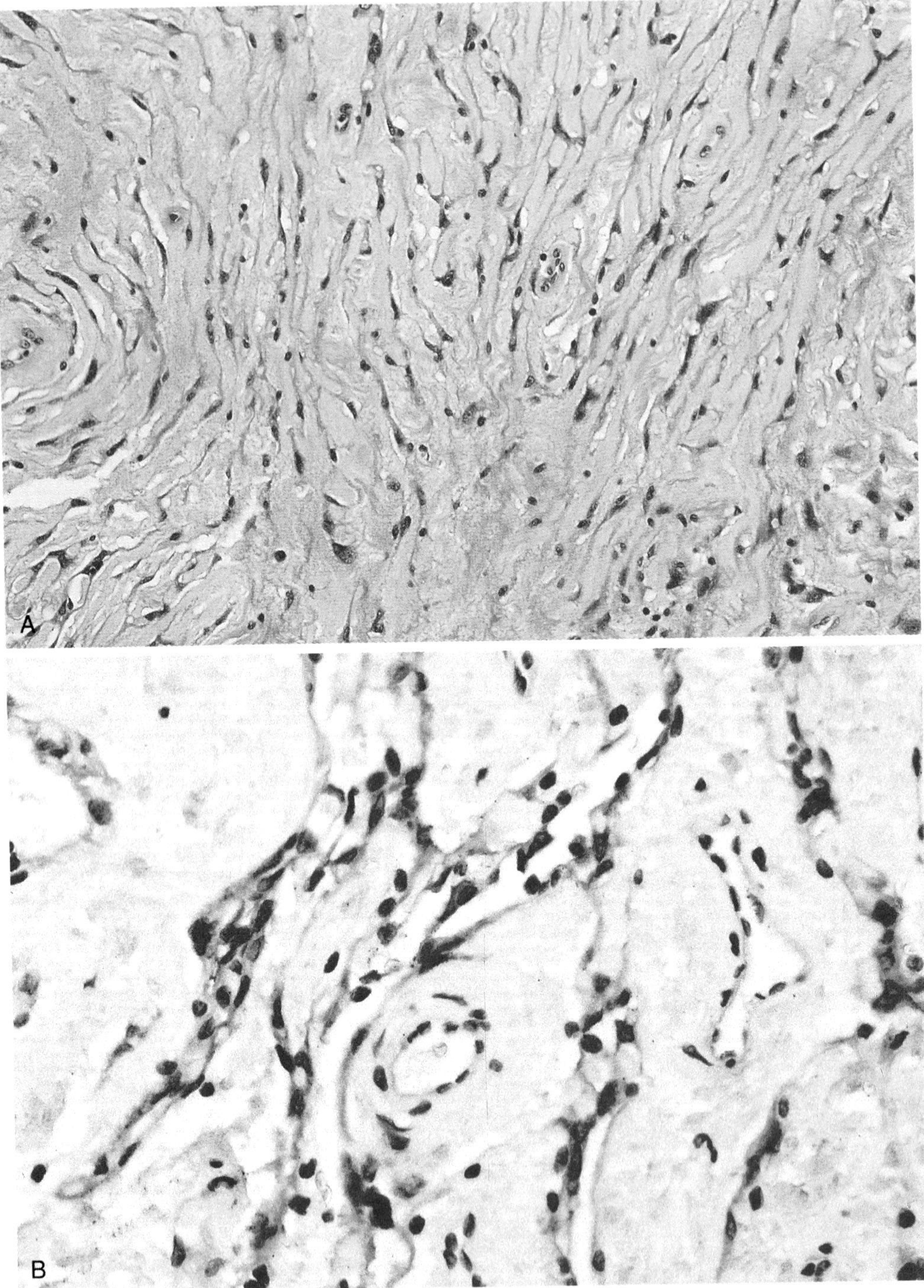


**FIGURE 8–8.** Malignant perineurioma (**A**) expressing epithelial membrane antigen (**B**).

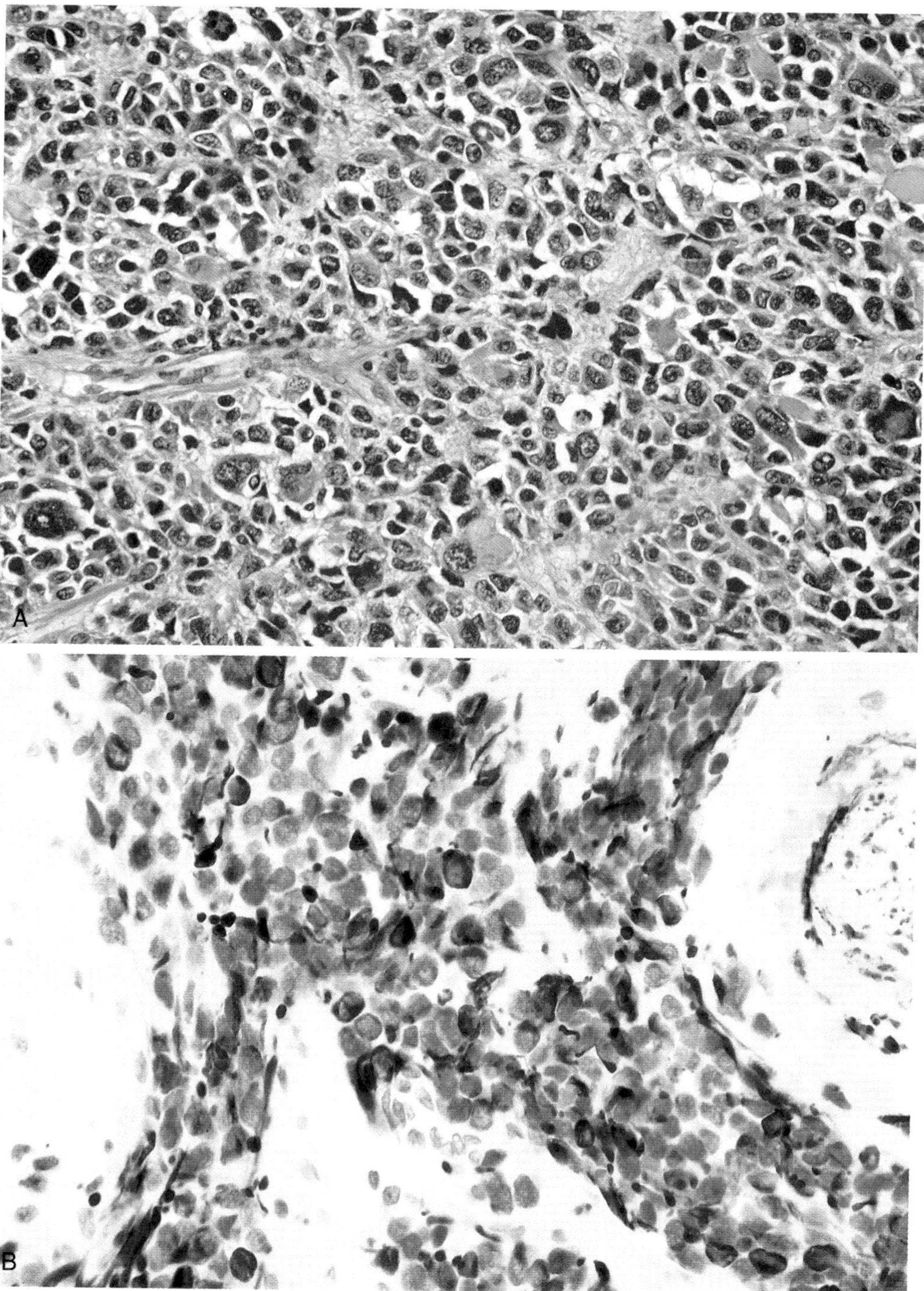

**FIGURE 8–9.** Alveolar rhabdomyosarcoma (**A**) demonstrating intense expression of desmin (**B**). Although desmin is a highly sensitive marker of myogenous sarcomas, it may also be expressed in a variety of nonmyogenous tumors. The most specific markers of rhabdomyosarcoma are antibodies to myogenic nuclear regulatory proteins, such as MyoD1

*Illustration continued on following page*

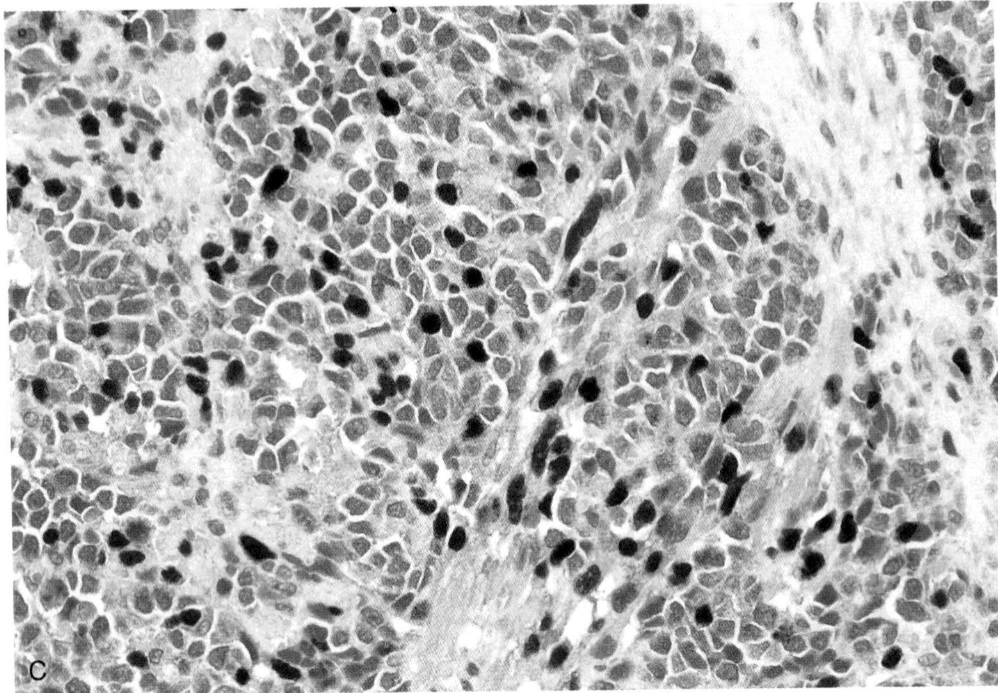


**FIGURE 8–9** (*Continued*). (**C**) or myogenin. Only a nuclear pattern of expression of these proteins should be accepted.

mors,[179] desmoplastic round cell tumors,[82,169] neuroblastoma,[211] mesothelial cells and tumors,[102] the blasternal component of Wilms' tumor,[73] and giant cell tumors of the tendon sheath[77]; in none of these contexts is there thought to be true muscle differentiation (Fig. 8–10). Desmin expression in the absence of other muscle markers is characteristic of angiomatoid fibrous histiocytomas[65,71] (Fig. 8–11).

## Actin

Actin, a ubiquitous protein, is expressed by all cell types; high concentrations of actins and unique isoforms, however, help make actin a marker of muscle differentiation. In general, actins can be grouped into muscle and nonmuscle isoforms, which differ by only a few amino acids in a protein with a molecular weight of 43,000. It has nevertheless been possible to generate antibodies specific to muscle actins versus nonmuscle actins and to specific actin isotypes with respect to the various muscle types (e.g. smooth muscle versus skeletal muscle).[135,206,207,225,226] Although an early body of literature speaks to the "specificity" of anti-actin polyclonal antibodies for muscle cells, in most of these studies it is a quantitative rather than a qualitative phenomenon: that is, muscle cells have far more actin than many other cells, and demonstration of positivity is determined on this basis alone. Whereas there are monoclonal antibodies that can identify all actin isoforms (i.e., the C4 clone[135]), given the sensitive immunohistochemical techniques available, this antibody cannot be used to distinguish muscle from nonmuscle actins. The antibody HHF35, which has been widely used to identify muscle cells and tumors, displays specificity for all muscle (versus nonmuscle) actins.[225,226] Antibody 1A4 is monoclonal and specifically identifies smooth muscle actin isoforms; it can thus distinguish smooth from skeletal muscle cells and tumors.[207] Smooth muscle actin isoforms are also expressed by myofibroblasts, and the characteristic pattern of actin expression in these cells may help distinguish them from true smooth muscle cells. In general, myofibroblasts show expression of smooth muscle actin only at the periphery of their cytoplasm ("tram-track" pattern); this is in contrast to the uniform cytoplasmic expression in smooth muscle (Fig. 8–12). On occasion this "tram-track" pattern is a clue that one is dealing with a myofibroblastic process (e.g., fasciitis) rather than a leiomyosarcoma. Antibody asr-1 is monoclonal and specifically identifies sarcomeric actins (skeletal, cardiac); it identifies rhabdomyosarcoma but not leiomyosarcoma.[206] One should be aware of the fact that some rhabdomyosarcomas, particularly the paratesticular spindle cell type, can express low levels of smooth muscle actins.[192]

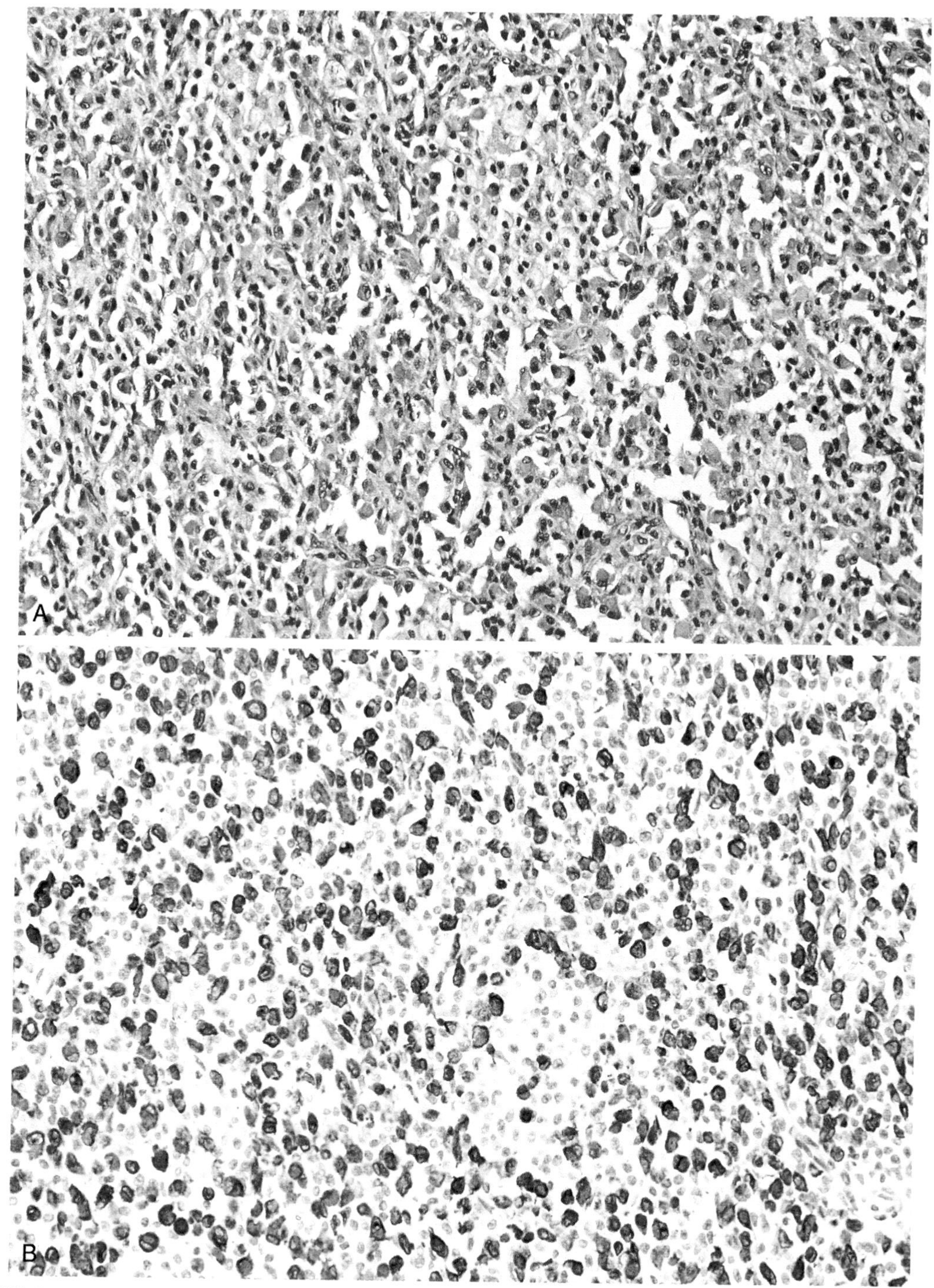


**FIGURE 8–10.** Diffuse-type tenosynovial giant cell tumor with a prominent population of large eosinophilic cells (**A**). These eosinophilic cells may show intense positivity with antibodies to desmin (**B**) and may result in an erroneous diagnosis of rhabdomyosarcoma. Such desmin-positive cells are present in approximately 40% of tenosynovial giant cell tumors.

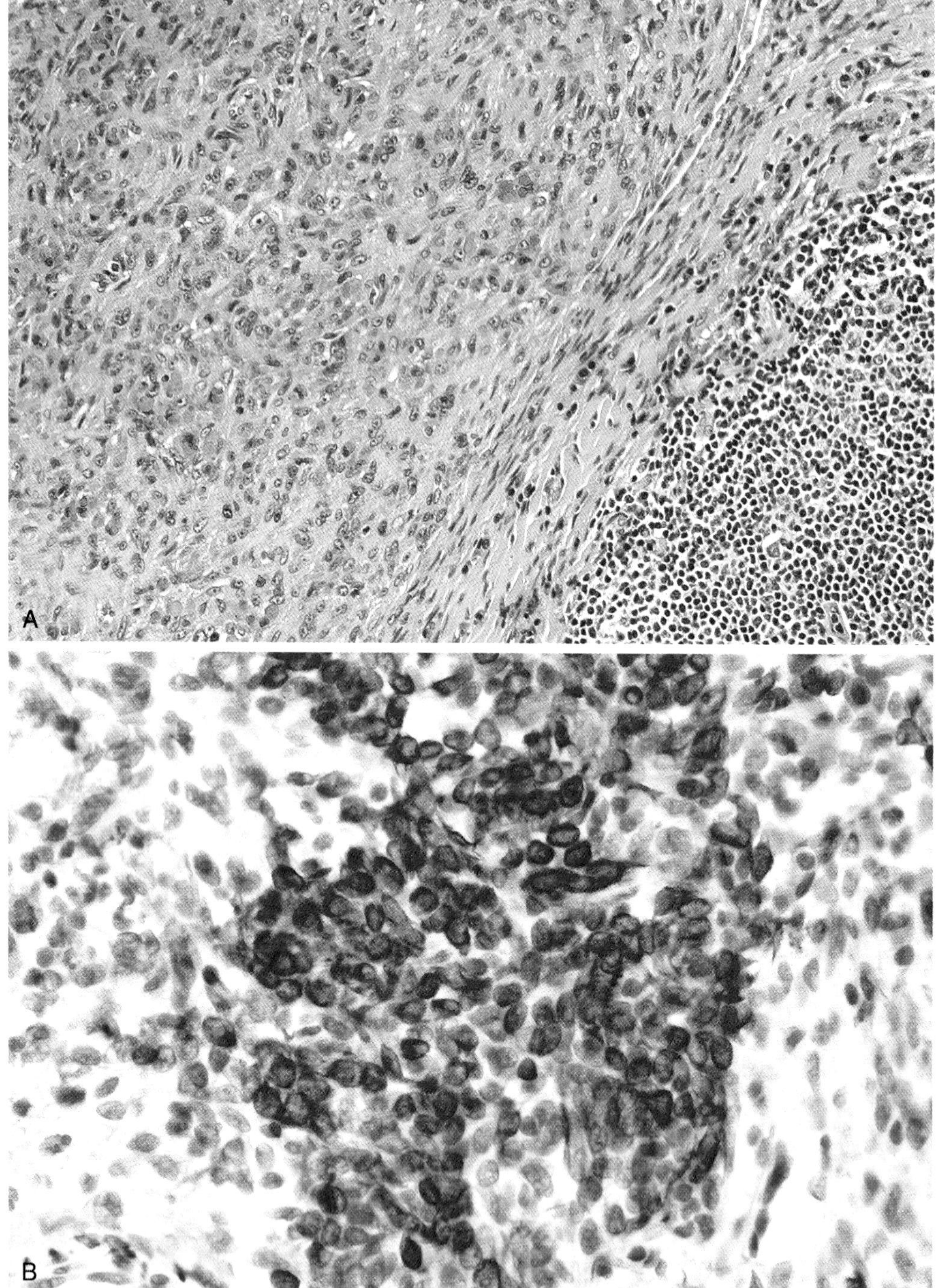

**FIGURE 8–11.** Angiomatoid fibrous histiocytoma (**A**) with strong expression of desmin (**B**). These tumors characteristically co-express desmin and CD68 but are negative for all other muscle-related markers.

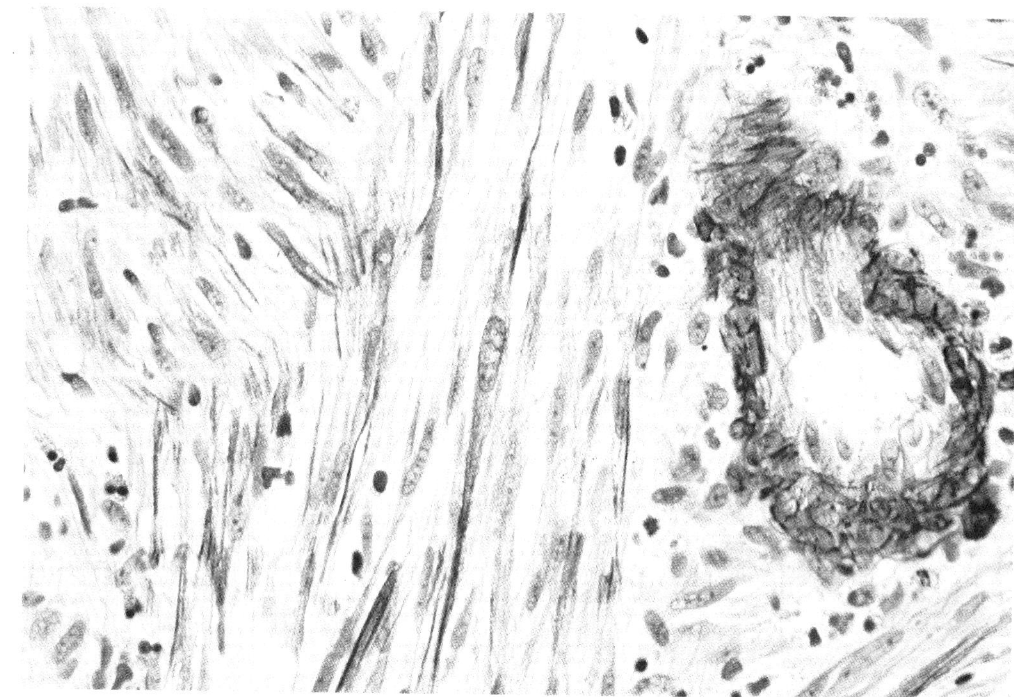

**FIGURE 8–12.** Immunostain for smooth muscle actin demonstrating the characteristic "tram-track" pattern of expression in myofibroblasts (left). This is in contrast to the uniform intracellular staining seen in true smooth muscle (right).

## Myogenic Transcription Factors

Myogenic regulatory proteins [i.e., transcription factors of the MyoD (*myo*genic *d*etermination) family] play a critical role in the commitment and differentiation of mesenchymal progenitor cells to the myogenic lineage and subsequent maintenance of the skeletal muscle phenotype. MyoD1 and myogenin are members of the basic helix–loop–helix family of DNA binding myogenic nuclear regulatory proteins; the other members include Myf5 and MRF4.[233,238] These genes encode transcription factors, whose introduction into nonmuscle cells in culture can initiate muscle-specific gene expression and muscle differentiation.[233] In addition, such regulatory factors are expressed much earlier in the normal skeletal muscle differentiation program than structural proteins such as desmin, actin, and myosin; indeed, expression of these myogenic regulatory proteins leads to activation of the latter.[63,64] Antibodies to both MyoD1 and myogenin, but not the other myogenic nuclear regulatory proteins, have been studied in terms of diagnosing rhabdomyosarcoma. Both MyoD1[52,53,73,236,243] and myogenin[73,236] are expressed in more than 90% of rhabdomyosarcomas. Antibodies to both MyoD1 and myogenin show excellent specificity (Fig. 8–9). There is only a single report of nuclear immunoreactivity for MyoD1 in formalin-fixed, paraffin-embedded sections: in a pleomorphic liposarcoma.[243] Four alveolar soft part sarcomas have been demonstrated to express MyoD1 by immunohistochemistry on frozen sections and by Western blot.[190] There have been no reports of myogenin immunoreactivity in nonrhabdomyosarcomas. Cytoplasmic immunoreactivity for MyoD1 has been reported in a small number of nonrhabdomyosarcomas, including primitive neuroectodermal tumor, Wilms' tumor, and undifferentiated sarcoma.[53] Only nuclear immunoreactivity for MyoD1 should be taken as evidence of skeletal muscle differentiation because the epitope recognized by the most commonly used antibody to MyoD1, 5.8A, includes amino acid sequences with close homology to the class 1 major histocompatibility antigen and transcription factors E2A and ITF-1,[52] suggesting that cytoplasmic immunoreactivity may represent a cross reaction rather than true MyoD1 expression. We routinely use antibodies to both MyoD1 and myogenin, as some rhabdomyosarcomas are positive for one of these proteins but not the other.

## Myoglobin and Other Less Commonly Used Markers

Antibodies to myoglobin, an oxygen-binding heme protein found in skeletal and cardiac muscle but not smooth muscle, were the first markers utilized in the immunohistochemical diagnosis of rhabdomyosarcoma.[21,120,160] Unfortunately, myoglobin is present in demonstrable amounts in fewer than 50% of rhabdomyosarcomas[107,180]; it may be identified in nonmyogenous tumor cells that are infiltrating skeletal muscle and phagocytosing myoglobin.[62] Commercially available myoglobin antibodies have a high level of nonspecific, "background" staining, which may be difficult to distinguish from true myoglobin expression. This is in distinct contrast to desmin and the myogenic regulatory protein, which do not diffuse. We do not use antibodies to myoglobin in our routine practice. Other muscle markers that have been used for diagnosing rhabdomyosarcoma include antibodies to myosin,[107] creatine kinase subunit M,[224] and titin.[176] In general, these markers suffer from a lack of sensitivity, and their use cannot be recommended.

### Recommendations for Use of Muscle Markers

In summary, for identifying skeletal muscle differentiation, the myogenic regulatory proteins myogenin and MyoD1 are the most specific; antibodies to desmin and muscle actins (i.e., HHF35) are of high sensitivity but are not skeletal muscle-specific. For identification of smooth muscle differentiation (e.g., in leiomyosarcomas), antibodies to desmin and muscle actins (i.e., antibody HHF35) or smooth muscle $\alpha$-actin (e.g., antibody 1A4) are the best markers of smooth muscle differentiation. For identifying myofibroblasts (e.g., the type of differentiation present in lesions such as nodular fasciitis), antibodies to desmin are useful only for distinguishing myofibroblasts from true smooth muscle cells; as the former (in contrast to the latter) generally do not express desmin.[104,124] Both cell types express smooth muscle actins, however, although myofibroblasts generally express the latter in a characteristic "wispy" or "tram-track" pattern of immunostaining that, upon higher resolution, can be demonstrated to correspond to the peripheral bundles of actin filaments, which are the hallmark of this cell type.

## MARKERS OF NERVE SHEATH DIFFERENTIATION

### S-100 Protein

The S-100 protein is a 20-kDa acidic calcium-binding protein, so named for its solubility in 100% ammonium sulfate. The protein is composed of two subunits, $\alpha$ and $\beta$, which combine to form three isotypes. The $\alpha$-$\alpha$ isotype is normally found in myocardium, skeletal muscle, and neurons; the $\alpha$-$\beta$ isotype is present in melanocytes, glia, chondrocytes, and skin adnexae; and the $\beta$-$\beta$ isotype is seen in Langerhans cells and Schwann cells.[216]

Immunohistochemically, S-100 protein can be demonstrated in a large number of normal tissues, including some neurons and glia; Schwann cells; melanocytes; Langerhans cells; interdigitating reticulum cells of lymph nodes; chondrocytes; myoepithelial cells and ducts of sweat glands, salivary glands, and the breast; serous glands of the lung; fetal neuroblasts; and sustentacular cells of the adrenal medulla and paraganglia[111] (Figs. 8–13, 8–14). In the immunohistochemical diagnosis of soft tissue neoplasms, S-100 protein is of most value as a marker of benign and malignant nerve sheath tumors and melanoma. S-100 protein is strongly and uniformly expressed in essentially all schwannomas.[106,240] The finding of uniform S-100 immunoreactivity may be a valuable clue to the diagnosis of cellular schwannoma,[27,245] as malignant peripheral nerve sheath tumors usually show only patchy, weak expression of S-100[99,141,144,240] and fibrosarcomas would not be expected to be S-100-positive (Fig. 8–15). S-100 protein expression is much more variable in neurofibromas than in schwannomas.[240] S-100 protein expression is seen in 40–80% of malignant peripheral nerve sheath tumors.[99,141,144,240] However, as may be inferred from the long list of normal tissues that express this protein, significant S-100 protein expression may be seen in a subset of nonneural tumors included in the differential diagnosis of malignant peripheral nerve sheath tumors: synovial sarcoma,[70,75,93] rhabdomyosarcoma,[36] leiomyosarcoma,[110] and myoepithelioma.[118] Other tumors that may express S-100 protein include adipocytic tumors, chondrocytic tumors, chordoma, and parachordoma. Malignant melanomas of all types, including the desmoplastic and sarcomatoid variants, are almost always strongly positive for S-100 protein.[161,162,240] Uniform, strong S-100 expression may be a valuable clue that one is dealing with a melanoma rather than a malignant peripheral nerve sheath tumor of skin or soft tissue because, as noted above, S-100 expression in malignant peripheral nerve sheath tumors tends to be weaker and more patchy. It has been our experience that approximately 2–3% of melanomas are negative for S-100; additional immunostaining for a melanosome-specific marker such as gp100 protein (identified by antibody HMB-45[89]) or Melan-A[25] is essential for arriving at the correct diagnoses in these cases.

### CD57

The 110-kDa protein CD57 is normally found on the surface of natural killer cells and T lymphocytes. An-

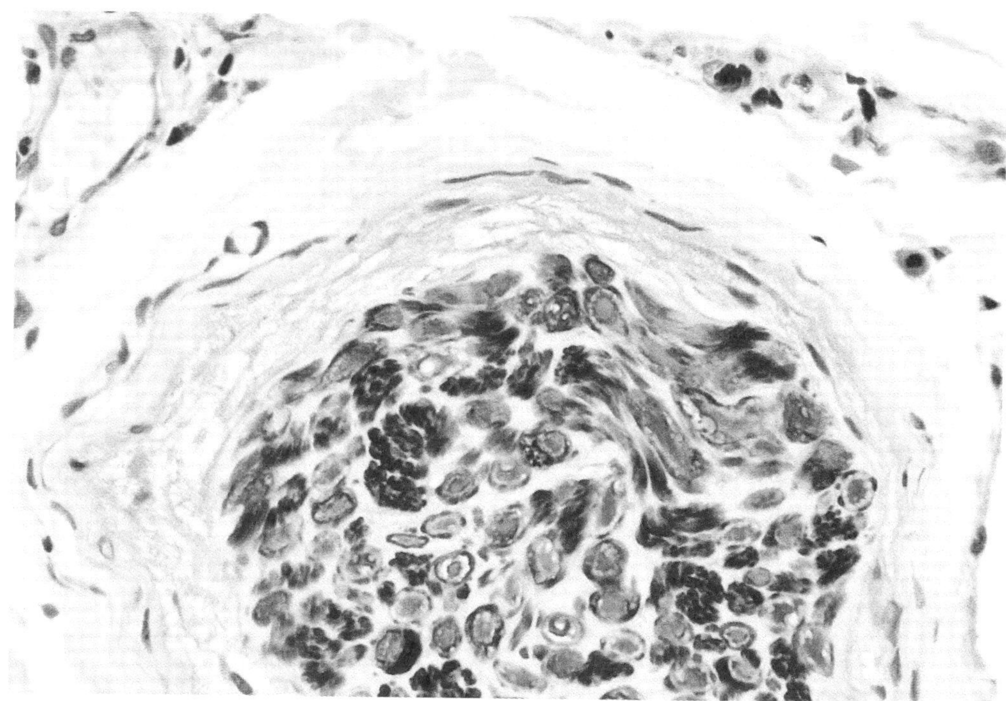

**FIGURE 8–13.** Nerve illustrating S-100 protein expression in schwann cells. Note that the perineurial cells do not express S-100.

tibodies to this protein, including Leu7 and HNK-1, have been found to react with myelin-associated glycoprotein,[142] and both central nervous system oligodendroglia and peripheral Schwann cells may be CD57-positive.[198] Although CD57 immunoreactivity is present in most malignant peripheral nerve sheath tumors,[7,214] a significant percentage of other sarcomas, including synovial sarcoma[7,75] and leiomyosarcoma,[214] are also positive. This lack of specificity limits the utility of CD57 in the immunohistochemical diagnosis of sarcomas. We recommend that antibodies to CD57 be used only in concert with antibodies to the S-100 protein for confirmation of suspected malignant peripheral nerve sheath tumors.

### p75NTR

The nerve growth factor receptor p75NTR, a low-affinity 75-kDa receptor, is normally expressed on neuronal axons, Schwann cells, perineurial cells, perivascular fibroblasts, outer follicular root sheath epithelium, and myoepithelium.[112,221] Expression of p75NTR has been reported in up to 80% of malignant peripheral nerve sheath tumors and nearly all schwannomas, granular cell tumors, and neurofibromas.[183] However, as with CD57, p75NTR expression is not limited to malignant peripheral nerve sheath tumors and may be seen in other sarcomas, including synovial sarcoma[75] and malignant melanoma.[112]

## MARKERS OF MELANOCYTIC DIFFERENTIATION

### HMB-45

Monoclonal antibody HMB-45 identifies the *Pmel 17* gene product gp100.[10] This gene product is a component of the premelanosomal/melanosomal melanogenic oxidoreductive enzymes and as such is melanosome-specific but not melanoma-specific.[113] HMB-45 is positive in the unusual myomelanocytic tumors that comprise the perivascular epithelioid cell family of tumors (angiomyolipoma, clear-cell tumor of lung, lymphangioleiomyomatosis)[10,18] but has not convincingly been shown to react with any tumor that does not contain melanosomes. Previous reports of HMB-45 positivity in carcinomas were based on the use of contaminated ascites fluid and have been retracted in the literature.[19] HMB-45 is generally negative in nevi and resting melanocytes but is expressed in approximately 85% of melanomas[10] (Fig. 8–16). Fewer than 10% of desmoplastic melanomas are HMB-45-positive.[138]

### Other Melanocytic Markers (Melan-A, Tyrosinase, Microphthalmia Transcription Factor)

The three most recently commercially available melanoma markers are Melan-A, tyrosinase, and microph-

*Text continued on page 222*

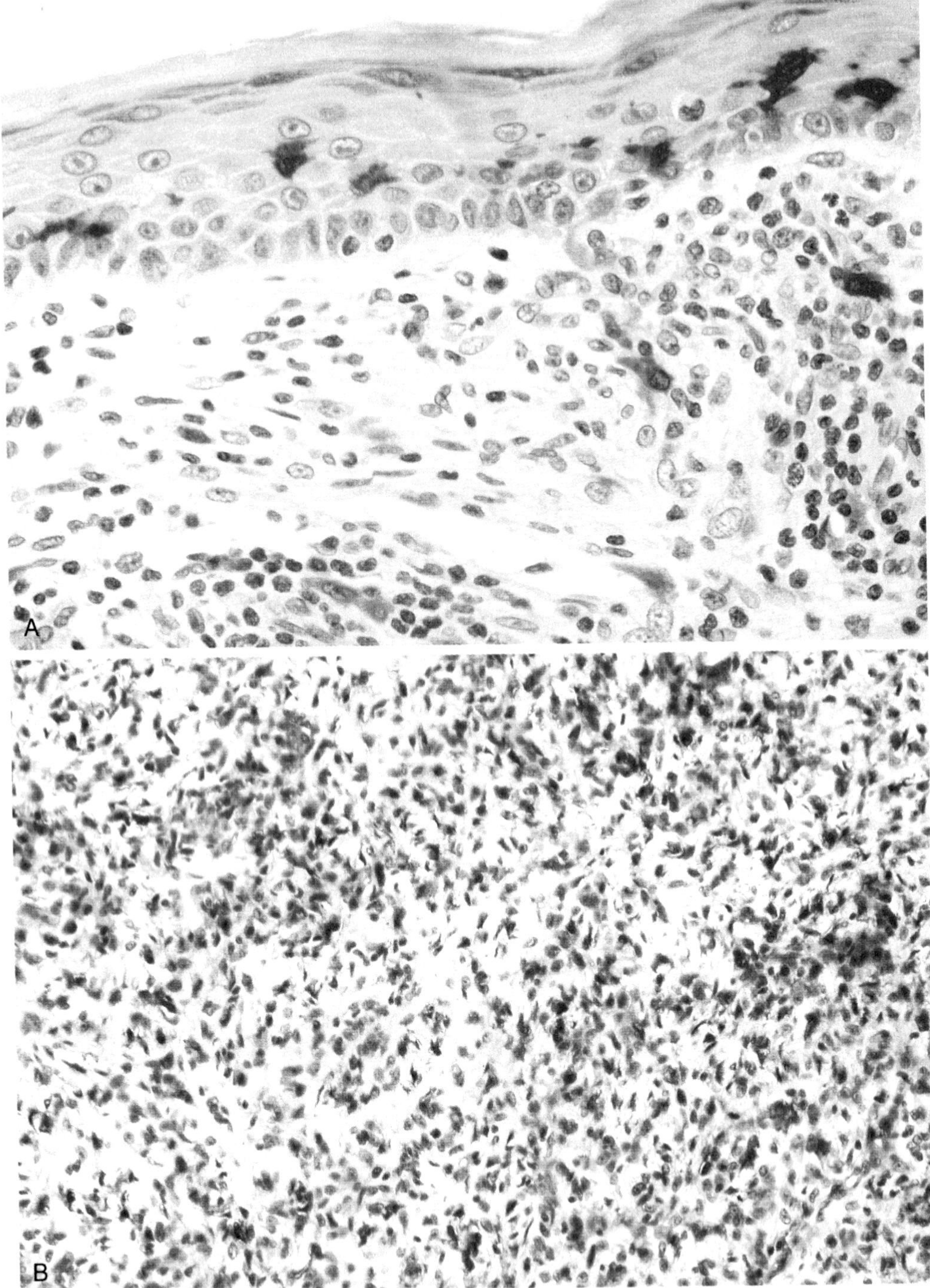


**FIGURE 8–14.** (**A**) Skin showing S-100 protein expression in both intraepidermal and dermal Langerhans cells. (**B**) Some dermal tumors, such as this benign fibrous histiocytoma, have a large number of infiltrating Langerhans cells. It is important to distinguish reactive from neoplastic subpopulations when interpreting immunostains of mesenchymal tumors.

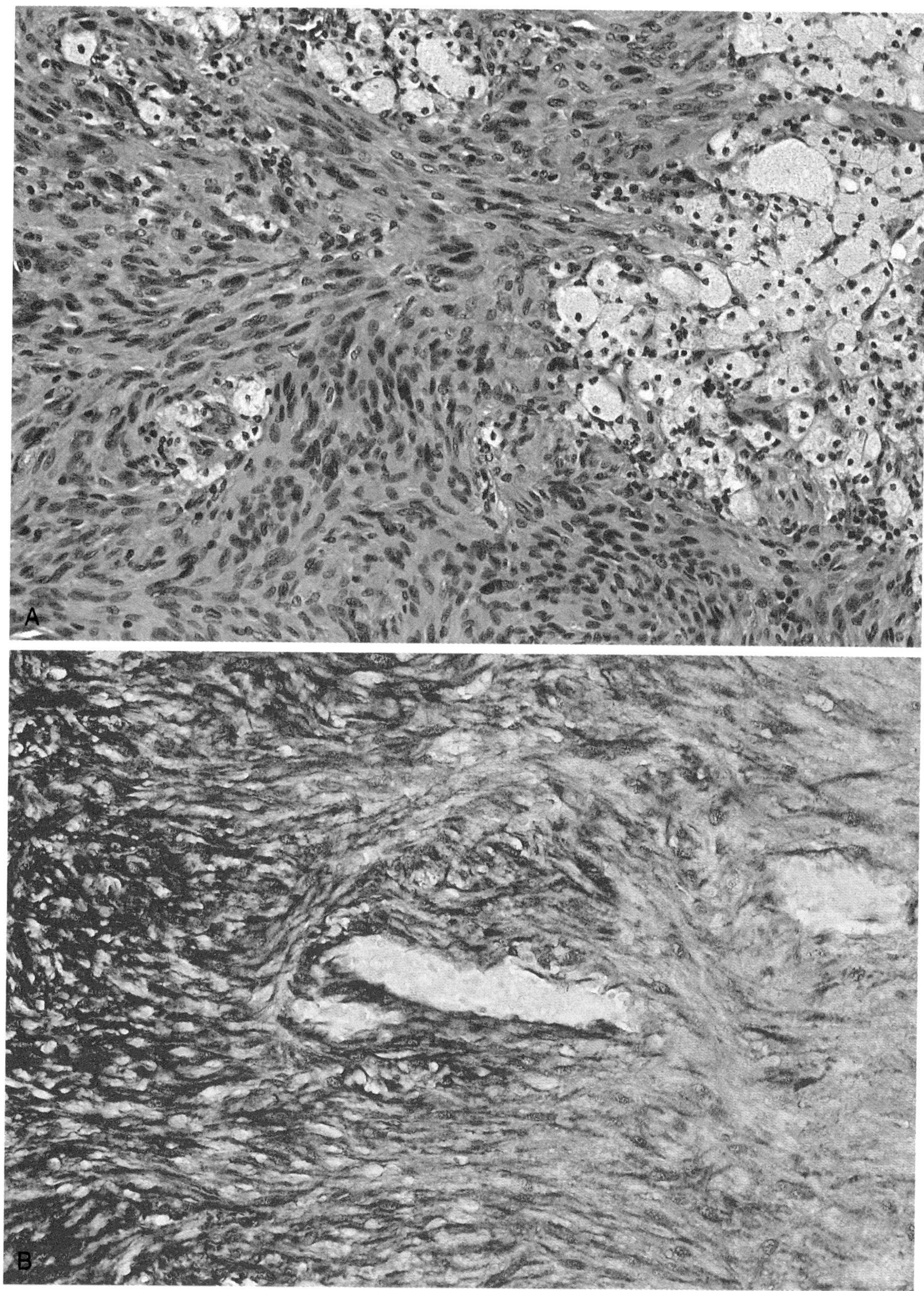


**FIGURE 8–15.** Cellular schwannoma (**A**) demonstrating uniform, intense S-100 protein expression (**B**). Such intense expression is characteristic of schwannomas and melanocytic tumors.

*Illustration continued on following page*

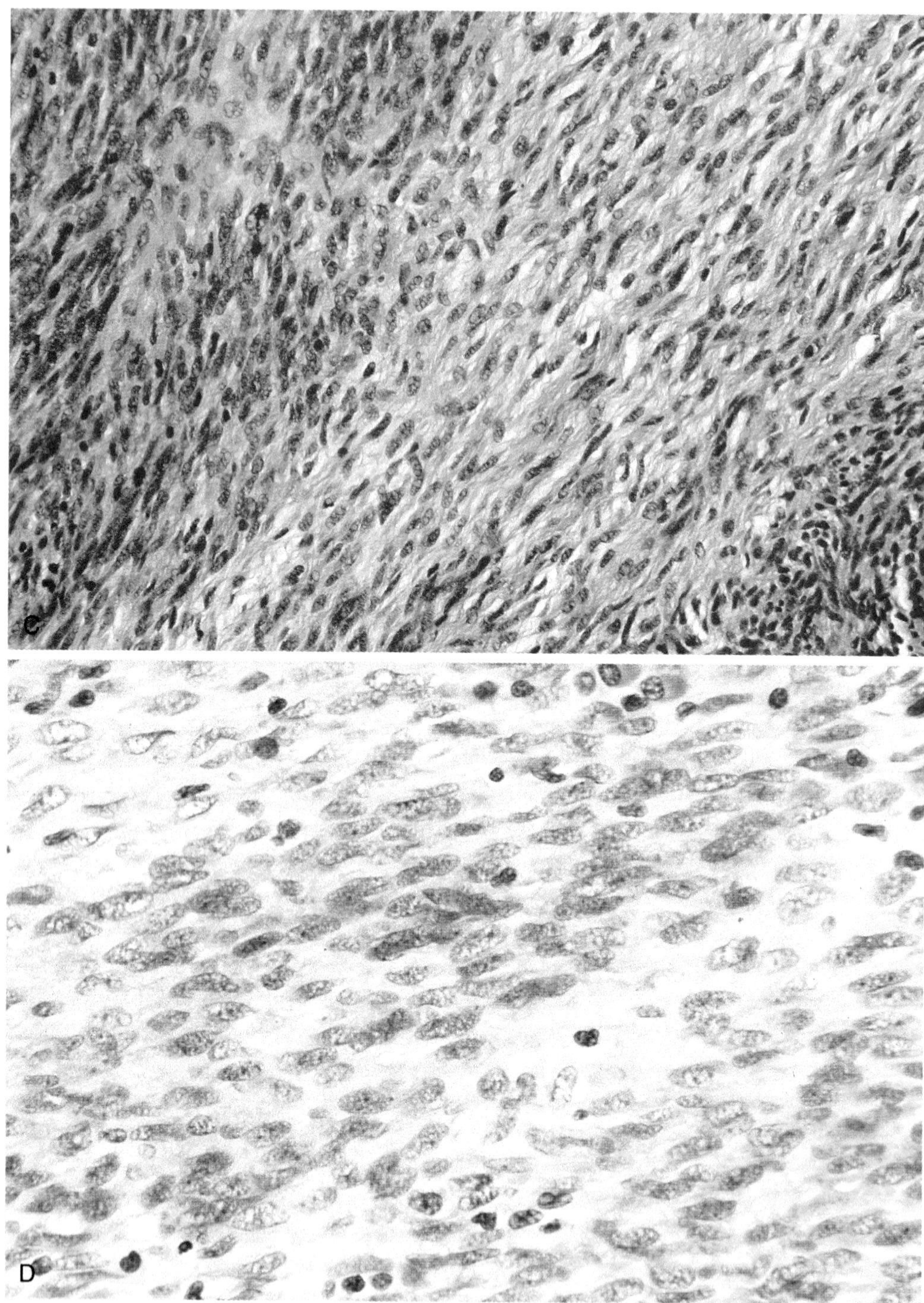


**FIGURE 8–15** (*Continued*). In contrast, malignant peripheral nerve sheath tumors (**C**) typically show only patchy, weak S-100 expression (**D**).

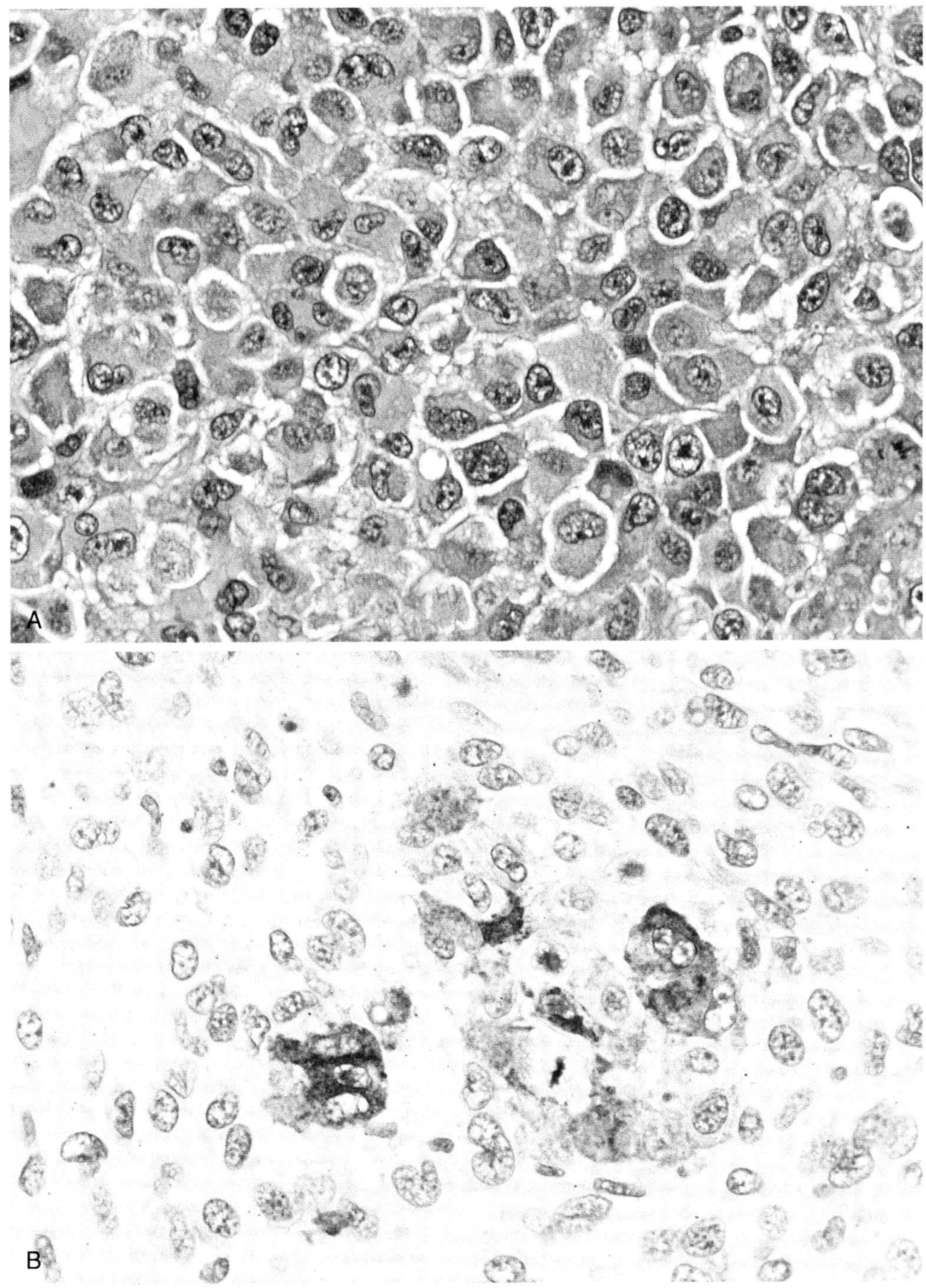


**FIGURE 8–16.** Malignant melanoma (**A**) immunostained with monoclonal antibody HMB-45 to gp100 protein (**B**). HMB-45 is positive in approximately 85% of epithelioid melanomas but in only a small fraction of spindled melanomas.

thalmia transcription factor. Melan-A, the product of the *MART-1* gene (melanoma antigen recognized by T cells), is a 20 to 22 kDa component of the premelanosomal membrane.[25,115] Its function is unknown. Like HMB-45, Melan-A is a marker of melanosomes, not melanomas: it is also present in perivascular epithelioid cell tumors (PEComas) (Fig. 8–17). Unlike HMB-45, Melan-A is positive in resting melanocytes and nevi. Melan-A is expressed by approximately 85% of epithelioid melanomas and has been reported to be present in upward of 50% of desmoplastic melanomas, although the true rate is almost certainly far lower and is probably the same as for HMB-45.[25,115] Melan-A is present in some HMB-45-negative melanomas and vice versa. One other interesting application of the most widely used antibody to Melan-A, A103, is for the diagnosis of adrenal cortical and other steroid-producing tumors. A103 has reproducible cross-reactivity with an unknown epitope present in these tumors, and it may be helpful for distinguishing adrenal cortical carcinomas from renal cell carcinoma.[26]

Tyrosinase is an enzyme involved in the synthesis of melanin. Antibodies to tyrosinase have recently been shown to have a sensitivity and specificity that is roughly equivalent to that of HMB-45 and Melan-A.[115] Although tyrosinase is potentially useful, we have not yet been impressed that it identifies melanomas that are negative with HMB-45 or A103.

Microphthalmia transcription factor is a recently characterized transcription factor that is critical in melanogenesis and in the expression of the tyrosinase gene.[121] Microphthalmia transcription factor has been shown to be expressed in close to 100% of epithelioid melanomas.[121] We have reported microphthalmia transcription factor in approximately 40% of desmoplastic melanomas and in more than 85% of clear-cell sarcomas[122] (Fig. 8–18).

## MARKERS OF ENDOTHELIAL DIFFERENTIATION

A number of markers have been used to demonstrate endothelial differentiation, paralleling the progression in our concept of spindle cell tumors manifesting endothelial differentiation. Endothelial markers include von Willebrand factor (factor VIII-associated protein, often erroneously referred to as factor VIII), CD34, and CD31. The pattern of expression of these three markers in endothelial tumors is much like an overlapping Venn diagram, in which most tumors express all three markers, but some express only one or two. Whereas early studies had suggested that markers such as von Willebrand factor (vWF) could differentially identify vascular versus lymphatic endothelium,[13,24,96] more recent studies have demonstrated that both vascular and lymphatic endothelium express all three markers; and novel markers such as podoplanin and vascular endothelial growth factor receptor-3 (positive on lymphatic endothelium and negative on vascular endothelium) are required to make this distinction.[20,76,109]

### von Willebrand Factor (Factor VIII-related Antigen)

The von Willebrand factor (vWF) was the first endothelium-specific marker employed in diagnostic immunohistochemical studies.[24] It was first used to identify the nature of the vinyl chloride-induced sarcomas of liver[78] and has subsequently been demonstrated to be a marker of vascular tumors of multiple sites, including but not limited to those of the central nervous system,[17] gastrointestinal tract,[175] and breast.[147] vWF is the least sensitive of the vascular markers and is positive in 50–75% of vascular tumors.[76] Although vWF expression is, in theory, absolutely specific for vascular tumors, technical problems limit its usefulness. vWF is not only produced by endothelial cells but circulates in the serum; and it therefore can be found often in zones of tumor necrosis and hemorrhage.

### CD34 (Human Hematopoietic Progenitor Cell Antigen)

The function of CD34, a 110-kDa transmembrane glycoprotein, is unknown. It is expressed on hematopoietic stem cells, endothelium, the interstitial cells of Cajal, and a group of interesting dendritic cells present in the dermis, around blood vessels, and in the nerve sheath.[230] CD34 is expressed in more than 90% of vascular tumors[155] and is the most sensitive marker of Kaposi's sarcoma.[76] As may be gathered from the above list of normal tissues, CD34 expression is not limited to vascular tumors. CD34 expression is well documented in dermatofibrosarcoma protuberans,[126] solitary fibrous tumors,[244] malignant peripheral nerve sheath tumors,[241] gastrointestinal stromal tumors,[119] and epithelioid sarcomas[152,230] (Fig. 8–19). CD34 is expressed by approximately 50–60% of epithelioid sarcomas, compared with fewer than 2% of carcinomas. CD34 expression may be valuable for distinguishing cytokeratin-positive epithelioid angiosarcomas and epithelioid sarcomas from carcinoma.[230]

### CD31 (Platelet Endothelial Cell Adhesion Molecule-1)

The newest of the vascular markers, CD31 is the most sensitive and specific marker.[44,155] It is expressed in more than 90% of angiosarcomas, hemangioendothe-

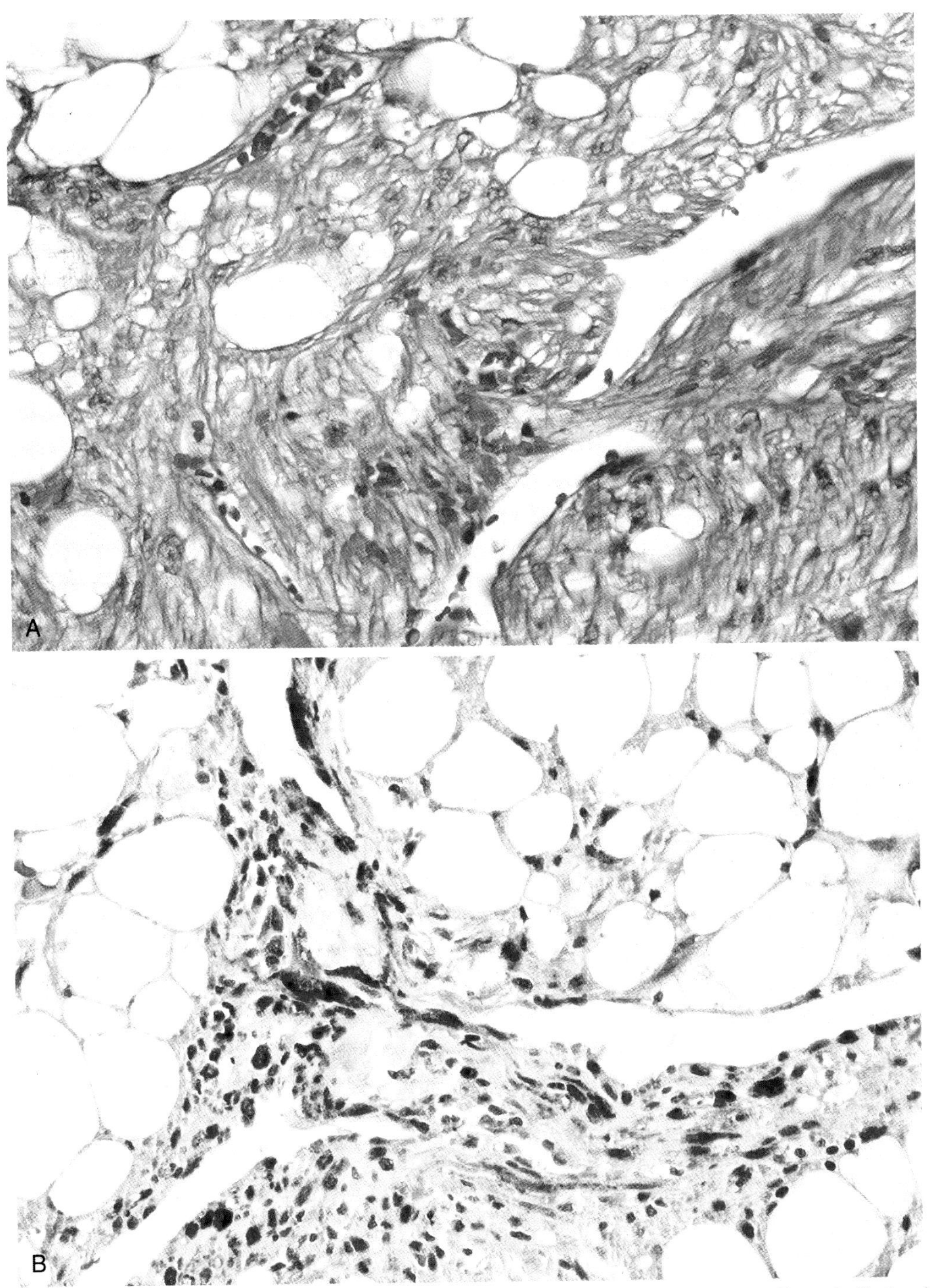

**FIGURE 8–17.** Angiomyolipoma (**A**), showing Melan-A expression in epithelioid cells, spindled cells and in the cytoplasm of lipid-distended cells ("adipocytes") (**B**). Co-expression of melanosome-related proteins, such as gp100 and Melan-A, with smooth muscle markers is characteristic of the perivascular epithelioid cell (PEComa) family of tumors.

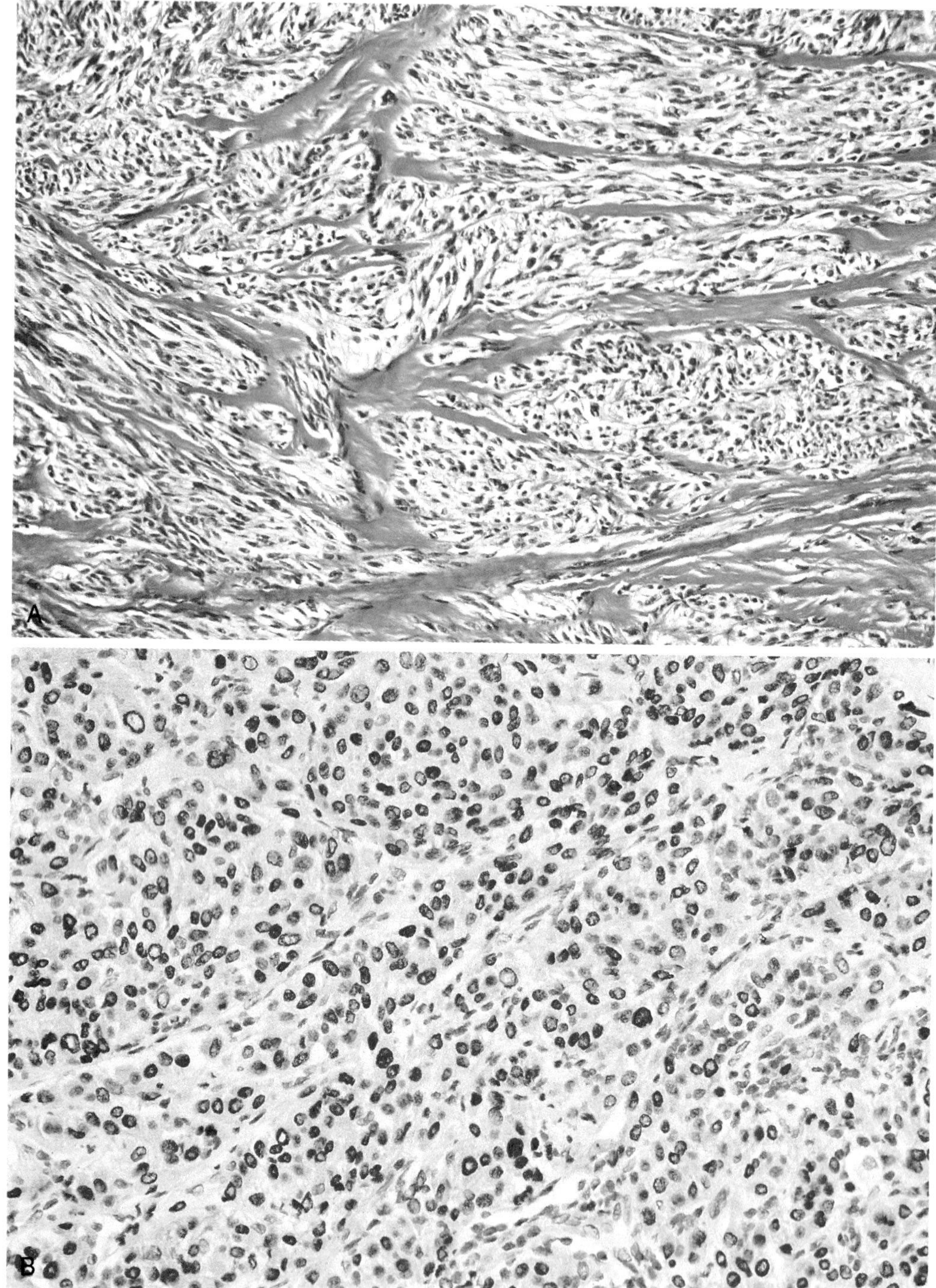

**FIGURE 8–18.** Clear-cell sarcoma (**A**) with uniform nuclear expression of microphthalmia transcription factor (**B**). Microphthalmia transcription factor is a highly sensitive marker of melanoma and of mesenchymal tumors with melanocytic differentiation.

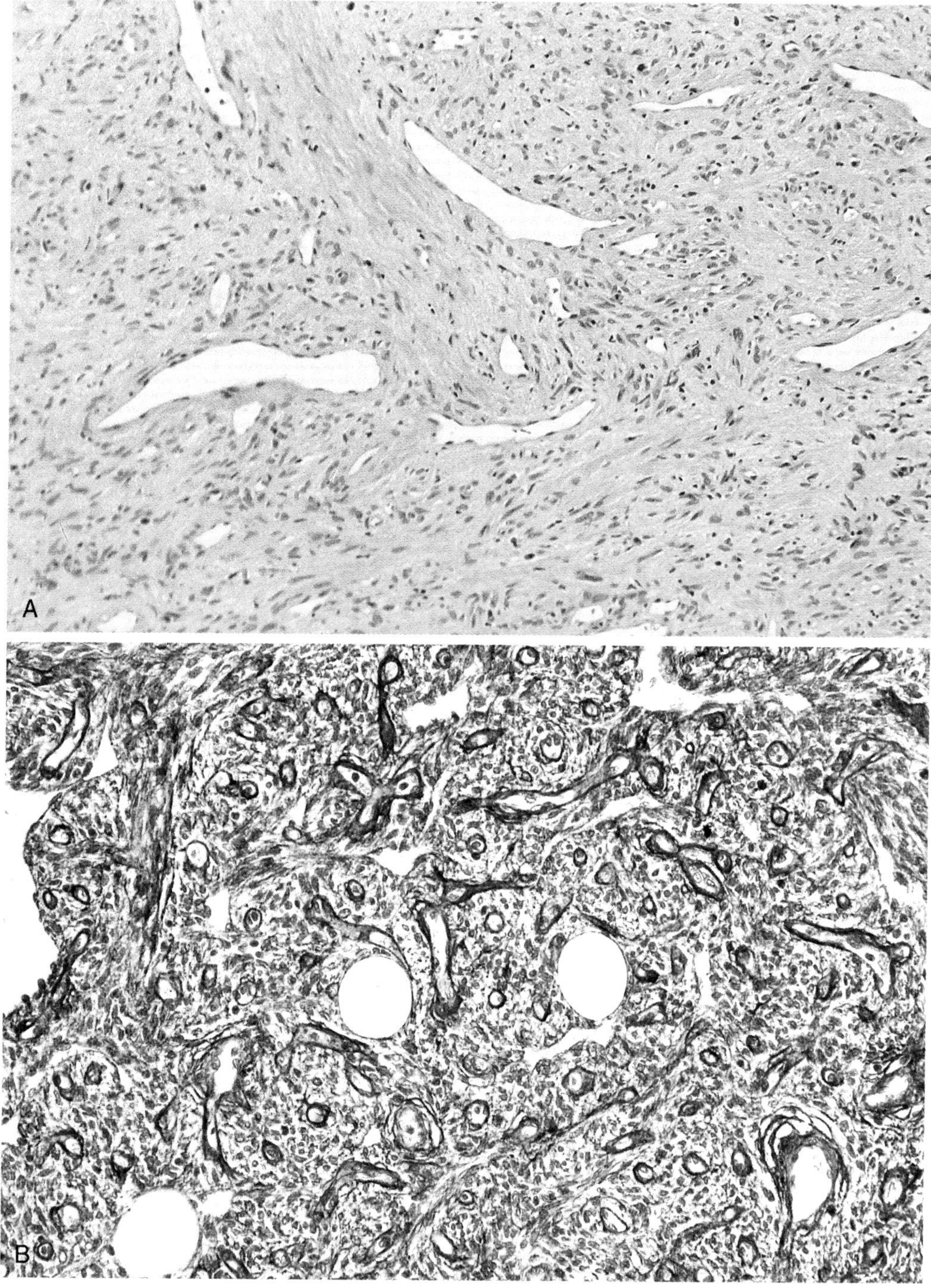


**FIGURE 8–19.** Solitary fibrous tumor (**A**) with uniform CD34 expression (**B**).

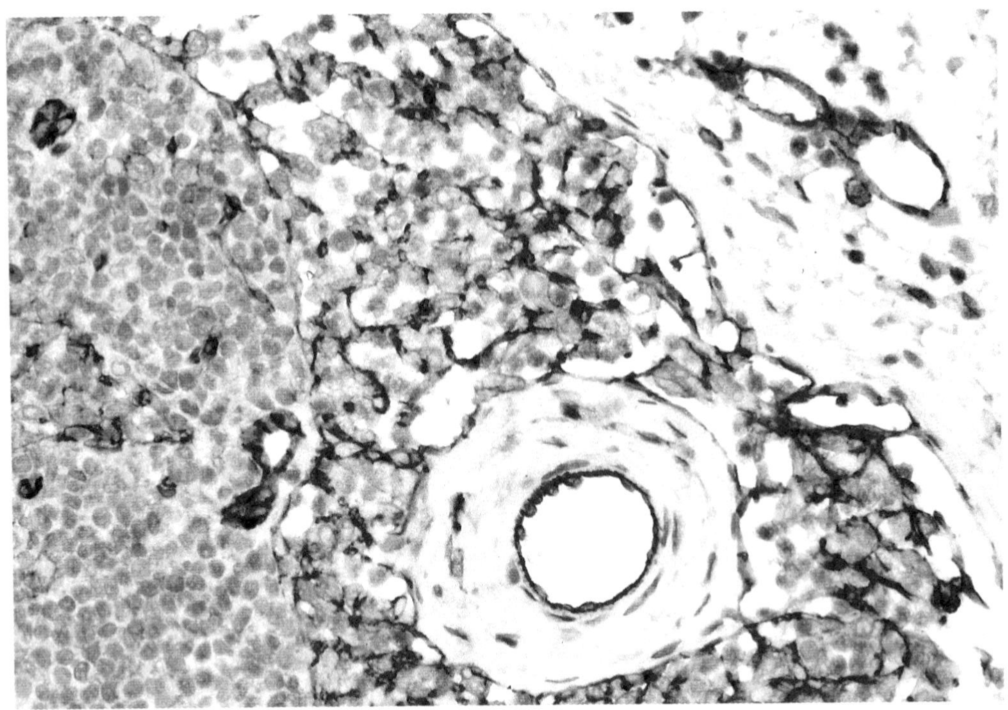

**FIGURE 8–20.** Granular, membranous CD31 expression in macrophages of the lymph node sinusoid. This granular expression in macrophages infiltrating a tumor may be mistaken for true expression by the tumor calls, leading to an erroneous diagnosis of angiosarcoma. CD31 expression in angiosarcomas is usually stronger and shows a linear, rather than granular, staining pattern (see also Figure 8–5).

liomas, hemangiomas, and Kaposi's sarcoma and in fewer than 1% of carcinomas (probably much less than 1%) (Fig. 8–5). CD31 expression is not seen in any nonendothelial tissue or tumor, with the notable exception of macrophages and platelets (Fig. 8–20). CD31 expression in macrophages is not well described in the pathology literature, and we have seen several cases in which a vascular sarcoma was misdiagnosed as a result. The CD31 expression seen in macrophages is distinctly granular, compared with the intense cytoplasmic and linear membranous staining of endothelium.

### Ulex Lectin

Ulex lectin was a popular alternative marker of endothelial cells and tumors.[153,235] Although it was initially praised for its great sensitivity for vascular tumors,[3,196] it was subsequently discovered that the sugar residue recognized by this lectin is also present on a wide range of epithelial tumors.[32,117,209] Ulex retains its high specificity for vascular tumors if its use is restricted to cytokeratin-negative tumors.

### Type IV Collagen

Type IV collagen, associated with basement membrane expression, is produced by smooth muscle, glomus cells, nerve sheath, and endothelial cells. In our experience, angiosarcomas demonstrate a characteristic pattern of type IV collagen expression in which the latter is present around clusters of cells rather than individual cells. This specific pattern of basement membrane deposition has been described.[134] Demonstration of uniform pericellular type IV collagen may also be a clue to the diagnosis of a glomus tumor (Fig. 8–21).

### Recommendations for Use of Vascular Markers

As a practical issue, it is best to employ a highly specific (e.g., antibodies to CD31) and a highly sensitive (e.g., antibodies to CD34) marker to assess the presence of endothelial differentiation in histologic and clinical settings in which the diagnosis of angiosarcoma is entertained. The endothelial markers are summarized in Table 8–3.

## IMMUNOHISTOCHEMICAL DISTINCTION OF MESOTHELIOMA AND CARCINOMA

Few subjects have generated the remarkable proliferation of studies, papers, seminars, review articles, and

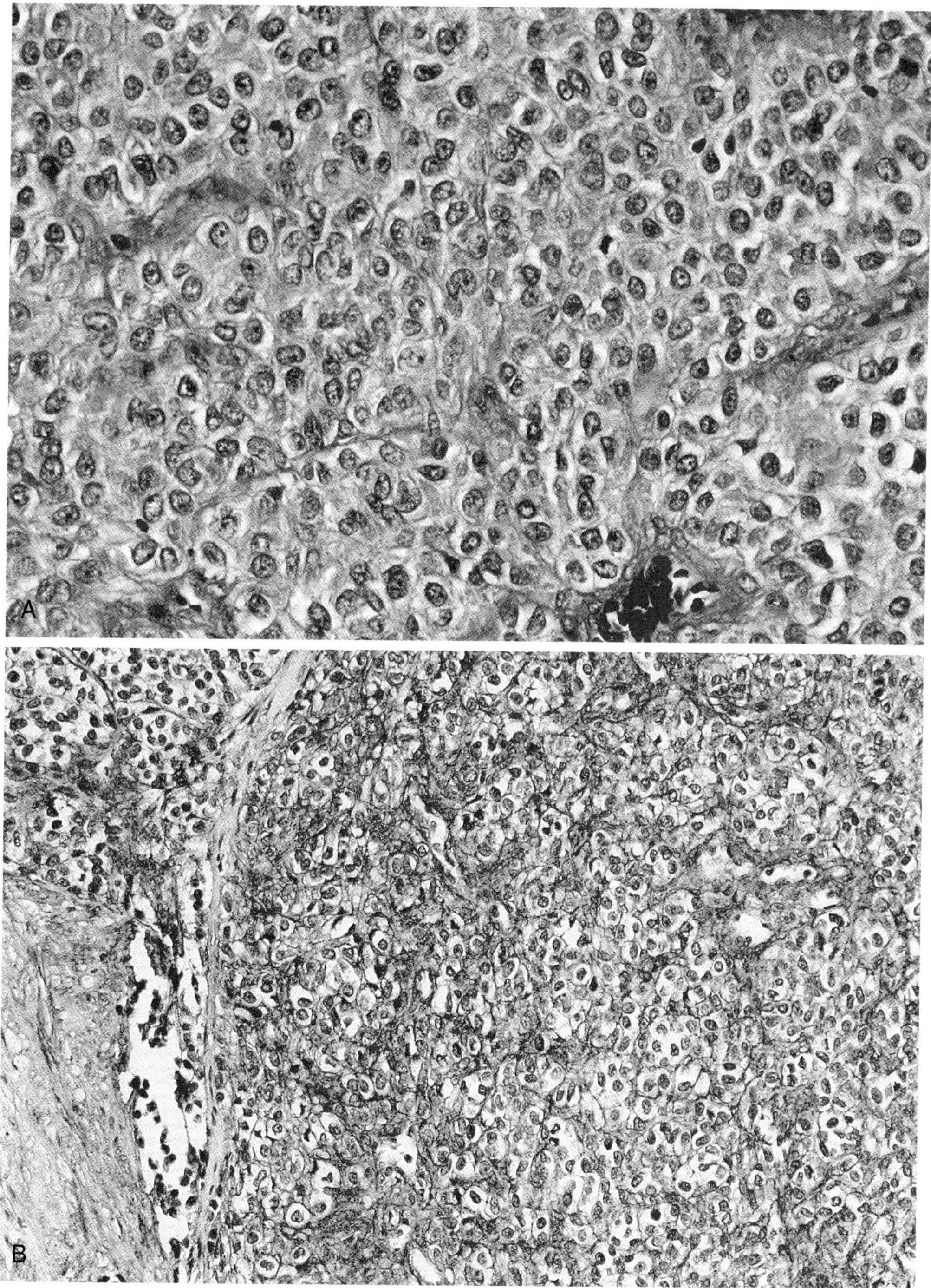

**FIGURE 8–21.** Malignant glomus tumor (**A**) with characteristic investment of individual cells by type IV collagen (**B**). Pericellular type IV collagen is characteristic of tumors with glomus cell, endothelial, schwannian, perineurial, and smooth muscle differentiation.

**TABLE 8–3 ENDOTHELIAL MARKERS**

| Marker | Specificity | Sensitivity | Also Identifies |
|---|---|---|---|
| vWF | High | Low | Megakaryocytes |
| Ulex lectin | High* | Moderate | Many epithelia |
| CD34 | Moderate | High | Epithelioid sarcoma, solitary fibrous tumor, DFSP, etc. |
| CD31 | High | High | Macrophages |
| Type IV collagen | Moderate* | Moderate | Nerve sheath tumors, smooth muscle tumors |

vWF, von Willebrand factor.
* In the soft tissue (i.e., nonepithelial) tumor group.

courses as has the differential diagnosis of mesothelioma and carcinoma. In large part, this is probably due to the legal implications of the diagnosis of mesothelioma in the United States. Along with this proliferation of studies has come a sometimes bewildering number of new antibodies, each touted as more specific or sensitive than the last. Historically, the immunohistochemical diagnosis of mesothelioma was one of exclusion in that there were no positive markers of mesothelial differentiation. The most widely used positive markers of adenocarcinoma/negative markers of mesothelioma include monoclonal antibodies to carcinoembryonic antigen (mCEA), monoclonal antibody LeuM1 to CD15, and monoclonal antibodies to the tumor-associated glycoproteins defined by antibodies B72.3 and Ber-EP4. We have close to 20 years of experience in the use of these antibodies, and their range of reactivities in various carcinomas and mesotheliomas has been studied extensively. The combination of these four antibodies alone can distinguish more than 90% of pulmonary adenocarcinomas from mesothelioma.[201] It is therefore critical always to interpret the newer positive mesothelial markers, with which we have much less experience, in the context of the findings with negative markers. Recommendations for the immunodiagnosis of mesothelioma are given in Table 8–4.

### Carcinoembryonic Antigen

Carcinoembryonic antigen is expressed in approximately 85–90% of carcinomas of lung, gastric, and pancreaticobiliary origin but in only 15–30% of breast and ovarian carcinomas.[23,170,171] Rare mesotheliomas that are rich in hyaluronic acid may show false positivity for CEA.[189] However, unlike in adenocarcinomas, which are usually diffusely positive, this false positivity is seen only in scattered cells.

### CD15 (LeuM1)

The CD15 marker is expressed by a somewhat smaller number of carcinomas (60–75%) than is CEA.[170] As with CEA, rare hyaluronic acid-rich mesotheliomas show granular cytoplasmic positivity, and rare mesotheliomas have been reported to show strong CD15 expression.[247]

### Tumor-associated Glycoproteins (B72.3, Ber-EP4)

The monoclonal antibodies B72.3 and Ber-EP4 are directed against different tumor-associated membrane glycoproteins. Of these two antibodies, B72.3 is the

**TABLE 8–4 RECOMMENDED IMMUNOHISTOCHEMICAL PANEL FOR MESOTHELIOMA**

| Antibodies To | Adenocarcinoma | Mesothelioma | Comments |
|---|---|---|---|
| Calretinin | 5–15% Positive | 75–95% Positive | Expressed by sarcomatoid mesothelioma |
| WT-1 or CK 5/6 | Rarely positive | 75–95% Positive | Experience limited; sensitivity for sarcomatoid mesothelioma unknown |
| CEA | Positive (except breast and ovary) | Negative | Rarely positive; hyaluronic acid-rich mesothelioma |
| CD15 | Positive | Negative | Rarely positive; hyaluronic acid-rich mesothelioma |
| Tumor-associated glycoproteins (B72.3 or Ber-EP4) | Positive | Negative | |

more sensitive marker of adenocarcinomas of all sites, except the ovary, where Ber-EP4 is more sensitive.[170,174] Mesotheliomas are not positive for either B72.3 or Ber-EP4.

### Positive Markers of Mesothelioma (Calretinin, Mesothelin, *WT-1*, Cytokeratin 5/6)

The diagnosis of mesothelioma has been greatly assisted by the development of new positive markers expressed by mesotheliomas but not carcinomas. At the moment, the most promising markers include those to calretinin, mesothelin, the Wilms' tumor gene product WT-1, and cytokeratins 5/6. As noted above, it is critical to remember that these markers are not absolutely specific for mesothelioma, and as such the results of these markers should always be interpreted in the context of the well established negative markers.

*Calretinin,* a calcium-binding protein originally identified in the retina, is probably the best studied of these new markers. Antibodies to calretinin recognize 75–95% of epithelial mesotheliomas and a smaller percentage of sarcomatoid mesotheliomas (about 50%)[54,172] (Fig. 8–22). A small percentage (5–15%) of carcinomas also express calretinin, including those of lung, colon, and ovarian origin.

*Mesothelin (CAK1),* a cell surface protein normally expressed by mesothelium, ovarian surface epithelium, and some squamous epithelium, is expressed by 50–75% of epithelial mesotheliomas.[30,31] The utility of mesothelin is somewhat limited by its total absence of expression in sarcomatoid mesotheliomas and by its even greater sensitivity for serous carcinomas of ovarian and peritoneal origin.

A tumor-suppressor gene located on chromosome 11p13, *WT-1* in contrast to other tumor-suppressor genes, is normally expressed only in certain tissues, including mesothelium. In paraffin sections 75–95% of mesotheliomas express this protein, compared with 25% of carcinomas metastatic to the pleura[125,165,170] (Fig. 8–23). The sensitivity and specificity of calretinin and *WT-1* are roughly equivalent. *WT-1* is also expressed by desmoplastic round cell tumors, which are characterize by t(11;22) (*EWS/WT-1*); expression of *WT-1* may be helpful for distinguishing these tumors from other primitive round cell sarcomas.[169]

The most recent addition to the family of positive mesothelioma markers is *cytokeratin 5/6.* Normal and neoplastic mesothelial cells express cytokeratins 4, 5, 6, 14, and 17, in addition to the cytokeratins (7, 8, 18 and 19) expressed by most glandular epithelium.[170] Cytokeratin 5/6 is expressed by 80–100% of mesotheliomas and only 15% of carcinomas, including those of lung and ovarian surface epithelial and endometrial origin.[35,173]

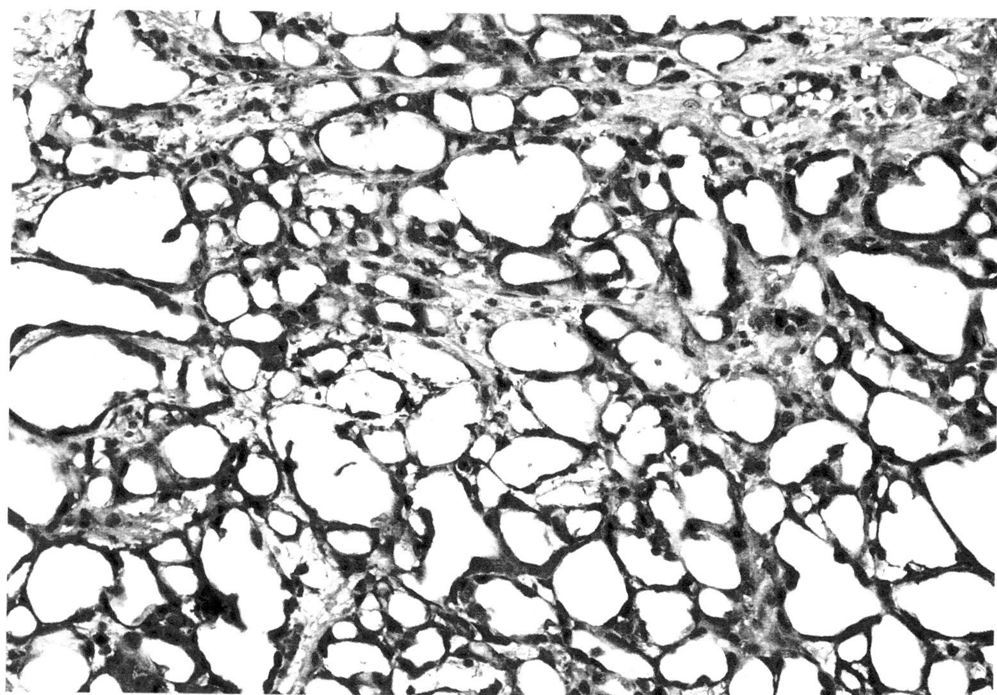

**FIGURE 8–22.** Intense nuclear and cytoplasmic calretinin expression in an adenomatoid tumor.

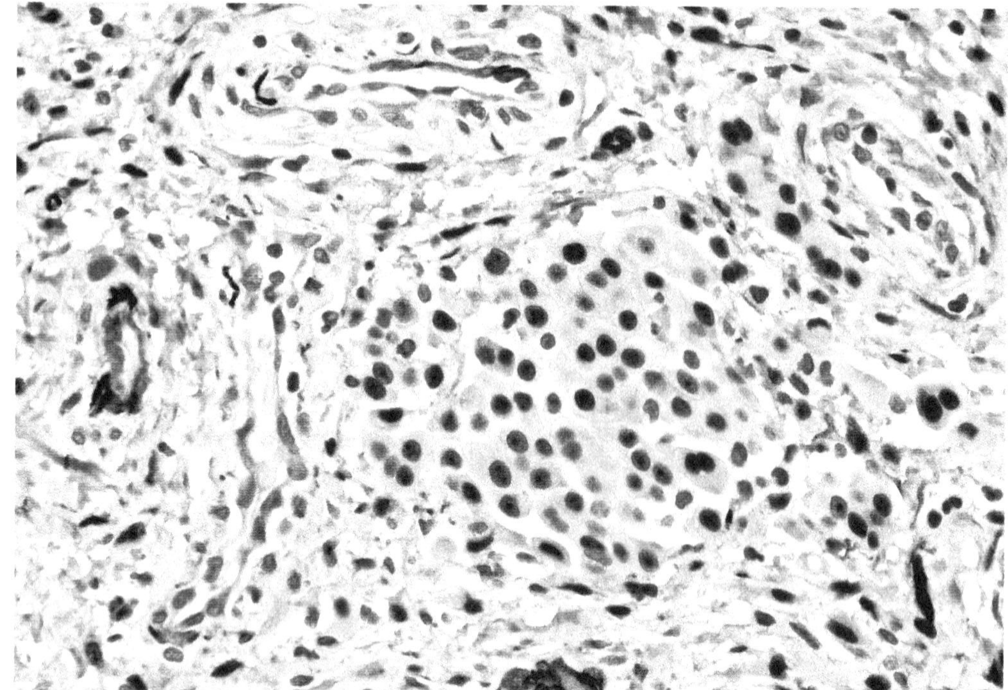

**FIGURE 8–23.** Nuclear WT-1 expression in an epithelioid mesothelioma. Note the typical cytoplasmic immunoreactivity of the endothelial cells. Only nuclear WT-1 expression should be accepted as positive.

# ADDITIONAL MARKERS

## CD117 (c-*kit*)

The c-*kit* proto-oncogene product (CD117), a transmembrane receptor for stem cell factor, is normally expressed by mast cells, melanocytes, germ cells, various subsets of hematopoietic cells, and the interstitial cells of Cajal of the gastrointestinal tract.[119] CD117 is expressed by 85–95% of gastrointestinal stromal tumors.[119,195] In the gastrointestinal tract CD117 is a highly specific marker of gastrointestinal stromal tumors; it is not expressed by tumors typically in the differential diagnosis of a gastrointestinal mesenchymal tumor, such as leiomyomas, leiomyosarcomas, and nerve sheath tumors[119,195] (Fig. 8–24). CD117 is expressed by melanocytic tumors, however, such as melanoma and clear-cell sarcoma.[195] CD117 is also expressed by mast cells, and care should be taken not to mistake mast cells in a tumor for scattered CD117-positive tumor cells (Fig. 8–25).

## CD68

The 110-kDa glycoprotein recognized by antibodies to CD68 (e.g., KP1, KI-M1P) is closely associated with, or a part of, lysosomes. Although CD68 has been thought of as a marker of histiocytes (owing to the presence of large numbers of lysosomes in these cells), it is important to remember that CD68 is organelle-specific rather than lineage-specific. Although CD68 expression is commonly seen in "fibrohistiocytic" soft tissue tumors, such as benign and malignant fibrous histiocytoma, it may also be seen in a variety of other sarcomas, melanomas, and carcinomas.[84,182,199] For this reason, antibodies to CD68 play only a limited role in the diagnosis of soft tissue tumors. CD68 is expressed at high levels by lysosome-rich tumors such as granular cell tumors and may also be useful in bringing out the sometimes subtle round cell population of plexiform fibrohistiocytic tumors (Fig. 8–26).

## CD99

The product of the pseudoautosomal *MIC2* gene,[86] CD99 is a transmembrane glycoprotein of 30–32 kDa (p30/32).[66] Its exact function is unknown, although it appears to play a role in cellular adhesion and regulation of cellular proliferation.[81,94] The *MIC2* gene is expressed; and the CD99 antigen is produced in nearly all human tissues, although the level of expression varies significantly. Normal tissues that commonly display strong CD99 expression include cortical thymocytes and Hassall's corpuscles, granulosa and Sertoli cells, endothelium, pancreatic islets, adenohypophysis, ependyma, and some epithelium, including urothelium, squamous epithelium, and columnar epithelium.[67,210]

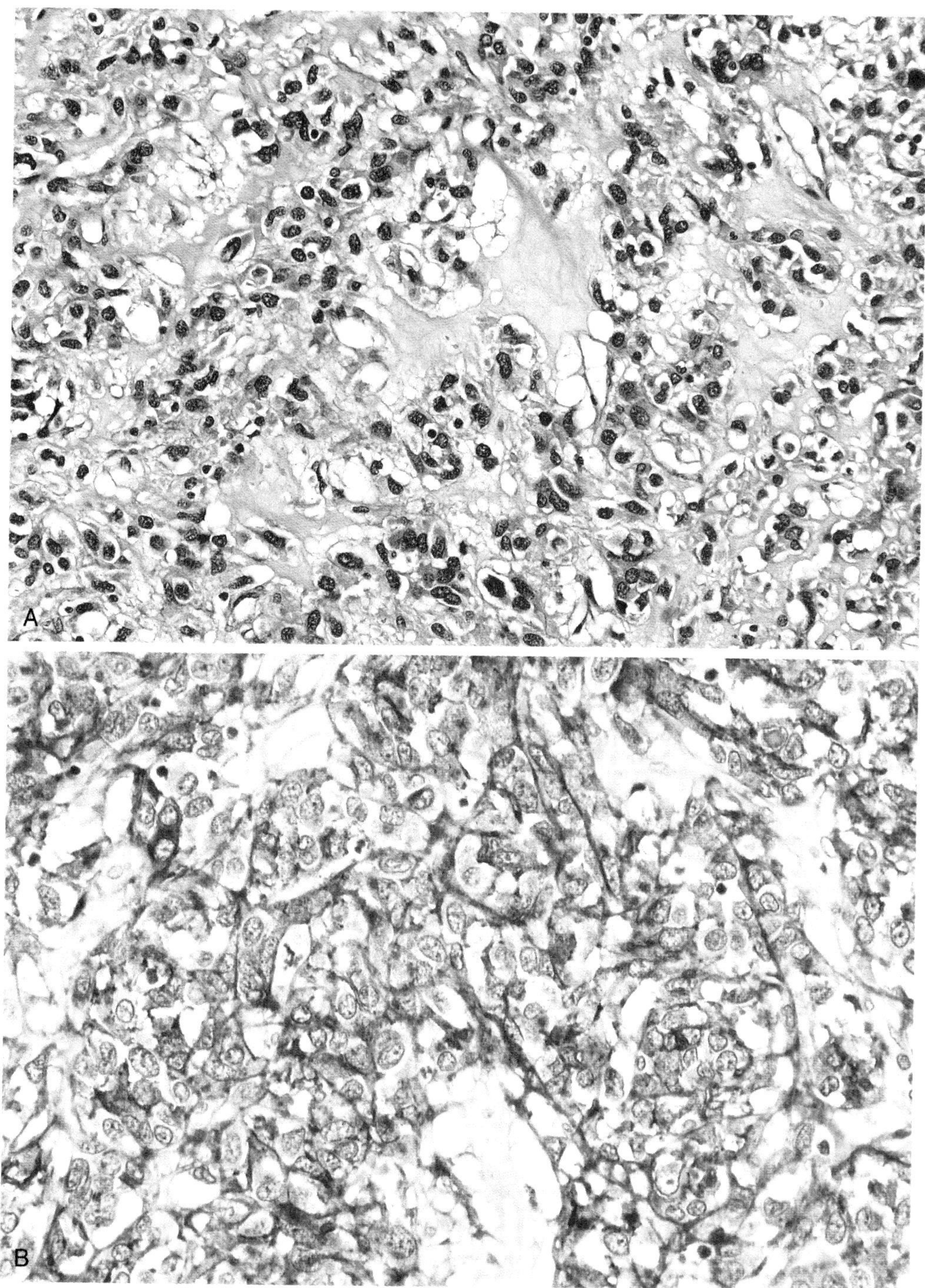


**FIGURE 8–24.** Gastrointestinal stromal tumor (**A**) with characteristic CD117 (c-*kit*) expression (**B**). Such expression distinguishes stromal tumors from leiomyosarcomas and nerve sheath tumors.

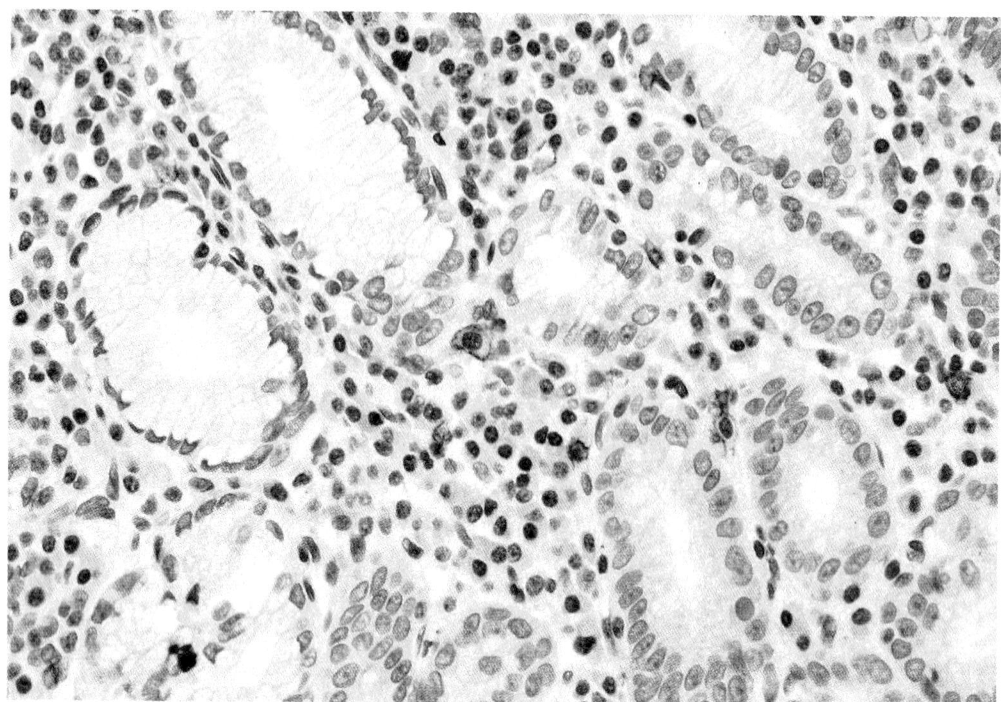

**FIGURE 8–25.** Mast cells in the lamina propria of the gut, demonstrating C117 (c-*kit*) expression. Failure to distinguish CD117 expression by mast cells infiltrating a nongastrointestinal stromal tumor from expression by tumor cells is a potential pitfall.

The most important use of antibodies to CD99 is for immunohistochemical diagnosis of Ewing's sarcoma/primitive neuroectodermal tumor (ES/PNET). Many studies have shown that well over 90% of ES/PNETs express CD99, with a characteristic membranous pattern[5,67,187,188,200,210,237] (Fig. 8–27). Despite early claims that CD99 expression was also specific for ES/PNET,[5,67,187,237] it has become increasingly obvious that this is not true. It is particularly important to recognize that a significant subset of other small, blue, round cell tumors considered in the differential diagnosis of ES/PNET may express this antigen. CD99 expression is seen in more than 90% of lymphoblastic lymphomas,[186] 20–25% of primitive rhabdomyosarcomas,[210] more than 75% of poorly differentiated synovial sarcomas,[47,75,229] approximately 50% of mesenchymal chondrosarcomas,[49,90] and in rare cases of small-cell osteosarcomas[50] and intraabdominal desmoplastic round cell tumor.[168,169] CD99 expression has never been reported in neuroblastomas[5,67,74,187,210,237] and has been seen in only a single esthesioneuroblastoma.[51,74]

Immunohistochemical analysis of CD99 expression plays a limited role in the diagnosis of pleomorphic or spindle cell soft tissue neoplasms. As noted above, many synovial sarcomas express CD99, which may be helpful in discriminating them from malignant peripheral nerve sheath tumors and fibrosarcomas.[47,75,229] Expression of CD99 may also be seen in solitary fibrous tumors, mesotheliomas, leiomyosarcomas, and malignant fibrous histiocytomas.[210,228]

## CD56 (Neural Cell Adhesion Molecule)

The 140-kDa isoform of the neural cell adhesion molecule, CD56, is an integral membrane glycoprotein that mediates calcium-independent homophilic cell–cell binding.[39,59] CD56 is expressed by many normal cells and tissues, including neurons, astrocytes and glia of the cerebral cortex and cerebellum, adrenal cortex and medulla, renal proximal tubules, follicular epithelium of the thyroid; gastric parietal cells; cardiac muscle; regenerating and fetal skeletal muscle; pancreatic islet cells, and peripheral nerve.[205] CD56 is also ubiquitously expressed on human natural killer cells and on a subset of T lymphocytes.[29,129]

As might be expected from this long list of CD56-positive normal tissues, CD56 expression is widespread among sarcomas. Soft tissue tumors that often express CD56 include synovial sarcoma, malignant peripheral nerve sheath tumor, schwannoma, rhabdomyosarcoma, leiomyosarcoma, leiomyoma, chondrosarcoma, and osteosarcoma.[80,143,151] For this reason, examination of CD56 expression is not helpful when evaluating spindle cell soft tissue tumors. CD56 expression may, however, be useful for evaluating

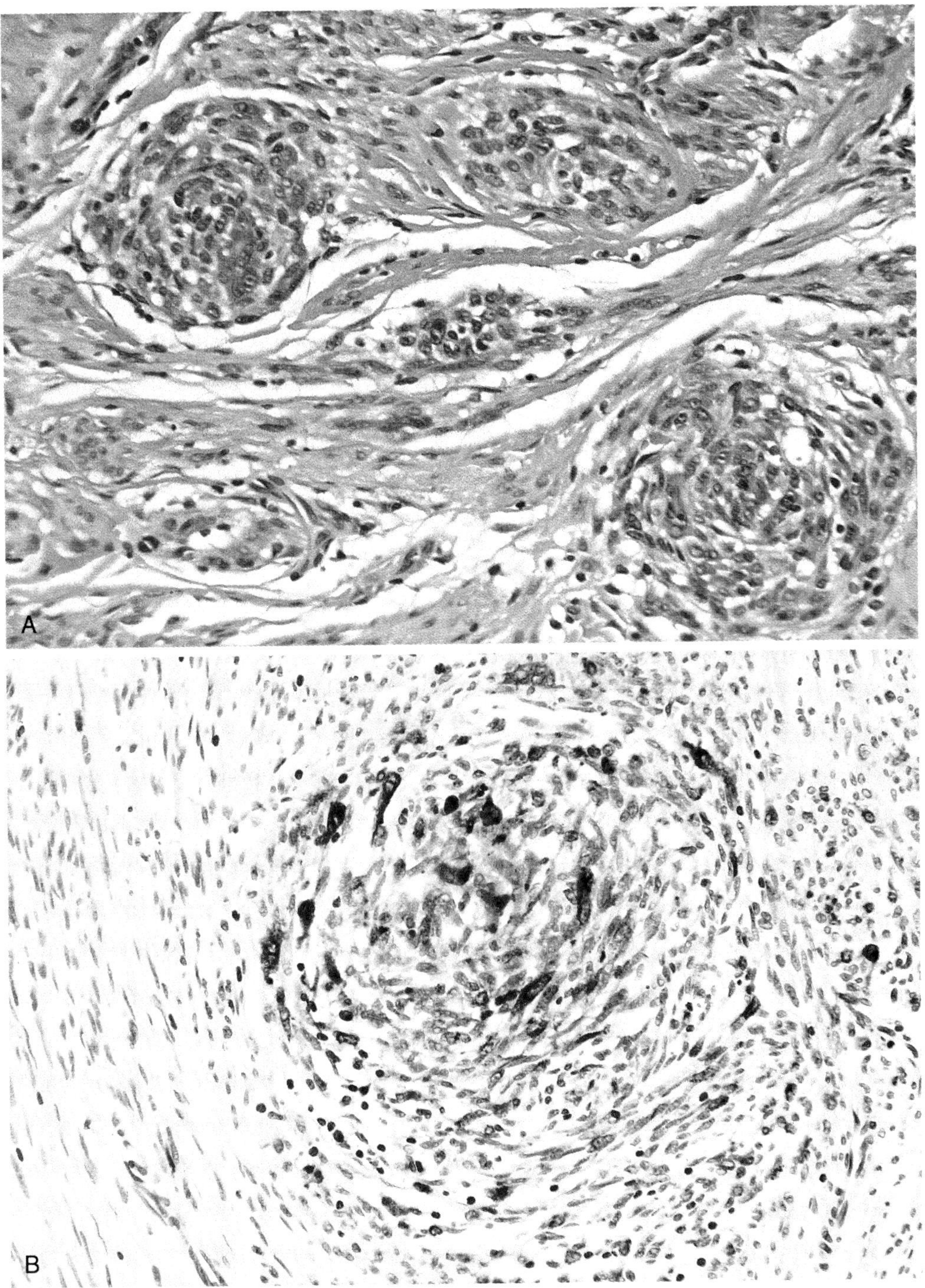


**FIGURE 8–26.** Plexiform fibrohistiocytic tumor (**A**) with strong CD68 expression in the histiocytoid nodules but not in the surrounding fibroblastic fascicles (**B**).

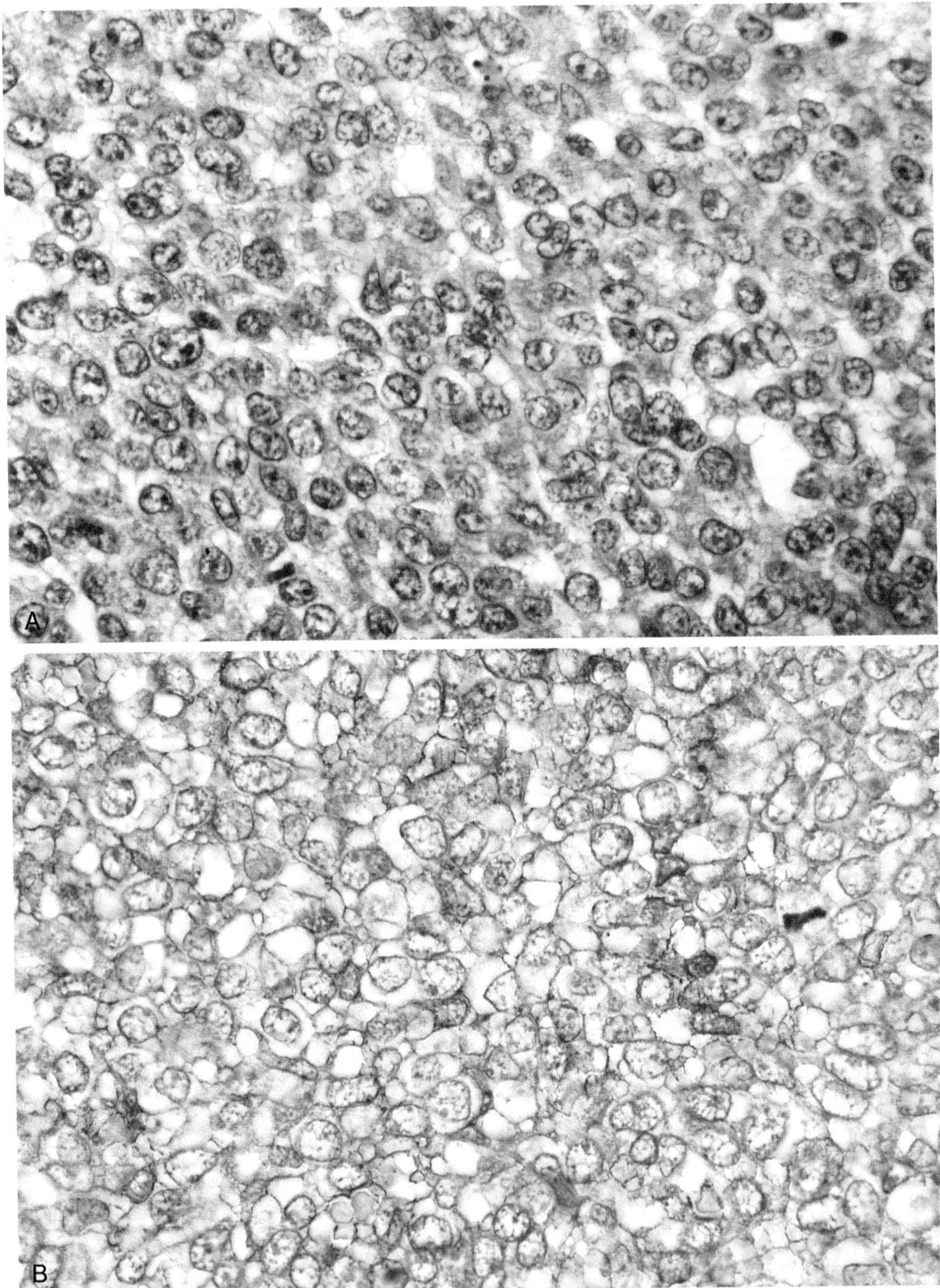


**FIGURE 8–27.** Ewing's sarcoma/primitive neuroectodermal tumor (**A**) with intense membranous expression of CD99 (*MIC2*) (**B**). Although CD99 expression is highly characteristic of Ewing's family tumors, it is not specific.

*Illustration continued on opposite page*

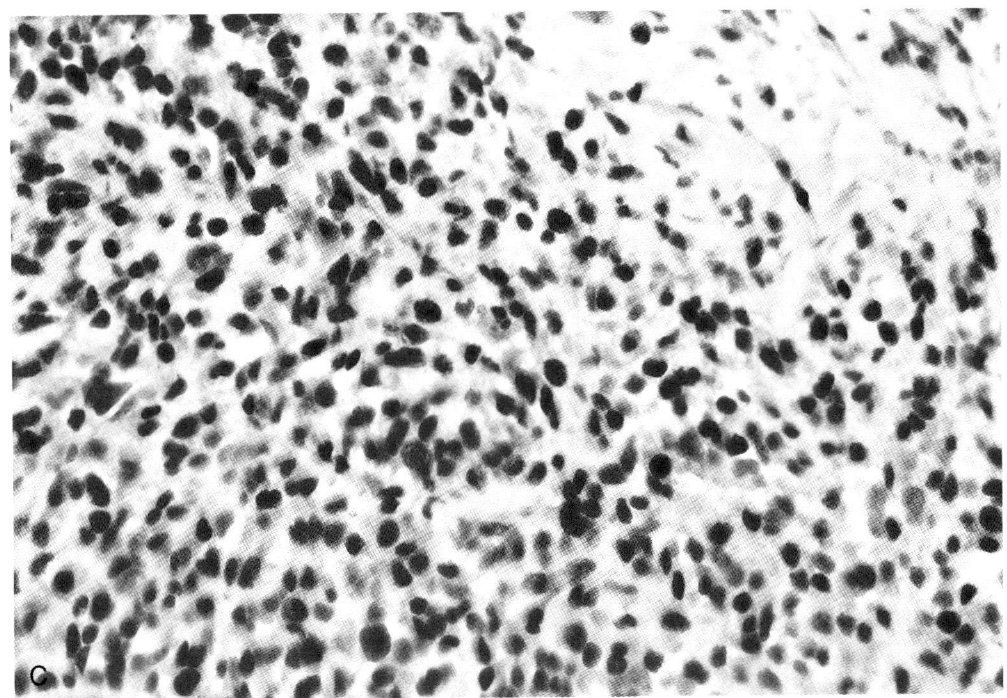


**FIGURE 8–27** *(Continued)*. Detection of nuclear expression of the carboxy-terminus of FLI-1 protein, expressed as a result of the Ewing's sarcoma-specific *EWS/FLI-1* gene fusion, is a much more specific marker of these tumors (**C**).

primitive "small, blue, round cell tumors," particularly in combination with CD99. CD56 expression is seen in only 10–25% of ES/PNETs and in rare lymphoblastic lymphomas, compared with nearly 100% of neuroblastomas, poorly differentiated synovial sarcomas, alveolar and primitive embryonal rhabdomyosarcomas, small-cell carcinomas, Wilms' tumors, and mesenchymal chondrosarcomas.[75,80,151] The absence of CD56 expression may be a clue to the diagnosis of ES/PNET in cases where results with more specific positive markers such as CD99, CD45, cytokeratin, and desmin are equivocal.

### NB-84

A recently developed monoclonal antibody raised against two neuroblastoma cell lines, NB-84 recognizes an as yet uncharacterized 57-kDa molecule.[220] NB-84 is a highly sensitive marker of neuroblastoma, being positive in more than 95% of cases, including undifferentiated and poorly differentiated subtypes.[74,150,220] It is relatively specific for neuroblastoma, although 16–25% of ES/PNETs react with NB-84, as do a small number of rhabdomyosarcomas, esthesioneuroblastomas, Wilms' tumors, desmoplastic round cell tumors, and small-cell osteosarcomas.[74,150,169,220] NB-84 antigen expression has not been examined in spindle cell soft tissue neoplasms.

### FLI-1

The ES/PNET family of tumors is characterized by a specific translocation, t(11;22)(q24;q12), in approximately 90% of cases.[43,127] This translocation results in fusion of the *EWS* gene on chromosome 22 with the *FLI-1* gene on chromosome 11. It has recently been shown that detection of the carboxy-terminus of FLI-1 protein by immunohistochemistry is a more specific, if somewhat less sensitive, marker of ES/PNET than are antibodies to CD99[72,163] (Fig. 8–27). Care should be taken with the use of the FLI-1 protein in the immunodiagnosis of round cell tumors, as it is expressed in a subset of normal lymphocytes and in nearly all lymphoblastic lymphomas.[72]

## PROGNOSTIC MARKERS

### Ki-67

A 395-kDa nuclear antigen, Ki-67 is encoded by a single gene on chromosome 10, the expression of which is confined to late $G_1$, S, M, and $G_2$ growth phases.[83] It appears to be localized to the nucleolus and may be a component of nucleolar preribosomes.[103] In formalin-fixed tissue the most widely used antibody against this antigen is MIB-1. Several studies have documented a correlation between a high Ki-67 labeling index and poor prognostic features in soft tissue sarcomas.[34,55,136,227] Most recently, significant associations have been shown between a Ki-67 labeling index of more than 20% with high grade, shortened overall survival and the development of metastatic disease.[193] In high grade sarcomas of the extremities, a recent study showed a Ki-67 labeling index of more than 20% to be an independent predictor of distant metastases and tumor mortality.[97]

### p53

The *TP53* gene product, p53, is a nuclear phosphoprotein that appears to regulate transcription by arresting cells with damaged DNA in $G_1$ phase.[68,114,128,185] Mutations of the *TP53* gene produce a mutant protein that loses its tumor-suppressing ability and has a longer half-life than wild-type p53[68]; this allows immunohistochemical detection of mutated p53. Overexpression of p53 has been examined in a variety of soft tissue sarcomas, with the incidence ranging from 9% to 41%.[28,38,85,97,116,130,222] Most studies of p53 expression in sarcomas have shown a correlation between p53 overexpression, high tumor grade, and worse outcome; however, p53 overexpression has not been shown to have prognostic significance independent of grade.[55,97,116,130,222,249]

### mdm2

A nuclear phosphoprotein whose transcription is activated by the *p53* gene, mdm2 binds the *p53* gene and removes its block on the cell cycle at the $G_1$/S checkpoint.[45,46] The mdm2 marker has also been shown to exert an inhibitory effect through binding RB protein[248] and a stimulatory effect on the E2F family of transcription factors.[140] Although overexpression of mdm2 has been previously documented in 33–37% of sarcomas, it has not yet been shown to be of prognostic significance.[38,131,167]

### *P21*$^{WAF1}$

A downstream effector of *p53*, *p21*$^{WAF1}$ is an inhibitor of the cyclin/cyclin-dependent kinase complexes.[202] Loss of normal p21$^{WAF1}$ expression has been documented in a subset of liposarcomas, including dedifferentiated, myxoid, and round cell liposarcomas, but has not yet been shown to be of prognostic significance.[45,46]

### *p16* and *p27*$^{kip}$

The p16 and p27$^{kip}$ markers are cyclin-dependent kinase inhibitors (CKIs) of the INK4 and KIP families, respectively. These CKIs have been most extensively studied in malignant peripheral nerve sheath tumors. Loss of p16 expression, secondary to homozygous deletion of CDKN2A/*p16*, has been shown to be present in malignant peripheral nerve sheath tumors but not neurofibromas from patients with neurofibromatosis 1. Lose of p27$^{kip}$ constitutive expression has been implicated in the malignant transformation of neurofibromas.[123]

## APPLICATION OF IMMUNOHISTOCHEMISTRY TO SARCOMA DIAGNOSIS: CLINICAL SCENARIOS

In general, it is advisable to have an initial panel of antibodies to analyze a sarcoma that is of uncertain differentiation histologically, including at least a representative of each of the antibody "groups" listed in Table 8–5. Of course, depending on the histologic setting of the tumor, it may or may not be necessary to include a member of each of the four groups.

In addition to the antibodies listed in the table, we sometimes find it useful to include antibodies to the basement membrane related protein, type IV collagen, in initial investigations of undefined soft tissue tumors. Although not specific for a cell or tumor type, the presence and even pattern of expression of type IV collagen can be helpful in identifying specific soft tissue tumor subtypes, such as vascular tumors or tumors of glomus cells.[134]

Several common histologic scenarios of soft tissue tumors, in which immunohistochemistry can provide valuable clues to the correct diagnosis, are described below. These histologic settings include "the undifferentiated round cell tumor", "the monomorphic spindle cell tumor" and "the poorly differentiated epithelioid tumor".

A basic principle in diagnostic immunohistochemistry that is illustrated in each of the four scenarios is the utilization of panels of antibodies, rather than single antibodies directed against markers of the suspected "correct" diagnosis. In general, such a panel should include not only antibodies that one would expect to be positive in a given tumor, but also antibodies that would be expected to be negative. This

**TABLE 8–5 BASIC ANTIGEN GROUPS FOR SARCOMA IMMUNODIAGNOSIS**

| Tumor Group | Markers |
|---|---|
| Synovial sarcoma, epithelioid sarcoma | Cytokeratin |
| Nerve sheath group | CD57, S-100, NGF receptor |
| Muscle group | Desmin, muscle actins, myogenic regulatory proteins |
| Endothelial group | vWF, UEA, CD34, CD31 |

approach is essential for several reasons. First, many, if not most, antigens are expressed by more than one type of tumor. Second, for technical reasons, antibodies may show false negative, and occasionally, false positive results. Lastly, malignant cells may show unexpected or anomalous expression of antigens, and this may be very confusing if not interpreted within the context of other results.

## The Undifferentiated Round Cell Tumor

The differential diagnosis of this case includes both sarcomas and non-sarcomas. As with all of our other diagnostic scenarios, the first task is to exclude a non-sarcoma. Non-sarcomatous neoplasms that might be legitimately included in this differential diagnosis include lymphoma, melanoma, and in an older patient, small cell carcinoma. Sarcomas that should be included in the differential diagnosis include primitive neuroectodermal tumor/extraosseous Ewing's sarcoma (PNET), rhabdomyosarcoma (RMS), poorly differentiated synovial sarcoma (PDSS), and desmoplastic round cell tumor (DRCT). Table 8–6 presents a screening panel of antibodies and the expected results for these tumors. The results of this panel dictate what additional studies are needed to confirm a specific diagnosis.

- *Small-cell carcinoma (poorly differentiated neuroendocrine carcinoma):* Confirm with antibodies to chromogranin A or synaptophysin.
- *Melanoma:* Confirm with antibodies to melanosome-specific proteins (HMB-45, Melan-A, tyrosinase, micropthalmia transcription factor). As noted above, a small number of melanomas may be S-100 protein-negative, and occasional melanomas express cytokeratin or desmin.
- *Lymphoma:* Lymphoblastic lymphoma in children may be CD45-negative and CD99-positive, which can result in a misdiagnosis as PNET. If the clinical or histologic features are suggestive of lymphoma, immunohistochemistry for terminal deoxyribonucleotide transferase (TDT) may be helpful. In adults and children, anaplastic large-cell lymphomas (which have a small-cell variant) may also be CD45-negative. In this setting, antibodies to CD30 may be useful.
- *Primitive neuroectodermal tumor:* As noted above, PNETs are unique among small blue round-cell tumors in that they do not usually express CD56. This negative finding may be useful in cases where CD99 is equivocal, or where there is anomalous expression of cytokeratin or desmin. Demonstration of FLI-1 protein expression may also be helpful.
- *Rhabdomyosarcoma:* Confirm with myogenin or MyoD1.
- *Poorly differentiated synovial sarcoma:* Cytokeratin expression is patchy or absent in some poorly differentiated synovial sarcomas. The addition of antibodies to EMA and high-molecular-weight cytokeratins may allow detection of scattered positive cells. Antibodies to type IV collagen also sometimes reveal nested growth, or "occult" glandular differentiation.
- *Desmoplastic round cell tumor:* Confirm with antibodies to neuron-specific enolase and WT-1.

## Monomorphic Spindle Cell Tumors

The differential diagnosis of monomorphic spindle cell tumors often includes such entities as fibrosarcoma, monophasic fibrous synovial sarcoma, malignant peripheral nerve sheath tumor, and malignant solitary fibrous tumor. Table 8–7 presents a screening immunohistochemical panel and the expected result for each tumor.

The following comments should also be borne in mind when immunostaining monomorphic spindle cell tumors.

- *Synovial sarcoma:* As noted above, cytokeratin and EMA expression may be focal in synovial sarcomas. Synovial sarcomas have never been reported to express CD34.
- *Malignant peripheral nerve sheath tumor:* S-100 protein expression is often weak and focal. EMA expression may be seen in tumors with perineurial differentiation. Confirm with CD57 and p75NTR.
- *Fibrosarcoma:* It may show limited actin expression (myofibrosarcoma).

**TABLE 8–6** SCREENING PANEL FOR UNDIFFERENTIATED ROUND CELL TUMOR

| Antibody To | Small-cell Carcinoma | Melanoma | Lymphoma | PNET | RMS | PDSS | DRCT |
|---|---|---|---|---|---|---|---|
| Pan-cytokeratin | Positive | Negative | Negative | Variable | Negative | Positive | Positive |
| S-100 protein | Negative | Positive | Negative | Negative | Variable | Variable | Negative |
| CD45 | Negative | Negative | Positive | Negative | Negative | Negative | Negative |
| Desmin | Negative | Negative | Negative | Rare | Positive | Variable | Positive |
| CD99 | Negative | Negative | Variable | Positive | Variable | Positive | Rare |

PNET, primitive neuroectodermal tumor; RMS, rhabdomyosarcoma; DRCT, dismoplastic round cell tumor; PDSS, poorly differentiated synovial sarcoma.

**TABLE 8-7 SCREENING PANEL FOR MONOMORPHIC SPINDLE CELL TUMORS**

| Antibody To | Synovial Sarcoma | MPNST | Fibrosarcoma | Leiomyosarcoma |
|---|---|---|---|---|
| Pan-cytokeratin | Positive | Negative | Negative | Negative |
| S-100 protein | Variable | Positive | Negative | Negative |
| CD34 | Negative | Variable | Negative | Variable |
| Desmin | Negative | Negative | Negative | Positive |
| Type IV collagen | Positive | Positive | Negative | Positive |

MPNST, malignant peripheral nerve sheath tumor.

### Poorly Differentiated Epithelioid Tumor

The differential diagnosis of poorly differentiated epithelioid tumors includes carcinoma, melanoma, lymphoma (including anaplastic large-cell lymphoma), and epithelioid soft tissue tumors such as epithelioid sarcoma and angiosarcoma. The recommended panel of antibodies and their expected reactivities are presented in Table 8–8. This initial screening panel can make a specific diagnosis of melanoma, lymphoma, or anaplastic large-cell lymphoma, but generally it is not able to discriminate carcinoma from epithelioid sarcoma or epithelioid angiosarcoma. These tumors can be reliably distinguished with the additional panel of antibodies listed in Table 8–9.

### "Orphan Sarcomas"

It should be noted, the above notwithstanding, that there remain "orphan sarcomas" without specific markers. This group include tumors for which there is no known normal cell counterpart (e.g., malignant fibrous histiocytoma) and those for which there is a known cell counterpart (e.g., liposarcoma, osteogenic sarcoma, chondrosarcoma) but for which there are no reliable, useful specific markers at present. Whereas markers for osteosarcoma have been developed, such as osteocalcin and osteonectin, they have not proved to be more sensitive markers than is the histologic identification of tumor osteoid.[63]

## CONCLUSIONS

Immunohistochemistry is a young, evolving science, with new techniques and new markers continually coming to the fore. The introduction of new techniques, such as heat-induced epitope retrieval ("antigen retrieval"), and new detection systems, such as tyramine-based amplification techniques, can result in revisions of previously recognized sensitivity and specificities of particular markers.[194,203,204] The history of immunohistochemistry also suggests that the introduction of new antibody-based markers can dramatically alter immunohistochemical approaches to the identification of specific tumor types.

It is anticipated that a new class of markers will have a significant impact in the field of soft tissue tumors. This class includes markers of lineage-specific nuclear regulatory proteins, such as myogenin and MyoD1 for skeletal muscle. Basic research into mesen-

**TABLE 8-8 SCREENING PANEL FOR EPITHELIOID TUMORS IN SOFT TISSUE**

| Antibody To | Carcinoma | Melanoma | B or T Cell Lymphoma | Anaplastic Large Cell (Ki-1) Lymphoma | Epithelioid Sarcoma | Epithelioid Angiosarcoma |
|---|---|---|---|---|---|---|
| Cytokeratin | Positive | Negative | Negative | Negative | Positive | Variable |
| S-100 protein | Variable | Positive | Negative | Negative | Negative | Negative |
| CD45 | Negative | Negative | Positive | Variable | Negative | Negative |
| CD30 | Negative | Negative | Negative | Positive | Negative | Negative |
| Vimentin | Variable | Positive | Variable | Variable | Positive | Positive |

**TABLE 8-9 DISCRIMINATION OF CARCINOMA, EPITHELIOID SARCOMA, AND EPITHELIOID ANGIOSARCOMA**

| Antibody To | Carcinoma | Epithelioid Sarcoma | Epithelioid Angiosarcoma |
|---|---|---|---|
| High-molecular-weight cytokeratin | Variable | Variable | Negative |
| CD34 | Negative | Positive | Positive |
| CD31 | Negative | Negative | Positive |

chymal development has already identified nuclear regulatory proteins expressed during osteoblastic differentiation (e.g., CBFA-1[57,178]) and chondroblastic differentiation (e.g., SOX-9[16,133]), and it is anticipated that monoclonal antibodies to these proteins will become available. The reader is cautioned to integrate the recommendations found in this chapter with new information appearing in the literature.

## REFERENCES


1. Abramovici LC, Steiner GC, Bonar F. Myxoid chondrosarcoma of soft tissue and bone: a retrospective study of 11 cases. Hum Pathol 26:1215, 1995.
2. Akhtar M, Tulbah A, Kardar AH, Ali MA. Sarcomatoid renal cell carcinoma: the chromophobe connection. Am J Surg Pathol 21:1188, 1997.
3. Alles JU, Bosslet K. Immunocytochemistry of angiosarcomas: a study of 19 cases with special emphasis on the applicability of endothelial cell specific markers to routinely prepared tissues. Am J Clin Pathol 89:463, 1988.
4. Altmannsberger M, Weber K, Droste R, Osborn M. Desmin is a specific marker for rhabdomyosarcomas of human and rat origin. Am J Pathol 118:85, 1985.
5. Ambros IM, Ambros PF, Strehl S, et al. MIC2 is a specific marker for Ewing's sarcoma and peripheral primitive neuroectodermal tumors: evidence for a common histogenesis of Ewing's sarcoma and peripheral primitive neuroectodermal tumors from MIC2 expression and specific chromosome aberration. Cancer 67:1886, 1991.
6. Andriko JW, Kaldjian EP, Tsokos M, et al. Reticulum cell neoplasms of lymph nodes: a clinicopathologic study of 11 cases with recognition of a new subtype derived from fibroblastic reticular cells. Am J Surg Pathol 22:1048, 1998.
7. Arber DA, Weiss LM. CD57: a review. Appl Immunohistochem 3:137, 1995.
8. Azumi N, Battifora H. The distribution of vimentin and keratin in epithelial and nonepithelial neoplasms: a comprehensive immunohistochemical study on formalin- and alcohol-fixed tumors. Am J Clin Pathol 88:286, 1987.
9. Azumi N, Ben-Ezra J, Battifora H. Immunophenotypic diagnosis of leiomyosarcomas and rhabdomyosarcomas with monoclonal antibodies to muscle-specific actin and desmin in formalin-fixed tissue. Mod Pathol 1:469, 1988.
10. Bacchi CE, Bonetti F, Pea M, et al. HMB-45: a review. Appl Immunohistochem 4:73, 1996.
11. Bacchi CE, Zarbo RJ, Jiang JJ, Gown AM. Do glioma cells express cytokeratin? Appl Immunohistochem 3:45, 1995.
12. Battifora H. Misuse of the term "expression"[letter]. Am J Clin Pathol 92:708, 1989.
13. Beckstead JH, Wood GS, Fletcher V. Evidence for the origin of Kaposi's sarcoma from lymphatic endothelium. Am J Pathol 119:294, 1985.
14. Ben-Izhak O, Auslander L, Rabinson S, et al. Epithelioid angiosarcoma of the adrenal gland with cytokeratin expression: report of a case with accompanying mesenteric fibromatosis. Cancer 69:1808, 1992.
15. Ben-Izhak O, Stark P, Levy R, et al. Epithelial markers in malignant melanoma: a study of primary lesions and their metastases. Am J Dermatopathol 16:241, 1994.
16. Bi W, Deng JM, Zhang Z, et al. Sox9 is required for cartilage formation. Nat Genet 22:85, 1999.
17. Bohling T, Paetau A, Ekblom P, Haltia M. Distribution of endothelial and basement membrane markers in angiogenic tumors of the nervous system. Acta Neuropathol (Berl) 62:67, 1983.
18. Bonetti F, Pea M, Martignoni G, et al. Clear cell ("sugar") tumor of the lung is a lesion strictly related to angiomyolipoma—the concept of a family of lesions characterized by the presence of the perivascular epithelioid cells (PEC). Pathology 26:230, 1994.
19. Bonetti F, Pea M, Martignoni G, et al. False-positive immunostaining of normal epithelia and carcinomas with ascites fluid preparations of antimelanoma monoclonal antibody HMB45. Am J Clin Pathol 95:454, 1991.
20. Breiteneder-Geleff S, Matsul K, Soleiman A, et al. Podoplanin, novel 43-kd membrane protein of glomerular epithelial cells, is down-regulated in puromycin nephrosis. Am J Pathol 151:1141, 1997.
21. Brooks JJ. Immunohistochemistry of soft tissue tumors: myoglobin as a tumor marker for rhabdomyosarcoma. Cancer 50:1757, 1982.
22. Brown DC, Theaker JM, Banks PM, et al. Cytokeratin expression in smooth muscle and smooth muscle tumours. Histopathology 11:477, 1987.
23. Brown RW, Campagna LB, Dunn JK, Cagle PT. Immunohistochemical identification of tumor markers in metastatic adenocarcinoma: a diagnostic adjunct in the determination of primary site. Am J Clin Pathol 107:12, 1997.
24. Burgdorf WH, Mukal K, Rosai J. Immunohistochemical identification of factor VIII-related antigen in endothelial cells of cutaneous lesions of alleged vascular nature. Am J Clin Pathol 75:167, 1981.
25. Busam KJ, Chen YT, Old LJ, et al. Expression of melan-A (MART1) in benign melanocytic nevi and primary cutaneous malignant melanoma. Am J Surg Pathol 22:976, 1998.
26. Busam KJ, Iversen K, Coplan KA, et al. Immunoreactivity for A103, an antibody to melan-A (Mart-1), in adrenocortical and other steroid tumors. Am J Surg Pathol 22:57, 1998.
27. Casadei GP, Scheithauer BW, Hirose T, et al. Cellular schwannoma: a clinicopathologic, DNA flow cytometric, and proliferation marker study of 70 patients. Cancer 75:1109, 1995.
28. Castresana JS, Rubio MP, Gomez L, et al. Detection of TP53 gene mutations in human sarcomas. Eur J Cancer 5:735, 1995.
29. Chan JK, Sin VC, Wong KF, et al. Nonnasal lymphoma expressing the natural killer cell marker CD56: a clinicopathologic study of 49 cases of an uncommon aggressive neoplasm. Blood 89:4501, 1997.
30. Chang K, Pai LH, Pass H, et al. Monoclonal antibody K1 reacts with epithelial mesothelioma but not with lung adenocarcinoma. Am J Surg Pathol 16:259, 1992.
31. Chang K, Pastan I, Willingham MC. Isolation and characterization of a monoclonal antibody, K1, reactive with ovarian cancers and normal mesothelium. Int J Cancer 50:373, 1992.
32. Ching CK, Black R, Helliwell T, et al. Use of lectin histochemistry in pancreatic cancer. J Clin Pathol 41:324, 1988.
33. Cho J, Gong G, Choe G, et al. Extrafollicular reticulum cells in pathologic lymph nodes. J Korean Med Sci 9:9, 1994.
34. Choong PF, Akerman M, Willen H, et al. Prognostic value of Ki-67 expression in 182 soft tissue sarcomas: proliferation—a marker of metastasis? APMIS 102:915, 1994.
35. Clover J, Oates J, Edwards C. Anti-cytokeratin 5/6: a positive marker for epithelioid mesothelioma. Histopathology 31:140, 1997.
36. Coindre JM, de Mascarel A, Trojani M, et al. Immunohistochemical study of rhabdomyosarcoma: unexpected staining with S100 protein and cytokeratin. J Pathol 155:127, 1988.
37. Connell ND, Rheinwald JG. Regulation of the cytoskeleton in mesothelial cells: reversible loss of keratin and increase in vimentin during rapid growth in culture. Cell 34:245, 1983.
38. Cordon-Cardo C, Latres E, Drobnjak M, et al. Molecular ab-

normalities of mdm2 and p53 genes in adult soft tissue sarcomas. Cancer Res 54:794, 1994.
39. Cunningham BA, Hemperly JJ, Murray BA, et al. Neural cell adhesion molecule: structure, immunoglobulin-like domains, cell surface modulation, and alternative RNA splicing. Science 236:799, 1987.
40. Dahl D. The vimentin-GFA protein transition in rat neuroglia cytoskeleton occurs at the time of myelination. J Neurosci Res 6:741, 1981.
41. Damjanov I. Antibodies to intermediate filaments and histogenesis. Lab Invest 47:215,1982.
42. Dardick I, Schatz JE, Colgan TJ. Osteogenic sarcoma with epithelial differentiation. Ultrastruct Pathol 16:463, 1992.
43. De Alava E, Kawai A, Healey JH, et al. EWS-FLI1 fusion transcript structure is an independent determinant of prognosis in Ewing's sarcoma. J Clin Oncol 16:1248, 1998.
44. De Young BR, Frierson HF Jr, Ly MN, et al. CD31 immunoreactivity in carcinomas and mesotheliomas. Am J Clin Pathol 110:374, 1998.
45. Dei Tos AP, Doglioni C, Piccinin S, et al. Molecular abnormalities of the p53 pathway in dedifferentiated liposarcoma. J Pathol 181:8, 1997.
46. Dei Tos AP, Piccinin S, Doglioni C, et al. Molecular aberrations of the G1-S checkpoint in myxoid and round cell liposarcoma. Am J Pathol 151:1531, 1997.
47. Dei Tos AP, Wadden C, Calonje E, et al. Immunohistochemical demonstration of glycoprotein p30/32(MIC2) (CD99) in synovial sarcoma: a potential cause of diagnostic confusion. Appl Immunohistochem 3:168, 1995.
48. Denk H, Krepler R, Artileb U, et al. Proteins of intermediate filaments: an immunohistochemical and biochemical approach to the classification of soft tissue tumors. Am J Pathol 110:193, 1983.
49. Devaney K, Abbondanzo SL, Shekitka KM, et al. MIC2 detection in tumors of bone and adjacent soft tissues. Clin Orthop 310:176, 1995.
50. Devaney K, Vinh TN, Sweet DE. Small cell osteosarcoma of bone: an immunohistochemical study with differential diagnostic considerations. Hum Pathol 24:1211, 1993.
51. Devaney K, Wenig BM, Abbondanzo SL. Olfactory neuroblastoma and other round cell lesions of the sinonasal region. Mod Pathol 9:658, 1996.
52. Dias P, Parham DM, Shapiro DN, et al. Monoclonal antibodies to the myogenic regulatory protein MyoD1: epitope mapping and diagnostic utility. Cancer Res 52:6431, 1992.
53. Dias P, Parham DM, Shapiro DN, et al. Myogenic regulatory protein (MyoD1) expression in childhood solid tumors: diagnostic utility in rhabdomyosarcoma. Am J Pathol 137: 1283,1990.
54. Doglioni C, Tos AP, Laurino L, et al. Calretinin: a novel immunocytochemical marker for mesothelioma. Am J Surg Pathol 20:1037, 1996.
55. Drobnjak M, Latres E, Pollack D, et al. Prognostic implications of p53 nuclear overexpression and high proliferation index of Ki-67 in adult soft-tissue sarcomas. J Natl Cancer Inst 86:549, 1994.
56. Droz D, Rousseau-Merck MF, Jaubert F, et al. Cell differentiation in Wilms' tumor (nephroblastoma): an immunohistochemical study. Hum Pathol 21:536, 1990.
57. Ducy P, Zhang R, Geoffroy V, et al. Osf2/Cbfa1: a transcriptional activator of osteoblast differentiation. Cell 89:747, 1997.
58. Eckert F, de Viragh PA, Schmid U. Coexpression of cytokeratin and vimentin intermediate filaments in benign and malignant sweat gland tumors. J Cutan Pathol 21:140, 1994.
59. Edelman GM. Cell adhesion molecules in the regulation of animal form and tissue pattern. Annu Rev Cell Biol 2:81, 1986.
60. Elias JM. Immunohistopathology: A Practical Approach to Diagnosis. ASCP Press, American Society of Clinical Pathologists, Chicago, 1990.
61. Erlandson RA. The enigmatic perineurial cell and its participation in tumors and in tumorlike entities. Ultrastruct Pathol 15: 335, 1991.
62. Eusebi V, Bondi A, Rosai J. Immunohistochemical localization of myoglobin in nonmuscular cells. Am J Surg Pathol 8:51, 1984.
63. Fanburg-Smith JC, Bratthauer GL, Miettinen M. Osteocalcin and osteonectin immunoreactivity in extraskeletal osteosarcoma: a study of 28 cases. Hum Pathol 30:32, 1999.
64. Fanburg-Smith JC, Hengge M, Hengge UR, et al. Extrarenal rhabdoid tumors of soft tissue: a clinicopathologic and immunohistochemical study of 18 cases. Ann Diagn Pathol 2:351, 1998.
65. Fanburg-Smith JC, Miettinen M. Angiomatoid "malignant" fibrous histiocytoma: a clinicopathologic study of 158 cases and further exploration of the myoid phenotype. Hum Pathol 30: 1336, 1999.
66. Fellinger EJ, Garin-Chesa P, Su SL, et al. Biochemical and genetic characterization of the HBA71 Ewing's sarcoma cell surface antigen. Cancer Res 51:336, 1991.
67. Fellinger EJ, Garin-Chesa P, Triche TJ, et al. Immunohistochemical analysis of Ewing's sarcoma cell surface antigen p30/32MIC2. Am J Pathol 139:317, 1991.
68. Finley CA, Hinds PW, Tan TH, et al. Activating mutations for transformation by p53 produce a gene product that forms an hsc70-p53 complex with an altered half-life. Mol Cell Biol 8: 531, 1988.
69. Fisher C, Carter RL, Ramachandra S, Thomas DM. Peripheral nerve sheath differentiation in malignant soft tissue tumours: an ultrastructural and immunohistochemical study. Histopathology 20:115, 1992.
70. Fisher C, Schofield JB. S-100 protein positive synovial sarcoma. Histopathology 19:375, 1991.
71. Fletcher CD. Angiomatoid "malignant fibrous histiocytoma": an immunohistochemical study indicative of myoid differentiation. Hum Pathol 22:563, 1991.
72. Folpe A, Hill C, Parham D, et al. Immunohistochemical detection of FLI-1 protein expression: a study of 132 round cell tumors, with emphasis on CD99-positive mimics of Ewing's sarcoma/primitive neuroectodermal tumors. Am J Surg Pathol (in press).
73. Folpe AL, Patterson K, Gown AM. Antibodies to desmin identify the blastemal component of nephroblastoma. Mod Pathol 10:895, 1997.
74. Folpe AL, Patterson K, Gown AM. Antineuroblastoma antibody NB-84 also identifies a significant subset of other small blue round cell tumors. Appl Immunohistochem 5:239, 1997.
75. Folpe AL, Schmidt RA, Chapman D, Gown AM. Poorly differentiated synovial sarcoma: immunohistochemical distinction from primitive neuroectodermal tumors and high-grade malignant peripheral nerve sheath tumors. Am J Surg Pathol 22:673, 1998.
76. Folpe AL, Veikkola T, Valtola R, Weiss SW. Vascular endothelial growth factor receptor-3 (VEGFR-3): a marker of vascular tumors with presumed lymphatic differentiation, including Kaposi's sarcoma, kaposiform and Dabska-type hemangioendotheliomas, and a subset of angiosarcomas. Mod Pathol 13: 180, 2000.
77. Folpe AL, Weiss SW, Fletcher CDM, Gown AM. Tenosynovial giant cell tumors: evidence for a desmin-positive dendritic cell subpopulation. Mod Pathol 11:939, 1998.
78. Fortwengler HP Jr, Jones D, Espinosa E, Tamburro CH. Evidence for endothelial cell origin of vinyl chloride-induced hepatic angiosarcoma. Gastroenterology 80:1415, 1981.
79. Franquemont DW, Frierson HF Jr, Mills SE. An immunohisto-

chemical study of normal endometrial stroma and endometrial stromal neoplasms: evidence for smooth muscle differentiation. Am J Surg Pathol 15:861, 1991.

80. Garin-Chesa P, Fellinger EJ, Huvos AG, et al. Immunohistochemical analysis of neural cell adhesion molecules: differential expression in small round cell tumors of childhood and adolescence. Am J Pathol 139:275, 1991.
81. Gelin C, Aubrit F, Phalipon A, et al. The E2 antigen, a 32 kd glycoprotein involved in T-cell adhesion processes, is the MIC2 gene product. EMBO J 8:3253, 1989.
82. Gerald WL, Miller HK, Battifora H, et al. Intra-abdominal desmoplastic small round-cell tumor: report of 19 cases of a distinctive type of high-grade polyphenotypic malignancy affecting young individuals. Am J Surg Pathol 15:499, 1991.
83. Gerdes J, Li L, Schlueter C, et al. Immunobiochemical and molecular biologic characterization of the cell proliferation-associated nuclear antigen that is defined by monoclonal antibody Ki-67. Am J Pathol 138:867, 1991.
84. Gloghini A, Rizzo A, Zanette I, et al. KP1/CD68 expression in malignant neoplasms including lymphomas, sarcomas, and carcinomas. Am J Clin Pathol 103:425, 1995.
85. Golouh R, Bracko M, Novak J. Predictive value of proliferation-related markers, p53, and DNA ploidy for survival in patients with soft tissue spindle-cell sarcomas. Mod Pathol 9: 919, 1996.
86. Goodfellow PN, Pym B, Pritchard C, et al. MIC2: a human pseudoautosomal gene. Philos Trans R Soc Lond B Biol Sci 322:145, 1988.
87. Gown AM, Boyd HC, Chang Y, et al. Smooth muscle cells can express cytokeratins of "simple" epithelium: immunocytochemical and biochemical studies in vitro and in vivo. Am J Pathol 132:223, 1988.
88. Gown AM, Vogel AM. Monoclonal antibodies to human intermediate filament proteins. III. Analysis of tumors. Am J Clin Pathol 84:413, 1985.
89. Gown AM, Vogel AM, Hoak D, et al. Monoclonal antibodies specific for melanocytic tumors distinguish subpopulations of melanocytes. Am J Pathol 123:195, 1986.
90. Granter SR, Renshaw AA, Fletcher CD, et al. CD99 reactivity in mesenchymal chondrosarcoma. Hum Pathol 27:1273, 1996.
91. Gray MH, Rosenberg AE, Dickersin GR, Bhan AK. Cytokeratin expression in epithelioid vascular neoplasms. Hum Pathol 21: 212, 1990.
92. Grieshammer T, Zimmer C, Vogeley KT. Immunohistochemistry of primitive neuroectodermal tumors in infants with special emphasis on cytokeratin expression. Acta Neuropathol (Berl) 82:494, 1991.
93. Guillou L, Wadden C, Kraus MD, et al. S-100 protein reactivity in synovial sarcomas: a potentially frequent diagnostic pitfall; immunohistochemical analysis of 100 cases. Appl Immunohistochem 4:167, 1996.
94. Hamilton G, Mallinger R, Hofbauer S, Havel M. The monoclonal HBA-71 antibody modulates proliferation of thymocytes and Ewing's sarcoma cells by interfering with the action of insulin-like growth factor I. Thymus 18:33, 1991.
95. Hasegawa T, Seki K, Yang P, et al. Differentiation and proliferative activity in benign and malignant cartilage tumors of bone. Hum Pathol 26:838, 1995.
96. Hashimoto H, Muller H, Falk S, Stutte HJ. Histogenesis of Kaposi's sarcoma associated with AIDS: a histologic, immunohistochemical and enzyme histochemical study. Pathol Res Pract 182:658, 1987.
97. Heslin MJ, Cordon-Cardo C, Lewis JJ, et al. Ki-67 detected by MIB-1 predicts distant metastasis and tumor mortality in primary, high grade extremity soft tissue sarcoma. Cancer 83:490, 1998.
98. Heyderman E, Steele K, Ormerod MG. A new antigen on the epithelial membrane: its immunoperoxidase localization in normal and neoplastic tissue. J Clin Pathol 32:35, 1979.
99. Hirose T, Hasegawa T, Kudo E, et al. Malignant peripheral nerve sheath tumors: an immunohistochemical study in relation to ultrastructural features. Hum Pathol 23:865, 1992.
100. Hirose T, Scheithauer BW, Sano T. Perineurial malignant peripheral nerve sheath tumor (MPNST): a clinicopathologic, immunohistochemical, and ultrastructural study of seven cases. Am J Surg Pathol 22:1368, 1998.
101. Hoefler H, Kerl H, Rauch HJ, Denk H. New immunocytochemical observations with diagnostic significance in cutaneous neuroendocrine carcinoma. Am J Dermatopathol 6:525, 1984.
102. Hurlimann J. Desmin and neural marker expression in mesothelial cells and mesotheliomas. Hum Pathol 25:753, 1994.
103. Isola J, Helin H, Kallioniemi OP. Immunoelectron-microscopic localization of a proliferation-associated antigen Ki-67 in MCF-7 cells. Histochem J 22:498, 1990.
104. Iwasaki H, Isayama T, Ichiki T, Kikuchi M. Intermediate filaments of myofibroblasts: immunochemical and immunocytochemical analyses. Pathol Res Pract 182:248, 1987.
105. Jahn L, Fouquet B, Rohe K, Franke WW. Cytokeratins in certain endothelial and smooth muscle cells of two taxonomically distant vertebrate species, Xenopus laevis and man. Differentiation 36:234, 1987.
106. Johnson MD, Glick AD, Davis BW. Immunohistochemical evaluation of Leu-7, myelin basic-protein, S100-protein, glial-fibrillary acidic-protein, and LN3 immunoreactivity in nerve sheath tumors and sarcomas. Arch Pathol Lab Med 112:155, 1988.
107. Jong AS, van Vark M, Albus-Lutter CE, et al. Myosin and myoglobin as tumor markers in the diagnosis of rhabdomyosarcoma: a comparative study. Am J Surg Pathol 8:521, 1984.
108. Judkins AR, Montone KT, LiVoisi VA, van de Rijn M. Sensitivity and specificity of antibodies on necrotic tumor tissue. Am J Clin Pathol 110:641, 1998.
109. Jussila L, Vaitola R, Partanen TA, et al. Lymphatic endothelium and Kaposi's sarcoma spindle cells detected by antibodies against the vascular endothelial growth factor receptor-3. Cancer Res 58:1599, 1998.
110. Kaddu S, Beham A, Cerroni L, et al. Cutaneous leiomyosarcoma. Am J Surg Pathol 21:979, 1997.
111. Kahn HJ, Marks A, Thom H, Baumal R. Role of antibody to S100 protein in diagnostic pathology. Am J Clin Pathol 79:341, 1983.
112. Kanik AB, Yaar M, Bhawan J. P75 nerve growth factor receptor staining helps identify desmoplastic and neurotropic melanoma. J Cutan Pathol 23:205, 1996.
113. Kapur RP, Bigler SA, Skelly M, Gown AM. Anti-melanoma monoclonal antibody HMB45 identifies an oncofetal glycoconjugate associated with immature melanosomes. J Histochem Cytochem 40:207, 1992.
114. Kastan MB, Onyekwere O, Sidransky D, et al. Participation of p53 protein in the cellular response to DNA damage. Cancer Res 51:6304, 1991.
115. Kaufmann O, Koch S, Burghardt J, et al. Tyrosinase, melan-A, and KBA62 as markers for the immunohistochemical identification of metestatic amalanotic melanomas on paraffin sections. Mod Pathol 11:740, 1998.
116. Kawai A, Noguchi M, Beppu Y, et al. Nuclear immunoreaction of p53 protein in soft tissue sarcomas: a possible prognostic factor. Cancer 73:2499, 1994.
117. Khalifa MA, Sesterhenn IA. Tumor markers of epithelial ovarian neoplasms. Int J Gynecol Pathol 9:217, 1990.
118. Kilpatrick SE, Hitchcock MG, Kraus MD, et al. Mixed tumors and myoepitheliomas of soft tissue: a clinicopathologic study

of 19 cases with a unifying concept. Am J Surg Pathol 21:13, 1997.

119. Kindblom LG, Remotti HE, Aidenborg F, Meis-Kindblom JM. Gastrointestinal pacemaker cell tumor (GIPACT): gastrointestinal stromal tumors show phenotypic characteristics of the interstitial cells of Cajal. Am J Pathol 152:1259, 1998.
120. Kindblom LG, Seidal T, Karisson K. Immuno-histochemical localization of myoglobin in human muscle tissue and embryonal and alveolar rhabdomyosarcoma. Acta Pathol Microbiol Immunol Scand [A] 90:167, 1982.
121. King R, Weilbaecher KN, McGill G, et al. Microphthalmia transcription factor: a sensitive and specific melanocyte marker for melanoma diagnosis. Am J Pathol 155:731, 1999.
122. Koch M, Arbiser Z, Weiss S, et al. Melanoma cell adhesion molecule (Mel-CAM, CD146) and microphthalmia transcription factor (MITF) expression distinguish desmoplastic/sarcomatoid melanoma from morphologic mimics. Mod Pathol 13: 63A, 2000.
123. Kourea HP, Orlow I, Scheithauer BW, et al. Deletions of the INK4A gene occur in malignant peripheral nerve sheath tumors but not in neurofibromas. Am J Pathol 155: 1855, 1999.
124. Kuhn C, McDonald JA. The roles of the myofibroblast in idiopathic pulmonary fibrosis: ultrastructural and immunohistochemical features of sites of active extracellular matrix synthesis. Am J Pathol 138:1257, 1991.
125. Kumar-Singh S, Segers K, Rodeck U, et al. WT1 mutation in malignant mesothelioma and WT1 immunoreactivity in relation to p53 and growth factor receptor expression, cell-type transition, and prognosis. J Pathol 181:67, 1997.
126. Kutzner H. Expression of the human progenitor cell antigen CD34 (HPCA-1) distinguishes dermatofibrosarcoma protuberans from fibrous histiocytoma in formalin-fixed, paraffin-embedded tissue. J Am Acad Dermatol 28:613, 1993.
127. Ladanyi M. The emerging molecular genetics of sarcoma translocations. Diagn Mol Pathol 4:162, 1995.
128. Lane DP. Cancer: p53, guardian of the genome. Nature 358:15, 1992.
129. Lanier LL, Le AM, Civin CI, et al. The relationship of CD16 (Leu-11) and Leu-19 (NKH-1) antigen expression on human peripheral blood NK cells and cytotoxic T lymphocytes. J Immunol 136:4480, 1986.
130. Latres E, Drobnjak M, Pollack D, et al. Chromosome 17 abnormalities and TP53 mutations in adult soft tissue sarcomas. Am J Pathol 145:345, 1994.
131. Leach FS, Tokino T, Meltzer P, et al. p53 Mutation and MDM2 amplification in human soft tissue sarcomas. Cancer Res 53 (Supp 10):2231, 1993.
132. Leader M, Collins M, Patel J, Henry K. Desmin: its value as a marker of muscle derived tumours using a commercial antibody. Virchows Arch [Pathol Anat] 411:345, 1987.
133. Lefebvre V, Huang W, Harley VR, et al. SOX9 is a potent activator of the chondrocyte-specific enhancer of the pro alpha1(II) collagen gene. Mol Cell Biol 17:2336, 1997.
134. Leong ASY, Vinyuvat S, Suthipintawong C, Leong FJ. Patterns of basal lamina immunostaining in soft-tissue and bony tumors. Appl Immunohistochem 5:1, 1997.
135. Lessard JL. Two monoclonal antibodies to actin: one muscle selective and one generally reactive. Cell Motil Cytoskeleton 10:349, 1988.
136. Levine EA, Holzmayer T, Bacus S, et al. Evaluation of newer prognostic markers for adult soft tissue sarcomas. J Clin Oncol 15:3249, 1997.
137. Litzky LA, Brooks JJ. Cytokeratin immunoreactivity in malignant fibrous histiocytoma and spindle cell tumors: comparison between frozen and paraffin-embedded tissues. Mod Pathol 5: 30, 1992.
138. Longacre TA, Egbert BM, Rouse RV. Desmoplastic and spindle-cell malignant melanoma: an immunohistochemical study. Am J Surg Pathol 20:1489, 1996.
139. Lopez-Beltran A, Escudero AL, Cavazzana AO, et al. Sarcomatoid transitional cell carcinoma of the renal pelvis: a report of five cases with clinical, pathological, immunohistochemical and DNA ploidy analysis. Pathol Res Pract 192:1218, 1996.
140. Martin K, Trouche D, Hagemeier C, et al. Stimulation of E2F1/DP1 transcriptional activity by MDM2 oncoprotein. Nature 375:691, 1995.
141. Matsunou H, Shimoda T, Kakimoto S, et al. Histopathologic and immunohistochemical study of malignant tumors of peripheral nerve sheath (malignant schwannoma). Cancer 56: 2269, 1985.
142. McGarry RC, Helfand SL, Quaries RH, Roder JC. Recognition of myelin-associated glycoprotein by the monoclonal antibody HNK-1. Nature 306:376, 1983.
143. Mechtersheimer G, Staudter M, Moller P. Expression of the natural killer cell-associated antigens CD56 and CD57 in human neural and striated muscle cells and in their tumors. Cancer Res 51:1300, 1991.
144. Meis JM, Enzinger FM, Martz KL, Neal JA. Malignant peripheral nerve sheath tumors (malignant schwannomas) in children. Am J Surg Pathol 16:694, 1992.
145. Meis JM, Ordoñez NG, Gallager HS. Sarcomatoid carcinoma of the breast: an immunohistochemical study of six cases. Virchows Arch [Pathol Ana] 410:415, 1987.
146. Meis-Kindblom JM, Kindblom LG. Angiosarcoma of soft tissue: a study of 80 cases. Am J Surg Pathol 22:683, 1998.
147. Merino MJ, Carter D, Berman M. Angiosarcoma of the breast. Am J Surg Pathol 7:53, 1983.
148. Miettinen M. Immunoreactivity for cytokeratin and epithelial membrane antigen in leiomyosarcoma. Arch Pathol Lab Med 112:637, 1988.
149. Miettinen M. Keratin subsets in spindle cell sarcomas: keratins are widespread but synovial sarcoma contains a distinctive keratin polypeptide pattern and desmoplakins. Am J Pathol 138:505, 1991.
150. Miettinen M, Chatten J, Paetau A, Stevenson A. Monoclonal antibody NB84 in the differential diagnosis of neuroblastoma and other small round cell tumors. Am J Surg Pathol 22:327, 1998.
151. Miettinen M, Cupo W. Neural cell adhesion molecule distribution in soft tissue tumors. Hum Pathol 24:62, 1993.
152. Miettinen M, Fanburg-Smith JC, Virolainen M, et al. Epithelioid sarcoma: an immunohistochemical analysis of 112 classical and variant cases and a discussion of the differential diagnosis. Hum Pathol 30:934, 1999.
153. Miettinen M, Holthofer H, Lehto VP, et al. Ulex europaeus I lectin as a marker for tumors derived from endothelial cells. Am J Clin Pathol 79:32, 1983.
154. Miettinen M, Lehto VP, Virtanen I, et al. Neuroendocrine carcinoma of the skin (Merkel cell carcinoma): ultrastructural and immunohistochemical demonstration of neurofilaments. Ultrastruct Pathol 4:219, 1983.
155. Miettinen M, Lindenmayer AE, Chaubal A. Endothelial cell markers CD31, CD34, and BNH9 antibody to H- and Y-antigens: evaluation of their specificity and sensitivity in the diagnosis of vascular tumors and comparison with von Willebrand factor. Mod Pathol 7:82, 1994.
156. Miettinen M, Rapola J. Immunohistochemical spectrum of rhabdomyosarcoma and rhabdomyosarcoma-like tumors: expression of cytokeratin and the 68-kD neurofilament protein. Am J Surg Pathol 13:120, 1989.
157. Miettinen M, Sioni Y. Malignant fibrous histiocytoma: heterogeneous patterns of intermediate filament proteins by immunohistochemistry. Arch Pathol Lab Med 113:1363, 1989.

158. Miettinen M, Virtanen I. Synovial sarcoma: a misnomer. Am J Pathol 117:18, 1984.
159. Moll R, Lee I, Gould VE, et al. Immunocytochemical analysis of Ewing's tumors: patterns of expression of intermediate filaments and desmosomal proteins indicate cell type heterogeneity and pluripotential differentiation. Am J Pathol 127:288, 1987.
160. Mukai K, Schollmeyer JV, Rosai J. Immunohistochemical localization of actin: applications in surgical pathology. Am J Surg Pathol 5:91, 1981.
161. Nakajima T, Watanabe S, Sato Y, et al. Immunohistochemical demonstration of S100 protein in human malignant melanoma and pigmented nevi. Gann 72:335, 1981.
162. Nakajima T, Watanabe S, Sato Y, et al. Immunohistochemical demostration of S100 protein in malignant melanoma and pigmented nevus, and its diagnostic application. Cancer 50:912, 1982.
163. Nilsson G, Wang M, Wejde J, et al. Detection of EWS/FLI-1 by immunostaining: an adjunctive tool in diagnosis of Ewing's sarcoma and primitive neuroectodermal tumor on cytological samples and paraffin-embedded archival material. Sarcoma 3: 25, 1999.
164. Norton AJ, Thomas JA, Isaacson PG. Cytokeratin-specific monoclonal antibodies are reactive with tumours of smooth muscle derivation: an immunocytochemical and biochemical study using antibodies to intermediate filament cytoskeletal proteins. Histopathology 11:487, 1987.
165. Oates J, Edwards C. HBME-1, MOC-31, WT1 and calretinin: an assessment of recently described markers for mesothelioma and adenocarcinoma. Histopathology 36:341, 2000.
166. O'Connell JX, Kattapuram SV, Mankin HJ, et al. Epithelioid hemangioma of bone: a tumor often mistaken for low-grade angiosarcoma or malignant hemangioendothelioma. Am J Surg Pathol 17:610, 1993.
167. Oliner JD, Kinzler KW, Meltzer PS, et al. Amplification of a gene encoding a p53-associated protein in human sarcomas. Nature 358:80, 1992.
168. Ordi J, de Alava E, Torne A, et al. Intraabdominal desmoplastic small round cell tumor with EWS/ERG fusion transcript. Am J Surg Pathol 22:1026, 1998.
169. Ordoñez NG. Desmoplastic small round cell tumor: II. An ultrastructural and immunohistochemical study with emphasis on new immunohistochemical markers. Am J Surg Pathol 22: 1314, 1998.
170. Ordoñez NG. Role of immunohistochemistry in differentiating epithelial mesothelioma from adenocarcinoma: review and update. Am J Clin Pathol 112:75, 1999.
171. Ordoñez NG. The immunohistochemical diagnosis of epithelial mesothelioma. Hum Pathol 30:313, 1999.
172. Ordoñez NG. Value of calretinin immunostaining in differentiating epithelial mesothelioma from lung adenocarcinoma. Mod Pathol 11:929, 1998.
173. Ordoñez NG. Value of cytokeratin 5/6 immunostaining in distinguishing epithelial mesothelioma of the pleura from lung adenocarcinoma. Am J Surg Pathol 22:1215, 1998.
174. Ordoñez NG. Value of the Ber-EP4 antibody in differentiating epithelial pleural mesothelioma from adenocarcinoma: the M.D. Anderson experience and a critical review of the literature. Am J Clin Pathol 109:85, 1998.
175. Ordoñez NG, del Junco GW, Ayala AG, Ahmed N. Angiosarcoma of the small intestine: an immunoperoxidase study. Am J Gastroenterol 78:218, 1983.
176. Osborn M, Hill C, Altmannsberger M, Weber K. Monoclonal antibodies to titin in conjunction with antibodies to desmin separate rhabdomyosarcomas from other tumor types. Lab Invest 55:101, 1988.
177. Osborn M, Weber K. Tumor diagnosis by intermediate filament typing: a novel tool for surgical pathology. Lab Invest 48:372, 1983.
178. Otto F, Thornell AP, Crompton T, et al. Cbfa1, a candidate gene for cleidocranial dysplasia syndrome, is essential for osteoblast differentiation and bone development. Cell 89:765, 1997.
179. Parham DM, Dias P, Kelly DR, et al. Desmin positivity in primitive neuroectodermal tumors of childhood. Am J Surg Pathol 16:483, 1992.
180. Parham DM, Webber B, Holt H, et al. Immunohistochemical study of childhood rhabdomyosarcomas and related neoplasms: results of an intergroup rhabdomyosarcoma study project. Cancer 67:3072, 1991.
181. Parkash V, Gerald WL, Parma A, et al. Desmoplastic small round cell tumor of the pleura. Am J Surg Pathol 19:659, 1995.
182. Pemick NL, DaSilva M, Gangl MD, et al. "Histiocytic markers" in melanoma. Mod Pathol 12:1072, 1999.
183. Perosio PM, Brooks JJ. Expression of nerve growth factor receptor in paraffin-embedded soft tissue tumors. Am J Pathol 132:152, 1988.
184. Pinkus GS, Kurtin PJ. Epithelial membrane antigen: a diagnostic discriminant in surgical pathology; immunohistochemical profile in epithelial, mesenchymal, and hematopoietic neoplasms using paraffin sections and monoclonal antibodies. Hum Pathol 16:929, 1985.
185. Pollock RE. Molecular determinants of soft tissue sarcoma proliferation. Semin Surg Oncol 10:315, 1994.
186. Ramaekers FC, Pruszczynski M, Smedts F. Cytokeratins in smooth muscle cells and smooth muscle tumours. Histopathology 12:558, 1988.
187. Ramani P, Rampling D, Link M. Immunocytochemical study of 12E7 in small round-cell tumours of childhood: an assessment of its sensitivity and specificity. Histopathology 23:557, 1993.
188. Riopel M, Dickman PS, Link MP, Perlman EJ. MIC2 analysis in pediatric lymphomas and leukemias. Hum Pathol 25:36, 1994.
189. Robb JA. Mesothelioma versus adenocarcinoma: false-positive CEA and Leu-M1 staining due to hyaluronic acid [Letter]. Hum Pathol 20:400, 1989.
190. Rosai J, Dias P, Parham DM, et al. MyoD1 protein expression in alveolar soft part sarcoma as confirmatory evidence of its skeletal muscle nature. Am J Surg Pathol 15:974, 1991.
191. Rosenberg AE, O'Connell JX, Dickersin GR, Bhan AK. Expression of epithelial markers in malignant fibrous histiocytoma of the musculoskeletal system: an immunohistochemical and electron microscopic study. Hum Pathol 24:284, 1993.
192. Rubin BP, Hasserjian RP, Singer S, et al. Spindle cell rhabdomyosarcoma (so-called) in adults: report of two cases with emphasis on differential diagnosis. Am J Surg Pathol 22:459, 1998.
193. Rudolph P, Kellner U, Chassevent A, et al. Prognostic relevance of a novel proliferation marker, Ki-S11, for soft- tissue sarcoma: a multivariate study. Am J Pathol 150:1997, 1997.
194. Sanno N, Teramoto A, Sugiyama M, et al. Application of catalyzed signal amplification in immunodetection of gonadotropin subunits in clinically nonfunctioning pituitary adenomas. Am J Clin Pathol 106:16, 1996.
195. Sariomo-Rikala M, Kovatich AJ, Barusevicius A, Miettinen M. CD117: a sensitive marker for gastrointestinal stromal tumors that is more specific than CD34. Mod Pathol 11:728, 1998.
196. Schelper RL, Olson SP, Carroll TJ, et al. Studies of the endothelial origin of cells in systemic angioendotheliomatosis and other vascular lesions of the brain and meninges using Ulex europaeus lectin stains. Clin Neuropathol 5:231, 1986.
197. Schnitt SJ, Vogel H. Meninglomas: diagnostic value of immunoperoxidase staining for epithelial membrane antigen. Am J Surg Pathol 10:640, 1986.

198. Schuller-Petrovic S, Gebhart W, Lassmann H, et al. A shared antigenic determinant between natural killer cells and nervous tissue. Nature 306:179, 1983.
199. Shah IA, Gani OS, Wheler L. Comparative immunoreactivity of CD-68 and HMB-45 in malignant melanoma, neural tumors and nevi. Pathol Res Pract 193:497, 1997.
200. Shanfeld RL, Edelman J, Willis JE, et al. Immunohistochemical analysis of neural markers in peripheral primitive neuroectodermal tumors (pPNET) without light microscopic evidence of neural differentiation. Appl Immunohistochem 5:78, 1997.
201. Sheibani K, Esteban JM, Balley A, et al. Immunopathologic and molecular studies as an aid to the diagnosis of malignant mesothelioma. Hum Pathol 23:107, 1992.
202. Sherr CJ. Cancer cell cycles. Science 274:1672, 1996.
203. Shi SR, Cote RJ, Chaiwun B, et al. Standardization of immunohistochemistry based on antigen retrieval technique for routine formalin-fixed tissue sections. Appl Immunohistochem 6:89, 1998.
204. Shi SR, Key ME, Kaira KL. Antigen retrieval in formalin-fixed, paraffin-embedded tissues: an enhancement method for immunohistochemical staining based on microwave oven heating of tissue sections. J Histochem Cytochem 39:741, 1991.
205. Shipley WR, Hammer RD, Lennington WJ, Macon WR. Paraffin immunohistochemical detection of CD56, a useful marker for neural cell adhesion molecule (NCAM), in normal and neoplastic fixed tissues. Appl Immunohistochem 5:87, 1997.
206. Skalli O, Gabbiani G, Babal F, et al. Intermediate filament proteins and actin isoforms as markers for soft tissue tumor differentiation and origin. II. Rhabdomyosarcomas. Am J Pathol 130:515, 1988.
207. Skalli O, Ropraz P, Trzeciak A, et al. A monoclonal antibody against alpha-smooth muscle actin: a new probe for smooth muscle differentiation. J Cell Biol 103:2787, 1986.
208. Smith KJ, Skelton HGD, Morgan AM, et al. Spindle cell neoplasms coexpressing cytokeratin and vimentin (metaplastic squamous cell carcinoma). J Cutan Pathol 19:286, 1992.
209. Soderstrom KO. Lectin binding to prostatic edenocarcinoma. Cancer 60:1823, 1987..
210. Stevenson A, Chatten J, Bertoni F, Miettinen M. CD99 (p30/32MIC2) neuroectodermal/Ewing's sarcoma antigen as an immunohistochemical marker: review of more than 600 tumors and the literature experience. Appl Immunohistochem 2:231, 1994.
211. Sugimoto T, Ueyama H, Hosoi H, et al. Alpha-smooth-muscle actin and desmin expressions in human neuroblastoma cell lines. Int J Cancer 48:277, 1991.
212. Swanson PE. Heffalumps, jagulars, and cheshire cats: a commentary on cytokeratins and soft tissue sarcomas. Am J Clin Pathol 95:S2, 1991.
213. Swanson PE. HIERanarchy: the state of the art in immunohistochemistry [editorial]. Am J Clin Pathol 107:139, 1997.
214. Swanson PE, Manivel JC, Wick MR. Immunoreactivity for Leu-7 in neurofibrosarcoma and other spindle cell sarcomas of soft tissue. Am J Pathol 126:546, 1987.
215. Tauchi K, Tsutsumi Y, Yoshimura S, Watanabe K. Immunohistochemical and immunoblotting detection of cytokeratin in smooth muscle tumors. Acta Pathol Jpn 40:574, 1990.
216. Taylor CR. Immunomicroscopy: A Diagnostic Tool for the Surgical Pathologist. WB Saunders, Philadelphia, 1986.
217. Theaker JM, Fletcher CD. Epithelial membrane antigen expression by the perineurial cell: further studies of peripheral nerve lesions. Histopathology 14:581,1989.
218. Theaker JM, Gatter KC, Esiri MM, Fleming KA. Epithelial membrane antigen and cytokeratin expression by meningiomas: an immunohistological study. J Clin Pathol 39:435, 1986.
219. Theaker JM, Gatter KC, Puddle J. Epithelial membrane antigen expression by the perineurium of peripheral nerve and in peripheral nerve tumours. Histophatology 13:171, 1988.
220. Thomas JO, Nijjar J, Turley H, et al. NB84: a new monoclonal antibody for the recognition of neuroblastoma in routinely processed material. J Pathol 163:69, 1991.
221. Thompson SJ, Schatteman GC, Gown AM, Bothwell M. A monoclonal antibody against nerve growth factor receptor: immunohistochemical analysis of normal and neoplastic human tissue. Am J Clin Pathol 92:415, 1989.
222. Toffoli G, Doglioni C, Cernigoi C, et al. P53 overexpression in human soft tissue sarcomas: relation to biological aggressiveness. Ann Oncol 5:167, 1994.
223. Tsokos M. The role of immunocytochemistry in the diagnosis of rhabdomyosarcoma [editorial]. Arch Pathol Lab Med 110: 776, 1986.
224. Tsokos M, Howard R, Costa J. Immunohistochemical study of alveolar and embryonal rhabdomyosarcoma. Lab Invest 48: 148, 1983.
225. Tsukada T, McNutt MA, Ross R, Gown AM. HHF35, a muscle actin-specific monoclonal antibody. II. Reactivity in normal, reactive, and neoplastic human tissues. Am J Pathol 127:389, 1987.
226. Tsukada T, Tippens D, Gordon D, et al. HHF35, a muscle-actin-specific monoclonal antibody. I. Immunocytochemical and biochemical characterization. Am J Pathol 126:51, 1987.
227. Ueda T, Aozasa K, Tsujimoto M, et al. Prognostic significance of Ki-67 reactivity in soft tissue sarcomas. Cancer 63:1607, 1989.
228. Vallat-Decouvelaere AV, Dry SM, Fletcher CD. Atypical and malignant solitary fibrous tumors in extrathoracic locations: evidence of their comparability to intra-thoracic tumors. Am J Surg Pathol 22:1501, 1998.
229. Van de Rijn M, Barr FG, Xiong QB, et al. Poorly differentiated synovial sarcoma: an analysis of clinical, pathologic, and molecular genetic features. Am J Surg Pathol 23:106, 1999.
230. Van de Rijn M, Rouse R. CD34: a review. Appl Immunohistochem 2:71, 1994.
231. Van Haelst UJ, Pruszczynski M, ten Cate LN, Mravunac M. Ultrastructural and immunohistochemical study of epithelioid hemangioendothelioma of bone: coexpression of epithelial and endothelial markers. Ultrastruct Pathol 14:141, 1990.
232. Van Muijen GN, Rulter DJ, Wamaar SO. Coexpression of intermediate filament polypeptides in human fetal and adult tissues. Lab Invest 57:359, 1987.
233. Venuti JM, Morris JH, Vivian JL, et al. Myogenin is required for late but not early aspects of myogenesis during mouse development. J Cell Biol 128:563, 1995.
234. Virtanen I, Lehto VP, Lehtonen E, et al. Expression of intermediate filaments in cultured cells. J Cell Sci 50:45, 1981.
235. Walker RA. Ulex europeus I: peroxidase as a marker of vascular endothelium: its application in routine histopathology. J Pathol 146:123, 1985.
236. Wang NP, Marx J, McNutt MA, et al. Expression of myogenic regulatory proteins (myogenin and MyoD1) In small blue round cell tumors of childhood. Am J Pathol 147:1799, 1995.
237. Weidner N, Tjoe J. Immunohistochemical profile of monoclonal antibody O13: antibody that recognizes glycoprotein p30/32MIC2 and is useful in diagnosing Ewing's sarcoma and peripheral neuroepithelioma. Am J Surg Pathol 18:486, 1994.
238. Weintraub H. The MyoD family and myogenesis: redundancy, networks, and thresholds. Cell 75:1241, 1993.
239. Weiss SW, Bratthauer GL, Morris PA. Postirradiation malignant fibrous histiocytoma expressing cytokeratin: implications for the immunodiagnosis of sarcomas. Am J Surg Pathol 12: 554, 1988.
240. Weiss SW, Langloss JM, Enzinger FM. Value of S-100 protein in the diagnosis of soft tissue tumors with particular reference

to benign and malignant Schwann cell tumors. Lab Invest 49: 299, 1983.

241. Weiss SW, Nickoloff BJ. CD-34 is expressed by a distinctive cell population in peripheral nerve, nerve sheath tumors, and related lesions. Am J Surg Pathol 17:1039, 1993.
242. Wenig BM, Abbondanzo SL, Heffess CS. Epithelioid angiosarcoma of the adrenal glands: a clinicopathologic study of nine cases with a discussion of the implications of finding "epithelial-specific" markers. Am J Surg Pathol 18:62, 1994.
243. Wesche WA, Fletcher CD, Dias P, et al. Immunohistochemistry of MyoD1 in adult pleomorphic soft tissue sarcomas. Am J Surg Pathol 19:261, 1995.
244. Westra WH, Gerald WL, Rosal J. Solitary fibrous tumor: consistent CD34 immunoreactivity and occurrence in the orbit. Am J Surg Pathol 18:992, 1994.
245. White W, Shiu MH, Rosenblum MK, et al. Cellular schwannoma: a clinicopathologic study of 57 patients and 58 tumors. Cancer 66:1266, 1990.
246. Wick MR, Manivel C, O'Leary TP, Cherwitz DL. Nephroblastoma: a comparative immunocytochemical and lectin-histochemical study. Arch Pathol Lab Med 110:630, 1986.
247. Wirth PR, Legier J, Wright GL Jr. Immunohistochemical evaluation of seven monoclonal antibodies for differentiation of pleural mesothelioma from lung adenocarcinoma. Cancer 67: 655, 1991.
248. Xiao ZX, Chen J, Levine AJ, et al. Interaction between the retinoblastoma protein and the oncoprotein MDM2. Nature 375:694, 1995.
249. Yang P, Hirose T, Hasegawa T, et al. Prognostic implication of the p53 protein and KI-67 antigen immunohistochemistry in malignant fibrous histiocytoma. Cancer 76:618, 1995.
250. Zamecnik M, Michal M. Malignant peripheral nerve sheath tumor with perineurial cell differentiation (malignant perineurioma). Pathol Int 49:69, 1999.
251. Zarbo RJ, Gown AM, Nagle RB, et al. Anomalous cytokeratin expression in malignant melanoma: one- and two-dimensional Western blot analysis and immunohistochemical survey of 100 melanomas. Mod Pathol 3:494, 1990.

# CHAPTER 9

# BENIGN FIBROUS TISSUE TUMORS

*Fibrous connective tissue* consists principally of fibroblasts and an extracellular matrix containing fibrillary structures (collagen, elastin) and nonfibrillary extracellular matrix, or ground substance. Dense fibrous connective tissue, such as that found in tendons, aponeuroses, and ligaments, is composed predominantly of fibrillar collagen, whereas loose fibrous connective tissue contains a relative abundance of nonfibrillary ground substance.

*Fibroblasts* are the predominant cells in fibrous connective tissue. These cells are spindle-shaped with pale-staining, smoothly contoured oval nuclei, one or two minute nucleoli, and eosinophilic to basophilic cytoplasm, depending on the state of synthetic activity. The cytoplasmic borders are usually indistinct, although fibroblasts deposited in a rich myxoid stroma tend to assume a more stellate shape with multiple slender cytoplasmic extensions. Ultrastructurally, fibroblasts typically contain numerous, often dilated cisternae of rough endoplasmic reticulum, a large Golgi complex associated with small vesicles filled with granular or flocculent material, scattered mitochondria typically in a perinuclear location, many free ribosomes, occasional fat droplets, and slender microfilaments. Fibroblasts are responsible for the intracellular assembly of various extracellular fibrillary and nonfibrillary products such as procollagen, protoelastin, and glycosaminoglycans, which form the ground substance of connective tissue. The term *fibrocytes* is used for relatively quiescent cells that are less active than fibroblasts and are mainly engaged in maintenance of the extracellular matrix. The cells tend to have smaller nuclei and scantier amounts of cytoplasm than typical fibroblasts.

*Myofibroblasts* share morphologic features with both fibroblasts and smooth muscle cells (Table 9–1). Gabbiani et al. initially described these cells in granulation tissue[6] and later in Dupuytren's contracture.[5] Since this initial description, these cells have been described in such processes as responses to injury and repair phenomena, in quasineoplastic proliferative conditions, as part of the stromal response to neoplasia, and in a variety of benign and malignant neoplasms composed, at least in part, of myofibroblasts.[1,9,14,16] Ultrastructurally, myofibroblasts are characterized by indented nuclei with numerous, long cytoplasmic extensions. In the cytoplasm, bundles of microfilaments which are usually arranged parallel to the long axis of the cell are present with interspersed dense bodies. Subplasmalemmal plaques and pinocytotic vesicles are also numerous. The cells are partly enveloped by a basal lamina.[14] The fibronexus, transmembrane complexes of intracellular microfilaments in continuity with the extracellular matrix, are also characteristic of this cell type.[18,19] Immunohistochemically, myofibroblasts may have a variable phenotype, including those that express (1) only vimentin (V type); (2) vimentin, smooth muscle $\alpha$-actin, and desmin (VAD type); (3) vimentin and smooth muscle $\alpha$-actin (VA type); and (4) vimentin and desmin (VD type) (Fig. 9–1).[11,15,20] These immunophenotypes differ depending on the type of myofibroblastic proliferation encountered.

*Collagen* is the main product of fibroblasts and the major constituent of the extracellular matrix. Up to 11 closely related but genetically distinct types of collagen are found in connective tissue, differing in the amino acid composition of their $\alpha$ chains.[4] Collagen chain polypeptides are synthesized on the ribosomes of the rough endoplasmic reticulum of fibroblasts and a variety of other cell types.[8] These precursor pro-$\alpha$ chains are then transported to the Golgi apparatus, where they coil into a triple helix, forming procollagens. After release from the Golgi apparatus, they are discharged into the pericellular matrix by exocytosis.[3] Following enzymatic cleavage by procollagen peptidases, tropocollagen filaments spontaneously aggregate in a staggered fashion, resulting in the formation

**TABLE 9–1** ULTRASTRUCTURAL FEATURES OF MYOFIBROBLASTS COMPARED TO FIBROBLASTS AND SMOOTH MUSCLE CELLS

| Feature | Fibroblasts | Myofibroblasts | Smooth Muscle Cells |
|---|---|---|---|
| Cell shape | Bipolar/tapered | Bipolar/stellate | Wider |
| Nucleus | Smooth | Deep marginations | Cigar-shaped |
| Golgi | + | + | Scanty |
| Rough endoplasmic reticulum | ++ | + | Scanty |
| Pinocytosis | − | + | ++ |
| Attachment plaques | − | + | ++ |
| Dense bodies | − | + | ++ |
| External lamina | − | Interrupted | Continuous |
| Cell–cell attachments | − | Gap, adherens | Gap, adherens |
| Cell–stroma attachments (fibronexus) | − | ++ | Attenuated |

Modified from Fisher C. IAP presentation, Nice, France, October 1998.

of typical banded collagen fibrils with 64 nm periodicity. Long-spacing collagen with 240 nm periodicity is occasionally encountered in both normal and neoplastic tissues.

*Type I collagen* is ubiquitous and consists of parallel arrays of thick, closely packed banded fibrils. This type of collagen is found in the dermis, tendons, ligaments, bone, fascia, corneal tissue, and dentin. It is strongly birefringent and consists of two $\alpha_1$ chains and one $\alpha_2$ chain entwined in a helical configuration. *Type II collagen,* synthesized by chondroblasts, is found in the extracellular matrix of cartilage and in the notochord, nucleus pulposus, embryonic cornea, and vitreous body of the eye. *Type III collagen* is often associated with type I collagen, characteristically in loose connective tissue, including the dermis, blood vessel walls, and various glands and parenchymal organs. *Type IV collagen* is the major component of basal lamina. This collagen type is nonfibrillar and does not undergo any changes following secretion from the cell. *Type V collagen* is primarily found in blood vessels and smooth muscle tissue. Other types of collagen (*types VII, VIII, IX*) are less common and less well defined. Reticular fibers form a delicate network of fibers that have the same cross-banding as collagen (67 nm) but differ from collagen fibers by their small size (approximately 50 nm in diameter) and their argyrophilia. They are composed mainly of type III collagen.[21] "Amianthoid" fibers are fused, abnormally thick collagen fibers with a typical periodicity but measuring up to 1000 nm in diameter.

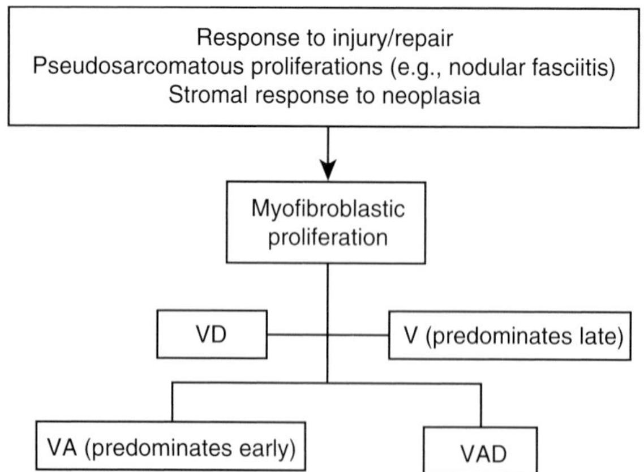


**FIGURE 9–1.** Immunophenotypes of myofibroblasts. V, vimentin; A, actin; D, desmin.

*Elastic fibers* are usually closely associated with collagen fibers and are important components of the extracellular matrix of the dermis, large vessels, and internal organs such as the heart and the lung. Light microscopy reveals them to be slender, branching, highly refractile, weakly birefringent structures that stain with Weigert's resorcin-fuchsin, Verhoeff's, and aldehyde-fuschin stains. Ultrastructurally, they have no cross-striations or banding. Elastic fibers are composed of two distinct components: *elastin,* a large amorphous homogeneous or finely granular structure of low electron density and peripherally located *microfibrils* which are 10- to 12-nm in length.[7,13] Elastin, the main component of elastic fibers, is synthesized and secreted as tropoelastin by fibroblasts; it typically contains large amounts of glycine, alanine, valine, and desmosine but little hydroxyproline. It is resistant to trypsin digestion but is hydrolyzed by elastase. Altered elastic fibers are found in a variety of heritable and acquired diseases and in the extracellular matrix of both benign and malignant neoplasms.

The extracellular matrix is also composed in part of *glycoproteins,* including fibronectin and laminin. *Fibronectin* is a high-molecular-weight glycoprotein synthesized by fibroblasts and a variety of other cells. It affects cell-to-cell cohesion and the interaction between cells and the extracellular matrix, serving as a "molecular glue."[10,22] *Laminin* is a large glycoprotein distributed throughout the lamina lucida and lamina densa of the basement membrane.[2,12]

*Glycosaminoglycans* (*mucopolysaccharides*) form the ground substance of connective tissue. They are intimately associated with fibroblasts and collagen fibers, play an important role in salt and water distribution, and serve as a link in various cellular interactions. These substances are synthesized in fibroblasts or chondroblasts, where they are polymerized and sulfated in the Golgi complex. Chemically, they are linear polysaccharide chains of hexosamines (glycosamino-) and various sugars (-glycans) that are (with the exception of hyaluronic acid) bound to proteins. They have a high molecular weight, are negatively charged, and are capable of binding large amounts of fluids. These substances do not stain with hematoxylin and eosin but stain well with alcian blue, colloidal iron, and toluidine blue.

One of the most important glycosaminoglycans is *hyaluronic acid,* a nonsulfated disaccharide chain composed of glucosamine and glucuronic acid. This substance is abundant in fibrous connective tissue and is the major component of synovial fluid. Histochemically, it is depolymerized and decolorized by hyaluronidase. *Chondroitin sulfates* (types 4 and 6) combine galactosamine and glucuronic acid, and these substances predominate in hyaline and elastic cartilage, nucleus pulposus, and intervertebral discs. Other glycosaminoglycans are *dermatin sulfate* and *heparin sulfate.* Dermatin sulfate is found predominantly in the dermis, tendons, and ligaments, whereas heparin sulfate is found in various structures rich in reticular fibers.[17]

## BENIGN FIBROUS PROLIFERATIONS

Fibrous tumors and tumor-like lesions form a large, diverse group of distinct entities that differ greatly in their clinical behavior. Some are completely benign and rarely if ever recur, even after incomplete excision. Others are poorly circumscribed and infiltrate the surrounding soft tissues, with a tendency to recurrence unless they are widely excised initially. Others are frankly malignant tumors that frequently recur and metastasize. On the basis of distinct clinical and histologic features, four categories of fibrous proliferation are distinguished: (1) benign fibrous proliferations, (2) fibromatoses, (3) fibrosarcomas, and (4) fibrous proliferations of infancy and childhood. The fourth category is included as a separate category because most fibrous lesions that occur during the first years of life have a characteristic structure, and their histologic picture and behavior differ from those in older children and adults.

The *benign fibroblastic proliferations* constitute a heterogeneous group of well defined entities that are predominantly reactive rather than true neoplasms. This category includes entities such as nodular fasciitis, proliferative fasciitis, and proliferative myositis, all of which may be mistaken for sarcomas, given their rapid clinical growth and rich cellularity. Despite the sometimes worrisome histologic features, these lesions rarely recur, even after incomplete excision, and they never metastasize.

Other entities included in this group differ by their slow, insidious growth and large size. As a rule, they are much less cellular and contain considerable amounts of collagen. Their incidence varies; fibroma of the tendon sheath, for example, is a comparatively common tumor but is still poorly recognized. Elastofibroma and nasopharyngeal angiofibroma, on the other hand, are well recognized, clearly defined entities, although they occur much less frequently than fibroma of the tendon sheath. There are still other, less well defined fibroma-like lesions in the soft tissues, but they are rare and most likely constitute the richly collagenous end-stage of a reparative fibroblastic proliferation. Nonetheless, the term *fibroma* is often loosely applied to these lesions. One of these lesions is a small, often pedunculated fibrous growth of the corium that is found chiefly on the trunk and seldom reaches a size of more than 1 cm; traditionally, it has been classified as *fibroma durum* or *molle,* depending on its relative content of collagen and fat. The term *fibroepithelial polyp* is usually applied to similar but pedunculated cutaneous nodules consisting of a mixture of dense fibrous tissue and fat covered by hyperplastic squamous epithelium. There are also fibromas with a prominent vascular component (*angiofibroma*), focal smooth muscle differentiation (*myofibroma*), and bone formation (*osteofibroma*), and fibroma-like pseudotumors that arise from the testicular tunic and other sites. *Pleomorphic fibroma* is a richly collagenous, polypoid growth marked by large pleomorphic and hyperchromatic nuclei occurring chiefly in the extremities of adults. Cutaneous fibroma-like lesions may be an occasional feature of Gardner syndrome and the tuberous sclerosis complex (*periungual, subungual,* and *gingival angiofibromas*).

There are also collagen-producing tumors that may mimic a fibroma. Fibrous histiocytoma, neurofibroma, and solitary fibrous tumor are the most common. The diagnosis of neurofibroma, in particular, is often used indiscriminantly as a convenient label for any benign collagen-forming tumor that arises in soft tissue.

Diagnostic confusion is frequently caused by reactive or reparative fibroblastic proliferations that are poorly defined and occur in association with chronic inflammation, wound healing, and organizing hemorrhage. These lesions can usually be recognized if attention is paid to the cellular polymorphism and the zonal variations in the histologic picture. In many such lesions, the presence of inflammatory infiltrates, siderophages, and hemorrhagic foci indicates the correct diagnosis.

## NODULAR FASCIITIS

Nodular fasciitis is a pseudosarcomatous, self-limiting reactive process composed of fibroblasts and myofibroblasts. Described by Kornwaler et al. in 1955 as "subcutaneous pseudosarcomatous fibromatosis,"[53] subsequent reports confirmed the benign nature of this proliferation.[33,52,57,73,77] Nodular fasciitis is probably the most common reactive or benign mesenchymal lesion that is misdiagnosed as a sarcoma given its characteristic rapid growth, rich cellularity, and mitotic activity. It is one of the most common soft tissue lesions and exceeds in frequency any other tumor or tumor-like lesion of fibrous tissue, which is attested to by the more than 1000 cases reviewed at the Armed Forces Institute of Pathology (AFIP) for a 20-year period and the large number of cases reported in the literature.

Although nodular fasciitis is clearly a benign process, the precise cause of this proliferation is unknown. Histologically, it bears a close resemblance to organizing granulation tissue, supporting a reactive proliferation that may be due to trauma, inconspicuous or otherwise. Morphologic variants of nodular fasciitis have been described, including intravascular, cranial, and ossifying fasciitis, all of which have overlapping histologic features unified by a proliferation of cytologically bland fibroblasts and myofibroblasts. It is the differences in clinical, gross, and light microscopic features that warrant retention of these specific designations.

### Clinical Findings

Most patients give a history of a rapidly growing mass or nodule that has been present for only 1–2 weeks. In about half of the cases there is associated soreness, tenderness, or slight pain. Numbness, paresthesia, or shooting pain is rare and develops only when the rapidly growing nodule exerts pressure on a peripheral nerve. Practically all lesions are solitary; among the AFIP cases there were only three in which two or more nodules were found at the same site. We have never encountered nodular fasciitis at multiple sites as was reported by Hutter et al.[49]

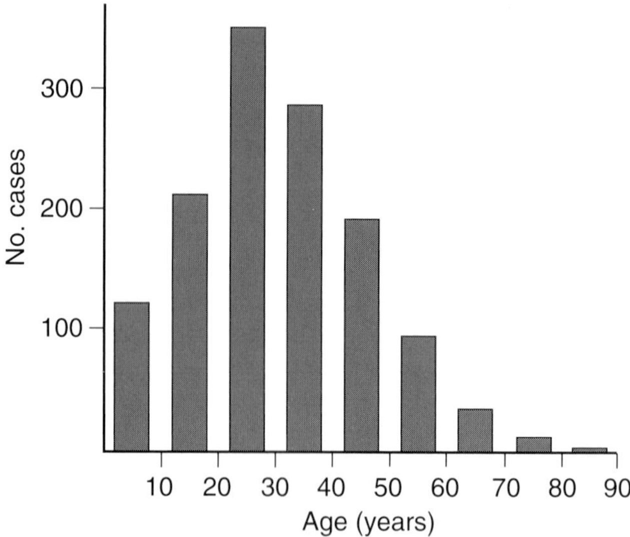

**FIGURE 9–2.** Age distribution for 1317 cases of nodular fasciitis.

Although nodular fasciitis may occur in patients of any age, it is most common in adults 20–40 years of age (Fig. 9–2). In the series by Allen, only 14% of patients were less than 10 or more than 60 years of age.[25] Males and females are about equally affected. Most of the lesions grow rapidly and have a preoperative duration of 1 month or less. Although nodular fasciitis may occur virtually anywhere on the body, there is a distinct predilection for certain sites, the most common being the upper extremities, especially the volar aspect of the forearm, followed by the trunk, particularly the chest wall and back. Nodular fasciitis in the head and neck is next in frequency and is the most common site in infants and children.[26,36,76,77] Nodular fasciitis is less common in the lower extremities and infrequent in the hands and feet (Table 9–2). This lesion has also been reported in a variety of unusual locations, including the parotid gland (Fig. 9–3),[23] urinary bladder,[71] vulva,[61] and lymph node capsule (Fig. 9–4).

**TABLE 9–2** ANATOMIC DISTRIBUTION OF NODULAR FASCIITIS (1319 CASES)

| Anatomic Location | No. of Patients | % |
|---|---|---|
| Lower extremities | 610 | 46 |
| Head, neck | 269 | 20 |
| Trunk | 235 | 18 |
| Lower extremities | 205 | 16 |
| *Total* | 1319 | 100 |

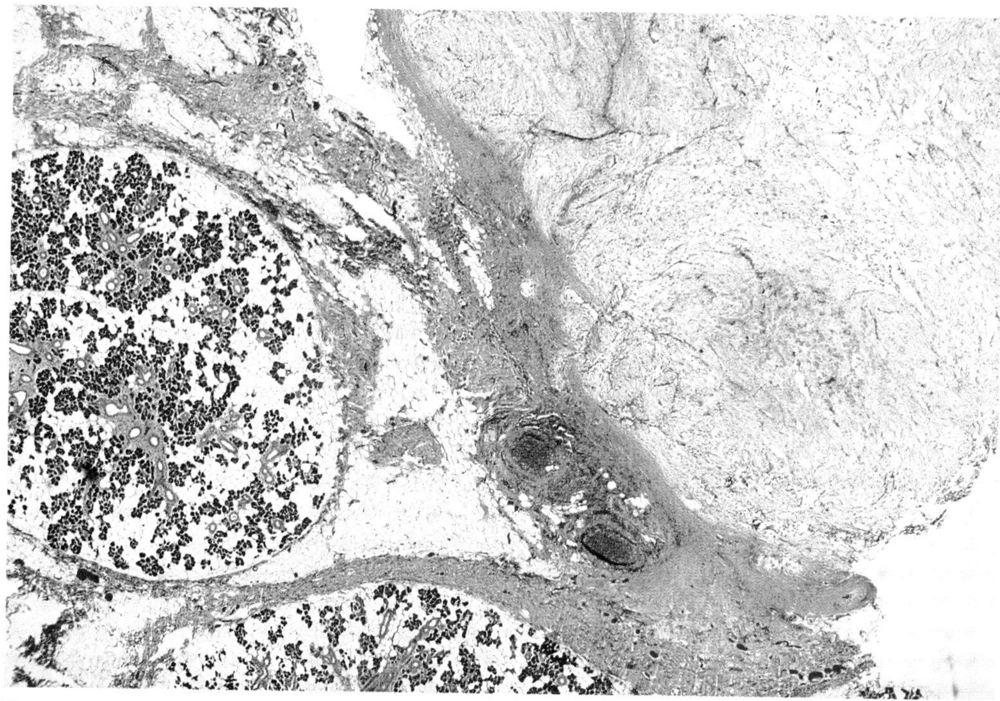

**FIGURE 9–3.** Nodular fasciitis involving the parotid gland. Note the circumscription and profuse myxoid change in the central portion of the lesion.

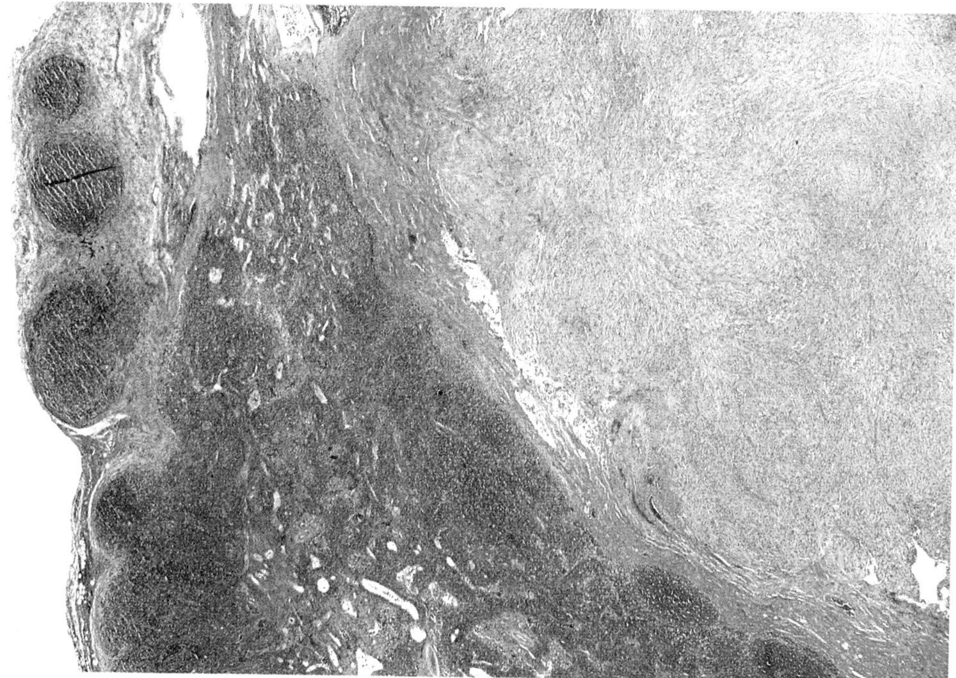

**FIGURE 9–4.** Rare example of nodular fasciitis involving the lymph node capsule.

## Gross Findings

The gross appearance of nodular fasciitis is highly dependent on the relative amounts of myxoid and fibrous stroma and the cellularity of the lesion. Most are relatively well circumscribed albeit nonencapsulated lesions, although some, particularly those centered about the deep fascia, are poorly circumscribed and appear to infiltrate the surrounding soft tissues. Most of the lesions are 2 cm or less in greatest dimension when they are excised[25,27,63,72,73]; intramuscular lesions tend to be slightly larger than those found in the subcutaneous tissue.[63] Although quite unusual, lesions as large as 10.5 cm have been described.[78] The appearance of the cut surface depends on the relative amounts of myxoid and collagenous material. Those with a predominantly myxoid matrix are soft and gelatinous and grossly may resemble other soft tissue lesions such as myxoma, ganglion, or benign peripheral nerve sheath tumors. Those with a pronounced collagenous stroma are firm and may resemble other fibrous lesions such as fibromatosis or fibrosarcoma. Although extravasated erythrocytes are a frequent microscopic feature, these lesions are rarely grossly hemorrhagic.

## Microscopic Findings

In general, nodular fasciitis can be grouped into three subtypes based on their relation with the fascia. The *subcutaneous type,* which is the most common form of nodular fasciitis, is typically a well circumscribed spherical nodule in the subcutis and based along the fascia (Fig. 9–5). The *intramuscular* type is superficially attached to the fascia; it grows as an ovoid intramuscular mass and is often larger than the subcutaneous type (Fig. 9–6). The *fascial* type, which is centered along the fascia, is less well circumscribed than the other forms, growing along the interlobular septa of the subcutaneous fat, resulting in a ray-like or stellate growth pattern (Fig. 9–7). Although Bernstein and Lattes cautioned against making a diagnosis of nodular fasciitis in skin,[27] rare examples of dermal nodular fasciitis have been reported.[45,55,64]

Several authors have grouped the various forms of fasciitis based on their predominant cellular features. Price et al. distinguished between myxomatous, fibromatous, and intermediate types (Figs. 9–8, 9–9),[63] but this approach is of little practical value and in fact many lesions have overlapping features. Regardless of the subtype, all nodular fasciitis lesions are composed predominantly of plump, immature-appearing fibroblasts that bear a close resemblance to the fibroblasts found in tissue culture or granulation tissue (Fig. 9–10). In general, the fibroblasts vary little in size and shape and have oval, pale-staining nuclei with prominent nucleoli. Mitotic figures are fairly common, but atypical mitoses are virtually never seen (Fig. 9–11).

Characteristically, the fibroblasts are arranged in short, irregular bundles and fascicles and are accompanied by a dense reticulin meshwork and only small amounts of mature birefringent collagen. The intervening matrix is rich in mucopolysaccharides which

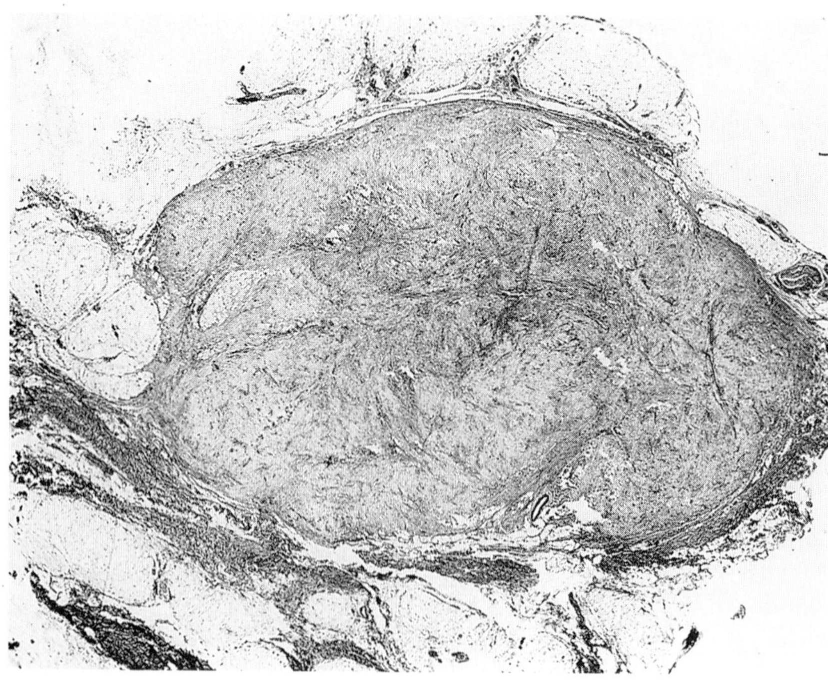

**FIGURE 9–5.** Nodular fasciitis involving the subcutis. Note circumscription of the lesion and attachment to the superficial fascia.

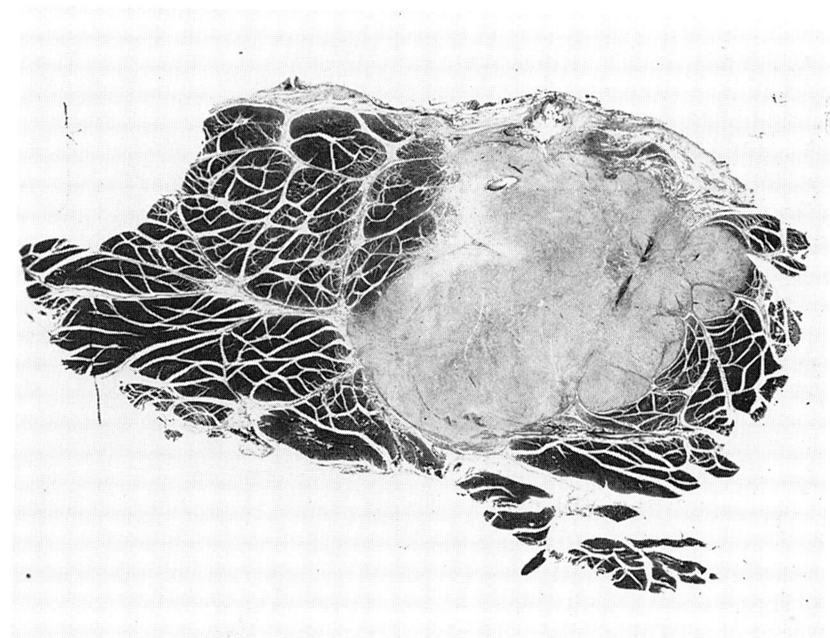

**FIGURE 9–6.** Intramuscular nodular fasciitis. Like the subcutaneous type, the nodule is well circumscribed and seems to arise from the fascia.

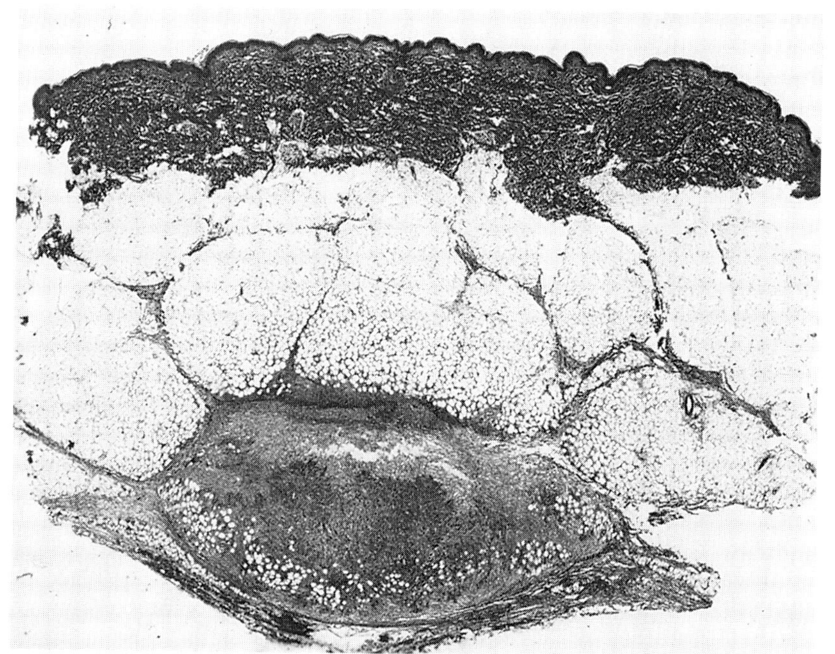

**FIGURE 9–7.** Fascial-type nodular fasciitis. This lesion is usually less well circumscribed and tends to extend along the interlobular septa into the surrounding subcutis.

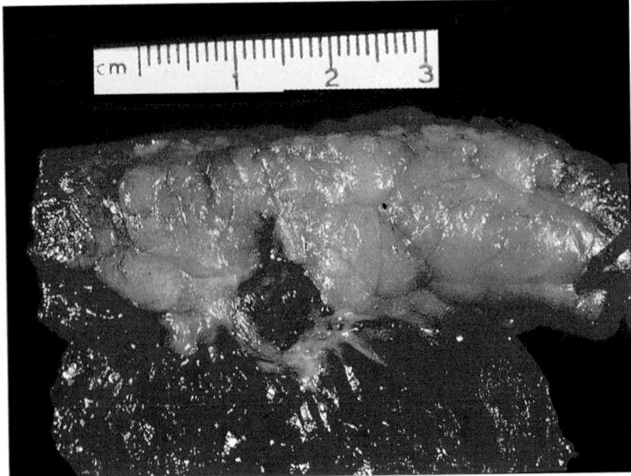


**FIGURE 9–8.** Gross appearance of the subcutaneous form of nodular fasciitis. The lesion is small and well circumscribed; it is superficially attached to the fascia.

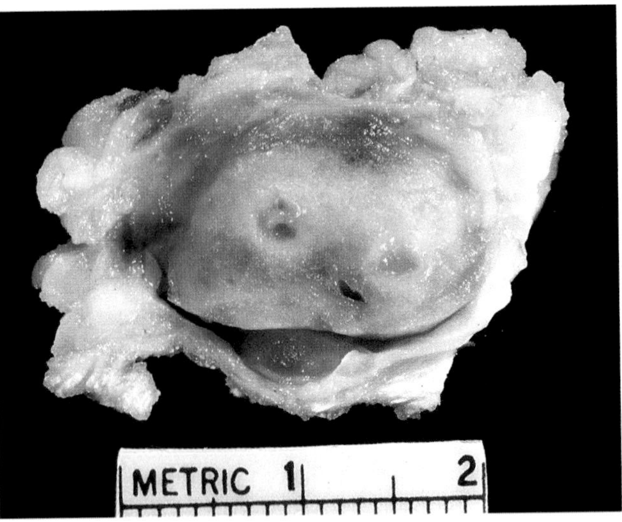


**FIGURE 9–9.** Nodular fasciitis with central cyst-like spaces, with accumulation of myxoid ground substance.

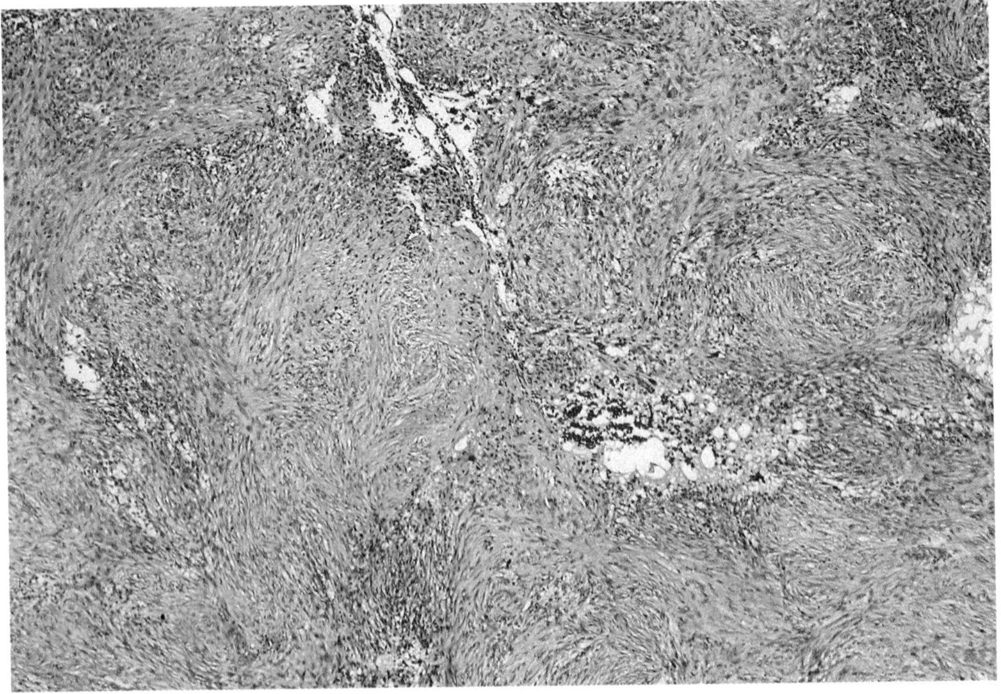

**FIGURE 9–10.** Nodular fasciitis showing varying cellularity with hypercellular spindle cell areas admixed with less cellular hyalinized zones.

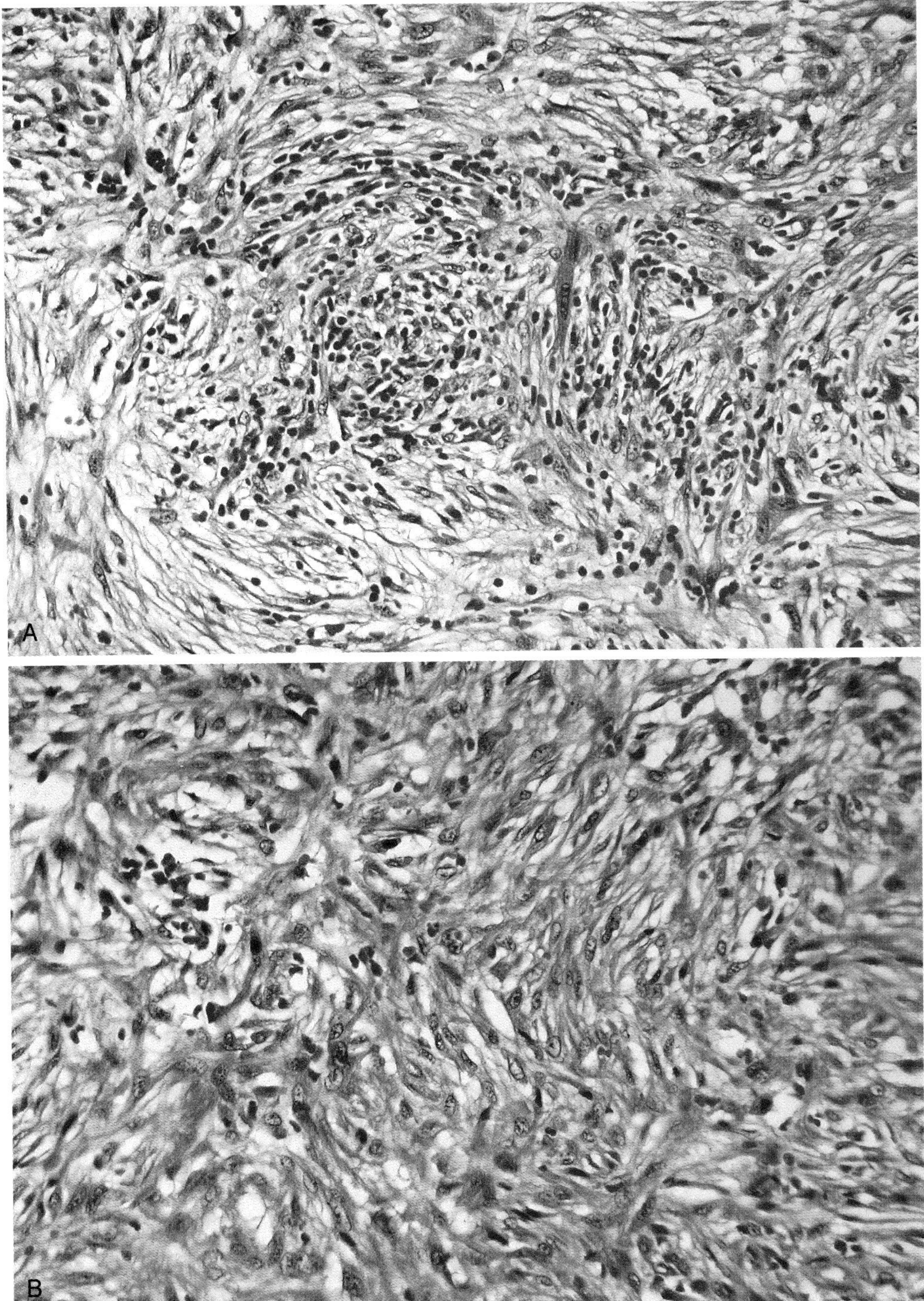


**FIGURE 9–11.** Nodular fasciitis. (**A**) Microhemorrhages between bundles of fibroblasts. (**B**) Bland cytologic features of cells in nodular fasciitis. There is an absence of nuclear hyperchromasia and variably sized nucleoli.

stain readily with alcian blue preparation and are depolymerized by hyaluronidase. The abundance of ground substance in most cases is responsible for the characteristic loosely textured, "feathery" pattern of nodular fasciitis; there are also cellular forms with only small amounts of interstitial myxoid material. Intermixed with the fibroblasts are scattered lymphoid cells and erythrocytes and, in the more central portion of the lesion, a small number of lipid macrophages and multinucleated giant cells. Occasionally, there are associated areas of microhemorrhage, but siderophages are rare (Fig. 9–12).

There are minor variations in the histologic picture; sometimes the intramuscular form of nodular fasciitis contains residual muscle fibers and muscle giant cells; this feature, however, is much less pronounced in nodular fasciitis than in fibromatosis. Sometimes in the fascial type of nodular fasciitis the fibroblasts are arranged in a radial fashion around a central, poorly cellular, edematous area containing a mixture of mucoid material and fibrin. In this type the fibroblasts are closely associated with newly formed vessels of narrow caliber; they have considerable mitotic activity, exceeding the average mitotic activity of the subcutaneous and intramuscular forms.

There is a close correlation between the microscopic picture and the preoperative duration of the lesion. Lesions of short duration tend to have a predominantly myxoid appearance (Fig. 9–13A,B), whereas those of longer duration are characterized by hyaline fibrosis (Fig. 9–13C,D), tissue shrinkage, and formation of minute fluid-filled spaces, or microcysts, a sequence closely paralleling the cicatrization of granulation tissue. In cases of long duration, the microcysts sometimes fuse and form a large centrally located cystic space (*cystic nodular fasciitis*).[35,72]

## Ossifying Fasciitis

On rare occasions a nodular fasciitis-like lesion has metaplastic bone, a condition described as *ossifying fasciitis*[37] or *fasciitis ossificans*[54] and, when arising from the periosteum, as *parosteal fasciitis* (Fig. 9–14).[48] Most of these lesions have features of both nodular fasciitis and myositis ossificans, but they are less well circumscribed than nodular fasciitis and lack the zonal maturation of myositis ossificans. Occasionally, small foci of metaplastic bone are also found in morphologically typical nodular fasciitis nodules. *Panniculitis ossificans* and *fibroosseous pseudotumor of the digits*[38] are closely related lesions that have a more irregular pattern and are somewhat akin to myositis ossificans. Rare cases of proliferative fasciitis,[31] proliferative myositis,[40] and cranial fasciitis[56] may also contain foci of metaplastic bone.

## Intravascular Fasciitis

Intravascular fasciitis is a rare variant of nodular fasciitis characterized by involvement of small or me-

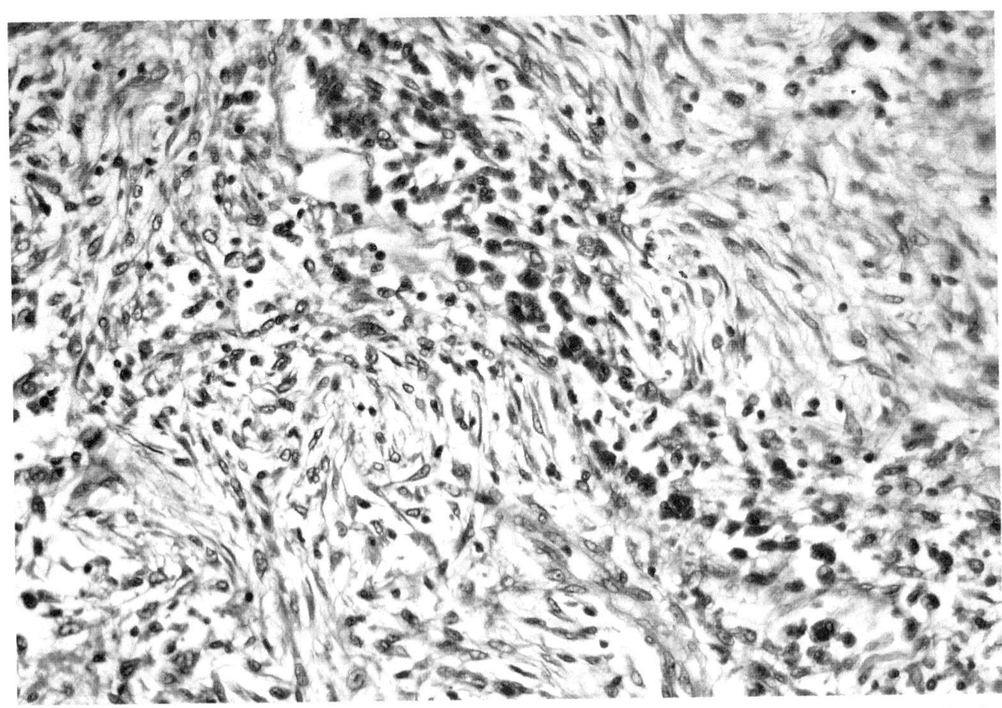

**FIGURE 9–12.** Nodular fasciitis with focal hemosiderin deposition, a feature rarely seen in this lesion.

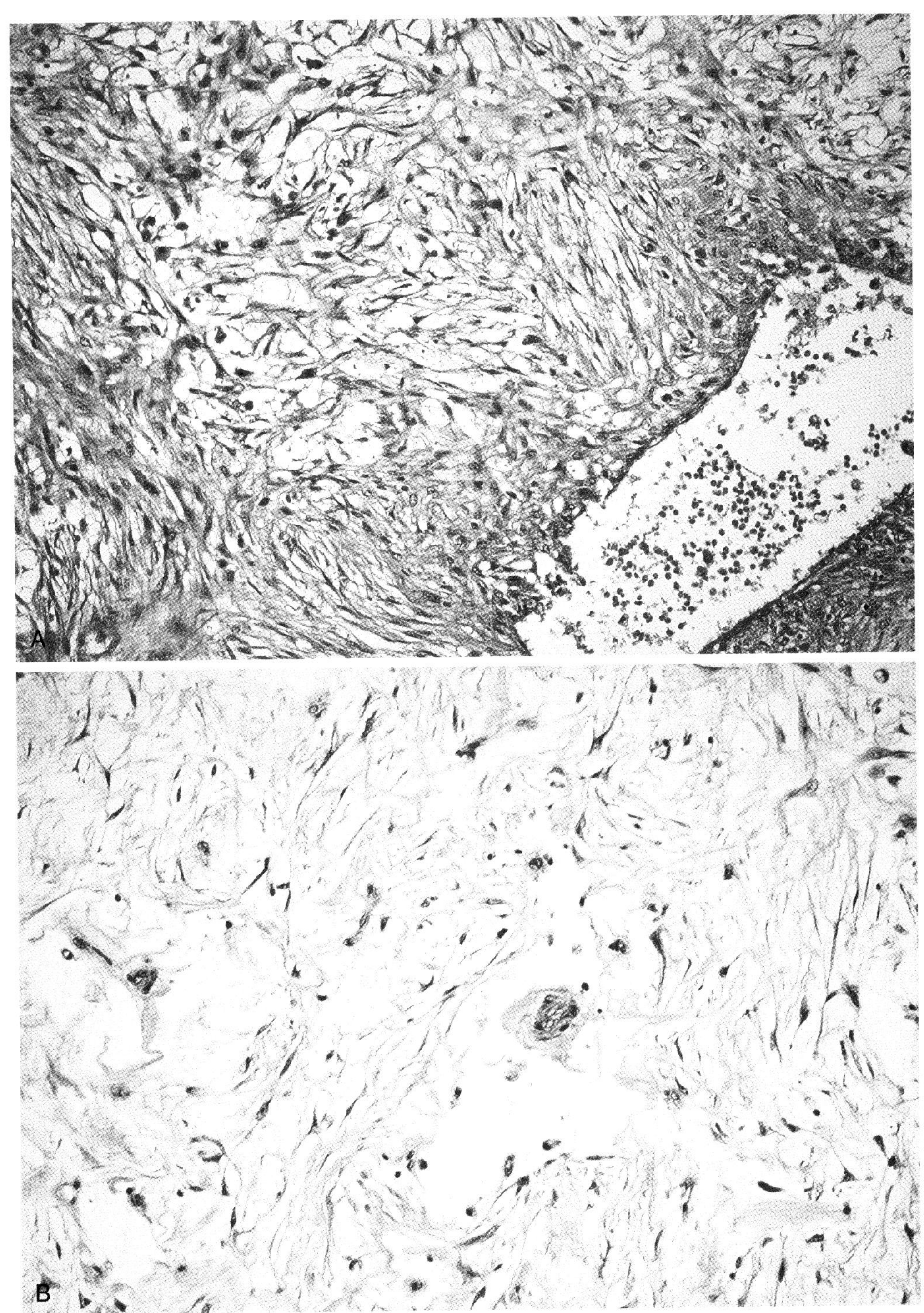


**FIGURE 9–13.** Nodular fasciitis. (**A**) Small area of myxoid breakdown imparting a loosely textured arrangement of fibroblasts. (**B**) More pronounced myxoid matrix with cells widely spaced by mucoid pools.

*Illustration continued on following page*

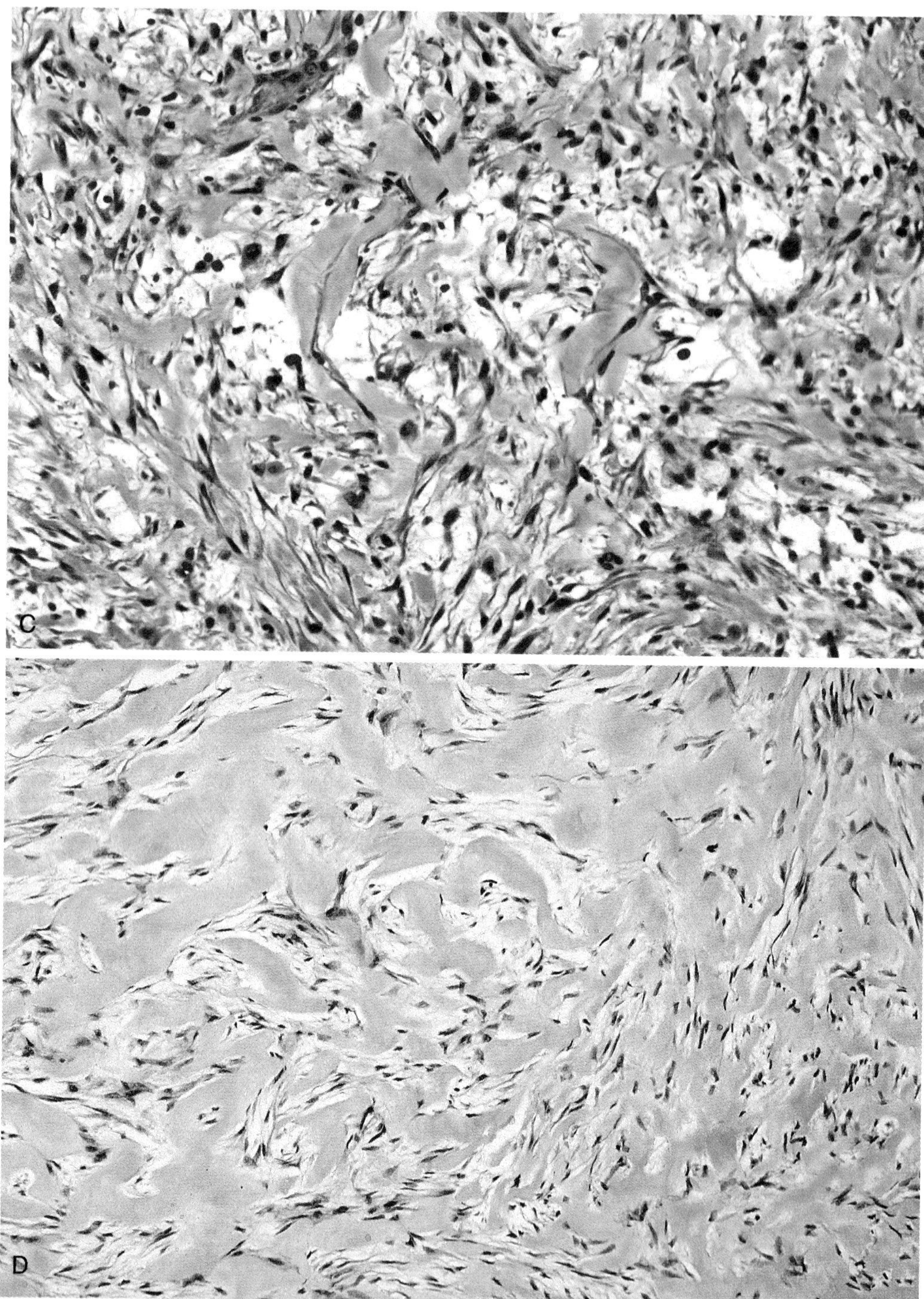


**FIGURE 9–13.** (*Continued*) (**C**) Nodular fasciitis showing hyaline fibrosis between fibroblasts. (**D**) Nodular fasciitis showing marked hyaline fibrosis, a feature usually encountered in lesions of long duration.

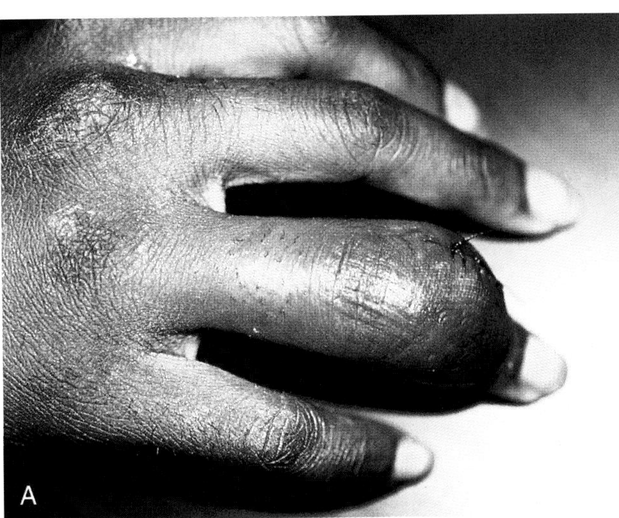


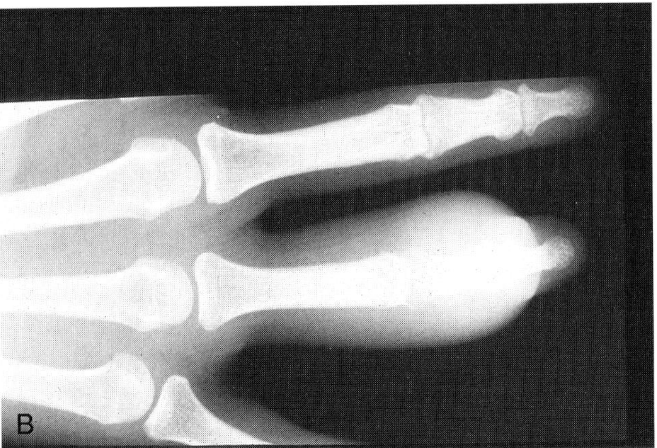


**FIGURE 9–14.** Juxtacortical fasciitis, (**A**) Gross appearance. (**B**) Accompanying radiograph of juxtacortical fasciitis.

dium-size veins or arteries.[62] Males and females are equally affected, and most patients are young, with only rare patients 30 years or older.[42,62,65] The typical presentation is that of a slowly growing, painless, solitary subcutaneous mass usually 2 cm or smaller. The upper extremity is the most common site, followed closely by the head and neck.[42,50] Less common sites are the trunk and lower extremities.[75] Grossly, the lesions may be round or oval; or they may be elongated, multinodular, or plexiform, particularly those that grow as a predominantly intravascular mass (Fig. 9–15). Small to medium-size veins are most commonly affected, but some lesions involve arteries alone or are seen in conjunction with venous structures. In most cases there is involvement of the intima, media, adventitia, and perivascular soft tissue, frequently with a predominantly extravascular component, although some grow as an intraluminal polypoid mass (Fig. 9–16). The association with a vessel may be obscured by the proliferation such that special stains are required to highlight the involved vessel. Histologically, the intravascular growth closely resembles nodular fasciitis, but it has a less prominent mucoid matrix and a conspicuous number of multinucleated giant cells resulting in a close resemblance to a benign fibrous histiocytoma or a giant cell tumor of soft parts (Figs. 9–17, 9–18). Clefts are often present in areas where the proliferation has separated from the vessel wall. Because of the vessel involvement, this lesion may be confused with a malignancy: 6 of 15 of the original lesions reported were initially confused with a sarcoma.[62] Despite the intravascular growth, there is no evidence of aggressive clinical behavior, recurrence, or metastasis.

## Cranial Fasciitis

Cranial fasciitis is a rapidly growing, nodular fasciitis-like fibroblastic proliferation of varying size.[24,56,63,66,68] It occurs chiefly, but not exclusively, in infants during the first year of life and involves the soft tissues of the scalp and the underlying skull. It usually erodes the outer table of the cranium but not infrequently also penetrates the inner table, infiltrating the dura and sometimes even the leptomeninges.[70] Radiographically, those that involve the underlying cranium create a lytic defect, often with a sclerotic rim.[29] Histologically, cranial fasciitis exhibits the broad morphologic spectrum of nodular fasciitis; it is composed of a proliferation of fibroblasts and myofibroblasts deposited in a variably myxoid and hyalinized matrix, occasionally with foci of osseous metaplasia (Fig. 9–19). The circumscription and the prominent myxoid matrix help distinguish the lesion from infantile fibromatosis or myofibromatosis.

Birth trauma may play a role in the development of the lesions[47]; several of the affected children had been delivered by forceps.[32,56] Cranial fasciitis is a benign, probably reactive process that seems to arise from the galea aponeurotica or the epicranial aponeurosis; it infiltrates the incompletely formed cranial bone.

There is no relation between cranial fasciitis and the *"headbanger's tumor,"* a fibrosing lesion of the forehead with pigmentation of the overlying skin. Neither is there any association with an inherited fibrosing lesion of the scalp (*cutis verticis gyrata*) that occurs in adults and is associated with clubbing of the digits, enlargement of the distal extremities, and periosteal bone formation (pachydermoperiostosis).

*Text continued on page 264*

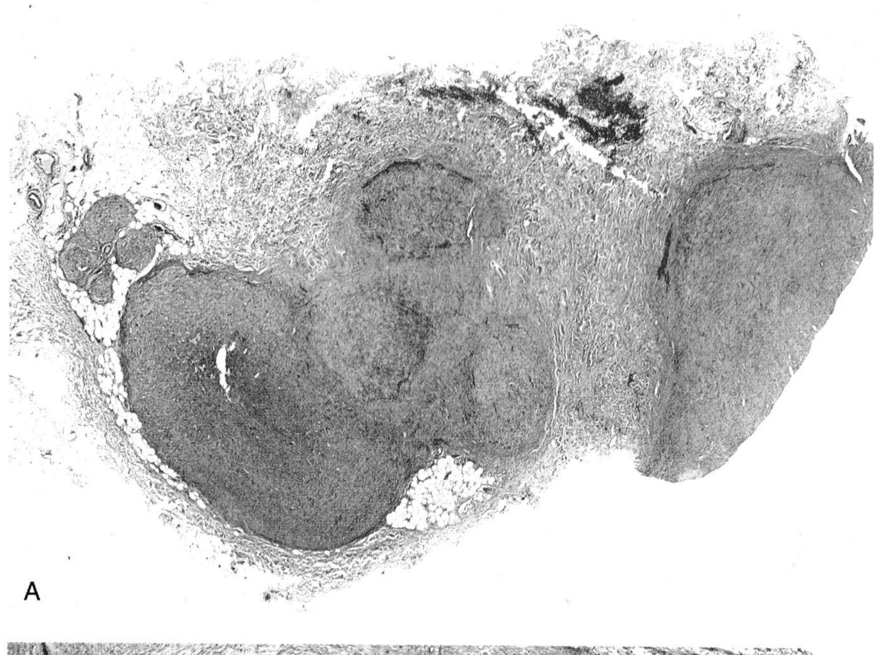


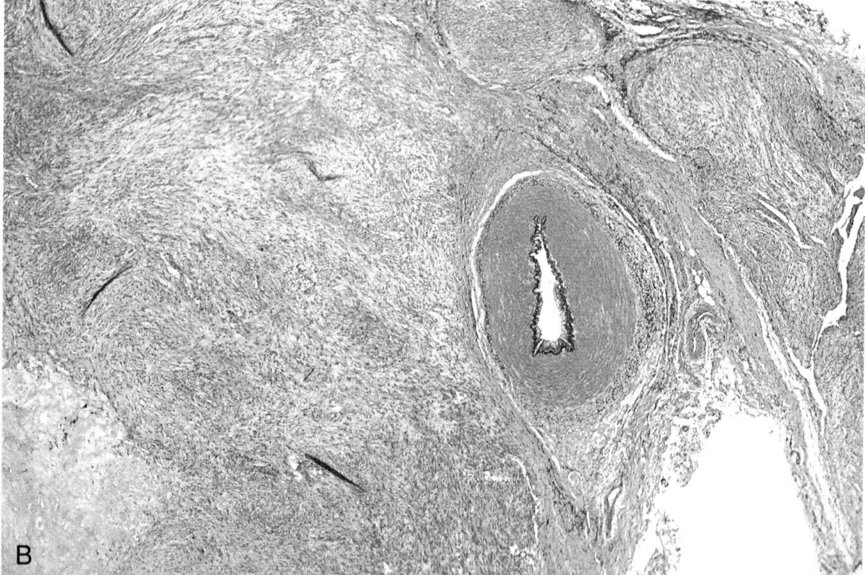


**FIGURE 9–15.** Intravascular fasciitis. (**A**) Low-power picture showing multinodular growth in several markedly dilated veins. (**B**) Movat stain of intravascular fasciitis outlining intravascular growth of the spindle cell proliferation.

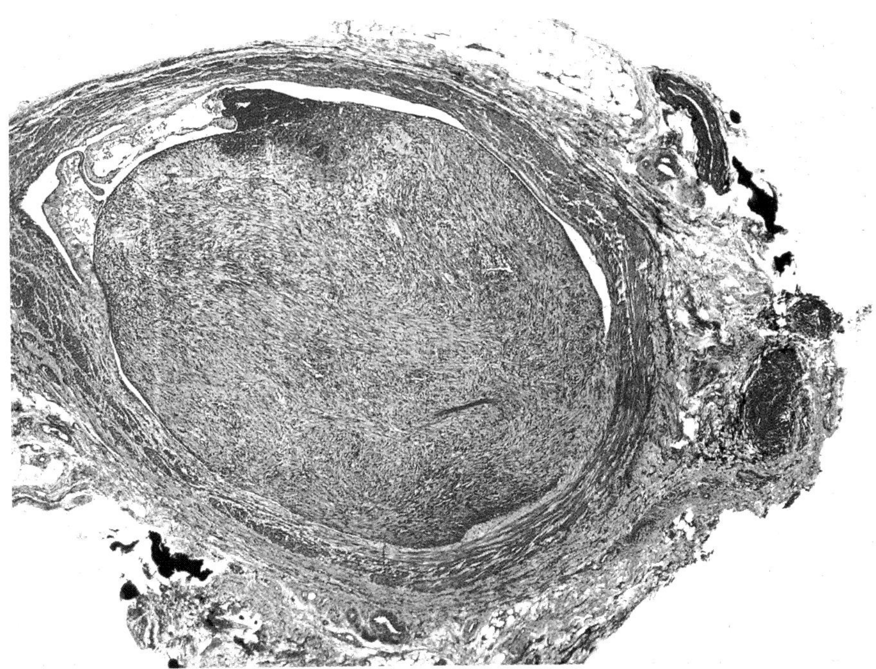

**FIGURE 9–16.** Movat stain of intravascular fasciitis highlighting the intravascular growth in a markedly dilated vein.

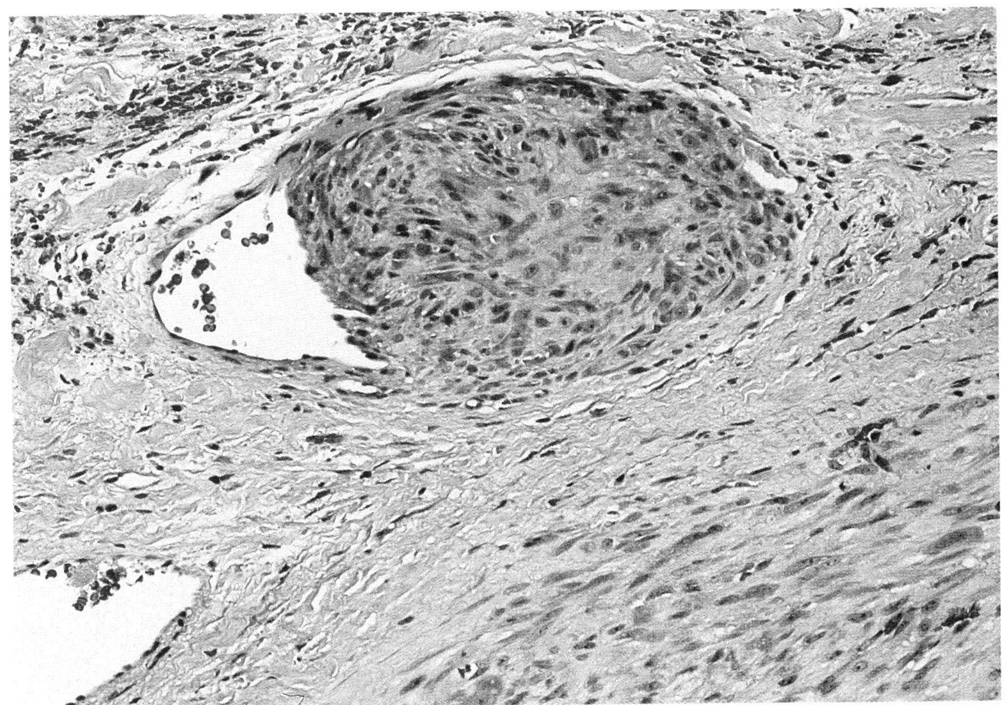

**FIGURE 9–17.** Small satellite nodule of intravascular fasciitis.

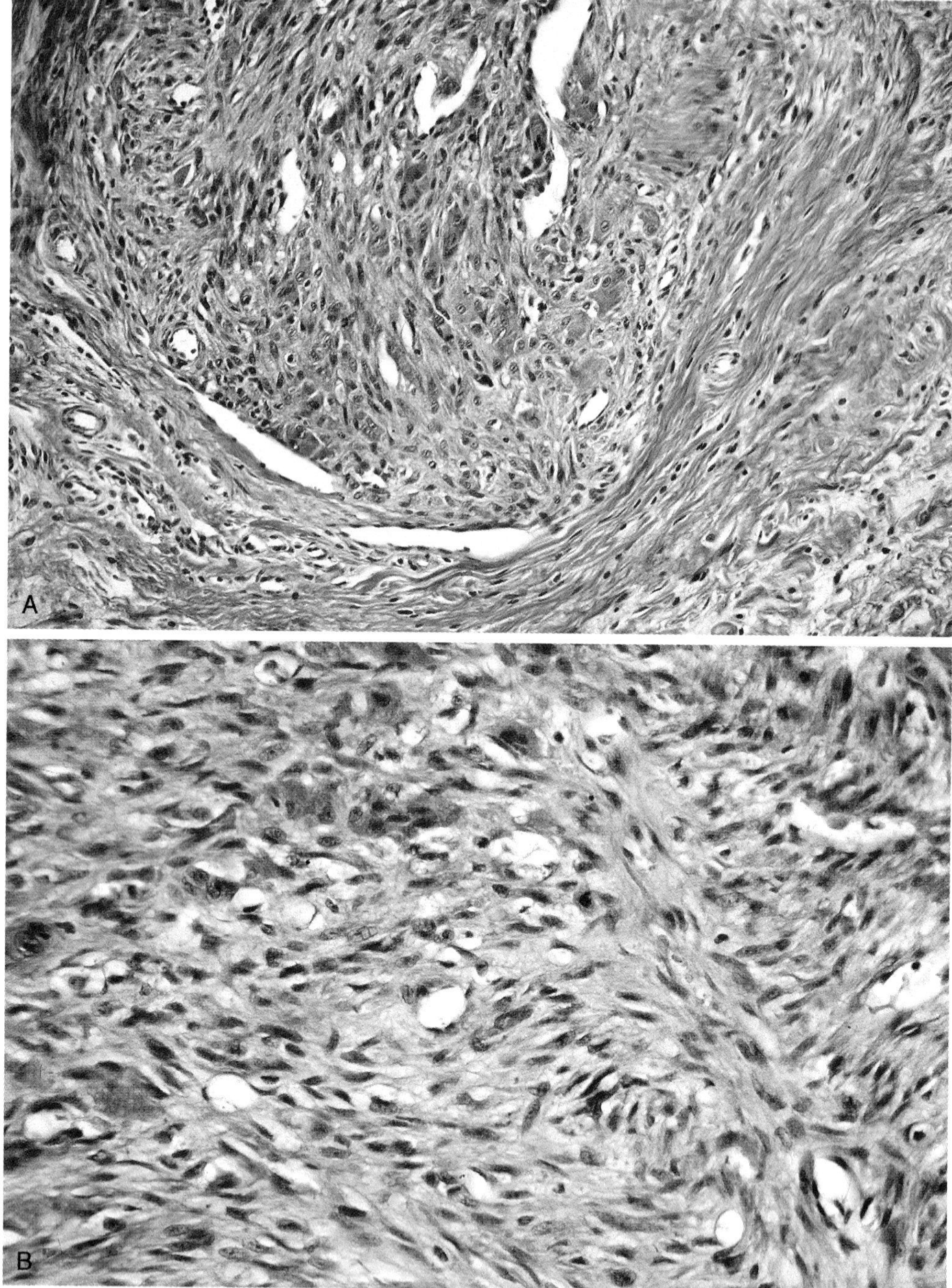


**FIGURE 9–18.** Intravascular fasciitis. (**A**) Intravascular proliferation of spindle-shaped cells with a conspicuous number of multinucleated giant cells. (**B**) Intravascular fasciitis composed of cytologically bland spindle cells similar to those found in nodular fasciitis.

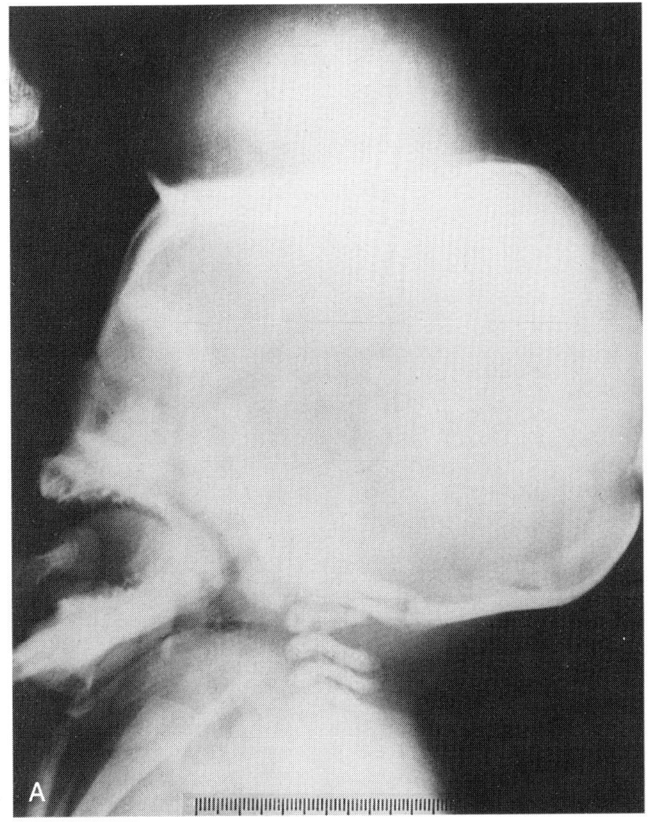


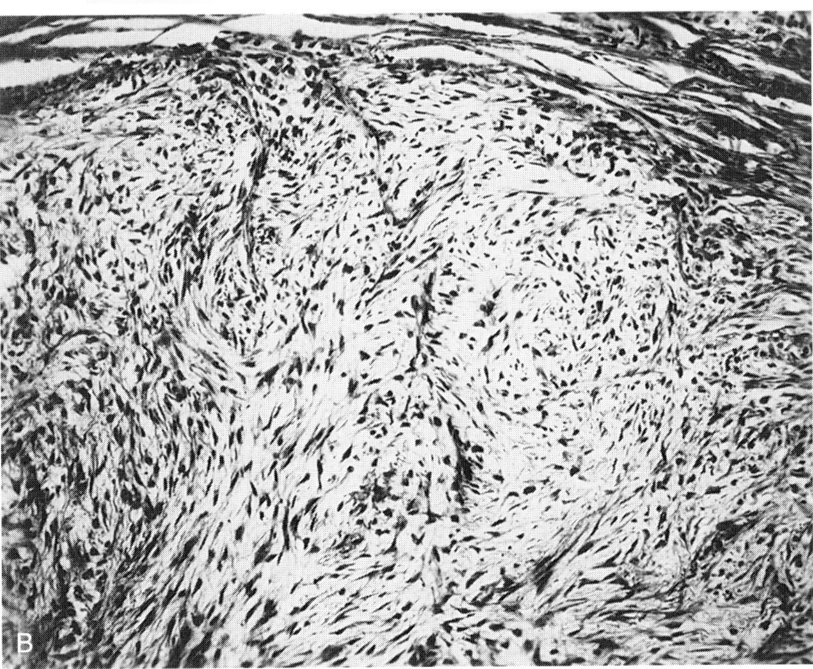


**FIGURE 9–19.** Cranial fasciitis. (**A**) Radiograph of large soft tissue mass attached to the inner table of the skull in an infant. (**B**) Histologic picture exhibiting proliferation of plump fibroblasts in a richly mucoid matrix.

### Immunohistochemical Findings

As one would expect in a lesion composed predominantly of myofibroblasts, most cells stain for smooth muscle actin and muscle-specific actin (Fig. 9–20). Although rare, desmin-positive cases have been reported.[46] This antigen, however, was not detected in any of the 53 cases of nodular fasciitis reported by Montgomery and Meis.[58] CD68 (KP1), a marker of lysosomes, is identified in macrophages and giant cells in these lesions and in a small number of the spindle cells, indicative of the acquisition of phagocytic properties.[58] Immunostains for cytokeratin and S-100 protein are typically negative.

### Ultrastructural Findings

Ultrastructurally, nodular fasciitis consists of elongated bipolar cells containing abundant intracytoplasmic rough endoplasmic reticulum, often with cisternae filled with finely granular, electron-dense material. The nuclei have a smooth nuclear membrane and finely dispersed chromatin. In many of the cells there are also intracytoplasmic bundles of electron-dense microfilaments with focal condensation, pinocytotic vesicles, and occasional desmosomes.[46,79] Collagen fibers and areas of basal lamina-like material surround many of the cells. All of these features are typical of myofibroblasts, a cell type that has been demonstrated in a variety of benign and malignant fibroblastic proliferations and appears to play a role in cellular contraction and motility.[43]

### Ancillary Findings

As suggested by the numerous mitotic figures that are typically present, nodular fasciitis has higher proliferative activity (as detected by antibodies to proliferating cell nuclear antigen) than other benign and malignant fibroblastic lesions.[60] However, the utility of these proliferative markers has not been established for distinguishing between these lesions for diagnostic purposes.

Few cases of nodular fasciitis have been evaluated cytogenetically. A reciprocal t(3;15)(q21;q22) and interstitial deletion (13)(q14q21),[69] loss of material from chromosomes 2 and 13, and a large acrocentric chromosome characterized as der (15)t(2;15)(q31;q26)[28] have been reported, confirming that karyotypic abnormalities may be found in reactive lesions as well as benign and malignant neoplasms.

### Differential Diagnosis

Nodular fasciitis may be confused with numerous benign and malignant mesenchymal lesions, and the differential diagnosis depends on the relative amounts of myxoid and fibrous stroma and the cellularity of the lesion in question. In fact, nodular fasciitis is the most common benign mesenchymal lesion misdiagnosed as a sarcoma. Hence many cases of nodular fasciitis have been treated by unnecessary and overly radical surgery.

Although nodular fasciitis and *myxoma* may display a prominent myxoid matrix, the latter lesion is readily recognized by its paucity of cells and its poor vascularization. Cellular nodular fasciitis may be confused with *fibrous histiocytoma,* and in a small number of cases distinction of these two lesions may be difficult if not somewhat arbitrary. The typical fibrous histiocytoma is dermis-based, less well circumscribed, and composed of a more polymorphous proliferation of spindle-shaped and round cells arranged in a more consistent storiform pattern. Secondary elements such as chronic inflammatory cells, xanthoma cells, siderophages, and Touton-type giant cells are also common. Peripherally located dense collagen fibers are typical; but similar-appearing fibers may occur in the central portion of nodular fasciitis, particularly in lesions of longer duration. Immunohistochemistry may play an ancillary role in distinguishing between these lesions, as most fibrous histiocytomas stain strongly for factor XIIIa,[44] in contrast to nodular fasciitis. Although smooth muscle actin can be focally present in a few cases of fibrous histiocytoma,[30] most nodular fasciitis lesions stain diffusely for this antigen.[58] In general, however, the distinction between the two lesions is best made on histologic sections rather than on minor differences in immunophenotype.

Some cases of nodular fasciitis resemble *fibromatosis.* Grossly, fibromatosis is a large, poorly circumscribed lesion that typically infiltrates the surrounding soft tissue, in contrast to the circumscribed nodular fasciitis lesion. Histologically, it is characterized by slender spindle-shaped fibroblasts arranged in long sweeping fascicles and separated by abundant collagen. Mitotic figures occur in both lesions, but they are much less frequent in musculoaponeurotic fibromatosis than in nodular fasciitis.

Distinction from *fibrosarcoma* is primarily a matter of growth pattern and cellularity. The cells in fibrosarcoma are nearly always densely packed and are arranged in interweaving bundles resulting in the characteristic "herringbone" pattern. Moreover, the individual cells are marked by a greater variation in size and shape, hyperchromatic nuclei, and a more pronounced mitotic rate, including atypical mitotic figures. The deep location, large size, and long duration of most fibrosarcomas also aid in the differential diagnosis.

Of the malignant myxoid lesions, *myxoid malignant fibrous histiocytoma (myxofibrosarcoma)* may closely re-

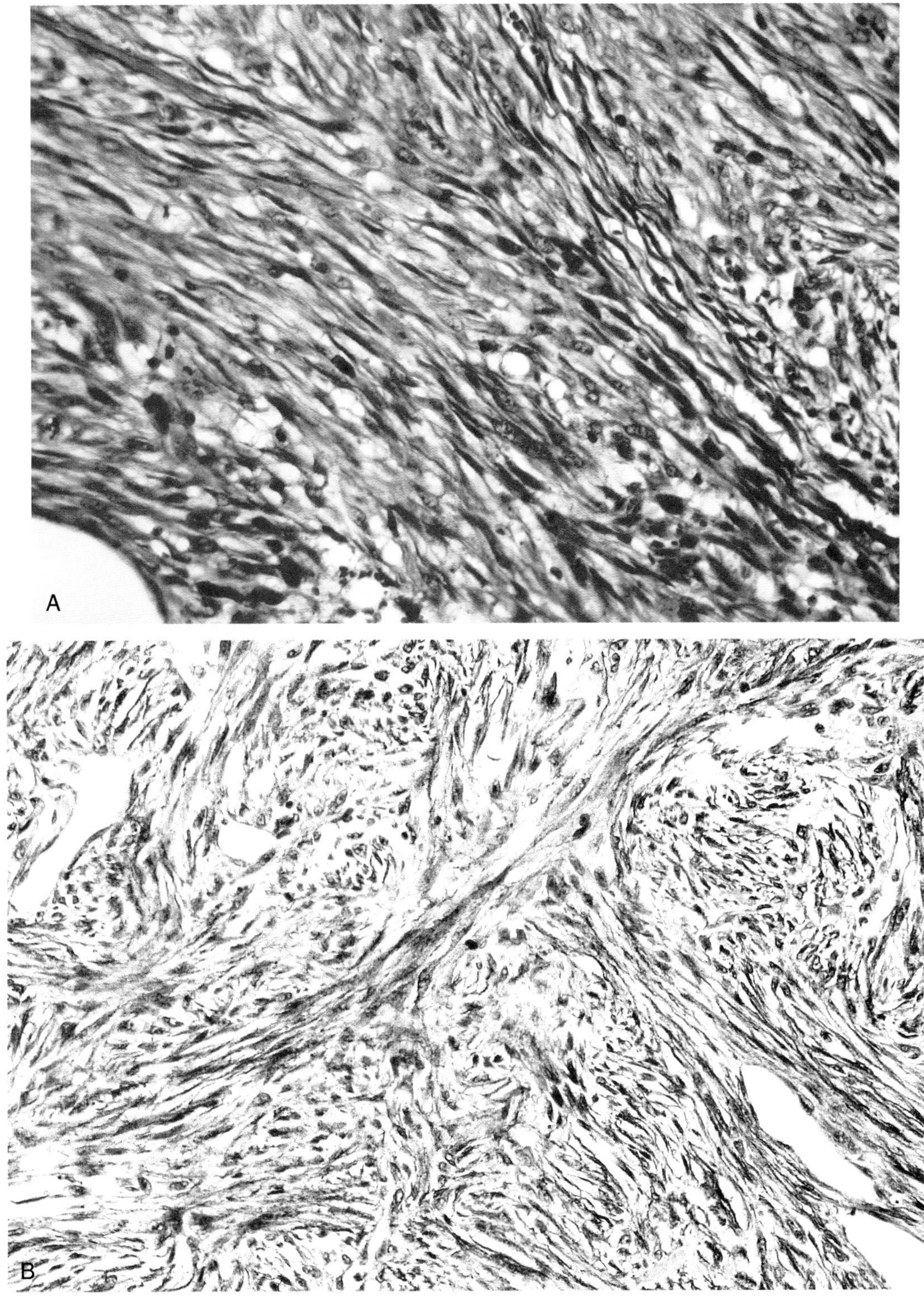

**FIGURE 9–20.** Nodular fasciitis. (**A**) Masson trichrome stain reveals fuchsinophilia of spindle cells. (**B**) Nodular fasciitis with diffuse smooth muscle actin immunoreactivity.

semble nodular fasciitis. This lesion occurs principally in patients older than 50 years and usually measures more than 3 cm when first excised. Microscopically, the cells show more nuclear pleomorphism, and there is typically a regular arborizing vasculature composed of coarse vessels, often invested with tumor cells. Atypical mitotic figures may be seen, as may areas of transition to high-grade pleomorphic-storiform malignant fibrous histiocytoma.

### Discussion

Although a well documented history of trauma is present in a small number of cases, nodular fasciitis is clearly a benign, reactive process that is likely triggered by local injury or in response to a localized inflammatory process. Bernstein and Lattes noted the presence of a central region containing residual fibrin clot, often surrounded by a radial proliferation of capillaries, raising the possibility that nodular fasciitis is an atypical form of granulation tissue brought about by minor trauma.[27] Regardless of the precise cause, histologic recognition of this reactive pattern is important to avoid misdiagnosing a sarcoma and unnecessary radical surgical treatment. The benign nature and excellent prognosis of nodular fasciitis has been well documented by numerous large clinicopathologic studies (Table 9–3). In the series of 895 cases reported by Allen,[25] only 9 (1%) reappeared after attempted complete surgical excision. Even those lesions that are incompletely excised rarely recur. Of the 18 cases of recurrent nodular fasciitis in the series by Bernstein and Lattes,[27] a review of the histology and clinical course led to revision of the original diagnosis in all 18 cases. In fact, these authors stated that recurrence of a lesion initially diagnosed as nodular fasciitis should lead to reappraisal of the original pathologic findings.

Several authors have reported the utility of fine-needle aspiration cytology for diagnosing nodular fasciitis.[34,41,51,74] However, this technique is limited by sampling error, and the aspirate must be interpreted in a clinical correlative fashion. In keeping with its benign nature, most cases of nodular fasciitis have been found to have a diploid DNA content.[39,59]

**TABLE 9–3 RECURRENCE RATES IN LARGE SERIES OF NODULAR FASCIITIS**

| First Author | Recurrence | % |
|---|---|---|
| Bernstein[27] | 18/134* | 13 |
| Shimizu[72] | 1/139 | 1 |
| Price[63] | 0/32 | 0 |
| Allen[25] | 9/895 | 1 |

*Upon re-review, all recurrent lesions were reclassified as something other than nodular fasciitis.

## PROLIFERATIVE FASCIITIS

Proliferative fasciitis, a term coined by Chung and Enzinger in 1975,[84] is the subcutaneous counterpart of proliferative myositis. Both of these lesions are pseudosarcomatous myofibroblastic proliferations characterized by the presence of unusual giant cells resembling ganglion cells. The microscopic appearance of the lesion is highly suggestive of a sarcoma, and many cases of this type have been misinterpreted in the past as embryonal rhabdomyosarcoma, ganglioneuroblastoma, or some other type of malignant neoplasm.[98]

### Clinical Findings

Proliferative fasciitis is a lesion of adult life, with most patients being 40–70 years of age (mean 54 years).[84,98] Thus as a group, patients with proliferative fasciitis tend to be older than those with nodular fasciitis. It is uncommon for patients younger than 15 years of age to develop proliferative fasciitis.[101] There is no gender or race predilection, and most of the lesions occur in the subcutaneous tissues of the extremities, with the upper extremity (especially the forearm) affected more commonly than the lower extremity. The lesion also occurs with some frequency on the trunk and rarely on the head and neck.

Clinically, most patients present with a firm, palpable subcutaneous nodule that is freely movable and unattached to the overlying skin, although about two-thirds of patients also have complaints of pain or tenderness. Most lesions measure less than 5 cm in greatest diameter, with a median size of 2.5 cm. Like nodular fasciitis, these lesions are typically rapidly growing, most being excised 2–6 weeks after their initial discovery. A history of trauma in the vicinity of the mass is elicited in about one-third of cases.[84]

### Pathologic Findings

Grossly, the lesion is usually poorly circumscribed, forming an elongated or discoid-shaped mass that predominantly involves the subcutaneous tissue, although some involve the superficial fascia. Rare lesions also involve the superficial skeletal muscle, making it difficult to distinguish it from proliferative myositis. The rare cases that arise during childhood tend to be more circumscribed and vaguely lobular, with only occasional extension along fascial planes.[101]

Microscopically, like nodular fasciitis, proliferative

fasciitis is composed of tissue culture-like fibroblastic and myofibroblastic spindle cells that have bland cytologic features and are deposited in a variably myxoid and collagenous stroma. This proliferation typically extends along the interlobular septa of the subcutaneous tissue, with some extension along the superficial fascia (Figs. 9–21, 9–22). The lesion is characterized by the presence of large basophilic cells with one or two vesicular nuclei and prominent nucleoli. The cells have abundant basophilic, slightly granular cytoplasm but lack cross-striations typical of rhabdomyoblasts (Figs. 9–23, 9–24, 9–25). Some cells have intracytoplasmic inclusions of collagen. These ganglion-like cells may be packed together or loosely arranged in aggregates. Multinucleated giant cells of the type seen in nodular fasciitis are rare in proliferative fasciitis. In children, the lesions tend to be more cellular (Fig. 9–26), have numerous mitoses, and have foci of acute inflammation and necrosis, features that are distinctly unusual in the typical adult form.[101] Childhood cases also tend to have less collagen and a less conspicuous myxoid matrix than their adult counterparts. Some lesions, particularly those that have been present for a long duration prior to excision, may have abundant hyalinized collagen that surrounds the ganglion-like cells, which could cause confusion with neoplastic osteoid and a misdiagnosis of osteosarcoma.

The immunohistochemical findings of proliferative fasciitis are similar to those of nodular fasciitis. The spindle and stellate-shaped cells stain for vimentin and both muscle-specific and smooth muscle actin. Some cells stain for CD68 (KP1); immunostains for cytokeratins, S-100 protein, and desmin are usually negative.[89,97,99,101] The ganglion-like cells may also stain for actin, although the staining is often focal and weak and may be membranous in distribution.[99,101]

Ultrastructurally, the spindle- and stellate-shaped cells have the typical features of fibroblasts and myofibroblasts.[85,88,107,108] The ganglion-like cells are characterized by abundant rough endoplasmic reticulum with dilated cisternae, some of which may contain short-spacing collagen fibrils.[67,93] Cell junctions and Z-line formations are not seen.

## PROLIFERATIVE MYOSITIS

Proliferative myositis is the intramuscular counterpart of proliferative fasciitis. Although Kern is credited with the original description of proliferative myositis,[96] Ackerman probably reported the first cases in his study of "extraosseous nonneoplastic localized bone and cartilage formation."[80] Like proliferative fasciitis, it is a rapidly growing lesion that infiltrates muscle tissue in a diffuse manner. It is characterized by bizarre giant cells bearing a close resemblance to ganglion cells.

### Clinical Findings

The symptoms are nonspecific, and the diagnosis always rests on the histologic examination of tissue obtained by biopsy or excision. In most cases the lesion is first noted as a palpable, more or less discrete, solitary nodular mass that measures 1–6 cm in diameter. It rarely causes tenderness or pain, even though it may double in size within a period of a few days. The duration between onset and excision is usually less than 3 weeks.[91,94]

The patients tend to be older than those with nodular fasciitis, with a median age of 50 years.[91] Rare cases of proliferative myositis have been described in children.[101,103,104] There seems to be no predilection for either gender or any particular race. The lesion mainly affects the flat muscles of the trunk and shoulder girdle, especially the pectoralis, latissimus dorsi, or serratus anterior muscle. Occasionally, tumors are also found in the muscles of the thigh. Involvement of the head and neck is rare.[82,87]

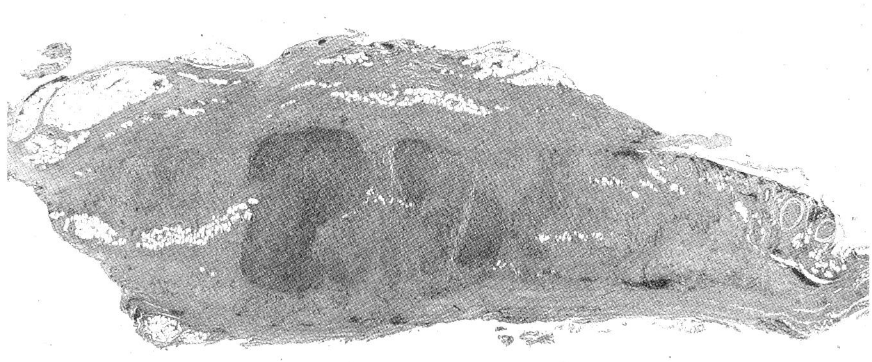

**FIGURE 9–21.** Proliferative fasciitis involving the subcutis.

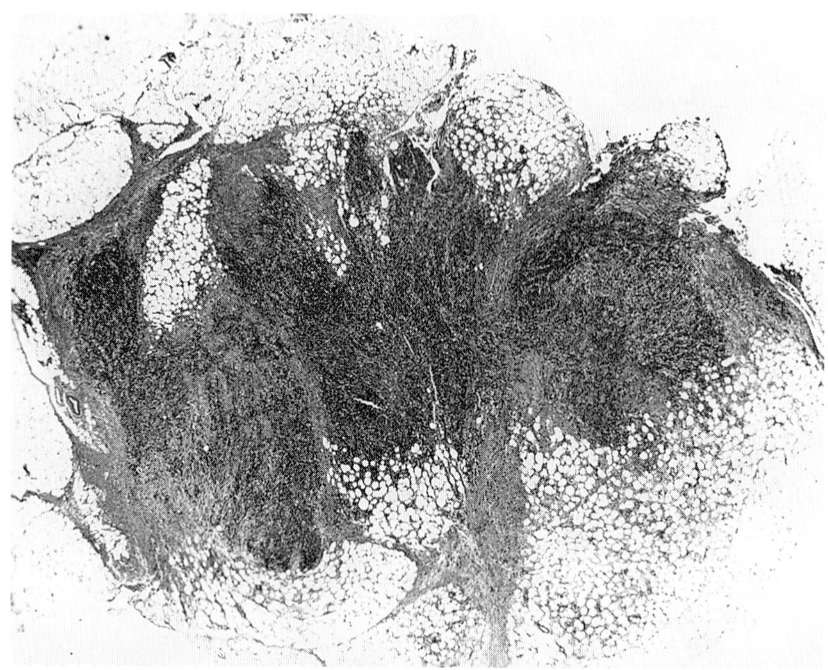

**FIGURE 9–22.** Proliferative fasciitis with an irregular stellate appearance.

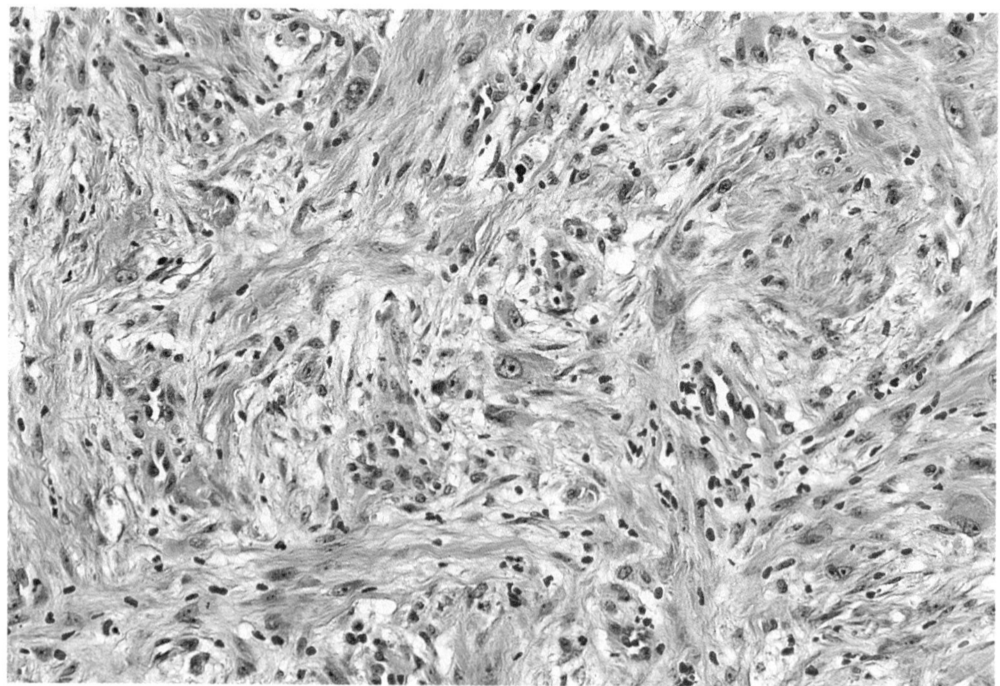

**FIGURE 9–23.** Proliferative fasciitis composed of a mixture of fibroblasts and giant cells with abundant basophilic cytoplasm bearing some resemblance to ganglion cells.

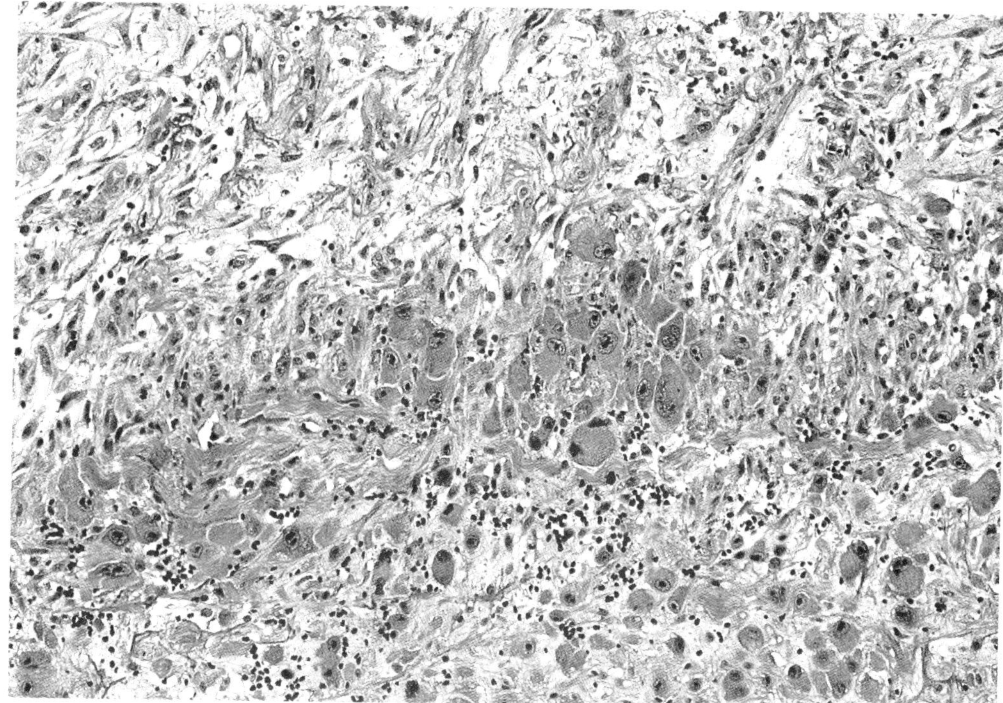

**FIGURE 9–24.** Peripheral portion of proliferative fasciitis with numerous ganglion-like giant cells.

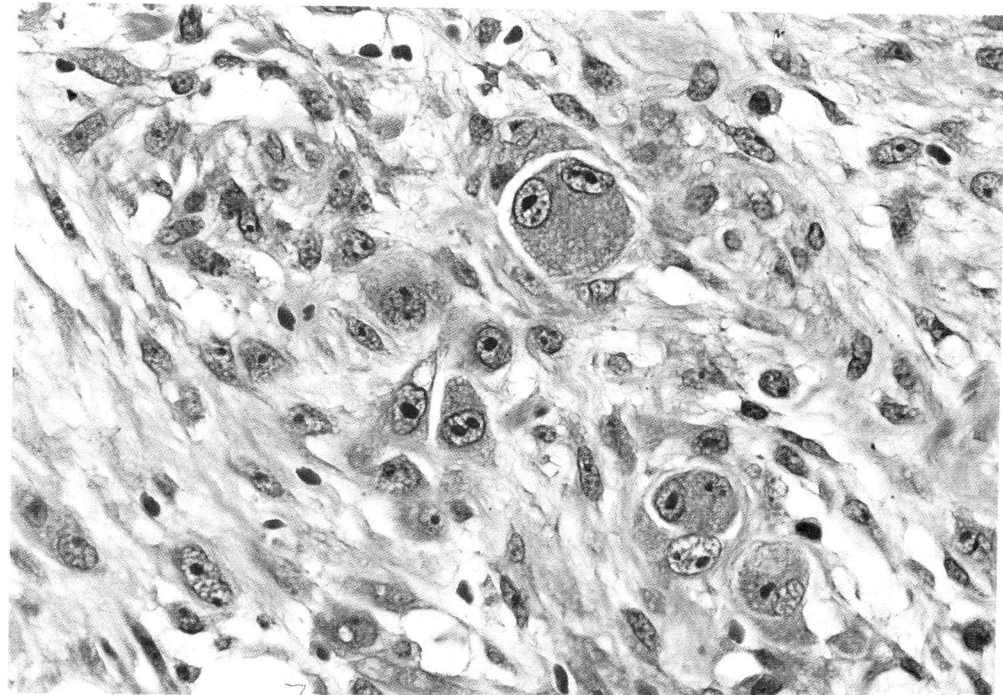

**FIGURE 9–25.** Proliferative fasciitis with large ganglion-like cells, some of which are multinucleated.

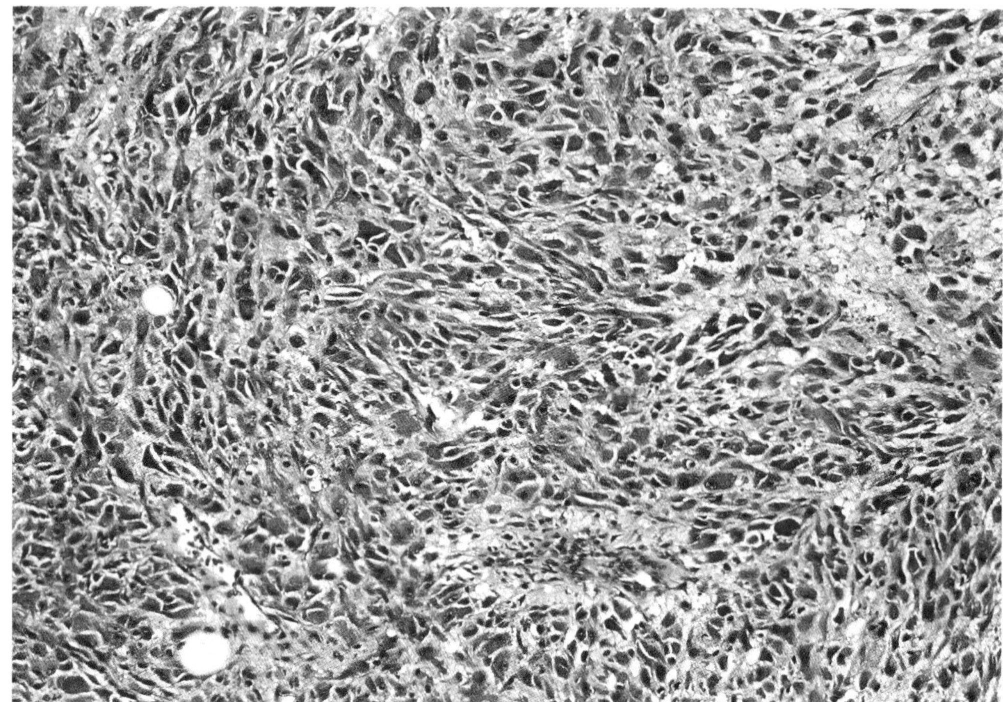

**FIGURE 9–26.** Proliferative fasciitis of childhood composed of round and polygonal cells with abundant cytoplasm and prominent nucleoli.

## Gross Findings

Similar to proliferative fasciitis, proliferative myositis typically appears pale gray or scar-like, resulting in induration of the involved skeletal muscle (Fig. 9–27). When present in small or flat muscles, it often replaces most or all of the involved musculature. When involving large muscles, there is preferential involvement of the skeletal muscle immediately underneath the fascia with a progressive decrease in the central portion of the muscle in a wedge-like fashion.

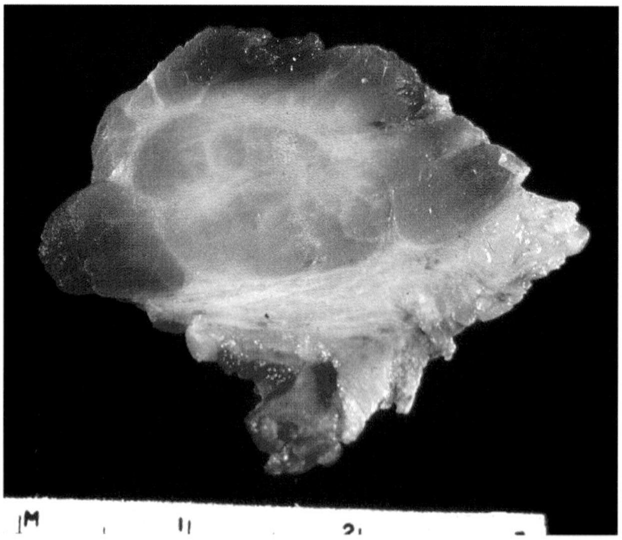

**FIGURE 9–27.** Proliferative myositis characterized by a poorly circumscribed scar-like fibrosing process involving muscle and muscle fascia.

## Microscopic Findings

The cellular components of proliferative myositis are identical to those found in proliferative fasciitis. There is a poorly demarcated proliferation of fibroblast-like cells that involve the epimysium, perimysium, and endomysium. Unlike the intramuscular form of nodular fasciitis and musculoaponeurotic fibromatosis, this cellular proliferation rarely completely replaces large areas of the involved muscle but, rather, is most striking in the subfascial region and interfascicular connective tissue septa. The skeletal muscle fibers are relatively unaffected except for the presence of secondary atrophy, with neither sarcolemmal proliferation nor any evidence of skeletal muscle regeneration. This alternation of proliferating fibrous tissue with persistent atrophic skeletal muscle fibers results in a typical "checkerboard" pattern that is apparent at low magnification (Fig. 9–28). The other conspicuous histologic feature of proliferative myositis is the presence of large basophilic ganglion-like cells, identical to those found in proliferative fasciitis (Figs. 9–29, 9–30). Occasional giant cells contain eosinophilic collagen inclusions. Mitotic figures are often easily identi-

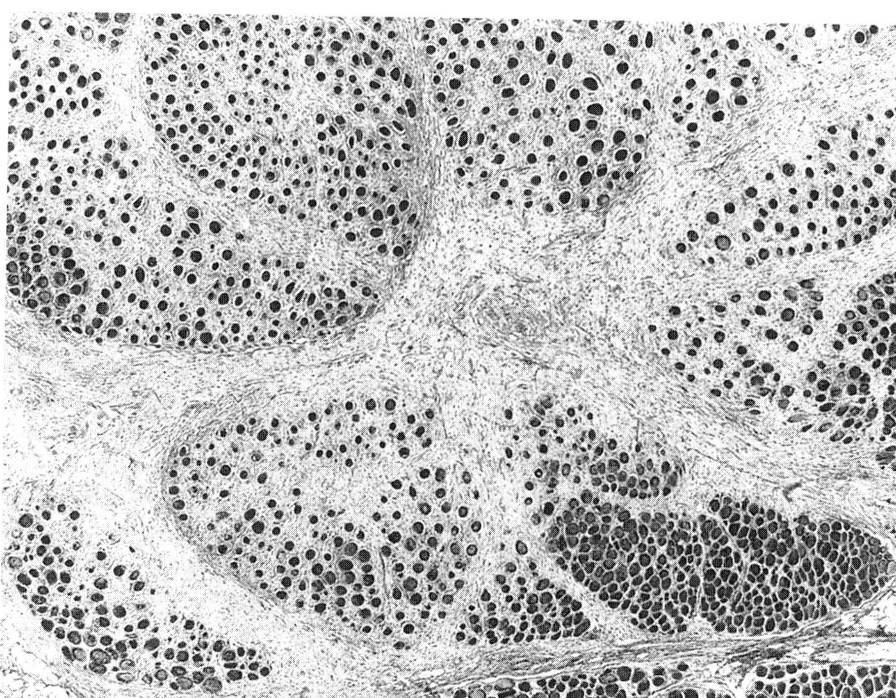

**FIGURE 9–28.** Low-power view of proliferative myositis. The muscle bundles are separated by endomysial and epimysial proliferation of fibrous connective tissue in a checkerboard-like fashion.

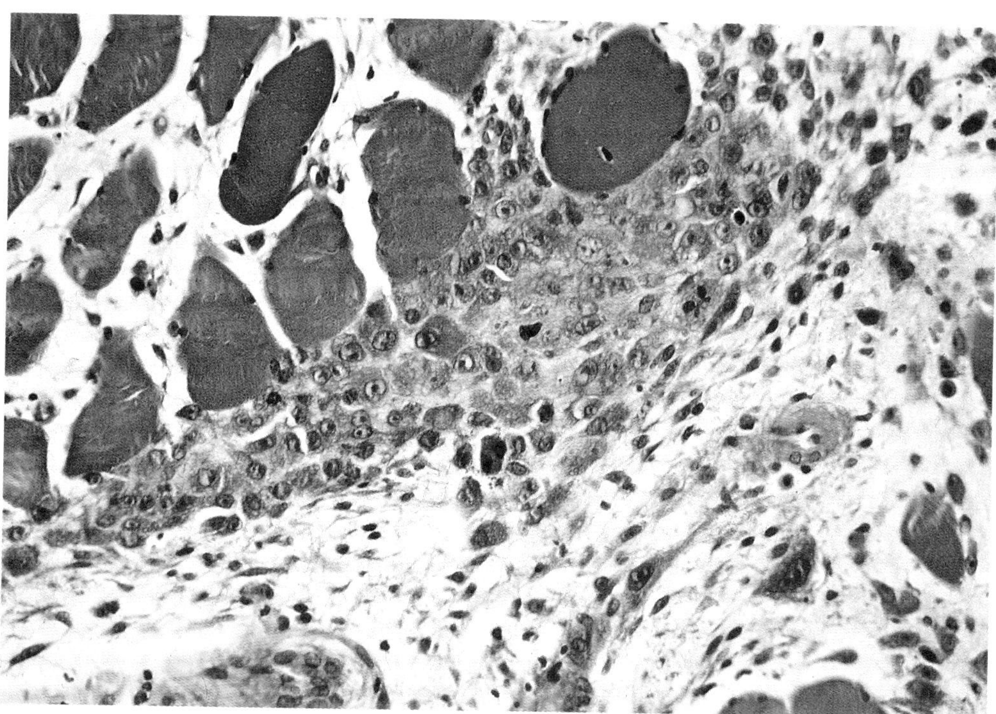

**FIGURE 9–29.** Proliferative myositis. Ganglion-like giant cells are seen immediately adjacent to and infiltrating skeletal muscle fibers.

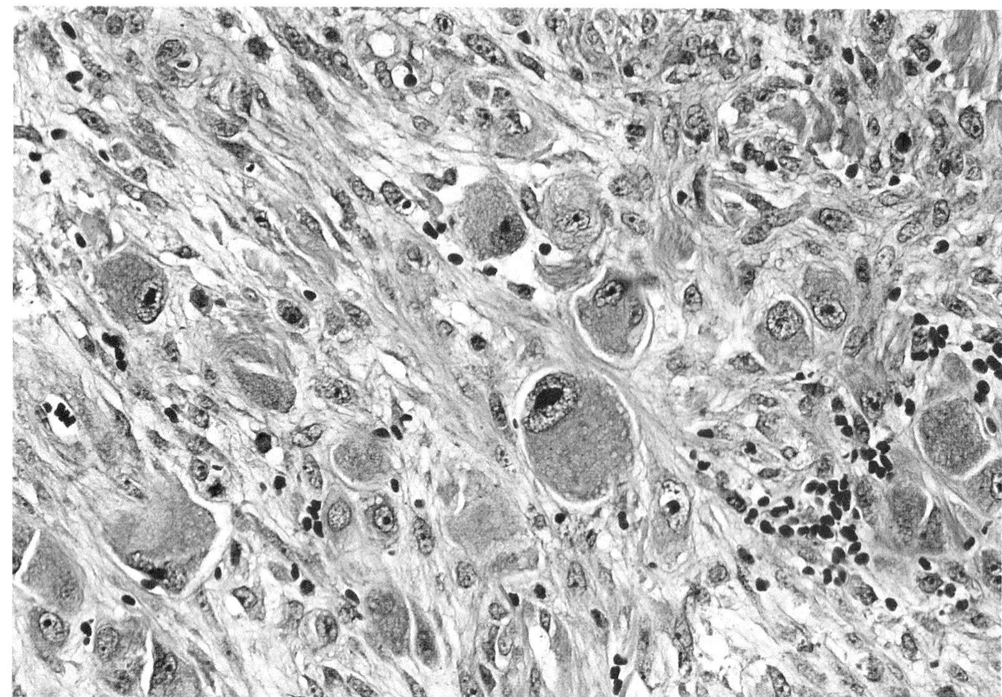

**FIGURE 9–30.** High-power view of ganglion-like giant cells in proliferative myositis.

fied in both the spindle and giant cells, although atypical mitoses are not seen. Rare lesions contain foci of metaplastic bone (Fig. 9–31).

The immunohistochemical and ultrastructural features of proliferative myositis are identical to those of proliferative fasciitis, with most cells showing evidence of myofibroblastic differentiation.[94,106] Both the spindle and giant cells express vimentin, muscle-specific actin, and smooth muscle actin (Fig. 9–32); immunostains for desmin and myoglobin are typically negative.[81,89,92]

Trisomy 2 has been described in both proliferative fasciitis[86] and proliferative myositis,[102] and t(6;14) was described in a single case of proliferative myositis.[100] Flow cytometric DNA analysis of these lesions has revealed a uniformly diploid pattern.[90,99]

## Differential Diagnosis

Proliferative fasciitis and myositis may be mistaken for a variety of malignant neoplasms, most commonly *rhabdomyosarcoma* or *ganglioneuroblastoma*. In the series of 53 cases of proliferative fasciitis by Chung and Enzinger, 16 were originally diagnosed as a sarcoma.[84] Similarly, 14 of 33 cases of proliferative myositis reported by Enzinger and Dulcey were believed to be some type of sarcoma.[91] Errors are most likely to occur with proliferative fasciitis or myositis during childhood, where rhabdomyosarcoma is a strong diagnostic consideration. The history of a rapidly growing mass of short duration that typically attains a maximum size of less than 3 cm is more consistent with a reactive process than a sarcoma. Histologically, the ganglion-like cells lack cross-striations and show more cytoplasmic basophilia than is seen in rhabdomyoblasts. Although the immunohistochemical profiles may overlap, stains for desmin and myoglobin are usually negative in the ganglion-like cells, in contrast to the staining found in true rhabdomyoblasts. Although ganglioneuroblastoma is also a consideration, proliferative fasciitis and myositis lack a fibrillary background, and the ganglion-like cells may express actin, unlike true ganglion cells.

## Discussion

Proliferative fasciitis and myositis, like nodular fasciitis, are self-limiting, benign, reactive processes that are probably preceded by some type of fascial or muscular injury resulting in a proliferation of myofibroblasts. However, only a small number of patients report a preceding injury in the exact location of the lesion, raising the possibility that causes other than mechanical trauma play a role in the development of proliferative fasciitis and myositis. Although some have reported the diagnosis of these lesions by fine-needle aspiration cytology,[83,95,99,105] the unusual histologic features of these lesions warrant caution with this technique. The lesions are adequately treated by local excision, and recurrence is rare.[84]

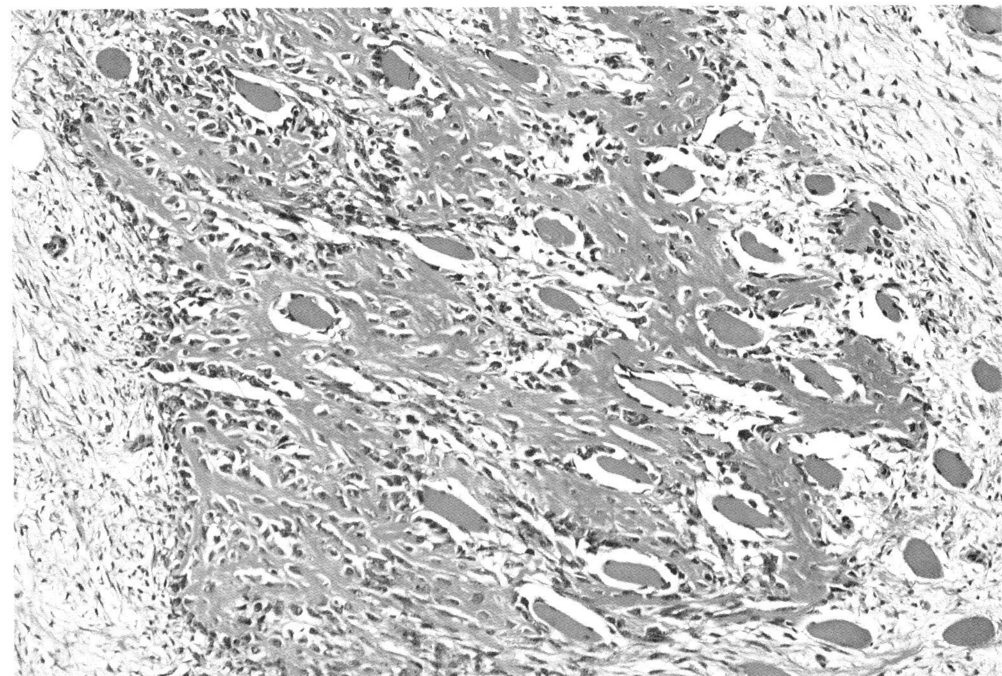

**FIGURE 9–31.** Unusual case of proliferative myositis with extensive metaplastic bone formation.

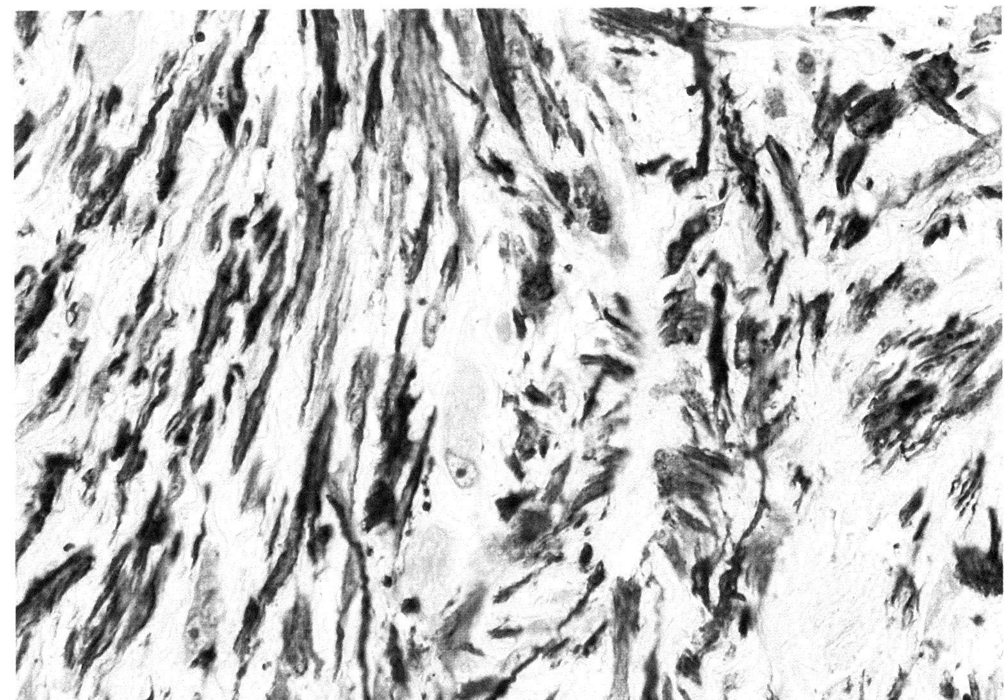

**FIGURE 9–32.** Proliferative myositis stained for smooth muscle actin. Most spindle cells stain for this antigen, but the ganglion-like cells in this case are negative.

## ORGAN-ASSOCIATED PSEUDOSARCOMATOUS MYOFIBROBLASTIC PROLIFERATIONS

Organ-associated pseudosarcomatous myofibroblastic proliferations, most of which arise in the genitourinary tract, have been described under a variety of names, including *inflammatory pseudotumor*,[111,113,116,120,123,127,133] *pseudosarcomatous fibromyxoid tumor*,[130,132] *atypical myofibroblastic tumor*,[114] *atypical fibromyxoid tumor*,[115] *pseudosarcomatous myofibroblastic proliferation*,[109] *plasma cell granuloma*,[121] and *nodular fasciitis*.[112] They probably represent an exuberant reparative reaction, although not all are associated with previous biopsy or surgical trauma. They have overlapping clinical and morphologic features with the so-called *postoperative spindle cell nodule*, a lesion that has the propensity to develop in the genitourinary tract soon after surgical trauma.[110,119,122,124,126,128,129,134,136] The discussion below centers on those pseudosarcomatous lesions that appear to arise spontaneously (inflammatory pseudotumor) and those associated with surgical trauma (postoperative spindle cell nodule).

### Clinical Findings

Inflammatory pseudotumors of the genitourinary tract are most common in the urinary bladder, but they have also been described in the prostate,[27,137] urethra,[137] and ureter.[118] These lesions seem to arise spontaneously, most commonly in children or young adults, although the age range is broad. Females are affected about twice as often as males. When they arise in the urinary bladder, most patients present with hematuria, dysuria, or recurrent cystitis.[135]

The postoperative spindle cell nodule typically arises in the vagina, vulva, urinary bladder, or prostatic urethra 5–12 weeks following a surgical procedure. Unlike inflammatory pseudotumor, males and females are equally affected.

### Pathologic Findings

Grossly, most lesions present as exophytic, nodular or polypoid intramural lesions that may extend deeply into the visceral organ from which they arise. They range in size from 1.5 to 9.0 cm, although most are 3–5 cm. The lesion may be firm or soft, depending on the amount of myxoid stroma present; and it has a gray-tan appearance that may be due to focal hemorrhage.

On microscopic examination, the lesion is characterized by a spindle cell proliferation in a loose, edematous, myxoid stroma associated with granulation tissue-type vessels and a mixed acute and chronic inflammatory infiltrate (Fig. 9–33). The spindle cells are arranged in a haphazard fashion and bear close resemblance to the cells seen in nodular fasciitis; they lack cytologic atypia or nuclear hyperchromasia and have bipolar or stellate-shaped cytoplasmic processes (Fig. 9–34). Most commonly, spindle cells are widely separated and haphazardly distributed in a myxoid stroma composed predominantly of hyaluronic acid. Some are characterized by more cellular areas in

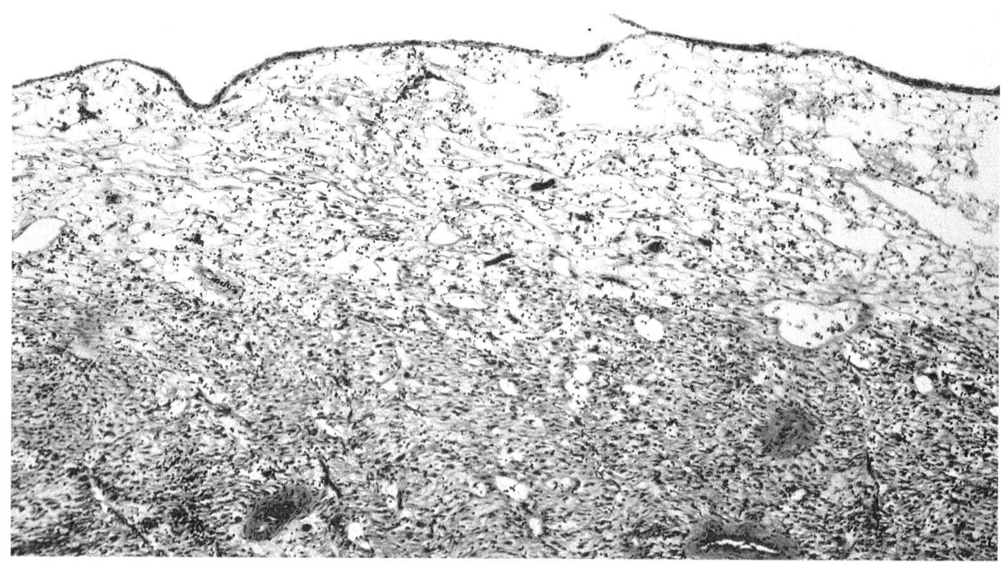

**FIGURE 9–33.** Inflammatory pseudotumor (pseudosarcomatous fibromyxoid tumor) of the urinary bladder. Proliferation of spindle cells in a loose, edematous, myxoid stroma with mixed acute and chronic inflammatory cells.

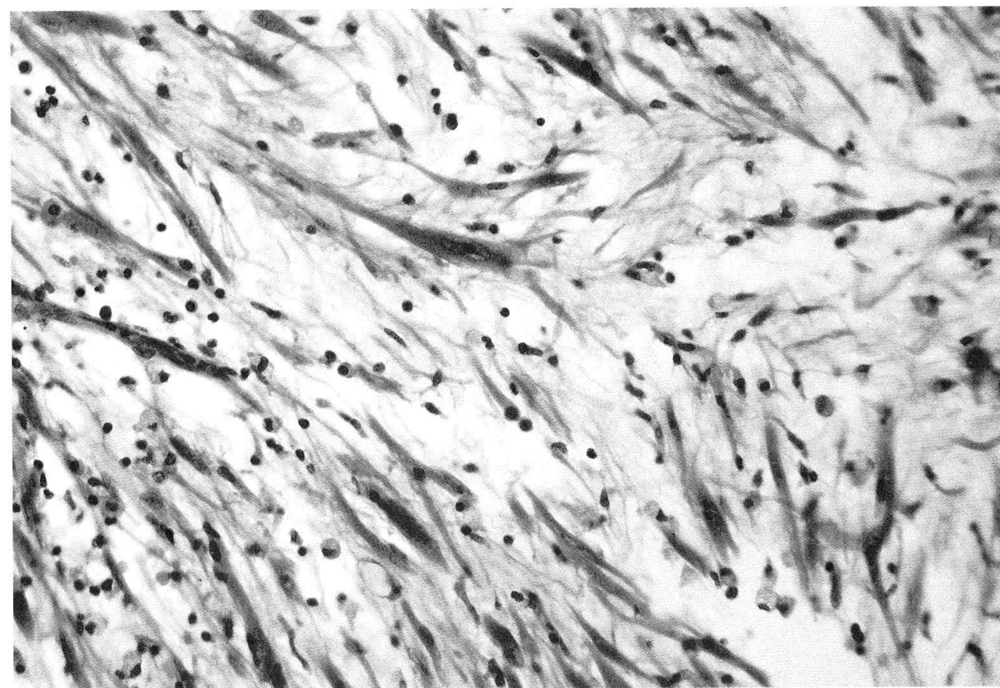

**FIGURE 9–34.** High-power view of inflammatory pseudotumor (pseudosarcomatous fibromyxoid tumor) of the urinary bladder. Haphazard arrangement of spindle cells with bipolar or stellate-shaped cytoplasmic processes deposited in a myxoid stroma with scattered chronic inflammatory cells.

which the cells are arranged in irregular fascicles with variable amounts of intercellular collagen. The cells have oval to spindle-shaped nuclei with open chromatin, variably sized nucleoli, and eosinophilic to amphophilic cytoplasm. Mitotic figures are present, usually with fewer than 1–2 mitoses/10 high-power fields (HPF), and they are not atypical. In the more myxoid areas, there is a prominent capillary network often associated with extravasated erythrocytes. A mixed inflammatory infiltrate composed of lymphocytes, plasma cells, eosinophils, and occasional mast cells is usually conspicuous. When present, neutrophils are associated with areas of mucosal ulceration.

A postoperative spindle cell nodule is composed of a compact spindle cell proliferation with easily identifiable mitotic figures deposited in a less conspicuous myxoid background than that found in inflammatory pseudotumors. Cytologic atypia is minimal or mild, and necrosis is found only near the ulcerated surface.

Immunohistochemical tests reveal that the spindle cells stain strongly for vimentin and various muscle markers, including muscle-specific actin, smooth muscle actin, and desmin. In addition, it is not uncommon to find scattered cells that stain for cytokeratin, epithelial membrane antigen, or both, although the tumor cells are negative for myoglobin and S-100 protein.[117,119,125,131]

Ultrastructurally, the cells show prominent myofibroblastic features, with bipolar cytoplasmic processes containing abundant rough endoplasmic reticulum and peripheral bundles of thin filaments with focal densities.[120] The immunohistochemical and ultrastructural features of a postoperative spindle cell nodule overlap those found in inflammatory pseudotumor.

## Differential Diagnosis

Although inflammatory pseudotumor should be suspected when one encounters a spindle cell lesion in a young patient with no history of surgery at that site, numerous other benign and malignant spindle cell proliferations should be considered (Table 9–4). *Myxoid leiomyosarcoma* may be difficult to distinguish from inflammatory pseudotumor. This tumor tends to occur in older patients and is rare before the age of 20 years. Microscopically, the tumor is composed of spindle to epithelioid cells with eosinophilic fibrillar cytoplasm, often with a perinuclear vacuole, deposited in a myxoid stroma. Inflammatory pseudotumors are characterized by a more prominent vasculature, more variable cellularity, and a more conspicuous inflammatory component. Ultrastructural features suggesting smooth muscle differentiation are useful, as myxoid leiomyosarcoma and inflammatory pseudotumor have overlapping immunophenotypes, with the expression of actin and desmin.

The *botryoid-type rhabdomyosarcoma* is a diagnostic consideration but it is characterized by the presence

**TABLE 9–4** DIFFERENTIAL DIAGNOSTIC FEATURES OF INFLAMMATORY PSEUDOTUMOR OF THE GENITOURINARY TRACT

| Feature | IP | PSCN | ML | RMS | SC |
|---|---|---|---|---|---|
| Cellularity | + | ++ | +/++ | +/++ | ++ |
| Growth pattern | Loose | Intersecting | Loose | Botryoid | Biphasic |
| Pleomorphism | + | + | +/++ | ++ | +++ |
| Mitoses | −/+ | ++ | ++ | ++ | ++ |
| Electron microscopy | Fibroblasts/myofibroblasts | Fibroblasts/myofibroblasts | Smooth muscle | Striated muscle | Epithelial |
| Keratin | −/+ | −/+ | −/+ | −/+ | + |
| Desmin | −/+ | −/+ | + | + | −/+ |
| SMA | + | + | + | − | −/+ |

Modified from Ro JY, El-Naggar AK, Amin MB, et al. Pseudosarcomatous fibromyxoid tumor of the urinary bladder and prostate: immunohistochemical, ultrastructural and DNA flow cytometric analyses of nine cases. Hum Pathol 24:1203, 1993, with permission.

IP, inflammatory pseudotumor; PSCN, postoperative spindle cell nodule; ML, myxoid leiomyosarcoma; RMS, rhabdomyosarcoma; SC, sarcomatoid carcinoma; SMA, smooth muscle actin.

of a cambium layer under the epithelium composed of atypical hyperchromatic cells, occasionally with rhabdomyoblastic differentiation. Immunohistochemical and ultrastructural analysis reveal evidence of skeletal muscle differentiation.

The immunohistochemical detection of epithelial markers in some inflammatory pseudotumors raises concern about a *sarcomatoid carcinoma*. However, the latter lesion tends to arise in elderly patients and presents as a bulky mass with hemorrhage and necrosis. Recognizing a typical in situ or invasive carcinomatous component is useful for recognizing this tumor.

### Discussion

All available evidence indicates that inflammatory pseudotumors arising in this location are a nonneoplastic, reparative process.[131] Although this lesion is not clearly related to trauma, it may represent a chronic response or a delayed presentation related to remote or undetected trauma.[120]

Genitourinary inflammatory pseudotumors arising in this location typically follow a benign course[109,117,120,125,131] with only rare reports of local recurrence, presumably due to incomplete excision (Table 9–5).[116] Thus far there have been no reported metastases. Most authors advocate conservative local excision.[117,120] Almost all cases have a diploid DNA content and a low S-phase fraction in keeping with the benign nature of this lesion.[117,120,125,131]

## ISCHEMIC FASCIITIS (ATYPICAL DECUBITAL FIBROPLASIA)

*Ischemic fasciitis* and *atypical decubital fibroplasia* are synonyms for a pseudosarcomatous fibroblastic proliferation that predominantly involves soft tissues overlying bony prominences and occurs primarily in elderly and physically debilitated or immobilized patients.[138,141–143] Most of the patients are elderly, with a peak incidence during the eighth and ninth decades of life, although this lesion has rarely been described in adolescents (Table 9–6).[139] Females are affected slightly more commonly than males. Most patients present with a painless mass of short duration, usually less than 6 months; many but not all are debilitated or immobilized, bedridden, or wheelchair-bound. The soft tissues in the region of the shoulder are most commonly affected, followed by the soft tis-

**TABLE 9–5** SUMMARY OF DATA FROM LARGEST STUDIES OF INFLAMMATORY PSEUDOTUMOR OF THE URINARY BLADDER

| First Author | No. of Cases | Mean Age (Years) | Outcome | Follow-up |
|---|---|---|---|---|
| Albores-Saavedra et al.[109] | 10 | 8.0 | No recurrence | 18 months to 6 years |
| Jones et al.[120] | 13 | 35.4 | No recurrence | 6–64 months |
| Ro et al.[131] | 9 | 48.7 | No recurrence | 2–7 years |
| Lundgren et al.[125] | 12 | 49.5 | No recurrence | 1 month to 15 years |
| Hojo et al.[117] | 11 | 9.4 | No recurrence | 2 weeks to 3.5 years |

Modified from Chan JKC. Inflammatory pseudotumor: A family of lesions of diverse nature and etiologies. Adv Anat Pathol 3:156, 1996.

**TABLE 9-6 AGE DISTRIBUTION OF 34 PATIENTS WITH ISCHEMIC FASCIITIS REPORTED IN THE LITERATURE**

| Age Range (Years) | No. of Patients |
|---|---|
| 0–10 | 0 |
| 11–20 | 1 |
| 21–30 | 2 |
| 31–40 | 1 |
| 41–50 | 0 |
| 51–60 | 1 |
| 61–70 | 3 |
| 71–80 | 13 |
| 81–90 | 11 |
| 91–100 | 2 |
| *Total* | 34 |

sues of the chest wall overlying the ribs, those overlying the sacrococcygeal region, or the greater trochanter.

## Pathologic Findings

Grossly, the lesion is poorly circumscribed and vaguely multinodular, often with a myxoid quality; it ranges from 1.0 to 8.5 cm in greatest diameter. It typically involves the subcutaneous tissue but may extend into the overlying dermis, with infrequent epidermal ulceration. In addition, the proliferation can involve the underlying skeletal muscles or adjacent periosteum.

Microscopically, ischemic fasciitis has a zonal pattern, often with a central zone of liquefactive or focally coagulative necrosis surrounded by a fringe of proliferating vessels and fibroblasts (Figs. 9–35, 9–36). The peripheral vessels are usually small, thin-walled, and ectatic; they are lined by prominent, occasionally atypical endothelial cells (Fig. 9–37). In addition, a proliferation of plump fibroblasts form perivascular clusters or merge imperceptibly with the peripheral vessels. The fibroblasts may be cytologically atypical, with large, eccentric, often smudgy hyperchromatic nuclei, prominent nucleoli, and abundant basophilic cytoplasm. Rare cells closely resemble the ganglion-like cells seen in proliferative fasciitis or myositis. The proliferation is usually paucicellular; although mitotic figures may be numerous, they are not atypical. The peripheral vessels may contain fibrin thrombi and secondary acute inflammation with perivascular hyalinization. Rare multivacuolated muciphages can be seen in the myxoid zones and may mimic the lipoblasts of myxoid liposarcoma.

Immunohistochemically, the atypical fibroblast-like cells stain strongly and diffusely for vimentin but may also stain focally for both actin and CD68 (KP1).[141] In addition, some cells also express CD34, possibly suggesting early endothelial differentiation.

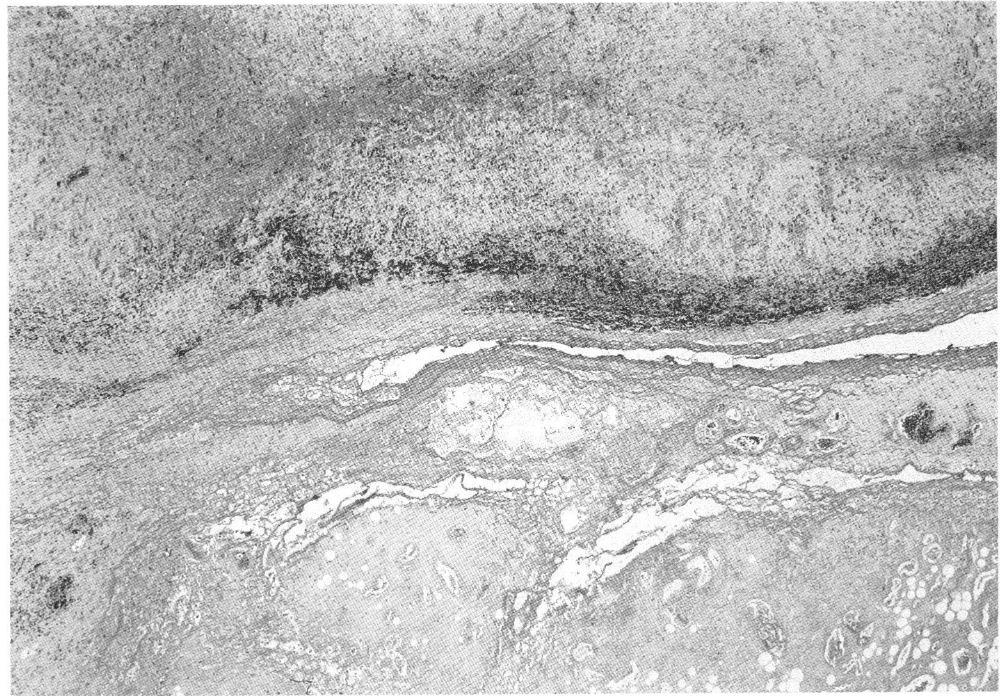

**FIGURE 9–35.** Low-power view of ischemic fasciitis showing a central zone of liquefactive necrosis with a proliferating fringe of fibroblasts and vessels.

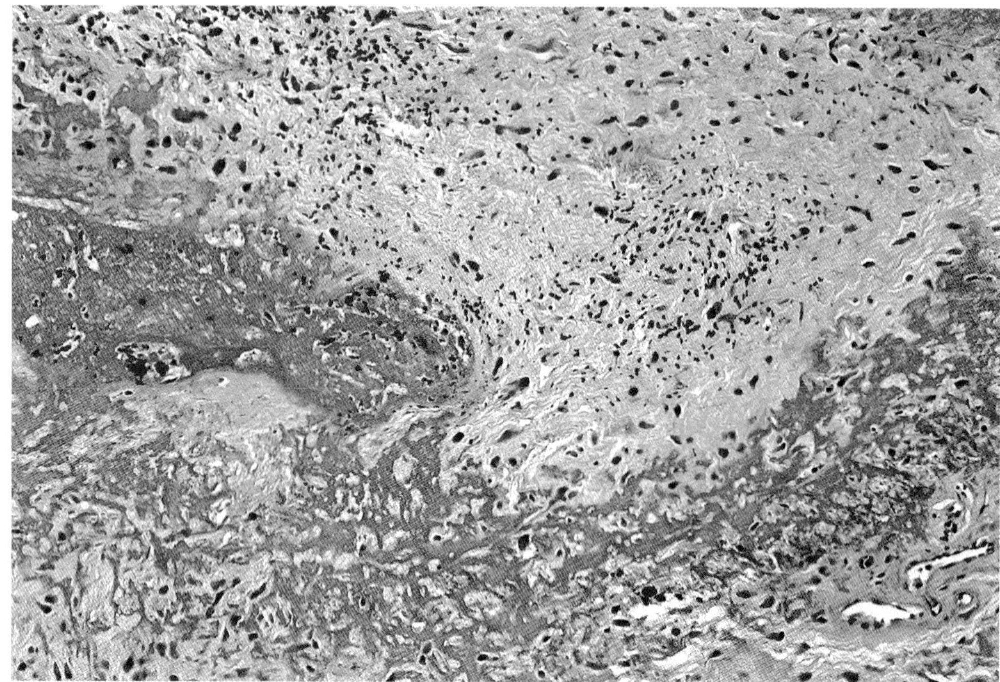

**FIGURE 9–36.** Interface between a liquefactive zone with fibrinous material and a reactive zone with atypical-appearing fibroblasts.

### Differential Diagnosis

In more than one-third of reported cases of ischemic fasciitis, a malignant diagnosis was seriously considered.[140–144] Although the multinodular appearance with central necrosis is reminiscent of *epithelioid sarcoma,* the latter typically occurs on the distal extremity of young patients and is composed of cells with prominent cytoplasmic eosinophilia and cytokeratin immunoreactivity. *Myxoid liposarcoma* is also a consideration, but ischemic fasciitis lacks the organized plexiform vasculature typical of myxoid liposarcoma. Furthermore, although multivacuolated muciphages may be seen, true lipoblasts are not identified. *Myxoid malignant fibrous histiocytoma* lacks the zonation of ischemic fasciitis and the degenerative and reactive features, such as cells with smudgy chromatin, fat necrosis, hemosiderin deposition, and fibrin thrombi.

### Discussion

Ischemic fasciitis is probably related to intermittent ischemia with subsequent tissue breakdown and regenerative changes. Most lesions develop in areas where the subcutaneous tissue lies in close apposition to bone, and they arise in patients with a clinical history of prolonged immobilization or trauma at that site. Histologically, the zonal quality is similar to that seen in other reactive fibroblastic and myofibroblastic proliferations. As suggested by Perosio and Weiss, the pathogenesis is probably similar to that of a decubitus ulcer, except that the ischemia may be less severe or of an intermittent nature, and it does not lead to breakdown of the overlying skin.[142] Although local recurrences have been described,[141] most patients are cured by conservative excision, supporting its benign nature. Awareness of this entity should allow the pathologist to avert a misdiagnosis of sarcoma and allow the clinical measures necessary to prevent subsequent recurrence or progression.

## FIBROMA OF THE TENDON SHEATH

Whether fibroma of the tendon sheath is a reactive fibrosing process or a neoplasm is not clear, but it is a distinct entity of characteristic location and histologic appearance. It consists of a slowly growing, dense, fibrous nodule that is firmly attached to the tendon sheath and is found most frequently in the hands and feet. Its lobular configuration resembles that of a giant cell tumor of the tendon sheath, but it is much less cellular and lacks the polymorphic features of the latter lesion.

The chief complaint is a small mass that has been present for some time and has increased slowly in size, often over many years. It is found most com-

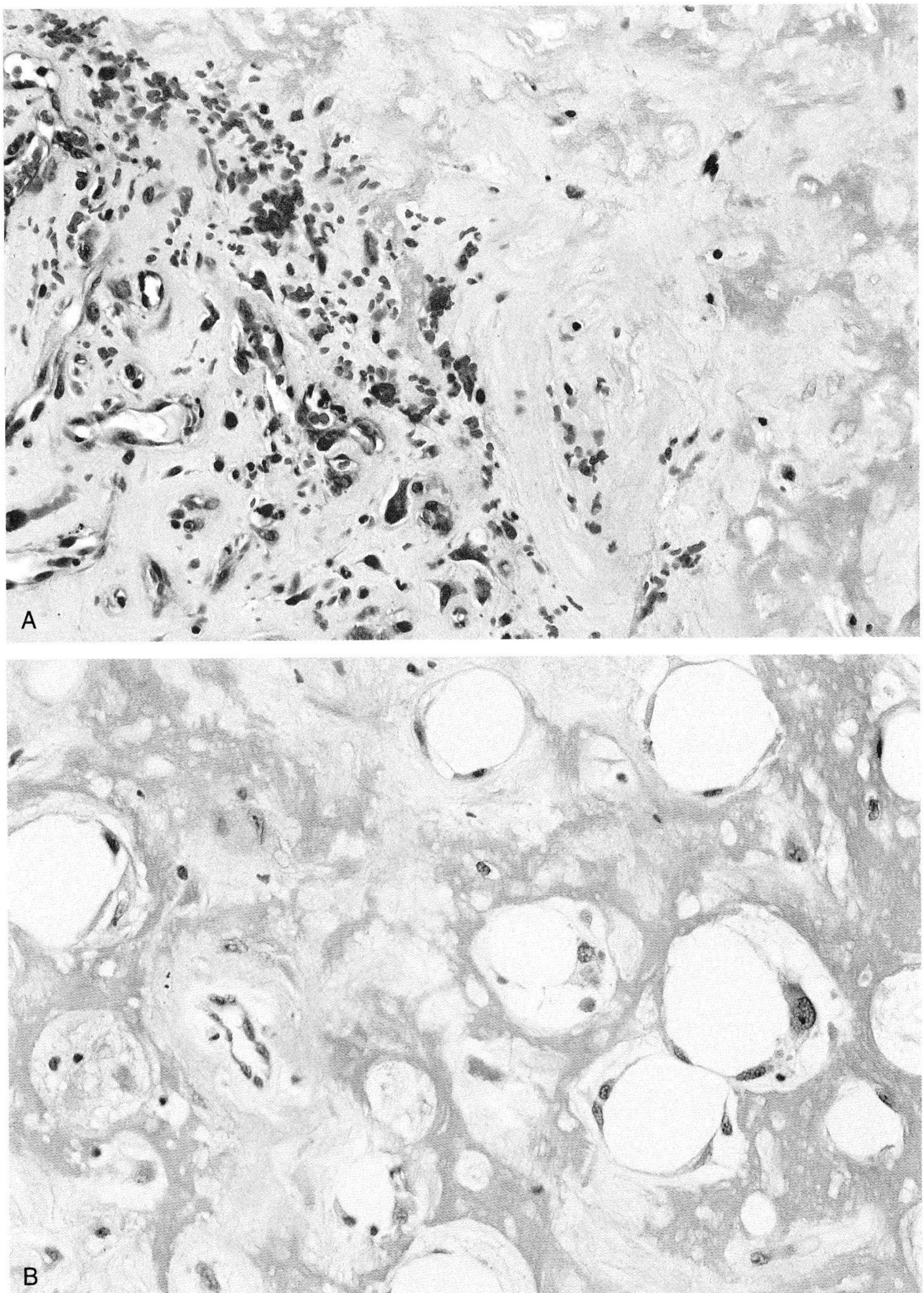


**FIGURE 9–37.** Ischemic fasciitis. (**A**) Interface between a zone of liquefactive necrosis and reactive fibroblastic and vascular proliferation. (**B**) High-power view of residual "ghosted" fat cells in a zone of coagulative necrosis.

*Illustration continued on following page*

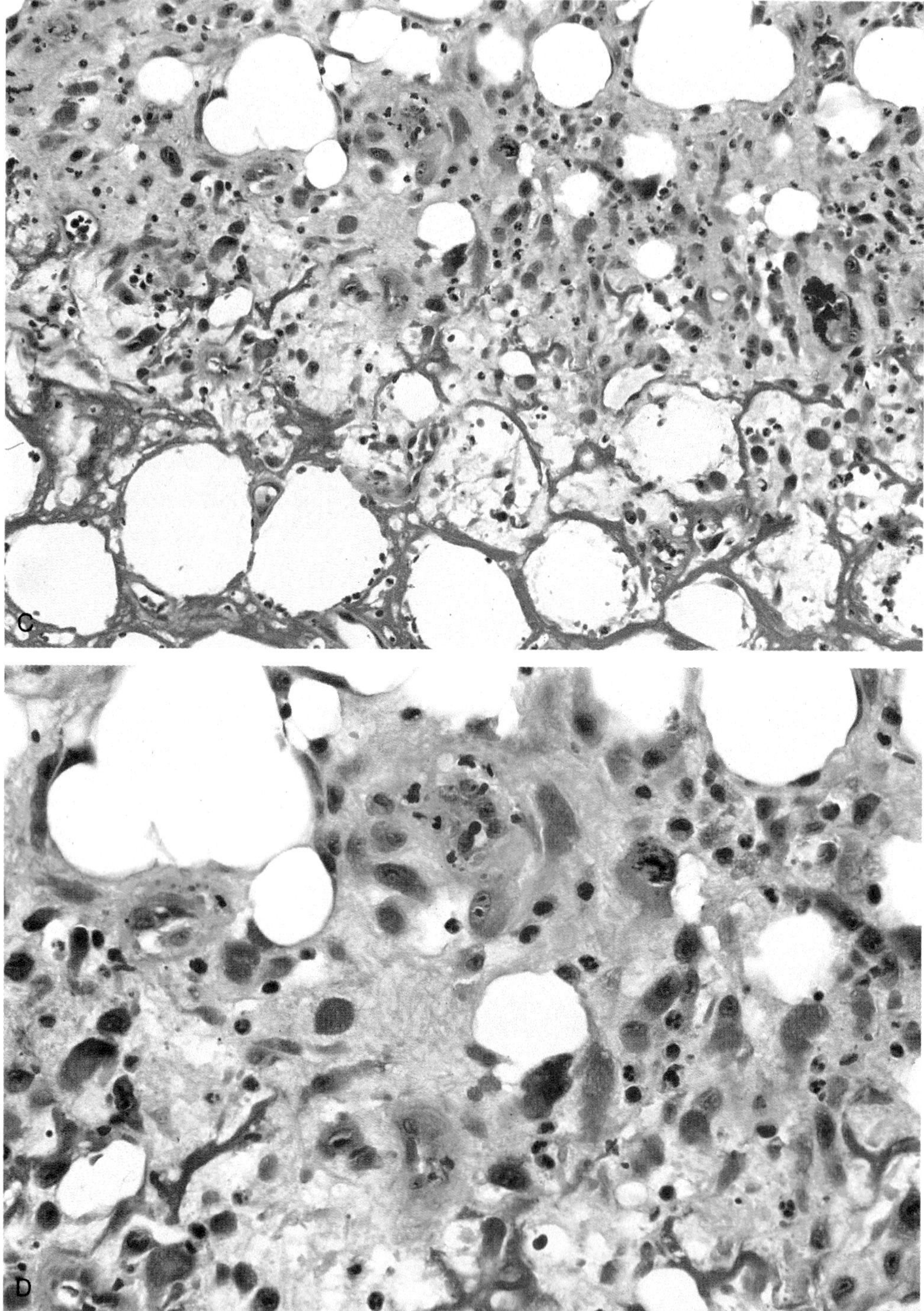

**FIGURE 9–37.** (*Continued*) (**C**) Fibrinous material with an adjacent reactive fibroblastic zone. Some of the fibroblasts are round and similar to those seen in proliferative fasciitis. (**D**) High-power view of atypical fibroblasts in a reactive zone of ischemic fasciitis.

monly in adults 20–50 years of age and is more than twice as common in men as in women.[146,147] Almost all of these tumors arise in the extremities, with the upper extremity being affected much more commonly than the lower extremity (Table 9–7). The most common sites of involvement in the upper extremity are the fingers, hand, and wrist, with only rare involvement of the forearm, elbow, or upper arm. Sites of involvement in the lower extremity are the knee, foot, ankle, and rarely the toe or leg. The mass is usually less than 2 cm in greatest diameter; as many as one-third of patients have slight tenderness, pain, or limited range of motion of the affected digit. A history of trauma related to the development of the lesion has been reported in approximately 9% of cases.[146,156]

### Gross Findings

Most lesions are well circumscribed and have a lobular configuration, similar to that found with giant cell tumor of the tendon sheath. Attachment to a tendon or tendon sheath is visible in most but not all cases. On cut section, the lesions are usually uniform in appearance, with a gray or pearly white color. Occasionally, grossly myxoid and cystic areas are seen.

### Microscopic Findings

Microscopically, the lesion appears well circumscribed and lobulated or multilobulated. There is a predominant proliferation of spindle-shaped cells resembling fibroblasts with elongated nuclei, diffusely stippled chromatin, and small basophilic nucleoli. Most lesions lack cytologic atypia, although striking nuclear pleomorphism has been described (so-called pleomorphic fibroma of the tendon sheath).[153] In these rare cases, the mitotic index is not commensurate with the degree of nuclear pleomorphism, suggesting a degenerative phenomenon. Scattered stellate-shaped cells may also be present, particularly in myxoid zones. Most lesions are hypocellular, with widely spaced cytologically bland spindle-shaped cells deposited in a densely eosinophilic hyalinized collagenous stroma. However, some have zones of increased cellularity in which the cells are arranged in either a storiform or fascicular growth pattern resembling nodular fasciitis (Figs. 9–38, 9–39). These cellular areas always blend with less cellular collagenous areas. Not uncommonly, small myxoid zones are interspersed between the densely collagenized zones. Characteristically, elongated cleft-like spaces lined by flattened cells are found throughout the lesion, imparting a lobular arrangement.[147,151] These cells have been reported to stain for factor VIII-related antigen, suggesting that the spaces are truly vascular.[145,152] Rare lesions contain multinucleated giant cells, but xanthoma cells and hemosiderin deposits are not present.

**TABLE 9–7 ANATOMIC DISTRIBUTION OF 165 CASES OF FIBROMA OF THE TENDON SHEATH**

| Site | No. | % |
|---|---|---|
| Upper extremities | 145 | 88 |
| Fingers | 79 | |
| Hands | 41 | |
| Wrist | 17 | |
| Forearm | 4 | |
| Elbow | 3 | |
| Upper arm | 1 | |
| Lower extremities | 18 | 11 |
| Knee | 7 | |
| Foot | 5 | |
| Ankle | 3 | |
| Toes | 2 | |
| Leg | 1 | |
| Trunk | 2 | 1 |
| Chest | 1 | |
| Back | 1 | |

Data are from Chung and Enzinger[146] and Pulitzer et al.[156]

### Immunohistochemical and Electron Microscopic Findings

There are relatively limited data on the immunohistochemical features of fibroma of the tendon sheath. Maluf et al. found these lesions to co-express vimentin and muscle markers, including muscle-specific and smooth muscle actin, without staining for desmin.[155] In addition, stains for markers (albeit relatively nonspecific) of monocytic-histiocytic differentiation, including CD68 (KP1) and HAM 56, were also positive in some cases. Given an overlapping immunophenotype with giant cell tumor of the tendon sheath, these authors proposed that fibroma and giant cell tumor of the tendon sheath probably represent histogenetically related lesions that are the extremes in a spectrum of histiocytic-fibroblastic-myofibroblastic differentiation, as suggested by others.[158,160] In addition, Silverman and Knapik found the cells of fibroma of the tendon sheath to express both factor XIIIa and CD34, which they interpreted as evidence of dendritic histiocytic differentiation.[159]

Ultrastructurally, fibroma of the tendon sheath is composed of fibroblasts and myofibroblasts.[150,156,157] Cells with fibroblastic features (including abundant rough endoplasmic reticulum with dilated cisternae) predominate in the less cellular collagenized zones, whereas cells with myofibroblastic features (including actin-type intermediate filaments and dense bodies) predominate in the more cellular and myxoid zones.[154,161]

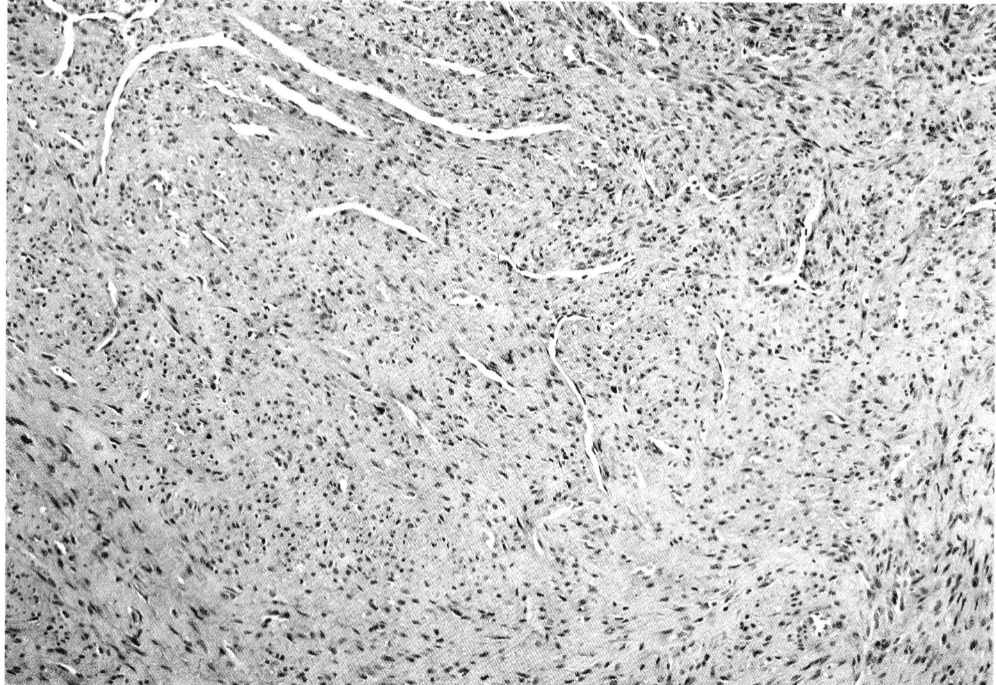

**FIGURE 9–38.** Cellular zone of a fibroma of the tendon sheath, including cleft-like spaces.

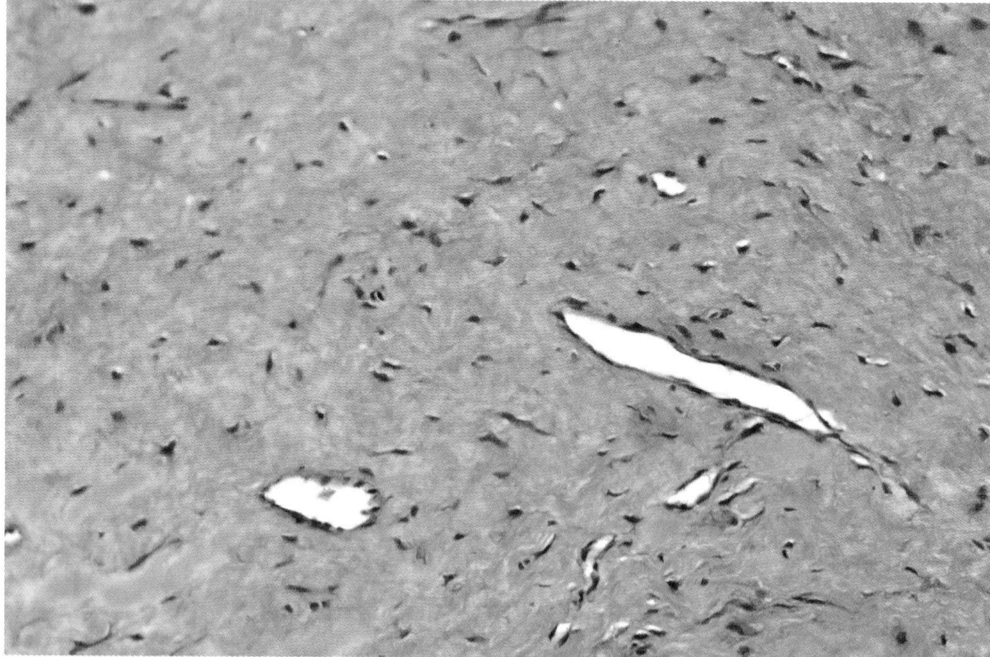

**FIGURE 9–39.** Fibroma of the tendon sheath composed of scattered spindle to stellate-shaped fibroblasts in a sparsely cellular and richly collagenous stroma.

### Differential Diagnosis

The typical fibroma of the tendon sheath, composed of a hypocellular proliferation of bland spindle cells deposited in a densely collagenized stroma, is characteristic and unlikely to be confused with other entities, although lesions that show more cellular zones may be confused with *fibrous histiocytoma* or *nodular fasciitis*. Pulitzer et al. reported that up to one-fourth of their cases had areas that were indistinguishable from nodular fasciitis.[156] However, nodular fasciitis typically presents as a more rapidly growing lesion that reaches its maximum size in a short time and rarely affects the hands or feet. In addition, it is usually less well circumscribed, typically has a more pronounced myxoid stroma, and is more mitotically active.

Although fibroma of the tendon sheath and *giant cell tumor of the tendon sheath* arise in similar locations and are grossly similar, giant cell tumor of the tendon sheath is composed of a proliferation of round cells (in contrast to spindle-shaped cells) and usually contains more multinucleated giant cells as well as xanthoma cells and hemosiderin deposits. Interestingly, translocations involving the long arm of chromosome 2 have been described in both fibromas[148] and giant cell tumors[149] of the tendon sheath, but the breakpoints were found to be different (2q31-32 and 2q35-36, respectively).

Rare fibromas of the tendon sheath show striking nuclear pleomorphism and may be confused with a pleomorphic sarcoma, such as *malignant fibrous histiocytoma* (MFH). Pleomorphic MFH, though, is characterized by greater cellularity and more mitotic activity, including atypical mitoses, as well as a more pronounced storiform growth pattern.

### Discussion

Fibroma of the tendon sheath is a benign process that can recur but does not metastasize. In the series by Chung and Enzinger, 13 of 54 patients (24%) with follow-up information developed local recurrences, including three patients with two recurrences.[146] In most cases the lesions recurred 1–4 months after the initial surgery. Local excision and reexcision of recurrences appears to be the treatment of choice.

The exact nature of this lesion is not clear. It is likely that there is an initial, transient cellular phase that resembles nodular fasciitis or fibrous histiocytoma and a collagenous phase that predominates and is typical and diagnostic of this entity. Friction inherent in the location of the tumor or vascular impairment may account for the early onset of the sclerosing process.

## PLEOMORPHIC FIBROMA OF SKIN

Pleomorphic fibroma involving the skin is a relatively rare entity that shares some histologic features with pleomorphic fibroma of the tendon sheath, particularly the presence of large pleomorphic, hyperchromatic cells deposited in a collagenized stroma. Clinically, most patients present with a slowly growing, asymptomatic, solitary lesion that appears as a flesh-colored, nonulcerated, dome-shaped papule. These lesions most commonly involve the papillary and reticular dermis of the extremities, followed by the trunk and the head and neck.[162–166] Most lesions appear in adults, with a peak incidence during the fifth decade of life; and women are affected slightly more commonly than men. The lesion is 0.5–2.0 cm and clinically is often mistaken for a nevus, neurofibroma, or hemangioma.

Grossly, the mass is well circumscribed and involves the papillary and reticular dermis, resulting in a dome-shaped or polypoid lesion covered by a thin, nonulcerated epidermis. Histologically, it is sparsely cellular and composed predominantly of thick, haphazardly arranged collagen. The characteristic feature is the presence of scattered spindle-shaped or stellate cells, including multinucleated giant cells with large pleomorphic, hyperchromatic nuclei and small nucleoli (Fig. 9–40). Mitotic figures are rare, but occasionally an atypical mitotic figure is seen.[164,165] The stroma may show focal or (rarely) diffuse myxoid change.[166] Adnexal structures are generally not found, and there may be a sparse lymphoplasmacytic infiltrate in the lesion.

Immunohistochemically, the cells stain diffusely for vimentin, and variable numbers of cells also stain for muscle-specific actin, suggesting myofibroblastic differentiation.[163] Immunostains for S-100 protein, desmin, and cytokeratin are negative. Ultrastructurally, the fibroblast-like cells have complex nuclear contours and abundant rough endoplasmic reticulum.[162,165]

The differential diagnosis includes other cutaneous neoplasms characterized by the presence of pleomorphic cells. *Atypical fibroxanthoma* most commonly occurs as a rapidly growing lesion on sun-damaged skin of the face of elderly patients. It is characterized by higher cellularity, cells with foamy cytoplasm, and a large number of typical and atypical mitotic figures. *Dermatofibroma with atypical cells*, also referred to as *dermatofibroma with monster cells, atypical cutaneous fibrous histiocytoma, pseudosarcomatous dermatofibroma*, and *atypical (pseudosarcomatous) cutaneous histiocytoma*, is a more densely cellular proliferation of pleomorphic cells, including cells with hemosiderin and foamy cytoplasm. In addition, most lesions have foci

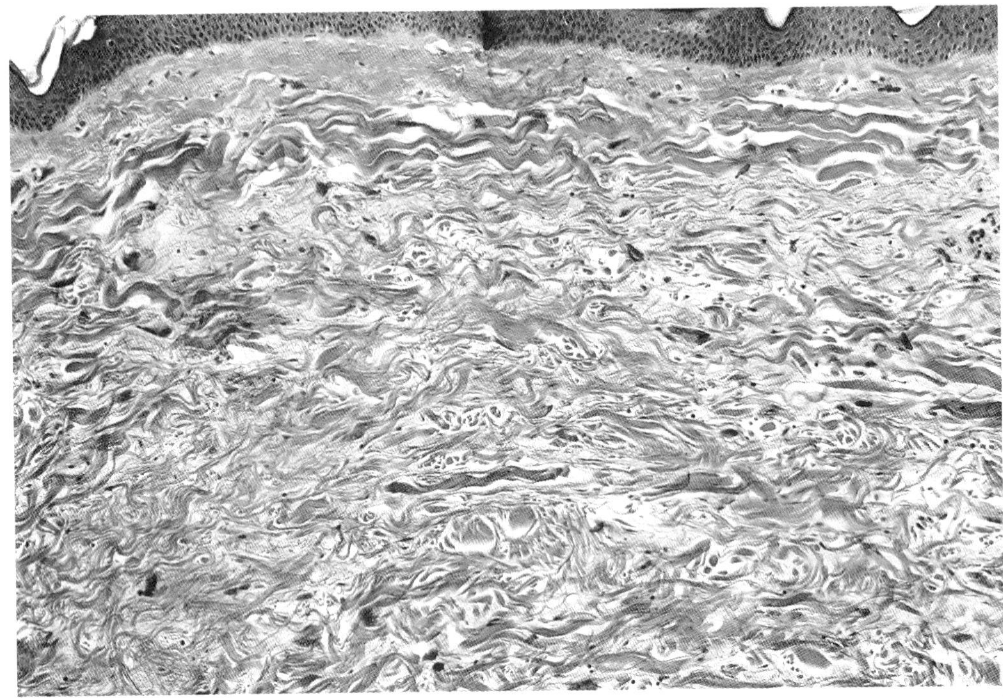

**FIGURE 9–40.** Pleomorphic fibroma of skin with scattered floret-like giant cells deposited in a densely collagenized dermis.

of typical fibrous histiocytoma. *Giant cell fibroblastoma* most commonly occurs as an infiltrative lesion on the trunk or extremities of patients less than 10 years of age. It is characterized by pseudovascular or angiectoid spaces lined by atypical spindle cells and floret-like giant cells. The absence of S-100 protein in pleomorphic fibroma of skin helps distinguish it from benign peripheral nerve sheath tumors with atypia (*ancient schwannoma* and *neurofibroma with atypia*).

In general, simple excision of this lesion is curative, as there has been only one reported case of local recurrence.[164]

## NUCHAL FIBROMA

Nuchal fibroma is a rare fibrocollagenous proliferation that typically arises in the cervicodorsal region in adults. The lesion is significantly more common in men, with a peak incidence during the third through fifth decades of life.[167,168,170] Patients typically present with a solitary unencapsulated subcutaneous mass in the cervicodorsal region, although cases have also been described in extranuchal sites including the extremities,[170] buttock,[172] and lumbosacral area.[168] The process appears to be strongly associated with diabetes mellitus[170] and may also be linked to Gardner syndrome.[170]

Grossly, the lesions are unencapsulated and arise in the subcutaneous tissue, with minimal extension into the deep dermis. Rare lesions also infiltrate the superficial skeletal muscle.[170] Most are 2.5–8.0 cm in greatest diameter, and the mass is usually present for several years prior to excision. Lipoma is the most common preoperative diagnosis.

Microscopically, nuchal fibroma is a hypocellular or almost completely acellular densely collagenized mass with scattered mature fibroblasts and islands of mature adipose tissue of varying size (Fig. 9–41). The mass is ill-defined, with some radiation of collagenous septa into the subcutaneous fat and deep dermis. Small nerves are frequently entrapped by this fibrous proliferation. Occasionally, altered elastic fibers similar to those seen in elastofibromas are identified.

Probably the most difficult distinction is from *fibrolipoma*. Unlike nuchal fibroma, fibrolipoma is typically well circumscribed and encapsulated, has a greater proportion of the lesion composed of mature adipose tissue, and lacks entrapped nerves. The subcutaneous location and the paucity of cells permit exclusion of *extraabdominal fibromatosis*. The *nuchal fibrocartilaginous pseudotumor* arises in the posterior aspect of the base of the neck at the junction of the nuchal ligament and the deep cervical fascia and probably develops as a reaction to soft tissue injury.[169,171] Unlike the former lesion, nuchal fibroma lacks an association with ligaments, occurs superficial to the fascia, and lacks cartilaginous metaplasia. *Elastofibroma* typically occurs in the deep soft tissue in the vicinity of the inferomedial portion of the scapula. Given the finding of altered

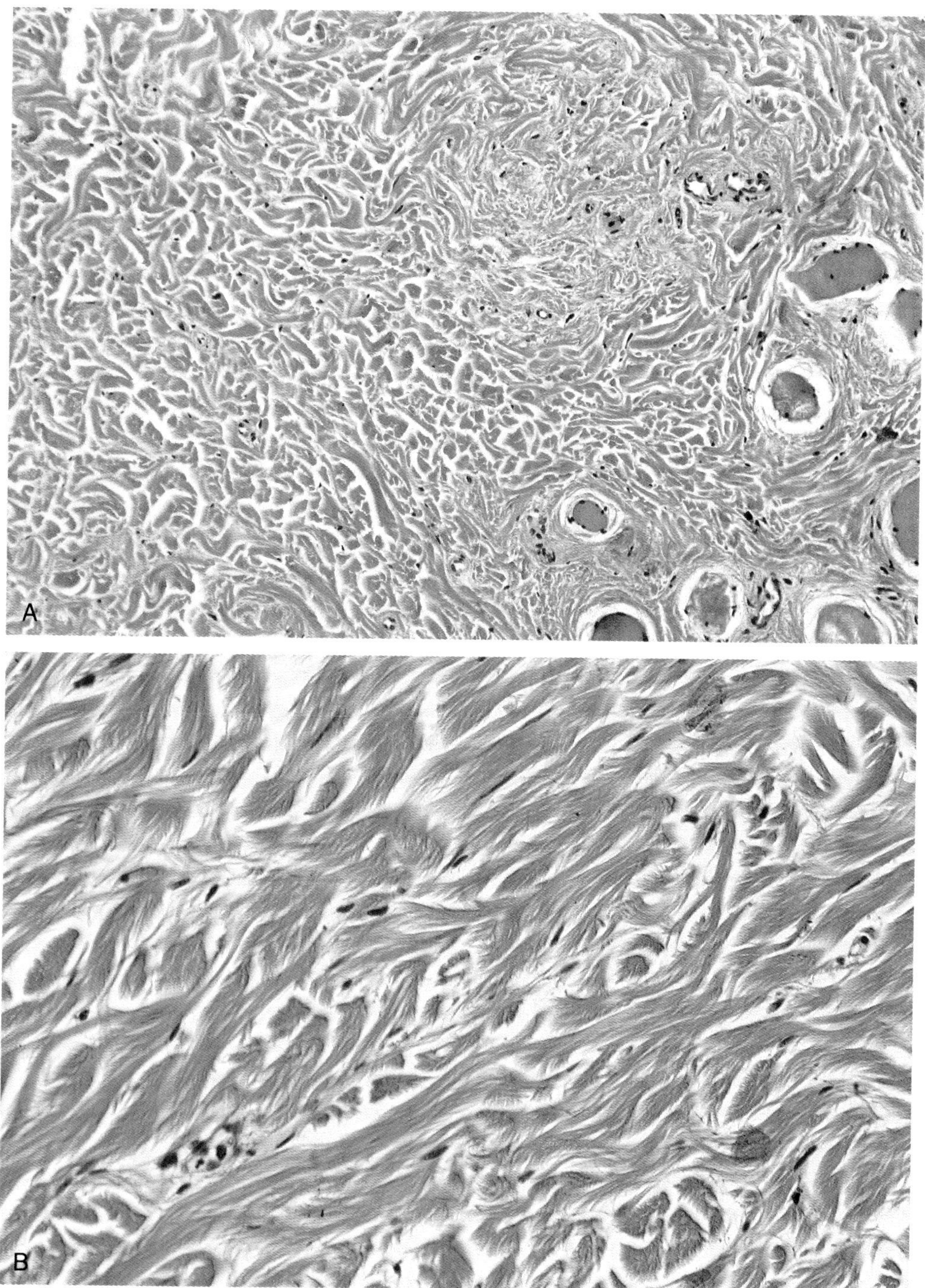


**FIGURE 9–41.** Nuchal fibroma. (**A**) Low-power view of nuchal fibroma, characterized by a hypocellular, densely collagenized mass with scattered fibroblasts among skeletal muscle fibers. (**B**) Scattered fibroblasts deposited in densely collagenized stroma.

elastic fibers in the nuchal fibroma, it is possible that these two lesions are closely related entities. Nuchal fibroma is benign but may recur if incompletely excised.[170]

## ELASTOFIBROMA

Elastofibroma, an unusual fibroelastic pseudotumor, is most commonly encountered in elderly persons; it arises chiefly from the connective tissue between the inferomedial portion of the scapula and the chest wall. Originally described by Järvi and Saxén in 1961 as elastofibroma dorsi,[189] it has become increasingly apparent that rare lesions are found in extrascapular locations; thus the term elastofibroma is preferred.

### Clinical Findings

Most patients are elderly, with a peak incidence during the sixth and seventh decades of life. Only rare tumors have been described in children.[179,196] Women are affected more commonly than men. Most but not all patients have a history of intensive, often repetitive manual labor. Although originally considered a rare lesion, several autopsy studies have shown elastofibroma and pre-elastofibroma-like changes in 13–17% of elderly individuals.[183,188] The most common presentation is that of a slowly growing, deep-seated mass that only rarely causes pain or tenderness or limits movement. Most arise from the connective tissue between the lower portion of the scapula and the chest wall, deep to the rhomboid major and latissimus dorsi muscles, with attachment to the periosteum and ligaments in the region of the sixth, seventh, and eighth ribs. Although most are unilateral, bilateral elastofibromas have been described[181,186] and in fact may be more common than previously recognized. Naylor et al. described the radiologic findings in 12 patients with elastofibroma; all patients in whom both sides of the chest wall were imaged had bilateral elastofibromas, suggesting subclinical bilateral involvement in many cases.[201] This lesion has been increasingly recognized by radiologists on computed tomography (CT) scans and magnetic resonance imaging (MRI) as a poorly circumscribed, heterogeneous soft tissue mass with attenuation of signal intensity similar to that of skeletal muscle; it is interlaced with fat, allowing a presumptive diagnosis.[193,197,208] Numerous extrascapular sites have been reported, including the small bowel, tracheobronchial tree,[203] colon (resulting in a colonic polyp),[185] greater omentum,[206] deltoid region,[198] greater trochanter,[174] foot,[177] cornea,[187] stomach (in the region of a peptic ulcer),[181] and rectal submucosa.[184]

### Pathologic Findings

The mass is usually ill-defined, oblong or spherical, firm, and ranges from 5–10 cm. The cut surface has a variegated appearance with small areas of adipose tissue interposed between gray-white fibrous areas, occasionally with cystic change (Fig. 9–42). Not infrequently, the surgeon is concerned about the possibility of a sarcoma, given the irregular margins and infiltration of skeletal muscle or periosteum.

On microscopic examination, the tumor-like mass consists of a mixture of intertwining swollen, eosinophilic collagen and elastic fibers in about equal proportions associated with occasional fibroblasts, small amounts of interstitial mucoid material, and variably sized aggregates of mature fat cells. Typically, the elastic fibers have a degenerated beaded appearance or are fragmented into small flower-like, serrated disks or globules (chenille bodies) with a distinct linear arrangement (Fig. 9–43).

Elastic stains (Verhoeff, Weigert, Gomori) reveal deeply staining, branched and unbranched fibers that have a central dense core and an irregular moth-eaten or serrated margin (Figs. 9–44, 9–45, 9–46). The elastin-like material is removed by prior treatment of the sections with pancreatic or bacterial elastase and pepsin; collagenase or trypsin has no effect.[195,200,204] These altered elastic fibers can be recognized by specific antibodies to elastin,[194] and they exhibit a green fluorescence under ultraviolet light.

Ultrastructurally, the interspersed spindle cells have features of fibroblasts and myofibroblasts; some cells contain abundant rough endoplasmic reticulum and dilated cisternae, and others have cytoplasmic microfilaments and pinocytotic vesicles.[192,202] Non-membrane-bound dense granular bodies with an intensity similar to that of extracellular elastin and measuring 200–350 nm are present in the cytoplasm of fibroblasts, suggesting that these cells produce the abnor-

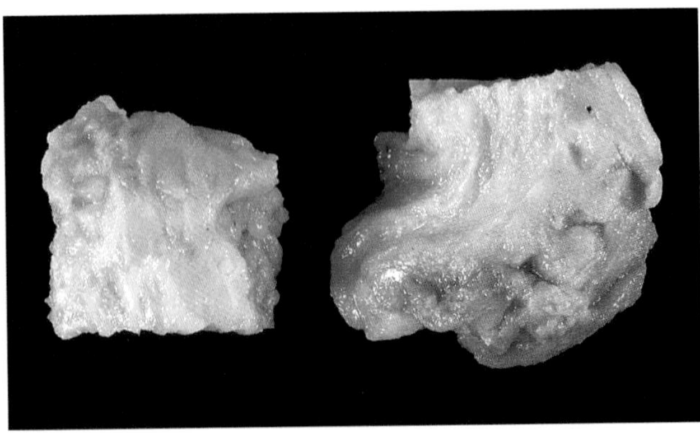

**FIGURE 9–42.** Elastofibroma. There is an intimate admixture of firm collagenous tissue with fat.

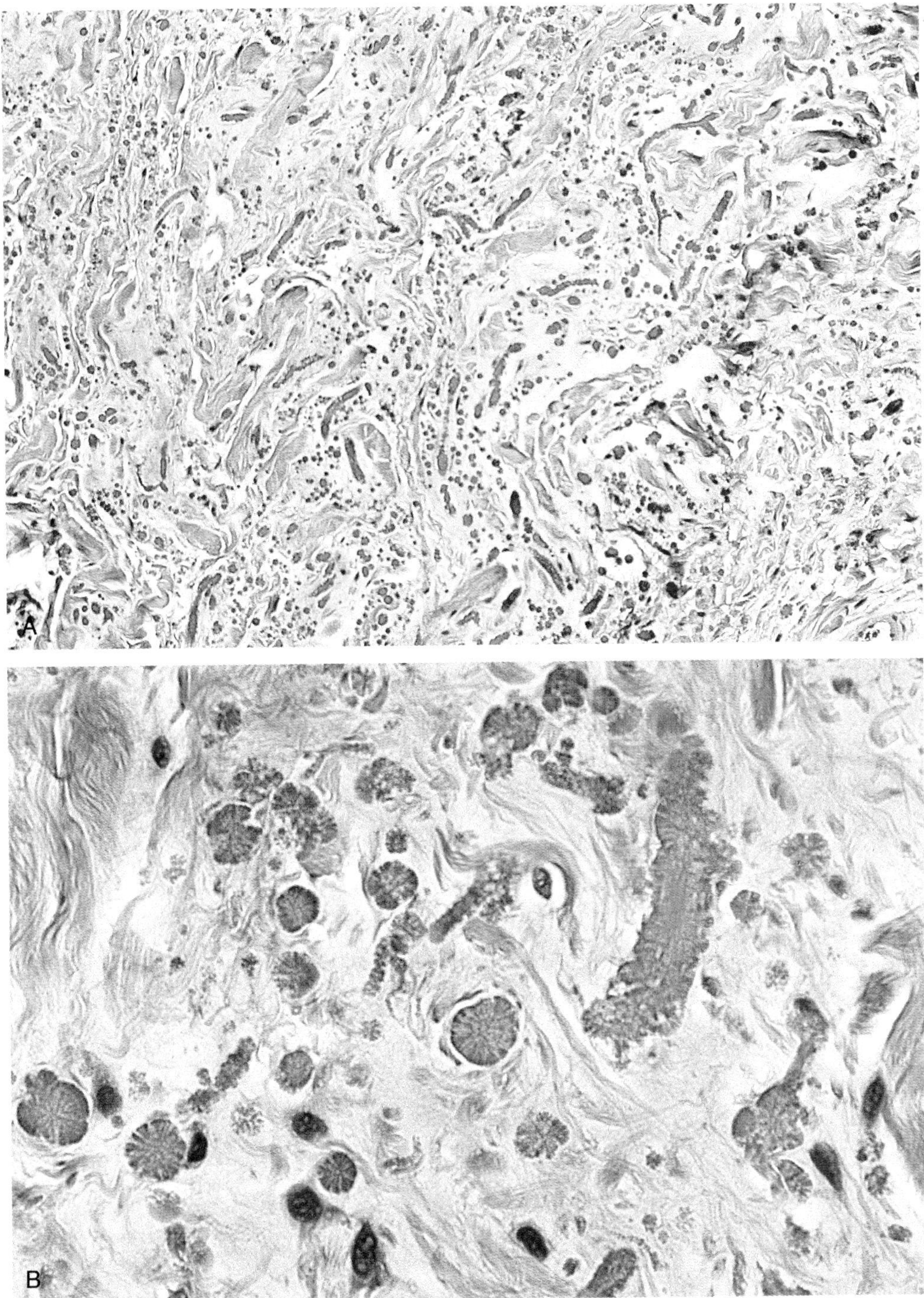


**FIGURE 9–43.** Elastofibroma. (**A**) Altered elastic fibers in a collagenous matrix. (**B**) Elastic fibers in cross section showing a characteristic serrated edge (petaloid globules).

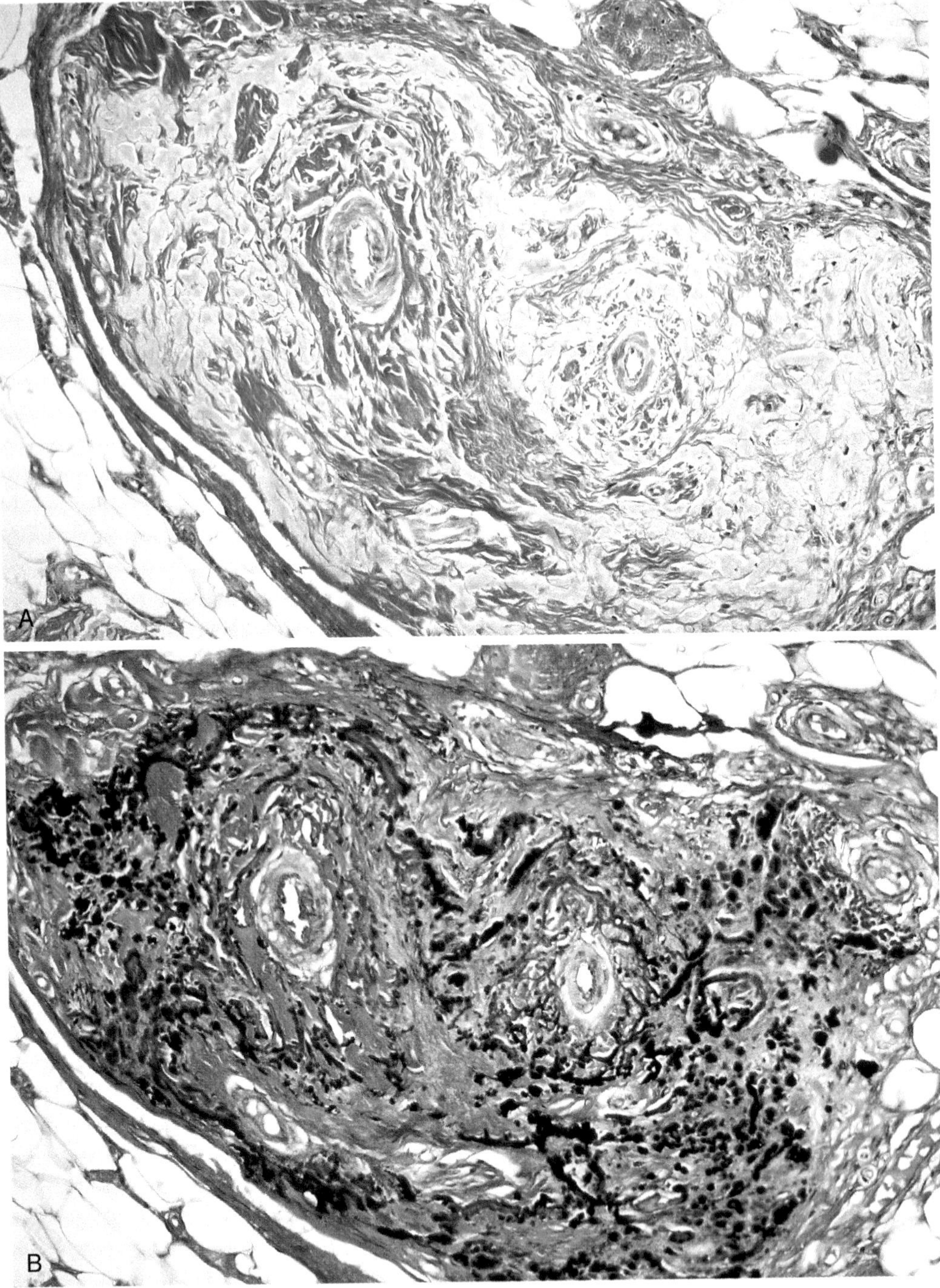


**FIGURE 9–44.** Elastofibroma. (**A**) Masson trichrome stain of elastofibroma outlining the collagen surrounding the abnormal elastic fibers. (**B**) Verhoeff elastin stain shows the mirror image, accentuating the abnormal elastic fibers.

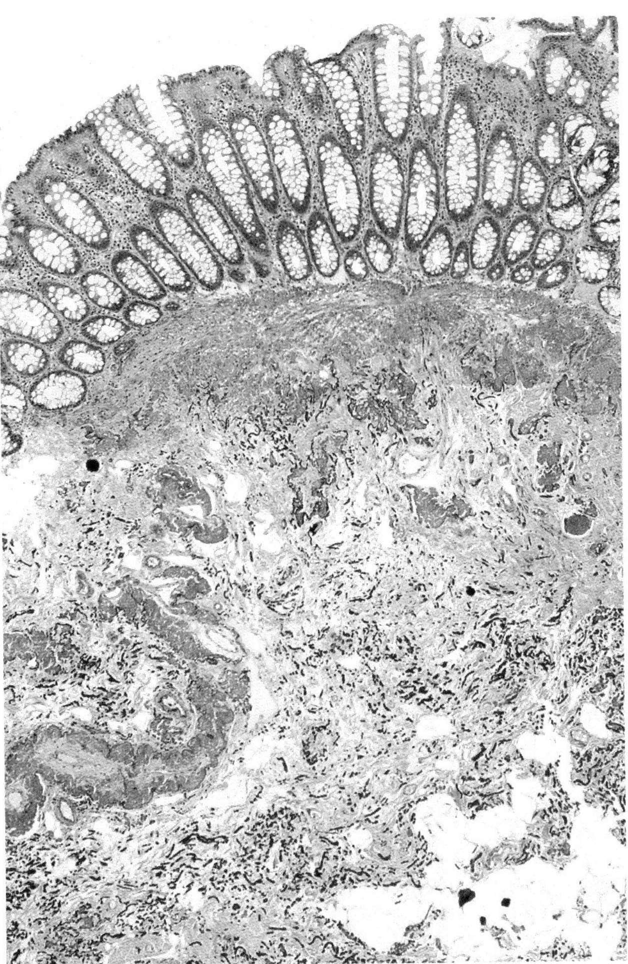

**FIGURE 9–45.** Verhoeff elastin stain shows elastic fibers in the submucosa of the rectum. This patient had a history of radiation therapy to this area.

mal extracellular elastic tissue.[180] Numerous electron-dense elongated and globular masses corresponding to the elastinophilic material seen on light microscopy are present in collagenous stroma. A central core of more electron-lucent material resembling mature elastic tissue is surrounded by granular or fibrillary aggregations of electron-dense material resembling immature elastin or preelastin. The proximity of these aggregates to fibroblasts further supports a process of abnormal elastogenesis by these cells.[175] At high magnification, the outer zones are seen to consist of compactly and randomly arranged elastic microfibrils measuring approximately 12 nm in diameter.[182]

### Differential Diagnosis

The clinical and histologic features of elastofibroma are characteristic and are unlikely to be confused with those of other fibroblastic proliferations. De Nictolis et al. described a case of an *elastofibrolipoma* arising in the mediastinum.[178] Unlike elastofibroma, the elastofibrolipoma is well circumscribed, is surrounded by a fibrous capsule, and has a more conspicuous adipose component in both the central and peripheral portions of the tumor. In a report of elastofibromatous change of the rectal submucosa,[184] the lesion closely mimicked amyloidosis, although elastic and congo red stains allowed this distinction.

### Discussion

The etiology of the abnormal elastic fibers has been debated since its initial description by Järvi and Saxén.[189] Whereas some have suggested that these fibers are derived from the elastotic degeneration of collagen fibers,[174,204,205] others believe they are derived from degeneration of preexisting elastic fibers[207] or from disturbed elastic fibrillogenesis.[173,180,191,192] The preponderance of evidence suggests that elastofibroma is a degenerative pseudotumor that is the result of excessive formation of collagen and abnormal elastic fibers. Although friction between the inferior edge of the scapula and the underlying chest wall has been implicated as the cause of this abnormal elastogenesis, other factors such as radiation therapy have been implicated,[184] particularly for lesions arising in extrascapular sites. Interestingly, Nagamine et al. reported that about one-third of the patients with this lesion in Okinawa occurred in patients with a family history of elastofibroma, suggesting a genetic predisposition.[199] A unique elastofibromatous lesion of the stomach at the base of a peptic ulcer has been described in a 69-year-old woman with bilateral subscapular elastofibromas, raising the possibility of an underlying systemic enzymatic defect.[181] Whether the central core of mature elastic tissue represents maturation of newly formed elastin fibers[173,180] or serves as a structural skeleton for newly formed elastin[190,192] is uncertain. Although most believe that fibroblasts and myofibroblasts serve as the source of the abnormal elastic fibers, some have proposed that elastofibromas arise from periosteum-derived cells in response to repeated physical irritation in susceptible individuals.[194]

Elastofibroma, a benign lesion, is best treated by conservative excision given that local recurrence is rare.[199] One regressed elastofibroma has been described.[176] There are no reports of malignant transformation.

## NASOPHARYNGEAL ANGIOFIBROMA

Nasopharyngeal angiofibroma, a relatively rare, histologically benign fibrovascular tumor, occurs in the nasopharynx, predominantly in adolescent boys. Although originally referred to as juvenile nasopha-

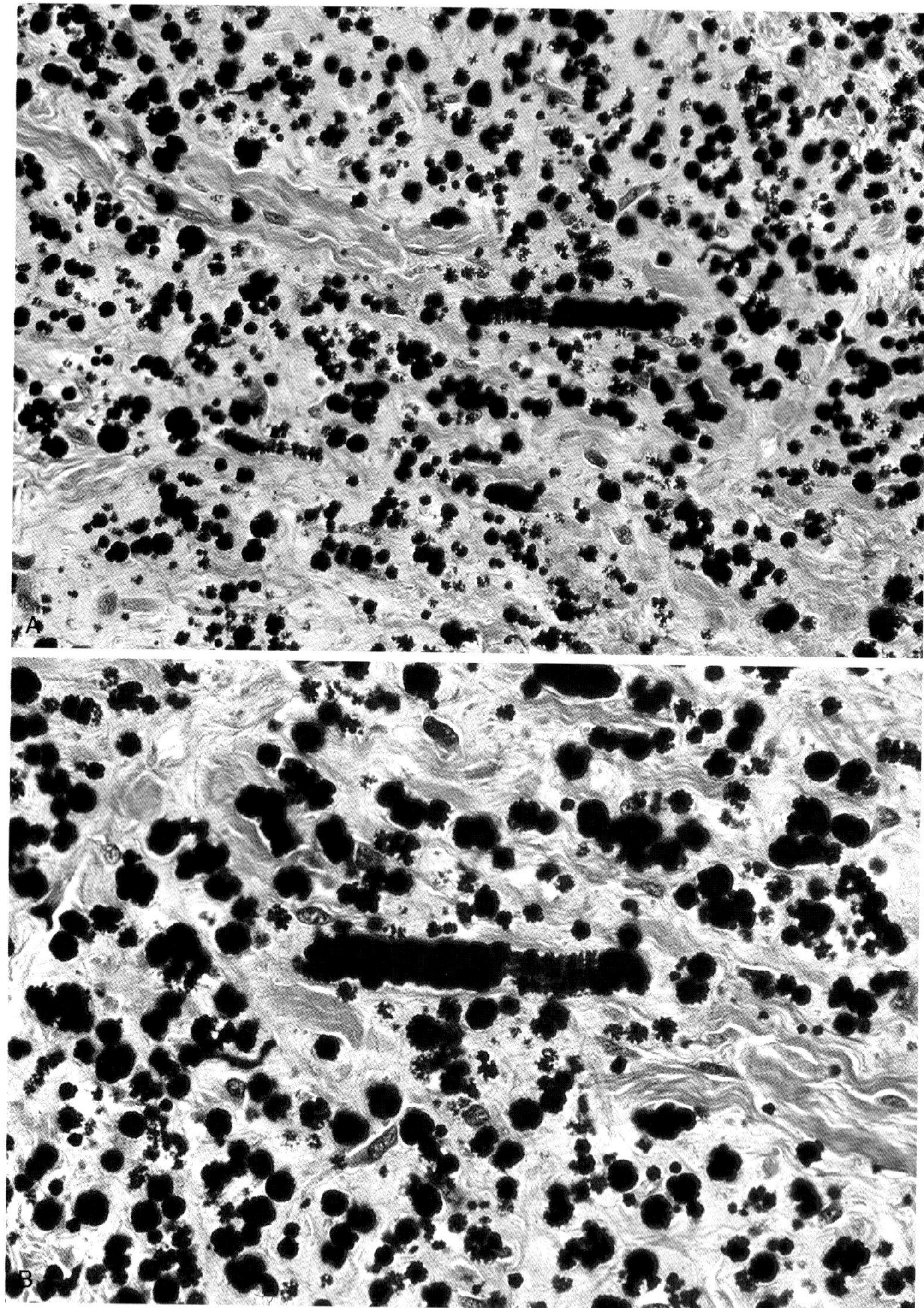

**FIGURE 9–46.** Elastofibroma. (**A**) Verhoeff elastin stain shows elongated and globoid elastic fibers. (**B**) High-power view of Verhoeff elastin stain showing elastic fibers with a dense core.

ryngeal angiofibroma, some occur in adults, so this lesion is best referred to simply as nasopharyngeal angiofibroma.

## Clinical Findings

Most of these lesions occur in adolescent boys and young men 10–20 years of age, although it has also been reported in older patients.[216,232] Almost all of these tumors occur in males, with only a few having been found in females.[216,235,236] Rare patients with nasopharyngeal angiofibroma have also been found to have familial adenomatous polyposis (FAP).[219,222] Along with desmoids, nasopharyngeal angiofibroma has been proposed to be a "fibroblastic misdemeanor" associated with FAP, possibly related to a mutation in the adenomatous polyposis coli (*APC*) gene on the long arm of chromosome 5.[222] The common presenting symptoms are nasal obstruction, facial deformity, and repeated epistaxis. In some cases, excessive hemorrhage requires blood transfusions and hospitalization and on rare occasions is life-threatening. Other symptoms include headache, sinusitis, otitis media, mastoiditis, and dacrocystitis.[209,216,228] Facial deformity of the temporal and cheek region is not uncommon.[220,231]

Physical examination typically reveals a variably sized, red or red-blue, lobulated or polypoid mass that can be easily seen through the nose or underneath the palate with a nasopharyngeal mirror. Most lesions appear to originate from the superolateral nasopharyngeal area and, with growth, extend into the posterior aspect of the nasal cavity and superiorly into the sphenoid sinus.[214] As the tumor enlarges, it extends through the pterygopalatine foramen and grows laterally into the pterygomaxillary and infratemporal fossae. It can extend into the soft tissues of the cheek and the orbit and often erodes bone with extension into the middle or anterior cranial fossae.

Radiologic techniques are useful for diagnostic and staging purposes. MRI and CT scans usually show a well demarcated soft tissue mass in the nasopharynx with or without extension into the nasal cavity or paranasal sinuses, anterior bowing of the posterior wall of the maxillary sinus, and erosion of adjacent bony structures (Fig. 9–47). MRI appears to be superior to CT scans for demarcating the margin of the tumor from the surrounding soft tissue.[244] Angiography is useful for demonstrating the tumor's vascularity; transarterial embolization can be performed at the same time.[243,248] For cases in which the diagnosis remains in question following radiographic evaluation, a transnasal biopsy may be used to confirm the diagnosis. It should be performed in an operating room, as significant hemorrhage requiring nasal packing or cautery may be encountered.[237]

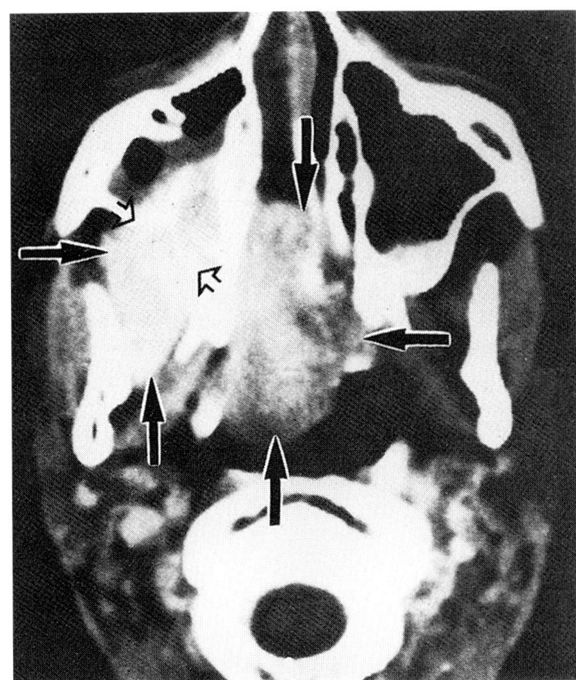

**FIGURE 9–47.** Nasopharyngeal angiofibroma involving the nasopharynx, nasal cavity, and right infratemporal fossa (arrows) and eroding through the posterior wall of the right maxillary antrum (small arrows). (From Chandler JR, Goulding R, Moskowitz L, et al. Nasopharyngeal angiofibromas: staging and management. Ann Otol Rhinol Laryngol 93:322, 1984.)

## Gross Findings

The tumor is typically well circumscribed with a lobulated, smooth, glistening mucosal surface that may be focally ulcerated. The tissue is firm and rubbery; on cut section it has a spongy appearance owing to the presence of numerous vascular spaces characteristic of this lesion.

## Microscopic Findings

The tumor is characterized by numerous vascular channels surrounded by dense paucicellular fibrous tissue (Fig. 9–48). The cells in the fibrous tissue are cytologically bland and may be spindle or stellate in shape with nuclei that lack hyperchromasia and have small nucleoli (Fig. 9–49). Mitotic figures are rare. The dense fibrous stroma may show hyalinization or focal myxoid change, often with collagen fibers arranged in a parallel fashion.[240] The vascular channels vary in number and configuration. They are slit-like or dilated, with significant variation in thickness. Some vessels are surrounded by few if any smooth muscle cells, whereas others show focal pad-like thickenings.[211] Peripherally located vessels are often larger and of the arterial type with visible elastic lam-

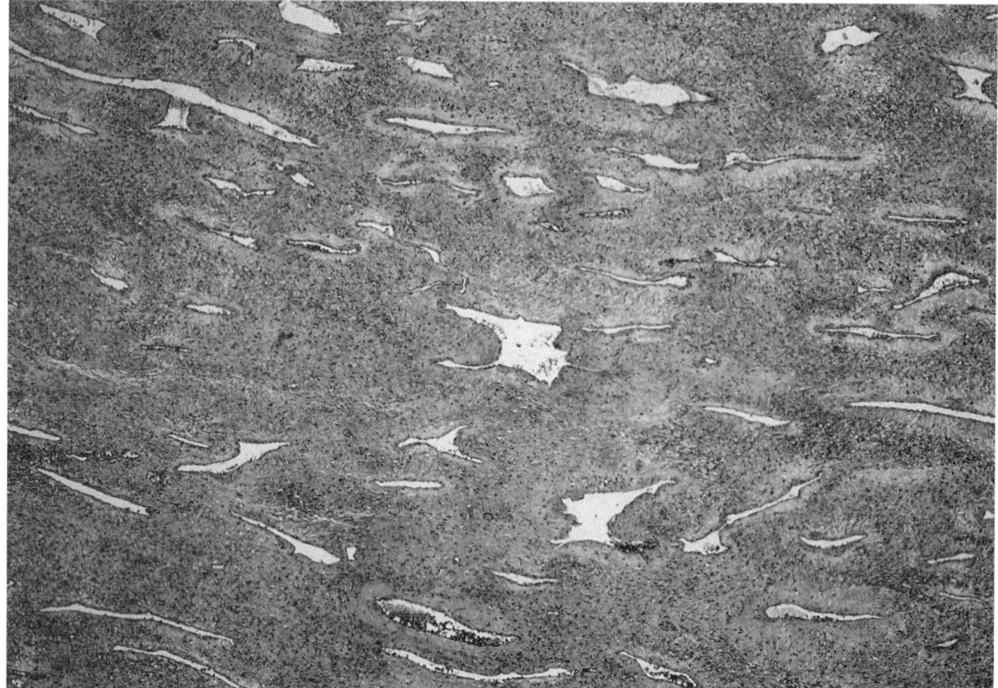

**FIGURE 9–48.** Nasopharyngeal angiofibroma consisting of dense fibrocollagenous tissue with interspersed vascular channels of varying caliber.

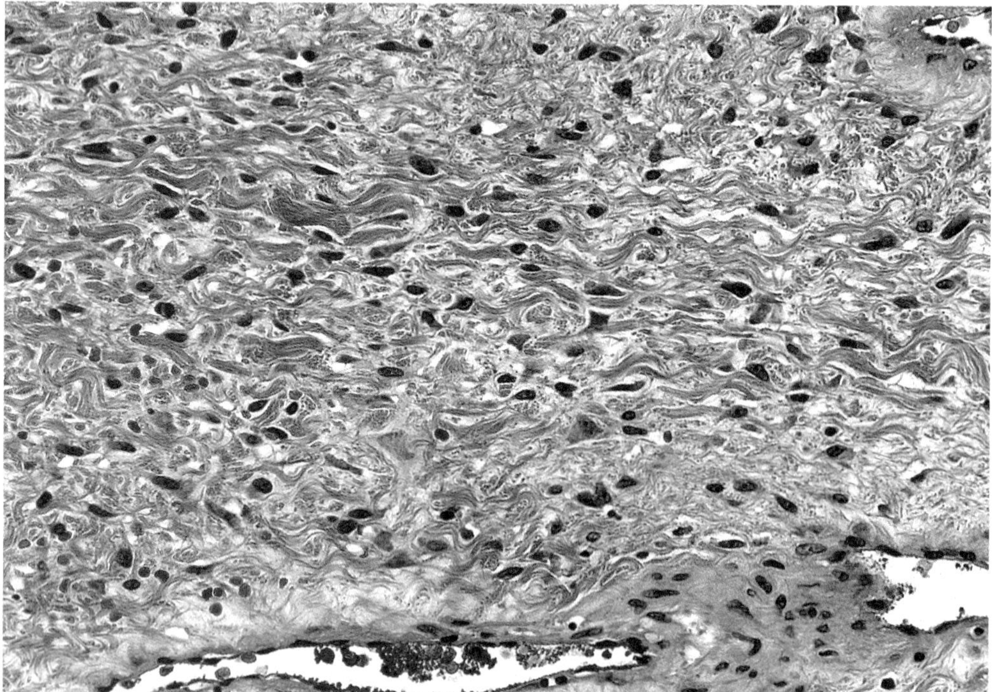

**FIGURE 9–49.** Nasopharyngeal angiofibroma composed of cytologically bland fibroblasts deposited in a dense collagenous stroma.

inae. However, the smaller vessels in the central portion of the tumor typically lack elastic laminae, which may explain the propensity for spontaneous or surgically induced hemorrhage.[211] The nature and organization of the vessels has suggested to some that this lesion could represent a vascular malformation as opposed to a neoplastic process.[212a]

### Immunohistochemical and Electron Microscopic Findings

Immunohistochemically, the endothelial cells lining the slit-like or dilated vessels stain for endothelial markers, including factor VIII-related antigen, CD31, and CD34. The immediate perivascular cells show variable staining for smooth muscle actin, depending on the amount of perivascular smooth muscle.[211] The spindle and stellate-shaped cells deposited in the dense fibrous stroma stain for vimentin, although some also stain for smooth muscle actin.[211,212] Recently, androgen receptors have been detected in the nuclei of endothelial and stromal cells using immunohistochemical techniques.[221,226]

Several ultrastructural studies have attempted to evaluate the nature of the spindle and stellate-shaped cells. Some authors have found these cells to have the features of fibroblasts, containing variable amounts of rough endoplasmic reticulum and intracytoplasmic filaments.[241,246] Taxy suggested that these cells have myofibroblastic features, with bundles of intracellular filaments with focal densities, pinocytotic vesicles, and hemidesmosomes.[242] Many of these cells also harbor electron-dense granular intranuclear inclusions which are less common and of smaller diameter in cells that exhibit myofibroblastic differentiation.[242] The nature of these peculiar intranuclear granular inclusions remains unknown. Walike and Mackay evaluated the ultrastructural features of a tumor before and after stilbestrol treatment and found increased synthetic activity in the cells, with increased collagen production and more widely spaced vascular channels with flattened endothelial cells in the posttreatment tumor.[246]

### Prognosis and Treatment

Although nasopharyngeal angiofibroma is histologically benign, it may act in an aggressive fashion characterized by recurrences that may extend into and destroy adjacent bony structures. The likelihood of recurrence is most closely related to the adequacy of the initial surgical excision, which in turn depends on the tumor stage.[237] The type of surgical approach depends on the extent of the tumor, as determined by preoperative radiographic studies. For low-stage tumors, some propose a transnasal[229,244] or intranasal[218,233] endoscopic approach. A transcranial approach may be more appropriate for tumors that have intracranial extension.[224–227,245] Preoperative transarterial embolization has been reported to result in decreased blood loss[234] and a decreased rate of local recurrence.[238,245] Hormone therapy has generally been ineffective.[213,240] Some authors advocate the use of radiation therapy, particularly for tumors with intracranial extension,[217,230,245,247] but radiation may cause osteonecrosis,[216] and there have been several reports of postradiation sarcomatous transformation into lesions that resemble fibrosarcoma[210,215,223] or malignant fibrous histiocytoma.[239] Rare squamous cell carcinomas[216] and papillary thyroid carcinomas[217] have also been related to prior irradiation of nasopharyngeal angiofibromas.

## GIANT CELL ANGIOFIBROMA

Giant cell angiofibroma is a distinctive tumor that most commonly arises in the orbital region of adults and shares morphologic features with giant cell fibroblastoma and solitary fibrous tumor. Although all seven tumors in the original report by Dei Tos et al. were located in the soft tissues of the orbit,[250] extraorbital tumors have also been described.[252,253a,255,256] There is a male predilection, and the peak incidence is during the fourth decade of life, although the age range is broad. Tumors arising in the orbit most commonly are found in the eyelid close to or involving the lacrimal gland. Most patients present with swelling of the eyelid, but some have proptosis or diplopia. Extraorbital tumors arise as slow-growing, painless, well circumscribed lesions.

On microscopic examination, the lesions may be circumscribed or ill-circumscribed, but they do not frankly infiltrate the surrounding soft tissues. The tumor has moderate to high cellularity and is composed of haphazardly arranged round to spindle-shaped cells deposited in a predominantly collagenized stroma that may exhibit myxoid change. There is typically a prominent vasculature with congested vessels of varying size, often with perivascular hyalinization (Fig. 9–50). At low magnification, a helpful diagnostic clue is the presence of pseudovascular spaces filled with granular material and surrounded by multinucleated floret-like giant cells.

At high magnification, the round and spindle-shaped cells have plump nuclei, inconspicuous nucleoli, and scanty pale eosinophilic cytoplasm. Multinucleated giant cells with a wreath-like configuration of hyperchromatic nuclei are scattered between the round and spindle-shaped cells and line the pseudovascular spaces (Fig. 9–51). Mitotic figures are rare, generally with fewer than 2 mitoses/10 HPF. Scattered inflammatory cells, including lymphocytes and

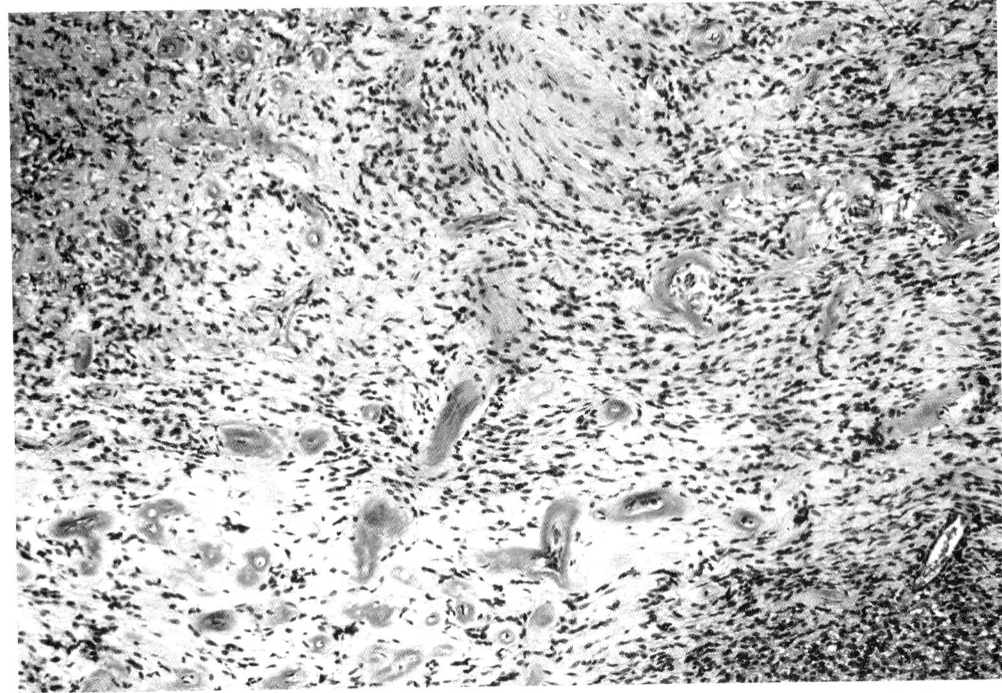

**FIGURE 9–50.** Giant cell angiofibroma with cellular proliferation of spindle-shaped cells between small blood vessels with marked perivascular hyalinization.

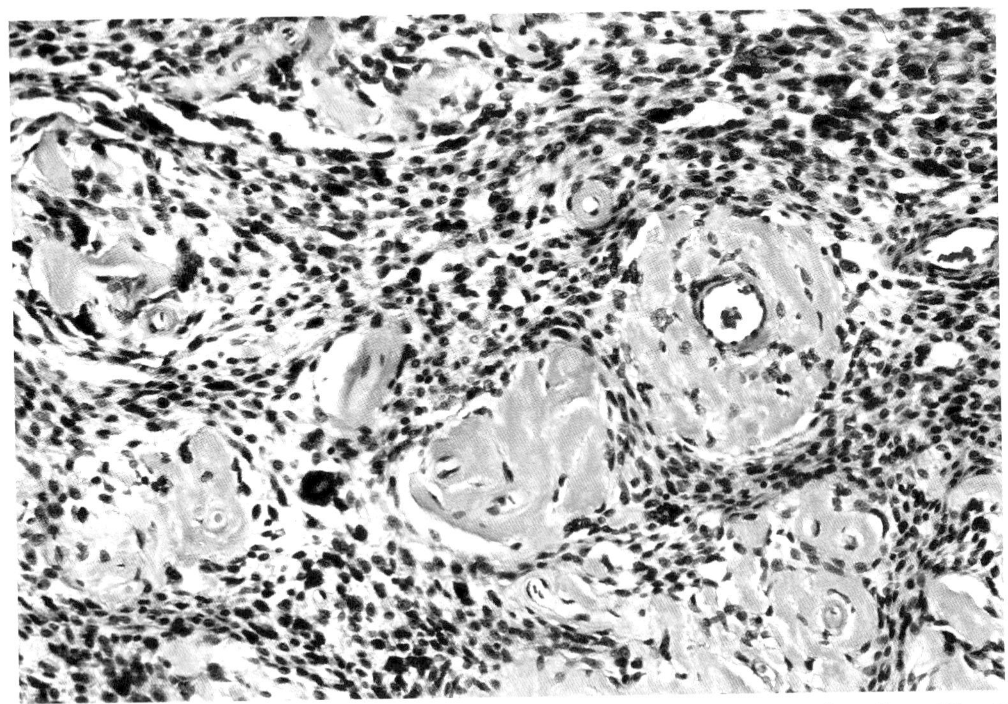

**FIGURE 9–51.** High-power view of a giant cell angiofibroma with cellular spindle cell proliferation between hyalinized blood vessels and scattered multinucleated floret-like giant cells.

plasma cells, are rare. Hemosiderin-laden macrophages may be present.

Immunohistochemically, the cells, including the giant cells, stain diffusely for vimentin and CD34 but do not stain for actin, desmin, S-100 protein, cytokeratin, epithelial membrane antigen, or vascular markers.[250,253,255] Few cases have been studied by electron microscopy, but most show fibroblastic features, with numerous rough endoplasmic reticulum, free ribosomes, and an absence of external lamina.[250]

The differential diagnosis includes a wide spectrum of mesenchymal lesions that occur in the orbit, including benign fibrous histiocytoma, hemangioma, hemangiopericytoma, meningioma, and benign peripheral nerve sheath tumors. This lesion is most easily confused with giant cell fibroblastoma and solitary fibrous tumor (Table 9–8).

*Giant cell fibroblastoma* generally occurs in much younger patients, typically during the first decade of life, and is usually a poorly circumscribed lesion that involves the dermis and subcutis of the somatic soft tissues, most commonly the trunk. This tumor has not been described in the orbit. Histologically, both tumors are characterized by the presence of $CD34^+$ cells (including multinucleated floret-like giant cells) and pseudovascular spaces lined by these giant cells. Giant cell fibroblastoma is more infiltrative than giant cell angiofibroma, has a less conspicuous vasculature, and is typically less cellular. Up to 50% of giant cell fibroblastomas recur, a rate that is apparently higher than that found with giant cell angiofibroma. Although there are no cytogenetic data yet available on giant cell angiofibroma, giant cell fibroblastoma is characterized by a balanced 17;22 translocation.[249]

*Solitary fibrous tumor* is a distinctive neoplasm that occurs predominantly in the pleura, although it has been increasingly recognized at other sites, including the orbit.[251,254,257] Characteristically, this lesion is well circumscribed and composed of a patternless array of uniform $CD34^+$ spindle-shaped cells, typically deposited in a matrix with prominent wire-like collagen. There is often a hemangiopericytomatous vascular pattern; unlike giant cell angiofibroma, pseudovascular spaces and multinucleated giant cells are not a feature of solitary fibrous tumor. It has recently been proposed that giant cell angiofibroma is a giant cell-rich variant of solitary fibrous tumor.[253a]

Thus far, most giant cell angiofibromas have been treated by local excision. The lesion appears to be benign, although the follow-up periods have been relatively short. In the study by Dei Tos et al.,[250] one patient showed persistent tumor after incomplete excision and another patient developed a local recurrence 60 months after the initial excision.

## KELOID

Keloid is a benign overgrowth of scar tissue occurring primarily in the dermis of persons 15–45 years of age. It may be solitary or multiple and has a predilection for dark-skinned individuals, especially Blacks. Keloid (Greek: claw-like) was named for its multiple extensions, which bestow on the lesion an imaginary crab-like appearance. There are, in addition to its common cicatricial forms, "spontaneous" or "idiopathic" forms of the condition, but these too are likely the result of some minor infection or injury in areas with increased skin tension. *Hypertrophic scars,* lesions that remain confined to the original wound site, should be distinguished from keloids because of their substantially lower recurrence rate.

**TABLE 9–8** HISTOLOGIC FEATURES OF GIANT CELL ANGIOFIBROMA COMPARED TO SOLITARY FIBROUS TUMOR AND GIANT CELL FIBROBLASTOMA

| Feature | Giant Cell Angiofibroma | Giant Cell Fibroblastoma | Solitary Fibrous Tumor |
|---|---|---|---|
| Age | Adults | Early childhood | Predominantly adults |
| Sites | Orbit | Trunk | Ubiquitous |
| Cellularity | ++ | + | Variable |
| Floret cells | + | + | Absent |
| Margins | Less infiltrative | Infiltrative | Well circumscribed |
| Vessels | Thick-walled, congested | Inconspicuous | Hemangiopericytomatous |
| Pseudovascular spaces | + | + | Absent |
| Myxoid stroma | Variable | Present | Absent |
| CD34 | + | + | + |
| Local recurrence | Rare | 50% | Rare |

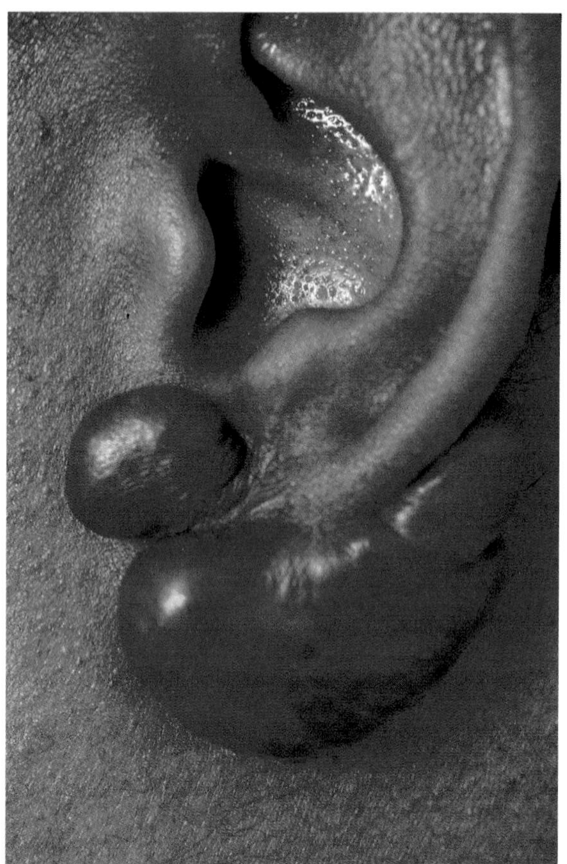

**FIGURE 9–52.** Keloid in a 25-year-old African American woman. It appeared after the earlobes were pierced for earrings.

## Clinical Findings

Keloids usually manifest as well circumscribed round, oval, or linear elevations of the skin and often extend with multiple processes into the surrounding areas. They may be asymptomatic but more often are described by the patient as being itchy, tender, or painful. In their earlier phase, keloids tend to be soft and erythematous; later they become increasingly indurated and turn white. They are found more commonly above than below the waist and have a predilection for the face, shoulders, forearms, and hands. About half of the "spontaneous" keloids occur as a transverse band in the presternal region, probably the result of minor infection and increased skin tension in this region. In some patients keloids are limited to one portion of the body; thus they may develop after piercing the earlobes for earrings but are absent in an appendectomy scar (Figs. 9–52, 9–53, 9–54).[279,280,286]

Keloids are induced by minor infections (especially acne and furuncles), smallpox and other vaccinations, tattooing and cautery, and laparotomies and various other surgical procedures. Sometimes even minor injuries, such as needle marks or mosquito bites, produce small keloids of pinhead size. In some African countries, keloidal scarification is produced deliberately in a special design and is considered an adornment and mark of beauty. The condition occurs mainly during the late teens and early adult life. It is found rarely in infants, small children, or the aged. Although originally reported to be more common in women than men, more recent studies have found no significant difference in incidence between the genders.[297]

Keloids are more commonly encountered in dark-skinned persons, particularly those of African descent.[269,270,284] Individuals of Chinese descent also appear to be at increased risk.[260] Several authors have found a distinct familial predisposition, with inheritance in an autosomal recessive or dominant pattern,[267,299] and those with a family history are more likely to have large, multiple keloids.[269] Keloid formation has been reported in association with numerous dermatologic disorders, particularly acne vulgaris,[291] and some connective tissue diseases, including Ehlers-

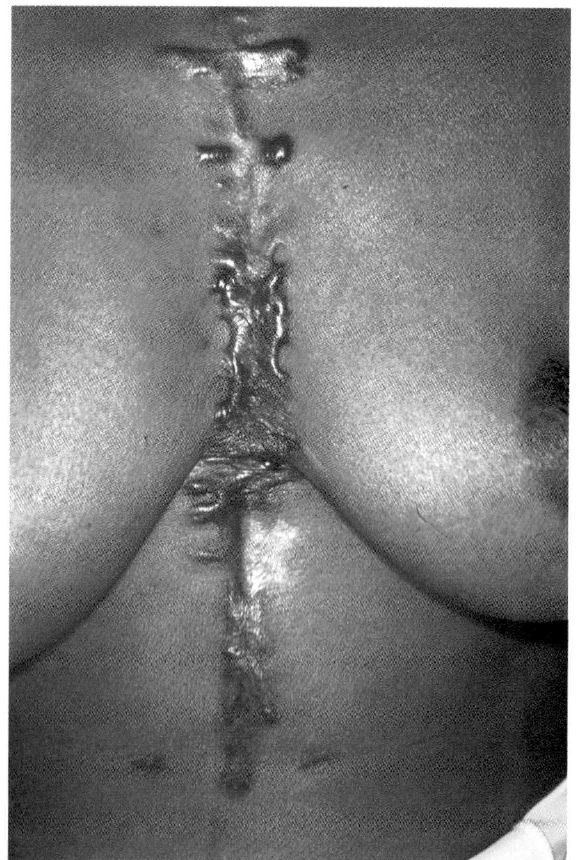

**FIGURE 9–53.** Keloid in the presternal region. These lesions may develop as the result of minor infection in an area of increased skin tension.

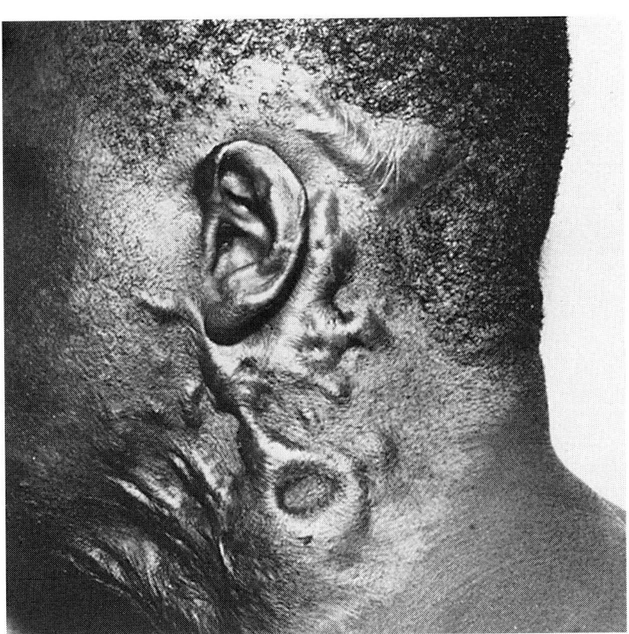

**FIGURE 9–54.** Keloid following thermal injury.

Danlos syndrome,[268] scleroderma,[259] and Rubinstein-Taybi syndrome.[277] An association of keloids with palmar, plantar, and penile fibromatosis has also been observed.[273]

## Pathologic Findings

Keloids are characterized by a fibrocollagenous proliferation of the dermis, with haphazardly arranged, thick, glassy, deeply acidophilic collagen fibers (Fig. 9–55). During the early phase the lesions tend to be vascular, particularly at their periphery, accounting for the clinical appearance of an erythematous lesion. Later lesions show decreased vascularity and more prominent hyalinization, which may undergo focal calcification or osseous metaplasia. Bland spindle-shaped cells are scattered throughout this hypocellular lesion. As the lesion grows, there is progressive displacement of the normal skin appendages, often with flattening or even atrophy of the overlying epidermis. Immunohistochemically, the spindle cells stain for vimentin. Although smooth muscle actin decorates the spindle cells of hypertrophic scars, the cells of keloids show minimal or no staining for this antigen.[271,305] Ultrastructurally, the constituent cells have the features of active fibroblasts, with abundant rough endoplasmic reticulum and prominent Golgi apparatus,[294] although some cells are described as having myofibroblastic features.[281,292]

*Hypertrophic scars* share the macroscopic features of keloids during the early phase of the lesion, but at later stages they flatten and have less mucoid matrix and few or no glassy collagen fibers. The initial cellular phase is also marked by a larger proportion of myofibroblasts, which may play a role in the contraction and elevation of the scar tissue.[263,278] In contrast to keloids, the changes are strictly limited to the area of injury.[266,283]

*Collagenoma,* a "connective tissue nevus," is an intradermal fibrocollagenous nodule that microscopically resembles a hypertrophic scar or keloid but there is no history of acne or dermal injury. The condition presents clinically as multiple discrete, asymptomatic, skin-colored, small nodules that affect mainly the regions of the trunk and the proximal portion of the upper extremities. In general, they make their first appearance during the postpubertal period and are frequently found in two or more members of the same family. Their number is significantly increased during pregnancy.[276,301,306]

*Circumscribed storiform collagenoma (sclerotic fibroma)* and *fibrous papules of the face* are two other morphologically related lesions. The former presents as a solitary dermal nodule composed of glassy, thickened collagen fibers arranged in a storiform pattern, occasionally with bizarre multinucleated giant cells.[303] It is identical to the fibrous nodules that occur in the multiple hamartoma syndrome or Cowden's disease.[293,296] The term *fibrous papules of the face* has been applied to a small dome-shaped fibrous nodule of the nose and face with an "onionskin" periadnexal or perivascular collagen pattern. This lesion has also been described as perifollicular fibroma and melanocytic angiofibroma.[274,295,300,302,308]

*Scleroderma (morphea)* is characterized by thickening and altered staining characteristics of existing collagen fibers. There is no new fiber formation and consequently no elevation of the skin.

*Keloidal dermatofibroma* is a recently described variant of dermatofibroma that may also histologically resemble a keloid.[288] Clinically, these lesions appear similar to ordinary dermatofibromas but are characterized by the presence of keloid-like collagen admixed with elements typically present in the usual dermatofibroma.

## Treatment

Numerous treatment modalities have been attempted to minimize local recurrence of keloids. The rate of local recurrence for surgical excision alone is high: 45–100%.[265] Surgery combined with topical injection of corticosteroids reduces the local recurrence rate to less than 50%.[289] Postoperative radiation therapy has also been reported to have good results, with local recurrence rates of less than 10%.[287,304] Numerous other therapeutic modalities, including laser therapy,[261] cryosurgery,[309] application of pressure pads,[290]

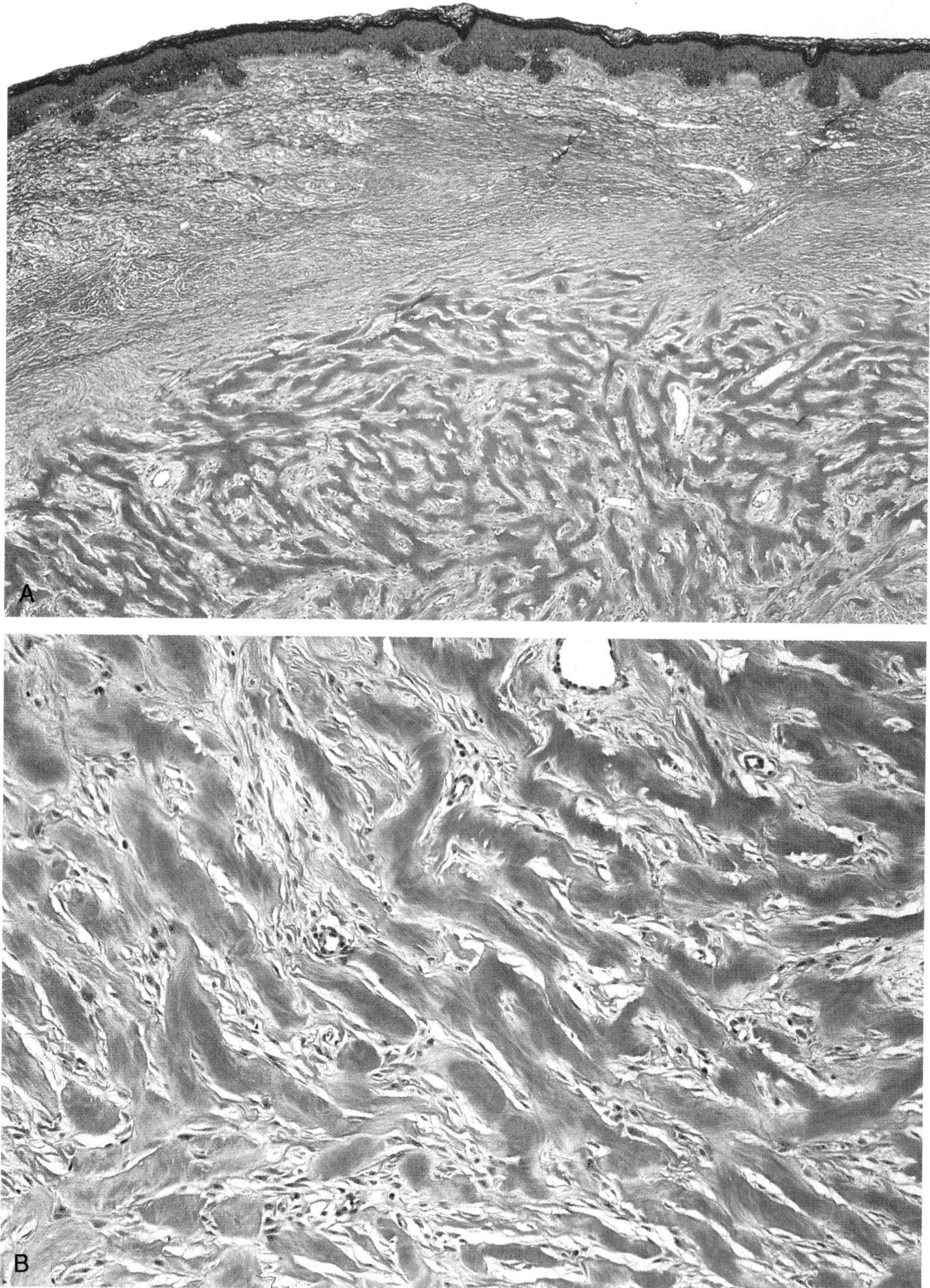


**FIGURE 9–55.** Keloid. (**A**) Low-power view. (**B**) Keloid displaying thick, glassy eosinophilic fibers in fibroblastic tissue.

and silicone gel or occlusive sheeting,[282] may also be effective. Patients who have a history of keloid formation should also avoid elective cosmetic procedures.

### Discussion

Unlike hypertrophic scars, keloids remain stationary or grow slowly and do not regress spontaneously. Although these lesions have a distinct tendency for local recurrence, the rate is highly dependent on the treatment. Immunohistochemical analyses of the proliferative activity of keloids using antibodies to Ki-67 or proliferating cell nuclear antigen have consistently found keloids to have a greater proliferative activity than is found in hypertrophic scars or normal skin, accounting for their tendency for continued growth.[262,272,298]

Keloids are composed predominantly of type I collagen. Compared with normal skin, in which type I collagen constitutes approximately 75% of the collagen, this type of collagen represents approximately 95% of the total collagen in keloids.[265] In addition, keloids have been reported to contain increased histamine,[285] fibronectin,[264] and proline hydroxylase[258] compared to that in hypertrophic scars or normal skin. Numerous growth factors appear to be important in the pathogenesis of this lesion by inducing increased collagen synthesis by fibroblasts, including epidermal growth factor,[285] platelet-derived growth factor receptors,[275] and transforming growth factor-$\beta$1.[307]

## DESMOPLASTIC FIBROBLASTOMA (COLLAGENOUS FIBROMA)

The desmoplastic fibroblastoma is a distinctive fibrous soft tissue tumor that typically occurs in the subcutaneous tissue or skeletal muscle of adults.[310–313] Most patients are in their fifth or sixth decade of life and present with a slowly growing, painless mass. Men are affected three to four times more commonly than women.[312] The most common site is the upper extremities, including the shoulder, upper arm, and forearm, followed by the lower extremity and the head and neck region. Most are predominantly subcutaneous, but some involve skeletal muscle exclusively. Although most are 4 cm or smaller, tumors as large as 20 cm have been described.[312]

Grossly, the desmoplastic fibroblastoma appears as a well circumscribed, firm mass with a white to gray cut surface, without hemorrhage or necrosis. Microscopically, the tumor is more or less circumscribed but not infrequently infiltrates the surrounding soft tissues. The lesion is hypocellular and consists of widely spaced bland spindle to stellate-shaped cells embedded in a collagenous or myxocollagenous stroma (Figs. 9–56, 9–57). Mitotic figures are rare or absent, and necrosis is not present. Blood vessels are

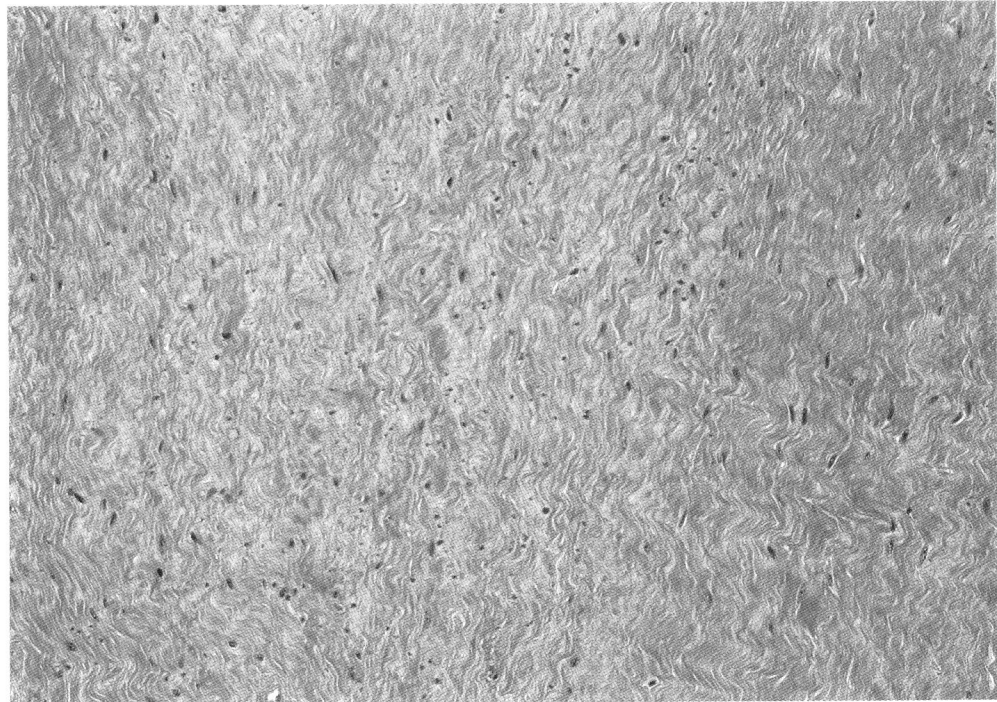

**FIGURE 9–56.** Low-power view of desmoplastic fibroblastoma. The lesion is hypocellular, with widely spaced bland cells embedded in a fibromyxoid stroma.

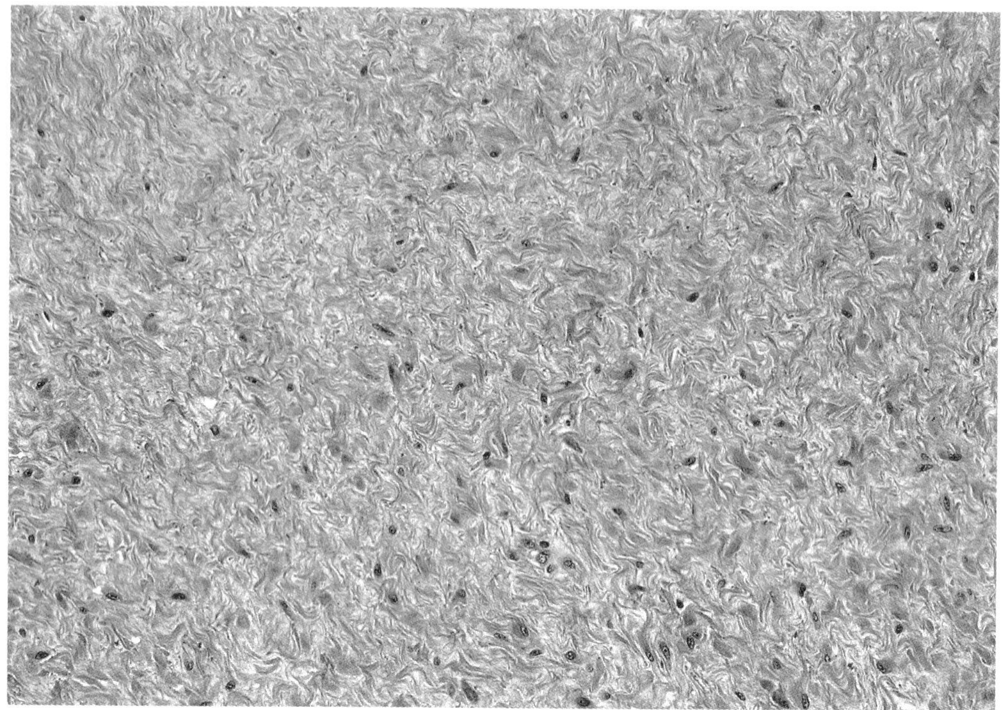

**FIGURE 9–57.** Desmoplastic fibroblastoma with bland spindle and stellate-shaped cells deposited in a fibromyxoid stroma.

inconspicuous but may exhibit perivascular hyalinization.

Immunohistochemically, the cells stain for vimentin, and most show focal staining for smooth muscle actin or muscle-specific actin. In addition, rare cells may stain for cytokeratin.[312] Immunostains for desmin, CD34, and S-100 protein are typically negative. Ultrastructurally, the neoplastic cells have the features of fibroblasts and myofibroblasts, with dilated rough endoplasmic reticulum and few cells with pinocytotic vesicles and focal myofilaments with dense bodies.

The differential diagnosis includes a variety of benign or low-grade, predominantly fibrous lesions. *Neurofibroma* is composed of cells with a wavy configuration deposited in a myxocollagenous stroma, often with wire-like bundles of collagen. Unlike desmoplastic fibroblastoma, S-100 protein is typically strongly positive in neurofibromas. *Fibromatosis,* even when hypocellular, is more cellular than desmoplastic fibroblastoma, and the cells tend to be arranged in broad fascicles. *Calcifying fibrous pseudotumor,* which affects children and young adults, is characterized by psammomatous calcifications and a lymphoplasmacytic infiltrate. *Low-grade fibromyxoid sarcoma* is typically more cellular, with cells arranged in whorls and deposited in a variably fibromyxoid stroma. *Elastofibroma,* usually found in the subscapular area, is characterized by wavy elastic fibers that are not present in desmoplastic fibroblastoma. *Nodular fasciitis* of long duration can also resemble this lesion but usually has areas of increased cellularity and other features typical of nodular fasciitis, even if present focally.

Most of the patients have been treated by conservative simple excision, and neither local recurrence nor metastasis has been reported. Because of the bland hypocellular appearance, it is not certain whether these lesions are the end-stage of a reactive process or a true neoplasm, although we favor the latter. Sciot et al.[314] reported two such tumors with aberrations of 11q12, similar to those described for fibroma of the tendon sheath.

## REFERENCES

### Fibrous Connective Tissue: Structure and Function

1. Bhawan J. The myofibroblast. Am J Dermatopathol 3:73, 1981.
2. Campbell JH, Terranova VP. Laminin: molecular organization and biological function. Oral Pathol 17:309, 1988.
3. Cox RW, Grant RA, Horne RW. The structure and assembly of collagen fibrils. I. Native collagen fibrils and their formation from tropocollagen. J R Microsc Soc 87:123, 1967.
4. Erlandson RE. Extracellular constituents. In: Diagnostic Transmission Electron Microscopy of Tumors. Raven, New York, 1994, p 221.
5. Gabbiani G, Majno G. Dupuytren's contracture: fibroblast contraction? An ultrastructural study. Am J Pathol 66:131, 1972.
6. Gabbiani G, Ryan GB, Majno G. Presence of modified fibroblasts in granulation tissue and their possible role in wound contraction. Experientia 27:549, 1971.

7. Hashimoto K, DiBella RJ. Electron microscopic studies of normal and abnormal elastic fibers of the skin. J Invest Dermatol 48:405, 1967.
8. Leblond CP. Synthesis and secretion of collagen by cells of connective tissue, bone and dentin. Anat Rec 224:123, 1989.
9. Majno G. The story of the myofibroblasts. Am J Surg Pathol 3: 535, 1979.
10. McDonagh J. Fibronectin: a molecular glue. Arch Pathol Lab Med 105:393, 1981.
11. Mentzel T, Fletcher CDM. The emerging role of myofibroblasts in soft tissue neoplasia. Am J Clin Pathol 107:2, 1997.
12. Olsen D, Nagayoshi T, Fazio M, et al. Human laminin: cloning and sequence analysis of cDNAs encoding A, B1 and B2 chains, and expression of the corresponding genes in human skin and cultured cells. Lab Invest 60:772, 1989.
13. Rosenbloom J. Elastin: relation of protein and gene structure to disease. Lab Invest 51:605, 1984.
14. Schürch W, Seemayer TA, Gabbiani G. The myofibroblast: a quarter century after its discovery. Am J Surg Pathol 22:141, 1998.
15. Schürch W, Seemayer DA, Lagace R, et al. The intermediate filament cytoskeleton of myofibroblasts: an immunofluorescence and ultrastructural study. Virchows Arch [Pathol Anat] 403:323, 1984.
16. Seemayer TA, Schurch W, Lagace R, et al. Myofibroblasts in the stroma of invasive and metastatic carcinoma. Am J Surg Pathol 3:575, 1979.
17. Silbert JE. Structure and metabolism of proteoglycans and glycosaminoglycans. J Invest Dermatol 79(Suppl 1):31, 1982.
18. Singer II. The fibronexus: a transmembrane association of fibronectin-containing fibres in hamster and human fibroblasts. Cell 16:675, 1979.
19. Singer II, Kawka DW, Kazazis DN, et al. In vivo co-distribution of fibronectin and actin fibers in granulation tissue: immunofluorescence and electron microscope studies of the fibronexus at the myofibroblast surface. J Cell Biol 98:2091, 1984.
20. Skalli O, Schürch W, Seemayer T, et al. Myofibroblasts from diverse pathologic settings are heterogeneous in their content of actin isoforms and intermediate filament proteins. Lab Invest 60;275, 1989.
21. Snodgrass MJ. Ultrastructural distinction between reticular and collagenous fibers with an ammoniacal silver stain. Anat Rec 187:191, 1977.
22. Stenman S, Vaheri A. Distribution of a major connective tissue protein, fibronectin, in normal human tissues. J Exp Med 147: 1054, 1978.

## Nodular Fasciitis

23. Abendroth CS, Frauenhoffer EE. Nodular fasciitis of the parotid gland: report of a case with presentation in an unusual location and cytologic differential diagnosis. Acta Cytol 39:530, 1995.
24. Adler R, Wang CA. Cranial fasciitis simulating histiocytosis. J Pediatr 109:85, 1996.
25. Allen PW. Nodular fasciitis. Pathology 4:9, 1972.
26. Batsakis JG, El-Naggar AK. Pseudosarcomatous proliferative lesions of soft tissues. Ann Otol Rhinol Laryngol 103:578, 1994.
27. Bernstein KE, Lattes R. Nodular (pseudosarcomatous) fasciitis, a non-recurrent lesion: clinicopathologic study of 134 cases. Cancer 49:1668, 1982.
28. Birdsall SH, Shipley JM, Summersgill BM, et al. Cytogenetic findings in a case of nodular fasciitis of the breast. Cancer Genet Cytogenet 81:166, 1995.
29. Boddie DE, Distante S, Blaiklock CT. Cranial fasciitis of childhood: an incidental finding of a lytic skull lesion. Br J Neurosurg 11:445, 1997.
30. Calonje E, Mentzel T, Fletcher CDM. Cellular benign fibrous histiocytoma: clinicopathologic analysis of 74 cases of a distinctive variant of cutaneous fibrous histiocytoma with frequent recurrence. Am J Surg Pathol 18:668, 1994.
31. Chung EB, Enzinger FM. Proliferative fasciitis. Cancer 36:1450, 1975.
32. Clapp CG, Dodson EE, Pickett BP, et al. Cranial fasciitis presenting as an external auditory canal mass. Arch Otolaryngol Head Neck Surg 123:223, 1997.
33. Culberson JD, Enterline HT. Pseudosarcomatous fasciitis: a distinctive clinical-pathologic entity: report of five cases. Am Surg 151:235, 1960.
34. Dahl I, Akerman M. Nodular fasciitis: a correlative cytologic and histologic study of 13 cases. Acta Cytol 25:215, 1981.
35. Dahl I, Angervall L, Magnusson S, et al. Classical and cystic nodular fasciitis. Pathol Eur 7:211, 1972.
36. Dahl I, Jarlstedt J. Nodular fasciitis in the head and neck: a clinicopathological study of 18 cases. Acta Otolaryngol 90:152, 1980.
37. Daroca PJ, Pulitzer DR, LoCicero J. Ossifying fasciitis. Arch Pathol Lab Med 106:682, 1982.
38. Dupree WB, Enzinger FM. Fibro-osseous pseudotumor of the digits. Cancer 58:2103, 1986.
39. El-Jabbour JN, Wilson GD, Bennett MH, et al. Flow cytometric study of nodular fasciitis, proliferative fasciitis and proliferative myositis. Hum Pathol 22:1146, 1991.
40. Enzinger FM, Dulcey F. Proliferative myositis: report of thirty-three cases. Cancer 20:2213, 1967.
41. Fernando SS, Gune S, George S, et al. Nodular fascitiis: a case with unusual clinical presentation initially diagnosed by aspiration cytology. Cytopathology 4:305, 1993.
42. Freedman PD, Lumerman H. Intravascular fasciitis: report of two cases and review of the literature. Oral Surg 62:549, 1986.
43. Gabbiani G, Ryan GB, Majno G. Presence of modified fibroblasts in granulation tissue and their possible role in wound contraction. Experientia 27:549, 1971.
44. Goldblum JR, Tuthill RJ. CD34 and factor-XIIIa immunoreactivity in dermatofibrosarcoma protuberans and dermatofibroma. Am J Dermatopathol 19:147, 1997.
45. Goodlad JR, Fletcher CDM. Intradermal variant of nodular fasciitis. Histopathology 17:569, 1990.
46. Hasegawa T, Hirose T, Kudo E, et al. Cytoskeletal characteristics of myofibroblasts in benign neoplastic and reactive fibroblastic lesions. Virchows Arch [Pathol Anal] 416:375, 1990.
47. Hoya K, Usui M, Sugiyama Y, et al. Cranial fasciitis. Childs Nerv Syst 12:556, 1996.
48. Hutter RVP, Foote FW Jr, Francis KC, et al. Parosteal fasciitis: a self-limited benign process that simulates a malignant neoplasm. Am J Surg 104:800, 1962.
49. Hutter RVP, Stewart FW, Foote FW Jr. Fasciitis: a report of 70 cases with follow-up proving the benignity of the lesion. Cancer 15:992, 1962.
50. Kahn MA, Weathers DR, Johnson DN. Intravascular fasciitis: a case report of an intraoral location. J Oral Pathol Med 16:308, 1987.
51. Kaw YT, Cuesta RA. Nodular fasciitis of the orbit diagnosed by fine needle aspiration cytology: a case report. Acta Cytol 37:957, 1993.
52. Kleinstiver BJ, Rodriguez HA. Nodular fasciitis: a study of forty-five cases and review of the literature. J Bone Joint Surg [Am] 50:1204, 1968.
53. Kornwaler BE, Keasbey L, Kaplan L. Subcutaneous pseudosarcomatous fibromatosis (fasciitis). Am J Clin Pathol 25:241, 1955.
54. Kwittken J, Branche M. Fasciitis ossificans. Am J Clin Pathol 51:251, 1969.

55. Lai FMM, Lam WY. Nodular fasciitis of the dermis. J Cutan Pathol 20:66, 1993.
56. Lauer DH, Enzinger FM. Cranial fasciitis of childhood. Cancer 45:401, 1980.
57. Meister P, Buckmann FW, Konrad E. Nodular fasciitis: analysis of 100 cases and review of the literature. Pathol Res Pract 162:133, 1978.
58. Montgomery EA, Meis JM. Nodular fasciitis: its morphologic spectrum and immunohistochemical profile. Am J Surg Pathol 15:942, 1991.
59. Ooe M, Ishiguro N, Kawashima M. Nuclear DNA content and distribution of Ki-67 positive cells in nodular fasciitis. J Dermatol 20:214, 1993.
60. Oshiro Y, Fukuda T, Tsuneyoshi M. Fibrosarcoma versus fibromatoses and cellular nodular fasciitis: a comparative study of their proliferative activity using proliferating cell nuclear antigen, DNA flow cytometry and p53. Am J Surg Pathol 18: 712, 1994.
61. O'Connell JX, Young RH, Nielsen GP, et al. Nodular fasciitis of the vulva: a study of six cases and literature review. Int J Gynecol Pathol 16:117, 1997.
62. Patchefsky AS, Enzinger FM. Intravascular fasciitis: a report of 17 cases.. Am J Surg Pathol 5:29, 1981.
63. Price EB Jr, Silliphant WM, Shuman R. Nodular fasciitis: a clinicopathologic analysis of 65 casess. Am J Clin Pathol 35: 122, 1961.
64. Price SK, Kahn LB, Saxe N. Dermal and intravascular fasciitis: unusual variants of nodular fasciitis. Am J Dermatopathol 15: 539, 1993.
65. Samaratunga H, Searle J, O'Loughlin B. Intravascular fasciitis: a case report and review of the literature. Pathology 28:8, 1996.
66. Sarangarajan R, Dehner LP. Cranial and extracranial fasciitis of childhood: a clinicopathologic and immunohistochemical study. Hum Pathol 30:87, 1999.
67. Sasano H, Yamaki H, Ohashi Y, et al. Proliferative fasciitis of the forearm: case report with immunohistochemical, ultrastructural and DNA ploidy studies and a review of the literature. Pathol Int 48:486, 1998.
68. Sato Y, Kitamura T, Suganuma Y, et al. Cranial fasciitis of childhood: a case report. Eur J Pediatr Surg 3:107, 1993.
69. Sawyer JR, Sammartino G, Baker GF, et al. Clonal chromosome aberrations in a case of nodular fasciitis. Cancer Genet Cytogenet 76:154, 1994.
70. Sayama P, Morioka T, Baba T, et al. Cranial fasciitis with massive intracranial extension. Childs Nerv Syst 11:242, 1995.
71. Senoh H, Nonomura N, Akai H, et al. A case of nodular fasciitis of the bladder. Acta Urol Jpn 40:427, 1994.
72. Shimizu S, Hashimoto H, Enjoji M. Nodular fasciitis: an analysis of 250 patients. Pathology 16:161, 1984.
73. Soule EH. Proliferative (nodular) fasciitis. Arch Pathol 73:437, 1962.
74. Stanley MW, Skoog L, Tani EM, et al. Nodular fasciitis: spontaneous resolution following diagnosis by fine-needle aspiration. Diagn Cytopathol 9:322, 1993.
75. Sticha RS, Deacon JS, Wertheimer SJ, et al. Intravascular fasciitis in the foot. J Foot Ankle Surg 36:95, 1997.
76. Stiller D, Katenkamp D. Die nodulare fasziitiz. Zentrabl Chir 98:885, 1973.
77. Stout AP. Pseudosarcomatous fasciitis in children. Cancer 14: 1216, 1961.
78. Stout AP, Lattes R. Tumors of the soft tissues, second series. In: Atlas of Tumor Pathology. Armed Forces Institute of Pathology, Washington, DC, 1967.
79. Wirman JA. Nodular fasciitis, a lesion of myofibroblasts: an ultrastructural study. Cancer 38:2378, 1976.

**Proliferative Fasciitis and Myositis**

80. Ackerman LV. Extra-osseous localized non-neoplastic bone and cartilage formation (so-called myositis ossificans): clinical and pathological confusion with malignant neoplasms. J Bone Joint Surg [Am] 40:279, 1958.
81. Brooks JSJ. Immunohistochemistry of proliferative myositis. Arch Pathol Lab Med 105:682, 1981.
82. Choi SS, Myer CM. Proliferative myositis of the mylohyoid muscle. Am J Otolaryngol 11:198, 1990.
83. Chow LPC, Chow WH, Lee JCK. Fine needle aspiration (FNA) cytology of proliferative fasciitis: report of a case with immunohistochemical study. Cytopathology 6:349, 1995.
84. Chung EB, Enzinger FM. Proliferative fasciitis. Cancer 36:1450, 1975.
85. Craver JL, McDivitt RW. Proliferative fasciitis: ultrastructural study of two cases. Arch Pathol Lab Med 105:542, 1981.
86. Dembinski A, Bridge JA, Neff JR, et al. Trisomy 2 in proliferative fasciitis. Cancer Genet Cytogenet 60:27, 1992.
87. Dent CD, DeBoom GW, Hanlin ML. Proliferative myositis of the head and neck: report of a case and review of the literature. Oral Surg Oral Med Oral Pathol 78:354, 1994.
88. Diaz-Flores L, Martin-Harrera AI, Garcia Montelongo R, et al. Proliferative fasciitis: ultrastructure and histogenesis. J Cutan Pathol 16:85, 1989.
89. El-Jabbour JN, Bennett MH, Burke MM, et al. Proliferative myositis: an immunohistochemical and ultrastructural study. Am J Surg Pathol 15:654, 1991.
90. El-Jabbour JN, Wilson GD, Bennett MH, et al. Flow cytometric study of nodular fasciitis, proliferative fasciitis and proliferative myositis. Hum Pathol 22:1146, 1991.
91. Enzinger FM, Dulcey F. Proliferative myositis: report of thirty-three cases. Cancer 20:2213, 1967.
92. Fujiwara K, Watanabe T, Katsuki T, et al. Proliferative myositis of the buccinator muscle: a case report with immunohistochemical and electron microscopic analysis. Oral Surg Oral Med Oral Pathol 63:963, 1987.
93. Ghadially FN, Thomas MJ, Jabi M, et al. Intracisternal collagen fibrils in proliferative fasciitis and myositis of childhood. Ultrastruct Pathol 17:161, 1993.
94. Gokel JM, Meister P, Hübner G. Proliferative myositis: a case report with fine structural analysis. Virchows Arch [Pathol Anat Histol] 367:345, 1975.
95. Jacobs JC. Aspiration cytology of proliferative myositis: a case report. Acta Cytol 39:535, 1995.
96. Kern WH. Proliferative myositis; a pseudosarcomatous reaction to injury: a report of seven cases. Arch Pathol 69:209, 1960.
97. Kiryu H, Takeshita H, Hori Y. Proliferative fasciitis: report of a case with histopathologic and immunohistochemical studies. Am J Dermatopathol 19:396, 1997.
98. Kitano M, Iwasaki H, Enjoji M. Proliferative fasciitis: a variant of nodular fasciitis. Acta Pathol Jpn 27:485, 1977.
99. Lundgren L, Kindblom LG, Willems J, et al. Proliferative myositis and fasciitis: a light and electron microscopic, cytologic, DNA-cytometric and immunohistochemical study. APMIS 100:437, 1992.
100. McComb EN, Neff JR, Johansson SL, et al. Chromosomal anomalies in a case of proliferative myositis. Cancer Genet Cytogenet 98:142, 1997.
101. Meis JM, Enzinger FM. Proliferative fasciitis and myositis of childhood. Am J Surg Pathol 16:364, 1992.
102. Ohjimi Y, Iwasaki H, Ishiguro M, et al. Trisomy 2 found in proliferative myositis cultured cell. Cancer Genet Cytogenet 76:157, 1994.
103. Pasquel P, Salazar M, Marvan E. Proliferative myositis in an infant: report of a case with electron microscopic observations. Pediatr Pathol 8:545, 1988.

104. Pollock L, Fullilove S, Shaw DG, et al. Proliferative myositis in a child: a case report. J Bone Joint Surg [Am] 77:132, 1995.
105. Reif RM. The cytologic picture of proliferative myositis. Acta Cytol 26:376, 1982.
106. Rose AG. An electron microscopic study of the giant cells in proliferative myositis. Cancer 33:1543, 1974.
107. Stiller D, Katenkamp D. The subcutaneous fascial analogue of myositis proliferans: electron microscopic examination of two cases and comparison with myositis ossificans localisata. Virchows Arch [Pathol Anat Histol] 368:361, 1975.
108. Ushigome S, Takakuwa T, Takagi M, et al. Proliferative myositis and fasciitis: report of five cases with an ultrastructural and immunohistochemical study. Acta Pathol Jpn 36:963, 1986.

### Organ-Associated Pseudosarcomatous Myofibroblastic Proliferations

109. Albores-Saavedra J, Manivel JC, Essenreid H, et al. Pseudosarcomatous myofibroblastic proliferations in the urinary bladder of children. Cancer 66:1234, 1990.
110. Clement CB. Postoperative spindle cell nodule of the endometrium. Arch Pathol Lab Med 112:566, 1988.
111. Coyne JD, Wilson G, Sandhu D, et al. Inflammatory pseudotumor of the urinary bladder. Histopathology 18:261, 1991.
112. Das S, Upton JD, Amar AD. Nodular fasciitis of the bladder. J Urol 140:1532, 1988.
113. Dietrick DD, Kabalain JN, Daniels GF, et al. Inflammatory pseudotumor of the bladder. J Urol 148:141, 1992.
114. Forrest JB, King GS, Pittman GR. An atypical myofibroblastic tumor of the bladder resembling a sarcoma. J Okla State Med Assoc 81:222, 1988.
115. Goussot JF, Coindre JM, Merlio JP, et al. An adult atypical fibromyxoid tumor of the urinary bladder. Tumori 75:79, 1989.
116. Gugliada K, Nardi PM, Borenstein MS, et al. Inflammatory pseudosarcoma (pseudotumor) of the bladder. Radiology 1779: 66, 1991.
117. Hojo H, Newton WA Jr, Hamoudi AB, et al. Pseudosarcomatous myofibroblastic tumor of the urinary bladder in children: a study of 11 cases with review of the literature; an Intergroup Rhabdomyosarcoma Study. Am J Surg Pathol 19:1224, 1995.
118. Horn L-C, Reuter S, Biesold M. Inflammatory pseudotumor of the ureter and the urinary bladder. Pathol Res Pract 193:607, 1997.
119. Huang WL, Ro JY, Grignon DJ, et al. Postoperative spindle cell nodule of the prostate and bladder. J Urol 143:824, 1990.
120. Jones EC, Clement PB, Young RH. Inflammatory pseudotumor of the urinary bladder: a clinicopathological, immunohistochemical, ultrastructural and flow cytometric study of 13 cases. Am J Surg Pathol 17:264, 1993.
121. Jufe R, Molinolo AA, Feffer SA, et al. Plasma cell granuloma of the bladder: a case report. J Urol 131:1175, 1984.
122. Kay S, Schneider V. Reactive spindle cell nodule of the endocervix simulating uterine sarcoma. Int J Gynecol Pathol 4:255, 1985.
123. Lamovec J, Zidar A, Trsinar B, et al. Sclerosing inflammatory pseudotumor of the urinary bladder in a child. Am J Surg Pathol 16:1233, 1992.
124. Lo JW, Fung CHK, Yonan T, et al. Postoperative spindle-cell nodule of urinary bladder with unusual intracytoplasmic inclusions. Diagn Cytopathol 8:171, 1992.
125. Lundgren L, Aldenborg F, Angervall L, et al. Pseudomalignant spindle-cell proliferafions of the urinary bladder. Hum Pathol 25:181, 1994.
126. Manson CM, Hirsch PJ, Coyne JD. Post-operative spindle cell nodule of the vulva. Histopathology 26:571, 1995.
127. Nochomovitz LE, Orenstein JM. Inflammatory pseudotumor of the urinary bladder: possible relationship to nodular fasciitis: two case reports, cytologic observations, and ultrastructural observations. Am J Surg Pathol 9:366, 1985.
128. Papadimitriou JC, Drachenberg CB. Posttraumatic spindle cell nodules: immunohistochemical and ultrastructural study of two scrotal lesions. Arch Pathol Lab Med 118:709, 1994.
129. Proppe KH, Scully RE, Rosai J. Postoperative spindle cell nodules of genitourinary tract resembling sarcomas: a report of eight cases. Am J Surg Pathol 8:101, 1984.
130. Ro JY, Ayala AG, Ordonez NG, et al. Pseudosarcomatous fibromyxoid tumor of the urinary bladder. Am J Clin Pathol 86: 583, 1986.
131. Ro JY, El-Naggar AK, Amin MB, et al. Pseudosarcomatous fibromyxoid tumor of the urinary bladder and prostate: immunohistochemical, ultrastructural and DNA flow cytometric analyses of nine cases. Hum Pathol 24:1203, 1993.
132. Sahin AA, Ro JY, El-Naggar AK, et al. Pseudosarcomatous fibromyxoid tumor of the prostate. Am J Clin Pathol 96:253, 1991.
133. Stark GL, Feddersen R, Lowe BA, et al. Inflammatory pseudotumor (pseudosarcoma) of the bladder. J Urol 141:610, 1989.
134. Vekemans K, Vanneste A, Van Oyen P, et al. Postoperative spindle cell nodule of bladder. Urology 35:342, 1990.
135. Weidner N. Inflammatory (myofibroblastic) pseudotumor of the bladder: a review in differential diagnosis. Adv Anat Pathol 2:362, 1995.
136. Wick MR, Brown BA, Young RH, et al. Spindle-cell proliferations of the urinary tract: an immunohistochemical study. Am J Surg Pathol 12:379, 1988.
137. Young RH, Scully RE. Pseudosarcomatous lesions of the urinary bladder, prostate gland, and urethra: a report of three cases and review of the literature. Arch Pathol Lab Med 111: 354, 1987.

### Ischemic Fasciitis (Atypical Decubital Fibroplasia)

138. Baldassano MF, Rosenberg AE, Flotte TJ. Atypical decubital fibroplasia: a series of three cases. J Cutan Pathol 25:149, 1998.
139. Baranzelli MC, Leconte-Houcke M, De Saint Maur P, et al. Atypical decubitus fibroplasia: a recent entity; report of a case in an adolescent girl. Bull Cancer 83:81, 1996.
140. Kendall BS, Liang CY, Lancaster KJ, et al. Ischemic fasciitis: report of a case with fine needle aspiration findings. Acta Cytol 41:598, 1997.
141. Montgomery EA, Meis JM, Mitchell MS, et al. Atypical decubital fibroplasia: a distinctive fibroblastic pseudotumor occurring in debilitated patients. Am J Surg Pathol 16:708, 1992.
142. Perosio PM, Weiss SW. Ischemic fasciitis: a juxta-skeletal fibroblastic proliferation with a predilection for elderly patients. Mod Pathol 6:69, 1993.
143. Yamamoto M, Ishida T, Machinami R. Atypical decubital fibroplasia in a young patient with melaorheostosis. Pathol Int 48:160, 1998.
144. Zamecnik M, Michal M, Patrikova J. Atypical decubital fibroplasia (ischemic fasciitis): a new pseudosarcomatous entity. Cesk Patol 30:130, 1994.

### Fibroma of the Tendon Sheath

145. Azzopardi JG, Tanda F, Salm R. Tenosynovial fibroma. Diagn Histopathol 6:59, 1983.
146. Chung EB, Enzinger FM. Fibroma of tendon sheath. Cancer 44:1945, 1979.
147. Cooper PH. Fibroma of tendon sheath. J Am Acad Dermatol 11:625, 1984.
148. Dal Cin P, Sciot R, de Smet L, et al. Translocation 2;11 in a fibroma of tendon sheath. Histopathology 32:433, 1998.
149. Dal Cin P, Sciot R, Samson I, et al. Cytogenetic characterization of tenosynovial giant cell tumors (nodular tenosynovitis). Cancer Res 54:3986, 1994.

150. Hashimoto H, Tsuneyoshi M, Daimaru Y, et al. Fibroma of tendon sheath: a tumor of myofibroblasts; a clinicopathologic study of 18 cases. Acta Pathol Jpn 35:1099, 1985.
151. Humphreys S, McKee PH, Fletcher CDM. Fibroma of tendon sheath: a clinicopathologic study. J Cutan Pathol 13:331, 1986.
152. Jablokow VR, Kathuria S. Fibroma of tendon sheath. J Surg Oncol 19:90, 1982.
153. Lamovec J, Brako M, Vonina D. Pleomorphic fibroma of tendon sheath. Am J Surg Pathol 15:1202, 1991.
154. Lundgren LG, Kindblom LG. Fibroma of tendon sheath: a light and electron microscopic study of 6 cases. Acta Pathol Microbiol Immunol Scand 92:401, 1984.
155. Maluf HM, DeYoung BR, Swanson PE, et al. Fibroma and giant cell tumor of tendon sheath: a comparative histological and immunohistological study. Mod Pathol 8:155, 1995.
156. Pulitzer DR, Martin PC, Reed RJ. Fibroma of tendon sheath: a clinicopathologic study of 32 cases. Am J Surg Pathol 13:472, 1989.
157. Sarma DP, Weilbaecher TG, Rodriguez FH Jr. Fibroma of tendon sheath. J Surg Oncol 32:230, 1986.
158. Satti MB. Tendon sheath tumors: a pathological study of the relationships between giant cell tumor and fibroma of tendon sheath. Histopathology 20:213, 1992.
159. Silverman JS, Knapik M. Fibroma of tendon sheath is rich in factor XIIIa positive dendrocytes [abstract]. Am J Clin Pathol 105:519, 1994.
160. Silverman JS, Knapik M. Letter to the editor. Mod Pathol 9:82, 1996.
161. Smith PS, Pieterse AS, McClure J. Fibroma of tendon sheath. J Clin Pathol 35:842, 1982.

### Pleomorphic Fibroma of Skin

162. Ahn SK, Won JH, Lee SH, et al. Pleomorphic fibroma of scalp. Dematology 191:245, 1995.
163. Garcia-Doval I, Casas L, Toribio J. Pleomorphic fibroma of the skin, a form of sclerotic fibroma: an immunohistochemieal study. Clin Exp Dermatol 23:22, 1998.
164. Kamino H, Lee JY-Y, Berke A. Pleomorphic fibroma of the skin: a benign neoplasm with cytologic atypia; a clinicopathologic study of eight cases. Am J Surg Pathol 13:107, 1989.
165. Layfield LJ, Fain JS. Pleomorphic fibroma of skin: a case report and immunohistochemical study. Arch Pathol Lab Med 115: 1046, 1991.
166. Miliauskas JR. Myxoid cutaneous pleomorphic fibroma. Histopathology 24:179, 1994.

### Nuchal Fibroma

167. Abraham Z, Rozenbaum M, Rosner I, et al. Nuchal fibroma. J Dermatol 24:262, 1997.
168. Balachandran K, Allen PW, MacCormac LB. Nuchal fibroma: a clinicopathological study of 9 cases. Am J Surg Pathol 19:313, 1995.
169. Laskin WB, Fetsch JF, Miettinen M. Nuchal fibrocartilaginous pseudotumor: a clinicopathologic study of five cases and review of the literature. Mod Pathol 12:663, 1999.
170. Michal M, Fetsch JF, Hes O, et al. Nuchal-type fibroma: a clinicopathologic study of 52 cases. Cancer 85:156, 1999.
171. O'Connell JX, Janzen DL, Hughes TR. Nuchal fibrocartilaginous pseudotumor: a distinctive soft-tissue lesion associated with prior neck injury. Am J Surg Pathol 21:836, 1987.
172. Shek TWH, Chan ACL, Ma L. Extranuchal nuchal fibroma. Am J Surg Pathol 20:902, 1996.

### Elastofibroma

173. Akhtar M, Miller RM. Ultrastructure of elastofibroma. Cancer 40:728, 1977.
174. Barr JR. Elastofibroma. Am J Clin Pathol 45:679, 1966.
175. Benisch B, Peison B, Marquet E, et al. Pre-elastofibroma and elastofibroma (the continuum of elastic-producing fibrous tumors): a light and ultrastructural study. Am J Clin Pathol 80: 88, 1983.
176. Brown GW. Elastofibroma dorsi: report of two cases and literature review. Wis Med J 90:281, 1991.
177. Cross DL, Mills SE, Kulund DN. Elastofibroma arising in the foot. South Med J 77:1194, 1984.
178. De Nictolis M, Goteri G, Campanati G, et al. Elastofibrolipoma of the mediastinum: a previously undescribed benign tumor containing abnormal elastic fibers. Am J Surg Pathol 19:364, 1995.
179. Devaney D, Livesley P, Shaw D. Elastofibroma dorsi: MRI diagnosis in a young girl. Pediatr Radiol 25:282, 1995.
180. Dixon AY, Lee SH. An ultrastructural study of elastofibromas. Hum Pathol 11:257, 1980.
181. Enjoji M, Sumiyoshi K, Sueyoshi K. Elastofibromatous lesion of the stomach in a patient with elastofibroma dorsi. Am J Surg Pathol 9:233, 1985.
182. Fukuda Y, Miyake H, Masuda Y, et al. Histogenesis of unique elastinophilic fibers of elastofibroma: ultrastructural and immunohistochemical studies. Hum Pathol 18:424, 1987.
183. Giebel GD, Bierhoff E, Vogel J. Elastofibroma and pre-elastofibroma: a biopsy and autopsy study. Eur J Surg Oncol 22:93, 1996.
184. Goldblum JR, Beals T, Weiss SW. Elastofibromatous change of the rectum: a lesion mimicking amyloidosis. Am J Surg Pathol 16:793, 1992.
185. Hayashi K, Ohtsuki Y, Sonobe H, et al. Pre-elastofibroma-like colonic polyp: another cause of colonic polyp. Acta Med Okayama 45:49, 1991.
186. Hoffman JK, Klein MH, Mclnerney VK. Bilateral elastofibroma: a case report and review of the literature. Clin Orthop 325:245, 1996.
187. Hsu JK, Cavanagh HD, Green WR. An unusual case of elastofibroma oculi. Cornea 16:112, 1997.
188. Järvi OH, Lansimies PH. Subclinical elastofibromas in the scapular region in an autopsy series. Acta Pathol Microbiol Scand [A] 83:87, 1975.
189. Järvi OH, Saxén AE. Elastofibroma dorsi. Acta Pathol Microbiol Scand 51:83, 1961.
190. Järvi OH, Saxén AE, Hopsu-Havu VK, et al. Elastofibroma: a degenerative pseudotumor. Cancer 23:42, 1969.
191. Kahn HJ, Hanna VM. Aberrant elastic in elastofibroma: an immunohistochemical and ultrastructural study. Ultrastract Pathol 19:45, 1995.
192. Kindblom LG, Spicer SS. Elastofibroma: a correlated light and electron microscopic study. Virchows Arch [Pathol Anat] 396: 127, 1982.
193. Kransdorf MJ, Meis JM, Montgomery E. Elastofibroma: MR and CT appearance with radiologic-pathologic correlation. AJR 159:575, 1992.
194. Kumaratilake JS, Krishnan R, Lomax-Smith J, et al. Elastofibroma: disturbed elastic fibrillogenesis by periosteal-derived cells? An immunoelectron microscopic and in situ hybridization study. Hum Pathol 22:1017, 1991.
195. Madri JA, Dise CA, LiVolsi VA, et al. Elastofibroma dorsi: an immunochemical study of collagen content. Hum Pathol 12: 186, 1981.
196. Marin ML, Perzin KH, Markowitz AM. Elastofibroma dorsi: benign chest wall tumour. J Thorac Cardiovasc Surg 98:234, 1989.
197. Massengill AD, Sundaram M, Kathol MH, et al. Elastofibroma dorsi: a radiological diagnosis. Skeletal Radiol 22:121, 1993.
198. Mirra JM, Straub LR, Järvi OH. Elastofibroma of the deltoid: a case report. Cancer 33:234, 1974.

199. Nagamine M, Nohara Y, Ito E. Elastofibroma in Okinawa: a clinicopathologic study in 170 cases. Cancer 50:1794, 1982.
200. Nakamura Y, Okamoto K, Tanimura A, et al. Elastase digestion and biochemical analysis of the elastin from an elastofibroma. Cancer 58:1070, 1986.
201. Naylor MF, Nascimento AG, Sherrick AD, et al. Elastofibroma dorsi: radiologic findings in 12 patients. AJR 167:683, 1996.
202. Ramos CV, Gillespie W, Narconis RJ. Elastofibroma: a pseudotumor of myofibroblasts. Arch Pathol Lab Med 102:538, 1978.
203. Schiffman R. Elastofibromatous lesion [letter]. Am J Surg Pathol 17:951, 1993.
204. Stemmerman GN, Stout AP. Elastofibroma dorsi. Am J Clin Pathol 37:499, 1962.
205. Tighe JR, Clark AE, Turvey DJ. Elastofibroma dorsi. J Clin Pathol 21:463, 1968.
206. Tsutsumi A, Kawabata K, Taguchi K, et al. Elastofibroma of the greater omentum. Acta Pathol Jpn 35:233, 1988.
207. Waisman J, Smith DW. Fine structure of an elastofibroma. Cancer 22:671, 1968.
208. Yu JS, Weis LD, Vaughan LM, et al. MRI of elastofibroma dorsi. J Comp Assist Tomogr 19:601, 1995.

### Nasopharyngeal Angiofibroma

209. Batsakis JG. Tumor of the Head and Neck. Williams & Wilkins, Baltimore, 1979, pp 296–300.
210. Batsakis JG, Klopp CT, Newman W. Fibrosarcoma arising in a juvenile nasopharyngeal angiofibroma following extensive radiation therapy. Am Surg 21:786, 1976.
211. Beham A, Fletcher CDM, Kainz J, et al. Nasopharyngeal angiofibroma: an immunohistochemical study of 32 cases. Virchows Arch [Pathol Anat] 423:281, 1993.
212. Beham A, Kainz J, Stammberger H, et al. Immunohistochemical and electron microscopical characterization of stromal cells in nasopharyngeal angiofibromas. Eur Arch Otorhinolaryngol 254:196, 1997.
212a. Beham A, Beham-Schmid C, Regauer S, et al. Nasopharyngeal angiofibroma: True neoplasm or vascular malformation? Adv Anat Pathol 7:36, 2000.
213. Briant TDR, Fitzpatrick PJ, Book H. The radiological treatment of juvenile nasopharyngeal angiofibroma. Ann Otolaryngol 79: 1108, 1970.
214. Chandler JR, Goulding R, Moskowitz L, et al. Nasopharyngeal angiofibromas: staging and management. Ann Otol Rhinol Laryngol 93:322, 1984.
215. Chen KTK, Bauer FW. Sarcomatous transformation of nasopharyngeal angiofibroma. Cancer 49:369, 1982.
216. Conley J, Healey WV, Blaugrund SM, et al. Nasopharyngeal angiofibroma in the juvenile. Surg Gynecol Obstet 126:825, 1968.
217. Cummings BJ, Blend R, Keane T, et al. Primary radiation therapy for juvenile nasopharyngeal angiofibroma. Laryngoscope 94:1599, 1984.
218. Fagan JJ, Snyderman CH, Carrau RL, et al. Nasopharyngeal angiofibromas: selecting a surgical approach. Head Neck 19: 391, 1997.
219. Ferouz AS, Mohar RM, Paul P. Juvenile nasopharyngeal angiofibroma and familial adenomatous polyposis: an association? Head Neck Surg 113:435, 1995.
220. Fu YS, Perzin KH. Non-epithelial tumors of the nasal cavity, paranasal sinuses and nasopharynx: a clinicopathologic study. I. General features and vascular tumors. Cancer 33:1275, 1974.
221. Gatalica Z. Immunohistochemical analysis of steroid hormone receptors in nasopharyngeal angiofibromas. Cancer Lett 127: 89, 1998.
222. Giardiello FM, Hamilton SR, Krush AJ, et al. Nasopharyngeal angiofibroma in patients with familial adenomatous polyposis. Gastroenterology 105:1550, 1993.
223. Gisslesson L, Lindgren M, Stenram W. Sarcomatous transformation of a juvenile nasopharyngeal angiofibroma. Acta Pathol Microbiol Scand 42:305, 1958.
224. Goel A, Bhayani R, Sheide J. Technique of extended transcranial approach for massive nasopharyngeal angiofibroma. Br J Neurosurg 8:593, 1994.
225. Hazarika P, Nayak RG, Chandran M. Extra-nasopharyngeal extension of juvenile angiofibroma. J Laryngol Otol 99:813, 1985.
226. Hwang HC, Mills SE, Patterson K, et al. Expression of androgen receptors in nasopharyngeal angiofibroma: an immunohistochemical study of 24 cases. Mod Pathol 11:1122, 1998.
227. Iannetti G, Belli E, DePonte F, et al. The surgical approaches to nasopharyngeal angiofibroma. J Craniomaxillofac Surg 22: 311, 1994.
228. Jamal MN. Imaging and management of angiofibroma. Eur Arch Otorhinolaryngol 251:241, 1994.
229. Kamel RH. Transnasal endoscopic surgery in juvenile nasopharyngeal angiofibroma. J Laryngol Otol 110:962, 1996.
230. Kasper ME, Parsons JT, Mancuso AA, et al. Radiation therapy for juvenile angiofibroma: evaluation by CT and MRI, analysis of tumor regression, and selection of patients. Int J Radiat Oncol 25:689, 1993.
231. McDaniel RK, Houston GD. Juvenile nasopharyngeal angiofibroma with lateral extension into the cheek: report of case. J Oral Maxillofacial Surg 53:473, 1995.
232. McGavran MH, Sessions DG, Dorfman RF, et al. Nasopharyngeal angiofibroma. Arch Otolaryngol 90:68, 1969.
233. Mitskavich MT, Carrau RL, Snyderman CH, et al. Intranasal endoscopic excision of a juvenile angiofibroma. Auris Nasus Larynx 25:39, 1998.
234. Moulin G, Chagnaud C, Gras R, et al. Juvenile nasopharyngeal angiofibroma: comparison of blood loss during removal in embolized group versus non-embolized group. Cardiovasc Intervent Radiol 18:158, 1995.
235. Osborn DA, Sokolovski A. Juvenile nasopharyngeal angiofibroma in a female: report of a case. Arch Otolaryngol 82:629, 1965.
236. Peloquin L, Klossek JM, Basso-Brusa F, et al. A rare case of nasopharyngeal angiofibroma in a pregnant woman. Otolaryngol Head Neck Surg 117:S111, 1997.
237. Radkowski D, McGill T, Healy GB, et al. Angiofibroma: changes in staging and treatment. Arch Otolaryngol Head Neck Surg 122:122, 1996.
238. Siniluoto TM, Luotonen JP, Tikkakoski TA, et al. Value of preoperative embolization and surgery for nasopharyngeal angiofibroma. J Laryngol Otol 107:514, 1993.
239. Spagnolo DV, Papadimitriou JM, Archer M. Postirradiation malignant fibrous histiocytoma arising in juvenile nasopharyngeal angiofibroma and producing alpha-1-antitrypsin. Histopathology 8:339, 1984.
240. Sternberg SS. Pathology of juvenile nasopharyngeal angiofibroma: a lesion of adolescent males. Cancer 7:15, 1954.
241. Svoboda DJ, Kirchner F. Ultrastructure of nasopharyngeal angiofibromas. Cancer 19:1949, 1966.
242. Taxy JB. Juvenile nasopharyngeal angiofibroma: an ultrastructural study. Cancer 39:1044, 1977.
243. Tranbahuy P, Borsik M, Herman P, et al. Direct intratumoral embolization of juvenile angiofibroma. Am J Otolaryngol 15: 429, 1994.
244. Tseng HZ, Chao WY. Transnasal endoscopic approach for juvenile nasopharyngeal angiofibroma. Am J Otolaryngol 18:151, 1997.
245. Ungkamont K, Byers RM, Weber RS, et al. Juvenile nasopharyngeal angiofibroma: an update of therapeutic management. Head Neck 18:60, 1996.
246. Walike JW, Mackay B. Nasopharyngeal angiofibroma: light

and electron microscopic changes after stilbestrol therapy. Laryngoscope 80:1109, 1970.

247. Wiatrak BJ, Koopman CF, Turrisi AT. Radiation therapy as an alternative to surgery in the management of intracranial juvenile nasopharyngeal angiofibroma. Int J Pediatr Otorhinolaryngol 28:51, 1993.
248. Zicot AF, Daele J. Endoscopic surgery for nasal and sinusal vascular tumors. Acta Otorhinolaryngol Belg 50:177, 1996.

### Giant Cell Angiofibroma

249. Craver RD, Correa H, Kao YS, et al. Aggressive giant cell fibroblastoma with a balanced 17;22 translocation. Cancer Genet Cytogenet 80:20, 1995.
250. Dei Tos AP, Seregard S, Calonje E, et al. Giant cell angiofibroma: a distinctive orbital tumor in adults. Am J Surg Pathol 19:1286, 1995.
251. Dorfman DM, To K, Dickersin GR, et al. Solitary fibrous tumor of the orbit. Am J Surg Pathol 18:281, 1994.
252. Fukunaga M, Ushigome S. Giant cell angiofibroma of the mediastinum. Histopathology 32:187,1998.
253. Ganesan R, Hammond CJ, Van Der Walt JD. Giant cell angiofibroma of the orbit. Histopathology 30:93, 1997.
253a. Guillou L, Gebhard S, Coindre J-M. Orbital and extraorbital giant cell angiofibroma: A giant cell-rich variant of solitary fibrous tumor? Clinicopathologic and immunohistochemical analysis of a series in favor of a unifying concept. Am J Surg Pathol 24:971, 2000.
254. Lucas DR, Campbell RJ, Fletcher CDM, et al. Solitary fibrous tumor of the orbit. Int J Surg Pathol 2:193, 1995.
255. Mikami Y, Shimizu M, Hirokawa M, et al. Extraorbital giant cell angiofibromas. Mod Pathol 10:1082, 1997.
256. Sigel JE, Fisher C, Vogt D, et al. Giant cell angiofibroma of the inguinal region. Ann Diagn Pathol 4:1, 2000.
257. Westra WH, Gerald WL, Rosai J. Solitary fibrous tumor, consistent CD34 immunoreactivity and occurrence in the orbit. Am J Surg Pathol 18:992, 1994.

### Keloids

258. Aiba S, Tagami H. Inverse correlation between CD34 expression and proline-4-hydroxylase immunoreactivity on spindle cells noted in hypertrophic scars and keloids. J Cutan Pathol 24:65, 1997.
259. Akintewe TA, Alabi GO. Scleroderma presenting with multiple keloids. BMJ 291:448, 1985.
260. Alhady SMA, Sivanantharajah K. Keloids in various races: a review of 175 cases. Plast Reconstr Surg 44:564, 1969.
261. Alster TS, Williams CM. Treatment of keloid sternotomy scars with 585 nm flashlamp-pumped pulsed-dye laser. Lancet 345: 1198, 1995.
262. Appleton I, Brown NJ, Willoughby DA. Apoptosis, necrosis and proliferation: possible implications in the etiology of keloids. Am J Pathol 149:1441, 1996.
263. Arnold H Jr, Grauer F. Keloids, etiology and management by excision and intensive prophylactic radiation. Arch Dermatol 80:772, 1959.
264. Babu M, Diegelmann R, Oliver N. Fibronectin is overproduced by keloid fibroblasts during abnormal wound healing. Mol Cell Biol 9:1642, 1989.
265. Berman B, Bieley HC. Adjunct therapies to surgical management of keloids. Dermatol Surg 22:126, 1996.
266. Blackburn WR, Cosman B. Histologic basis of keloid and hypertrophic scar differentiation: clinicopathologic correlation. Arch Pathol 82:65, 1966.
267. Bloom D. Heredity of keloids: review of the literature and report of a family with multiple keloids in five generations. NY State J Med 56:511, 1956.
268. Char F. Ehlers-Danlos syndrome. Birth Defects 8:300, 1972.
269. Cosman B, Crikelair GF, Gaulin JS, et al. The surgical treatment of keloids. Plast Reconstr Surg 27:335, 1961.
270. Datubo-Brown DD. Keloids: a review of the literature. Br J Plast Surg 43:70, 1990.
271. Ehrlich HP, Desmouliere A, Diegelmann RF, et al. Morphological and immunohistochemical differences between keloid and hypertrophic scar. Am J Pathol 145:105, 1994.
272. Ghazizadeh M, Miyata N, Sasaki Y, et al. silver-stained nucleolar organizer regions in hypertrophic and keloid scars. Am J Dermatopathol 19:468, 1997.
273. Gonzalez-Martinez R, Marin-Bertolin S, Amorrortu-Velayos J. Association between keloids and Dupuytren's disease: case report. Br J Plast Surg 48:47, 1995.
274. Graham JH, Sanders JB, Johnson WC, et al. Fibrous papule of the nose. J Invest Dermatol 45:194, 1965.
275. Haisa M, Okochi H, Grotendorst GR. Elevated levels of PDGF alpha receptors in keloid fibroblasts contribute to an enhanced response to PDGF. J Invest Dermatol 103:560, 1994.
276. Hegedus SI, Schorr WF. Familial cutaneous collagenoma. Cutis 10:283, 1972.
277. Hendrix JD Jr, Greer KE. Rubinstein-Taybi syndrome with multiple flamboyant keloids. Cutis 57:346, 1996.
278. Holmstrand K, Longacre JJ, DeStefano GA. The ultrastructure of collagen in skin, scar and keloids. Plast Reconstr Surg 27: 597, 1961.
279. Hutchinson J. On keloids. Arch Surg 4:233, 1983.
280. Inalsingh CH. An experience in treating 501 patients with keloids. Johns Hopkins Med J 134:284, 1974.
281. James WD, Besancenez DC, Odom RB. The ultrastructure of a keloid. J Am Acad Dermatol 3:50, 1980.
282. Katz BE. Silicone gel sheeting in scar therapy. Cutis 56:65, 1995.
283. Kemble JV. Scanning electronmicroscopy of hypertrophic and keloid scar. Postgrad Med J 52:219, 1976.
284. Ketchum LD, Cohen IK, Masters FW. Hypertrophic scars and keloids: a collective review. Plast Reconstr Surg 53:140, 1974.
285. Kikuchi K, Kadono T, Takehara K. Effects of various growth factors and histamine on cultured keloid fibroblasts. Dermatology 190:4, 1995.
286. King TD, Salzman FA. Keloid scars: analysis of 89 patients. Surg Clin North Am 50:595, 1970.
287. Klumpar DI, Murray JC, Anscher M. Keloids treated with excision followed by radiation therapy. J Am Acad Dermatol 31:225, 1994.
288. Kuo TT, Hu S, Chan HL. Keloidal dermatofibroma: report of 10 cases of a new variant. Am J Surg Pathol 22:564, 1998.
289. Lawrence WT. In search of the optimal treatment of keloids: report of a series and review of the literature. Ann Plast Surg 27:164, 1991.
290. Lawrence WT. Treatment of earlobe keloids with surgery plus adjuvant intralesional verapamil and pressure earrings. Ann Plast Surg 37:167, 1996.
291. Layton AN, Yip J, Cunliffe WJ. A comparison of intralesional triamcinolone and cryosurgery in the treatment of acne keloids. Br J Dermatol 130:498, 1994.
292. Lee YS, Vijayasingam S. Mast cells and myofibroblasts in keloid: a light microscopic, immunohistochemical and ultrastructural study. Ann Acad Med 24:902, 1995.
293. Maize J, Leidel G, Mullins S, et al. Circumscribed storiform collagenoma [abstract] Am J Dermatopathol 11:287, 1989.
294. Matsuoka LY, Uitto J, Wortsman J, et al. Ultrastructural characteristics of keloid fibroblasts. Am J Dermatopathol 10:505, 1988.
295. Meigel WN, Ackerman AB. Fibrous papule of the face. Am J Dermatopathol 1:329, 1979.
296. Metcalf JS, Maize JC, LeBoit PE. Circumscribed storiform col-

lagenoma (sclerosing fibroma). Am J Dermatopathol 13:122, 1991.
297. Murray JC. Scars and keloids. Dermatol Clin 11:697, 1993.
298. Nakaoka H, Miyauchi S, Miki Y. Proliferating activity of dermal fibroblasts in keloids and hypertrophic scars. Acta Derm Venereol 75:102, 1995.
299. Omo-Dare P. Genetic studies on keloids. J Natl Med Assoc 76: 428, 1975.
300. Reed RJ, Hariston MA, Pelomieque FE. The histologic identity of adenoma sebaceum and solitary melanocytic angiofibroma. Dermatol Int 5:3, 1966.
301. Rocha G, Winkelman RK. Connective tissue nevus. Arch Dermatol 85:722, 1962.
302. Rosen LB, Suster S. Fibrous papules: a light microscopic and immunohistochemical study. Am J Dermatopathol 10:109, 1988.
303. Rudolph P, Schubert C, Harms D, et al. Giant cell collagenoma: a benign dermal tumor with distinctive multinucleate cells. Am J Surg Pathol 22:557, 1998.
304. Sallstrom K-O, Larson O, Heden P, et al. Treatment of keloids with surgical excision and post operative x-ray radiation. Scand J Plast Surg 23:211, 1989.
305. Santucci M, Borgognoni L, Reali UM, et al. Hypertrophic scars and keloids: a histologic, immunohistochemical and ultrastructural study. Clin Exp Pathol 46:303A, 1998.
306. Smith AD, Weissman M. Connective tissue nevi. Arch Dermatol 102:390, 1970.
307. Younai S, Nichter LS, Wellisz T, et al. Modulation of collagen synthesis by transforming growth factor-beta in keloid and hypertrophic scar fibroblasts. Ann Plast Surg 33:148, 1994.
308. Zackheim MS, Pinkus H. Perifollicular fibroma. Arch Dermatol 82:913, 1960.
309. Zouboulis CC, Blume U, Buttner P, et al. Outcomes of cryosurgery in keloids and hypertrophic scars: a prospective consecutive trial of case series. Arch Dermatol 129:1146, 1993.

### Desmoplastic Fibroblastoma

310. Evans HL. Desmoplastic fibroblastoma: a report of 7 cases. Am J Surg Pathol 19:1077, 1995.
310a. Fukunaga M, Ushigome S. Collagenous fibroma (desmoplastic fibroblastoma): A distinctive fibroblastic soft tissue tumor. Adv Anat Pathol 6:275, 1999.
311. Hasegawa T, Shimoda T, Hirohashi S, et al. Collagenous fibroma (desmoplastic fibroblastoma): report of four cases and review of the literature. Arch Pathol Lab Med 122:455, 1998.
312. Miettinen M, Fetsch JF. Collagenous fibroma (desmoplastic fibroblastoma): a clinicopathologic analysis of 63 cases of a distinctive soft tissue lesion with stellate-shaped fibroblasts. Hum Pathol 29:676, 1998.
313. Nielsen GP, O'Connell JX, Dickersin GR, Rosenberg AE. Collagenous fibroma (desmoplastic fibroblastoma): a report of 7 cases. Mod Pathol 9:781, 1996.
314. Sciot R, Samson I, van den Berghe H, et al. Collagenous fibroma (desmoplastic fibroblastoma): genetic link with fibroma of tendon sheath? Mod Pathol 12:565, 1999.

# CHAPTER 10

# FIBROMATOSES

Fibromatoses, as proposed by Stout,[229] comprise a broad group of benign fibrous tissue proliferations of similar microscopic appearance whose biologic behavior is intermediate between that of benign fibrous lesions and fibrosarcoma. Like fibrosarcoma, the fibromatoses are characterized by infiltrative growth and a tendency toward recurrence, but unlike this tumor they never metastasize.

The various entities that constitute this group occur predominantly in adults and consist of highly differentiated fibrous tissue that forms a firm, nonencapsulated, poorly circumscribed nodular mass that may be solitary or multiple and has a predilection for certain anatomic sites. The term *fibromatosis* should not be applied to nonspecific reactive fibrous proliferations that are part of an inflammatory process or are secondary to injury or hemorrhage and have no tendency toward infiltrative growth or recurrence.

The fibromatoses can be divided into two major groups with several subdivisions (Table 10–1). *Superficial (fascial) fibromatoses* are slowly growing and of small size. These lesions arise from the fascia or aponeurosis and only rarely involve deep structures. The clinical course usually can be divided into an early, rather cellular proliferative phase and a late, richly collagenous regressive or contractile phase. *Deep (musculoaponeurotic) fibromatoses* are rapidly growing tumors that often attain a large size. Their biologic behavior tends to be more aggressive than that of the superficial (fascial) fibromatoses; they have a high recurrence rate; and as their name indicates, they principally involve deep structures, particularly the musculature of the trunk and the extremities. The descriptive term *desmoid tumor,* coined by Mueller in 1838 to emphasize the band-like or tendon-like consistency of the lesions, is still widely used in the literature as a synonym for this type of fibromatosis. Other, less common synonyms such as *nonmetastasizing fibrosarcoma* and *grade I fibrosarcoma* should be discouraged, as both give the impression that fibromatosis is a sarcoma, and the latter implies metastatic potential.

Although all fascial and musculoaponeurotic fibromatoses are capable of recurrence after excision, the recurrence rate of the individual entities varies substantially. The risk of recurrence is governed less by the histologic picture than by the anatomic location of the lesion, the age of the patient, and of course the mode of therapy. In fact, histologic examination alone does not permit accurate prediction of the clinical course. Moreover, occasional fibromatoses do regress spontaneously, but the incidence and likelihood of regression, like that of recurrence, is unpredictable. Malignant transformation of fibromatosis was reported in one case many years after radiation therapy.[228]

## PALMAR FIBROMATOSIS

Palmar fibromatosis, better known as *Dupuytren's disease* or *Dupuytren's contracture,* is by far the most common type of fibromatosis. Although it is named for Baron Guillaime Dupuytren[20] who reported this condition in 1831, Felix Plater was probably the first to describe the lesion in 1614.[67] This form of superficial fibromatosis is characterized by a nodular fibroblastic proliferation that occurs in the volar surface of the hand and histologically closely resembles other forms of fibromatosis. The lesion appears to progress through a series of clinical and histologic stages, ultimately resulting in flexion contracture of the fingers, a complication that usually necessitates surgical therapy.

### Clinical Findings

Palmar fibromatosis is a relatively common condition that tends to affect adults, with a rapid increase in incidence with advancing age. It has been estimated that almost 20% of the general population is affected by 65 years of age. Patients younger than 30 years of age, particularly children, are seldom affected.[80] The condition is about three or four times more frequent in men than in women[56,84] and occurs most com-

**TABLE 10–1 CLASSIFICATION OF FIBROMATOSES**

Superficial (fascial) fibromatoses
- Palmar fibromatosis (Dupuytren's disease)
- Plantar fibromatosis (Ledderhose's disease)
- Penile fibromatosis (Peyronie's disease)
- Knuckle pads

Deep (musculoaponeurotic) fibromatoses
- Extraabdominal fibromatosis (extraabdominal desmoid)
- Abdominal fibromatosis (abdominal desmoid)
- Intraabdominal fibromatosis (intraabdominal desmoid)
  - Pelvic fibromatosis
  - Mesenteric fibromatosis
  - Mesenteric fibromatosis in Gardner syndrome

monly in northern Europe and in those parts of the world now settled by northern Europeans.[31] Although well documented, the disease is rare in the black population.[56,58,74]

The onset of the disease is slow and insidious, and the initial manifestation is typically an isolated, usually asymptomatic, firm nodule in the palmar surface of the hand. Because of the lack of symptoms at this stage, many patients ignore the presence of the nodule and do not seek medical therapy. There is a slight predilection for the right palmar surface, but almost 50% of cases are bilateral. Although clinical progression does not invariably occur, in many patients several months or years after the original appearance of the fibrous nodules, cord-like indurations or bands develop between nodules and adjacent fingers, often causing puckering and dimpling of the overlying skin (Fig. 10–1). These changes are usually most prominent on the ulnar side of the palm and are accompanied by flexion contractures that principally affect the fourth and fifth fingers of the hand. The thumb and index finger are least often affected. With increasing severity of the contractures, normal function of the hand becomes greatly impaired, and it is at this point that therapy is usually sought.

## Concurrence of Palmar Fibromatosis with Other Diseases

Palmar fibromatosis has been linked with numerous other disease processes, including other forms of fibromatosis. Approximately 5–20% of cases of palmar fibromatosis are associated with plantar fibromatosis, and about 2–4% of patients also have penile fibromatosis (Peyronie's disease).[13,27,48,81] Knuckle pads (fibrous thickenings on the dorsal aspect of the proximal interphalangeal or metacarpophalangeal joints) have also been associated with palmar fibromatosis.[27,35,57,73] Rare patients have been described with polyfibromatosis syndrome, a condition characterized by the occurrence of several cutaneous fibroproliferative lesions, including Dupuytren's contracture and keloids.[25,44]

Palmar fibromatosis has been consistently linked with seemingly unrelated diseases, including types I and II diabetes mellitus.[5,6,30,38,64,65] Arkkila et al. found that 14% of patients with type I or II diabetes mellitus had palmar fibromatosis.[6] Although there is a marked male predilection for palmar fibromatosis in the general population, gender differences are not observed in patients with diabetes. Several studies have found that the development of palmar fibromatosis is associated with increasing age and duration of diabetes.[6,64,65] Noble et al. noted that the fibromatosis tends to be milder with a lower rate of local recurrence in patients with diabetes than in the general population.[64] These patients also seem to have an increased frequency of bilateral disease[65] and a predilection for

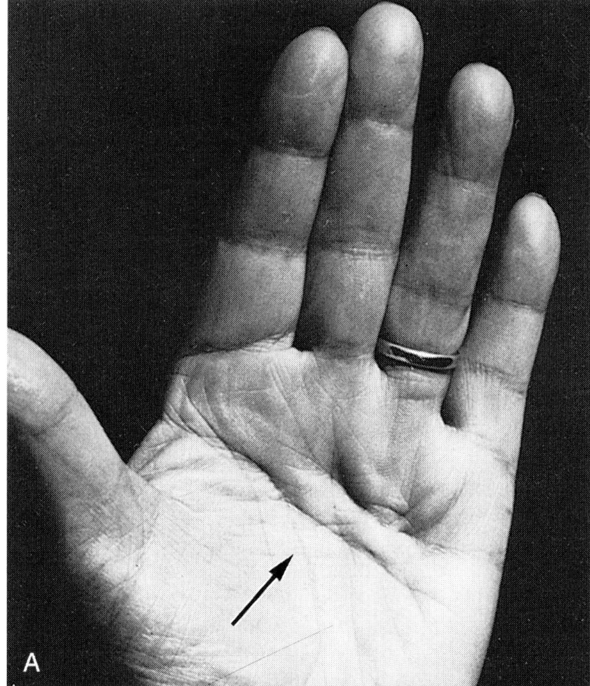


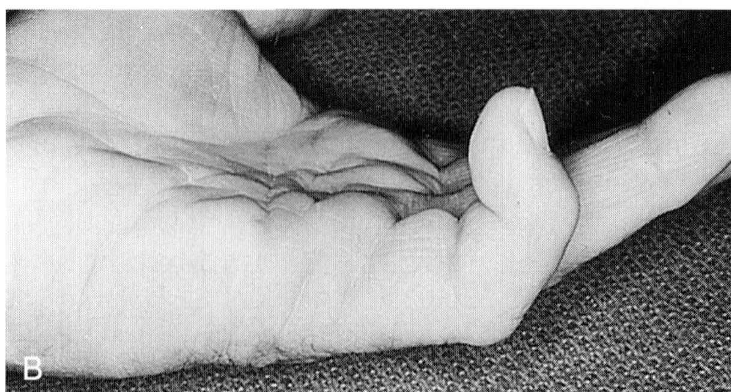


**FIGURE 10–1.** (**A**) Palmar fibromatosis with firm cord-like indurations and nodules causing puckering and dimpling (arrow) of the overlying skin. (**B**) Flexion contracture of the fifth finger (Dupuytren's contracture).

contractures to develop in the middle and ring fingers.[43] Although some have found palmar fibromatosis to be associated with diabetic complications, such as chronic peripheral neuropathy[23,38,75] or diabetic retinopathy,[38] others have found a lack of association with diabetic complications when controlled for age and duration of disease.[5]

There is also an increased incidence in epileptics.[3,4,21,48,68,73] Lund initially postulated a role for antiepileptic drugs, particularly phenobarbitone, in the etiology of palmar fibromatosis in these patients.[48] Although this observation has been supported by several authors,[18,68,73] others have not found it to be the case.[26,34] Alcoholics also have a high prevalence of Dupuytren's contracture.[7,15,32,61,63,68,82] The prevalence of palmar fibromatosis is higher in alcoholics with liver disease than in those without liver disease, suggesting it is alcohol's effect on the liver (rather than the direct effects of alcohol) that is the causative factor.[63,82] The condition is also more common in patients with increased serum cholesterol and triglyceride levels[71] and in those who smoke cigarettes.[2,15]

## Gross Findings

The excised tissue consists of a single small nodule, usually measuring less than 1 cm in diameter, or an ill-defined conglomerate of several nodular masses intimately associated with a thickened palmar aponeurosis and subcutaneous fat. The tissue is firm and scar-like on palpation and on cut section reveals a gray-yellow to gray-white surface, although the color depends on the collagen content, which in turn depends on the age of the lesion. The gross specimen may also contain excised skin, and occasionally these nodular masses adhere to the overlying skin.

## Microscopic Findings

The microscopic findings depend on the age of the lesion. The earliest or proliferative phase of the disease is characterized by a strikingly cellular proliferation of plump, immature-appearing spindle-shaped fibroblasts that form one or more nodules (Figs. 10–2, 10–3). The fibroblasts are uniform in size and shape, with normochromatic nuclei and small, pinpoint nucleoli (Fig. 10–4). Mitotic figures may be identified but are usually not numerous. The cells are intimately associated with small to moderate amounts of collagen suspended in a mucopolysaccharide-rich matrix. Microhemorrhages with small deposits of hemosiderin and scattered chronic inflammatory cells may be present. The fibrous nodules originate within the palmar aponeurosis and extend into and replace the overlying subcutaneous fat.

Nodules that have been present for long periods of time are considerably less cellular and contain markedly increased amounts of dense birefringent colla-

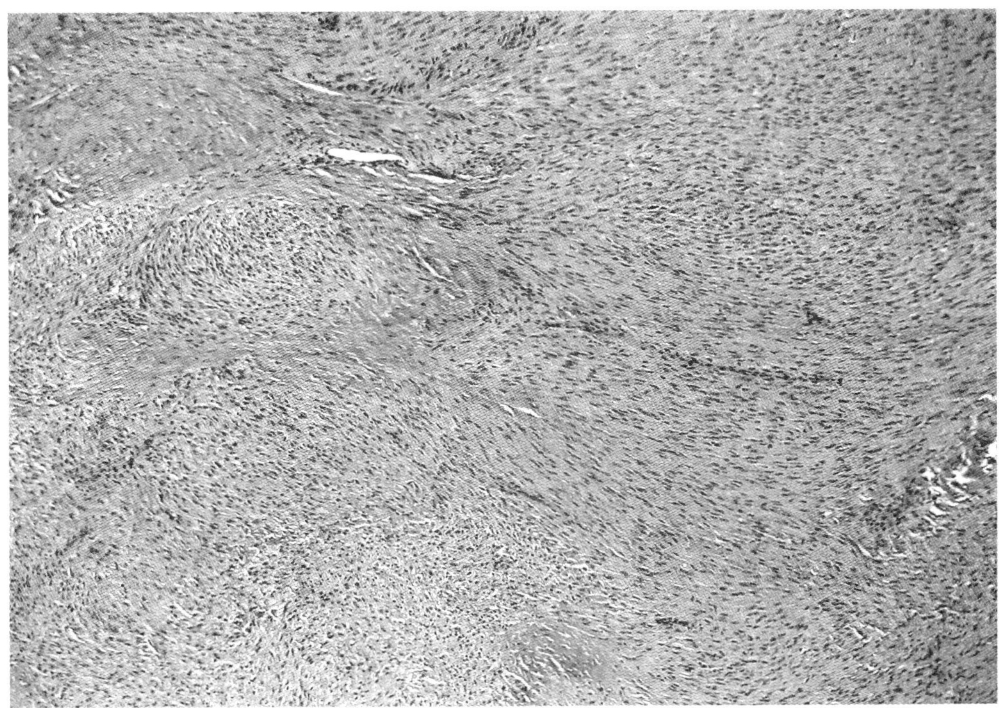

**FIGURE 10–2.** Palmar fibromatosis composed of parallel fascicles of slender fibroblasts separated by variable amounts of collagen.

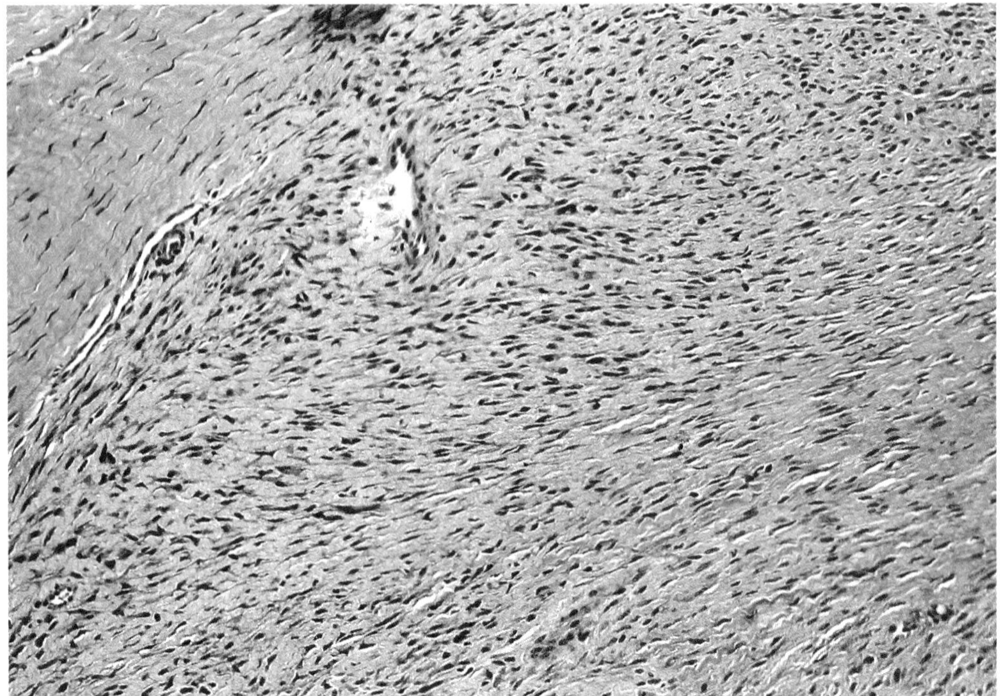

**FIGURE 10–3.** Uniform fibroblastic proliferation in palmar fibromatosis.

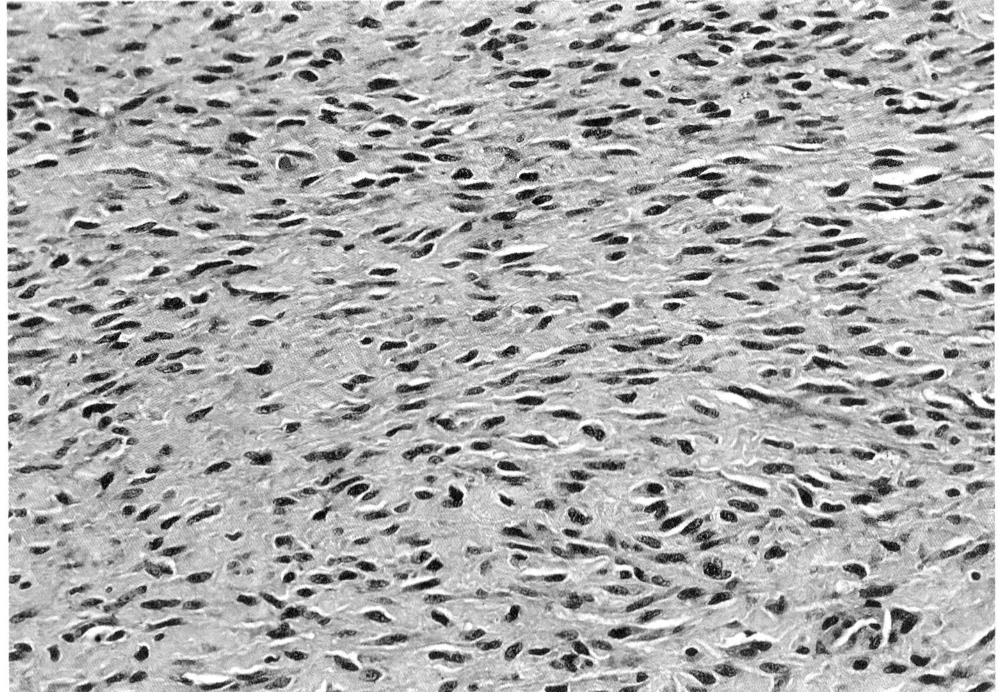

**FIGURE 10–4.** Early, rather cellular form of palmar fibromatosis showing uniform spindled cells separated by collagen.

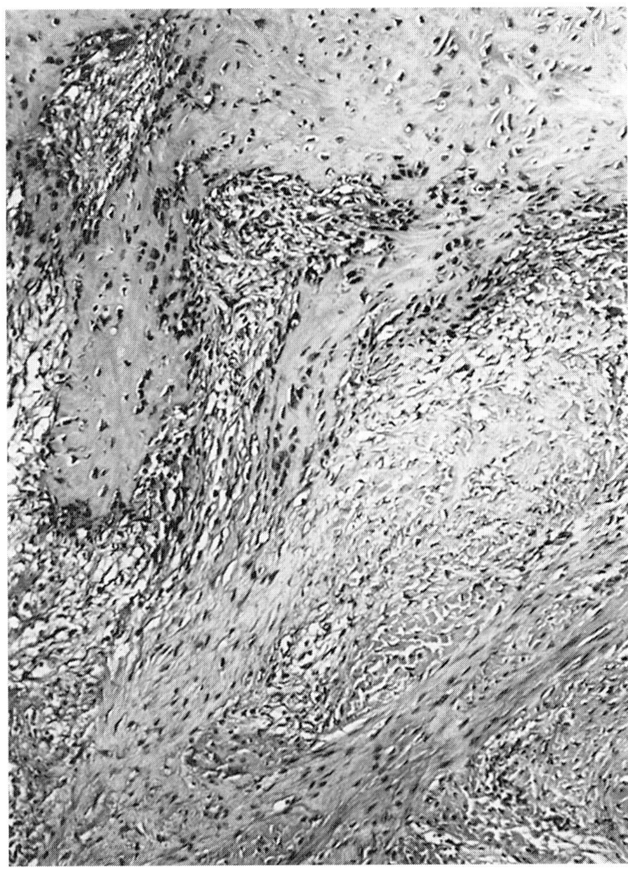

**FIGURE 10–5.** Cartilaginous metaplasia in a late, rare form of palmar fibromatosis.

gen. The fibroblasts are smaller and more slender in appearance, and the fascial or aponeurotic cords between nodules and fingers are composed of dense fibrocollagenous tissue that bears a close resemblance to that of tendons. Osseous and cartilaginous metaplasia of the fibrous nodules may be seen (Fig. 10–5).

### Electron Microscopic and Immunohistochemical Findings

Gabbiani and Majno, the first to emphasize the presence of myofibroblasts in palmar fibromatosis, suggested that these cells played a role in the pathogenesis of the contraction observed clinically.[22] Since then, numerous reports have confirmed the role of myofibroblasts in this disease.[36,37,54] Ultrastructurally, the cells are characterized by deeply indented nuclei and cytoplasm with well-developed rough endoplasmic reticulum, longitudinally arranged microfilaments with interspersed dense bodies, subplasmalemmal plaques, partial envelopment by basal lamina, and the presence of fibronexus (Fig. 10–6). Several ultrastructural studies have shown progression from a predominantly fibroblastic proliferative stage to an involutional stage composed predominantly of myofibroblasts, followed by a residual fibrocytic stage.[24,47] Throughout these stages there is a progressive decrease in cellularity with increased deposition of mature collagen, ultimately resulting in tendon-like structures.[36]

Immunohistochemically, the spindle-shaped cells stain for vimentin and variably for smooth muscle actin and muscle-specific actin, depending on the stage and the degree of myofibroblastic differentiation.[52,78,79] In addition, smooth muscle actin-positive cells are often numerous in apparently uninvolved dermis and may provide a pool of progenitor cells from which new foci develop, accounting for the high rate of local recurrence.[53]

Other constituents of the extracellular matrix have also been identified by immunohistochemical means. Types III and VI collagen predominate during the early proliferative phase, whereas type I collagen increases during the involutional and residual phases.[50,79] Similarly, laminin and fibronectin appear to follow the distribution of myofibroblasts and decrease in quantity with increasing duration of the lesion.[29,51] Numerous growth factors, including transforming growth factor-$\beta$,[9,11,12] platelet-derived growth factor,[1,77,87] and basic fibroblast growth factor,[1,11] have been implicated in the pathogenesis of this disease, as these growth factors are potent stimulators of collagen production. Badalamente et al.[8] found significantly increased amounts of prostaglandins $PGE_2$ and $PGF_{2\alpha}$ in the myofibroblasts of Dupuytren's contracture when compared to control fascia and suggested that prostaglandins influence the contractile behavior of myofibroblasts in this disease.

### Differential Diagnosis

In its most cellular phase, palmar fibromatosis may closely resemble *fibrosarcoma.* However, the cells of fibrosarcoma tend to be arranged in long fascicles or a herringbone pattern and show a greater degree of nuclear hyperchromasia, pleomorphism, and mitotic activity and occasionally necrosis. Furthermore, fibrosarcoma of the hand is rare, and when it does occur it is usually a deep-seated tumor that affects the aponeurosis and subcutaneous tissue only secondarily; whereas the cellular nodules in palmar fibromatosis arise within the aponeurosis and infiltrate the subcutaneous tissue.

### Treatment

Surgical extirpation remains the treatment of choice in patients with severe flexion contractures that impair

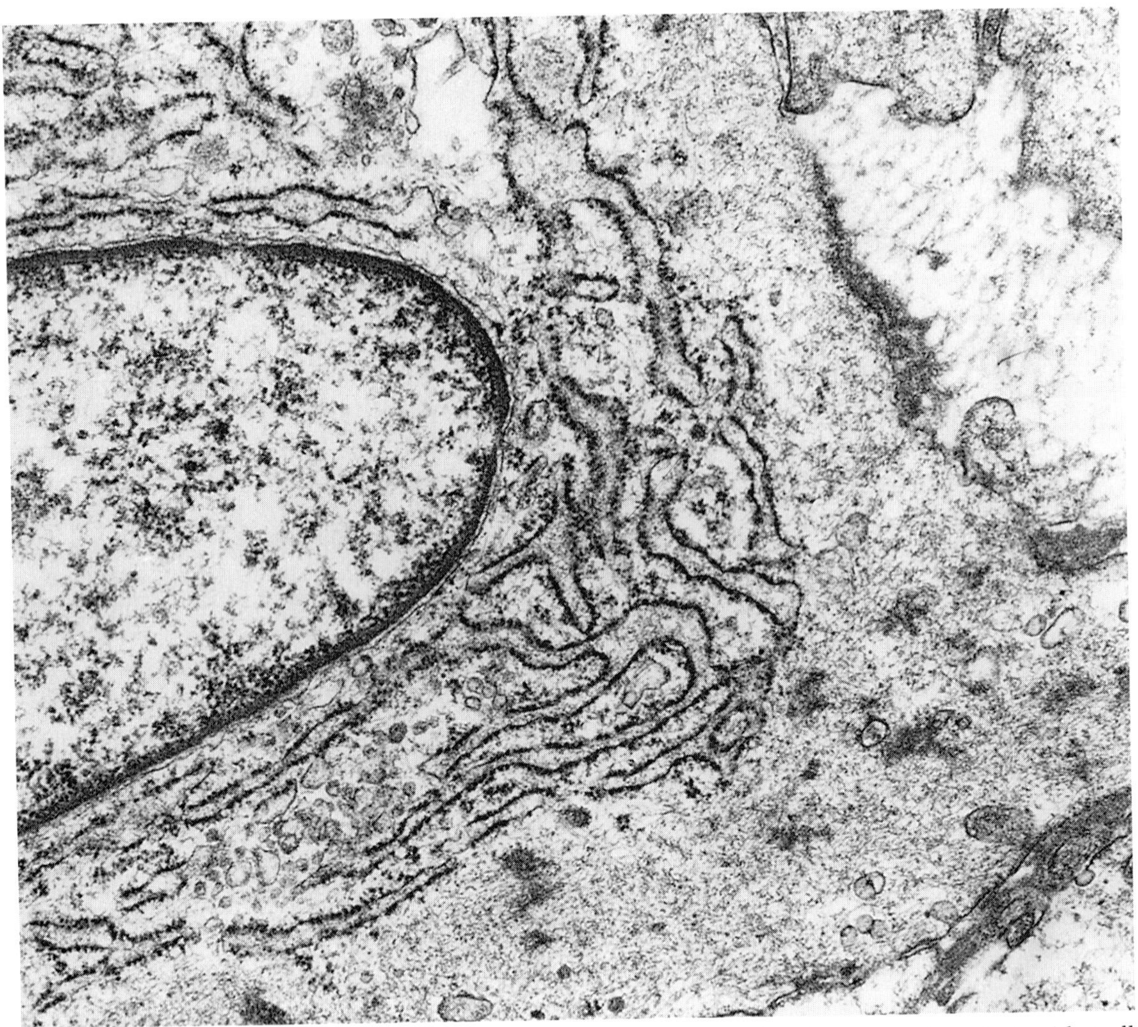

**FIGURE 10–6.** Electron microscopic picture of palmar fibromatosis showing a myofibroblast with well-developed rough endoplasmic reticulum, interspersed and focally condensed microfilaments, and partial basal lamina.

normal hand function. Fasciotomy (subcutaneous division of the fibrous bands) leads to good immediate improvement of contractures of the metacarpophalangeal joints. This procedure has no effect on the progression of the disease, as it affects the proximal interphalangeal joint; thus long-term results are only marginal.[70] Furthermore, this procedure may result in injury to the digital arteries or nerves. Fasciotomy may be the preferred therapy for those who can tolerate only minor surgical procedures or those who have only limited palmar involvement.[33] More extensive surgical procedures, including subtotal or total fasciectomy or aponeurosectomy, are associated with a lower rate of local recurrence and better long-term results than are obtained with fasciotomy.[59,70,72] Dermofasciectomy followed by skin grafting is associated with the lowest rate of local recurrence (<10%).[14,28] This technique has been advocated for cases of recurrent Dupuytren's contracture requiring reoperation and as a primary procedure when there is significant skin involvement.[14,28] Keilholz et al. found radiotherapy to be effective in preventing disease progression for early-stage Dupuytren's contracture, thereby helping to avoid unnecessary surgical procedures for more advanced stages of this disease.[40] Potential nonsurgical therapies include the use of collagenase[76] and calcium channel blockers,[69] but these agents have only been tested in vitro. Radiologic evaluation, particularly with magnetic resonance imaging (MRI), may be useful for determining the extent of the disease process, thereby facilitating the most appropriate surgical therapy.[83]

### Discussion

The pathogenesis of palmar fibromatosis is multifactorial. It has been well established that there is a genetic component. Ling found that 68% of 50 index cases had a family history of the disease.[45] The presence of Dupuytren's contractures in identical twins had been reported on several occasions.[17,39] Lyall argued that an appropriate genetic background is inadequate by itself for the development of this disease: He reported two pairs of identical twins, in each of which only one twin had evidence of palmar fibromatosis.[49] Cytogenetic aberrations including loss of the Y chromosome and trisomies of chromosomes 7 and 8 have been reported.[16,19]

In addition to a genetic predisposition, other factors have been implicated, including trauma and microtrauma.[42,85] Dupuytren himself suggested that repetitive minor trauma may be the major causative factor in this disease. Skoog proposed that minor trauma causes injury to the aponeurosis followed by reparative fibroblastic proliferation and subsequent contracture.[73] Liss and Stock reviewed 10 previously published studies and found good support for an association between hand vibration exposure and development of palmar fibromatosis.[46] Others have denied such a causative relation, pointing out that the disease is equally common in clerical workers and manual laborers, occurs at a site (the ulnar portion of the palm) that is least exposed to traumatic injury, and develops predominantly in older persons at a stage of life in which manual labor is normally greatly reduced.[60,84]

Kischer and Speer have proposed that microvascular changes are a major etiologic factor in the development of palmar fibromatosis and other fibrosing lesions.[41] These authors observed microvascular occlusion in and around areas involved by the fibromatosis and proposed that hypoxia stimulates the excessive collagen production, possibly through generation of oxygen-free radicals. Such a hypothesis would be attractive for linking hyperlipidemia, diabetes mellitus, and cigarette smoking, all of which affect the microvasculature.

Finally, some have proposed an immunologic basis for this disease. Several studies have found circulating serum antibodies to collagen in some patients with palmar fibromatosis,[55,66] and others have found an increased prevalence of HLA-DR3,[62] a major histocompatibility complex class II antigen that is associated with autoimmune diseases. Although inflammation is usually not a conspicuous component of this disease, most of the inflammatory cells present are $CD3^+$ lymphocytes and express HLA-DR antigen, suggesting a T cell-mediated autoimmune disorder.[10]

## PLANTAR FIBROMATOSIS

Plantar fibromatosis, sometimes referred to as *Ledderhose's disease,* is characterized by a nodular fibrous proliferation arising within the plantar aponeurosis, usually in non-weight-bearing areas. Although Dupuytren recognized that a process similar to that occurring with palmar aponeurosis could involve plantar aponeurosis, it was Madelung who reported the first isolated case of plantar fibromatosis in 1875,[97] described in more detail by Ledderhose in 1897.[96] This condition appears to occur much less frequently than its palmar counterpart, as Yost et al. found only one case (0.23%) in a series of 430 consecutive patients.[106]

### Clinical Findings

Like palmar fibromatosis, its incidence increases progressively with advancing age,[89] although there is a much higher incidence in children and young persons. Allen et al.[86] found that 35% of the patients were 30 years of age or younger, including two in whom the lesion was noted at birth. Several other series have noted a fairly high incidence in children and adolescents compared to that of palmar fibromatosis.[89,98,102] Although men are affected more commonly than women, the gender difference is not as great as that found with palmar fibromatosis. The frequency of bilaterality ranges from 20%[89] to up to 50%[98] of cases. In such cases the lesions are usually metachronous, with one lesion preceding the other by an interval of 2–7 years.[89]

Not infrequently, palmar and plantar fibromatoses affect the same patient, but the two lesions rarely occur at the same time; usually one precedes the other by 5–10 years. The reported incidence of palmar fibromatosis in patients with plantar fibromatosis ranges from 9%[89] to up to 69%[86] of cases. The association with penile fibromatosis (Peyronie's disease) is much less common. In a review of the literature by Pickren et al.,[102] only 1 of 104 patients with plantar fibromatosis had penile fibromatosis. Coexistence with dorsal knuckle pads has also been noted in up to 42% of cases.[103] Like palmar fibromatosis, this disease appears to be more common among epileptics, diabetics, and alcoholics with liver disease.

The lesion first appears as a single firm subcutaneous thickening or nodule that adheres to the skin and is typically located in the middle and medial portion of the sole of the foot. Cases arising in children tend to occur in the anteromedial portion of the heel pad.[94] It may be entirely asymptomatic but not infrequently causes mild pain after prolonged standing or walking.[95,105] Rarely, paresthesia of the distal portion of the sole of the foot and the undersurface of one or more toes may result when there is entrapment of the superficial plantar nerve.[91] Unlike its palmar counterpart, plantar fibromatosis only exceptionally results in contraction of the toes,[93] presumably because the distal extensions of the plantar aponeurosis to the toes are much less well developed than in the hand. In patients with symptoms, plantar fibromatosis is often biopsied or excised at an earlier, more cellular stage than palmar fibromatosis and may cause serious diagnostic concern that a sarcoma is present, particularly fibrosarcoma.

### Pathologic Findings

Grossly and microscopically, the lesions are virtually indistinguishable from those found with palmar fibromatosis, although they are less often multinodular and only rarely contain the thick cords of fibrocollagenous tissue extending distally from the nodular growth (Fig. 10–7). Many of the lesions are highly cellular, but the cells lack nuclear hyperchromasia or pleomorphism and have small, pinpoint nucleoli (Figs. 10–8, 10–9). Mitotic figures may also be identified but are few in number and are not atypical. Occasionally, one encounters mild perivascular chronic inflammation and deposits of hemosiderin; and in lesions of long duration, focal chondroid or osseous metaplasia may be present.

Immunohistochemically, as with palmar fibromatosis, this lesion is characterized by cells that stain for vimentin and in many cases for smooth muscle actin, indicating focal myofibroblastic differentiation. In addition, many of the growth factors identified in cases of palmar fibromatosis are also present in the plantar lesions and likely play an important role in stimulating collagen production by fibroblasts.[85,107]

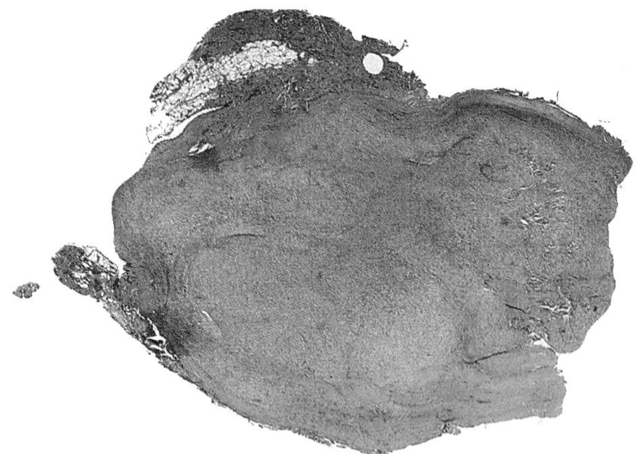

**FIGURE 10–7.** Plantar fibromatosis showing the characteristic nodular growth pattern.

The differential diagnosis is usually with *fibrosarcoma.* Although well-documented cases of fibrosarcoma in the foot have been reported,[90] they are rare and histologically are characterized by more hyperchromatic nuclei that show more nuclear pleomorphism and a higher degree of mitotic activity than that found with plantar fibromatosis.

### Treatment

In most cases, surgical therapy is not required unless the nodules cause discomfort or disability. Although intralesional steroid injections have been effective in some cases,[101] surgical excision is the treatment of choice. Radiologic evaluation, particularly with MRI, may be useful for determining the extent of the disease process, thereby facilitating the most appropriate surgical therapy.[99,100] Simple excision of the lesion is associated with a high rate of local recurrence.[86,102] Fasciectomy, with or without skin grafting, is associated with a much lower rate of recurrence. Most lesions recur less than 1 year after initial excision.[88] There appears to be an increased risk of local recurrence in patients with multiple nodules, bilateral lesions, a positive family history, and those who develop a postoperative neuroma.[88,104]

### Discussion

The etiology of plantar fibromatosis, like palmar fibromatosis, is probably multifactorial; and there seems to be a genetic predisposition. Like its palmar counterpart, cytogenetic aberrations have been reported in these lesions, including trisomies of chromosomes 8 and 14.[92] Trauma has frequently been considered an important factor in the pathogenesis of this disease. Certainly, the sole of the foot suffers a great variety of minor injuries over the years, and it is not surprising that a history of trauma can be elicited in many cases. There does not appear to be any occupational predilection, and most of these lesions arise in the medial portion of the plantar arch, an area least exposed to traumatic injury. The coexistence of the disease with epilepsy, diabetes, and alcohol-induced liver disease makes it likely that factors other than trauma are etiologically important.

## PENILE FIBROMATOSIS (PEYRONIE'S DISEASE)

Although François de la Peyronie is generally credited with describing the disease that bears his name,[127] descriptions of this disease date back at least as far as the mid-sixteenth century.[119] It is considered

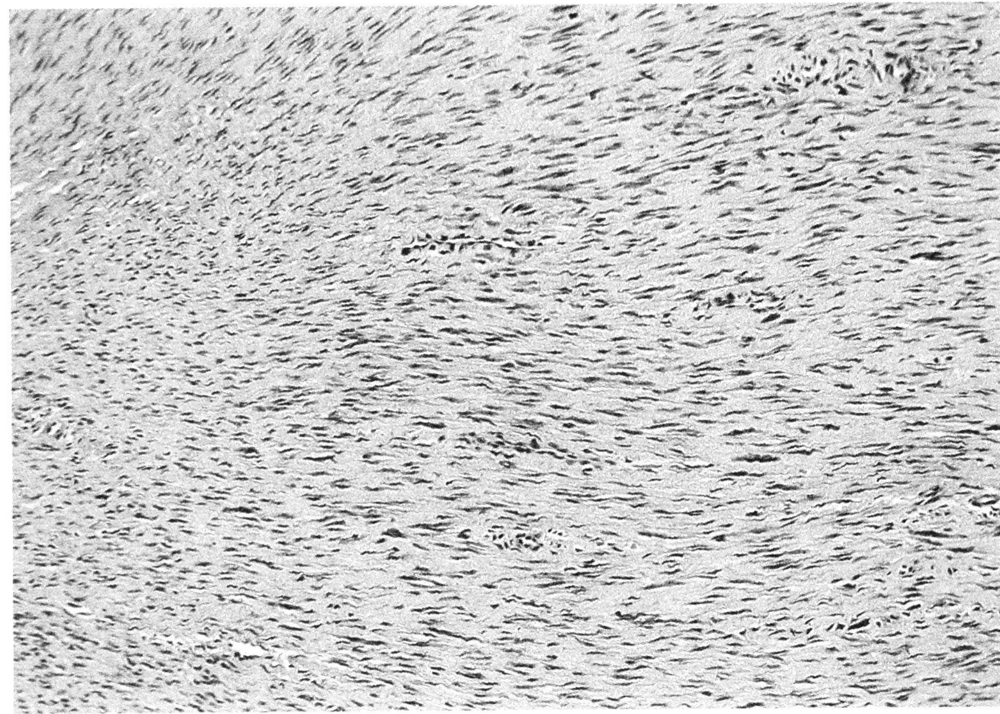

**FIGURE 10–8.** Plantar fibromatosis composed of uniform spindle-shaped cells arranged in long fascicles.

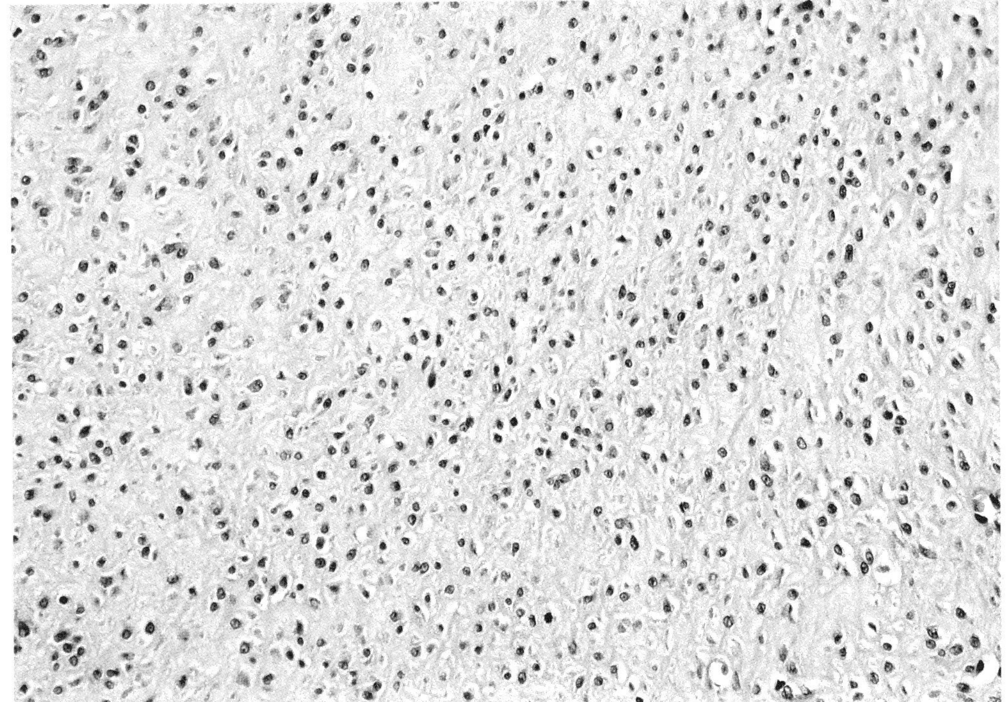

**FIGURE 10–9.** Plantar fibromatosis. Round-cell pattern caused by cross section of spindle-shaped fibroblasts.

a superficial form of fibromatosis that results in an ill-defined fibrous thickening or plaque-like mass in the shaft of the penis, frequently resulting in curvature of the erect penis. Despite numerous studies of the disease, its exact cause and pathogenesis are still unknown. The condition is also referred to in the literature as *plastic induration of the penis,*[124,131,146] *fibrous sclerosis of the penis,*[140] and *fibrous cavernositis.*[113]

## Clinical Findings

Although once considered rare, one study has found an approximately 1% incidence of symptomatic Peyronie's disease in two populations of male physicians.[117] It is seen primarily in men 45–60 years of age; it rarely affects young adults. There are no reports of cases in children. Most patients are white; the disease uncommonly affects Blacks or Orientals.[117]

The main complaint is a palpable plaque-like induration typically located on the dorsal or lateral aspect of the shaft of the penis causing the penis to curve toward the affected side. This curvature is the result of the relatively inelastic plaque-like scar tissue in the normally compliant tunica albuginea of the erectile body of the penis. It restricts expansion of the involved aspect of the penis during tumescence, limiting the extension of that segment of the penile shaft and causing the erection to be bent.[122] Associated symptoms include pain on erection and painful intercourse. Some patients who have penile curvature may have difficulty achieving an erection, presumably because the plaque-like induration impairs the venoocclusive function of the tunica albuginea.[108,130,145]

Penile fibromatosis is more common in patients with palmar and plantar fibromatosis than in the general population; its incidence varies from 2% to 4% in palmar fibromatosis and from 1% to 2% in plantar fibromatosis. Chilton et al. found that 15% of patients with Peyronie's disease have palmar fibromatosis,[115] whereas Williams and Thomas found that 10 of 17 patients with Peyronie's disease had palmar fibromatosis.[147] There is also an increased incidence in epileptic and diabetic patients. Bivens et al. reported Peyronie's disease as a presenting complaint of patients with carcinoid syndrome.[112] There have also been reports of an association between penile fibromatosis and Cogan syndrome (a vasculitis characterized by interstitial keratitis and vestibuloauditory symptoms[135]) and Paget's disease of bone.[132]

## Gross Findings

The fibrous mass chiefly involves fascial structures, corpus cavernosum, and rarely corpus spongiosum. It consists of dense, pearly white to gray-brown tissue that glistens on section; it averages 2 cm in greatest diameter.

## Microscopic Findings

There are relatively few descriptions of the pathologic features of Peyronie's disease.[140] The most consistent histologic abnormality is the irregular orientation and character of the collagen within the tunica albuginea.[116] There is an increased number of cytologically bland fibroblasts associated with haphazardly arranged collagen bands, irregular collagen plates, or nodules (Fig. 10–10). There is also a marked reduction of elastic fibers in affected areas as demonstrated by elastic stains. Fibrin may or may not be present. Inflammatory cells, particularly lymphocytes and plasma cells, may be present in early lesions, predominantly in a perivascular location, both within and external to the tunica albuginea.[114,116] As the lesions persist, there tends to be a decrease in the amount of chronic inflammation with a progressive increase in the amount of fibrosis, often with focal calcification or ossification. Metaplastic cartilage has also been described.[110]

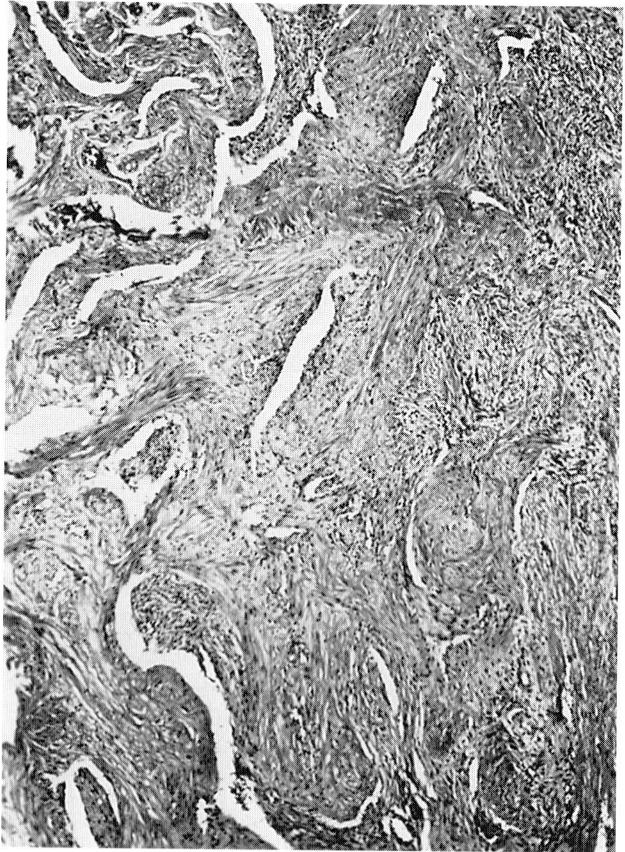

**FIGURE 10–10.** Penile fibromatosis of the corpus cavernosum with narrowing of the vascular spaces by extensive fibrosis.

### Treatment

The optimal therapy for Peyronie's disease remains unresolved. Many nonsurgical therapies have been attempted, including vitamin E,[139] potassium aminobenzoate,[150] colchicine,[109] intralesional injections of corticosteroids,[144] calcium channel blockers,[129] and collagenase,[123] all with limited success. Surgery appears to be the most effective treatment, although the best surgical technique is controversial. Surgical candidates include patients who have erectile dysfunction and those whose penile curvature precludes intercourse.[111] Straightening the penis usually requires at least partial excision of the plaque with surgery or laser therapy,[121,126] coupled with some type of grafting procedure.[120] There is a significant rate of postoperative erectile dysfunction, so some patients also require placement of a penile prosthesis.[149] Given that about one-third of patients who remain untreated have spontaneous resolution of their symptoms,[122, 147] many urologists choose to observe these patients for a period of time before embarking on definitive therapy.

### Discussion

The exact cause of Peyronie's disease is still not clear. As with palmar and plantar fibromatoses, a genetic component has been suggested,[125] perhaps requiring some environmental trigger. An inflammatory/infectious etiology has also been suggested. Smith found evidence of urethritis and fibrosis in 23 of 100 penises obtained at routine autopsies and concluded that penile fibromatosis is preceded by an inflammatory phase. They proposed the concept of "subclinical Peyronie's disease."[141]

There is also some evidence to support an autoimmune etiology, as this disease has been associated with several HLA tissue types, including the B7 cross-reactive group (HLA-B7, B22, B27, and B40),[134,136,148,151] HLA-DQ5,[133] DR3, and Dqw2.[138] Ralph et al. found that patients with early Peyronie's disease had immunoglobulin M (IgM) antibody deposition and a marked T lymphocytic infiltrate with increased expression of HLA class II antigens.[137]

Trauma may also be an important etiologic factor. Devine et al. suggested that repetitive microvascular injury results in the deposition of fibrin followed by fibroblast activation and proliferation and subsequent collagen deposition.[118] A similar observation was made by Somers and Dawson.[142] It is possible that Peyronie's disease does not represent a single distinct entity but a common morphologic appearance that is secondary to a variety of insults.[128] As with other forms of superficial and deep fibromatoses, multiple chromosome abnormalities have been described in Peyronie's disease,[125, 143] particularly abnormalities of the Y chromosome.

## KNUCKLE PADS

The term knuckle pads was coined by Jones in 1923 to describe flat or dome-shaped noninflammatory fibrous thickenings that occur on the dorsal aspect of the proximal interphalangeal or metacarpophalangeal joints and the paratenon of the extensor tendons (Fig. 10–11).[156] Most patients are asymptomatic, although some have mild tenderness or pain; the lesions rarely require surgical intervention. Knuckle pads comprise another fibrous proliferation not infrequently encountered in conjunction with palmar or plantar fibromatosis.[152,154,155,158,161,162] In Weckesser's series[162] 6% of patients with palmar fibromatosis also had knuckle pads, whereas in the study by Skoog 44% had the lesion.[161] The knuckle pads may precede the onset of palmar or plantar fibromatosis and may disappear spontaneously after these lesions are excised. Like palmar and plantar fibromatosis, the knuckle pad chiefly affects patients during the fourth, fifth, and sixth decades of life and is observed more commonly in men than in women. *Pachydermodactyly* is a rare variant of this condition that occurs mainly in adolescent boys.[160] Microscopically, it resembles palmar fibromatosis, but digital contractures do not occur.[153,157,159] Grossly, knuckle pads may be confused with pad-like hyperkeratoses that occur secondary to occupational trauma or self-manipulation. There is

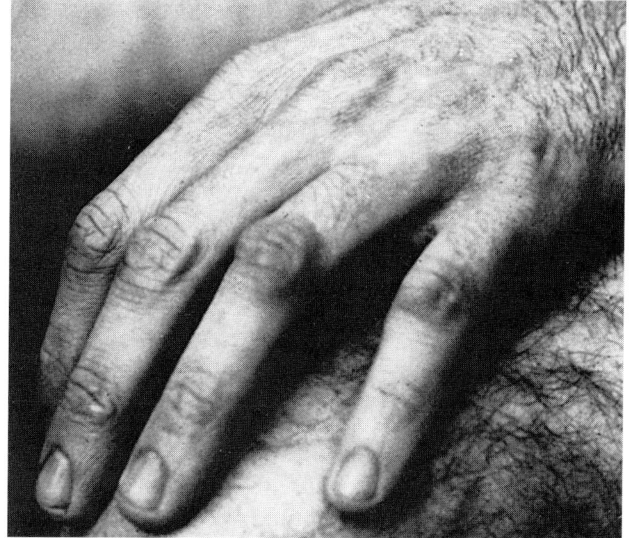

**FIGURE 10–11.** Knuckle pads, a lesion marked by fibrous thickening over the extensor surfaces of the interphalangeal joints. It may be associated with both palmar and plantar fibromatosis.

also some resemblance to Heberden's nodes of osteoarthritis.[159]

## EXTRAABDOMINAL FIBROMATOSIS (EXTRAABDOMINAL DESMOID)

Extraabdominal fibromatosis arises principally from the connective tissue of muscle and the overlying fascia or aponeurosis (*musculoaponeurotic fibromatosis*); it chiefly affects the muscles of the shoulder and pelvic girdles and the thigh of adolescents and young adults. Other terms used to describe this condition include *extraabdominal desmoid, desmoid tumor,* and *well-differentiated nonmetastasizing fibrosarcoma* or *grade I fibrosarcoma*. The term *aggressive fibromatosis* is often employed to emphasize its frequently aggressive behavior.

Extraabdominal fibromatosis is one of the more common soft tissue lesions. It is estimated that approximately 700–900 new cases (3–4 cases per million) occur in the United States annually.[173] Despite its relatively common occurrence, this tumor continues to present a problem in recognition and management, especially because of the striking discrepancy between its deceptively harmless microscopic appearance and its propensity to recur locally and infiltrate neighboring soft tissues.

### Clinical Findings

Extraabdominal fibromatosis is most common in patients between puberty and 40 years of age, with a peak incidence between the ages of 25 and 35 years. Children are sometimes affected. In the series by Rock et al., 5% of the patients were 10 years of age or less, the youngest being 9 months old.[223] Women are more commonly affected than men.[166,171,177,178,219,220,223] Reitamo et al.[221] reported 89 cases of desmoid tumor and demonstrated four major age groups where the site of the tumor, the gender of the patient, or both were nonrandomly distributed. "Juvenile" tumors occurred predominantly in an extraabdominal location, with a distinct predilection for girls younger than 15 years of age. "Fertile" tumors occurred nearly exclusively as abdominal desmoid tumors in fertile females. "Menopausal" tumors also occurred predominantly in the abdomen, with an approximately equal number of men and women affected. "Senescent" tumors were equally distributed between abdominal and extraabdominal locations and were equally frequently encountered in both genders.

Most patients present with a deep-seated, firm, poorly circumscribed mass that has grown insidiously and causes little or no pain. Decreased mobility of an adjacent joint may occur. Neurologic symptoms, including numbness, tingling, a "stabbing" or "shooting" pain, or motor weakness, may occur when the lesion compresses nearby nerves.

### Radiographic Findings

The lesion presents as a soft tissue mass that interrupts the adjacent intermuscular and soft tissue planes. The mass may encroach on adjacent bone and cause pressure erosion or superficial defects of the cortex. Occasionally, there is a periosteal reaction consisting of "frond-like" spicules of bone that extend deep into the tumor.[164] Häyry et al.[190] found that up to 80% of affected patients have multiple minor bony anomalies of the mandible, chest, and long bones. These abnormalities include cortical thickening, exostoses, and areas of cystic translucence or compact islands in the femur (or both). The frequency of these bony anomalies was similar in the group of patients with abdominal fibromatosis, and they occur in all age groups.

Radiographic studies, including computed tomography (CT) scans, MRI, and scintigraphy,[201, 231] are helpful in the diagnosis and assessment of tumor extent prior to surgery. Pritchard et al. found a lower local recurrence rate after the introduction of these improved imaging techniques compared to the recurrence rate prior to their routine use.[220]

### Anatomic Location

Extraabdominal fibromatosis may be located in a variety of anatomic locations. Most studies have found the principal site of the tumor to be the musculature of the shoulder, followed by the chest wall and back, thigh, and head and neck (Table 10–2).

In the shoulder and neck region, the growth presents most often in the deltoid, scapular region (Fig. 10–12), supraclavicular fossa, or posterior cervical triangle where it may extend into the anterior or posterior portion of the axilla and upper arm. Because of the numerous vital structures in this location, including nerves of the brachial plexus and large vessels, complete surgical excision of tumors in this location is often difficult if not impossible.

Fibromatoses in the region of the pelvic girdle primarily affect the gluteus muscle, whereas those in the region of the thigh affect the quadriceps muscle and muscles of the popliteal fossa. The hands and feet are rarely affected.[223]

The head and neck is not an unusual location for these lesions. As many as 23% of all extraabdominal fibromatoses occur in this location.[172,175,179,207,219] In

**TABLE 10–2 ANATOMIC DISTRIBUTION OF 367 CASES OF EXTRAABDOMINAL (DESMOID) FIBROMATOSIS**

| Anatomic Site | No. Patients | % |
|---|---|---|
| Head | 7 | 1.9 |
| Neck | 28 | 7.6 |
| Shoulder | 81 | 22.1 |
| Upper arm | 21 | 5.7 |
| Forearm | 13 | 3.5 |
| Hand | 4 | 1.1 |
| Chest wall; back | 63 | 17.2 |
| Mesentery | 38 | 10.4 |
| Buttock; hip | 21 | 5.7 |
| Thigh | 46 | 12.5 |
| Knee | 27 | 7.4 |
| Lower leg | 17 | 4.6 |
| Foot | 1 | 0.3 |
| *Total* | 367 | 100.0 |

children, more than one-third of extraabdominal fibromatoses are located in the head and neck.[185] At this site the soft tissue of the neck is most commonly involved, followed by the face, oral cavity, scalp, paranasal sinuses, and orbit.[172,179,185] Clinically, fibromatoses arising in the head and neck are more aggressive than extraabdominal fibromatoses arising elsewhere and are capable of massive destruction of adjacent bone and erosion of the base of the skull; they occasionally encroach on the trachea, sometimes with a fatal outcome.[172,212,229,239]

Fibromatosis of the breast may arise in the mammary gland or from extension of a lesion arising in the aponeurosis of the chest wall or shoulder girdle.[216,224,234] The differential diagnosis in this location includes metaplastic carcinoma, fibrosarcoma, and benign reactive processes such as nodular fasciitis and keloid.

## Multicentric Fibromatoses

Extraabdominal fibromatoses are not infrequently multicentric.[180,208,225] Fong et al. found almost 5% of these lesions to be multicentric, typically involving one anatomic region of the body.[182] In most cases the second growth develops proximal to the primary lesion. Rarely, coexistence of abdominal and extraabdominal fibromatoses has been observed in the same patient.[197,210]

## Gross Findings

The tumor is almost always confined to the musculature and the overlying aponeurosis or fascia. Large tumors may extend along the fascial plane or infiltrate the overlying subcutaneous tissue. Occasional lesions involve the periosteum and may lead to bone erosion, thereby closely resembling desmoplastic fibroma of bone.[170,193,230]

Most tumors measure 5–10 cm in greatest dimension, although rare lesions as large as 20 cm have been reported. The tumor is firm, cuts with a gritty sensation, and on cross section reveals a glistening white, coarsely trabeculated surface resembling scar tissue (Figs. 10–13, 10–14). Surgeons may have particular difficulty distinguishing recurrent fibromatosis from scar tissue related to prior excision.

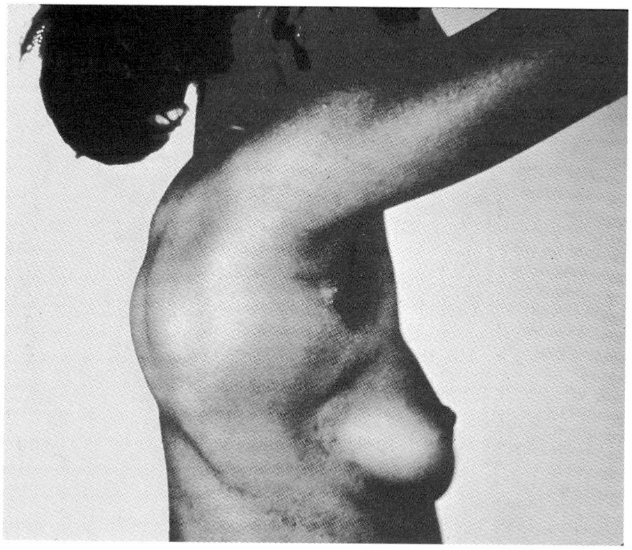

**FIGURE 10–12.** Mass in the scapular region in a patient with extraabdominal fibromatosis.

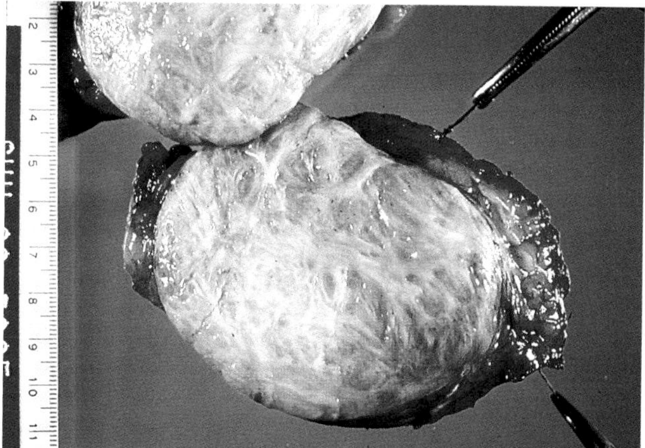

**FIGURE 10–13.** Extraabdominal fibromatosis (desmoid tumor) involving the chest wall. The cut surface reveals a trabecular appearance reminiscent of that seen in uterine leiomyomas.

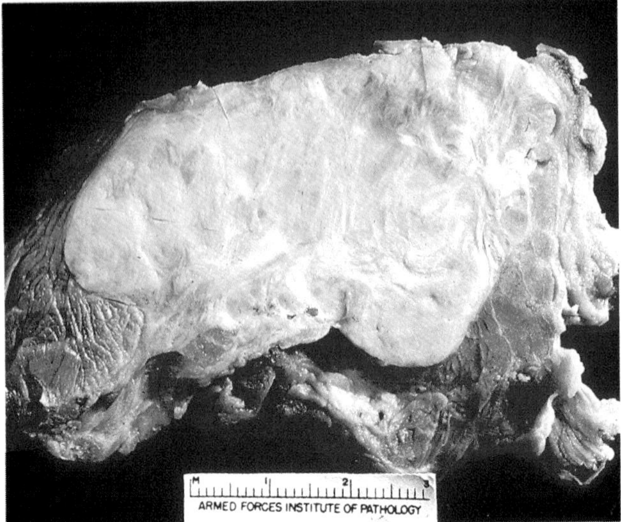


**FIGURE 10–14.** Extraabdominal fibromatosis (desmoid tumor) involving the pectoralis muscle.

## Microscopic Findings

Characteristically, the lesion is poorly circumscribed and infiltrates the surrounding tissue, usually striated musculature (Fig. 10–15). The proliferation consists of elongated, slender, spindle-shaped cells of uniform appearance surrounded and separated from one another by abundant collagen, with little or no cell-to-cell contact (Fig. 10–16). The cells lack hyperchromasia or atypia, but the cellularity varies from area to area within the lesion (Fig. 10–17). The constituent nuclei are small, pale-staining, and sharply defined, with one to three minute nucleoli (Figs. 10–18, 10–19). Clearly defined cellular boundaries can be discerned only in cases with a prominent mucoid matrix and relatively small amounts of collagen (Fig. 10–20).[178]

Cells and collagen fibers are usually arranged in sweeping bundles that are less well defined than those in fibrosarcoma. Glassy keloid-like collagen fibers or extensive hyalinization may be present and may obscure the basic pattern of the lesion (Fig. 10–21). Reticulin preparation and Masson trichrome stain clearly reveal the abundance of collagen between the individual tumor cells. Immunohistochemically, the spindle cells stain with vimentin and smooth muscle, and muscle-specific actin. Rare cases also stain with polyclonal or monoclonal antibodies to desmin.[191]

At the periphery of the growth where the tumor has infiltrated muscle tissue, remnants of striated muscle fibers are frequently entrapped and undergo atrophy (Fig. 10–22) or form multinucleated giant cells that may be mistaken for malignancy. Microhemorrhages and focal aggregates of lymphocytes are common. In rare instances there is calcification or chondroid or osseous metaplasia, but this is never a prominent feature of the tumor.[213]

## Ultrastructural Findings

Musculoaponeurotic fibromatosis consists of a uniform population of elongated fibroblast-like cells often terminating in long, slender processes. Most nuclei are rounded or oval, but some cells show prominent nuclear indentations or clefts. There is a prominent rough endoplasmic reticulum that is partly dilated and contains granular or fibrillary material within the dilated spaces. The cytoplasm has a small number of mitochondria, a prominent Golgi apparatus, free ribosomes, and occasional pinocytotic vesicles and microtubules (Fig. 10–23). Some cells contain intracytoplasmic bundles of actin-type microfilaments measuring about 60 nm in diameter, often with areas of condensation (dense bodies).[181,186,189,199,215] Some cells contain incomplete or clumped basal lamina along the cell borders, all features characteristic of myofibroblasts. Intranuclear inclusions of collagen

*Text continued on page 327*

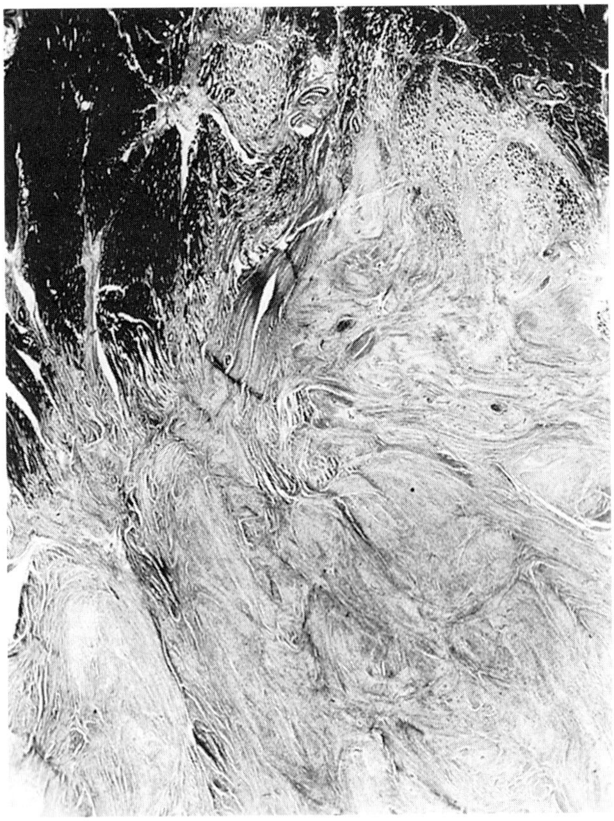

**FIGURE 10–15.** Extraabdominal fibromatosis (extraabdominal desmoid) invading striated muscle tissue. (Masson trichrome stain)

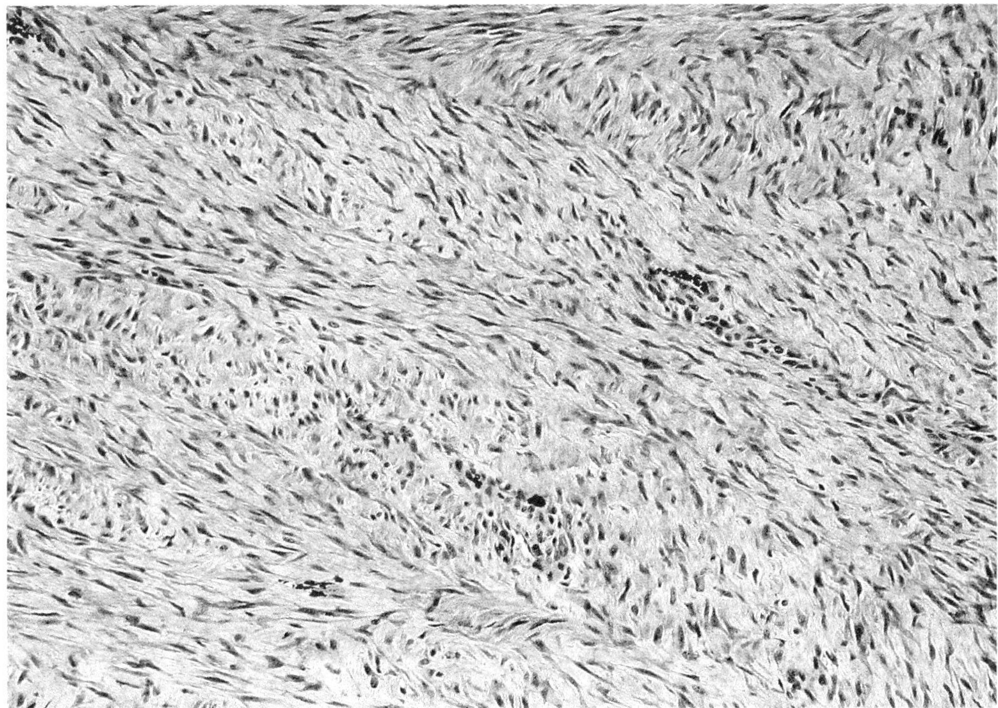

**FIGURE 10–16.** Interlacing bundles of fibroblasts separated by variable amounts of collagen in extraabdominal fibromatosis.

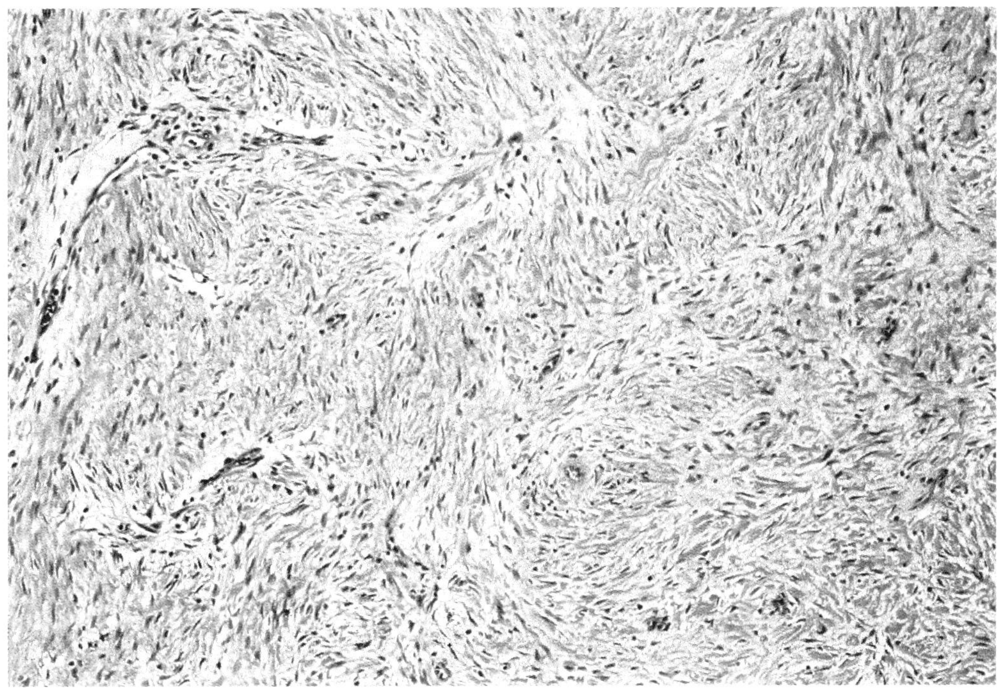

**FIGURE 10–17.** Extraabdominal fibromatosis in which the cells are arranged in a focal storiform growth pattern.

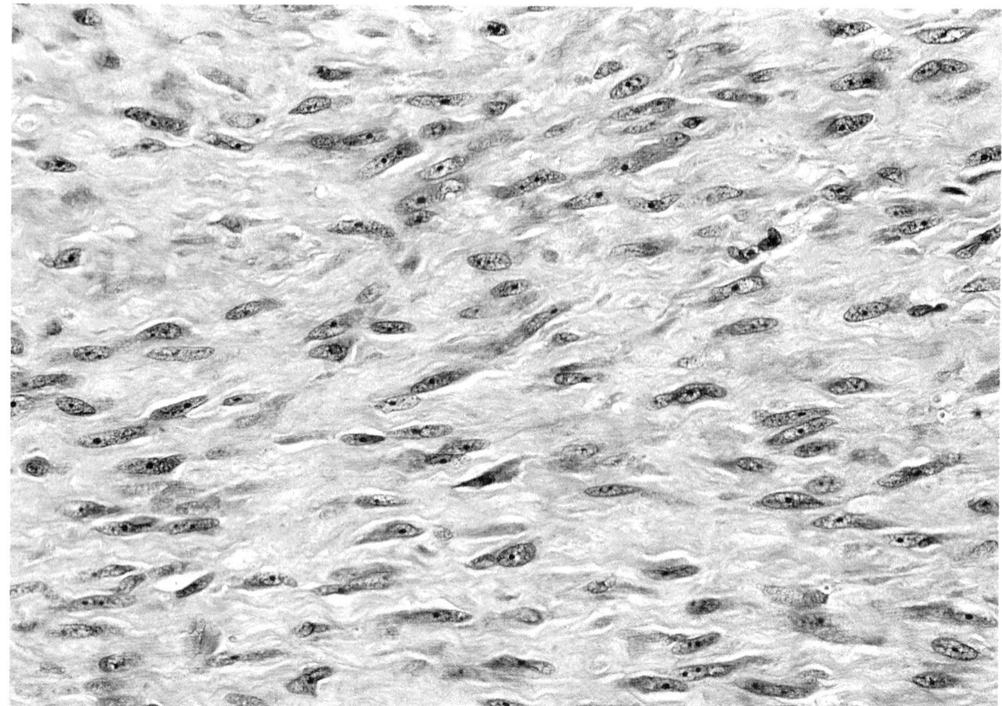

**FIGURE 10–18.** High-power view of extraabdominal fibromatosis showing vesicular nuclei with minute nucleoli, rather indistinct cytoplasm, and interstitial collagen.

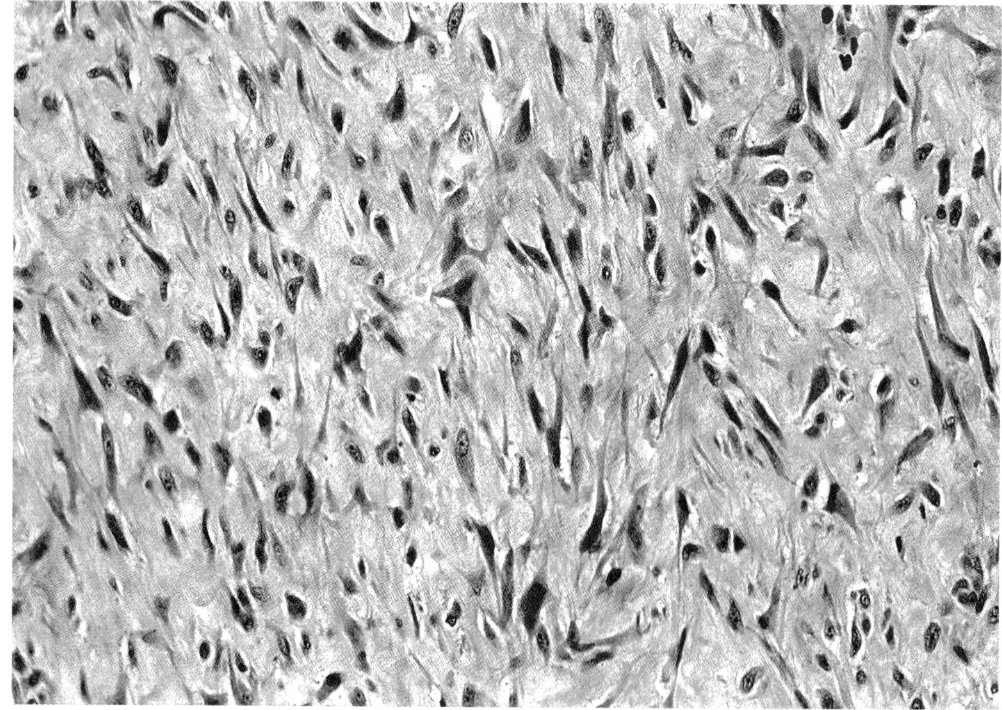

**FIGURE 10–19.** Stellate-shaped cells with uniform cytologic features in extraabdominal fibromatosis.

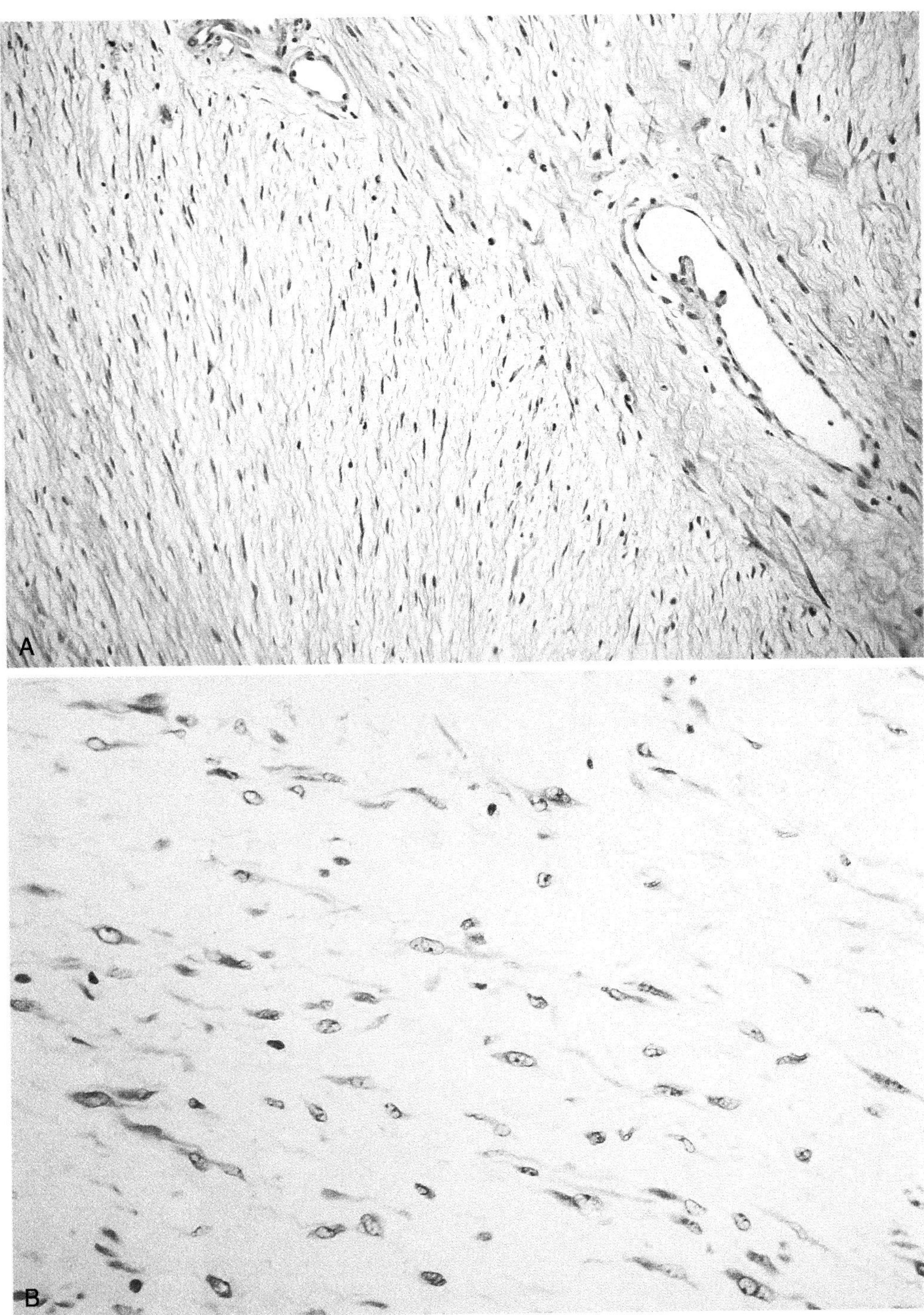


**FIGURE 10–20.** (**A**) Extraabdominal fibromatosis with relatively small amounts of collagen and a pronounced mucoid matrix. (**B**) High-power view of bland-appearing spindle-shaped cells in extraabdominal fibromatosis with abundant mucoid matrix.

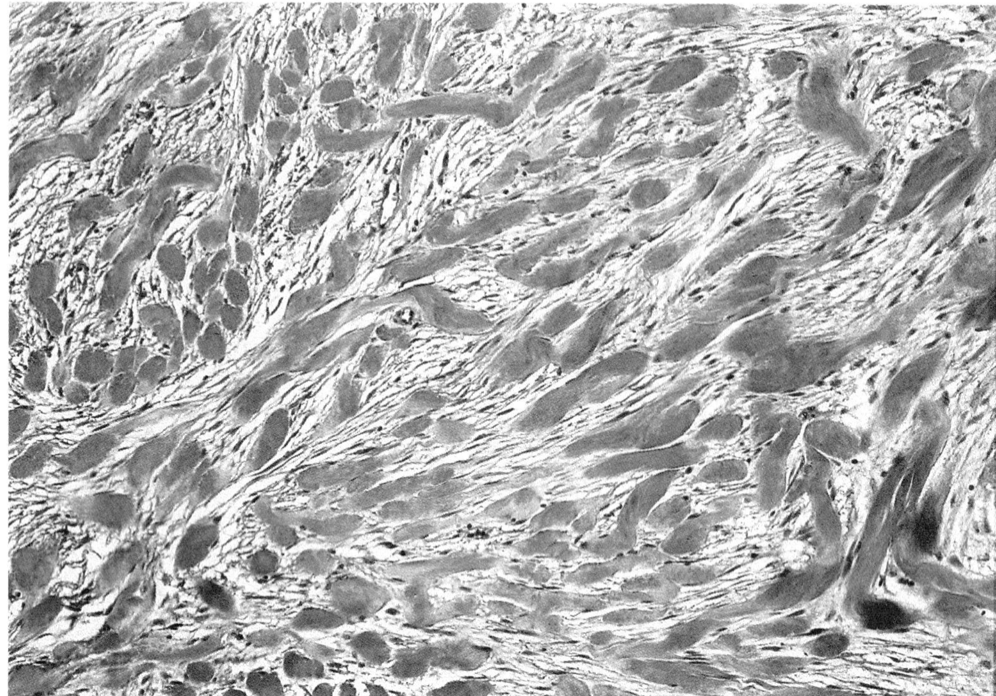

**FIGURE 10–21.** Fibromatosis with glassy hyalinized collagen fibers reminiscent of keloid, a rare feature of this tumor.

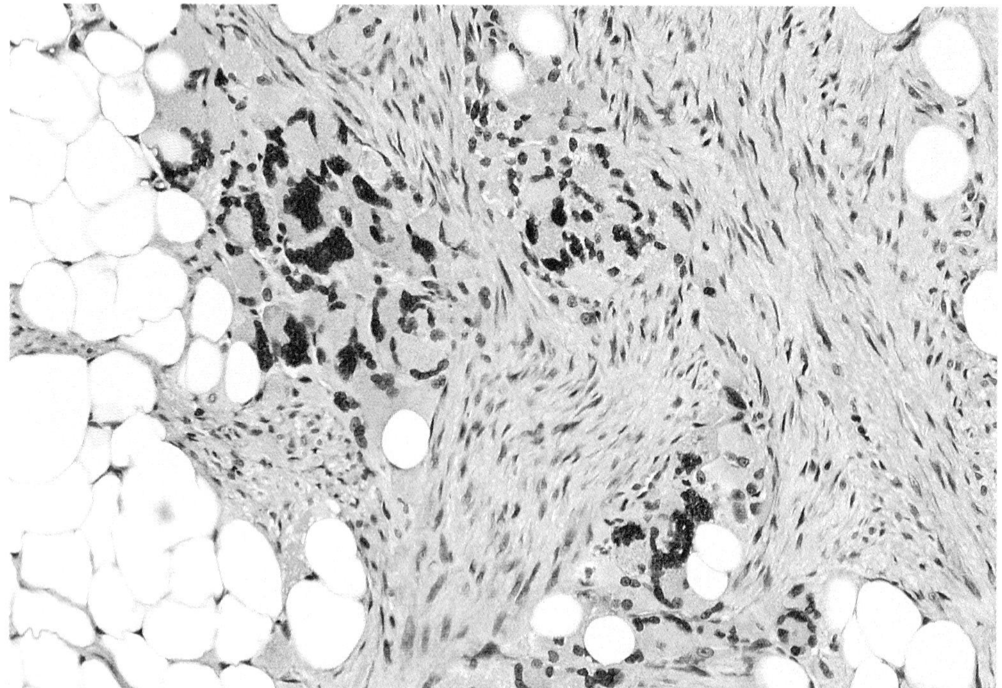

**FIGURE 10–22.** Peripheral portion of extraabdominal fibromatosis with entrapped muscle giant cells.

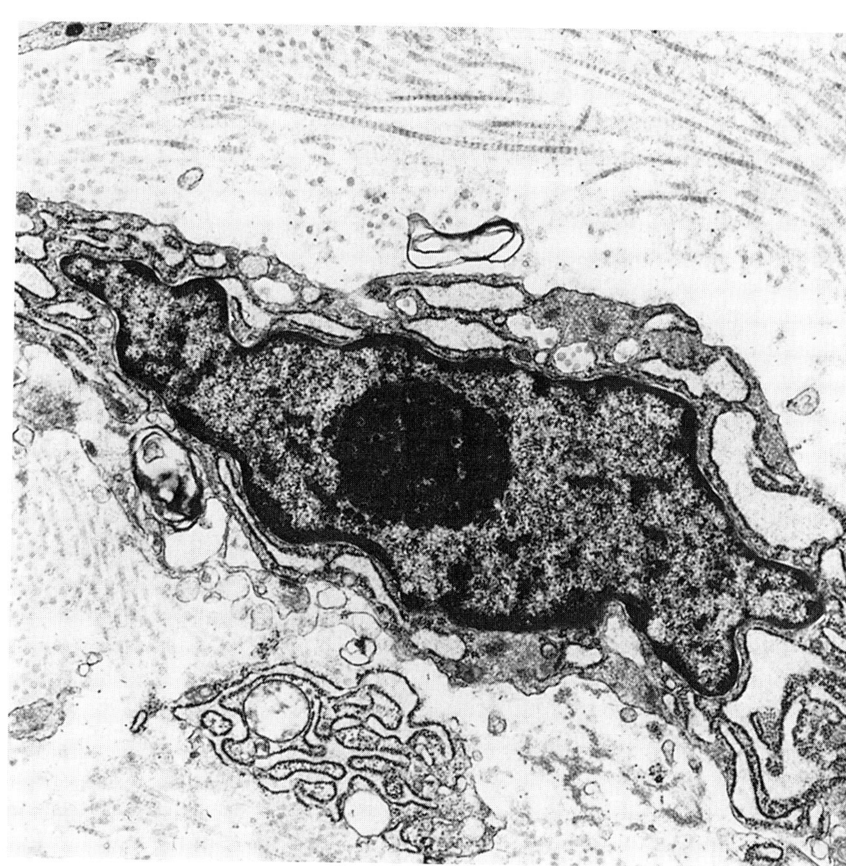

**FIGURE 10–23.** Fibroblast from typical extraabdominal fibromatosis. Note the prominent rough endoplasmic reticulum and mature collagen fibrils in the extracellular space. (From Taxy JB, Battifora H. The electron microscope in the study and diagnosis of soft tissue tumors. In: Trump BF, Jones RT (eds) Diagnostic Electron Microscopy. Wiley, New York, 1980.)

may be seen.[236] The stroma contains considerable amounts of collagen and ground substance.

## Differential Diagnosis

Fibromatosis most closely resembles fibrosarcoma and reactive fibrosis. *Fibrosarcoma* is usually more uniformly cellular than fibromatosis, and the cells are arranged in a more consistent sweeping fascicular (herringbone) growth pattern. Unlike fibromatosis, the cells are often overlapping and separated by less collagen. The nuclei are more hyperchromatic and atypical and have more prominent nucleoli than those found in fibromatosis. Although it is important to remember that there can be considerable overlap in levels of mitotic activity between fibromatosis and well-differentiated fibrosarcoma, high mitotic counts [>1 per 10 high-power fields (HPF)] throughout a tumor should arouse suspicion of fibrosarcoma. A small biopsy specimen may lead to a misdiagnosis, as some examples of fibrosarcoma have areas that are indistinguishable from fibromatosis and vice versa.

Fibromatosis can also be difficult to distinguish from *reactive fibroblastic proliferations* following injuries such as trauma, minor muscle tear, or intramuscular injection. Cytologically, these reactive proliferations are composed of cells indistinguishable from those found in fibromatosis. Thus, the low-magnification appearance is more useful for distinguishing these two entities. Reactive processes have a more variable growth pattern and frequently have focal hemorrhage or hemosiderin deposition, often situated along vascular structures. In some cases iron stains are useful for highlighting hemosiderin that is difficult to identify on hematoxylin and eosin (HE)-stained sections. In addition, an infiltrative growth pattern is much more characteristic of fibromatosis.

*Desmoplastic fibroma* of bone is indistinguishable from fibromatosis, especially when it presents as a soft tissue mass after breaking through the thinned or expanded cortex of the involved bone.[170,193] This lesion predominates in the metaphyseal or diaphyseal portions of long bones (e.g., the femur) or in the jaw, and radiographic studies are useful for distinguishing between these lesions.

Confusion with *myxoma* or *nodular fasciitis* is possible, particularly if only a small amount of tissue (or needle biopsy) is available for examination. Myxoma is usually paucicellular, with the cells separated from one another by abundant myxoid matrix. In contrast, fibromatosis always displays a greater degree of cellularity and more interstitial collagen than myxoma.

Although fibromatosis may show a focal whorled or feathery cellular pattern, this feature is never as prominent or as uniform as in nodular fasciitis.

*Fibrosarcomatous transformation of fibromatosis* is rare. Soule and Scanlon described and illustrated a case of typical fibromatosis of the inguinal region that evolved into a fibrosarcoma 10 years after initial excision and 9 years after radiotherapy.[228] Mooney et al. reported a case of metastasizing fibrosarcoma of the thigh that appeared 28 years after excision of a fibromatosis from the same region.[213] Following review of the slides from this reported case, Allen thought that the cells from the initial excision had too much nuclear hyperchromasia and atypia for fibromatosis and believed the lesion was a low-grade fibrosarcoma at the time of initial excision.[165] He went on to state that, "In my experience, all cases of metastasizing 'desmoid tumors' have proved to differ histologically from aggressive fibromatosis when the sections have been reviewed." In general, malignant transformation of fibromatosis may be erroneously suggested by occasional foci of increased cellularity and by exceptionally well-differentiated fibromatosis-like areas in some fibrosarcomas.

## Clinical Behavior

Despite its bland microscopic appearance, the tumor frequently behaves in an aggressive manner. Although incapable of metastasizing, extraabdominal fibromatoses often recur; they can rarely cause death when they invade or compress a vital structure, such as occurs with tumors in the root of the neck and within the abdomen.[166] In most studies, the 5-year survival rate is better than 90%.[171,219,220,223]

The recurrence rate recorded in the literature is variable, ranging from as low as 19%[195] to as high as 77%,[214] with an average of approximately 40%. In the study by Enzinger and Shiraki with a minimum 10 years of follow-up, 57% of tumors recurred.[178] In the largest series of extraabdominal desmoid tumors reported, Rock et al. found that 68% of patients experienced a recurrence an average 1.4 years after the initial treatment.[223] These authors found a greater tendency for recurrence in female patients, patients who were more than 30 years of age, and most importantly after treatment by intralesional or marginal excision. Only 50% of tumors recurred following wide local excision, compared to a recurrence rate of 90% following incomplete excision. Numerous other studies have found the extent of initial excision to be prognostically significant.[175,177,211,212,220] Old age[204] and large tumor size[178] have also been reported to be adverse prognostic factors.

Spontaneous regression of these tumors has been observed in sporadic cases, particularly in menarchal and menopausal patients. McDougall and McGarrity reported two cases of extraabdominal fibromatoses that spontaneously regressed after menopause,[210] and several other authors have confirmed this observation.[173,192,205] Enzinger and Shiraki reported a 36-year-old man with an extensive tumor involving the supraclavicular fossa, scalenus muscles, and brachial plexus that apparently resolved 9.5 years after the initial presentation.[178] A second patient, an elderly man with a large recurrent tumor of the axilla and chest wall, declined further treatment; 15 years later the tumor had substantially decreased in size and was no longer palpable.

## Treatment

Because the microscopic picture does not reliably reflect the growth potential of the tumor, therapy is predicated on its extent and anatomic relations. Most authors recommend wide local excision unless there is a risk of significant compromise of function, as there is a lower rate of recurrence when excision includes a wide margin of uninvolved structures around the grossly visible tumor. In view of the excellent prognosis for survival, amputation or other mutilating procedures should be done only for palliative purposes if the tumor recurs repeatedly and does not respond to adjuvant irradiation or endocrine therapy or if the extent of the tumor or threat of complications leaves no other choice.

In situations where a wide local excision cannot be performed, postoperative radiation therapy seems to be indicated for primary tumors that are incompletely excised. Karakousis et al. reported local control in 96% of patients treated with surgical resection supplemented by postoperative radiation therapy.[195] McCollough and colleagues[209] reported local control in 79% of patients treated with radiation postoperatively for known or presumed microscopic residual disease and in 88% of patients treated for known grossly apparent residual disease. In addition, these authors found radiation therapy alone to be an effective alternative to radical operation or when resection was not feasible. Similar results were achieved by Kamath et al.[194] and Kiel and Suit.[196] Interstitial brachytherapy, with surgical resection and postoperative iridium 192 implantation, has also been found to be effective therapy for patients with desmoid tumors.[240] There is no reliable information about the risk of malignant transformation following radiation therapy, but long-term follow-up is advisable.

Cytotoxic and noncytotoxic drug therapy has also been attempted for the treatment of these tumors. Chemotherapeutic agents, including doxorubicin,[217,227] vinblastine,[235] vincristine,[200] and colchicine[176] have been found to be effective in some cases. Nonsteroidal antiinflammatory prostaglandin-inhibiting drugs such as sulindac and indomethacin have been reported to cause stabilization or regression of both primary and recurrent tumors.[168,203,232,233] The efficacy of antiestrogen therapy, including tamoxifen, progesterone, or the luteinizing hormone-releasing hormone analogue goserelin acetate is not fully established but appears to be promising.[167,198,203,238]

### Discussion

Like other forms of fibromatosis, the etiology of extraabdominal fibromatosis is probably multifactorial, as genetic, endocrine, and physical factors seem to play an important role in its pathogenesis. Features suggesting an underlying genetic basis are the rare association of extraabdominal and abdominal fibromatosis in the same patient,[197] the occasional occurrence in siblings,[183] the presence of multiple bony abnormalities (in up to 80% of patients[190]), and the rare occurrence of extraabdominal fibromatosis in patients with familial adenomatous polyposis,[184,188,205] described in greater detail below. Recently, Lucas et al.[206] reported a uniform pattern of X chromosome inactivation, suggesting that this lesion is a true neoplasm. Although clearly implicated in the development of abdominal fibromatosis (discussed below), endocrine factors may also play a role in the development and growth of extraabdominal fibromatoses. Physical factors such as trauma or irradiation may also serve as a trigger mechanism. Cases of extraabdominal fibromatosis have been reported in the chest wall following trauma[237] and following reconstructive mammoplasty.[163,174,226] There have also been several reports of these lesions developing following radiation therapy for Hodgkin's disease.[169,187] Large studies of extraabdominal fibromatosis have reported an antecedent history of trauma in 16–28% of cases.[204,220,223]

## ABDOMINAL FIBROMATOSIS (ABDOMINAL DESMOID)

Although abdominal fibromatosis is indistinguishable grossly, microscopically, and by its infiltrative growth from extraabdominal fibromatosis, it deserves separate consideration because of its characteristic location and its tendency to occur in women of childbearing age during or following pregnancy. The tumor arises from musculoaponeurotic structures of the abdominal wall, especially the rectus and internal oblique muscles and their fascial coverings. Identical tumors originating from the pelvic wall have been described as pelvic fibromatosis or intraabdominal desmoid.

### Clinical Findings

Abdominal fibromatosis occurs in young, gravid or parous women during gestation or, more frequently, during the first year following childbirth. Pack and Ehrlich found that seven of ten patients with this disease are women 20–30 years of age.[274] Pfeiffer found that 87% of cases occurred in young women and 94% in women who had had one or more children.[275] Rare cases have been reported in children of both genders, especially boys[242,246,280] and adult men.[249]

The relative frequency of abdominal and extraabdominal desmoid tumors varies from one study to another. In a study carried out in Finland by Reitamo et al.,[277] abdominal fibromatoses (49%) outnumbered extraabdominal (43%) and mesenteric (8%) fibromatoses. The muscle most often involved is the rectus abdominis. Most lesions are solitary, but patients with both abdominal and extraabdominal fibromatoses have been described.[262,269]

### Pathologic Findings

The gross and microscopic appearances are similar to those described for extraabdominal fibromatosis, except that the average tumor is smaller and behaves less destructively than those in an extraabdominal location. Most tumors measure 3–10 cm in greatest dimension; and when arising in the rectus muscle or its fascia, they usually remain at the site of origin and do not cross the abdominal midline.

Microscopically, these lesions are variably cellular and often predominantly hypocellular; they are composed of cells with normochromatic nuclei with small, pinpoint nucleoli. The cells lack nuclear pleomorphism, and only rare mitotic figures can be identified. Cells are arranged into ill-defined fascicles with dense collagen separating the individual tumor cells. Characteristically, there is infiltration of the muscle tissue.

### Clinical Behavior and Therapy

As with all forms of fibromatosis, these lesions have a propensity to recur locally, although the rate of local recurrence (15–30%) is slightly lower than that of extraabdominal fibromatosis (35–65%). In most cases the lesions recur within the first 2 years after the initial excision or in connection with subsequent gestations or deliveries. Multiple recurrences are not uncommon. As with extraabdominal fibromatosis, wide local excision with ample margins is the therapy of choice to limit the rate of local recurrence, and adjuvant radiation therapy may help achieve control of inoperable or recurrent tumors. There are relatively few data regarding the efficacy of cytotoxic and noncytotoxic agents, although Hutchinson et al. reported eradication of a nonresectable fibromatosis in the lower abdomen of a 15-year-old boy following treatment with dactinomycin, vincristine, and cyclophosphamide.[259]

### Discussion

Like extraabdominal fibromatosis, genetic, endocrine, and physical factors seem to play an important role in the development of these tumors. Some arise in the setting of a polyposis syndrome, often at the site of previous abdominal surgery.[257,279] Endocrine factors are clearly implicated by the frequent occurrence of this tumor during or after pregnancy. In addition, there are reports of these tumors regressing with menopause.[259] Lipschutz and coworkers described the formation of desmoids in guinea pigs after prolonged estrogen administration and the prevention of these tumors by administration of testosterone, progesterone, and desoxycorticosterone.[261,267] Lim et al.[266] found estrogen receptors in one-third of desmoid tumors and antiestrogen binding sites in 79% of cases, including some without detectable estrogen receptors. The reported inhibitory effect of antiestrogenic agents such as tamoxifen supports the role of hormonal factors in the development of this disease.

Trauma may serve as a contributory cause, as some tumors have been reported to arise in the scars of appendectomies,[248] laparotomies,[245,251] and other abdominal operations (*cicatricial fibromatosis*).[218] Because most patients with abdominal fibromatosis have no history of gross injury to this region, minor and undetected trauma such as minute muscle tears may conceivably serve as a contributing etiologic factor that triggers the fibrous growth in a hormonally or genetically predisposed individual.

## INTRAABDOMINAL FIBROMATOSIS (INTRAABDOMINAL DESMOID)

The intraabdominal fibromatoses are a group of closely related lesions (rather than a single entity) that pose similar problems for the histologic diagnosis but can be distinguished from one another by the clinical setting and location. This category includes pelvic fibromatosis, mesenteric fibromatosis, and the fibromatosis of Gardner syndrome.

### Pelvic Fibromatosis

Pelvic fibromatosis is a variant of abdominal fibromatosis, differing from the latter by its location in the iliac fossa and lower portion of the pelvis, where it manifests as a slowly growing palpable mass that is asymptomatic or causes only slight pain. Clinically, it is often mistaken for an ovarian neoplasm or a mesenteric cyst. Large tumors in this location may encroach on the urinary bladder, vagina, or rectum; or they may cause hydronephrosis or compress the iliac vessels.[250,254,258,264]

As with fibromatosis of the abdominal wall, the tumor arises from the aponeurosis or muscle tissue and occurs chiefly in young women 20–35 years of age; in most cases it is unrelated to gestation or childbirth. Grossly and microscopically, the tumor is indistinguishable from other forms of extraabdominal or abdominal fibromatosis and requires similar modes of therapy. Several studies have reported some success with noncytotoxic therapy, such as tamoxifen, nonsteroidal antiinflammatory agents, and corticosteroids.[260,271]

### Mesenteric Fibromatosis

Fibromatosis is the most common primary tumor of the mesentery.[287] Most cases are sporadic, but some are associated with Gardner syndrome, trauma, or hyperestrogenic states. Most commonly, these tumors are located in the mesentery of the small bowel, but some originate from the ileocolic mesentery, gastrocolic ligament, omentum, or retroperitoneum. In the absence of a history of polyposis, distinguishing this lesion from other fibrosing processes that occur in this location such as idiopathic retroperitoneal fibrosis or sclerosing mesenteritis, may be difficult.

As with pelvic fibromatosis, most patients present with an asymptomatic abdominal mass, although some have mild abdominal pain. Less commonly, patients present with gastrointestinal bleeding or an acute abdomen secondary to bowel perforation. Occasionally, the tumor is found incidentally at laparotomy performed for some other reason, including patients undergoing bowel resection for Crohn's disease.[252,283] Data on age and gender vary: Kim et al.[264] reported nine intraabdominal desmoid tumors in eight females and one male who ranged in age from 15 to 62 years (mean 34 years). Yannopoulos and Stout reported that males and females were affected with equal frequency.[287] In the largest series reported to date, Burke et al.[247] noted that the tumor was more commonly encountered in males; and the mean age was slightly higher (41 years) in their series than in that reported by Kim et al. (35 years).[264]

Like many other neoplasms in the abdomen and retroperitoneum, most mesenteric fibromatoses are large, with the majority measuring 10 cm or more in greatest diameter. Many have an initial phase of rapid growth; and complications may be caused by compression of the ureter, development of a ureteral fistula,[278] or compression of the small or large intestines, sometimes complicated by intestinal perforation.[247,273,284] Grossly, most lesions are fairly well circumscribed, although microscopically there is typically infiltration into the surrounding soft tissues, including the bowel wall.

Microscopically, the lesions are composed of cytologically bland spindle-shaped or stellate cells evenly deposited in a densely collagenous stroma. Typically, there is variable cellularity, with some areas showing almost complete replacement by dense fibrous tissue. In others, the stroma shows marked myxoid change. Scattered keloid-type collagen fibers may be present, as are prominent dilated thin-walled veins and muscular hyperplasia of small arteries.[247] Inflammation is usually inconspicuous except in cases associated with bowel perforation.

The differential diagnosis includes *sclerosing (retractile) mesenteritis*,[263,285] a lesion that appears to be related to *mesenteric panniculitis*[241] and *mesenteric lipodystrophy*.[253,265] In general, these conditions are characterized by fibrosis and a more prominent chronic inflammatory infiltrate that abuts, but does not penetrate, the bowel wall.[253] *Inflammatory fibrosarcoma* of the mesentery and retroperitoneum is more cellular, has more pronounced cytologic atypia, and is less fibrotic and more inflamed than mesenteric fibromatosis.[270] *Idiopathic retroperitoneal fibrosis* (described below), a condition associated with methysergide administration[256] and inflammatory abdominal aortic aneurysms,[255] is usually more densely hyalinized and inflamed than fibromatosis.

Like other forms of fibromatosis, tumors arising in this location have a propensity for local recurrence, although data on the recurrence rate differ greatly. In the study by Burke et al.[247] 23% of all tumors recurred, although there was a striking difference in recurrence rates between patients with (90%) and without (12%) Gardner syndrome. In fact, none of the patients without Gardner syndrome had more than one recurrence, and none of these patients died as a direct result of their tumor. In contrast, most of the patients with Gardner syndrome had more than one recurrence, and four patients died of tumor. In the study by Kim et al.,[264] two of the seven patients (29%) without Gardner syndrome developed local recurrence.

Treatment is similar to that for extraabdominal fibromatosis, but excision is often difficult because of the irregular growth pattern and intestinal attachment of the tumor. Other modes of therapy, including treatment with antiestrogenic agents,[244] steroids,[272] cytotoxic chemotherapy,[268, 281] and postoperative irradiation,[276] have been met with variable success.

As with pelvic fibromatosis, the most likely cause appears to be tissue injury in a patient with a genetic predisposition to excessive fibrous growth. Of the patients without polyposis in the series by Burke et al.,[247] 12 (11%) had had abdominal surgery prior to detection of the fibromatosis. In some cases a second, morphologically similar lesion developed in the scar of the abdominal incision.[242,282] Rare cases of mesenteric fibromatosis have been reported following radiation therapy for Hodgkin's disease[243] or testicular seminoma.[286] Mesenteric fibromatosis may develop spontaneously in patients without polyposis or without prior surgical intervention. Although much less common than the association with abdominal fibromatosis, some mesenteric fibromatoses occur in patients with elevated serum estrogens. Of the 130 cases reported by Burke et al., 6 were associated with hyperestrogenic states, including 4 patients in whom the tumor developed during pregnancy, 1 in whom the tumor developed 6 months postpartum, and 1 who was a male alcoholic with bilateral gynecomastia.[247]

## Mesenteric Fibromatosis in Gardner Syndrome

Nichols was the first to recognize the association of desmoid tumors and familial adenomatous polyposis.[327] In 1951 Gardner reported the familial occurrence of intestinal polyposis, osteomas, fibromas, and epidermal or sebaceous cysts[301]; the term *Gardner syndrome* was coined by Smith in 1958.[332]

Gardner syndrome is inherited as an autosomal dominant trait that occurs in approximately half of the children of afflicted parents. It is more common in women than in men and is usually diagnosed in adults 25–35 years of age. Cutaneous cysts are present in 40–50% of patients, and osteomas can be detected in 35–50% of patients. The incidence of osteomas may be even higher, as a skeletal survey was done in only a few cases.[311,338,339] Osteomas may occur anywhere in the skeleton but are usually found in the skull and facial bones, especially the maxilla, mandible, sphenoid, and frontal bone. Cortical thickening is more common in long bones.[294,304,325,340] As a rule, the cutaneous cysts and osteomas occur during childhood or the teenage years and precede the onset of polyposis and fibromatosis by 10–15 years.

Early cases tend to be asymptomatic or manifest with mild diarrhea and passage of small amounts of mucus or blood. At age 20–25 years, radiographic examination reveals numerous discrete filling defects in the colon characteristic of multiple polyposis in about one-half of cases (Fig. 10–24). The intestinal adenomatous polyps are indistinguishable from those seen with other forms of polyposis and are found throughout the intestinal tract; the colon and rectum are the two major sites, although adenomas may also occur in the ileum, duodenum, and stomach. Colorectal adenocarcinoma, often at multiple sites, usually

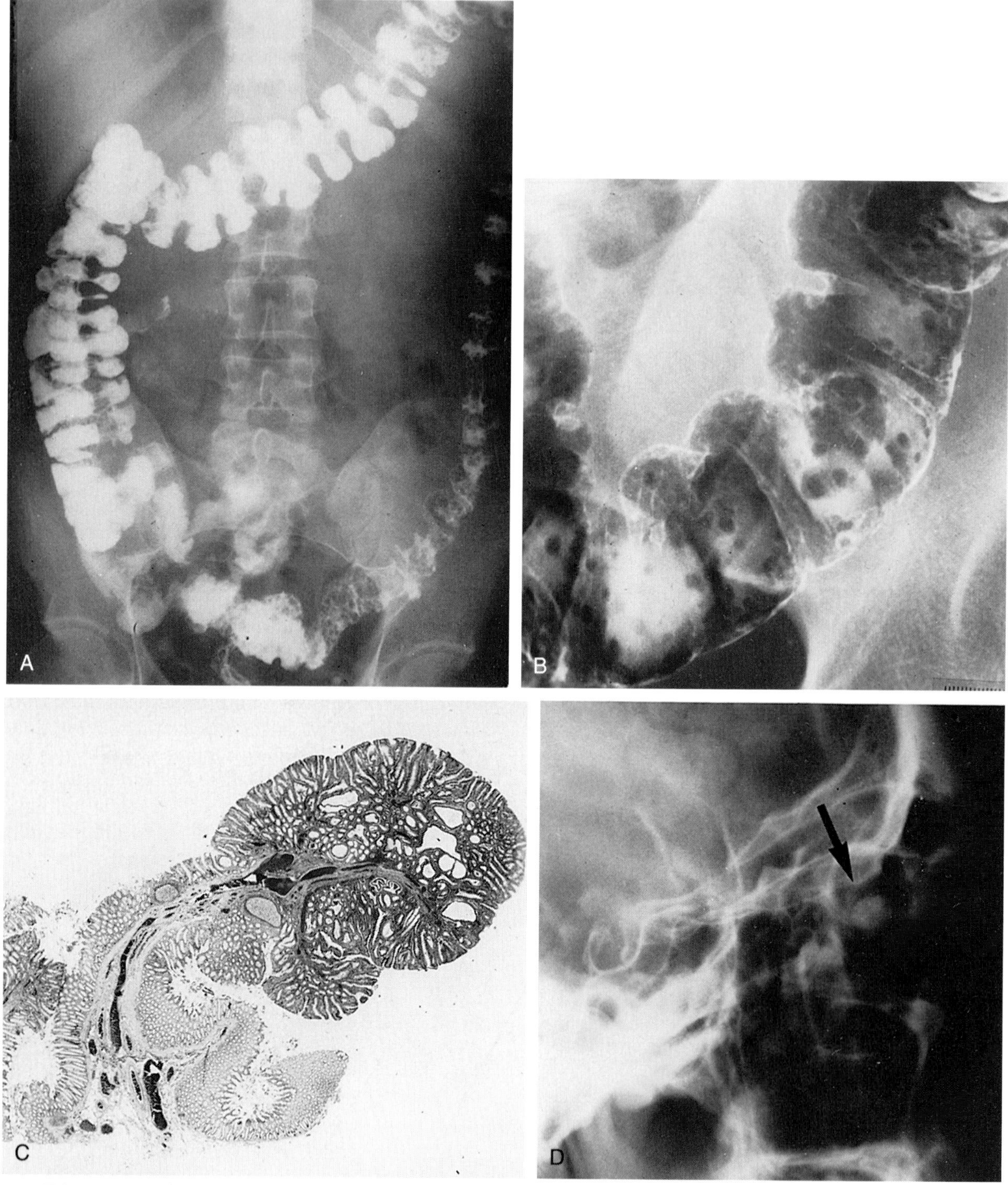


**FIGURE 10–24.** Gardner syndrome. (**A, B, C**) Familial polyposis of the colon. (**D**) Osteoma of the frontal sinus (arrow).

occurs 10–15 years after the onset of polyposis, as most patients are diagnosed with carcinoma by 40 years of age, approximately 25 years earlier than the onset of colorectal carcinoma in the general population. Early detection of the disease permits proper surgical therapy before malignant transformation of the polyps takes place. Because the lesion usually does not manifest before the patient reaches reproductive age, genetic counseling and lifelong surveillance are important parts of therapy in patients with a positive family history.[295] Many patients choose to undergo prophylactic colectomy, an operation that has been made more palatable by the advent of the ileal pouch–anal anastomotic procedure, which allows maintenance of fecal continence.

This syndrome may also be associated with a variety of other neoplasms, including adrenal cortical carcinoma,[333,337] ampulla of Vater carcinoma,[322] and thyroid carcinoma.[289,310,314] Various soft tissue and bone sarcomas, including fibrosarcoma,[302,304] osteosarcoma,[300] chondrosarcoma,[305] and liposarcoma,[300] as well as brain tumors (Turcot syndrome),[319] have also been described.

Mesenteric or retroperitoneal fibromatosis usually has its onset 1–2 years after excision of the diseased portion of the intestinal tract. Most large studies have found the incidence of fibromatosis in patients with polyposis to be in the vicinity of 10%.[306,309,330] Gurbuz et al. estimated the absolute risk of desmoids in polyposis patients to be 852 times that of the general population.[306] In this series, 68% of the patients had had abdominal surgery prior to discovery of the tumor (Fig. 10–25). Rarely, a similar-appearing tumor arises in the abdominal wall scar of the preceding laparotomy. Not all cases of fibromatosis develop as a result of surgical trauma; a small number have been noted prior to surgical intervention.[308,321,326,329] Kawashima et al.[313] found that tumors arising in association with Gardner syndrome were more likely to be multicentric, mesenteric, and smaller than those arising in patients without polyposis. Several studies have found that the female predominance is less striking than in nonpolyposis cases.[290,312,323]

Clinically, the fibromatosis may be asymptomatic or may cause mild abdominal pain or intestinal obstruction as a result of infiltrative growth into the wall of the small or large bowel. Although most tumors grow slowly, Gold and Mucha reported mesenteric fibromatosis in a 40-year-old man that increased in size from 4 cm to 27 cm in greatest diameter over a period of 1 year.[303]

Histologically, the fibromatosis is virtually indistinguishable from those at other sites, and one cannot distinguish polyposis-related cases from sporadic cases by morphology alone. These tumors tend to have a prominent myxoid matrix. (Figs. 10–26 to 10–

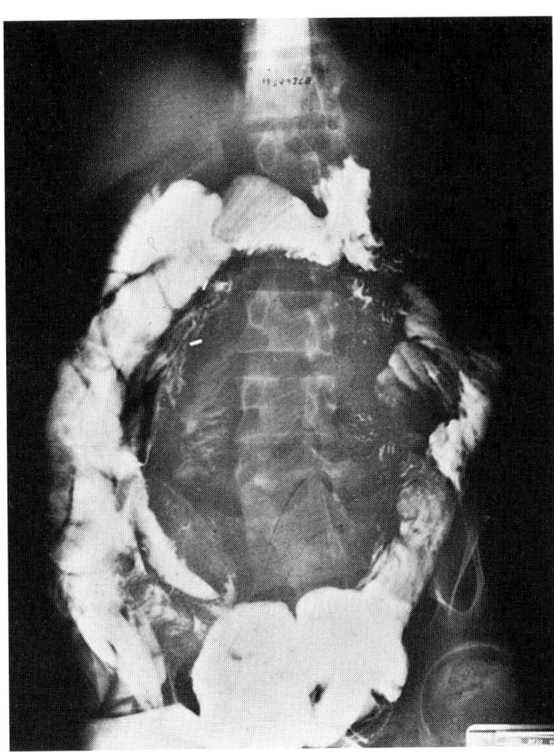

**FIGURE 10–25.** Plain film of the abdomen of a patient with mesenteric fibromatosis in Gardner syndrome following total colectomy. Loops of small bowel are displaced by mesenteric fibromatosis.

29), and the cells may be arranged in a vague storiform pattern that resembles benign or malignant fibrous histiocytoma.

As with mesenteric fibromatosis without polyposis, complete excision of the tumor is often difficult and necessitates removal of a sizable segment of the intestine together with the fibrous growth. For rapidly growing tumors, excision must be attempted to prevent complications caused by the presence of a massive, expanding intraabdominal growth. Recurrence is common, and several studies have found a higher rate of recurrence in polyposis-related fibromatosis than in sporadic cases.[292,293,318] In addition, fatal complications are more frequent than with nonpolyposis fibromatoses.[293,307,330] Endocrine therapy (tamoxifen and prednisolone), noncytotoxic drug therapy (sulindac and indomethacin), and chemotherapy have been reported to be efficacious for treating recurrent or inoperable tumors.[316,317,334–336]

## Discussion

Gardner syndrome is a genetically determined autosomal dominant disease caused by a germline abnormality of the adenomatous polyposis coli (*APC*) gene on the long arm of chromosome 5.[315] Several cytoge-

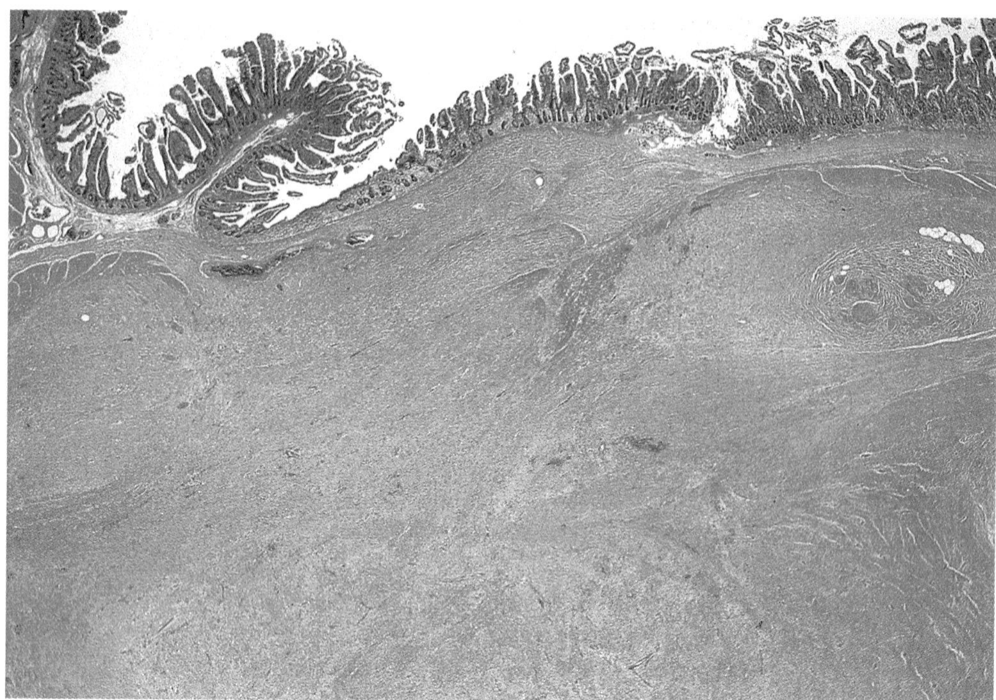

**FIGURE 10–26.** Low-power view of mesenteric fibromatosis in Gardner syndrome showing uniform fibrocollagenous growth infiltrating the wall of the small bowel.

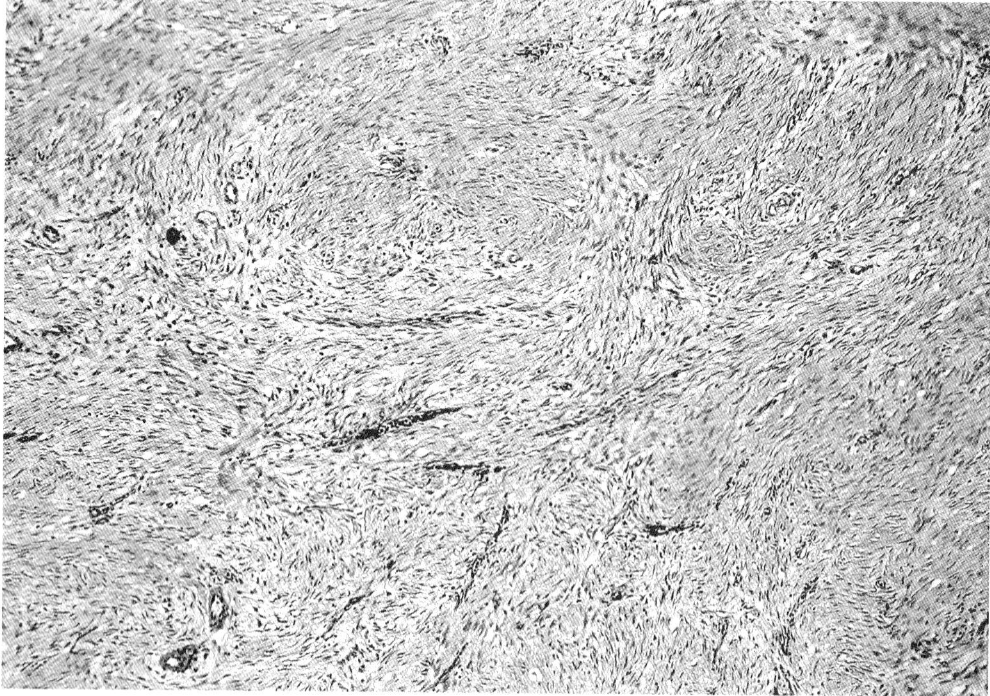

**FIGURE 10–27.** Orderly arrangement of uniform fibroblasts associated with moderate amounts of collagen and mucoid material in mesenteric fibromatosis.

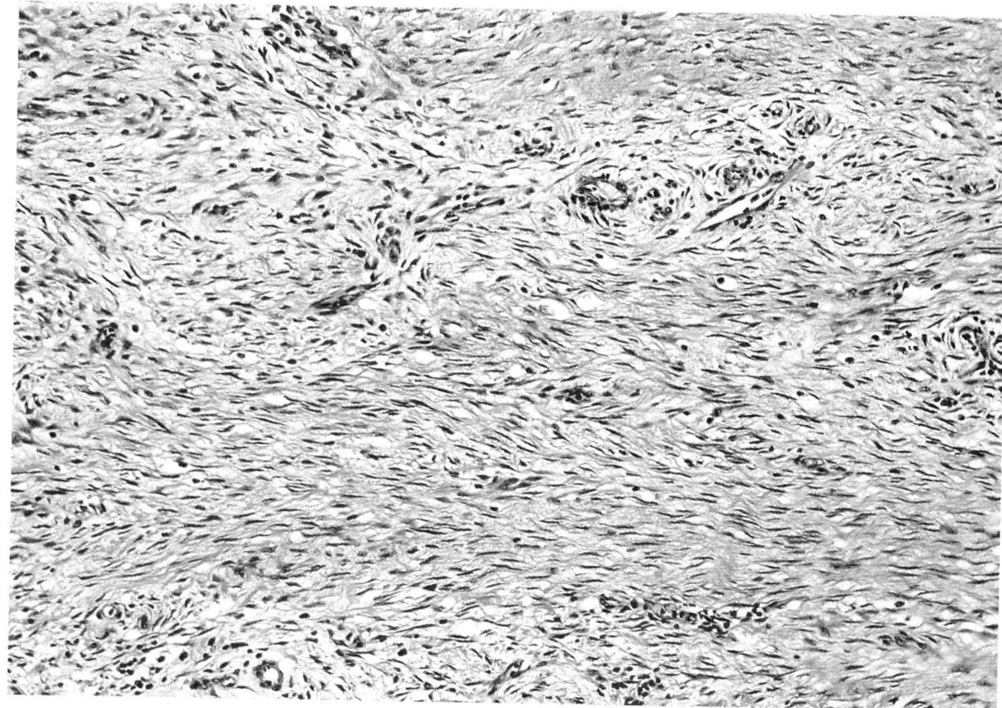

**FIGURE 10–28.** Uniform spindled proliferation in mesenteric fibromatosis.

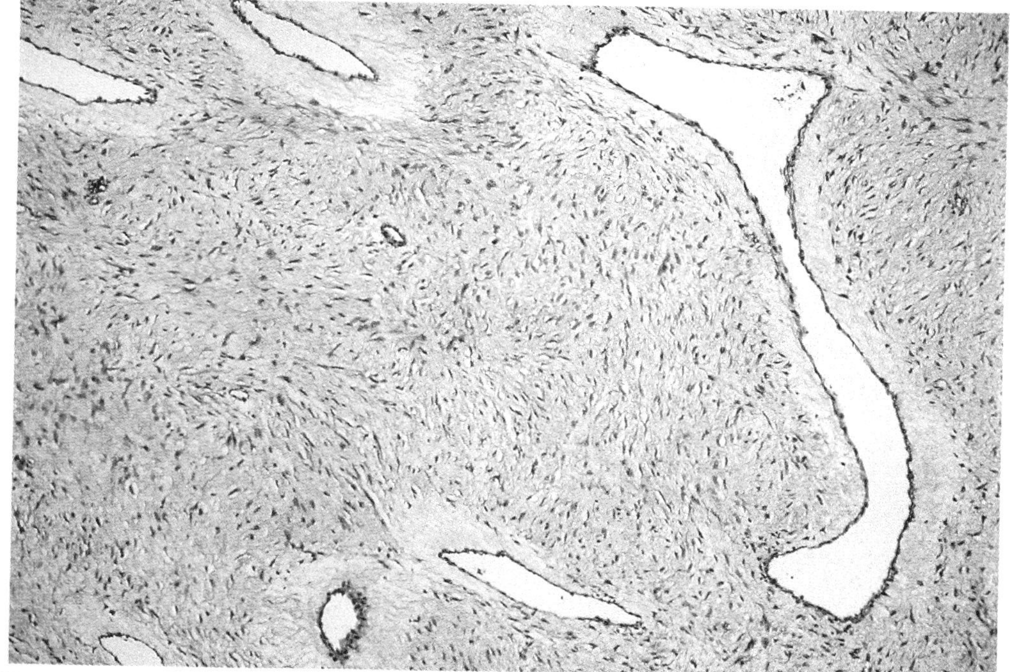

**FIGURE 10–29.** Prominent dilated blood vessels with perivascular hyalinization, a common feature of intraabdominal fibromatosis.

netic and molecular genetic studies have reported abnormalities of this locus in desmoid tumors.[298,324,328,340] Studies suggest that mutations of the *APC* gene result in a protein product that loses the ability to degrade $\beta$-catenin, resulting in an elevated $\beta$-catenin protein level, which in turn promotes fibroblastic proliferation.[288,320,331] Other cytogenetic abnormalities include loss of the Y chromosome,[291] trisomy 8,[296,299] and trisomy 20.[297]

## IDIOPATHIC RETROPERITONEAL FIBROSIS (ORMOND'S DISEASE)

Idiopathic retroperitoneal fibrosis is a rare fibrosing reactive process that may be confused with mesenteric fibromatosis. Although originally described in 1905 by the French urologist Albarran,[341] it was not until the publication of two cases in the English literature by Ormond in 1948 that this disease became more widely recognized.[385] It is characterized by diffuse or localized fibroblastic proliferation and a chronic lymphoplasmacytic infiltrate in the retroperitoneum causing compression or obstruction of the ureters, aorta, or other vascular structures.

The disease is two to three times more common in men, and most patients present during the fifth or sixth decade of life.[346,358,369] It is unusual before age 20 or over age 70, although several cases have been reported in children.[348,352,395] Most patients present with vague nonspecific abdominal symptoms, including dull, poorly localized back or flank pain. Other common symptoms include weight loss, nausea or vomiting, malaise, anorexia, fever, and hypertension.[370] The cause of the pain is probably related to ureteral obstruction or abnormal ureteral peristalsis.[406] Patients uncommonly present with colonic obstruction.[371] Laboratory abnormalities include anemia, azotemia, elevated erythrocyte sedimentation rate, hypergammaglobulinemia, and serum autoantibodies.[351,372] Although most cases are idiopathic, some have been associated with administration of methysergide, an ergot derivative used to treat migraine headaches.[363] It has been estimated that approximately 1% of patients taking this drug develop retroperitoneal fibrosis,[369] and symptoms are often relieved upon withdrawal of the drug.[361] Other cases of retroperitoneal fibrosis occur secondary to an exuberant desmoplastic response to a malignancy at this location.[398] The tumors that are most frequently implicated include Hodgkin's disease and other types of lymphoma, retroperitoneal sarcomas, carcinoid tumors, and a variety of carcinomas, including those in the breast, lung, stomach, colon, kidney, bladder, prostate, and cervix.[353,391,407] Approximately 5–25% of abdominal aortic aneurysms are associated with perianeurysmal fibrosis, and it may represent an early or mild form of retroperitoneal fibrosis.[370]

### Pathologic Findings

Grossly, the mass is dense, grayish-white, and plaque-like, usually arising at or just below the level of the aortic bifurcation.[370] As it progresses, the plaque surrounds the aorta and inferior vena cava and spreads through the retroperitoneum in a perivascular distribution; it may extend into the pelvis to surround the iliac and gonadal vessels. In some cases the plaque extends anteriorly along the celiac axis and superior mesenteric artery.[383] Typically, one or both ureters, usually in the middle one-third, are encased by this fibrous proliferation, often resulting in hydronephrosis.

Microscopic examination reveals a fibrous proliferation, broad anastomosing bands of hyalinized collagen, and a lymphoplasmacytic infiltrate of variable density, with occasional germinal centers (Fig. 10–30). Macrophages and eosinophils may also be conspicuous, but neutrophils are generally absent. Several studies have found a progression from active inflammation to fibrosis through serial biopsies.[369,383] The aorta that is surrounded by the fibrous proliferation typically shows severe atherosclerosis with protrusion of atherosclerotic debris through the media into the adventitia with chronic inflammation within the aortic wall.[384,386–388]

### Clinical Behavior and Therapy

Although spontaneous regression has been observed in some cases,[364,365,399,401] most patients require some form of treatment. Patients taking methysergide should stop the drug immediately, after which there is often relief of symptoms and regression of the fibrosis within a short time.[361] Surgical intervention is required in some patients. Multiple deep biopsies should be obtained to exclude the possibility of malignancy, as there may be a few malignant cells admixed within the fibrosis and inflammatory infiltrate.[343] Ureterolysis (dissection of the ureters from the surrounding fibrosis) is often required to relieve the ureteral obstruction and restore normal renal function.[405] Several authors have reported success with laparoscopic ureterolysis and ureteral intraperitonealization.[349,368,377,378] Although ureterolysis successfully relieves ureteral obstruction in approximately 90% of cases,[382] recurrent obstruction occurs in up to 22% of patients treated with ureterolysis alone.[404] The antiinflammatory action of corticosteroids appears to be effective for treating this disease,[342,360,396] although there is less benefit during the later fibrotic stages.[370] Variable success has been achieved with azathio-

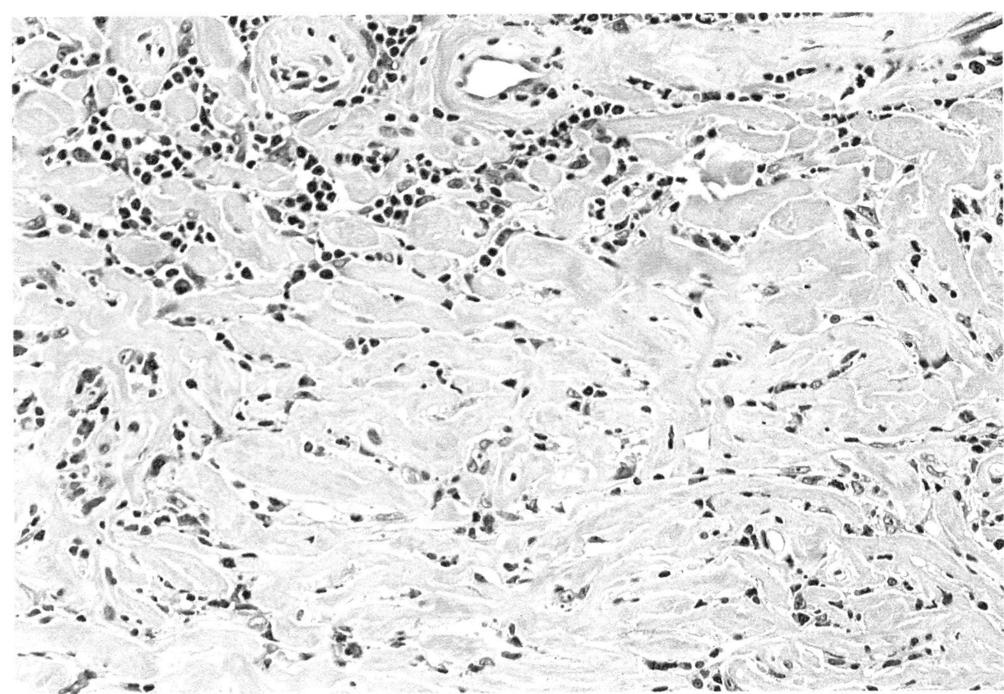

**FIGURE 10–30.** Anastomosing bands of hyalinized collagen admixed with a lymphoplasmacytic infiltrate in idiopathic retroperitoneal fibrosis.

prine,[355,380] cyclophosphamide,[376] tamoxifen,[354,397,400] and methotrexate.[394] The prognosis for patients with malignant retroperitoneal fibrosis is exceedingly poor,[344] but patients with the idiopathic form generally have a good prognosis with only rare reports of death due to the disease.

## Discussion

The exact cause of the idiopathic form of retroperitoneal fibrosis is unclear; some have suggested a central role for chronic fibrosing periaortitis.[376] Early periaortic fibrosis is localized around that portion of the aorta with the most severe atherosclerotic disease.[357] There is often inflammation of the aortic wall, not only in the area of fibrosis but in portions of the aorta where there is no periaortic fibrosis, suggesting that the aortitis precedes the fibrosis.[383] Ceroid, an inflammatory antigen that is an insoluble polymer of oxidized lipoproteins, has been demonstrated in macrophages within atherosclerotic plaques and extracellular periaortic tissues.[384,386] It has been speculated that rupture of an atherosclerotic plaque results in the release of ceroid, stimulating a chronic fibrosing inflammatory process, a hypothesis supported by the finding of antibodies to ceroid in patients with severe chronic periaortitis.[396]

Retroperitoneal fibrosis has been associated with a variety of other immune-mediated connective tissue diseases including systemic lupus erythematosus,[374] polyarteritis nodosa,[366] systemic vasculitis,[375] and the major histocompatibility complex class II antigen HLA-B27.[345,403] In approximately 8–15% of patients a histologically similar fibrosing process occurs outside the retroperitoneum,[350] including fibrosing mediastinitis,[362,393,402] fibrous pseudotumor of the orbit,[373,379,392] primary sclerosing cholangitis,[347] and Reidel's thyroiditis.[356,359,390] Hughes and Buckley found that many of the spindle-shaped cells in this disease express the immunophenotype of a tissue macrophage, with expression of CD13, CD11c, CD68, HAM-56, and MAC 387.[367] Menke et al. found a similar immunophenotype of the cells in inflammatory pseudotumors of lymph nodes and suggested that these processes are related.[381] Ramshaw et al.[389] found increased levels of cytokine gene expression, including interleukins 1, 2, and 4, in aortic adventitial inflammatory cells associated with chronic periaortitis. Given the ability of these cytokines to induce collagen production, their increased gene expression may link chronic periaortitis to idiopathic retroperitoneal fibrosis.

## REFERENCES

### Palmar Fibromatosis

1. Alioto RJ, Rosier RN, Burton RI, et al. Comparative effects of growth factors on fibroblasts of Dupuytren's tissue and normal palmar fascia. J Hand Surg [Am] 19:442, 1994.
2. An HS, Southworth SR, Jackson WT, et al. Cigarette smoking and Dupuytren's contracture of the hand. J Hand Surg [Am] 13:872, 1988.

3. Arafa M, Noble J, Royle SG, et al. Dupuytren's and epilepsy revisited. J Hand Surg [Br] 17:221, 1992.
4. Arieff AJ, Bell J. Epilepsy and Dupuytren's contracture. Neurology 6:115, 1956.
5. Arkkila PET, Kantola IM, Viikari JSA. Dupuytren's disease: association with chronic diabetic complications. J Rheumatol 24:153, 1997.
6. Arkkila PET, Kantola IM, Viikari JSA, et al. Dupuytren's disease in type 1 diabetic patients: a five-year prospective study. Clin Exp Rheumatol 14:59, 1996.
7. Attali P, Ink O, Pelletier G, et al. Dupuytren's contracture, alcohol consumption and chronic liver disease. Arch Intern Med 147:1065, 1987.
8. Badalamente MA, Hurst LC, Sampson SP. Prostaglandins influence myofibroblast contractility in Dupuytren's disease. J Hand Surg [Am] 13:867, 1988.
9. Badalamente MA, Sampson SP, Hurst LC, et al. The role of transforming growth factor beta in Dupuytren's disease. J Hand Surg [Am] 21:210, 1996.
10. Baird KS, Alwan WH, Crossan JF, et al. T-cell-mediated response in Dupuytren's disease. Lancet 341:1622, 1993.
11. Baird KS, Crossan JF, Ralston SH. Abnormal growth factor and cytokine expression in Dupuytren's contracture. J Clin Pathol 46:425, 1993.
12. Berndt A, Kosmehl H, Mandel U, et al. TGF beta and BFGF synthesis and relocalization in Dupuytren's disease (nodular palmar fibromatosis) relative to cellular activity, myofibroblast phenotype and oncofetal variants of fibronectin. Histochem J 27:1014, 1995.
13. Billig R, Baker R, Imergut M, et al. Peyronie's disease. Urology 6:408, 1975.
14. Brotherston TM, Balakrishnan C, Milner RH, et al. Long term follow-up of dermofasciectomy for Dupuytren's contracture. Br J Plast Surg 47:440, 1994.
15. Burge P, Hoy G, Regan P, et al. Smoking, alcohol and the risk of Dupuytren's contracture. J Bone Joint Surg [Br] 79:206, 1997.
16. Casalone R, Mazzola D, Meroni E, et al. Cytogenetic and interphase cytogenetic analyses reveal chromosome instability but no clonal trisomy 8 in Dupuytren contracture. Cancer Genet Cytogenet 99:73, 1997.
17. Couch H. Identical Dupuytren's contracture in identical twins. Can Med Assoc J 39:225, 1948.
18. Critchley EMR, Vakil SD, Hayward HW, et al. Dupuytren's disease in epilepsy: result of prolonged administration of anticonvulsants. J Neurol Neurosurg Psychiatry 39:498, 1976.
19. Dal Cin P, De Smet L, Sciot R, et al. Trisomy 7 and trisomy 8 in dividing and nondividing tumor cells in Dupuytren's disease. Cancer Genet Cytogenet 108:137, 1999.
20. Dupuytren G. De la retraction des doigts par suite d'une affection de l'aponeurose palmaire: description de la maladie, operation chirurgical qui convient dans de cas. J Univ Med Chir Prat Paris 5:348, 1831 (translated in Lancet 2:222, 1834).
21. Early PE. Population studies in Dupuytren's contracture. J Bone Joint Surg Br 44:602, 1962.
22. Gabbiani G, Majno G. Dupuytren's contracture: fibroblast contraction. Am J Pathol 66:131, 1972.
23. Gamstedt A, Holm-Glad J, Ohlson C-G, et al. Hand abnormalities are strongly associated with the duration of diabetes mellitus. J Intern Med 234:189, 1993.
24. Gokel JM, Huebner G, Meister P, et al. Zur formalen pathogenese des morbus Dupuytren. Verh Dtsch Ges Pathol 60:474, 1976.
25. Gonzalez-Martinez R, Marin-Bertolin S, Amorrortu-Velayos J, et al. Association between keloids and Dupuytren's disease: a case report. Br J Plast Surg 48:47, 1995.
26. Gordon S. Dupuytren's contracture: the significance of various factors in its etiology. Ann Surg 140:683, 1954.
27. Gossrau G, Sell W. The coexistence of plastic induration of the penis, Dupuytren's contracture and knuckle pads. Dermatol Wochenschr 151:1039, 1965.
28. Hall PN, Fitzgerald A, Sterne GD, et al. Skin replacement in Dupuytren's disease. J Hand Surg [Br] 22:193, 1997.
29. Halliday NL, Rayan GM, Zardi L, et al. Distribution of ED-A and ED-B containing fibronectin isoforms in Dupuytren's disease. J Hand Surg [Am] 19:428, 1994.
30. Heathcote JG, Cohen H, Noble J. Dupuytren's disease in diabetes mellitus. Lancet 1:1420, 1981.
31. Hill MA. Current concepts review: Dupuytren's contracture. J Bone Joint Surg Am 67:1439, 1985.
32. Houghton S, Holdstock G, Cockerell R, et al. Dupuytren's contracture, chronic liver disease and IgA immune complexes. Liver 3:220, 1983.
33. Howard LD. Dupuytren's contracture: a guide for management. Clin Orthop 15:118, 1959.
34. Hueston JT. The incidence of Dupuytren's contracture. Med J Aust 6:999, 1960.
35. Hueston JT. Some observations on "knuckle pads." J Hand Surg [Br] 9:75, 1984.
36. Hunter JAA, Ogdon C. Dupuytren's contracture. II. Scanning electron microscopic observations. Br J Plast Surg 28:19, 1975.
37. Iwasaki H, Muller H, Stutt HJ, et al. Palmar fibromatosis (Dupuytren's contracture): ultrastructural and enzyme histochemical studies of 43 cases. Virchows Arch Pathol Anat 405:41, 1984.
38. Jennings AM, Milner PC, Ward JD. Hand abnormalities are associated with the complications of diabetes in type 2 diabetes. Diabet Med 6:43, 1989.
39. Jentsch FR. Zur erblichkeit der Dupuytrenschen kontraktur der erbarzt. Zentralbl Chir 4:85, 1937.
40. Keilholz L, Seegenschmiedt MH, Sauer R. Radiotherapy for prevention of disease progression in early-stage Dupuytren's contracture: initial and long-term results. Int J Radiat Oncol Biol Phys 36:891, 1996.
41. Kischer CW, Speer DP. Microvascular changes in Dupuytren's contracture. J Hand Surg [Am] 9:58, 1984.
42. Lanzetta M, Morrison WA. Dupuytren's disease occurring after a surgical injury to the hand. J Hand Surg [Br] 21:481, 1996.
43. Larkin JG, Frier BM. Limited joint mobility in Dupuytren's contracture in diabetic, hypertensive, and normal populations. BMJ 292:1494, 1986.
44. Lee YC, Chan HH, Black MM. Aggressive polyfibromatosis: a ten-year follow-up. Aust J Dermatol 37:305, 1996.
45. Ling RSM. The genetic factor in Dupuytren's disease. J Bone Joint Surg Br 45:709, 1963.
46. Liss GM, Stock SR. Can Dupuytren's contracture be worked-related? Review of the evidence. Am J Ind Med 29:521, 1996.
47. Luck JV. Dupuytren's contracture: a new concept of the pathogenesis correlated with surgical management. J Bone Joint Surg Am 41:635, 1959.
48. Lund M. Dupuytren's contracture and epilepsy: clinical connection between Dupuytren's contracture, fibroma plantae, periarthrosis humeri, helodermia, induratio penis plastica and epilepsy with attempt at pathogenetic evaluation. Acta Psychiatr Neurol 16:465, 1941.
49. Lyall HA. Dupuytren's disease in identical twins. J Hand Surg [Br] 18:368, 1983.
50. Magro G, Colombatti A, Lanzafane S. Immunohistochemical expression of type VI collagen in superficial fibromatoses. Pathol Res Pract 191:1023, 1995.
51. Magro G, Freggetta S, Colombatti A, et al. Myofibroblasts and extracellular matrix glycoproteins in palmar fibromatosis. Gen Diagn Pathol 142:185, 1997.
52. Magro G, Lanzafane S, Micali G. Coordinate expression of

alpha-5 beta 1 integrin and fibronectin in Dupuytren's disease. Acta Histochem 97:229, 1995.
53. McCann BG, Logan A, Belcher H, et al. The presence of myofibroblasts in the dermis of patients with Dupuytren's contracture: a possible source for recurrence. J Hand Surg [Br] 18:656, 1993.
54. Meister P, Gokel JM, Renberger A. Palmar fibromatosis "Dupuytren's contracture": a comparison of light, electron and immunofluorescence microscopic findings. Pathol Res Pract 164:402, 1979.
55. Menzel EJ, Piza H, Zielinsky C, et al. Collagen types and anticollagen-antibodies in Dupuytren's disease. Hand 11:243, 1979.
56. Mikkelsen OA. Dupuytren's disease: initial symptoms, age of onset and spontaneous course. Hand 9:11, 1977.
57. Mikkelsen OA. Knuckle pads in Dupuytren's disease. Hand 9: 301, 1977.
58. Mitra A, Goldstein RY. Dupuytren's contracture in the black population: a review. Ann Plast Surg 32:619, 1994.
59. Moermans JP. Long-term results after segmental aponeurectomy for Dupuytren's disease. J Hand Surg [Br] 21:797, 1996.
60. Moorehead JJ. Trauma and Dupuytren's contracture. Am J Surg 85:352, 1953.
61. Nazari B. Dupuytren's contracture associated with liver disease. J Mt Sinai Hosp 33:69, 1966.
62. Neumuller J, Menzel J, Millesci H. Prevalence of HLA-DR3 and autoantibodies to connective tissue components in Dupuytren's contracture. Clin Immunol Immunopathol 71:142, 1994.
63. Noble J, Arafa M, Royle SG, et al. The association between alcohol, hepatic pathology and Dupuytren's disease. J Hand Surg [Br] 17:71, 1992.
64. Noble J, Heathcote JG, Cohen H. Diabetes mellitus in the aetiology of Dupuytren's disease. J Bone Joint Surg Br 66:322, 1984.
65. Pal B, Griffiths J, Anderson J, et al. Association of limited joint mobility with Dupuytren's contracture in diabetes mellitus. J Rheumatol 14:582, 1987.
66. Pereira RS, Black CM, Turner SM, et al. Antibodies to collagen types I-VI in Dupuytren's contracture. J Hand Surg [Br] 11:58, 1986.
67. Plater F. Observationum Felici Plateri libri tres. Liber I. Johannis Ludovici Koenig and Johannis Brandmylleri, Basel, 1630.
68. Pojer J, Radivojevic M, Williams TF. Dupuytren's disease: its association with abnormal liver function in alcoholism and epilepsy. Arch Intern Med 129:561, 1972.
69. Rayan GM, Parizi M, Tomasek JJ. Pharmacologic regulation of Dupuytren's fibroblast contraction in vitro. J Hand Surg [Br] 21:1065, 1996.
70. Rodrigo JJ, Niebauer JJ, Brown RL, et al. Treatment of Dupuytren's contracture: long-term results after fasciotomy and fascial extension. J Bone Joint Surg Am 58:380, 1976.
71. Sanderson PL, Morris MA, Stanley JK, et al. Lipids and Dupuytren's disease. J Bone Joint Surg Br 74:923, 1992.
72. Shaw DL, Wise DI, Holms W. Dupuytren's disease treated by palmar fasciectomy and an open palm technique. J Hand Surg [Br] 21:484, 1996.
73. Skoog T. Dupuytren's contraction with special reference to aetiology and improved surgical treatment: its occurrence in epileptics: note on knuckle-pads. Acta Chir Scand 96 (Suppl 139):1, 1948.
74. Sladicka MS, Benfanti P, Raab M, et al. Dupuytren's contracture in the black population: a case report and review of the literature. J Hand Surg [Am] 21:898, 1996.
75. Spring M, Fleck H, Cohen BD. Dupuytren's contracture: warning of diabetes? NY State J Med 70:1037, 1970.
76. Starkweather KD, Lattuga S, Hurst LC, et al. Collagenase in the treatment of Dupuytren's disease: an in vitro study. J Hand Surg [Am] 21:490, 1996.
77. Terek IM, Jiranek WA, Goldberg MJ, et al. The expression of platelet-derived growth factor gene in Dupuytren's contracture. J Bone Joint Surg Am 77:1, 1995.
78. Tomasek J, Rayan GM. Correlation of alpha-smooth muscle actin expression and contraction in Dupuytren's disease fibroblasts. J Hand Surg [Am] 20:450, 1995.
79. Tomasek JJ, Schultz RJ, Episalla CW, et al. The cytoskeleton and extracellular matrix of the Dupuytren's disease "myofibroblast": an immunofluorescence study of a non-muscle cell type. J Hand Surg [Am] 11:365, 1986.
80. Urban M, Feldberg L, Janssen A, et al. Dupuytren's disease in children. J Hand Surg [Br] 21:112, 1996.
81. Williams JL, Thomas GG. The natural history of Peyronie's disease. J Urol 103:75, 1970.
82. Wolfe SJ, Summerskill WHJ, Davidson CS. Thickening and contraction of the palmar fascia (Dupuytren's contracture) associated with alcoholism and hepatic cirrhosis. N Engl J Med 255:559, 1956.
83. Yacoe ME, Bergman AG, Ladd AL, et al. Dupuytren's contracture: MR imaging findings and correlation between MR signal intensity and cellularity of lesions. AJR 160:813, 1993.
84. Yost J, Winters T, Fett HC. Dupuytren's contracture: a statistical study. Am J Surg 90:568, 1955.
85. Zachariae L. Dupuytren's contracture: the etiological role of trauma. Scand J Plast Reconstr Surg 5:116, 1971.

### Plantar Fibromatosis

86. Allen RA, Woolner LB, Ghormley RK. Soft tissue tumors of the sole: with special. reference to plantar fibromatosis. J Bone Joint Surg Am 37:14, 1955.
87. Alman BA, Naber SP, Terek RM, et al. Platelet-derived growth factor in fibrous musculoskeletal disorders: a study of pathologic tissue sections and in vitro primary cell cultures. J Orthop Res 13:67, 1995.
88. Aluisio FV, Mair SD, Hall RL. Plantar fibromatosis: treatment of primary and recurrent lesions and factors associated with recurrence. Foot Ankle Int 17:672, 1996.
89. Aviles E, Arlen M, Miller T. Plantar fibromatosis. Surgery 69: 117, 1971.
90. Blume PA, Niemi WJ, Courtright DJ, et al. Fibrosarcoma of the foot: a case presentation and review of the literature. J Foot Ankle Surg 36:51, 1997.
91. Boc SF, Kushner S. Plantar fibromatosis causing entrapment syndrome of the medial plantar nerve. J Am Podiatr Med Assoc 84:420, 1994.
92. Breiner JA, Nelson M, Bredthauer BD, et al. Trisomy 8 and trisomy 14 in plantar fibromatosis. Cancer Genet Cytogenet 108:176, 1999.
93. Classen DA, Hurst LN. Plantar fibromatosis and bilateral flexion contractures: a review of the literature. Ann Plast Surg 28: 475, 1992.
94. Godette GA, O'Sullivan M, Menelaus MB. Plantar fibromatosis of the heel in children: a report of 14 cases. J Pediatr Orthop 17:16, 1997.
95. Landers PA, Yu GV, White JM, et al. Recurrent plantar fibromatosis. J Foot Ankle Surg 32:85, 1993.
96. Ledderhose G. Zur Pathologie der Aponeurose des Fusses und der Hand. Arch Klin Chir 55:694,1897.
97. Madelung OW. Die Aetiologie und die operative Behandlung der Dupuytren'schen Fingerverkrumung. Berl Klin Wochenschr 12:191, 1875.
98. Meyerding HW, Shellito JG. Dupuytren's contracture of the foot. J Int Coll Surg 11:595, 1948.
99. Morrison WB, Schweitzer ME, Wapner KL, et al. Plantar fibro-

matosis: a benign aggressive neoplasm with a characteristic appearance on MR images. Radiology 193:841, 1994.
100. Pasternack WA, Davison GA. Plantar fibromatosis: staging by magnetic resonance imaging. J Foot Ankle Surg 32:390, 1993.
101. Pentland AP, Anderson TF. Plantar fibromatosis response to intralesional steroids. J Am Acad Dermatol 12:212, 1985.
102. Pickren JW, Smith AG, Stevenson TW Jr, et al. Fibromatosis of the plantar fascia. Cancer 4:846, 1951.
103. Snyder M. Dupuytren's contracture and plantar fibromatosis. J Am Podiatr Assoc 70:410, 1980.
104. Wapner KL, Ververeli PA, Moore JH Jr, et al. Plantar fibromatosis: a review of primary and recurrent surgical treatment. Foot Ankle Int 16:548, 1995.
105. Wu KK. Plantar fibromatosis of the foot. J Foot Ankle Surg 33: 99, 1994.
106. Yost J, Winters T, Fett HC. Dupuytren's contracture: a statistical study. Am J Surg 90:568, 1955.
107. Zamora RL, Heights R, Kraemer BA, et al. Presence of growth factors in palmar and plantar fibromatoses. J Hand Surg [Am] 19:435, 1994.

### Penile Fibromatosis (Peyronie's Disease)

108. Akkus E, Carrier S, Baba K, et al. Structural alterations in the tunica albuginea of the penis: impact of Peyronie's disease, aging and impotence. Br J Urol 79:47, 1997.
109. Akkus E, Carrier S, Rehman J, et al. Is colchicine effective in Peyronie's disease? A pilot study. Urology 44;291, 1994.
110. Anafarta K, Beduk Y, Uluoglu O, et al. The significance of histopathological changes of the normal tunica albuginea in Peyronie's disease. Int Urol Nephrol 26:71, 1994.
111. Benson GS. Peyronie's disease [editorial]. J Urol 149:1326, 1993.
112. Bivens CH, Marecek RL, Feldman JM. Peyronie's disease: a presenting complaint of the carcinoid syndrome. N Engl J Med 289:844, 1973.
113. Burford CE, Gleen JE, Burford EH. Fibrous cavernositis. J Urol 56:118, 1946.
114. Bystrom J, Rubio C. Induratio penis plastica (Peyronie's disease): clinical features and etiology. Scand J Urol Nephrol 10: 12, 1976.
115. Chilton CP, Castle WM, Westwood CA, et al. Factors associated in the aetiology of Peyronie's disease. Br J Urol 54:748, 1982.
116. Davis CJ. The microscopic pathology of Peyronie's disease. J Urol 157:282, 1997.
117. Devine CJ. Introduction: international conference on Peyronie's disease. J Urol 157:272, 1997.
118. Devine CJ, Somers KD, Jordan GH, et al. Proposal: trauma as the cause of the Peyronie's lesion. J Urol 157:285, 1997.
119. Dunsmuir WD, Kirby RS. François de la Peyronie (1678–1747): the man and the disease he described. Br J Urol 78:613, 1996.
120. Faerber GJ, Connak JW. Results of combined nesbit penile plication with plaque incision and placement of Dacron patch in patients with severe Peyronie's disease. J Urol 149:1319, 1993.
121. Fournier GR, Lue TF, Tanagho EA. Peyronie's plaque: surgical treatment with the carbon dioxide laser and a deep dorsal vein patch graft. J Urol 149:1321, 1993.
122. Gelbard MK, Dorey F, James K. The natural history of Peyronie's disease. J Urol 144:1376, 1990.
123. Gelbard MK, James K, Riach P, et al. Collagenase versus placebo in the treatment of Peyronie's disease: a double-blind study. J Urol 149:56, 1993.
124. Gossrau G, Sell W. The coexistence of plastic induration of the penis, Dupuytren contracture and knuckle pads. Dermatol Wochenschr 151:1039, 1965.
125. Gueneri S, Stioui S, Mantovani F, et al. Multiple chromosome abnormalities in Peyronie's disease. Cancer Genet Cytogenet 52:181, 1991.
125. Hinman F Jr. Etiologic factors in Peyronie's disease. Urol Int 35:407, 1980.
126. Kim ED, McVary KT. Long-term follow-up of treatment of Peyronie's disease with plaque incision, carbon dioxide laser plaque ablation and placement of a deep dorsal vein patch graft. J Urol 153:1843, 1995.
127. La Peyronie F. Sur quelques obstacles qui s'opposent a l'ejaculation naturelle de la semence. In: Mein de l'Academie Royale de Chir. Paris, 1743, p 425.
128. Leffell MS. Is there an immunogenetic basis for Peyronie's disease? J Urol 157:295, 1997.
129. Levine LA, Merrick PF, Lee RC. Intralesional verapamil injection for the treatment of Peyronie's disease. J Urol 151:1522, 1994.
130. Lopez JA, Jarrow JP. Penile vascular evaluation of men with Peyronie's disease. J Urol 149:53, 1993.
131. Lund M. Dupuytren's contracture and epilepsy: clinical connection between Dupuytren's contracture, fibroma plantae, periarthrosis humeri, helodermia, induratio penis plastica and epilepsy with attempt at pathogenetic evaluation. Acta Psychiatr Neurol 16:465, 1971.
132. Lyles KW, Gold DT, Newton RA, et al. Peyronie's disease is associated with Paget's disease of bone. J Bone Miner Res 12: 929, 1997.
133. Nachtsheim DA, Reardon A. Peyronie's disease is associated with an HLA class II antigen, HLA-DQ5, implying an autoimmune etiology. J Urol 156:1330, 1996.
134. Nyberg LM, Bias WB, Hochberg MC, et al. Identification of an inherited form of Peyronie's disease with autosomal dominant inheritance and association with Dupuytren's contracture and histocompatibility B7 cross-reacting antigens. J Urol 128:48, 1982.
135. Ollivaud L, Godeau B, Lionnet F, et al. Cogan's syndrome and Peyronie's disease: a non-fortuitous association. Br J Rheumatol 32:1111, 1993.
136. Ralph DJ, Mirakian R, Pryor JP, et al. The immunological features of Peyronie's disease. J Urol 155:159, 1996.
137. Ralph DJ, Schwartz G, Moore W, et al. The genetic and bacteriological aspects of Peyronie's disease. J Urol 157:291, 1997.
138. Rompel R, Mueller-Eckhardt G, Schroeder-Printzen I, et al. HLA antigens in Peyronie's disease. Urol Int 52:34, 1994.
139. Scardino PL, Scott WW. The use of tocopherols in the treatment of Peyronie's disease. Ann NY Acad Sci 52:390, 1949.
140. Smith BH. Peyronie's disease. Am J Clin Pathol 45:670, 1966.
141. Smith BH. Subclinical Peyronie's disease. Am J Clin Pathol 52: 385, 1969.
142. Somers KD, Dawson DM. Fibrin deposition in Peyronie's disease plaque. J Urol 157:311, 1997.
143. Somers KD, Winters BA, Dawson DM, et al. Chromosome abnormalities in Peyronie's disease. J Urol 137:672, 1987.
144. Teasley GH. Peyronie's disease: a new approach. J Urol 71:611, 1954.
145. Weidner W, Schroeder-Printzen I, Weiske WH, et al. Sexual dysfunction in Peyronie's disease: an analysis of 222 patients without previous local plaque therapy. J Urol 157:325, 1997.
146. Wesson MB. Peyronie's disease (plastic induration), cause and treatment. J Urol 49:350, 1943.
147. Williams JL, Thomas GG. The natural history of Peyronie's disease. J Urol 103:75, 1970.
148. Willscher MK, Cwazka WF, Novicki DE. The association of histocompatibility antigens of the B7 cross-reacting group with Peyronie's disease. J Urol 122:34, 1979.
149. Wilson SK, Delk JR. A new treatment for Peyronie's disease: modeling the penis over an inflatable penile prosthesis. J Urol 152:1121, 1994.

150. Zarfonetis CJD, Horrax TM. Treatment of Peyronie's disease with potassium p-aminobenzoate (POTABA). J Urol 81:770, 1959.
151. Ziegelbaum M, Thomas A, Zachary AA. The association of Peyronie's disease with HLA B7 cross-reacting antigens: a case report of identical twins. Cleve Clin J Med 54:427, 1987.

### Knuckle Pads

152. Allen PW. The fibromatoses: a clinicopathologic classification based on 140 cases. Part I. Am J Surg Pathol 1:255, 1977.
153. Allison JR Jr, Allison JR Sr. Knuckle pads. Arch Dermatol 93: 311, 1966.
154. Gossrau G, Sell W. The coexistence of plastic induration of the penis, Dupuytren contracture and knuckle pads. Dermatol Wochenschr 151:1039, 1965.
155. Hueston JT. Some observations on "knuckle pads." J Hand Surg [Br] 9b:75, 1984.
156. Jones HW. Two cases of "knuckle pads." BMJ 1:759, 1923.
157. Lagier R, Meinecke R. Pathology of "knuckle pads." Virchows Arch Pathol Anat 365:185, 1975.
158. Mikkelsen OH. Knuckle pads in Dupuytren's disease. Hand 9: 301, 1977.
159. Morginson WJ. Discrete keratodermas over the knuckle and finger articulations. Arch Dermatol 71:349, 1955.
160. Reichert CM, Costa J, Barsky SH, et al. Pachydermodactyly. Clin Orthop 194:252, 1985.
161. Skoog T. Dupuytren's contraction with special reference to aetiology and improved surgical treatment: its occurrence in epileptics: note on knuckle-pads. Acta Chir Scand 96 (Suppl 139):1, 1948.
162. Weckesser EC. Results of wide excision of palmar fascia for Dupuytren's contracture: special reference to factors which adversely affect prognosis. Ann Surg 160:1007, 1964.

### Extraabdominal Fibromatosis (Extraabdominal Desmoid)

163. Aaron AD, O'Mara JW, Legendre KE, et al. Chest wall fibromatosis associated with silicone breast implants. Surg Oncol 5: 93, 1996.
164. Abramowitz D, Zornoza J, Ayala AG, et al. Soft tissue desmoid tumors: radiographic bone changes. Radiology 146:11, 1983.
165. Allen PW. Desmoids with sarcomatous change and metastases. Histopathology 27:199, 1995.
166. Allen PW. The fibromatoses: a clinicopathologic classification based on 140 cases. Part I. Am J Surg Pathol 1:255, 1977.
167. Bauernhofer T, Stöger H, Schmid M, et al. Sequential treatment of recurrent mesenteric desmoid tumor. Cancer 77:1061, 1996.
168. Belliveau P, Graham AM. Mesenteric desmoid tumor and Gardner's syndrome treated by sulindac. Dis Colon Rectum 27:53, 1984.
169. Ben-Izhak O, Kuten A, Pery M, et al. Fibromatosis (desmoid tumor) following radiation therapy for Hodgkin's disease. Arch Pathol Lab Med 118:815, 1994.
170. Bohm P, Krober S, Greschniok A, et al. Desmoplastic fibroma of the bone: a report of two patients, review of the literature and therapeutic implications. Cancer 78:1011, 1996.
171. Brodsky JT, Gordon MS, Hajdu SI, et al. Desmoid tumors of the chest wall: a locally recurrent problem. J Thorac Cardiovasc Surg 104:900, 1992.
172. Conley J, Healey WV, Stout AP. Fibromatosis of the head and neck. Am J Surg 112:609, 1966.
173. Dahn I, Jonsson N, Lundh G. Desmoid tumors: a series of 33 cases. Acta Chir Scand 126:305, 1963.
174. Dale PS, Wardlaw JC, Wooton DG, et al. Desmoid tumor occurring after reconstruction mammoplasty for breast carcinoma. Ann Plast Surg 35:515, 1995.
175. Das Gupta TK, Brasfield RD, O'Hara J. Extraabdominal desmoids: a clinico-pathologic study. Ann Surg 170:109, 1969.
176. Dominguez-Malagon HR, Alfeiran-Ruiz A, Chavarria-Xicotencatl P, et al. Clinical and cellular effects of colchicine in fibromatosis. Cancer 69:2478, 1992.
177. Easter DW, Halasz NA. Recent trends in the management of desmoid tumors: summary of 19 cases and review of the literature. Ann Surg 210:765, 1989.
178. Enzinger FM, Shiraki M. Musculo-aponeurotic fibromatosis of the shoulder girdle (extraabdominal desmoid): analysis of 30 cases followed up for 10 or more years. Cancer 21:1131, 1967.
179. Fasching MC, Saleh J, Woods JE. Desmoid tumors of the head and neck. Am J Surg 156:327, 1988.
180. Faulkner LB, Hajdu SI, Kher U, et al. Pediatric desmoid tumor: Retrospective analysis of 63 cases. J Clin Oncol 13:2813, 1995.
181. Feiner H, Kaye GI. Ultrastructural evidence of myofibroblasts in circumscribed fibromatosis. Arch Pathol 100:265, 1976.
182. Fong Y, Rosen PP, Brennan MF. Multifocal desmoids. Surgery 114:902, 1993.
183. Gaches C, Burke J. Desmoid tumor (fibroma of the abdominal wall) occurring in siblings. Br J Surg 58:495, 1971.
184. Gardner EJ. A genetic and clinical study of intestinal polyposis, a predisposing factor for carcinoma of the colon and rectum. Am J Hum Genet 3:167, 1951.
185. Gnepp DR, Henley J, Weiss SW, et al. Desmoid fibromatosis of the sinonasal tract and nasopharynx: a clinicopathologic study of 25 cases. Cancer 78:2572, 1996.
186. Goellner JR, Soule EH. Desmoid tumors: an ultrastructural study of eight cases. Hum Pathol 11:43, 1980.
187. Gunther T, Buhtz P, Forgbert K, et al. Extraabdominal aggressive fibromatosis after treatment of a Morbus Hodgkin: a case report. Gen Diagn Pathol 141:161, 1995.
188. Gurbuz AK, Giardiello FM, Petersen GM, et al. Desmoid tumors in familial adenomatous polyposis. Gut 35:377, 1994.
189. Hasegawa T, Hirose T, Kudo E, et al. Cytoskeletal characteristics of myofibroblasts in benign neoplastic and reactive fibroblastic lesions. Virchows Arch Pathol Anat 416:375, 1990.
190. Häyry P, Reitamo JJ, Tötterman S, et al. The desmoid tumor. II. Analysis of factors possibly contributing to the etiology and growth behavior. Am J Clin Pathol 77:674, 1982.
191. Häyry P, Reitamo JJ, Vihko R, et al. The desmoid tumor. III. A biochemical and genetic analysis. Am J Clin Pathol 77;681, 1982.
192. Humar A, Chou S, Carpenter B. Fibromatosis in infancy and childhood: the spectrum. J Pediatr Surg 28:1446, 1993.
193. Inwards CY, Unni KK, Beabout JW, et al. Desmoplastic fibroma of bone. Cancer 68:1978, 1991.
194. Kamath SS, Parsons JT, Marcus RB, et al. Radiotherapy for local control of aggressive fibromatosis. Int J Radiat Oncol Biol Phys 36:325, 1996.
195. Karakousis CP, Mayordomo J, Zografos GC, et al. Desmoid tumors of the trunk and extremity. Cancer 72:1637, 1993.
196. Kiel KD, Suit HD. Radiation therapy in the treatment of aggressive fibromatoses (desmoid tumors). Cancer 54:2051, 1984.
197. Kim DH, Goldsmith HS, Quan SH, et al. Intraabdominal desmoid tumor. Cancer 27:1041, 1971.
198. Kinzbrunner B, Ritter S, Domingo J, et al. Remission of rapidly growing desmoid tumors after tamoxifen therapy. Cancer 52: 2201, 1983.
199. Kiryu H, Tsuneyoshi M, Enjoji M. Myofibroblasts in fibromatoses: an electron microscopic study. Acta Pathol Jpn 35:533, 1985.
200. Kitamura A, Kanagawa T, Yamada S, et al. Effective chemotherapy for abdominal desmoid tumor in a patient with Gardner's syndrome: report of a case. Dis Colon Rectum 34:822, 1991.

201. Kobayashi H, Kotoura Y, Hosono M, et al. MRI and scintigraphic features of extraabdominal desmoid tumors. Clin Imaging 21:35, 1997.
202. Lackner H, Urban C, Kerbl R, et al. Noncytotoxic drug therapy in children with unresectable desmoid tumors. Cancer 80: 334, 1997.
203. Lee Y-S, Sen BK. Dystrophic and psammomatous calcifications in a desmoid tumor: a light microscopic and ultrastructural study. Cancer 55:84, 1985.
204. Lopez R, Kemalyan N, Moseley S, et al. Problems in diagnosis and management of desmoid tumors. Am J Surg 159:450, 1990.
205. Lotfi AM, Dozois RR, Gordon H, et al. Mesenteric fibromatosis complicating familial adenomatous polyposis: predisposing factors and results of treatment. Int J Colorectal Dis 4:30, 1989.
206. Lucas DR, Shroyer KR, McCarthy PJ, et al. Desmoid tumor is a clonal cellular proliferation: PCR amplification of HUMARA for analysis of patterns of X-chromosome inactivation. Am J Surg Pathol 21:306, 1997.
207. Masson JK, Soule EH. Desmoid tumors of the head and neck. Am J Surg 112:615, 1966.
208. Maurer F, Horst F, Pfannenberg C, et al. Multifocal extraabdominal desmoid tumor—diagnostic and therapeutic problems. Arch Orthop Trauma Surg 115:359, 1996.
209. McCollough WM, Parsons JT, van der Griend R, et al. Radiation therapy for aggressive fibromatosis: the experience at the University of Florida. J Bone Joint Surg Am 73:717, 1991.
210. McDougall A, McGarrity G. Extraabdominal desmoid tumors. J Bone Joint Surg Br 61:373, 1979.
211. McKinnon JG, Niefield JP, Kay S, et al. Management of desmoid tumors. Surg Gynecol Obstet 169:104, 1989.
212. Miralbell R, Suit HD, Mankin HJ, et al. Fibromatoses: from postsurgical surveillance to combined surgery and radiation therapy. Int J Radiat Oncol Biol Phys 18:535, 1990.
213. Mooney EE, Meagher P, Edwards GE, et al. Fibrosarcoma of the thigh 28 years after excision of fibromatosis. Histopathology 23:498, 1993.
214. Musgrove JE, McDonald JR. Extraabdominal desmoid tumors: their differential diagnosis and treatment. Arch Pathol 45:513, 1948.
215. Navas-Palacios JJ. The fibromatoses: an ultrastructural study of 31 cases. Pathol Res Pract 176:158, 1983.
216. Ng WH, Lee JS, Poh WT, et al. Desmoid tumor (fibromatosis) of the breast: a clinician's dilemma—a case report and review. Arch Surg 132:444, 1997.
217. Patel SR, Evans HL, Benjamin RS. Combination chemotherapy in adult desmoid tumors. Cancer 72:3244, 1993.
218. Penick RM. Desmoid tumors developing in operative scars. Int Surg Dig 23:323, 1937.
219. Posner MC, Shiu MH, Newsome JL, et al. The desmoid tumor: not a benign disease. Arch Surg 124:191, 1989.
220. Pritchard DJ, Nascimento AG, Petersen IA. Local control of extraabdominal desmoid tumors. J Bone Joint Surg Am 78:848, 1996.
221. Reitamo JJ, Häyry P, Nykyri E, et al. The desmoid tumor. I. Incidence, sex, age and anatomical distribution in the Finnish population. Am J Clin Pathol 77:665, 1982.
222. Ritter MA, Marshall JL, Straub LR. Extraabdominal desmoid of the hand: a case report. J Bone Joint Surg Am 51:1641, 1969.
223. Rock MG, Pritchard DJ, Reiman HM, et al. Extraabdominal desmoid tumors. J Bone Joint Surg Am 66:1369, 1984.
224. Rosen PP, Ernsberger D. Mammary fibromatosis: a benign spindle-cell tumor with significant risk for local recurrence. Cancer 63:1363, 1989.
225. Sabate JM, Parellada JA, Franquet T, et al. Metachronous multicentric aggressive fibromatosis with mediastinal involvement. Eur Radiol 6:207, 1996.
226. Schiller VL, Arndt RD, Brenner RJ. Aggressive fibromatosis of the chest associated with a silicone breast implant. Chest 108: 1466, 1995.
227. Seiter K, Kemeny N. Successful treatment of a desmoid tumor with doxorubicin. Cancer 71:2242, 1993.
228. Soule EH, Scanlon PW. Fibrosarcoma arising in an extraabdominal desmoid tumor: report of a case. Mayo Clin Proc 37: 443, 1962.
229. Stout AP. Fibrosarcoma, well-differentiated (aggressive fibromatosis). Cancer 7:953, 1954.
230. Taconis WK, Schutte HE, van der Heul RO. Desmoplastic fibroma of bone: a report of 18 cases. Skeletal Radiol 23:283, 1994.
231. Terui S, Terauchi T, Abe H, et al. Role of technetium-99m pertechnetate scintigraphy in the management of extraabdominal fibromatosis. Skeletal Radiol 24:331, 1995.
232. Tsukada K, Church JM, Jagelman DG, et al. Noncytotoxic drug therapy for intraabdominal desmoid tumor in patients with familial adenomatous polyposis. Dis Colon Rectum 35:29, 1992.
233. Waddell WR, Kirsch WM. Testolactone, sulindac, warfarin, and vitamin $K_1$ for unresectable desmoid tumors. Am J Surg 161:416, 1991.
234. Wargotz ES, Norris HJ, Austin RM, et al. Fibromatosis of the breast: a clinical and pathological study of 28 cases. Am J Surg Pathol 11:38, 1987.
235. Weiss AJ, Lackman RD. Low-dose chemotherapy of desmoid tumors. Cancer 64:1192, 1989.
236. Welsh RA. Intracytoplasmic collagen formation in desmoid fibromatosis. Am J Pathol 49:515, 1966.
237. Wiel Marin A, Romagnoli A, Carlucci I, et al. Thoracic desmoid tumors: a rare evolution of rib fracture; etiopathogenesis and therapeutic considerations. G Chir 16:341, 1995.
238. Wilcken N, Tattersall MHN. Endocrine therapy for desmoid tumors. Cancer 68:1384, 1991.
239. Wilkins SA, Waldron CA, Mathews WH, et al. Aggressive fibromatosis of the head and neck. Am J Surg 130:412, 1975.
240. Zelefsky MJ, Harrison LB, Shui MH, et al. Combined surgical resection and iridium 192 implantation for locally advanced and recurrent desmoid tumors. Cancer 67:380, 1991.


### Abdominal, Intraabdominal, and Mesenteric Fibromatoses


241. Adachi Y, Mori M, Enjoji M, et al. Mesenteric panniculitis of the colon: review of the literature and report of two cases. Dis Colon Rectum 30:962, 1987.
242. Bach C. Desmoid tumors of the abdominal wall in children. Ann Pediatr 11:239, 1964.
243. Bar-Maor JA, Shabshin U. Mesenteric fibromatosis. J Pediatr Surg 28:1618, 1993.
244. Bauernhofer T, Stöger H, Schmid M, et al. Sequential treatment of recurrent mesenteric desmoid tumor. Cancer 77:1061, 1996.
245. Berardi RS, Canlas M. Desmoid tumor and laparotomy scars. Int Surg 58:253, 1973.
246. Brockman DD. Congenital desmoid of the abdominal wall. J Pediatr 31:217, 1947.
247. Burke AP, Sobin LH, Shekitka KM, et al. Intraabdominal fibromatosis: a pathologic analysis of 130 tumors with comparison of clinical subgroups. Am J Surg Pathol 14:335, 1990.
248. Cahn A. Ein Fall von Fibrom der Bauchdecken in einer Appendektomienarbe. Zentralbl Chir 49:110, 1922.
249. Caldwell EH. Desmoid tumor: musculoaponeurotic fibrosis of the abdominal wall. Surgery 79:104, 1976.
250. Cormio G, Cormio L, Marzullo A, et al. Fibromatosis of the female pelvis. Ann Chir Gynaecol 86:84, 1997.
251. Danforth WC. Occurrence of new growths in abdominal wall after laparotomy. Surg Gynecol Obstet 29:175, 1919.
252. DiGiacomo JC, Lazenby AJ, Salloum LJ. Mesenteric fibromato-

sis associated with Crohn's disease. Am J Gastroenterol 89: 1103, 1994.
253. Emory TS, Monihan JM, Carr NJ, et al. Sclerosing mesenteritis, mesenteric panniculitis and mesenteric lipodystrophy: a single entity? Am J Surg Pathol 21:392, 1997.
254. Fishman A, Girtanner RE, Kaplan AL. Aggressive fibromatosis of the female pelvis: a case report and review of the literature. Eur J Gynaecol Oncol 17:208, 1996.
255. Goldstone J, Malone JM, Moore WS. Inflammatory aneurysms of the abdominal aorta. Surgery 83:425, 1978.
256. Graham JR. Methysurgide for the prevention of headaches: experience in 500 patients over three years. N Engl J Med 270: 67, 1964.
257. Gurbuz AK, Giardiello FM, Petersen GM, et al. Desmoid tumors in familial adenomatous polyposis. Gut 35:377, 1994.
258. Häyry P, Reitamo JJ, Tötterman S, et al. The desmoid tumor. II. Analysis of factors possibly contributing to the etiology and growth behavior. Am J Clin Pathol 77:674, 1982.
259. Hutchinson JR, Norris DG, Schnaufer L. Chemotherapy: a successful application in abdominal fibromatosis [letter to the editor]. Pediatrics 63:157, 1979.
260. Izes JK, Zinman LN, Larsen CR. Regression of large pelvic desmoid tumor by tamoxifen and sulindac. Urology 47:756, 1996.
261. Jadrijevic D, Mardones E, Lipschutz A. Antifibromatogenic activity of 19-nor-$\alpha$-ethinyltestosterone in the guinea pig. Proc Soc Exp Biol Med 91:38, 1956.
262. Keely J, DeRosario J, Schairer A. Desmoid tumors of the abdominal and thoracic walls in a child. AMA Arch Surg 80:144, 1960.
263. Kelly JK, Huang W-S. Idiopathic retractile (sclerosing) mesenteritis and its differential diagnosis. Am J Surg Pathol 13:513, 1989.
264. Kim DH, Goldsmith HS, Quan SH, et al. Intraabdominal desmoid tumor. Cancer 27:1041, 1971.
265. Kipfer RE, Moertel CG, Dahlin DC. Mesenteric lipodystrophy. Ann Intern Med 80:582, 1974.
266. Lim CL, Walker MJ, Mehta RR, et al. Estrogen and antiestrogen binding sites in desmoid tumors. Eur J Cancer Clin Oncol 22:583, 1986.
267. Lipschutz A, Grismali J. On the antifibromatogen activity of synthetic progesterone in experiments with the 17-caprylic and dipropionic esters of estradiol. Cancer Res 4:186, 1944.
268. Lynch HT, Fitzgibbons R Jr, Chong S, et al. Use of doxorubicin and dacarbazine for the management of unresectable intraabdominal desmoid tumors in Gardner's syndrome. Dis Colon Rectum 37:260, 1994.
269. McDougall A, McGarrity G. Extraabdominal desmoid tumors. J Bone Joint Surg Br 61:373, 1979.
270. Meis JM, Enzinger FM. Inflammatory fibrosarcoma of the mesentery and retroperitoneum: a tumor closely simulating inflammatory pseudotumor. Am J Surg Pathol 15:1146, 1991.
271. Mukherjee A, Malcolm A, de la Hunt M, et al. Pelvic fibromatosis (desmoid)—treatment with steroids and tamoxifen. Br J Urol 75:559, 1995.
272. Nakada I, Ubukata H, Goto Y, et al. Prednisolone therapy for intraabdominal desmoid tumors in a patient with familial adenomatous polyposis. J Gastroenterol 32:255, 1997.
273. Newmark H III, Ching G, Halls J. An abdominal mass caused by mesenteric fibromatosis. Am J Gastroenterol 77:885, 1982.
274. Pack GT, Ehrlich HE. Neoplasms of the anterior abdominal wall with special consideration of desmoid tumors: experience with 391 cases and collective review of the literature. Surgery 45:77, 1959.
275. Pfeiffer C. Die Desmoide der Bauchdecken und ihre Prognose. Beitr Klin Chir 44:334, 1904.
276. Plukker JT, van Oort I, Vermey A, et al. Aggressive fibromatosis (non-familial desmoid tumor): therapeutic problems and the role of adjuvant radiotherapy. Br J Surg 82:510, 1995.
277. Reitamo JJ, Häyry P, Nykyri E, et al. The desmoid tumor. I. Incidence, sex, age and anatomical distribution in the Finnish population. Am J Clin Pathol 77:665, 1982.
278. Richard HM III, Thall EH, Mitty H, et al. Desmoid tumor—ureteral fistula in Gardner's syndrome. Urology 49:135, 1997.
279. Rodriguez-Bigas MA, Mahoney MC, Karakousis CP, et al. Desmoid tumors in patients with familial adenomatous polyposis. Cancer 74:1270, 1994.
280. Salmon M. Desmoid tumor of the abdominal wall in a young boy. Ann Chir Infant 5:107, 1964.
281. Schnitzler M, Cohen Z, Blackstein M, et al. Chemotherapy for desmoid tumors in association with familial adenomatous polyposis. Dis Colon Rectum 40:798, 1997.
282. Schweitzer RJ, Robbins GF. A desmoid tumor of multicentric origin. AMA Arch Surg 80:488, 1960.
283. Slater G, Greenstein AJ. Mesenteric fibromatosis in Crohn's disease. J Clin Gastroenterol 22:147, 1996.
284. Stout AP, Hendry J, Purdie FJ. Primary solid tumors of the omentum. Cancer 16:231, 1963.
285. Tedeschi CG, Botta GC. Retractile mesenteritis. N Engl J Med 266:1035, 1962.
286. Wegner HE, Fleige B, Dieckmann KP. Mesenteric desmoid tumor 19 years after radiation therapy for testicular seminoma. Urol Int 53:48, 1994.
287. Yannopoulos K, Stout AP. Primary solid tumors of the mesentery. Cancer 16:914, 1963.

### Gardner Syndrome

288. Alman BA, Li C, Pajerski ME, et al. Increased $\beta$-catenin protein and somatic APC mutations in sporadic aggressive fibromatoses (desmoid tumors). Am J Pathol 151:329, 1997.
289. Bell B, Mazzaferri EL. Familial adenomatous polyposis (Gardner's syndrome) and thyroid carcinoma: a case report and review of the literature. Dig Dis Sci 38:185, 1993.
290. Bochetto JF, Raycroft JF, DeInnocentes LW. Multiple polyposis, exostosis and soft tissue tumors. Surg Gynecol Obstet 117:489, 1963.
291. Bridge JA, Sreekantaiah C, Mouron B, et al. Clonal chromosomal abnormalities in desmoid tumors: implications for histopathogenesis. Cancer 69:430, 1992.
292. Bruce JM, Bradley EL, Satchidanand SK. A desmoid tumor of the pancreas: sporadic intraabdominal desmoids revisited. Int J Pancreatol 19:197, 1996.
293. Burke AP, Sobin LH, Shekitka KM, et al. Intraabdominal fibromatosis: a pathologic analysis of 130 tumors with comparison of clinical subgroups. Am J Surg Pathol 14:335, 1990.
294. Chang CH, Platt ED, Thomas KE, et al. Bone abnormalities in Gardner's syndrome. AJR 103:645, 1968.
295. Coli RD, Moore JP, Lamarche PH, et al. Gardner's syndrome: a revisit to a previously described family. Am J Dig Dis 15: 551, 1970.
296. Dal Cin P, Sciot R, Aly MS, et al. Some desmoid tumors are characterized by trisomy 8. Genes Chromosomes Cancer 10: 131, 1994.
297. Dal Cin P, Sciot R, Van Damme B, et al. Trisomy 20 characterizes a second group of desmoid tumors. Cancer Genet Cytogenet 79:189, 1995.
298. Dangel A, Meloni AM, Lynch HT, et al. Deletion (5q) in a desmoid tumor of a patient with Gardner's syndrome. Cancer Genet Cytogenet 78:94, 1994.
299. Fletcher JA, Naeem R, Xiao S, et al. Chromosome aberrations in desmoid tumors: trisomy 8 may be a predictor of recurrence. Cancer Genet Cytogenet 79:139, 1995.
300. Fraumeni JF Jr, Vogel CL, Easton JM. Sarcomas and multiple

polyposis in a kindred: a genetic variety of hereditary polyposis? Arch Intern Med 121:57, 1968.
301. Gardner EJ. A genetic and clinical study of intestinal polyposis, a predisposing factor for carcinoma of the colon and rectum. Am J Hum Genet 3:167, 1951.
302. Gardner EJ. Follow-up study of a family group exhibiting dominant inheritance for a syndrome including intestinal polyps, osteomas, fibromas and epidermal cysts. Am J Hum Genet 14:376, 1962.
303. Gold RS, Mucha SJ. Unique case of mesenteric fibrosis in multiple polyposis. Am J Surg 130:366, 1975.
304. Gorlin RJ, Chaudhry AP. Multiple osteomatosis, fibromas, lipomas and fibrosarcomas of the skin and mesentery, epidermoid inclusion cysts of the skin, leiomyomas and multiple intestinal polyposis: a heritable disorder of connective tissue. N Engl J Med 263:1151, 1960
305. Greer JA Jr, Devine KD, Dahlin DC. Gardner's syndrome and chondrosarcoma of the hyoid bone. Arch Otolaryngol 103:425, 1977.
306. Gurbuz AK, Giardiello FM, Petersen GM, et al. Desmoid tumors in familial adenomatous polyposis. Gut 35:377, 1994.
307. Haggitt RC, Reid BJ. Hereditary gastrointestinal polyposis syndromes. Am J Surg Pathol 10:871, 1986.
308. Halata MS, Miller J, Stone RK. Gardner syndrome: early presentation with a desmoid tumor; discovery of multiple colonic polyps. Clin Pediatr 28:538, 1989.
309. Heiskanen I, Jarvinen HJ. Occurrence of desmoid tumors in familial adenomatous polyposis and results of treatment. Int J Colorectal Dis 11:157, 1996.
310. Hizawa K, Iida M, Aoyagi K, et al. Thyroid neoplasia and familial adenomatous polyposis/Gardner's syndrome. J Gastroenterol 32:196, 1997.
311. Jarvinen HJ. Desmoid disease as a part of familial adenomatous polyposis coli. Acta Chir Scand 153:379, 1987.
312. Jones IT, Jagelman DG, Fazio VW, et al. Desmoid tumors in familial polyposis. Ann Surg 204:94, 1986.
313. Kawashima A, Goldman SM, Fishman EK, et al. CT of intraabdominal desmoid tumors: is the tumor different in patients with Gardner's disease? AJR 162:339, 1994.
314. Kelly MD, Hugh TB, Field AS, et al. Carcinoma of the thyroid gland and Gardner's syndrome. Aust N Z J Surg 63:505, 1993.
315. Kinzler KW, Nilbert MC, Su LK, et al. Identification of FAP locus genes on chromosome 5q21. Science 253:661, 1991.
316. Kitamura A, Kanagawa T, Yamada S, et al. Effective chemotherapy for abdominal desmoid tumor in a patient with Gardner's syndrome: report of a case. Dis Colon Rectum 34:822, 1991.
317. Klein WA, Miller HH, Anderson M, et al. The use of indomethacin, sulindac and tamoxifen for the treatment of desmoid tumors associated with familial polyposis. Cancer 60: 2863, 1987.
318. Lambroza A, Tighe MK, DeCosse JJ, et al. Disorders of the rectus abdominis muscle and sheath: a 22-year experience. Am J Gastroenterol 90:1313, 1995.
319. Lewis JH, Ginsberg AL, Toomey KE. Turcot's syndrome: evidence of autosomal dominant inheritance. Cancer 51:524, 1983.
320. Li C, Bapat B, Alman BA. Adenomatous polyposis coli gene mutation alters proliferation through its β-catenin-regulatory function in aggressive fibromatosis (desmoid tumor). Am J Pathol 153:709, 1998.
321. Lotfi AM, Dozois RR, Gordon H, et al. Mesenteric fibromatosis complicating familial adenomatous polyposis: predisposing factors and results of treatment. Int J Colorectal Dis 4:30, 1989.
322. Mao C, Huang Y, Howard JM. Carcinoma of the ampulla of Vater and mesenteric fibromatosis (desmoid tumor) associated with Gardner's syndrome: problems in management. Pancreas 10:239, 1995.
323. McAdam WA, Goligher JC. The occurrence of desmoids in patients with familial polyposis coli. Br J Surg 57:618, 1970.
324. Miyaki M, Konishi M, Kikuchi-Yanoshita R, et al. Coexistence of somatic and germ-line mutations of APC gene in desmoid tumors from patients with familial adenomatous polyposis. Cancer Res 53:5079, 1993.
325. Neal CJ Jr. Multiple osteomas of the mandible associated with polyposis of the colon (Gardner's syndrome). Oral Surg Oral Med Oral Pathol 28:628, 1969.
326. Neale HW, Pickrell KL, Quinn GW. Extraabdominal manifestations of Gardner's syndrome. Plast Reconstr Surg 56:92, 1975.
327. Nichols RW. Desmoid tumors: a report of 31 cases. Arch Surg 7:227, 1923.
328. Okamoto M, Sato C, Kohno Y, et al. Molecular nature of chromosome 5q loss in colorectal tumors and desmoids from patients with familial adenomatous polyposis. Hum Genet 85: 595, 1990.
329. Richards RC, Rogers SW, Gardner EJ. Spontaneous mesenteric fibromatosis in Gardner's syndrome. Cancer 47:597, 1981.
330. Rodriguez-Bigas MA, Mahoney MC, Karakousis CP, et al. Desmoid tumors in patients with familial adenomatous polyposis. Cancer 74:1270, 1994.
331. Rubinfeld B, Albert I, Porfiri E, et al. Loss of β-catenin regulation by the APC tumor suppressor protein correlates with loss of structure due to common somatic mutations of the gene. Cancer Res 15:4624, 1997.
332. Smith WG. Multiple polyposis, Gardner's syndrome and desmoid tumors. Dis Colon Rectum 1:323, 1958.
333. Traill Z, Tuson J, Woodham C. Adrenal carcinoma in a patient with Gardner's syndrome: imaging findings. AJR 165:1460, 1995.
334. Tsukada K, Church JM, Jagelman DG, et al. Systemic cytotoxic chemotherapy and radiation therapy for desmoid and familial adenomatous polyposis. Dis Colon Rectum 34:1090, 1991.
335. Tsukada K, Church JM, Jagelman DG, et al. Noncytotoxic drug therapy for intraabdominal desmoid tumor in patients with familial adenomatous polyposis. Dis Colon Rectum 35:29, 1992.
336. Umemoto S, Makuuchi H, Amemiya T, et al. Intraabdominal desmoid tumors in familial polyposis coli: a case report of tumor regression by prednisolone therapy. Dis Colon Rectum 34:89, 1991.
337. Wakatsuki S, Sasano H, Matsui T, et al. Adrenocortical tumor in a patient with familial adenomatous polyposis: a case associated with a complete inactivating mutation of the APC gene and unusual histological features. Hum Pathol 29:302, 1998.
338. Weary PE, Linthicum A, Cawley EP, et al. Gardner's syndrome: a family group study and review. Arch Dermatol 90: 20, 1964.
339. Witkop CJ Jr. Gardner's syndrome and other osteognathodermal disorders with defects in parathyroid functions. J Oral Surg 26:639, 1968.
340. Yoshida MA, Ikeuchi T, Iwama T, et al. Chromosome changes in desmoid tumors developed in patients with familial adenomatous polyposis. Jpn J Cancer Res 82:16, 1991.

### Idiopathic Retroperitoneal Fibrosis (Ormond's Disease)

341. Albarran J. Retention renale par peri-ureterite: liberation externe de l'uretere. Assoc Fr Urol 9:511, 1905.
342. Alexopoulos E, Memmos D, Bakatselos S. Idiopathic retroperitoneal fibrosis: a long-term follow-up study. Eur Urol 13:313, 1987.
343. Amis ES Jr. Retroperitoneal fibrosis. Urol Radiol 12;135, 1990.
344. Arrivé L, Hricak H, Tavares NJ, et al. Malignant versus nonmalignant retroperitoneal fibrosis: differentiation with MR imaging. Radiology 172:139, 1989.

345. Aylward GW, Sullivan TJ, Garner A, et al. Orbital involvement in multifocal sclerosis. Br J Ophthalmol 79:246, 1995.
346. Baker LR, Mallinson WJ, Gregory MC, et al. Idiopathic retroperitoneal fibrosis: a retrospective analysis of 60 cases. Br J Urol 60:497, 1987.
347. Bartholomew LG, Cain JC, Woolner LB, et al. Sclerosing cholangitis: its possible association with Reidel's struma and fibrous retroperitonitis: a report of two cases. N Engl J Med 269:8, 1963.
348. Birnberg FA, Vinstein AL, Gorlick G, et al. Retroperitoneal fibrosis in children. Radiology 145:59, 1982.
349. Boeckmann W, Wolff JM, Adam G, et al. Laparoscopic bilateral ureterolysis in Ormond's disease. Urol Int 56:133, 1996.
350. Buff DD. The etiology of retroperitoneal fibrosis. NY State J Med 91:336, 1991.
351. Buff DD, Bogin MB, Faltz LL. Retroperitoneal fibrosis: a report of selected cases and review of the literature. NY State J Med 89:511, 1989.
352. Calder HL, McArthur JE, Allan DG, et al. Retroperitoneal fibrosis in childhood: case report and review. NZ Med J 94:213, 1981.
353. Chordia ML, Ockuly EA, Ockuly JJ, et al. Ureteral and vesical metastases from parenchymal renal cell carcinoma: case report and review of the literature. J Urol 102:298, 1969.
354. Clark CP, Vanderpool D, Preskitt JT. The response of retroperitoneal fibrosis to tamoxifen. Surgery 109:502, 1991.
355. Cogan E, Fastrez R. Azothiaprine: an alternative treatment for recurrent idiopathic retroperitoneal fibrosis. Arch Intern Med 145:753, 1985.
356. De Boer WA, van Coevorden F, Wiersinga WM. A rare case of Reidel's thyroiditis, six years after retroperitoneal fibrosis: two diseases with one pathogenesis? Neth J Med 40:190, 1992.
357. Debrand-Passard A, Wilhelm H. Ormond's disease or aortic aneurysm? Case reports. Int Urol Nephrol 28:295, 1996.
358. Dehner LP, Coffin CM. Idiopathic fibrosclerotic disorders and other inflammatory pseudotumors. Semin Diagn Pathol 15:161, 1998.
359. Elewaut D, Rubens R, Elewaut A, et al. Lusoria dysphagia in a patient with retroperitoneal fibrosis and Reidel's thyroiditis. J Intern Med 239:75, 1996.
360. Feldberg MAM, Hene RJ. Perianeurysmal fibrosis and its response to corticosteroid treatment: a computerized tomography follow-up in one case. J Urol 130:1163, 1983.
361. Gelford GJ, Wilets AJ, Nelson D, et al. Retroperitoneal fibrosis and methysergide: report of three cases. Radiology 88:976, 1967.
362. Graal MB, Lustermans FA. A patient with combined mediastinal, mesenteric and retroperitoneal fibrosis. Neth J Med 44:214, 1994.
363. Graham JR. Methysergide for the prevention of headaches: experience in 500 patients over three years. N Engl J Med 270: 67, 1964.
364. Hache L, Utz DC, Woolner LB. Idiopathic fibrous retroperitonitis. Surg Gynecol Obstet 115:737, 1962.
365. Hawk WA, Hazard JB. Sclerosing retroperitonitis and sclerosing mediastinitis. Am J Clin Pathol 32:321, 1959.
366. Hollingworth P, Denman AN, Gumpel JM. Retroperitoneal fibrosis and polyarteritis nodosa successfully treated by intensive immunosuppression. J R Soc Med 73:61, 1980.
367. Hughes D, Buckley PJ. Idiopathic retroperitoneal fibrosis is a macrophage-rich process: implications for its pathogenesis and treatment. Am J Surg Pathol 17:482, 1993.
368. Kavoussi LR, Clayman RV, Brunt LM, et al. Laparoscopic ureterolysis. J Urol 147:426, 1992.
369. Koep L, Zuidema GD. The clinical significance of retroperitoneal fibrosis. Surgery 81:250, 1977.
370. Kottra JJ, Dunnick NR. Retroperitoneal fibrosis. Radiol Clin North Am 34:1259, 1996.
371. Leone JP, Nguyen-Minh NC, Lee DA, et al. Retroperitoneal fibrosis: a report of complete colonic obstruction. Am Surg 63: 475, 1997.
372. Lepor H, Walsh PC. Idiopathic retroperitoneal fibrosis. J Urol 122:1, 1979.
373. Levine MR, Kaye L, Mair S, et al. Multifocal fibrosclerosis: report of a case of bilateral idiopathic sclerosing pseudotumor and retroperitoneal fibrosis. Arch Ophthalmol 111:841, 1993.
374. Lichon FS, Sequeira W, Pilloff A, et al. Retroperitoneal fibrosis associated with systemic lupus erythematosis: a case report and brief review. J Rheumatol 11:373, 1984.
375. Littlejohn GO, Keystone EC. The association of retroperitoneal fibrosis with systemic vasculitis and HLA-B27: a case report and review of the literature. J Rheumatol 8:665, 1981.
376. Martina FB, Nuesch R, Gasser TC. Retroperitoneal fibrosis and chronic periaortitis: a new hypothesis. Eur Urol 23:371, 1993.
377. Matsuda T, Arai Y, Muguruma K, et al. Laparoscopic ureterolysis for idiopathic retroperitoneal fibrosis. Eur Urol 26:286, 1994.
378. Mattelaer P, Boeckmann W, Brauers A, et al. Laparoscopic ureterolysis in retroperitoneal fibrosis. Acta Urol Belg 64:15, 1996.
379. McCarthy JM, White VA, Harris G, et al. Idiopathic sclerosing inflammation of the orbit: immunohistologic analysis and comparison with retroperitoneal fibrosis. Mod Pathol 6:581, 1993.
380. McDougal WS, MacDonell RC Jr. Treatment of idiopathic retroperitoneal fibrosis by immunosuppression. J Urol 145:112, 1991.
381. Menke DM, Griesser H, Araujo I, et al. Inflammatory pseudotumors of lymph node origin show macrophage-derived spindle cells and lymphocyte-derived cytokine transcripts without evidence of T-cell receptor gene rearrangements. Am J Clin Pathol 105:430, 1996.
382. Mikkelsen D, Lepor H. Innovative surgical management of idiopathic retroperitoneal fibrosis. J Urol 141:1192, 1989.
383. Mitchinson MJ. The pathology of idiopathic retroperitoneal fibrosis. J Clin Pathol 23:681, 1970.
384. Mitchinson MJ. Retroperitoneal fibrosis revisited. Arch Pathol Lab Med 110:784, 1986.
385. Ormond JK. Bilateral ureteral obstruction due to envelopment and compression by an inflammatory retroperitoneal process. J Urol 59:1072, 1948.
386. Parums DV, Brown DL, Mitchinson MJ. Serum antibodies to oxidized low-density lipoprotein and ceroid in chronic periaortitis. Arch Pathol Lab Med 114:383, 1990.
387. Parums DV, Choudhoury RP, Shields SA, et al. Characterisation of inflammatory cells associated with "idiopathic retroperitoneal fibrosis." Br J Urol 67:564, 1991.
388. Parums DV. The spectrum of chronic periaortitis. Histopathology 16:423, 1990.
389. Ramshaw AL, Roskell DE, Parums DV. Cytokine gene expression in aortic adventitial inflammation associated with advanced atherosclerosis (chronic periaortitis). J Clin Pathol 47: 721, 1994.
390. Rao CR, Ferguson GC, Kyle VN. Retroperitoneal fibrosis associated with Reidel's struma. Can Med Assoc J 108:1019, 1973.
391. Reiner I, Yachia D, Nissim F, et al. Retroperitoneal fibrosis in association with urothelial tumor. J Urol 132:115, 1984.
392. Richards AB, Shalka HW, Roberts FJ, et al. Pseudotumor of the orbit and retroperitoneal fibrosis: a form of multifocal fibrosclerosis. Arch Ophthalmol 98:1617, 1980.
393. Salmon HW. Combined mediastinal and retroperitoneal fibrosis. Thorax 23:158, 1968.
394. Scavalli AS, Spadaro A, Riccieri V, et al. Long-term follow-up

of low-dose methotrexate therapy in one case of idiopathic retroperitoneal fibrosis. Clin Rhematol 14:481, 1995.
395. Sherman C, Winchester P, Brill PW, et al. Childhood retroperitoneal fibrosis. Pediatr Radiol 18:245, 1988.
396. Smith SJ, Bosniak MA, Megibow AJ, et al. CT demonstration of rapid improvement of retroperitoneal fibrosis in response to steroid therapy. Urol Radiol 8:104, 1986.
397. Spillane RM, Whitman GJ. Treatment of retroperitoneal fibrosis with tamoxifen. AJR 164:515, 1995.
398. Thomas MH, Chisholm GD. Retroperitoneal fibrosis associated with malignant disease. Br J Cancer 28:453, 1973.
399. Tiptaft RC, Costello AJ, Paris AMI, et al. The long-term follow-up of idiopathic retroperitoneal fibrosis. Br J Urol 54:620, 1982.
400. Tonietto G, Agresta F, Della Libera D, et al. Treatment of idiopathic retroperitoneal fibrosis by tamoxifen. Eur J Surg 163:231, 1997.
401. Utz DC, Rooke ED, Spittel JA Jr, et al. Retroperitoneal fibrosis in patients taking methysergide. JAMA 194:983, 1965.
402. Van Bommel EF, Bouvy ND, Liem E, et al. Coexistent idiopathic retroperitoneal and mediasinal fibrosis presenting with portal hypertension. Neth J Med 44:174, 1994.
403. Vital-Durand D, Pouthier D, Brette R. Could the HLA-B27 antigen be a predisposing factor in the development of fibrotic changes? J Urol 124:162, 1980.
404. Wagenknecht LV, Hardy JC. Value of various treatments for retroperitoneal fibrosis. Eur Urol 7:193, 1981.
405. Webb AJ, Dawson-Edwards P. Non-malignant retroperitoneal fibrosis. Br J Surg 54:508, 1967.
406. Wicks IP, Robertson MR, Murnaghan GF, et al. Idiopathic retroperitoneal fibrosis presenting with back pain. J Rheumatol 15:1572, 1988.
407. Young IS. Ureteral implant from renal adenocarcinoma: report of a case and review of the literature. J Urol 98:661, 1967.

# CHAPTER 11

# FIBROUS TUMORS OF INFANCY AND CHILDHOOD

Fibrous tumors of infancy and childhood can be divided into two large groups. The first group consists of lesions that correspond to similar lesions in adults in terms of clinical setting, microscopic picture, and behavior. Typical examples of such lesions are nodular fasciitis, palmar or plantar fibromatosis, and abdominal or extraabdominal fibromatosis. The second group consists of fibrous lesions that are peculiar to infancy and childhood and generally have no clinical or morphologic counterpart in adult life. The latter are less common; because of their unusual microscopic features, they pose a special problem in diagnosis. In fact, in this group of tumors the microscopic picture often fails to reflect the biologic behavior accurately, and features such as cellularity and rapid growth may be mistaken for evidence of malignancy, sometimes leading to unnecessary and excessive therapy. Accurate interpretation and diagnosis of these lesions are therefore of utmost importance for predicting clinical behavior and for selecting the proper forms of therapy (Table 11–1).

## FIBROUS HAMARTOMA OF INFANCY

Fibrous hamartoma of infancy is a distinctive, benign, fibrous growth that most frequently occurs during the first 2 years of life. This lesion was first reported by Reye in 1956 as *subdermal fibromatous tumor of infancy*.[15] In 1965 Ensinger reviewed a series of 30 cases from the files of the Armed Forces Institute of Pathology (AFIP) and suggested the term *fibrous hamartoma of infancy* to emphasize its organoid microscopic appearance and its frequent occurrence at birth and during the immediate postnatal period.[3]

### Clinical Findings

As a rule, the lesion develops during the first 2 years of life (median age 10 months) as a small, rapidly growing, soft to firm mass in the subcutis or reticular dermis. Rare lesions have been reported in older infants and children. About 15–25% of cases are present at birth.[1,3,13] Like other fibrous tumors in children, it is more common in boys than in girls, with boys affected two to three times more often.[13] Usually the mass is freely movable; occasionally it is fixed to the underlying fascia but only rarely involves the superficial portion of the musculature. These lesions grow rapidly from the outset up to the age of about 5 years. The growth of the lesion then slows but does not cease or regress spontaneously.[2]

Most occur above the waist, with the most common location being the anterior or posterior axillary fold, followed in frequency by the upper arm, thigh, inguinal and pubic region, shoulder, back, and forearm. This lesion has also been described in unusual locations, including the scrotum,[9,11,14,16,17,19] labium majus,[14,18] scalp,[4,12] and gluteal region.[13] Few cases have been described in the feet or hands,[6,7] a feature that helps distinguish this lesion from digital fibromatosis and calcifying aponeurotic fibroma. Virtually all cases are solitary, with only rare reports of multiple lesions in the same patient.[3] There is no evidence of increased familial incidence or of associated malformations or other neoplasms. Antecedent trauma is occasionally reported at the time of presentation.[7,13]

### Gross Findings

The excised lesion tends to be poorly circumscribed and consists of an intimate mixture of firm gray-white tissue and fat (Fig. 11–1). In some cases the fatty component is inconspicuous, whereas in others it occupies a large portion of the tumor, thereby resembling a fibrolipoma. Most measure 3–5 cm in greatest diameter, but tumors as large as 15 cm have been reported.

**TABLE 11–1 CLINICOPATHOLOGIC CHARACTERISTICS OF FIBROUS TUMORS OF INFANCY AND CHILDHOOD**

| Histologic Diagnosis | Age (Years) | Location | Solitary | Multiple | Regression |
|---|---|---|---|---|---|
| Fibrous hamartoma | B–2 | Axilla, inguinal area | + | – | – |
| Digital fibromatosis | B–2 | Fingers, toes | + | + | + |
| Myofibromatosis | B–A | Soft tissue, bone, viscera | + | + | + |
| Hyalin fibromatosis | 2–A | Dermis, subcutis | – | + | – |
| Gingival fibromatosis | B–A | Gingiva, hard palate | + | + | + |
| Fibromatosis colli | B–2 | Sternocleidomastoid muscle | + | Bilateral | + |
| Infantile fibromatosis | B–4 | Musculature | + | – | – |
| Infantile fibrosarcoma | B–2 | Musculature | + | – | – |
| Calcifying aponeurotic fibroma | 2–A | Hands, feet | + | – | + |

A, adult life; B, birth.

## Microscopic Findings

Fibrous hamartoma of infancy is characterized by three distinct components forming a vague, irregular, "organoid" pattern (Figs. 11–2, 11–3): (1) well defined intersecting trabeculae of fibrous tissue of varying size and shape and composed of well oriented spindle-shaped cells (predominantly myofibroblasts) separated by varying amounts of collagen (Figs. 11–4, 11–5); (2) loosely textured areas consisting chiefly of immature small, round or stellate cells in a mucoid matrix that stains well with the alcian blue preparation and is removed by prior treatment with hyaluronidase (Figs. 11–6, 11–7, 11–8); and (3) varying amounts of interspersed mature fat, which may be present only at the periphery of the lesion or may be the major component. Despite the lack of clear boundaries between the fat in the tumor and that in the surrounding subcutis, there is little doubt that the fat is an integral part of the lesion. In fact, in many cases its total amount exceeds many times the amount of fat normally present in the surrounding panniculus.[3] In some cases the immature small round cells in the myxoid foci are oriented around small veins.[5,8]

Some tumors show an additional tissue component, a peculiar fibrosing process that has a superficial resemblance to a neurofibroma.[3] It consists of thick collagen fibers and scattered fibroblasts and chiefly replaces the fat in the loosely textured mesenchymal areas; sometimes it is the principal component of the tumor.

## Immunohistochemical and Electron Microscopic Findings

Immunohistochemically, staining for vimentin is positive in both the trabecular and loosely cellular areas.

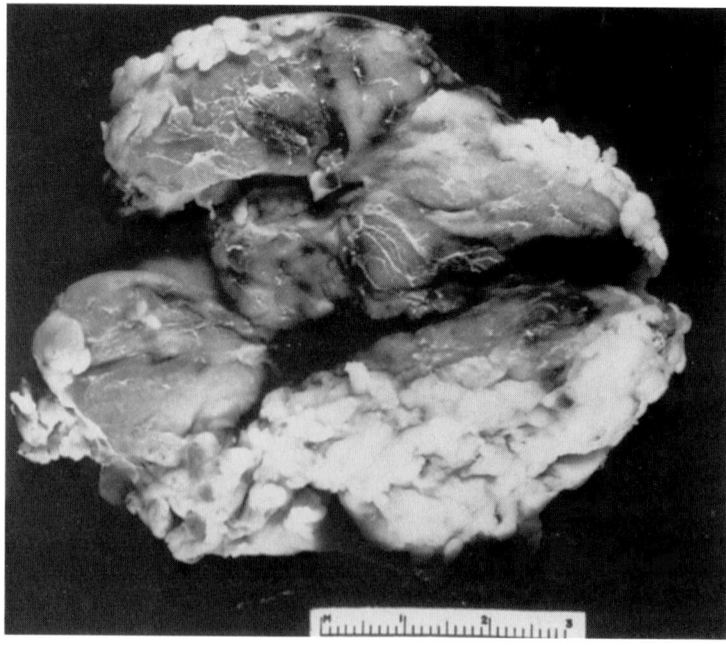

**FIGURE 11–1.** Fibrous hamartoma of infancy of the right axilla in a 9-month-old girl. The lesion, which had been present for 4 months, is for the most part poorly circumscribed and blends with the surrounding subcutaneous fat.

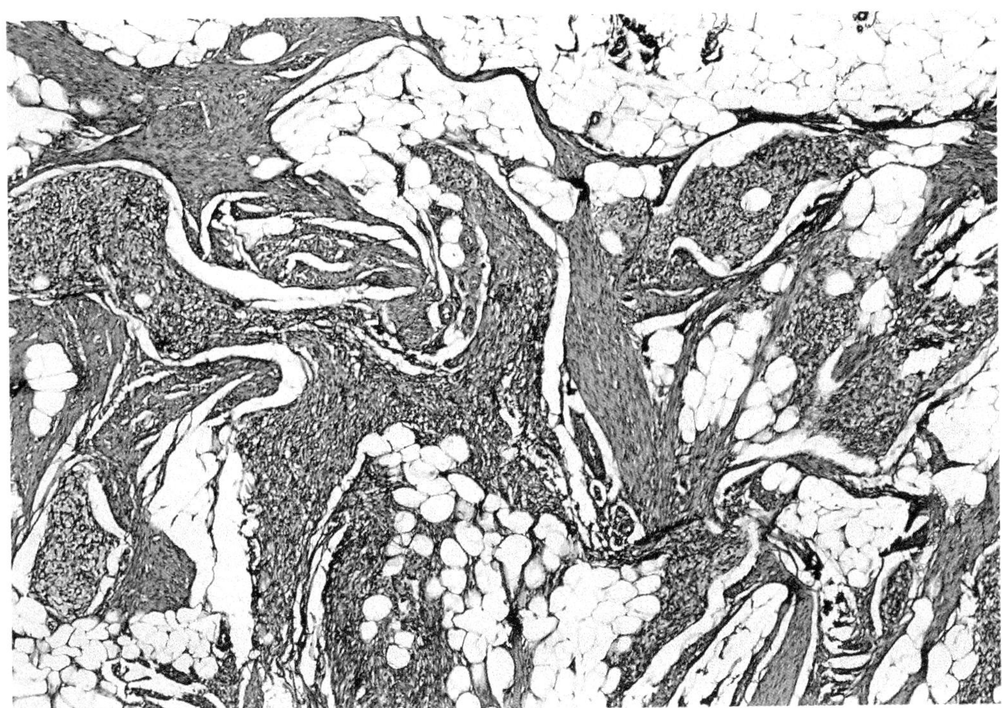

**FIGURE 11–2.** Fibrous hamartoma of infancy showing a characteristic organoid pattern composed of interlacing fibrous trabeculae, islands of loosely arranged spindle-shaped cells, and mature adipose tissue.

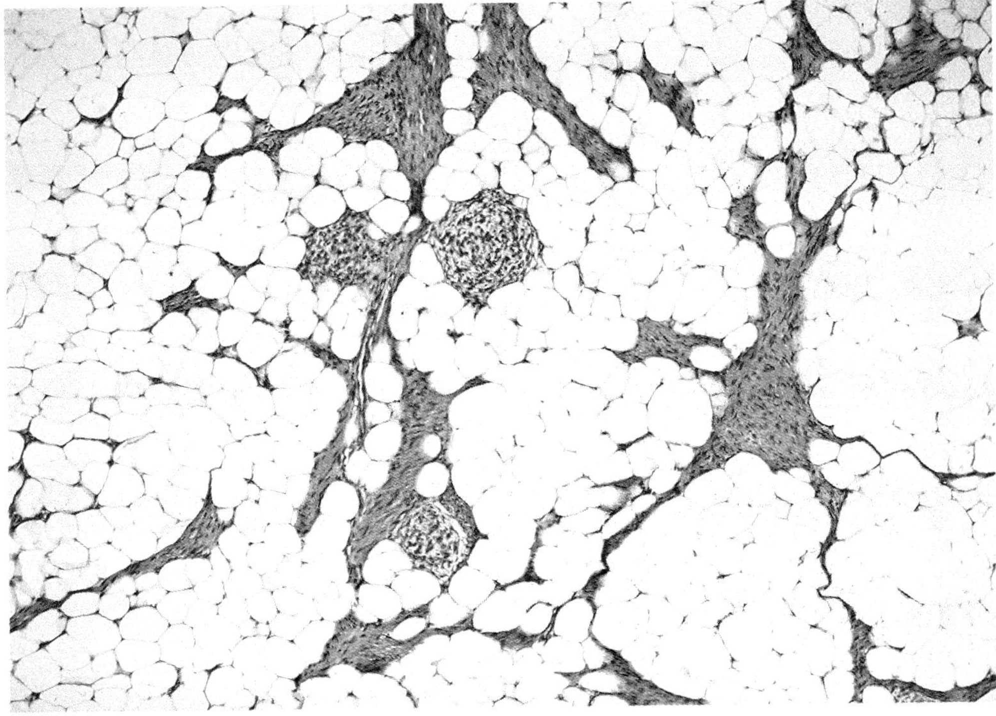

**FIGURE 11–3.** Fibrous hamartoma of infancy with an organoid pattern but composed predominantly of mature adipose tissue.

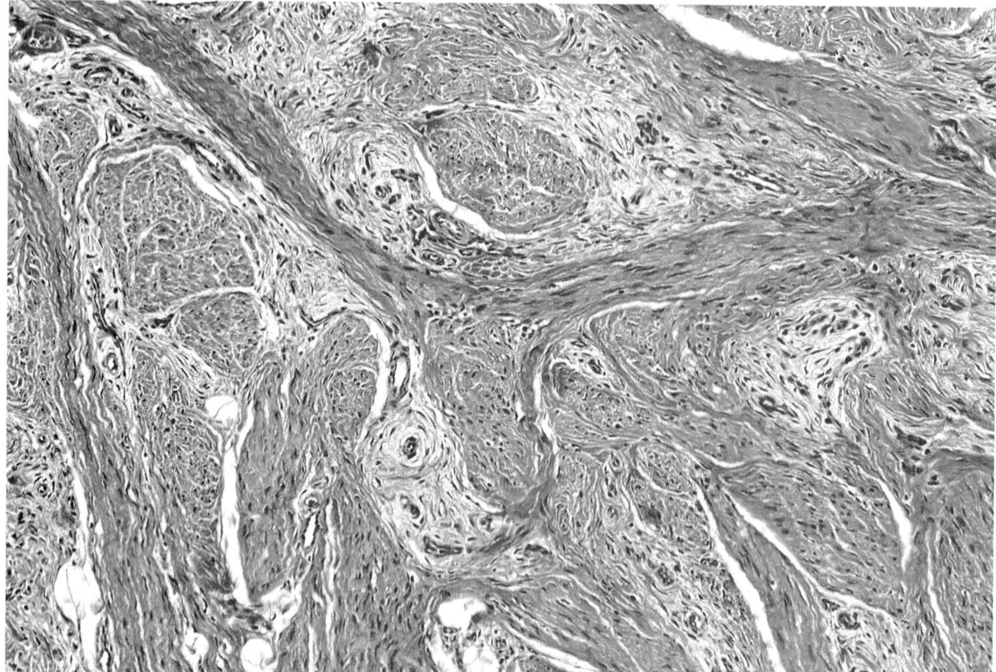

**FIGURE 11–4.** Fibrous hamartoma of infancy with interlacing fibrous trabeculae and interspersed myxoid zones.

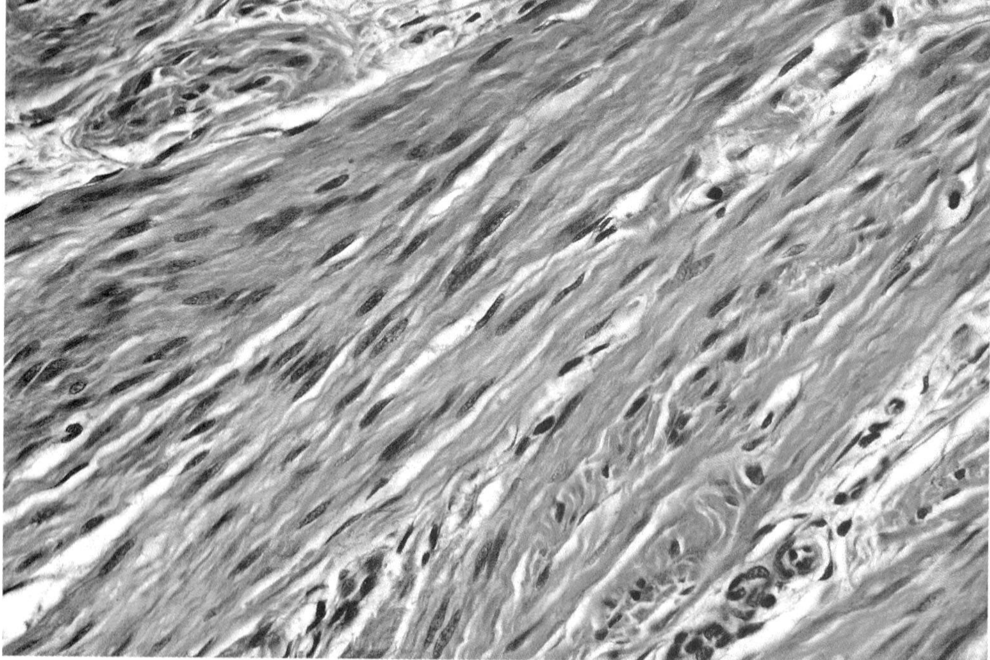

**FIGURE 11–5.** High-power view of spindle-shaped cells in fibrous trabeculae of a fibrous hamartoma of infancy.

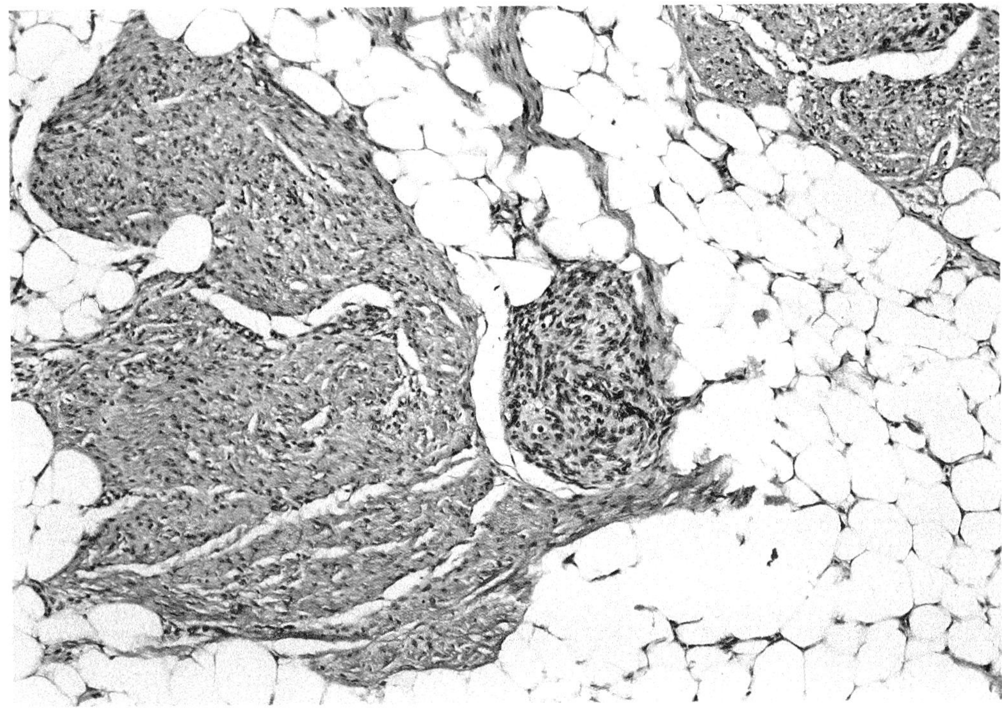

**FIGURE 11–6.** Fibrous hamartoma of infancy showing an admixture of mature adipose tissue, fibrous trabeculae, and a nodule of spindle-shaped cells.

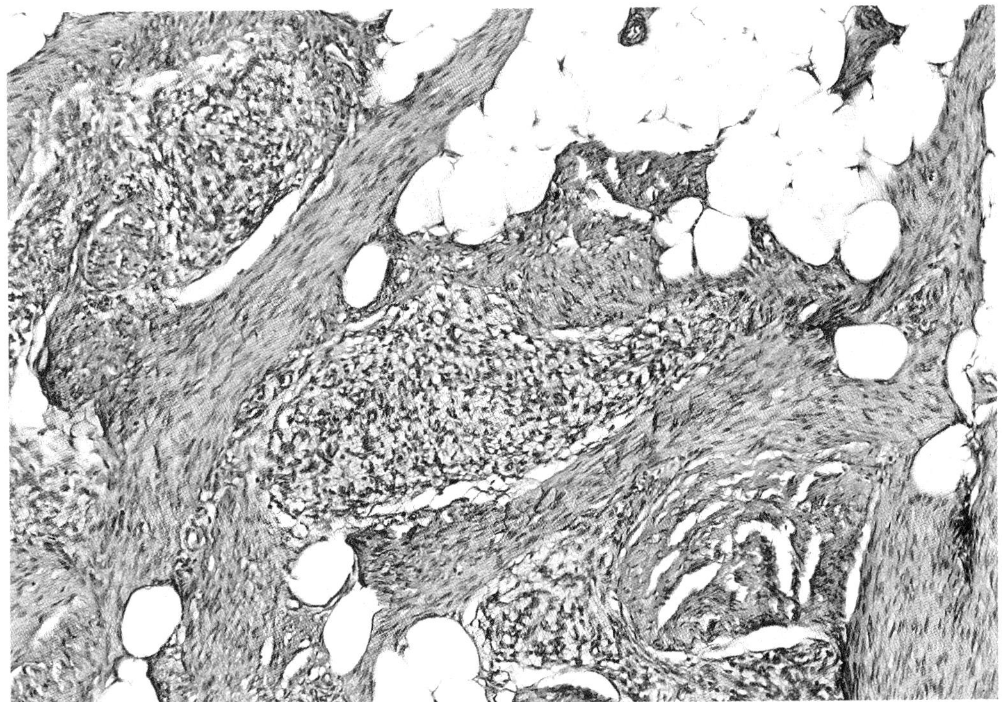

**FIGURE 11–7.** Organoid pattern with a characteristic arrangement of the three distinct components typical of fibrous hamartoma of infancy.

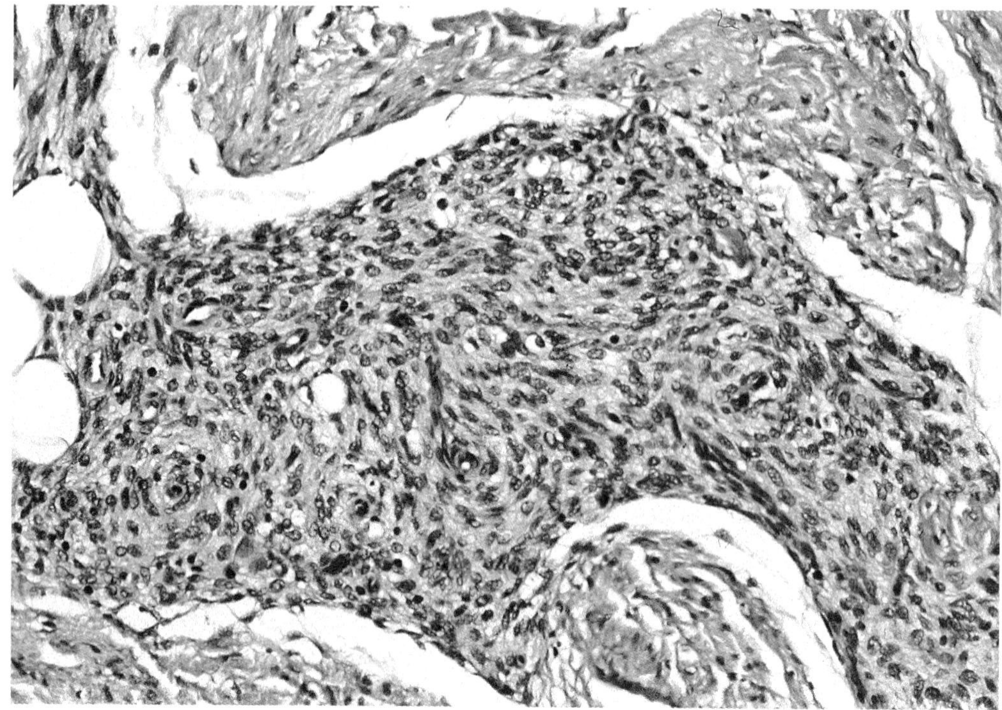

**FIGURE 11–8.** High-power view of cytologically bland spindle-shaped cells deposited in a myxoid stroma in a fibrous hamartoma of infancy.

Actin immunoreactivity is present only in the trabecular component.[5,10] Although some have also reported desmin staining in the trabecular component,[10] others have not found this to be the case.[5,14]

Electron microscopically, the lesion is seen to consist of a mixture of fibroblasts and myofibroblasts, with some cells showing partial envelopment by basal lamina, pinocytotic vesicles, myofilaments with focal dense bodies, and occasional subplasmalemmal densities.[10,12] The immature-appearing cells resemble immature mesenchymal cells with few intracytoplasmic organelles.

## Differential Diagnosis

In most cases the "organoid" pattern characteristic of fibrous hamartoma of infancy is readily recognized, so the lesion is not difficult to distinguish from other entities. On occasion, when the myofibroblastic areas predominate, the lesion may be difficult to distinguish from infantile fibromatosis, diffuse myofibromatosis, and calcifying aponeurotic fibroma. *Infantile fibromatosis* may encroach on the subcutis in a similar trabecular manner, but this tumor arises primarily in muscle rather than in the subcutis and lacks the "organoid" pattern of fibrous hamartoma. *Diffuse myofibromatosis,* typically nodular or multinodular, is characterized by light-staining nodules separated by or associated with hemangiopericytoma-like vascular areas. *Calcifying aponeurotic fibroma* may grow in the same trabecular manner, especially during its earliest phase, when there is still little or no calcification. However, the older age of the children and the location of the tumor in the palm of the hand permit an unequivocal diagnosis.

Awareness of the characteristic "organoid" pattern also facilitates distinction from *infantile fibrosarcoma* and *embryonal rhabdomyosarcoma.* Because some fibrous hamartomas of infancy occur in the scrotal region, the *spindle cell form of embryonal rhabdomyosarcoma* enters the differential diagnosis, but this lesion generally occurs in older children and is composed of cells with more cytologic atypia.[16]

## Discussion

It is important to recognize and distinguish fibrous hamartoma of infancy from other forms of fibromatosis because it is a benign lesion that, despite its focal cellularity, is usually cured by local excision. As many as 16% locally recur,[1,3,14,17] but recurrences are nondestructive and are generally cured by local reexcision.

The true nature of fibrous hamartoma of infancy remains obscure. Although Reye suggested that it might be a reparative process,[15] there are no histologic features that suggest the lesion is a response to local injury. As its name implies, most have advocated the hamartomatous nature of this lesion, but it is not possible to exclude the possibility that it is a benign neoplasm.

## INFANTILE DIGITAL FIBROMATOSIS

Infantile digital fibromatosis (or infantile digital fibroma) is a distinctive fibrous tumor of infancy characterized by its occurrence in the fingers and toes, a marked tendency for local recurrence, and the presence of characteristic inclusion bodies in the cytoplasm of the proliferated fibroblasts.[34,52] In 1957, Jensen et al. reported seven patients whose presentations were consistent with this entity but referred to these lesions as *digital neurofibrosarcoma in infancy*.[42] Enzinger also reported seven cases in 1965 as *infantile dermal fibromatosis*.[32]

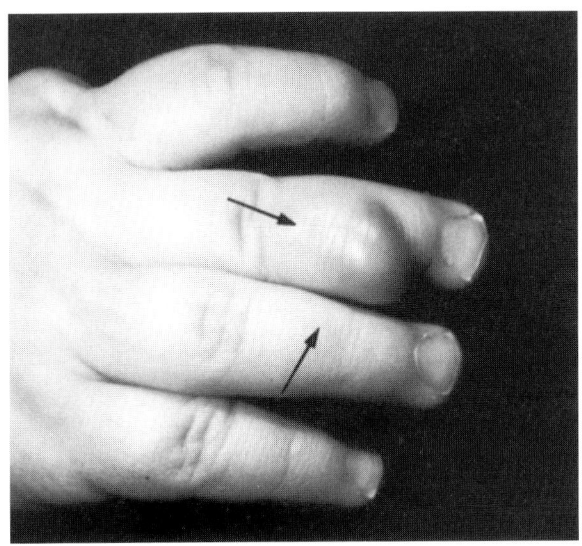

**FIGURE 11-9.** Infantile digital fibromatosis of the middle finger of the right hand of a 7½-month-old boy.

### Clinical Findings

Most patients present with a firm, broad-based, hemispheric or dome-shaped, nontender nodule with a smooth, glistening surface that is skin-colored or pale red. They are usually small, rarely exceeding 2 cm in greatest diameter. Almost all of these lesions are noted within the first 3 years of life, with most recognized by 1 year of age. Up to one-third of cases are already present at birth. Some lesions have been described in older children, adolescents, and rarely in adults.[21,24,36,53,56] Unlike most other forms of fibromatosis, the condition seems to be slightly more common in girls than in boys, but there is no evidence of any familial tendency.

The nodules are more often found in the fingers than the toes and in most instances are located on the sides or dorsum of the distal or middle phalangeal joints, especially of the third, fourth, and fifth digits (Fig. 11-9). Although rare cases have been described involving the thumb,[27] none involving the great toe have been reported. The lesions may be single or multiple and often affect more than one digit of the same hand or foot. Occasionally they involve both the fingers and toes of the same patient. Rare cases have been described as occurring outside the hands and feet. Purdy and Colby reported a case with typical eosinophilic perinuclear inclusions that occurred in the upper arm of a 2½-year-old child near an old injection site.[51] Pettinato et al. described two cases of "extradigital inclusion body fibromatosis" in the breasts of 24- and 53-year-old women.[49]

Although pain and tenderness are not typical symptoms, associated functional impairment or joint deformities may be present, such as lateral deviation or flexion deformities of the adjacent joints.[27,28] These deformities typically remain unchanged following surgical removal of the lesions.

### Pathologic Findings

The excised lesions are small, firm masses that are covered on one side by intact skin and have a solid white cut surface (Fig. 11-10). They show little variation in their microscopic appearance; like the desmoid form of infantile fibromatosis, they consist of a uniform proliferation of fibroblasts surrounded by a dense collagenous stroma (Fig. 11-11). They are poorly circumscribed and extend from the epidermis into the deeper portions of the dermis and subcutis, typically surrounding the dermal appendages. The overlying epidermis is usually minimally altered, with slight hyperkeratosis or acanthosis.

The most striking feature of the tumor is the presence of small, round inclusions in the cytoplasm of the fibroblasts. The number of inclusions varies from case to case. In some they are numerous and easily detected, whereas in others they are scarce and difficult to find with hematoxylin and eosin-stained slides. Typically, these inclusions are situated close to the nucleus from which a narrow clear zone (Fig. 11-12) often separates them. They are eosinophilic and resemble erythrocytes except for their more variable size (3–15$\mu$m), intracytoplasmic location, and lack of refringence. Numerous histochemical preparations can be used to highlight these inclusions. They stain a deep red with Masson trichrome stain (Fig. 11-13), purple with phosphotungstic acid hematoxylin (PTAH) bright red with Lendrum's phloxine tartrazine stain, and black with iron-hematoxylin prepara-

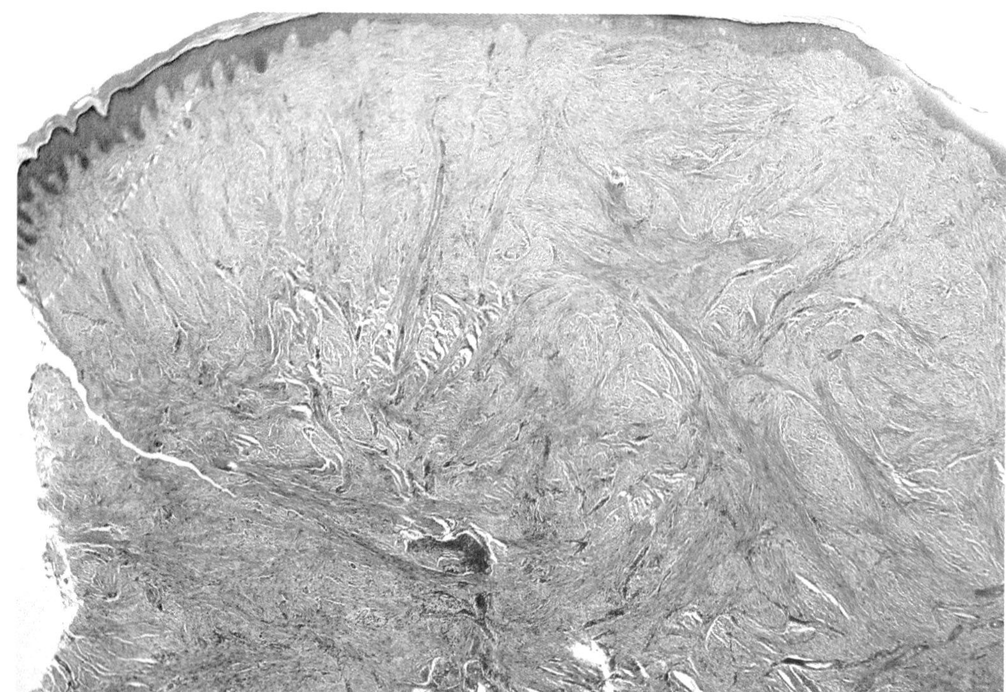

**FIGURE 11–10.** Low-power view of a broad-based hemispheric dermal nodule composed of spindle-shaped cells, characteristic of infantile digital fibromatosis.

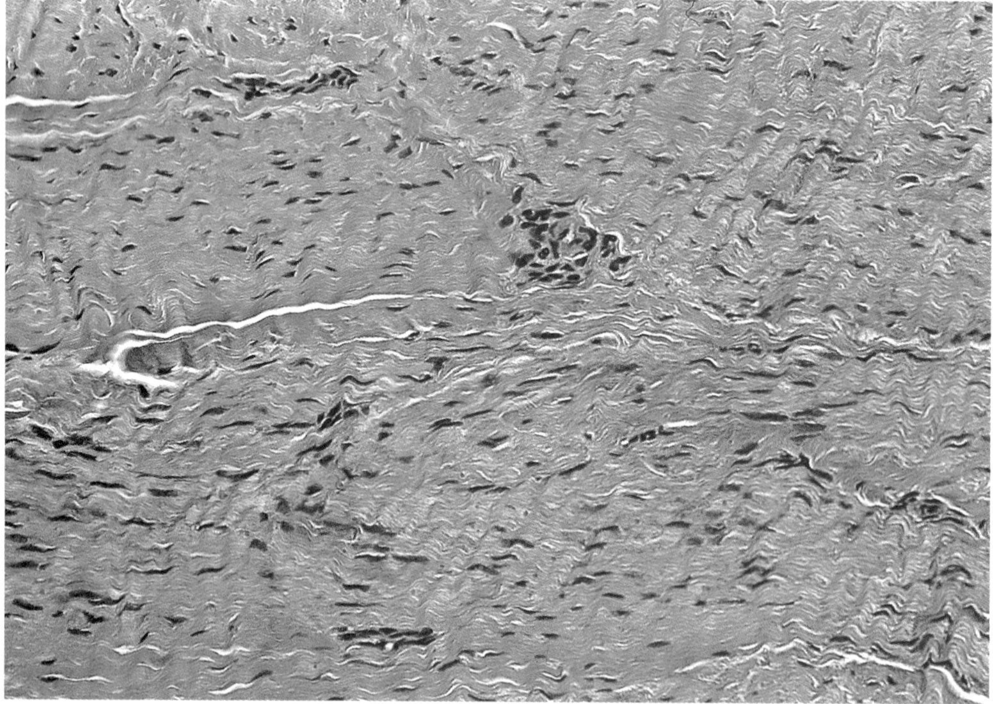

**FIGURE 11–11.** Infantile digital fibromatosis, composed of a uniform proliferation of fibroblasts surrounded by a dense collagenous stroma.

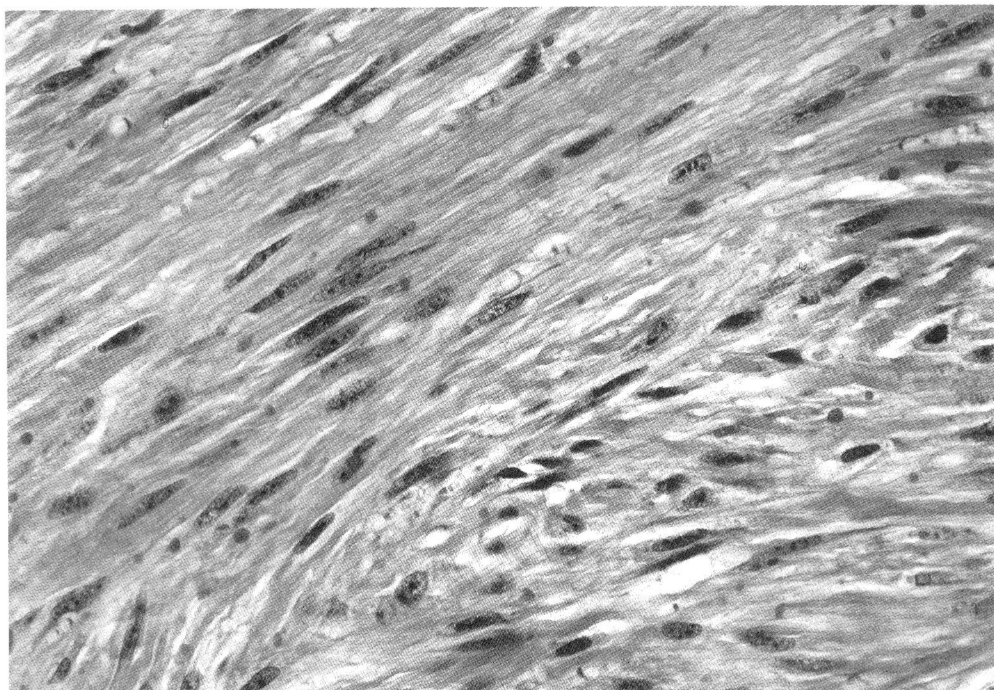

**FIGURE 11–12.** Infantile digital fibromatosis. Fibroblasts with characteristic intracytoplasmic inclusions separated by a narrow clear zone.

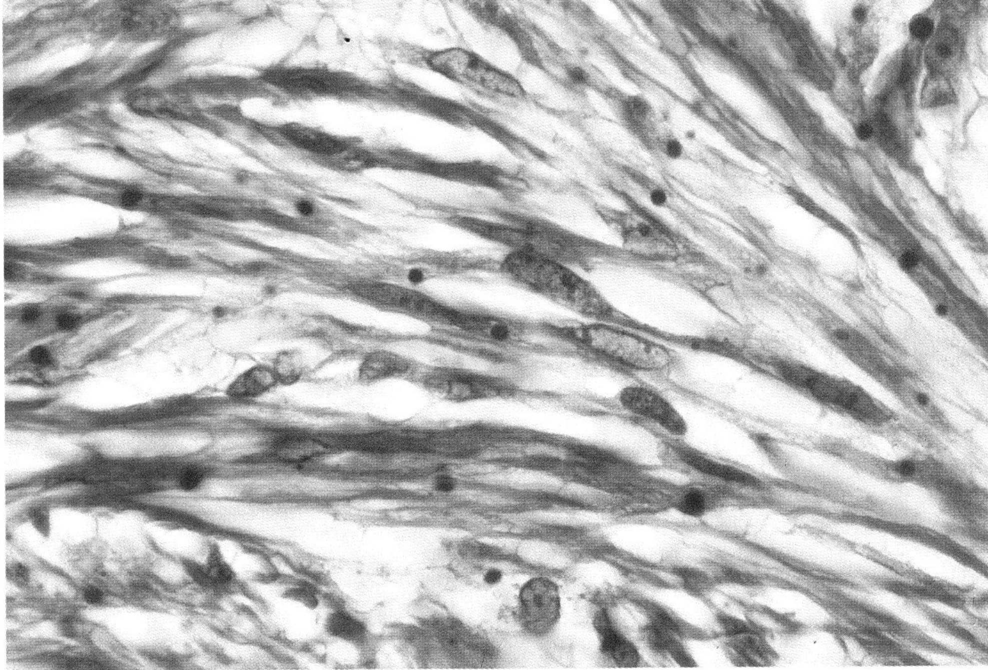

**FIGURE 11–13.** Masson trichrome stain demonstrating intracytoplasmic inclusions characteristic of infantile digital fibromatosis.

tions; they do not stain with periodic acid-schiff (PAS), alcian blue, or colloidal iron stains. Some have found these inclusions to stain with methyl green-pyronine,[52,54] but others have not found this to be the case.[20,41,44]

## Immunohistochemical and Electron Microscopic Findings

Immunohistochemically, most authors have noted actin positivity in the cytoplasm of the spindle cells, but variable results have been obtained with respect to actin immunoreactivity of the inclusion bodies. Most of the earlier studies using formalin-fixed tissues were unable to demonstrate actin staining of the inclusion bodies.[47,56–59] However, actin staining of the inclusion bodies has been demonstrated using alcohol-fixed tissue as well as KOH and trypsin-pretreated formalin-fixed tissue.[31,35,46]

Bhawan et al. were the first to emphasize the myofibroblastic nature of many of the cells in infantile digital fibromatosis and proposed the alternate term *infantile digital myofibroblastoma*.[25] Many other studies have confirmed that this lesion is composed mainly of fibroblasts and myofibroblasts.[39,47] The myofibroblasts contain narrow intracellular bundles of 5- to 7-nm microfilaments with interspersed dense bodies and occasional patches of basal lamina. These strap-like bundles of filaments are continuous with the juxtanuclear inclusion bodies, which also consist of fibrillary and granular material that has no limiting membrane and seems to originate in the endoplasmic reticulum (Fig. 11–14). Identical intracellular inclusions were also observed in cultured spindle cells obtained from patients with digital fibromatosis.[40,57] Small membrane-bound vesicles may also be found in the inclusion bodies and are probably derived from entrapped cell organelles.[36,40,57]

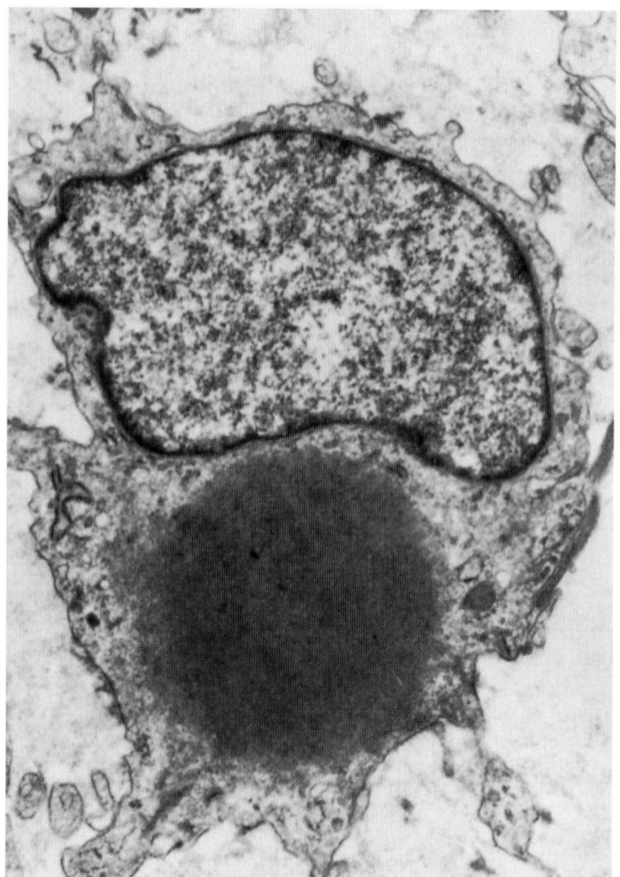

**FIGURE 11–14.** Infantile digital fibromatosis. Electron microscopy shows an inclusion within the fibroblast. (From Taxy JB, Battifora H. The electron microscope in the study and diagnosis of soft tissue tumors. In: Trump BF, Jones RT (eds) Diagnostic Electron Microscopy. Wiley, New York, 1980.)

## Prognosis and Therapy

Although 60% of these lesions recur locally, the ultimate prognosis is excellent. Recurrences appear at the same site within a few weeks or months after the initial excision, or a second tumor develops in an adjacent finger or toe.[27] Although there is an initial period of growth, if watched for a long enough time many lesions regress spontaneously.[22,38,44] Most authors advocate conservative treatment.[28,33] Because there is no evidence of aggressive behavior or malignant transformation, only surgical excision is needed, although some advocate a "watch and wait" approach following a diagnosis, given the high rate of spontaneous regression. Deformities and contractures develop in some cases regardless of whether the lesions are removed surgically, and surgical correction of contractures and functional changes is sometimes necessary.

## Discussion

The exact nature of the inclusions is not clear. Because of the resemblance of these inclusions to the viroplasm of fibroblasts infected with SHOPE fibroma virus, Battifora and Hines proposed a possible viral etiology.[23] Pohjanpelto et al. isolated a filterable cell-transforming agent from nodules of infantile digital fibromatosis,[50] although this finding has never been reproduced. The immunohistochemical and ultrastructural findings strongly suggest that the inclusions are related to the intracellular bundles of microfilaments and represent densely packed masses of actin microfilaments.[31,39,46] The occurrence of extradigital posttraumatic lesions that are histologically indistinguishable from those on the digits[45,51] and antecedent trauma related to digital lesions[36,43] suggests that trauma may stimulate development of the lesion.

Inclusion bodies identical to those found in infantile digital fibromatosis have also been described in a variety of tumors including a fibrous tumor of the tongue,[30] a dermal fibrous lesion in the toxic oil epidermic syndrome,[48] an endocervical polyp,[29,58] a vulvar angioleiomyoma,[55] a fibroepithelial tumor of the breast,[26] and a phyllodes tumor of the breast.[37]

## MYOFIBROMA AND MYOFIBROMATOSIS

Myofibromatosis was initially described in 1951 by Williams and Schrum, who designated the lesions *congenital fibrosarcoma*.[106] Three years later, Stout renamed the entity *congenital generalized fibromatosis*.[102] His patients were two male infants who died soon after birth and had multiple fibrous nodules in soft tissues and internal organs. Subsequent reports emphasized the multicentricity of this disorder, for which a variety of terms have been applied, including benign mesenchymoma,[68] generalized hamartomatosis,[91] and multiple mesenchymal hamartomas.[64] In 1965 Kauffman and Stout grouped their cases of congenital fibromatosis into two categories: (1) a multiple form, with lesions restricted to skin, subcutaneous tissue, skeletal muscle, and bone and characterized by a good prognosis; and (2) a generalized form, with visceral lesions and a poor prognosis.[86] Following recognition of the myofibroblastic nature of the constituent cells,[64] Chung and Enzinger reported 61 cases of this entity and renamed it *infantile myofibromatosis*.[71] We prefer the terms *myofibroma* and *myofibromatosis* for the solitary and multiple lesions, respectively, not only because these lesions occur in infants, children, and adults and have a prominent myofibroblastic component but also because their behavior distinguishes them from other, more aggressive types of fibromatosis.

### Clinical Findings

*Myofibroma* manifests as a single swelling or mass most commonly in the dermis and subcutis. It measures a few millimeters to several centimeters in diameter. The more superficially located nodules are freely movable, and when skin is involved, the lesion may manifest as a purplish macule giving the impression of a hemangioma. Some lesions are more deeply seated and appear to be fixed. Although Chung and Enzinger found the solitary lesions to be almost three times as common as the multicentric form,[71] in a review of the literature of 170 cases by Wiswell et al. solitary lesions were half as common as the multicentric form.[107]

Solitary nodules are found most commonly in the general region of the head and neck, including the scalp, forehead, orbit, parotid region, and oral cavity.[62,85,88,89] The trunk is the second most commonly affected site, followed by the lower and upper extremities. Rare cases of the multicentric form of this disease have been limited to the skeleton.[81,92] There have also been several reports of solitary intraosseous myofibromas[79,83,87] most of which have involved the craniofacial bones. Solitary lesions involving the viscera are rare.[69,80,99] The condition is almost twice as common in males as in females and occurs not only in infants and children but also in adults; solitary[63,71,72,93,98] and multifocal[77,78] lesions have been reported in adults.

In patients with multiple lesions (*myofibromatosis*) the individual nodules have essentially the same appearance as the solitary nodules; they occur not only in dermis and subcutis but also in muscle, the internal organs, and the skeleton. Up to 40% of patients have visceral lesions that are invariably present at birth[107] (Fig. 11–15). The nodules may be numerous,

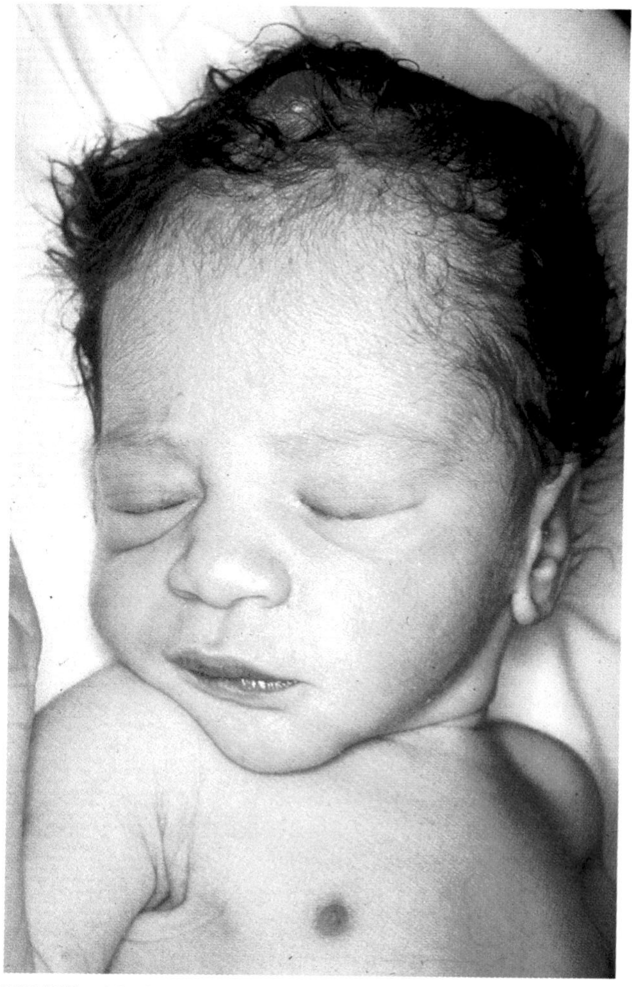

**FIGURE 11–15.** Newborn infant with myofibromatosis, with numerous dermal and subcutaneous nodules of the head and neck region.

especially when they are in the subcutis, lung, or skeleton; in several patients more than 50 nodules were counted. For example, Schaffzin et al. reported a newborn girl who had 59 subcutaneous nodules noted at birth.[97] Heiple et al. also described an infant who had more than 100 lesions in the skeleton that involved both flat and long bones.[81] In the latter case, the nodules were recognized only after the infant suffered a fracture in a minor fall and underwent a radiographic examination of the injured leg.

Apart from the soft tissues and the skeleton, the most common sites of the nodules are the lung, heart, gastrointestinal tract, and pancreas[94,101,107] and rarely the central nervous system.[60,95,96] Internal lesions often cause symptoms such as severe respiratory distress, vomiting, or diarrhea, which often fail to respond to therapy and prove fatal within a few days or weeks after birth. Others cause few symptoms, making it likely that some internal lesions remain unrecognized. The nodules grow principally during the immediate perinatal period. Growth is not restricted to this period, and continued enlargement or formation of new lesions may be observed during infancy or even later in life.[66,82]

Radiographically, the bone lesions are circumscribed lytic areas with marginal sclerosis and without penetration of the cortex in most cases.[79,83] Occasionally, however, a soft tissue lesion may extend into the underlying bone. Extraosseous lesions may show weak radiodensity as a result of focal calcification[67,70,83] (Figs. 11–16, 11–17).

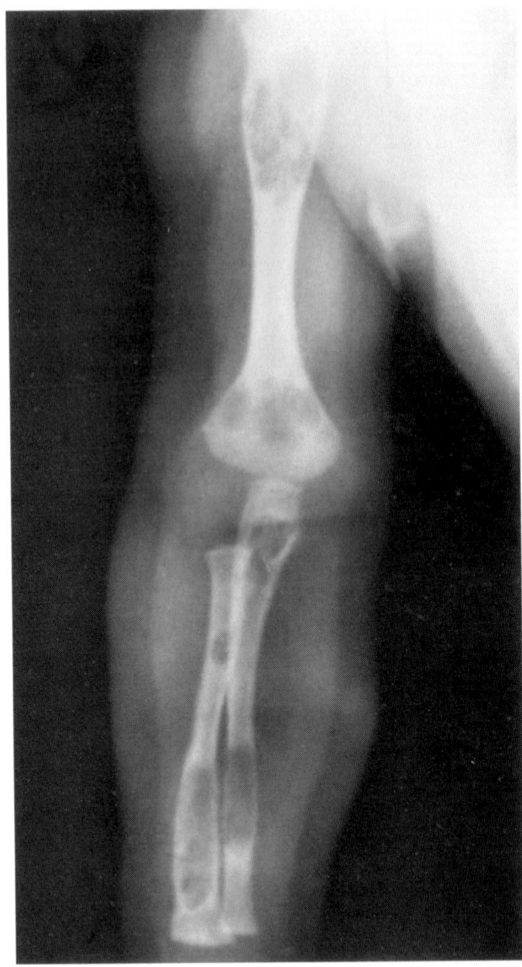

**FIGURE 11–16.** Infantile myofibromatosis, multicentric type, with extensive bone involvement of the right arm. (From Brill PW, Yandow DR, Langer LO, et al. Congenital generalized fibromatosis: case report and literature review. Pediatr Radiol 12:269, 1982, with permission.)

## Pathologic Findings

As a rule, the nodules in the dermis and subcutis are better delineated than those in the muscle, bone, or viscera (Fig. 11–18). They are rubbery or firm and scar-like in consistency and typically have a white-gray or pink surface; they vary greatly in size, averaging 0.5–1.5 cm in greatest diameter. Large lesions may ulcerate the overlying epidermis.[84]

Microscopically, *myofibroma* and *myofibromatosis* have similar features. At low magnification, there is typically a nodular or multinodular growth pattern that appears biphasic owing to the alternation of light- and dark-staining areas. The light-staining areas consist mainly of plump myoid spindle cells with eosinophilic cytoplasm arranged in nodules, short fascicles, or whorls (Fig. 11–19). The nuclei are elongated and tapering or cigar-shaped and lack nuclear atypia. Some areas have extensive hyalinization. These areas are usually located more peripherally although in some cases they are distributed haphazardly throughout the lesion. Immunohistochemically, the cells are immunoreactive for vimentin and actin but do not stain for desmin or S-100 protein, consistent with myofibroblastic differentiation.[63,90]

The dark-staining areas of the lesion, usually centrally located, are composed of round or polygonal cells with slightly pleomorphic hyperchromatic nuclei or small spindle cells typically arranged around a distinct hemangiopericytoma-like vascular pattern (Figs. 11–20 to 11–23). These primitive cells have vesicular nuclei, small amounts of eosinophilic cytoplasm, and indistinct cell margins. Mitotic figures are usually rare, although as many as 8 mitoses/10 high-power fields may be seen.[71] In some cases focal hemorrhage, cystic degeneration, or coagulative necrosis is present, often with foci of calcification. Peripherally located chronic inflammatory cells, including lymphocytes and plasma cells, may be present. Because of these cellular and richly vascular areas and the exten-

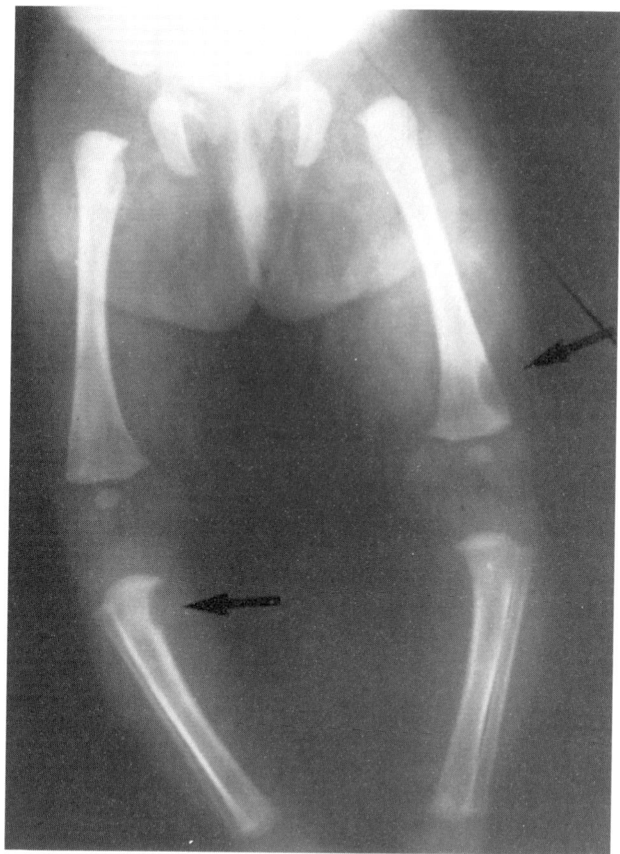

**FIGURE 11–17.** Infantile myofibromatosis, multicentric type, with multiple bone involvement (arrows). These osseous lesions tend to regress spontaneously and usually are no longer demonstrable after a few years.

sive necrosis, some tumors have been mistaken for sarcoma. In addition, the presence of intravascular growth, a feature that is present in up to one-fifth of cases, may also be worrisome but does not seem to have any prognostic significance. Some cases are composed almost exclusively of these cellular areas (so-called monophasic cellular variant of infantile myofibromatosis) and may represent the earliest stage of the disease.[108]

## Immunohistochemical and Electron Microscopic Findings

Immunohistochemically, the primitive-appearing cells stain focally and weakly for actin.[63,90] Fletcher et al. thought these cells had smooth muscle differentiation based on the immunohistochemical expression of desmin.[75] However, a study by the same authors several years later found an absence of desmin staining in these primitive cells, and they proposed that the different results were obtained because of the the use of an outdated polyclonal anti-chicken antibody.[63] Ultrastructurally, there is general agreement that the predominant cells are fibroblasts and myofibroblasts, with prominent endoplasmic reticulum, intracytoplasmic microfilaments, dense bodies, focal basal lamina, and occasional intercellular attachment sites[64,65,74] (Fig. 11–24).

## Differential Diagnosis

The differential diagnosis of this lesion depends in part on whether the eosinophilic myofibroblasts or more primitive small cells predominate in a given lesion. The peripheral areas of myofibroma can resemble nodular fasciitis, fibrous histiocytoma, neurofibroma, or infantile fibromatosis. *Nodular fasciitis* is a rare lesion in newborns and infants but certainly should be considered in the differential diagnosis in adults. Nodular fasciitis arises from the fascia, has a more prominent myxoid matrix, and usually contains scattered chronic inflammatory cells and occasional erythrocytes. The hemangiopericytoma-like pattern characteristic of myofibroma is absent in nodular fas-

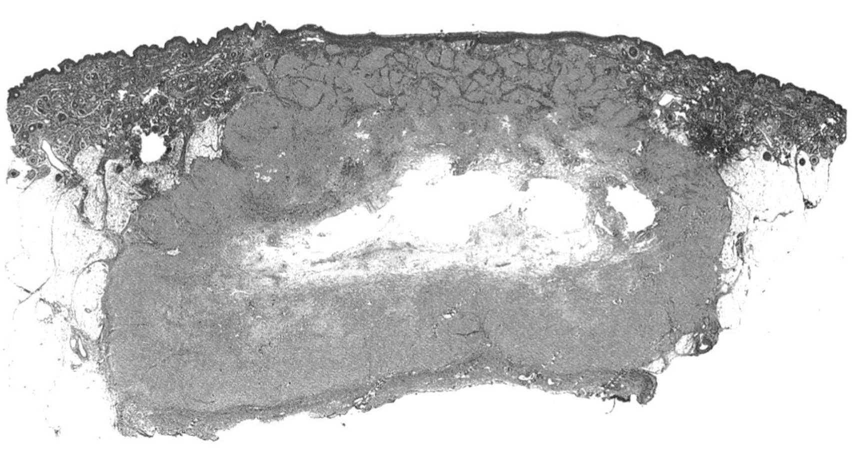

**FIGURE 11–18.** Low-power view of a solitary myofibroma involving the dermis and subcutis.

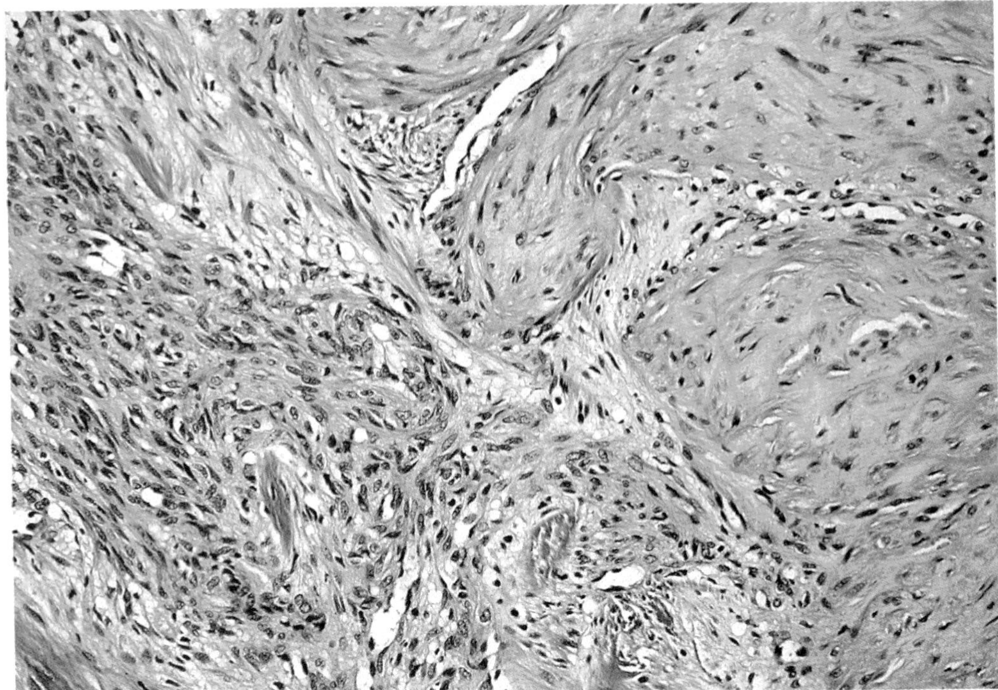

**FIGURE 11–19.** Infantile myofibromatosis, solitary type, consisting of broad bundles of plump myoid spindle cells with eosinophilic cytoplasm.

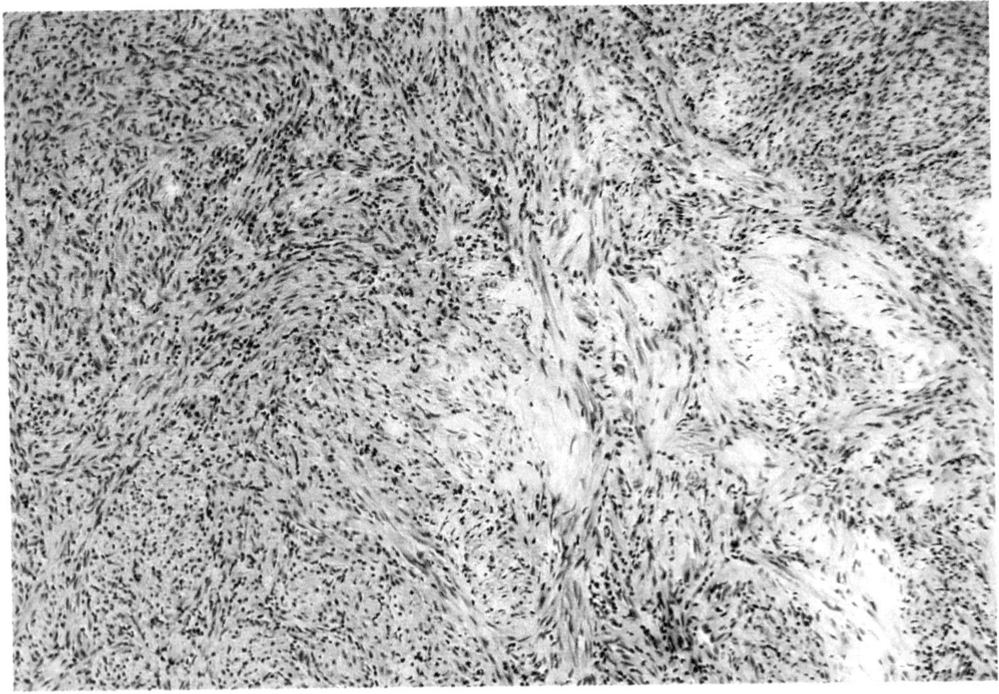

**FIGURE 11–20.** Infantile myofibromatosis, solitary type, composed predominantly of darkly staining spindle-shaped cells with intermixed plumper myoid-like cells.

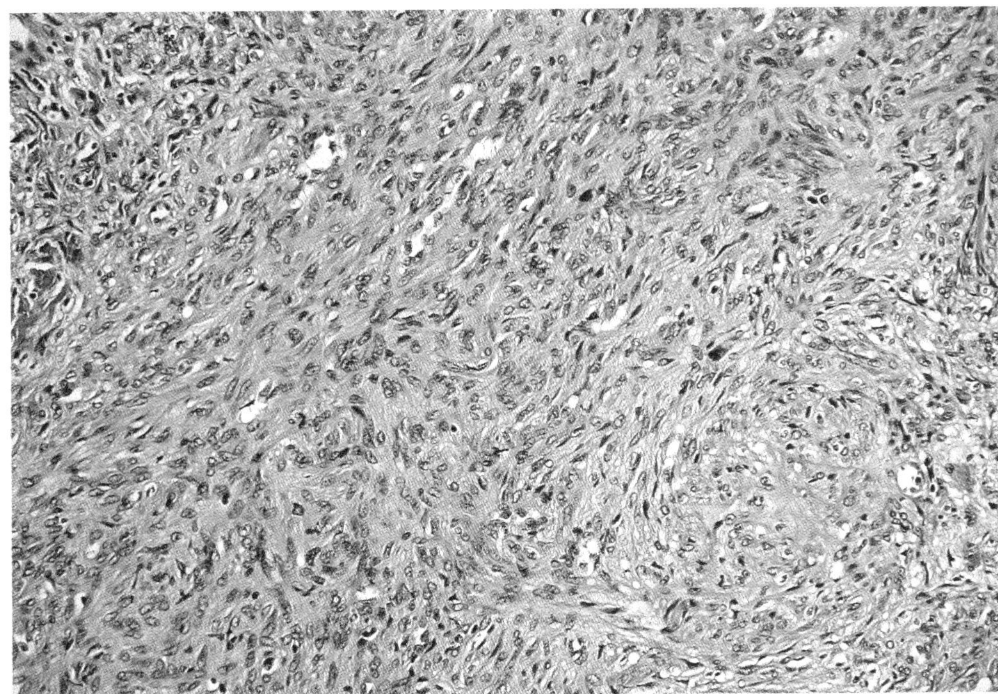

**FIGURE 11–21.** Infantile myofibromatosis with cellular proliferation of ovoid cells without cytologic atypia.

ciitis. The peripheral areas may also resemble *neurofibroma,* but the myofibroblastic cells lack S-100 protein. Clinically, *myofibromatosis* should not be confused with *neurofibromatosis,* as myofibromatosis manifests with multiple nodules at birth or within the first few weeks of life, whereas neurofibromatosis affects older children with evidence of multiple café au lait spots and in about one-half of cases a history of familial involvement. *Fibrous histiocytoma* is composed of a polymorphous proliferation of cells arranged in a more pronounced storiform pattern. Although smooth muscle actin may be found in fibrous histiocytoma, the staining is usually focal. Furthermore, the cells of fibrous histiocytomas usually express factor XIIIa. Solitary forms of the disease may be mistaken for *infantile fibromatosis.* In the latter process, however, the tumors tend to be less well circumscribed, arise in muscle, and show a more uniform spindle cell pattern. In addition, infantile fibromatosis shows neither central necrosis nor a central hemangiopericytoma-like vascular pattern.

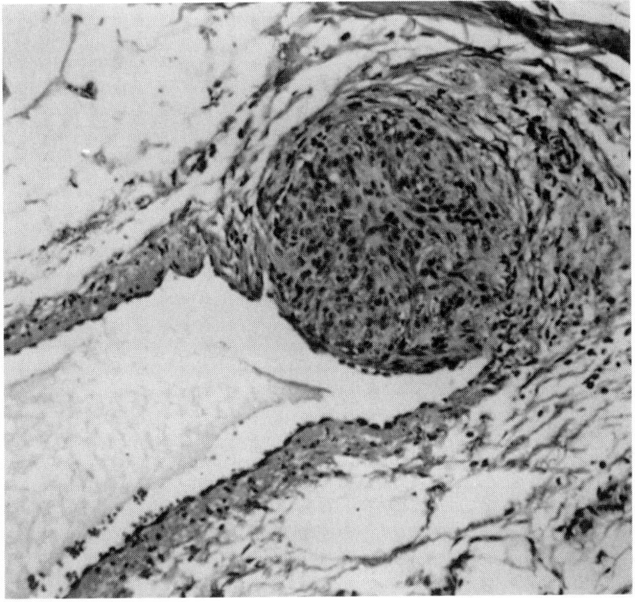

**FIGURE 11–22.** Intravascular growth in solitary-type infantile myofibromatosis. Despite this feature, these lesions are uniformly benign and are cured by simple local excision.

Infantile myofibromatosis has a number of clinical and morphologic similarities with *infantile hemangiopericytoma.*[90] As in infantile myofibromatosis, most infantile hemangiopericytomas are present at birth or occur early in life, with a predilection for boys. Although most are solitary subcutaneous lesions, both multicentricity and visceral involvement have been described. In addition, the main affected sites are similar between these lesions. Histologically, the central immature-appearing areas of infantile myofibromatosis are indistinguishable from those of infantile he-

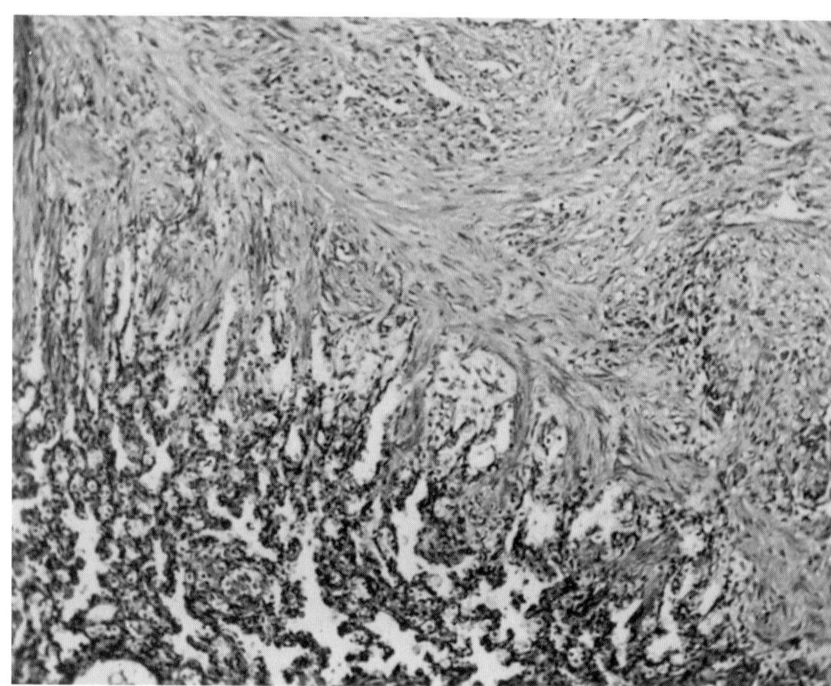

**FIGURE 11–23.** Infantile myofibromatosis (multicentric type) involving lung.

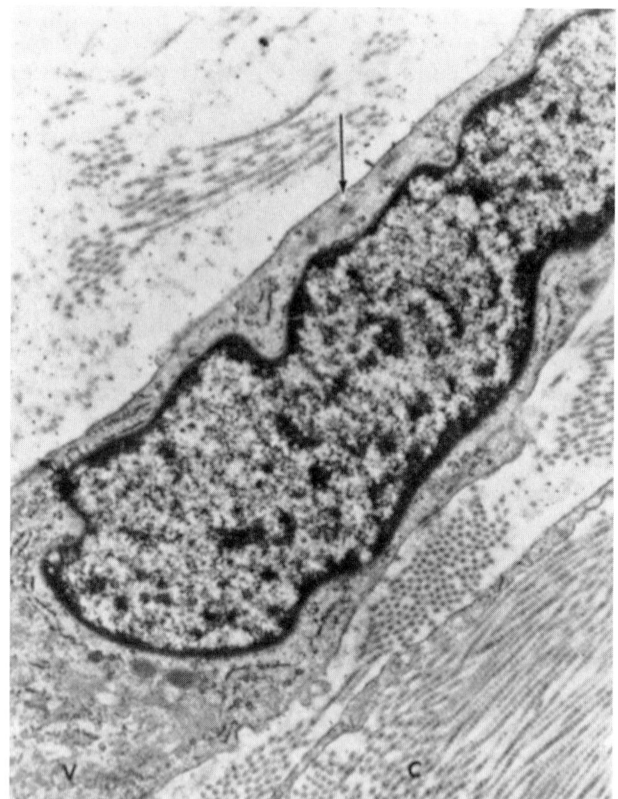


**FIGURE 11–24.** Infantile myofibromatosis. Myofibroblasts with condensed filamentous material (arrow). (From Benjamin SP, Mercer RD, Hawk W. Myofibroblastic contraction in spontaneous regression of multiple congenital mesenchymal hamartomas. Cancer 40:2343, 1977, with permission.)

mangiopericytoma. Upon review of 11 cases originally diagnosed as infantile hemangiopericytoma, Mentzel et al. found focal mature-appearing, actin-positive, spindle-shaped smooth muscle cells similar to those seen in infantile myofibromatosis in all cases.[90] These authors proposed that infantile hemangiopericytoma and infantile myofibromatosis represent different stages of maturation of a single entity. Other authors have also proposed a relation between these two tumors.[73,104]

Finally, biopsy specimens obtained from the central portion of this lesion may have features that resemble various types of sarcoma, particularly those composed of small round cells arranged around a hemangiopericytoma-like vasculature. Such lesions include peripheral primitive neuroectodermal tumor, mesenchymal chondrosarcoma, malignant hemangiopericytoma, and poorly differentiated synovial sarcoma. A battery of immunostains, including those for cytokeratins, S-100 protein, and CD99, can assist in the differential diagnosis. Although not always present, identifying peripheral myoid-appearing cells is the most useful feature for recognizing infantile myofibromatosis.

## Discussion

The clinical course seems to be largely determined by the extent of the disease. Solitary and multiple lesions confined to soft tissues and bone carry an excellent prognosis; they tend to regress spontaneously and rarely require more than a diagnostic biopsy.[62,64,71] In the review by Wiswell et al., only 5 of 54 (9%) solitary lesions recurred locally following excision (with many of the excisions incomplete).[107] In addition, in 11 of 18 patients with multicentric lesions without visceral involvement and follow-up of more than 1 year there was spontaneous regression. Chung and Enzinger found that only 3 of 28 solitary lesions (11%) locally recurred, and several of the multicentric lesions showed spontaneous regression.[71] Fukasawa et al. documented massive apoptosis in two cases of infantile myofibromatosis and proposed that this mechanism may account for the high rate of spontaneous regression of these lesions.[76] On the other hand, the prognosis is much less favorable in newborns and infants with multiple visceral lesions, and as many as 75% of them die with signs of respiratory distress or diarrhea soon after birth.[71,107] There are exceptions, however. Teng et al.[103] described a 4-month-old boy with a large mass in the kidney and multiple bony lesions who was well 18 months after excision of the renal tumor. Radiographic examination of the skeleton revealed spontaneous regression of the bony lesions. Similarly, Zeller et al.[109] reported an unusual case of an 8-month-old boy with numerous osteolytic lesions throughout the skeleton that resulted in a softened thoracic wall and respiratory failure. Supportive therapy was given, and many of the lesions subsequently regressed. Likewise, Dimmick and Wood[74] reported a case of congenital myofibromatosis that involved numerous sites and caused respiratory distress and quadriplegia. They noted regression of the lesions, neurologic improvement, and disappearance of most of the lesions within 9 months. Occasionally, new lesions develop years after the primary tumor has regressed.[66,82] Although Dictor et al. reported a myofibromatosis-like hemangiopericytoma that metastasized as a "myosarcoma," this lesion seems to be more akin to malignant hemangiopericytoma than myofibroma.[73]

Myofibroma and myofibromatosis are clearly expressions of a benign, self-limiting, localized or generalized process that consists to a large degree of cells with the characteristics of myofibroblasts and sometimes of pericytes. The exact cause of this condition is not clear. Several studies have documented a familial occurrence, including the presence of this lesion in siblings,[61,66,71,105] suggesting an autosomal recessive pattern of inheritance. Jennings et al. reported infantile myofibromatoses in a neonate and the father and proposed an autosomal dominant mode of inheritance.[84] A single solitary myofibroma has been described with a cytogenetic abnormality: del (6)(q12;q15).[100]

## JUVENILE HYALIN FIBROMATOSIS

Juvenile hyalin fibromatosis is another rare hereditary disease that bears a superficial resemblance to myofibromatosis but differs by its cutaneous distribution of the tumor nodules and the histologic picture. The latter is characterized by a paucity of cells, a fibrillary matrix, and complete absence of mature collagen fibers. The condition was first described by Murray in 1873 as *molluscum fibrosum in children*, an early synonym of neurofibromatosis.[137] Whitfield and Robinson offered a follow-up report of these three cases in 1903.[150] No further reports occurred until 1962, when Puretic et al. reported a case under the name *mesenchymal dysplasia*.[142] A variety of terms were used in subsequent reports, including systemic hyalinosis[110] and disseminated painful fibromatosis.[138] Kitano et al. coined "juvenile hyalin fibromatosis," and it has become the preferred term.[133] This entity appears to be rare, as fewer than 50 cases of the disease have been recorded.[110–154]

### Clinical Findings

Clinical onset is usually noted from birth to 5 years of age. Boys are affected slightly more commonly than girls.[121] The condition is characterized by multiple cutaneous papules, nodules, or tumor masses, gingival hypertrophy, joint contractures, and osteolytic defects. The skin lesions have been grouped into three types: (1) small, pearly papules on the face and neck; (2) small nodules and large plaques with a translucent appearance and a gelatinous consistency developing on fingers and ears and around the nose; and (3) firm, large, subcutaneous tumors with a predilection for the scalp, trunk, and limbs[119] (Fig. 11–25). The tumor masses vary in size from 1 mm to about 5 cm; they are slow-growing and painless and have a tendency to recur following excision. The number of cutaneous lesions varies from case to case, but some patients have been found to have more than 100 tumors in various parts of the body.[153] Occasional patients also have perianal papillomatous lesions.[114,120,130,141] Most patients have extracutaneous findings. Gingival hypertrophy and painful flexion contractures of the major joints are present in most patients, and these findings may precede the development of skin lesions.[139] Although poorly developed musculature and muscle weakness have been reported, the nature of the muscle disorder has not been well characterized.[126,132,133] More than 60% of patients reveal multiple osteolytic defects on radiographic examination.[121] Puretic et al. described osteolysis of the distal phalanges of the toes and fingers that progressed to almost complete destruction.[142] Atherton et al. reported osteolytic lesions in the distal phalanges of the great toes and lateral malleolus.[111] Ishikawa and Hori found that tissue obtained from one of these bony defects revealed infiltration of hyalin material similar to that seen in the skin and muscle.[126] Most patients report painful, debilitating flexion contractures of large joints, often resulting in marked deformity and generalized stiffness.[112,119,147]

## Pathologic Findings

The tumors are poorly circumscribed and consist of cords of spindle-shaped cells embedded in a homogeneous eosinophilic matrix (Figs. 11–26 to 11–30). They are often found in the dermis, subcutis, and gingiva, although the bone and joints may also be involved.[126,148] Deposition of this amorphous eosinophilic matrix is widespread in some patients, as Kitano et al. reported a patient with autopsy-proven deposition of this substance in the tongue, esophagus, stomach, intestine, thymus, spleen, and lymph nodes.[133] Early lesions show increased cellularity and less prominent stroma, whereas the large, older lesions are less cellular and contain more ground substance.[135] The matrix stains positively with PAS and alcian blue but does not stain with toluidine blue or congo red. Elastic tissue is completely absent. Occasional nodules reveal marked calcification.[135,148]

Electron microscopic examination reveals scattered fibroblast-like cells with enlarged rough endoplasmic reticulum and a prominent Golgi apparatus containing cystic vesicles filled with a fibrillar and granular material as well as aggregates of microfilaments or fibril-filled balls of varying size.[132,144,149,152,154] Large amounts of microfibrillary material are present in the interstices, with occasional alignment of the fibrils to mature normal and long-spaced collagen fibers.

## Differential Diagnosis

*Multicentric infantile myofibromatosis* is composed of multiple nodules that are almost always present at birth or appear during the first year of life. In general, the nodules are better circumscribed and are found not only in the subcutis but also in muscle, bone, and viscera. Microscopically, they consist of broad, interlacing bundles of plump myofibroblasts, often with a central hemangiopericytoma-like area composed of primitive-appearing cells. The gums or joints are never involved. *Neurofibromatosis* tends to make its first appearance in slightly older children and is associated with café au lait spots; the tumors are composed of hyperchromatic serpentine nuclei in a fibrillary eosinophilic matrix and are positive for S-100 protein. *Gingival fibromatosis,* a lesion with a similar hereditary pattern, is limited to the gums of the upper and lower jaws and consists of dense, scar-like connective tissue rich in collagen. *Cylindromas,* or turban tumors, are confined to the head.

*Winchester syndrome,* a rare autosomal hereditary disease, is characterized by densely cellular, poorly demarcated fibrous proliferations in the dermis, subcutis, and joints without deposition of a hyalin matrix; periarticular thickening and limited motion in the limbs and the spine, corneal opacities and radiographic changes of bones and joints are also part of this disorder.[151] The precise relation between juvenile hyalin fibromatosis, Winchester syndrome, and *infantile systemic hyalinosis* is unclear, and some believe that these conditions represent different expressions of the same disorder.[122,146]

## Discussion

Although most lesions in this condition are formed during childhood, new lesions may continue to ap-

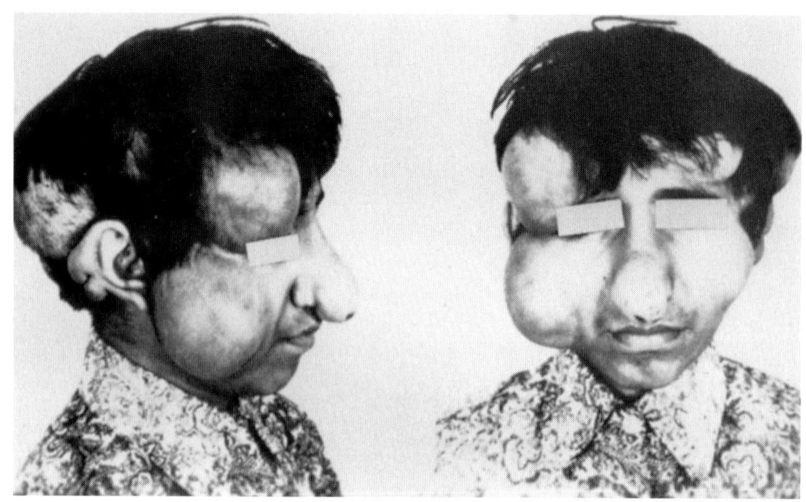

**FIGURE 11–25.** Juvenile hyalin fibromatosis. Multiple masses involve the scalp and face. (Courtesy of Prof. Dr. Eduardo Carceres, Director, Instituto Nacional de Enfermades Neoplasicas, Lima, Peru.)

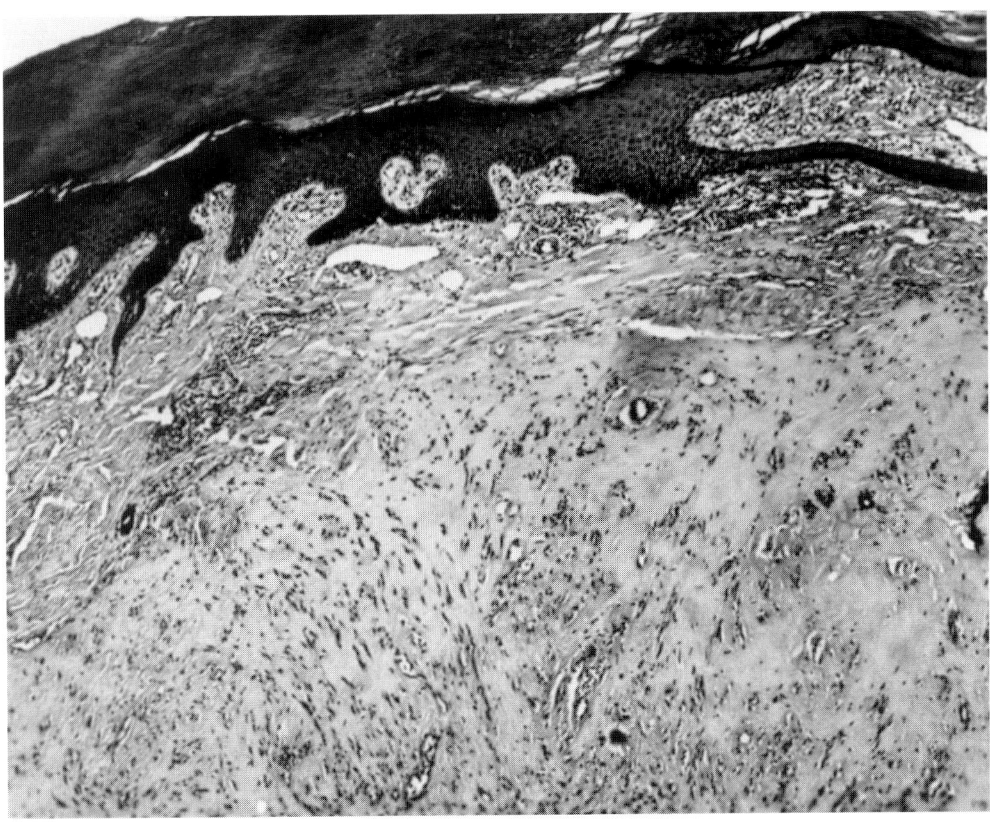

**FIGURE 11–26.** Juvenile hyalin fibromatosis. Dermal nodule shows characteristic association of fibroblasts and large amounts of inspissated hyalinized material.

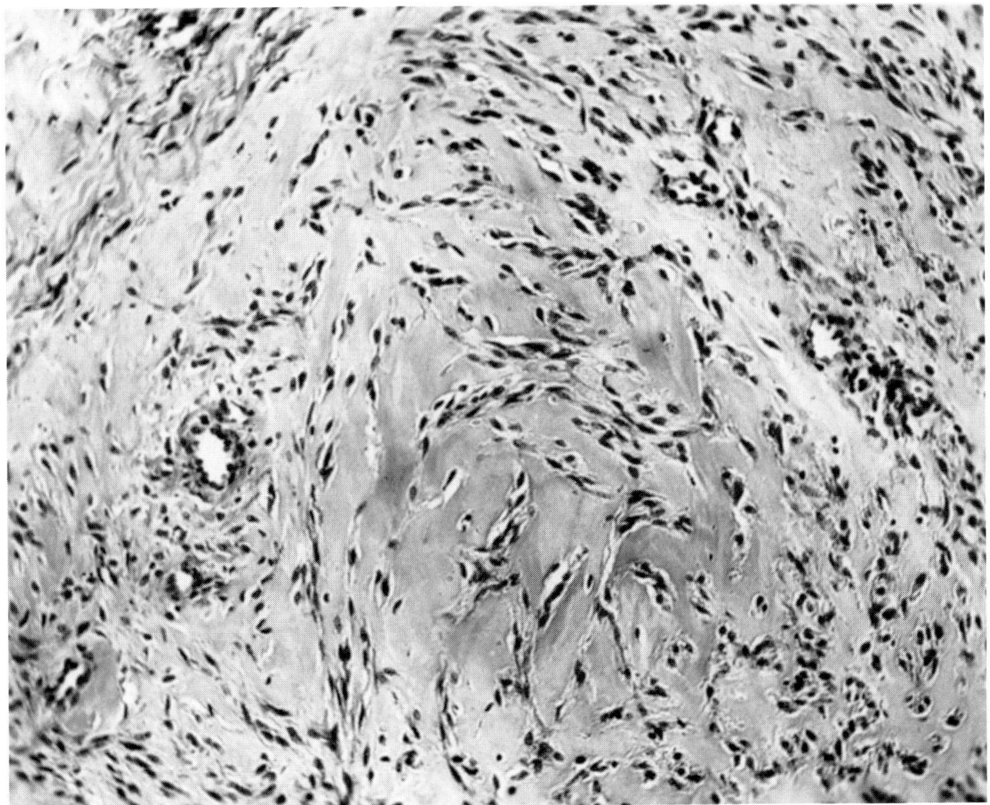

**FIGURE 11–27.** Juvenile hyalin fibromatosis. Cords of fibroblasts are associated with large amounts of hyalinized collagen-like material.

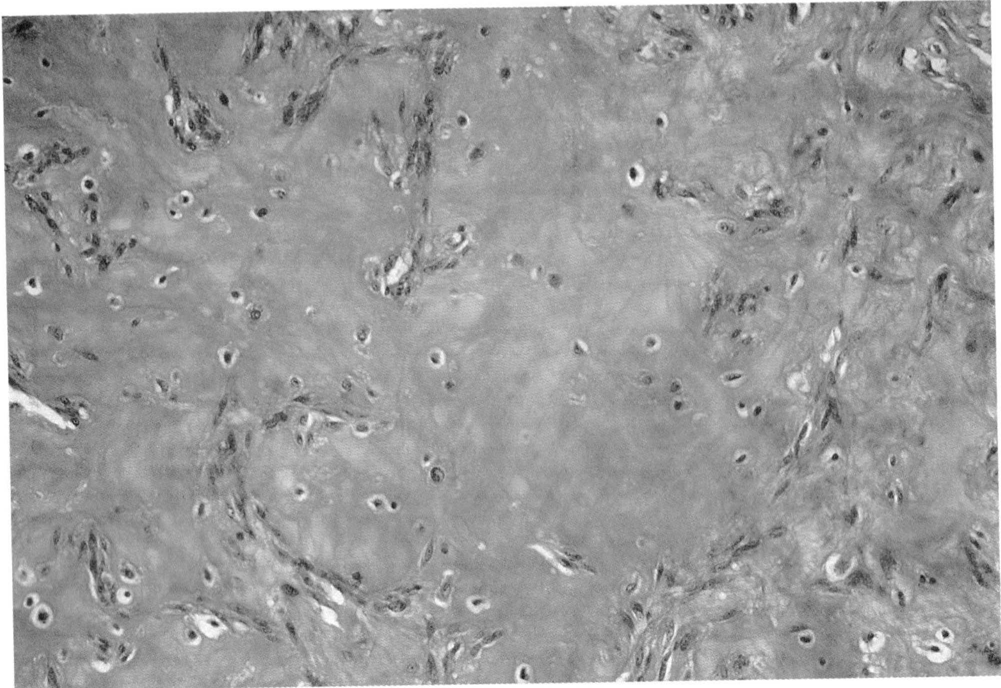

**FIGURE 11–28.** Less cellular area of juvenile hyalin fibromatosis than in Figure 11–27, with only scattered cells deposited in densely hyalinized stroma.

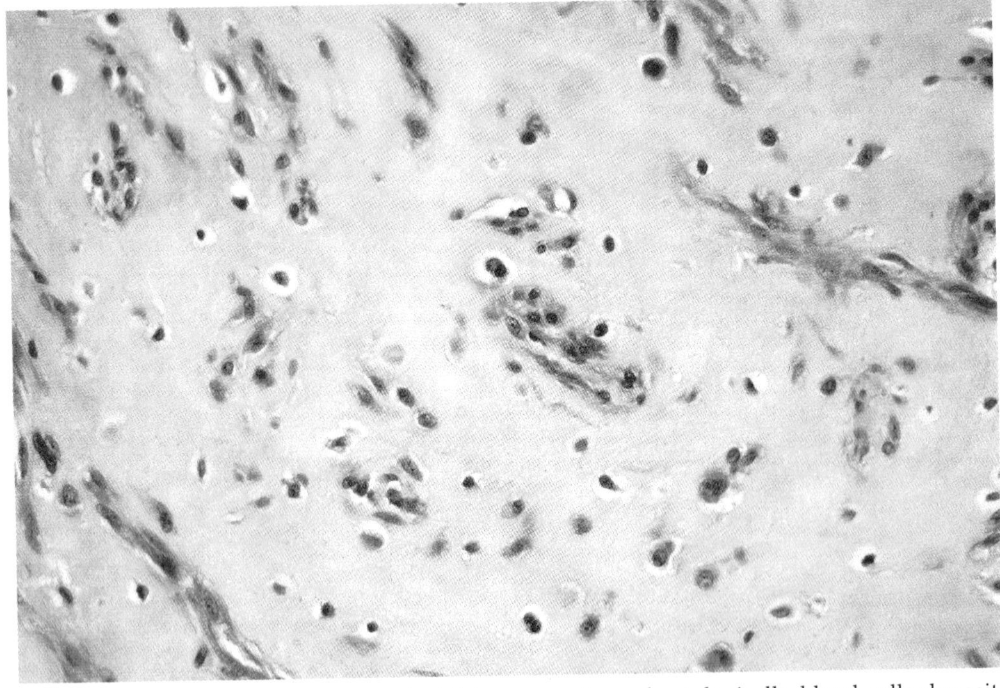

**FIGURE 11–29.** Juvenile hyalin fibromatosis. High-power view of cytologically bland cells deposited in a densely hyalinized stroma.

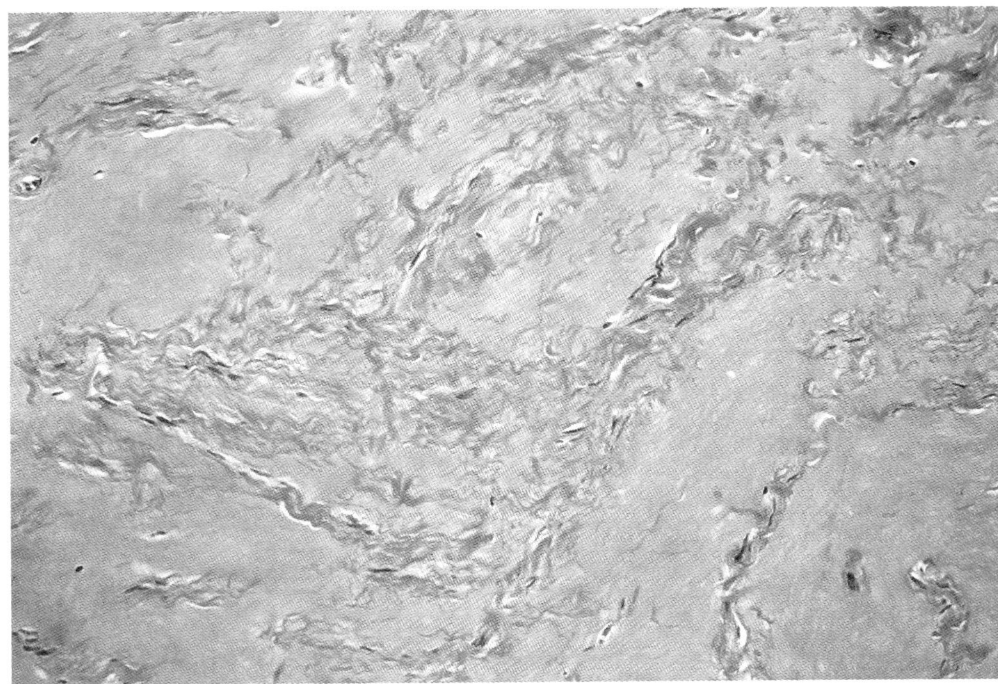

**FIGURE 11–30.** Juvenile hyalin fibromatosis. This lesion of long duration is almost completely acellular.

pear into adult life. The nodules continue to grow slowly and may ulcerate the overlying skin.[133] Spontaneous regression of the lesions has been reported only rarely.[116,141] Although local recurrence does occur, Woyke et al. reported a patient who underwent successful surgical removal of more than 100 tumors over a period of 19 years with good cosmetic results.[153] Hence these authors advocate surgical excision of all newly discovered tumors and hypertrophic gingival tissue. On the other hand, Quintal and Jackson reported a patient who had numerous surgical excisions over a period of 34 years and found that the therapy was as mutilating as the disease.[143] The tumors do not appear to respond to radiotherapy.[143,153] Most patients with long-term follow-up are severely physically handicapped by joint contractures, although there may be slight joint improvement with cortisone, adrenocortisotropic hormone (ACTH) therapy, and physiotherapy.[119]

The condition is inherited as an autosomal recessive trait. It usually affects more than one sibling of the same family. Although we are not aware that it has ever been observed in more than one generation, consanguinuity of the parents of the afflicted children has been reported.[113]

It has been hypothesized that juvenile hyalin fibromatosis is a connective tissue disorder characterized by aberrant synthesis of glycosaminoglycans by fibroblasts.[117] The matrix is composed predominantly of chondroitin sulfate[128,135] with significant amounts of type VI collagen and dermatan sulfate.[131]

## GINGIVAL FIBROMATOSIS

Gingival fibromatosis is a rare benign fibroproliferative disorder that has been described under various names, including *idiopathic* or *hereditary gingival fibromatosis*,[156,161,185] *hereditary gingival hyperplasia*,[163] *congenital macrogingivae*,[159] *generalized hypertrophy of the gums*,[168] and *gingival elephantiasis*.[181] It is a clinically distinct entity that chiefly affects young persons of both genders and has a tendency for recurrent local growth. Lesions may be idiopathic or familial, and some are associated with a heterogeneous group of hereditary syndromes. Takagi et al.[179] classified gingival fibromatosis into six categories: (1) isolated familial gingival fibromatosis; (2) isolated idiopathic gingival fibromatosis; (3) gingival fibromatosis associated with hypertrichosis; (4) gingival fibromatosis associated with hypertrichosis and mental retardation or epilepsy (or both); (5) gingival fibromatosis with mental retardation, epilepsy, or both; and (6) gingival fibromatosis associated with hereditary syndromes.

### Clinical Findings

The principal complaint is of a slowly growing, ill-defined enlargement or swelling of the gingivae, causing little pain but considerable difficulty in speaking and eating. The gingival overgrowth may be to such a degree that the teeth are completely covered and the lips are prevented from closing.[161] The lesions may also extend over the hard palate, resulting in a deformity of the contour of the palate.[179] Some patients also have marked swelling of the jaw bone. In some cases the swelling is minimal and is limited to a small portion of the gum (*localized type*), but in most cases it is extensive and bilateral, involving the gingival tissues of both the upper and lower jaws and the hard palate (*generalized type*). Idiopathic cases are slightly more common than familial cases. Among the idiopathic cases, the generalized type outnumbers the localized type by almost 2:1.[179] Most familial cases are generalized, as relatively few localized familial cases have been documented.[169,175,178] The condition occurs at any age, most at the time of eruption of the deciduous or permanent teeth. In fact, it has been postulated that the erupting teeth trigger the fibrous growth, as evidenced by effective treatment with tooth extraction alone in some cases. Patients with the familial form of the disease tend to be younger than those with the idiopathic form. Up to 8% of cases are found at birth or immediately after delivery.[179]

Hypertrichosis is found in almost 10% of patients with this condition. Some patients also have mental retardation or epilepsy (or both), although the latter features may be present in the absence of hypertrichosis. The gingival fibromatosis associated with these conditions generally occurs at a younger age than in the idiopathic form and is more common in females.

This condition may also be associated with a variety of syndromes. *Zimmerman-Laband syndrome* is a rare autosomal dominant disorder characterized by gingival fibromatosis, various skeletal anomalies including dysplasia of the distal phalanges of thumbs and halluces, vertebral defects, and hepatosplenomegaly.[160,170,171,180] Gingival fibromatosis has also been found to be associated with cherubism (*Ramon syndrome*),[173,174,183] hearing loss and supernumerary teeth,[182] *Klippel-Trenaunay-Weber syndrome*,[166] *Cowden's disease*,[156,179] and prune-belly syndrome.[167]

### Pathologic Findings

Grossly, the growth consists of dense scar-like tissue that cuts with difficulty and has a gray-white glistening surface. On microscopic examination, the specimens (which vary little in appearance) consist of poorly cellular, richly collagenous fibrous connective tissue underneath a normal or acanthotic squamous epithelium. Mild perivascular chronic inflammation and small foci of dystrophic calcification may be present.[165,169] The histologic features of the familial and idiopathic forms are indistinguishable. Ultrastructurally, the lesion is composed mainly of fusiform fibroblast-like cells with scattered myofibroblast-like cells with dilated endoplasmic reticulum; these cells are surrounded by abundant collagen and an interspersed finely granular substance.[179]

### Differential Diagnosis

There is a striking resemblance between gingival fibromatosis and hypertrophy of the gums following prolonged therapy with diphenylhydantoin sodium (Dilantin, phenytoin sodium).[155,162] In epileptic patients treated with this drug, it is difficult if not impossible to determine the cause of the gingival overgrowth. However, patients with gingival fibromatosis and epilepsy were described prior to the use of phenytoin, indicating that the changes are not entirely drug-induced. Lesions of similar appearance may also be found during pregnancy and as the result of chronic gingivitis. In most of these cases, a detailed clinical and family history permits the correct diagnosis. *Juvenile hyalin fibromatosis,* a hereditary lesion that may involve the gingiva in a similar manner, can be distinguished by its association with multiple cutaneous tumors and the characteristic microscopic appearance, especially the prominent PAS-positive hyaline matrix.

### Discussion

Surgical excision of the hyperplastic tissue is frequently followed by local recurrence.[161] However, the overgrowth may recede or disappear with tooth extraction. Thus many authors recommend excision of the excess tissue and removal of all teeth in severe cases.[161,184] Others have reported success with $CO_2$ laser excision.[158,172,176]

Approximately 35% of cases of gingival fibromatosis are familial. Most appear to be inherited in an autosomal dominant manner,[157,165,169] but others are inherited in an autosomal recessive manner.[177] Although Takagi et al. did not identify any cytogenetic defects in two patients with gingival fibromatosis,[179] Fryns identified partial duplication of the short arm of chromosome 2 in a case of gingival fibromatosis.[164]

## FIBROMATOSIS COLLI

Fibromatosis colli has long been recognized as a peculiar benign fibrous growth of the sternocleidomastoid muscle that usually appears during the first weeks of life and is often associated with muscular torticollis, or wryneck. It bears a close resemblance to other forms of infantile fibromatosis but is sufficiently different in its microscopic appearance and behavior to warrant separation as a distinct entity. According to Coventry et al., it occurs in 0.4% of newborns.[192] The finding of torticollis is not synonymous with the presence of fibromatosis colli, as nearly 80 entities have been reported to cause torticollis (acquired torticollis).[202]

## Clinical Findings

Characteristically, the lesion manifests between the second and fourth weeks of life as a mass lying in or replacing the mid to lower portion of the sternocleidomastoid muscle, especially its sternal or clavicular portion. The lesion is movable only in a horizontal plane and never affects the overlying skin. Rare cases also simultaneously involve the trapezius muscle.[203] The lesion is rarely noted at birth or before the second week of life. Most commonly, a 1–3 cm long, hard mass or "bulb" is palpable at the base of the sternocleidomastoid muscle 2–4 weeks after birth. Although the lesion may be first noted in older patients, fewer than one-fifth give a history of a mass during the neonatal period.[203] Almost all cases are unilateral, with a slight predilection for the right side of the neck; rare cases of bilateral fibromatosis colli have been described.[208] Most authors have found a slight predilection for this lesion to occur in boys.[186,191,196,212]

Initially the mass grows rapidly, but after a few weeks or months the growth slows and becomes stationary. In many cases, spontaneous regression occurs by the age of 1–2 years, and the lesion may no longer be palpable. During the initial growth period, torticollis (rotation and tilting of the head to the affected side) occurs in only about one-fourth to one-third of cases and usually is mild and transient. In addition, the face and skull on the affected side may begin to appear smaller, resulting in facial asymmetry and plagiocephaly; there is flattening of the affected side of the face with posterior displacement of the ipsilateral ear.[188] A number of patients with this lesion present with torticollis later in life, as the affected sternocleidomastoid muscle is incapable of keeping pace with the growth and elongation of the sternocleidomastoid muscle on the opposite side, causing functional imbalance and torticollis.[207]

Fibromatosis colli is associated with a high incidence of difficult deliveries. Specifically, breech deliveries have been reported in up to 60% of these patients,[190,191,195,197,206] and a significant number have also been associated with forceps delivery.[190,203] Several reports have noted an association with other congenital anomalies, including rib cage anomalies[190] and ipsilateral congenital dysplasia of the hip.[187,190,198]

Rare cases of fibromatosis colli appear to be familial. A hereditary component to this disease was first proposed by Joachimsthal in 1905,[200] and since that time there have been numerous reports of familial muscular torticollis.[189,214,216,219,220] Isigkeit reported that 11.2% of 1388 patients with fibromatosis colli had a positive family history[199] and concluded that this condition is a hereditary disease that is influenced by environmental factors.

## Pathologic Findings

When the growth is excised at an early stage, the operative specimen consists of a small mass of firm tissue averaging 1–2 cm in diameter. The cut surface is gray-white and glistening and blends imperceptibly with surrounding skeletal muscle. Microscopic examination of the lesion discloses partial replacement of the sternocleidomastoid muscle by a diffuse fibroblastic proliferation of varying cellularity (Figs. 11–31, 11–32). The constituent cells lack significant nuclear hyperchromasia, pleomorphism, and mitotic activity. Scattered throughout the lesion are residual muscle fibers that have undergone atrophy or degeneration with swelling, loss of cross-striations, and proliferation of sarcolemmal nuclei. This intimate mixture of proliferated fibroblasts and residual atrophic skeletal muscle fibers is fully diagnostic of the lesion and should not be confused with the infiltrative growth of a malignant neoplasm. Lesions of longer duration typically show less cellularity and more stromal collagen, but there does not appear to be a correlation between the histologic picture and the age of the patient. Although hemosiderin deposits are present in some cases, they are never a prominent feature. Unlike *fibrosing myositis,* there is no inflammatory infiltrate; unlike *fibrodysplasia ossificans progressiva,* there are no associated malformations of the hands or feet. Numerous reports have advocated the reliability of fine-needle aspiration for diagnosing this lesion, with the aspirate characterized by bland spindle-shaped fibroblasts of low cellularity admixed with degenerating skeletal muscle fibers.[210,211,213,215,221]

## Prognosis and Treatment

After a stationary period of several months, the growth slowly subsides and spontaneously resolves in up to 70% of cases by 1 year of age without surgical treatment.[187,192,197] It never recurs and at no time behaves aggressively, although some patients develop a compensatory thoracic scoliosis, persistent head tilt, or obvious cosmetic deformity.[190] Recommendations as to the best type of therapy differ. Most advocate a conservative approach for patients younger than 1 year of age, often with implementation of an exercise program.[190,203–205] Surgery is a more effective mode of therapy for patients more than 1 year of age.[190,205] Features predictive of a poor outcome include the

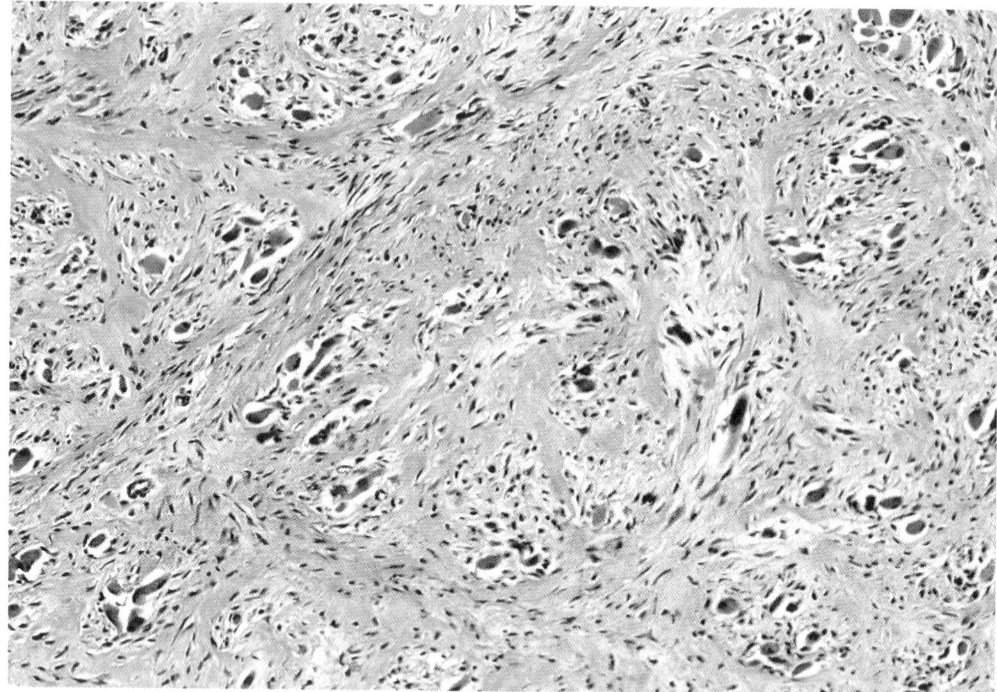

**FIGURE 11–31.** Fibromatosis colli in a 4-month-old boy. Note the intimate mixture of fibrous tissue and entrapped and partly atrophic muscle fibers.

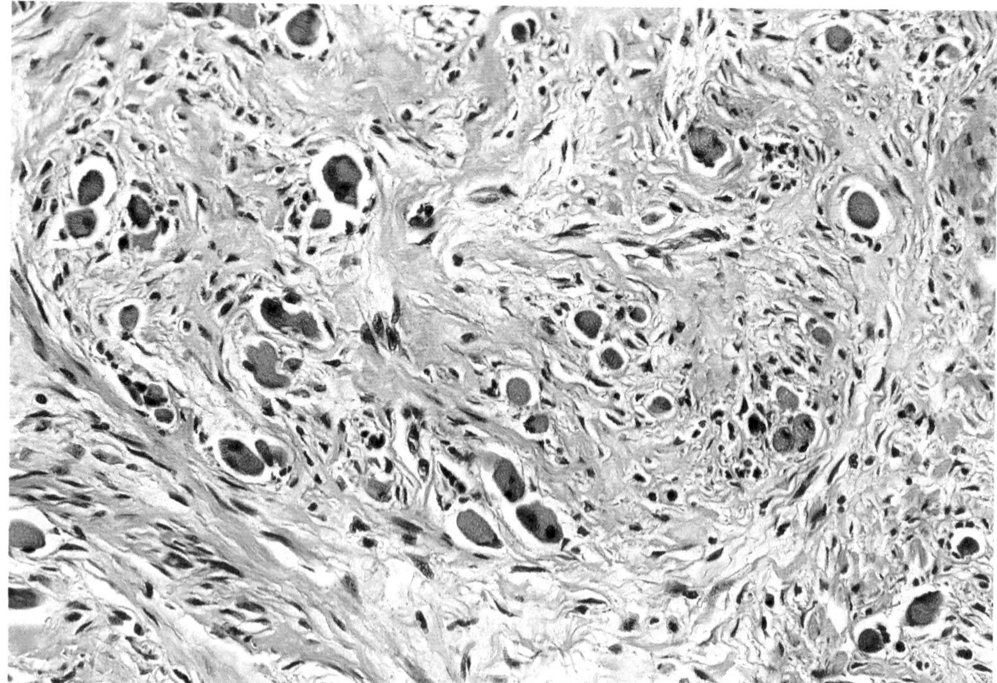

**FIGURE 11–32.** Fibromatosis colli. Separation of atrophic muscle fibers by dense fibrous tissue.

presence of severe facial asymmetry, significant limitation of neck rotation,[190] and delayed treatment.[203] Ferkel et al.[194] reported better surgical results with release of the sternal and clavicular heads of the sternocleidomastoid muscle, but most have not found that one surgical approach is better than another.

### Discussion

The cause of the growth has been the subject of considerable debate in the literature. In view of the unusually high incidence of breech and forceps deliveries, birth injury may play a role in the pathogenesis.[218] Stromeyer proposed that rupture of the sternocleidomastoid muscle during birth results in formation of a hematoma with subsequent fibrous replacement of the sternocleidomastoid muscle.[217] However, microscopic examination reveals little evidence of an organizing hematoma, and few cases exhibit deposition of hemosiderin. The fact that coexistent facial deformities are often present at birth and the development of these lesions in patients following cesarean section[201] casts doubt on this hypothesis. Several authors have proposed that intrauterine trauma results in torticollis that subsequently predisposes to an increased incidence of complicated deliveries.[192,193] Others have postulated that abnormal intrauterine positioning results in occlusion of the sternocleidomastoid branch of the superior thyroid artery, resulting in ischemic necrosis of the sternocleidomastoid muscle.[209] Middleton proposed that venous occlusion during labor could result in a similar mechanism of injury.[207] Certainly, contributing genetic factors are suggested by the reports of familial fibromatosis colli and association of the growth with certain congenital malformations.

## INFANTILE FIBROMATOSIS

Infantile fibromatosis, which represents the childhood counterpart of musculoaponeurotic fibromatosis (abdominal or extraabdominal desmoid), usually arises as a solitary mass in skeletal muscle or in the adjacent fascia, aponeurosis, or periosteum. It chiefly affects children from birth to 8 years of age and is slightly more common in boys than girls. There are considerable variations in its morphologic appearance, depending on the stage of differentiation of the constituent fibroblasts. The lesion ranges from a tumor composed of primitive mesenchymal cells (diffuse or mesenchymal type) to those that closely resemble adult desmoids (desmoid type), except perhaps for a less uniform pattern and a greater degree of cellularity.

Stout was the first to identify and describe the childhood form of fibromatosis as a distinct entity,[253] but since his report relatively few cases have been added to the literature and some of those were without detailed information as to their histologic picture or clinical behavior.

### Clinical Findings

Most patients present with a solitary firm mass that is poorly circumscribed and deep-seated and that usually has grown rapidly during the preceding weeks or months. In almost all cases, the mass is noted during the first 8 years of life, most commonly before age 2. Although most patients are asymptomatic, some report pain or tenderness of the involved site.[246] Most originate in skeletal muscle, especially the muscles of the head and neck, shoulder and upper arm, and thigh.[226,230,233,234] In the head and neck region the preferred sites are the tongue, mandible, maxilla, and mastoid process.[225,237,243,251,254–256] Unusual sites in the head and neck region include the paranasal sinuses[239,242] and parotid gland.[244] As the region progresses, it may infiltrate adjacent muscles and grow around vessels and nerves, with resultant tenderness, pain, or functional disturbances. Involvement of the joint capsule may lead to contracture and restriction of movement.

Radiographic examination shows a soft tissue mass sometimes associated with bowing or deformation of bone, especially in cases in which the onset was during the first 2–3 years of life and has been present for several months or years.[230] Lesions in the regions of the mandible, maxilla, or mastoid frequently involve bone; it may be difficult to determine whether the lesion arose in the soft tissues, periosteum, or bone,[227,241,247,257] thereby making distinction from desmoplastic fibroma of bone difficult in some cases.[238] Eady et al. described an unusual case in which congenital bowing of the ulna and dislocation of the radial head preceded the onset of fibromatosis.[231]

### Pathologic Findings

Grossly, the tumor is a firm, ill-defined scar-like mass of gray-white tissue measuring 1–10 cm in greatest diameter, although some may be as large as 19 cm.[226] The tumor is not encapsulated and usually is excised together with portions of the involved muscle and subcutaneous fat (Figs. 11–33, 11–34).

Microscopically, infantile fibromatosis has a wide morphologic spectrum reflecting progressive stages in the differentiation of the fibroblasts. The more common form of infantile fibromatosis is the *diffuse* (*mesenchymal*) type. This form, found chiefly in infants during the first few months of life, is characterized by small, haphazardly arranged round or oval cells in a

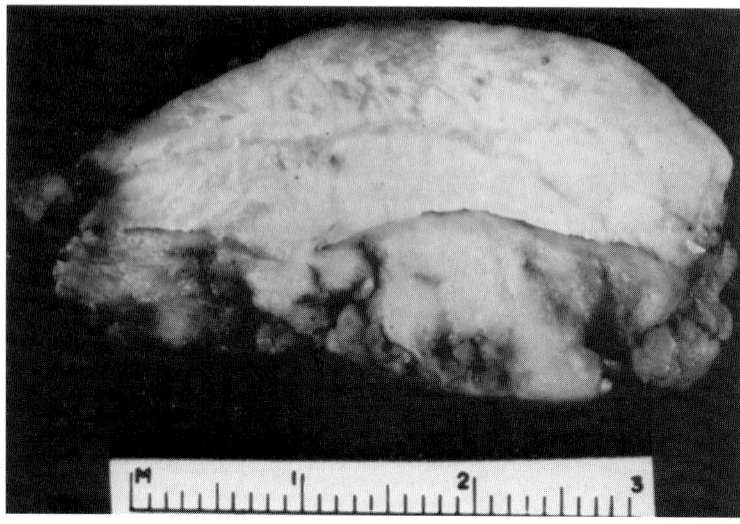

**FIGURE 11–33.** Infantile fibromatosis. Replacement of muscle tissue by fibrous tissue and mature fat bearing a superficial resemblance to a lipomatous tumor. The lesion was excised from the right arm of a 2-year-old girl.

myxoid background (Figs. 11–35 to 11–40). The cells are intermediate in appearance between primitive mesenchymal cells and fibroblasts, and they are often intimately associated with residual muscle fibers and lipocytes. The interspersed lipocytes are probably the result of ex vacuo fatty proliferation secondary to muscular atrophy of the infiltrated and immobilized muscle tissue. Peripherally located lymphocytic inflammation may be present. These areas blend with a more cellular proliferation composed chiefly of plump and spindle-shaped fibroblasts arranged in distinct bundles and fascicles. It may be highly cellular, and mitotic figures may be found, making distinction from infantile fibrosarcoma rather difficult and somewhat arbitrary in some cases. This lesion goes by several names, including cellular fibromatosis,[249] fibrosarcoma-like fibromatosis, and aggressive infantile fibromatosis.[224]

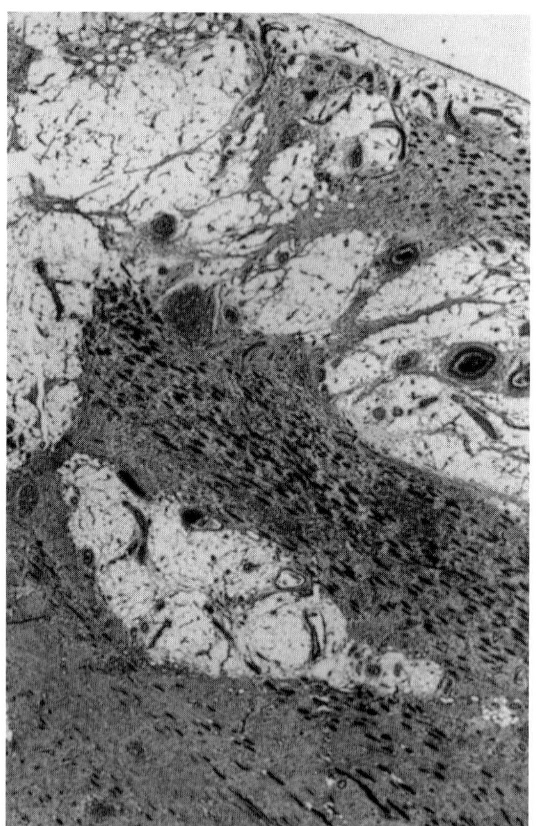

**FIGURE 11–34.** Photomicrograph of the infantile fibromatosis shown in Figure 11–33.

The less common form of infantile fibromatosis (*desmoid type*) is virtually indistinguishable from the adult form of fibromatosis or desmoid tumor. This form usually occurs in children older than 5 years of age, and its behavior appears to be similar to that of the adult form of fibromatosis.[250] Rare cases show focal calcification[230] or ossification.[235]

Like other forms of fibromatosis, infantile fibromatosis is composed of a mixture of fibroblasts and myofibroblasts with prominent, often dilated endoplasmic reticulum and bundles of peripherally located microfilaments in some cells.[247] Immunohistochemically, the more primitive-appearing cells characteristic of the diffuse type and the plump spindle-shaped cells of both the diffuse and desmoid types stain for vimentin, with variable staining for muscle markers including muscle-specific actin, smooth muscle actin, and desmin.[248]

## Differential Diagnosis

The differential diagnosis depends on the type of infantile fibromatosis encountered. The diffuse (mesenchymal) type of this tumor frequently causes diagnos-

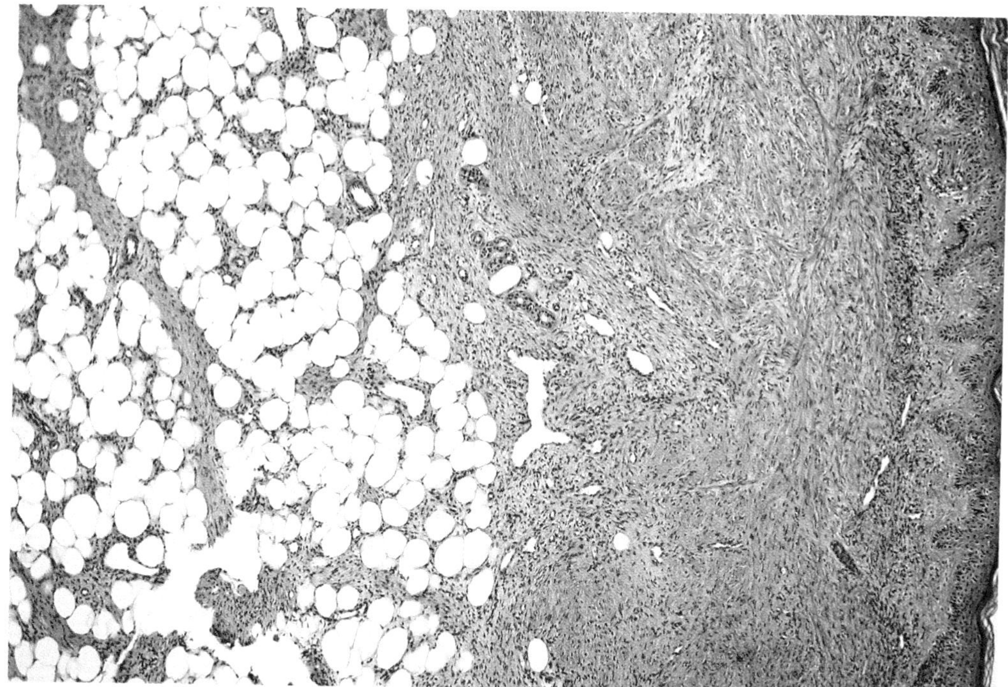

**FIGURE 11–35.** Infantile fibromatosis, diffuse type, with infiltration of small ovoid cells in the dermis and subcutis.

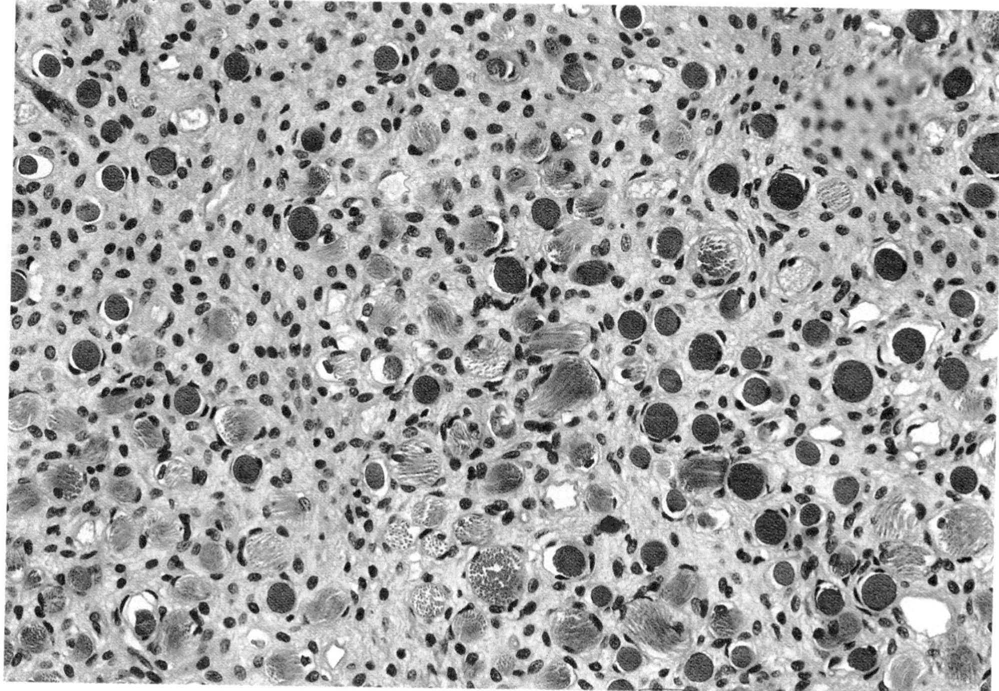

**FIGURE 11–36.** Infantile fibromatosis, diffuse type, removed from the trapezius muscle of a 5½-month-old girl. The absence of digital malformations helps distinguish it from an early nonossifying stage of fibrodysplasia ossificans progressiva.

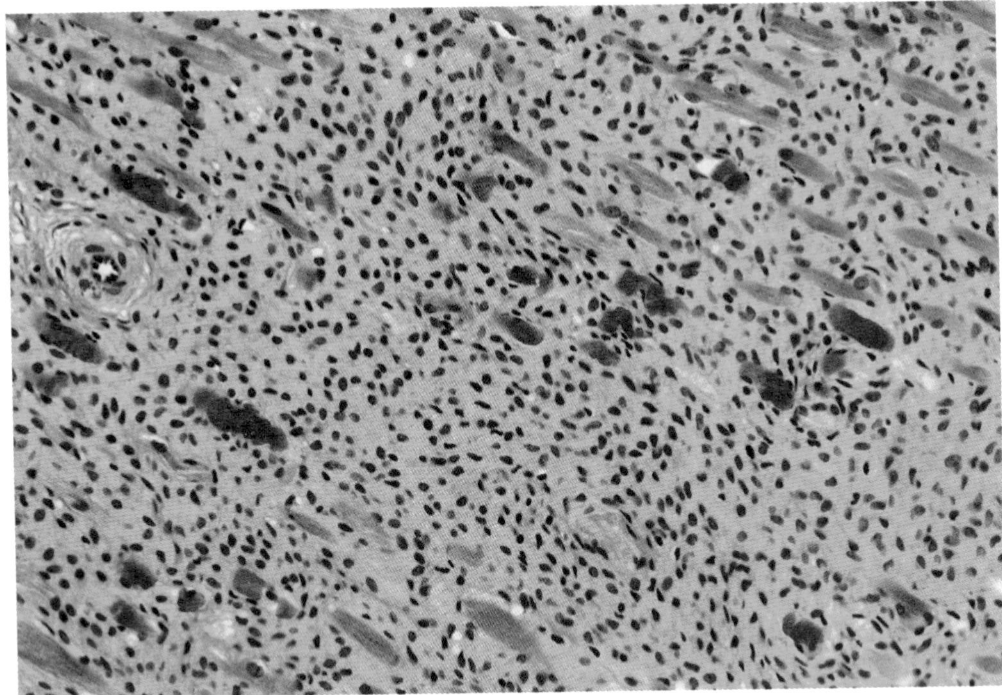

**FIGURE 11–37.** Infantile fibromatosis, diffuse type. Note the separation of striated muscle fibers by primitive fibroblasts with little variation in size and shape.

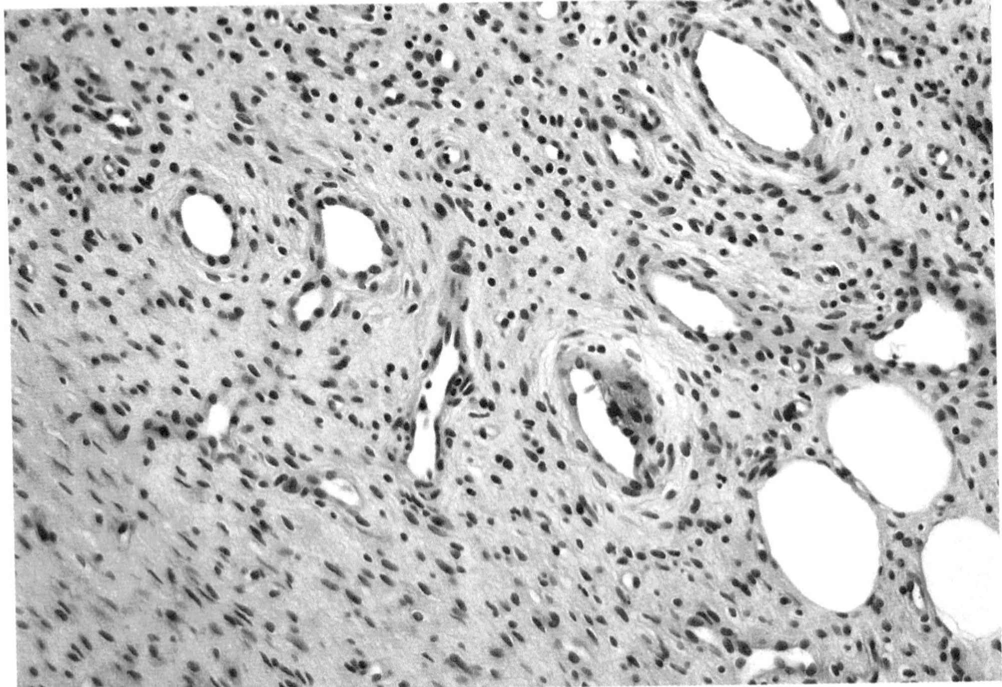

**FIGURE 11–38.** Infantile fibromatosis, diffuse type. Immature fibroblasts are deposited in a myxoid background.

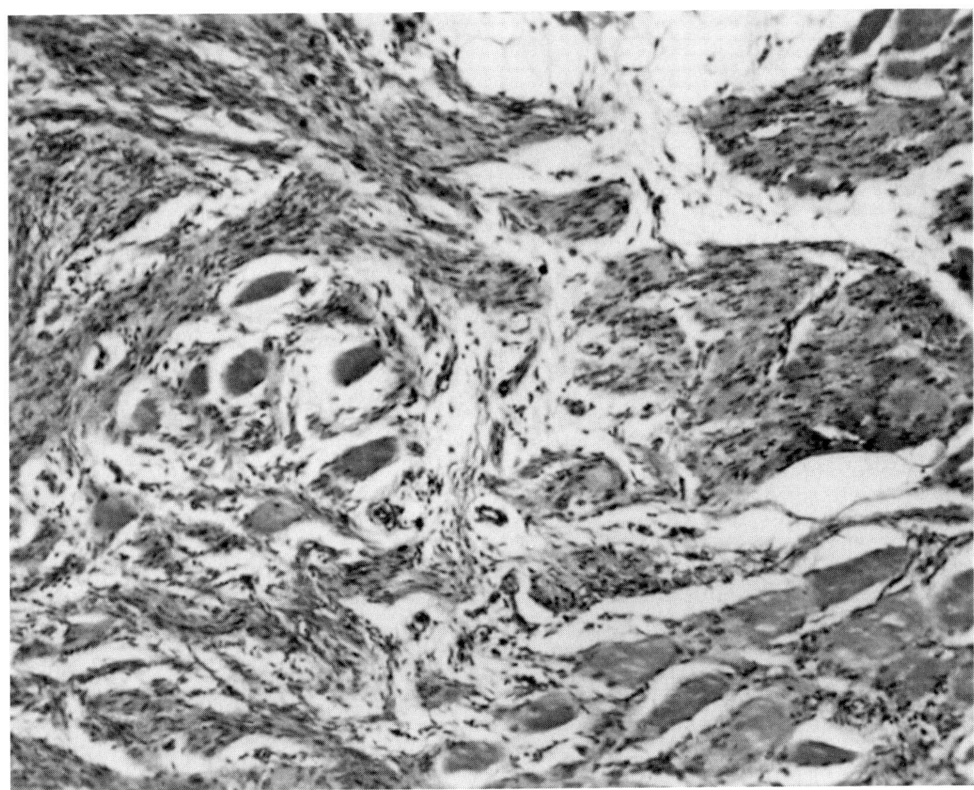

**FIGURE 11–39.** Infantile fibromatosis showing a more cellular picture and greater amounts of collagen than in Figures 11–37 and 11–38. This type prevails in children 1–3 years of age.

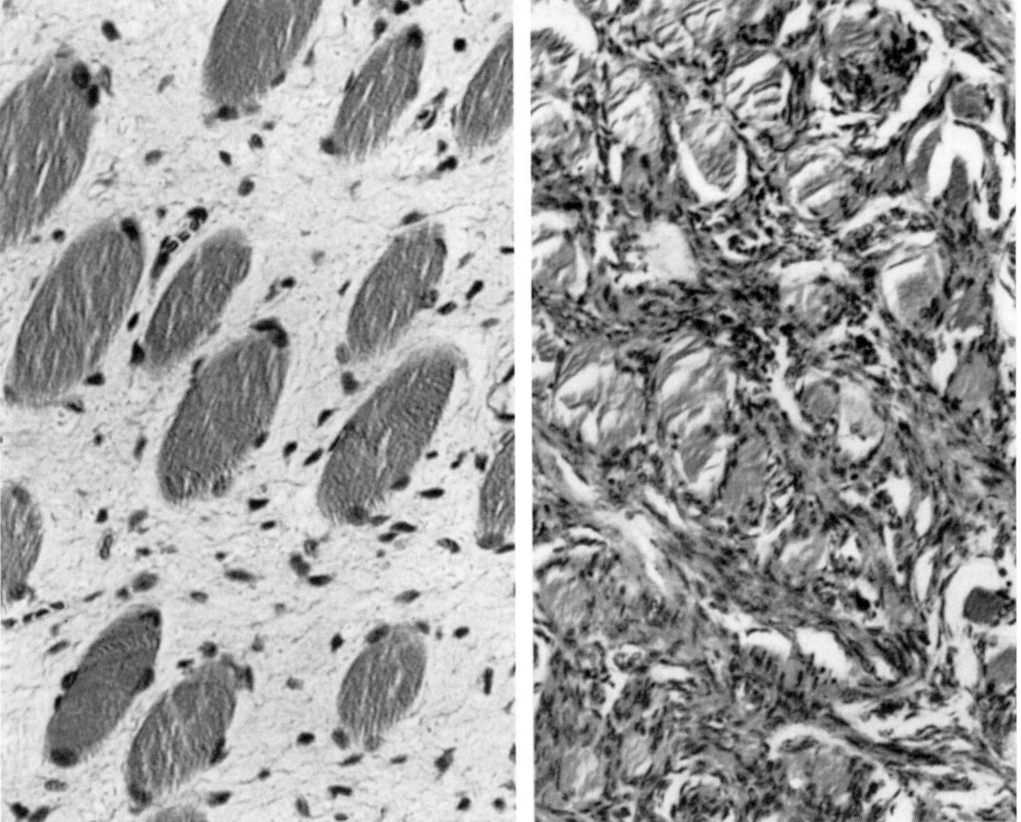

**FIGURE 11–40.** Infantile fibromatosis, diffuse type, with ovoid cells deposited in a myxoid stroma infiltrating residual skeletal muscle fibers.

tic problems, as it may be confused with a wide variety of myxoid or lipomatous lesions because of the large amounts of glycosaminoglycans (mucopolysaccharides) in its stroma and the partial replacement of the infiltrated muscle by lipocytes. *Myxoid liposarcoma* is rare in children younger than 5 years of age and is characterized by the presence of a uniform plexiform capillary pattern and variable numbers of typical lipoblasts. *Lipoblastomatosis,* the infantile counterpart of lipoma, can be distinguished by its distinctly lobular pattern and the uniform appearance of the constituent lipoblasts. There may be some resemblance to *botryoid rhabdomyosarcoma,* which has a similar age incidence; but this lesion is uncommon in the musculature and nearly always occurs in the wall of mucosa-lined cavities such as the urinary bladder or vagina. *Fibrodysplasia ossificans progressiva* bears some resemblance to the diffuse form of infantile fibromatosis, but patients with this disorder have bilateral malformations and shortening of fingers and toes (microdactylia).[228] Confusion may also occur with the early stages of *calcifying aponeurotic fibroma,* although the lesion is characterized by its location in the palmar and plantar regions as well as foci of linear calcifications and chondroid metaplasia.

Perhaps the most difficult problem in the differential diagnosis is distinguishing the more cellular variants of infantile fibromatosis from *infantile fibrosarcoma* (Table 11–2). Although infantile fibrosarcoma has a more favorable prognosis than adult fibrosarcoma, most of these tumors resemble the adult form of fibrosarcoma, with characteristic high cellularity, arrangement in a uniform herringbone pattern, and a high mitotic rate. In addition, zones of hemorrhage and necrosis are not uncommon. In our experience, distinction between infantile fibromatosis and infantile fibrosarcoma is usually feasible if one pays attention to the infiltrative growth pattern of fibromatosis and its variation in the degree of cellularity, often with alternating cellular and more collagenous areas, resembling the desmoid form. Yet in some cases reliable distinction between these entities is difficult if not impossible. Several authors have proposed that the relative number and distribution of nucleolar organizer regions (AgNORs) are useful parameters for distinguishing infantile fibromatosis from infantile fibrosarcoma.[232,248] Cytogenetics may also be useful in this regard, as infantile fibrosarcoma is characterized by gains of chromosomes 8, 11, 17, and 20,[222,223,229,240,249] whereas these changes are not present in infantile fibromatosis. Transitions from fibromatosis to fibrosarcoma have not been clearly established, and the recorded metastasizing cases of fibromatosis may actually be infantile fibrosarcoma.[252]

**TABLE 11–2 SUMMARY OF FEATURES DISTINGUISHING INFANTILE FIBROMATOSIS AND INFANTILE FIBROSARCOMA**

| Feature | Infantile Fibromatosis | Infantile Fibrosarcoma |
|---|---|---|
| Cellularity | Variable | Moderate to high |
| Herringbone pattern | Absent | Usually present |
| Mitotic figures | Rare | Few to many |
| Hemorrhage | Absent | Often present |
| Necrosis | Absent | Often present |
| Karyotype (+8,11,17,20) | Absent | Present |

## Discussion

Although the tumor does not metastasize, it may reach a large size and tends to recur locally when inadequately excised. In the series by Faulkner et al.,[233] none of the patients developed metastatic disease or died as a direct result of their tumor, but 41 of 63 patients (65%) developed local recurrences, with 51% of them appearing less than 1 year after the initial excision, and 90% occurring within 3 years. The status of the resection margins was the only significant prognostic factor, as those patients who had undergone a wide local excision with tumor-free margins were significantly less likely to develop local recurrence. Histologic features do not allow accurate prediction of the clinical course,[226,227,233] although Schmidt et al.[248] and Yokoyama et al.[258] found that the tendency to recur locally was correlated with a large number of slit-like blood vessels and increased numbers of undifferentiated mesenchymal cells. In rare cases, encroachment on critical structures, particularly those of the head and neck, may result in the patient's death.[224,246]

Complete excision with ample margins is the treatment of choice, although it is difficult in some anatomic locations and may be impossible without disfigurement or dysfunction. There is relatively little information as to the efficacy of adjuvant chemotherapy or radiotherapy. Raney et al. obtained local control in five of six patients treated with chemotherapy, radiation therapy, or both.[245] Goepfert et al. found objective improvement in all six patients treated with pre- or postoperative chemotherapy.[236]

The cause of the lesion is not clear. As with other forms of this disease, trauma has been implicated. In the series by Faulkner et al., 17% of patients had a history of antecedent trauma in the vicinity of the lesion.[233] Coffin and Dehner reported two cases that arose at sites of previous surgery.[226] Unlike many other fibrous lesions, increased familial incidence has not been observed with this type of fibromatosis.

## CONGENITAL AND INFANTILE FIBROSARCOMA

Fibrosarcoma in newborns, infants, and small children bears a close morphologic resemblance to adult fibrosarcoma, but it must be considered a separate entity because of its markedly different clinical behavior. On one hand, it must be distinguished from richly cellular forms of infantile fibromatosis, a lesion that lacks metastatic capability; on the other hand, it must be distinguished from more aggressive childhood sarcomas (e.g., embryonal rhabdomyosarcoma) that behave more aggressively, are prone to metastasize, and require more radical therapy. Fibrosarcomas in older children behave similar to those seen in adults.

Congenital or infantile fibrosarcoma is relatively rare. The first detailed clinicopathologic study of this entity was reported by Stout in 1962.[303] He reviewed 31 cases from the literature and added 23 cases of "juvenile fibrosarcoma," 11 of which developed during the first 5 years of life and 4 of which were present at birth. He suggested that fibrosarcomas arising in this group of patients were more indolent than their adult counterparts, as only 1 of the 11 patients died of metastasis. Although several subsequent smaller series of congenital and infantile fibrosarcoma were reported,[261,270,271,281] it was not until 1976 that Chung and Enzinger reported their series of 53 congenital and infantile fibrosarcomas, supporting the contention of Stout that this tumor should be considered a distinct entity.[266] Similar conclusions were reached by Soule and Pritchard in their report of 110 cases, including 70 reports from the literature and 40 from the files of the Mayo Clinic.[299]

### Clinical Findings

The principal manifestation of the disease is a nontender, painless swelling or mass that ranges from 1 to 20 cm. The tumor tends to grow steadily, although some grow rapidly; Chung and Enzinger reported one case in which the tumor "doubled in size within a period of 2.5 weeks."[266] Up to one-third of the tumors are present at birth; in most cases the mass becomes evident during the first year of life. In the series by Chung and Enzinger, 20 of 53 tumors (38%) were present at birth, and 27 (51%) were noted before 3 months of life.[266] Similarly, 40 of the 110 (36%) cases reported by Soule and Pritchard were congenital.[299] Males are affected slightly more commonly than females. The principal sites of involvement are the extremities, especially the regions of the foot, ankle, and lower leg and the hand, wrist, and forearm. The next most common sites of involvement are the trunk and head and neck regions, although these tumors have also been reported in such locations as the retroperitoneum,[269,279,280] mesentery,[268] and orbit.[308]

Radiographic examination may show, in addition to a soft tissue mass, cortical thickening, bending deformities, and rarely extensive destruction of the underlying bone[266] (Fig. 11–41).

### Gross Findings

The tumors vary considerably in size. Some are only a few centimeters when first detected, whereas others are extremely large and may replace the entire distal portion of the involved limb. Some patients present with a large exophytic mass that ulcerates the overlying skin. Most are poorly circumscribed, are fusiform or disk-shaped, and have a gray-white or pale pink cut surface. Large tumors may be markedly distorted by central necrosis or hemorrhage (Fig. 11–42), whereas others show extensive myxoid or cystic change.[282]

### Microscopic Findings

Most of these tumors closely resemble their adult counterparts and are composed of sheets of solidly packed spindle-shaped cells that are relatively uniform in appearance and arranged in bundles or fascicles, imparting a herringbone appearance. The cells show little nuclear pleomorphism and are mitotically active, but their numbers vary from area to area in the same tumor. Tumors with abundant collagen tend to be more fasciculated and often approach the appearance of an adult fibrosarcoma. Tumors with minimal amounts of collagen, on the other hand, show a lesser degree of cellular polarity and consist of small, more rounded, immature-appearing cells with only focal evidence of fibroblastic differentiation (Figs. 11–43, 11–44, 11–45). Dahl et al. distinguished between the "medullary" type, characterized by a compact arrangement of monomorphous ovoid cells with a less conspicuous fascicular arrangement and scant stromal collagen, and the "desmoplastic" type, composed of uniform spindle-shaped cells arranged in a distinct fascicular pattern with more prominent stromal collagen[271] (Fig. 11–46).

As in the adult fibrosarcoma, multinucleated giant cells are rare. Scattered chronic inflammatory cells, particularly lymphocytes, are another common, sometimes striking feature that helps distinguish infantile from adult fibrosarcoma. Some tumors are characterized by a prominent hemangiopericytoma-like vascular pattern (Fig. 11–47) that may cause confusion with infantile hemangiopericytoma.

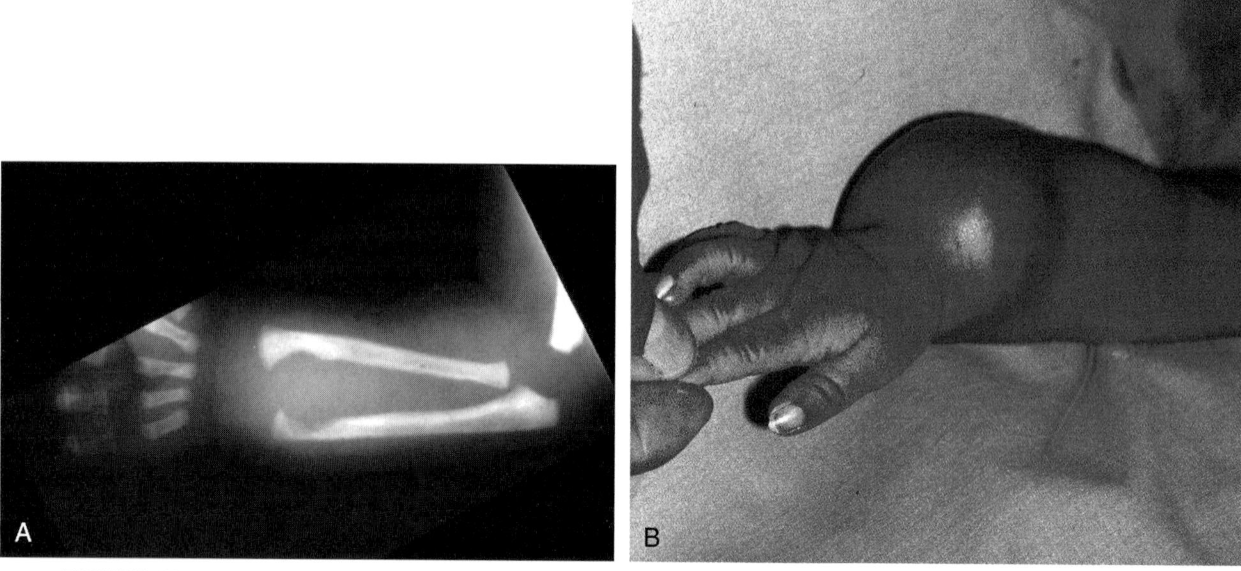


**FIGURE 11–41.** Radiograph (**A**) and gross photomicrograph (**B**) of a congenital fibrosarcoma in a 1-day-old infant.

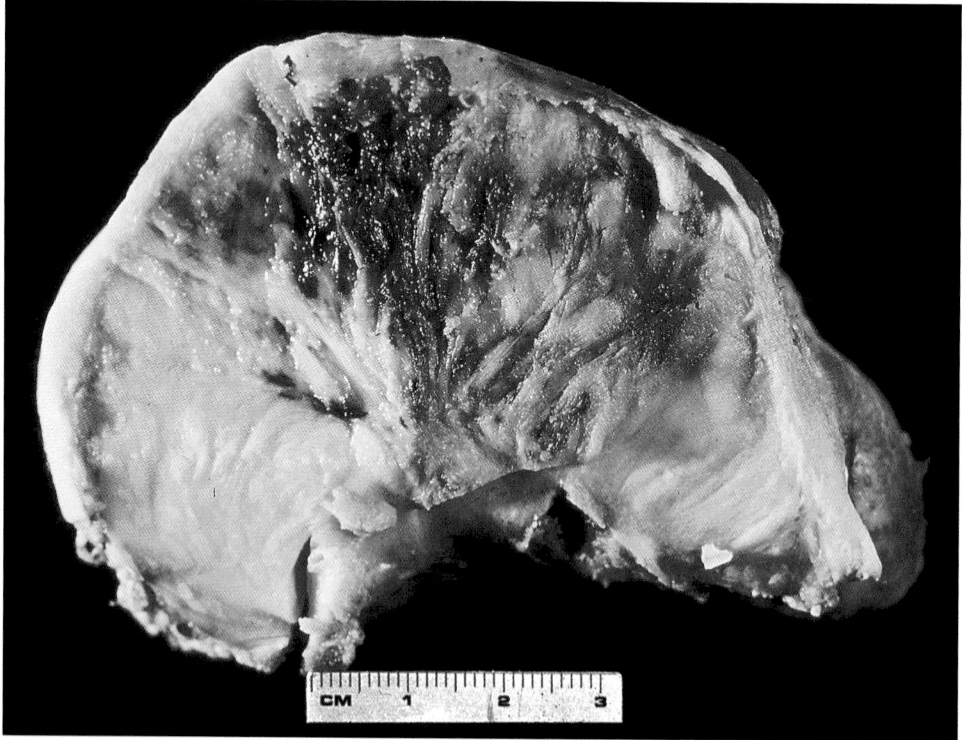


**FIGURE 11–42.** Infantile fibrosarcoma of the right shoulder in a 1-month-old boy, showing marked interstitial hemorrhage.

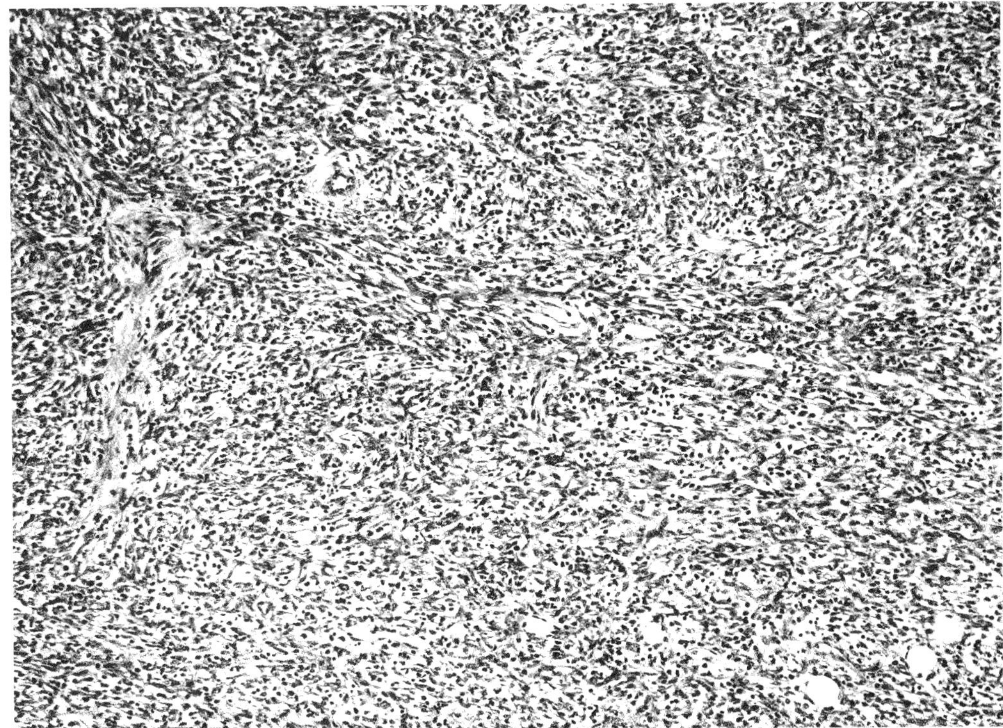

**FIGURE 11–43.** Infantile fibrosarcoma composed of uniform, well oriented fibroblasts arranged in a fascicular growth pattern.

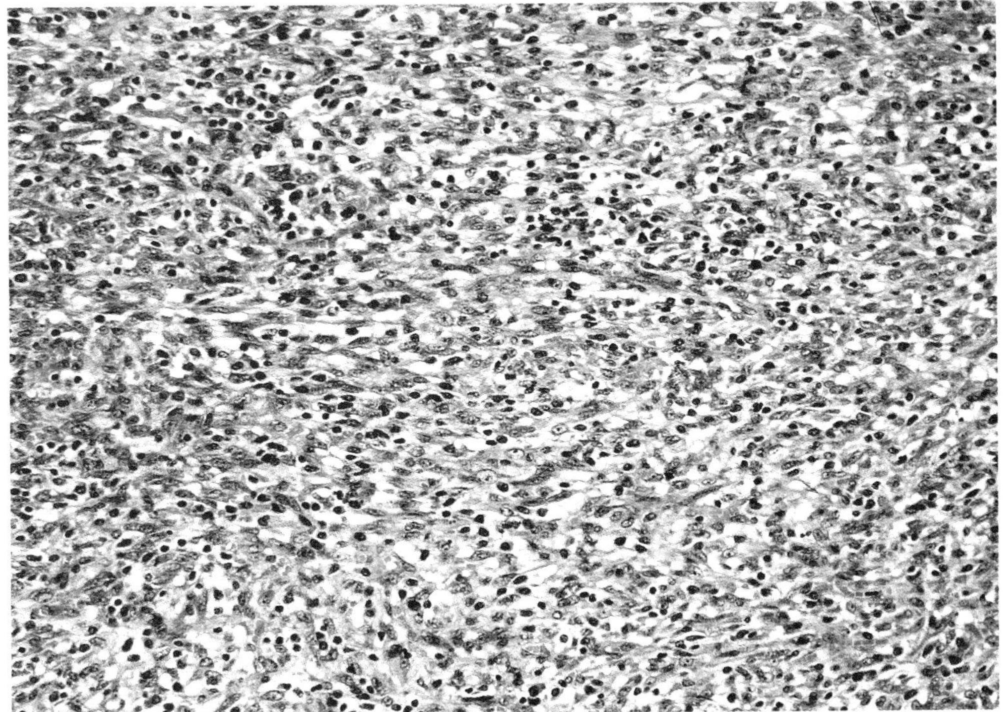

**FIGURE 11–44.** Characteristic microscopic view of an infantile fibrosarcoma with immature-appearing fibroblasts associated with small round cells, probably lymphocytes.

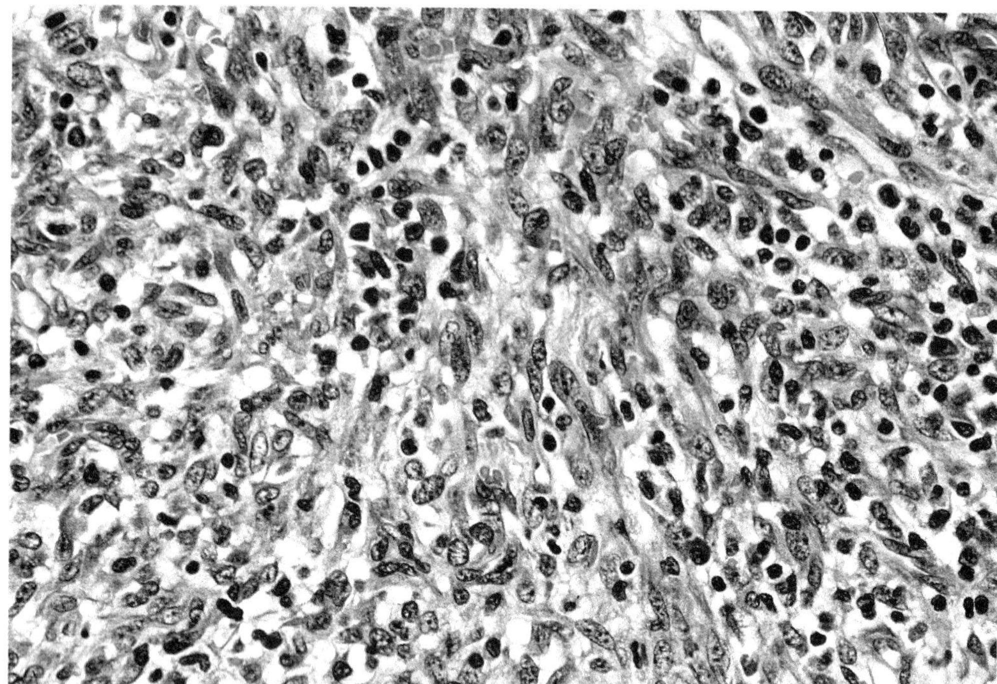

**FIGURE 11–45.** High-power view of immature-appearing fibroblasts with a prominent lymphocytic infiltrate, characteristic of infantile fibrosarcoma.

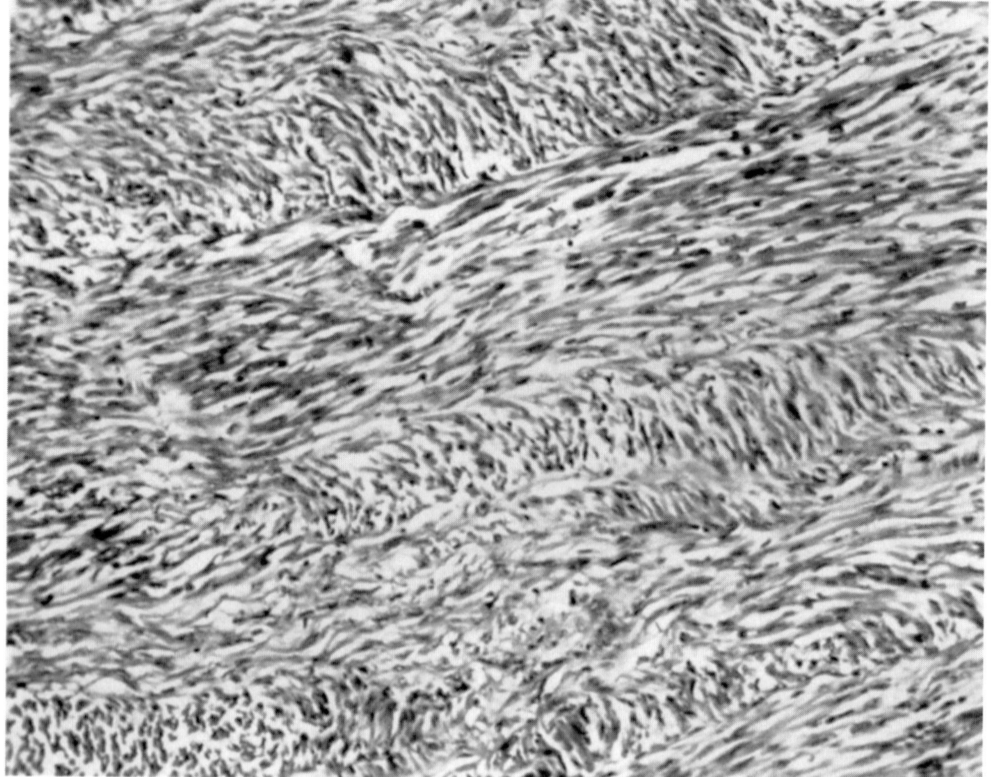

**FIGURE 11–46.** Well differentiated infantile fibrosarcoma with large amounts of interstitial collagen.

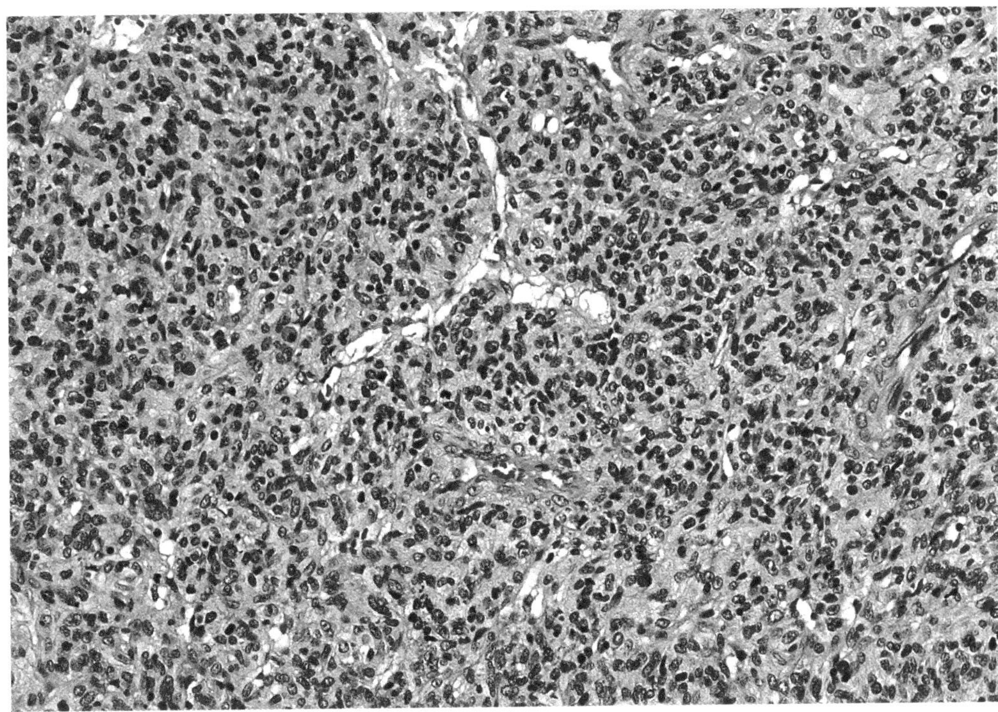

**FIGURE 11–47.** Infantile fibrosarcoma composed of immature-appearing fibroblasts arranged around a prominent hemangiopericytoma-like vascular pattern.

## Immunohistochemical and Electron Microscopic Findings

Immunohistochemically, the spindle cells of infantile fibrosarcoma stain for vimentin and variably for muscle markers including muscle-specific and smooth muscle actin.[268,287,307] The more primitive-appearing ovoid cells tend not to express these muscle markers. Stains for desmin, myoglobin, S-100 protein, and factor VIII are generally negative.[309]

Ultrastructural examination reveals fibroblast-like cells with large irregular nuclei, one or two nucleoli, free ribosomes, a well developed Golgi apparatus, and a prominent, often dilated rough endoplasmic reticulum, sometimes containing amorphous material.[271,276] Bundles of thin filaments characteristic of myofibroblastic differentiation may be present.[287] Some authors have reported cells with histiocyte-like features.[277,279]

## Cytogenic Findings

Numerous studies have noted a nonrandom gain of chromosomes 11, 20, 17, and 8 (in descending order of frequency) in infantile fibrosarcomas.[259,260,262,272,292,296,300] Using fluorescence in situ hybridization techniques, Schofield et al. found gains of these chromosomes (in various combinations) in 11 of 12 infantile fibrosarcomas in patients less than 2 years of age.[298] In contrast, alterations of these chromosomes were not found in four fibrosarcomas in patients 6–17 years of age. Interestingly, one of three cases of "cellular fibromatosis" also showed the above cytogenetic abnormalities, suggesting that "these two entities are on a spectrum and that their distinction may not be clear-cut."[298] The authors proposed that all cellular fibrous neoplasms in children less than 2 years of age be classified as "cellular fibrous tumors of infancy."[298]

More recently, it has been found that most infantile fibrosarcomas and cellular mesoblastic nephromas have the same diagnostic chromosomal translocation: t(12;15)(p13;q25).[285,295] This translocation results in fusion of the *ETV6* gene (also known as *TEL*) on chromosome 12 with the neurotrophin-3 receptor *NTRK3* (also known as *TRKC*) gene on chromosome 15. Although this translocation is difficult to detect by conventional cytogenetic means, it can be readily demonstrated by the reverse transcriptase-polymerase chain reaction or fluorescence in situ hybridization using frozen or paraffin-embedded tissue.[259a,264a] Given the similar histologic and cytogenetic findings in infantile fibrosarcoma and cellular mesoblastic nephroma,[288,297,306] it has been suggested that these two lesions are histogenetically related entities arising in soft tissue or renal locations. Other cytogenetic abnormalities noted in infantile fibrosarcomas include deletions of the short arm of chromosome 17[278] and t(12; 13).[304]

## Differential Diagnosis

The microscopic picture may be confused with that of other mesenchymal neoplasms, but in most cases the uniformity of the spindle-shaped tumor cells, the solid growth pattern, the fascicular arrangement, and the lack of any other form of cellular differentiation seen by electron microscopy and immunohistochemistry permit a reliable diagnosis.

*Spindle cell type of rhabdomyosarcoma* is a subtype of embryonal rhabdomyosarcoma that may be difficult to distinguish from infantile fibrosarcoma. This tumor is most often encountered in the paratesticular region and the head and neck, but it may also be present at other sites, including the extremities.[265,274,289] The tumor is composed of uniform spindle cells with eosinophilic fibrillary cytoplasm and elongated hyperchromatic nuclei separated by abundant, partly hyalinized collagen. Immunohistochemically, this tumor characteristically expresses desmin, which is usually absent in infantile fibrosarcoma.

In 1993, Lundgren et al. described three cases of *infantile rhabdomyofibrosarcoma,* each of which was initially diagnosed as infantile fibrosarcoma.[290] This tumor, which was observed in three children 3 months to 3 years of age, has the features of a spindle cell rhabdomyosarcoma and desmoplastic portions reminiscent of infantile fibrosarcoma. Immunohistochemically, the cells express vimentin, smooth muscle actin, and desmin but not myoglobin; they have the ultrastructural features of rhabdomyoblasts, fibroblasts, and myofibroblasts. By cytogenetics, 2 of the 3 cases reported by Lundgren et al.[290] showed monosomy of chromosome 19 and 22, among other abnormalities; a case reported by Miki et al. showed der (2) t(2; 11)(q37;q13).[292a] Two of the patients developed metastases and died within 2 years of the primary operation; the third patient was alive with a local recurrence. The exact nature of this tumor is still not clear. It may represent an intermediate form between an infantile fibrosarcoma and a spindle cell rhabdomyosarcoma. The authors also raised the possibility that some tumors reported as infantile fibrosarcoma that have metastasized and followed a fatal course may actually be this entity.

Infantile fibrosarcoma with a marked degree of vascularity may be difficult to distinguish from *infantile hemangiopericytoma.* The latter is marked by a distinct lobulated arrangement and more regularly distributed dilated vascular channels that form a branching, or "staghorn," pattern. In some cases, clear distinction is difficult and mandates examination of multiple sections from different portions of the tumor. Some authors have reported tumors with overlapping histologic features and have proposed that these two entities represent a histologic continuum.[307]

Perhaps the most difficult lesion to distinguish from infantile fibrosarcoma is the cellular form of *infantile fibromatosis* (Table 11–2). Some authors have reported cases in which the primary tumor had the appearance and growth pattern of infantile fibromatosis, whereas the recurrent tumor showed more cellularity and was virtually indistinguishable from fibrosarcoma.[266] On the other hand, we have also observed tumors with a fibrosarcoma-like appearance in the primary neoplasm and a fibromatosis-like appearance in the recurrence. Egan et al. found a significantly larger number of nucleolar organizer regions (AgNORs) in infantile fibrosarcoma than in infantile fibromatosis.[275] In addition, cytogenetic and molecular genetic analysis may be useful for distinguishing between these entities.

## Discussion

Compared with adult fibrosarcoma, the clinical course of infantile fibrosarcoma is a favorable one. Of the 48 patients with follow-up in the study by Chung and Enzinger, 8 (17%) developed one or more local recurrences 6 weeks to 10 years after the initial excision.[266] Only 4 (8%) of the 48 patients died of metastatic disease, and one patient was living 6.5 years after lobectomy for metastatic tumor. The 5-year survival rate in this series was 84%. The recurrent and nonrecurrent groups showed no demonstrable differences in regard to tumor site, age at onset, or size of the tumor. However, the initial therapy was more radical for the tumors that neither recurred nor metastasized.

Although Dahl et al. found that the more primitive ("medullary") tumors carried a more favorable prognosis than the more collagenous ("desmoplastic") tumors,[271] other studies have found that cellularity, mitotic counts, and the extent of tumor necrosis do not correlate well with clinical behavior.[266,267,299] Blocker et al. found that tumors located in the axial skeleton behaved more aggressively than those found peripherally.[263] There are reports of incompletely excised infantile fibrosarcomas that have not recurred or metastasized after several years,[309] as well as sporadic reports of spontaneous regression.[291,301]

Despite rapid growth and a high degree of cellularity, most infantile fibrosarcomas are cured by wide local excision. In some cases, amputation is necessary if the extent or large size of the tumor precludes surgical therapy.[279] A number of reports have indicated that preoperative chemotherapy is useful for decreasing tumor bulk, enabling a more conservative surgical approach.[280,283,293,302,305] There are also reports of success with postoperative chemotherapy[293,294] and with chemotherapy alone as a mode of treatment for inoperable tumors.[273,279] The value of radiotherapy is difficult to assess, as it has been used only in selected cases.[287,299] In view of the generally favorable clinical course, it appears that adjuvant radiotherapy and chemotherapy should be reserved for infantile fibrosarcomas that are unresectable or have recurred or metastasized.[293]

Most studies have found infantile fibrosarcomas to be diploid,[268,287,298] in keeping with the low-grade behavior. When compared to adult fibrosarcomas, the infantile form has a higher apoptotic index and a lower proliferative index using antibodies to the Ki-67 antigen.[284] In addition, *p53* gene mutations are rare in fibrous tumors of infancy and childhood, including infantile fibrosarcoma.[264]

## INFLAMMATORY MYOFIBROBLASTIC TUMOR

Inflammatory myofibroblastic tumor is a distinctive pseudosarcomatous lesion that occurs primarily in the viscera and soft tissue of children and young adults. The lesion has a distinctive histologic appearance and usually pursues a benign clinical course. Although original descriptions of this lesion focused on their occurrence in the lung,[350,356,359] subsequent reports described this lesion in virtually every anatomic location. This entity has been called many names, including plasma cell granuloma,[350] plasma cell pseudotumor,[339] inflammatory myofibrohistiocytic proliferation,[353] omental-mesenteric myxoid hamartoma.[323] and most commonly inflammatory pseudotumor.[341,344,362] The term inflammatory myofibroblastic tumor is preferred, as "inflammatory pseudotumor" has been applied to diverse entities,[315] including reparative pseudosarcomatous lesions of the lower genitourinary tract,[310,325,328,340,342] infectious lesions, including those secondary to *Mycobacterium avium intracellulare* infection,[357,361] and Epstein-Barr virus-associated follicular dendritic cell tumors usually found in the liver or spleen[312,345,347] (Fig. 11–48). The discussion that follows focuses on inflammatory myofibroblastic tumors that occur in an extrapulmonary location.

### Clinical Findings

Inflammatory myofibroblastic tumors have been reported in many sites, including the skin,[326,363] soft tissues,[319,341] breast,[338] mediastinum,[354] gastrointestinal tract,[314,329,336,337,353] pancreas,[331,358] oral cavity,[313] nerve,[360] bone,[343] and central nervous system.[311,315,332] The most common sites of extrapulmonary inflammatory myofibroblastic tumor are the mesentery and omentum.[318] In a study by Coffin et al.,[319] 36 of 84 tumors (43%) arose at these sites. Although the age range is broad, extrapulmonary tumors show a predilection for children, with a mean age of approximately 10 years. Females are affected slightly more commonly than males.

Presenting symptoms depend on the site of primary tumor involvement. Patients with intraabdominal tumors most commonly complain of abdominal pain or an abdominal mass with increased girth, occasionally with signs and symptoms of gastrointestinal obstruction. Some patients have prominent systemic manifestations, including fever, night sweats, weight loss, and malaise. Laboratory abnormalities are present in a small number of patients and include an elevated erythrocyte sedimentation rate, anemia, thrombocytosis, and hypergammaglobulinemia, which often resolve when the lesion is excised.[319,349,351]

### Gross Findings

Grossly, most lesions are lobular, multinodular, or bosselated with a hard or rubbery cut surface that may appear white, gray, tan-yellow, or red (Fig. 11–49). Some cut with a gritty sensation due to the presence of calcifications. Although most are solitary tumors, multiple nodules generally restricted to the same anatomic location are found in almost one-third of cases.[319,333] The tumors range in size from 2 to 20 cm, but most are 5–10 cm.

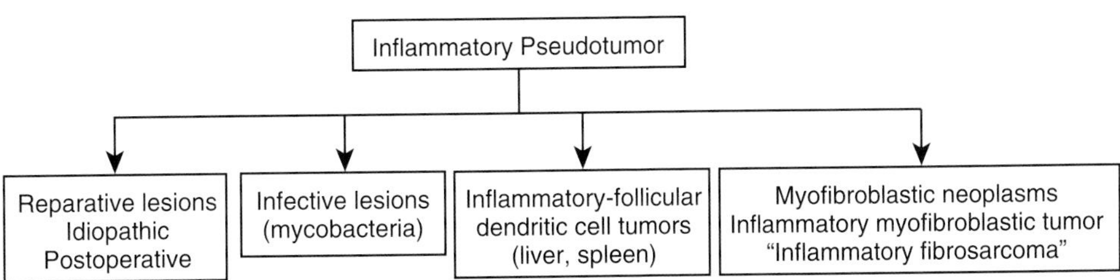


**FIGURE 11–48.** Inflammatory pseudotumor. A variety of lesions of differing etiologies have been referred to as inflammatory pseudotumor. (Modified from Chan JKC. Inflammatory pseudotumor: a family of lesions of diverse nature and etiologies. Adv Anat Pathol 3:156, 1996.)

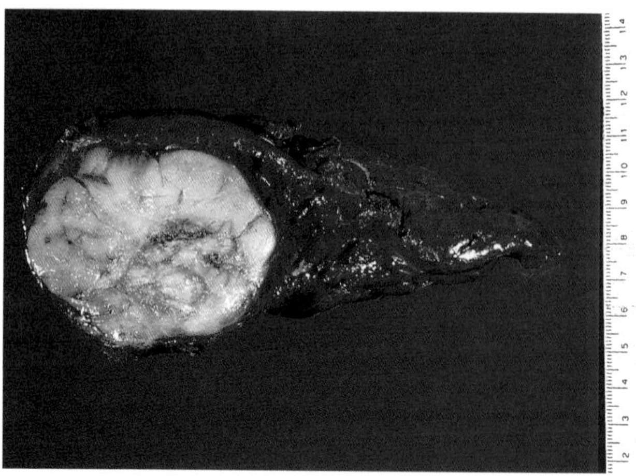

**FIGURE 11–49.** Gross appearance of an inflammatory myofibroblastic tumor in the left upper lobe of the lung of a 21-year-old woman.

## Microscopic Findings

A variety of histologic patterns may be seen, and different patterns may be found in the same tumor. Some tumors are composed predominantly of cytologically bland spindle- or stellate-shaped cells loosely arranged in a myxoid or hyaline stroma with scattered inflammatory cells, somewhat resembling nodular fasciitis. Others are composed of a compact proliferation of spindle-shaped cells arranged in a storiform or fascicular growth pattern (Figs. 11–50 to 11–53). In these foci, the nuclei tend to be elongated but lack significant hyperchromasia or cytologic atypia. Mitotic figures are variable but not atypical. These foci are usually associated with a prominent lymphoplasmacytic infiltrate, occasionally with formation of germinal centers. Other foci may be sparsely cellular, with cytologically bland cells deposited in a sclerotic stroma resembling a scar. Lymphocytes and plasma cells are often seen in these foci, and small punctate areas of calcification or metaplastic bone may be observed.

In some lesions there is pronounced cytologic atypia, with cells containing large nuclei and distinct nucleoli. Some tumors have large histiocytoid cells resembling ganglion cells or Reed-Sternberg cells.[335]

## Immunohistochemical and Electron Microscopic Findings

In most cases there is strong, diffuse staining of tumor cells with vimentin and less commonly with myogenic markers including smooth muscle actin, muscle-specific actin, and desmin. Focal cytokeratin immunoreactivity is found in more than one-third of cases, and CD68 is detected in up to 25% of cases.[319] Immunostains for myoglobin and S-100 protein are typically negative.

Ultrastructurally, most cells have features of fibroblasts with a well developed Golgi apparatus, abundant rough endoplasmic reticulum, and extracellular collagen. Some cells have evidence of myofibroblastic differentiation, with intracytoplasmic thin filaments and dense bodies.[319,333]

## Differential Diagnosis

The differential diagnosis of this lesion depends on the clinicopathologic setting, including the patient's age, gender, tumor location, and number of lesions. *Inflammatory malignant fibrous histiocytoma* is characterized by bizarre pleomorphic cells that may be obscured by numerous xanthomatous and inflammatory cells. For tumors composed of elongated spindle cells with eosinophilic cytoplasm arranged in a focal fascicular growth pattern, differentiation from *leiomyosarcoma* may pose a problem. However, the nuclei in leiomyosarcoma are cigar-shaped and arranged in a more regular fascicular growth pattern. In addition, leiomyosarcoma is not typified by a conspicuous inflammatory infiltrate. Rare inflammatory myofibroblastic tumors have a conspicuous population of large multinucleated tumor cells with prominent nucleoli bearing a resemblance to the Reed-Sternberg cells of *Hodgkin's disease*.[335] The immunohistochemical reactivity of the spindle and ganglion-like cells for actins and negativity for CD15 and CD30 assist in distinguishing these two entities. *Inflammatory fibroid polyp* is a benign, probably reactive lesion that most often occurs in the stomach and ileum as a solitary submucosal polyp. Histologically, this lesion is dominated by stellate-shaped cells deposited in a myxoid stroma with reactive blood vessels and mixed inflammatory cells, particularly eosinophils. *Inflammatory cell-rich gastrointestinal autonomic nerve tumor* may closely resemble an inflammatory myofibroblastic tumor,[346] but these tumors show evidence of neural differentiation immunohistochemically and ultrastructurally. Although they share some histologic similarities, inflammatory myofibroblastic tumor can be distinguished from the group of inflammatory fibrosclerosing lesions, including *sclerosing mediastinitis, idiopathic retroperitoneal fibrosis,* and *Riedel's thyroiditis,* by paying close attention to the clinical setting and gross and microscopic findings. These lesions tend to occur in older patients and, although mass-forming, are usually ill-defined, entrapping the normal tissues in the vicinity. They tend to have more prominent sclerosis and phlebitis than the typical inflammatory myofibroblastic tumor. Other fibroinflammatory processes that occur in this location, including *xanthogranuloma-*

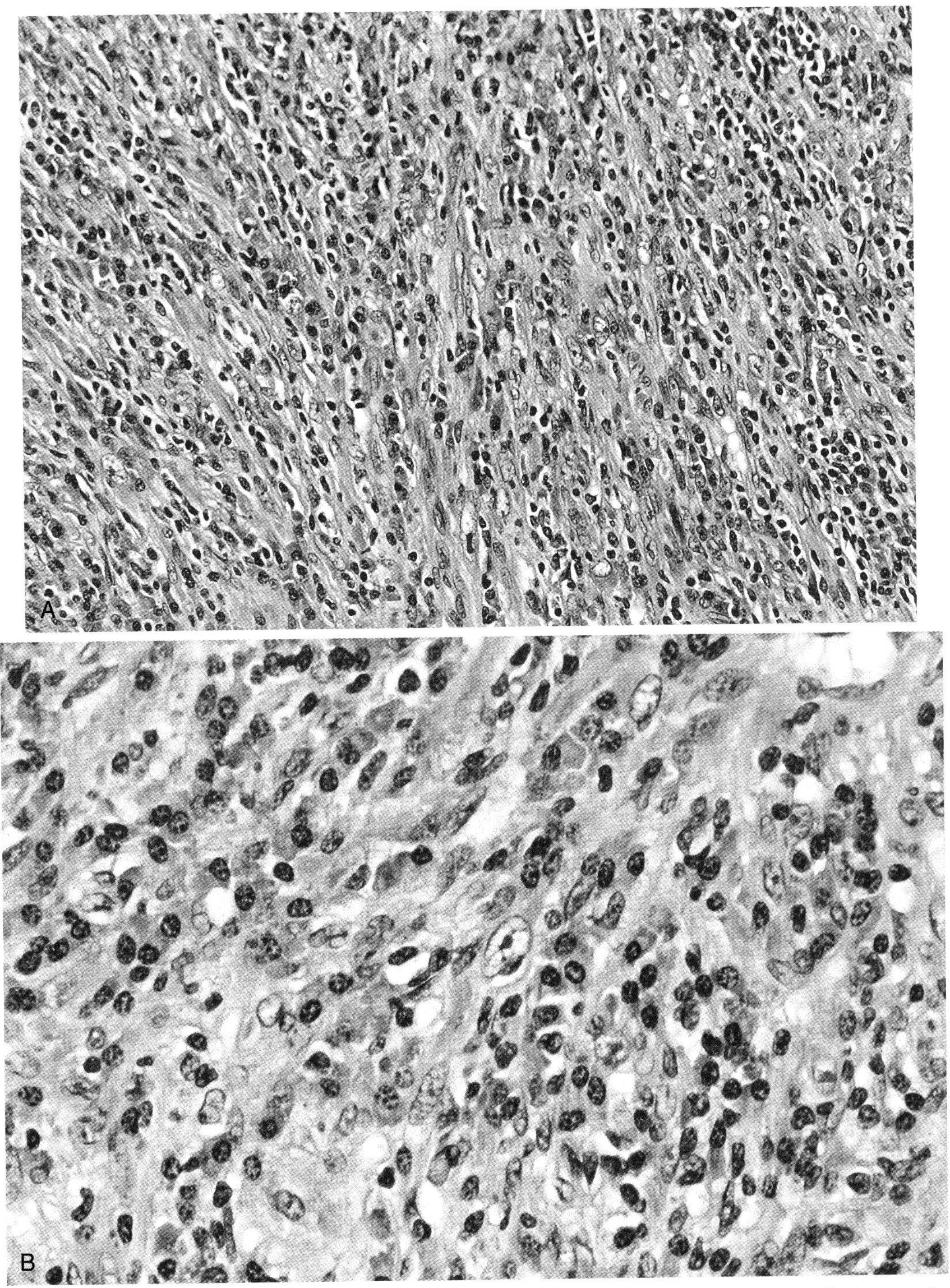


**FIGURE 11–50.** Inflammatory myofibroblastic tumor. (**A**) Low-power view showing an admixture of spindle-shaped and ovoid cells with a prominent inflammatory infiltrate. (**B**) High-power view of an inflammatory myofibroblastic tumor. Note the conspicuous admixture of lymphocytes and plasma cells.

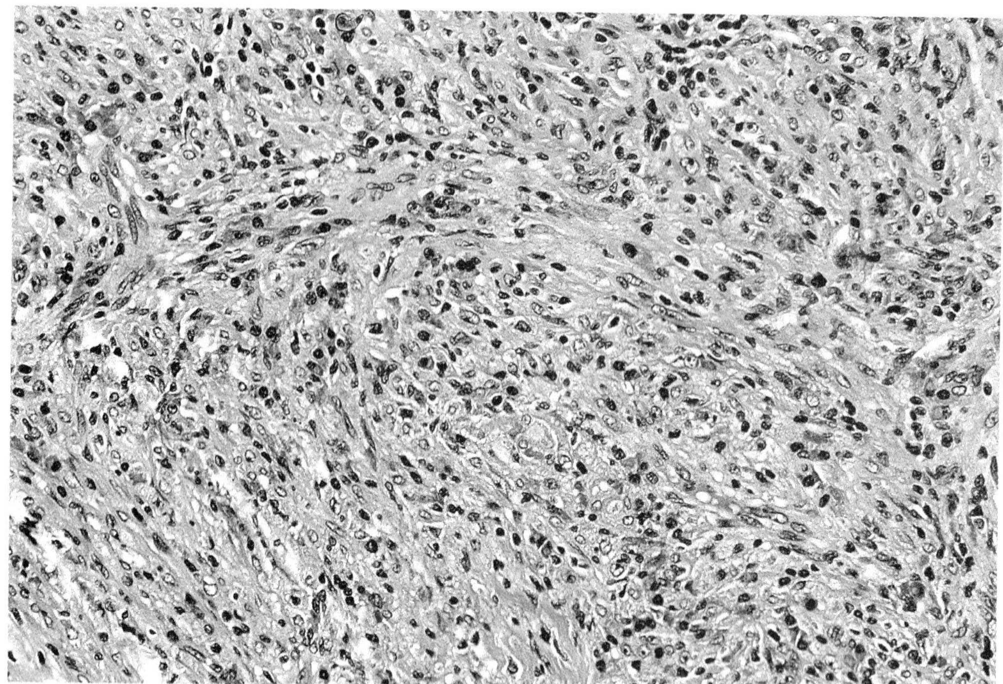

**FIGURE 11–51.** Inflammatory myofibroblastic tumor. Cytologically bland spindle-shaped cells are intimately admixed with a predominantly plasmacytic infiltrate.

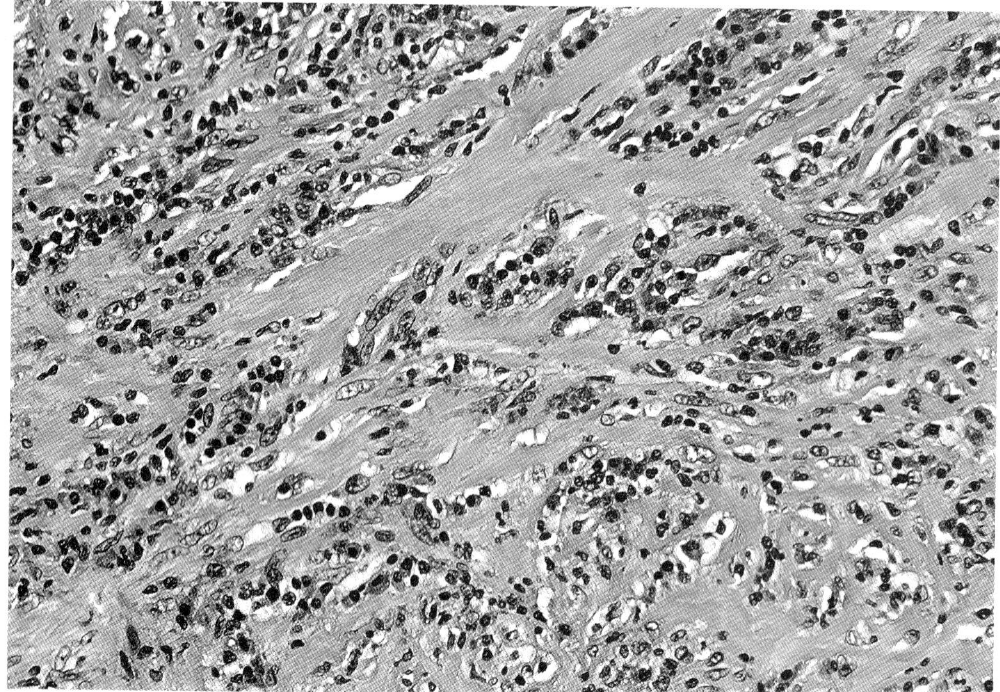

**FIGURE 11–52.** Less cellular inflammatory myofibroblastic tumor than that depicted in Figures 11–50 and 11–51. Plate-like collagen is present.

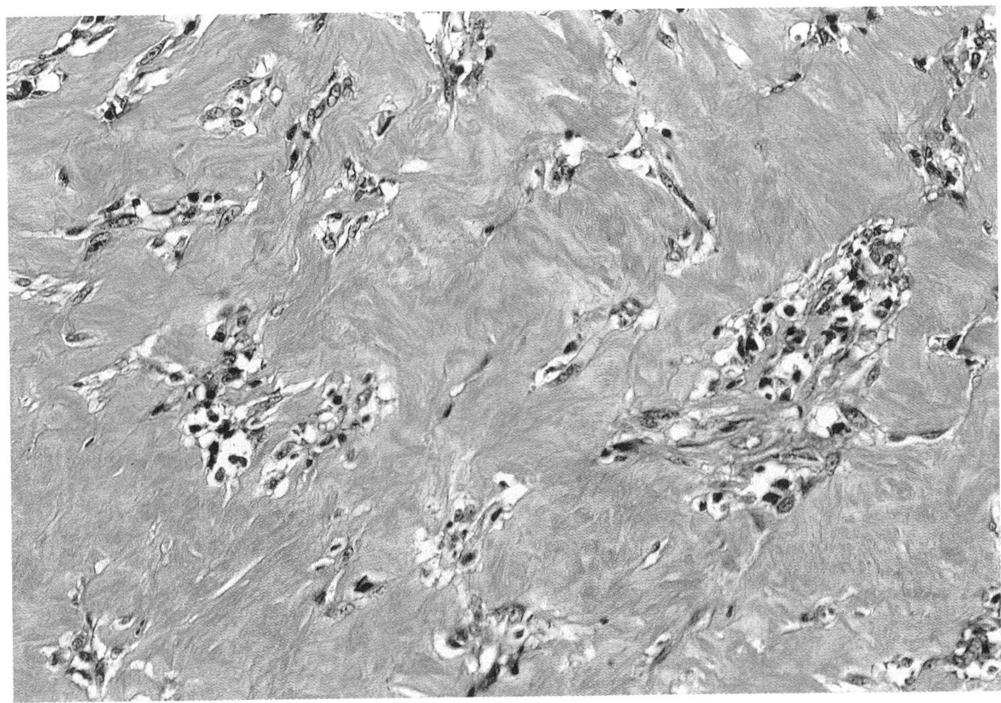

**FIGURE 11–53.** Hypocellular inflammatory myofibroblastic tumor composed predominantly of sclerotic fibrous tissue with scattered spindle-shaped and inflammatory cells.

*tous inflammation secondary to Erdheim-Chester disease*[322] and *pseudotumor resulting from atypical mycobacterial infection,*[357,361] also may be in the differential diagnosis and can be distinguished by virtue of their distinct clinicopathologic setting.

Finally, the question as to whether inflammatory myofibroblastic tumor and *inflammatory fibrosarcoma* are the same tumor, distinct entities, or represent a spectrum separated by the degree of cytologic atypia remains unresolved.[317] Certainly, these two entities share clinical and pathologic features; as stated by Coffin et al., the distinction of inflammatory fibrosarcoma "from inflammatory myofibroblastic tumor may be more semantic than real."[319] Some inflammatory myofibroblastic tumors do exhibit more pronounced cytologic atypia but given the generally benign clinical behavior of this group of lesions, we prefer to group all of these tumors under the term "inflammatory myofibroblastic tumor."

## Discussion

There have been a number of controversial issues with respect to these lesions over the years, such as whether the lesions are a homogeneous entity, if they are neoplastic, and, if neoplastic, their level of malignancy. It seems reasonably certain that the lesions reported under the various terms noted above indeed refer to the same process, although the features of any given lesion may vary somewhat depending on the degree of inflammation, sclerosis, and cellularity. In our opinion, it is not possible to make histologic distinctions between lesions reported by some authors as inflammatory fibrosarcoma and by others as inflammatory myofibroblastic tumor. In support of this statement is the fact that there is overlap in case material reported in the two largest studies under the two preceding terms.[319,333] There is also compelling evidence that these lesions are true neoplasms rather than pseudotumors. Presenting as large, discrete lesions, many have been associated with aggressive local behavior that has resulted in some deaths. In addition, a number of inflammatory myofibroblastic tumors have been studied cytogenetically and found to have clonal abnormalities, especially at 2p22-24, supportive of a neoplastic process.[324,325,348,352,355] The anaplastic lymphoma kinase (ALK) gene, located on 2p23, has been implicated in the pathogenesis of this lesion, and a significant percentage of intraabdominal inflammatory myofibroblastic tumors which have been studied show immunohistochemical expression of ALK.[319a,331a] A fusion gene involving the tropomyosin (TPM) N-terminal coiled-coil domains and the ALK C-terminal kinase domain likely play a central pathogenetic role.[331a] Also in support of a neoplastic process, Biselli et al. found that almost 50% of pediatric inflammatory myofibroblastic tumors are aneuploid.[314]

Based on the two largest studies of abdominal and retroperitoneal lesions, it is clear that tumors in this location have a propensity for more aggressive behavior than their extraabdominal counterparts, with recurrence rates of 23–37%.[319,333] The major question seems to be whether these lesions have metastatic potential or whether multiple lesions in a single patient represent multifocal disease. Coffin et al.,[319] in a series of 53 cases with follow-up, reported no instances of metastasis, whereas 3 of 27 patients reported by Meis and Enzinger[333] developed metastasis to lung and brain. The reasons for this discrepancy are not clear. In at least one case reported by Meis and Enzinger (case 26), the simultaneous presentation of histologically bland mediastinal and cerebral lesions with no evidence of disease nearly 4 years after surgery raises the possibility that these lesions are multifocal. It would be extremely interesting to see if different lesions in the same patient had identical clonal abnormalities, supporting the contention that they represent metastasis. Finally, there are rare reports of inflammatory myofibroblastic tumors merging into frankly malignant-appearing neoplasms.[319,321,334,350,364]

The mainstay of therapy is surgical resection with reexcision of recurrent tumors. The benefit of chemotherapy and radiation therapy remains to be proven.[320] Cellularity, mitotic counts, and extent of inflammation do not appear to be prognostic markers; in contrast, cytologic atypia, ganglion-like cells, *p53* expression, and DNA aneuploidy may be useful for identifying tumors that are more likely to pursue an aggressive clinical course.[327,330]

## CALCIFYING APONEUROTIC FIBROMA

Originally described as *juvenile aponeurotic fibroma* by Keasbey in 1953,[372] fewer than 100 cases of calcifying aponeurotic fibroma have been recorded in the literature. Although initially reported in children and adolescents between birth and 16 years of age,[367,372] it has subsequently become apparent that this lesion affects a much wider age range than other forms of juvenile fibromatosis and may occur in young adults and rarely in older adults. Keasbey described its characteristic histologic picture, its predilection for the palm and fingers of the hand, and its propensity to locally recur after excision. In view of the wide age range of patients, the term juvenile aponeurotic fibroma was changed to aponeurotic fibroma[373] and *calcifying aponeurotic fibroma*.[370]

### Clinical Findings

Most patients present with a slowly growing, painless mass in the hands or feet of several months' or even years' duration. In most cases the mass is poorly circumscribed and causes neither discomfort nor limitation of movement, although rare patients do have complaints of mild tenderness.[366] Grossly, lesions that have been present for several years are often more sharply circumscribed and distinctly nodular than those of shorter duration.

Most lesions occur in children, with a peak incidence at ages 8–14 years,[366,372] although this lesion has also been described in young and middle-aged adults.[369,373,375] Although most small series have not reported a distinct gender predilection, 70% of the patients in the series by Allen and Enzinger were male.[366] There is no record of increased familial incidence. The two principal sites of growth are the hands and the feet. In the hand, the most common sites are the palm and fingers with only rare lesions having been described on the dorsum of the hand.[365] Fewer lesions occur on the plantar surface of the foot or ankle region and rarely the toes. Isolated tumors have been observed at other sites, including the neck, forearm, thigh, popliteal fossa, knee, and soft tissues of the lumbosacral region.[366,368,377–379] They may be found in the subcutaneous tissue or attached to the aponeurosis, tendons, or fascia. Moskovich and Posner observed a lesion in the flexor pollicis longus tendon.[376] Preoperative radiographic examination reveals a faint mass, frequently with calcific stippling, especially in the more heavily calcified tumors.

### Gross Findings

Most lesions are ill-defined, firm or rubbery, and gray-white and most are less than 3 cm in greatest diameter. Older lesions appear to be more grossly well circumscribed, although there is typically microscopic infiltration of the surrounding soft tissues even in these cases. Portions of the surrounding fat, skeletal muscle, and fibrous tissue frequently merge with the tumor. In some tumors, calcifications are evident as small white flecks (Fig. 11–54), although in heavily calcified cases they may be more grossly apparent. On sectioning, the lesion often has a gritty sensation due to these calcifications.

### Microscopic Findings

The histologic picture varies little from case to case. It reveals a fibrous growth that extends with multiple processes into the surrounding tissue with more centrally located foci of calcification and cartilage formation. The cellularity of the lesion varies from region to region and is composed of plump fibroblasts with round or ovoid nuclei and indistinctly outlined cytoplasm separated by a densely collagenous stroma (Figs. 11–55 to 11–62). Despite the focal cellularity of

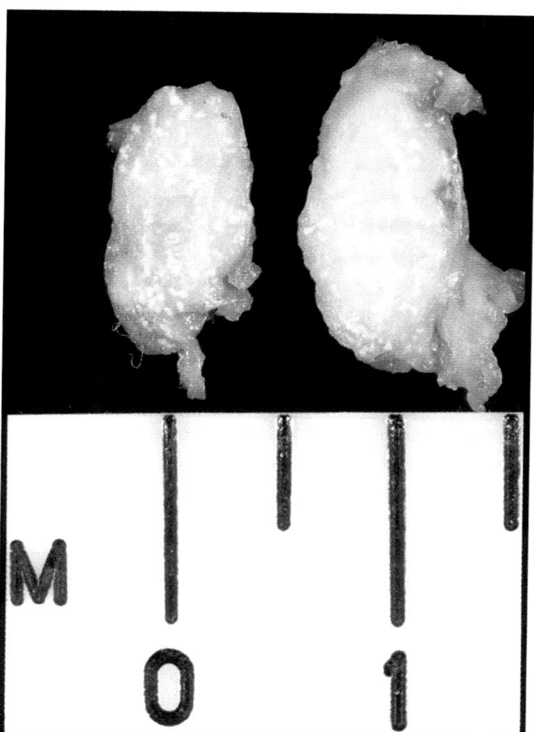


**FIGURE 11–54.** Calcifying aponeurotic fibroma in the palm of a 4-year-old-boy. Note the small white flecks, indicative of calcification.

the lesion, mitotic figures are scarce. Not infrequently, the fibrous growth is attached to a tendon or aponeurosis and encircles blood vessels and nerves. Unlike other forms of fibromatosis, there tends to be orientation of the stromal cells. There may be a vague cartwheel or whorled pattern, or the nuclei may line up in columns, occasionally resulting in marked nuclear palisading.[366]

Focal calcification is invariably present except in lesions in infants or small children. Calcification and cartilage formation are much more pronounced in lesions removed from older children and young adults. The calcifications are usually small and vary from fine granules or string-like deposits to large amorphous masses. In many cases these calcified foci are surrounded by radiating columns of cells that resemble chondrocytes, with rounded nuclei lying in lacunae (Fig. 11–63). These cartilage-like cells are often aligned in linear columns that radiate from the center of the calcified areas, although there may be a circumferential arrangement as well.[366] Occasionally, multinucleated giant cells resembling osteoclasts are present adjacent to the calcific foci (Fig. 11–64), but they may also be seen adjacent to noncalcified fibrocartilage-like tissue. Ossification occurs but is rare.

## Differential Diagnosis

The differential diagnosis differs from case to case, depending on the age of the patient at the time the lesion is excised. In infants and small children, when there is still little or no calcification, this lesion may be difficult to distinguish from *infantile* or *juvenile forms of fibromatosis*. However, infantile fibromatosis most commonly presents as a soft tissue mass in the head and neck and the proximal extremities; involve-

*Text continued on page 394*

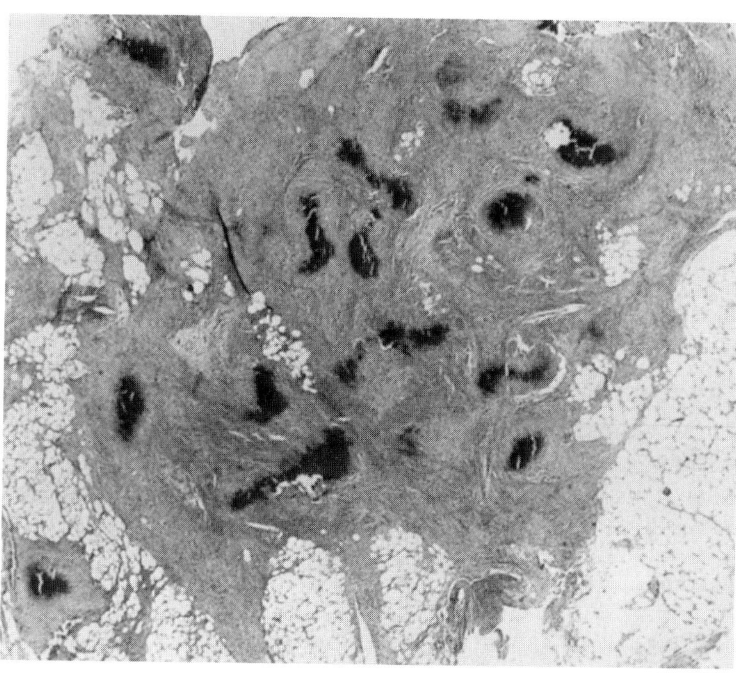

**FIGURE 11–55.** Calcifying aponeurotic fibroma in the palm of a 1-year-old boy. Note the poor circumscription of the lesion and multiple short bands of calcification in the proliferated fibrous tissue.

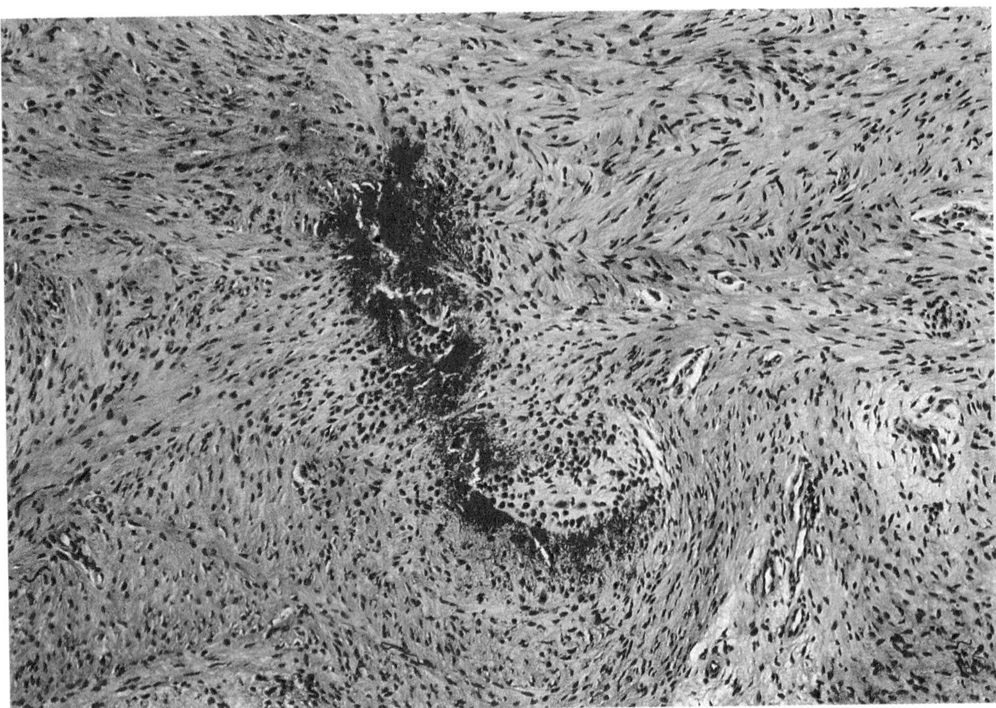

**FIGURE 11–56.** Calcifying aponeurotic fibroma with early focal calcification.

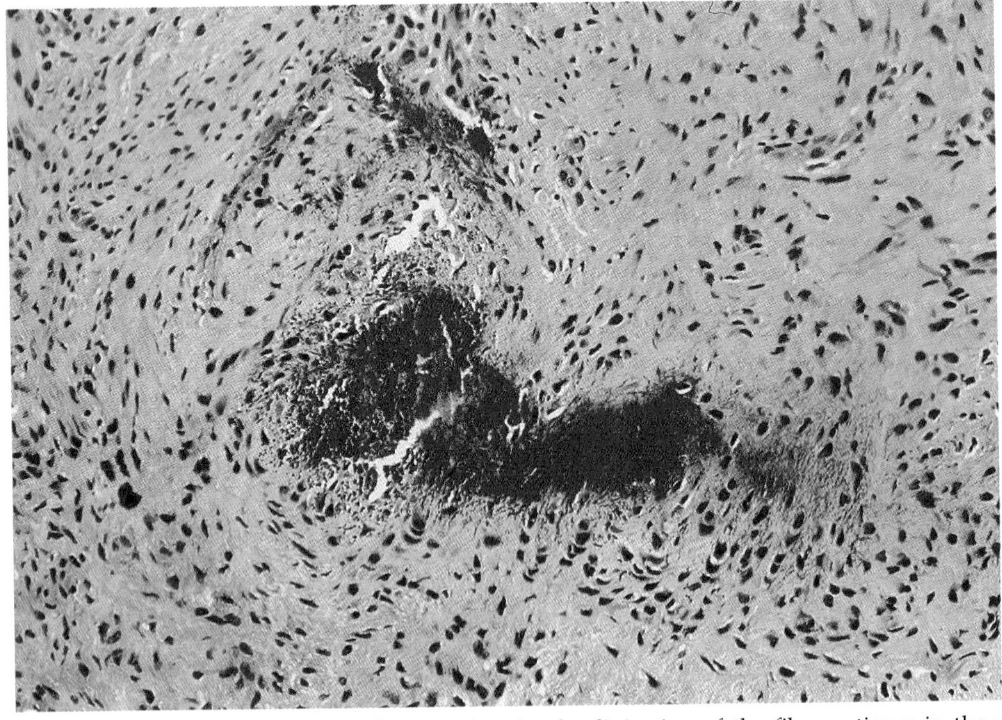

**FIGURE 11–57.** Calcifying aponeurotic fibroma showing hyalinization of the fibrous tissue in the vicinity of heavily calcified areas.

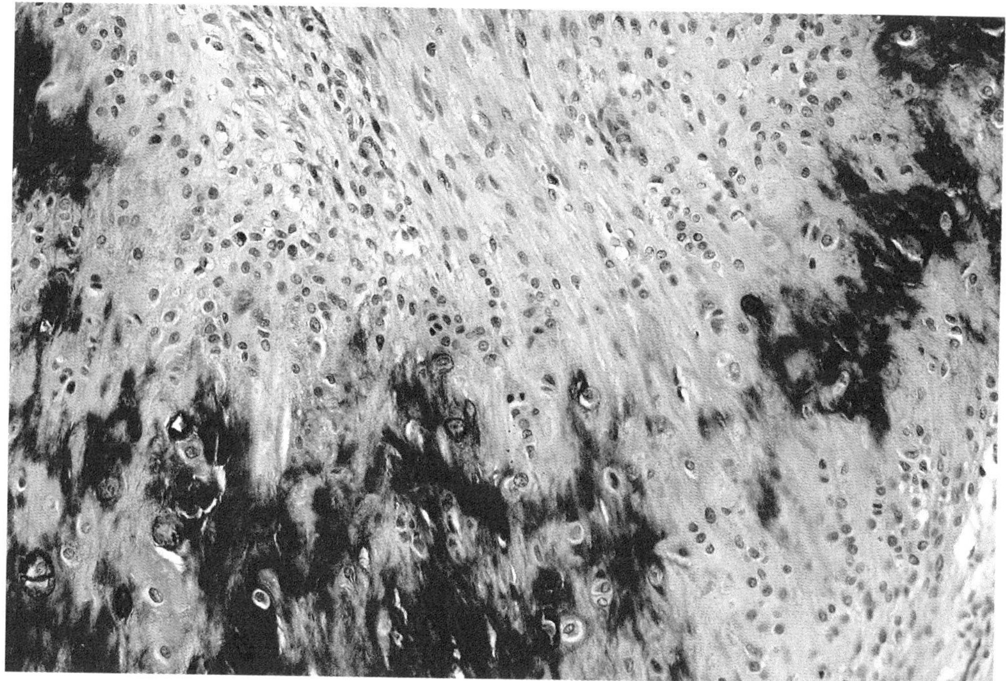

**FIGURE 11–58.** Calcifying aponeurotic fibroma with small round cells radiating from the calcified areas and arranged in linear arrays.

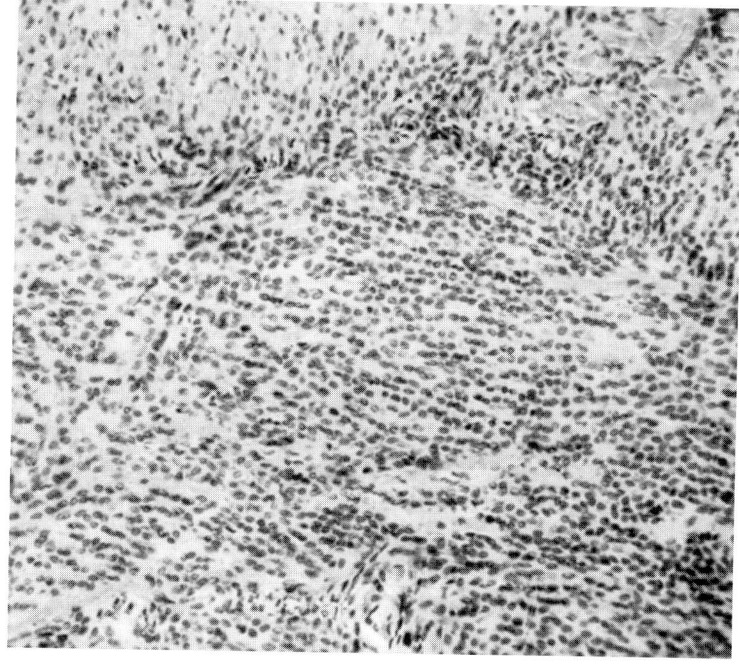

**FIGURE 11–59.** Calcifying aponeurotic fibroma. Peripheral fibrous portion with a characteristic arrangement of fibroblasts in parallel cords.

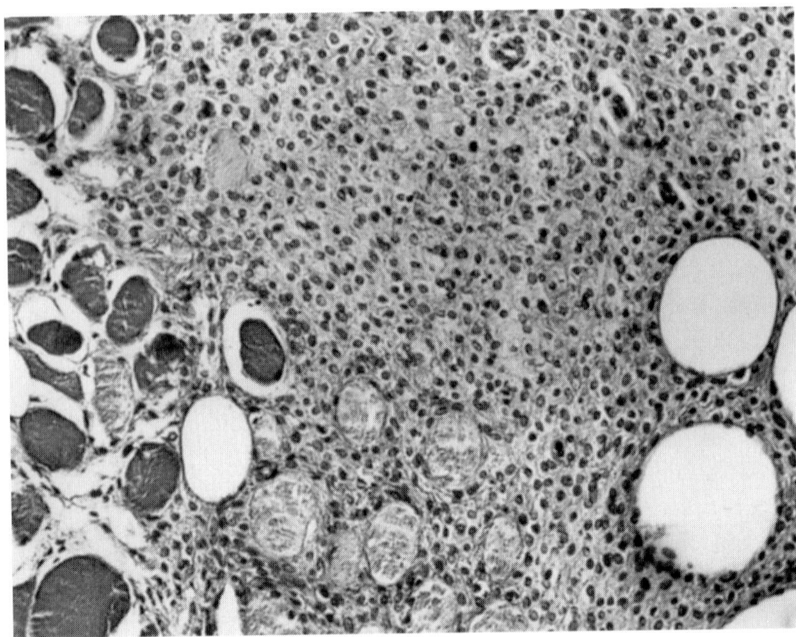

**FIGURE 11–60.** Fibrous portion of a calcifying aponeurotic fibroma with infiltration of muscle tissue and subcutaneous fat.

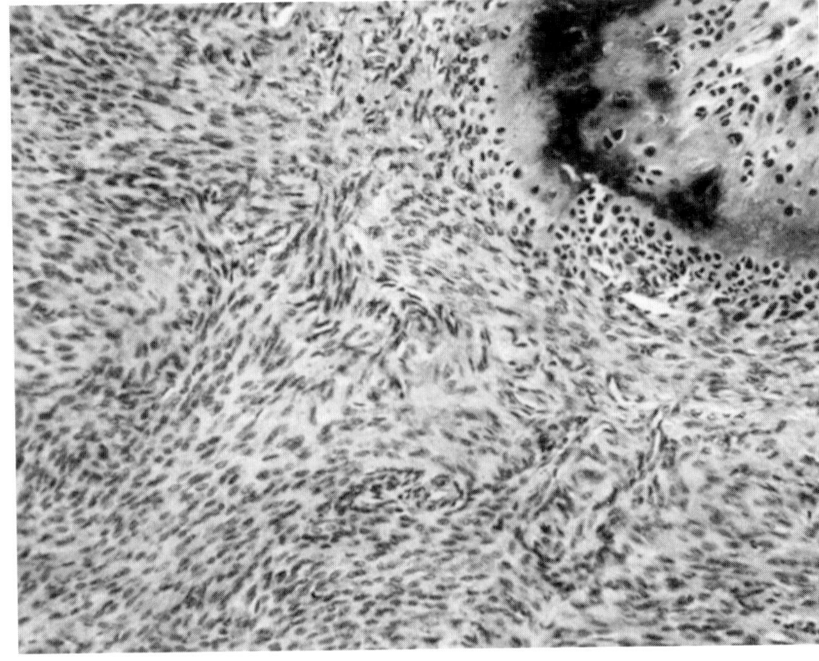

**FIGURE 11–61.** Calcifying aponeurotic fibroma. The cellular fibrous portion resembles fibrosarcoma.

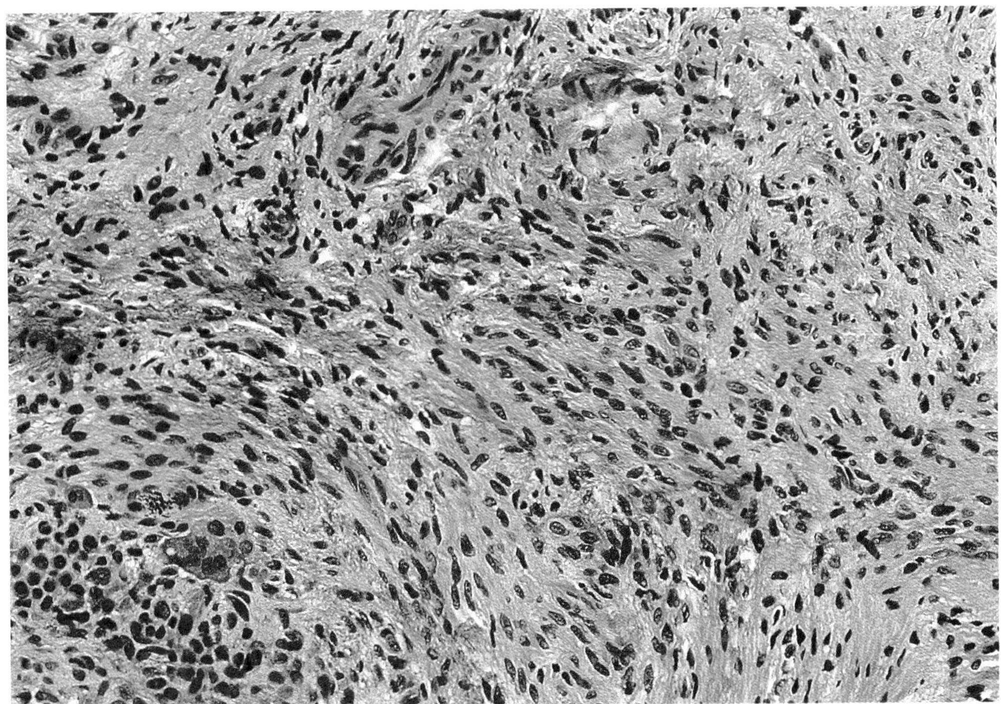

**FIGURE 11–62.** High-power view of the cellular fibrous portion of a calcifying aponeurotic fibroma.

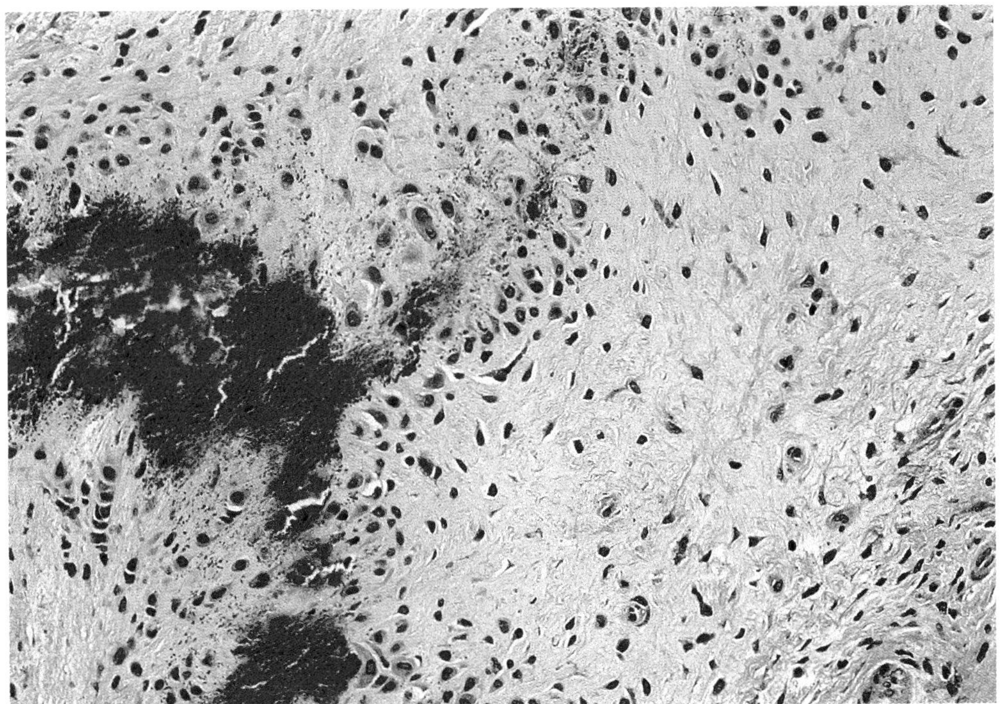

**FIGURE 11–63.** Calcifying aponeurotic fibroma with focal cartilaginous metaplasia in an area of calcification.

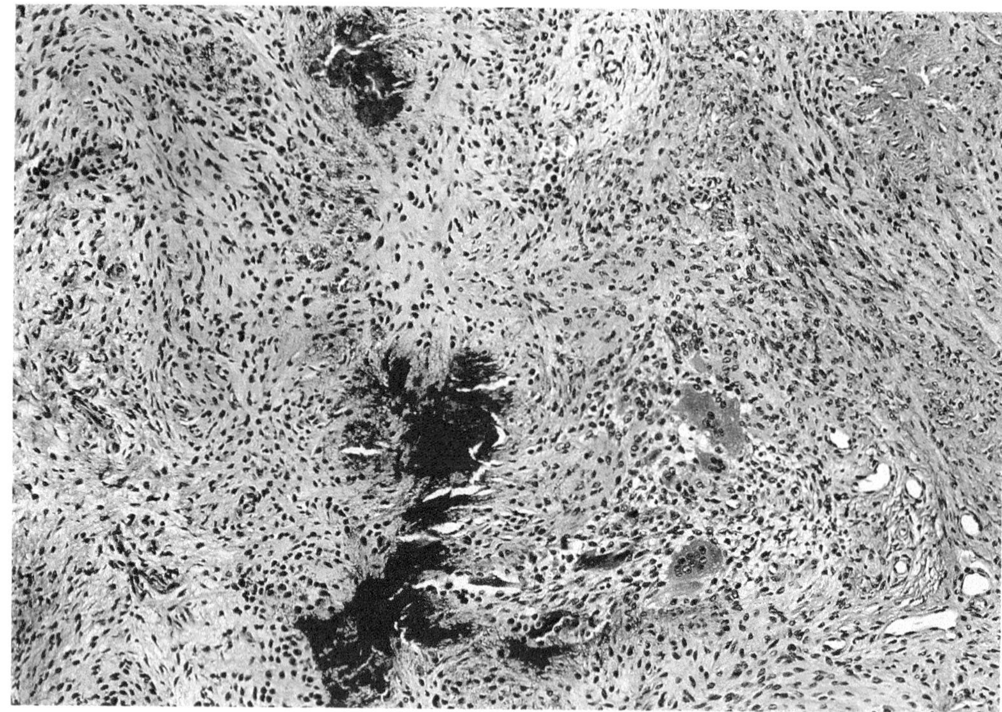

**FIGURE 11–64.** Calcifying aponeurotic fibroma with multinucleated giant cells adjacent to an area of calcification.

ment of the distal extremities is rare. Moreover, the fibroblasts of infantile fibromatosis are more elongated and are often deposited in a myxoid background, and foci of calcification and ossification are rare. Giant cells, as are frequently seen in calcifying aponeurotic fibroma, are not typical of fibromatosis. *Palmar* and *plantar fibromatoses* are rare in children, are more nodular in appearance, and lack calcification or chondroid differentiation. Malignant spindle cell tumors, such as *monophasic fibrous-type synovial sarcoma,* may rarely be mistaken for calcifying aponeurotic fibroma with a prominent spindle cell pattern. Immunoreactivity for epithelial markers is useful for this distinction.

In older patients, distinction of the growth from a *soft part chondroma* may cause considerable difficulty, especially because both calcifying aponeurotic fibromas and soft part chondromas occur in similar locations and are most common in the hands. However, soft part chondromas more frequently affect older adults and have a lower rate of local recurrence than aponeurotic fibromas. Histologically, soft part chondromas are well circumscribed lobulated masses that are sharply demarcated from the surrounding soft tissues. Furthermore, the extent of chondroid differentiation is more well developed in soft tissue chondromas than aponeurotic fibromas.

## Electron Microscopic Findings

Calcifying aponeurotic fibromas have a biphasic pattern consisting of fibroblasts and occasional myofibroblasts and cartilage cells, with a well developed granular endoplasmic reticulum, a prominent Golgi complex, and multiple microvilli.[371] These cells are surrounded by an intercellular matrix containing fine fibrils and spherical granules.

## Prognosis and Treatment

Because of its infiltrative nature, the calcifying aponeurotic fibroma is characterized by a high rate of local recurrence. In the series by Allen and Enzinger, 10 of 19 lesions recurred 1 month to 11 years after the initial excision.[366] The authors did not identify any histologic features that were likely to predict recurrence but did note that, based on their study and a review of the literature, young patients, particularly those under 5 years of age, had a higher risk of recurrence.[366] Rare cases of malignant transformation have been reported. Lafferty et al. reported a calcifying aponeurotic fibroma of the palm in a 3-year-old girl that metastasized as a metastatic fibrosarcoma to the lungs and bones 5 years after a second local excision.[374] One of us (S.W.W.) has also reviewed a single case of malignant transformation of a calcifying aponeurotic fibroma.

Surgical management should be conservative for all tumors with the typical appearance of a calcifying aponeurotic fibroma. In fact, excision and reexcision, if necessary, appear to be preferable to radical or mutilating surgical procedures to maintain function of the extremity.[380] Radical surgical therapy, of course, is required in those rare cases that display evidence of malignant transformation.

### Discussion

There seem to be two phases in the development of this tumor: (1) an initial phase, which is more common in infants and small children, in which the tumor grows diffusely, often lacks calcification, and bears a close resemblance to infantile fibromatosis; and (2) a late phase, in which the tumor is more compact and nodular and shows a more prominent degree of calcification and cartilage formation. In some of the latter cases, calcification and cartilage formation are so prominent it may be difficult to distinguish this lesion from a calcifying soft part chondroma. For this reason, Lichtenstein and Goldman suggested the term "the cartilage analog of fibromatosis" for this lesion.[375]

## CONGENITAL AND ACQUIRED MUSCULAR FIBROSIS

Muscular fibrosis was first defined as an entity by Hnevkovsky in 1961 as *progressive fibrosis of vastus intermedius muscle in children*.[391] Since 1961 numerous examples of this condition have been reported in the literature; most affected the quadriceps muscle,[382,385,386,389,394,396,402] although a few have been reported in the gluteus[383,395,398,400] and deltoid[381,387,390,403] muscles. Rare cases have also been reported in the triceps[384,401] and gastrocnemius[395] muscles. Both congenital and acquired lesions of this type have been described.

### Clinical Findings

Although the onset of the lesion usually dates back to the first year of life, the mass develops slowly and often does not become apparent before the second or third year of life. Clinically, most patients present with a progressive painless mass or cord-like induration of the involved muscle. Lesions are generally poorly circumscribed and may occur on one or both sides.[400] Progressive fibrosis results in shortening and contracture of the involved muscle, which leads to various functional disturbances depending on the extent of the fibrosis and the muscle involved. Concomitant dimpling or depressions of the overlying skin are observed occasionally; they are most likely a result of fatty atrophy and extension of the fibrosing process into the adjacent fascia and subcutaneous fat.

The fibrosing process is most commonly encountered in the quadriceps muscle, where it usually affects the distal portion of the vastus intermedius and vastus lateralis. It severely limits the range of active and passive flexion of the knee joint and causes difficulty squatting and sitting straight as well as an abnormal gait. In some cases the patella dislocates laterally every time the knee is flexed. Involvement of the gluteus muscle may lead to external rotation and abduction contracture of the hip in a seated position and a waddling gait. Napiontek and Ruszkowski reported a case of gluteal fibrosis following intramuscular injection that resulted in paralytic footdrop secondary to sciatic nerve injury and external rotation contracture of the hip.[397] Involvement of the deltoid muscle may cause abduction contracture of the shoulder and lateral elevation of the arms.[388]

### Pathologic Findings

Grossly, the involved muscle shows patchy, firm, scar-like, gray or gray-yellow areas that consist microscopically of a conglomerate of collagenous fibrous tissue, residual partly degenerated atrophic muscle fibers, and replacement of atrophic muscle by mature fat. Not infrequently, the fibrosis extends into the muscle fascia or aponeurosis and even into the subcutaneous fat. There is no evidence of foreign body reaction or significant inflammation.

### Discussion

Various concepts have been suggested as to the most likely cause of the fibrosing process. Lloyd-Roberts et al.[394] and Gunn[389] were the first to recognize the association of this lesion with multiple intramuscular injections. In many cases the patients have a history of severe illness during infancy and treatment with multiple intramuscular injections of antibiotics or other medications. No single drug has been incriminated as the cause of the fibrosis, although antibiotics appear to be the most frequently injected medication. It has been proposed that the intramuscular injection results in chemical myositis or pressure ischemia with subsequent fibrosis.[388] Given the fact that only a small number of infants who undergo this type of therapy develop intramuscular fibrosis, other predisposing factors have been suggested. Peiro et al. noted scar puncture marks and keloid formation at the sites of injection in some cases.[398] There are also some reports of muscle fibrosis in children who are said to have had the lesions since birth with no history of intramuscular injections.[382,386,393,399] There is no clear hereditary pattern, but the condition has been observed in four pairs of siblings[400] and several pairs of identical twins.[382,385]

To regain a normal range of function, tenotomy (rather than physical therapy or other conservative measures) is the treatment of choice. Most patients regain full range of motion, although a subset of patients continue to have functional impairment of the involved extremity.[396]

## CEREBRIFORM FIBROUS PROLIFERATION (PROTEUS SYNDROME)

Proteus syndrome, a rare entity, is included here because the cerebriform or gyriform fibrous proliferation characteristically found on the volar surfaces may be mistaken for fibromatosis. Although isolated or localized cerebriform fibrous proliferations have been described,[404,414,417,418] more commonly they occur in conjunction with the complex group of lesions involving the skin, soft tissue, and skeleton. Proteus syndrome was first described by Wiedemann et al. in 1983[420] and was named after the Greek ocean deity, Proteus (the polymorphous), because of the broad range of its features. Although "the elephant man," Joseph Merrick, was originally believed to have neurofibromatosis, evidence indicates that he suffered from Proteus syndrome.[405,415]

Patients with the Proteus syndrome exhibit a constellation of congenital and developmental defects that cannot be classified into previously defined disorders, and these patients demonstrate wide morphologic variability.[413] Manifestations include gigantism of the hands or feet (macrodactyly), asymmetry, skeletal abnormalities including hemihypertrophy and exostoses (particularly cranial exostoses), and a variety of cutaneous abnormalities including epidermal nevi and lipomatous and hemangiomatous tumors. The lipomatous proliferations may be present in the subcutis but may also affect the abdomen, pelvis, and mesentery.[407,408,416] The cerebriform fibrous changes affect the plantar surfaces and to a lesser degree the palmar surfaces, and they are associated with unilateral or bilateral macrodactyly or hypertrophy of long bones (partial gigantism). Grossly, there is marked thickening of the skin in the volar areas resulting in a coarse cerebriform or gyriform pattern (Fig. 11–65).

Microscopically, the plantar and palmar lesions consist of dense fibrosis involving both the dermis and subcutis, with hyperkeratosis of the overlying skin[413,419] (Figs. 11–66, 11–67, 11–68). Uitto et al. showed that these lesions consist almost exclusively of type I collagen and suggested an underlying defect in the production of collagenase,[417] possibly related to disturbed production of insulin-like growth factors.[412]

The cause of the Proteus syndrome is unknown. There is no gender predilection, and all reported cases appear to be sporadic.[405,419,420] Cytogenetic studies have shown normal karyotypes.[419] Happle suggested that the underlying defect is a somatic mutation that is lethal in the nonmosaic state.[409] Other studies have lent support to the hypothesis of somatic mosaicism as a cause of Proteus syndrome.[406,410,411,414]

## CALCIFYING FIBROUS PSEUDOTUMOR

Originally reported as *childhood fibrous tumor with psammoma bodies,*[430] calcifying fibrous pseudotumor is a rare entity; it is a hypocellular fibrous lesion that

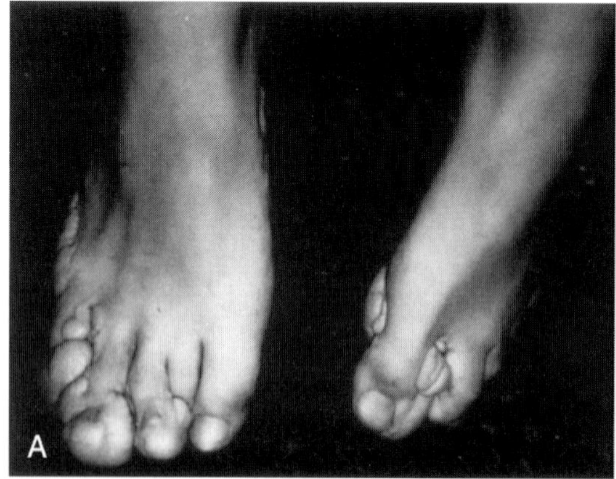


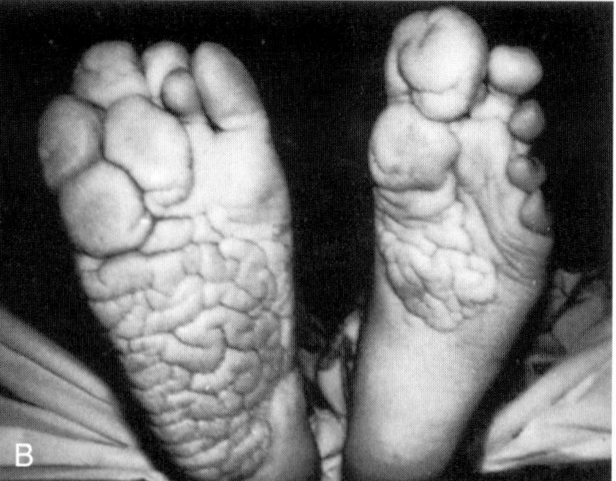


**FIGURE 11–65.** Bilateral cerebriform (gyriform) fibrous proliferation of toes (**A**) and plantar surfaces (**B**). This process may occur alone or in conjunction with lipomatous and hemangiomatous tumors and various skeletal changes, including scoliosis, multiple exostoses, and craniofacial asymmetry (Proteus syndrome).

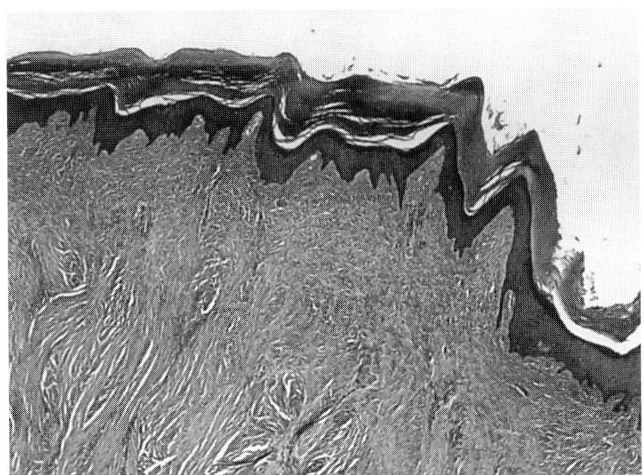

**FIGURE 11–66.** Proteus syndrome. The lesions contain extensive dermal fibrosis with acanthosis and hyperkeratosis of the overlying epithelium.

most often affects patients during the second or third decade of life.[421–433] Females are affected slightly more commonly than males. Most patients present with a slowly growing, painless mass in the subcutaneous or deep soft tissues that is associated with systemic symptoms. The lesions most commonly arise in the extremities, followed by the trunk, inguinal and scrotal regions, and head and neck. Rare lesions have also been described in the mediastinum,[421] pleura,[424,428] and visceral peritoneum.[425,427,432] The tumors range in size from 2.5 to 15.0 cm, but most are 3–5 cm. Most have been treated by simple local excision, and there has been a report of only a single recurrence that occurred 7.5 years after the initial excision.[422] There have been no reports of metastasis.

On gross examination, the mass is well circumscribed, somewhat lobulated, and solid or firm; it has a uniform gray-white fibrous cut appearance. It often cuts with a gritty sensation due to the extensive calcifications typically present. Histologically, the mass is well circumscribed, nonencapsulated, and composed chiefly of hyalinized birefringent fibrosclerotic tissue with a variable inflammatory infiltrate composed of lymphocytes and plasma cells, with the formation of occasional germinal centers. The lesions are hypocellular, with scattered cytologically bland, fibroblastic or myofibroblastic spindle cells.[426] Immunohistochemically, these cells stain diffusely for vimentin and focally and weakly for smooth muscle actin.[423] A characteristic feature is the presence of dystrophic, frequently psammomatous calcifications that may be focally present or comprise most of the tumor (Fig. 11–69).

The differential diagnosis includes inflammatory myofibroblastic tumor, fibromatosis, nodular fasciitis, fibroma of the tendon sheath, calcifying aponeurotic fibroma, and amyloidoma. *Inflammatory myofibroblastic tumor* is generally more cellular, less hyalinized, and typically lacks calcifications. However, clearly there is histologic overlap of these lesions, and it has been proposed that calcifying fibrous pseudotumor represents a late sclerosing phase of inflammatory myofi-

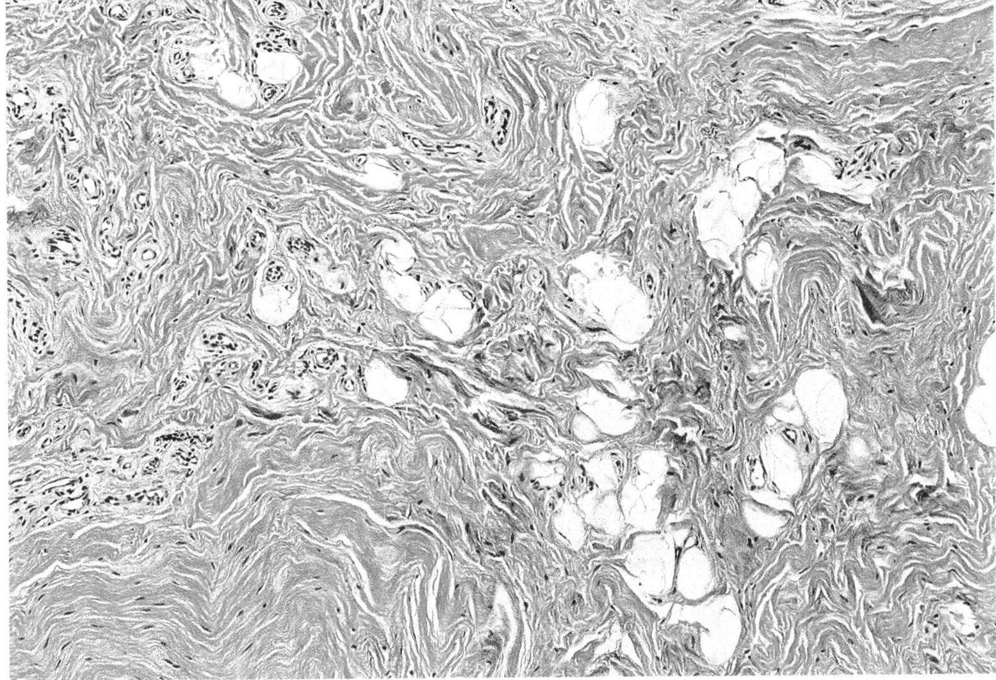

**FIGURE 11–67.** Proteus syndrome. Hypocellular dense collagen with admixed adipocytes.

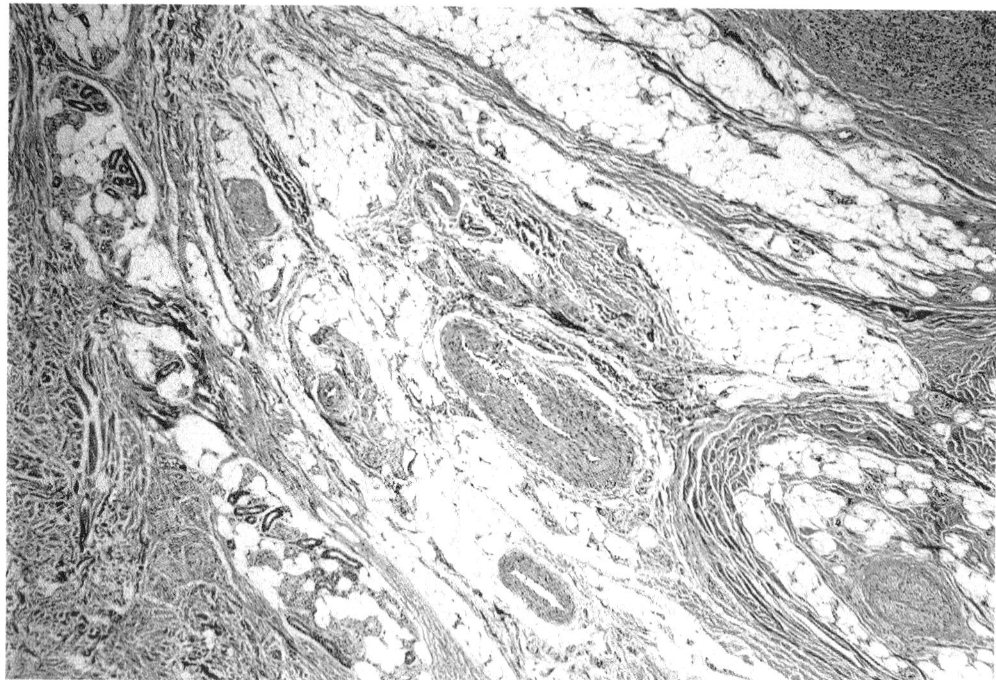

**FIGURE 11–68.** Benign lipomatous lesion in a patient with Proteus syndrome.

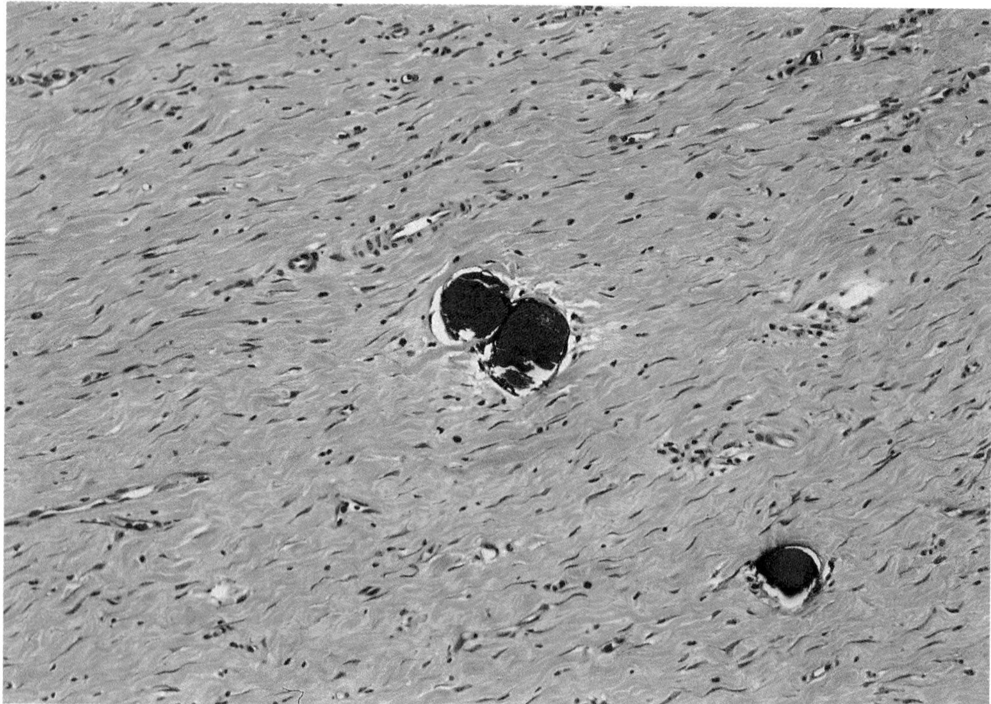

**FIGURE 11–69.** Calcifying fibrous pseudotumor chiefly composed of a uniform dense collagenous matrix with psammomatous calcifications and scattered spindle-shaped and inflammatory cells.

broblastic tumor.[422,431] *Fibromatosis* is less well circumscribed, and histologically the spindle cells typically infiltrate the surrounding soft tissues. In addition, fibromatosis is characterized by more cellularity in which the cells are frequently arranged in a prominent fascicular growth pattern. Microcalcifications have only rarely been described in fibromatosis. *Nodular fasciitis* is composed of tissue culture-like spindle cells deposited in a myxoid stroma that lacks microcalcifications. *Fibroma of the tendon sheath* is also well circumscribed and composed chiefly of densely sclerotic collagen, but there are frequently areas of increased cellularity, some of which resemble nodular fasciitis. In addition, elongated slit-like spaces are typical, and calcifications are not present. *Calcifying aponeurotic fibroma* usually arises in the hands or feet, is less well circumscribed than calcifying fibrous pseudotumor, and is characterized by band-like calcifications frequently surrounded by cartilaginous metaplasia and multinucleated giant cells. Unlike amyloid tumor (*amyloidoma*), calcifying fibrous pseudotumor is devoid of giant cells or demonstrable amyloid, as congo red stains are negative.

The exact nature of this lesion is uncertain. It could represent the end-stage of an inflammatory myofibroblastic tumor. Van Dorpe et al. described an intra-abdominal tumor which arose in a 17-year-old female with features overlapping those seen in these two entities, as well as transitional stages between calcifying fibrous pseudotumor and inflammatory myofibroblastic tumor.[431] There are no cytogenetic data reported on calcifying fibrous pseudotumor and thus it is not known whether the ALK gene is involved as it is in inflammatory myofibroblastic tumor. We have been unable to demonstrate ALK1 immunoreactivity in a small group of deep soft tissue calcifying fibrous pseudotumors.[430a]

## REFERENCES

### Fibrous Hamartoma of Infancy


1. Dickey GE, Sotelo-Avila C. Fibrous hamartoma of infancy: current review. Pediatr Dev Pathol 2:236, 1999.
2. Efem SE, Ekpo MD. Clinicopathological features of untreated fibrous hamartoma of infancy. J Clin Pathol 46:522, 1993.
3. Enzinger FM. Fibrous hamartoma of infancy. Cancer 18:241, 1965.
4. Eppley BL, Harruff R, Shah M, et al. Fibrous hamartomas of the scalp in infancy. Plast Reconstr Surg 94:195, 1994.
5. Fletcher CDM, Powell G, van Noorden S, et al. Fibrous hamartoma of infancy: a histochemical and immunohistochemical study. Histopathology 12:65, 1988.
6. Jebson PJ, Louis DS. Fibrous hamartoma of infancy in the hand: a case report. J Hand Surg [Am] 22:740, 1997.
7. German DS, Paletta CE, Gabriel K. Fibrous hamartoma of infancy. Orthopedics 19:258, 1996.
8. Greco MA, Schinella RA, Vuletin JC. Fibrous hamartoma of infancy: an ultrastructural study. Hum Pathol 15:717, 1984.
9. Groisman G, Kerner H. A case of fibrous hamartoma of infancy in the scrotum, including immunohistochemical findings. J Urol 144:340, 1990.
10. Groisman G, Lichtig C. Fibrous hamartoma of infancy: an immunohistochemical and ultrastructural study. Hum Pathol 22:914, 1991.
11. Harris CJ, Das S, Vogt PJ. Fibrous hamartoma of infancy in the scrotum. J Urol 127:781, 1982.
12. Mitchell ML, Di Sant'Agnese PA, Gerber JE. Fibrous hamartoma of infancy. Hum Pathol 13:586, 1982.
13. Paller AS, Gonzalez-Crussi F, Sherman JO. Fibrous hamartoma of infancy: eight additional cases and a review of the literature. Arch Dermatol 125:88, 1989.
14. Popek EJ, Montgomery EA, Fourcroy JL. Fibrous hamartoma of infancy in the genital region: findings in 15 cases. J Urol 152:990, 1994.
15. Reye RDK. Considerations of certain subdermal "fibromatous tumors" of infancy. J Pathol 72:149, 1956.
16. Ritchie EL, Gonzalez-Crussi F, Zaontz MR. Fibrous hamartoma of infancy masquerading as a rhabdomyosarcoma of the spermatic cord. J Urol 140:800, 1988.
17. Sotelo-Avila C, Bale PM. Subdermal fibrous hamartoma of infancy: pathology of 40 cases and differential diagnosis. Pediatr Pathol 14:39, 1994.
18. Stock JA, Niku SD, Packer MG, et al. Fibrous hamartoma of infancy: a report of two cases in the genital region. Urology 45:130, 1995.
19. Thami GP, Jaswal R, Kanwar AJ. Fibrous hamartoma of infancy in the scrotum. Pediatr Dermatol 15:326, 1998.


### Infantile Digital Fibromatosis


20. Allen PW. Recurring digital fibrous tumors of childhood. Pathology 4:215, 1972.
21. Arundell FD. Proceedings: recurring digital fibrous tumor of childhood, case 1. Arch Dermatol 111:1372, 1975.
22. Azam SH, Nicholas JL. Recurring infantile digital fibromatosis: report of two cases. J Pediatr Surg 30:89, 1995.
23. Battifora H, Hines JR. Recurrent digital fibromas of childhood: an electron microscope study. Cancer 27:1530, 1971.
24. Beckett JH, Jacobs AH. Recurring digital fibrous tumors of childhood: a review. Pediatrics 59:401, 1977.
25. Bhawan J, Bacchetta C, Joris I, et al. A myofibroblastic tumor: infantile digital fibroma (recurrent digital fibrous tumor of childhood). Am J Pathol 94:19, 1979.
26. Bittesini L, Dei Tos AP, Doglioni C, et al. Fibroepithelial tumor of the breast with digital fibroma-like inclusions in the stromal component: case report with immunocytochemical and ultrastructural analysis. Am J Surg Pathol 18:296, 1994.
27. Bloem JJ, Vuzevski VD, Huffstadt AJC. Recurring digital fibroma of infancy. J Bone Joint Surg Br 56:746, 1974.
28. Burgert S, Jones DH. Recurring digital fibroma of childhood. J Hand Surg [Br] 21:400, 1996.
29. Cachaza JA, Caballero JJL, Fernandez JA, et al. Endocervical polyp with pseudosarcomatous pattern and cytoplasmic inclusions: an electron microscopic study. Am J Clin Pathol 85:633, 1986.
30. Canioni D, Richard S, Rambaud C, et al. Lingual localization of an inclusion body fibromatosis (Reye's tumor). Pathol Res Pract 187:886, 1991.
31. Choi KC, Hashimoto K, Setoyama M, et al. Infantile digital fibromatosis: immunohistochemical and immunoelectron microscopic studies. J Cutan Pathol 17:225, 1990.
32. Enzinger FM. Dermal fibromatosis. In: Tumors of Bone and Soft Tissue. Year Book, Chicago, 1965, pp 375–396.
33. Falco NA, Upton J. Infantile digital fibromas. J Hand Surg [Am] 20:1014, 1995.
34. Frank A. Ein Fall von angeborenen Fibromen am Finger nebst

Beitraegen zur Kasuistic der Fingertumoren. Wien Klin Rundschau 22:659, 1908.

35. Fringes B, Thais H, Bohm N, et al. Identification of actin microfilaments in the intracytoplasmic inclusions present in recurring infantile digital fibromatosis (Reye tumor). Pediatr Pathol 6:311, 1986.
36. Hayashi T, Tsuda N, Chowdhury PR, et al. Infantile digital fibromatosis: a study of the development and regression of cytoplasmic inclusion bodies. Mod Pathol 8:548, 1995.
37. Hiraoka N, Mukai M, Hosada Y, et al. Phyllodes tumor of the breast containing the intracytoplasmic inclusion bodies identical with infantile digital fibromatosis. Am J Surg Pathol 18: 506, 1994.
38. Ishii N, Matsui K, Ichiyama S, et al. A case of infantile digital fibromatosis showing spontaneous regression. Br J Dermatol 121:129, 1989.
39. Iwasaki H, Kikuchi M, Mori R, et al. Infantile digital fibromatosis: ultrastructural, histochemical and tissue culture observations. Cancer 46:2238, 1980.
40. Iwasaki H, Kikuchi M, Ohtsuki I, et al. Infantile digital fibromatosis: identification of actin filaments in cytoplasmic inclusions by heavy meromyosin binding. Cancer 52:1653, 1983.
41. Iwasaki H, Tsuneyoshi M, Enjoji M. Infanfile digital fibromatosis: histopathological and electron microscopic study with a review of the literature. Acta Pathol Jpn 24:717, 1974.
42. Jensen AR, Martin LW, Longino LA. Digital neurofibrosarcoma in infancy. J Pediatr 51:566, 1957.
43. Kawabata H, Masada K, Aoki Y, et al. Infantile digital fibromatosis after web construction in syndactyly. J Hand Surg [Am] 11:741, 1986.
44. McKenzie AW, Innes FLF, Rack JM, et al. Digital fibrous swellings in children. Br J Dermatol 83:446, 1970.
45. Miyamoto T, Mihara M, Hagari Y, et al. Posttraumatic occurrence of infantile digital fibromatosis: a histologic and electron microscopic study. Arch Dermatol 122:915, 1986.
46. Mukai M, Torikata C, Iri H, et al. Immunohistochemical identification of aggregated actin filaments in formalin-fixed, paraffin-embedded sections. I. A study of infantile digital fibromatosis by a new pretreatment. Am J Surg Pathol 16:110, 1992.
47. Mukai M, Torikata C, Iri H, et al. Infantile digital fibromatosis: an electron microscopic and immunohistochemical study. Acta Pathol Jpn 36:1605, 1986.
48. Navas-Palacios JJ, Conde-Zurita JM. Inclusion body myofibroblasts other than those seen in recurring digital fibroma of childhood. Ultrastruct Pathol 7:109, 1984.
49. Pettinato G, Manival JC, Gould EW, et al. Inclusion body fibromatosis of the breast: two cases with immunohistochemical and ultrastructural findings. Am J Clin Pathol 101:714, 1994.
50. Pohjanpelto P, Ahlqvist J, Hurme K, et al. Recurring digital fibrous tumor of childhood. II. Isolation of a cell transforming agent. Acta Pathol Microbiol Scand 70:297, 1967.
51. Purdy LJ, Colby TV. Infantile digital fibromatosis occurring outside the digit. Am J Surg Pathol 8:787, 1984.
52. Reye RDK. Recurring digital fibrous tumors of childhood. Arch Pathol 80:228, 1965.
53. Rimareix F, Bardot J, Andrac L, et al. Infantile digital fibroma: report on eleven cases. Eur J Pediatr Surg 7:345, 1997.
54. Shapiro HL. Infantile digital fibromatosis and aponeurotic fibroma. Acta Derm Venereol 99:37, 1969.
55. Terada S, Suzuki N, Uchide K, et al. Vulvar angioleiomyoma. Arch Gynecol Obstet 253:51, 1993.
56. Viale G, Doglioni C, Iuzzolino P, et al. Infantile digital fibromatosis-like tumor (inclusion body fibromatosis) of adulthood: report of two cases with ultrastructural and immunocytochemical findings. Histopathology 12:415, 1988.
57. Yun K. Infantile digital fibromatosis: immunohistochemical and ultrastructural observations of cytoplasmic inclusions. Cancer 61:500, 1988.
58. Yusoff KL, Spagnolo DV, Digwood KI. Atypical cervical polyp with intracytoplasmic inclusions. Pathology 30:215, 1998.
59. Zina AM, Rampini E, Fulcheri E, et al. Recurrent digital fibromatosis of childhood: an ultrastructural and immunohistochemical study of two cases. Am J Dermatopathol 8:22, 1986.

### Myofibroma and Myofibromatosis

60. Altemani AM, Amstalden EI, Martins FJ. Congenital generalized fibromatosis causing spinal cord compression. Hum Pathol 16:1063, 1985.
61. Baird PA, Worth AJ. Congenital generalized fibromatosis: an autosomal recessive condition. Clin Genet 9:488, 1976.
62. Beck JC, Devaney KO, Weatherly RA, et al. Pediatric myofibromatosis of the head and neck. Arch Otolaryngol Head Neck Surg 125:39, 1999.
63. Beham A, Badve S, Suster S, et al. Solitary myofibroma in adults: clinicopathological analysis of a series. Histopathology 22:335, 1993.
64. Benjamin SP, Mercer RD, Hawk WA. Myofibroblastic contraction in spontaneous regression of multiple congenital mesenchymal hamartomas. Cancer 40:2343, 1977.
65. Boman F, Foliguet B, Metaizeau JP, et al. Myofibromatosis in children: histopathologic and ultrastructural study of a localized form with a spontaneously regressive course. Ann Pathol 4:211, 1984.
66. Bracko M, Cindro L, Golouh R. Familial occurrence of infantile myofibromatosis. Cancer 69:1294, 1992.
67. Brill PW, Yandow DR, Langer LO, et al. Congenital generalized fibromatosis: case report and literature review. Pediatr Radiol 12:269, 1982.
68. Bures C, Barnes L. Benign mesenchymomas of the head and neck. Arch Pathol Lab Med 102:237, 1978.
69. Chang WW, Griffith KM. Solitary intestinal fibromatosis: a rare cause of intestinal obstruction in neonate and infant. J Pediatr Surg 26:1406, 1991.
70. Chateil JF, Brun M, Lebail B, et al. Infantile myofibromatosis. Skeletal Radiol 24:629, 1995.
71. Chung EB, Enzinger FM. Infantile myofibromatosis. Cancer 48: 1807, 1981.
72. Daimaru Y, Hashimoto H, Enjoji M. Myofibromatosis in adults (adult counterpart of infantile myofibromatosis). Am J Surg Pathol 13:859, 1989.
73. Dictor M, Elner A, Andersson T, et al. Myofibromatosis like hemangiopericytoma metastasizing as differentiated vascular smooth muscle and myosarcoma: myopericytes as a subset of "myofibroblasts." Am J Surg Pathol 16:1239, 1992.
74. Dimmick JE, Wood WS. Congenital multiple fibromatosis. Am J Dermatopathol 5:289, 1983.
75. Fletcher CD, Achu P, Van Noorden S, et al. Infantile myofibromatosis: a light microscopic, histochemical and immunohistochemical study suggesting true smooth muscle differentiation. Histopathology 11:245, 1987.
76. Fukasawa Y, Ishikura H, Takada A, et al. Massive apoptosis in infantile myofibromatosis: a putative mechanism of tumor regression. Am J Pathol 144:480, 1994.
77. Giannini C, Wright A, Dyck PJ. Polyneuropathy associated with nerve angiomatosis and multiple soft tissue tumors. Am J Surg Pathol 19:1325, 1995.
78. Granter SR, Badizadegan K, Fletcher CDM. Myofibromatosis in adults, glomangiopericytoma, and myopericytoma: a spectrum of tumors showing perivascular myoid differentiation. Am J Surg Pathol 22:513, 1998.
79. Hasegawa T, Hirose T, Seki K, et al. Solitary infantile myofibromatosis of bone: an immunohistochemical and ultrastructural study. Am J Surg Pathol 17:308, 1993.

80. Hastier P, Caroli-Bose FX, Harris AG, et al. Solitary hepatic infantile myofibromatosis in a female adolescent. Dig Dis Sci 43:1124, 1998.
81. Heiple KG, Perrin E, Aikawa M. Congenital generalized fibromatosis: a case limited to osseous lesions. J Bone Joint Surg Am 54:663, 1972.
82. Hogan SF, Salassa JR. Recurrent adult myofibromatosis: a case report. Am J Clin Pathol 97:810, 1992.
83. Inwards CY, Unni KK, Beabout JW, et al. Solitary congenital fibromatosis (infantile myofibromatosis) of bone. Am J Surg Pathol 15:935, 1991.
84. Jennings T, Duray PH, Collins FS, et al. Infantile myofibromatosis: evidence for an autosomal-dominant disorder. Am J Surg Pathol 8:529, 1984.
85. Jones AC, Freedman PD, Kerpel SM. Oral myofibromas: a report of 13 cases and review of the literature. J Oral Maxillofac Surg 52:870, 1994.
86. Kauffman SL, Stout AP. Congenital mesenchymal tumors. Cancer 18:460, 1965.
87. Kindblom LG, Angervall L. Congenital solitary fibromatosis of the skeleton: case report of a variant of congenital generalized fibromatosis. Cancer 41:636, 1978.
88. Lingen MW, Mostofi RS, Solt DB. Myofibromas of the oral cavity. Oral Surg Oral Med Oral Pathol Oral Radiol Endod 80: 297, 1995.
89. Lo LJ, Hsueh C, Noordhoff MS, et al. Infantile myofibromatosis: a solitary lesion involving the upper lip. Ann Plast Surg 39:624, 1997.
90. Mentzel T, Calonje E, Nascimento AG, et al. Infantile hemangiopericytoma versus infantile myofibromatosis: study of a series suggesting a continuous spectrum of infantile myofibroblastic lesions. Am J Surg Pathol 18:922, 1994.
91. Morettin LB, Mueller E, Schreiber M. Generalized hamartomatosis (congenital generalized fibromatosis). AJR 114:722, 1972.
92. Present DA, Abdelwahab IF, Zwass A, et al. Case report 575. Skeletal Radiol 18:557, 1989.
93. Requena L, Kutzner H, Hugel K, et al. Cutaneous adult myofibroma: a vascular neoplasm. J Cutan Pathol 23:445, 1996.
94. Roggli VL, Kim HS, Hawkins E. Congenital generalized fibromatosis with visceral involvement: a case report. Cancer 45: 954, 1980.
95. Rutigliano MJ, Pollack IF, Ahdab-Barmada M, et al. Intracranial infantile myofibromatosis. J Neurosurg 81:539, 1994.
96. Salamah MM, Haammoudi SM, Sadi ARM. Infantile myofibromatosis. J Pediatr Surg 23:975, 1988.
97. Schaffzin EA, Chung SMK, Kaye R. Congenital generalized fibromatosis with complete spontaneous regressions. J Bone Joint Surg Am 54:657, 1972.
98. Smith KJ, Skelton HG, Barrett TL, et al. Cutaneous myofibroma. Mod Pathol 2:603, 1989.
99. Srigley JR, Mancer K. Solitary intestinal fibromatosis with perinatal bowel obstruction. Pediatr Pathol 2:249, 1984.
100. Stenman G, Nadal N, Persson S, et al. del (6)(q12;q15) as the sole cytogenetic anomaly in a case of solitary infantile myofibromatosis. Oncol Rep 6:1101, 1999.
101. Stenzel P, Fitterer S. Gastrointestinal multicentric infantile myofibromatosis: characteristic histology on rectal biopsy. Am J Gastroenterol 84:1115, 1989.
102. Stout AP. Juvenile fibromatosis. Cancer 7:953, 1954.
103. Teng P, Warden MJ, Cohn WI. Congenital generalized fibromatosis (renal and skeletal) with complete spontaneous regression. J Pediatr 62:748, 1963.
104. Variend S, Bax NMA, Van Gorp J. Are infantile myofibromatosis, congenital fibrosarcoma and congenital hemangiopericytoma histogenetically related? Histopathology 26:57, 1995.
105. Venencie PY, Bigel P, Desgruelles C, et al. Infantile myofibromatosis: report of two cases in one family. Br J Dermatol 117: 255, 1987.
106. Williams JO, Schrum D. Congenital fibrosarcoma: report of a case in a newborn infant. AMA Arch Pathol 51:548, 1951.
107. Wiswell TE, Davis J, Cunningham BE, et al. Infantile myofibromatosis: the most common fibrous tumor of infancy. J Pediatr Surg 23:314, 1988.
108. Zelger BWH, Calonje E, Sepp N, et al. Monophasic cellular variant of infantile myofibromatosis: an unusual histopathologic pattern in two siblings. Am J Dermatopathol 17:131, 1995.
109. Zeller B, Storm-Mathisen I, Smevik B, et al. Cure of infantile myofibromatosis with severe respiratory complications without antitumour therapy. Eur J Pediatr 156:841, 1997.

### Juvenile Hyalin Fibromatosis

110. Alfi OS, Heuser ET, Landing BA, et al. A syndrome of systemic hyalinosis, short-limbed dwarfism and possible thymic dysplasia. Earth Rep 5:57, 1975.
111. Atherton DJ, Lake BD, Wells RS. Juvenile hyaline fibromatosis. Br J Dermatol 19:61, 1981.
112. Bedford CD, Sills JA, Sommelet-Olive D, et al. Juvenile hyaline fibromatosis: a report of two severe cases. J Pediatr 119:404, 1991.
113. Castro DJ, Hoover L, Lufkin RB, et al. Multicentric fibromatosis of familial inheritance. Arch Pathol Lab Med 111:867, 1987.
114. Costa OG, Costa PB. Fibromatosis hialina juvenil. Med Cutan Iber Lat Am 5:331, 1975.
115. De Rosa G, Tornillo L, Orabona P, et al. Juvenile hyaline fibromatosis: a case report of a localized form? Am J Dermatopathol 16:624, 1994.
116. Drescher E, Woyke S, Markiewicz C, et al. Juvenile fibromatosis in siblings (fibromatosis hyalinica multiplex juvenilis). J Pediatr Surg 2:427, 1967.
117. Enjoji M, Kato N, Kamikozuru K, et al. Juvenile fibromatosis of the scalp in siblings. Acta Med Univ Kagoshima 10:145, 1968.
118. Fayad MN, Yacoub A, Salman S, et al. Juvenile hyaline fibromatosis: two new patients and review of the literature. Am J Med Genet 26:123, 1987.
119. Finlay AY, Ferguson SD, Holt PJA. Juvenile hyaline fibromatosis. Br J Dermatol 108:609, 1983.
120. Gianotti F, Ermacora E, Magrini U. Fibromatosis hyaline juvenile. Ann Dermatol Venereol 104:152, 1977.
121. Gilaberte Y, Gonzalez-Mediero I, Lopez-Barrantes V, et al. Juvenile hyaline fibromatosis with skull-encephalic anomalies: a case report and review of the literature. Dermatology 187:144, 1993.
122. Glover MT, Lake VD, Atherton DJ. Infantile systemic hyalinosis: newly recognized disorder of collagen? Pediatrics 878: 228, 1991.
123. Hallock GG. An adult with juvenile hyaline fibromatosis of the foot. Foot Ankle Int 15:634, 1994.
124. Hallock GG. Juvenile hyaline fibromatosis of the hand in an adult. J Hand Surg [Am] 18:614, 1993.
125. Hutchinson I. Juvenile systemic hyalinosis: a rare cause of gingival hypertrophy: a case report. Int J Paediatr Dent 6:39, 1996.
126. Ishikawa H, Hori Y. Systematisierte hyalinose im zusammenhang mit epidermalysis bullosa polydystraphica und hyalinosis cutis et mucosae. Arch Klin Dermatol 218:30, 1964.
127. Ishikawa H, Maeda H, Takamuatsu H, et al. Systemic hyalinosis (juvenile hyaline fibromatosis): ultrastructure of the hyaline with particular reference to the cross-ended structure. Arch Dermatol Res 265:195, 1979.
128. Iwata S, Horiuchi R, Maeda H, et al. Systemic hyalinosis or

juvenile hyaline fibromatosis: ultrastructural and biochemical study. Arch Dermatol Res 267:115, 1980.
129. Jacyk WK, Wentzel LF. Juvenile hyaline fibromatosis in two South African black children. Int J Dermatol 35:740, 1996.
130. Kan AE, Rogers M. Juvenile hyaline fibromatosis: an expanded clinicopathologic spectrum. Pediatr Dermatol 6:868, 1989.
131. Katagiri K, Takasaki S, Fujiwara S, et al. Purification and structural analysis of extracellular matrix of a skin tumor from a patient with juvenile hyaline fibromatosis. J Dermatol Sci 13: 37, 1996.
132. Kitano Y. Juvenile hyalin fibromatosis. Arch Dermatol 112:86, 1976.
133. Kitano Y, Horiki M, Aoki T, et al. Two cases of juvenile hyalin fibromatosis: some histological, electron microscopic and tissue culture observations. Arch Dermatol 106:877, 1972.
134. Mancini GM, Stojanov L, Willemsen R, et al. Juvenile hyaline fibromatosis: clinical heterogeneity in three patients. Dermatology 198:18, 1999.
135. Mayer-da-Silva A, Poiares-Baptista A, Guerra-Rodrigo F, et al. Juvenile hyaline fibromatosis: a histologic and histochemical study. Arch Pathol Lab Med 112:928, 1988.
136. Miyake I, Tokumaru H, Sugino H, et al. Juvenile hyaline fibromatosis: case report with five years follow-up. Am J Dermatopathol 17:584, 1995.
137. Murray J. On three peculiar cases of molluscum fibrosum in children. Med Chir Trans 38:235, 1873.
138. Nezelof C, Letourneux-Toromanoff B, Griscelli C, et al. La fibromatose disseminee douloureuse hyalinose systemique. Arch Fr Pediatr 35:1063, 1978.
139. O'Neill DB, Kasser JR. Juvenile hyaline fibromatosis: a case report and review of musculoskeletal manifestations. J Bone Joint Surg Am 71:941, 1989.
140. Piattelli A, Scarano A, Di Bellucci A, et al. Juvenile hyaline fibromatosis of gingiva: a case report. J Periodontol 67:451, 1996.
141. Poiares Baptista A, Foseca M, Gancalo S. Fibromatose hyaline juvenile. Ann Dermatol Venereol 110:751, 1983.
142. Puretic S, Puretic B, Fiser-Herman M. A unique form of mesenchymal dysplasia. Br J Dermatol 74:8, 1962.
143. Quintal D, Jackson R. Juvenile hyaline fibromatosis: a 15-year follow-up. Arch Dermatol 121:1062, 1985.
144. Remberger K, Krieg T, Kunze D, et al. Fibromatosis hyalinica multiplex (juvenile hyaline fibromatosis): light microscopic, electron microscopic, immunohistochemical and biochemical findings. Cancer 56:614, 1985.
145. Sezaki H, Kiyozuka Y, Uemura Y, et al. Juvenile hyaline fibromatosis: a report of two unrelated adult sibling cases and a literature review. Pathol Int 48:230, 1998.
146. Shehab ZP, Raafat S, Proops DW. Juvenile hyaline fibromatosis. Int J Pediatr Otorhinolaryngol 33:179, 1995.
147. Stringer DA, Hall CM. Juvenile hyaline fibromatosis. Br J Radiol 54:473, 1981.
148. Török E, Jellinek K, Schneider F, et al. Juvenile hyaline fibromatose. Akttuelle Dermatol 10:6, 1984.
149. Wang NS, Knaack T. Fibromatosis hyalinica multiplex juvenilis. Ultrastruct Pathol 3:153, 1982.
150. Whitfield A, Robinson AH. A further report of a remarkable series of cases of molluscum fibrosum in children. Med Chir Trans 86:293, 1903.
151. Winchester P, Grossman H, Lim WN, et al. A new acid mucopolysaccharidosis with skeletal deformities simulating rheumatoid arthritis. AJR 106:121, 1969.
152. Winik BC, Boente MC, Asial R. Juvenile hyaline fibromatosis: ultrastructural study. Am J Dermatopathol 20:373, 1998.
153. Woyke S, Domagala W, Markiewicz D. A 19-year follow-up of multiple juvenile fibromatosis. J Pediatr Surg 19:302, 1984.
154. Woyke S, Domagala W, Olszewski W. Ultrastructure of a fibromatosis hyalinica multiplex juvenilis. Cancer 26:1157, 1970.

## Gingival Fibromatosis

155. Angelopoulos AP, Goaz P. Incidence of diphenylhydantoin gingival hyperplasia. Oral Surg Oral Med Oral Pathol 34:898, 1972.
156. Bakaeen G, Scully C. Hereditary gingival fibromatosis in a family with the Zimmerman-Laband syndrome. J Oral Pathol Med 20:457, 1991.
157. Bozzo L, de Almedia OP, Scully C, et al. Hereditary gingival fibromatosis: report of an extensive four-generation pedigree. Oral Surg Oral Med Oral Pathol 78:452, 1994.
158. Brown RS, Trejo PM, Weltman R, et al. Treatment of a patient with hereditary gingival fibromatosis: a case report. Spec Care Dentist 15:149, 1995.
159. Byars LT, Jurkiewicz N. Congenital macrogingivae and hypertrichosis with subsequent giant fibroadenoma of the breasts. J Plast Reconstr Surg 27:608, 1961.
160. Chadwick B, Hunter B, Hunter L, et al. Laband syndrome: report of two cases, review of the literature, and identification of additional manifestations. Oral Surg Oral Med Oral Pathol 78:57, 1994.
161. Cuestas-Carnero R, Bornancini CA. Hereditary gingival fibromatosis associated with hypertrichosis: report of five cases in one family. J Oral Maxillofac Surg 46:415, 1988.
162. Dreyer WP, Thomas CJ. Diphenylhydantoinate-induced hyperplasia of the masticatory mucosa in an edentulous epileptic patient. Oral Surg Oral Med Oral Pathol 45:701, 1978.
163. Emerson TG. Hereditary gingival hyperplasia: a familial pedigree of four generations. Oral Surg Oral Med Oral Pathol 19:1, 1965.
164. Fryns JP. Gingival fibromatosis and partial duplication of the short arm of chromosome 2 (dup(2)(p13-p21)). Ann Genet 39: 54, 1996.
165. Gunhan O, Gardner DG, Bostanci H, et al. Familial gingival fibromatosis with unusual histologic findings. J Periodontol 66: 1008, 1995.
166. Hallett KD, Bankier A, Chow CW, et al. Gingival fibromatosis and Klippel-Trenaunay-Weber syndrome: case report. Oral Surg Oral Med Oral Pathol Oral Radiol Endod 79:578, 1995.
167. Harrison M, Odell EW, Agarwal M, et al. Gingival fibromatosis with prune-belly syndrome. Oral Surg Oral Med Oral Pathol Oral Radiol Endod 86:304, 1998.
168. Heath C. Two cases of hypertrophy of the gums and alveoli treated by operation. Trans Odont Soc Great Britain 11:18, 1878.
169. Jorgenson RJ, Cocker ME. Variation in the inheritance and expression of gingival fibromatosis. J Periodontol 45:472, 1974.
170. Laband PF, Habib G, Humphreys GS. Hereditary gingival fibromatosis: report of an affected family with associated splenomegaly and skeletal and soft tissue abnormalities. Oral Surg Oral Med Oral Pathol 17:339, 1964.
171. Lacombe D, Bioulac-Sage P, Sibout M, et al. Congenital marked hypertrichosis and Laband syndrome in a child: overlap between the gingival fibromatosis-hypertrichosis and Laband syndromes. Genet Couns 5:251, 1994.
172. Mason C, Hopper C. The use of $CO_2$ laser in the treatment of gingival fibromatosis: a case report. Int J Paediatr Dent 4:105, 1994.
173. Pina-Neto JM, Moreno AFC, Silva MLR, et al. Cherubism, gingival fibromatosis, epilepsy and mental deficiency (Ramon syndrome) with juvenile rheumatoid arthritis. Am J Med Genet 25:433, 1986.
174. Ramon Y, Berman W, Bubis JJ. Gingival fibromatosis combined with cherubism. Oral Surg Oral Med Oral Pathol 24:435, 1967.

175. Redman RS, Ward CC, Patterson RH. Focus of epithelial dysplasia arising in hereditary gingival fibromatosis. J Periodontol 56:158, 1985.
176. Roed-Petersen B. The potential use of $CO_2$-laser gingivectomy for phenytoin-induced gingival hyperplasia in mentally retarded patients. J Clin Periodontol 20:729, 1993.
177. Singer SL, Goldblatt J, Hallam LA, et al. Hereditary gingival fibromatosis with a recessive mode of inheritance. Aust Dent J 38:427, 1993.
178. Srsen S, Mosik A. Hereditary gingival fibromatosis. Acta Univ Carol 56:141, 1973.
179. Takagi M, Yamamoto H, Mega H, et al. Heterogeneity in the gingival fibromatoses. Cancer 68:2202, 1991.
180. Van Buggenhout GJ, Brunner HG, Trommelen JC, et al. Zimmerman-Laband syndrome in a patient with severe mental retardation. Genet Couns 6:321, 1995.
181. Weski H. Elephantiasis gingivae hereditaria. Dtsch Monatsschr Zahnh 38:557, 1920.
182. Wynne SE, Aldred MJ, Bartold PM. Hereditary gingival fibromatosis associated with hearing loss and supernumerary teeth: a new syndrome. J Periodontol 66:75, 1995.
183. Yalcin S, Yalcin F, Soydinc M, et al. Gingival fibromatosis combined with cherubism and psychomotor retardation: a rare syndrome. J Periodontol 70:201, 1999.
184. Zackin SJ, Weisberger D. Hereditary gingival fibromatosis. Oral Surg 14:828, 1961.
185. Zegarelli EV, Kutcher AH, Lichtenthal R. Idiopathic gingival fibromatosis: report of 20 cases. Am J Digest Dis 8:782, 1962.

### Fibromatosis Colli

186. Armstrong D, Pickrell K, Fetter B, et al. Torticollis: analysis of 271 cases. Plast Reconstr Surg 35:14, 1965.
187. Binder H, Eng GD, Gaiser JF, et al. Congenital muscular torticollis: results of conservative management with long-term follow-up in 85 cases. Arch Phys Med Rehabil 68:222, 1987.
188. Blythe WR, Logan TC, Holmes DK, et al. Fibromatosis colli: a common cause of neonatal torticollis. Am Fam Physician 54: 1965, 1996.
189. Campbell CJ, Padre G. Sternomastoid tumor in an identical twin. J Bone Joint Surg Am 38:350, 1956.
190. Canale ST, Griffin DW, Hubbard CN. Congenital muscular torticollis: a long-term follow-up. J Bone Joint Surg Am 64:810, 1982.
191. Chandler FA, Altenberg A. "Congenital" muscular torticollis. JAMA 125:476, 1944.
192. Coventry MB, Harris LE, Bianco AJ Jr, et al. Congenital muscular torticollis (wry neck). Postgrad Med 28:383, 1960.
193. Dunn PN. Congenital sternomastoid torticollis: an intrauterine postural deformity. J Bone Joint Surg Br 55:877, 1973.
194. Ferkel RD, Westin GW, Dawson EG, et al. Muscular torticollis: a modified surgical approach. J Bone Joint Surg Am 65:894, 1983.
195. Fitzsimmons HJ. Congenital torticollis: review of the pathological aspects. N Engl J Med 209:66, 1933.
196. Gruhn J, Hurwitt ES. Fibrous sternomastoid tumor of infancy. Pediatrics 8:522, 1951.
197. Hulbert KF. Congenital torticollis. J Bone Joint Surg Br 32:50, 1950.
198. Hummer CD Jr, MacEwen GD. The coexistence of torticollis and congenital dysplasia of the hip. J Bone Joint Surg Am 54: 1255, 1972.
199. Isigkeit E. Untersuchungen uber die Hereditat orthopadischer Leiden. Arch Orthop Unfallchir 30:459, 1931.
200. Joachimsthal G. Handbuch der orthopadischen Chirurgie, vol 1, sect 2. Gustav Fischer, Jena, 1905, p 234.
201. Kiesewetter WB, Nelson PK, Palladino VS, et al. Neonatal torticollis. JAMA 157:1281, 1955.
202. Kiwak KJ. Establishing an etiology for torticollis. Postgrad Med 75:126, 1984.
203. Lawrence WT, Azizkhan RG. Congenital muscular torticollis: a spectrum of pathology. Ann Plast Surg 23:523, 1989.
204. Ling CM. The influence of age on the results of open sternomastoid tenotomy in muscular torticollis. Clin Orthop 116:142, 1976.
205. Ling CM, Low YS. Sternomastoid tumor in muscular torticollis. Clin Orthop 86:144, 1972.
206. MacDonald D. Sternomastoid tumor and muscular torticollis. J Bone Joint Surg Br 51:432, 1969.
207. Middleton DS. Pathology of congenital torticollis. Br J Surg 18: 188, 1930.
208. Muralt RH. Bilateral occurrence of congenital muscular torticollis. Helv Paediatr Acta 1:349, 1946.
209. Nové-Josserand G, Viannay C. Pathogenie du Torticollis congenital. Rev Orthop 7:397, 1906.
210. Pereira S, Tani E, Skoog L. Diagnosis of fibromatosis colli by fine needle aspiration (FNA) cytology. Cytopathology 10:25, 1999.
211. Raab SS, Silverman JF, McLeod DL, et al. Fine needle aspiration biopsy of fibromatoses. Acta Cytol 37:323, 1993.
212. Radtke J. Fibromatosis colli: a benign tumor of the neck in diagnosis and therapy. Dtsch Z Mund Kiefer Ges 15:248, 1991.
213. Sauer T, Selmer L, Freng A. Cytologic features of fibromatosis colli of infancy. Acta Cytol 41:633, 1997.
214. Schmid W. L'etiologie du torticollis musculaire. Presse Med 45:1189, 1937.
215. Schwartz RA, Powers CN, Wakeley PE, et al. Fibromatosis colli: the utility of fine-needle aspiration in diagnosis. Arch Otolaryngol Head Neck Surg 123:301, 1997.
216. Stevens AE. Congenital torticollis in identical twins. Lancet 2: 378, 1948.
217. Stromeyer GF. Beitrage zur operativen orthopadik oder Erfahrungen uber die subcutane Durchschneidung berkurzter Muskeln und deren Schnen. Helwing, Hannover, 1838.
218. Suzuki S, Yamamuro T, Fujita A. The aetiological relationship between congenital torticollis and obstetrical paralysis. Int Orthop 8:175, 1984.
219. Thompson F, McManus S, Colville J. Familial congenital muscular torticollis: case report and review of the literature. Clin Orthop 202:193, 1986.
220. Von Lackum HL. Torticollis: removal in early life of the fibrous mass from the sternomastoid muscle. Surg Gynecol Obstet 48:691, 1929.
221. Wakeley PE, Price WG, Frable WJ. Sternomastoid tumor of infancy (fibromatosis colli): diagnosis by aspiration cytology. Mod Pathol 2:378, 1989.

### Infantile Fibromatosis

222. Adam LR, Davison EV, Malcolm AJ, et al. Cytogenetic analysis of a congenital fibrosarcoma. Cancer Genet Cytogenet 51: 37, 1991.
223. Argyle JC, Tomlinson GE, Stewart D, et al. Ultrastructural, immunocytochemical and cytogenetic characterization of a large congenital fibrosarcoma. Arch Pathol Lab Med 116:972, 1992.
224. Ayala AG, Ro JY, Goepfert H, et al. Desmoid fibromatosis: a clinicopathologic study of 25 children. Semin Diagn Pathol 3: 138, 1986.
225. Carr RJ, Zaki GA, Leader MB, et al. Infantile fibromatosis with involvement of the mandible. Br J Oral Maxillofac Surg 30:257, 1992.
226. Coffin CM, Dehner LP. Fibroblastic-myofibroblastic tumors in children and adolescents: a clinicopathologic study of 108 examples in 103 patients. Pediatr Pathol 11:559, 1991.

227. Connoly NK. Juvenile fibromatosis: a case report showing invasion of bone. Arch Dis Child 36:171, 1961.
228. Cramer SF, Ruehl A, Mandel MA. Fibrodysplasia ossificans progressiva: a distinct bone-forming lesion of soft tissue. Cancer 48:1016, 1991.
229. Dal Cin P, Rao BN, Brock P, et al. Cytogenetic characterization of congenital or infantile fibrosarcoma. Eur J Pediatr 15:579, 1991.
230. Dehner LP, Askin FB. Tumors of fibrous tissue origin in childhood: a clinicopathologic study of cutaneous and soft tissue neoplasms in 66 children. Cancer 38:888, 1976.
231. Eady JL, Lundquist JE, Grant RE, et al. Congenital bowing of the ulna in aggressive fibromatosis. J Natl Med Assoc 83:978, 1991.
232. Egan M, Raafat F, Crocker J, et al. Nucleolar organizer regions in fibrous proliferations of childhood and infantile fibrosarcoma. J Clin Pathol 41:31, 1988.
233. Faulkner LD, Hajdu SI, Kher U, et al. Pediatric desmoid tumor: retrospective analysis of 63 cases. J Clin Oncol 13:2813, 1995.
234. Fisher C. Fibromatosis and fibrosarcoma in infancy and childhood. Eur J Cancer 32A:2094, 1996.
235. Fromowitz FB, Hurst LC, Nathan J, et al. Infantile (desmoid type) fibromatosis with extensive ossification. Am J Surg Pathol 11:66, 1987.
236. Goepfert H, Cangir A, Ayala AG, et al. Chemotherapy of locally aggressive head and neck tumors in the pediatric age group: desmoid fibromatosis and nasopharyngeal angiofibroma. Am J Surg 144:437, 1982.
237. Hidayat AA, Font RL. Juvenile fibromatosis of the periorbital region and eyelid: a clinicopathologic study of six cases. Arch Ophthalmol 98:280, 1980.
238. Inwards CY, Unni KK, Beabout JW, et al. Desmoplastic fibroma of bone. Cancer 68:1978, 1991.
239. Maillard AAJ, Kountakis SE. Pediatric sino-orbital desmoid fibromatosis. Ann Otol Rhinol Laryngol 105:463, 1996.
240. Mandahl N, Heim S, Rydholm A, et al. Nonrandom numerical chromosome aberrations (+8, +11, +17, +20) in infantile fibrosarcoma. Cancer Genet Cytogenet 40:137, 1989.
241. Melrose JR, Abrams AM. Juvenile fibromatosis affecting the jaws: report of three cases. Oral Surg Oral Med Oral Pathol 49:317, 1980.
242. Naidu RK, Aviv JE, Lawson W, et al. Aggressive juvenile fibromatosis involving the paranasal sinuses. Otolaryngol Head Neck Surg 104:549, 1991.
243. Peede LF Jr, Epker BN. Aggressive juvenile fibromatosis involving the mandible: surgical excision with immediate reconstruction. Oral Surg Oral Med Oral Pathol 43:651, 1977.
244. Ramanathan RC, Thomas JM. Infantile (desmoid-type) fibromatosis of the parotid gland. J Laryngol Otol 111:669, 1997.
245. Raney B, Evans A, Granowetter L, et al. Nonsurgical management of children with recurrent or unresectable fibromatosis. Pediatrics 79:394, 1987.
246. Rao BN, Horowitz ME, Parham DM, et al. Challenges in the treatment of childhood fibromatosis. Arch Surg 122:1296, 1987.
247. Rodu B, Weathers DR, Campbell WG Jr. Aggressive fibromatosis involving the paramandibular soft tissues: a study with the aid of electron microscopy. Oral Surg Oral Med Oral Pathol 52:395, 1981.
248. Schmidt D, Klinge P, Leuschner I, et al. Infantile desmoid-type fibromatosis: morphological features correlate with biologic behavior. J Pathol 164:315, 1991.
249. Schofield DE, Fletcher JA, Grier AG, et al. Fibrosarcoma in infants and children: application of new techniques. Am J Surg Pathol 18:14, 1994.
250. Scougall P, Staheli LT, Chew DE, et al. Desmoid tumors in childhood. Orthop Rev 16:481, 1987.
251. Shah AC, Katz RI. Infantile aggressive fibromatosis of the base of the tongue. Otolaryngol Head Neck Surg 98:346, 1988.
252. Shankwiler RA, Athey PA, Lamki N. Aggressive infantile fibromatosis: pulmonary metastases documented by plain film and computed tomography. Clin Imaging 13:127, 1989.
253. Stout AP. Juvenile fibromatoses. Cancer 7:953, 1954.
254. Tagawa T, Ohse S, Hirano Y, et al. Aggressive infantile fibromatosis of the submandibular region. Int J Oral Maxillofac Surg 18:264, 1989.
255. Takagi M, Ishikawa G. Fibrous tumor of infancy: report of a case originating in the oral cavity. J Oral Pathol 2:293, 1973.
256. Thompson DH, Khan A, Gonzalez C, et al. Juvenile aggressive fibromatosis: report of three cases and review of the literature. Ear Nose Throat J 70:462, 1991.
257. Wilkins SA, Waldron CA, Mathews WH, et al. Aggressive fibromatosis of the head and neck. Am J Surg 130:412, 1975.
258. Yokoyama R, Shinohara M, Tsuneyoshi M, et al. Extraabdominal desmoid tumors: correlation between histologic features and biologic behavior. Surg Pathol 2:29, 1989.

### Infantile Fibrosarcoma

259. Adam LR, Davison EV, Malcolm AJ, et al. Cytogenetic analysis of a congenital fibrosarcoma. Cancer Genet Cytogenet 52: 37, 1991.
259a. Argani P, Fritsch M, Kadkol SS, et al. Detection of the ETV6-NTRK3 chimeric RNA of infantile fibrosarcoma/cellular congenital mesoblastic nephroma in paraffin-embedded tissue: Application to challenging pediatric stromal tumors. Mod Pathol 13:29, 2000.
260. Argyle JC, Tomlinson GE, Stewart D, et al. Ultrastructural, immunocytochemical and cytogenetic characterization of a large congenital fibrosarcoma. Arch Pathol Lab Med 116:972, 1992.
261. Balsaver AM, Butler JJ, Martin RC. Congenital fibrosarcoma. Cancer 20:1607, 1967.
262. Bernstein R, Zeltzer PM, Lin F, et al. Trisomy 11 and other nonrandom trisomies in congenital fibrosarcoma. Cancer Genet Cytogenet 78:82, 1994.
263. Blocker S, Koenig J, Ternberg J. Congenital fibrosarcoma. J Pediatr Surg 22:665, 1987.
264. Boman F, Peters J, Ragge N, et al. Infrequent mutation of the p53 gene in fibrous tumors of infancy and childhood. Diagn Mol Pathol 2:14, 1993.
264a. Bourgeois JM, Knezevich SR, Mathers JA, et al. Molecular detection of the ETV6-NTRK3 gene fusion differentiates congenital fibrosarcoma from other childhood spindle cell tumors. Am J Surg Pathol 24:937, 2000.
265. Cavazzana AO, Schmidt D, Ninfo V, et al. Spindle cell rhabdomyosarcoma: a prognostically favorable variant of rhabdomyosarcoma. Am J Surg Pathol 16:229, 1992.
266. Chung EB, Enzinger FM. Infanfile fibrosarcoma. Cancer 38:729, 1976.
267. Cofer BR, Vescio PJ, Wiener ES. Infanfile fibrosarcoma: complete excision is the appropriate treatment. Ann Surg Oncol 3: 159,1996.
268. Coffin CM, Jaszcz W, O'Shea PA, et al. So-called congenital-infantile fibrosarcoma: does it exist and what it is? Pediatr Pathol 14:133, 1994.
269. Corsi A, Boldrini R, Bosman C. Congenital-infantile fibrosarcoma: study of two cases and review of the literature. Tumori 80:392, 1994.
270. Dahl I, Angervall L, Save-Soderbergh J. Atypical fibroblastic tumors in early infancy. Acta Pathol Microbiol Scand 81A:224, 1973.
271. Dahl I, Save-Soderbergh J, Angervall L. Fibrosarcoma in early infancy. Pathol Eur 8:193, 1973.
272. Dal Cin P, Brock P, Casteels-Yan Daele M, et al. Cytogenetic

characterization of congenital or infantile fibrosarcoma. Eur J Pediatr 150:579, 1991.
273. Delepine N, Cornille H, Desbois JC, et al. Complete response of congenital fibrosarcoma to chemotherapy. Lancet 2:1453, 1986.
274. Edel G, Wuisman P, Erlenmann R. Spindle cell (leiomyomatous) rhabdomyosarcoma, a rare variant of embryonal rhabdomyosarcoma. Pathol Res Pract 189:102, 1993.
275. Egan MJ, Raafat F, Crocker J, et al. Nucleolar organiser regions in fibrous proliferations of childhood and infantile fibrosarcoma. J Clin Pathol 41:31, 1988.
276. Gonzalez-Crussi F. Ultrastructure of congenital fibrosarcoma. Cancer 26:1289, 1970.
277. Gonzalez-Crussi F, Wiederhold ND, Sotelo-Avila C. Congenital fibrosarcoma: presence of a histiocytic component. Cancer 46:77, 1980.
278. Gorman PA, Malone M, Pritchard J, et al. Deletion of part of the short arm of chromosome 17 in a congenital fibrosarcoma. Cancer Genet Cytogenet 48:193, 1990.
279. Grier HE, Perez-Atayde AR, Weinstein AJ. Chemotherapy for inoperable infantile fibrosarcoma. Cancer 56:1507, 1985.
280. Hamm CN, Pyesmany A, Resch L. Case report: congenital retroperitoneal fibrosarcoma. Med Pediatr Oncol 28:65, 1997.
281. Hays DM, Mirabal VQ, Karlan MS, et al. Fibrosarcomas in infants and children. J Pediatr Surg 5:176, 1970.
282. Hayward PG, Orgill BP, Mulliken JB, et al. Congenital fibrosarcoma masquerading as lymphatic malformation: report of two cases. J Pediatr Surg 30:84, 1995.
283. Kanaston JA, Malcolm AJ, Craft AW, et al. Chemotherapy in the management of infantile fibrosarcoma. Med Pediatr Oncol 21:488, 1993.
284. Kihara S-I, Nehlsen-Cannarella S, Kirsch WM, et al. A comparative study of apoptosis and cell proliferation in infantile and adult fibrosarcomas. Am J Clin Pathol 106:493, 1996.
285. Knezevich SR, Garnett MJ, Pysher TJ, et al. ETV6-NTRK3 gene fusions and trisomy 11 establish a histogenetic link between mesoblastic nephroma and congenital fibrosarcoma. Cancer Res 58:5046, 1998.
286. Knezevich SR, McFadden DE, Tao W, et al. A novel ETV6-NTRK3 gene fusion in congenital fibrosarcoma. Nat Genet 18: 184, 1998.
287. Kodet R, Stejskal J, Pilat D, et al. Congenital-infantile fibrosarcoma: a clinicopathological study of five patients entered on the Prague Children's Tumor Registry. Pathol Res Pract 192: 845, 1996.
288. Kovacs G, Szucs S, Maschek H. Two chromosomally different cell populations in a partly cellular congenital mesoblastic nephroma. Arch Pathol Lab Med 111:383, 1987.
289. Leuschner I, Newton WA Jr, Schmidt D, et al. Spindle cell variants of embryonal rhabdomyosarcoma in the paratesticular region: a report of the Intergroup Rhabdomyosarcoma Study. Am J Surg Pathol 17:221, 1993.
290. Lundgren L, Angervall L, Stenman G, et al. Infantile rhabdomyofibrosarcoma: a high-grade sarcoma distinguishable from infantile fibrosarcoma and rhabdomyosarcoma. Hum Pathol 24:785, 1993.
291. Madden NP, Spicer RD, Allibore EB, et al. Spontaneous regression of neonatal fibrosarcoma. Br J Cancer 18 (Suppl):S72, 1992.
292. Mandahl N, Heim S, Rydholm A, et al. Nonrandom numerical chromosome aberrations (+8, +11, +17, +20) in infantile fibrosarcoma. Cancer Genet Cytogenet 40:137, 1989.
292a. Miki H, Kobayashi S, Kushida Y, et al. A case of infantile rhabdomyofibrosarcoma with immunohistochemical, electron microscopical, and genetic analyses. Hum Pathol 30:1519, 1999.
293. Ninane J, Gosseye S, Panteon E, et al. Congenital fibrosarcoma: preoperative chemotherapy and conservative therapy. Cancer 58:1400, 1986.
294. Robinson W, Crawford AH. Infantile fibrosarcoma. J Bone Joint Surg Am 72:291, 1990.
295. Rubin BP, Chen CJ, Morgan TW, et al. Congenital mesoblastic nephroma t(12;15) is associated with ETV6-NTRK3 gene fusion: cytogenetic and molecular relationship to congenital (infantile) fibrosarcoma. Am J Pathol 153:1451, 1998.
296. Sankary S, Dickman PS, Wiener E, et al. Consistent numerical chromosome aberrations in congenital fibrosarcoma. Cancer Genet Cytogenet 65:152, 1993.
297. Schofield D, Yunis J, Fletcher JA. Chromosome aberrations in mesoblastic nephromas. Am J Pathol 143:714, 1993.
298. Schofield DE, Fletcher JA, Grier HE, et al. Fibrosarcoma in infants and children: application of new techniques. Am J Surg Pathol 18:14, 1994.
299. Soule EH, Pritchard DJ. Fibrosarcoma in infants and children: a review of 110 cases. Cancer 40:1711, 1977.
300. Speleman F, Dal Cin P, De Potter K, et al. Cytogenetic investigation of a case of congenital fibrosarcoma. Cancer Genet Cytogenet 39:21, 1989.
301. Spicer RD. Neonatal fibrosarcoma. Med Pediatr Oncol 18:427, 1990.
302. Spicer RD. Chemotherapy for infantile fibrosarcoma [letter]. Med Pediatr Oncol 21:80, 1993.
303. Stout AP. Fibrosarcoma in infants and children. Cancer 15: 1028, 1962.
304. Strehl S, Ladenstein R, Wrba F, et al. Translocation (12;13) in a case of infantile fibrosarcoma. Cancer Genet Cytogenet 71:94, 1993.
305. Tay Y-K, Morelli JG, Weston WL. Congenital palmar nodule in infants. Pediatr Dermatol 14:241, 1997.
306. Teyssier JR, Ferre D. Frequent clonal chromosomal changes in human non-malignant tumors. Int J Cancer 44:828, 1989.
307. Variend S, Bax NMA, Van Gorp J. Are infantile myofibromatosis, congenital fibrosarcoma and congenital hemangiopericytoma histogenetically related? Histopathology 26:57, 1995.
308. Weiner JM, Hidayat AA. Juvenile fibrosarcoma of the orbit and eyelid: a study of five cases. Arch Ophthalmol 101:253, 1983.
309. Wilson MB, Stanley W, Sens D, et al. Infantile fibrosarcoma: a misnomer? Pediatr Pathol 10:901, 1993.

### Inflammatory Myofibroblastic Tumor

310. Albores-Saavedra J, Manivel JC, Essenfeld H, et al. Pseudosarcomatous myofibroblastic proliferations in the urinary bladder of children. Cancer 66:1234, 1990.
311. Al-Sarraj S, Wasserberg J, Bartlett R, et al. Inflammatory pseudotumor of the central nervous system: clinicopathologic study of one case and review of the literature. Br J Neurosurg 9:57, 1995.
312. Arber DA, Weiss LM, Chang KL. Detection of Epstein-Barr virus in inflammatory pseudotumor. Semin Diagn Pathol 15: 155, 1998.
313. Ballesteros E, Osborne BM, Matsushima AY. Plasma cell granuloma of the oral cavity: a report of two cases and review of the literature. Mod Pathol 11:60, 1998.
314. Biselli R, Ferlini C, Fattorossi A, et al. Inflammatory myofibroblastic tumor (inflammatory pseudotumor): DNA flow cytometric analysis of nine pediatric cases. Cancer 77:778, 1996.
315. Chan JKC. Inflammatory pseudotumor: a family of lesions of diverse nature and etiologies. Adv Anat Pathol 3:156, 1996.
316. Chan YF, White J, Brash H. Metachronous pulmonary and cerebral inflammatory pseudotumors in a child. Pediatr Pathol 14:805, 1994.
317. Coffin CM, Dehner LP, Meis-Kindblom JM. Inflammatory myofibroblastic tumor, inflammatory fibrosarcoma, and related

lesions: an historical review with differential diagnostic considerations. Semin Diagn Pathol 15:102, 1998.

318. Coffin CM, Humphrey PA, Dehner LP. Extrapulmonary inflammatory myofibroblastic tumor: a clinical and pathological survey. Semin Diagn Pathol 15:85, 1998.
319. Coffin CM, Watterson J, Priest JR, et al. Extrapulmonary inflammatory myofibroblastic tumor (inflammatory pseudotumor): a clinicopathologic and immunohistochemical study of 84 cases. Am J Surg Pathol 19:859, 1995.
319a. Coffin CM, Hussong J, Perkins S, et al. ALK and p80 expression in inflammatory myofibroblastic tumor. Mod Pathol 13: 8A, 1999.
320. Conte M, Milanaccio C, Nantron M, et al. Multiple inflammatory fibrosarcoma of the abdominal cavity in a child. Med Pediatr Oncol 27:198, 1996.
321. Donner LR, Trompler RA, White RR. Progression of inflammatory myofibroblastic tumor (inflammatory pseudotumor) of soft tissue into sarcoma after several recurrences. Hum Pathol 27:1095, 1996.
322. Eble JN, Rosenberg AE, Young RH. Retroperitoneal xanthogranuloma in a patient with Erdheim-Chester disease. Am J Surg Pathol 18:843, 1994.
323. Gonzales-Crussi F, de Mello DE, Sotelo-Avila C. Omental-mesenteric myxoid hamartomas: infantile lesions simulating malignant tumors. Am J Surg Pathol 7:567, 1983.
324. Griffin CA, Hawkins AL, Dvorak C, et al. Recurrent involvement of 2p23 in inflammatory myofibroblastic tumors. Cancer Res 59:2776, 1999.
325. Hojo H, Newton WA, Hamoudi AB, et al. Pseudosarcomatous myofibroblastic tumor of the urinary bladder in children: a study of 11 cases with review of the literature—an intergroup rhabdomyosarcoma study. Am J Surg Pathol 19:1224, 1995.
326. Hurt MA, Santa Cruz DJ. Cutaneous inflammatory pseudotumor: lesions resembling "inflammatory pseudotumor" or "plasma cell granulomas" of extracutaneous sites. Am J Surg Pathol 14:764, 1990.
327. Hussong J, Brown M, Perkins S, et al. Comparison of histology, DNA ploidy and immunohistochemistry with clinical outcome in inflammatory myofibroblastic tumors. Mod Pathol 12:279, 1999.
328. Jones EC, Clement PB, Young RH. Inflammatory pseudotumor of the urinary bladder: a clinicopathological, immunohistochemical, ultrastructural, and flow cytometric study of 13 cases. Am J Surg Pathol 17:264, 1993.
329. Kohimahra KI, Mukai M, Yamazaki K, et al. Inflammatory pseudotumor of the stomach: report of a highly infiltrative case with electron microscopic and immunohistochemical study. Acta Pathol Jpn 43:65, 1993.
330. Kovarik P, Pyle J, Chou PM. Ploidy, proliferative activity, and p53 as biologic markers in inflammatory myofibroblastic tumors. Mod Pathol 11:43A, 1998.
331. Kroft SH, Stryker SJ, Winter JN, et al. Inflammatory pseudotumor of the pancreas. Int J Pancreatol 18:277, 1995.
331a. Lawrence B, Perez-Atayde A, Hibbard MK, et al. TPM3-ALK and TPM4-ALK oncogenes in inflammatory myofibroblastic tumors. Am J Pathol 157:377, 2000.
332. Marc'hadour FL, Laveille JP, Guilcher C, et al. Coexistence of plasma cell granulomas of lung and central nervous system, a case report. Pathol Res Pract 191:1038, 1995.
333. Meis JM, Enzinger FM. Inflammatory fibrosarcoma of the mesentery and retroperitoneum: a tumor closely simulating inflammatory pseudotumor. Am J Surg Pathol 15:1146, 1991.
334. Meis-Kindblom JM, Kjellström C, Kindblom L-G. Inflammatory fibrosarcoma: update, reappraisal, and perspective on its place in the spectrum of inflammatory myofibroblastic tumors. Semin Diagn Pathol 15:133, 1998.
335. Mirra M, Falconieri G, Zanconati F, et al. Inflammatory fibrosarcoma: another imitator of Hodgkin's disease? Pathol Res Pract 192:474, 1996.
336. Myint MA, Medeiros LF, Sulaiman RA, et al. Inflammatory pseudotumor of the ileum: a report of a multifocal, transmural lesion with regional lymph node involvement. Arch Pathol Lab Med 118:1138, 1994.
337. Pettinato G, Manivel JC, De Rosa N, et al. Inflammatory myofibroblastic tumor (plasma cell granuloma): clinicopathologic study of 20 cases with immunohistochemical and ultrastructural observations. Am J Clin Pathol 94:538, 1990.
338. Pettinato G, Manivel JC, Insabato L, et al. Plasma cell granuloma (inflammatory pseudotumor) of the breast. Am J Clin Pathol 90:627, 1988.
339. Pisciotto PT, Gray GF, Miller VR. Abdominal plasma cell pseudotumor. J Pediatr 93:628, 1978.
340. Proppe KH, Scully RE, Rosai J. Postoperative spindle cell nodules of genitourinary tract resembling sarcomas: a report of eight cases. Am J Surg Pathol 8:101, 1984.
341. Ramachandra S, Hollowood K, Cisceglia M, et al. Inflammatory pseudotumor of soft tissues: a clinicopathological and immunohistochemical analysis of 18 cases. Histopathology 27: 313, 1995.
342. Ro JY, El-Naggar AK, Amin MB, et al. Pseudosarcomatous fibromyxoid tumor of the urinary bladder and prostate: immunohistochemical, ultrastructural and DNA flow cytometric analysis of nine cases. Hum Pathol 24:1203, 1993.
343. Sciot R, Dal Cin P, Fletcher CDM, et al. Inflammatory myofibroblastic tumor of bone: report of two cases with evidence of clonal chromosomal changes. Am J Surg Pathol 21:1166, 1997.
344. Scully RE, Mark EJ, McNeely BU. Case records of the Massachusetts General Hospital; case 13-1984: cellular inflammatory pseudotumor, involving ileal mesentery. N Engl J Med 310: 839, 1984.
345. Selves J, Meggetto F, Brousset P, et al. Inflammatory pseudotumor of the liver: evidence for follicular dendritic reticulum cell proliferation associated with clonal Epstein-Barr virus. Am J Surg Pathol 20:747, 1996.
346. Shek TW, Luck IS, Loong F, et al. Inflammatory cell-rich gastrointestinal autonomic nerve tumor: an expansion of its histologic spectrum. Am J Surg Pathol 20:325, 1996.
347. Shek TWH, Ho FCS, Ng IOL, et al. Follicular dendritic cell tumor of the liver: evidence for an Epstein-Barr virus-related clonal proliferation of follicular dendritic cells. Am J Surg Pathol 20:313, 1996.
348. Snyder CS, Aquila MD, Haghighi P, et al. Clonal changes in inflammatory pseudotumor of the lung: a case report. Cancer 76:1545, 1995.
349. Souid AK, Ziemba MC, Dubansky AS, et al. Inflammatory myofibroblastic tumor in children. Cancer 72:1042, 1993.
350. Spencer H. Pulmonary plasma cell/histiocytoma complex. Histopathology 8:903, 1984.
351. Stringer MD, Ramani P, Yeung CK, et al. Abdominal inflammatory myofibroblastic tumors in children. Br J Surg 79:1357, 1992.
352. Su LD, Atayde-Perez A, Sheldon S, et al. Inflammatory myofibroblastic tumor: cytogenetic evidence supporting clonal origin. Mod Pathol 11:364, 1998.
353. Tang TT, Segura AD, Oechler HW, et al. Inflammatory myofibrohistiocytic proliferation simulating sarcoma in children. Cancer 65:1626, 1990.
354. Tong TR, Gil J, Batheja N, et al. Inflammatory pseudotumor of the mediastinum associated with azacytidine therapy, acute myeloid leukemia, and previous chemotherapy for astrocytoma: case report and review of the literature. Int J Surg Pathol 3:49, 1995.

355. Treissman SP, Gillis DA, Lee TLY, et al. Omental-mesenteric inflammatory pseudotumor: cytogenetic demonstration of genetic changes and monoclonality of one tumor. Cancer 73: 1433, 1994.
356. Umiker WO, Iverson L. Postinflammatory "tumors" of the lung: report of four cases simulating xanthoma, fibroma, or plasma cell granuloma. J Thorac Cardiovasc Surg 28:55, 1954.
357. Umlas J, Federman M, Crawford C, et al. A spindle cell pseudotumor due to Mycobacterium avium-intracellulare in patients with acquired immunodeficiency syndrome (AIDS). Am J Surg Pathol 15:1181, 1991.
358. Walsh SV, Evangelista F, Khettry U. Inflammatory myofibroblastic tumor of pancreaticobiliary region: morphologic and immunocytochemical study of three cases. Am J Surg Pathol 22:412, 1998.
359. Warter A, Satge D, Roeslin N. Angioinvasive plasma cell granuloma of the lung. Cancer 59:435, 1987.
360. Weiland TL, Scheithauer BW, Rock MG, et al. Inflammatory pseudotumor of nerve. Am J Surg Pathol 20:121, 1996.
361. Wood C, Nickoloff BJ, Todes-Taylor NR. Pseudotumor resulting from atypical mycobacterial infection: a "histoid" variety of Mycobacteria avium-intracellular complex infection. Am J Clin Pathol 83:524, 1985.
362. Wu JP, Yunis EJ, Fetterman G, et al. Inflammatory pseudotumors of the abdomen: plasma cell granulomas. J Clin Pathol 26:943, 1973.
363. Yang M. Cutaneous inflammatory pseudotumor: a case report with immunohistochemical and ultrastructural studies. Pathology 25:405, 1993.
364. Zavaglia C, Barberis M, Gelosa F, et al. Inflammatory pseudotumor of the liver with malignant transformation: report of two cases. Ital J Gastroenterol 28:152, 1996.

### Calcifying Aponeurotic Fibroma

365. Adeyemi-Doro HO, Olude O. Juvenile aponeurotic fibroma. J Hand Surg [Br] 10:127, 1985.
366. Allen PW, Enzinger FM. Juvenile aponeurotic fibroma. Cancer 26:857, 1970.
367. Booher RJ, McPeak CJ. Juvenile aponeurotic fibromas. Surgery 46:924, 1959.
368. Fetsch JF, Miettinen M. Calcifying aponeurotic fibroma: a clinicopathologic study of 22 cases arising in uncommon sites. Hum Pathol 29:1504, 1998.
369. Goldman RL. The cartilage analog of fibromatosis (aponeurotic fibroma): further observations based on seven new cases. Cancer 26:1325, 1970.
370. Iwasaki H, Enjoji M. Calcifying aponeurotic fibroma. Fukuoka Acta Med 64:52, 1973.
371. Iwasaki H, Kikuchi M, Eimoto T, et al. Juvenile aponeurotic fibroma: an ultrastructural study. Ultrastract Pathol 4:75, 1983.
372. Keasbey LE. Juvenile aponeurotic fibroma (calcifying fibroma): a distinctive tumor arising in the palms and soles of young children. Cancer 6:338, 1953.
373. Keasbey LE, Fanselau HA. The aponeurotic fibroma. Clin Orthop 19:115, 1961.
374. Lafferty KA, Nelson LE, Demuth RJ, et al. Juvenile aponeurotic fibroma with disseminated fibrosarcoma. J Hand Surg [Am] 11:737, 1986.
375. Lichtenstein L, Goldman RL. The cartilage analog of fibromatosis: a reinterpretation of the condition called "juvenile aponeurotic fibroma." Cancer 17:810, 1964.
376. Moskovich R, Posner MA. Intratendinous aponeurotic fibroma. J Hand Surg [Am] 13:563, 1988.
377. Murphy BA, Kilpatrick SE, Panella MJ, et al. Extra-acral calcifying aponeurotic fibroma: a distinctive case with 23-year follow-up. J Cutan Pathol 23:369, 1996.
378. Rios-Dalenz JL, Kim JS, McDowell FW. The so-called "juvenile aponeurotic fibroma." Am J Clin Pathol 44:632, 1965.
379. Sharma R, Punia RS, Sharma A, et al. Juvenile (calcifying) aponeurotic fibroma of the neck. Pediatr Surg Int 13:295, 1998.
380. Specht EE, Konkin LA. Juvenile aponeurotic fibroma: the cartilage analog of fibromatosis. JAMA 234:626, 1975.

### Congenital and Acquired Muscular Fibrosis

381. Bhattacharyya S. Abduction contractures of the shoulder from contracture of the intermediate part of the deltoid: report of three cases. J Bone Joint Surg Br 48:127, 1966.
382. Chiu SS, Furuya K, Arai T, et al. Congenital contracture of the quadriceps muscle: four case reports in identical twins. J Bone Joint Surg Am 56:1054, 1974.
383. Duran-Sacristan H, Sanchez-Barba A, Lopez-Duran Stern L, et al. Fibrosis of the gluteal muscles: report of three cases. J Bone Joint Surg Am 56:1510, 1974.
384. Esteban Mugica B, Gutierrez de la Cuesta S, Martinez-Sanchez R. Fibrosis muscular progressiva. Rev Esp Cir Osteoartic 5:321, 1970.
385. Fairbank TJ, Barrett AM. Vastus intermedius contracture in early childhood: case report in identical twins. J Bone Joint Surg Br 43:326, 1961.
386. Gammie WFP, Taylor JH, Urich H. Contracture of the vastus intermedius in children (a report of two cases). J Bone Joint Surg Br 45:370, 1963.
387. Goodfellow JF, Nade S. Flexion contracture of the shoulder joint from fibrosis of the anterior part of the deltoid muscle. J Bone Joint Surg Br 51:356, 1969.
388. Groves RJ, Goldner JL. Contracture of the deltoid muscle in the adult after intramuscular injections. J Bone Joint Surg Am 56:817, 1974.
389. Gunn DR. Contracture of the quadriceps muscle: a discussion on the etiology and relationship to recurrent dislocation of the patella. J Bone Joint Surg Br 46:492, 1964.
390. Hill NA, Liebler WA, Wilson HJ, et al. Abduction contracture of both glenohumeral joints and extensor contracture of one knee joint secondary to partial muscle fibrosis: a case report. J Bone Joint Surg Am 49:961, 1967.
391. Hnevkovsky O. Progressive fibrosis of the vastus intermedius muscle in children. J Bone Joint Surg Br 43:318, 1961.
392. Howard RC. Iatrogenic quadriceps and gluteal fibrosis. J Bone Joint Surg Br 53:354, 1971.
393. Karlen A. Congenital fibrosis of the vastus intermedius muscle. J Bone Joint Surg Br 46:488, 1964.
394. Lloyd-Roberts GC, Thomas TG. The etiology of quadriceps contracture in children. J Bone Joint Surg Br 46:498, 1964.
395. Matsusue Y, Yamamuro T, Ohta H, et al. Fibrotic contracture of the gastrocnemius muscle: a case report. J Bone Joint Surg Am 76:739, 1994.
396. Mukherjee PK, Das AK. Injection fibrosis in the quadriceps fermoris muscle in children. J Bone Joint Surg Am 62:453, 1980.
397. Napiontek M, Ruszkowski K. Paralytic foot drop and gluteal fibrosis after intramuscular injections. J Bone Joint Surg Br 75: 83, 1993.
398. Peiro A, Fernandez CI, Gomar F. Gluteal fibrosis. J Bone Joint Surg Am 57:987, 1975.
399. Saunders FP, Hoefnagel D, Staples OS. Progressive fibrosis of the quadriceps muscle. J Bone Joint Surg Am 47:380, 1965.
400. Shen YSH. Abduction contracture of the hip in children. J Bone Joint Surg Br 57:463, 1975.
401. Varma BP, Chandra U. Bilateral ankylosis of the elbows in extension due to contracture of the triceps: a case report. Int Surg 52:337, 1969.

402. Williams PF. Quadriceps contracture. J Bone Joint Surg Br 50: 278, 1968.
403. Wolbrink AJ, Shu Z, Bianco AJ. Abduction contracture of the shoulders and hips secondary to fibrous bands. J Bone Joint Surg Am 55:844, 1973.


## Cerebriform Fibrous Proliferation (Proteus Syndrome)


404. Botella-Estrada R, Alegra V, Sanmartin O, et al. Isolated plantar cerebriform collagenoma. Arch Dermatol 127:1589, 1991.
405. Clark RD, Donnai D, Rogers J, et al. Proteus syndrome: an expanding phenotype. Am J Med Genet 27:99, 1987.
406. Cohen MM Jr. Proteus syndrome: clinical evidence for somatie mosaicism and selected review. Am J Med Genet 47:645, 1993.
407. Costa T, Fitch N, Azouz EM. Proteus syndrome: report of two cases with pelvic lipomatosis. Pediatrics 76:984, 1985.
408. Fitch N, Azouz EM. Proteus syndrome: report of two cases with pelvic lipomatosis. Pediatrics 76:984, 1985.
409. Happle R. Cutaneous manifestation of lethal genes. Hum Genet 72:280, 1986.
410. Haramoto U, Kobayashi S, Ohmari K. Hemifacial hyperplasia with meningeal involvement: a variant of Proteus syndrome? Am J Med Genet 59:164, 1995.
411. Rizzo R, Pavone L, Micali G, et al. Encephalocraniocutaneous lipomatosis, Proteus syndrome and somatic mosaicism. Am J Med Genet 47:653, 1993.
412. Rudolph G, Blum WF, Genne EW, et al. Growth hormone, insulin-like growth factors, an IGF-binding protein-3 in a child with Proteus syndrome. Am J Med Genet 50:204, 1994.
413. Samlaska RP, Levin SW, Janes WD, et al. Proteus syndrome. Arch Dermatol 125:1109, 1989.
414. Smeets E, Frins JP, Cohen MM Jr. Regional Proteus syndrome and somatic mosaicism. Am J Med Genet 51:29, 1994.
415. Tibbles JAR, Cohen MM Jr. Proteus syndrome: the elephant man diagnosed. BMJ 293:683, 1996.
416. Tihan T, Okun J. Pathology of lipomatous lesions in Proteus syndrome. Pediatr Dev Pathol 1:443, 1998.
417. Uitto J, Bauer EA, Santa Cruz DJ, et al. Decreased collagenase production by regional fibroblasts cultured from skin of a patient with connective tissue nevi of the collagen type. J Invest Dermatol 78:136, 1982.
418. Van Bever Y, Hennekam RC. Isolated macrodactyly or extremely localized Proteus syndrome? Clin Dysmorphol 3:351, 1994.
419. Viljoen DL, Saxe N, Temple-Camp C. Cutaneous manifestations of the Proteus syndrome. Pediatr Dermatol 5:14, 1988.
420. Wiedemann HR, Burgio GR, Aldenhoff P. The Proteus syndrome. Eur J Pediatr 140:5, 1983.


## Calcifying Fibrous Pseudotumor


421. Dumont P, de Muret A, Skrobala D, et al. Calcifying fibrous pseudotumor of the mediastinum. Ann Thorac Surg 63:543, 1997.
422. Fetsch JF, Montgomery EA, Meis JM. Calcifying fibrous pseudotumor. Am J Surg Pathol 17:502, 1993.
423. Fukunaga N, Kikuchi Y, Endo Y, et al. Calcifying fibrous pseudotumor: case report. Pathol Int 47:60, 1997.
424. Hainaut P, Lesage V, Weynand B, et al. Calcifying fibrous pseudotumor: a patient presenting with multiple pleural lesions. Acta Clin Belg 54:162, 1999.
425. Kocova L, Michal M, Sulc M, et al. Calcifying fibrous pseudotumor of visceral peritoneum. Histopathology 31:182, 1997.
426. Maeda T, Hirose T, Furuya K, et al. Calcifying fibrous pseudotumor: an ultrastructural study. Ultrastruct Pathol 23:189, 1999.
427. Najat M, Dominque W, Rolland P, et al. Intraabdominal calcifying fibrous pseudotumor: a clinicopathologic review of three cases. Clin Exp Pathol 46:47A, 1998.
428. Pinkard NB, Wilson RW, Lawless N, et al. Calcifying fibrous pseudotumor of pleura: a report of three cases of a newly described entity involving the pleura. Am J Clin Pathol 105: 189, 1996.
429. Reed MK, Margraf LR, Nikaidoh H, et al. Calcifying fibrous pseudotumor of the chest wall. Ann Thorac Surg 62:873, 1996.
430. Rosenthal NS, Abdul-Karim FW. Childhood fibrous tumor with psammoma bodies: clinicopathologic features in two cases. Arch Pathol Lab Med 112:798, 1988.
430a. Sigel JE, Smith TA, Reith JD, et al. Immunohistochemical analysis of ALK expression in deep soft tissue calcifying fibrous pseudotumor: Evidence of a late sclerosing stage of inflammatory myofibroblastic tumor? Ann Diagn Pathol (in press).
431. Van Dorpe J, Ectors N, Geboes K, et al. Is calcifying fibrous pseudotumor a late sclerosing stage of inflammatory myofibroblastic tumor? Am J Surg Pathol 23:329, 1999.
432. Weynand B, Draguet AP, Bernard P, et al. Calcifying fibrous pseudotumour: first case report in the peritoneum with immunostaining for CD34. Histopathology 34:86, 1999.
433. Zámecník M, Dorociak F, Veselý L. Calcifying fibrous pseudotumor after trauma. Pathol Int 47:812, 1997.

# CHAPTER 12

# FIBROSARCOMA

Traditionally, fibrosarcoma has been defined as a malignant mesenchymal tumor, the cells of which recapitulate the appearance of the normal fibroblast. This admittedly broad definition has resulted in a great deal of subjectivity as to which spindle cell, collagen-forming tumors were appropriately termed fibrosarcoma and which were better classified as another form of sarcoma. Depending on the era and the criteria in vogue at that time, the incidence and behavior of this neoplasm have varied greatly. This trend is well illustrated by a series of studies from the Mayo Clinic over a period of 50 years. In 1936 Meyerding et al.[51] reported that 65% of soft tissue sarcomas were fibrosarcoma, a figure revised to 12% in 1974 by Pritchard et al.[59] and to even less by Scott et al. in 1989.[66]

On closer scrutiny, several factors are probably responsible for the apparent decline in the incidence of fibrosarcoma. Most important has been the general acceptance of the concept that pleomorphic spindle cell tumors that produce collagen are better classified as malignant fibrous histiocytomas. Thus, by convention many previously diagnosed high-grade fibrosarcomas became malignant fibrous histiocytomas. Second, refinement of histologic criteria resulted in the segregation of fibromatosis (desmoid tumors) as a unique group of tumors distinct from fibrosarcoma. Lastly, with the advent of immunohistochemistry and cytogenetics it became possible to recognize monophasic fibrous synovial sarcomas and malignant peripheral nerve sheath tumors with a greater degree of diagnostic accuracy. Despite much progress in this area, the differential diagnosis of spindle cell tumors remains a difficult, challenging, sometimes inextricable problem, especially when only a small biopsy specimen is available for microscopic examination.

As a result of the foregoing trends, a number of general statements can be made concerning the diagnosis of fibrosarcoma.

1. Fibrosarcoma has become, in large part, a diagnosis of exclusion. It presupposes that diagnoses such as monophasic fibrous synovial sarcoma and malignant peripheral nerve sheath tumor have been excluded by the appropriate immunohistochemical, ultrastructural, or cytogenetic studies.
2. Fibrosarcomas, like other fibroblastic tumors (e.g., fibromatosis), may have a variable component of neoplastic cells with features of myofibroblasts. Therefore the finding of various actin isoforms within these tumors does not mitigate against the diagnosis of fibrosarcoma.
3. Collagen-forming spindle cell tumors of high nuclear grade by convention are classified as malignant fibrous histiocytomas. Consequently, lesions diagnosed as fibrosarcoma, for the most part, occupy the low-grade end (grades 1 and 2) of a spectrum that includes malignant fibrous histiocytoma at the high-grade end.

Despite the fact that the incidence of fibrosarcoma has markedly diminished in recent years, there have been renewed efforts to identify unique subsets or variants within this group of lesions. Although it is still not clear to what extent these variants are biologically different from one another, they certainly have distinct histologic features that allow their identification in a more or less consistent fashion. These variants include myxoid fibrosarcoma (myxofibrosarcoma), low-grade fibromyxoid sarcoma/hyalinizing spindle cell tumor with giant rosettes, and sclerosing epithelioid fibrosarcoma, all of which are discussed in this chapter (Table 12–1). Juvenile/infantile-type fibrosarcoma is discussed in Chapter 11, given its distinctive clinical features. "Inflammatory fibrosarcoma" is also discussed in Chapter 11 under the heading inflammatory myofibroblastic tumor.

## CLINICAL FINDINGS

Like most other sarcomas, fibrosarcoma causes no characteristic symptoms and is difficult to diagnose clinically. Most patients present with a solitary palpable mass ranging from 3 to 8 cm in greatest dimension; it rarely becomes larger than 10 cm. In general, it is slow-growing and during the initial phase causes

**TABLE 12–1 CLASSIFICATION OF FIBROSARCOMA**

Adult-type fibrosarcoma
  Myxoid type (myxofibrosarcoma, low-grade myxoid malignant fibrous histiocytoma)
  Fibromyxoid type (low-grade fibromyxoid type/fibromyxoid type with giant rosettes)
  Sclerosing epithelioid type
Juvenile/infantile-type fibrosarcoma

pain in only about one-third of cases. In fact, pain is encountered more commonly with synovial sarcoma and malignant peripheral nerve sheath tumor than with fibrosarcoma.

The skin overlying the tumor is generally intact, although more superficially located neoplasms that grow rapidly or have been traumatized may result in ulceration of the skin. Such tumors, particularly when clinically neglected, may form large fungating masses in the areas of ulceration. The preoperative duration of symptoms varies greatly and ranges from as little as a few weeks to as long as 20 years. In the study by Pritchard et al.,[58] the average preoperative duration was 3 years 4 months.

Fibrosarcoma may occur at any age but is most common at 30–55 years. The average age in the literature ranges from 39.4[56] to 47.7[58] years, although the mean age reported prior to 1955 is closer to the mid-fifties presumably because of the inclusion of cases of malignant fibrous histiocytoma. Most studies have reported a slightly higher incidence of the tumor in men than in women. For instance, Scott et al.,[66] in a series of 132 cases, noted that 61% of the patients were men.

The tumor may occur in any soft tissue site but is most common in the deep soft tissues of the lower extremities, particularly in the thigh and knee followed by the upper extremities and trunk (Table 12–2). There are numerous reports of fibrosarcoma in the head and neck, including the nasal cavity, paranasal sinuses, and nasopharynx.[13,24,30,31,47] Rare examples of this tumor have also been reported in the breast,[35] thyroid,[67] heart,[1,40] lung,[43] liver,[57] and central nervous system.[18,25,44]

**TABLE 12–2 ANATOMIC LOCATIONS OF FIBROSARCOMA ($N$ = 695)**

| Anatomic Location | No. Patients | % |
|---|---|---|
| Lower extremities | 313 | 45 |
| Upper extremities | 195 | 28 |
| Trunk | 118 | 17 |
| Head, neck | 69 | 10 |
| *Total* | 695 | 100 |

Data are from the Armed Forces Institute of Pathology.

Fibrosarcoma predominantly involves deep structures, where it tends to originate from the intramuscular and intermuscular fibrous tissue, fascial envelopes, aponeuroses, and tendons. Deeply situated tumors may even encircle bone and cause radiographically demonstrable periosteal and cortical thickening; in such cases distinction from parosteal sarcoma may be difficult. Other radiographic findings, in addition to a soft tissue mass, include occasional foci of calcification and ossification, although this feature is much more common with synovial sarcoma than fibrosarcoma. Fibrosarcomas arising from the subcutis, excluding those that arise in dermatofibrosarcoma protuberans, are rare and tend to originate in tissues damaged by radiation, heat, or scarring.

Most patients lack systemic manifestations except weight loss in those with tumors of large size and long duration and in cases where tumors have metastasized widely. Hypoglycemia, presumably owing to the production of insulin-like substances excreted from the tumor,[39] has been reported.[39,56]

## GROSS FINDINGS

Generally, the excised tumor consists of a solitary, soft to firm, fleshy, rounded or lobulated mass that is gray-white to tan-yellow and measures 3–8 cm in greatest dimension (Figs. 12–1, 12–2). The small tumors tend to be well circumscribed and frequently are partly or completely encapsulated. Large tumors are less well defined; they often extend with multiple processes into the surrounding tissues or grow in a diffusely invasive or destructive manner. The frequent circumscription of small fibrosarcomas can be misleading and may result in an erroneous diagnosis of a benign tumor and inadequate surgical therapy.

## MICROSCOPIC FINDINGS

Although there are minor variations in the histologic picture, most fibrosarcomas have in common a rather uniform fasciculated growth pattern consisting of fusiform or spindle-shaped cells that vary little in size and shape, have scanty cytoplasm with indistinct cell borders, and are separated by interwoven collagen fibers arranged in a parallel fashion. In fact, the amount and orientation of the intervening collagen fibers seem largely to determine the shape of the tumor cells and reflect the degree of cellular differentiation. Mitotic activity varies, but caution should be exercised when diagnosing fibrosarcoma in the absence of mitotic figures. Multinucleated giant cells or giant cells of bizarre size and shape are rarely a feature of this tumor.

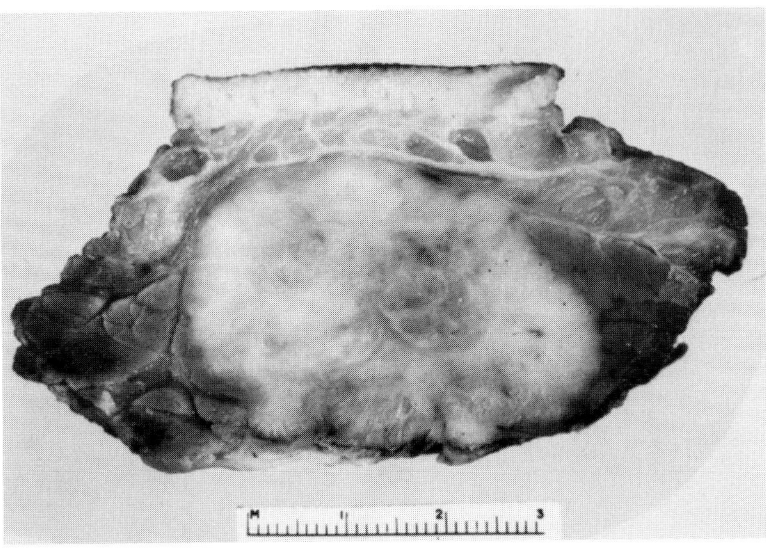

**FIGURE 12–1.** Fibrosarcoma involving the musculature of the shoulder in a 63-year-old man.

There are no sharply defined morphologic subdivisions as, for example, in liposarcoma and rhabdomyosarcoma; and histologic grading of fibrosarcomas is mainly based on the degree of cellularity, degree of cellular differentiation, number of mitotic figures, amount of collagen produced by the tumor cells, and extent of necrosis.

*Well-differentiated fibrosarcomas* are characterized by a uniform, orderly appearance of the spindle cells that typically exhibit marked fibrogenesis (Fig. 12–3).

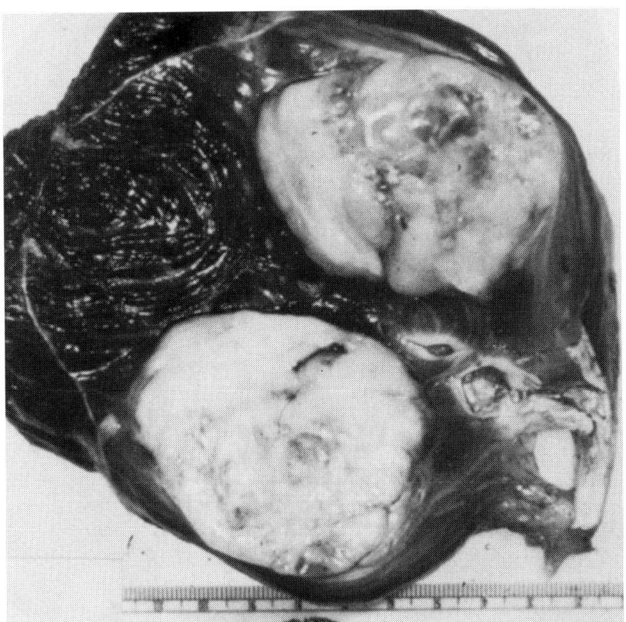

**FIGURE 12–2.** Fibrosarcoma of the posterior thigh in a 37-year-old man. Despite the circumscription of the lesion and treatment by wide local excision, the tumor metastasized to the lung.

In some cases the cells are oriented in curving or interlacing fascicles, forming a classic herringbone pattern (Figs. 12–4 to 12–7). In others, the cells are separated by thick, wire-like collagen fibers that may be hyalinized (Fig. 12–8). Some tumors are characterized by more rounded cells with small nuclei and clear cytoplasm that are surrounded, individually or in groups or cords, by dense, often hyalinizing collagen fibers, a variant referred to as *sclerosing epithelioid fibrosarcoma* (described below).

*Poorly differentiated fibrosarcomas* are characterized by closely packed, less well oriented tumor cells that are small, ovoid or rounded, and associated with less collagen (Fig. 12–9). The fascicular or herringbone growth pattern is less distinct, mitotic figures are more numerous, and there are areas of necrosis or hemorrhage. Although the cells show some variation in size and shape, marked nuclear pleomorphism is more suggestive of malignant fibrous histiocytoma than fibrosarcoma. In some cases, distinction of poorly differentiated fibrosarcoma from monophasic fibrous synovial sarcoma or malignant peripheral nerve sheath tumor may be difficult or impossible without the use of immunohistochemistry, electron microscopy, or cytogenetics.

Secondary features are common. Well-differentiated fibrosarcomas, which are rich in mature collagen, may focally show osseous or, less frequently, cartilaginous metaplasia. Some tumors have areas that are less cellular or extensively myxoid (Fig. 12–10) and closely mimic portions of fibromatosis (desmoid tumor), thereby making distinction of these two lesions difficult, particularly when only a small sample is available for evaluation.

As seen by immunohistochemistry, the cells are marked with antibodies for vimentin, but they do not

*Text continued on page 415*

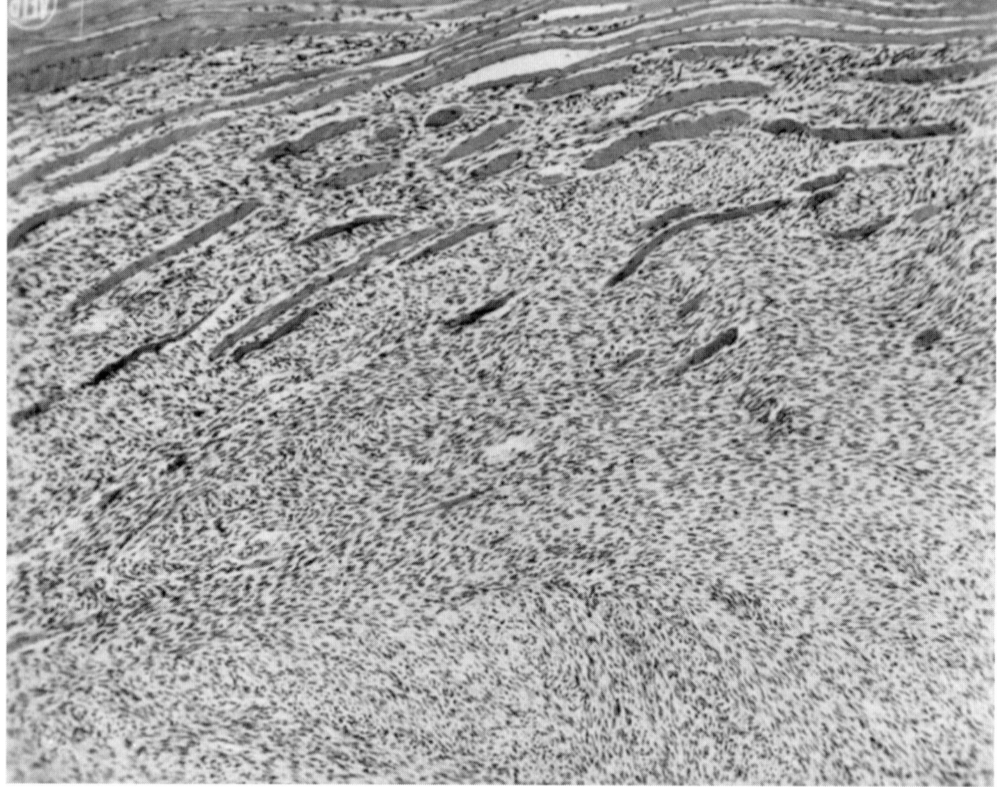

**FIGURE 12–3.** Fibrosarcoma invading muscle tissue. Note the orderly arrangement of spindle cells and lack of cellular pleomorphism.

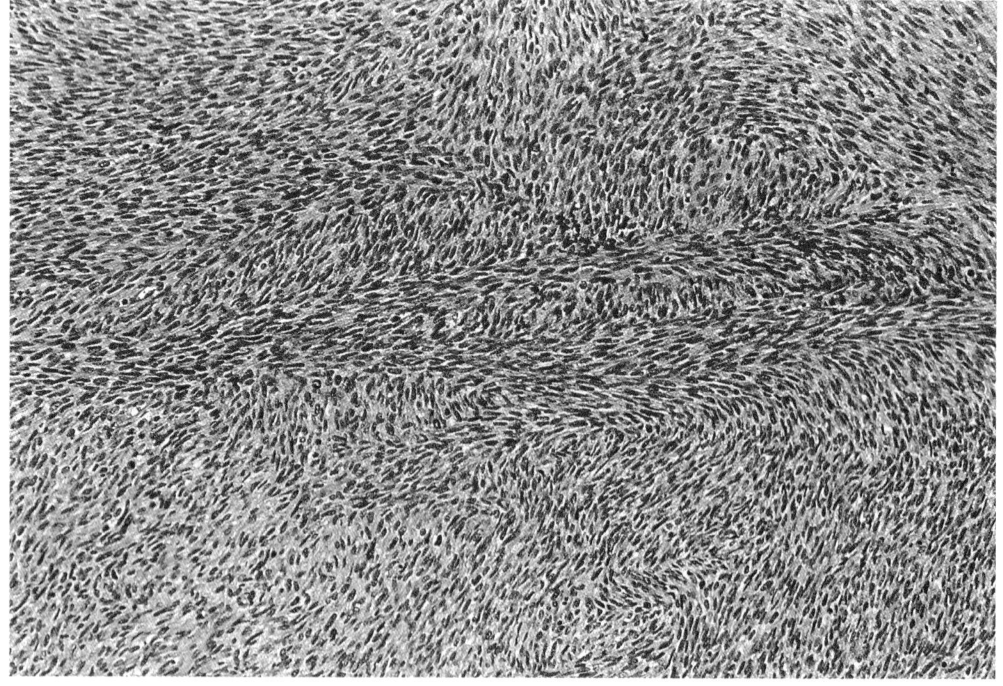

**FIGURE 12–4.** Low-power view of a fibrosarcoma exhibiting a distinct fascicular ("herringbone") pattern.

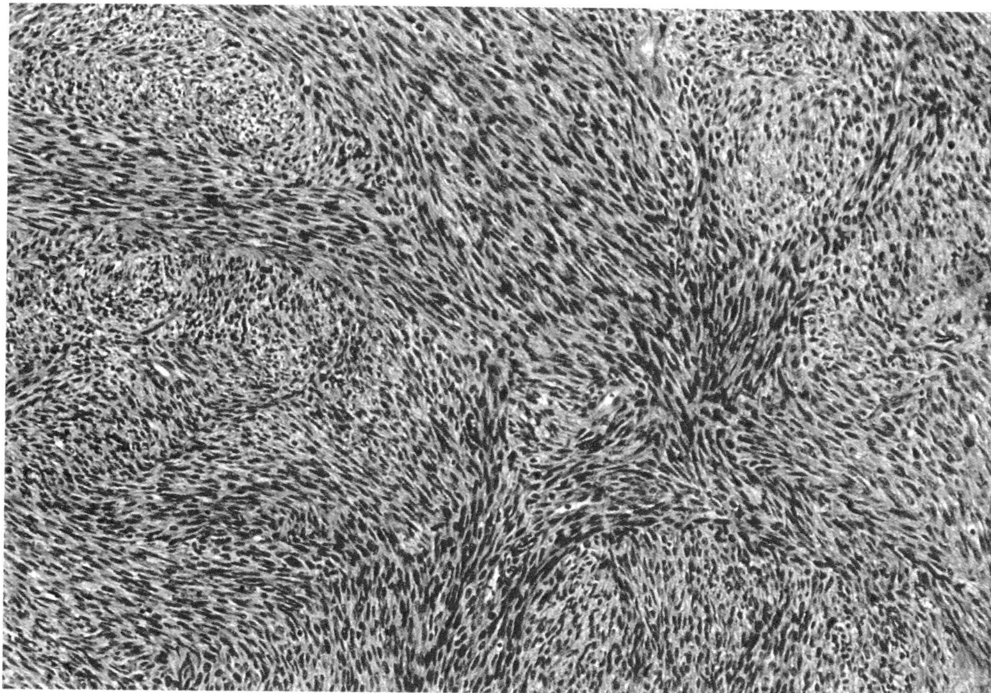

**FIGURE 12–5.** Fibrosarcoma consisting of uniform spindle cells showing little variation in size and shape and a distinct fascicular pattern.

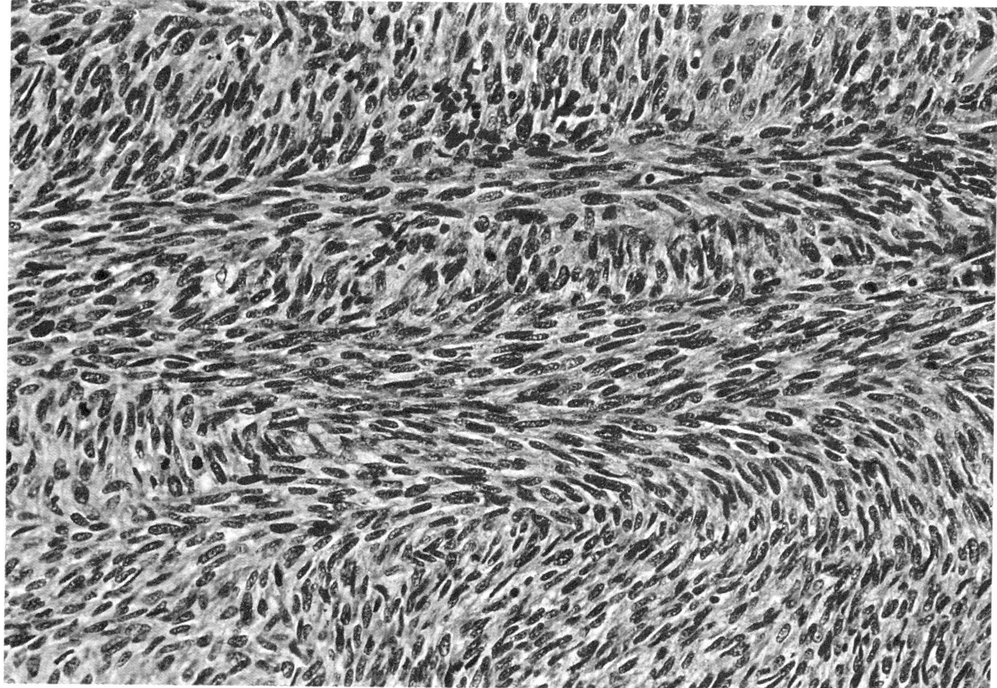

**FIGURE 12–6.** Fibrosarcoma showing arrangement of the fibroblasts in distinct intersecting fascicles ("herringbone" pattern).

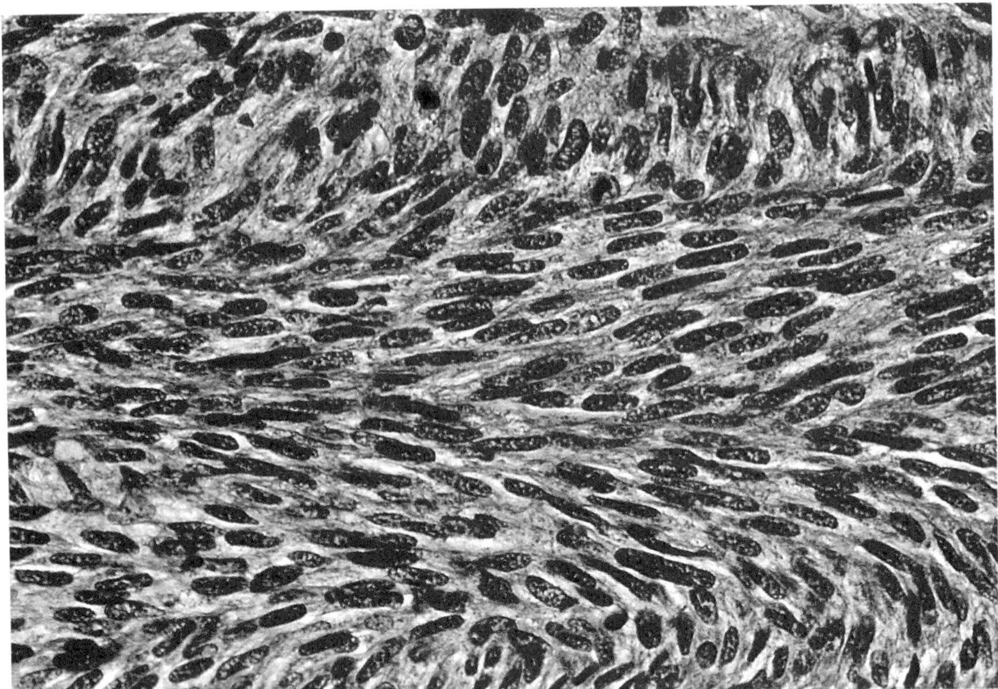

**FIGURE 12–7.** High-power view of fibrosarcoma showing uniformity of the tumor cells and the characteristic fascicular pattern.

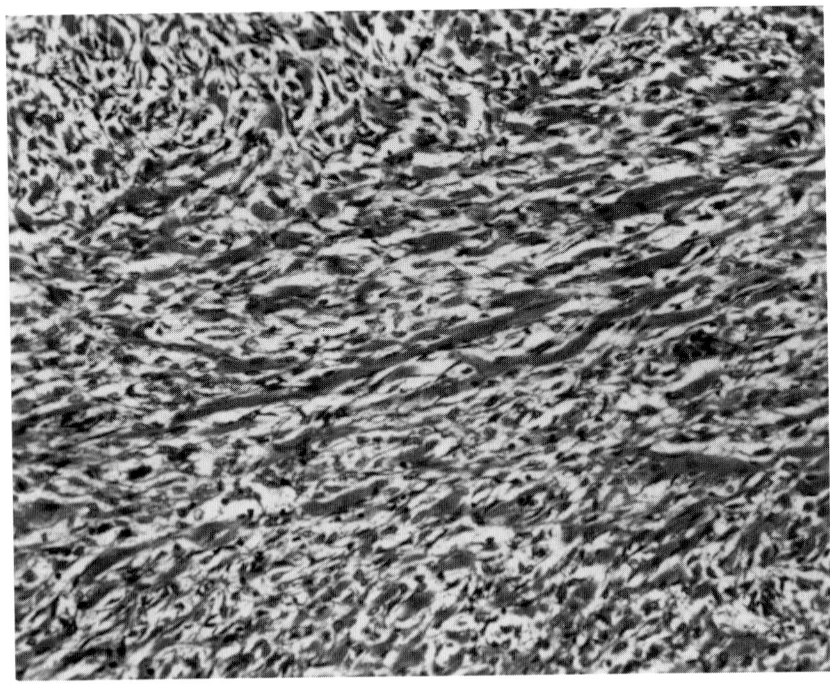

**FIGURE 12–8.** Postirradiation fibrosarcoma with thick, wire-like collagen fibers between tumor cells.

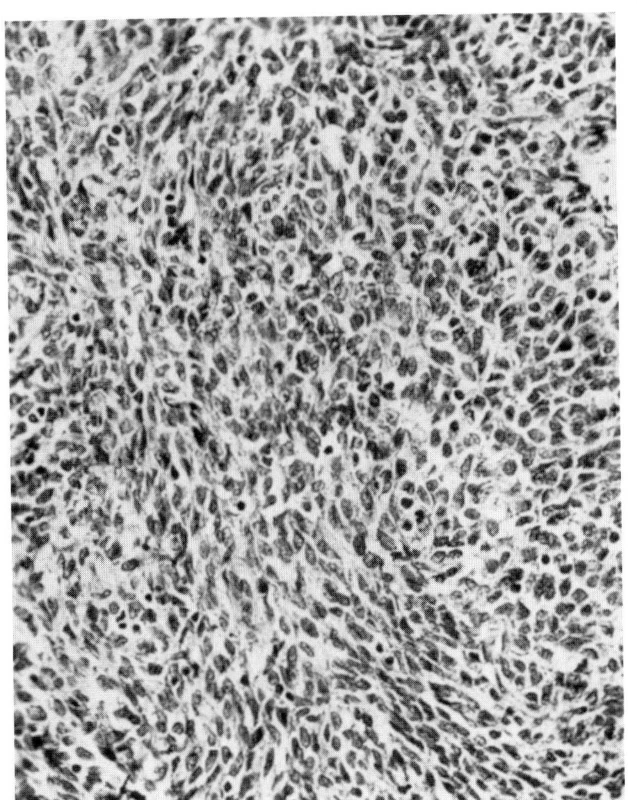

**FIGURE 12–9.** Poorly differentiated fibrosarcoma with a focal round cell pattern.

exhibit any other specific line of cellular differentiation, as the cells do not stain for epithelial markers or S-100 protein. The lack of cytokeratin immunoreactivity aids in distinction from monophasic fibrous synovial sarcoma. Negative immunostaining for S-100 protein distinguishes fibrosarcoma from spindle cell or desmoplastic malignant melanomas but not necessarily from malignant peripheral nerve sheath tumors, as only 50–60% of the latter stain focally for this antigen. In some fibrosarcomas scattered cells stain for smooth muscle or muscle-specific actin.

## ELECTRON MICROSCOPIC FINDINGS

As might be anticipated from the light microscopic features, the tumors are largely composed of elongated fibroblast-like cells with irregularly outlined or indented nuclei, infrequent nucleoli, and prominent rough endoplasmic reticulum that is often dilated and contains granular or amorphous material. Some cells contain, in addition, intracytoplasmic bundles of microfilaments measuring up to 60 nm in diameter, focal condensations or dense bodies, and sometimes basal lamina material, features characteristic of myofibroblasts. Suh et al.[70] studied the ultrastructural features of 60 fibrosarcomas and found myofibroblastic

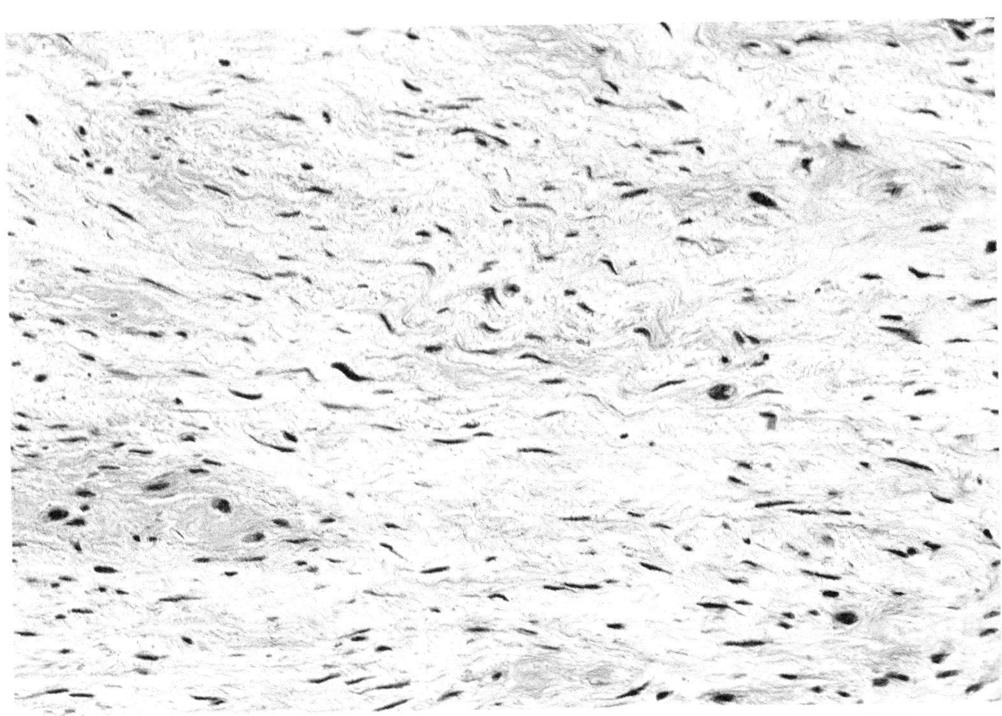

**FIGURE 12–10.** Fibrosarcoma with extensive myxoid change. The fibroblasts are widely separated by abundant myxoid stroma, making the fascicular pattern less conspicuous.

differentiation in scattered cells in 33 of the tumors. Infrequently, there are also scattered, round, histiocyte-like cells with multiple processes and a small number of lysosomes. The extracellular spaces contain a varying number of collagen fibers.

## MYOFIBROBLASTIC SARCOMA

As noted above, scattered cells in typical cases of fibrosarcoma may stain for smooth muscle or muscle-specific actin, and ultrastructural data support the presence of cells with myofibroblastic differentiation in otherwise typical fibrosarcoma. The issue as to whether there are sarcomas composed predominantly or exclusively of myofibroblasts remains a contentious one, primarily because the diagnostic criteria for recognizing such tumors remain obscure. According to Schürch and colleagues, most benign and malignant neoplasms composed of myofibroblasts reported in the literature lack specific myofibroblastic features.[37,62,64] According to these authors, myofibroblasts can be recognized by the ultrastructural identification of stress fibers, well-developed microtendons (fibronexuses), and intercellular intermediate-type end-gap junctions.[21,63] Because of the heterogeneous immunophenotype of myofibroblasts with regard to intermediate filaments and actin isoforms, these authors argued that categorizing a cell as a myofibroblast by its immunohistochemical staining pattern alone is imprecise.[37] Others have argued that myofibroblastic sarcomas are recognizable even in the absence of the aforementioned ultrastructural features.[23,50] Mentzel et al.[50] reported a series of 18 low-grade myofibroblastic sarcomas that generally behaved in an indolent fashion. However, inclusion criteria for this study were not specifically stated, and ultrastructural examination was performed in only five cases. In our opinion, myofibroblastic sarcomas do exist but are rare. Although one may suspect myofibroblastic sarcoma on the basis of routine morphology, we believe that confirmation of myofibroblastic differentiation usually requires ultrastructural analysis, although the minimal ultrastructural criteria required for recognizing such cells are yet to be well defined.

## DIFFERENTIAL DIAGNOSIS

It is often difficult to distinguish fibrosarcoma from other spindle cell tumors, and in many instances only careful examination of multiple sections and ancillary studies permit a correct diagnosis. *Benign processes* likely to be mistaken for fibrosarcoma range from nodular fasciitis to fibrous histiocytoma and fibromatosis. *Malignant neoplasms* considered in the differential diagnosis are much more numerous and include foremost malignant peripheral nerve sheath tumor, malignant fibrous histiocytoma, and monophasic fibrous synovial sarcoma. Other tumors that tend to simulate fibrosarcoma include sarcomatoid mesothelioma, clear cell sarcoma, epithelioid sarcoma, dermatofibrosarcoma protuberans, desmoplastic leiomyosarcoma, spindle cell forms of rhabdomyosarcoma, liposarcoma, malignant melanoma, and spindle cell carcinoma. Because the differential diagnosis of most of these tumors is discussed elsewhere, the following comments are limited to lesions most frequently confused with fibrosarcoma.

*Nodular fasciitis,* a pseudosarcomatous reactive fibroblastic/myofibroblastic proliferation that grows rapidly and is marked by its cellularity and immature cellular appearance, differs from fibrosarcoma by its smaller size and microscopically by its more irregular growth pattern; characteristically, its cells are arranged in short bundles—never in long, sweeping fascicles or a herringbone pattern as in fibrosarcoma. Moreover, there is usually a prominent myxoid matrix and scattered chronic inflammatory cells.

*Fibrous histiocytoma (dermatofibroma)* may also show a distinct spindle cell pattern but never exhibits the cellular polarity and regular fascicular arrangement seen in fibrosarcoma. In fact, the cells are often arranged in a storiform pattern with interspersed collagen fibers (collagen trapping) at the periphery. In addition to the spindle cells, secondary elements such as histiocyte-like cells, siderophages, xanthoma cells, multinucleated giant cells, and chronic inflammatory cells are common. In most cases fibrous histiocytoma is situated in the dermis or subcutis; unlike fibrosarcoma and malignant fibrous histiocytoma, it is rarely found in deep soft tissue structures. Mitotic figures are present in fibrous histiocytoma (and nodular fasciitis), but the presence of atypical mitotic figures lends strong support to a diagnosis of malignancy.

*Musculoaponeurotic fibromatosis (desmoid tumor)* has a growth pattern similar to that of fibrosarcoma but is less cellular and contains more collagen. The cells are uniformly spindled, with delicate chromatin and one or two minute nucleoli. In general, the cells do not touch one another but, rather, are separated by collagen, whereas the cells of fibrosarcoma frequently overlap with closely spaced nuclei. Mitotic figures are rare, and the presence of more than one mitotic figure per high-power field (HPF) in such a tumor should raise a suspicion of fibrosarcoma (Table 12–3). Low levels of mitotic activity may be present in fibromatosis such that considerable overlap in mitotic activity between fibromatosis and fibrosarcoma may be encountered. Montgomery et al.[52] documented a range in mitotic activity of 0/50 to 21/50 HPF in fibromatosis, compared to 0/50 to 40/50 HPF in low-grade fibrosarcoma. Thus mitotic activity is not a reliable discriminant between fibromatosis and fibrosarcoma

**TABLE 12–3 COMPARISON OF HISTOLOGIC FEATURES OF LOW-GRADE FIBROSARCOMA AND FIBROMATOSIS**

| Parameter | Low-grade Fibrosarcoma | Fibromatosis |
|---|---|---|
| Cellularity | Low to moderate | Low to moderate |
| Nuclear overlap | Present | Usually absent |
| Nuclear hyperchromasia | Present | Absent |
| Nucleoli | More prominent | Inconspicuous |
| Mitotic figures | 1+ to 3+ | 1+ |
| Necrosis | Rare | Absent |
| Vessel wall infiltration | Rare | Absent |

when dealing with low levels of mitotic activity (<50/50 HPF) but might become useful when higher levels of mitotic activity (>50/50 HPF) are encountered. Because fibromatosis-like areas may be present in well-differentiated fibrosarcoma, careful sampling of the tumor is mandatory for a reliable diagnosis. Clinical considerations are of little help for distinguishing these tumors because they may occur at the same location and in patients of similar age.

*Malignant fibrous histiocytoma* has been included in many of the earlier reports of poorly differentiated or pleomorphic fibrosarcomas. Clinically, malignant fibrous histiocytoma is principally a tumor of elderly persons, with a peak during the seventh decade; microscopically, it can be recognized by its storiform pattern and the presence of multinucleated bizarre giant cells, often with eosinophilic cytoplasm and containing delicate droplets of lipid material. Siderophages and xanthoma cells are also common features that assist in the diagnosis. Transitions between malignant fibrous histiocytoma and fibrosarcoma do occur; but on close examination, most malignant spindle cell tumors with abundant hyalinized, intensely eosinophilic collagen turn out to be variants of malignant fibrous histiocytoma.

*Malignant peripheral nerve sheath tumor* (MPNST) may display areas that are virtually indistinguishable from fibrosarcoma, but in most of these cases specific features can be found that point toward a tumor with neural differentiation. In general, the cells of MPNST have a wavy or buckled appearance, rather than the finely tapered fibroblasts of fibrosarcoma. Although the cells may be arranged into an irregular fascicular growth pattern, the long sweeping fascicles characteristic of fibrosarcoma are usually not present. Moreover, the cells of MPNST tend to show perivascular cuffing and may be arranged in distinct whorls or palisades. In addition, there is a more prominent myxoid matrix, and there are often transitions between malignant and benign neurofibroma-like areas. Cartilaginous metaplasia is also more frequent than in fibrosarcoma or any other noncartilaginous neoplasm. The finding of S-100 protein in scattered tumor cells supports a diagnosis of MPNST, although up to 40% of cases do not stain for this antigen.

*Monophasic fibrous synovial sarcoma* may also closely simulate a fibrosarcoma, although it is generally composed of more ovoid-appearing cells arranged in an irregular fascicular growth pattern. Moreover, many of these sarcomas have areas in which the cells contain more eosinophilic cytoplasm with a suggestion of cellular cohesion, even if well-formed glands are not present. Immunohistochemically, almost all cases of synovial sarcoma express at least one epithelial marker, a feature not found in fibrosarcoma. The identification of t(X;18) by fluorescence in situ hybridization (FISH) or reverse transcriptase-polymerase chain reaction (RT-PCR) is a highly sensitive and specific method for identifying a tumor as a synovial sarcoma.

## CLINICAL BEHAVIOR

It is difficult to compare the results of many of these published studies, as many of the tumors probably represent entities other than fibrosarcoma. Few studies have utilized immunohistochemistry to exclude other lesions in the differential diagnosis. As such, the rate of local recurrence varies significantly among studies. For example, Mackenzie noted a recurrence in 93 (49%) of 190 cases[46] and Pritchard et al. in 113 (57%) of 199 cases.[59] In the study by Scott et al.[66] the overall rate of recurrence was 42% at 5 years. In that study, although neither tumor grade nor tumor stage was associated with an increased risk of local recurrence, the status of the surgical margins was strongly predictive, as the 5-year cumulative probability of local recurrence was 79% in tumors with inadequate surgical margins and 18% in tumors treated by wide or radical excision. In a study of low-grade fibrosarcomas, Montgomery et al.[52] found a recurrence rate of 12%, with a mean interval of 69 months prior to recurrence.

Metastasis of fibrosarcoma occurs almost exclusively by way of the bloodstream. The lung is the principal metastatic site, followed by the skeleton, especially the vertebrae and skull. Most metastases are noted within the first 2 years after diagnosis, although some patients, particularly those with low-grade fibrosarcomas, develop metastasis late in their course.[52] Therefore a 5-year follow-up is too short, and "5-year cure rates" are misleading.

Lymph node metastasis is rare, occurring in 0.5%[59] to 8.0%[68,69] of cases; the relative incidence is, of course, influenced by the number of autopsy cases in the reported material because lymph nodes tend to be more often involved in the terminal phase of the disease. Therefore it seems that regional lymph node excision is not a necessary part of the initial therapeutic regimen.

The rate of metastasis varies widely among studies. Scott et al.[66] found 1-, 2-, and 5-year metastasis rates to be 34%, 52%, and 63%, respectively. Using a four-grade classification scheme, these authors noted an increased risk of metastasis with increasing tumor grade, as those patients with grade 1 or 2 tumors had a 5-year metastasis rate of 43% compared to 82% for those patients with grade 4 tumors. In their study of low-grade fibrosarcomas, Montgomery et al.[52] reported that 9% of patients developed metastases at a mean interval of 124 months after the initial excision.

Survival rates also vary considerably, especially in earlier descriptions of the tumor. In more recent reports, however, the 5-year survival rates are more uniform, ranging from 39.0%[66] to 54.4%.[46] These data differ considerably from those of Castro et al.,[9] who reported a 5-year survival rate of 70% and a 10-year rate of 60%. In the latter series, however, it is not clear whether fibromatoses were included as grade 1 fibrosarcomas.

Most studies have found a significant relation between the degree of differentiation and survival. This point was clearly established as early as 1939 by Broders et al.,[7] who demonstrated close parallels between prognosis and histologic features. Their work has been amply confirmed by most authors who attempted to correlate histologic grade and prognosis.[58,66] Mackenzie, employing a three-grade classification, reported 5-year survival rates of 82.2% for grade 1, 55.0% for grade 2, and 35.5% for grade 3 tumors.[46] Scott et al.,[66] using a four-grade classification, noted 58% survival for grades 1 or 2, 34% for grade 3, and 21% for grade 4 (Table 12–4). It is evident from these data that prognosis in regard to recurrence and metastasis is least favorable with tumors that are richly cellular, have more than two mitotic figures per high-power field, contain little collagen, and show evidence of necrosis.

A second and equally important factor when determining prognosis is the adequacy of the initial excision. Bizer reported a 5-year survival rate of 30% for patients treated by local excision and 78% for those treated by radical excision.[4] Likewise, Scott et al.[66] found a 29% five-year survival rate for the group treated with inadequate margins and a 40% rate for those treated with adequate margins. In the latter series the incidence of recurrence was even more closely related to the extent of surgery, as those with positive margins were more than four times as likely to develop a recurrence than those treated with wide margins. There was no clear relation between the extent of surgery and metastasis.

## TREATMENT

Once the diagnosis of fibrosarcoma is established by biopsy, the tumor should be promptly excised with a wide margin of normal tissue. Because tumors in the extremities are prone to extend proximally along the neurovascular bundle, a wider proximal than distal margin is advisable. As with other sarcomas, enucleation or shelling out of the tumor invites recurrent growth because this procedure does not take into account the frequent presence of small satellite nodules around the main tumor mass. When adequate margins cannot be obtained, as is often the case with tumors situated near large vessels, nerves, or joints, amputation or excision with supplementary radiotherapy is mandatory. Lymph node metastasis is a rare event, and removal of regional lymph nodes is generally unnecessary unless there is strong clinical evidence of lymph node involvement. Similar to other

**TABLE 12–4** RELATION BETWEEN HISTOLOGIC GRADE AND 5-YEAR SURVIVAL FOR FIBROSARCOMA

| | 5-Year Survival Rate (%) | | | | | |
|---|---|---|---|---|---|---|
| ***Study*** | ***Grade 1*** | ***Grades 1 & 2*†** | ***Grade 2*** | ***Grade 3*** | ***Grades 3 & 4*‡** | ***Grade 4*** |
| Mackenzie[46]* | 82.0 | | 55.0 | 35.5 | | — |
| Scott et al.[66] | | 58.0 | | 34.0 | | 21.0 |
| Castro et al.[9] | | 82.0 | | | 68.0 | |

* Used only a three-grade scale.
† Grouped grades 1 and 2 together.
‡ Grouped grades 3 and 4 together.

sarcomas, adjuvant radiation therapy seems to be beneficial for those whose tumors are incompletely excised.[42,47] Adjuvant systemic chemotherapy is indicated for high-grade fibrosarcomas because with these tumors subclinical or microscopic metastases may exist at the time of the initial surgery.[71]

## DISCUSSION

Little is known about the cytogenetic and molecular genetic alterations in fibrosarcoma. In contrast to congenital and infantile fibrosarcoma,[61] adult fibrosarcoma does not appear to have a characteristic cytogenetic abnormality. Dal Cin et al.[14] reported a case of fibrosarcoma with complex karyotypic alterations, whereas Limon et al.[41] reported a nonrandom chromosomal change involving t(2;19). Klein and Bauck[36] suggested the presence of a tumor-suppressor gene on the distal region of the long arm of chromosome 1 that may be important in the development of this tumor. Alterations of the *p53* tumor-suppressor gene are relatively rare but have been reported to correlate with poor survival.[54]

Considering the prominent role of fibroblasts in posttraumatic repair, it is not surprising that trauma has been implicated repeatedly as a possible and even likely causative factor.[16] Stout, for example, reported 36 cases of fibrosarcoma arising in scar tissue *(cicatricial fibrosarcoma)* or at the site of a former injury.[68] One patient had suffered an injury at age 9 years and developed a fibrosarcoma in the scar at age 35; it recurred when the patient was 65 years old; and the patient was well and free of recurrence at age 91. Ivins et al.[34] noted a history of preceding trauma in 19 of 78 cases of fibrosarcoma but concluded that "only in one an etiologic significance was remotely possible." Heller and Sieber[32] observed the appearance of a fibrosarcoma in the right thigh 4 months after a sledgehammer injury at the same site. Melzner[49] and Stout[68] described a fibrosarcoma that developed in a healed shotgun wound in close vicinity to the bullet; in both cases the tumor made its first clinical appearance after a latent period of 11 years. Several authors have reported the development of fibrosarcoma in a draining sinus of long duration.[10,17] Evaluation of the significance of these cases is difficult. In some of them trauma may be a contributing factor, whereas in others trauma may merely serve to alert the patient or the physician to the presence of the disease and may be an incidental finding rather than a tumor-provoking factor.

Factors other than trauma have also been implicated to induce or contribute to the development of fibrosarcoma. Burns et al.[8] reported a tumor arising in a 31-year-old man 10 years after a plastic Teflon-Dacron prosthetic vascular graft was placed for a lacerated femoral artery; a similar case was described by O'Connell et al.[53] Eckstein et al.[19] reported a fibrosarcoma that arose in the vicinity of a total knee joint prosthesis. There is another report of a fibrosarcoma arising at the site of a penicillin-sesame oil injection.[28]

## FIBROSARCOMA VARIANTS

### Sclerosing Epithelioid Type

Sclerosing epithelioid fibrosarcoma is an unusual variant of fibrosarcoma composed of cytologically bland epithelioid cells deposited in a densely hyalinized collagenous matrix. Since the initial description of this tumor by Meis-Kindblom et al.,[48] few reports of this neoplasm have appeared in the literature.[12,20,60] Unlike other forms of fibrosarcoma, this tumor may express a number of specific antigens, raising the possibility that it is a unique form of sarcoma best distinguished from other types of fibrosarcoma. We currently prefer to continue to classify this unusual neoplasm as a variant of fibrosarcoma.

#### *Clinical Findings*

Most patients present with a deep-seated mass that is painful in up to one-third of cases. The age range is wide, with a median age of approximately 45 years; the tumor is slightly more common in males.[48] The most common location is the deep soft tissues of the lower extremity or limb girdle followed by the trunk, upper extremities and limb girdle, and neck.

#### *Pathologic Findings*

Grossly, the tumor is usually well circumscribed and lobulated, bosselated, or multinodular; most are 5–10 cm in greatest diameter. Occasional tumors show cystic or myxoid change, and some have a gritty sensation upon sectioning owing to the presence of focal calcifications. Most arise within the skeletal muscles of the extremities, deep fascia, or periosteum; some invade adjacent bone or the deep subcutaneous tissue.

Although grossly well circumscribed, there is characteristically infiltration of the surrounding soft tissues. At low magnification, the tumor is hypocellular with extensive areas of densely hyalinized stroma (Fig. 12–11A). The neoplastic cells are predominantly epithelioid in appearance and are arranged in a variety of patterns, including nests, cords, strands, and occasionally acinar or alveolar patterns. The cells have oval to round angulated nuclei with finely stippled or vesicular chromatin, small basophilic nucleoli, and scanty cleared-out or faintly eosinophilic cytoplasm (Fig. 12–11B). Mitotic figures are generally in-

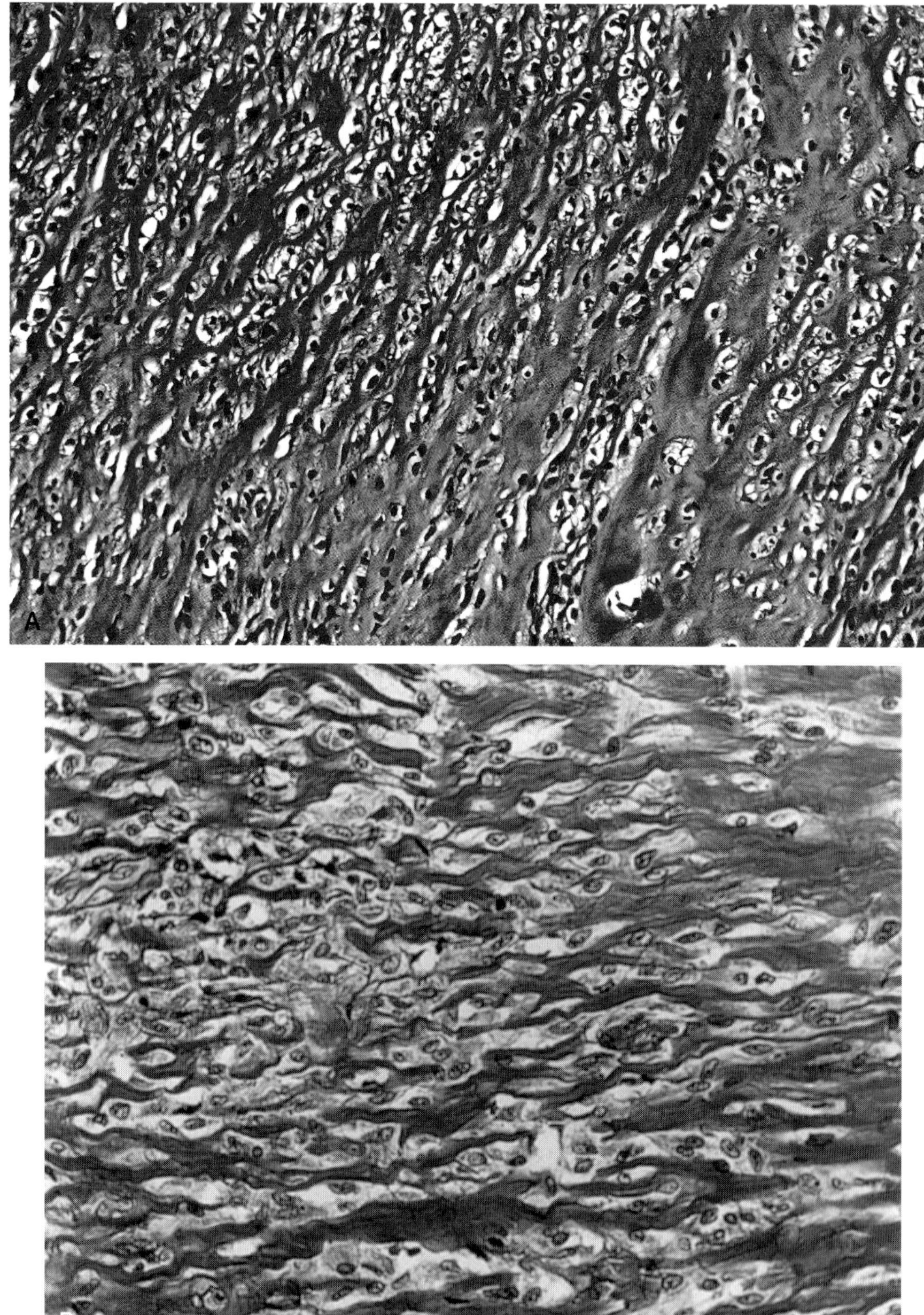


**FIGURE 12–11.** (**A**) Sclerosing epithelioid fibrosarcoma characterized by abundant hyalinized collagen between small, rounded tumor cells with clear cytoplasm. (**B**) Another example of sclerosing epithelioid fibrosarcoma.

conspicuous, but occasional tumors are characterized by a high mitotic rate (more than 5 mitoses per 10 HPF). The stroma is composed predominantly of deeply acidophilic collagen, which in some foci nearly completely obliterates the neoplastic cells resulting in paucicellular occasionally calcified zones. Myxoid areas and foci exhibiting chondroosseous differentiation may be present. In some portions of the tumor, branching vessels that are frequently hyalinized and organized in a hemangiopericytoma-like pattern are present. Peripherally located cleft-like spaces filled with tumor, suggesting true angiolymphatic invasion, may be seen. In almost all cases the tumor shows foci of spindle-shaped sarcoma similar to conventional fibrosarcoma.

### *Immunohistochemical and Electron Microscopic Findings*

As seen by immunohistochemistry, almost all tumors stain strongly and diffusely for vimentin. Up to one-half have a membranous pattern of immunoreactivity using antibodies to epithelial membrane antigen, contributing to confusion with carcinoma, epithelioid sarcoma, and synovial sarcoma. In addition, neural markers including S-100 protein and neuron-specific enolase are positive in a small number of cases, making distinction from a malignant peripheral nerve sheath tumor difficult. Stains for desmin, smooth muscle actin, HMB-45, CD68, and leukocyte common antigen are negative.

Ultrastructural analysis can be helpful in tumors without conventional fibrosarcoma and in those for which the immunohistochemical results are confounding. The neoplastic cells have the features of fibroblasts and myofibroblasts, with abundant rough endoplasmic reticulum, usually arranged in parallel arrays, and often dilated and filled with granular or fibrillar material.[48,60] Intermediate filaments, sometimes arranged in perinuclear whorls, are present. Intracytoplasmic collagen may be seen, and most cells contain particulate glycogen. The tumor cells are intimately associated with dense bundles or irregular whorls of stromal collagen.

### *Differential Diagnosis*

The differential diagnosis includes a wide range of both benign and malignant lesions composed, at least in part, of epithelioid cells. In the series by Meis-Kindblom et al.,[48] many of the cases were submitted in consultation with a diagnosis of a benign lesion, including nodular fasciitis, fibrous histiocytoma, myositis ossificans, hyalinized leiomyoma, or desmoid tumor, perhaps accounting for the large number of cases treated with inadequate surgical excision in that series.

The most difficult differential diagnostic considerations are other malignant neoplasms, particularly *infiltrating lobular carcinoma* and *infiltrating signet ring adenocarcinoma.* Distinction is made more difficult by the immunohistochemical expression of epithelial membrane antigen in up to one-half of cases of sclerosing epithelioid fibrosarcoma. Identification of conventional areas of fibrosarcoma and ultrastructural features indicative of fibroblastic or myofibroblastic differentiation allow this distinction. The absence of leukocyte common antigen is helpful for distinguishing this tumor from a *sclerosing lymphoma. Clear cell sarcoma* is characterized by a more uniform pattern of nested cells with vesicular nuclei and macronucleoli. Although S-100 protein is present in a few cases of sclerosing epithelioid fibrosarcoma, the absence of HMB-45 helps distinguish between these lesions. The more nested and cord-like areas of sclerosing epithelioid fibrosarcoma may resemble *ossifying fibromyxoid tumor of soft parts,* but the latter entity is characterized by a peripherally located incomplete shell of lamellar bone in most cases and is composed of cells of lower nuclear grade. *Synovial sarcoma,* particularly those with poorly differentiated areas, may be composed of round cells often arranged around a hemangiopericytoma-like vascular pattern, with the immunohistochemical expression of epithelial markers. All of these features are similar to those of sclerosing epithelioid fibrosarcoma, and thus the recognition of lower-grade biphasic or monophasic synovial sarcoma is useful for this distinction. Although only limited cytogenetic data have been reported on sclerosing epithelioid fibrosarcoma,[27] cytogenetic or molecular genetic identification of the t(X;18) characteristic of synovial sarcoma is helpful. Finally, distinguishing it from *malignant peripheral nerve sheath tumor* may be difficult, particularly because both tumors may express S-100 protein and neuron-specific enolase. Recognizing that it originated from a nerve or a surrounding benign peripheral nerve sheath tumor is useful in this regard. In equivocal cases, ultrastructural analysis may be the best way to arrive at a definitive diagnosis.

### *Discussion*

Comparing the clinical behavior of this variant of fibrosarcoma to conventional fibrosarcoma is difficult, particularly because fibrosarcoma has essentially become a diagnosis of exclusion. In the study by Meis-Kindblom et al.,[48] 8 of 15 (53%) patients in whom follow-up information was available developed local recurrence a median 4.8 years after diagnosis. Metastases, most commonly to the lungs, followed by the pleura/chest wall, bones, and brain, were detected in 43% of patients. Of the six patients with metastatic disease, four died and two were alive with pulmonary metastases 14 years after the initial diagnosis. Although the data are limited, patients with tumors on the trunk, those with large tumors, and those of male gender may have a worse prognosis. Wide surgical excision appears to be the mainstay of therapy, and long-term follow-up is indicated as some patients develop local recurrence or metastatic disease late in their course.

## Myxoid Type (Myxofibrosarcoma or Low-grade Myxoid Malignant Fibrous Histiocytoma)

The term *myxofibrosarcoma* was originally proposed by Angervall et al. to describe a group of fibroblastic lesions that show a spectrum of cellularity, nuclear pleomorphism, and mitotic activity ranging from a hypocellular lesion with minimal cytologic atypia to a more cellular lesion with features similar to those of pleomorphic-storiform malignant fibrous histiocytoma.[74] These tumors have been subdivided into three[78] or four[74,78] grades based on the degree of cellularity, nuclear pleomorphism, and mitotic activity. There is a continuum between low- and high-grade variants, as indicated by the presence of low-grade areas in high-grade lesions and a histologic progression of low-grade to high-grade tumors in recurrences.[74,75,78] Comparing data among these studies is somewhat difficult, as the proportion of myxoid areas in the tumor required for inclusion has varied. For example, all of the tumors reported by Merck et al.[79] and Angervall et al.[74] were "wholly, or almost wholly, myxomatous in appearance," whereas Mentzel et al.[78] required only 10% of the tumor to show prominent myxoid change to be included in their study. In their initial description of the *myxoid variant of malignant fibrous histiocytoma,* Weiss and Enzinger required at least 50% of the tumor to be composed of myxoid areas.[80] In our opinion, the term *myxofibrosarcoma* should be used only for tumors that are predominantly (>50%) myxoid and of low nuclear grade. Failure to adhere to these guidelines results in a heterogeneous group of lesions of variable biologic course that overlap considerably with malignant fibrous histiocytoma and its myxoid variant. The following discussion focuses on the low-grade tumors in the myxofibrosarcoma spectrum.

### Clinical Findings

The tumor most commonly arises as a slowly enlarging painless mass in the extremities of elderly patients. Although the age range is broad, most patients are in their fifth to seventh decades of life, and men and women are about equally affected. The most common site is the extremities, with a slight predilection for the lower extremities. The tumor is found less commonly on the trunk, head, and neck region and rarely in the retroperitoneum and pelvis.

### Pathologic Findings

The tumor typically is located in the subcutaneous tissue and is composed of multiple gelatinous nodules that have a tendency to spread in a longitudinal manner. In almost one-third of cases the tumor involves underlying skeletal muscle. Deep-seated lesions tend to be less nodular, demonstrate a more infiltrative growth pattern, and are usually larger than their superficial counterparts.[78]

Histologically, low magnification reveals a multinodular tumor of low cellularity (Fig. 12–12). The constituent cells are generally spindle or stellate-shaped and are deposited in a prominent myxoid matrix composed predominantly of hyaluronic acid. The cells have slightly eosinophilic cytoplasm and indistinct cell borders; the nuclei are hyperchromatic, are mildly pleomorphic, and have only rare mitotic figures (Fig. 12–13). Occasional tumor cells show cytoplasmic vacuolation, but true lipoblasts are not seen. Most tumors have elongated, curvilinear capillaries; there is a tendency for the tumor cells to align themselves along the vessel periphery.

Immunohistochemically, the cells stain strongly and diffusely for vimentin, although focal staining for muscle-specific actin and smooth muscle actin may be seen, indicative of myofibroblastic differentiation.[75,78] Electron microscopically, the cells are seen to have prominent, sometimes dilated rough endoplasmic reticulum, a well-developed Golgi apparatus, and moderate numbers of mitochondria.[76,77] Rare cells show myofibroblastic features, with intracytoplasmic bundles of microfilaments with focal densities. Some cells have prominent cytoplasmic vacuolation.

### Differential Diagnosis

The differential diagnosis includes myriad benign and malignant myxoid soft tissue neoplasms. In fact, tumors without a transition to higher-grade areas may be mistaken for a benign lesion. *Nodular fasciitis* is characterized by a proliferation of fibroblasts and myofibroblasts that lack nuclear hyperchromasia, although mitotic figures are often easily seen. Other features, such as the presence of slit-like spaces, extravasated erythrocytes, and keloid-like collagen, help distinguish nodular fasciitis from myxofibrosarcoma. *Myxoma* typically presents as a large, painless, fluctuant intramuscular mass composed of oval-shaped and

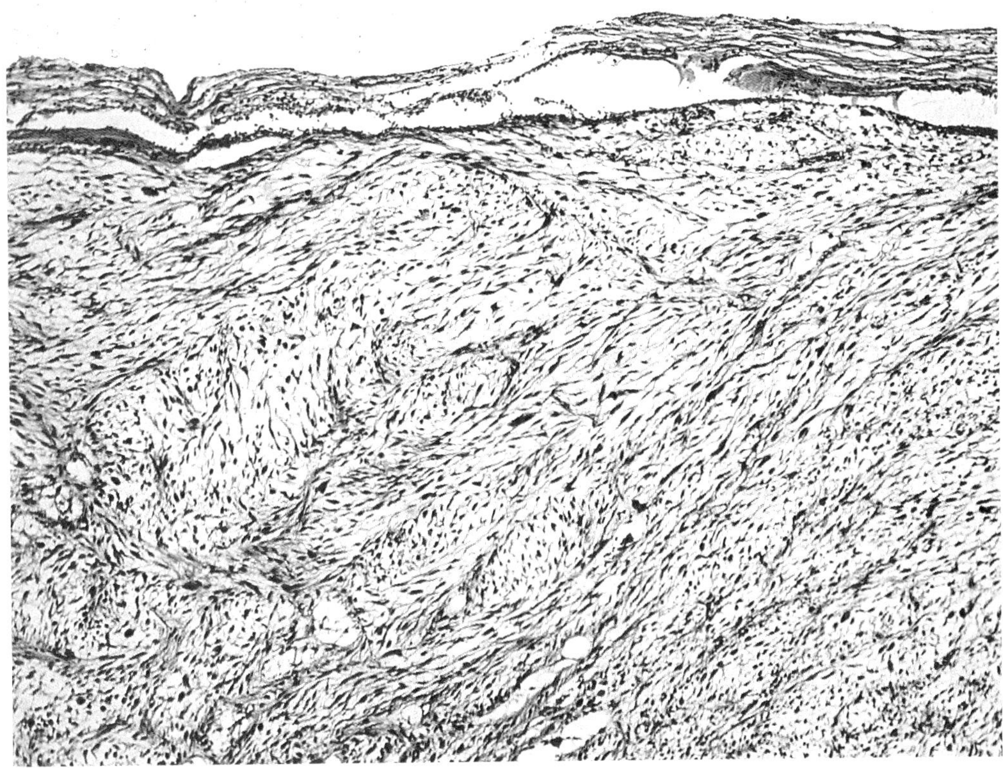

**FIGURE 12–12.** Myxofibrosarcoma. The spindle cells are minimally pleomorphic and separated by copious amounts of myxoid stroma.

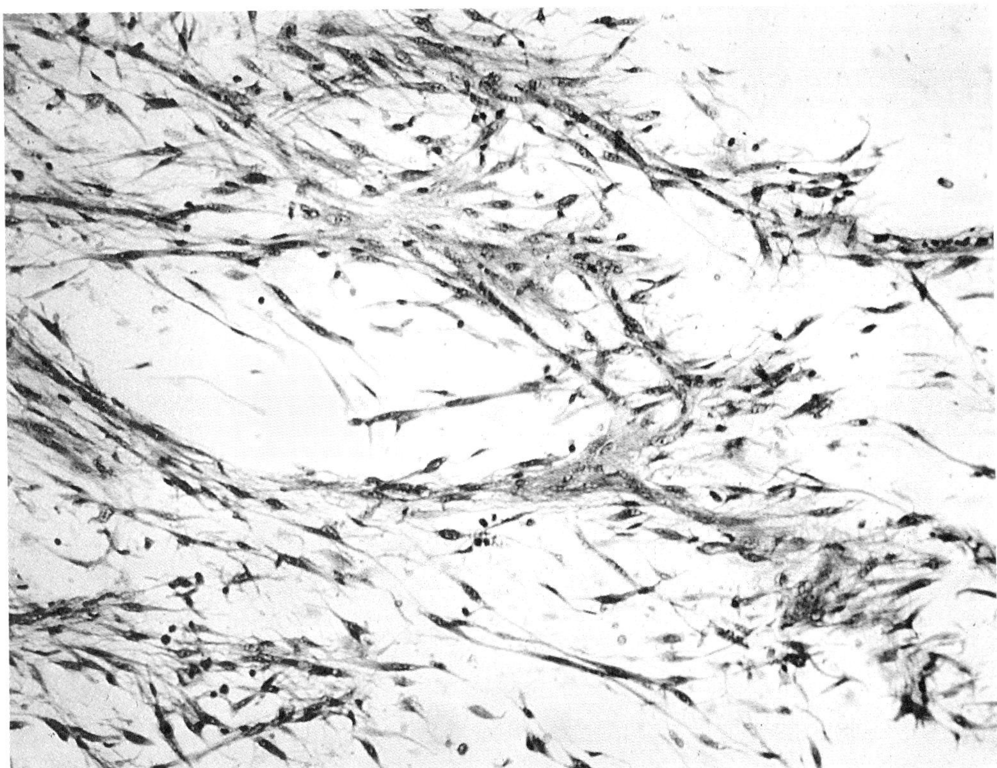

**FIGURE 12–13.** High-power view of myxofibrosarcoma. The spindle-shaped cells tend to arrange themselves around a curvilinear vasculature.

**TABLE 12–5 DISTINCTION OF LOW-GRADE FIBROMYXOID SARCOMA FROM MYXOFIBROSARCOMA**

| Feature | LGFMS | Myxofibrosarcoma |
|---|---|---|
| Peak age | Young to middle age | Elderly |
| Depth | Skeletal muscle | Subcutaneous tissue |
| Stroma | Alternating myxoid and fibrous | Usually uniformly myxoid |
| Atypia | Absent to minimal | More prominent |
| Metastasis | Up to 50% of cases | Rare |

LGFMS, low-grade fibromyxoid sarcoma.

stellate cells deposited in an abundant hyaluronic acid-rich myxoid matrix. Although the cellularity of a myxoma may be similar to that of myxofibrosarcoma, the cells show less atypia and mitotic activity. Furthermore, myxoma is hypovascular and lacks the curvilinear vessels characteristically found in myxofibrosarcoma. *Spindle cell lipoma* is a benign lipomatous tumor typically found in the subcutaneous tissue of the posterior neck, shoulder, or back region of elderly people, mostly men. The spindle cells lack cytologic atypia and mitotic activity, and they stain for CD34. Mature lipocytes and ropey collagen fibers are also characteristic of this lesion. *Nerve sheath myxoma* or *neurothekeoma* is typically a small, solitary, intradermal or subcutaneous multinodular tumor often located on the fingers. Although some show nuclear pleomorphism, most are composed of cells with less atypia than those found in myxofibrosarcoma; this tumor also lacks the curvilinear vessels found in the latter lesion. In addition, most of the myxoid variants of this tumor contain cells that stain for S-100 protein.

Myxofibrosarcoma must also be distinguished from other myxoid sarcomas that tend to be more clinically aggressive. *Myxoid liposarcoma* has less cytologic atypia; has a fine plexiform vascular pattern without perivascular tumor cell condensation, and contains scattered lipoblasts. Clinically, myxoid liposarcoma is almost always deep-seated and occurs predominantly in the thigh or popliteal fossa of middle-aged adults. *Extraskeletal myxoid chondrosarcoma* is a multinodular neoplasm composed of rounded cells arranged in strands and cords deposited in a chondroitin sulfate-rich myxoid stroma. These lesions tend to show prominent hemorrhage and lack the curvilinear vessels of myxofibrosarcoma.

Perhaps the most difficult distinction is from the more aggressive *low-grade fibromyxoid sarcoma* (Table 12–5). Clinically, this tumor occurs in young patients and has a tendency for multiple recurrences, with a risk of metastasis. Histologically, it is composed of cytologically bland spindle cells arranged in a whorled pattern and deposited in a variably myxoid and fibrous stroma. In contrast, myxofibrosarcoma is always predominantly myxoid, and the cells show more cytologic atypia than those found in low-grade fibromyxoid sarcoma.

### Discussion

The clinical behavior of myxofibrosarcoma appears to be closely related to the tumor grade. For example, Merck et al. found the risk of local recurrence to be 38%, 48%, 51%, and 61% for grade 1, 2, 3, and 4 tumors, respectively.[79] In contrast, in the study by Mentzel et al.,[78] the rate of local recurrence was independent of histologic grade, as 6 of 12 (50%) low-grade lesions recurred; one patient developed eight recurrences (Table 12–6). Two subcutaneous low-grade lesions recurred as higher-grade lesions with increased cellularity, nuclear pleomorphism, and mitotic activity. Thus it is clear that adequate initial surgical therapy is necessary to limit the rate of local

**TABLE 12–6 RELATION BETWEEN HISTOLOGIC GRADE AND RATE OF LOCAL RECURRENCE FOR MYXOFIBROSARCOMA**

| | Local Recurrence | | | |
|---|---|---|---|---|
| **Study** | **Grade 1** | **Grade 2** | **Grade 3** | **Grade 4** |
| Mentzel et al.[78]* | 6/12 (50%) | 9/13 (69%) | 18/33 (55%) | — |
| Angervall et al.[74] | 0/2 | 2/7 (29%) | 6/10 (60%) | 7/11 (64%) |
| Merck et al.[79] | 3/8 (38%) | 13/27 (48%) | 21/41 (51%) | 17/28 (61%) |

* Used only a three-grade scale.

**TABLE 12–7 RELATION BETWEEN HISTOLOGIC GRADE AND RATE OF METASTASIS FOR MYXOFIBROSARCOMA**

| | Metastasis | | | |
|---|---|---|---|---|
| ***Study*** | ***Grade 1*** | ***Grade 2*** | ***Grade 3*** | ***Grade 4*** |
| Mentzel et al.[78]* | 0/12 | 5/13 (38%) | 10/34 (29%) | — |
| Angervall et al.[74] | 0/2 | 2/7 (29%) | 2/11 (18%) | 3/11 (27%) |
| Merck et al.[79] | 0/8 | 6/28 (21%) | 21/45 (47%) | 11/29 (38%) |

* Used only a three-grade scale.

recurrence and the subsequent risk of histologic progression. The risk of metastasis is minimal for pure low-grade tumors. In the study by Merck et al.,[79] although 35% of patients developed metastases none of the eight patients with grade 1 tumors did so. Similarly, Angervall et al.[74] found that no patient with a grade 1 tumor developed metastatic disease, although two of seven patients with grade 2 tumors eventually did so. (Tables 12–7, 12–8).

## Fibromyxoid Type (Low-grade Fibromyxoid Sarcoma)

The low-grade fibromyxoid sarcoma was first recognized by Evans in 1987, when he reported bland fibromyxoid neoplasms arising in the deep soft tissue of two young women.[83] Although initially diagnosed as benign, both tumors eventually metastasized; subsequent reports have verified the metastatic potential of this histologically deceptive neoplasm. Although fewer than 35 cases had been reported as of 1998, low-grade fibromyxoid sarcoma is probably more common than the literature would lead one to believe, as some have undoubtedly been diagnosed as myxofibrosarcoma, low-grade myxoid sarcoma, not otherwise specified, or a variety of other benign or malignant fibrous or myxoid neoplasms.

### *Clinical Findings*

Most patients are young to middle-aged adults, but this tumor may arise in patients as young as 3 years and as old as 78 years.[85] Males are affected more commonly than females. The usual presentation is that of a slowly growing, painless, deep soft tissue mass that ranges from 1 to 18 cm in greatest diameter, although most are 8–10 cm. The tumor most commonly arises in the deep soft tissue of the lower extremities, particularly the thigh, followed, in decreasing order of frequency, by the chest wall/axilla, shoulder region, inguinal region, buttock, and neck. Rare cases have also been described in unusual sites including the retroperitoneum[87] and small bowel mesentery.[84]

**TABLE 12–8 RATES OF LOCAL RECURRENCE AND METASTASIS FOR GRADE 1 (LOW-GRADE) MYXOFIBROSARCOMA**

| Study | Recurrence | Metastasis |
|---|---|---|
| Mentzel et al.[78] | 6/12 (50%) | 0/12 |
| Angervall et al.[74]* | 0/2 | 0/2 |
| Merck et al.[79]* | 3/8 (38%) | 0/8 |

* Used a four-grade scale; data include only tumors designated grade 1.

### *Gross Findings*

Most tumors arise in the skeletal muscle, although some appear to be centered in the subcutaneous tissue, with minimal or no muscle involvement. Although the tumor is grossly well circumscribed, there is often extensive microscopic infiltration into the surrounding soft tissues. On cut section, the tumor has a yellow-white appearance with focal areas with a glistening appearance secondary to the accumulation of myxoid ground substance. Neither necrosis nor hemorrhage is present.

### *Microscopic Findings*

Characteristically, this tumor is of low or moderate cellularity composed of bland spindle-shaped cells with small hyperchromatic oval nuclei, finely clumped chromatin, and one to several small nucleoli. The cells have indistinct pale eosinophilic cytoplasm and show only mild nuclear pleomorphism with little mitotic activity. The cells are deposited in a variably fibrous and myxoid stroma that tends to alternate in different areas of the tumor (Figs. 12–14, 12–15, 12–16). In general, the lesions appear more fibrous than myxoid. The myxoid zones may abut abruptly with the fibrous zones, or there may be a gradual transition between these areas. Cells with a stellate configuration are often present in the myxoid zones, and the cells are generally arranged in a whorled or random

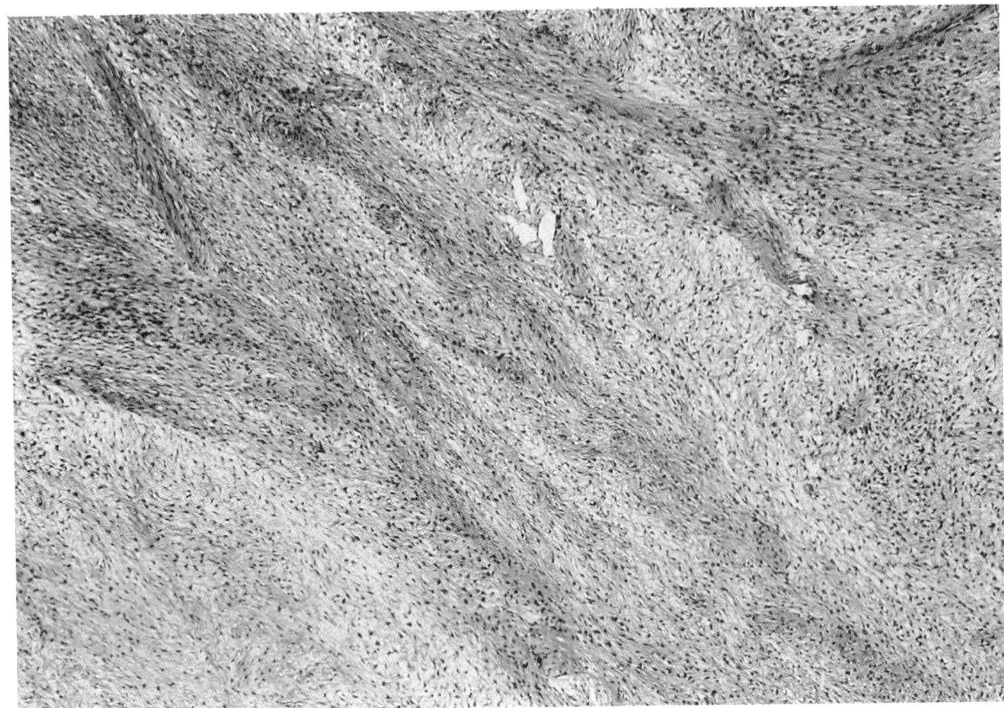

**FIGURE 12–14.** Low-grade fibromyxoid sarcoma. At low power, alternating areas with a fibrous and myxoid stroma are apparent.

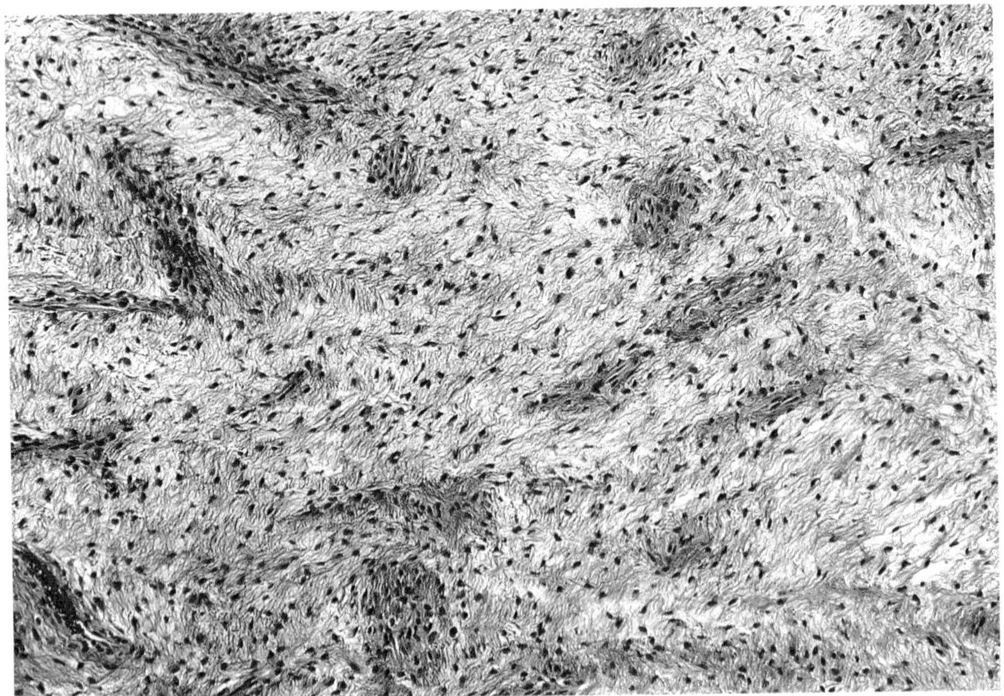

**FIGURE 12–15.** Low-grade fibromyxoid sarcoma with alternating fibrous and myxoid areas. The cells commonly show a whorled pattern of growth.

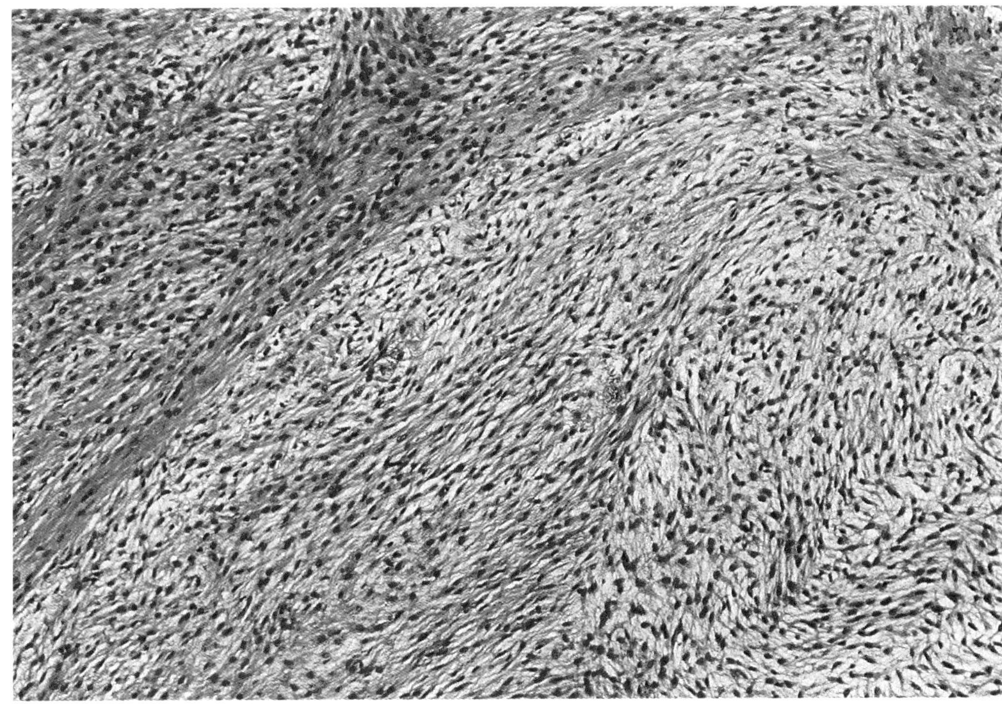

**FIGURE 12–16.** Junction between fibrous and myxoid zones in low-grade fibromyxoid sarcoma.

fashion (Figs. 12–17, 12–18). There is often a prominent network of curvilinear and branching capillary-size blood vessels in the myxoid zones, somewhat reminiscent of that seen in myxoid liposarcoma (Fig. 12–19),[84,87] sometimes with perivascular hypercellularity. The stroma stains with alcian blue, which is completely removed by pretreatment with hyaluronidase.[89,91] Epithelioid cells may also be present focally, and there are areas of intermediate-grade fibrosarcoma in about 15–20% of cases.[85]

Although this neoplasm is characterized by a deceptively bland appearance, recurrences may show areas of increased cellularity and mitotic activity, sometimes with the formation of hypercellular nodules (Figs. 12–20, 12–21).[82,87] Transition to a high-grade sarcoma resembling malignant fibrous histiocytoma has not been described, but Evans reported one case that "dedifferentiated" into a neoplasm composed of sheets of anaplastic round cells 30 years after the initial excision.[84] In most cases, recurrences and metastases resemble the primary lesions, although we have seen a case in which the metastasis had a predominantly primitive round-cell appearance.

### Immunohistochemical and Electron Microscopic Findings

Immunohistochemically, the neoplastic cells stain strongly and diffusely for vimentin. Focal immunoreactivity for muscle markers including smooth muscle actin and muscle-specific actin may be present, suggesting myofibroblastic differentiation in at least some of the cells. Rare cases show focal staining for desmin and cytokeratins. Although CD34 was not detected in the nine cases cited by Goodlad et al.,[87] Nichols and Cooper reported one case with diffuse CD34 staining.[89]

Ultrastructurally, the neoplastic cells are spindle-shaped with delicate and irregular cytoplasmic processes. The cytoplasm is rich in rough endoplasmic reticulum and has a well-developed Golgi apparatus. Intracytoplasmic intermediate-sized filaments are conspicuous, as are pinocytotic vesicles, but basal lamina-like material is not seen.[81,86,88,90,91a]

### Differential Diagnosis

The differential diagnosis of low-grade fibromyxoid sarcoma includes numerous benign and malignant soft tissue lesions characterized by a variably fibrous and myxoid stroma. *Myxoid neurofibroma* is composed of cells with more slender and wavy nuclei that consistently express S-100 protein. *Perineurioma* may resemble the fibrous whorled areas seen in low-grade fibromyxoid sarcoma, but the immunohistochemical detection of epithelial membrane antigen allows its distinction. Some areas of low-grade fibromyxoid sarcoma may resemble *nodular fasciitis,* but the latter le-

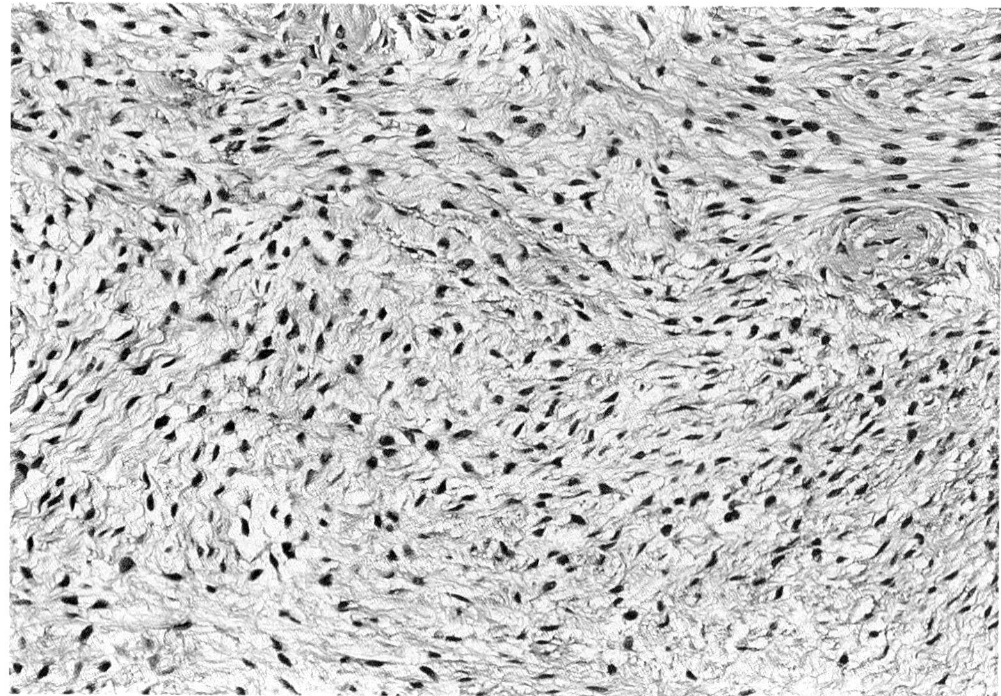

**FIGURE 12–17.** Myxoid zone of low-grade fibromyxoid sarcoma. The lesion is of low cellularity and composed of bland spindle-shaped cells.

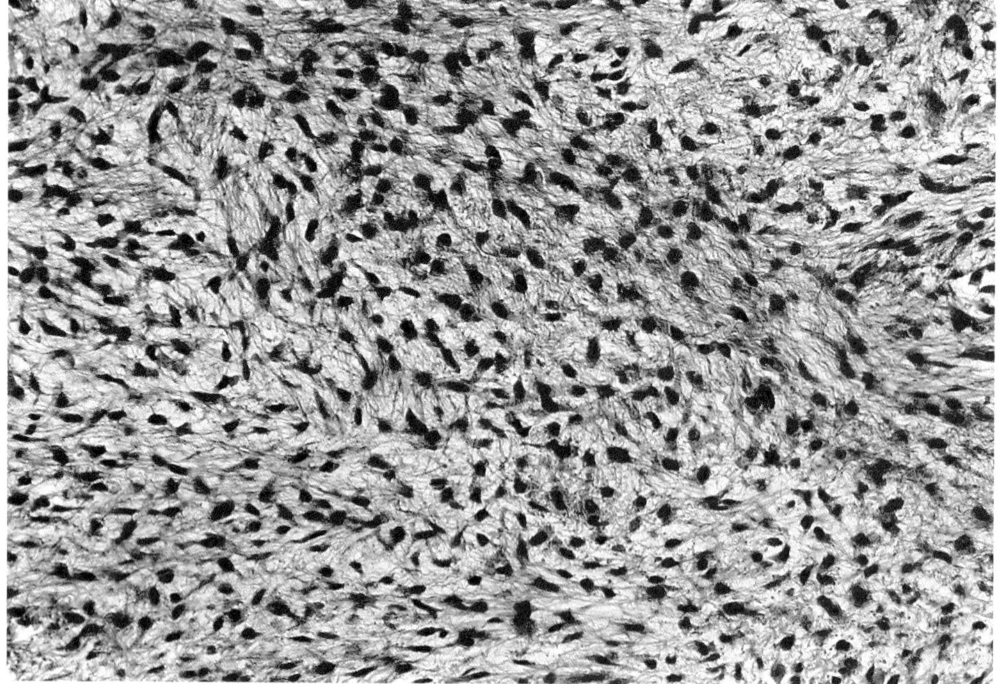

**FIGURE 12–18.** More cellular area of a low-grade fibromyxoid sarcoma. The cells have a stellate appearance and are evenly distributed within a fibromyxoid stroma.

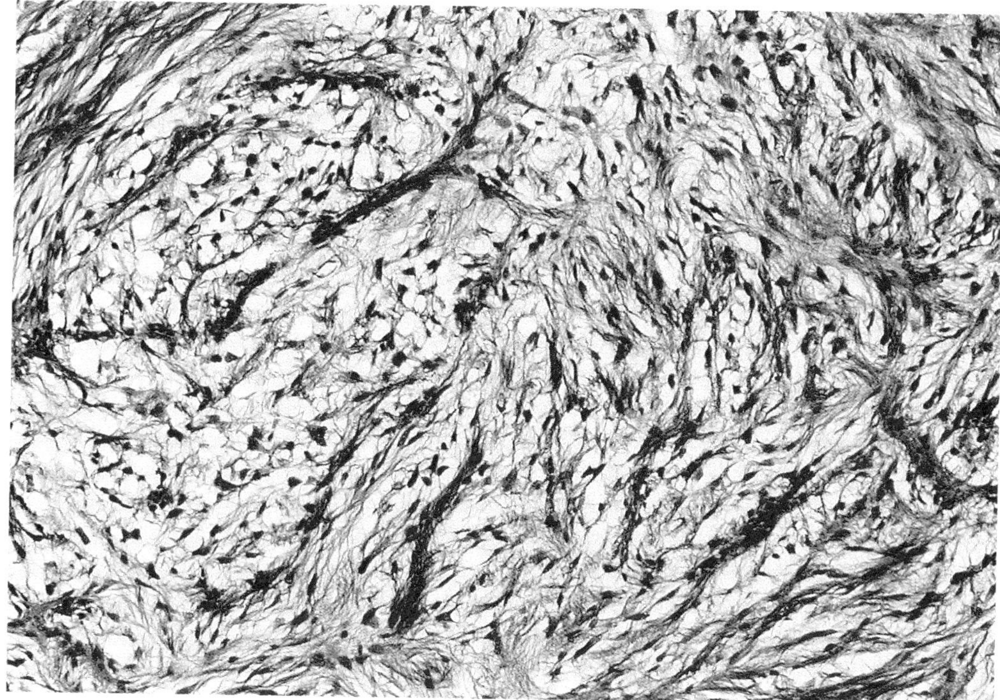

**FIGURE 12–19.** Low-grade fibromyxoid sarcoma showing a prominent network of branching capillary-sized blood vessels reminiscent of myxoid liposarcoma.

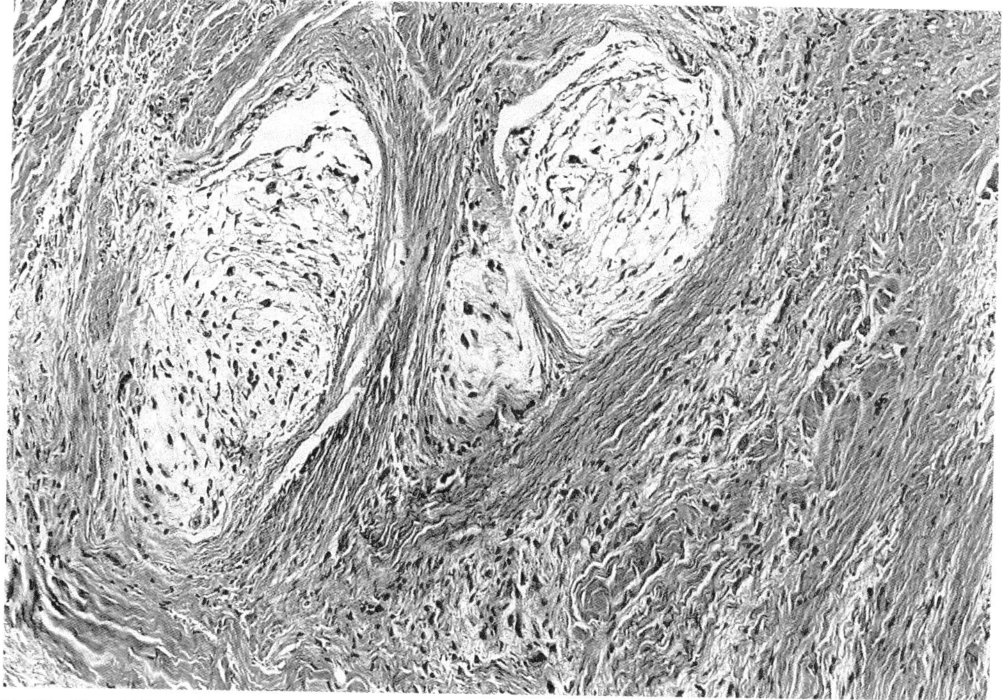

**FIGURE 12–20.** Although grossly well circumscribed, low-grade fibromyxoid sarcoma often shows microscopic infiltration of the surrounding soft tissues by small myxoid nodules.

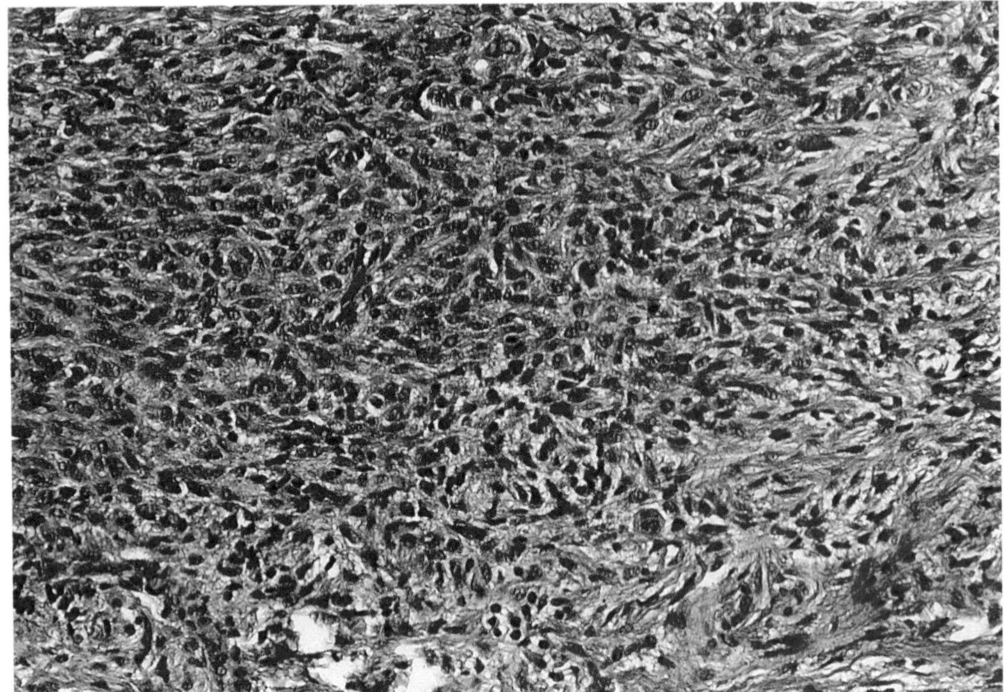

**FIGURE 12–21.** Recurrent low-grade fibromyxoid sarcoma showing an area of increased cellularity and nuclear pleomorphism.

sion is characterized by cells that resemble tissue culture fibroblasts. Other features of fasciitis, such as cleft-like spaces, extravasation of erythrocytes, and the presence of multinucleated giant cells, are not found in low-grade fibromyxoid sarcoma. *Desmoid fibromatoses* are composed of nuclei that tend to be plumper and more vesicular and are arranged in a fascicular growth pattern. The *myxoid variant of dermatofibrosarcoma protuberans* may resemble the myxoid zones of low-grade fibromyxoid sarcoma, but this lesion tends to be more superficial, predominantly involving the dermis and subcutaneous tissue; moreover, the cells are arranged in a more uniform storiform growth pattern with diffuse staining for CD34.

*Malignant peripheral nerve sheath tumors* may contain myxoid foci, but the cells are more elongated or wavy, are typically arranged in an irregular fascicular growth pattern, and stain for S-100 protein in up to 60% of cases. In addition, ultrastructural analysis reveals evidence of schwannian differentiation. *Spindle cell liposarcoma* usually arises in the subcutaneous tissue of adults and always contains an atypical lipomatous component that includes the presence of lipoblasts. The myxoid zones of low-grade fibromyxoid sarcoma may also resemble *myxoid liposarcoma*, particularly the cases with a well-developed plexiform vascular pattern. However, low-grade fibromyxoid sarcoma lacks lipoblasts, and adequate sampling always reveals fibrous areas. Cytogenetically, myxoid liposarcoma is characterized by t(12;16)(q13;p11), which is not present in low-grade fibromyxoid sarcoma.[81]

The lesion with which low-grade fibromyxoid sarcoma is most easily confused is *myxofibrosarcoma* (Table 12–5), a lesion at the lower end of the spectrum that overlaps with myxoid malignant fibrous histiocytoma. Unlike low-grade fibromyxoid sarcoma, which typically arises in the skeletal muscle of young patients, myxofibrosarcoma commonly arises in the subcutaneous tissues of the extremities of elderly patients. Histologically, myxofibrosarcoma is uniformly myxoid, lacks alternating fibrous zones, and always has a greater degree of nuclear pleomorphism and hyperchromasia. The distinction between these two entities is of clinical importance, as myxofibrosarcoma rarely metastasizes, in contrast to low-grade fibromyxoid sarcoma.

### Discussion

Despite its deceptively bland histologic appearance, low-grade fibromyxoid sarcoma is characterized by a high rate of local, often repeated recurrence and by pulmonary metastases in a significant percentage of cases. Approximately 65% of cases reported in the literature have recurred locally 6 months to 50 years after the initial excision, with most patients developing multiple recurrences. Evans reported one case in which the patient developed 17 recurrences over a period of 29 years.[84] Metastases may be present at the time of initial excision or may develop late in the clinical course. Evans described one case that metastasized 45 years after the initial presentation.[84] The lung has been involved in all cases with metastatic disease. Thus far, fewer than 20% of patients have died as a direct result of their tumor, and most patients have a protracted, indolent course, with some surviving 10–15 years after detection of metastases.[84,87] Folpe et al.[85] reported follow-up data on 43 patients (median follow-up 24 months), only two of whom (5%) developed metastases. Importantly, most of these patients had been treated by wide excision with tumor-free margins either on initial excision or at the first reexcision. Given the small number of patients treated with chemotherapy or radiotherapy, the effects of these adjuvant therapies remain unknown.

## Fibromyxoid Type (Hyalinizing Spindle Cell Tumor) with Giant Rosettes

Hyalinizing spindle cell tumor with giant rosettes is an unusual fibrous tumor of deep soft tissues that was first delineated in 1997 by Lane et al.[95] in 19 cases. Virtually all reported cases have behaved in an indolent fashion,[99] although rare examples exhibit aggressive clinical behavior. There is significant histologic overlap with low-grade fibromyxoid sarcoma, and we believe this tumor represents a variant of the latter.

### *Clinical Findings*

Most patients are in their third or fourth decade of life, and men are affected twice as often as women. The most common presenting symptom is a painless, deep-seated, slowly enlarging mass that may be present months to years prior to presentation. The tumor may arise at a variety of locations but is most common in the extremities, particularly the thigh. Other sites of involvement are the chest wall, axilla, buttock, and neck.

### *Pathologic Findings*

Grossly, the tumor is an oval, multilobulated mass that ranges from 2 to 20 cm in greatest diameter, although most are 5–10 cm. Typically, the lesion is well circumscribed and surrounded by a thin, fibrous pseudocapsule. The cut surface has a whorled white-tan appearance; it may exhibit cystic degeneration but no necrosis.

Despite the gross circumscription, most tumors extensively infiltrate the surrounding soft tissues. Aside from the presence of the characteristic rosettes, the stroma of this neoplasm is virtually identical to that of low-grade fibromyxoid sarcoma. The tumor is characterized by spindle-shaped cells arranged into a variety of patterns and deposited in a densely hyalinized stroma punctuated by large collagen rosettes (Figs. 12–22, 12–23, 12–24). Cellularity varies from case to case and in different areas of the same tumor. In most areas, the cells are arranged in irregular crisscrossing fascicles separated by moderate amounts of collagen (Fig. 12–25), often with a "cracking" artifact around the elongated fibroblastic cells. In some areas there is extensive stromal hyalinization with a paucity of neoplastic cells, whereas in others the cells are deposited in a myxoid stroma that may have a delicate arborizing vasculature (Figs. 12–26, 12–27). The tumor cells have irregular or wavy nuclei with a mild degree of nuclear atypia. Mitotic figures are difficult to find, usually with fewer than one mitosis per 50 HPF. Like ordinary fibromyxoid sarcoma, areas of an intermediate-grade fibrosarcoma may be present.

The most characteristic feature is the presence of a variable number of large rosette-like structures that merge abruptly or imperceptibly with the surrounding hyalinized or spindled stroma. The rosettes, which tend to cluster together, are composed of a central core of brightly eosinophilic birefringent collagen arranged centrifugally from the center surrounded by rounded to ovoid cells that have clear to eosinophilic cytoplasm and little to no nuclear atypia or mitotic activity. Occasional cells show intranuclear cytoplasmic inclusions (Fig. 12–28). Other features include the presence of hemosiderin deposition, cystic degeneration, calcification, and osseous and chondroid metaplasia.[98] Immunohistochemically, both the spindle-shaped and ovoid cells comprising the rosettes stain strongly for vimentin. S-100 protein, Leu-7, and neuron-specific enolase are frequently present in the rounded cells but are less often identified in the spindle-shaped cells.[95–97] Electron microscopically, the neoplastic cells are characterized by irregular nuclei with clumped chromatin and occasional nucleoli. The cytoplasm contains intermediate filaments and numerous, often markedly dilated rough endoplasmic reticulum; the cells are surrounded by abundant extracellular matrix consisting of banded collagen fibers.[92,98,99] Although Nielsen et al.[98] noted that the cells surrounding the collagen rosettes exhibited ultrastructural features similar to those of the spindle-shaped cells, de Pinieux et al.[92] found that the rounded cells surrounding the collagen rosettes had schwannian features.

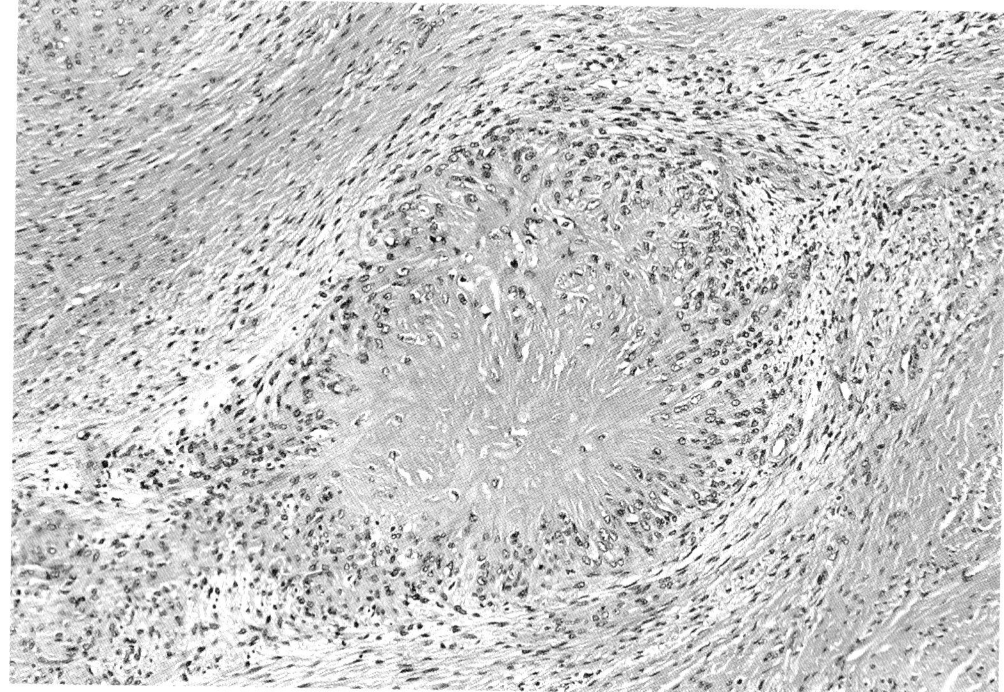

**FIGURE 12–22.** Hyalinizing spindle cell tumor with giant rosettes. The most characteristic feature is the presence of large collagen rosettes.

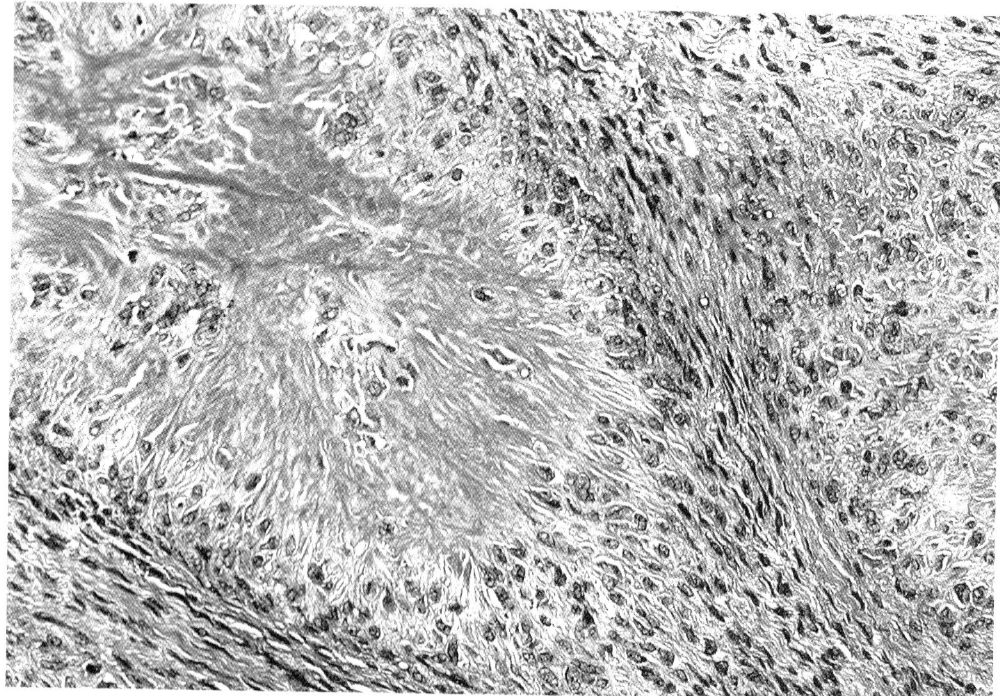

**FIGURE 12–23.** Trichrome stain of collagen rosette in a case of hyalinizing spindle cell tumor demonstrating that the central eosinophilic portion of the rosette is composed of collagen.

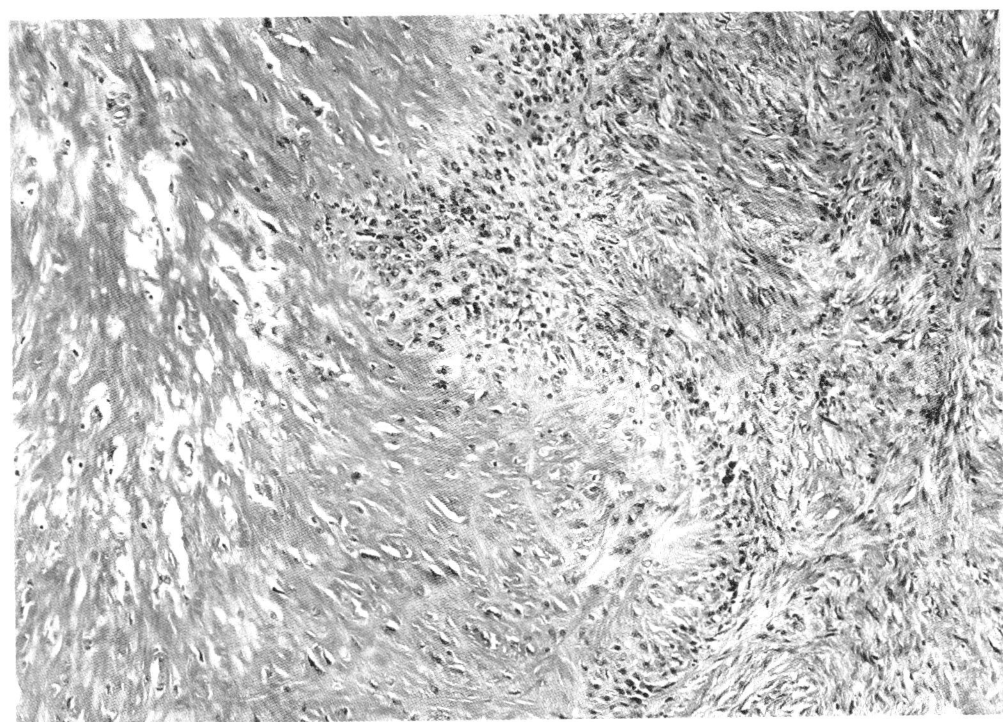

**FIGURE 12–24.** Hyalinizing spindle cell tumor with giant rosettes showing transition between a collagen rosette and a more cellular fibrosarcoma-like area.

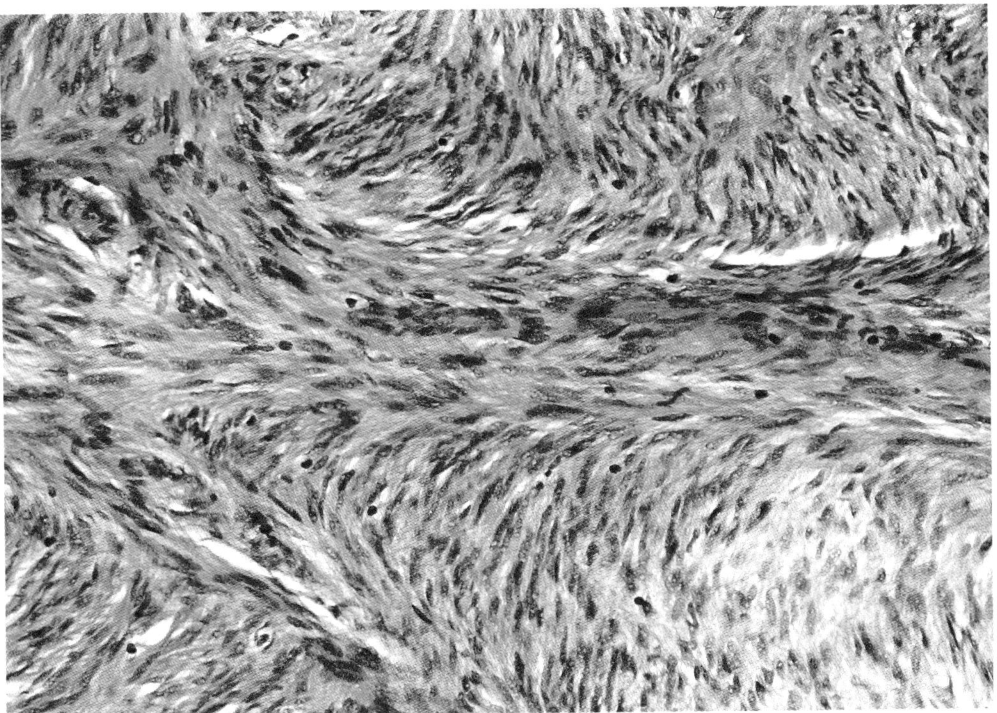

**FIGURE 12–25.** Fibrosarcoma-like area in a case of hyalinizing spindle cell tumor with giant rosettes. The cells are arranged into irregular crisscrossing fascicles.

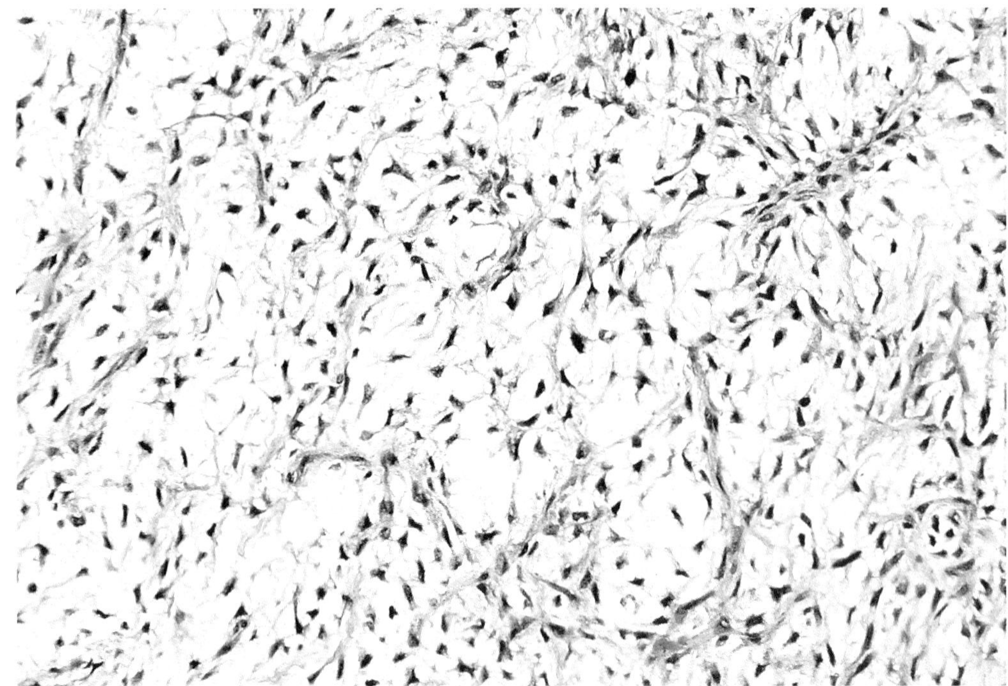

**FIGURE 12–26.** Myxoid zone of hyalinizing spindle cell tumor with giant rosettes. The neoplastic cells are widely separated by myxoid stroma, and a plexiform vasculature is apparent.

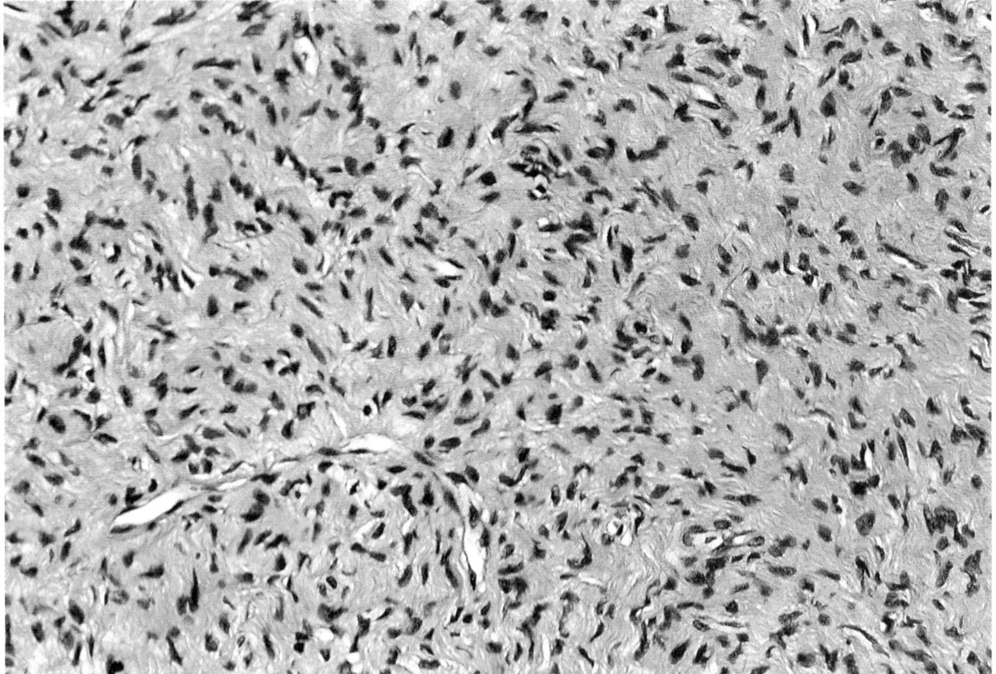

**FIGURE 12–27.** Hyalinizing spindle cell tumor with giant rosettes. Spindled stroma shows greater cellularity than in Figure 12–26. Cells have an irregular wavy shape somewhat reminiscent of cells in neurofibroma.

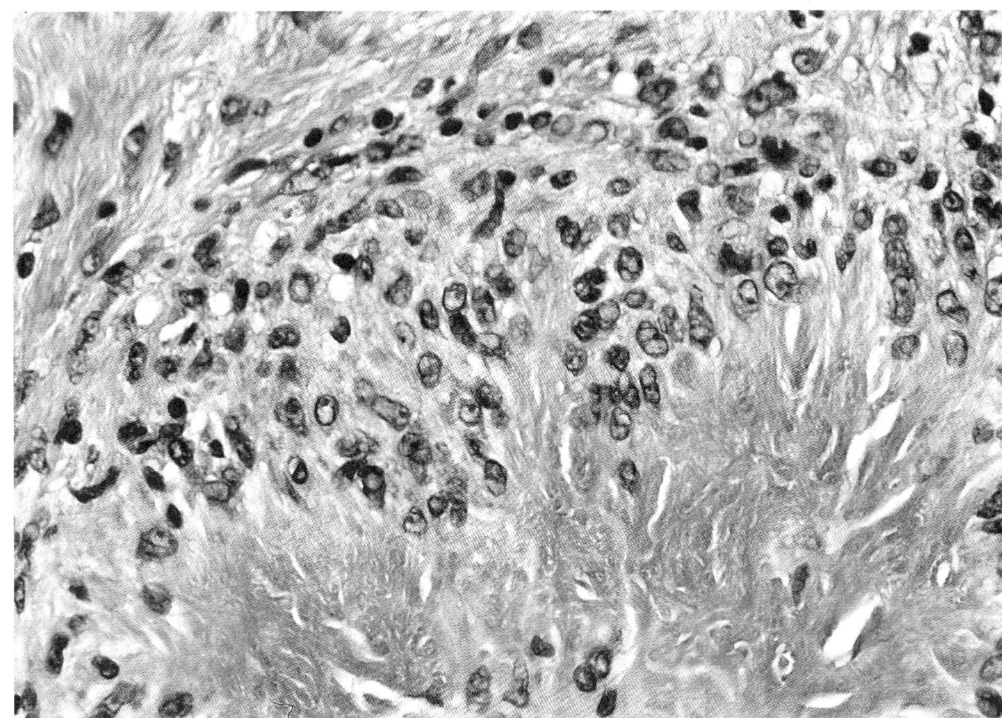

**FIGURE 12–28.** Rounded cells comprising the periphery of a rosette in a case of hyalinizing spindle cell tumor with giant rosettes. A few of the cells have intranuclear cytoplasmic inclusions.

### *Differential Diagnosis*

Similar appearing giant collagen-containing rosettes may be seen in other mesenchymal tumors, including *neuroblastoma-like neurilemmoma,* in which the rosettes are made up of a core of collagen flanked by small, rounded, differentiated Schwann cells.[93] Rare cases of *osteosarcoma* have been reported to contain similar rosettes, but in these cases the central core is composed of an osteoid-like material, often with central calcification, and surrounded by cells with more nuclear pleomorphism than those encountered in the hyalinizing spindle cell tumor.[94] The spindle-shaped areas may also resemble *fibromatosis,* but the latter lesion is characterized by more uniform cellularity with arrangement into a distinct fascicular growth pattern and an absence of rosette-like structures.

### *Discussion*

Although originally considered a distinctive entity, these lesions are now regarded as fibromyxoid sarcomas with rosettes. The reasons for believing them to be the same are as follows: similarity in age and location, virtual identity of the spindled stroma (Fig. 12–29) including the occasional presence of intermediate-grade fibrosarcoma, and the ability of this lesion to metastasize like low-grade fibromyxoid sarcoma.

In the original report by Lane et al.,[95] follow-up information was available for 12 of the 19 patients, with a mean follow-up of 39 months. Of the 12 patients, 7 were treated by simple local excision and 5 by wide excision. Although one of the patients treated by simple excision developed a local recurrence 20 months after the initial surgery, none of the remaining patients developed recurrent or metastatic disease within the follow-up period. Woodruff et al.,[99] however, reported a tumor that arose in the arm of a 28-year-old woman that had the typical features of hyalinizing spindle cell tumor with giant rosettes; it ultimately metastasized to the lung 4 years after presentation. Farinha et al.[92a] reported a patient with prolonged survival following detection of pulmonary metastases from an 11 cm thigh mass. We too have reviewed a case in consultation that produced metastasis 8 years after the initial resection. Therefore this lesion is best considered a low-grade sarcoma, and wide surgical excision is the treatment of choice.

## FIBROSARCOMATOUS CHANGE ARISING IN DERMATOFIBROSARCOMA PROTUBERANS

A small number of cases of dermatofibrosarcoma protuberans show areas with increased cellularity, cells with increased nuclear pleomorphism and mitotic ac-

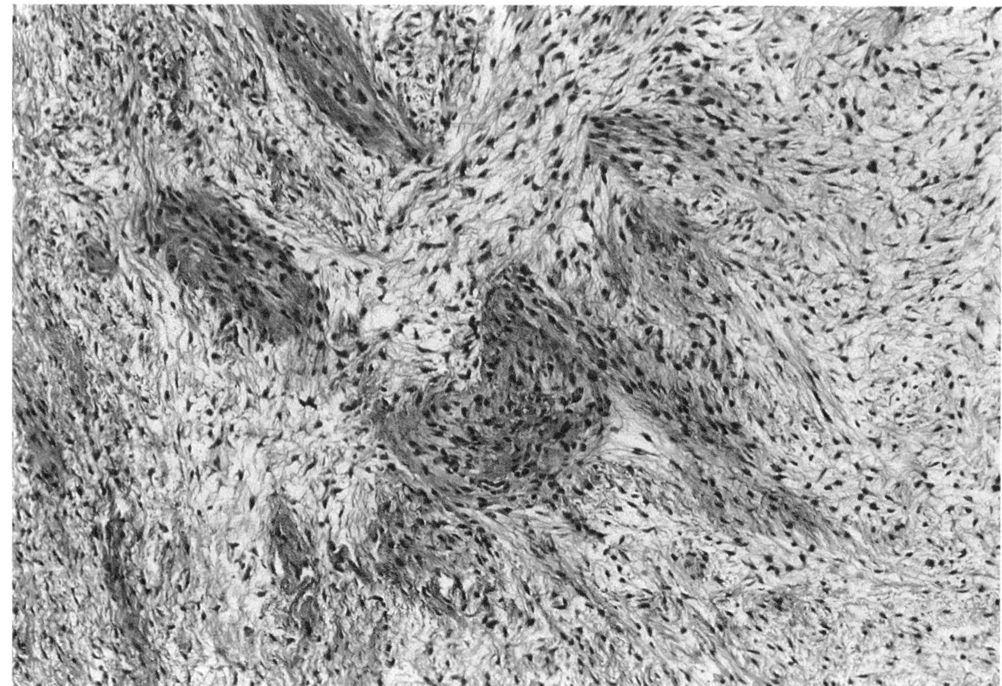

**FIGURE 12–29.** Alternating fibrous and myxoid zones in a hyalinizing spindle cell tumor with giant rosettes. Such zones are reminiscent of low-grade fibromyxoid sarcoma.

tivity, and arrangement in a fascicular growth pattern resembling conventional soft tissue fibrosarcoma. The significance of fibrosarcomatous change in dermatofibrosarcoma protuberans is discussed in greater detail in Chapter 14.

## POSTRADIATION FIBROSARCOMA

Although malignant fibrous histiocytoma is by far the most common postradiation sarcoma, there is clearly a higher incidence of fibrosarcoma in patients who have been exposed to radiation than in the general population. There are numerous reports in which a fibrosarcoma or fibrosarcoma-like tumor originated at the site of therapeutic irradiation for various benign[29,38,45] and malignant[3,5,6,11,15,65,72,73] neoplasms and for nonneoplastic disorders such as psoriasis and hypertrichosis.[68]

The latency period between irradiation and tumor development is of significance when evaluating these cases. The tumor usually develops 4–15 years following irradiation, although periods as short as 15 months have been reported.[2] Tumors appearing less than 2 years following irradiation are unlikely to be radiation-induced. Opinions vary as to the significance of the radiation dose for tumor development, and both small and large doses have been implicated as being more likely to produce radiation-related neoplasms. In general, the prognosis for patients developing postradiation fibrosarcoma is poor, as most patients die within 2 years of the development of the tumor. Ito et al.[33] implicated rearrangements of the *RET* oncogene in the development of postradiation fibrosarcoma.

## FIBROSARCOMA ARISING IN BURN SCARS

Although less common than postradiation fibrosarcoma, there are rare cases of fibrosarcoma arising in scars formed at sites of thermal injury. Nearly all of the affected patients have suffered extensive burns as children and developed tumors after an interval of 30 years or more.[55] For example, Fleming and Rezek reported a patient who had fallen into a bonfire at age 5 and developed a fibrosarcoma at age 54.[22] Similarly, Pack and Ariel described a 53-year-old man who developed a fibrosarcoma arising in a burn scar suffered at age 6.[56] Wilson and Brunschwig described an unusual case of a 15-year-old girl who developed a fibrosarcoma only 5 years after an extensive burn involving the right neck and cheek and after irradiation of the resulting cicatricial contractures and keloids.[73] Carcinomas are more common than sarcomas as a late sequence of thermal injury (Marjolin's ulcer) and usually develop after a 30- to 40-year latent period.[26] Thus immunohistochemical analysis with cytokeratins, including high-molecular-weight cytokeratins, is useful for excluding the possibility of a desmoplastic or spindle cell carcinoma before rendering a diagnosis of fibrosarcoma arising in a burn scar.

## REFERENCES

### Fibrosarcoma


1. Anand A, Anand N, Anand A. Primary cardiac fibrosarcoma. Am Heart J 132:1320, 1996.
2. Aydin F, Ghatak NR, Leshner RT. Possible radiation-induced dural fibrosarcoma with an unusual short latent period: case report. Neurosurgery 36:591, 1995.
3. Bhattacharyya N, Nadol JB, Curtin HD, et al. Vertigo produced by petrous extension of a radiation-induced fibrosarcoma of the anterior skull base. Ann Otol Rhinol Laryngol 107:898,1998.
4. Bizer LS. Fibrosarcoma: report of 64 cases. Am J Surg 121:586, 1971.
5. Borman H, Safak T, Ertoy D. Fibrosarcoma following radiotherapy for breast carcinoma: a case report and review of the literature. Ann Plast Surg 41:201,1998.
6. Brady MS, Garfein CF, Petrek JA, et al. Post-treatment sarcoma in breast cancer patients. Ann Surg Oncol 1:66, 1994.
7. Broders AC, Hargrave R, Meyerding HW. Pathological features of soft tissue fibrosarcoma: with special reference to the grading of its malignancy. Surg Gynecol Obstet 69:267, 1939.
8. Burns WA, Kanhouwa S, Tillman L, et al. Fibrosarcoma occurring at the site of a plastic vascular graft. Cancer 29:66, 1972.
9. Castro EB, Hajdu SI, Fortner JG. Surgical therapy of fibrosarcoma of extremities. Arch Surg 107:284, 1973.
10. Cayley FE, Bijapur HI. Fibrosarcoma occurring in draining sinus. J Bone Joint Surg Am 45:384, 1963.
11. Chang SM, Barker FG II, Larson DA, et al. Sarcoma subsequent to cranial irradiation. Neurosurgery 36:685, 1995.
12. Christensen DR, Ramsamooj R, Gilbert TJ. Sclerosing epithelioid fibrosarcoma: short T2 on MR imaging. Skeletal Radiol 26:619, 1997.
13. Conley J, Stout AP, Healey WV. Clinico-pathologic analysis of eighty-four patients with an original diagnosis of fibrosarcoma of the head and neck. Am J Surg 114:564, 1967.
14. Dal Cin P, Pauwels P, Sciot R, et al. Multiple chromosome rearrangements in a fibrosarcoma. Cancer Genet Cytogenet 87: 176, 1996.
15. De Boer MF, Deron PB, Eijkenboom WM, et al. Radiation-induced fibrosarcoma of the tongue. Clin Otolaryngol 20:323, 1995.
16. Delpla PA, Rouge D, Durroux R, et al. Soft tissue tumors following traumatic injury: two observations of interest for the medicolegal causality. Am J Forensic Med Pathol 19:152, 1998.
17. Denham RH, Dingley F. Fibrosarcoma occurring in a draining sinus. J Bone Joint Surg Am 45:384, 1963.
18. Donnet A, Figarella-Branger D, Grisoli F. Primary meningeal fibrosarcoma: a particular neuroradiological presentation. J Neurooncol 42:79, 1999.
19. Eckstein FS, Vogel U, Mohr W. Fibrosarcoma in association with a total knee joint prosthesis. Virchous Arch Pathol Anat 421:175, 1992.
20. Eyden BP, Manson C, Banerjee SS, et al. Sclerosing epithelioid fibrosarcoma: a study of five cases emphasizing diagnostic criteria. Histopathology 33:354, 1998.
21. Eyden BP, Ponting J, Davies H, et al. Defining the myofibroblasts: normal tissues, with special reference to the stroma cells of the Warton's jelly in human umbilical cord. J Submicrosc Cytol Pathol 26:347, 1994.
22. Fleming RM, Rezek PR. Sarcoma developing in an old burn scar. Am J Surg 54:457, 1941.
23. Fletcher CDM. Myofibroblastic sarcoma [letter to the editor]. Am J Sug Pathol 23:1433, 1999.
24. Fu YS, Perzin KH. Nonepithelial tumors of the nasal cavity, paranasal sinuses, and nasopharynx. VI. Fibrous tissue tumors (fibroma, fibromatosis, fibrosarcoma). Cancer 37:2912, 1976.
25. Gaspar LE, Mackenzie IRA, Gilbert JJ, et al. Primary cerebral fibrosarcomas: clinicopathologic study and review of the literature. Cancer 72:3277, 1993.
26. Giblin T, Pickrell K, Pitts W, et al. Malignant degeneration in burn scars: Marjolin's ulcer. Ann Surg 162:291, 1965.
27. Gisselsson D, Andreasson P, Meis-Kindblom JM, et al. Amplification of 12q13 and 12q15 sequences in a sclerosing epithelioid fibrosarcoma. Cancer Genet Cytogenet 107:102, 1998.
28. Goldenberg IS. Pencillin in sesame oil and fibrosarcoma: a report of two cases. Cancer 7:905, 1954.
29. Gray GR. Fibrosarcoma: a complication of interstitial radiation therapy for benign hemangioma occurring after 18 years. Br J Radiol 47:60, 1974.
30. Greager JA, Reichard K, Campana JP, et al. Fibrosarcoma of the head and neck. Am J Surg 167:437, 1994.
31. Heffner DK, Gnepp DR. Sinonasal fibrosarcomas, malignant schwannomas and "Triton" tumors: a clinicopathologic study of 67 cases. Cancer 70:1089, 1992.
32. Heller EL, Sieber WK. Fibrosarcoma: a clinical and pathological study of 60 cases. Surgery 27:539, 1950.
33. Ito T, Seyama T, Iwamoto KS, et al. In vitro irradiation is able to cause RET oncogene rearrangement. Cancer Res 53:2940, 1993.
34. Ivins JC, Dockerty MB, Ghormley RK. Fibrosarcoma of the soft tissues of the extremities: a review of 78 cases. Surgery 28:492, 1950.
35. Jones MW, Norris HJ, Wargotz ES, et al. Fibrosarcoma—malignant fibrous histiocytoma of the breast: a clinicopathological study of 32 cases. Am J Surg Pathol 16:667, 1992.
36. Klein KG, Bauck NP. The distal region of the long arm of human chromosome 1 carries tumor suppressor activity for a human fibrosarcoma line. Cancer Genet Cytogenet 73:109, 1994.
37. Lagace R, Seemayer TA, Gabbiani G, et al. Myofibroblastic sarcoma [letter to the editor]. Am J Surg Pathol 23:1432, 1999.
38. Lalwani AK, Jackler RK, Gutin PH. Lethal fibrosarcoma complicating radiation therapy for benign glomus jugulare tumor. Am J Otol 14:398, 1993.
39. Lengle FJ, Hecht ST, Link DP, et al. Palliative embolization of fibrosarcoma for control of tumor-induced hypoglycemia. Cardiovasc Intervent Radiol 18:255, 1995.
40. Lim YT, Lee CN, Chia BI. Images in cardiology: fibrosarcoma of the heart. Heart 80:369, 1998.
41. Limon J, Szadowska A, Iliszko M, et al. Recurrent chromosome changes in two adult fibrosarcomas. Genes Chromosomes Cancer 21:119, 1998.
42. Lindberg RD, Martin RG, Romsdahl MM. Surgery and postoperative radiotherapy in the treatment of soft tissue sarcomas in adults. AJR 123:123, 1975.
43. Logrono R, Filipowicz EA, Eyzaguirre FJ, et al. Diagnosis of primary fibrosarcoma of the lung by fine-needle aspiration and core biopsy. Arch Pathol Lab Med 123:731, 1999.
44. Lopes MB, Lanzino G, Cloft HJ, et al. Primary fibrosarcoma of the sella unrelated to previous radiation therapy. Mod Pathol 11:579, 1998.
45. Lustig LR, Jackler RK, Lanser MJ. Radiation-induced tumors of the temporal bone. Am J Otol 18:230, 1997.

46. Mackenzie DH. Fibroma: a dangerous diagnosis: a review of 205 cases of fibrosarcoma of soft tissues. Br J Surg 51:607, 1964.
47. Mark RJ, Sercarz JA, Tran L, et al. Fibrosarcoma of the head and neck: the UCLA experience. Arch Otolaryngol Head Neck Surg 117:396, 1991.
48. Meis-Kindblom JM, Kindblom LG, Enzinger FM. Sclerosing epithelioid fibrosarcoma: a variant of fibrosarcoma simulating carcinoma. Am J Surg Pathol 19:979, 1995.
49. Melzner E. Über Sarkonentstehung nich Kregsverletzung. Arch Klin Chir 147:153, 1927.
50. Mentzel T, Dry S, Katenkamp D, et al. Low-grade myofibroblastic sarcoma: analysis of 18 cases in the spectrum of myofibroblastic tumors. Am J Surg Pathol 22:1228, 1998.
51. Meyerding HW, Broders AC, Hargrave RL. Clinical aspects of fibrosarcoma of the soft tissues of the extremities. Surg Gynecol Obstet 62:1010, 1936.
52. Montgomery EA, Devaney KO, Weiss SW. Low-grade fibroblastic sarcomas and their distinction from deep fibromatoses. Mod Pathol 9:42A, 1996.
53. O'Connell TX, Fee HJ, Golding A. Sarcoma associated with Dacron prosthetic material: case report and review of the literature. J Thorac Cardiovasc Surg 72:94, 1976.
54. Oshiro Y, Fukuda T, Tsuneyoshi M. Fibrosarcoma versus fibromatoses and cellular nodular fasciitis: a comparative study of their proliferative activity using proliferating cell nuclear antigen, DNA flow cytometry and p53. Am J Surg Pathol 18:712, 1994.
55. Ozyazgan I, Kontas O. Burn scar sarcoma. Burns 25:455, 1999.
56. Pack GT, Ariel IM. Fibrosarcoma of the soft somatic tissues: a clinical and pathologic study. Surgery 31:443, 1952.
57. Pinson CW, Lopez RR, Ivancez K, et al. Resection of primary hepatic malignant fibrous histiocytoma, fibrosarcoma and leiomyosarcoma. South Med J 87:384, 1994.
58. Pritchard DJ, Sim FH, Ivins JC. Fibrosarcoma of bone and soft tissues of the trunk and extremities. Orthop Clin North Am 8: 869, 1977.
59. Pritchard DJ, Soule EH, Taylor WF, et al. Fibrosarcoma—a clinicopathologic and statistical study of 199 tumors of the soft tissues of the extremities and trunk. Cancer 33:888, 1974.
60. Reid R, Barrett A, Hamblen DL. Sclerosing epithelioid fibrosarcoma. Histopathology 28:451, 1996.
61. Schofield DE, Fletcher JA, Grier HE, et al. Fibrosarcoma in infants and children: application of new techniques. Am J Surg Pathol 18:14, 1994.
62. Schürch W. The myofibroblast in neoplasia. In: Desmouliere A, Tuchweber B (eds) Tissue Repair and Fibrosis. Springer-Verlag, Berlin, 1999, p 135.
63. Schürch W, Seemayer TA, Gabbiani G. Myofibroblast. In: Sternberg SS (ed) Histology for Pathologists, 2nd ed. Lippincott-Raven, Philadelphia, 1997, p 129.
64. Schürch W, Seemayer TA, Gabbiani G. The myofibroblast: a quarter century after its discovery [editorial]. Am J Surg Pathol 22:141, 1998.
65. Schwartz EE, Rothstein JD. Fibrosarcoma following radiation therapy. JAMA 203:296, 1968.
66. Scott SM, Reiman HM, Pritchard DJ, et al. Soft tissue fibrosarcoma: a clinicopathologic study of 132 cases. Cancer 64:925, 1989.
67. Sichel JY, Wygoda M, Dano I, et al. Fibrosarcoma of the thyroid in a man exposed to fallout from the Chernobyl accident. Ann Otol Rhinol Laryngol 105:832, 1996.
68. Stout AP. Fibrosarcoma: the malignant tumor of fibroblasts. Cancer 1:30, 1948.
69. Stout AP. The fibromatoses and fibrosarcoma. Bull Hosp Joint Dis 12:126, 1951.
70. Suh C-H, Ordonez NG, Mackay B. Fibrosarcoma: observations on the ultrastructure. Ultrastruct Pathol 17:221, 1993.
71. Weiss SW. Proliferative fibroblastic lesions: from hyperplasia to neoplasia. Am J Surg Pathol 10:14, 1986.
72. Wiklund TA, Blomquist CP, Raety J, et al. Postirradiation sarcoma: analysis of a nationwide cancer registry material. Cancer 68:524, 1991.
73. Wilson H, Brunschwig A. Irradiation sarcoma. Surgery 2:607, 1937.

### Myxofibrosarcoma

74. Angervall L, Kindblom LG, Merck C. Myxofibrosarcoma: a study of 30 cases. Acta Pathol Microbiol Scand [A] 85:127, 1977.
75. Fukunaga M, Fukunaga N. Low-grade myxofibrosarcoma: progression in recurrence. Pathol Int 47:161, 1997.
76. Hirose T, Sano T, Hizawa K. Ultrastructural study of the myxoid area of malignant fibrous histiocytomas. Ultrastruct Pathol 12:621, 1988.
77. Kindblom LG, Merck C, Angervall L. The ultrastructure of myxofibrosarcoma: a study of 11 cases. Virchous Arch A Pathol Anat Histol 381:121, 1979.
78. Mentzel T, Calonje E, Wadden C, et al. Myxofibrosarcoma: clinicopathologic analysis of 75 cases with emphasis on the low-grade variant. Am J Surg Pathol 20:391, 1996.
79. Merck C, Angervall L, Kindblom LG, et al. Myxofibrosarcoma: a malignant soft tissue tumor of fibroblastic-histiocytic origin: a clinicopathologic and prognostic study of 110 cases using a multivariate analysis. Acta Pathol Microbiol Scand [A] 91(Suppl 282):1, 1983.
80. Weiss SW, Enzinger FM. Myxoid variant of malignant fibrous histiocytoma. Cancer 39:1672, 1977.

### Low-grade Fibromyxoid Sarcoma

81. Aoki T, Hisaoka M, Kouho H, et al. Interphase cytogenetic analysis of myxoid soft tissue tumors by fluorescence in-situ hybridization and DNA flow cytometry using paraffin-embedded tissue. Cancer 79:284, 1997.
82. Dvornik G, Barbareschi M, Gallotta P, et al. Low-grade fibromyxoid sarcoma. Histopathology 30:274, 1997.
83. Evans HL. Low-grade fibromyxoid sarcoma: a report of two metastasizing neoplasms having a deceptively benign appearance. Am J Clin Pathol 88:615, 1987.
84. Evans HL. Low-grade fibromyxoid sarcoma: a report of 12 cases. Am J Surg Pathol 17:595, 1993.
85. Folpe AL, Lane KL, Paull G, et al. Low grade fibromyxoid sarcoma: a study of 72 cases with particular reference to high-grade areas and its relationship to "hyalinizing spindle cell tumor with giant rosettes" [abstract]. Mod Pathol 13:2000.
86. Fukunaga M, Ushigome S, Fukunaga N. Low-grade fibromyxoid sarcoma. Virchows Arch Pathol Anat 429:301, 1996.
87. Goodlad JR, Mentzel T, Fletcher CDM. Low-grade fibromyxoid sarcoma: clinicopathological analysis of eleven new cases in support of a distinct entity. Histopathology 26:229, 1995.
88. Lindberg GM, Maitra A, Gokaslan ST, et al. Low grade fibromyxoid sarcoma: fine-needle aspiration cytology with histologic, cytogenetic, immunohistochemical and ultrastructural correlation. Cancer 87:75,1999.
89. Nichols GE, Cooper PH. Low-grade fibromyxoid sarcoma: case report and immunohistochemical study. J Cutan Pathol 21:356, 1994.
90. Sidham VB, Ayala GE, Lahaniatis JE, et al. Low-grade fibromyxoid sarcoma: clinicopathologic case report with review of the literature. Am J Clin Oncol 22:150, 1999.
91. Ugai K, Kizaki T, Morimoto K, et al. A case of low-grade fibromyxoid sarcoma of the thigh. Pathol Int 44:793, 1994.
91a. Zamecnik M, Michal M. Low-grade fibromyxoid sarcoma: A report of eight cases with histologic, immunohistochemical, and ultrastructural study. Ann Diagn Pathol 4:207, 2000.

### Fibrosarcoma, Low-grade Fibromyxoid type, with Giant Rosettes


92. De Pinieux G, Anract P, le Charpentier M, et al. A case of hyalinizing spindle cell tumor with giant rosettes in the presacral region: immunohistochemical and ultrastructural study. Ann Pathol 18:488, 1998.

92a. Farinha P, Oliveira P, Soares J. Metastasizing hyalinizing spindle cell tumour with giant rosettes: report of a case with long survival (letter to the editor). Histopathology 36:92, 2000.

93. Goldblum JR, Beals T, Weiss SW. Neuroblastoma-like neurilemmoma. Am J Surg Pathol 18:266, 1994.

94. Kim H, Park C, Lee YP, et al. Case report 643. Skeletal Radiol 19:609, 1990.

95. Lane KL, Shannon RJ, Weiss SW. Hyalinizing spindle cell tumor with giant rosettes: a distinctive tumor closely resembling low-grade fibromyxoid sarcoma. Am J Surg Pathol 21:1481, 1997.

96. Ludvikova M, Michal M, Zamecnik M. Hyalinizing spindle cell tumor with giant rosette-like structures. Pathol Res Pract 194: 577, 1998.

97. Magro G, Fraggetta F, Manusia M, et al. Hyalinizing spindle cell tumor with giant rosettes: a previously undescribed lesion of the lung [letter to the editor]. Am J Surg Pathol 22:1431, 1998.

98. Nielsen GP, Selig MK, O'Connell JX, et al. Hyalinizing spindle cell tumor with giant rosettes: a report of three cases with ultrastructural analysis. Am J Surg Pathol 23:1227, 1999.

99. Woodruff JM, Antonescu CR, Erlandson RA, et al. Low-grade fibrosarcoma with palisaded granulomalike bodies (giant rosettes): report of a case that metastasized. Am J Surg Pathol 23: 1423, 1999.

# CHAPTER 13

# BENIGN FIBROHISTIOCYTIC TUMORS

The so-called benign fibrohistiocytic tumors are a diverse group of lesions that have in common certain morphologic features but the pathogenesis of which differs significantly. Xanthoma is a "pseudotumor" that usually arises in response to a disturbance in serum lipids. Fibrous histiocytoma is a true neoplasm with definite growth potential but a limited capacity for aggressive behavior. Between these extremes are lesions of an indeterminate nature, exemplified by juvenile xanthogranuloma. Although juvenile xanthogranuloma resembles a tumor morphologically, it usually regresses with time, thereby raising the question of its proper position in the spectrum between hyperplasia and neoplasia. The present classification represents a practical, rather than a conceptual, approach aimed at defining differences among several histologically similar lesions.

In the past, fibrohistiocytic tumors were so named to imply their origin from a tissue histiocyte that could assume fibroblastic properties. The histiocytic origin has now been questioned, and in the case of the malignant fibrous histiocytoma a fibroblastic origin has been proposed (see Chapter 15). For that reason, use of the term "fibrohistiocytic" is descriptive and merely denotes a lesion composed of cells that resemble normal histiocytes and fibroblasts.

## FIBROUS HISTIOCYTOMA

Fibrous histiocytoma is a benign tumor composed of a mixture of fibroblastic and histiocytic cells that are often arranged in a cartwheel or storiform pattern and accompanied by varying numbers of inflammatory cells, foam cells, and siderophages. Most commonly this tumor occurs in the dermis and superficial subcutis, but it is also found in deep soft tissue and sporadically in parenchymal organs. When located in the skin, fibrous histiocytoma has also been referred to as dermatofibroma,[33,44] histiocytoma cutis,[10,33] nodular subepidermal fibrosis,[35,40] and sclerosing hemangioma.[15,28] Although many of these terms are now obsolete, some authors continue to subdivide cutaneous fibrous histiocytomas into dermatofibroma and histiocytoma,[44] the former being characterized by large amounts of collagen and the latter by numerous phagocytic cells containing lipid and hemosiderin. Such a sharp distinction is not always possible because of the intrinsic variability of a given tumor. When similar tumors are encountered in deep soft tissue, the use of some of these terms is obviously inappropriate. We use the all-inclusive *fibrous histiocytoma* to refer to both cutaneous and deep lesions regardless of collagen content or proportion of histiocytic and fibroblastic cells.

### Clinical Findings

Cutaneous fibrous histiocytoma is a solitary, slowly growing nodule that usually makes its appearance during early or mid adult life. Although any part of the skin surface may be affected, it is most common on the extremities.[27] Roughly one-third of these tumors are multiple and present metachronously. Synchronous development can occur in the setting of immunosuppression,[42] but these lesions are not associated with human herpes virus 8 (HHV8),[21] as has been demonstrated for other multifocal tumors such as Kaposi's sarcoma.[27] Cutaneous fibrous histiocytomas are elevated or pedunculated lesions measuring a few millimeters to a few centimeters in diameter (Figs. 13–1, 13–2, 13–3). Rarely, they result in a depressed area in the skin ("atrophic dermatofibroma").[11] They impart a red or red-brown color to the overlying skin but occasionally appear blue or black as a result of excessive deposits of hemosiderin. Such lesions may be confused clinically with malignant melanoma. The presence of a central dimple on lateral compression is regarded as a useful clinical sign for distinguishing it from melanoma.[20] Deeply situated fibrous histiocytomas are less common than

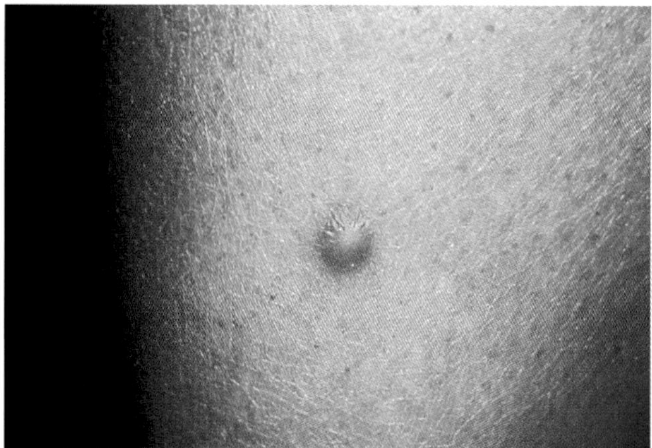

**FIGURE 13–1.** Red nodular appearance of a benign fibrous histiocytoma. (Case courtesy of Dr. John T. Headington.)

cutaneous ones. The relative incidence is difficult to determine because the latter are less likely to be subjected to biopsy or excised than the former. In a study by Fletcher,[22] only three cases of fibrous histiocytoma involving skeletal muscle were culled from more than 1000 fibrohistiocytic tumors. Like their cutaneous counterparts, they present as painless masses, usually on an extremity. Although they develop at any age, most occur between the ages of 20 and 40 years. They tend to be larger than the cutaneous tumors. Nearly half of these tumors are 5 cm or more when excised, in contrast to most cutaneous fibrous histiocytomas, which are less than 3 cm in our experience. Grossly, they are circumscribed, yellow or white masses that may have focal areas of hemorrhage.

## Microscopic Findings

The cutaneous fibrous histiocytoma consists of a nodular cellular proliferation involving dermis and occasionally subcutis (Fig. 13–4). The lateral margins are not sharply defined (Fig. 13–5), and the overlying epidermis frequently shows some degree of hyperplasia including acanthosis or elongation and widening of the rete pegs[29] (Fig. 13–6). The presence of a rim of normal dermis between epidermis and tumor is variable. At the deep margin the tumor extends small tentacles for short distances into the subcutis (Fig. 13–7) or, less commonly, has a smoothly contoured margin (Fig. 13–8). Both types contrast with the deeply penetrating border of dermatofibrosarcoma protuberans. Most cutaneous fibrous histiocytomas consist of short, intersecting fascicles of fibroblastic cells (Figs. 13–9 to 13–15) The fascicles usually form a loose crisscross pattern or a vague storiform pattern (Fig. 13–9). Occasional rounded "histiocytic" cells accompany the spindle cells, but they rarely predominate. Multinucleated giant cells of the foreign body or Touton type are a typical feature of this form of fibrous histiocytoma and often contain phagocytosed lipid and hemosiderin (Fig. 13–14). Inflammatory cells, particularly lymphocytes and xanthoma cells, are scattered randomly throughout the tumors but vary greatly in number. The stroma consists of a delicate collagen network surrounding individual cells. In a small number of cases the vessels and stroma exhibit striking hyalinization, a feature that has led to use of the misnomer "sclerosing hemangioma" (Figs. 13–12, 13–13). This term conveyed the earlier belief that the cells of these tumors were derived from endothelium that was pinched off obliterated vessels.[28] Cystic areas of hemorrhage are common (see Figs. 13–30 to 13–32) and, when prominent, result in large accumulations of hemosiderin in the tumor cells. When this feature is striking, some have employed the term "aneurysmal"[13,37,46] fibrous histiocytoma (see below). A number of other unusual features are seen in these lesions, including clear-cell change, granular cell change, nuclear palisading, extensive hyalinization, and lipidization (see below). Recently it was pointed out that fibrous histiocytomas occasionally evoke an unusual mesenchymal response around them usually in the form of proliferation of mature smooth muscle.[36]

Deep fibrous histiocytomas are similar to their cutaneous counterparts, but they usually have a more prominent storiform pattern and fewer secondary elements such as xanthoma cells (Figs. 13–16, 13–17, 13–18). The stroma often undergoes myxoid change (Fig. 13–17) or hyalinization. In unusual cases, dense bundles of collagen (amianthoid fibers) and even metaplastic osteoid are detected. Not infrequently, deep fibrous histiocytomas blend with areas indistinguishable from a benign hemangiopericytoma (Fig. 13–18).

*Text continued on page 451*

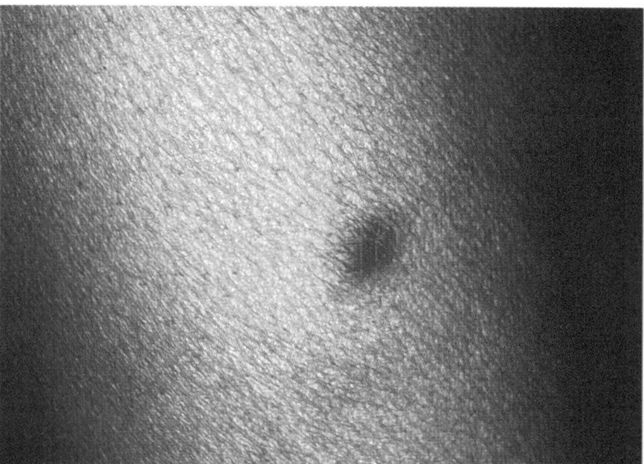

**FIGURE 13–2.** Benign fibrous histiocytoma with a pigmented appearance. (Case courtesy of Dr. John T. Headington.)

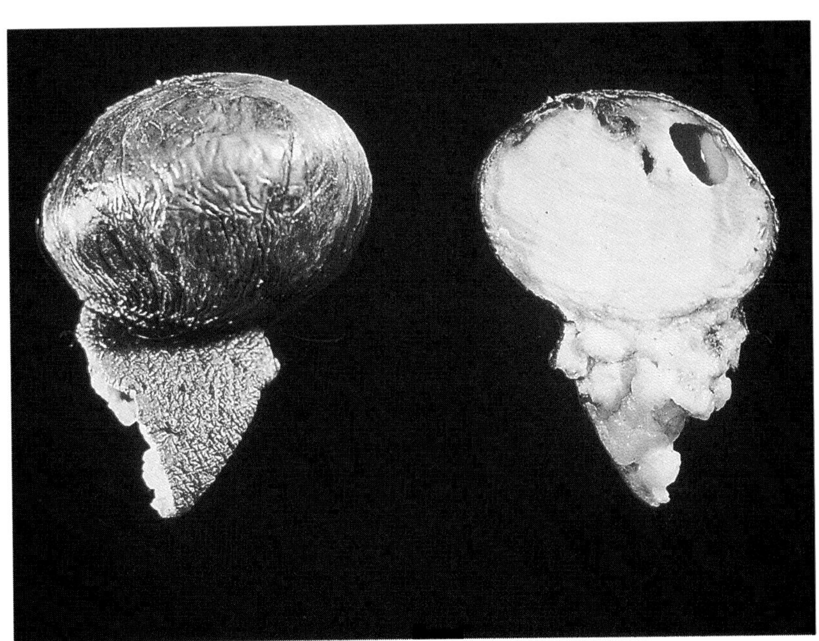

**FIGURE 13–3.** Gross appearance of a pedunculated cutaneous fibrous histiocytoma. The light color of the lesion is a result of the presence of large amounts of lipid. Focal cyst formation is also present.

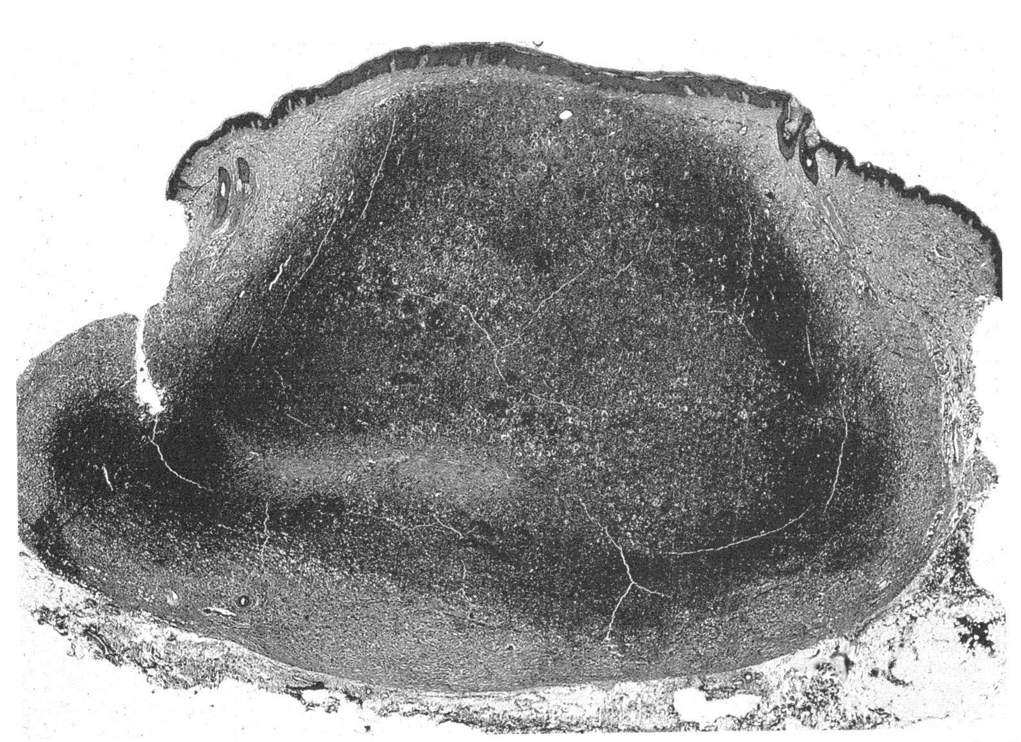

**FIGURE 13–4.** Low-power view of a cutaneous fibrous histiocytoma. The lesion is confined to the dermis and has a smooth, bulging deep margin.

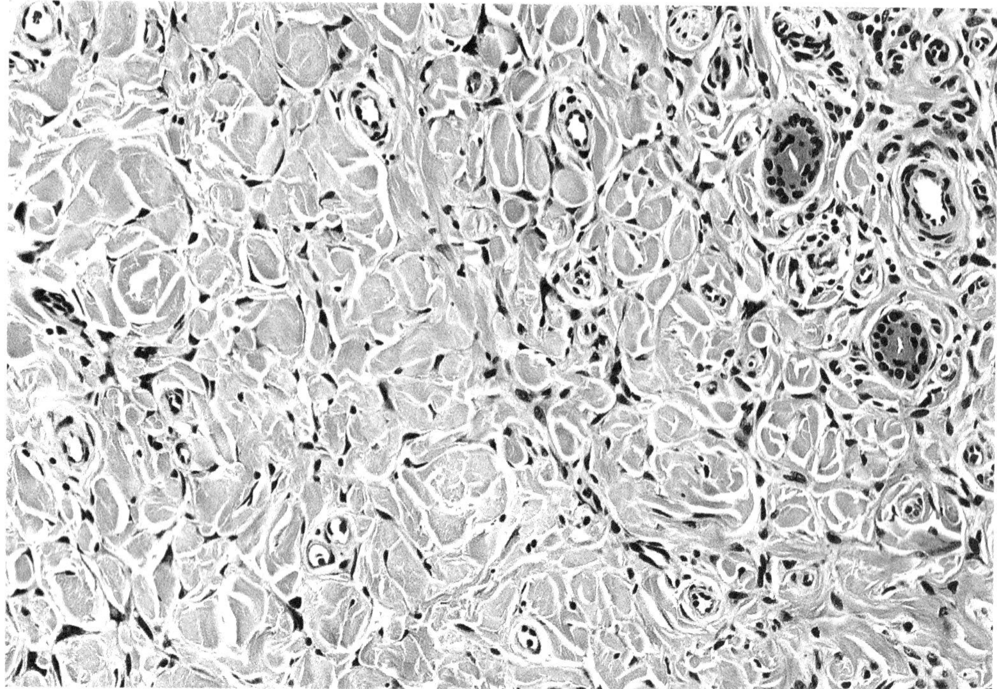

**FIGURE 13–5.** Lateral border of a fibrous histiocytoma illustrating entrapment of collagen.

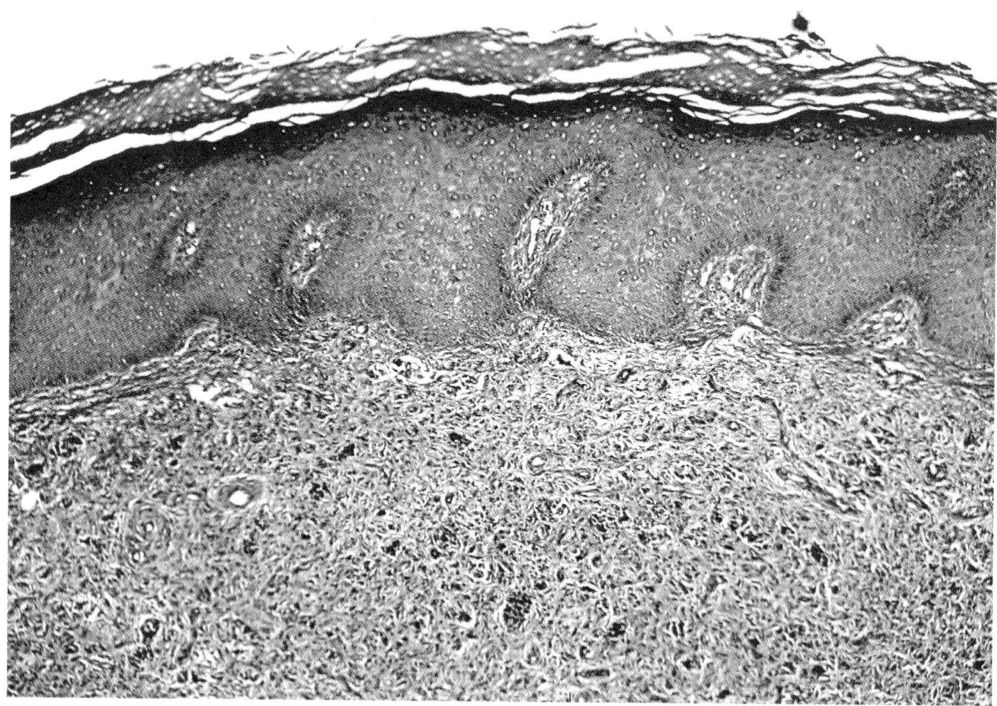

**FIGURE 13–6.** Epithelial hyperplasia overlying a fibrous histiocytoma.

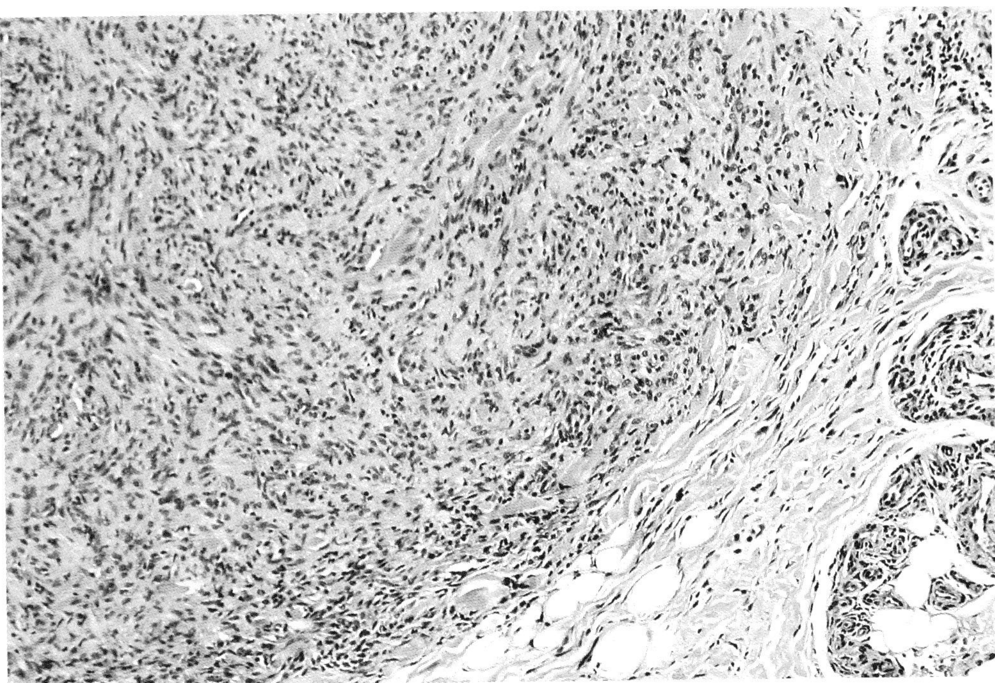

**FIGURE 13–7.** Smoothly contoured deep border of a benign fibrous histiocytoma.

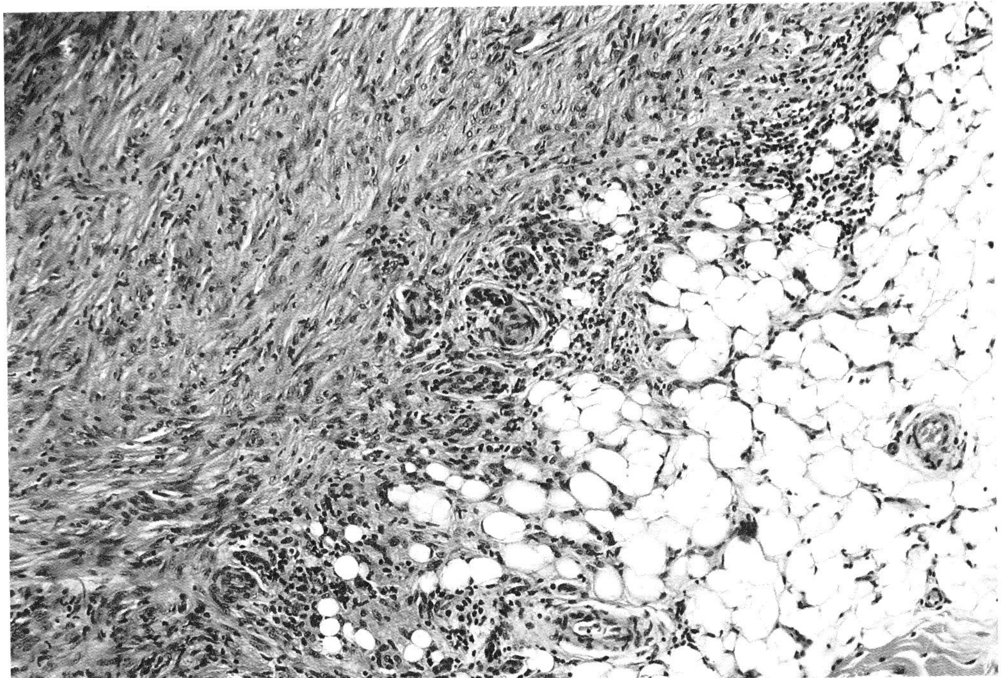

**FIGURE 13–8.** Minimal irregular penetration of the subcutis at the deep border of a fibrous histiocytoma contrasts with a more-infiltrative border of dermatofibrosarcoma protuberans.

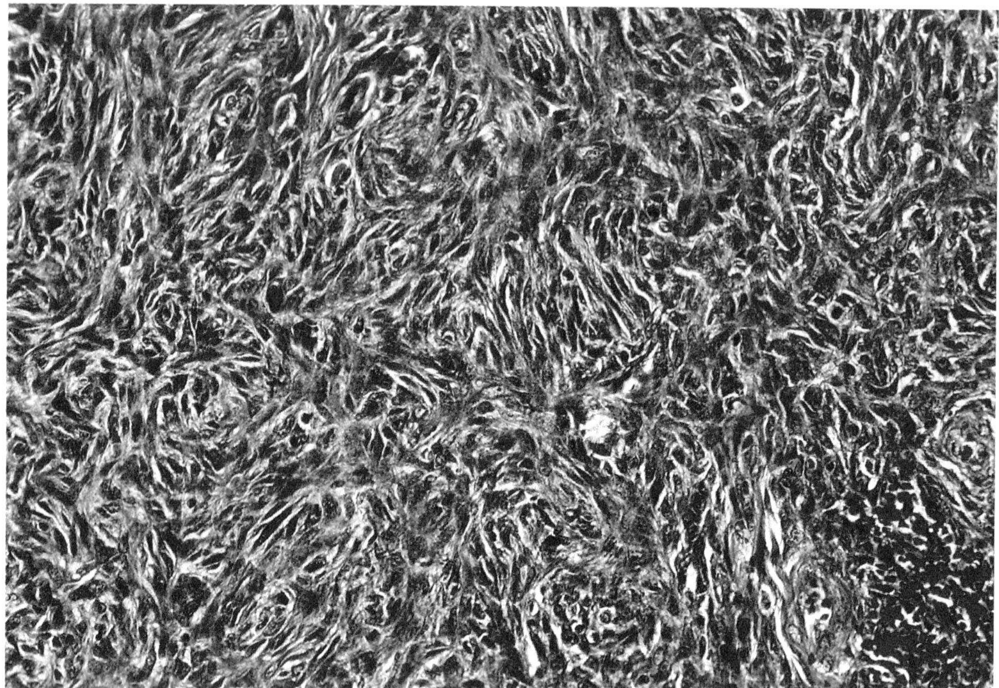

**FIGURE 13–9.** Fibrous histiocytoma with a predominantly spindled appearance.

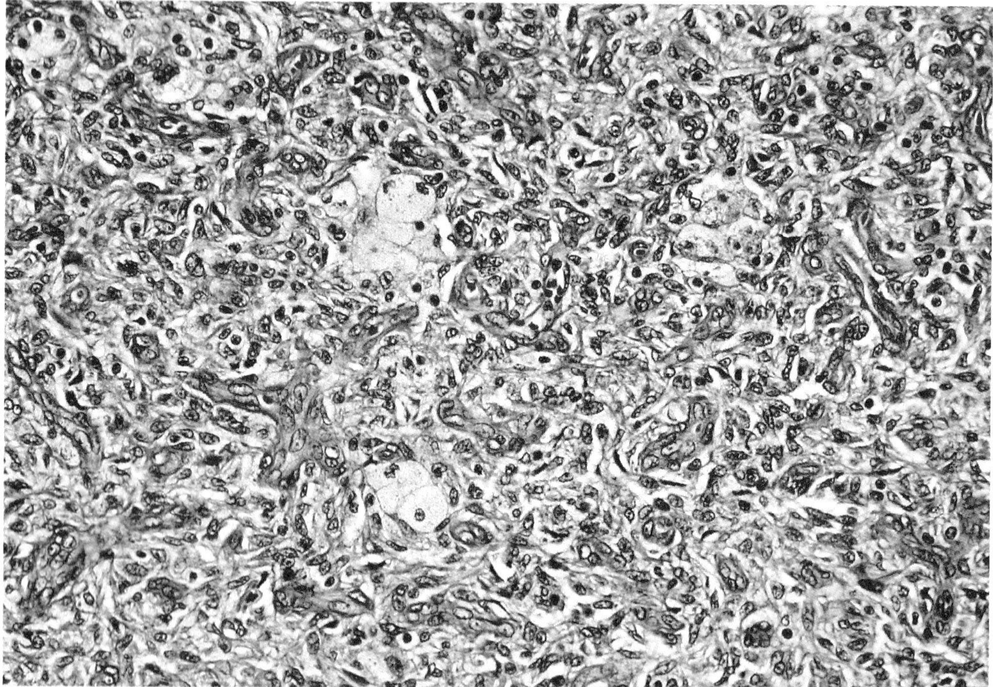

**FIGURE 13–10.** Fibrous histiocytoma with a mixture of spindled and xanthomatous cells.

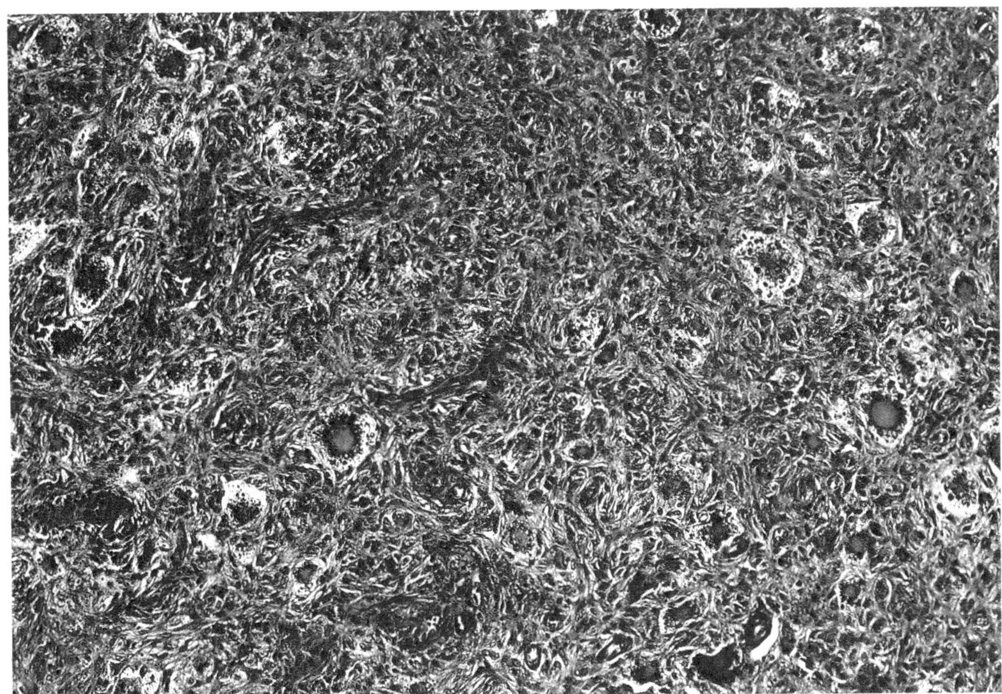

**FIGURE 13–11.** Fibrous histiocytoma with numerous Touton giant cells.

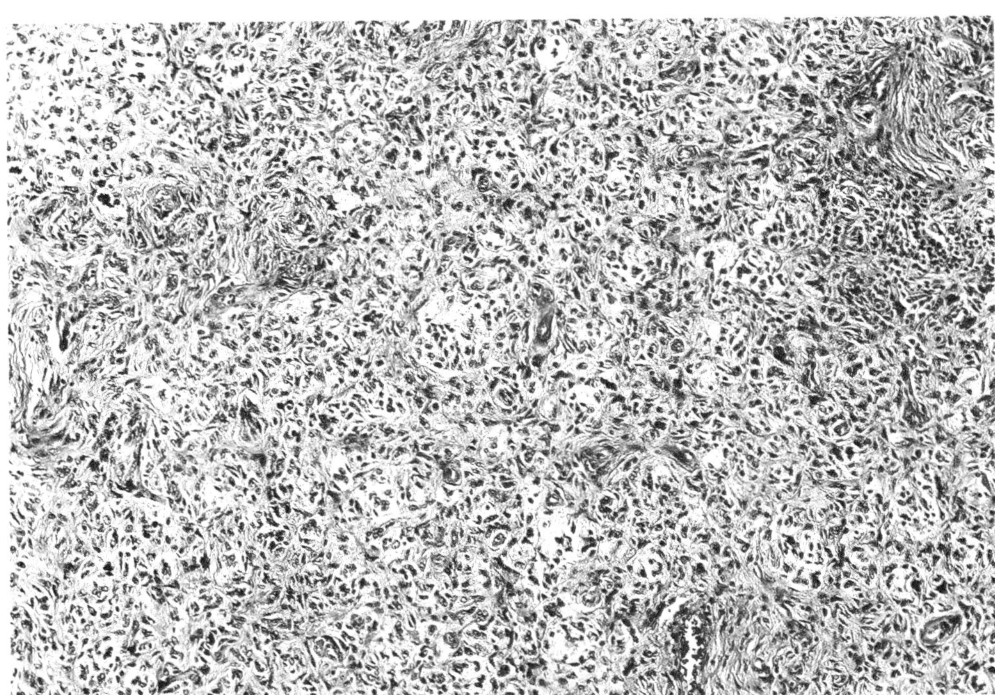

**FIGURE 13–12.** Fibrous histiocytoma with a lipidized appearance and some nuclear atypia.

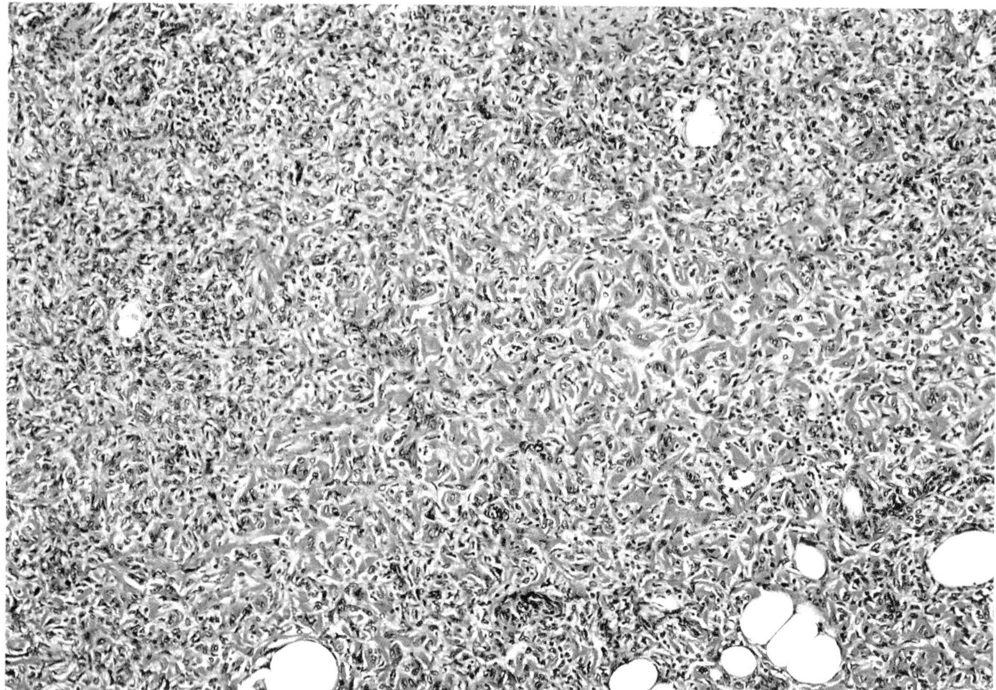

**FIGURE 13–13.** Fibrous histiocytoma with interstitial and perivascular hyalinization.

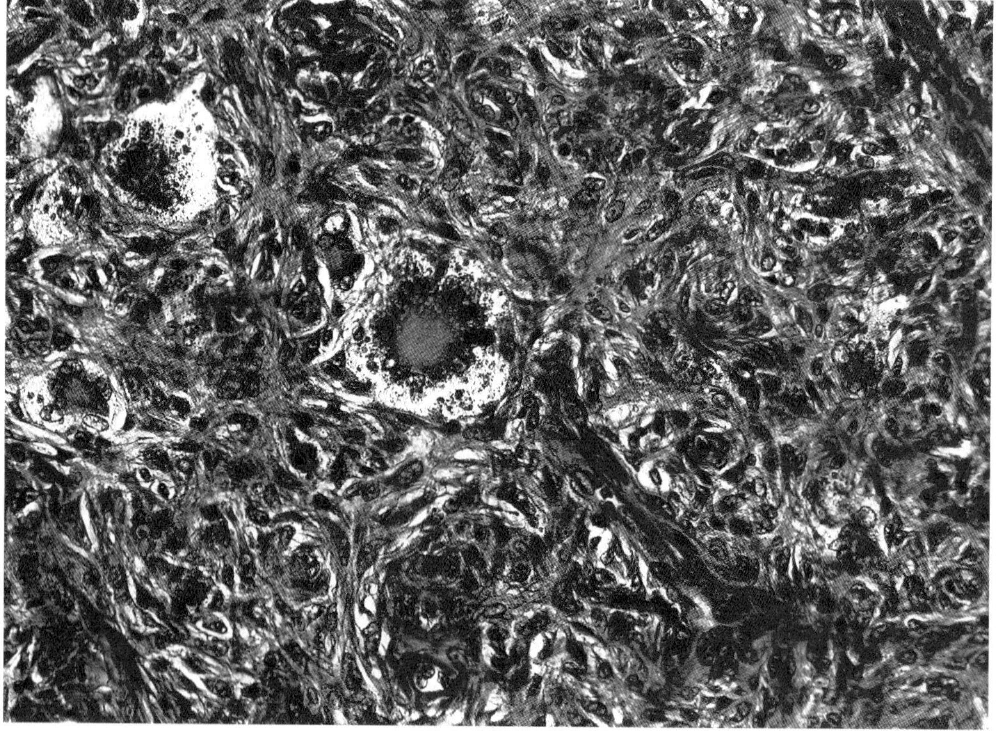

**FIGURE 13–14.** Touton giant cells containing lipid and hemosiderin.

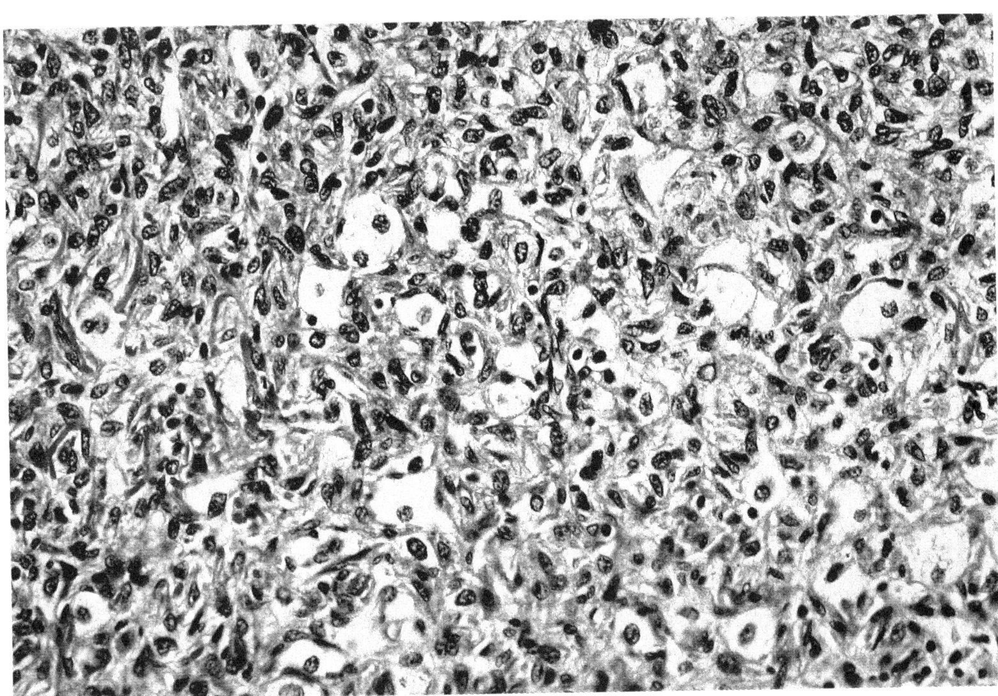

**FIGURE 13–15.** Xanthoma cells within fibrous histiocytoma.

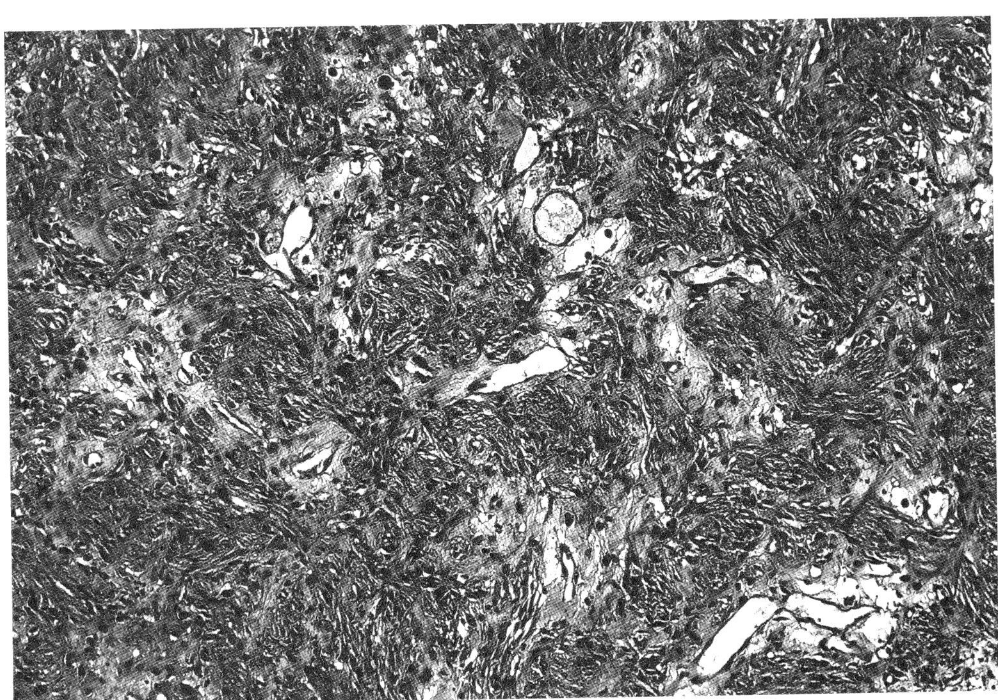

**FIGURE 13–16.** Fibrous histiocytoma of soft tissue. In contrast to cutaneous fibrous histiocytomas, these lesions have a more distinct storiform pattern but lack the variety of secondary elements such as xanthoma cells and siderophages.

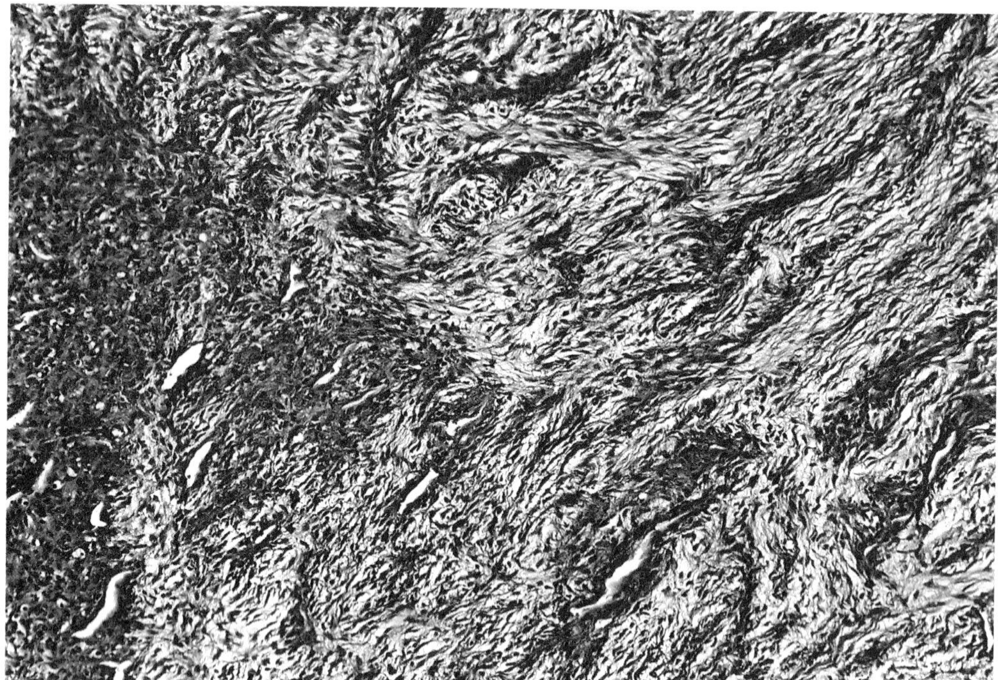

**FIGURE 13–17.** Fibrous histiocytoma of soft tissue with myxoid areas.

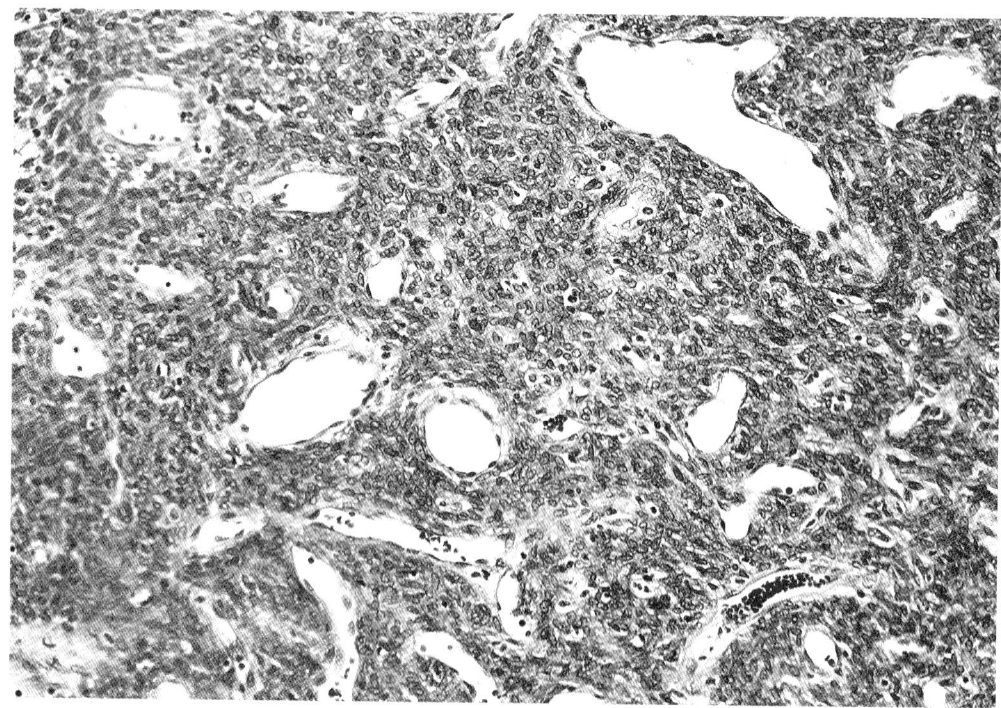

**FIGURE 13–18.** Hemangiopericytoma-like area within a fibrous histiocytoma of soft tissue.

This combination of hemangiopericytic and fibrohistiocytic areas is particularly characteristic of fibrous histiocytomas of the orbit.

The benign nature of fibrous histiocytoma is usually apparent histologically. The cells are well differentiated and exhibit little pleomorphism and usually little or no mitotic activity (Fig. 13–19). The occasional pleomorphic cells with hyperchromatic nuclei and clear to eosinophilic cytoplasm (Fig. 13–20), referred to by some as "monster cells,"[52] seem to be a degenerative phenomenon and do not affect the prognosis adversely.[12,52] However, the presence of both pleomorphism and mitotic activity suggest malignancy (see below). A small subset of fibrous histiocytomas known as "cellular fibrous histiocytomas" are characterized by somewhat longer, cellular fascicles of spindle cells bereft of other cellular elements. Although benign, these lesions may have a high local recurrence rate and are discussed below.

Histochemical, immunohistochemical, and electron microscopic studies have contributed little to the practical diagnosis of these tumors, but they have extended the observations made by conventional microscopy.[24] Lysosomal (acid phosphatase, nonspecific esterase) and oxidative (succinate dehydrogenase) enzymes can be demonstrated consistently in these tumors[35,44] and are present in greater quantities in the cells resembling histiocytes rather than fibroblasts. This is in keeping with the prevalence of these enzymes in normal histiocytes. One-fourth to three-fourths of cutaneous fibrous histiocytomas contain immunoreactive $\alpha_1$-antitrypsin. Although this finding has been used to support a histiocytic origin, the specificity of these proteolytic enzymes as markers of histiocytic differentiation has been questioned (see Chapter 8). Most recently, factor XIIIa[45] and tinascin have been demonstrated in a significant portion of cells in fibrous histiocytomas, leading some to conclude that these tumors arise from dermal dendrocytes[16] (Fig. 13–21). Whether factor XIIIa stains tumor elements or reactive dermal dendrocytes that populate benign fibrous histiocytomas is a matter of debate.[1] Electron microscopic studies have shown a spectrum of cell types in these tumors. Cells resembling fibroblasts represent one end of this spectrum.[19] They contain organized lamellae of rough endoplasmic reticulum but few or no lipid droplets and no phagolysosomes.[19,41] Depending on the functional state of these cells, they may acquire features of myofibroblasts.[2,6,9] The other end of the spectrum is represented by rounded cells resembling histiocytes with numerous cell processes, mitochondria, and phagolysosomes.[19] Transitions between the histiocytic and fibroblastic cells have been documented[19] and have led to conflicting views as to whether the tumor is of histiocytic or fibroblastic origin. Only one ultrastructural study has suggested that the tumor is of vascular origin because of the presence of Weibel-Palade bodies,[15] which are tubular organelles characteristic of endothelium.[8] However, in this study most stromal

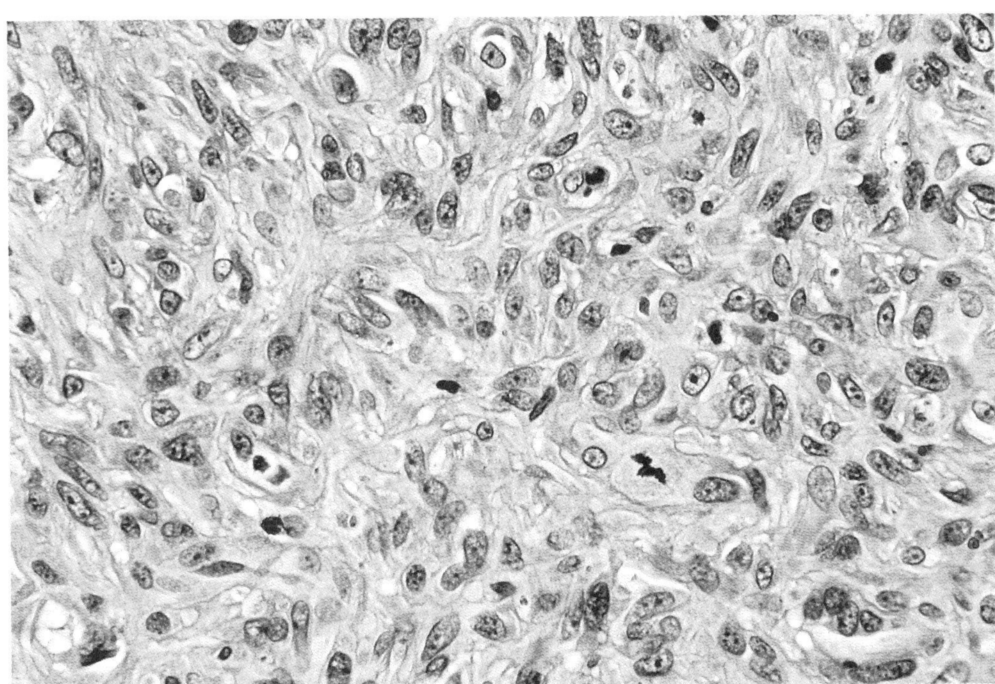

**FIGURE 13–19.** Plump spindle cells with benign fibrous histiocytoma displaying an occasional mitotic figure.

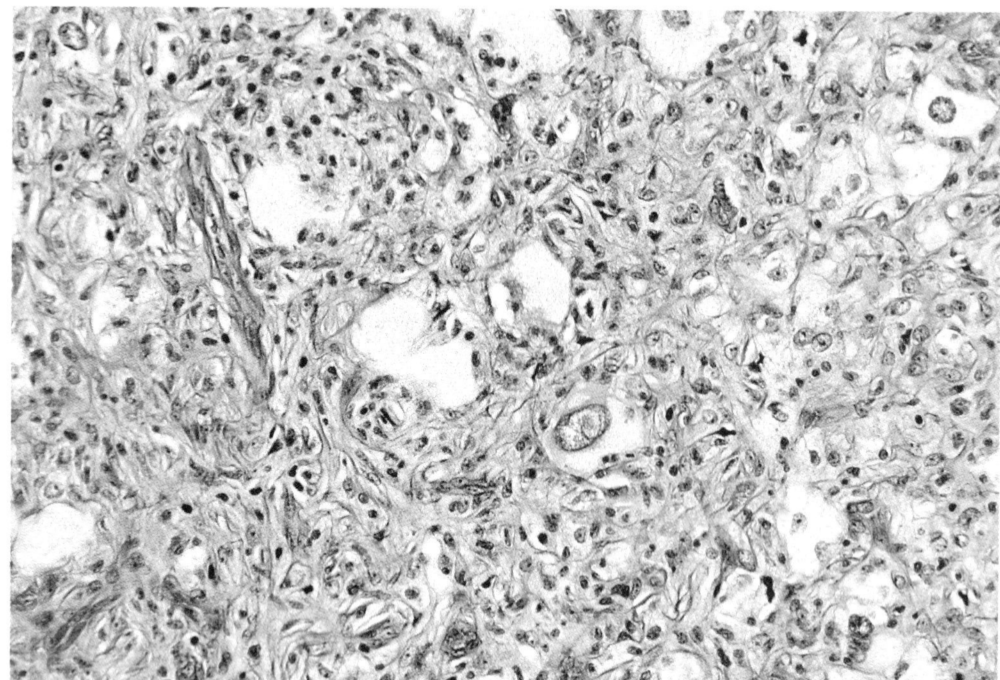

**FIGURE 13–20.** Pleomorphic (monster) cell within an otherwise benign fibrous histiocytoma of the skin.

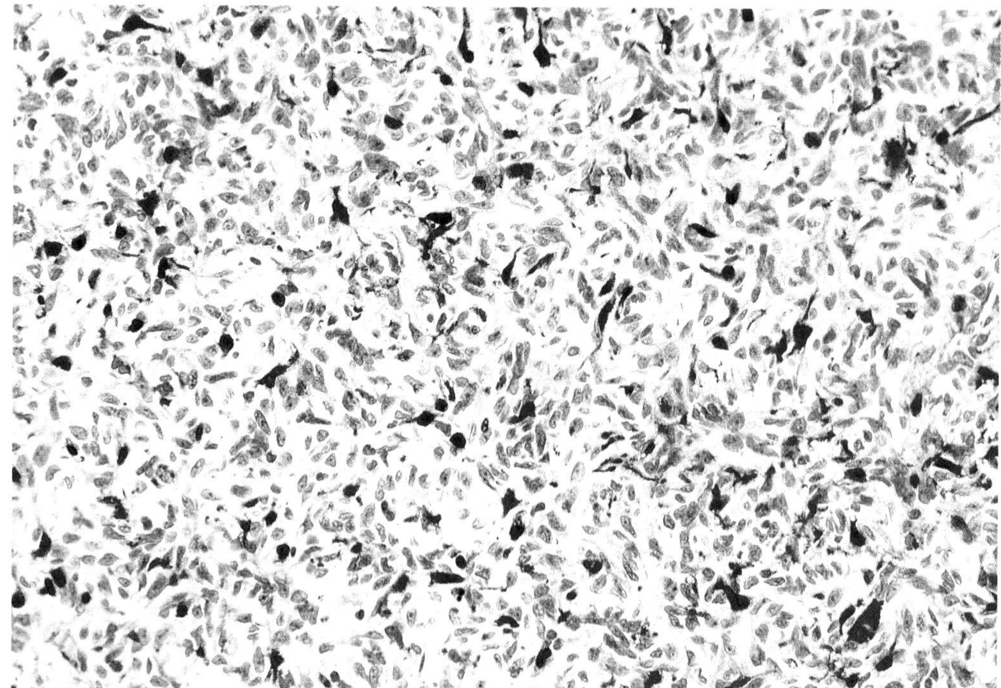

**FIGURE 13–21.** Factor XIIIa immunostain of a fibrous histiocytoma showing numerous postively staining dendritic cells.

cells did not contain this marker, and other studies have failed to confirm the presence of these bodies in any tumor cells.

## Differential Diagnosis

Fibrous histiocytomas are most frequently confused with other benign lesions, notably nodular fasciitis, neurofibroma, and leiomyoma. Although *nodular fasciitis* may display a storiform pattern, it is distinguished from fibrous histiocytoma by its loosely arranged bundles of fibroblasts. Cellular areas containing proliferating fibroblasts alternate with loose myxoid zones containing extravasated red blood cells and inflammatory cells. The vasculature in fasciitis is seldom as orderly or as uniform as that of fibrous histiocytoma. Finally, because most cases of fasciitis are excised during the period of active growth, they usually manifest much more mitotic activity than a fibrous histiocytoma of comparable cellularity. In our experience it is difficult if not impossible to distinguish the early (cellular phase) of nodular fasciitis from a benign fibrous histiocytoma. Fortunately, from a practical point of view this diagnostic imprecision has little adverse effect on patient care. The distinction between a fibrous histiocytoma and a *neurofibroma* is usually not difficult. Neurofibromas contain a population of schwann cells expressing S-100 protein and having serpentine nuclei. Additional features of neural differentiation may include organoid structures reminiscent of sensory receptors or vague nuclear palisading. The usual lack of any storiform pattern or significant inflammation in the neurofibroma further underscores the difference between the two tumors. Sclerotic forms of *leiomyoma* may resemble a fibrous histiocytoma. However, smooth muscle tumors have a more distinct fascicular growth pattern. Their blunt-ended nuclei are plumper, and the cytoplasm typically has longitudinal striations corresponding to the presence of myofilamentous material, which can be accentuated with Masson trichrome stain. They strongly express smooth muscle actin and muscle-specific actin in a diffuse pattern, unlike the focal immunoreactivity noted in benign fibrous histiocytomas reflective of myofibroblastic differentiation.

The most important diagnostic distinction for this tumor is from aggressive forms of fibrohistiocytic neoplasms including dermatofibrosarcoma protuberans and malignant fibrous histiocytoma. Like fibrous histiocytoma, *dermatofibrosarcoma protuberans* occurs in the dermis and subcutis but typically displays extensive subcutaneous involvement in the form of long, penetrating tentacles of tumor. It is also characterized by a more uniform cellular population and lacks giant cells, inflammatory cells, and xanthomatous elements. Its fascicles, composed of slender attenuated cells, are longer and arranged in a distinct storiform pattern, unlike the short curlicue fascicles of fibrous histiocytoma. Its margins are infiltrative, in contrast to the better defined margins of fibrous histiocytoma. Immunostaining reveals distinct differences in the cellular composition of these tumors as well. Fibrous histiocytomas contain a significant population of factor XIIIa-positive cells, although it has been debated whether these cells represent a population of neoplastic cells or a peculiar infiltrate that accompanies the tumor. Dermatofibrosarcoma protuberans contains only scattered factor XIIIa-positive cells but, in striking contrast to benign fibrous histiocytoma, expresses CD34 in a significant portion of neoplastic cells (Fig. 13–22). The combination of these two stains, in our experience, has proved to be highly reliable for distinguishing these two lesions, which often cause diagnostic problems, particularly when only a superficial biopsy specimen is available for review.

The difference between benign and frankly *malignant fibrous histiocytomas* is usually obvious because the latter is a pleomorphic, deeply situated tumor with numerous typical and atypical mitotic figures and prominent areas of hemorrhage and necrosis. Less obvious is the difference between this tumor and the *angiomatoid form of fibrous histiocytoma*. The latter is a tumor of childhood characterized by sheets of histiocytic cells interrupted by cystic areas of hemorrhage. They are surrounded by a dense cuff of lymphocytes and plasma cells but almost never have giant cells or xanthoma cells like the fibrous histiocytoma.

## Discussion

Fibrous histiocytomas in general are considered benign tumors.[38] Fewer than 5% of cutaneous fibrous histiocytomas recur following local excision.[1,44] In our unpublished experience, the overall recurrence rate of cutaneous and soft tissue fibrous histiocytomas is approximately 10% following conservative therapy. Those located in deep soft tissue have a recurrence rate that is somewhat higher and is reflective of the larger size and incompleteness of the surgical excision. In this regard, Franquemont et al.[25] reported a recurrence rate of nearly 50% for fibrous histiocytomas (8 cases) that extended into the subcutis or grew in a multinodular fashion, (or both); and Font and Kidaya[23] noted that 57% of orbital fibrous histiocytomas with infiltrative margins or hypercellular zones (or both) recurred compared with 31% of those without these features. It should be pointed out that nearly every histologic feature used to assess malignancy of tumors in general has been recorded in clinically benign fibrous histiocytomas as an isolated finding (i.e., increased cellularity,[14] necrosis,[22] vascular

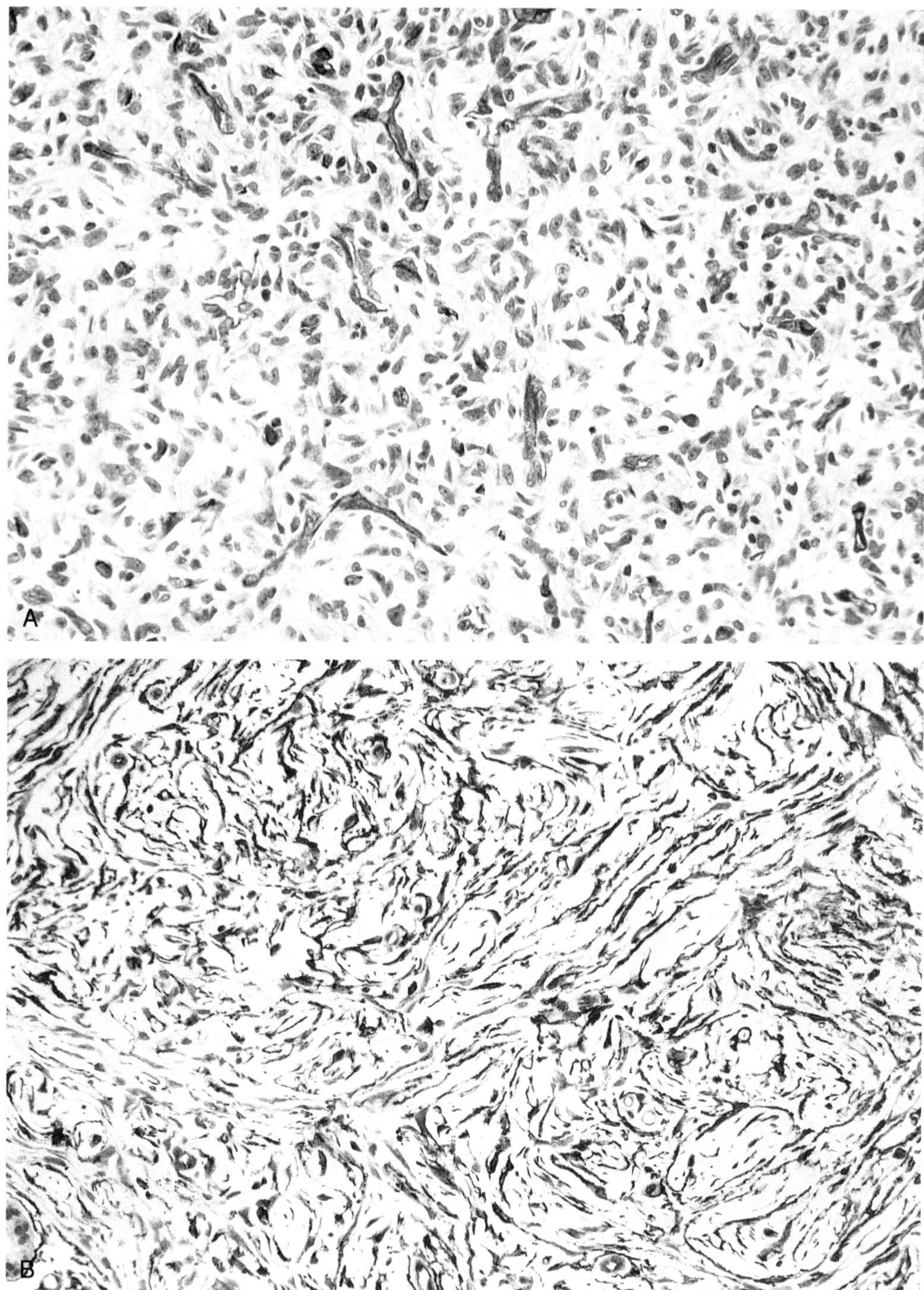


**FIGURE 13–22.** CD34 immunostains of benign fibrous histiocytoma and dermatofibrosarcoma protuberan. (**A**) CD34 immunostain of fibrous histiocytoma decorates normal vessels. (**B**) CD34 immunostain of a dermatofibrosarcoma protuberans in which majority of tumor cells are decorated.

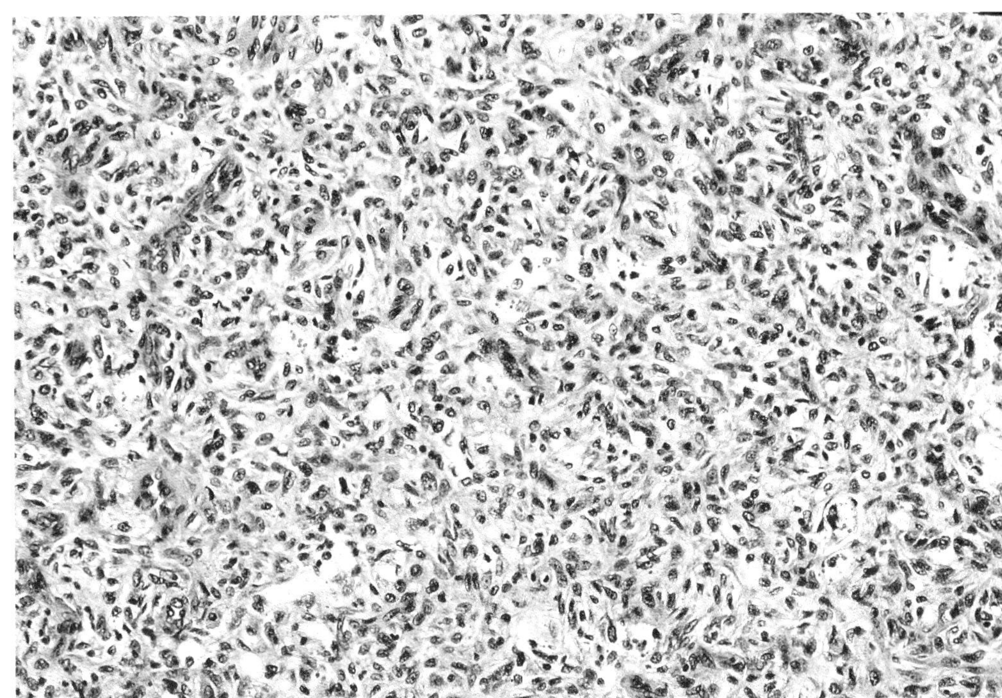

**FIGURE 13–23.** Benign fibrous histiocytoma that produced pulmonary metastasis.

invasion,[22,43] mitotic activity, atypia[12,52]) and sometimes even in company with one another without adverse consequences. Therefore it is important to recognize the underlying nature of the lesion to know what significance to place on many of these features. A useful guideline is that benign fibrous histiocytomas may show enhanced cellularity and some level of mitotic activity (e.g., cellular fibrous histiocytoma) and still be considered benign. Likewise, benign fibrous histocytomas may display nuclear atypia on a degenerative basis in the form of large "monster cells" set amidst the typical backdrop of banal neoplastic cells. Such lesions also are clinically benign. The presence of both mitotic activity and atypia (especially atypical mitotic figures) in the same lesion should be a cause for concern and raise the question of an atypical fibroxanthoma or superficial malignant fibrous histiocytoma. Having said this, there are anecdotal examples of histologically benign fibrous histiocytomas that have produced metastases. Two cases were recently reported by Colome-Grimmer and Evans.[17] Both were small (2 cm) cutaneous lesions that recurred, producing regional lymph node (and ultimately pulmonary) metastasis. The metastases appeared similar to the primary lesions, and both patients were alive 4 and 8 years after resection of the pulmonary deposits. We too have seen an instance of pulmonary metastasis from a benign cutaneous fibrous histiocytoma in which the metastasis also appeared benign (Fig. 13–23). Fortunately, such cases are rare and should not alter the approach to patients with these tumors.

The most controversial aspect of this tumor is its histogenesis. Although a reactive process (nodular subepidermal fibrosis)[40] is no longer a tenable concept, the lesion has been variably interpreted as a histiocytic or fibroblastic tumor. The presence of lysosomal and proteolytic enzymes in these tumors[18,34,35] and the phagocytic activity of the tumor following colloidal iron injection[48] have been interpreted as evidence favoring a histiocytic origin. The predominantly fibroblastic appearance of the cells ultrastructurally[40] and the lack of a histiocytic marker (Langerhans' granules)[32] have been used in support of a fibroblastic origin. Cell marker studies in malignant fibrous histiocytomas currently support a fibroblastic origin for this tumor (see Chapter 15), but comparable studies have not been carried out on benign fibrous histiocytomas.

## VARIANTS OF BENIGN FIBROUS HISTIOCYTOMA

A number of histologic variations may occur in benign fibrous histiocytomas, and they are seldom worthy of a separate designation, with the possible exception of the cellular and epithelioid forms of fibrous histiocytoma. The former appears to have a higher risk of local recurrence and often poses a diagnostic challenge to distinguish it from more aggressive lesions such as fibrosarcoma, whereas the epithelioid fibrous histiocytoma can be confused with tumors of melanocytic lineage.

## Cellular Fibrous Histiocytoma

Cellular fibrous histiocytoma is a designation used for lesions characterized by increased cellularity and a more fasicular (and less storiform) growth pattern. Some cases of "dermatofibroma with subcutaneous extension"[30,56] and "dermatofibroma with potential for local recurrence"[25] are examples of this variant. Occurring in an age range and anatomic location similar to those for ordinary benign fibrous histiocytoma, these lesions are composed of a relatively monomorphic population of plump spindle cells arranged in longer fascicles with fewer inflammatory cells and giant cells. (Figs. 13–24, 13–25) In addition, mitotic activity is usually somewhat higher [mean 3 mitoses/10 high-power fields (HPF)], and subcutaneous extension more common (30%), than in the usual fibrous histiocytoma. About 10% undergo spontaneous central necrosis. Although the local recurrence rate of 25% for this form of fibrous histiocytoma seemingly contrasts with that of the ordinary form, it has not been demonstrated that cellularity is an independent predictor of recurrence. The high incidence of extension into the subcutis by this form of fibrous histiocytoma suggests that this feature might be equally significant. Nonetheless, we believe it is still useful for recognizing the cellular form of fibrous histiocytoma as a distinct variant, but we think it is also important to comment on extensive subcutaneous extension when present in fibrous histiocytomas of the usual type as a possible predictor of recurrence. Recently a distinct chromosomal translocation [t(4;17)] has been identified in this form of fibrous histiocytoma,[53] but it is not clear whether it uniquely identifies this variant or is a feature of all fibrous histiocytomas[53]

## Epithelioid Fibrous Histiocytoma

Epithelioid fibrous histiocytoma is defined as a fibrous histiocytoma in which one-half or more of the cells assume a rounded epithelioid shape.[26,49,54] It presents as solitary, red cutaneous nodules with an epidermal collarette similar to that of a pyogenic granuloma. The cells, large and polygonal with abundant eosinophilic cytoplasm, are somewhat similar to those of a reticulohistiocytoma. Transitions to areas of conventional fibrous histiocytoma are frequent (Figs. 13–26, 13–27, 13–28) The principal significance of this form of fibrous histiocytoma is that it may be mistaken for a variety of other tumors, particularly a Spitz nevus. The cells within epithelioid fibrous histiocytoma are variably factor XIIIa-positive but lack S-100 protein.[49]

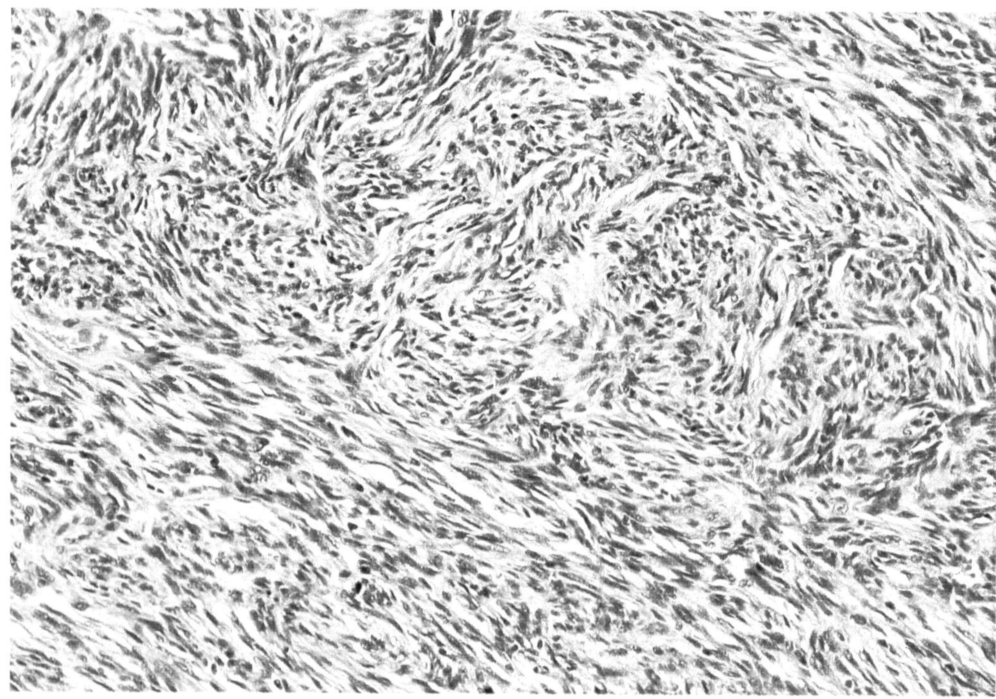

**FIGURE 13–24.** Cellular fibrous histiocytoma illustrating monomorphic spindle cells arranged in short and long fascicles.

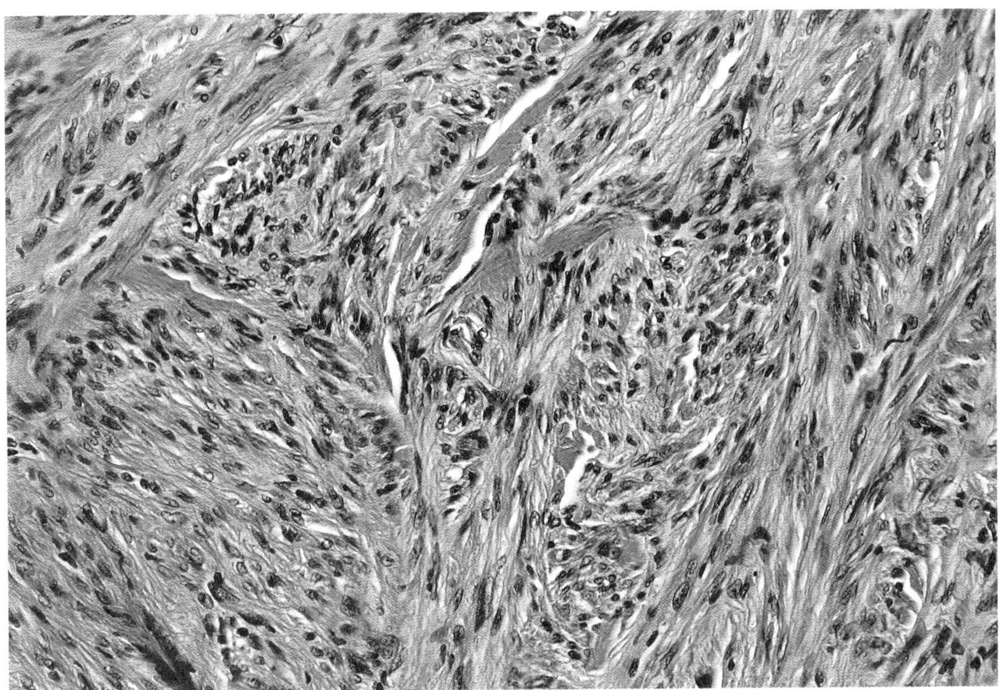

**FIGURE 13–25.** Cellular fibrous histiocytoma.

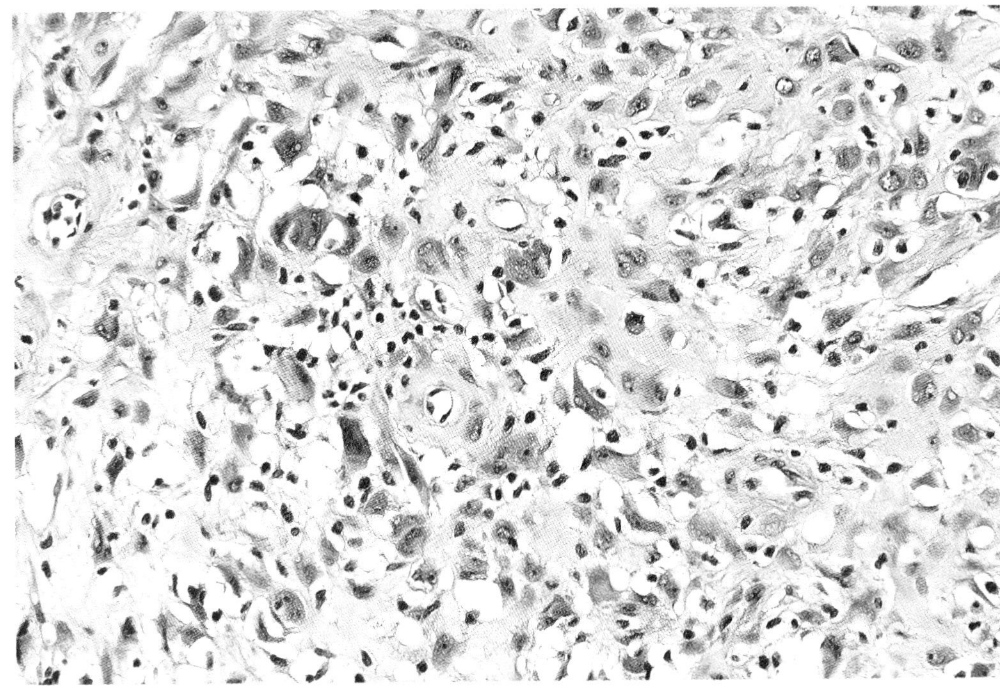

**FIGURE 13–26.** Epithelioid fibrous histiocytoma.

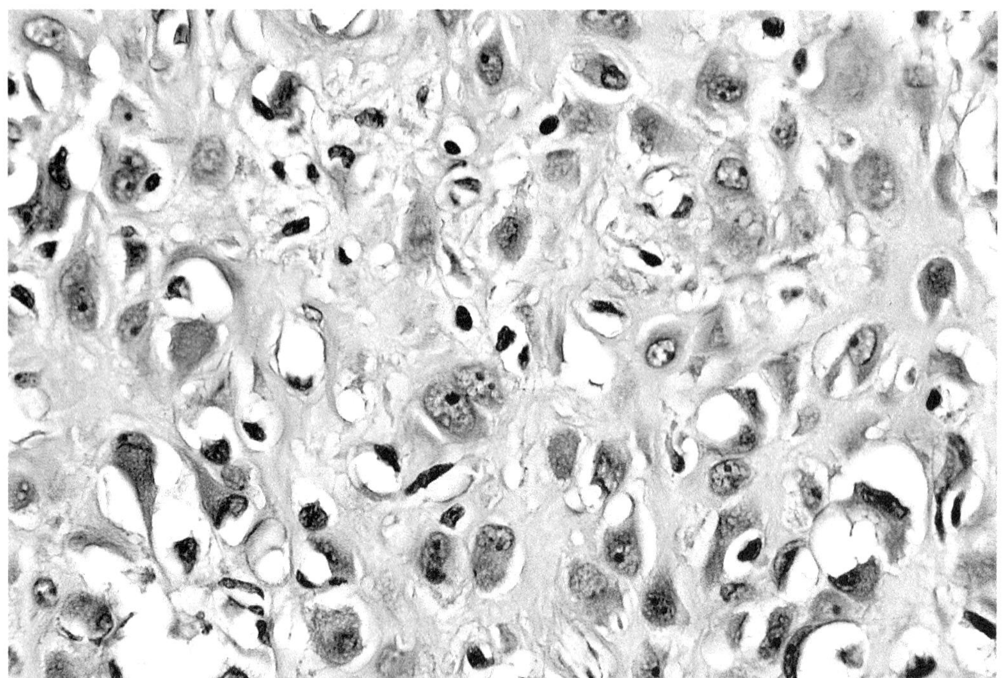

**FIGURE 13–27.** High power view of an epithelioid fibrous histiocytoma.

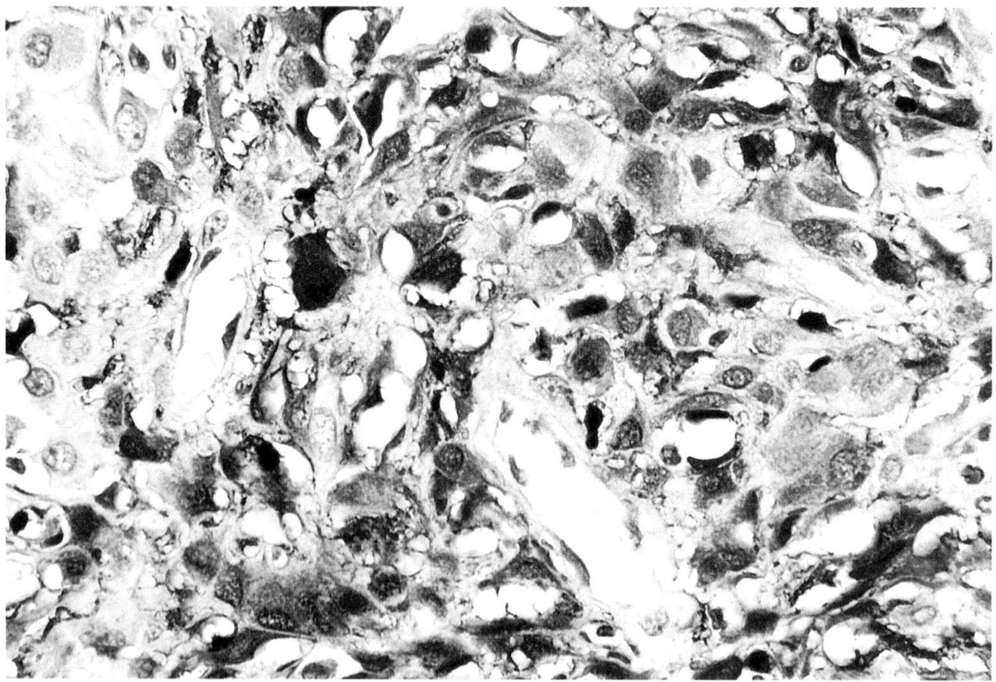

**FIGURE 13–28.** Factor XIIIa immunostain decorate cells of an epithelioid fibrous histiocytoma.

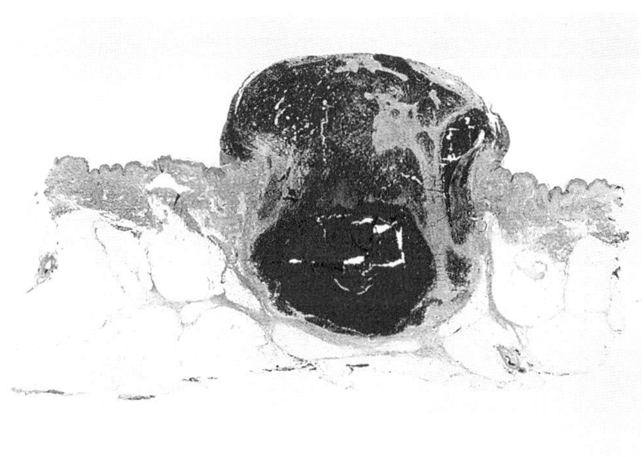

**FIGURE 13–29.** Aneurysmal fibrous histiocytoma.

## Aneurysmal Fibrous Histiocytoma

Approximately 1–2% of benign fibrous histiocytomas undergo extensive cystic hemorrhage. Dubbed "aneurysmal fibrous histiocytomas," their significance resides in the fact that they can evolve rapidly as a result of of spontaneous intralesional hemorrhage.[13,37,46,58] Their blue to black color suggests the clinical diagnosis of a vascular or melanocytic tumor. At low power these lesions are seen to contain large blood-filled spaces lined by discohesive fragments of tumor rather than endothelium (Figs. 13–29 to 13–32). Hemosiderin may be abundant, and mitotic activity is often noted in the immediate vicinity of the hemorrhage. A 20% recurrence rate has been reported for these tumors, but there are too few cases to know if this is meaningful. Despite the similarity of names, the aneurysmal fibrous histiocytoma should be clearly distinguished from the angiomatoid (malignant) fibrous histiocytoma of childhood, a subcutaneous lesion often associated with systemic symptoms (see Chapter 14).

## Minor Histologic Variations

There are a number of rare and minor variations of benign fibrous histiocytoma.[31,39,47,52,55] They are principally important in that they evoke a somewhat different list of diagnostic considerations. Zelger et al. recently described a "clear cell dermatofibroma" in which most of the cells underwent a translucent clear-cell change[57] (Fig. 13–33). This lesion must be distinguished from clear-cell carcinomas or melanocytic tumors involving the skin. The cells are positive for factor XIII but not for melanocytic antigens. Fortuitous palisading of nuclei ("palisaded fibrous histiocytoma"[47]), extensive myxoid change ("myxoid dermatofibroma"[55]) or lipidization ("lipidized fibrous histiocytoma"[1]) (Fig. 13–34), and granular cell change have also been noted in fibrous histiocytomas.

# JUVENILE XANTHOGRANULOMA

Juvenile xanthogranuloma is a stable or regressing histiocytic lesion that usually occurs during child-

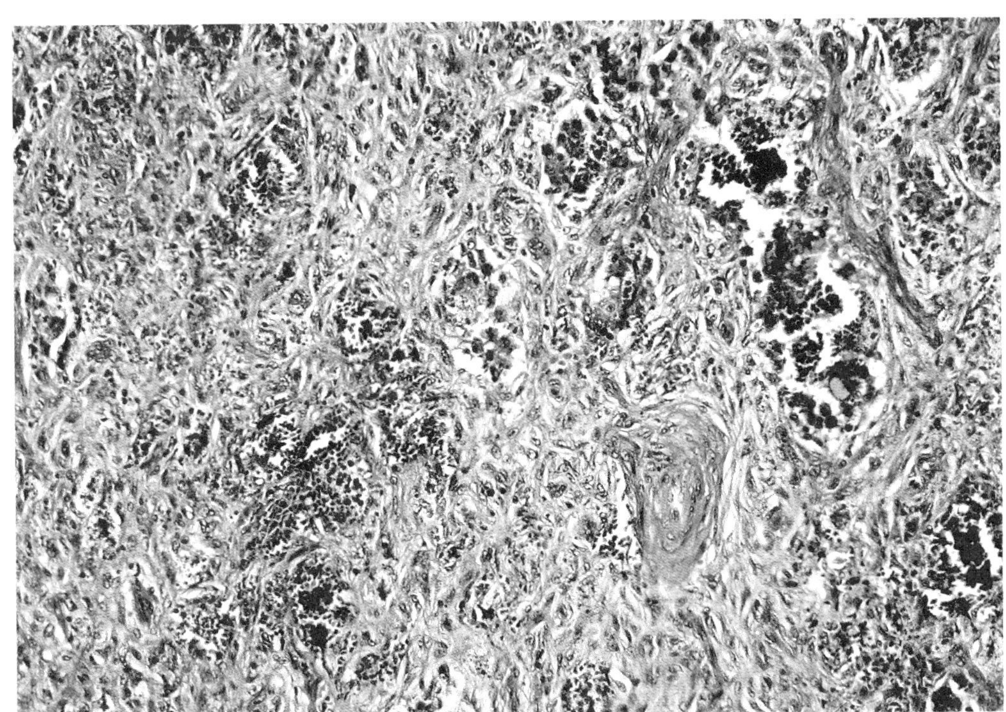

**FIGURE 13–30.** Cystic hemorrhage in an aneurysmal fibrous histiocytoma.

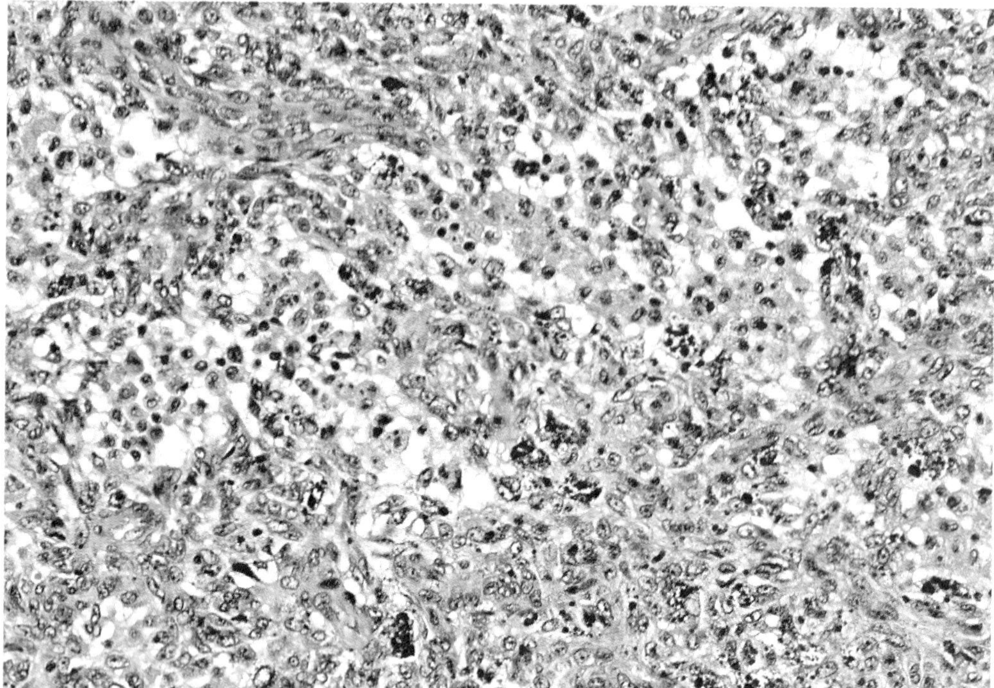

**FIGURE 13–31.** Hemosiderin deposits in an aneurysmal fibrous histiocytoma.

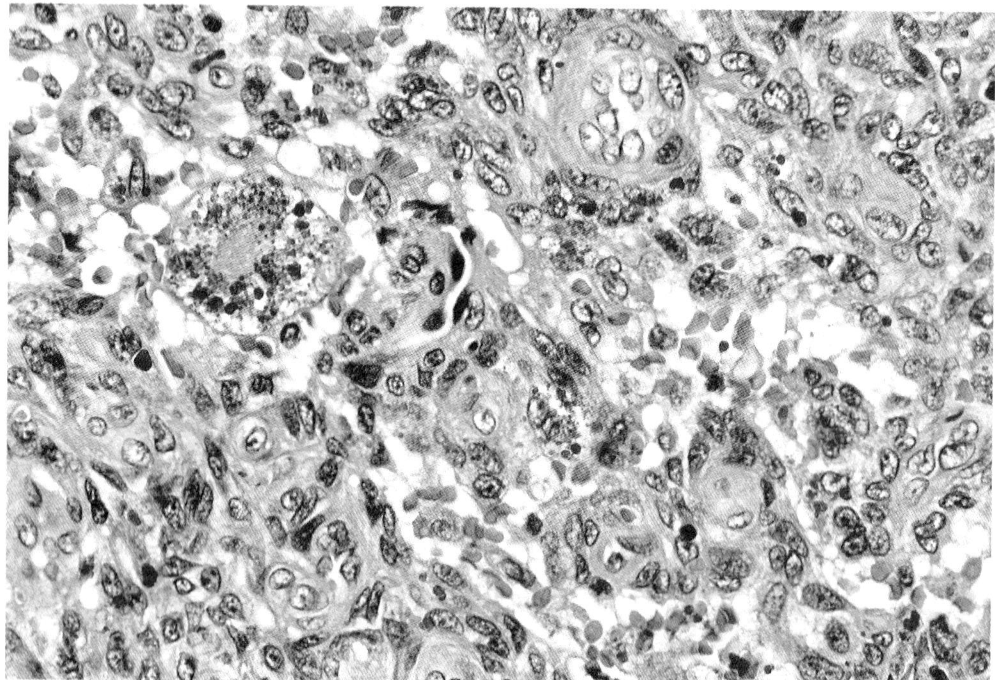

**FIGURE 13–32.** Hemosiderin deposits and cystic hemorrhage in an aneurysmal fibrous histiocytoma.

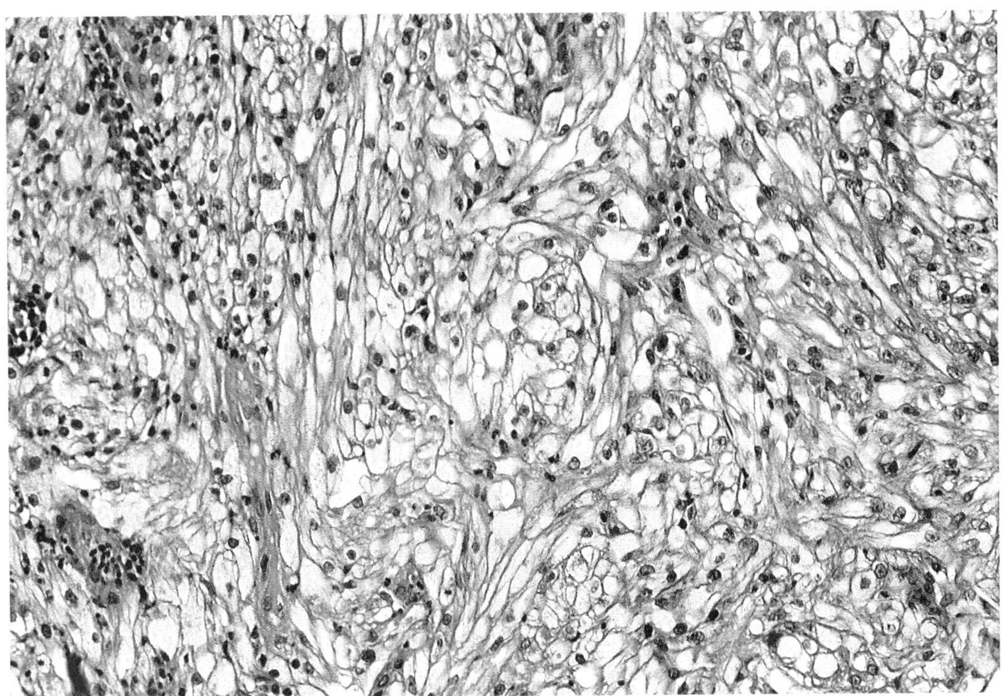

**FIGURE 13–33.** Clear-cell fibrous histiocytoma (dermatofibroma).

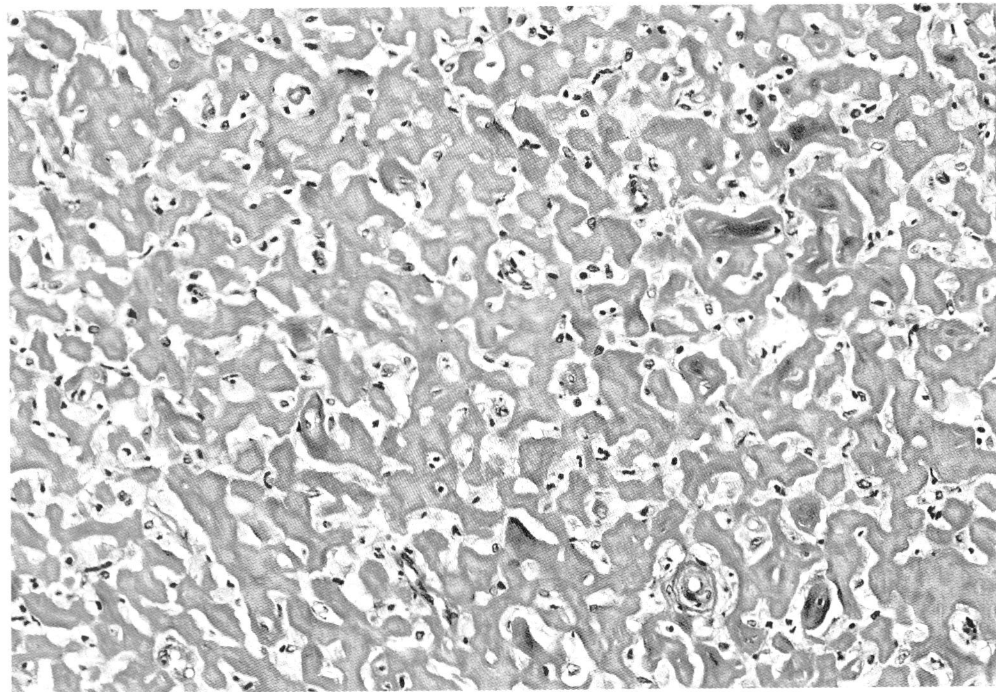

**FIGURE 13–34.** Lipidized fibrous histiocytoma.

**TABLE 13–1 CLASSIFICATION OF HISTIOCYTIC SYNDROMES IN CHILDREN**

**Class I:** Langerhans cell histiocytosis
  Forms of histiocytosis X (including eosinophilic granuloma and Hand-Schüller-Christian disease, among others)
**Class II:** mononuclear phagocytes other than Langerhans cells
  Hemophagocytic lymphohistiocytosis
  Infection-associated hemophagocytic syndrome
  Sinus histiocytosis with massive lymphadenopathy
  Juvenile xanthogranuloma
  Reticulohistiocytoma
**Class III:** malignant histiocytic disorders
  Acute monocytic leukemia
  Malignant histiocytosis
  True histiocytic lymphomas

Data are from the Writing Group of the Histiocyte Society.[87]

hood.[59,68,69,77,81] It is clearly distinct from the Langerhans cell histiocytosis and for that reason is grouped with the non-X (class II) forms of histiocytosis of childhood, which includes a number of other non-Langerhans cell histiocytic processes (Table 13–1).[87] The lesion(s) usually develop during infancy and is (are) characterized by one or more cutaneous nodules and less often by additional lesions in deep soft tissue or organs.[60,63,65,70,72,74,79,86] As a rule, those that develop after the age of 2 years or in adults are usually solitary.[88] These lesions have also been referred to as congenital xanthoma multiplex or nevoxanthoendothelioma.[75] Because the lesions are distinct from ordinary xanthomas and have no relation to endothelial cells, the term *juvenile xanthogranuloma* has been used for the past three decades. Tahan et al.[85] suggested that it be changed to xanthogranuloma because 15–30% of these lesions occur in individuals older than 20 years of age. Use of this term alone, we believe, could be problematic, as xanthogranuloma has been used for a variety of tumorous and reactive conditions whose pathogenesis varies.

## Clinical Findings and Gross Appearance

This disease may occur exclusively as a cutaneous lesion or a disease affecting deep soft tissue or parenchymal organs. In the more common cutaneous form, one or more nodules develop shortly after birth, although approximately one-fifth of the patients have lesions at birth. Two-thirds of patients develop the lesions by age 6 months. Depending on the series, 10–40% of patients develop the lesion after the age of 20 years.[71,73,79] There is no underlying lipid abnormality, and no well established familial incidence, although rare reports have documented the disease in parent and offspring. A finding of uncertain significance is the association of this disease with neurofibromatosis[71,73,79] and urticaria pigmentosa.[64]

About half of the lesions develop on the head and neck, followed by the trunk and extremities. They measure a few millimeters to a few centimeters in diameter. The early lesions are red papules (Fig. 13–35), and the older lesions are brown or yellow. Following a limited period of growth most nodules regress spontaneously, leaving a depressed, sometimes hyperpigmented area of skin. In patients with numerous skin nodules the tumors may appear in crops. Older lesions begin to regress as new ones emerge, so lesions of various ages may be present simultaneously. Although most lesions subside by adolescence, those that develop after age 20 may persist in a stable form.[62]

In the less common form of the disease, cutaneous lesions may be accompanied by similar lesions in other sites, such as the eye,[82] lung,[73,74] epicardium,[65,80,86] oral cavity,[73] and testis.[68] In a large series of referral cases, 5% of juvenile xanthogranulomas oc-

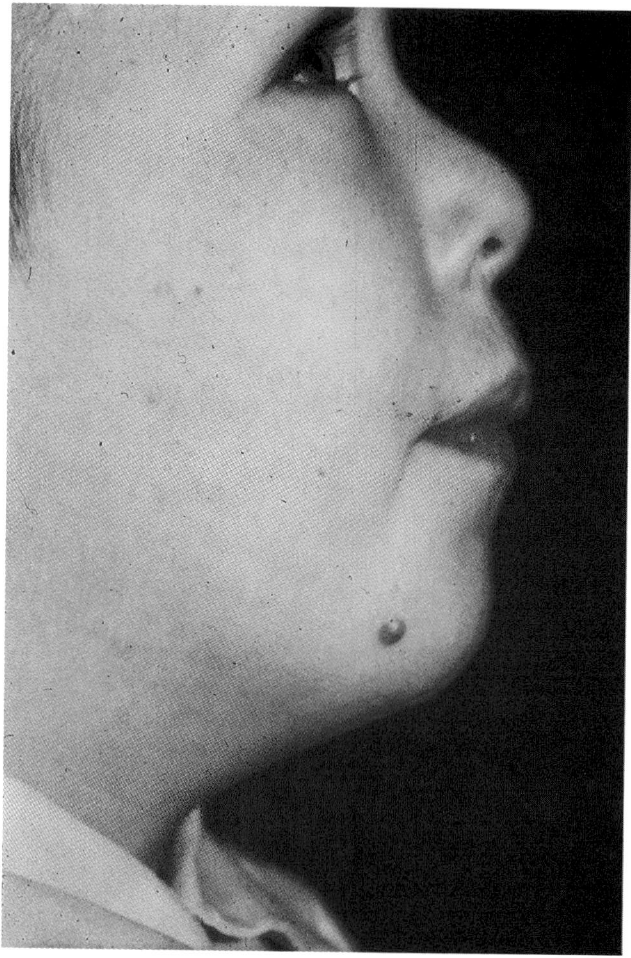

**FIGURE 13–35.** Clinical appearance of a juvenile xanthogranuloma. (Case courtesy of Dr. Elson Helwig.)

curred in deep soft tissue (usually skeletal muscle) or parenchymal organs.[69] In such patients the presenting symptoms are often referable to the extracutaneous tumor, and the skin lesions may be overlooked or appear later. The eye is the most common extracutaneous site, and patients may present with anterior chamber hemorrhage and glaucoma. An unusual presentation was that of profound cyanosis in a 3-month-old child with a tumor of the epicardium.[65,80,86]

## Microscopic Findings

Juvenile xanthogranulomas are similar whether they occur in children or adults.[88] There is a tendency, however, for deep lesions to appear more monomorphic and less lipidized[76] (Figs. 13–36, 13–37). The cutaneous lesions consist of sheets of histiocytes involving the dermis and extending to, but not invading, the flattened epidermis (Fig. 13–36). The infiltrate closely apposes adnexal structures and extends into the subcutis. Deeply situated juvenile xanthogranulomas appear circumscribed but blend with or infiltrate skeletal muscle at their periphery (Fig. 13–37). In both forms of the disease the histiocytes are well differentiated and exhibit little pleomorphism and only rare mitoses. The cytoplasm varies, depending on the amount of lipid present. Early lesions have little lipid; hence the cells have a homogeneous amphophilic or eosinophilic cytoplasm (Fig. 13–38). In older lesions the cells have a finely vacuolated or even xanthomatous cytoplasm (Figs. 13–39, 13–40).[3] Giant cells, including Touton giant cells, are typical of this lesion (Figs. 13–41, 13–42) but may vary considerably in number from one area to another or from lesion to lesion. Usually a modest number of inflammatory cells are present, consisting of both acute and chronic inflammatory cells, especially eosinophils. Longstanding or regressive lesions eventually develop an interstitial fibrosis and even a vague storiform pattern (Fig. 13–43), so they may resemble the more conventional fibrous histiocytoma seen in adults.

Electron microscopic studies show that the cells have characteristics of histiocytes.[66,67] They have numerous pseudopodia, lipid droplets, and lysosomes. Lipid, however, is not present to any extent within vessel walls,[66] in contrast to certain types of eruptive xanthoma. Langerhans' granules, tubular organelles associated with forms of histiocytosis X,[5,7] have not been demonstrated.[67] The cells have a phenotypic profile indicative of a histiocyte of the non-Langerhans type. They express CD68, $\alpha_1$-antitrypsin, $\alpha_1$-antichymotrypsin, lysozyme,[76,88] and CD31. Factor XIIIa can be demonstrated peripherally and to a lesser extent in the central portions of the lesion.

## Differential Diagnosis

Juvenile xanthogranuloma must be differentiated from forms of *Langerhans cell histiocytosis* involving skin.[89] Juvenile xanthogranuloma does not generally

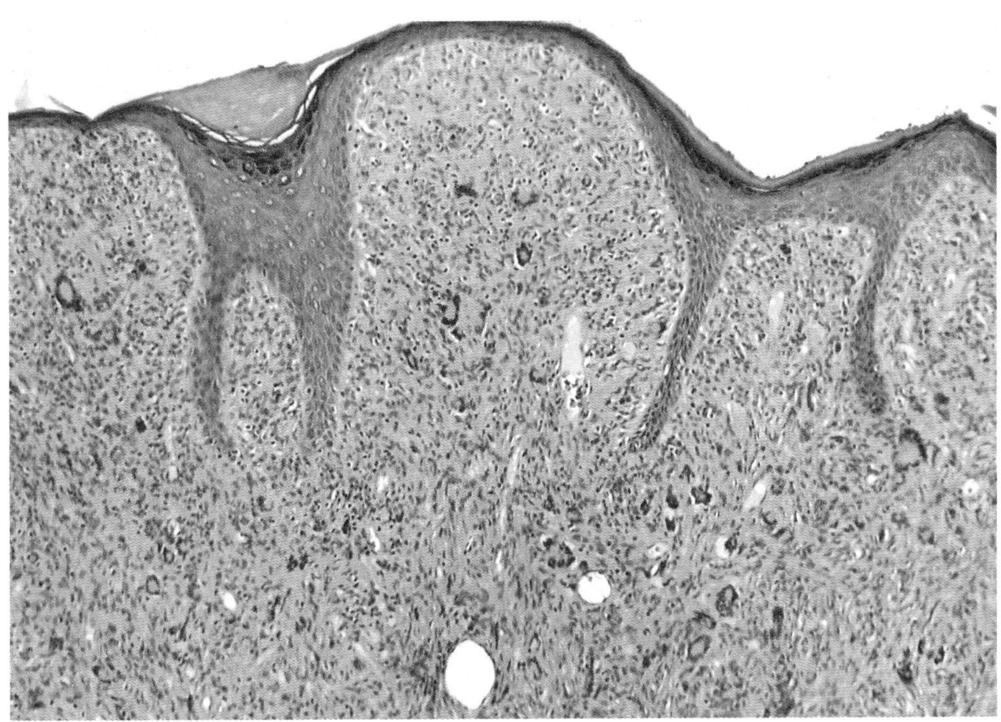

**FIGURE 13–36.** Juvenile xanthogranuloma.

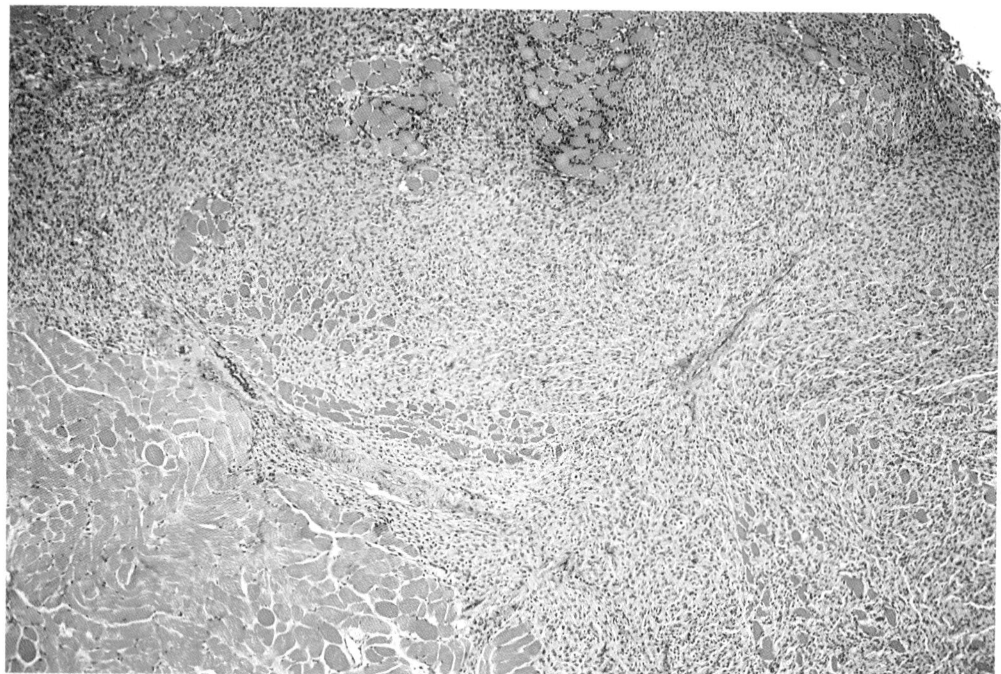

**FIGURE 13–37.** Deep juvenile xanthogranuloma infiltrating muscle.

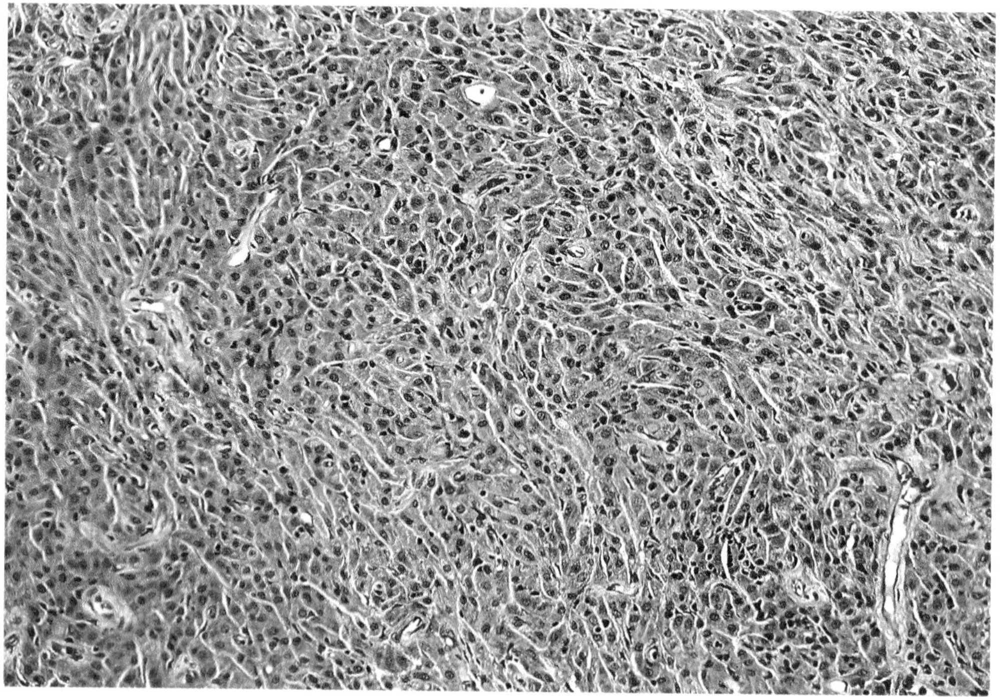

**FIGURE 13–38.** Early juvenile xanthogranuloma composed of nonlipidized histiocytes.

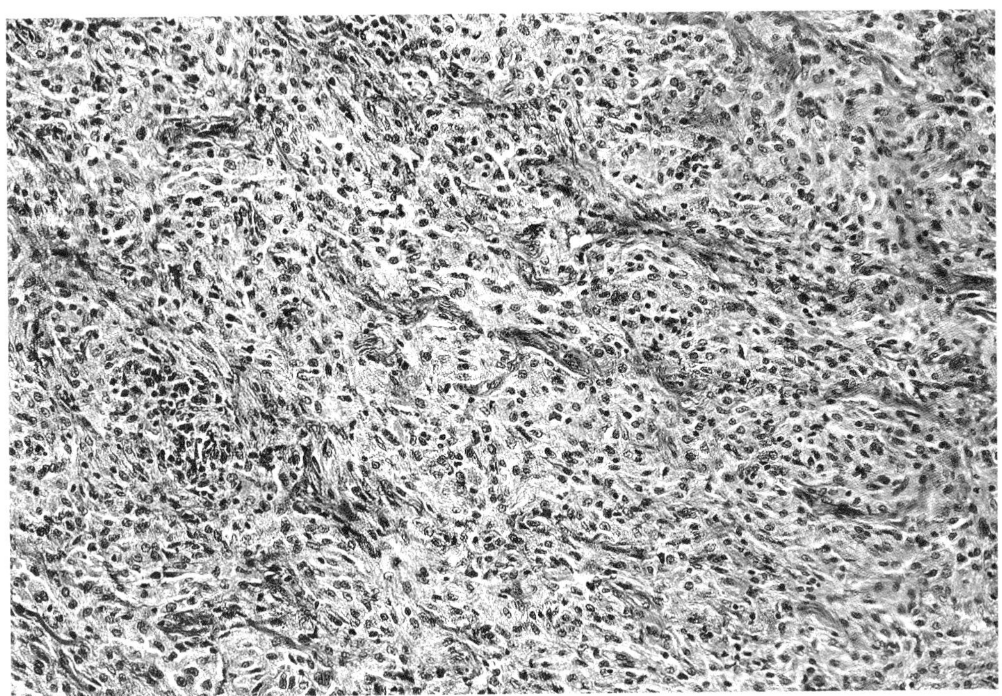

**FIGURE 13–39.** Lipidized juvenile xanthogranuloma.

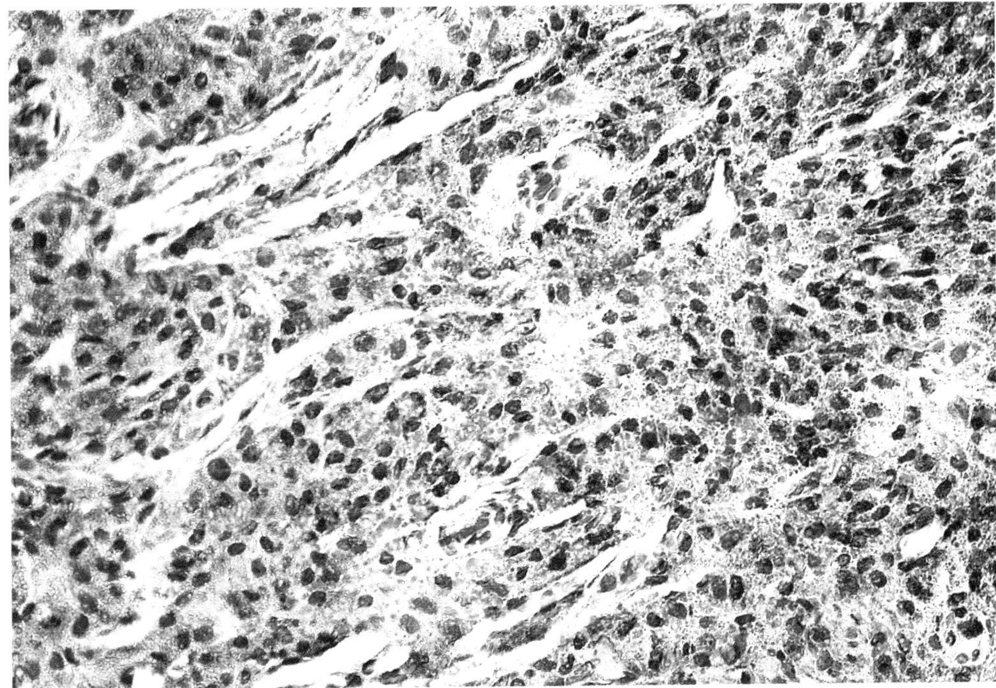

**FIGURE 13–40.** Fat stain showing extensive lipid within a juvenile xanthogranuloma.

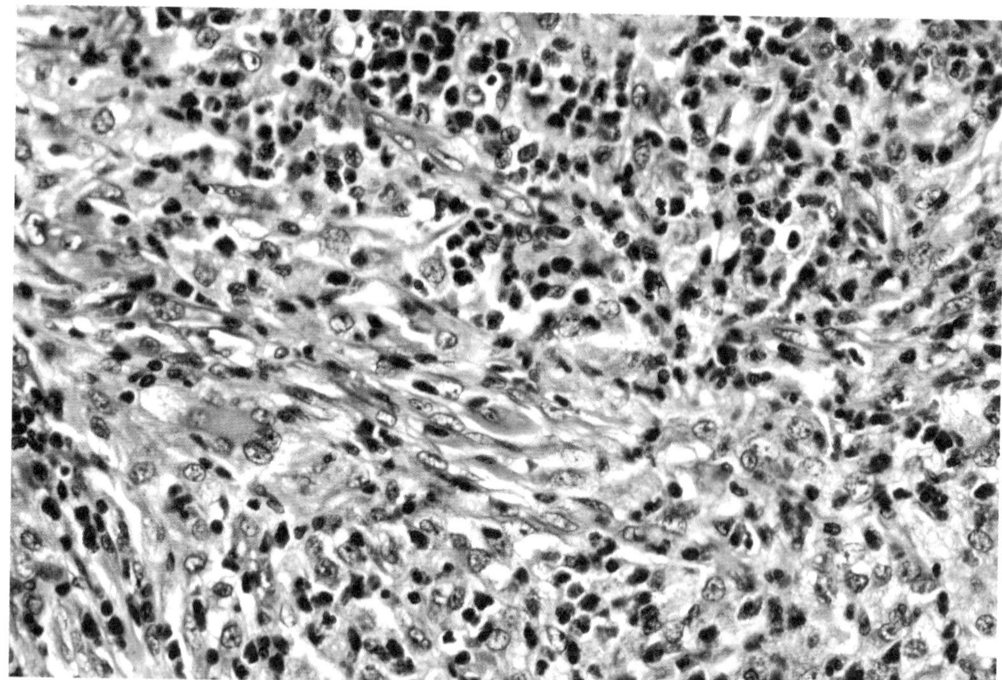

**FIGURE 13-41.** Juvenile xanthogranuloma with an eosinophilic infiltrate.

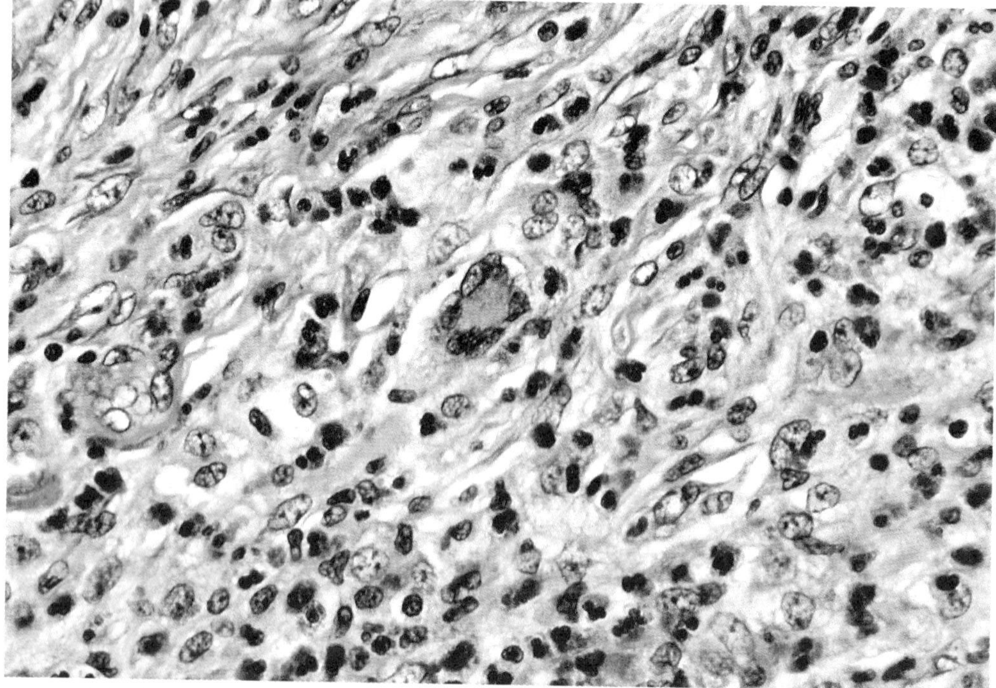

**FIGURE 13-42.** Juvenile xanthogranuloma with eosinophils and Touton giant cells.

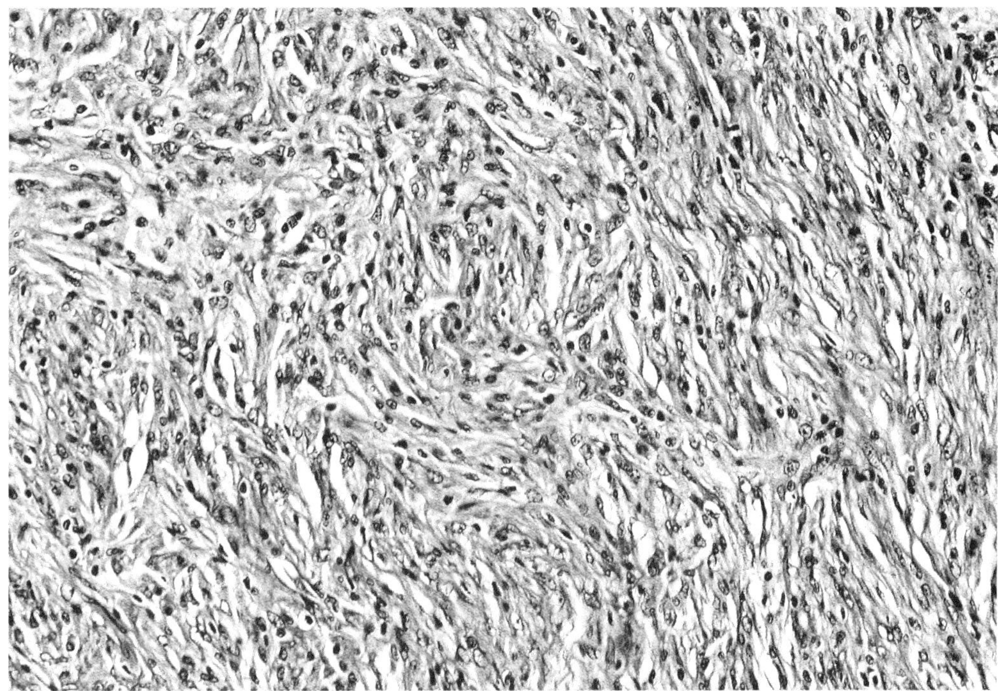

**FIGURE 13–43.** Late juvenile xanthogranuloma with fibrosis.

invade the epidermis and shows greater cellular cohesion and fewer eosinophils than Langerhans cell histiocytosis. Touton giant cells, a feature of juvenile xanthogranuloma, are typically absent in Langerhans cell histiocytosis; but when these cells are scarce, distinction of the two diseases may be difficult. In these situations, ultrastructural studies documenting the presence or absence of Langerhans' granules and immunostaining for S-100 protein may be required. The latter is stongly positive in Langerhans cell histiocytosis but is negative or present in scattered cells juvenile xanthogranuloma. Usually juvenile xanthogranuloma can be easily distinguished from *xanthomas* histologically because the latter contain a more uniform population of foamy cells and lack Touton giant cells and acute inflammation. Moreover, xanthomas associated with hypercholesterolemia often have large extracellular cholesterol deposits. The greater uniformity of juvenile xanthogranuloma, the usual lack of a storiform pattern, and the distinctive clinical setting distinguish it from *solitary fibrous histiocytoma of adults.*

## Discussion

The prognosis for patients with this disease is excellent. The skin lesions usually regress or at least stabilize with time, and even large, deeply located tumors pursue a favorable course. One patient with a large epicardial tumor was alive 13 months following excision.[65,80,86] Another child with skin lesions of juvenile xanthogranuloma proved on biopsy and pulmonary nodules presumed to be juvenile xanthogranulomas was well with no therapy at 4 years of age.[74] Therefore conservative therapy is indicated. Only one patient died with the disease and had lesions of the lung and testes at autopsy,[68] but death was due to other causes.[68] Radiotherapy has been employed for lesions in inaccessible locations such as the eye.[65]

Although the exact nature of this disease is unsettled, theories concerning its histogenesis have undergone considerable revision since the early description by McDonagh in 1912.[75] He coined the term nevoxanthoendothelioma because he believed that the tumor emanated from the vascular endothelium and that the Touton giant cells were small vessels with diminished or obliterated lumens. Others failed to confirm the continuity of the tumor cells and the endothelium and suggested the term juvenile xanthogranuloma.[68] This term not only underscores the histiocytic properties of the lipid-filled tumor cells, it distinguishes this disease from other xanthomatous lesions of childhood. Unlike the usual forms of pediatric xanthomas, juvenile xanthogranulomas occur at a younger age and are not associated with lipid abnormalities.

The question remains as to whether these lesions represent a true neoplasm or an unusual reactive process. The involutional nature of the disease, although not completely excluding a neoplasm with limited growth potential, argues for a reactive process. It has been suggested that the disease represents a response to viral infection. Circumstantial evidence for this idea is derived from an unusual case of juvenile xanthogranuloma that occurred in a parotid gland positive for the presence of cytomegalovirus[60] and by induction of similar tumors experimentally.[61,78,84] Viral studies in a group of patients with juvenile xanthogranuloma were negative.[76]

## SOLITARY RETICULOHISTIOCYTOMA

Reticulohistiocytoma is a distinctive but rare lesion of adult life. It consists of nodules of eosinophilic histiocytes, often exhibiting multinucleation. It has been suggested that the solitary forms of reticulohistiocytoma are similar to adult xanthogranulomas, the distinction being largely based on whether there is a predominance of multinucleated eosinophilic histiocytes. On the other hand, solitary reticulohistiocytoma appears to be a fundamentally different disease from multicentric reticulohistiocytomas, both clinically and immunophenotypically.[108]

Solitary reticulohistiocytoma is a nodular dermatosis (reticulohistiocytoma, reticulohistiocytic granuloma)[103,108] that develops at any body site. Most patients are adult men, and fewer than one-fifth have multiple tumors.[108] The lesions are yellow-brown papules composed of dense circumscribed dermal nodules of deeply eosinophilic histiocytes (Figs. 13–44, 13–45, 13–46). Multinucleated forms, often 20–30 times larger than their mononuclear counterparts, with abundant nuclei are common. The so-called oncocytic histiocytes may display some degree of nuclear atypia, and occasionally mitotic figures are noted. In some areas there is a subtle degree of spindling of the histiocytes, although frankly spindled areas and Touton giant cells such as are seen in fibrous histiocytomas are absent. Occasional lymphocytes are present. Immunohistochemically, the lesions express several markers associated with the non-X forms of histiocytosis. They consistently express CD68, variably $\alpha_1$-antitrypsin, and lysozyme; but they lack S-100 protein.[112] They also express muscle-specific actin, an antigen that has been identified in the mononuclear cells of giant cell tumors of bone and in the mononuclear cells of soft tissue giant cell tumors of low malignant potential (see Chapter 14).

Isolated cutaneous lesions with some degree of pleomorphism must be distinguished from *superficial forms of malignant fibrous histiocytoma* (malignant giant cell tumor of soft parts), *carcinoma,* and *melanoma.* In contrast to superficial forms of malignant fibrous histiocytoma, these tumors are smaller and have fewer mitotic figures, less prominent spindling, and no necrosis. Unlike melanoma, there is no junctional activity, more interstitial collagen, and a less distinct organoid growth pattern. The frequent accompaniment of acute inflammatory cells and numerous multinucleated cells also aids in this distinction.

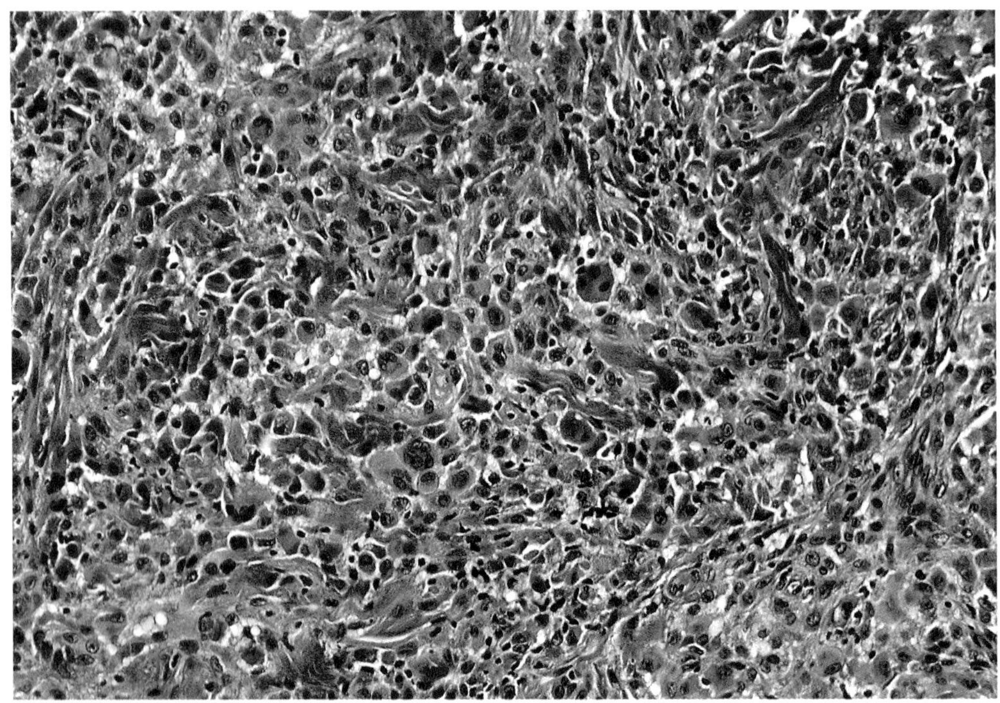

**FIGURE 13–44.** Reticulohistiocytoma.

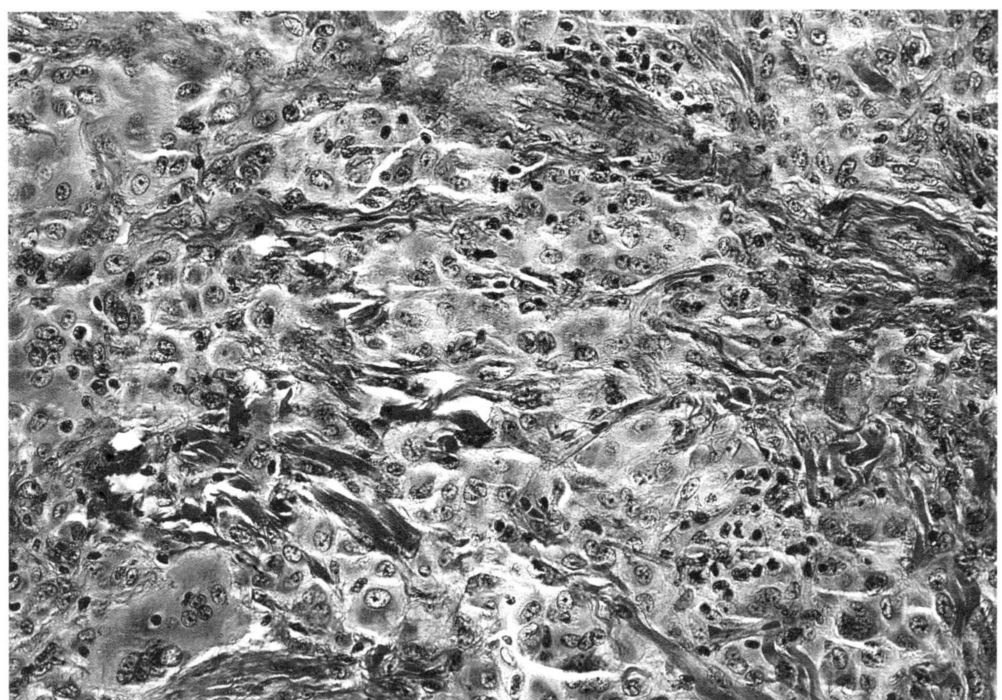

**FIGURE 13–45.** Reticulohistiocytoma.

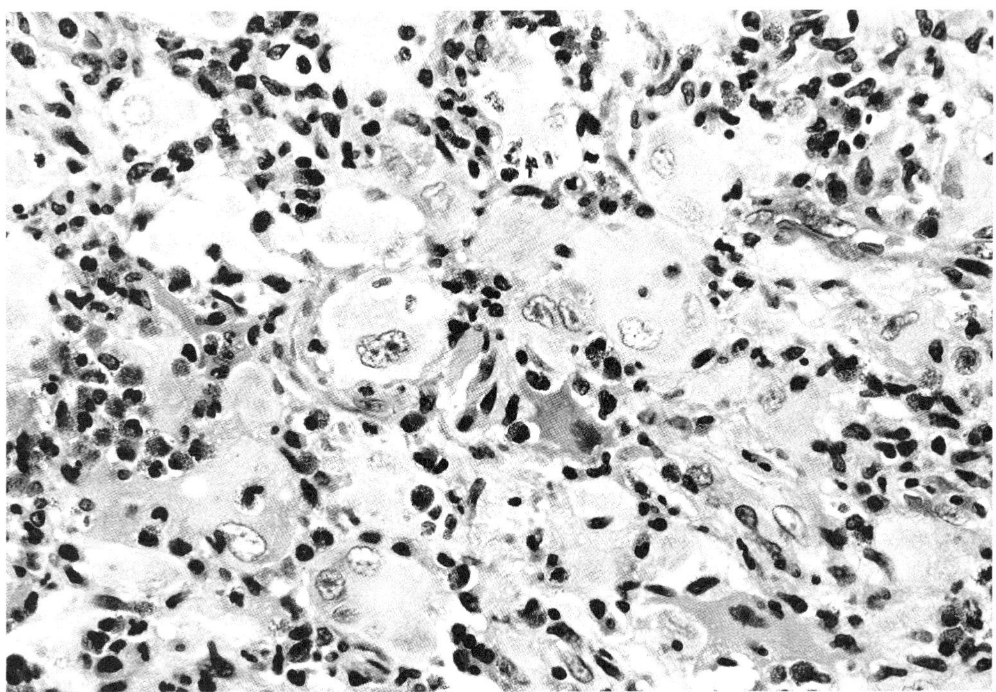

**FIGURE 13–46.** High-power view of a reticulohistiocytoma.

The lesions pursue a benign or self-limiting course. In one study[108] most patients with follow-up information were cured by simple excision; two patients developed a recurrence, and three had a nodule elsewhere. Several patients with multiple nodules noted spontaneous regression of a lesion.

## MULTICENTRIC RETICULOHISTIOCYTOSIS

In contrast to the cutaneous disease, multicentric reticulohistiocytosis is a systemic, occasionally paraneoplastic disease characterized by myriad symptoms including progressive symmetric, erosive arthritis, episodes of pyrexia, and weight loss.[90–93,95,106,109,111] Multiple cutaneous and mucosal nodules follow the arthritis within a period of months to years, although occasionally the skin lesions initiate the disease. The disease may be associated with a number of other conditions including tuberculosis, diabetes, Sjögren syndrome, hypothyroidism, Wegener's granulomatosis, polyarteritis,[90,105,110] celiac disease, and systemic lupus erythematosus.[113] In addition, malignancies of various types (carcinoma of the colon, breast, lung, ovary, and cervix; sarcoma; lymphoma) develop in about 30% of patients.[90,99] In one dramatic case, the constitutional symptoms regressed when the underlying neoplasm was treated.[103] Despite the fact that the various lipid materials accumulate within lesion cells, no consistent or specific serum lipid abnormality has been identified in the disease. The disease is usually marked by a waxing and waning course over a period of several years, eventually leaving most patients with a disfiguring, crippling arthritis that most severely affects the distal interphalangeal joint and bears some similarity to rheumatoid arthritis (Fig. 13–47).

### Pathologic Findings

The cutaneous lesions consist of circumscribed collections of histiocytes confined to the dermis or extending to the epidermis and subcutis (Fig. 13–21). Delicate reticulin fibers are present around individual cells, and occasionally acute and chronic inflammatory cells are present. Although multinucleated eosinophilic histiocytes characterize both this disease and the solitary reticulohistiocytoma, these histiocytes tend to be smaller, are less eosinophilic, and show only a minor degree of multinucleation. Similar deposits may be seen in other involved organs such as synovium, bone, and lymph nodes. In most cases they stain strongly with Sudan black B fat stain, oil red O, and periodic acid-Schiff (PAS) after diastase digestion and are believed to contain a mixture of phospholipid, mucoprotein or glycoprotein, and neutral fat.[90] Immunohistochemically, these cells contrast slightly with those of solitary reticulohistiocytoma in that they lack muscle-specific actin and factor XIIIa; but they express CD68, $\alpha_1$-antitrypsin, and lysozyme. Electron microscopy shows that the histiocytes have numerous lipid droplets and a dilated rough endoplasmic reticulum filled with granular material.[94] Langerhans' granules, tubular structures present in certain normal and neoplastic[5] histiocytes, are usually not identified in multicentric reticulohistiocytosis,[100,102] although there have been some reports to the contrary.[94,97]

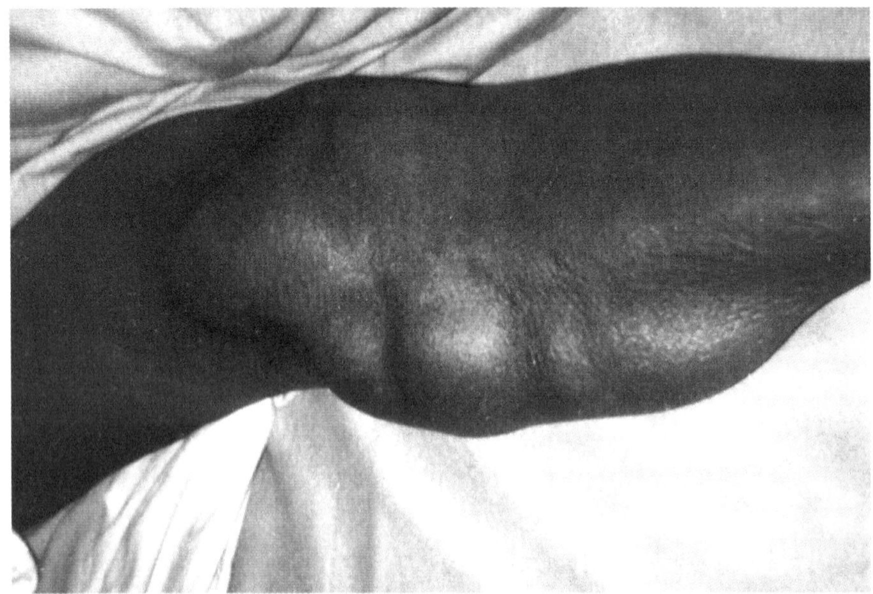

**FIGURE 13–47.** Deforming arthritis of the elbow in a patient with multicentric reticulohistiocytosis.

**TABLE 13–2 PLASMA LIPOPROTEIN PHENOTYPES**

| Disorder | I | IIa | IIb | III | IV | V |
|---|---|---|---|---|---|---|
| **Lipoprotein elevation** | Chylomicrons | LDL | LDL, VLDL | Chylomicrons, VLDL remnants | VLDL | Chylomicrons, VLDL |
| **Xanthoma** | Eruptive | Tendon, tuberous | None | Palmar, tuberous, eruptive | None | Eruptive |
| **Molecular defect** | Lipoprotein lipase, apoC-II | LDL receptor, apoB-100 | Unknown | ApoE | Unknown | Unknown |

* Modified from Rader DJ. Disorders of lipid metabolism. In: Kelley WN (ed) Textbook of Internal Medicine, 3rd ed. Lippincott-Raven, Philadelphia, 1997.
LDL, low density lipoproteins; VLDL, very low density lipoproteins; apo/Apo, apolipoprotein.

### Discussion

Usually this disease poses few diagnostic problems for the pathologist because evaluation of the skin lesions is aided immeasurably by the clinical history and in some cases by a confirmatory biopsy of synovium or other tissue. The etiology of this condition remains obscure, however. Because a disproportionately large number of patients with multicentric reticulohistiocytosis have associated malignancies or other systemic disease, some have suggested that the disease is a reflection of an altered immune state. It furthermore appears that the histiocytes in these lesions have the ability to secrete a wide variety of substances that may be responsible for many of the manifestations of the disease.[102,104,112] β-Interleukin-1β and platelet-derived growth factor-β, both of which promote synovial proliferation, can be identified immunohistochemically in the histiocytes.[104] Urokinase is elevated in synovial tissue and could, by activation of collagenase, account for the destruction of articular tissue. Although in the past there was little or no therapy for the disease, a number of reports have attested to alleviation of the condition with the use of chemotherapeutic agents, including alkylating agents.[96,98,101]

## XANTHOMA

Xanthoma is a localized collection of tissue histiocytes containing lipid.[114,120,123,131,142,143] It is not a true tumor but, rather, a reactive histiocyte proliferation that occurs in response to alterations in serum lipids. Xanthomas may develop in most primary and some secondary (primary biliary cirrhosis, diabetes mellitus) hyperlipoproteinemias and occasionally in the normolipemic state. A brief synopsis of the various primary hyperlipidemias and their associated defects is provided in Table 13–2. Usually xanthomas occur in the skin and subcutis,[116,119,133,134] but occasionally they involve deep soft tissue such as tendons (xanthoma of the tendon sheath)[119,122,124,125,132] or synovium.[121]

### Clinical Findings and Gross Appearance

Cutaneous xanthomas are designated according to their gross appearance and clinical presentation (Table 13–3). Eruptive xanthomas are small, yellow papules with a predilection for the gluteal surfaces. They develop in individuals with hyperlipoproteinemia types I, III, and V. Tuberous xanthomas, large plaque-like lesions of the subcutis, are usually located on the

**TABLE 13–3 COMPARISON OF CLINICAL TYPES OF XANTHOMA**

| Type of Xanthoma | Association with Lipoprotein Phenotype | Location | Histologic Appearance |
|---|---|---|---|
| **Eruptive** | I, III, V | Predilection for buttocks | Foamy and nonfoamy histiocytes |
| **Tuberous** | IIa, III | Elbows, buttocks, knees, fingers | Foamy histiocytes, extracellular cholesterol deposits, fibrosis, inflammation |
| **Tendinous** | IIa, cerebrotendinous xanthomatosis | Tendons of hands and feet, Achilles tendon | Similar to tuberous xanthoma |
| **Xanthelasma** | IIa, III | Eyelids | Foamy histiocytes |
| **Plane** | Primary biliary cirrhosis III, normolipemic states | Skin creases of palms | Foamy histiocytes |

buttocks, elbows, knees, and fingers and are seen with type IIa or III hyperlipoproteinemia. Plane xanthomas occur in skinfolds, such as the palmar creases, and are characteristic of type III hyperlipoproteinemia; or they are associated with primary biliary cirrhosis. Occasionally they occur in normolipemic persons, and in this setting they have a high association with reticuloendothelial malignancies.[130,133] Xanthelasmas are xanthomas of the eyelid and usually are observed in normolipemic persons,[3] although they also occur in those with type IIa or III hyperlipoproteinemia. The last three types of xanthoma contain large amounts of cholesterol and its esters, which may be demonstrated under polarized light in fresh tissue as birefringent crystals.

Deep xanthomas occur most frequently in tendon[119,122,124,125,132] or synovium[121] and rarely bone.[127,139] Most tendinous xanthomas occur in the setting of hypercholesterolemia associated with type IIa hyperlipoproteinemia (Fig. 13–48). Usually the severity of the xanthoma is roughly proportional to the severity and duration of the increased cholesterol levels. A rare inherited disease known as cerebrotendinous xanthomatosis is now also recognized as a cause of bilateral xanthomas occurring exclusively in the Achilles tendon.[128,129,140] This disease is an autosomal recessive disorder caused by mutations in the gene for sterol 27-hydroxylase, an enzyme important for hepatic bile acid synthesis. As a result, bile acids are synthesized to the end-product cholestanol, which accumulates systemically, producing multiple signs and symptoms including dementia, ataxia, cataracts, and tendinous xanthomas. Recognition of this disease is important, as early treatment with chenodeoxycholic acid can prevent progression of clinical symptoms.

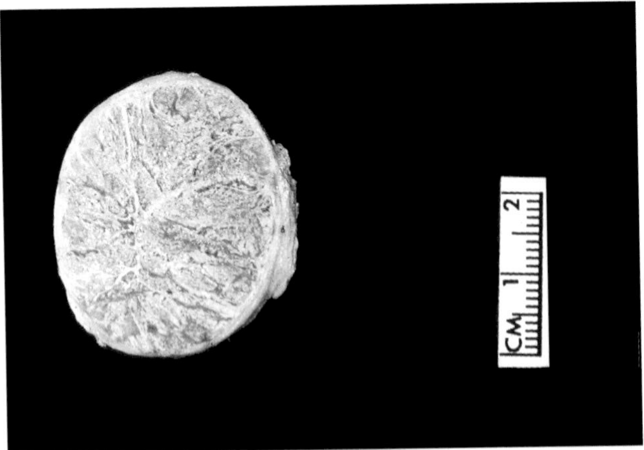


**FIGURE 13–48.** Xanthoma of the Achilles tendon cut in cross section. White bands correspond to residual tendinous tissue that has been spread apart by xanthomatous infiltration.

Most tendinous xanthomas present as painless, slowly growing masses that produce few symptoms unless joint function is compromised. The lesions may be solitary or multiple, and they occur in sites subjected to minor trauma such as the finger, wrist, and ankle. They are usually a few centimeters in diameter, although large lesions in excess of 20 cm have been reported in the Achilles tendon (Fig. 13–48). Xanthomas may be circumscribed or diffuse and are firmly attached to tendon but not to overlying skin. On cut section they have a variegated color ranging from yellow to brown to white, depending on the amount of lipid, hemorrhage, and fibrosis present from area to area. Like tuberous and plane xanthomas, they also have a high cholesterol content.

## Microscopic Findings

The various types of xanthoma differ in histologic appearance. Eruptive xanthoma, which represents an acute, evanescent lesion, contains a large proportion of nonfoamy histiocytes in addition to occasional foam cells and inflammatory cells. Tuberous and tendinous xanthomas are essentially identical (Figs. 13–49, 13–50, 13–51). Although in their early stages they may contain some nonfoamy histiocytes, the typical appearance is that of sheets of foamy histiocytes interspersed with occasional inflammatory cells. The histiocytes are bland with small pyknotic nuclei. Some cells contain fine granules of hemosiderin. Collections of extracellular cholesterol (cholesterol clefts) flanked by giant cells are conspicuous. Varying amounts of fibrosis may be present but are most marked in long-standing lesions. Plane xanthoma and xanthelasma are characterized by sheets of xanthoma cells, but they rarely exhibit the degree of fibrosis present in the foregoing two lesions.[3] Ultrastructurally, xanthoma cells of all of these lesions are similar and contain numerous clear vacuoles, presumably representing cholesterol or its esters.[115,144] Eruptive xanthomas, in addition, have fat in the vessel walls[135] and tissue macrophages.

## Discussion

Cutaneous xanthomas usually present few problems in diagnosis or management. The superficial location, gross appearance, and associated clinical findings leave little doubt as to the diagnosis. Xanthomas of the tendon sheath may be more problematic. The deep location and slow, persistent growth occasionally raise the question of sarcoma. When a biopsy is done, such lesions should be adequately sampled because giant cell tumors of the tendon sheath, diffuse villonodular synovitis, or sarcomas with xanthomatous change may focally resemble this lesion. The di-

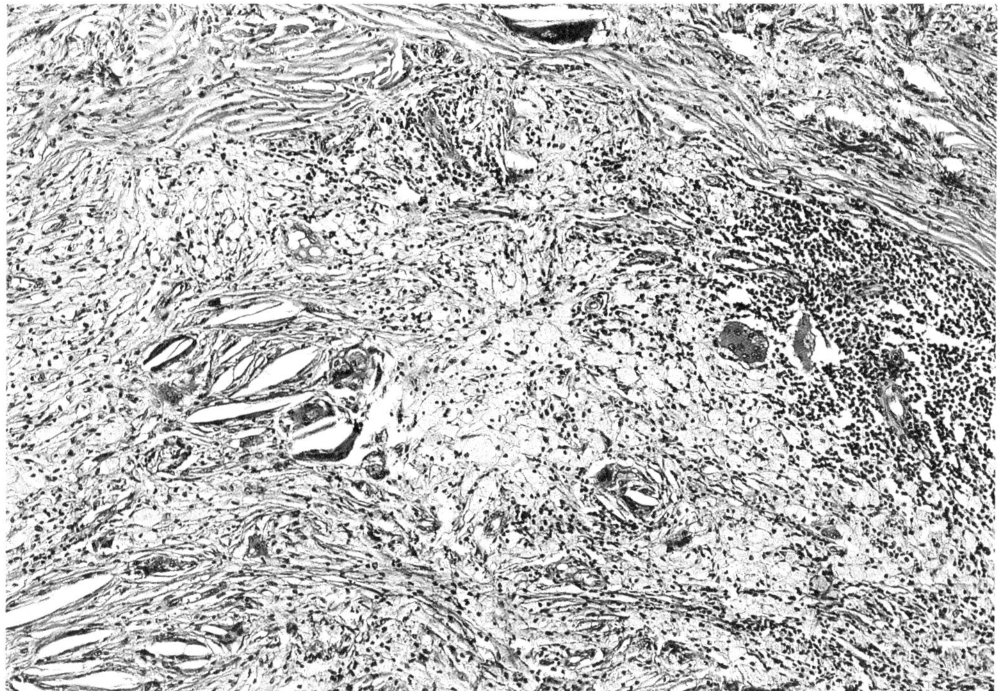

**FIGURE 13–49.** Tuberous xanthoma of the leg consisting of xanthoma cells admixed with inflammatory cells and giant cells surrounding cholesterol-containing clefts.

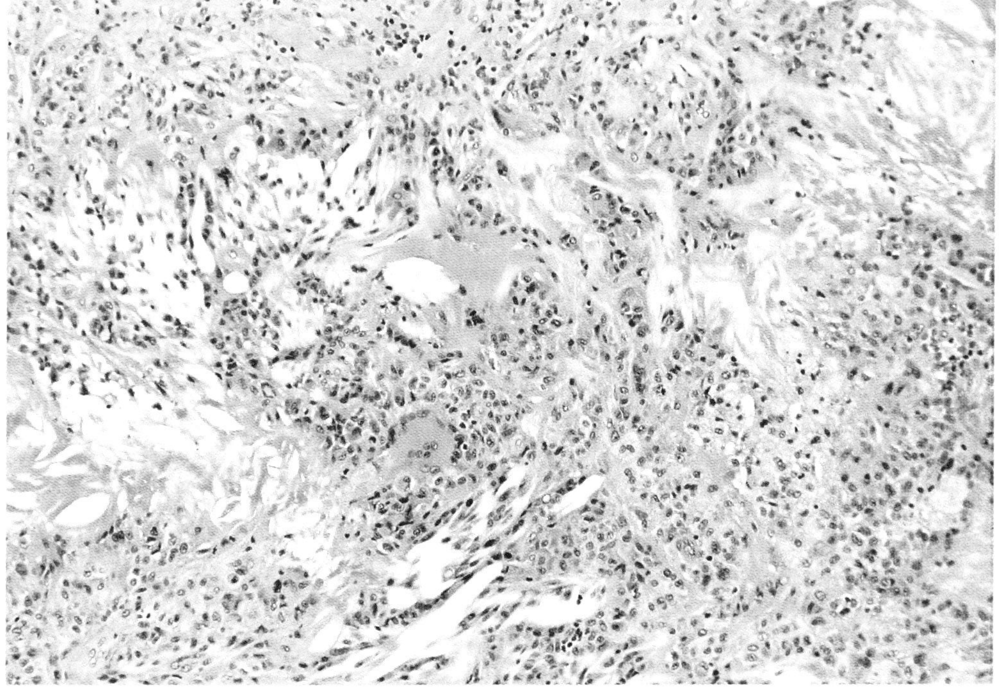

**FIGURE 13–50.** Tuberous xanthoma with xanthoma cells but without fibrosis or inflammation.

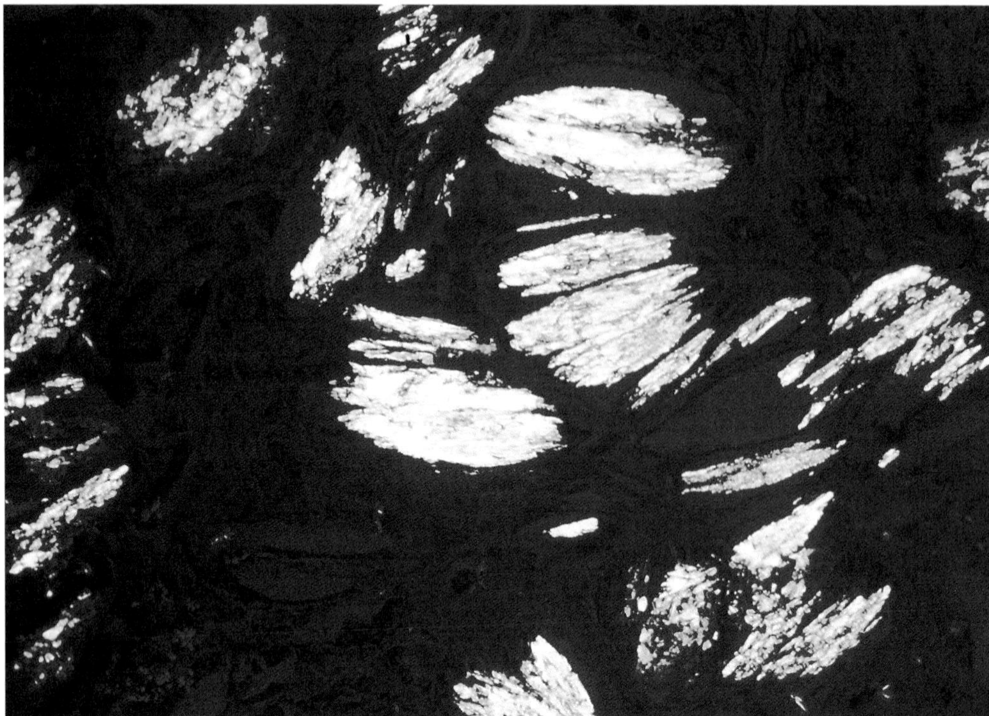

**FIGURE 13–51.** Frozen section of a xanthoma viewed under polarized light to illustrate numerous birefringent cholesterol crystals.

agnosis of xanthoma of the tendon sheath should always be considered in a patient with hypercholesterolemia, especially if the lesions are multiple.

Because of the nonneoplastic nature of these lesions, conservative therapy is generally recommended. In fact, xanthelasmas and tuberous xanthomas have regressed on medical therapy alone,[118,134] although months or years may be required before tangible benefits are appreciated. Soft tissue radiographs may be helpful for serial assessment of tendinous xanthomas under treatment.[126] Surgery, including excision with tendon reconstruction, has been reserved for large or symptomatic xanthomas. Surgically treated xanthomas may slowly recur, although generally reoperation is not necessary.[122] Irradiation has also been employed as therapy for these lesions, but there are few data to support its efficacy. Long-term treatment of cerebrotendinous xanthomatosis with chenodeoxycholic acid has resulted in alleviation of some of the neurologic symptoms but has not affected the tendinous xanthomas.[117]

Although xanthomas were formerly considered neoplastic, their association with hyperlipidemic states leaves little doubt that they are reactive lesions. Current evidence suggests that the lipid in them is derived from blood.[136,137,141] It has been demonstrated experimentally that serum lipoproteins leave the vascular compartment, traverse small vessels, and enter the macrophages of soft tissue.[137] This series of events can be confirmed ultrastructurally by the sequential finding of lipoprotein between endothelium and basement membrane and finally in the pericytes. Once ingested by macrophages the lipoprotein is degraded to lipid, and the lipid is released to the extracellular space. The fibrosis characteristic of mature or long-standing xanthomas is believed to be related to the fibrogenic properties of extracellular cholesterol.[113] Although xanthomas can potentially occur at any soft tissue site, the localization stimulus seems directly related to the vascular permeability, as agents that increase permeability (e.g., histamine) can accelerate xanthoma formation at a given site.[137] Likewise, minor trauma or injury that results in histamine release also accelerates xanthoma formation.[138] This observation provides an explanation for the common occurrence of such lesions in the tendons of the hands and feet.

## ATYPICAL FIBROXANTHOMA

Atypical fibroxanthoma is a pleomorphic spindle cell tumor that occurs principally on the actinic-damaged skin of the head and neck area of elderly persons. Conventionally, it has been classified among the benign fibrohistiocytic tumors because of its almost uniformly excellent prognosis following conservative therapy. The tumor is histologically indistinguishable from pleomorphic forms of malignant fibrous histiocytoma. For this reason, it seems best regarded conceptually as a superficial form of that tumor and is discussed in greater detail in Chapter 15. Its small size and superficial location probably account for the benign clinical course.

## RETROPERITONEAL XANTHOGRANULOMA

In 1935 Oberling described several patients with large retroperitoneal tumors consisting predominantly of xanthoma and inflammatory cells. Because of the polymorphic population of cells in these lesions, he believed they did not represent malignant tumors but, rather, variants of Hand-Schüller-Christian disease. The persistence of the term retroperitoneal xanthogranuloma has conveyed the general impression that such lesions are benign. However, in a critical review by Kahn of cases with adequate follow-up information, it was shown that almost three-fourths of patients either died of the tumor or were alive with persistent recurrent disease, and one-fourth had metastatic disease at autopsy (see Chapter 15). There is little doubt now that most retroperitoneal xanthogranulomas are malignant neoplasms and are probably best classified among the malignant fibrohistiocytic tumors. They are therefore discussed more fully in Chapter 15. Although there may be exceptional cases of "benign retroperitoneal xanthogranuloma," this diagnosis should be assigned with extreme caution. It should be considered only in cases that have been carefully sampled and display little or no atypia of the constituent cells.

## MISCELLANEOUS HISTIOCYTIC REACTIONS RESEMBLING NEOPLASM

Histiocytic reactions may be difficult to distinguish from neoplasms when they are localized lesions with few inflammatory cells. In these cases it is necessary to obtain detailed clinical data, perform special staining procedures for microorganisms, and examine the specimen under polarized light for foreign material before rendering a diagnosis. Even under the best circumstances, the etiology of some histiocytic proliferations remains enigmatic. The more distinctive histiocytic reactions with known etiologies are discussed below.

### Infectious Disease

Gram-positive and gram-negative bacteria can induce inflammatory changes similar to those of xanthogranuloma. The lesions are composed of sheets of foamy histiocytes set against a mixed background of inflammatory cells. They differ from a neoplastic xanthogranuloma by the presence of focal abscesses and numerous microorganisms in the histiocytes. We have seen several cases of chronic staphylococcal infection with this appearance, and we are aware of a similar lesion of the retroperitoneum secondary to *Arizona hinshawii*, a gram-negative bacillus.[155]

Histoid leprosy, a rare form of lepromatous leprosy described by Wade[157,162] in 1963, grossly and microscopically resembles fibrous histiocytoma (Figs. 13–52, 13–53, 13–54). Unlike the usual type of lepromatous leprosy, which spreads in an infiltrative manner, this disease develops as an expansile nodule of the subcutis and dermis. The cells resemble fibroblasts rather than histiocytes and are often arranged in a storiform pattern. Although the similarity of this disease to a true fibrous histiocytoma is striking, numerous intracellular acid-fast bacilli can be demonstrated with special stains (Fite-Feraco) (Fig. 13–54). Because this form of leprosy occurs in patients with long-standing lepromatous leprosy treated with sulfones, it has been suggested that these lesions are the result of emergence of sulfone-resistant bacilli.

### Malacoplakia

Malacoplakia is a rare inflammatory disease believed to represent an unusual host response to infection with a variety of organisms, including *Escherichia coli*, *Klebsiella*, and acid-fast bacilli. The reaction results in the formation of yellow plaque-like lesions on the mucosal surface of the affected organs.[147] The disease typically develops in the genitourinary tract, particularly the bladder, although it may affect the soft tissues of the retroperitoneum as well. It is characterized by sheets of pale, slightly granular, or vacuolated histiocytes (von Hansemann's cells) containing PAS-positive, diastase-resistant inclusions in the cytoplasm (Fig. 13–55). Lymphocytes, plasma cells, and neutrophils are typically abundant. The distinctive Michaelis-Gutmann bodies, small calcospherites that consist of a mixture of organic and inorganic materials including calcium and phosphate, can be identified within the histiocytes and extracellularly (Fig. 13–56). Electron microscopic studies show that the von Hansemann histiocytes contain numerous phagolysosomes, occasional bacterial forms, and lamellated crystalline bodies representing the early stage of Michaelis-Gutmann bodies.[149]

### Extranodal (Soft Tissue) Rosai-Dorfman Disease

Since the original description of sinus histiocytosis with massive lymphadenopathy (SHML) by Rosai

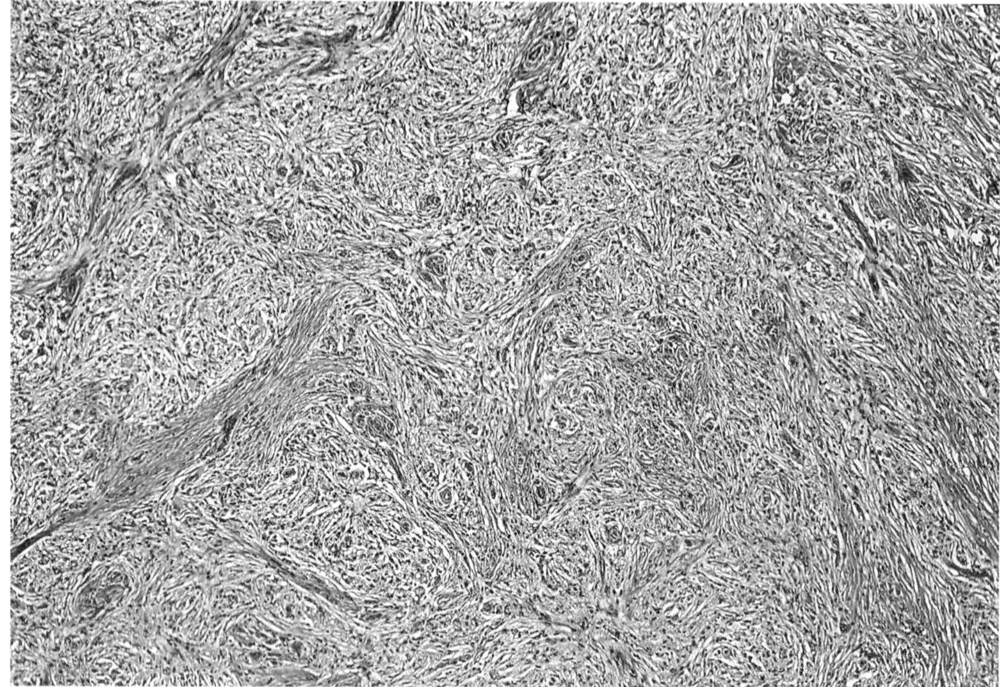

**FIGURE 13–52.** Histoid leprosy with a pattern similar to that of a fibrous histiocytoma.

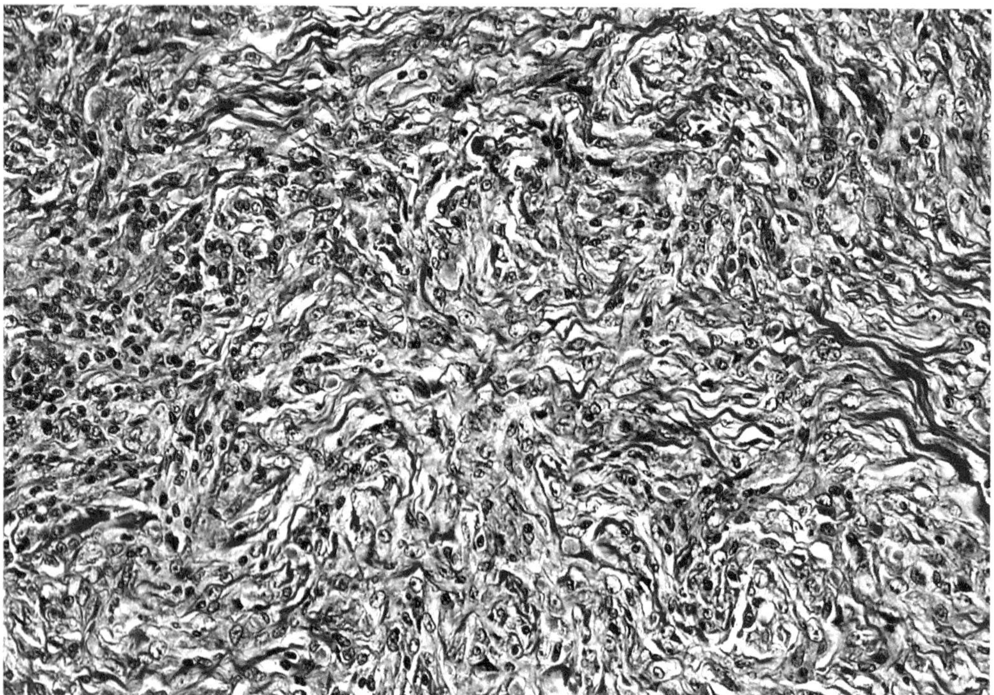

**FIGURE 13–53.** Medium-power view of histoid leprosy.

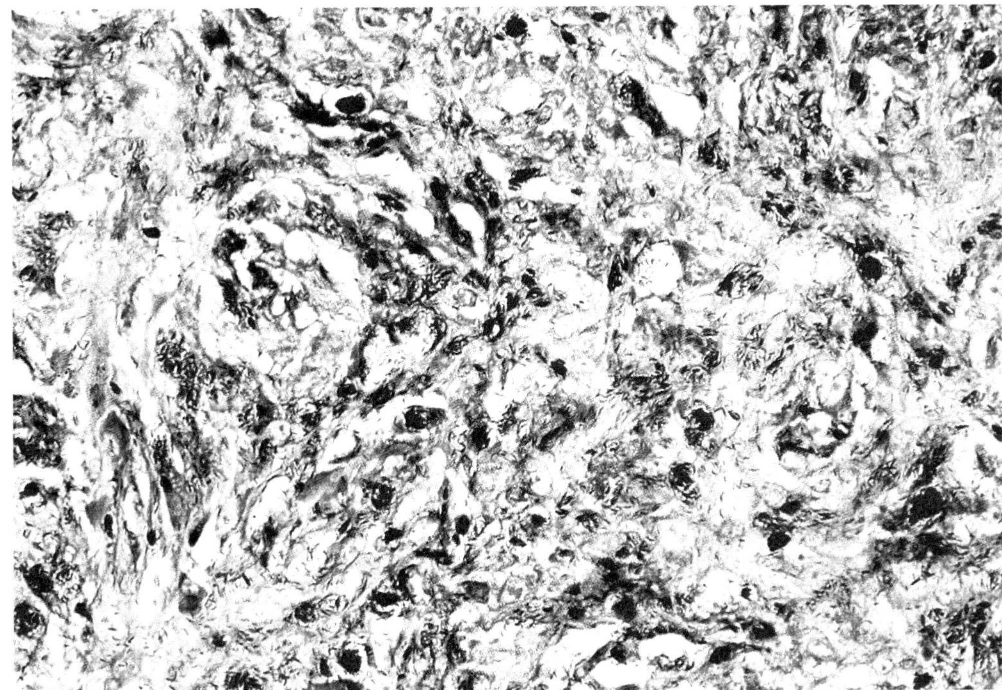

**FIGURE 13–54.** Fite-Feraco stain demonstrates numerous intracellular acid-fast bacilli in histoid leprosy.

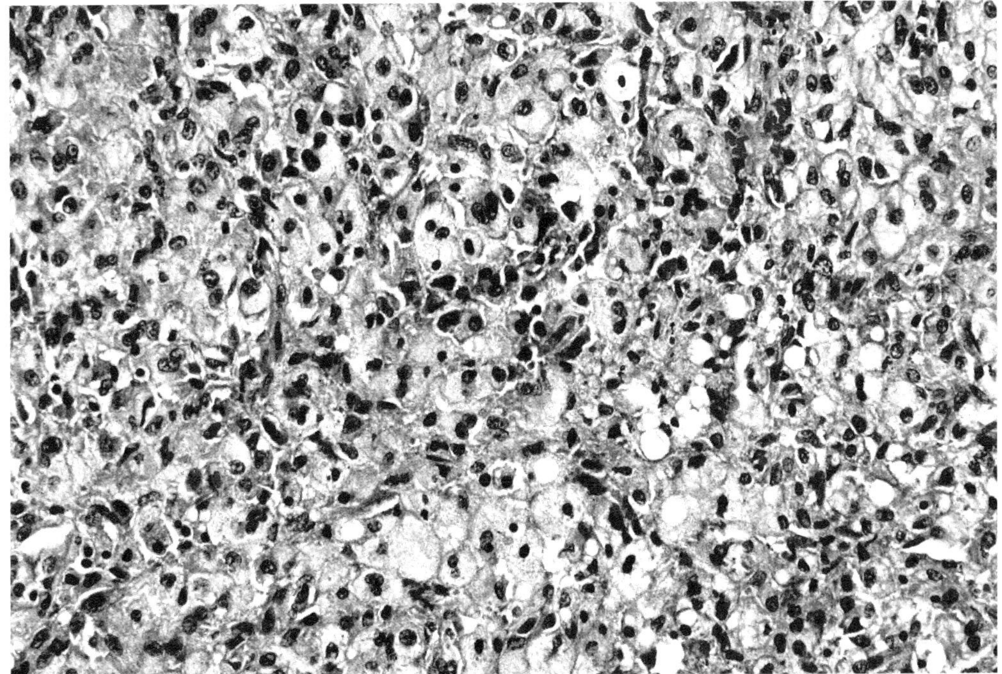

**FIGURE 13–55.** Malacoplakia of the retroperitoneum with solid sheets of histiocytes admixed with inflammatory cells.

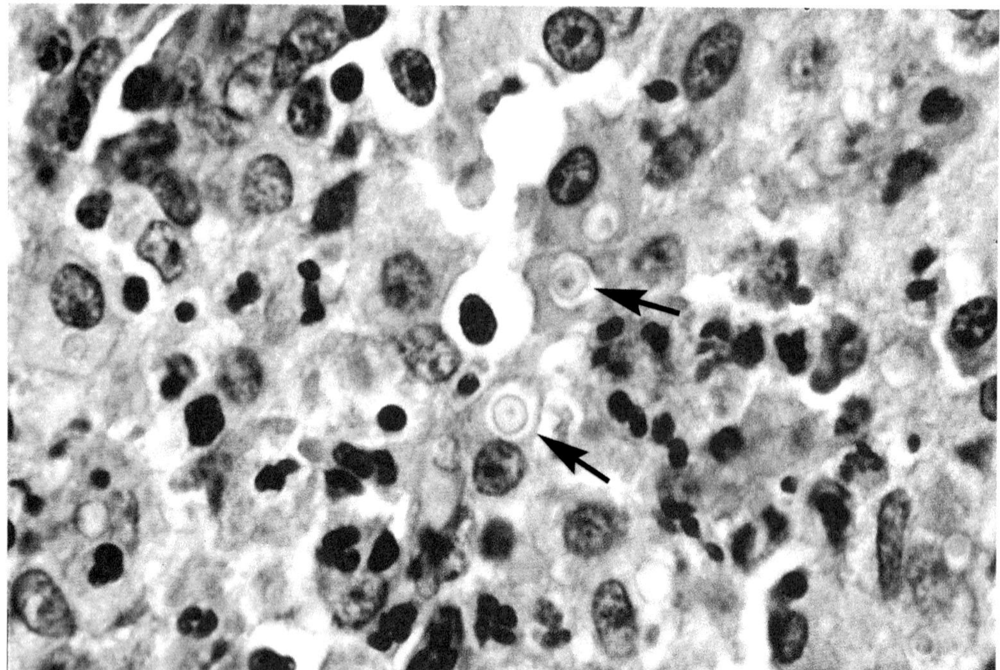

**FIGURE 13–56.** High-power view of malacoplakia showing Michaelis-Gutmann bodies (arrows) in occasional cells.

and Dorfman in 1972,[160] it has been recognized that this disease may occur in extranodal sites, often without any involvement of lymph nodes. Approximately 10% of all cases of Rosai-Dorfman disease are associated with soft tissue involvement, and in some cases it is the sole manifestation of the disorder.[150,158] However, the actual incidence of associated lymphadenopathy in patients with soft tissue lesions depends greatly on the bias of the study. In the study by Foucar et al.[150] most had lymphadenopathy, whereas in the study by Montgomery et al.[158] only a few did (4 of 23). The former study was based on a referral of all cases to the National SHML Registry at Yale University, whereas the latter represented referral cases to the Soft Tissue Registry of the Armed Forces Institute of Pathology (AFIP). Patients with soft tissue Rosai-Dorfman disease tend to be older than those with lymph node-based disease.

Microscopically, the lesions consist of sheets or syncytia of large, pale histiocytes with large, round, vesicular nuclei with some degree of atypia (Figs. 13–57, 13–58). Mitotic figures are usually difficult to detect or are absent altogether. The cytoplasm of the histiocytes may contain lymphocytes (emperipolesis), although this is seldom as striking as in the lesions of lymph nodes. Microabscesses, when present, suggest the possibility of an infectious process. The feature that tends to complicate the diagnosis of these unusual lesions is the presence of fibrosis, which distorts the sheet-like growth pattern, creating instead a storiform pattern. Predictably, the latter pattern, in association with atypical histiocytes, is often construed as evidence that one is dealing with a fibrohistiocytic tumor. The histiocytes of Rosai-Dorfman disease strongly express S-100 protein in virtually all cases and often a number of other histiocytic antigens.[148] The presence of S-100 protein is useful for discriminating these lesions from malignant fibrous histiocytomas and histiocytic proliferations of infectious etiology. Obviously this antigen does not discriminate examples of soft tissue Rosai-Dorfman disease from Langerhans' cell histiocytosis, although usually the cytologic differences between the proliferating histiocytes in the two conditions and the differences in the inflammatory cells accompanying them readily permit this distinction. The data, at present, suggest that the prognosis of soft tissue Rosai-Dorfman disease is good overall. Most patients with isolated soft tissue masses appeared well following surgery, although some developed recurrent disease.

## Histiocytic Reactions to Endogenous and Exogenous Material

### *Silica Reaction*

Although the usual response to silica in soft tissue is a localized foreign body reaction, exuberant reactions to the material simulate a fibrohistiocytic neoplasm (Figs. 13–59, 13–60). In our experience the latter form

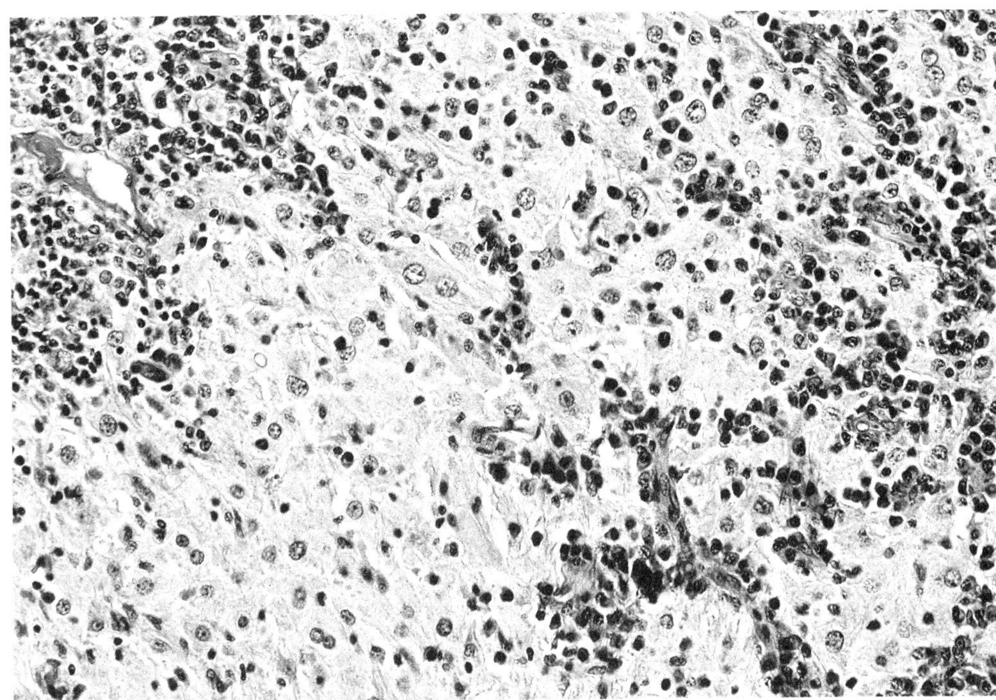

**FIGURE 13–57.** Extranodal Rosai-Dorfman disease characterized by sheets of pale histiocytes with voluminous cytoplasm.

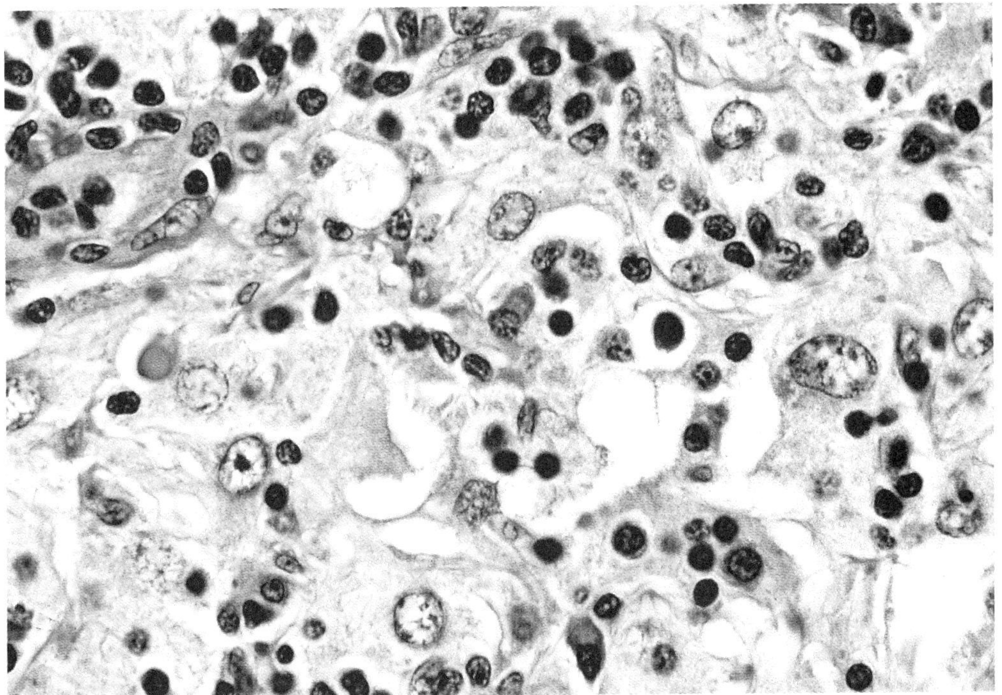

**FIGURE 13–58.** High-power view of Rosai-Dorfman disease illustrating mild nuclear atypia and emperipolesis.

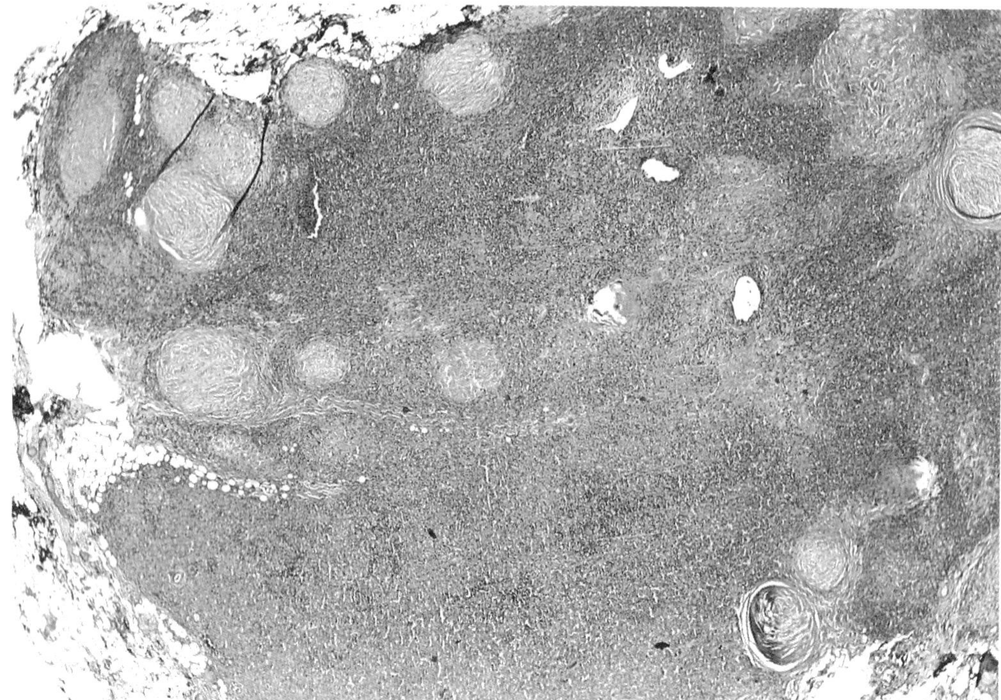

**FIGURE 13–59.** Silica reaction in the inguinal region. Lesion is composed of sheets of well-differentiated histiocytes interlaced with fibrous bands.

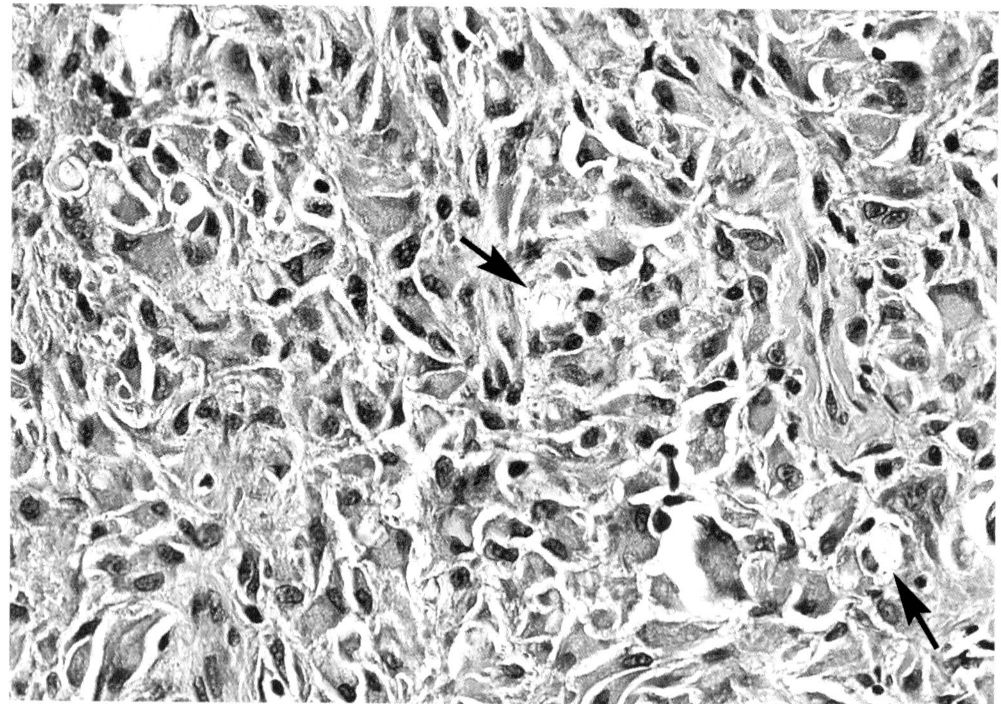

**FIGURE 13–60.** Silica reaction in the inguinal region showing well-differentiated histiocytes. Spicules of foreign material can be seen in the cytoplasm of some histiocytes, but full elucidation requires polarization.

of soft tissue silicosis is probably related to the presence of large amounts of silica. It seems principally to be an iatrogenic disease secondary to the now obsolete injection therapy for hernias.[163] Clinically, these lesions present as slowly enlarging tumorous masses, usually in the inguinal region or abdominal wall. Typically they occur many years after the injection of silica so the causal relation of the injection is minimized or overlooked. Grossly, the lesions are ill-defined, gray-yellow masses with a gritty consistency on cutting. They consist of sheets of histiocytes with a clear or amphophilic cytoplasm. Although usually well differentiated, the histiocytes occasionally display moderate pleomorphism. Mitotic figures are rare. PAS-positive, diastase-resistant bodies may be present in the histiocytes and probably represent large phagolysosomes, organelles involved in the intracellular storage of silica. Numerous silica crystals can be identified under polarized light. A striking feature of the lesion is the large amount of fibrosis. The collagen varies from delicate interstitial or perivascular fibers in the early stages to broad bands and finally mats or large nodules. The presence of silica, extensive fibrosis, scarcity of mitotic figures, and poorly developed vasculature all serve to distinguish these lesions from benign or malignant fibrous histiocytomas.

### Polyvinylpyrrolidone Granuloma

Polyvinylpyrrolidone (PVP) is a polymer of vinylpyrrolidone, which was used notably as a plasma expander during wartime and until recently was utilized in various intravenous preparations in Asia. It has been marketed under various names, including Plasgen, Periston, Plasmagel, Biseko, Blutogen, and Subplasm. Because of its hydroscopic properties it has also been used as a retardant in various injectable medicines (hormones, antihypertensives, local anesthetics), as a clarifier in fruit juices, and as a resin in hair sprays.[164] The molecular weight of PVP varies depending on its chain length (MW 10,000–200,000 daltons). Low-molecular-weight PVP is filtered by the glomerulus and cleared by the kidney, whereas high-molecular-weight PVP (MW 50,000 daltons or more) is retained indefinitely by the body and is stored throughout the reticuloendothelial system. The common appearance of PVP disease following intravenous injection of the substance is that of blue-gray histiocytes lining the sinusoids of the liver, spleen, and lymph nodes. A second form of PVP disease presumably occurs following inhalation of the substance from hair spray.[145] The alveolar walls are thickened, and macrophages fill the alveolar spaces. An uncommon form of PVP disease is a localized pseudotumor,[146,153,159] presumably caused by local injection of the material. Cases reported in the literature have documented PVP pseudotumors secondary to the anesthetic Depot-Impletol[151] and vasopressin.[159]

Histologically, these lesions are composed of numerous histiocytes massively engorged with PVP (Figs. 13–61, 13–62, 13–63). The material appears glassy blue or blue-gray in sections stained with hematoxylin-eosin. The histiocytes form sheets or small clusters in a matrix containing copious amounts of foreign material. Giant cells are occasionally present and may be helpful in suggesting the diagnosis of a foreign body reaction. Another feature suggesting a reactive process is the manner in which the histiocytes "percolate" around the adnexal structures, nerves, and vessels. Typically there are few if any inflammatory cells and no necrosis. The tinctoral properties of PVP have been well documented and serve to distinguish this lesion from other myxoid lesions (Table 13–4).[156] PVP characteristically does not stain with alcian blue and therefore stains differently from all myxoid tumors of soft tissue, such as liposarcoma, chondrosarcoma, and chordoma. It does not stain blue with Giemsa stain and should therefore not be confused with the syndrome of sea-blue histiocytes. PVP is carminophilic, and this fact should be kept in mind, as occasional cases of PVP granuloma have been mistaken for infiltrating carcinomas of the signet-ring type.[156] The best stains for demonstrating the cytoplasmic material are Congo red or Sirius red. Ultrastructurally, the material is contained in large membrane-limited vacuoles believed to be distended lysosomes. Dense bodies, probably composed of ferritin, are condensed at the periphery of the vacuoles.

### Granular Cell Reaction

Collections of histiocytes with granular eosinophilic cytoplasm occasionally accumulate at the site of surgical trauma.[161] These peculiar histiocytic reactions bear a close similarity to granular cell tumor (Figs. 13–64, 13–65, 13–66) but can usually be differentiated from the foregoing by the fact that the nuclei in these reactions are rather small and inconspicuous and the granules are large and coarsely textured (Fig.

*Text continued on page 486*

**TABLE 13–4 STAINING REACTIONS OF POLYVINYLPYRROLIDONE**

| |
|---|
| **Positive** |
| Congo red |
| Sirius red |
| Mucicarmine |
| Colloidal iron |
| **Negative** |
| Periodic acid-Schiff (PAS) |
| Alcian blue |

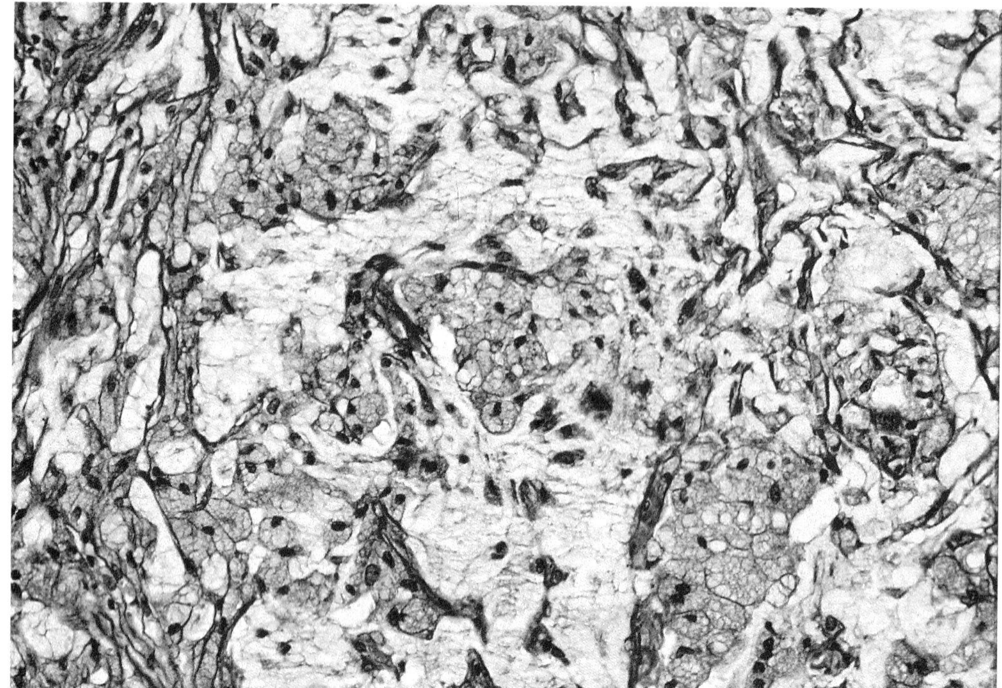

**FIGURE 13–61.** Polyvinylpyrrolidone (PVP) granuloma. Clusters of bubbly histiocytes are suspended in pools of basophilic-appearing PVP.

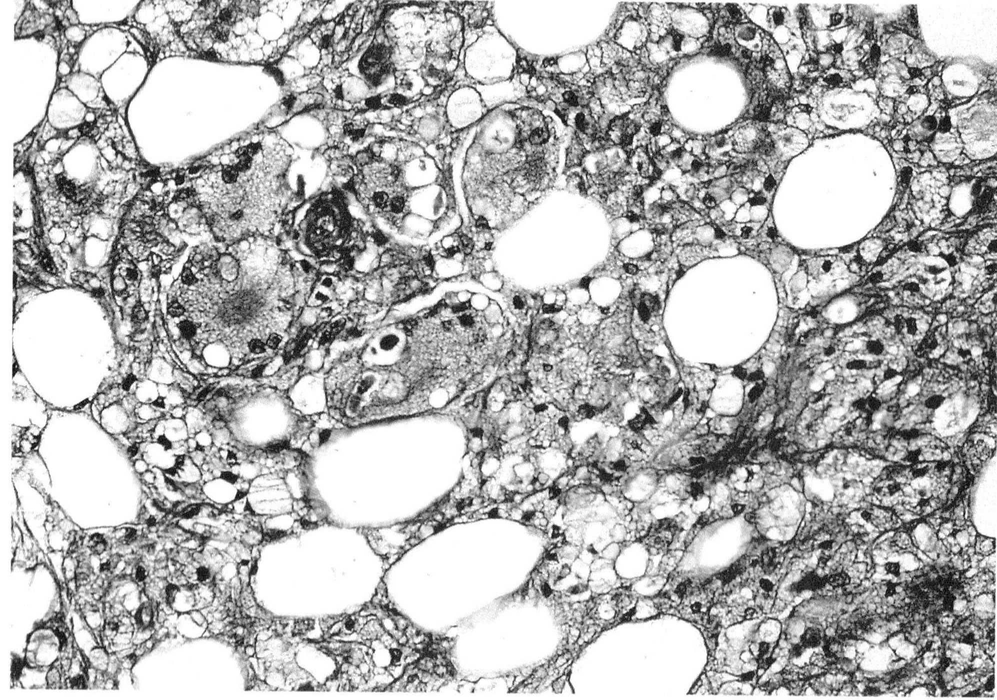

**FIGURE 13–62.** Multinucleated histiocytes filled with PVP.

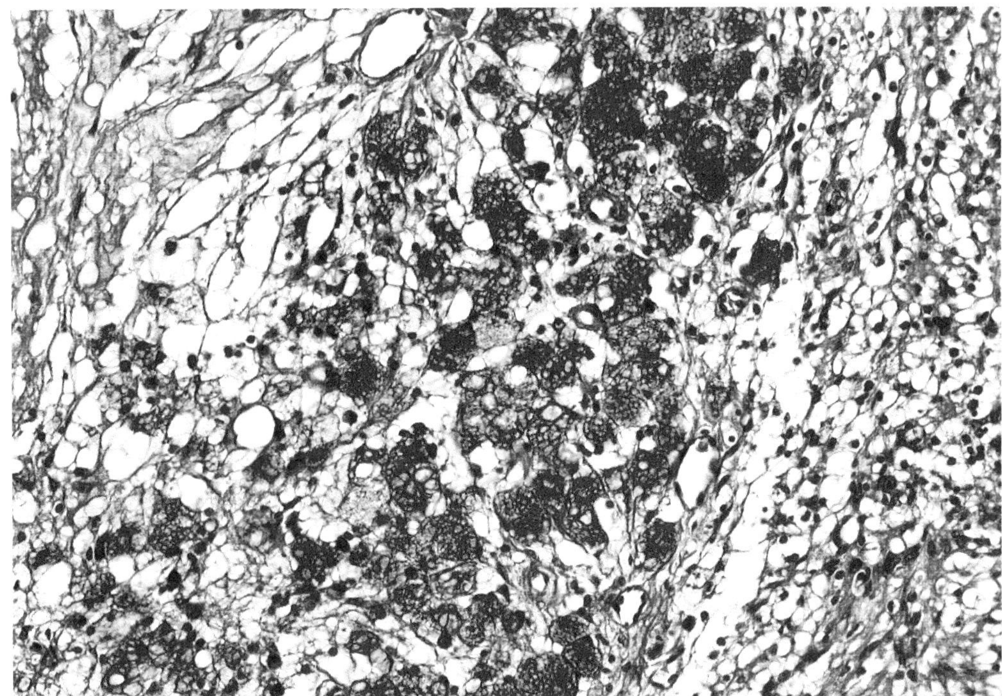

**FIGURE 13–63.** Congo red staining of PVP.

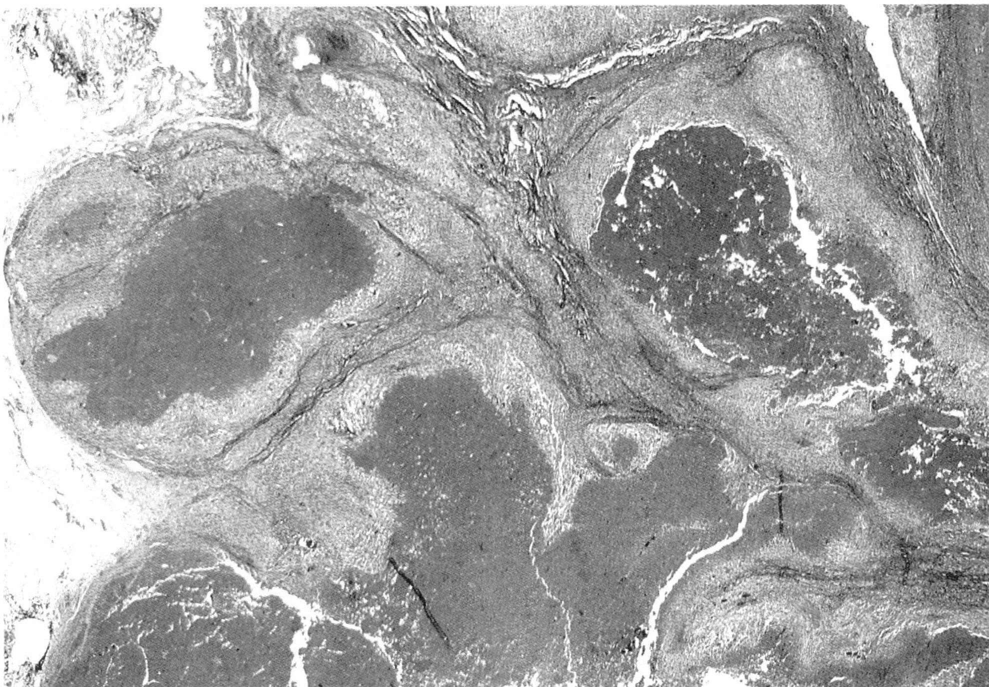

**FIGURE 13–64.** Granular cell reaction showing a fringe of histiocytes surrounding the core of the granuloamorphous material.

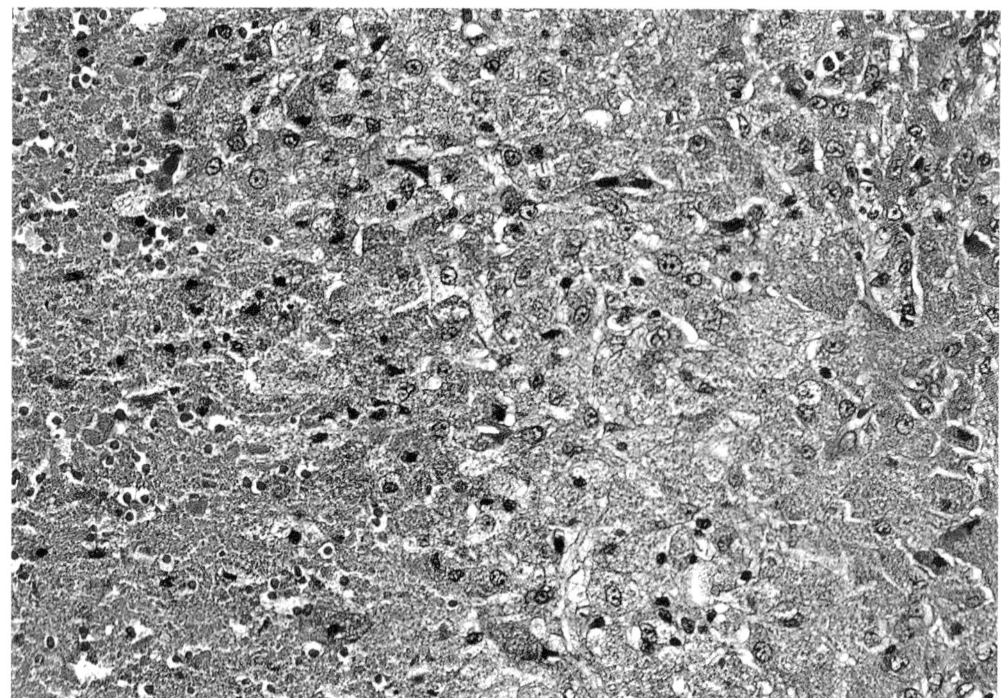

**FIGURE 13–65.** Histiocytic reaction with "granular cell" features at the site of previous surgery.

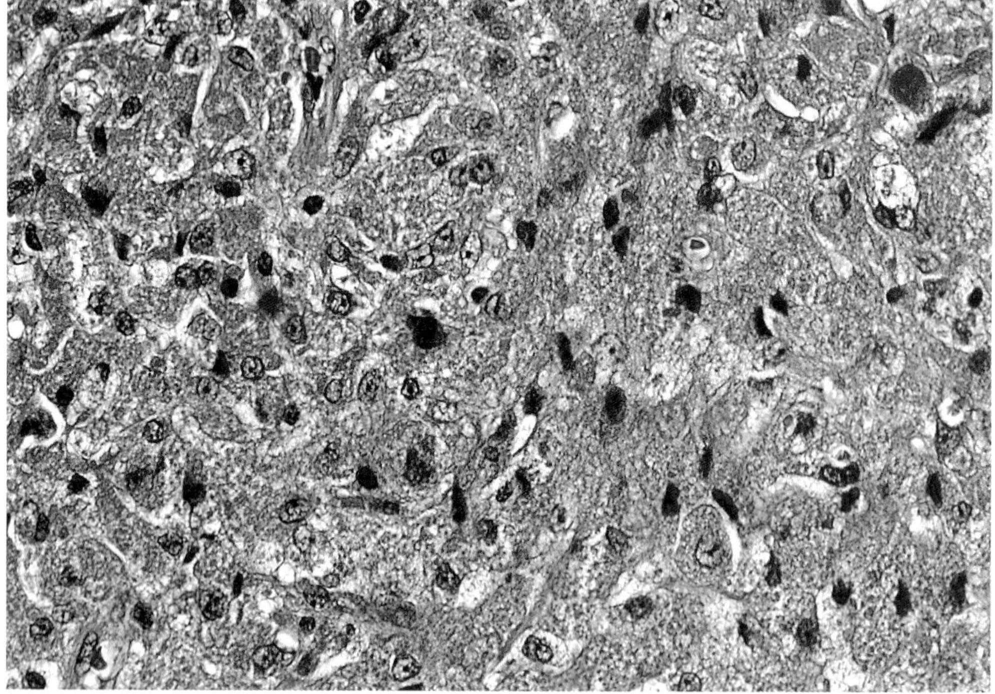

**FIGURE 13–66.** High-power view of granular-appearing histiocytes in granular cell reactions.

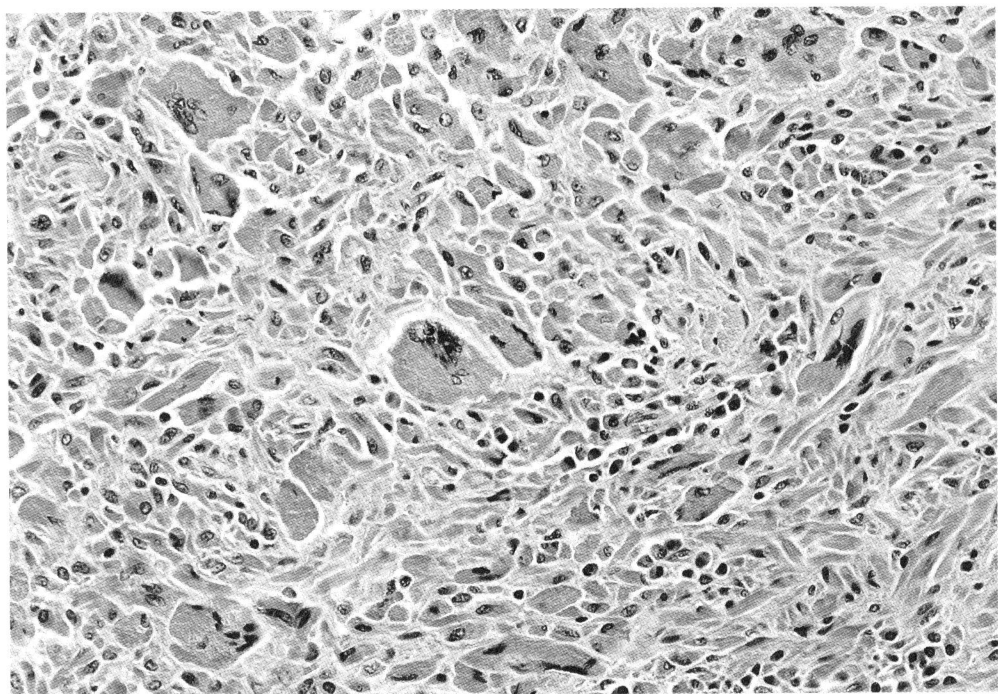

**FIGURE 13–67.** Crystalline-bearing histiocytosis in a patient with lymphoplasmatic lymphoma.

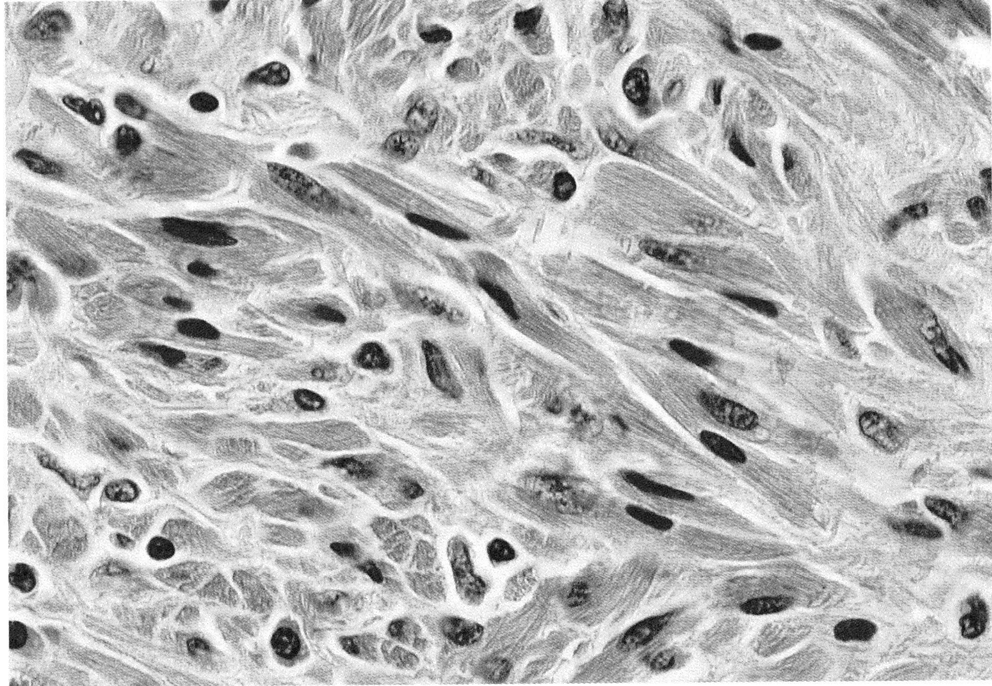

**FIGURE 13–68.** High-power view of crystal-containing histiocytes from Figure 13–67 showing massive distortion and spindling as a result of intracytoplasmic crystalline immunoglobulin.

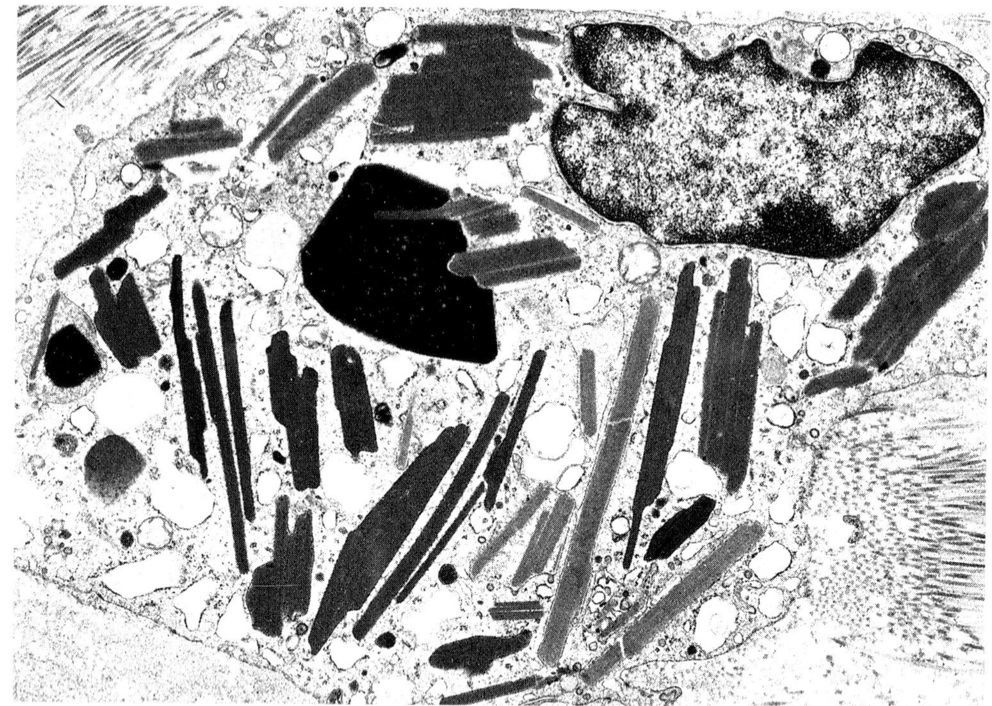

**FIGURE 13–69.** Electron micrograph of crystalline immunoglobulin from Figure 13–68 showing periodicity.

13–66). Furthermore, the cells often surround nodules of granuloamorphous debris similar to the cytoplasmic granular material (Figs. 13–64, 13–65). Sobel et al.[161] pointed out that the staining reactions serve to distinguish the two lesions. The ceroid-lipofuscin substance in these histiocyte reactions is usually acid-fast and autofluorescent compared with that of the granular cell tumor.

### *Crystal-storing Histiocytosis Resembling Rhabdomyoma*

Crystal-storing histiocytosis is a rare condition in which tumorous deposits of histiocytes containing crystalline immunoglobulin occur in soft tissue.[152,154] A small number of cases have been reported, all of which were associated with a lymphoplasmacytic neoplasm and monoclonal immunglobulin production. It appears that the immunoglobulin is crystallized locally and phagocytosed by histiocytes, which become massively distorted by the material. The histiocytes are large, rounded to angular cells that occasionally appear multinucleated (Figs. 13–67, 13–68). The crystalline material varies in size, but the largest deposits can be visualized easily by light microscopy. The histiocytic cells can be few in number or so abundant that the underlying lymphoplasmatic neoplasm is overlooked, resulting in an erroneous diagnosis of rhabdomyoma.[154] However, the cells can be clearly identified as histiocytic by strong immunostaining for CD68. Ultrastructurally, the crystalline material displays a lattice pattern with a periodicity of 45–60 Å, consistent with immunoglobulin (Fig. 13–69).

## REFERENCES

### General


1. Calonje E, Fletcher CDM. Cutaneous fibrohistiocytic tumors: an update. Adv Anat Pathol 1:2, 1994.
2. Gabbiani G, Ryan GB, Majno G. Presence of modified fibroblasts in granulation tissue and their possible role in wound contraction. Experientia 27:549, 1971.
3. Lever WF, Schaumburg-Lever G. Histopathology of the Skin, 5th ed. Lippincott, Philadelphia, 1975.
4. Rader DJ. Disorders of lipid metabolism. In: Kelley WN (ed) Textbook of Internal Medicine, 3rd ed. Lippincott-Raven, Philadelphia, 1997.
5. Shamoto M. Langerhans' cell granule in Letterer-Siwe disease. Cancer 26:1102, 1970.
6. Taxy JB. Juvenile nasopharyngeal angiofibroma: an ultrastructural study. Cancer 39:1044, 1977.
7. Vernon ML, Fountain L, Krebs HM, et al. Birbeck granules (Langerhans' cell granules) in human lymph nodes. Am J Clin Pathol 160:771, 1973.
8. Weibel ER, Palade GE. New cytoplasmic components in arterial endothelia. J Cell Biol 23:101, 1964.
9. Wirman JA. Nodular fasciitis: an ultrastructural study. Cancer 38:2378, 1976.


### Fibrous Histiocytoma


10. Arnold HL, Tilden IL. Histiocytoma cutis: a variant of xanthoma. Arch Dermatol Syph 47:498, 1943.

11. Beer M, Eckert F, Schmoeckel C. The atrophic dermatofibroma. J Am Acad Dermatol 25:1081, 1991.
12. Beham A, Fletcher CD. Atypical "pseudosarcomatous" variant of cutaneous benign fibrous histiocytoma: report of eight cases. Histopathology 17:167, 1990.
13. Calonje E, Fletcher CDM. Aneurysmal benign fibrous histiocytoma: clincopathological analysis of 40 cases of a tumor frequently misdiagnosed as a vascular neoplasm. Histopathology 26:323, 1995.
14. Calonje E, Mentzel T, Fletcher CDM. Cellular benign fibrous histiocytoma: clinicopathologic analysis of 74 cases of a distinctive variant of cutaneous fibrous histiocytoma with frequent recurrence. Am J Surg Pathol 18:668, 1994.
15. Carstens PHB, Schrodt GR. Ultrastructure of sclerosing hemangioma. Am J Pathol 77:377, 1974.
16. Cerio R, Spaull J, Wilson Jones E. Histiocytoma cutis: a tumour of dermal dendrocytes (dermal dendrocytoma). Br J Dermatol 120:197, 1989.
17. Colome-Grimmer MI, Evans HL. Metastasizing cellular dermatofibroma: a report of two cases. Am J Surg Pathol 20:1361, 1996.
18. Du Boulay CEH. Demonstration of alpha-1-antitrypsin and alpha-1-antichymotrypsin in fibrous histiocytomas using immunoperoxidase technique. Am J Surg Pathol 6:559, 1982.
19. Fine G, Morales MD, Pardo V. Ultrastructure of histiocytomas [abstract]. Am J Clin Pathol 67:214, 1977.
20. Fitzpatrick TB, Gilchrest BA. Dimple sign to differentiate benign from malignant pigmented cutaneous lesions. N Engl J Med 296:1518, 1977.
21. Foreman K, Bonish BMS, Nickoloff B. Absence of human herpesvirus 8 DNA sequences in patients with immunosuppression associated dermatofibroma. Arch Dermatol 133:108, 1997.
22. Fletcher CD. Benign fibrous histiocytoma of subcutaneous and deep soft tissue: a clinicopathologic analysis of 21 cases. Am J Surg Pathol 14:801, 1990.
23. Font RL, Kidayat AA. Fibrous histiocytoma of the orbit: a clinicopathologic study of 150 cases. Hum Pathol 13:199, 1982.
24. Franchi A, Santucci M. Tenascin, expression in cutaneous fibrohistiocytic tumors: immunohistochemical investigation of 24 cases. Am J Dermatopathol 18:454, 1996.
25. Franquemont DW, Cooper PH, Shmookler BM, et al. Benign fibrous histiocytoma of the skin with potential for local recurrence: a tumor to be distinguished from dermatofibroma. Mod Pathol 3:58, 1990.
26. Glusac EJ, Barr RJ, Everett MA, et al. Epithelioid cell histiocytoma: a report of 10 cases including a new cellular variant. Am J Surg Pathol 18:583, 1994.
27. Gonzalez S, Duarte I. Benign fibrous histiocytoma of the skin: a morphologic study of 290 cases. Pathol Res Pract 174:379, 1982.
28. Gross RE, Wolbach SB. Sclerosing hemangiomas: their relationship to dermatofibroma, histiocytoma, xanthoma, and certain pigmented lesions of the skin. Am J Pathol 19:533, 1943.
29. Halpryn JH, Allen AC. Epidermal changes associated with sclerosing hemangiomas. Arch Dermatol 80:160, 1959.
30. Kamino H, Jacobson M. Dermatofibroma extending into the subcutaneous tissue: differential diagnosis from dermatofibrosarcoma protuberans. Am J Surg Pathol 14:1156, 1990.
31. Kamino H, Reddy VB, Gero M, Greco MA. Dermatomyofibroma: a benign cutaneous plaque like proliferation of fibroblasts in young adults. J Cutan Pathol 19:85, 1992.
32. Kamino H, Salcedo E. Histopathologic and immunohistochemical diagnosis of benign and malignant fibrous and fibrohistiocytic tumors of the skin. Dermatol Clin 17:487, 1999.
33. Katenkamp D, Stiller D. Cellular composition of the so-called dermatofibroma (histiocytoma cutis). Virchows Arch [Pathol Anat] 367:325, 1975.
34. Kindblom LG, Jacobsen GK, Jacobsen M. Immunohistochemical investigation of tumours of supposed fibroblastic-histiocytic origin. Hum Pathol 13:834, 1982.
35. Klaus SN, Winkelmann RK. The enzyme histochemistry of nodular subepidermal fibrosis. Br J Dermatol 78:398, 1966.
36. LeBoit PE, Barr RJ. Smooth muscle proliferation in dermatofibromas. Am J Dermatopathol 16:155, 1994.
37. McKenna DB, Kavanagh GM, McLaren KM, Tidman MJ. Aneurysmal fibrous histiocytoma: an unusual variant of cutaneous fibrous histiocytoma. J Eur Acad Dermatol Venereol 12: 238, 1999.
38. Meister P, Konrad E, Krauss F. Fibrous histiocytoma: a histological and statistical analysis of 155 cases. Pathol Res Pract 162:361, 1978.
39. Mentzel T, Calonje E, Fletcher CDM. Dermatomyofibroma: additional observations on a distinctive cutaneous myofibroblastic tumour with emphasis on differential diagnosis. Br J Dermatol 129:69, 1993.
40. Michelson HE. Nodular subepidermal fibrosis. Arch Dermatol Syph 27:812, 1933.
41. Mihatsch-Konz B, Schaumburg-Lever G, Lever WR. Ultrastructure of dermatofibroma. Arch Derm Forsch 246:181, 1973.
42. Newman DM, Walter JB. Multiple dermatofibromas in patients with systemic lupus erythematosus on immunosuppressive therapy. N Engl J Med 289:842, 1973.
43. Nguyen G-K, Johnson ES. Invasive benign histiocytoma. Am J Surg Pathol 11:487, 1987.
44. Niemi KM. The benign fibrohistiocytic tumours of the skin. Acta Dermatol Venereol 50(Suppl 63):1, 1970.
45. Reid MB, Bray C, Gear JD, et al. Immunohistochemical demonstration of factors XIIIa and XIIIs in reactive and neoplastic fibroblastic fibrohistiocytic lesions. Histopathology 10:1171, 1986,
46. Santa Cruz DJ, Kyriakos M. Aneurysmal ("angiomatoid") fibrous histiocytoma of the skin. Cancer 47:2053, 1981.
47. Schwob VS, Santa Cruz DJ. Palisading cutaneous fibrous histiocytoma. J Cutan Pathol 13:403, 1986
48. Senear FE, Caro MR. Histiocytoma cutis. Arch Dermatol Syph 33:209, 1936.
49. Singh GAC, Calonje E, Fletcher CDM. Epithelioid benign fibrous histiocytoma of skin: clinicopathological analysis of 20 cases of a poorly known variant. Histopathology 24:123, 1994.
50. Smith NM, Davies JB, Shrimankar JS, et al. Deep fibrous histiocytoma with giant cells and bone metaplasia. Histopathology 17:365, 1990.
51. Soini Y, Miettinen M. Alpha 1-antichymotrypsin and lysozyme: their limited significance in fibrohistiocytic tumors. Am J Clin Pathol 91:515, 1989.
52. Tamada S, Ackerman AB. Dermatofibroma with monster cells. Am J Dermatopathol 9:380, 1987.
53. Vanni R, Marras S, Faa G, et al. Cellular fibrous histiocytoma of the skin: evidence of a clonal process with different karyotype from dermatofibrosarcoma. Genes Chromosomes Cancer 18:314, 1997.
54. Wilson Jones E, Cerio R, Smith NP. Epithelioid cell histiocytoma: a new entity. Br J Dermatol 120:185, 1989.
55. Zelger BG, Calonje E, Zelger B. Myxoid dermatofibroma. Histopathology 34:357, 1999.
56. Zelger B, Sidoroff A, Stanzl U, et al. Deep penetrating dermatofibroma versus dermatofibrosarcoma protuberans: a clinicopathologic comparison. Am J Surg Pathol 18:677, 1994.
57. Zelger B, Steiner H, Kutzner H. Clear cell dermatofibroma. Am J Surg Pathol 20:483, 1996.
58. Zelger BW, Zelger BG, Steiner H, Ofner D. Aneurysmal and hemangiopericytoma-like fibrous histiocytoma. J Clin Pathol 49:313, 1996.

### Juvenile Xanthogranuloma

59. Adamson HG. Society intelligence: the Dermatologic Society of London. Br J Dermatol 17:222, 1905.
60. Balfour H, Speicher C. Juvenile xanthogranuloma associated with cytomegalovirus infection. Am J Med 50:380, 1971.
61. Bearcroft WBC, Jamieson MF. An outbreak of subcutaneous tumours in rhesus monkeys. Nature 182:195, 1958.
62. Cohen BA, Hood A. Xanthogranuloma: report on clinical and histologic findings in 64 patients. Pediatr Dermatol 6:262, 1989.
63. De Graaf JH, Timens W, Tamminga RY, Molenaar WM. Deep juvenile xanthogranuloma: a lesion related to dermal indeterminate cells. Hum Pathol 23:905, 1992.
64. DeVillex RL, Limmer BL. Juvenile xanthogranuloma and urticaria pigmentosa. Arch Dermatol 111:365, 1975.
65. Eller JL. Roentgen therapy for visceral juvenile xanthogranuloma, including a case with involvement of the heart. AJR 95: 52, 1965.
66. Esterly NB, Sahihi T, Medenica M. Juvenile xanthogranuloma: an atypical case with a study of ultrastructure. Arch Dermatol 105:99, 1972.
67. Gonzalez-Crussi F, Campbell RJ. Juvenile xanthogranuloma: ultrastructural study. Arch Pathol 89:65, 1970.
68. Helwig EB. Histiocytic and fibrocytic disorders. In: Graham JH, Johnson WC, Helwig EG (eds) Dermal Pathology. Harper & Row, New York, 1972.
69. Helwig EB, Hackney VC. Juvenile xanthogranuloma (nevoxantho-endothelioma). Am J Pathol 30:625, 1954.
70. Janney CG, Hurt MA, Santa Cruz DJ. Deep juvenile xanthogranuloma: subcutaneous and intramuscular forms. Am J Surg Pathol 15:150, 1991.
71. Jensen NE. Naevoxanthoendothelioma and neurofibromatosis. Br J Dermatol 85:326, 1971.
72. Kjaerheim A, Stokke T. Juvenile xanthogranuloma of the oral cavity. Oral Surg Oral Med Oral Pathol 38:414, 1974.
73. Lamb JH, Lain ES. Nevo-xantho-endothelioma. South Med J 30: 585, 1937.
74. Lottsfeldt F, Good R. Juvenile xanthogranuloma with pulmonary lesions: a case report. Pediatrics 33:233, 1964.
75. McDonagh JER. A contribution to our knowledge of the naevoxanthoendotheliomata. Br J Dermatol 24:85, 1912.
76. Nascimento AG. A clinicopathologic and immunohistochemical comparative study of cutaneous and intramuscular forms of juvenile xanthogranuloma. Am J Surg Pathol 21:645, 1997.
77. Newell GB, Stone OJ, Mullins JF. Juvenile xanthogranuloma and neurofibromatosis. Arch Dermatol 107:262, 1973.
78. Niven JSF, Armstrong JA, Andrewes CH. Subcutaneous "growths" in monkeys produced by a poxvirus. J Pathol Bacteriol 81:1, 1961.
79. Nomland R. Nevoxantho-endothelioma: a benign xanthomatous disease of infants and children. J Invest Dermatol 22:207, 1954.
80. Pois AJ, Johnson LA. Multiple congenital xanthogranuloma of skin and heart: report of a case. Dis Chest 50:325, 1966.
81. Senear FE, Caro MR. Nevo-xantho-endothelioma or juvenile xanthoma. Arch Dermatol Syph 34:195, 1936.
82. Smith ME, Sanders TE, Bresnick GH. Juvenile xanthogranuloma of the ciliary body in an adult. Arch Ophthalmol 81:813, 1969.
83. Sonoda T, Hashimoto H, Enjoji M. Juvenile xanthogranuloma: clinicopathologic analysis and immunohistochemical study of 57 patients. Cancer 56:2280, 1985.
84. Sproul EE, Metzgar RS, Grace JT Jr. The pathogenesis of Yaba virus-induced histiocytomas in primates. Cancer Res 23:671, 1963.
85. Tahan SR, Pastel-Levy C, Bhan AK, et al. Juvenile xanthogranuloma: clinical and pathologic characterization. Arch Pathol Lab Med 113:1057, 1989.
86. Webster SB, Reister HC, Harman LE. Juvenile xanthogranuloma with extra-cutaneous lesions: a case report and review of the literature. Arch Dermatol 93:71, 1966.
87. Writing Group of the Histiocyte Society. Histiocytosis syndromes in children. Lancet 1:208, 1987.
88. Zelger B, Cerio R, Orchard G, Wilson-Jones E. Juvenile and adult xanthogranuloma: a histological and immunohistochemical comparison. Am J Surg Pathol 18:126, 1994.
89. Zelger BW, Sidoroff A, Orchard G, Cerio R. Non-Langerhans cell histiocytoses: a new unifying concept. Am J Dermatopathol 18:490, 1996.

### Reticulohistiocytoma

90. Barrow MV, Holubar K. Multicentric reticulohistiocytosis. Medicine 48:287, 1969.
91. Conaghan P, Miller M, Dowling JP, et al. A unique presentation of multicentric reticulohistiocytosis in pregnancy. Arthritis Rheum 36:269, 1993.
92. Davies BT, Wood SR. The so-called reticulohistiocytoma of the skin: a comparison of two distinct types. Br J Dermatol 67:205, 1955.
93. Davies NEJ, Roenigk HH, Hawk WA, et al. Multicentric reticulohistiocytosis: report of a case with histochemical studies. Arch Dermatol 97:543, 1968.
94. Ehrlich GE, Young I, Nosheny SZ, et al. Multicentric reticulohistiocytosis (lipoid dermatoarthritis). Am J Med 52:830, 1972.
95. Flam M, Ryan SC, Mah-Poy GL, et al. Multicentric reticulohistiocytosis: report of a case with atypical features and electron microscopic study of skin lesions. Am J Med 52:841, 1972.
96. Ginsburg WW, O'Duffy JD, Morris JL, et al. Multicentric reticulohistiocytosis: response to alkylating agents in six patients. Ann Intern Med 11:384, 1989.
97. Hashimoto K, Pritzker MS. Electron microscopic study of reticulohistiocytoma. Arch Dermatol 107:263, 1973.
98. Kenik JG, Fok F, Huerter CJ, et al. Multicentric reticulohistiocytosis in a patient with malignant melanoma: a response to cyclophosphamide and a unique cutaneous feature. Arthritis Rheum 33:1047, 1990.
99. Kuramoto Y, Iizawa O, Matsunaga J. Development of Ki-1 lymphoma in a child suffering from multicentric reticulohistiocytosis. Acta Dermatol Venereol 71:448, 1991.
100. Kuwabara H, Uda H, Tanaka S. Multicentric reticulohistiocytosis: report of a case with electron microscopic studies. Acta Pathol Jpn 42:130, 1992.
101. Lambert CM, Nuki G. Multicentric reticulohistiocytosis with arthritis and cardiac infiltration: regression following treatment for underlying malignancy. Ann Rheum Dis 51:815, 1992.
102. Lotti T, Santucci M, Casigliani R, et al. Multicentric reticulohistiocytosis: report of three cases with evaluation of tissue proteinase activity. Am J Dermatopathol 10:497, 1988.
103. Montgomery H, Polley HF, Pugh DG. Reticulohistiocytoma (reticulohistiocytic granuloma). Arch Dermatol 77:61, 1958.
104. Nakajima Y, Sato K, Morita H, et al. Severe progressive erosive arthritis in multicentric reticulohistiocytosis: possible involvement of cytokines in synovial proliferation. J Rheumatol 19:1643, 1992.
105. Oliver GF, Umbert I, Winkelmann RK, et al. Reticulohistiocytoma cutis: review of 15 cases and an association with systemic vasculitis in two cases. Clin Exp Dermatol 15:1, 1990.
106. Orkin M, Goltz RW, Good RA, et al. A study of multicentric reticulohistiocytosis. Arch Dermatol 89:640, 1964.
107. Perrin C, Lacour JP, Michiels JF, et al. Multicentric reticulohistiocytosis: immunohistochemical and ultrastructural study: a pathology of dendritic cell lineage. Am J Dermatopathol 14: 418, 1992.
108. Purvis WE, Helwig EB. Reticulohistiocytic granuloma ("reticulohistiocytoma") of the skin. Am J Clin Pathol 24:1005, 1954.

109. Salisbury JR, Hall PAS, Williams HC, et al. Multicentric reticulohistiocytosis. Am J Surg Pathol 14:687, 1990.
110. Shiokawa S, Shingu M, Nishimura M, et al. Multicentric reticulohistiocytosis associated with subclinical Sjögren's syndrome. Clin Rheumatol 10:201, 1991.
111. Taylor DR. Multicentric reticulohistiocytosis. Arch Dermatol 113:330, 1977.
112. Zagala A, Guyot A, Bensa JC, et al. Multicentric reticulohistiocytomas: a case with enhanced interleukin-1, prostaglandin $E_2$, and interleukin-2 secretion. J Rheumatol 15:136, 1988.
113. Zelger B, Cerio R, Soyer HP, et al. Reticulohistiocytoma and multicentric reticulocytosis: histopathologic and immunophenotypic distinct entities. Am J Dermatopathol 16:577, 1994.

### Xanthoma

114. Adams CWM, Bayliss LB, Ibrahim MZM, et al. Phospholipids in atherosclerosis: the modification of the cholesterol granuloma by phospholipid. J Pathol Bacteriol 86:43, 1963.
115. Anderson DR. Ultrastructure of xanthelasma. Arch Ophthalmol 81:692, 1969.
116. Beerman H. Lipid diseases as manifested in the skin. Med Clin North Am 35:433, 1951.
117. Berginer VM, Salen G, Shefer S. Long-term treatment of cerebrotendinous xanthomatosis with chenodeoxycholic acid. N Engl J Med 311:1649, 1984.
118. Buxtorf JC, Beaumont V, Jacotot B, et al. Regression de xanthomes et medicaments hypolipidemiants. Atherosclerosis 19:1, 1974.
119. Cristol DS, Gill AB. Xanthoma of tendon sheath. JAMA 122: 1013, 1943.
120. Crocker AC. Skin xanthomas in childhood. Pediatrics 8:573, 1951.
121. DeSanto DA, Wilson PD. Xanthomatous tumors of joints. J Bone Joint Surg 21:531, 1939.
122. Fahey JJ, Stark HH, Donovan WF, et al. Xanthoma of the Achilles tendon: seven cases with familial hyperbetalipoproteinemia. J Bone Joint Surg Am 55:1197, 1973.
123. Fredrickson DS, Lees RS. A system for phenotyping hyperlipoproteinemia. Circulation 31:321, 1965.
124. Friedman MS. Xanthoma of the Achilles tendon. J Bone Joint Surg 29:760, 1947.
125. Galloway JDB, Broders AC, Ghormley RK. Xanthoma of tendon sheaths and synovial membranes: a clinical and pathologic study. Arch Surg 40:485, 1940.
126. Gattereau A, Davignon J, Levesque HP. Roentgenological evaluation of Achilles-tendon xanthomatosis. Lancet 2:705, 1971.
127. Hamilton WC, Ramsey PL, Hanson SM, et al. Osseous xanthoma and multiple hand tumors as a complication of hyperlipidemia. J Bone Joint Surg Am 57:551, 1975.
128. Hughes JD, Meriwether TW. Familial pseudohypertrophy of tendoachillis with multisystem disease. South Med J 64:311, 1971.
129. Kearns WP, Wood WS. Cerebrotendinous xanthomatosis. Arch Ophthalmol 94:148, 1976.
130. Lynch PJ, Winkelmann RK. Generalized plane xanthoma and systemic disease. Arch Dermatol 93:639, 1966.
131. Marcoval J, Moreno A, Bordas X, et al. Diffuse plane xanthoma: clinicopathologic study of 8 cases. J Am Acad Dermatol 39:439, 1998.
132. McWhorter JE, Weeks C. Multiple xanthoma of the tendons. Surg Gynecol Obstet 40:199, 1925.
133. Montgomery H. Cutaneous xanthomatosis. Ann Intern Med 13:671, 1939.
134. Montgomery H, Osterberg AE. Xanthomatosis: correlation of clinical histopathologic and chemical studies of cutaneous xanthoma. Arch Dermatol Syph 37:373, 1938.
135. Palmer AJ, Blacket R. Regression of xanthomata of the eyelids with modified fat diet. Lancet 1:67, 1972.
136. Parker F, Odland GF. Electron microscopic similarities between experimental xanthoma and human eruptive xanthomas. J Invest Dermatol 52:136, 1969.
137. Parker F, Odland GF. Experimental xanthoma: a correlative biochemical, histologic, histochemical, and electron microscopic study. Am J Pathol 53:537, 1968.
138. Scott PJ, Winterbourn CC. Low density lipoprotein accumulation in actively growing xanthomas. J Atheroscler Res 7:207, 1967.
139. Siegelman SS, Schlossberg I, Becker NH, et al. Hyperlipoproteinemia with skeletal lesions. Clin Orthop 87:228, 1972.
140. Sloan HR, Frederickson DS. Rare familial diseases with neutral lipid storage: Wolman's disease, cholesterol ester storage disease, and cerebrotendinous xanthomatosis. In: Stanbury JB, Wyngaarden JB, Frederickson DS (eds) Metabolic Basis of Inherited Disease, 3rd ed. McGraw-Hill, New York, 1972.
141. Walton KW, Thomas C, Dunkerley DJ. The pathogenesis of xanthomata. J Pathol 109:271, 1973.
142. Wilkes LL. Tendon xanthoma in type IV hyperlipoproteinemia. South Med J 70:254, 1977.
143. Wilson DE, Flowers CM, Hershgold EJ, et al. Multiple myeloma, cryoglobulinemia, and xanthomatosis: distinct clinical and biochemical syndromes in two patients. Am J Med 59:721, 1975.
144. Zemel H, Deeken J, Asel N, et al. The ultrastructural features of normolipemic plane xanthoma. Arch Pathol 89:111, 1970.

### Miscellaneous Histiocytic Reactions Resembling Tumor

145. Bergman M, Flance IJ, Cruz PT, et al. Thesaurosis due to inhalation of hair spray: report of twelve new cases including three autopsies. N Engl J Med 266:750, 1962.
146. Bubis JJ, Cohen S, Dinbar J, et al. Storage of polyvinylpyrrolidone mimicking a congenital mucolipid storage disease in a patient with Munchhausen's syndrome. Isr J Med Sci 11:999, 1975.
147. Damjanov I, Katz SM. Malakoplakia. Pathol Annu 16:103, 1981.
148. Eisen RN, Buckley PJ, Rosai J. Immunophenotypic characterization of sinus histiocytomas with massive lymphadenopathy (Rosai-Dorfman disease). Semin Diagn Pathol 7:74, 1990.
149. Font RL, Bersani TA, Eagle RC. Malakoplakia of the eyelid: clinical, histopathologic and ultrastructural characteristics. Ophthalmology 95:61, 1988.
150. Foucar E, Rosai J, Dorman RF. Sinus histiocytosis with massive lymphadenopathy (Rosai-Dorfman disease): review of the entity. Semin Diagn Pathol 7:19, 1990.
151. Gille J, Brandau H. Fremdkorpergranulation in der Brusdruse nach Injektion eines polyvinylpyrrolidonhaltigen Praparats: eine Fallbeobactung. Geburtsch Frauenheilkd 35:799, 1975.
152. Harada M, Shimada M, Fuhayama M, et al. Crystal-storing histiocytosis associated with lymphoplasmacytic lymphoma mimicking Weber-Christian disease: immunohistochemical, ultrastructural and gene-rearrangment studies. Hum Pathol 27: 84, 1996.
153. Hizawa K, Inaba H, Nakanishi S, et al. Subcutaneous pseudosarcomatous polyvinylpyrrolidone granuloma. Am J Surg Pathol 8:393, 1984.
154. Kapadia SB, Enzinger FM, Heffner DK, et al. Crystal-storing histiocytosis associated with lymphoplasmacytic neoplasm: report of three cases mimicking adult rhabdomyoma. Am J Surg Pathol 17:461, 1993.
155. Keren DF, Rawlings W, Murray HW, et al. Arizona hinshawii osteomyelitis with antecedent enteric fever and sepsis: a case report and review of the literature. Ann J Med 60:577, 1976.
156. Kuo TT, Hsueh S. Mucicarminophilic histiocytosis: a polyvi-

nylpyrrolidone (PVP) storage disease simulating signet ring carcinoma. Am J Surg Pathol 8:419, 1984.
157. Mansfield RE. Histoid leprosy. Arch Pathol 87:580, 1969.
158. Montgomery EA, Meis JM, Frizzera G. Rosai-Dorfman disease of soft tissue. Am J Surg Pathol 16:122, 1992.
159. Reske-Nielsen E, Bojsen-Moller M, Vetner M, et al. Polyvinylpyrrolidone-storage disease: light and microscopical, ultrastructural, and chemical verification. Acta Pathol Microbiol Scand 84A:397, 1976.
160. Rosai J, Dorfman RF. Sinus histiocytosis with massive lymphadenopathy: a pseudolymphomatous benign disorder: analysis of 34 cases. Cancer 30:1174, 1972.
161. Sobel H, Arvin E, Marquet E, et al. Reactive granular cells in sites of trauma: a cytochemical and ultrastructural study. Am J Clin Pathol 61:223, 1974.
162. Wade HW. Histoid variety of lepromatous leprosy. Int J Leprosy 31:129, 1963.
163. Weiss SW, Enzinger FM, Johnson FB. Silica reaction simulating fibrous histiocytoma. Cancer 42:2738, 1978.
164. Wessel W, Schoog M, Winkler E. Polyvinylpyrrolidone (PVP): its diagnostic, therapeutic, and technical application and consequences thereof. Arzneim Forsch 21:1468, 1971.

CHAPTER 14

# FIBROHISTIOCYTIC TUMORS OF INTERMEDIATE MALIGNANCY

Fibrohistiocytic tumors of intermediate malignancy originally included dermatofibrosarcoma protuberans and the closely related giant cell fibroblastoma. They now embrace a number of other lesions such as the plexiform fibrohistiocytic tumor and angiomatoid fibrous histiocytoma. All are characterized by a significant risk of local recurrence but a limited risk of regional and distant metastasis. They differ from the malignant fibrous histiocytoma in this important respect. They also occur in a decidedly younger population; indeed, some seem to occur almost exclusively in children. As with malignant fibrous histiocytoma, there seems to be a general consensus that most of these lesions do not display true histiocytic differentiation despite earlier reports.[60] Their present classification, therefore, is considered a tentative one pending a general consensus on reclassification. On one hand, the dermatofibrosarcoma and its juvenile counterpart, giant cell fibroblastoma, seem to be most closely related to a fibroblast; and indeed the discovery of CD34 immunoreactivity in these two lesions provides a linkage to the $CD34^+$ dendritic cells that populate the dermis. On the other hand, the plexiform fibrohistiocytic tumor seems to most closely approach the spirit of the term "fibrohistiocytic." It has a bimodal population of cells, one of which has the histologic and immunophenotypic properties of a histiocyte and the other resembling a myofibroblast. The cells of many angiomatoid fibrous histiocytomas have a striking "histiocytic" appearance, contain phagocytosed particles of hemosiderin, and occasionally express the histiocytic marker CD68 but more frequently express various myoid markers.

## DERMATOFIBROSARCOMA PROTUBERANS

Dermatofibrosarcoma protuberans, first described in 1924 by Darier and Ferrand[15] as "progressive and recurring dermatofibroma," is a nodular cutaneous tumor characterized by a prominent storiform pattern. Over the years it has been considered a fibroblastic, histiocytic, and neural tumor. It bears some histologic similarity to benign fibrous histiocytoma; and on this basis it, along with its pigmented counterpart (Bednar tumor), was classified with the fibrohistiocytic neoplasms. In contrast to fibrous histiocytoma, dermatofibrosarcoma protuberans grows in a more infiltrative fashion and has a greater capacity for local recurrence. Moreover, in unusual instances it metastasizes, although distant metastasis is usually a late event.

### Clinical Findings

Dermatofibrosarcoma protuberans typically presents during early or middle adult life as a nodular cutaneous mass. Although early studies reflected its rarity in children,[16,17,42,63,78] there are an increasing number of reports of its appearing in the pediatric age group. In fact, given the indolent growth and long preclinical duration, it is likely that many begin during childhood and become apparent only during young adulthood.[41,42] Males are affected more frequently than females. Although these tumors occur at almost any site, they are seen most frequently on the trunk and proximal extremities (Table 14–1). Unusual sites for this tumor are the vulva[4,8,39] and parotid.[37] Anteced-

**TABLE 14–1 ANATOMIC DISTRIBUTION OF DERMATOFIBROSARCOMA PROTUBERANS (1960–1979)**

| Anatomic Location | No. of Cases | % |
|---|---|---|
| Head and neck | 124 | 14.5 |
| Upper extremity | 155 | 18.2 |
| Trunk | 404 | 47.4 |
| Lower extremity | 170 | 19.9 |
| *Total* | 853 | 100 |

Data are from the Armed Forces Institute of Pathology (AFIP).

ent trauma, reported in about 10–20% of cases, is probably coincidental,[61,63,78] although several striking cases reporting the origin of this tumor in a previous burn or surgical scar raise the question of a causal relation.[36,44] Other interesting features of the disease include association with acanthosis nigricans,[45] chronic arsenic exposure,[71] bacille Calmette Guérin (BCG) vaccination site,[43] acrodermatitis enteropathica,[69] regression following topical administration of a wild plant,[36] and rapid enlargement during pregnancy.[78] The first two cases, however, are not well documented and must be interpreted accordingly.

In most cases this tumor is characterized by slow but persistent growth over a long period, often several years. The clinical and gross appearances then are determined to a great extent by the stage of the disease. The initial manifestation is usually the development of a firm, plaque-like lesion of the skin, often with surrounding red to blue discoloration.[78] These lesions have been compared with the morphea of scleroderma or morphea-like basal cell carcinoma.[38] Rarely the lesions appear as an area of atrophy.[3,41] Less often, multiple small subcutaneous nodules appear initially rather than a plaque. The plaque may grow slowly or remain stationary for a variable period, eventually entering a more rapid growth phase and giving rise to one or more nodules. Thus only in the fully developed lesion is the typical "protuberant" appearance manifested. Neglected tumors may achieve enormous proportions and have multiple satellite nodules. Despite the large size of many of these tumors, though, the patients appear surprisingly well and lack the signs of cachexia associated with malignancies.

## Gross Findings

Most of these tumors are biopsied during the nodular stage; therefore the specimen consists of a solitary, protuberant, gray-white mass involving subcutis and skin (Figs. 14–1, 14–2, 14–3). The average size at surgery is approximately 5 cm.[78] Multiple discrete masses are usually not seen in the original tumor but are more characteristic of recurrent lesions (Fig. 14–4).[78] The skin overlying these tumors is taut or even ulcerated. Skeletal muscle extension is uncommon except in large or recurrent lesions. We and others have found that in rare cases this tumor is confined to the subcutis and lacks dermal involvement altogether.[19] Occasionally, areas of the tumor have a translucent or gelatinous appearance corresponding microscopically to myxoid change. Hemorrhage and cystic change are sometimes seen in the tumors, but necrosis, a common feature of malignant fibrous histiocytoma, is rare.

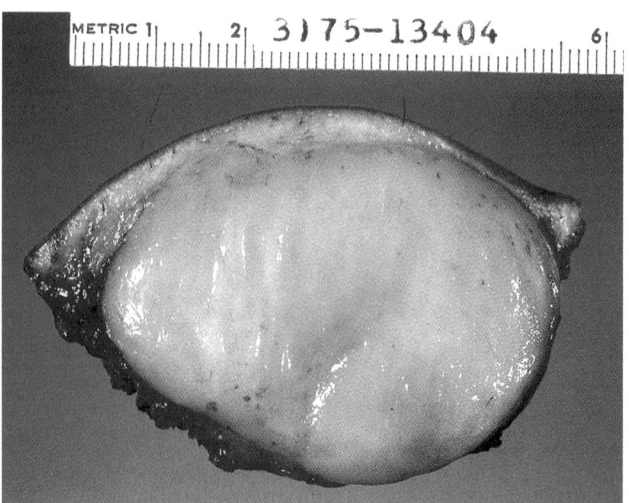


**FIGURE 14–1.** Typical dermatofibrosarcoma protuberans involving the dermis and subcutis in a nodular fashion.

## Microscopic Findings

Despite the apparent gross circumscription of these lesions, the tumor diffusely infiltrates the dermis and

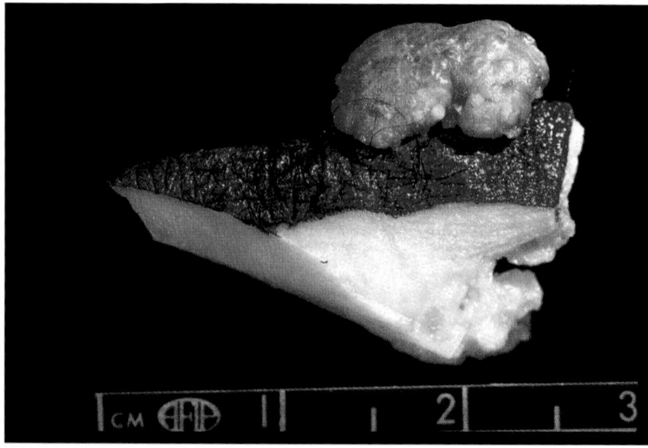


**FIGURE 14–2.** Small dermatofibrosarcoma displaying protuberant growth.

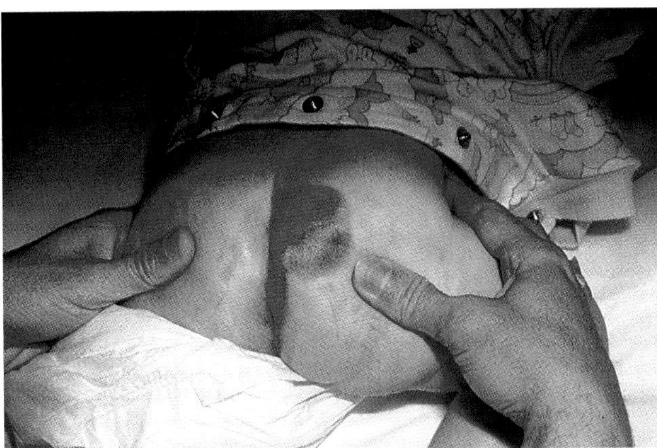

**FIGURE 14–3.** Dermatofibrosarcoma protuberans from the buttock of young child. It has the red color that some of these lesions exhibit.

subcutis (Fig. 14–5). The tumor may reach the epidermis or leave an uninvolved zone of dermis just underneath the epidermis. In either event, the overlying epidermis does not usually display the hyperplasia that characterizes some cutaneous fibrous histiocytomas (dermatofibromas).[78] The peripheral portions of the tumor have a deceptively bland appearance due in part to the marked attenuation of the cells at their advancing edge. This is especially true in superficial areas, where the spread of slender cells between preexisting collagen is easily mistaken for cutaneous fibrous histiocytoma (dermatofibroma) (Fig. 14–6A). In the deep regions the tumor spreads along connective tissue septa and between adnexae (Fig. 14–7), or it intricately interdigitates with lobules of subcutaneous fat, creating a lace-like or honeycomb effect (Fig. 14–6B).

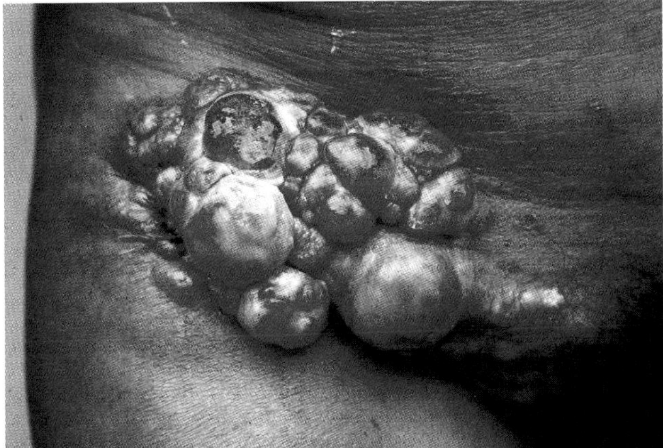

**FIGURE 14–4.** Gross appearance of an advanced case of dermatofibrosarcoma protuberans with multiple tumor nodules.

The central or main portion of the tumor is composed of a uniform population of slender fibroblasts arranged in a distinct, often monotonous storiform pattern around an inconspicuous vasculature (Figs. 14–8, 14–9). There is usually little nuclear pleomorphism and only low to moderate mitotic activity. Secondary elements such as giant cells, xanthoma cells, and inflammatory elements are few in number or absent altogether. In this respect, dermatofibrosarcoma protuberans displays remarkable uniformity compared with other fibrohistiocytic neoplasms. Although most tumors are characterized by these highly ordered cellular areas, occasional tumors contain myxoid areas (Fig. 14–10). These myxoid areas were initially believed to be a feature of recurrent lesions,[78] but recent reports indicate they may also be seen in the primary tumor.[25] Myxoid areas are characterized by the interstitial accumulation of ground substance material. As myxoid change of the stroma becomes more pronounced, the storiform pattern becomes less distinct and the vascular pattern more apparent. By virtue of these features, such tumors can resemble myxoid liposarcoma (Fig. 14–10B).

Giant cells, similar to those in giant cell fibroblastoma, can be identified in a small percentage of otherwise typical dermatofibrosarcomas. An unusual feature of dermatofibrosarcoma protuberans is the myoid nodule (Fig. 14–11). Originally construed as evidence of myofibroblastic differentiation,[13] these structures seem to be centered for the most part around blood vessels.[51,68] and likely represent an unusual nonneoplastic vascular response to the tumor. Infrequently, dermatofibrosarcoma protuberans contains areas that are indistinguishable from fibrosarcoma (Figs. 14–12, 14–13, 14–14). Characterized by long fascicles of spindle cells with more nuclear atypia and mitotic activity, these areas usually sharply abut conventional low-grade areas. Mitotic activity usually averages more than 5 mitotic figures/10 high-power fields (HPF), in contrast to areas of conventional dermatofibrosarcoma protuberans, which usually have fewer than 5 mitotic figures/10 HPF. In exceptional instances, dermatofibrosarcoma protuberans contains areas resembling malignant fibrous histiocytoma (Figs. 14–15, 14–16).[31,56] Fibrosarcomatous areas were originally believed to be more common in recurrent lesions, but recent studies have documented that the contrary is true.[31] The biologic significance of sarcomatous areas in dermatofibrosarcoma protuberans is discussed below. Metastatic deposits from this tumor occur most commonly in the lung and secondly in regional lymph nodes, where they may resemble the parent tumor or may appear more pleomorphic, like a fibrosarcoma (Fig. 14–17).

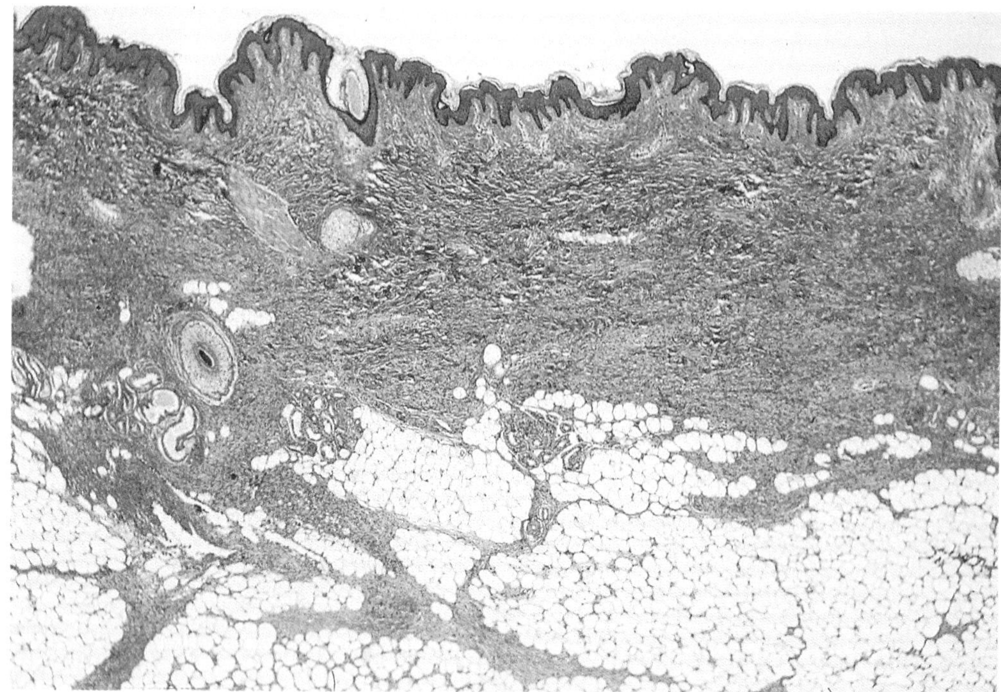

**FIGURE 14–5.** Plaque form of dermatofibrosarcoma protuberans illustrating the expansion of the interface between dermis and subcutis and the extension into subcutaneous fat.

## Immunohistochemical and Ultrastructural Findings

Dermatofibrosarcoma protuberans is characterized by the nearly consistent presence of CD34 (Fig. 14–18), the human progenitor cell antigen, in a significant proportion of its cells.[31,32,100] Although this antigen has been identified in a growing number of soft tissue tumors, its presence in dermatofibrosarcoma protuberans suggests a close linkage to the normal CD34$^+$ dendritic cells of the dermis, including those that ensheath the adnexa, nerves, and vessels.[100] The nearly consistent expression of this antigen has also proved useful for distinguishing dermatofibrosarcoma protuberans from benign fibrous histiocytoma, especially when dealing with small biopsies. Only occasional benign fibrous histiocytomas express this antigen.[31] Caution should be used when interpreting CD34 immunostains in spindle cell tumors of the skin, being certain that positively staining cells are neoplastic, not entrapped normal dermal dendritic cells. Because of the sensitivity of CD34 in the diagnosis of dermatofibrosarcoma protuberans, there has been little recent interest in studying these lesions ultrastructurally. Earlier studies indicated that the cells resemble fibroblasts,[33] although some have noted certain modifications that suggest perineural differentiation.[2,35] These features included convoluted nuclei, elaborate cell processes, moderate numbers of desmosomes, and incomplete basal lamina (Fig. 14–19).

## Cytogenetic Analysis

Both dermatofibrosarcoma and giant cell fibroblastoma are characterized by the presence of a supernumerary ring chromosome 11, 15 consisting of amplified sequences from chromosomes 17 and 22.[40,72] This genetic event fuses the platelet-derived growth factor $\beta$-chain (PDGF$\beta$) gene to the collagen type 1 $\alpha$1 gene (*COL1A1*) resulting in a fusion transcript that places PDGF$\beta$ under the control of the *COL1A1* promotor.[54,72] The fusion protein can be processed to an end-product that is indistinguishable from normal PDGF$\beta$.[70] It has been suggested that overproduction of PDGF$\beta$ by dermatofibrosarcoma results in autocrine stimulation and cell proliferation. This proposed sequence of events implies that inhibition of the PDGF receptor by specific blocking agents could be incorporated in pharmacologic agents to retard the growth of dermatofibrosarcoma protuberans, as has been demonstrated in nude mice.[70]

## Differential Diagnosis

The most common problem in the differential diagnosis is distinguishing this tumor from other fibrohistiocytic neoplasms. In general, dermatofibrosarcoma protuberans has a more uniform appearance and smaller cells, and it displays a more distinct storiform pattern with fewer secondary elements (giant cells, inflamma-

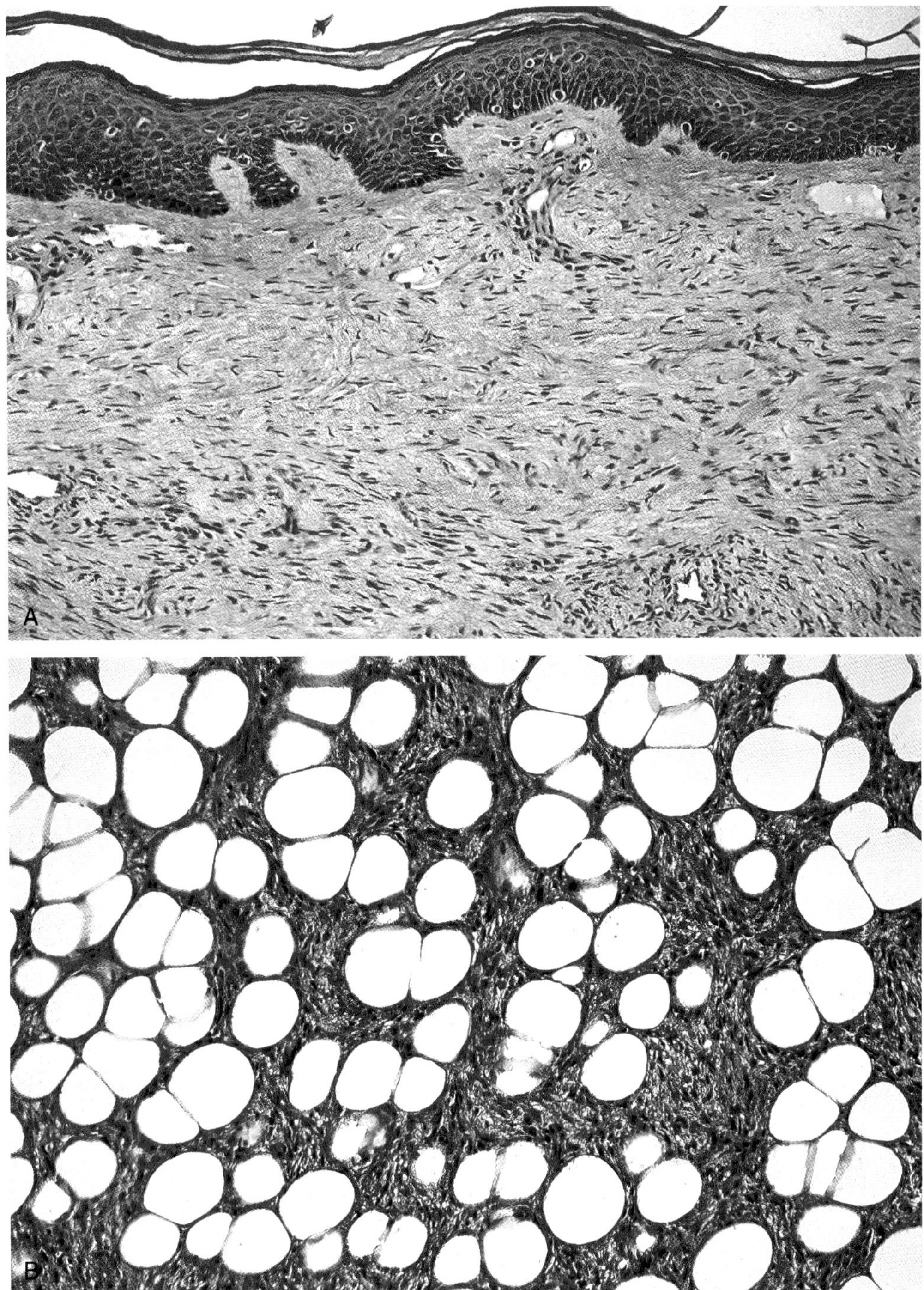

**FIGURE 14–6.** Superficial (**A**) and deep (**B**) extensions of dermatofibrosarcoma protuberans. Spread of the tumor between preexisting collagen of the dermis may simulate the appearance of a cutaneous fibrous histiocytoma (**A**). At the deep margin the tumor intricately interdigitates with normal fat (**B**).

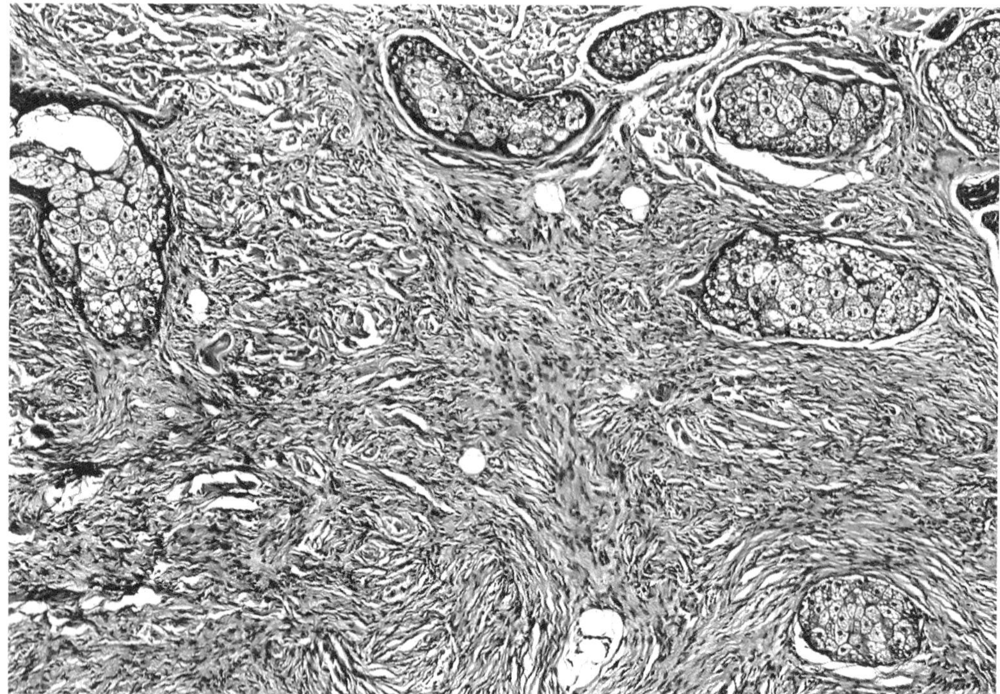

**FIGURE 14–7.** Dermatofibrosarcoma protuberans infiltrating between adnexal structures.

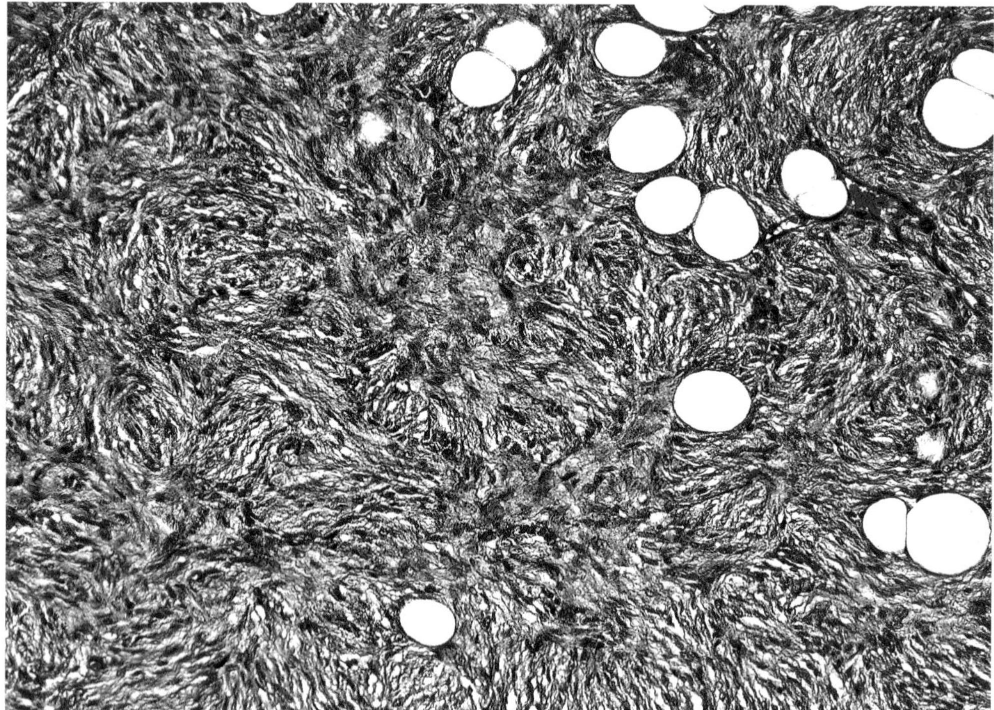

**FIGURE 14–8.** Slender spindle cells arranged in a distinct storiform pattern characterize most of these tumors.

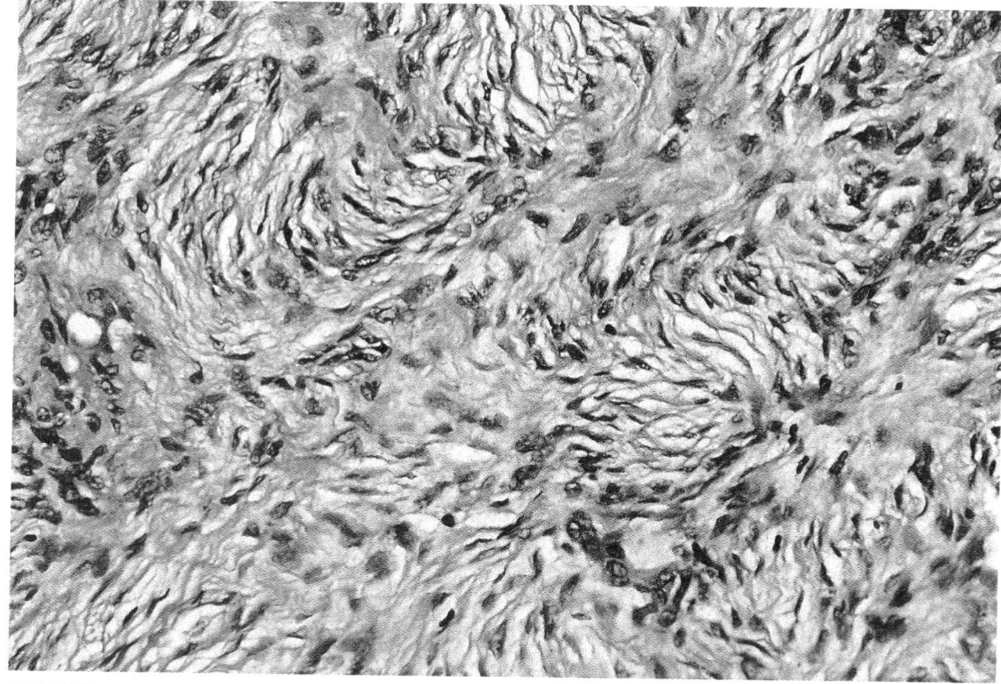

**FIGURE 14–9.** Dermatofibrosarcoma protuberans showing greater interstitial collagenization.

tory cells) than either a benign or malignant fibrous histiocytoma. The distinction between *benign fibrous histiocytoma* and dermatofibrosarcoma occasionally proves difficult when only the superficial portion of the dermatofibrosarcoma is present in a biopsy specimen, because these areas appear so well differentiated (Table 14–2). Under these circumstances, knowledge of the size and configuration of the lesion in question suggests the diagnosis, and biopsy of a deeper portion confirms it. In addition, because CD34 is almost always expressed by dermatofibrosarcoma and far less so by benign fibrous histiocytoma, CD34 is an extremely useful antigen for analyzing this problem.[32,100] *Malignant fibrous histiocytoma* is not often confused with this tumor because it is characterized by far more pleomorphism, mitotic activity, and necrosis. Moreover, its typical deep location in muscle and more rapid growth are at variance with the indolent course of this tumor. Rarely, one encounters dermatofibrosarcoma protuberans with areas of malignant fibrous histiocytoma (Figs. 14–15, 14–16). As indicated earlier, when such areas represent more than just a microscopic focus, they should be diagnosed as "sarcoma arising in dermatofibrosarcoma protuberans."

*Text continued on page 503*

**TABLE 14–2** COMPARISON OF FIBROUS HISTIOCYTOMA AND DERMATOFIBROSARCOMA PROTUBERANS

| Parameter | Benign Fibrous Histiocytoma | Dermatofibrosarcoma |
|---|---|---|
| Common locations | Extremities | Trunk, groin |
| Size | Usually small | Small to large |
| Growth pattern | Short fascicles, haphazard | Monotonous storiform |
| Cell population | Plump spindle cells often admixed with inflammatory cells, siderophages, giant cells | Slender spindle cells with few if any secondary elements |
| Hemorrhage | Occasional | No |
| Subcutaneous extension | Occasional and limited | Consistent and extensive |
| CD34 | Focal staining in occasional cases | Diffuse and extensive staining in most cases |
| Local recurrence | 5–10% | 20–50% |
| Metastasis | Anecdotal cases only | Rare in conventional form; potentially higher if fibrosarcoma present with inadequate local control |
| Malignant transformation | Anecdotal cases only | Fibrosarcoma in occasional cases |

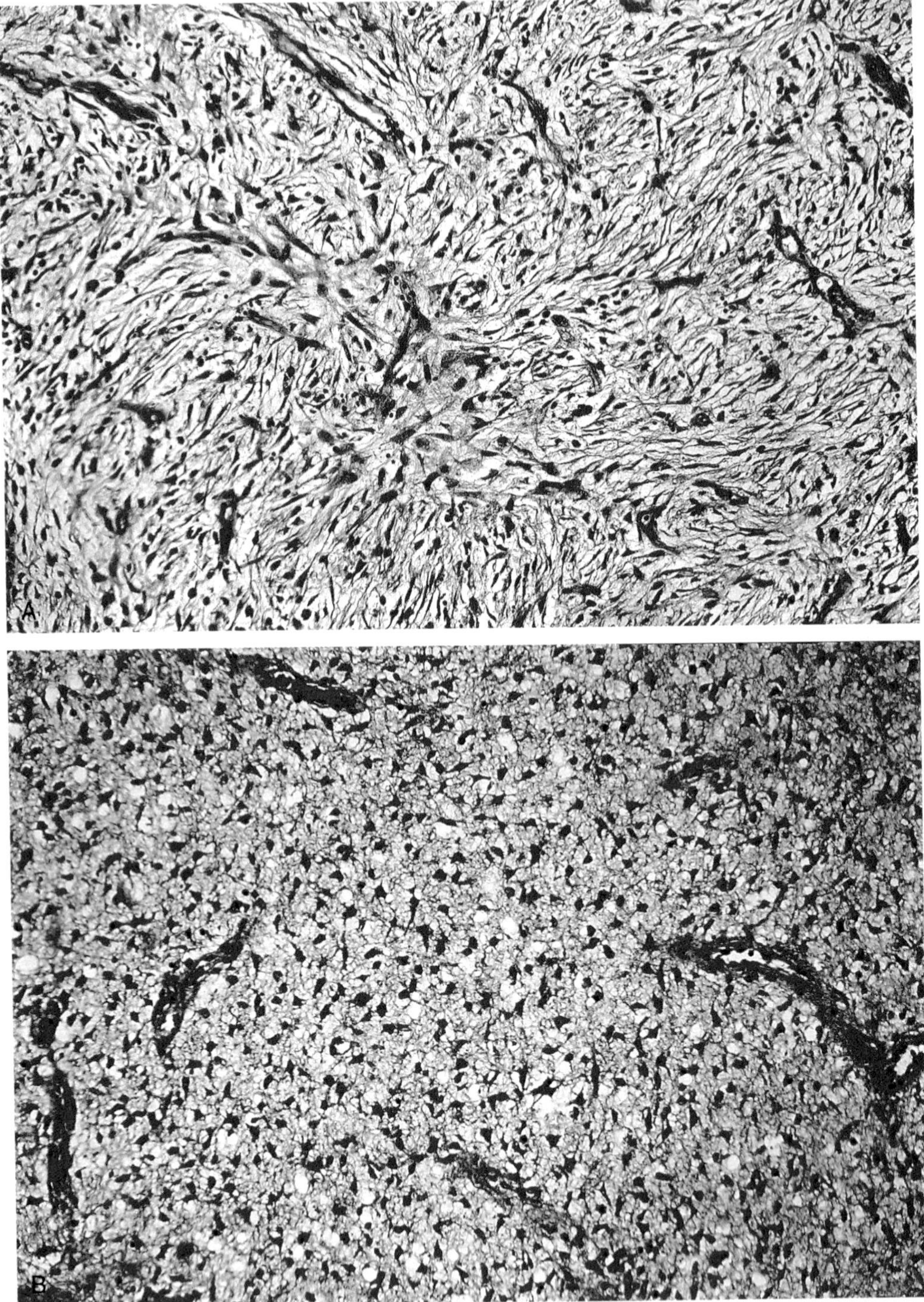


**FIGURE 14–10.** (**A**) Myxoid change in dermatofibrosarcoma protuberans. (**B**) When the myxoid change is prominent, the storiform pattern may be lacking altogether, and the tumor may resemble a myxoid liposarcoma.

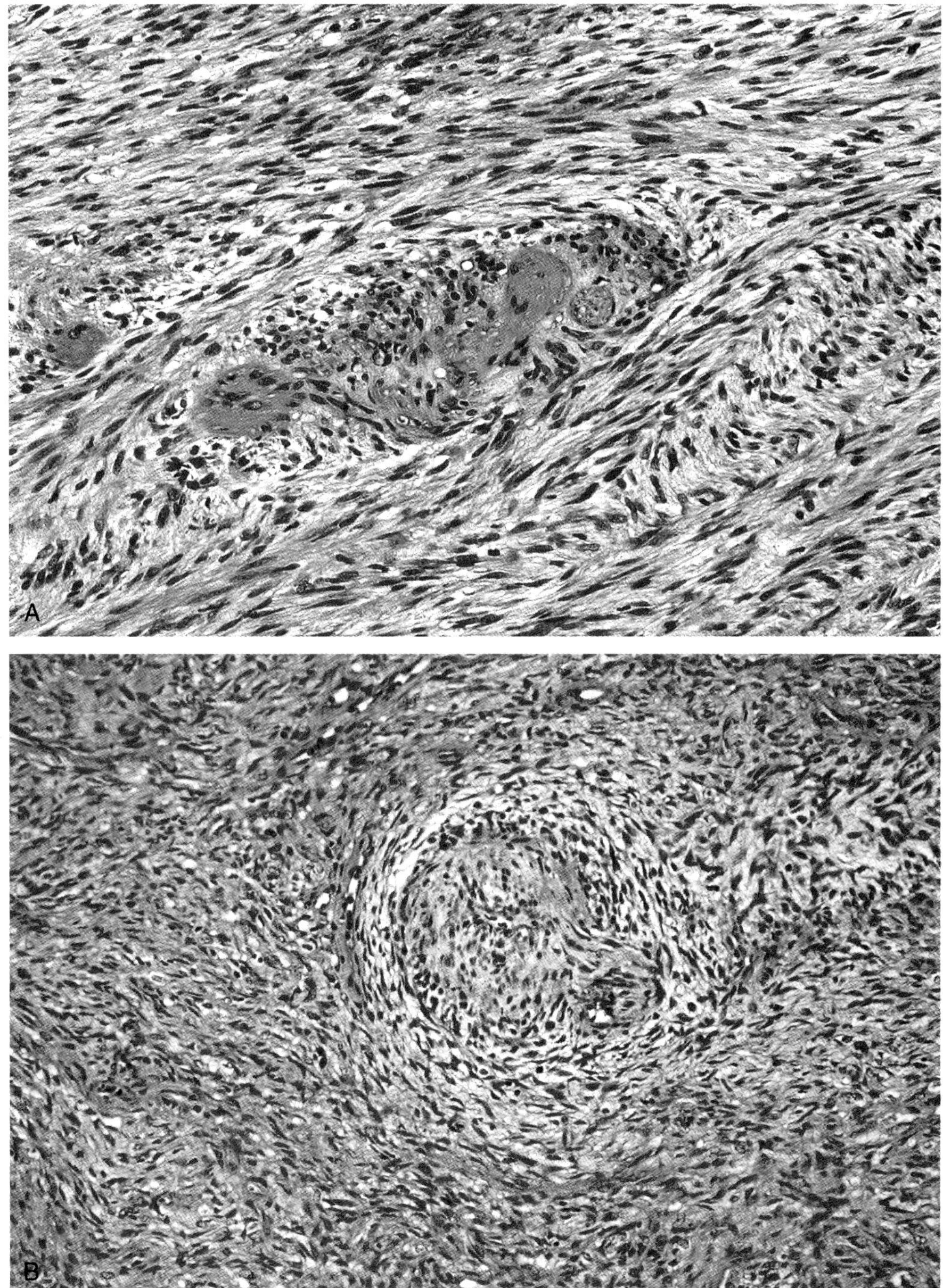

**FIGURE 14–11.** (**A**) Myoid balls within dermatofibrosarcoma protuberans. (**B**) Myoid ball centered around a small vessel.

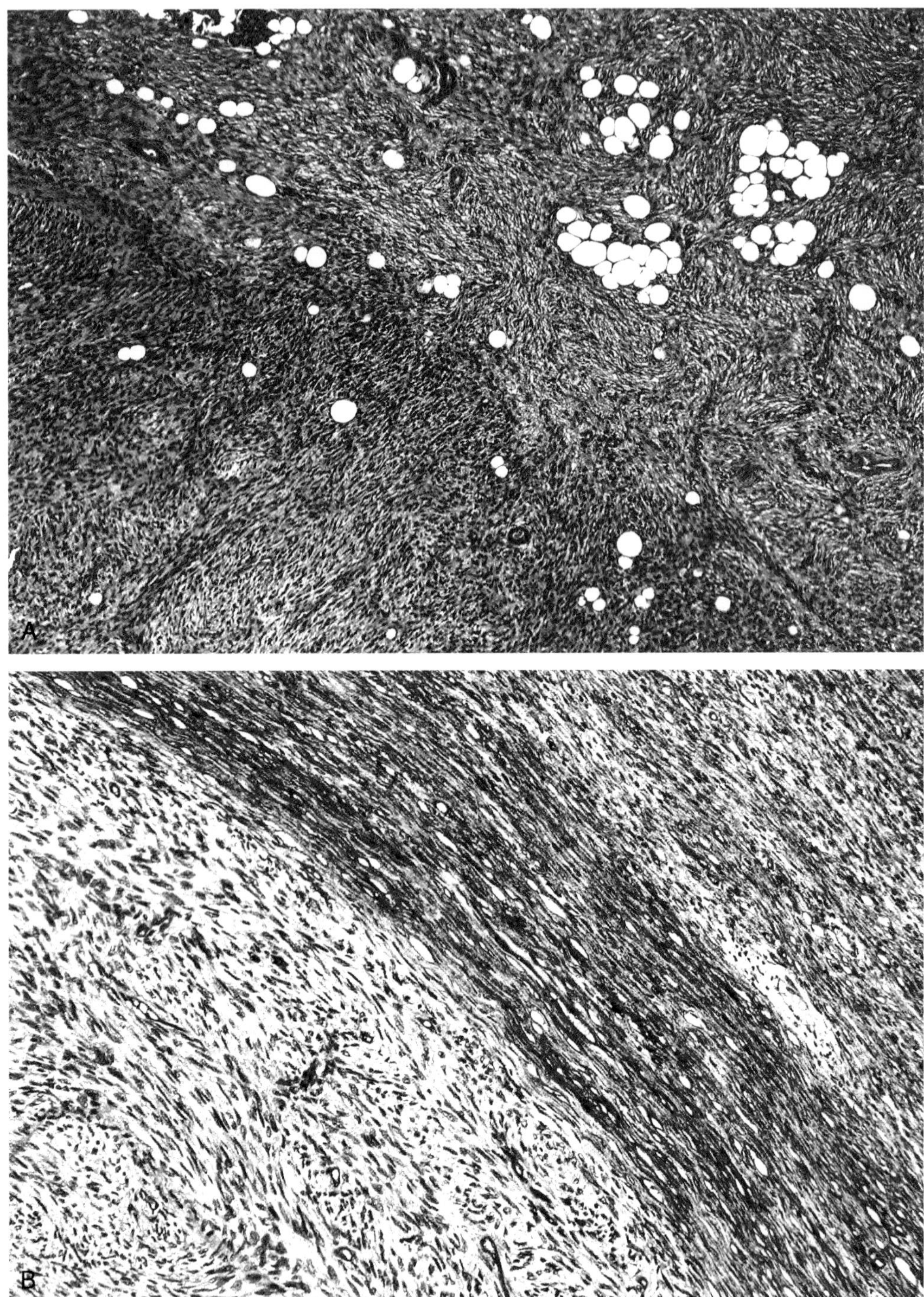


**FIGURE 14–12.** (**A**) Dermatofibrosarcoma protuberans showing the transition to fibrosarcoma (lower left corner). (**B**) CD34 immunostain in a dermatofibrosarcoma (upper right) with fibrosarcomatous areas. Note the marked diminution of CD34 immunostain in the fibrosarcomatous portion of the tumor (lower left).

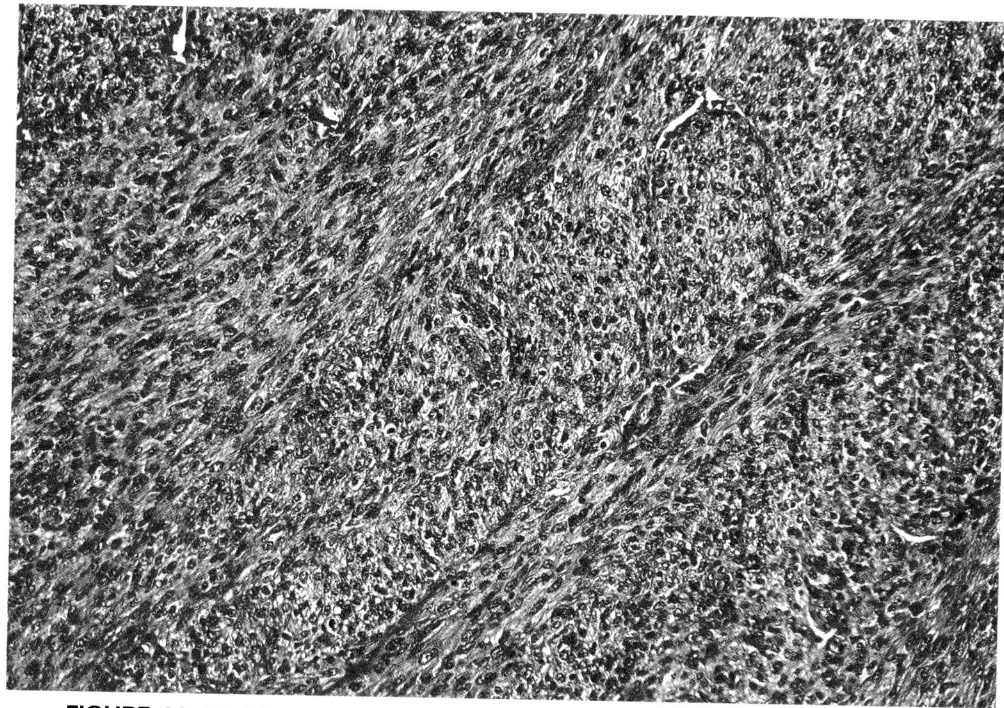

**FIGURE 14–13.** Fibrosarcomatous areas within dermatofibrosarcoma protuberans.

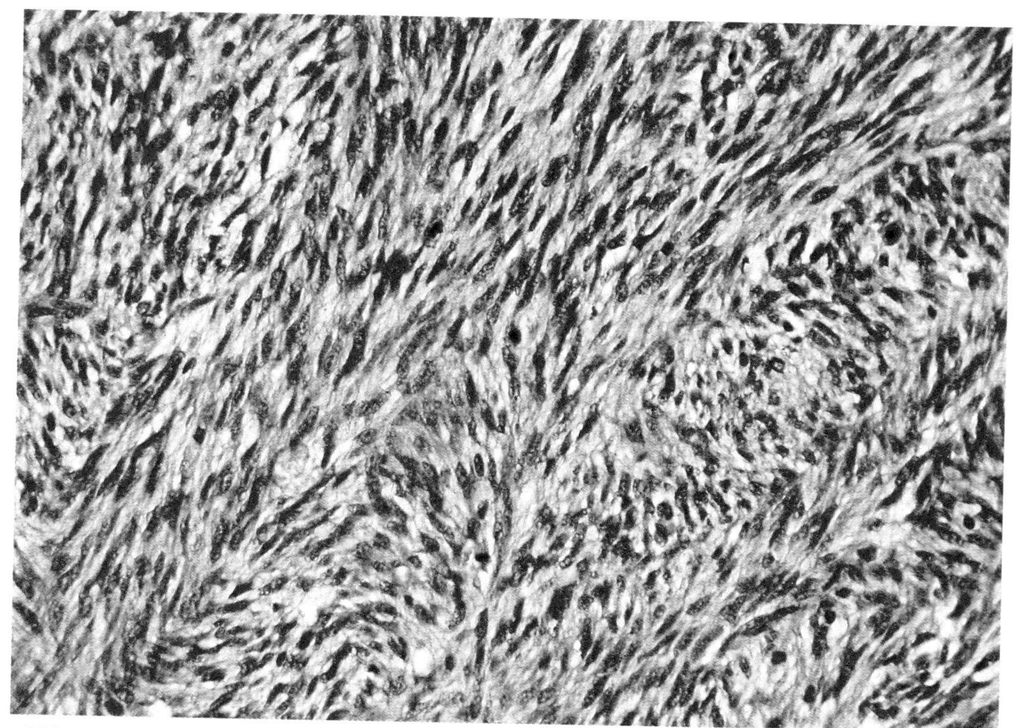

**FIGURE 14–14.** Fibrosarcomatous areas showing increased cellularity and mitotic activity.

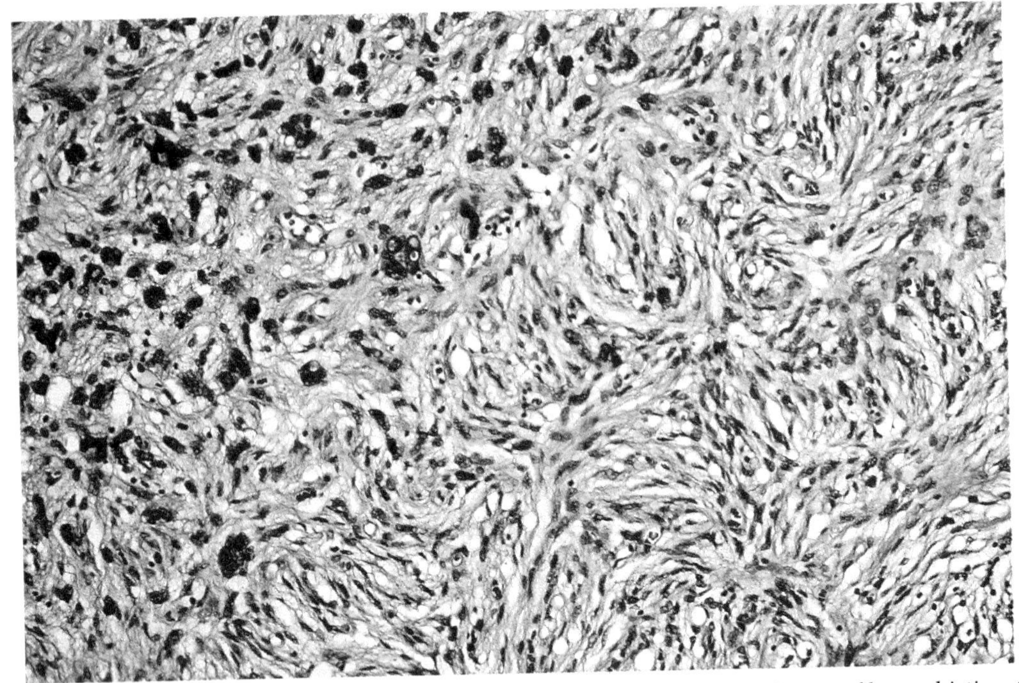

**FIGURE 14–15.** Dermatofibrosarcoma protuberans with transformation to malignant fibrous histiocytoma.

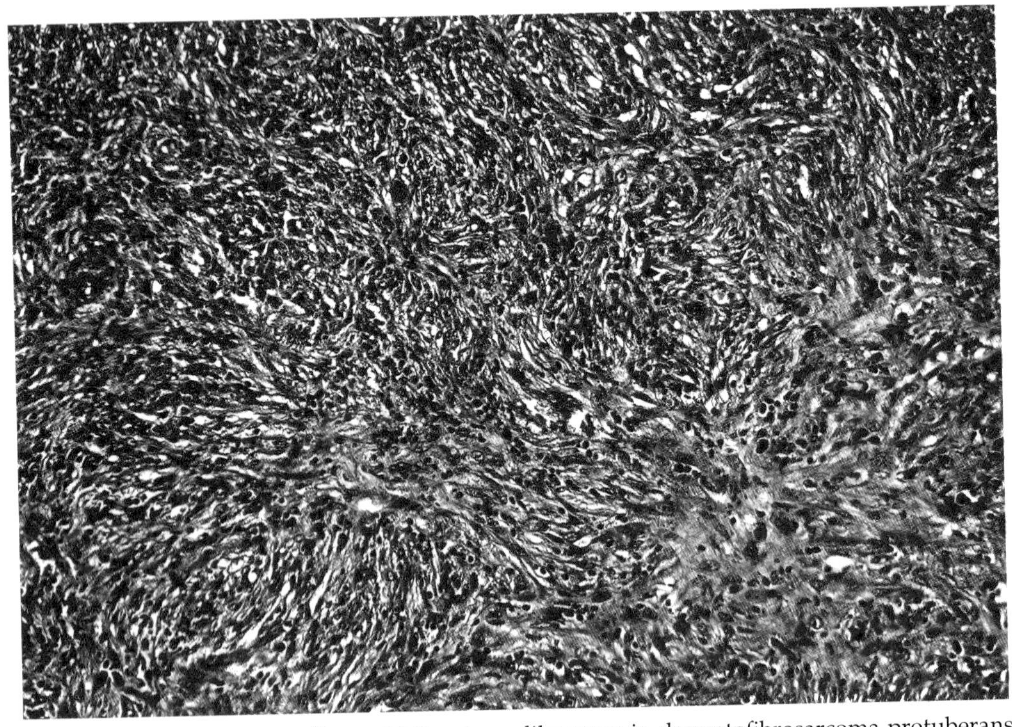

**FIGURE 14–16.** Malignant fibrous histiocytoma-like areas in dermatofibrosarcoma protuberans.

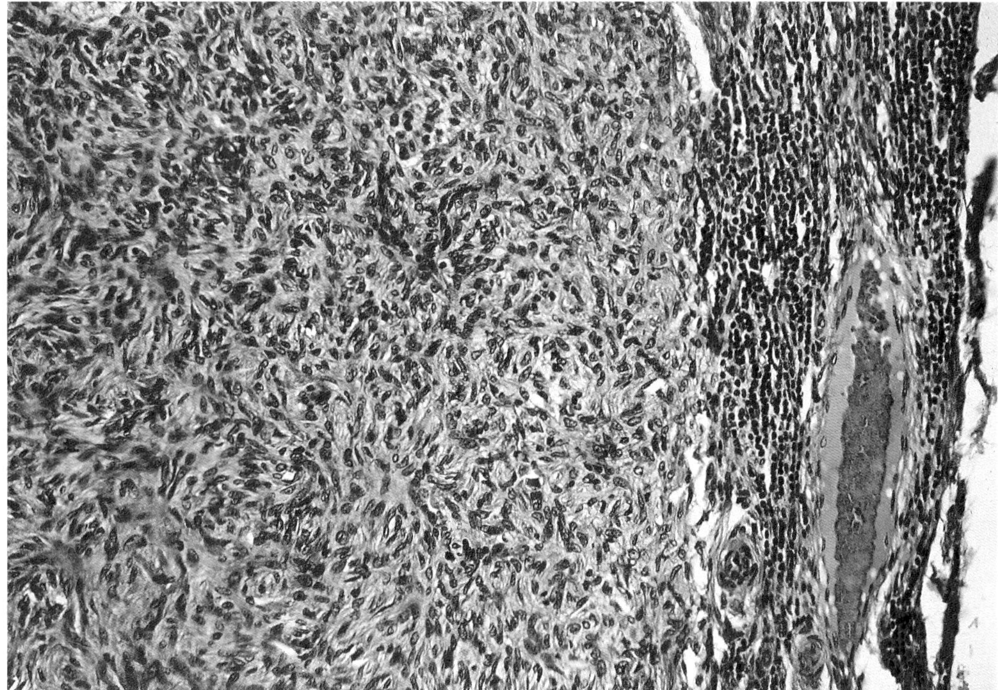

**FIGURE 14–17.** Lymph node metastasis from dermatofibrosarcoma protuberans.

A second common problem is the confusion of this tumor with benign neural tumors, specifically a diffuse form of *neurofibroma*. This is most likely to occur when dermatofibrosarcoma is in the plaque stage or when a biopsy is done on only the periphery of the tumor. However, neurofibroma usually contains tactoid structures or other features of neural differentiation, and it lacks the highly cellular areas with mitotic figures that characterize the central portion of a dermatofibrosarcoma. The presence of S-100 protein in virtually all neurofibromas and its absence in dermatofibrosarcoma is an additional contrasting point.

Finally, highly myxoid forms of dermatofibrosarcoma may resemble *myxoid liposarcoma* by virtue of the prominent vasculature and bland stellate or fusiform cells. However, the superficial location, gross configuration, CD34 immunoreactivity, and complete absence of lipoblasts should raise serious questions concerning the diagnosis of liposarcoma. In such cases additional sampling of the tumor or review of the original material in a recurrent lesion may reveal the diagnostic cellular areas.

## Discussion

Unlike the benign fibrous histiocytoma it resembles, dermatofibrosarcoma protuberans is a locally aggressive neoplasm that recurs in up to half of the patients.[44,78] The high recurrence rate in part reflects the extensive infiltration of the tumor compared with fibrous histiocytoma and failure to appreciate this phenomenon at the time of surgery. It is clear that prompt wide local excision (2–3 cm), the standard of practice for this lesion, can markedly alter the recurrence rate. Recurrence rates reported in the literature for patients treated by wide local excision average 18% compared to 43% when the excision was undefined or conservative.[30] In addition, recurrence rates in cases treated primarily at large referral centers are low (1.75%–33%),[12,61,63] again suggesting that adequate initial surgery is essential for minimizing recurrences. The risk of local recurrence, furthermore, correlates well with the extent of the wide excision. If the excision margin is 3 cm or more, the recurrence rate is 20%, compared with 41% if the margin is 2 cm or less.[67] If local recurrence develops it is usually within 3 years of the initial surgery,[44] although recurrences after several years have been reported, attesting to the need for long-term follow-up. In patients who develop multiple recurrences, progressively shorter intervals between successive recurrences have been noted.[78]

Moh's micrographic surgery has been met with growing enthusiasm for treatment of this disease.[66] Those who advocate this approach point out that dermatofibrosarcoma protuberans occasionally grows in an asymmetric fashion from its epicenter such that a traditional wide local excision fails to remove all tumor in a subset of cases.[65] Moh's surgery offers the potential to achieve clear margins with minimum re-

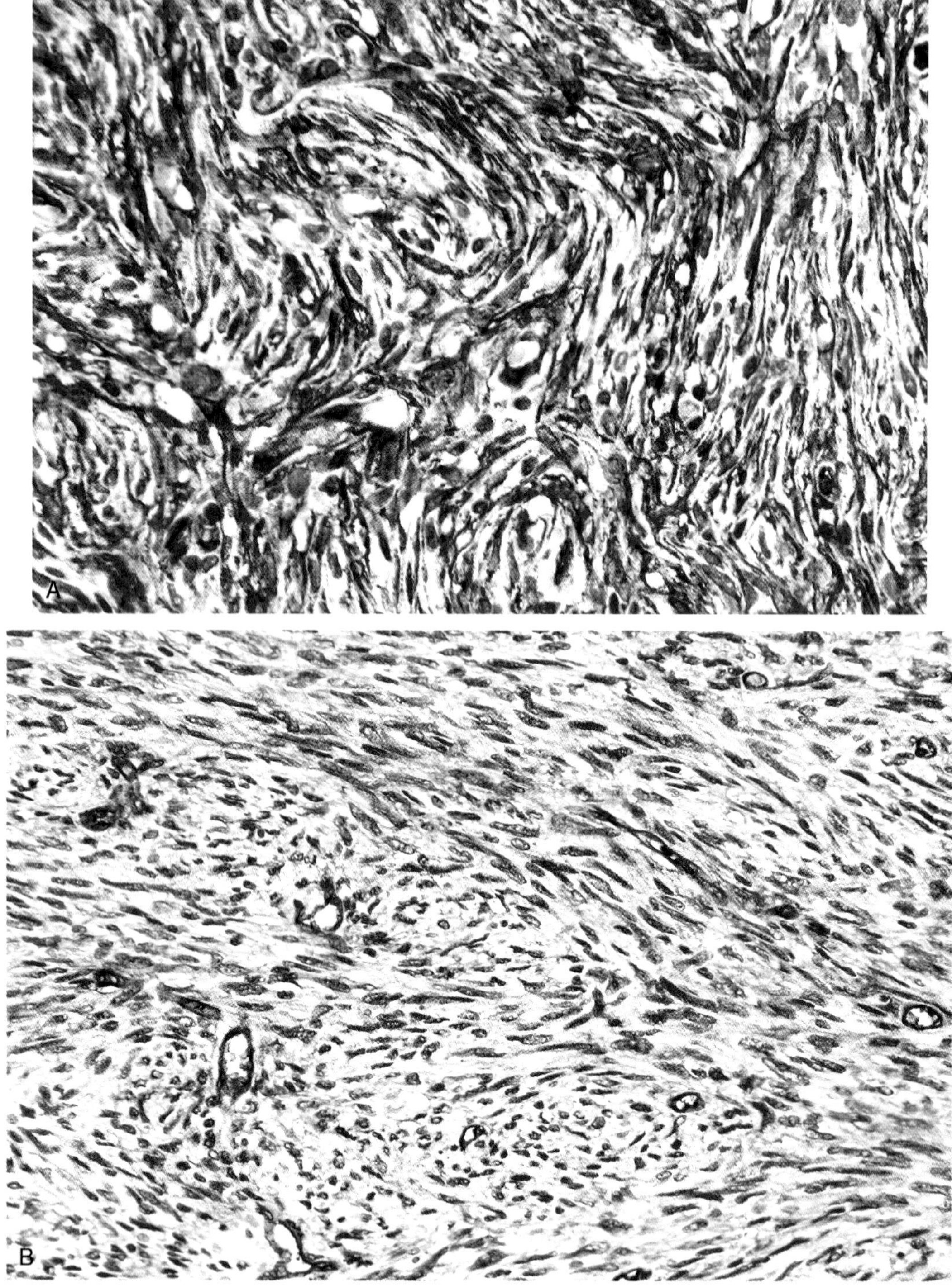


**FIGURE 14–18.** CD34 immunoreactivity within a conventional dermatofibrosarcoma (**A**) compared to markedly reduced immunoreactivity within a fibrosarcomatous area of dermatofibrosarcoma protuberans (**B**).

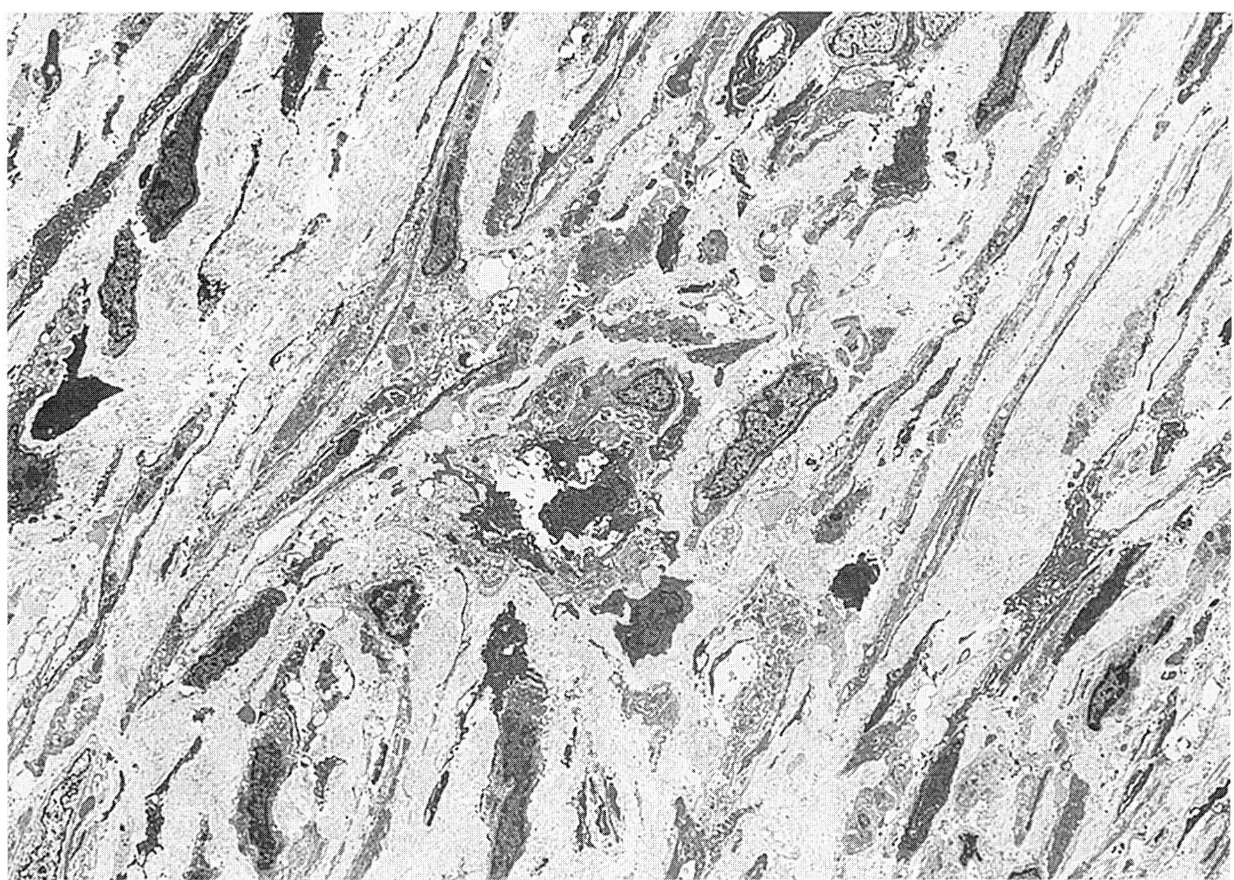

**FIGURE 14–19.** Electron micrograph of dermatofibrosarcoma protuberans showing the center of a storiform area occupied by a small vessel. Fibroblast-like cells spin out from the vessel and have numerous slender processes that may join each other by means of specialized cell contacts. (From Taxy JB, Battifora H. The electron microscope in the study and diagnosis of soft tissue tumors. In: Trump BF, Jones RT (eds) Diagnostic Electron Microscopy. Wiley, New York, 1980.)

moval of normal tissue, an advantage particularly attractive for sites such as the head and neck. In a review of the literature by Gloster et al.,[30] recurrence rates following Moh's surgery were 6–7% compared to 18% with standard wide excision.

Despite its locally aggressive behavior, this tumor infrequently metastasizes and therefore should be clearly distinguished from conventional sarcomas. The incidence of metastasis is difficult to assess because of the bias introduced when selectively reporting metastasizing tumors, the inability to determine if sarcomatous areas were noted in a subset of reported cases, and the lack of uniform treatment. In general, however, for the ordinary dermatofibrosarcoma protuberans uncomplicated by areas of fibrosarcoma, metastasis appears to be an uncommon event. In one large study of 115 patients no metastases were observed,[78] whereas in two other studies 5 of 86 patients[44] and 4 of 96 patients[63] developed metastases. In the latter study the follow-up period was 15 years. Thus long-term follow-up may indicate higher metastatic rates than previously accepted. Of the 471 patients reported in the literature, 16 (3.4%) developed metastatic disease.[63] About three-fourths of patients with metastases have hematogenous spread to the lungs, and one-fourth have lymphatic spread to regional lymph nodes. Metastases to other sites, such as the brain, bones, and heart, have also been documented. Although some metastasizing cases have clearly originated from tumors with areas of "sarcoma" (see below), some have not.[1,38]

Metastasizing lesions share some common clinical features: They are almost always recurrent lesions, and there is usually an interval of several years between diagnosis and metastasis. The low incidence of regional lymph node metastasis and the negative findings in a small series of blind lymph node dissections do not warrant routine node dissection. Resection of isolated pulmonary metastases has been advocated because of the overall low-grade behavior of the tumor.[1] Radiotherapy has been recommended for large, unresectable tumors or postoperatively for margin-positive tumors.[76]

## SARCOMA ARISING IN DERMATOFIBROSARCOMA PROTUBERANS (FIBROSARCOMATOUS VARIANT OF DERMATOFIBROSARCOMA PROTUBERANS)

There has been increasing awareness that a small subset of dermatofibrosarcoma may contain areas indistinguishable from conventional fibrosarcoma (and rarely malignant fibrous histiocytoma).[31,34,46,51,56,81] This had led to the use of the term "fibrosarcomatous variant of dermatofibrosarcoma" and the suggestion that these lesions pursue a more aggressive course, although the risk of distant metastasis is debated. These tumors share the same general clinical properties as ordinary dermatofibrosarcoma protuberans, and in most cases the sarcomatous foci are noted in the original tumor.

Criteria for the diagnosis of sarcoma arising in dermatofibrosarcoma protuberans have never been precisely defined. We have generally used a constellation of features to establish the diagnosis: The "sarcomatous" foci should constitute at least 5–10% of the tumor, in contrast to simply a rare to occasional microscopic focus. These zones are characterized by a fascicular (rather than storiform) architectural pattern and are composed of plump spindle cells of high nuclear grade. Mitotic activity is usually increased in these areas, whereas CD34 immunoreactivity is diminished (Fig. 14–19B), compared to the surrounding dermatofibrosarcoma. Although we have never required an absolute level of mitotic activity to diagnose sarcomatous change, mitotic activity within these sarcomatous averages 7–15/10 HPF[31,46] compared to 1–3/10 HPF in the dermatofibrosarcoma. CD34 immunoreactivity is usually reduced in these areas as well.

The significance of sarcomatous forms of dermatofibrosarcoma protuberans has been the subject of a number of studies. Although it seems logical that high-grade areas within a low-grade lesion would affect behavior adversely, early studies failed to confirm this hypothesis in a statistically meaningful fashion.[20,80] Ding and Enjoji suggested that fibrosarcomatous areas within dermatofibrosarcoma protuberans are associated with a higher local recurrence rate and thus a more aggressive course, but the status and adequacy of surgical excisions in these cases was not made clear.[20] Connelly and Evans[14] reported no difference in the local recurrence rate or in time to recurrence compared with conventional dermatofibrosarcoma protuberans but noted that two of their six patients with fibrosarcomatous areas developed metastatic disease. Two large studies by Mentzel et al.[46] and Pizarro et al.,[64] on the other hand, revealed higher local recurrence rates (58% and 42%, respectively) and metastatic rates (13.7% and 33.0%, respectively) (Table 14–3). In neither study, however, did it appear that wide local excision with clear margins was achieved in most cases. Because the ability to eradicate tumor locally arguably affects the risk of subsequent dissemination, neither of these studies addressed the behavior of this neoplasm in the context of the current standard of practice. In our experience with 18 patients treated by wide local excision and clear margins and with a minimum follow-up of 5 years, local recurrence rates are essentially identical to those of ordinary dermatofibrosarcoma protuberans; and we noted no instance of metastasis. Similarly, culling cases from the literature of sarcomatous dermatofibrosarcoma in which wide local excisions were performed, only one instance of metastasis was noted (Table 14–4).

In summary, although dermatofibrosarcoma protuberans containing fibrosarcoma may well be an inherently more aggressive neoplasm, this behavior can be favorably influenced by wide local excision to the extent that there may be little increased risk of distant metastasis over that of conventional dermatofibrosarcoma protuberans. Thus wide local excision should be

**TABLE 14–3 SARCOMA ARISING IN DERMATOFIBROSARCOMA PROTUBERANS**

| Study | No. of Patients* | Recurrence Rate (%) | Metastatic Rate (%) |
|---|---|---|---|
| Mentzel et al.[46] | 34 | 58 | 14.7 |
| Pizarro et al.[64] | 19 | 42 | 33.0 |
| Goldblum et al.[31] | 18 | 22 | 0 |

*Patients with follow-up information.

**TABLE 14–4 SARCOMAS ARISING IN DERMATOFIBROSARCOMA PROTUBERANS TREATED WITH WIDE LOCAL EXCISION, WITH FOLLOW-UP INFORMATION**

| Study | No. of Patients | Metastasis |
|---|---|---|
| Goldblum et al.[31] | 18 | 0/18 |
| Mentzel et al.[46] | 6 | 0/6 |
| Diaz-Cascajo et al.[18] | 3 | 1/3 |
| O'Connell et al.[55] | 2 | 0/2 |
| *Total* | 29 | 1/30 |

even more forcefully encouraged than for conventional dermatofibrosarcoma protuberans.

## BEDNAR TUMORS (PIGMENTED DERMATOFIBROSARCOMA PROTUBERANS, STORIFORM NEUROFIBROMA)

In 1957 Bednar[6] described a group of nine cutaneous tumors characterized by indolent growth and a prominent storiform pattern and in four cases by the presence of melanin pigment. He regarded these tumors as variants of neurofibroma (*storiform neurofibroma*) and cited as evidence the presence of similar areas within neural nevi[5] and the presence of melanin. We reserve the term *Bednar tumor* for tumors that resemble dermatofibrosarcoma protuberans but that, in addition, have melanin pigment. These tumors are uncommon,[6,20,21,23,26,79] as evidenced by the fact that Bednar gleaned only four cases from among 100,000 biopsy specimens; in our experience these tumors account for fewer than 5% of all cases of dermatofibrosarcoma protuberans. Although, as suggested by Bednar, these tumors may represent neural lesions, their nonpigmented portions are virtually identical to dermatofibrosarcoma protuberans. Moreover, their clinical and gross features are similar. Most are slowly growing cutaneous masses that extend to the epidermis and advance into the deep subcutis. The number of melanin-bearing cells varies widely within these tumors. In some, large numbers of melanin-containing cells cause black discoloration of the tumor (Fig. 14–20), whereas in others melanin is so sparse it can be appreciated only microscopically. These cells are scattered irregularly throughout the tumor (Fig. 14–21A). Their tentacle-like processes emanating from a central nucleus-containing zone give them a characteristic bipolar or multipolar shape, depending on the plane of the section (Fig. 14–21B). They stain with conventional melanin stains and ultrastructurally contain mature membrane-bound melanosomes. Electron microscopic studies reveal that most areas of Bednar tumors are composed of slender fibroblastic cells arranged in a delicate collagen matrix (Fig. 14–22), although other areas have cells more suggestive of Schwann cell differentiation (Fig. 14–23). The cells have numerous interlocking processes elaborately invested with basal laminae. Mature and immature melanosomes can be identified within the tumor cells. We have suggested that this finding indicates that the tumor synthesizes rather than phagocytoses melanin (Fig. 14–24), whereas others have suggested that the tumor is simply colonized by melanin-bearing cells.[26] On the other hand, we have not been able to identify S-100 protein,[49] which is present in certain neural tumors,[22,28,52,53] in Bednar tumors or their nonpigmented counterparts.

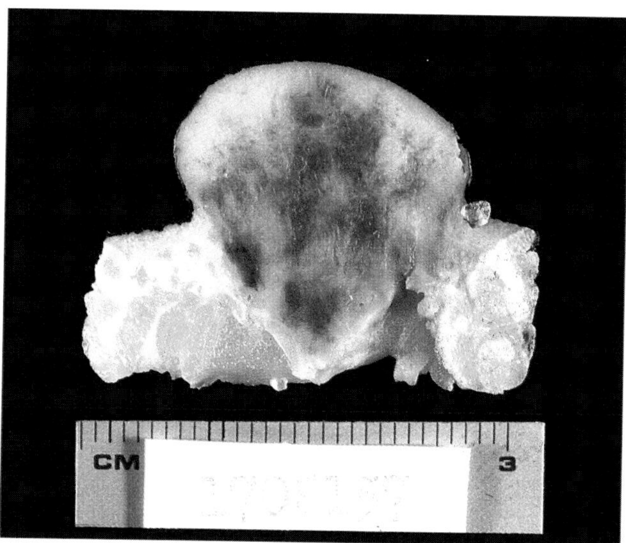

**FIGURE 14–20.** Bednar tumor. Gross appearance of the tumor is identical to conventional dermatofibrosarcoma protuberans, but the substance of the tumor is flecked with melanin pigment.

Because of the rarity of this tumor, there are few collective data in the literature concerning its behavior, although overall it appears to be similar to dermatofibrosarcoma protuberans. In addition, these tumors may display fibrosarcomatous areas.[7] There are also rare examples of metastasis, some with areas of fibrosarcoma,[7,58] including one report in the literature of a Bednar tumor with pulmonary metastasis.[59]

## GIANT CELL FIBROBLASTOMA

Giant cell fibroblastoma was first described in 1982 by Shmookler and Enzinger, who suggested that it represents a juvenile form of dermatofibrosarcoma protuberans, a view reinforced in their seminal publication in 1989.[99] Subsequent reports reaffirmed it as an entity[83,86,88,91,93,94,96–98] and embraced this notion for describing tumors with hybrid features or lesions that evolved from one pattern to the other.[83–85,87,88,90,91,95]

Most recently this lesion has been shown to have the same cytogenetic abnormality (supernumerary ring chromosome derived from chromosomes 17 and 22)[89] and fusion transcript as dermatofibrosarcoma protuberans, leaving little doubt that the giant cell fibroblastoma is a histologic variant of dermatofibrosarcoma.

### Clinical Findings

Giant cell fibroblastoma develops as a painless nodule or mass in the dermis or subcutis, with a predilection for the back of the thigh, inguinal region, and chest

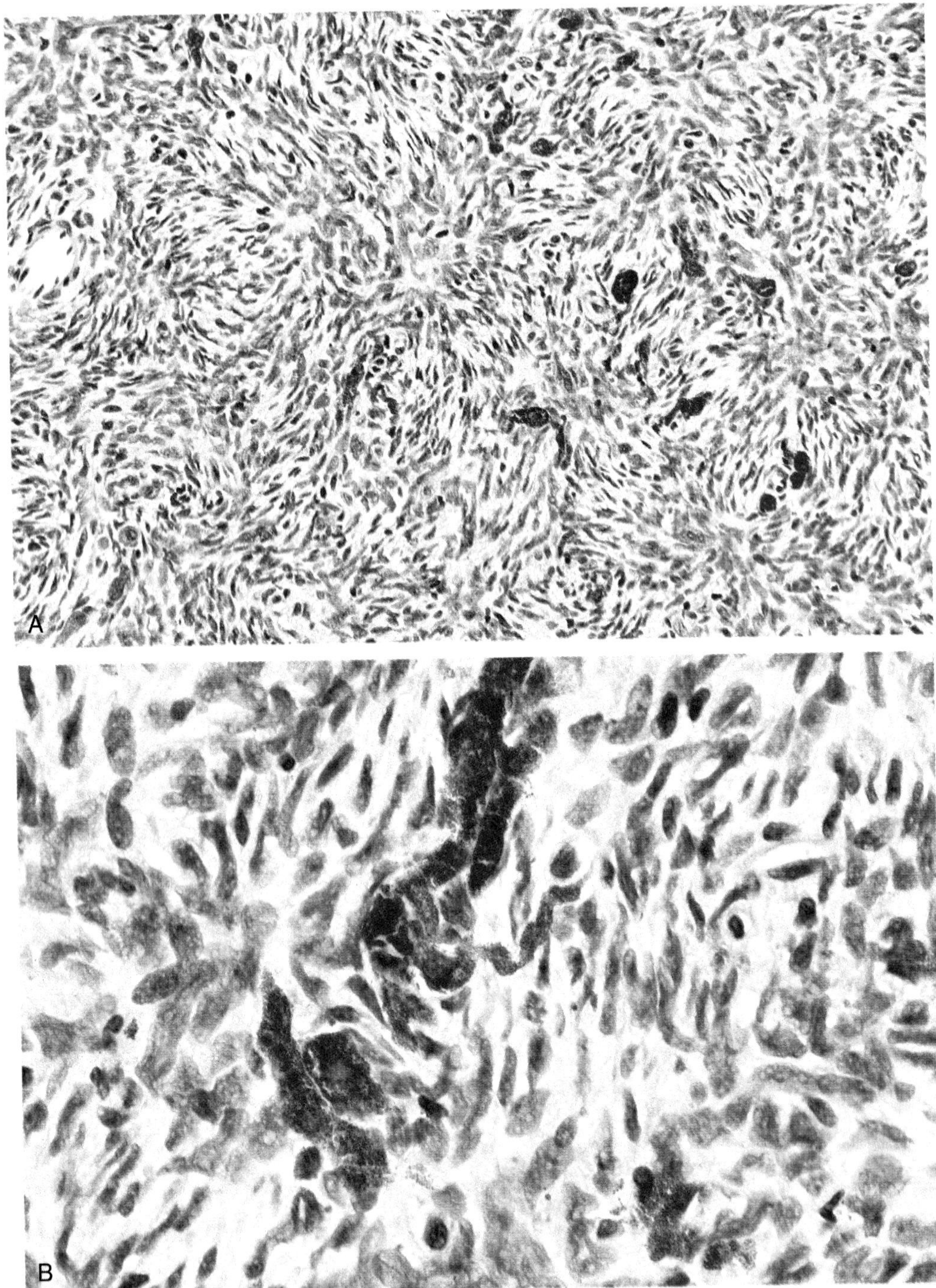


**FIGURE 14–21.** Pigmented dermatofibrosarcoma protuberans (Bednar tumor) (**A**) showing dendritic pigmented cells (**B**).

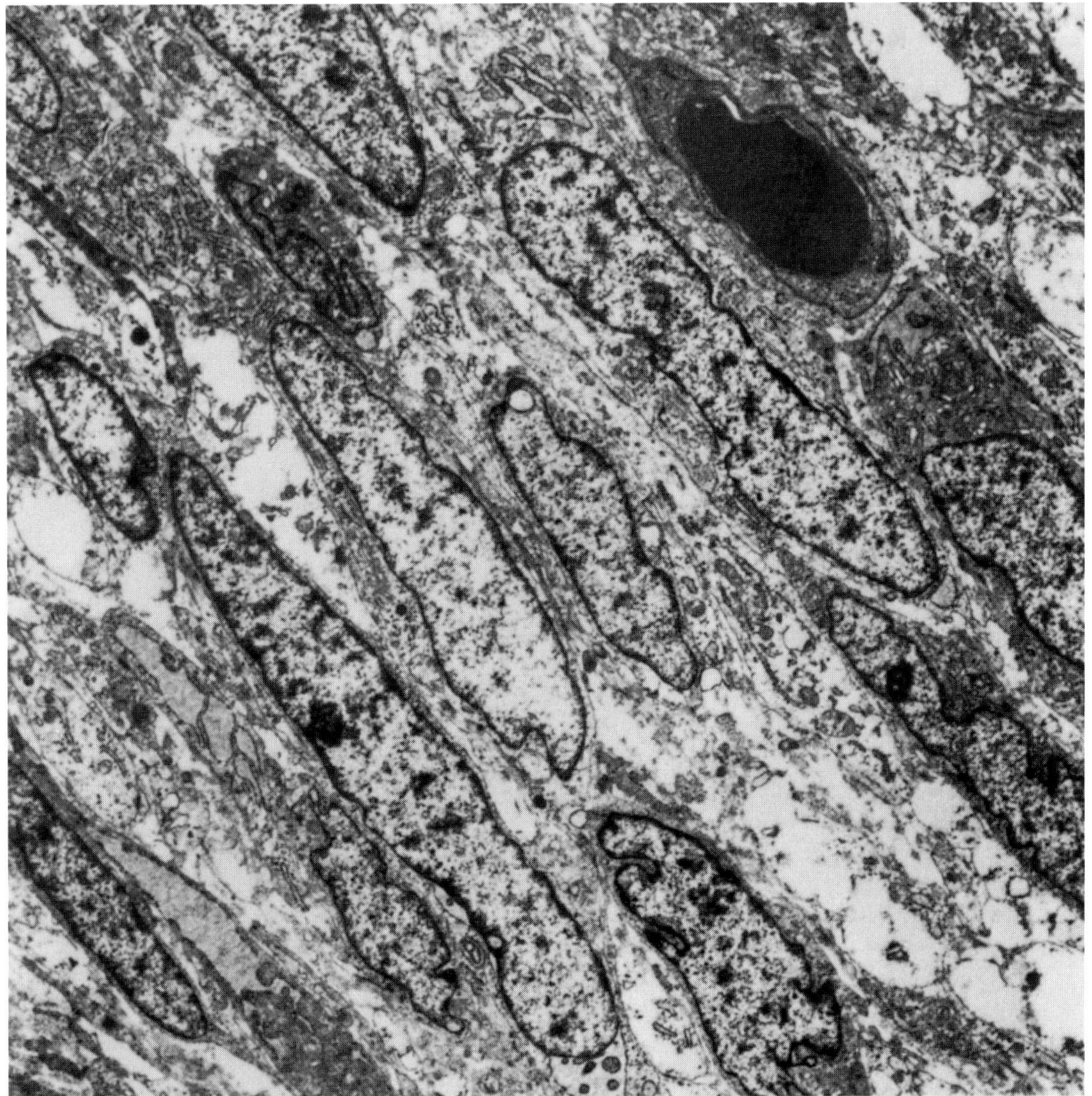

**FIGURE 14–22.** Predominant cells in a Bednar tumor have features of fibroblasts. (×5700) (From Dupree SB, Langloss JM, Weiss SW. Pigmented dermatofibrosarcoma protuberans (Bednar tumor): a pathologic, ultrastructural, and immunohistochemical study. Am J Surg Pathol 9:630, 1985, with permission.)

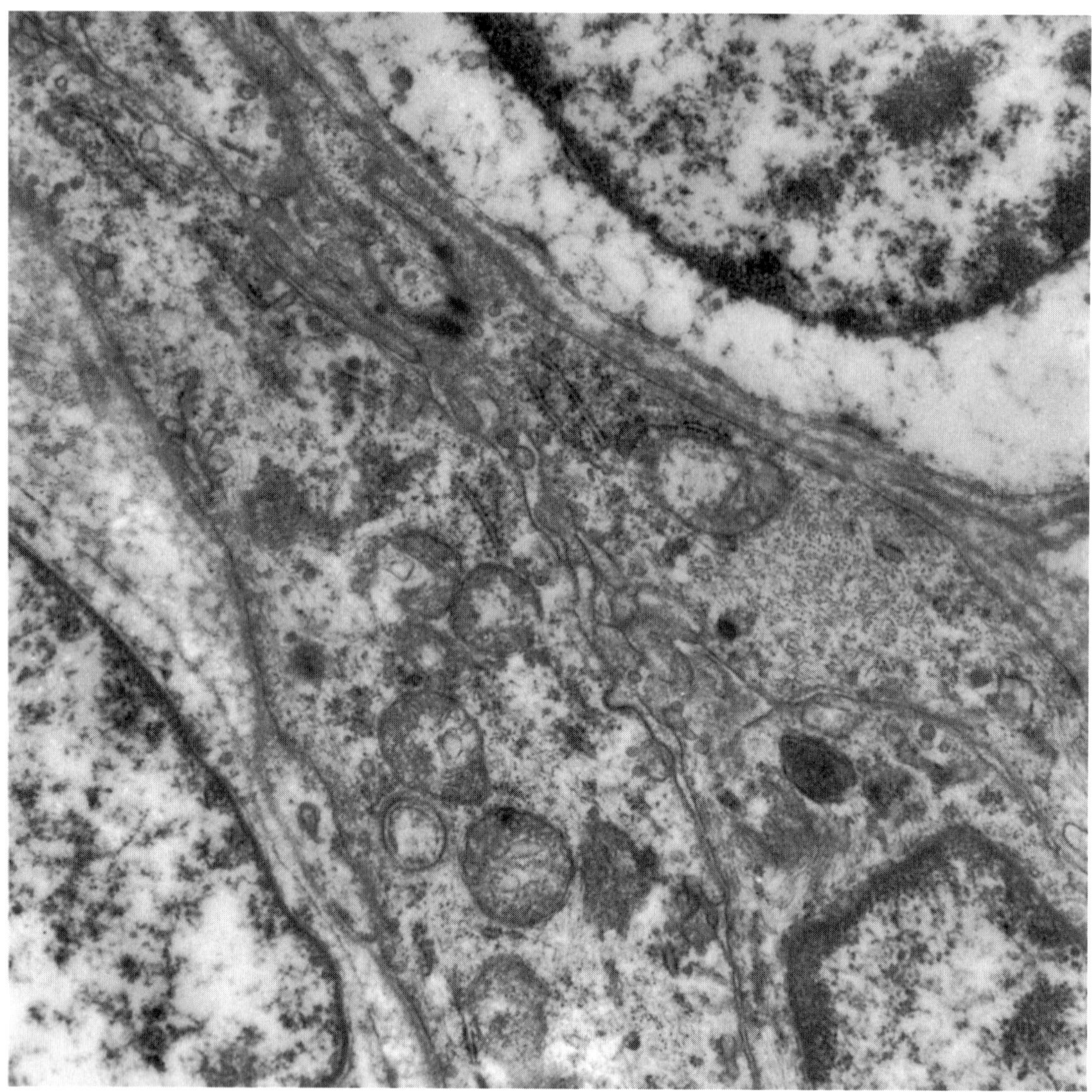

**FIGURE 14–23.** Schwann cell-like areas of a Bednar tumor where cells have interlacing processes, junctions, and basal lamina. (×24,800) (From Dupree WB, Langloss JM, Weiss SW. Pigmented dermatofibrosarcoma protuberans (Bednar tumor): a pathologic, ultrastructural, and immunohistochemical study. Am J Surg Pathol 9:630, 1985, with permission.)

wall. It affects predominantly infants and children, being encountered only infrequently in adults.[86,92] In our experience, about two-thirds of the children were younger than 5 years of age when brought to medical attention, and the median age was 3 years. About two-thirds of patients are male.

## Pathologic Findings

Grossly, the lesions consist of gray to yellow mucoid masses that are poorly circumscribed and measure 1–8 cm. They are composed of loosely arranged, wavy spindle cells with a moderate degree of nuclear pleomorphism that infiltrate the deep dermis and subcutis and encircle adnexal structures in a fashion similar to dermatofibrosarcoma protuberans (Figs. 14–25 to 14–32). The tumors vary in cellularity from those approximating the cellularity of dermatofibrosarcoma protuberans (Figs. 14–27, 14–31) to those that are hypocellular with a myxoid or hyaline stroma (Figs. 14–28, 14–29, 14–30). The characteristic feature of the tumor is the peculiar pseudovascular spaces, which seem to reflect a loss of cellular cohesion. Large and irregular in shape, the pseudovascular spaces are lined by a discontinuous row of multinucleated cells that represent variants of the basic proliferating tumor cell (Figs. 14–26, 14–32). Although these cells appear to contain multiple overlapping nuclei, as seen by light microscopy, they actually represent multiple sausage-like lobations of a single nucleus when studied ultrastructurally (Fig. 14–33).[99] Immunohistochemical studies indicate that these tu-

*Text continued on page 516*

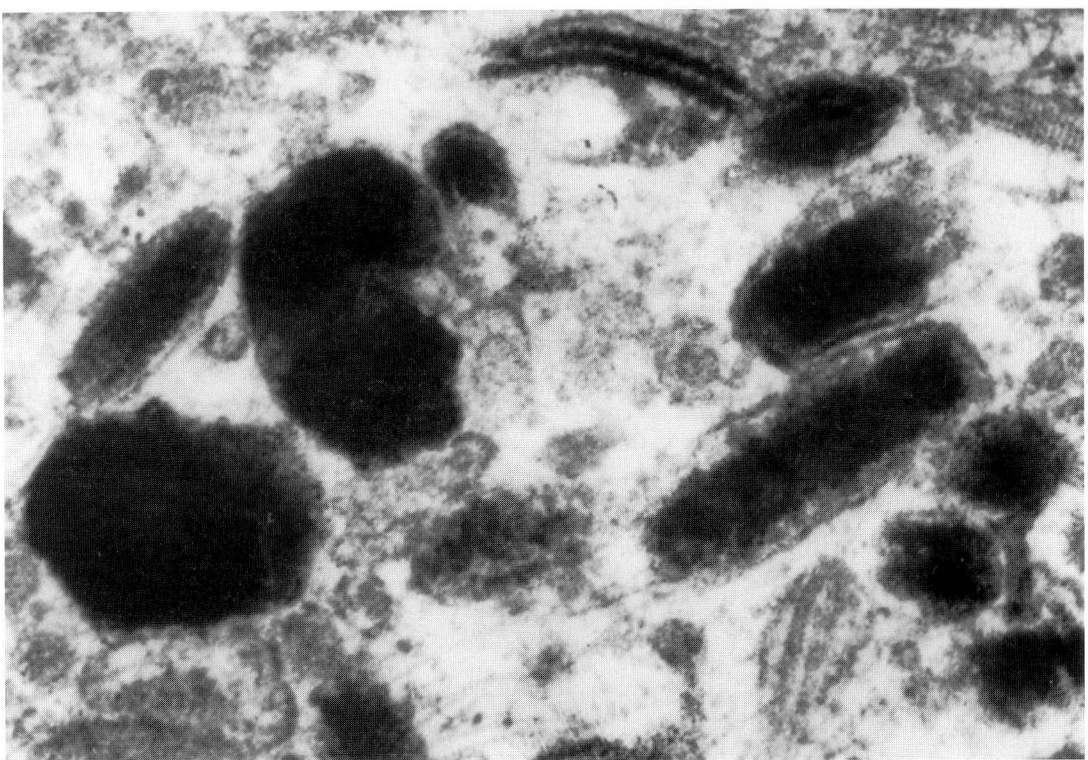

**FIGURE 14–24.** Mature and immature melanosomes in a Bednar tumor. (×93,900) (From Dupree WB, Langloss JM, Weiss SW. Pigmented dermatofibrosarcoma protuberans (Bednar tumor): a pathologic, ultrastructural, and immunohistochemical study. Am J Surg Pathol 9:630, 1985, with permission.)

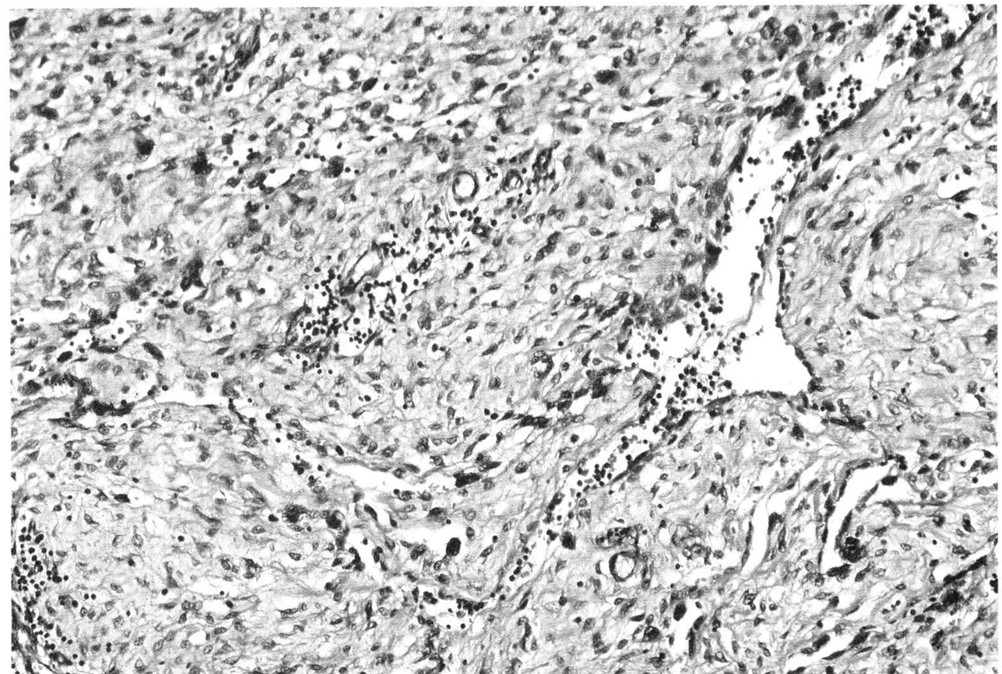

**FIGURE 14–25.** Classic appearance of a giant cell fibroblastoma showing pseudovascular spaces lined by giant cells.

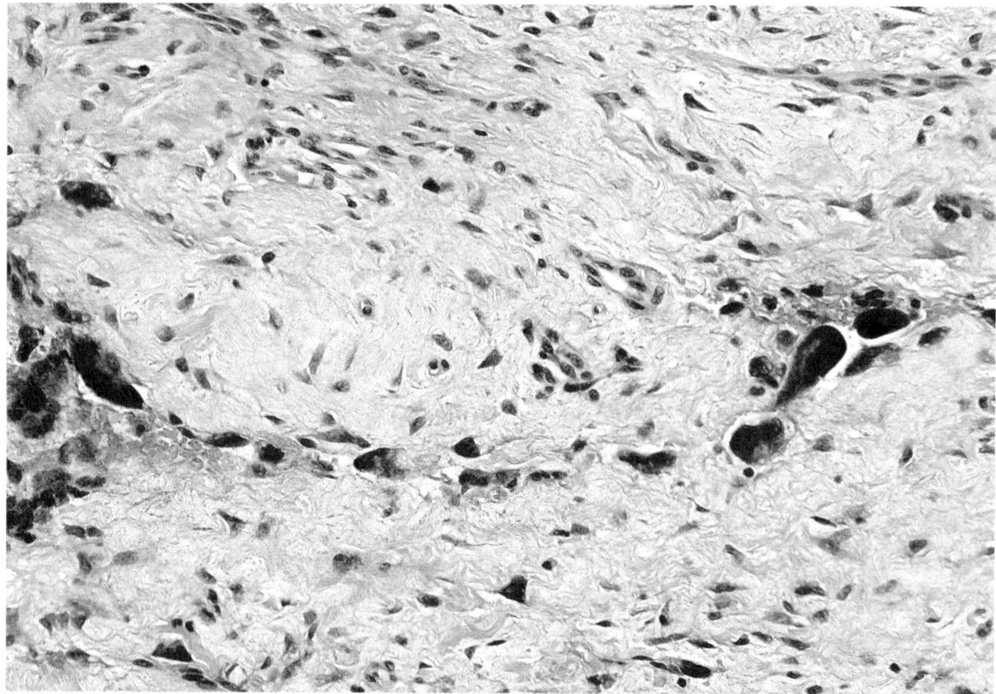

**FIGURE 14–26.** Hyperchromatic giant cells lining pseudovascular spaces in a giant cell fibroblastoma.

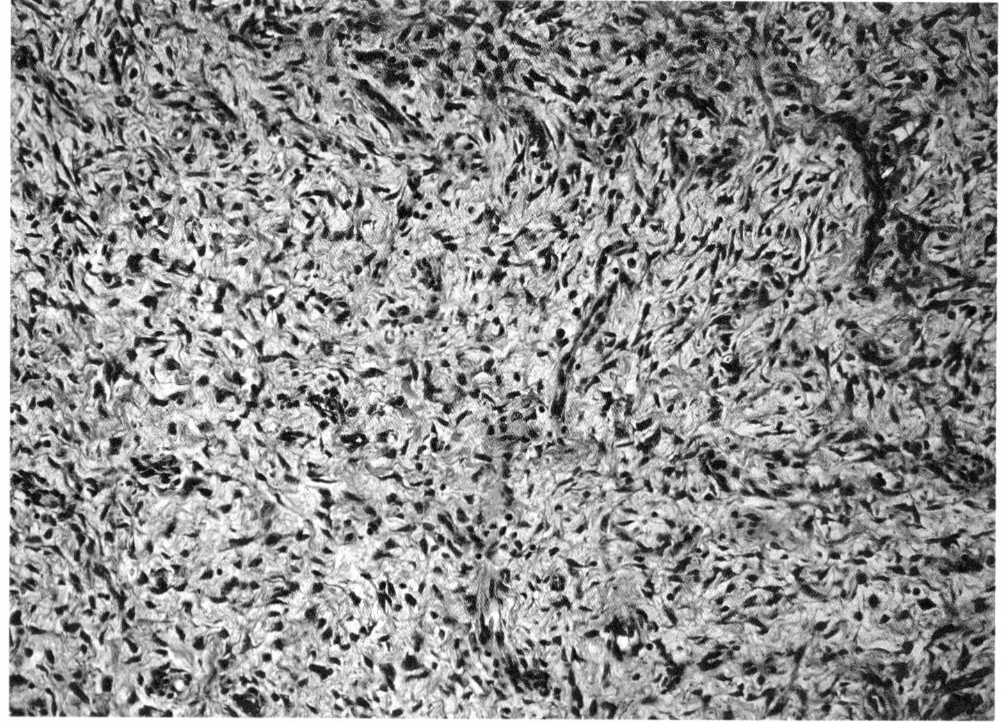

**FIGURE 14–27.** Cellular areas in a giant cell fibroblastoma. (×160)

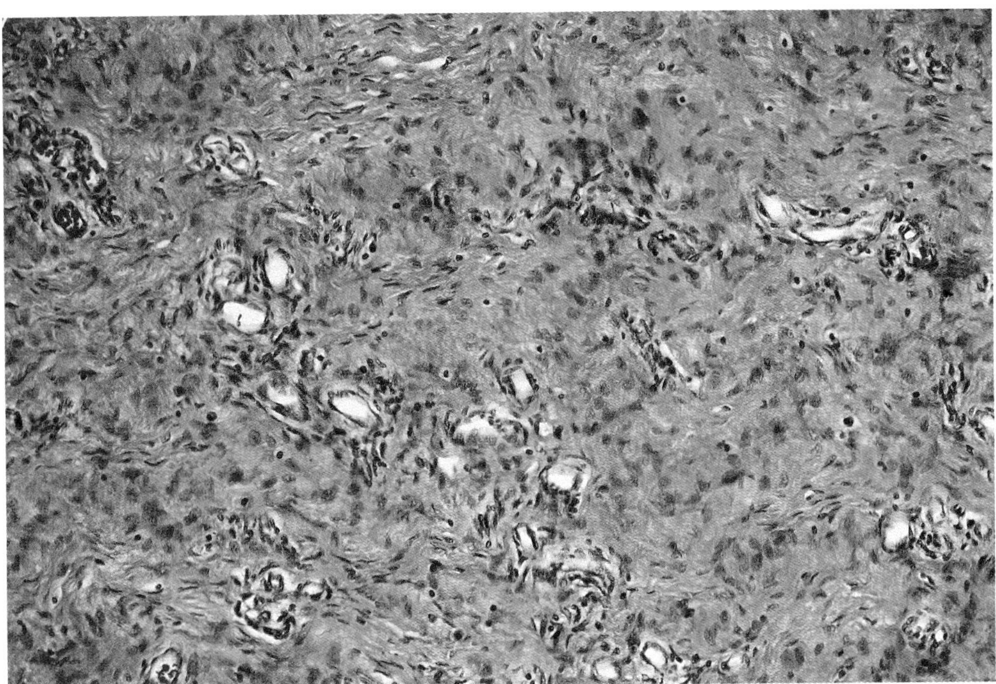

**FIGURE 14–28.** Hypocellular hyalinized zones in a giant cell fibroblastoma. (×160)

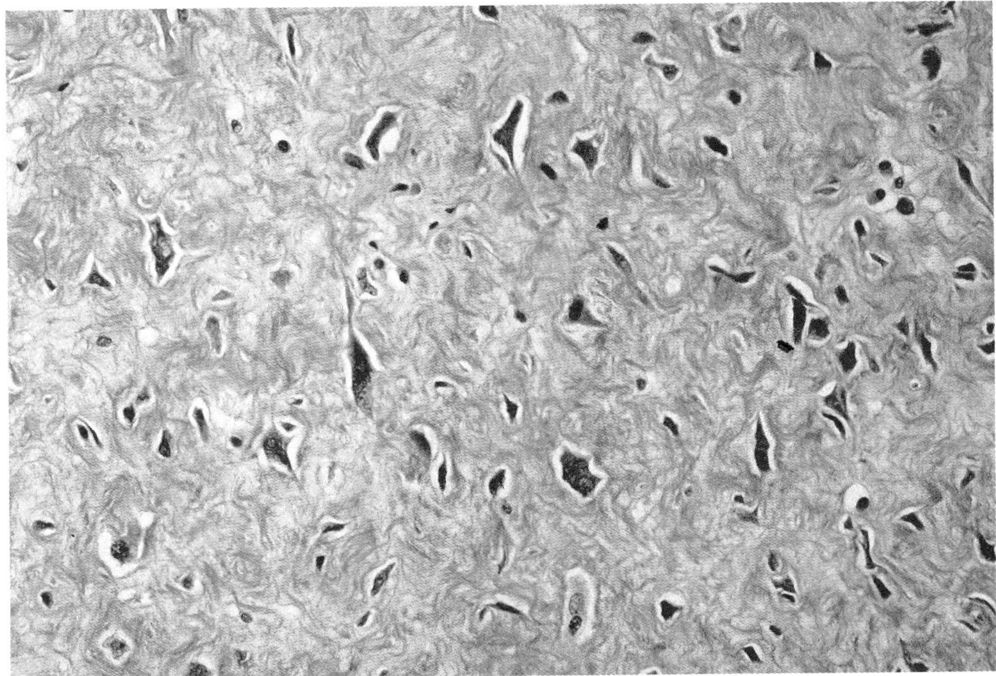

**FIGURE 14–29.** Markedly hyalinized area in a giant cell fibroblastoma.

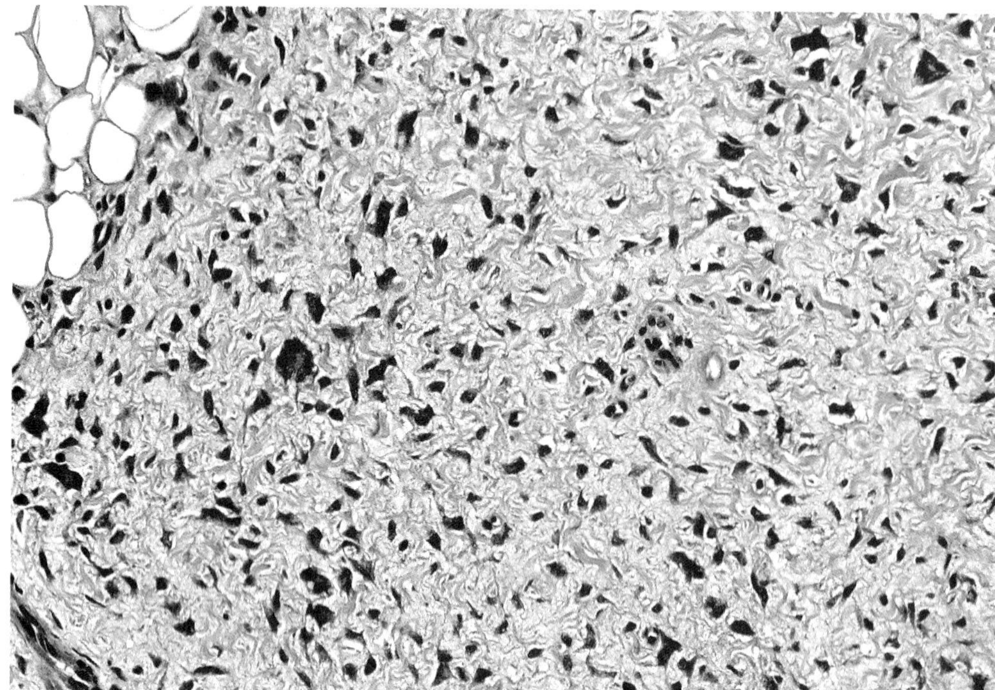

**FIGURE 14–30.** Hypocellular area in a giant cell fibroblastoma with giant cells not associated with pseudovascular spaces.

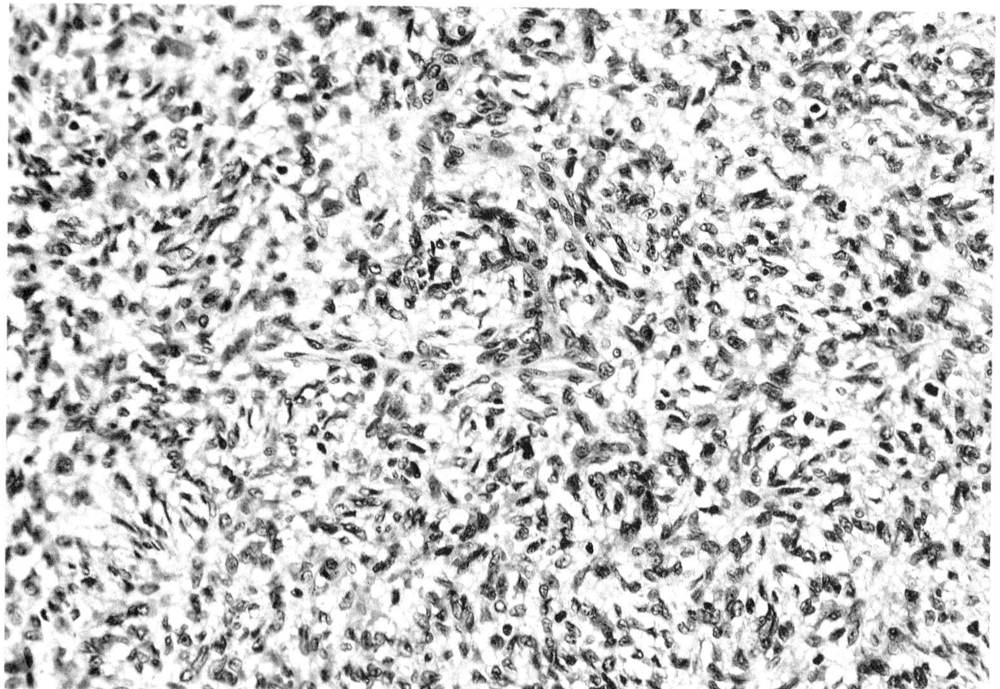

**FIGURE 14–31.** Dermatofibrosarcoma protuberans-like area in a giant cell fibroblastoma.

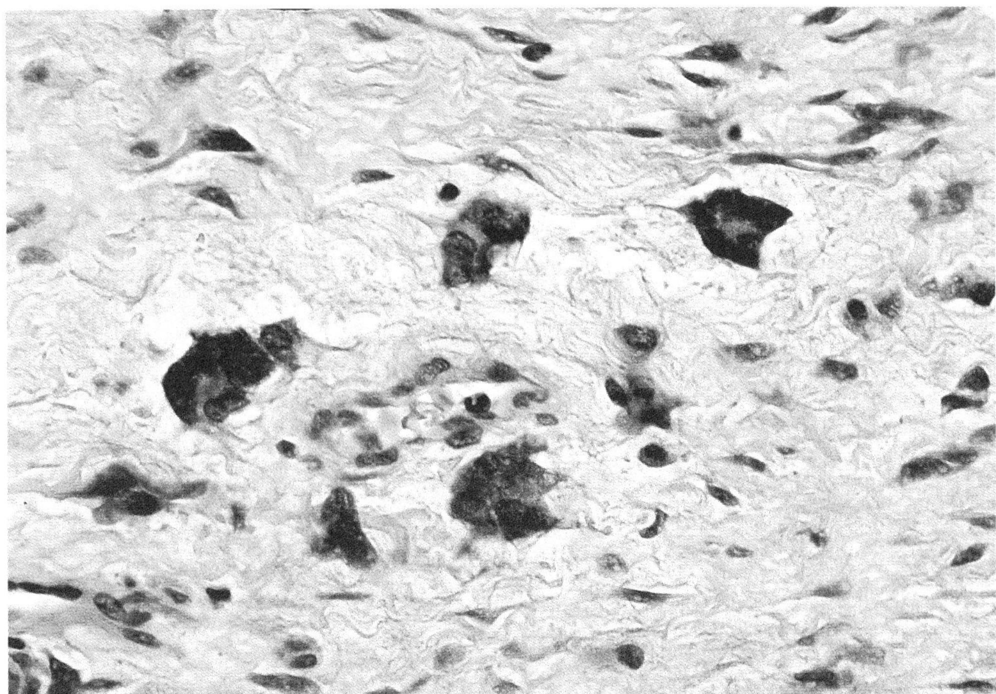

**FIGURE 14–32.** Giant cells in a giant cell fibroblastoma.

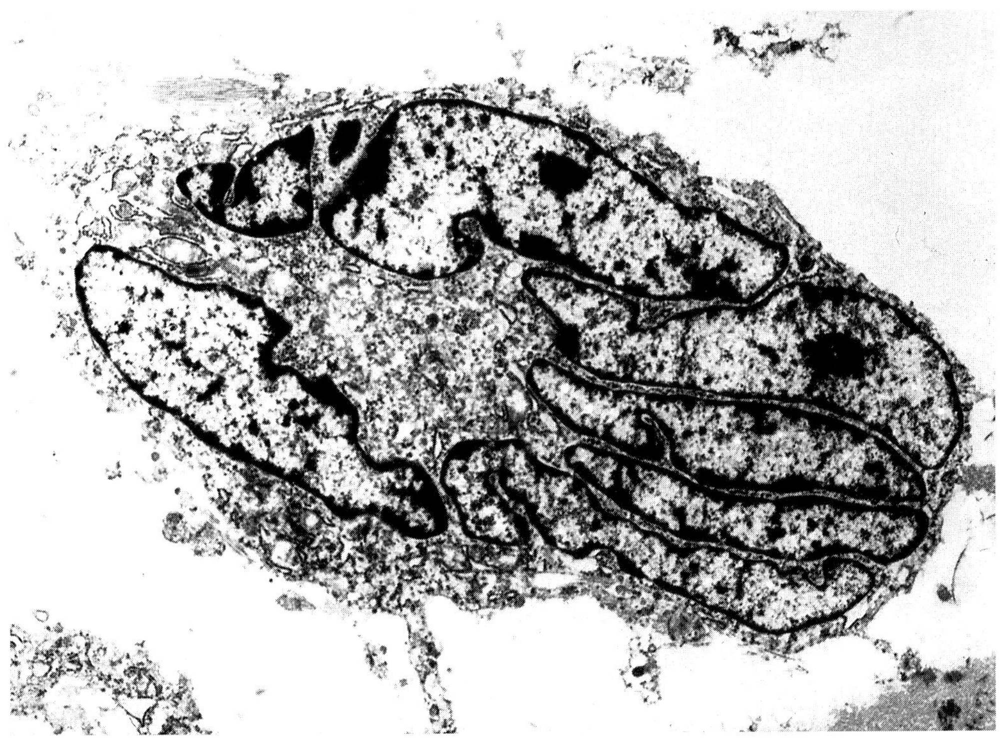

**FIGURE 14–33.** Electron micrograph of giant cells illustrating a hypersegmented nucleus. (Courtesy of Dr. Barry Schmookler.)

mors express vimentin but lack S-100 protein and vascular markers.[92] Some giant cell fibroblastomas express CD34, a feature they share with dermatofibrosarcoma protuberans.

### Differential Diagnosis

In our early experience about 40% of giant cell fibroblastomas were misdiagnosed as *sarcoma.* Because of the myxoid areas and hyperchromatic giant cells, there is a tendency to assume they represent examples of myxoid liposarcoma or myxoid malignant fibrous histiocytoma occurring in an unusually young individual. Important clues to the diagnosis include the superficial location, lack of an intricate vasculature, and the presence of hyperchromatic cells lying preferentially along the pseudovascular spaces.

### Discussion

There have been fewer reports of giant cell fibroblastoma than dermatofibrosarcoma protuberans in the literature. Recurrences have developed in about one-half of cases, but metastases have not been reported. Treatment of these tumors ideally is wide local excision. If less therapy is contemplated, conscientious follow-up is advisable to document and treat recurrences.

It is well accepted that giant cell fibroblastoma and dermatofibrosarcoma are slightly different expressions of the same neoplasm. Like dermatofibrosarcoma protuberans, giant cell fibroblastoma occurs in superficial soft tissues, with a strong predilection for the abdominal wall, back, and groin. Even more compelling is the observation that hybrid tumors occur. For example, occasional dermatofibrosarcomas of adults contain giant cells or foci similar to those of giant cell fibroblastoma,[87]; less frequently, otherwise typical giant cell fibroblastomas of childhood contain areas of dermatofibrosarcoma protuberans.[114] There have also been a number of recorded instances in which either dermatofibrosarcoma protuberans or giant cell fibroblastoma has recurred and recapitulated the pattern of the other tumor in the recurrence.[84,85,90] Finally, the giant cell fibroblastoma displays a cytogenetic abnormality identical to that of dermatofibrosarcoma protuberans (see above).

## ANGIOMATOID FIBROUS HISTIOCYTOMA

Previously termed *angiomatoid malignant fibrous histiocytoma,*[104] this distinctive tumor of children and young adults has been renamed *angiomatoid fibrous histiocytoma* by the World Health Organization Committee for the Classification of Soft Tissue Tumors. This designation reflects the relative rarity of metastasis and the overall excellent clinical course.

### Clinical Findings

Angiomatoid fibrous histiocytoma, a tumor that occurs primarily in children and young adults, is therefore rarely encountered in adults over age 40. It develops as a slowly growing nodular, multinodular, or cystic mass of the hypodermis or subcutis. It most often occurs on the extremities. Local symptoms such as pain and tenderness are uncommon, but systemic symptoms such as anemia, pyrexia, and weight loss are occasionally encountered and suggest the production of cytokines by the neoplasm.

### Gross and Microscopic Findings

The tumors are firm, circumscribed lesions that usually measure a few centimeters in diameter and vary in color from gray-tan to red-brown, depending on the amount of hemosiderin present. One of the most characteristic features is the presence of irregular blood-filled cystic spaces best appreciated on cross section (Fig. 14–34). This feature may be so striking as to give the impression of a hematoma, hemangioma, or a thrombosed vessel.

These lesions are characterized by three features: irregular solid masses of histiocyte-like cells, cystic areas of hemorrhage, and chronic inflammation. In general, the solid masses of histiocyte-like cells interspersed with areas of hemorrhage occupy the central portion of the tumor, and the inflammatory cells form a dense peripheral cuff that blends with the surrounding pseudocapsule (Figs. 14–35 to 14–43).

*Text continued on page 521*

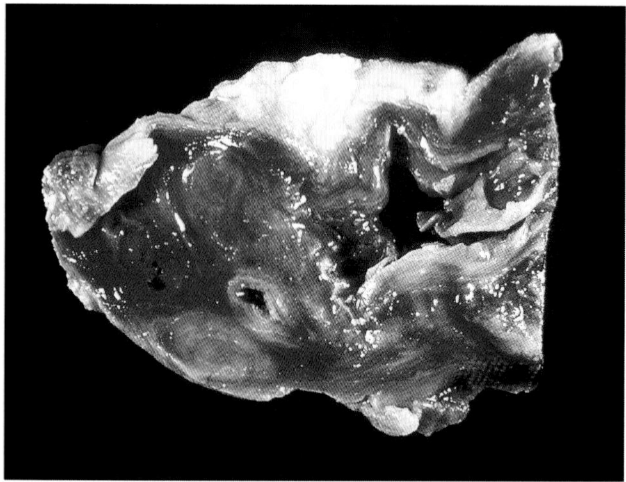

**FIGURE 14–34.** Gross specimen of an angiomatoid fibrous histiocytoma illustrating cystic change and a hemosiderin-stained tumor. Normal fat is present at the periphery.

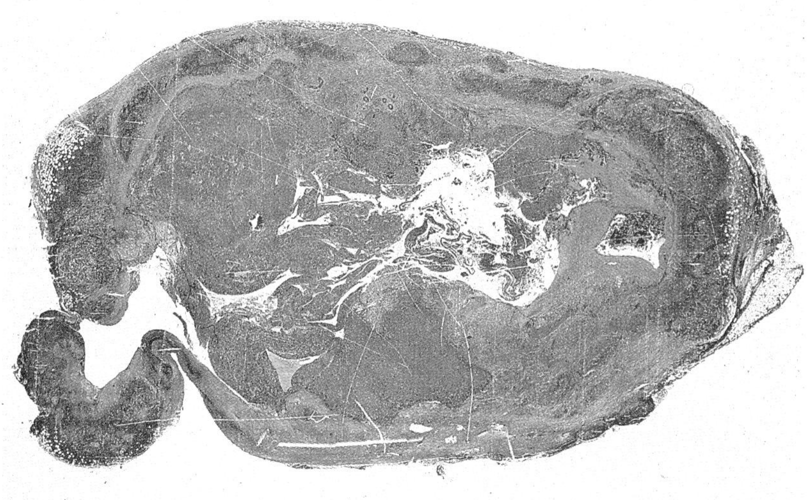

**FIGURE 14–35.** Angiomatoid fibrous histiocytoma shows a partially cystic tumor mass surrounded by a dense fibrous pseudocapsule and prominent lymphoid cuff.

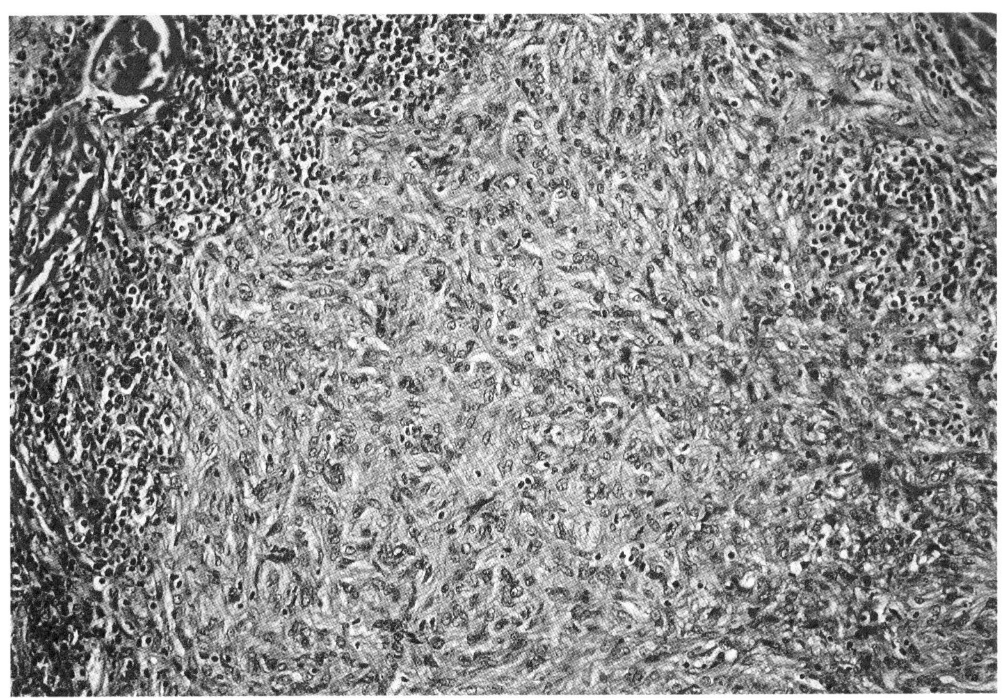

**FIGURE 14–36.** Angiomatoid fibrous histiocytoma. Histiocyte-like cells are arranged in solid sheets. Lymphoid infiltrate surrounds the tumor nodule.

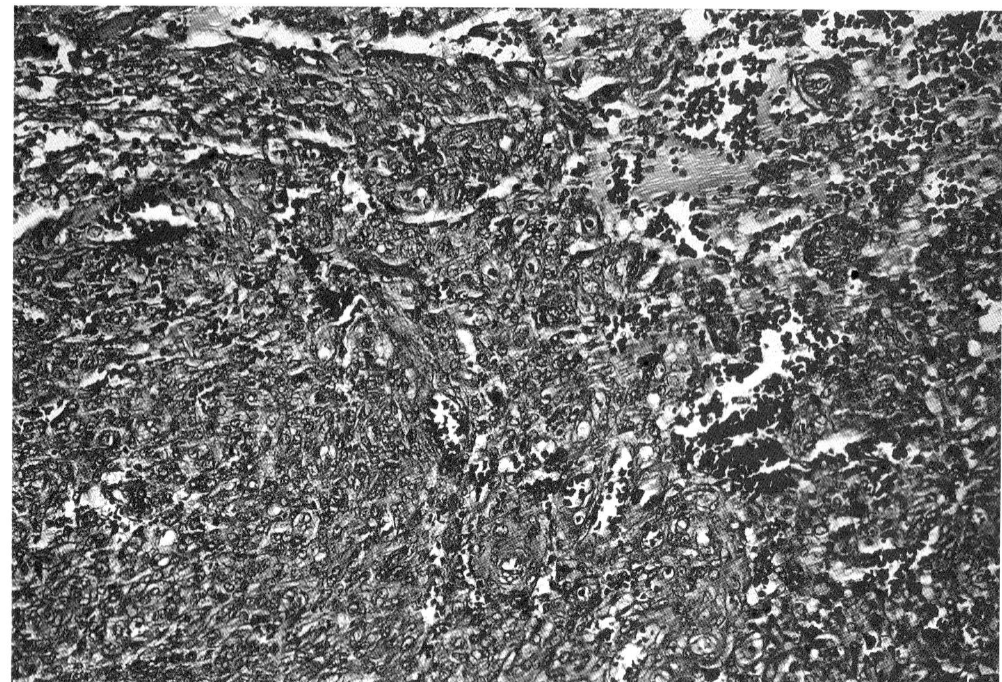

**FIGURE 14–37.** Areas of microscopic hemorrhage and cystic change in an angiomatoid fibrous histiocytoma.

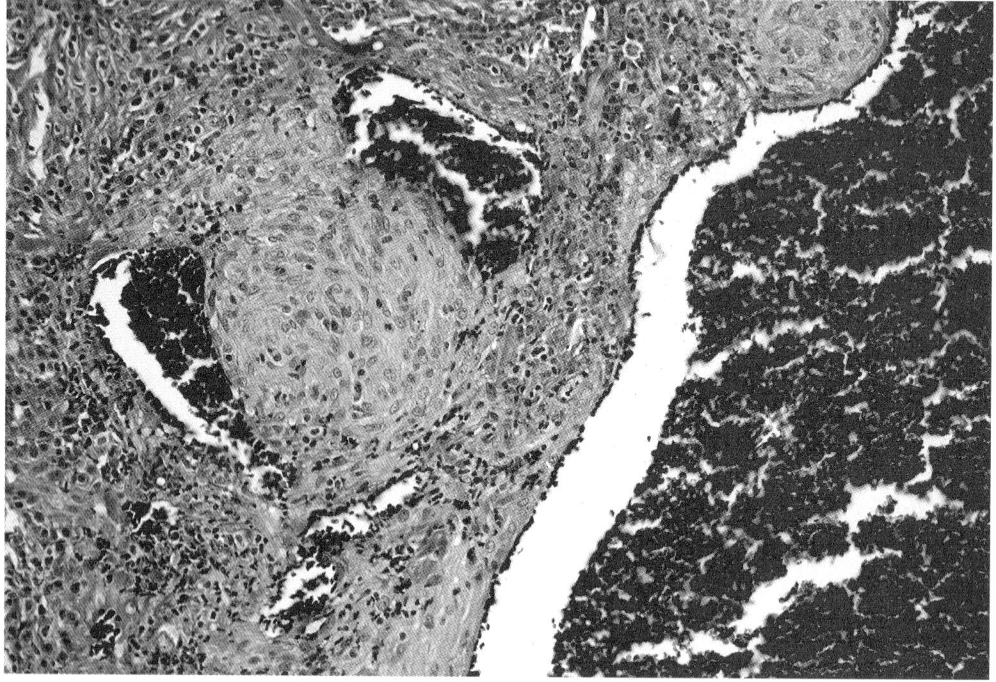

**FIGURE 14–38.** Cystic hemorrhage in an angiomatoid fibrous histiocytoma.

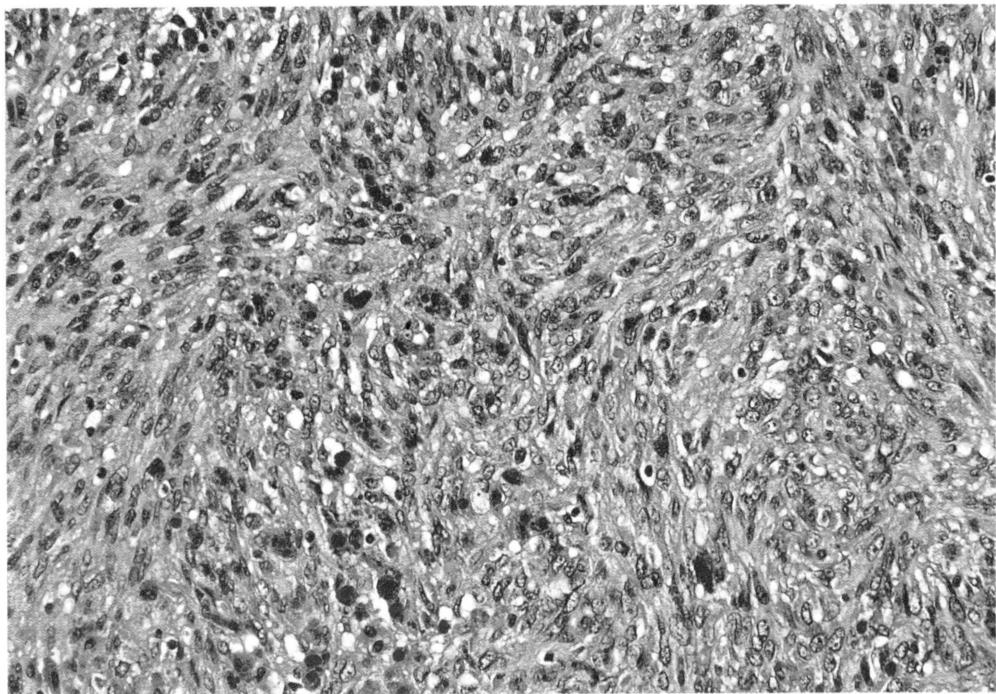

**FIGURE 14–39.** Spindle cell area in an angiomatoid fibrous histiocytoma.

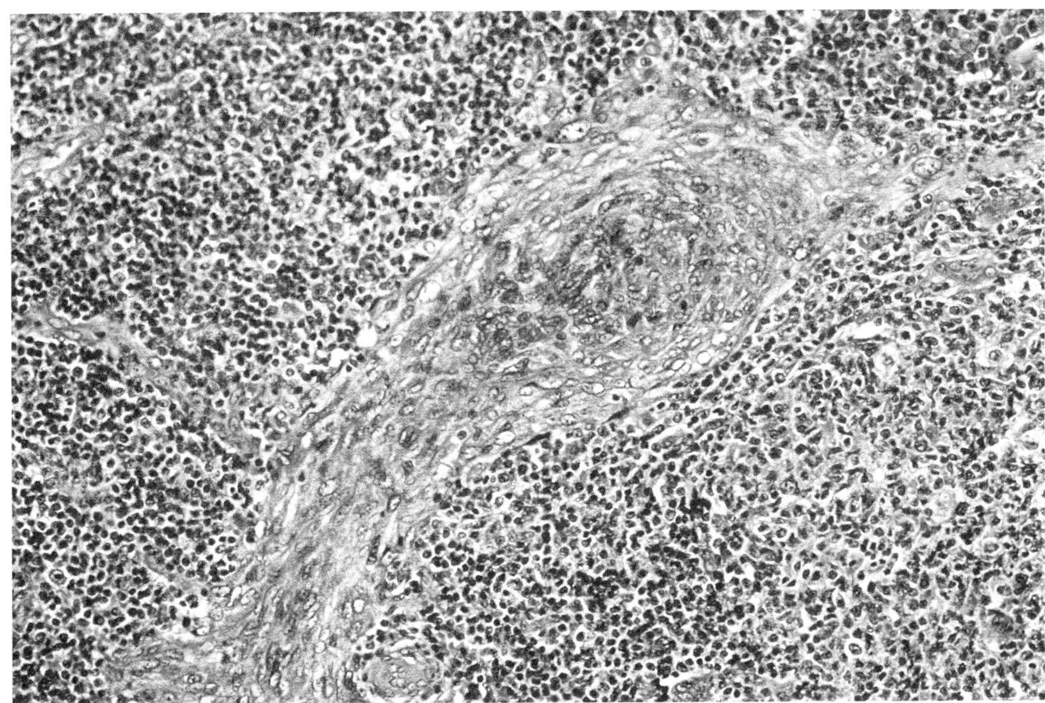

**FIGURE 14–40.** Tentacle-like extension of tumor in an angiomatoid fibrous histiocytoma surrounded by a chronic inflammatory response.

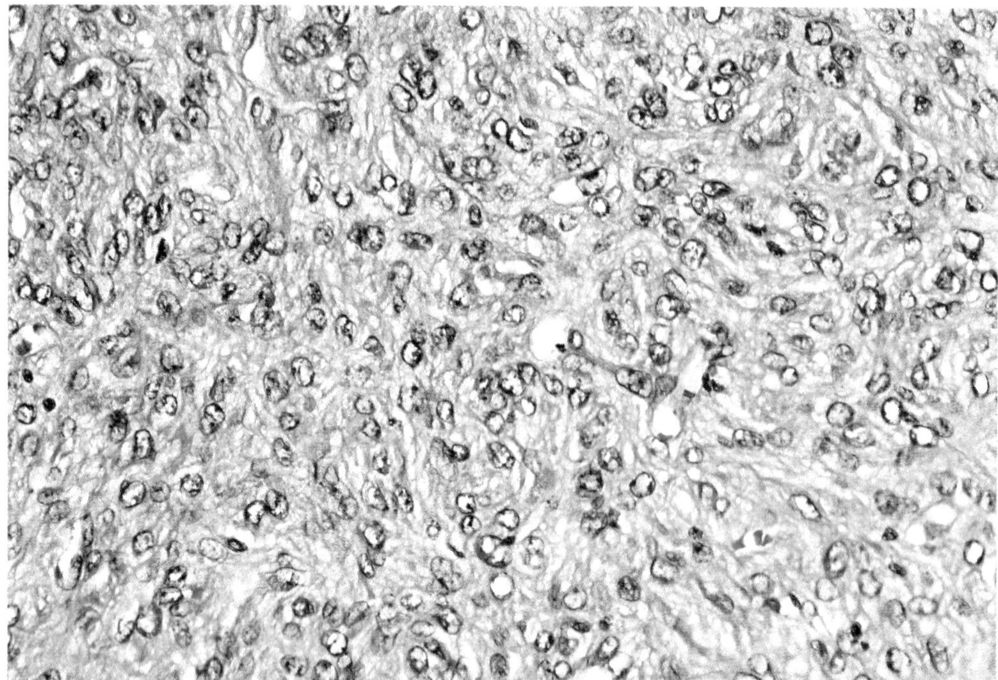

**FIGURE 14–41.** Histiocyte-like cells in an angiomatoid fibrous histiocytoma.

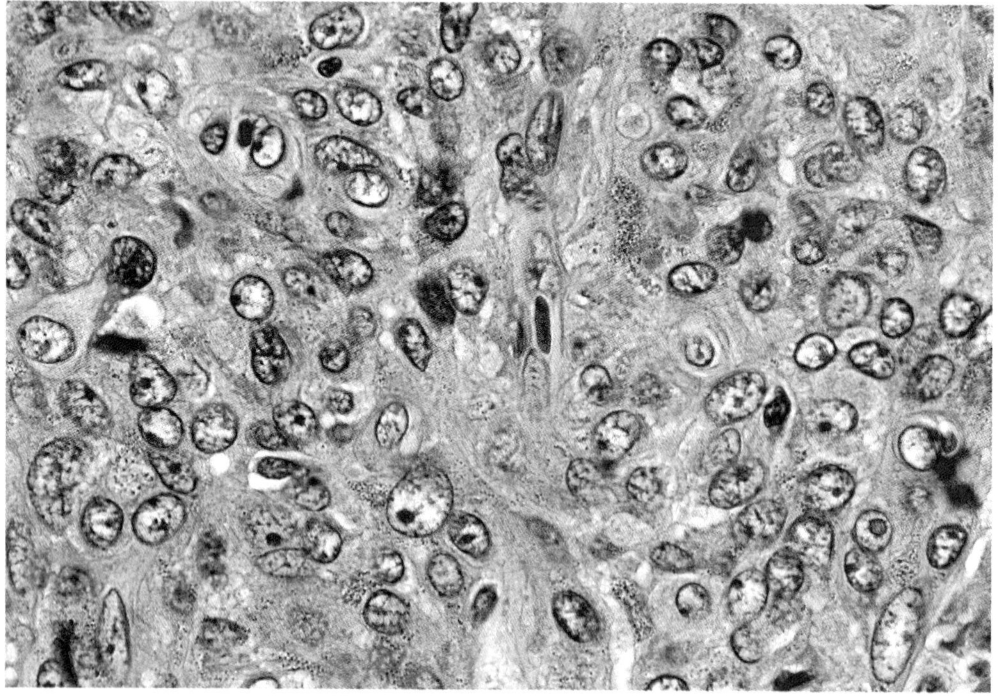

**FIGURE 14–42.** Histiocyte-like cells in an angiomatoid fibrous histiocytoma.

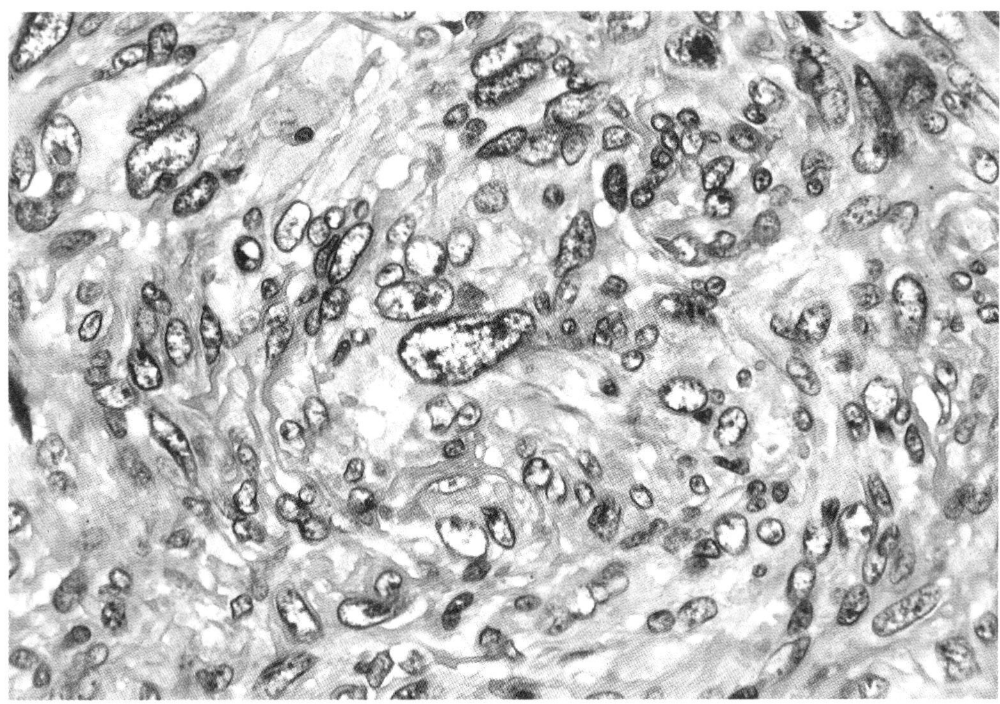

**FIGURE 14–43.** Cellular atypia in angiomatoid fibrous histiocytoma.

The histiocyte-like cells are usually quite uniform; they have a round or oval nucleus and a faintly staining eosinophilic cytoplasm often containing finely particulate hemosiderin. In most instances the cells are bland, such that some may be confused with the histiocytes of granulomas (Figs. 14–41, 14–42). In about one-fifth of cases significant nuclear atypia or hyperchromatic giant cells are present (Fig. 14–43), a feature that does not correlate with aggressive behavior.[102] In a small number of cases, myxoid change may develop in the tumor. Lipid and especially hemosiderin are present in the cells, but xanthoma cells are usually absent. Multifocal hemorrhage is a striking feature in all cases and results in the formation of irregular cystic spaces (Figs. 14–37, 14–38). Although these spaces resemble vascular spaces, they are not lined by endothelium but, rather, by flattened tumor cells. Small vessels may be present at the periphery of the nodules, but they do not seem to be the major components of these tumors. Inflammatory cells consist of a mixture of lymphocytes and plasma cells. Germinal center formation is occasionally observed, a feature suggesting lymph node metastasis, especially if the tumor represents a recurrence. The resemblance to a lymph node is further heightened by the thick pseudocapsule, a structure often interpreted as a lymph node capsule. However, unlike a true lymph node, there are no subcapsular or medullary sinuses, and germinal center formation occurs randomly around the tumor, without a predilection for the subcapsular zone. Differentiation of these tumors from hemorrhagic fibrous histiocytomas is discussed in Chapter 13.

## Discussion

Angiomatoid fibrous histiocytoma was originally believed to be a reasonably aggressive neoplasm based on follow-up of a small number of cases ascertained retrospectively.[104] Evaluation of a large number of cases diagnosed and treated adequately indicates that the tumor has a relatively good prognosis, however.[102] Among more than 100 patients evaluated, only 20% developed local recurrence and fewer than 1% (one patient) developed distant metastatic disease. A number of factors can be correlated with the risk of local recurrence, including infiltrating margins, location on the head and neck, and involvement of skeletal muscle rather than the subcutis.[102] Complete surgical excision without adjuvant therapy is the appropriate treatment for these low-grade tumors.

Since the original description of this tumor in 1979, a number of views have been espoused concerning the line of differentiation.[106,110,111] Early views endorsing the belief that these lesions were endothelial[106] are not supported by immunohistochemical data showing that the lesions do not express any of the well known vascular markers.[108] Although the lesions have a decidedly histiocytic appearance and show ample evidence of phagocytosis of hemosiderin, immunohistochemical analysis of histiocytic antigens has likewise been disappointing.[108] The tumors do not express muramidase, L-1, or Leu-M. About half express CD68 (KP-1),[108] probably because of acquisition of this antigen by cells that are phagocytic and have a high density of phagolysosomes. An intriguing observation is the finding of desmin within half of these cases[103,105] and other muscle markers within a smaller percent (muscle specific and smooth muscle actin, and calponin). The close association of these tumors with lymphoid tissue as well as this myoid phenotype has led to the postulate that these cells may be related to the desmin positive stromal cells of lymph node.[104a] Although desmin has also been construed as evidence of myoid differentiation,[105] the presence of this antigen in occasional tumors that are clearly not myoid urges a conservative interpretation at present.

## PLEXIFORM FIBROHISTIOCYTIC TUMOR

### Clinical Findings

Plexiform fibrohistiocytic tumor, like giant cell fibroblastoma and angiomatoid fibrous histiocytoma, occurs almost exclusively in children and young adults and is rarely encountered after the age of 30 years.[113] It typically presents as a slowly growing mass of the deep dermis and subcutaneous tissues. In our experience, the most common location is the upper extremity (63%) followed by the lower extremity (14%).

### Gross and Microscopic Findings

The lesions are relatively small (1–3 cm), ill-defined masses with a gray-white trabecular appearance. In its most typical form (about 40% of cases) the lesion contains a mixture of two components: a differentiated fibroblastic component and a round cell histiocytic component containing multinucleated giant cells. At low-power microscopy one is impressed by the numerous tiny cellular nodules that occupy the dermis and subcutaneous tissue (Figs. 14–44, 14–45). These nodules are composed of nests of histiocytic cells that often contain multinucleated, osteoclast-like giant cells and occasionally undergo focal hemorrhage (Figs. 14–46 to 14–50). The cells in these nodules are well differentiated and do not display atypia or significant levels of mitotic activity. The nodules, in turn, are circumscribed by short fascicles of fibroblastic cells (Figs. 14–47, 14–48, 14–49) that intersect slightly or ramify in the soft tissue, creating a plexiform growth pattern. The fascicles of spindle cells to some extent resemble fibromatosis, except that the cells are usually plumper and the fascicles shorter than those of fibromatosis. In the less typical case, the two components described above may not be equally represented. For example, in a few cases the nodules of giant cells are rare or absent, and only short intersecting fascicles of plump spindle cells are seen. In other cases there may be a blending of the nodules and fascicles; and the cells in these two zones may appear

*Text continued on page 527*

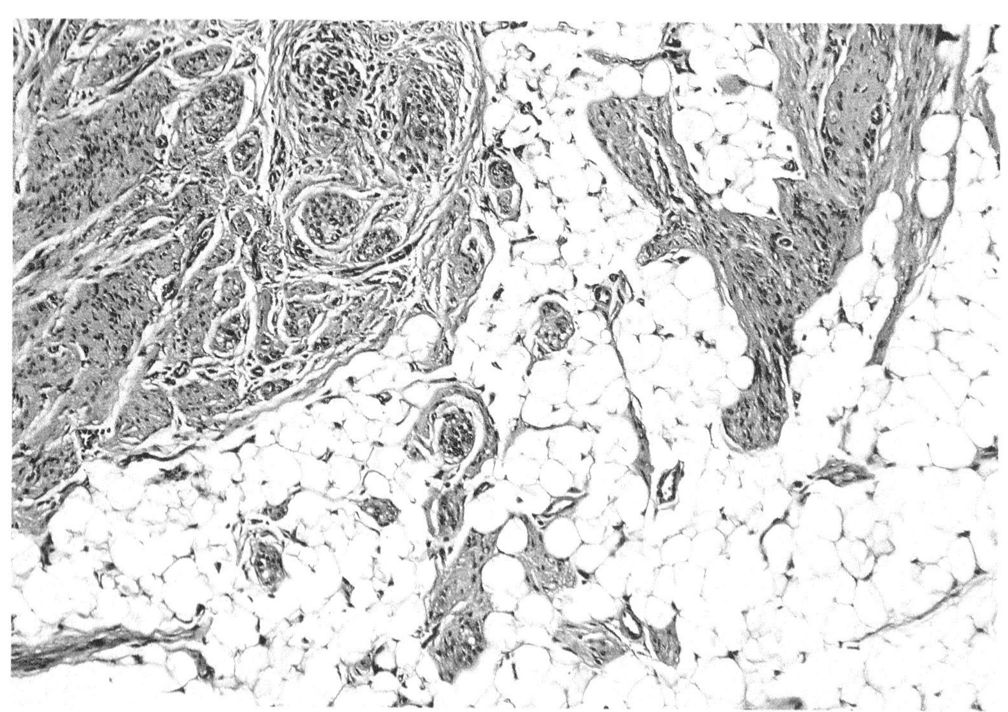

**FIGURE 14–44.** Plexiform fibrohistiocytic tumor showing ramifying fascicles of tumor in the subcutis.

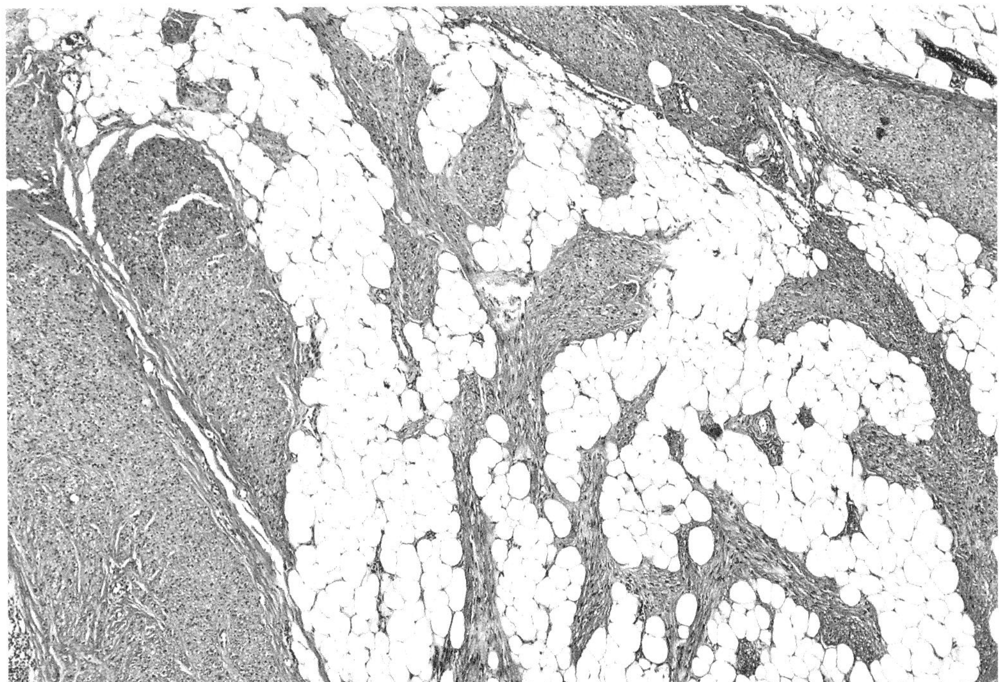

**FIGURE 14–45.** Plexiform fibrohistiocytic tumor showing relatively acellular ramifying fascicles in the subcutis.

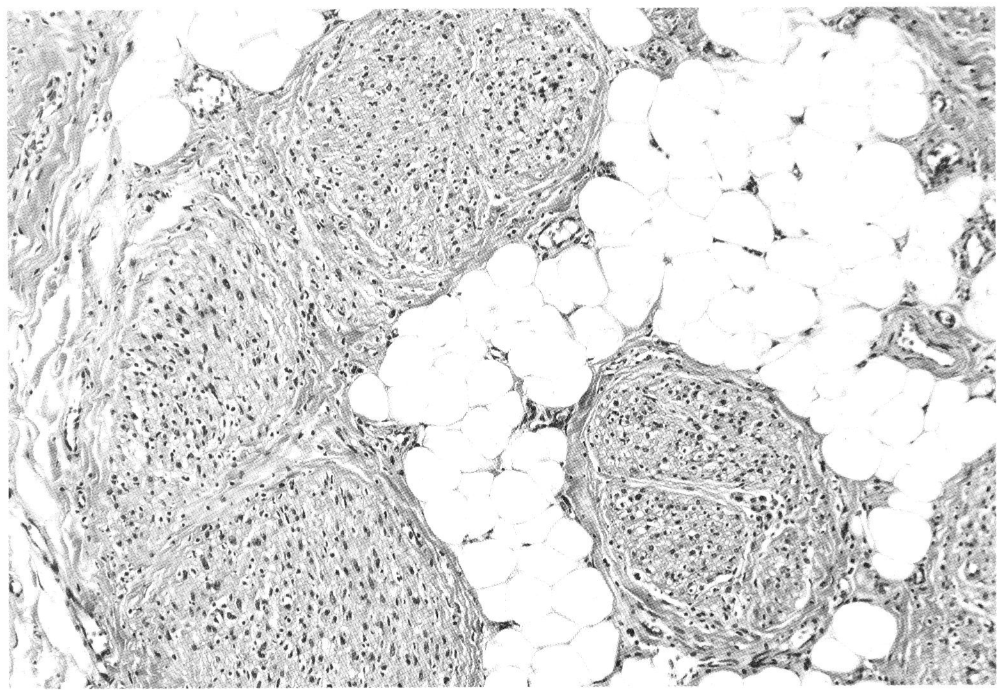

**FIGURE 14–46.** Irregular fascicles and nodules of a plexiform fibrohistiocytic tumor.

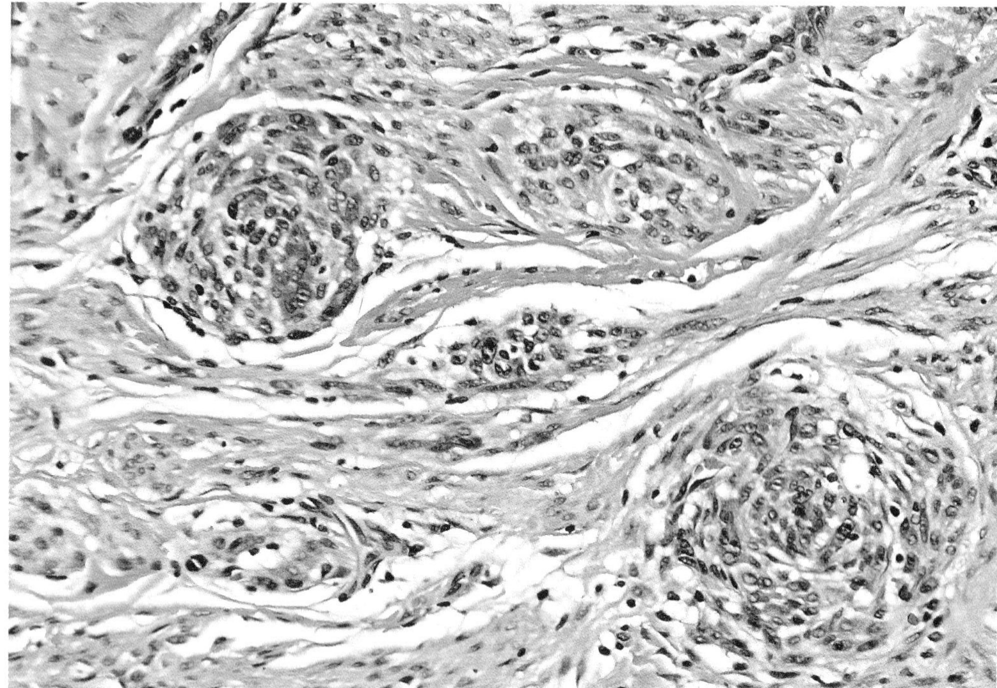

**FIGURE 14–47.** Typical "biphasic" appearance of a plexiform fibrohistiocytic tumor. Histiocyte-like nodules circumscribed by fibromatosis-like areas.

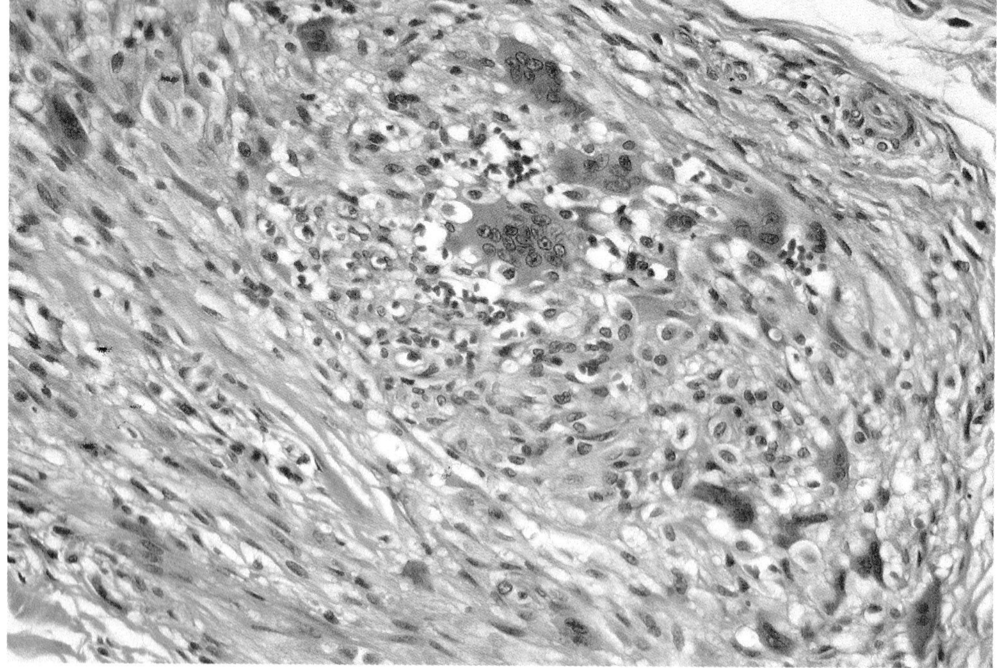

**FIGURE 14–48.** Nodules of histiocyte-like cells in a plexiform fibrohistiocytic tumor.

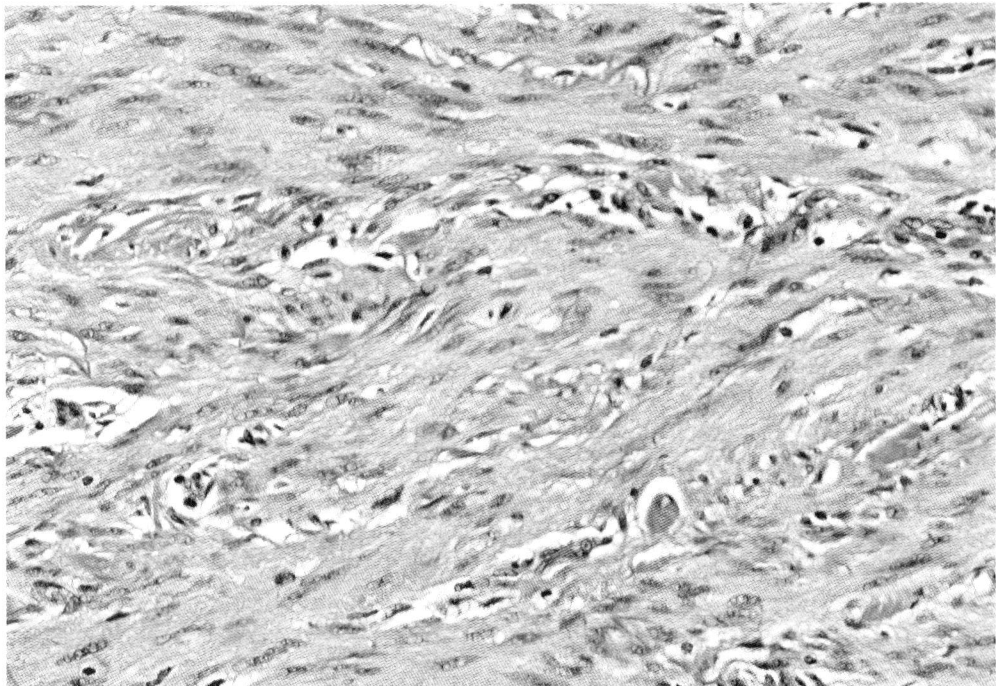

**FIGURE 14–49.** Plexiform fibrohistiocytic tumor with areas of short, ramifying fascicles of fibroblasts without histiocytes.

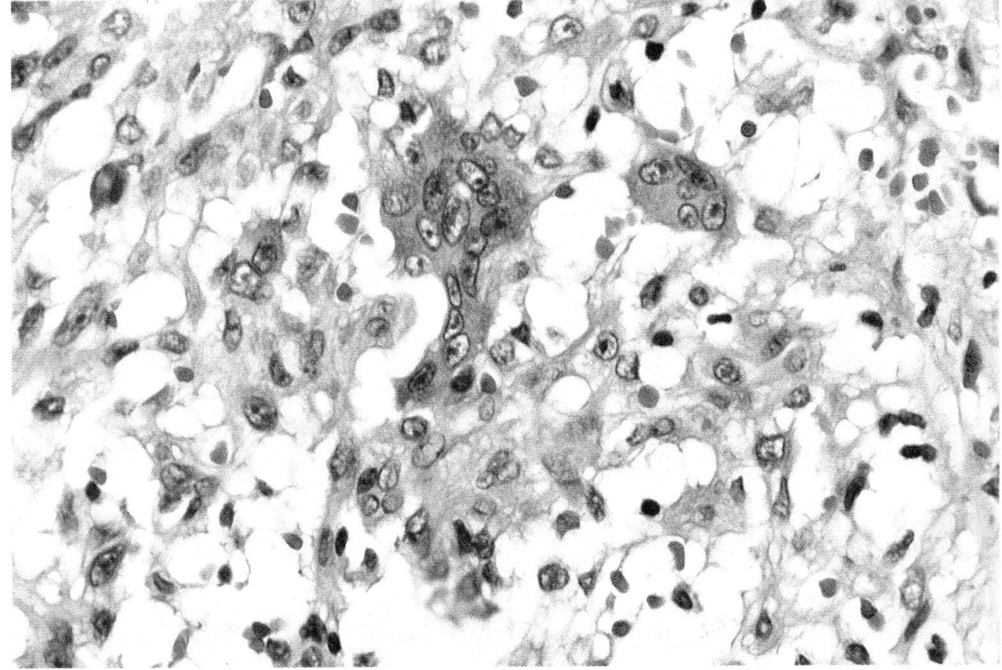

**FIGURE 14–50.** Plexiform fibrohistiocytic tumor with a high-power view of histiocyte-like cells comprising tumor nodules.

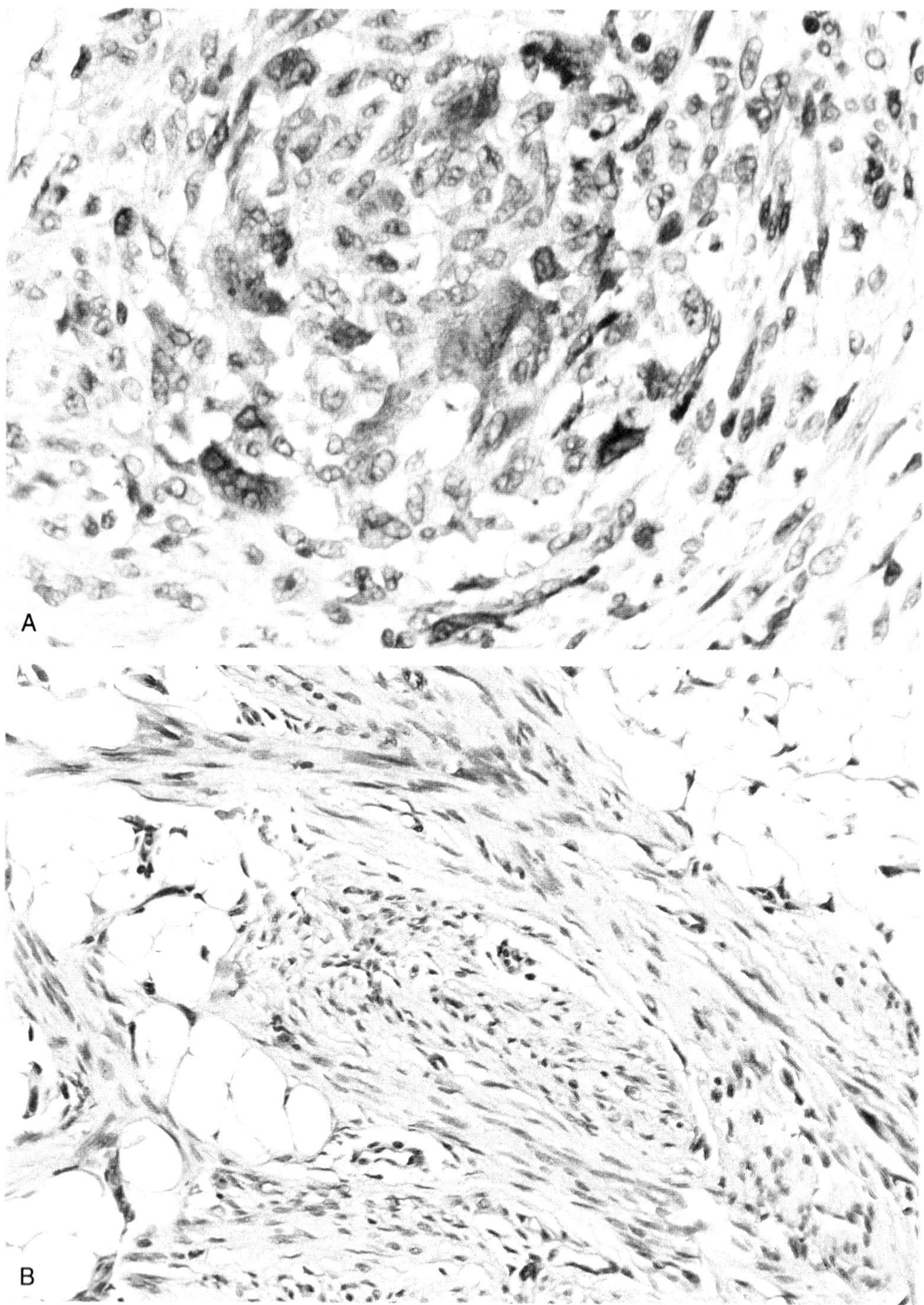


**FIGURE 14–51.** CD68 immunostain of a plexiform fibrohistiocytic tumor showing positivity of histiocytic giant cell nodules (**A**) and no positivity of fibroblastic areas (**B**).

to be in an intermediate stage between fibroblasts and histiocytes.

### Ancillary Studies

Immunohistochemically, the multinucleated giant cells and many of the mononuclear cells express CD68, suggesting true histiocytic differentiation, whereas the spindle cells express smooth muscle actin, as one would expect of myofibroblasts (Fig. 14–51). The cells do not contain other histiocytic markers such as HLA-DR, lysozyme, or L-2; nor are S-100 protein, keratin, desmin, and factor XIIIa present.

Ultrastructural studies have identified cells with features of histiocytes and myofibroblasts.[115] In a large series reported by Remstein et al., all cases were diploid with an S-phase fraction of 0.93–7.22%.[117] Cytogenetic analysis has been carried out in a few cases. One patient had a complex karyotype with numerous deletions, whereas the other had a t(4;15)(q21;q15).[116,119]

### Differential Diagnosis

A variety of benign diagnoses that include granuloma, fibrous hamartoma, fibrous histiocytoma, giant cell tumor, and fibromatosis are entertained in these cases. The most important distinctions are those that materially affect the management of the patient. It is essential to distinguish the lesion from an infectious granulomatous process. In the typical case the presence of associated fibroblastic cuffing of the histiocytic nodules is usually sufficient to suggest an alternative diagnosis. In tumors that are predominantly histiocytic, the important observations include the fact that these tumors do not have a surrounding inflammatory infiltrate, nor do the histiocytic nodules undergo central necrosis. Predominantly fibroblastic forms of plexiform fibrohistiocytic tumor may resemble fibromatosis; but in fibromatosis the fascicles are wider, longer, and composed of more slender fibroblastic cells.

### Discussion

Based on three series, these tumors appear to be low-grade neoplasms that frequently recur (12.5–40%) within 1–2 years of the original diagnosis.[112,114,116] Lymph node metastases have been observed in only two cases,[112,116] and only three patients in the literature have had histologically proven pulmonary metastases, one of whom died of the disease. It should be noted that there may be pulmonary metastases at the time of presentation, emphasizing the need for careful initial evaluation. Unfortunately, no histologic parameters (e.g., mitotic activity, vascular invasion) have been correlated with aggressive behavior. Ideally, these lesions are completely, if not widely, excised. It does not seem appropriate to commit the patient to adjuvant therapy based on the limited risk of regional or distant disease.

## SOFT TISSUE GIANT CELL TUMOR OF LOW MALIGNANT POTENTIAL

In 1999 we proposed the term "soft tissue giant cell tumors of low malignant potential" for a group of lesions that represent the benign end of the spectrum of malignant giant cell tumor of soft parts (malignant fibrous histiocytoma, giant cell type) and that seem to be the soft tissue analogue of giant cell tumor of bone.[121] These lesions were first described in two nearly simultaneous publications during the 1970s.[122,124] Salm and Sissons reported a group of 10 giant cell tumors of soft parts that they likened to giant cell tumors of bone[124]; and Guccion and Enzinger noted a subset of malignant giant cell tumors of soft parts characterized by "less atypia and mitotic activity" and that did not give rise to metastatic disease.[122] Interest in this group of lesions was rekindled by Nascimento in 1993, who reported 10 cases in abstract form.[123] Two additional studies have also appeared.[122a,b]

Although seemingly a new entity, these lesions were probably grouped with a number of other lesions in the past, such as tenosynovial giant cell tumor, malignant giant cell tumor of soft parts, plexiform fibrohistiocytic tumor, and even epithelioid sarcoma. Although to date there has not been an instance of metastasis from any of these lesions, logically one might expect to encounter rare instances of metastasis similar to those seen with giant cell tumor of bone.

### Clinical and Pathologic Features

These lesions tend to occur in all age groups and may develop in superficial or deep soft tissue, most commonly on the arm or hand. They consist of multiple tumor nodules that diffusely infiltrate soft tissue. The nodules are composed of bland mononuclear cells, short spindle cells, and osteoclasts (Figs. 14–52, 14–53, 14–54). By definition, the mononuclear and giant cells in these lesions lack the striking atypia that is the hallmark of giant cell forms of malignant fibrous histiocytoma (Fig. 14–53). Despite the lack of nuclear atypia, they often have brisk mitotic activity; about one-half display vascular invasion (as may be seen with giant cell tumor of bone), although necrosis is not seen. Metaplastic bone and angiectatic spaces

*Text continued on page 531*

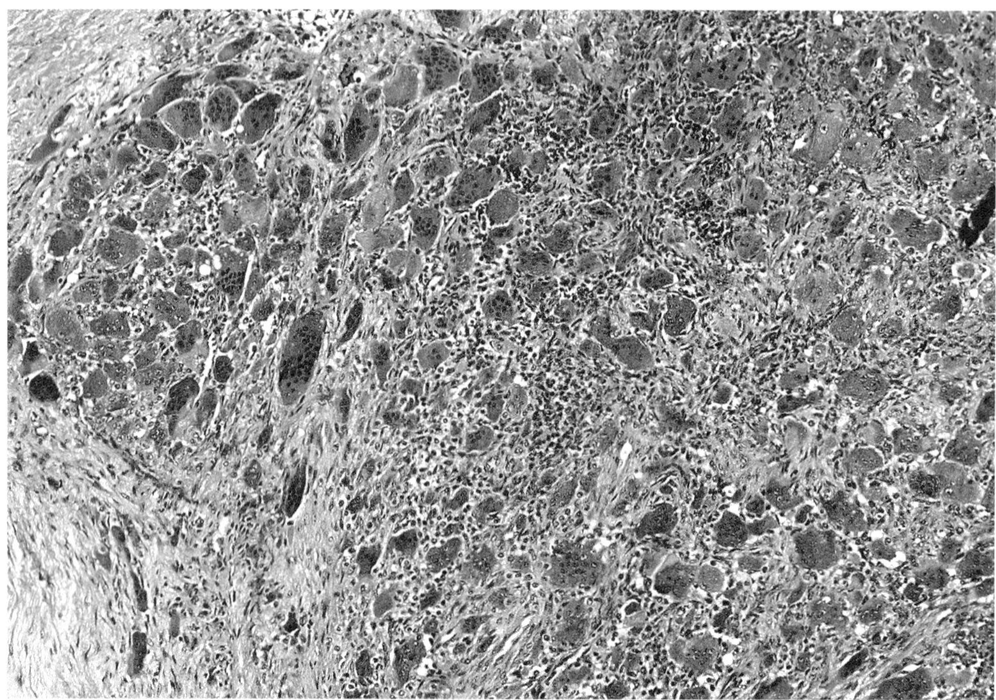

**FIGURE 14–52.** Giant cell tumor of low malignant potential with coarse nodular architecture.

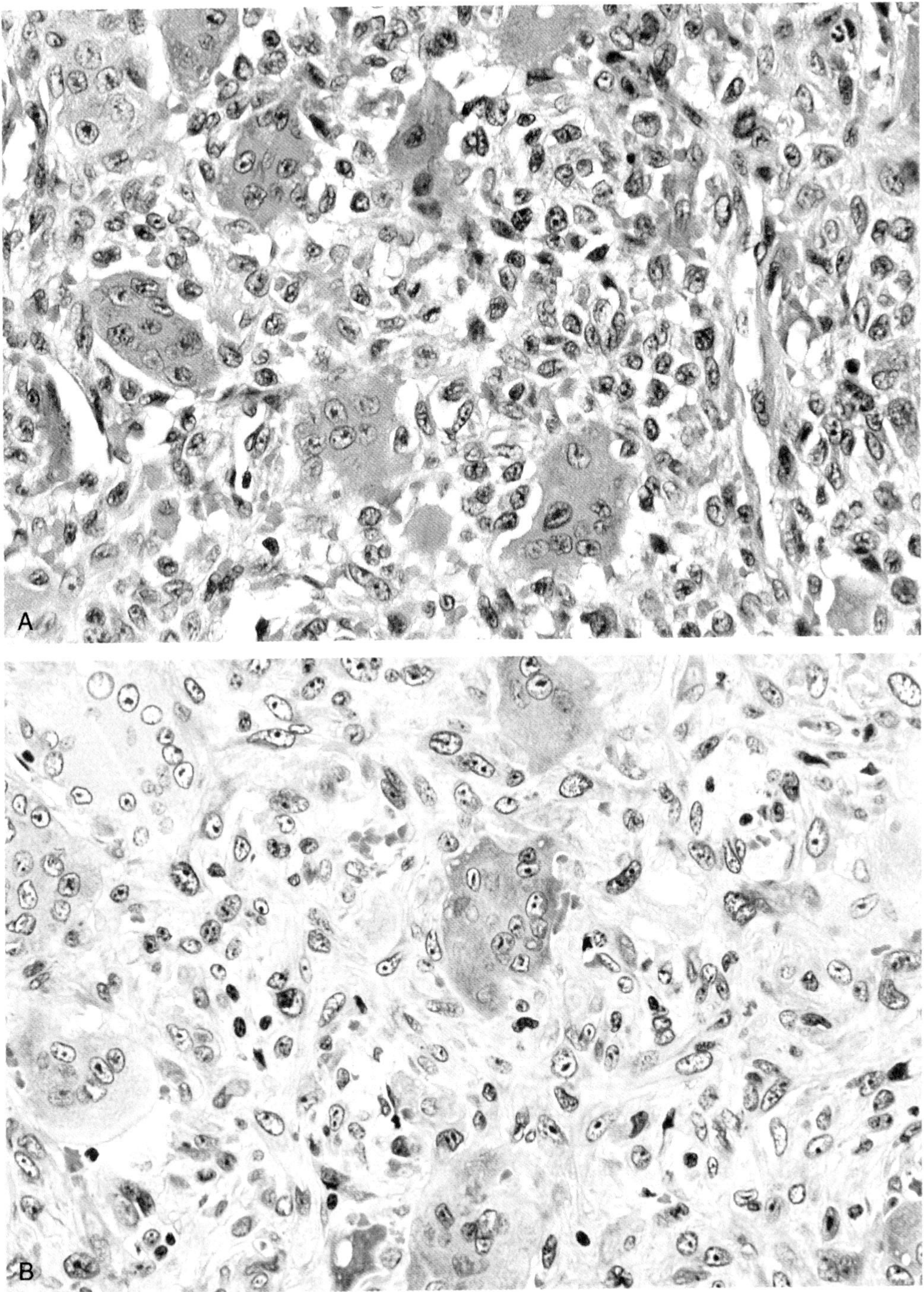


**FIGURE 14–53.** Giant cell tumor of low malignant potential with mild (**A**) and moderate (**B**) atypia of the mononuclear tumor cells. This contrasts with the marked atypia of classic malignant fibrous histiocytoma, giant cell type.

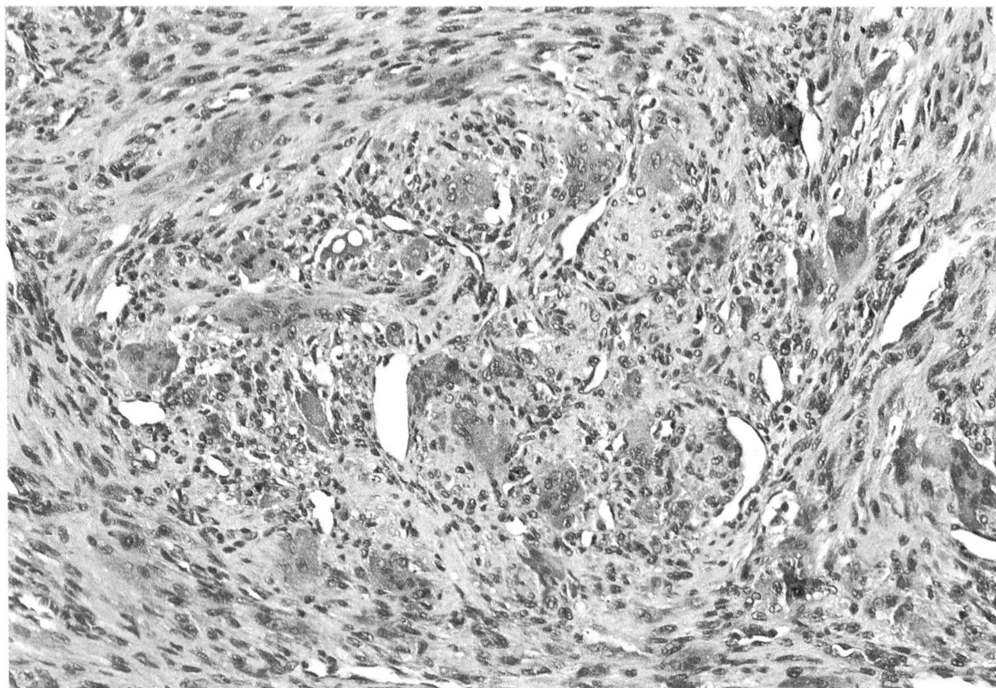

**FIGURE 14–54.** Giant cell tumor of low malignant potential showing spindling of cells.

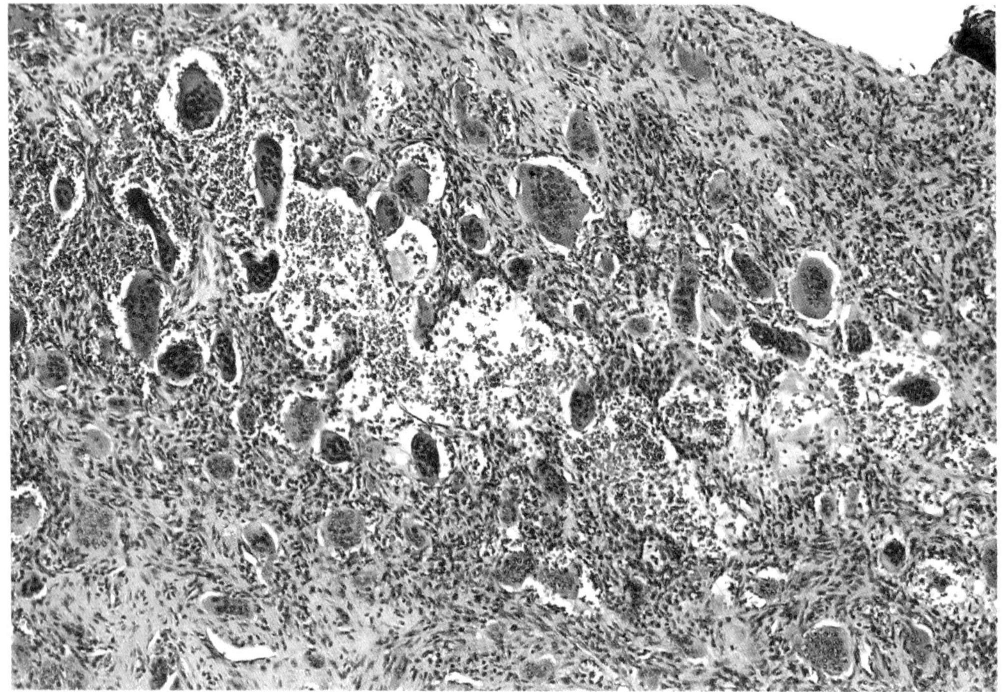

**FIGURE 14–55.** Aneursymal bone cyst-like changes in a giant cell tumor of low malignant potential.

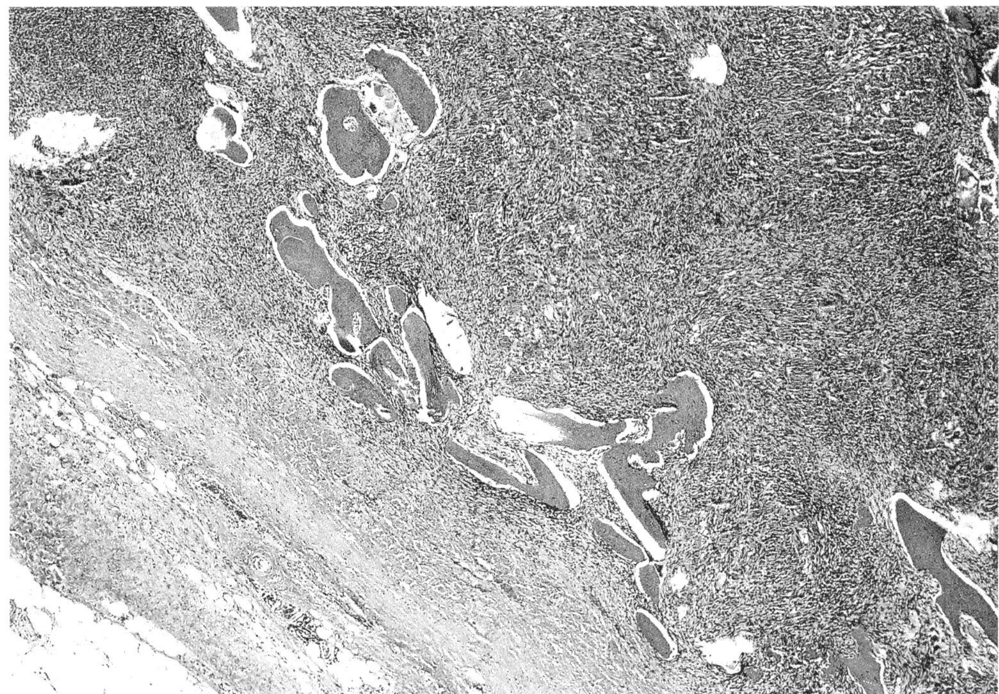

**FIGURE 14–56.** Metaplastic bone formation in a giant cell tumor of low malignant potential.

reminiscent of the changes of aneurysmal bone cysts can be seen (Figs. 14–55, 14–56). Soft tissue giant cell tumors have an immunophenotypic profile similar to that of giant cell tumor of bone in that they express CD68 and smooth muscle actin, and the osteoclastic giant cells express the osteoclast-specific marker tartrate-resistant acid phosphatase (TRAP). However, they lack CD45, S-100 protein, desmin, and lysozyme.

## Differential Diagnosis

In our experience these tumors are most often confused with tenosynovial giant cell tumor or malignant giant cell tumor of soft parts (malignant fibrous histiocytoma, giant cell type). Apart from the rather significant difference in location, *tenosynovial giant cell tumor* usually has prominent stromal hyalinization and a more heterogeneous population of cells, including xanthoma cells, siderophages, and lymphocytes. Giant cell forms of malignant fibrous histiocytoma, by definition, contain mononuclear and giant cells with significant levels of atypia. In addition, necrosis and atypical mitotic figures are often present. Areas of *plexiform fibrohistiocytic tumor* bear a startling resemblance to these tumors. Clearly identification of the bimodal population of cells and the dermal/subcutaneous location aid in the distinction. Lastly, *epithelioid sarcomas* and *nodular fasciitis with giant cells* should always be excluded before diagnosing a soft tissue giant cell tumor of low malignant potential. Keratin, present in epithelioid sarcoma, is absent in these tumors.

## Clinical Behavior

The clinical behavior of this group of tumors is considerably better than that reported for malignant giant cell tumor of soft parts. Of our 17 patients, 4 developed recurrences but none had metastasis. Although one of the original lesions reported by Nascimento allegedly metastasized, that case was later reclassified as a plexiform fibrohistiocytic tumor of childhood.

## REFERENCES

### Dermatofibrosarcoma Protuberans and Bednar Tumor


1. Adams JT, Salzstein SL. Metastasizing dermatofibrosarcoma protuberans. Am Surg 29:879, 1963.
2. Alguacil-Garcia A, Unni KK, Goellner JR. Histogenesis of dermatofibrosarcoma protuberans: an ultrastructural study. Am J Clin Pathol 69:427, 1978.
3. Ashack RJ, Tejada E, Parker C, et al. A localized atrophic plaque on the back: dermatofibrosarcoma protuberans (DFSP) (atrophic variant). Arch Dermatol 128:1549, 1990.
4. Barnhill DR, Boling R, Nobles W, et al. Vulvar dermatofibrosarcoma protuberans. Gynecol Oncol 30:149, 1988.
5. Bednar B. Storiform neurofibroma in core of naevocellular naevi. J Pathol 101:199, 1970.
6. Bednar B. Storiform neurofibromas of the skin, pigmented and nonpigmented. Cancer 10:368, 1957.

7. Bisceglia M, Vairo M, Calonje E, Fletcher CD. Pigmented fibrosarcomatous dermatofibrosarcoma protuberans (Bednar tumor): 3 case reports, analogy with conventional type and review of the literature. Pathologica 89:264, 1997.
8. Bock JE, Andreasson B, Thorn A, et al. Dermatofibrosarcoma protuberans of the vulva. Gynecol Oncol 20:129, 1985.
9. Bonnabeau RC, Stoughton WB, Armanious AW, et al. Dermatofibrosarcoma protuberans: report of a case with pulmonary metastasis and multiple intrathoracic recurrences. Oncology 29:1, 1974.
10. Brenner W, Schaefler K, Chhabra H, et al. Dermatofibrosarcoma protuberans metastatic to a regional lymph node. Cancer 36:1897, 1975.
11. Bridge JA, Neff JR, Sandberg AA. Cytogenetic analysis of dermatofibrosarcoma protuberans. Cancer Genet Cytogenet 49: 199, 1990.
12. Burkhardt BR, Soule EH, Winkelmann RK. Dermatofibrosarcoma protuberans: study of 56 cases. Am J Surg 111:638, 1966.
13. Calonje E, Fletcher CDM. Myoid differentiation in dermatofibrosarcoma protuberans and its fibrosarcomatous variant: clinicopathologic analysis of 5 cases. J Cutan Pathol 23:30, 1996.
14. Connelly JH, Evans HL. Dermatofibrosarcoma protuberans: a clinicopathologic review with emphasis on fibrosarcomatous areas. Am J Surg Pathol 16:921, 1992.
15. Darier J, Ferrand M. Dermatofibromas progressifs et recidivants ou fibrosarcomes de la peau. Ann Dermatol Syph 5:545, 1924.
16. David MMV, Preaux J. Dermatofibrosarcome de Darier-Ferrand chez l'enfant. Bull Soc Fr Derm Syph 75:187, 1968.
17. Degos R, Mouly R, Civatte J, et al. Dermatofibro-sarcome de Darier-Ferrand, datant de 70 ans, opere au stade ultime de tumeur monstrueuse. Bull Soc Fr Derm Syph 74:190, 1967.
18. Diaz-Cascajo C, Weyers W, Borrego L, et al. Dermatofibrosarcoma protuberans with fibrosarcomatous areas: a clinicopathologic and immunohistochemical study in four cases. Am J Dermatopathol 19:562, 1997.
19. Diaz-Cascajo C, Weyers W, Rey-Lopes A, Borghi S. Deep dermatofibrosarcoma protuberans. Histopathology 32:552, 1998.
20. Ding JA, Enjoji M. Dermatofibrosarcoma protuberans with fibrosarcomatous areas: a clinicopathologic study of nine cases and a comparison with allied tumors. Cancer 64:7212, 1989.
21. Ding JA, Hashimoto H, Sugimoto T, et al. Bednar tumor (pigmented dermatofibrosarcoma protuberans): an analysis of six cases. Acta Pathol Jpn 40:744, 1990.
22. Dohan FC, Kornblith PL, Wellum GR. S-100 protein and 2, 3-cyclic nucleotide 3′ phosphohydrolase in human brain tumors. Acta Neuropathol (Berl) 40:123, 1977.
23. Dupree WB, Langloss JM, Weiss SW. Pigmented dermatofibrosarcoma protuberans (Bednar tumor): a pathologic, ultrastructural, and immunohistochemical study. Am J Surg Pathol 9: 630, 1985.
24. Fekete E, From L, Kahn HJ. Tenascin differentiates dermatofibrosarcom protuberans from dermatofibroma: comparison with CD34 and factor XIIIa. Lab Invest 78:49, 1998.
25. Fletcher CDM, Evans BJ, Macartney JC, et al. Dermatofibrosarcoma protuberans: a clinicopathological and immunohistochemical study with a review of the literature. Histopathology 9:921, 1985.
26. Fletcher CD, Theaker JM, Flanagan A, et al. Pigmented dermatofibrosarcoma protuberans (Bednar tumour): melanocytic colonization or neuroectodermal differentiation? A clinicopathological and immunohistochemical study. Histopathology 13: 631, 1988.
27. Franchi A, Santucci M. Tenascin expression in cutaneous fibrohistiocytic tumors: Immunohistochemical investigation of 24 cases. Am J Dermatopathol 18:454, 1996.
28. Gaynor R, Irie R, Morton D, et al. S-100 protein: a marker for human malignant melanomas. Lancet 1:869, 1981.
29. Gaynor SM, Lewis JE, McCaffrey TV. Effect of resection margins on dermatofibrosarcoma protuberans of the head and neck. Arch Otolaryngol Head Neck Surg 123:430, 1997.
30. Gloster HM, Harris KR, Roenigk RK. A comparison between Mohs micrographic surgery and wide surgical excsion for the treatment of dermatofibrosarcoma protuberans. J Am Acad Dermatol 35:82, 1996.
31. Goldblum JR, Reith JD, Weiss SW. Sarcomas arising in dermatofibrosarcoma protuberans: a reappraisal of biologic behavior in eighteen cases treated by wide local excision with extended clinical follow up. Am J Surg Pathol 24:1125, 2000.
32. Goldblum JR, Tuthill RJ. CD34 and factor XIIIa immunoreactivity in dermatofibrosarcoma protuberans and dermatofibroma. Am J Dermatopathol 19:147, 1997.
33. Gutierrez G, Ospina JE, de Baez NE, et al. Dermatofibrosarcoma protuberans. Int J Dermatol 23:396, 1984.
34. Hagedorn M, Thomas C, von Kannen W. Dermatofibrosarcoma protuberans mit Ubergang in ein sogenanntes Fibrosarkom. Dermatologica 149:84, 1974.
35. Hashimoto K, Brownstein MH, Jakobiec FA. Dermatofibrosarcoma protuberans. Arch Dermatol 110:874, 1974.
36. Holm J. Dermatofibrosarcoma protuberans: report of a case with review of the literature. Acta Chir Stand 134:303, 1968.
37. Junaid TA, Ani AN, Ejeckam GC. Dermatofibrosarcoma protuberans in the parotid gland: a case report. Br J Oral Surg 12: 298, 1975.
38. Kahn LB, Saxe N, Gordon W. Dermatofibrosarcoma protuberans with lymph node and pulmonary metastases. Arch Dermatol 114:599, 1978.
39. Leake JF, Buscema J, Cho KR, et al. Dermatofibrosarcoma protuberans of the vulva. Gynecol Oncol 41:245, 1991.
40. Mandahl N, Heim S, Willen H, et al. Supernumerary ring chromosome as the sole cytogenetic abnormality in a dermatofibrosarcoma protuberans. Cancer Genet Cytogenet 49:273, 1990.
41. Martin L, Combemale P, Dupin M, et al. The atrophic variant of dermatofibrosarcoma protuberans in childhood: a report of six cases. Br J Dermatol 139:719, 1998.
42. McKee PH, Fletcher CD. Dermatofibrosarcoma protuberans presenting in infancy and childhood. J Cutan Pathol 18:241, 1991.
43. McLeiland J, Chu T. Dermatofibrosarcoma protuberans arising in a BCG vaccination scar. Arch Dermatol 124:496, 1988.
44. McPeak CJ, Cruz T, Nicastri AD. Dermatofibrosarcoma protuberans: an analysis of 86 cases—five with metastasis. Ann Surg 166(Suppl 12):803, 1967.
45. Melezer M, Dvorszky C. Acanthosis nigricans bei Dermatofibrosarcoma protuberans mit multiplen Hautmetastasen. Hautarzt 8:54, 1957.
46. Mentzel T, Beham A, Katemkamp D, et al. Fibrosarcomatous ("high grade") dermatofibrosarcoma protuberans: clinicopathologic and immunohistochemical study of a series of 41 cases with emphasis on prognostic significance. Am J Surg Pathol 22:576, 1998.
47. Michelson HE. Dermatofibrosarcoma protuberans. Surgery 31: 705, 1952.
48. Miyamoto Y, Morimatsu M, Nakashima T. Pigmented storiform neurofibroma. Acta Pathol Jpn 34:821, 1984.
49. Moore BW. A soluble protein characteristic of the nervous system. Biochem Biophys Res Commun 19:739, 1965.
50. Mopper C, Pinkus H. Dermatofibrosarcoma protuberans: report of two cases. Am J Clin Pathol 20:171, 1950.
51. Morimitsu Y, Hisaoka M, Okamoto S, et al. Dermtofibrosarcoma protuberans and its fibrosarcomatous variant with areas

of myoid differentiation: a report of three cases. Histopathology 32:547, 1998.
52. Nakajma T, Watanabe S, Sato Y, et al. Immunohistochemical demonstration of S100 protein in human malignant melanoma and pigmented nevi. Gan 72:335, 1981.
53. Nakazato Y, Ishizeki J, Takahashi KN, et al. Immunohistochemical localization of S100 protein in granular cell myoblastoma. Cancer 49:1624, 1982.
54. O'Brien KP, Seroussi E, Dal Cin P, et al. Various regions within the alpha-helical domain of the COL1A1 gene are fused to the second exon of the PDGFB gene in dermatofibrosarcomas and giant-cell fibroblastoma. Genes Chromosomes Cancer 23:187, 1998.
55. O'Connell JX, Trotter MJ. Fibrosarcomatous dermatofibrosarcoma protuberans: a variant. Mod Pathol 9:273, 1996.
56. O'Dowd J, Laidler P. Progression of dermatofibrosarcoma protuberans to malignant fibrous histiocytoma: report of a case with implications for tumour histogenesis. Hum Pathol 19:368, 1988.
57. Oku T, Takigawa M, Fukamizu H, et al. Tissue cultures of benign and malignant fibrous histiocytomas: SEM observations. J Cutan Pathol 11:534, 1984.
58. Onoda N, Tsutsumi Y, Kakudo K, et al. Pigmented dermatofibrosarcoma protuberans (Bednar tumor): an autopsy case with systemic metastasis. Acta Pathol Jpn 40:935, 1990.
59. Ozawa A, Niizuma K, Onkido M, et al. Pigmented dermatofibrosarcoma protuberans: an analysis of six cases. Acta Pathol Jpn 40:935, 1990.
60. Ozzello L, Hamels J. The histiocytic nature of dermatofibrosarcoma protuberans: tissue culture and electron microscopic study. Am J Clin Pathol 65:136, 1976.
61. Pack GT, Tabah EJ. Dermatofibrosarcoma protuberans. Arch Surg 62:391, 1951.
62. Parker TL, Zitelli JA. Surgical margins for excision of dermatofibrosarcoma protuberans. J Am Acad Dermatol 32:233, 1995.
63. Petoin DS, Verola O, Banzet P, et al. Dermatofibrosarcome de Darier et Ferrand: etude de 96 cas sur 15 ans. Chirurgie 111: 132, 1985.
64. Pizarro GB, Fanburg JC, Miettinen M. Dermatofibrosarcoma protuberans (DFSP) with fibrosarcomatous transformation: reexplored. Mod Pathol 10:13A, 1997.
65. Ratner D, Thomas CO, Johnson TM, et al. Mohs micrographic surgery for the treatment of dermatofibrosarcoma protuberans. J Am Acad Dermatol 37:600, 1997.
66. Robinson JK. Dermatofibrosarcoma protuberans resected by Mohs' surgery (chemosurgery): a 5-year prospective study. J Am Acad Dermatol 12:1093, 1985.
67. Roses DF, Valensi Q, Latrenta G, et al. Surgical treatment of dermatofibrosarcoma protuberans. Surg Gynecol Obstet 162: 449, 1986.
68. Sanz-Trelles A, Ayala-Carbonero A, Rodrigo-Fernandex I, Weil-Lara B. Leiomyomatous nodules and bundles of vascular origin in the fibrosarcomatous variant of dermatofibrosarcoma protuberans. J Cutan Pathol 25:44, 1998.
69. Shelley WB. Malignant melanoma and dermatofibrosarcoma in a 60-year-old patient with lifelong acrodermatitis enteropathica. J Am Acad Dermatol 6:63, 1982.
70. Shimizu A, O'Brien KP, Sjoblom T, et al. The dermatofibrosarcoma protubernas associated collagen type I/platelet derived growth factor (PDGF) $\beta$ chain fusion gene generates a transforming protein that is processed to functional PDGF-$\beta\beta$. Cancer Res 59:3719, 1999.
71. Shneidman D, Belizaire R. Arsenic exposure followed by the development of dermatofibrosarcoma protuberans. Cancer 58: 1585, 1986.
72. Simon M-P, Pedeutour F, Sirbent N, et al. Deregulation of the platelet-derived growth factor $\beta$-chain gene via fusion with collagen gene COL1A1 in dermatofibrosarcoma protuberans and giant cell fibroblastoma. Nat Genet 15:95, 1997.
73. Simstein NL, Tuthill RJ, Sperber EE, et al. Dermatofibrosarcoma protuberans: case reports and review of literature. South Med J 70:487, 1977.
74. Smola MG, Soyer HP, Scharnagl E. Surgical treatment of dermatofibrosarcoma protuberans: a retrospective study of 20 cases with review of the literature. Eur J Surg Oncol 17:44, 1991.
75. Stephenson CF, Berger CS, Leong SP, et al. Ring chromosome in a dermatofibrosarcoma protuberans. Cancer Genet Cytogenet 58:52, 1992.
76. Suit H, Sprior I, Mankin HJ, et al: Radiation in management of patients with dermatofibrosarcoma protuberans. J Clin Oncol 145:2365, 1996.
77. Talib VH, Sultana Z, Patil SK, et al. Dermatofibrosarcoma protuberans: report of four cases with review of literature. Indian J Cancer 11:200, 1974.
78. Taylor HB, Helwig EB. Dermatofibrosarcoma protuberans: a study of 115 cases. Cancer 15:717, 1962.
79. Tsuneyoshi M, Enjoji M. Bednar tumor (pigmented dermatofibrosarcoma protuberans): an analysis of six cases. Acta Pathol Jpn 40:744, 1990.
80. Wooldridge WE. Dermatofibrosarcoma protuberans: a tumor too lightly considered. Arch Dermatol 75:132, 1957.
81. Wrotnowski U, Cooper PH, Shmookler BM. Fibrosarcomatous change in dermatofibrosarcoma protuberans. Am J Surg Pathol 12:287, 1988.
82. Yosida H, Matsui K, Hashimoto K, et al. Dermatofibrosarcoma protuberans and its tissue culture study: ultrastructural, enzyme, histochemical, and immunological study. Acta Pathol Jpn 32:83, 1982.

### Giant Cell Fibroblastoma

83. Abdul-Karim FW, Evans HL, Silva EG. Giant cell fibroblastoma: a report of three cases. Am J Clin Pathol 83:165, 1985.
84. Alguacil-Garcia A. Giant cell fibroblastoma recurring as a dermatofibrosarcoma protuberans. Am J Surg Pathol 15:798, 1991.
85. Allen PW, Zwi J. Giant cell fibroblastoma transforming into dermatofibrosarcoma protuberans [letter]. Am J Surg Pathol 15:1127, 1992.
86. Barr RJ, Young EM, Liao SY. Giant cell fibroblastoma: an immunohistochemical study. J Cutan Pathol 13:301, 1986.
87. Beham A, Fletcher CD. Dermatofibrosarcoma protuberans with areas resembling giant cell fibroblastoma: report of two cases. Histopathology 17:165, 1990.
88. Chou P, Gonzalez-Crussi F, Mangkornkanok M. Giant cell fibroblastoma. Cancer 63:756, 1989.
89. Cin PD, Sciot R, De Wever I, et al. Cytogenetic and immunohistochemical evidence that giant cell fibroblastoma is related to dermatofibrosarcoma protuberans. Genes Chromosomes Cancer 15:73, 1996.
90. Coyne J, Kaftan SM, Craig RD. Dermatofibrosarcoma protuberans recurring as a giant cell fibroblastoma. Histopathology 21:184, 1992.
91. Dymock RB, Allen PW, Stirling JW, et al. Giant cell fibroblastoma: a distinctive recurrent tumor of childhood. Am J Surg Pathol 11:263, 1987.
92. Fletcher CD. Giant cell fibroblastoma of soft tissue: a clinicopathologic and immunohistochemical study. Histopathology 13:499, 1988.
93. Hirose T, Sasaki M, Shintaku M. Giant cell fibroblastoma. Acta Pathol Jpn 40:540, 1990.
94. Kanai Y, Mukai M, Sugiura H, et al. Giant cell fibroblastoma:

a case report and immunohistochemical comparison with ten cases of dermatofibrosarcoma protuberans. Acta Pathol Jpn 41: 552, 1991.
95. Maeda T, Hirose T, Furuya K, et al. Giant cell fibroblastoma associated with dermatofibrosarcoma protuberans: a case report. Mod Pathol 11:491, 1998.
96. Michal M, Zamecnik M. Giant cell fibroblastoma with a dermatofibrosarcoma protuberans component. Am J Dermatopathol 14:549, 1992.
97. Nair R, Kane SV, Borges A, et al. Giant cell fibroblastoma. J Surg Oncol 53:136, 1993.
98. Rosen LB, Amazon K, Weitzner J, et al. Giant cell fibroblastoma: a report of a case and review of the literature. Am J Dermatopathol 11:242, 1989.
99. Shmookler BM, Enzinger FM, Weiss SW. Giant cell fibroblastoma: a juvenile form of dermatofibrosarcoma protuberans. Cancer 15:2154, 1989.
100. Weiss SW, Nickoloff BJ. CD34 is expressed by a distinctive cell population in peripheral nerve, nerve sheath tumors, and related lesions. Am J Surg Pathol 17:1039, 1993.

### Angiomatoid Fibrous Histiocytoma

101. Chow LT, Allen P, Kumata SM, et al. Angiomatoid malignant fibrous histiocytoma: report of an unusual case with highly aggressive clinical course. J Foot Ankle Surg 37:235, 1998.
102. Costa MJ, Weiss SW. Angiomatoid malignant fibrous histiocytoma: a follow-up study of 108 cases with evaluation of possible histologic predictors of outcome. Am J Surg Pathol 14: 1126, 1990.
103. El-Naggar AK, Ro JY, Ayala AG, et al. Angiomatoid malignant fibrous histiocytoma: flow cytometric DNA analysis of six cases. Surg Oncol 40:201, 1989.
104. Enzinger FM. Angiomatoid malignant fibrous histiocytoma: a distinct fibrohistiocytic tumor of children and young adults simulating a vascular neoplasm. Cancer 44:2147, 1979.
104a. Fanburg-Smith JC, Miettinen M. Angiomatoid "malignant" fibrous histiocytoma a clinicopathologic study of 158 cases and further exploration of the myoid phenotype. Hum Path 30: 1336, 1999.
105. Fletcher CD. Angiomatoid "malignant fibrous histiocytoma": an immunohistochemical study indicative of myoid differentiation. Hum Pathol 22:563, 1991.
106. Kay S. Angiomatoid malignant fibrous histiocytoma: report of two cases with ultrastructural observations of one case. Arch Pathol Lab Med 109:934, 1985.
107. Leu HJK, Makek M. Angiomatoid malignant fibrous histiocytoma. Arch Pathol Lab Med 110:2010, 1977.
108. Pettinato G, Manivel JC, De Rosa G, et al. Angiomatoid malignant fibrous histiocytoma: cytologic, immunohistochemical, ultrastructural, and flow cytometric study of 20 cases. Mod Pathol 3:479, 1990.
109. Smith ME, Costa MJ, Weiss SW. Evaluation of CD68 and other histiocytic antigens in angiomatoid malignant fibrous histiocytoma. Am J Surg Pathol 15:757, 1991.
110. Sun CC Jr, Toker C, Breitenecker R. An ultrastructural study of angiomatoid fibrous histiocytoma. Cancer 40:2103, 1982.
111. Wegmann W, Heitz PU. Angiomatoid malignant fibrous histiocytoma: evidence for the histiocytic origin of tumor cells. Virchows Arch [Pathol Anat] 406:59, 1985.

### Plexiform Fibrohistiocytic Tumor

112. Angervall L, Kindsblom LG, Lindholm K, et al. Plexiform fibrohistiocytic tumor: report of a case involving preoperative aspiration cytology and immunohistochemical and ultrastructural analysis of surgical specimens. Pathol Res Pract 188:350, 1992.
113. Enzinger FM, Zhang RY. Plexiform fibrohistiocytic tumor presenting in children and young adults: an analysis of 65 cases. Am J Surg Pathol 12:818, 1988.
114. Giard F, Bonneau R, Raymond GP. Plexiform fibrohistiocytic tumor. Dermatologica 183:290, 1991.
115. Hollowood K, Holley MP, Fletcher CD. Plexiform fibrohistiocytic tumour: clinicopathological, immunohistochemical and ultrastructural analysis in favour of a myofibroblastic lesion. Histopathology 19:503, 1991.
116. Redlich GC, Montgomery KD, Allgood GA, Joste NE. Plexiform fibrohistiocytic tumor with a clonal cytogenetic anomaly. Cancer Genet Cytogenet 108:141, 1999.
117. Remstein E, Arndt CA, Nascimento AG. Plexiform fibrohistiocytic tumor: clinicopathologic analysis of 22 cases. Am J Surg Pathol 23:662, 1999.
118. Salomao DR, Nascimento AG. Plexiform fibrohistiocytic tumor with systemic metastases: a case report. Am J Surg Pathol 21: 469, 1997.
119. Smith S, Fletcher CD, Smith MA, et al. Cytogenetic analysis of a plexiform fibrohistiocytic tumor. Cancer Genet Cytogenet 48: 31, 1990.
120. Zelger B, Weinlich G, Steiner H, et al. Dermal and subcutaneous variants of plexiform fibrohistiocytic tumor. Am J Surg Pathol 21:235, 1997.

### Soft Tissue Giant Cell Tumor of Low Malignant Potential

121. Folpe AL, Morris RJ, Weiss SW. Soft tissue giant cell tumor of low malignant potential: a proposal for the reclassification of malignant giant cell tumor of soft parts. Mod Pathol 12:894, 1999.
122. Guccion JG, Enzinger FM. Malignant giant cell tumor of soft parts: an analysis of 32 cases. Cancer 29:1518, 1972.
122a. O'Connell JX, Wehrli BM, Nielsen GP, Rosenberg HE. Giant cell tumors of soft tissue: a clinicopathologic study of 18 benign and malignant tumors. Am J Surg Pathol 24:386, 2000.
122b. Oliviera AM, Dei Tos AP, Fletcher CDM, Nascimento AG. Primary giant cell tumor of soft tissues: a study of 22 cases. Am J Surg Pathol 24:248, 2000.
123. Nascimento AG. Giant cell tumors of soft parts. Lab Invest 68: 32, 1993.
124. Salm R, Sissons HA. Giant cell tumors or soft tissues. J Pathol 107:27, 1972.

# CHAPTER 15

# MALIGNANT FIBROHISTIOCYTIC TUMORS

The term *malignant fibrous histiocytoma* was first introduced in 1963 to refer to a group of soft tissue tumors characterized by a storiform, or cartwheel-like, growth pattern. Although the tumors initially described by Ozzello et al.[105] and later by O'Brien and Stout[103] had a predominantly fibroblastic appearance, it was postulated that they were derived from histiocytes that could assume the appearance and function of fibroblasts ("facultative fibroblasts"). This theory was based principally on tissue culture studies of tumor explants[105] in which the cultured tumor cells initially resembled histiocytes and exhibited ameboid movement and phagocytosis. Later the cells assumed bipolar shapes resembling fibroblasts. The versatility of the histiocyte became an accepted means of explaining the bimodal population of cells often encountered in these tumors. The large number of early ultrastructural studies has both endorsed and refuted the histiocytic origin of these tumors while at the same time raising fundamental questions concerning structure and function.

The advent of immunohistochemistry and the accessibility of numerous monoclonal antibodies directed against various structural proteins of specific cell types have answered some questions and raised new ones. The debate as to whether malignant fibrous histiocytoma represents a true histiocytic neoplasm has largely subsided. Most studies have failed to confirm monocyte and macrophage differentiation but, rather, have established a closer phenotypic link with the fibroblast. The more contentious issue has been whether malignant fibrous histiocytoma represents a homogeneous entity or a collection of sarcomas of diverse type in which subtle differentiation has been overlooked. Clearly the extent to which this represents a homogeneous versus a heterogeneous entity depends, in part, on the degree of sampling and the number of ancillary studies a pathologist is willing to devote to a given case, as well as the definitional criteria for making alternative diagnoses. A large retrospective study of tumors diagnosed as pleomorphic sarcoma indicated that approximately one-fourth fulfilled current diagnostic criteria for malignant fibrous histiocytoma.[48] Undoubtedly, "interlopers" can be found in the category of malignant fibrous histiocytoma from time to time, but this category is still useful, provided a modicum of care is taken when establishing the diagnosis. Specific issues related to diagnostic criteria are discussed later in the chapter. There is little pressing need to change the term malignant fibrous histiocytoma, even though it is a taxonomically inaccurate term: It is well accepted in the clinical literature, and it implies a pleomorphic high grade sarcoma, usually of adults, with no specific light microscopic features of differentiation apart from collagen production.

The ambiguity concerning the behavior of these tumors expressed in the early work of O'Brien and Stout has been clarified by several large clinical studies[31,72,85,106,114,127,128,133] indicating the malignant nature of the lesions and the fact that the prognosis can be related to various factors, including size, depth, location, and clinical stage. There is also preliminary evidence that specific cytogenetic abnormalities of malignant fibrous histiocytomas may represent independent prognostic factors for this disease.

The spectrum of malignant fibrohistiocytic tumors includes atypical fibroxanthoma, a cutaneous form that carries an excellent prognosis because of its small size and superficiality, as well as the conventional or more deeply situated malignant fibrous histiocytoma, which is divided into several subtypes (storiform-pleomorphic, myxoid, giant cell, inflammatory). Angiomatoid malignant fibrous histiocytoma, a distinctive tumor of childhood, which was formerly classified with the conventional malignant fibrous histiocytomas of adults, has been grouped with the fibrohistiocytic tumors of low grade malignancy (see Chapter 14) because of its associated excellent rate of survival.

Although malignant fibrous histiocytoma has been defined classically as a soft tissue sarcoma, it may arise from supporting structures of various parenchymal organs. Indeed, it has been described in bone[40,96,99,100] and other organs. At these sites its incidence, biologic potential, and diagnostic criteria are not fully defined (subjects beyond the scope of this chapter).

## ATYPICAL FIBROXANTHOMA

Atypical fibroxanthoma is a pleomorphic tumor that usually occurs on actinic-damaged skin of the elderly.[3,6,7,14,16,19,23–25] It has been referred to in the past as *pseudosarcoma of the skin*,[8,26] *paradoxical fibrosarcoma*,[4] *pseudosarcomatous dermatofibroma*,[18] and *pseudosarcomatous reticulohistiocytoma*.[10] It is histologically indistinguishable from pleomorphic forms of malignant fibrous histiocytoma. From a conceptual point of view, we regard it as a superficial form of that tumor, which by virtue of its superficial location almost invariably pursues a benign course. However, from a practical point of view, we have retained the term *atypical fibroxanthoma* to distinguish it from deep forms of malignant fibrous histiocytoma, which require more radical therapy and carry a less favorable prognosis. Unfortunately, the term atypical fibroxanthoma has also been loosely used to refer to borderline or even malignant-appearing fibrohistiocytic tumors not occurring in the skin. This nonrestrictive use of this term is confusing and should be discouraged.

### Clinical Findings

Atypical fibroxanthomas occur in two clinical settings.[9] The more common form of the disease presents on the exposed surface of the head and neck, particularly the nose, cheek, and ear. Elderly persons are afflicted with this form of the disease. The less common form, which accounts for about one-fourth of cases, occurs on the limbs and trunk of young persons. Both forms of the disease are characterized by a solitary nodule or ulcer that produces few symptoms aside from bleeding; it is often present several months before biopsy.

Solar radiation is probably a predisposing factor in the pathogenesis of this disease, supported by the common occurrence of the tumor on actinic-damaged skin and its frequent association with other actinic-related lesions (e.g., basal cell carcinoma, squamous carcinoma). Occupational and therapeutic irradiation may also be etiologic factors, but this source is less well documented. The incidence of previous irradiation varies from less than 5% in some series[9] to more than 50% in others.[12] In most instances the latent period between the previous radiation exposure and the appearance of the atypical fibroxanthoma is more than 10 years and thus well in keeping with the accepted interval for a radiation-induced tumor. Indeed, many early reported sarcoma-like lesions of skin following irradiation were probably atypical fibroxanthomas.[21]

### Gross Appearance

Grossly, the lesions are solitary nodules or ulcers usually measuring less than 2 cm in diameter (Figs. 15–1, 15–2). Their appearance is not distinctive, and for this reason a variety of preoperative diagnoses are considered, including basal cell carcinoma, squamous carcinoma, pyogenic granuloma, and sebaceous cyst.[9]

### Microscopic Findings

These tumors are expansile dermal nodules that abut the epidermis, causing pressure atrophy or ulceration (Fig. 15–3). Alternatively, a *grenz* zone of uninvolved dermis is present. The tumor compresses the skin appendages laterally and extends into the subcutis. By definition, the tumor does not extensively involve the subcutis, nor does it invade deeper structures such as fascia or muscle. Areas adjacent to these lesions may display solar elastosis, vascular dilatation, and capillary proliferation.

Histologically, these tumors resemble pleomorphic forms of malignant fibrous histiocytoma. They are characterized by bizarre cells arranged in a haphaz-

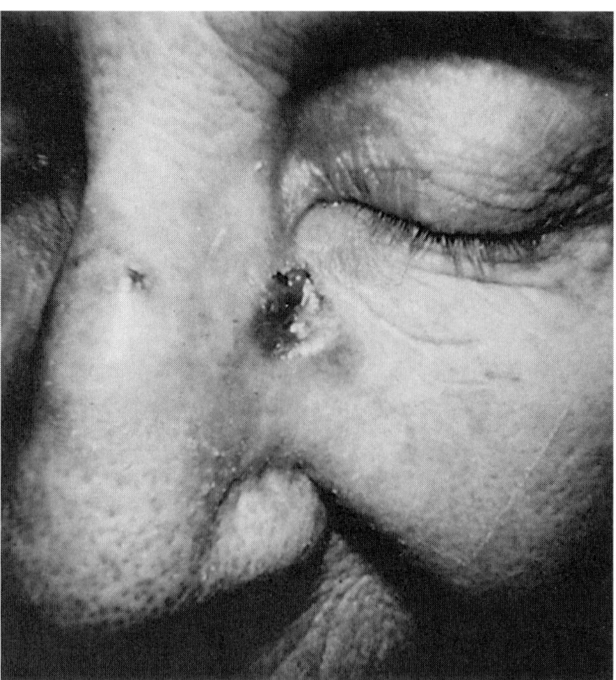

**FIGURE 15–1.** Ulcerating atypical fibroxanthoma from the nose of an 80-year-old woman. Grossly, the tumor resembled a basal cell carcinoma. (From Fretzin DF, Helwig EB. Atypical fibroxanthoma of the skin. Cancer 31:1541, 1973.)

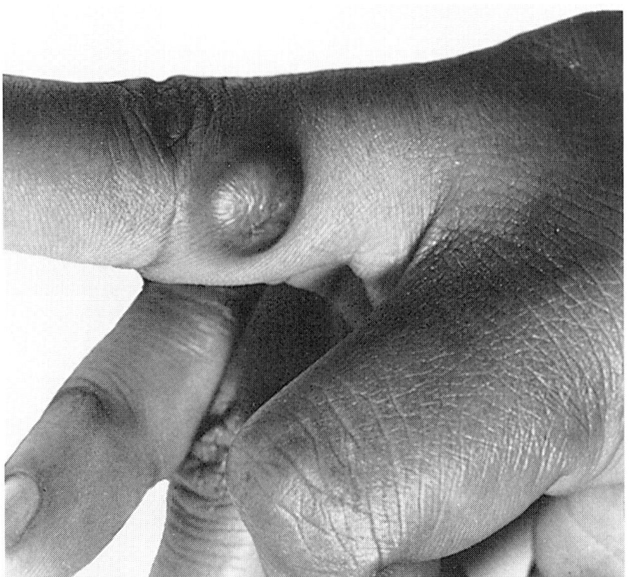

**FIGURE 15–2.** Nodular atypical fibroxanthoma from the finger of a 36-year-old woman. Atypical fibroxanthomas in young patients typically occur on the extremities, in contrast to those in elderly patients, which are located on sun-exposed or actinic-damaged surfaces. (From Fretzin DF, Helwig EB. Atypical fibroxanthoma of the skin. Cancer 31: 1541, 1973.)

ard or vague fascicular pattern (Fig. 15–4). Rarely, a storiform pattern is evident. The cells are spindle-shaped or round, and they exhibit multinucleation, pleomorphism, and numerous typical and atypical mitotic figures. The cells occasionally have small droplets of neutral fat and periodic acid-Schiff (PAS)-positive, diastase-resistant material, two features that probably reflect, in part, degenerative changes. Occasional inflammatory cells are present; and rarely osteoclastic giant cells[15] or osteoid[5] are seen. Clear-cell[22] and granular cell variants[20] of atypical fibroxanthoma have been reported but are rare. Necrosis, a common feature of malignant fibrous histiocytoma, is rare; if it is present in significant degree, it should raise serious questions about the diagnosis of atypical fibroxanthoma (see discussion).

Overall, the ultrastructural features of this tumor are similar to those of malignant fibrous histiocytoma. Cells with characteristics of fibroblasts,[2] myofibroblasts, and histiocytes[1,2] have been reported. In no atypical fibroxanthomas have there been prominent intercellular junctions, tonofibrils, or other features specifically suggesting epithelial differentiation. Electron microscopy has confirmed the light microscopic impression that atypical fibroxanthoma is a mesenchymal lesion rather than a spindled carcinoma or melanoma.

## Differential Diagnosis

The most common problem in the differential diagnosis is distinguishing atypical fibroxanthoma from spindled carcinoma or melanoma. Although generally atypical fibroxanthoma is more pleomorphic, we have seen many cases of both primary and metastatic epi-

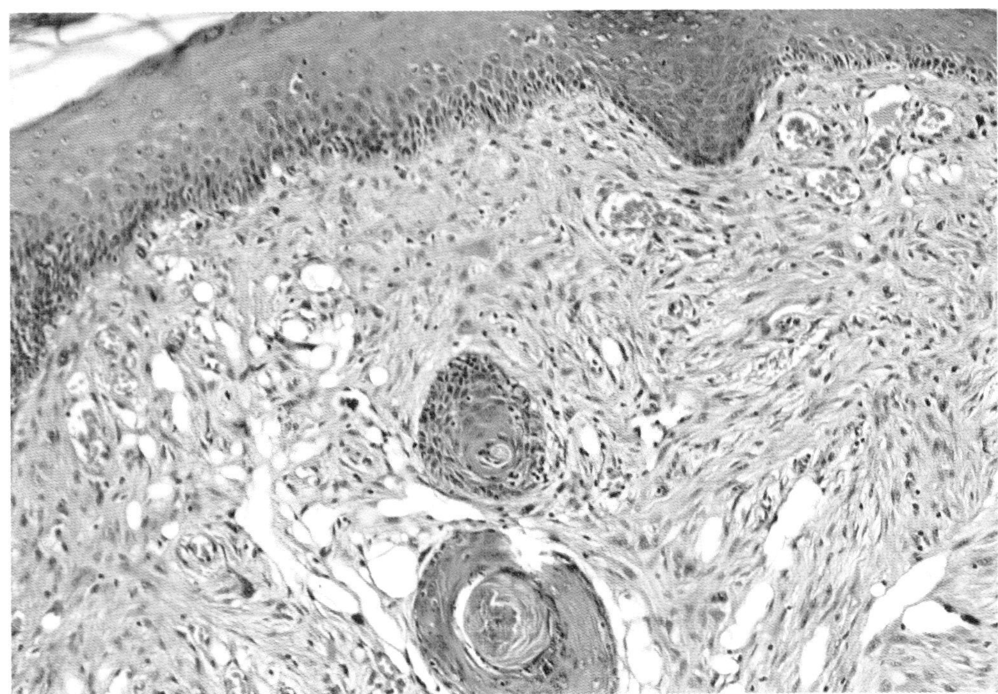

**FIGURE 15–3.** Atypical fibroxanthoma abutting epidermis. Dilated capillaries are commonly seen adjacent to and in the tumor.

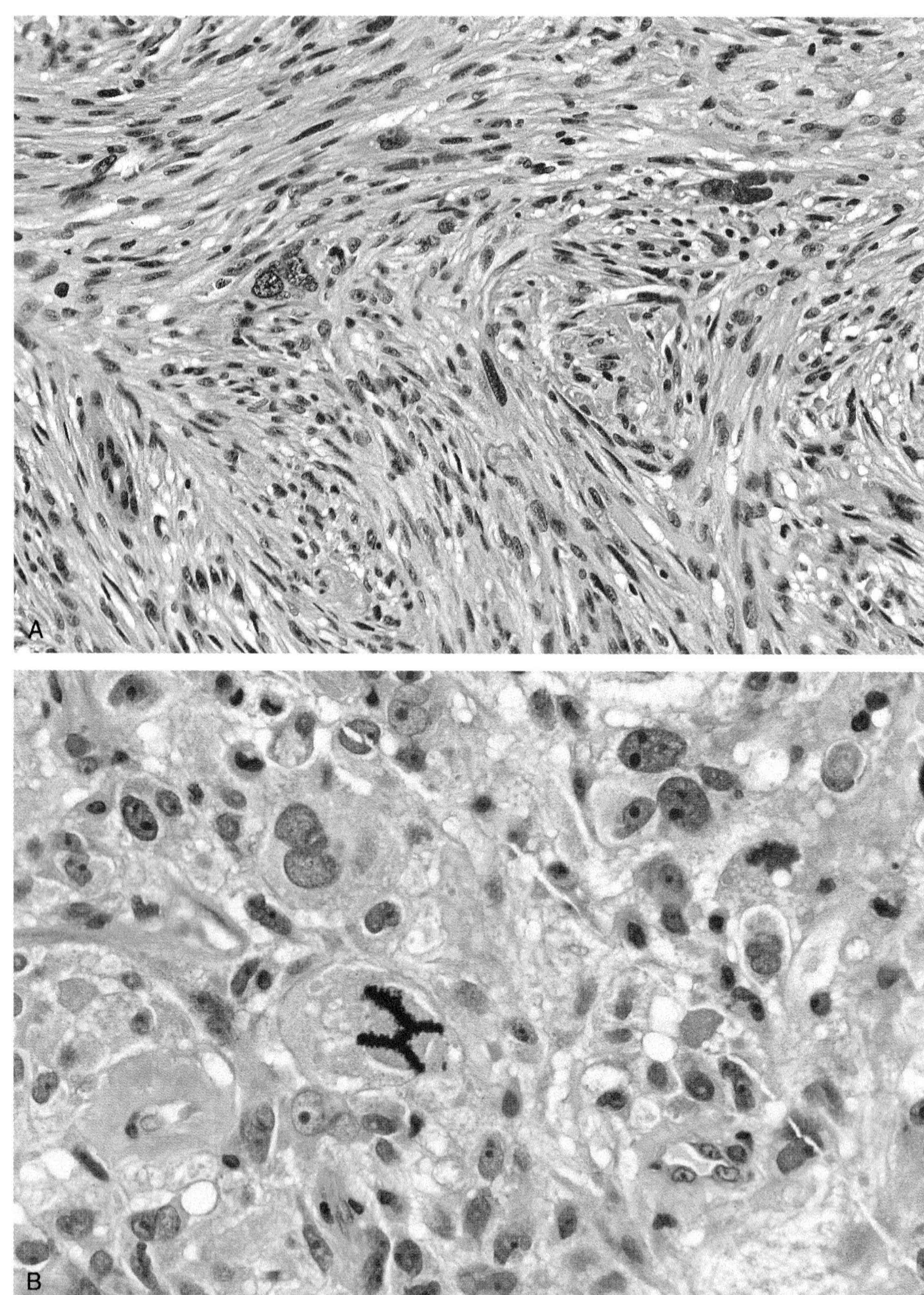


**FIGURE 15–4.** Bizarre cells comprising atypical fibroxanthoma vary from plump spindled cells to large round cells. (**A**) Pleomorphism is marked; and mitotic figures, including atypical forms, are common (**B**).

thelial neoplasms that in areas have exactly mimicked atypical fibroxanthoma. Therefore there is no substitute for extensively sampling a given tumor, particularly when a presumptive atypical fibroxanthoma presents in an unusual setting. The tumor should be examined to make certain there is neither junctional activity nor focal epithelial differentiation. Immunostains for cytokeratin, S-100 protein, and various melanin-associated antigens (HMB-45, Melan-A, microphthalmia transcription factor) are helpful and in some cases mandatory for excluding the other diagnoses.

Atypical fibroxanthoma must also be distinguished from other mesenchymal tumors, most commonly malignant fibrous histiocytoma. Because we currently regard atypical fibroxanthoma as a superficial or even an early form of malignant fibrous histiocytoma, the distinction of the two is for the most part one of size and depth, although one report suggests that CD74 may discriminate malignant fibrous histiocytoma from atypical fibroxanthoma.[17] The more selective one is when diagnosing atypical fibroxanthoma, the better is the resultant behavior. In our opinion, if a tumor extensively involves the subcutis, penetrates fascia and muscle, or displays necrosis or vascular invasion, it should be diagnosed as malignant fibrous histiocytoma, as such tumors run a definite risk of recurrence and metastasis. The tumors reported by Helwig and May[11] as atypical fibroxanthoma with metastases we would have designated malignant fibrous histiocytoma because most displayed deep invasion, necrosis, or vascular invasion.

An atypical fibroxanthoma is sometimes mistaken for leiomyosarcoma, but leiomyosarcomas have distinct fascicles containing cells with characteristic blunt-ended nuclei, and cytoplasmic glycogen is often abundant. Trichrome stains, furthermore, demonstrate distinct longitudinal striations corresponding ultrastructurally to myofilamentous material dispersed throughout the cytoplasm. From a practical point of view, the distinction of dermal (primary) leiomyosarcoma and atypical fibroxanthoma may simply be an act of discipline because of the similarity in therapy and prognosis. Rarely, leiomyosarcomas (particularly of the retroperitoneum) present as cutaneous metastases.

### Discussion

Although this tumor is histologically indistinguishable from some forms of malignant fibrous histiocytoma, it deserves a special designation because of its almost uniformly excellent prognosis following conservative therapy. In the largest series in the literature, only 9 of 140 patients had a recurrence, and none developed metastasis.[9] It is now recognized that in exceptional instances this tumor does metastasize. One such case, characterized by vascular invasion, was mentioned by Fretzin and Helwig[9] but was not included in their series. A second case was reported by Jacobs et al.[13] Although this tumor, located on the nose, was histologically typical, it recurred, involved the nasal cartilage, and ultimately metastasized to a cervical lymph node. We have seen similar cases in which an atypical fibroxanthoma recurred, grew deeply, and eventually metastasized. As mentioned above, the lesions reported by Helwig and May[11] as metastatic atypical fibroxanthoma, in our opinion, would have been better classified as superficial forms of malignant fibrous histiocytoma. In view of the rarity of metastases, conservative therapy is initially indicated. However, when atypical fibroxanthoma recurs as a large deeply situated mass, it should be considered malignant fibrous histiocytoma and must be treated accordingly.

Despite the widespread use of the term atypical fibroxanthoma, some have suggested it is not an entity but, rather, a heterogeneous group of mesenchymal and epithelial lesions arising in a common clinical setting.[1] Because the diagnosis of atypical fibroxanthoma is to some extent an exclusionary one, it is inevitable that certain cases are misdiagnosed. By thoroughly sampling such tumors and by selectively applying electron microscopy and immunohistochemistry in ambiguous cases, we believe that heterogeneity is minimal and that the term refers to a relatively homogeneous group of superficial fibrohistiocytic neoplasms.

## MALIGNANT FIBROUS HISTIOCYTOMA

Malignant fibrous histiocytoma is the most common soft tissue sarcoma of late adult life.[45,128] It manifests a broad range of histologic appearances, and for this reason we have found it necessary to divide it into the following subtypes[126]: storiform-pleomorphic, myxoid (myxofibrosarcoma), giant cell (malignant giant cell tumor of soft parts), and inflammatory (xanthosarcoma, malignant xanthogranuloma).

Most malignant fibrous histiocytomas are cellular neoplasms with a mixture of storiform and pleomorphic areas; they have been descriptively termed the *storiform-pleomorphic type.* Depending on the relative proportions of these areas, the tumor may appear well differentiated and resemble dermatofibrosarcoma protuberans, or it may appear highly anaplastic. This subtype serves as the prototype for much of our thinking concerning the behavior of this group of neoplasms. The *myxoid type,* which accounts for roughly one-fourth of malignant fibrous histiocytomas, is the second most common variety.[129] It is characterized by prominent myxoid change of the stroma and contains cellular areas indistinguishable from the foregoing type. It is distinguished form the storiform-pleomorphic type not only because of its distinctive appearance but also because of its better prognosis. The last two types are less common. The *giant cell type* (malignant giant cell tumor of soft parts)[52] contains numerous osteoclast-type giant cells, and the *inflammatory type* is characterized by a predominance of xanthoma cells and acute inflammatory cells. The latter group has also been called *malignant xanthogranuloma, xanthosarcoma,*[65,66,69] and *inflammatory fibrous histiocytoma.*[71,79] Although formerly grouped with malignant fibrohistiocytic tumors, the angiomatoid fibrous histiocytoma has been reclassified as a fibrohistiocytic tumor of low malignant potential (see Chapter 14).

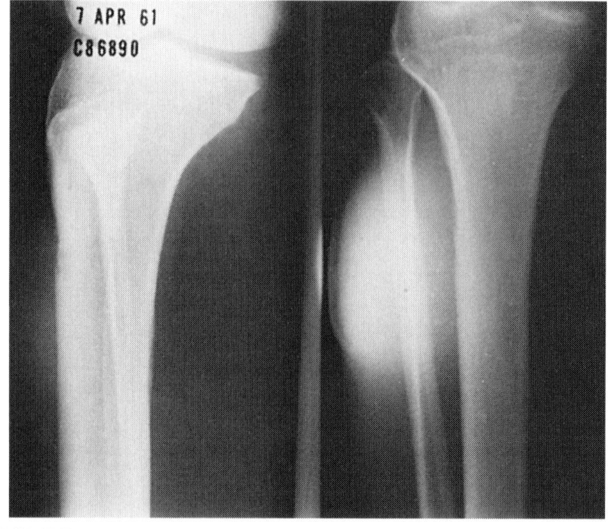


**FIGURE 15–6.** Radiograph showing a malignant fibrous histiocytoma of the lower leg (same case as in Figure 15–5). Ill-defined soft tissue mass has eroded a portion of the tibial cortex.

## Clinical Findings

The clinical features of the various subtypes are similar and are considered together. Malignant fibrous histiocytoma is characteristically a tumor of late adult life, with most cases occurring in persons between the ages of 50 and 70 years.[128] Tumors in children with the same histologic features as the adult forms of malignant fibrous histiocytoma are rare, and this diagnosis should always be made with caution in patients under 20 years of age. Approximately two-thirds of malignant fibrous histiocytomas occur in men, and Whites are affected more often than Blacks or Asians. The tumor occurs most frequently on the lower extremity (Figs. 15–5, 15–6), especially the thigh, followed by the upper extremity and retroperitoneum (Fig. 15–7). A notable exception is inflammatory malignant fibrous histiocytoma, which is most often located in the retroperitoneum; relatively few are found in the extremities.

When on an extremity, the tumor presents as a painless, enlarging mass usually of several months' duration. The duration is greatly influenced by the

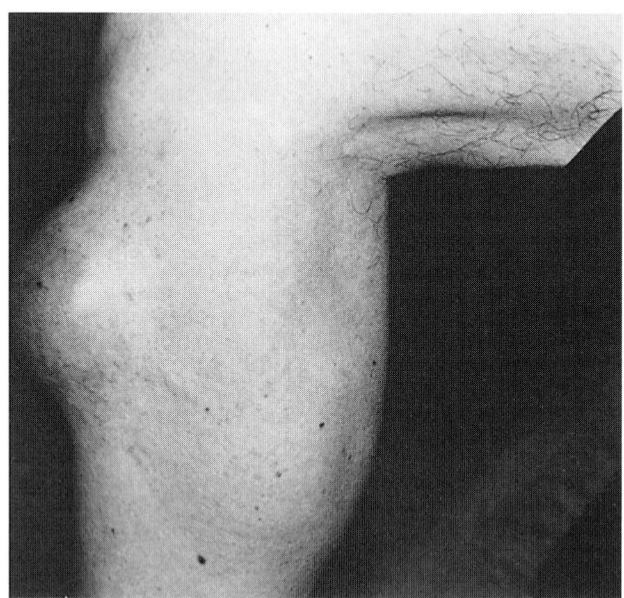

**FIGURE 15–5.** Malignant fibrous histiocytoma of the lower leg of a 62-year-old man. (From Guccion JG, Enzinger FM. Malignant giant cell tumor of soft parts: an analysis of 32 cases. Cancer 29:1518, 1972.)

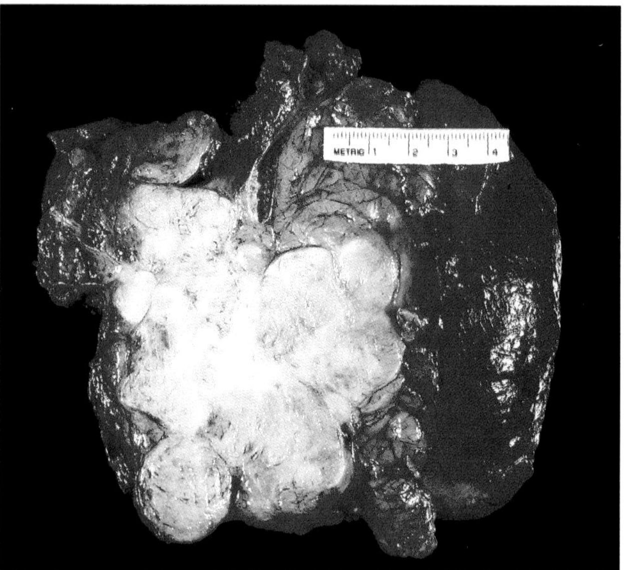


**FIGURE 15–7.** Gross appearance of a malignant fibrous histiocytoma of the retroperitoneum. The tumor is a multinodular white mass arising adjacent to the tumor.

growth rate. For instance, we have seen several slowly growing myxoid tumors for which 2 years or more have elapsed before the patient sought medical attention.[129] Rapid acceleration of the growth rate prompts the patient to seek medical attention quickly. As with other sarcomas, growth rate acceleration has been observed during pregnancy.[128] In contrast to patients with lesions of the extremity, patients with retroperitoneal tumors develop constitutional symptoms including anorexia, malaise, weight loss, and signs of increasing abdominal pressure.[128]

Occasionally, fever and leukocytosis with neutrophilia or eosinophilia dominate the clinical presentation of this disease. This unusual constellation of symptoms has been documented for the inflammatory type of malignant fibrous histiocytoma,[79] although rarely it occurs with the other subtypes.[53] These paraneoplastic signs and symptoms appear to be the result of tumor-related production of cytokines,[60] which have included interleukins (IL-6, IL-8)[53] and tumor necrosis factor. The symptoms usually remit following removal of the tumor. Rarely, hypoglycemia occurs in association with this disease.[79,128] The mechanism of this abnormality is not clearly defined, but in one of our cases there was some evidence of secretion of an insulin-like substance by the tumor.[128] Malignant fibrous histiocytoma rarely presents as a metastatic tumor without a clinically evident primary lesion,[128] although a small percentage of patients present with synchronous primary and metastatic disease.[111] A number of cytogenetic abnormalities have been identified in malignant fibrous histiocytomas.[35,38,82,89,92,104,112] Emerging evidence suggests that certain chromosomes appear to be structurally rearranged more consistently than others in this disease.

## Etiologic Factors

Like atypical fibroxanthomas, there is excellent circumstantial evidence that some of these tumors are radiation-induced. We have seen malignant fibrous histiocytomas following irradiation of breast carcinoma, retinoblastoma, Hodgkin's disease, and multiple myeloma.[128] In each instance malignant fibrous histiocytoma occurred in the irradiated area after an appropriately long interval of several years. Similar reports have been mentioned in the literature.[29] In fact, it seems likely that some postirradiation pleomorphic sarcomas are actually malignant fibrous histiocytomas. Aside from these sporadic iatrogenic tumors, there are few data on etiologic factors for this disease. About 10% of patients with malignant fibrous histiocytoma have had or subsequently develop a second neoplasm. This does not seem statistically meaningful in view of the generally older age of these patients and the accepted risk of a second neoplasm complicating the course of a first. Several malignant fibrous histiocytomas have occurred in patients exposed to phenoxy acids, although a direct causal relation has not been established.[46] The tumor has also been reported in a patient with Lynch II syndrome.[36] The tumor has been induced in experimental animals with tea extracts[68] and with macrophages transformed with SV40 virus.[132] Intraosseous malignant fibrous histiocytomas have occurred in preexisting bone infarcts[96,99,100] and at the site of shrapnel injury.[87]

## Gross Findings

Typically, the lesions are solitary, multilobulated, fleshy masses 5–10 cm in diameter when first detected (Fig. 15–7), although retroperitoneal lesions are much larger than lesions in the extremities.[106] About two-thirds of these tumors are located in skeletal muscle, and fewer than 10% are confined to the subcutis. Tumors located adjacent to bone may induce mild degrees of periosteal reaction or cortical erosion, which can be detected radiographically. Although malignant fibrous histiocytoma has a circumscribed appearance grossly, it often spreads for a considerable distance along fascial planes (Fig. 15–8) or between muscle fibers microscopically, which accounts for its high rate of local recurrence.

On cut section most tumors are gray to white (Fig. 15–9), but this pattern may be modified by an abundance of one or more elements. For example, the inflammatory form of malignant fibrous histiocytoma (*malignant xanthogranuloma, xanthosarcoma*) may have a yellow hue because of the predominance of xanthoma cells (see Fig. 15–33, below), whereas hemorrhagic tumors appear brown. Myxoid malignant fibrous histiocytoma typically has a translucent mucoid appearance (see Fig. 15–20, below) and in this respect cannot be distinguished grossly from other myxoid sarcomas, such as myxoid liposarcoma. In contrast to less aggressive fibrohistiocytic tumors, hemorrhage and necrosis are common features of this tumor. In fact about 5% of malignant fibrous histiocytomas undergo such extensive hemorrhage that they present clinically as fluctuant masses and are diagnosed as cystic hematomas.[128] Nonetheless, residual tumor cells can be identified microscopically in the wall of such "cysts," leaving no doubt as to the correct diagnosis.

## Malignant Fibrous Histiocytoma: Storiform-pleomorphic Type

Microscopically, the storiform-pleomorphic form of malignant fibrous histiocytoma has a highly variable morphologic pattern[128] and shows frequent transitions

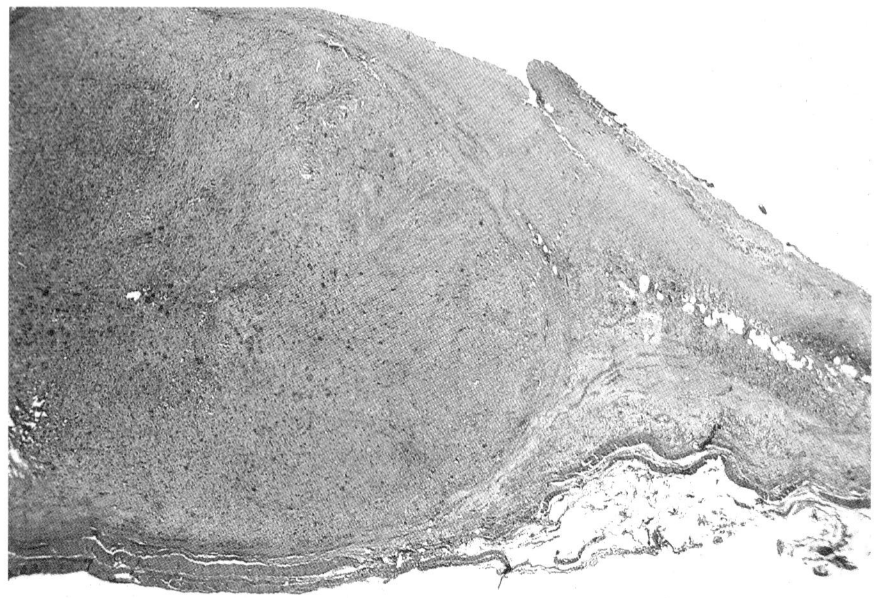

**FIGURE 15–8.** Malignant fibrous histiocytoma arising in and extending along superficial fascia.

from storiform to pleomorphic areas (Figs. 15–10 to 15–17). In its classic form the tumor consists of plump spindle cells arranged in short fascicles in a cartwheel, or storiform, pattern around slit-like vessels. The spindle cells are well differentiated and resemble fibroblasts. Although such tumors resemble dermatofibrosarcoma protuberans, they differ by a less distinctive storiform pattern and by the presence of occasional plump histiocytic cells, numerous typical and atypical mitotic figures, and secondary elements including xanthoma cells and modest numbers of chronic inflammatory cells. Although this pattern of malignant fibrous histiocytoma is easily recognized, it is seldom seen throughout the entire tumor.

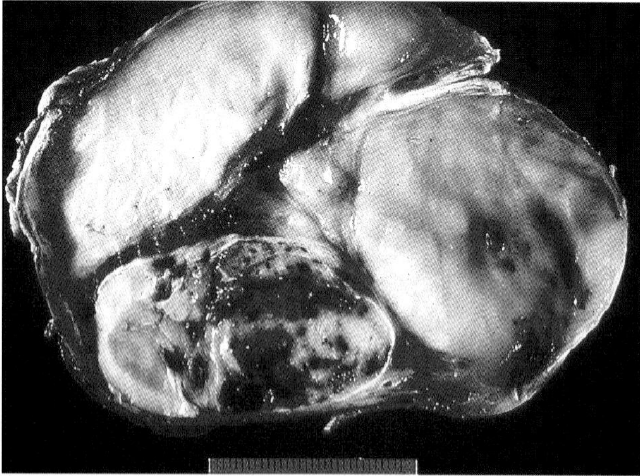

**FIGURE 15–9.** Typical gross appearance of a malignant fibrous histiocytoma showing a multinodular white mass with areas of hemorrhage and necrosis.

Instead, most tumors have a combination of storiform and pleomorphic areas, with an emphasis on the latter. Least often tumors have a fascicular growth pattern and resemble fibrosarcomas, except for scattered giant cells. In contrast to the storiform areas, pleomorphic areas contain plumper fibroblastic cells and more round histiocytic cells arranged haphazardly with no particular orientation to vessels. Pleomorphism and mitotic activity are usually more prominent. A characteristic feature of these areas is the presence of large numbers of giant cells with multiple hyperchromatic irregular nuclei. The intense eosinophilia of these giant cells often suggests cells with myoblastic differentiation (Fig. 15–14), but they consistently lack myofibrils, as demonstrated by special stains. Although small droplets of neutral fat and PAS-positive, diastase-resistant droplets may be seen in mononuclear cells in this tumor, they are especially prominent in the giant cells and probably reflect degenerative changes.

The stroma and secondary elements vary considerably in the storiform and pleomorphic areas. Usually the stroma consists of delicate collagen fibrils encircling individual cells. Occasionally, the collagenization becomes marked and widely separates cells. Focal myxoid change is also a common phenomenon and consists of localized collections of hyaluronidase-sensitive acid mucopolysaccharide (Fig. 15–13). When this change becomes especially prominent, the tumors are classified as myxoid variants of malignant fibrous histiocytoma. Rarely, the stroma contains metaplastic osteoid or chondroid. We have even seen one case in which mature lamellar bone with marrow elements was present in a pleomorphic malignant fibrous histiocytoma.

*Text continued on page 547*

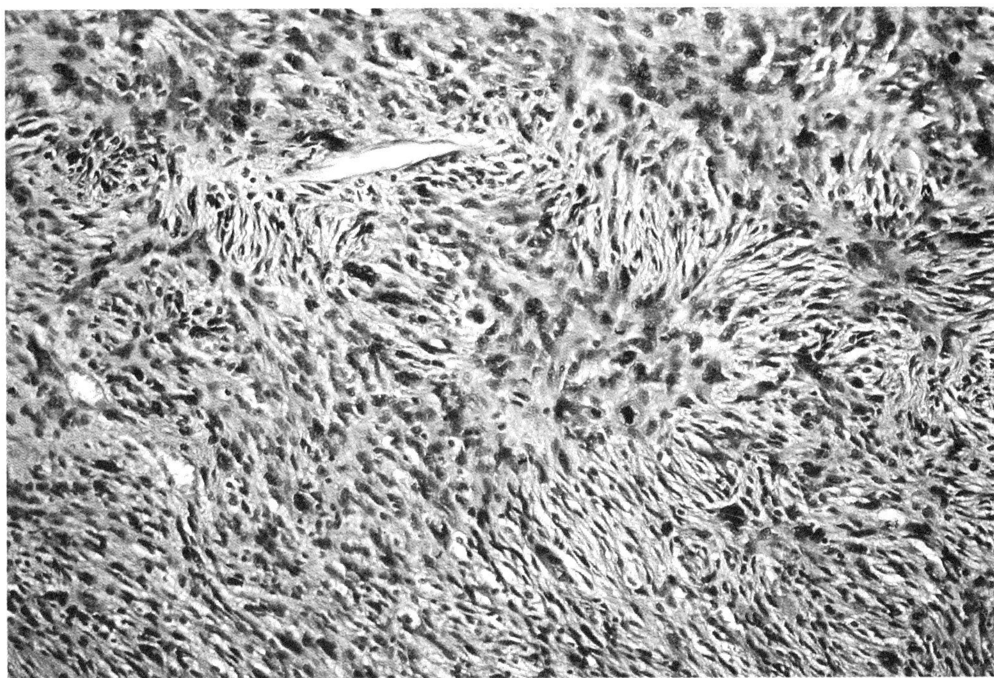

**FIGURE 15–10.** Malignant fibrous histiocytoma, storiform-pleomorphic type, with a predominantly storiform pattern. Tumors may resemble dermatofibrosarcoma at low power but are distinguished from them by the greater degree of nuclear atypia and mitotic activity.

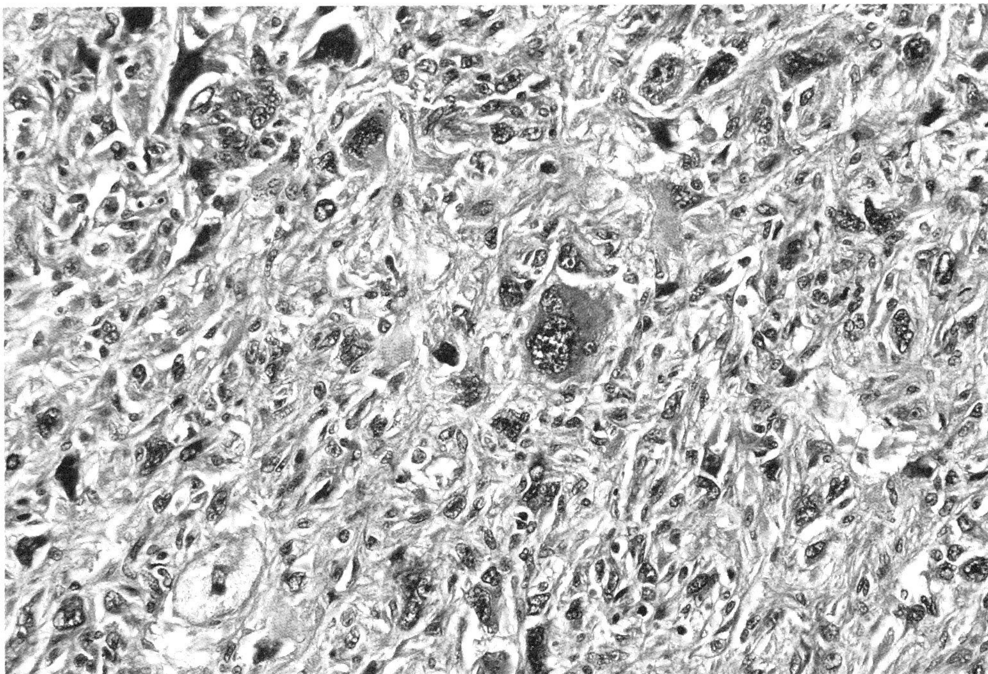

**FIGURE 15–11.** Malignant fibrous histiocytoma, storiform-pleomorphic type, with a pleomorphic pattern. Anaplastic tumor cells are arranged haphazardly in sheets.

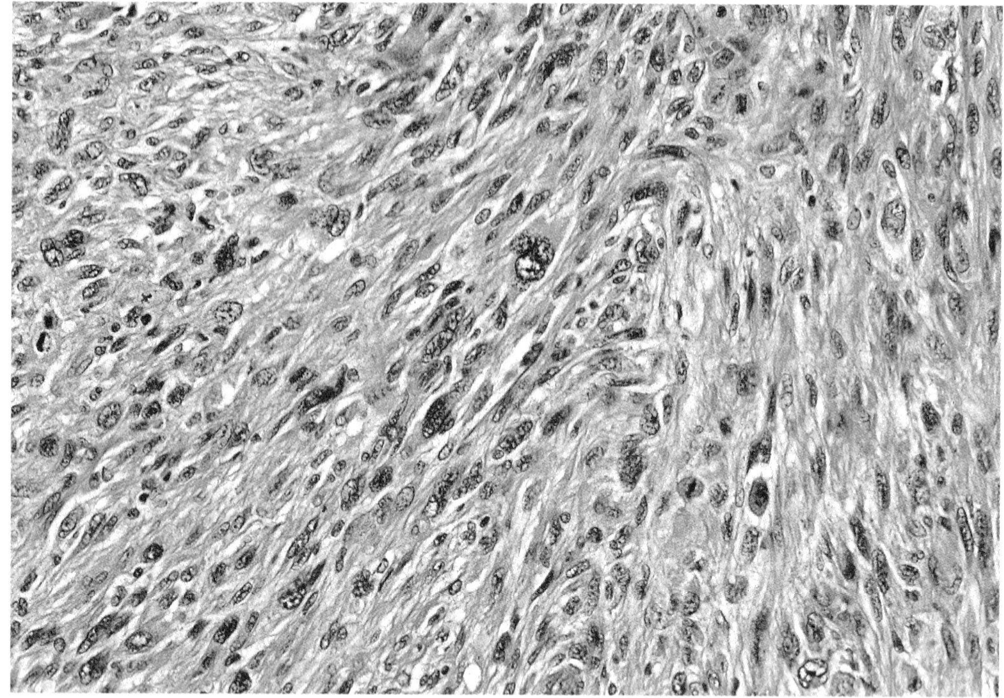

**FIGURE 15–12.** Malignant fibrous histiocytoma, storiform-pleomorphic type, with a predominantly fascicular pattern. Tumors of this type are classified by some as pleomorphic (high grade) fibrosarcomas.

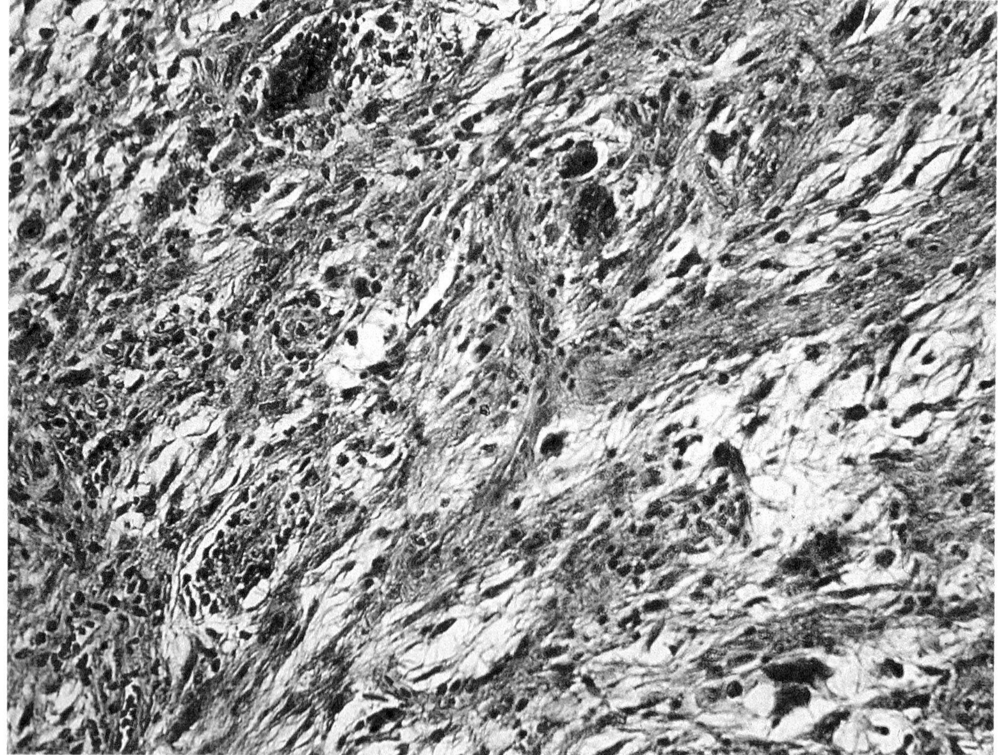

**FIGURE 15–13.** Malignant fibrous histiocytoma, storiform-pleomorphic type, with focal (microscopic) areas of myxoid change. Myxoid forms of malignant fibrous histiocytoma, in contrast, should have a predominantly (>50%) myxoid pattern.

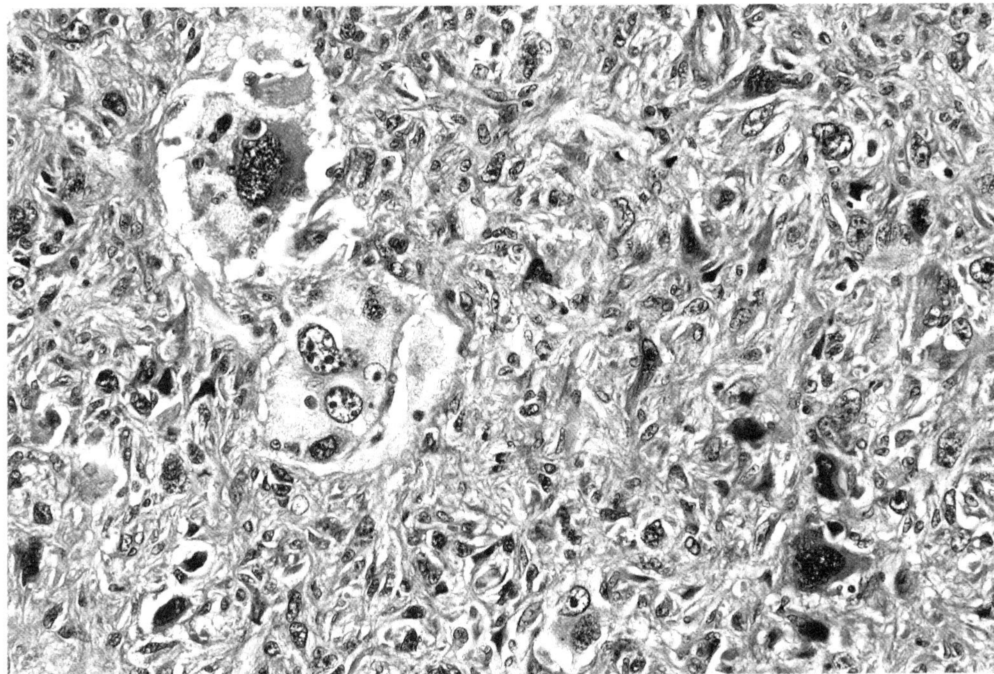

**FIGURE 15–14.** Cells in a malignant fibrous histiocytoma are characterized by an extreme degree of pleomorphism and occasional multinucleation. Bizarre cells may vary from deeply eosinophilic to xanthomatous. In the past, pleomorphic eosinophilic cells in these tumors were confused with rhabdomyoblasts, and the lesions were regarded as pleomorphic rhabdomyosarcomas.

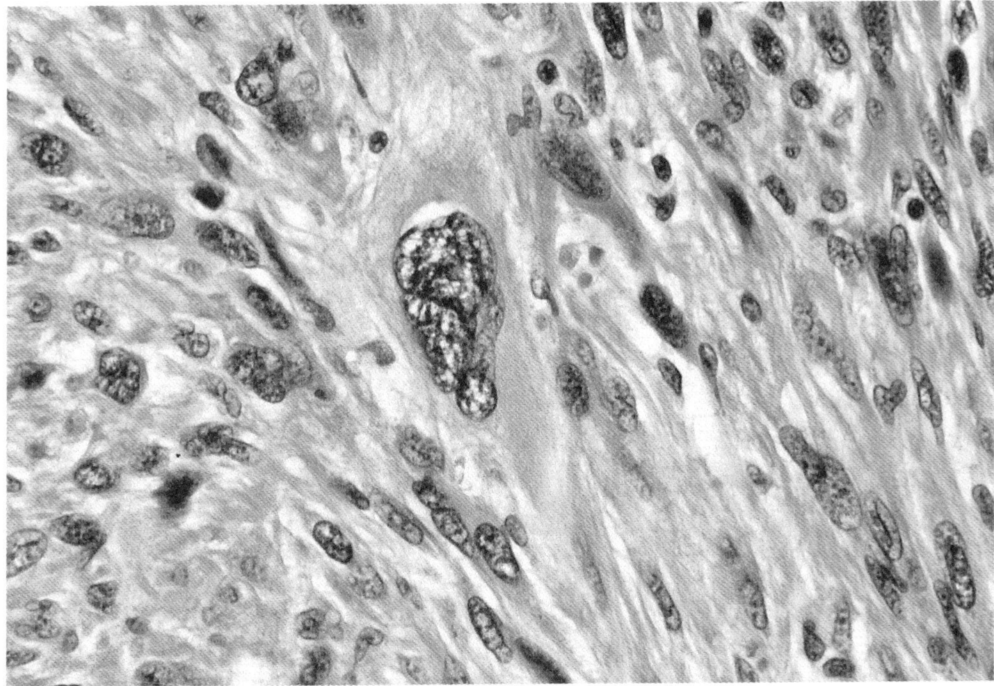

**FIGURE 15–15.** Bizarre spindled cells in a malignant fibrous histiocytoma.

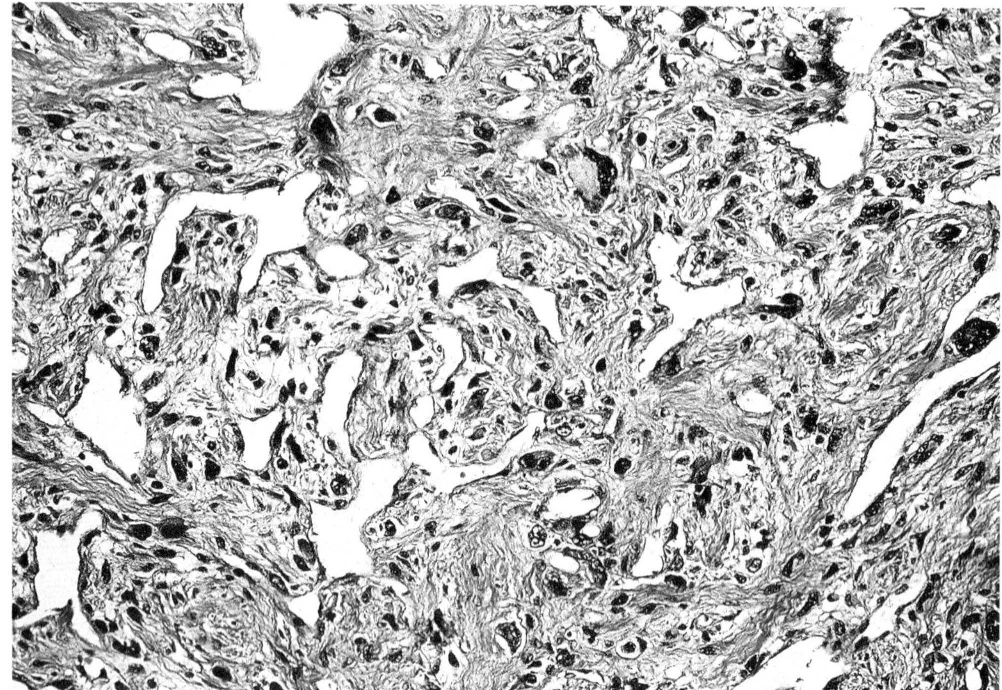

**FIGURE 15–16.** Hemangiopericytoma-like vascular pattern in a malignant fibrous histiocytoma.

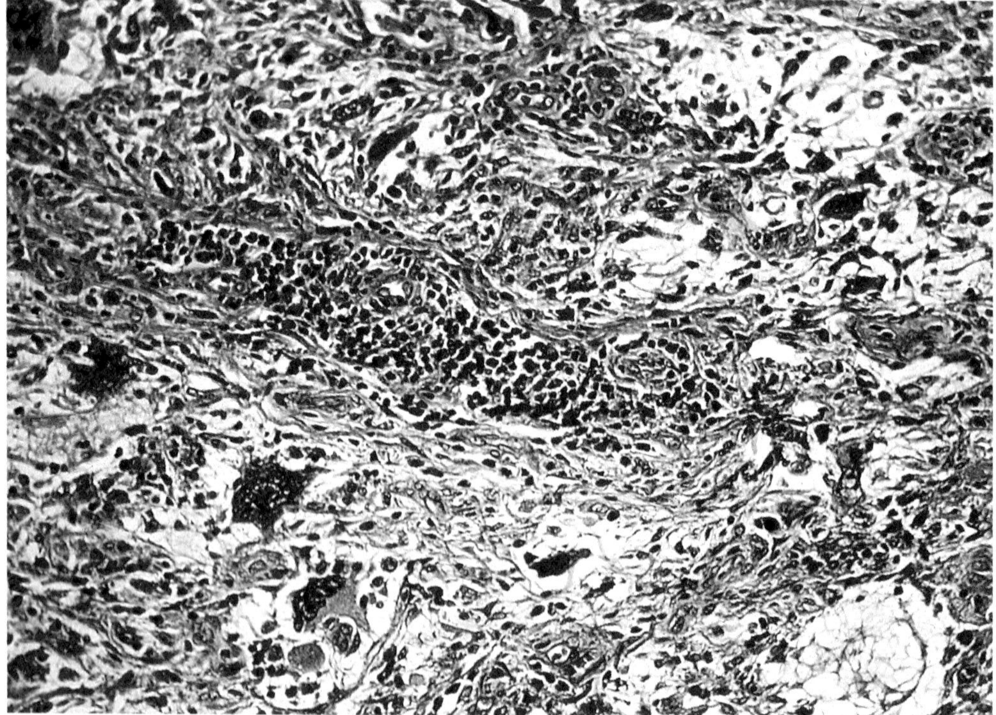

**FIGURE 15–17.** Malignant fibrous histiocytoma with a focally dense lymphocytic infiltrate. Chronic inflammation is a common feature in many malignant fibrous histiocytomas.

The vasculature, although elaborate, is seldom appreciated with routine hematoxylin-eosin staining. Sometimes the vessels become dilated, and the close apposition of the tumor cells to their walls simulate the pattern of hemangiopericytoma (Fig. 15–16).

Modest numbers of lymphocytes or plasma cells characterize most of these tumors. In about one-fifth of them, inflammatory cells are numerous, usually with a predominance of acute or chronic inflammatory cells rather than equal mixtures of the two. The inflammatory cells are scattered throughout the tumor, with some predilection for the periphery of the lesion and the immediate perivascular zones (Fig. 15–17). Occasionally the intermingling of bizarre histiocytic cells and lymphocytes at the periphery closely simulate lymphoma, particularly Hodgkin's disease. The significance and mechanism of a prominent inflammatory component in these tumors is not clear but possibly relates to cytokine production by the tumor cells.

Metastatic deposits from malignant fibrous histiocytoma involve organs in a nodular fashion. In rare instances metastatic lesions to lymph nodes are diffuse and consist of nests of cells scattered throughout a lymph node, thereby resembling lymphoma. However, usually adjacent nodes can be found with the more typical solid pattern of involvement. Metastatic lesions in general resemble the original tumor, although they are less likely to manifest a storiform pattern.

## Immunohistochemical Findings

The role of immunohistochemistry in the diagnosis of malignant fibrous histiocytoma has traditionally been an ancillary one, primarily serving as a means to exclude other pleomorphic tumors such as anaplastic carcinoma and sarcoma, which may bear a resemblance to malignant fibrous histiocytoma. Thus the diagnosis of malignant fibrous histiocytoma continues to presuppose excellent sampling and evaluation of hematoxylin-eosin stained sections. Despite the limited diagnostic applications of immunohistochemistry, they have provided ample evidence that these tumors are not derived from cells of monocyte or macrophage lineage[34,110,130] but, rather, from fibroblasts. Although several workers earlier suggested that the presence of two histiocytic enzymes $\alpha_1$-antitrypsin and $\alpha_1$-antichymotrypsin, in these tumors supported their histiocytic origin,[76,101] it has been shown that these enzymes are present inconsistently and that they may be present in sarcomas of diverse types and carcinomas, possibly as a result of endocytosis from plasma.[37,43,110] More reliable histiocytic markers such as Leu-3 and Leu-M3 have not been identified in these tumors.[130] Likewise, CD68, a panhistiocytic marker detected by the monoclonal antibody KP-1, cannot be identified in these tumors in our experience, despite one report to the contrary.[32] Moreover, cells of malignant fibrous histiocytoma do not express CD45.[130] Although malignant fibrous histiocytomas express HLA-DR, a major histocompatibility antigen present on most histiocytes, this substance is not specific for histiocytes and is also present on endothelial cells and on certain stimulated fibroblasts.[130] Fibroblast-associated antigens can be identified on the surface of the cells,[61,130] whereas laminin is detected in the cytoplasm.[115] Mutant *p53* is detected immunohistochemically in about 30% of cases, although the significance of this finding in terms of prognosis is not clear.[116]

With the widespread use of monoclonal antibodies, a number of interesting questions have been raised regarding the diagnostic criteria for this neoplasm. It has been repeatedly observed that tumors that qualify by light microscopy as malignant fibrous histiocytomas may express a number of intermediate filaments such as keratin, desmin, and neurofilament protein.[57,84,88,97,108,109] Under these circumstances the immunoreactivity is usually focal. Initially, such findings were dismissed as technical artifacts or unusual patterns of cross-reactivity. It is clear, however, that true expression of some intermediate filaments, specifically keratin, occurs in the malignant fibrous histiocytoma,[108,127] and that the incidence of this immunoreactivity increases as the sensitivity of the method is enhanced.[88] This has been confirmed by immunoblotting studies and by the fact that immunostaining can be reproduced on a given tumor by a number of antibody preparations. Moreover, recognition that normal mesenchymal cells may express certain types of keratin seems to have paved the way toward a growing acceptance that their neoplastic counterparts may also do so. The issue then becomes whether minor patterns of immunoreactivity in an otherwise typical malignant fibrous histiocytoma should be considered sufficient evidence of specific differentiation and, accordingly, alter the diagnosis. We have adopted the approach that focal immunostaining for substances such as keratin and desmin in otherwise typical malignant fibrous histiocytomas is not sufficient in itself to alter the diagnosis but should be corroborated by other light microscopic or ultrastructural features. On the other hand, diffuse, intense immunoreactivity for one of these antigens is more likely reflective of specific differentiation. For example, rare desmin-positive cells in a malignant fibrous histiocytoma can probably be ascribed to focal myofibroblastic differentiation, whereas large areas of desmin immunoreactivity are more likely indicative of pleomorphic rhabdomyosarcoma or leiomyosarcoma masquerading as malignant fibrous histiocytoma. In ambiguous situations, one can take solace in the fact that the choice between two or more forms of pleomorphic sarcoma is an academic one and does not, in current therapy protocols, usually alter the fundamental approach to the patient. Obviously, however, the distinction between anaplastic carcinoma and pleomorphic sarcoma is usually a therapeutically important distinction that materially affects the management of the patient.

## Ultrastructural Findings

With widespread use of immunohistochemistry, electron microscopic studies have assumed a diminished role in the diagnosis of malignant fibrous histiocytoma. It should be regarded as a confirmatory procedure that is best applied when the differential diagnosis has been narrowed by light microscopy. The limited role of electron microscopy reflects the fact that no ultrastructural features are ultimately specific for malignant fibrous histiocytoma, and cells with similar characteristics can be found in other tumors.[55,56,80,81] Thus electron microscopy is used principally to establish the absence of certain organelles that would indicate a higher order of differentiation. Three cell types can be identified in the tumors[27,49,59,64,122]: 1) a fibroblastic cell with elongated nuclei, prominent nucleoli, and abundant lamellae of rough endoplasmic reticulum (Fig. 15–18).[1,49,121] Some of these fibroblastic cells have nuclear clefting and contain wispy actin-like filaments underneath the cytoplasmic membrane[39]; they resemble "myofibroblasts" seen in a variety of conditions. 2) round cells, resembling "histiocytes," contain oval or lobated nuclei, cytoplasmic processes, a prominent Golgi zone, and numerous lysosomes, phagosomes, and lipid droplets (Fig. 15–19).[1,49,121] Langerhans' granules, structures present in certain alleged histiocytic tumors, are almost always absent. Occasionally, filamentous material is present in a perinuclear location. 3) Primitive mesenchymal cells with a narrow rim of cytoplasm largely devoid of organelles except for free ribosomes are present in small numbers.[1,49]

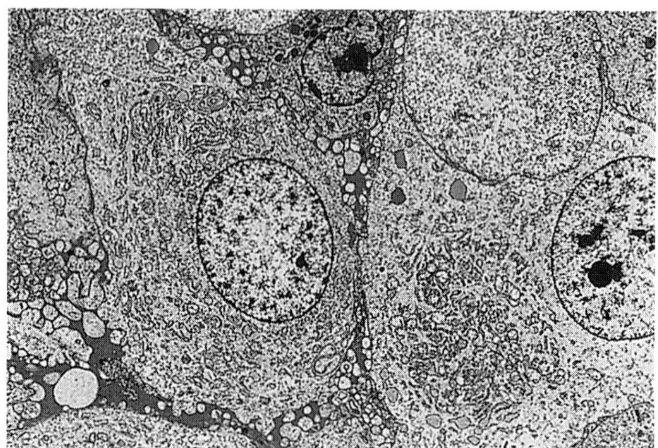

**FIGURE 15–19.** Electron micrograph of malignant cells with histiocyte-like features. They contain numerous phagolysosomes in the cytoplasm. (×6300) (Courtesy of Dr. Bruce Mackay, M.D. Anderson Cancer Hospital.)

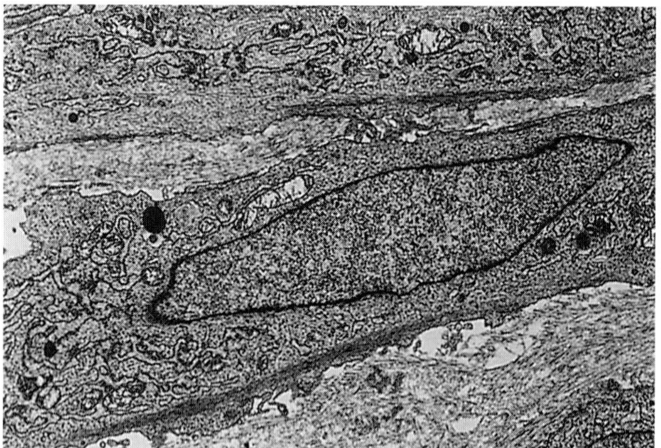

**FIGURE 15–18.** Electron micrograph showing fibroblast-like cells comprising a malignant fibrous histiocytoma. Cells are elongated with numerous profiles of rough endoplasmic reticulum. Actin-like filaments are often clustered underneath the cytoplasmic membrane. (×17,000) (Courtesy of Dr. Bruce Mackay, M.D. Anderson Cancer Hospital.)

## Differential Diagnosis

The most common and difficult problem in the differential diagnosis is distinguishing this form of malignant fibrous histiocytoma from other malignant neoplasms with a comparable degree of cellular pleomorphism. Pleomorphic liposarcoma, in particular, may have areas that closely simulate malignant fibrous histiocytoma. It usually lacks a distinct whorled or storiform pattern, contains less stromal collagen, and most importantly shows evidence of specific cellular differentiation (i.e., lipoblasts of typical form and structure). Intracellular fat in varying amounts is generally present in both tumors, but the lipid in malignant fibrous histiocytoma is more finely dispersed or irregularly distributed; and as a rule it does not displace or indent the nucleus as in typical lipoblasts. Intracellular lipid, of course, may also be encountered in various other mesenchymal neoplasms, especially in areas of cellular degeneration and at the margin of the tumor where it has infiltrated the surrounding normal fat. Only rarely have we encountered sarcomas with areas of "dedifferentiation" that exactly mimic malignant fibrous histiocytomas. Such tumors have included liposarcoma, extraosseous osteosarcoma, chondrosarcoma, malignant schwannoma, and leiomyosarcoma. By convention, however, we have classified such tumors by the area showing the more specific form of differentiation.

Distinction from pleomorphic rhabdomyosarcoma may also cause difficulty. Traditionally, the deeply eosinophilic giant cells of malignant fibrous histiocytoma were thought to be rhabdomyoblasts; consequently, many malignant fibrous histiocytomas were classified and reported as pleomorphic rhabdomyosarcoma. In our experience, pleomorphic rhabdomyosarcoma is rare in adult patients, and most tumors so diagnosed are actually malignant fibrous histiocytomas. In contrast to malignant fibrous histiocytoma, pleomorphic rhabdomyosarcoma usually is composed of cells that have more uniformly and deeply eosinophilic cytoplasm, display more cell-to-cell molding, and usually have less interstitial collagenization. The presence of longitudinal striations in some of these cells is not sufficient evidence of rhabdomyoblastic differentiation. By electron microscopy, longitudinal striations correspond to cells containing actin-like filaments, organelles now known to be present in a variety of neoplastic mesenchymal and epithelial cells. Therefore the diagnosis of adult or pleomorphic rhabdomyosarcoma should be restricted to those rare sarcomas with cross-striations by light microscopy, typical thin (6–8 nm) and thick (12–15 nm) filaments or Z-band material ultrastructurally, or specific muscle protein (e.g., MyoD1, myogenin) detected by immunohistochemistry. As mentioned above, however, focal or weak desmin immunoreactivity is probably not sufficient by itself to warrant a diagnosis of myosarcoma, as myofibroblasts may express this antigen, and occasional sarcomas of diverse type express the antigen anomalously.

Distinction between malignant fibrous histiocytoma and pleomorphic carcinoma may also pose a problem for the pathologist. This is especially true for pleomorphic forms of malignant fibrous histiocytoma composed chiefly of haphazardly arranged round or polygonal cells without a storiform pattern. Such pleomorphic tumors, therefore, when occurring in visceral organs or in patients known to have an epithelial malignancy, should be carefully sampled for evidence of epithelial differentiation. Stains for mucin and glycogen and immunostains for cytokeratin may prove helpful. As noted above, keratin is expressed in a small percentage of malignant fibrous histiocytomas but almost invariably with focal, weak staining. Electron microscopy may also aid in the distinction by detecting minor degrees of epithelial differentiation not readily apparent by light microscopy, such as numerous large intercellular junctions or tonofibrils. For most malignant fibrous histiocytomas distinction from benign fibrous histiocytoma or dermatofibrosarcoma protuberans is not difficult because the latter two usually have conspicuous storiform patterns and lack pleomorphic cells and necrosis. Occasional tumors have borderline histologic features. As pointed out in Chapter 13, when such lesions are large and deeply situated they should be regarded as potentially malignant. Likewise, the distinction between malignant fibrous histiocytoma and atypical fibroxanthoma is principally one of size and clinical extent, as discussed earlier in the chapter.

Rarely, malignant fibrous histiocytoma resembles Hodgkin's disease. This resemblance occurs most often with tumors in which histiocyte-like cells intermingle with chronic inflammatory cells. The extranodal location and finding cohesive groups of spindle cells usually aid in the distinction. In exceptional instances when metastatic malignant fibrous histiocytoma involves a lymph node diffusely, the resemblance to Hodgkin's disease may be so striking that histologic distinction is not possible without employing immunostains for markers such as Leu-M1, which identifies Reed-Sternberg cells but not cells of a malignant fibrous histiocytoma. Because malignant fibrous histiocytoma rarely presents as lymphadenopathy without a known primary soft tissue mass, clinical information is helpful.

## Discussion

Since the original description of malignant fibrous histiocytoma during the early 1960s, there has been a gradual, diametric change in our views of this tumor. It is no longer believed to show histiocytic differentiation but, rather, fibroblastic differentiation; and it has come to represent the prototype of the high grade pleomorphic sarcoma of adult life. An emerging question, however, has been whether the tumor exists at all or represents a potpourri of various mesenchymal and nonmesenchymal tumors with certain superficial similarities.[41] To be sure, failure to examine a tumor fully may result in the inclusion of other lesions in this group.

Fletcher analyzed 159 cases that had been diagnosed as pleomorphic sarcoma over a more than 30-year period at his hospital and addressed this issue.[48] Only about 100 would qualify as malignant fibrous histiocytoma by current light microscopic criteria. Careful analysis of the entire group by means of extensive tissue sampling, immunohistochemistry, or electron microscopy indicated that 42 lesions would continue to meet the diagnostic criteria of malignant fibrous histiocytoma (in large part these criteria are defined as the absence of differentiation). Thus his study indicated that slightly fewer than half of cases that might be diagnosed by pathologists as malignant fibrous histiocytoma would continue to fulfill the criteria when studied extensively. This figure varies depending on the experience of the pathologist making

**TABLE 15–1** BEHAVIOR OF MALIGNANT FIBROUS HISTIOCYTOMA

| Study | No. of Patients | Local Recurrence (%) | Metastasis (%) | 5 Year Survival (%) |
|---|---|---|---|---|
| Salo et al.[114] | 239 | 19 | 35 | 65 |
| Le Doussal et al.[85] | 216 | 31 | 33 | 70 |
| Zagars et al.[133] | 271 | 21 | 31 | 68 |

the initial diagnosis. Based on this study and our own experience, we believe that the diagnosis continues to serve a useful purpose when identifying an undifferentiated pleomorphic sarcoma, although in time it may become intellectually more forthright to consider a change in nomenclature.

This tumor is a fully malignant sarcoma, although previous large retrospective studies indicating a local recurrence rate and metastatic rate of nearly 50% have been superceded by more recent studies from large cancer centers indicating far lower rates, probably because of more immediate efficacious therapy. In fact, recent studies from the same institution disclose an improvement in survival in this disease based on data derived from the three most recent and largest series from Memorial Sloan Kettering Cancer Center, M.D. Anderson Cancer Center, and the French Federation of Cancer Centers; the tumor has a local recurrence rate of 19–31%, a metastatic rate of 31–35%, and a 5-year survival of 65–70% (Table 15–1).[85,113,114] Both local recurrence and distant metastases develop within 12–24 months of diagnosis, with the common metastatic sites being lung (90%), bone (8%), and liver (1%). Regional lymph node metastasis, formerly believed to be common, is quite uncommon. In our series of 20 regional lymph node dissections or biopsies[128] seven samples (35%) contained tumor, but this figure is falsely high because it represents a preselected group of patients. The true incidence of regional lymph node metastases lies closer to 12%, the overall incidence of lymph node metastases in our series. Bertoni et al.[31] and Kearney et al.[72] reported the incidence of lymph node metastasis to be 4% and 17%, respectively.

The factors that seem to correlate consistently with metastasis, survival, or both are depth, tumor size, grade, and histologic subtype, although they are not necessarily independent variables. For example, size and depth appear to co-vary[114] because large tumors tend to be deep tumors, and highly myxoid forms of malignant fibrous histiocytoma tend to be smaller and more superficial than nonmyxoid forms (Table 15–2). The new staging system for soft tissue sarcomas takes into account size, grade, and depth, so it has become a useful means for predicting outcome[114] (Table 15–3).

There has been recent interest in correlating various cytogenetic abnormalities in malignant fibrous histiocytoma with clinical parameters.[38,82,89,92,95] More than 80% of malignant fibrous histiocytomas show gains affecting 1p31, 9q31, 5p14-pter, and 7q32 by comparative genomic hybridization. Gains at 7q32 are a predictor of a worse metastasis-free and overall survival in a multivariate analysis with tumor size and grade.[82] Because this chromosomal region is seldom amplified in other cancers, the authors have suggested that it represents a unique prognostic marker of malignant fibrous histiocytoma. There is some preliminary evidence that breakpoints and rearrangements of chromosome 19p correlate with an increased propensity for local recurrence, but the number of cases studied was small.[38] There have been sporadic studies relating aneuploidy,[107] nuclear shape factor,[30] and heat shock protein 27 (HSP-27)[123] to prognosis in malignant fibrous histiocytomas. Analysis of proliferating antigens in these tumors correlates with the mitotic rate and nuclear grade but does not provide prognostic information with respect to survival over and above the histologic grade.[134]

## Malignant Fibrous Histiocytoma: Myxoid Type

The myxoid type of malignant fibrous histiocytoma is characterized by myxoid areas in association with cellular areas indistinguishable from ordinary malignant fibrous histiocytoma (Figs. 15–20 to 15–24).[129] Al-

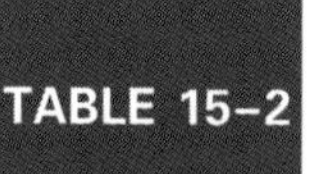
**TABLE 15–2** INDEPENDENT FAVORABLE PROGNOSTIC FACTORS WITH RESPECT TO DISEASE-SPECIFIC SURVIVAL IN MALIGNANT FIBROUS HISTIOCYTOMA

UICC/AJCC stage I or II
Freedom from gross disease following initial treatment
Superficial location
Myxoid subtype
Age <50 years

From Le Doussal V, Coindre J-M, Leroux A, et al. Prognostic factors for patients with localized primary malignant fibrous histiocytoma. Cancer 77: 1823, 1996, with permission.

**TABLE 15–3** DISEASE-SPECIFIC SURVIVAL FOR MALIGNANT FIBROUS HISTIOCYTOMA BY STAGE

| Stage | No. of Patients | Disease-specific Survival (%) | |
|---|---|---|---|
| | | *5 Years* | *10 Years* |
| Stage I | | | |
| Low grade (<5 cm) | 17 | 100 | 100 |
| Stage II | | | |
| Low grade (>5 cm deep) | 100 | 83 | 79 |
| Stage III | | | |
| High grade (5–10 cm deep) | 55 | 59 | 48 |
| High grade (>10 cm deep) | 59 | 34 | 31 |

From Salo JC, Lewis JJ, Woodruff JM, et al. Malignant fibrous histiocytoma of the extremity. Cancer 85:1765, 1999, with permission.

though the proportion of myxoid and cellular areas can vary in these tumors, at least half of the tumor should appear myxoid before it is designated a "myxoid variant."

The myxoid areas appear either as small foci blending with the adjacent cellular areas or as large areas abutting cellular areas with little transition (Fig. 15–22). In the extreme case an entire nodule of a tumor may appear myxoid and an adjacent nodule cellular. Qualitatively, the myxoid zones are similar to the cellular zones; they differ principally in their interstitial accumulation of hyaluronidase-sensitive acid mucopolysaccharide. As a result, the storiform pattern becomes less evident and the vasculature more prominent (Fig. 15–23A,B). The vessels typically form arcs along which tumor cells and inflammatory cells condense. Less often the vessels are extremely delicate and assume an intricate plexiform pattern similar to that of myxoid liposarcoma.

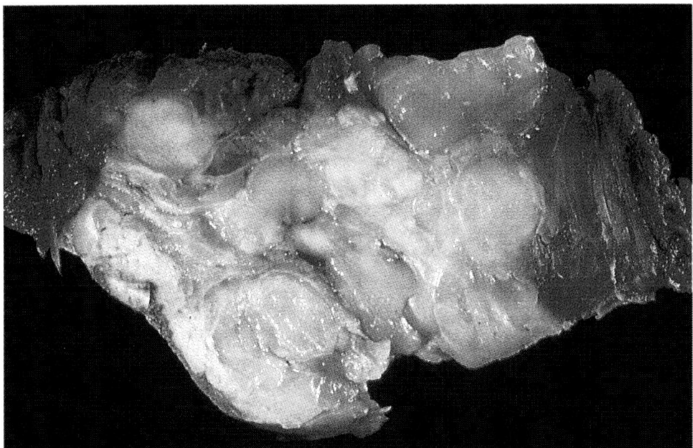

**FIGURE 15–20.** Gross specimen of myxoid malignant fibrous histiocytoma depicting the gelatinous appearance of several of the tumor nodules.

As in the cellular areas, the cells in the myxoid zones show a spectrum of differentiation, ranging from well differentiated fibroblasts to cells showing pleomorphism, mitotic activity, and multinucleation. Highly myxoid tumors with a predominance of the former cells may be bland enough to be confused with myxoma or nodular fasciitis (Fig. 15–23C,D). Such tumors have sometimes been designated myxofibrosarcoma.[77,93] Occasionally, cells in the myxoid zones contain coarse cytoplasmic vacuoles, thereby resembling lipoblasts (Fig. 15–24). However, unlike lipoblasts, these vacuoles contain acid mucin rather than neutral fat. There have been a number of ultrastructural studies of this tumor,[57,58,77,81,86,94] documenting cells with characteristics of fibroblasts[77] embedded in an electron-dense filamentous matrix (Fig. 15–25). The vacuolation of the cells is caused by dilatation of the endoplasmic reticulum and formation of "pseudocanaliculi" by delicate cytoplasmic processes.[80]

### *Differential Diagnosis*

The most important aspect of the differential diagnosis is the clear distinction of this lesion from benign myxoid lesions, such as nodular fasciitis and myxoma. Although nodular fasciitis may have focal myxoid change, it lacks the extensive orderly vasculature, bizarre cells, and atypical mitotic figures seen in myxoid malignant fibrous histiocytoma. Myxomas also lack the extensive vasculature of the malignant fibrous histiocytoma and usually have small cells with minimal atypia and few if any mitotic figures.

The sarcoma most nearly resembling this tumor is liposarcoma. Although myxoid liposarcoma resembles this tumor grossly, it consists of a more uniform population of small spindle cells embedded in a clear matrix with a delicate plexiform vasculature. Bizarre

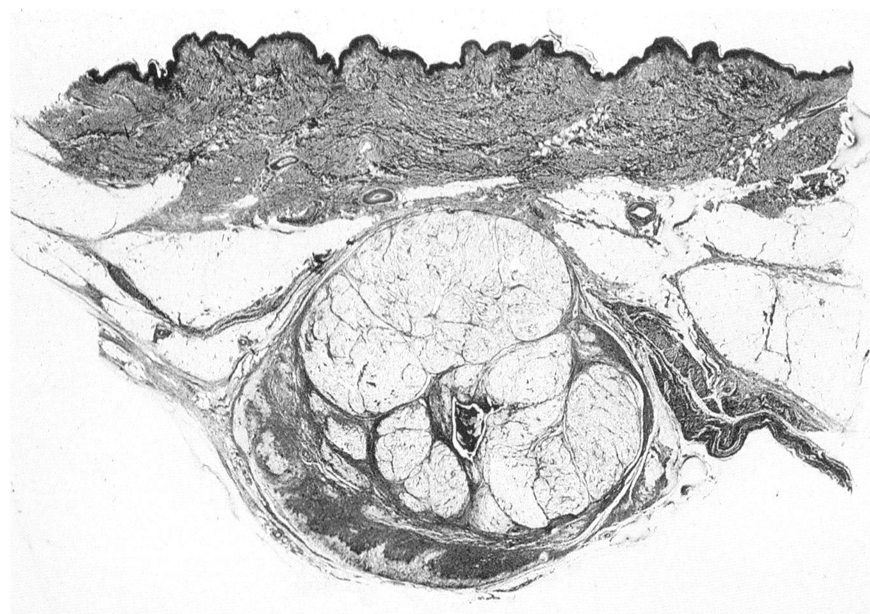

**FIGURE 15–21.** Low-power view of a superficial (subcutaneous) myxoid malignant fibrous histiocytoma. Most of the tumor is myxoid, but at the deep border there is a rim of typical (nonmyxoid) malignant fibrous histiocytoma.

cells are absent, and mitotic figures are infrequent. Lipoblasts are usually present. Pleomorphic liposarcoma, on the other hand, does have bizarre cells similar to myxoid malignant fibrous histiocytoma, but it has a cellular rather than a myxoid background, is more uniform in appearance, and contains lipoblasts.

### *Discussion*

The myxoid variant of malignant fibrous histiocytoma was proposed as a separate subgroup by us in 1976 because of its distinctive appearance and better prognosis compared with the storiform-pleomorphic type. By definition, this tumor is composed of cells that qualitatively resemble those of an ordinary malignant fibrous histiocytoma, implying that the cells have a moderate or marked degree of nuclear atypia. In addition, at least one-half of the tumor should be characterized by an abundant myxoid background. Defined in this fashion, the lesions can be shown to have a better prognosis than the ordinary forms of malignant fibrous histiocytoma.

This tumor recurs in almost two-thirds of cases but metastasizes in only about one-fourth. The indolent course of the tumor is, furthermore, underscored by the longer interval between the time of diagnosis and metastasis. Although in part the better prognosis is due to the fact that such lesions tend to segregate more often to the superficial soft tissues and to be smaller, it has been shown by multivariate analysis that the myxoid subtype is by itself an independent prognostic factor.

There has been a trend to popularize use of the term "myxofibrosarcoma" orginally used during the 1970s instead of "myxoid malignant fibrous histiocytoma" because of the belief that the lesions are fibroblastic rather than fibrohistiocytic. Unfortunately, the term "myxofibrosarcoma" has been employed by some to refer to a spectrum of myxoid sarcomas that range in appearance from low grade, myxoid-appearing fibrosarcomas to high grade storiform-pleomorphic malignant fibrous histiocytomas in which as little as 10% of the tumor displays a myxoid background.[93] Use of this term in an unqualified manner is of dubious clinical value, as it can refer to lesions that vary from grade I to grade III. Because all data derived from large studies indicating the improved outcome of myxoid forms of malignant fibrous histiocytoma use stringent criteria for diagnosis (a tumor > 50% myxoid), acceptance of loose diagnostic criteria inevitably erode the prognostic importance of this subtype and lead to general confusion regarding its behavior. For these reasons we have adopted the approach shown in Figure 15–26. Highly myxoid fibroblastic/fibrohistiocytic sarcomas (>50% myxoid) can be divided into two groups depending on the level of atypia. We refer to those with minimal atypia as "myxoid fibrosarcoma" or "myxofibrosarcoma," grade I (Fig. 15–27A), whereas those with signifcant atypia are designated myxoid malignant fibrous histiocytoma, grade II (Figs. 15–23A,B, 15–27B). Predominantly nonmyxoid lesions (<50% myxoid) are designated fibrosarcoma or malignant fibrous histiocytoma depending on the level of atypia and are graded accordingly. These lesions usually range in grade from II to III. Of course, an equally acceptable approach is to refer to all as "myxoid fibroblastic/fibrohistiocytic sarcomas" with an appended grade.

*Text continued on page 557*

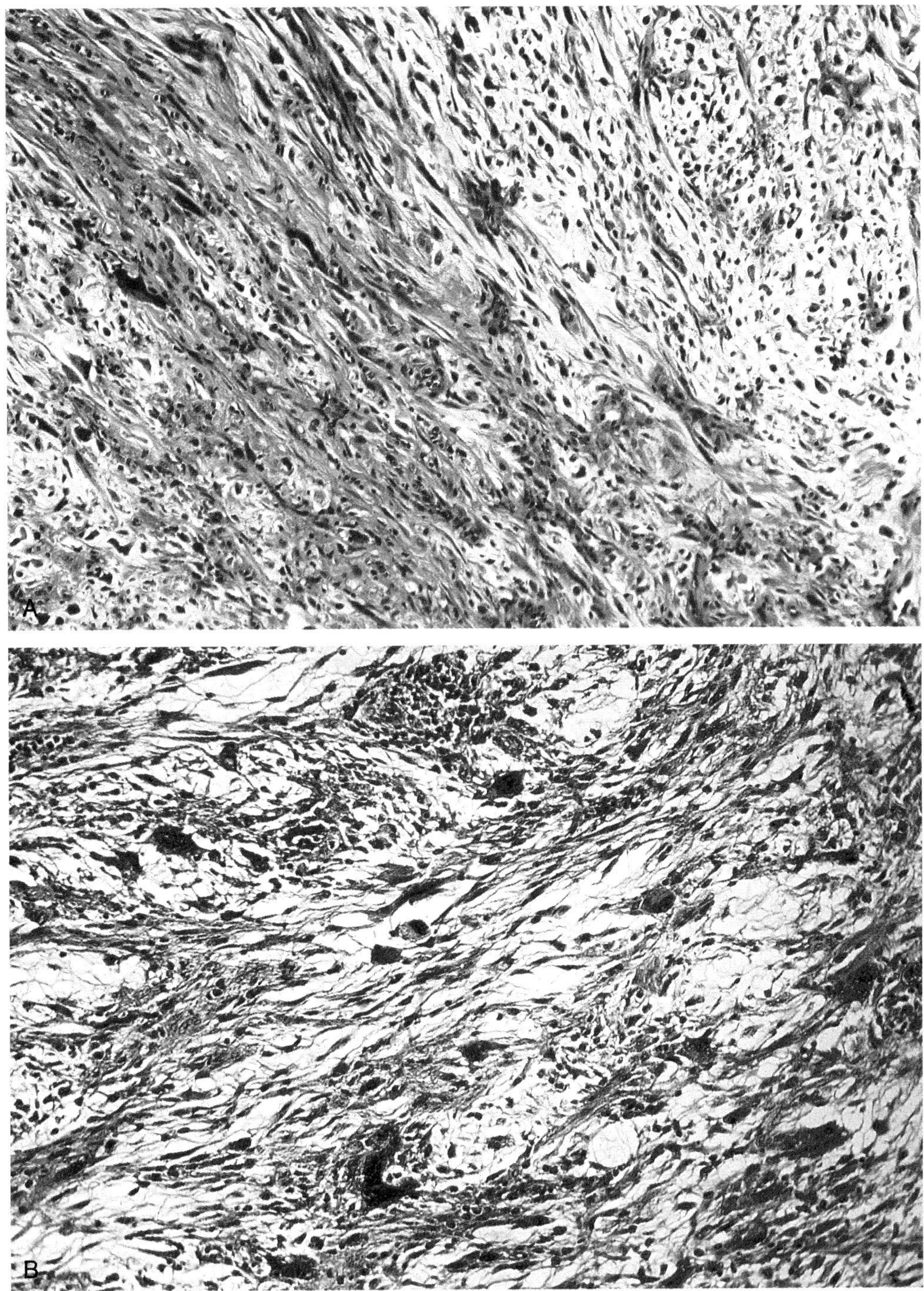


**FIGURE 15–22.** Broad myxoid zones may abut sharply on cellular areas (**A**) or may be scattered on small microscopic foci throughout the myxoid malignant fibrous histiocytoma (**B**).

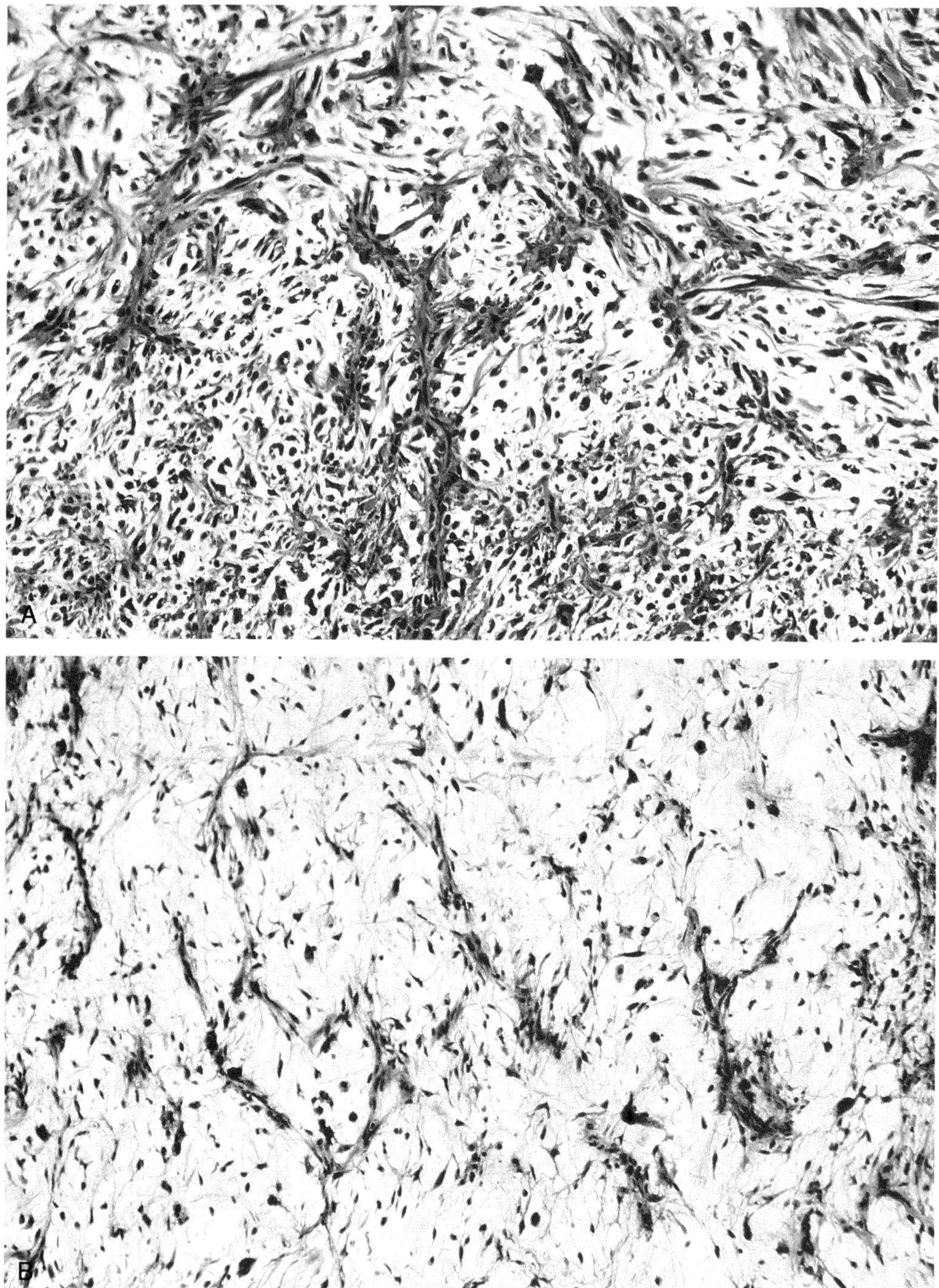

**FIGURE 15–23.** Range of cellularity that may be encountered in myxoid malignant fibrous histiocytoma/myxofibrosarcoma spectrum of lesions from most cellular (**A**) to least cellular (**D**). (**A, B**) Easily recognized pleomorphic lesions fall in the spectrum of malignant fibrous histiocytoma.

*Illustration continued on opposite page*

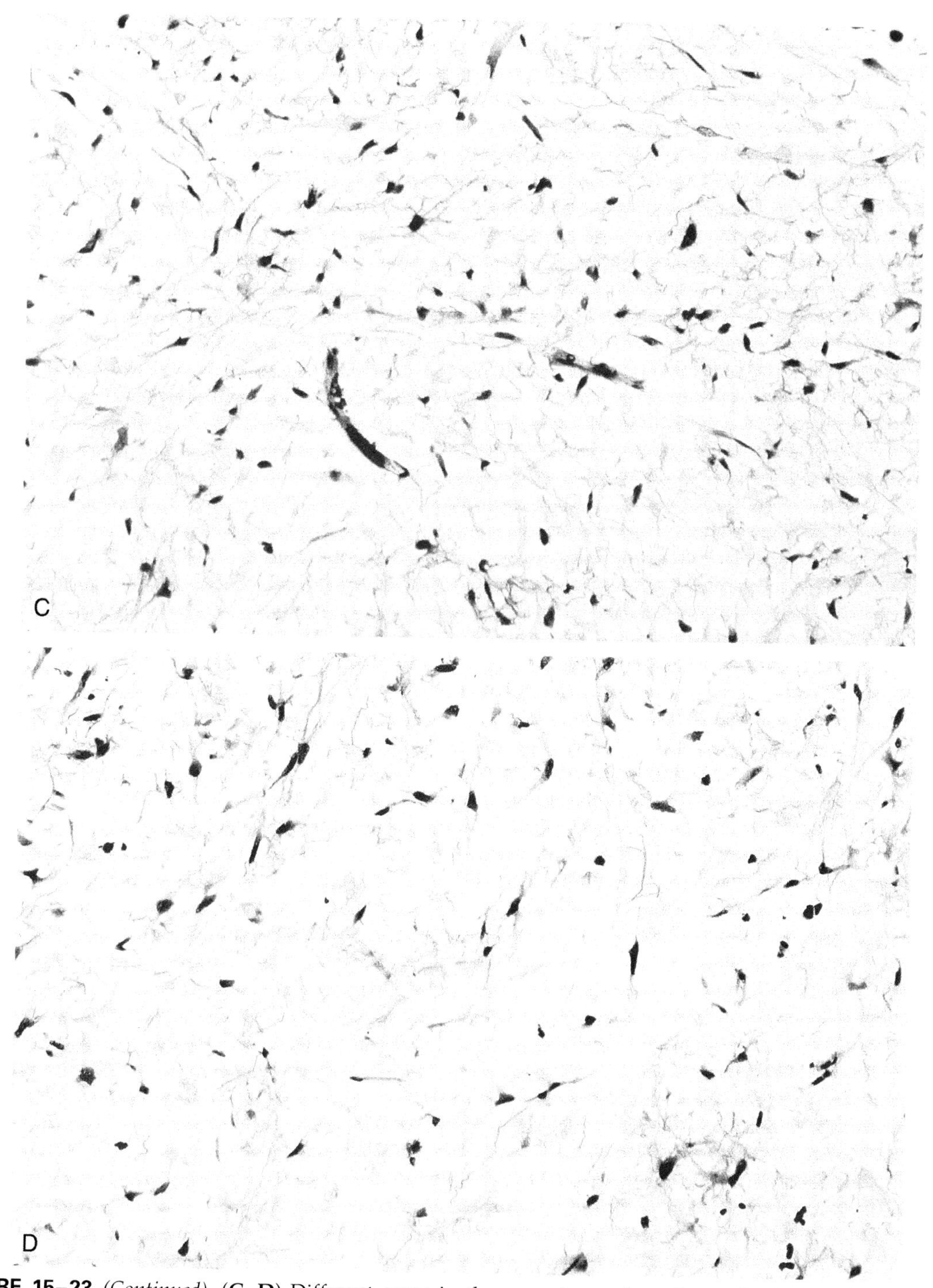


**FIGURE 15–23** *(Continued).* (**C, D**) Different areas in the same tumor have less cellularity and atypia and might be classified as "low grade myxofibrosarcoma." (**D**) Note the lack of vascularity. It superficially resembles a myxoma except for the greater degree of nuclear atypia.

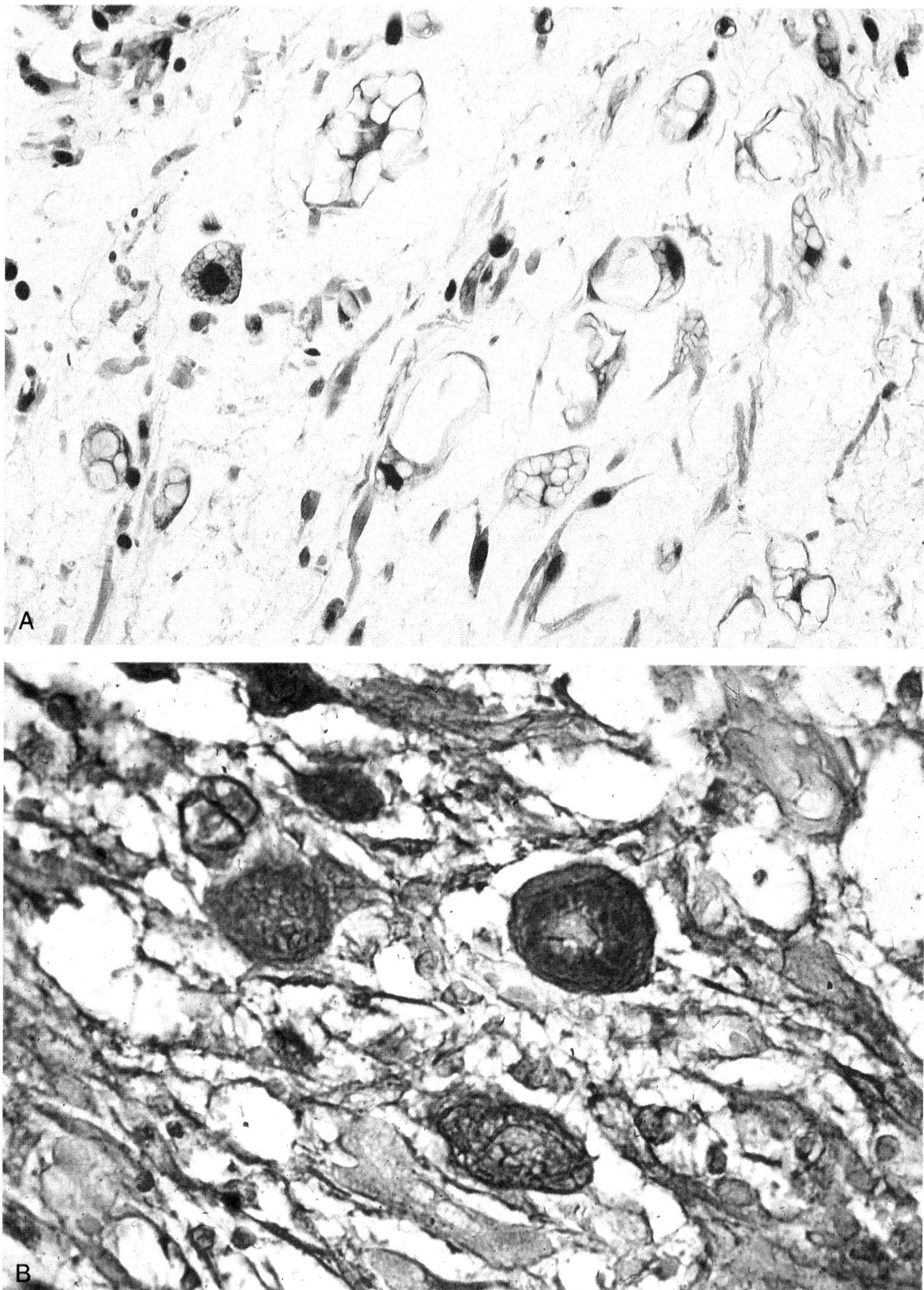


**FIGURE 15–24.** Pseudolipoblasts in a myxoid malignant fibrous histiocytoma. Tumor cells become distended with hyaluronic acid and resemble lipoblasts. Note, however, that the vacuoles are ill-defined and do not cause the sharp indentation of the nucleus seen in true lipoblasts (**A**). Vacuoles stain positively for hyaluronic acid with alcian blue (**B**).

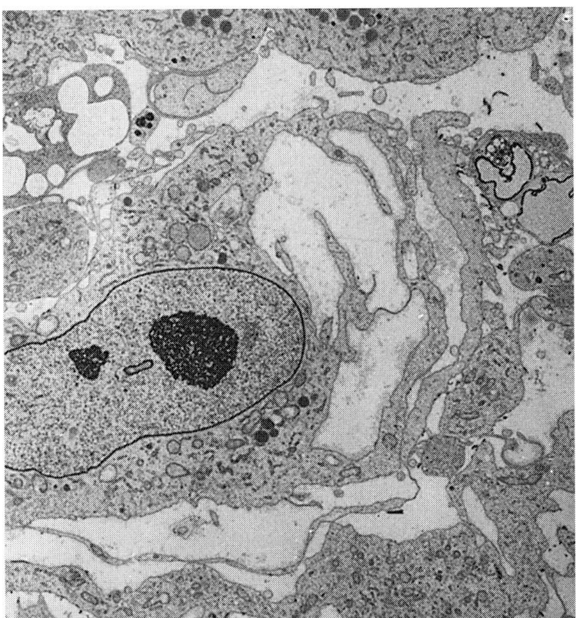

**FIGURE 15–25.** Electron micrograph of a myxoid malignant fibrous histiocytoma. Cells are surrounded by abundant ground substance. Vacuolation of cells is caused by numerous invaginations of the cytoplasmic membrane, trapping ground substance around the nucleus, and by dilatation of the endoplasmic reticulum. (Courtesy of Dr. Bruce Mackay.)

Despite its better prognosis, the myxoid form of malignant fibrous histiocytoma should be treated by wide local excision or amputation. All previous comments concerning metastatic sites, therapy, and prognostic criteria for the storiform-pleomorphic type are equally applicable to this type. The significance of myxoid change in these tumors is not entirely clear. It is unlikely that it is a degenerative feature because other features of degeneration are lacking. Viewed simplistically, it might be regarded as an area in which the cells multiply more slowly but produce abundant mucoid matrix as a form of differentiation. This would explain the better prognosis most myxoid tumors have compared to their cellular counterparts (e.g., myxoid liposarcoma, myxoid chondrosarcoma).

## Malignant Fibrous Histiocytoma: Giant Cell Type

The giant cell type of malignant fibrous histiocytoma, also termed malignant giant cell tumor of soft parts,[28,52] is a multinodular tumor composed of a mixture of histiocytes, fibroblasts, and osteoclast-type giant cells. Dense, fibrous bands containing vessels encircle the nodules of tumor, and secondary hemorrhage and necrosis are commonly present in them (Fig. 15–28). As in other fibrohistiocytic tumors, the relative amounts of the three cell types vary. Most tumors contain all three cell types arranged randomly, with some tendency for the fibroblasts to aggregate at the periphery of a nodule (Figs. 15–29 to 15–32). The fibroblasts and histiocytes are similar to those in other malignant fibrous histiocytomas. They display pleomorphism and mitotic activity and often contain ingested material such as lipid and hemosiderin. The hallmark of this tumor is the giant cell. Although these cells resemble normal osteoclasts, they are usually not found in association with osteoid, and their nuclei tend to be of high nuclear grade. Hemorrhage tends to be common in these lesions (Fig. 15–32) and occasionally forms large cystic hemorrhagic spaces.

Focal osteoid or mature bone is present (Fig. 15–29) in approximately half of the cases. This material is usually located at the periphery of a tumor nodule and appears to be produced by neoplastic cells. In view of this feature, the question can legitimately be raised as to whether this tumor is one of bone-forming mesenchyme. Ultrastructural studies have presented divergent views on this point. One study documented the same spectrum of cell types as have been seen in other forms of malignant fibrous histiocytoma and have regarded it as a variant thereof.[1] Another study described a population of cells with

*Text continued on page 562*

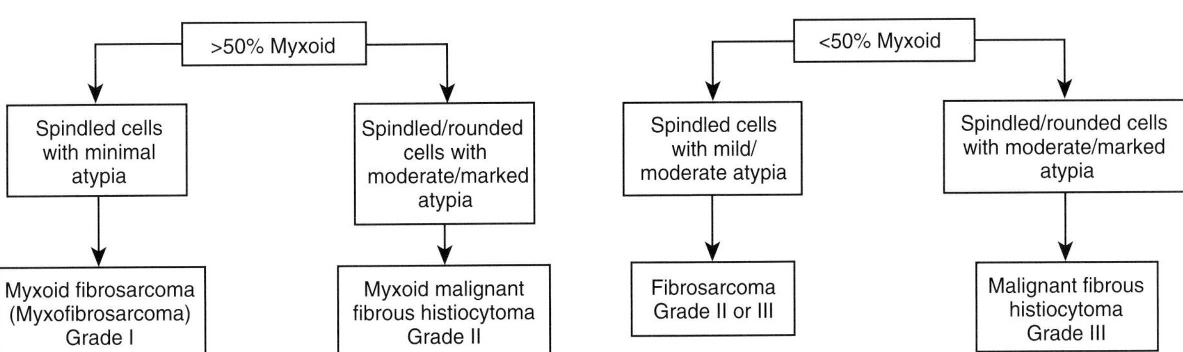


**FIGURE 15–26.** Proposed nomenclature for myxoid fibroblastic and fibrohistiocytic neoplasms.

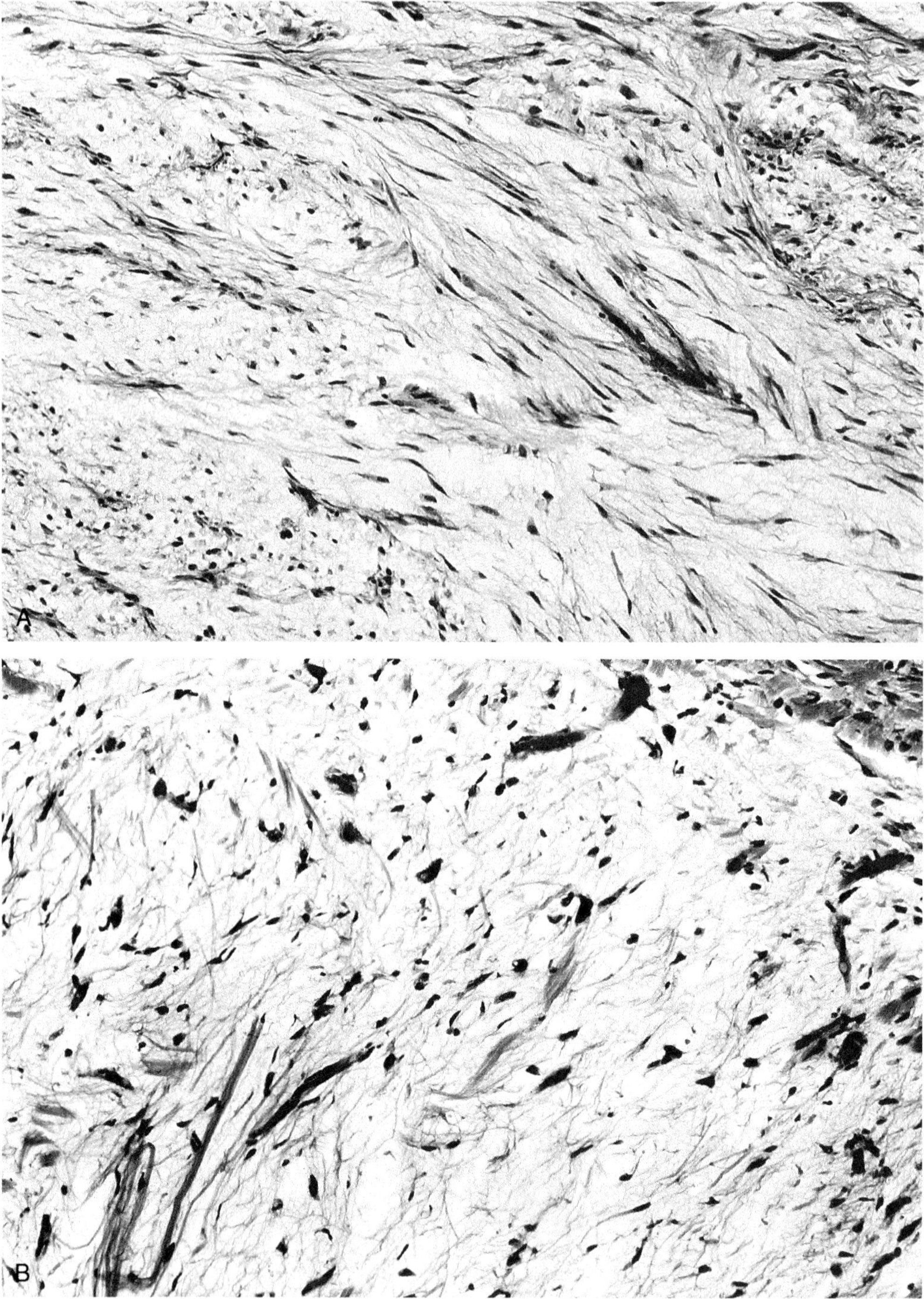


**FIGURE 15–27.** Comparison of a classic "low-grade myxofibrosarcoma" or fibrosarcoma, myxoid type, grade I (**A**) with a myxoid malignant fibrous histiocytoma, grade II (**B**). Although both are predominantly myxoid, myxofibrosarcomas are composed of differentiated spindled cells arranged in fascicles, whereas myxoid fibrous histiocytomas are composed of stellate, spindled, and pleomorphic cells arranged haphazardly.

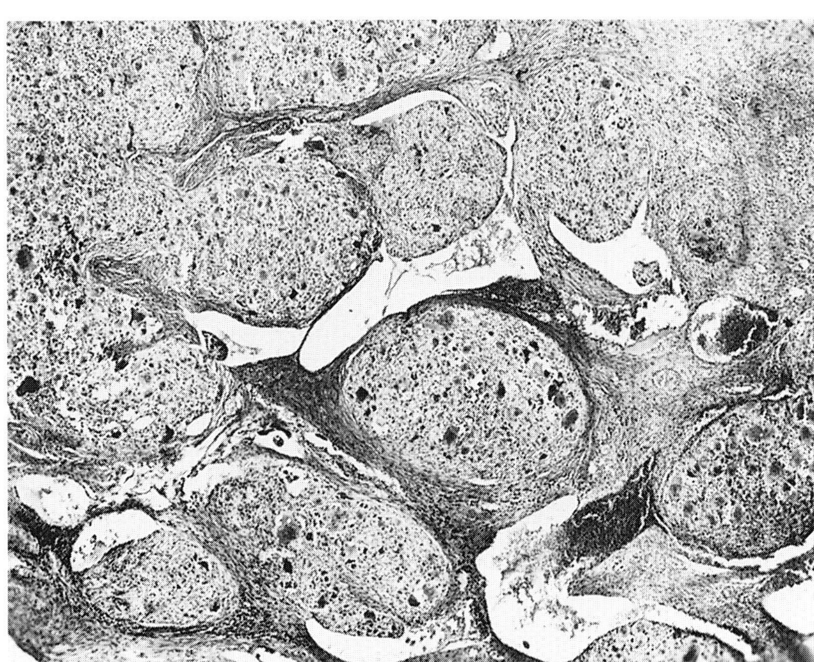

**FIGURE 15–28.** Characteristic multinodular pattern of the giant cell type of malignant fibrous histiocytoma. (×38) (From Guccion JG, Enzinger FM. Malignant giant cell tumor of soft parts: an analysis of 32 cases. Cancer 29:1518, 1972.)

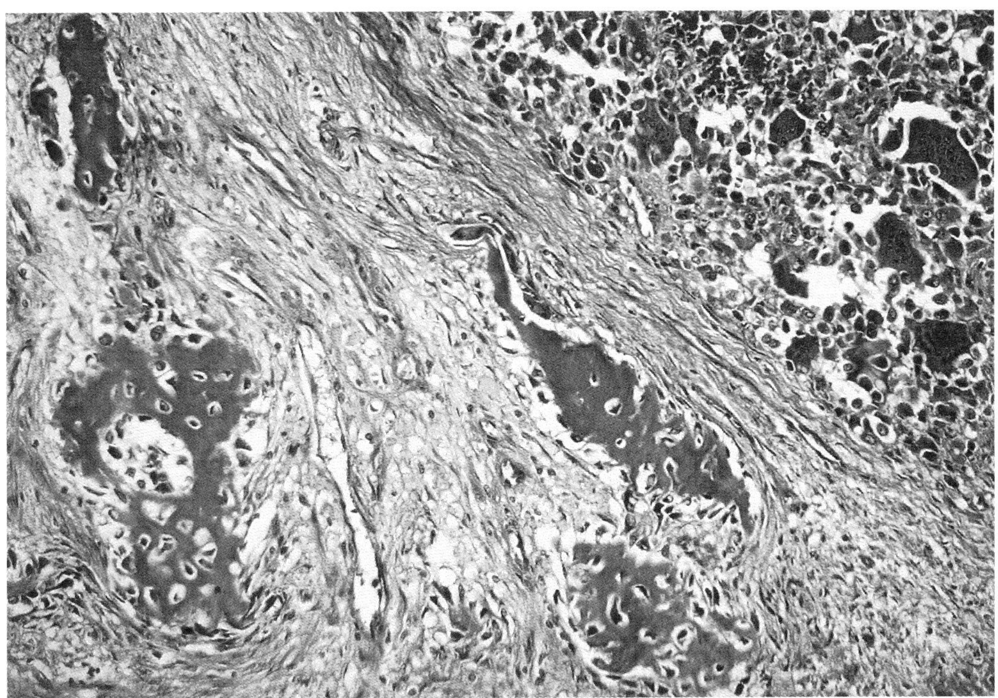

**FIGURE 15–29.** Giant cell form of malignant fibrous histiocytoma showing a shell of lamellar bone at the periphery.

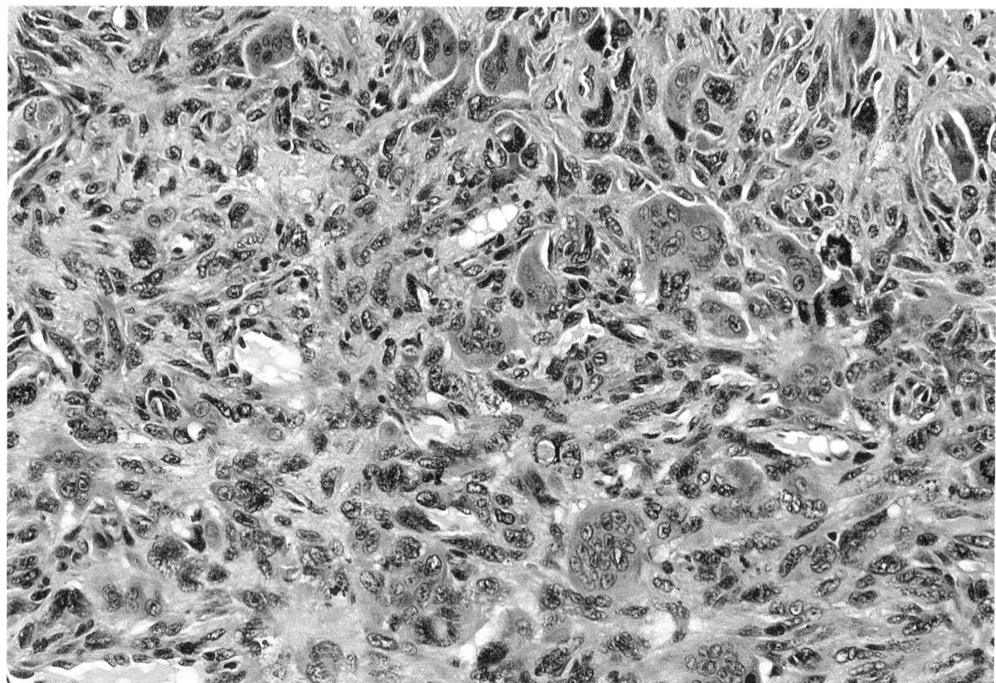

**FIGURE 15–30.** Giant cell form of malignant fibrous histiocytoma.

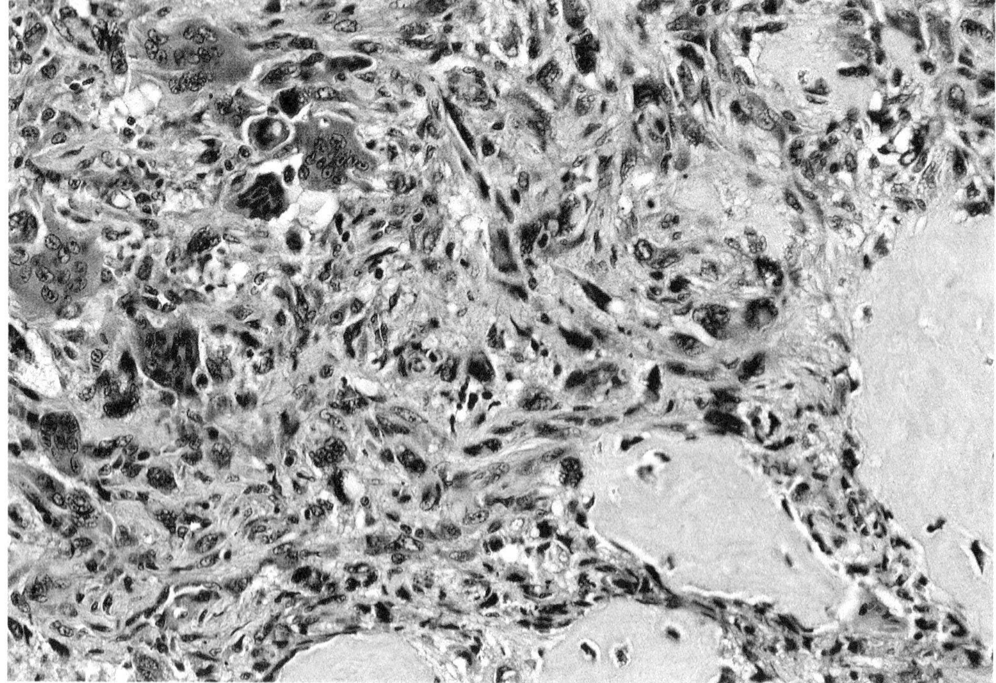

**FIGURE 15–31.** Giant cell form of malignant fibrous histiocytoma containing less mature bone in the tumor.

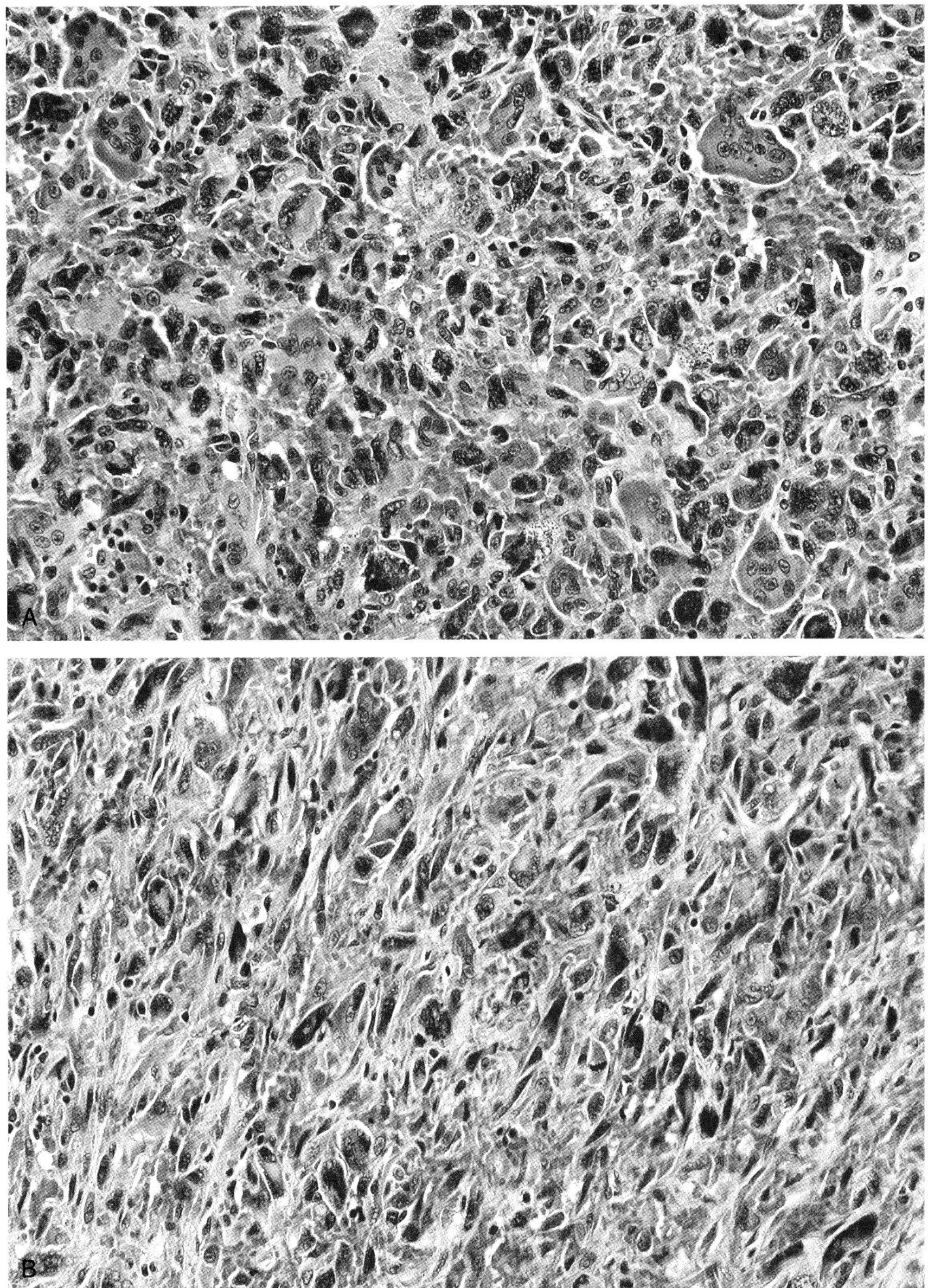


**FIGURE 15–32.** Hemorrhagic areas in a giant cell form of malignant fibrous histiocytoma that vary from having a predominantly round cell population with numerous osteoclast-like giant cells with high-grade nuclear atypia (**A**) to a spindled population (**B**).

features of primitive osteoblasts or chondroblasts[124] and matrix material similar to osteoid.

It has been recognized that a subset of giant cell tumors of soft parts are composed of cells lacking significant nuclear atypia but with mitotic activity and vascular invasion. These lesions appear to be the soft tissue counterpart of giant cell tumor of bone. Because they produce metastasis infrequently, they are referred to as "soft tissue giant cell tumors of low malignant potential" and are discussed in Chapter 14.

We believe, for the most part, that this tumor has more in common with other forms of malignant fibrous histiocytoma. On occasion, the neoplastic cells acquire some of the properties of osteoblasts or chondroblasts. So long as osteoid is relatively focal and mature, we classify these tumors as giant cell forms of malignant fibrous histiocytoma. When osteoid is prominent, a diagnosis of extraosseous osteosarcoma seems justified. This approach implies a close histogenetic relation of the two tumors.

### Differential Diagnosis

The distinctive appearance of this neoplasm usually causes few problems with the diagnosis. Deeply situated tumors may raise the question of a giant cell tumor of bone involving soft tissue. This tumor, however, has a degree of multinodularity not generally encountered in giant cell tumors of bone and does not create major osseous defects as would be expected in a bone tumor.

### Discussion

Although there are considerably fewer data concerning this form of malignant fibrous histiocytoma compared with data for the foregoing types, the original study of 32 cases[52] indicates the same general tendencies as discussed previously. Superficial tumors involving the subcutis or fascia have a much better prognosis than deeply situated tumors. Two-thirds of superficial tumors recur, but only about one-sixth metastasize. On the other hand, about 40% of deep tumors recur, and about half metastasize, a proportion roughly comparable to the ordinary forms of malignant fibrous histiocytoma. This tumor should also be treated by prompt radical surgery.

## Malignant Fibrous Histiocytoma: Inflammatory Type

One of the earliest complete descriptions of this tumor was that of Oberling[102] in 1935. He presented three cases of his own and three from the literature under the name "retroperitoneal xanthogranuloma." These tumors were bulky infiltrating retroperitoneal masses that contained a polymorphic population of xanthoma cells and inflammatory cells. Despite his astute observations, Oberling concluded that these lesions were not malignant but were variants of Hand-Schüller-Christian disease, a view subsequently endorsed by others.[125] Unfortunately, since Oberling's early description the term *xanthogranuloma* has been applied inappropriately to a variety of retroperitoneal lesions characterized by xanthoma cells. These processes probably have included conditions such as retroperitoneal fibrosis, xanthogranulomatous pyelonephritis, and nonspecific inflammatory conditions. Thus it is not surprising that "retroperitoneal xanthogranuloma" has remained an elusive diagnostic and biologic concept for the pathologist and clinician. The heterogeneity of such lesions probably accounts in part for the earlier belief that they were not only benign but also nonneoplastic.

It is clear that lesions similar to that described by Oberling occasionally occur outside the retroperitoneum, rarely metastasize, and frequently contain a fibroblastic element similar to other forms of malignant fibrous histiocytoma. In fact, lesions comparable to that of Oberling have been reported under the rubric *inflammatory fibrous histiocytoma*.[79,93] We have modified this term to *inflammatory malignant fibrous histiocytoma* to emphasize the aggressive nature of the tumor. In some respects this term fails to convey fully the difference between this tumor and the other forms of malignant fibrous histiocytoma. Although acute inflammatory cells are striking, so too are the xanthoma cells; and it is the latter that give the tumor its almost invariable yellow color (Fig. 15–33A). Analysis of tumor extracts has documented eosinophilic and neutrophilic chemotactic activity along with myelopoietic activity, suggesting that production of specific cytokines by the tumor could explain all of the unusual associated blood manifestations.[60,118]

Histologically, the tumor is composed of benign- and malignant-appearing xanthoma cells, the latter often assuming a gigantic size with bizarre nuclei. Typically, these neoplastic cells display phagocytosis of neutrophils, a feature that helps distinguish them from anaplastic lymphoma in which inflammatory cells typically are not internalized by the neoplastic lymphoid cells (Figs. 15–34 to 15–38). The neoplastic cells in malignant fibrous histiocytomas express vimentin but not various leukocyte lineage markers (CD15, CD20, CD45), although they may contain CD68 as a reflection of their phagocytic activity. The inflammatory component is characteristically prominent and usually consists of a mixture of acute and chronic inflammatory cells with marked emphasis on the former. A delicate vasculature is sometimes appreciated throughout the tumor, creating a superficial resemblance to granulation tissue. There are frequent

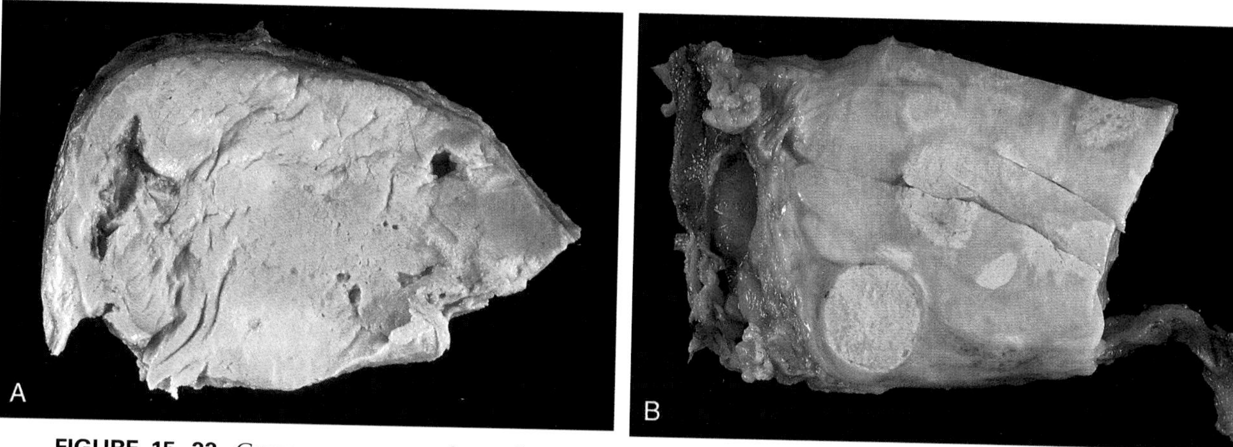


**FIGURE 15–33.** Gross appearance of a malignant fibrous histiocytoma with a tawny yellow color (**A**). In some portions of the tumor there were areas of conventional malignant fibrous histiocytoma. (**B**) Interface of conventional malignant fibrous histiocytoma (white areas) with the inflammatory areas.

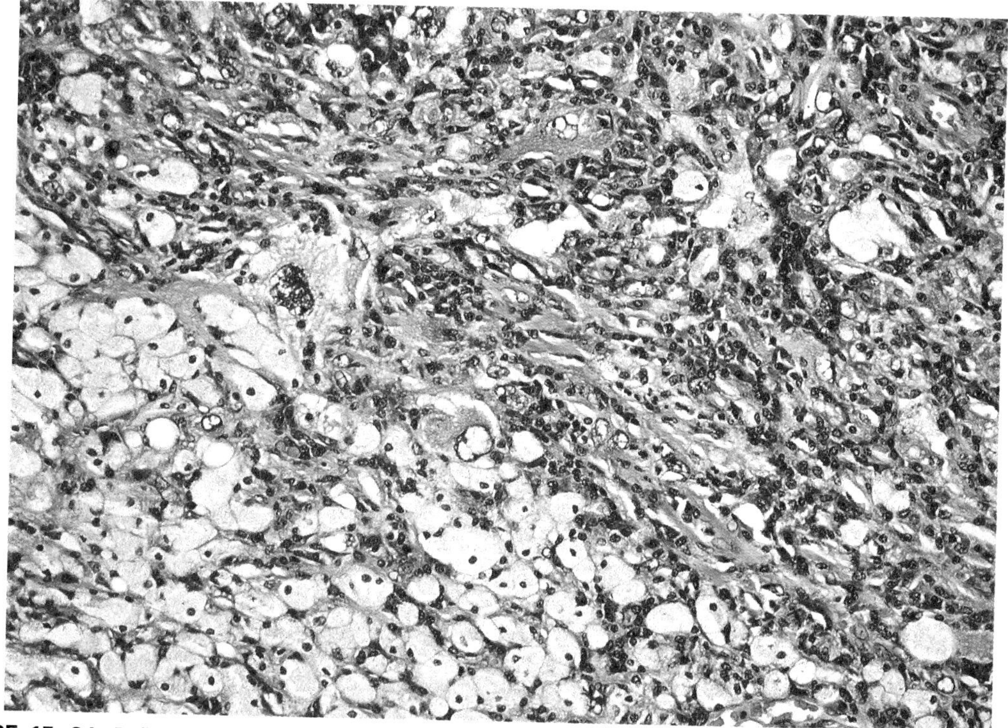

**FIGURE 15–34.** Inflammatory malignant fibrous histiocytoma showing transition to a conventional malignant fibrous histiocytoma (top right).

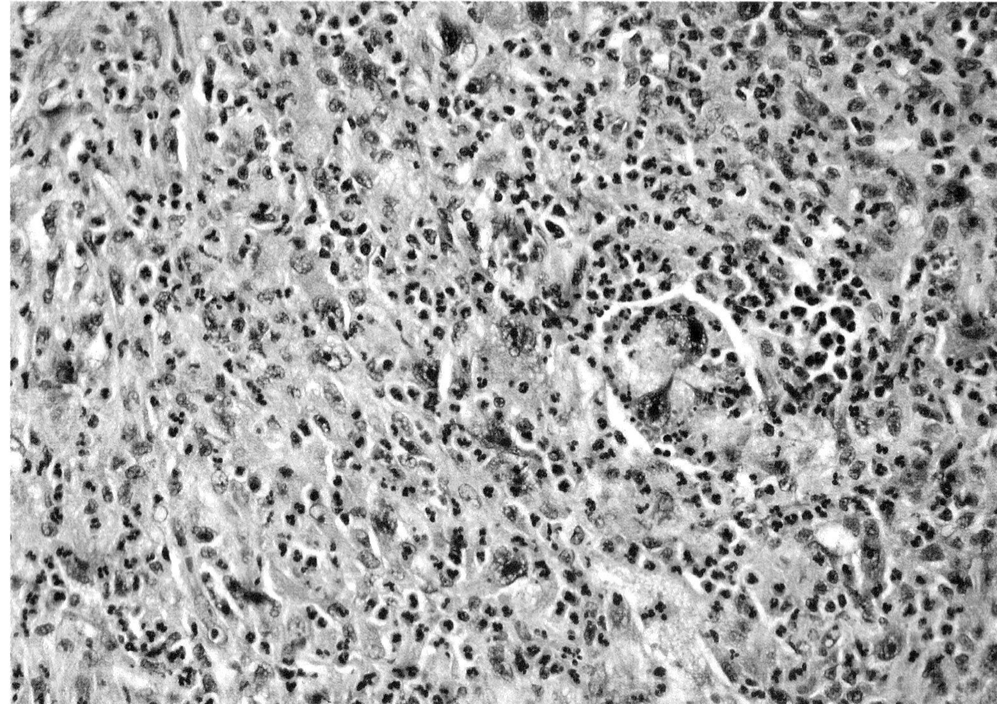

**FIGURE 15–35.** Inflammatory malignant fibrous histiocytoma with a predominance of neutrophils, some in tumor cells.

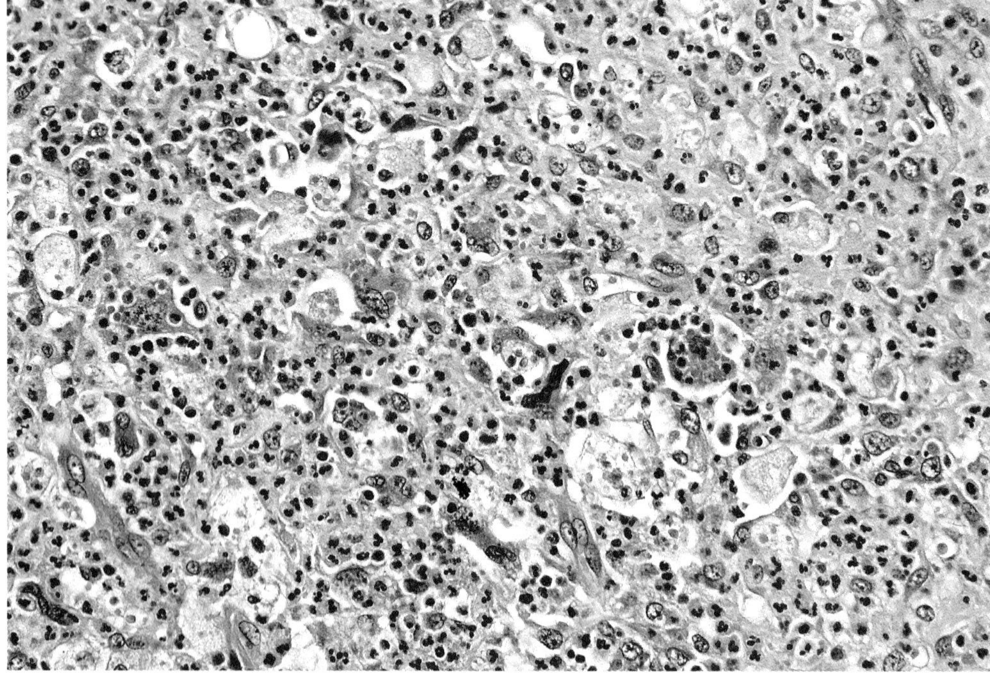

**FIGURE 15–36.** Inflammatory malignant fibrous histiocytoma.

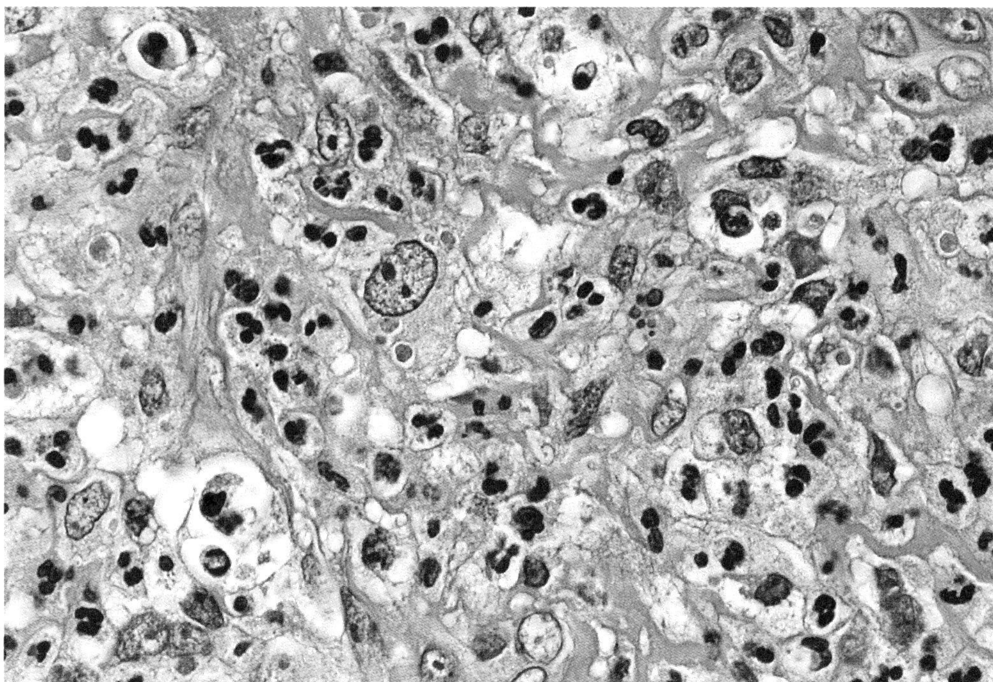

**FIGURE 15–37.** High-power view of cells in an inflammatory malignant fibrous histiocytoma. The round neoplastic cells sometimes resemble the cells in anaplastic large cell lymphomas or Hodgkin's disease.

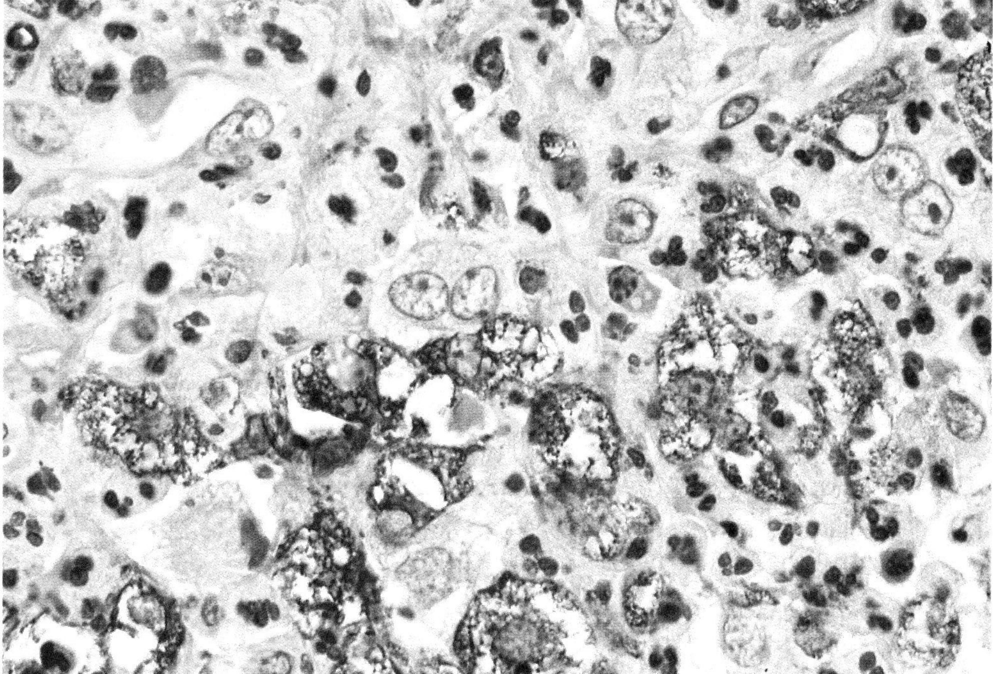

**FIGURE 15–38.** CD68 stain of an inflammatory malignant fibrous histiocytoma with staining of benign xanthoma cells. Some phagocytic tumor cells also stain. Other leukocyte lineage markers are not present in the neoplastic cells in the tumor.

transitions to spindled areas with a fascicular or even a storiform growth pattern (Fig. 15–33B). These areas resemble the more typical malignant fibrous histiocytomas and are therefore of great help in establishing a diagnosis. Metastases from this tumor usually resemble the parent lesion; when the metastases are different, they usually appear to be less xanthomatous and more fibroblastic.

### Differential Diagnosis

The differential diagnosis consists primarily of distinguishing this tumor from nonneoplastic xanthomatous processes. Although xanthogranulomatous pyelonephritis may involve the retroperitoneal soft tissue, it first and foremost affects the kidneys and is accompanied by the usual constellation of symptoms of urinary tract infection. Xanthogranulomatous inflammatory processes may also be seen in other settings,[74,98] some of which are related to infectious agents. Thus culture of these lesions and bacterial stains are mandatory. Ultimately, the distinction of this tumor from xanthogranulomatous inflammation rests on the documentation of atypia or mitotic activity in the xanthoma cells or fibroblastic areas resembling the usual form of malignant fibrous histiocytoma. Therefore careful sampling of large xanthomatous lesions, especially in the retroperitoneum, is of the utmost importance.

The malignant tumor most often confused with inflammatory malignant fibrous histiocytoma is lymphoma. Small biopsy specimens or peripheral sampling of large tumors may result in close intermingling of rounded histiocyte-like cells with inflammatory cells simulating the pattern of lymphoma. Although the clinical symptoms of fever and leukemoid reaction, which occasionally characterize inflammatory malignant fibrous histiocytoma, are rare with lymphoma, it is often necessary to perform a number of immunostaining procedures to establish the diagnosis. Negative immunostaining for leukocyte common antigen, Leu-M1, and other leukocyte lineage markers are helpful for distinguishing the two lesions particularly when only a small needle biopsy is available. In our experience leukocyte lineage markers are not identified in the neoplastic cells of inflammatory malignant fibrous histiocytoma, although CD68 may be identified in neoplastic cells that have evidence of phagocytosis (Fig. 15–38).[75]

### Discussion

In the past it has been difficult to characterize the behavior of these tumors because of the uncertainty of the diagnosis in some cases and the limited follow-up information in others. In a review of 29 acceptable cases from the literature[66] approximately half of the patients had persistent or recurrent disease, and about one-third developed distant metastases in such sites as the liver, lung, and lymph nodes. The aggressive nature of the tumor is corroborated by another report of seven cases[79] in which virtually all patients suffered severe effects of local disease, and four eventually developed metastases. Although it is obvious that these lesions are malignant, it is not clear to what extent they should be regarded as comparable to the other forms of malignant fibrous histiocytoma. The deep location of most of these tumors, the surgical inaccessibility, and the therapeutic delays resulting from diagnostic errors adversely affect the prognosis of these cases. As a result, it has thus far not been possible to find properly matched groups for comparison.

Radical surgery is indicated for these tumors. Radiotherapy and chemotherapy have generally been used as adjunctive or palliative measures. In a case reported by Kyriakos and Kempson,[79] reduction of the tumor was noted following a single high dose of nitrogen mustard.

Although it is sometimes claimed that inflammatory forms of malignant fibrous histiocytoma are, in effect, lymphomas that are misdiagnosed, this is an overstatement. It is true that failure to exclude other tumors that legitimately enter the differential diagnosis can lead to overdiagnosis, but application of immunohistochemistry to this problem area helps considerably. When evaluating small needle biopsy specimens with a presumptive diagnosis of inflammatory malignant fibrous histiocytoma, immunostains for leukocyte lineage markers and for cytokeratin serve to rule out retroperitoneum-based carcinomas and lymphomas (including Hodgkin's disease), which occasionally have a striking inflammatory infiltrate.

## REFERENCES

### Atypical Fibroxanthoma

1. Alguacil-Garcia A, Unni KK, Goellner JR, et al. Atypical fibroxanthoma of the skin. Cancer 40:1471, 1977.
2. Barr RJ, Wuerker RB, Graham JH. Ultrastructure of atypical fibroxanthoma. Cancer 40:736, 1977.
3. Berschadsky M, Gianetti CO, David A. Atypical fibroxanthoma in the pharynx. Plast Reconstr Surg 52:443, 1973.
4. Bourne RB. Paradoxical fibrosarcoma of the skin (pseudosarcoma): a review of 13 cases. Med J Aust 50:504, 1963.
5. Chen KTK. Atypical fibroxanthoma of the skin with osteoid production. Arch Dermatol 116:113, 1980.
6. Dahl L. Atypical fibroxanthoma of the skin: a clinicopathological study of 57 cases. Acta Pathol Microbiol Scand 84:183, 1976.
7. Evans HL, Smith JL. Spindle cell squamous carcinoma and sarcoma-like tumors of the skin: a comparative study of 38 cases. Cancer 45:2687, 1980.
8. Finlay-Jones LR, Nicoll P, ten Seldam REJ. Pseudosarcoma of the skin. Pathology 3:215, 1971.

9. Fretzin DF, Helwig EB. Atypical fibroxanthoma of the skin. Cancer 31:1541, 1973.
10. Gordon HW. Pseudosarcomatous reticulohistiocytoma: a report of four cases. Arch Dermatol 90:319, 1964.
11. Helwig EB, May D. Atypical fibroxanthoma of the skin with metastases. Cancer 57:368, 1986.
12. Hudson AW, Winkelmann RK. Atypical fibroxanthoma of the skin: a reappraisal of 19 cases in which the original diagnosis was spindle-cell squamous carcinoma. Cancer 29:413, 1972.
13. Jacobs DS, Edwards WD, Ye RC. Metastatic atypical fibroxanthoma of the skin. Cancer 35:457, 1975.
14. Kempson RL, McGavran MH. Atypical fibroxanthomas of the skin. Cancer 17:1463, 1964.
15. Khan ZM, Cockerell CJ. Atypical fibroxanthoma with osteoclast-like multinucleated giant cells. Am J Dermatopathol 19: 174, 1997.
16. Kroe DJ, Pitcock JA. Atypical fibroxanthoma of the skin: report of 10 cases. Am J Clin Pathol 51:487, 1969.
17. Lazova R, Moynes R, Scott G. CD-74: a useful marker to distinguish atypical fibroxanthoma from malignant fibrous histiocytoma. J Cutan Pathol 23:54, 1996.
18. Levan NE, Hirsch P, Kwong MQ. Pseudosarcomatous dermatofibroma. Arch Dermatol 88:908, 1963.
19. Mandard AM, Herline P, Chasle J, et al. Cutaneous pseudosarcomas: electron microscopic study of three tumors. J Submicrosc Cytol Pathol 10:441, 1978.
20. Orosz Z. Atypical fibroxanthoma with granular cells. Histopathology 33:88, 1998.
21. Rachmaninoff N, McDonald JR, Cook JC. Sarcoma-like tumors of the skin following irradiation. Am J Clin Pathol 36:427, 1961.
22. Requena L, Sangueza OP, Sanchez YE, Furio V. Clear cell atypical fibroxanthoma. J Cutan Pathol 24:176, 1997.
23. Ricci A, Cartun RW, Zakowski MF. Atypical fibroxanthoma: a study of 14 cases emphasizing the presence of Langerhans' histiocytes with implications for differential diagnosis by antibody panels. Am J Surg Pathol 12:591, 1988.
24. Vargas-Cortes F, Winkelmann RK, Soule EH. Atypical fibroxanthomas of the skin: further observations with 19 additional cases. Mayo Clin Proc 48:211, 1973.
25. Westermann FN, Langlois NE, Simpson JC. Apoptosis in atypical fibroxanthoma and pleomorphic malignant fibrous histiocytoma. Am J Dermatopathol 19:228, 1997.
26. Woyke S, Momagala W, Olszewski W, et al. Pseudosarcoma of the skin: an electron microscopic study and comparison with the fine structure of the spindle cell variant of squamous carcinoma. Cancer 33:970, 1974.

### Malignant Fibrous Histiocytoma

27. Alguacil-Garcia A, Unni KK, Goellner JR. Malignant fibrous histiocytoma: an ultrastructural study of six cases. Am J Clin Pathol 69:121, 1978.
28. Alguacil-Garcia A, Unni KK, Goellner JR. Malignant giant cell tumor of soft parts: ultrastructural study of four cases. Cancer 40:244, 1977.
29. Angervall L, Johnsson S, Kindblom LG, et al. Primary malignant fibrous histiocytoma of bone after radiation. Acta Pathol Microbiol Scand [A] 87:437, 1979.
30. Becker RL Jr, Venzon D, Lack EE, et al. Cytometry and morphometry of malignant fibrous histiocytoma of the extremities: prediction of metastasis and mortality. Am J Surg Pathol 15: 957, 1991.
31. Bertoni F, Capanna R, Biagini R, et al. Malignant fibrous histiocytoma of soft tissue: an analysis of 78 cases located and deeply seated in the extremities. Cancer 56:356, 1985.
32. Binder SW, Said JW, Shintaku IP, et al. A histiocyte-specific marker in the diagnosis of malignant fibrous histiocytoma: use of monoclonal antibody KP-1 (CD68). Am J Clin Pathol 97:759, 1992.
33. Bonfiglio TA, Patten SF, Woodworth FE. Fibroxanthosarcoma of the uterine cervix: cytopathologic and histopathologic manifestations. Acta Cytol 20:501, 1976.
34. Brecher ME, Franklin WA. Absence of mononuclear phagocyte antigens in malignant fibrous histiocytoma. Am J Clin Pathol 86:344, 1986.
35. Bridge JA, Sanger WG, Shaffer B, et al. Cytogenetic findings in malignant fibrous histiocytoma. Cancer Genet Cytogenet 29:97, 1987.
36. Buckley C, Thomas V, Cros J, et al. Cancer family syndrome associated with multiple malignant melanomas and a malignant fibrous histiocytoma. Br J Dermatol 126:83, 1992.
37. Burgdorf WHC, Duray P, Rosai J. Immunohistochemical identification of lysozyme in cutaneous lesions of alleged histiocytic nature. Am J Clin Pathol 75:162, 1981.
38. Choong PF, Mandahl N, Mertens F, et al. 19p+ Marker chromosome correlates with relapse in malignant fibrous histiocytoma. Genes Chromosomes Cancer 16:88, 1996.
39. Churg AM, Kahn LB. Myofibroblasts and related cells in malignant fibrous and fibrohistiocytic tumors. Hum Pathol 8:205, 1977.
40. Dahlin DC, Unni KK, Matsuno T. Malignant (fibrous) histiocytoma of bone: fact or fancy? Cancer 39:1508, 1977.
41. Dehner LP. Malignant fibrous histiocytoma: nonspecific morphologic pattern, specific pathologic entity, or both [editorial]? Arch Pathol Lab Med 112:236, 1988.
42. Diaz-Cascajo C, Borghi S, Bonczkowitz M. Pigmented atypical fibroxanthoma. Histopathology 33:537, 1998.
43. DuBoulay CEH. Demonstration of alpha-1-antitrypsin and alpha-1-antichymotrypsin in fibrous histiocytomas using immunoperoxidase technique. Am J Surg Pathol 6:559, 1982.
44. Enjoji M, Hashimoto H, Iwasaki H. Malignant fibrous histiocytoma: a clinicopathologic study of 130 cases. Acta Pathol Jpn 30:727, 1980.
45. Enzinger FM. Malignant fibrous histiocytoma 20 years after Stout. Am J Surg Pathol 10 (Suppl 1):43, 1986.
46. Eriksson M, Hardell L, Berg NO, et al. Soft tissue sarcomas and exposure to chemical substances: a case referent study. Br J Ind Med 38:27, 1981.
47. Fanburg-Smith JC, Spiro IJ, Katapuram SV, et al. Infiltrative subcutaneous malignant fibrous histiocytoma: a comparative study with deep malignant fibrous histiocytoma and an observation of biologic behavior. Ann Diagn Pathol 3:1, 1999.
48. Fletcher CD. Pleomorphic malignant fibrous histiocytoma: fact or fiction? A critical reappraisal based on 159 tumors diagnosed as pleomorphic sarcoma. Am J Surg Pathol 16:213, 1992.
49. Fu Y-S, Gabbiani G, Kaye GI, et al. Malignant soft tissue tumors of probable histiocytic origin (malignant fibrous histiocytoma): general considerations and electron microscopic and tissue culture studies. Cancer 35:176, 1975.
50. Fukuda T, Tsuneyoshi M, Enjoji M. Malignant fibrous histiocytoma of soft parts: an ultrastructural quantitative study. Ultrastruct Pathol 12:117, 1988.
51. Genberg M, Mark J, Hakelius L, et al. Origin and relationship between different cell types in malignant fibrous histiocytoma. Am J Pathol 135:1185, 1989.
52. Guccion JG, Enzinger FM. Malignant giant cell tumor of soft parts: an analysis of 32 cases. Cancer 29:1518, 1972.
53. Hamada T, Komiya S, Hiraoka K, et al. IL-6 in a pleomorphic type of malignant fibrous histiocytoma presenting high fever. Hum Pathol 29:758, 1998.
54. Hatano H, Tokunaga K, Ogose A, et al. Origin of histiocyte-like cells and multinucleated giant cells in malignant fibrous histiocytoma: neoplastic or reactive. Pathol Int 49:14, 1999.

55. Hayashi Y, Kikuchi-Tada A, Jitsukawa K, et al. Myofibroblasts in malignant fibrous histiocytoma: histochemical, immunohistochemical, ultrastructural and tissue culture studies. Clin Exp Dermatol 13:402, 1988.
56. Hirose T, Kudo E, Hasegawa T, et al. Expression of intermediate filaments in malignant fibrous histiocytomas. Hum Pathol 20:871, 1989.
57. Hirose T, Sano T, Hizawa K. Ultrastructural study of the myxoid area of malignant fibrous histocytomas. Ultrastruct Pathol 12:621, 1988.
58. Huang WL, Ordonez NG, Mackay B. Myxoid malignant fibrous histiocytoma with erythrophagocytosis. Ultrastruct Pathol 13:315, 1989.
59. Inada O, Yumoto T, Furuse K, et al. Ultrastructural features of malignant fibrous histiocytoma. Acta Pathol Jpn 26:491, 1976.
60. Isoda M, Yasumoto S. Eosinophil chemotactic factor derived from a malignant fibrous histiocytoma. Clin Exp Dermatol 11: 253, 1986.
61. Iwasaki H, Isayama T, Johzaki H, et al. Malignant fibrous histiocytoma: evidence of perivascular mesenchymal cell origin immunocytochemical studies with monoclonal anti-MFH antibodies. Am J Pathol 128:528, 1987.
62. Iwasaki H, Isayama T, Ohjimi Y, et al. Malignant fibrous histiocytoma: a tumor of facultative histiocytes showing mesenchymal differentiation in cultured cell lines. Cancer 69:437, 1992.
63. Iwasaki H, Yoshitake K, Ohjimi Y, et al. Malignant fibrous histiocytoma: proliferative compartment and heterogeneity of "histiocytic" cells. Am J Surg Pathol 16:735, 1992.
64. Jabi M, Jeans D, Dardick I. Ultrastructural heterogeneity in malignant fibrous histiocytoma of soft tissue. Ultrastruct Pathol 11:583, 1987.
65. Kahn LB. Retroperitoneal xanthogranuloma and xanthosarcoma. S Afr Med J 46:1767, 1972.
66. Kahn LB. Retroperitoneal xanthogranuloma and xanthosarcoma (malignant fibrous xanthoma). Cancer 31:411, 1973.
67. Kanzaki T, Kitajima S, Suzomori K. Biological behavior of cloned cells of human malignant fibrous histiocytoma in vivo and in vitro. Cancer Res 51:2133, 1991.
68. Kapadia GJ, Paul BD, Chung EB, et al. Carcinogenicity of Camelia sinesis (tea) and some tannin-containing fold medicinal herbs administered subcutaneously in rats. J Natl Cancer Inst 57:207, 1976.
69. Kaplan G, Sarino EF. Malignant fibrohistiocytoma (fibroxanthoma): case report. Radiology 100:155, 1971.
70. Kato T, Takeya M, Takagi K, et al. Chemically induced transplantable malignant fibrous histiocytoma of the rat: analyses with immunohistochemistry, immunoelectron microscopy and [$^3$H] thymidine autoradiography. Lab Invest 62:635, 1990.
71. Kay S. Inflammatory fibrous histiocytoma (xanthogranuloma). Report of two cases with ultrastructural observations in one. Am J Surg Pathol 2:313, 1978.
72. Kearney MM, Soule EH, Ivins JC. Malignant fibrous histiocytoma: a retrospective study of 167 cases. Cancer 45:167, 1980.
73. Kempson RL, Kyriakos M. Fibroxanthosarcoma of the soft tissue: a type of malignant fibrous histiocytoma. Cancer 29:961, 1972.
74. Keren DF, Rawlings W, Murray HW, et al. Arizona hinshawii osteomyelitis with antecedent enteric fever and sepsis. Am J Med 60:577, 1976.
75. Khalidi H, Singleton T, Weiss SW. Inflammatory malignant fibrous histiocytoma: distinction from Hodgkin's disease and non-Hodgkin's lymphoma by a panel of leukocyte markers. Mod Pathol 10:438, 1997.
76. Kindblom LG, Jacobsen GK, Jacobsen M. Immunohistochemical investigations of tumours of supposed fibroblastic-histiocytic origin. Hum Pathol 13:834, 1982.
77. Kindblom LG, Merck C, Svendsen P. Myxofibrosarcoma: a pathological-anatomical, microangiopathic and angiographic correlative study of eight cases. Br J Radiol 50:876, 1977.
78. Klugo RC, Farah RN, Cerny JC. Renal malignant histiocytoma. J Urol 112:727, 1974.
79. Kyriakos M, Kempson RL. Inflammatory fibrous histiocytoma: an aggressive and lethal lesion. Cancer 37:1584, 1976.
80. Lagace R. The ultrastructural spectrum of malignant fibrous histiocytoma. Ultrastruct Pathol 11:153, 1987.
81. Lagace R, Delage C, Seemayer TA. Myxoid variant of malignant fibrous histiocytoma: ultrastructural observations. Cancer 43:526, 1979.
82. Lararamendy ML, Tarkkanen M, Blomqvist C, et al. Comparative genomic hybridization of malignant fibrous histiocytoma reveals a novel prognostic marker. Am J Pathol 151:1153, 1997.
83. Laskin WB, Conklin RC, Enzinger FM. Malignant fibrous histiocytoma associated with hyperlipoproteinemia. Am J Surg Pathol 12:727, 1988.
84. Lawson CW, Fisher C, Garter KC. An immunohistochemical study of differentiation in malignant fibrous histiocytoma. Histopathology 11:375, 1987.
85. Le Doussal V, Coindre J-M, Leroux A, et al. Prognostic factors for patients with localized primary malignant fibrous histiocytoma. Cancer 77:1823, 1996.
86. Leak LV, Caufield JB, Burke JF, et al. Electron microscopic studies on a human fibromyxosarcoma. Cancer Res 27:261, 1967.
87. Lindeman G, McKay MJ, Taubman KL, et al. Malignant fibrous histiocytoma developing in bone 44 years after shrapnel trauma. Cancer 66:2229, 1990.
88. Litzky LA, Brooks JJ. Cytokeratin immunoreactivity in malignant fibrous histiocytoma and spindle cell tumors: comparison between frozen and paraffin-embedded tissues. Mod Pathol 5: 30, 1992.
89. Mairal A, Terrier P, Chibon F, et al. Loss of chromosome 13 is the most frequent genomic imbalance in malignant fibrous histiocytoma: a comparative genomic hybridization analysis of a series of 30 cases. Cancer Genet Cytogenet 111:134, 1999.
90. Mandahl N, Heim S, Willen H, et al. Characteristic karyotypic anomalies identify subtypes of malignant fibrous histiocytoma. Genes Chromosomes Cancer 1:9, 1989.
91. Meister P, Nathrath W. Immunohistochemical markers of histiocytic tumors. Hum Pathol 11:300, 1980.
92. Meloni-Ehrig AM, Chen Z, Guan XY, et al. Identification of a ring chromosome in a myxoid malignant fibrous histiocytoma with chromosome microdissection and fluroescence in situ hybridization. Cancer Genet Cytogenet 109:81, 1999.
93. Mentzel T, Calonje E, Wadden C, et al. Myxofibrosacroma: clinicopathologic analysis of 75 cases with emphasis on the low grade variant. Am J Surg Pathol 20:391, 1996.
94. Merkow LP, Frich JC, Sliekin M, et al. Ultrastructure of a fibroxanthosarcoma (malignant fibroxanthoma). Cancer 28:372, 1971.
95. Mertens F, Fletcher CDM, Dal Cin P, et al. Cytogenetic analysis of 46 pleomorphic sarcomas and correlation with morphological and clinical features: a report of the CHAMP Study Group. Genes Chromosomes Cancer 22:16, 1998.
96. Michael RH, Dorfman HD. Malignant fibrous histiocytoma associated with bone infarcts. Clin Orthop 118:180, 1976.
97. Miettinen M, Soini Y. Malignant fibrous histiocytoma: heterogeneous patterns of intermediate filament proteins by immunohistochemistry. Arch Pathol Lab Med 113:1363, 1989.
98. Minkowitz S, Friedman F, Henniger G. Xanthogranuloma of the ovary. Arch Pathol 80:209, 1965.
99. Mirra JM, Bullough PG, Marcove RC, et al. Malignant fibrous histiocytoma and osteosarcoma in association with bone infarcts. J Bone Joint Surg Am 56:932, 1974.

100. Mirra JM, Gold RH, Marafiote R. Malignant (fibrous) histiocytoma arising in association with a bone infarct in sickle cell disease: coincidence or cause-and-effect? Cancer 39:186, 1977.
101. Nemes Z, Thomazy V. Factor XIIIa and the classic histiocytic markers in malignant fibrous histiocytoma: a comparative immunohistochemical study. Hum Pathol 19:822, 1988.
102. Oberling C. Retroperitoneal xanthogranuloma. Am J Cancer 23:477, 1935.
103. O'Brien JE, Stout AP. Malignant fibrous xanthomas. Cancer 17: 1445, 1964.
104. Orndal C, Mandahl N, Carlen B, et al. Near-haploid clones in a malignant fibrous histiocytoma. Cancer Genet Cytogenet 60: 147, 1992.
105. Ozzello L, Stout AP, Murray MR. Cultural characteristics of malignant histiocytomas and fibrous xanthomas. Cancer 16: 331, 1963.
106. Pezzi CM, Rawlings MS Jr, Esgro JJ, et al. Prognostic factors in 227 patients with malignant fibrous histiocytoma. Cancer 69: 2098, 1992.
107. Radio SJ, Wooldridge TN, Linder J. Flow cytometric DNA analysis of malignant fibrous histiocytoma and related fibrohistiocytic tumors. Hum Pathol 19:74, 1988.
108. Roholl PJ, Kleyne J, Elbers J, et al. Characterization of tumour cells in malignant fibrous histiocytomas and other soft tissue tumours in comparison with malignant histiocytes. I. Immunohistochemical study on paraffin sections. J Pathol 147:87, 1985.
109. Roholl PJM, Kleyne J, Van Unnik JAM. Characterization of tumour cells in malignant fibrous histiocytomas and other soft tissue tumors, in comparison with malignant histiocytes. II. Immunoperoxidase study on cryostat sections. Am J Pathol 121:269, 1985.
110. Roholl PJ, Prinsen I, Rademakers LP, et al. Two cell lines with epithelial cell-like characteristics established from malignant fibrous histiocytomas. Cancer 68:1963,1991.
111. Rooser B, Willen H, Gustafson P, et al. Malignant fibrous histiocytoma of soft tissue: a population-based epidemiologic and prognostic study of 137 patients. Cancer 67:499, 1991.
112. Rydholm A, Mandahl N, Heim S, et al. Malignant fibrous histiocytomas with a 19p+ marker chromosome have increased relapse rate. Genes Chromosomes Cancer 2:296, 1990.
113. Rydholm A, Syk I. Malignant fibrous histiocytoma of soft tissue: correlation between clinical variables and histologic malignancy grade. Cancer 57:2323, 1986.
114. Salo JC, Lewis JJ, Woodruff JM, et al. Malignant fibrous histiocytoma of the extremity. Cancer 85:1765, 1999.
115. Soini Y, Miettinen M. Immunohistochemistry of markers of histiomonocytic cells in malignant fibrous histiocytomas: a monoclonal antibody study. Pathol Res Pract 186:759, 1990.
116. Soini Y, Vahakangas K, Nuorva K, et al. P53 immunohistochemistry in malignant fibrous histiocytomas and other mesenchymal tumours. J Pathol 168:29, 1992.
117. Szymanska J, Tarkkanen M, Wiklung T, et al. A cytogenetic study of malignant fibrous histiocytoma. Cancer Genet Cytogenet 85:91, 1995.
118. Takahashi K, Kimura Y, Naito M, et al. Inflammatory fibrous histiocytoma presenting leukemoid reaction. Pathol Res Pract 184:498, 1989.
119. Takeya M, Yoshimura T, Leonard EJ, et al. Production of monocyte chemoattractant protein-1 by malignant fibrous histiocytoma: relation to the origin of histiocyte-like cells. Exp Mol Pathol 54:61, 1991.
120. Taniuchi K, Yamada Y, Nonomura A, Takehara K. Immunohistochemical analysis of platelet-derived growth factor and its receptors in fibrohistiocytic tumors. J Cutan Pathol 24:393, 1997.
121. Taxy JB, Battifora H. Malignant fibrous histiocytoma: a clinicopathologic and ultrastructural study. Cancer 40:254, 1977.
122. Taxy JB, Battifora H. The electron microscope in the study and diagnosis of soft tissue tumors. In: Trump BF, Jones RT (eds) Diagnostic Electron Microscopy, vol 3. Wiley, New York, 1980.
123. Tetu B, Lacasse B, Bouchard HL, et al. Prognostic influence of HSP-27 expression in malignant fibrous histiocytoma: a clinicopathological and immunohistochemical study. Cancer Res 52:2325, 1992.
124. Van Haelst UJGM, de Haas van Dorsser AH. Giant cell tumor of soft parts: an ultrastructural study. Virchows Arch [Pathol Anat] 371:199, 1976.
125. Waller JI, Hellwig CA, Barbosa E. Retroperitoneal xanthogranuloma associated with visceral eosinophilic granuloma. Cancer 10:388, 1957.
126. Weiss SW. Malignant fibrous histiocytoma: a reaffirmation. Am J Surg Pathol 6:773, 1982.
127. Weiss SW, Bratthauer GL, Morris PA. Postirradiation malignant fibrous histiocytoma expressing cytokeratin: implications for the immunodiagnosis of sarcomas. Am J Surg Pathol 12: 554, 1988.
128. Weiss SW, Enzinger FM. Malignant fibrous histiocytoma: an analysis of 200 cases. Cancer 41:2250, 1978.
129. Weiss SW, Enzinger FM. Myxoid variant of malignant fibrous histiocytoma. Cancer 39:1672, 1977.
130. Wood GS, Beckstead JH, Turner RR, et al. Malignant fibrous histiocytoma tumor cells resemble fibroblasts. Am J Surg Pathol 10:323, 1986.
131. Yamamoto I, Oshiro Y, Fukuda T, Tsuneyoshi M. Pleomorphic leiomyosarcoma of the soft parts: a reassessment by histology and immunohistochemistry of pleomorphic soft tissue sarcomas. Oncol Rep 6:533, 1999.
132. Yumoto T, Morimoto K. Experimental approach to fibrous histiocytoma. Acta Pathol Jpn 30:767, 1980.
133. Zagars GK, Mullen JR, Pollack A. Malignant fibrous histiocytoma: outcome and prognostic factors following conservation surgery and radiotherapy. Int J Oncol Biol Phys 34:983, 1996.
134. Zehr RJ, Bauer TW, Marks KE, et al. Ki-67 and grading of malignant fibrous histiocytomas. Cancer 66:1984, 1990.

# CHAPTER 16

# BENIGN LIPOMATOUS TUMORS

Although adipose tissue has been the subject of intensive investigation in recent years, its significance and multiple functions are not always fully appreciated. Fat serves not only as one of the principal and most readily available sources of energy in the body, it functions as a barrier for the conservation of heat and as mechanical protection of the underlying tissues against physical injury.

## ADIPOSE TISSUE

Two basic forms of adipose tissue can be distinguished, *white fat* and *brown fat*.

### White Fat

White fat makes it first appearance at a relatively late stage of development; it is rarely encountered before the third or fourth month of intrauterine life. In its earliest stages, after 10–14 weeks' gestation, it consists of aggregates of mesenchymal cells that are condensed around proliferating primitive blood vessels.[14] Following this stage, the stellate-shaped preadipocytes are organized into lobules that contain a rich network of proliferating capillaries. At later stages (14–24 weeks' gestation), small oil red O-positive and sudanophilic lipid droplets appear in these cells, gradually converting them to rounded or spherical, multivacuolated lipoblasts (Figs. 16–1, 16–2). Intracellular glycogen is usually present at this stage of development. The multiple lipid droplets then fuse to form a single vacuole and displace the nucleus marginally, forming the mature fat cell, or lipocyte. Small aggregates of lipocytes form small lobules that make their first appearance in the regions of the face, neck, breast, and abdominal wall followed by the back and shoulders. The lobules multiply and enlarge, and by the end of the fifth month a continuous subcutaneous layer of fat is formed in the extremities.[15]

Postnatally, white fat cells enlarge significantly during the first 6 months of life without a significant increase in cell number.[15] This phase is followed by a progressive increase in adipocyte number, although the cell size remains fairly constant. At puberty there is a marked increase in both adipocyte size and number. After puberty, new adipocytes may continue to form throughout adult life, although at a much slower rate.[8]

White fat serves several functions, including thermal insulation and mechanical protection. Its main role is the uptake, synthesis, and storage of lipid and the release of free fatty acids in response to hormonal and neural stimuli.[3] This function is mediated by lipoprotein lipase, an enzyme synthesized by adipocytes and transferred to the luminal surface of endothelial cells.

Histologically, differentiated white fat consists of spherical or polygonal cells in which most of the cytoplasm has been replaced by a single large lipid droplet, leaving only a narrow rim of cytoplasm at the periphery. The eccentrically placed nucleus is flattened and is crescent-shaped on cross section; not infrequently it contains one small lipid invagination (Lochkern). The white fat cells (lipocytes) measure up to 120$\mu$m in diameter. Like any metabolically active tissue, white fat is highly vascularized, a feature that is more evident in atrophic fat than in normal fat. In the subcutis and to a lesser extent in deeper tissues, the fat cells are arranged in distinct lobules separated by a thin membrane of fibrous connective tissue. The lobular architecture of white fat is most prominent in areas subjected to pressure and probably has a cushioning effect.[18,20]

According to Napolitano's[11,12] classic description, the ultrastructure of adipose tissue cells during the earliest stage of development closely resembles that of fibroblasts: the cells are spindle-shaped, have slender cytoplasmic extensions, and contain small spherical mitochondria and abundant highly organized endo-

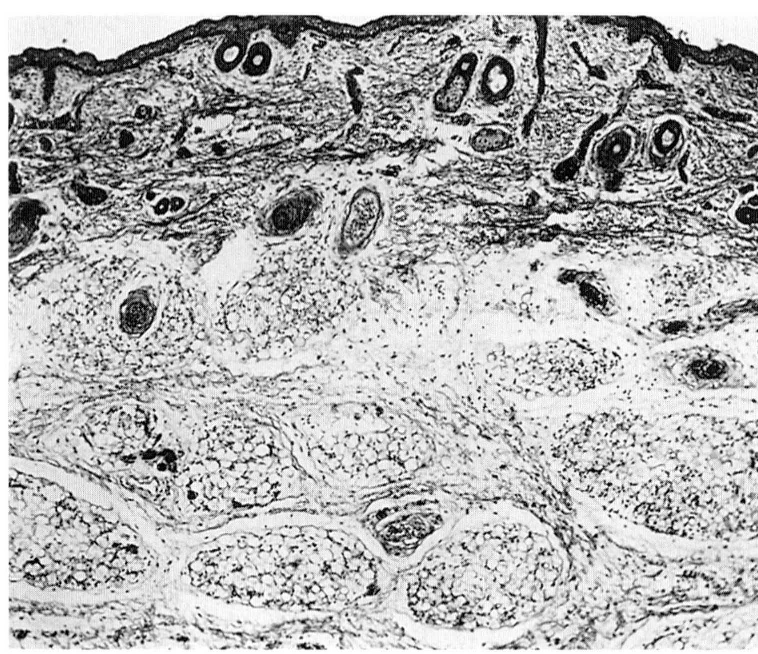

**FIGURE 16–1.** Subcutaneous fat at the sixth month of intrauterine development. Note the lobulated growth, the "primitive fat organs" of Wassermann.

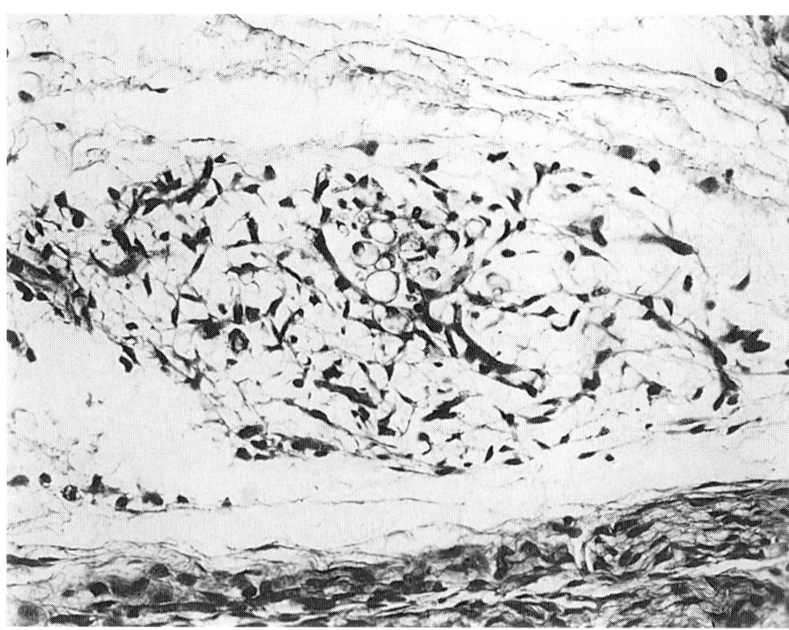

**FIGURE 16–2.** Subcutaneous fat at the sixth month of intrauterine development consisting of delicate branching capillaries surrounded by a "cloud" of spindle and stellate-shaped mesenchymal cells gradually being transformed into lipoblasts.

plasmic reticulum. At later stages of development the endoplasmic reticulum becomes less conspicuous, and one or more inclusions of non-membrane-bound lipid make their appearance in the cytoplasm, usually adjacent to the nucleus. There are also irregular, smooth-surfaced, membrane-limited vesicles, a rather poorly developed Golgi apparatus, and glycogen granules (in close association with the lipid inclusions). An amorphous basal lamina sets the cells apart from the surrounding collagen and occasional nonmyelinated nerves; the basal lamina is present at all stages of cellular differentiation and helps distinguish preadipocytes from fibroblasts.

Continued accumulation of cytoplasm and increasing amounts of intracellular lipid lead to more rounded cells, which are characterized by a large, centrally located lipid droplet, a thin rim of cytoplasm, and a peripherally placed, flattened or crescent-shaped nucleus. There is a membrane separating the central lipid inclusion from the surrounding cytoplasm. This "signet ring" stage of cellular development represents the lipocyte of mature adipose tissue.

## Brown Fat

The precursors of brown fat are spindle-shaped cells that are closely related to a network of capillaries.[13] Subsequently, there is proliferation of capillaries and brown adipocytes, with organization into lobules by fibrous connective tissue septa. As the cells accumulate lipid, they are initially unilocular; but with further lipid accumulation, multiple cytoplasmic lipid vacuoles appear.[3] Brown fat is found mainly in infants and children and gradually disappears from most sites with increasing age. In children, brown fat deposits are most conspicuous in the interscapular region, around the blood vessels and muscles of the neck, around the structures of the mediastinum, adjacent to the lung hila, on the anterior abdominal wall, and surrounding intraabdominal and retroperitoneal structures including the kidneys, pancreas, and spleen. During adulthood, deposits of brown fat persist around the kidneys, adrenal glands, and aorta and within the mediastinum and neck.

The principal function of brown fat is heat production.[7] It has been estimated that even small quantities of brown fat are capable of increasing heat production by more than 20%.[16] This process is principally controlled by the release of norepinephrine from sympathetic nerves. Thermotenin, a mitochondrial uncoupling protein unique to brown fat, uncouples oxidation of fatty acids to form adenosine triphosphate (ATP),[4] which is dissipated as heat. Brown fat may also play a role in weight regulation in adults.[3] Santos et al.[17] found an increased amount of periadrenal fat in malnourished people at autopsy, suggesting a compensatory increase in nonshivering thermogenesis to maintain body temperature in those with diminished subcutaneous fat.

The term brown fat refers to its gross appearance, which results from its abundant vascularity and numerous mitochondria. Compared to white fat, brown fat tends to have a more prominent lobulated growth pattern. Its cells are smaller (25–40 $\mu$m in diameter), are round or polygonal, and contain a large amount of cytoplasm that stains deeply eosinophilic with hematoxylin-eosin. The cells are mostly multivacuolated, with distinctly granular cytoplasm between the individual lipid droplets. Intermixed with these cells are nonvacuolated, purely granular cells and cells with a single large lipid vacuole, resembling lipocytes. The nuclei are rounded and situated in a central position, although the nucleus may be displaced to the periphery in cells with large lipid vacuoles as in white fat. The cells are arranged in distinct lobular aggregates and are intimately associated with a prominent vascular network and numerous nerves (Fig. 16–3).

There are apparent transitions between brown and white fat in both humans and animals, but brown fat can be clearly identified by electron microscopy. The brown fat cell is smaller and can be recognized by small lipid inclusions with mitochondria that are both numerous and more complex in structure. There are also scattered ribosomes, variable amounts of glycogen, and a poorly developed endoplasmic reticulum.

## Molecular Biology

The *CHOP* gene, also known as *GADD153*, appears to be involved in adipocytic differentiation.[9] This gene encodes a member of the CCAAT/enhancer binding protein family (C/EBP), which may be an inhibitor of other C/EBP transcription factors known to be important in cell proliferation. Members of the C/EBP group are highly expressed in fat and are involved in the growth arrest of terminally differentiated adipocytes.[1] In myxoid/round cell liposarcoma, the t(12;16)(q13;p11) results in a fusion gene involving *CHOP* and *TLS* (translocated in liposarcoma), a gene that shows great structural and functional similarity to the *EWS* gene of Ewing's sarcoma.

## Immunohistochemistry

Adipocytes and benign and malignant fatty tumors stain positively for vimentin and stain variably for S-100 protein.[5,6,10,19] More recently, an antibody to the adipocyte lipid-binding protein p422 (also known as aP2), a protein expressed exclusively in preadipocytes late in adipogenesis, has been found to stain only lipoblasts and brown fat cells, as well as liposarco-

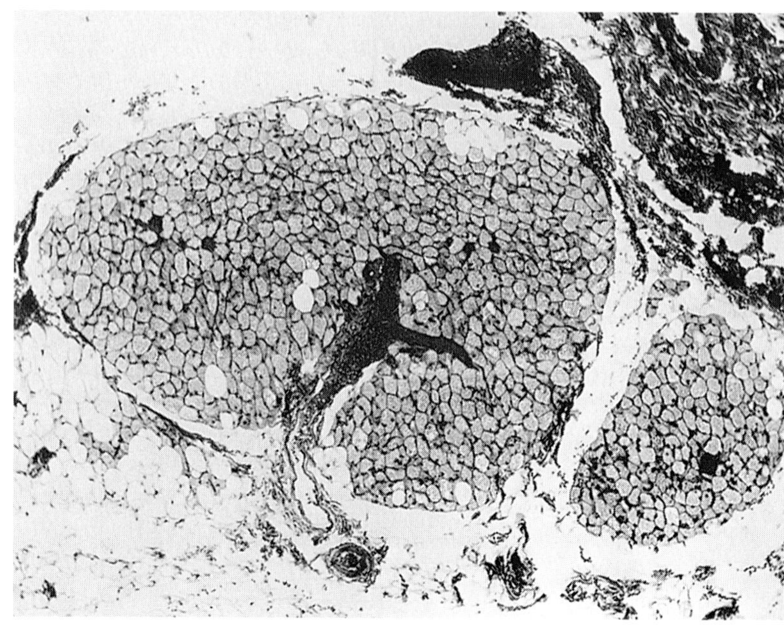

**FIGURE 16–3.** Brown fat from the neck region of a 1-year-old child. The cells are arranged in lobular aggregates and have a distinctly granular appearance.

mas.[2] The diagnostic utility of this antibody has yet to be proven.

## CLASSIFICATION OF BENIGN LIPOMATOUS TUMORS

It is widely assumed that benign lipomatous tumors represent a common group of neoplasms that cause few complaints or complications and present little diagnostic difficulty. This may be largely true for the ordinary subcutaneous lipoma, but it does not take into account the great variety of benign tumors and tumor-like lesions of adipose tissue that are well defined but often have received little attention in the medical literature.

The bulk of benign lipomatous tumors may be grouped into five categories, each of which may be further divided.

1. *Lipoma,* a tumor composed of mature fat, represents by far the most common mesenchymal neoplasm. It may be single or multiple and may occur as a superficial (subcutaneous) or deep-seated tumor.
2. *Variants of lipoma* are much less common and differ from ordinary lipoma by a characteristic microscopic picture and specific clinical setting. This group is chiefly represented by angiolipoma, myolipoma, angiomyolipoma, myelolipoma, chondroid lipoma, spindle cell and pleomorphic lipoma, and benign lipoblastoma. "Atypical lipoma" is a term applied to superficial (subcutaneous) forms of well-differentiated liposarcoma. It is discussed in Chapter 17.
3. *Lipomatous tumors* or *hamartomatous lesions* arise from or are intimately associated with specific tissue other than adipose tissue. The main subdivisions of this group are angiomyolipoma, intramuscular and intermuscular lipoma, lipoma of the tendon sheath, neural fibrolipoma with and without macrodactyly (fibrolipomatous hamartoma), and lumbosacral lipoma.
4. *Infiltrating* or *diffuse neoplastic* or *nonneoplastic proliferations of mature fat* may cause compression of vital structures or may be confused with well-differentiated liposarcoma. This group is composed of six entities: diffuse lipomatosis, pelvic lipomatosis, symmetric lipomatosis (Madelung's disease), adiposis dolorosa (Dercum's disease), steroid lipomatosis, and nevus lipomatosus.
5. *Hibernoma* is a benign tumor of brown fat.

When describing these entities, we have made no attempt to distinguish between true neoplasms, hamartomatous processes, and localized overgrowth of fat, as it would be largely speculative and of little practical consequence. Cytogenetic data have contributed to our understanding of the pathogenesis of both benign and malignant lipomatous tumors. Although cytogenetic analysis is of limited diagnostic utility in this group of benign lipomatous tumors, the knowledge gained by such analyses has allowed a better understanding of how these lipomatous tumors are related to one another (Table 16–1).

## LIPOMA

Solitary lipomas, consisting entirely of mature fat, have stirred little interest in the past and have been

**TABLE 16–1 PRINCIPAL CHROMOSOMAL ABERRATIONS OF BENIGN LIPOMATOUS TUMORS**

| Tumor | Chromosomal Aberration |
|---|---|
| Lipoma (ordinary) | Translocations involving 12q13–15<br>Interstitial deletions of 13q<br>Rearrangements involving 6p21–23 |
| Angiolipoma | None |
| Spindle cell/pleomorphic lipoma | Loss of 16q13<br>Unbalanced 13q alterations |
| Lipoblastoma/lipoblastomatosis | Translocations involving 8q11–13 |
| Hibernoma | Translocations involving 11q13<br>Translocations involving 10q22 |

largely ignored in the literature. This continued neglect is not surprising, considering that most lipomas grow insidiously and cause few problems other than those of a localized mass. Many lipomas remain unrecorded or are brought to the attention of a physician only if they reach a large size or cause cosmetic problems or complications because of their anatomic site. As a consequence, the reported incidence of lipoma is probably much lower than the actual incidence. Even if we consider only the recorded data, however, lipomas outnumber other benign or malignant soft tissue tumors by a considerable margin and undoubtedly represent the most common soft tissue tumor. This is true for the solitary subcutaneous lipoma and for lipomas in general, regardless of histologic type.

### Age and Gender Incidence

Lipoma is rare during the first two decades of life and usually makes its appearance when fat begins to accumulate in inactive individuals. Most become apparent in patients 40–60 years of age. When not excised, they persist for the remainder of life, although they hardly increase in size after the initial growth period. Statistics as to gender incidence vary, but most report a higher incidence in men.[66,74] There seems to be no difference in regard to race; and in the United States, Whites and African Americans are affected in proportion to their distribution in the general population.

### Localization

Two types of solitary lipoma can be distinguished. *Subcutaneous,* or *superficial, lipomas* are most common in the regions of the upper back and neck, shoulder, and abdomen, followed in frequency by the proximal portions of the extremities, chiefly the upper arms, buttocks, and upper thigh. They are seldom encountered in the face, hands, lower legs, or feet.[28,32,45]

*Deep lipomas* are rare in comparison. They are often detected at a relatively late stage of development and consequently tend to be larger than more superficial lipomas. Numerous sites may be involved. When in the extremities they often arise from the subfascial tissues of the hands and feet, where they may be mistaken for ganglion cysts.[24,58] They may also arise from juxtaarticular regions or the periosteum *(parosteal lipoma)*,[25,31,39,57] sometimes causing nerve compression, erosion of bone, or focal cortical hyperostosis. There may also be secondary bone and cartilage formation in the tumor[80] or an association with congenital skeletal anomalies.[70] Deep lipomas in the region of the head occur chiefly in the forehead and scalp[42]; those in the trunk are found principally in the thorax and mediastinum,[27,41,44,59,73] chest wall and pleura,[54] pelvis and retroperitoneum,[21,29] and paratesticular region.[23,33]

In the gastrointestinal tract, lipomas are mainly seen in the submucosa and subserosa of the small and large intestines, often as an incidental finding at endoscopy.[26,38,78] They are solitary or multiple and present as a sessile or pedunculated mass; sometimes they are associated with ulceration and bleeding, intussusception, Crohn's disease, or malignancy.[72,78]

Deep or subfascial lipomas tend to be less well circumscribed than superficial ones, and their contours are usually determined by the space they occupy. Intrathoracic lipomas, for instance, may extend from the upper mediastinum, neck, or subpleural region *(cervicomediastinal lipoma)* into the subcutis of the chest wall, sometimes assuming an hourglass configuration *(transmural lipoma)*. Deep-seated lipomas of the hand or wrist form irregular masses with multiple processes underneath fascia or aponeurosis; they may attain a large size and, on rare occasions, extend from the palm to the dorsal surface of the hand. These tumors must be distinguished from lipomas growing in the tendon sheath *(endovaginal lipomas)* and those involving major nerves in the regions of the hand and wrist *(neural fibrolipomas)*, which usually occur in young patients.

There are also rare lipoma-like fatty proliferations in the region of the umbilicus and inguinal ring *(hernial lipoma)* that may be associated with direct or indirect hernias or merely simulate a hernia clinically. A similar overgrowth of fat arising from surgical scars has been termed *incisional lipoma.*

### Clinical Findings

The usual clinical history of lipoma is that of an asymptomatic, slow-growing, round or discoid mass with a soft or doughy consistency. The fact that the mass hardens after application of ice has been used by some clinicians as a diagnostic criterion. There is usually good mobility, with dimpling of the skin on movement. Pain is rare with ordinary lipomas; when it occurs it is a late symptom generally confined to large angiolipomas or lipomas that compress peripheral nerves. Rarely nerve compression leads to sensory and motor disturbances and carpal or tarsal tunnel syndrome.[28] Lipomas are more common in obese persons and often increase in size during a period of rapid weight gain. In contrast, severe weight loss in cachectic patients or during periods of prolonged starvation rarely affects the size of lipoma, suggesting that the fatty tissue of lipomas (or liposarcomas) is largely unavailable for general metabolism.

Deep or subfascial lipomas may cause a variety of symptoms, depending on their site and size. The symptoms range from a feeling of fullness and discomfort on motion and, rarely, restriction of movement with lipomas of the hand to dyspnea or palpitation with mediastinal tumors. Although some benign lipomatous tumors have been described in the retroperitoneum, most reported in the early literature probably represent well-differentiated liposarcomas rather than lipomas.

Radiographs are most helpful for diagnosis; lipomas present as globular radiolucent masses clearly outlined by the greater density of the surrounding tissue. On computed tomography (CT) scans lipomas have the appearance of subcutaneous fat and, like fat, have a much more uniform density than liposarcomas. On magnetic resonance imaging (MRI) both benign and malignant lipomatous tumors exhibit a high signal intensity on T1-weighted images. Furthermore, MRI does not permit their distinction from old hematomas.[43,56]

## Gross Findings

Subcutaneous lipoma usually manifests as a soft, well-circumscribed, thinly encapsulated, rounded mass varying in size from a few millimeters to 5 cm or more (median 3 cm); lipomas larger than 10 cm are rare (Fig. 16–4). On cross section the lipoma is pale yellow to orange and has a uniform greasy surface and an irregular lobular pattern (Fig. 16–5A). Lipomas of deeper structures vary much more in shape, but they also tend to be well delineated from the surrounding tissues by a thin capsule. Focal discoloration caused by hemorrhage or fat necrosis occurs, but it is much less common than in liposarcomas. Chemical analysis of normal adipose tissue and lipomas has revealed quantitative rather than qualitative differences, such as increased lipoprotein lipase, indicating merely more lipid synthesis and triglyceride accumulation than mobilization.[60]

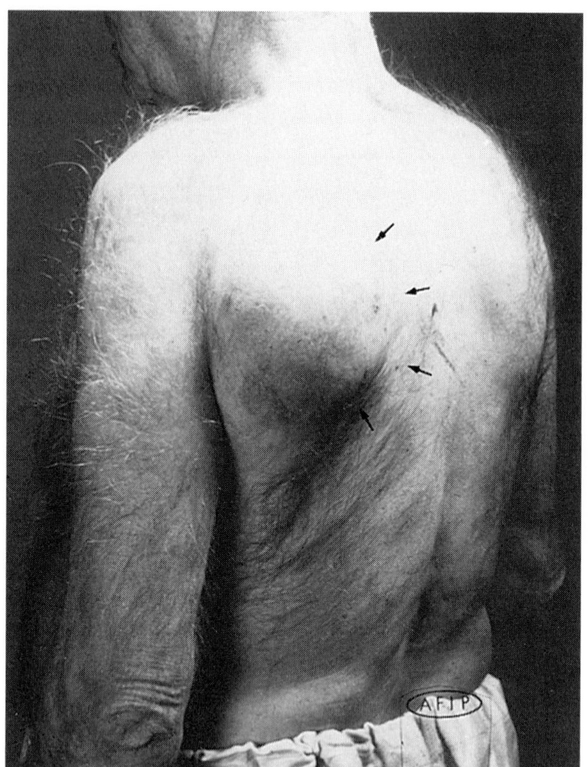


**FIGURE 16–4.** Large lipoma (arrows) of the left shoulder region in a 65-year-old man.

## Microscopic Findings

Lipomas differ little in microscopic appearance from the surrounding fat. Like fat they are composed of mature fat cells, but the cells vary slightly in size and shape and are somewhat larger, measuring up to 200 μm in diameter (Fig. 16–5B) The nuclei are fairly uniform, but the presence of a rare cell with mild atypia is still compatible with a benign diagnosis. Subcutaneous lipomas are usually thinly encapsulated and have distinct lobular patterns. Deep-seated lipomas have a more irregular configuration, largely depending on the site of origin. All are well vascularized, but under normal conditions the vascular network is compressed by the distended lipocytes and is not clearly discernible. The rich vascularity of these tumors becomes apparent in atrophic lipomas in which the markedly reduced volume of the lipocytes reveals the intricate vascular network in the interstitial spaces.

Lipomas are occasionally altered by the admixture of other mesenchymal elements that comprise an intrinsic part of the tumor. The most common of these elements is fibrous connective tissue, which is often hyalinized and may or may not be associated with the capsule or the fibrous septa. Lipomas with these features are often classified as *fibrolipomas*.[68] *Sclerotic*

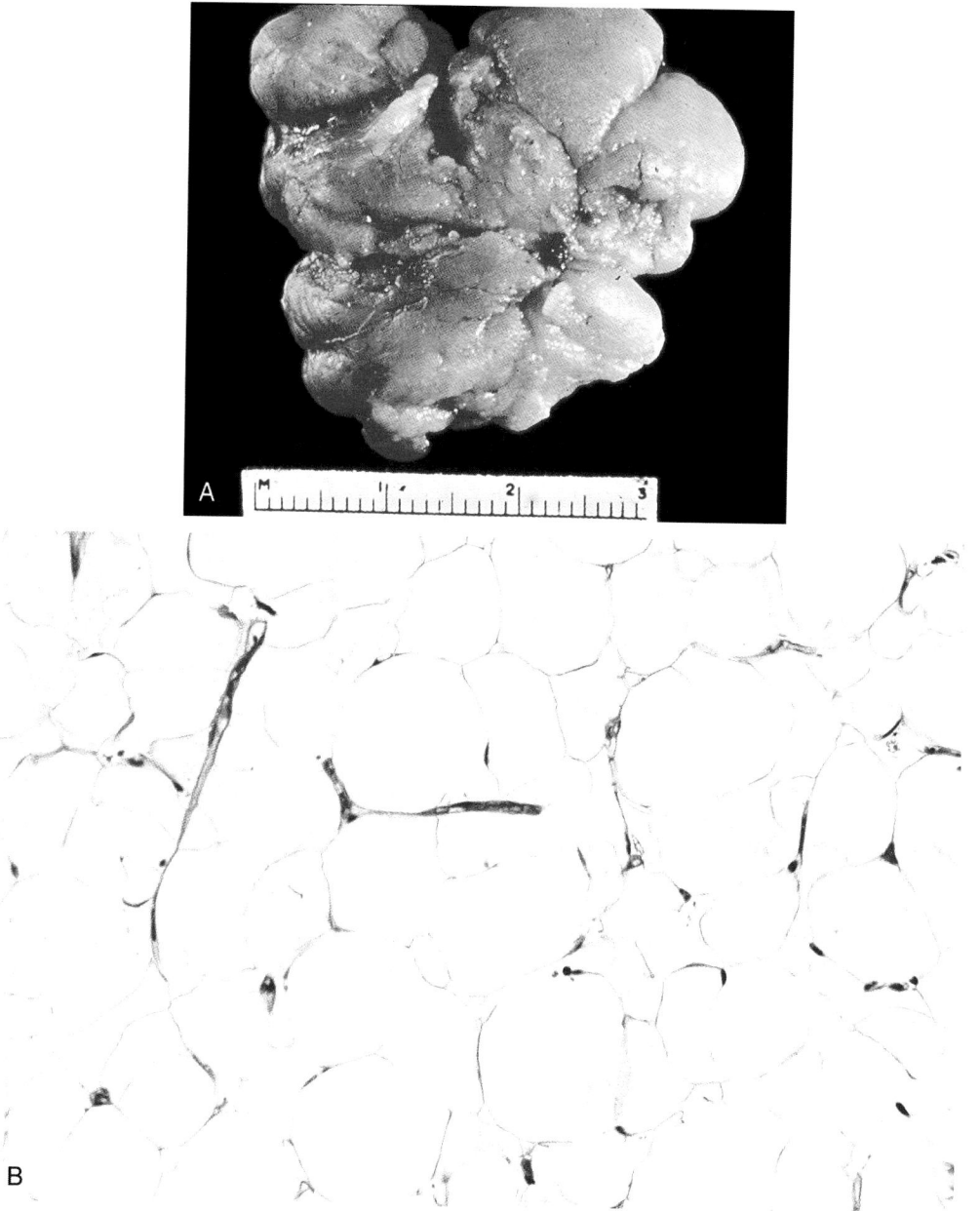

**FIGURE 16–5.** (**A**) Lipoma showing a distinct multilobular pattern and uniform yellow color. (**B**) Lipoma consisting throughout of mature fat cells has only a slight variation in cellular size and shape.

*lipomas* have a predilection to occur on the scalp or hands of young men and are composed predominantly of sclerotic fibrous tissue with only focal lipocytic areas.[82] In *myxolipomas* portions of the tumor are replaced by mucoid substances that stain well with alcian blue and are removed or depolymerized by prior treatment of the sections with testicular hyaluronidase (Fig. 16–6).[77] Some of these lesions have an abundance of thin- and thick-walled blood vessels and have been termed *vascular myxolipoma* or *angiomyxolipoma*.[48] Distinction of these tumors from *myxomas* and *myxoid liposarcomas* may be difficult. In general, however, the presence of transitional zones between fat and myxoid areas helps rule out myxoma, and the absence of lipoblasts and a plexiform capillary pattern militates against myxoid liposarcoma. Atypical vacuolated cells containing mucoid material are occasionally seen in myxolipomas and angiomyxolipomas; but unlike neoplastic lipoblasts, these cells lack hyperchromatic nuclei and distinctly outlined lipid droplets within the cytoplasm. Like normal fat cells, the cytoplasmic rim of the fat cells of lipoma is immunoreactive for S-100 protein.

Cartilaginous or osseous metaplasia (*chondrolipoma, osteolipoma*) is rare and is mainly encountered in lipomas of large size and long duration.[37,47] Some pathologists prefer to classify these variants of lipoma as *benign mesenchymomas. Myolipoma,* which has a distinct smooth muscle component, and *chondroid lipoma,* a tumor displaying features of both chondrolipoma and hibernoma, are discussed below as separate entities.

Secondary changes occur occasionally as the result of impaired blood supply or traumatic injury. Prolonged ischemia may lead to infarction, hemorrhage, and calcification[63] and may terminate in cyst-like changes. Similarly, infection or trauma may cause fat necrosis and local liquefaction of fat, a process marked by phagocytic activity and formation of lipid cysts. Characteristically, nests of foamy macrophages are found in the intercellular spaces or around lipocytes that have been ruptured or traumatized (Fig. 16–7). This process is sometimes accompanied by multinucleated giant cells and scattered inflammatory elements, chiefly lymphocytes or plasma cells. As for lipogranuloma, hyaline fibrosis and calcification may become prominent features during the late stages of this process. Rarely there is a nodular pattern caused by encapsulation of the necrotic lobules of fat. In some cases cystic spaces are lined by an eosinophilic, hyaline membrane with pseudopapillary luminal projections (membranous fat necrosis).[62]

### Ultrastructure

Like normal white fat, lipomas are composed of mature lipocytes with a single centrally positioned large lipid vacuole and peripherally placed cytoplasm and

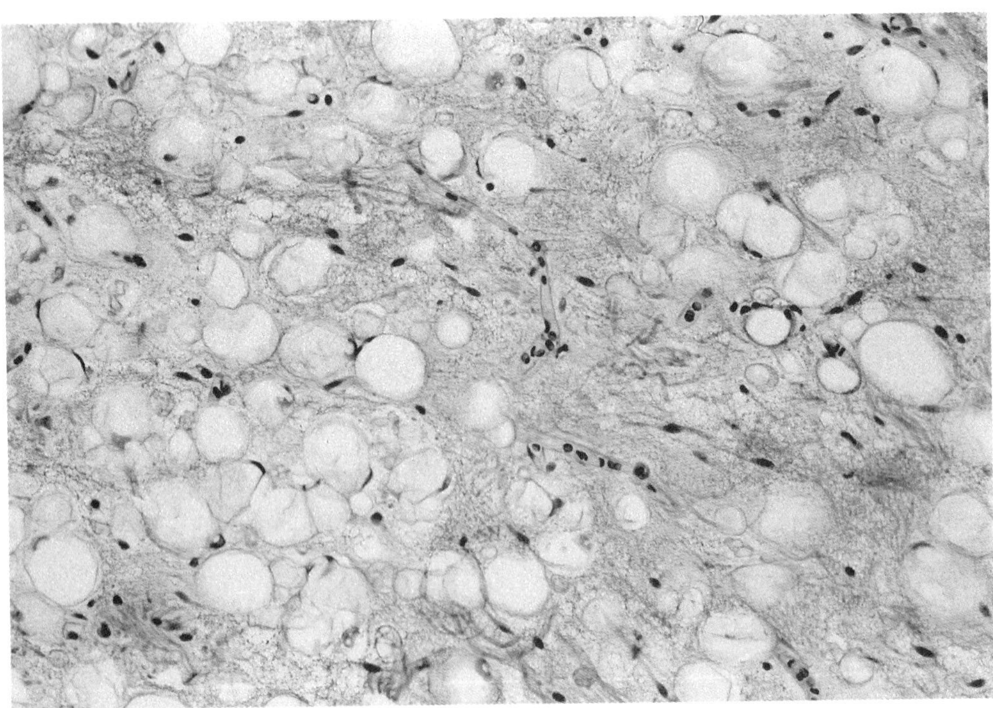

**FIGURE 16–6.** Lipoma with myxoid change.

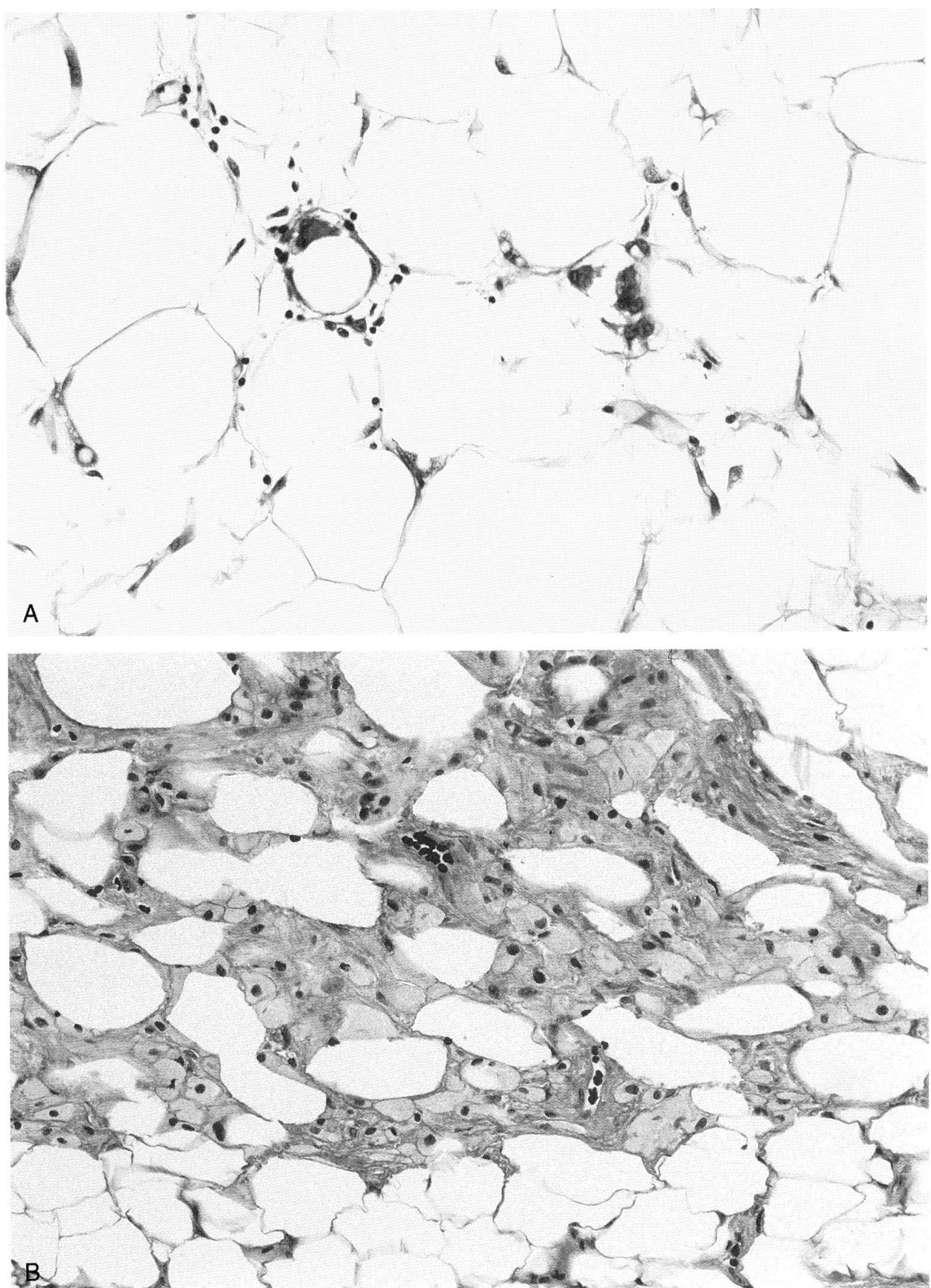


**FIGURE 16–7.** (**A**) Lipoma with focal fat necrosis with rare macrophage nuclei and vacuolated cytoplasm between mature fat cells. (**B**) Lipoma with a more extensive area of fat necrosis. Numerous macrophage nuclei with granular cytoplasm are seen between mature adipocytes.

*Illustration continued on following page*

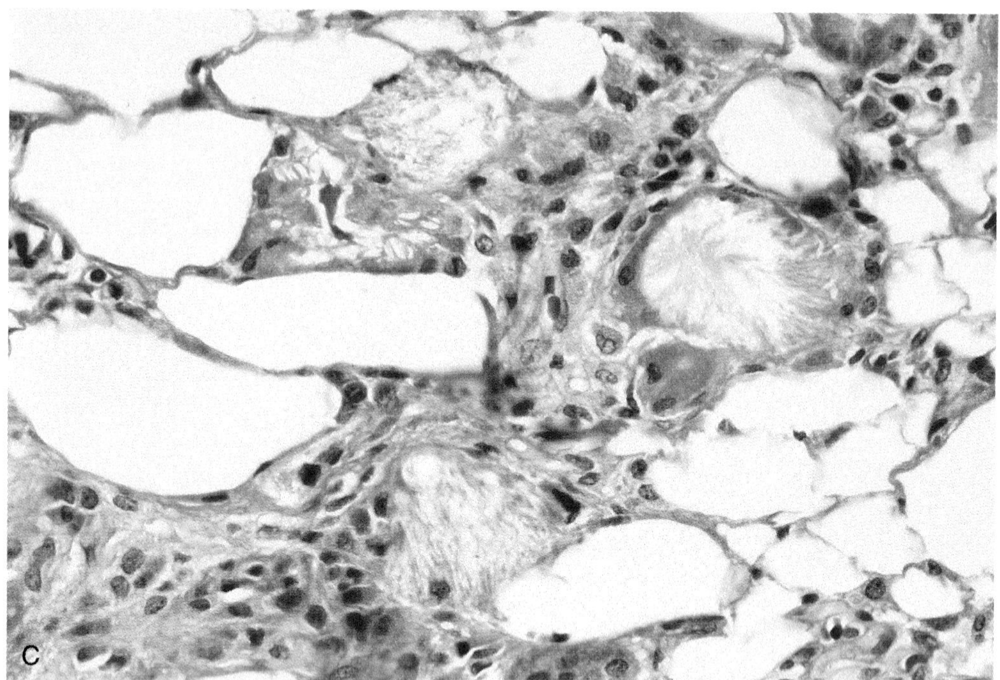

**FIGURE 16–7** *(Continued).* **(C)** Rare example of fat necrosis in a newborn infant.

nucleus. The cytoplasm consists of smooth membrane-bound vesicles, ribosomes, and round or oval mitochondria, together with small amounts of glycogen, rough endoplasmic reticulum, and an inconspicuous Golgi apparatus. The nuclei display peripheral condensation of chromatin and prominent nucleoli. There are also numerous pinocytotic vesicles and a well developed basal lamina.[40] Small spindle cells with occasional lipid vacuoles are often situated along the interstitial capillaries and are probably potential precursors of adipocytes (preadipocytes).[74]

## Behavior and Treatment

Lipomas are benign. They may recur locally, but following local excision the recurrence rate is less than 5% for all tumors.[81] Malignant changes in a lipoma are rare, and only a few cases have been reported in the literature. It is likely, however, that some of them are pleomorphic lipomas, and others are well-differentiated liposarcomas in which the malignant characteristics were absent or missed when the tumor was first examined. Deep lipomas have a greater tendency to recur, presumably because of the difficulty with complete surgical removal.

## Etiologic Factors

Aside from the relatively small number of patients in whom an increased familial incidence of lipomas can be demonstrated, little is known about the pathogenesis of these tumors. Certainly lipomas are more common in obese than in slender persons and perhaps as a consequence are more frequently encountered in patients older than 45 years. An increased incidence of lipomas is also claimed for diabetic patients and those with elevated serum cholesterol. It is doubtful, however, whether the stated association of lipoma with rheumatoid arthritis or with a family history of cancer is more than a mere coincidence.[74]

Trauma or irradiation may lead to overgrowth of fat indistinguishable from a lipoma. In particular, such lesions, often exceeding 10 cm in diameter, have been observed to develop secondary to blunt, bruising injuries, often preceded by a large hematoma.[53,61,69]

Clonal cytogenetic abnormalities have been identified in 50–80% of solitary lipomas.[34,35,49–51,76,79] The most common aberration involves translocations between 12q13–15 and various other chromosomes, most commonly chromosomes 1, 2, 3, and 21.[65] The breakpoint on chromosome 12 has been shown to be distinct from that found in myxoid liposarcoma (12q13.3).[55] The *HMGI-C* gene, which has been mapped to 12q15, is a member of the high mobility group protein gene family[22,36,71] and has been implicated as playing a central role in the development of lipomas. Other less common cytogenetic abnormalities in lipomas include interstitial deletions of 13q[51,76] and translocations involving chromosome 6p21–

23.[51,67] Supernumerary ring or giant marker chromosomes derived from 12q13–15 are found in virtually all atypical lipomas/well-differentiated liposarcomas, including tumors with few atypical cells.[30,52,64,75] Rosai et al. argued that finding ring or giant marker chromosomes in a well-differentiated lipomatous tumor helps distinguish atypical lipomas/well-differentiated liposarcomas with few atypical cells from ordinary lipoma.[64]

## MULTIPLE LIPOMAS

Approximately 5–8% of all patients with lipomas have multiple tumors that are indistinguishable grossly and microscopically from solitary lipomas.[83] The term "lipomatosis" has been used to describe this lesion, but we prefer to use this name for a diffuse neoplastic proliferation of fat.

Multiple lipomas vary in number from a few to several hundred lesions, and they occur predominantly in the upper half of the body, with a predilection for the back, shoulder, and upper arms (Fig. 16–8). Not infrequently the lipomas are arranged in a symmetric distribution, with a slight predilection for the extensor surfaces of the extremities. They are about three times as common in men as in women.[74] Most have their onset during the fifth and sixth decades, although occasional lesions appear as early as puberty. Hyperlipidemia with high serum levels of cholesterol was reported in some cases.[92,94] Local excision and suction lipectomy have been recommended as the treatments of choice.[90]

There is a definite hereditary trait in about one-third of patients with this condition (*familial multiple lipomas*).[96] For instance, in one of our cases multiple lipomas were observed in members of the same family during three successive generations. In most reports both males and females are affected, suggesting simple dominant inheritance.[74,95]

There is no evidence of any chemical differences in the composition of solitary and multiple lipomas. Associated hypercholesterolemia, however, was noted repeatedly.[92] An increased incidence of multiple lipomas has also been reported in diabetic patients at the site of insulin injections,[97] in patients with psoriasis and arthritis,[88] and during pregnancy.[87] According to our material, myocardial infarction is slightly more common in patients with solitary or multiple lipomas, but it may be related to the age incidence and male predominance of these tumors.

The question of a relation between multiple lipomas and neurofibromatosis has been raised repeatedly in the literature, but to our knowledge there is no convincing proof of this association, including Alsberg's[84] much cited case of "neurolipoma." In fact, given the frequency of lipomas and the relative frequency of neurofibromatosis, these entities probably occur together fortuitously.

There are several syndromes with multiple lipomatous lesions: *Bannayan-Zonana syndrome* is characterized by the congenital association of multiple lipomas (including lipomatosis of the thoracic and abdominal cavity in some cases), hemangiomas, and macrocephaly.[85,86,99] *Cowden syndrome* consists of multiple lipomas and hemangiomas associated with goiter and lichenoid, papular, and papillomatous lesions of the skin and mucosae.[91,93,98] *Frohlich syndrome* is defined by multiple lipomas, obesity, and sexual infantilism. *Proteus syndrome* is marked by multiple lipomatous lesions, including pelvic lipomatosis, fibroplasia of the

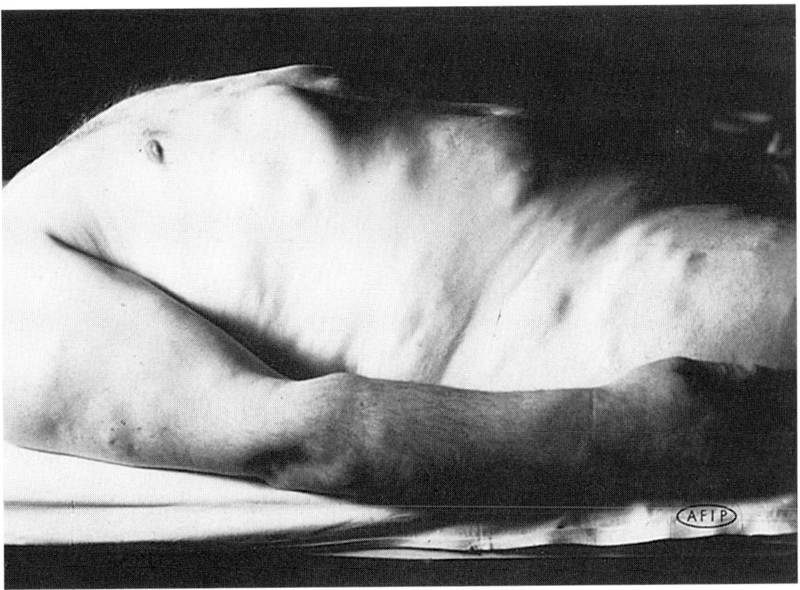


**FIGURE 16–8.** Patient with multiple lipomas affecting the arm, trunk, and thigh.

feet and hands, skeletal hypertrophy, exostoses and scoliosis, and various pigmented lesions of the skin.[89]

## ANGIOLIPOMA

Angiolipoma occurs chiefly as a subcutaneous nodule in young adults, often making its first appearance when the patient is in the late teens or early twenties; it is rare in children and, unlike solitary or multiple subcutaneous lipomas, in patients older than 50 years. The forearm is by far the most common site, and almost two-thirds of all angiolipomas are found in this location. Next in frequency are the trunk and upper arm. Like all lipomas it seldom occurs in the face, scalp, hands, and feet. Spinal angiolipoma is a specific entity that should be distinguished from cutaneous angiolipoma.[116] Rare tumors have also been reported in the stomach,[106,113] bone,[112] and cranium.[114]

Multiple angiolipomas are much more common than solitary ones and account for about two-thirds of all angiolipoma.[105] Belcher et al.,[100] for example, reported a 31-year-old man who developed no fewer than 204 angiolipomas over a 15-year period.

Characteristically, angiolipomas are tender to painful (often only on touch or palpation) particularly during the initial growth period; frequently pain becomes less severe or ceases entirely when the tumor reaches its final size, which is rarely more than 2 cm. There seems to be no correlation between the degree of vascularity and the occurrence or intensity of pain,[102] nor is the pain intensified by heat, cold, or venous occlusion. Increased familial incidence has been recorded; but as with ordinary lipomas, familial incidence does not exceed 5% of all cases.[104,109] Angiolipomas have also been described as occurring as part of unusual syndromes,[101,103,119,120] although there is little evidence that the tumors reported in these cases are true angiolipomas. Trauma has been implicated as a possible contributing or causative factor.[117]

At operation angiolipomas are always located in the subcutis, where they present as encapsulated yellow nodules with a more or less pronounced reddish tinge (Fig. 16–9). Microscopy reveals these nodules to consist of mature fat cells separated by a branching network of small vessels (Fig. 16–10); the proportion of fatty tissue and vascular channels varies, but usually the vascularity is slightly more prominent in the subcapsular areas (Fig. 16–11). Late forms of this tumor frequently undergo perivascular and interstitial fibrosis. Characteristically, the vascular channels contain fibrin thrombi (Fig. 16–12), a feature that is absent in ordinary lipomas.[102] Dixon and McGregor[102] demonstrated fluorescein-labeled antihuman fibrinogen in the thrombi and, to a lesser degree, in the surrounding endothelial cells. Mast cells are often conspicuous in angiolipomas, another feature that distinguishes this tumor from the usual lipoma. Some tumors are highly cellular and composed almost entirely of vascular channels (cellular angiolipoma) (Fig. 16–13).[107,108,121]

Ultrastructurally, the angiolipoma consists of adipocytes and interspersed vascular structures lined by

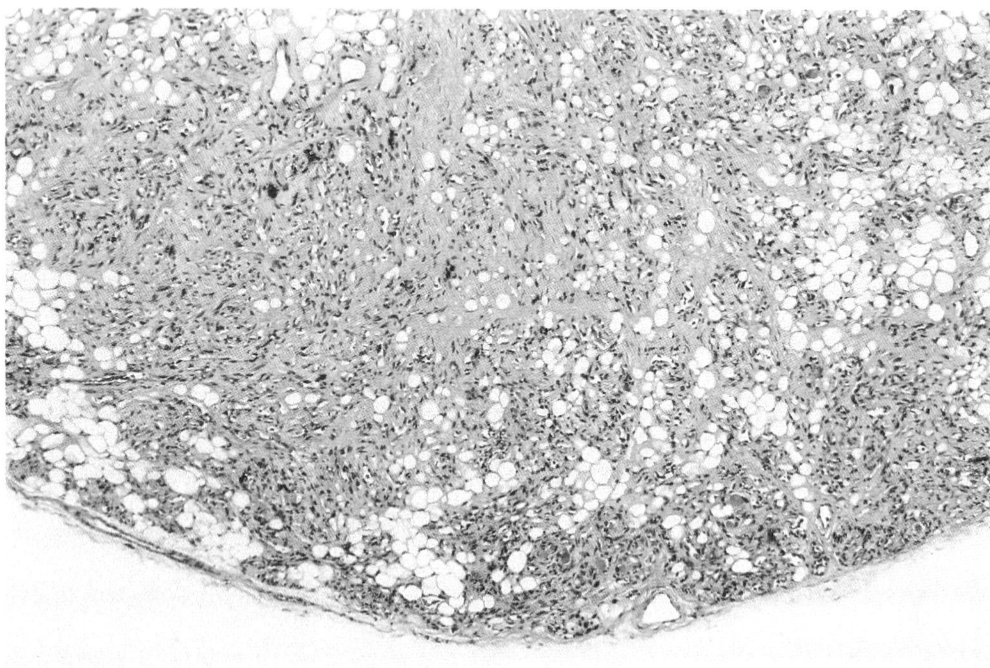

**FIGURE 16–9.** Angiolipoma showing sharp circumscription and proliferation of numerous vascular channels between mature fat cells.

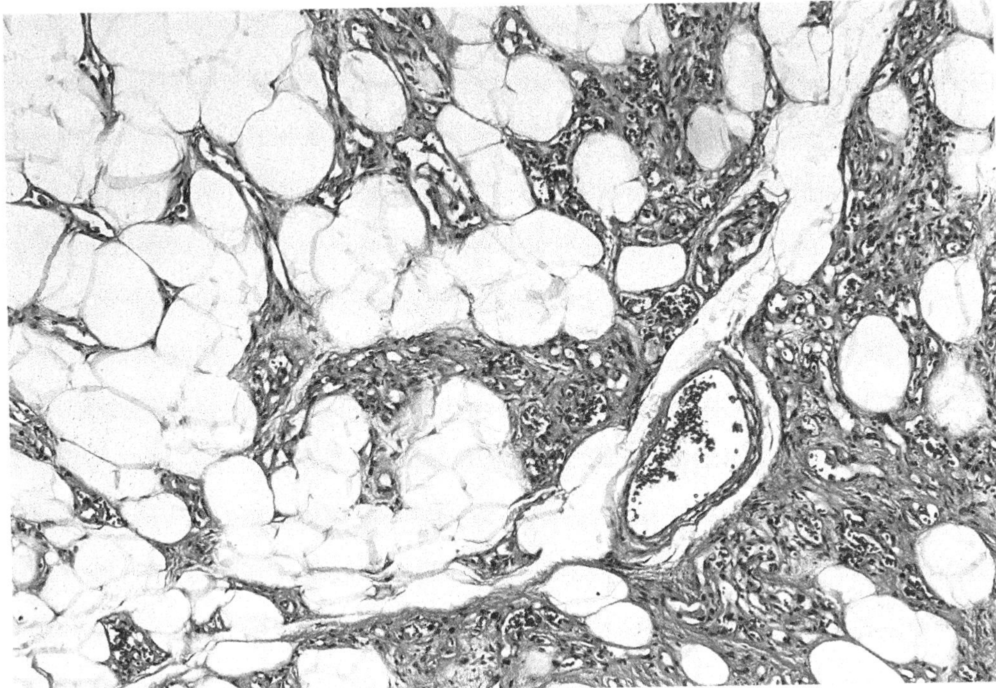

**FIGURE 16–10.** Angiolipoma consisting of a mixture of fat cells and narrow vascular channels. The vascularity is more prominent in the subcapsular areas.

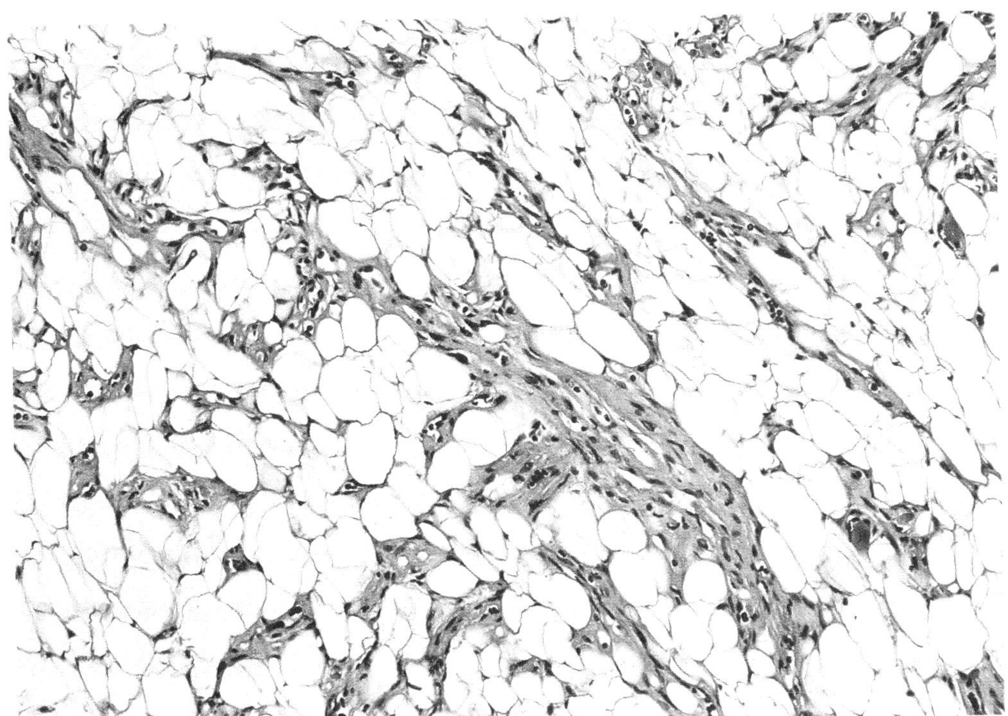

**FIGURE 16–11.** Angiolipoma with small vessels with an infiltrative-like appearance between mature fat cells.

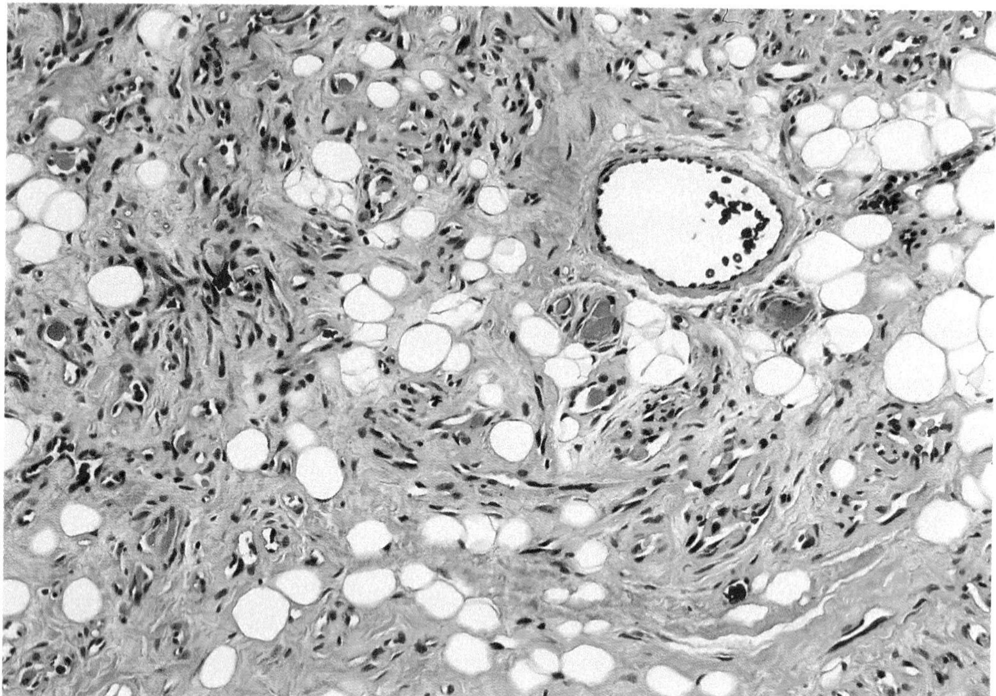

**FIGURE 16–12.** Angiolipoma with fibrin thrombi, a characteristic feature of this tumor.

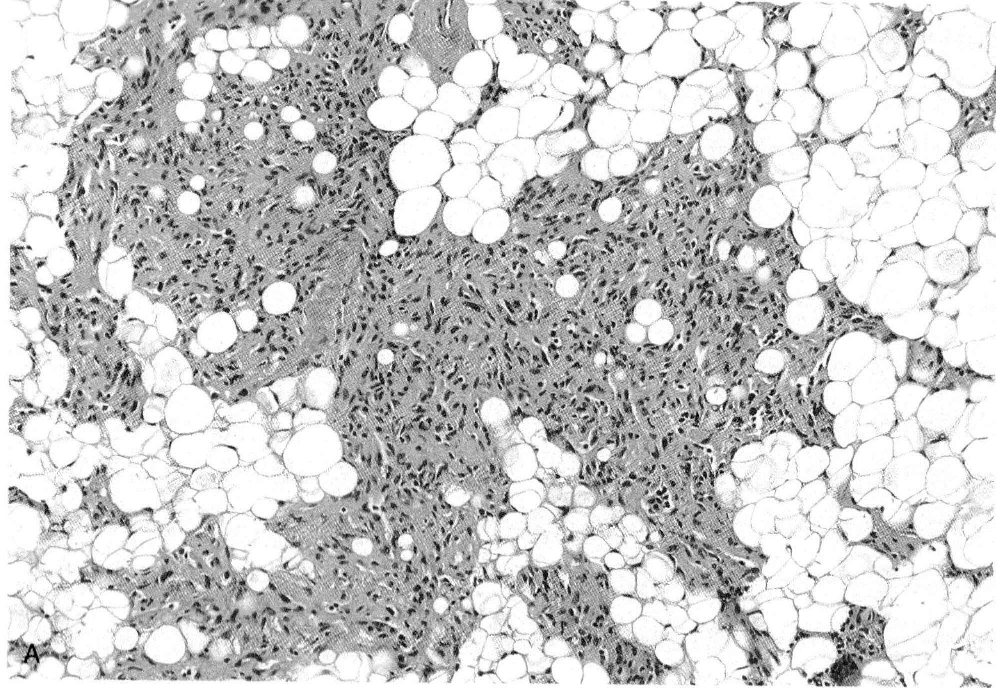


**FIGURE 16–13.** (**A**) Low-power appearance of an angiolipoma with increased cellularity.

*Illustration continued on opposite page*

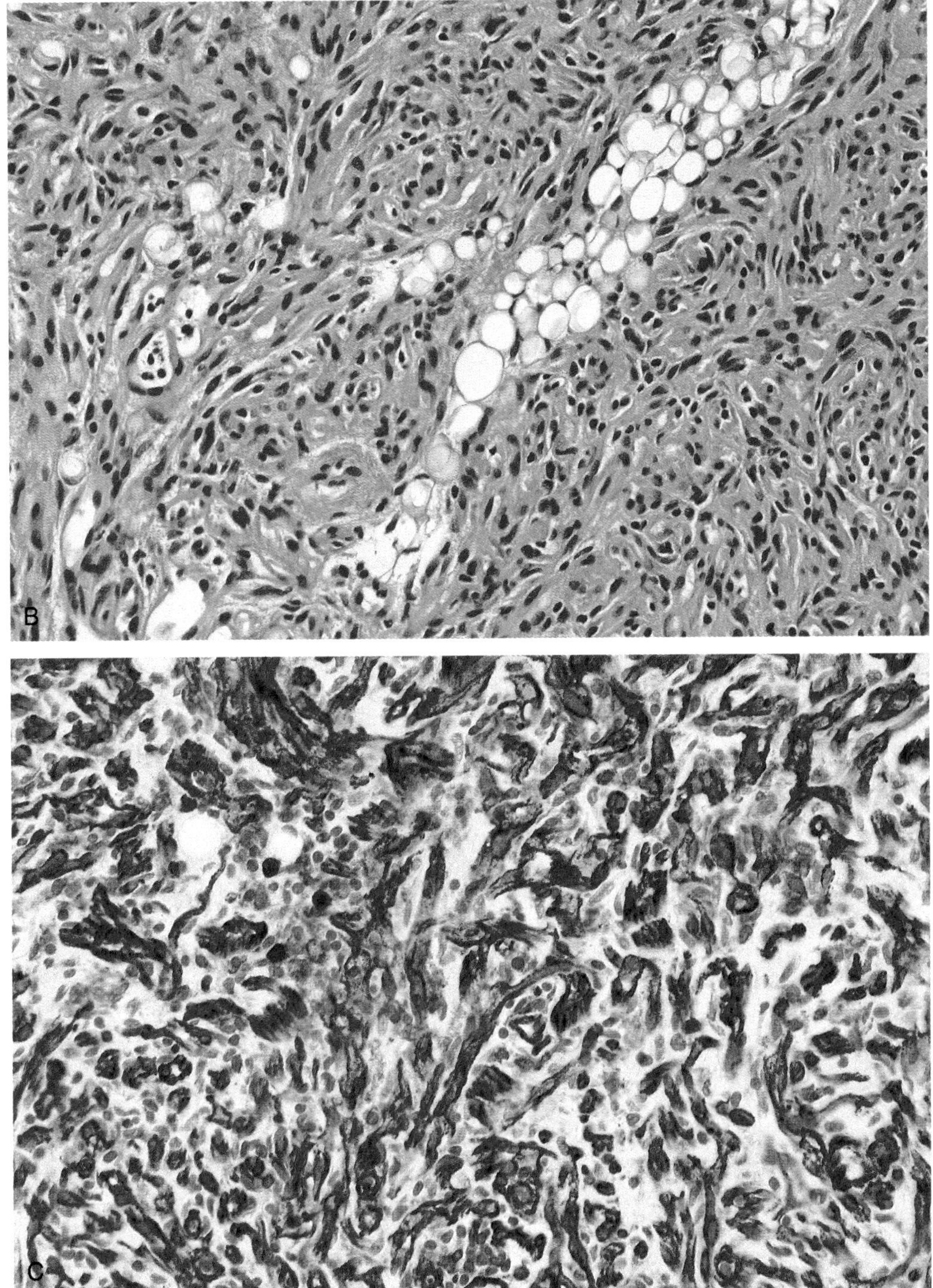


**FIGURE 16–13** *(Continued).* (**B**) High-power view of a cellular area of the angiolipoma, with virtually complete replacement by proliferating small vessels. Lesions of this type have been mistaken for Kaposi's sarcoma or spindle cell angiosarcoma. (**C**) Cellular angiolipoma stained for CD31, indicating that virtually all of the spindle cells are endothelial cells.

elongated endothelial cells with irregular finger-like extensions, basal lamina, and long tight junctions, and surrounded by pericytes. Compared with normal endothelium, Weibel-Palade bodies are scarce. The fibrin thrombi are associated with disrupted endothelial cells.

Unlike ordinary lipomas, which usually have karyotypic abnormalities involving 12q, 6p, and 13q, all karyotyped angiolipomas, except one, have been reported to show a normal karyotype.[111,118] The only exception was a single case reported by Mandahl et al., which showed t (X;2) as the sole anomaly.[111] Sciot et al. argued that the normal karyotype characteristic of this tumor is more in keeping with a nonneoplastic lesion that is reactive or hamartomatous.[118] Furthermore, because benign hemangiomas also usually have a normal karyotype, it raises the possibility that a vascular proliferation is the primary component of this tumor.

The differential diagnosis of this lesion in part depends on the density of vessels. The hypovascular lesions may be difficult to distinguish from *ordinary lipomas,* although the identification of microthrombi allows this distinction. *Intramuscular hemangioma,* a tumor that also has been reported under the name *cellular* or *infiltrating angiolipoma,*[110,115] may be difficult to distinguish from angiolipoma, although the latter can be correctly diagnosed if attention is paid to the encapsulation of the lesion, the presence of microthrombi, and the small size, multiplicity, and subcutaneous location of the lesion. The cellular angiolipoma may be difficult to distinguish from *Kaposi's sarcoma.* Like cellular angiolipoma, Kaposi's sarcoma can be found as multiple subcutaneous nodules in young men. However, Kaposi's sarcoma has slit-like vascular spaces and periodic acid-Schiff (PAS)-positive globules in the cytoplasm of some of the cells, and it lacks microthrombi.

Angiolipomas are benign. There is no evidence that these lesions ever undergo malignant transformation.

## MYOLIPOMA

Myolipoma is a rare variant of lipoma marked by the proliferation of fat and smooth muscle tissue. The tumor occurs in adults, most commonly during the fifth and sixth decades of life, with a predilection for women. Most commonly, myolipoma is found in the retroperitoneum, abdomen, pelvis, or abdominal wall, with only rare cases arising in the subcutaneous tissue.[122,126,127,130] Most patients present with a mass, but in some cases the tumor is found incidentally because of its propensity to arise in deep locations. Most of the reported tumors are large, with a median size of 17 cm.

Grossly, the tumors are completely or partially encapsulated with a glistening, yellow-white cut surface, although some have large areas of white or gray firm tissue with a whorled appearance. Histologically, myolipoma consists of a variable admixture of mature adipose tissue and bundles or sheets of well-differentiated smooth muscle, both of which lack nuclear atypia. Generally, the smooth muscle component is regularly interspersed with the adipose tissue, imparting a sieve-like appearance at low magnification. The smooth muscle bundles are typically arranged in short interweaving fascicles and are characterized by cytologically bland oval nuclei with longitudinally oriented eosinophilic fibrillar cytoplasm. The adipose tissue component is entirely mature, and lacks floret-like giant cells or lipoblasts. Some lesions have prominent stromal sclerosis and chronic inflammation. Medium-caliber arteries with thick muscular walls, characteristic of angiomyolipoma, are absent.

The smooth muscle element stains well with Masson trichrome preparation, and the cells are immunoreactive for smooth muscle actin and desmin (Figs. 16–14, 16–15). Electron microscopy confirms the coexistence of mature smooth muscle and adipocytic differentiation.

The differential diagnosis includes spindle cell lipoma, angiolipoma, angiomyolipoma, leiomyoma with fatty degeneration, and dedifferentiated liposarcoma. *Spindle cell lipoma* is composed of cytologically bland spindle-shaped cells that do not have smooth muscle differentiation. The spindle cells stain for CD34 but not for smooth muscle markers. Furthermore, spindle cell lipoma is rare in the retroperitoneum, abdomen, and pelvis. *Angiomyolipoma* often presents as a large retroperitoneal mass, as does myolipoma. It differs from myolipoma by the presence of medium-sized arteries with thick muscular walls, as well as HMB-45 epithelioid smooth muscle cells. Unlike angiomyolipoma, myolipoma is not associated with tuberous sclerosis. *Leiomyoma with fatty degeneration* lacks the regular distribution of fat that is present in myolipoma (Fig. 16–16). Furthermore, fatty degeneration of smooth muscle tumors of soft tissue is rare. Finally, *dedifferentiated liposarcoma* can be distinguished from myolipoma by the presence of atypical hyperchromatic cells in the adipocytic component and cytologic atypia with mitotic activity in the dedifferentiated component.

Myolipoma, despite its frequently large size and occurrence in deep soft tissue locations, is a benign neoplasm, with no reported recurrence or metastasis. Tumors of similar appearance have been described in the uterus and the soft tissues as "fibrolipoleiomyoma" or "lipoleiomyoma."[123–125,128,129]

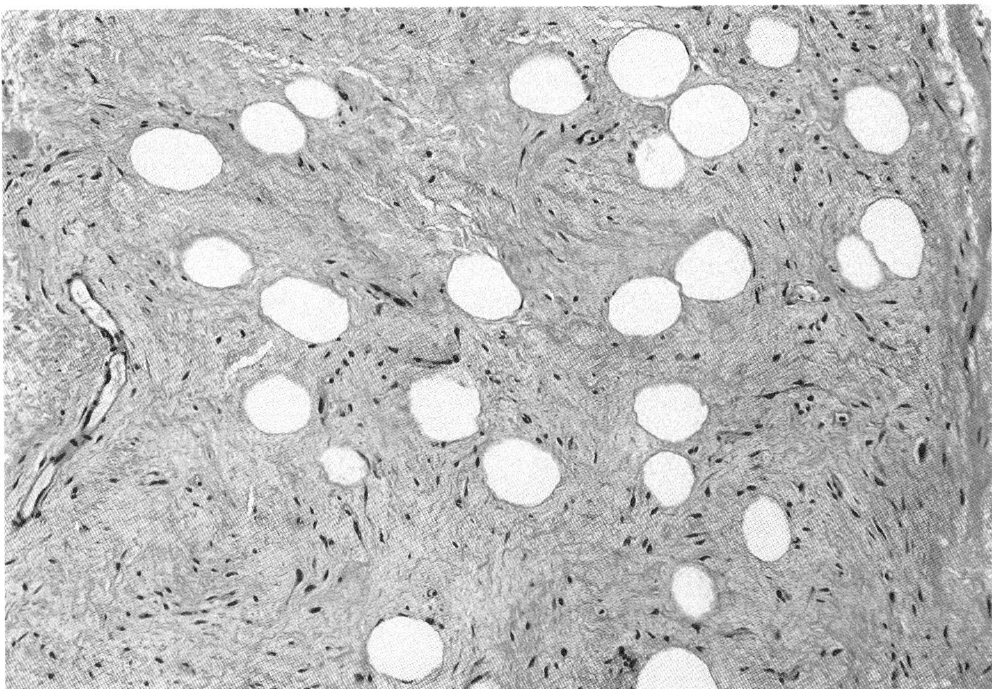

**FIGURE 16–14.** Myolipoma with a mixture of elongated eosinophilic smooth muscle cells and adipocytes.

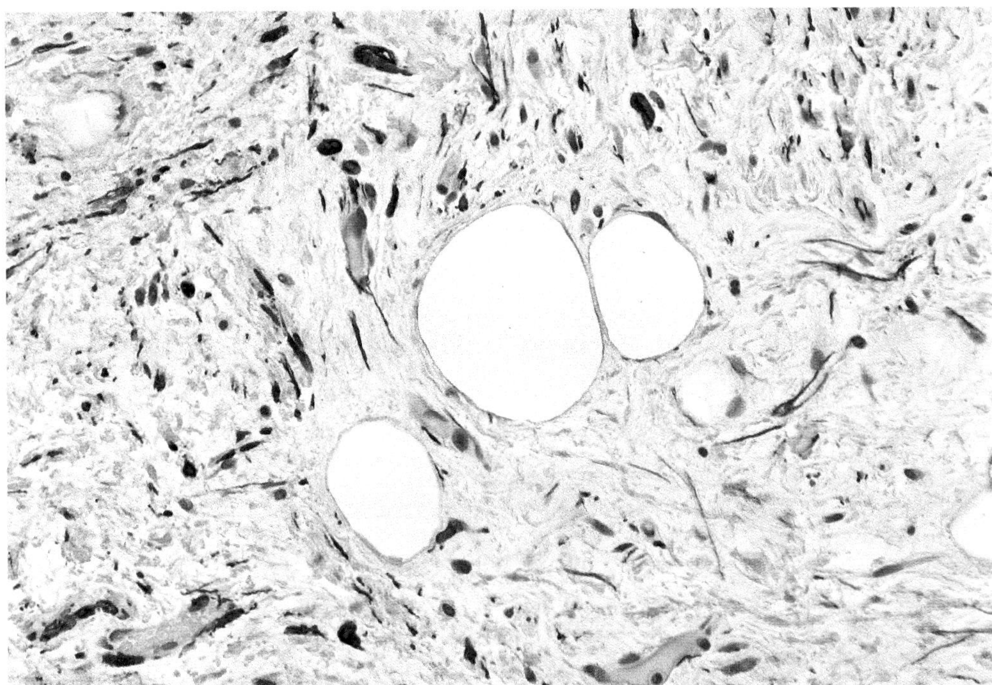

**FIGURE 16–15.** Myolipoma stained for desmin, showing that virtually all of the spindle cells are smooth muscle cells.

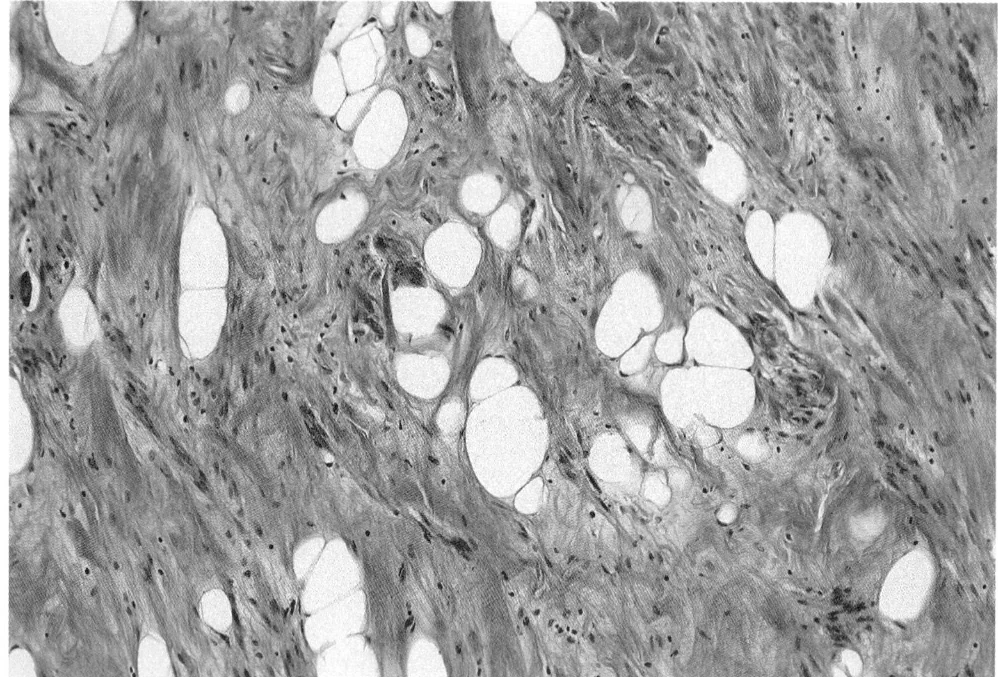

**FIGURE 16–16.** Uterine leiomyoma with fatty degeneration. This lesion is composed predominantly of mature smooth muscle cells, with only focal areas of mature fat cells. Fatty degeneration of smooth muscle tumors of soft tissue is rare.

## CHONDROID LIPOMA

The chondroid lipoma is a rare, benign fatty tumor found in the subcutaneous tissue or in deeper soft tissues predominantly in the limbs and limb girdles of adult women. Although it is clinically benign, it is another example of a pseudosarcoma, in that it may be mistaken for a myxoid liposarcoma or chondrosarcoma. Although first recognized as a distinct entity in 1993 by Meis and Enzinger,[135] it was probably first described by Chan et al. as an "extraskeletal chondroma with lipoblast-like cells."[131]

### Clinical Findings

Although the age range is broad, most patients are in the third or fourth decade of life, and there is a striking predilection for this tumor to occur in women. Most patients present with a slowly growing painless mass that is often present for several years prior to excision. Most commonly, this lesion arises in the proximal extremity or limb girdle followed by the leg, trunk, and head and neck region.[133] Rare cases also have been documented on the feet and hands.

### Pathologic Findings

Grossly, the tumor is well demarcated and often encapsulated with a yellow, white, or pink-tan cut surface. The tumor ranges in size from 1 to 11 cm (mean 4 cm). Some lesions are located entirely within the subcutaneous tissue, whereas others involve the superficial fascia or skeletal muscle, and some are entirely intramuscular.

Microscopically, chondroid lipoma has a lobular pattern and consists of strands and nests of round cells deposited in a myxochondroid or hyalinized fibrous background. Some cells have eosinophilic, granular cytoplasm, whereas others have lipid vacuoles closely simulating lipoblasts (Figs. 16–17, 16–18). Most commonly these multivacuolated cells predominate, although in some cases they may be less conspicuous. The cells are not pleomorphic, nor do they show significant mitotic activity. They stain positively with oil red O and PAS stains, consistent with the presence of intracytoplasmic neutral fat and glycogen. A mature adipose tissue component may be present only focally, or it may be the predominant component of the tumor. The extracellular matrix is often extensively myxoid and may be intermingled with zones of hyalinization and fibrin deposition reminiscent of serous atrophy of fat. The matrix is stained with alcian blue or colloidal iron stains and is usually partially or completely resistant to hyaluronidase digestion. Most lesions are vascular, with thick-walled blood vessels and cavernous thin-walled vascular spaces. Other changes include the presence of hemorrhage, hemosiderin deposition, focal calcification, and hyalinized zones.

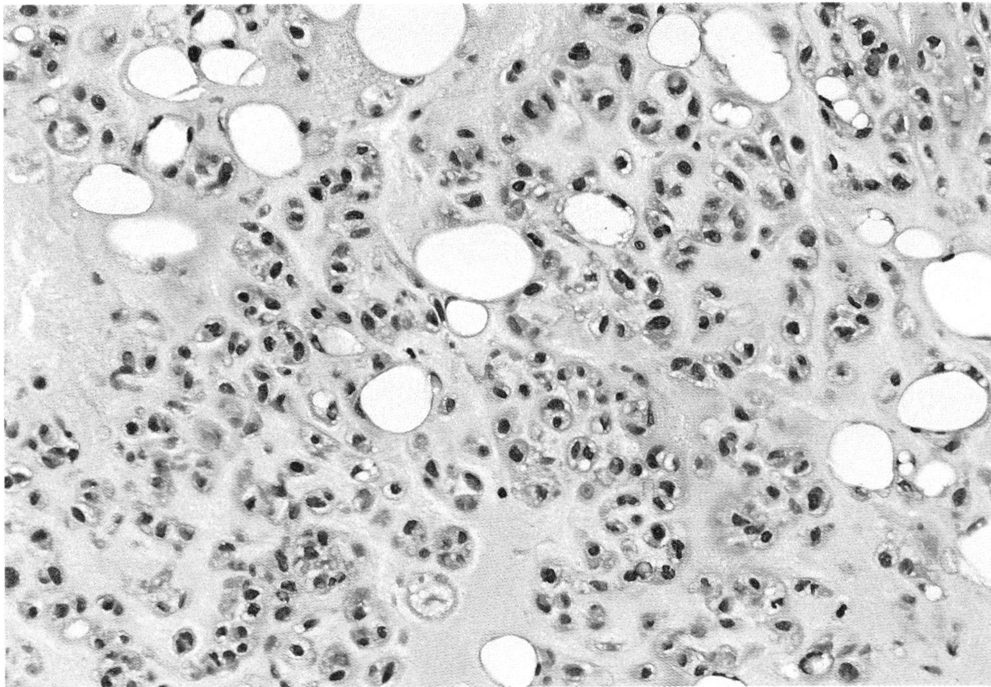

**FIGURE 16–17.** Chondroid lipoma showing nests of vacuolated cells deposited in a chondroid-like matrix associated with mature fat cells.

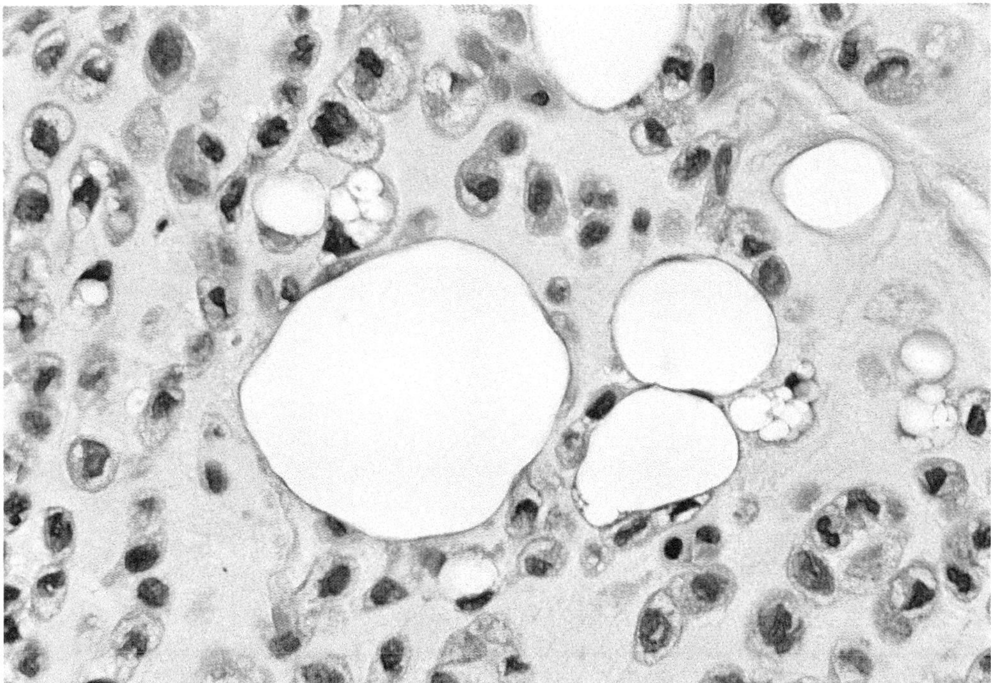

**FIGURE 16–18.** High-power view of a chondroid lipoma showing vacuolated cells associated with mature fat cells. Some of the vacuolated cells closely simulate lipoblasts.

By immunohistochemistry, the tumor cells stain positively for vimentin and S-100 protein, with focal staining for CD68 in the vacuolated tumor cells. Some lesions also show focal cytokeratin immunoreactivity, although immunostains for epithelial membrane antigen are negative. Ultrastructurally, the cells have abundant cytoplasmic glycogen and relatively little undilated rough endoplasmic reticulum. Peripherally located mitochondria and pinocytotic vesicles are also present.[134,136] According to Nielsen et al., the cells have the features of white adipocytes, without evidence of brown fat or true chondroblastic differentiation.[136] Others have found that the cells have ultrastructural features of embryonal fat and, to a lesser extent, embryonal cartilage[134,138] (Table 16–2).

### Differential Diagnosis

The differential diagnosis of chondroid lipoma is broad and includes myxoid liposarcoma, extraskeletal myxoid chondrosarcoma, soft tissue chondroma, and myoepithelial tumors. *Myxoid liposarcoma* may have hibernoma-like cells deposited in a myxoid matrix that on occasion show chondroid metaplasia. However, unlike chondroid lipoma, this tumor is characterized by a delicate, plexiform vascular pattern and true lipoblasts. *Extraskeletal myxoid chondrosarcoma* typically has fibrous septa that impart a distinct lobulated appearance. The chondroblasts of extraskeletal myxoid chondrosarcoma are more uniformly round or oval and have few if any intracytoplasmic vacuoles. *Soft tissue chondroma* occurs in the hands and feet and often contains multinucleated giant cells and true hyaline cartilage. *Myoepithelial tumors,* including mixed tumor, tend to be more superficially located and typically display epithelial areas. The myoepithelial cells may have cytoplasmic vacuoles, but they are usually not multivacuolated. Immunohistochemically, myoepithelial cells stain more uniformly for cytokeratins and are marked with antibodies to epithelial membrane antigen and actins.

### Discussion

Chondroid lipoma, despite its worrisome histologic appearance, is clearly benign; the lesion does not recur, nor does it metastasize. All available evidence supports a neoplastic, not a reactive, origin. Several cases of chondroid lipoma have been reported with t(11;16), both involving 11q13.[132,137] It is of interest that 11q13 aberrations have been reported in hibernomas,[488,490] raising the possibility of a histogenetic link between these two entities.

## SPINDLE CELL LIPOMA

Originally described by Enzinger and Harvey in 1975, spindle cell lipoma is a histologically distinct lesion characterized by replacement of mature fat by collagen-forming spindle cells.[148] Despite its cellularity, it is a benign lesion that is readily cured by local excision.

### Clinical Findings

The lesion occurs in a characteristic clinical setting, arising mainly in men 45–60 years of age in the subcutaneous tissue of the posterior neck, shoulder, and back (Fig. 16–19).[139,155] In general, the tumor is not encountered in adolescents or children, although

**TABLE 16–2 ULTRASTRUCTURAL FEATURES OF CHONDROID LIPOMA AND COMPARISON WITH EARLY LIPOBLASTS/PREADIPOCYTES AND CHONDROBLASTS/EARLY CHRONDROCYTES**

| Feature | Chondroid Lipoma | Early Lipoblasts/Preadipocytes | Chondroblasts/Early Chondrocytes |
|---|---|---|---|
| Nuclear shape | Irregular clefts | Smooth-scalloped | Multilobulated |
| Nucleoli | Small to medium size; central or peripheral | Small and central | Small and central |
| Rough endoplasmic reticulum | Sparse to abundant | Decreasing with maturation | Abundant |
| Mitochondria | Moderate | Moderate | Abundant |
| Intermediate filaments | Sparse | Bundles | Diffuse network |
| Lipid droplets | Many small, few large or single | Many small to few large | Few and small |
| Glycogen | Sparse to abundant | Little or none | Abundant |
| External lamina | None | Present | None |
| Pinocytotic vesicles | None to sparse | Prominent | None to few |
| Cell membrane | Smooth | Smooth | Spike-like projections |
| "Protruding bodies" | Prominent | None | None |
| Matrix | Abundant, cartilaginous | Myxoid early | Abundant, cartilaginous |

Modified from Kindblom L-G, Meis-Kindblom JM. Chondroid lipoma: an ultrastructural and immunohistochemical analysis with further observations regarding its differentiation. Hum Pathol 26:706, 1995.

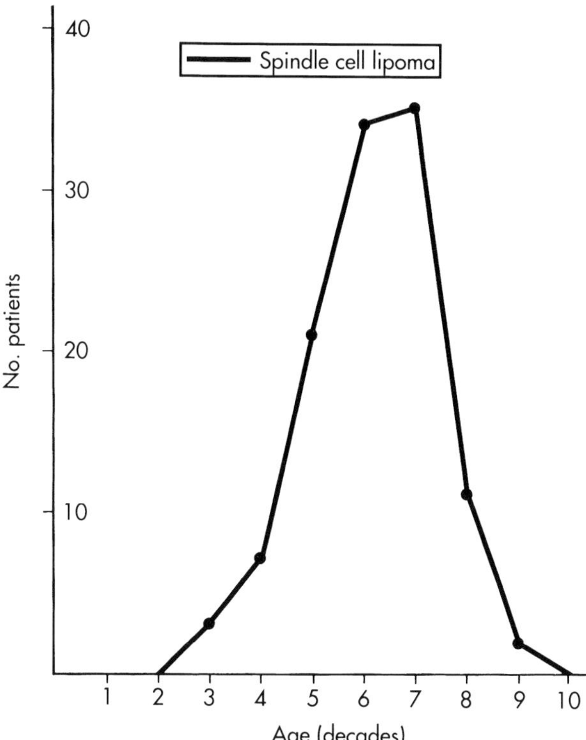


**FIGURE 16–19.** Age distribution of 114 patients with spindle cell lipoma ranges from 25 to 89 years (median 56 years). Of these patients, 91% were men.

there is one report of it arising in a 14-month-old girl.[146] There is a striking predilection for men. In the study from the Armed Forces Institute of Pathology (AFIP), 91% of the patients were men.[148] Although most tumors arise in the neck, shoulders, or back, the tumor has also been described in unusual sites, including the oral cavity,[173] larynx,[162] bronchus,[160] breast,[169] orbit,[142] and extremities.[152] Like ordinary lipomas, it manifests as a slowly growing solitary, circumscribed or encapsulated, painless, firm nodule in the subcutaneous tissue; and it is often present for years prior to excision. Rare cases involve the dermis or have predominantly dermal involvement[176], others involve the superficial skeletal muscle or are located exclusively in an intramuscular location.[139] Multiple lesions are rare.[150,158] Fanburg-Smith et al. reported 18 patients with multiple spindle cell lipomas, including seven familial cases.[150] Most patients present with the initial tumors on the posterior neck or back, with subsequent lesions developing bilaterally on the upper neck, shoulders, arms, chest, and then axillae; spread is in a predominantly caudal direction.

## Pathologic Findings

Grossly, the nodule resembles a lipoma except for gray-white gelatinous foci, representing the areas of spindle cell proliferation (Fig. 16–20). Although some tumors are large (up to 14 cm), most are 3–5 cm. The tumor is usually well circumscribed and easily distinguished from the surrounding subcutaneous tissue (Fig. 16–21). Rare tumors have a plexiform architecture and are composed of multiple small nodules separated by collagen.[176]

Microscopically, spindle cell lipomas vary in appearance depending on the relative amounts of mature fat and spindle cells. Although either component may predominate, almost to the exclusion of the other component, most cases consist of a relative equal mixture of mature fat and spindle cells. The spindle cells are uniform, with a single elongated nucleus and narrow, bipolar cytoplasmic processes (Fig. 16–22). Nucleoli are inconspicuous, as are mitotic figures. The cells may be haphazardly distributed but tend to be arranged in short parallel bundles, often with striking nuclear palisading reminiscent of a neural tumor.[139,148] In some cases scattered multinucleated floret-like giant cells, typical of those found in pleomorphic lipomas, are present, supporting the concept of a histologic spectrum between these tumors (Fig. 16–23). The cells are deposited in a mucoid matrix composed of hyaluronic acid and mixed with a varying number of birefringent collagen fibers (Fig. 16–24). In some cases the tumors are highly myxoid and hypocellular, with haphazardly arranged cells; such cases may be confused with myxoma (Fig. 16–25). The vascular pattern is usually inconspicuous and consists of a few small or intermediate-size thick-walled vessels, although some tumors have a prominent plexiform vascular pattern reminiscent of myxoid liposarcoma[152] and others a prominently hemangiopericytoma-like vascular pattern.[174] A pseudoangiomatous variant,

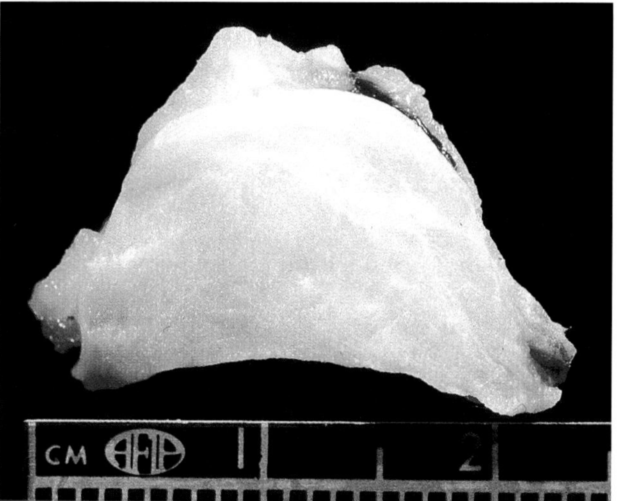


**FIGURE 16–20.** Gross appearance of a spindle cell lipoma showing a well-circumscribed mass with gray-white foci between areas that resemble the usual type of lipoma.

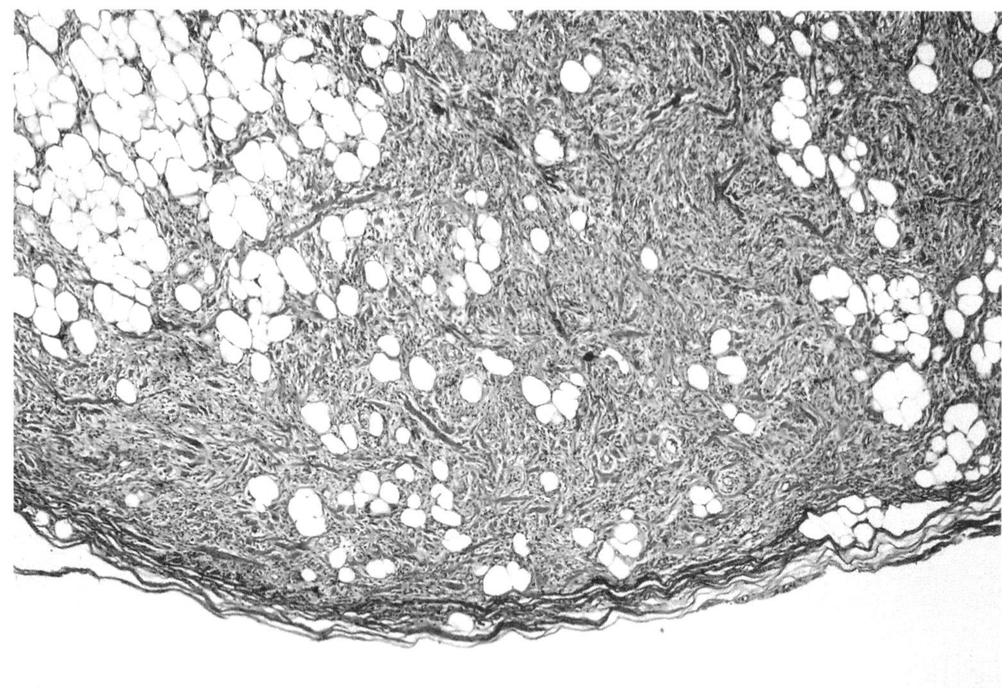

**FIGURE 16–21.** Spindle cell lipoma. Note the circumscription of the lesion and irregular distribution of the spindle cell areas between mature fat cells.

characterized by irregular branching spaces with well formed connective tissue projections, has also been described (Figs. 16–26, 16–27).[154,164] The lipocytic component consists of mature fat that in some cases may be present only focally, thereby obscuring the lipomatous nature of the neoplasm. Mast cells are a conspicuous feature in almost all cases. Rare tumors show small foci of osseous or cartilaginous metaplasia.[152]

Immunohistochemically, the spindle cells stain strongly for vimentin. S-100 protein does not mark the spindle cells, but mature lipocytes show strong peripheral immunoreactivity for this antigen.[143] Almost all tumors are strongly positive for CD34 (Fig. 16–28),[170–172] but they are not immunoreactive for actins, desmin, laminin, or the monocyte/macrophage antigen MAC-387.[143] Ultrastructurally, the cells have abundant rough endoplasmic reticulum, a well-formed Golgi apparatus, and non-membrane-bound lipid vacuoles (Fig. 16–29).[144,163] An interrupted basal lamina has been noted by some authors.[163]

Recent studies have found that both spindle cell and pleomorphic lipomas have characteristic cytogenetic abnormalities, with loss of 16q material and less frequently 13q.[145,151,157] These unique cytogenetic abnormalities coupled with the usual absence of giant marker and ring chromosomes, which are frequently seen in association with atypical lipoma/well-differentiated liposarcoma, supports the relation between spindle cell and pleomorphic lipomas and their distinction from atypical lipoma/well-differentiated liposarcoma.[159,165,166]

## Differential Diagnosis

The differential diagnosis of spindle cell lipoma includes a variety of benign and malignant entities characterized by spindle cells deposited in a myxoid stroma. *Dermatofibrosarcoma protuberans* is composed of a relatively uniform population of CD34$^+$ spindle cells arranged in a tight storiform pattern. However, dermatofibrosarcoma protuberans tends to occur in young patients, has a predilection to arise in the trunk and extremities, and histologically infiltrates the subcutaneous tissue in a characteristic lace-like pattern. *Nodular fasciitis* has a more variable appearance with tissue culture fibroblast-like cells characterized by smooth muscle actin positivity and an absence of CD34 staining. Spindle cell lipoma has pathologic features that overlap those of *angiomyofibroblastoma*,[153] a superficially located vulvar tumor, and *angiomyofibroblastoma-like tumor of the male genital tract*,[156] including CD34 immunoreactivity. Although these tumors differ with respect to site, the morphologic overlap between these tumors is striking; Laskin et al. proposed a CD34$^+$ perivascular stem cell with a capacity for lipocytic and myofibroblastic differentiation as the progenitor cell for these neoplasms.[156] Given the striking

*Text continued on page 597*

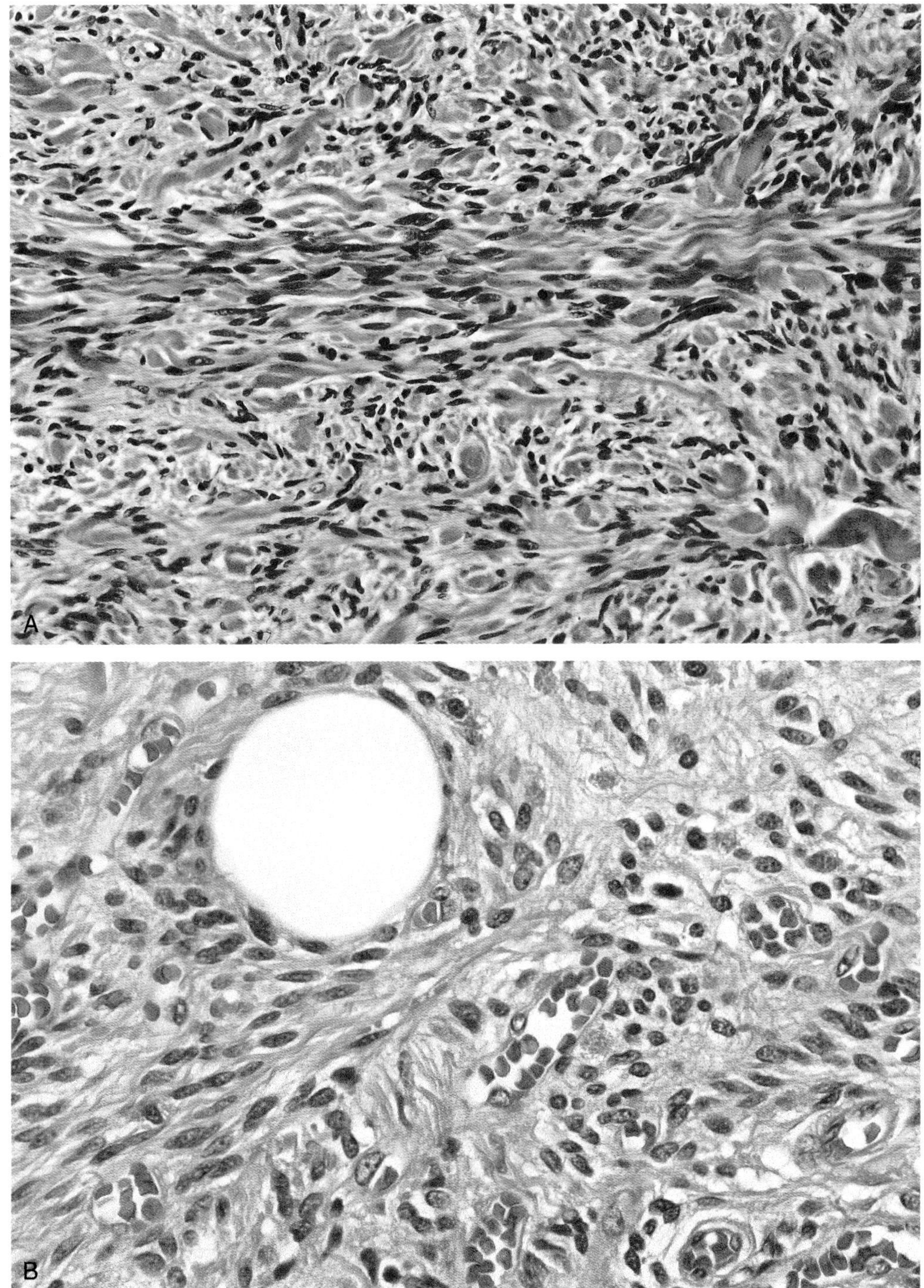


**FIGURE 16–22.** (**A**) Cellular area of a spindle cell lipoma showing spindle cells arranged in short bundles and separated by dense collagen. (**B**) High-power view of cytologically bland spindle cells in a spindle cell lipoma. The cells are uniform, with an elongated nucleus and bipolar cytoplasmic processes.

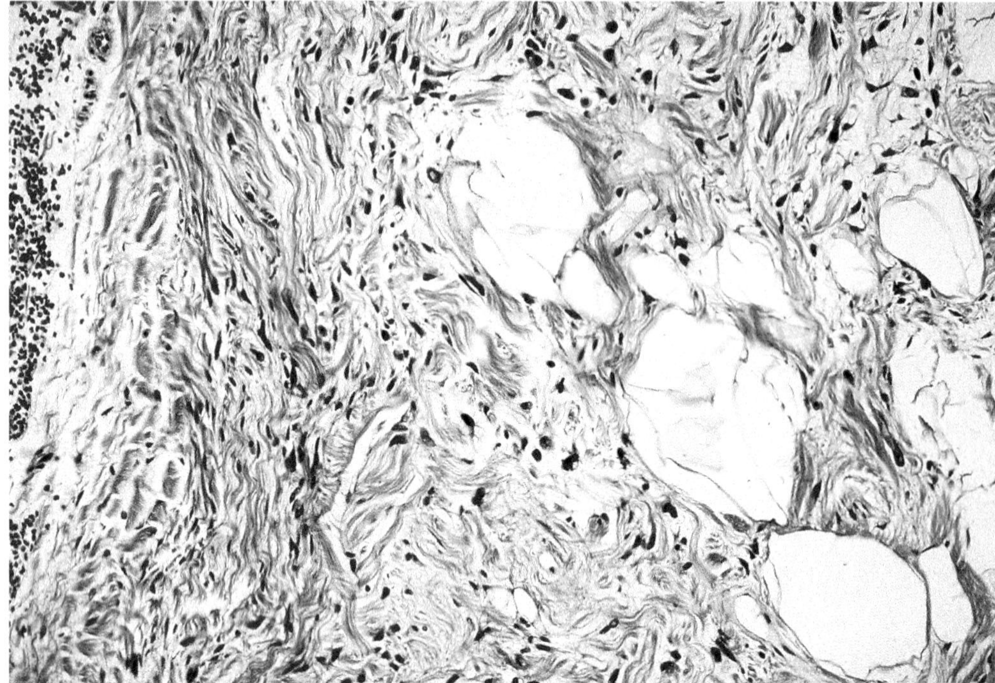

**FIGURE 16–23.** Spindle cell lipoma with transitional features between a spindle cell lipoma and a pleomorphic lipoma. The cells have more cytologic atypia than that seen in the usual spindle cell lipoma, but multinucleated floret-like giant cells are not seen.

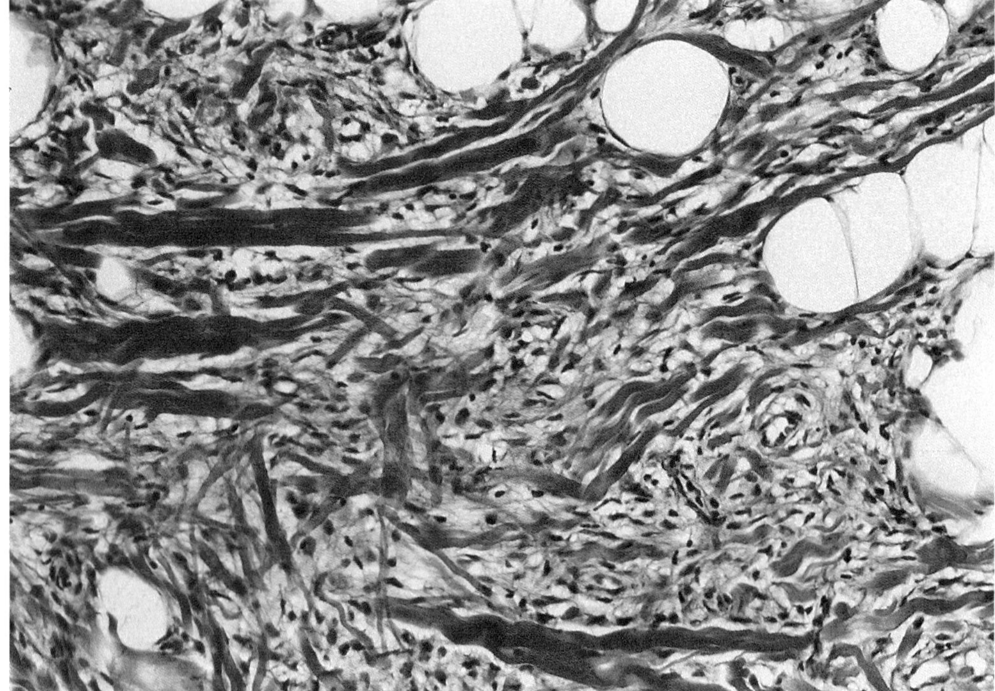

**FIGURE 16–24.** Spindle cell lipoma with characteristic ropey collagen bundles between bland spindle cells.

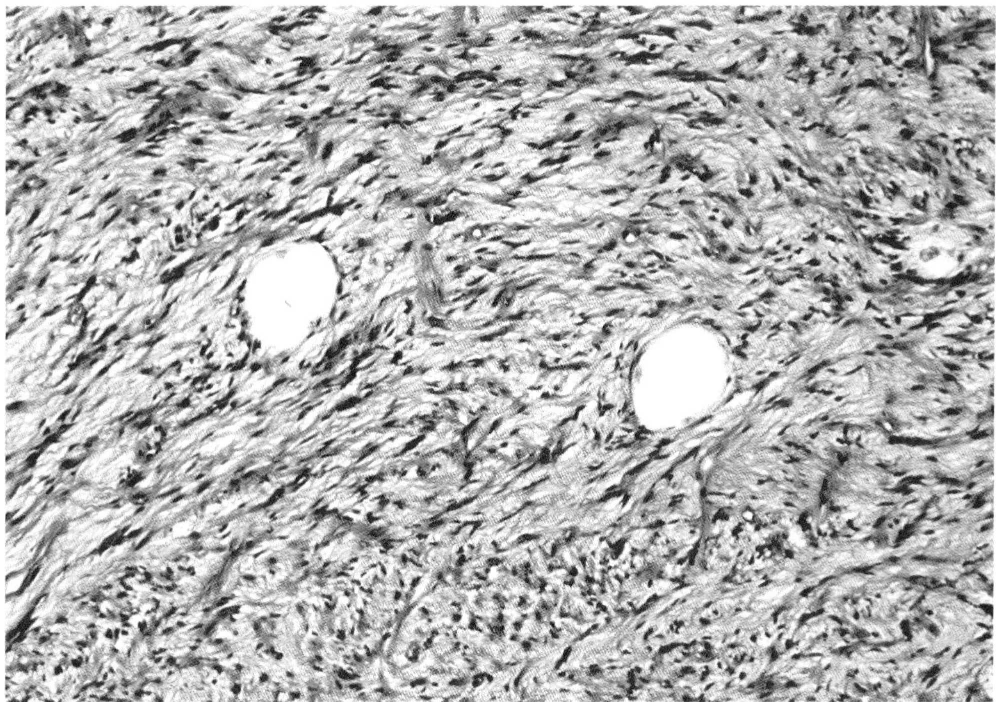

**FIGURE 16–25.** Spindle cell lipoma with extensive myxoid change. Such areas may resemble myxoid liposarcoma.

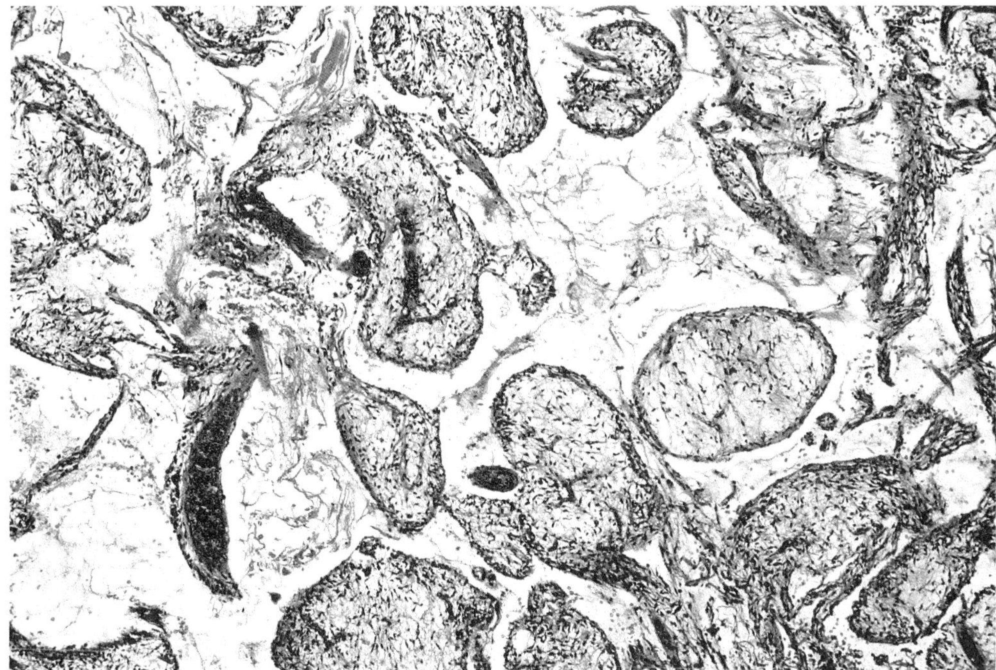

**FIGURE 16–26.** Spindle cell lipoma with pseudoangiomatous features characterized by irregular branching spaces with well formed connective tissue projections.

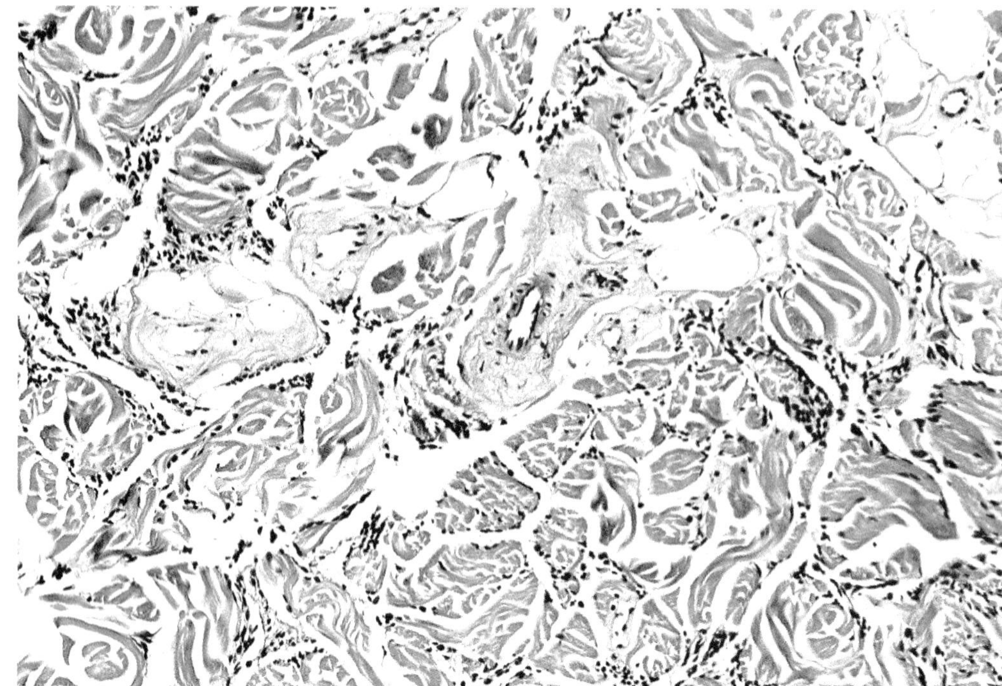

**FIGURE 16–27.** Pseudoangiomatous variant of a spindle cell lipoma closely resembling angiosarcoma. Short bundles of cytologically bland spindle cells are separated by dense connective tissue projections, simulating the dissecting pattern of angiosarcoma.

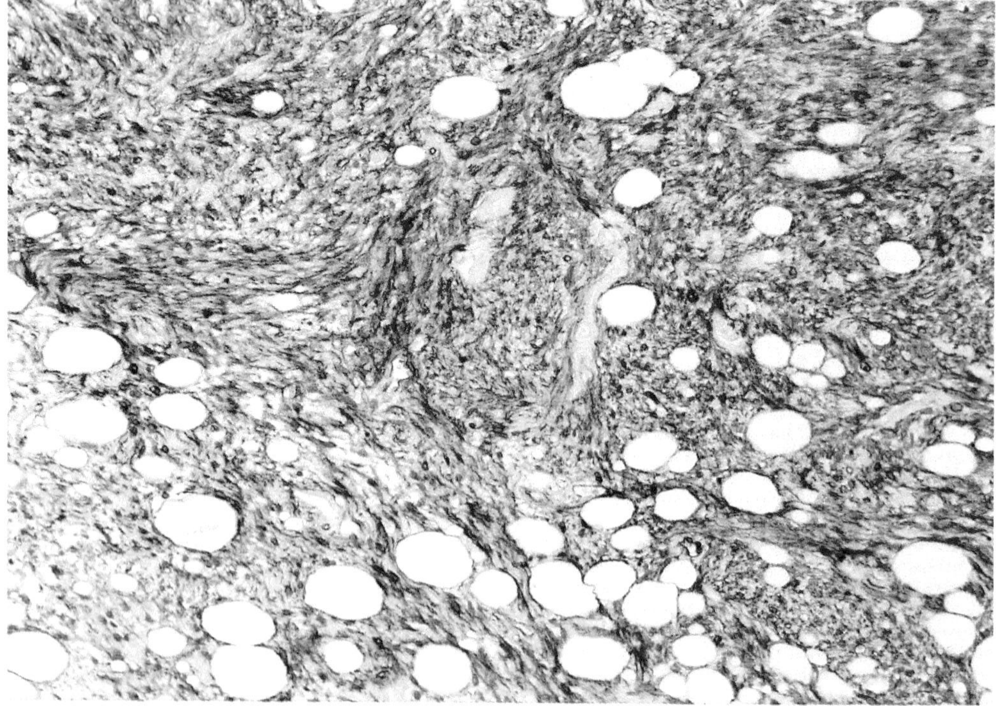

**FIGURE 16–28.** Diffuse CD34 immunoreactivity in a spindle cell lipoma.

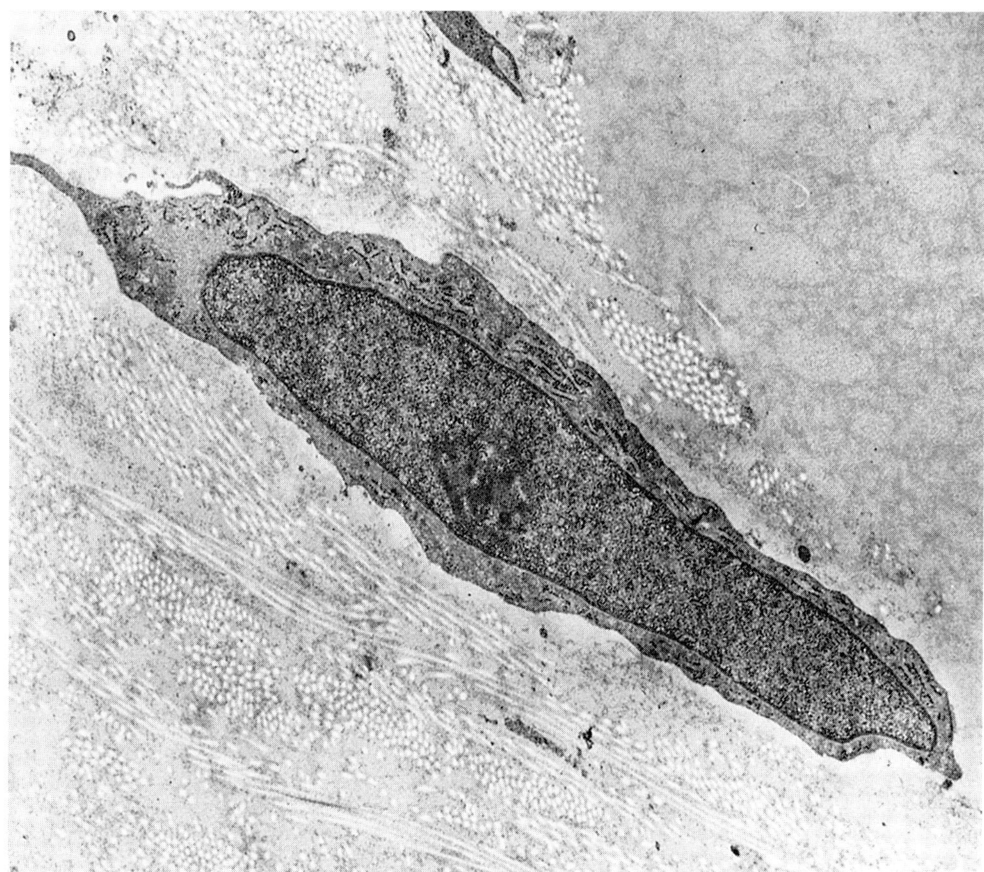

**FIGURE 16–29.** Electron micrograph of a spindle cell lipoma. Note the close resemblance to a fibroblast and the presence of collagen fibrils in the extracellular space.

nuclear palisading present in some spindle cell lipomas and the conspicuous mast cell infiltrate, *schwannoma* and *neurofibroma* are diagnostic considerations. The cells of these benign peripheral nerve sheath tumors tend to be more wavy or buckled in appearance; although both lesions may express CD34, they more commonly express S-100 protein, a marker that is negative in spindle cell lipoma. *Myxoid liposarcoma* is a consideration, as some spindle cell lipomas have a prominent plexiform vascular pattern in the myxoid areas. However, spindle cell lipoma is more circumscribed and superficially located than myxoid liposarcoma, lacks lipoblasts, and is characterized by ropey collagen bundles. Similarly, *spindle cell liposarcoma,* an uncommon variant of liposarcoma, is characterized by relatively bland spindle cells, mature fat, scattered lipoblasts, and only rare cells that may stain for CD34.

### Discussion

Spindle cell lipoma, as the name indicates, is a benign lesion; and local excision usually effects lasting relief. Although recurrences are rare, metastases have not been reported. The exact nature of the spindle cells is uncertain, as it is difficult to distinguish early fibroblasts and prelipoblasts by electron microscopy.[148] Based on finding CD34 immunoreactivity in spindle cell lipomas, Suster and Fisher suggested that this lesion is a dendritic interstitial cell neoplasm located in fat, rather than a true lipogenic neoplasm.[171]

## PLEOMORPHIC LIPOMA

The term *pleomorphic lipoma* has been applied to a neoplasm that closely simulates a sclerosing or pleomorphic liposarcoma but represents an extremely pleomorphic variant of spindle cell lipoma.[141,147,161,167] Although spindle cell and pleomorphic lipomas at one time were grouped under the term "atypical lipoma" by some authors,[140,149] we believe that both of these lesions are sufficiently characteristic to justify consideration as entities distinct from atypical lipoma on clinical, histologic, and cytogenetic grounds. The term atypical lipoma is used by most to refer to a well-differentiated liposarcoma of the subcutis.

Like spindle cell lipoma, pleomorphic lipoma oc-

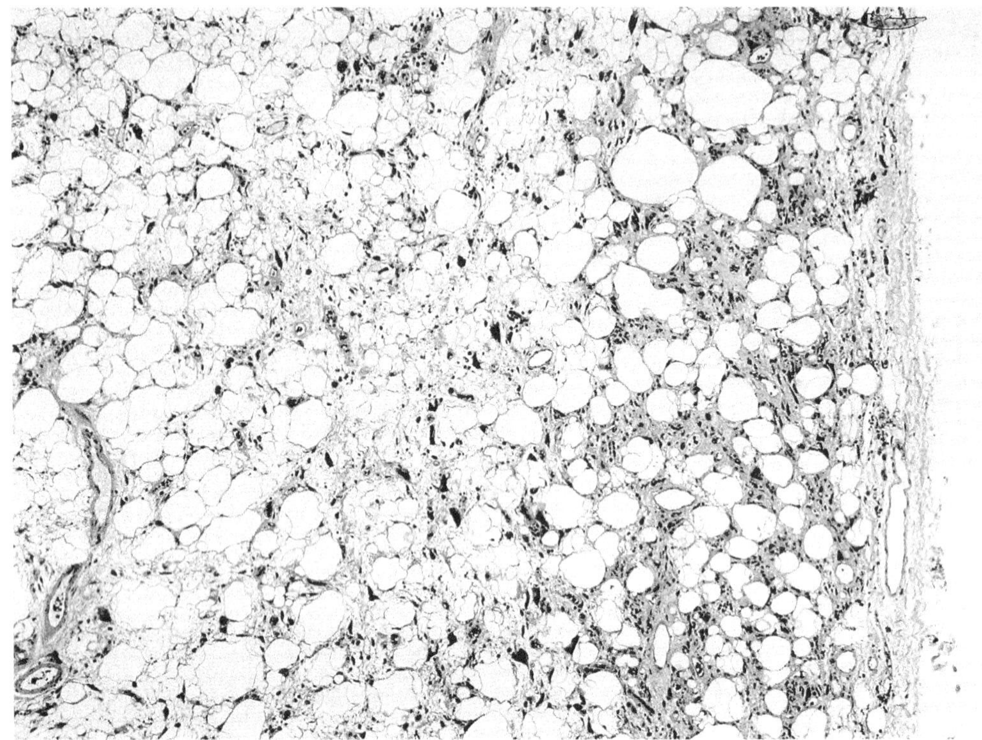

**FIGURE 16–30.** Pleomorphic lipoma. The lesion is typically well circumscribed and separated from the surrounding subcutaneous tissue.

curs as a circumscribed subcutaneous mass most commonly found in the posterior neck, shoulder, and back region of men older than 45 years (Fig. 16–30; Table 16–3).[167] It is characterized by the presence of scattered, bizarre giant cells that frequently have a concentric floret-like arrangement of multiple hyperchromatic nuclei about a deeply eosinophilic cytoplasm (Figs. 16–31, 16–32). Ropey collagen bundles similar to those found in spindle cell lipoma are also characteristic. The mature adipocytic component may predominate, but in some cases only small amounts of mature fat are present, making recognition of this tumor difficult. Some tumors also have extensive myxoid change and may be associated with numerous mast cells. Transitional forms between spindle cell and pleomorphic lipomas are not uncommon. Like spindle cell lipoma, the atypical and multinucleated giant cells of pleomorphic lipoma also stain for CD34 (Fig. 16–33).

Distinction from *sclerosing liposarcoma* may be difficult but usually can be accomplished on the basis of the typical setting of the lesion on the shoulder or head and neck region, its location in subcutaneous tissue, and its circumscription. Although the multinucleated floret-like giant cells are characteristic of this lesion, they are not pathognomonic, as such cells are occasionally also seen in sclerosing liposarcomas and a variety of nonlipogenic neoplasms (Table 16–4). Like spindle cell lipoma, this lesion is characterized by aberrations of the long arms of chromosomes 16 and 13.[145,151,157] Some have proposed a potential role for karyotypic analysis when distinguishing it from atypical lipoma/well-differentiated liposarcoma, which harbors genetic abnormalities different from those seen in spindle cell/pleomorphic lipomas.[165]

**TABLE 16–3** ANATOMIC DISTRIBUTION OF PLEOMORPHIC LIPOMA

| Anatomic Location | No. of Patients | % |
|---|---|---|
| Neck | 27 | 48 |
| Shoulder | 7 | 13 |
| Back | 6 | 11 |
| Head | 5 | 9 |
| Upper extremity | 4 | 7 |
| Lower extremity | 3 | 5 |
| Chest wall/axilla | 3 | 5 |
| Buttock | 1 | 2 |
| *Total* | 56 | 100 |

Data from Azzopardi JG, Iocco J, Salm R. Pleomorphic lipoma: a tumour simulating liposarcoma. Histopathology 7:511, 1983; and Shmookler BM, Enzinger FM. Pleomorphic lipoma: a benign tumor simulating liposarcoma: a clinicopathologic analysis of 48 cases. Cancer 47:126, 1981.

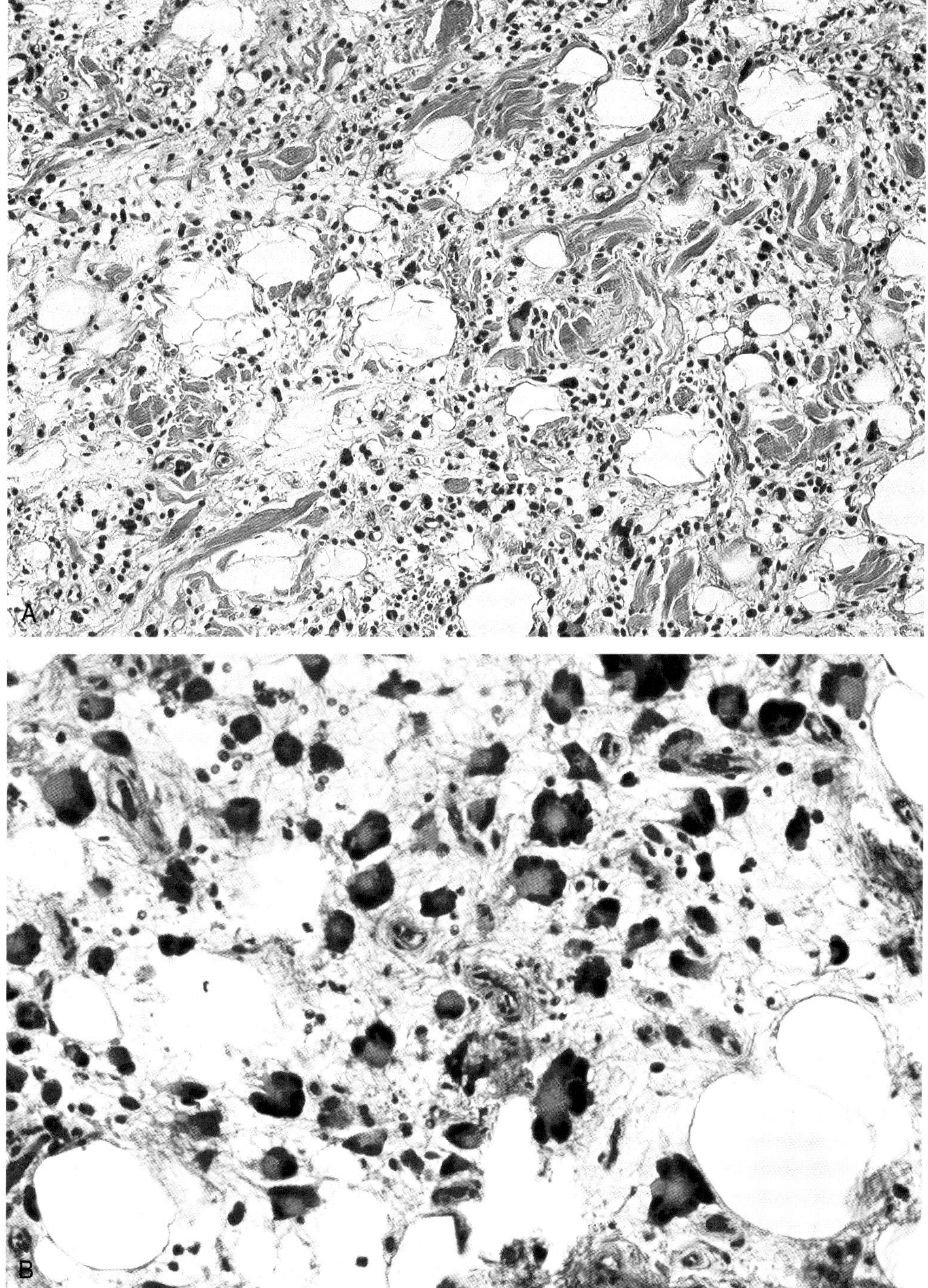


**FIGURE 16–31.** (**A**) Pleomorphic lipoma, characterized by a mixture of mature fat cells, multinucleated giant cells, and ropey collagen bundles similar to those found in spindle cell lipoma. (**B**) Pleomorphic lipoma with numerous multinucleated floret-like giant cells deposited in a myxoid stroma.

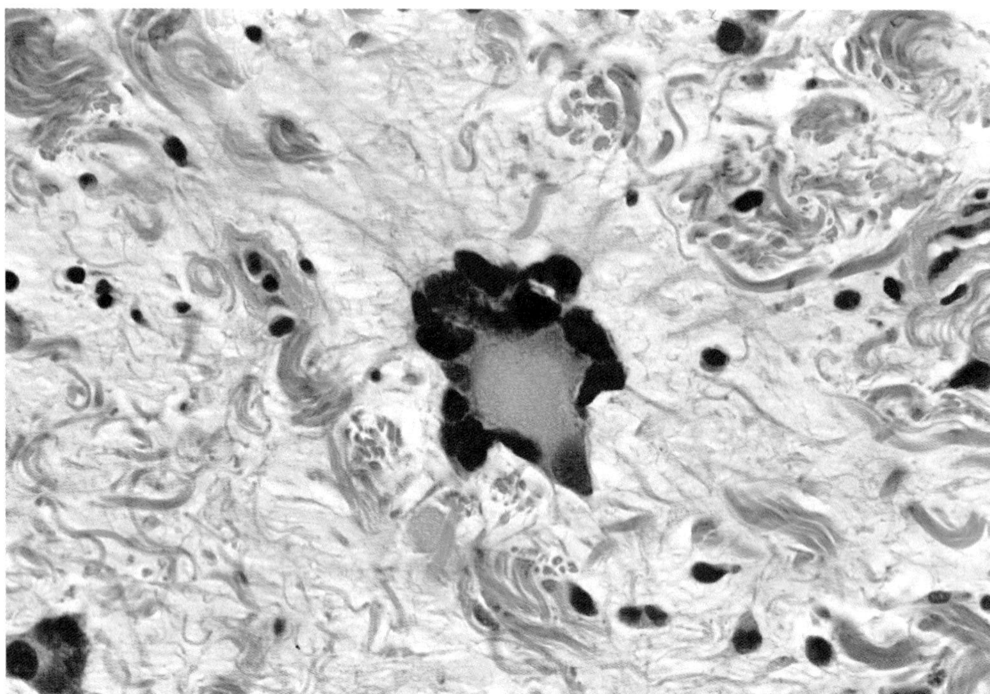

**FIGURE 16–32.** High-power view of a typical multinucleated floret-like giant cell as seen in pleomorphic lipomas. There is a wreath-like arrangement of hyperchromatic nuclei about a deeply eosinophilic cytoplasm.

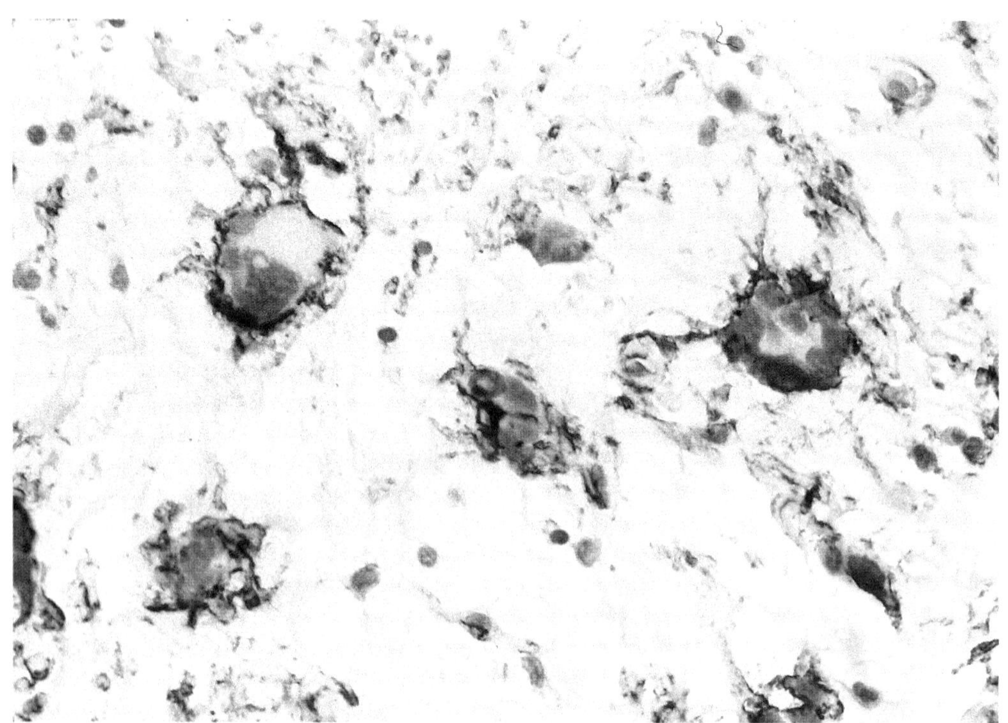

**FIGURE 16–33.** CD34 immunoreactivity in the multinucleated giant cells of a pleomorphic lipoma.

**TABLE 16–4 COMPARISON OF PLEOMORPHIC LIPOMA, WELL-DIFFERENTIATED LIPOSARCOMA, AND PLEOMORPHIC LIPOSARCOMA**

| Feature | Pleomorphic Lipoma | Well-differentiated Liposarcoma | Pleomorphic Liposarcoma |
|---|---|---|---|
| Favored site(s) | Subcutis of posterior neck, back, and shoulders | Deep soft tissue of extremities, retroperitoneum | Extremities |
| Peak age (years) | 45–60 | 50–70 | 50–70 |
| Floret-like cells | Characteristic | Present | Rare |
| Pleomorphic lipoblasts | Absent | Present | Characteristic |
| Cytogenetics | Loss of 16q, 13q | Giant marker and ring chromosomes | Varied complex abnormalities |
| Metastasis | None | Extremely rare, except in dedifferentiated cases | Common |

Despite the bizarre cellular features and the occasional presence of lipoblast-like cells with atypical mitotic figures, the prognosis is excellent; and local excision is nearly always adequate for cure. Although Shouzhu et al.[168] reported a case of a retroperitoneal pleomorphic lipoma that subsequently progressed to a high-grade pleomorphic sarcoma,[175] this case in our opinion most likely represented a well-differentiated liposarcoma that subsequently underwent dedifferentiation. There are no other reports of histologic progression or metastasis.

## BENIGN LIPOBLASTOMA AND LIPOBLASTOMATOSIS

Benign lipoblastoma and lipoblastomatosis refer, respectively, to the circumscribed and diffuse forms of the same tumor. This tumor is a peculiar variant of lipoma and lipomatosis occurring almost exclusively during infancy and early childhood. The lesions differ from lipoma and lipomatosis by their cellular immaturity and their close resemblance to the myxoid form of liposarcoma.

Lipoblastomatosis was named by Vellios et al.[201] in 1958, who reported an infiltrating lipoblastoma in the regions of the anterior chest wall and axilla and the supraclavicular region of an 8-month-old girl. The tumor had not recurred after 30 months. Earlier, Van Meurs[200] reported a similar tumor as "embryonic lipoma." He demonstrated its transformation to a common lipoma with repeated biopsies.

### Clinical Findings

Lipoblastoma is a tumor of infancy. It is usually noted during the first 3 years of life and occasionally at birth.[182,184,194] Sporadic examples have also been described in older children[193] (Table 16–5). Most studies have found a predilection for this tumor to occur in boys. Most commonly, it is found in the upper and lower extremities as a painless nodule or mass (Fig. 16–34). Less common sites of involvement include the head and neck area, trunk, mediastinum, mesentery, and retroperitoneum[177,186,192,202] (Table 16–6). Two types of lipoblastoma have been described; circumscribed (*benign lipoblastoma*) and diffuse (*diffuse lipoblastomatosis*). The more common circumscribed form, located in the superficial soft tissues, clinically simulates a lipoma. The diffuse type tends to infiltrate not only the subcutis but also the underlying muscle tissue, it has an infiltrative growth pattern and a greater tendency to recur.[183] Most patients present with a slowly growing soft tissue mass, although some report tumors with a rapid period of growth.[178] Depending on the tumor size and location, the mass may compress adjacent structures and interfere with function, such as in a head and neck location where it may cause airway obstruction and respiratory insufficiency.[196] Radiologic studies typically show a well delineated soft tissue mass with the density of adipose tissue, although neither CT nor MRI reliably distinguishes this lesion from lipoma or liposarcoma.[198]

**TABLE 16–5 AGE DISTRIBUTION OF LIPOBLASTOMA/ LIPOBLASTOMATOSIS PATIENTS AT THE TIME OF OPERATION**

| Age (Months) | No. of Patients | % |
|---|---|---|
| 0–11 | 26 | 36 |
| 12–23 | 19 | 26 |
| 24–35 | 10 | 14 |
| 36–47 | 4 | 5 |
| 48–59 | 5 | 7 |
| 60–70 | 3 | 4 |
| 71–83 | 2 | 3 |
| ≥84 | 4 | 5 |
| *Total* | 73 | 100 |

Data are from refs. 182,184,194.

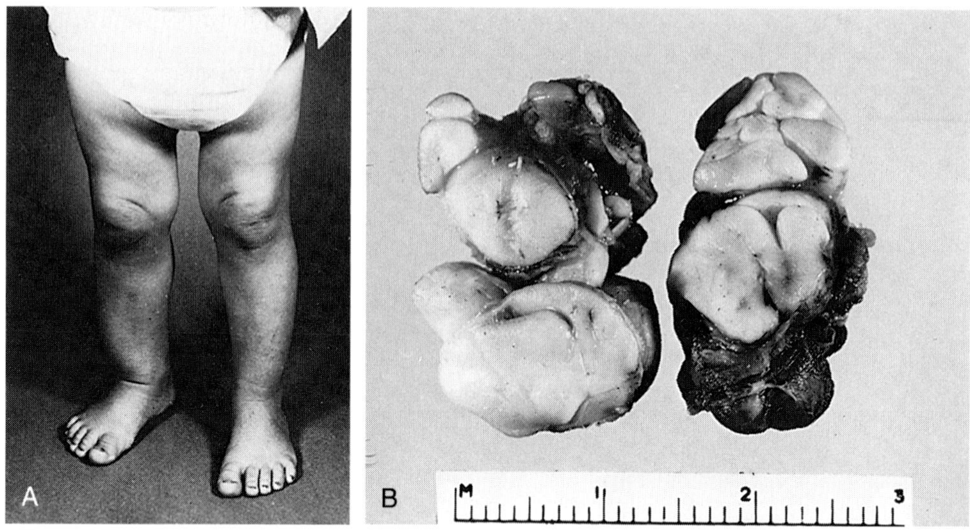

**FIGURE 16–34.** Lipoblastoma of the right lower leg of a 2-year-old boy. Clinical (**A**) and multilobular gross appearance (**B**).

## Pathologic Findings

On section, lipoblastoma is more pale staining than the ordinary lipoma, and its cut surfaces are distinctly myxoid or gelatinous (Fig. 16–35). Most tumors are 3–5 cm in diameter, although some are much larger, occasionally as large as 1 kg.[179,181]

Microscopy shows that it consists of irregular small lobules of immature fat cells separated by connective tissue septa of varying thickness and mesenchymal areas with a loose myxoid appearance (Fig. 16–36).[182] The individual lobules are composed of lipoblasts in different stages of development, ranging from primitive, stellate, and spindle-shaped mesenchymal cells (preadipocytes) to lipoblasts approaching the univacuolar "signet ring" picture of a mature fat cell (Fig. 16–37). The degree of cellular differentiation may be the same throughout the tumor, or it may vary in different tumor lobules. There are occasional examples in which the cells are more rounded and finely vacuolated with intracellular eosinophilic granules, resembling the cells of brown fat.[194] Characteristically, the lipoblasts are surrounded by mucinous material rich in hyaluronic acid, the amount of which is inversely proportional to the degree of cellular differentiation. The cellular composition is the same regardless of whether the tumor is circumscribed or diffuse. Diffuse tumors (*diffuse lipoblastomatosis*), however, have a less pronounced lobular pattern and usually contain an admixture of residual muscle fibers similar to intramuscular lipoma. Cases with sheets of primitive mesenchymal cells or broad fibrous septa may be mistaken for infantile fibromatosis. Cellular maturation of lipoblastoma has been observed with multiple biopsies (Fig. 16–38).[184,200]

Ultrastructural studies disclose a variable picture. As in normal developing fat, the cells display a wide morphologic spectrum ranging from immature mesenchymal cells and preadipocytes to multivacuolar lipoblasts and univacuolar lipocytes. The lipoblasts contain numerous vesicles, round to oval mitochondria, and well developed Golgi membranes.[190] Pinocytotic vesicles are abundant along the plasma membrane. Stellate mesenchymal cells with prominent rough endoplasmic reticulum may be present in the

**TABLE 16–6** ANATOMIC DISTRIBUTION OF LIPOBLASTOMA/ LIPOBLASTOMATOSIS

| Anatomic Site | No. of Patients | % |
|---|---|---|
| Head and neck | 10 | 14 |
| Mediastinum | 1 | 2 |
| Upper extremity | 19 | 26 |
| Hand | 8 | |
| Elbow | 1 | |
| Upper arm | 2 | |
| Shoulder | 3 | |
| Axilla | 4 | |
| Forearm | 1 | |
| Lower extremity | 29 | 40 |
| Buttock | 8 | |
| Groin | 4 | |
| Thigh | 11 | |
| Lower leg | 6 | |
| Trunk | 10 | 14 |
| Back | 5 | |
| Labia | 2 | |
| Chest wall | 3 | |
| Retroperitoneum | 3 | 4 |
| *Total* | 72 | 100 |

Data are from refs. 182,184,194.

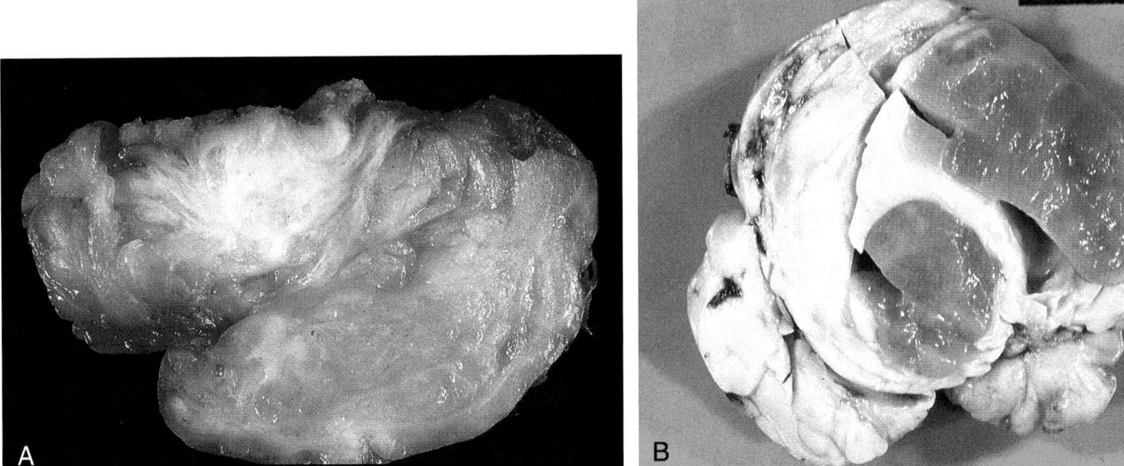


**FIGURE 16–35.** (**A**) Gross appearance of a lipoblastoma. This lesion is well circumscribed and has a predominantly fatty appearance, although focal cartilaginous metaplasia (white to gray area) is present. (**B**) Lipoblastoma with multinodular appearance and foci with extensive myxoid change.

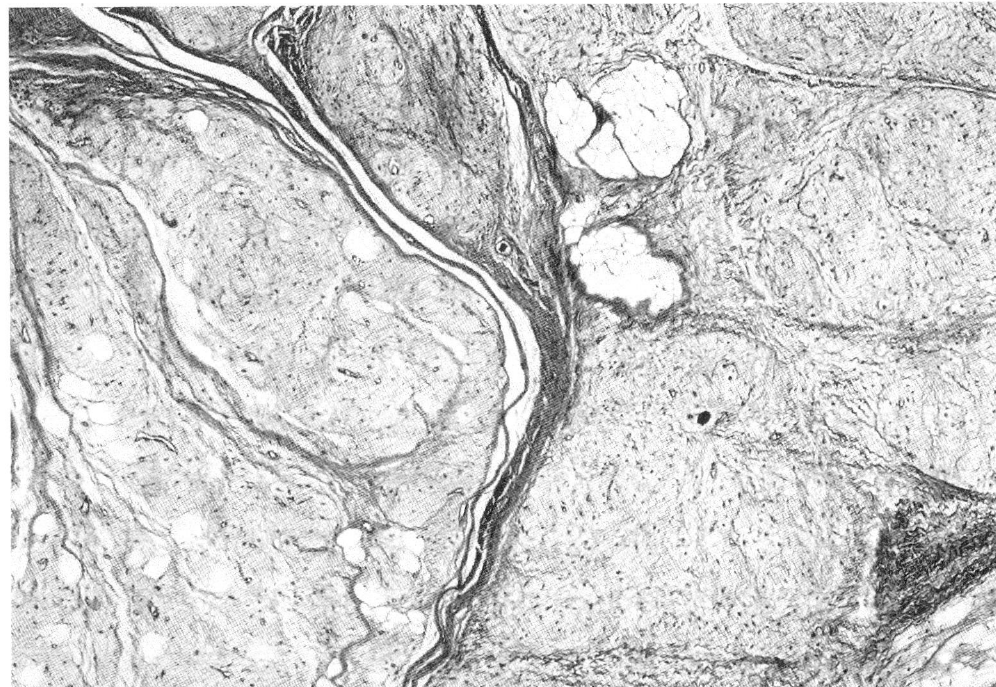

**FIGURE 16–36.** Lipoblastoma with the characteristic multilobular pattern. Many of the nodules show extensive myxoid change.

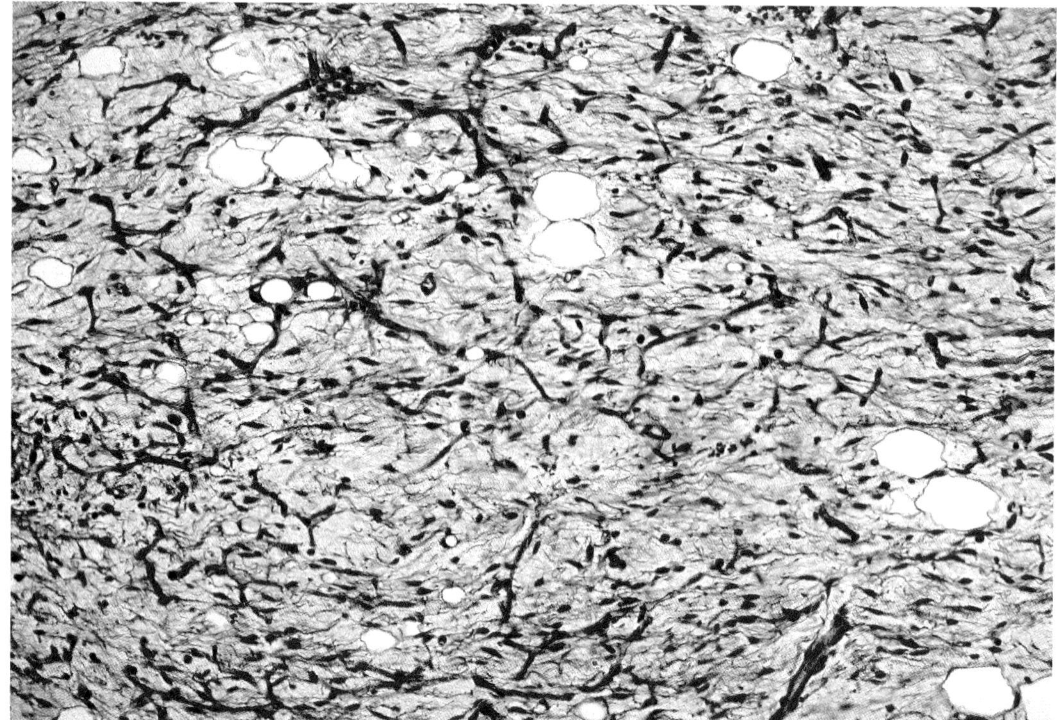

**FIGURE 16–37.** Lipoblastoma of a 1-year-old child composed of lipoblasts and a prominent mucoid matrix. A plexiform vasculature reminiscent of myxoid liposarcoma is also apparent.

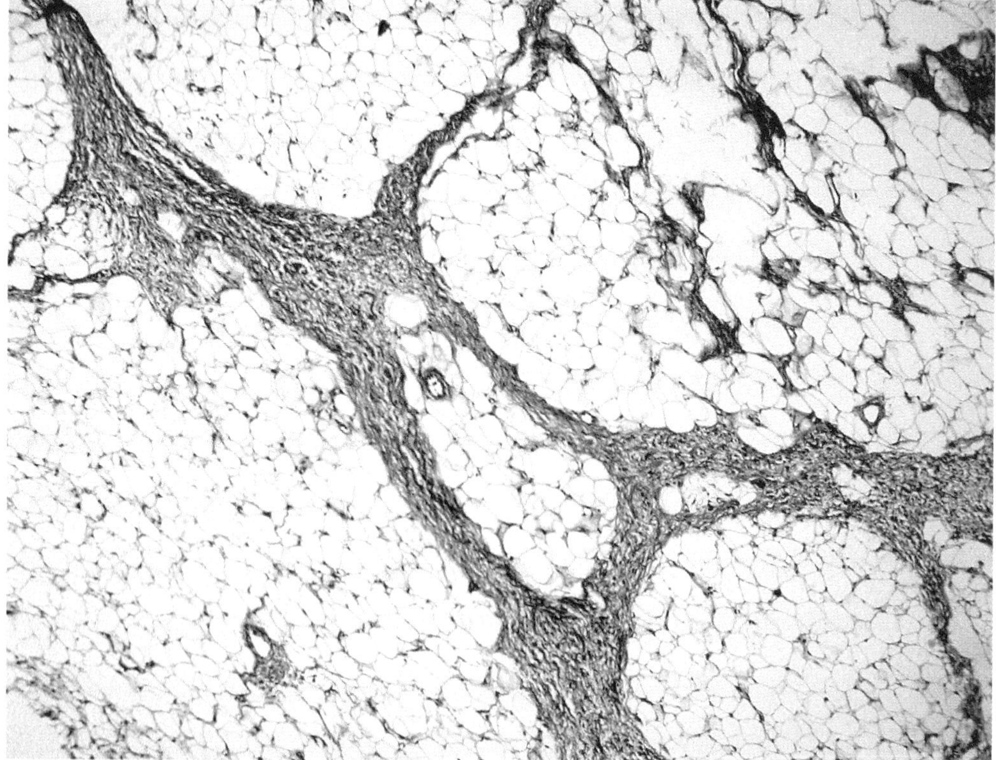

**FIGURE 16–38.** Recurrent lipoblastoma composed of multiple lobules of mature-appearing fat cells separated by fibrous septa. Some examples of lipoblastoma show maturation in recurrent lesions.

peripheral portions of the lobules.[180] The extracellular matrix contains fibrillar material and collagen fibers.[191]

### Differential Diagnosis

The principal differential diagnostic consideration is *myxoid liposarcoma*. Unlike lipoblastoma, which is a tumor of infancy and early childhood predominantly occurring in patients less than 5 years of age, myxoid liposarcoma has a peak incidence during the third through sixth decades of life. Occasional myxoid liposarcomas have been reported during adolescence, although such cases are rare under the age of 10 years. Histologically, both lesions may be lobulated, contain lipoblasts, and spindled cells deposited in a myxoid stroma with a prominent plexiform capillary network. However, lipoblastoma has a more pronounced lobulation than that typically seen in myxoid liposarcoma. Although myxoid liposarcoma lacks marked nuclear atypia or hyperchromasia, such features are usually present focally, whereas lipoblastoma lacks any degree of nuclear atypia. Foci of hypercellularity may be found in myxoid liposarcoma but are not found in extraseptal loci in the lipoblastoma.[184] Microcystic spaces may be present in lipoblastoma but are more often found and are more pronounced in myxoid liposarcoma. Finally, the lipoblastoma is characterized cytogenetically by deletions of 8q11–13[185,187–189,195,197] but lacks the characteristic t(12;16) translocation in myxoid liposarcoma.[199]

Lipoblastoma may also be confused with other benign adipose tissue tumors, including *ordinary lipoma* and *hibernoma*. Ordinary lipoma is less cellular than lipoblastoma and lacks lipoblasts, whereas hibernoma consists almost entirely of brown fat cells with mitochondria-rich, eosinophilic, granular cytoplasm. The latter two entities have cytogenetic abnormalities distinct from those found in lipoblastoma.

### Discussion

The prognosis is excellent. The reported rate of local recurrence ranges from 9%[184] to 22% in the series reported by Mentzel et al.[194] Recurrence is not related to any morphologic features such as lobulation, myxoid change, or degree of adipocytic differentiation; for the most part it is restricted to patients with the diffuse type, rather than the circumscribed type, particularly those whose tumors are incompletely excised. Therefore wide local excision of the diffuse or infiltrating type of lipoblastomatosis is well advised. The neoplasm has been viewed by some as a blastoma of soft tissue,[183] supported by the ultrastructural similarity to white fat and the observation of maturation to lipoma in sequential biopsy specimens or in recurrent tumors. Detection of a clonal chromosomal abnormality supports its classification as a neoplasm rather than a hamartoma.[183]

## ANGIOMYOLIPOMA

The term *angiomyolipoma* should be reserved for a specific lesion arising most commonly in one or both kidneys as a solitary or multicentric mass; rarely, the mass is a pedunculated growth or presents as a satellite nodule outside the renal capsule. Multiple and bilateral lesions are less common than solitary ones and are more often encountered in patients with tuberous sclerosis.[248]

### Clinical Findings

Angiomyolipoma occurs more commonly in women than men, with a median age of 46 years. In about two-thirds of cases it causes symptoms such as abdominal or flank pain, hematuria, or chills and fever. Less commonly it is asymptomatic and is discovered as an incidental finding at operation for some unrelated cause or at autopsy. Rarely, sudden, severe flank pain and shock are caused by rupture of the tumor and massive perirenal or retroperitoneal hemorrhage.[204,251] Rare instances of associated hypertension have been recorded.[220,223] Although most lesions occur in the kidney, extrarenal sites of angiomyolipoma include the liver,[250,266,267,270] nasal cavity,[225] oral cavity,[273] heart,[259] colon,[245] lung,[228] and skin.[268]

Approximately one-third of patients with angiomyolipoma present with manifestations of the tuberous sclerosis complex, ranging from hyperpigmented spots, shagreen patches, periungual fibromas, and angiofibromas to renal cysts, cardiac rhabdomyoma, and gliosis and calcification of the cerebral cortex with mental deficiency.[257,265] There are also rare cases in which the tumor is associated with lymphangiomyoma and lymphangiomyomatosis of the lung,[208,240] renal cell carcinoma,[262,269] and neurofibromatosis.[263] CT scans and MRI reveal a fatty mass with intermixed soft tissue densities, except in those cases in which the absence of fat or hemorrhage obscures the radiologic findings.[261] Ultrasonography seems to be less reliable and does not always permit ruling out renal cell carcinoma, especially in the absence of a significant fatty component.[260,264] Aspiration or needle biopsy has been employed successfully to confirm the diagnosis.[209,258]

### Pathologic Findings

Grossly, the lesion presents as a yellow to gray mass, varying in size from a few centimeters to 20 cm or more (average 9 cm). Large lesions may become attached to the diaphragm or liver.[231,239] Focal hemorrhage is present in about half of the cases. The tumor is usually well delineated from the surrounding renal parenchyma (Fig. 16–39). Some tumors extend into the inferior vena cava,[241] and others involve perirenal lymph nodes,[203,216] both of which may contribute to a diagnosis of malignancy.

Microscopically, angiomyolipoma is composed of three tissue components that vary greatly in distribution: (1) mature adipose tissue with some variations in cellular size and nuclear appearance; (2) convoluted thick-walled blood vessels with little or abnormal elastica and frequent hyalinization of the media; and (3) irregularly arranged sheets and interlacing bundles of smooth muscle often with a prominent perivascular arrangement (Figs. 16–40, 16–41). In some cases the smooth muscle element displays a striking degree of cellular pleomorphism, with hyperchromatic nuclei, occasional multinucleated giant cells, and necrotic foci (Fig. 16–42). Additionally, there may be epithelioid smooth muscle cells containing spherical granules and dense PAS-positive needle-shaped or rhomboid crystals similar to those in juxtaglomerular tumors, but the cells do not stain for renin (Fig. 16–43).[212,219,246]

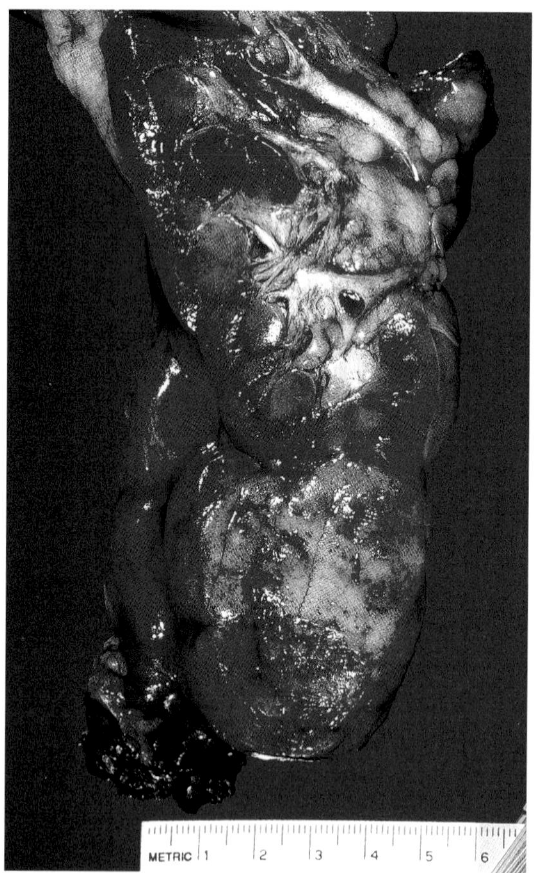


**FIGURE 16–39.** Angiomyolipoma of the kidney. The lesion, well circumscribed, is broadly attached to one pole of the kidney. Focal hemorrhage within the nodule is apparent.

Immunohistochemically, the smooth muscle cells of angiomyolipoma are not only immunoreactive for actin and desmin but also, unlike other smooth muscle tumors, express the melanoma-associated antigen HMB-45 (Fig. 16–44).[235,237,254,271] This antigen, which recognizes a peptide involved in the process of melanogenesis,[206] has been found in other tumors that coexpress markers of melanogenesis and muscle differentiation, including lymphangioleiomyomatosis,[211,215] clear cell "sugar" tumor of the lung,[212,224] and extrapulmonary "sugar" tumor.[255,274] Pea et al. reevaluated five tumors previously reported as renal cell carcinoma arising in patients with the tuberous sclerosis complex.[253] Based on the immunohistochemical expression of HMB-45, the authors proposed that these tumors were monotypic epithelioid variants of angiomyolipoma, casting doubt on the real frequency of renal cell carcinoma in these patients. Such monotypic epithelioid angiomyolipomas may also be found in patients without tuberous sclerosis.[247] In addition to HMB-45, other markers of melanocytic differentiation including MART-1 have been identified in these lesions.[222,236] A significant percentage of cases also stain for progesterone receptors.[232]

Ultrastructurally, many of these muscle cells contain myofilaments, glycogen particles, and electron-dense granules. Some have transverse striations, similar to melanosomes.[214,243,249]

## Differential Diagnosis

Although the histologic appearance of the tumor is characteristic and should not cause difficulty with the diagnosis, rare cases of angiomyolipoma are mistaken for *sarcomas* or *carcinomas.* Those tumors that have a prominent fatty component may be mistaken for *liposarcoma.* The presence of convoluted thick-walled blood vessels and immunoreactivity for HMB-45 in the smooth muscle cells allows their distinction. Angiomyolipomas with an inconspicuous fatty component may be confused with *leiomyosarcoma,* particularly those that are large, hypercellular, and pleomorphic. This distinction may be particularly challenging on a needle biopsy specimen. The smooth muscle cells of angiomyolipoma tend to be plumper and paler than those found in leiomyosarcoma, and HMB-45 immunoreactivity can be extremely useful in this setting. Given that both renal cell carcinoma and angiomyolipoma are associated with the tuberous sclerosis complex, some epithelioid angiomyolipomas are confused with renal cell carcinoma and vice versa. The use of cytokeratin and HMB-45 immunostains should allow the distinction of these two lesions.

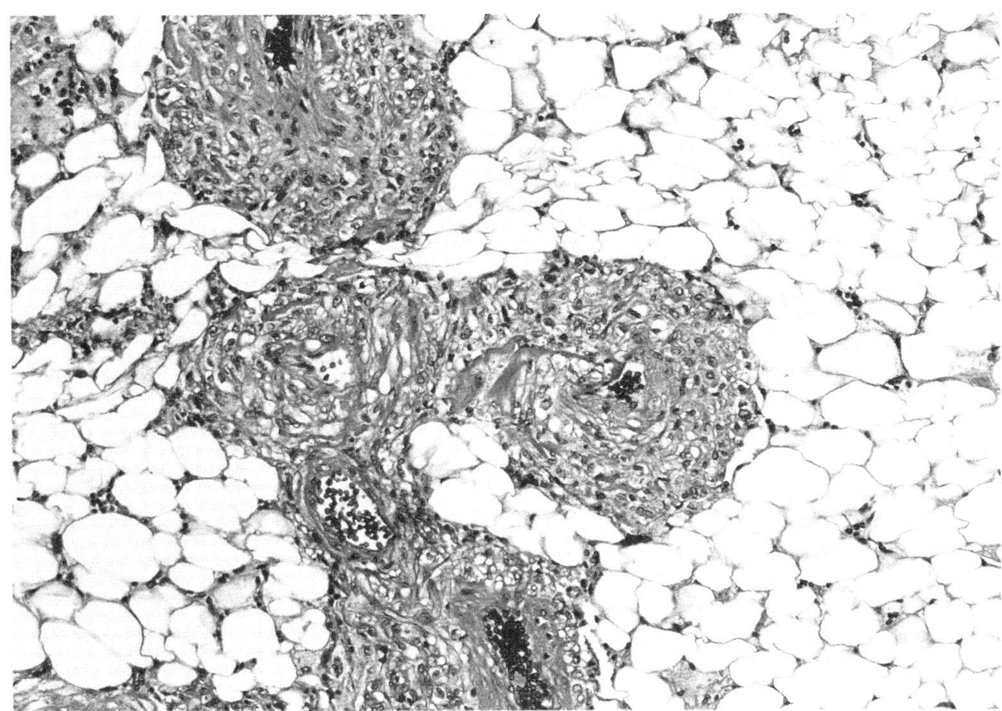

**FIGURE 16–40.** Angiomyolipoma with the basic components of the tumor: mature adipose tissue and smooth muscle surrounding thick-walled, medium-sized vascular channels.

## Discussion

Despite the presence of atypical features in some angiomyolipomas, nearly all of these tumors seem to pursue a benign clinical course. In fact, there is no evidence that the presence of regional or systemic lymph node involvement, perirenal satellite tumors, or angiomyolipomatous growth in other organs reflects malignant potential.[210,213]

Malignant transformation, if it occurs, must be rare. Cellular pleomorphism and intravascular growth have been interpreted as evidence of malignancy,[207,244] but marked cellular pleomorphism is not uncommon in angiomyolipomas, and intravascular growth may be found in perfectly benign tumors. There are, however, reports of leiomyosarcomatous transformation of pleomorphic angiomyolipomas, with subsequent metastasis. In a case described by Lowe et al.,[244] multiple sarcomatous lesions were found in various organs 18 months after removal of a pleomorphic renal angiomyolipoma. In another case reported by Ferry et al.,[221] the patient developed multiple pulmonary lesions that were diagnosed by fine-needle biopsy as metastatic angiomyolipoma, but it is possible this case represents multifocal disease. An "angiolipomyosarcoma" reported by Hartveit and Hallerbraker[231] is likely a bilateral angiomyolipoma in which the pleomorphic tumor in the opposite kidney was interpreted as a metastasis. Several of the cases reported by Pea et al.[253] of "renal cell carcinoma," which they reclassified as monotypic epithelioid angiomyolipoma, were characterized by multifocality and an aggressive clinical course, prompting the authors to propose the term "monotypic epithelioid malignant angiomyolipoma" for these tumors. Similarly, L'Hostis et al.[242] reported a case of a "monophasic epithelioid pleomorphic" angiomyolipoma that metastasized to the liver and perivertebral region resulting in the patient's death 2 years after presentation.

Angiomyolipomas grow slowly and are adequately treated by partial nephrectomy. Small, asymptomatic tumors may require only careful follow-up, although total nephrectomy may be necessary for large tumors. Cases have also been treated successfully by therapeutic embolization[229,230] or cryotherapy.[218] Although most believe that this lesion represents a hamartomatous proliferation, others have suggested a neoplastic origin, based on the detection of monoclonality.[226,238,252] Although relatively few of these lesions have been studied by cytogenetics, some have been found to show trisomy 7[217,272] and others loss of heterozygosity of the tuberous sclerosis complex genes on chromosomes 9q34 (*TSC1*) and 16p13 (*TSC2*).[205,227,233,234] Loss of hamartin and tuberin expression, the products of *TSC1* and *TSC2* genes, respectively, can be detected in angiomyolipomas with *TSC1* and *TSC2* mutations.[256]

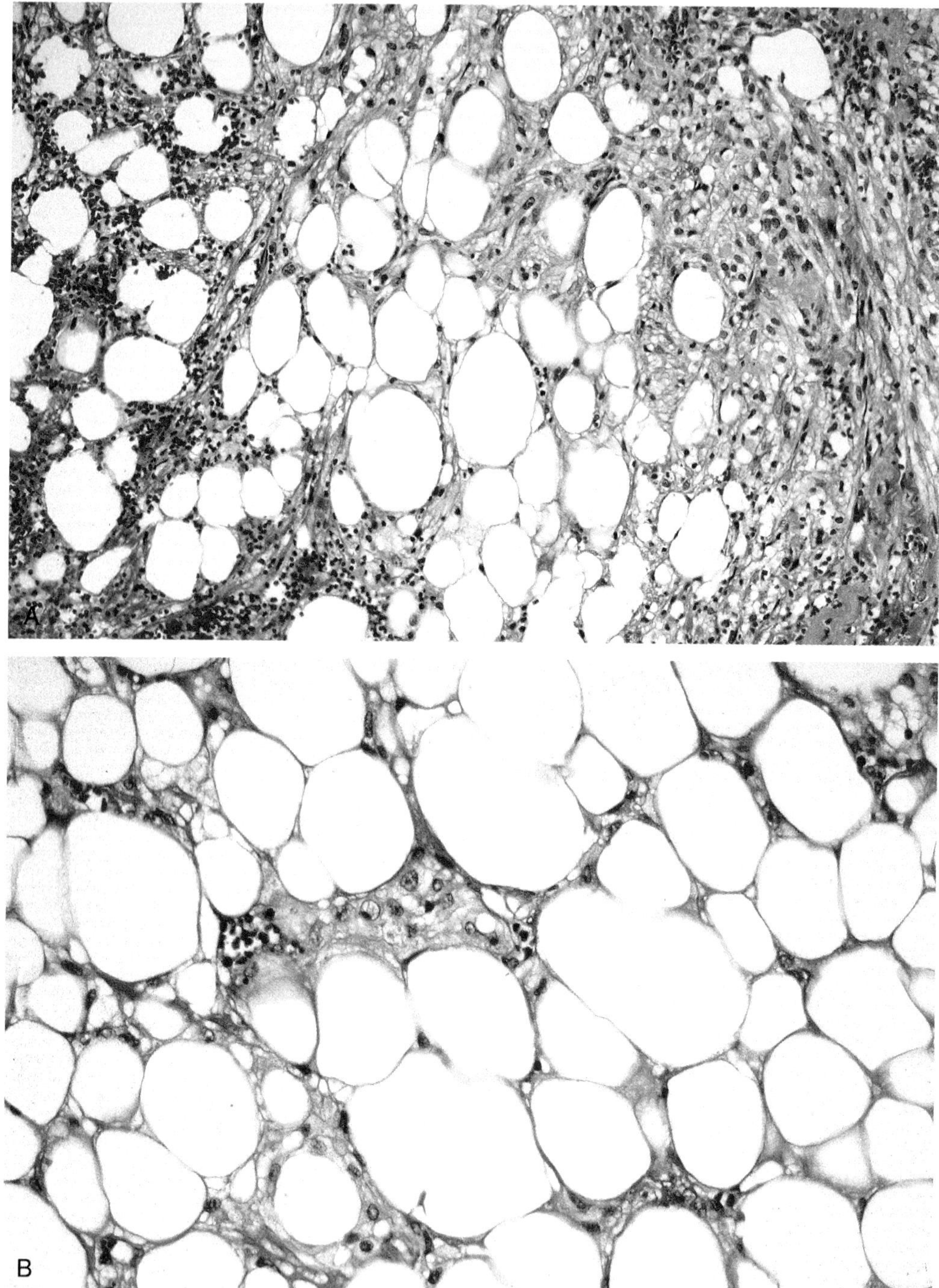


**FIGURE 16–41.** (**A**) Angiomyolipoma exhibiting an admixture of mature fat cells and vacuolated smooth muscle cells. (**B**) Isolated vacuolated smooth muscle cells in an angiomyolipoma. Areas such as this could be mistaken for liposarcoma, particularly when the cells show cytologic atypia.

*Illustration continued on opposite page*

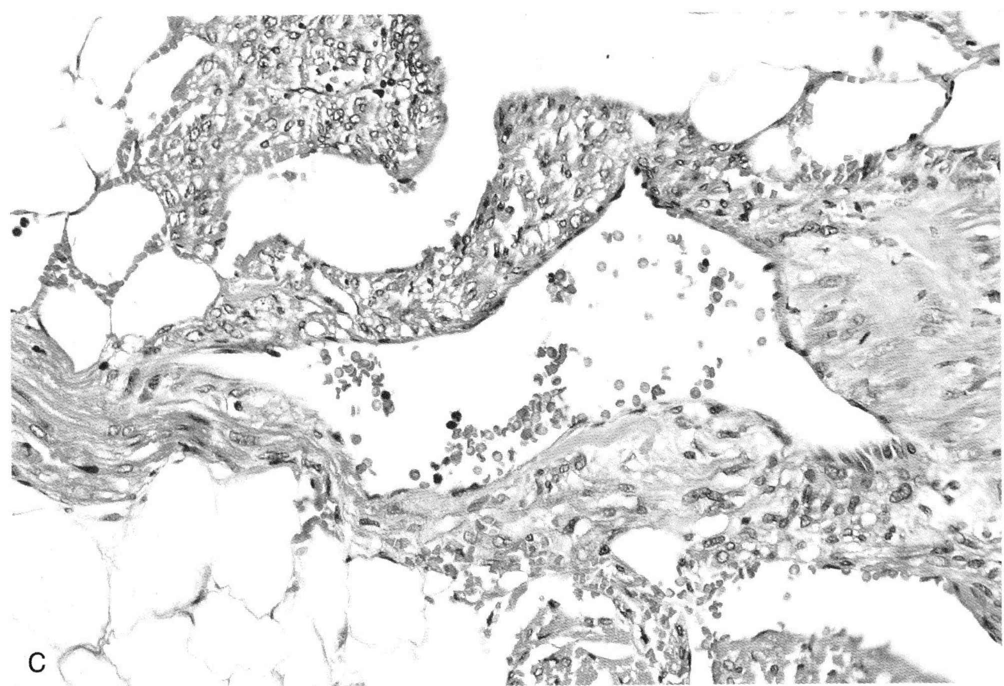


**FIGURE 16–41** *(Continued).* (**C**) Angiomyolipoma with collections of vacuolated smooth muscle cells arranged around dilated vascular spaces.

## MYELOLIPOMA

Although myelolipoma, a tumor-like growth of mature fat and bone marrow elements, is most common in the adrenal glands,[276,285,291,295] it also occurs as an isolated soft tissue mass, especially in the retroperitoneum or pelvic region, in patients without hepatosplenomegaly and with no evidence of hematopoietic disorders.[293,296,298,303] Rare extraadrenal myelolipomas have also been described in numerous other locations, including the mesentery,[278] spleen,[282] testis,[275] and mediastinum.[300] It must be distinguished from *extramedullary hematopoietic tumors,* which are more often multiple than solitary, are frequently associated with splenomegaly and hepatomegaly, and are secondary to severe anemia (thalassemia, hereditary spherocytosis), various myeloproliferative diseases, myelosclerosis, and skeletal disorders.[279,286]

Myelolipomas are rare in young patients, and most are encountered in persons older than 40 years. Small tumors tend to be asymptomatic and often are detected as incidental findings during surgery for some unrelated disease or at autopsy. Large tumors may cause abdominal pain, constipation, or nausea.[277,297,299] Rare tumors may also rupture spontaneously and cause massive retroperitoneal hemorrhage.[281,289]

On radiography myelolipoma presents as a well-circumscribed radiolucent mass, usually in the pelvis or retroperitoneum. When it occurs in the adrenal gland, it causes inferior renal displacement, seen on intravenous urography. It is avascular on arteriography and echodense on ultrasonography.[301] A confidant diagnosis can often be made using CT and MRI scans,[283] but ultrasonography or CT-guided needle biopsy of the lesion may be required.[278,287]

Grossly, myelolipoma has the features of a lipoma; but when the myeloid elements prevail, the tumor assumes a more grayish or grayish-red appearance. The lesion rarely measures more than 5 cm in diameter, although a few large tumors ("giant myelolipomas") are on record.[280,294] Damjanov et al.,[284] for example, reported a myelolipoma that arose in an ectopic adrenal gland and was 15 cm in diameter. Microscopically, the lesion is composed of a mixture of bone marrow elements and lipocytes in varying proportions (Fig. 16–45). Some exhibit extensive myxoid change.[296]

The nature and histogenesis of this lesion are not clear. Many of the reported tumors have been associated with hormonally active neoplasms, including adrenocortical adenomas,[288] adrenocortical carcinomas,[288] and pheochromocytomas.[302] Others have been described in association with adrenocortical hyperplasia,[290] 21-hydroxylase deficiency,[292] and Conn syndrome.[304] It has been proposed that these lesions arise by hormonally driven metaplasia of undifferentiated adrenal stromal cells or, in the case of extraadrenal myelolipomas, from choristomatous hematopoietic stem cell rests.[286]

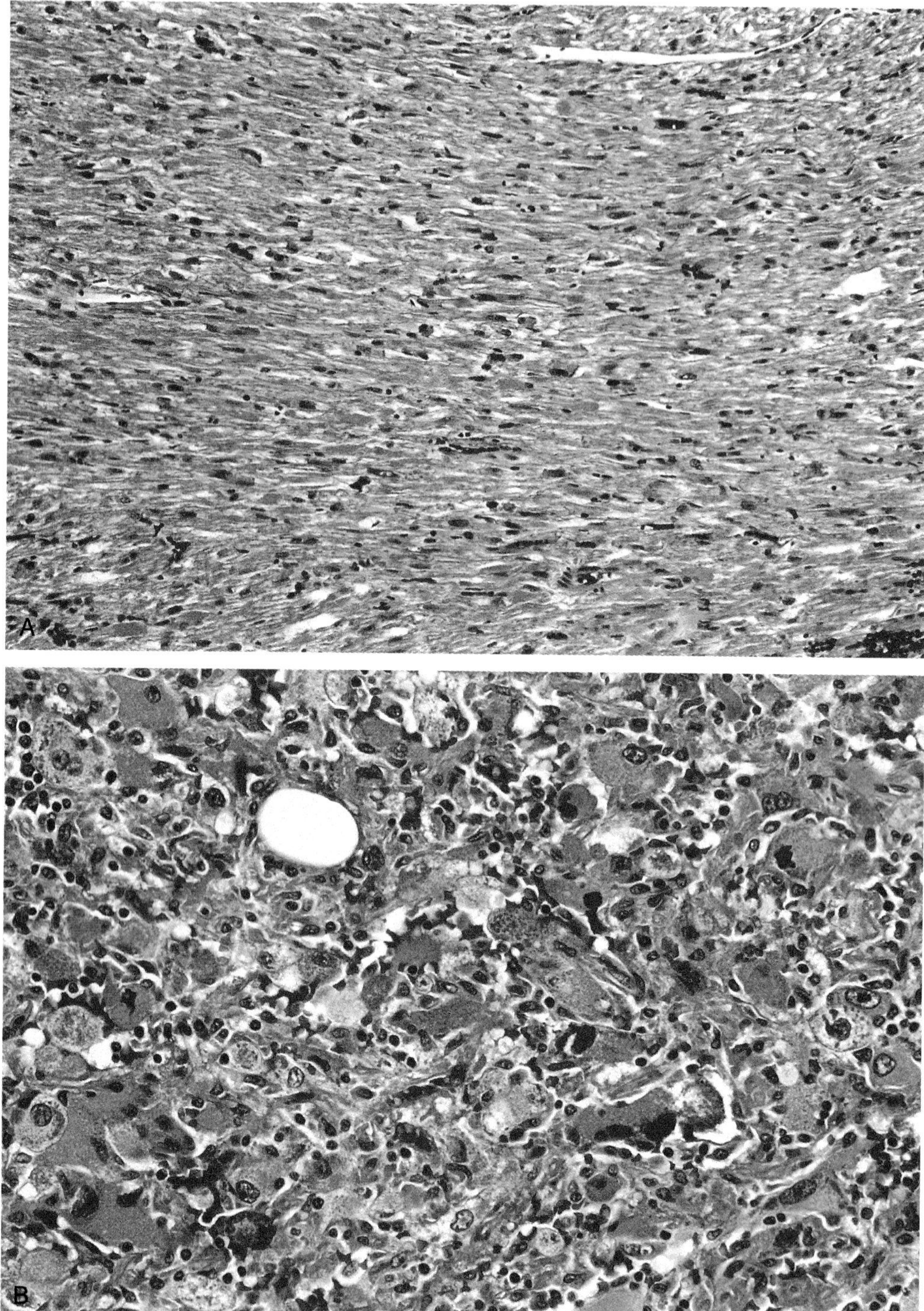

**FIGURE 16–42.** (**A**) Angiomyolipoma with an area composed of atypical spindle-shaped smooth muscle cells arranged in fascicles. Such areas could be confused for leiomyosarcoma or dedifferentiated liposarcoma with divergent leiomyosarcomatous differentiation. (**B**) Angiomyolipoma exhibiting striking variation in the size and shape of smooth muscle elements, with rare cells showing marked cytologic atypia, a feature that has been mistaken for evidence of malignancy.

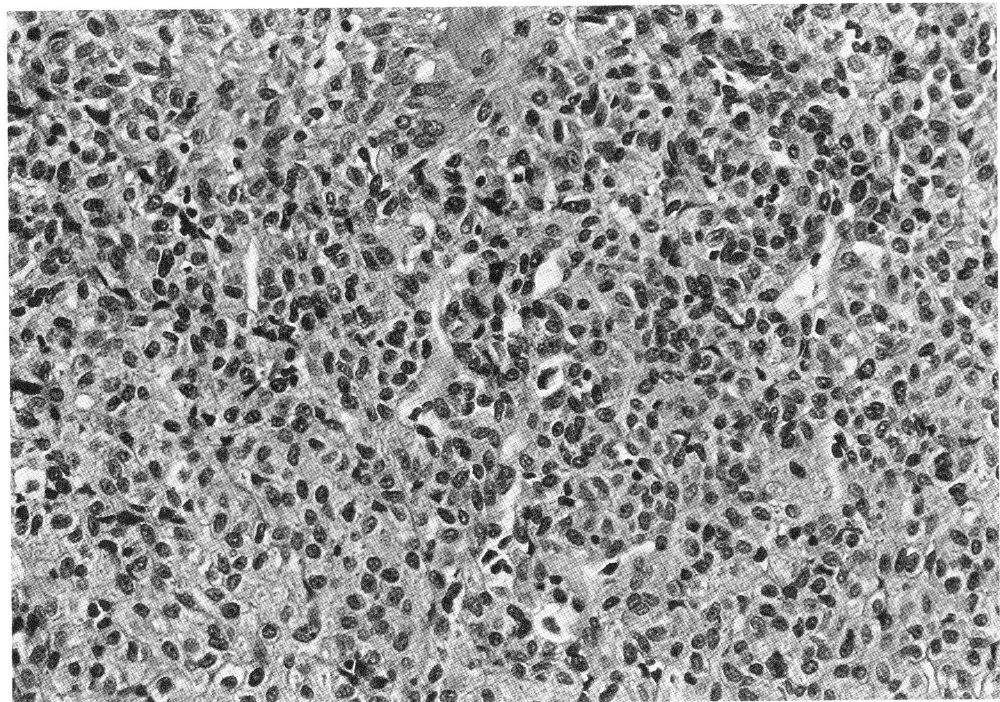

**FIGURE 16–43.** Angiomyolipoma composed of uniform small epithelioid smooth muscle cells, a feature that could be mistaken for renal cell carcinoma, particularly in patients with tuberous sclerosis.

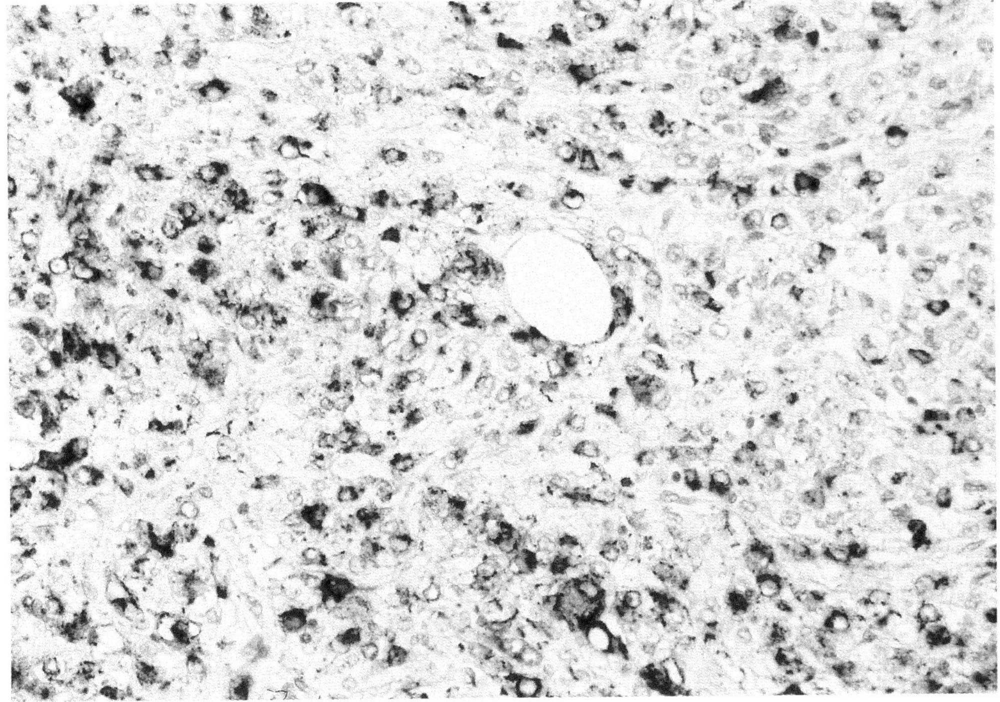

**FIGURE 16–44.** HMB-45 immunoreactivity in the smooth muscle cells of an angiomyolipoma.

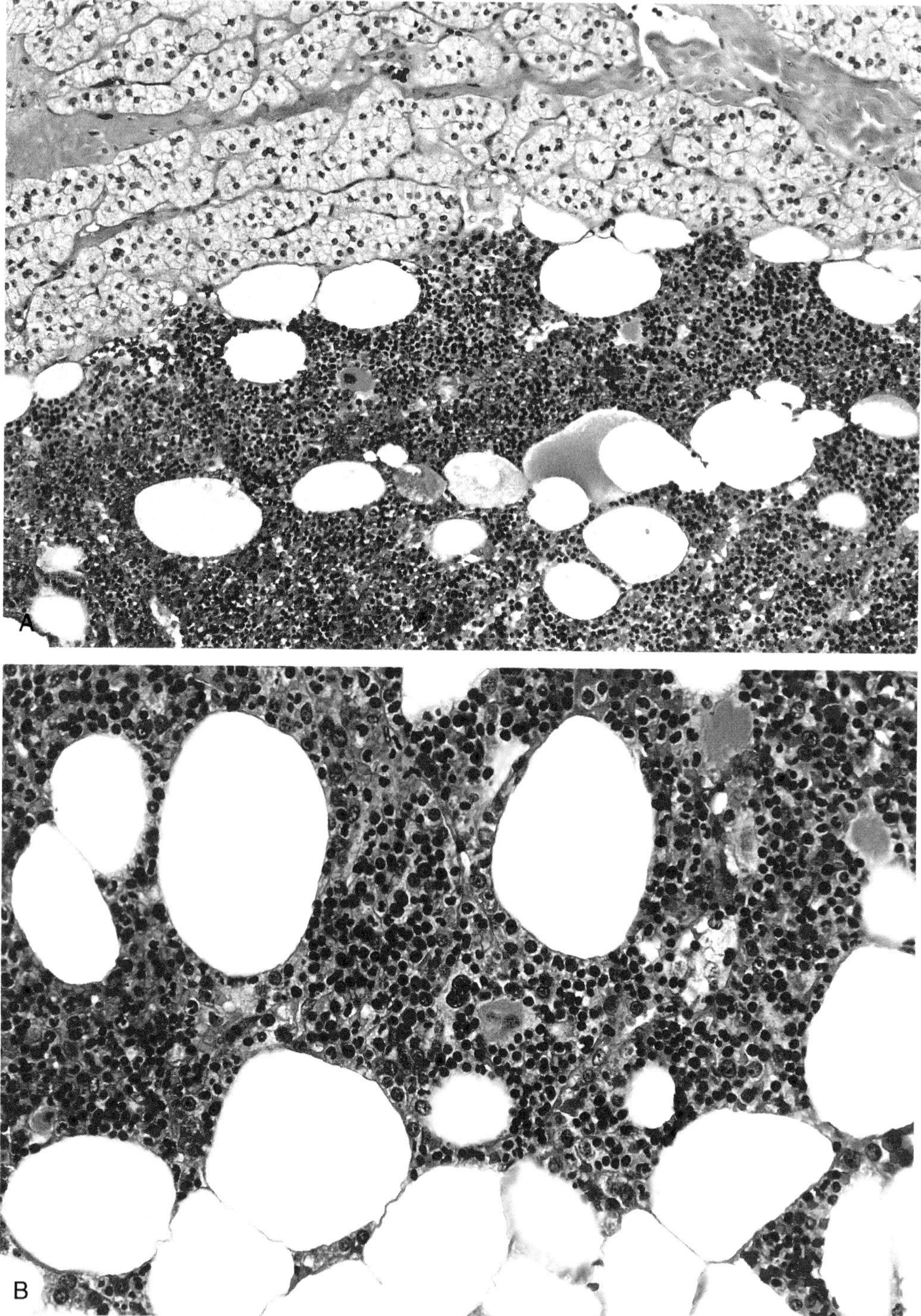


**FIGURE 16–45.** (**A**) Low-power view of a myelolipoma with an admixture of adrenal cortical cells, mature fat cells, and myeloid elements. (**B**) High-power view of a myelolipoma with a mixture of mature fat cells and bone marrow elements, including megakaryocytes.

## INTRAMUSCULAR AND INTERMUSCULAR LIPOMAS

Intramuscular and intermuscular lipomas are relatively common. They concern both clinicians and pathologists because of their large size, deep location, and infiltrating growth. Intramuscular lipomas outnumber intermuscular lipomas by a considerable margin, but many lesions involve both muscular and intermuscular tissues.[305,310,315] The condition has also been described in the literature as an *infiltrating lipoma*.[309,311,314]

The tumor arises at all ages, but most occur in adults 30–60 years of age. Occasionally it is encountered in children.[313] In such cases, distinction from diffuse lipomatosis and lipoblastomatosis may be difficult. There is general agreement that men are more often afflicted than women and that the most important sites are the large muscles of the extremities, especially those of the thigh, shoulder, and upper arm. Unusual cases have also been described in the paraspinal muscles[307] and larynx.[306,308] Most tumors are slow-growing and painless, and they often become apparent only during muscle contraction when the tumor is converted to a firm spherical mass. Sometimes movement causes aching or pain,[316] but the pain is rarely severe. Their size varies considerably, ranging from minute lesions to tumors 20 cm or more in diameter. Occasional tumors are found on routine radiologic examination because intramuscular lipomas, like other forms of lipoma, are radiolucent and are readily demonstrated radiographically (Fig. 16–46). Microangiographically, the intramuscular lipoma is much less vascular than the surrounding muscle tissue.[312]

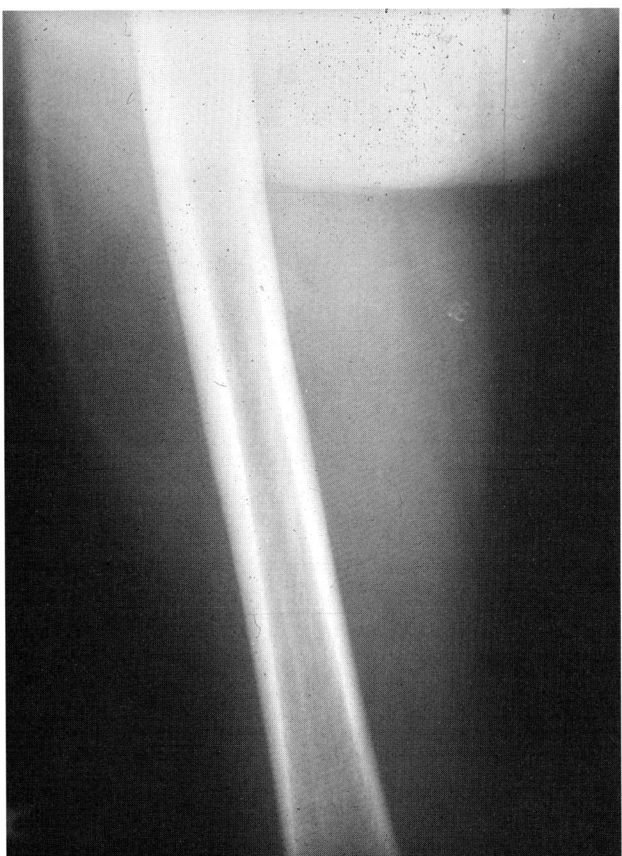

**FIGURE 16–46.** Radiograph of an intramuscular lipoma involving the muscles of the thigh. Note the sharply circumscribed radiolucent mass surrounded by a rim of muscle tissue.

Cross sections of the intramuscular lipoma reveal gradual replacement of the muscle tissue by fat that may extend beyond the muscle fascia into the intermuscular connective tissue spaces. On longitudinal section it often assumes a striated appearance owing to the proliferation of fat cells between muscle fibers (Fig. 16–47).

Microscopic examination reveals lipocytes that infiltrate muscle in a diffuse manner. The entrapped muscle fibers usually show few changes other than various degrees of muscular atrophy (Figs. 16–48, 16–49). Characteristically, the lipocytes are mature; there are no lipoblasts or cells with atypical nuclei as in *well-differentiated liposarcoma*. Nonetheless, careful sampling of these tumors is mandatory because portions of well-differentiated intramuscular liposarcoma may be indistinguishable from those of intramuscular lipoma. *Diffuse lipoblastomatosis and lipomatosis*, lesions that occur mostly in infants and children, affect the subcutis *and* muscle; and generally more than one muscle is involved. Furthermore, these lesions tend to be more distinctly lobulated than intramuscular lipoma, with connective tissue septa of varying thickness and lobules composed of lipoblasts in different stages of development. In some *intramuscular hemangiomas*, "ex vacuo" growth of fat may simulate the picture of an intramuscular lipoma; such cases have been misinterpreted as "angiolipoma."

The prospect of cure is excellent if the tumor is completely removed. In the AFIP series 85% of patients remained well following the initial excision; the tumor recurred in the other 15%.[310] Overall, the recurrence rate reported in the literature has varied from as little as 3.0%[312] to as much as 62.5%,[309] probably depending on the completeness of the excision and doubtlessly on the criteria employed for diagnosis and distinction from well-differentiated intramuscular liposarcoma.

## LIPOMAS OF TENDON SHEATHS AND JOINTS

Lipomas of the tendon sheaths and joints are rare. There are two types: (1) solid fatty masses that extend

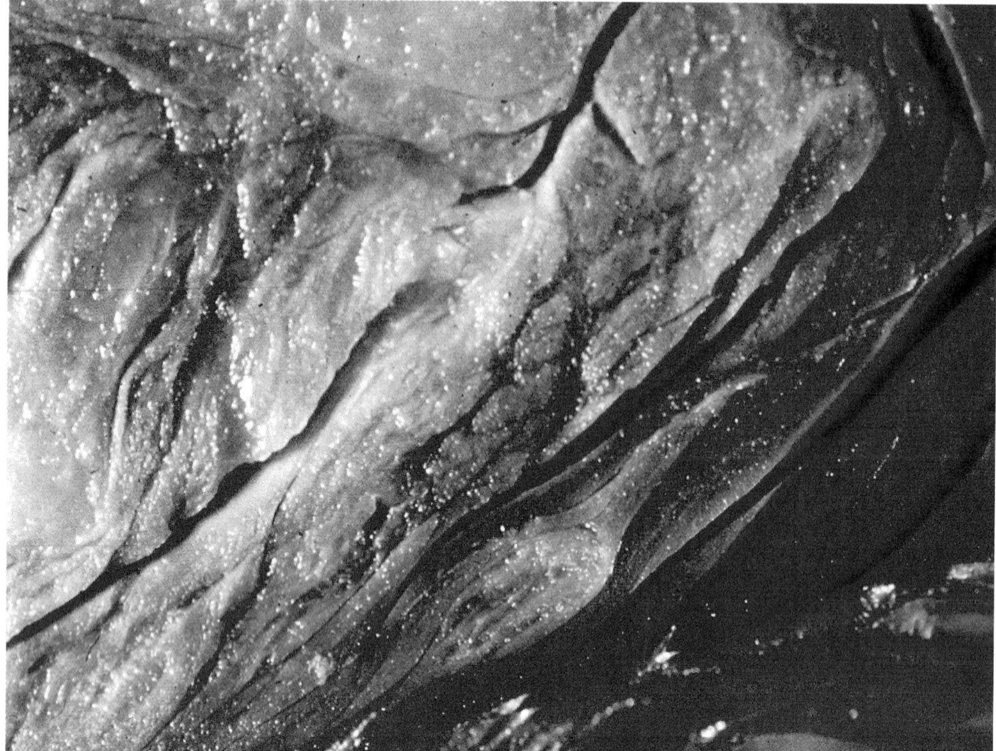

**FIGURE 16–47.** Partial replacement of muscle tissue by fat in an intramuscular lipoma.

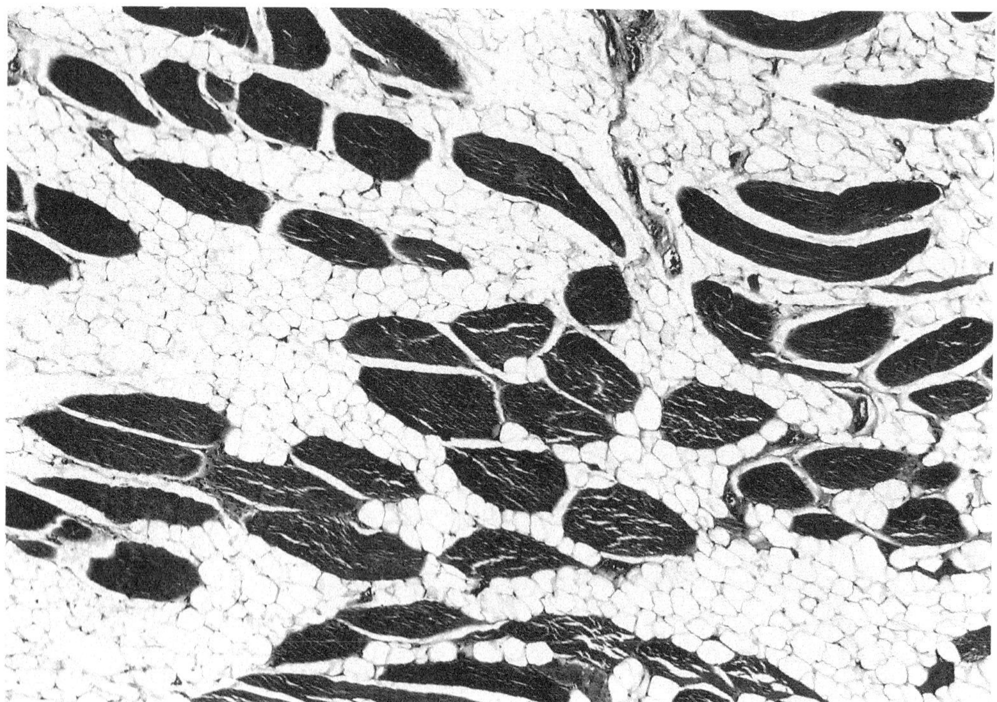

**FIGURE 16–48.** Intramuscular lipoma with entrapped striated muscle fibers in cross section. There is some atrophy of the fat cells but no lipoblasts or cells with hyperchromatic nuclei as in well-differentiated liposarcoma.

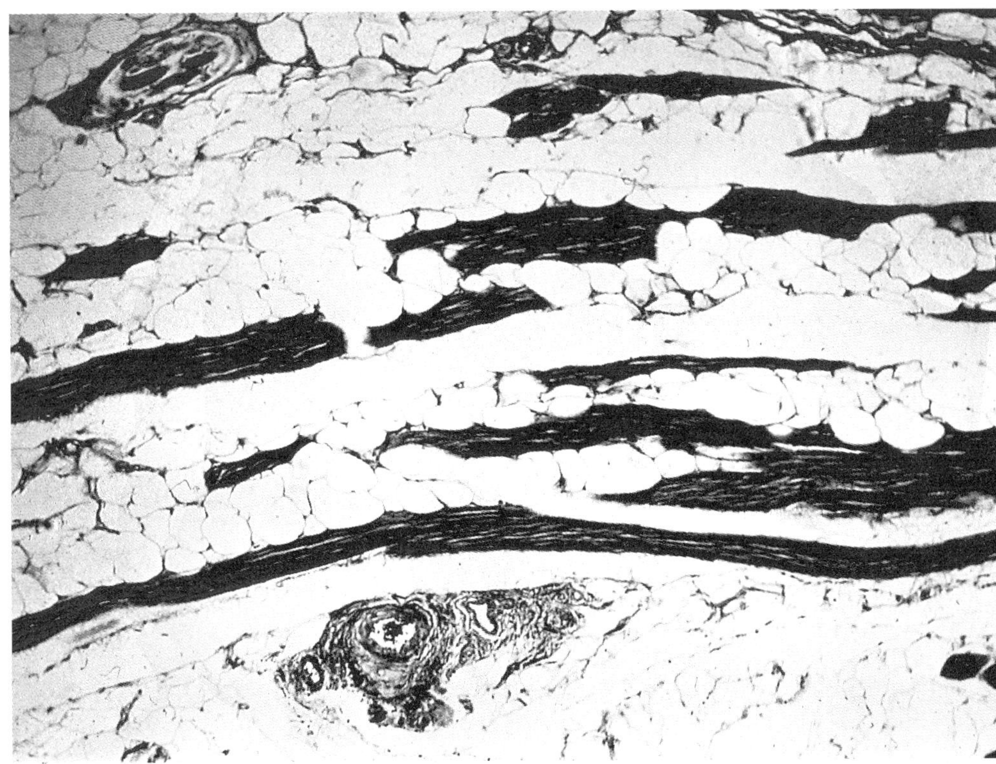

**FIGURE 16–49.** Intramuscular lipoma with striated muscle fibers in longitudinal section. Note the complete absence of cellular atypism.

along tendons for varying distances; and (2) *lipoma-like* lesions that consist chiefly of hypertrophic synovial villi distended by fat, most commonly seen in the region of the knee joint (*lipoma arborescens*). When they occur in tendon sheaths, these lesions have been described as *endovaginal* tumors, in contrast to *epivaginal* tumors (e.g., deep lipomas arising outside the tendon sheath).

According to Sullivan et al.,[338] lipoma of the tendon sheath occurs with about equal frequency in both genders and chiefly in young persons (15–35 years); it affects the wrist and hand and less commonly the ankle and foot. About half are bilateral and show a symmetric distribution. Occasionally they involve both the hands and feet of the same individual. By the time the patient seeks treatment most of the lesions have been present for several years, and many cause pain that may be severe. Other patients develop a trigger finger[334] or symptoms of carpal tunnel syndrome.[329] Rupture of a tendon secondary to lipoma of the tendon sheath has been reported. As with other types of lipoma, radiologic examination shows a mass of less density than the surrounding tissue, which may be helpful for the diagnosis.[320]

Lipoma in joints (*lipoma arborescens*) is more common than lipoma of the tendon sheath. The condition most commonly affects the knee joint, particularly the suprapatellar pouch,[317,324,332] although rare cases occur in the glenohumeral joint,[331] subdeltoid bursa,[321] hip,[333] and elbow.[339] Most patients are adults, although there are some reports of this tumor in children.[322] Men are affected more commonly than women. The typical presentation is insidious swelling of the knee with intermittent effusions followed by progressive pain and debilitation.[318,325] Arthrography reveals irregular, nonspecific filling defects, most commonly in the posteromedial aspect of the suprapatellar pouch.[319] Both CT and MRI are useful for a preoperative diagnosis.[320,323,335,337] Grossly and microscopically, the lesion consists of fibrofatty tissue or thickened, grape-like or finger-like villi infiltrated by fat and lined by synovium (Figs. 16–50, 16–51). Some cases are associated with osseous or chondroid metaplasia.[330,336]

Lipoma arborescens is probably a reactive process; it is found in association with joint trauma, meniscal lesions, chronic synovitis, and diabetes mellitus.[317,327] Hallel et al.[325] proposed the term "villous lipomatous proliferation of the synovial membrane" to avoid confusion with a neoplastic process. It is likely some of the symmetric lipoma arborescens-like lesions of the tendon sheath are also reactive hyperplastic lesions associated with various forms of chronic tenosynovitis. Traumatic proliferation of fatty tissue in the retropatellar portion of the knee joint is sometimes referred to as *Hoffa's disease*.[326,328]

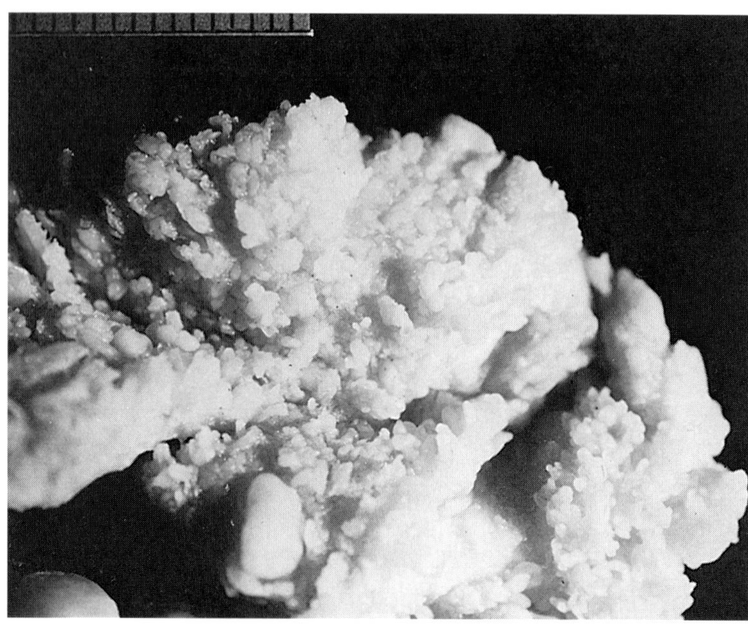

**FIGURE 16–50.** "Lipoma arborescens," a reactive, lipoma-like lesion caused by overgrowth of fat in hypertrophied synovial villi.

## LUMBOSACRAL LIPOMA

Lumbosacral lipoma is another curious type of lipomatous growth that deserves recognition because of its close relation to the spinal cord and its coverings. It is characterized by a diffuse proliferation of mature fat overlying the lower portion of the spine in the lumbosacral region. The lesion is always associated with spina bifida or a similar laminar defect (lipomyeloschisis), and there is a stalk-like connection (tethered cord) between the fatty growth and a portion of the spinal cord that often also harbors an intradural or extradural lipoma. The stalk may cause traction and ischemia. Lipomas extending from the middle to one side are more likely to contain a meningocele or a myelocele.[344] According to Rickwood et al.,[353] its overall incidence is slightly less than 1 in 10,000 live births.

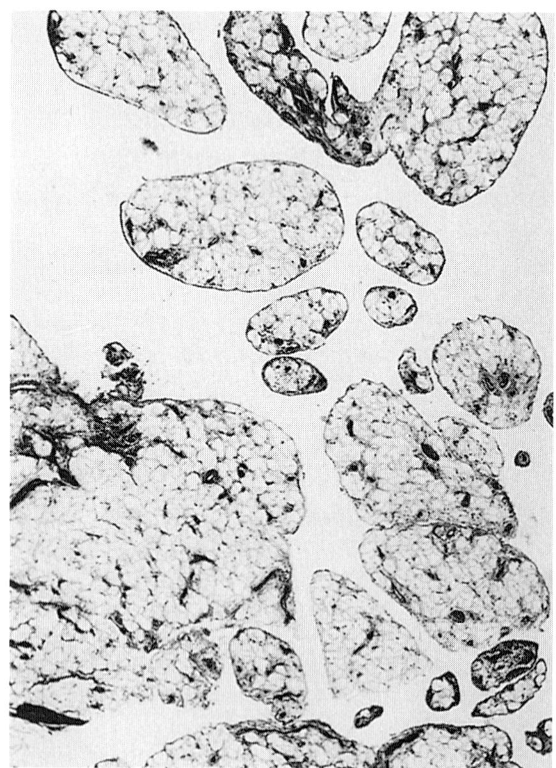

**FIGURE 16–51.** Cross section of synovial villi in "lipoma arborescens" showing stromal deposition of mature fat.

Clinically, lumbosacral lipoma tends to be asymptomatic initially and often is noted only because of the presence of a large soft tissue mass or because of a sinus, skin tag, hemangioma, or excessive hair associated with a soft swelling in the lumbosacral region. Later, in about two-thirds of cases progressive myelopathy or radiculopathy causes motor or sensory disturbances in the lower legs, bladder, or bowel.[350,351]

The lesion affects females almost twice as often as males and is encountered chiefly in infants or children between birth and 10 years of age. Occasional cases in adults have been reported[342,348,349]; Loeser and Lewin[348] described such a case in a 34-year-old man who complained of weakness of 4–5 years' duration in both legs, associated with a spina bifida at L4–5 and an intradural filling defect. In the series of Lassman and James[347] all 19 patients had evidence of spina bifida, and 9 had evidence of progressive neuropathy. The authors also found 26 cases of lumbosacral lipoma among 100 cases of occult spina bifida.

Sonography, CT scans, or MRI is essential for diagnosis and for planning therapy; these procedures show not only the exact position of the cord and its relation to the lipoma but also the association of the mass with spina bifida or some degree of sacral dysgenesis[341]; on myelography there is frequently blockage of the spinal canal.[354]

At operation the lipomatous growth is usually unencapsulated and consists of lobulated adipose tissue microscopically indistinguishable from lipoma. In some cases vascular proliferation and smooth muscle tissue are present in addition to the adipocytes. Rarely, islets of neuroglia, ependyma-lined tubular structures, and primitive neural tissue are found near the spinal defect.[340]

Surgical exploration—laminectomy and division of the stalk and fibrous bands that have formed at the upper margin of the spinal defect—should be performed as early as possible, preferably prior to the onset of neurologic symptoms.[343] Early treatment, however, does not always prevent the development of leg paralysis and neurogenic bladder.[345,346,352]

## NEURAL FIBROLIPOMA (LIPOFIBROMATOUS HAMARTOMA OF NERVES)

The neural fibrolipoma is a tumor-like lipomatous process that involves principally the volar aspects of the hands, wrists, and forearms of young persons. It usually manifests as a soft slowly growing mass consisting of proliferating fibrofatty tissue surrounding and infiltrating major nerves and their branches.[365,367] Other terms applied to this condition are *lipofibromatous hamartoma of nerves*[369,373] and *neurolipomatosis.*[355] About one-third of neural fibrolipomas are associated with overgrowth of bone and macrodactyly.[363,366] In the series of 26 cases reported by Silverman and Enzinger,[374] 7 were associated with macrodactyly. Lesions of this type have also been described as *macrodystrophia lipomatosa,*[358,375] but it is preferable to refer to them as *neural fibrolipoma with macrodactyly.*

The lesion is almost always seen during the first three decades of life, usually because of increasing pain, tenderness, diminished sensation, or paresthesias associated with a gradually enlarging mass causing compression neuropathy. There may also be some loss of strength. Growth is usually slow and in most patients has been noted for years. Lesions present at birth or infancy far outnumber those recognized later in childhood or adult life. Males are more often affected than females, and the left hand is more often involved than the right. There may be a genetic disposition, but there is no history of any hereditary disorders. The onset is linked to trauma in some cases. Carpal tunnel syndrome is a late complication of some lesions.[359,361] Findings on MRI scans are characteristic, and it can usually be diagnosed preoperatively.[360,364]

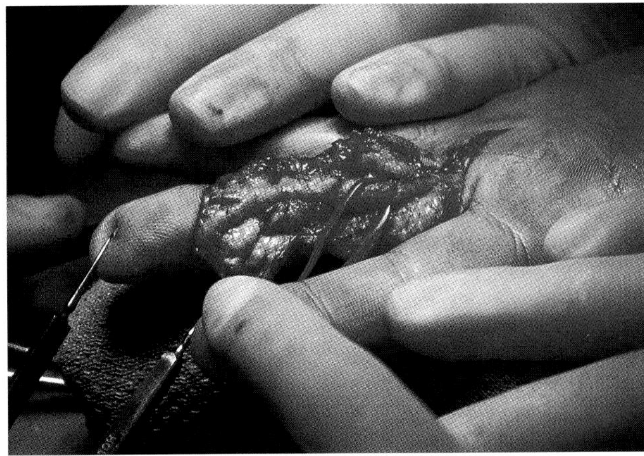

**FIGURE 16–52.** Neural fibrolipoma with a fusiform, sausage-shaped mass caused by diffuse infiltration of a digital nerve.

At operation neural fibrolipoma presents as a soft, gray-yellow, fusiform, sausage-shaped mass that has diffusely infiltrated and replaced portions of a large nerve and its branches (Figs. 16–52, 16–53). The median nerve is affected in most cases. Rarely, the lesion is found in other nerves, such as the ulnar,[370] radial,[371] peroneal,[357] and cranial nerves.[356] It consists of fibrofatty tissue that grows along epi- and perineurium and surrounds and infiltrates the nerve trunk (Figs. 16–54, 16–55, 16–56). Prolonged duration and compression of nerves by the fatty tissue result in neural degeneration and atrophy, which accounts for the usual late appearance of symptoms. Rare cases

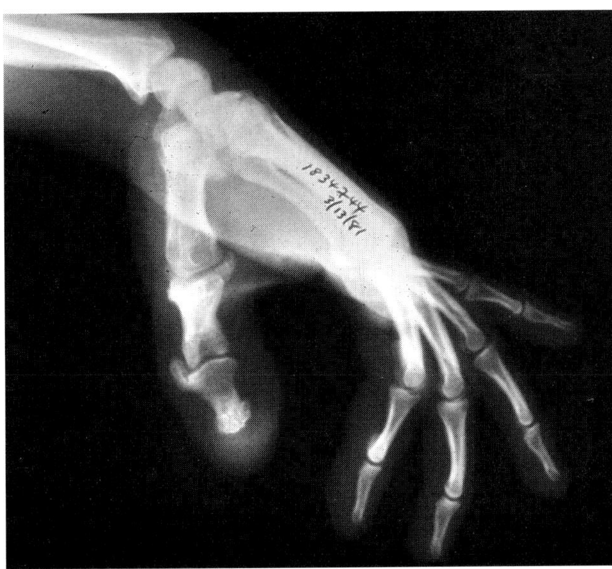

**FIGURE 16–53.** Radiograph displaying macrodactyly in a patient with an associated neural fibrolipoma.

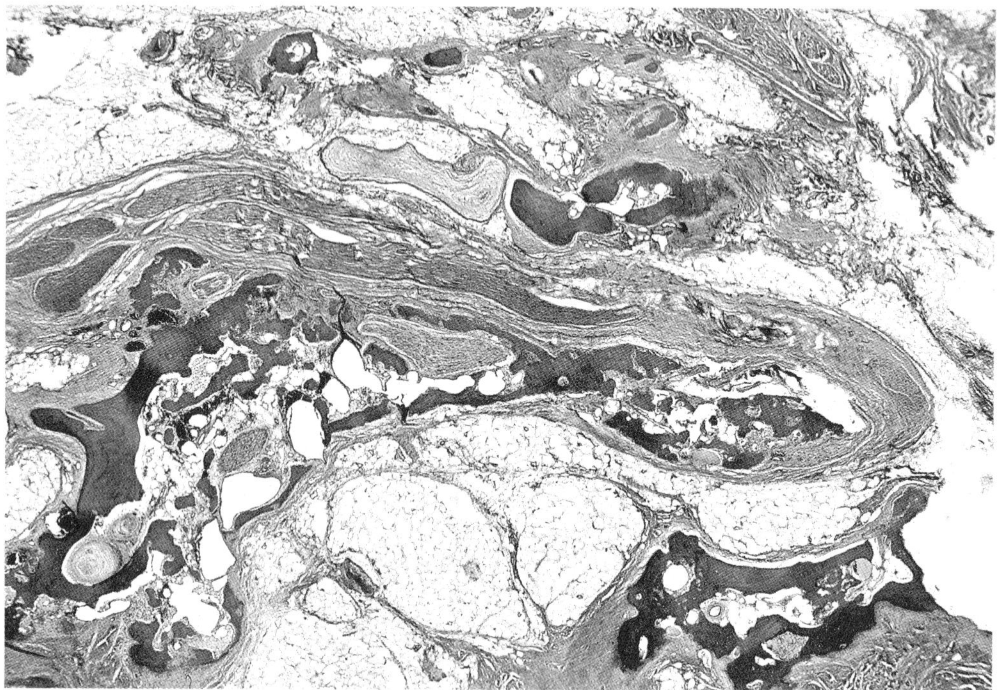

**FIGURE 16–54.** Low-power view of a neural fibrolipoma with extensive osseous metaplasia.

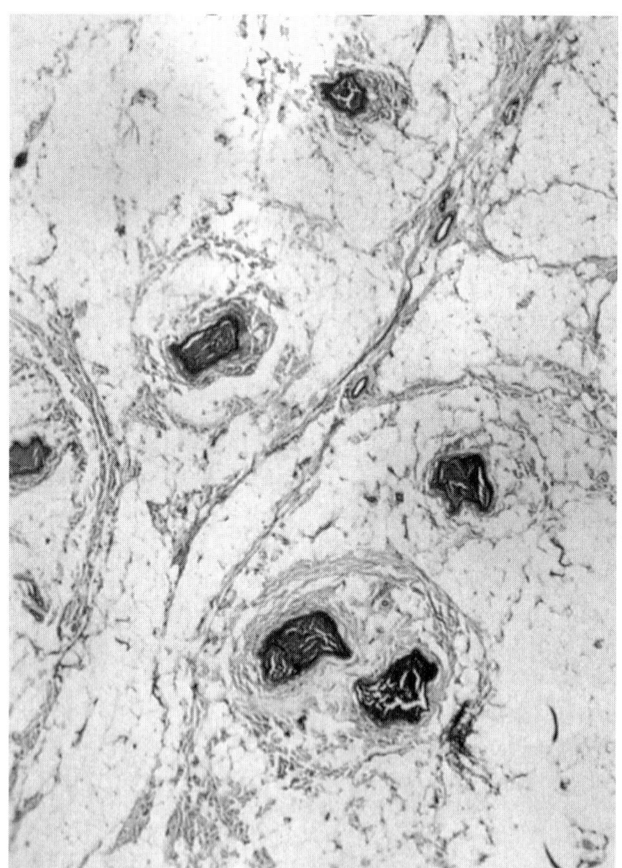

**FIGURE 16–55.** Neural fibrolipoma (fibrolipomatous hamartoma of nerves) with fat tissue surrounding and splaying apart peripheral nerves.

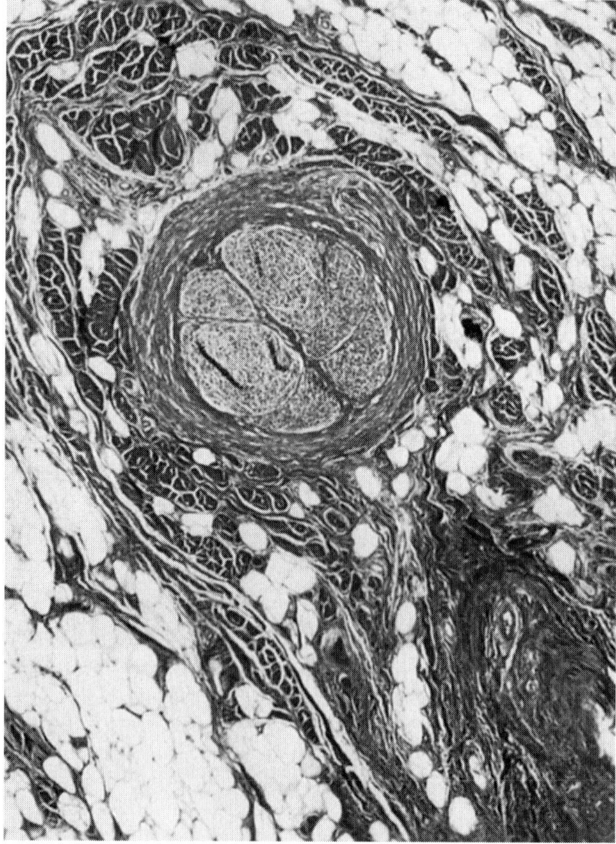

**FIGURE 16–56.** Neural fibrolipoma (fibrolipomatous hamartoma of nerves) with fibrosis of the nerve sheath and perineural fibrofatty growth.

show foci of metaplastic bone.[362,374] Masses of fibrofatty tissue may also be found outside the involved nerves, unattached to either the overlying skin or neighboring tendons and indistinguishable from a deep-seated lipoma. There is also marked thickening of the perineurium and the perivascular fibrous tissue. The diffuse infiltrative character of the lesion distinguishes it from localized and circumscribed lipomas of nerves occurring elsewhere in the body, including lipomas originating in the spinal canal. Unlike *neuromas* and *neurofibromas,* there is atrophy rather than proliferation of neural elements. Clear distinction from *diffuse lipomatosis with overgrowth of bone* is not always possible, but diffuse lipomatosis is primarily a lesion of the subcutis and muscle and only secondarily affects nerves.

There is no effective therapy for neural fibrolipoma. Complete excision of the fibrofatty growth is contraindicated because it may cause severe sensory or motor disturbances. If necessary, biopsy of a small cutaneous nerve can establish the diagnosis.[373] Pain and sensory loss may be partially or completely relieved by dividing the transverse carpal ligament and decompressing the median nerve.[368,372,376]

## DIFFUSE LIPOMATOSIS

Diffuse lipomatosis may be defined as a rare, diffuse overgrowth of mature adipose tissue that usually affects large portions of an extremity or the trunk. Although it simulates liposarcoma by its size and aggressive growth, it is indistinguishable from lipoma microscopically. Like lipoma, it consists entirely of adult-type fat; and despite its frequently rapid enlargement, there is no evidence of lipoblastic activity or cellular pleomorphism.

The condition is not limited to the panniculus, and in nearly all cases subcutis and muscle are diffusely involved. Many lesions are associated with osseous hypertrophy, leading to macrodactyly or giantism of a digit or limb (Fig. 16–57).[378,382,384] Unlike perineural fibrolipoma, there is no involvement of nerves, and the process is not limited to the extremities. Association with lipomas or angiomas in other portions of the body is by no means rare. In addition to the extremities and trunk, the lesion occurs in the head and neck, intestinal tract, abdominal cavity, and pelvis.[379] There are also reports of symmetric lipomatosis of the hands[377] and diffuse lipomatosis of the leg following poliomyelitis.[380] Most cases have their onset during the first 2 years of life, but we and others have also observed typical examples of this tumor in adolescents and adults (Figs. 16–58, 16–59).[381,383,385]

The differential diagnosis may be difficult. *Intramuscular lipomas* may exhibit a similar microscopic picture, but these tumors are always confined to muscle or intermuscular tissue spaces and usually contain a larger number of entrapped muscle fibers. *Diffuse angiomatosis* may be accompanied by considerable fatty and osseous overgrowth, but it is always recognizable by its more pronounced vascular pattern. *Well-differentiated liposarcoma* is usually less of a problem if the tumor is carefully sampled for evidence of lipoblastic activity and cellular pleomorphism. Distinction is also facilitated by the age of the patient. Liposarcomas are rare during infancy, and virtually all lipoblastic tumors seen during this period are benign lipoblastomas or lipoblastomatosis.

Diffuse lipomatosis tends to recur, often repeatedly over many years. It may reach a large size and in rare instances causes severely impaired function, necessitating drastic surgery.

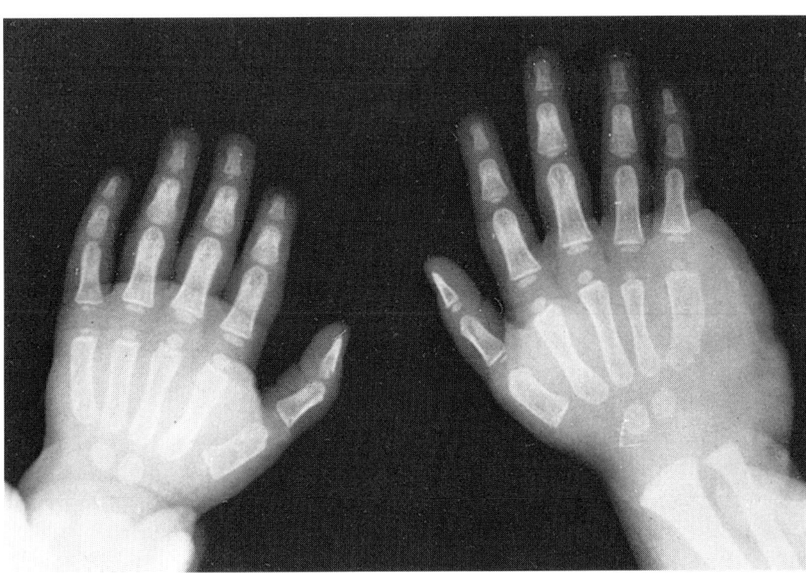

**FIGURE 16–57.** Diffuse lipomatosis of the right hand with slight overgrowth of phalangeal bones.

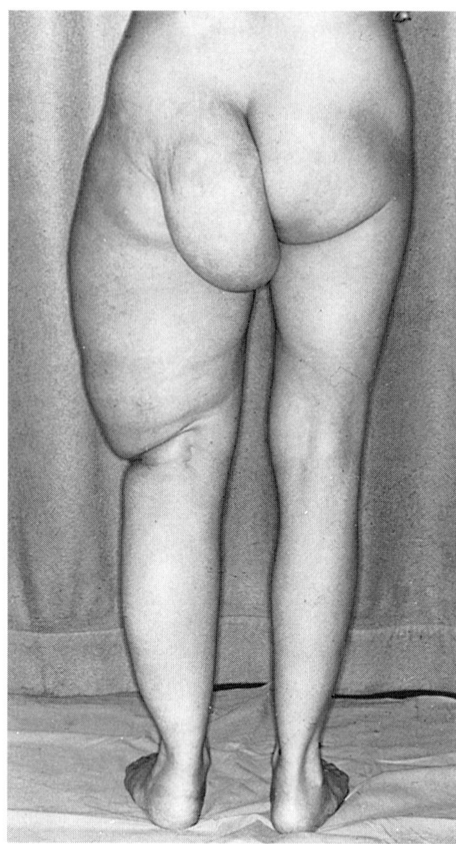

**FIGURE 16–58.** Diffuse lipomatosis confined mainly to the left buttock and thigh.

## SYMMETRIC LIPOMATOSIS

Symmetric lipomatosis is a rare, fascinating disease that has also been described under the eponyms *Madelung's disease* and *Launois-Bensaude syndrome.*[403,404,409] Originally described by Brodie in 1846,[392] the disease was not well described until Madelung reported a series of cases with "horse collar" cervical involvement by adipose tissue.[404] It was further described in 1889 by Launois and Bensaude in a report of 65 cases.[403] Patients with this condition suffer from massive symmetric deposition of mature fat in the region of the neck, so the head appears to be pushed forward by a hump that has been likened to a horse collar or doughnut-shaped ring (*lipoma annulare colli*) (Fig. 16–60).

The disease affects middle-aged men almost exclusively, particularly those of Mediterranean origin.[396] Excessive alcohol intake or liver disease has been reported in 60–90% of patients in various series,[410] although the precise role of these factors in the development of the lipomatosis is unclear. The fatty deposits grow insidiously, frequently over many years; and in contrast to Dercum's disease (adiposis dolorosa), they are nontender and painless. They are chiefly located bilaterally in the region of the neck but also may involve the cheeks, breast, upper arm, and axilla. The distal portions of the forearm and leg remain unaffected. Up to 86% of patients have a predominantly axonal sensorimotor neuropathy,[397,407,408] and up to 50% have central nervous system involvement, including hearing loss, atrophy of the optic nerve, and cerebellar ataxia.[389] Most cases are sporadic, but a few are familial,[394] with some suggesting an autosomal dominant mode of inheritance.[402,411] It has also been suggested that occult malignancy is found with increased frequency in patients with symmetric lipomatosis.[410]

The fatty deposits are poorly circumscribed and affect both the subcutis and deep soft tissue spaces, frequently extending in tongue-like projections between the cervical and thoracic muscles. Massive deposits in the deep portion of the neck, larynx, and

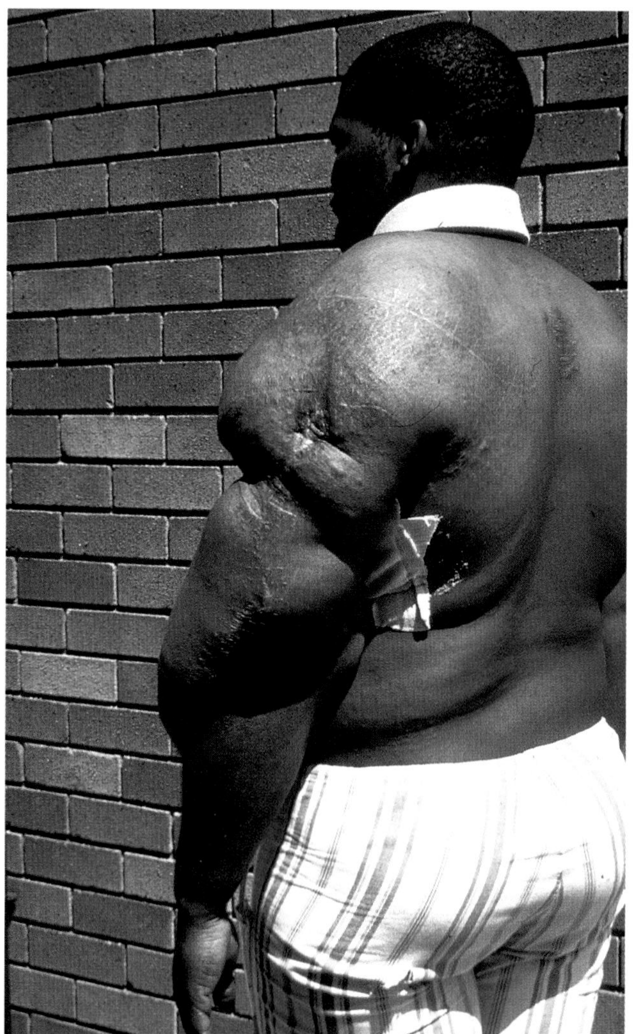

**FIGURE 16–59.** Diffuse lipomatosis confined to the left arm.

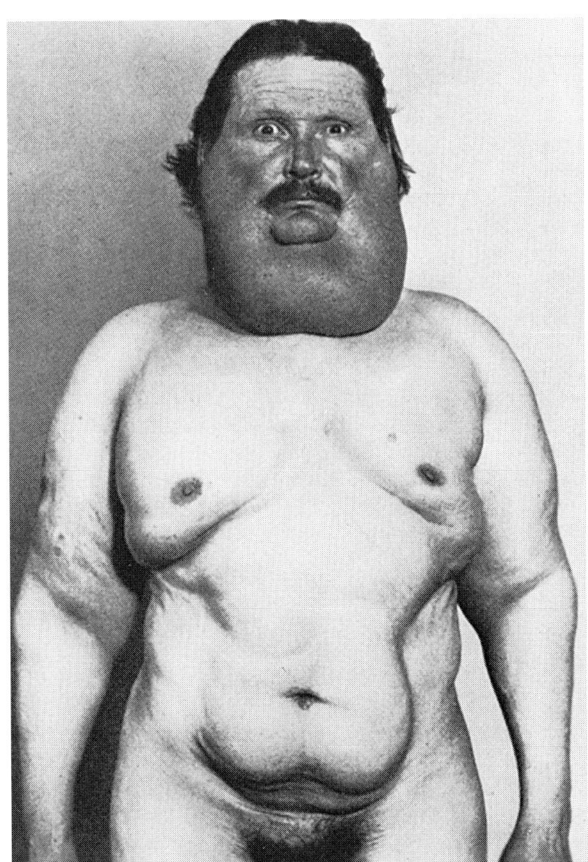

**FIGURE 16–60.** Symmetric lipomatosis (Madelung's disease). (From Saalfeld E, Saalfeld U. Klinic der gutartigen Tumoren; Handbuch der Haut und Geschlechtskrankheiten, Geschwuelst der Haut. Julius Springer, Berlin, 1932, with permission.)

mediastinum may cause dysphagia, stridor, and respiratory embarrassment[386,390] or progressive vena caval compression.[396] As a rule, patients with this condition are not particularly obese, a fact that adds to the striking appearance of the fatty deposits in the neck. Both CT and MRI are useful for determining the extent of fat accumulation, particularly in the deep soft tissue sites.[398,414] Grossly and microscopically, the accumulated fat is indistinguishable from mature fat, except for varying degrees of fibrosis and, rarely, calcification and ossification.

The exact cause of the condition remains obscure. A variety of metabolic disturbances such as hyperuricemia and gout,[405] hyperlipidemia,[399] and diabetes[395] have been associated with symmetric lipomatosis, but these findings are inconsistent. It has been suggested that the increased synthesis of fat is the result of a defect in catecholamine-stimulated lipolysis.[396] Others have proposed that functional sympathetic denervation results in the hypertrophy of embryologic brown fat.[401] Zancanaro et al. found that the adipose tissue in symmetric lipomatosis ultrastructurally resembles brown fat.[415] More recently, a mitochondrial cytopathy, with point mutations at the MERRF (myoclonus epilepsy and ragged-red fibers syndrome) locus of the human mitochondrial genes[388,400,406] has been implicated in the pathogenesis.

Although conservative surgery and liposuction have been used effectively to treat the disease,[391,412] it may not be necessary, as in some cases the deposited fat recedes with abstinence from alcohol and correction of nutritional deficiencies.[387]

Symmetric lipomatosis must be distinguished from *adiposis dolorosa (Dercum's disease)*.[393,413] This condition is marked by tender or painful, diffuse or nodular accumulation of subcutaneous fat. It occurs predominantly in postmenopausal women and affects primarily the regions of the pelvic girdle and the thigh. The lesion is associated with marked asthenia (e.g., loss of strength and fatigue with the least amount of effort), depression, and psychic disturbances. As with symmetric lipomatosis, there is no evidence of a hormonal abnormality.

## PELVIC LIPOMATOSIS

Pelvic lipomatosis, first described by Engels[423] in 1959, is characterized by an overgrowth of fat in the perirectal and perivesical regions, causing compression of the lower urinary tract and rectosigmoid colon. The lesion is probably more common than is implied by the relatively small number of cases so far described.[417,424,426,434]

The condition chiefly affects black men during the third and fourth decades of life. Women are rarely affected.[431,433] In a review of the literature, Heyns found a male/female ratio of 18:1.[428] In this same review, 67% of patients were black and 78% were 20–60 years old. The only clinical complaints during the early stages of the disease are mild perineal pain and increased urinary frequency. At later stages, patients often complain of hematuria, constipation, nausea, lower abdominal pain, or backache of increasing severity and sometimes edema of the lower extremities.[437] Rarely, pelvic lipomatosis causes venous obstruction resulting in recurrent deep venous thrombosis.[435] Hypertension is present in about one-third of patients. The condition is associated with cystitis cystica or cystitis glandularis in up to 75% of cases,[428,436] and rare cases have been associated with adenocarcinoma of the urinary bladder.[422,425,429,432]

Radiographically (excretory urography and CT scan), the typical findings include a pear- or gourd-shaped urinary bladder with an elevated base, a high-lying prostate gland, and straightening and tubular narrowing of the rectosigmoid as the result of extrin-

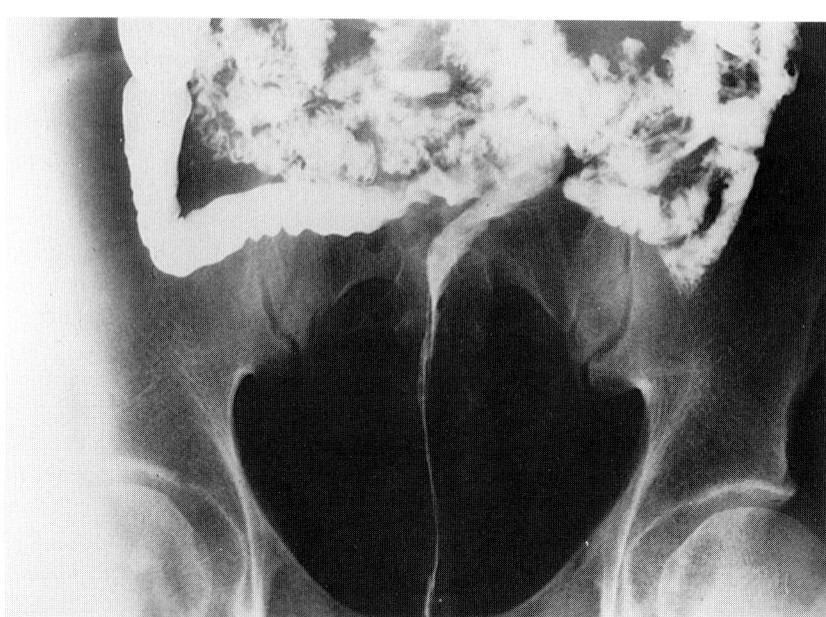

**FIGURE 16–61.** Radiograph of pelvic lipomatosis with marked compression of the rectum by the accumulated radiolucent fat.

sic pressure by a radiolucent mass (Fig. 16–61). The mass may cause dilatation and medial displacement of one or both ureters and occasionally unilateral or bilateral hydronephrosis. CT and MRI reveal a homogeneous perivesical mass with linear densities, reflecting fibrous bands within the proliferated fatty tissue.[416,419]

Pelvic lipomatosis is the result of massive overgrowth of fat in the perivesical and perirectal portions of the pelvic retroperitoneum. The fatty growth is diffuse rather than nodular and consists entirely of mature fat indistinguishable grossly and microscopically from fatty tissue elsewhere in the body. Increased vascularity, fibrosis, and inflammatory changes may be present but are rare.

The cause of this overgrowth is unknown, but it appears that it is a hyperplastic rather than a neoplastic process that almost always is limited to the pelvic region. Cases with associated multiple lipomas[426] and manifestations of Proteus syndrome[418,421] have been reported, however. *Lipomatosis of the ileocecal region* (submucosal, polypoid fatty infiltration of the ileocecal valve[420]) and *renal replacement lipomatosis* (secondary to long-standing inflammation and calculi with severe atrophy and destruction of the renal parenchyma[430]) should not be confused with this lesion. The symmetric diffuse growth and absence of atypical nuclei help rule out liposarcoma.

Prediction of the clinical course is difficult in the individual case. Frequently, pelvic lipomatosis is a slowly progressive process that may cause vesicoureteric obstruction, hydronephrosis, and uremia requiring surgical intervention, mainly urinary diversion and attempts to excise the accumulated fat.[427,434]

## STEROID LIPOMATOSIS

The term *steroid lipomatosis* is used here to describe a benign, diffuse fatty overgrowth caused by prolonged stimulation by adrenocortical hormones. The condition may be endogenous, as in Cushing's disease and adrenal cortical hyperplasia, or the result of prolonged corticosteroid therapy or steroid immunosuppression in transplant patients. As with Cushing's disease, the newly formed fat is unevenly distributed and tends to be concentrated in certain portions of the body. Thus in some cases the accumulation of fat is found mainly in the face (moon face), episternal region (dewlap), or interscapular region (buffalo hump); in others it is limited to the mediastinum,[448,449] pericardium,[444,452] paraspinal region,[442,451] mesentery,[450] retroperitoneum,[441] or epidural space.[439,440,445,454] Symptoms vary depending on the location but are usually the result of compression in a confined space, such as compression of the trachea in the mediastinum or the spinal cord in the spinal canal.[446] In rare cases, spinal compression results in paraplegia.[443] CT or MRI scans and demonstration of increased serum and urine cortisol levels are essential for diagnosis.[438,447] Steroid lipomatosis tends to resolve when the steroid concentration is lowered.[453]

## NEVUS LIPOMATOSUS CUTANEOUS SUPERFICIALIS

First described by Hoffman and Zurhelle in 1921,[463] nevus lipomatosus cutaneous superficialis is a relatively rare disease characterized by groups of ectopic fat cells in the papillary or reticular dermis. Two clinical forms have been identified. The multiple form (classic type) is characterized by multiple soft nontender skin-colored or yellow papules, nodules, or plaques that usually develop shortly after birth or during the first two decades of life (Figs. 16–62, 16–63).[457,458] The distribution of these lesions is usually linear or along the lines of the skinfolds with a predilection for the pelvic girdle, most commonly the buttock, sacrococcygeal region, and upper portion of the posterior thigh.[458,464] Rare cases of this form have also been described in the scalp,[457] shoulder,[460] abdomen,[458] thorax,[471] and back.[459] Less commonly, these lesions arise as solitary nodules that usually develop after the age of 20 years.[457,464] There is no site predilection for the solitary form; and the lesions have been reported to occur on the scalp,[470] forehead,[467] back,[462] and extremities.[471] There is no gender prevalence, and patients are otherwise in good health.

Microscopically, the nodules are composed of aggregates of mature fat cells in the mid and upper dermis, sometimes with keratotic plugs, increased vascularity, and scattered lymphocytes, mast cells, and histiocytes (Fig. 16–64).

Like other connective tissue nevi, this lesion should be considered a developmental anomaly or hamartomatous growth. Several electron microscopic studies[458,465] have suggested that the adipose tissue is derived from precursor cells arising from or in close proximity to dermal blood vessels. Treatment is not necessary other than for cosmetic reasons, and the lesion does not generally recur following simple excision.[471]

Another peculiar variant of this condition is marked by excessive symmetric, circumferential folds of skin with underlying nevus lipomatosus that affects the neck, forearms, and lower legs and resolves

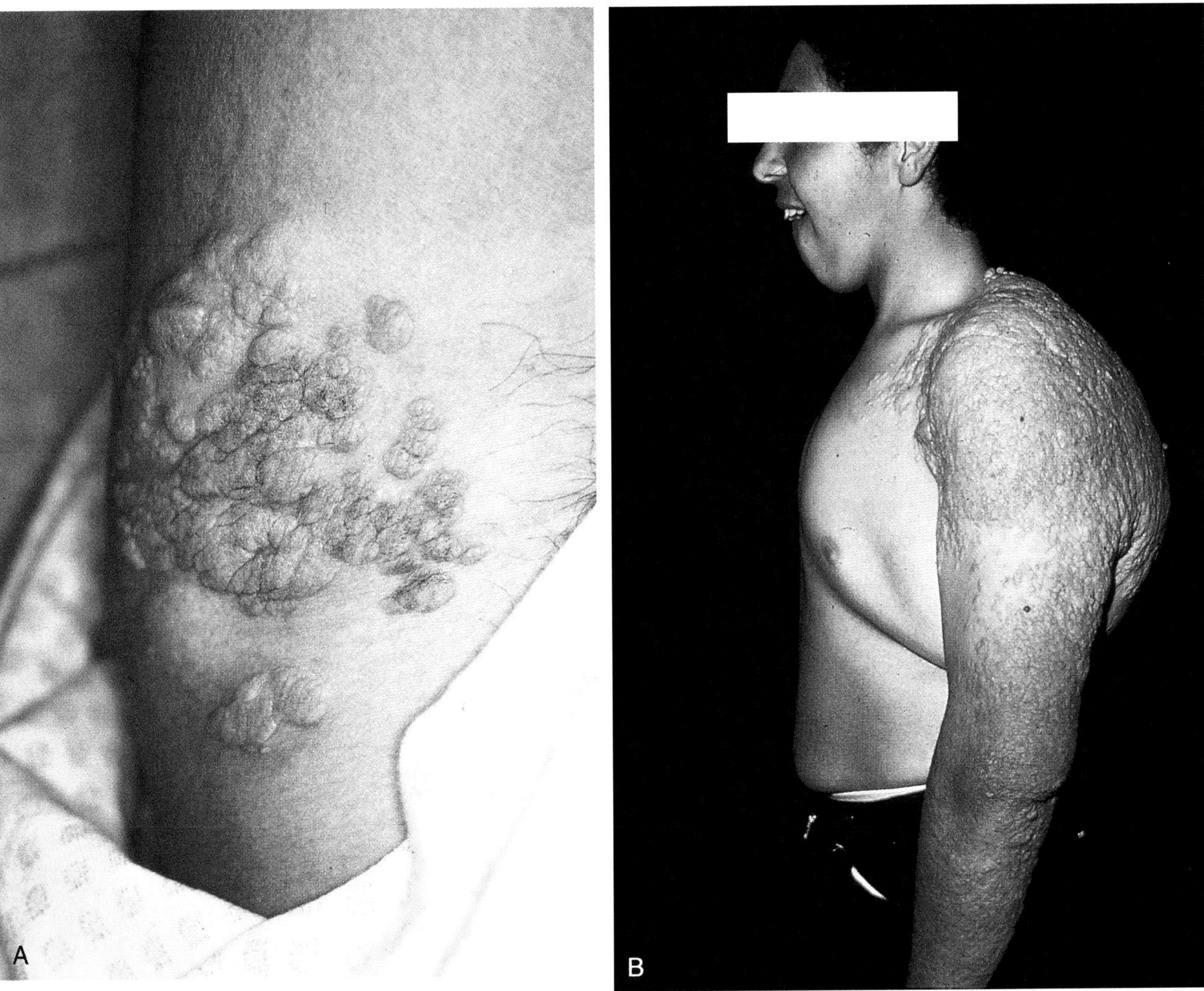


**FIGURE 16–62.** (**A**) Classic type of nevus lipomatosus cutaneous superficialis, characterized by multiple skin-colored papules, nodules, and plaques. (**B**) Unusual form of nevus lipomatosus cutaneous superficialis, with numerous lesions localized to the middle to upper back and proximal portion of the left arm.

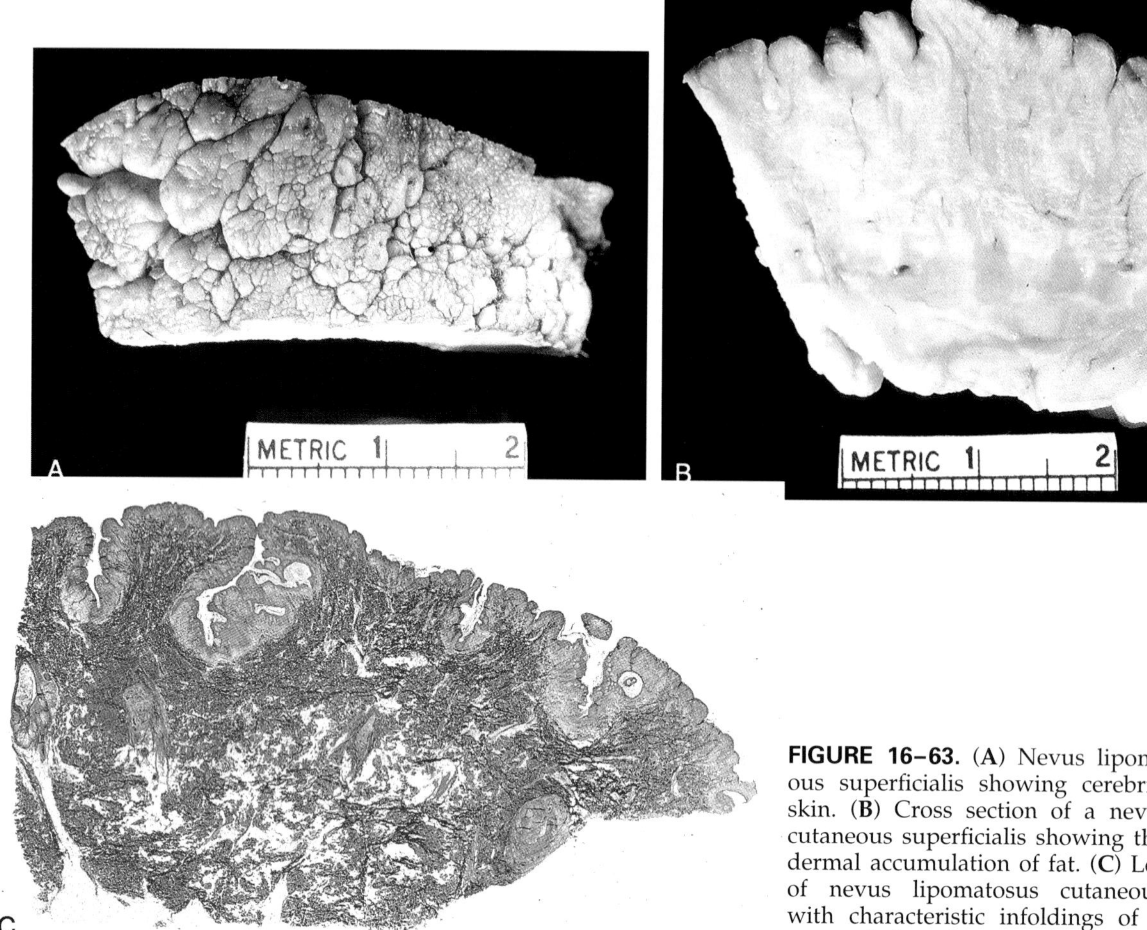


**FIGURE 16–63.** (**A**) Nevus lipomatosus cutaneous superficialis showing cerebriform wrinkled skin. (**B**) Cross section of a nevus lipomatosus cutaneous superficialis showing the characteristic dermal accumulation of fat. (**C**) Low-power view of nevus lipomatosus cutaneous superficialis with characteristic infoldings of epidermis and accumulation of mature fat in the dermis.

spontaneously during childhood; it has been aptly described as the *Michelin tire baby syndrome*.[456] The syndrome is inherited as an autosomal dominant trait and, according to Bass et al.[455] and others,[461,466,469] is characterized by deletion of chromosome 11. Association with smooth muscle hamartomas and multiple anomalies has been described.[468]

## HIBERNOMA

The term *hibernoma* was coined by Gery in 1914[481] and should be retained even though not all hibernomas occur at the few sites in which brown fat is encountered in humans. Such terms as *lipoma of immature adipose tissue, lipoma of embryonic fat*, and *fetal lipoma* were also proposed by some authors because brown fat bears a close resemblance to early stages in the development of white fat.

Hibernomas occur chiefly in adults, with a peak incidence during the third decade of life; but patients with hibernomas are on average considerably younger than those with lipoma. There is only one report of a hibernoma in a small child[478]; in this case, a tumor of the mediastinum and neck in a 6-week-old infant, probably represents a variant of lipoblastomatosis simulating hibernoma. In the AFIP series and in the literature, the tumor predominates in the scapular and interscapular regions, mediastinum, and upper thorax,[472,480,484] although a number of cases have originated in the thigh and popliteal fossa, sites normally devoid of brown fat.[474,486,495] Less common locations are the neck, chest wall, and retroperitoneum and the axillary and inguinal regions.[483,489,492,496]

Clinically, hibernomas are slowly growing painless tumors that occur in the subcutis or rarely in muscle; they are often noted several years before they are excised.[485] They are usually well defined, soft, and mobile and are 5–10 cm in diameter, although hibernomas as large as 20 cm have been reported.[492] Their color varies from tan to a deep red-brown (Fig. 16–65). CT and MRI scans reveal a lipomatous tumor but are unreliable for distinguishing hibernoma from liposarcoma.[476,477,491]

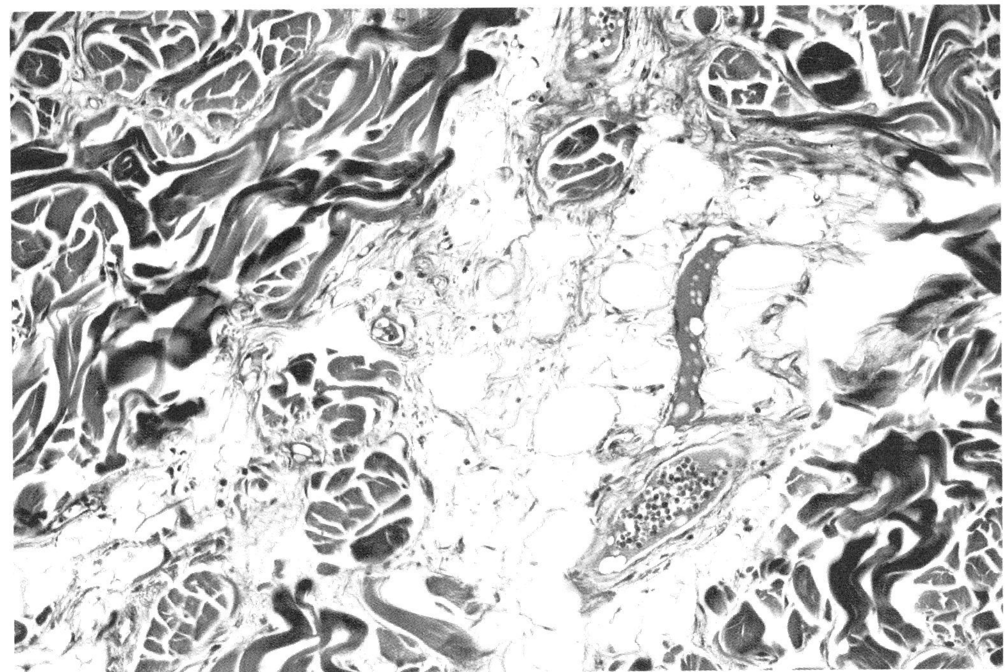

**FIGURE 16–64.** Nevus lipomatosus cutaneous superficialis with separation of dermal collagen by mature fat.

Microscopically, hibernomas display a distinct lobular pattern and are composed of cells that show varying degrees of differentiation, ranging from uniform, round to ovoid, granular eosinophilic cells with a distinct cellular membrane to multivacuolated cells with multiple, small, oil red O-positive lipid droplets and centrally placed nuclei (Figs. 16–66 to 16–69). There are also intermixed univacuolar cells with one or more large lipid droplets and peripherally placed nuclei resembling lipocytes. In cases with numerous univacuolar cells, microscopic distinction from lipoma may be difficult. Less commonly there are myxoid changes and infiltration of the underlying muscle tissue (Fig. 16–70). The vascular supply is considerably more prominent in hibernomas than in lipomas, a fact demonstrated angiographically by Angervall et al.[475] and others.[493] In fact, the distinct brown color of hibernoma is due to the prominent vascularity and profusion of mitochondria in the tumor.

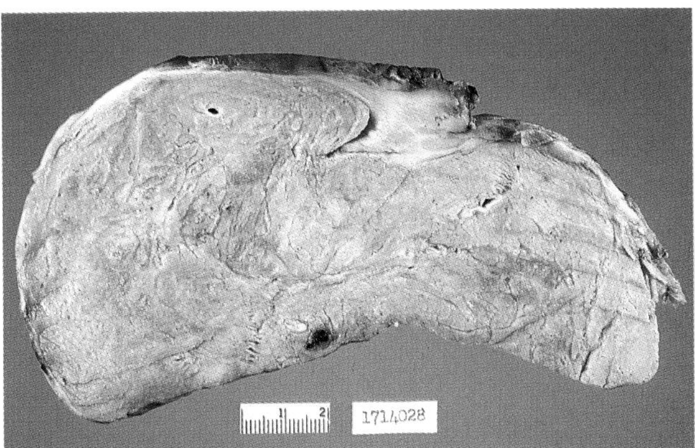

**FIGURE 16–65.** Gross appearance of a hibernoma of the retroperitoneum.

Ultrastructural studies[482,494,497] reveal multivacuolated and univacuolated cells packed with round to tubular mitochondria with parallel transverse cristae, a varying number of well defined lipid droplets, and occasional lysosomes with a well formed limiting membrane. In addition, there are pinocytotic vesicles and a well defined basal lamina. The nucleus contains uniformly distributed chromatin condensed under a well defined nuclear membrane. The scarcity of rough endoplasmic reticulum and a prominent Golgi apparatus distinguish the cells from the preadipocytes of white fat. In perisinusoidal cells of a hibernoma Allegra et al.[473] noted "endoplasmacrine" lipid granule secretion, rows of pedunculated plasmalemmal granules, and periodic plasmalemmal densities, resembling secretory features present in the cortical cells of the adrenal gland.

The likelihood of confusion with other tumors is minimal. *Adult rhabdomyoma* is composed of similar eosinophilic cells, but its cells are larger and contain considerable amounts of glycogen and, on careful search, crystals and cross-striations. *Granular cell tu-*

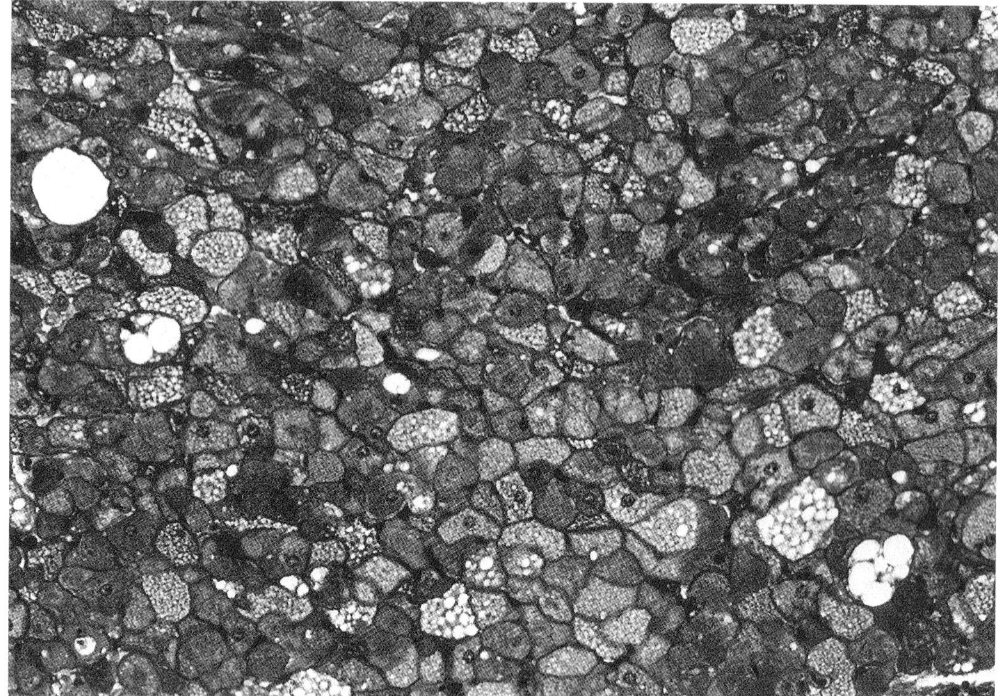

**FIGURE 16–66.** Hibernoma composed predominantly of vacuolated granular eosinophilic cells.

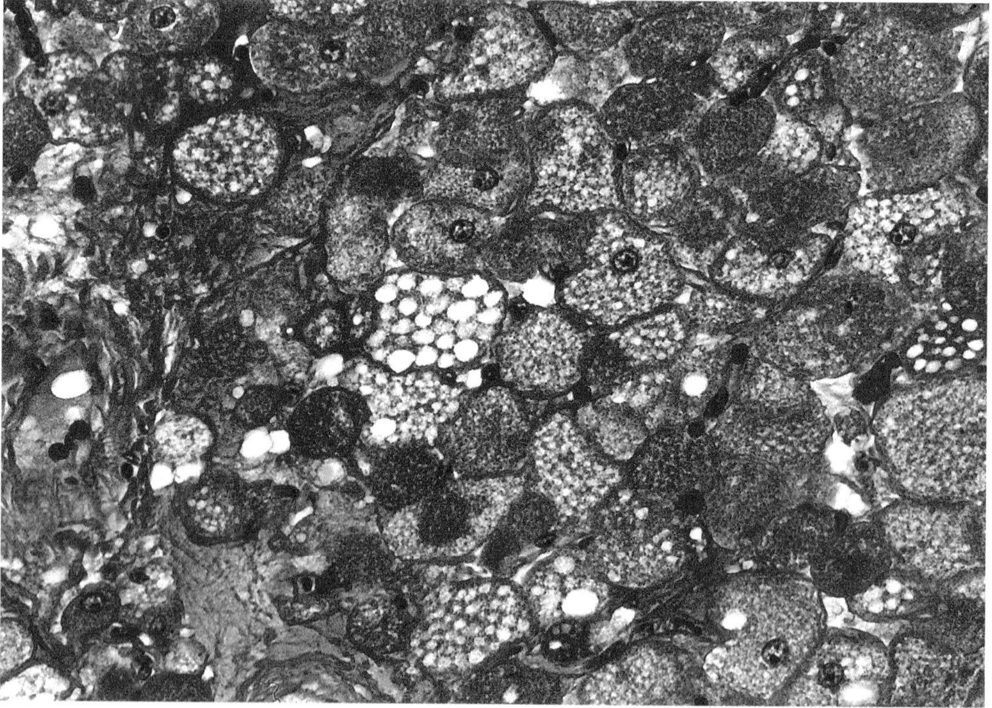

**FIGURE 16–67.** High-power view of granular and multivacuolated cells in a hibernoma.

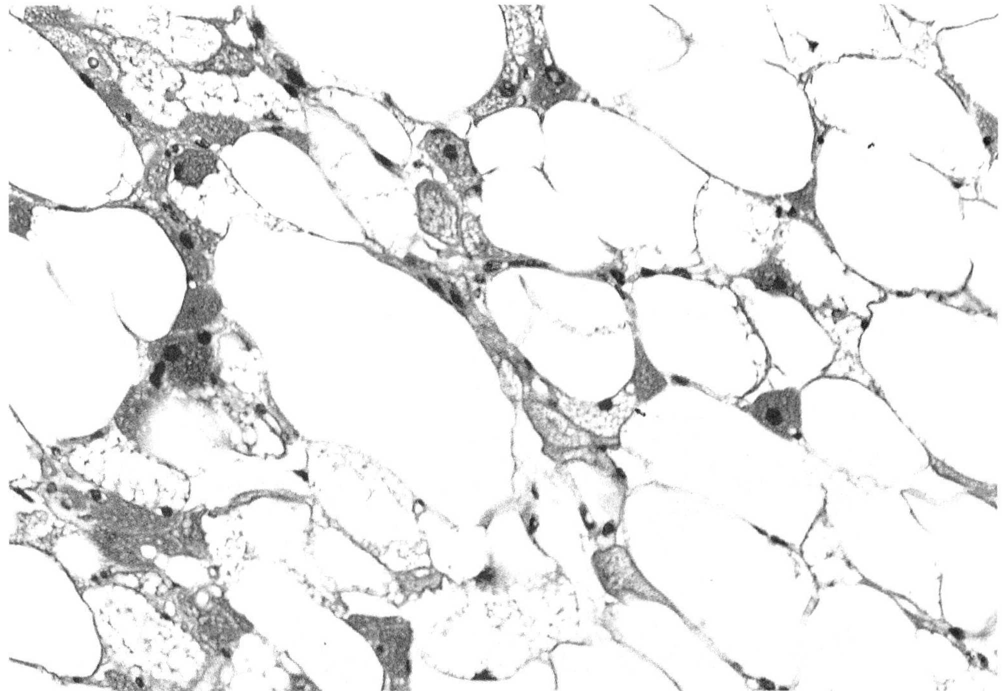

**FIGURE 16–68.** Hibernoma showing gradual transition between brown and white fat cells.

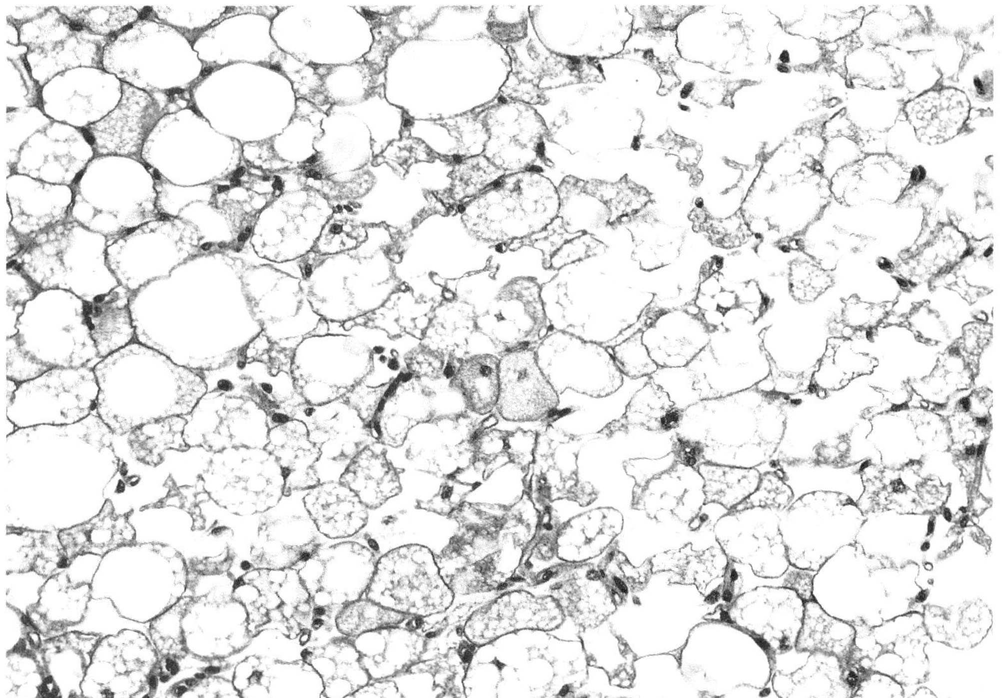

**FIGURE 16–69.** Hibernoma composed predominantly of fat cells with multiple cytoplasmic vacuoles.

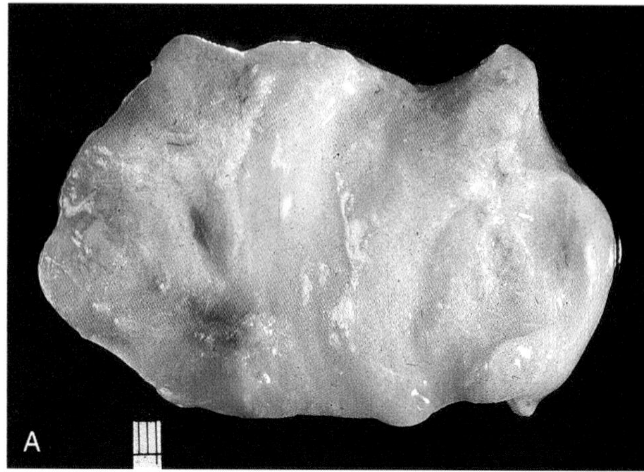


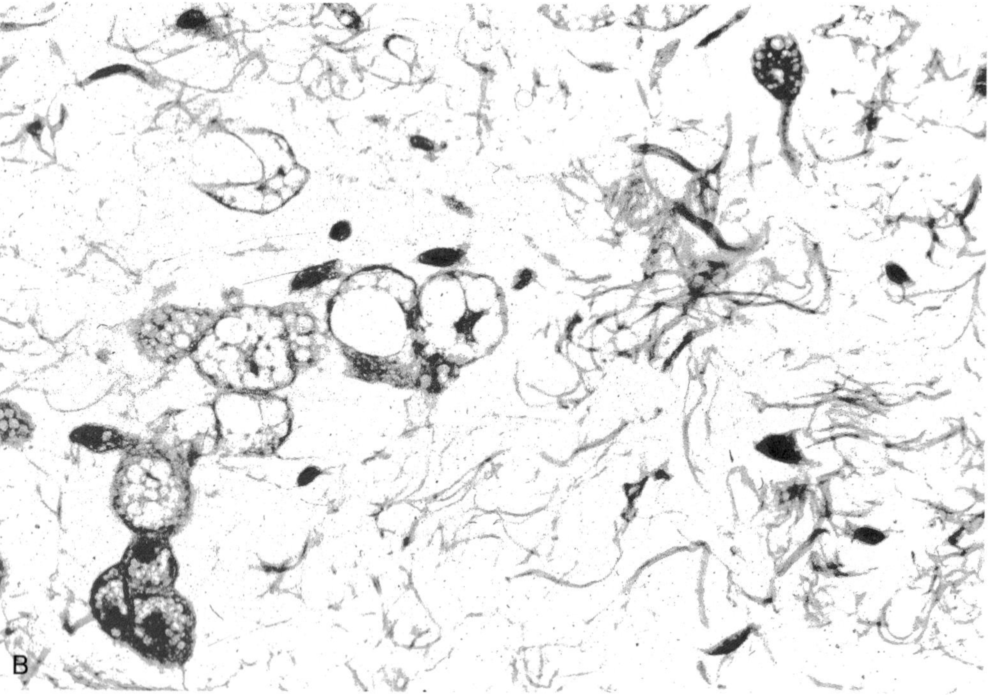


**FIGURE 16–70.** (**A**) Gross appearance of a hibernoma with extensive myxoid change. (**B**) Hibernoma with extensive myxoid change, with multivacuolated fat cells deposited in a mucoid matrix.

*mors* bear a superficial resemblance to hibernoma but are readily distinguished by the complete absence of intracellular oil red O-positive lipid vacuoles. We are uncertain as to the existence of malignant hibernoma. We have encountered possible cases but have interpreted them microscopically as variants of round cell liposarcoma with multivacuolar eosinophilic lipoblasts. An accurate diagnosis of these cases would require ultrastructural or possibly even cytogenetic analysis.

Like many other benign lipomatous tumors, hibernoma has a characteristic cytogenetic abnormality, that is, abnormalities of the long arm of chromosome 11 (11q13–21) and 10q22.[479,487,488,490]

## REFERENCES

### Adipose Tissue: Histology and Ultrastructure

1. Aman P, Ron D, Mandahl N, et al. Rearrangement of the transcription factor gene CHOP in myxoid liposarcomas with t(12;16)(q13;p11). Genes Chromosomes Cancer 5:278, 1992.
2. Bennett JH, Shousha S, Puddle B, et al. Immunohistochemical identification of tumours of adipocytic differentiation using an antibody to aP2 protein. J Clin Pathol 48:950, 1995.
3. Brooks JJ, Perosio PM. Adipose tissue. In: Histology for Pathologists, 2nd ed. Lippincott-Raven, Philadelphia, 1997, p 167.
4. Cunningham S, Leslie P, Hopwood D. The characterization and energetic potential of brown adipose tissue in man. Clin Sci 69:343, 1985.
5. Haimoto H, Kato K, Suzuki F, et al. The ultrastructural changes of S-100 protein localization during lipolysis in adipo-

cytes: an immunoelectron-microscopic study. Am J Pathol 121: 185, 1985.

6. Hashimoto H, Daimaru Y, Enjoji M. S-100 protein distribution in liposarcoma: an immunoperoxidase study with special reference to the distinction of liposarcoma from myxoid malignant fibrous histiocytoma. Virchows Arch [A] 405:1, 1984.
7. Heaton JM. The distribution of brown adipose tissue in the human. J Anat 112:35, 1972.
8. Hirsch J, Batchelor B. Adipose tissue cellularity in human obesity. Clin Endocrinol Metab 5:299, 1976.
9. Ladanyi M. The emerging molecular genetics of sarcoma translocations. Diagn Mol Pathol 4:162, 1995.
10. Michetti F, Dell'Anna E, Tiberio G, et al. Immunochemical and immunocytochemical study of S-100 protein in rat adipocytes. Brain Res 262:352, 1983.
11. Napolitano L. The differentiation of white adipose tissue cells: an electron microscope study. J Cell Biol 18:663, 1963.
12. Napolitano L. The fine structure of adipose tissues. In: Handbook of Physiology, sect 5: Adipose Tissue. American Physiological Society, Washington, DC, 1965, p 109.
13. Nnodim JO. Development of adipose tissue. Anat Rec 219:331, 1987.
14. Poissonnet CM, Burdie AR, Bookstein FI. Growth and development of human adipose tissue during early gestation. Early Hum Dev 8:1, 1983.
15. Poissonet CM, La Velle M, Bordi AR. Growth and development of adipose tissue. J Pediatr 113:1, 1988.
16. Rothwell NJ, Stock MJ. Brown adipose tissue. In: Baker PF (ed) Recent Advances in Physiology. Churchill Livingstone, Edinburgh, 1984, p 349.
17. Santos GC, Aroujo MR, Silveira TC, et al. Accumulation of brown adipose tissue and nutritional status: a prospective study of 366 consecutive autopsies. Arch Pathol Lab Med 116: 1152, 1992.
18. Sigwart U, Tedeschi LG, Tedeschi CG. Factors in adipogenesis. Hum Pathol 1:399, 1970.
19. Weiss SW, Langloss JM, Enzinger FM. Value of S-100 protein in the diagnosis of soft tissue tumors with particular reference to benign and malignant Schwann cell tumors. Lab Invest 49: 299, 1983.
20. Wells HG. Adipose tissue: a neglected subject. JAMA 114:2117, 2284, 1940.

## Lipoma

21. Acheson A, McIlrath E, Barros D'Sa AA. Pelvic lipoma causing venous obstruction syndrome. Eur J Vasc Endovasc Surg 14:149, 1997.
22. Ashar HR, Schoenberg F, Tkachenko M, et al. Disruption of the architectural factor HMGI-C: DNA-binding AT hook motifs fused in lipomas to distinct transcriptional regulatory domains. Cell 82:57, 1995.
23. Ashby BS, MacGillivray JB. Paratesticular lipoma. Br J Surg 53: 828, 1966.
24. Booher R. Lipoblastic tumors of the hands and feet: review of the literature and report of 33 cases. J Bone Joint Surg Am 47: 727, 1965.
25. Bridge JA, DeBoer J, Walker CW, et al. Translocation t(3;12)(q28;q14) in parosteal lipoma. Genes Chromosomes Cancer 12: 70, 1995.
26. Buetow PC, Buck JL, Carr NJ, et al. Intussuscepted colonic lipomas: loss of fat attenuation on CT with pathologic correlation in 10 cases. Abdom Imaging 21:153, 1996.
27. Cicciarelli RE, Soule EH, McGoon DC. Lipoma and liposarcoma of the mediastinum: a report of 14 tumors including lipomas of the thymus. J Thorac Cardiovasc Surg 47:411, 1964.
28. De Smet L, Bande S, Fabry G. Giant lipoma of the deep palmar space, mimicking persistent carpal tunnel syndrome. Acta Orthop Belg 60:334, 1994.
29. De Weerd JH, Dockerty MB. Lipomatous retroperitoneal tumors. Am J Surg 84:397, 1952.
30. Fletcher CDM, Akerman M, Dal Cin P, et al. Correlation between clinicopathological features and karyotype in lipomatous tumors: a report of 178 cases from the chromosomes and the morphology (CHAMP) collaborative study group. Am J Pathol 148:623, 1996.
31. Goldman AB, DiCarlo EF, Maxcove RC. Case report 774: coincidental parosteal lipoma with osseous excresence and intramuscular lipoma. Skeletal Radiol 22:138, 1993.
32. Goodman HJ, Richards AM, Klaassen MF. Use of magnetic resonance imaging on a large lipoma of the hand: a case report. Aust N Z J Surg 67:489, 1997.
33. Greeley DJ Jr, Sullivan JG, Wolfe GR. Massive primary lipoma of the scrotum. Am Surg 61:954, 1995.
34. Heim S, Mandahl N, Kristoffersson U, et al. Reciprocal translocation t(3;12)(q27;q13) in lipoma. Cancer Genet Cytogenet 23: 301, 1986.
35. Heim S, Mandahl N, Rydholm A, et al. Different karyotypic features characterize different clinicopathologic subgroups of benign lipogenic tumors. Int J Cancer 42:863, 1988.
36. Hess JL. Chromosomal translocations in benign tumors: the HMGI proteins. Am J Clin Pathol 109:251, 1998.
37. Hietanen J, Makinen J. Chondrolipoma of the tongue: a case report. Int J Oral Maxillofac Surg 26:127, 1997.
38. Kabaalioglu A, Gelen T, Aktan S, et al. Acute colonic obstruction caused by intussusception and extrusion of a sigmoid lipoma through the anus after barium enema. Abdom Imaging 22:389, 1997.
39. Kawashima A, Magid D, Fishman EK, et al. Parosteal ossifying lipoma: CT and MR findings. J Comput Assist Tomogr 17: 147, 1993.
40. Kim YH, Reiner L. Ultrastructure of lipoma. Cancer 50:102, 1982.
41. Kitami A, Suzuki T. A case report of cervical mediastinal lipoma. Nippon Kyobu Geka Gakkai Zasshi 45:624, 1997.
42. Koopman RJ, van der Wey LP, van Rappard JH. Subfascial lipoma of the forehead. Ned Tijdschr Geneeskd 136:844, 1992.
43. Kransdorf MJ, Moser RP, Meis JM, et al. Fat containing soft tissue masses of the extremities. Radiographics 11:81, 1991.
44. Lang-Lazdunski L, Rooudji M, Pansard Y, et al. Successful resection of giant intrapericardial lipoma. Ann Thorac Surg 58: 238, 1994.
45. Leffert RD. Lipomas of the upper extremity. J Bone Joint Surg Am 54:1262, 1972.
46. Liessi G, Pavanello M, Cesari S, et al. Large lipomas of the colon: CT and MR findings in three symptomatic cases. Abdom Imaging 21:150, 1996.
47. Mackenzie IR, Girvin JP, Lee D. Symptomatic osteolipoma of the tuber cinereum. Clin Neuropathol 15:60, 1996.
48. Mai KT, Yazdi HM, Collins JP. Vascular myxolipoma ("angiomyxolipoma") of the spermatic chord. Am J Surg Pathol 20: 1145, 1996.
49. Mandahl N, Heim S, Arheden K, et al. Three major cytogenetic subgroups can be identified among chromosomally abnormal solitary lipomas. Hum Genet 79:203, 1988.
50. Mandahl N, Heim S, Johansson B, et al. Lipomas have characteristic structural chromosomal rearrangements of 12q13-q14. Int J Cancer 39:685, 1987.
51. Mandahl N, Hoglund M, Mertens F, et al. Cytogenetic aberrations in 188 benign and borderline adipose tissue tumors. Genes Chromosomes Cancer 9:207, 1994.
52. Mandahl N, Merten F, Willen H, et al. Nonrandom pattern of telomeric associations in atypical lipomatous tumors with ring

and giant marker chromosomes. Cancer Genet Cytogenet 103: 25, 1998.
53. Meggit BF. The battered buttock syndrome: a report of a group of traumatic lipomata. Br J Surg 59:165, 1972.
54. Millward S, Escott N, Masood K. The diagnosis of a pleural lipoma by CT and fine needle biopsy to avoid thoracotomy. Can Assoc Radiol J 39:57, 1988.
55. Mrozek K, Karakousis CP, Bloomfield CD. Chromosome 12 breakpoints are cytogenetically different in benign and malignant lipogenic tumors: localization of breakpoints in lipoma to 12q15 and in myxoid liposarcoma to 12q13.3. Cancer Res 53: 1670, 1993.
56. Munk PL, Lee MJ, Janzen DL, et al. Lipoma and liposarcoma: evaluation using CT and MR imaging. AJR 169:589, 1997.
57. Murphy MD, Johnson DL, Bhatia PS, et al. Parosteal lipoma: MR imaging characteristics. AJR 162:105, 1994.
58. Oster LH, Blair WF, Steyers CM. Large lipomas in the deep palmar space. J Hand Surg [Am] 14:700, 1989.
59. Pachter MR, Lattes R. Mesenchymal tumors of the mediastinum. I. Tumors of fibrous tissue, adipose tissue, smooth muscle and striated muscle. Cancer 16:74, 1963.
60. Park JW, Yang JY, Rhee SR, et al. Glycosylation of lipoprotein lipase in human subcutaneous lipomas. Horm Metab Res 28:7, 1996.
61. Penoff JH. Traumatic lipomas/pseudolipomas. J Trauma 22:63, 1982.
62. Ramdial PK, Madaree A, Singh B. Membranous fat necrosis in lipomas. Am J Surg Pathol 21:841, 1997.
63. Robson PN. A large calcified lipoma of the thigh. J Bone Joint Surg Br 32:384, 1950.
64. Rosai J, Akerman M, Dal Cin P, et al. Combined morphologic and karyotypic study of 59 atypical lipomatous tumors: evaluation of their relationship in differential diagnosis with other adipose tissue tumors (a report of the CHAMP Study Group). Am J Surg Pathol 20:1182, 1996.
65. Rubin BP, Fletcher CDM. The cytogenetics of lipomatous tumors. Histopathoiogy 30:507, 1997.
66. Rydholm A, Berg NO. Size, site and clinical incidence of lipoma: factors in differential diagnosis of lipoma and sarcoma. Acta Orthop Scand 54:929, 1983.
67. Sait SNJ, Dal Cin P, Sandberg AA, et al. Involvement of 6p in benign lipomas: a new cytogenetic entity? Cancer Genet Cytogenet 37:281, 1989.
68. Saitoh Y, Hama T, Ishizaka S, et al. Fibrolipoma of the parotid in a child. Am J Otolaryngol 16:433, 1995.
69. Sasaki M, Harada K, Nakanuma Y, et al. Pseudolipoma of Glisson's capsule: report of six cases and review of the literature. J Clin Gastroenterol 19:75, 1994.
70. Sauer JM, Ozonoff MB. Congenital bone anomalies associated with lipomas. Skeletal Radiol 13:276, 1985.
71. Schoenmakers EFPM, Wanschura S, Mols R, et al. Recurrent rearrangements in the high-mobility-group protein gene, HMGI-C, in benign mesenchymal tumours. Nat Genet 10:436, 1995.
72. Siegal A, Witz M. Gastrointestinal lipoma and malignancies. J Surg Oncol 47:170, 1991.
73. Solsona-Norbon B, Sanchez-Paris O, Bernal-Sprekelsen JC, et al. Hourglass thoracic lipoma of infancy: case report and review of the literature. J Pediatr Surg 32:785, 1997.
74. Solvonuk PF, Taylor GP, Hancock R, et al. Correlation of morphologic and biochemical observations in human lipomas. Lab Invest 51:469, 1984.
75. Sreekantaiah C, Karakousis CP, Leong SPL, et al. Cytogenetic findings in liposarcoma correlate with histopathologic subtypes. Cancer 69:2484, 1992.
76. Sreekantaiah C, Leong SPL, Karakousis CP, et al. Cytogenetic profile of 109 lipomas. Cancer Res 51:422, 1991.
77. Tokumaru S, Kudo S, Mihara M, et al. Myxolipoma mimicking a cystic tumor. Skeletal Radiol 25:573, 1996.
78. Urbano J, Serantes A, Hernandez L, et al. Lipoma-induced jejunojejunal intussusception: US and CT diagnosis. Abdom Imaging 21:522, 1996.
79. Willen H, Akerman M, Dal Cin P, et al. Comparison of chromosomal patterns with clinical features in 165 lipomas: a report of CHAMP study group. Cancer Genet Cytogenet 102:46, 1998.
80. Wittig H, Casper U, Warich-Kirches M, et al. Hypothalamic osteolipoma: a case report. Gen Diagn Pathol 142:361, 1997.
81. Wurlitzer F, Bedrossian C, Ayala A, et al. Problems of diagnosis and treating lipomas. Ann Surg 39:240, 1973.
82. Zelger BG, Zelger B, Steiner H, et al. Sclerotic lipoma: lipomas simulating sclerotic lipoma. Histopathology 31:174, 1997.

## Multiple Lipomas

83. Adair FE, Pack GT, Farrior JH. Lipomas. Am J Cancer 16:1104, 1932.
84. Alsberg A. Ueber Neurolipome, inaugural dissertation. Gustav Schade, Berlin, 1892.
85. Arch EM, Goodman BK, Van Wesep RA, et al. Deletion of PTEN in a patient with Bannayan-Riley-Ruvalcaba syndrome suggests allelism with Cowden disease. Am J Med Genet 71: 489, 1997.
86. Bannayan GA. Lipomatosis, angiomatosis, and macrocephalia: a previously undescribed congenital syndrome. Arch Pathol 92:1, 1971.
87. Benny PS, Macvicar J. Multiple lipomas in pregnancy. BMJ 1: 1679, 1979.
88. Buschke A, Mattissohn L. Symmetrische Lipomatosis (Uebersicht nebst Mitteilung von 2 Fallen, kombiniert mit Psoriasis and Arthritis). Arch Dermatol 120:537, 1914.
89. Costa T, Fitch N, Azouz EM. Proteus syndrome: report of two pelvic lipomatosis. Pediatrics 76:994, 1985.
90. Ersek RA, Lele E, Surak GS, et al. Hereditary progressive nodular lipomatosis: a report and selective review of a new syndrome. Ann Plast Surg 23:450, 1989.
91. Frayling IM, Bodmer WF, Tomlinson IP. Allele loss in colorectal cancer at the Cowden disease/juvenile polyposis locus on 10q. Cancer Genet Cytogenet 97:64, 1997.
92. Kurzweg FT, Spencer R. Familial multiple lipomatosis. Am J Surg 82:726, 1951.
93. Marsh DJ, Zheng Z, Zedenius J, et al. Differential loss of heterozygosity in the region of the Cowden locus within 10q22-23 in follicular thyroid adenomas and carcinomas. Cancer Res 57:500, 1997.
94. Rubinstein A, Goor Y, Gazit E, et al. Non symmetric subcutaneous lipomatosis associated with familial combined hyperlipidaemia. Br J Dermatol 120:689, 1989.
95. Shanks JA, Paranchych W, Tuba J. Familial multiple lipomatosis. Can Med Assoc J 77:881, 1957.
96. Stoll C, Alembik Y, Truttmann M. Multiple familial lipomatosis with polyneuropathy, an inherited dominant condition. Ann Genet 39:193, 1996.
97. Traquada RE. Subcutaneous lipomas at sites of insulin injection. Diabetes 15:807, 1966.
98. Weary PE, Gorlin RJ, Gentry WC, et al. Multiple hamartoma syndrome (Cowden's disease). Arch Dermatol 106:682, 1972.
99. Zigman AF, Lavine JE, Jones MC, et al. Localization of the Bannayan-Riley-Ruvalcaba syndrome gene to chromosome 10q23. Gastroenterology 113:1433, 1997.

## Angiolipoma

100. Belcher RW, Czarnetzki BM, Carney IF, et al. Multiple (subcutaneous) angiolipomas: clinical, pathologic and pharmacologic studies. Arch Dermatol 110:583, 1974.

101. Chung JY, Ramos-Caro FA, Beers B, et al. Multiple lipomas, angiolipomas, and parathyroid adenomas in a patient with Birt-Hogg-Dube syndrome. Int J Dermatol 35:365, 1996.
102. Dixon AY, McGregor DH. Angiolipomas: an ultrastructural and clinicopathological study. Hum Pathol 12:739, 1981.
103. Halal F, Silver K. Slowly progressive macrocephaly with hamartomas: a new syndrome? Am J Med Genet 33:182, 1989.
104. Heymann WR, Fiorillo A, Simons J. Eruptive familial angiolipomas occurring during pregnancy. Cutis 42:525, 1988.
105. Howard WR, Helwig EB. Angiolipoma. Arch Dermatol 82:924, 1960.
106. Hunt J, Tindal D. Solitary gastric Peutz-Jeghers polyp and angiolipoma presenting as acute hemorrhage. Aust N Z J Surg 66:713, 1996.
107. Hunt SJ, Santa Cruz DJ, Barr RJ. Cellular angiolipoma. Am J Surg Pathol 14:75, 1990.
108. Kanik A, Oh CH, Bhawan J. Cellular angiolipoma. Am J Dermatopathol 17:312, 1995.
109. Kanter, WR, Wolfort FG. Multiple familial angiolipomatosis: treatment by liposuction. Ann Plast Surg 20:277, 1988.
110. Lin JJ, Lin F. Two entities in angiolipoma: a study of 459 cases of lipomas with review of literature on infiltrating angiolipomas. Cancer 34:720, 1974.
111. Mandahl N, Höglund M, Mertens F, et al. Cytogenetic aberrations in 188 benign and borderline adipose tissue tumors. Genes Chromosomes Cancer 9:207, 1994.
112. Manganaro AM, Hammond HL, Williams TP. Intraosseous angiolipomas of the mandible: a case report and review of the literature. J Oral Maxillofac Surg 52:767, 1994.
113. McGregor DH, Kerley SW, McGregor MS. Case report: gastric angiolipoma with chronic hemorrhage and severe anemia. Am J Med Sci 305:229, 1993.
114. Prabu SS, O'Donovan DG, Gurusinghe NT. Intracranial angiolipoma: report of two cases. Br J Neurosurg 9:793, 1995.
115. Pribyl C, Burke SW, Roberts JM, et al. Infiltrating angiolipoma or intramuscular hemangioma? A report of five cases. J Pediatr Orthop 6:172, 1986.
116. Provenzale JM, McLendon RE. Spinal angiolipomas: MR features. Am J Neuroradiol 17:713, 1996.
117. Rasanen O, Nohteri H, Dammert K. Angiolipoma and lipoma. Acta Chir Scand 133:461, 1974.
118. Sciot K, Akerman M, Dal Cin P, et al. Cytogenetic analysis of subcutaneous angiolipoma: further evidence supporting its difference from ordinary pure lipomas: a report of the CHAMP Study Group. Am J Surg Pathol 21:441, 1997.
119. Skovby F, Graham JM, Sonne-Holm S, et al. Compromise of the spinal canal in proteus syndrome. Am J Med Genet 47:656, 1993.
120. Stevenson JC, Choksey MS, McMahon J, et al. Multiple cerebral aneurysms, multiple meningiomas and multiple subcutaneous angiolipomas: a case report. Br J Neurosurg 8:477, 1994.
121. Yu GH, Fishman SJ, Brooks JS. Cellular angiolipoma of the breast. Mod Pathol 6:497, 1993.

### Myolipoma

122. Ben-Izhak O, Elmalach I, Kerner H, et al. Pericardial myolipoma: a tumour presenting as a mediastinal mass and containing oestrogen receptors. Histopathology 29:184, 1996.
123. Honore LH. Uterine fibrolipoleiomyoma: report of a case with discussion of histogenesis. Am J Obstet Gynecol 132:635, 1978.
124. Jacobs DS, Cohen H, Johnson JS. Lipoleiomyomas of the uterus. Am J Clin Pathol 44:45, 1965.
125. Lehrman BJ, Nisenbaum HL, Glasser SA, et al. Uterine myolipoma: magnetic resonance imaging, computed tomographic, and ultrasound appearance. J Ultrasound Med 9:665, 1990.
126. Liang EY, Cooper JE, Lam WWM, et al. Case report: myolipoma or liposarcoma—a mistaken identity in the retroperitoneum. Clin Radiol 51:295, 1996.
127. Meis JM, Enzinger FM. Myolipoma of soft tissue. Am J Surg Pathol 15:121, 1991.
128. Michal M. Retroperitoneal myolipoma: a tumour mimicking retroperitoneal angiomyolipoma and liposarcoma with myosarcomatous differentiation. Histopathology 25:86, 1994.
129. Scurry JP, Carey MP, Targett CS, et al. Soft tissue lipoleiomyoma. Pathology 23:360, 1991.
130. Sonobe H, Ontsuki Y, Iwata J, et al. Myolipoma of the round ligament: report of a case with a review of the English literature. Virchows Arch 427:455, 1995.

### Chondroid Lipoma

131. Chan JKC, Lee KC, Saw D. Extraskeletal chondroma with lipoblast-like cells. Hum Pathol 17:1285, 1986.
132. Gisselsson D, Domanski HA, Hoglund M, et al. Unique cytological features and chromosome aberrations in chondroid lipoma: a case report based on fine-needle aspiration cytology, histopathology, electron microscopy, chromosome banding, and molecular cytogenetics. Am J Surg Pathol 23:1300, 1999.
133. Gomez-Ortega JM, Rodilla IG, Basco Lopez de Lerma JM. Chondroid lipoma: a newly described lesion that may be mistaken for malignancy. Oral Surg Oral Med Oral Pathol Oral Radiol Endod 81:586, 1996.
134. Kindblom L-G, Meis-Kindblom JM. Chondroid lipoma: an ultrastructural and immunohistochemical analysis with further observations regarding its differentiation. Hum Pathol 26:706, 1995.
135. Meis JM, Enzinger FM. Chondroid lipoma: a unique tumor simulating liposarcoma and myxoid chondrosarcoma. Am J Surg Pathol 17:1103, 1993.
136. Nielsen GP, O'Connell JX, Dickersin GR, et al. Chondroid lipoma, a tumor of white fat cells: a brief report of two cases with ultrastructural analysis. Am J Surg Pathol 19:1272, 1995.
137. Thomson TA, Horsman D, Bainbridge TC. Cytogenetic and cytologic features of chondroid lipoma of soft tissue. Mod Pathol 12:88, 1999.
138. Zamecnik M, Michal M, Fakan F. Chondroid lipoma. Cesk Patol 32:115, 1996.

### Spindle Cell and Pleomorphic Lipoma

139. Angervall L, Dahl I, Kindblom LG, et al. Spindle cell lipoma. Acta Pathol Microbiol Scand 84:477, 1976.
140. Azumi N, Curtis J, Kempson R, et al. Atypical and malignant neoplasms showing lipomatous differentiation: a study of 111 cases. Am J Surg Pathol 11:161, 1987.
141. Azzopardi JG, Iocco J, Salm R. Pleomorphic lipoma: a tumour simulating liposarcoma. Histopathology 7:511, 1983.
142. Bartley GB, Yeatts RP, Garrity JA, et al. Spindle cell lipoma of the orbit. Am J Ophthalmol 100:605, 1985.
143. Beham A, Schmid C, Hödl S, et al. Spindle cell and pleomorphic lipoma: an immunohistochemical study and histogenetic analysis. J Pathol 158:219, 1989.
144. Bolen JW, Thorning D. Spindle-cell lipoma: a clinical, light and electron microscopical study. Am J Surg Pathol 5:435, 1981.
145. Dal Cin P, Sciot R, Polito P, et al. Lesions of 13q may occur independently of deletion of 16q in spindle cell/pleomorphic lipomas. Histopathology 31:222, 1997.
146. Diau GY, Chu CC, Chou GS, et al. Spindle cell lipoma in a 14-month old girl. J Pediatr Surg 30:1603, 1995.
147. Digregorio F, Barr RJ, Fretzin D. Pleomorphic lipoma: case report and review of the literature. J Dermatol Surg Oncol 18: 197, 1992.
148. Enzinger, FM, Harvey, DA. Spindle cell lipoma. Cancer 36: 1852, 1975.
149. Evans HL, Soule EH, Winkelman RK. Atypical lipoma, atypi-

cal intramuscular lipoma and well differentiated liposarcoma. Cancer 43:574, 1979.
150. Fanburg-Smith JC, Devaney KO, Miettinen M, et al. Multiple spindle cell lipomas: a report of seven familial and 11 nonfamilial cases. Am J Surg Pathol 22:40, 1998.
151. Fletcher CDM, Akerman M, Dal Cin P, et al. Correlation between clinicopathological features and karyotype in lipomatous tumors: a report of 178 cases from the Chromosomes and Morphology (CHAMP) Collaborative Study Group. Am J Pathol 148:623, 1996.
152. Fletcher CDM, Martin-Bates E. Spindle cell lipoma: a clinicopathological study with some original observations. Histopathology 11:803, 1987.
153. Fletcher CDM, Tsang WYW, Fisher C, et al. Angiomyofibroblastoma of the vulva: a benign neoplasm distinct from aggressive angiomyxoma. Am J Surg Pathol 16:373, 1992.
154. Hawley IC, Krausz T, Evans DJ, et al. Spindle cell lipoma: a pseudoangiomatous variant. Histopathology 24:565, 1994.
155. Kitano M, Enjoji M, Iwasaki H. Spindle cell lipoma—a clinicopathologic analysis of 12 cases. Acta Pathol Jpn 29:891, 1979.
156. Laskin WB, Fetsch JF, Mostofi FK. Angiomyofibroblastoma-like tumor of the male genital tract: analysis of 11 cases with comparison to female angiomyofibroblastoma and spindle cell lipoma. Am J Surg Pathol 22:6, 1998.
157. Mandahl N, Mertens F, Willen H, et al. A new cytogenetic subgroup in lipomas: loss of chromosome 16 material in spindle cell and pleomorphic lipomas. J Cancer Res Clin Oncol 120:707, 1994.
158. Mehregan DR, Mehregan DA, Mehregan AH, et al. Spindle cell lipomas: a report of two cases: one with multiple lesions. Dermatol Surg 21:796, 1995.
159. Mentzel T, Fletcher CDM. Lipomatous tumors of soft tissues: an update. Virchows Arch Pathol Anat 427:353, 1995.
160. Moran CA, Suster S, Koss MN. Endobronchial lipomas: a clinicopathologic study of four cases. Mod Pathol 7:212, 1994.
161. Muenchow T, Senitz D, Goertchen R. Pleomorphic lipoma. Zentralbl Allg Pathol 130:13, 1985.
162. Nonaka S, Enomoto K, Kawabori S, et al. Spindle cell lipoma within the larynx: a case report with correlated light and electron microscopy. J Otorhinolaryngol Relat Spec 55:147, 1993.
163. Pitt MA, Roberts ISD, Curry A. Spindle cell and pleomorphic lipoma: an ultrastructural study. Ultrastruct Pathol 19:475, 1995.
164. Richmond I, Banerjee SS. Spindle cell lipoma: a pseudoangiomatous variant. Histopathology 27:199, 1995.
165. Rosai J, Akerman M, Dal Cin P, et al. Combined morphologic and karyotypic study of 59 atypical lipomatous tumors: evaluation of their relationship and differential diagnosis with other adipose tissue tumors (a report of the CHAMP Study Group). Am J Surg Pathol 20:1182, 1996.
166. Rubin BP, Fletcher CDM. The cytogenetics of lipomatous tumors. Histopathology 30:507, 1997.
167. Shmookler BM, Enzinger FM. Pleomorphic lipoma: a benign tumor simulating liposarcoma: a clinicopathologic analysis of 48 cases. Cancer 47:126, 1981.
168. Shouzhu Z, Xinhua Y, Xumin L, et al. Giant retroperitoneal pleomorphic lipoma. Am J Surg Pathol 11:557, 1997.
169. Smith DN, Denison CM, Lester SC. Spindle cell lipoma of the breast: a case report. Acta Radiol 37:893, 1996.
170. Smith TA, Goldblum JR. CD34 immunoreactivity in the spindle cells of benign and malignant lipomatous tumors. Am J Clin Pathol 106:405, 1996.
171. Suster S, Fisher C. Immunoreactivity for the human hematopoietic progenitor cell antigen (CD34) in lipomatous tumors. Am J Surg Pathol 21:195, 1997.
172. Templeton SF, Solomon AR Jr. Spindle cell lipoma is strongly CD34 positive: an immunohistochemical study. J Cutan Pathol 23:546, 1996.
173. Tosios K, Papanicolaou SI, Kapranos N, et al. Spindle cell lipoma of the oral cavity. Int J Oral Maxillofac Surg 24:363, 1995.
174. Warkel RL, Rehme CG, Thompson WH. Vascular spindle cell lipoma. J Cutan Pathol 9:113, 1982.
175. Yue XH, Liu YQ. Pleomorphic lipoma [letter]. Am J Surg Pathol 20:898, 1996.
176. Zelger BWH, Zelger BG, Plörer A, et al. Dermal spindle cell lipoma: plexiform and nodular variants. Histopathology 27: 533: 1995.

### Lipoblastoma and Lipoblastomatosis

177. Adams RJ, Drwiega PJ, Rivera CA. Congenital orbital lipoblastoma: a pathologic and radiologic study. J Pediatr Ophthalmol Strabismus 34:194, 1997.
178. Al-Qattan MM, Weinberg M, Clarke HM. Two rapidly growing fatty tumors of the upper limb in children: lipoblastoma and infiltrating lipoma. J Hand Surg [Am] 20:20, 1995.
179. Beebe MM, Smith MD. Omental lipoblastoma. J Pediatr Surg 28:162, 1993.
180. Bolen JW, Thorning D. Benign lipoblastoma and myxoid liposarcoma: a comparative light and electron-microscopic study. Am J Surg Pathol 4:163, 1980.
181. Cacciaguerra S, Lebet M, DiCataldo A, et al. An unusual intrathoracic tumor: giant lipoblastoma. Eur J Pediatr Surg 5:40, 1995.
182. Chung EB, Enzinger FM. Benign lipoblastomatosis: an analysis of 35 cases. Cancer 32:482, 1973.
183. Coffin CM. Lipoblastoma: an embryonal tumor of soft tissue relating to organogenesis. Semin Diagn Pathol 11:98, 1994.
184. Collins MH, Chatten J. Lipoblastoma/lipoblastomatosis: a clinicopathologic study of 25 tumors. Am J Surg Pathol 21:1131, 1997.
185. Dal Cin P, Sciot R, De Wever I, et al. New discriminative chromosomal marker in adipose tissue tumors: the chromosome 8q11-q13 region in lipoblastoma. Cancer Genet Cytogenet 78:232, 1994.
186. Enghardt MH, Warren RC. Congenital palpebral lipoblastoma: first report of a case. Am J Dermatopathol 12:408, 1990.
187. Fletcher CD, Akerman M, Dal Cin P, et al. Correlation between clinicopathological features and karyotype in lipomatous tumors: a report of 178 cases from the Chromosomes and Morphology (CHAMP) Collaborative Study Group. Am J Pathol 148:623, 1996.
188. Fletcher JA, Kozakewich HP, Schoenberg ML, et al. Cytogenetic findings in pediatric adipose tumors: consistent rearrangement of chromosome 8 in lipoblastoma. Genes Chromosomes Cancer 6:24, 1993.
189. Francois A, Bodenant C, Rives N, et al. Lipoblastome mésentérique avec remaniement du chromosome 8. Ann Pathol 17:406, 1997.
190. Gaffney EF, Vellios F, Hargreaves HK. Lipoblastomatosis: ultrastracture of two cases and relationship to human fetal white adipose tissue. Pediatr Pathol 5:207, 1986.
191. Greco MA, Garcia RL, Vuletin JC. Benign lipoblastomatosis: ultrastructure and histogenesis. Cancer 45:511, 1980.
192. Krempl GA, McGuff HS, Pulitzer DR, et al. Lipoblastoma in the parotid gland of an infant. Otolaryngol Head Neck Surg 117:S234, 1997.
193. Mahour GH, Bryan BJ, Isaacs H. Lipoblastoma and lipoblastomatosis: a report of six cases. Surgery 104:577, 1988.
194. Mentzel T, Calonje E, Fletcher CDM. Lipoblastoma and lipoblastomatosis: a clinicopathologic study of 14 cases. Histopathology 23:527, 1993.

195. Panarello C, Rosanda C, Morerio C, et al. Lipoblastoma: a case with t(7;8)(q31;q13). Cancer Genet Cytogenet 102:12, 1998.
196. Rasmussen IS, Kirkegaard J, Kaasbol M. Intermittent airway obstruction in a child caused by a cervical lipoblastoma. Acta Anaesthesiol Scand 41:945, 1997.
197. Sawyer JR, Parsons EA, Crowson ML, et al. Potential diagnostic implications of breakpoints in the long arm of chromosome 8 in lipoblastoma. Cancer Genet Cytogenet 76:39, 1994.
198. Schultz E, Rosenblatt R, Mitsudo S, et al. Detection of a deep lipoblastoma by MRI and ultrasound. Pediatr Radiol 23:409, 1993.
199. Tallini G, Akerman M, Dal Cin P, et al. Combined morphologic and karyotypic study of 28 myxoid liposarcomas: implications for a revised morphologic typing (a report from the CHAMP group). Am J Surg Pathol 20:1047, 1996.
200. Van Meurs DP. The transformation of an embryonic lipoma to a common lipoma. Br J Surg 34:282, 1947.
201. Vellios F, Baez JM, Shumacker HB. Lipoblastomatosis: a tumor of fetal fat different from hibernoma: report of a case, with observations on the embryogenesis of human adipose tissue. Am J Pathol 34:1149, 1958.
202. Zanetti G. Benign lipoblastoma: first case report of a mesenteric origin. Tumori 74:495, 1988.

## Angiomyolipoma

203. Agarwal R, Agarwal PK, Dalela D. Renal angiomyolipoma with nodal involvement: a 20 year follow-up. Br J Urol 76:517, 1995.
204. Antonopoulos P, Drossos C, Triantopoulou C, et al. Complications of renal angiomyolipomas: CT evaluation. Abdom Imaging 21:357, 1996.
205. Au K-S, Rodriguez JA, Finch JL, et al. Germ-line mutational analysis of the TSC 2 gene in 90 tuberous-sclerosis patients. Am J Hum Genet 62:286, 1998.
206. Baachi CE, Bonetti F, Pea M, et al. HMB 45: a review. Appl Immunohistochem 4:73, 1996.
207. Berg JW. Angiolipomyosarcoma of kidney (malignant hamartomatous angiolipomyoma) in a case with solitary metastasis from bronchogenic carcinoma. Cancer 8:759, 1955.
208. Bernstein SM, Newell JD Jr, Adamczyk D, et al. How common are renal angiomyolipomas in patients with pulmonary lymphangiomyomatosis? Am J Respit Crit Care Med 152:2138, 1995.
209. Blasco A, Vargas J, de Agustin P, et al. Solitary angiomyolipoma of the liver: report of a case with diagnosis by fine needle aspiration biopsy. Acta Cytol 39:813, 1995.
210. Bloom DA, Scardino P, Ehrlich RM. The significance of lymph node involvement in renal angiomyolipoma. J Urol 128:1292, 1982.
211. Bonetti F, Chiodera P, Pea M, et al. Transbronchial biopsy in lymphangioleiomyomatosis of the lung: HMB45 for diagnosis. Am J Surg Pathol 17:1092, 1993.
212. Bonetti F, Pea M, Martignoni G, et al. Clear cell ("sugar") tumor of the lung is a lesion strictly related to angiomyolipoma: the concept of a family of lesions characterized by the presence of the perivascular epithelioid cell (PEC). Pathology 26:230, 1994.
213. Brecher ME, Gill WB, Straus FH. Angiomyolipoma with regional lymph node involvement and long-term follow-up study. Hum Pathol 17:962, 1986.
214. Bryant DA, Gaudin PB, Hutchinson JB, et al. Angiomyolipoma of the kidney: a histologic and immunohistochemical study of 39 cases. Mod Pathol 11:442A, 1998.
215. Chan JKC, Tsang WYW, Pau MY, et al. Lymphangiomyomatosis and angiomyolipoma: closely related entities characterized by hamartomatous proliferation of HMB 45-positive smooth muscle. Histopathology 22:445, 1993.
216. Csanaky G, Szereday Z, Magyarlaki T, et al. Renal angiomyolipoma: report of three cases with regional lymph node involvement and/or with renal cell carcinoma. Tumori 81:469, 1995.
217. De Jong B, Castedo SM, Oosterhuis JW, et al. Trisomy 7 in a case of angiomyolipoma. Cancer Genet Cytogenet 34:219, 1988.
218. Delworth MG, Pisters LL, Fornage BD, et al. Cryotherapy for renal cell carcinoma and angiomyolipoma. J Urol 155:252, 1996.
219. Eble JN, Amin MB, Young RH. Epithelioid angiomyolipoma of the kidney: a report of five cases with a prominent and diagnostically confusing epithelioid smooth muscle component. Am J Surg Pathol 21:1123, 1997.
220. Farrow GM, Harrison EG Jr, Utz DC, et al. Renal angiomyolipoma: a clinicopathologic study of 32 cases. Cancer 22:564, 1968.
221. Ferry JA, Malt RA, Young RH. Renal angiomyolipoma with sarcomatous transformation and pulmonary metastases. Am J Surg Pathol 15:1083, 1991.
222. Fetsch PA, Fetsch JF, Marincola FM, et al. Comparison of melanoma antigen recognized by T cells (MART-1) to HMB-45: additional evidence to support a common lineage for angiomyolipoma, lymphangiomyomatosis, and clear cell sugar tumor. Mod Pathol 11:699, 1998.
223. Futter NG, Collins WE. Renal angiomyolipoma causing hypertension. Br J Urol 46:485, 1974.
224. Gaffey MJ, Mills SE, Zarbo RJ, et al. Clear cell tumor of the lung: immunohistochemical and ultrastructural evidence of melanogenesis. Am J Surg Pathol 15:644, 1991.
225. Gatalica Z, Lowry LD, Petersen RO. Angiomyolipoma of the nasal cavity: case report and review of the literature. Head Neck 16:278, 1994.
226. Green AJ, Sepp T, Yates JR. Clonality of tuberous sclerosis hamartomas shown by non-random X-chromosome inactivation. Hum Genet 97:240, 1996.
227. Green AJ, Smith M, Yates JRW. Loss of heterozygosity on chromosome 16pl3.3 in hamartomas from tuberous sclerosis patients. Nat Genet 6:193, 1994.
228. Guinee DG Jr, Thornberry DS, Azumi N, et al. Unique pulmonary presentation of an angiomyolipoma: analysis of clinical, radiographic, and histopathologic features. Am J Surg Pathol 19:476, 1995.
229. Hamlin JA, Smith DC, Taylor FC, et al. Renal angiomyolipomas: long-term follow-up of embolization for acute hemorrhage. Can Assoc Radiol J 48:191, 1997.
230. Han YM, Kim JK, Roh BS, et al. Renal angiomyolipoma: selective arterial embolization: effectiveness and changes in angiomyogenic components in long-term follow-up. Radiology 204:65, 1997.
231. Hartveit F, Hallerbraker B. A report of three angiomyolipomata and one angiomyoliposarcoma. Acta Pathol Microbiol Scand 49:329, 1960.
232. Henske EP, Ao X, Short MP, et al. Frequent progesterone receptor immunoreactivity in tuberous sclerosis-associated renal angiomyolipomas. Mod Pathol 11:665, 1998.
233. Henske EP, Neumann HPH, Scheithauer BW, et al. Loss of heterozygosity in the tuberous sclerosis (TSC 2) region of chromosome band 16p13 occurs in sporadic as well as TSC-associated renal angiomyolipoma. Genes Chromosomes Cancer 13:295, 1995.
234. Henske EP, Scheithauer BW, Short MP, et al. Allelic loss is frequent in tuberous sclerosis kidney lesions but rare in brain lesions. Am J Hum Genet 59:400, 1996.

235. Hoon V, Thung SN, Kaneko M, et al. HMB-45 reactivity in renal angiomyolipoma and lymphangioleiomyomatosis. Arch Pathol Lab Med 118:732, 1994.
236. Jungbluth AA, Busam KJ, Gerald WL, et al. A103: an anti-melan-A monoclonal antibody for the detection of malignant melanoma in paraffin embedded tissues. Am J Surg Pathol 22: 595, 1998.
237. Kaiserling E, Krober S, Xiao JC, et al. Angiomyolipoma of the kidney: immunoreactivity with HMB45; light and electron-microscopic findings. Histopathology 25:41, 1994.
238. Kattar MM, Grignon DJ, Eble JN, et al. Chromosomal analysis of renal angiomyolipoma by comparative genomic hybridization: evidence for clonal origin. Hum Pathol 30:295, 1999.
239. Kragel PJ, Toker C. Infiltrating recurrent renal angiomyolipoma with fatal outcome. J Urol 133:90, 1985.
240. Lack E, Dolan MF, Finisio J, et al. Pulmonary and extrapulmonary lymphangioleiomyomatosis: report of a case with bilateral renal angiomyolipomas: multifocal lymphangioleiomyomatosis and a glial polyp of the endocervix. Am J Surg Pathol 10:650, 1986.
241. Leder RA. Genitourinary case of the day: angiomyolipoma of the kidney with fat thrombus in the inferior vena cava. AJR 165:198, 1995.
242. L'Hostis H, Deminiere C, Ferriere JM, et al. Renal angiomyolipoma: a clinicopathologic, immunohistochemical, and follow-up study of 46 cases. Am J Surg Pathol 23:1011, 1999.
243. Liwnicz BH, Weeks DA, Zuppan CW. Extrarenal angiomyolipoma with melanocytic and hibernoma-like features. Ultrastruct Pathol 18:443, 1994.
244. Lowe BA, Brewer J, Houghton DC, et al. Malignant transformation of angiomyolipoma. J Urol 147:1356, 1992.
245. Maesawa C, Tamura G, Sawada H, et al. Angiomyolipoma arising in the colon. Am J Gastroenterol 91:1852, 1996.
246. Mai TK, Perkins DG, Collins JB. Epithelioid cell variant of renal angiomyolipoma. Histopathology 28:277, 1996.
247. Martignoni G, Pea M, Bonetti F, et al. Carcinoma-like monotypic epithelioid angiomyolipoma in patients without evidence of tuberous sclerosis: a clinicopathologic and genetic study. Am J Surg Pathol 22:663, 1998.
248. Monteforte WJ, Kohnen PW. Angiomyolipomas in a case of lymphangiomyomatosis syndrome: relationship to tuberous sclerosis. Cancer 34:317, 1974.
249. Mukai M, Torikata C, Iri H, et al. Crystalloids in angiomyolipoma: a previously unnoticed phenomenon of renal angiomyolipoma occurring at a high frequency. Am J Surg Pathol 16:1, 1992.
250. Nonomura A, Mizukami Y, Muraoka K, et al. Angiomyolipoma of the liver with pleomorphic histological features. Histopathology 24:279, 1994.
251. O'Donnell M, Fleming S. Angiomyolipoma of kidney: a cause of recurrent retroperitoneal haemorrhage. Br J Urol 76:521, 1995.
252. Paradis V, Laurendeau I, Vieillefond A, et al. Clonal analysis of renal sporadic angiomyolipomas. Hum Pathol 29:1063, 1998.
253. Pea M, Bonetti F, Martignoni G, et al. Apparent renal cell carinomas in tuberous sclerosis are heterogeneous: the identification of malignant epithelioid angiomyolipoma. Am J Surg Pathol 22:180, 1998.
254. Pea M, Bonetti F, Zamboni G, et al. Melanocyte marker HMB-45 is regularly expressed in angiomyolipoma of the kidney. Pathology 23:185, 1991.
255. Pea M, Martignoni G, Zamboni G, et al. Perivascular epithelioid cell. Am J Surg Pathol 20:1409, 1996.
256. Plank TL, Logginidou H, Klein-Szanto A, et al. The expression of hamartin, the product of the TSC1 gene, in normal human tissues and in TSC1- and TSC2- linked angiomyolipomas. Mod Pathol 12:539, 1999.
257. Price EB, Mostofi FK. Symptomatic angiomyolipoma of the kidney. Cancer 18:761, 1965.
258. Sempoux C, Weynand B, van Beers BE, et al. Angiomyolipoma of the liver: an unusual benign tumor identifiable on cytological material. Cytopathology 8:196, 1997.
259. Shimizu M, Manabe T, Tazelaar HD, et al. Intramyocardial angiomyolipoma. Am J Surg Pathol 18:1164, 1994.
260. Siegel CL, Middleton WD, Teefey SA, et al. Angiomyolipoma and renal cell carcinoma: US differentiation. Radiology 198: 789, 1996.
261. Silverman SG, Pearson GD, Seltzer SE, et al. Small hyperechoic renal masses: comparison of helical and conventional CT for diagnosis of angiomyolipoma. AJR 167:877, 1996.
262. Stillwell TJ, Gomez MR, Kelalis PP. Renal lesions in tuberous sclerosis. J Urol 138:477, 1987.
263. Stone NN, Atlas I, Kim US, et al. Renal angiomyolipoma associated with neurofibromatosis and primary carcinoid of mesentery. Urology 41:66, 1993.
264. Taniguchi N, Itoh K, Nakamura S, et al. Differentiation of renal cell carcinomas from angiomyolipomas by ultrasonic frequency dependent attenuation. J Urol 157:1242, 1997.
265. Taylor RS, Joseph DB, Kohaut EC, et al. Renal angiomyolipoma associated with lymph node involvement and renal cell carcinoma in patients with tuberous sclerosis. J Urol 141:930, 1989.
266. Terris B, Flejou JF, Picot R, et al. Hepatic angiomyolipoma: a report of four cases with immunohistochemical and DNA-flow cytometric studies. Arch Pathol Lab Med 120:68, 1996.
267. Tsui WMS, Colombari R, Portmann BC, et al. Hepatic angiomyolipoma: a clinicopathologic study of 30 cases and delineation of unusual morphologic variants. Am J Surg Pathol 23:34, 1999.
268. Val-Bernal JF, Mira C. Cutaneous angiomyolipoma. J Cutan Pathol 23:364, 1996.
269. Washecka R, Hanna M. Malignant renal tumors in tuberous sclerosis. Urology 37:340, 1991.
270. Weeks DA, Chase DR, Malott RL, et al. HMB-45 staining in angiomyolipoma, cardiac rhabdomyoma, other mesenchymal processes, and tuberous sclerosis-associated brain lesions. Int J Surg Pathol 1:191, 1994.
271. Weeks DA, Malott RL, Arnesen M, et al. Hepatic angiomyolipoma with striated granules and positivity with melanoma-specific antibody (HMB-45): a report of two cases. Ultrastruct Pathol 15:563, 1991.
272. Wullich B, Henn W, Siemer S, et al. Clonal chromosome aberrations in three of five sporadic angiomyolipomas of the kidney. Cancer Genet Cytogenet 96:42, 1997.
273. Yamamoto K, Nakamine H, Osaki T. Angiomyolipoma of the oral cavity: report of two cases. J Oral Maxillofac Surg 53:459, 1995.
274. Zamboni G, Pea M, Martignoni G, et al. Clear cell "sugar" tumor of the pancreas: a novel member of the family of lesions characterized by the presence of perivascular epithelioid cells (PEC). Am J Surg Pathol 9:399, 1996.

## Myelolipoma

275. Adesokan A, Adegboyega PA, Cowan DF, et al. Testicular "tumor" of the adrenogenital syndrome: a case report of an unusual association with myelolipoma and seminoma in cryptorchidism. Cancer 80:2120, 1997.
276. Bennett BD, McKenna TJ, Hough AJ, et al. Adrenal myelolipoma associated with Cushing's disease. Am J Clin Pathol 73: 443, 1980.
277. Bishoff JT, Waguespack RL, Lynch SC, et al. Bilateral symptomatic adrenal myelolipoma. J Urol 158:1517, 1997.
278. Bryan JA, Sykes CH, Garvin DF. Fine needle aspiration diag-

nosis of a mesenteric myelolipoma: a case report. Acta Cytol 40:592, 1996.
279. Burrows S, Drake WM Jr, Singley TL. Large retroperitoneal myelolipoma associated with acute myelogenous leukemia. Am J Clin Pathol 52:733, 1969.
280. Casey LR, Cohen AJ, Wile AG, et al. Giant adrenal myelolipomas: CT and MRI findings. Abdom Imaging 19:165, 1994.
281. Catalano O. Retroperitoneal hemmorhage due to a ruptured adrenal myeloplipoma: a case report. Acta Radiol 37:688, 1996.
282. Cina SJ, Gordon BM, Curry NS. Ectopic adrenal myelolipoma presenting as a splenic mass. Arch Pathol Lab Med 119:561, 1995.
283. Cyran KM, Kenney PJ, Memel DS, et al. Adrenal myelolipoma. AJR 166:395, 1996.
284. Damjanov I, Katz SM, Catalano E, et al. Myelolipoma in a heterotopic adrenal gland: light and electron microscopic findings. Cancer 44:1350, 1979.
285. El-Mekresh MM, Abdel-Gawad M, El-Diasty T, et al. Clincial, radiological and histological features of adrenal myelolipoma: review and experience with a further eight cases. Br J Urol 78: 345, 1996.
286. Fowler MR, Williams RB, Alba JM, et al. Extra-adrenal myelolipomas compared with extramedullary hematopoietic tumors: a case of presacral myelolipoma. Am J Surg Pathol 6:363, 1982.
287. Fujiwara R, Onishi T, Shimada A, et al. Adrenal myelolipoma: comparison of diagnostic imaging and pathological findings: Intern Med 32:166, 1993.
288. Goetz SP, Niemann TH, Robinson RA, et al. Hematopoietic elements associated with adrenal glands: a study of the spectrum of change in nine cases. Arch Pathol Lab Med 118:895, 1994.
289. Goldman HB, Howard RC, Patterson AL. Spontaneous retroperitoneal hemmorhage from a giant adrenal myelolipoma. J Urol 155,639, 1996.
290. Jenkins PJ, Chew SL, Lowe DG, et al. Adrenocorticotrophin-independent unilateral macronodular adrenal hyperplasia occurring with myelolipoma: an unusual cause of Cushing's syndrome. Clin Endocrinol (Oxf) 41:827, 1994.
291. Noble MJ, Montague DK, Levin HS. Myelolipoma: an unusual surgical lesion of the adrenal gland. Cancer 49:952, 1982.
292. Oliva A, Duarte B, Hammadeah R, et al. Myelolipoma and adrenal dysfunction. Surgery 103:711, 1988.
293. Prahlow JA, Loggie BW, Cappellari JO, et al. Extra-adrenal myelolipoma: a report of two cases. South Med J 88:639, 1995.
294. Reynard JM, Newman ML, Pollock L, et al. Giant adrenal myelolipoma. Br J Urol 75:802, 1995.
295. Sanders R, Bissada N, Curry N, et al. Clinical spectrum of adrenal myelolipoma: analysis of 8 tumors in 7 patients. J Urol 153:1791, 1995.
296. Shapiro JL, Goldblum JR, Dobrow DA, et al. Giant bilateral extra-adrenal myelolipoma. Arch Pathol Lab Med 119:283, 1995.
297. Sharma MC, Kashyap S, Sharma R, et al. Symptomatic adrenal myelolipoma: clinicopathologic analysis of 7 cases and a brief review of the literature. Urol Int 59:119, 1997.
298. Sneiders A, Zhang G, Gordon BE. Extra-adrenal perirenal myelolipoma. J Urol 150:1496, 1993.
299. Spinelli C, Materazzi G, Berti P, et al. Symptomatic adrenal myelolipoma: therapeutic considerations. Eur J Surg Oncol 21: 403, 1995.
300. Strimlan CV, Khasnabis S. Primary mediastinal myelolipoma. Cleve Clin J Med 60:69, 1993.
301. Sutker B, Balthazar EJ, Fazzini E. Presacral myelolipoma: CT findings. J Comput Assist Tomogr 9:1128, 1985.
302. Ukimura O, Inui E, Ochiai A, et al. Combined adrenal myelolipoma and pheochromocytoma. J Urol 154:1470, 1995.
303. Wagner JR, Kleiner DE, Walther MM, et al. Perirenal myelolipoma. Urology 49:128, 1997.
304. Whaley D, Becker S, Presbrey T, et al. Adrenal myelolipoma associated with Conn's syndrome: CT evaluation. J Comput Assist Tomogr 9:959, 1985.

### Intramuscular and Intermuscular Lipomas

305. Austin RM, Mack GR, Townsend CM, et al. Infiltrating (intramuscular) lipomas and angiolipomas. Arch Surg 115:281, 1980.
306. Cauchois R, Laccourreye O, Rotenberg M, et al. Intrinsic infiltrating intramuscular laryngeal lipoma. Otolaryngol Head Neck Surg 112:777, 1995.
307. Dattolo RA, Nesbit GM, Kelly KE, et al. Infiltrating intramuscular lipoma of the paraspinal muscles. Ann Otol Rhinol Laryngol 104:582, 1995.
308. Deschler DG, Lee K, Tami TA. Laryngeal infiltrating intramuscular lipoma. Otolaryngol Head Neck Surg 108:374, 1993.
309. Dionne GP, Seemayer TA. Infiltrating lipomas and angiolipomas revisited. Cancer 33:732, 1974.
310. Enzinger FM. Benign lipomatous tumors stimulating a sarcoma. In: Management of Primary Bone and Soft Tissue Tumors. Year Book, Chicago, 1977.
311. Greenberg SD, Isensee C, Gonzalez-Angulo A, et al. Infiltrating lipomas of the thigh. Am J Clin Pathol 39:66, 1963.
312. Kindblom LG, Angervall L, Stener B, et al. Intermuscular and intramuscular lipomas and hibernomas: a clinical, roentgenologic, histologic and prognostic study of 46 cases. Cancer 33: 754, 1974.
313. Kubota M, Nagasaki A, Ohgami H, et al. An infantile case of infiltrating lipoma in the buttock. J Pediatr Surg 26:230, 1991.
314. Regan JM, Bickle WH, Broders AC. Infiltrating benign lipomas of the extremities. West J Surg 54:87, 1946.
315. Seemayer TA, Dionne PC. Infiltrating lipomas of soft tissue. Lab Invest 30:304, 1974.
316. Warner JJ, Madsen N, Gerber C. Intramuscular lipoma of the deltoid causing shoulder pain: report of two cases. Clin Orthop 253:110, 1990.

### Lipoma of Tendon Sheaths and Joints

317. Armstrong SJ, Watt I. Lipoma arborescens of the knee. Br J Radiol 62:178, 1989.
318. Blais RE, LaPrade RF, Chaljub G, et al. The arthroscopic appearance of lipoma arborescens of the knee. Arthroscopy 11: 623, 1995.
319. Burgan DW. Lipoma arborescens of the knee: another cause of filling defects on a knee arthrogram. Radiology 101:583, 1971.
320. Chaljub G, Johnson PR. In vivo MRI characteristics of lipoma arborescens utilizing fat suppression and contrast administration. J Comput Assist Tomogr 20:85, 1996.
321. Dawson JS, Dowling F, Preston BJ, et al. Case report: lipoma arborescens of the sub-deltoid bursa. Br J Radiol 68:197, 1995.
322. Donnelly LF, Bisset GS, Passo MH. MRI findings of lipoma arborescens of the knee in a child: case report. Pediatr Radiol 24:258, 1994.
323. Feller JF, Rishi M, Hughes EC. Lipoma arborescens of the knee: MR demonstration. AJR 163:162, 1994.
324. Grieten M, Buckwalter KA, Cardinal E, et al. Case report 873: lipoma arborescens (villous lipomatous proliferation of the synovial membrane). Skeletal Radiol 23:652, 1994.
325. Hallel T, Lew S, Israel K-S, et al. Villous lipomatous proliferation of the synovial membrane (lipoma arborescens). J Bone Joint Surg Am 70:264, 1988.
326. Hoffa A. Zur Bedeutung des Fettgewebes fur die Pathologie des Kniegelenks. Dtsch Med Wochenschr 30:337, 1904.
327. Hubscher O, Costanza E, Elsner B. Chronic monoarthritis due to lipoma arborescens. J Rheumatol 17:861, 1990.
328. Krebs VE, Parker RD. Arthroscopic resection of an extrasyno-

vial ossifying chondroma of the infrapatellar fat pad: end-stage Hoffa's disease? Arthroscopy 10:301, 1994.
329. Kremchek TE, Kremchek EJ. Carpal tunnel syndrome caused by flexor tendon sheath lipoma. Orthop Rev 17:1083, 1988.
330. Kurihashi A, Yamaguchi T, Tamal K, et al. Lipoma arborescens with osteochondral metaplasia: a case mimicking synovial osteochondromatosis in a lateral knee bursa. Acta Orthop Scand 68:304, 1997.
331. Laorr A, Peterfy CG, Tirman PF, et al. Lipoma arborescens of the shoulder: magnetic resonance imaging findings. Can Assoc Radiol J 46:311, 1995.
332. Martinez D, Millner PA, Coral A, et al. Case report 745: synovial lipoma arborescens. Skeletal Radiol 21:393, 1992.
333. Noel ER, Tebib JG, Dumontet C, et al. Synovial lipoma arborescens of the hip. Clin Rheumatol 6:92, 1987.
334. Pampliega T, Arenas AJ. An unusual trigger finger. Acta Orthop Belg 63:132, 1997.
335. Ryu KN, Jaovisidha S, Schweitzer M, et al. MR imaging of lipoma arborescens of the knee joint. AJR 167:1229, 1996.
336. Shih WJ, Banks ER, Purcell M, et al. Multiple imagings to diagnose the chondrosseous metaplasia within a lipoma near the knee. Arch Orthop Trauma Surg 116:181, 1997.
337. Sola JB, Wright RW. Arthroscopic treatment for lipoma arborescens of the knee. J Bone Joint Surg Am 80:99, 1998.
338. Sullivan CR, Dahlin DC, Bryan RS. Lipoma of the tendon sheath. J Bone Joint Surg Am 38:1275, 1956.
339. Weston WJ. The intra-synovial fatty masses in chronic rheumatoid arthritis. Br J Radiol 46:213, 1973.

### Lumbosacral Lipoma

340. Alston SR, Fuller GN, Boyko OB, et al. Ectopic immature renal tissue in a lumbosacral lipoma: pathologic and radiologic findings. Pediatr Neurosci 15:100, 1989.
341. Brown E, Matthes JC, Bazan C, et al. Prevalence of incidental intraspinal lipoma of the lumbosacral spine as determined by MRI. Spine 19:833, 1994.
342. Harrison MJ, Mitnick RJ, Rosenblum BR, et al. Leptomyelolipoma: analysis of 20 cases. J Neurosurg 73:360, 1990.
343. Kanev PM, Bierbrauer KS. Reflections on the natural history of lipomyelomeningocele. Pediatr Neurosurg 22:137, 1995.
344. Kieck C, Villiers J. Subcutaneous lumbosacral lipomas. S Afr Med J 49:1563, 1975.
345. Koyanagi I, Iwasaki Y, Hida K, et al. Surgical treatment of syringomyelia associated with spinal dysraphism. Childs Nerv Syst 13:194, 1997.
346. Koyanagi I, Iwasaki Y, Hida K, et al. Surgical treatment supposed natural history of the tethered cord with occult spinal dysraphism. Childs Nerv Syst 13:268, 1997.
347. Lassman LP, James CCM. Lumbosacral lipomas: critical survey of 26 cases submitted to laminectomy. J Neurol Neurosurg Psychol 30:174, 1967.
348. Loeser JD, Lewin RD. Lumbosacral lipoma in an adult. J Neurosurg 29:405, 1968.
349. Maiuri F, Corriero G, Gallichio B, et al. Late neurological dysfunction in adult lumbosacral lipoma. J Neurosurg Sci 31:7, 1987.
350. Naidich TP, McLone DG, Mutluer S. A new understanding of dorsal dysraphism with lipoma (lipomyeloschisis). AJR 140: 1065, 1983.
351. Pasternak JF, Volpe JJ. Lumbosacral lipoma with acute deterioration during infancy. Pediatrics 66:125, 1980.
352. Pierre-Kahn A, Zerah M, Renier D, et al. Congenital lumbosacral lipomas. Childs Nerv Syst 13:298, 1997.
353. Rickwood AMK, Hemalatha V, Zachary RB. Lipoma of the cauda equina (lumbosacral lipoma): a study of 74 cases operated in childhood. Z Kinderchir 27:159, 1979.
354. Taviere V, Brunelle F, Baraton J, et al. MRI study of lumbosacral lipoma in children. Pediatr Radiol 19:316, 1989.

### Neural Fibrolipoma

355. Adair FE, Pack GT, Farrior JH. Lipomas. Am J Cancer 16:1104, 1932.
356. Berti E, Roncaroli F. Fibrolipomatous hamartoma of a cranial nerve. Histopathology 24:391, 1994.
357. Bibbo C, Warren AM. Fibrolipomatous hamartoma of nerve. J Foot Ankle Surg 33:64, 1994.
358. Boren WL, Henry RE Jr, Wintch K. MR diagnosis of fibrolipomatous hamartoma of nerve: association with nerve territory-oriented macrodactyly (macrodystrophia lipomatosa). Skeletal Radiol 24:296, 1995.
359. Cavallaro MC, Taylor JAM, Gorman JD, et al. Imaging findings in a patient with fibrolipomatosis hamartoma of the median nerve. AJR 161:837, 1993.
360. Declercq H, De Man R, Van Herek G, et al. Case report 814: fibrolipoma of the median nerve. Skeletal Radiol 22:610, 1993.
361. De Maeseneer M, Jaovisidha S, Lenchik L, et al. Fibrolipomatous hamartoma: MR imaging findings. Skeletal Radiol 26:155, 1997.
362. Drut R. Ossifying fibrolipomatous hamartoma of the ulnar nerve. Pediatr Pathol 8:179, 1988.
363. Erichsen B, Medgyesi S. Congenital lipoma imitating giantism of the toe. Scand J Plast Reconstr Surg 17:77, 1983.
364. Evans HA, Donnelly LF, Johnson ND, et al. Fibrolipoma of the median nerve: MKI. Clin Radiol 52:304, 1997.
365. Friedlander HL, Rosenberg NJ, Graubard DJ. Intraneural lipoma of the median nerve. J Bone Joint Surg Am 51:352, 1969.
366. Gupta SK, Sharma OP, Sharma SV, et al. Macrodystrophia lipomatosa: radiographic observations. Br J Radiol 65:769, 1992.
367. Haverbush TJ, Kendrick JL, Nelson CL. Intraneural lipoma of the median nerve: report of two cases. Cleve Clin Q 37:145, 1970.
368. Houpt P, Storm van Leeuwen JB, Van Den Bergen HA. Intraneural lipofibroma of the median nerve. J Hand Surg [Am] 14: 706, 1989.
369. Johnson RJ, Bonfiglio M. Lipofibromatous hamartoma of the median nerve. J Bone Joint Surg Am 51:984, 1969.
370. Meyer BU, Roricht S. Fibrolipomatous hamartoma of the proximal ulnar nerve associated with macrodactyly and macrodystrophia lipomatosa as an unusual cause of cubital tunnel syndrome. J Neurol Neurosurg Psychiatry 63:808, 1997.
371. Oleaga L, Florencio MR, Ereno C, et al. Fibrolipomatous hamartoma of the radial nerve: MR imaging findings. Skeletal Radiol 24:559, 1995.
372. Paletta FX, Rybka FJ. Treatment of hamartomas of the median nerve. Ann Surg 176:217, 1972.
373. Patel ME, Silver JW, Lipton DE, et al. Lipofibroma of the median nerve in the palm and digits of the hand. J Bone Joint Surg Am 61:393, 1979.
374. Silverman TA, Enzinger FM. Fibrolipomatous hamartoma of nerve: a clinicopathologic analysis of 26 cases. Am J Surg Pathol 9:7, 1985.
375. Soler R, Rodriguez E, Bargiela A, et al. MR findings of macrodystrophia lipomatosa. Clin Imaging 21:135, 1997.
376. Sondergaard G, Mikkelsen S. Fibrolipomatous hamartoma of the median nerve. J Hand Surg [Br] 12:224, 1987.

### Diffuse Lipomatosis

377. Findlay GH, Duvenage M. Acquired symmetric lipomatosis of the hands: a distal form of Madelung-Launois-Bensaude syndrome Clin Exp Dermatol 14:58, 1989.
378. Greiss ME, Williams DH. Macrodystrophia lipomatosis in the

foot: a case report and review of the literature. Arch Orthop Trauma Surg 110:220, 1991.
379. Karademir M, Kocak M, Usal A, et al. A case of infiltrating lipomatosis with diffuse, symmetrical distribution. Br J Clin Pract 44:728, 1990.
380. Kindblom L, Moller-Nielson J. Diffuse lipomatosis of the leg after poliomyelitis. Acta Pathol Microbiol Stand 83:339, 1975.
381. Lippit DH, Johnston JR. Diffuse lipomatosis of a lower extremity: report of case. Bull Ayer Clin Lab 4:55, 1954.
382. McCarthy DM, Dorr CA, Mackintosh CE. Unilateral localized giantism of the extremities with lipomatosis, arthropathy and psoriasis. J Bone Joint Surg Br 51:348, 1969.
383. Nixon HH, Scobie WG. Congenital lipomatosis: a report of four cases. J Pediatr Surg 6:742, 1971.
384. Oosthuizen SF, Barnetson J. Two cases of lipomatosis involving bone. Br J Radiol 20:426, 1947.
385. Schlicht D. Recurrent lipoblastomatosis in a child. Med J Austr 2:959, 1965.

## Symmetric Lipomatosis

386. Agrez M, Heller A, Barrie P. Benign symmetric lipomatosis. Aust NZ J Surg 65:616, 1995.
387. Basse P, Lohmann M, Hovgard C, et al. Multiple symmetric lipomatosis: combined surgical treatment and liposuction: case report. Scand J Plast Reconstr Surg Hand Surg 26:111, 1992.
388. Berkovic SF, Andermann F, Schoubridge EA. Mitochondrial dysfunction in multiple symmetric lipomatosis. Ann Neurol 29:566, 1991.
389. Berkovic SF, Schoubridge EA, Andermann F, et al. Clinical spectrum of mitochondrial DNA mutation at base pair 8344. Lancet 338:457, 1991.
390. Borges A, Torrinha F, Lufkin RB, et al. Laryngeal involvement in multiple symmetrical lipomatosis (the role of computed tomography in diagnosis). Am J Otolaryngol 18:127, 1997.
391. Brackenbury ET, Morgan WE. Surgical management of Launois-Bensaude syndrome. Thorax 52:834, 1997.
392. Brodie BC. Clinical Lectures on Surgery Delivered at St. George's Hospital. Lea & Blanchard, Philadelphia, 1846, p 275.
393. Brodovsky S, Westreich M, Leibowitz A, et al. Adiposis dolorosa (Dercum's disease): 10 year follow-up. Ann Plast Surg 33: 664, 1994.
394. Chalk CH, Mills KR, Jacobs JM, et al. Familial multiple symmetric lipomatosis with peripheral neuropathy. Neurology 40: 1246, 1990.
395. Colwell JA, Cruz SR. Effects of reception of adipose tissue on the diabetes and hyperinsulinism of benign symmetrical lipomatosis. Diabetes 21:13, 1972.
396. Enzi G. Multiple symmetrical lipomatosis: an updated clinical report. Medicine 63:56, 1984.
397. Enzi G, Angelini C, Negrin P, et al. Sensory, motor and autonomic neuropathy in patients with multiple symmetrical lipomatosis. Medicine 64:388, 1986.
398. Feldman DR, Schabel SI. Multiple symmetrical lipomatosis: computed tomographic appearance. South Med J 88:681, 1995.
399. Greene ML, Glueck CJ, Fujimoto WY, et al. Benign symmetrical lipomatosis (Launois-Bensaude adenolipomatosis) with gout and hyperlipoproteinemia. Am J Med 48:239, 1970.
400. Klopstock T, Naumann M, Seibel P, et al. Mitochondrial DNA mututations in multiple symmetrical lipomastosis. Mol Cell Biochem 174:271, 1997.
401. Kodish ME, Alsever RN, Block MB. Benign symmetric lipomatosis: functional sympathetic denervation of adipose tissue and possible hypertrophy of brown fat. Metabolism 23:937, 1974.
402. Kurzweg FT, Spencer R. Familial multiple lipomatosis. Am J Surg 82:762, 1951.
403. Launois PE, Bensaude R. De l'adenolipomatose symmetrique. Soc Med Hosp Paris Bull Mem 15:298, 1889.
404. Madelung OW. Ueber den Fetthals. Arch Klin Chir 37:106, 1888.
405. Müller MM, Frank O. Lipid and purine metabolism in benign symmetric lipomatosis. Adv Exp Med Biol 41:509, 1974.
406. Naumann M, Kiefer R, Toyka KV, et al. Mitochondrial dysfunction with myoclonus epilepsy and ragged-red fibers point mutation in nerve, muscle, and adipose tissue of a patient with multiple symmetric lipomatosis. Muscle Nerve 20:833, 1997.
407. Naumann M, Schalke B, Klopstock T, et al. Neurological multisystem manifestation in multiple symmetric lipomatosis: a clinical and electrophysiological study. Muscle Nerve 18:693, 1995.
408. Pollock M, Nicholson GI, Nukada H, et al. Neuropathy in multiple symmetrical lipomatosis. Brain 111:1157, 1988.
409. Ross M, Goodman MM. Multiple symmetric lipomatosis (Launois-Bensaude syndrome). Int J Dermatol 31:80, 1992.
410. Ruzicka T, Vieluf D, Landthaler M, et al. Benign symmetric lipomatosis (Launois-Bensaude): report of ten cases and review of literature. J Am Acad Dermatol 17:663, 1987.
411. Stoll C, Alembik Y, Truttmann M. Multiple familial lipomatosis with polyneuropathy, an inherited dominant condition. Ann Genet 39:193, 1996.
412. Stravropoulos PG, Zouboulis CC, Trautmann C, et al. Symmetric lipomatoses in female patients. Dermatology 194:26, 1997.
413. Whol MG, Pastor N. Adiposis dolorosa (Dercum's disease). JAMA 110:1261, 1938.
414. Williams DW, Ginsberg LE, Moody DM, et al. Madelung disease: MR findings. Am J Neuroradiol 14:107, 1993.
415. Zancanaro C, Sbarbati A, Morroni M, et al. Multiple symmetrical lipomatosis: ultrastructural investigation of the tissue and preadipocytes in primary culture. Lab Invest 63:253, 1990.

## Pelvic Lipomatosis

416. Allen FJ, De Kock ML. Pelvic lipomatosis: the nuclear magnetic resonance appearance and associated vesicoureteral reflux. J Urol 138:1228, 1987.
417. Becker JA, Weiss RM, Schiff M Jr, et al. Pelvic lipomatosis: a consideration in the diagnosis of intrapelvic neoplasms. Arch Surg 100:94, 1970.
418. Beluffi G, DiGiulio G, Fiori P. Pelvic lipomatosis in the Proteus syndrome: a further diagnostic sign. Eur J Pediatr 149: 866, 1990.
419. Berens BM, Azarvan A. Bladder outlet obstruction due to pelvic lipoma: computerized tomography, magnetic resonance imaging and radiographic evaluation. J Urol 145:138, 1991.
420. Boquist L, Bergdahl L, Andersson A. Lipomatosis of the ileocecal valve. Cancer 29:136, 1972.
421. Costa T, Fitch N, Azouz EM. Proteus syndrome: report of two cases with pelvic lipomatosis. Pediatrics 76:984, 1985.
422. Duffis AW, Weinberg B, Diakoumakis EE. A case of cystitis glandularis with associated pelvic lipomatosis: ultrasound evaluation. J Clin Ultrasound 18:733, 1990.
423. Engels EP. Sigmoid colon and urinary bladder in high fixation: roentgen changes simulating pelvic tumor. Radiology 72:419, 1959.
424. Fogg LB, Smyth JW. Pelvic lipomatosis: a condition simulating pelvic neoplasm. Radiology 90:558, 1968.
425. Gordon NSI, Sinclair RA, Snow RM. Pelvic lipomatosis with cystitis cystica, cystitis glandularis and adenocarcinoma of the bladder: first reported case. Aust N Z J Surg 60:229, 1990.
426. Grimmett GM, Hall MG, Aird CC, et al. Pelvic lipomatosis. Am J Surg 125:347, 1973.
427. Halachmi S, Moskovitz B, Calderon N, et al. The use of an ultrasonic assisted lipectomy device for the treatment of obstructive pelvic lipomatosis. Urology 48:128, 1996.

428. Heyns CF. Pelvic lipomatosis: a review of its diagnosis and management. J Urol 146:267, 1991.
429. Heyns CF, De Kock ML, Kirsten PH, et al. Pelvic lipomatosis associated with cystitis glandularis and adenocarcinoma of the bladder. J Urol 145:364, 1991.
430. Honda H, McGuire CW, Barloon TJ, et al. Replacement lipomatosis of the kidney: CT features. J Comput Assist Tomogr 14:229, 1990.
431. Honecke K, Butz M. Pelvic lipomatosis in a female: diagnosis and initial therapy. Urol Int 46:93, 1991.
432. Johnston OL, Bracken RB, Ayala AG. Vesical adenocarcinoma occurring in patient with pelvic lipomatosis. Urology 15:280, 1980.
433. Joshi KK, Wise HA. Pelvic lipomatosis: 9-year follow-up in a woman. J Urol 129:1233, 1983.
434. Klein FA, Vernon-Smith MJ, Kasenetz I. Pelvic lipomatosis: 35 year experience. J Urol 139:998, 1988.
435. Van Heurn LW, Varekamp AP. A rare case of iliac vein obstruction: pelvic lipomatosis. Neth J Surg 42:58, 1990.
436. Yalla SV, Ivker M, Burros HM, et al. Cystitis glandularis with perivesical lipomatosis: frequent association of two unusual proliferative conditions. Urology 5:383, 1975.
437. Yamaguchi T, Shimizu Y, Ono N, et al. A case of pelvic lipomatosis presenting with edema of the lower extremities. Jpn J Med 30:559, 1991.

### Steroid Lipomatosis

438. Benamou PH, Hilliquen P, Chemla N, et al. Epidural lipomatosis not induced by corticosteroid therapy: three cases including one in a patient with primary Cushing's disease (review of the literature). Rev Rhum Engl Ed 63:207, 1996.
439. Fessler RG, Johnson DL, Brown FD, et al. Epidural lipomatosis in steroid treated patients. Spine 17:183, 1992.
440. George WE Jr, Wilmot M, Greenhouse A, et al. Medical management of steroid-induced epidural lipomatosis. N Engl J Med 308:316, 1983.
441. Gilsanz V, Brill PW, Wolf BS. Increased retroperitoneal fat: a sign of corticosteroid therapy. Radiology 123:147, 1977.
442. Glickstein MF, Miller WT, Dalinka MK, et al. Paraspinal lipomatosis: a benign mass. Radiology 163:79, 1987.
443. Kaplan JG, Barasch E, Hirschfeld A, et al. Spinal epidural lipomatosis: a serious complication of iatrogenic Cushing's syndrome. Neurology 39:1031, 1989.
444. Mulrow CD, Corey GR. Pericardial pseudoeffusion due to steroid-induced lipomatosis. NC Med J 46:179, 1985.
445. Noel P, Pepersack T, Vanbinst A, et al. Spinal epidural lipomatosis in Cushing's syndrome secondary to adrenal tumor. Neurology 42:1250, 1992.
446. Perling LH, Laurent JP, Cheek WR. Epidural hibernoma as a complication of corticosteroid treatment. J Neurosurg 69:613, 1988.
447. Roy-Camille R, Mazel C, Husson JL, et al. Symptomatic spinal epidural lipomatosis induced by a long-term steroid treatment: review of the literature and report of two additional cases. Spine 16:1365, 1991.
448. Shukla LW, Katz JA, Wagner ML. Mediastinal lipomatosis: a complication of high dosed steroid therapy in children. Pediatr Radiol 19:57, 1988.
449. Shuman BM. Mediastinal lipomatosis complicating steroid therapy of regional enteritis. Gastroenterology 61:244, 1971.
450. Siskind BN, Weiner FR, Frank M, et al. Steroid induced mesenteric lipomatosis. Comput Radiol 8:175, 1984.
451. Streiter ML, Schneider HJ, Proto AV. Steroid induced thoracic lipomatosis: paraspinal involvement. AJR 139:679, 1982.
452. Van de Putte LBA, Wagenaar JPM. Pericardiac lipomatosis in exogenous Cushing syndrome. Thorax 28:653, 1973.
453. Vazquez L, Ellis A, Saint-Jenez D, et al. Epidural lipomatosis after renal transplantation: complete recovery without surgery. Transplantation 46:773, 1988.
454. Zentner J, Buchbender K, Vahlensieck M. Spinal epidural lipomatosis as a complication of prolonged corticosteroid therapy. J Neurosurg Sci 39:81, 1995.

### Nevus Lipomatosus Cutaneous Superficialis

455. Bass HN, Caldwell S, Brooks BS. Michelin tire baby syndrome: familial constriction bands during infancy and early childhood in four generations. Am J Med Genet 45:370, 1993.
456. Burgdorf WH, Doran CK, Worret WI. Folded skin with scarring: Michelin tire baby syndrome? J Am Acad Dermatol 7:90, 1982.
457. Chanoki M, Sugamoto I, Suzuki S, et al. Nevus lipomatosus cutaneous superficialis of the scalp. Cutis 43:143, 1989.
458. Dotz W, Prioleau PG. Nevus lipomatosus cutaneous superficialis: a light and electron microscopic study. Arch Dermatol 120:376, 1984.
459. Eyre SP, Hebert AA, Rapini RP. Rubbery zosteriform nodules on the back: nevus lipomatosus cutaneous superficialis (Hoffman-Zurhelle). Arch Dermatol 128:1395, 1992.
460. Finley AG, Musso LA. Naevus lipomatosus cutaneus superficialis (Hoffman-Zurhelle). Br J Dermatol 87:557, 1972.
461. Gardner EW, Miller HM, Lowney ED. Deletion of chromosome 11 in babies with Michelin tire syndrome. Arch Dermatol 116:622, 1980.
462. Hann SK, Yang DS, Lee SH. Giant nevus lipomatosus superficialis associated with cavernous hemangioma. J Dermatol 15: 543, 1988.
463. Hoffman E, Zurhelle E. Ueber einen Naevus lipomatosus cutaneous superficialis der linken Glutaealgegend. Arch Dermatol 130:327, 1921.
464. Park HJ, Park CJ, Yi JY, et al. Nevus lipomatosus superficialis on the face. Int J Dermatol 36:435, 1997.
465. Reymond JL, Stoebner P, Amblard P. Nevus lipomatosus cutaneous superficialis: an electron microscopic study of four cases. J Cutan Pathol 7:295, 1980.
466. Sato M, Ishikawa O, Miyachi Y, et al. Michelin tire syndrome: a congenital disorder of elastic fibre formation? Br J Dermatol 136:583, 1997.
467. Sawada Y. Solitary nevus lipomatosus superficialis on the forehead. Ann Plast Surg 16:356, 1986.
468. Schnur RE, Herzberg AJ, Spinner N, et al. Variability in the Michelin tire syndrome: a child with multiple anomalies, smooth muscle hamartoma, and familial paracentric inversion of chromosome 7q. J Am Acad Dermatol 28:364, 1993.
469. Schnur RE, Zackai EH. Circumferential ringed creases ("Michelin tire babies") with specific histologic findings and/or karyotype abnormalities: clues to molecular pathogenesis? Am J Med Genet 69:221, 1997.
470. Weitzner S. Solitary nevus lipomatosus cutaneus superficialis of scalp. Arch Dermatol 97:540, 1968.
471. Wilson-Jones E, Marks R, Pongshirun D. Naevus superficialis lipomatosus. Br J Dermatol 93:121, 1975.

### Hibernoma

472. Ahn C, Harvey JC. Mediastinal hibernoma, a rare tumor. Ann Thorac Surg 50:828, 1990.
473. Allegra SR, Gmuer C, O'Leary GP Jr. Endocrine activity in a large hibernoma. Hum Pathol 14:1044, 1983.
474. Alvine G, Rosenthal H, Murphey M, et al. Hibernoma. Skeletal Radiol 25:493, 1996.
475. Angervall L, Nilsson L, Stener B. Microangiographic and histologic studies in two cases of hibernoma. Cancer 17:685, 1964.
476. Atilla S, Eilenberg SS, Brown JJ. Hibernoma: MRI appearance of a rare tumor. Magn Reson Imaging 13:335, 1995.

477. Cook MA, Stern M, De Silva RD. MRI of a hibernoma. J Comput Assist Tomogr 20:333, 1996.
478. Cox RW. "Hibernoma": the lipoma of immature adipose tissue. J Pathol Bacteriol 68:511, 1954.
479. Dal Cin P, Van Damme B, Hoogmartens M, et al. Chromosome changes in a case of hibernoma. Genes Chromosomes Cancer 5:178, 1992.
480. Gaffney EF, Hargreaves HK, Semple E, et al. Hibernoma: distinctive light and electron microscopic features and relationship to brown adipose tissue. Hum Pathol 14:677, 1983.
481. Gery L. Discussions. Bull Mem Soc Anat (Paris) 89:111, 1914.
482. Gould VE, Jao W, Gould NS, et al. Electron microscopy of adipose tissue tumors: comparative features of hibernomas, myxoid and pleomorphic liposarcomas. Pathobiol Annu 9:339, 1979.
483. Gulmez I, Dogan A, Balkanli S, et al. The first case of periureteric hibernoma: case report. Scand J Urol Nephrol 31:203, 1997.
484. Heifetz SA, Parikh SR, Brown JW. Hibernoma of the pericardium presenting as pericardial effusion in a child. Pediatr Pathol 10:575, 1990.
485. Kindblom G, Angervall L, Stener B, et al. Intermuscular and intramuscular lipomas and hibernomas. Cancer 33:754, 1974.
486. Lewandowski PJ, Weiner SD. Hibernoma of the medial thigh: case report and literature review. Clin Orthop 330:198, 1996.
487. Meloni AM, Spanier SS, Bush CH, et al. Involvement of 10q22 and 11q13 in hibernoma. Cancer Genet Cytogenet 72:59, 1994.
488. Mertens F, Rydholm A, Brosjo O, et al. Hibernomas are characterized by rearrangements of chromosome bands 11p13-21. Int J Cancer 58:503, 1994.
489. Minic AJ. Hibernoma: unusual location in the submental space. J Craniomaxillofac Surg 20:264, 1992.
490. Mrozek K, Karakousis CP, Bloomfield CD. Band 11q13 is nonrandomly rearranged in hibernomas. Genes Chromosomes Cancer 9:145, 1994.
491. Peer S, Kuhberger R, Dessl A, et al. MR imaging findings in hibernoma. Skeletal Radiol 26:507, 1997.
492. Rigor VU, Goldstone SE, Jones J, et al. Hibernoma: a case report and discussion of a rare tumor. Cancer 57:2207, 1986.
493. Rossi P, Francone A, Martini S, et al. Multiple imaging modalities in a case of hibernoma. Eur J Radiol 8:125, 1988.
494. Seemayer TA, Knaack J, Wang NS, et al. On the ultrastructure of hibernoma. Cancer 36:1785, 1975.
495. Seynaeve P, Mortelmans L, Kockx M, et al. Case report 813: hibernoma of the left thigh. Skeletal Radiol 23:137, 1994.
496. Worsey J, McGuirt W, Carrau RL, et al. Hibernoma of the neck: a rare cause of neck mass. Am J Otolaryngol 15:152, 1994.
497. Zancanaro C, Pelosi G, Accordini C, et al. Immunohistochemical identification of the uncoupling protein in human hibernoma. Biol Cell 80:75, 1994.

# CHAPTER 17

# LIPOSARCOMA

Liposarcoma is one of the most common soft tissue sarcomas of adult life, with an annual incidence estimated to be 2.5 per million in a Swedish population[23] and the relative incidence among other sarcomas ranging from 9.8% to 16.0%.[20,32] Included in the general category of liposarcoma are a number of subtypes that are histologically, biologically, cytogenetically, and by molecular analyses[7,11–13,20,28,31,55] distinct from one another (Table 17–1). These subtypes range in behavior from nonmetastasizing neoplasms (e.g., well differentiated liposarcoma) to high grade sarcomas with full metastatic potential (e.g., round cell liposarcoma, pleomorphic liposarcoma). So impressed were Enzinger and Winslow by the diversity of this group of lesions that they wrote in their seminal work on liposarcoma in 1962, "Among mesenchymal tumors, liposarcomas are probably unsurpassed by their wide range in structure and behavior. In fact the variations are striking that it seems more apt [sic] to regard them as groups of closely related tumors rather than as a well defined entity."[11] In no other group of sarcomas does the pathologist receive such a strong mandate to subclassify these lesions accurately, as accurate subtyping translates into grade and biologic behavior.

Although the World Health Organization (WHO) divides liposarcomas into five subtypes (well differentiated, myxoid, round cell, dedifferentiated, pleomorphic[36]), it is useful to think of liposarcomas as three large groups from a conceptual point of view. Well differentiated and dedifferentiated liposarcomas comprise one subgroup. Widely disparate in terms of biologic behavior, they are closely related from a pathogenetic point of view, as with time a subset of well differentiated liposarcomas histologically progress to dedifferentiated sarcomas. With dedifferentiation the tumor acquires metastatic potential, a phenomenon accompanied by more cytogenetic abnormalities. A second group comprises the myxoid and round cell liposarcomas. This continuum of lesions ranges from pure myxoid liposarcoma at one extreme to round cell (poorly differentiated myxoid) liposarcomas at the other. Pleomorphic liposarcomas are rare poorly characterized tumors. Many, but not all, are virtually indistinguishable from malignant fibrous histiocytoma except for the presence of pleomorphic lipoblasts. Finally, a small number of liposarcomas exhibit unusual features or combine patterns not accounted for in the above classification (liposarcomas of mixed type). Such lesions are best individualized and diagnosed as liposarcomas of mixed or miscellaneous type until refinements in the current classification account for these nosologic oddities.

Certain generalizations should be kept in mind when considering the diagnosis of liposarcoma. First, most liposarcomas occur in deep soft tissue, in contrast to lipomas, which occur in superficial soft tissue. This implies that subcutaneous well differentiated liposarcomas are rare and that the diagnosis should be made only after the more common mimics (e.g., spindle cell lipoma, pleomorphic lipoma, chondroid lipoma, cellular forms of angiolipoma) are excluded from the differential diagnosis. On the other hand, when true liposarcomas develop in superficial tissues they have an excellent prognosis and are designated "atypical lipoma" rather than well differentiated liposarcoma. Second, there is little if any evidence that lipomas undergo malignant transformation to liposarcomas, an axiom that derives strong support from the marked difference in location of lipomas and liposarcomas. Most likely, lesions suggesting malignant transformation of a lipoma are in reality liposarcomas in which inadequate sampling led to underdiagnosis of malignancy in the original material. Third, liposarcomas rarely occur in children. Liposarcoma-like lesions in this age group are apt to represent lipoblastoma, a fetal form of lipoma.

There have been great strides in our understanding of liposarcomas during the last several years largely as a result of cytogenetic studies. The reciprocal translocation between chromosomes 12 and 16, which characterizes most myxoid/round cell liposarcomas, results in expression of a number of fusion transcripts, which appear to play a direct role in oncogenesis. The large group of well differentiated liposarcomas (atypical lipoma), on the other hand, have an

**TABLE 17–1 COMPARISON OF LIPOSARCOMA SUBTYPES**

| Liposarcoma Type | Age (Years) | Location | Cytogenetic Abnormality | Behavior |
|---|---|---|---|---|
| WDL | 50–70 | Extremity (75%); retroperitoneum | Giant marker + ring chromosome | Local recurrence high; no metastasis 5–15% dedifferentiated |
| DL | 50–70 | Retroperitoneum (75%) | Giant marker + ring + additional abnormalities | High local recurrence; metastasis |
| MRCL | 25–45 | Extremity (75%) | t(12;16) | Recurrence + metastasis (determined by round cell component) |

WDL, well differentiated liposarcoma; DL, dedifferentiated liposarcoma; MRCL, myxoid/round cell liposarcoma.

entirely different abnormality in the form of giant and ring chromosomes, derived at least in part from chromosome 12, resulting in amplification of a number of genes (e.g., *MDM2, SAS, GLI*) which represent a recurring motif in a number of mesenchymal tumors. Liposarcoma cells have recently been shown to express the peroxisome proliferator-activated receptor gamma (PPAR gamma) which when bound to its ligand pioglitazone terminally differentiate.[34a] Binding is associated with withdrawal from the cell cycle, induction of adipocyte specific genes, and intracellular accumulation of lipid. In three patients with high grade liposarcoma use of this ligands also resulted in differentiation of the tumors.[7a] This suggests that pharmacologically induced differentiation may be a viable approach to treatment of some sarcomas.

Interestingly, liposarcomas are seldom induced by radiation. We have never encountered such a case in our consultation experience, although anecdotal reports following irradiation for carcinoma of the mouth and breast[2,10] are on record. Like other sarcomas, liposarcoma may also be associated with various signs and symptoms. Dedifferentiated liposarcomas have been associated with a leukemoid blood reaction,[63] and there has been one unillustrated report of an acquired factor VII deficiency associated with a pleural liposarcoma that vanished and then reappeared with remission and relapse of the tumor, respectively.[8]

## CRITERIA AND IMPORTANCE OF LIPOBLASTS

Traditionally, great emphasis has been placed on the identification of lipoblasts for diagnosing liposarcoma. Although it is certainly an appropriate task for pathologists to search for these cells in some situations, their importance in other situations has been overemphasized. For example, well differentiated sclerosing liposarcomas usually have few lipoblasts; and in such cases the overall pattern and cellular components become more important determinants when making the diagnosis. On the other hand, imprecise criteria for the recognition of lipoblasts often lead to an erroneous diagnosis of liposarcoma.

Defined in the context of liposarcoma, the lipoblast is a neoplastic cell that to some extent recapitulates the differentiation cascade of normal fat. The earliest cells arise as pericapillary adventitial cells that closely resemble fibroblasts. These spindled cells, endowed with ample endoplasmic reticulum, slowly acquire fat droplets first at the poles of the cell and later throughout the cytoplasm. As fat accumulates in the cytoplasm, the cell loses its endoplasmic reticulum and assumes a round shape. Gradually the nucleus becomes indented and pushed to one side of the cell. A similar range of changes can be identified in lipoblasts of some liposarcomas, notably the myxoid/round cell type (Fig. 17–1). In addition, pleomorphic cells with the features of lipoblasts can be identified in well differentiated and pleomorphic liposarcomas (Fig. 17–2), but these cells have no equivalent in the differentiation sequence of normal fat. The task for the pathologist is to decide at what point in the differentiation scheme the cell becomes sufficiently diagnostic to warrant the designation "lipoblast."

Criteria that have proved useful for identifying *diagnostic* lipoblasts include the following: (1) a hyperchromatic indented or sharply scalloped nucleus; (2) lipid-rich (neutral fat) droplets in the cytoplasm; and (3) an appropriate histologic background. The importance of the last criterion cannot be overemphasized, as lipoblast-like cells may be seen in a variety of conditions, and failure to take into consideration the overall appearance of a lesion can lead to an erroneous diagnosis of liposarcoma. For example, lipomas with fat necrosis (Fig. 17–3), fat with atrophic changes (Fig. 17–4), hibernomatous change in lipomas (Fig. 17–5), foreign body reaction to silicone (Fig. 17–6), nonspecific accumulation of intracytoplasmic

*Text continued on page 648*

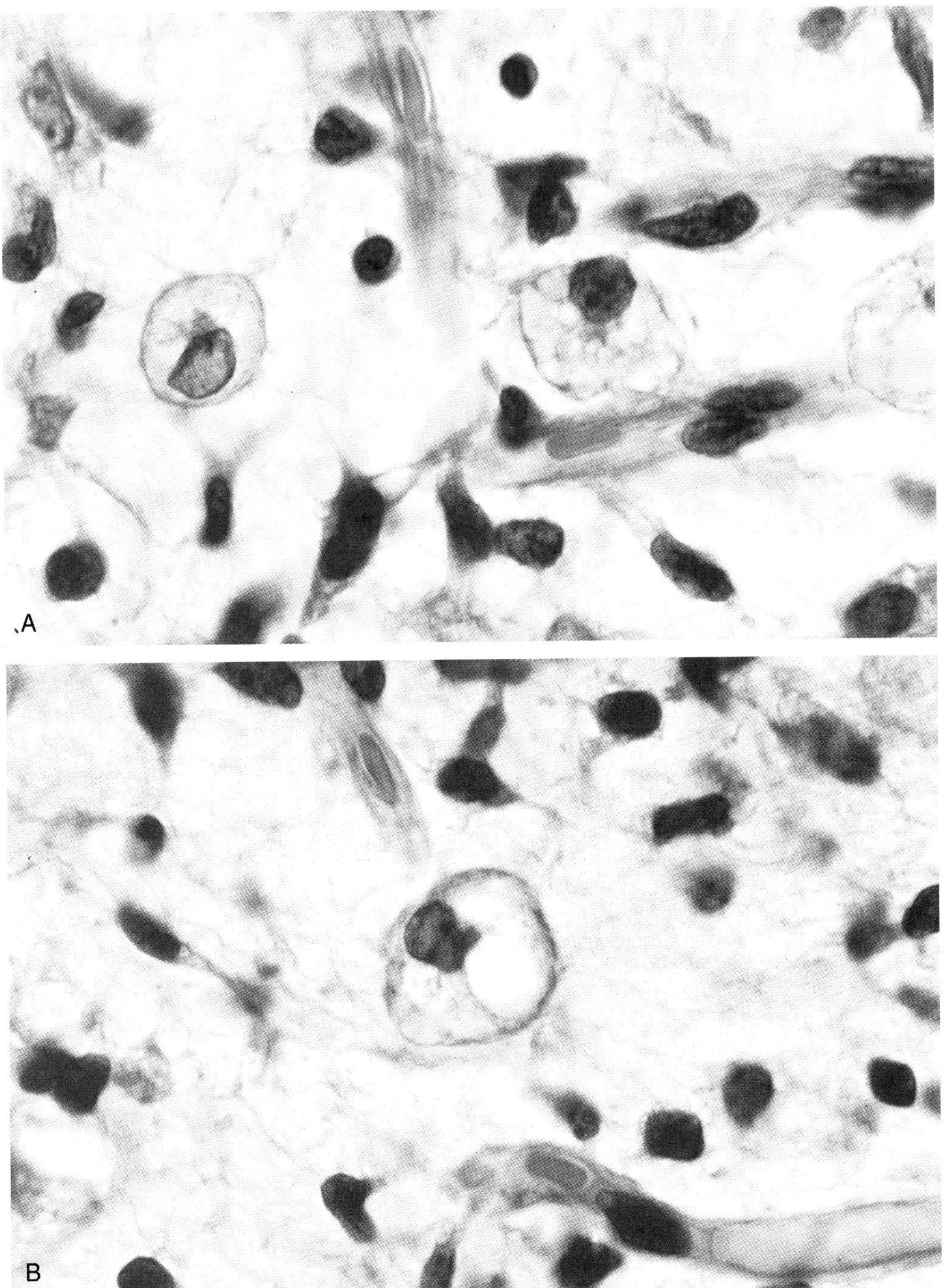


**FIGURE 17–1.** Developing lipoblasts from a myxoid liposarcoma, with an early stage (**A**) with fine vacuoles, an intermediate stage (**B, C**), and a late stage (**D**) resembling mature white fat.

*Illustration continued on following page*

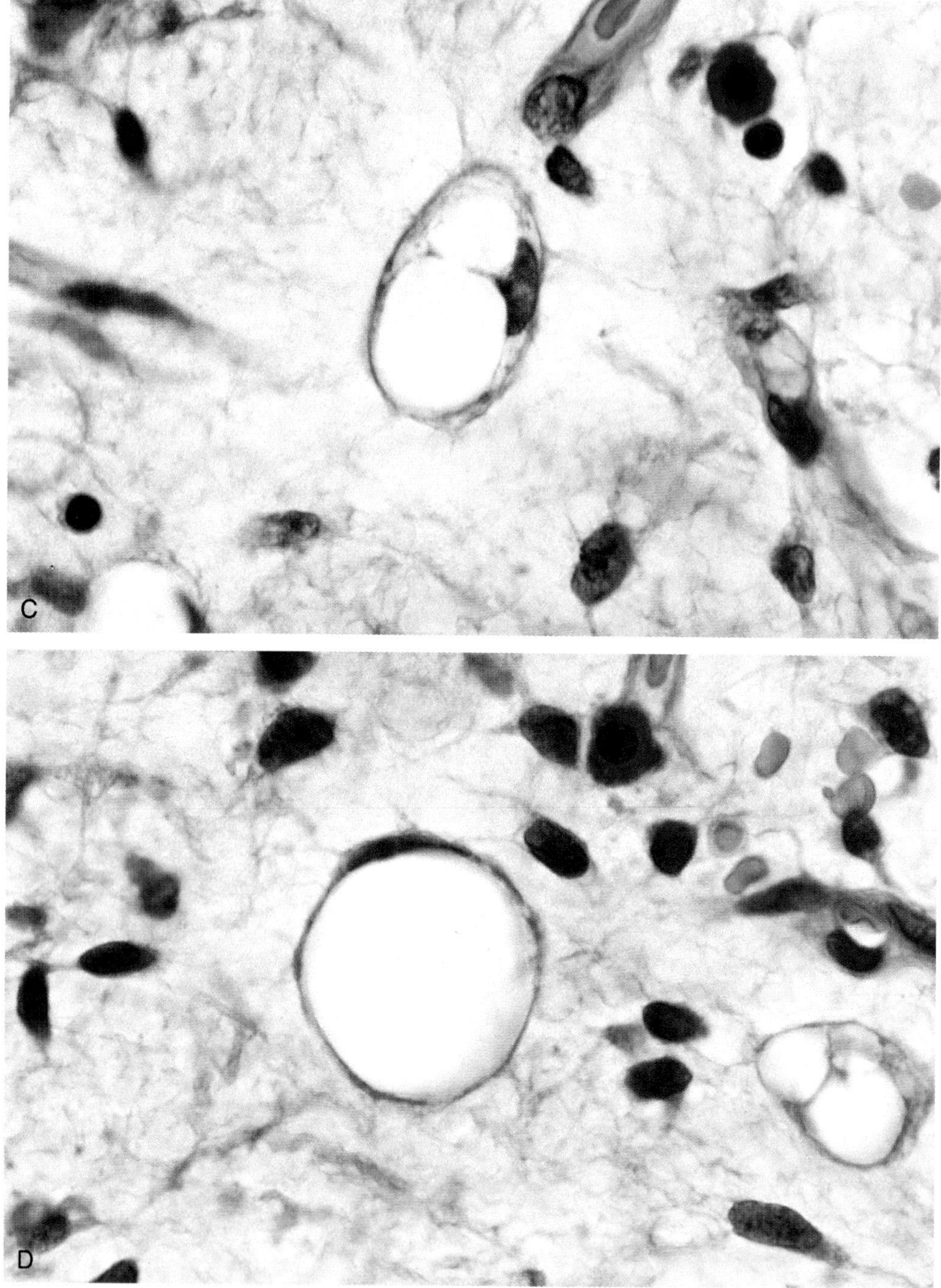


**FIGURE 17–1** *(Continued).*

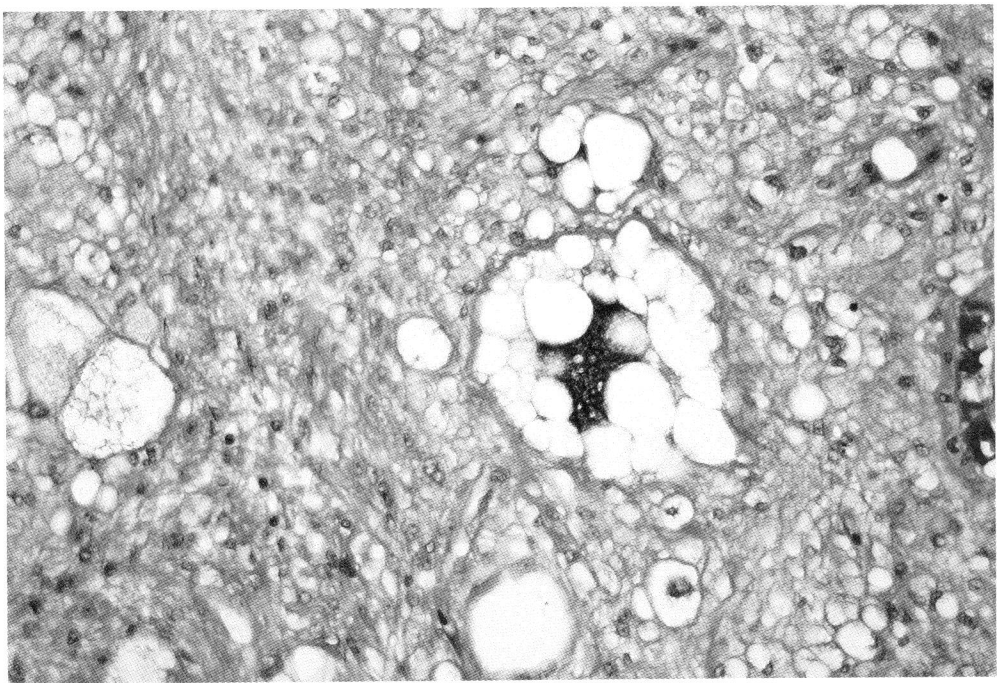

**FIGURE 17–2.** Pleomorphic lipoblast from a pleomorphic liposarcoma.

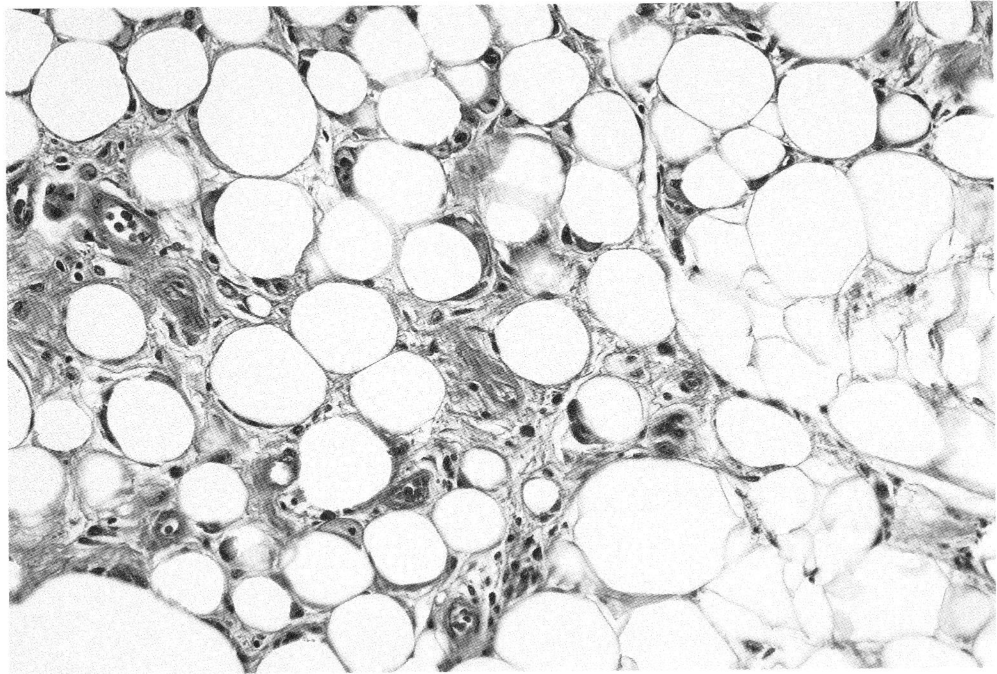

**FIGURE 17–3.** Fat necrosis in a lipoma. Scattered macrophages may be confused with atypical stromal cells of liposarcoma.

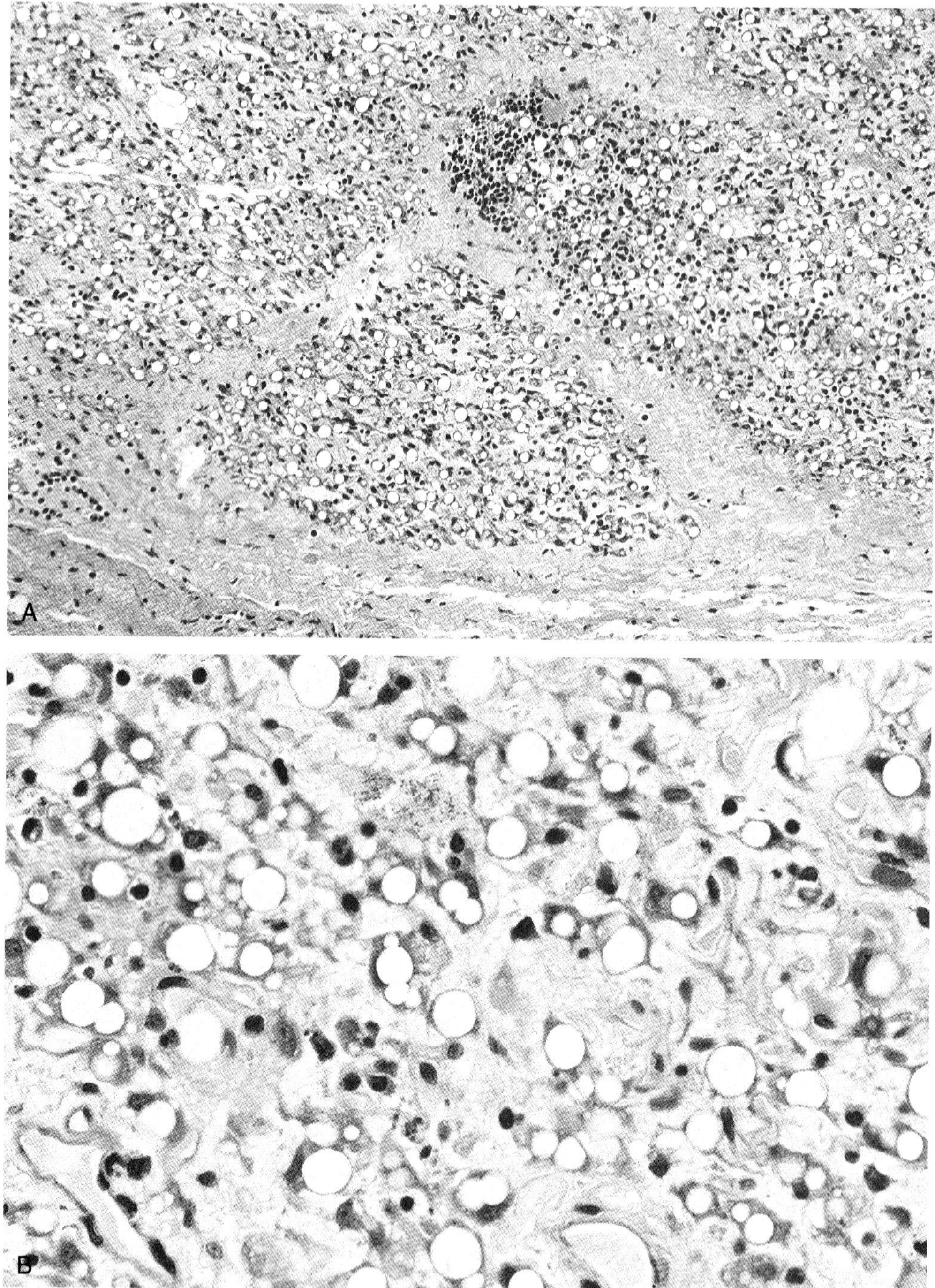

**FIGURE 17–4.** Atrophic fat occurring with malnutrition. Cell are arranged in lobules (**A**) and are uniformly small with lipofuscin pigment in the cytoplasm (**B**).

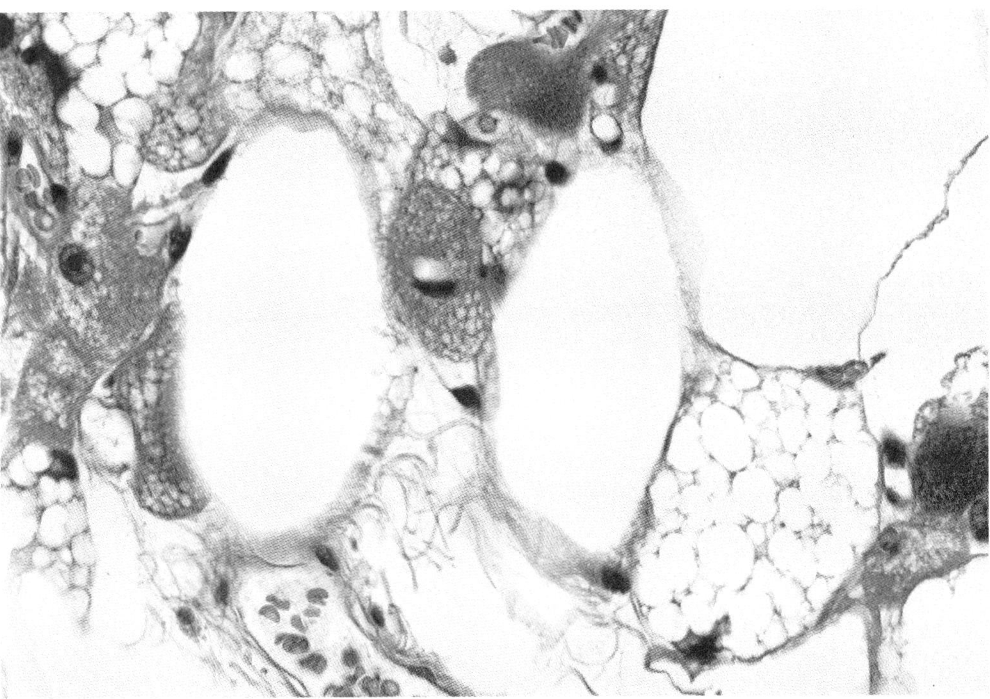

**FIGURE 17–5.** Finely vacuolated brown fat cells in a lipoma with hibernomatous changes mimicking lipoblasts.

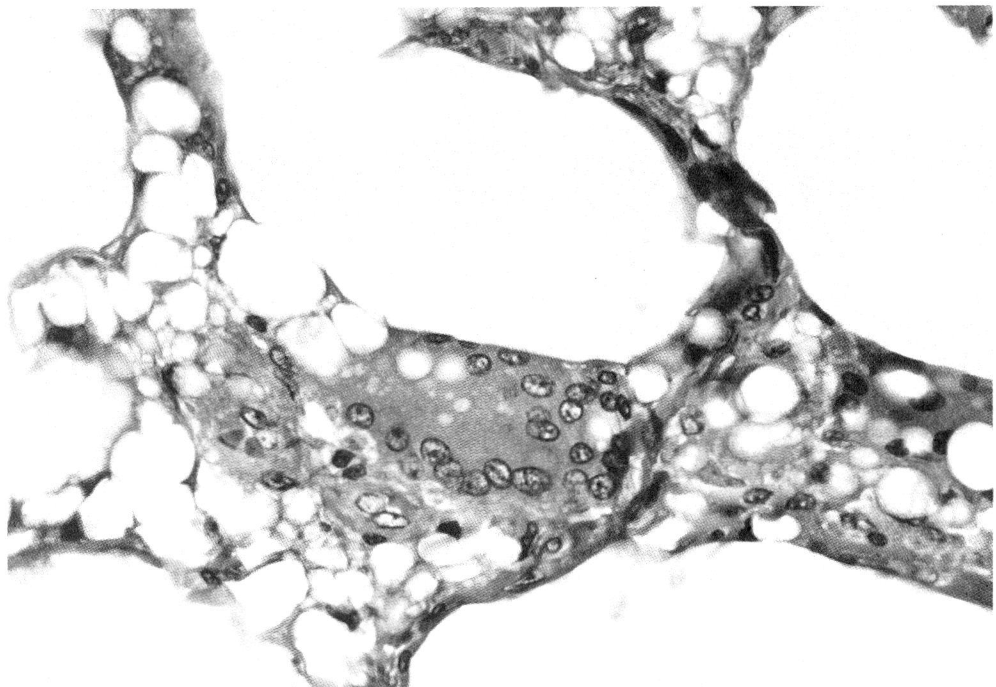

**FIGURE 17–6.** Silicone granuloma with multivacuolated histiocytes resembling lipoblasts.

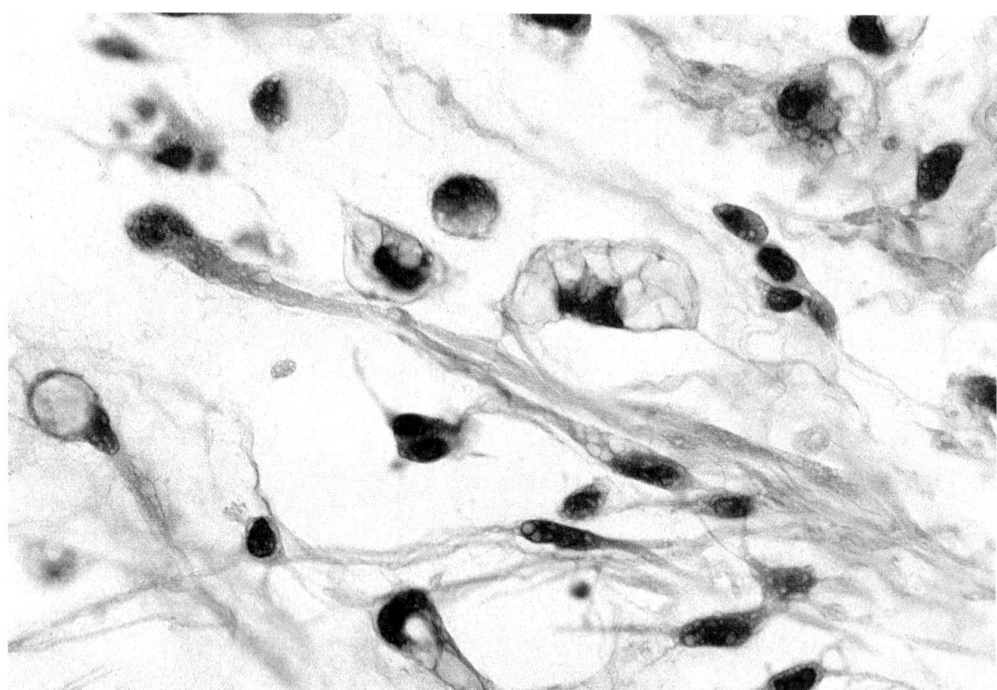

**FIGURE 17–7.** Cells of a myxoid malignant fibrous histiocytoma distended with hyaluronic acid. These cells are commonly misidentified as lipoblasts.

stromal mucin (Fig. 17–7), fixation artifact (Fig. 17–8), or signet ring melanoma, carcinoma and lymphoma (Fig. 17–9)[18,22] all have cells that to some extent resemble lipoblasts. In each instance, other features indicate that the diagnosis of liposarcoma is not appropriate. Silicone reactions, for example, exhibit numerous multivacuolated histiocytes that fulfill some of the criteria of lipoblasts, yet the histologic background of foreign body giant cells and inflammation should alert the pathologist to the fact that the lesion is not a liposarcoma.

## WELL DIFFERENTIATED LIPOSARCOMA (ATYPICAL LIPOMA, ATYPICAL LIPOMATOUS TUMOR)

### Clinical Findings

Well differentiated liposarcoma is the most common form of this tumor encountered during late adult life. It reaches a peak incidence during the sixth and seventh decades of life. Men and women are equally affected, although at certain sites (e.g., groin) there appears to be a predilection for men. In the collective experience of the Armed Forces Institute of Pathology (AFIP) and the Mayo Clinic, 75% of cases develop in the deep muscles of the extremities and 20% in the retroperitoneum, with the remainder divided between the groin, spermatic cord, and miscellaneous sites.[51,57] Rarely do these tumors develop in the subcutis, and issues regarding the nomenclature of such lesions is discussed below. Well differentiated liposarcomas at sites such as the oral cavity, larynx,[1,37] breast,[4] and mediastinum[16,25] are largely curiosities.

Symptoms related to these tumors are dependent on the exact site. Those in the extremities develop as slowly growing masses that are present months or even several years before the patient seeks medical attention, whereas those in the retroperitoneum are associated with the usual symptoms of an intraabdominal mass. Because well differentiated liposarcomas contain a significant component of mature fat, they present as fat density masses,[3,9,21] with mottled or streaky zones of higher density corresponding to the fibrous or sclerotic zones. They also tend to have less well defined borders than lipomas (Fig. 17–10).

### Gross and Microscopic Features

Grossly, well differentiated liposarcomas are large multilobular lesions that range in color from deep yellow to ivory (Figs. 17–11, 17–12). Many could be mistaken for a lipoma except for their extremely large size and their tendency to have more fibrous bands, gelatinous zones, or punctate hemorrhage.

Well differentiated liposarcomas have traditionally been divided into three subtypes: (1) lipoma-like; (2)

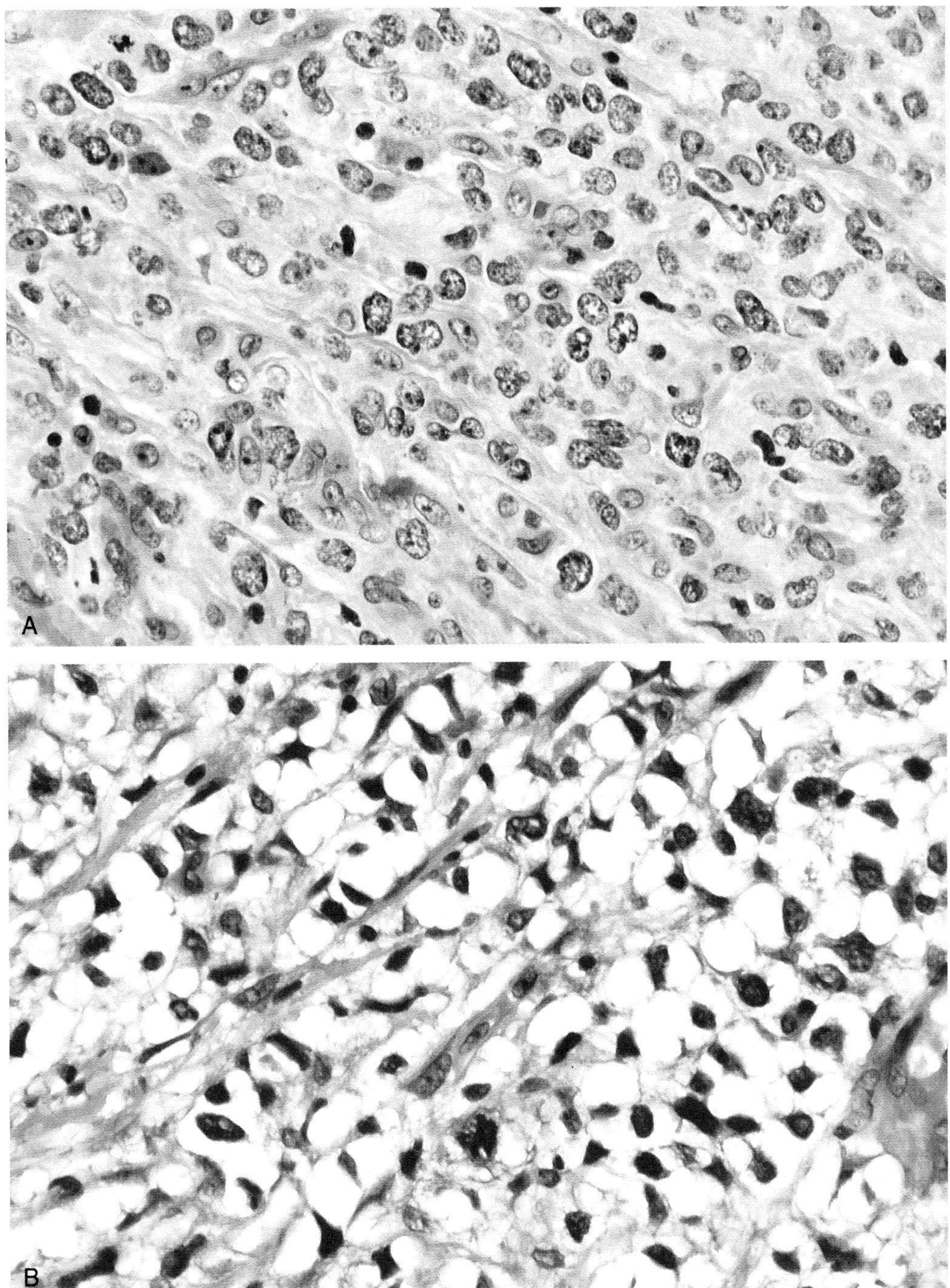


**FIGURE 17–8.** Large-cell lymphoma (**A**) with poorly fixed areas (**B**) in which the retraction artifact led to an erroneous diagnosis of liposarcoma.

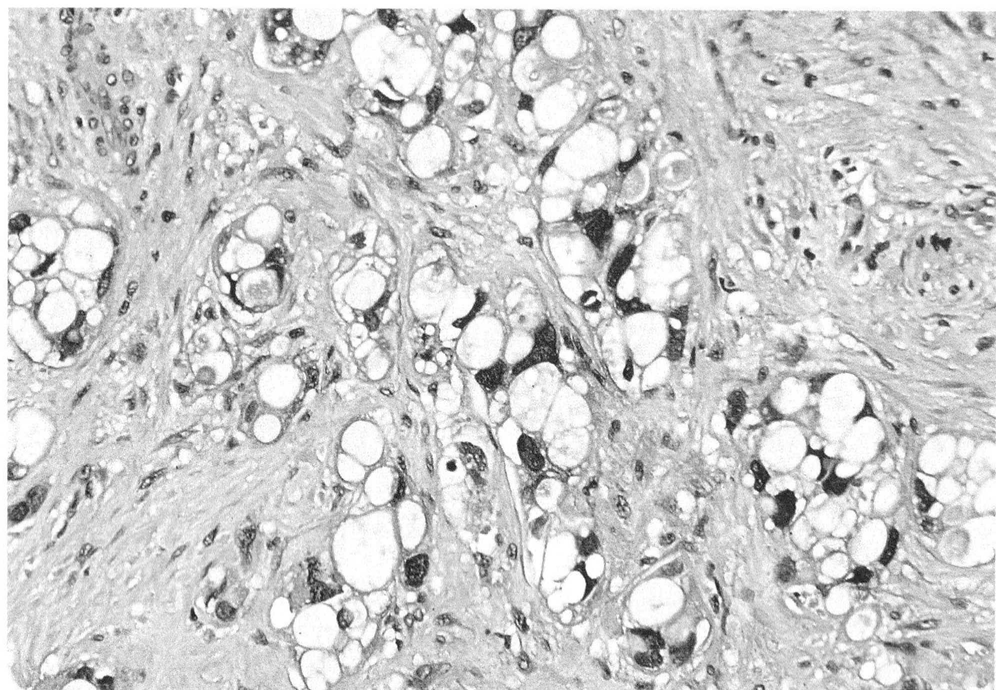

**FIGURE 17–9.** Adenocarcinoma arising in Barrett's mucosa showing a treatment effect with pseudolipoblasts.

sclerosing; and (3) inflammatory. Because many liposarcomas combine features of both lipoma-like and sclerosing subtypes, the distinction between these two types is often arbitrary and of limited practical importance. We rarely subclassify well differentiated liposarcomas in our daily practice, although these designations serve to draw attention to the range of appearances these tumors may assume. In the typical lipoma-like liposarcoma the tumor consists predominantly of mature fat with a variable number of spindled cells with hyperchromatic nuclei and multivacuolated lipoblasts (Figs. 17–13, 17–14, 17–15). In some cases these atypical spindle cells are numerous, whereas in other cases the cells are so rare as to require extensive sampling of the tissue. Sclerosing forms of well differentiated liposarcoma, prevailing in the groin and retroperitoneum, have dense fibrotic zones alternating with mature adipocytes (Figs. 17–16 to 17–20). In some cases the fibrotic zones consist of trabeculae intersecting fat, and in others the fibrous areas consist of broad sheets (Figs. 17–17, 17–19). The fibrotic areas contain collagen fibrils of varying thickness in which are embedded scattered spindle and multipolar stromal cells with hyperchromatic nuclei. Similar cells may also be present between the mature adipocytes. Although lipoblasts may be present, they are usually rare. Thus the diagnosis for this pattern of liposarcoma is more dependent on the identification of stromal cells with a requisite degree of atypia than on the identification of diagnostic lipoblasts. The inflammatory form of well differentiated liposarcoma occurs almost exclusively in the retroperitoneum and consists of a dense lymphocytic or plasmacytic infiltrate superimposed on a lipoma-like or sclerosing form of well differentiated liposarcoma[39,49] (Fig. 17–21). Because of the intense inflammatory infiltrate these tumors may be confused with

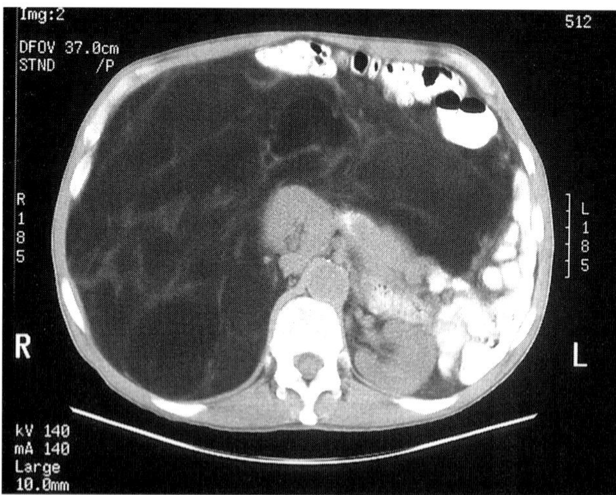


**FIGURE 17–10.** Computer tomography (CT) scan of well differentiated liposarcoma of the abdominal cavity and retroperitoneum. The mass, with a low attenuation value, replaces abdominal contents.

*Text continued on page 657*

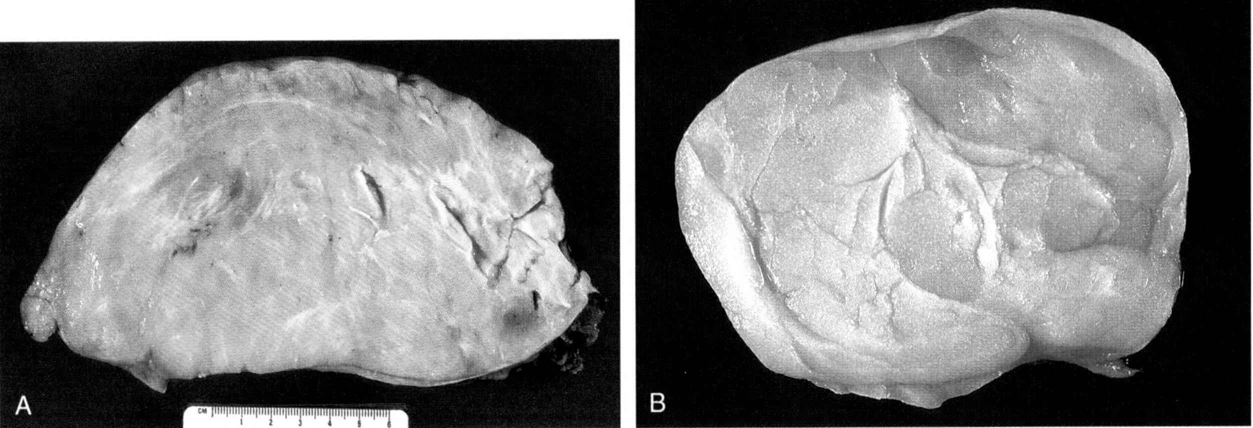


**FIGURE 17–11.** Well differentiated liposarcoma closely resembling normal fat except for fibrous bands (**A**). Others have a more gelatinous appearance (**B**).

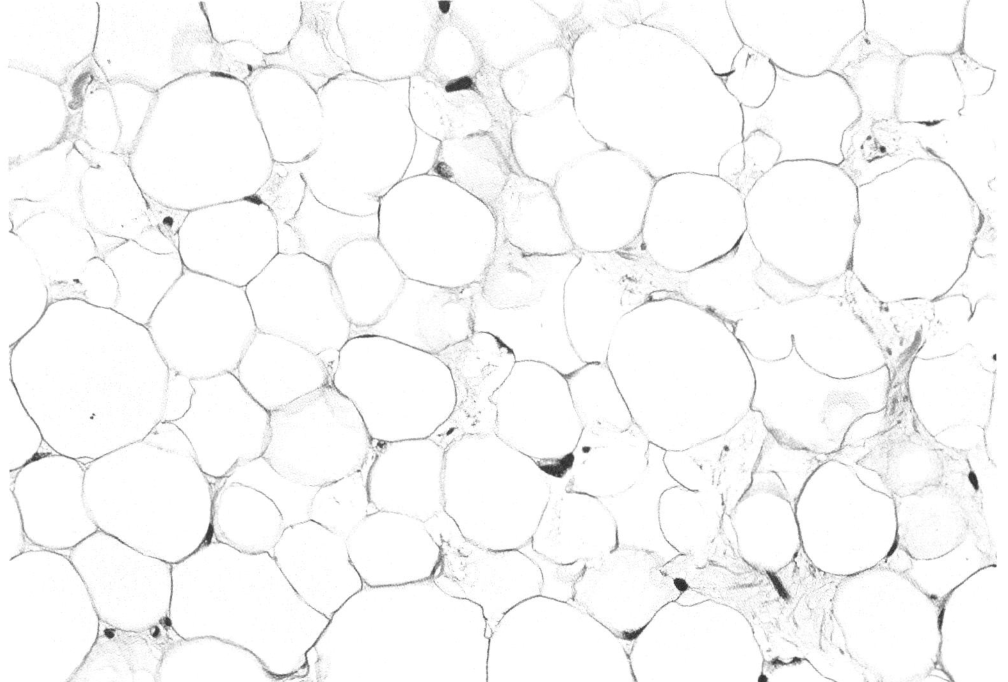

**FIGURE 17–12.** Well differentiated (lipoma-like) liposarcoma showing only a rare atypical stromal cell amid a mature lipomatous backdrop.

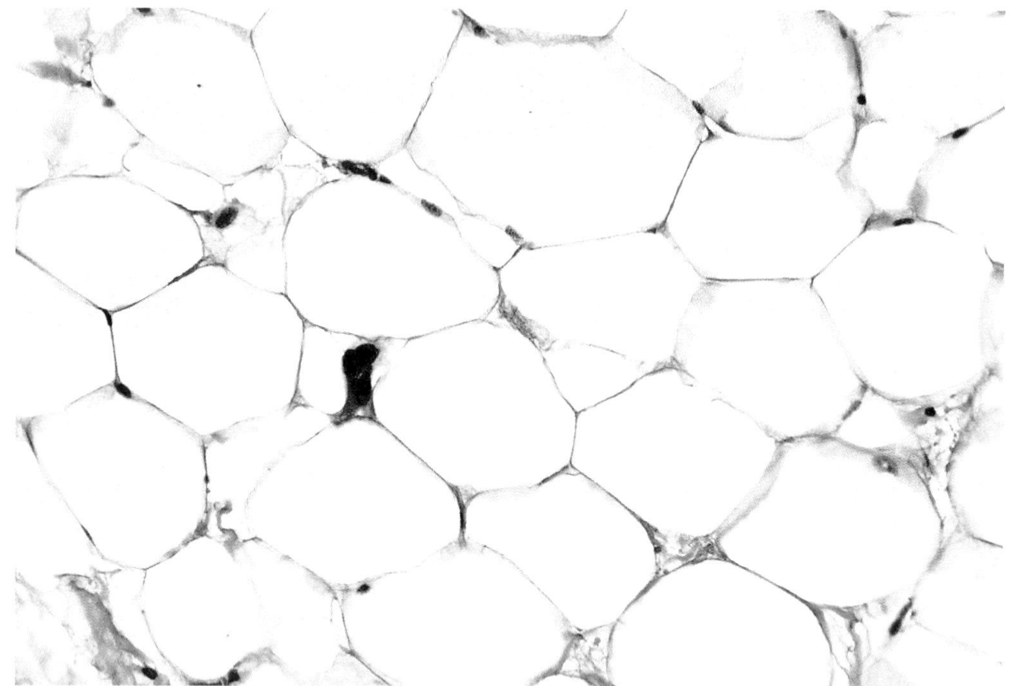

**FIGURE 17–13.** Atypical stromal cell in a well differentiated liposarcoma illustrating nuclear hyperchromatism.

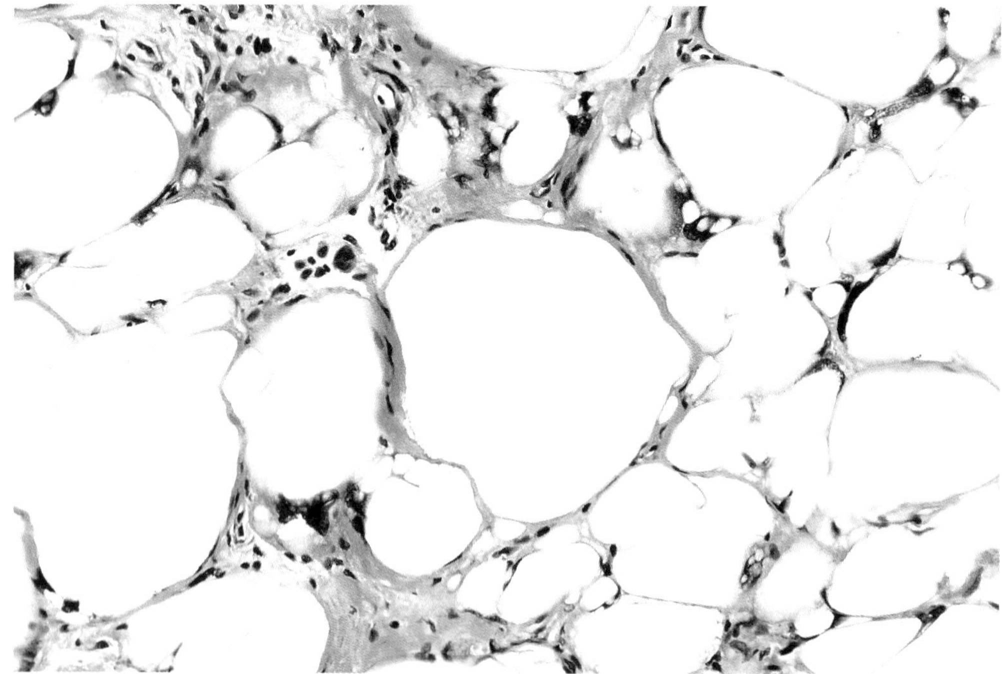

**FIGURE 17–14.** Well differentiated liposarcoma with a larger number of atypical stromal cells and lipoblasts than in Figure 17–13.

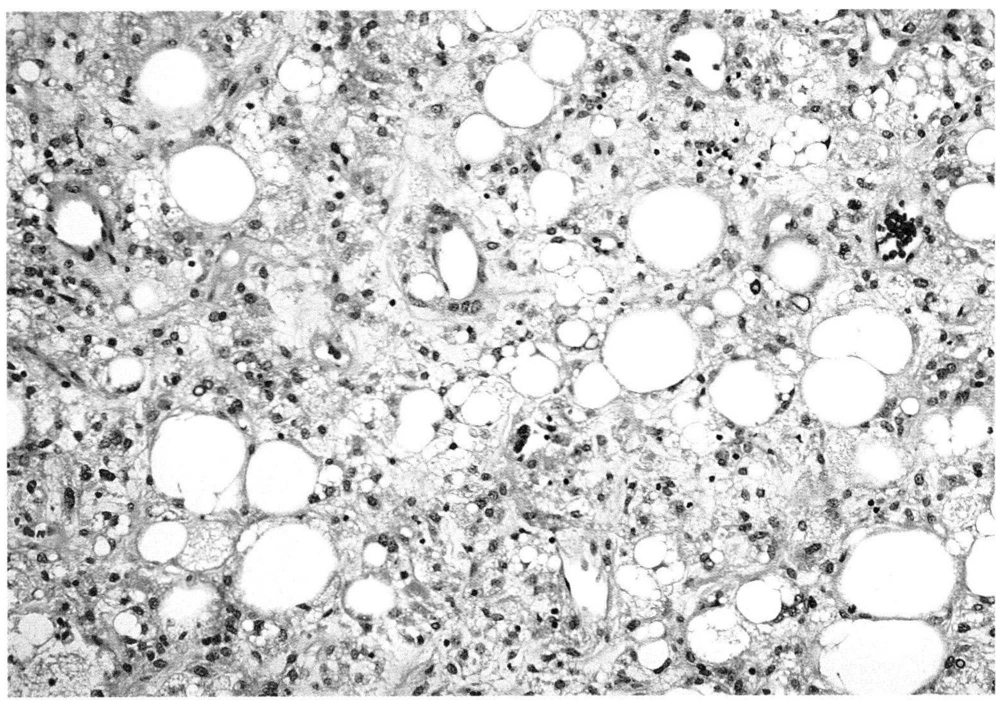

**FIGURE 17–15.** Well differentiated (lipoma-like) liposarcoma with numerous lipoblasts.

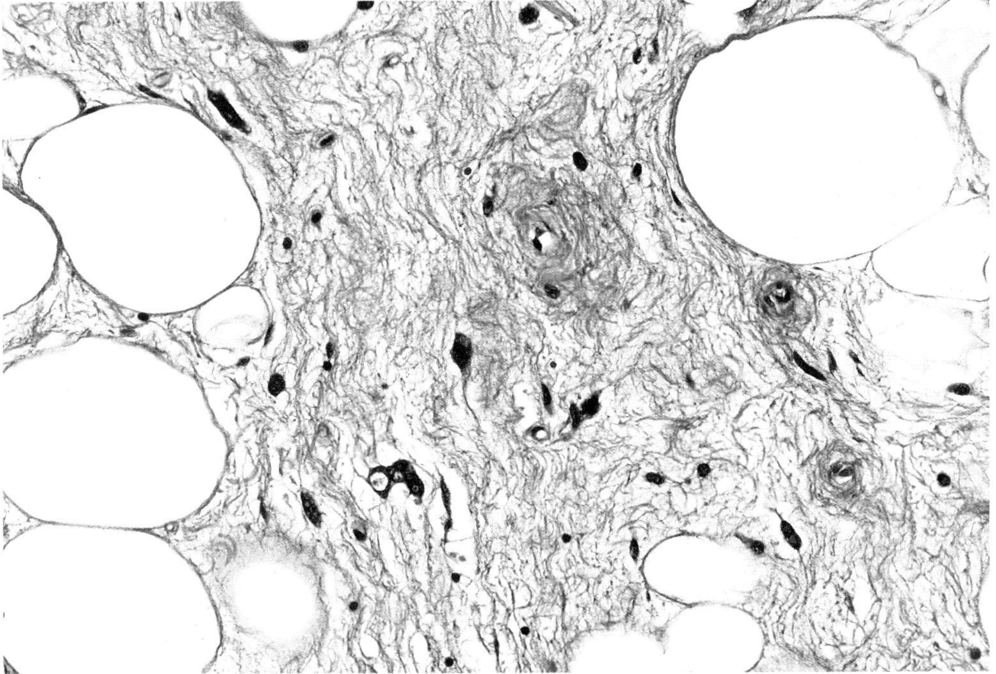

**FIGURE 17–16.** Sclerosing well differentiated liposarcoma.

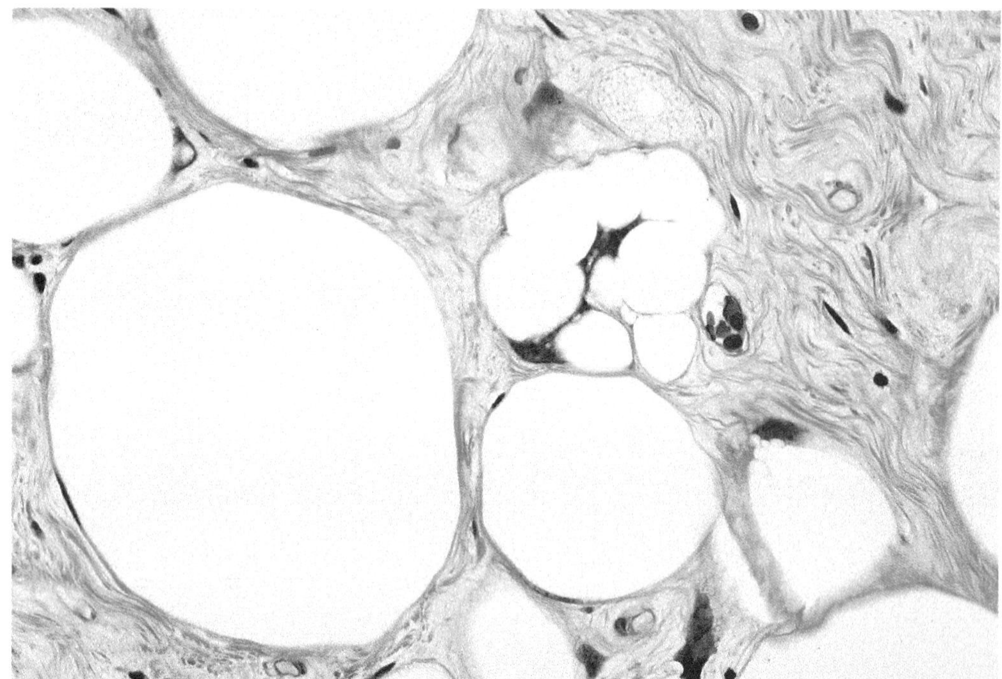

**FIGURE 17–17.** Well differentiated (sclerosing) liposarcoma showing sheet-like areas of collagen and fat. Note the multivacuolated lipoblast in this lesion. Such cells are typically rare.

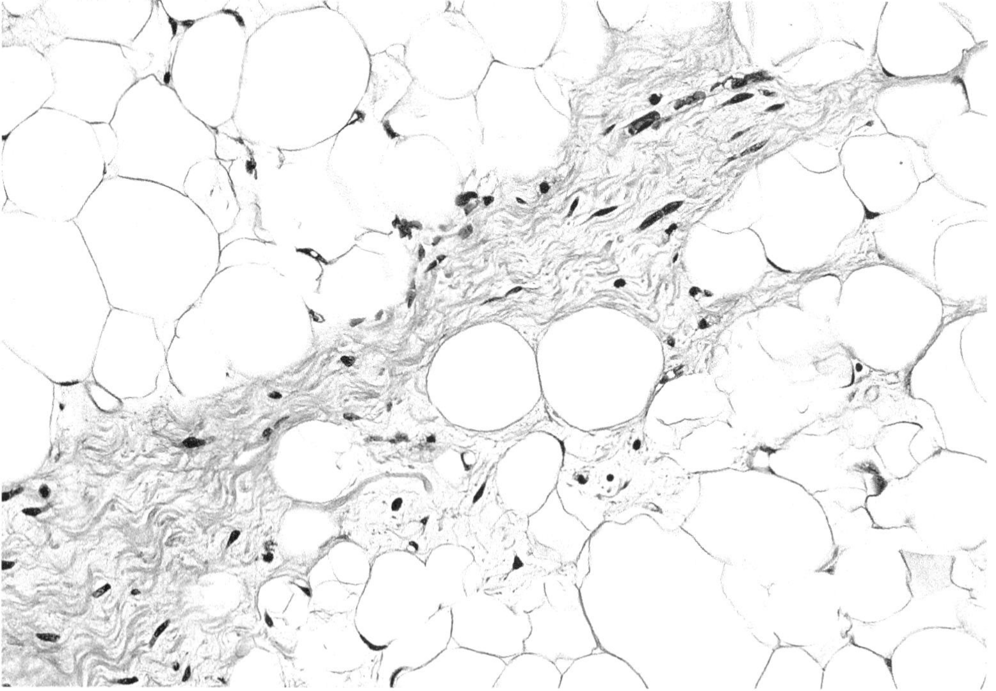

**FIGURE 17–18.** Well differentiated (sclerosing) liposarcoma with fibrous bands containing atypical cells.

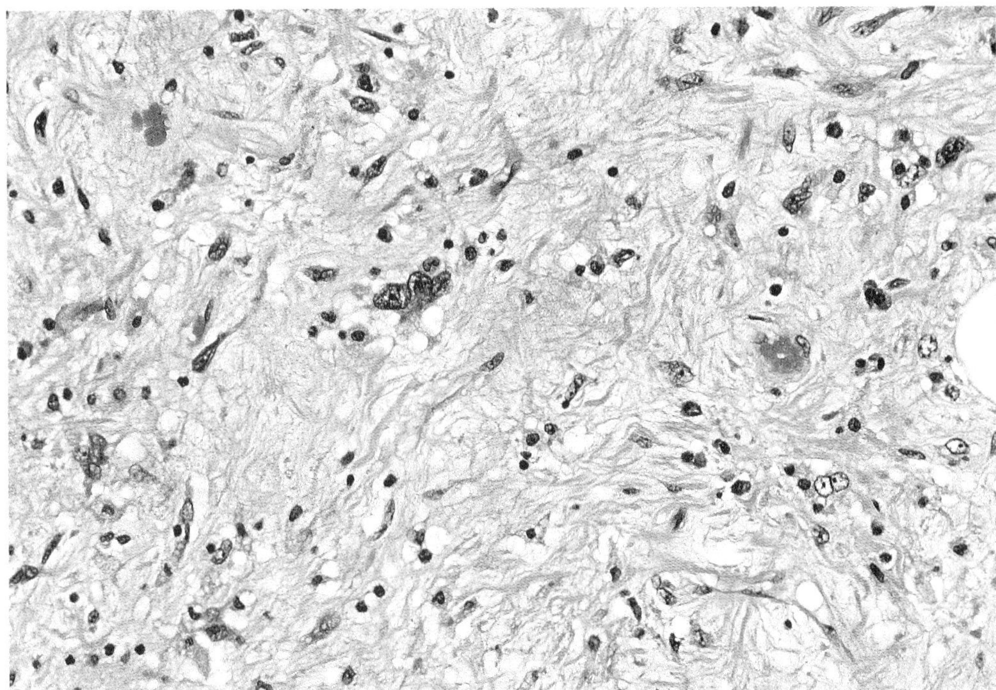

**FIGURE 17–19.** Nonlipogenic zone in a well differentiated (sclerosing) liposarcoma. Note that the cellularity is far less than in nonlipogenic zones of dedifferentiated liposarcoma. Small-needle biopsies providing specimens from such areas can lead to the erroneous conclusion that the tumor is not a liposarcoma.

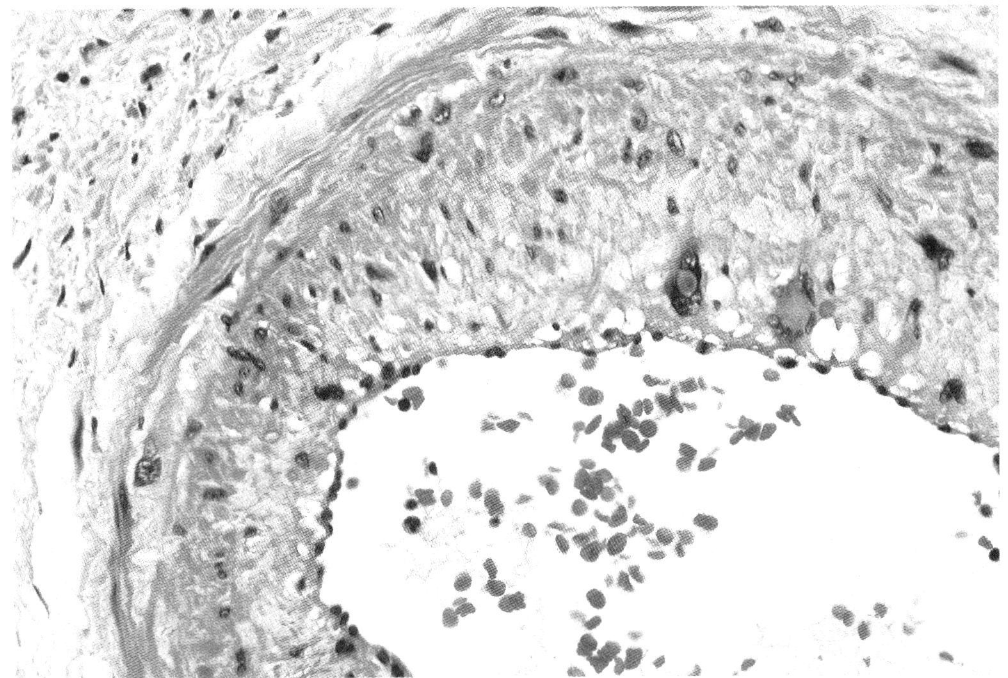

**FIGURE 17–20.** Well differentiated liposarcoma with involvement of the vessel wall.

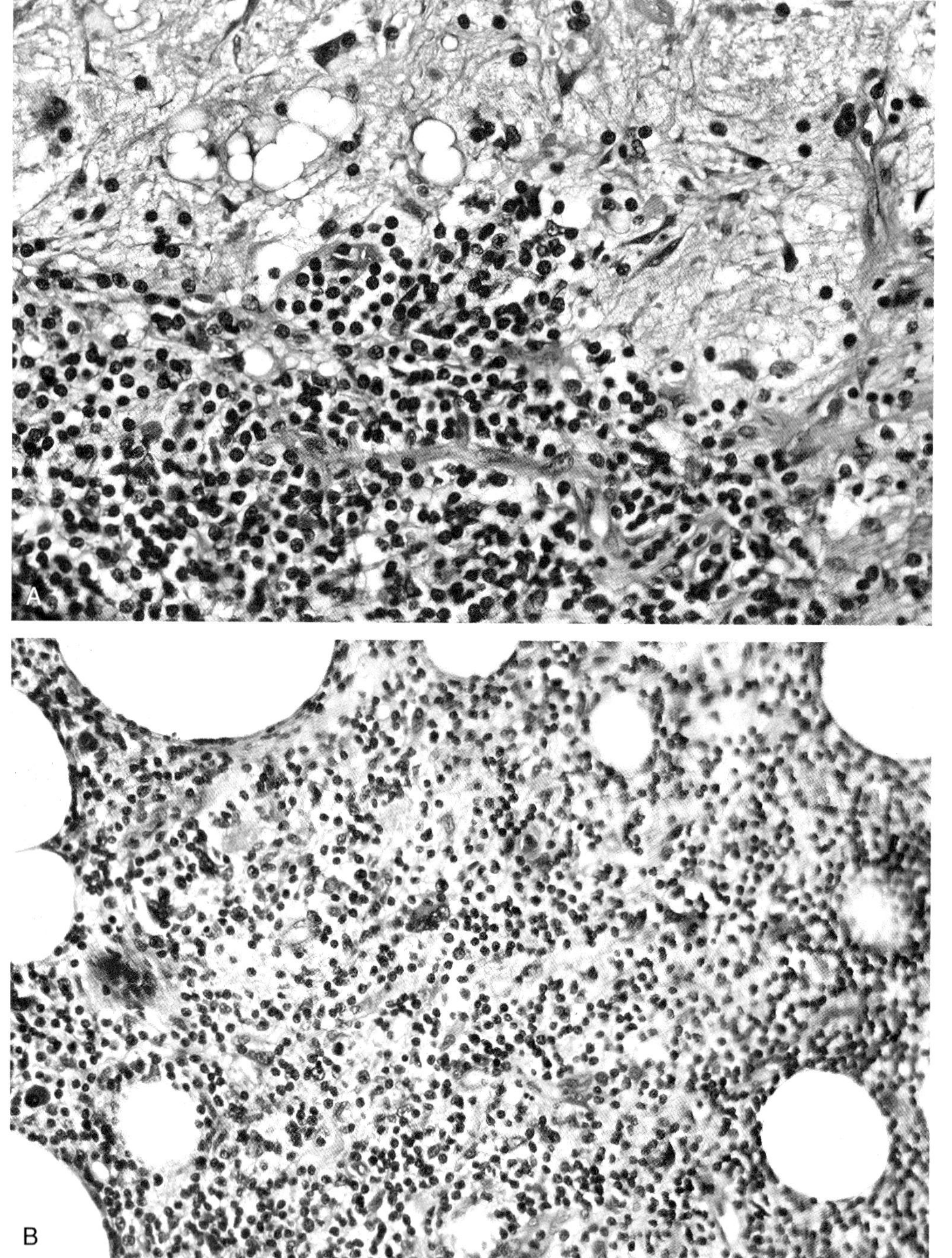

**FIGURE 17–21.** Well differentiated liposarcoma of the inflammatory type with a dense lymphocytic infiltrate (**A**) and areas of lipoblastic differentiation (**B**).

lipogranulomatous inflammation. An unusual feature that has received recent attention is the coexistence of mature or malignant-appearing smooth muscle tissue in well differentiated liposarcomas[43,47,54,56] (Fig. 17–22). There are too few cases to determine whether this feature has any biologic or clinical significance.

## Differential Diagnosis

Various neoplastic and nonneoplastic lesions enter the differential diagnosis of well differentiated liposarcoma (Table 17–2). For most of these conditions none of the available histochemical or immunohistochemical stains is useful. Rather, careful sampling of the material and thin, well stained hematoxylin and eosin sections comprise the mainstay of accurate diagnosis. Lipid stains, although obviously positive in well differentiated liposarcomas, also disclose lipid-positive deposits in the vast panorama of reactive lesions in fat and a variety of tumors.

**Normal Fat with *Lochkern*.** Normal white fat consists of spherical cells containing one large lipid vacuole that displaces the thin oval nucleus to one side. On routine sections the nucleus of most fat cells is barely perceptible. From time to time, a section grazes an adipocyte nucleus such that it is viewed en face, displaying its characteristic central vacuole, termed *lochkern* (German: hole in the nucleus) (Fig. 17–23). Nuclei *lochkern* are viewed more frequently in thick sections and therefore are sometimes misinterpreted as evidence of lipoblastic differentiation and hence a liposarcoma.

**Fat Necrosis.** In areas of fat necrosis, finely granular or vacuolated macrophages are located in the vicinity of damaged fat characterized by diminished cell size, dropout of adipocytes, and chronic inflammation (Fig. 17–3). Unlike lipoblasts, these macrophages are of uniform size and have small, evenly dispersed vacuoles that do not indent the nucleus. The nucleus has a rounded shape with delicate staining. In thick sections the nuclei of macrophages may overlap one another, giving the impression of hyperchromatism, which typifies the atypical stromal cells in well differentiated liposarcoma. It is important when making such distinctions to have suitably thin histologic sections.

**TABLE 17–2 LESIONS SIMULATING WELL DIFFERENTIATED LIPOSARCOMA**

| |
|---|
| Lipoma with fat necrosis |
| Lipoma with *lochkern* |
| Fatty atrophy |
| Silicone reaction |
| Diffuse lipomatosis |
| Spindle cell lipoma/pleomorphic lipoma |
| Myolipoma |
| Cellular angiolipoma |
| Angiomyolipoma |
| Lipomatous hemangiopericytoma |

**Atrophy of Fat.** Starvation, malnutrition, and local trauma result in atrophy of fat. Atrophy is accompanied by a loss of intracellular lipid such that the cell shrinks dramatically and assumes an epithelioid shape (Fig. 17–4). With loss of lipid the nuclei become more prominent, and the cells superficially resemble lipoblasts. Important observations include the fact that such cells appear to be of uniform size and maintain their arrangement in lobules. With extreme atrophy the cells may contain lipofuscin. Such changes are particularly noticeable in subcutaneous tissue and omentum.

**Localized Massive Lymphedema.** Massive forms of lymphedema restricted to a portion of the body may be confused clinically and histologically with well differentiated liposarcoma.[45] These lesions develop in morbidly obese individuals and appear to be the result of lymphedema secondary to chronic dependence of a fatty panniculus. Not surprisingly, these lesions develop in the proximal extremities and may be aggravated by underlying factors such as lymphadenectomy. Grossly and microscopically, the lesions exhibit the changes of lymphedema, including thickening of overlying skin, dermal fibrosis, ectasia and proliferation of lymphatics with focal cysts, and expansion of connective tissue septa (Fig. 17–24). A misdiagnosis of liposarcoma is attributable to the fact that the expanded connective tissue septa are believe to be part of a sclerosing liposarcoma. The septa contain mild to moderately atypical fibroblasts and delicate collagen fibrils separated by edema. In addition, there is often striking vascular proliferation at the interface between the expanded connective tissue septa and lobules of fat.

**Silicone Reaction.** Injection of silicone for various therapeutic and cosmetic purposes results in sheets of massively distended multivacuolated histiocytes that are disarming replicas of lipoblasts (Fig. 17–6). Lipoblasts of such quality and number are rarely encountered in true liposarcomas. Silicone reactions are also accompanied by a modest inflammatory and giant cell reaction and a large cyst with eosinophilic borders. Most silicone reactions in clinical practice are encountered around silicone breast implants but occasionally are seen on the face and in the abdomen. Free silicone can also migrate under gravitational effect and therefore is found at sites distant from the original introduction site.

**Intramuscular Lipoma with Atrophic Muscle.** Infrequently, atrophic skeletal muscle fibers are seen in

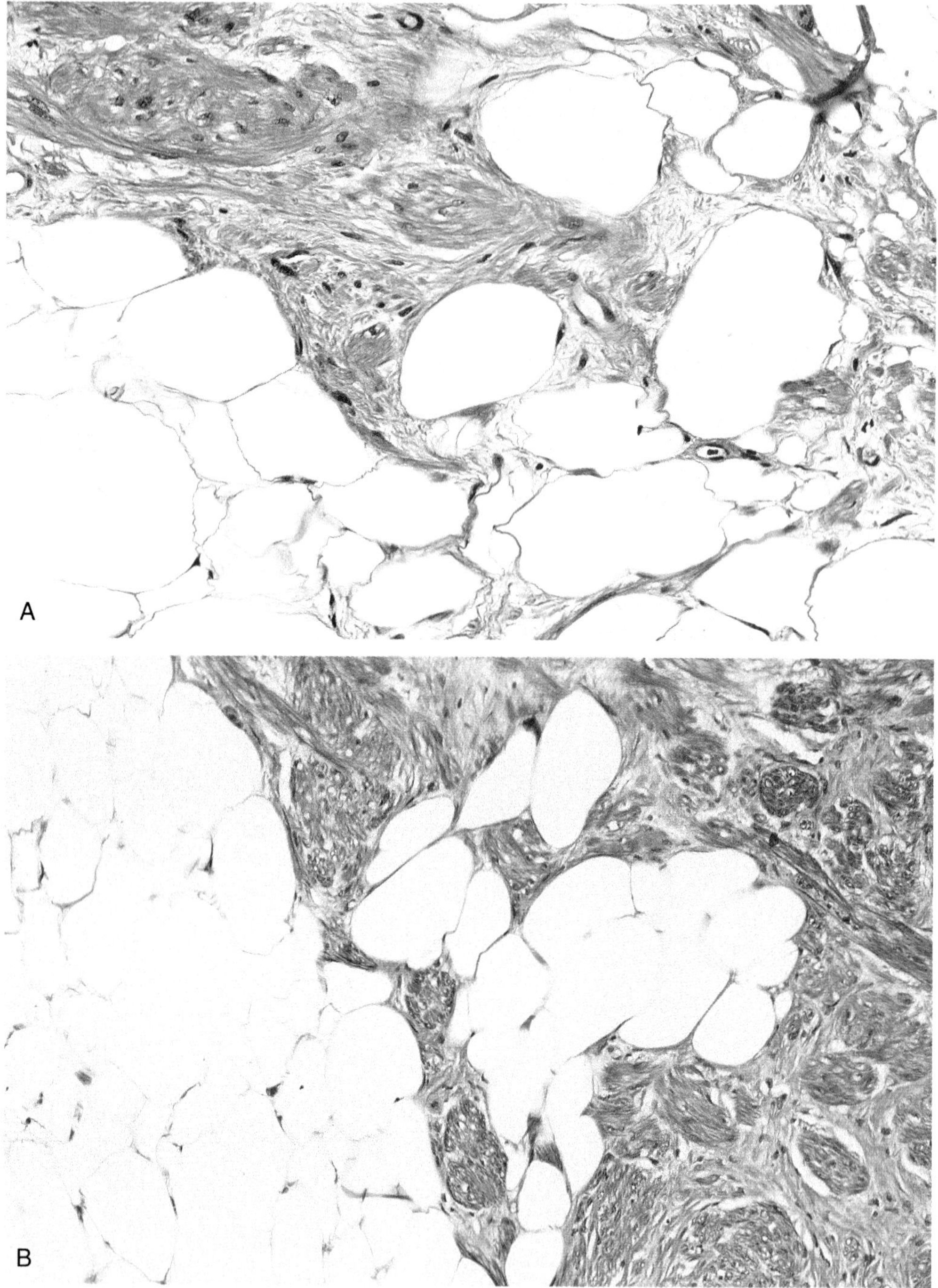


**FIGURE 17–22.** Well differentiated liposarcoma with mature smooth muscle (**A**) stained with Masson trichrome (**B**).

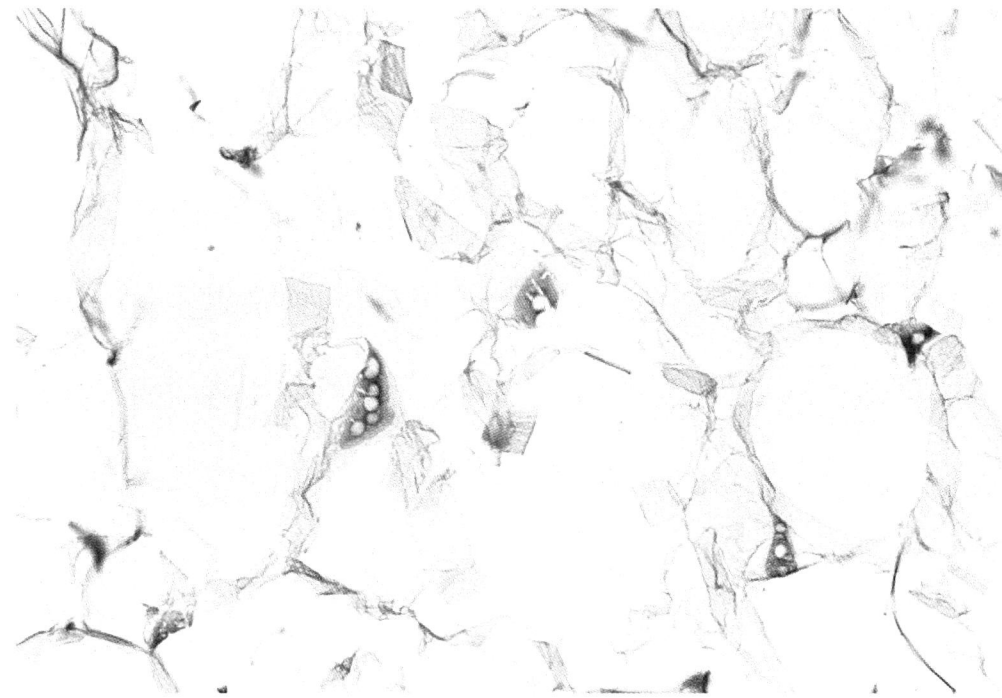

**FIGURE 17–23.** Nuclear vacuoles *(lochkern)* in normal fat.

intramuscular lipomas (Fig. 17–25). When these collections retain a clustered arrangement and have identifiable eosinophilic cytoplasm, this phenomenon is easily recognized. Isolated degenerating myofibers with barely perceptible cytoplasm understandably can be misidentified as atypical stromal cells of a well differentiated liposarcoma. Positive identification can be accomplished with desmin immunostains.

## Cytogenetic Studies

Well differentiated liposarcomas are characterized by giant marker and ring chromosomes.[14,53] Analysis of 59 well differentiated liposarcomas, termed atypical lipomatous tumors by the CHAMP Study Group, has shown that 93% display clonal abnormalities, and in 63% it consists of ring or giant marker chromosomes (RGCs). There appears to be a significant correlation between RGCs and the presence of lipoblasts, marked cytologic atypia, large size (> 11 cm), and retroperitoneal location. RGCs appear to be a rather consistent, specific finding of the well differentiated liposarcoma regardless of site and are present or retained even in those that have undergone dedifferentiation. On the other hand, they are rarely encountered in lipomas. One can infer from the data generated by this group that finding an RGC in an apparent lipoma suggests that additional sampling of the lesion might well reveal changes diagnostic of liposarcoma.

The role of RGCs in oncogenesis in these tumors is not clear. Although they contain consistently amplified sequences of 12q13-q15, a region known to contain a number of genes (e.g., *GLI1, SAS, MDM2, HMGI-C*) amplified in mesenchymal tumors, they receive variable contributions from other chromosomes (e.g., chromosomes 1, 4, and 16).[52] HMGI-C protein can be detected immunohistochemically in well differentiated liposarcomas.[55] Unfortunately, there is considerable overlap between its expression in ordinary lipomas and well differentiated liposarcomas such that it does not now appear to be useful diagnostically for distinguishing the two.[37]

## Clinical Behavior

Well differentiated liposarcomas are for all practical purposes nonmetastasizing lesions that are accorded a grade I rating in grading schemes, but their rate of local recurrence and disease-related mortality are strongly influenced by location.[10,44,51,57] As depicted in Table 17–3, tumors in the extremities have significantly lower rates of local recurrence than those in the retroperitoneum. Extremity lesions recur in nearly one-half of cases, whereas in the retroperitoneum recurrence rates approach 100%.[57] One could legitimately argue that well differentiated liposarcoma of the retroperitoneum is an incurable lesion. About one-third of patients die as a direct result of their

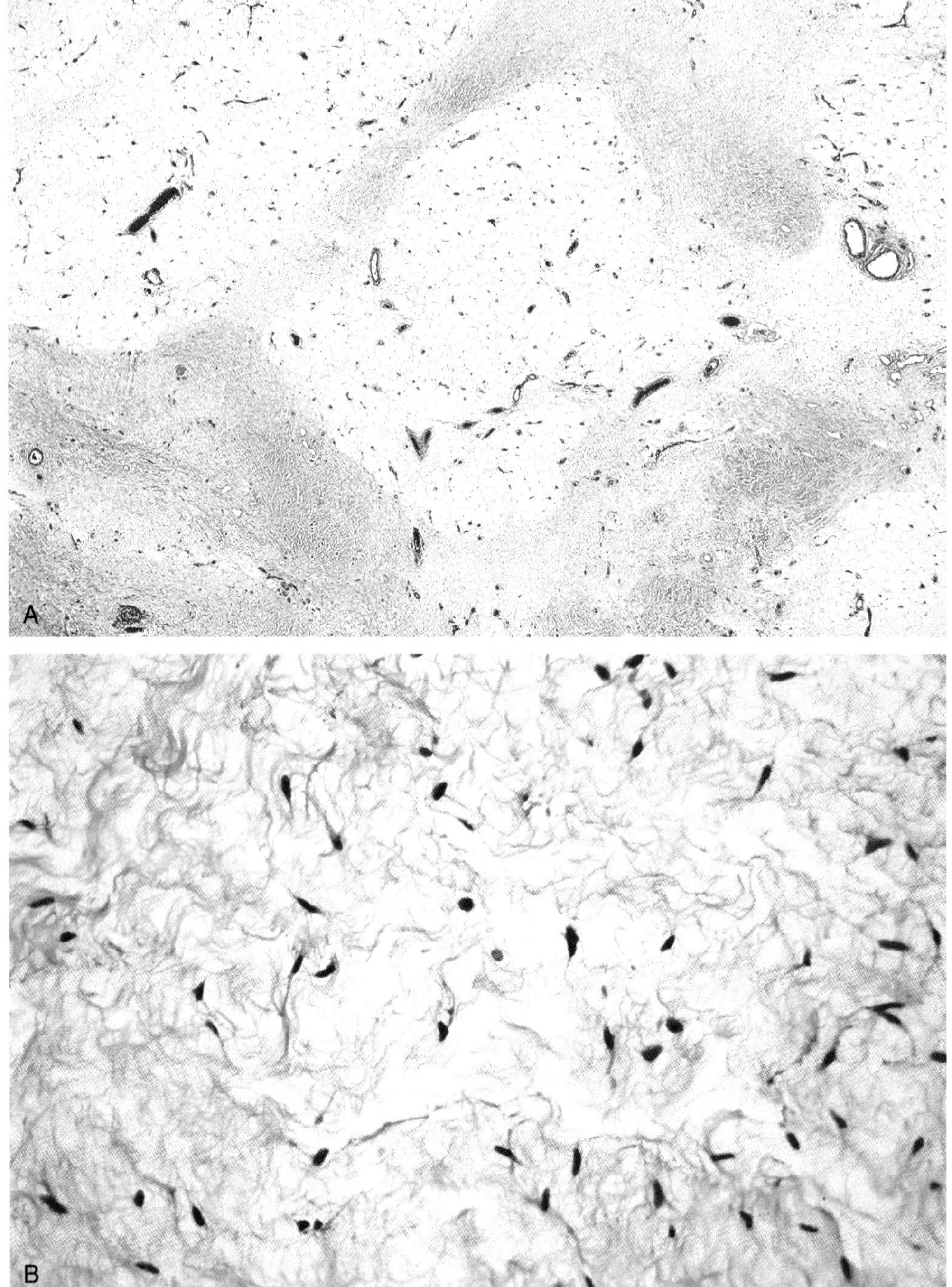


**FIGURE 17–24.** Changes of lymphedema that may mimic a well differentiated liposarcoma. Connective tissue septa are expanded (**A**), with mildly atypical fibroblasts in the septa (**B**).

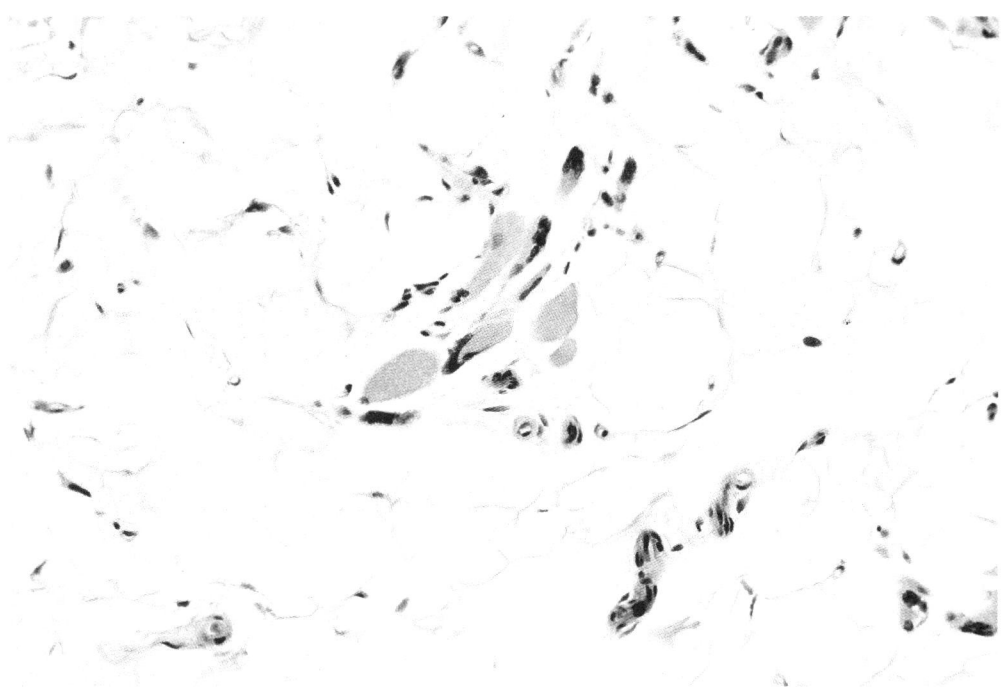

**FIGURE 17–25.** Atrophic muscle in an intramuscular lipoma. Degenerating myofibers are occasionally mistaken for atypical cells in liposarcomas.

disease, but this figure increases with longer follow-up periods owing to the indolent growth of these lesions. On the other hand, those rare well differentiated liposarcomas that occur in the subcutaneous tissues are generally cured by limited excisions. Although the data reported by Azumi et al.[40] and Evans et al.[44] indicate essentially no recurrences of well differentiated liposarcomas of the subcutis, it should be noted that some of the tumors included in this group were spindle cell and pleomorphic lipomas, which are known to have a benign course. Nonetheless, the thrust of their collective data appears accurate.

Lest well differentiated liposarcomas be dismissed as little more than benign but locally aggressive lesions, a small percentage of these tumors over time dedifferentiate or progress histologically to high grade lesions (dedifferentiated liposarcoma).[42,51,57] Although this phenomenon occurs most frequently with retroperitoneal liposarcomas, it also occurs with deep extremity lesions; it is rare in subcutaneous tumors. It therefore does not appear to be a site-specific phenomenon as was formerly believed but a time-dependent phenomenon encountered in those locations in which there is a high likelihood of clinical persistence of disease. With retroperitoneal tumors, for which complete excision is a veritable impossibility, there is a substantial risk of dedifferentiation (about 10–15%); it is somewhat lower for extremity lesions (5%). In well differentiated liposarcomas that have been followed longitudinally, dedifferentiation occurs after an average of 7–8 years but may be seen as long as 17–20 years after the original diagnosis. Once dedifferentiation occurs, the lesions can usually be considered fully malignant sarcomas. An exception is the rare

**TABLE 17–3** BEHAVIOR OF 92 WELL DIFFERENTIATED LIPOSARCOMAS

| Site | Recurrence (%) | Died of Disease (%) | Dedifferentiation (%) | Years of Follow-Up: Range and Median |
|---|---|---|---|---|
| Extremity | 43 | 0 | 6 | 2–25 (9) |
| Retroperitoneum | 91 | 33 | 17 | 1–35 (10) |
| Groin | 79 | 14 | 28 | 2–25 (8) |
| *Total* | 63 | 11 | 13 | |

From Weiss SW, Rao VK. Well differentiated liposarcoma (atypical lipoma) of deep soft tissue of the extremities, retroperitoneum and miscellaneous sites: a follow-up study of 92 cases with analysis of the incidence of "dedifferentiation." Am J Surg Pathol 16:1051, 1992.

tumor in which dedifferentiation is restricted to an extremely small focus (see Minimal Dedifferentiation, below).

Because of site-dependent differences in behavior of well differentiated liposarcomas, "atypical lipoma" was a term originally introduced in 1979 by Evans et al. and used by others[48] for well differentiated liposarcomas of the subcutis and deep muscles of the extremity.[44] At that time they endorsed retention of the term "well differentiated liposarcoma" for lesions in the retroperitoneum. Modifying this approach slightly, Evans later embraced the term "atypical lipomatous tumor" to replace "well differentiated liposarcoma" altogether (Fig. 17–26).[13] A similar approach has been used by the international CHAMP Study Group.[53]

We believe that broad usage of the terms "atypical lipoma" and "atypical lipomatous tumor" has potential drawbacks. Most importantly, use of terms that downplay the life-threatening nature of these tumors in the retroperitoneum run the risk of denying the patient adequate therapy and follow-up care or giving clinicians the impression that there is uncertainty about the diagnosis. Second, use of these terms does not take into account that some of these tumors dedifferentiate over time. The World Health Organization (WHO) has suggested that "atypical lipoma" be used only for subcutaneous lesions for which the morbidity is negligible and dedifferentiation virtually nonexistent; but it endorsed retention of the term "well differentiated liposarcoma" for lesions at other sites (Fig. 17–27). Implied in the foregoing statements is the understanding that **choice of these terms is determined solely by the location of the tumor and not by some subtle constellation of histologic features.** In fact, the cytogenetic abnormalities, specifically RGCs, that characterize these tumors irrespective of site provide one of the strongest lines of evidence linking these lesions. Similar conclusions have been reached on the basis of image analysis data.[41] Regardless of which set of labels one adopts, it

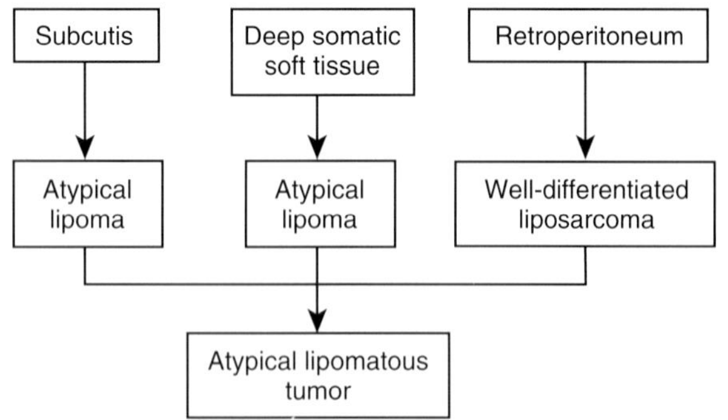


**FIGURE 17–26.** Nomenclature for well differentiated liposarcomas/atypical lipomas as proposed by Evans.[13]

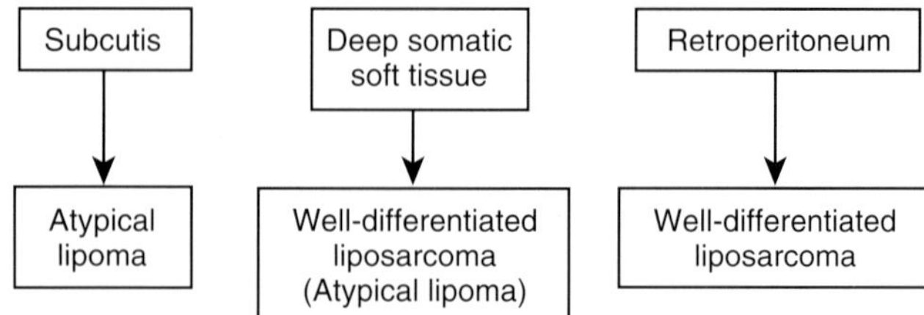


**FIGURE 17–27.** Nomenclature of well differentiated liposarcomas/atypical lipomas as proposed by the World Health Organization (WHO).

is most important to convey to the clinician the anticipated behavior of the lesion and the long-term risk of dedifferentiation.

Unfortunately, it has not been possible to predict in the individual case which rumors will dedifferentiate. Immunohistochemical analysis of *p53* mutations in well differentiated liposarcomas that had dedifferentiated compared to those that had not has identified no differences.[46] Analysis of *p53* mutations by molecular methods disclosed abnormalities in this gene in fewer than 10% of cases, but there were *MDM2* gene abnormalities in well over half of the dedifferentiated liposarcomas in both the well differentiated and nonlipogenic areas, suggesting that *p53* inactivation occurs via the *MDM2* pathway.[60] Although cytogenetic abnormalities might be a promising approach in this regard, there has been no large study correlating cytogenetic data with outcome. For the moment, all well differentiated liposarcomas of deep soft tissues should be considered at risk to dedifferentiate, although that risk varies with the location and duration of disease.

## DEDIFFERENTIATED LIPOSARCOMA

Dedifferentiation or histologic progression to a higher-grade, less well differentiated neoplasm was first described by Dahlin as a late complication in the natural history of well differentiated chondrosarcoma, but it is now known to occur in other low grade mesenchymal tumors including parosteal osteosarcoma, chordoma, and well differentiated liposarcoma.[59,62,65] Traditionally, dedifferentiated liposarcomas were defined as well differentiated liposarcoma juxtaposed to areas of high grade nonlipogenic sarcoma, usually resembling either a fibrosarcoma or malignant fibrous histiocytoma. Dedifferentiation was believed to occur after a latent period of several years. These views have now been modified. Whereas most dedifferentiated liposarcomas display high grade dedifferentiation, a small number contain exclusively low grade areas or a combination of low and high grade areas.[61,62] Second, in most dedifferentiated liposarcomas encountered in clinical practice, the dedifferentiated foci are seen at the original excision (primary dedifferentiation, dedifferentiation ab initio). Arguably, they could be examples of secondary dedifferentiation that were biopsied late in their course.

## Clinical Features

Dedifferentiated liposarcomas develop in approximately the same age group as well differentiated liposarcomas, reaching a peak during the early seventh decade.[59,61,62,65] The genders are affected approximately equally. Unlike well differentiated liposarcomas, a location in the retroperitoneum is favored over deep soft tissues of the extremities by a margin of nearly 3:1. Fewer than 20% of dedifferentiated liposarcomas occur collectively in the head, neck, trunk, and spermatic cord and fewer than 1% in subcutaneous sites.[67] Radiographically, they have areas characteristic of well differentiated liposarcoma but have, in addition, mass-like areas of nonfatty tissue. The latter have imaging characteristics similar to other sarcomas, with prolonged T1 and T2 relaxation by magnetic resonance imaging (MRI) and attenuation coefficients higher than that for normal fat on computed tomography (CT) scans.[64]

## Gross and Microscopic Features

The lesions present as large multinodular masses ranging in color from yellow to yellow-tan admixed with firm tan-gray areas that correspond to the dedifferentiated foci. Microscopically, the lesions consist of areas of well differentiated liposarcoma that display the range of changes described above and a nonlipogenic (dedifferentiated) component. The interface between the two zones is typically abrupt (Fig. 17–28), although in some cases there is a gradual transition between the two (Fig. 17–29). Rarely, the two patterns co-mingle, giving the impression of mosaicism (Fig. 17–30).

In about 90% the dedifferentiated zones have the appearance of a high grade fibrosarcoma or malignant fibrous histiocytoma (Figs. 17–31, 17–32). Those areas resembling malignant fibrous histiocytoma may display the full range of subtypes, from the common storiform pleomorphic and myxoid to the less common giant cell and inflammatory forms.

Those with dedifferentiated areas resembling an inflammatory malignant fibrous histiocytoma have been associated with leukemoid blood reactions.[63] Some dedifferentiated liposarcomas contain areas that, out of context, resemble a low grade fibrosarcoma or fibromatosis. Usually these areas coexist with areas of high grade dedifferentiation, but in about 10% of cases only low grade areas are present (Fig. 17–33). A number of unusual patterns are seen in dedifferentiated zones (Figs. 17–34 to 17–38). They include undifferentiated large round cells in areas resembling a carcinoma or melanoma (Fig. 17–35), spindled cells areas containing whorled structures reminiscent of a meningioma or nerve sheath tumor[61a,62,65a] (Fig. 17–

*Text continued on page 670*

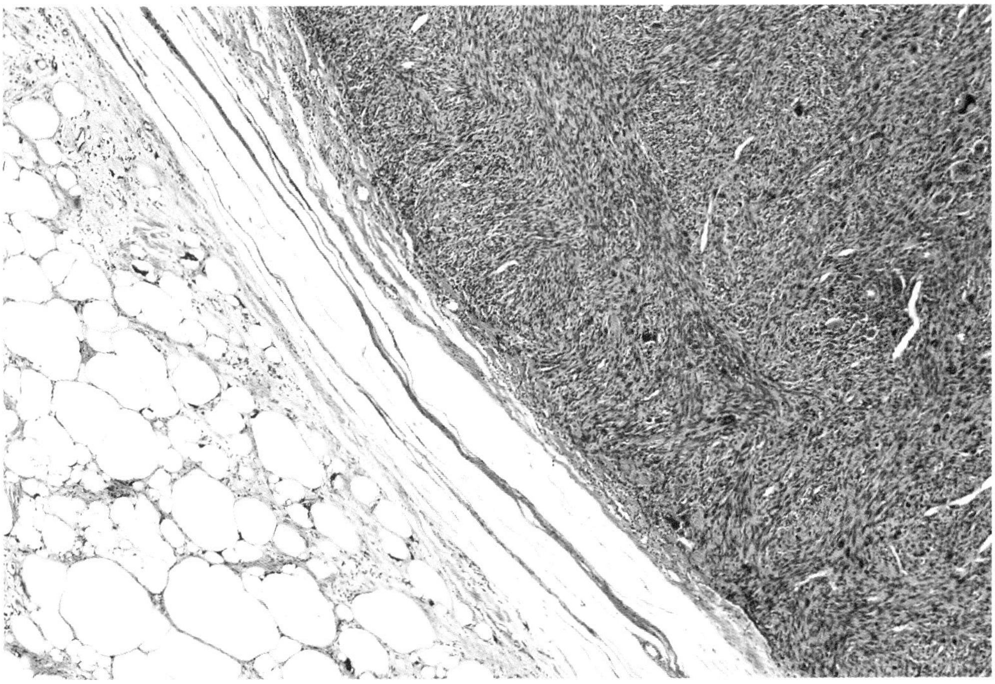

**FIGURE 17–28.** Dedifferentiated liposarcoma with sharp abutment of two zones.

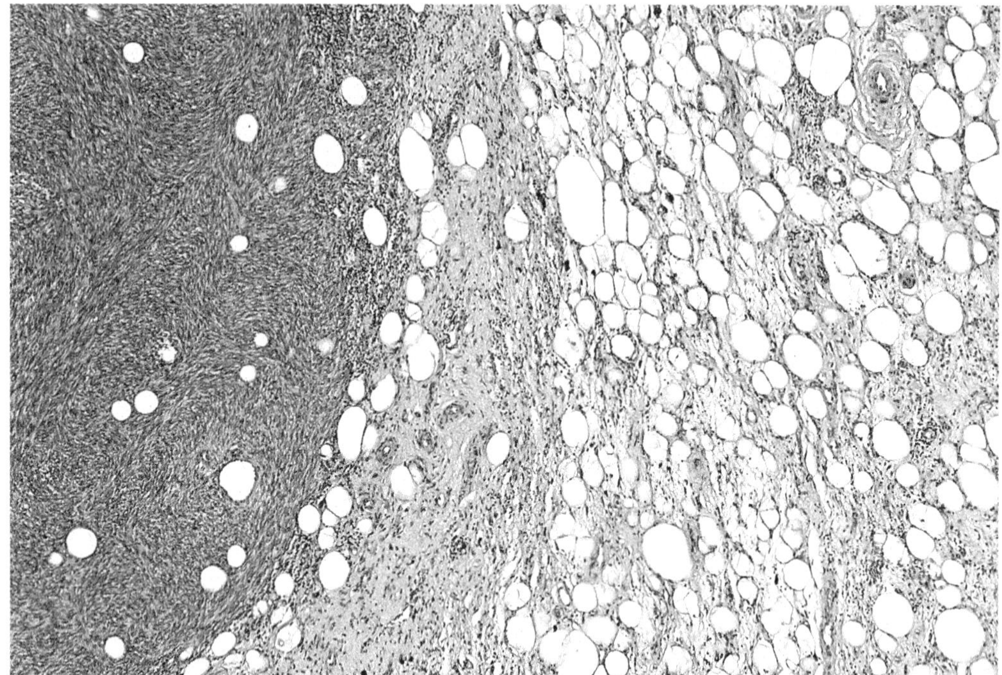

**FIGURE 17–29.** Dedifferentiated liposarcoma with an indistinct margin between well differentiated and dedifferentiated zones.

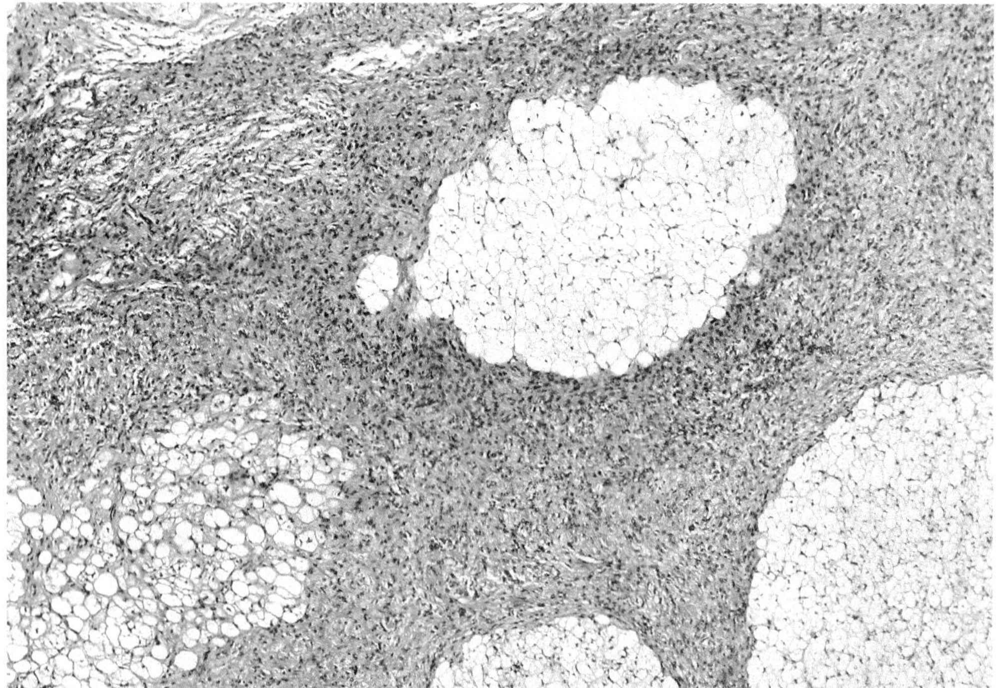

**FIGURE 17–30.** Mosaic pattern of a dedifferentiated liposarcoma.

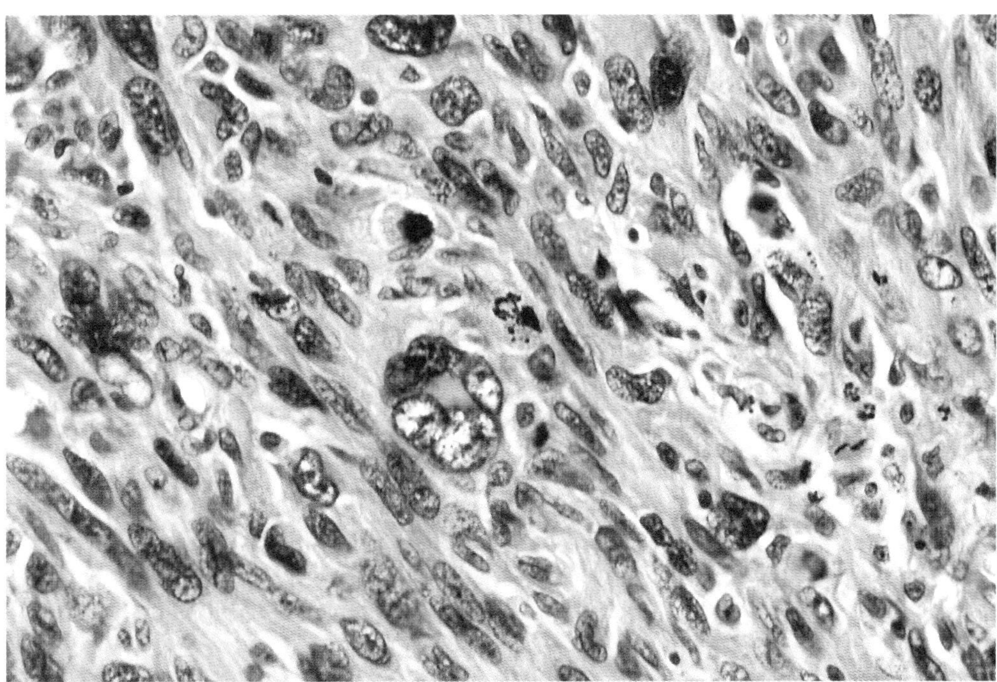

**FIGURE 17–31.** Dedifferentiated liposarcoma with areas resembling high grade malignant fibrous histiocytoma.

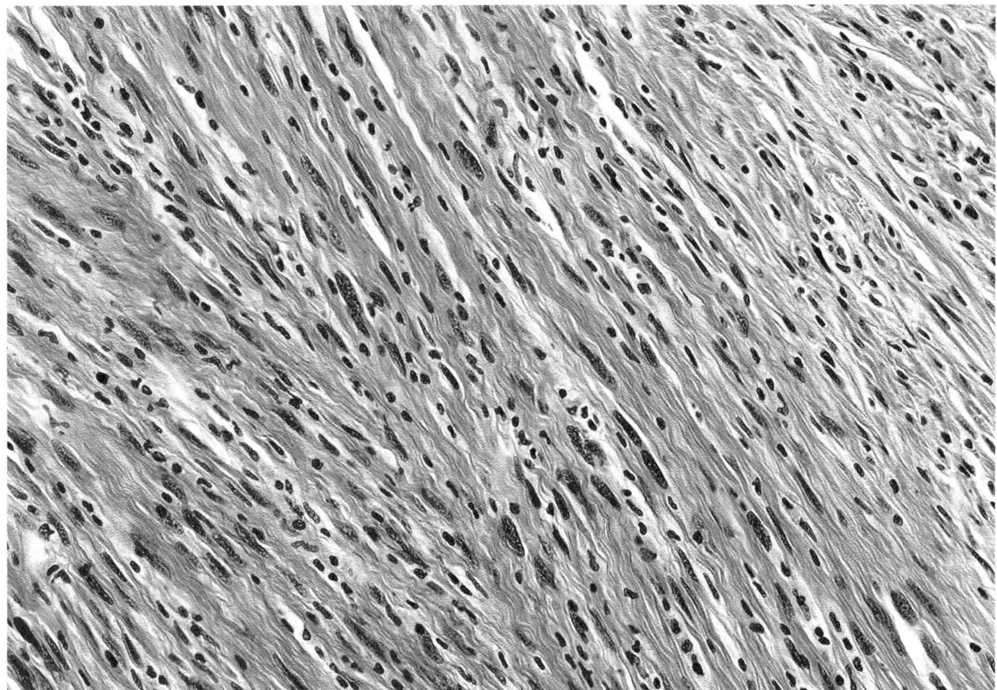

**FIGURE 17–32.** Dedifferentiated liposarcoma with areas having the appearance of a fibrosarcoma.

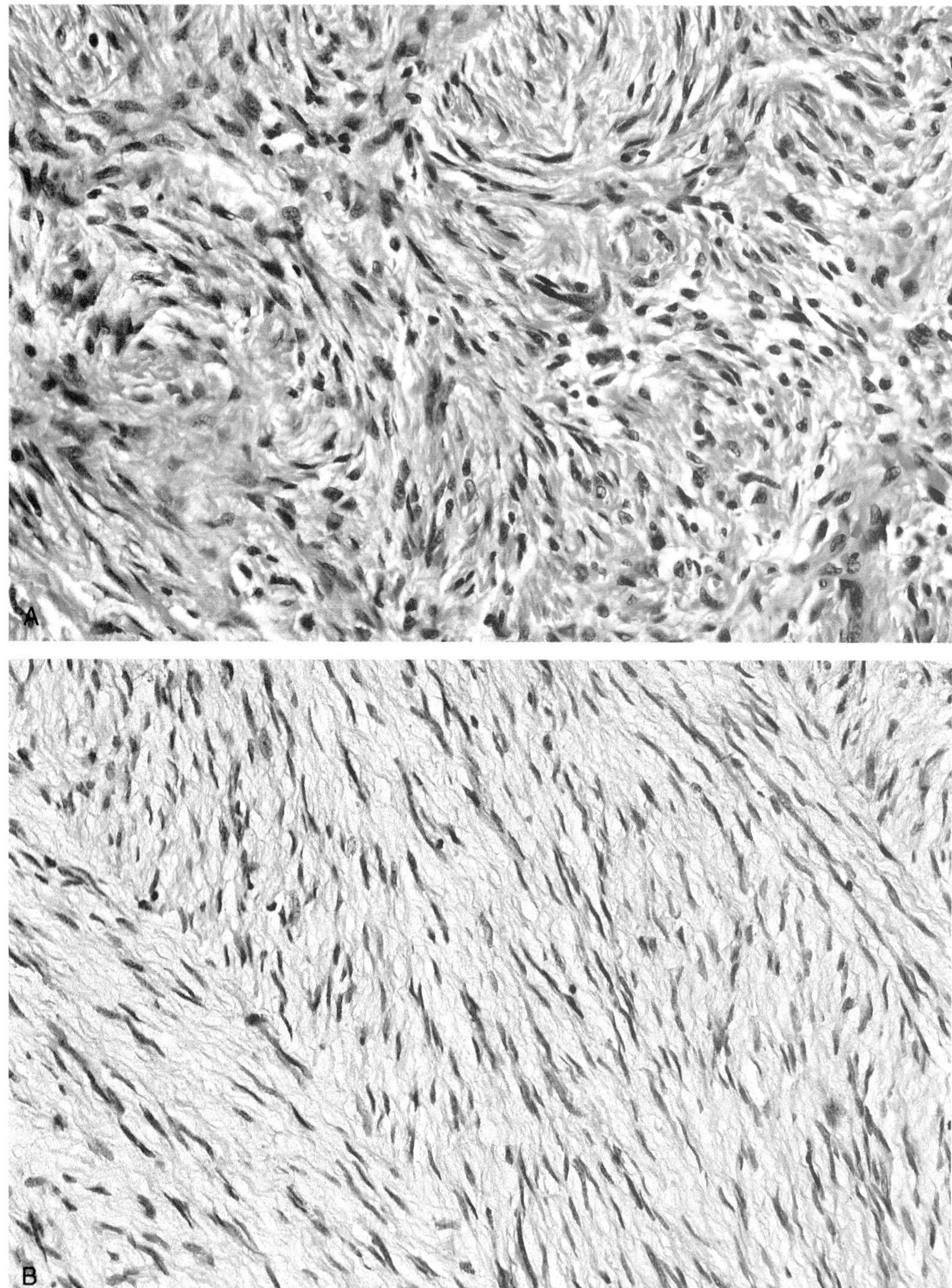


**FIGURE 17–33.** Dedifferentiated liposarcoma with low grade dedifferentiation, ranging from grade II (**A**) to grade I (**B, C**).

*Illustration continued on opposite page*

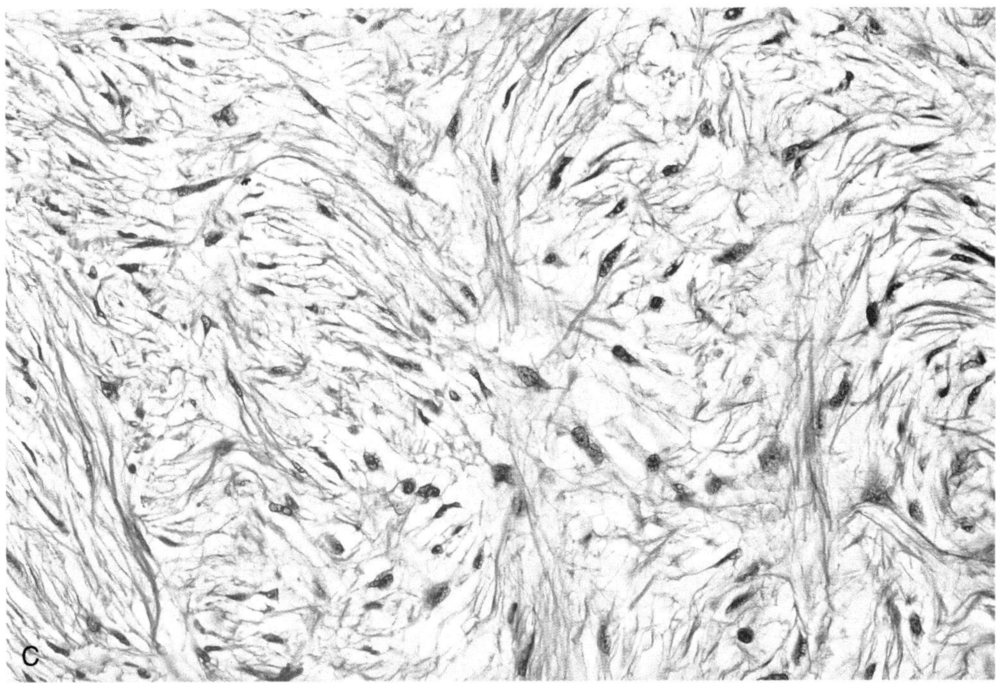


**FIGURE 17–33** *(Continued).*

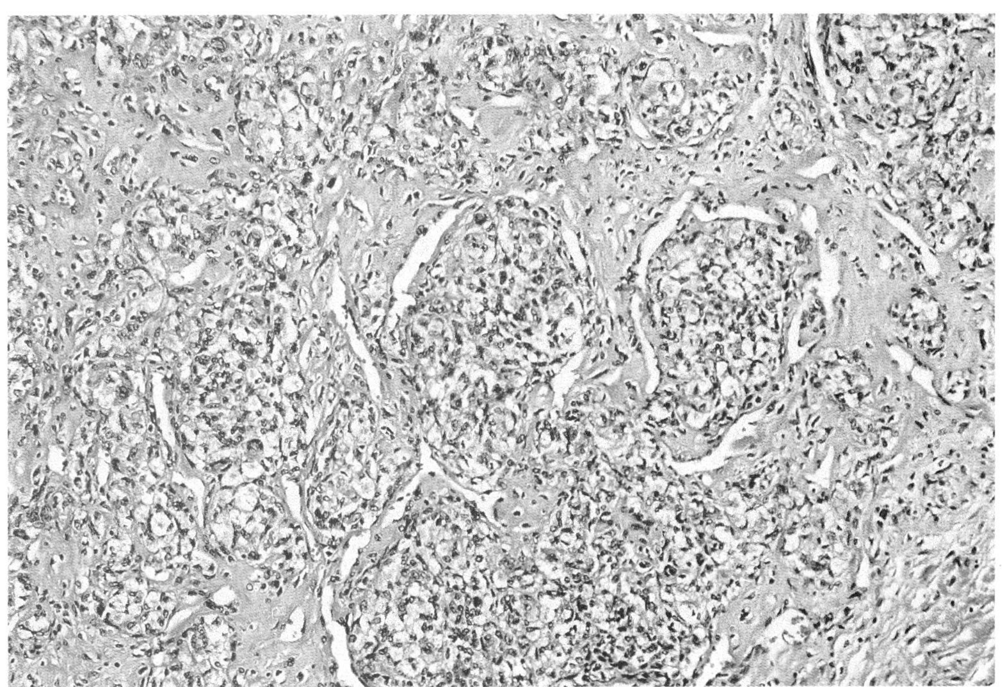

**FIGURE 17–34.** Dedifferentiated liposarcoma with areas of whorled structures.

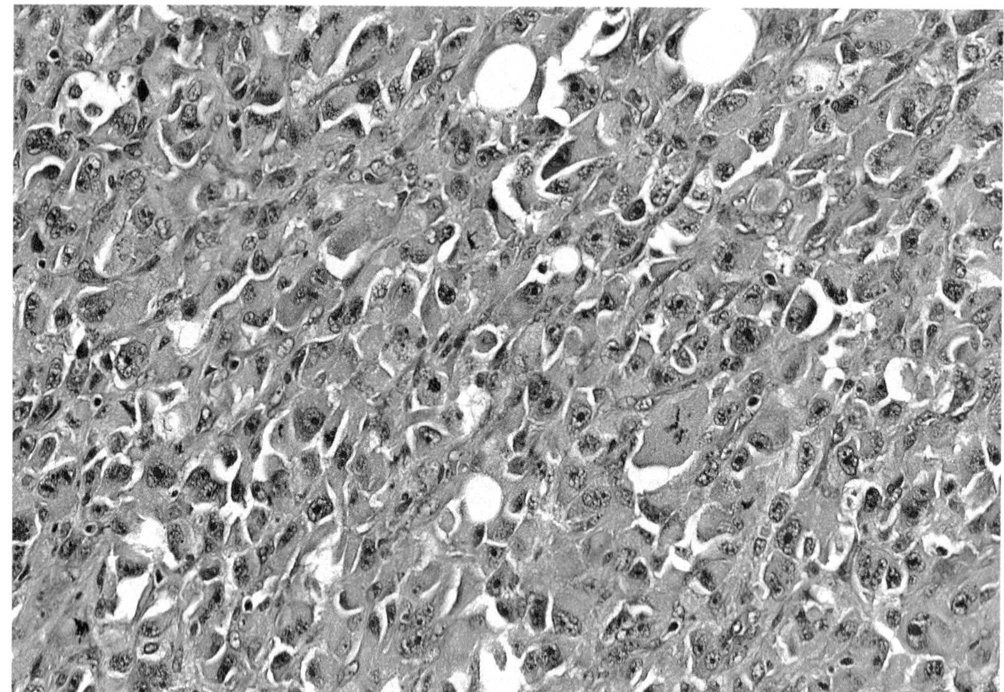

**FIGURE 17–35.** Dedifferentiated liposarcoma composed of undifferentiated large round cells.

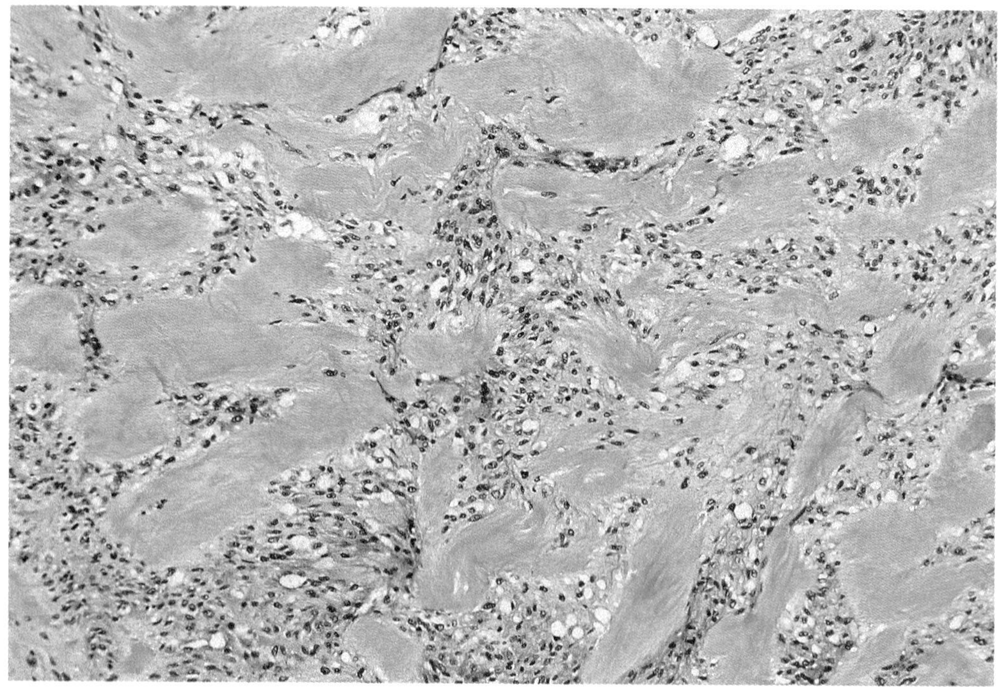

**FIGURE 17–36.** Dedifferentiated liposarcoma with amianthoid fibers.

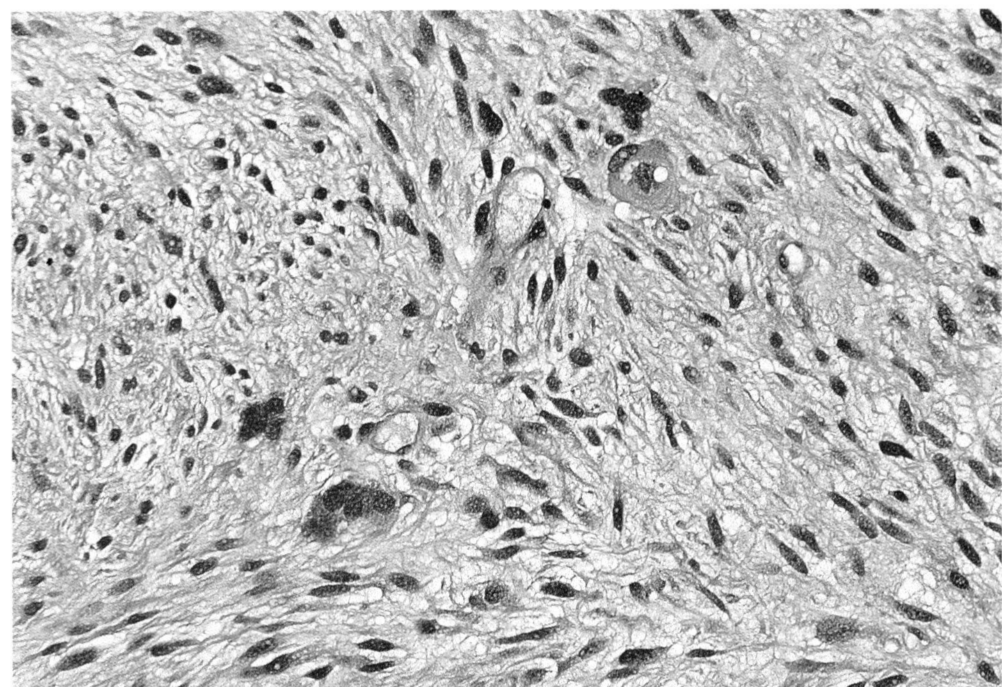

**FIGURE 17–37.** Dedifferentiated liposarcoma with rhabdomyosarcomatous differentiation in dedifferentiated areas.

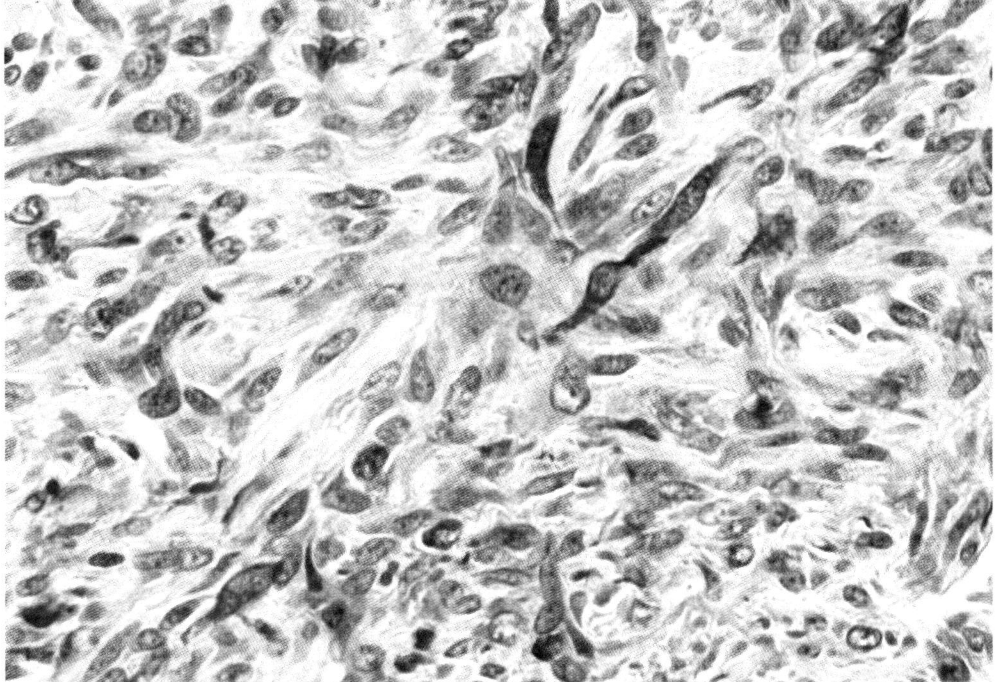

**FIGURE 17–38.** Dedifferentiated liposarcoma with rhabdomyosarcomatous differentiation in dedifferentiated areas. Desmin immunostain decorates rhabdomyoblasts.

34), areas with a pericytic pattern, amianthoid fibers (Fig. 17–36), and divergent rhabdomyosarcomatous,[66] osteosarcomatous, or leiomyosarcomatous elements (Figs. 17–37, 17–38).[62]

Ultrastructurally, the dedifferentiated zones display little lipogenic differentiation. The cells have well developed rough endoplasmic reticulum, primitive cell junctions, and prominent lysosomes. Occasional cells have a small amount of cytoplasmic lipid.[58]

### Differential Diagnosis

**Sarcoma Infiltrating Fat.** The most common problem with the differential diagnosis is distinguishing between a pleomorphic sarcoma infiltrating fat and a dedifferentiated liposarcoma. We believe there should clear-cut evidence of well differentiated liposarcoma some distance from the dedifferentiated areas for the diagnosis of dedifferentiated liposarcoma. Evaluating a high grade sarcoma at its interface with normal fat results in an inappropriately low threshold for the diagnosis of dedifferentiated liposarcoma.

**Minimal Dedifferentiation.** A relatively rare problem with the diagnosis is finding a microscopic focus of dedifferentiation in an otherwise typical well differentiated liposarcoma. We have adopted the position that dedifferentation ought to be macroscopically visible (>1.0 cm) before the label "dedifferentiated liposarcoma" is applied. Even so, it is likely that small foci of dedifferentiation (1–2 cm), which we have termed "minimal" or "early" dedifferentiation, are associated with a prolonged clinical course. For example, we have followed a patient with a 3-cm focus of dedifferentation that evolved into a fully dedifferentiated tumor over a 25-year course. Nonetheless, the above case serves to illustrate the fact that even tumors with minimal dedifferentiation can progress to full-fledged dedifferentiated liposarcomas. We believe such cases should be individualized and signed out in a descriptive fashion, indicating the size of the dedifferentiated focus, until additional data are available.

### Clinical Behavior

The behavior of dedifferentiated liposarcomas appears to be similar to that of other pleomorphic high grade sarcomas in adults.[62] Altogether, 41% of patients experience local recurrences and 17% metastasis, with 28% dying of their tumors. These figures reflect the accelerated tempo of the disease once dedifferentiation occurs. Whereas the metastatic rate might appear low compared to that of some high grade sarcomas, two points should be emphasized. First, most patients die of the local effects of their tumor before distant metastasis become apparent; and second, it is difficult to determine accurately what criteria differentiate between local (contiguous) intraabdominal spread and local metastasis. For these reasons the metastatic rate, determined with an average follow-up of 3 years, represents a conservative estimate of metastatic potential.[62]

Among the various prognostic factors, site appears to be the most significant. As with well differentiated liposarcomas, the dedifferentiated liposarcomas located in the retroperitoneum have the worst prognosis. Although one might anticipate that the extent and grade of dedifferentiation would affect outcome, it does not appear to be true for the range of tumors commonly encountered in clinical practice.[62] What this seems to imply is that once these tumors are clinically apparent the amount of dedifferentiation is already so significant that quantitating and grading these zones does not provide any additional stratification that can identify good and poor prognosis subgroups. Furthermore, the fact that patients with low grade dedifferentiation may suffer the same untoward consequences as those with high grade dedifferentiation indicates that the traditional definition of dedifferentiation (high grade nonlipogenic sarcoma) should be expanded to include low grade nonlipogenic sarcomas as well.

## MYXOID/ROUND CELL LIPOSARCOMA

Myxoid and round cell liposarcomas, although given separate designations in the WHO classification of soft tissue tumors, actually occupy two ends of a common spectrum. Evidence supporting the congruency of these two tumors is derived from their similarity in terms of age, location, and cytogenetic abnormalities and by the identification of tumors with transitional or hybrid features.[73,79,87] To emphasize their similarity, some prefer the designation "poorly differentiated myxoid" instead of "round cell" liposarcoma. Regardless of the nomenclature, it is imperative that the clinician be given some indication as to the level of malignancy (in the form of a grade) and the risk of metastatic disease.

### Clinical Features

Myxoid/round cell liposarcomas account for one-half of all liposarcomas. Unlike well differentiated and dedifferentiated liposarcomas, this form occurs in a younger age group, with a peak incidence during the fifth decade. It develops preferentially in the lower extremity (75%), particularly the medial thigh and popliteal area, and less frequently in the retroperitoneum (Fig. 17–39). Radiographically, these lesions are

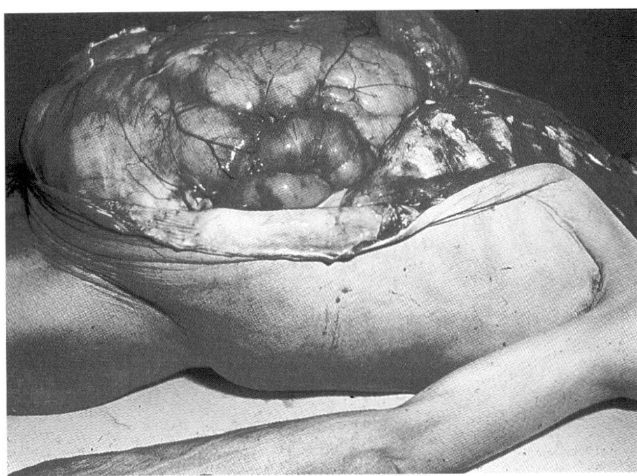

**FIGURE 17–39.** Myxoid liposarcoma massively replacing the abdominal contents.

quite varied. Typically they appear as nonhomogeneous masses on CT scans. The attenuation values of highly myxoid lesions exceed those of normal fat but are less than that of the surrounding soft tissue. Less differentiated round cell areas have attenuation values similar to those of other soft tissue sarcomas.[3]

## Gross and Microscopic Features

Grossly, pure or predominantly myxoid liposarcomas are multinodular, gelatinous masses usually devoid of necrosis, although occasionally hemorrhage is encountered (Fig. 17–40). Those tumors with discrete areas of round cell liposarcoma have corresponding opaque white nodules situated in the myxoid mass, whereas those that are predominantly round cell have a white fleshy appearance similar to that of other high grade sarcomas.

Histologically pure myxoid liposarcomas bear a marked similarity to developing fetal fat (Figs. 17–41 to 17–46). At low power, the lesion is a multinodular mass of low cellularity with enhanced cellularity at the periphery (Fig. 17–42). Each nodule is composed of bland fusiform or round cells that lie suspended individually in a myxoid matrix composed of hyaluronic acid. Mitotic figures are typically rare or absent altogether. A delicate plexiform capillary vascular network is present throughout these tumors and provides an important clue for distinguishing them from myxomas. The proliferating neoplastic cells recapitulate, albeit imperfectly, the sequence of adipocyte differentiation. Immature spindled cells lacking obvious lipogenesis may be seen next to multivacuolar and univacuolar lipoblasts. Although lipoblasts are usually easy to identify in these liposarcomas, they may be especially prominent at the periphery of the tumor nodules (Fig. 17–43).

The hyaluronic acid-rich (alcian blue-positive; hyaluronidase-sensitive)[38] stroma (Figs. 17–47 to 17–49) is present primarily in the extracellular space but may also be found in individual tumor cells. Frequently, the extracellular mucin forms large pools, creating a cribriform or lace-like pattern in the tumor and infrequently gross cysts (Figs. 17–47 to 17–49). The cellular condensation at the rim of these pools produces a pseudoacinar pattern. In others the weak staining of accumulated mucin and the flattened tumor cells mimic a lymphangioma. Interstitial hemorrhage is common and may be so prominent that the tumor is confused with a hemangioma. Focal cartilaginous[71,84] leiomyomatous, or osseous differentiation occurs in

*Text continued on page 676*

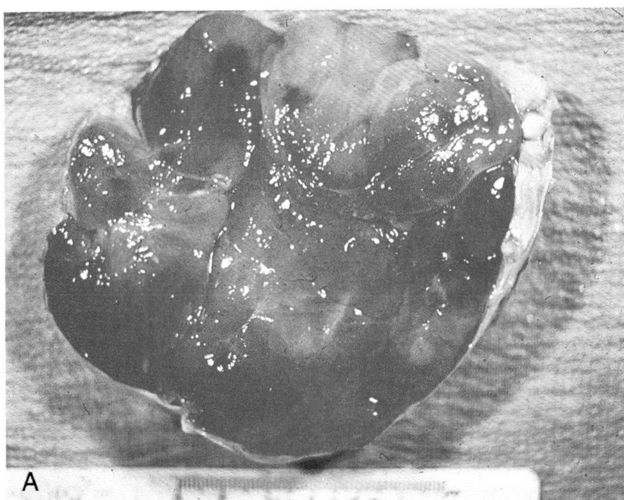


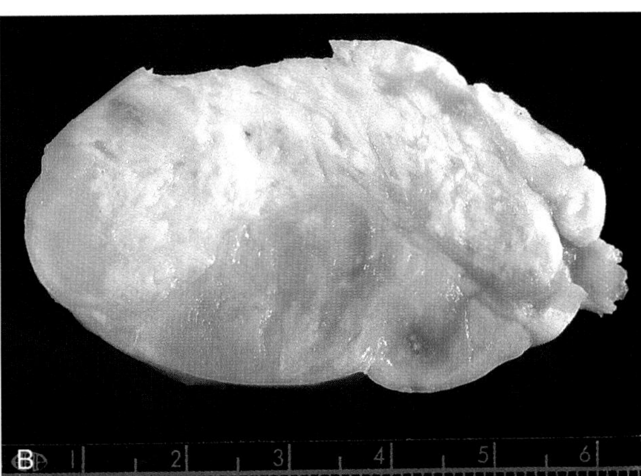


**FIGURE 17–40.** Gross specimen of a pure myxoid liposarcoma with a gelatinous cut surface (**A**) compared to a liposarcoma that contains myxoid (gelatinous) and round cell (opaque) areas (**B**).

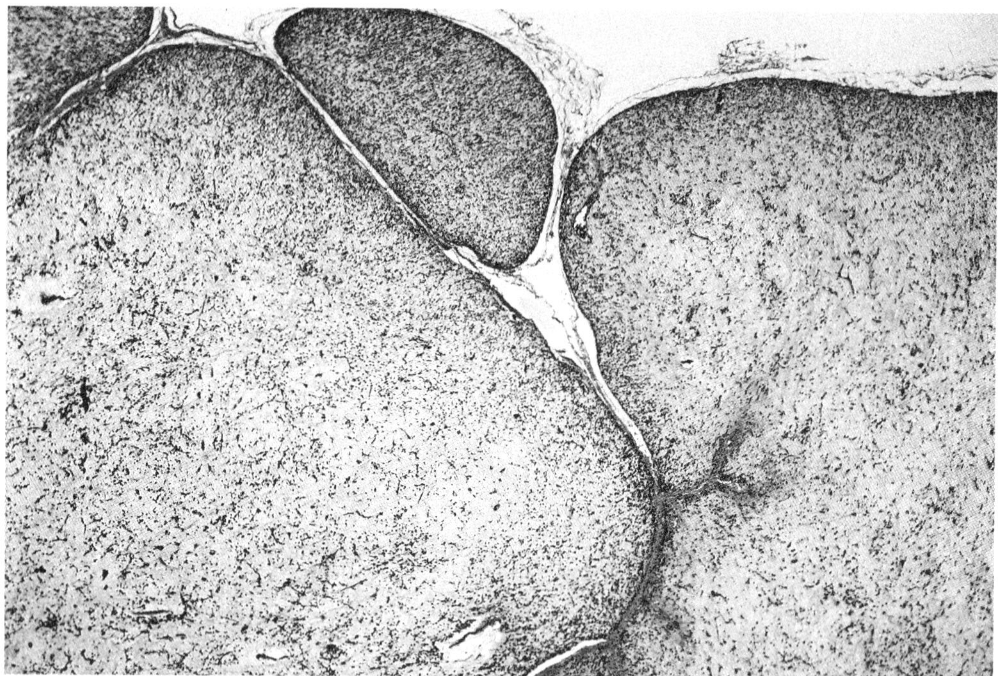

**FIGURE 17–41.** Multinodular appearance of a myxoid liposarcoma.

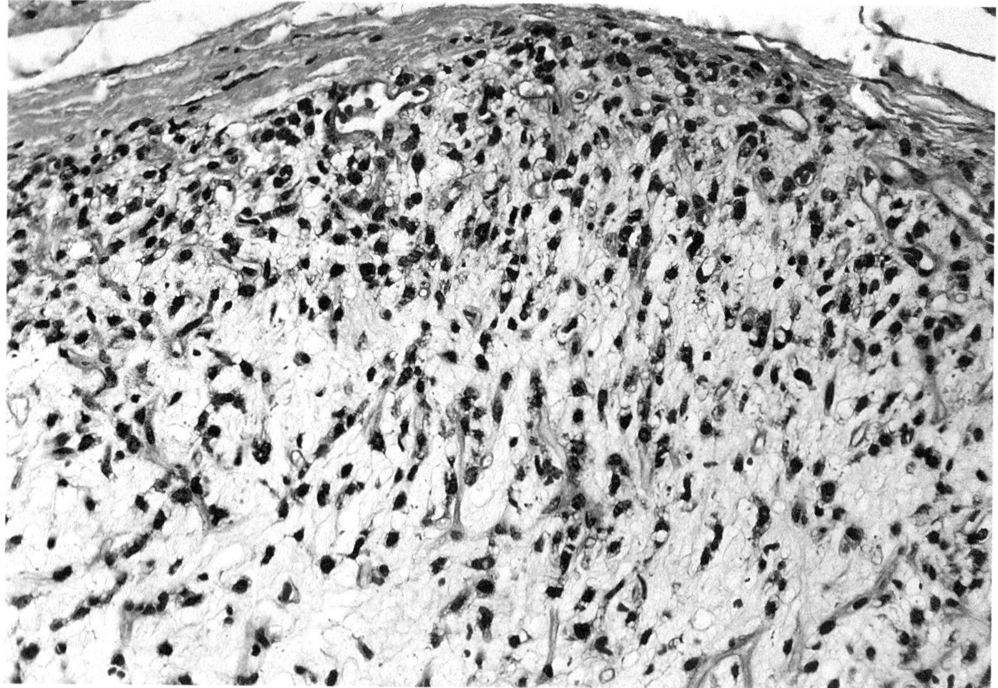

**FIGURE 17–42.** Enhanced cellularity at the periphery of nodules in a myxoid liposarcoma.

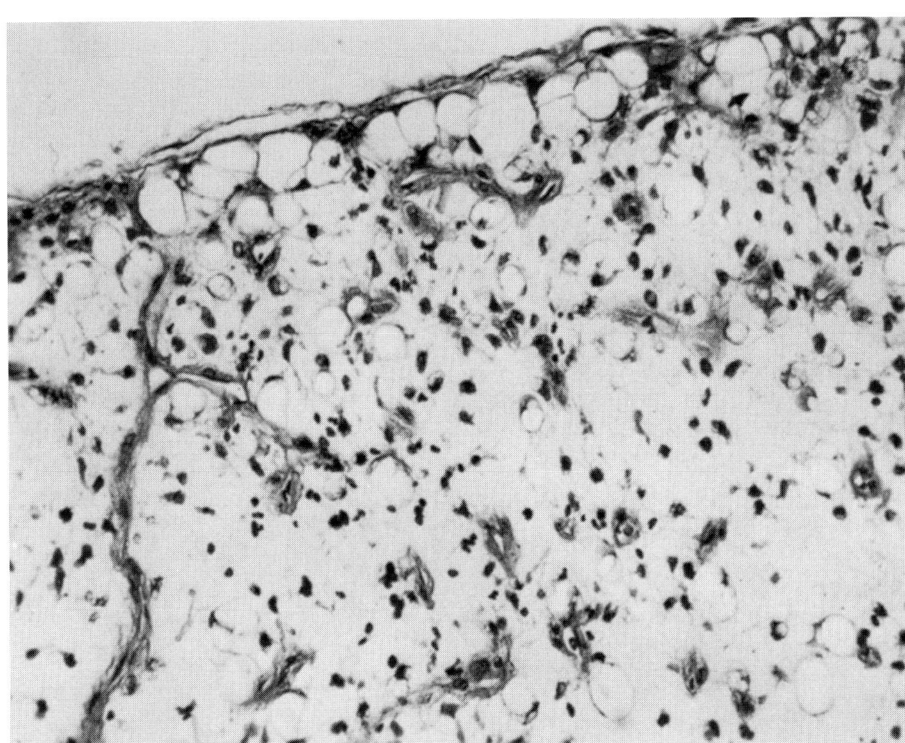

**FIGURE 17–43.** Myxoid liposarcoma with characteristic lipoblastic differentiation at the periphery.

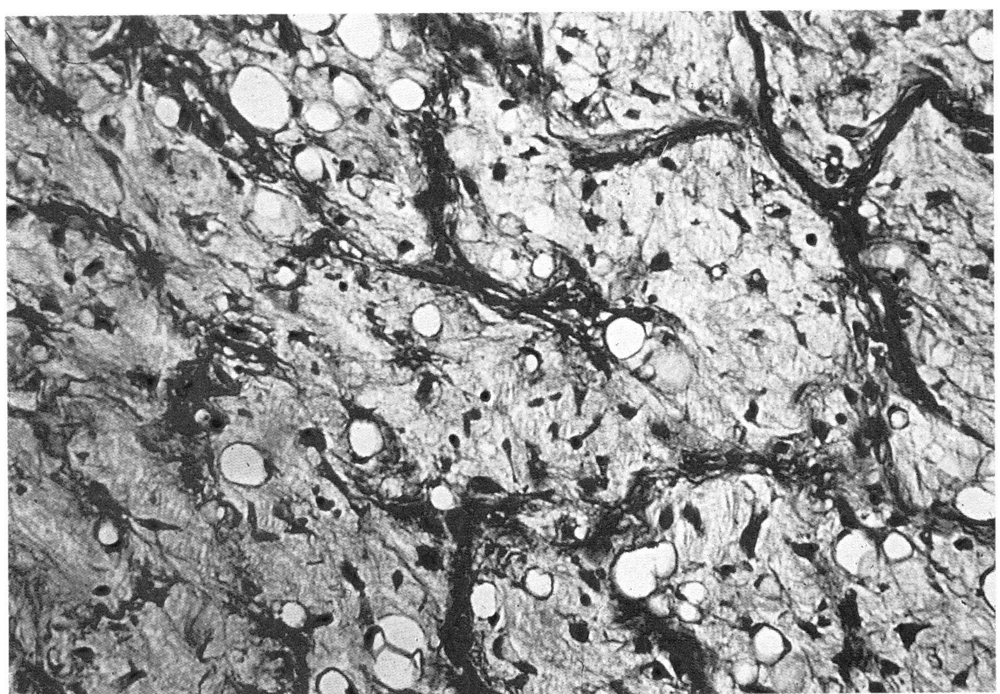

**FIGURE 17–44.** Typical appearance of a myxoid liposarcoma.

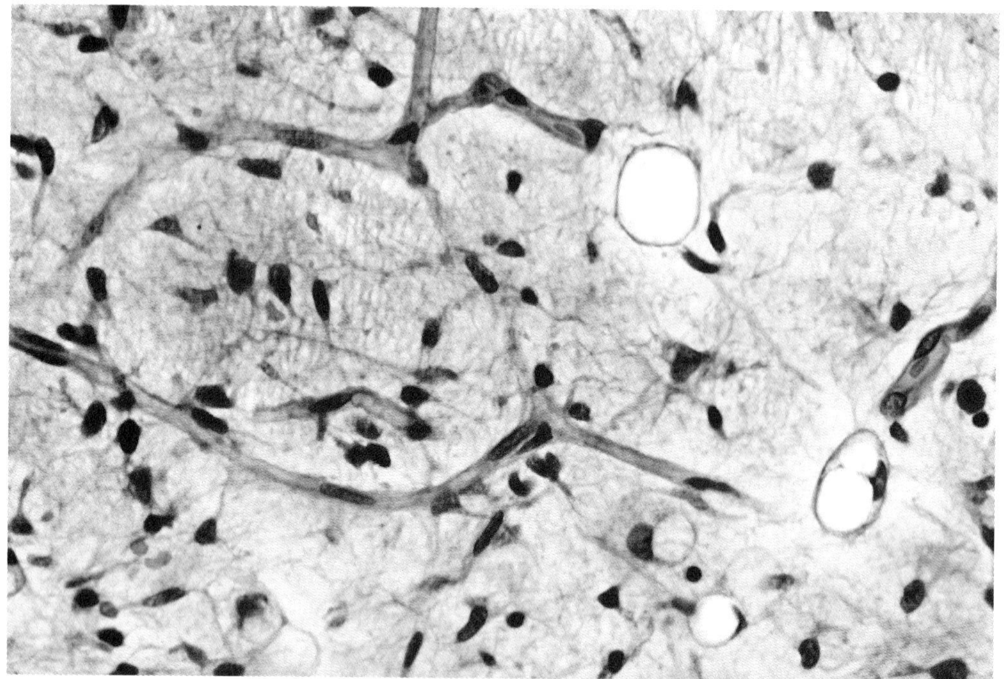

**FIGURE 17–45.** Myxoid liposarcoma with arborizing vasculature and lipoblasts at varying stages.

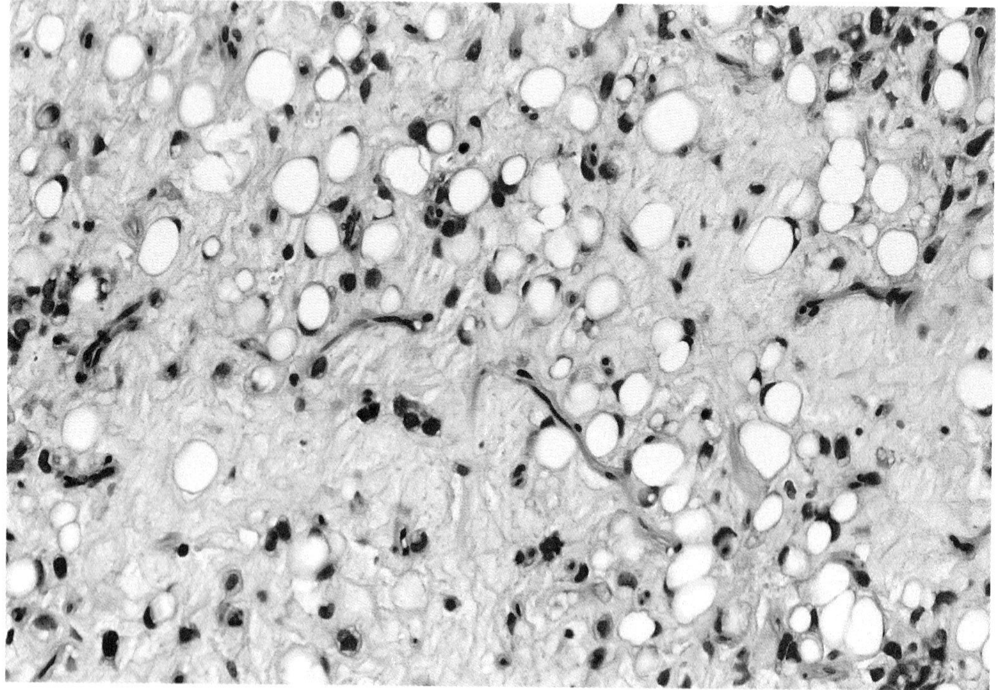

**FIGURE 17–46.** Myxoid liposarcoma with a larger number of mature lipoblasts than seen in Figure 17–45.

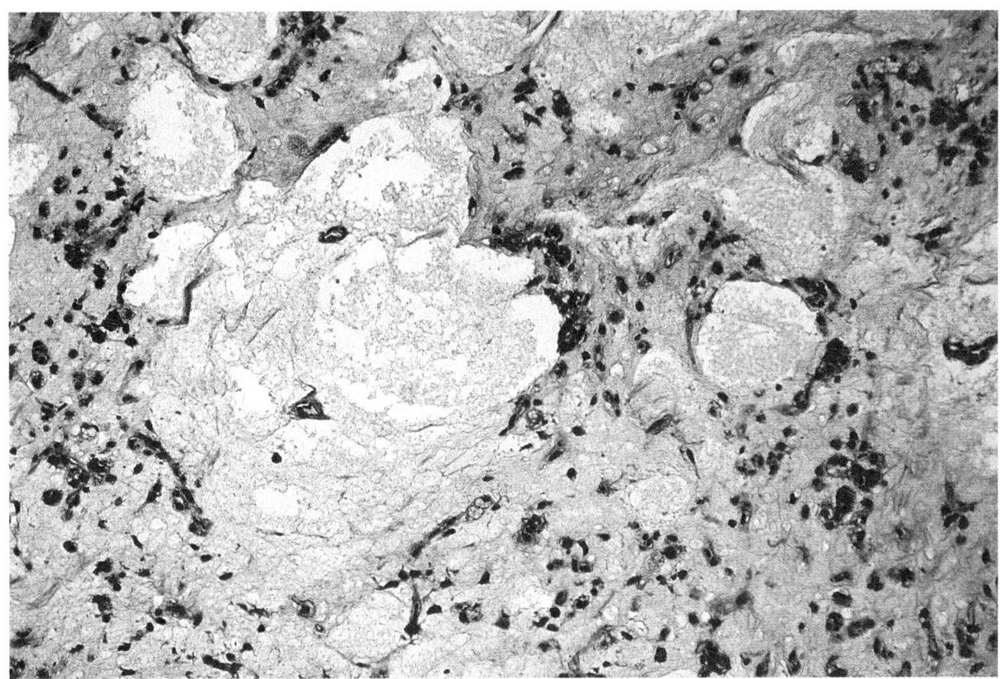

**FIGURE 17–47.** Small pools of stromal mucin in myxoid liposarcoma.

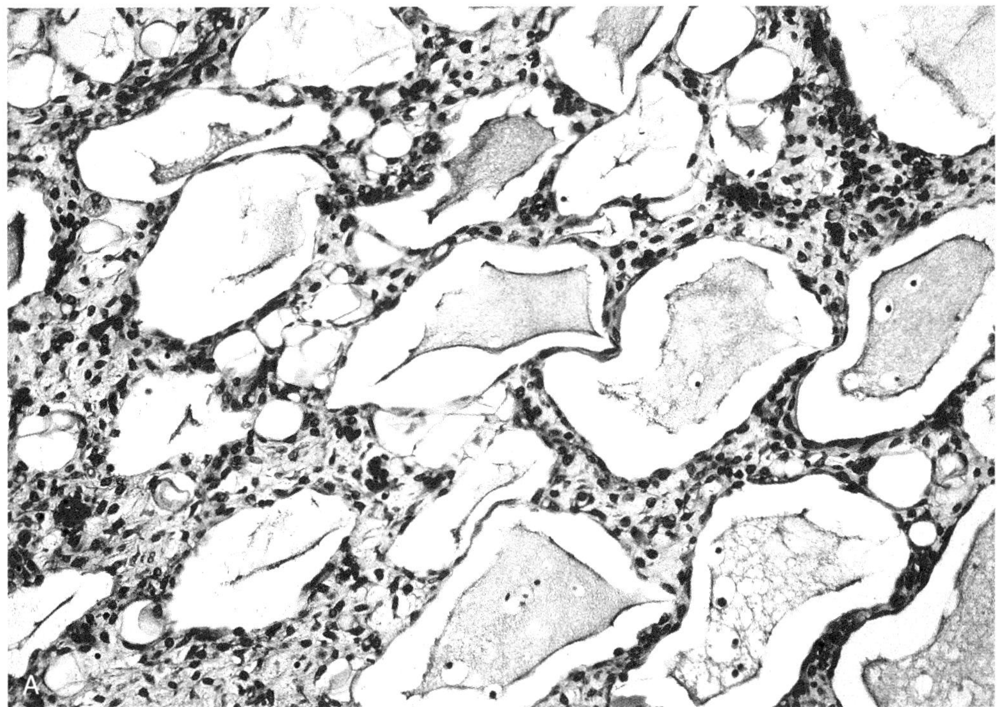


**FIGURE 17–48.** **(A)** Pools of stromal mucin in a myxoid liposarcoma forming a sieve pattern. **(B)** Pools of stromal mucin forming cysts.

*Illustration continued on following page*

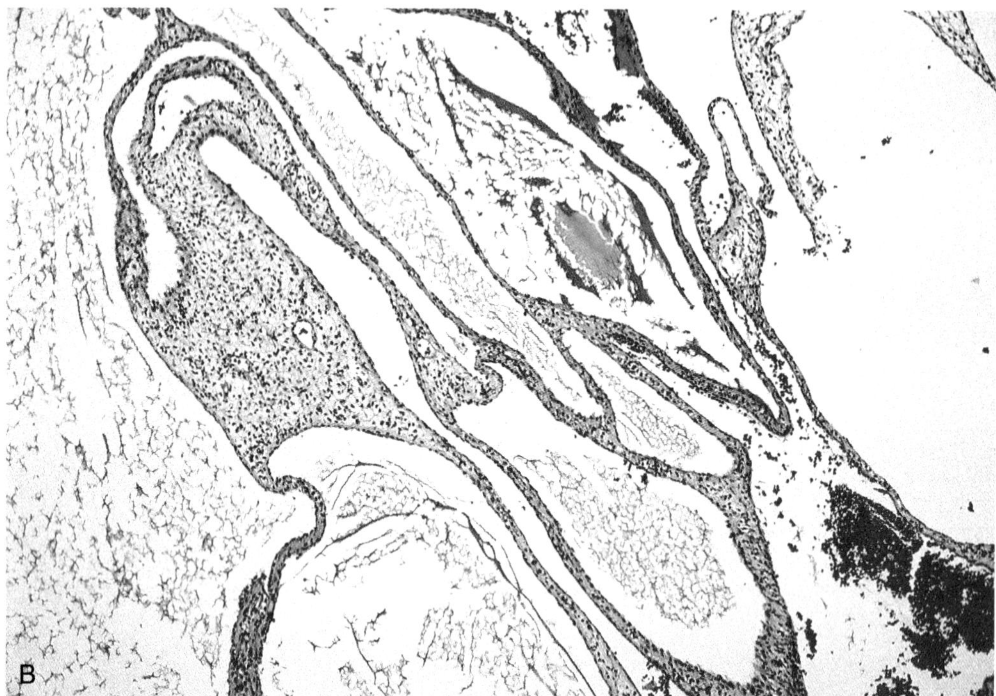


**FIGURE 17–48** *(Continued).*

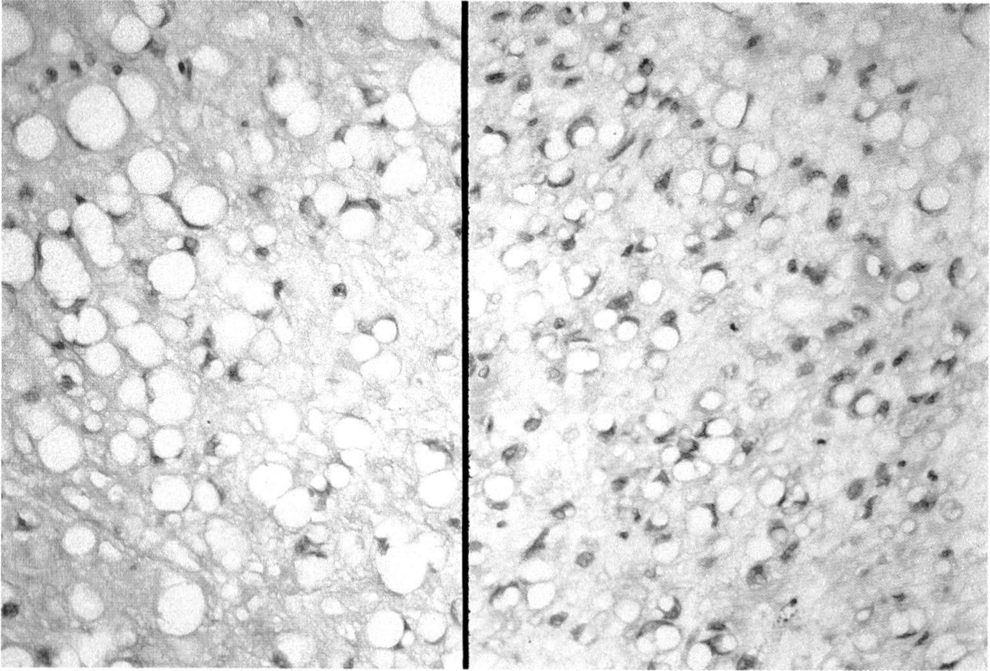

**FIGURE 17–49.** Alcian blue staining of myxoid liposarcoma before (left) and after (right) hyaluronidase digestion. Stromal mucin staining is abolished following enzyme treatment, indicating the presence of hyaluronic acid.

myxoid liposarcomas. These elements do not appear to affect the prognosis. The significance of rhabdomyosarcomatous differentiation (Figs. 17–50, 17–51, 17–52), which we have encountered once and which has been reported anecdotally in the literature, is uncertain.[83]

A peculiar subtype of myxoid liposarcoma consists almost entirely of loosely arranged fibroblast-like spindle cells oriented along a single plane and surrounded by a delicate reticulin meshwork. The uniformity of the spindle cells and their parallel orientation distinguishes this tumor from the more irregularly shaped and distributed cells of well differentiated sclerosing liposarcoma (Figs. 17–53, 17–54, 17–55). Recently termed "spindle cell liposarcoma,"[69] and regarded as variants of well differentiated liposarcoma, we regard them as variants of myxoid liposarcoma because of transitional or hybrid cases.

As myxoid liposarcomas lose their differentiation, they acquire features of round cell liposarcoma, which is expressed in one of two ways. Amid a backdrop of myxoid liposarcoma one may encounter a nodule of pure round cell liposarcoma (Fig. 17–56). The latter areas are characterized by sheets of primitive round cells with a high nuclear/cytoplasmic ratio and a prominent nucleolus. In these areas the cells are so numerous that essentially they lie back to back with no intervening myxoid stroma; and the capillary vascular pattern, though present, cannot be visualized easily. More commonly, however, the progression toward round cell liposarcoma is reflected in a more gradual fashion; and, instead, one encounters areas with transitional features (Fig. 17–57). In these areas the cellularity is clearly greater, and the cells are usually larger with a more rounded shape. At what point one applies the label "round cell liposarcoma" has been problematic. Smith et al. suggested that for a threshold definition for round cell differentiation there should be areas in which the cells acquired a rounded shape and had overlapping nuclei such that one can easily identify clusters of cells sitting back to back.[85] On the other hand, they did not regard areas of enhanced cellularity with cells lying individually in a myxoid background as sufficient for a diagnosis of round cell differentiation, as these "transitional areas" did not correlate with an adverse outcome (Fig. 17–57A).

Occasionally, areas of round cell liposarcoma are characterized by branching cords and rows of primitive round cells (Figs. 17–58, 17–59) or large cells with an eosinophilic granular or multivacuolar cytoplasm resembling malignant brown fat cells (Fig. 17–60). Solidly cellular round cell areas, out of context, can be difficult to recognize as a liposarcoma unless an occasional lipoblast is identified. In fact, in the absence of a lipoblast one might entertain a diagnosis of another round cell sarcoma or a lymphoma. Finally, there have been a few exceptional myxoid/

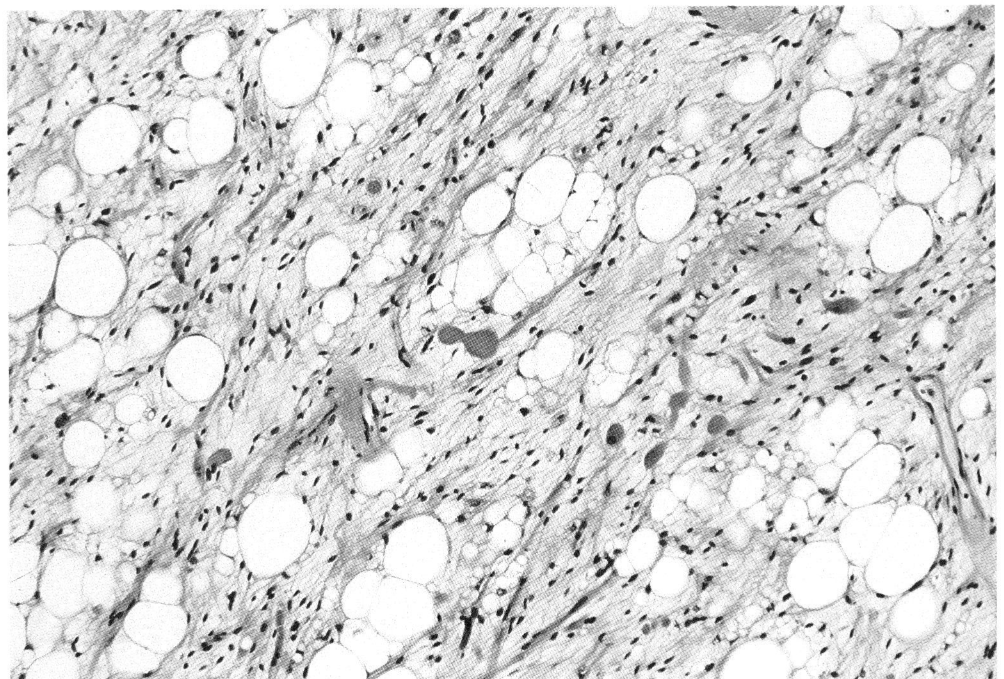

**FIGURE 17–50.** Unusual myxoid liposarcoma with rhabdomyoblastic differentiation.

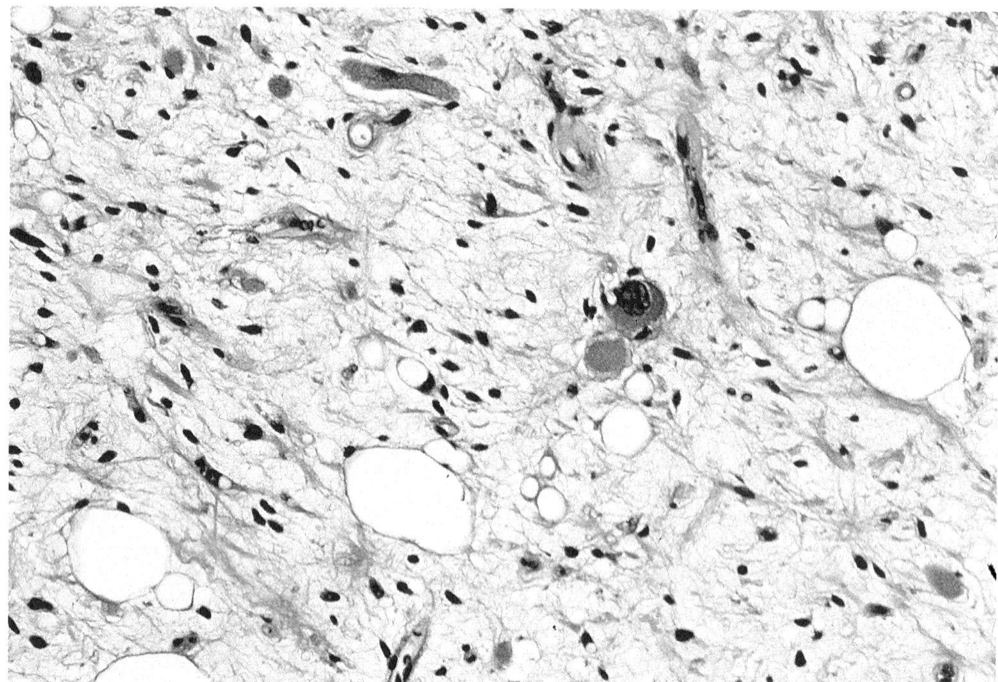

**FIGURE 17–51.** Rhabdomyoblasts in a myxoid liposarcoma.

**FIGURE 17–52.** Desmin positive rhabdomyoblasts in myxoid liposarcoma.

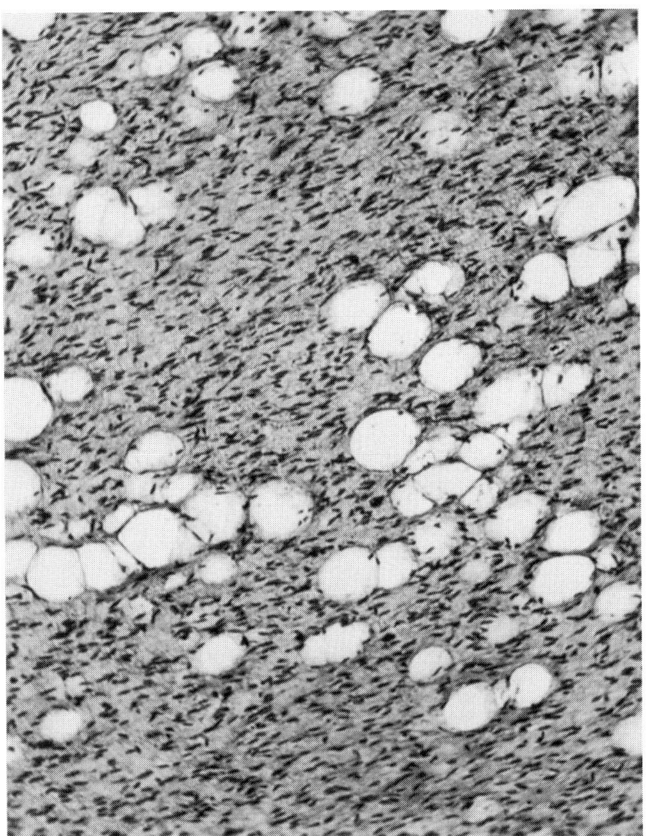

**FIGURE 17–53.** Spindle cell liposarcoma with prominent spindled tumor cells.

round cell liposarcomas that have displayed dedifferentiated areas similar to those seen in well differentiated liposarcomas.[27]

## Ancillary Studies

The diagnosis of myxoid/round cell liposarcoma continues to be based primarily on review of routine histologic sections, although ultrastructural studies effectively demonstrate lipogenic differentiation. The cells in myxoid and round cell liposarcomas display a range of differentiation from primitive mesenchymal cells with high nuclear/cytoplasmic ratios, few organelles, and discontinuous basal lamina to identifiable lipoblasts containing non-membrane-bound lipid. In the less differentiated round cell areas the cells tend have more mitochondria, numerous polyribosomes, and fewer lipid vacuoles[5,15,17,24,30] (Figs. 17–61, 17–62). Recently antibodies to aP2 protein (adipocyte lipid-binding protein) have been used effectively to mark prelipoblasts in a variety of lipomatous lesions.[6] This antibody decorates many of the cells in myxoid/round cell liposarcomas and some cells in pleomorphic liposarcomas, hibernomas, and brown fat. It does not decorate mature lipoblasts or mature fat and thus provides some specificity in distinguishing various histologic forms of lipomatous tumors. It has not yet been widely applied diagnostically.

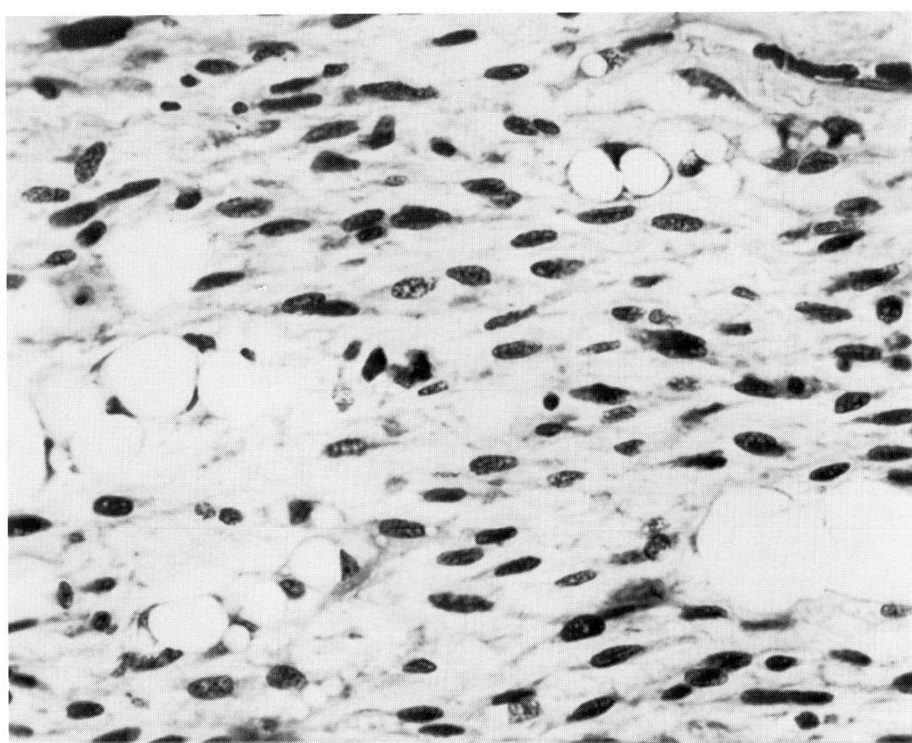

**FIGURE 17–54.** Spindle cell liposarcoma with scattered lipoblasts. The presence of lipoblasts and the variably sized spindle cells with hyperchromatc nuclei help distinguish this tumor from spindle cell lipoma.

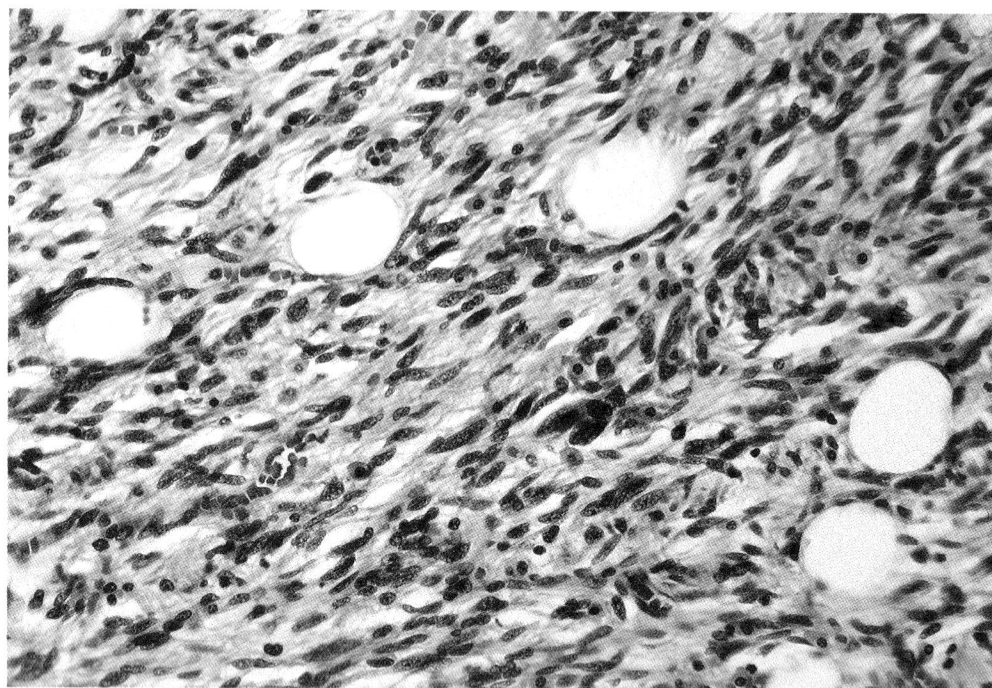

**FIGURE 17–55.** Spindle cell liposarcoma with more atypia of spindled cells than in Figure 17–54. Note the presence of mast cells.

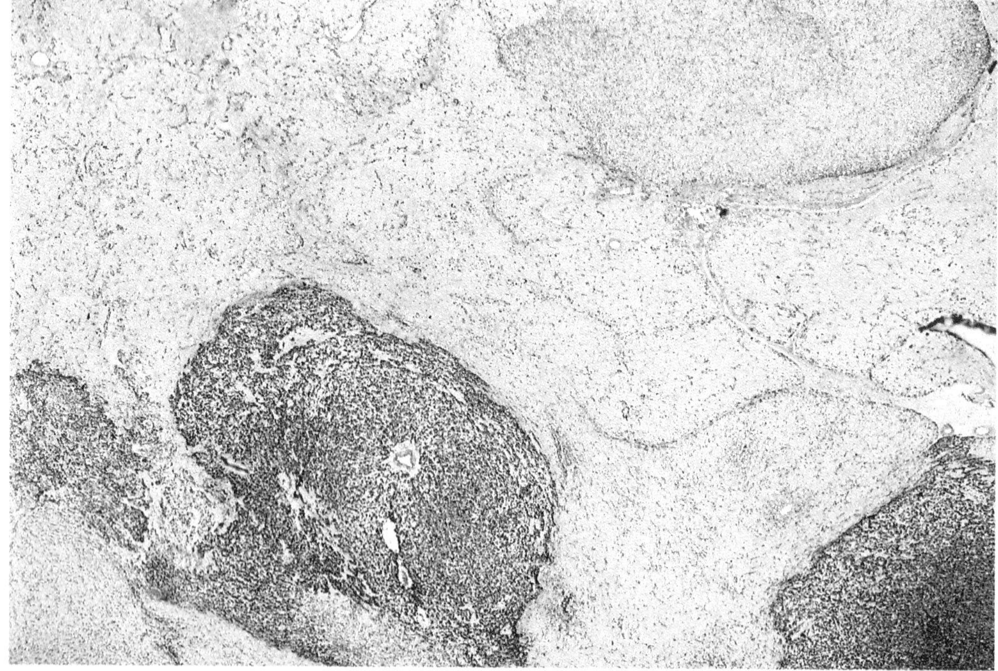

**FIGURE 17–56.** Myxoid liposarcoma with sharply demarcated nodules of round cell liposarcoma.

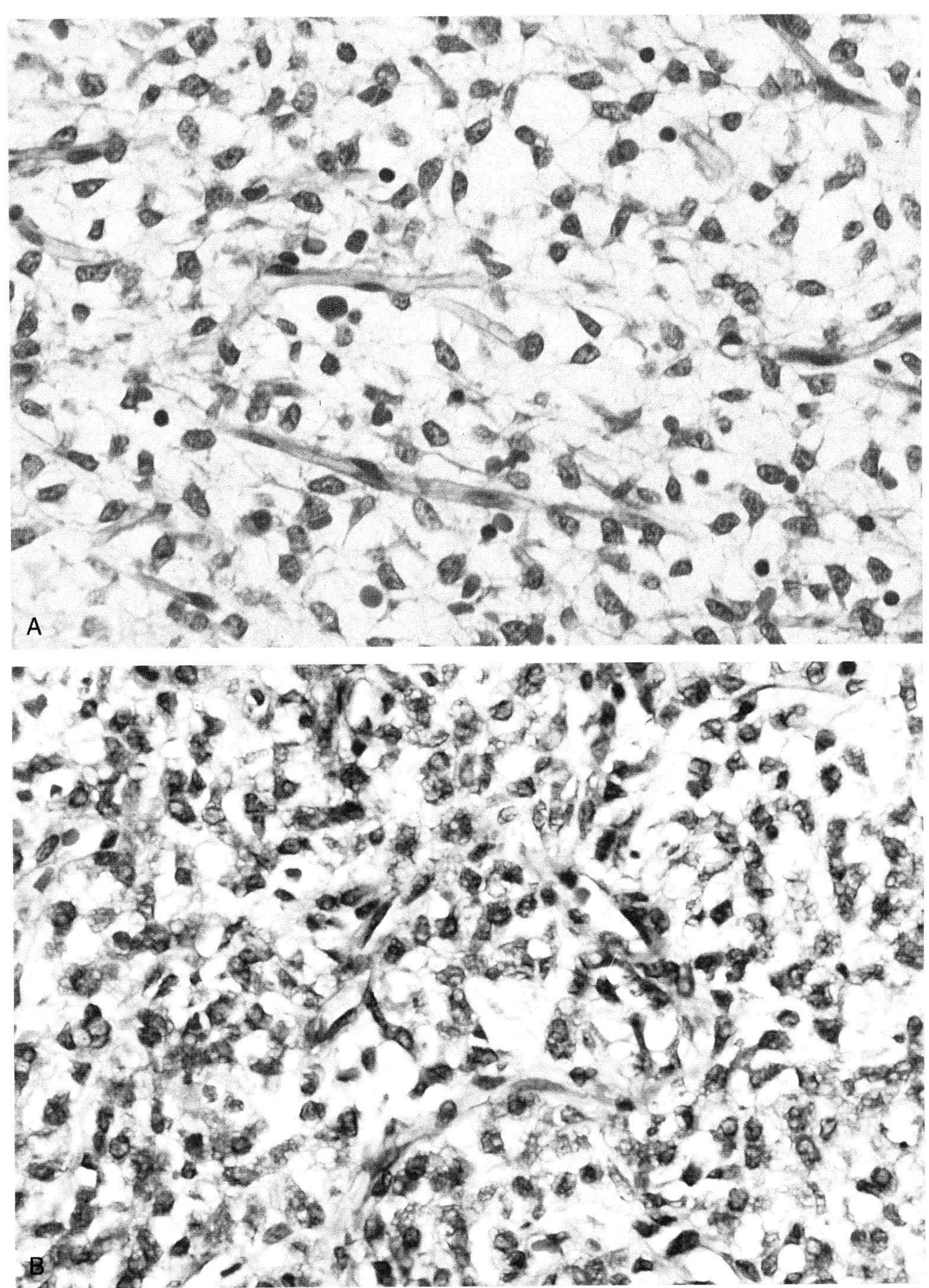


**FIGURE 17–57.** Myxoid/round cell liposarcoma with progressive transition, from somewhat cellular myxoid areas (**A**) to borderline areas (**B**) to round cell liposarcoma

*Illustration continued on following page*

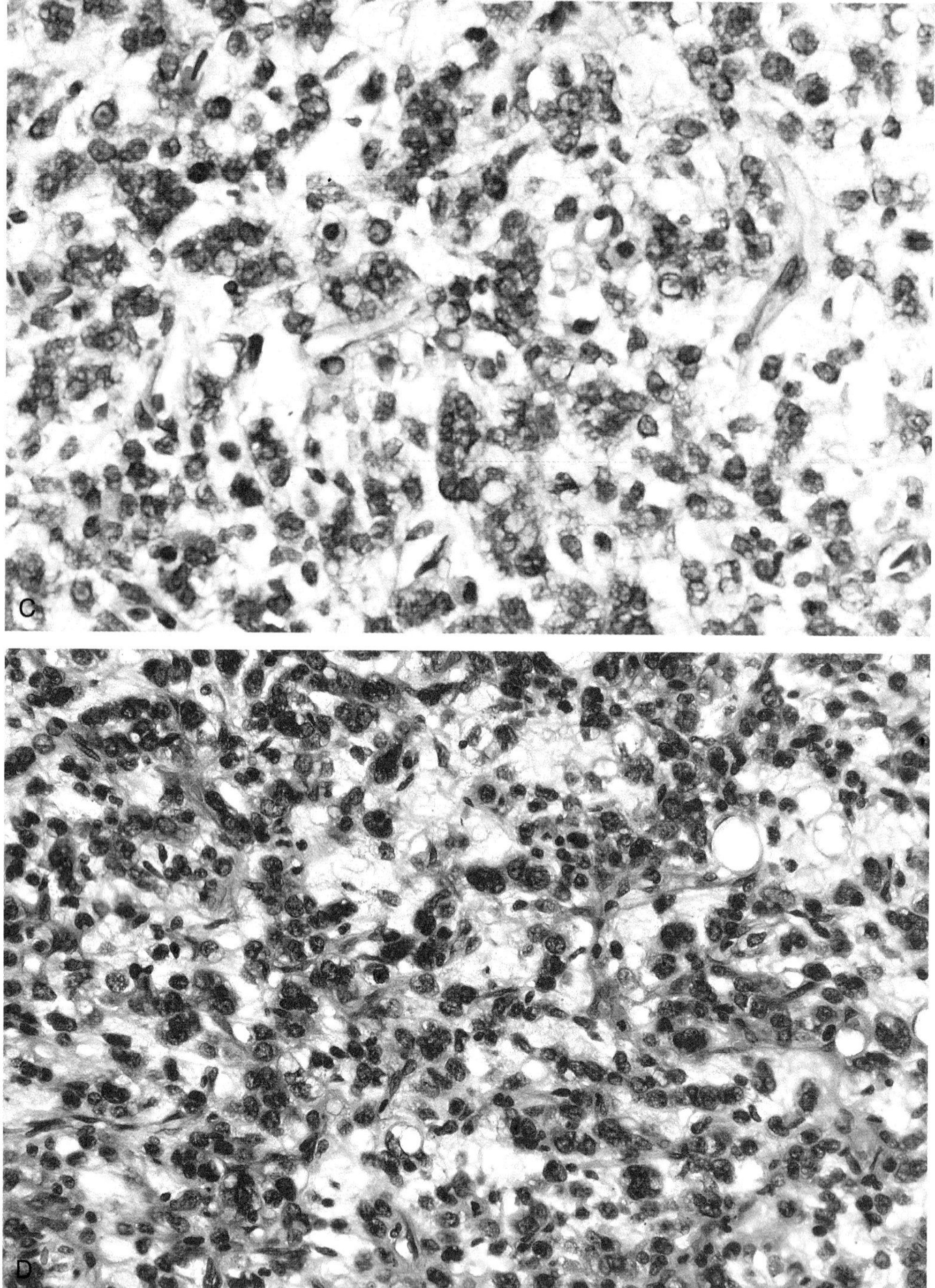


**FIGURE 17–57** *(Continued).* (**C, D**) where cells have overlapping nuclei and some residual myxoid stroma.

*Illustration continued on opposite page*

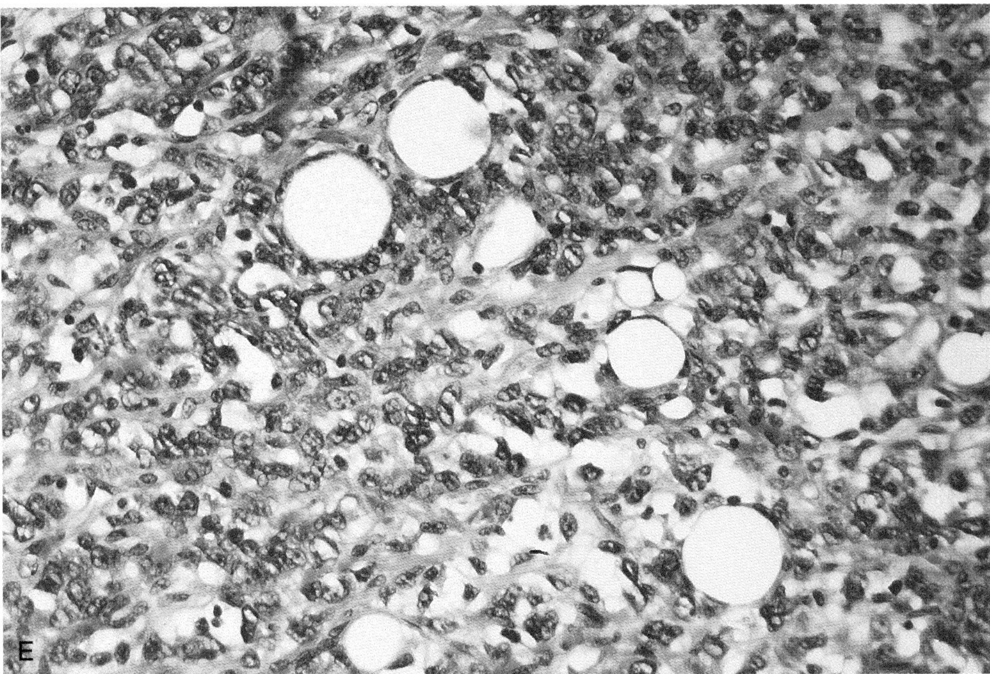


**FIGURE 17–57** *(Continued).* Round cell areas without myxoid stroma (**E**) may be impossible to diagnose as liposarcoma.

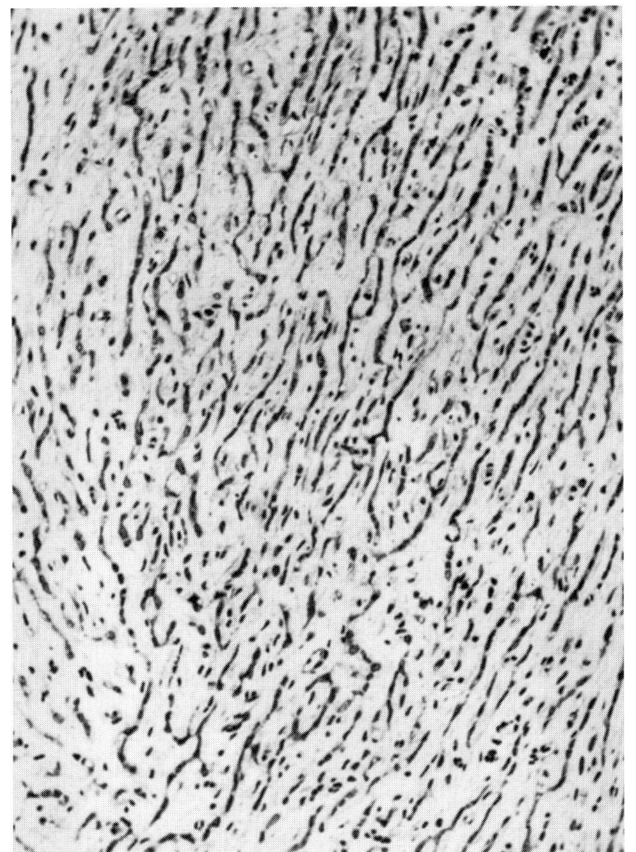

**FIGURE 17–58.** Cord-like pattern in a round cell liposarcoma.

## Differential Diagnosis

The differential diagnosis of myxoid liposarcoma includes a wide range of lesions that appear myxoid (Table 17–4), whereas round cell liposarcomas evoke the differential diagnosis of round cell tumors. The two most common myxoid sarcomas of adults that are confused with myxoid liposarcoma are myxoid malignant fibrous histiocytoma and myxoid chondrosarcoma. The former is characterized by a significant degree of nuclear atypia and a coarser vasculature than is encountered in myxoid liposarcomas. It is tempting to interpret the pleomorphic vacuolated cells encountered in these tumors as lipoblasts and to draw the erroneous conclusion that the tumor is a liposarcoma (Fig. 17–7). The vacuoles of these pseudolipoblasts are large, poorly defined, and filled with hyaluronic acid rather than lipid. Myxoid chondrosarcomas are composed of small, distinctly eosinophilic

**TABLE 17–4 LESIONS SIMULATING MYXOID LIPOSARCOMA**

Myxoma (intramuscular and cutaneous forms)
Angiomyxoma
Myxoid dermatofibrosarcoma protuberans
Myxoid chondrosarcoma
Myxoid malignant fibrous histiocytoma, low grade (myxofibrosarcoma)

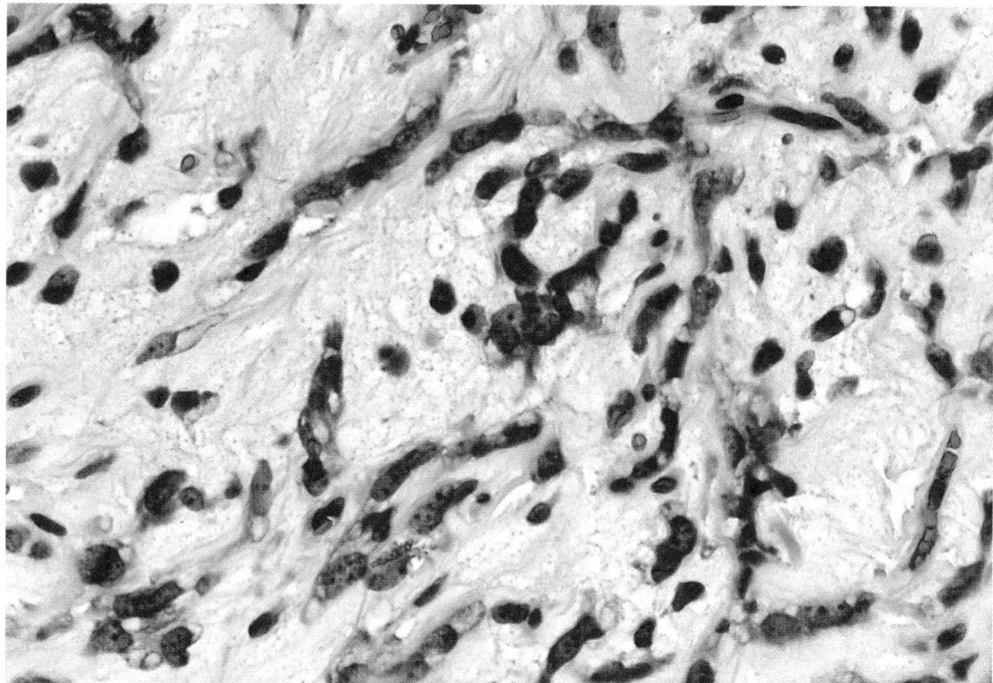

**FIGURE 17–59.** Cord-like pattern and stromal hyalinization in a round cell liposarcoma.

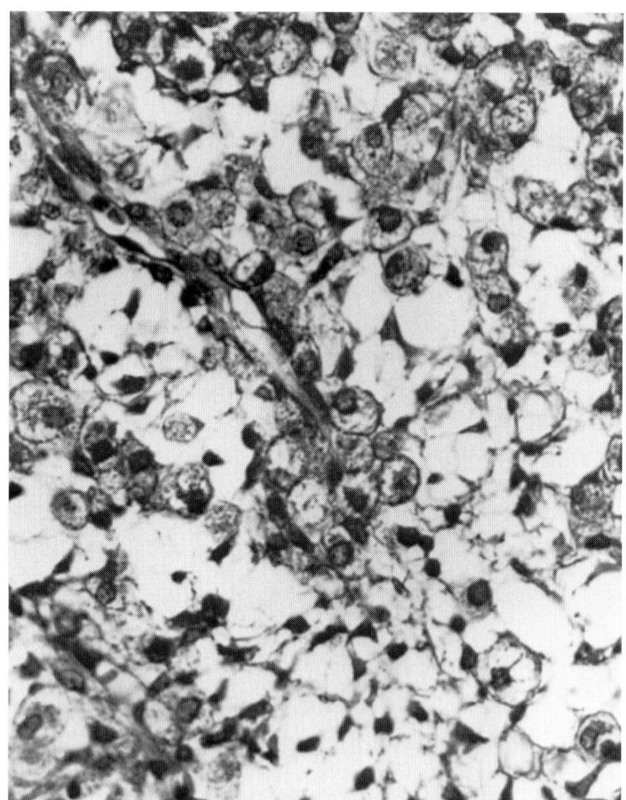

**FIGURE 17–60.** Transitional form between myxoid and round cell liposarcoma with numerous rounded granular cells resembling brown fat.

cells typically arranged in small clusters, cords, or pseudoacini, unlike the single-cell arrangement in pure myxoid liposarcomas. The myxoid background in well stained hematoxylin and eosin sections usually has a pale blue appearance in contrast to the clear appearance of the stroma in myxoid liposarcomas. Extremely myxoid forms of dermatofibrosarcoma protuberans occasionally closely mimic myxoid liposarcoma, but the superficial location of such lesions and the lack of lipoblastic differentiation are important observations that alert one to the correct diagnosis.

The diagnosis of round cell liposarcomas fundamentally rests on finding unequivocal areas of myxoid liposarcoma or lipoblasts in the lesion. Fortunately, pure round cell liposarcomas are extraordinarily rare, and one can almost always find at least a few more differentiated diagnostic zones. Obviously, ancillary studies to exclude other round cell sarcomas such as rhabdomyosarcoma, poorly differentiated (round cell) synovial sarcoma, and Ewing's sarcoma/primitive neuroepithelial tumors are important in selected cases (see Chapter 32).

## Cytogenetic and Molecular Studies

Nearly all myxoid/round cell liposarcomas are characterized by a reciprocal translocation between chro-

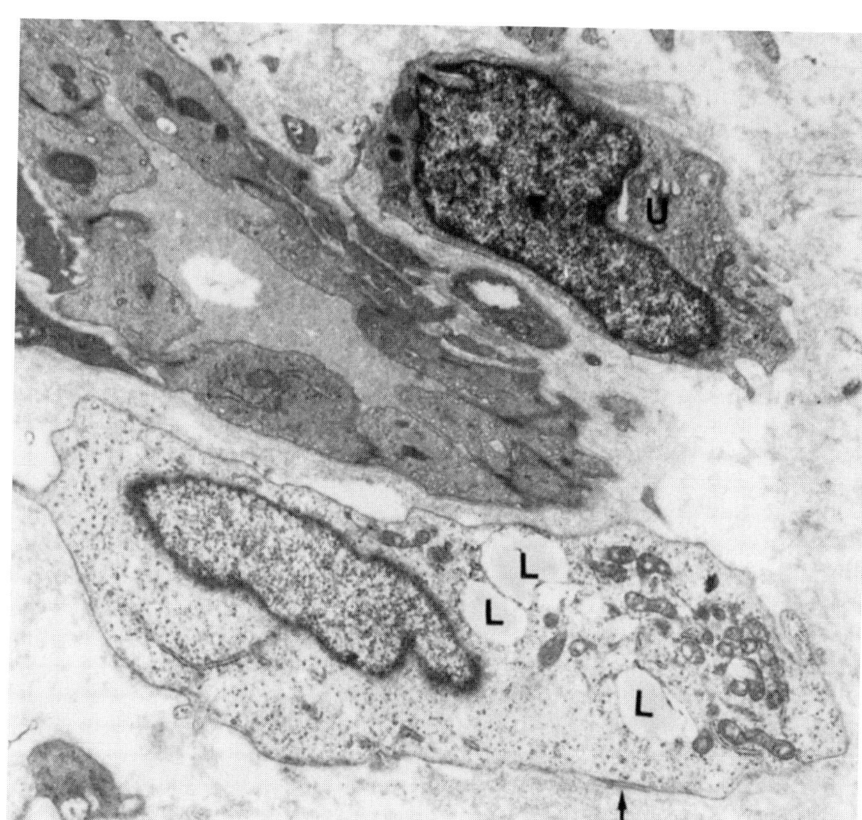


**FIGURE 17–61.** Electron micrograph of a myxoid liposarcoma showing an undifferentiated mesenchymal cell (U) and lipoblasts with multiple non-membrane-bound lipid inclusions (L). Note the basal lamina (arrow). (From Taxy JB, Battifora H. The electron microscope in the study and diagnosis of soft tissue tumors. In: Trump BF, Jones RT (eds) Diagnostic Electron Microscopy. Wiley, New York, 1980.)

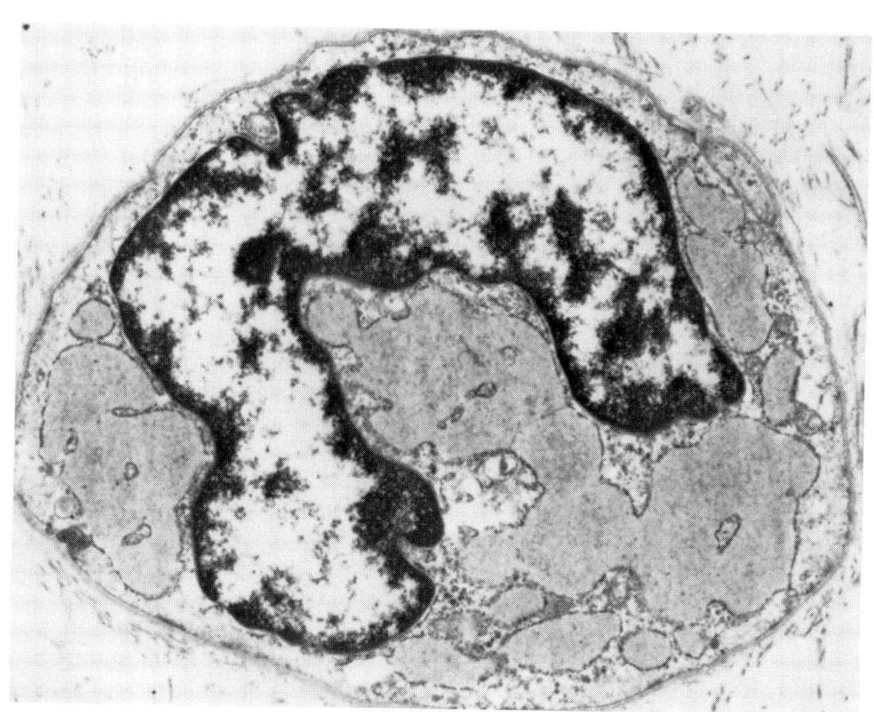

**FIGURE 17–62.** Electron micrograph of an undifferentiated mesenchymal cell from a myxoid liposarcoma. The cell has dilated endoplasmic reticulum filled with granular material suggestive of mucopolysaccharide and is surrounded by a basal lamina. (From Taxy JB, Battifora H. The electron microscope in the study and diagnosis of soft tissue tumors. In: Trump BF, Jones RT (eds) Diagnostic Electron Microscopy, Wiley, New York, 1980.)

mosomes 12 and 16: t(12;16)(q13;p11).[71,72,74,79,81] This molecular event results in fusion of the *CHOP* gene on chromosome 12 with the *TLS* (translocated in liposarcoma) gene on chromosome 16. Rarely translocation between chromosomes 12 and 22,[68,80] t(12;22)(q13; p11), or an insertion between chromosomes 12 and 16, (12;16)(q13;p11.2p13), occurs.[78] The normal *CHOP* gene encodes a DNA transcription factor, whereas the *TLS* gene encodes an RNA binding protein with an affinity for steroid, thyroid hormone, and retinoid receptors.[82] The chimeric *CHOP-TLS* gene gives rise to at least three fusion transcripts,[75,76,89] one of which (type II) has been identified in most myxoid/round cell liposarcomas. When introduced experimentally into preadipocyte cell lines, this transcript makes them unresponsive to adipogenic stimulation and adipocytic genes.[76] These cells also lose the property of contact inhibition and are capable of generating tumors in nude mice. Interestingly, it has also been possible to detect chimeric *CHOP/TLS* DNA in peripheral blood of patients with myxoid/round cell liposarcoma by means of the polymerase chain reaction. Detection of genomic DNA in peripheral blood has not been correlated with clinical outcome on the basis of the few cases studied, however.[80]

A number of studies have focused on the integrity of the *p53* pathway in this group of neoplasms.[70,86] Unlike well differentiated liposarcoma, in which only a small percentage demonstrate aberrations in this pathway, about 30% of myxoid/round cell liposarcomas have mutations in this gene, indicating differences among subsets of liposarcoma in terms of molecular oncogenic events.

## Clinical Course

In the past it has been difficult to compare the behavior of myxoid/round cell liposarcomas because of the lack of common criteria for making the diagnosis, the failure of some to distinguish clearly the pure myxoid forms of the tumor from the remainder, and the inability to compare outcome based on common therapeutic strategies.[35] For example, Enzinger and Winslow reported a 77% five-year survival rate for patients with myxoid liposarcoma in 1962 based on consultation material referred to the AFIP,[11] whereas Reszel et al. reported a survival of 47.3% for patients with all myxoid liposarcomas treated at the Mayo Clinic but included in this category lesions ranging from grade I to III.[29] This group may well have contained both round cell liposarcomas and myxoid forms of malignant fibrous histiocytoma. Considering only grade I myxoid liposarcomas, they reported a 15% mortality rate due to disease at 5 years. More recently, Evans reported metastases in about 50% of myxoid liposarcomas.[13]

Evans suggested dividing this family of lesions into three subgroups depending on the relative amount of round cell differentiation (< 10%, 10–25%, > 25%) and showed that this system correlates well with survival.[13] Tumors should be well sampled (utilizing one section per centimeter tumor diameter) and the proportion of round cell component qualitatively estimated. We have generally labeled those with < 10% round cell differentiation as grade I (and designated them "myxoid liposarcoma"), those with 10–25% as grade II (and designated them "mixed myxoid and round cell liposarcoma"), and the remainder as grade III (and designated them "round cell liposarcoma") Although the Evans system seems to be the best advanced to date, there are still imprecise areas when evaluating these tumors. For example, the Evans system deals only with the percentage of a tumor with a round cell component, not the absolute amount of round cell differentiation. Thus it does not allow for disparities that might occur between a small liposarcoma that contains a large proportion of round cells and a large liposarcoma containing a low percentage of round cells.

The largest series of patients to date treated at one institution showed excellent correlation with survival and metastasis using this system, although it was modified slightly using 5% as the lower threshold for myxoid liposarcoma (Table 17–5). Overall, 35% of patients with these lesions developed metastasis, and 31% died of their tumors. Using a multivariate analysis, age (> 45 years), the percent of round cell differentiation, and the presence of spontaneous necrosis were significantly associated with a poor prognosis (Table 17–6).[73] These authors also analyzed ploidy status in these tumors. Most of the tumors were diploid, and there was no correlation between round cell differentiation and aneuploidy.

Although myxoid/round cell liposarcoma metastasizes to usual sites, such as lung and bone, it displays a curious tendency, unlike all other liposarcomas, to metastasize to other soft tissue sites. Of the 16 metastatic myxoid liposarcomas reported by Evans, 12 me-

**TABLE 17–5 MYXOID/ROUND CELL LIPOSARCOMA: CORRELATION OF ROUND CELL DIFFERENTIATION WITH CLINICAL OUTCOME**

| Round Cell Population (%) | Metastasis |
|---|---|
| 0–5 | 11/48 (23%) |
| 5–10 | 5/14 (35%) |
| >25% | 14/24 (58%) |

From Kilpatrick SE, Doyon J, Choong PF, et al. The clinicopathologic spectrum of myxoid and round cell liposarcoma: a study of 95 cases. Cancer 77: 1450, 1996.

**TABLE 17-6 MYXOID/ROUND CELL LIPOSARCOMA: CORRELATION OF CLINICAL AND HISTOLOGIC FEATURES WITH SURVIVAL**

| Feature | 5-Year Survival (%) | 10-Year Survival (%) |
|---|---|---|
| Age (years) | | |
| <45 | 88 | 80 |
| >45 | 72 | 50 |
| Necrosis | | |
| Yes | 25 | 0 |
| No | 90 | 70 |
| Round cell (%) | | |
| <25 | 89 | 66 |
| >25 | 79 | 40 |

From Kilpatrick SE, Doyon J, Choong PF, et al. The clinicopathologic spectrum of myxoid and round cell liposarcoma: a study of 95 cases. Cancer 77: 1450, 1996, with permission.

tastasized to soft tissue sites, 7 to lung, and 8 to bone.[13]

## PLEOMORPHIC LIPOSARCOMA

Pleomorphic liposarcoma is the least common and consequently the least well understood of the various liposarcomas. It represents about 10–15% of all liposarcomas,[10,11,19,23] develops during late adult life, and is equally distributed between the retroperitoneum and deep somatic soft tissues of the extremities. We have seen an occasional lesion develop as a solitary subcutaneous mass.

Pleomorphic liposarcomas include two related but clearly distinguishable histologic forms: They share a disorderly growth pattern and an extreme degree of cellular pleomorphism, including bizarre giant cells; but they differ in their content of intracellular lipid material. The first, more common form resembles a malignant fibrous histiocytoma but contains, in addition, giant lipoblasts with bizarre hyperchromatic, scalloped nuclei, many of which have a deeply acidophilic cytoplasm with eosinophilic hyaline droplets (Fig. 17–63). In the absence of these characteristic univacuolated or multivacuolated lipoblasts (which may require careful sampling to identify), these lesions are routinely diagnosed as malignant fibrous histiocytoma or rhabdomyosarcoma.

The second form of pleomorphic liposarcoma is less common. It consists mainly of sheets of large pleomorphic giant cells associated with smaller mononuclear forms (Fig. 17–64). Both cell types are highly vacuolated and lipid-rich, and lipoblasts are easy to identify (in contrast to those in the first type of pleomorphic liposarcoma). Depending on the relative proportions of the two cell populations, this form of liposarcoma can be a highly anaplastic tumor or a small round clear-cell tumor resembling a carcinoma or melanoma. Miettinen and Enzinger suggested that tumors with a plethora of small round clear cells be distinguished as a third form of liposarcoma and termed it the "epithelioid" variant. We doubt that this distinction is warranted, as these lesions clearly represent a histologic continuum with those having a plethora of giant cells. Thus until cytogenetic or molecular evidence clearly establishes the separateness of these lesions, we regard pleomorphic liposarcoma as having only two subgroups.

There are few collective data concerning pleomorphic liposarcoma. A 21% five-year survival was reported in the early seminal work of Enzinger and Winslow.[11] Five of eight patients died in the series reported by Miettinen and Enzinger.[90]

## LIPOSARCOMA OF MIXED AND MISCELLANEOUS TYPE

Approximately 5% of liposarcomas do not fit easily into any of the foregoing categories,[26] or they exhibit an unusual combination of patterns. For example, myxoid liposarcomas occasionally display areas of well differentiated liposarcoma, dedifferentiated liposarcoma, or rhabdomyosarcoma. Some liposarcomas, although appearing highly myxoid, display an inordinate degree of nuclear atypia such that they resemble a myxoid malignant fibrous histiocytoma. The WHO has recommended that these unusual cases be diagnosed as liposarcomas of mixed type. More importantly, the combination of patterns along with their relative proportions and grade should be noted so their biologic behavior can be assessed.

## LIPOSARCOMA IN CHILDREN

Although most liposarcomas occur in patients older than 15 years, rare bone fide liposarcomas in patients 10–15 years of age are on record.[92a,97] Liposarcomas in infants and children are vanishingly uncommon, and nearly all such tumors are lipoblastomas or lipoblastomatosis,[93,94] We have encountered unequivocal examples in an 8-month-old boy with a massive tumor in the scapular region and a 3-year-old girl with a tumor of the knee. The former had a tumor of the round cell type and the latter one of the myxoid type. It is remarkable that both were well over 2 years of age at the initial diagnosis. In fact, the youngest patient in a series of 17 children with liposarcoma who died of the disease was an 11-year-old boy with a myxoid liposarcoma of the right axilla that was treated by local excision and postoperative radiotherapy.[97] Many of the reported cases are poorly illustrated and difficult to evaluate.[95,96] Castleberry et

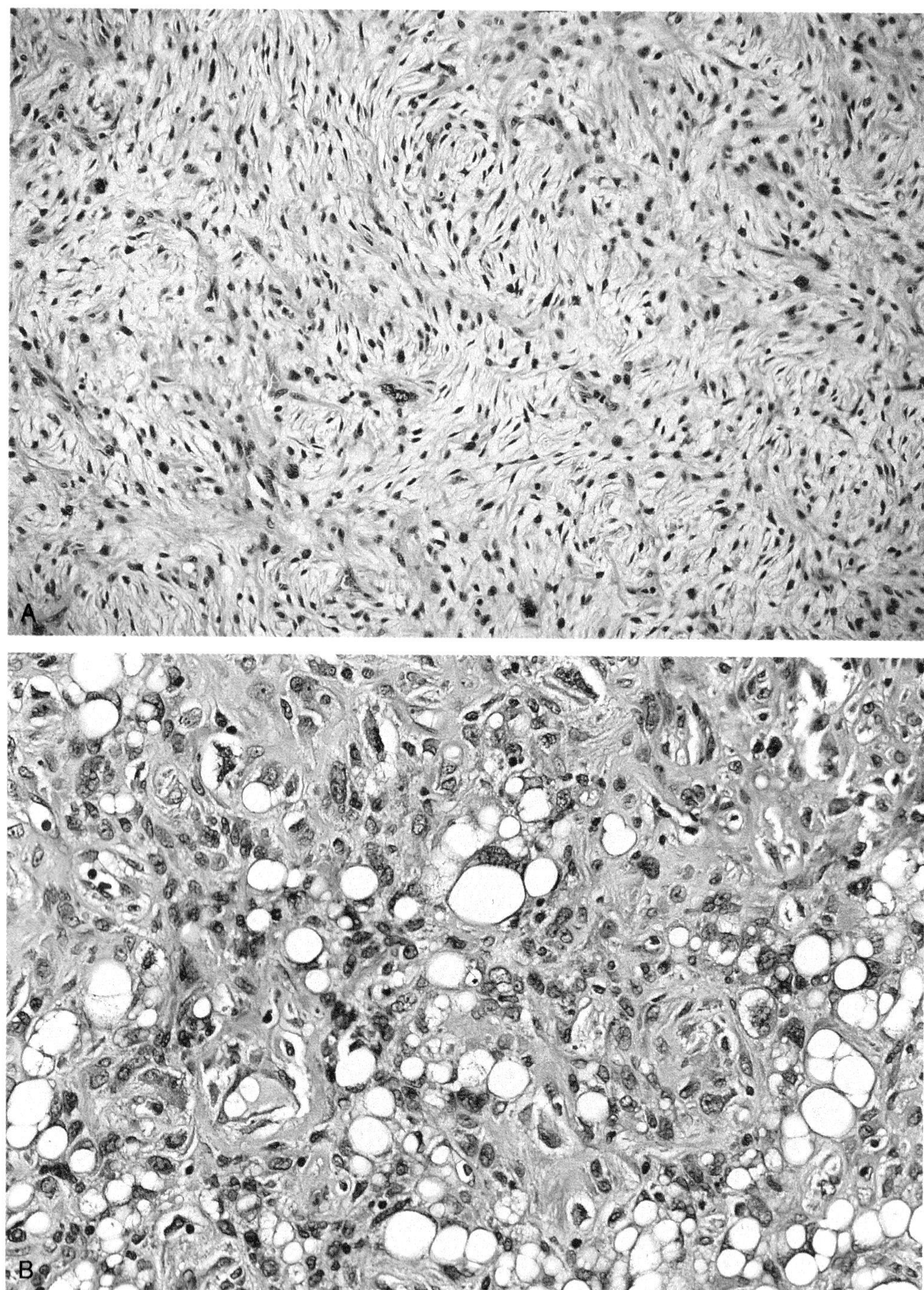


**FIGURE 17–63.** Pleomorphic liposarcoma with areas of undifferentiated pleomorphic sarcoma (**A**) and areas containing pleomorphic lipoblasts (**B**).

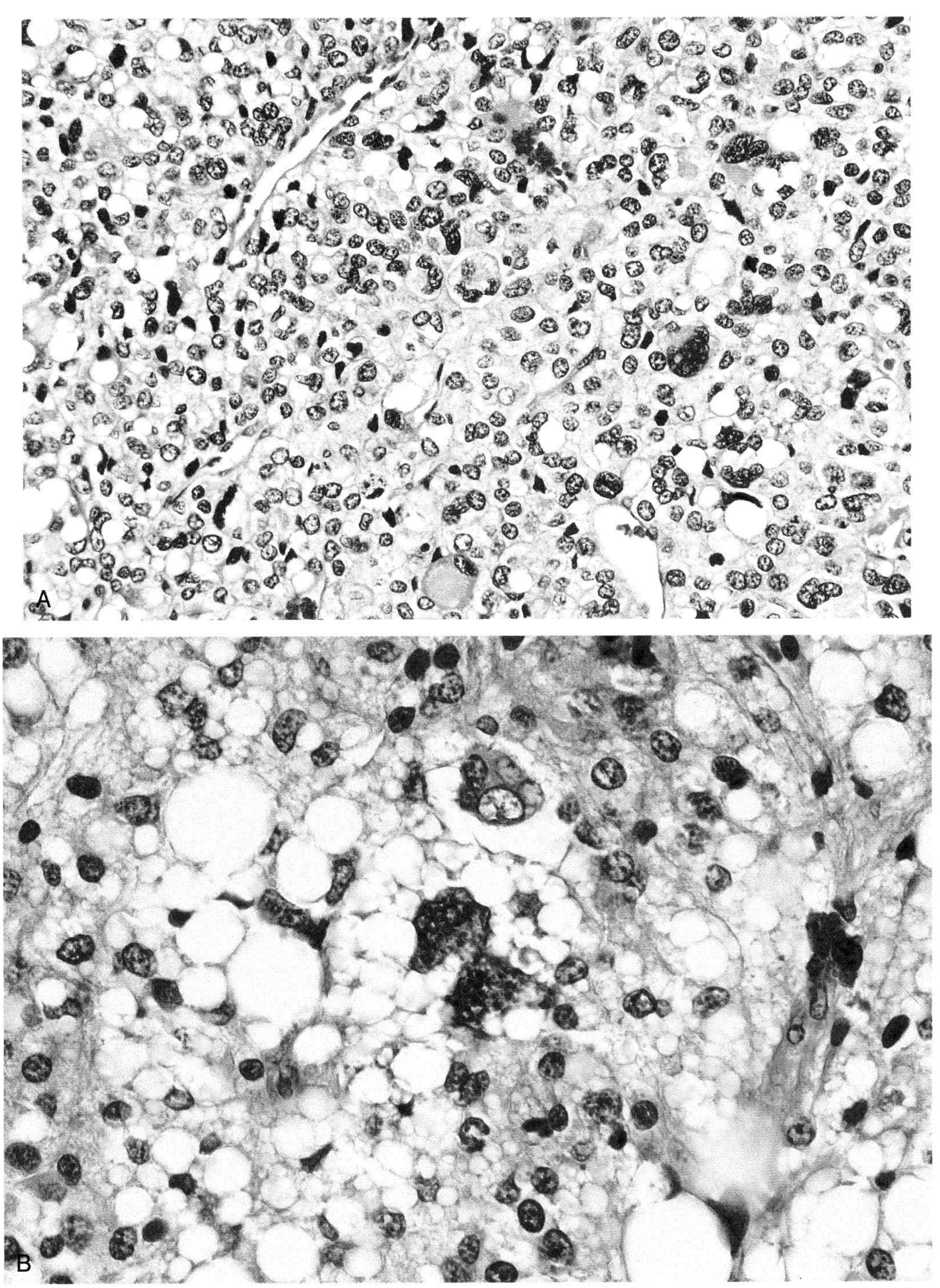


**FIGURE 17–64.** Pleomorphic liposarcoma with sheets of round and pleomorphic cells (**A**) along with pleomorphic lipoblasts (**B**). Tumors may resemble carcinomas of adrenal or renal origin.

al. reviewed the reported cases of childhood liposarcoma in 1984.[92]

## SO-CALLED MULTICENTRIC LIPOSARCOMA

Drawing a sharp line between multicentric and metastatic liposarcoma in the past has been difficult. In favor of the existence of multicentric liposarcomas was the frequent occurrence of another liposarcoma at sites in which metastasis normally does not occur, as well as the long interval between the appearance of the first and second neoplasms.[98,99] Evidence against this concept, however, was the frequent similarity in the histologic pictures of these tumors and the fact that many so-called multicentric liposarcomas develop outright metastases to the lung or other visceral organs at a later stage of the disease.

Recently the ability to study the rearranged portion of the CHOP gene in myxoid liposarcoma presenting in 2 or more locations has indicated clonality of the lesions within a given patient.[98a] This provides a persuasive argument that "multicentric" liposarcomas are in effect metastatic liposarcomas.

## LIPOSARCOMA ARISING IN A LIPOMA

In general, the concept that lipomas give rise to liposarcomas is not accepted. The fact that the two tumors are segregated in terms of location provides circumstantial evidence in support of their distinctness. Based on consultation material reviewed at the AFIP over several decades, we never encountered a clear-cut example of malignant transformation of lipoma, although a few possible cases have been reported in the literature.[100–103] When assessing those cases it is well to remember the histologic variability of some well differentiated liposarcomas and the fact that poor sampling is probably the most common reason well differentiated liposarcomas are underdiagnosed as lipomas. It is possible that cytogenetic analysis of differentiated lipomatous lesions will allow more precise evaluation of this issue.

### REFERENCES

#### General

1. Allsbrook WC, Harmon JD, Congchitnan N, et al. Liposarcoma of the larynx. Arch Pathol Lab Med 109:294, 1985.
2. Arbabi L, Warhol MJ. Pleomorphic liposarcoma following radiotherapy for breast carcinoma. Cancer 49:878, 1982.
3. Arkun R, Memis A, Akalin T, et al. Liposarcoma of soft tissue: MRI findings with pathologic correlation. Skeletal Radiol 26: 167, 1997.
4. Austin RM, Dupree WB. Liposarcoma of the breast: a clinicopathologic study of 20 cases. Hum Pathol 17:906, 1986.
5. Battifora H, Nunez-Alonso C. Myxoid liposarcoma: study of 10 cases. Ultrastruct Pathol 1:157, 1980.
6. Bennett JH, Shousha S, Puddle B, Athanasou NA. Immunohistochemical identification of tumours of adipocytic differentiation using an antibody to a P2 protein. J Clin Pathol 48:950, 1995.
7. Bolen JW, Thorning D. Liposarcomas: a histogenetic approach to the classification of adipose tissue neoplasms. Am J Surg Pathol 8:3, 1984.
7a. Demetri GD, Fletcher CD, Mueller F, et al. Induction of solid tumor differentiation by the peroxisome proliferator-activator receptor-gamma ligand troglitazone in patients with liposarcoma. Proc Natl Acad Sci 96:3951, 1999.
8. de Raucourtz E, Dumont MD, Tourani JM, et al. Acquired factor VII deficiency associated with pleural liposarcoma. Blood Coagul Fibrinolysis 5:833, 1994.
9. Ehara S, Rosenberg AE, Kattapuram SV. Atypical lipomas, liposarcomas, and other fat containing sarcomas: CT analysis of the fat element. Clin Imaging 19:50, 1995.
10. Enterline HT, Culberson JD, Rochlin DB, et al. Liposarcoma: a clinical and pathological study of 53 cases. Cancer 13:932, 1960.
11. Enzinger FM, Winslow DJ. Liposarcoma: a study of 103 cases. Virchows Arch [Pathol Anat] 335:367, 1962.
12. Evans HL. Liposarcoma: a study of 55 cases with a reassessment of its classification. Am J Surg Pathol 3:507, 1979.
13. Evans HL. Liposarcomas and atypical lipomatous tumors: a study of 66 cases followed for a minimum of 10 years. Surg Pathol 1:41, 1988.
14. Fletcher CDM, Akerman M, Dal Cin P, et al. Correlation between clinicopathological features and karyotype in lipomatous tumors: a report of 178 cases from the chromosomes and morphologic (CHAMP) collabortive study group. Am J Pathol 148:623, 1996.
15. Fu YS, Parker FG, Kaye GI, et al. Ultrastructure of benign and malignant adipose tissue tumors. Pathol Annu 15:67, 1980.
16. Golledge J, Fisher C, Rhys-Evans PH. Head and neck liposarcoma. Cancer 76:1051, 1995.
17. Gould VE, Wellington J, Gould NS. Electron microscopy of adipose tissue tumors: comparative features of hibernomas, myxoid and pleomorphic liposarcomas. Pathobiol Annu 9:339, 1979.
18. Hanna W, Kahn HJ, From L. Signet ring lymphoma of the skin: ultrastructural and immunohistochemical features. J Am Acad Dermatol 14:344, 1986.
19. Hashimoto H, Daimaru Y, Enjoji M. S-100 protein distribution in liposarcoma: an immunoperoxidase study with special reference to the distinction of liposarcoma from myxoid malignant fibrous histiocytoma. Virchows Arch [Pathol Anat] 405:1, 1984.
20. Hashimoto H, Enjoji M. Liposarcoma: a clinicopathologic subtyping of 52 cases. Acta Pathol Jpn 32:933, 1982.
21. Jelinek JS, Kransdorf MJ, Schmookler BM, et al. Liposarcoma of the extremities: MR and CT findings in the histologic subtypes. Radiology 186:455, 1993.
22. Kim H, Dorfman RF, Rappaport H. Signet ring cell lymphoma: a rare morphological and functional expression of nodular (follicular) lymphoma. Am J Surg Pathol 2:119, 1978.
23. Kindblom LG, Angervall L, Svendsen P. Liposarcoma: a clinicopathologic, radiographic and prognostic study. Acta Pathol Microbiol Scand 253:1, 1975.
24. Kindblom LG, Save-Soderbergh J. The ultrastructure of liposarcoma: a study of 10 cases. Acta Pathol Microbiol Scand [A] 87:109, 1979.

25. Klimstra DS, Moran CA, Perino G, et al. Liposarcoma of the anterior mediastinum and thymus: a clinicopathologic study of 28 cases. Am J Surg Pathol 119:782, 1995.
26. Menon M, Velthoven PM. Liposarcoma of the breast. Arch Pathol 98:370, 1974.
27. Mentzel T, Fletcher CD. Dedifferentiated myxoid liposarcoma: a clincopathological study suggesting a closer relationship between myxoid and well-differentiated liposarcoma. Histopathology 30:457, 1997.
28. Pilotti S, Della Torre G, Lavarino C, et al. Distinct mdm2/p53 expression patterns in liposarcoma subgroups: implications for different pathogenetic mechanisms. J Pathol 181:14, 1997.
29. Reszel PA, Soule EH, Coventry MB. Liposarcoma of the extremities and limb girdles: a study of 222 cases. J Bone Joint Surg Am 48:229, 1966.
30. Rossouw DJ, Cinti S, Dickersin GR. Liposarcoma: an ultrastructural study of 15 cases. Am J Clin Pathol 85:649, 1985.
31. Rubin BP, Fletcher CDM. The cytogenetics of lipomatous tumours. Histopathology 30:507, 1997.
32. Russell WO, Cohen J, Enzinger FM, et al. A clinical and pathological staging system for soft tissue sarcomas. Cancer 40: 1562, 1977.
33. Suster S, Fisher C. Immunoreactivity for the human hematopoietic progenitor cell antigen (CD34) in lipomatous tumors. Am J Surg Pathol 21:195, 1997.
34. Taxy JB, Battifora H. The electron microscope in the study and diagnosis of soft tissue tumors. In: Trump BF, Jones RT (eds) Diagnostic Electron Microscopy. Wiley, New York, 1980, p 147.
34a. Tontonoz P, Singer S, Forman BM, et al. Terminal differentiation of human liposarcoma cells induced by ligands for peroxisome proliferator-activator receptor gamma and the retinoid X receptor. Proc Natl Acad Sci 94:237, 1997.
35. Weiss SW. Lipomatous tumors. In: Weiss SW, Brooks JJ (eds) Soft Tissue Tumors. Williams & Wilkins, Baltimore, 1996.
36. Weiss SW, Sobin LH. Histological Typing of Soft Tissue Tumours, Springer Verlag, Berlin, 1994.
37. Wenig BM, Heffner DK. Liposarcomas of the larynx and hypopharynx: a clinicopathologic study of eight new cases and a review of the literature. Laryngoscope 105:747, 1995.
38. Winslow DJ, Enzinger FM. Hyaluronidase-sensitive acid mucopolysaccharides in liposarcomas. Am J Pathol 37:497, 1960.


### Well Differentiated Liposarcoma (Atypical Lipoma; Atypical Lipomatous Tumor)


39. Argani P, Facchetti F, Inghirami G, Rosai J. Lymphocyte-rich well-differentiated liposarcoma: report of nine cases. Am J Surg Pathol 21:884, 1997.
40. Azumi N, Curtis J, Kempson RL, et al. Atypical and malignant neoplasms showing lipomatous differentiation: a study of 111 cases. Am J Surg Pathol 11:161, 1987.
41. Berthe JV, Goldschmidt D, Salmon I, et al. Image cytometry analysis of Feulgen-stained nuclei in 72 lipomatous lesions including atypical lipomas and well-differentiated liposarcomas. Am J Clin Pathol 106:289, 1996.
42. Brooks JJ, Connor AM. Aypical lipoma of the extremities and peripheral soft tissues with dedifferentiation: implications for management Surg Pathol 3:169, 1990.
43. Evans HL. Smooth muscle in atypical lipomatous tumors: a report of three cases. Am J Surg Pathol 14:714, 1990.
44. Evans HL, Soule EH, Winkelman RK. Atypical lipoma, atypical intramuscular lipoma, and well differentiated retroperitoneal liposarcoma. Cancer 43:574, 1979.
45. Farshid G, Weiss SW. Massive localized lymphedema in the morbidly obese simulating liposarcoma. Mod Pathol 10:9A, 1997.
46. Goldblum JR, Poy ES, Frank TS, Weiss SW. p53 mutations and histologic progression in well-differentiated liposarcoma and dermatofibrosarcoma protuberans. Int J Surg Pathol 3:35, 1995.
47. Gomez-Roman JJ, Val-Bernal JF. Lipoleiomyosarcoma of the mediastinum. Pathology 29:428, 1997.
48. Kindblom LG, Angervall L, Fassina AS. Atypical lipoma. Acta Pathol Microbiol Scand 90A:27, 1982.
49. Kraus MD, Guillou L, Fletcher CD. Well-differentiated inflammtory liposarcoma: an uncommon and easily overlooked variant of a common sarcoma. Am J Surg Pathol 21:518, 1997.
50. Lazarus SS, Trombetta LD. Ultrastructure and histochemical identification of sclerosing liposarcoma. Histopathology 5:223, 1981.
51. Lucas DR, Nascimento AG, Sanjay KSS, Rock MG. Well-differentiated liposarcoma: the Mayo Clinic experience with 58 cases. Am J Clin Pathol 102:677, 1994.
52. Pedeutour F, Suijkerbuijk RF, Forus A, et al. Complex composition and co-amplification of SAS and MDM2 in ring and giant rod marker chromosomes in well- differentiated liposarcoma. Genes Chromosomes Cancer 10:85, 1994.
53. Rosai J, Akerman M, Dal Cin P, et al. Combined morphologic and karyotypic study of 59 atypical lipomatous tumors: evaluation of their relationship and differential diagnosis with other adipose tissue tumors (a report of the CHAMP study group). Am J Surg Pathol 20:1182, 1996.
54. Suster S, Wong TY, Moran CA. Sarcomas with combined features of liposarcoma and leiomyosarcoma: study of two cases of an unusual soft-tissue tumor showing dual lineage differentiation. Am J Surg Pathol 17:905, 1993.
55. Tallini G, Dal Cin P, Rhoden KJ, et al. Expression of HMGI-C and HMG(Y) in ordinary and atypical lipomatous tumors: immunohistochemical reactivity correlates with karyotypic alterations. Am J Pathol 151:37, 1997.
56. Tallini G, Erlandson RA, Brennan MF, et al. Divergent myosarcomatous differentiation in retroperitoneal liposarcoma. Am J Surg Pathol 17:546, 1993.
57. Weiss SW, Rao VK. Well differentiated liposarcoma (atypical lipoma) of deep soft tissue of the extremities, retroperitoneum and miscellaneous sites: a follow-up study of 92 cases with analysis of the incidence of "dedifferentiation." Am J Surg Pathol 16:1051, 1992.


### Dedifferentiated Liposarcoma


58. Chorneyko K. The ultrastructure of liposarcomas with attention to "dedifferentiation." Ultrastruct Pathol 21:545, 1997.
59. Coindre JM, de Loynes B, Bui NB, et al. Dedifferentiated liposarcoma: a clinicopathologic study of 6 cases. Ann Pathol 12: 20, 1992.
60. Dei Tos AP, Doglioni C, Piccinin S, et al. Molecular abnormalities of the p53 pathway in dedifferentiated liposarcoma. J Pathol 181:8, 1997.
61. Elgar F, Goldblum JR. Well-differentiated of the retroperitoneum: a clinicopathologic analysis of 20 cases, with particular attention to the extent of low grade dedifferentiation. Mod Pathol 10:113, 1997.
61a. Fanburg-Smith JC, Miettinen M. Liposarcoma with meningothelial like whorls: a study of 17 cases of a distinctive histological pattern associated with dedifferentiated liposarcoma. Histopathol 33:414, 1998.
62. Henricks WH, Chu Y-C, Goldblum JR, Weiss SW. Dedifferentiated liposarcoma: a clinicopathological analysis of 155 cases with a proposal for an expanded definition of dedifferentiation. Am J Surg Pathol 21:271, 1997.
63. Hisaoka M, Tsuji S, Hashimoto H, et al. Dedifferentiated liposarcoma with an inflammatory malignant fibrous histiocytoma-like component presenting a leukemoid reaction. Pathol Int 47:642, 1997.

64. Kransdorf MJ, Meis JM, Jelinek JS. Dedifferentiated liposarcoma of the extremities: imaging findings in four patients. AJR 161:127, 1993.
65. McCormick D, Mentzel T, Beham A, Fletcher CDM. Dedifferentiated liposarcoma: clinicopathologic analysis of 32 cases suggesting a better prognostic group among pleomorphic sarcomas. Am J Surg Pathol 18:1213, 1994.
65a. Nascimento AG, Kurtin PJ, Guillou L, Fletcher CDM. Dedifferentiated liposarcoma: a report of nine cases with a peculiar neurallike whorling pattern associated with metaplastic bone formation. Am J Surg Path 22:945, 1998.
66. Salzano RP, Tomkiewicz Z, Africano WA. Dedifferentiated liposarcoma with features of rhabdomyosarcoma. Conn Med 55: 200, 1991.
67. Yoshikawa H, Ueda T, Mori S, et al. Dedifferentiatied liposarcoma of the subcutis. Am J Surg Pathol 20:1525, 1996.

### Myxoid/Round Cell Liposarcoma

68. Dal Cin P, Sciot R, Panagopoulos I, et al. Additional evidence of a variant translocation t(12;22) with EWS/CHOP fusion in myxoid liposarcoma: clinicopathologic features. J Pathol 182: 437, 1997.
69. Dei Tos AP, Mentzel T, Newman PL, Fletcher CDM. Spindle cell liposarcoma: a hitherto unrecognized variant of well-differentiated liposarcoma: an analysis of six cases. Am J Surg Pathol 18:913, 1994.
70. Dei Tos AP, Piccinin S, Doglioni C, et al. Molecular aberrations of the $G_1$-S checkpoint in myxoid and round cell liposarcoma. Am J Pathol 151:1531, 1997.
71. Dijkhuizen T, Molenaar WM, Hoekstra HJ, et al. Cytogenetic analysis of a case of myxoid liposarcoma with cartilaginous differentiation. Cancer Genet Cytogenet 92:141, 1996.
72. Gibas Z, Miettinen M, Limon J, et al. Cytogenetic and immunohistochemical studies were performed in nine myxoid liposarcomas: Am J Clin Pathol 103:20, 1995.
73. Kilpatrick SE, Doyon J, Choong PF, et al. The clinicopathologic spectrum of myxoid and round cell liposarcoma: a study of 95 cases. Cancer 77:1450, 1996.
74. Knight JC, Renwick PJ, Cin PD, et al. Translocation t(12; 16)(q13;p11) in myxoid liposarcoma and round cell liposarcoma: molecular and cytogenetic analysis. Cancer Res 55:24, 1995.
75. Kuroda M, Ishida T, Horiuchi H, et al. Chimeric TLS/FUS-CHOP gene expression and the heterogeneity of its junction in human myxoid and round cell liposarcoma. Am J Pathol 147: 1221, 1995.
76. Kuroda M, Ishida T, Takanashi M, et al. Oncogenic transformation and inhibition of adipocytic conversion of preadipocytes by TLS/FUS-CHOP type II chimeric protein. Am J Pathol 151:735, 1997.
77. Lagace R, Jacob S, Seemayer TA. Myxoid liposarcoma: an electron microscopic study: biological and histogenic considerations. Virchows Arch [Pathol Anat] 384:159, 1979.
78. Mrozek K, Szumigala J, Brooks JS, et al. Round cell liposarcoma with the insertion (12;16)(q13;p11.2p13). Am J Clin Pathol 108:35, 1997.
78a. Oliveira AM, Nascimento AG, Okuno SH, Lloyd RV. p27(kip1) protein expression correlates with survival in myxoid and round-cell liposarcoma. J Clin Oncol 18:2888, 2000.
79. Orndal C, Mandahl N, Rydholm A, et al. Chromosomal evolution and tumor progression in a myxoid liposarcoma. Acta Orthop Scand 61:99, 1990.
80. Panagopoulos I, Aman P, Mertens F, et al. Genomic PCR detects tumor cells in peripheral blood from patients with myxoid liposarcoma. Genes Chromosomes Cancer 17:102, 1996.
81. Panagopoulos I, Hoglund M, Mertens F, et al. Fusion of the EWS and CHOP genes in myxoid liposarcoma. Oncogene 12: 489, 1996.
81a. Pearlstone DB, Pisters PW, Bold RJ, et al. Patterns of recurrence in extremity liposarcoma: implications for staging and follow-up. Cancer 85:85, 1999.
82. Powers CS, Mathur M, Raaka BM, et al. TLS (translocated-in-liposarcoma) is a high affinity interactor for steroid, thyroid hormone, and retinoid receptors. Mol Endocrinol 12:4, 1998.
83. Shanks JH, Banerjee SS, Eyden BP. Focal rhabdomyosarcomatous differentition in primary liposarcoma. J Clin Pathol 49: 770, 1996.
84. Siebert JDS, Williams RP, Pulitzer DR. Myxoid liposarcoma with cartilaginous differentiation. Mod Pathol 9:249, 1996.
85. Smith TA, Easley KA, Goldblum JR. Myxoid/round cell liposarcoma of the extremities: a clinicopathologic study of 29 cases with particular attention to the extent of round cell liposarcoma. Am J Surg Pathol 17:171, 1996.
86. Smith TA, Goldblum JR. Immunohistochemical analysis of p53 protein in myxoid/round cell liposarcoma of the extremities. Appl Immunohistochem 4:228, 1996.
87. Tallini G, Akerman M, Dal Cin P, et al. Combined morphologic and karyotypic study of 28 myxoid liposarcomas: implications for a revised morphologic typing (a report from the CHAMP Group). Am J Surg Pathol 20:1047, 1996.
88. Tsuneyoshi M, Hashimoto H, Enjoji M. Myxoid malignant fibrous histiocytoma versus myxoid liposarcoma: a comparative ultrastructural study. Virchows Arch [Pathol Anat] 400:187, 1983.
89. Yang X, Nagasaki K, Egawa S, et al. FUS/TLS-CHOP chimeric transcripts in liposarcoma tissues. Jpn J Clin Oncol 25:234, 1995.

### Pleomorphic Liposarcoma

89a. Downes KA, Goldblum JR, Montgomery E, Fisher C. Pleomorphic liposarcoma: a clinicopathologic analysis of 19 cases. Mod Pathol 13:9A (Abst 29), 2000.
90. Miettinen M, Enzinger FM. Epithelioid variant of pleomorphic liposarcoma: a study of 12 cases of a distinctive variant of high-grade liposarcoma. Mod Pathol 12:722, 1999.
91. Suzuki T. Ultrastructural characteristics of a pleomorphic liposarcoma: a possible involvement of myofibroblasts. Acta Pathol Jpn 37:843, 1987.

### Liposarcoma in Children

92. Castleberry RP, Kelly DR, Wilson ER, et al. Childhood liposarcoma: report of a case and review of the literature. Cancer 54: 579, 1984.
92a. Ferrari A, Casanova M, Spreafico F, et al. Childhood liposarcoma: a single institutional twenty year experience. Pediatric Hematology & Oncology 16:415, 1999.
93. Hanada M, Tokuda R, Ohnishi Y, et al. Benign lipoblastoma and liposarcoma in children. Acta Pathol Jpn 36:605, 1986.
94. Kauffman SL, Stout AP. Lipoblastic tumors of children. Cancer 12:912, 1959.
95. Kretschmer HL. Retroperitoneal lipofibrosarcoma in a child. J Urol 43:61, 1940.
96. Peeples WJ, Hazra T. Retroperitoneal liposarcoma in a child. Urology 7:89, 1976.
97. Shmookler BM, Enzinger FM. Liposarcoma occurring in children: an analysis of 17 cases and review of the literature. Cancer 52:567, 1983.

### So-Called Multicentric Liposarcoma

98. Ackerman LV. Multiple primary liposarcomas. Am J Pathol 20:789, 1944.

98a. Antonescu CR, Humphrey H, Elahi A, et al. Monoclonality of multifocal myxoid liposarcoma: molecular confirmation by analysis of TLS-CHOP or EWS-CHOP rearrangements. Mod Pathol 13:7A (Abst 21), 2000.
99. Barkhof F, Melkert P, Meyer S, et al. Derangement of adipose tissue: a case report of multicentric retroperitoneal liposarcoma, retroperitoneal lipomatosis, and multiple subcutaneous lipomas. Eur J Oncol 17:547, 1991.

### Liposarcoma Arising in Lipoma

100. Sampson CC, Saunders EH, Green WE, et al. Liposarcoma developing in a lipoma. Arch Pathol 69:506, 1960.
101. Schiller H. Lipomata in sarcomatous transformation. Surg Gynecol Obstet 27:218, 1918.
102. Sternberg SS. Liposarcoma arising within a subcutaneous lipoma. Cancer 5:975, 1952.
103. Wright CJE. Liposarcoma arising in a simple lipoma. J Pathol Bacteriol 60:483, 1948.

# CHAPTER 18

# BENIGN TUMORS OF SMOOTH MUSCLE

To a large extent the distribution of benign smooth muscle tumors parallels the distribution of smooth muscle tissue in the body. The tumors tend to be relatively common in the genitourinary and gastrointestinal tracts, less frequent in the skin, and rare in deep soft tissue. In the experience of Farman,[1] based on 7748 leiomyomas, approximately 95% occurred in the female genital tract, and the remainder were scattered over various sites, including the skin (230 cases), gastrointestinal tract (67 cases), and bladder (5 cases). This study, based on surgical material, probably underestimates the large number of asymptomatic gastrointestinal and genitourinary lesions documented only in autopsy material. In general, soft tissue leiomyomas cause little morbidity; hence, there are few studies in the literature concerning their presentation, diagnosis, and therapy. For purposes of classification these tumors can be divided into several groups.

Cutaneous leiomyomas (leiomyoma cutis) comprise the most common group and are of two types. Those arising from the pilar arrector muscles of the skin are often multiple and associated with significant pain. Those arising from the network of muscle fibers that lie in the deep dermis of the scrotum (dartoic muscles), labia majora, and nipple are almost always solitary and are collectively referred to as genital leiomyomas.[24–26,28] The second group of benign smooth muscle tumors includes the angiomyomas (vascular leiomyomas),[33–38] which are distinctive, painful, subcutaneous tumors composed of a conglomerate of thick-walled vessels associated with smooth muscle tissue. They differ from cutaneous leiomyomas in their anatomic distribution, predominantly subcutaneous location, and predilection for women. The leiomyomas of deep soft tissue[39–48] comprise the third group of benign smooth muscle tumors. These tumors are much larger than their superficial counterparts, usually display a greater spectrum of histologic changes, and must be clearly distinguished from leiomyosarcomas, which are statistically more common in deep soft tissue. Some deep leiomyomas probably arise from blood vessels, but their large size at the time of diagnosis makes it difficult to establish this point with certainty. Leiomyomatosis peritonealis disseminata[59–82] and intravenous leiomyomatosis[49–58] are also included, although they are not strictly soft tissue tumors. The first can be conceptualized as a diffuse metaplastic response of the peritoneal surfaces in which multiple smooth muscle nodules form. The second is a uterine tumor that extends into the uterine or pelvic veins. Both may be confused with metastatic leiomyosarcoma because of their unusual growth patterns. Lastly, a number of newly described lesions are discussed in this chapter (palisaded myofibroblastoma,[83–94] myofibroblastoma of the breast,[95–101] angiomyofibroblastoma),[102,106] which are composed of modified smooth muscle cells.

## STRUCTURE AND FUNCTION OF SMOOTH MUSCLE CELLS

Smooth muscle cells are widely distributed throughout the body and contribute to the wall of the gastrointestinal, genitourinary, and respiratory tracts. They constitute the muscles of the skin, erectile muscles of the nipple and scrotum, and iris of the eye. Their characteristic arrangements in these organs determine the net effect of contraction. For instance, the circumferential arrangement in blood vessels results in narrowing of the lumen during contraction, whereas contraction of the longitudinal and circumferential muscle layers in the gastrointestinal tract causes the propulsive peristaltic wave.

Smooth muscle cells are fusiform in shape and have centrally located cylindrical nuclei with round ends that develop deep indentations during contraction. The length of the muscle cell varies depending on the organ, achieving its greatest length in the gravid uterus, where it may measure as much as 0.5 mm. The cells are usually arranged in fascicles in which the nuclei are staggered so the tapered end of one cell lies in close association with the thick nuclear region of an adjacent cell. Typically there are no connective tissue cells between individual muscle fibers, although a delicate basal lamina and small connective tissue fibers, presumably synthesized by the muscle cells,[6] can be seen as a delicate periodic acid-Schiff (PAS)-positive rim around individual cells in light microscopic preparations.

Ultrastructurally, the cells are characterized by clusters of mitochondria, rough endoplasmic reticulum, and free ribosomes, which occupy the zone immediately adjacent to the nucleus. The remainder of the cytoplasm (sarcoplasm) is filled with myofilaments oriented parallel to the long axis of the cell.[2–5] There are three types of filament in the cell. Thick myosin filaments (12 nm) are surrounded by seven to nine thin actin filaments (6–8 nm). Thick and thin filaments are aggregated into larger groups, or units, which correspond by light microscopy to linear myofibrils. In addition to the contractile proteins, intermediate filaments, measuring 10 nm and forming part of the cytoskeleton, are centered around the dense bodies or plaques, which are believed to be the smooth muscle analogue of the Z-band. The plasma membrane is dotted with tiny pinocytotic vesicles; and overlying the surface of the cell is a delicate basal lamina. Although the basal lamina separates individual cells, limited areas exist between cells in which the substance is lacking and in which the plasma membranes lie in close proximity, separated by a space of about 2 nm. This area, known as a gap junction or nexus, may allow spread of electrical impulses between adjacent cells.

Smooth muscle cells display diversity in their content of contractile and intermediate filament proteins, depending on their location and function. It is useful to be aware of some of the regional variations when evaluating neoplasms. For example, the gamma isoform of muscle actin is present along with desmin in most smooth muscle cells, whereas in vascular smooth muscle the alpha isoform of muscle actin and vimentin predominate.

## CUTANEOUS LEIOMYOMA (LEIOMYOMA CUTIS)

Superficial, or cutaneous, leiomyomas are of two types. Those arising from the pilar arrector muscles of the skin may be solitary or multifocal and are often associated with considerable pain and tenderness.[20] The other form, the genital leiomyoma, arises from the diffuse network of muscle in the deep dermis of the genital zones (e.g., scrotum, nipple, areola, vulva). In the scrotum they arise from the dartoic muscles (dartoic leiomyoma) and in the nipple from the muscularis mamillae and areolae. This form is nearly always solitary and rarely causes significant pain.

### Leiomyoma of Pilar Arrector Origin

Although formerly believed to be the more common form of cutaneous leiomyoma,[16,27] leiomyomas of pilar arrector origin are probably far less common than previously thought[32] and are probably outnumbered by those arising in genital sites. They may be solitary or multiple. Most develop during adolescence or early adult life, although occasional cases appear at birth or during early childhood. Some of these lesions occur on a familial basis[11,17,21,31] seemingly inherited as an autosomal dominant trait with variable penetrance.[21] The distribution of lesions among affected family members does not always follow a similar pattern.[11] Multiple cutaneous leiomyomas have also been associated with dermatitis herpetiformis and HLA-B8,[19] premature uterine leiomyomas,[14,15] increased erythropoietin activity,[13,30] and multiple endocrine adenomatosis (type I).[12] Typically the lesions develop as small brown-red to pearly discrete papules that in the incipient stage can be palpated more readily than they can be seen (Fig. 18–1). Eventually they form nodules that coalesce into a fine linear pattern following a dermatome distribution. The extensor surfaces of the extremities are most often affected. The lesions often produce significant pain that can be triggered by exposure to cold. In one unusual case reported by Fisher and Helwig,[16] the patient claimed that strong emotions evoked pain in the lesions. It is not clear whether the pain produced by these tumors is the result of contraction of the muscle tissue or compression of nearby nerves by the tumors. Usually the tumors grow slowly over a period of years, with new lesions forming as older lesions stabilize. The slowly progressive nature of the disease probably accounts for the fact that patients often seek medical attention only after a number of years.

Most pilar leiomyomas are 1–2 cm in diameter. They lie in the dermal connective tissue and are separated from the overlying atrophic epidermis by a grenz zone. The lesions are less well defined than the angiomyoma and blend in an irregular fashion with the surrounding dermal collagen and adjacent pilar muscle (Fig. 18–2). The central portions of the lesions are usually devoid of connective tissue and consist exclusively of packets or bundles of smooth muscle fibers. They usually intersect in an orderly fashion and often create the impression of hyperplasia or overgrowth of the pilar arrector muscle. The cells resemble normal smooth muscle cells, and myofibrils can be easily demonstrated with special stains such as the Masson trichrome stain, in which they appear as red linear streaks traversing the cytoplasm in a longi-

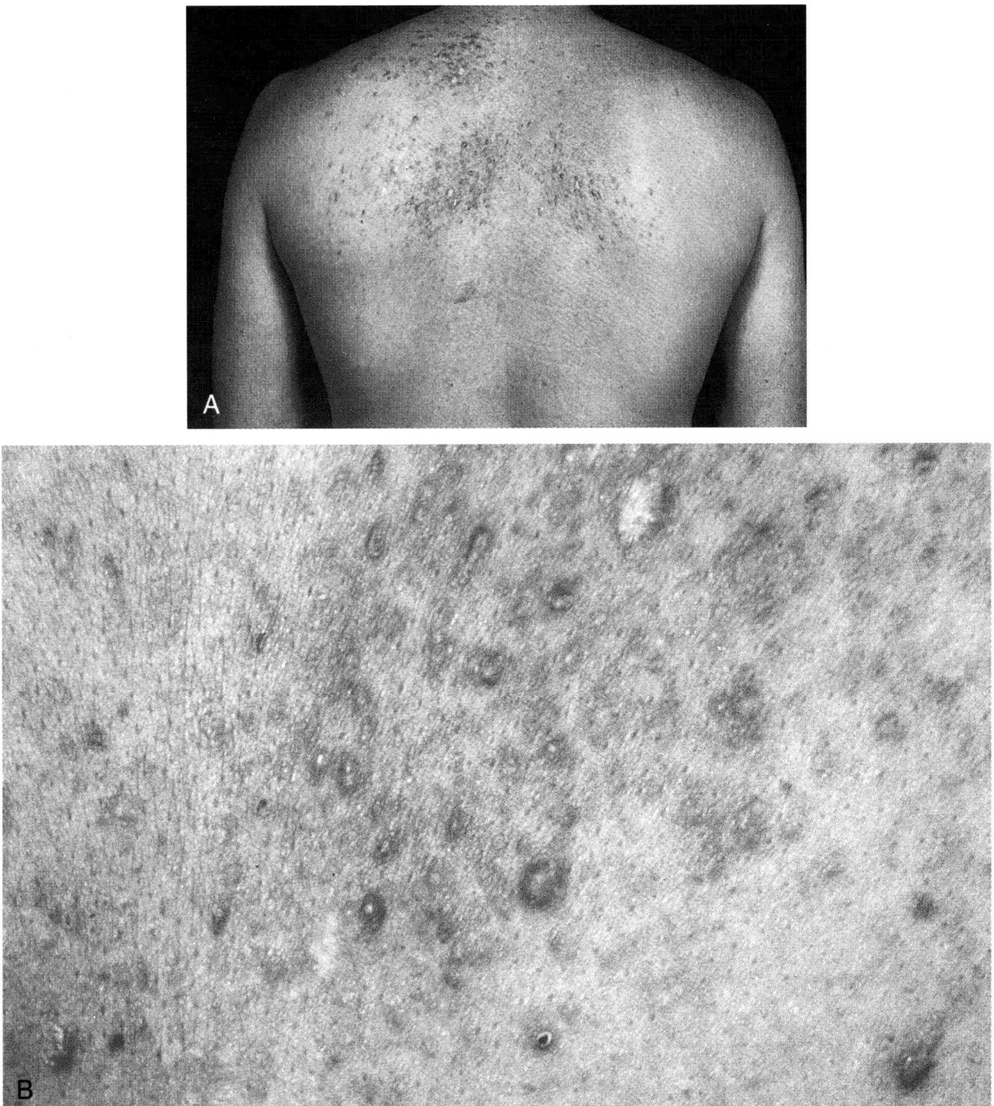


**FIGURE 18–1.** (**A, B**) Clinical appearance of multiple cutaneous leiomyomas.

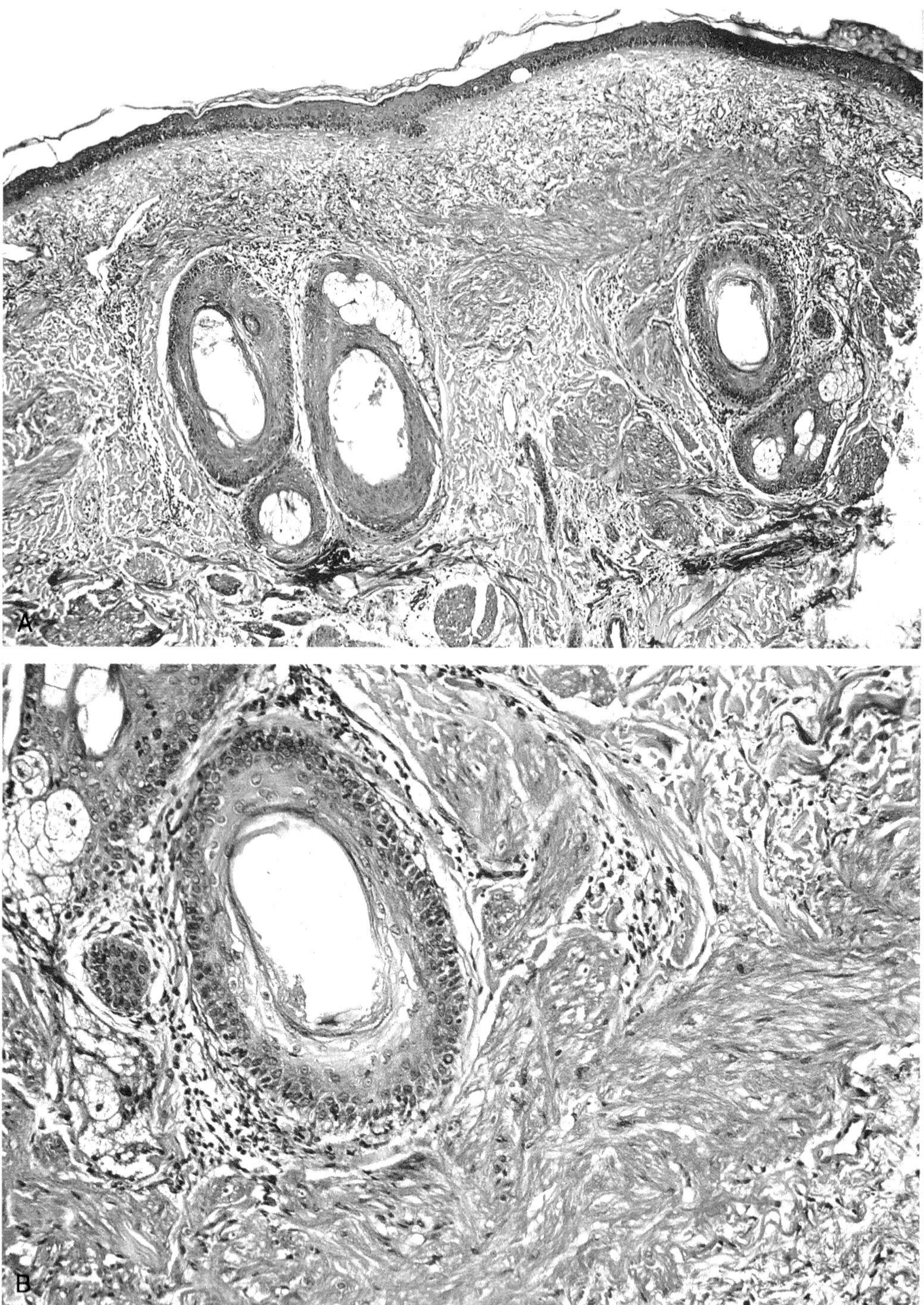


**FIGURE 18–2.** (**A**) Cutaneous leiomyoma of pilar arrector origin. (**B**) Smooth muscle bundles are closely associated with hair follicles and consist of well-differentiated, highly oriented cells.

tudinal fashion. Muscle antigens are readily identified by immunohistochemistry (Fig. 18–3). Ultrastructurally, the cells have myofilaments, surface pinocytotic vesicles, and investing basal laminae.[22]

Diagnosis is rarely difficult in the typical case, particularly one with a characteristic history. Occasionally solitary forms of the disease are mistaken for other benign tumors such as the cutaneous fibrous histiocytoma (dermatofibroma). The cells in the fibrous histiocytoma are slender, less well ordered, and lack myofibrils. Secondary elements such as inflammatory cells, giant cells, and xanthoma cells, common to the cutaneous fibrous histiocytoma, are lacking in the cutaneous leiomyoma. Distinction of cutaneous leiomyomas from lesions reported as smooth muscle hamartomas of the skin is less clear-cut and may relate more to differences in clinical presentation than histologic features. Smooth muscle hamartomas are typically described as a single lesion measuring several centimeters in diameter and occurring in the lumbar region during childhood or early adult life.[18]

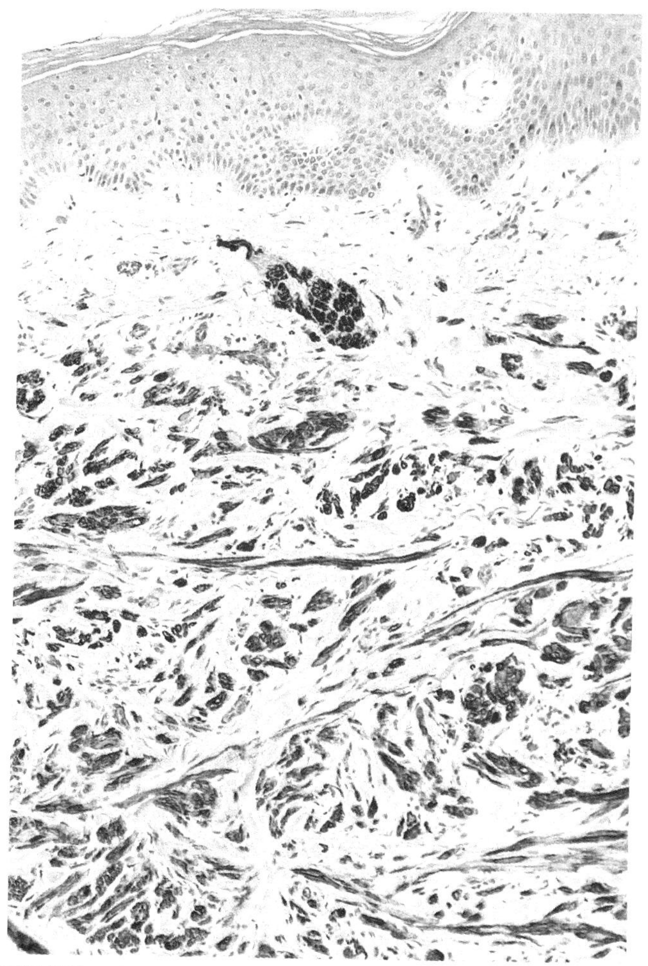

**FIGURE 18–3.** Actin immunostain of a cutaneous leiomyoma showing irregular packets and fascicles of spindle cells.

Consisting of well defined smooth muscle bundles in the dermis, these lesions are sometimes associated with hyperpigmentation and hypertrichosis (Becker's nevus).[29]

Cutaneous leiomyomas do not undergo malignant transformation; nonetheless, they may be difficult to treat. The lesions are often so numerous total surgical excision is not possible; furthermore, half of the patients who undergo surgery develop recurrences or new lesions in the same area.[16] When multiple, surgery has been recommended for large lesions, with symptomatic management for small lesions. In a few patients the pain may be so severe as to be incapacitating. Nitroglycerin has been used successfully to abort attacks,[14] and phenoxybenzamine along with hyoscine hydrobromide has been used to decrease pain.[10,30]

### Genital Leiomyomas

Early studies based on referred consultations suggested that genital leiomyomas were far less common than those of pilar arrecti origin.[16] Judging from more recent hospital-based series, genital leiomyomas may outnumber pilar ones by a margin of 2:1.[32] Affected sites include the areola of the nipple, scrotum, labium, penis, and vulva. The tumors are small, seldom exceeding 2 cm, and pain is not a prominent symptom. Histologically, genital leiomyomas, with the exception of the nipple lesions, differ from pilar leiomyomas in that they tend to be more circumscribed and more cellular, and they display a greater range of histologic appearances.[16,25] For example, Tavassoli and Norris,[28] in a review of 32 vulvar leiomyomas, noted myxoid change and an epithelioid phenotype of the cells, features not encountered in pilar leiomyomas.

## ANGIOMYOMA (VASCULAR LEIOMYOMA)

The angiomyoma, a solitary form of leiomyoma that usually occurs in the subcutis, is composed of numerous thick-walled vessels. In the early literature little attempt was made to distinguish these lesions from cutaneous leiomyomas, and the two were collectively termed tuberculum dolorosum because of their pain-producing properties. Stout[27] later designated them vascular leiomyomas to contrast them with the cutaneous leiomyoma that has inconspicuous thin-walled vessels. These lesions account for about 5% of all benign soft tissue tumors[38] and one-fourth[23] to one-half[27] of all superficial leiomyomas. They occur more frequently in women,[35] except for those in the oral cavity where the reverse is true.[37] Unlike cutaneous leiomyomas, these tumors develop later in life, usually between the fourth and sixth decades, as solitary lesions.[35,38] They occur preferentially on the extremities, particularly the lower leg. In the series reported by Hachisuga et al., 375 of 562 occurred in the lower extremity, 125 on the upper extremity, 48 on the head, and 14 on the trunk.[38] Most were less than 2 cm in diameter. Isolated cases of angiomyoma have been associated with paraproteinemia, myomas of the uterus, and astrocytoma.[33]

Affected patients complain most often of a small, slowly enlarging mass usually of several years' duration. Pain is a prominent feature in about half of the patients,[35] and in some cases it is exacerbated by pressure, change in temperature, pregnancy,[35,38] or menses.[33] The prevalence of pain has led some to suggest that these tumors are probably derived from arteriovenous anastomoses, similar to the glomus tumor.[36] They differ in appearance from the glomus tumor and are almost never encountered in a subungual location, however. The tumors are usually located in the subcutis and less often in the deep dermis, where they produce overlying elevations of the skin but without surface changes of the epidermis. Grossly, the tumors are circumscribed, glistening, white-gray nodules. Occasional they are blue or red, and rarely calcium flecks are visible grossly. The leiomyomas that visibly contract or writhe when touched or surgically manipulated are probably of this type.

Microscopically, the tumors have a characteristic appearance that varies little from case to case. The usual appearance is of a well demarcated nodule of smooth muscle tissue punctuated with thick-walled vessels with partially patent lumens (Figs. 18–4, 18–5). Typically the inner layers of smooth muscle of the vessel are arranged in an orderly circumferential fashion, and the outer layers spin or swirl away from the vessel, merging with the less well ordered peripheral muscle fibers. Areas of myxoid change (Fig. 18–6), hyalinization, calcification, and fat are seen. The vessels in these tumors are difficult to classify because they are not altogether typical of veins or arteries. Their thick walls and small lumens are reminiscent of arteries, but they consistently lack internal and external elastic laminae. In the experience of Hachisuga et al., a small number of angiomyomas are composed of predominantly cavernous-type vessels.[38] Nerve fibers are usually difficult to demonstrate but undoubtedly are present, accounting for the exquisite sensitivity of these lesions to manipulation. Rarely, angiomyomas display degenerative nuclear atypia similar to that seen in symplastic leiomyomas.[34] The angiomyoma is a benign tumor, causing few problems apart from pain. Simple excision is adequate. None of the patients reported by Duhig and Ayer[35] developed recurrence following excision. In the series of Hachisuga et al.,[38] only two patients had a recurrence, although their follow-up data were incomplete.

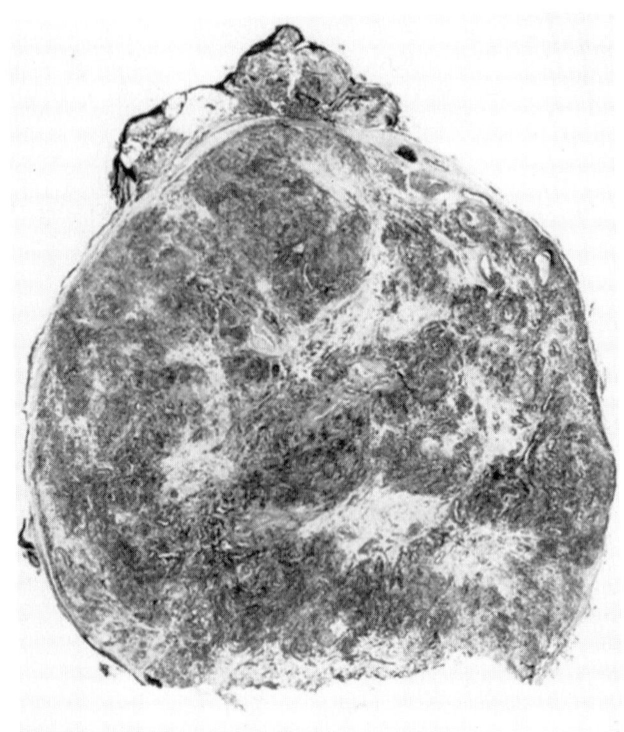

**FIGURE 18–4.** Angiomyoma of subcutaneous tissue. Congeries of thick-walled vessels constitute a major portion of the lesion and blend with surrounding smooth muscle tissue and focal myxoid stroma. (Masson trichrome)

## LEIOMYOMA OF DEEP SOFT TISSUE

Compared with the foregoing tumors, leiomyomas of deep soft tissue are uncommon, and until recently only sporadic cases were reported in the literature. Those occurring in the somatic soft tissues affect the sexes equally, whereas those in the body cavity/retroperitoneum occur almost exclusively in women. They tend to be much larger than those of the skin, probably because they produce few symptoms and are therefore discovered at a relatively late stage. Many are calcified, so they may be detected radiographically (Fig. 18–7), leading to diagnoses such as "calcifying schwannoma," "synovial sarcoma," or "myositis ossificans." Others are highly vascular, giving the radiologist the impression of malignancy.[43] Grossly, they are well circumscribed, gray-white lesions. Some have a gelatinous appearance when significant myxoid change has occurred. Histologically, these tumors are similar to their cutaneous counterparts, except they are likely to undergo degenerative or regressive changes. Most are easily recognized as smooth muscle

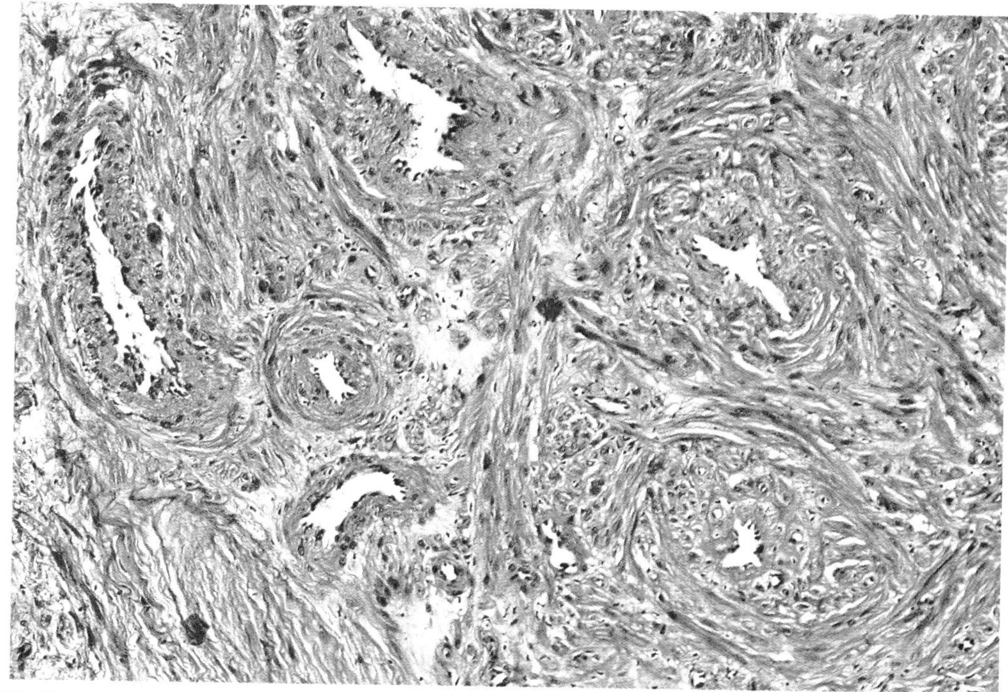

**FIGURE 18–5.** Thick-walled vessel of an angiomyoma. Inner layer of muscle is usually arranged circumferentially, and outer layer blends with less well ordered smooth muscle tissue of tumors.

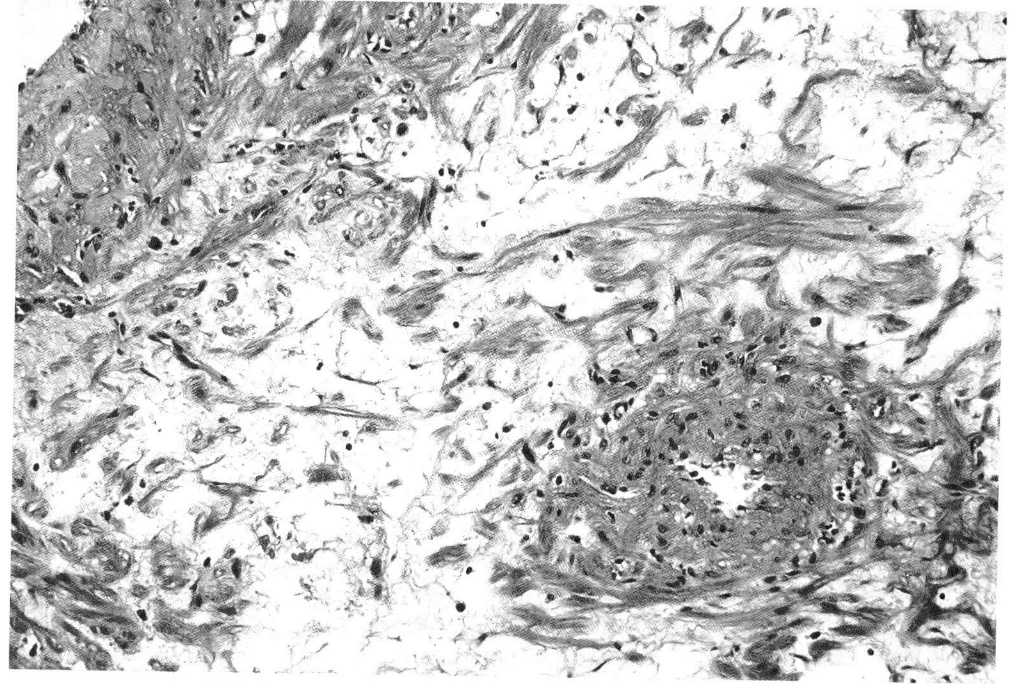

**FIGURE 18–6.** Focal myxoid change in an angiomyoma.

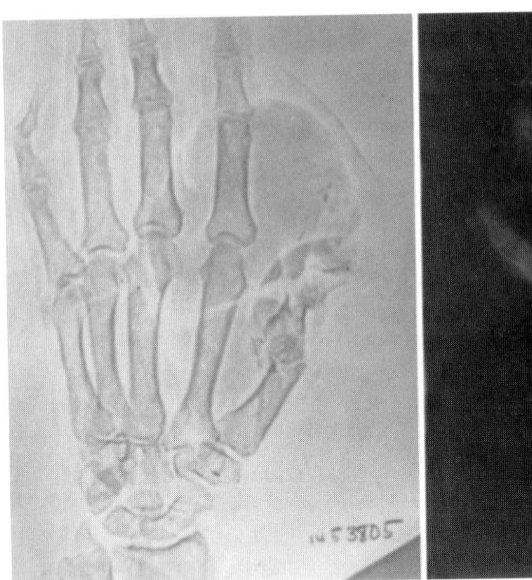


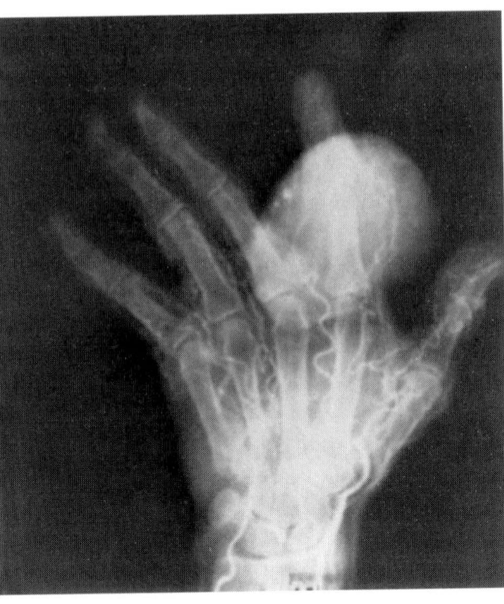

**FIGURE 18–7.** Radiograph showing calcification of a soft tissue leiomyoma.

tumors because of the orderly pattern of intersecting fascicles of deeply acidophilic cells with blunt-ended nuclei without significant cellular pleomorphism or mitotic activity (Fig. 18–8). In occasional cases nuclear palisading is noted.

Leiomyomas with nuclear palisading can be distinguished from schwannomas in that the former tumor has significant amounts of cytoplasmic glycogen, cytoplasmic fuchsinophilia, and longitudinal striations (Fig. 18–9). Some leiomyomas of soft tissue accumulate large amounts of myxoid ground substance between the cells, resulting in loss of the fascicular pattern. These tumors vaguely resemble the myxoid zones of nodular fasciitis or myxoma (Fig. 18–10) but can be distinguished from both by the cellular staining characteristics elaborated earlier.

Mature fat may be seen in smooth muscle tumors of all types, including angiomyomas, intravenous leiomyomatosis, and deep leiomyomas. In the uterus these mixed lesions have been termed "lipoleiomyoma," whereas in deep soft tissue they have been referred to as "lipoleiomyoma"[48] and "myolipoma"[46] (see Chapter 16), depending on the emphasis the authors have chosen to give to the two elements (Fig. 18–11). Although in the past, these retroperitoneal leiomyomas were considered autoamputated uterine leiomyomas, our recent experience (showing origin at sites clearly distinct from uterus) suggests that they are more likely soft tissue lesions arising from hormally sensitive smooth muscle cells. The principal significance of these lesions is that the intermingling of wisps of smooth muscle cells between lobules of mature fat suggest alternative diagnoses, such as well-differentiated liposarcoma or spindle cell lipoma. Recognition that the spindled element consists of mature smooth muscle, rather than the atypical, hyperchromatic spindle cells of liposarcomas, is a critical observation for arriving at the correct diagnosis.

Another uncommon feature in leiomyomas is "clear-cell change" (Fig. 18–12) of the cytoplasm. When this change is extreme, a variety of diagnoses may be entertained, including clear-cell carcinoma, balloon cell melanoma, or adnexal tumor. Careful sampling to document typical smooth muscle cells is usually sufficient to establish the correct diagnosis. Immunostaining for desmin may also be helpful (see Chapter 18).

Regressive changes are common in large leiomyomas, particularly those of long duration. Most commonly these changes include fibrosis, calcification,[39,40,42,44,47] and in rare cases ossification. Calcium is usually laid down in distinct spherules reminiscent of psammoma bodies (Fig. 18–13), which sometimes invokes a surrounding giant cell reaction (Fig. 18–14). Focal epithelioid change (Fig. 18–15) and cording of smooth muscle cells is occasionally encountered as well (Fig. 18–16).

Evaluation for malignancy in deeply situated smooth muscle tumors is difficult. Because leiomyosarcomas are more common in deep soft tissue than leiomyomas, it is mandatory that smooth muscle tumors in this location be carefully sampled. In general, mitotic activity is the principal criterion used to evaluate malignancy in these lesions and is discussed in detail in Chapter 19. Although most can agree that above certain levels a smooth muscle tumor should be considered malignant, it is difficult to ensure a benign state when a lesion has an exceptionally low number of mitotic figures. This was well illustrated in a series of deep soft tissue leiomyomas reported by

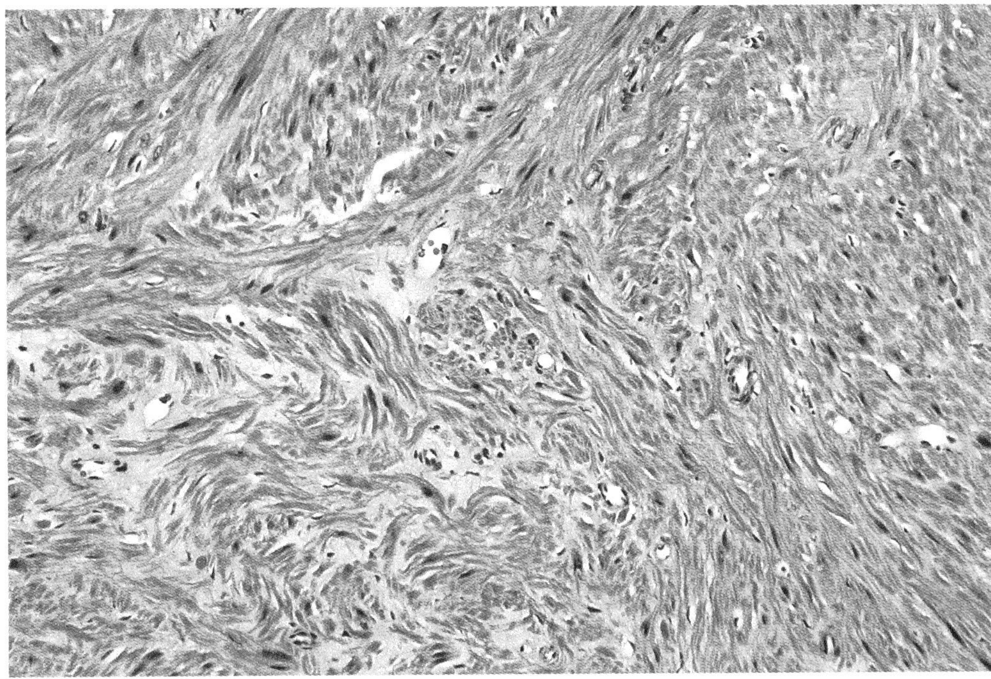

**FIGURE 18–8.** Leiomyoma of deep soft tissue. Fascicles of smooth muscle tend to be less well oriented than in cutaneous leiomyomas.

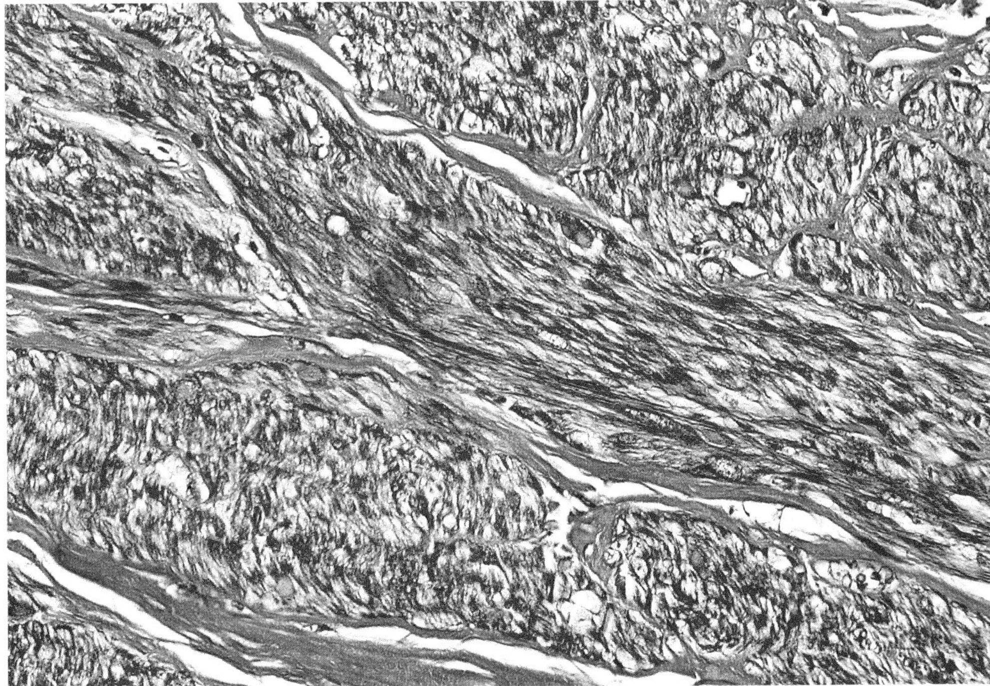

**FIGURE 18–9.** Masson trichrome stain of a deep leiomyoma. Cells are deeply fuchsinophilic with linear striations.

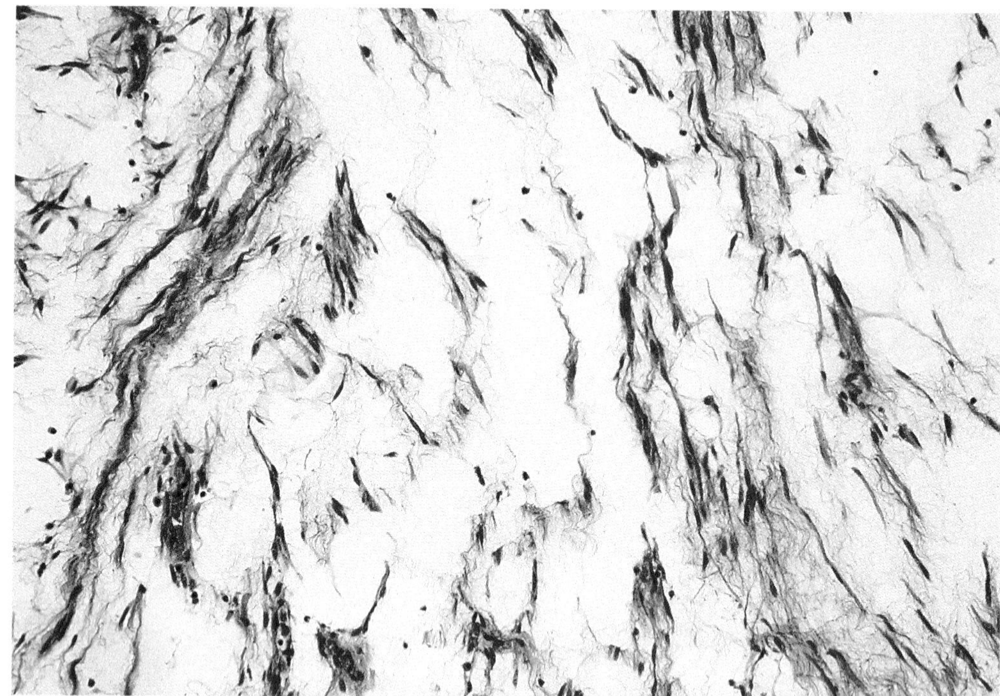

**FIGURE 18–10.** Myxoid change within a leiomyoma simulating the appearance of a myxoma. In contrast to a myxoma, these cells are more parallel.

Kilpatrick et al.[44] Eight of eleven tumors had no detectable mitotic activity following careful sampling. Three cases had levels estimated at ≥1 mitoses/50 high-power fields (HPF). One of these cases recurred within 16 months and at that time displayed 4 mitoses/10 HPF. In our opinion, deeply situated smooth muscle tumors that can be confidently labeled benign are those that are mitotically inactive, Such lesions usually also have areas of hyalinization, myxoid degeneration, and calcification.[38a] Although nuclear atypia can occur in deep leiomyomas, (Fig. 18–17) it should be accepted as a degenerative phenomenon in smooth muscle tumors only when the lesions are reasonably hypocellular and amitotic. In this setting it is analogous to the nuclear atypia in long-standing schwannomas (ancient schwannomas). In contrast, leiomyosarcomas are characterized by nuclear atypia in the context of cellularity and mitotic activity.

Although assessment of mitotic activity remains the cornerstone for determining malignancy in smooth muscle tumors of soft tissue, information regarding location in certain circumstances is invaluable as well. For example, leiomyomas of the pelvic retroperitoneum in perimenopausal woman are a distinct subgroup of soft tissue leiomyomas which occasionally display low levels of mitotic activity and possess estrogen and progesterone receptor protein. Despite low levels of mitotic activity, they appear to have a good prognosis suggesting a close kinship to uterine leiomyomas.[38a] In rare instances we have even seen uterine leiomyomas that extended through the sacral notch into the buttock and that, without the benefit of radiographic studies, would have been interpreted as a well-differentiated leiomyosarcoma because of low levels of mitotic activity.

True leiomyomas of soft tissue are benign lesions that require complete excision with a small cuff of surrounding normal tissue. In the one series comprising 11 tumors with a median follow-up of 4.5 years, 10 lesions neither recurred nor metastasized.[44] The other lesion (see above) recurred and displayed elevated mitotic activity during the recurrence.[41] In our experience with 36 cases, 1 recurred and none metastasized within a follow-up period that averaged about 4 years.[38a]

## INTRAVENOUS LEIOMYOMATOSIS

Intravenous leiomyomatosis is a rare condition in which gross nodules of benign smooth muscle tissue grow in the veins of the myometrium and occasionally extend for a variable distance into the uterine

*Text continued on page 709*

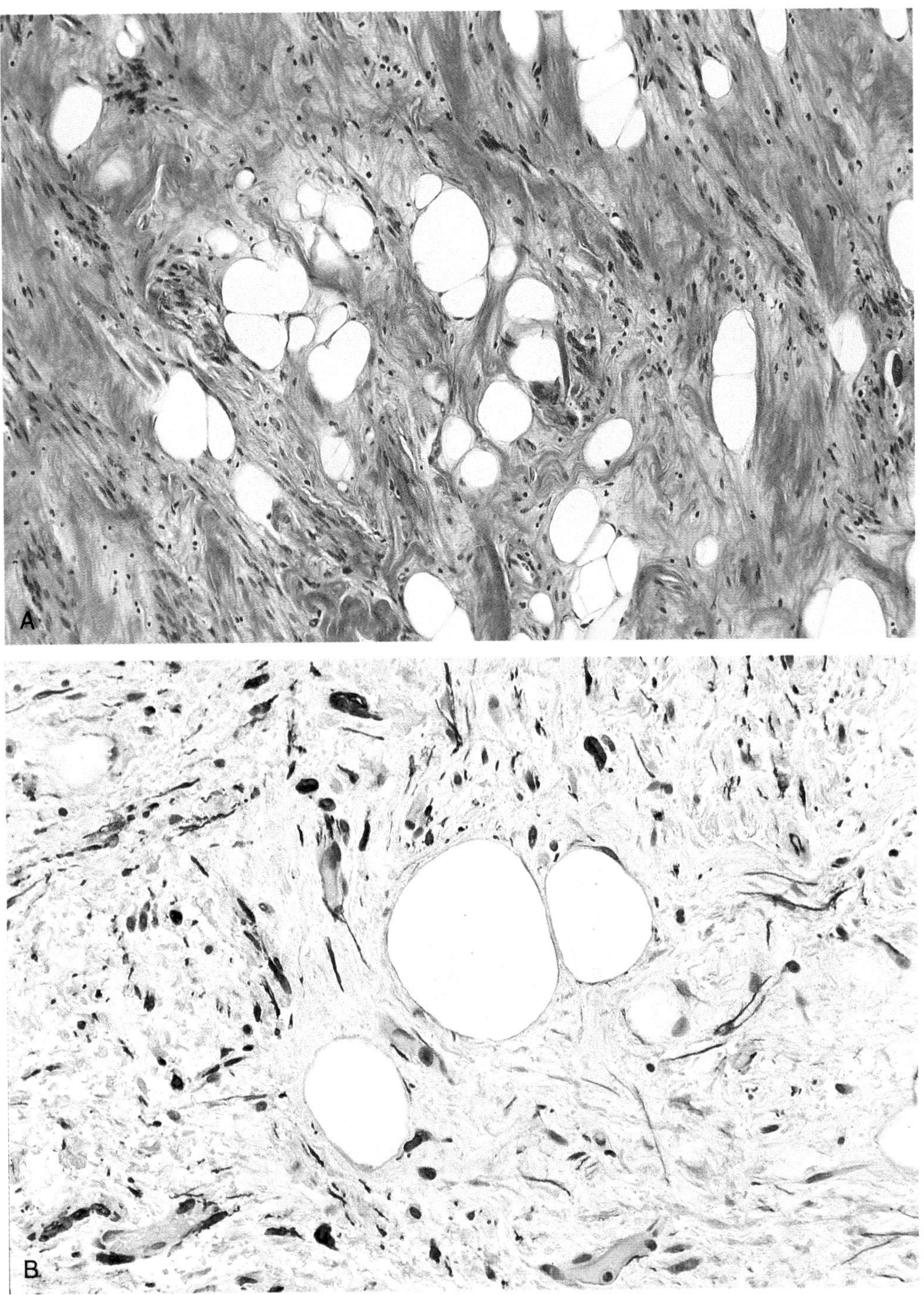

**FIGURE 18–11.** Leiomyoma with fat (myolipoma) (**A**). Desmin immunostain illustrates muscle cells between adipocytes (**B**).

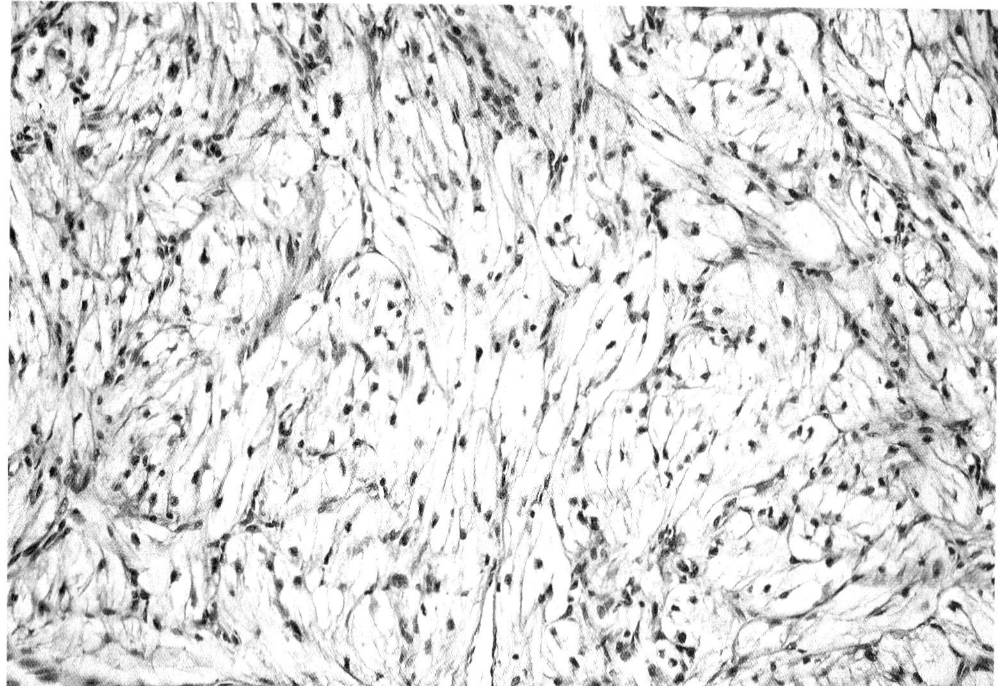

**FIGURE 18–12.** Clear-cell change of the cytoplasm in a leiomyoma of soft tissue.

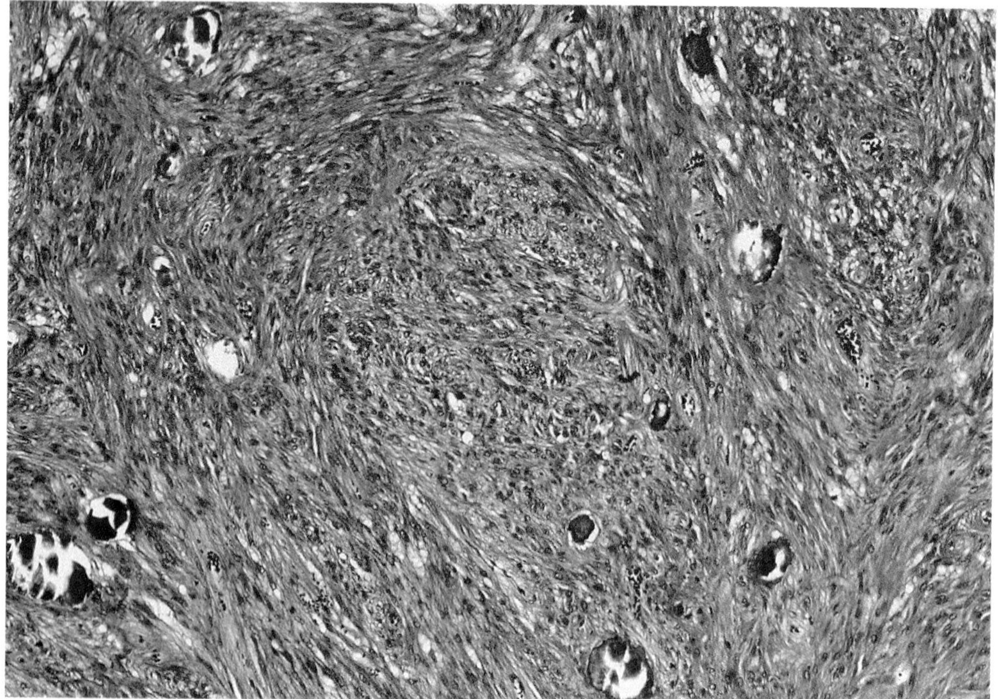

**FIGURE 18–13.** Leiomyoma with psammomatous calcification.

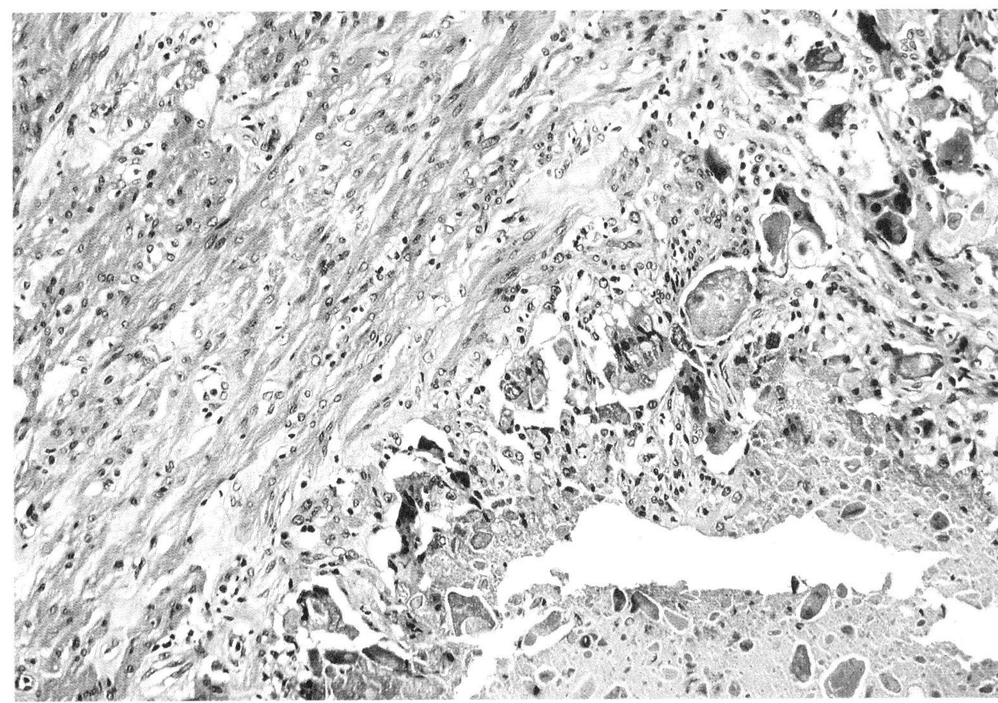

**FIGURE 18–14.** Leiomyoma with extensive calcification and a surrounding giant cell reaction.

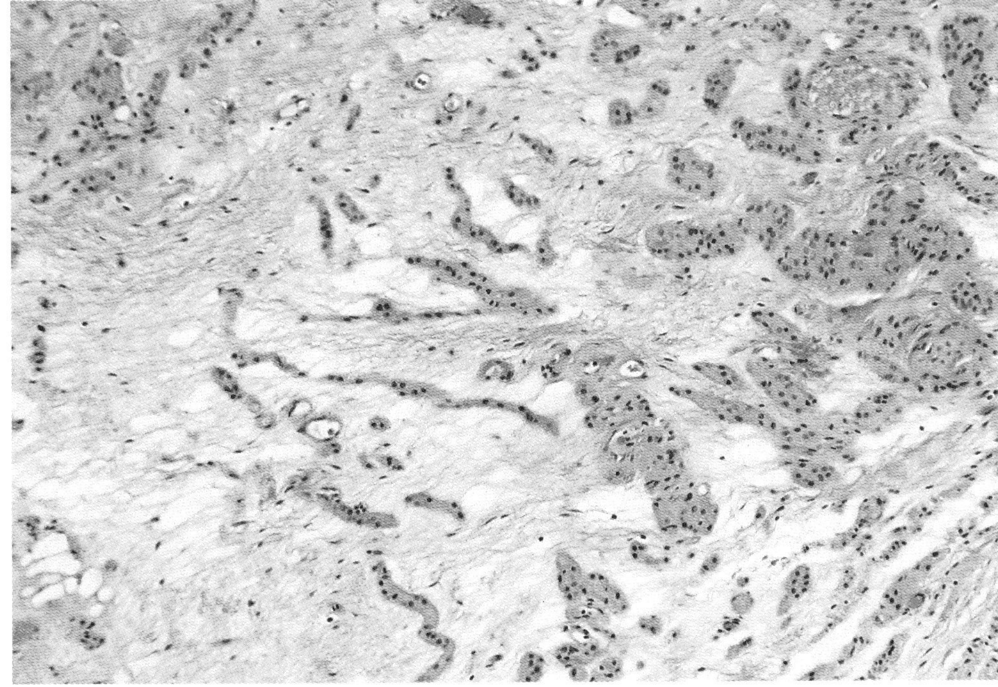

**FIGURE 18–15.** Focal epithelioid change in a leiomyoma.

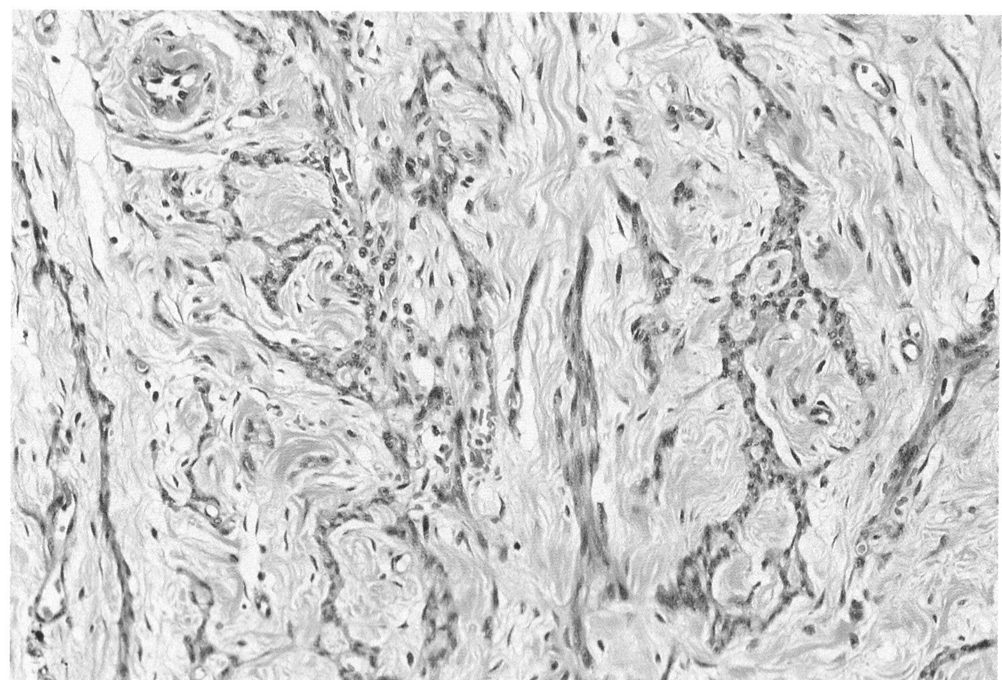

**FIGURE 18–16.** Cord-like arrangement of smooth muscle cells in a leiomyoma.

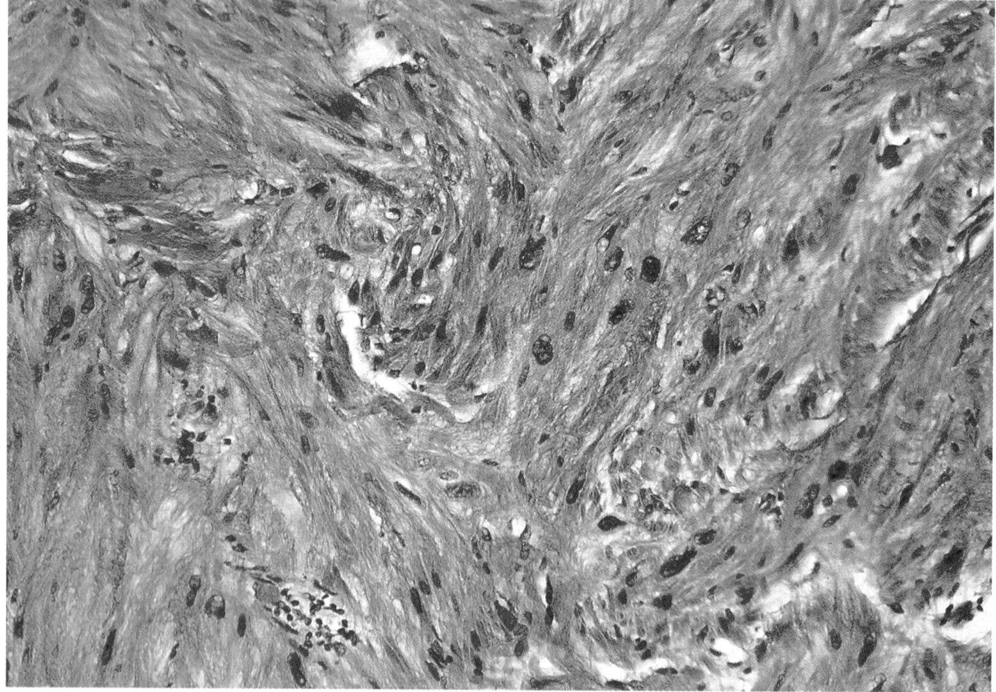

**FIGURE 18–17.** Leiomyoma of soft tissue showing mildly degenerative nuclear atypia. Note that the lesion is hypocellular and amitotic; and it has areas of hyalinization.

and hypogastric veins. In about 10% of patients cardiac symptoms predominate owing to the presence of tumor in the vena cava and heart. This condition may develop as a result of extensive vascular invasion by a leiomyoma or by de novo origin from the uterine veins.[52]

The lesion develops primarily in premenopausal middle-aged women, and prior pregnancy is noted in about half of the patients. The common presenting symptoms are abnormal vaginal bleeding and pelvic pain. In more than half of the patients the uterus is enlarged. Grossly, the lesion is distinctive, characterized by coiled masses in the myometrium and in some cases by serpiginous extensions of the process into the uterine veins of the broad ligament (Fig. 18–18). The masses have a rubbery texture and a pink to white-gray color similar to an ordinary uterine myoma. Histologically, the smooth muscle proliferations in leiomyomatosis may show the same spectrum of changes as those in ordinary leiomyomas (Figs. 18–19, 18–20, 18–21). The lesions may vary from highly cellular smooth muscle proliferations to less cellular ones marked by fibrosis, hydropic change, and perivascular hyalinization. A characteristic feature is the presence of thick-walled vessels in the plugs of intravascular smooth muscle tissue, creating a "vessel within a vessel" appearance (Fig. 18–19). Unusual features in this condition include epithelioid change of the cells, fat, or endometrial glands in association with smooth muscle cells[50] and bizarre nuclear changes similar to those of symplastic leiomyoma.[50] Despite the intravascular location, the smooth muscle cells are well differentiated, showing

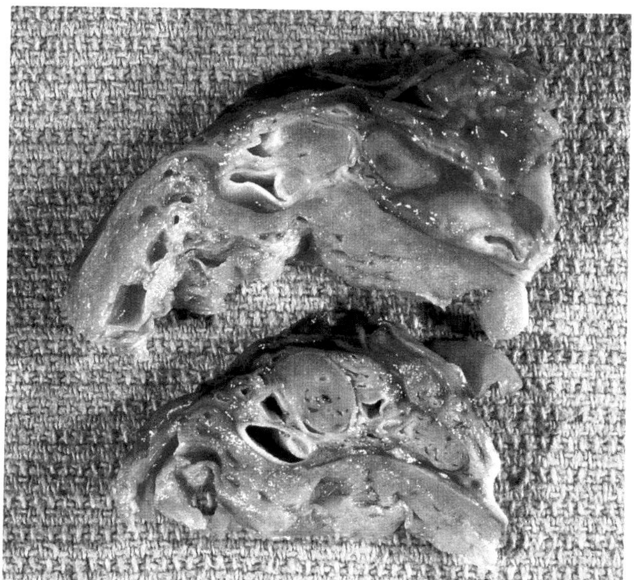

**FIGURE 18–18.** Gross specimen of intravenous leiomyomatosis showing intravascular growth of the neoplasm.

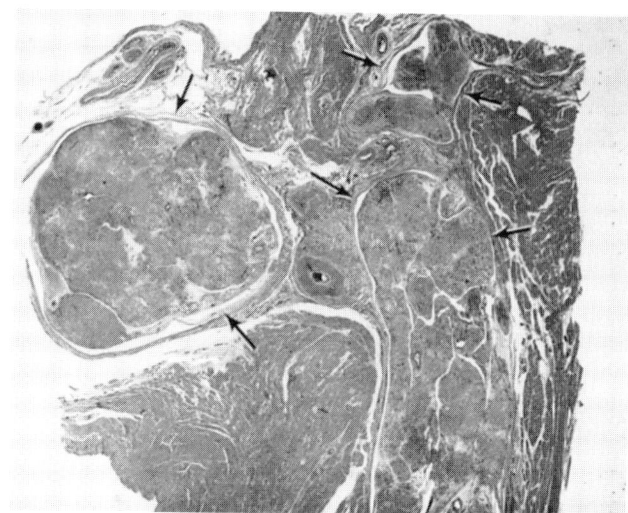

**FIGURE 18–19.** Intravenous leiomyomatosis with plugs of smooth muscle tissue in uterine veins. (×60) (Courtesy of Dr. H.J. Norris.)

in nearly all cases no or only a modest degree of nuclear hyperchromatism. Mitotic figures are rare, with an incidence well below that associated with borderline (5–9 mitoses/10 HPF) or malignant (≥10 mitoses/10 HPF) smooth muscle tumors of the uterus (see Chapter 18). Thus from a purely morphologic point of view, the tumor would be classified as "leiomyoma."

The pathogenesis of these tumors has been debated; current evidence suggests that two mechanisms are operational.[52] In most cases there are associated uterine leiomyomas, supporting the notion that extensive angioinvasion by one or more myometrial tumors results in this condition (Fig. 18–15). In a few instances, however, the smooth muscle proliferation appears to be entirely intravascular, indicating direct origin from the venous wall (Fig. 18–16). In fact, as pointed out by Norris and Parmley,[52] women may be particularly susceptible to the development of intravascular smooth muscle proliferation, as evidenced by the inordinately high incidence of leiomyosarcomas of the vena cava in women and the peculiar intimal changes of vessels that develop secondary to reproductive steroid use.

Despite the intravascular location, the prognosis in most cases is good. About 70% of patients can be cured by hysterectomy; the remaining 30% have persistence or recurrence of the disease.[49] Unfortunately, recurrence rates have not correlated well with the presence of extrauterine extension noted at the time of the original surgery. In a small percentage of patients the disease may be fatal because of extension into the hepatic veins, the heart, and even the lungs.[49,52–55] Resection of these cardiac and caval ex-

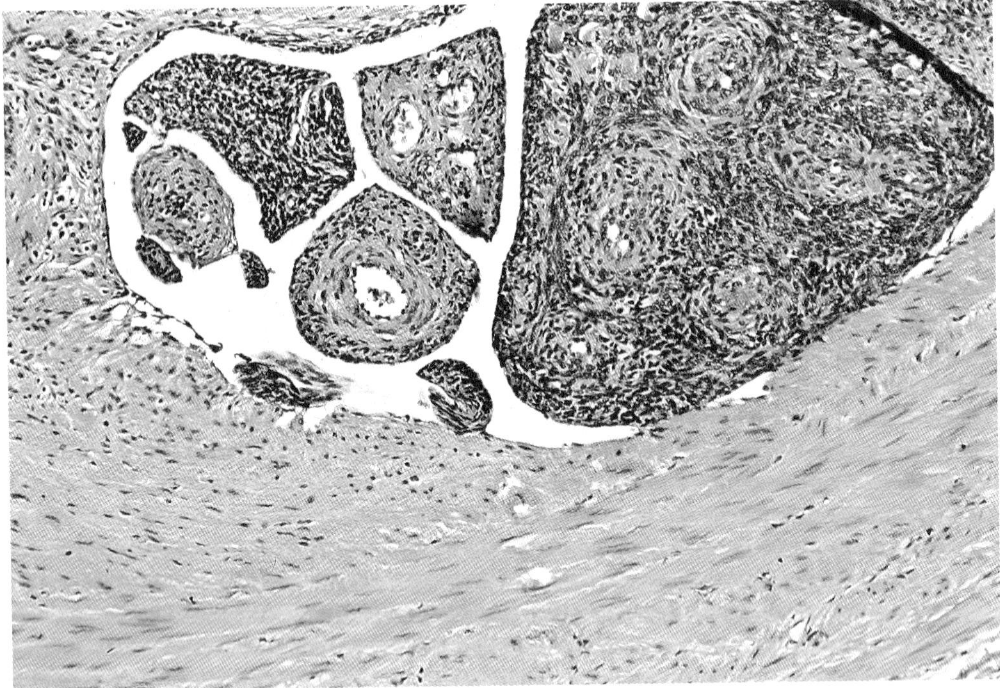

**FIGURE 18–20.** Intravenous leiomyomatosis with intraluminal protrusions or growths.

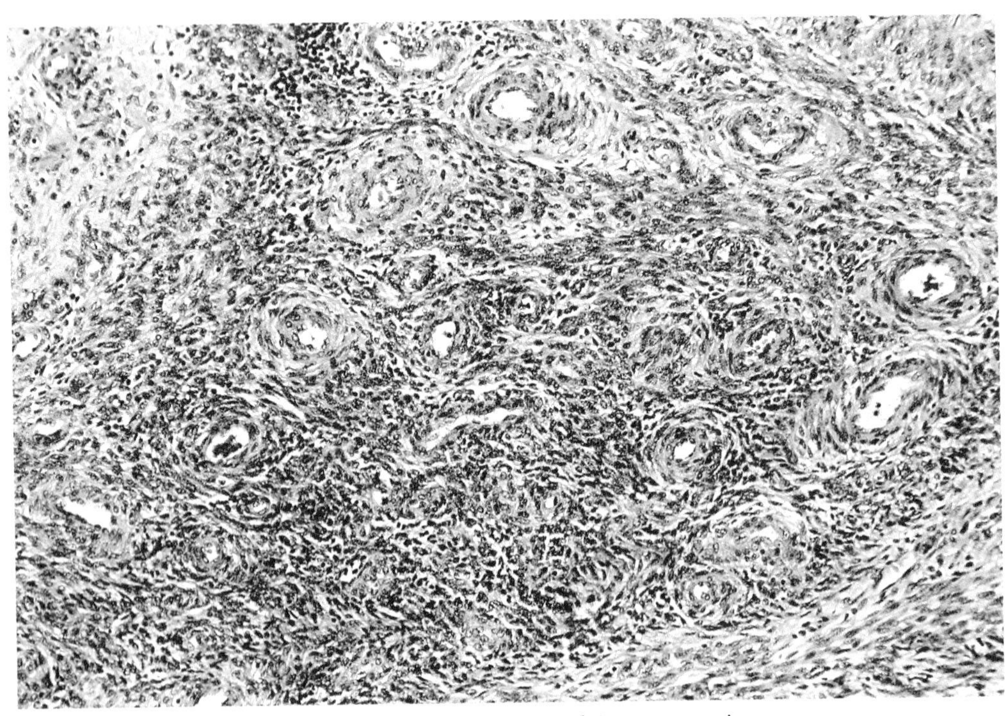

**FIGURE 18–21.** Intravenous leiomyomatosis.

tensions, if technically feasible, is compatible with prolonged survival.[49,50,54,55] Because some patients with intravenous leiomyomatosis have steroid receptors,[51,56] it has been suggested that oophorectomy or estrogen antagonists can play a therapeutic role in those in whom tumor excision has been incomplete. It is likely that some "benign metastasizing leiomyomas" of the lung evolve by way of "intravenous leiomyomatosis."[52] Others may evolve as a result of microscopic showers of tumor emboli occurring at the time of myomectomy; and still others may represent well-differentiated leiomyosarcomas in which the original tumor or the metastasis was misdiagnosed as a leiomyoma.[58]

The best name for this condition is debatable, as the ability of a tumor to invade the bloodstream and grow in foreign tissue satisfies a minimum definition of malignancy for some. On the other hand, the condition is compatible with long survival and differs histologically from most leiomyosarcomas of venous origin. The latter are usually high-grade tumors composed of smooth muscle cells with easily recognized mitotic figures. They arise preferentially in the vena cava, particularly the upper portion, and are usually associated with a poor prognosis because of their unresectability (see Chapter 19).

## LEIOMYOMATOSIS PERITONEALIS DISSEMINATA

Leiomyomatosis peritonealis disseminata is a rare condition in which multiple smooth muscle or smooth muscle-like nodules develop in a subperitoneal location throughout the abdominal cavity. The lesion occurs exclusively in women, usually during the childbearing years. Most cases reported in the United States have been in African American women. More than half have occurred in pregnant women. Others have occurred in women taking oral contraceptives, and one patient had a functioning ovarian tumor.[81] These observations and the fact that the lesion regresses following pregnancy[64] provide circumstantial evidence for the involvement of hormonal factors in its pathogenesis. The rarity of the condition suggests that other unknown factors must also be important. In most instances leiomyomatosis is discovered incidentally at the time of surgery for other medical or obstetric conditions, although vague abdominal pain is often an accompanying symptom.

Grossly, the disease has an alarming appearance. The peritoneal surfaces, including the surfaces of the bowel, urinary bladder, and uterus, are studded with firm white-gray nodules of varying size (Fig. 18–22). The smallest nodules may be only a few millimeters in diameter whereas the largest are several centimeters. Although the diffuseness of the process initially suggests an intraabdominal malignancy, the lesions lack hemorrhage and necrosis. Moreover, they do not violate the parenchyma of the affected organs, nor are they found in extraabdominal sites such as the lung or in lymph nodes. Leiomyomas of the uterus have been identified in some but not all cases of leiomyomatosis, indicating that the lesions do not represent localized spread of an intrauterine lesion.

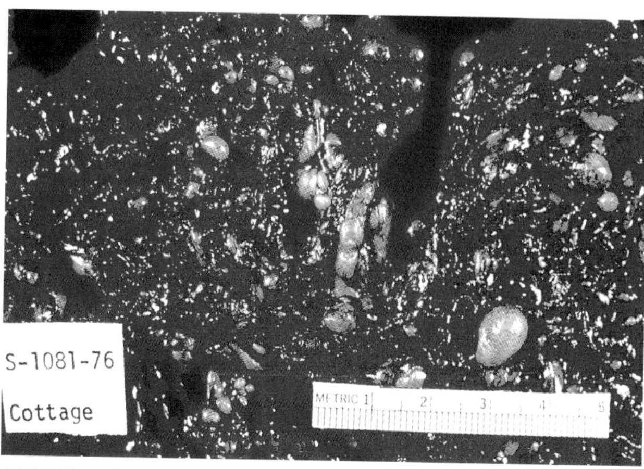

**FIGURE 18–22.** Gross appearance of leiomyomatosis peritonealis disseminata.

### Microscopic Findings

Although the term leiomyomatosis indicates the similarity to normal smooth muscle and to benign leiomyomas, reports in the literature coupled with cases reviewed at the Armed Forces Institute of Pathology (AFIP)[80] suggest that there is a range of histologic changes perhaps not fully appreciated when the term was coined. In the classic case the earliest nodules develop as small microscopic foci of proliferating smooth muscle immediately subjacent to the peritoneum (Figs. 18–23, 18–24, 18–25). With progressive growth they may remain nodular or may, in addition, dissect through the underlying soft tissue in a more permeative fashion. The slender cells are arranged in close, compact fascicles oriented perpendicular to each other. The cells may show a minimal degree of nuclear pleomorphism that falls far short of being a leiomyosarcoma. Mitotic figures may be seen, but they are infrequent. Bundles of longitudinally oriented myofibrils can be identified in the cells by means of conventional special stains (Masson trichrome). In some cases endometriosis has been present in the smooth muscle nodules.[69,71]

In a significant number of cases the histologic appearance of these subperitoneal nodules is more fibroblastic or "myofibroblastic." Cases of this type have been described by Parmley et al.,[76] Winn et al.,[82] and Pieslor et al.[77] The proliferating cell is usually large,

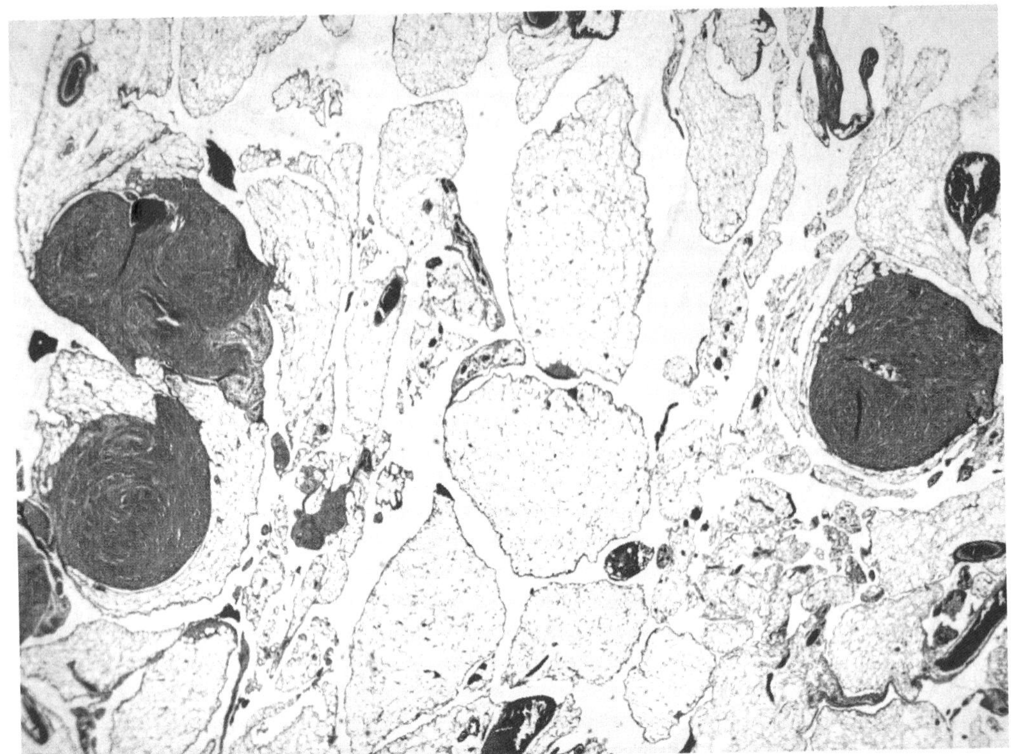

**FIGURE 18–23.** Leiomyomatosis peritonealis disseminata with numerous smooth muscle nodules of varying size arising underneath the peritoneal surface and involving underlying fat. Early nodules are present as small microscopic foci.

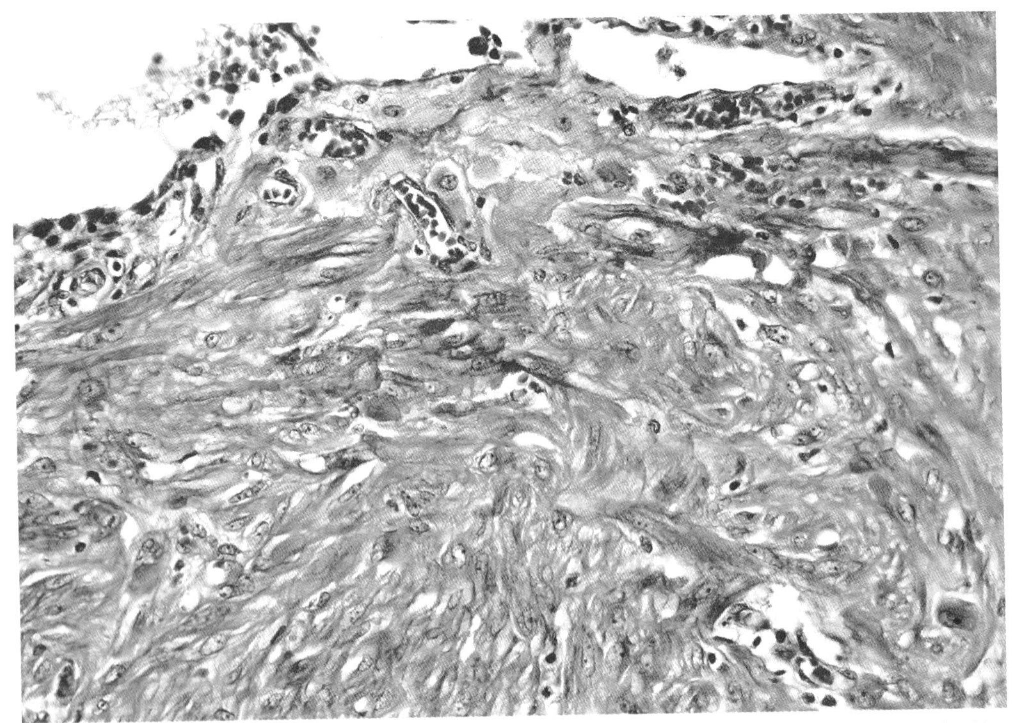

**FIGURE 18–24.** Subperitoneal nodule of leiomyomatosis peritonealis disseminata with decidualization.

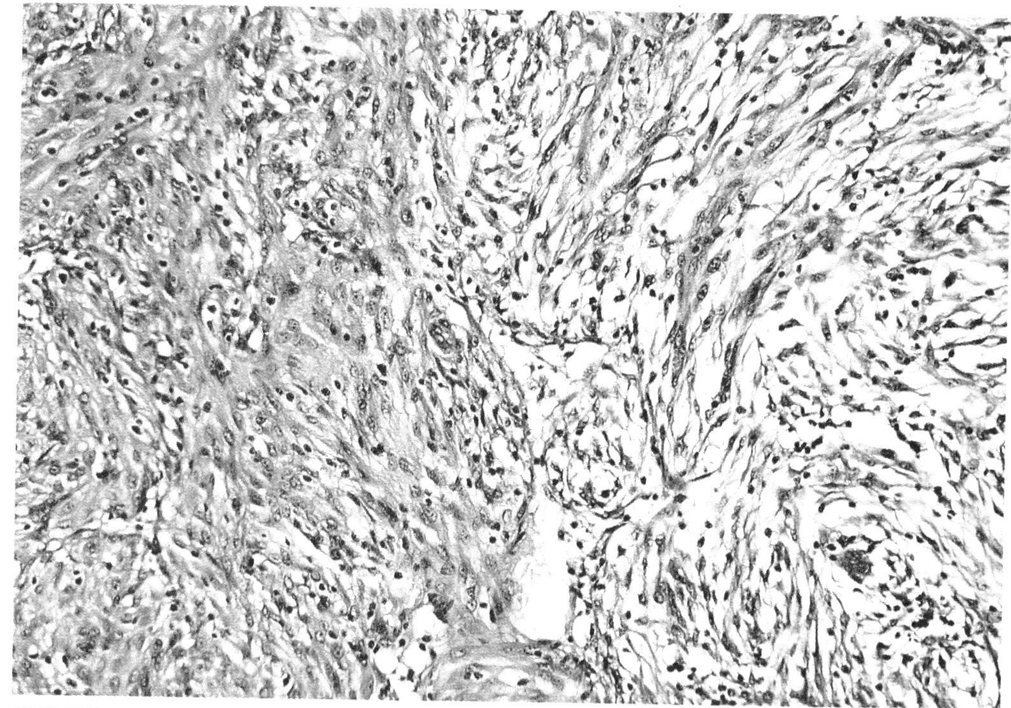

**FIGURE 18–25.** Leiomyomatosis peritonealis disseminata with a myofibroblastic appearance.

has a plump eosinophilic cytoplasm, and is usually not arranged in well defined fascicles. Round decidual cells with an eosinophilic or foamy cytoplasm are usually scattered amid the spindled cells; and at times it is impossible to delimit these cells clearly from spindle cells by light microscopy. In such cases the cells lack distinct longitudinal striations, as are seen in the foregoing type. Hyalinization of the nodules is seen in cases of regressing or regressed leiomyomatosis (Fig. 18–26). The one case in the literature allegedly representing lipomatous differentiation in the cells is dubious, judging from the photomicrographs.[70] Glandular inclusions or sex cord-like structures may be seen infrequently in these lesions.[63,73]

## Ultrastructural Findings

In view of the range of changes observed by light microscopy, it is not surprising that electron microscopy has produced conflicting reports regarding the histogenesis of this condition. In the studies of Nogales et al.,[74] Kuo et al.,[71] and Goldberg et al.,[65] most of the cells resembled mature smooth muscle cells and had an investiture of basal lamina, surface-oriented pinocytotic vesicles, and abundant longitudinally oriented myofilaments. In contrast, Parmley et al.[76] and Winn et al.[82] believed the predominant cells were fibroblastic and, based on the close relation with the decidual cells, suggested that leiomyomatosis is a reparative fibrosis occurring in a preexisting decidual reaction (fibrosing deciduosis). Others have documented a variety of cell types, including fibroblasts, myofibroblasts, and smooth muscle cells[77,80] and suggested a close interrelation of all three.[80] The theory that leiomyomatosis represents metaplasia or differentiation of pluripotential cells of the serosa or subserosal tissue along several closely related cell lines is supported by the experimental work of Fujii et al.[66] Estrogen administered to guinea pigs induces peritoneal nodules similar to those of leiomyomatosis peritonealis. These nodules are composed of fibroblasts and myofibroblasts in animals receiving estrogen only, whereas smooth muscle differentiation and decidualization occurs if estrogen plus progesterone are administered.

## Behavior and Treatment

In view of the benign nature of this condition, no particular therapy is warranted once the diagnosis has been firmly secured. In fact, there seems to be some evidence that the lesions regress following pregnancy or removal of the estrogenic source,[77] although with subsequent pregnancy progression or recrudescence occurs.[72] The case reported by Aterman et al.[61] documented partial regression of lesions 5 months after the initial surgery without any intervening therapy and regression of another lesion within 12 weeks.[68] Recently, gonadotropin-releasing hormone antagonists (e.g., leuprolide acetate) and megestrol ac-

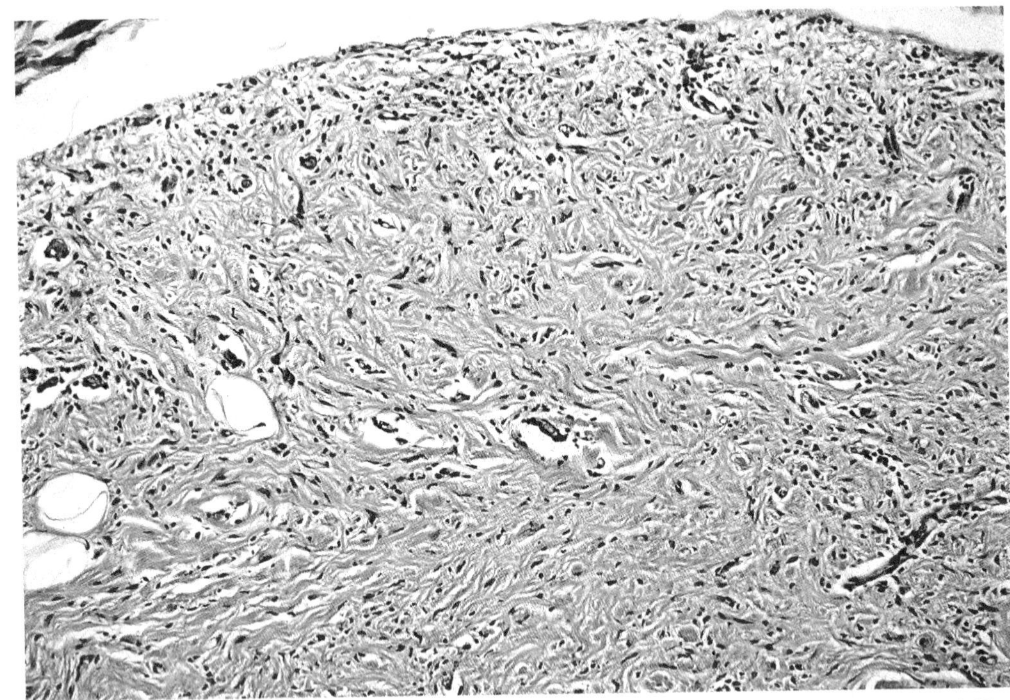

**FIGURE 18–26.** End stage of leiomyomatosis peritonealis disseminata with extensive interstitial fibrosis.

etate[75] have been used with some success to treat this disease.[75] There have been a few cases purporting to show malignant degeneration of the condition. The cases reported by Akkersdijk et al.[60] and Abulafia et al.[59] are scantily illustrated, and autopsies were not performed in either case. The case reported by Rubin et al.[79] is better documented.

In the past leiomyomatosis peritonealis disseminata was regarded as a diffuse metaplastic process of the peritoneum. Recently, however, Quade et al. demonstrated clonality of multiple lesions in a given patient using X-linked inactivation of the androgen receptor gene human androgen receptor (HUMARA).[78] Although the authors believe that this indicates metastasis from a unicentric disease, they are careful to point out that their data are also consistent with multicentric clones selected for an X-linked gene.

## PALISADED MYOFIBROBLASTOMA OF LYMPH NODES (INTRANODAL HEMORRHAGIC SPINDLE CELL TUMOR WITH AMIANTHOID FIBERS)

Reported simultaneously by Weiss et al.[94] and Suster and Rosai,[93] the palisaded myofibroblastoma is a distinctive benign spindle cell tumor arising exclusively from the lymph nodes and bearing an unmistakable similarity to a schwannoma. In fact, so striking is the resemblance that these lesions were originally regarded as schwannoma of the lymph node[89] and reported as such in the first two editions of this textbook. However, with the advent of immunohistochemistry it has become clear that the tumor is more closely related to a myofibroblast or modified smooth muscle cell. The tumor may develop at any age but typically presents as a localized swelling in the region of the groin. A few cases have been reported in submandibular lymph nodes,[83,88] and one of us (S.W.W.) reviewed a case (in consultation) in the mediastinal nodes.

On cut section the tumors are gray-white, focally hemorrhagic masses that usually obscure the nodal landmarks (Fig. 18–27). It is usually possible to identify a rim of residual node at the periphery of the tumor (Fig. 18–28). The tumors are composed of differentiated spindle cells arranged in short intersecting or crisscrossed fascicles with vaguely palisaded nuclei focally (Figs. 18–29, 18–30). In some areas the cells form broad sheets with slit-like extracellular spaces containing erythrocytes similar to those of Kaposi's sarcoma (Fig. 18–31). The cells usually have little atypia and only a rare mitotic figure. They seem to represent an unusual myofibroblastic (or myoid) cell in that they strongly express actin and vimentin but not desmin. Linear striations, which are easily identi-

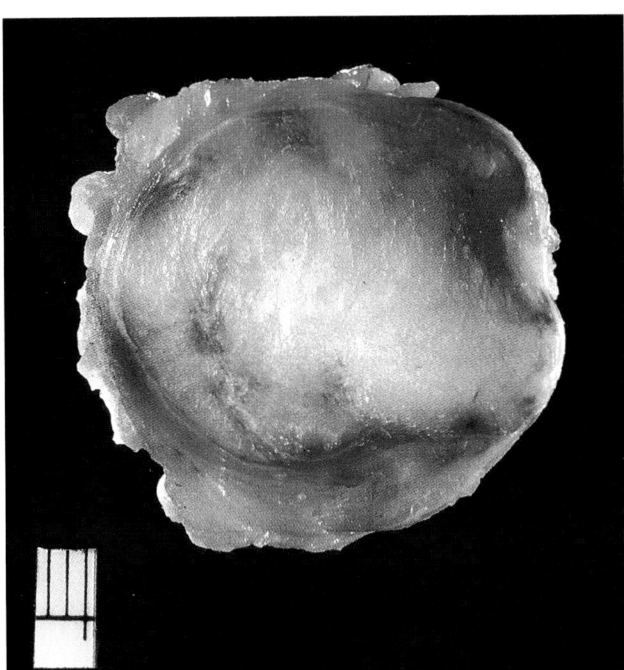

**FIGURE 18-27.** Gross specimen of a palisaded myofibroblastoma. Note the focal hemorrhages.

fied in conventional benign smooth muscle cells, cannot be demonstrated with Masson trichrome stain, although in many cases fuchsinophilic bodies, representing accumulations of actin, are prominent.

The most distinctive feature of the tumor is the amianthoid fibers or thick collagen mats that are nearly always present. These structures appear as broad eosinophilic bands, ellipses, or circular profiles, depending on the plane of the section. They contain a central collagen-rich zone surrounded by a paler collagen-poor zone containing actin and other materials extruded from nearby degenerating cells. Immunohistochemically, type I collagen can be identified throughout the amianthoid fibers, and type III collagen is localized peripherally.[92] Although the name "amianthoid" was used by Suster and Rosai for these distinctive bodies, it has recently been pointed out that these structures do not meet the strict definition of amianthoid fibers.[92] The latter are thick collagen fibers measuring 280–1000 nm, whereas the fibers in these structures have the width of normal collagen fibers. The mechanism of formation of these unusual bodies is not clear. Some have suggested that they represent a degenerative change around vessels[93] to which the tumor cells and their contents become adherent[85,94] These lesions appear to arise from modified smooth muscle cells that normally are found in the lymph node capsule and stroma. The predilection of this tumor to occur in the groin probably reflects the relative frequency with which smooth muscle cells are found in this location relative to other lymph node chains.[94]

All of the cases reported in the literature have behaved in a benign fashion, with no recurrence or metastasis.[93,94] It is important to recognize that this lesion represents a primary benign mesenchymal lesion and not a metastatic sarcoma. These tumors are quite well differentiated and have extremely low levels of mitotic activity, in contrast to most metastatic sarcomas. Moreover, sarcomas infrequently metastasize to lymph nodes, and when they do so it is usually an expression of disseminated disease and rarely an initial presentation.

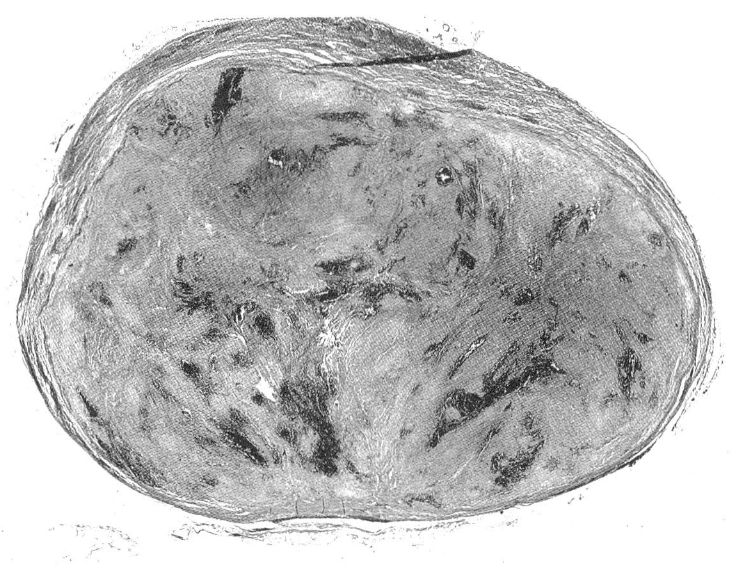

**FIGURE 18-28.** Palisaded myofibroblastoma with nearly complete effacement of a lymph node.

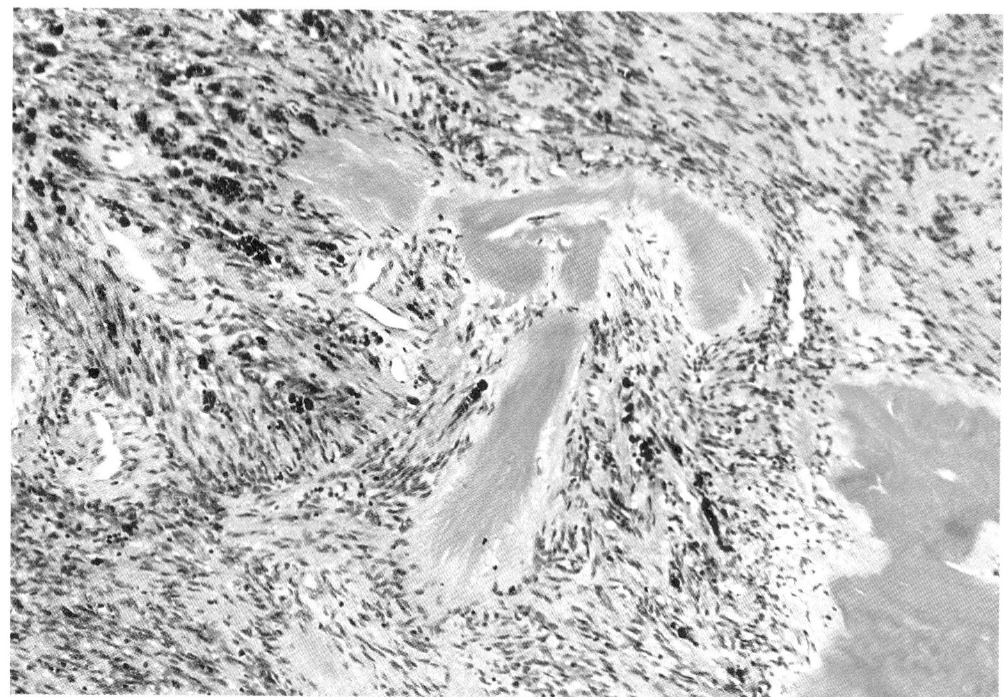

**FIGURE 18–29.** Palisaded myofibroblastoma with amianthoid fibers. It has a deeply eosinophilic core and lighter periphery.

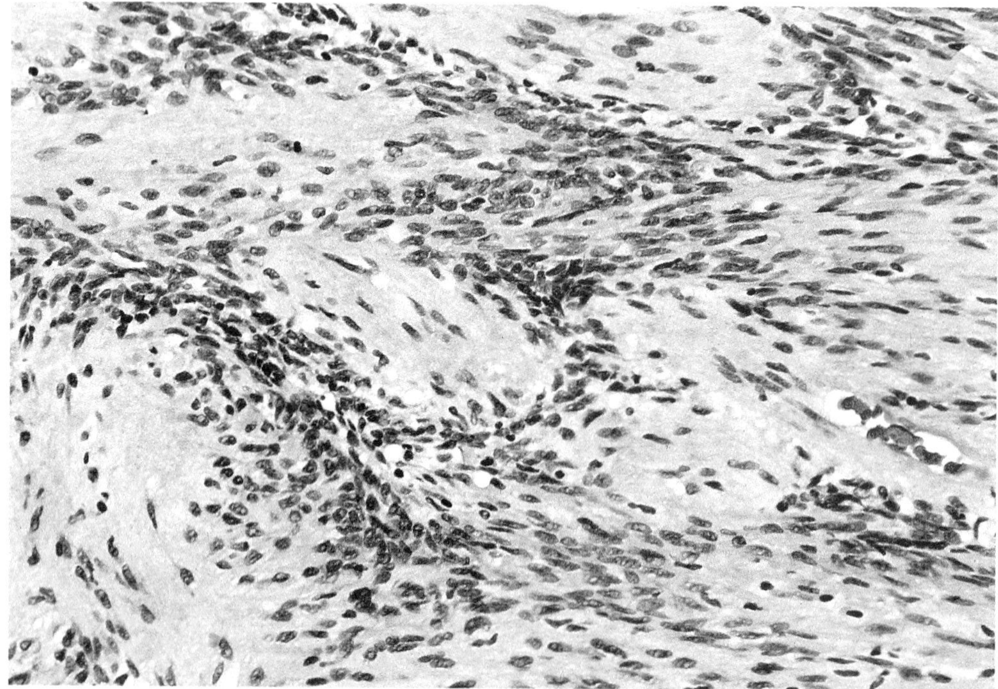

**FIGURE 18–30.** Palisaded myofibroblastoma with vague palisading of cells.

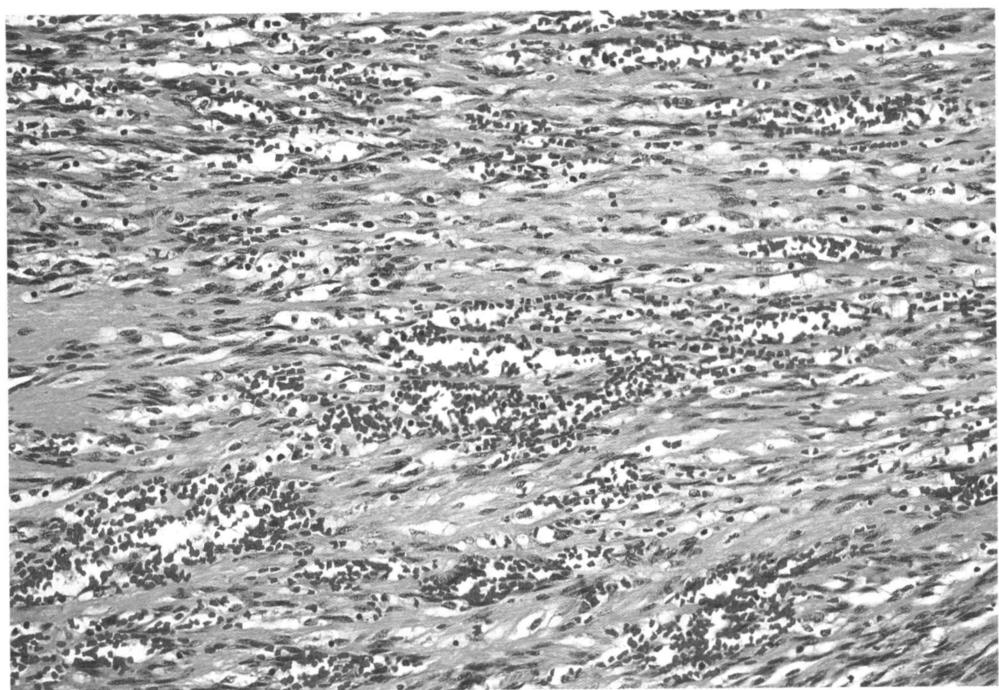

**FIGURE 18–31.** Kaposi-like areas in a palisaded myofibroblastoma.

## MYOFIBROBLASTOMA OF THE BREAST

Myofibroblastoma of the breast is an uncommon but highly characteristic mesenchymal tumor that occurs more frequently in men.[105,106] Of the 16 original cases reported by Wargotz et al.,[101] 11 were in men, with an average age of 63 years. Rare cases have occurred bilaterally.[98] The tumor develops as a discrete, well marginated mass that does not infiltrate the surrounding breast tissue (Fig. 18–32), although fat trapping may be seen in the middle of the tumor. The tumors contain slender fibroblast-like spindle cells arranged in sheets or short packets separated by thick collagen bundles. Mast cells may be scattered throughout the lesions (Figs. 18–33, 18–34). Rarely, chondroid metaplasia is seen. On electron microscopy and immunohistochemistry the proliferating cells seem most closely related to myofibroblasts. They express desmin[100,101] and actin and contain collections of actin filaments, dense bodies, basal lamina, and surface-oriented pinocytotic vesicles.[10] CD34 has recently been identified in these lesions, and some have suggested that they are variants of or closely related to solitary fibrous tumors,[97,100] a lesion that characteristically expresses this antigen. In our opinion the lesions are histologically different from solitary fibrous tumor, although they do have an unmistakable similarity to spindle cell lipoma, a lesion that may express CD34.

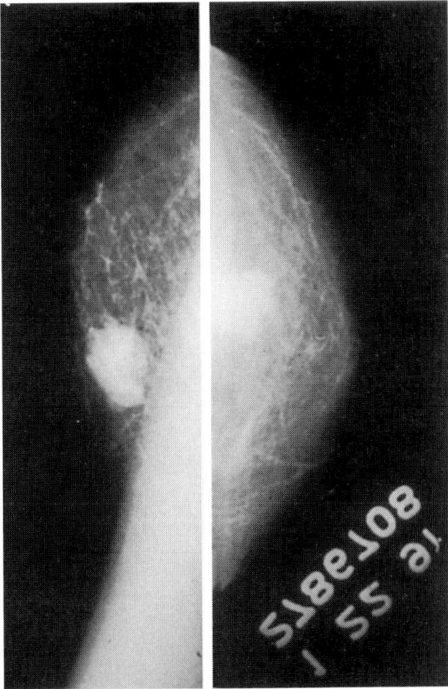

**FIGURE 18–32.** Mammogram showing a sharply marginated myofibroblastoma.

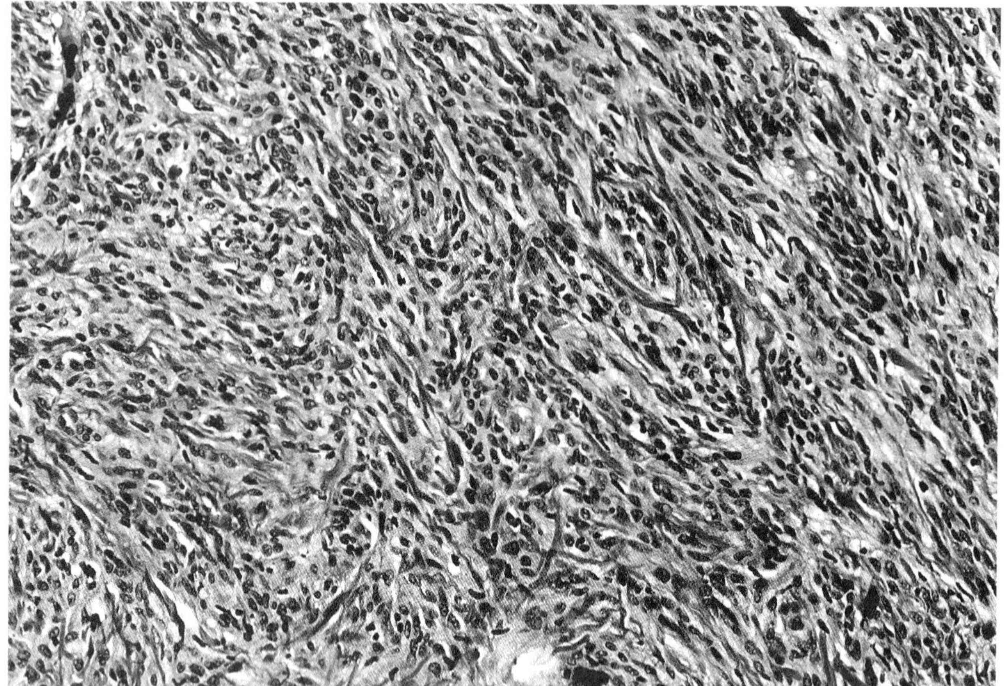

**FIGURE 18–33.** Mammary myofibroblastoma.

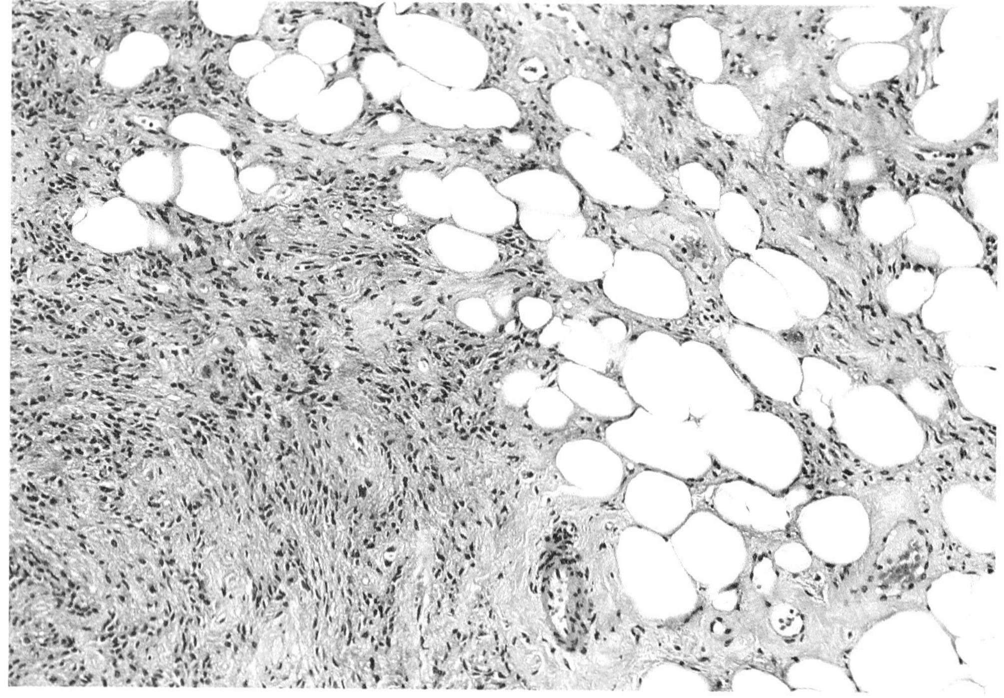

**FIGURE 18–34.** Fat trapping in a mammary myofibroblastoma.

Once familiar with the pattern of this tumor, most pathologists have little difficulty identifying it. Those unfamiliar with the lesion have a tendency to regard it as a well-differentiated metaplastic carcinoma of the breast or a stromal sarcoma. Perhaps the most helpful feature seen at low power is the impressive circumscription of this lesion compared to malignant spindle cell lesions of the breast. It is also helpful to note that the lesion does not insinuate itself in the substance of the breast, as one would see with carcinomas or stromal sarcomas. The presence of short fascicles of plump cells interrupted by collagen bundles is also at variance with fibromatosis, which consists of long, sweeping fascicles of attenuated fibroblastic cells.

These tumors are entirely benign. None of the original patients described by Wargotz et al.[101] developed recurrence or metastasis. Thus once the correct diagnosis is established, simple excision is adequate.

## ANGIOMYOFIBROBLASTOMA

Angiomyofibroblastoma is a distinctive tumor that usually involves the vulva[102–108] but can involve the vagina and rarely the scrotum. It is closely related to epithelioid forms of leiomyoma. These tumors develop as slowly growing, marginated masses in the subcutaneous tissues. Because of their preferential location on the vulva they may be confused with a Bartholin's cyst. The tumors contain prominent, sometimes ectatic vessels surrounded by clusters of eosinophilic epithelioid cells, some of which blend or fan out from the muscular walls of the vessels. The cells lie in small chains, cords, or singly in a matrix that varies from myxoid to hyaline (Figs. 18–35, 18–36). In some cases the cells spindle, and in others they separate from the stroma, creating pseudovascular spaces (Figs. 18–37, 18–38).

The tumors with a prominent myxoid matrix can be confused with the the so-called aggressive angiomyxoma, another highly vascularized lesion of the lower gynecologic tract. However, angiomyxoma is a uniformly myxoid tumor, unlike the angiomyofibroblastoma, which usually has at best only a partially myxoid appearance.

Immunohistochemically, the cells of angiomyofibroblastoma express vimentin and desmin but usually not actin. This immunophenotypic profile was originally thought to be a useful means for distinguishing angiomyofibroblastoma from aggressive angiomyxoma, which typically expresses vimentin and actin, although in some cases desmin has been reported as well. In our opinion, most of these lesions are best distinguished on the basis of the usual morphologic features rather than by resorting to immunohistochemistry. Although it has been suggested that they are part of the same spectrum,[103] we believe that for

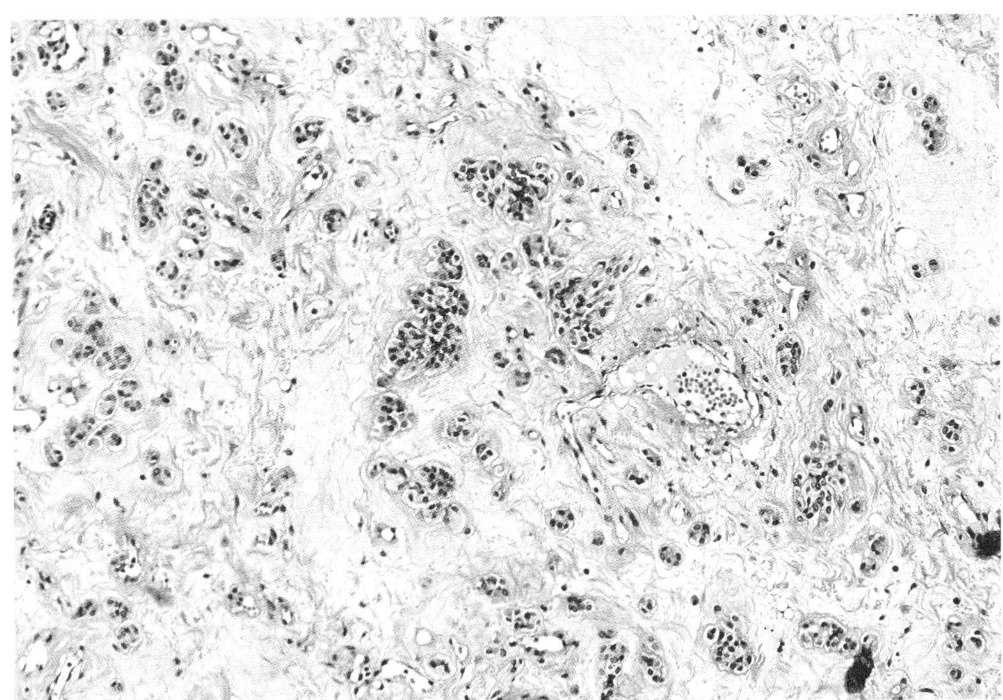

**FIGURE 18–35.** Angiomyofibroblastoma of the vulva.

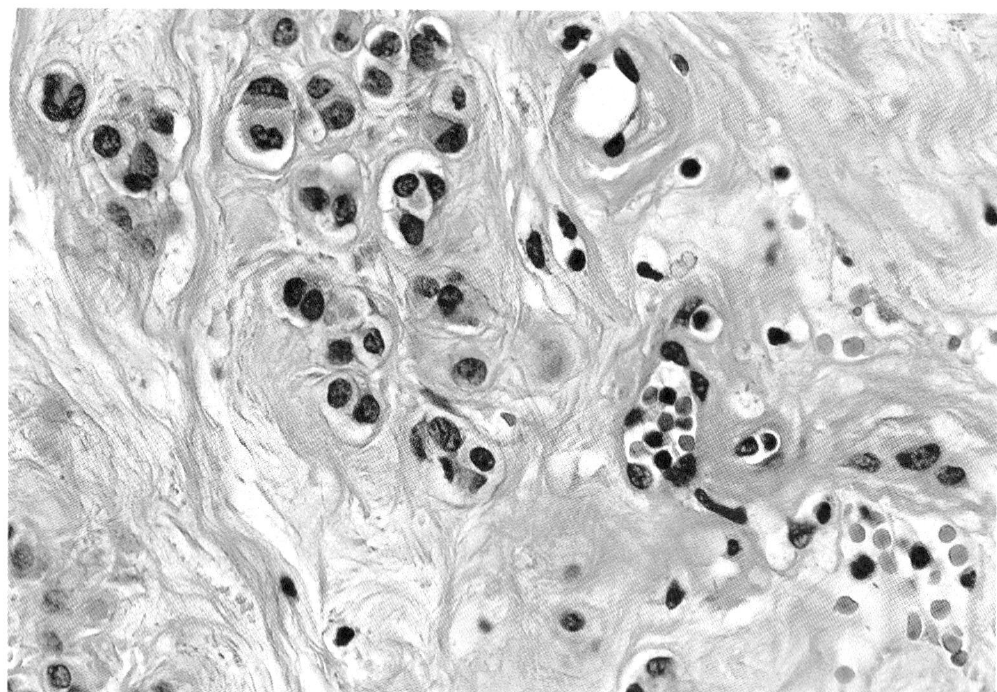

**FIGURE 18–36.** Epithelioid-appearing cells in an angiomyofibroblastoma.

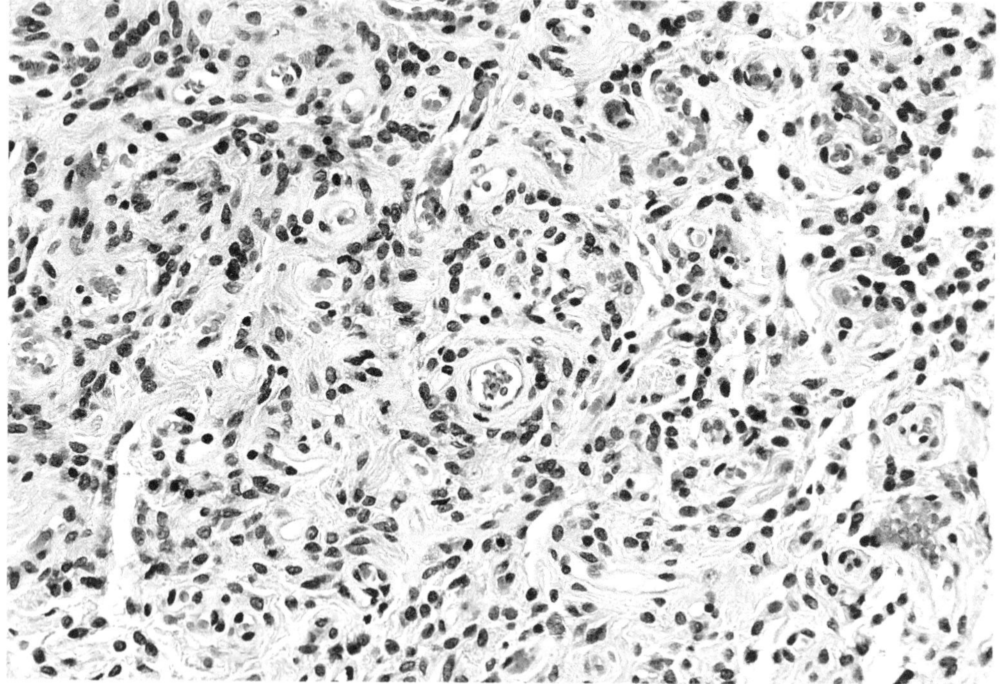

**FIGURE 18–37.** Angiomyofibroblastoma with more cellularity and spindling than is seen in Figure 18–36.

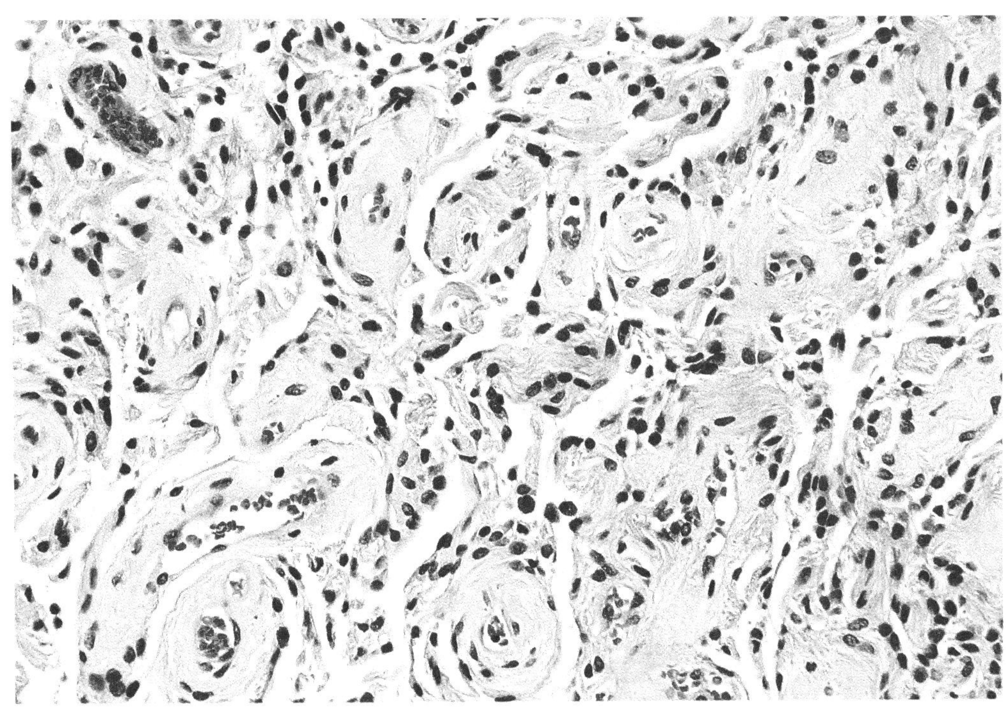

**FIGURE 18–38.** Pseudovascular spaces in an angiomyofibroblastoma.

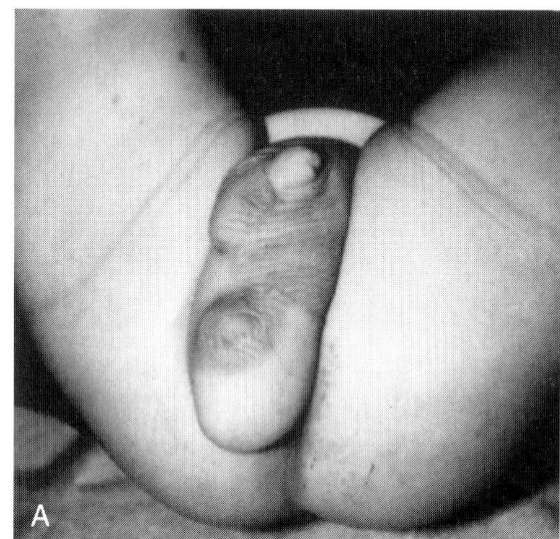

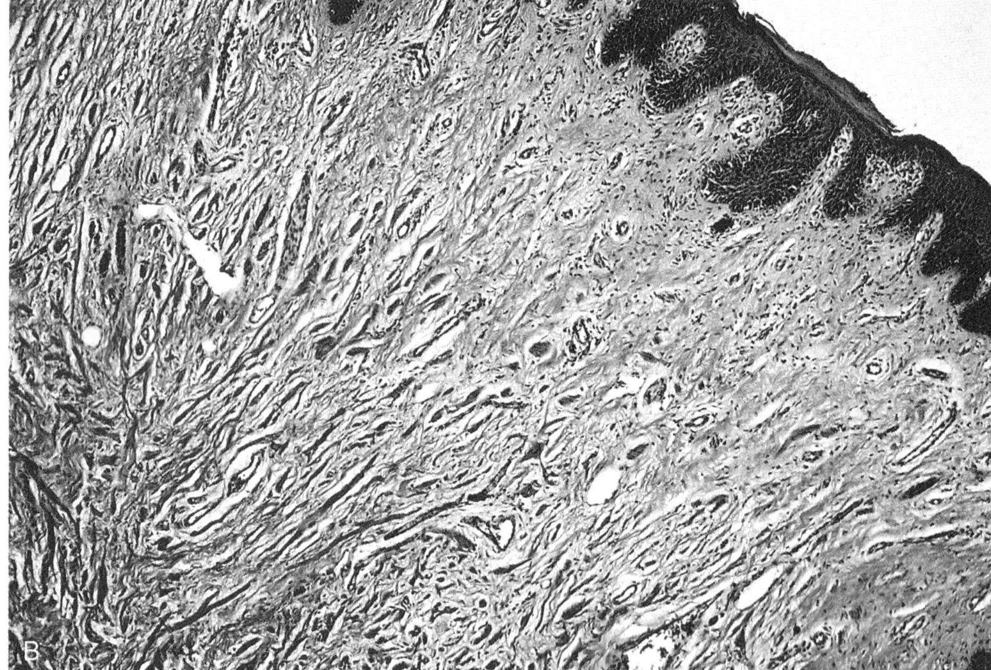

**FIGURE 18–39.** (**A**) Accessory scrotum in an infant. (**B**) Microscopic section shows well-differentiated smooth fibers oriented perpendicular to the skin surface.

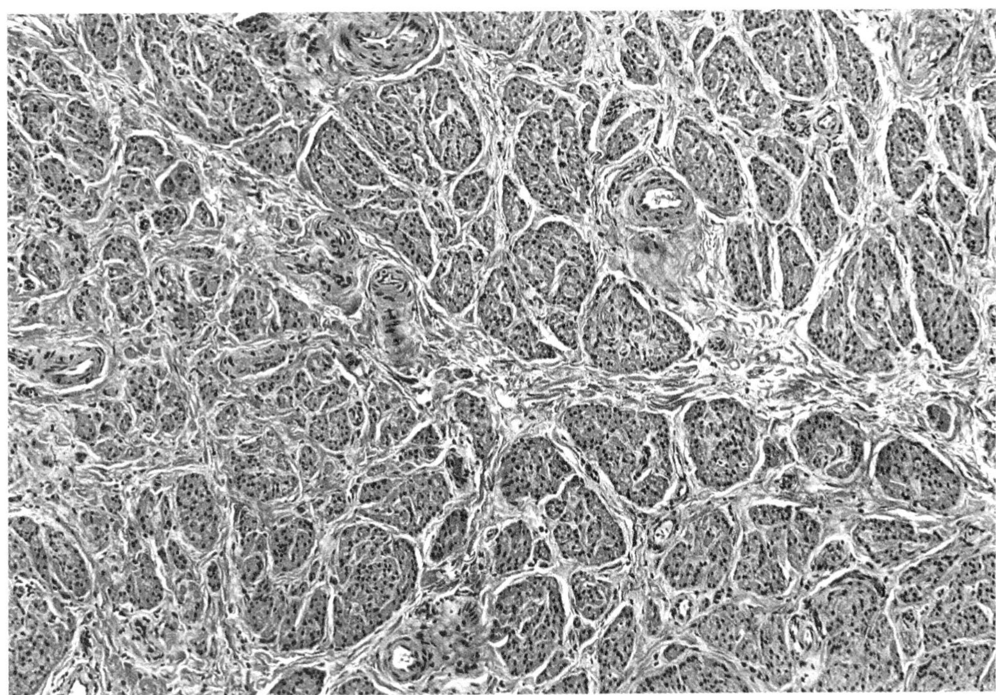

**FIGURE 18–40.** Round ligament removed at the time of inguinal herniorrhaphy. Cells are distinctly rounded with small centrally placed nuclei.

the most part these two lesions are separate entities capable of distinction in most instances.

Although none of the original 10 tumors reported by Fletcher et al.[102] recurred, we have encountered recurrences in our material. It appears to be more common when tumors are less sharply marginated and are therefore more difficult to excise completely. Moreover, along with Nielson et al., we have encountered angiomyofibroblastomas with sarcomatous areas. These tumors may either resemble an angiomyofibroblastoma with "malignant features" or they may display sarcomatous areas resembling leiomyosarcoma or undifferentiated sarcoma. None of these rare malignant tumors has metastasized to date.

## MISCELLANEOUS LESIONS CONFUSED WITH LEIOMYOMAS

Although the diagnosis of leiomyoma is seldom difficult, occasionally hamartomatous or choristomatous deposits of smooth muscle tissue suggest leiomyoma. Examples include accessory scrotal (Fig. 18–39) or areolar tissue. The clinical appearance and location of the lesions usually suggest the correct diagnosis. The round ligament, when removed incidentally during repair of an inguinal hernia, may also be misinterpreted as a leiomyoma. The round ligament is composed of distinctive, closely packed, polygonal muscle cells with small, dark, centrally placed nuclei (Fig. 18–40).

## REFERENCES

### General

1. Farman AG. Benign smooth muscle tumors. S Afr Med J 48: 1214, 1974.
2. Harman JW, O'Hegarty MT, Byrnes CK. The ultrastructure of human smooth muscle. I. Studies of cell surface and connections in normal and achalasia esophageal smooth muscle. Exp Mol Pathol 1:204, 1962.
3. Hashimoto H, Komori A, Kosaka M, et al. Electron microscopic studies on smooth muscle of the human uterus. J Jpn Obstet Gynecol Soc 7:115, 1960.
4. Morales AR, Fine G, Pardo V, et al. The ultrastructure of smooth muscle tumors with a consideration of the possible relationship of glomangiomas, hemangiopericytomas, and cardiac myxomas. Pathol Annu 10:65, 1975.
5. Rosenbluth J. Smooth muscle: an ultrastructural basis for the dynamics of its contraction. Science 148:1337, 1965.
6. Ross R. The smooth muscle cell. II. Growth of smooth muscle in culture and formation of elastic fibers. J Cell Biol 50:172, 1971.
7. Schuerch LW, Skalli O, Seemeyer TA, et al. Intermediate filament proteins and actin isoforms as markers for soft tissue tumour differentiation and origin. 1. Smooth muscle tumors. Am J Pathol 128:91, 1987.
8. Skalli O, Ropraz P, Trzeciak A, et al. A monoclonal antibody against alpha smooth muscle actin: a new probe for smooth muscle differentiation. J Cell Biol 103:2787, 1986.
9. Uehara Y, Campbell GR, Burnstock G. Cytoplasmic filaments in developing and adult vertebrate smooth muscle. J Cell Biol 50:484, 1971.

### Cutaneous Leiomyoma

10. Archer CB, Whittaker S, Greaves MW. Pharmacological modulation of cold-induced pain in cutaneous leiomyomata. Br J Dermatol 118:255, 1988.

11. Auckland G. Hereditary multiple leiomyoma of the skin. Br J Dermatol 79:63, 1967.
12. Burton JL, Hartog M. Multiple endocrine adenomatosis (type I) with cutaneous leiomyomata and cysts of Moll. Br J Dermatol 97(Suppl 15):75, 1977.
13. Eldor A, Even-Paz Z, Polliak A. Erythrocytosis associated with multiple cutaneous leiomyomata: report of a case with demonstration of erythropoietic activity in the tumour. Scand J Haematol 16:245, 1976.
14. Engelke H, Christophers E. Leiomyomatosis cutis et uteri. Acta Dermatol Venereol 59(Suppl 85):51, 1979.
15. Fernandez-Pugnaire MA, Delgado-Florencio V. Familial multiple cutaneous leiomyomas. Dermatology 191:295, 1995.
16. Fisher WC, Helwig EB. Leiomyomas of the skin. Arch Dermatol 88:510, 1963.
17. Fox SR. Leiomyomatosis cutis. N Engl J Med 263:1248, 1960.
18. Gagne, EJ, Su WPD. Congenital smooth muscle hamartoma of the skin. Pediatr Dermatol 10:142, 1993.
19. Grenier R, Rostas A, Wilkinson RD. Dermatitis herpetiformis and leiomyomas with HLA-B8, a marker of immune disease. Can Med Assoc J 115:882, 1976.
20. Jansen LH, Driessen FML. Leiomyoma cutis. Br J Dermatol 70: 446, 1958.
21. Kloepfer HW, Krafchuk J, Derbes V, et al. Hereditary multiple leiomyoma of the skin. Am J Hum Genet 10:48, 1958.
22. Mann PR. Leiomyoma cutis: an electron microscope study. Br J Dermatol 82:463, 1970.
23. Montgomery H, Winkelmann RK. Smooth muscle tumors of the skin. Arch Dermatol 79:32, 1959.
24. Nascimento AG, Karas M, Rosen PP, et al. Leiomyoma of the nipple. Am J Surg Pathol 3:151, 1979.
25. Newman PL, Fletcher CDM. Smooth muscle tumours of the external genitalia: clinicopathologic analysis of a series. Histopathology 8:523, 1991.
26. Siegel GP, Gaffey TA. Solitary leiomyomas arising from the tunica dartos scrotis. J Urol 116:69, 1976.
27. Stout AP. Solitary cutaneous and subcutaneous leiomyoma. Am J Cancer 24:435, 1937.
28. Tavassoli FA, Norris HJ. Smooth muscle tumors of the vulva. Obstet Gynaecol 53:213, 1979.
29. Urbanek RW, Johnson WC. Smooth muscle hamartoma associated with Becker's nevus. Arch Dermatol 114:104, 1978.
30. Venencie PY, Puissant A, Boffa GA, et al. Multiple cutaneous leiomyomata and erythrocytosis. Br J Dermatol 107:483, 1982.
31. Verma KC, Chawdhry SD, Rathi KS. Cutaneous leiomyomata in two brothers. Br J Dermatol 90:351, 1973.
32. Yokayama R, Hashimoto H, Daimaru Y, et al. Superficial leiomyomas: a clinicopathologic study of 34 cases. Acta Pathol Jpn 37:1415, 1987.

### Angiomyoma (Vascular Leiomyoma)

33. Bardach H, Ebner H. Das Angioleiomyoma der Haut. Hautarzt 26:638, 1975.
34. Carla TG, Filotico R, Filotico M. Bizarre angiomyomas of superficial soft tissues. Pathologica 83:237, 1991.
35. Duhig JJ, Ayer JP. Vascular leiomyoma: a study of 61 cases. Arch Pathol 68:424, 1959.
36. Ekestrom S. Comparison between glomus tumour and angioleiomyoma. Acta Pathol Microbiol Stand 27:86, 1950.
37. Gutmann J, Cifuentes C, Balzarini MA, et al. Angiomyoma of the oral cavity. Oral Surg Oral Med Oral Pathol 38:269, 1974.
38. Hachisuga T, Hashimoto H, Enjoji M. Angioleiomyoma: a clinicopathologic reappraisal of 562 cases. Cancer 54:126, 1984.

### Leiomyoma of Deep Soft Tissue

38a. Billings S, Folpe AL, Weiss SW. Do leiomyomas of deep soft tissue exist? An analysis of highly differentiated smooth muscle tumors of deep soft tissue supporting two distinct subtypes. Mod Pathol (in press).
39. Bulmer JH. Smooth muscle tumors of the limbs. J Bone Joint Surg Br 49:52, 1967.
40. Cooperman B, McAllister FF, Smith FM. Recurrent calcified leiomyoma of the pelvis and gluteal regions complicated by pregnancy. J Bone Joint Surg Am 40:1149, 1958.
41. Fletcher CDM, Kilpatrick SE, Mentzel T. The difficulty of predicting behavior of smoothmuscle tumors in deep soft tissue. Am J Surg Pathol 19:116, 1995.
42. Goodman AH, Briggs RC. Deep leiomyoma of an extremity. J Bone Joint Surg Am 47:529, 1965.
43. Herrin K, Willen H, Rydholm A. Deep-seated soft tissue leiomyomas: report of four cases. Skeletal Radiol 19:363, 1990.
44. Kilpatrick SE, Mentzel T, Fletcher CDM. Leiomyoma of deep soft tissue: clinicopathologic analysis of a series. Am J Surg Pathol 18:576, 1994.
45. Ledesma-Medina J, Oh KS, Girdany BR. Calcification in childhood leiomyoma. Radiology 135:339, 1980.
46. Meis JM, Enzinger FM. Myolipoma of soft tissue. Am J Surg Pathol 15:121, 1991.
47. Ross LS, Eckstein MR, Hirschhorn R, et al. Calcified leiomyoma: an unusual cause of large soft-tissue calcification of calf in childhood. NY State J Med 83:747, 1983.
48. Scurry JP, Carey MP, Targett CS, et al. Soft tissue lipoleiomyoma. Pathology 23:360, 1991.

### Intravenous Leiomyomatosis

49. Clement PH. Intravenous leiomyomatosis of the uterus. Pathol Annu 23:153, 1988.
50. Clement PH, Young RH, Scully RE. Intravenous leiomyomatosis of the uterus: a clinicopathological analysis of 16 cases with unusual histologic features. Am J Surg Pathol 12:932, 1988.
51. Heinonen PK, Taina E, Nerdrum T, et al. Intravenous leiomyomatosis. Ann Chir Gynaecol 73:100, 1984.
52. Norris HJ, Parmley TH. Mesenchymal tumors of the uterus. V. Intravenous leiomyomatosis: a clinical and pathologic study of 14 cases. Cancer 36:2164, 1975.
53. Ohmori T, Uraga N, Tavei R, et al. Intravenous leiomyomatosis: a case report emphasizing the vascular component. Histopathology 13:470, 1988.
54. Shida T, Yoshimura M, Chihara H, et al. Intravenous leiomyomatosis of the pelvis and re-extension into the heart. Ann Thorac Surg 42:104, 1986.
55. Suginami H, Kaura R, Ochi H, et al. Intravenous leiomyomatosis with cardiac extension: successful surgical management and histopathologic study. Obstet Gynecol 76:527, 1990.
56. Tierney WM, Ehrlich CE, Bailey JC, et al. Intravenous leiomyomatosis of the uterus with extension into the heart. Am J Med 69:471, 1980.
57. Tresukosol D, Kudelka AP, Malpica A, et al. Leuprolide acetate and intravascular leiomyomatosis. Obstet Gynecol 86:688, 1995.
58. Wolff M, Silva F, Kaye G. Pulmonary metastases (with admixed epithelial elements) from smooth muscle neoplasms: report of nine cases including three males. Am J Surg Pathol 3:325, 1979.

### Leiomyomatosis Peritonealis Disseminata

59. Abulafia O, Angel C, Sherer DM, et al. Computed tomography of leiomyomatosis peritonealis disseminata with malignant transformation. Am J Obstet Gynecol 169:52, 1993.
60. Akkersdijk GJ, Flu PK, Giard RW, et al. Malignant leiomyomatosis peritonealis disseminata. Am J Obstet Gynecol 163:591, 1990.
61. Aterman K, Fraser GM, Lea RH. Disseminated peritoneal leiomyomatosis. Virchows Arch [Pathol Anat] 374:13, 1977.
62. Buettner A, Baessler R, Theele C. Pregnancy-associated ectopic decidua (deciduosis) of the greater omentum: an analysis of 60

biopsies with cases of fibrosising deciduosis and leiomyomatosis peritonealis disseminata. Pathol Res Pract 189:352, 1993.
63. Chen KT, Hendricks EJ, Freeburg B. Benign glandular inclusion of the peritoneum associated with leiomyomatosis peritonealis disseminata. Diagn Gynecol Obstet 4:41, 1982.
64. Crosland DB. Leiomyomatosis peritonealis disseminata: a case report. Am J Obstet Gynecol 117:179, 1973.
65. Goldberg MF, Hurt WG, Frable WJ. Leiomyomatosis peritonealis disseminata: report of a case and review of the literature. Obstet Gynecol 49:46, 1977.
66. Fujii S, Nakashima N, Okamura H, et al. Progesterone-induced smooth muscle-like cells in subperitoneal nodules produced by estrogen: experimental approach to leiomyomatosis peritonealis disseminata. Am J Obstet Gynecol 139:164, 1981.
67. Hales HA, Peterson CM, Jones KP, et al. Leiomyomatosis peritonealis disseminata treated with a gonadotropin-releasing hormone agonist: a case report. Am J Obstet Gynecol 167:515, 1992.
68. Hovnck van Papendrecht HPCM, Gratam S. Leiomyomatosis peritonealis disseminata. Eur J Obstet Reprod Biol 14:251, 1983.
69. Kaplan C, Bernirschke K, Johnson KC. Leiomyomatosis peritonealis disseminata with endometrium. Obstet Gynecol 55: 119,1980.
70. Kitazawa S, Shiraishi N, Maeda S. Leiomyomatosis peritonealis disseminata with adipocytic differentiation. Acta Obstet Gynecol Scand 71:482, 1992.
71. Kuo T, London SN, Dinh TV. Endometriosis occurring in leiomyomatosis peritonealis disseminata: ultrastructural study and histogenetic consideration. Am J Surg Pathol 4:197, 1980.
72. Lim OW, Segal A, Ziel HK. Leiomyomatosis peritonealis disseminata associated with pregnancy. Obstet Gynecol 55:122, 1980.
73. Ma KF, Chow LT. Sex cord-like pattern leiomyomatosis peritonealis disseminata: a hitherto undescribed feature. Histopathology 21:389, 1992.
74. Nogales FF, Matilla A, Carrascal E. Leiomyomatosis peritonealis disseminata: an ultrastructural study. Am J Clin Pathol 69:452, 1978.
75. Parente JT, Levy J, Chinea F, et al. Adjuvant surgical and hormonal treatment of leiomyomatosis peritonealis disseminata: a case report. J Reprod Med 40:468, 1995.
76. Parmley TH, Woodruff JD, Winn K, et al. Histogenesis of leiomyomatosis peritonealis disseminata (disseminated fibrosing deciduosis). Obstet Gynecol 46:511, 1975.
77. Pieslor PC, Orenstein JM, Hogan DL, et al. Ultrastructure of myofibroblasts and decidualized cells in leiomyomatosis peritonealis disseminata. Am J Clin Pathol 72:875, 1979.
78. Quade BJ, McLachlin CM, Soto-Wright V, et al. Disseminated peritoneal leiomyomatosis: clonality analysis by X chromosome inactivation and cytogenetics of a clinically benign smooth muscle proliferation. Am J Pathol 150:2153, 1997.
79. Rubin SC, Wheeler JE, Mikuta JJ. Malignant leiomyomatosis peritonealis disseminata. Obstet Gynecol 68:126, 1986.
80. Tavassoli FA, Norris HJ. Peritoneal leiomyomatosis (leiomyomatosis peritonealis disseminata). Int J Gynecol Pathol 1:59, 1982.
81. Willson JR, Peale AR. Multiple peritoneal leiomyomas associated with a granulosa-cell tumor of the ovary. Am J Obstet Gynecol 64:204, 1952.
82. Winn KJ, Woodruff JD, Parmley TH. Electron microscopic studies of leiomyomatosis peritonealis disseminata. Obstet Gynecol 48:225, 1976.

### Palisaded Myofibroblastoma

83. Alguacil-Garcia A. Intranodal myofibroblastoma in a submandibular lymph node: a case report. Am J Clin Pathol 97:69, 1992.
84. Barbareschi M, Mariscotti C, Ferrero S, et al. Intranodal hemorrhagic spindle cell tumor: a benign Kaposi-like nodal tumor. Histopathology 17:93, 1990.
85. Bigotti G, Coli A, Mottolese M, et al. Selective location of palisaded myofibroblastoma with amianthoid fibres. J Clin Pathol 44:761, 1991.
86. Burns MK, Headington JT, Rasmussen JE. Palisaded myofibroblastoma simulating chronic primary lymphadenopathic Kaposi's sarcoma. J Am Acad Dermatol 25:566, 1991.
87. Deligdish L, Loewenthal M, Friedlaender E. Malignant neurilemoma (schwannoma) in the lymph nodes. Int Surg 49:226, 1968.
88. Fletcher CD, Stirling RW. Intranodal myofibroblastoma presenting in the submandibular region: evidence of a broader clinical and histological spectrum. Histopathology 16: 287, 1990.
89. Katz D. Neurilemoma with calcerosiderotic nodules. Isr J Med Sci 10:1156, 1974.
90. Lee JY-Y, Abell E, Shevechek GJ. Solitary spindle cell tumor with myoid differentiation of lymph node. Arch Pathol Lab Med 113:547, 1989.
91. Michal M, Chlumska A, Povysilova V. Intranodal "amianthoid" myofibroblastoma: report of six cases with immunohisochemical and electron microscopical study. Pathol Res Pract 188:199, 1992.
92. Skalova A, Michal M, Chlumska A, et al. Collagen composition and ultrastructure of the so-called amianthoid fibres in palisaded myofibroblastoma: ultrastructural and immunohistochemical study. J Pathol 167:335, 1992.
93. Suster S, Rosai J. Intranodal hemorrhagic spindle-cell tumor with "amianthoid" fibers: report of six cases of a distinctive mesenchymal neoplasm of the inguinal region that simulates Kaposi's sarcoma. Am J Surg Pathol 13:347, 1989.
94. Weiss SW, Gnepp DR, Bratthauer GL. Palisaded myofibroblastoma: a benign mesenchymal tumor of lymph node. Am J Surg Pathol 13:341, 1989.

### Myofibroblastoma of the Breast

95. Amin MB, Gottlieb CA, Fitzmaurice M, et al. Fine-needle aspiration cytologic study of myofibroblastoma of the breast: immunohistochemical and ultrastructural findings. Am J Clin Pathol 99:593, 1993.
96. Begin LR. Myogenic stromal tumor of the male breast (so-called myofibroblastoma). Ultrstruct Pathol 15:613, 1991.
97. Damiani S, Miettinen M, Peterse JL, Eusebi V. Solitary fibrous tumor (myofibroblastoma) of the breast. Virchows Arch 425: 89, 1994.
98. Hamele-Bena D, Cranor ML, Sciotto C, et al. Uncommon presentation of mammary myofibroblastoma. Mod Pathol 9:786, 1996.
99. Julien M, Trojani M, Coindre JM. Myofibroblastoma of the breast: report of 8 cases. Ann Pathol 14:143, 1994.
100. Lee AH, Sworn MJ, Theaker JM, et al. Myofibroblastoma of breast: immunohistochemical study. Histopathology 22:75, 1993.
101. Wargotz ES, Weiss SW, Norris HJ. Myofibroblastoma of the breast: sixteen cases of a distinctive benign mesenchymal tumor. Am J Surg Pathol 11:493, 1987.

### Angiomyofibroblastoma

102. Fletcher CD, Tsang WY, Fisher C, et al. Angiomyofibroblastoma of the vulva: a benign neoplasm distinct from aggressive angiomyxoma. Am J Surg Pathol 16:373, 1992.
103. Granter SR, Nucci MR, Fletcher CDM. Aggressive angiomyxoma: reappraisal of its relationship with angiomyofibroblastoma in a series of 16 cases. Histopathology 30:3, 1997.

104. Hiruki T, Thomas MJ, Clement PB. Vulvar angiomyofibroblastoma. Am J Surg Pathol 17:423, 1993.
105. Hisaoka M, Kouho H, Aoki T, et al. Angiomyofibroblastoma of the vulva: a clinicopathologic study of seven cases. Pathol Int 45:487, 1995.
106. Nielsen GP, Rosenberg AE, Young RH, et al. Angiomyofibroblastoma of the vulva and vagina: a clinicopathologic study of 12 cases. Mod Pathol 9:284, 1996.
107. Nielsen GP, Young RH, Dickersin GR, Rosenberg AE. Angiomyofibroblastoma of the vulva with sarcomatous transformation ("angiomyofibrosarcoma"). Am J Surg Pathol 21:1104, 1997.
108. Ockner DM, Sayadi H, Swanson PE, et al. Genital angiomyofibroblastoma: comparison with aggressive angiomyxoma and other myxoid neoplasms of skin and soft tissue. Am J Clin Pathol 107:36, 1997.

# CHAPTER 19

# LEIOMYOSARCOMA

Leiomyosarcomas account for 5–10% of soft tissue sarcomas.[10,33,46] They are principally tumors of adult life but are far outnumbered by the more common adult sarcomas such as liposarcoma and malignant fibrous life histiocytoma. Likewise, they are less common than leiomyosarcomas of uterine or gastrointestinal origin, and only some of the data gleaned from the collective experience with tumors in these two sites are directly applicable to the soft tissue counterpart. Few predisposing or etiologic factors are recognized for this disease. In general, these tumors are more common in women than men. About two-thirds of all retroperitoneal leiomyosarcomas[44,47,54] and more than three-fourths of all vena caval leiomyosarcomas occur in women.[84] The significance of this observation is not clear, although growth and proliferation of smooth muscle tissue in women have been noted to coincide with pregnancy and estrogenic stimulation (see Chapter 18). Children rarely develop these tumors,[2,38,42] and there is conflicting evidence as to whether leiomyosarcomas in children have a better prognosis.[2,5a,14,42] A recent study suggesting a better prognosis included a disproportionate number of superficial lesions.[5a]

Reports in the literature and in our experience at the Armed Forces Institute of Pathology (AFIP) indicate that leiomyosarcomas are rarely induced by irradiation.[12,15,32,33,60,61] Such tumors are largely curiosities, and it is much more common to see fibrosarcomas, osteosarcomas, and malignant fibrous histiocytomas induced by irradiation. Leiomyosarcomas may develop as a second malignancy in the setting of bilateral (hereditary) retinoblastoma.[9] Because these tumors may occur at sites distant from their irradiated site, it is clear that they are directly attributable to the *Rb1* mutation and not to irradiation. A study by Stratton et al. indicated that deletions or mutations of the *Rb1* locus can be identified in a small number of leiomyosarcomas that occur on a sporadic basis as well.[37]

There is little evidence that leiomyomas undergo malignant transformation with any degree of regularity. Well differentiated areas resembling leiomyoma are often found in a leiomyosarcoma, but this by no means proves that malignant transformation occurred. In fact, the predilection of leiomyosarcomas for deep soft tissue, in contrast to the superficial location of leiomyomas, provides some evidence to the contrary. Leiomyosarcomas have also been associated with the production of human $\beta$-chorionic gonadotropin.[19] Experimentally, the tumors may be induced in rabbits by intramuscular deposition of nickel subsulfide.[11] One alleged leiomyosarcoma occurred on the diaphragmatic surface of an asbestos worker, although the illustrations in this case cast some doubt on the diagnosis.[7]

Although all leiomyosarcomas of soft tissue are histologically similar, it is useful to divide them into site-related groups because of clinical and biologic differences. Leiomyosarcomas of soft tissue, particularly the retroperitoneum, are the most common group and serve as the prototype, as they best illustrate the range of histologic changes common to these tumors, the problems inherent in histologic evaluation, and occasionally the inability to predict biologic behavior from the histologic appearance alone. Some recent evidence suggests that a significant number of leiomyosarcomas of soft tissue arise from small vessels, and this relation may be important for defining the behavior and risk of metastasis. Although technically such lesions could be referred to as "vascular leiomyosarcomas," this designation usually refers to a tumor arising from a major vessel such that clinical symptoms, radiographic findings, or both suggest the relationship preoperatively. Cutaneous leiomyosarcomas are a second group and usually have a good prognosis because of their superficial location. They can be likened to atypical fibroxanthoma and superficial forms of malignant fibrous histiocytoma (see Chapter 15), which have a highly atypical appearance but a favorable clinical course because of their limited clinical stage. In the last group are leiomyosarcomas of vascular origin. As implied above, in this chapter we use this designation to refer to tumors arising from medium-size or large veins, in contrast to leiomyosarcomas in which the vascular origin is identified on the basis of microscopic examination. Defined in this fashion these tumors are rare.

## LEIOMYOSARCOMAS OF SOFT TISSUE

Leiomyosarcomas of soft tissue arise principally in the retroperitoneal space and abdominal cavity. According to Golden and Stout[44] and the Soft Tissue Task Force,[33] about half of all soft tissue leiomyosarcomas occur in the retroperitoneum, making it the single most common soft tissue site. Leiomyosarcomas also occur in intraabdominal locations such as the omentum and mesentery[57,58] and infrequently in soft tissues of the extremities and trunk. Mediastinal leiomyosarcomas are even less common.[50] Smooth muscle tumors presenting as pedunculated masses attached to the serosal surfaces of the viscera, particularly the stomach, are traditionally considered gastrointestinal tract lesions and are not included in the present discussion.

### Clinical Findings

About two-thirds of retroperitoneal leiomyosarcomas occur in women.[54] The median age at the time of presentation is 60 years,[54] which is roughly comparable to other retroperitoneal sarcomas such as liposarcomas and malignant fibrous histiocytomas. This contrasts with the younger age of patients with gastrointestinal leiomyosarcomas, which probably become symptomatic at an earlier stage. The presenting signs and symptoms are relatively nonspecific and include an abdominal mass or swelling, pain, weight loss, nausea, or vomiting. Computed tomography (CT) and angiography can localize the lesions to the retroperitoneal space, although they cannot be distinguished from other retroperitoneal sarcomas.[45] They appear to be hypovascular or moderately vascular and derive their main arterial supply from the lumbar arteries, with an ancillary supply from vessels such as the celiac, superior mesenteric, inferior mesenteric, and renal arteries. Displacement and distortion of normal vessels are common findings, and in some cases neovascularization is observed.[45] The use of indium 111-antimyosin, which is taken up by neoplastic muscle cells, has been suggested as a means of identifying these tumors preoperatively.[5] At surgery the masses are usually large and often unresectable. In the AFIP experience with 36 leiomyosarcomas of the retroperitoneum, the mean size was about 16 cm, (range 7.5–35.0 cm), and the average weight was approximately 1600 g.[54] They commonly involve other structures, such as the kidney, pancreas, and vertebral column by direct extension. Some tumors have a white-gray whorled appearance resembling a leiomyoma on cut section (Fig. 19–1). More often the tumors are fleshy white-gray masses with foci of hemorrhage and necrosis and are therefore indistinguishable from other sarcomas (Fig. 19–2). Cysts may be present and occasionally are so striking that these tumors are mistaken on gross inspection for cystic neurilemomas.

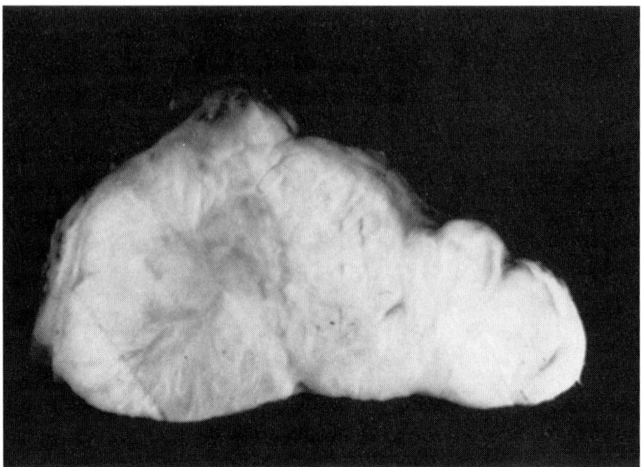

**FIGURE 19–1.** Well-differentiated leiomyosarcoma with a whorled appearance similar to that of a leiomyoma on cut section.

Compared with retroperitoneal lesions, tumors arising from the soft tissues of the extremities and trunk are far less common and seem to affect the genders

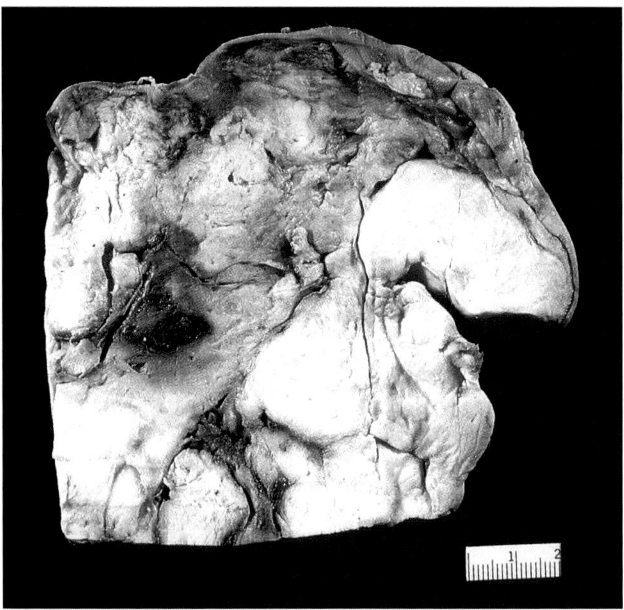

**FIGURE 19–2.** Poorly differentiated leiomyosarcoma characterized by fleshy white tissue with hemorrhage and necrosis.

equally. Only 48 cases were identified by Gustafson et al.[10] in a 22-year review of a Swedish population in Lund, and we have studied 42 cases largely based on referred consultations. These tumors present as an enlarging mass, usually in the lower extremity. About half develop in the subcutis and the remainder in muscle. They have a circumscribed multinodular appearance and are significantly smaller (6 cm) than those in the retroperitoneum. In our experience at least one-third arise from a small vein when examined microscopically.[43] Such lesions may be surrounded by the adventitia of the vessel, giving them a discrete appearance, leading to simple enucleation by the surgeon.

## Microscopic Findings

As a group, retroperitoneal and deep soft tissue leiomyosarcomas probably display the greatest variety of patterns of any of the soft tissue leiomyosarcomas. The typical cell of the leiomyosarcoma is elongated and has an abundant cytoplasm that varies tinctorially from pink to deep red in sections stained with hematoxylin-eosin. The nucleus is usually centrally located and blunt-ended or "cigar-shaped" (Fig. 19–3). In some smooth muscle cells a vacuole is seen at one end of the nucleus, causing a slight indentation, so the nucleus assumes a concave rather than a convex contour (Fig. 19–3). In less well differentiated tumors the nucleus is larger and more hyperchromatic and often loses its central location. Multinucleated giant cells are common. Likewise, depending on the degree of differentiation, the appearance of the cytoplasm varies. Differentiated cells have numerous well oriented myofibrils that are demonstrable as deep red, longitudinally placed parallel lines running the length of the cell on staining with Masson trichrome (Fig. 19–4). With phosphotungstic acid-hematoxylin (PTAH) staining, the striations are purple. In poorly differentiated cells the longitudinal striations are less numerous, poorly oriented, and therefore more difficult to identify. In some tumors the cytoplasm has a "clotted" appearance as a result of clumping of the myofilamentous material (Fig. 19–5). When this phenomenon occurs it may be difficult to identify linear striations. Glycogen can usually be demonstrated by periodic acid-Schiff stain (PAS) in the cytoplasm of the leiomyosarcomas. As a rule, most retroperitoneal and soft tissue leiomyosarcomas are moderately differentiated tumors, often displaying sharply marginated borders. They are composed of slender or slightly plump cells arranged in fascicles of varying size (Figs. 19–6 to 19–9). In well-differentiated areas the fascicles intersect at right angles so it is possible to see transverse and longitudinal sections side by side, similar to the pattern of a uterine myoma. In many areas the pattern is not that orderly, however, and it more closely resembles the intertwining fascicular growth of a fibrosarcoma (Fig. 19–10). In occasional leiomyosarcomas the nuclei align them-

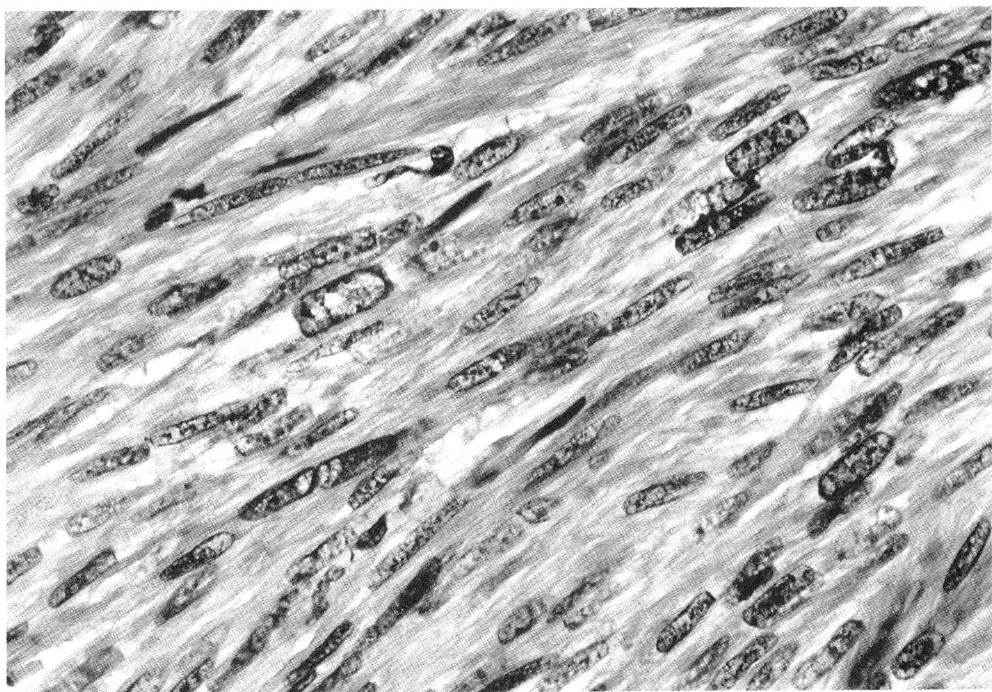

**FIGURE 19–3.** Cytologic features of leiomyosarcoma showing eosinophilic cytoplasm and blunt-ended nuclei. Occasional cells have perinuclear vacuoles.

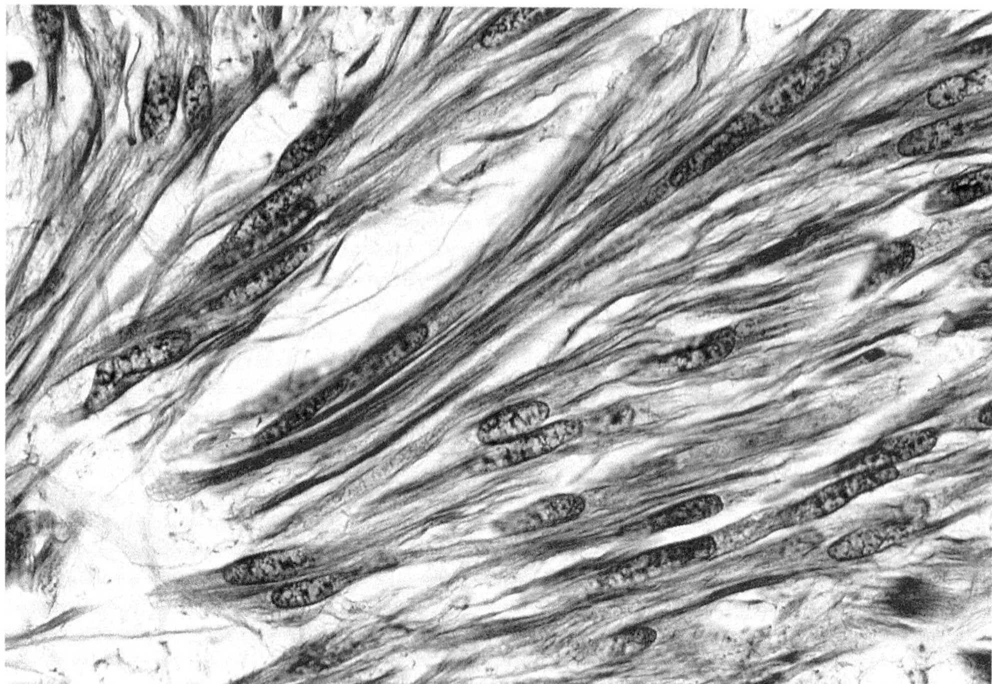

**FIGURE 19–4.** Masson trichrome stain illustrating longitudinal striations in a leiomyosarcoma. Striations appear as red hair-like streaks in the cytoplasm.

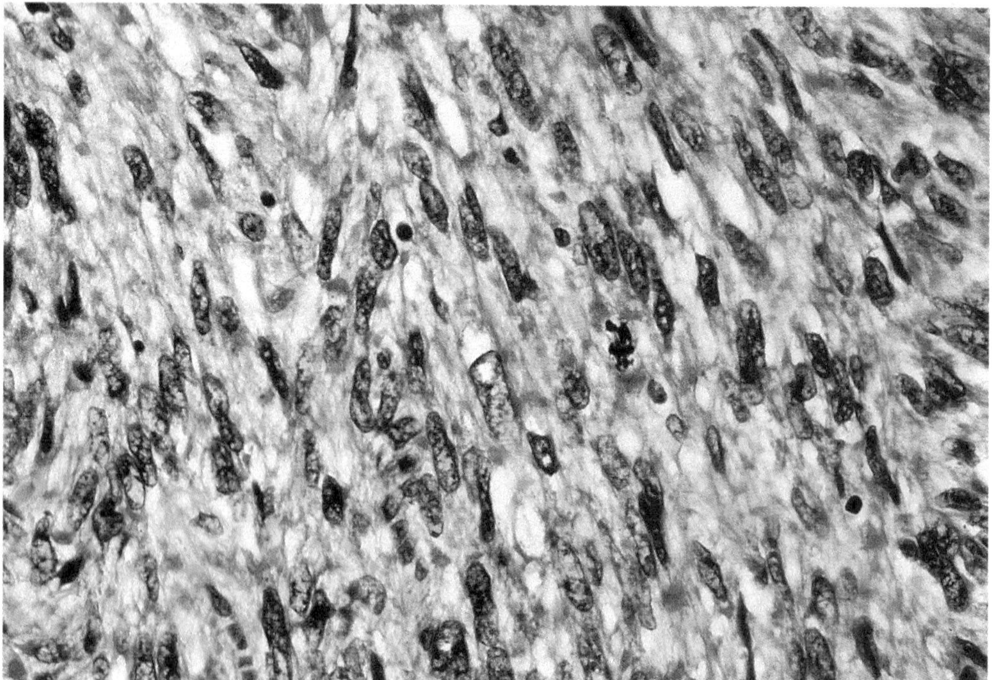

**FIGURE 19–5.** Leiomyosarcoma with "clotted" or clumped myofilamentous material in the cytoplasm.

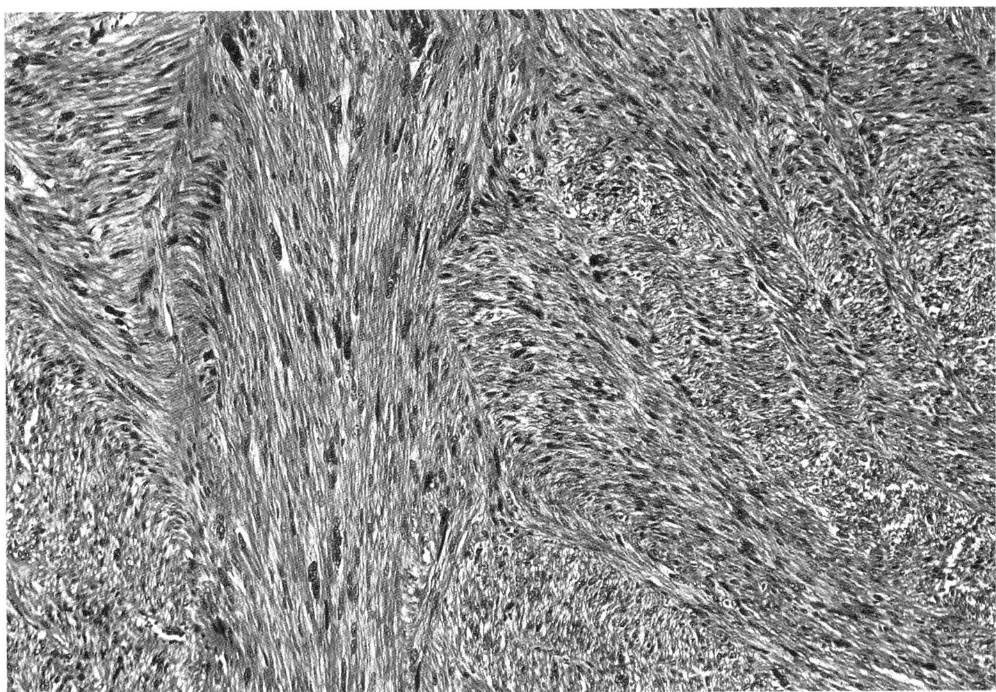

**FIGURE 19–6.** Moderately differentiated leiomyosarcoma composed of deeply eosinophilic fascicles intersecting at right angles.

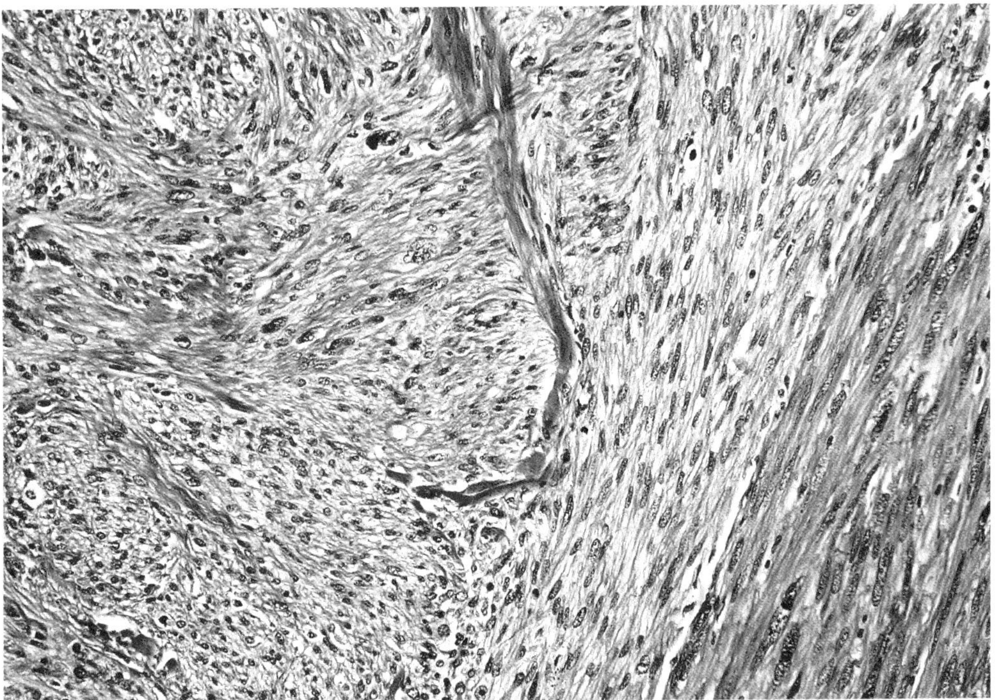

**FIGURE 19–7.** Moderately differentiated leiomyosarcoma composed of intersecting fascicles, some having a deeply eosinophilic hue and others a clear-cell appearance.

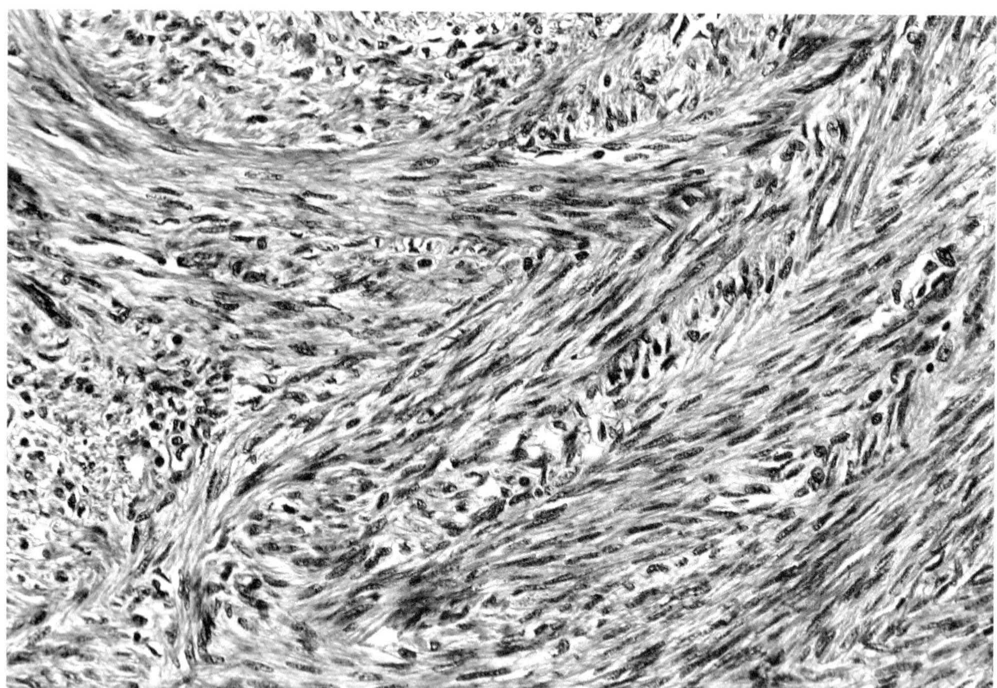

**FIGURE 19–8.** Well-differentiated leiomyosarcoma with a fascicular growth pattern.

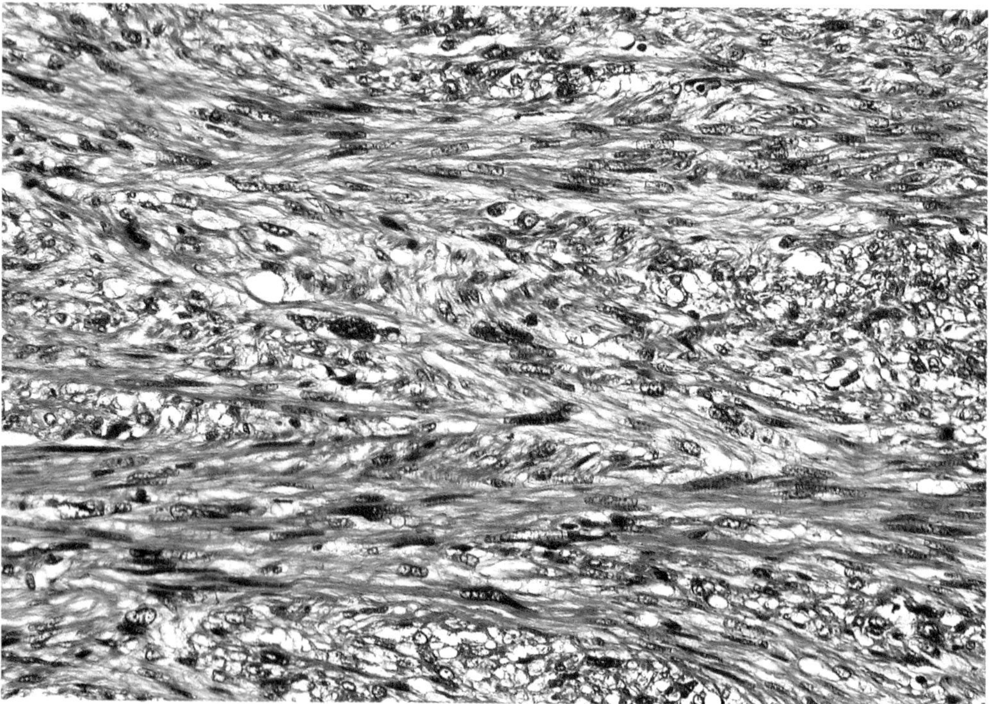

**FIGURE 19–9.** Moderately differentiated leiomyosarcoma with a fascicular growth pattern.

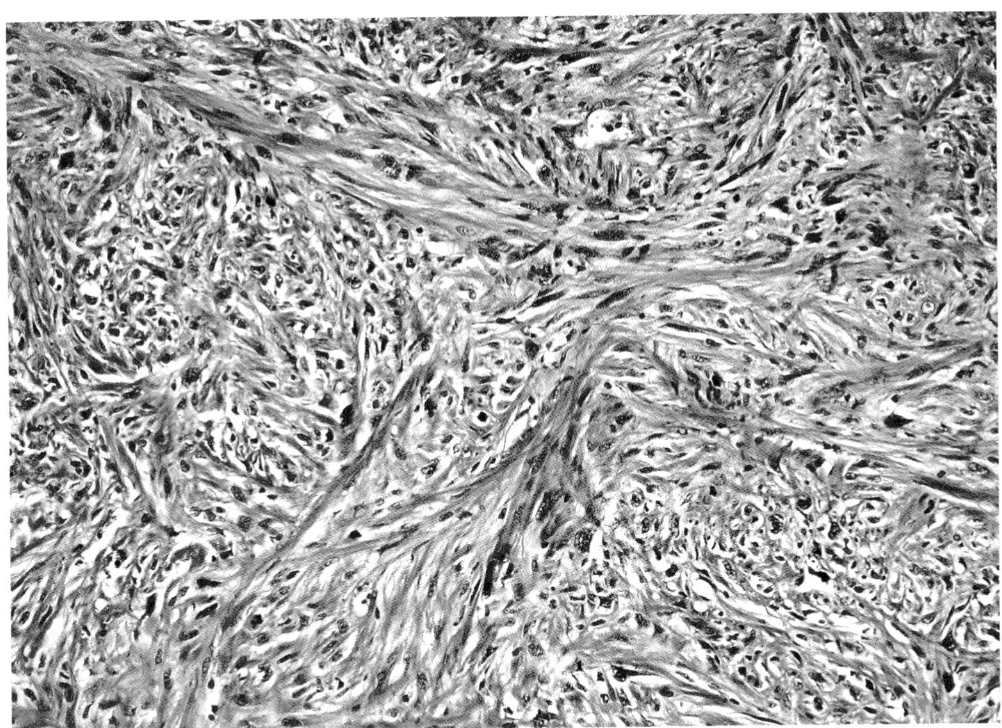

**FIGURE 19–10.** Leiomyosarcoma with a pattern of short intersecting fascicles.

selves to create palisades, similar to a schwannoma (Fig. 19–11).

These tumors can pose considerable problems with the differential diagnosis. The staining characteristics of the cells, including the presence of cytoplasmic glycogen and linear striations and the absence of S-100 protein, figure significantly in distinguishing well-differentiated leiomyosarcomas with palisading from schwannomas. Hyalinization is a relatively common, but usually focal, feature of many leiomyosarcomas (Fig. 19–12).[64] The number of mitotic figures varies greatly, but more than 80% of retroperitoneal leiomyosarcomas average ≥5 mitoses/10 high-power fields (HPF)[54] (see Criteria of Malignancy, below). A small number of retroperitoneal leiomyosarcomas are anaplastic tumors (Figs. 19–13, 19–14), which in the extreme case resemble a malignant fibrous histiocytoma. They contain numerous pleomorphic giant cells with deeply eosinophilic cytoplasm intimately admixed with a complement of more uniform-appearing spindle and round cells (Figs. 19–15, 19–16, 19–17). In contrast to malignant fibrous histiocytoma, these tumors have less interstitial collagen, few inflammatory cells, and at least some cytoplasmic glycogen. In addition, it is usually possible to document myogenic differentiation in the less pleomorphic areas. Necrosis, hemorrhage, and mitotic figures are frequent in these pleomorphic tumors. Osteoclastic giant cells, with histiocytic (CD68) but not myogenic markers[49] are an uncommmon feature of leiomyosarcomas.[16,17,40,49] Based on their distinct immunophenotypic profile they may well represent an unusual host response to the tumor, rather than an intrinsic part of the lesion. Unusually, leiomyosarcomas with liposarcoma[56] or rhabdomyosarcomas have been reported.[52]

## Epithelioid Leiomyosarcoma

There are several distinctly uncommon features of leiomyosarcomas. "Epithelioid changes" may occur in smooth muscle tumors.[55] The cells become rounded, and there is often a concomitant "vacuolar" or "clear cell" change in the cytoplasm. This feature may be seen focally in otherwise typical smooth muscle tumors. These tumors may occur in superficial[55] or deep soft tissue, although in the latter location they are usually considered to be extragastrointestinal stromal tumors (leiomyoblastoma) (see Chapter 20). Suster has reported a group of superficial epithelioid leiomyosarcomas that expressed actin in the absence of desmin. Relying in part on ultrastructural features of smooth muscle differentiation (thin filaments with dense bodies, surface pinocytotic vesicles, and basal lamina), he emphasized the fact that the superficial location suggests the diagnosis of a metastatic neoplasm or malignant melanoma.[55]

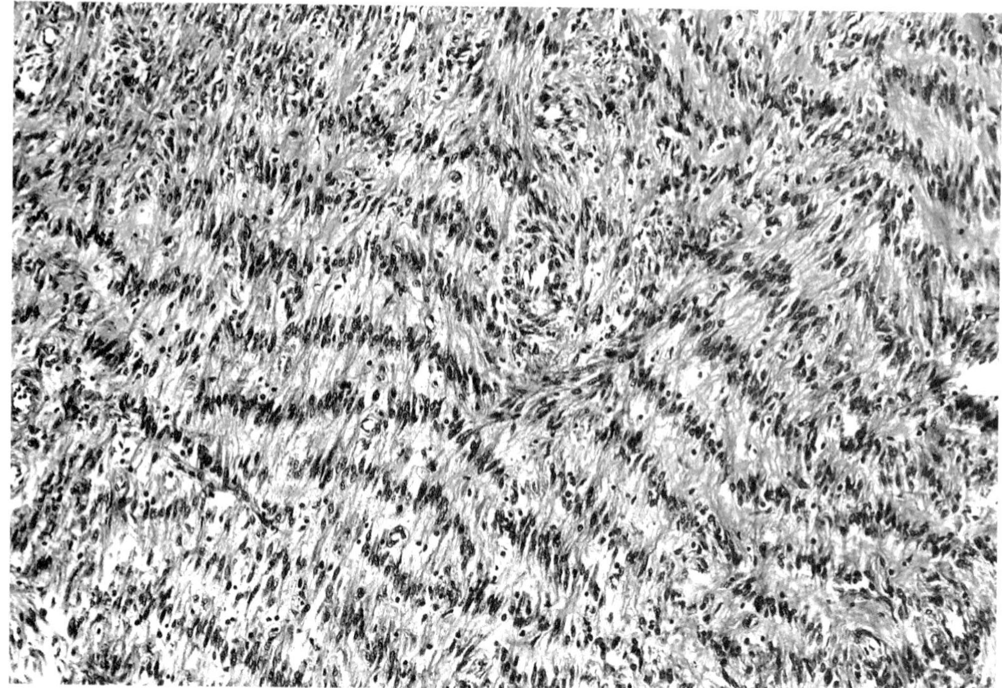

**FIGURE 19–11.** Leiomyosarcoma with nuclear palisading.

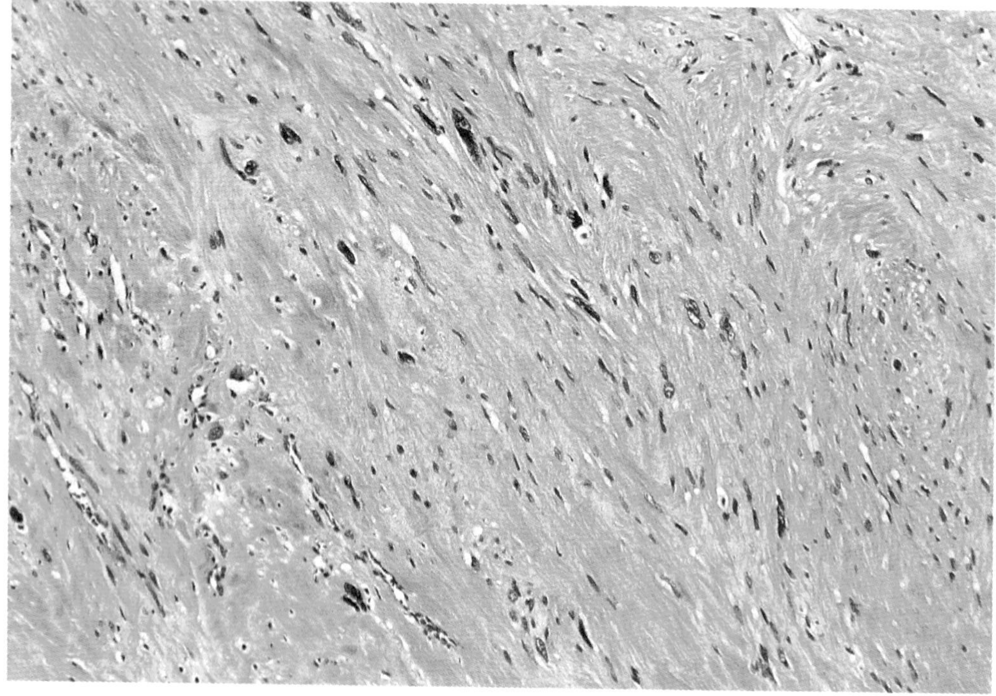

**FIGURE 19–12.** Hyalinization in a leiomyosarcoma.

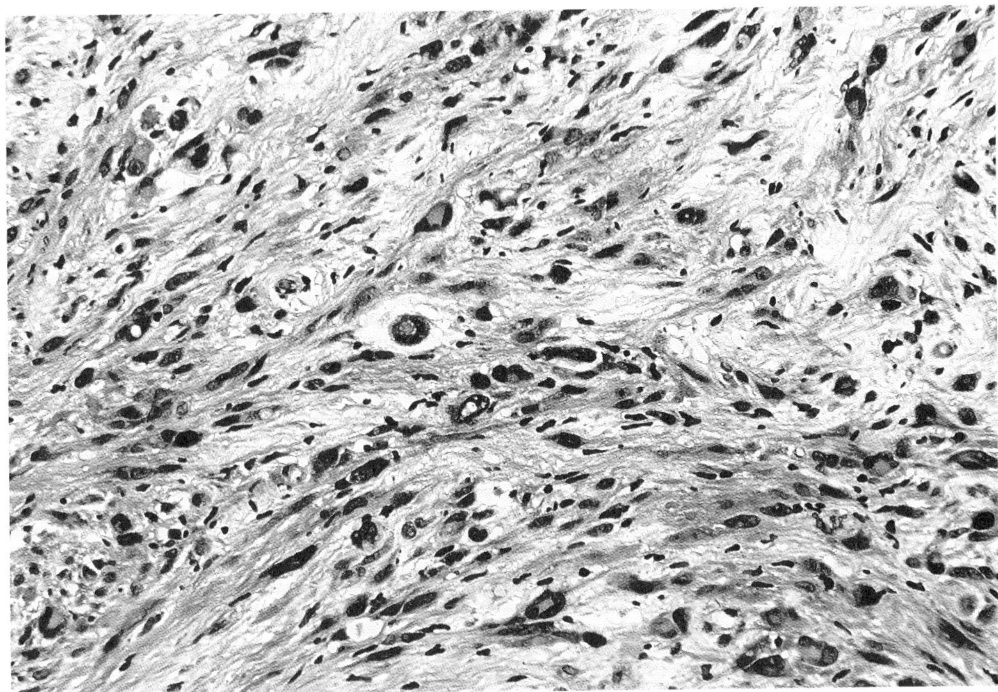

**FIGURE 19–13.** Pleomorphism in a leiomyosarcoma.

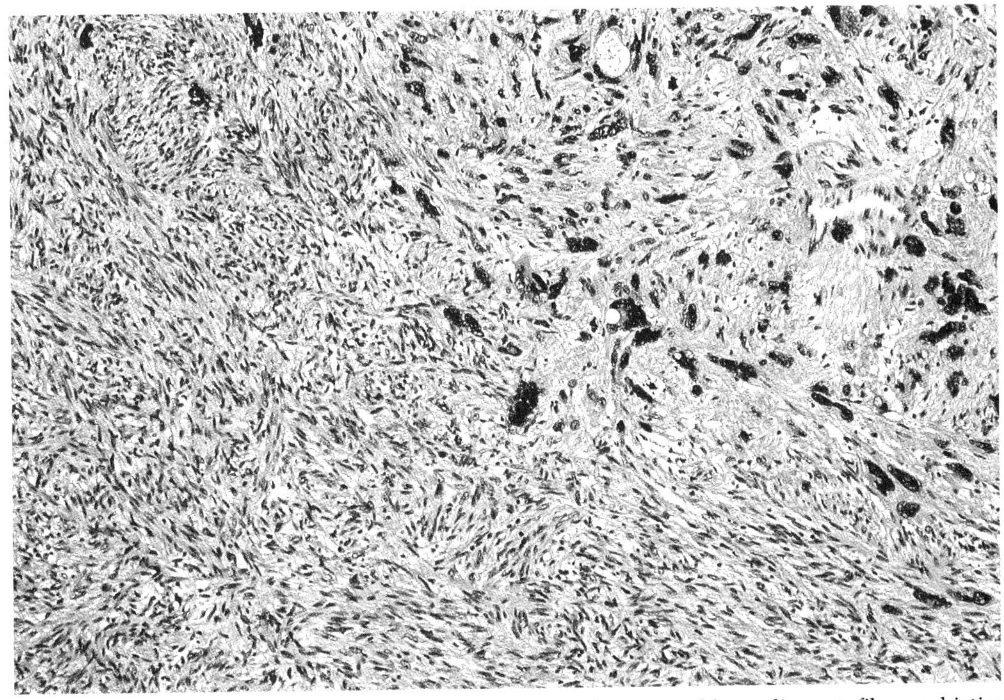

**FIGURE 19–14.** Leiomyosarcoma with pleomorphic areas that resemble malignant fibrous histiocytoma (top right).

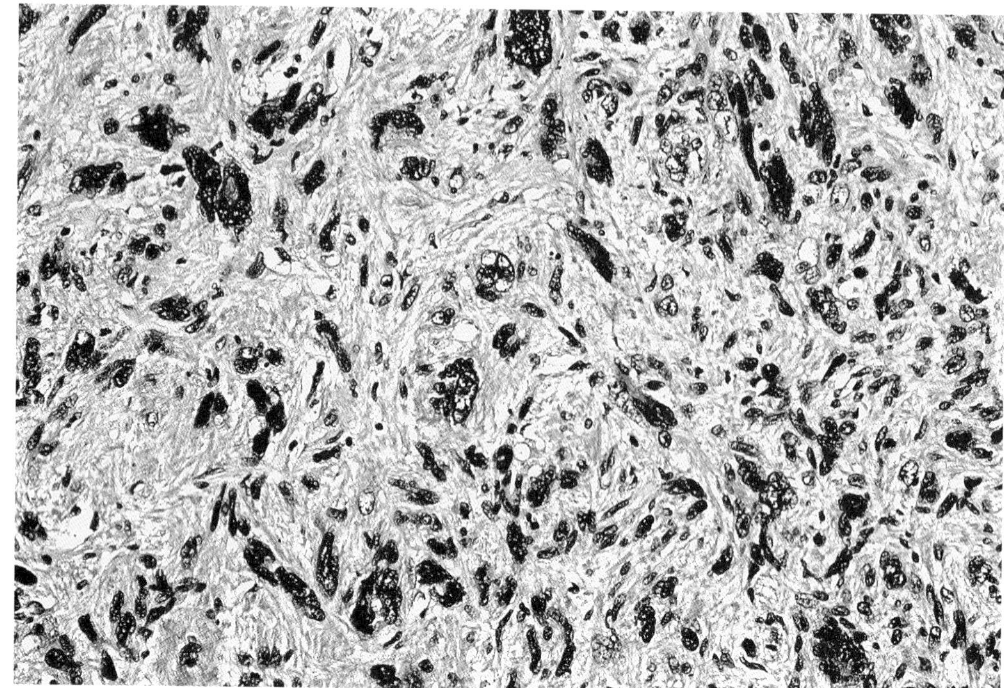

**FIGURE 19–15.** Pleomorphism area in leiomyosarcoma resembling malignant fibrous histiocytoma.

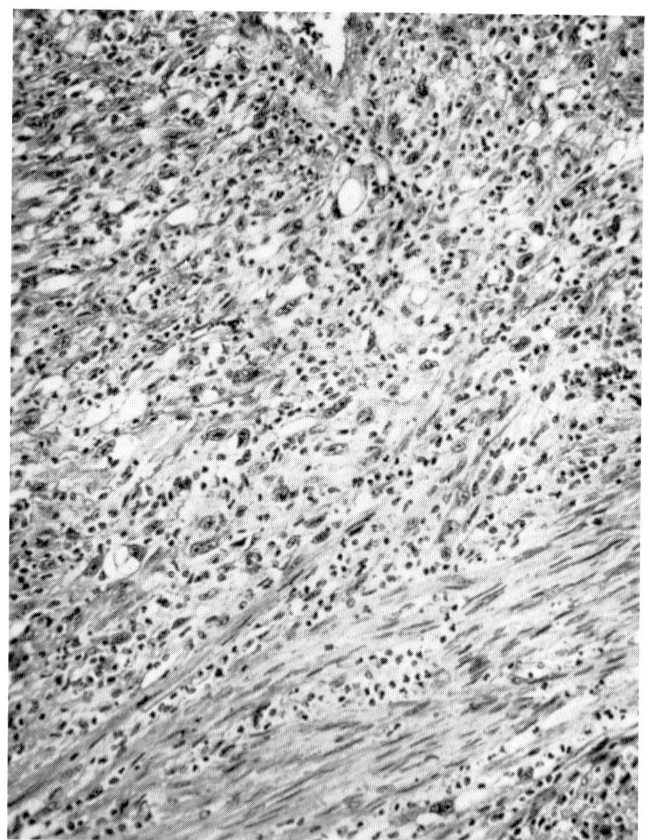

**FIGURE 19–16.** Leiomyosarcoma with pleomorphic areas resembling the inflammatory form of malignant fibrous histiocytoma. (×160)

## Myxoid Leiomyosarcoma

Myxoid change may occur in leiomyosarcomas. It is occasionally so extensive the tumors appear grossly gelatinous. Although these so-called myxoid leiomyosarcomas have been reported most commonly in the uterus,[48,53] they develop in conventional soft tissue locations as well. The spindled muscle cells are separated by pools of hyaluronic acid, and in cross section the fascicles may resemble the cords of tumor seen in a myxoid chondrosarcoma (Figs. 19–18, 19–19). Because these tumors are quite hypocellular relative to conventional leiomyosarcomas, mitotic rates estimated by counting high-power fields are usually deceptively low, giving the false impression of a benign state. In the experience of King et al.,[48] tumors averaging 0–2 mitoses/10 HPF have proved to be aggressive. Four of their six patients died of disease, one was alive with disease, and one died of other causes but was known to have residual tumor at death. Hence these tumors must be considered fully malignant. It is quite possible that spillage of the gelatinous matrix at the time of surgery contributes to the common phenomenon of local recurrence.

## Inflammatory Leiomyosarcoma

Leiomyosarcomas containing xanthoma cells and a prominent inflammatory infiltrate (usually lymphocytes but occasionally neutrophils) have been desig-

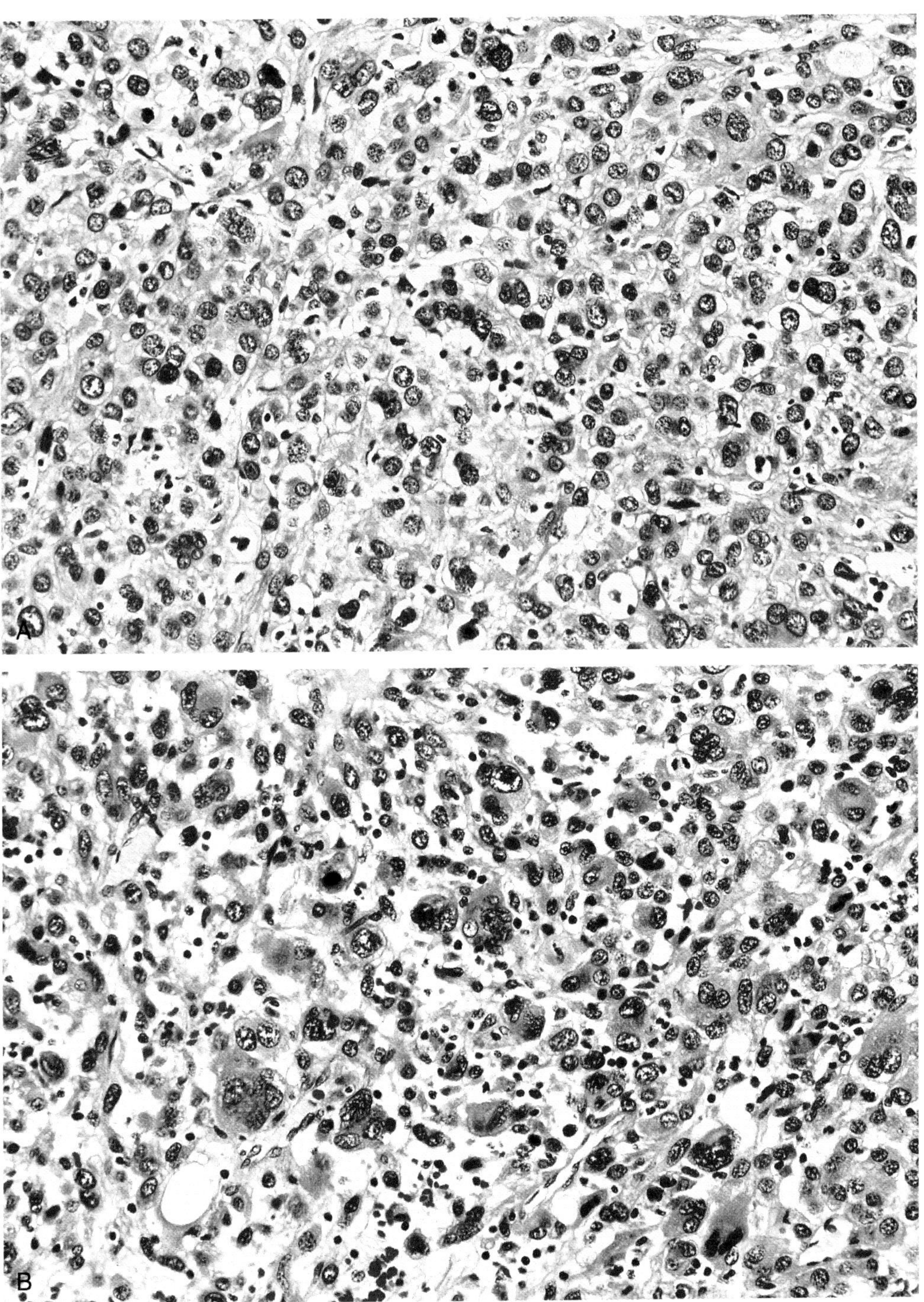


**FIGURE 19–17.** Leiomyosarcoma with round cell (**A**), and pleomorphic (**B**) areas.

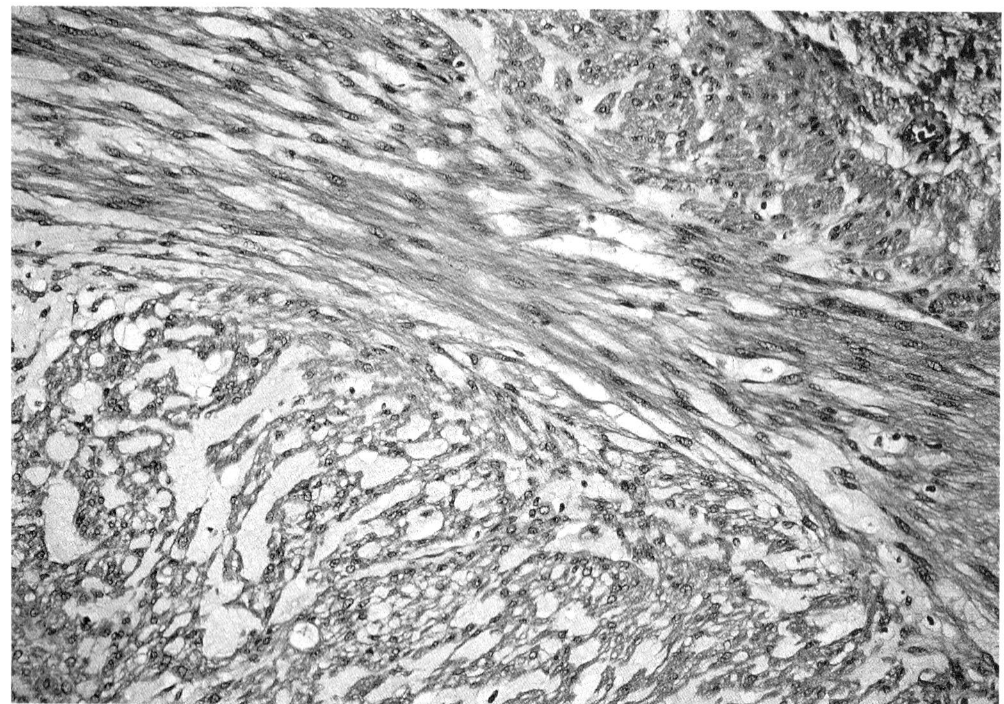

**FIGURE 19–18.** Myxoid leiomyosarcoma.

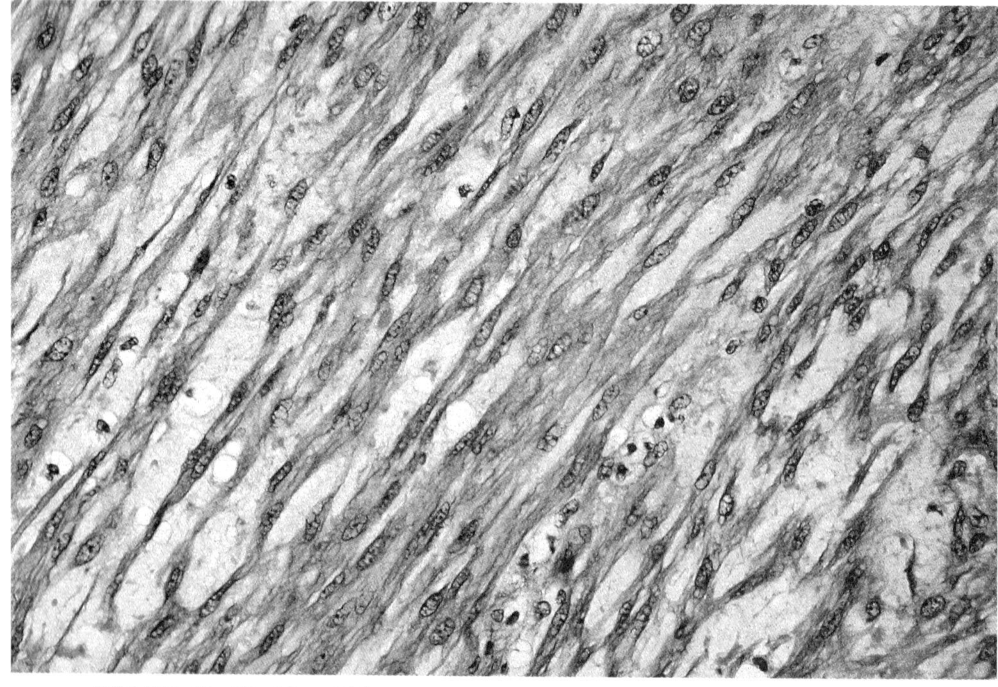

**FIGURE 19–19.** Myxoid leiomyosarcoma showing separation of spindle cells.

nated "inflammatory leiomyosarcoma" (Fig. 19–16).[18] They do not occur in any specific location, nor are they associated with the systemic symptoms that characterize "inflammatory fibrosarcoma" and "inflammatory malignant fibrous histiocytoma." The principal significance of this variant of leiomyosarcoma resides in the fact that it may be misdiagnosed as an inflammatory malignant fibrous histiocytoma.

## Granular Cell Leiomyosarcoma

Rarely, leiomyosarcomas contain cells with granular eosinophilic cytoplasm.[24] This change corresponds to the presence of numerous granules that stain positively with PAS and are resistant to diastase. Ultrastructurally, they are similar to the phagolysosomes seen in granular cell tumors.

## Criteria of Malignancy

Determining suitable criteria of malignancy for smooth muscle tumors is difficult because these tumors represent a biologic continuum for which one is forced to draw arbitrary lines when designating some "benign" and others "malignant." Although a number of features, such as size, cellularity, atypia, and necrosis, correlate to some extent with malignancy, mitotic activity has been used as the most reliable parameter.[51,54] Consequently, it is this feature that we rely on most heavily when evaluating these tumors.

The importance of a representative mitotic rate implies that smooth muscle tumors of soft tissue be carefully sampled, as has been recommended for uterine lesions. The levels of mitotic activity that seem suitable when evaluating uterine tumors are not valid for soft tissue tumors, as they would result in a significant number of underdiagnoses. For instance, uterine lesions with 5–9 mitoses/10 HPF are considered borderline lesions,[84] but in soft tissue this level of mitotic activity almost always signifies a tumor that is capable of metastasis.[54] In our experience, retroperitoneal smooth muscle tumors with 5 mitoses/10 HPF should be considered malignant, as most patients with tumors of this type succumb to the disease. Tumors with 1–4 mitoses/10 HPF are best considered potentially malignant, especially if they are large and have areas of necrosis or nuclear atypia. The most problematic lesions of deep soft tissue are those with extremely low levels of mitotic activity in the range of 0-5/50 HPF. We still regard such lesions as potentially malignant if there is any degree of nuclear atypia present. In the absence of nuclear atypia the diagnosis of "leiomyomas" can be made provisionally. However, it is important to emphasize that those smooth muscle tumors in deep somatic soft tissue which behave in a benign fashion usually also have significant areas of hyalinization or calcification. Likewise, smooth muscle tumors in the retroperitoneum that behave in a benign fashion occur nearly exclusively in the pelvic retroperitoneum of women and closely resemble uterine leiomyomas. Although in the past many were considered auto-amputated leiomyomas, recent evidence suggest that some arise within soft tissue. (see Chapter 18).

## Ultrastructural and Immunohistochemical Findings

Leiomyosarcomas are characterized by many of the same features as normal smooth muscle cells, but in general they are less developed. Differentiated leiomyosarcomas have deeply clefted nuclei and numerous well oriented, thin (6–8 nm) myofilaments and dense bodies that occupy a large portion of the cell (Fig. 19–20). Pinocytotic vesicles and intercellular connections are conspicuous, and basal lamina invests the entire cell membrane. The presence of these features is diagnostic of smooth muscle differentiation even without the benefit of light microscopic findings. On the other hand, poorly differentiated tumors show a loss of myofilaments as rough endoplasmic reticulum, and free ribosomes assume greater prominence.[8] Pinocytotic vesicles and intercellular attachments are sparse, and basal lamina may be incomplete or lacking altogether. All of these features must be evaluated in toto in these tumors and interpreted in conjunction with the light microscopic findings for diagnostic pur-

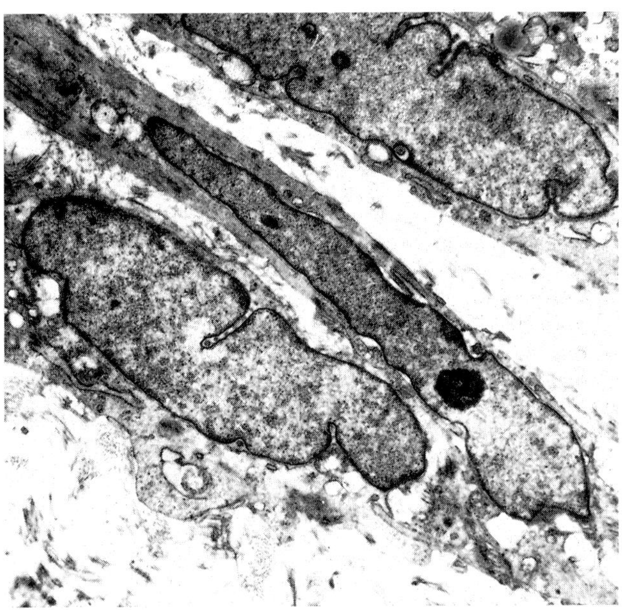

**FIGURE 19–20.** Electron micrograph of metastatic leiomyosarcoma. Cells are characterized by an elongated shape, deeply grooved nuclei, and numerous thin filaments with dense bodies.

poses. The importance of the light microscopic findings should not be minimized in these situations because some leiomyosarcomas assume "a diagnostic growth pattern at the light microscopic level prior to or possibly without developing the specific organelles of smooth muscle cells."[22] On the other hand, it should be emphasized that the mere presence of thin myofilaments with dense bodies does not identify a smooth muscle cell. Thin myofilaments are a nonspecific finding and can be seen in a variety of tumors where they typically occur underneath the cytoplasmic membrane.

Localization of muscle antigens by means of immunohistochemistry has become an increasingly popular adjunctive procedure for diagnosing these neoplasms. Over the last several years issues have been raised concerning the specificity and sensitivity of various muscle antigens and their related antibodies in terms of diagnosis. The appearance of commercially available antibodies that perform well on formalin-fixed tissues has, to a large extent, ameliorated the situation; yet it is imperative that the pathologist be aware of the distribution of various muscle antigens in normal nonmuscle tissues to avoid serious errors in diagnosis. Muscle-specific actin (HHF35)[39] can be detected in most leiomyosarcomas.[1,30,38,68] Desmin, more variable, has been documented in one-half[1] to nearly 100% of tumors,[68] depending on the series. Although there seems to be general agreement that the presence of desmin diffusely throughout a tumor is usually indicative of myoid differentiation, the presence of actin or desmin focally should not necessarily be equated with myoid lineage, as myofibroblasts in a variety of neoplastic and nonneoplastic conditions also display this phenotype.[34,35] It has also been demonstrated that tumors with definite ultrastructural features of leiomyosarcomas may lack both antigens. Smooth muscle tumors comprise one of the mesenchymal lesions in which keratin immunoreactivity has been reported.[3,19–21,26] The immunoreactivity is usually localized to a perinuclear zone and coexists with desmin. This immunoreactivity is due to the presence of keratins 8 and 18,[20] which are present in simple (nonstratified) epithelium and some mesenchymal tissues. Other antigens sporadically identified in leiomyosarcomas are S-100 protein, Leu-7, myelin basic protein, epithelial membrane antigen, and cathepsin B.[68]

## Differential Diagnosis

The differential diagnosis of leiomyosarcomas traditionally includes other sarcomas composed of fascicles of moderately differentiated spindle cells, such as fibrosarcoma and malignant peripheral nerve sheath tumor. Although the low-power appearance of all three can be similar, there is a greater tendency to see a close juxtaposition of longitudinally and transversely cut fascicles in a leiomyosarcoma. The cytologic features play a more important role in the differential diagnosis. Compared with the cells of leiomyosarcoma, those of a fibrosarcoma tend to be tapered, and those of a malignant peripheral nerve sheath tumor are wavy, buckled, and distinctly asymmetric. Usually neither malignant peripheral nerve sheath tumors nor fibrosarcomas contain glycogen; and although both occasionally display fuchsinophilia of the cytoplasm, neither has longitudinal striations. There are, in addition to the above lesions, reactive fibroblastic lesions in the submucosa of various parenchymal organs that are commonly confused with leiomyosarcomas or even rhabdomyosarcomas. Many of these lesions have been reported in the bladder, where some have been associated with prior instrumentation. We have also encountered them in the vagina, endometrium, larynx, and oral cavity. They have been termed postoperative spindle cell nodule,[29] inflammatory pseudotumor,[25] and pseudosarcomatous fibromyxoid tumor.[31] They are composed of bipolar or stellate fibroblasts with bizarre nuclei and a light basophilic cytoplasm set in a myxoid stroma containing inflammatory cells (see Chapter 9). Mitotic figures may be encountered, although atypical mitotic figures are not seen. The principal features we have found helpful for distinguishing these bizarre reactive lesions from leiomyosarcoma are the less-ordered arrangement of the cells with respect to one another, the basophilic hue of the cytoplasm, and the absence of distinct linear striations. In the limited number of cases we have studied, the cells have been strongly positive for vimentin but negative for desmin; interestingly, they may express cytokeratin.

## Behavior and Treatment

Retroperitoneal leiomyosarcomas are a highly aggressive group of tumors that are often so large total resection is impossible. Consequently, they may cause death not only by distant metastasis but also by local extension. The survival figures differ among series and are obviously influenced by the criteria of malignancy, proportion of high-grade versus low-grade tumors, and length of the follow-up. Wile et al.[57] reported a survival of 6%, Ranchod and Kempson[51] 16% (with a 2-year follow-up), and Shmookler and Lauer 29% (from 5-year actuarial data).[54] In the study by Shmookler and Lauer of 30 patients with follow-up data, 17 developed distant metastasis, with the liver and the lung being the two most common sites.[54] Other sites include the skin, soft tissue, and bone.

The behavior of soft tissue leiomyosarcomas exclusive of retroperitoneal lesions has been poorly defined owing to the relatively small number of reported cases. Our experience,[43] combined with that of Gustafson et al.[10] for a total of 90 cases, indicates that these lesions are aggressive but do not have nearly the accelerated disease tempo as do retroperitoneal lesions. Local recurrence rates range from 10% to 25% and metastatic rates from 44% to 45%, with a 5-year survival of 64%. Most metastases develop in lung and rarely in lymph nodes.

A number of variables seem to affect the prognosis in this subgroup of leiomyosarcomas, but their relative importance differs depending on the study. Gustafson et al. found that age over 60 years and vascular invasion were independent risk factors for death from the tumor,[10] whereas Hashimoto et al. reported depth as a significant determinant.[46] In our experience factors which were predictive of metastasis at 36 months in a multivariate analysis were grade (FNCLCC system) and whether the tumor had been violated surgically (i.e. disruption). However, disruption also correlated with size and depth and therefore could represent a surrogate marker of metastasis. On the other hand group of soft tissue sarcomas requires special scrutiny, as their frequent origin from vessels may grant them greater accessibility to the bloodstream and hematogenous dissemination. This phenomenon was underscored by Berlin et al., who reported metastasis from all six extremity leiomyosarcomas that originated from veins.[70] One patient with a small (3 cm) mass arising from the saphenous vein died 1 month after surgery with liver and lung metastases.

Attempts to utilize various molecular and proliferation markers to predict the behavior of leiomyosarcomas have met with limited success. Mutations of *p53* have been detected in about 15–50% of leiomyosarcomas[13,27,28] depending of the methods and the study cited. Although *p53* mutations have been shown by some to be associated with a worse prognosis for deep-seated lesion,[13] others have found no statistical correlation between *p53* mutations and clinical behavior.[27] It appears that alterations of the *Rb-cyclin* pathway, which are detected in 90% of leiomyosarcomas, may be more significant mutagenic events than those associated with *p53*.[6] Until a sufficiently large enough number of tumors of similar size and depth are studied utilizing precise molecular analyses, the relative prognostic significance of these molecular markers will not be clear.

## CUTANEOUS LEIOMYOSARCOMAS

Although in the past the term cutaneous leiomyosarcoma referred to tumors arising in the dermis or subcutis, we believe this designation should be restricted to lesions that arise from the dermis and only secondarily invade the subcutis. The reason for this change resides in the fact that leiomyosarcomas based exclusively in the subcutis, in many instances, arise from vessels and therefore have far more in common with soft tissue leiomyosarcomas with respect to their origin, access to the bloodstream, and ultimate prognosis. Unfortunately, this definition has not been routinely employed in the past, and so the distinction between these two potentially different diseases has been blurred.

Cutaneous leiomyosarcomas occur at almost any age but are most common between the fifth and seventh decades. Although Stout and Hill[67] originally commented on the predilection of the tumors for women, more recent reports indicate that the disease is far more common in men, by a ratio of 2:1 or 3:1.[60] Like their benign counterparts, they usually occur on the extremities and show a predilection for the hair-bearing extensor surfaces.[60] Unlike subcutaneous leiomyomas, most are solitary lesions; and the presence of multiple superficial leiomyosarcomas always suggests the possibility of metastasis from another soft tissue site such as the retroperitoneum.[46] In a few cases the tumor has developed at a site of previous irradiation.[60,61]

Cutaneous tumors are usually small, averaging less than 2 cm when first detected.[62] They often produce surface changes in the overlying epidermis such as discoloration, umbilication, and ulceration. Because of their rarity these lesions are seldom correctly diagnosed preoperatively.

### Gross and Microscopic Findings

Grossly, these leiomyosarcomas usually have a gray-white whorled appearance and a varying degree of circumscription. Those in the dermis appear ill-defined by virtue of the intricate blending of tumor fascicles with the surrounding collagen and pilar arrector muscle. Those with extensions into the subcutis, in contrast, appear more circumscribed owing to the fact that they compress the surrounding tissue, creating a pseudocapsule. Most superficial leiomyosarcomas resemble retroperitoneal leiomyosarcomas in basic organization (Fig. 19–21).

Most are moderately well-differentiated tumors, differing principally by a lack of regressive or degenerative change. Hemorrhage, necrosis, hyalinization, and myxoid change are rarely encountered, which is probably a reflection of the smaller size of these lesions. Giant cells may be present, but, as in retroperitoneal tumors, it is uncommon to encounter a tumor that has a predominantly pleomorphic appearance. Mitotic figures, including atypical forms, are easily identified in these tumors. In the largest series, re-

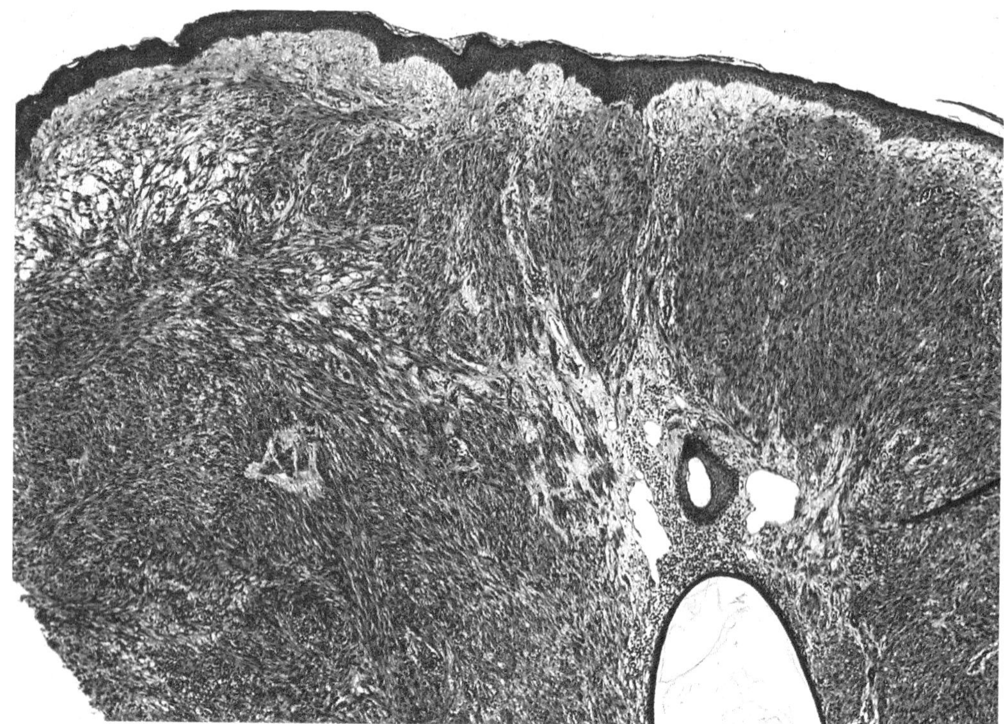

**FIGURE 19–21.** Superficial leiomyosarcoma arising from dermis.

ported by Fields and Helwig,[60] 80% of these tumors had more than 2 mitoses/10 HPF. We have generally employed the same criteria of histologic malignancy for these tumors as was proposed earlier for retroperitoneal tumors, recognizing that the better course of these tumors is directly attributable to the superficial location and small size, rather than to intrinsic histologic differences. Muscle actin is present in virtually all tumors, although desmin is variably expressed and when present may be seen only focally.[62,63] A small number of cutaneous leiomyosarcomas contain cytokeratin.[62]

### Behavior and Treatment

The behavior of this tumor is good, and its outcome is analogous to that of other sarcomas restricted to the superficial soft tissue (see Chapter 15): It has a favorable prognosis. Although recurrences develop in almost half of the patients,[60] metastases are infrequent and seem to correlate well with the depth of the original tumor. Tumors confined to the dermis do not metastasize,[59,60,62] whereas those involving the subcutis metastasize in approximately 30–40% of cases[59,60,62] The high rate of metastasis (50%) noted in the early report of Stout and Hill[67] reflects the fact that most of their cases were subcutaneous lesions, and some even penetrated deep soft tissue, a phenomenon that substantially alters the outcome for the worse. As indicated above, tumors of this type are better classified as soft tissue leiomyosarcomas rather than cutaneous ones. Other factors that correlate with outcome include the size of the tumor and the histologic grade. Both of these parameters correlate with depth. For example, nearly all intradermal leiomyosarcomas are small (<2 cm) and are of low histologic grade (I–II), although even those unusual intradermal leiomyosarcomas that are high grade have behaved in a benign fashion.[62] Metastatic spread occurs hematogenously to the lung, although regional lymph nodes were noted in about 25% of Stout and Hill's cases[67] and have been noted in sporadic case reports.[66,67]

Because many of these lesions are potentially curable, every effort should be made to eradicate the tumor initially with wide excision. Lesions allowed to recur run an increased risk of eventual metastasis because there is a distinct tendency for recurrent lesions to be larger and to involve deeper structures.[60] Radiotherapy has been employed, but it has not been particularly efficacious.[65]

## LEIOMYOSARCOMAS OF VASCULAR ORIGIN

Leiomyosarcomas of vascular origin comprise a seemingly rare group of tumors illustrated by the fact that only a few hundred cases have been reported in the literature since the initial report by Perl in 1871, and only isolated instances are recorded in several large autopsy series. Hallock et al.[78] noted one case in 34,000 autopsies from the University of Minnesota; Abell[69] reported two in 14,000 autopsies at the University of Pennsylvania; and Dorfman and Fisher[74] found none in 30,000 autopsies at the Johns Hopkins Hospital. Yet it should be emphasized that several features of this disease probably significantly affect its detection, diagnosis, and incidence. Lesions arising from major vessels such as the vena cava are likely to produce symptoms leading to their detection. Conversely, tumors arising from small vessels, vessels subserved by ancillary tributaries, or vessels in deep locations probably go unrecognized in a significant percentage of cases. It is difficult, therefore, to be certain what percentage of leiomyosarcomas of the retroperitoneum or other deep soft tissue sites may actually be of vascular origin. Hashimoto et al.[46] recently documented that at least one-fourth of leiomyosarcomas of peripheral soft tissue in their experience arose from or involved a vessel; and we have observed this in at least one-third of cases.[43] Thus the recorded experience with vascular leiomyosarcomas is a biased one, which probably underestimates the true incidence and possibly also conveys a false impression concerning clinical behavior.

## Clinical Findings

The frequency distribution of vascular leiomyosarcomas parallels in a crudely inverse fashion the pressure in the vascular bed. Leiomyosarcomas are most common in large veins such as the vena cava, far less common in the pulmonary artery, and rare in systemic arteries. In an extensive review by Kevorkian and Cento[84] of cases reported up to the early 1970s, a total of 33 cases arose in the inferior vena cava, and 35 collectively affected other medium-size or large veins; 10 occurred in the pulmonary artery alone, and 8 arose in systemic arteries. One report has indicated the unique occurrence of a leiomyosarcoma in a surgically created arteriovenous fistula.[97] The symptoms related to these tumors are diverse and are determined by the location of the tumor, rate of growth, and degree of collateral blood flow or drainage in an affected part.

## Inferior Vena Cava Leiomyosarcoma

Inferior vena cava leiomyosarcoma occur during middle or late adult life, at an average age of about 50 years; 80–90% of patients are women.[73,75,83] The location of the tumor in the vessel is significant because it determines the symptoms and surgical resectability. Based on material submitted to the International Registry of Inferior Vena Cava Leiomyosarcomas, most tumors arise in the lower (44.2%) or middle (50.8%) portion, with only a small number (4.2%) arising from the upper third or suprahepatic region.[88] Patients with upper segment tumors develop Budd-Chiari syndrome, with hepatomegaly, jaundice, and massive ascites. Nausea, vomiting, and lower extremity edema may also be present. These tumors are surgically unresectable. Tumors of the middle segment involve the region between the renal veins and hepatic veins; they produce symptoms of right upper quadrant pain and tenderness, frequently mimicking biliary tract disease. Extension into the hepatic veins may cause some of the symptoms of the Budd-Chiari syndrome, whereas extension into the renal veins results in varying degrees of renal dysfunction, from mild elevation of blood urea nitrogen to nephrotic syndrome. Some of these lesions are surgically resectable. Lesions arising below the renal veins cause lower leg edema; but unless they have spread extensively beyond the confines of the vessel, they are often amenable to surgical excision. In a few cases of vena cava leiomyosarcoma, abnormalities of red blood cell morphology and consumption coagulopathy have been observed.[96] Although previously an antemortem diagnosis of these lesions was difficult, selective arteriography and vena cavography can now be used to define the presence and extent of the mass.[71]

To date, the long-term outlook for this disease is poor. A large study comparing the effect of caval wall resection with more extended segmental resection of the vessel demonstrated no significant difference in either 5-year (55% vs. 37%) or 10-year (42% vs. 23%) survival. This seems to indicate that at the time of clinical detection the disease is relatively advanced and not curable by surgery. This conjecture is supported by the relatively large size of these tumors and the predominantly extraluminal growth in both groups. Metastatic disease is seen most commonly in lung, kidney, pleura, chest wall, liver, and bone.[72]

## Leiomyosarcomas of Other Veins

Unlike vena cava lesions, those in other veins affect the sexes equally and most often arise in the veins of the lower extremity, including the saphenous, iliac, and femoral veins. They usually present as mass lesions of variable duration that occasionally produce lower leg edema. Pressure on nerves coursing close to the affected vessel may produce additional symptoms of numbness. Angiographically, the lesions are highly vascular and create compression of the accompanying artery. The compression appears to be the result of entrapment of the artery that resides in the same preformed fibrous sheath (conjunctiva vasorum) as the vein. Because incisional biopsy of intravascular sarcomas can give rise to considerable seeding of tumor by hemorrhage, it has been suggested that thorough radiographic evaluation be followed by needle biopsy in selected cases. The behavior of this group of leiomyosarcomas has been a controversial topic.[85] Although one series suggested that small intravascular leiomyosarcomas might have a relatively good prognosis,[85] all six patients reported by Berlin et al.[70] developed metastases, even those with relatively low mitotic rates. However, all but one of the tumors exceeded 4 cm in diameter.

### Pulmonary Artery Leiomyosarcoma

Pulmonary artery leiomyosarcomas are the most common form of arterial leiomyosarcoma. They occur in adults and display no predilection for either sex. Their symptoms are referable to decreased pulmonary outflow and include chest pain, dyspnea, palpitations, dizziness, syncopal attacks, and eventual right heart failure. Until recently the diagnosis was inevitably made at autopsy. Most of these tumors arise at the base of the heart and grow distally into the left and right main pulmonary arteries.

### Gross and Microscopic Findings

In almost all reported cases, vascular leiomyosarcomas are described as polypoid or nodular masses that are firmly attached to the vessel at some point and have spread for a variable extent along its surface (Fig. 19–22). The rare cases describing extensive spread along the vena cava into the right heart, however, may represent intravenous leiomyomatosis that was originally misdiagnosed[82] (see Chapter 17). In the case of thin-walled veins extension to the adventitial surfaces and adjacent structures is a relatively early event, whereas in arteries the integrity of the internal elastic lamina is often preserved so there is no spread outside the vessel. Histologically, the tumors are basically similar to those in the retroperitoneum, although they usually do not exhibit as prominent a degree of hemorrhage or necrosis (Fig. 19–23). Mitoses, in our experience, are rather easy to identify in these tumors; and the histologic criteria of malignancy previously discussed are equally applicable to these lesions. In fact, in our experience true leiomyomas arising from vessels are rare, and this diagnosis should be made with extreme caution and only after the lesion has been sampled extensively.

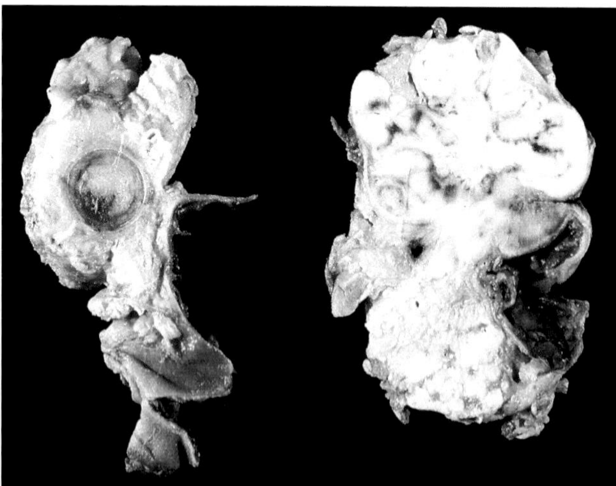

**FIGURE 19–22.** Leiomyosarcoma arising from the vena cava. Tumor occludes the lumen and extends into soft tissue (left). Adjacent section of tumor shows a close relation to the duodenal wall (right).

### Behavior and Treatment

The morbidity and mortality associated with these tumors are primarily a result of direct extension of the tumor along vessels, compromising the circulation. In only about half of the patients are metastases documented at the time of surgery or autopsy; they occur mainly in the liver or lung and less often in regional lymph nodes or intraabdominal organs. Unfortunately, owing to the fact that only about half of the cases were diagnosed antemortem in the past, there is little information concerning the results of therapy. It may be anticipated that more sophisticated angiographic techniques leading to earlier diagnosis and therapy will improve survival rates, which thus far have been poor. In 1973 Stuart and Baker,[93] analyzed 10 such tumors in the vena cava that were treated surgically; they noted that all five patients who were followed longer than 1 year died. In a more recent series by Burke and Virmani,[72] only 7 of 13 inferior vena cava sarcomas developed metastases.

One of the greatest problems when treating this disease is that the location itself may preclude surgical resection. This is true of suprahepatic lesions, where ligation of the cava and partial hepatectomy have never been accomplished. Middle caval lesions may be resected with difficulty but require removal of one kidney and pelvic transplantation of the other if irradiation is contemplated.

## MISCELLANEOUS SARCOMAS OF VASCULAR ORIGIN

Nonmyogenic sarcomas arising from vessels are a veritable potpourri of lesions that are difficult to classify.[69,76,79,81,87,91,98,100] In contrast to the foregoing group, most of these peculiar hybrid lesions occur more often in the arterial system, particularly the pulmonary artery, where they tend to present during middle age

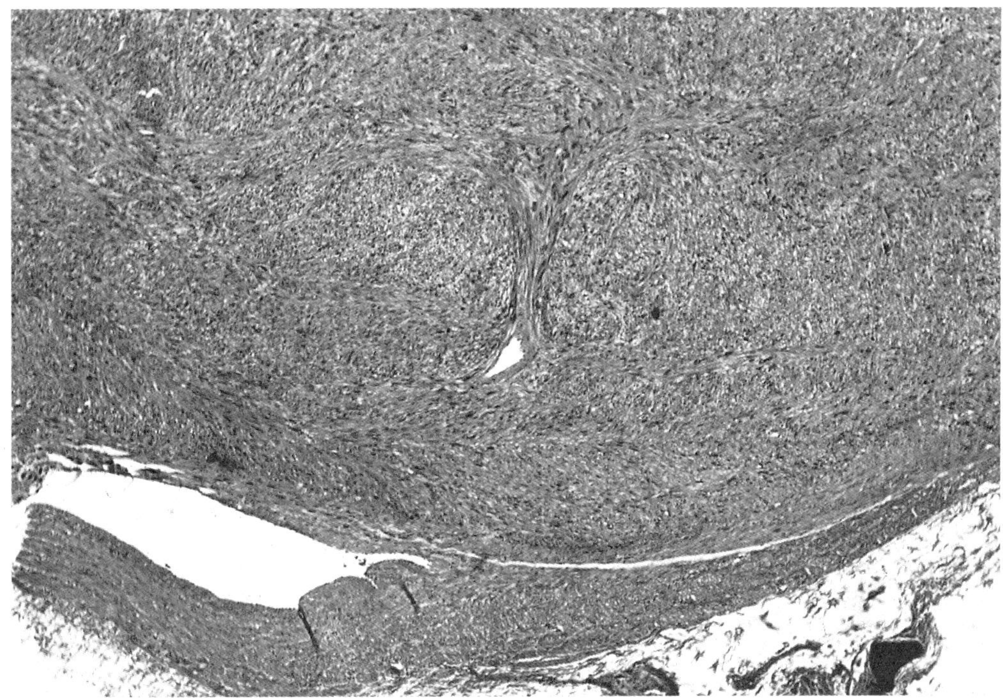

**FIGURE 19–23.** Leiomyosarcoma arising from a vein. Tumor protrudes into the vessel lumen.

with a constellation of symptoms associated with right ventricular outflow obstruction or pulmonary emboli.[72] Most of the tumors in this location probably arise from the base of the heart, although it is difficult to exclude an origin from the valve or even the heart itself. Aortic sarcomas tend to develop in older patients and involve the lower portion of the vessel. They are associated with myriad symptoms related to systemic embolization.[72] Arterial sarcomas grow in an intraluminal fashion similar to leiomyosarcomas, but there is a tendency for such lesions to creep along the vessel wall, splitting apart the layers of intima and media in their paths. This form of spreading was termed intimal sarcomatosis by Hedinger.[80] Histologically, a variety of terms have been applied to these tumors, including pleomorphic sarcoma, intimal sarcoma, undifferentiated sarcoma,[92] fusocellular sarcoma, malignant mesenchymoma,[77] chondrosarcoma,[81] and osteosarcoma.[86,88,89] The terms serve to emphasize the fact that these tumors are, in general, highly pleomorphic tumors composed of haphazardly arranged giant cells and spindle cells.

The largest institutional review of arterial sarcomas reported recently by the AFIP analyzed 11 and 16 cases from the aorta and pulmonary artery, respectively.[72] Histologically, the sarcomas in both locations were for the most part pleomorphic, intima-based lesions. Of the 17 cases reported, 3 had the pattern of angiosarcoma and 3 osteosarcoma; the remainder were pleomorphic sarcomas that were difficult to classify. Other reports have documented the presence of cartilage or skeletal muscle differentiation in these tumors.[77,87]

The fact that these tumors occur in a different set of vessels, exhibit a strikingly different histologic appearance, and often remain confined to the superficial portions of the vessel suggests the possibility that they are intimal sarcomas, in contrast to the previous group, which are more properly considered sarcomas of medial or adventitial origin. Because of their location the diagnosis is rarely made antemortem, and death from local tumor extension, particularly to the lungs, is the rule.

## SMOOTH MUSCLE TUMORS IN IMMUNOCOMPROMISED PATIENTS

Smooth muscles tumors, predominantly leiomyosarcomas, occur in immunocompromised patients with greater frequency than in the general population. Reported initially as a complication of renal transplantation and immunosuppression during the 1970s,[108,109] these smooth muscle tumors have been associated more recently with acquired immunodeficiency syndrome (AIDS)[99,101–104,107] and with cardiac[105] and liver[106] transplantation. Most occur in children and involve parenchymal organs such as the gastrointestinal tract, liver, and lung, often in a multifocal fashion. Although most reported tumors are scantily illustrated and have been variously diagnosed as "leiomyoma," "leiomyosarcoma," and "smooth muscle tumor of uncertain malignant potential," they are mitotically active lesions that qualify as leiomyosarcomas in soft tissue. Furthermore, many patients have developed extensive or disseminated disease documented at autopsy, leaving little doubt as to their malignancy.

Clonal Epstein-Barr virus (EBV) DNA has been demonstrated in these tumors[105,107] along with EBV surface receptor protein (CD21).[106,107] In a few cases the tumors have been biclonal for EBV.[107] Interestingly, in some cases different episomal EBV clones were identified in separate tumors in the same patient, indicating distinct monoclonal EBV-related tumors.[107] These findings suggest that multiple tumors in some patients are reflective of multifocal disease, in contrast to metastatic disease in the traditional sense.

## REFERENCES

### General

1. Azumi N, Ben-Ezra J, Battifora H. Immunophenotypic diagnosis of leiomyosarcomas and rhabdomyosarcomas with monoclonal antibodies to muscle-specific actin and desmin in formalin-fixed tissue. Mod Pathol 1:469, 1988.
2. Botting AJ, Soule EH, Brown AL. Smooth muscle tumors in children. Cancer 18:711, 1965.
3. Brown DC, Theaker JM, Banks PM, et al. Cytokeratin expression in smooth muscle and smooth muscle tumours. Histopathology 11:477, 1987.
4. Cavazzana AO, Ninfo V, Tirabosco R, et al. Leiomyosarcoma. Curr Top Pathol 89:313, 1995.
5. Cox PH, Verweij J, Pillay M, et al. Indium 111 antimyosin for the detection of leiomyosarcoma and rhabdomyosarcoma. Eur J Nucl Med 14:50, 1988.
5a. De Saint Aubain Somerhausen N, Fletcher CDM. Leiomyosarcoma of soft tissue in children: clinicopathologic analysis of 20 cases. Am J Surg Pathol 23:755, 1999.
6. Dei Tos AP, Maestro R, Doglioni C, et al. Tumor suppressor genes and related molecules in leiomyosarcoma. Am J Pathol 148:1037, 1996.
7. Dionne GP, Beland JE, Wang N-S. Primary leiomyosarcoma of the diaphragm of an asbestos worker. Arch Pathol Lab Med 100:398, 1976.
8. Ferenczy A, Richart RM, Okagaki T. A comparative ultrastructural study of leiomyosarcoma, cellular leiomyoma, and leiomyoma of the uterus. Cancer 28:1004, 1971.
9. Font RL, Jurco S, Brechner RJ. Postradiation leiomyosarcoma of the orbit complicating bilateral retinoblastoma. Arch Ophthalmol 101:1557, 1983.
10. Gustafson P, Willen H, Baldetorp B, et al. Soft tissue leiomyosarcoma: a population-based epidemiologic and prognostic study of 48 patients, including cellular DNA content. Cancer 70:114, 1992.
11. Hildebrand HF, Biserte G. Nickel subsulphide-induced leiomyosarcoma in rabbit white skeletal muscle. Cancer 43:1358, 1979.
12. Hutton KA, Swift RI, Urban M, et al. Leiomyosarcoma of the chest wall following treatment of Hodgkin's disease. Eur J Surg Oncol 18:388, 1992.
12a. Hwang ES, Gerald W, Wollner N, et al. Leiomyosarcoma in childhood and adolescence. Ann Surg Oncol 4:223, 1997.
13. Konomoto T, Fukuda T, Hayashi K, et al. Leiomyosarcoma in soft tissue: examination of p53 status and cell proliferating factors in different locations. Hum Pathol 29:74, 1988.
14. Lack EE. Leiomyosarcomas in childhood: a clinical and pathologic study of 10 cases. Pediatr Pathol 6:181, 1986.
15. Laskin WB, Silverman TA, Enzinger FM. Postradiation soft tissue sarcomas: an analysis of 53 cases. Cancer 62:2330, 1988.
16. Matthews TJ, Fisher C. Leiomyosarcoma of soft tissue and pulmonary metastasis, both with osteoclast-like giant cells. J Clin Pathol 47:370, 1994.
17. Mentzel T, Calonje E, Fletcher CD. Leiomyosarcoma with prominent osteoclast-like giant cells: analysis of eight cases closely mimicking the so-called giant cell variant of malignant fibrous histiocytoma. Am J Surg Pathol 18:258, 1994.
18. Merchant W, Calonje E, Fletcher CD. Inflammatory leiomyosarcoma: a morphological subgroup within the heterogeneous family of so-called inflammatory malignant fibrous histiocytoma. Histopathology 27:525, 1995.
19. Meredith RF, Wagman LD, Piper JA, et al. Beta-chain human chorionic gonadotropin-producing leiomyosarcoma of the small intestine. Cancer 58:131, 1986.
20. Miettinen M. Immunoreactivity for cytokeratin and epithelial membrane antigen in leiomyosarcomas. Arch Pathol Lab Med 112:637, 1988.
21. Miettinen M. Keratin subsets in spindle cell sarcomas: keratins are widespread but synovial sarcoma contains a distinctive keratin polypeptide pattern and desmoplakins. Am J Pathol 138:505, 1991.
22. Morales AR, Fine G, Pardo V, et al. The ultrastructure of smooth muscle tumors with a consideration of the possible relationship of glomangioma, hemangiopericytomas, and cardiac myxomas. Pathol Annu 10:65, 1975.
23. Mukai K, Schollmeyer JV, Rosai J. Immunohistochemical localization of actin. Am J Surg Pathol 5:91, 1981.
24. Nistal M, Raniagua R, Picazo ML, et al. Granular changes in vascular leiomyosarcoma. Virchows Arch [Pathol Anat] 386: 239, 1980.
25. Nochomovitz LE, Orenstein JM. Inflammatory pseudotumor of the urinary bladder: possible relationship to nodular fasciitis: two case reports, cytologic observations, and ultrastructural observations. Am J Surg Pathol 9:366, 1985.
26. Norton AJ, Thomas JA, Isaacson PG. Cytokeratin-specific monoclonal antibodies are reactive with tumours of smooth muscle derivation: an immunohistochemical and biochemical study using antibodies to intermediate filament cytoskeletal proteins. Histopathology 11:487, 1987.
27. O'Reilly PE, Raab SS, Niemann TH, et al. p53, proliferating cell nuclear antigen, and Ki-67 expression in extrauterine leiomyosarcomas. Mod Pathol 10:91, 1997.
28. Patterson H, Gill S, Fisher C, et al. Abnormalities of the p53, MDM2 and DCC genes in human leiomyosarcomas. Br J Cancer 69:1052, 1994.
29. Proppe KH, Scully RE, Rosai J. Postoperative spindle cell nodules of genitourinary tract resembling sarcomas: a report of eight cases. Am J Surg Pathol 8:101, 1984.
30. Rangdaeng S, Truong LD. Comparative immunohistochemical staining for desmin and muscle-specific actin: a study of 576 cases. Am J Clin Pathol 96:32, 1991.
31. Ro JY, Ayala AG, Ordonez NG, et al. Pseudosarcomatous fibromyxoid tumor of the urinary bladder. Am J Clin Pathol 86: 583, 1986.
32. Robinson E, Neugut AI, Wylie P. Clinical aspects of postirradiation sarcomas. J Natl Cancer Inst 80:233, 1988.
33. Russell WO, Cohen J, Enzinger FM, et al. A clinical and path-

ological staging system for soft tissue sarcomas. Cancer 40: 1562, 1977.
34. Schuerch W, Skalli O, Seemayer TA, et al. Intermediate filament proteins and actin isoforms as markers for soft tissue tumor differentiation and origin. I. Smooth muscle tumors. Am J Pathol 128:91, 1987.
35. Skalli O, Schuerch W, Seemayer T, et al. Myofibroblasts from diverse pathologic settings are heterogeneous in their content of actin isoforms and intermediate filament proteins. Lab Invest 60:275, 1989.
36. Stevens GN, Tattersall MH, Stalley P. Leiomyosarcoma following therapeutic irradiation for ankylosing spondylitis. Br J Radiol 63:730, 1990.
37. Stratton MR, Williams S, Fisher C, et al. Structural alterations of the RB1 gene in human soft tissue tumours. Br J Cancer 60: 202, 1989.
38. Swanson PE, Wick MR, Dehner LP. Leiomyosarcoma of somatic soft tissues in childhood: an immunohistochemical analysis of six cases with ultrastructural correlation. Hum Pathol 22:569, 1991.
39. Tsukada T, Tippens D, Mar H, et al. HHF35, a muscle-actin-specific monoclonal antibody. I. Immunocytochemical and biochemical characterization. Am J Pathol 126:51, 1987.
40. Wilkinson N, Fitzmaurice RJ, Turner PG, et al. Leiomyosarcoma with osteoclast-like giant cells. Histopathology 20:446, 1992.
41. Wolff M, Silva F, Kaye G. Pulmonary metastases (with admixed epithelial elements) from smooth muscle neoplasms: report of nine cases, including three males. Am J Surg Pathol 3:325, 1979.
42. Yannopoulos K, Stout AP. Smooth muscle tumors in children. Cancer 15:958, 1962.

### Leiomyosarcomas of Retroperitoneum and Deep Soft Tissues

43. Farshid G, Goldblum J, Weiss SW. Leiomyosarcomas of somatic soft tissue: a tumor of vascular origin with multivariate analysis of outcome. Mod Pathol (abst), in press.
44. Golden T, Stout AP. Smooth muscle tumors of the gastrointestinal tract and retroperitoneal tissues. Surg Gynecol Obstet 73: 784, 1941.
45. Granmayeh M, Jonsson K, McFarland W, et al. Angiography of abdominal leiomyosarcoma. AJR 130:725, 1978.
46. Hashimoto H, Daimaru Y, Tsuneyoshi M, et al. Leiomyosarcoma of the external soft tissues. Cancer 57:2077, 1986.
47. Hashimoto H, Tsuneyoshi M, Enjoji M. Malignant smooth muscle tumors of the retroperitoneum and mesentery: a clinicopathologic analysis of 44 cases. J Surg Oncol 28:177, 1985.
48. King ME, Dickersin GR, Scully RE. Myxoid leiomyosarcoma of the uterus: a report of six cases. Am J Surg Pathol 6:589, 1982.
49. Mentzel T, Calonje E, Fletcher CD. Leiomyosarcoma with prominent osteoclast-like giant cells. Am J Surg Pathol 19:487, 1995.
50. Moran C, Suster S, Periono G, et al. Malignant smooth muscle tumors presenting as mediastinal soft tissue masses. Cancer 74:2251, 1994.
51. Ranchod M, Kempson RL. Smooth muscle tumors of the gastrointestinal tract and retroperitoneum. Cancer 39:255, 1977.
52. Roncaroli F, Eusebi V. Rhabdomyoblastic differentiation in a leiomyosarcoma of the retroperitoneum. Hum Pathol 27:310, 1996.
53. Salm R, Evans DJ. Myxoid leiomyosarcoma. Histopathology 9: 159, 1985.
54. Shmookler BM, Lauer DH. Retroperitoneal leiomyosarcoma: a clinicopathologic analysis of 36 cases. Am J Surg Pathol 7:269, 1983.
55. Suster S. Epithelioid leiomyosarcoma of the skin and subcutaneous tissue: clinicopathologic, immunohistochemical and ultrastructural study of five cases. Am J Surg Pathol 18:232, 1994.
56. Suster S, Wong TY, Moran CA. Sarcomas with combined features of liposarcoma and leiomyosarcoma: study of two cases of an unusual soft-tissue tumor showing dual lineage differentiation. Am J Surg Pathol 17:905, 1993.
57. Wile AG, Evans HL, Romsdahl MM. Leiomyosarcoma of soft tissue: a clinicopathologic study. Cancer 48:1022, 1981.
58. Yannopoulos K, Stout AP. Primary solid tumor of the mesentery. Cancer 16:914, 1963.

### Cutaneous and Subcutaneous Leiomyosarcomas

59. Dahl I, Angervall L. Cutaneous and subcutaneous leiomyosarcoma: a clinicopathologic study of 47 patients. Pathol Eur 9: 307, 1974.
60. Fields JP, Helwig EB. Leiomyosarcoma of the skin and subcutaneous tissue. Cancer 47:156, 1981.
61. Hietanen A, Sakai Y. Leiomyosarcoma in an old irradiated lupus lesion. Acta Dermatol Venereol 40:167, 1960.
62. Jensen ML, Myhre Jensen O, Michalski W, et al. Intradermal and subcutaneous leiomyosarcoma: a clinicopathological and immunohistochemical study of 451 cases. J Cutan Pathol 23: 458, 1996.
63. Kaddu S, Beham A, Cerroni L, et al. Cutaneous leiomyosarcoma. Am J Surg Pathol 21:979, 1997.
64. Karroum JE, Zappi EG, Cockerell CJ. Sclerotic primary cutaneous leiomyosarcoma. Am J Dermatopathol 17:292, 1995.
65. Phelan JT, Sherer W, Mesa P. Malignant smooth muscle tumors (leiomyosarcomas) of soft tissue origin. N Engl J Med 266:1027, 1962.
66. Rising JA, Booth E. Primary leiomyosarcoma of the skin with lymphatic spread. Arch Pathol 81:94, 1966.
67. Stout AP, Hill WT. Leiomyosarcoma of the superficial soft tissue. Cancer 11:844, 1964.
68. Swanson PE, Stanley MW, Scheithauer BW, et al. Primary cutaneous leiomyosarcoma: a histologic and immunohistochemical study of 9 cases with ultrastructural correlations. J Cutan Pathol 15:129, 1988.

### Vascular Leiomyosarcomas and Related Lesions

69. Abell MR. Leiomyosarcoma of inferior vena cava: review of literature and report of two cases. Am J Clin Pathol 28:272, 1957.
70. Berlin O, Stener B, Kindblom L, et al. Leiomyosarcomas of venous origin in the extremities: a correlated clinical, roentgenologic, and morphologic study with diagnostic and surgical implications. Cancer 54:2147, 1984.
71. Brewster DC, Athanasoulin CA, Darling RC. Leiomyosarcoma of the inferior vena cava: diagnosis and surgical management. Arch Surg 111:1081, 1976.
72. Burke AP, Virmani R. Sarcomas of the great vessels: a clinicopathologic study. Cancer 71:1761, 1993.
73. Demers ML, Curley SA, Romsdahl MM. Inferior vena cava leiomyosarcoma. J Surg Oncol 51:89, 1992.
74. Dorfman HD, Fisher ER. Leiomyosarcoma of the greater saphenous vein. Am J Clin Pathol 39:73, 1963.
75. Griffin AS, Sterchi JM. Primary leiomyosarcoma of the inferior vena cava: a case report and review of the literature. J Surg Oncol 34:53, 1987.
76. Haber IM, Truong L. Immunohistochemical demonstration of the endothelial nature of aortic intimal sarcoma. Am J Surg Pathol 12:798, 1988.
77. Hagstrom L. Malignant mesenchymoma in pulmonary artery and right ventricle. Acta Pathol Microbiol Scand 51:87, 1961.

78. Hallock P, Watson CJ, Berman L. Primary tumor of inferior vena cava with clinical features suggestive of Chari's disease. Arch Intern Med 66:50, 1940.
79. Hayata T, Sato I. Primary leiomyosarcoma arising in the trunk of pulmonary artery: a case report and review of the literature. Acta Pathol Jpn 27:137, 1977.
80. Hedinger E. Ueber Intima Sarkomatose von Venen und Arterien in sarkomatoesen Strumen. Virchows Arch [Pathol Anat] 164:199, 1901.
81. Hohbach C, Mall W. Chondrosarcoma of the pulmonary artery. Beitr Pathol 160:298, 1977.
82. Jonasson D, Pritchard J, Long L. Intraluminal leiomyosarcoma of the inferior vena cava. Cancer 19:1311, 1966.
83. Jurayj MN, Midell AJ, Bederman S, et al. Primary leiomyosarcoma of the inferior vena cava: report of a case and review of the literature. Cancer 26:1349, 1970.
84. Kevorkian J, Cento JP. Leiomyosarcoma of large arteries and veins. Surgery 73:39, 1973.
85. Leu HJ, Makek M. Intramural venous leiomyosarcomas. Cancer 57:1395, 1986.
86. McConnel TH. Bony and cartilaginous tumor of the heart and great vessels. Cancer 25:611, 1970.
87. McGlennen RC, Manivel JC, Stanley SJ, et al. Pulmonary artery trunk sarcoma: a clinicopathological, ultrastructural, and immunohistochemical study of four cases. Mod Pathol 2:486, 1989.
88. Mingoli A, Sapienza P, Cavallaro A, et al. The effect of extent of caval resection in the treatment of inferior vena cava leiomyosarcoma. Anticancer Res 17:3877, 1997.
89. Murphy MSN, Meckstroth GV, Merkel BH, et al. Primary intimal sarcoma of pulmonary valve and trunk with osteogenic sarcomatous elements. Arch Pathol Lab Med 100:649, 1976.
90. Navarra G, Occhionorelli S, Mascoli F, et al. Primary leiomyosarcoma of the aorta: report of a case and review of the literature. J Cardiovasc Surg 35:333, 1994.
91. Nonomura A, Kurumaya H, Kono J, et al. Primary pulmonary artery sarcomas: report of two autopsy cases studied by immunohistochemistry and electron microscopy, and review of 110 cases reported in the literature. Acta Pathol Jpn 38:883, 1988.
92. Shmookler BM, Marsh HB, Roberts WC. Primary sarcoma of the pulmonary trunk and of left main pulmonary artery: a rare cause of obstruction to right ventricular outflow. Am J Med 63:263, 1977.
93. Stuart FP, Baker WH. Palliative surgery for leiomyosarcoma of the inferior vena cava. Ann Surg 177:237, 1973.
94. Thomas MA, Fine G. Leiomyosarcoma of the veins: report of two cases and review of literature. Cancer 13:96, 1960.
95. Varela-Duran J, Oliva H, Rosai J. Vascular leiomyosarcoma: the malignant counterpart of vascular leiomyoma. Cancer 44:1684, 1979.
96. Wackers FJT, Vander Schoot JB, Hampe JF. Sarcoma of the pulmonary trunk associated with hemorrhagic tendency: a case report and review of the literature. Cancer 23:339, 1969.
97. Weinreb W, Steinfeld A, Rodil J, et al. Leiomyosarcoma arising in an arteriovenous fistula. Cancer 52:390, 1983.
98. Wright EP, Virmani R, Glick AD, et al. Aortic intimal sarcoma with embolic metastasis. Am J Surg Pathol 9:890, 1985.

### Smooth Muscle Tumors Occurring in Immunocompromised Patients

99. Bluhm JM, Yi ES, Diaz G, et al. Multicentric endobronchial smooth muscle tumors associated with the Epstein-Barr virus in an adult patient with the acquired immunodeficiency syndrome. Cancer 80:1910, 1997.
100. Boman F, Gultekin H, Dickman PS. Latent Epstein-Barr virus infection demonstrated in low grade leiomyosarcomas of adults with acquired immunodeficiency syndrome, but not in adjacent Kaposi's lesion or smooth muscle tumors in immunocompetent patients. Arch Pathol Lab Med 121:834, 1997.
101. Chadwick EG, Connor EJ, Guerra Hanson C, et al. Tumors of smooth-muscle origin in HIV infected children. JAMA 263:3182, 1990.
102. Kingma DW, Shad A, Tsokos M, et al. Epstein-Barr virus (EBV)-associated smooth muscle tumor arising in a post-transplant patient treated successfully for two PT-EBV associated large-cell lymphomas: case report. Am J Surg Pathol 20:1511, 1996.
103. Lee E, Locker J, Nalesnik M, et al. The association of Epstein-Barr virus with smooth muscle tumors occurring after organ transplantation. N Engl J Med 332:19, 1995.
104. McClain KL, Leach CT, Jenson HB, et al. Association of Epstein-Barr virus with leiomyosarcomas in young people with AIDS. N Engl J Med 332:12, 1995.
105. McLoughlin LC, Nord KS, Joshi VV, et al. Disseminated leiomyosarcma in a child with acquired immune deficiency syndrome. Cancer 67:2618, 1991.
106. Pritzker KPH, Huang SN, Marshall KG. Malignant tumors following immunosuppressive therapy. Can Med Assoc J 103:1362, 1970.
107. Ross JS, Del Rosario A, Bui HX, et al. Primary hepatic leiomyosarcoma in a child with the acquired immunodeficiency syndrome. Hum Pathol 23:69, 1992.
108. Shen SC, Yunis EJ. Leiomyosarcoma developing in a child during remission of leukemia. J Pediatr 89:780, 1976.
109. Walker D, Gill TJ III, Corson JM. Leiomyosarcoma in a renal allograft recipient treated with immunosuppressive drugs. JAMA 215:2084, 1971.

# CHAPTER 20

# EXTRAGASTROINTESTINAL STROMAL TUMORS

Mesenchymal tumors arising from the wall of the gastrointestinal tract have attracted a great deal of attention in recent years. Continued debate over their histogenesis or line of differentiation has resulted in a vast, rather confusing literature. Originally there was an unquestioned belief that most mesenchymal tumors of the gastrointestinal tract were derived from smooth muscle cells and therefore could be viewed as analogous to smooth muscle tumors in other organs such as the uterus.[1,30] With time it became evident that only a small number of gastrointestinal tumors faithfully recapitulated the appearance of a traditional smooth muscle cell. Such lesions were usually small, incidental lesions in the esophagus or rectum (i.e., leiomyomatous polyp).[15,30] The remainder displayed various cytologic and architectural peculiarities not entirely typical of smooth muscle. Stout[48] and Martin et al.[33] alluded to this phenomenon in their early papers describing smooth muscle tumors of the stomach characterized by round or epithelioid cells. Coining the term leiomyoblastoma for these unusual tumors, Stout believed they were derived from primitive or immature smooth muscle cells.[48] Unfortunately, this term implied little about biologic behavior, making a large body of early literature difficult to interpret, and contributed to the impression that malignancy was difficult if not impossible to predict. With refined criteria of malignancy, the terms "epithelioid leiomyoma" and "epithelioid leiomyosarcoma" supplanted the term "leiomyoblastoma" for these lesions in the gastrointestinal tract and analogous lesions in soft tissue. These terms were used in earlier editions of this textbook and in the *World Health Organization Classification of Soft Tissue Tumors*.[61]

A significant nomenclature change occurred in 1983 when Mazur and Clark published a seminal paper documenting the absence of muscle markers in most of these lesions and the unexpected finding of neural markers in some detected by immunohistochemistry.[35] They postulated that these lesions displayed different lines of differentiation, reflecting the various elements of the gut wall (e.g., muscle, autonomic nerve), and proposed the unifying term "stromal tumor," which has since been modified to "gastrointestinal stromal tumor" (GIST) to ensure distinction from stromal tumors of other sites (e.g., uterus, breast). Numerous papers followed attesting to the wide range in histologic appearance, immunophenotype, and criteria of malignancy.[18,21,23,28,38,50,52] To some extent the lack of agreement among studies has been the result of case bias. Some studies, for example, included all mesenchymal lesions of the gastrointestinal tract as "stromal tumors," whereas others specifically excluded smooth muscle lesions from this umbrella term. Moreover, the earlier trend of treating stromal tumors from all gastrointestinal sites as a common entity has been supplanted by a more site-specific analysis because of embryologic and biologic differences of these lesions from site to site (e.g., stomach versus small intestine).[3,19,30] The trend to subclassify gastrointestinal stromal tumors by immunohistochemical and ultrastructural analyses[11] has led to recognition of a subset of gastrointestinal stromal tumors that exhibit autonomic differentiation (gastrointestinal autonomic tumor, or GANT).

Most recently it has been shown that gastrointestinal stromal tumors have a phenotype similar to that of the intersititial cells of Cajal[24] (gastrointestinal pacemaker cell). Developing from smooth muscle cell precursors, interstitial cells of Cajal form a ramifying network in Auerbach's plexus and are responsible for generation of the slow-wave activity of the gut musculature. They can be recognized immunohistochemically by expression of the tyrosine kinase receptor kit (CD117), which is important for their development and function. CD117 has also been identified in virtually all gastrointestinal stromal tumors[24,37,43] but not in smooth muscle tumors. Based on this observation Kindblom et al. suggested the term "gastrointestinal pacemaker cell tumor (GIPACT)" for these lesions.[24]

This chapter discusses stromal tumors that arise in the soft tissues of the abdomen, alluding to gastrointestinal tumors only as necessary. Tumors with smooth muscle differentiation (i.e., leiomyomas and leiomyosarcomas) are excluded from this category and are dealt with in Chapters 18 and 19. Extragastrointestional stromal tumors, by definition, originate from the soft tissues of the abdomen and retroperitoneum but display no connection, however tenuous, to the wall or serosal surface of the viscera.

## CLINICAL FINDINGS

Extragastrointestinal stromal tumors are uncommon compared to their gastrointestinal counterparts. In the early study of Pizzimbono et al., fewer than 5% of leiomyoblastomas arose in the soft tissues of the abdomen,[42] whereas in a recent study from the Armed Forces Institute of Pathology (AFIP) of 1004 cases 7% of tumors arose in the soft tissues of the omentum, mesentery, and retroperitoneum.[12] The latter study, however, makes no clear-cut distinction between tumors with true smooth muscle differentiation and those with features of a stromal tumor. Putative cases have been reported in the neck, vulva, and skin[49]; but in our experience tumors with all the histologic and immunophenotypic features of gastrointestinal stromal tumors occurring outside the abdomen and retroperitoneum are so rare that the diagnosis should be questioned or the possibility of a metastasis from an intraabdominal primary tumor be raised. Although gastrointestinal stromal tumors have been associated with Carney's triad (multiple gastric stromal tumors, pulmonary chondroma, paraganglioma)[6,7] and neurofibromatosis 1,[25,27] such an association has not yet been noted with extragastrointestinal variants. In addition familial forms of gastrointestinal stromal tumors occur secondary to germlike mutation of the c-kit gene.[22b,40a,40b]

Extragastrointestinal stromal tumors usually present during adult life as enlarging masses of variable duration, although occasionally such tumors are discovered incidentally at the time of laparotomy. Approximately 80% are located in the omentum or mesentery, and the remainder develop in the retroperitoneum (Fig. 20–1) Unlike their gastrointestinal counterpart, these lesions tend to be large when first detected, with most measuring more than 10 cm.[43] Most are firm, fleshy gray-red masses lacking the whorled appearance that is often seen with conventional smooth muscle tumors (Fig. 20–2). A significant subset undergo cystic change as a result of extensive hemorrhage or necrosis.

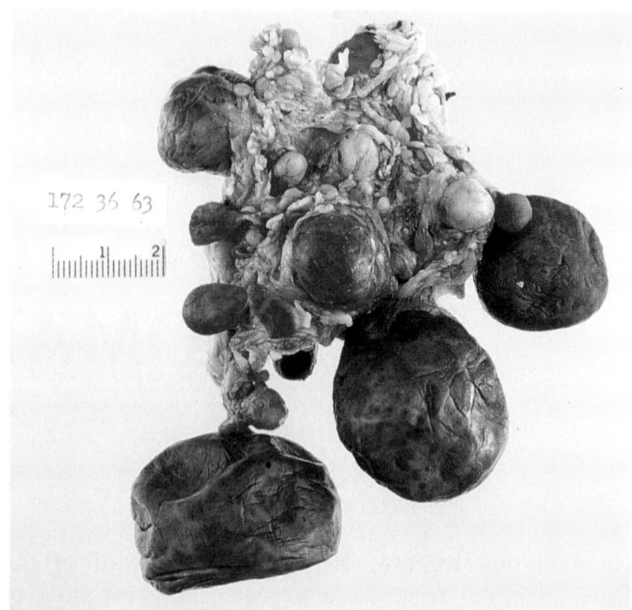

**FIGURE 20–1.** Stromal tumor of the omentum, presenting as multiple pedunculated masses.

## MICROSCOPIC FINDINGS

The histologic appearance of extragastrointestinal stromal tumors is variable, but in general there are two patterns: epithelioid and spindle cell. In a given tumor one pattern usually predominates, although in about 10% of cases the patterns coexist in roughly equal proportions. The epithelioid pattern corresponds to most of the older descriptions of leiomyoblastoma in which the tumor is composed of round cells that vary from small uniform cells to large pleomorphic cells with eosinophilic cytoplasm (Figs. 20–3 to 20–6). In some cases there is a striking population of epithelioid cells with multiple peripherally oriented nuclei (Fig. 20–6). Although the hyperchromatism of

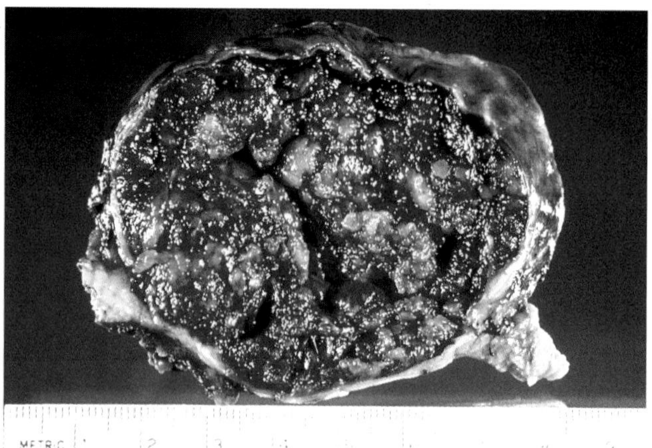

**FIGURE 20–2.** Stromal tumor of the omentum with a partially hemorrhagic red-gray appearance.

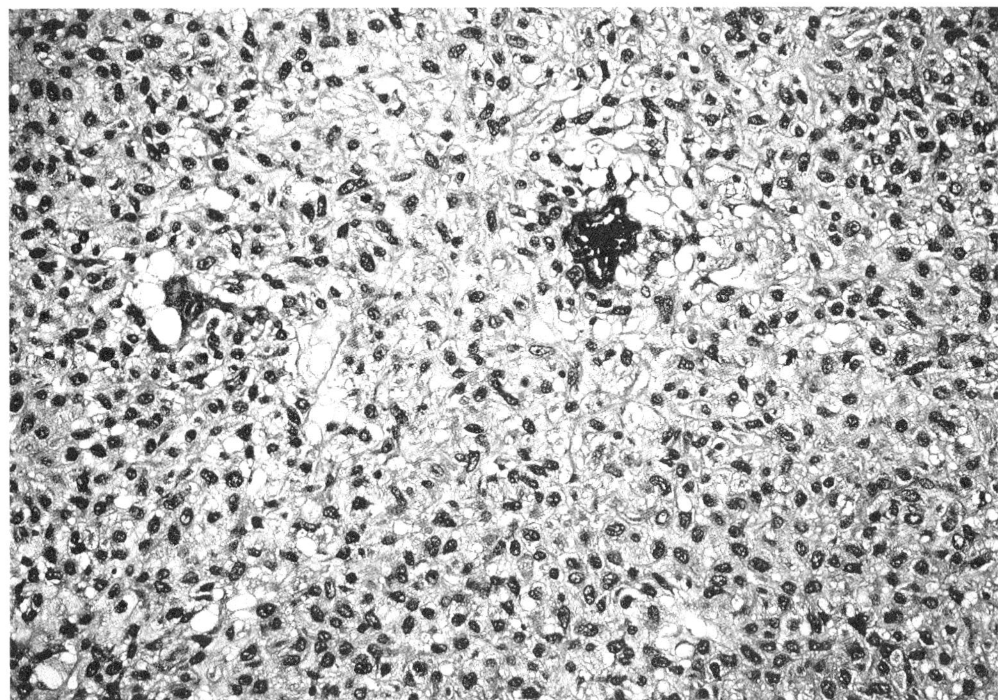

**FIGURE 20–3.** Stromal tumor composed of sheets of dispersed epithelioid cells.

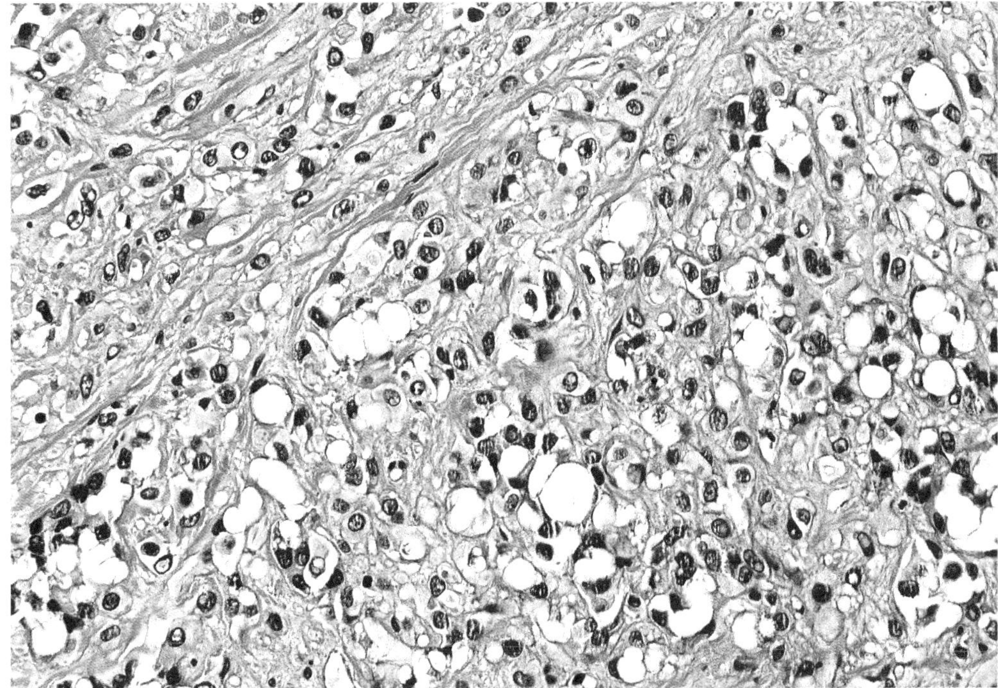

**FIGURE 20–4.** Stromal tumor composed of epithelioid cells with focal vacuolar (signet ring) change.

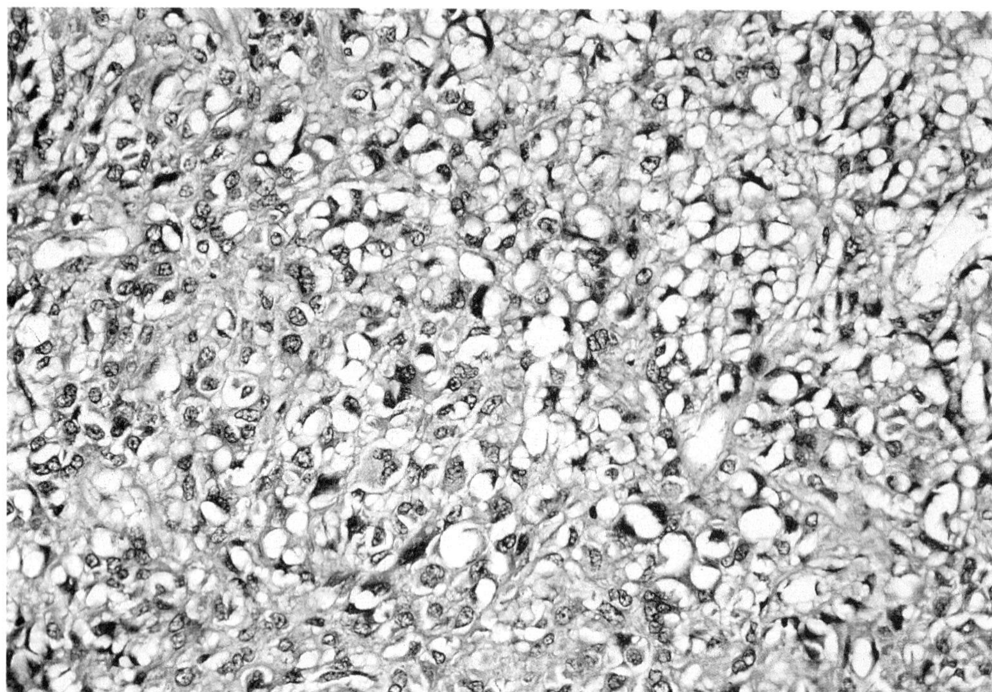

**FIGURE 20–5.** Stromal tumor with epithelioid cells with extensive signet ring change.

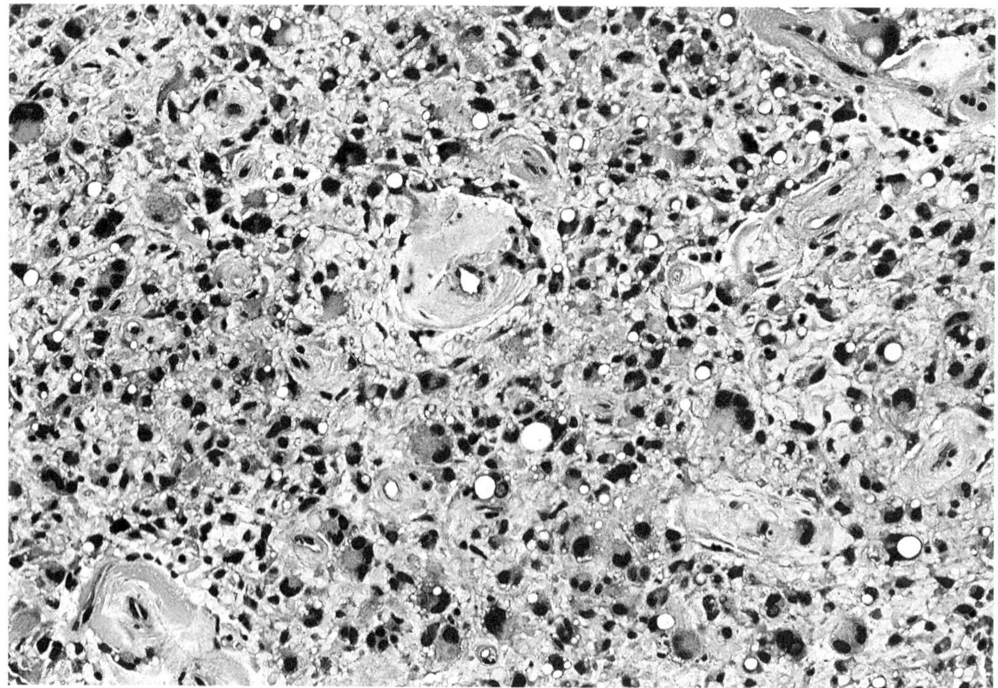

**FIGURE 20–6.** Stromal tumor with numerous hyperchromatic cells with multiple peripherally oriented nuclei. These cells are typically seen in benign stromal tumors.

the nuclei sometimes suggests malignancy, these multinucleated cells are more likely to be encountered in benign than malignant stromal tumors.[30] Another characteristic feature of these tumors is the prominent cytoplasmic vacuole, which in extreme instances results in a signet ring cell.[51] (Figs. 20–4, 20–5) Tumors composed of a predominance of signet ring cells may be mistaken for liposarcoma or mucinous carcinoma by those unfamiliar with their appearance. As emphasized originally by Stout, the vacuoles of these signet ring cells do not stain for fat, mucosubstances, or glycogens and therefore can be readily distinguished from those of liposarcoma or carcinoma. In fact, these vacuoles seem to represent an artifact of formalin fixation because they are not present in frozen sections or in material fixed for electron microscopy. The cells in epithelioid stromal tumors are commonly arranged in small groups or nests separated by a matrix of dense or fibrillary collagen, pools of stromal mucin, or both (Figs. 20–7, 20–8, 20–9). In some instances mucin collections are striking enough to form microscopic cysts.

Tumors with a spindled pattern more closely resemble conventional smooth muscle tumors but nonetheless can be distinguished from them by the fact that the cells usually have a short fusiform shape in contrast to the elongated cells of leiomyomas and leiomyosarcomas (Figs. 20–10 to 20–14). They have an oval, centrally placed nucleus and lightly staining cytoplasm in which it is usually not possible to identify distinct myofibrils with hematoyxlin-eosin or trichrome stain. At best, a few wisps of fuchsinophilic material may be seen. The neoplastic cells, furthermore, are not arranged in long well oriented fascicles like a smooth muscle tumor but consist of short ill-defined fascicles, sometimes in a storiform pattern. Nuclear palisading is occasionally seen and in some cases is so striking as to suggest the diagnosis of a schwannoma (Figs. 20–13, 20–14). The stroma is typically composed of mats of fine hair-like collagen interrupted by a delicate vasculature. As in epithelioid stromal tumors, microcystic change is also observed.

A number of features may be encountered in these tumors independent of pattern. Extensive hyaline change is seen in about 20% of cases and can result in striking perivascular hyalinization as in a hemangiopericytoma (Fig. 20–15), extensive intratumoral hyaline change as in uterine leiomyomas, or bands of hyaline material creating a secondary trabecular pattern (Fig. 20–16). Skeinoid fibers (extracellular collagen-containing eosinophilic blobs),[34,39] reported occasionally in small intestinal stromal tumors and originally believed to reflect neural differentiation, are usually absent in extragastrointestinal stromal tumors (Fig. 20–17).

Usually metastases from extragastrointestinal stromal tumors resemble the parent growth, although mitotic rates sometimes differ. Occasionally isolated metastases in the liver or lymph node are difficult to diagnose because of their similarity to metastatic car-

*Text continued on page 759*

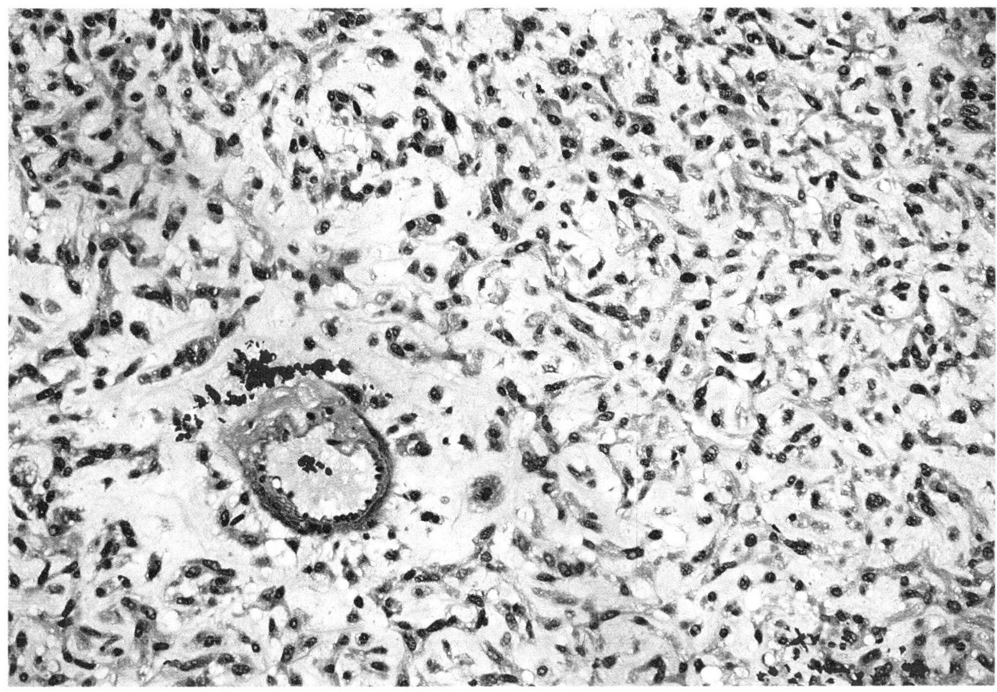

**FIGURE 20–7.** Stromal tumor with myxoid change.

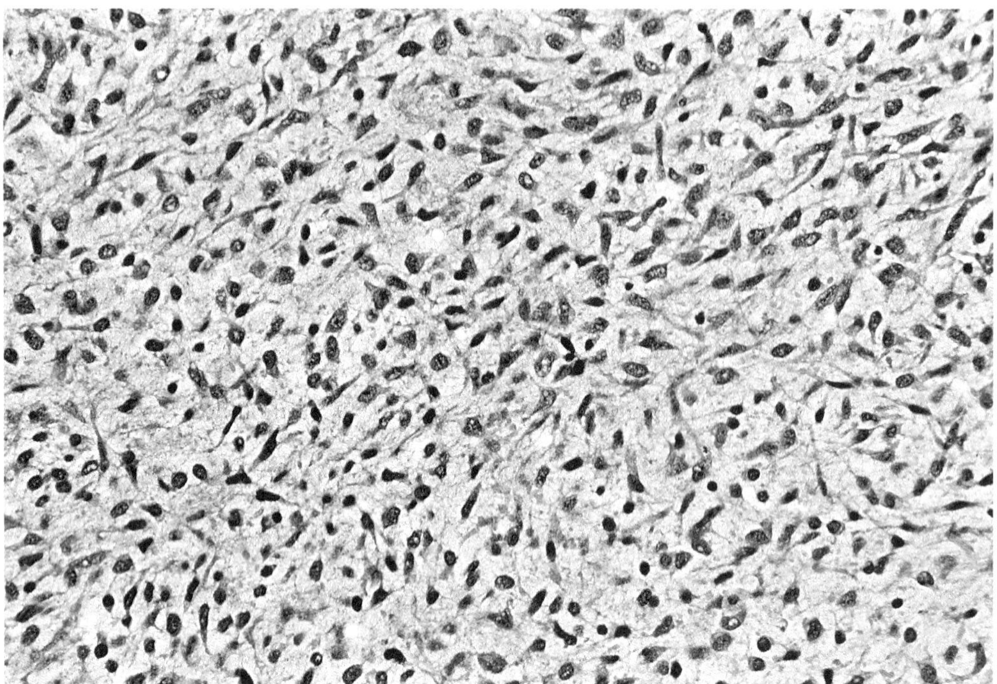

**FIGURE 20–8.** Stromal tumor with myxoid change.

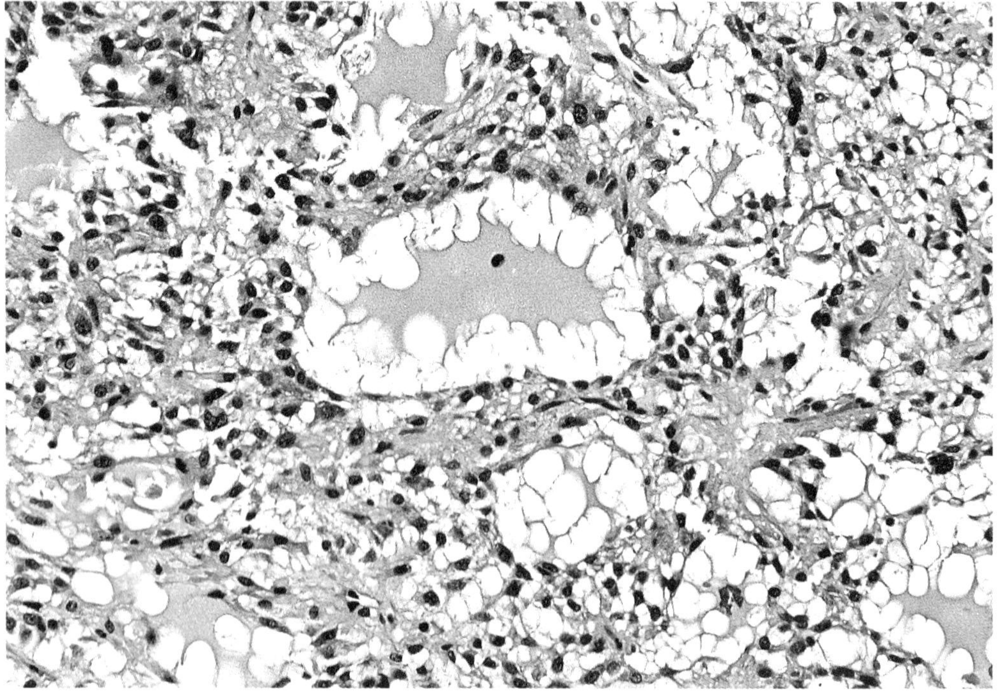

**FIGURE 20–9.** Stromal tumor with microcysts.

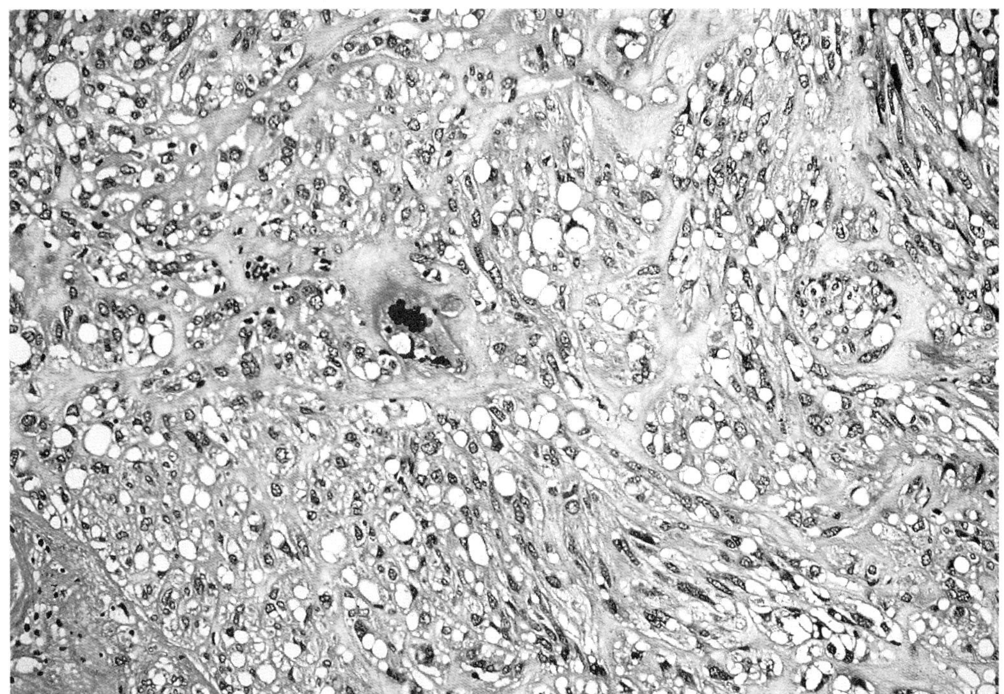

**FIGURE 20–10.** Stromal tumor with transition between epithelioid and spindled areas.

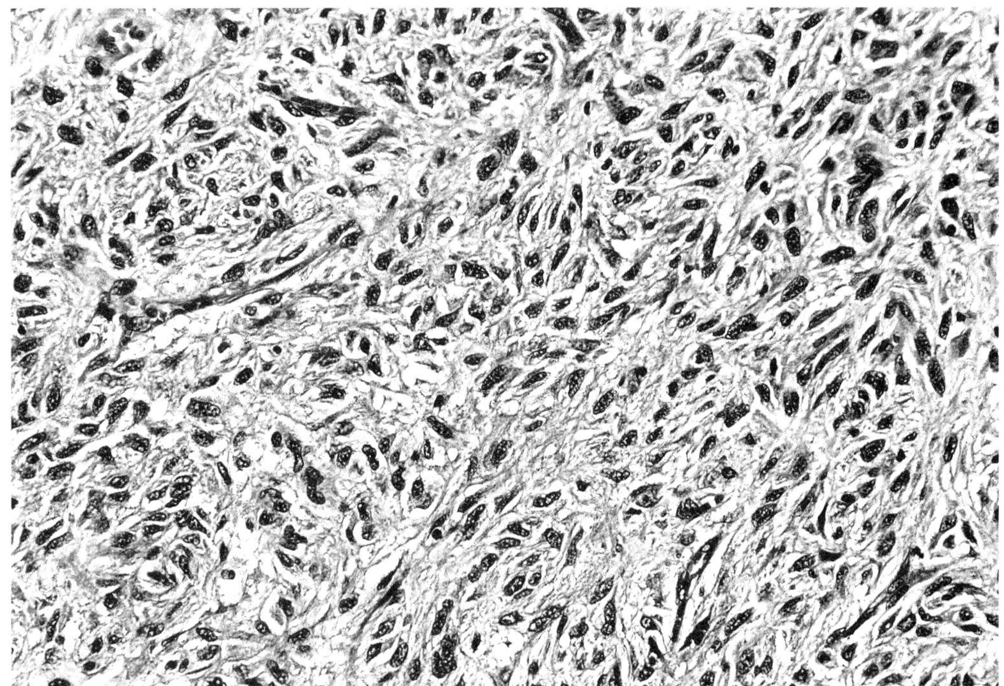

**FIGURE 20–11.** Stromal tumor with a spindled pattern composed of short fusiform cells in a fine fibrillary background.

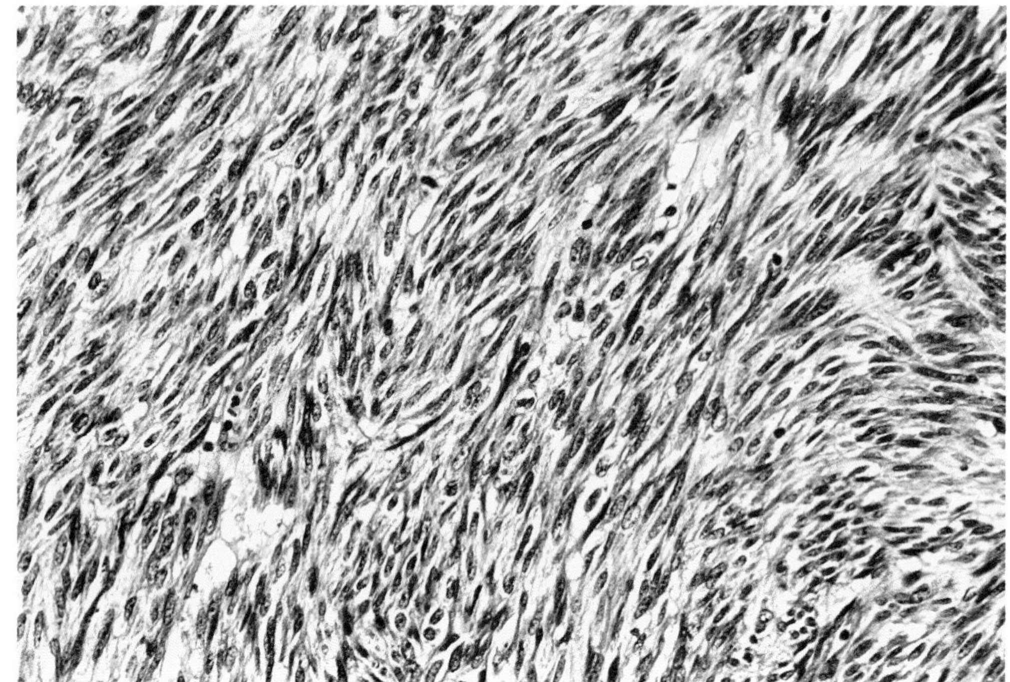

**FIGURE 20–12.** Stromal tumor with a spindled pattern composed of cells arranged in distinct fascicles.

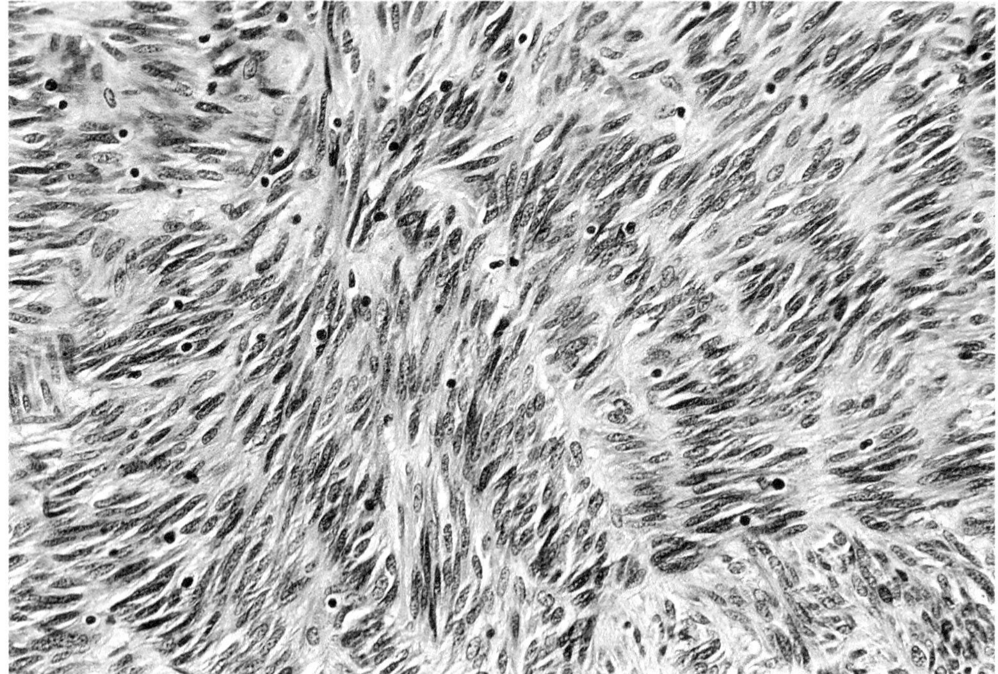

**FIGURE 20–13.** Stromal tumor with nuclear palisading.

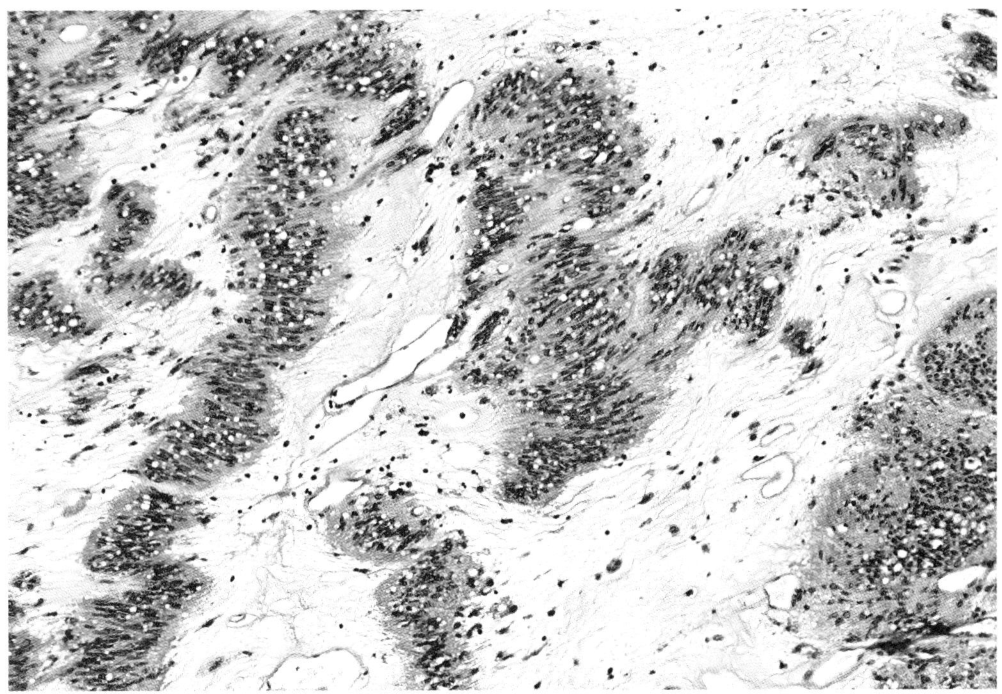

**FIGURE 20–14.** Stromal tumor with nuclear palisading.

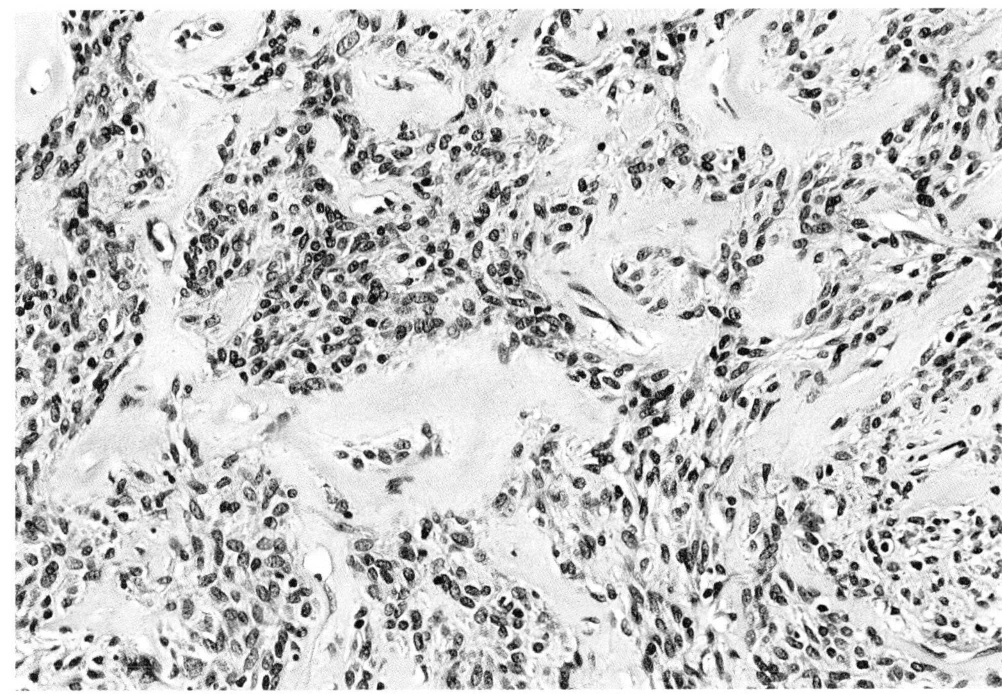

**FIGURE 20–15.** Stromal tumor with prominent hyalinization.

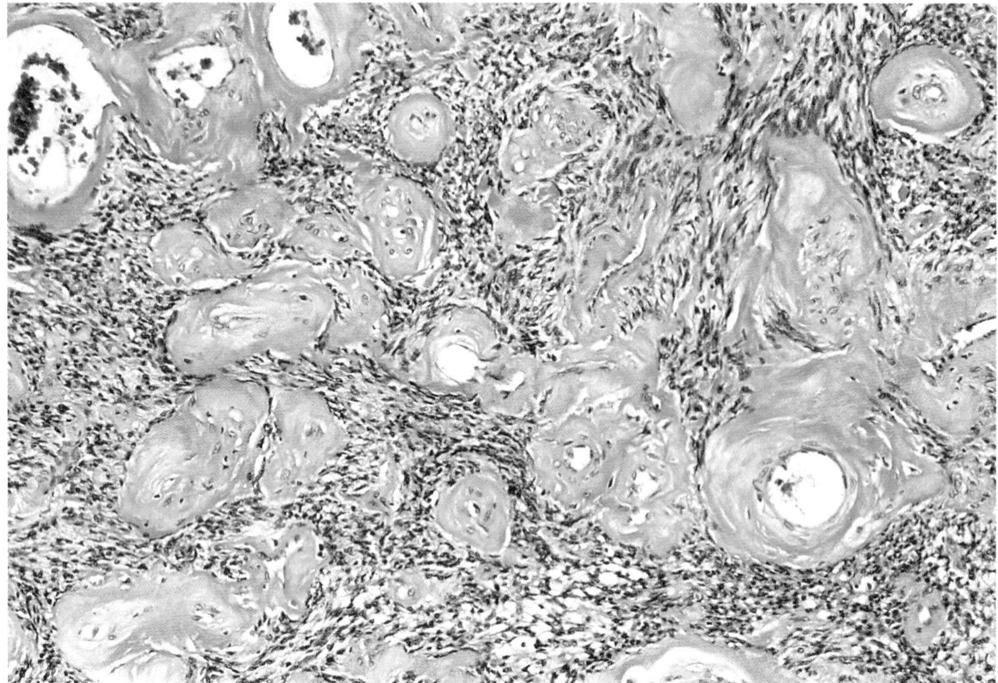

**FIGURE 20–16.** Stromal tumor with perivascular hyalinization.

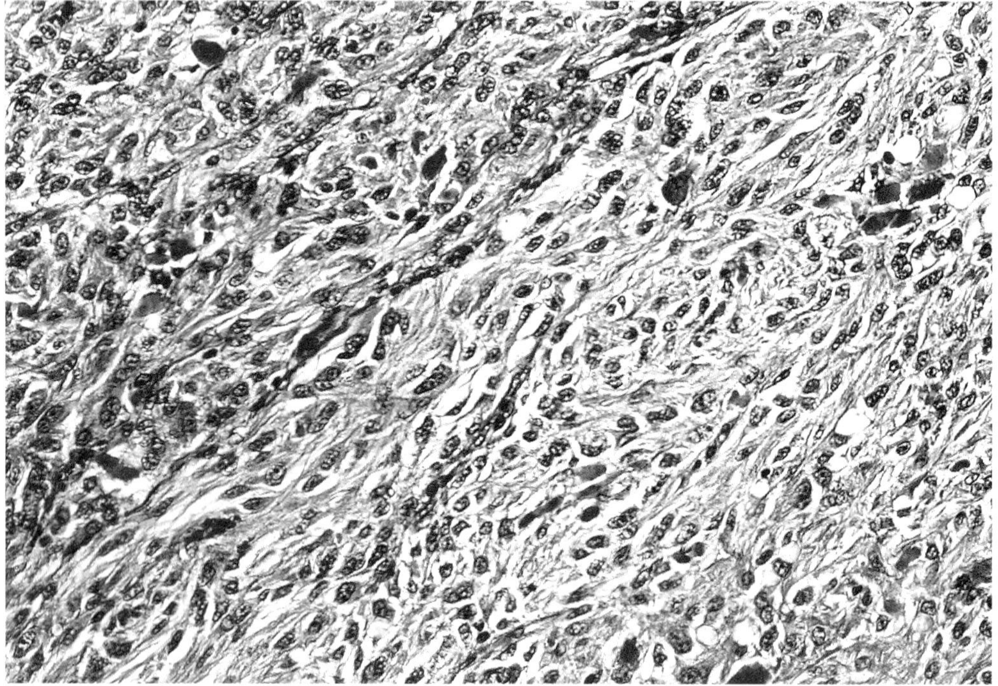

**FIGURE 20–17.** Skeinoid fibers in a stromal tumor appear as interstitial eosinophilic blobs.

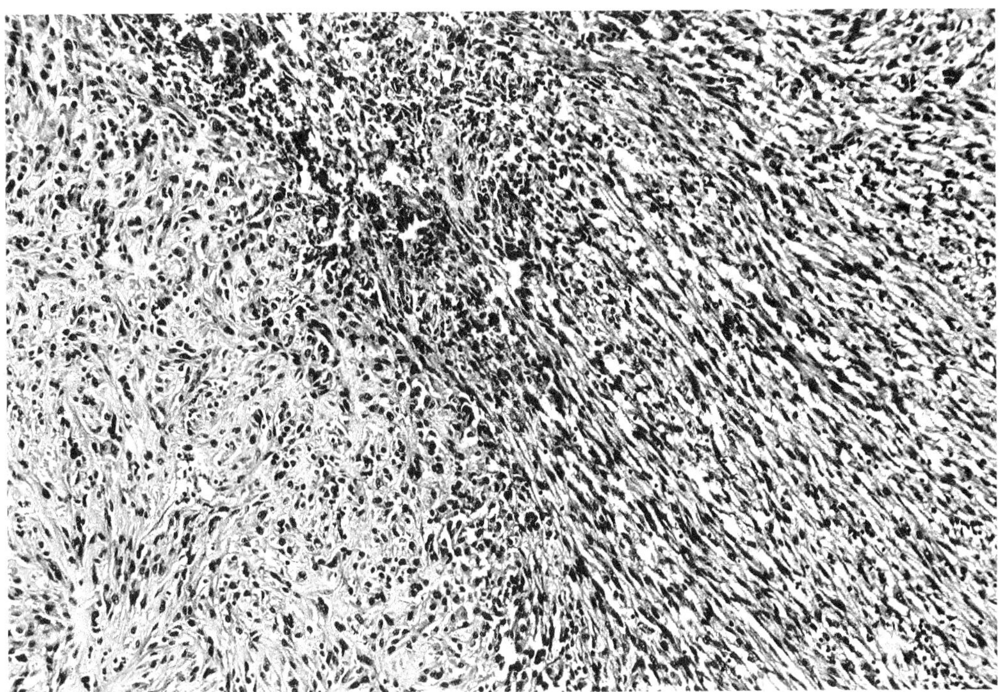

**FIGURE 20–18.** Stromal tumor with a transition between more differentiated (left) and more aggressive (right) appearing areas.

cinoma or metastatic neuroendocrine tumors. This situation most frequently arises in patients from whom tumors were resected previously and in whom metastatic disease supervenes years later.

Distinguishing benign from malignant extragastrointestinal tumors depends on evaluation of a number of parameters independent of the pattern or immunophenotypic profile.[43] In our experience, the most important criteria of malignancy are cellularity, mitotic activity, and necrosis (Figs. 20–18 to 20–21). Lesions at high risk to produce metastasis have high cellularity (as defined by areas with frequent overlapping nuclei), mitotic activity in excess of 2 mitoses/50 high-power fields (HPF), and any amount of coagulative necrosis. Such lesions can comfortably be labeled malignant. Lesions lacking these features have a lower risk of metastasis, although it is not possible to guarantee benignancy.

## IMMUNOHISTOCHEMICAL FINDINGS

Numerous studies have dealt with the immunohistochemical profile of gastrointestinal stromal tumors,[3,19,31,36,37,39–41,45,46,53–58] but it is nearly impossible to compare data from one study to another for various reasons. First, many studies blur the distinction between conventional smooth muscle tumors of the gastrointestinal tract and those with the unique features of stromal tumors. Second, the precise location in the gastrointestinal tract, which has a bearing on both histologic appearance and immunophenotype, is frequently not reported. Third, the sensitivity of various antibodies, type of fixation, and preparations (fixed versus frozen) differ from study to study. Even so there is general agreement that gastrointestinal stromal tumors do not express muscle antigens to the same extent as conventional smooth muscle tumors. A similar trend is noted for extragastrointestinal lesions (Table 20–1). Desmin is rarely noted in these lesions, although a significant subset express smooth muscle actin[37,43] (Fig. 20–22). Like the gastrointestinal counterpart, c-*kit* (CD117) expression can be identified in virtually all lesions and CD34 in about half, making these two antigens the most reliable ones for diagnosis (Fig. 20–23). These findings are similar to those reported by Kindblom et al. in gastrointestinal stromal tumors from all sites[24] but contrast slightly with those of Erlandson et al., who reported a higher incidence of neural markers (neuron-specific enolase, NFP).[11] Possibly this is a reflection of the authors' interest in gastrointestinal autonomic nerve tumors and selective inclusion in their series.

The presence of c-kit in these tumors has been used as evidence to suggest they have a close kinship with the interstitial cell of Cajal. CD34 in stromal tumors is less easily explained. Interstitial cells of Cajal do not express this antigen, whereas fibroblasts within Auer-

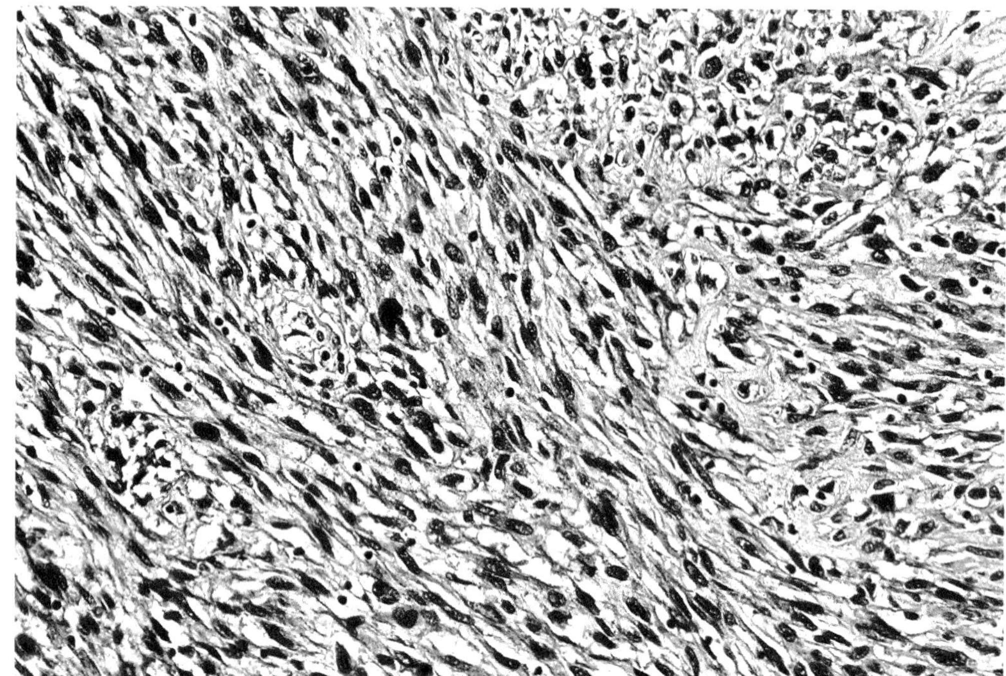

**FIGURE 20–19.** Stromal tumor with malignant features. Tumor is highly cellular with significant atypia.

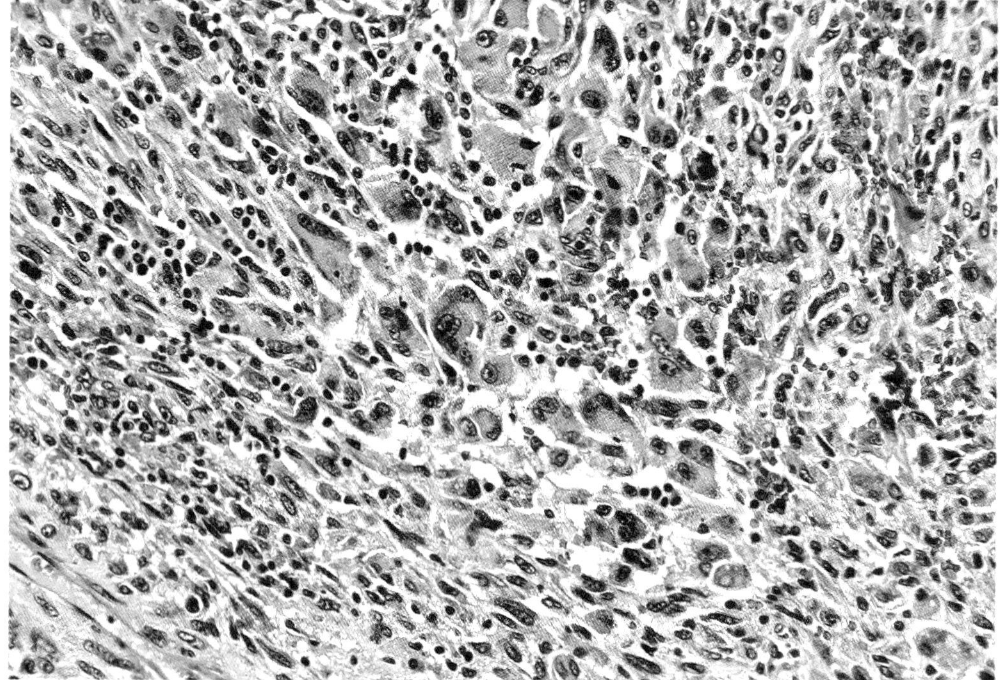

**FIGURE 20–20.** Stromal tumor with malignant features. Tumor is highly cellular with marked atypia.

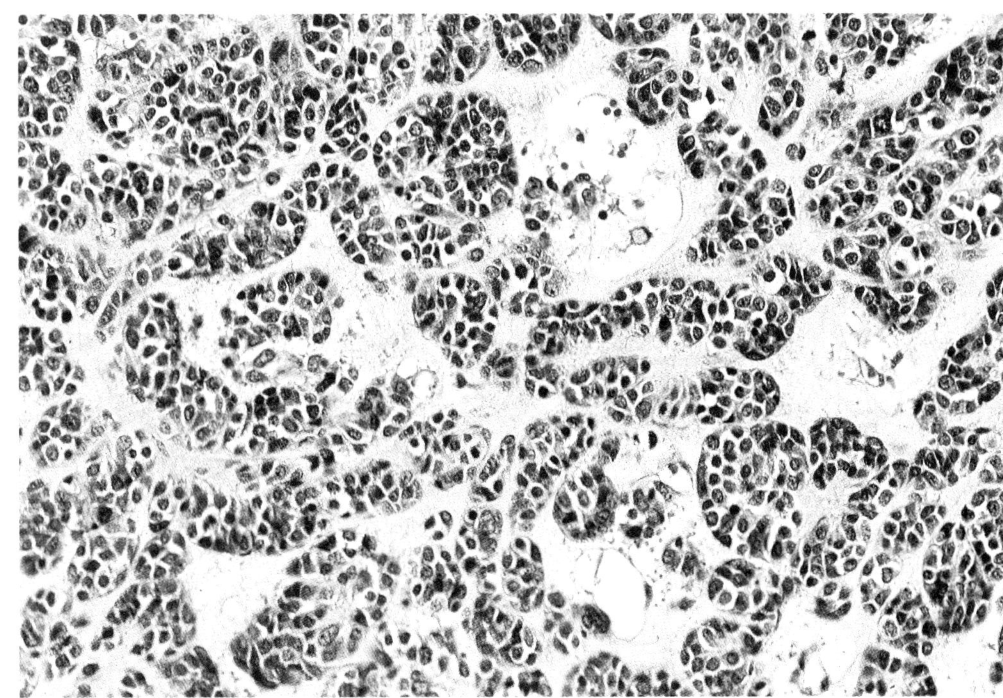

**FIGURE 20–21.** Stromal tumor with malignant features. Tumor is composed of nests of small, round, primitive-appearing cells.

bach's plexus do.[59] Thus stromal tumors share immunophenotypic similarities with two normal, but distinct, cell populations in the gut wall.

## ULTRASTRUCTURAL FINDINGS

These tumors may have features of smooth muscle cells [evidenced by parallel arrays of intracytoplasmic thin (actin) filaments with or without dense bodies, micropinocytotic vesicles, and discontinuous basal lamina] or neural cells (with thin interdigitating cytoplasmic processes connected by primitive junctions and containing microtubules and dense-core granules).[11] By convention, stromal tumors with neural (synaptic) differentiation are classified as autonomic nerve tumors (GANT).[63–75] Still other tumors display few if any features of specific differentiation, having cytoplasmic processes without any diagnostic structures.[11]

The range of features noted in these tumors has led to an elaborate system of subclassifying them.[11] Oth-

**TABLE 20–1** STROMAL TUMORS: IMMUNOHISTOCHEMICAL FINDINGS

| Immunohistochemical Profile | Extragastrointestinal (%) | Gastrointestinal (%) | |
|---|---|---|---|
| | *Reith et al.*[43] *(25 cases)* | *Kindblom et al.*[24] *(78 cases)* | *Erlandson et al.*[11] *(56 cases)* |
| c-kit | 100 | 100 | ND |
| CD34 | 48 | 75 | 59 |
| SMA | 24 | 15 | 23 |
| Desmin | 4 | 0 | 16 |
| S-100 Protein | 8 | 0 | 9 |
| MSA | ND | 0 | 50 |
| NSE | 31 | 0 | 59 |
| NFP | ND | 0 | 3 |
| Chromogranin | 0 | 0 | 3 |
| Synaptophysin | ND | ND | ND |
| Keratin | 0 | ND | 2 |

NSE, neuron-specific enolase; SMA, smooth muscle actin; MSA, muscle-specific actin; ND, not done.

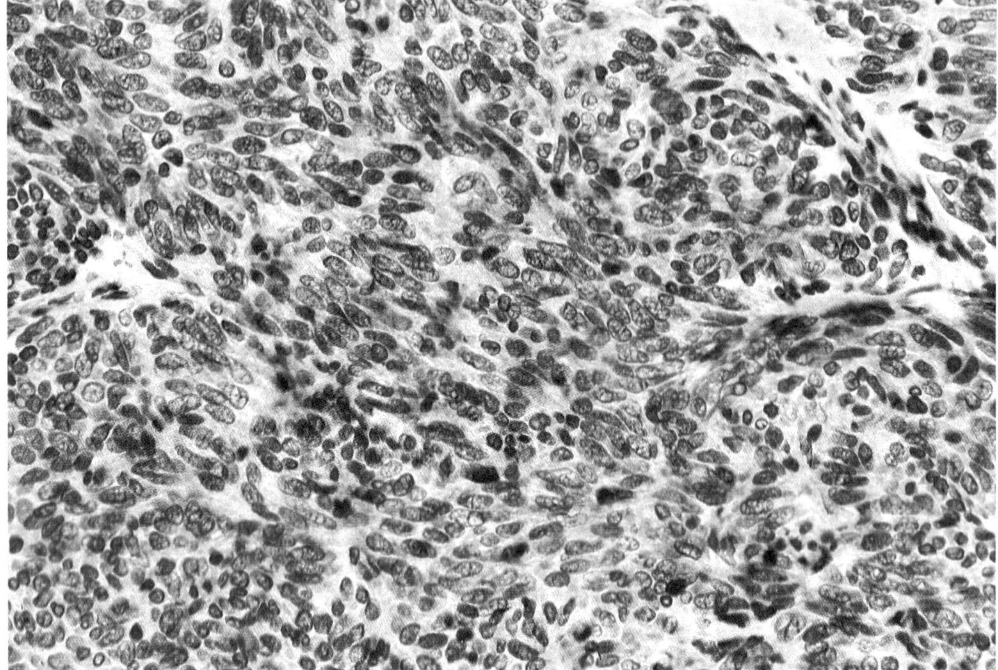

**FIGURE 20–22.** Immunostaining of stromal tumor for smooth muscle actin. Rare to occasional cells are positive.

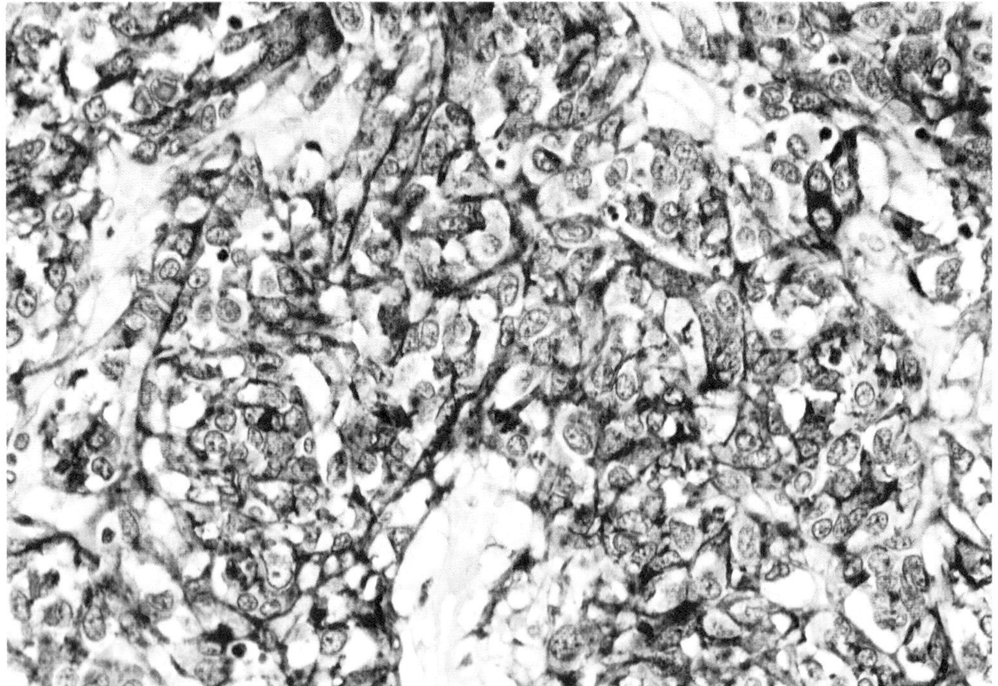

**FIGURE 20–23.** Immunostain for c-kit receptor in a stromal tumor. The tumor displays strong immunoreactivity in the cytoplasm and along the surface membrane.

ers, noting the presence of c-kit receptor in all tumors regardless of the type of ultrastructural differentiation, have suggested that these lesions exhibit the same range of differentiation as the interstitial cell of Cajal, which may display both neural and smooth muscle features.[24]

## CYTOGENETIC AND MOLECULAR FINDINGS

Gain-of-function mutations in the c-kit gene appear to be an important molecular event in the tumorigenesis of gastrointestinal stromal tumors,[13,22a,39a,44] and these observations will likely pertain to the extragastrointestinal forms as well. There are three principal lines of evidence to support this statement: First, approximately 50% of gastrointestinal stromal tumors have mutations in exon 11 of the *kit* gene resulting in alteration of juxtamembrane portion of the kit (tyrosine kinase) receptor (kit gene product). This mutation leads to ligand-independent phosphorylation and perpetuation of the kit signaling pathway to the nucleus. Other mutations in the kit gene have been described but appear to be relatively infrequent.[31a] Although correlation between mutational status and biologic behavior is not fully delineated, c-kit mutations are more common in large or malignant lesions.[28] Second, introduction of mutant c-kit cDNA into murine lymphoid cell lines results in constitutive activation of the kit receptor, and, in turn, these cells produce tumors when transplanted into nude mice. Third, patients with multiple gastrointestinal stromal and autonomic tumors have germline gain-of-function mutations of the c-kit gene. These patients also manifest a striking hyperplasia of the interstitial cells of Cajal within the gut suggesting this is a precursor (premalignant) lesion.[22b,40a,40b]

A number of other cytogenetic abnormalities have been noted in gastrointestinal stromal tumors but their role is less well defined than that of c-kit. For example, alterations of chromosomes 14 and 22[4,10,32] have been identified in virtually all tumors regardless of biologic or histologic features suggesting an early molecular event. Loss of heterozygosity of 1p36.3 is noted in nearly one half of tumors and is proposed as the site of a tumor suppressor gene.[14]

## BEHAVIOR AND TREATMENT

Numerous studies have attempted to define the clinical behavior of stromal tumors based on a combination of pathologic and clinical features. Early studies typically assigned a label of benign or malignant to a given lesion based on a predetermined set of histologic criteria devised by the author or validated by earlier studies.[61] Although this approach usually distinguishes lesions with high metastatic potential from those with low potential, it is at best imperfect. Often lesions designated benign proved to have metastatic potential, whereas not all of those labeled malignant proved fatal. More recently the trend has shifted to one of "risk assessment,"[17,43,55–57] a method that analyzes a number of features independently and correlates them with an adverse or nonadverse outcome. By combining features, high risk versus low risk groups can be identified.

It is well accepted that the behavior of stromal tumors is strongly influenced by site. Gastric lesions appear to have the best prognosis,[12,58] whereas those arising in the small bowel or soft tissues of the abdomen have the worst.[12] In view of this observation it is not surprising that the criteria of malignancy have also been strongly influenced by location.[3,22,37a,37b,55–57] The features generally accorded prognostic significance in various studies are size, nuclear grade, mitotic activity, cellularity, and necrosis, although the relative importance of these features varies from site to site and from study to study. The level of cellularity has been one of the most consistent prognostic indicators (Table 20–2). Tumors with high cellularity,

**TABLE 20–2** ADVERSE PROGNOSTIC INDICATORS IN STROMAL TUMORS

| | Indicator, by Tumor Site | | | | | |
|---|---|---|---|---|---|---|
| **Parameter** | ***Stomach***[2,30] | ***Duodenum***[19] | ***Jejunum/ileum***[55] | ***Colon***[56] | ***Rectum***[57] | ***Soft Tissues***[43] |
| High cellularity | + | + | + | + | | + |
| Mitoses | >10/50 HPF, 100% metastasis | >2/50 HPF | >5/50 HPF | High | | >2/50 HPF |
| Size | >6 cm | >4.5 cm | >9 cm | | >5 cm | |
| Necrosis | | | | | | + |
| Mucosal invasion | + | | + | + | | |
| Growth pattern | | Nonorganoid | Epithelioid (>50%) | | | |
| Infiltration of muscularis propria | | | | + | | |

as defined by frequent areas with overlapping nuclei, have been associated with a statistically higher risk of an adverse outcome in several studies of both gastrointestinal and extragastrointestinal lesions. Likewise, mitotic activity is usually an important prognostic indicator, although the threshold level reported from site to site differs with threshold levels as low as 2 mitoses/50 HPF in the duodenum.[19]

To date only one study has dealt exclusively with extragastrointestinal stromal tumors.[43] In other studies extragastrointestinal lesions are either absent or comprise only a small proportion.[12] In view of the site-dependent criteria of malignancy, it may not be appropriate to apply data gleaned from the gastrointestinal experience to stromal tumors arising from the omentum, mesentery, and retroperitoneum. In our experience of 32 patients with follow-up information, 41% developed metastasis or died of tumor during a follow-up period of 24 months. Because the follow-up was relatively short, it is expected that this figure may increase significantly with time. In a univariate analysis cellularity (high versus low), mitotic activity (<2 or >2 mitoses/50 HPF), and necrosis (present or absent) correlated with an adverse outcome as defined by metastasis or death due to the tumor. In a multivariate analysis both mitotic activity and necrosis displayed a trend toward an independent predictive value. Despite this, stratification of patients with extragastrointestinal stromal tumors into those with more or one adverse histologic factor versus those with two or three factors offers the advantage of grouping patients into two categories with markedly different risk of an adverse outcome in the short term (Table 20–3). No correlation was noted between tumor type (spindled versus epithelioid appearance) or immunophenotypic profile. Miettinen et al. suggested that omental lesions are associated with a better prognosis than mesenteric lesions, but the number of cases in each group was small.[37]

More sophisticated analyses such as the proliferating cell nuclear antigen (PCNA) index and DNA ploidy, which have been advocated by some for analyzing gastrointestinal stromal tumors,[5,8,9,16,20,26,29,41,45,47,62] have not been evaluated for extragastrointestinal lesions. Rudolph et al. proposed a grading system for stromal tumors modeled after the FNCLCC system for sarcomas; it is based on differentiation, mitotic activity, and necrosis. Dividing lesions into benign, grade I, grade II, and grade III, a good correlation was noted between these subgroups and survival.[45]

Nearly 50% of patients with extragastrointestinal stromal tumors develop metastases or die of their tumors. Therefore these lesions should be viewed as highly aggressive lesions[43] that are associated with a high risk of malignant behavior; and they should be treated as any other high grade intraabdominal sarcoma. Because the follow-up care information of soft tissue stromal tumors is limited, it seems prudent to consider long-term follow-up even for histologically benign lesions.

## GASTROINTESTINAL AUTONOMIC NERVE TUMOR

First described in 1984 by Herrera et al. as "plexosarcoma," the gastrointestinal autonomic nerve tumor is a variant of gastrointestinal stromal tumor that exhibits evidence of neuronal differentiation by electron microscopy.[65] Although originally believed to be rare, it appears that approximately 40% of gastrointestinal stromal tumors, when carefully analyzed, fall into this category.[11] The tumor occurs at all ages but has a peak incidence during the sixth decade. Most occur in the stomach and small intestine, but they infrequently appear in the esophagus, colon, and abdominal soft tissues. In the experience reported from Memorial–Sloan Kettering Cancer Hospital, 3 of 21 autonomic nerve tumors arose outside the gastrointestinal tract, suggesting that this variant may have a somewhat greater predilection for soft tissue.[11] Like other gastrointestinal stromal tumors, they too have been associated with Carney syndrome and neurofibromatosis 1.[60,75]

**TABLE 20–3** EXTRAGASTROINTESTINAL STROMAL TUMOR: INCIDENCE OF ADVERSE OUTCOME BY NUMBER OF HISTOLOGIC RISK FACTORS

| Risk Factors (No.) | Patients with Adverse Outcome/Total in Group (No.) | Incidence of Adverse Outcomes Per Person-year* |
|---|---|---|
| 0–1 | 1/19 (5%) | 0.02 |
| 2–3 | 11/12 (92%) | 0.54 |

Data from Reith J, Goldblum JR, Weiss SW. Extragastrointestinal (soft tissue) stromal tumors: an analysis of 48 cases with emphasis on histologic predictors of outcome. Mod Pathol 13:577, 2000.
* Risk factors are cellularity, necrosis, and mitotic activity (>2 mitoses/10 HPF).

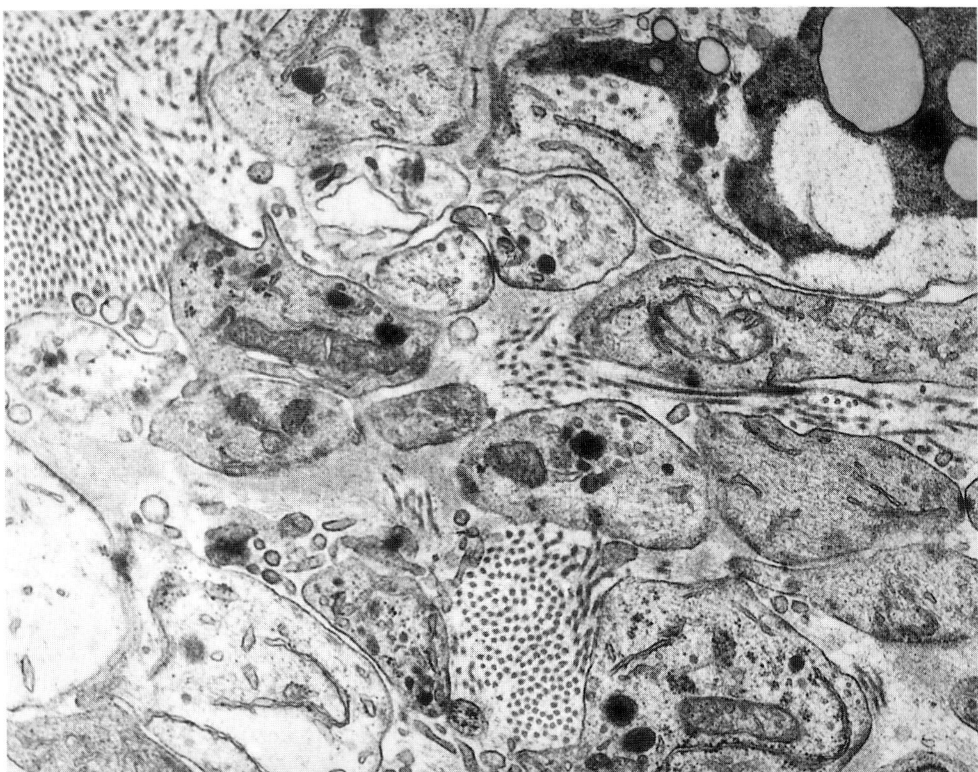

**FIGURE 20–24.** Electron micrograph of a gastrointestinal autonomic nerve tumor with neurites and synapse-like structures containing dense-core neurosecretory granules and microtubules. (×17,700) (Courtesy of Dr. Robert Erlandson.)

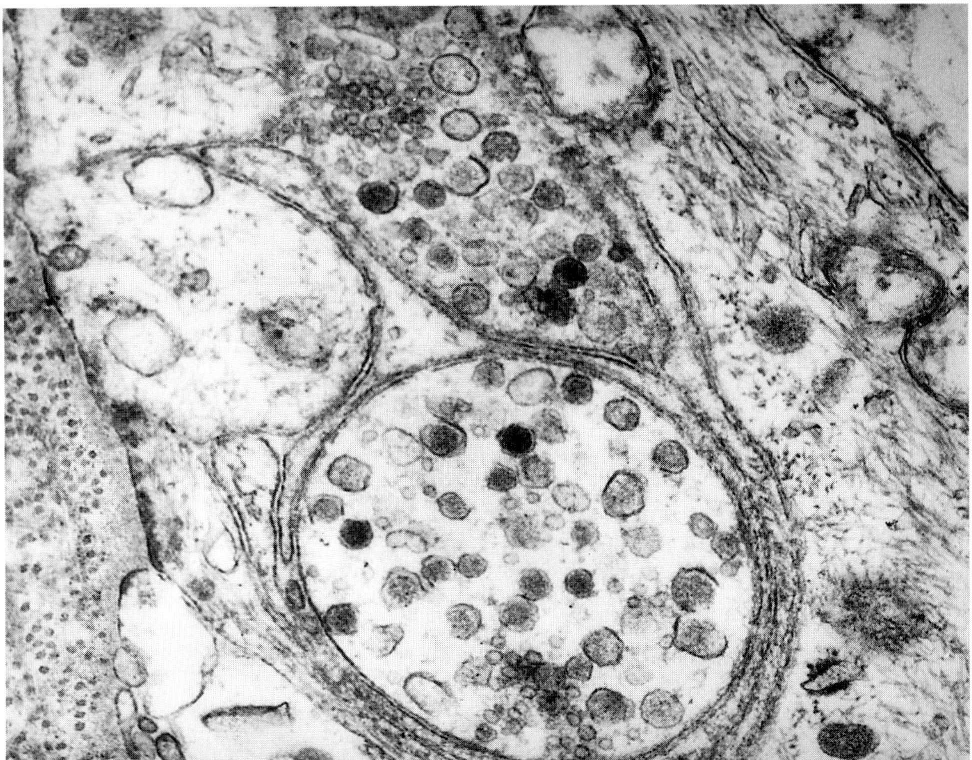

**FIGURE 20–25.** Electron micrograph of a gastrointestinal autonomic nerve tumor illustrating details of the synapse-like structures. Note the neurosecretory granules and vesicles. A portion of a neurite is also present. (×35,700) (Courtesy of Dr. Robert Erlandson.)

Grossly and microscopically, the lesions resemble gastrointestinal stromal tumors and display a range of appearances, from a predominantly spindle cell lesion to an epithelioid one. Most have a spindle cell pattern, but tumors composed predominantly of epithelioid cells are also observed. Within the spindled areas the pattern may be fascicular, storiform, or even palisaded. Myxoid change, hyalinization, skeinoid fibers, and prominent inflammatory cells (including plasma cells, lymphocytes, and eosinophils)[74] have been reported. The tumors virtually all express vimentin, and most express neuron-specific enolase. CD34 and synaptophysin are seen in about one-half of cases,[11] whereas a far smaller percent express chromogranin, S-100 protein, and NFP. Although the presence of one or more of these markers suggests an autonomic nerve tumor, a conclusive diagnosis is dependent on ultrastructural analysis. The tumor has elongated processes containing dense-core neurosecretory granules, microtubules, intermediate filaments, and a bulbous synapse-like structure (Figs. 20–24, 20–25).

Although most autonomic nerve tumors have a rather low-grade appearance, they exhibit aggressive behavior. About one-half of the patients reviewed by Lam et al. developed metastatic disease.[67] There is no clear-cut evidence that autonomic nerve tumors behave significantly differently from the overall group of gastrointestinal nerve tumors if one matches cases by size, location, and other relevant parameters. Until such time as important behavioral or therapeutic differences exist, it is not practical to advocate ultrastructural analysis of every stromal tumor to identify the occasional one with autonomic differentiation.

## REFERENCES


1. Appelman HD. Smooth muscle tumors of the gastrointestinal tract: what we know that Stout didn't know. Am J Surg Pathol 10(Suppl):83, 1986.
2. Appelman HD, Helwig EB. Gastric epithelioid leiomyoma and leiomyosarcoma (leiomyoblastoma). Cancer 38:708, 1976.
3. Brainard JA, Goldblum JR. Stromal tumors of the jejunum and ileum: a clinicopathologic study of 39 cases. Am J Surg Pathol 21:407, 1997.
4. Breiner JA, Meis-Kindblom J, Kindblom L-G, et al. Loss of 14q and 22q in gastrointestional pacemaker cell tumors (GIPACTs) Mod Pathol 12:72A, 1999.
5. Carillo R, Candia A, Rodriquez-Peralto JL, et al. Prognostic significance of DNA ploidy and proliferative index (MIB-1 index) in gastrointestinal stromal tumors. Hum Pathol 28:160, 1997.
6. Carney JA. The triad of gastric epithelioid leiomyosarcoma, functioning extraadrenal paraganglioma, and pulmonary chondroma. Cancer 43:374, 1979.
7. Carney JA. The triad of gastric epithelioid leiomyosarcoma, pulmonary chondroma, and functioning extraadrenal paraganglioma: a five year review. Medicine 62:159, 1983.
8. Cooper PN, Hardy GJ, Dixon MF. A flow cytometric, clinical, and histological study of stromal neoplasms of the gastrointestinal tract. Am J Surg Pathol 16:163, 1992.
9. El-Naggar AK, McLemore D, Garnsey L, et al. Gastrointestinal stromal tumors: DNA flow-cytometric study of 58 patients with at least five years of follow-up. Mod Pathol 2:511, 1988.
10. El-Rifai W, Sarlomo-Rikala M, Miettinen M, et al. DNA copy number losses in chromosome 14: an early change in gastrointestinal stromal tumors. Cancer Res 56:3230, 1996.
11. Erlandson RA, Klimstra DS, Woodruff JM. Subclassification of gastrointestinal stromal tumors based on evaluation by electron microscopy and immunohistochemistry. Ultrastruct Pathol 20: 373, 1996.
12. Emory TS, Sobin LH, Lukes L, et al. Prognosis of gastrointestinal smooth-muscle (stromal) tumors. Am J Surg Pathol 23:82, 1999.
13. Ernst S, Hubbs A, Przygodzki T, et al. *kit* mutation portends poor prognosis in gastrointestinal stromal/smooth muscle tumors. Mod Pathol 12:75A, 1999.
14. Ernst S, Przygodzki T, Emory L, et al. Loss of heterozygosity on chromosome 1 in gastrointestinal stromal/smooth mucle tumors: implications for pathogenesis and prognosis. Mod Pathol 12:75A, 1999.
15. Evans HL. Smooth muscle tumors of the gastrointestinal tract: a study of 56 cases followed for a minimum of 10 years. Cancer 56:2242, 1985.
16. Flint A, Appelman HD, Beckwith AL. DNA analysis of gastric stromal neoplasm: correlation with pathologic features. Surg Pathol 2:117, 1989.
17. Franquemont DW. Differentiation and risk assessment of gastrointestinal stromal tumors. Am J Clin Pathol 103:41, 1995.
18. Franquemont DW, Frierson HF. Muscle differentiation and clinicopathologic features of gastrointestinal stromal tumors. Am J Surg Pathol 16:947, 1992.
19. Goldblum JR, Appelman HD. Stromal tumors of the duodenum: a histologic and immunohistochemical study of 20 cases. Am J Surg Pathol 19:71, 1995.
20. Goldblum JR, Mandell SH, Appelman HD, et al. Proliferating cell nuclear antigen and p53 antigen expression in gastrointestinal stromal tumors. Am J Clin Pathol 98:351, 1992.
21. Hajdu SI, Erlandson RA, Paglia MA. Light and electron microscopic studies of a gastric leiomyoblastoma. Arch Pathol 93:36, 1972.
22. Haque S, Dean PJ. Stromal neoplasms of the rectum and anal canal. Hum Pathol 23:762, 1992.

22a. Hirota S, Isozaki K, Moriyama Y, et al. Gain-of-function mutations of c-kit in human gastrointestinal stromal tumors. Science 279:577, 1998.

22b. Hirota S, Okazaki T, Kitamura Y, et al. Cause of familial and multiple autonomic nerve tumors with hyperplasia of interstitial cells of Cajal is germline mutation of the c-kit gene. Am J Surg Pathol 24:326, 2000.

23. Hjermstad BM, Sobin LH, Helwig EB. Stromal tumors of the gastrointestinal tract: myogenic or neurogenic. Am J Surg Pathol 11:383, 1987.
24. Kindblom LG, Remotti HE, Aldenborg F, Meis-Kindblom JM. Gastrointestinal pacemaker cell tumor (GIPACT): gastrointestinal stromal tumors show phenotypic characteristics of the interstitial cells of Cajal. Am J Pathol 152:12459, 1998.
25. Kindblom LG, Remotti HE, Angervall L, Meis-Kindblom JM. Gastrointestinal pacemaker cell tumor—a manifestation of neurofibromatosis 1 (NF1). Mod Pathol 12:77A, 1999.
26. Kiyabu MT, Bishop PC, Parker JW, et al. Smooth muscle tumors of the gastrointestinal tract: flow cytometric quantitation of DNA and nuclear antigen content and correlation with histologic grade. Am J Surg Pathol 12:954, 1988.
27. Langel D, Grotte DA, Batts KP. Multiple gastrointestinal tumors arising from the interstitial cells of Cajal (ICCs): a potential

association with neurofibromatosis type 1 (NF1). Mod Pathol 12:78A, 1999.

28. Lasota J, Jasinski M, Sarlomo-Rikala M, Miettinen M. Mutations in exon 11 of c-kit occur preferentially in malignant versus benign gastrointestinal stromal tumors and do not occur in leiomyomas and leiomyosarcomas. Am J Pathol 154:53, 1999.
29. Lerma E, Oliva E, Tugues D, Prat J. Stromal tumors of the gastrointestinal tract: a clinicopathological and ploidy analysis of 33 cases. Virchows Arch 424:19, 1994.
30. Lewin K, Appelman HD. Tumors of the stomach. In: Atlas of Tumor Pathology, Armed Forces Institute of Pathology, Washington, DC, 1996.
31. Ma CK, Amin MB, Kintanar E, et al. Immunohistochemical characterization of gastrointestinal stromal tumors: a study of 82 cases compared with 11 cases of leiomyomas. Mod Pathol 6: 139, 1993.
31a. Lux M, Rubin BP, Biase TL. KIT extracellular and kinase domain mutations in gastrointestinal stromal tumors. Am J Pathol 156:791, 2000.
32. Marci V, Casorzo L, Sarotto I, et al. Gastrointestinal stromal tumor, uncommitted type, with monosomies 14 and 22 as the only chromosomal abnormalities. Cancer Genet Cytogenet 102: 135, 1998.
33. Martin JF, Bazin P, Feroldi J, et al. Tumeurs myoides intramurales de l'estomac: considerations microscopiques a propos de 6 cas. Ann Anat Pathol (Paris) 5:484, 1960.
34. Matsukuma S, Doi M, Suzuki M, et al. Numerous eosinophilic globules (skeinoid fibers) in a duodenal stromal tumor: an exceptional case showing smooth muscle differentiation. Pathol Int 47:789, 1997.
35. Mazur MT, Clark HB. Gastric stromal tumors: reappraisal of histogenesis. Am J Surg Pathol 7:507, 1983.
36. Miettinen M. Gastrointestinal stromal tumors: an immunohistochemical study of cellular differentiation. Am J Clin Pathol 89: 601, 1988.
37. Miettinen M, Monihan JM, Sarlomo-Rikala M, et al. Gastrointestinal stromal tumors/smooth muscle tumors (GISTs) primary in the omentum and mesentery: clinicopathologic and immunohistochemical study of 26 cases. Am J Surg Pathol 23:1109, 1999.
37a. Miettinen M, Sarlomo-Rikala M, Lasota J. Gastrointestinal stromal tumors: new findings on their biology: a review. Hum Pathol 23:1209, 1999.
37b. Miettinen M, Sarlomo-Rikala M, Sobin LH, Lasota J. Esophageal stromal tumors: a clinicopathologic, immunohistochemical, and molecular genetic study of 17 cases and comparison with esophageal leiomyomas and leiomyosarcomas. Am J Surg Pathol 245:211, 2000.
38. Miettinen M, Virolainen M, Maarit-Sarlomo-Rikala M. Gastrointestinal stromal tumors: value of CD 34 antigen in their identification and separation from true leiomyomas and schwannomas. Am J Surg Pathol 19:207, 1995.
39. Min K-W. Small intestinal stromal tumors with skeinoid fibers: clinicopathological, immunohistochemical, and ultrastructural investigations. Am J Surg Pathol 16:145, 1992.
39a. Nakahara M, Isozaki K, Hirota S, et al. A novel gain of function mutation of c-kit gene in gastrointestinal stromal tumors. Gastroenterology 115:1090, 1998.
40. Newman PL, Wadden C, Fletcher CDM. Gastrointestinal stromal tumors: correlation of immunophenotype with clinicopathologic features. J Pathol 164:107, 1991.
40a. Nishida T, Hirota S, Taniguchi M, et al. Familial gastrointestinal stromal tumours with germline mutation of the KIT gene. Nature Genet 19:323, 1998.
40b. O'Brien P, Kapusta L, Dardick I, et al. Multiple familial gastrointestinal autonomic nerve tumors and small intestinal neuronal dysplasia. Am J Surg Pathol 23:198, 1999.
41. Pike AM, Lloyd RV, Appelman HD. Cell markers in gastrointestinal stromal tumors. Hum Pathol 19:830, 1988.
42. Pizzimbono CA, Higa E, Wise L. Leiomyoblastoma of the lesser sac: case report and review of the literature. Am Surg 39:692, 1973.
43. Reith J, Goldblum JR, Weiss SW. Extragastrointestinal (soft tissue) stromal tumors: an analysis of 48 cases with emphasis on histologic predictors of outcome. Mod Pathol 13:577, 2000.
44. Rubin BP, Lux M, Singer S, et al. Correlation of c-kit mutations status with c-kit protein expression in gastrointestinal stromal tumors. Mod Pathol 12:83A, 1999.
45. Rudolph P, Gloeckner K, Parwaresch R, et al. Immunophenotype, proliferation, DNA ploidy, and biological behavior of gastrointestinal stromal tumors: a multivariate clinicopathologic study. Hum Pathol 29:791, 1998.
46. Saul SH, Rast ML, Brooks JJ. The immunohistochemistry of gastrointestinal stromal tumors: evidence supporting origin from smooth muscle. Am J Surg Pathol 11:464, 1987.
47. Sbasachinig RIJ, Cunningham RE, Sobin LH, O'Leary TJ. Proliferating-cell nuclear antigen immunocytochemistry in the evaluation of gastrointestinal smooth muscle tumors. Mod Pathol 7: 780, 1994.
48. Stout AP. Bizarre smooth muscle tumors of the stomach. Cancer 15:400, 1962.
49. Suster S. Epithelioid leiomyosarcoma of the skin and subcutaneous tissue: clinicopathologic, immunohistochemical, and ultrastructural study of five cases. Am J Surg Pathol 18:232, 1994.
50. Suster S. Gastrointestinal stromal tumors. Semin Diagn Pathol 13:297, 1996.
51. Suster S, Fletcher CD. Gastrointestinal stromal tumors with prominent signet ring cell features. Mod Pathol 9:609, 1996.
52. Suster S, Sorace D, Moran CA. Gastrointestinal stromal tumors with prominent myxoid matrix: clinicopathologic, immunohistochemical, and ultrastructural study of nine cases of a distinctive morphologic variant of myogenic stromal tumor. Am J Surg Pathol 19:1444, 1995.
53. Thompson EM, Evans DJ. The significance of PGP 9.5 in tumours: an immunohistochemical study of gastrointestinal stromal tumours. Histopathology 17:175, 1990.
54. Tirabosco R, Cavazzana AO, Santeusanio G, Spagnoli LG. Gastrointestinal stromal tumor: evidence for a smooth-muscle origin. Mod Pathol 8:193, 1995.
55. Tworek JA, Appelman HD, Singleton TP, Greenson JK. Stromal tumors of the jejunum and ileum. Mod Pathol 10:200, 1997.
56. Tworek JA, Goldblum JR, Weiss SW, et al. Stromal tumors of the abdominal colon: a clinicopathologic study of 20 cases. Am J Surg Pathol 23:937, 1999.
57. Tworek JA, Goldblum JA, Weiss SW, et al. Stromal tumors of the anorectum: a clinicopathologic study of 22 cases. Am J Surg Pathol 23:946, 1999.
58. Ueyama T, Guo K-J, Hashimoto H, et al. A clinicopathologic and immunohistochemical study of gastrointestinal stromal tumors. Cancer 69:947, 1992.
59. Vanderwinden J-M, Rumessen JJ, De Laet M-H, et al. $CD34^+$ cells in human intestine are fibroblasts adjacent to, but distinct from, interstitial cells of Cajal. Lab Invest 79:59, 1999.
60. Walsh NMG, Bodurtha A. Auerbach's myenteric plexus: a possible site of origin for gastrointestinal stromal tumors in von Recklinghusens neurofibromatosis. Arch Pathol Lab Med 114: 522, 1990.
61. Weiss SW, Sobin LH. World Health Organization Classification of Soft Tissue Tumors. Springer-Verlag, Berlin, 1994.
62. Yu CC-W, Fletcher CDM, Newman PL, et al. A comparison of proliferating cell nuclear antigen (PCNA) immunostaining, nucleolar organizer region (AgNOR) staining, and histological grading in gastrointestinal stromal tumors. J Pathol 166:147, 1992.

### Gastrointestinal Autonomic Nerve Tumor

63. Dhimes P, Lopez-Carreira M, Ortega-Serrano MP, et al. Gastrointestinal autonomic nerve tumours and their separation from other gastrointestinal stromal tumours: an ultrastructural and immunohistochemical study of seven cases. Virchows Arch 426: 27, 1995.
64. Donner LR. Gastrointestinal autonomic nerve tumor: a common type of gastrointestinal stromal neoplasm. Ultrastruct Pathol 21: 419, 1997.
65. Herrera GA, Pinto de Moraes H, Grizzle WE, Han SG. Malignant small bowel neoplasm of enteric plexus derivation (plexosarcoma): light and electron microscopic study confirming the origin of the neoplasm. Dig Dis Sci 29:275, 1984.
66. Kodet R, Snajdauf J, Smelhous V. Gastrointestinal autonomic nerve tumor: a case report with electron microscopic and immunohistochemical analysis and review of the literature. Pediatr Pathol 14:1005, 1994.
67. Lam KY, Law SY, Chu KM, Ma LT. Gastrointestinal autonomic nerve tumor of the esophagus: a clinicopathologic immunohistochemical, ultrastructural, study of a case and review of the literature. Cancer 79:1651, 1996.
68. Lauwers GY, Erlandson RA, Casper ES, et al. Gastrointestinal autonomic nerve tumor: a clinicopathologic, immunohistochemical, and ultrastructural study of 12 cases. Am J Surg Pathol 17: 887, 1993.
69. MacLeod CB, Tsokos M. Gastrointesntial autonomic nerve tumor. Ultrastruct Pathol 15:49, 1991.
70. Matsumoto K, Min W, Yamada N, Asano G. Gastrointestinal autonomic nerve tumors: immunohistochemical and ultrastructural studies in cases of gastrointestinal nerve tumors. Pathol Int 47:308, 1997.
71. Ojanguren I, Ariza A, Navas-Palacios JJ. Gastrointestinal autonomic nerve tumor: further observations regarding an ultrastructural and immunohistochemical analysis of six cases. Hum Pathol 27:1311, 1996.
72. Segal A, Carello S, Carterina P, et al. Gastrointestinal autonomic nerve tumors: a clinicopathological, immunohistochemical and ultrastructural study of 10 cases. Pathology 26:439, 1994.
73. Shanks JH, Harris M, Banerjee SS, Eyden BP. Gastrointestinal autonomic nerve tumours: a report of nine cases. Histopathology 29:111, 1996.
74. Shek TW, Luk IS, Loong F, et al. Inflammatory cell-rich gastrointestinal autonomic nerve tumor: an expansion of its histologic spectrum. Am J Surg Pathol 20:325, 1996.
75. Tortella BJ, Matthews JB, Antonioli DA, et al. Gastric autonomic nerve (GAN) tumor and extra-adrenal paraganglioma in Carney's triad: a common origin. Ann Surg 205:221, 1987.

# CHAPTER 21

# RHABDOMYOMA

## STRIATED MUSCLE TISSUE: DEVELOPMENT AND STRUCTURE

Skeletal muscle is formed primarily within myotomes, which are arranged in segmental pairs along the spine and make their first appearance in the cephalic region during the third week of intrauterine life. In the region of the anterior head and neck, skeletal muscle may also develop from mesenchyme derived from the neural crest (mesectoderm).

At the earliest stage of muscle development, primitive mesenchymal cells differentiate along two lines: (1) as fibroblasts, which are loosely arranged spindle-shaped cells with the capacity to form collagen; and (2) as myoblasts, which are round or oval cells with single, centrally positioned nuclei and granular eosinophilic cytoplasm. Over the next few weeks the individual myoblasts assume a more elongated bipolar shape with slender, symmetrically arranged processes and nonstriated longitudinal myofibrils that are laid down first in the peripheral portion of the cytoplasm; this phase is followed by successive alignment and fusion of the individual myoblasts into myotubes with multiple centrally placed nuclei (myotubular stage) (Figs. 21–1, 21–2). During the seventh to tenth weeks of intrauterine development, as differentiation progresses, the myofibrils become thicker and more numerous by longitudinal division, and they develop increasingly distinct cross-striations. Finally, during the eleventh to fifteenth weeks the nucleus is moved from its initial central position toward the periphery of the muscle fiber. Muscles derived from the cervical and thoracic myotomes mature earlier than those arising more distally.

Ultrastructurally, the individual myofibrils are composed of two types of myofilaments: thin (actin) filaments measuring 50–70 nm in diameter and thick (myosin) filaments measuring 140–160 nm in diameter. The thin filaments are laid down first in a random fashion, but later they become rearranged and form parallel bundles together with thick filaments and polyribosomes. In cross section the thin filaments are seen to surround the thick filaments in distinct, evenly spaced hexagonal patterns.

Mature striated muscle consists of parallel arrays of closely packed myofibrils embedded within sarcoplasm and enveloped by a thin sarcolemmal sheath. Each of the myofibrils shows distinct cross-banding, light and dark bands caused by the periodic arrangement and interdigitation of the thin and thick myofilaments. In this arrangement, isotropic (I) bands, anisotropic (A) bands, and H bands can be distinguished. The I band consists solely of thin (actin) filaments and is divided at its center by the Z line or disc, which is thought to serve as an attachment site for the sarcomeres, the repeating individual units of the muscle fiber. The adjacent A band is a zone of overlapping thin and thick (actin and myosin) filaments; it is separated by the H band, which consists only of thick myofilaments. The width of the individual bands and sarcomeres varies and depends on the state of muscle contraction (Fig. 21–3).

Closely associated with the parallel arrays of myofilaments and the surrounding sarcoplasm are mitochondria, a canalicular network of endoplasmic reticulum, a small Golgi complex, ribosomes, and glycogen and lipid granules. These organelles are confined by a sarcolemmal membrane that measures approximately 70 nm in thickness and is covered by a basal lamina. The sarcolemmal nuclei measure 6–12 mm in greatest diameter and contain one or two small nucleoli; they are located at the periphery of the myofibrils underneath the sarcolemmal membrane. Satellite cells—reserve cells and possible precursors of myoblasts that play a role in the regeneration of striated muscle tissue—are situated in the endomysium between the sarcolemmal membrane and basal lamina.

## CLASSIFICATION OF RHABDOMYOMAS

Although as a general rule benign soft tissue neoplasms outnumber malignant neoplasms by a sizable

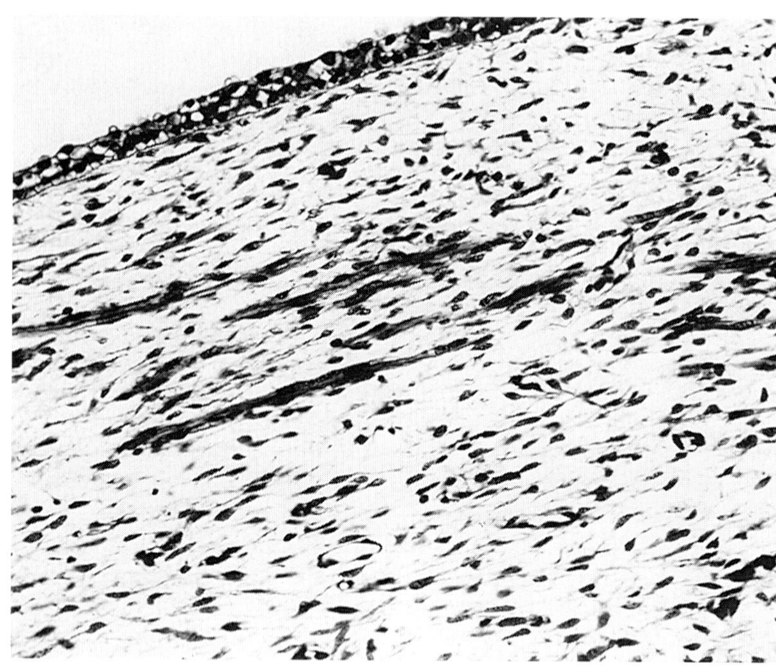

**FIGURE 21–1.** Developing striated muscle in the soft tissue of a 9-week-old fetus. Note the close resemblance to botryoid-type embryonal rhabdomyosarcoma.

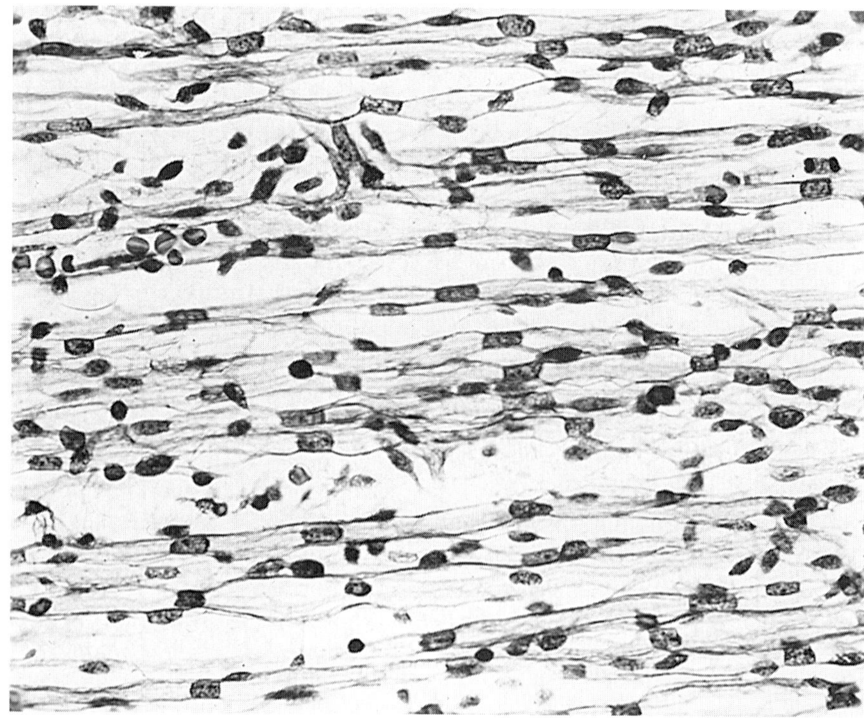

**FIGURE 21–2.** Myotube stage in the development of striated muscle bearing a close resemblance to both fetal rhabdomyoma and the "tubular" type of embryonal rhabdomyosarcoma.

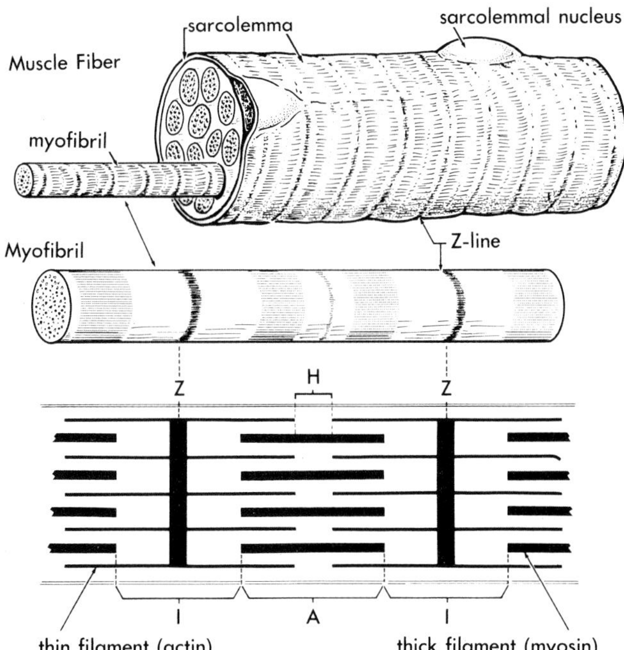


**FIGURE 21–3.** Muscle fiber, myofibril, and sliding actin and myosin filaments during the rest phase of muscle contraction.

margin, this does not hold true for the neoplasms of striated muscle tissue. In this particular group of neoplasms, rhabdomyomas (benign tumors of striated muscle tissue) are considerably less common than rhabdomyosarcomas, accounting for no more than 2% of all striated muscle tumors.

Among the extracardiac rhabdomyomas, four clinically and morphologically different types can be distinguished: (1) the *adult type,* a slowly growing lesion that is nearly always found in the head and neck area of elderly persons; (2) the *fetal type,* a rare process that also affects mainly the head and neck region but occurs in both children and adults; (3) the *genital type,* a tumor-like polypoid mass found almost exclusively in the vagina and vulva of middle-aged women; and (4) the *rhabdomyomatous mesenchymal hamartoma,* a peculiar striated muscle proliferation that occurs chiefly in the periorbital and perioral region of infants and young children (Table 21–1).

*Rhabdomyoma of the heart (cardiac rhabdomyoma)* is a well established lesion that occurs almost exclusively in the hearts of infants and young children, often as multiple intramural lesions in the right and left ventricles, although the interventricular septum and atria may be involved as well.[2,14] It often occurs in association with other congenital abnormalities, including tuberous sclerosis of the brain, sebaceous adenomas, and renal angiomyolipomas. Bosi et al. studied 33 patients with cardiac rhabdomyoma, 30 of whom (91%) had tuberous sclerosis.[1] In studies that have examined patients with tuberous sclerosis by repeated echocardiograms, 47%[7] to up to 67%[4,11,12] of patients have been found to harbor one or more cardiac rhabdomyomas.

Clinically, the lesion may be asymptomatic or may cause cardiac arrhythmia,[5,10,17] tachycardia, ventricular outflow obstruction,[15] Wolff-Parkinson-White syndrome,[1] or even sudden death.[6,13] To our knowledge, the concurrence of cardiac and extracardiac rhabdomyomas in the same patient has not been observed, although rare examples of adult rhabdomyoma may occur in the heart.[18] Furthermore, extracardiac rhabdomyoma has not been found in association with manifestations of the tuberous sclerosis complex.

Histologically, the lesions are usually small and are composed predominantly of large polygonal "spider cells" with large cytoplasmic vacuoles secondary to loss of glycogen during processing (Figs. 21–4, 21–5). The cells stain for muscle markers, including muscle-specific actin, desmin, and myoglobin.[2] Some authors have also reported HMB-45 immunoreactivity,[16] supporting a relation with angiomyolipoma and lymphangioleiomyomatosis as components of the tuberous sclerosis complex composed of cells with both myogenic and melanocytic features.

**TABLE 21–1** CLINICAL FEATURES OF VARIOUS RHABDOMYOMAS

| Parameter | Cardiac Type | Adult Type | Fetal Myxoid Type | Fetal Intermediate Type | Genital Type | RHM |
|---|---|---|---|---|---|---|
| Peak age | Infants | >40 years | Infants | Children and adults | Young to middle-aged adults | Newborns |
| Gender (M/F) | 1:1 | 3:1 | 3:1 | 3:1 | Almost all female | Almost all male |
| Favored site(s) | Ventricles | Head and neck | Head and neck | Head and neck | Vagina, vulva | Chin |
| Associated conditions | Tuberous sclerosis | None | Nevoid BCC syndrome | Nevoid BCC syndrome | None | Congenital anomalies |
| Spontaneous regression | Yes | No | No | No | No | No |

RHM, rhabdomyomatous mesenchymal hamartoma; BCC: basal cell carcinoma.

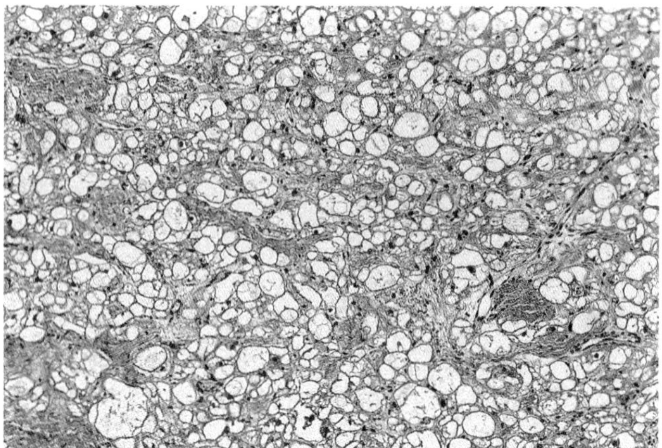

**FIGURE 21–4.** Cardiac rhabdomyoma. The lesion is composed predominantly of large polygonal "spider cells" with large cytoplasmic vacuoles.

Treatment of this lesion is generally reserved for those with life-threatening obstructive symptoms or arrhythmias refractory to medical therapy.[3,8,9] The lesions have a tendency to regress spontaneously over time. DiMario et al. found that most lesions in patients followed with serial echocardiograms were undetectable by the age of 6 years.[4]

## ADULT RHABDOMYOMA

The adult type of rhabdomyoma, also sometimes referred to as *rhabdomyoma purum*,[33,51] is a rare but morphologically characteristic lesion; fewer than 150 cases have been reported in the literature. There is no etiologic relation between adult rhabdomyoma and *granular cell tumor* (*granular cell myoblastoma* or *Abrikossoff's tumor*).[19]

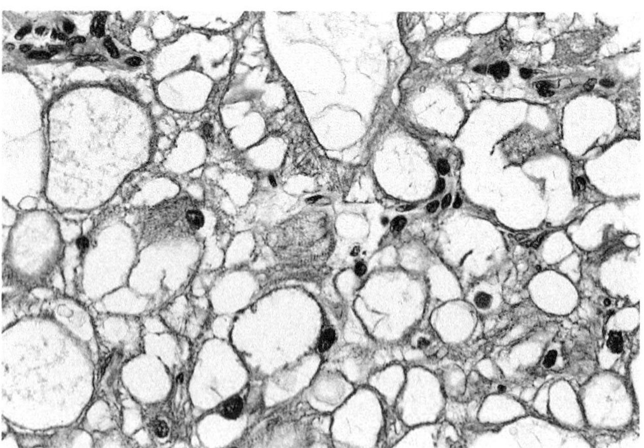

**FIGURE 21–5.** Cardiac rhabdomyoma with vacuolated spider cells. Cross-striations are rare but can be identified.

### Clinical Findings

The process usually presents as a solitary round or polypoid mass in the head and neck region that causes neither tenderness nor pain; it may compress or displace the tongue or may protrude into and partially obstruct the pharynx or larynx. As a consequence, it may cause hoarseness or progressive difficulty with breathing or swallowing.[31,42,44,56,66] It has also been reported as an incidental finding at autopsy or during radical neck dissection for an unrelated cause. It is a slowly growing process, and several of the reported cases have been known to be present for many years. Parsons and Puro,[55] for instance, reported a 74-year-old patient who had had a rhabdomyoma of the sternohyoid muscle for no less than 55 years that eventually grew to be 10 cm. Most cases occur in adults older than 40 years (median age 60 years), with few reports of these lesions arising in children.[61] Men are affected three to four times more commonly than women,[21,44] but apparently there is no predilection for any particular race. The principal site of involvement is the neck, where the tumor seems to arise from the branchial musculature of the third and fourth branchial arches. It is found most frequently in the region of the pharynx,[24,37,41,44] oral cavity including the floor of the mouth[28,45] or base of the tongue,[64] and the larynx.[48,67,71] It may also involve the soft palate and the uvula,[26,30] usually as an extension of a pharyngeal rhabdomyoma. Isolated examples have been encountered in the somatic muscles of the lateral neck,[20,57] the lower lip and cheek,[23,49,62,70] and the orbit.[46] Rare tumors have been described outside the head and neck region, including the stomach,[63] esophagus,[54] and mediastinum.[27,50] Yu et al.[69] described a typical adult rhabdomyoma that arose in the right atrium of a 42-year-old woman. It was not until very recently that a case of adult rhabdomyoma was described arising in the deep soft tissue of the extremities.[29a]

Most adult rhabdomyomas are solitary, but about 20% are multifocal, mostly involving the general area of the neck.[25,34,35,39,53,58,59] For example, the patient reported by Parsons and Puro[55] and Goldman,[38] who had an adult rhabdomyoma of the left neck, developed a second tumor of similar appearance in the left vocal cord, which was found at autopsy. Gardner and Corio reported one patient with separate tumors in the larynx and submandibular region.[35]

### Pathologic Findings

As a rule, the tumor is well defined, rounded, or coarsely lobulated and ranges from 0.5 to 10.0 cm in greatest diameter (median 3.0 cm). Some are multi-

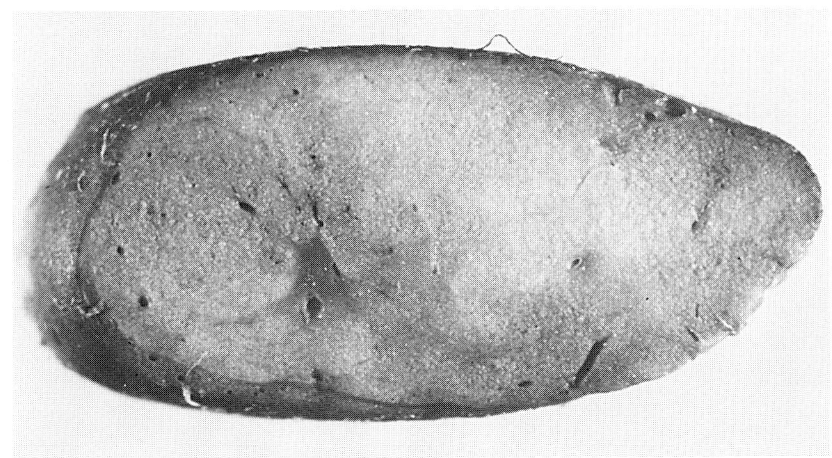

**FIGURE 21–6.** Adult rhabdomyoma in cross section showing a well vascularized, finely granular surface.

nodular, and others form sessile or pedunculated polypoid submucosal masses. On cut section it has a finely granular, gray-yellow to red-brown appearance (Fig. 21–6).

Microscopically, it is composed of tightly packed, large, round or polygonal cells 15–150 μm in diameter and separated from one another by thin fibrous septa and narrow vascular channels. The cells have deeply acidophilic, finely granular cytoplasm, one or (rarely) two centrally or peripherally placed vesicular nuclei, and one or more prominent nucleoli (Figs. 21–7, 21–8). Many of the cells are vacuolated because intracellular glycogen has been removed during processing; some of the vacuolated cells, in fact, contain merely a small central acidophilic cytoplasmic mass connected by thin strands of cytoplasm to a condensed rim of cytoplasm at the periphery (spider cells), but these cells are much more conspicuous in cardiac than extracardiac rhabdomyomas. Mitotic figures are nearly always absent.[32,44] Cross-striations can be discerned in most cases, but sometimes they are detected only after a prolonged search; additional features present in many cases are intracytoplasmic rodlike or "jackstraw"-like crystalline structures (Figs. 21–9, 21–10), first described by Moran and Enterline[52] in 1964. Both cross-striations and crystalline structures are identified much more readily with the phosphotungstic acid-hematoxylin (PTAH) stain than with hematoxylin-eosin; moreover, many cells contain intracellular lipid demonstrable with oil red O. Immunohistochemically, the cells also stain positively for myoglobin, desmin (Fig. 21–11), and muscle-specific actin; they are positive less commonly for vimentin, S-100 protein, and Leu-7.[40,44] Some cases also show focal staining for smooth muscle actin.[44]

Gibas and Miettinen,[36] in a cytogenetic study of a recurrent peripharyngeal rhabdomyoma in a 64-year-old man, found a reciprocal translocation of chromo-

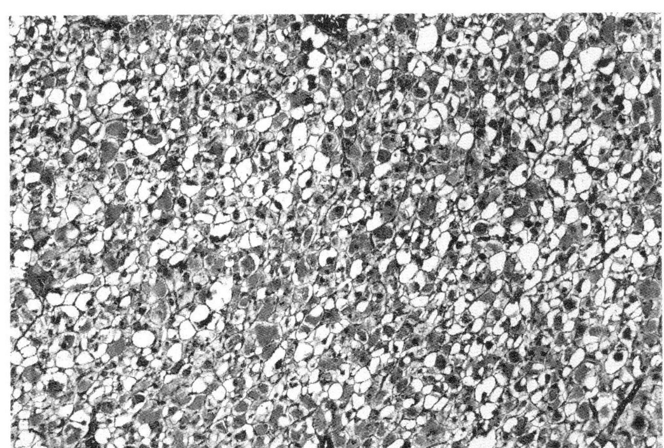

**FIGURE 21–7.** Low-power view of adult rhabdomyoma composed of an admixture of deeply eosinophilic polygonal cells and cells with vacuolated cytoplasm.

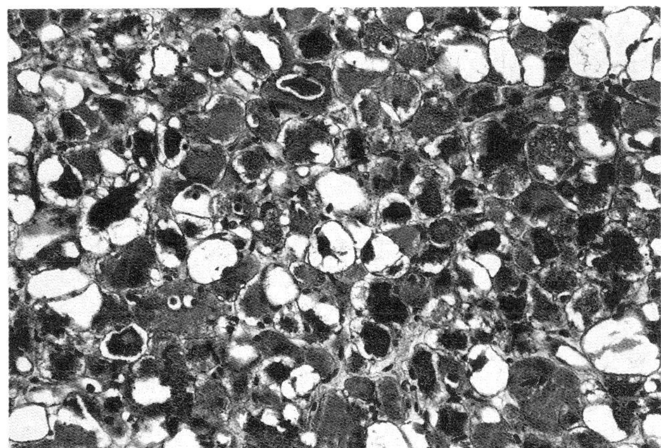

**FIGURE 21–8.** Adult rhabdomyoma composed of variously sized, deeply eosinophilic polygonal cells with small, peripherally placed nuclei and occasional intracellular vacuoles.

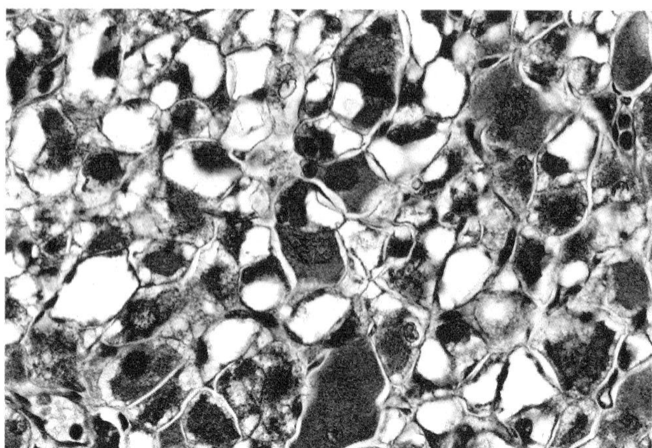

**FIGURE 21–9.** Adult rhabdomyoma with rare "jackstraw"-like crystalline structures within the cytoplasm of some of the eosinophilic polygonal cells.

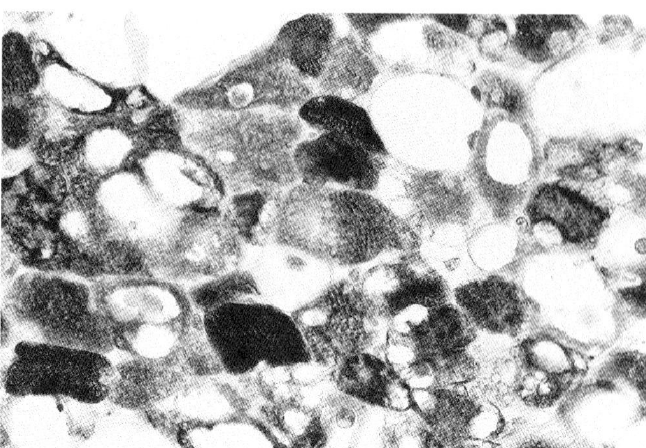

**FIGURE 21–11.** Adult rhabdomyoma showing immunoreactivity for desmin. Note accentuation of cross-striations.

somes 15 and 17 and miscellaneous abnormalities in the long arm of chromosome 10. They concluded that this finding lends support to the notion that the adult rhabdomyoma is a true neoplasm rather than a hamartoma.

## Ultrastructural Findings

There is agreement among most observers as to the ultrastructure of adult rhabdomyoma.[60] The cytoplasm contains, in addition to a variable number of mitochondria with linear cristae and deposits of glycogen, thin and thick myofilaments showing a varying degree of differentiation and measuring 50–70 nm and 135–150 nm in diameter, respectively. Distinct Z lines are readily discernible within the I band, but sometimes A, H, M, and N bands are also apparent (Fig. 21–12). Cornog and Gonatas[29] identified the crystalline intracytoplasmic inclusions as hypertrophied Z bands and pointed out their close resemblance to structures found in nemaline myopathy. There are also "triads," trigonal arrays of actin and myosin filaments that can be seen in cross section,[65] and parallel rows of electron-dense particles within the mitochondria.[25,47,68] The individual cells are surrounded by a thin basal lamina with focal infoldings of the plasma membrane in some of the cells.[26] Kay et al.[45] compared the ultrastructure of cardiac rhabdomyoma and adult rhabdomyoma and noted better organization and more prominent Z lines in cardiac rhabdomyoma.

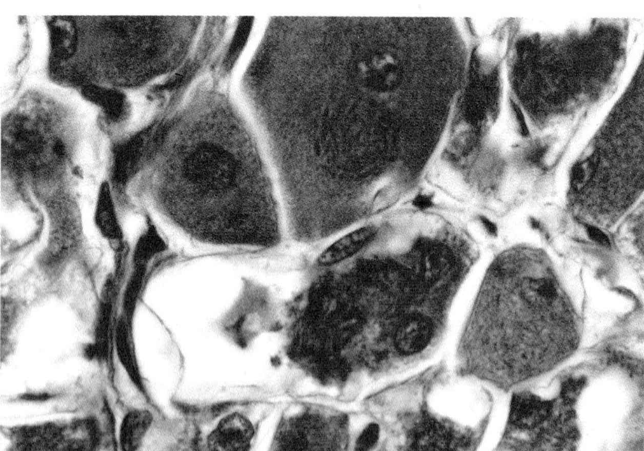

**FIGURE 21–10.** High-power view of adult rhabdomyoma with crystalline intracellular structures, probably representing Z-band material.

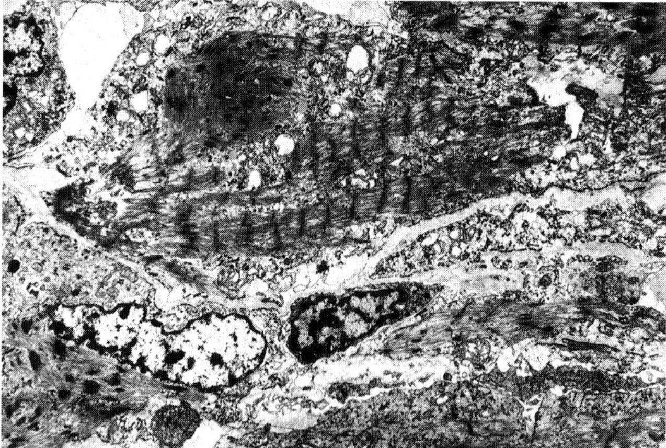

**FIGURE 21–12.** Electron micrograph of adult rhabdomyoma. Clearly discernible Z-lines are present, along with bundles of actin and myosin filaments.

## Differential Diagnosis

Problems in diagnosis are unlikely for anyone familiar with the characteristic picture of the tumor (Table 21–2). Yet in the earlier literature, *granular cell tumor* (granular cell myoblastoma)[19] and adult rhabdomyoma were often confused. Granular cell tumor, of Schwann cell origin, most often involves the skin, tongue, or larynx. The cells of a granular cell tumor tend to be less well defined and lack the characteristic vacuolation caused by intracellular glycogen; they are also devoid of cross-striations and usually are associated with more collagen. Moreover, the cells of granular cell tumors contain numerous periodic acid-Schiff (PAS)-positive, diastase-resistant granules that are related to the numerous intracytoplasmic phagolysosomes. Although S-100 protein is focally expressed in some cases of adult rhabdomyoma, its expression is more constant and diffuse in granular cell tumors.

*Hibernoma* also enters the differential diagnosis because of its frequent intracytoplasmic vacuoles and the presence of intracellular lipid. This tumor, however, is composed of small deeply eosinophilic granular cells that frequently contain distinct, variably sized lipid droplets in the cytoplasm. Clinically, hibernoma is most often found in the interscapular region of patients who are usually younger than 40 years of age. *Reticulohistiocytoma,* another lesion that must be included in the differential diagnosis, usually consists of an intimate mixture of deeply acidophilic histiocytes and fibroblasts intermingled with xanthoma cells, multinucleated giant cells, and chronic inflammatory elements. Typically, none of these cells contains glycogen, and the cells do not express myogenic antigens.

*Crystal-storing histiocytosis associated with lymphoplasmacytic neoplasms* may also simulate adult rhabdomyoma. In this lesion, however, the crystal-storing cells and histiocytes stain positively for CD68 (KP1) but are negative for skeletal muscle markers and S-100 protein.[43] Moreover, the associated lymphoplasmacytic infiltrate demonstrates monoclonality with immunostains for kappa and lambda chains.

*Cardiac rhabdomyoma* bears a close resemblance to adult rhabdomyoma, but its cells show a greater number of vacuolated spider cells and a more prominent population of giant cells. Cardiac rhabdomyoma is frequently encountered in association with tuberous sclerosis of the brain, sebaceous adenomas, and various other hamartomatous lesions of the kidney and other organs. Unlike adult rhabdomyomas, it has a propensity for spontaneous regression.

*Rhabdomyosarcoma,* always less well defined, characteristically is composed of poorly differentiated and pleomorphic round or spindle-shaped cells associated with varying numbers of rhabdomyoblasts. Mitotic figures are common in rhabdomyosarcomas but are absent or rare in adult rhabdomyomas. *Oncocytoma* is an epithelial neoplasm of salivary gland origin composed of mitochondria-rich polyhedral cells with finely granular, eosinophilic cytoplasm. The cells stain for epithelial markers but do not express actin or desmin. *Paraganglioma* is a neuroendocrine neoplasm composed of cells arranged in an organoid pattern (Zellballen). As seen by immunohistochemistry, the cells express neuroendocrine markers, including neuron-specific enolase, synaptophysin, and chromogranin. S-100 protein outlines the sustentacular cells, and the cells lack myogenic antigens. Neurosecretory granules can be demonstrated by electron microscopy.

## Prognosis and Therapy

The tumor is readily amenable to therapy but may recur locally if incompletely excised. In one series of 19 cases with follow-up information, the tumor recurred in 8 (42%) of the cases.[44] Examples of multiple and late recurrences have also been described.[31,44] Andersen and Elling[22] reported three recurrences within 35 years. Spontaneous regression, as is seen with some cardiac rhabdomyomas, has not been observed.

# FETAL RHABDOMYOMA

Fetal rhabdomyoma is even rarer in our experience than adult-type rhabdomyoma, and only a small

**TABLE 21–2** DIFFERENTIAL DIAGNOSIS OF ADULT-TYPE RHABDOMYOMA

| Parameter | Adult Rhabdomyoma | Granular Cell Tumor | Hibernoma | Paraganglioma |
|---|---|---|---|---|
| Favored site | Head and neck | Skin, tongue | Interscapular | Extra-adrenal ganglia |
| Electron microscopy | Thin/thick filaments | Phagolysosomes | Mitochondria | Neurosecretory granules |
| S-100 protein | Rare, focal | Diffuse | Diffuse | Sustentacular cells |
| Muscle-specific actin | Diffuse | Negative | Negative | Negative |
| Chromogranin | Negative | Negative | Negative | Diffuse |

number of cases have been recorded in the medical literature. Awareness of the existence of this tumor, however, is of considerable importance because of its close similarity to embryonal rhabdomyosarcoma; in fact, failure to recognize this lesion as a benign process may lead to excessive and unnecessary therapy. Diagnosis of this tumor may be difficult, as it is marked by a variable histological pattern, with a spectrum of skeletal muscle differentiation that ranges from immature, predominantly myxoid tumors to those showing a high degree of cellular differentiation and hardly any myxoid matrix. The former have been described as *myxoid*[77] or *classic*[83] *fetal rhabdomyomas;* the latter are variously described as *intermediate,*[83] *cellular,*[77] or *juvenile*[74] *fetal rhabdomyomas.* Intermediate forms between these two types are not uncommon. There is also a third, still ill-defined morphologic variant of this tumor that is marked by prominent neural involvement showing some similarities to neuromuscular hamartoma.[81,91]

## Clinical Features

The age incidence varies slightly according to the prevailing histologic type. Tumors of the predominantly *myxoid type* mainly affect boys during the first year of life and are rare in older patients. In the series of Kapadia et al.,[83] for instance, six of the eight patients with this type of tumor were infants younger than 1 year of age. The favorite sites of the myxoid type are the subcutaneous tissue and the submucosa of the head and neck, especially the pre- and postauricular regions.[76,83,90] The *intermediate type* affects adults more often than children. It occurs almost exclusively in the region of the head and neck, including the orbit, tongue, nasopharynx, and soft palate.[72,73,79,82] Rare cases of fetal rhabdomyoma have been described outside the head and neck region, including the chest wall/axilla,[89] abdominal wall,[86] retroperitoneum,[93] and perianal region.[87] For both types, males outnumber females by a ratio of approximately 3:1.

There are only a few reports in the literature of fetal rhabdomyomas associated with the nevoid basal cell carcinoma syndrome.[75,78,80,81,84,88] This syndrome is an autosomal dominant disorder characterized by multiple basal cell carcinomas that appear early during childhood, various skeletal abnormalities, and odontogenic keratocysts, among other findings. Schweisguth et al.[88] were the first to report an association between fetal rhabdomyomas and this syndrome, and others have confirmed this observation. In one case, described by Dahl et al.,[75] two fetal rhabdomyomas in the left thigh and the chest wall were associated with multiple basal cell carcinomas and anomalies of the eye and rib (bifurcated rib). In another case reported by Di Santo et al.,[78] a large fetal rhabdomyoma, extending from the mediastinum to the retroperitoneum, was removed from a 6-year-old girl who had multiple osseous anomalies and a family history of nevoid basal cell carcinoma.

## Pathologic Findings

On gross examination the tumors are well to moderately well circumscribed and average 2–6 cm in greatest diameter, although lesions as large as 12.5 cm have been reported.[83] Mucosal lesions tend to be smooth and polypoid or pedunculated. On sectioning they are gray-white to pink, often with a mucoid, glistening surface. Unlike rhabdomyosarcoma, fetal rhabdomyoma is primarily a superficial tumor and is found more often in the subcutis or submucosa than in muscle. Most are solitary, but multicentric fetal rhabdomyomas have been reported in association with the nevoid basal cell carcinoma syndrome.[75,84]

Two closely related types can be distinguished by microscopy. The *myxoid type* is chiefly composed of primitive oval or spindle-shaped cells with indistinct cytoplasm, interspersed immature skeletal muscle fibers reminiscent of fetal myotubes seen during the seventh to tenth weeks of intrauterine life,[76] and a richly myxoid matrix (Figs. 21–13, 21–14). The immature skeletal muscle cells have small uniform nuclei with delicate chromatin and inconspicuous nucleoli with bipolar or sometimes unipolar, finely tapered eosinophilic cytoplasmic processes. Cross-striations are rare and often difficult to discern; they are best seen with PTAH or Masson trichrome stains or with immunohistochemical stains for desmin, muscle-specific actin, or myoglobin. The cells may be arranged in short bundles or isolated within the myxoid ma-

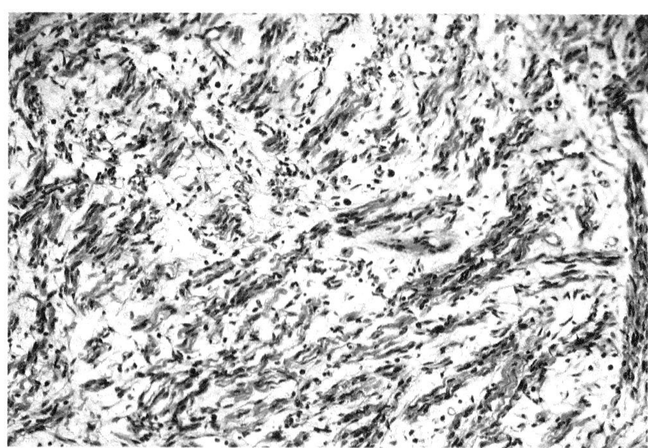

**FIGURE 21–13.** Fetal rhabdomyoma, myxoid type. The lesion is composed of an intimate mixture of primitive, round and spindle-shaped mesenchymal cells and differentiated myofibrils within a richly myxoid background.

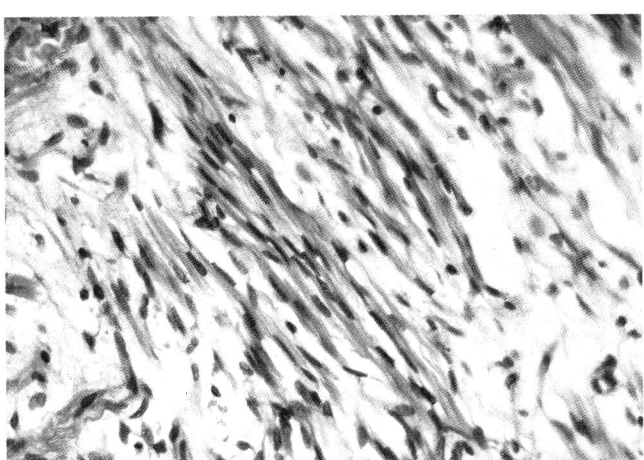

**FIGURE 21–14.** Fetal rhabdomyoma, myxoid type. Unlike embryonal rhabdomyosarcoma, the muscle cells vary little in size and shape, and there is no mitotic activity. The cells are deposited in an abundant myxoid matrix.

trix. Sometimes focal proliferation of abundant muscle fibers makes it difficult to draw a sharp line between tumor and normal muscle tissue (Fig. 21–15). The primitive undifferentiated cells have oval nuclei with slight nuclear hyperchromasia and scanty, indistinct cytoplasm.

The *intermediate type* is characterized by the presence of numerous differentiated muscle fibers, less conspicuous or absent spindle-shaped mesenchymal cells, and little or no myxoid stroma. In any given case, there may be a wide spectrum of skeletal muscle differentiation. The predominant cells are broad, strap-shaped muscle cells with abundant eosinophilic cytoplasm, centrally located vesicular nuclei, and frequent cross-striations reminiscent of the cells seen in adult rhabdomyomas; many of the cells contain glycogen and are often vacuolated (Figs. 21–16, 21–17). Others have prominent ganglion-like rhabdomyoblasts with large vesicular nuclei and prominent nucleoli. Kapadia et al. noted that mucosa-based lesions tend to have the widest spectrum of rhabdomyoblastic differentiation and the most mature-appearing cells.[83] In some cases there is mild cellular pleomorphism, but marked cellular atypia is not a feature of the disease, as it is with embryonal rhabdomyosarcoma. Transitional forms between the myxoid and intermediate types are not rare.[83,93] In fact, age and duration may play a role in the maturation of some tumors, as suggested by the older mean age of patients with the intermediate (cellular) type and the reported long duration of some cases. Mitotic figures are rare or absent. No mitotic figures were found in 19 of 24 fetal rhabdomyomas described by Kapadia et al.,[83] although in one case 14 mitoses were found per 50 high power fields.

In addition to the myxoid and intermediate types there are sporadic fetal rhabdomyoma-like tumors that are intimately associated with peripheral nerves reminiscent of neuromuscular choristoma (benign Triton tumor). We have seen two such cases in the head and neck region; others have reported similar lesions associated with the trigeminal nerve,[94] facial nerve,[91] or in association with the nevoid basal cell carcinoma syndrome.[81] By immunohistochemistry, the muscle cells stain positively for myoglobin, desmin, and muscle-specific actin, with only rare and focal staining for vimentin, S-100 protein, Leu-7, glial fibrillary acidic protein, and smooth muscle actin.[83,89]

Ultrastructurally, the differentiated muscle cells consist of organized bundles of thick (myosin) and thin (actin) myofilaments with the characteristic banding in some of the more differentiated muscle cells. Rod-like cytoplasmic inclusions or hypertrophied Z-band materials have been described but seem to be much less common than with adult rhabdomyoma.[74,86,92] The differentiated cells also contain considerable amounts of intracellular glycogen and a small number of mitochondria. The intervening small spindle cells are devoid of any specific cellular differentiation.

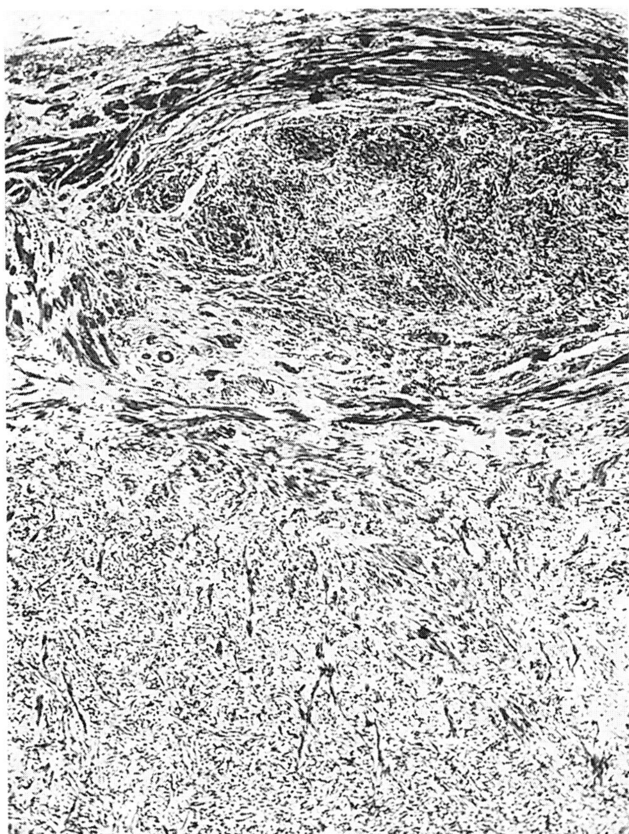

**FIGURE 21–15.** Fetal rhabdomyoma. The better differentiation of the muscle tissue at the periphery helps distinguish it from embryonal rhabdomyosarcoma. (Masson trichrome)

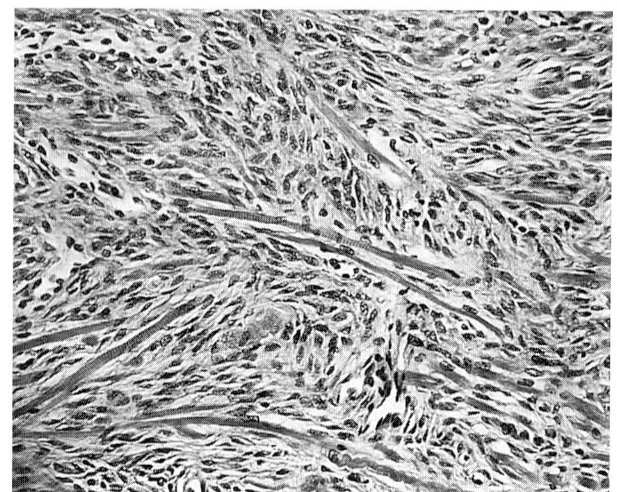

**FIGURE 21–16.** Fetal rhabdomyoma, intermediate (cellular) type. Prominent spindle cell pattern with interspersed differentiated eosinophilic myofibrils containing cross-striations.

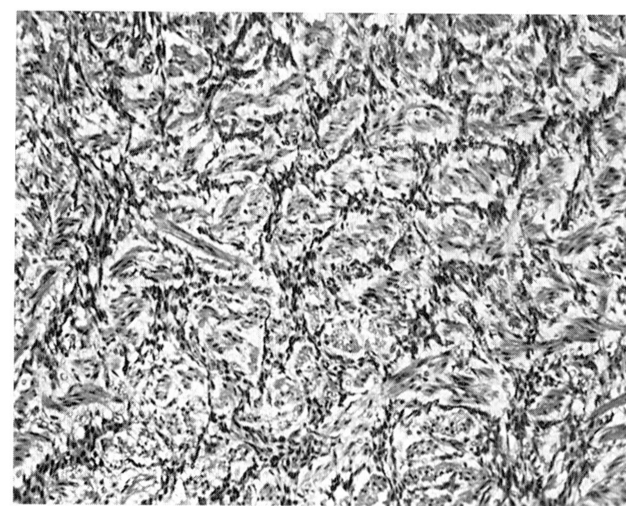

**FIGURE 21–17.** Fetal rhabdomyoma, intermediate (cellular) type consisting of intersecting bundles of differentiated myofibrils separated by strands of small undifferentiated spindle cells.

## Differential Diagnosis

Distinction from *embryonal* and *spindle cell rhabdomyosarcomas* is the principal problem with a diagnosis of fetal rhabdomyoma (Table 21–3); unlike rhabdomyosarcoma, fetal rhabdomyoma tends to be fairly well circumscribed and is superficially located. Mitotic figures are rare, and the tumor lacks a significant degree of cellular pleomorphism and areas of necrosis; considerable cellularity, a mild degree of cellular pleomorphism, and occasional mitotic figures do not rule out this diagnosis.[83]

Caution must also be exercised in the differential diagnosis because of the possible malignant transformation of fetal rhabdomyoma. We have encountered one case in which the initial lesion, biopsied at 3 weeks of age, seemed to be characteristic of fetal rhabdomyoma, whereas the recurrent tumor, excised at 23 months, showed a much greater degree of cellularity and mitotic activity and was indistinguishable from embryonal rhabdomyosarcoma. Another possible case of "cellular fetal rhabdomyoma with malignant transformation" was reported by Kodet et al.[85] in the tongue of an 18-month-old infant.

*Infantile (desmoid-type) fibromatosis* may bear a close resemblance to fetal rhabdomyoma, especially if the tumor diffusely infiltrates muscle tissue and contains numerous residual muscle fibers that have been entrapped by the proliferating fibroblasts. Fetal rhabdomyoma, however, is better circumscribed than fibromatoses, is situated in the subcutis rather than in muscle tissue, and lacks the fasciculated spindle cell pattern. In addition, interspersed fat cells, a frequent feature of diffuse infantile fibromatosis, are absent in fetal rhabdomyoma. The "neural variant of fetal rhabdomyoma"[81] may be difficult to distinguish from a neuromuscular choristoma (benign Triton tumor). However, the latter tends to be more lobular and has a more distinct mature skeletal muscle and Schwann cell population, with clear macroscopic attachment to a nerve.

**TABLE 21–3** DISTINGUISHING FEATURES OF FETAL RHABDOMYOMA AND EMBRYONAL RHABDOMYOSARCOMA

| Parameter | Fetal Rhabdomyoma | Embryonal Rhabdomyosarcoma |
|---|---|---|
| Gross appearance | Well circumscribed | Infiltrative |
| Depth | Superficial | Deep |
| Mitotic figures | Absent or rare | Easily identified |
| Pleomorphism | Absent or slight | Moderate or marked |
| Necrosis | Absent | Often present |

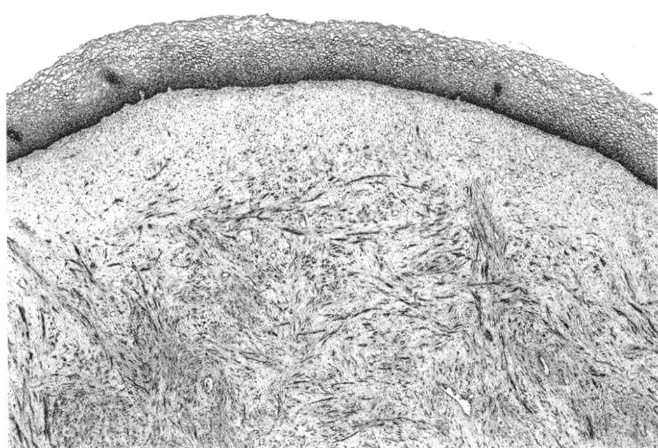

**FIGURE 21–18.** Genital (vaginal) rhabdomyoma. Submucosal proliferation of striated muscle cells separated by varying amounts of myxoid material and collagen.

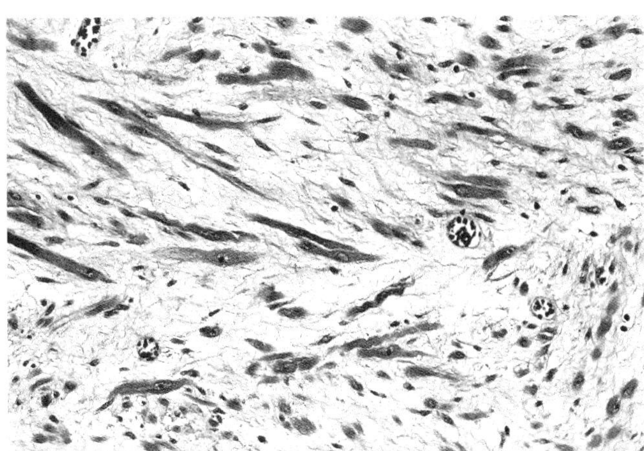

**FIGURE 21–19.** Genital rhabdomyoma composed of loosely arranged striated muscle cells and fibroblasts.

### Prognosis and Therapy

Fetal rhabdomyoma, a benign condition, is readily curable by local excision, with only rare reports of local recurrence.[83,86] It is a slowly growing process, and several lesions are known to have been present for years with little change in size or histologic picture except for interstitial fibrosis. The exact pathogenesis of fetal rhabdomyoma is still obscure; it may be a hamartomatous growth, as suggested by association of the lesion with the nevoid basal cell carcinoma syndrome, or it may be a true neoplasm. There is no valid support for the contention that fetal rhabdomyoma is an early stage in the development of adult rhabdomyoma.

## GENITAL RHABDOMYOMA

Although genital rhabdomyoma bears some resemblance to both adult and fetal rhabdomyomas, it is sufficiently different in its clinical and microscopic manifestations to qualify as a separate entity. So far only a small number of cases have been described,[95–107] including some that were reported as fetal rhabdomyoma.[77] Almost all arose as a slowly growing "polypoid" mass or "cyst" in the vagina or vulva of young or middle-aged women.[101,103] Rare cases have been described in the cervix,[107] labia majora,[97] prostate[104] and testicular tunica vaginalis.[106] Most are asymptomatic and are found on routine physical examination; some cause dyspareunia or vaginal bleeding secondary to mucosal erosion.

Microscopically, the excised tumor usually forms a polypoid or cauliflower-like mass covered by epithelium and rarely measuring more than 3 cm in greatest diameter. Under the microscope it is seen to consist of scattered, more or less mature muscle fibers showing distinct cross-striations and a matrix containing varying amounts of collagen and mucoid material (Figs. 21–18, 21–19, 21–20). As with other rhabdomyomas, the cells are immunoreactive with desmin, myoglobin, actin, and myosin antibodies.[103] Electron microscopic examination of the lesion reveals a large nucleus with a prominent dense nucleolus and arrays of thick and thin myofilaments with Z lines and A and I bands, together with intracytoplasmic bodies and basal lamina. There are also attachment plaques or peripheral couplings.[96,100]

The differential diagnosis includes benign *vaginal polyps* and *botryoid embryonal rhabdomyosarcoma (sarcoma botryoides)*. Benign vaginal polyps are characterized by atypical single or multinucleated stromal cells, but they lack classic strap cells with cross-striations. Botryoid embryonal rhabdomyosarcoma usually occurs in young children who present with a rapidly

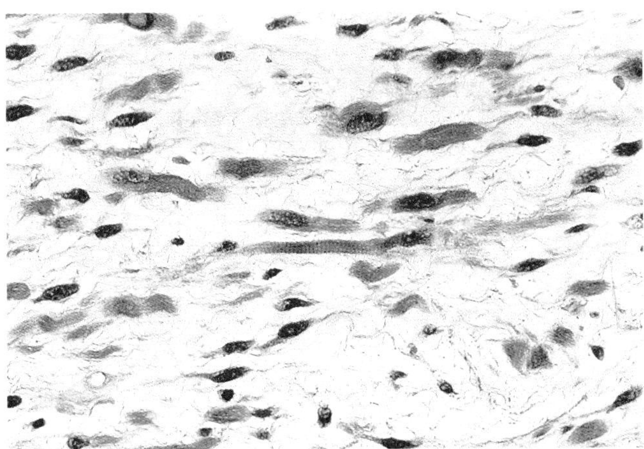

**FIGURE 21–20.** High-power view of genital rhabdomyoma showing rare striated muscle cells with cross-striations.

**TABLE 21–4 DISTINGUISHING FEATURES OF GENITAL RHABDOMYOMA AND BOTRYOID RHABDOMYOSARCOMA**

| Parameter | Genital Rhabdomyoma | Botryoid Rhabdomyosarcoma |
|---|---|---|
| Peak age | Young to middle-aged adults | Birth to 15 years |
| Gender (M/F) | Almost all females | 1:1 |
| Growth | Slowly growing | Rapidly growing |
| Epithelial ulceration | Absent | Often present |
| Cambium layer | Absent | Present |
| Mitotic figures | Absent or rare | Easily identified |
| Pleomorphism | Absent or slight | Moderate or marked |

growing lesion that frequently ulcerates the overlying epithelium. In contrast, genital rhabdomyoma usually occurs in middle-aged women and is generally a slowly growing tumor associated with an intact overlying epithelium. The subepithelial "cambium layer" characteristic of botryoid embryonal rhabdomyosarcoma is not found in genital rhabdomyomas. In addition, nuclear pleomorphism and mitotic figures are more prominent in rhabdomyosarcomas than in rhabdomyomas (Table 21–4).

The lesion, which pursues a benign course, is adequately treated by local excision. As with other types of rhabdomyoma, it is still undecided whether the lesion is a hamartomatous growth or a neoplasm.

## RHABDOMYOMATOUS MESENCHYMAL HAMARTOMA OF SKIN

Originally described in 1986 by Hendrick et al. as *striated muscle hamartoma*,[113] rhabdomyomatous mesenchymal hamartoma of skin, which occurs principally in the face and neck of newborns, is rare, with fewer than 15 cases reported in the literature.[108–118] The lesion typically presents as a small dome-shaped papule or a polypoid pedunculated lesion in newborns ranging in size from a few millimeters to 1–2 cm. The most common location appears to be the chin, followed by the periorbital, periauricular, and anterior mid-neck region. Cases have also been described on the upper lip[113] and nares.[111] Almost all lesions have arisen in males, with only rare cases having been described in females.[111,112] Most are solitary, but Sahn et al. described multiple pedunculated lesions arising in the periorbital and periauricular region in a newborn boy.[117] Some patients have associated congenital anomalies. One of the patients described by Hendrick et al. had a cleft lip and cleft gum as well as circumferential amniotic bands around the head and distal left leg.[113] Sahn et al. described one patient with bilateral diffuse sclerocorneas with probable retinal dysplasia.[117]

Grossly, most lesions are polypoid and attached to the skin by a long stalk, with circumferential constriction of the distal attachment site. Other lesions are more globular in shape, occasionally with central umbilication.[117] Histologically, the lesions are covered by normal-appearing squamous epithelium. More centrally, single or small groups of mature-appearing skeletal muscle fibers are found within the subcutaneous tissue and dermis. The fibers frequently are deposited in a collagenous stroma admixed with mature adipose tissue and adnexal structures, often aligned perpendicular to the surface epithelium. Blood vessels and nerves may also be found admixed among the mature skeletal muscle fibers. Rare cases show central calcification or ossification.[117]

The differential diagnosis includes *nevus lipomatosis superficialis*, which shows mature adipose tissue within the dermis but lacks skeletal muscle elements. Similarly, *fibrous hamartoma of infancy* contains an admixture of mature adipose tissue, collagenous bundles, and more cellular areas deposited in a myxoid stroma but lacks the skeletal muscle fibers. *Benign Triton tumor* (neuromuscular choristoma), a rare subcutaneous lesion found in association with peripheral nerves, is composed of mature skeletal muscle fibers and neural tissue. Finally, rhabdomyomatous mesenchymal hamartoma must be distinguished from the rare and much less differentiated *cutaneous embryonal rhabdomyosarcoma*.[109] This congenital hamartomatous lesion is adequately treated by local excision, and recurrences have not been described. The identification of these lesions in female patients suggests that this entity is not an X-linked disorder, as previously suggested.[116]

## MISCELLANEOUS LESIONS MIMICKING BENIGN STRIATED MUSCLE TUMORS

Various benign lesions of striated muscle may be confused with benign rhabdomyoma. Durm[119] described supernumerary muscles in the popliteal fossa and ankle region of young adults that presented as tumor-like masses and were identified as accessory hamstring and soleus muscles. Similar accessory muscles may occur in the hand, fingers, and other portions of the body. Some are bilateral. Likewise, unilateral or bilateral hypertrophy of the masseter muscle may be mistaken for a muscle tumor.[121] According to Waldhart and Lynch,[119] this condition occurs chiefly in young adults and is often accompanied by bony overgrowth or a spur at the angle of the mandible. Benign skeletal muscle differentiation has also been observed in the uterus and in a uterine leiomyoma.[120]

## REFERENCES


### Cardiac Rhabdomyoma

1. Bosi G, Lintermans JP, Pellegrino PA, et al. The natural history of cardiac rhabdomyoma with and without tuberous sclerosis. Acta Paediatr 85:928, 1996.
2. Burke AP, Virmani R. Cardiac rhabdomyoma: a clinicopathologic study. Mod Pathol 4:70, 1992.
3. Demkow M, Sorensen K, Whitehead BF, et al. Heart transplantation in an infant with rhabdomyoma. Pediatr Cardiol 16:204, 1995.
4. DiMario FJ Jr, Diana D, Leopold H, et al. Evolution of cardiac rhabdomyoma in tuberous sclerosis complex. Clin Pediatr 35: 615, 1996.
5. Enbergs A, Borggrefe M, Kurleman NG, et al. Ventricular tachycardia caused by cardiac rhabdomyoma in a young adult with tuberous sclerosis. Am Heart J 132:1263, 1996.
6. Grellner W, Henssge C. Multiple cardiac rhabdomyoma with exclusively histological manifestation. Forensic Sci Int 78:1, 1996.
7. Jozwiak S, Kawalec W, Dluzewska J, et al. Cardiac tumors in tuberous sclerosis: their incidence and course. Eur J Pediatr 153:155, 1994.
8. Lee ST, Hung CR, Wu MH, et al. Surgical treatment of infantile cardiac tumor: report of a case. J Formos Med Assoc 92: 288, 1993.
9. Luciani GB, Faggian G, Consolaro G, et al. Pulmonary valve origin of pedunculated rhabdomyoma causing moderate right ventricular outflow obstruction: surgical implications. Int J Cardiol 41:233, 1993.
10. Muhler EG, Kienast W, Turniski-Harder V, et al. Arrhythmias in infants and children with primary cardiac tumors. Eur Heart J 15:915, 1994.
11. Muhler EG, Turniski-Harder V, Engelhardt W, et al. Cardiac involvement in tuberous sclerosis. Br Heart J 72:584, 1994.
12. Nir A, Tajik AJ, Freeman WK, et al. Tuberous sclerosis and cardiac rhabdomyoma. Am J Cardiol 76:420, 1995.
13. Schenkman KA, O'Rourke PP, French JW. Cardiac rhabdomyoma with cardiac arrest. West J Med 162:460, 1995.
14. Silverman NA. Primary cardiac tumors. Ann Surg 191:127, 1980.
15. Stellingwerff GC, Hess J, Bogers AJ. Left ventricular rhabdomyoma: a case report. J Cardiovasc Surg 40:131, 1999.
16. Weeks DA, Chase DR, Malott RL, et al. HMB-45 staining in angiomyolipoma, cardiac rhabdomyoma, other mesenchymal processes, and tuberous sclerosis-associated brain lesions. Int J Surg Pathol 1:191, 1994.
17. Wu CT, Chen MR, Hou SH. Neonatal tuberous sclerosis with cardiac rhabdomyomas presenting as fetal supraventricular tachycardia. Jpn Heart J 38:133, 1997.
18. Yu GH, Kussmaul WG, DiSesa VJ, et al. Adult intracardiac rhabdomyoma resembling the extracardiac variant. Hum Pathol 24:448, 1993.

### Adult Rhabdomyoma

19. Abrikossoff A. Über: Myome, ausgehend von der quergestreiften willkurlichen Muskulatur. Virchows Arch [Pathol Anat] 260:215, 1926.
20. Adickes ED, Neumann T, Anderson RJ. Sternomastoid rhabdomyoma mimicking a thyroid nodule. Nebr Med J 81:359, 1996.
21. Agamanolis DP, Dau S, Krill CE. Tumors of skeletal muscle. Hum Pathol 17:778, 1986.
22. Andersen CB, Elling F. Adult rhabdomyoma of the oropharynx recurring three times within thirty-five years. Acta Pathol Microbiol Immunol Scand 94A:281, 1986.
23. Bastian BC, Bröcker EB. Adult rhabdomyoma of the lip. Am J Dermatopathol 20:61, 1998.
24. Bizakis J, Segas J, Tsardis M, et al. Pathologic quiz case one: adult rhabdomyoma of the parapharyngeal space. Arch Otolaryngol Head Neck Surg 119:350, 1993.
25. Blaauwgeers JL, Troost D, Dingemans KP, et al. Multifocal rhabdomyoma of the neck: report of a case studied by fine-needle aspiration, light and electron microscopy, histochemistry and immunohistochemistry. Am J Surg Pathol 13:791, 1989.
26. Bock D, Bock P. Rhabdomyoma of the soft palate: fine structural details of a highly differentiated muscle tumor. Histol Histopathol 2:285, 1987.
27. Box JC, Newman CL, Anastasiades KD, et al. Adult rhabdomyoma: presentation as a cervicomediastinal mass (case report and review of the literature). Am Surg 61:271, 1995.
28. Cleveland DB, Chen S-Y, Allen CM, et al. Adult rhabdomyoma: a light microscopic, ultrastructural, virologic, and immunologic analysis. Oral Surg Oral Med Oral Pathol 77:147, 1994.
29. Cornog JL Jr, Gonatas NK. Ultrastructure of rhabdomyoma. J Ultrastruct Res 20:433, 1967.

29a. Cronin CT, Keel SB, Grabbe J, et al. Adult rhabdomyoma of the extremity: A case report and review of the literature. Hum Pathol 31:1074, 2000.

30. Czernobilsky B, Cornog JL, Enterline HT. Rhabdomyoma: report of a case with ultrastructural and histochemical studies. Am J Clin Pathol 49:782, 1968.
31. Di Sant'Agnese PA, Knowles DM. Extracardiac rhabdomyoma: a clinicopathologic study and review of the literature. Cancer 46:780, 1980.
32. Enzinger FM. Adult rhabdomyoma: letter to the case. Pathol Res Pract 183:512, 1988.
33. Ferlito A, Frugoni P. Rhabdomyoma purum of the larynx. J Laryngol Otol 89:1131, 1975.
34. Fortson JK, Prunes FS, Lang AG. Adult multifocal extracardiac rhabdomyoma. J Natl Med Assoc 85:147, 1993.
35. Gardner DG, Corio RL. Multifocal adult rhabdomyoma. Oral Surg Oral Med Oral Pathol 56:76, 1983.
36. Gibas Z, Miettinen M. Recurrent parapharyngeal rhabdomyoma: evidence of neoplastic nature of the tumor from cytogenetic study. Am J Surg Pathol 16:721, 1992.
37. Goldfarb D, Lowry LD, Keane WM. Recurrent rhabdomyoma of the parapharyngeal space. Am J Otolaryngol 17:58, 1996.
38. Goldman L. Multicentric benign rhabdomyoma of skeletal muscle. Cancer 16:1609, 1963.
39. Golz R. Multifocal adult rhabdomyoma: case report and literature review. Pathol Res Pract 183:512, 1988.
40. Helliwell TR, Sissons MC, Stoney PJ, et al. Immunochemistry and electron microscopy of head and neck rhabdomyoma. J Clin Pathol 41:1058, 1988.
41. Helmberger RC, Stringer SP, Mancuso AA. Rhabdomyoma of the pharyngeal musculature extending into the prestyloid parapharyngeal space. Am J Neuroradiol 17:1115, 1996.

42. Johansen EC, Illum P. Rhabdomyoma of the larynx: a review of the literature with a summary of previously described cases of rhabdomyoma of the larynx and a report of a new case. J Laryngol Otol 109:147, 1995.
43. Kapadia SB, Enzinger FM, Heffner DK, et al. Crystal-storing histiocytosis associated with lymphoplasmacytic neoplasms: report of three cases mimicking adult rhabdomyoma. Am J Surg Pathol 17:461, 1993.
44. Kapadia SB, Meis JM, Frisman DM, et al. Adult rhabdomyoma of the head and neck: a clinicopathologic and immunophenotypic study. Hum Pathol 24:608, 1993.
45. Kay S, Gerszten E, Dennison S. Light and electron microscopic study of a rhabdomyoma arising in the floor of the mouth. Cancer 23:708, 1969.
46. Knowles DM, Jakobiec FA. Rhabdomyoma of the orbit. Am J Ophthalmol 80:1011, 1975.
47. Konrad EA, Meister P, Hubner G. Extracardiac rhabdomyoma: report of different types with light microscopic and ultrastructural studies. Cancer 49:898, 1982.
48. LaBagnara J, Hitchcock E, Spitzer T. Rhabdomyoma of the true vocal cord. J Voice 13:289, 1999.
49. Liapi-Avgeri G, Zachariades N, Karabela-Bouropoulou V. Adult-type of rhabdomyoma of the cheek: a case report with emphasis on the histological and immunohistochemical features. Arch Anat Cytol Pathol 42:321, 1994.
50. Miller R, Kurtz SM, Powers JM. Mediastinal rhabdomyoma. Cancer 42:1983, 1978.
51. Misch KA. Rhabdomyoma purum: a benign rhabdomyoma of tongue. J Pathol Bacteriol 75:105, 1958.
52. Moran JJ, Enterline HT. Benign rhabdomyoma of the pharynx: a case report, review of the literature, and comparison with cardiac rhabdomyoma. Am J Clin Pathol 42:174, 1964.
53. Neville BW, McConnel FMS. Multifocal adult rhabdomyoma: report of a case and review of the literature. Arch Otolaryngol 177:175, 1991.
54. Pai GK, Pai PK, Kamath SM. Adult rhabdomyoma of the esophagus. J Pediatr Surg 22:991, 1987.
55. Parsons HG, Puro HE. Rhabdomyoma of skeletal muscle: report of a case. Am J Surg 89:1187, 1955.
56. Roberts DN, Corbett MJ, Breen D, et al. Rhabdomyoma of the larynx: a rare cause of stridor. J Laryngol Otol 108:713, 1994.
57. Ross CF. Rhabdomyoma of sternomastoid. J Pathol Bacteriol 95:556, 1968.
58. Scrivner D, Meyer JS. Multifocal recurrent adult rhabdomyoma. Cancer 46:790, 1980.
59. Shemen L, Spiro R, Tuazon R. Multifocal adult rhabdomyomas of the head and neck. Head Neck 14:395, 1992.
60. Silverman JF, Kay S, Chang CH. Ultrastructural comparison between skeletal muscle and cardiac rhabdomyomas. Cancer 42:189, 1978.
61. Solomon MP, Tolete-Velcek F. Lingual rhabdomyoma (adult variant) in a child. J Pediatr Surg 14:91, 1979.
62. Tandler B, Rossi EP, Stein M, et al. Rhabdomyoma of the lip: light and electron microscopical observations. Arch Pathol 89: 118, 1970.
63. Tuazon R. Rhabdomyoma of the stomach. Am J Clin Pathol 52:37, 1969.
64. Walker WP, Laszewski MJ. Recurrent adult rhabdomyoma diagnosed by fine-needle aspiration cytology: report of a case and review of the literature. Diagn Cytopathol 6:354, 1990.
65. Warner TF, Goell W, Sundharades M, et al. Adult rhabdomyoma: ultrastructure and immunocytochemistry. Arch Pathol Lab Med 105:608, 1981.
66. Willis J, Abdul-Karim FW, di Sant'Agnese PA. Extracardiac rhabdomyomas. Semin Diagn Pathol 11:15, 1994.
67. Wood GS, Brammer R, Durham JC, et al. Adult rhabdomyoma of the larynx. Ear Nose Throat J 72:296, 1993.
68. Wyatt RB, Schochet SS Jr, McCormick WF. Rhabdomyoma: light and electron microscopic study of a case with intranuclear inclusions. Arch Otolaryngol 92:32, 1970.
69. Yu GH, Kussmaul WG, DiSesa VJ, et al. Adult intracardiac rhabdomyoma resembling the extracardiac variant. Hum Pathol 24:448, 1993.
70. Zachariades N, Skora C, Sourmelis A, et al. Recurrent twin adult rhabdomyoma of the cheek. J Oral Maxillofac Surg 52: 1324, 1994.
71. Zbaren P, Lang H, Becker M. Rare benign neoplasms of the larynx: rhabdomyomas and lipoma. J Otorhinolaryngol Relat Spec 57:351, 1995.

**Fetal Rhabdomyoma**

72. Bozic C. Fetal rhabdomyoma of the parotid gland in an infant: histological, immunohistochemical, and ultrastructural features. Pediatr Pathol 6:139, 1986.
73. Corio RL, Lewis DM. Intraoral rhabdomyomas. Oral Surg Oral Med Oral Pathol 48:525, 1979.
74. Crotty PL, Nakleh RE, Dehner LP. Juvenile rhabdomyoma: an intermediate form of skeletal muscle tumor in children. Arch Pathol Lab Med 117:43, 1993.
75. Dahl I, Angervall L, Save-Soderbergh J. Foetal rhabdomyoma. Acta Pathol Microbiol Scand 84:107, 1976.
76. Dehner LP, Enzinger FM, Font RL. Fetal rhabdomyoma: an analysis of nine cases. Cancer 30:160, 1972.
77. Di Sant'Agnese PA, Knowles DM. Extracardiac rhabdomyoma: a clinicopathologic study and review of the literature. Cancer 46:780, 1980.
78. Di Santo S, Abt AB, Boal DK, et al. Fetal rhabdomyoma and nevoid basal cell carcinoma syndrome. Pediatr Pathol 12:441, 1992.
79. Gardner DG, Corio RL. Fetal rhabdomyoma of the tongue, with a discussion of the two histologic variants of this tumor. Oral Surg Oral Med Oral Pathol 56:293, 1983.
80. Gordlin RJ. Nevoid basal-cell carcinoma syndrome. Dermatol Clin 13:113, 1995.
81. Hardisson D, Jimenez-Heffernan JA, Nistal M, et al. Neural variant of fetal rhabdomyoma and naevoid basal cell carcinoma syndrome. Histopathology 29:247, 1996.
82. Hatsukawa Y, Furukawa A, Kawamura H, et al. Rhabdomyoma of the orbit in a child. Am J Ophthalmol 123:142, 1997.
83. Kapadia SB, Meis JM, Frisman DM, et al. Fetal rhabdomyoma of the head and neck: a clinicopathologic and immunophenotypic study of 24 cases. Hum Pathol 24:754, 1993.
84. Klijanienko J, Caillaud JM, Micheau C, et al. Naevomatose basocellulaire associee a un rhabdomyome foetal multifocal: une observation. Presse Med 17:2247, 1988.
85. Kodet R, Fajstavr J, Kabelka Z, et al. Is fetal cellular rhabdomyoma an entity or a differentiated rhabdomyosarcoma? A study of patients with rhabdomyoma of the tongue and sarcoma of the tongue enrolled in the intergroup rhabdomyosarcoma studies I, II, and III. Cancer 67:2907, 1991.
86. Konrad EA, Meister P, Hübner G. Extracardiac rhabdomyoma: report of different types with light microscopic and ultrastructural studies. Cancer 49:898, 1982.
87. Lapner PC, Chou S, Jimenez C. Perianal fetal rhabdomyoma: case report. Pediatr Surg Int 12:544, 1997.
88. Schweisguth O, Gerard-Marchant R, Lemerle J. Naevomatose basocellulaire; association à un rhabdomyosarcoma congénital. Arch Fr Pediatr 25:1083, 1968.
89. Seidal T, Kindblom L-G, Angervall L. Myoglobin, desmin and vimentin in ultrastructually proven rhabdomyomas and rhabdomyosarcomas. Appl Pathol 5:201, 1987.
90. Simha M, Doctor V, Dalal S, et al. Postauricular fetal rhabdomyoma: light and electron microscopic study. Hum Pathol 13: 673, 1982.

91. Vandewalle G, Brucher JM, Michotte A. Intracranial facial nerve rhabdomyoma: case report. J Neurosurg 38:919, 1995.
92. Walter P, Guerbaoui M. Rhabdomyoma foetal: etude histologique et ultrastructurale d'une nouvelle observation. Virchows Arch [Pathol Anat] 371:59, 1976.
93. Whitten RO, Benjamin DR. Rhabdomyoma of the retroperitoneum: a report of a tumor with both adult and fetal characteristics: a study by light and electron microscopy, histochemistry, and immunochemistry. Cancer 59:818, 1987.
94. Zwick DL, Livingston K, Clapp L, et al. Intracranial trigeminal nerve rhabdomyoma/choristoma in a child: a case report and discussion of possible histogenesis. Hum Pathol 20:390, 1989.

### Genital Rhabdomyoma

95. Ceremsak RJ. Benign rhabdomyoma of the vagina. Am J Clin Pathol 52:604, 1969.
96. Chabrel CM, Beilby JOW. Vaginal rhabdomyoma. Histopathology 4:645, 1980.
97. De MN, Tribedi BP. Skeletal muscle tissue tumour. Br J Surg 28:17, 1940.
98. Gad A, Eusebi V. Rhabdomyoma of the vagina. J Pathol 115: 179, 1975.
99. Gee DC, Finckh ES. Benign vaginal rhabdomyoma. Pathology 9:263, 1977.
100. Gold JH, Bossen EH. Benign vaginal rhabdomyoma: a light and electron microscopic study. Cancer 37:2283, 1976.
101. Iversen UM. Two cases of benign vaginal rhabdomyoma: case reports. Acta Pathol Microbiol Immunol Scand 104:575, 1996.
102. Leone PG, Taylor HB. Ultrastructure of a benign polypoid rhabdomyoma of the vagina. Cancer 31:1414, 1973.
103. Lopez Varela C, Lopez de la Riva M, La Cruz Pelea C. Vaginal rhabdomyomas. Int J Gynaecol Obstet 47:169, 1994.
104. Morra MN, Manson AL, Gavrell GJ, et al. Rhabdomyoma of prostate. Urology 39:271, 1992.
105. Suarez Vilela D, Gimenez Pizarro A, Rio Suarez M. Vaginal rhabdomyoma and adenosis. Histopathology 16:393, 1990.
106. Tanda F, Cossu Rocca P, Bosincu L, et al. Rhabdomyoma of the tunica vaginalis of the testis: a histologic, immunohistochemical, and ultrastructural study. Mod Pathol 10:608, 1997.
107. Urbanke A. Reines Rhabdomyom der Gebärmutter. Zbl Allg Pathol 103:241, 1962.

### Rhabdomyomatous Mesenchymal Hamartoma of Skin

108. Ashfaq R, Timmons CF. Rhabdomyomatous mesenchymal hamartoma of skin. Pediatr Pathol 12:731, 1992.
109. Chang Y, Dehner LP, Egbert B. Primary cutaneous rhabdomyosarcoma. Am J Surg Pathol 14:977, 1990.
110. Elgart GW, Patterson JW. Congenital midline hamartoma: case report with histochemical and immunohistochemical findings. Pediatr Dermatol 7:199, 1990.
111. Farris PE, Manning S, Vuitch F. Rhabdomyomatous mesenchymal hamartoma. Am J Dermatopathol 16:73, 1994.
112. Hayes M, van der Westhuizen N. Congenital rhabdomyomatous mesenchymal hamartoma [letter]. Am J Dermatopathol 14:64, 1992.
113. Hendrick SJ, Sanchez RL, Blackwell SJ, et al. Striated muscle hamartoma: description of two cases. Pediatr Dermatol 3:153, 1986.
114. Katsumata M, Keong CH, Satoh T. Rhabdomyomatous mesenchymal hamartoma of skin. J Dermatol 17:384, 1990.
115. Mills AE. Rhabdomyomatous mesenchymal hamartoma of skin. Am J Dermatopathol 11:58, 1989.
116. Mills E. Congenital rhabdomyomatous mesenchymal hamartoma [letter]. Am J Dermatopathol 13:429, 1991.
117. Sahn EE, Garen PD, Pai GS, et al. Multiple rhabdomyomatous mesenchymal hamartomas of the skin. Am J Dermatopathol 12:485, 1990.
118. White G. Congenital rhabdomyomatous mesenchymal hamartoma [letter]. Am J Dermatopathol 12:539, 1990.

### Miscellaneous Lesions Mimicking Benign Striated Muscle Tumors

119. Durm AW. Anomalous muscle simulating soft tissue tumors on the lower extremities. J Bone Joint Surg Am 47:1397, 1965.
120. Martin-Reay DG, Christ ML, LaPata RE. Uterine leiomyoma with skeletal muscle differentiation: report of a case. Am J Clin Pathol 96:344, 1991.
121. Wade MW, Roy EW. Idiopathic masseter muscle hypertrophy. J Oral Surg 29:196, 1971.
122. Waldhart E, Lynch JB. Benign hypertrophy of the masseter muscles and mandibular angles. Arch Surg 102:115, 1971.

# CHAPTER 22

# RHABDOMYOSARCOMA

The concept of what constitutes rhabdomyosarcoma has been the subject of considerable change over the years. Sporadic tumors have been described since the early nineteenth century, but most were treated as curiosities or as striking examples of the close resemblance between sarcoma and developing normal tissue; and there were often lengthy debates as to their histogenesis.[173,177,242,310] In fact, in some of the earlier studies, Wilms' tumor and malignant mixed mesodermal tumors of the urogenital tract were included among the rhabdomyosarcomas.

Much later, during the 1930s and 1940s, the diagnosis of adult or pleomorphic rhabdomyosarcoma gained in popularity, and most of the rhabdomyosarcomas reported during this period were of this type.[96,206,275] These tumors occurred mainly in the muscles of the lower extremity and affected patients 50–70 years of age. They displayed a striking degree of cellular pleomorphism, but cells with cross-striations were absent in most instances. It was soon realized that most of these tumors were in fact other types of pleomorphic sarcoma. With the redefinition and acceptance of the fact that malignant fibrous histiocytoma was not a true histiocytic tumor but, rather, one with fibroblastic features, most lesions that had formerly been labeled "pleomorphic rhabdomyosarcoma" were placed in the broad group of malignant fibrous histiocytoma, such that the very existence of pleomorphic rhabdomyosarcoma was questioned.

It also became gradually evident that many childhood sarcomas formerly diagnosed merely as round or spindle cell sarcomas were rhabdomyosarcomas of the embryonal or alveolar type. Knowledge of these tumors was fostered by the introduction of newer, more effective modes of therapy. Before 1960, childhood rhabdomyosarcoma was known as an almost uniformly fatal neoplasm that recurred and metastasized in a high percentage of cases. During the last three decades, however, it has been shown that this tumor responds well to multidisciplinary therapy—encompassing biopsy or conservative surgery, multiagent chemotherapy, and radiotherapy—and that most children treated by these modalities remain free of recurrent and metastatic disease. The many reports of the Intergroup Rhabdomyosarcoma Studies have greatly contributed to our understanding of childhood rhabdomyosarcomas and especially the effect of the various treatment modalities on the survival of patients with this tumor.[44,45,93,175,176,199]

As with other sarcomas, there is little to suggest that rhabdomyosarcoma arises from differentiated cells (i.e., skeletal muscle). These tumors arise at sites in which striated muscle tissue is normally absent, as in the common bile duct and urinary bladder, or in areas in which striated muscle is scant, as in the nasal cavity, middle ear, and vagina.

Little is known about the underlying cause of the rhabdomyoblastic proliferations and the stimulus that induces such growth. Genetic factors are implicated by the rare occurrence of the disease in siblings,[125] the occasional presence of the tumor at birth, and the association of the disease with other neoplasms in the same patient. Rhabdomyosarcoma has been described in conjunction with a rhabdomyosarcomatous tumor of the kidney,[141] congenital retinoblastoma,[103,130,160] familial polyposis,[8] multiple lentigines syndrome,[113] and a variety of congenital anomalies.[246] One of our patients, a 41-year-old man with rhabdomyosarcoma of the lower leg, had suffered from familial muscular dystrophy of the scapulohumeral type and bilateral cataracts since the age of 18 years. Li and Fraumeni[161] found among 418 reported cases of rhabdomyosarcoma, five families in which a second child (three siblings and two cousins) had a soft tissue sarcoma and in which the parents, grandparents, and other relatives of these children had a high incidence of carcinoma. There appears to be an increased risk of a familial cancer syndrome when embryonal rhabdomyosarcoma (or other soft tissue sarcoma) is diagnosed during the first 2 years of life, especially in a male child.[24,38,235] Priest et al.[220] reported an association between the familial pleuropulmonary blastoma syndrome and embryonal rhabdomyosarcoma and synovial sarcoma in family members during childhood. Genetic factors, of course, are also implicated by the described cytogenetic anomalies, especially in alveolar rhabdomyosarcoma.[68] Savasan et al.[251] reported two children with alveolar rhabdomyosarcoma with constitutional balanced translocations, with peripheral blood lymphocytes harboring the same cytogenetic abnormality as that of the tumor cells.

## INCIDENCE

Rhabdomyosarcoma is not only the most common soft tissue sarcoma in children under 15 years of age but also one of the most common soft tissue sarcomas of adolescents and young adults. It is rare in persons older than 45 years. There were 234 rhabdomyosarcomas (19%) among 1215 sarcomas reviewed and staged by the Task Force of Soft Tissue Tumors,[245] and there were 379 rhabdomyosarcomas (19%) among 2000 malignant soft tissue tumors collected at the Mayo Clinic.[174] Enjoji and Hashimoto[74] reported 89 rhabdomyosarcomas (12%) among 752 malignant soft tissue tumors.

## HISTOLOGIC CLASSIFICATION

Arthur Purdy Stout was the first to delineate rhabdomyosarcoma as a distinct entity,[275] and Horn and Enterline devised the first classification scheme based on the clinical and pathologic features of these tumors.[123] From their review of earlier reports of embryonal,[274] alveolar,[237] and botryoid[124,190] rhabdomyosarcomas, as well as 39 cases of their own, this scheme, also known as the "conventional scheme," recognized embryonal, botryoid, alveolar, and pleomorphic subtypes. Most patients in that series died of rhabdomyosarcoma, and the authors were unable to identify any prognostic differences among the four histologic subtypes. This scheme was adopted by the World Health Organization (WHO) Classification of Soft Tissue Tumors in 1969[76] and served as the basis for the classification scheme of the Intergroup Rhabdomyosarcoma Study (IRS)[44,45,175,176] with minor modifications (Table 22–1). During subsequent decades the results from the IRS-I[175] and IRS-II[176] studies suggested that patients whose tumors had an alveolar architecture had a more aggressive clinical course than those whose tumors were of the embryonal subtype.[109]

During the IRS-I study, Palmer et al.[208,209] devised a classification scheme based on tumor cytology rather than tumor architecture. This scheme, known as the cytohistologic scheme, identified two major unfavorable histologic subtypes: the monomorphous round cell type and the anaplastic type. This was the only classification that was not based on the Horn and Enterline scheme but, rather, based solely on nuclear morphology.

**TABLE 22–1 MODIFIED CONVENTIONAL (HORN AND ENTERLINE) CLASSIFICATION USED BY INTERGROUP RHABDOMYOSARCOMA STUDIES I AND II**

Embryonal
Botryoid
Alveolar
Pleomorphic
Sarcoma, not classified
Small round-cell sarcoma, type indeterminate
Extraosseous Ewing's sarcoma

In 1989, the International Society for Pediatric Oncology (SIOP), including collaborators from 30 European countries, developed a classification scheme that emphasized the relation between clinical behavior and cellular differentiation in rhabdomyosarcoma subtypes with and without alveolar morphology (Table 22–2).[29] Based on a review of 513 rhabdomyosarcomas from the SIOP tumor registry, they found that an alveolar architecture was not independently prognostically significant. Loose botryoid and dense well differentiated rhabdomyosarcomas had a better prognosis than loose nonbotryoid and dense poorly differentiated and alveolar rhabdomyosarcomas. This group also delineated "embryonal sarcoma" as a spindle cell tumor composed of primitive mesenchymal cells with no evidence of myoblastic differentiation.

In 1992, collaborators at the Pediatric Branch at the National Cancer Institute (NCI) developed a modification of the conventional scheme based on their review of 159 rhabdomyosarcomas (Table 22–3).[288] This scheme recognized the favorable prognosis of conventional embryonal rhabdomyosarcomas and three subtypes (pleomorphic, leiomyomatous, and those with aggressive histologic features) and the unfavorable

**TABLE 22–2 INTERNATIONAL SOCIETY FOR PEDIATRIC ONCOLOGY CLASSIFICATION FOR RHABDOMYOSARCOMA**

Embryonal sarcoma
Embryonal rhabdomyosarcoma
- Loose
  - Botryoid
  - Nonbotryoid
- Dense
  - Well differentiated
  - Poorly differentiated

Alveolar rhabdomyosarcoma
Adult (pleomorphic) rhabdomyosarcoma
Other specified soft tissue tumors
Sarcoma, not otherwise specified

**TABLE 22-3 NATIONAL CANCER INSTITUTE CLASSIFICATION OF RHABDOMYOSARCOMA**

Embryonal rhabdomyosarcoma (favorable)
- Conventional
- Pleomorphic
- Leiomyomatous
- Aggressive histologic features

Alveolar rhabdomyosarcoma (unfavorable)
- Conventional
- Solid alveolar

Pleomorphic rhabdomyosarcoma

Rhabdomyosarcoma, "other"

prognosis of alveolar rhabdomyosarcomas. It also delineated the "solid alveolar rhabdomyosarcoma," composed of round tumor cells identical to those in conventional alveolar rhabdomyosarcomas but lacking the characteristic alveolar architecture. They found that tumors with any degree of alveolar architecture or cytology had an unfavorable prognosis, regardless of extent.

From 1987 to 1991 the IRS committee conducted a comparative study of the various rhabdomyosarcoma classification systems to determine the reproducibility and prognostic significance of each of these systems.[9] Eight hundred representative rhabdomyosarcomas were reviewed by 16 pathologists and classified using the conventional, SIOP, NCI, and cytohistologic classification systems; survival rates for all subtypes were studied. The highest degree of interobserver and intraobserver reproducibility was achieved using a modification of the conventional system, with fair to good observer agreement (Table 22–4). In addition, the histologic subtypes of the modified conventional system demonstrated a highly significant relation to survival. Based on the reproducibility and prognostic significance of this system, this group proposed a classification scheme, known as the International Classification of Rhabdomyosarcoma (ICR), which essentially was a modification of the conventional scheme with elements of the SIOP and NCI systems (Table 22–5).[198] The botryoid and spindle cell variants of embryonal rhabdomyosarcoma were found to have a superior prognosis, conventional embryonal rhabdomyosarcoma an intermediate prognosis, and alveolar rhabdomyosarcoma and undifferentiated sarcoma a poor prognosis. In addition, this classification scheme included those rhabdomyosarcoma subtypes in which the prognosis was yet to be determined (rhabdomyosarcoma with rhabdoid features). Similar to the NCI scheme, the ICR classified a tumor as the alveolar subtype if there was any degree of alveolar architecture or cytology. Pleomorphic rhabdomyosarcoma was excluded from the ICR given its extreme rarity in children.

**TABLE 22-4 INTEROBSERVER AND INTRAOBSERVER VARIATION IN THE DIAGNOSIS OF RHABDOMYOSARCOMA SUBTYPES**

| System | Interobserver Average Kappa *(K)* | Intraobserver Average Kappa *(K)* |
|---|---|---|
| Modified conventional | 0.451 | 0.605 |
| SIOP | 0.406 | 0.573 |
| NCI | 0.384 | 0.579 |
| Cytohistologic | 0.328 | 0.508 |
| ICR | 0.525 | 0.625 |

Modified from Asmar L, Gehan EM, Newton WA Jr, et al. Agreement among and within groups of pathologists in the classification of rhabdomyosarcoma and related childhood sarcomas: report of an international study of four pathology classifications. Cancer 74:2579, 1994.

SIOP, International Society for Pediatric Oncology; NCI, National Cancer Institute; ICR, International Classification of Rhabdomyosarcoma.

## AGE AND GENDER INCIDENCE

Despite the striking diversity in location, clinical presentation, and histologic picture, rhabdomyosarcoma has a fairly uniform age incidence; it occurs predominantly in infants and children and somewhat less frequently in adolescents and young adults. In the series of Ragab et al.,[222] 5% of 1561 patients with rhabdomyosarcomas were younger than 1 year of age. About 2% of tumors are present at birth.[164] As discussed below, each of the rhabdomyosarcoma subtypes occurs in a characteristic age group. For example, embryonal rhabdomyosarcomas and the botryoid and spindle cell subtypes affect mainly, but not exclusively, children between birth and 15 years of age. On the other hand, alveolar rhabdomyosarcoma tends to affect older patients, with a peak age of 10–25 years. The median age of 440 patients with embryonal rhabdomyosarcomas diagnosed at the Armed Forces Insti-

**TABLE 22-5 INTERNATIONAL CLASSIFICATION OF RHABDOMYOSARCOMA**

Superior prognosis
- Botryoid rhabdomyosarcoma
- Spindle cell rhabdomyosarcoma

Intermediate prognosis
- Embryonal rhabdomyosarcoma

Poor prognosis
- Alveolar rhabdomyosarcoma
- Undifferentiated sarcoma

Subtypes whose prognosis is not presently evaluable
- Rhabdomyosarcoma with rhabdoid features

tute of Pathology (AFIP) during a 10-year period was 8 years; the median age of 118 patients with alveolar rhabdomyosarcomas seen during the same period was 16 years (Fig. 22–1).

Rhabdomyosarcomas are rare in patients older than 40 years.[122,182,188,265] Most rhabdomyosarcomas in adults are of the pleomorphic subtype, with a reported median age range of 50–56 years,[92,122,162] although sporadic rhabdomyosarcoma subtypes that typically arise in children may also be found in adults.[98,163,196] There is also some correlation between tumor location and age; for example, rhabdomyosarcomas of the urinary bladder, prostate, vagina, and middle ear tend to occur at a younger age (median 4 years) than those in the paratesticular region (median 14 years) or the extremities (median 14 years).

Males are affected more commonly than females by a ratio of approximately 1.3:1.0, but the male preponderance is less pronounced during adolescence and young adulthood and for rhabdomyosarcomas of the alveolar type. African Americans are less commonly involved than Caucasians, but this may be a sampling error and further data in this regard are needed.[309]

## CLINICAL FEATURES

Although rhabdomyosarcomas may arise anywhere in the body, they occur predominantly in three regions: the head and neck, genitourinary tract and retroperitoneum, and upper and lower extremities. Each rhabdomyosarcoma histologic subtype may occur in virtually any location, but each subtype has a site predilection. Table 22–6 shows the anatomic distribution of rhabdomyosarcomas reviewed and diagnosed at the AFIP during a 10-year period. Table 22–7

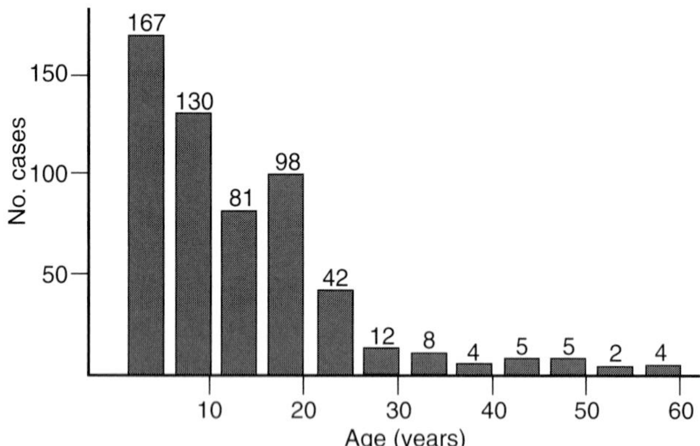


**FIGURE 22–1.** Age distribution of 558 rhabdomyosarcomas reviewed at the Armed Forces Institute of Pathology (AFIP) during a 10-year period. More than half of the cases occurred during the first 10 years of life, and most of these tumors were of the embryonal type. The second peak lies at 15–20 years of age, a result of the preponderance of alveolar rhabdomyosarcomas in this age group.

**TABLE 22–6** ANATOMIC DISTRIBUTION OF RHABDOMYOSARCOMA: AFIP, 558 CASES)

| Anatomic Location | No. | % |
|---|---|---|
| Head and neck | 246 | 44.0 |
| Orbit, eyelid, skull | 109 | 19.5 |
| Nasal cavity, nasopharynx, palate, mouth, pharynx | 73 | 13.1 |
| Sinuses, cheek, neck | 47 | 8.4 |
| Ear, mastoid | 17 | 3.1 |
| Trunk | 231 | 41.4 |
| Paratesticular region | 114 | 20.4 |
| Retroperitoneum, pelvis | 46 | 8.2 |
| Chest wall, back, flank, abdominal wall | 41 | 7.3 |
| Urinary bladder, prostate | 25 | 4.5 |
| Vagina, vulva | 5 | 0.9 |
| Extremities | 81 | 14.6 |
| Upper extremity | 41 | 7.4 |
| Lower extremity | 40 | 7.2 |
| *Total* | 558 | 100.0 |

AFIP, Armed Forces Institute of Pathology.

shows the anatomic distribution of these tumors from the IRS-I, IRS-II, and IRS-III studies between 1972 and 1991.[45,175,176]

The head and neck is the principal location of rhabdomyosarcoma; 246 (44%) of 558 AFIP tumors occurred in this general region. Similarly, 970 (35%) of 2747 tumors from the IRS-I, IRS-II, and IRS-III studies occurred in this location. In the head and neck, parameningeal tumors are the most common, accounting for 16% of all tumors in the IRS studies. Parameningeal rhabdomyosarcomas are distinguished from the other rhabdomyosarcomas arising in the head and neck because of their potential intracranial extension and seeding—hence their less favorable clinical course.[19,175,176,199,211,230]

**TABLE 22–7** ANATOMIC DISTRIBUTION OF RHABDOMYOSARCOMA FROM INTERGROUP RHABDOMYOSARCOMA GROUP STUDIES (IRS-I, IRS-II, IRS-III), 1972–1991

| Anatomic Location | No. | % |
|---|---|---|
| Head and neck | 970 | 35 |
| Parameningeal | 437 | 16 |
| Miscellaneous sites | 276 | 10 |
| Orbit | 257 | 9 |
| Genitourinary | 650 | 24 |
| Extremities | 511 | 19 |
| Other sites | 616 | 22 |
| *Total* | 2747 | 100 |

Modified from Pappo AS, Shapiro DN, Crist WM, et al. Biology and therapy of pediatric rhabdomyosarcoma. J Clin Oncol 13:2123, 1995.

The orbit is the second most common site of rhabdomyosarcoma in the head and neck, accounting for 9% of cases from the IRS series. As a rule, the neoplasm manifests as a rapidly enlarging, painless mass in the upper, inner quadrant of the orbit and causes protrusion and displacement of the globe usually in a downward or temporal direction, blurred vision, and diplopia; in general, there is little change in visual acuity. Extension into the eyelids, a common occurrence, is associated with marked edema of the lid and conjunctivae, ptosis, and sometimes conjunctival ulceration. The expanding orbital tumor may also erode into the paranasal sinuses and the base of the skull, where it may spread along the meningeal membranes. Most rhabdomyosarcomas in this location are of the embryonal subtype.[100,120,144,300] For example, 221 (90%) of 245 orbital tumors from the IRS-I through IRS-IV studies were of the embryonal subtype, although rare botryoid-type embryonal rhabdomyosarcomas and alveolar rhabdomyosarcomas also arise in the orbit.[144]

Rhabdomyosarcoma may also involve a variety of other sites in the head and neck, including the nasal cavity and nasopharynx,[90] followed in frequency by the ear and ear canal, paranasal sinuses, soft tissues of the face and neck, and the oral cavity including the tongue, lip, and palate.[30,34,62,65,216,278] As a rule, the tumors in this general region grow rapidly, often in an infiltrative and destructive manner, particularly if the initial treatment is inadequate or delayed. Many invade bone, and computed tomography (CT) or magnetic resonance imaging (MRI) is indicated to obtain a clear picture of the size and spatial relations of the tumor and the extent of bone destruction.[158,308] Tumors of the nasal cavity and nasopharyngeal region may be confused clinically with enlarged adenoids, nasopharyngeal angiofibroma, or a protracted infection that has failed to respond to conventional therapy. Patients may present with an enlarging growth that causes increasing difficulty breathing or swallowing, hoarseness, or alteration of voice. It may fill the nasal cavity and protrude from one or both nostrils as a gelatinous or hemorrhagic polypoid mass. Tumors of the middle ear, ear canal, and mastoid are often misdiagnosed initially as otitis media. Patients with tumors in this location present with a history of hearing loss, otalgia, and hemorrhagic or purulent discharge from the ear canal. Physical examination usually reveals a gray to purple, fleshy, friable polypoid mass in the ear canal that has penetrated the tympanum and infiltrated the surrounding soft tissue, causing diffuse swelling in the periauricular region. Radiologic examination may demonstrate destruction of the petrous portion of the temporal bone, bony labyrinth, osseous wall of the auditory canal, and portions of the sphenoid bone.[299]

After the head and neck, the genitourinary tract is the second most common site for rhabdomyosarcoma. In the IRS series, 650 (24%) of 2747 cases arose in this general region. Histologically, most tumors here are of the embryonal subtype. For example, 71% of patients in the IRS-I and IRS-II studies with tumors in the genitourinary tract were of this subtype, and 20% were of the botryoid subtype; there were only rare alveolar rhabdomyosarcomas.[199] The tumors in this region most commonly arise in a paratesticular location and occur predominantly in adolescents. The spindle cell subtype of embryonal rhabdomyosarcoma has a propensity to arise in the paratesticular region.[32,159] Generally, tumors at this site manifest as unilateral, firm, painless masses that have been present for a few weeks or months and are usually located at the upper pole of the testis. They may also involve the spermatic cord and epididymis but usually are separate from the testis proper. There is a high incidence of retroperitoneal or paraaortic lymph node involvement.[228] Clinically, the condition must be distinguished from hernia, hydrocele, spermatocele, and adenomatoid tumor.

The retroperitoneum and pelvis are not uncommon sites of involvement. Approximately 45% of tumors in these sites are of the embryonal subtype, although up to 15% are alveolar rhabdomyosarcomas.[199] In general, effective therapy of rhabdomyosarcomas in the retroperitoneum and pelvic region is more difficult than that of paratesticular rhabdomyosarcomas.[82,106,126]

Approximately 5% of rhabdomyosarcomas arise in the urinary bladder or prostate. In fact, rhabdomyosarcoma is the most common bladder tumor in children under 10 years of age, and it is also the most common rhabdomyosarcoma during infancy. Almost all tumors arising in this location are embryonal or botryoid rhabdomyosarcomas.[132,283] For example, of 109 tumors arising in the urinary bladder or prostate in the IRS-I and IRS-II studies, 69 (63%) were embryonal and 32 (29%) had botryoid features.[227] Most bladder tumors originate in the submucosa of the posterior wall, with a particular preference for the bladder neck and trigone. Those with a botryoid histology typically grow into the lumen of the urinary bladder as a grape-like, richly mucoid, multinodular or polypoid mass with a broad base that not infrequently causes obstruction of the internal urethral orifice and prostatic urethra. This in turn results in incontinence and difficulty with urination, and when the mucosa becomes necrotic or ulcerated there is gross hematuria. Retention of urine ultimately leads to hydroureter and hydronephrosis. The tumor may also spread diffusely along the submucosa or may penetrate the bladder wall and invade the perivesical region, displacing the rectum and sigmoid colon. Excretory cystograms usually reveal a vesical filling defect. Prostatic tumors may cause bilateral ureteral obstruction and renal failure.

Rarely, rhabdomyosarcomas arise in other genitourinary sites, including the fallopian tube,[28] uterus,[102,226,268] cervix,[11,51,310] vagina,[1,42,160] labium and vulva,[42,226,279] and the perineum and perianal region.[224,272] Tumors in these locations are often of the botryoid subtype, but embryonal and alveolar rhabdomyosarcoma have also been reported.

Unlike adult soft tissue sarcomas, rhabdomyosarcomas involve the extremities much less commonly. As shown in Table 22–6, only 14.6% of cases from the AFIP series occurred in this location, with a similar incidence in the upper and lower extremities. A similar percentage (19%) of extremity tumors have been reported in the IRS series.[211] In the material from the AFIP, the forearms, hands, and feet were more often involved than other portions of the extremities; alveolar rhabdomyosarcomas outnumbered embryonal rhabdomyosarcomas by a ratio of 4:3, similar to that found in the IRS-I and IRS-II studies.[199] Although rare, most pleomorphic rhabdomyosarcomas arise in the deep soft tissues of the extremities of adults.

Most of the neoplasms in the limbs present as enlarging masses that usually are deep-seated and intimately associated with striated muscle tissue. As a rule, they are neither painless nor tender despite evidence of rapid growth during the preoperative period. Large lesions may cause pain or other neurologic disturbances as a result of pressure exerted by the tumor on peripheral nerves. Erosion of bone is rare and is associated mainly with rhabdomyosarcomas of the hands and feet. Radiographs show no specific features that would permit a reliable diagnosis as to the type of tumor.

Unusual rhabdomyosarcomas arise outside the head and neck, the genitourinary tract and retroperitoneum, and extremities. Tumors originating in the hepatobiliary tract have been described and usually arise from the submucosa of the common bile duct.[128,169,195,240,247] Some extend into the porta hepatis or the ampulla of Vater. Most are rhabdomyosarcomas of the botryoid type, with typical myxoid grapelike gross and microscopic appearances. Rare rhabdomyosarcomas of virtually all subtypes have also been described in the anterior mediastinum,[277] lung,[221] bone,[167,202] and skin.[41,253,305]

## GROSS FINDINGS

Macroscopically, there is little that is characteristic of this tumor; as with other rapidly growing sarcomas, the gross appearance reflects the degree of cellularity, the relative amounts of collagenous or myxoid stroma, and the presence and extent of secondary changes such as hemorrhage, necrosis, and ulceration. In general, tumors growing into body cavities, such as those in the nasopharynx and urinary bladder, are fairly well circumscribed, multinodular, or distinctly polypoid with a glistening, gelatinous, gray-white surface that on cross section often shows patchy areas of hemorrhage or cyst formation. Deep-seated tumors involving or arising in the musculature, like most rhabdomyosarcomas in the extremities, are usually less well defined and nearly always infiltrate the surrounding tissues. They are more firm and rubbery and have a mottled gray-white to pink-tan, smooth or finely granular, often bulging surface. They rarely become large, averaging 3–4 cm in greatest diameter. There are often areas of focal necrosis and cystic degeneration.

## RHABDOMYOSARCOMA SUBTYPES

### Embryonal Rhabdomyosarcoma

The embryonal subtype of rhabdomyosarcoma (without other distinguishing features) accounts for approximately 49% of all rhabdomyosarcomas.[198] It mostly affects children younger than 10 years of age, but it also occurs in adolescents and young adults; it is rare in patients older than 40 years of age. The mean age of patients with this subtype of rhabdomyosarcoma enrolled in the IRS-I and IRS-II studies was 7.2 years.[199] Overall, the most common site of embryonal rhabdomyosarcoma is the head and neck, particularly the orbit and parameninges (Table 22–8). After the head and neck, this tumor is most commonly found in the genitourinary tract, followed by the deep soft tissues of the extremities and the pelvis and retroperitoneum.

Histologically, embryonal rhabdomyosarcoma bears a close resemblance to various stages in the embryogenesis of normal skeletal muscle, but its pattern is much more variable, ranging from poorly differentiated tumors that are difficult to diagnose without immunohistochemical or electron microscopic examination to well differentiated neoplasms that resemble fetal muscle. Features common to most are (1) varying degrees of cellularity with alternating densely packed, hypercellular areas and loosely textured myxoid areas (Figs. 22–2 to 22–5); (2) a mixture of poorly oriented, small, undifferentiated, hyperchromatic round or spindle-shaped cells (Fig. 22–6) and a varying number of differentiated cells with eosinophilic cytoplasm characteristic of rhabdomyoblasts; and (3) a matrix containing little collagen and varying amounts of myxoid material. Cross-striations are discernible in 50–60% of cases. Schmidt et al.[254] distinguished primitive (<10% rhabdomyoblasts), intermediate (10–50% rhabdomyoblasts), and well

**TABLE 22–8** DISTRIBUTION OF ANATOMIC SITES OF RHABDOMYOSARCOMA SUBTYPES FOR 1626 IRS-I AND IRS-II PATIENTS

| Site | Embryonal | Alveolar | Botryoid | Pleomorphic | Other | Total No. |
|---|---|---|---|---|---|---|
| Head and neck | 411 (71%) | 76 (13%) | 13 (2%) | — | 77 (13%) | 577 |
| Genitourinary | 246 (71%) | 8 (2%) | 70 (20%) | 1 (<1%) | 23 (7%) | 348 |
| Extremities | 76 (24%) | 156 (50%) | — | 5 (2%) | 74 (24%) | 311 |
| Trunk | 27 (19%) | 43 (30%) | — | 3 (2%) | 71 (49%) | 144 |
| Pelvis | 45 (48%) | 19 (20%) | — | — | 29 (31%) | 93 |
| Retroperitoneum | 44 (59%) | 14 (19%) | — | 1 (1%) | 16 (21%) | 75 |
| Perineum/anus | 13 (33%) | 19 (48%) | 1 (2%) | 1 (2%) | 6 (15%) | 40 |
| Other sites | 15 (39%) | 9 (24%) | 4 (11%) | — | 10 (26%) | 38 |

Modified from Newton WA Jr, Soule EH, Hamoudi AB, et al. Histopathology of childhood sarcomas, Intergroup Rhabdomyosarcoma Studies I and II: clinicopathologic correlation. J Clin Oncol 6:67, 1988.

differentiated (>50% rhabdomyoblasts) forms of embryonal rhabdomyosarcoma.

The least well differentiated examples of this tumor correspond in appearance to developing muscle at 5–8 weeks' gestation. They consist for the most part of small, round or spindle-shaped cells with darkly staining hyperchromatic nuclei and indistinct cytoplasm. The nuclei vary slightly in size and shape (more so than those of the solid form of alveolar rhabdomyosarcoma), have one or two small nucleoli, and usually exhibit a high rate of mitotic activity. Differentiated rhabdomyoblasts are either absent entirely or are confined to a few small areas, making it mandatory to examine multiple sections from different portions of the tumor; they also require adjunctive diagnostic procedures to confirm the diagnosis in most cases.

Better differentiated examples of the round cell and spindle cell types have, in addition to the primitive or undifferentiated cellular areas, larger round or oval eosinophilic cells characteristic of rhabdomyoblasts (Figs. 22–7 to 22–10); the cytoplasm of these cells contains granular material or deeply eosinophilic masses of stringy or fibrillary material concentrically

*Text continued on page 797*

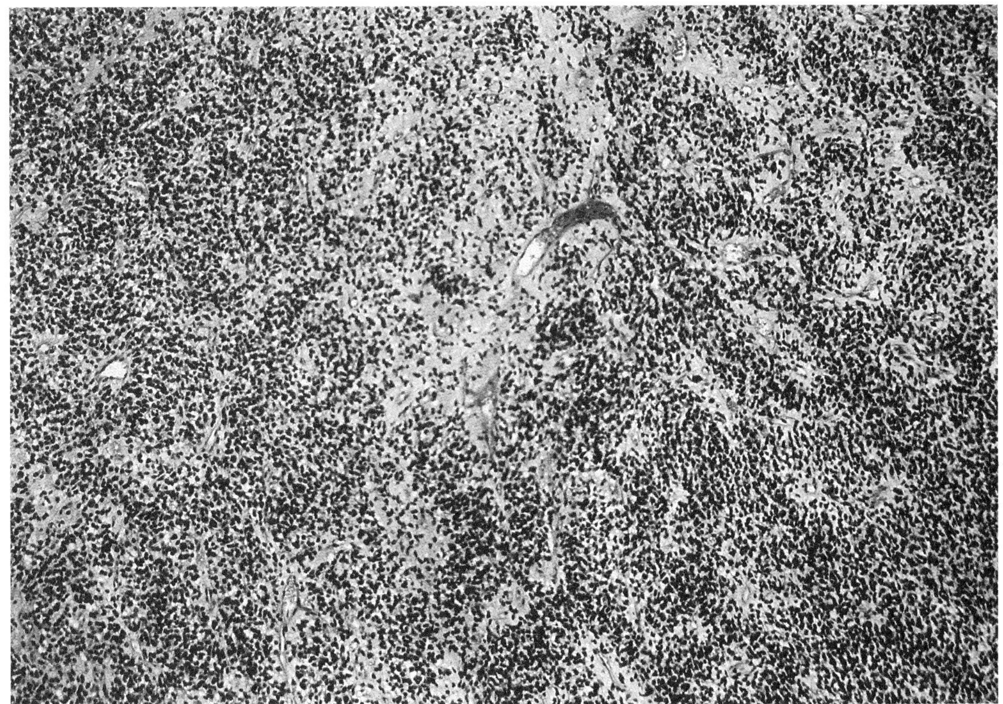

**FIGURE 22–2.** Low-power view of embryonal rhabdomyosarcoma with alternating cellular and myxoid areas, a characteristic feature of this tumor.

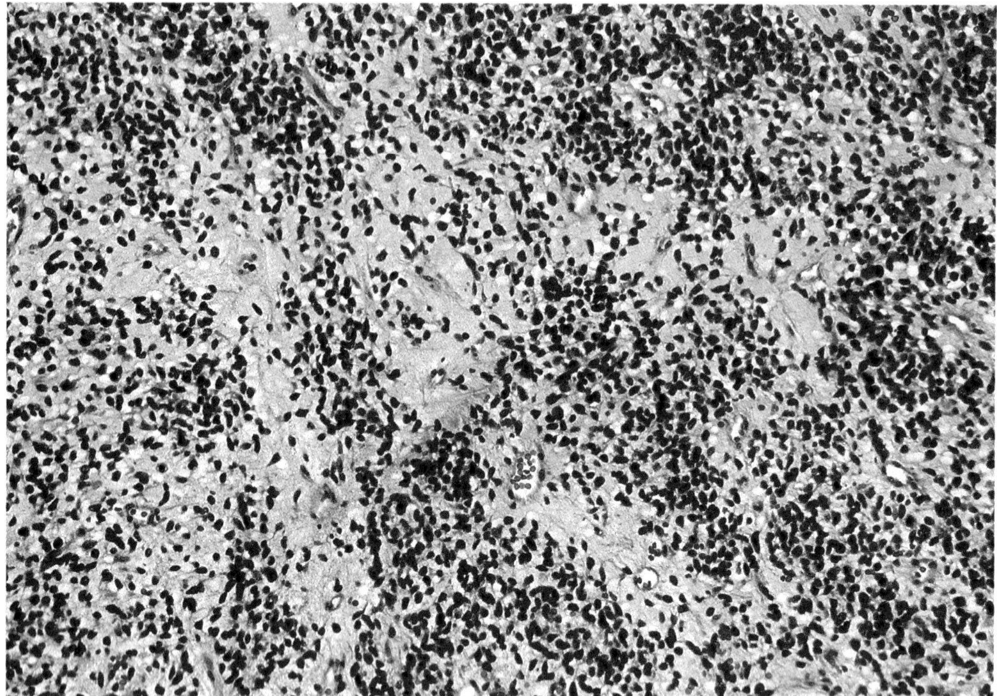

**FIGURE 22–3.** Alternating cellular and myxoid zones in an embryonal rhabdomyosarcoma.

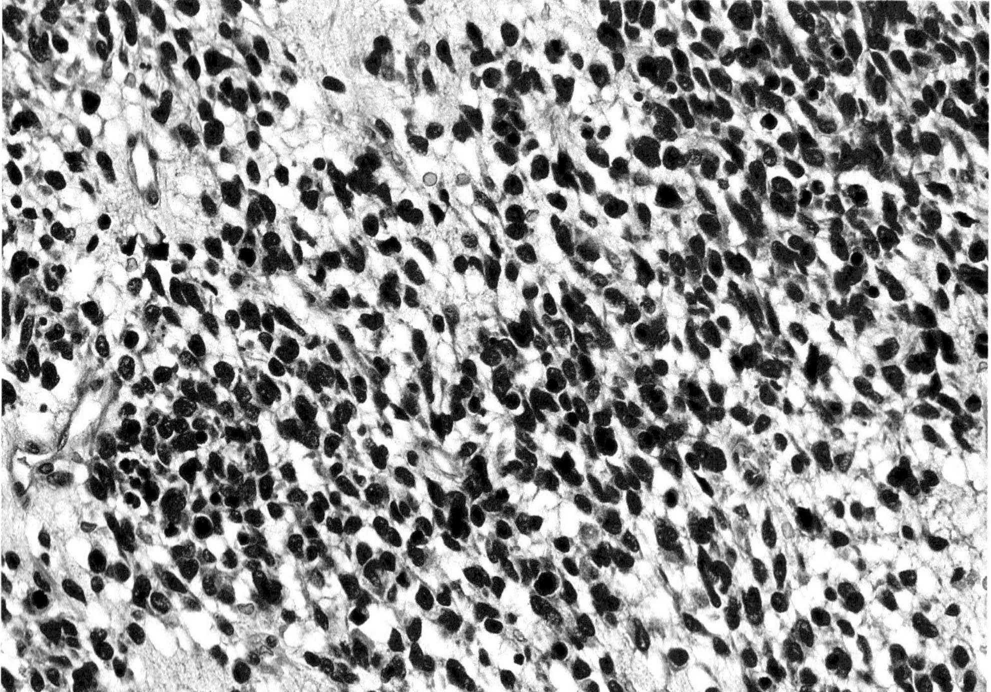

**FIGURE 22–4.** High-power view of an embryonal rhabdomyosarcoma composed predominantly of primitive ovoid cells.

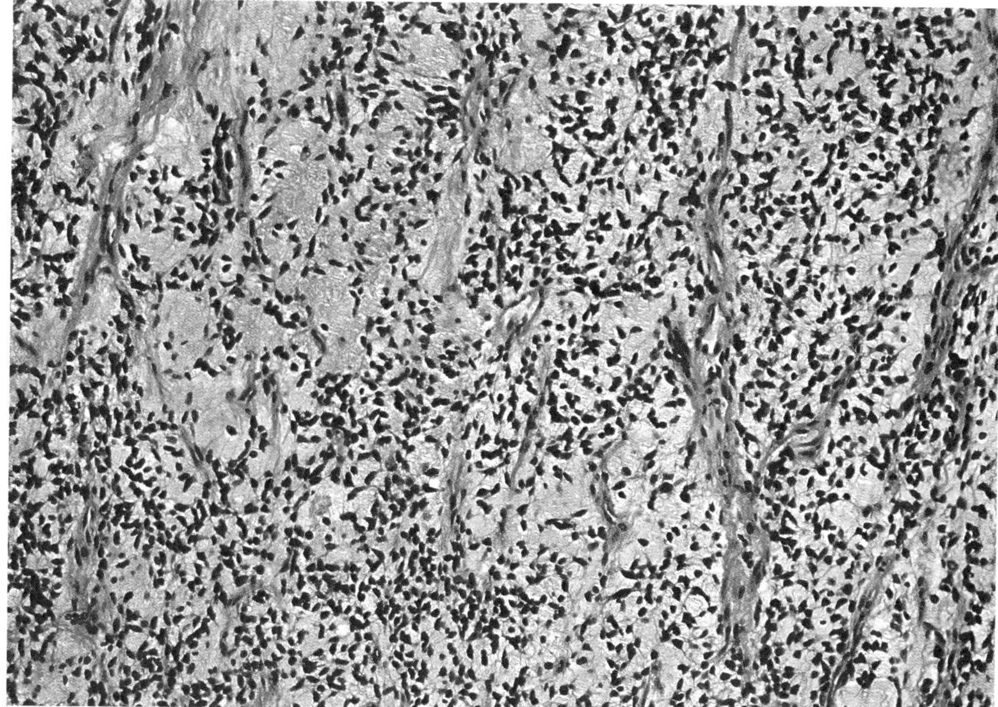

**FIGURE 22–5.** Primitive spindle-shaped cells deposited in an abundant myxoid stroma in an embryonal rhabdomyosarcoma.

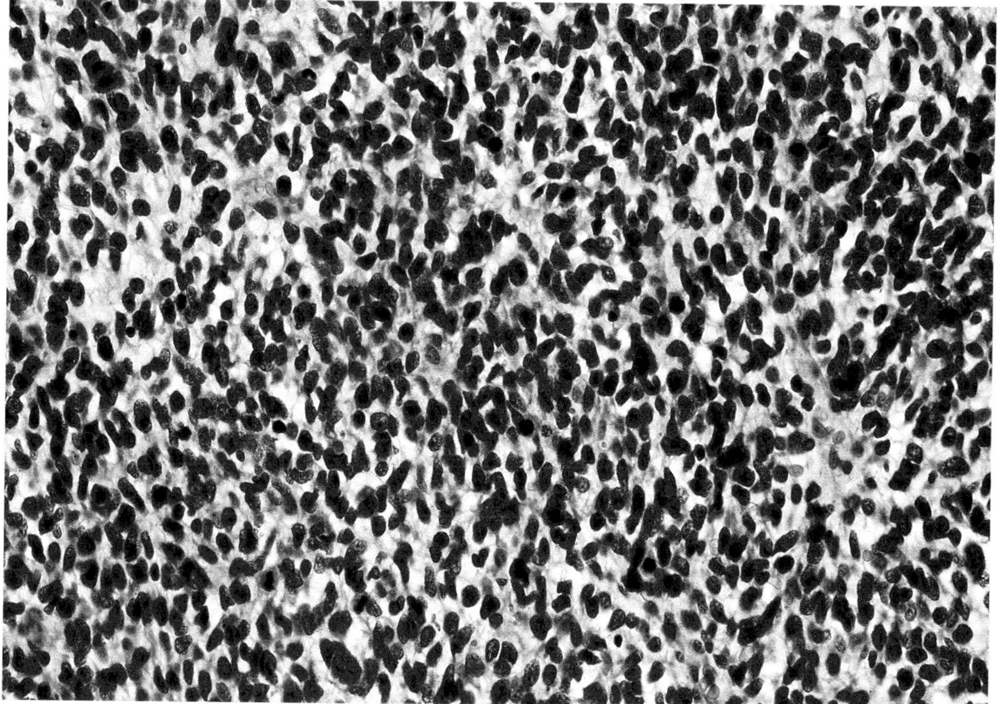

**FIGURE 22–6.** Embryonal rhabdomyosarcoma composed almost exclusively of primitive cells devoid of rhabdomyoblastic differentiation.

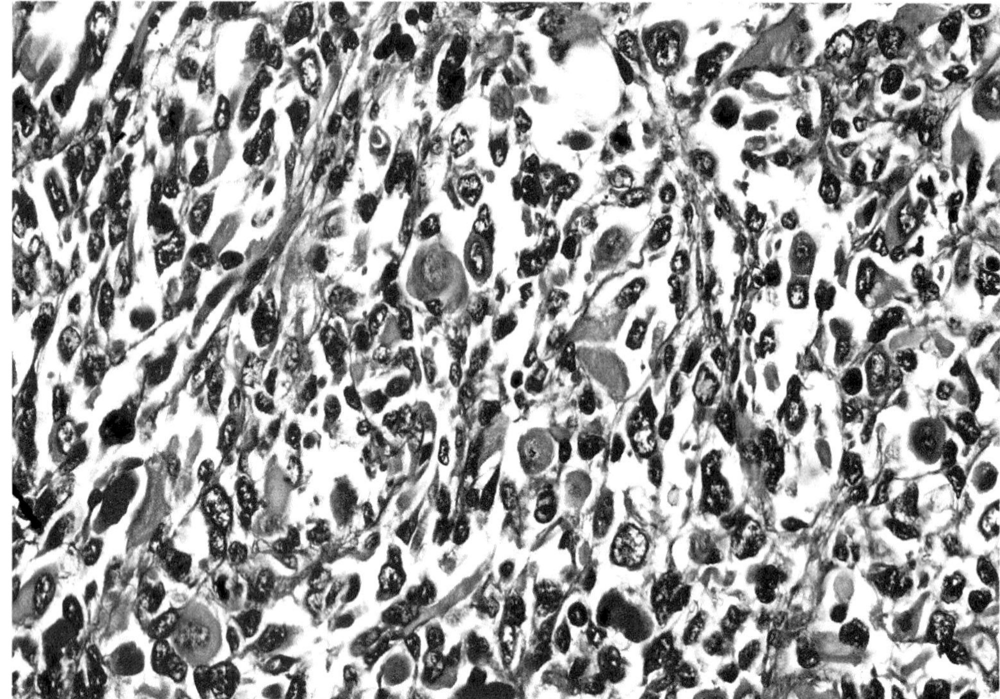

**FIGURE 22–7.** Embryonal rhabdomyosarcoma. Note the scattered cells with eosinophilic cytoplasm.

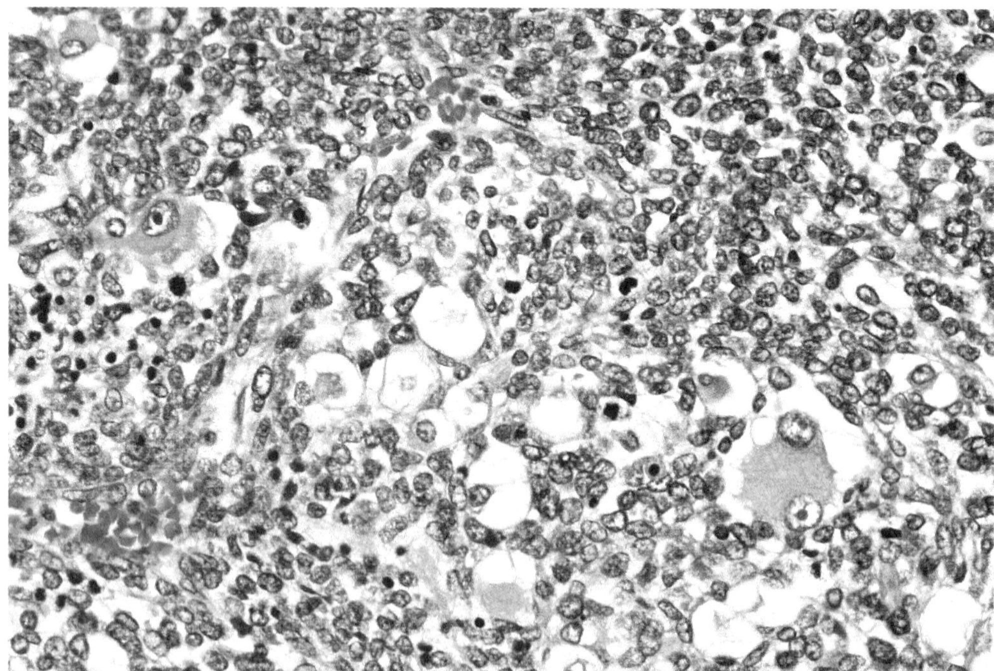

**FIGURE 22–8.** Embryonal rhabdomyosarcoma composed predominantly of primitive ovoid cells with scattered rhabdomyoblasts. The rhabdomyoblasts in this case have eccentric vesicular nuclei and abundant densely eosinophilic cytoplasm.

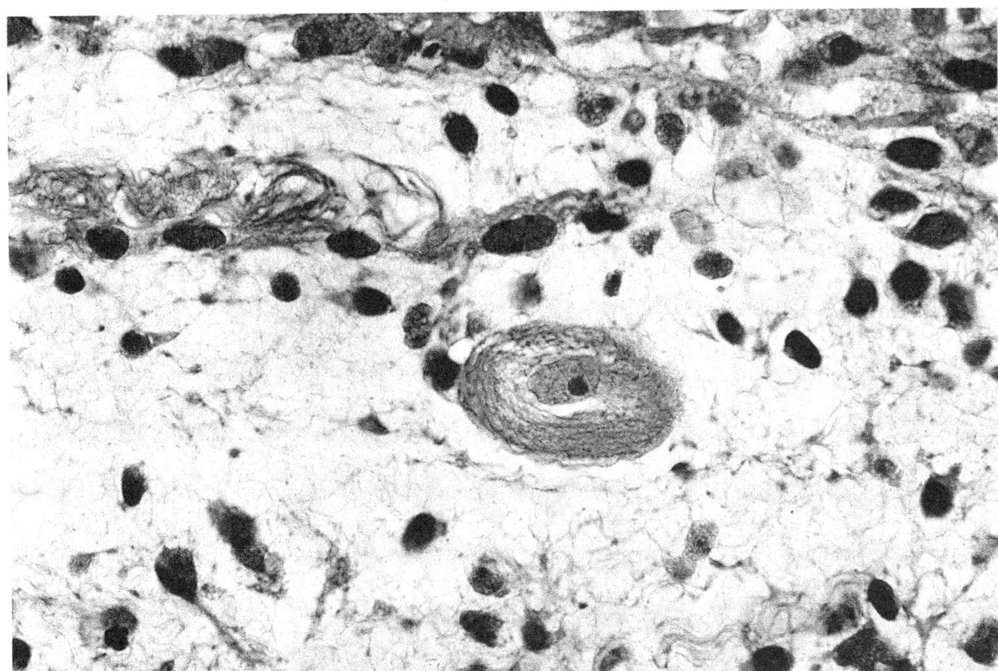

**FIGURE 22–9.** Characteristic rhabdomyoblast in an embryonal rhabdomyosarcoma. Deeply eosinophilic fibrillar material is concentrically arranged around the nucleus.

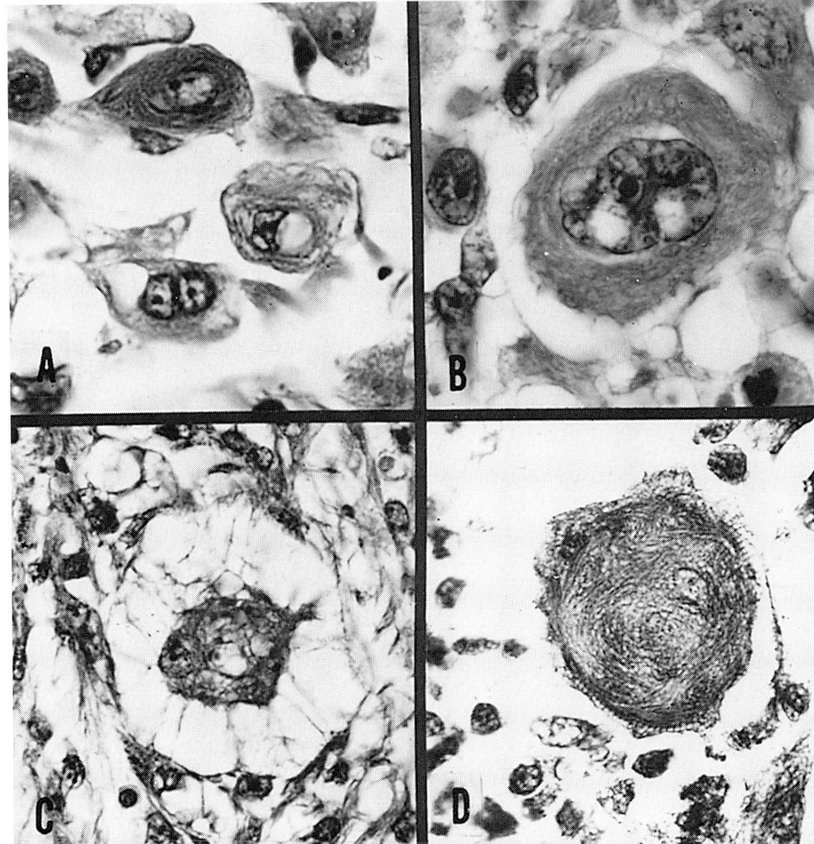


**FIGURE 22–10.** Rhabdomyoblasts with filamentous stringy material surrounding the nucleus and occasional juxtanuclear vacuoles (**A**), perinuclear bundles of myofilaments (**B**), vacuolated cytoplasm secondary to removal of glycogen ("spider web" cell) (**C**), and radiating cross-striations at the periphery (**D**).

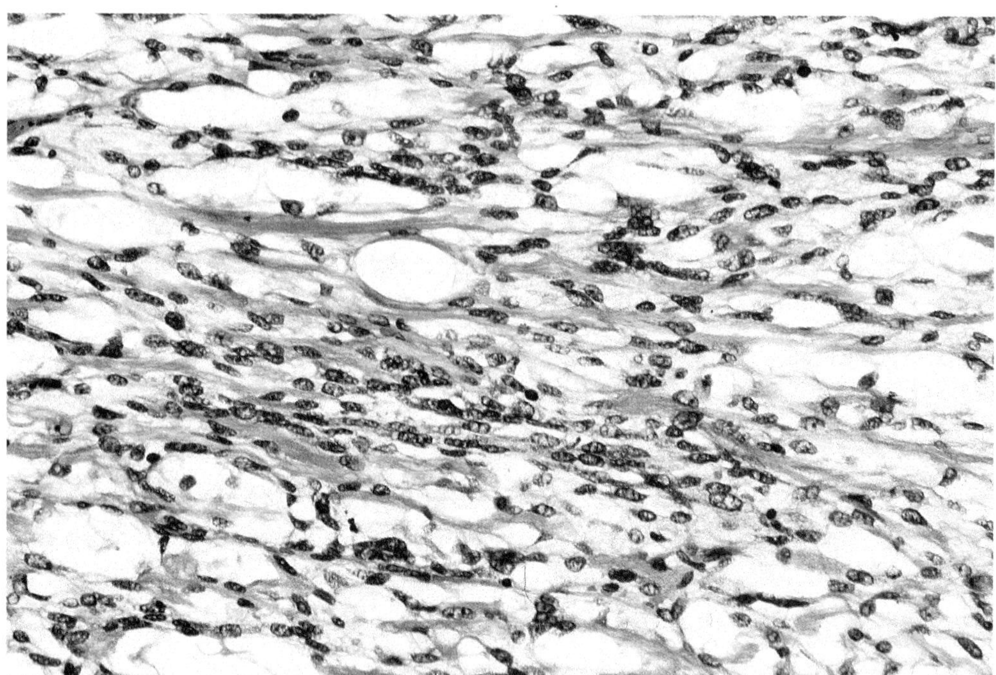

**FIGURE 22–11.** Embryonal rhabdomyosarcoma composed predominantly of atypical spindle-shaped cells with scattered elongated rhabdomyoblasts.

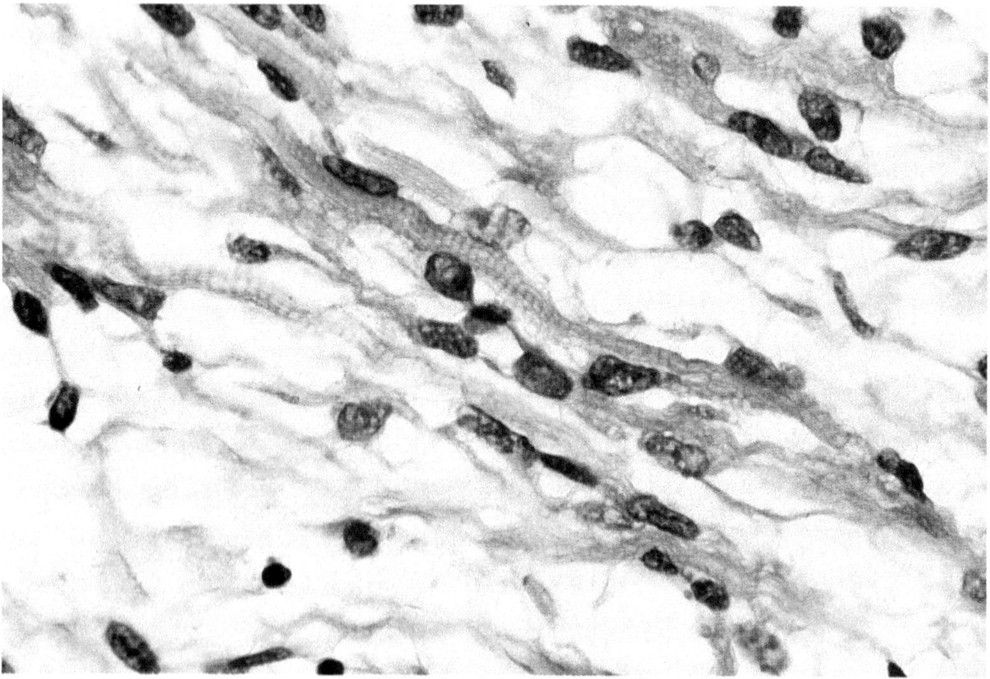

**FIGURE 22–12.** High-power view of elongated rhabdomyoblasts with distinct cross-striations in an embryonal rhabdomyosarcoma.

arranged near or around the nucleus. Cross-striations are rare in the round cells, and if present they are usually confined to narrow bundles of concentrically arranged myofibrils at the circumference of the rhabdomyoblast. Degenerated rhabdomyoblasts with a glassy or hyalinized deeply eosinophilic cytoplasm and pyknotic nuclei but without cross-striations are a frequent feature of this tumor.

Cross-striations are more readily discernible in embryonal rhabdomyosarcomas with a more prominent spindle cell component (Figs. 22–11, 22–12), tumors that might be regarded as the morphologic equivalent of normal muscle at 9–15 weeks of intrauterine development; these neoplasms are composed mainly of a mixture of undifferentiated cells and differentiated fusiform or elongated cells that are readily identifiable as rhabdomyoblasts by light microscopy. The rhabdomyoblasts range from slender spindle-shaped cells with a small number of peripherally placed myofibrils to large eosinophilic cells with a strap, ribbon, tadpole, or racquet shape and one or two centrally positioned nuclei and prominent nucleoli, with or without cross-striations. Cross-striations in neoplastic cells differ from those in residual or entrapped muscle cells by their more irregular distribution and the fact that they often traverse only part of the tumor cell. Intracellular granules may be confused with cross-striations, but their granular nature is readily apparent after careful examination of the cell under oil immersion. Sometimes the strap-shaped cells are sharply angulated and form a diagnostically useful "zigzag," or "broken straw," pattern (Figs. 22–13, 22–14). Most of these tumors have only a moderate degree of cellular pleomorphism.

Embryonal rhabdomyosarcomas with a prominent degree of cellular pleomorphism are rare and, in some cases, are difficult to distinguish from adult pleomorphic rhabdomyosarcomas (Fig. 22–15), except for the more frequent occurrence of cross-striations in childhood tumors and the identification of areas of more typical embryonal rhabdomyosarcoma. According to Kodet et al.,[143] the cellular pleomorphism adversely affects the outcome only if it is diffuse and involves the entire neoplasm.

There are also extremely well differentiated embryonal rhabdomyosarcomas that consist almost entirely of well differentiated rounded, spindle-shaped, or polygonal rhabdomyoblasts with abundant eosinophilic cytoplasm and frequent cross-striations. Some of these differentiated tumors are found in recurrent or metastatic neoplasms after prolonged therapy (Fig. 22–16), possibly due to the "selective destruction of undifferentiated tumor cells."[186]

Glycogen is demonstrable in most rhabdomyosarcomas regardless of type; when the glycogen is removed during fixation, multivacuolated cells or "spider cells" result, which are large multivacuolated rhabdomyoblasts with narrow strands of cytoplasm connecting the center of the cell with its periphery.[173] The centrally located nuclei and the irregular shape of the cytoplasmic vacuoles help distinguish these cells from the more rounded lipid-filled vacuoles of lipoblasts. In contrast to alveolar rhabdomyosarcoma, multinucleated giant cells are rare in embryonal rhabdomyosarcomas.

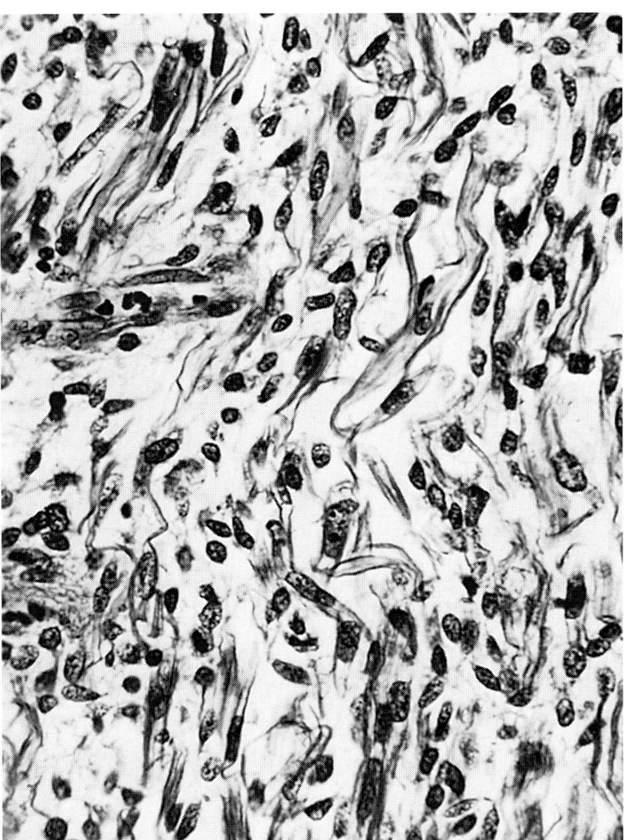

**FIGURE 22–13.** Embryonal rhabdomyosarcoma resembling the tubular stage in fetal muscle.

Occasionally, the embryonal rhabdomyosarcoma displays, in addition to its rhabdomyoblastic component, foci of immature cartilaginous (Fig. 22–17) or osseous tissue, or both. These tumors occur at any age and any location but seem to be more common in the genitourinary tract and the retroperitoneum. Daya and Scully[51] observed cartilaginous differentiation in 45% of rhabdomyosarcomas of the uterine cervix.

### *Cytogenetic Findings*

The cytogenetic abnormalities of embryonal and alveolar rhabdomyosarcomas are distinct. Embryonal rhabdomyosarcoma is characterized by a consistent loss of heterozygosity for multiple closely linked loci at chromosome 11p15.5.[20,21,147,148,165,260–262] This loss of

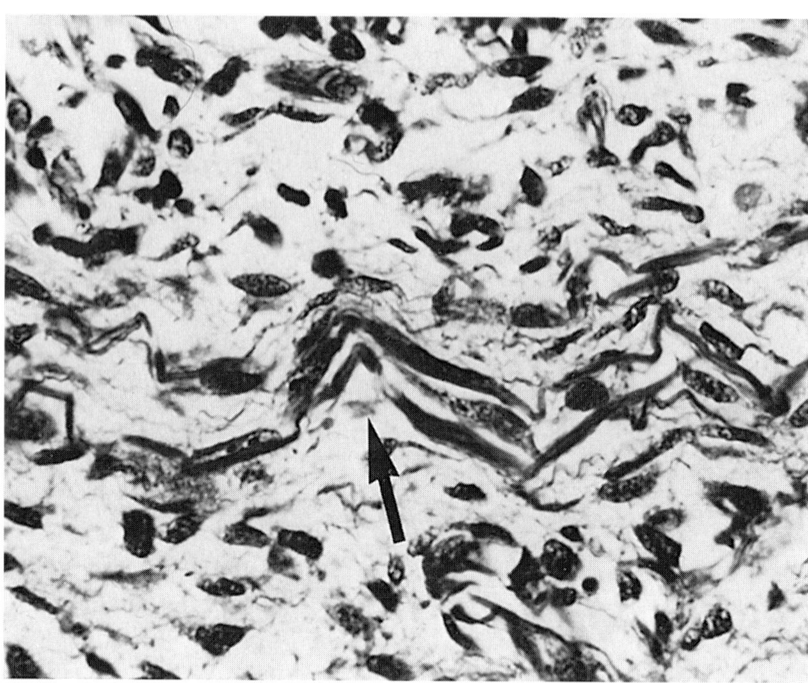

**FIGURE 22–14.** Embryonal rhabdomyosarcoma with elongated rhabdomyoblasts showing distinct angulation of the muscle fibers (arrow), a feature that may aid in the diagnosis ("broken straw" sign).

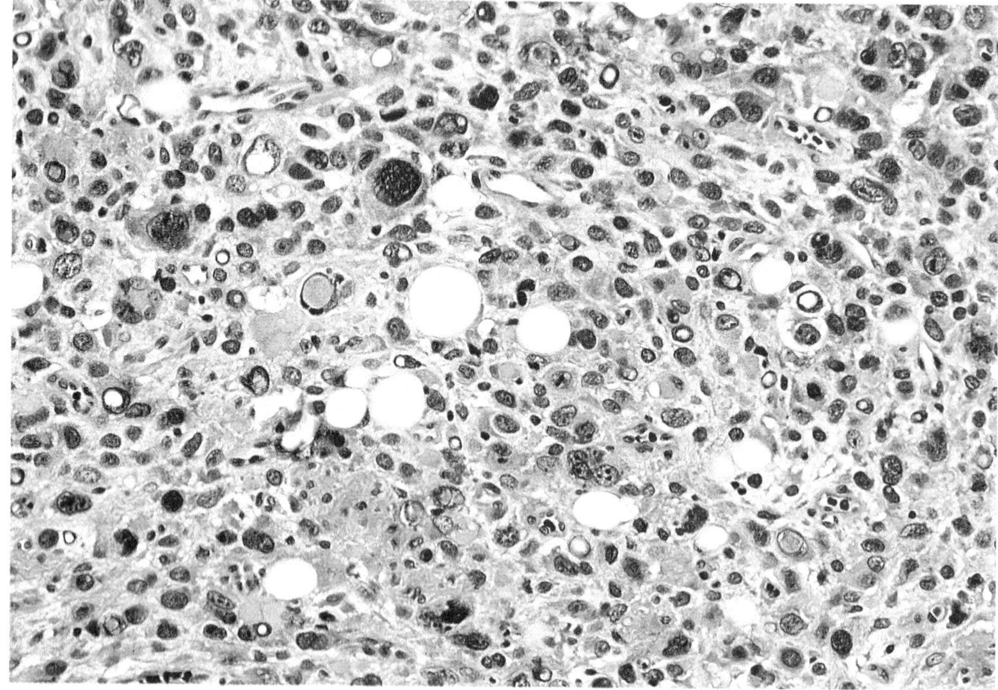

**FIGURE 22–15.** Embryonal rhabdomyosarcoma with anaplastic features arising in a 3-year-old child.

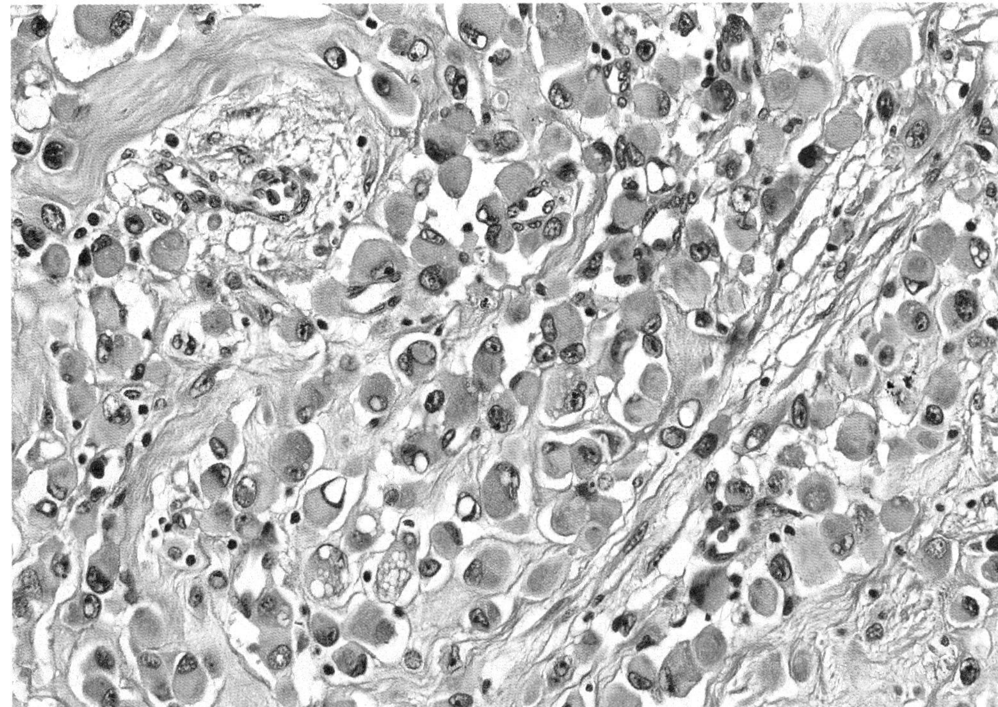

**FIGURE 22–16.** Embryonal rhabdomyosarcoma consisting almost entirely of differentiated rhabdomyoblasts, a feature occasionally encountered in recurrent tumors following therapy.

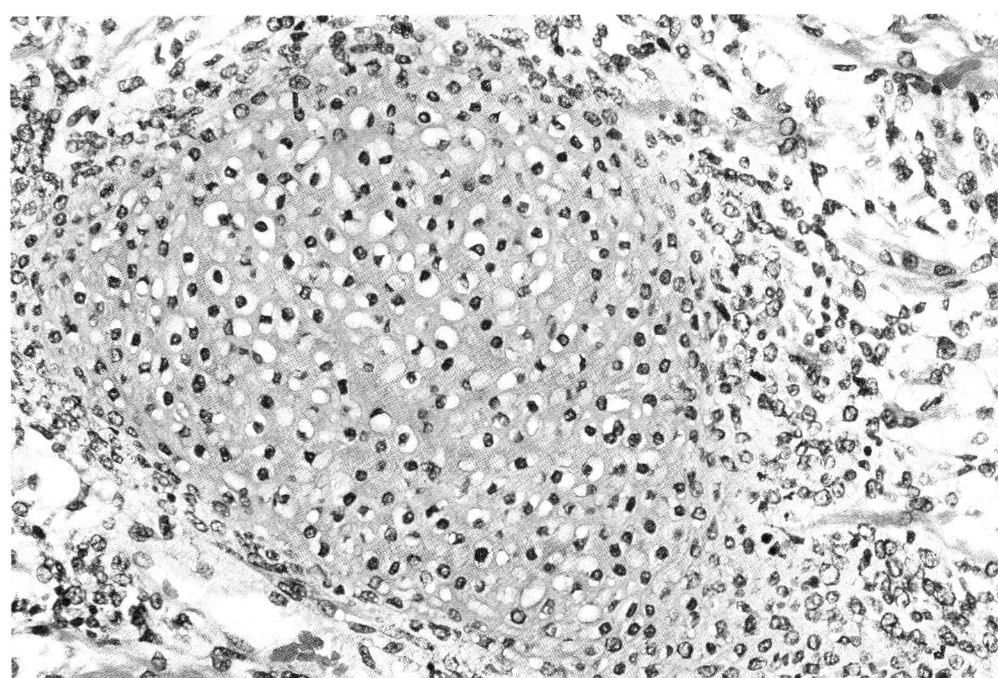

**FIGURE 22–17.** Embryonal rhabdomyosarcoma with foci of immature cartilage.

heterozygosity may result in activation of a tumor-suppressor gene or genes, including the human tyrosine hydroxylase gene,[20] or *GOK*.[248] Abnormalities of the short arm of chromosome 11 are also found in a number of small-cell pediatric neoplasms, including Wilms' tumor.[171,212,270] Others have reported trisomy 8 as a consistent finding in embryonal rhabdomyosarcomas.[1a,61]

### Embryonal Rhabdomyosarcoma, Spindle Cell Type

In 1992 Cavazzana et al.[32] reported 21 embryonal rhabdomyosarcomas that were composed predominantly (>80%) of elongated spindle cells mimicking fetal myotubes at a late stage of cellular differentiation. In this study, there was a striking predilection for this tumor to arise in males, particularly in a paratesticular location. By immunohistochemistry and electron microscopy, the cells showed a high degree of skeletal muscle differentiation. The authors coined the term *spindle cell rhabdomyosarcoma* to distinguish this entity from the usual embryonal rhabdomyosarcoma because of its more favorable clinical course. Subsequent studies have confirmed the distinctive clinical and pathologic features of this rhabdomyosarcoma subtype.[64,71,159]

Spindle cell rhabdomyosarcoma is a rare subtype of rhabdomyosarcoma, accounting for 21 (4.4%) of 471 rhabdomyosarcomas retrieved from the files of the German-Italian Cooperative Soft Tissue Sarcomas Study Group.[32] Of 800 randomly selected rhabdomyosarcomas from the International Rhabdomyosarcoma Study Group, this variant accounted for 3% of all rhabdomyosarcomas.[198] Like other forms of embryonal rhabdomyosarcoma, the spindle cell type tends to arise in young patients (mean age approximately 7 years), but rare cases have been described in adults.[244,290a] There appears to be a striking male predilection, as Cavazzana et al.[32,159] found males to be affected six times more commonly than females. The most common site of involvement is the paratesticular soft tissue (38%), followed by the head and neck (27%) (Table 22–9). This tumor has also been described in the urinary bladder, abdomen, retroperitoneum, and soft tissues of the extremities.

Grossly, the tumor is usually firm and well circumscribed but unencapsulated, and most range between 4 and 6 cm in greatest dimension. The cut surface reveals a distinctly nodular pattern, often with a whorled appearance.

Histologically, the tumor is composed almost exclusively of elongated fusiform cells with cigar-shaped nuclei and prominent nucleoli (Figs. 22–18, 22–19, 22–20). The tumor cells have eosinophilic fibrillar cytoplasm with distinct cellular borders, closely resembling late-stage fetal myoblasts. Cytoplasmic cross-striations may be observed. The collagen-rich form is characterized by spindle cells separated by abundant collagen fibers arranged in a storiform or whorled growth pattern. The collagen-poor form is a more cellular proliferation of cells arranged in bundles or fascicles, reminiscent of leiomyosarcoma.

Immunohistochemically, the tumor cells consistently express myogenic antigens, including muscle-specific actin, desmin, and myoglobin. However, this rhabdomyosarcoma subtype more consistently expresses myogenic antigens, which are generally expressed at a late stage of myogenesis, including titin[32] and troponin T,[159] supporting a greater degree of differentiation of these spindle-shaped cells.

There are essentially no data regarding the cytogenetic abnormalities found in the spindle cell type of embryonal rhabdomyosarcoma. Thus it cannot be determined whether such abnormalities might be responsible for the more favorable clinical behavior when compared to the conventional type of embryonal rhabdomyosarcoma.

**TABLE 22–9 ANATOMIC DISTRIBUTION OF SPINDLE CELL RHABDOMYOSARCOMAS**

| Anatomic Location | No. | % |
|---|---|---|
| Paratesticular | 30 | 38 |
| Head and neck | 21 | 27 |
| Extremities | 8 | 10 |
| Genitourinary | 8 | 10 |
| Other | 11 | 15 |
| *Total* | 78 | 100 |

Data are from refs. 32 and 159.

### Embryonal Rhabdomyosarcoma, Botryoid Type

Botryoid rhabdomyosarcoma accounts for approximately 6% of all rhabdomyosarcomas.[198] The word *botryoid* is derived from the Greek word for grapes, and this variant is characterized grossly by its polypoid (grape-like) growth and microscopically by its relative sparsity of cells and abundance of mucoid stroma, often resulting in a myxoma-like picture. Most botryoid rhabdomyosarcomas are found in mucosa-lined hollow organs, such as the nasal cavity, nasopharynx, bile duct, urinary bladder, and vagina (Figs. 22–21, 22–22; Table 22–8); tumors of this type may also be encountered in areas where the expanding neoplasm reaches the body surface, as in some rhabdomyosarcomas of the eyelid or the anal region. Obviously, its unrestricted growth in body cavities or

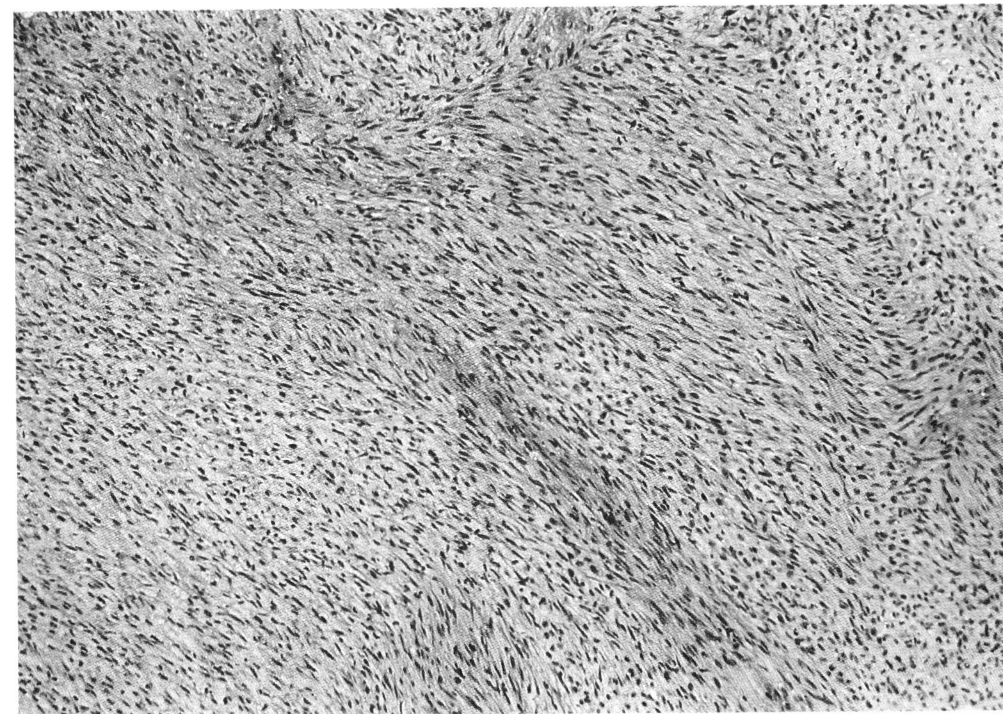

**FIGURE 22–18.** Low-power view of spindle cell type of embryonal rhabdomyosarcoma arising in the urinary bladder.

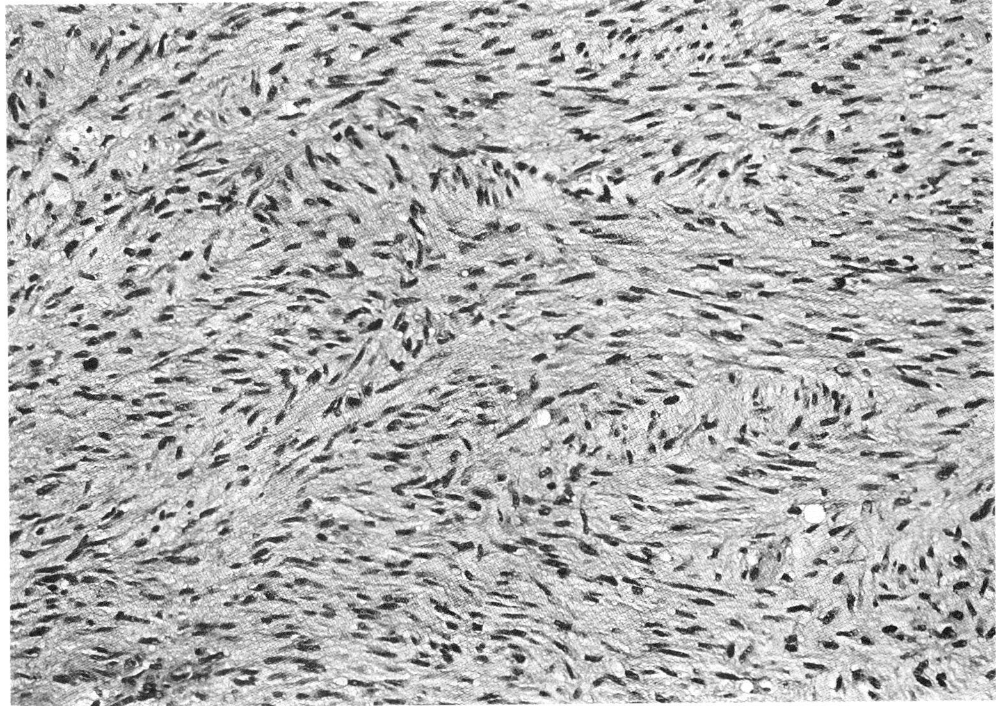

**FIGURE 22–19.** Spindle cell type of embryonal rhabdomyosarcoma composed of relatively uniform spindle-shaped cells deposited in a myxoid stroma. Cells are arranged in an irregular fascicular pattern reminiscent of leiomyosarcoma.

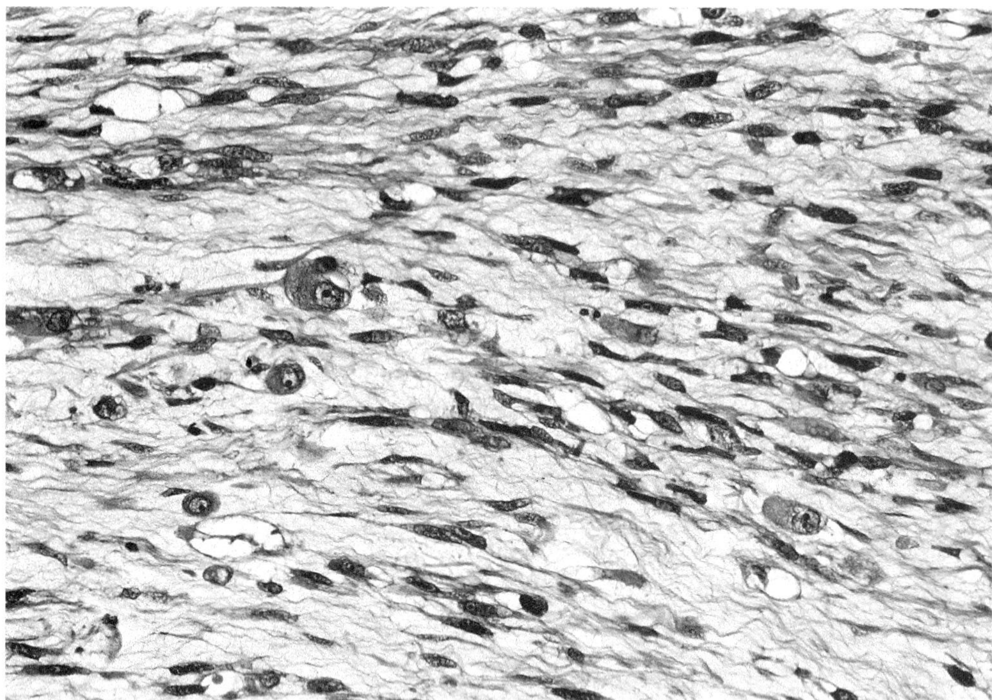

**FIGURE 22–20.** Scattered rhabdomyoblasts are apparent in this spindle cell type of embryonal rhabdomyosarcoma.

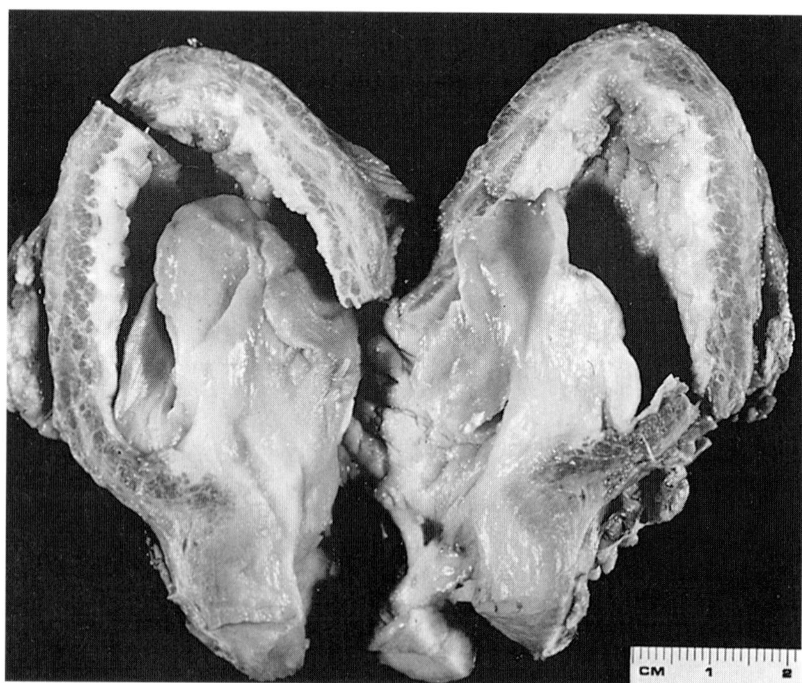


**FIGURE 22–21.** Botryoid-type embryonal rhabdomyosarcoma of the urinary bladder in a 3-year-old child. Note the polypoid and myxoid appearance of the tumor.

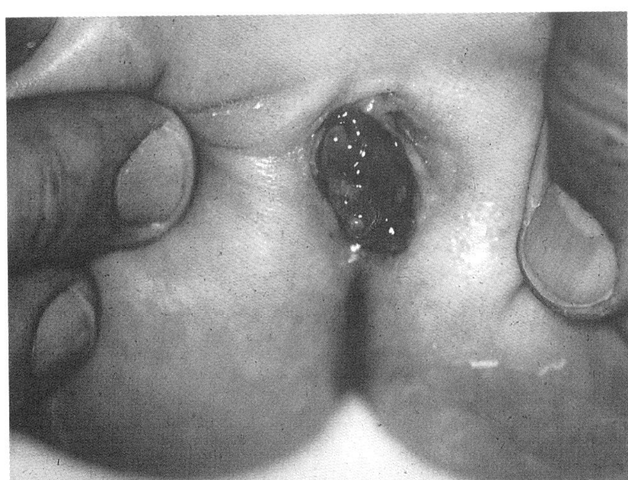

**FIGURE 22–22.** Botryoid-type embryonal rhabdomyosarcoma of the vagina.

on body surfaces accounts for its characteristic edematous and grape-like appearance.

Although a grape-like configuration has traditionally been a defining feature of the botryoid variant, the ICR scheme does not require this characteristic gross appearance.[198] According to the ICR criteria, a "cambium layer," characterized by a subepithelial condensation of tumor cells separated from an intact surface epithelium by a zone of loose stroma, must be present to recognize this variant (Figs. 22–23 to 22–26). The tumor cells should form a distinct zone that is several layers thick, although the thickness of this layer may vary in extent in different areas of the tumor. The tumor cells also vary in appearance, ranging from primitive small cells to cells with clear-cut myoblastic differentiation (Fig. 22–27). Cells with stellate cytoplasmic processes are often prominent. The stroma is typically loosely cellular with a myxoid appearance, including a hypocellular zone that separates the surface epithelium from an underlying cambium layer. The surface epithelium may be hyperplastic or may undergo squamous changes, sometimes mimicking a carcinoma.

Immunohistochemically, there is usually strong staining for myogenic antigens, particularly in cells showing light microscopic evidence of myoblastic differentiation. There are few data regarding cytogenetic abnormalities in botryoid rhabdomyosarcoma, although Palazzo et al. reported deletion of the short arm of chromosome 1 and trisomies of chromosomes 13 and 18.[207]

## Alveolar Rhabdomyosarcoma

Alveolar rhabdomyosarcoma is the second most common subtype, accounting for approximately 31% of all rhabdomyosarcomas.[198] The tumor tends to arise at a slightly older age than embryonal, botryoid, and spindle cell rhabdomyosarcomas, with a peak incidence at 10–25 years of age. It has a predilection for the deep soft tissues of the extremities (Figs. 22–28, 22–29) and accounts for approximately 50% of all extremity rhabdomyosarcomas,[199] although the tumor may arise in many other sites, including the head and neck, trunk, perineum, pelvis, and retroperitoneum (Table 22–8).

Histologically, the alveolar rhabdomyosarcoma is composed largely of ill-defined aggregates of poorly differentiated round or oval tumor cells that frequently show central loss of cellular cohesion and

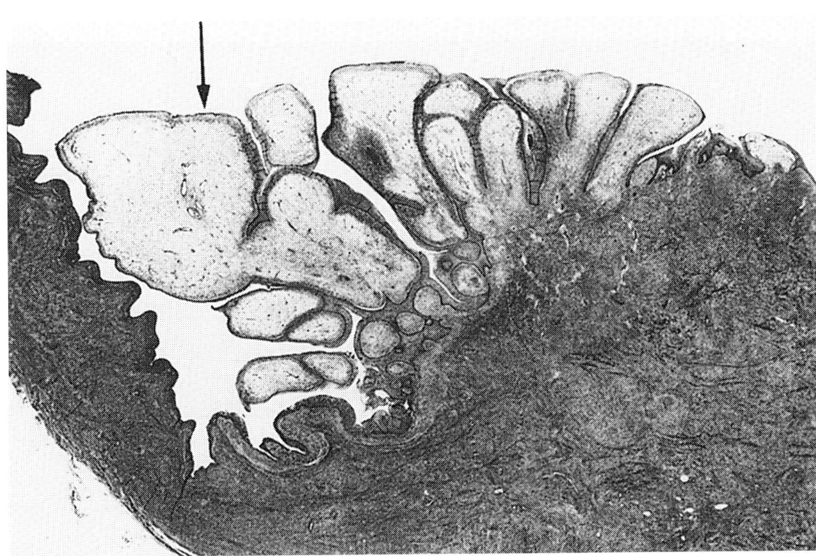

**FIGURE 22–23.** Botryoid-type embryonal rhabdomyosarcoma of the urinary bladder. Note the polypoid and myxoid appearance of the tumor and the submucosal hypercellular "cambium" layer (arrow).

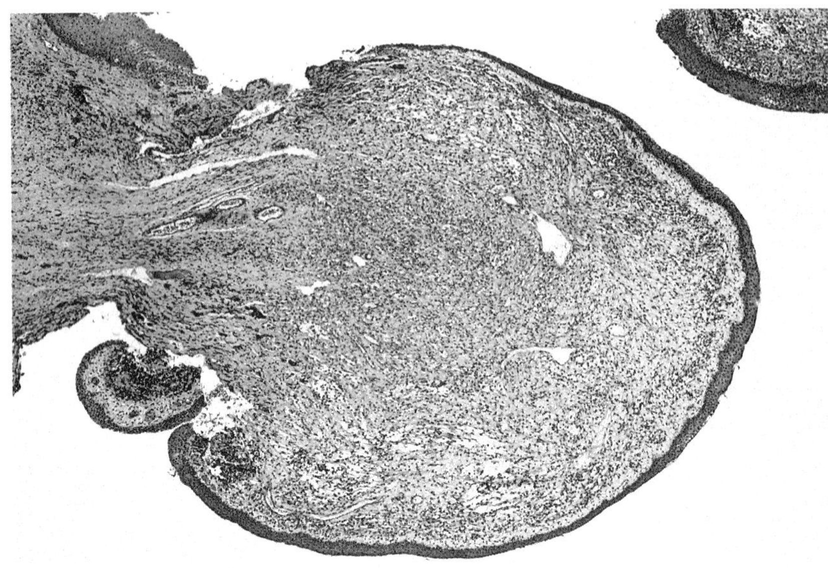

**FIGURE 22–24.** Polypoid fragment lined by squamous mucosa in a botryoid-type embryonal rhabdomyosarcoma of the vagina.

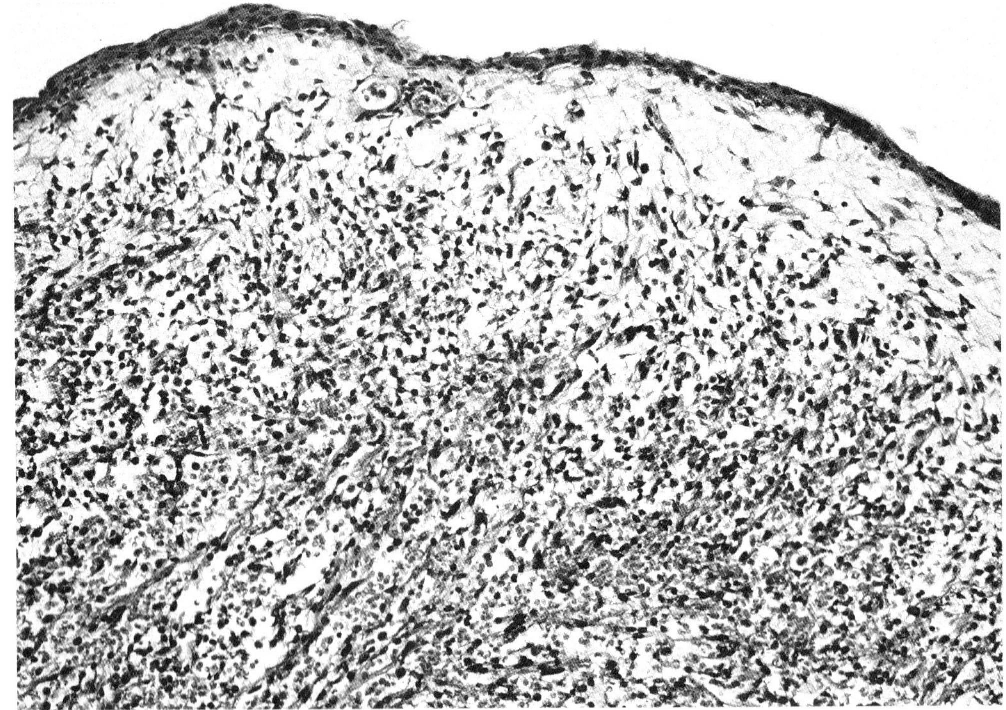

**FIGURE 22–25.** Botryoid-type embryonal rhabdomyosarcoma with the characteristic "cambium" layer, a submucosal zone of markedly increased cellularity.

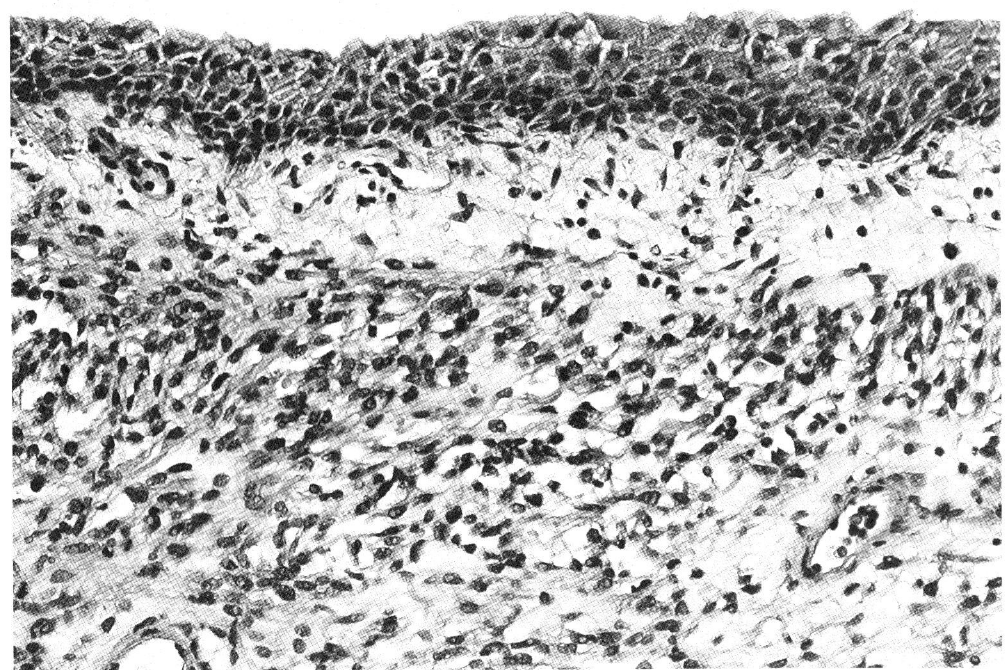

**FIGURE 22–26.** Primitive spindle-shaped and ovoid cells in the cambium layer of this botryoid-type embryonal rhabdomyosarcoma.

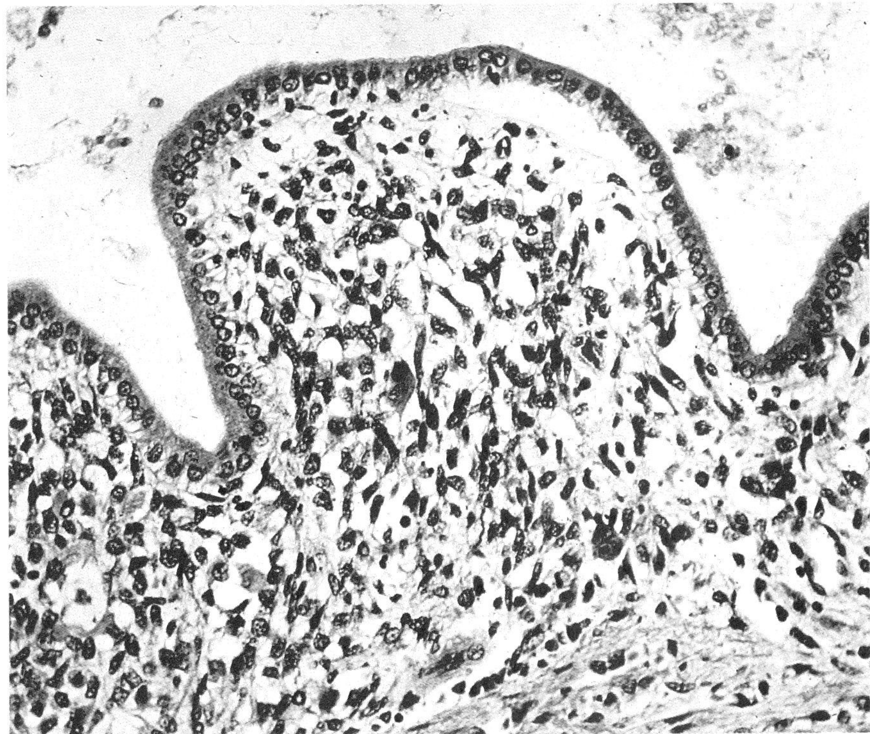

**FIGURE 22–27.** Embryonal rhabdomyosarcoma of the biliary tract with botryoid features. Scattered rhabdomyoblasts are apparent.

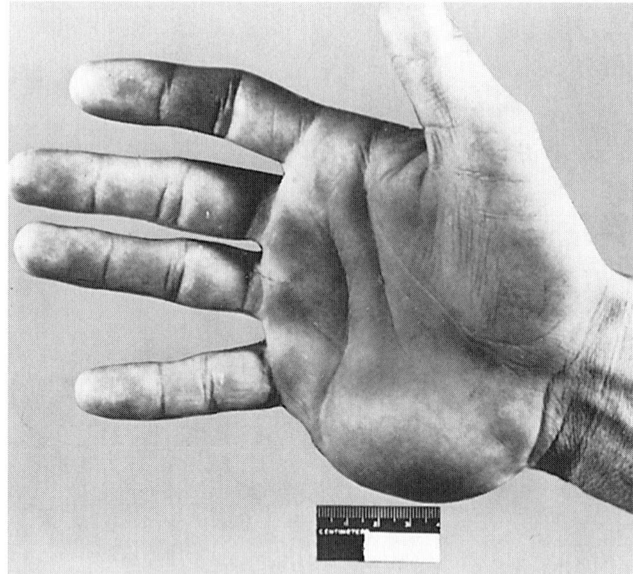

**FIGURE 22–28.** Alveolar rhabdomyosarcoma of the hypothenar eminence of the right hand in a 20-year-old man.

formation of irregular "alveolar" spaces (Figs. 22–30, 22–31, 22–32). The individual cellular aggregates are separated and surrounded by a framework of dense, frequently hyalinized fibrous septa that surround dilated vascular channels. Characteristically, the cells at the periphery of the alveolar spaces are well preserved and adhere in a single layer to the fibrous septa in a manner somewhat reminiscent of an adenocarcinoma or papillary carcinoma. The cells in the center of the alveolar spaces tend to be more loosely arranged, or "freely floating" (Fig. 22–33); they are often poorly preserved and show evidence of degeneration and necrosis. In rare instances viable cells are virtually absent, and the tumor consists merely of a coarse sieve-like or honeycomb-like meshwork of thick fibrous trabeculae surrounding small, loosely textured groups of severely degenerated cells with pyknotic nuclei and necrotic cellular debris.[77]

There are also "solid" forms of this tumor that lack an alveolar pattern entirely and are composed of densely packed groups or masses of tumor cells resembling the round cell areas of embryonal rhabdomyosarcoma but with a more uniform cellular picture with little or no fibrosis[249,288] (Fig. 22–34). These solidly cellular areas are more commonly encountered at the periphery of the tumor and probably represent the most active and most cellular stage of growth. It is important not to confuse the solid form of alveolar rhabdomyosarcoma with the undifferentiated form of embryonal rhabdomyosarcoma, as the former carries a less favorable prognosis. Distinction may be difficult; but in most cases examination of the solid tumors shows, in addition to the uniform cellular pattern, incipient alveolar features. Even in the solid areas there is a regular arrangement of fibrous septa that surround the primitive round cells. As discussed below, cytogenetic studies may aid in this distinction. There are also rare cases in which the cells have abundant pale-staining, glycogen-containing cytoplasm and vaguely resemble clear-cell carcinoma or clear-cell malignant melanoma (*clear-cell rhabdomyosarcoma*).[16,25]

The individual cells in both alveolar and solid portions of the tumor have round or oval hyperchromatic nuclei with scant amounts of indistinct cytoplasm. Bulbous or club-shaped cells, sometimes with deeply eosinophilic cytoplasm, are often seen pro-

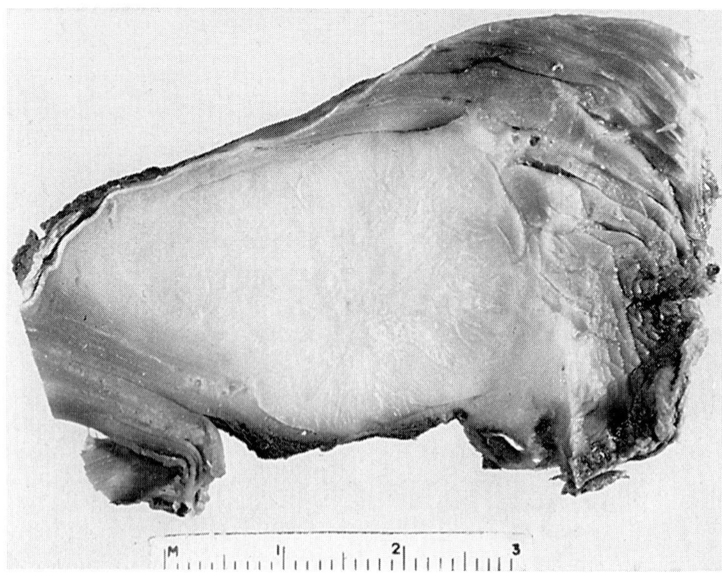

**FIGURE 22–29.** Cross section of alveolar rhabdomyosarcoma of the soleus muscle in a 35-year-old man.

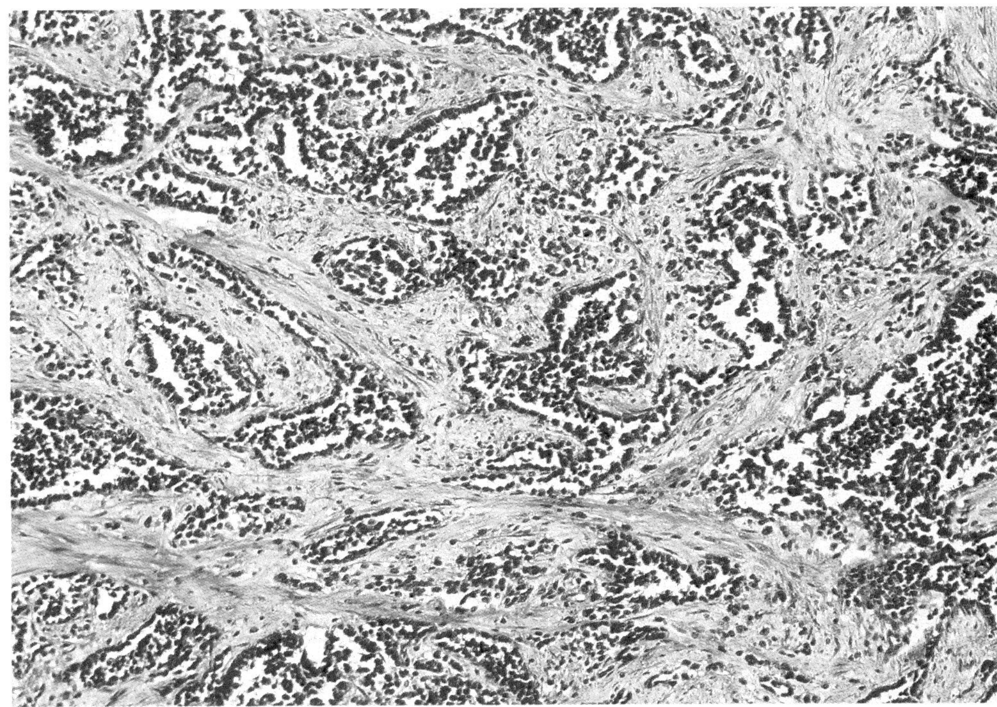

**FIGURE 22–30.** Alveolar rhabdomyosarcoma with the characteristic "alveolar" growth pattern.

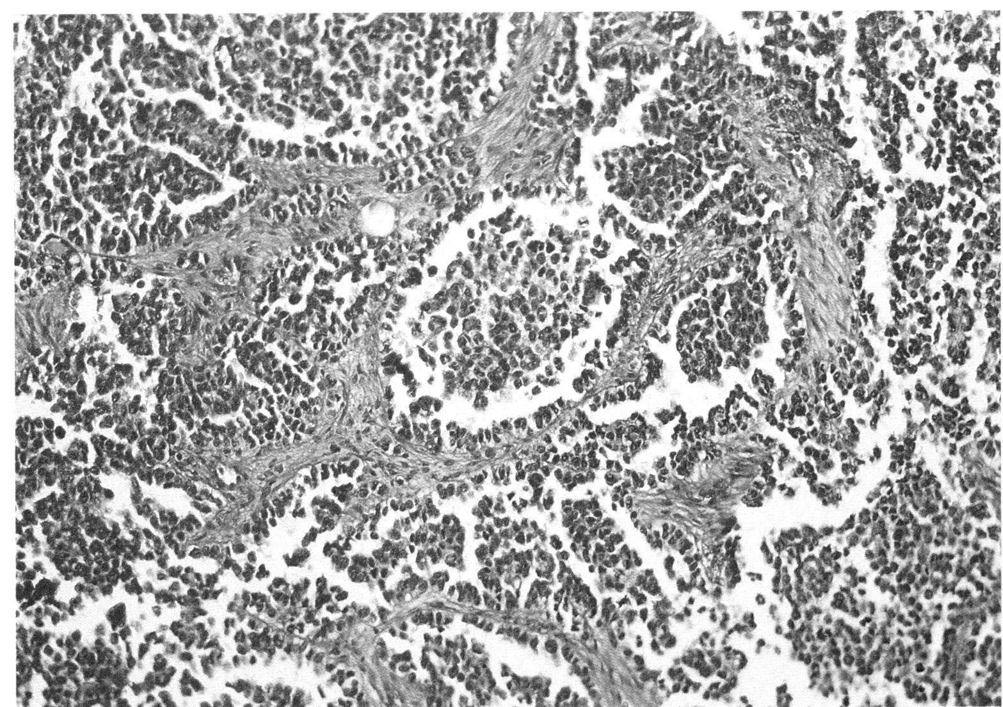

**FIGURE 22–31.** Alveolar rhabdomyosarcoma. A single layer of neoplastic cells adheres to dense fibrous septa with central loss of cellular cohesion.

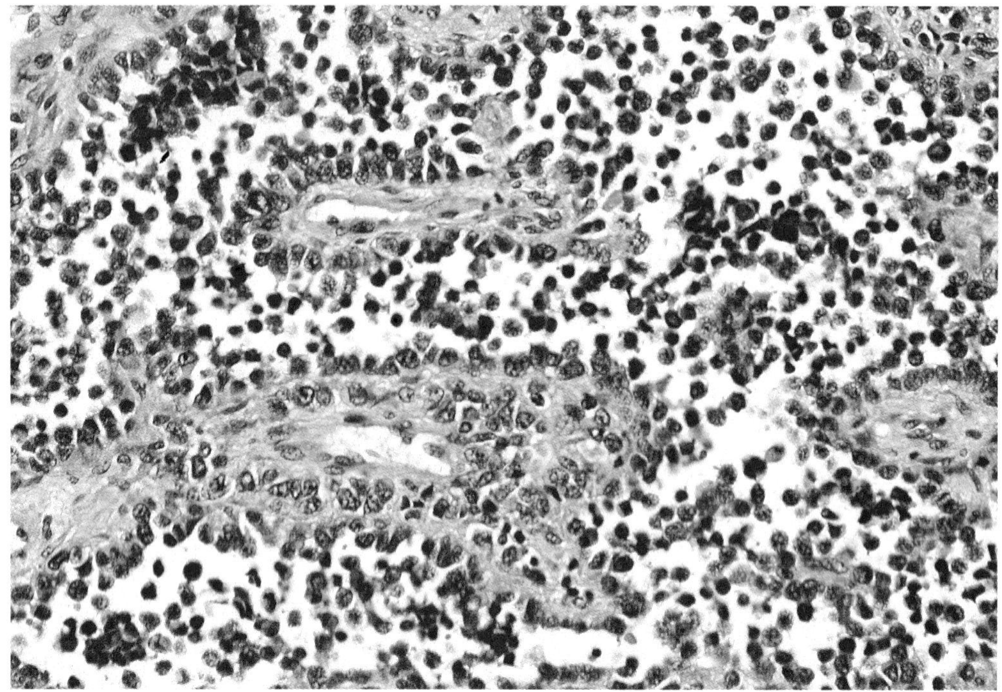

**FIGURE 22–32.** High-power view of alveolar rhabdomyosarcoma. Fibrovascular septa are lined by a single layer of round cells. There is loss of cellular cohesion and individual tumor cell necrosis between the fibrous septa.

truding from the fibrous walls into the lumen of the alveolar spaces. Mitotic figures are common.

Neoplastic rhabdomyoblasts with pronounced stringy or granular eosinophilic cytoplasm are less common in alveolar than in embryonal rhabdomyosarcomas and are present in no more than about 30% of cases. Most of the rhabdomyoblasts in the alveolar spaces have a round or oval configuration (Fig. 22–35); those located in or attached to the fibrous septa tend to be strap-shaped or spindle-shaped. If cross-striations are present, they are almost exclusively found in the spindle-shaped cells.

In contrast to embryonal rhabdomyosarcomas, multinucleated giant cells are a prominent and diagnostically important feature of alveolar rhabdomyosarcomas (Figs. 22–36, 22–37). Usually the giant cells have multiple, peripherally placed nuclei in a pale-staining or weakly eosinophilic cytoplasm. We have never been able to detect cross-striations in these cells; according to the ultrastructural studies of Churg and Ringus,[36] they do not contain myofilaments. Yet transitional forms between rhabdomyoblasts and giant cells suggest that the latter are formed by cellular fusion. Collagen formation is usually confined to the intervening septa, but occasionally large portions of the tumor are obliterated by extensive fibroplasia. As already mentioned, mixed types with embryonal and alveolar features should be classified as alveolar rhabdomyosarcomas.[198]

Most alveolar rhabdomyosarcomas seem to originate in muscle tissue, and entrapment of normal muscle fibers is common. These fibers are apt to be mistaken for neoplastic rhabdomyoblasts with cross-striations, a feature that sometimes results in the correct diagnosis for the wrong reason.

Metastatic alveolar rhabdomyosarcomas in lymph nodes, lung, and other viscera also display a distinct alveolar pattern (Fig. 22–38), making it unlikely that this pattern is merely the result of infiltrative growth along the fibrous framework of the involved musculature. Diffuse bone marrow metastases have been mistaken for leukemia.

The immune profile of alveolar rhabdomyosarcoma is similar to that for other rhabdomyosarcomas. Because the differential diagnosis includes numerous other "small round cell tumors," a large battery of immunostains is often required to exclude other entities, as discussed below.

Alveolar rhabdomyosarcoma is characterized by distinctive cytogenetic abnormalities that allow its distinction from other rhabdomyosarcoma subtypes and other round cell neoplasms in the differential diagnosis. Most of these tumors have a t(2;13)(q35;q14) translocation,[68,290] which results in the generation of

*Text continued on page 813*

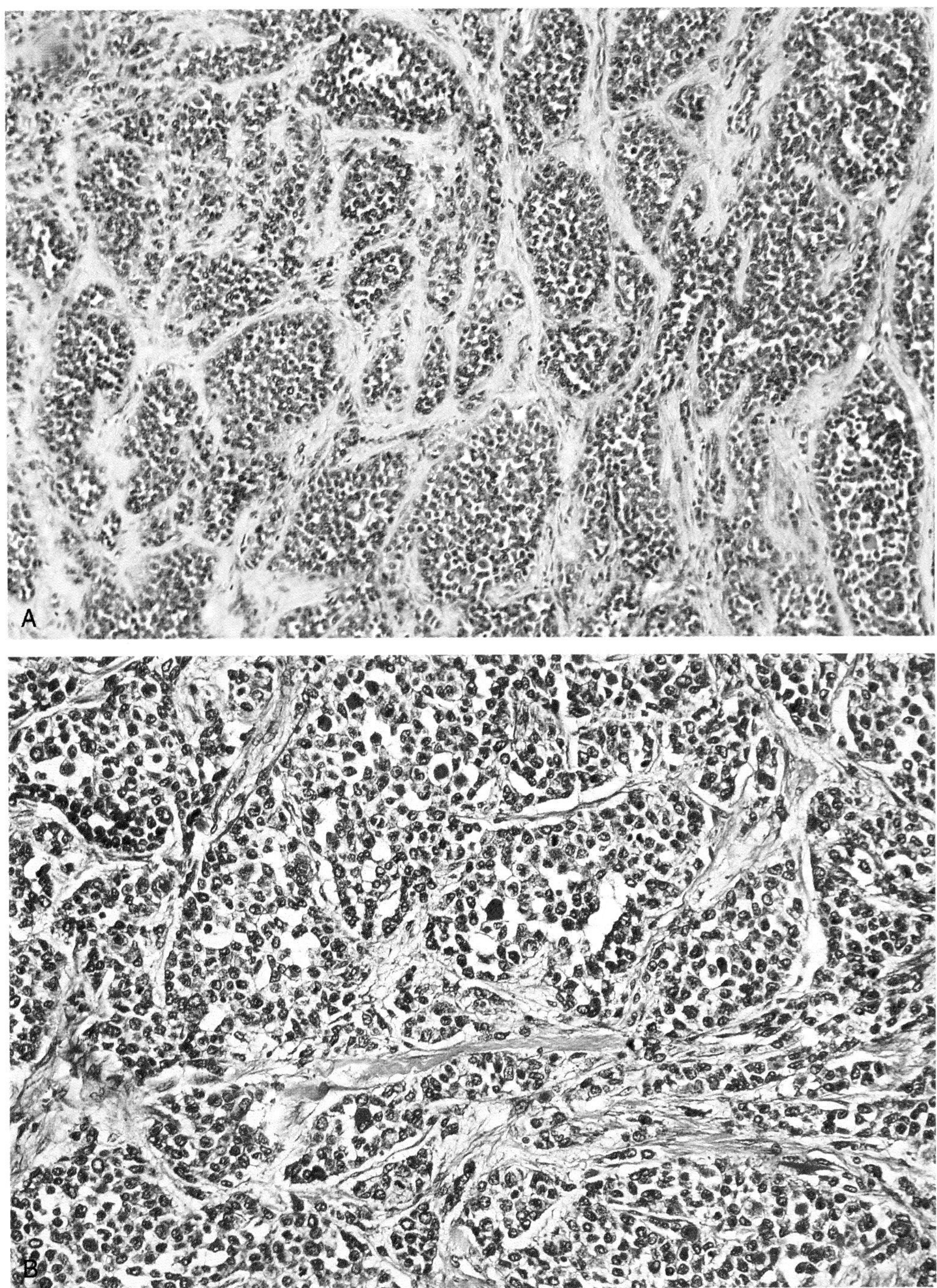


**FIGURE 22–33.** (**A**) Low-power view of alveolar rhabdomyosarcoma with incipient loss of cellular cohesion in cellular nests. (**B**) Masson trichrome-stained section of an alveolar rhabdomyosarcoma accentuating fibrous trabeculae between cellular nests.

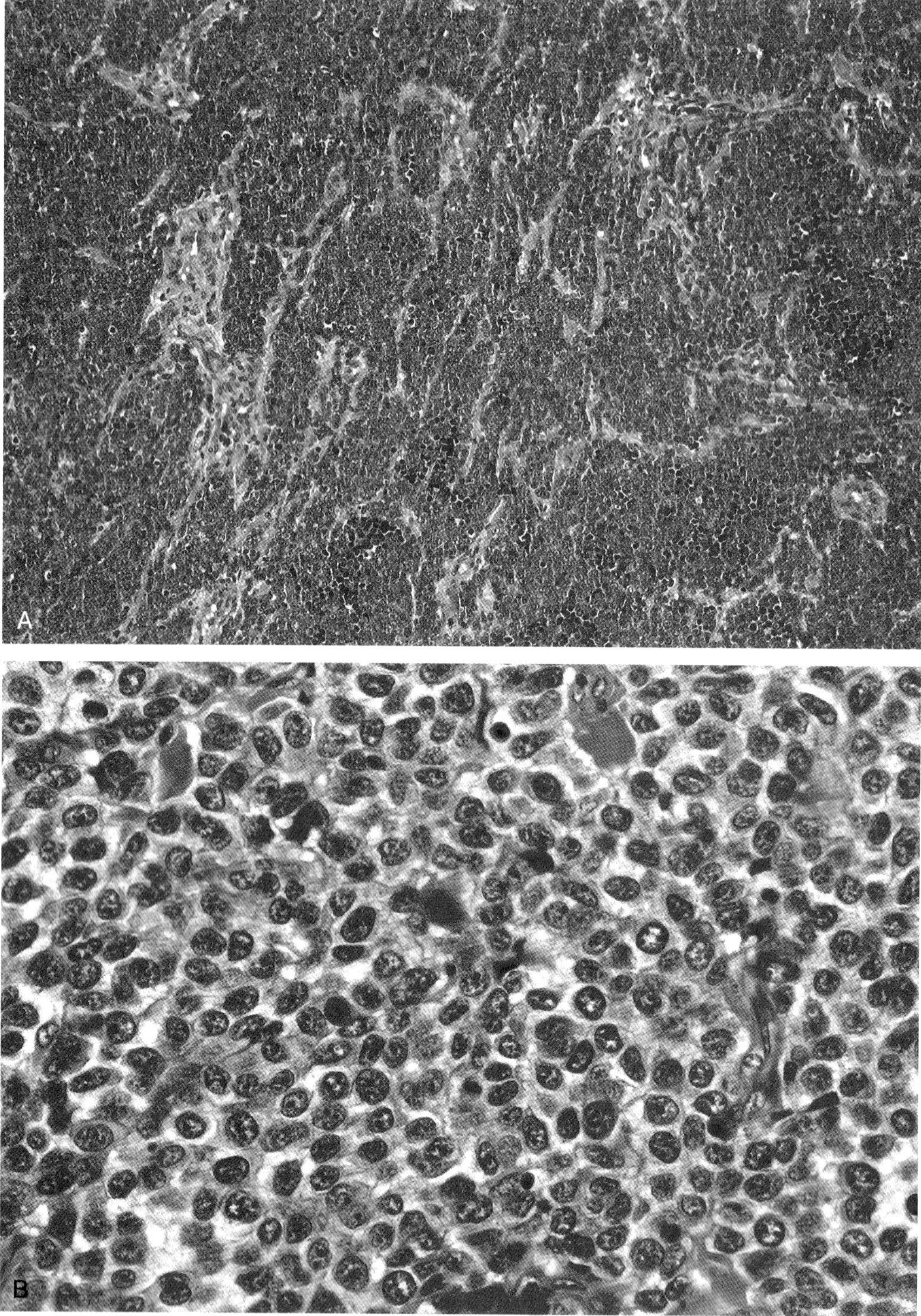

**FIGURE 22–34.** (**A**) Low-power view of a solid variant of alveolar rhabdomyosarcoma. Although the characteristic alveolar structures are not present, cellular nests are still separated by fibrovascular septa, characteristic of this tumor. (**B**) High-power view of a solid variant of alveolar rhabdomyosarcoma. The cytologic features are identical to those of the usual type of alveolar rhabdomyosarcoma. Cells are round with large nuclei and little cytoplasm.

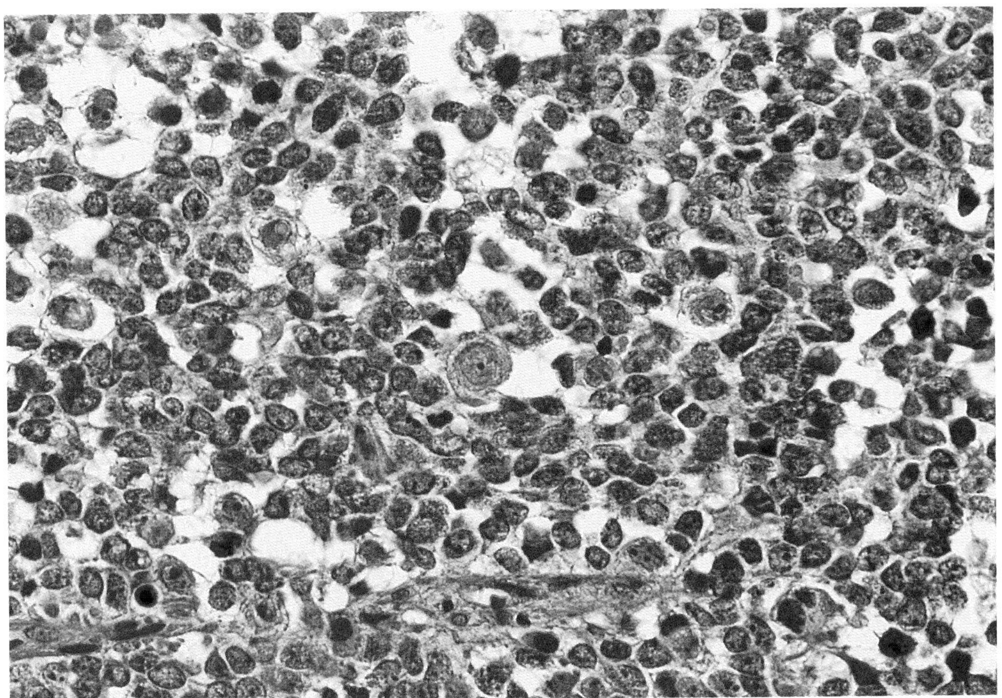

**FIGURE 22–35.** High-power view of an alveolar rhabdomyosarcoma with rare rhabdomyoblasts.

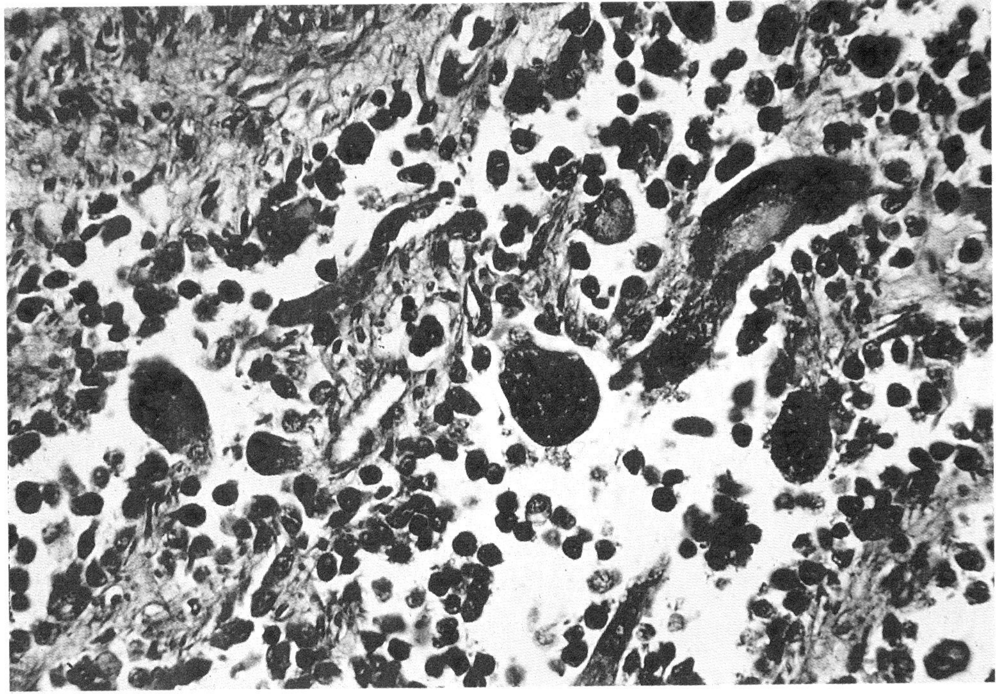

**FIGURE 22–36.** Multinucleated giant cells in an alveolar rhabdomyosarcoma.

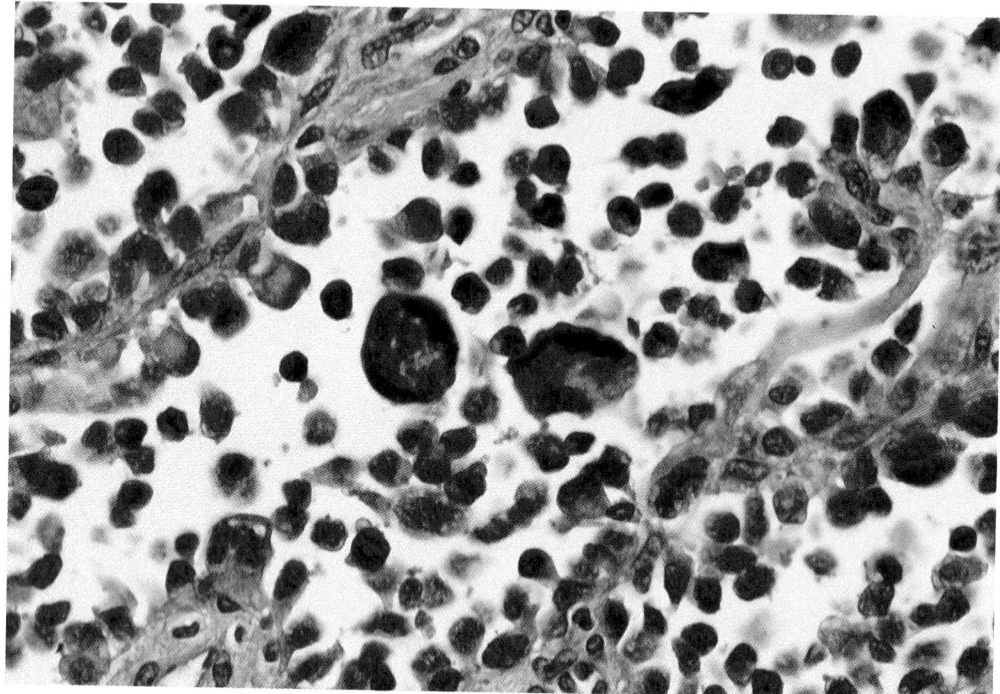

**FIGURE 22–37.** Alveolar rhabdomyosarcoma with multinucleated giant cells. These cells have peripherally placed "wreath-like" nuclei and are usually free-floating in alveolar structures.

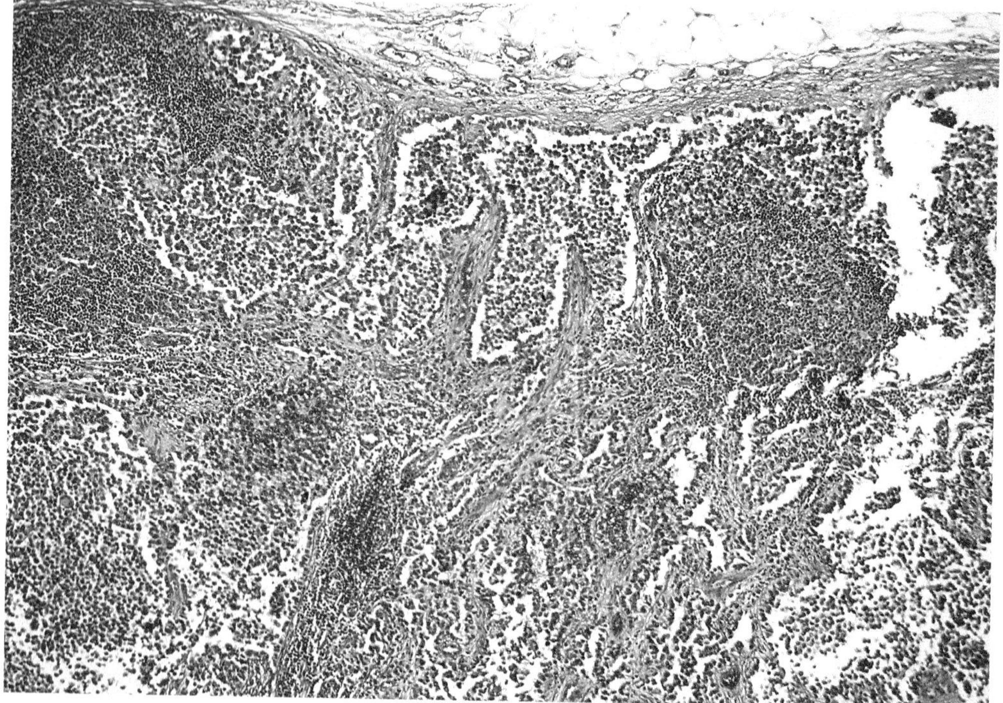

**FIGURE 22–38.** Metastatic alveolar rhabdomyosarcoma to a lymph node. The alveolar pattern is present in the metastasis as well.

two derivative chromosomes: a shortened chromosome 13 and an elongated chromosome 2. The breakpoints occur within the *PAX3* gene on chromosome 2 and the *FKHR* gene on chromosome 13[14,15,94,267] resulting in a *PAX3-FKHR* chimeric gene on chromosome 13 and a *FKHR-PAX3* chimeric gene on chromosome 2. Both of these genes encode transcription factors that regulate the expression of specific target genes. The chimeric gene that results from this translocation encodes for a chimeric protein that acts as an aberrant transcription factor that excessively activates expression of genes with *PAX3* binding sites.[18] The *PAX3-FKHR* transcript appears to be more sensitive and specific than the *FKHR-PAX3* transcript in detecting this tumor.[89] Scheidler et al. demonstrated that this chimeric fusion protein is capable of transforming fibroblasts in tissue culture.[252]

A subset of alveolar rhabdomyosarcomas is associated with a variant translocation, t(1;13)(p36;q14),[22,66] which juxtaposes the *PAX7* gene on 1p36 with the *FKHR* gene on 13q14.[49] There is a high degree of homology between *PAX3* and *PAX7*, and it is likely that the fusion proteins that result from the translocations involving these genes aberrantly regulate a common set of target genes involved in the pathogenesis of alveolar rhabdomyosarcoma.

In addition to cytogenetic examination,[67] these molecular abnormalities can be detected by the reverse transcriptase-polymerase chain reaction (RT-PCR)[7,13,52,69] or fluorescence in situ hybridization (FISH).[23,178] The high sensitivity of these techniques allows evaluation of small amounts of tissue; recent studies report success using fixed, paraffin-embedded tissues.[6,72]

Overall, 70–85% of tumors diagnosed histologically as alveolar rhabdomyosarcoma express either the *PAX3-FKHR* or *PAX7-FKHR* fusion transcripts (Table 22–10). Of the fusion-positive cases, 10–20% are *PAX7-FKHR*-positive, and the remainder are *PAX3-FKHR*-positive.[7,52,69] Kelly et al.[138] found that tumors with the *PAX7-FKHR* fusion transcript tend to arise in young patients, more often arise in the extremities, are usually localized, and are associated with significantly longer event-free survival. Rarely, these molecular abnormalities have been reported in tumors diagnosed histologically as embryonal rhabdomyosarcoma,[13,69] but this might be related to an unsampled alveolar component in these tumors. The detection of minimal residual disease following therapy might also be an important clinical application of these techniques.[137]

## Pleomorphic Rhabdomyosarcoma

Pleomorphic rhabdomyosarcoma is a rare variant of rhabdomyosarcoma that almost always arises in adults older than 45 years of age.[53,92,122] Given its extreme rarity in children,[143] this subtype was not included in the most recent ICR proposed by the Intergroup Rhabdomyosarcoma Study.[198] The concept of pleomorphic rhabdomyosarcoma has changed considerably since its inclusion in the Horn and Enterline classification scheme reported in 1958.[123] One-third of the 39 tumors in their study were designated pleomorphic rhabdomyosarcomas, most of which arose in the deep soft tissues of the extremities of adults. Numerous studies during the 1960s described the clinical and pathologic features of pleomorphic rhabdomyosarcoma,[2,162,206,215] and this tumor was reported to account for between 9%[276] and 14%[206] of all soft tissue sarcomas. However, with the emergence of the concept of malignant fibrous histiocytoma (MFH), many pleomorphic rhabdomyosarcomas were reclassified as storiform pleomorphic variants of MFH,[135,296] and this rhabdomyosarcoma variant subsequently became regarded as rare[75,295] or nonexistent.[265] Subsequently, with the advent of immunohistochemistry and refinement in recognizing tumors with skeletal muscle differentiation, several studies confirmed the existence of pleomorphic rhabdomyosarcoma[92,256] and delineated criteria by which this sarcoma could be distinguished from other pleomorphic sarcomas.

Most of these tumors arise in adults (mean age 56 years).[92] The youngest patient in a study by Gaffney et al. was 27 years of age,[92] although Hollowood and Fletcher recorded encountering this tumor in a 13-year-old.[122] Most series have shown a predilection for

**TABLE 22–10 FREQUENCY OF *PAX3-FKHR* AND *PAX7-FKHR* FUSION TRANSCRIPTS IN ALVEOLAR AND EMBRYONAL RHABDOMYOSARCOMAS**

| | Alveolar | | Embryonal | |
|---|---|---|---|---|
| **Study** | ***PAX3-FKHR*** | ***PAX7-FKHR*** | ***PAX3-FKHR*** | ***PAX7-FKHR*** |
| Barr[13] | 16/21 (76%) | 2/21 (10%) | 1/30 (3%) | 1/30 (3%) |
| De Alava[52] | 7/13 (54%) | 2/13 (15%) | 0/9 (0%) | 0/9 (0%) |
| Downing[69] | 20/23 (87%) | — | 2/12 (17%) | — |
| Arden[7] | 8/13 (62%) | 1/13 (8%) | 0/11 (0%) | 0/11 (0%) |
| *Total* | 51/70 (73%) | 5/47 (11%) | 3/62 (5%) | 1/50 (2%) |

this tumor to arise in males. For example, Gaffney et al. reported 10 of 11 patients with this tumor to be male.[92] The tumor most commonly arises in the skeletal muscle of the extremities, particularly the thigh,[92,256] although rare tumors arise in the chest wall musculature,[92,256] retroperitoneum,[92,256] and head and neck.[53] Most present with a rapidly growing, painless mass of several months' duration; some present with pulmonary metastases.[122]

The tumor is usually large (> 10 cm), and most are fleshy, well-circumscribed, intramuscular masses with focal hemorrhage and extensive necrosis. Histologically, pleomorphic rhabdomyosarcoma can be distinguished from embryonal and alveolar rhabdomyosarcoma by the association of loosely arranged, haphazardly oriented, large, round or pleomorphic cells with hyperchromatic nuclei and deeply eosinophilic cytoplasm (Figs. 22–39, 22–40). As in embryonal rhabdomyosarcomas, there are racket-shaped and tadpole-shaped rhabdomyoblasts, but they are generally larger with more irregular outlines. Cells with cross-striations are commonly found in embryonal rhabdomyosarcomas with focal pleomorphic features[143] but are rare in adult pleomorphic rhabdomyosarcomas.[92,188] The tumor cells may be arranged in a haphazard pattern, but arrangement in a storiform pattern suggestive of MFH or a fascicular pattern reminiscent of leiomyosarcoma may be present (Fig. 22–41). The most helpful light microscopic feature that suggests this diagnosis is the presence of large bizarre tumor cells with deeply eosinophilic cytoplasm (Fig. 22–42). Rare lesions have cells with a rhabdoid morphology characterized by the presence of a peripherally located vesicular nucleus, with a prominent nucleolus and an intracytoplasmic eosinophilic hyaline inclusion.[92,256] Other features include phagocytosis by tumor cells, the presence of intracytoplasmic glycogen, and a moderately dense lymphohistiocytic infiltrate.

Ancillary techniques are required to confirm the diagnosis of pleomorphic rhabdomyosarcoma. Immunohistochemical detection of sarcomeric differentiation using antibodies to desmin (Fig. 22–43), muscle-specific actin, myoglobin, and sarcomeric $\alpha$-actin, is extremely useful. Wesche et al.[298] reported the high sensitivity and specificity of the MyoD1 antibody in recognizing pleomorphic rhabdomyosarcoma and its distinction from other adult pleomorphic soft tissue sarcomas.

The ultrastructural features of pleomorphic rhabdomyosarcomas are similar to those of other rhabdomyosarcoma subtypes.[78] The tumor cells range from undifferentiated cells to those showing alternating thin and thick filaments with Z-band material to cells with well defined sarcomeres.[233,297]

The differential diagnosis includes a variety of other pleomorphic sarcomas and many other tumors that may simulate a pleomorphic sarcoma. First, the

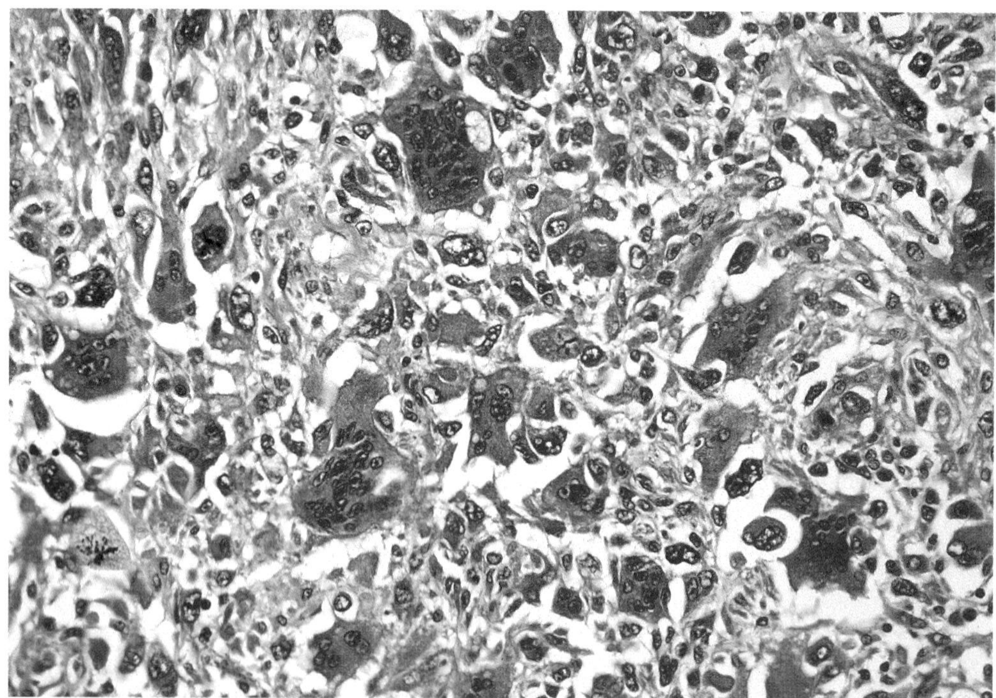

**FIGURE 22–39.** Pleomorphic rhabdomyosarcoma. This tumor was found in the deep soft tissues of the thigh in a 69-year-old man.

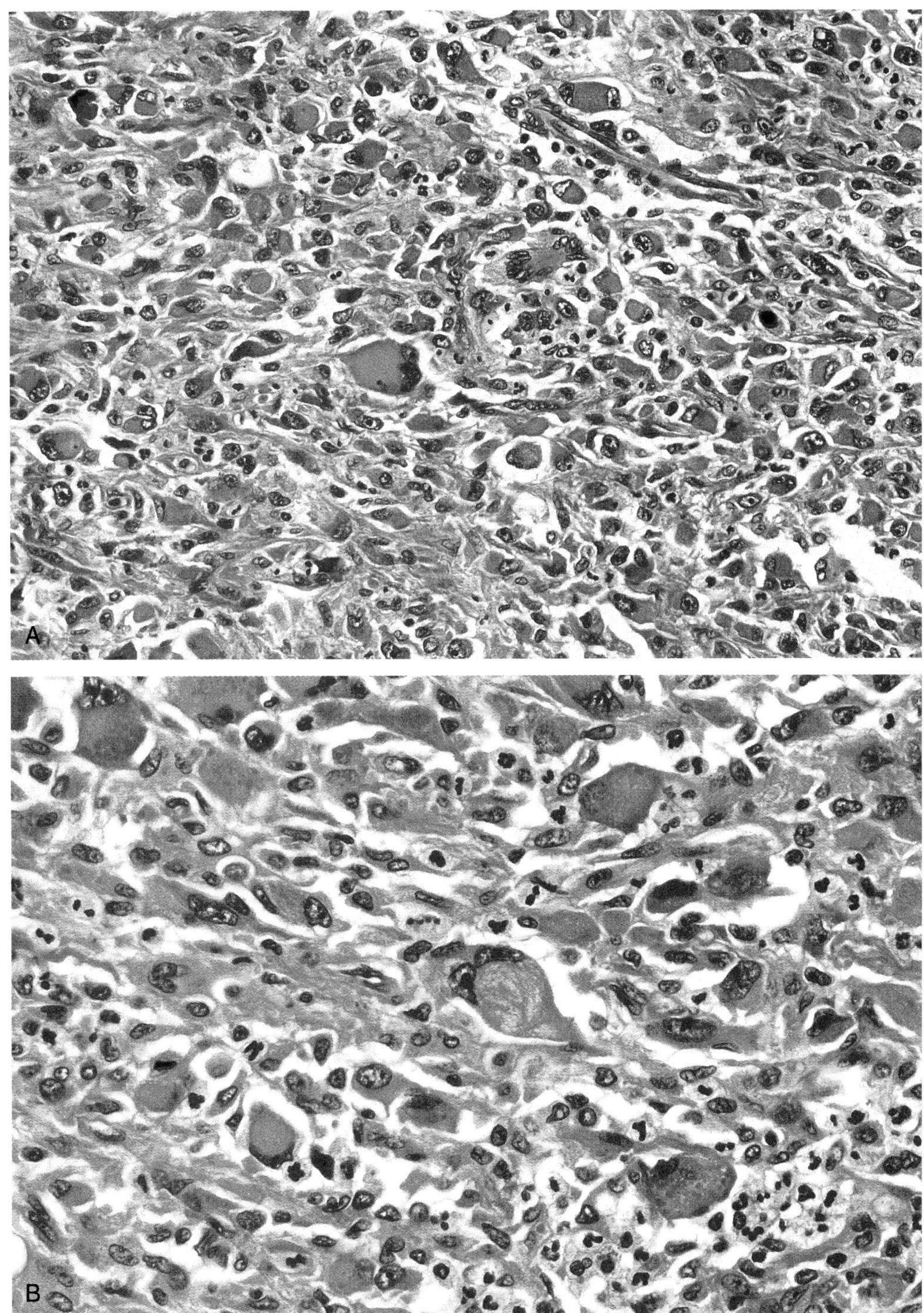


**FIGURE 22–40.** (**A**) Pleomorphic rhabdomyosarcoma composed predominantly of spindle-shaped cells with scattered large cells containing deeply eosinophilic cytoplasm. (**B**) Large cells with eosinophilic stringy cytoplasm in a pleomorphic rhabdomyosarcoma.

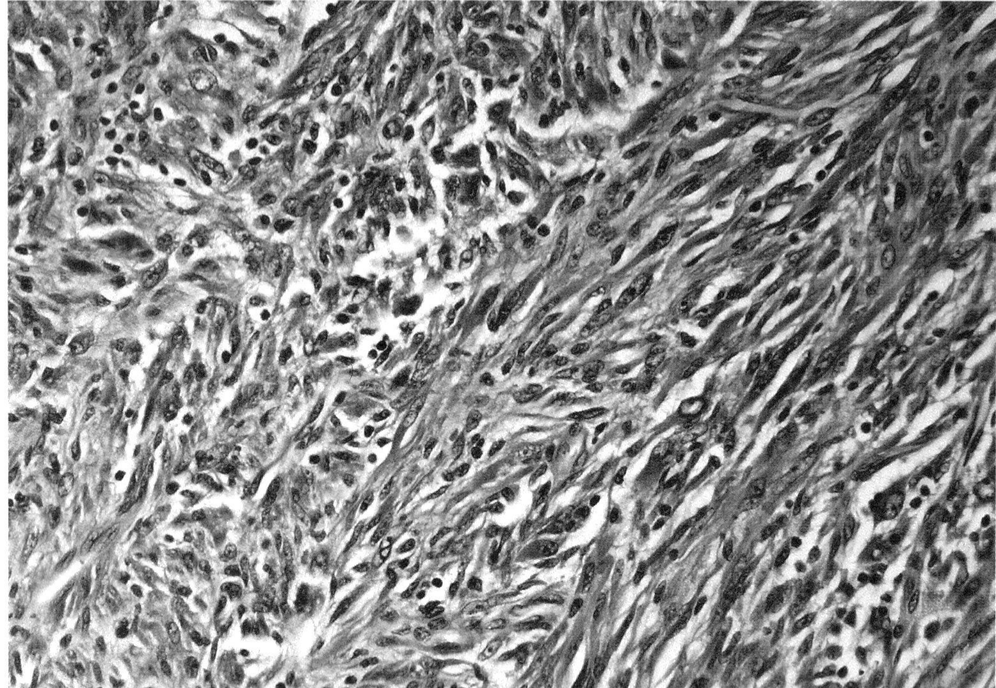

**FIGURE 22-41.** Pleomorphic rhabdomyosarcoma composed of spindle-shaped cells arranged in a fascicular pattern reminiscent of leiomyosarcoma.

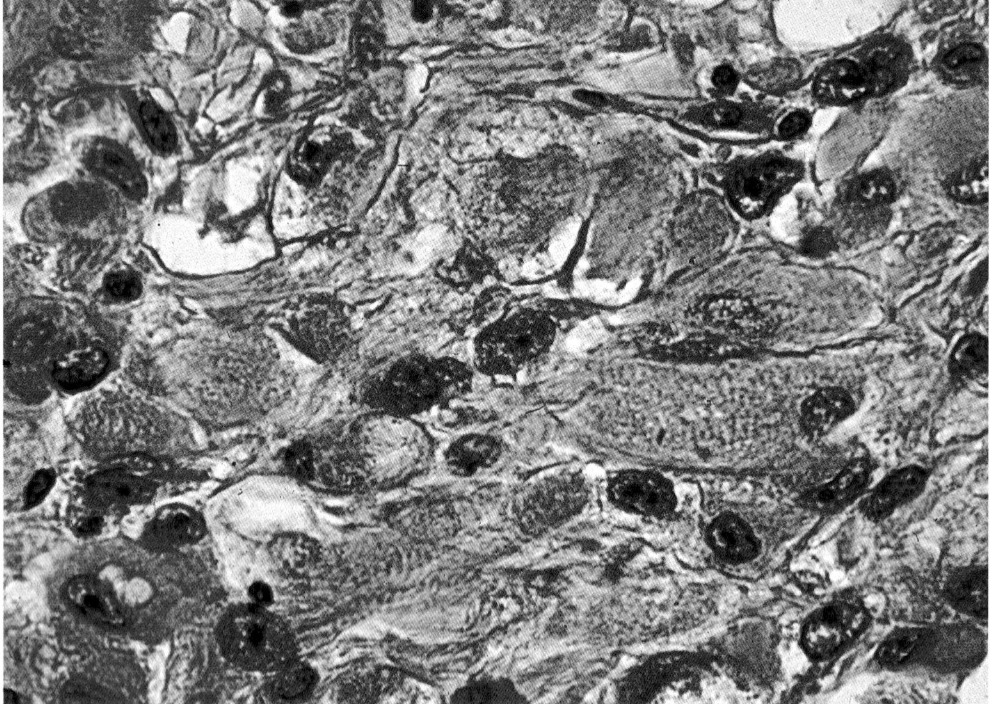

**FIGURE 22-42.** Unusual pleomorphic rhabdomyosarcoma. This focus was composed of numerous cells with eosinophilic fibrillar cytoplasm and cross-striations. Other portions of this tumor more closely resembled malignant fibrous histiocytoma.

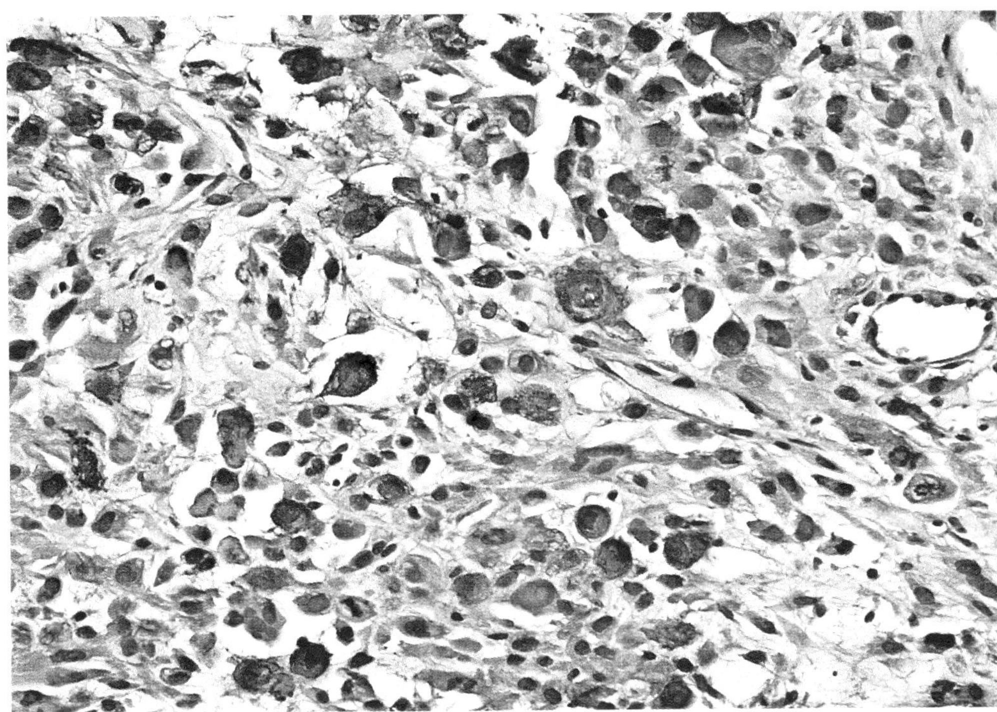

**FIGURE 22–43.** Desmin immunoreactivity in large eosinophilic cells in a pleomorphic rhabdomyosarcoma.

pleomorphic rhabdomyosarcoma should be distinguished from the other rhabdomyosarcoma subtypes, all of which may have foci of pleomorphic cells. Adequate sampling of these tumors usually reveals more typical areas of embryonal or alveolar rhabdomyosarcoma. Furthermore, pleomorphic rhabdomyosarcoma occurs in adults, whereas the other subtypes are seen mostly in children or adolescents and are rare in adults. Pleomorphic rhabdomyosarcoma may be arranged in a fascicular growth pattern reminiscent of that seen in *pleomorphic leiomyosarcoma.* However, most cases of pleomorphic leiomyosarcoma have lower-grade areas that display a well defined fascicular pattern composed of cells with typical smooth muscle features. Both tumors are immunoreactive for actin and desmin; but immunostains for myoglobin, fast myosin, MyoD1, and myogenin are useful for recognizing pleomorphic rhabdomyosarcomas. Ultrastructurally, the identification of ribosome–myosin complexes and hexagonal arrays of thick and thin filaments help identify a tumor as a pleomorphic rhabdomyosarcoma.

Although some have questioned the concept of *malignant fibrous histiocytoma* as a distinct entity,[88] there remains a group of pleomorphic sarcomas in which, following evaluation with immunohistochemical or electron microscopic techniques (or both), a specific line of cellular differentiation cannot be determined. It is these tumors that, by convention, have been termed MFH. They contain large eosinophilic giant cells often with a finely vacuolated cytoplasm (unlike the coarsely vacuolated "spider web" cells of rhabdomyosarcoma) and are associated with occasional xanthoma cells and a prominent inflammatory component. The distinction of pleomorphic rhabdomyosarcoma from MFH ultimately requires identification of sarcomeric differentiation, even if only focally present. Because of the lack of specificity of desmin and actin in various pleomorphic sarcomas,[121,156] this distinction is best made using more specific antibodies such as MyoD1 or myogenin,[280,298] or by electron microscopy.

Like other pleomorphic sarcomas, pleomorphic rhabdomyosarcoma is a clinically aggressive neoplasm that frequently metastasizes early in its course.[122] In the series by Gaffney et al.,[92] seven of eight patients for whom follow-up information was available died, including five within 8 months of diagnosis.

## SPECIAL DIAGNOSTIC PROCEDURES

### Special Stains

Although many rhabdomyosarcomas can be diagnosed with hematoxylin-eosin-stained sections on the basis of their histologic features or patterns, many poorly differentiated sarcomas masquerade as rhabdomyosarcomas, and ancillary diagnostic procedures are often essential for an objective and reliable diagnosis. During the past decade conventional special stains, such as the periodic acid-Schiff (PAS) preparation or the Masson trichrome stain, have become much less important for diagnosis and have been largely replaced by immunohistochemical procedures or electron microscopic study of the tumor. Despite the greatly diminished role of conventional stains, Masson trichrome stain, phosphotungstic acid hematoxylin (PTAH), and iron-hematoxylin stain complement the morphologic findings and facilitate scanning multiple sections for the presence of differentiated cells (rhabdomyoblasts) among poorly differentiated cellular elements. These stains, however, lack specificity and stain both myofibrils and other cellular and extracellular structures. Other stains, such as the PAS preparation with and without diastase, are useful for the differential diagnosis of small-cell tumors, as most rhabdomyosarcomas contain considerable amounts of intracellular PAS-positive glycogen; in many tumors the glycogen is irregularly distributed and as a rule is much more conspicuous in well differentiated than poorly differentiated tumor cells. Extracellular mucinous material stains positively with colloidal iron and alcian blue and is removed by prior treatment of the sections with hyaluronidase. Reticulin preparations usually reveal little interstitial collagen, but fibrosis may be marked in tumors of the alveolar type.

## Immunohistochemical Procedures

Many immunohistochemical markers have been applied to the diagnosis of rhabdomyosarcoma, but their diagnostic value, sensitivity, and specificity vary substantially (Table 22–11); not all of the reported markers are commercially available. Of the various markers, antibodies against desmin (for the muscle type of intermediate filaments),[3–5,10] muscle-specific actin (HHF35),[10,181,193,231,241] and myoglobin[43,79,140,192] have been the most widely used for diagnostic purposes. These markers can be used with frozen and alcohol-fixed material as well as with formalin-fixed tissue, even after years in paraffin.

Desmin is a particularly sensitive marker of rhabdomyosarcoma using frozen tissues,[187,214] although there is a loss of sensitivity with formalin fixation (Fig. 22–44).[10,157,214] Rhabdomyosarcomas composed predominantly of primitive cells may not stain for desmin,[258,269] and this marker is not useful for distinguishing rhabdomyosarcoma from leiomyosarcoma. The sensitivity of desmin can be increased using antigen retrieval techniques,[304] although desmin is not entirely specific: It has been detected in a number of nonmyogenic tumors, including primitive neuroectodermal tumors, neuroblastomas, and malignant mesotheliomas.[127,213] Similarly, muscle-specific actin, although a sensitive marker of rhabdomyosarcoma, is not useful for distinguishing this tumor from leiomyosarcoma. This antigen is more resistant to formalin fixation than desmin[255] but may also be negative in poorly differentiated rhabdomyosarcomas. Smooth muscle actin is an excellent marker of tumors with smooth muscle differentiation, but it may be found in up to 13% of rhabdomyosarcomas.[257,304]

Sarcomeric $\alpha$-actin has also been reported to be a specific marker of rhabdomyosarcoma.[31,55,257] Monoclonal antibodies recognize both cardiac and skeletal $\alpha$-actin; however, Schürch et al.[257] found that all variants of rhabdomyosarcoma express cardiac $\alpha$-actin transcripts but not skeletal $\alpha$-actin mRNA by Northern blot hybridization. Because cardiac $\alpha$-actin is present in embryonic skeletal muscle,[250] these authors suggested that rhabdomyosarcomas follow normal skeletal myogenesis but do not complete the final step of skeletal $\alpha$-actin mRNA expression.

Myoglobin, although a specific marker of skeletal muscle tumors, is not particularly sensitive.[80,214,262,285] For example, Parham et al.[214] reported staining for myoglobin in only 17 (46%) of 37 formalin-fixed rhabdomyosarcomas. Furthermore, staining tends to be re-

**TABLE 22–11** IMMUNOHISTOCHEMICAL EXPRESSION OF VARIOUS MYOGENIC MARKERS IN 95 RHABDOMYOSARCOMAS

| Rhabdomyosarcoma Subtype | Positive Staining (%) | | | | |
|---|---|---|---|---|---|
| | *Desmin* | *Actin (HHF-35)* | *Sarcomeric Actin* | *Troponin-T* | *Smooth Muscle Actin* |
| Embryonal ($n$ = 61) | 95 | 95 | 73 | 87 | 14 |
| Alveolar ($n$ = 19) | 100 | 100 | 61 | 67 | 11 |
| Botryoid ($n$ = 9) | 100 | 100 | 63 | 89 | 0 |
| Spindle cell ($n$ = 6) | 100 | 100 | 83 | 83 | 0 |

Modified from Wijnaendts LCD, van der Linden JC, van Unnik AJM, et al. The expression pattern of contractile and intermediate filament proteins in developing skeletal muscle and rhabdomyosarcoma of childhood: diagnostic and prognostic utility. Am J Pathol 174:283, 1994.

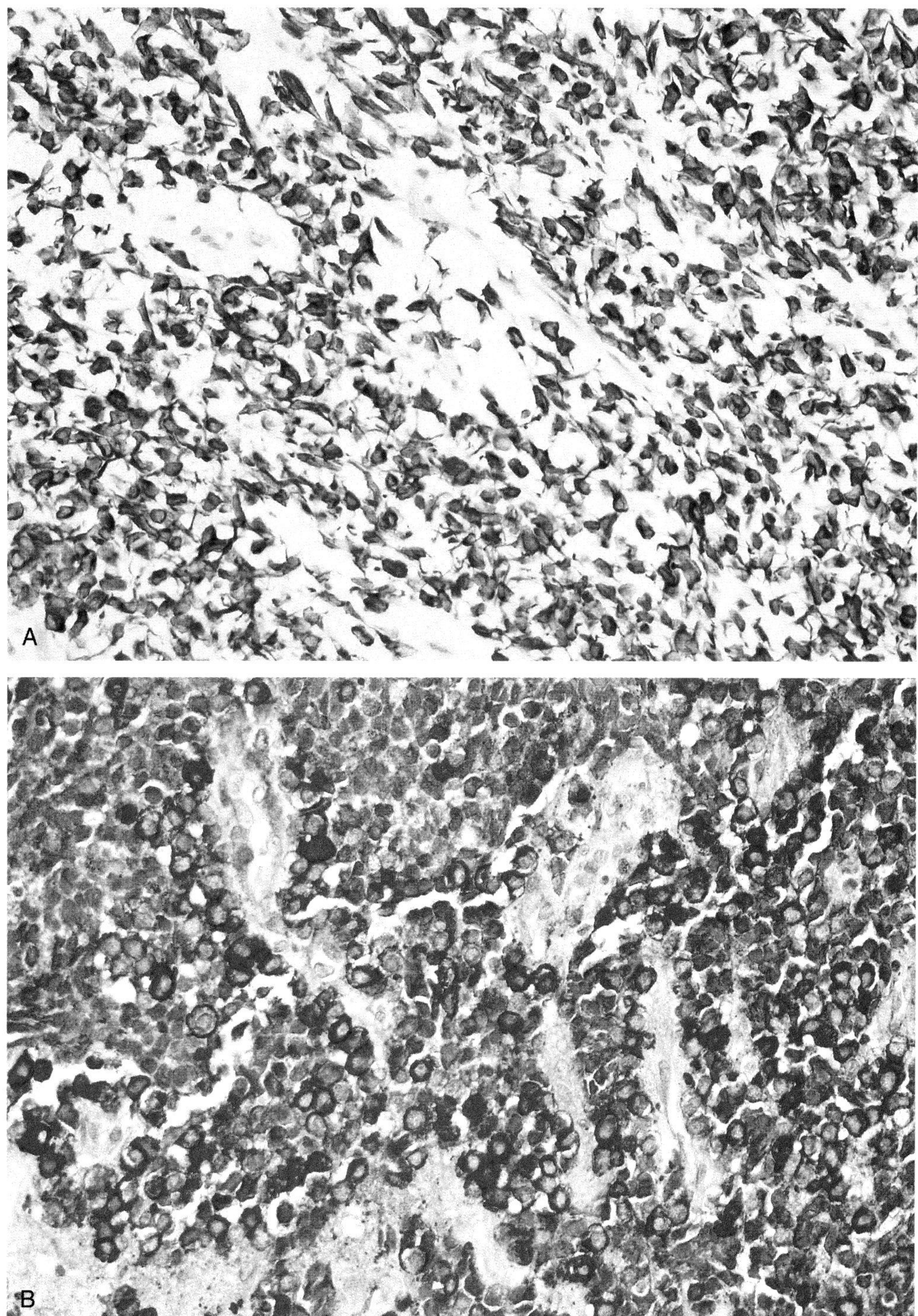

**FIGURE 22–44.** Diffuse, strong immunoreactivity for desmin in an embryonal rhabdomyosarcoma (**A**) and an alveolar rhabdomyosarcoma (**B**).

stricted to the more differentiated cells, and this antigen may also be detected in nonmuscle cells as a result of diffusion.[79]

Other, somewhat less sensitive markers that have been used in the diagnosis of rhabdomyosarcoma include antibodies for fast, slow, and fetal myosin,[56,81] creatine kinase (isoenzymes MM and BB),[54,287] $\beta$-enolase,[243] Z-protein,[191] titin,[32,204] and vimentin.[142,264] Vimentin is co-expressed in virtually all rhabdomyosarcomas but is more prominent in undifferentiated than well differentiated tumors. Primitive rhabdomyosarcomas may stain negatively for vimentin, however.[187] Because vimentin is present in a variety of sarcomas and carcinomas, its diagnostic utility is minimal. Cytokeratin and S-100 protein have also been demonstrated in occasional undifferentiated tumor cells and rhabdomyoblasts, respectively.[40,183] Of course, many malignant Triton tumors (malignant peripheral nerve sheath tumors with rhabdomyoblastic differentiation) contain, in addition to rhabdomyoblasts, nerve sheath elements that stain positively for S-100 protein. Neural cell adhesion molecules and isoforms of neurofilament protein have also been detected in some rhabdomyosarcomas.[185]

More recently, immunohistochemical expression of myoregulatory proteins has been found to be an excellent marker of all rhabdomyosarcoma subtypes, showing high sensitivity and specificity (Table 22–12). MyoD1, the best-studied member of a family of myogenic regulatory genes, which includes *myf-5* and *mrf-4-herculin/myf-6*, acts as a nodal point for the initiation of skeletal muscle differentiation by binding to enhancer sequences of muscle-specific genes.[48,91,293,294] These genes are expressed at an early stage of striated muscle differentiation[284] and are capable of converting multipotential murine fibroblasts into myoblasts.[50] The MyoD1 gene (*MYOD1*), located on the short arm of chromosome 11,[97] encodes a transcript and a 45-kDa nuclear phosphoprotein that can be detected by Northern blot analysis[37] and immunohistochemical analysis, respectively. Although originally detected only using frozen tissues,[59,60,281] antigen retrieval techniques have allowed detection of this antigen in formalin-fixed paraffin-embedded tissues.[73,286,292] Detection of this nuclear antigen is useful in the differential diagnosis of pediatric small round cell tumors[292] and for distinguishing pleomorphic rhabdomyosarcoma from other pleomorphic sarcomas of adulthood.[281,298] Wang et al.,[292] using formalin-fixed paraffin-embedded tissues and antigen retrieval techniques, detected nuclear expression of MyoD1 in 30 (91%) of 33 rhabdomyosarcomas, with no significant differences in sensitivity among the various histologic subtypes. Furthermore, none of the peripheral primitive neuroectodermal tumors or neuroblastomas demonstrated nuclear immunoreactivity for this antigen. Similarly, these authors found an equal percentage of lesions to stain with antibodies to myogenin. The anti-myogenin antibody was found to have technical advantages over the anti-MyoD1 antibody in that there was an absence of nonspecific cytoplasmic immunoreactivity, which was sometimes seen with the anti-MyoD1 antibody (Fig. 22–45). Expression of both MyoD1 and myogenin was reciprocally related to the degree of cellular differentiation, with more primitive-appearing cells staining and decreased or absent immunoreactivity in large differentiated rhabdomyoblasts.

## Ultrastructural Findings

The ultrastructure of rhabdomyosarcoma bears a striking resemblance to that of embryonal muscle tissue in varying stages of development, but there is a much wider spectrum in the appearance of the tumor cells. The tumor cells range from primitive undifferentiated cells with few organelles to highly differentiated cells with abundant but often incomplete sarcomeres. In the least differentiated cells the cytoplasm may contain only scattered or parallel bundles of thin (actin) myofilaments measuring 6–8 nm in diameter;

**TABLE 22–12 IMMUNOREACTIVITY FOR MYOGENIC MARKERS IN RHABDOMYOSARCOMA AND OTHER PEDIATRIC ROUND CELL TUMORS**

| Tumor | Myogenin | MyoD1 | Actin (HHF-35) | Sarcomeric Actin | Desmin | Myoglobin |
|---|---|---|---|---|---|---|
| Rhabdomyosarcomas | 30/33 | 30/33 | 30/33 | 21/33 | 33/33 | 8/28 |
| Embryonal | 22/25 | 23/25 | 22/25 | 18/25 | 25/25 | 6/20 |
| Spindle cell | 1/1 | 1/1 | 1/1 | 1/1 | 1/1 | 0/1 |
| Alveolar | 4/4 | 3/4 | 4/4 | 3/4 | 4/4 | 1/4 |
| Pleomorphic | 3/3 | 3/3 | 3/3 | 2/3 | 3/3 | 1/3 |
| pPNETs | 0/26 | 0/26 | 0/26 | 0/6 | 3/26 | 0/6 |
| Neuroblastomas | 0/12 | 0/12 | 0/12 | 0/12 | 0/12 | 0/12 |

Modified from Wang NP, Marx J, McNutt MA, et al. Expression of myogenic regulatory proteins (myogenin and MyoD1) in small blue round cell tumors of childhood. Am J Pathol 147:1799, 1995.
pPNET, peripheral primitive neuroectodermal tumors.

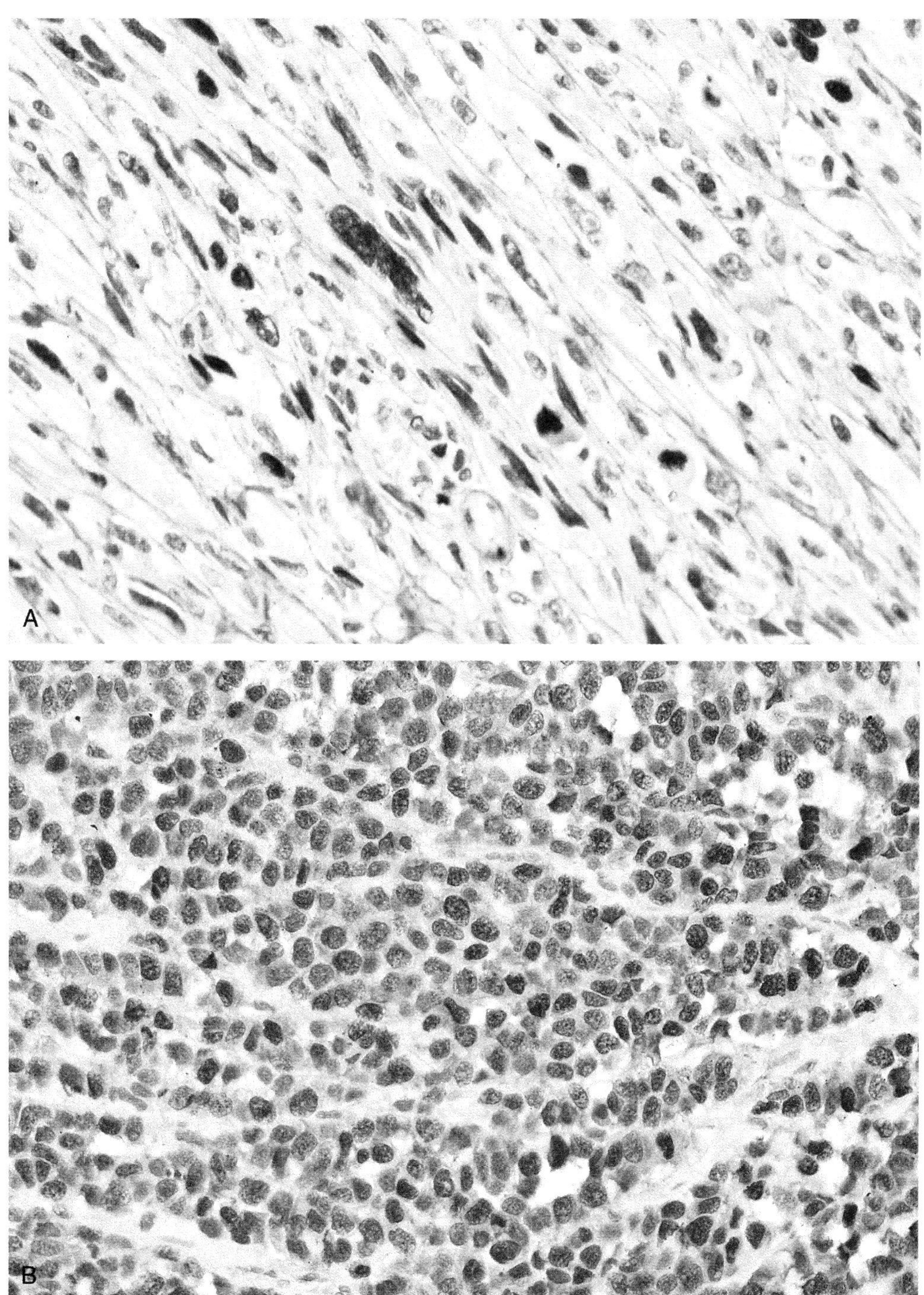


**FIGURE 22–45.** Nuclear staining for myogenin in an embryonal rhabdomyosarcoma (**A**) and an alveolar rhabdomyosarcoma (**B**).

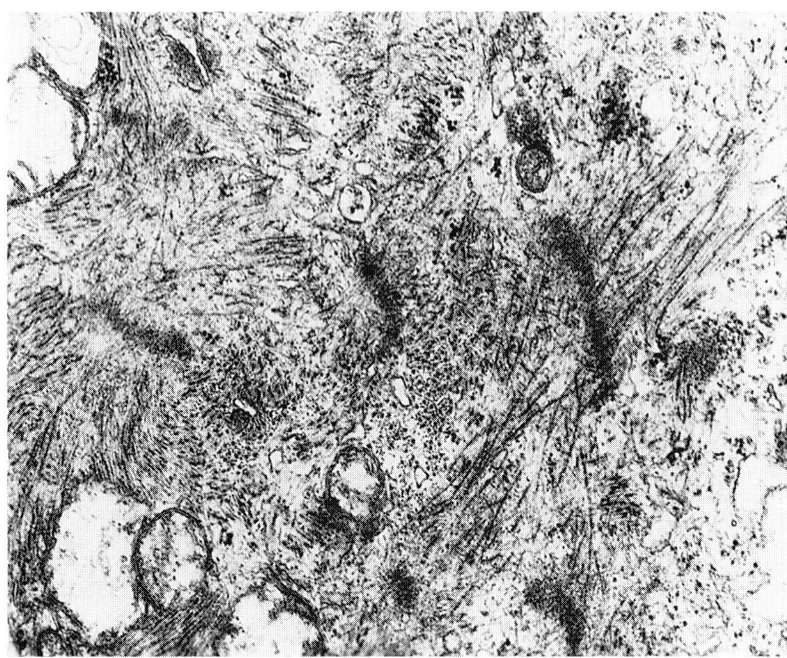

**FIGURE 22–46.** Ultrastructure of an embryonal rhabdomyosarcoma with a typical mixture of thick (myosin) and thin (actin) fibrils in longitudinal and cross section with distinct Z banding in several places.

this is a nonspecific finding that does not permit a reliable diagnosis of rhabdomyosarcoma; better differentiated cells are characterized by distinct bundles of thick (myosin) filaments 12–15 nm in diameter, with attached ribosomes having an Indian-file arrangement (ribosome and myosin complex), a feature characteristic of rhabdomyoblastic differentiation. Further cellular maturation is marked by alternating thin (actin) and thick (myosin) filaments in a parallel arrangement, with a characteristic hexagonal pattern seen on cross sections and rod-like structures or disks composed of Z-band material. In many tumors there are also well differentiated rhabdomyoblasts with distinct sarcomeres, including the characteristic A and I banding and clearly discernible Z lines (Fig. 22–46).[78,180,189] Entrapped degenerated muscle fibers can be recognized ultrastructurally by the presence of autolysosomes.[263]

In addition to the myofilaments, the cytoplasm of the rhabdomyoblasts contains a prominent Golgi apparatus and varying numbers of mitochondria and glycogen particles. There are also small lysosomes, droplets of lipid, occasional pinocytotic vesicles, and complete or incomplete basal lamina. The multinucleated giant cells, characteristic of the alveolar type, have neither myofilaments nor basal laminae.[36] Gaffney et al.,[92] examining six pleomorphic rhabdomyosarcomas, found the typical ultrastructural features of this tumor in only two cases. The remaining four tumors showed only collections of nonspecific filamentous material.

## DIFFERENTIAL DIAGNOSIS

Poorly differentiated round and spindle cell sarcomas, especially in children or young adults, constitute the most common problem for the differential diagnosis. Included in this group are neuroblastomas, peripheral primitive neuroectodermal tumors (including peripheral neuroepithelioma and extraskeletal Ewing's sarcoma), poorly differentiated angiosarcomas, synovial sarcomas, malignant melanomas, melanotic neuroectodermal tumors of infancy, granulocytic sarcomas, and malignant lymphomas. Small-cell carcinoma must also be considered when the tumor occurs in a patient older than 45 years. The differential diagnosis requires not only careful evaluation of the clinical data, the age of the patient, and the location of the lesion, but also painstaking examination of multiple sections for specific features such as rhabdomyoblasts, rosettes, biphasic cellular or vascular differentiation, and intracellular pigment, as well as immunohistochemical assessment of the tumor with multiple markers. Special stains may also help. For example, intracellular glycogen, which stains positively with PAS and can be removed by diastase, is demonstrable in most rhabdomyosarcomas, Ewing's sarcomas, and malignant melanomas but is absent in most synovial sarcomas and malignant lymphomas. Other stains useful in the differential diagnosis are the Leder stain for naphthol AS-D chloracetate esterase and Fontana's stain or Warthin-Starry preparation for melanin.

Immunohistochemical analysis using a battery of stains is indispensible in this broad differential diagnosis. As mentioned previously, immunostains for muscle markers, including desmin, muscle-specific actin, and myoglobin, are frequently used; but each of these markers lacks complete sensitivity and specificity. The recent introduction of monoclonal antibodies to more specific myogenic proteins (MyoD1 and myogenin) offers marked advantages over the aforementioned markers. It must also be kept in mind that the product of the *MIC2* gene (HBA71 or CD99), although a highly sensitive marker of the peripheral primitive neuroectodermal tumor family, is rarely found in cases of embryonal or alveolar rhabdomyosarcoma.[116,259,273] The distinction of rhabdomyosarcoma from peripheral primitive neuroectodermal tumors and other round cell neoplasms is discussed in further detail in Chapter 32.

*Infantile rhabdomyofibrosarcoma,* described by Lundgren et al. in 1993,[168] is a rare tumor that resembles infantile fibrosarcoma but has ultrastructural and immunocytochemical evidence of rhabdomyoblastic differentiation. The spindle-shaped cells in this tumor express vimentin, desmin, smooth muscle actin, and sarcomeric actin; electron microscopy reveals fibroblastic and myofibroblastic features. The tumor shows cytogenetic alterations (monosomy 19 and monosomy 22) distinct from those found in either infantile fibrosarcoma or embryonal or alveolar rhabdomyosarcoma.

Rare *rhabdomyosarcomas with rhabdoid features* have been described. These lesions have cells with cytoplasmic globular inclusions composed of intermediate filaments.[145,217] Many other mesenchymal and nonmesenchymal neoplasms also contain clusters of perinuclear intermediate filaments resulting in a rhabdoid morphology. A battery of immunostains is often necessary to distinguish among these tumors, including stains for cytokeratins and myoregulatory proteins.[146,271,289]

Problems in diagnosis may also be caused by benign reactive and neoplastic lesions such as polypoid cystitis, polyps and pseudosarcomas of the vagina and vulva with atypical stromal cells,[201,205] pseudosarcoma of the vagina during pregnancy, infectious granuloma, proliferative myositis, skeletal muscle regeneration,[99] granular cell tumor, and fetal rhabdomyoma. Conversely, we have also encountered sparsely cellular botryoid-type rhabdomyosarcomas that were initially misinterpreted as *myxomas.* In these cases consideration of age and location usually provides the correct diagnosis, as myxomas are virtually nonexistent in children and almost never occur in visceral organs. For the differential diagnosis from *fetal rhabdomyoma* see Chapter 21.

Some tumors have *heterologous rhabdomyoblastic components.* Focal rhabdomyoblastic differentiation occurs in a variety of malignant neoplasms, including those with only sarcomatous differentiation, those with epithelial or germ cell elements, and tumors of neuroectodermal derivation (Table 22–13).[307] Identification of such elements may be obvious on light microscopic examination alone, but in some cases the use of immunohistochemical or electron microscopic techniques is required to support rhabdomyoblastic differentiation.

A variety of sarcomas contain rhabdomyoblastic elements. Malignant mesenchymoma, a tumor characterized by at least two distinctive lines of malignant mesenchymal differentiation, may contain rhabdomyoblastic foci,[27,197,291] but it is rare in our experience, particularly if rhabdomyosarcomas with cartilaginous or osseous metaplasia are excluded and diagnosed as rhabdomyosarcomas rather than malignant mesenchymomas. In addition, sarcomas with a propensity for undergoing dedifferentiation, including chondrosarcomas and liposarcomas, may have areas of so-called divergent rhabdomyoblastic differentiation.[114,236,280]

Epithelial tumors may also exhibit rhabdomyoblastic differentiation, including malignant mixed mesodermal tumors of the uterus, cervix, or ovary, carcinosarcomas of the breast and stomach, pulmonary blastomas, nephroblastomas, and mixed-type hepatoblastomas.[112,129] In fact, in rare neoplasms the rhabdomyoblastic component dominates the microscopic picture. Rhabdomyoblastic differentiation is also encountered in malignant or immature teratomas but rarely as a major element. In most of these tumors the rhabdomyoblastic component is accompanied by

**TABLE 22–13 TUMORS WITH HETEROLOGOUS RHABDOMYOBLASTIC COMPONENTS**

Tumors with epithelial components
- Carcinosarcoma (especially of breast, stomach, urinary bladder)
- Malignant mixed müllerian tumor (uterus, cervix, ovary)
- Wilms' tumor
- Hepatoblastoma
- Pulmonary blastoma
- Thymoma

Tumors with germ cell or sex cord elements
- Germ cell tumors (seminoma, teratoma)
- Sertoli-Leydig cell tumor

Tumors with only sarcomatous elements
- Malignant mesenchymoma
- Dedifferentiated chondrosarcoma
- Dedifferentiated liposarcoma

Tumors of neuroectodermal derivation
- Malignant peripheral nerve sheath tumor (malignant Triton tumor)
- Ectomesenchymoma
- Medulloepithelioma
- Medulloblastoma
- Congenital pigmented nevus (giant nevus)

Modified from Woodruff JM, Perino G. Non-germ-cell or teratomatous malignant tumors showing additional rhabdomyoblastic differentiation, with emphasis on the malignant Triton tumor. Semin Diagn Pathol 11:69, 1994.

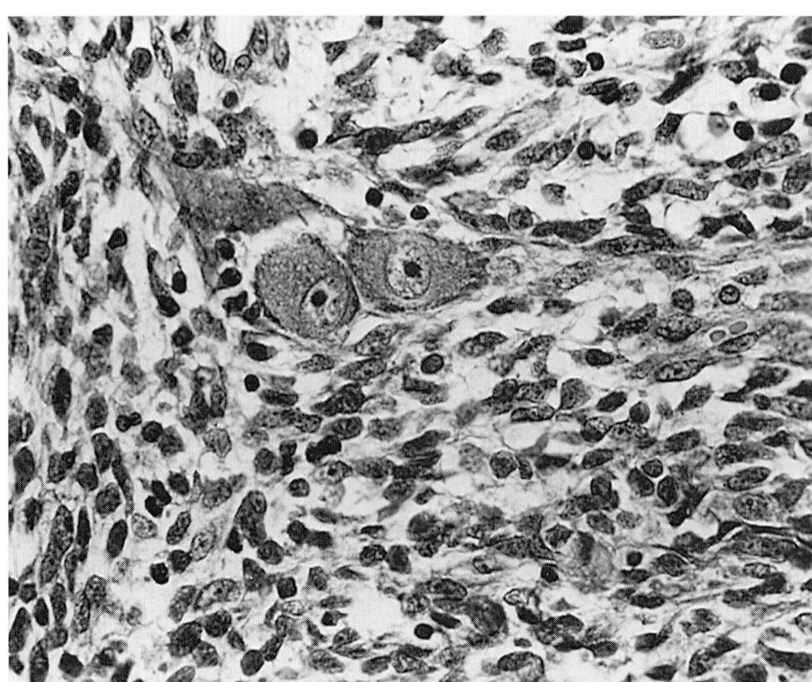

**FIGURE 22–47.** Malignant ectomesenchymoma of the scrotum in a 20-year-old man. Note the mature ganglion cells with a rhabdomyosarcoma-like tumor. Cells with cross-striations were present in another portion of this neoplasm.

malignant epithelial and other mesenchymal elements such as cartilage and bone. Rare ovarian Sertoli-Leydig cell tumors contain heterologous rhabdomyoblastic foci.[218]

Lastly, rhabdomyoblastic elements may be found in various neuroectodemal neoplasms, notably the malignant peripheral nerve sheath tumor (malignant Triton tumor and malignant glandular Triton tumor), ganglioneuroma (ectomesenchymoma), medulloepithelioma, and medulloblastoma. Malignant Triton tumors chiefly occur in patients older than 30 years who have manifestations of neurofibromatosis.[46,203,306] Malignant ectomesenchymoma is primarily a tumor of children and is not known to be associated with neurofibromatosis; it consists of a mixture of rhabdomyoblastic elements, mature ganglion cells, and neuroma-like structures (Fig. 22–47).[134] We have observed one case in which the initial tumor had features of an embryonal rhabdomyosarcoma and the recurrent tumor was indistinguishable from a ganglioneuroma save for a few peripherally located groups of rhabdomyoblasts (Fig. 22–48). We have also reviewed concurrent rhabdomyosarcoma of the retroperitoneum and pheochromocytoma in a 46-year-old woman.

## DISCUSSION

During the past 30–40 years the prognosis of rhabdomyosarcoma has improved dramatically. Prior to 1960 the prognosis was extremely poor, and there were few survivors even after radical, often destructive and disfiguring, surgical therapy. A 1963 follow-up study[76] based on 147 cases from the files of the AFIP showed that 90% of the patients died of the disease within a period of 5 years. In another AFIP study[77] devoted exclusively to alveolar rhabdomyosarcomas, the 5-year mortality rate was 98%. Others reported similar discouraging data: in 1965 Masson and Soule[174] reported a 5-year death rate of 88%, and in 1962 Dito and Batsakis[63] reported a 5-year death rate of 94% based on 170 rhabdomyosarcomas of the head and neck with an average survival time of 16 months.

Since the early 1960s there has been marked improvement in the survival rates of patients with rhabdomyosarcoma because of a multidisciplinary therapeutic approach that consists of biopsy or surgical removal of the neoplasm and multiagent chemotherapy with or without radiotherapy.[86,87,239] As a rule, treatment is carried out after biopsy or resection and careful, comprehensive assessment of tumor stage or tumor group with radiography, CT scans, MRI, and if necessary, angiograms. Recommendations for therapy chiefly depend on the stage or clinical group of the disease and the site of the tumor following accurate microscopic diagnosis. Because rhabdomyosarcomas tend to metastasize to bone marrow, bone marrow aspiration should be part of the staging process.

The IRS-II study, confined to patients younger than 21 years with a confirmed diagnosis of rhabdomyosarcoma, distinguished four clinical groups based on

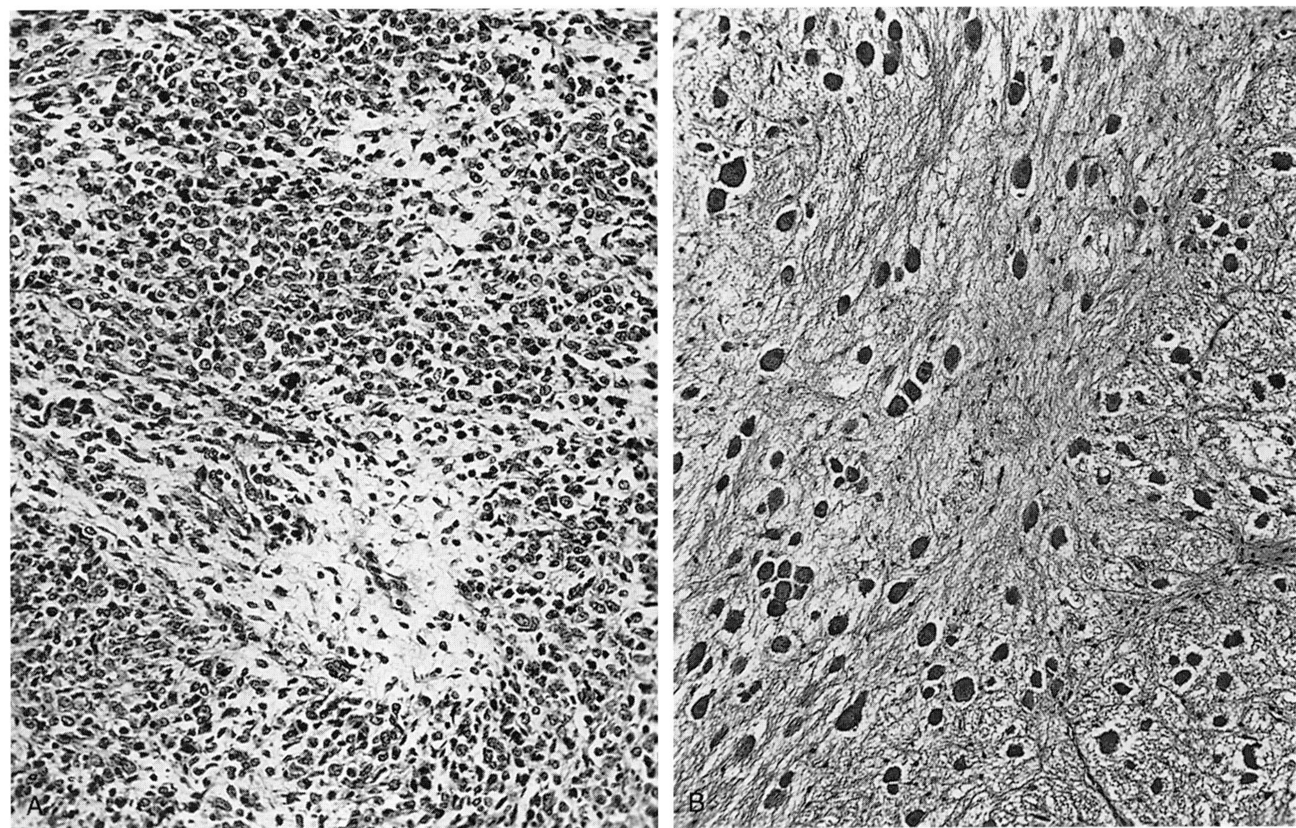


**FIGURE 22–48.** Malignant ectomesenchymoma of the pelvic retroperitoneum in a 1-year-old girl with rhabdomyosarcomatous features in the initial specimen (**A**) and a ganglioneuroma-like picture in the material obtained at autopsy (**B**). Rhabdomyoblasts with cross-striations and typical ganglion cells were present in the surgical material and occasional rhabdomyoblasts in the ganglioneuroma-like tumor removed at autopsy.

the amount of tumor remaining after initial surgery (Table 22–14). Because this approach is influenced by the variable approaches taken by surgeons, the IRS Committee adopted a modification of the tumor–node–metastasis (TNM) system,[154,238] which relies on pretreatment assessment of tumor extent.[211] This system includes evaluation of the site of the primary tumor, the maximum diameter of the tumor, determination of tumor invasion into adjacent structures, status of regional lymph nodes, and the presence or absence of distant metastases (Table 22–15). More recent studies of rhabdomyosarcoma rely on both the IRS clinical grouping system and the TNM stage to determine therapy. Both IRS clinical group and TNM stage have been found to have major prognostic significance (Table 22–16). According to the IRS-II study,[176] the prognosis is excellent for patients with groups I and II tumors, with 5-year survival rates of 85% and 88%, respectively (excluding alveolar rhabdomyosarcomas of the extremities); survival rates are less favorable for patients with group III tumors (66% five-year survival) (excluding some pelvic tumors) and poor for those with group IV tumors (26% five-year survival). Slightly better survival was obtained in each of the clinical groups in the IRS-III study.[45] Similarly, several studies have found a progressive decline in survival with increasing TNM stage.[155,238]

Additional factors that influence the clinical course of the disease and necessitate more intensive therapy include the anatomic site and histologic type of the tumor. According to data from the IRS-II study,[44,176,199] tumors of the orbit had the best prognosis (92% five-year survival) followed by tumors of the head and neck and nonbladder/prostate genitourinary tumors (about 80% five-year survival). A less favorable prognosis was found in patients whose tumors were located in a parameningeal location, bladder and prostate, and the extremities, with approximately 70% five-year survivals for each. The poorest prognosis was for patients with tumors at other sites, including the retroperitoneum, biliary tract, and peritoneum. In contrast to the findings of the IRS-II study, the data from the IRS-III study[45] found that patients with genitourinary bladder/prostate tumors

**TABLE 22–14 CLINICAL STAGING OF PATIENTS WITH RHABDOMYOSARCOMA (INTERGROUP RHABDOMYOSARCOMA STUDIES CLASSIFICATION)**

Group I
- Localized disease, completely resected (regional nodes not involved)
- Confined to muscle or organ of origin
- Contiguous involvement with infiltration outside the muscle or organ of origin, as through fascial planes

Group II
- Grossly resected tumor with microscopic residual disease
- No evidence of gross residual tumor; no evidence of regional node involvement
- Regional disease, completely resected (regional nodes involved, extension of tumor into an adjacent organ, or both); all tumor completely resected with no microscopic residual tumor
- Regional disease with involved nodes, grossly resected, but with evidence of microscopic residual disease

Group III
- Incomplete resection or biopsy with gross residual disease

Group IV
- Distant metastatic disease present at onset (lung, liver, bones, bone marrow, brain, distant muscle and nodes)

From Maurer HM, Beltangady M, Gehan EA, et al. The Intergroup Rhabdomyosarcoma Study I: a final report. Cancer 61:209, 1988, with permission.

fared approximately as well as those with head and neck tumors. Late detection and large tumor size, difficulties encountered during removal, extension into the meninges with or without spinal fluid spread, and an increased rate of lymph node metastasis are primarily responsible for the prognostic differences related to the anatomic sites.

Anatomic site is a major factor when determining the mode of therapy. For example, for rhabdomyosarcomas of the orbit, control is typically accomplished with biopsy, systemic chemotherapy, and irradiation alone.[120,144] In the few children with refractory orbital tumors, salvage surgery has also been found to be of some benefit.[172] Excellent results are achieved with rhabdomyosarcomas of the paratesticular region using radical orchiectomy with clear margins, radical retroperitoneal lymph node resection, and chemotherapy.[84,151,228] Tumors in parameningeal and paraspinal regions require extended irradiation and intrathecal chemotherapy to reduce local failure and spread of the disease.[17,230,234] Preoperative radiotherapy or chemotherapy for rhabdomyosarcomas of the urinary bladder and prostate usually allow less extensive surgical therapy and better functional preservation.[108,110,111,119,227] Total excision of the tumor is part of the recommended therapy for rhabdomyosarcomas in the trunk and extremities.[95,107,117,152]

Histologic subtype has been found to be an important independent prognostic variable by most investigators.[198,302,303] Patients with clinical group I alveolar rhabdomyosarcomas treated in the IRS-I and IRS-II studies fared worse than those with other rhabdomyosarcoma subtypes.[44] However, in the IRS-III study[45] alveolar histology did not adversely influence outcome in patients with localized tumors, probably owing to the more intensive therapy used for these patients. However, Newton et al.[198] found the histologic subtype to be strongly predictive of survival by multivariate analysis, in addition to the known prognostic factors of primary site, clinical group, and tumor size. The latter study established that the botryoid and spindle cell subtypes of embryonal rhabdomyosarcoma have a superior prognosis (95% and 88% five-year survivals, respectively); classic embryonal rhabdomyosarcoma has an intermediate prognosis (66% five-year survival); and the alveolar subtype, including solid alveolar rhabdomyosarcomas, has a poor prognosis, with a 54% five-year survival.

The degree of cellular differentiation (i.e., tumor cells resembling skeletal muscle cells) has been found by some to be of major prognostic significance.[254,303] Wijnaendts et al.[303] found that a greater degree of

**TABLE 22–15 TNM STAGING CLASSIFICATION FOR RHABDOMYOSARCOMA, AS MODIFIED BY THE IRS COMMITTEE**

| Stage | Sites | T* | Size* | N† | M‡ |
|---|---|---|---|---|---|
| 1 | Orbit, head and neck (excluding parameningeal sites); genitourinary (nonbladder/nonprostate) | T1 or T2 | a or b | N0 or N1 or Nx | M0 |
| 2 | Bladder/prostate; extremity; cranial parameningeal sites; other (e.g., trunk, retroperitoneum) | T1 or T2 | a | N0 or Nx | M0 |
| 3 | Bladder/prostate; extremity; cranial parameningeal sites; other (e.g., trunk, retroperitoneum) | T1 or T2 | a | N1 | M0 |
| | | | b | N0 or N1 or Nx | M0 |
| 4 | All | T1 or T2 | a or b | N0 or N1 | M1 |

Modified from Pappo AS, Shapiro DN, Crist WM, et al. Biology and therapy of pediatric rhabdomyosarcoma. J Clin Oncol 13:2123, 1995.

* Tumor: T (site) 1, confined to anatomic site of origin; (a) ≤5 cm, (b) >5 cm. T (site) 2, extension and/or fixation to surrounding tissue; (a) ≤5 cm, (b) >5 cm.

† Regional nodes: N0, regional nodes not clinically involved; N1, regional nodes clinically involved by neoplasm; Nx, status of regional nodes unknown.

‡ Metastasis: M0, no distant metastasis; M1, distant metastasis.

**TABLE 22-16 FAVORABLE AND UNFAVORABLE FACTORS FOR RHABDOMYOSARCOMAS**

Prognostically favorable factors
- Age: infants and children
- Orbital or genitourinary (nonbladder/prostate) location
- Small size (<5 cm)
- Botryoid or spindle cell type
- Localized noninvasive tumor without regional lymph node involvement or distant metastasis
- Complete initial resection

Prognostically unfavorable factors
- Age: adults
- Location in head and neck (nonorbital), paraspinal region, abdomen, biliary tract, retroperitoneum, perineum, or extremities
- Large size (>5 cm)
- Alveolar (especially *PAX3/FKHR* fusion transcript-positive) or pleomorphic type
- Diploid DNA content
- Local tumor invasion, especially parameningeal or paraspinal region, sinuses, or skeleton
- Local recurrence
- Local recurrence during therapy
- Regional lymph node involvement or distant metastasis
- Incomplete initial excision or unresectability

cellular maturation was associated with prolonged survival, independent of histologic subtype. In addition, it has been repeatedly documented that tumor cells may undergo therapy-induced cytodifferentiation.[39,47,179,186] Coffin et al.[39] found that botryoid and embryonal rhabdomyosarcoma subtypes were more likely to exhibit therapy-induced cytodifferentiation than other rhabdomyosarcoma subtypes. Furthermore, cytodifferentiation and decreased proliferative activity were associated with a favorable clinical course in patients with botryoid rhabdomyosarcoma.

Age at diagnosis is also an independent predictor of outcome in patients with rhabdomyosarocma.[44,153] Reboul-Marty et al.,[232] in a study of children with alveolar rhabdomyosarcomas, found a significantly lower disease-free survival in patients older than 10 years of age compared to that of younger patients. Age has its greatest prognostic effect on patients with invasive but nonmetastatic tumors.[153]

The mitotic rate is of little value for predicting therapeutic response and outcome of the disease, as it is elevated in most rhabdomyosarcomas.[12,104] Numerous studies have evaluated the possible prognostic value of flow cytometric DNA analysis in rhabdomyosarcomas.[26,35,139,149,184,194,210,266,301] Whereas some investigators have not found DNA ploidy to be of prognostic significance,[139] others claim that the technique is of independent prognostic value.[210,266] Tetraploidy is associated with alveolar morphology, whereas a hyperdiploid DNA content is associated with embryonal histology.[57,266] De Zen et al.[57] found a 73% five-year survival for patients with hyperdiploid tumors, compared to 33% and 25% five-year survivals for patients with diploid and tetraploid tumors, respectively. The MIB-1 index, measured by antibodies to the Ki-67 antigen, has not been found to correlate with histologic subtype or clinical outcome.[200]

The possible prognostic impact of various molecular alterations has been an area of intensive research in recent years. Accumulated intranuclear P53 protein has been detected by immunohistochemical techniques in a proportion of rhabdomyosarcomas.[83,136,194] Although some of these tumors harbor *p53* gene mutations, it appears that *MDM2* gene overexpression with subsequent *MDM2–p53* complex formation constitutes an alternative mechanism of inactivation of wild-type *p53* in some rhabdomyosarcomas.[136] The prognostic significance of *p53* alterations is still unknown. The *MYCN* oncogene, formerly known as N-*myc*, is amplified in up to 50% of alveolar rhabdomyosarcomas[58,70,101] but not in embryonal rhabdomyosarcomas. Thus far, *MYCN* gene amplification does not correlate with clinical behavior. P-glycoprotein, a product of the multiple drug resistance (*MDR*) gene, functions as a membrane transport system associated with chemotherapy resistance. P-glycoprotein immunoreactivity correlates with decreased survival of rhabdomyosarcoma patients in some studies[33] but not in others.[150] Finally, techniques such as RT-PCR and FISH to detect fusion transcripts may emerge as important tools for determining prognosis in this group of patients. Preliminary data suggest that in alveolar rhabdomyosarcomas the *PAX7/FKHR* fusion transcript is associated with a better prognosis than is the *PAX3/FKHR* fusion transcript.[138]

Long-term complications resulting from therapy depend on the location of the primary tumor. On occasion, treatment causes cataracts, xerophthalmia and craniofacial deformities, enteritis, acute or chronic diarrhea, intestinal obstruction, cystitis, hematuria, neutropenia, and excessive weight loss, among others.[225,230] Radiation therapy may affect growth and induce secondary tumors. There are also cases in which bone sarcoma or leukemia developed following successful treatment of rhabdomyosarcoma.[115,118,133] Occasionally, diffuse bone marrow involvement of an undifferentiated rhabdomyosarcoma leads to a mistaken diagnosis of leukemia.[85,131]

## RECURRENCE

Inadequately treated tumors grow in an infiltrative, destructive manner and recur in a high percentage of cases. Recurrence may herald metastasis, but by no means do all cases that recur metastasize. Bone does not constitute an effective barrier to growth of the tumor, and bone invasion is a frequent finding, particularly with rhabdomyosarcomas in the head and neck region and in the hands and feet. In the head and neck, the tumors tend to erode and destroy the bony walls of the orbit and sinuses, the temporal or mastoid bone, and the base of the skull; they may prove fatal because of extensive meningeal spread (parameningeal rhabdomyosarcomas) and spinal cord "drop metastases."[223,230] Tefft et al.[282] reported that 20 of 57 lesions located at parameningeal sites (nasopharynx, middle ear, paranasal sinuses) developed extension (or metastasis) to the meninges or subarachnoidal fluid. Meningeal spread may also occur with rhabdomyosarcomas at other sites.

## METASTASIS

Metastases develop during the course of the disease or, in about 20% of cases, are present at diagnosis.[154] Major metastatic sites are the lung, lymph nodes, and bone marrow followed by the heart, brain, meninges, pancreas, liver, and kidney. The lungs are involved in at least two-thirds of patients with metastasis.[229] The incidence of lymph node metastasis largely depends on the location of the tumor. It is higher with rhabdomyosarcomas of the prostate, paratesticular region, and extremities than with those of the orbit and head and neck.[154] In fact, exploration and biopsy of ipsilateral retroperitoneal lymph nodes is recommended when assessing paratesticular rhabdomyosarcomas.[228] It is also useful to keep in mind that alveolar rhabdomyosarcoma is one of the few soft tissue tumors in which lymph node metastasis may antedate discovery of the primary mass. Pratt et al.[219] reported a high incidence of metastasis to the heart; in their series of 23 fatal cases, 17 metastasized to the lung and 8 to both the bone marrow and the heart. There are also rare reports of multiple skin metastases as the primary manifestation of the disease.[105,253]

Microscopically, the recurrent and metastatic lesions may be less well differentiated than the primary growth; but unlike most other types of sarcoma, some recurrent or metastatic lesions for unknown reasons show a higher degree of differentiation. We have observed three cases where a positive diagnosis of rhabdomyosarcoma was possible only after rhabdomyoblasts with cross-striations were found in the pulmonary metastases. In addition, cytologic differentiation in rhabdomyosarcomas following polychemotherapy, probably due to "selective destruction of undifferentiated tumor cells,"[186] has been demonstrated in vitro[166] and in vivo.[39,47]

## REFERENCES


1. Adrassy RJ, Wiener ES, Raney RB, et al. Progress in the surgical management of vaginal rhabdomyosarcoma: a 25-year review from the Intergroup Rhabdomyosarcoma Study Group. J Pediatr Surg 34:731, 1999.

1a. Afify A, Mark HFL. Trisomy 8 in embryonal rhabdomyosarcoma detected by fluorescence in situ hybridization. Cancer Genet Cytogenet 108:127, 1999.

2. Albores-Saavedra J, Martin RG, Smith JL. Rhabdomyosarcoma: a study of 35 cases. Ann Surg 157:186, 1963.

3. Altmannsberger M, Dirk T, Osborn M, et al. Immunohistochemistry of cytoskeletal filaments in the diagnosis of soft tissue tumors. Semin Diagn Pathol 3:306, 1986.

4. Altmannsberger M, Osborn M, Treuner J, et al. Diagnosis of human childhood rhabdomyosarcoma by antibodies to desmin, the structural protein of muscle specific intermediate filaments. Virchows Arch [Cell Pathol] 39:203, 1982.

5. Altmannsberger M, Weber K, Droste R, et al. Desmin is a specific marker for rhabdomyosarcomas of human and rat origin. Am J Pathol 118:85, 1985.

6. Anderson J, Renshaw J, McManus A, et al. Amplification of the t(2;13) and t(1;13) translocations of alveolar rhabdomyosarcoma in small formalin-fixed biopsies using a modified reverse transcriptase polymerase chain reaction. Am J Pathol 150:477, 1997.

7. Arden KC, Anderson MJ, Finckenstein FG, et al. Detection of the t(2;13) chromosomal translocation in alveolar rhabdomyosarcoma using the reverse transcriptase-polymerase chain reaction. Genes Chromosomes Cancer 16:254, 1996.

8. Armstrong SJ, Duncan AW, Mott MG. Rhabdomyosarcoma with familial adenomatous polyposis. Pediatr Radiol 21:445, 1991.

9. Asmar L, Gehan EM, Newton WA Jr, et al. Agreement among and within groups of pathologists in the classification of rhabdomyosarcoma and related childhood sarcomas: report of an international study of four pathology classifications. Cancer 74: 2579, 1994.

10. Azumi N, Ben-Ezra J, Battifora H. Immunophenotypic diagnosis of leiomyosarcomas and rhabdomyosarcomas with monoclonal antibodies to muscle-specific actin and desmin in formalin-fixed tissue. Mod Pathol 1:469, 1988.

11. Balat O, Balat A, Verschraegen C, et al. Sarcoma botryoides of the uterine endocervix: long-term results of conservative surgery. Eur J Gynaecol Oncol 17:335, 1996.

12. Bale PM, Parsons RE, Stevens MM. Diagnosis and behavior of juvenile rhabdomyosarcoma. Hum Pathol 14:596, 1983.

13. Barr FG, Chatten J, D'Cruz CM, et al. Molecular assays for chromosomal translocations in the diagnosis of pediatric soft tissue sarcomas. JAMA 273:553, 1995.

14. Barr FG, Galili N, Holick J, et al. Rearrangement of the PAX 3 paired box gene in the paediatric solid tumour alveolar rhabdomyosarcoma. Nat Genet 3:113, 1993.

15. Barr FG, Holick J, Nycum L, et al. Localization of the t(2;13) breakpoint of alveolar rhabdomyosarcoma on a physical map of chromosome 2. Genomics 13:1150, 1992.

16. Bégin LR, Schürch W, Lacoste J, et al. Glycogen-rich clear cell rhabdomyosarcoma of the mediastinum: potential diagnostic pitfall. Am J Surg Pathol 18:302, 1994.

17. Benk V, Rodary C, Donaldson SS, et al. Paramaningeal rhabdomyosarcoma: results of an international workshop. Int J Radiat Oncol 36:533, 1996.

18. Bennicelli JL, Edwards RH, Barr FG. Mechanism for trancriptional gain of function resulting from chromosomal translocation in alveolar rhabdomyosarcoma. Proc Natl Acad Sci USA 93:5455, 1996.

19. Berry MP, Jenkin RDT. Parameningial rhabdomyosarcoma in the young. Cancer 48:281, 1981.

20. Besnard-Guérin C, Cavenee WK, Newsham I. A new highly polymorphic DNA restriction site marker in the 5′ region of the human tyrosine hydroxylase gene (TH) detecting the loss

of heterozygosity in human embryonal rhabdomyosarcoma. Hum Genet 93:349, 1994.
21. Besnard-Guérin C, Newsham I, Winqvist R, et al. A common region of loss of heterozygosity in Wilms' tumor and embryonal rhabdomyosarcoma distal to the d11S988 locus on chromosome 11p15.5. Hum Genet 97:163, 1996.
22. Biegel JA, Meek RS, Parmiter AH, et al. Chromosomal translocation t(1;13)(p36;q14) in a case of rhabdomyosarcoma. Genes Chromosomes Cancer 3:483, 1991.
23. Biegel JA, Nycum LM, Valentine V, et al. Detection of the t(2; 13)(q35;q14) and PAX 3-FKHR fusion in alveolar rhabdomyosarcoma by fluorescence in-situ hybridization. Genes Chromosomes Cancer 12:186, 1995.
24. Birch JM, Hartley AL, Blair V, et al. Cancer in the families of children with soft tissue sarcoma. Cancer 66:2239, 1990.
25. Boman F, Champigneulle J, Schmitt C, et al. Clear cell rhabdomyosarcoma. Pediatr Pathol Lab Med 16:951, 1996.
26. Boyle ET Jr, Reiman HM, Kramer SA, et al. Embryonal rhabdomyosarcoma of bladder and prostate: nuclear DNA patterns studied by flow cytometry. J Urol 140:1119, 1988.
27. Brady MS, Perino G, Tallini G, et al. Malignant mesechymoma. Cancer 77:467, 1996.
28. Buchwalter CL, Jenison EL, Fromm M, et al. Pure embryonal rhadomyosarcoma of the fallopian tube. Gynecol Oncol 67:95, 1997.
29. Caillaud JM, Gerard-Marchant R, Marsden HB, et al. Histopathological classification of childhood rhabdomyosarcoma: a report from the International Society of Pediatric Oncology Pathology Panel. Med Pediatr Oncol 17:391, 1989.
30. Callender TA, Reber RS, Janjan N, et al. Rhabdomyosarcoma of the nose and paranasal sinuses in adults and children. Otolaryngol Head Neck Surg 112:252, 1995.
31. Carter RL, Hall JM. A note on immunohistochemical staining for sarcomeric actin in rhabdomyosarcomas and other round cell tumors. Histopathology 21:575, 1992.
32. Cavazzana AO, Schmidt D, Ninfo V, et al. Spindle cell rhabdomyosarcoma: a prognostically favorable variant of rhabdomyosarcoma. Am J Surg Pathol 16:229, 1992.
33. Chan HFL, Thorner PS, Haddad G, et al. Immunohistochemical detection of P-glycoprotein: prognostic correlation in soft tissue sarcoma of childhood. J Clin Oncol 8:689, 1990.
34. Chen SY, Thakur A, Miller AS, et al. Rhabdomyosarcoma of the oral cavity: report of four cases. Oral Surg Oral Med Oral Pathol Oral Radiol Endod 80:192, 1995.
35. Chou P, Shen-Schwarz S, Crawford S, et al. DNA analysis of genitourinary rhabdomyosarcoma in children. Surg Pathol 4: 145, 1991.
36. Churg A, Ringus J. Ultrastructural observations on the histogenesis of alveolar rhabdomyosarcoma. Cancer 41:1355, 1978.
37. Clark J, Rocques PJ, Braun T, et al. Expression of members of the MYF gene family in human rhabdomyosarcomas. Br J Cancer 64:1039, 1991.
38. Coffin CM, Dehner LP. Pathologic evaluation of pediatric soft tissue tumors. Am J Clin Pathol 109 (Suppl 1):S38, 1998.
39. Coffin CM, Roulon J, Smith L, et al. Pathologic features of rhabdomyosarcoma before and after treatment: a clinicopathologic and immunohistochemical analysis. Mod Pathol 10:1175, 1997.
40. Coindre JM, de Mascarel A, Trojani M, et al. Immunohistochemical study of rhabdomyosarcoma: unexpected staining with S-100 protein and cytokeratin. J Pathol 155:127, 1988.
41. Colleoni M, Nelli P, Sgarbossa G, et al. Primary cutaneous rhabdomyosarcoma in adults: description of an uncommon aggressive disease. Acta Oncol 35:494, 1996.
42. Copeland LJ, Sneige N, Stringer A, et al. Alveolar rhadomyosarcoma of the female genitalia. Cancer 56:849, 1985.
43. Corson JM, Pinkus GS. Intracellular myoglobin: a specific marker for skeletal muscle differentiation in soft tissue sarcomas—an immunoperoxidase study. Am J Pathol 103:384, 1981.
44. Crist WM, Garnsey L, Beltangady MS, et al. Prognosis in children with rhabdomyosarcoma: a report of the Intergroup Rhabdomyosarcoma Studies I and II. J Clin Oncol 8:443, 1990.
45. Crist WM, Gehan EA, Ragab AH, et al. The Intergroup Rhabdomyosarcoma Study III. J Clin Oncol 13:610, 1995.
46. Daimaru Y, Hashimoto H, Enjoji M. Malignant "Triton" tumors: a clinicopathologic and immunohistochemical study of nine cases. Hum Pathol 15:768, 1984.
47. D'Amore EFG, Pollot M, Stracta-Pansa V, et al. Therapy associated differentiation in rhabdomyosarcomas. Mod Pathol 7:69, 1994.
48. Davis RL, Cheng PF, Lassar AB, et al. The MyoD DNA binding domain contains a recognition code for muscle-specific gene activation. Cell 60:733, 1990.
49. Davis RL, D'Cruz CM, Lovell MA, et al. Fusion of PAX 7 to FKHR by the variant t(1;13)(p36;q14) translocation in alveolar rhabdomyosarcoma. Cancer Res 54:2869, 1994.
50. Davis RL, Weintraub H, Lassar AB. Expression of a single transfected cDNA converts fibroblasts to myoblasts. Cell 51: 987, 1987.
51. Daya DA, Scully RE. Sarcoma botryoides of the uterine cervix in young women: a clinicopathologic study of 13 cases. Gynecol Oncol 229:290, 1988.
52. De Alava E, Ladanyi M, Rosai J, et al. Detection of chimeric transcripts in desmoplastic small round cell tumor and related developmental tumors by reverse transcriptase polymerase chain reaction: a specific diagnostic assay. Am J Pathol 147: 1584, 1995.
53. De Jong AS, van Kessel-van Vark M, Albus-Lutter CE. Pleomorphic rhabdomyosarcoma in adults: immunohistochemistry as a tool for its diagnosis. Hum Pathol 18:298, 1987.
54. De Jong AS, van Kessel-van Vark M, Albus-Lutter CE, et al. Creatine kinase subunits M and B as markers in the diagnosis of poorly differentiated rhabdomyosarcomas in children. Hum Pathol 16:924, 1985.
55. De Jong AS, van Kessel-van Vark M, Albus-Lutter CE, et al. Skeletal muscle actin as tumor marker in the diagnosis of rhabdomyosarcoma in childhood. Am J Surg Pathol 9:467, 1985.
56. De Jong AS, van Vark M, Albus-Lutter CE, et al. Myosin and myoglobin as tumor markers in the diagnosis of rhabdomyosarcoma: a comparative study. Am J Surg Pathol 8:521, 1984.
57. De Zen L, Sommaggio A, D'Amore ESG, et al. Clinical relevance of DNA ploidy and proliferative activity in childhood rhabdomyosarcoma: a retrospective analysis of patients enrolled onto the Italian Cooperative Rhabdomyosarcoma Study RMS 88. J Clin Oncol 15:11298, 1997.
58. Dias P, Kumar P, Marsden HB, et al. N-myc gene is amplified in alveolar rhadomyosarcomas (RMS) but not in embryonal rhabdomyosarcoma. Int J Cancer 45:593, 1990.
59. Dias P, Parham DM, Shapiro DN, et al. Monoclonal antibodies to the myogenic regulatory protein MyoD1: epitope mapping and diagnostic utility. Cancer Res 52:6431, 1992.
60. Dias P, Parham DM, Shapiro DN, et al. Myogenic regulatory protein (MyoD1) expression in childhood solid tumors: diagnostic utility in rhabdomyosarcoma. Am J Pathol 137:1283, 1990.
61. Dietrich CU, Jacobsen BB, Starklant H, et al. Clonal karyotypic evolution in an embryonal rhabdomyosarcoma with trisomy 8 as the primary chromosomal abnormality. Genes Chromosomes Cancer 7:240, 1993.
62. Dito WR, Batsakis JG. Intraoral, pharyngeal, and nasopharyngeal rhabdomyosarcoma. Arch Otolaryngol 77:123, 1963.
63. Dito WR, Batsakis JG. Rhabdomyosarcoma of the head and

neck: appraisal of biologic behavior in 170 cases. Arch Surg 84:582, 1962.

64. Don DM, Newman AN, Fu Y-S. Spindle cell variant of embryonal rhabdomyosarcoma. Otolaryngol Head Neck Surg 116: 529, 1997.
65. Donaldson SS, Castro JR, Wilbur JR, et al. Rhabdomyosarcoma of head and neck in children: combination treatment by surgery, irradiation, and chemotherapy. Cancer 31:26, 1973.
66. Douglass EC, Rowe ST, Valentine M, et al. Variant translocations of chromosome 13 in alveolar rhabdomyosarcoma. Genes Chromosomes Cancer 3:480, 1991.
67. Douglass EC, Shapiro DN, Valentine M, et al. Alveolar rhabdomyosarcoma with the t(2;13): cytogenetic findings and clinicopathologic correlations. Med Pediatr Oncol 21:83, 1993.
68. Douglass EC, Valentine M, Etcubanas E, et al. A specific chromosomal abnormality in rhabdomyosarcoma. Cytogenet Cell Genet 45:148, 1987.
69. Downing JR, Khandeker A, Shurtleff SA, et al. Multiplex RT-PCR assay for the differential diagnosis of alveolar rhabdomyosarcoma and Ewing's sarcoma. Am J Pathol 146:626, 1995.
70. Driman D, Thorner PS, Greenberg ML, et al. N-myc and gene amplification in rhabdomyosarcoma. Cancer 73:2231, 1994.
71. Edel G, Wuisman P, Erlemann R. Spindle cell (leiomyomatous) rhabdomyosarcoma, a rare variant of embryonal rhabdomyosarcoma. Pathol Res Pract 189:102, 1993.
72. Edwards RH, Chatten J, Xiong Q-B, et al. Detection of gene fusions in rhabdomyosarcoma by reverse transcriptase-polymerase chain reaction assay of archival samples. Diagn Mol Pathol 6:91, 1997.
73. Engel ME, Mouton SCE, Emms M. Paediatric rhabdomyosarcoma: MyoD1 demonstration in routinely processed tissue sections using wet heat pretreatment (pressure cooking) for antigen retrieval. J Clin Pathol 50:37, 1997.
74. Enjoji M, Hashimoto H. Diagnosis of soft tissue sarcomas. Pathol Res Pract 178:215, 1984.
75. Enzinger FM. Malignant fibrous histiocytoma 20 years after Stout. Am J Surg Pathol 10:43, 1986.
76. Enzinger FM, Lattes R, Torloni H. Histological typing of soft tissue tumours. In: International Histological Classification of Tumors, No. 3. World Health Organization, Geneva, 1969.
77. Enzinger FM, Shiraki M. Alveolar rhabdomyosarcoma: an analysis of 110 cases. Cancer 24:18, 1969.
78. Erlandson RA. The ultrastructural distinction between rhabdomyosarcoma and other undifferentiated sarcomas. Ultrastruct Pathol 11:83, 1987.
79. Eusebi V, Bondi A, Rosai J. Immunohistochemical localization of myoglobin in nonmuscular cells. Am J Surg Pathol 8:51, 1984.
80. Eusebi V, Cecarelli C, Gorca L, et al. Immunocytochemistry of rhabdomyosarcoma: the use of four different markers. Am J Surg Pathol 10:293, 1986.
81. Eusebi V, Rilke F, Ceccarelli C, et al. Fetal heavy chain skeletal myosin: an oncofetal antigen expressed by rhabdomyosarcoma. Am J Surg Pathol 10:680, 1986.
82. Exelby PR, Ghavimi F, Jereb B. Genitourinary rhabdomyosarcoma in children. J Pediatr Surg 13:746, 1978.
83. Felix CA, Kappel CC, Mitsudomi T, et al. Frequency and diversity of p53 mutations in childhood rhabdomyosarcoma. Cancer Res 52:2243, 1992.
84. Ferrari A, Casanova M, Massimino M, et al. The management of paratesticular rhabdomyosarcoma: a single institutional experience with 44 consecutive children. J Urol 159:1031, 1998.
85. Fitzmaurice RJ, Johnson PR, Yin JA, et al. Rhabdomyosarcoma presenting as "acute leukaemia." Histopathology 18:173, 1991.
86. Flamant F, Hill C. The improvement in survival associated with combined chemotherapy in childhood rhabdomyosarcoma: a historical comparison of 345 patients in the same center. Cancer 53:2417, 1984.
87. Flamant F, Rodary C, Voute PA, et al. Primary chemotherapy in the treatment of rhabdomyosarcoma in children: trial of international society of pediatric oncology (SIOP) preliminary results. Radiother Oncol 3:227, 1985.
88. Fletcher CDM. Pleomorphic malignant fibrous histiocytoma: fact or fiction? Am J Surg Pathol 16:213, 1992.
89. Frascella E, Toffolatti L, Rosolen A. Normal and rearranged PAX 3 expression in human rhabdomyosarcoma. Cancer Genet Cytogenet 102:104, 1998.
90. Fu YS, Perzin KH. Nonepithelial tumors of the nasal cavity, paranasal sinuses, and nasopharynx: a clinicopathological study. V. Skeletal muscle tumors (rhabdomyoma and rhabdomyosarcoma). Cancer 37:364, 1976.
91. Funk WD, Ouellette M, Wright WE. Molecular biology of myogenic regulatory factors. Mol Biol Med 8:185, 1991.
92. Gaffney EF, Dervan PA, Fletcher CDM. Pleomorphic rhabdomyosarcoma in adulthood: analysis of 11 cases with definition of diagnostic criteria. Am J Surg Pathol 17:601, 1993.
93. Gaiger AM, Soule EH, Hewton WA Jr, et al. Pathology of rhabdomyosarcoma: experience of the Intergroup Rhabdomyosarcoma Study, 1972–1978. Natl Cancer Inst Monogr 56:19, 1981.
94. Galili N, Davis RJ, Fredericks WJ, et al. Fusion of a forkhead domain gene to PAX 3 in the solid tumour alveolar rhabdomyosarcoma. Nat Genet 5:230, 1993.
95. Ghavimi F, Mandell LR, Heller G, et al. Prognosis in childhood rhabdomyosarcoma of the extremity. Cancer 64:2233, 1989.
96. Glasunow M. Ueber unreife, begrenzt und destruierend wachsende Rhabdomyoblastome. Frankfurt Z Pathol 45:328, 1933.
97. Gressler M, Hameister H, Henry I, et al. The human MyoD1 (MYF3) gene maps on the short arm of chromosome 11 but is not associated with WAGR locus on the region of the B-W syndrome. Hum Genet 86:135, 1990.
98. Gruchala A, Niezabitowski A, Wasilewska A, et al. Rhabdomyosarcoma: morphologic, immunohistochemical, and DNA study. Gen Diagn Pathol 142:175, 1997.
99. Guillou L, Coquet M, Chaubert P, et al. Skeletal muscle regeneration mimicking rhabdomyosarcoma: a potential diagnostic pitfall. Histopathology 33:136, 1998.
100. Gunalp I, Duruk K, Gunduz K. Orbital rhabdomyosarcoma: a twenty-year survey in Turkey. Jpn J Ophthalmol 37:499, 1993.
101. Hachitanda Y, Toyoshima S, Akazawa K, et al. N-myc gene amplification in rhabdomyosarcoma detected by fluorescence in-situ hybridization: its correlation with histologic features. Mod Pathol 11:1222, 1998.
102. Hart W, Craig JR. Rhabdomyosarcomas of the uterus. Am J Clin Pathol 170:217, 1978.
103. Hasegawa T, Matsuno Y, Niki T, et al. Second primary rhabdomyosarcomas in patients with bilateral retinoblastoma: a clinicopathologic and immunohistochemical study. Am J Surg Pathol 22:1351, 1998.
104. Hawkins HK, Cancho-Velasquez JV. Rhabdomyosarcoma in children: correlation of form and prognosis in one institution's experience. Am J Surg Pathol 11:531, 1987.
105. Hayashi K, Ohtsuki Y, Takahashi K, et al. Congenital alveolar rhabdomyosarcoma with multiple skin metastases: report of a case. Acta Pathol Jpn 38:241, 1988.
106. Hays DM. Pelvic rhabdomyosarcomas in childhood: diagnosis and concepts of management reviewed. Cancer 45:1810, 1980.
107. Hays DM. Rhabdomyosarcoma. Clin Orthop 289:36, 1993.
108. Hays DM, Lawrence W Jr, Crist WM, et al. Partial cystectomy in the management of rhabdomyosarcoma of the bladder: a report from the Intergroup Rhabdomyosarcoma Study. J Pediatr Surg 25:719, 1990.

109. Hays DM, Newton W Jr, Soule EH, et al. Mortality among children with rhabdomyosarcomas of alveolar histologic subtype. J Pediatr Surg 18:412, 1983.
110. Hays DM, Raney RB, Lawrence W Jr, et al. Primary chemotherapy in the treatment of children with bladder-prostate tumors in the Intergroup Rhabdomyosarcoma Study (IRS-II). J Pediatr Surg 17:812, 1982.
111. Hays DM, Raney RB, Wharam MD, et al. Children with vesical rhabdomyosarcoma treated by partial cystectomy with neoadjuvant or adjuvant chemotherapy, with or without radiotherapy. Am J Pediatr Hematol Oncol 17:44, 1995.
112. Heckman CJ, Truong LD, Cagle PT, et al. Pulmonary blastoma with rhabdomyosarcomatous differentiation: an electron microscopic and immunohistochemical study. Am J Surg Pathol 12:35, 1988.
113. Heney D, Lockwood L, Alliabone EB, et al. Nasopharyngeal rhabdomyosarcoma and multiple lentigines syndrome: a case report. Med Pediatr Oncol 20:227, 1992.
114. Henricks WH, Chou J, Goldblum JR, et al. Dedifferentiated liposarcoma: a clinicopathologic analysis of 155 cases with a proposal for an expanded definition of dedifferentiation. Am J Surg Pathol 21:271, 1997.
115. Hensley MF, Cangir A, Culbert SJ. Acute granulocytic leukemia following successful treatment of rhabdomyosarcoma. Am J Dis Child 131:1417, 1977.
116. Hess E, Cohen C, DeRose PB, et al. Nonspecificity of p30/32$^{MIC2}$ immunolocalization with the 013 monoclonal antibody in the diagnosis of Ewing's sarcoma: application of an algorithmic immunohistochemical analysis. Appl Immunohistochem 5:94, 1997.
117. Heyn R, Beltangady M, Hays D, et al. Results of intensive therapy in children with localized alveolar extremity rhabdomyosarcoma: a report from the Intergroup Rhabdomyosarcoma Study. J Clin Oncol 7:200, 1989.
118. Heyn R, Haeberlen V, Newton WA, et al. Second malignant neoplasms in children treated for rhabdomyosarcoma: Intergroup Rhabdomyosarcoma Study Committee. J Clin Oncol 11: 262, 1993.
119. Heyn R, Newton WA, Raney RB, et al. Preservation of the bladder in patients with rhabdomyosarcoma. J Clin Oncol 15: 69, 1997.
120. Heyn R, Ragab A, Raney RB, et al. Late effects of therapy in orbital rhabdomyosarcoma in children: a report from the Intergroup Rhabdomyosarcoma Study. Cancer 57:1738, 1986.
121. Hirose T, Kudo E, Hasegawa T, et al. Expression of intermediate filaments in malignant fibrous histiocytomas. Hum Pathol 20:871, 1989.
122. Hollowood K, Fletcher CDM. Rhabdomyosarcoma in adults. Semin Diagn Pathol 11:47, 1994.
123. Horn RC, Enterline HT. Rhabdomyosarcoma: a clinicopathological study of 39 cases. Cancer 11:181, 1958.
124. Horn RC, Yakovac WC, Kaye R, et al. Rhabdomyosarcoma (sarcoma botryoides) of common bile duct: report of a case. Cancer 8:468, 1955.
125. Howard GM, Casten VG. Rhabdomyosarcoma of the orbit in brothers. Arch Ophthalmol 70:319, 1963.
126. Huang CJ. Rhabdomyosarcoma involving the genitourinary organs, retroperitoneum, and pelvis. J Pediatr Surg 21:101, 1986.
127. Hurlimann J. Desmin and neural marker expression in mesothelial cells and mesotheliomas. Hum Pathol 25:753, 1994.
128. Isaacson C. Embryonal rhabdomyosarcoma of the ampulla of Vater. Cancer 41:365, 1978.
129. Ishak KG, Glunz PR. Hepatoblastoma and hepatocarcinoma in infancy and childhood: report of 47 cases. Cancer 20:396, 1967.
130. Jones IS, Reese AB, Krout J. Orbital rhabdomyosarcoma: an analysis of 62 cases. Trans Am Ophthalmol Soc 63:223, 1965.
131. Kahn DG. Rhabdomyosarcoma mimicking acute leukemia in an adult: report of a case with histologic, flow cytometric, cytogenetic, immunohistochemical, and ultrastructural studies. Arch Pathol Lab Med 122:375, 1998.
132. Kamat MR, Kulkarni JN, Tongaonkar HB, et al. Rhabdomyosarcoma of the bladder and prostate in children. J Surg Oncol 48:180, 1991.
133. Kaplinsky C, Frisch A, Cohen IJ, et al. T-cell acute lymphoblastic leukemia following therapy of rhabdomyosarcoma. Med Pediatr Oncol 20:229, 1992.
134. Kawamoto EH, Weidner N, Agostini RM Jr, et al. Malignant ectomesenchymoma of soft tissue: report of two cases and review of the literature. Cancer 59:1791, 1987.
135. Kearney MM, Soule DH, Ivans JT. Malignant fibrous histiocytoma: a retrospective study of 167 cases. Cancer 45:167, 1980.
136. Keleti J, Quezado MM, Abaza MM, et al. The MDM2 oncoprotein is overexpressed in rhabdomyosarcoma cell lines and stabilizes wild-type p53 protein. Am J Pathol 149:143, 1996.
137. Kelly KM, Womer RV, Barr FG. Minimal disease detection in patients with alveolar rhabdomyosarcoma using a reverse transcriptase-polymerase chain reaction method. Cancer 78: 1320, 1996.
138. Kelly KM, Womer RV, Sorensen PHB, et al. Common and variant gene fusions predict distinct clinical phenotypes in rhabdomyosarcoma. J Clin Oncol 15:1831, 1997.
139. Kilpatrick SP, Teot LA, Geisinger KR, et al. Relationship of DNA ploidy to histology and prognosis in rhabdomyosarcoma: comparison of flow cytometry and image analysis. Cancer 74:3227, 1994.
140. Kindblom L-G, Seidal T, Karlsson K. Immunohistochemical localization of myoglobin in human muscle tissue and embryonal and alveolar rhabdomyosarcoma. Acta Pathol Microbiol Immunol Scand 90A:167, 1982.
141. Kirk RC, Zimmerman LE. Rhabdomyosarcoma of the orbit in a survivor of rhabdomyosarcoma of the kidney. Arch Ophthalmol 81:559, 1969.
142. Kodet R. Rhabdomyosarcoma in childhood: an immunohistochemical analysis with myoglobin, desmin, and vimentin. Pathol Res Pract 185:207, 1989.
143. Kodet R, Newton WA Jr, Hamoudi AB, et al. Childhood rhabdomyosarcoma with anaplastic (pleomorphic) features: a report of the Intergroup Rhabdomyosarcoma Study. Am J Surg Pathol 17:443, 1993.
144. Kodet R, Newton WA Jr, Hamoudi AB, et al. Orbital rhabdomyosarcomas and related tumors in childhood: relationship of morphology to prognosis: an Intergroup Rhabdomyosarcoma Study. Med Pediatr Oncol 29:51, 1997.
145. Kodet R, Newton WA Jr, Hamoudi AB, et al. Rhabdomyosarcomas with intermediate-filament inclusions and features of rhabdoid tumors: light microscopic and immunohistochemical study. Am J Surg Pathol 15:257, 1991.
146. Kodet R, Newton WA Jr, Sachs N, et al. Rhabdoid tumors of soft tissues: a clinicopathologic study of 26 cases enrolled on the Intergroup Rhabdomyosarcoma Study. Hum Pathol 22:674, 1991.
147. Koi M, Johnson LA, Kalikin LM, et al. Tumor cell growth arrest caused by subchromosomal transferable DNA fragments from chromosome 11. Science 260:361, 1993.
148. Koufos A, Hansen MF, Copeland NG, et al. Loss of heterozygosity in three embryonal tumours suggests a common pathogenetic mechanism. Nature 316:330, 1985.
149. Kowal-Vern A, Gonzalez-Crussi F, Turner J, et al. Flow and image cytometric DNA analysis in rhabdomyosarcoma. Cancer Res 50:6023, 1990.
150. Kuttesch JF, Parham D, Schell M, et al. Lack of correlation of P-glygoprotein expression with treatment outcome in ad-

vanced rhabdomyosarcoma (RMS) [abstract]. Proc Am Soc Clin Oncol 11:367, 1992.
151. La Quaglia MP, Ghavimi F, Heller G, et al. Mortality in pediatric paratesticular rhabdomyosarcoma: a multivariate analysis. J Urol 142:473, 1989.
152. La Quaglia MP, Ghavimi F, Penenberg D, et al. Factors predictive of mortality in pediatric extremity rhabdomyosarcoma. J Pediatr Surg 25:238, 1990.
153. La Quaglia MP, Heller G, Ghavimi F, et al. The affect of age at diagnosis on outcome in rhabdomyosarcoma. Cancer 73:109, 1994.
154. Lawrence W, Gehan EA, Hays DM, et al. Prognostic significance of staging factors of the UICC staging system in childhood rhabdomyosarcoma: a report from the Intergroup Rhabdomyosarcoma Study (IRS-II). J Clin Oncol 5:46, 1987.
155. Lawrence W Jr, Anderson JR, Gehan EA, et al. Pretreatment TNM staging of childhood rhabdomyosarcoma: a report of the Intergroup Rhabdomyosarcoma Study Group. Cancer 80:1165, 1997.
156. Lawson CW, Fisher C, Gatter KC. An immunohistochemical study of differentiation in malignant fibrous histiocytoma. Histopathology 11:375, 1987.
157. Leader M, Collins M, Patel J, et al. Desmin: its value as a marker of muscle derived tumours using a commercial antibody. Virchows Arch [A] 411:345, 1987.
158. Lee JH, Lee MS, Lee BH, et al. Rhabdomyosarcoma of the head and neck in adults: MR and CT findings. Am J Neuroradiol 17:1923, 1996.
159. Leuschner I, Newton WA Jr, Schmidt D, et al. Spindle cell variants of embryonal rhabdomyosarcoma in the paratesticular region: a report of the Intergroup Rhabdomyosarcoma Study. Am J Surg Pathol 17:221, 1993.
160. Levene M. Congenital retinoblastoma and sarcoma botryoides of the vagina: report of a case. Cancer 13:532, 1960.
161. Li FP, Fraumeni JF Jr. Rhabdomyosarcoma in children: epidemiologic study and identification of a familial cancer syndrome. J Natl Cancer Inst 43:1365, 1969.
162. Linscheid RL, Soule EH, Henderson ED. Pleomorphic rhabdomyosarcomata of the extremities and limb girdles: a clinicopathological study. J Bone Joint Surg Am 47:715, 1965.
163. Lloyd RV, Hajdu SI, Knapper WH. Embryonal rhabdomyosarcoma in adults. Cancer 51:557, 1983.
164. Lobe TE, Wiener ES, Hays DM, et al. Neonatal rhabdomyosarcoma: the IRS experience. J Pediatr Surg 29:1167, 1994.
165. Loh WE Jr, Scrable HJ, Livanos E, et al. Human chromosome 11 contains two different growth suppressor genes for embryonal rhabdomyosarcoma. Proc Natl Acad Sci USA 89:1755, 1992.
166. Lollini PL, De Giovanni C, Del Re B, et al. Myogenic differentiation of human rhabdomyosarcoma cells induced in vitro by antineoplastic drugs. Cancer Res 49:3631, 1989.
167. Lucas DR, Ryan JR, Zalupski MM, et al. Primary embryonal rhabdomyosarcoma of long bone: case report and review of the literature. Am J Surg Pathol 20:239, 1996.
168. Lundgren L, Angervall L, Stenman G, et al. Infantile rhabdomyofibrosarcoma: a high grade sarcoma distinguishable from infantile fibrosarcoma and rhabdomyosarcoma. Hum Pathol 24:785, 1993.
169. Majmudar B, Kumar VS. Embryonal rhabdomyosarcoma (sarcoma botryoides) of the common bile duct. Hum Pathol 7:705, 1976.
170. Malek RS, Kelalis PP. Paratesticular rhabdomyosarcoma in childhood. J Urol 118:450, 1977.
171. Mannens MMAM, Devilee P, Bliek J, et al. Loss of heterozygosity in Wilms' tumors, studied for six putative tumor suppressor regions, is limited to chromosome 11. Cancer Res 50: 3279, 1990.
172. Mannor GE, Rose GE, Plowman PN, et al. Multidisciplinary management of refractory orbital rhabdomyosarcoma. Ophthalmology 104:1198, 1997.
173. Marchand F. Ueber eine Geschwulst aus quergestreiften Muskelfasern mit ungewohnlichem Gehalte an Glykogen nebst Bemerkungen ueber das Glycogen in einigen fotalen Geweben. Virchows Arch [Pathol Anat] 100:42, 1885.
174. Masson JK, Soule EH. Embryonal rhabdomyosarcoma of the head and neck: report of 88 cases. Am J Surg 110:585, 1965.
175. Maurer HM, Beltangady M, Gehan EA, et al. The Intergroup Rhabdomyosarcoma Study I: a final report. Cancer 61:209, 1988.
176. Maurer HM, Gehan EA, Beltangady M, et al. The Intergroup Rhabdomyosarcoma Study II. Cancer 71:1904, 1993.
177. Mayer L. Quergestreifte Muskelfasern inmitten einer Augenhohlengeschwulst. Virchows Arch [Pathol Anat] 37:417, 1866.
178. McManus AP, O'Reilly M-A, Pritchard-Jones K, et al. Interphase fluorescence in-situ hybridization detection of t(2; 13)(q35;q14) in alveolar rhabdomyosarcoma: a diagnostic tool in minimally invasive biopsies. J Pathol 178:410, 1996.
179. Melguizo C, Prados J, Aneiros J, et al. Differentiation of a human rhabdomyosarcoma cell line after antineoplastic drug treatment. J Pathol 175:23, 1995.
180. Mierau GW, Favara BE. Rhabdomyosarcoma in children: ultrastructural study of 31 cases. Cancer 46:2035, 1980.
181. Miettinen M. Antibodies specific to muscle actins in the diagnosis and classification of soft tissue tumors. Am J Pathol 130: 205, 1988.
182. Miettinen M. Rhabdomyosarcoma in patients older than 40 years of age. Cancer 62:2060, 1988.
183. Miettinen M, Rapola J. Immunohistochemical spectrum of rhabdomyosarcoma and rhabdomyosarcoma-like tumors: expression of cytokeratin and the 68-kd neurofilament protein. Am J Surg Pathol 13:120, 1989.
184. Molenaar WM, Dam-Meiring A, Kamps WA, et al. DNA-aneuploidy in rhabdomyosarcomas compared with other sarcomas of childhood and adolescence. Hum Pathol 19:573, 1988.
185. Molenaar WM, Muntinghe FLH. Expression of neural cell adhesion molecules and neurofilament protein isoforms in skeletal muscle tumors. Hum Pathol 29:1290, 1998.
186. Molenaar WM, Oosterhuis JW, Kamps WA. Cytological "differentiation" in childhood rhabdomyosarcoma following polychemotherapy. Hum Pathol 15:973, 1984.
187. Molenaar WM, Oosterhuis JW, Oosterhuis AM, et al. Mesenchymal and muscle-specific intermediate filaments (vimentin and desmin) in relation to differentiation in childhood rhabdomyosarcoma. Hum Pathol 16:838, 1985.
188. Molenaar WM, Oosterhuis AM, Ramaekers FCS. The rarity of rhabdomyosarcomas in the adult: a morphologic and immunohistochemical study. Pathol Res Pract 180:400, 1985.
189. Morales AR, Fine G, Horn RC Jr. Rhabdomyosarcoma: an ultrastructural appraisal. Pathol Annu 7:81, 1972.
190. Mostofi FK, Morse WH. Polypoid rhabdomyosarcoma (sarcoma botryoides) of bladder in children. J Urol 67:681, 1952.
191. Mukai M, Iri H, Torikata C, et al. Immunoperoxidase demonstration of a new muscle protein (Z-protein) in myogenic tumors as a diagnostic aid. Am J Pathol 114:164, 1984.
192. Mukai K, Rosai J, Hallaway BE. Localization of myoglobin in normal and neoplastic human skeletal muscle cells using an immunoperoxidase method. Am J Surg Pathol 3:373, 1979.
193. Mukai K, Schollmeyer J, Rosai J. Immunohistochemical localization of actin: applications in surgical pathology. Am J Surg Pathol 5:91, 1981.
194. Mulligan LM, Matlashewski GJ, Scrable HJ, et al. Mechanisms of p53 loss in human sarcomas. Proc Natl Acad Sci USA 87: 5963, 1990.

195. Nagaraj HS, Kmetz DR, Leitner C. Rhabdomyosarcoma of the bile ducts. J Pediatr Surg 12:1071, 1977.
196. Nakleh RE, Swanson PE, Dehner LP. Juvenile (embryonal and alveolar) rhabdomyosarcoma of head and neck in adults. Cancer 67:1019, 1991.
197. Newman PL, Fletcher CDM. Malignant mesenchymoma: clinicopathologic analysis of a series with evidence of low-grade behavior. Am J Surg Pathol 15:607, 1991.
198. Newton WA Jr, Gehan EA, Webber BL, et al. Classification of rhabdomyosarcomas and related sarcomas: pathologic aspects and proposal for a new classification—an Intergroup Rhabdomyosarcoma Study. Cancer 76:1073, 1995.
199. Newton WA Jr, Soule EH, Hamoudi AB, et al. Histopathology of childhood sarcomas, Intergroup Rhabdomyosarcoma Studies I and II: clinicopathologic correlation. J Clin Oncol 6:67, 1988.
200. Noguchi S, Tamiya S, Nagoshi M, et al. Nuclear morphometry and the MIB-1 index in rhabdomyosarcoma. Mod Pathol 9:253, 1996.
201. Norris HJ, Taylor HB. Polyps of the vagina: a benign lesion resembling sarcoma botryoides. Cancer 19:227, 1966.
202. Oda Y, Tsuneyoshi M, Hashimoto H, et al. Primary rhabdomyosarcoma of the iliac bone in an adult: a case mimicking fibrosarcoma. Virchows Arch [Pathol Anat] 423:65, 1993.
203. Ordoñez NG, Tornos C. Malignant peripheral nerve sheath tumor of the pleura with epithelial and rhabdomyoblastic differentiation: report of a case clinically simulating mesothelioma. Am J Surg Pathol 21:1515, 1997.
204. Osborn M, Hill C, Altmannsberger M, et al. Monoclonal antibodies to titin in conjunction with antibodies to desmin separate rhabdomyosarcomas from other tumor types. Lab Invest 55:101, 1986.
205. Ostor AG, Fortune DW, Riley CB. Fibroepithelial polyps with atypical stromal cells (pseudosarcoma botryoides) of vulva and vagina: a report of 13 cases. Int J Gynecol Pathol 7:351, 1988.
206. Pack GT, Eberhart WF. Rhabdomyosarcoma of skeletal muscle: report of 100 cases. Surgery 32:1023, 1952.
207. Palazzo JP, Gibas Z, Dunton CJ, et al. Cytogenetic study of botryoid rhabdomyosarcoma of the uterine cervix. Virchows Arch [A] 422:87, 1993.
208. Palmer NF, Sachs N, Foulkes M. Histopathology and prognosis in rhabdomyosarcoma [abstract] Proc Int Soc Pediatr Oncol 1:113, 1981.
209. Palmer NF, Sachs N, Foulkes M. Histopathology and prognosis in rhabdomyosarcoma (IRS-I) [abstract] Proc Am Soc Clin Oncol 1:170, 1982.
210. Pappo AS, Crist WM, Kuttesch J, et al. Tumor-cell DNA content predicts outcome in children and adolescents with clinical group III embryonal rhabdomyosarcoma. J Clin Oncol 11:1901, 1993.
211. Pappo AS, Shapiro DN, Crist WM, et al. Biology and therapy of pediatric rhabdomyosarcoma. J Clin Oncol 13:2123, 1995.
212. Parham DM. The molecular biology of childhood rhabdomyosarcoma. Semin Diagn Pathol 11:39, 1994.
213. Parham DM, Dias P, Kelly DR, et al. Desmin positivity in primitive neuroectodermal tumors of childhood. Am J Surg Pathol 16:483, 1992.
214. Parham DM, Webber B, Holt H, et al. Immunohistochemical study of childhood rhabdomyosarcomas and related neoplasms: results of an Intergroup Rhabdomyosarcoma Study project. Cancer 67:3072, 1991.
215. Patton RB, Horn RC Jr. Rhabdomyosarcoma: clinical and pathological features and comparison with human fetal and embryonal skeletal muscle. Surgery 52:572, 1962.
216. Pavrthran K, Doval DC, Mukherjee G, et al. Rhabdomyosarcoma of the oral cavity: report of eight cases. Acta Oncol 36: 819, 1997.
217. Perez-Ordonez B, Kandel RA, Bell R, et al. Rhabdomyosarcoma with rhabdoid-like features. Pathol Res Pract 194:357, 1998.
218. Prat J, Young RH, Scully RE. Ovarian Sertoli-Leydig cell tumors with heterologous elements: cartilage and skeletal muscle: a clinicopathological analysis of twelve cases. Cancer 50: 2465, 1982.
219. Pratt CB, Hustu HO, Kumar APM, et al. Treatment of childhood rhabdomyosarcoma at St. Jude Children's Research Hospital 1962–1978. Natl Cancer Inst Monogr 56:93, 1981.
220. Priest JR, McDermott MB, Bhatia S, et al. Pleuropulmonary blastoma: a clinicopathologic study of 50 cases. Cancer 80:147, 1997.
221. Przygodzki RM, Moran CA, Suster S, et al. Primary pulmonary rhabdomyosarcomas: a clinicopathologic and immunohistochemical study of three cases. Mod Pathol 8:658, 1995.
222. Ragab AH, Heyn R, Tefft M, et al. Infants younger than 1 year of age with rhabdomyosarcoma. Cancer 58:2606, 1986.
223. Raney RB. Spinal cord "drop metastases" from head and neck rhabdomyosarcoma: proceedings of the tumor board of the Children's Hospital of Philadelphia. Med Pediatr Oncol 4:3, 1978.
224. Raney RB Jr, Crist W, Hays D, et al. Soft tissue sarcoma of the perineal region in childhood: a report from the Intergroup Rhabdomyosarcoma Studies I and II, 1972 through 1984. Cancer 65:2787, 1990.
225. Raney RB Jr, Crist WM, Maurer HM, et al. Prognosis of children with soft tissue sarcoma who relapse after achieving a complete response: a report from the Intergroup Rhabdomyosarcoma Study I. Cancer 52:44, 1983.
226. Raney RB Jr, Gehan EA, Hays DM, et al. Primary chemotherapy with and without radiation therapy and/or surgery for children with localized sarcoma of the bladder, prostate, vagina, uterus, and cervix: a comparison of the results in Intergroup Rhabdomyosarcoma Studies I and II. Cancer 66:2072, 1990.
227. Raney RB Jr, Heyn R, Hays DM, et al. Sequelae of treatment in 109 patients followed for 5 to 15 years after diagnosis of sarcoma of the bladder and prostate: a report of the Intergroup Rhabdomyosarcoma Study Committee. Cancer 71:2387, 1993.
228. Raney RB Jr, Tefft M, Lawrence W, et al. Paratesticular sarcoma in childhood and adolescence. Cancer 60:2337, 1987.
229. Raney RB Jr, Tefft M, Maurer HM, et al. Disease pattern and survival rate in children with metastatic soft-tissue sarcoma: a report from the Intergroup Rhabdomyosarcoma Study (IRS) I. Cancer 62:1257, 1988.
230. Raney RB Jr, Tefft M, Newton WA, et al. Improved prognosis with intensive treatment of children with cranial soft tissue sarcomas arising in nonorbital parameningeal sites. Cancer 59: 147, 1987.
231. Rangdaeng S, Truong LD. Comparative immunohistochemical staining for desmin and muscle specific actin: a study of 576 cases. Am J Clin Pathol 96:32, 1991.
232. Reboul-Marty J, Quintana E, Mossed V, et al. Prognostic factors of alveolar rhabdomyosarcoma in childhood: an International Society of Pediatric Oncology Study. Cancer 68:493, 1991.
233. Reddick RL, Michelitch H, Triche PJ. Malignant soft tissue tumors (malignant fibrous histiocytoma, pleomorphic liposarcoma, and pleomorphic rhabdomyosarcoma): an electron microscopic study. Hum Pathol 10:327, 1979.
234. Regine WF, Fontanesi J, Kumar P, et al. A phase II trial evaluating selective use of altered radiation dose and fractionation

in patients with unresectable rhabdomyosarcoma. Int J Radiat Oncol 31:799, 1995.
235. Reich S, Overberg-Schmidt US, Leenan A, et al. Neurofibromatosis 1 associated with embryonal rhabdomyosarcoma of the urinary bladder. Pediatr Hematol Oncol 16:263, 1999.
236. Reith JD, Bauer TW, Fischler DF, et al. Dedifferentiated chondrosarcoma with rhabdomyosarcomatous differentiation. Am J Surg Pathol 20:293, 1996.
237. Riopelle JL, Theriault JP. Sur une forme meconnue de sarcome des parties molles: le rhabdomyosarcome alveolaire. Ann Anat Pathol (Paris) 1:88, 1956.
238. Rodary C, Flamant F, Donaldson SS. An attempt to use a common staging system in rhabdomyosarcoma: a report of an international workshop initiated by the International Society of Pediatric Oncology (SIOP). Med Pediatr Oncol 17:210, 1989.
239. Rodary C, Gehan D, Flamant S, et al. Prognostic factors in 951 nonmetastatic rhabdomyosarcomas in children: a report from the International Rhabdomyosarcoma Workshop. Med Pediatr Oncol 19:89, 1991.
240. Roebuck DJ, Yang WT, Lam WW, et al. Hepatobiliary rhabdomyosarcoma in children: diagnostic radiology. Pediatr Radiol 28:101, 1998.
241. Roholl PJM, Elbers HR, Prinsen I, et al. Distribution of actin isoforms in sarcomas: an immunohistochemical study. Hum Pathol 21:1269, 1990.
242. Rokitansky K. Ein aus quergestreiften Muskelfasern constituirtes Aftergebilde. Z Wien Aerzte 1849.
243. Royds JA, Variend S, Timperley WR, et al. An investigation of beta enolase as a histologic marker of rhabdomyosarcoma. J Clin Pathol 37:905, 1984.
244. Rubin BP, Hasserjian RP, Singer S, et al. Spindle cell rhabdomyosarcoma (so-called) in adults: report of two cases with emphasis on differential diagnosis. Am J Surg Pathol 22:459, 1998.
245. Russell WO, Cohen HJ, Enzinger FM, et al. A clinical and pathological staging system for soft tissue sarcomas. Cancer 40:1562, 1977.
246. Ruymann FB, Maddux HR, Ragab A, et al. Congenital anomalies associated with rhabdomyosarcoma: an autopsy study of 115 cases: a report from the Intergroup Rhabdomyosarcoma Study Group. Med Pediatr Oncol 16:33, 1988.
247. Ruymann FB, Raney B, Crist WM, et al. Rhabdomyosarcoma of the biliary tree in childhood: a report from the Intergroup Rhabdomyosarcoma Study. Cancer 56:575, 1985.
248. Sabbioni S, Barbanti-Brodano G, Croce CM, et al. GOK: a gene at 11p15 involved in rhabdomyosarcoma and rhabdoid tumor development. Cancer Res 57:4493, 1997.
249. Sartelet H, Lantuejoul S, Armari-Alla C, et al. Solid alveolar rhabdomyosarcoma of the thorax in a child. Histopathology 32:165, 1998.
250. Sassoon DA. Myogenic regulatory factors: dissecting their role in regulation during vertebrate embryogensis. Dev Biol 156:11, 1993.
251. Savasan S, Lorenzana A, Williams JA, et al. Constitutional balanced translocations in alveolar rhabdomyosarcoma. Cancer Genet Cytogenet 105:50, 1998.
252. Scheidler S, Fredericks WJ, Rauscher FJ, et al. The hybrid PAX3-FKHR fusion protein of alveolar rhabdomyosarcoma transforms fibroblasts in culture. Proc Natl Acad Sci USA 93: 9805, 1996.
253. Schmidt D, Fletcher CDM, Harms D. Rhabdomyosarcomas with primary presentation in the skin. Pathol Res Pract 189: 422, 1993.
254. Schmidt D, Reimann O, Treuner J, et al. Cellular differentiation and prognosis in embryonal rhabdomyosarcoma: a report from the Cooperative Soft Tissue Sarcoma Study 1981 (CWS 81). Virchows Arch [Pathol Anat] 409:183, 1986.
255. Schmidt RA, Cone R, Haas JE, et al. Diagnosis of rhabdomyosarcomas with HHF35, a monoclonal antibody directed against muscle actins. Am J Pathol 131:19, 1988.
256. Schürch W, Bégin LR, Seemayer TA, et al. Pleomorphic soft tissue myogenic sarcomas of adulthood: a reappraisal in the mid-1990s. Am J Surg Pathol 20:131, 1996.
257. Schürch W, Bochaton-Paillat ML, Teinoz A, et al. All histological types of primary human rhabdomyosarcoma express alpha-cardiac and not alpha-skeletal actin messenger RNA. Am J Pathol 144:836, 1994.
258. Schürch W, Skalli O, Seemayer TA, et al. Intermediate filament proteins and actin isoforms as markers for soft tissue tumor differentiation and origin. I. Smooth muscle tumors. Am J Pathol 128:91, 1987.
259. Scotlandi K, Serra M, Manara MC, et al. Immunostaining of the p30/32$^{MIC2}$ antigen and molecular detection of EWS rearrangements for the diagnosis of Ewing's sarcoma and peripheral neuroectodermal tumor. Hum Pathol 27:408, 1996.
260. Scrable HJ, Whitte DP, Lampkin BC, et al. Chromosomal location of the human rhabdomyosarcoma locus by mitotic recombination mapping. Nature 329:645, 1987.
261. Scrable H, Whitte D, Shimada H, et al. Molecular differential pathology of rhabdomyosarcoma. Genes Chromosomes Cancer 1:23, 1989.
262. Scupham R, Gilbert EF, Wilde J, et al. Immunohistochemical studies of rhabdomyosarcoma. Arch Pathol Lab Med 110:818, 1986.
263. Seidal T, Kindblom LG. The ultrastructure of alveolar and embryonal rhabdomyosarcoma: a correlative and electron microscopic study of 17 cases. Acta Pathol Microbiol Immunol Scand 92A:231, 1984.
264. Seidal T, Kindblom LG, Angervall L. Myoglobin, desmin, and vimentin in ultrastructurally proven rhabdomyomas and rhabdomyosarcomas: an immunohistochemical study utilizing a series of monoclonal and polyclonal antibodies. Appl Pathol 5: 201, 1987.
265. Seidal T, Kindblom LG, Angervall L. Rhabdomyosarcoma in middle-aged and elderly individuals. APMIS 97:236, 1989.
266. Shapiro DN, Parham DM, Douglass EC, et al. Relationship of tumor cell ploidy to histologic subtype and treatment outcome in children and adolescents with unresectable rhabdomyosarcoma. J Clin Oncol 9:159, 1991.
267. Shapiro DN, Sublett JE, Li B, et al. Fusion of PAX 3 to a member of the forkhead family of transcription factors in human alveolar rhabdomyosarcoma. Cancer Res 53:5108, 1993.
268. Shu WH, Chang TC, Hsueh S, et al. Embryonal rhabdomyosarcoma of the uterine corpus mistaken for small cell carcinoma: a case report. Chang Keng Hsueh 19:181, 1996.
269. Skalli O, Gabbiani G, Babai F, et al. Intermediate filament proteins and actin isoforms as markers for soft tissue differentiation and origin. II. Rhabdomyosarcomas. Am J Pathol 130: 515, 1988.
270. Slater RM, Mannens MMAM. Cytogenetics and molecular genetics of Wilms' tumor of childhood. Cancer Genet Cytogenet 61:111, 1992.
271. Sotello-Avila C, Gonzales-Crussi F, de Mello D, et al. Renal and extrarenal rhabdoid tumors in children: a clinicopathologic study of 14 patients. Semin Diagn Pathol 3:151, 1986.
272. Srouji MN, Donaldson MH, Chatten J, et al. Perianal rhabdomyosarcoma in childhood. Cancer 38:1008, 1976.
273. Stevenson AJ, Chatten J, Bertoni F, et al. CD99 (p30/32$^{MIC2}$) neuroectodermal/Ewing's sarcoma antigen as an immunohistochemical marker: review of more than 600 tumors and the literature experience. Appl Immunohistochem 2:231, 1994.
274. Stobbe GD, Dargeon HW. Embryonal rhabdomyosarcoma of head and neck in children and adolescents. Cancer 3:826, 1950.

275. Stout AP. Rhabdomyosarcoma of the skeletal muscles. Ann Surg 123:447, 1946.
276. Stout AP, Lattes R. Tumors of the soft tissues. In: Atlas of Tumor Pathology, Second Series, Fascicle 1. Armed Forces Institute of Pathology, Washington, DC, 1966.
277. Suster S, Moran CA, Koss MN. Rhabdomyosarcomas of the anterior mediastinum: report of four cases unassociated with germ cell, teratomatous or thymic carcinomatous components. Hum Pathol 25:349, 1994.
278. Sutow WW, Lindberg RD, Gehan EA, et al. Three-year relapse-free survival rates in childhood rhabdomyosarcoma of the head and neck: report from the Intergroup Rhabdomyosarcoma Study. Cancer 49:2217, 1982.
279. Talerman A. Sarcoma botryoides presenting as a polyp on the labium majus. Cancer 32:994, 1973.
280. Tallini G, Erlandson RA, Brennan MF, et al. Divergent myosarcomatous differentiation in retroperitoneal liposarcoma. Am J Surg Pathol 17:546, 1993.
281. Tallini G, Parham DM, Dias P, et al. Myogenic regulatory protein expression in adult soft tissue sarcomas: a sensitive and specific marker of skeletal muscle differentiation. Am J Pathol 144:693, 1994.
282. Tefft M, Fernandez C, Donaldson M, et al. Incidence of meningeal involvement by rhabdomyosarcoma of the head and neck in children: a report of the Intergroup Rhabdomyosarcoma Study (IRS). Cancer 42:253, 1978.
283. Timmons JW Jr, Burgert EO Jr, Soule EH, et al. Embryonal rhabdomyosarcoma of the bladder and prostate in childhood. J Urol 113:694, 1975.
284. Tonin RM, Scrable H, Shimada H, et al. Muscle-specific gene expression in rhabdomyosarcomas and stages of human fetal skeletal muscle development. Cancer Res 51:5100, 1991.
285. Tsokos M. The role of immunocytochemistry in the diagnosis of rhabdomyosarcoma. Arch Pathol Lab Med 110:776, 1986.
286. Tsokos M, Dias P, Jefferson J, et al. Detection of the MyoD1 gene product in paraffin sections of pediatric tumors. Mod Pathol 7:148A, 1994.
287. Tsokos M, Howard R, Costa J. Immunohistochemical study of alveolar and embryonal rhabdomyosarcoma. Lab Invest 48: 148, 1983.
288. Tsokos M, Webber BL, Parham DM, et al. Rhabdomyosarcoma: a new classification scheme related to prognosis. Arch Pathol Lab Med 116:847, 1992.
289. Tsuneyoshi M, Daimaru Y, Hashimoto H, et al. Malignant soft tissue neoplasms with the histologic features of renal rhabdoid tumors: an ultrastructural and immunohistochemical study. Hum Pathol 16:1235, 1985.
290. Turc-Carel C, Livard-Nacol S, Justrabo E, et al. Consistent chromosomal translocations in alveolar rhabdomyosarcoma. Cancer Genet Cytogenet 19:361, 1986.
290a. Val-Bernal J, Fernandez N, Gomez-Roman JJ. Spindle cell rhabdomyosarcoma in adults. A case report and literature review. Pathol Res Pract 196:67, 2000.
291. Van Dorpe J, Sciot R, Samson I, et al. Primary osteorhabdomyosarcoma (malignant mesenchymoma) of bone: a case report and review of the literature. Mod Pathol 10:1047, 1997.
292. Wang NP, Marx J, McNutt MA, et al. Expression of myogenic regulatory proteins (myogenin and MyoD1) in small blue round cell tumors of childhood. Am J Pathol 147:1799, 1995.
293. Weintraub H, Davis R, Tabscott S, et al. The MyoD gene family: nodal point during specification of the muscle cell lineage. Science 251:761, 1991.
294. Weintraub H, Tabscott SJ, Davis RL, et al. Activation of muscle-specific genes in pigment nerve, fat, liver and fibroblast cell lines by forced expression of MyoD. Proc Natl Acad Sci USA 86:5434, 1989.
295. Weiss SW. Malignant fibrous histiocytoma: a reaffirmation. Am J Surg Pathol 6:773, 1982.
296. Weiss SW, Enzinger FM. Malignant fibrous histiocytoma: an analysis of 200 cases. Cancer 41:2250, 1978.
297. Weiss LM, Warhol MJ. Ultrastructural distinctions between adult pleomorphic rhabdomyosarcomas, pleomorphic liposarcoma and pleomorphic fibrous histiocytomas. Hum Pathol 15: 1025, 1982.
298. Wesche WA, Fletcher CDM, Dias P, et al. Immunohistochemistry of Myo-D1 in adult pleomorphic soft tissue sarcomas. Am J Surg Pathol 19:261, 1995.
299. Wiatrak BJ, Pensak MI. Rhabdomyosarcoma of the ear and temporal bone. Laryngoscope 99:1188, 1989.
300. Wiener ES. Head and neck rhabdomyosarcoma. Semin Pediatr Surg 3:203, 1994.
301. Wijnaendts LCD, van der Linden JC, van Diest PJ, et al. Prognostic importance of DNA flow cytometric variables in rhabdomyosarcomas. J Clin Pathol 46:948, 1993.
302. Wijnaendts LCD, van der Linden JC, van Unnik AJM, et al. Histopathological classification of childhood rhabdomyosarcoma: relationship with clinical parameters and prognosis. Hum Pathol 25:900, 1994.
303. Wijnaendts LCD, van der Linden JC, van Unnik AJM, et al. Histopathological features and grading in rhabdomyosarcoma of childhood. Histopathology 24:303, 1994.
304. Wijnaendts LCD, van der Linden JC, van Unnik AJM, et al. The expression pattern of contractile and intermediate filament proteins in developing skeletal muscle and rhabdomyosarcoma of childhood: diagnostic and prognostic utility. J Pathol 174:283, 1994.
305. Wong T-Y, Suster S. Primary cutaneous sarcomas showing rhabdomyoblastic differentiation. Histopathology 26:25, 1995.
306. Woodruff JM, Christensen WN. Glandular peripheral nerve sheath tumors. Cancer 72:3618, 1993.
307. Woodruff JM, Perino G. Non-germ-cell or teratomatous malignant tumors showing additional rhabdomyoblastic differentiation, with emphasis on the malignant Triton tumor. Semin Diagn Pathol 11:69, 1994.
308. Yang WT, Kwan WH, Li CK, et al. Imaging of pediatric head and neck rhabdomyosarcomas with emphasis on magnetic resonance imaging and a review of the literature. Pediatr Hematol Oncol 14:243, 1997.
309. Young JL, Miller RW. Incidence of malignant tumors in U.S. children. J Pediatr 86:254, 1975.
310. Zanetta G, Rota SM, Lissoni A, et al. Conservative treatment followed by chemotherapy with doxorubicin and ifosfamide for cervical sarcoma botryoides in young females. Br J Cancer 80:403, 1999.

CHAPTER 23

# BENIGN TUMORS AND TUMOR-LIKE LESIONS OF BLOOD VESSELS

Hemangiomas are benign lesions that closely resemble normal vessels. So closely is this facsimile reproduced that it is difficult to distinguish clearly hamartomas, malformations, and tumors. These taxonomic distinctions have been made all the more difficult by the fact that classifications of vascular lesions as proposed by clinicians, pathologists, and radiologists vary because of the reliance on different parameters.[3,11] For example, clinicians emphasize clinical presentation and growth characteristics, contending that lesions present at birth are vascular malformations, whereas actively growing lesions presenting shortly after birth are neoplastic (e.g., cellular hemangioma of infancy). Although scientific evidence supports the idea that congenital and noncongenital lesions may be fundamentally different, there are problematic aspects to this generalization.[11] For example, it can be argued that some congenital malformations do not become apparent until later in life (e.g., angiomatosis) depending on their location and rate of growth, and that cellular hemangiomas of infancy, which nearly always regress with time, are not neoplasms at all. From the point of view of the pathologist, who frequently lacks detailed clinical and radiologic information, vascular lesions are usually classified by the type of vessel (e.g., capillary, venous) that predominates; and thus lesions with markedly different clinical or radiologic features might well earn the same pathologic designation. Most recently, some vascular lesions have been linked to specific genetic defects,[1,41,42,68] suggesting that with time the classification of vascular lesions will embrace an even more sophisticated level of information.

In this chapter we have retained the pathologic designations of vascular lesions but indicate in specific situations the unique clinical and radiographic features that accompany the lesion. "Hemangioma" is used in the broadest sense as a benign, nonreactive process in which there is an increase in the number of normal or abnormal-appearing vessels, recognizing that many of these lesions represent tissue malformations rather than true tumors.

Hemangiomas may be of two general types: those that are more or less localized to one area and those that involve large segments of the body, such as an entire extremity. The latter type, known as *angiomatosis,* deserves specific mention because of the inherent problems it poses in diagnosis and therapy. Localized hemangiomas, however, are far more common and account for most of the vascular tumors encountered in daily practice. Certain conditions, such as granuloma pyogenicum and angiolymphoid hyperplasia (epithelioid hemangioma), which in the past have been variably classified as reactions and tumors, are considered benign neoplasms.

## NORMAL STRUCTURE AND FUNCTION

### Vascular Development

*Vasculogenesis* refers to the de novo development of blood vessels from stem cells or primitive endothelial cells and contrasts with *angiogenesis,* a term that implies the formation of new microvessels from differentiated endothelium.[23] Vasculogenesis is largely restricted to early embryogenesis, whereas angiogenesis occurs during embryogenesis and in the postnatal state. Angiogenesis is also the mechanism whereby tumors derive their blood supply. The embryonic vascular system develops during the third week of fetal life from mesodermal cells of the "blood islands." Although initially located in the region of the yolk sac, these cells eventually populate the mesenchyme throughout the fetus; the peripheral cells of the islands give rise to endothelial tubes, and the central cells give rise to the hematopoietic elements.

On a molecular level, embryonic vasculogenesis and angiogenesis are the result of a series of genetic events that depend on the orderly expression of at least two sets of tyrosine kinase receptors, one set largely influencing endothelial differentiation and proliferation and the other governing vascular wall formation and vascular bed morphogenesis.[19] Initial events in vasculogenesis are dependent on fibroblast growth factor (FGF) and vascular endothelial growth factors A and B (VEGF A and B). Under their influence, endothelial cells differentiate from mesoderm of the blood islands, proliferate, and migrate. The pattern of endothelial differentiation is further determined by VEGF C, the receptor to which (VEGFR3) is expressed on endothelial cells destined to become veins and lymphatics.[19] Continued growth of endothelial cells and modeling of vascular walls is dependent on the expression of an additional set of tyrosine kinase receptors, tie1 and tie2. The binding of tie1 by its ligand, angiopoietin 1, plays a critical role in the induction of components of the vessel wall, as mutations in the genes for either result in defective vessels with poorly formed muscle walls and microaneurysms.

In contrast to formation of blood vessels in the embryo, new vessel formation in the postnatal state occurs largely as a result of microvessel formation from differentiated endothelial cells. Angiogenesis is governed by a complex interaction of proangiogenic and antiangiogenic factors[7,18] (Table 23–1) which are under tight control so that there is little, if any, increase in vessels in the normal state.[8,19] However, in response to stimuli such as tissue injury or hypoxia, this balance is perturbed and angiogenesis occurs. These substances therefore serve as "signals" that influence growth, migration, and the permeability of endothelial cells. During angiogenesis endothelial cells acquire protease, which permits them to digest basal lamina and move in the direction of the signal. Foremost among the signaling substances are VEGF and FGF. Once separated from a parent vessel, endothelial cells acquire small vacuoles or primitive lumens, which fuse with lumens of adjacent endothelium to form capillary channels. Although the mechanism by which these signals are processed by the endothelial cells is still the subject of intense inquiry, it appears that endothelial junctions (adherens junctions) play a pivotal role.[20] This specialized apparatus, consisting of a transmembrane protein VE (vascular endothelial) cadherin bound in its intracellular domain to catenin and in its extracellular domain to VE cadherins of adjacent cells, localizes or traps extracellular signaling molecules. The extracellular signals, in turn, alter the cadherin–catenin complex, thereby modifying the confluence and permeability of the endothelial cell. The cadherin–catenin complex is also involved in intracellular signaling from the cytoplasm to the nucleus such that gene expression is affected.

**TABLE 23–1 PROANGIOGENIC AND ANTIANGIOGENIC MOLECULES**

| |
|---|
| **Proangiogenic molecules** |
| Basic fibroblast growth factor (FGF) |
| Vascular endothelial growth factor (VEGF) |
| Prostaglandin $E_2$ |
| Hepatocyte growth factor |
| Nitric oxide |
| Integrins |
| Interleukin-8 |
| Platelet-derived growth factor |
| **Antiangiogenic molecules** |
| Angiostatin |
| Endostatin |
| Curcumin |
| Thalidomide |
| Nitric oxide inhibitors |
| Interferon-$\alpha$ |
| Glucocorticoids |
| Retinoids |

Modified from Arbiser JL. Angiogenesis: relevance for pathogenesis and treatment of dermatologic disease. Adv Dermatol 15:31, 1999.

## Normal Structure

The vasculature is divided into arterial and venous components joined by a network of capillaries. The arteries represent a system of dichotomously branching conduits that serve to regulate pressure and deliver blood to the capillary bed; the thin-walled veins return blood to the heart under lower pressures. The capillaries along with the terminal venules are the principal sites of gas exchange. Larger venules (postcapillary venules) are sensitive to vasoactive amines; hence they represent the most permeable portions of the vascular tree. The capillaries represent the smallest vessels, but it is often difficult to determine morphologically the exact point of transition between the smallest vein (or artery) and the capillary. Indeed, the current definition of *capillary* as a vessel, the diameter of which approximates that of the normal erythrocyte (8 mm), is based not only on morphologic but also physiologic observations.[25] The vessels are composed of a single flattened endothelial cell surrounded by basal lamina and occasional pericytes. The basal lamina is not appreciated by light microscopy but can be inferred by the periodic acid-Schiff (PAS)-positive staining material underneath the endothelium. Although this basic pattern pertains to all capillaries, electron microscopy has demonstrated various alterations from organ to organ. For instance, continuous capillaries consisting of a continuous layer of endothelium and basal lamina are typical of capillaries in skeletal and smooth muscle. Fenestrated capillaries, with small pores closed by flaps or diaphragms, are found in endocrine organs, the renal glomerulus, and other sites where there is rapid exchange of solute material.

Veins parallel the arterial system but are more numerous and appear as partially collapsed structures in tissue sections as a result of their inelasticity. In large and medium-size veins most of the wall is composed of adventitia made up of muscle fibers and elastic tissue arranged in a less orderly fashion than in the arteries. Small veins have no elastic tissue and only a small investiture of smooth muscle. The smallest veins are difficult to distinguish from small arteries, and the distinction at times is best made by the topographic relation to the capillary.

### Ultrastructure of the Vascular Membrane

The endothelial cell has an elongated shape and measures 25–50 mm in length. It is covered on its luminal aspect by a fine coat of carbohydrate-rich material. This nearly imperceptible covering was at one time thought to be the morphologic correlate for the nonthrombogenic property of the endothelium, although current evidence suggests that this probably is not true.[26] Underneath the fine cell coat the luminal surface is thrown into small folds or projections. Small micropinocytotic vesicles (60–70 nm) dot both the luminal and antiluminal surfaces of the cell and are believed important in the transport of fluid across the cell.[26] The cytoplasm usually contains a small amount of smooth and rough endoplasmic reticulum, free ribosomes, and mitochondria. A variety of filaments are present in the endothelium, including thin (actin), intermediate (vimentin), and thick (myosin) filaments. Rod-shaped bodies (Weibel-Palade bodies), a relatively specific feature of the endothelial cell, measure 0.1–0.3 mm in length and contain an internal structure of parallel tubules. They vary in number depending on the type of vessel; and on rare occasions they are also found in pericytes. Von Willebrand factor has been localized to these organelles by means of immunoelectron microscopy.[22] Intercellular attachments are typically prominent in the endothelial cell. Arterioles have elaborate attachments, whereas venules have less prominent ones, a feature that correlates with the observation that the venules represent preferred sites of permeability changes.

Vascular endothelium rests on a thin basal lamina (50 nm) of nonperiodic collagen, which is synthesized at least in part by the endothelial cells. In some areas in the vascular tree, the basal lamina may have a multilayered appearance. External to the endothelium but enveloped within the basal lamina are the pericytes. These mesenchymal cells have few distinguishing features apart from their branched processes, their close contacts with the endothelial cell, and their investiture by basal lamina. These cells are probably derived from fibroblasts of the surrounding connective tissue and in turn may differentiate into smooth muscle cells of the vessel wall.

### Normal Function

In additional to its traditional lining, or barrier, role the endothelium engages in a variety of other functions including vasoregulation, coagulation, and mediation of the immune response. The specific function and phenotype of a given endothelial cell are dependent on the tissue in question, the local microenvironment, and the activation by cytokines. Basic properties of endothelial metabolism include its ability to transport macromolecules through its system of pinocytotic vesicles, its receptor-mediated uptake of low density lipoproteins, and its uptake of sugars and amino acids. Endothelium has both procoagulant and anticoagulant properties, but under normal conditions it represents a nonthrombogenic surface. It synthesizes von Willebrand factor,[22] factor V, and plasminogen activator, which promote coagulation, whereas thrombomodulin, a surface endothelial protein, indirectly causes proteolyisis of von Willebrand factor and factor V. When appropriately stimulated, endothelial cells produce prostacyclin, a potent inhibitor of platelet aggregation. By virtue of its interactions with various mediators, the endothelium, particularly that of the microcirculation, is an important regulator of vascular tone and permeability. It produces both vasodilators (e.g., nitric oxide) and vasoconstrictors (e.g., angiotensin-converting enzyme and endothelin). Finally, endothelium participates in the immune and inflammatory responses by facilitating cell adhesion and transmigration. The selectins and the immunoglobulin gene superfamily are the two most important groups of cellular adhesion molecules expressed by endothelium. Many are constituitively expressed by endothelium but can also be upregulated by inflammatory cytokines. For example intercellular adhesion molecule-1 (ICAM-1) is normally expressed by endothelium but increases during the inflammatory response and is responsible for leukocyte adhesion and transendothelial migration.

## HEMANGIOMAS

Hemangioma is one of the most common soft tissue tumors (7% of all benign tumors) and is the most common tumor during infancy and childhood.[2,4,6,12,13,43]

**TABLE 23–2 DISTRIBUTION OF 570 HEMANGIOMAS**

| Location | No. of Cases |
|---|---|
| Cutaneous or mucosal hemangiomas | 370 |
| Oral cavity | 80 |
| Face | 75 |
| Arm | 60 |
| Leg | 50 |
| Scalp | 46 |
| Vulva and scrotum | 5 |
| Other | 54 |
| Liver | 109 |
| Central nervous system | 43 |
| Heart | 16 |
| Bone | 12 |
| Gastrointestinal tract, kidney, mesentery | 10 |
| Muscle | 10 |
| *Total* | 570 |

Data modified from Geshickter CF, Keasbey LE. Tumors of blood vessels. Am J Cancer 23:568, 1935.

Most hemangiomas are superficial lesions that have a predilection for the head and neck region, but they may also occur internally, notably in organs such as the liver (Table 23–2). The common capillary and cavernous hemangiomas of adults are more frequently encountered in women and may fluctuate in size with pregnancy and menarche; this suggests that the endothelial cells of these tumors may be responsive to circulating hormones. Although some vascular tumors regress altogether (e.g., juvenile hemangioma), most persist if untreated but have limited growth potential. Hemangiomas virtually never undergo malignant transformation; likewise, the concept of a benign metastasizing hemangioma is no longer accepted. Most prove to be angiosarcomas with well differentiated areas.

## Capillary Hemangioma

Capillary hemangiomas comprise the largest single group of hemangiomas. They usually appear during the first few years of life (with the notable exception of the senile or cherry angioma) and are located in the skin or subcutaneous tissue. Rare cases are familial; linkage analysis has localized the mutation to chromosome 5, where candidate genes include FGF and platelet-derived growth factor (PDGF).[67] Typically elevated and red to purple in color, they are composed of a proliferation of capillary-size vessels lined by flattened endothelium (Fig. 23–1). Architecturally, virtually all capillary hemangiomas are composed of nodules of small capillary-size vessels, each of which is subserved by a "feeder" vessel. This lobular or grouped arrangement of vessels is a helpful feature for distinguishing benign and malignant vascular proliferations.[16] The term *lobular hemangioma* has been employed as a generic designation for a number of hemangiomas characterized by this architectural

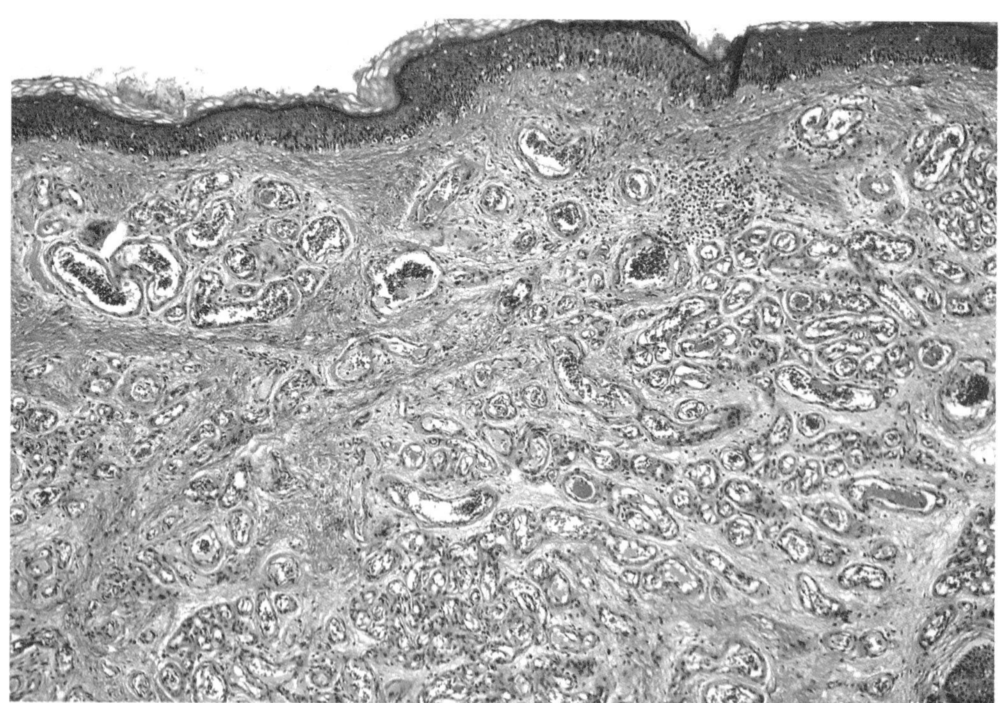

**FIGURE 23–1.** Adult form of capillary hemangioma consisting of small vessels lined by flattened mature endothelium.

pattern, including capillary hemangioma of infancy, pyogenic granuloma, and epithelioid hemangioma. Several clinical variants of capillary hemangiomas are discussed below, including the cellular hemangioma of infancy (strawberry nevus, nevus vasculosus, hypertrophic angioma of infancy, benign hemangioendothelioma of infancy). The cellular hemangioma of infancy is a form of capillary hemangioma.[48–53,56,57,59,64,65,67,69] It occurs during infancy at a rate of about 1 in every 200 live births.[108] About one-fifth of the cases are multiple. During the early stage it may resemble a common birthmark in that it is a flat, red lesion that intensifies in color when the infant strains or cries. With time it acquires an elevated, protruding appearance that distinguishes it from birthmarks and has earned it the fanciful designation of **strawberry nevus** (Fig. 23–2). Deeply situated lesions impart little color to the overlying skin and consequently may be misdiagnosed preoperatively. These tumors may be located on any body surface but are most common in the region of the head and neck, particularly the parotid, where they seemingly follow the distribution of cutaneous nerves and arteries.

The evolution of these lesions is characteristic. Although described as congenital they actually appear within a few weeks after birth[66] and rapidly enlarge over a period of several months, achieving the largest size in about 6–12 months; they regress over a period of a few years. Regression is usually accompanied by fading of the lesion from scarlet to dull red-gray and by concomitant wrinkling of the once-taut skin. It has been estimated that by age 7 years, 75–90% have involuted, leaving a small pigmented scar. In the lesions that have ulcerated, the cosmetic defect may be more significant. The clinical phases of cellular hemangioma have distinctive physiologic differences elegantly detailed by Takahashi et al.[63] (see below).

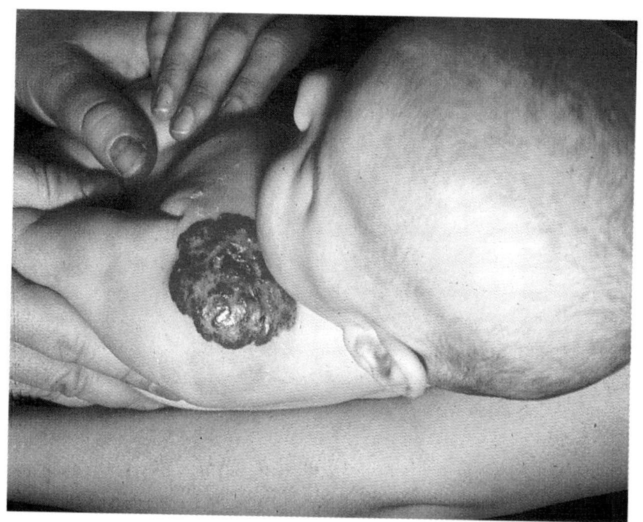

**FIGURE 23–2.** Clinical appearance of juvenile hemangioma.

The tumors are multinodular masses fed by a single normally occurring arteriole[66] (Fig. 23–3). Histologically, the tumor varies with its age. Early lesions are characterized by plump endothelial cells that line vascular spaces with small inconspicuous lumens (Figs. 23–4, 23–5, 23–6) Mitotic figures may be present in moderate numbers. Mast cells and factor XIII-positive interstitial cells are a consistent feature of these tumors. The former may be important in the production of angiogenic factors that regulate the growth of these tumors.[53] At this early stage of development the vascular nature of the tumor may not be readily apparent unless a reticulin preparation is done that demonstrates connective tissue fibers encircling myriad tiny vessels. As the lesions mature and blood flow through the lesion commences, the endothelium becomes flattened and resembles that seen in adult forms of capillary hemangioma (Fig. 23–5). Maturation usually begins at the periphery of the tumors but ultimately involves all zones. Regression of the juvenile hemangioma is accompanied by a progressive, diffuse interstitial fibrosis and is believed to be mediated by way of apoptosis. In unusual cases infarction of the tumor may occur, presumably as a result of thrombosis.

Electron microscopy and immunohistochemistry can be helpful for defining the vascular nature of these tumors.[59,60,64] Solid nests of endothelium are surrounded by basal lamina and are encircled by a cuff of pericytes (Fig. 23–6). More mature areas, of course, display canalization of the vessels. Weibel-Palade bodies may be present but tend to be scarce in less mature areas. A peculiar crystalline structure has been identified in the endothelium of these tumors.[55,60] Measuring about 0.5–2.0 mm, they have a substructure consisting of parallel lamellar bands with a periodicity of 18–30 nm. Their exact significance is unknown, although it is believed that they reflect the immaturity of the endothelium, as similar structures have been noted in human fetal endothelium.

The clinical phases of cellular hemangiomas have been correlated with a distinctive immunophenotypic profile.[47,61–63,65,69] During the early proliferative phase (0–12 months) the tumors can be shown immunohistochemically to express proliferating cell nuclear antigen (PCNA), VEGF, and type IV collagenase, the former two localized to both endothelium and pericytes and the last to endothelium. All of these substances are associated with proliferation and growth of vessels. The adjacent epidermis potentially contributes to the production of angiogenic factors.[47] During the involuting phase (1–5 years) these substances are dra-

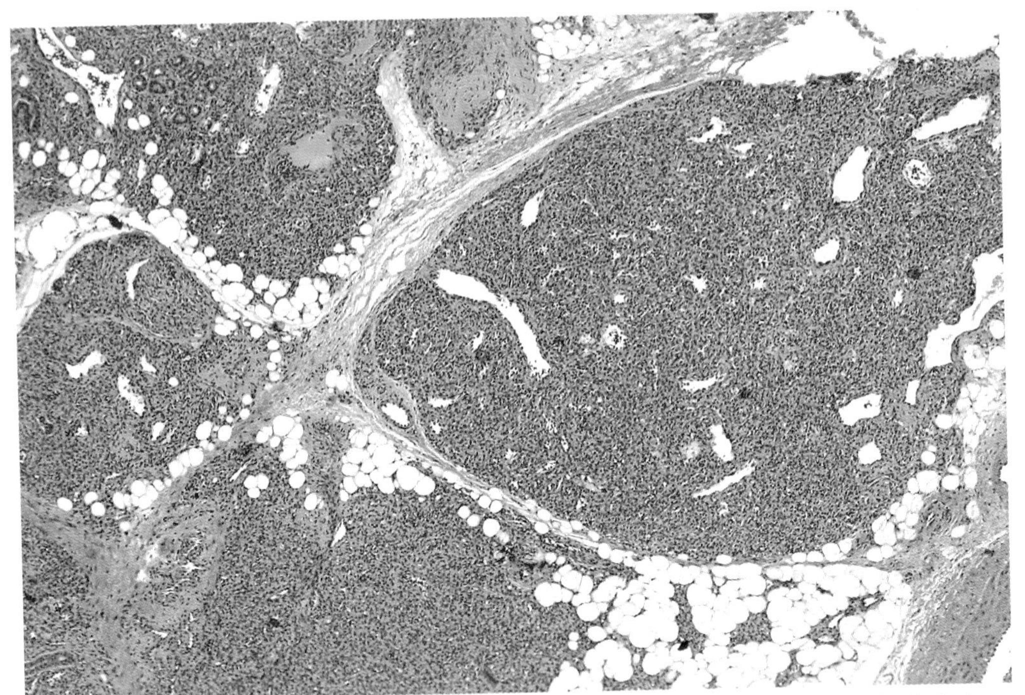

**FIGURE 23–3.** Low power view of juvenile hemangioma illustrating lobular growth. Lobules contain central "feeding" vessels.

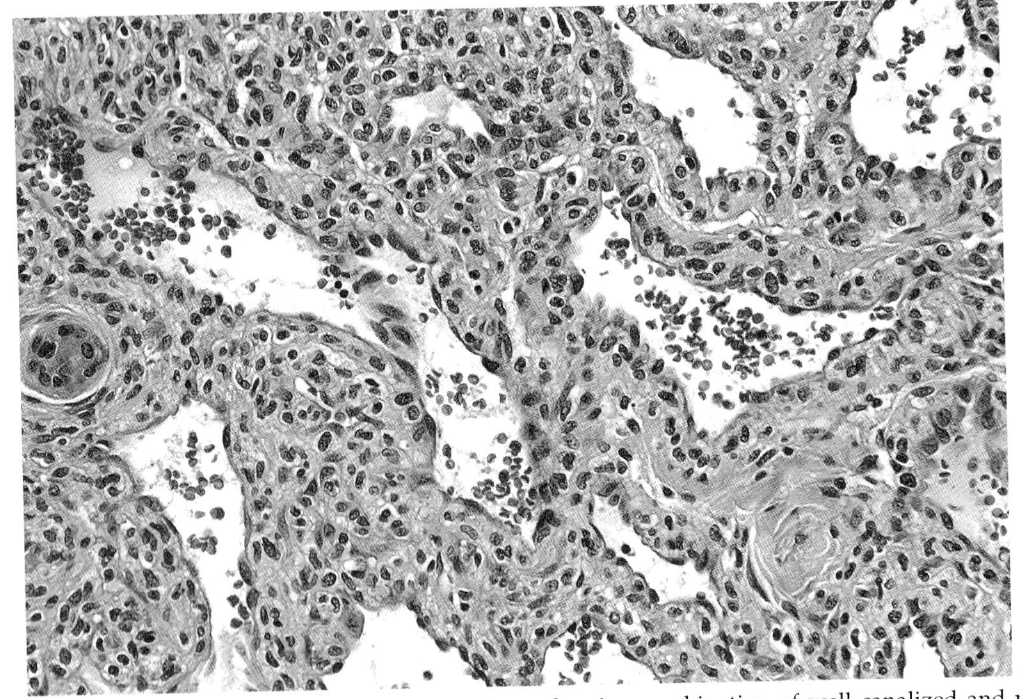

**FIGURE 23–4.** Juvenile form of capillary hemangioma showing combination of well canalized and poorly canalized vessels.

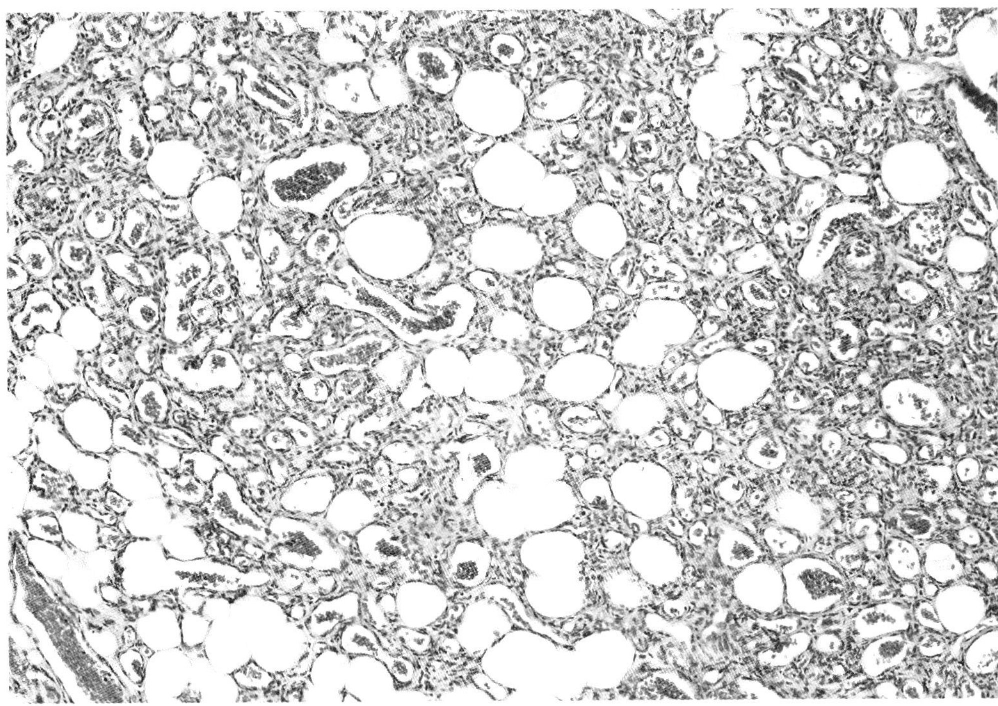

**FIGURE 23–5.** Juvenile hemangioma showing canalization of most vessels.

matically reduced, whereas the tissue inhibition of metalloproteinases (TIMP), an antiangiogenic factor, is markedly elevated. The traditional vascular markers CD31, von Willebrand factor (vWF), and smooth muscle actin are present during the proliferative and involuting phases but are lost after the lesion is fully involuted. These findings contrast with congenital vascular lesions and malformations, which remain static throughout their natural history, and do not express PCNA, VEGF, and type IV collagenase. Of interest is the observation that, independent of stage, all cellular hemangiomas of infancy express GLUT1, a glucose transport receptor.[58] The expression of this receptor is independent of proliferative activity and is not found in other forms of hemangioma, although it is present rarely in angiosarcomas.

Treatment of these lesions must be individualized and depends on factors such as the location or rate of growth. When this tumor is in the rapid growth phase, there is often a tendency to be overzealous in therapy. It has been suggested that these lesions be approached with a policy of masterful neglect. Most can be followed clinically with little or no intervention. Large, life-threatening lesions impinging on critical structures (e.g., airway) are usually treated with systemic glucocorticoids until a clinical response is achieved. A second option is interferon-$\alpha$ (INF$\alpha$) which retards endothelial proliferation. Both glucocorticoids[35] and INF$\alpha$ require long-term administration with some attendant side effects. INF$\alpha$, in particular, has been associated with spastic diplegia.[18]

### Acquired Tufted Angioma (Angioblastoma of Nakagawa)

First described by Wilson-Jones and Orkin,[73] the acquired tufted angioma shares some features of juvenile hemangioma,[71–73] but more likely represents a limited form of kaposiform hemangioendothelioma in an adult unassociated with Kasabach-Merritt syndrome. As implied by its name, it usually occurs in an older group of patients on an acquired basis and is characterized by slowly growing erythematous macules or plaques involving the dermis of the upper portions of the body. Histologically, the lesion is made up of nodules of capillary-sized vessels that grow in a "cannonball" fashion throughout the deep dermis. The capillary-size vessels may be imperfectly canalized, giving the impression of solid nests of endothelial cells (Fig. 23–7). At the periphery some of the vessels appear flattened or slit-like, somewhat reminiscent of Kaposi's sarcoma. Although the appearance of this tumor is perhaps most similar to that of cellular hemangioma of infancy, it is not arranged in distinct lobules but rather grows in an irregular fashion throughout the dermis. Moreover, with immunohistochemical procedures, most of the solid endothelial nests do not express factor VIII-associated

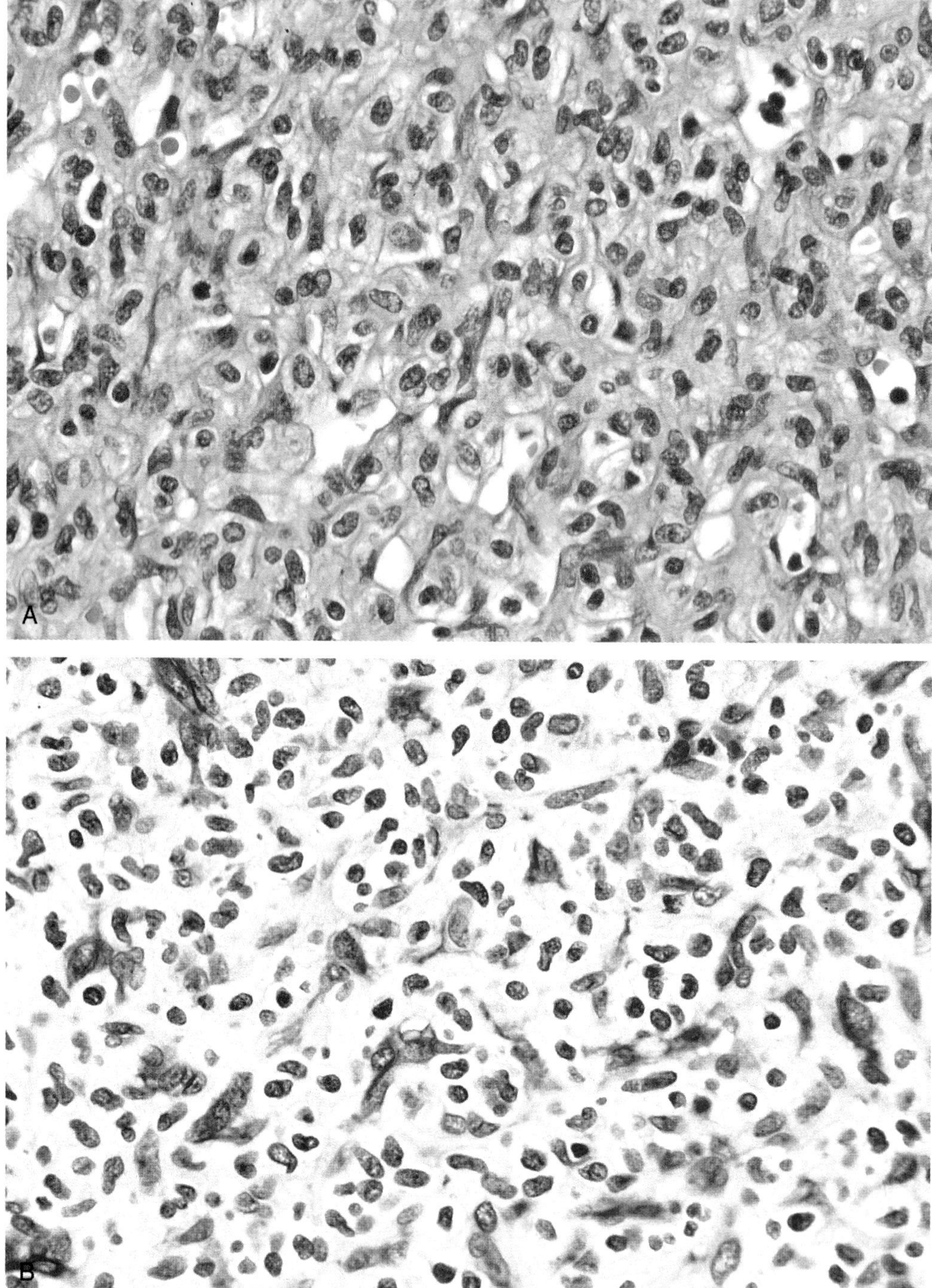

**FIGURE 23–6.** (**A**) High power view of cellular areas of juvenile hemangioma. (**B**) Immunostain for von Willebrand factor (vWF) illustrates a network of mature endothelial cells. Note the population of nonreactive cells representing a combination of immature endothelial cells and pericytes.

*Illustration continued on opposite page*

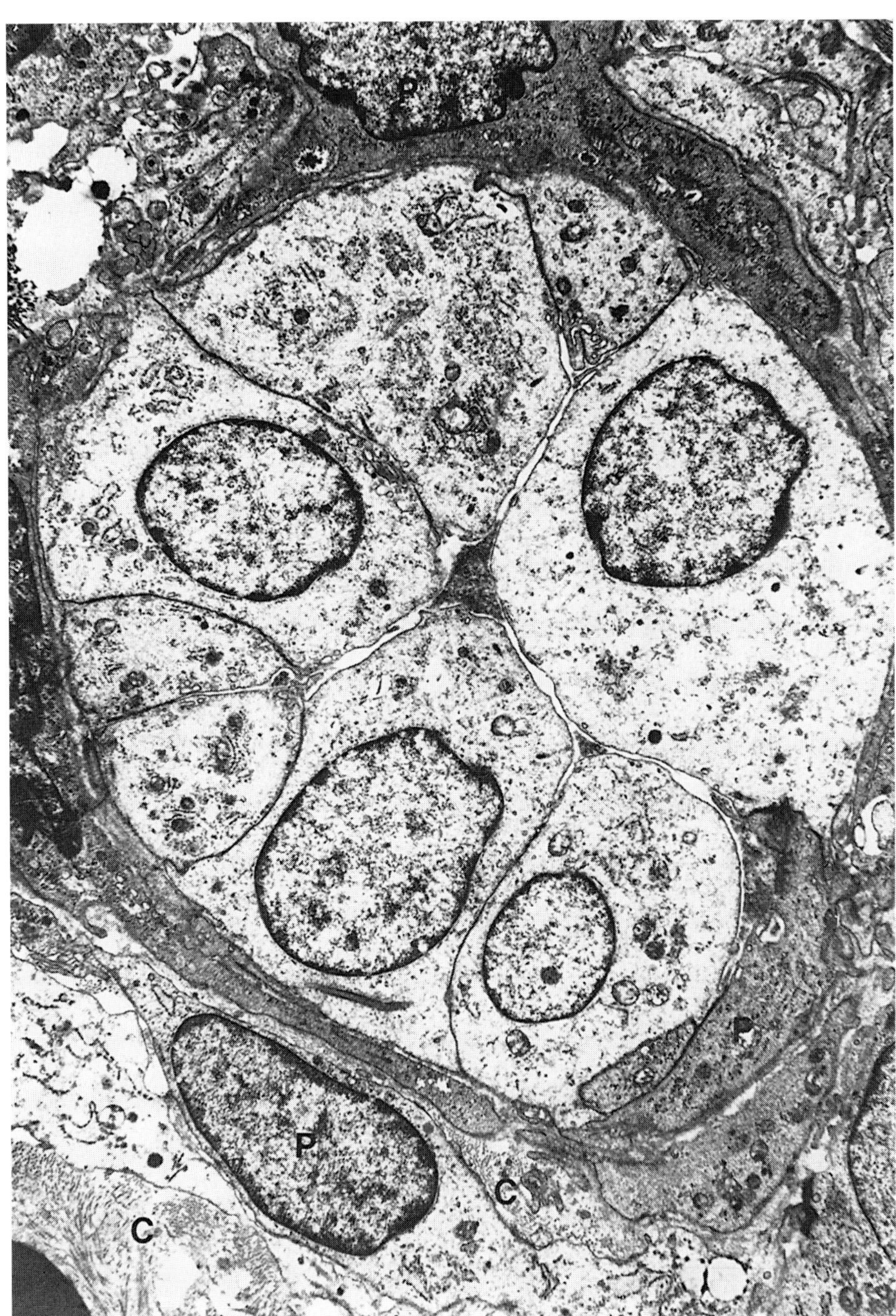


**FIGURE 23–6** *(Continued).* (**C**) Electron micrograph of juvenile hemangioma. Prominent endothelial cells eclipse the lumen. Vessels are surrounded by basal lamina, pericytes (P), and collagen (C). (From Taxy JB, Battifora H. In: Trump BF, Jones RT (eds) Diagnostic Electron Microscopy. Wiley, New York, 1980.)

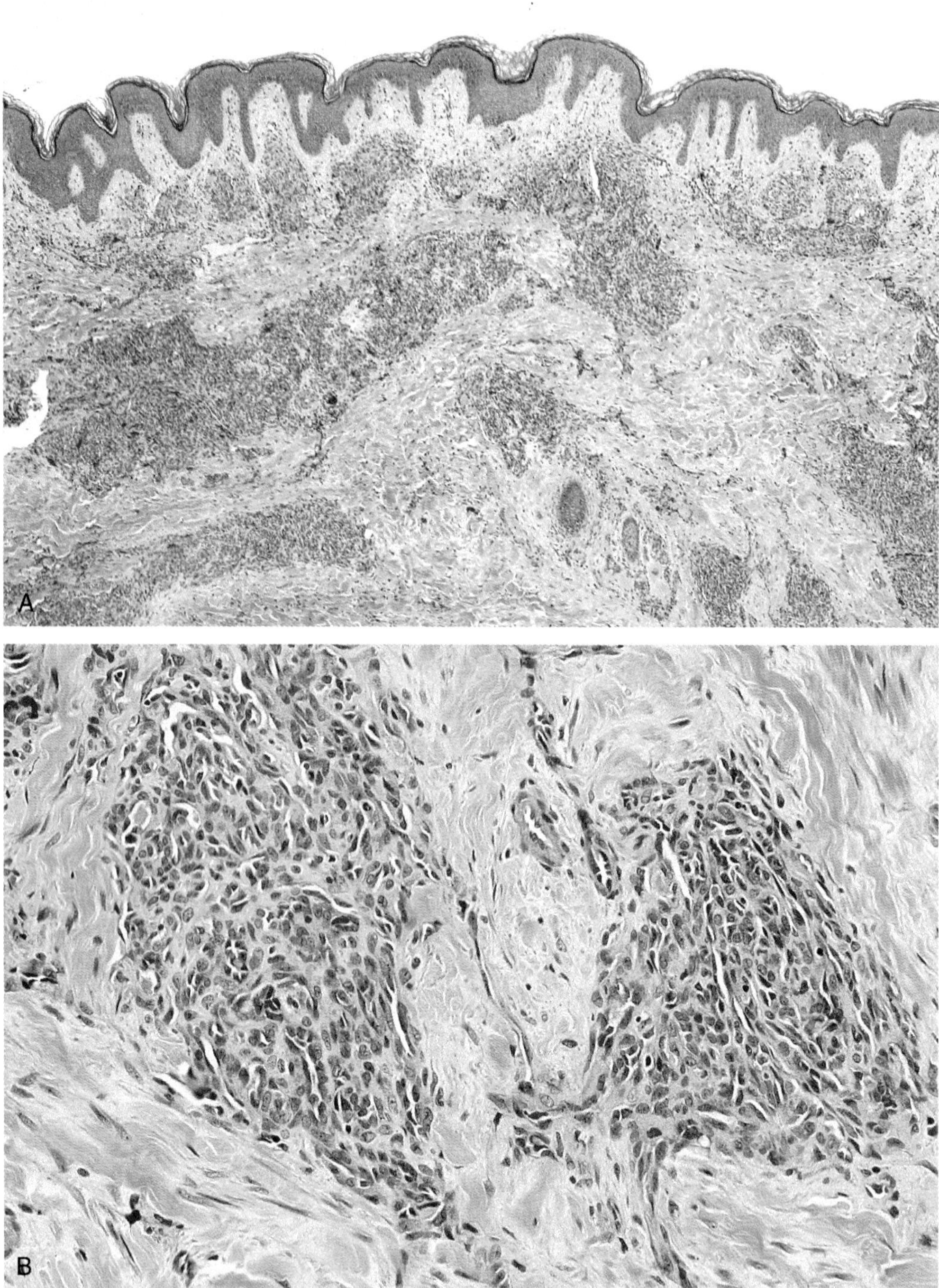


**FIGURE 23–7.** Acquired tufted hemangioma illustrating "cannonball" nests of tumor in the dermis (**A**). High power view depicts irregular groups of capillary-sized vessels (**B**). (Case courtesy of Dr. Philip Allen.)

antigen, although other endothelial markers can be identified, suggesting that the cells represent a more primitive form of endothelial cell. Ultrastructurally, endothelial crystalloids similar to those in capillary hemangiomas of infancy have been identified.[71] The usual course of this tumor is that of progressive spread with ultimate stabilization.

### Hobnail Hemangioma (Targetoid Hemosiderotic Hemangioma)

Hobnail hemangioma, described by Guillou et al.,[74] represents the benign counterpart of retiform hemangioendothelioma. It usually develops on the skin of the extremities in young adults as an angiomatous/pigmented or exophytic mass and has a distinctive biphasic appearance (Figs. 23–8, 23–9). The superficial portion of the lesion consists of dilated vessels lined by hobnail endothelial cells (see Chapter 25) containing occasional intraluminal papillary tufts similar to the Dabska tumor. The deep portion consists of attenuated, slit-like capillaries that ramify in the dermis. Although the pattern is somewhat suggestive of an angiosarcoma, vessels have a rather innocuous appearance. Hemorrhage, hemosiderin deposits, lymphocytes, and dermal sclerosis can accompany the lesions. The endothelial cells in hobnail hemangiomas are $CD31^+$ and $VEGFR3^+$, indicating a phenotypic similarity to those in hobnail hemangioendothelioma (retiform-type). The more than 50 cases that have been reported have had a benign clinical course.[74,75]

Hobnail hemangiomas correspond to some lesions originally termed targetoid hemosiderotic hemangioma by Santa Cruz and Aronberg.[77,78] However, targetoid hemosiderotic hemangioma is a clinical term referring to the presence of an ecchymotic halo surrounding a violaceous papule, and it is doubtful that these clinically defined lesions have a common pathologic appearance. The term hobnail hemangioma has therefore proven to be more useful to pathologists.

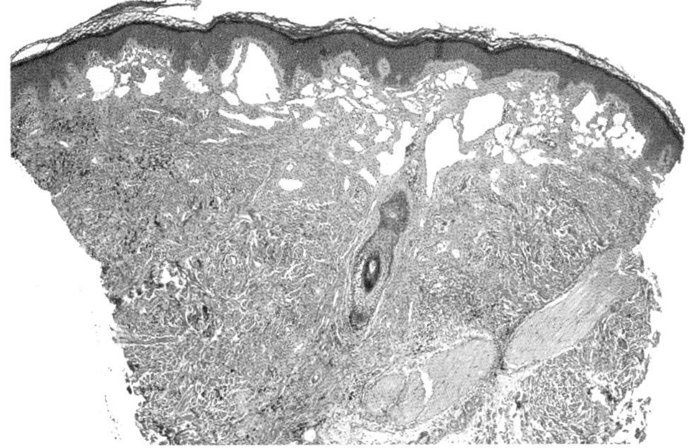

**FIGURE 23–8.** Hobnail hemangioma (targetoid hemosiderotic hemangioma).

### Verrucous Hemangioma

Verrucous hemangioma is a variant of capillary or cavernous hemangioma that undergoes reactive hyperkeratosis of the overlying skin and consequently may be confused with a wart or keratosis.[37] The lesions begin during childhood as unilateral lesions in the dermis of the lower extremity. Grossly and histologically, they resemble conventional hemangiomas during their early stage of development. With time the overlying epidermis displays hyperkeratosis, acanthosis, and papillomatosis, features that obscure the vascular nature of the lesions. These tumors have a propensity to recur locally and to develop satellite lesions if incompletely excised.

### Cherry Angioma (Senile Angioma, De Morgan's Spots).

Cherry angioma is a ruby red papule that measures a few millimeters in diameter and has a pale halo zone.[156] It may appear during adolescence but is most common in late adult life. The predilection for the trunk and extremity contrasts with the head and neck location for most childhood hemangiomas. The lesions are located in the superficial corium and consist of dilated thin-walled capillaries, which create an elevation and mild atrophy of the overlying skin.

### Cavernous Hemangioma

Cavernous hemangiomas are less frequent than capillary hemangiomas but share common age and anatomic distributions. They are most common during childhood and are located in the upper portion of the body. As a result, it has been suggested that they simply represent massively engorged capillary hemangiomas, a contention supported by the fact that some hemangiomas have a capillary component at the surface and a cavernous component in the deeper portion. They differ from capillary hemangiomas in several important respects. They are usually larger and less circumscribed, and they more frequently involve deep structures. They show essentially no tendency to regress and may even be locally destructive by virtue of the pressure they exert on neighboring structures. Consequently, most cavernous hemangiomas require surgery, in contrast to their capillary counterparts.

The color and surface appearance of these lesions relate to the location. Superficial lesions are blue, puffy masses with an irregular surface caused by dil-

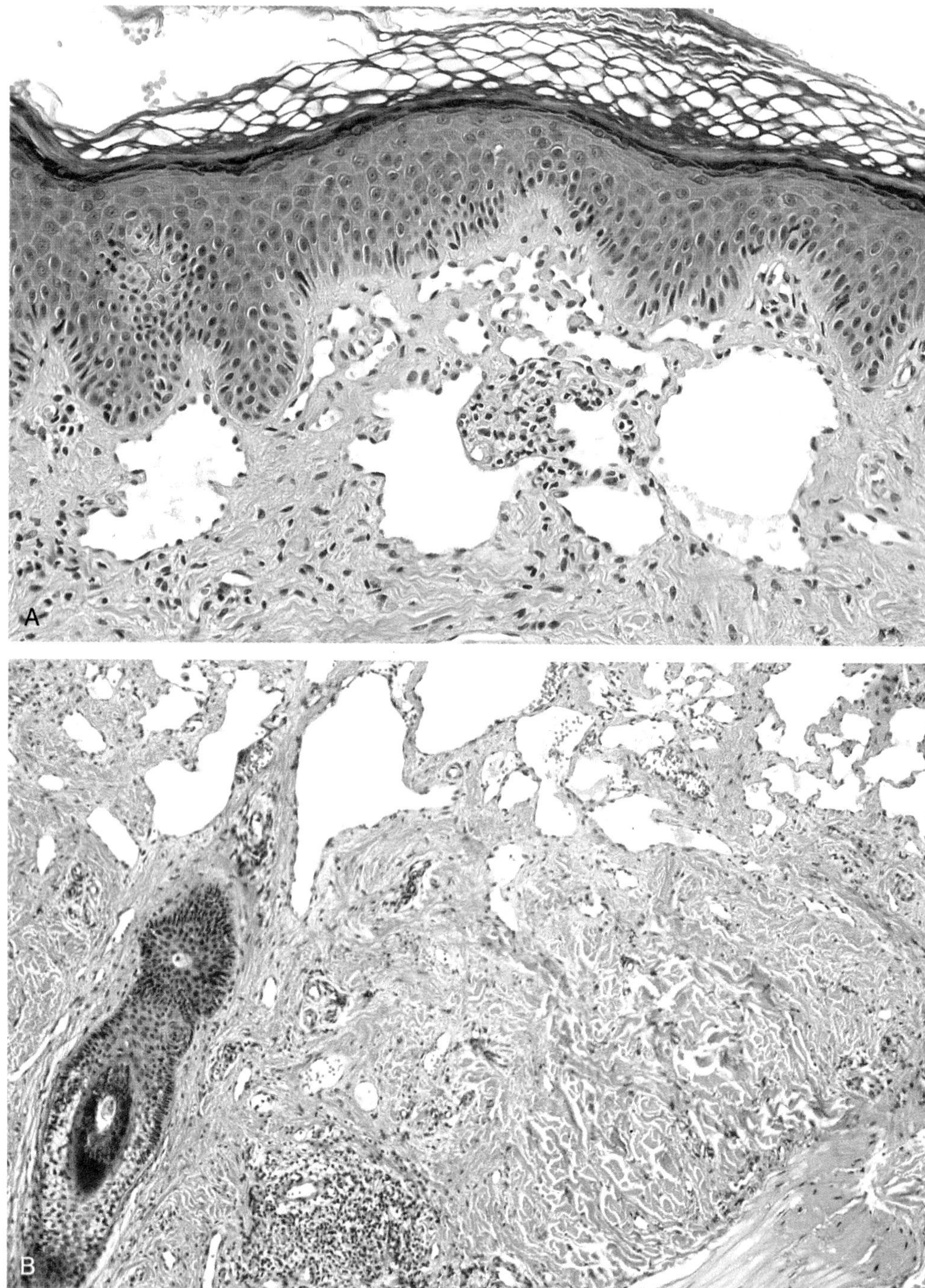


**FIGURE 23–9.** Hobnail hemangioma (targetoid hemosiderotic hemangioma) showing ectatic vessels at the surface (**A**) and in deeper regions illustrating the interface of ectatic vessels with attentuated slit-like vessels (**B**).

atation of the vessels (Fig. 23–10). Deep lesions may impart little or no color to the overlying skin. Radiographically, the large deep lesions appear as localized or diffuse nonhomogeneous water density masses. Tortuous water density channels representing the afferent and efferent blood supplies are occasionally seen in adjacent fat. Calcification is common and may be of several types (Fig. 23–11). Amorphous or curvilinear calcification is nonspecific, whereas phlebolith formation is not only more frequent but also a more specific finding. Both are the result of dystrophic calcification in organizing thrombi.[9] Cavernous hemangiomas are composed of large, dilated, blood-filled vessels lined by flattened endothelium (Fig. 23–12). The vessels may be arranged in a roughly lobular arrangement or in a diffuse haphazard pattern. The walls are occasionally thickened by an adventitial fibrosis, and inflammatory cells may be scattered throughout the stroma. Mature bone is occasionally present (Fig. 23–13).

*Sinusoidal hemangioma* is a variant of cavernous hemangioma that differs from the latter in several respects.[31] It occurs as a solitary acquired lesion in adults, usually women, and is relatively well demarcated (Figs. 23–14, 23–15). The thin-walled cavernous vessels ramify with one another to a much greater extent than in a conventional cavernous hemangioma. Papillary infoldings of the endothelium are usually identified; and in two cases reported by Calonje and Fletcher,[31] central infarction of the tumors occurred. Whether these lesions deserve to be considered a distinct entity is not clear, as sinuoidal patterns may be seen in hemangiomas of all types secondary to thrombosis and reorganization.

Several syndromes may be associated with cavernous hemangiomas. Thrombocytopenia purpura complicating giant hemangiomas is known as *Kasabach-Merritt syndrome*.[30,33,38,39] Most of these hemangiomas are large solitary cavernous lesions located on an extremity, although the syndrome occurs with kaposiform hemangioendothelioma,[14] angiomatosis, and rarely angiosarcoma. Typically the syndrome occurs during infancy, and the onset of purpura is heralded by rapid enlargement of the tumor. The patients develop numerous cutaneous petechiae and ecchymoses, not only in the skin but also in internal organs, due

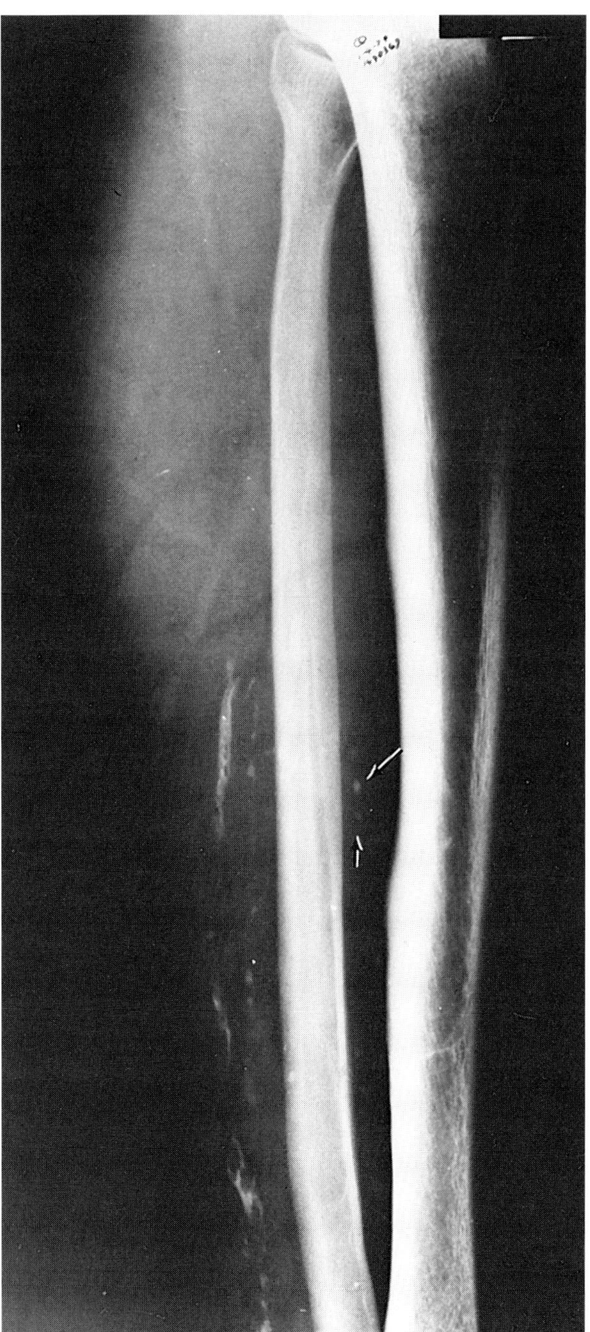

**FIGURE 23–11.** Radiograph of a hemangioma with both cavernous and venous features histologically. Note the long curvilinear calcifications in addition to phleboliths (arrows). The latter are highly characteristic of cavernous hemangiomas. (Courtesy of Dr. John Madewell.)

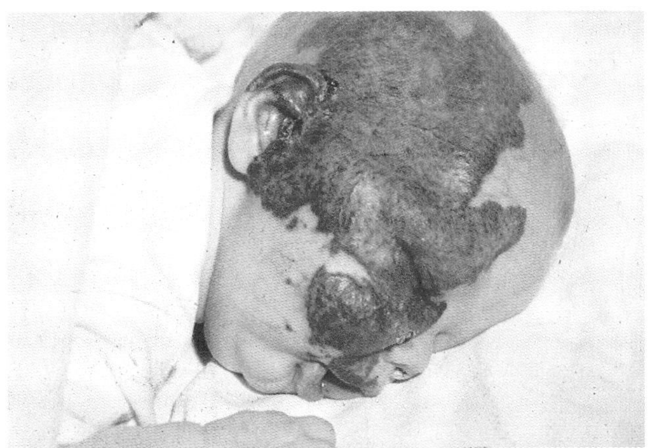

**FIGURE 23–10.** Cavernous hemangioma of the face.

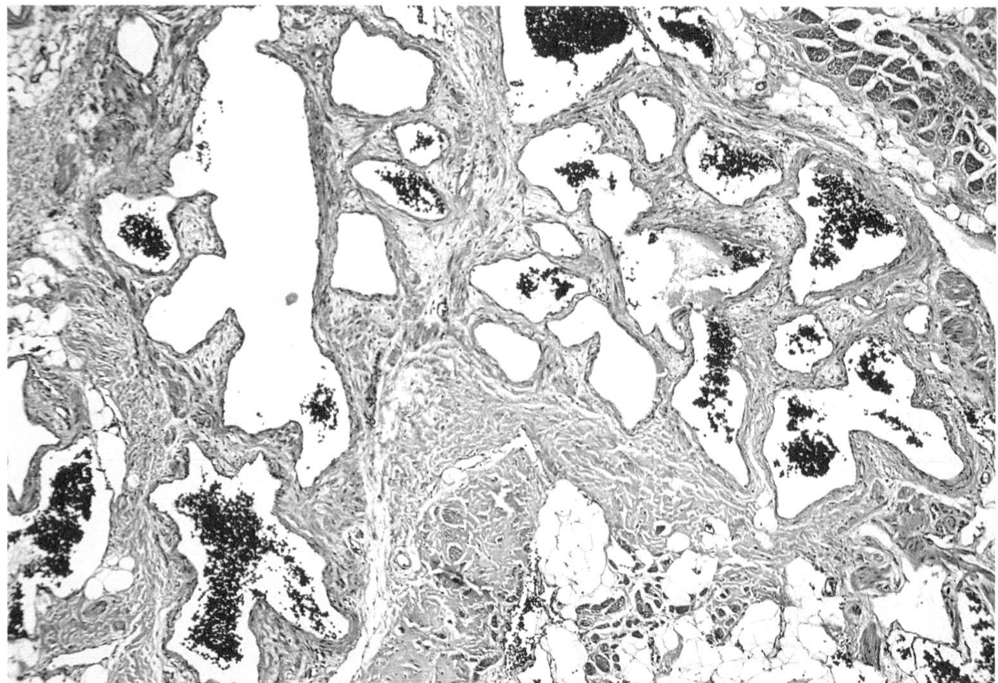

**FIGURE 23–12.** Cavernous hemangioma with large, thin-walled veins.

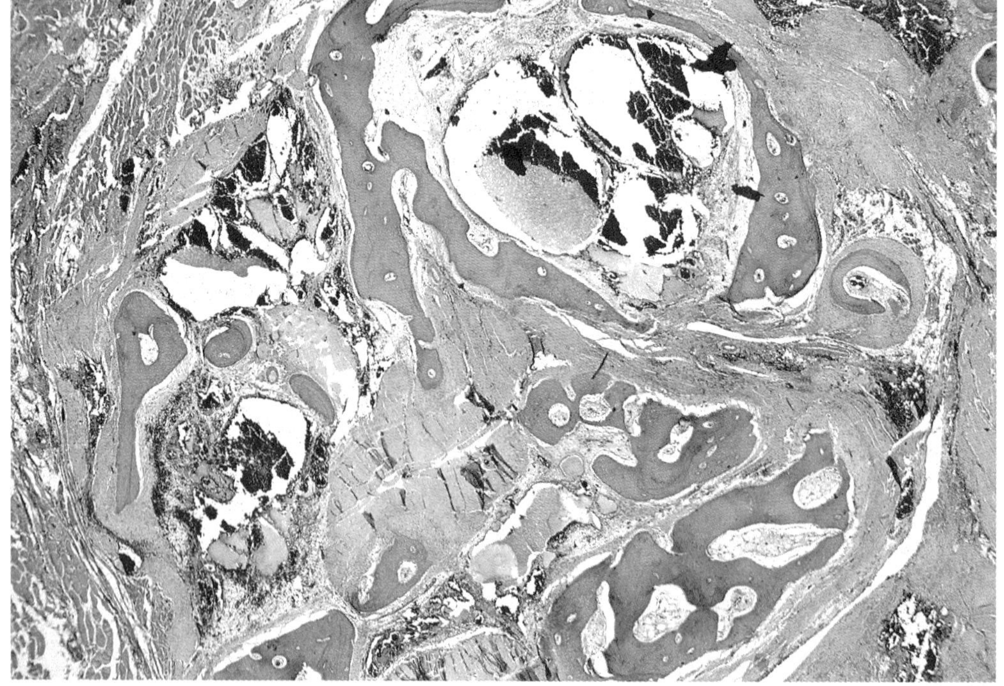

**FIGURE 23–13.** Cavernous hemangioma with bone.

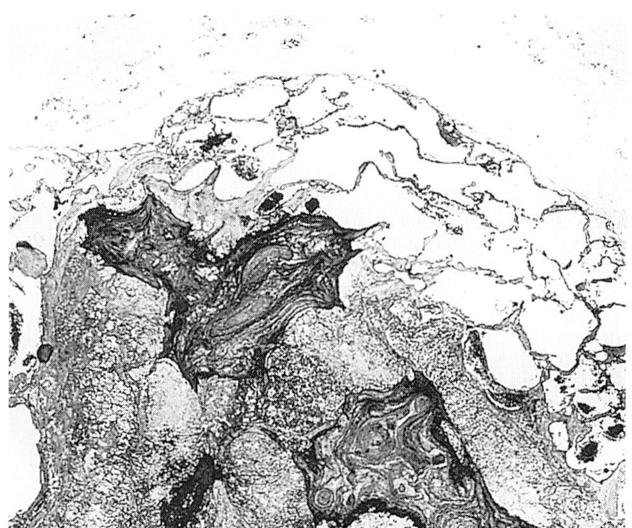

**FIGURE 23–14.** Sinusoidal hemangioma. (×25) (Case courtesy of Dr. C.D.M. Fletcher.)

to intravascular coagulation and sequestration of platelets in the tumor. Patients with this syndrome usually require therapy because death from hemorrhage and infection approaches 30%, and spontaneous regression of these tumors cannot be anticipated. In most cases surgery is not possible because of the precarious hematologic status of the patient and the large size of the tumor. In the past, steroids, irradiation, or both were the mainstay of treatment. Several new strategies include the administration of recombinant interferon alpha-2a[7,18] and pentoxifylline.[33]

A distinctive form of cavernous hemangioma of the skin in association with similar gastrointestinal tract lesions was delineated by Bean in 1958 as *blue rubber bleb nevus syndrome*.[156] The term aptly describes the blue cutaneous lesions, which look and feel like rubber nipples. They compress easily with pressure, leaving a flaccid wrinkled appearance to the skin, and then regain their shape with cessation of pressure. Hyperhidrosis may occur over these lesions probably as a result of increased surface termperature. In addition, most patients have gastrointestinal hemangiomas, usually in the small intestine. These internal lesions commonly bleed, so chronic anemia complicates the course of the disease. Some cases are inherited in an autosomal dominant fashion, although most appear to be sporadic. Because of the diffuse nature of the disease, therapy is aimed at resecting only bleeding lesions from the intestine.

*Maffucci syndrome (dyschondroplasia with vascular hamartomas)* is a rare mesodermal dysplasia characterized by multiple hemangiomas and enchondromas (Fig. 23–16). The vascular tumors are usually noted at birth and are of the cavernous type,[156] although the question has been raised as to whether many of these cavernous hemangiomas are really spindle cell hemangiomas. Other vascular lesions including lymphangiomas and phlebectasias may also be present.

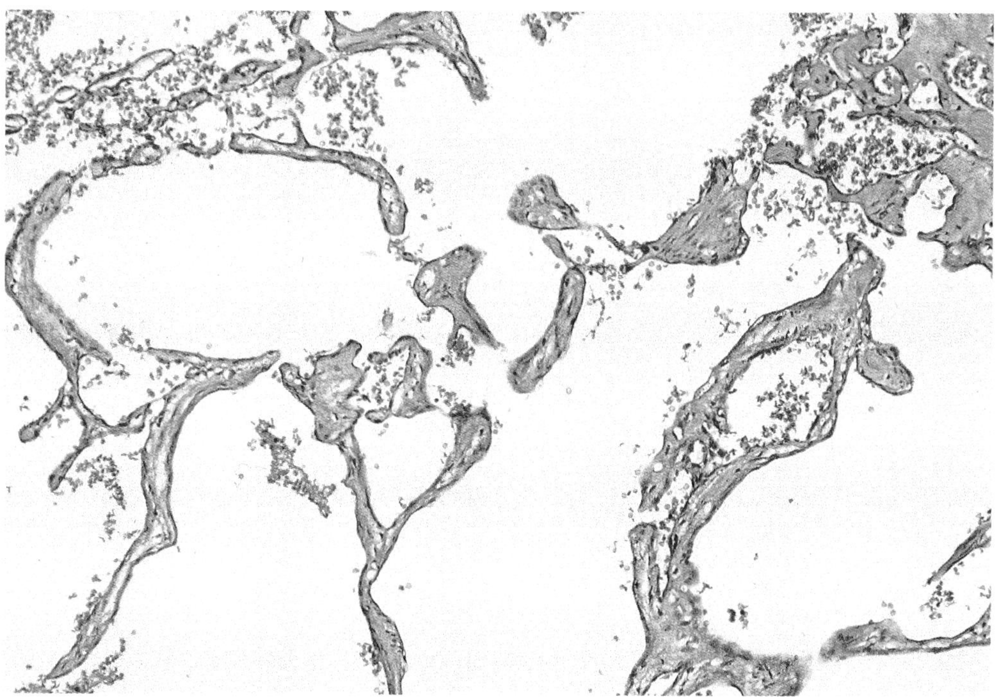

**FIGURE 23–15.** Sinusoidal hemangioma. (Case courtesy of Dr. C.D.M. Fletcher.)

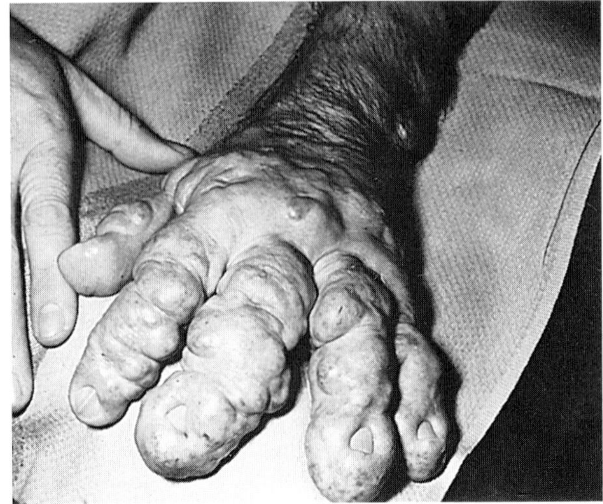

**FIGURE 23–16.** Multiple enchondromas in a patient with Maffucci syndrome. Patients also develop hemangiomas.

The cartilaginous tumors typically develop after the vascular lesions and are the result of a defect in endochondral ossification, so there is a marked overgrowth in the cartilage plates. The bones are shortened and have numerous enchondromas and exostoses. Pathologic fractures are common; and in about 20% of the patients malignant tumors, usually chondrosarcomas (or rarely angiosarcomas), develop.

## Arteriovenous Hemangioma (Arteriovenous Malformation)

Arteriovenous hemangioma is a term used in the past to describe deeply situated vascular lesions with a significant component of veins and arteries, often associated with arteriovenous shunting, documented radiologically or clinically (Fig. 23–17). We have largely abandoned this term because most of these lesions are now classified as intramuscular hemangioma, angiomatosis, or capillary hemangioma from a patho-

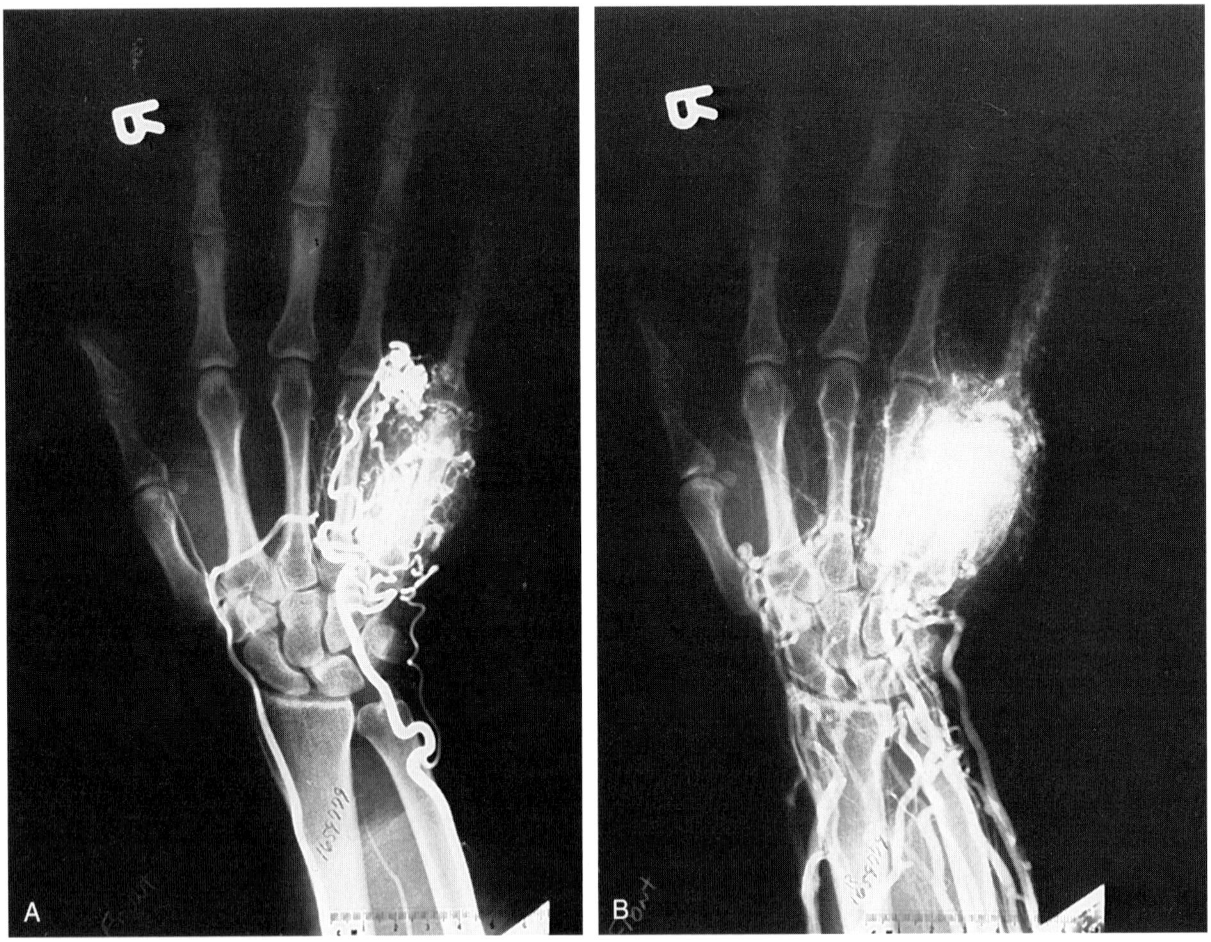

**FIGURE 23–17.** Arteriovenous hemangioma of hand. (**A**) Arteriogram shows filling of arterial vessels supplying tumor. (**B**) Opacification of tumor in the region of the fifth metacarpal and filling of draining veins while still in the arterial phase. (Courtesy of Dr. John Madewell.)

logic point of view. In passing, it should be noted that the cutaneous manifestations of arteriovenous malformations can crudely simulate the appearance of Kaposi's sarcoma (see Chapter 25). These changes have been referred to as *kaposiform angiodermatitis* or *pseudo-Kaposi's sarcoma*[79,80,82] These changes consist of a proliferation of small capillary-size vessels with thickened walls in association with fibroblasts and hemosiderin deposits (Fig. 23–18).

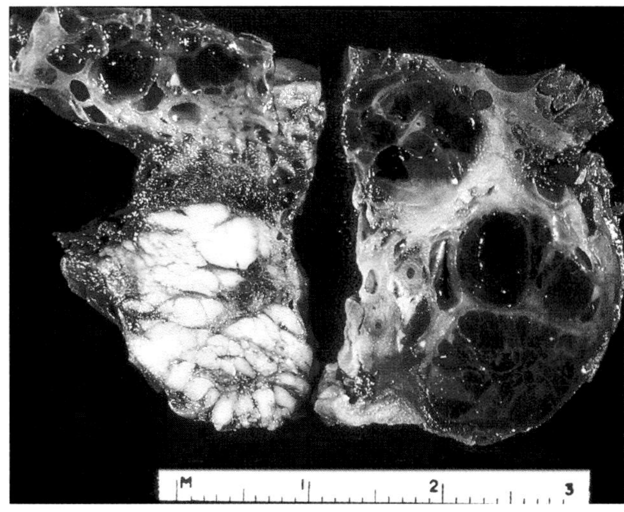

**FIGURE 23–19.** Gross specimen of a venous hemangioma.

## Venous Hemangioma (Venous Malformation)

Venous hemangiomas characteristically present during adult life and are most common in deep locations such as the retroperitoneum, mesentery, and muscles of the extremity, where they develop as large masses consisting of congeries of gaping venous vessels (Fig. 23–19). Blood flow is slow in these spaces, and the feeding vessels may be thrombosed. Consequently, these lesions are often not visualized on arteriography but require venography or direct injection to identify their presence and extent[9] (Fig. 23–20). Histologically, they are distinguished from capillary and cavernous hemangiomas by the fact that most of their vessels are thick-walled. The muscle in the vessel walls is less well organized than that of normal veins and appears irregularly attenuated or blends with surrounding soft tissue structures (Fig. 23–21). Calcification may also occur in these lesions and represents dystrophic calcification in organizing thrombus material just as it does in cavernous hemangiomas. Venous hemangiomas may also have areas that are indistinguishable from a cavernous hemangioma. Although we have designated such lesions "hemangiomas of mixed (cavernous and venous) type," they probably are best regarded as variations on the theme of venous hemangioma. It should also be noted that some cases of angiomatosis essentially have the appearance of a venous hemangioma. We have encountered two distinctive venous hemangiomas composed of thick-walled vessels that occurred on the dorsum of the feet in two children with Turner syndrome.[17] These rather distinctive forms of venous hemangioma may represent one of the various cardiovascular abnormalities associated with this genetic syndrome.

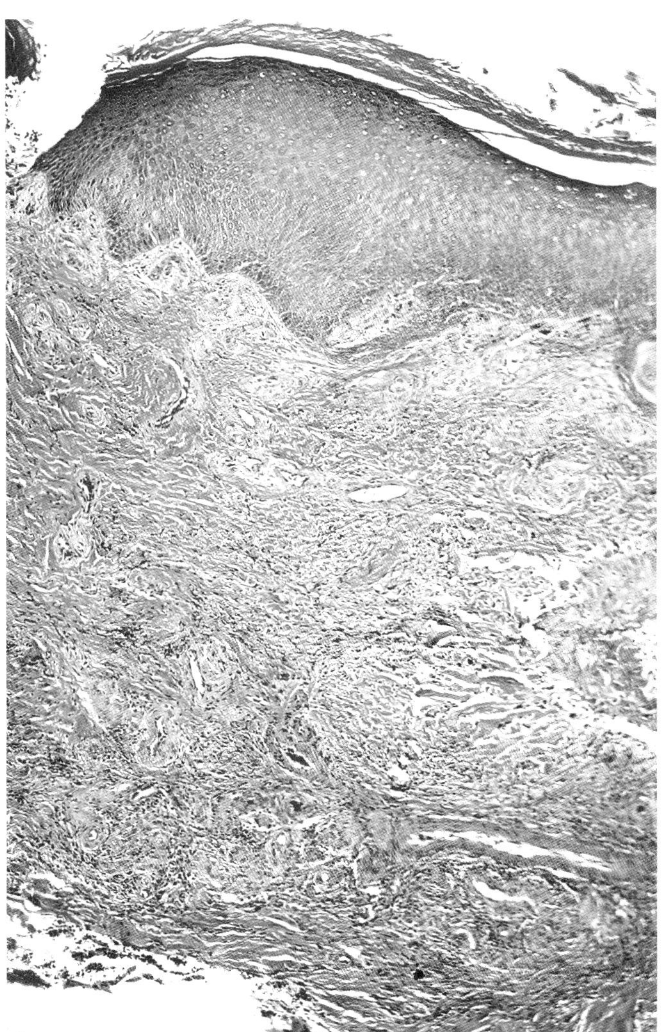
**FIGURE 23–18.** Kaposiform changes in skin overlying an arteriovenous fistula.

## Spindle Cell Hemangioma

First described in 1986 by Weiss and Enzinger as "spindle cell hemangioendothelioma,"[93] the spindle

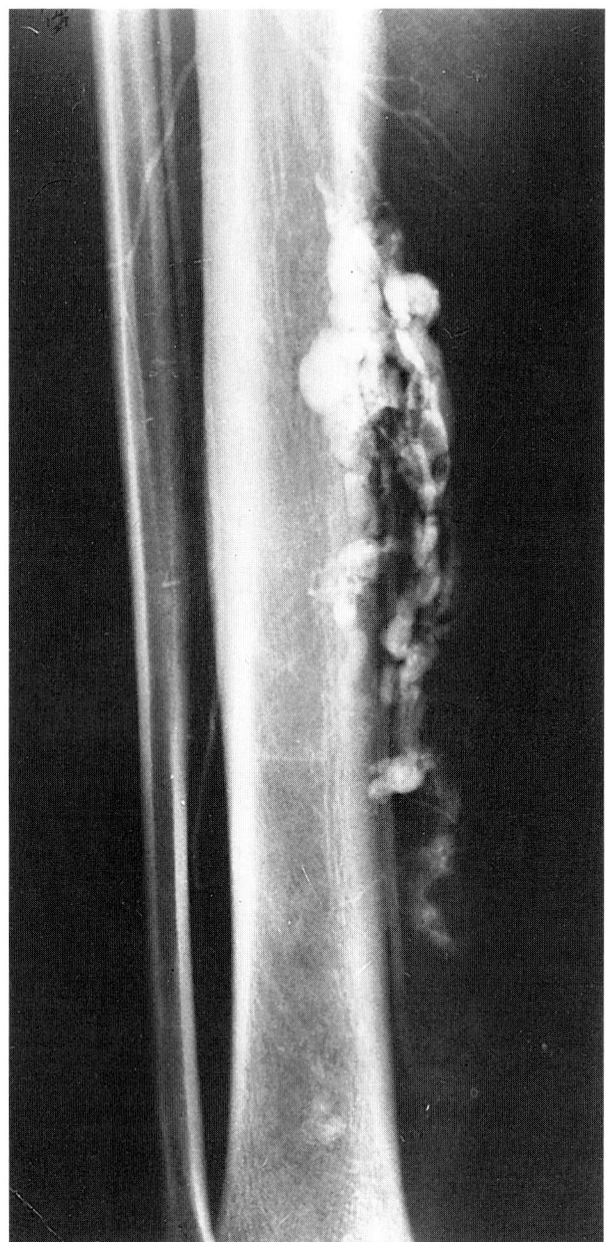

**FIGURE 23–20.** Hemangioma with venous and cavernous features (same case as in Fig. 23–8). Venous phase of the arteriogram portrays large saccular structures that correspond to tortuous thick-walled muscular veins. (Courtesy of Dr. John Madewell.)

cell hemangioma is an acral vascular tumor characterized by cavernous blood vessels and spindled areas reminiscent of Kaposi's sarcoma. Although originally believed to be a tumor with limited metastatic potential, it is regarded as a benign, frequently multifocal lesion. The tumor usually occurs in young adults and affects the subcutis of the distal extremities, particularly the hand. The lesions produce so few symptoms patients may delay seeking medical attention for several years. The tumor is occasionally associated with Maffucci syndrome[86] (Fig. 23–22); and it appears that many of the lesions originally described as cavernous hemangiomas in Maffucci syndrome may well be spindle cell hemangiomas. In addition, spindle cell hemangiomas are also seen in Klippel-Trenaunay syndrome,[86] early-onset varicosities, congenital lymphedema, and rarely in association with epithelioid hemangioendothelioma. Most begin as a solitary nodule but have a remarkable tendency to give rise to multiple lesions in the same general area (Figs. 23–23, 23–24). Approximately one-half of cases are intravascular; it appears that intravascular growth is the mechanism by which they give rise to multiple lesions in the same general area.

Histologically, the lesions are composed of thin-walled cavernous vessels lined by flattened endothelial cells and containing a mixture of erythrocytes and thrombi. Between the cavernous spaces are bland spindled areas reminiscent of Kaposi's sarcoma (Figs. 23–25, 23–26, 23–27). Unlike Kaposi's sarcoma, however, they contain distinctive round or epithelioid cells containing vacuoles or intracytoplasmic lumens similar to those in an epithelioid hemangioendothelioma (Fig. 23–28). In the extreme case, clusters of vacuolated cells lie in the spindled stroma and are easily mistaken for entrapped fat (Fig. 23–29). Von Willebrand factor can be identified in the endothelium lining of the cavernous spaces and in the epithelioid endothelium of the stroma. The spindled areas appear to be made up of collapsed vessels, pericytes, and fibroblastic cells, indicating that architecturally they are complex and have all the elements of the vessel wall.

About 60% of spindle cell hemangiomas recur,[91] although as stated above the mechanism of recurrence appears to be growth in vessels to discontinuous regional sites in contrast to true local regrowth or local metastasis. There is no evidence that these lesions have the ability to metastasize either distantly or regionally, however. There has been considerable debate as to whether these lesions are reactive or neoplastic. We do not believe these lesions can be explained as a purely reactive process, as has been suggested. The lesions arise in the vicinity of what are clearly abnormal vessels, supporting the idea that the spindle cell hemangioma is most likely a vascular malformation in which variation in blood flow gives rise to alternating areas of vascular expansion and collapse. The fact that the cellular zones appear to have all the elements of the vessel wall suggest that they are fundamentally similar to the cavernous areas but represent areas of vascular collapse.

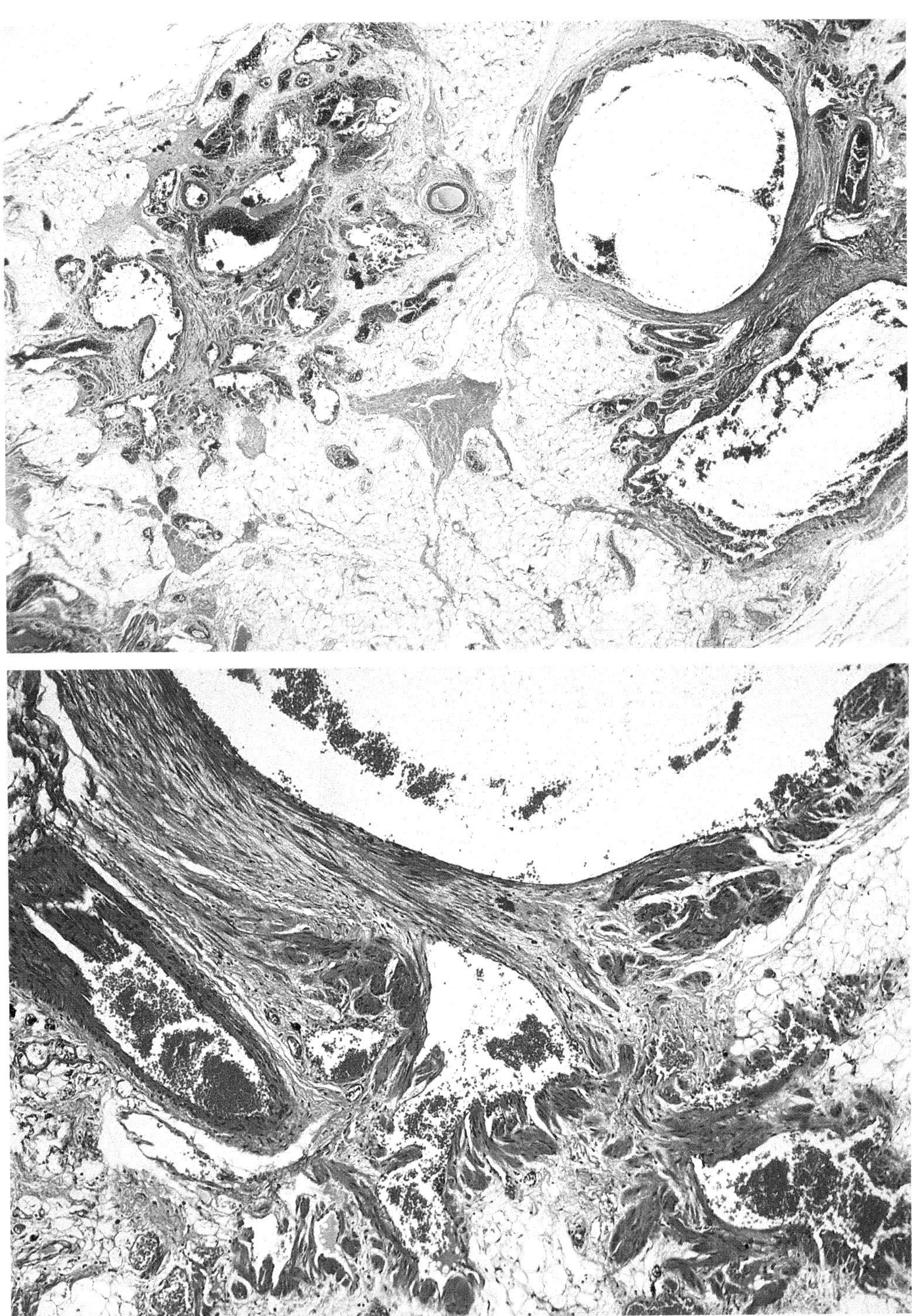

**FIGURE 23–21.** Large thick-walled veins of a venous hemangioma.

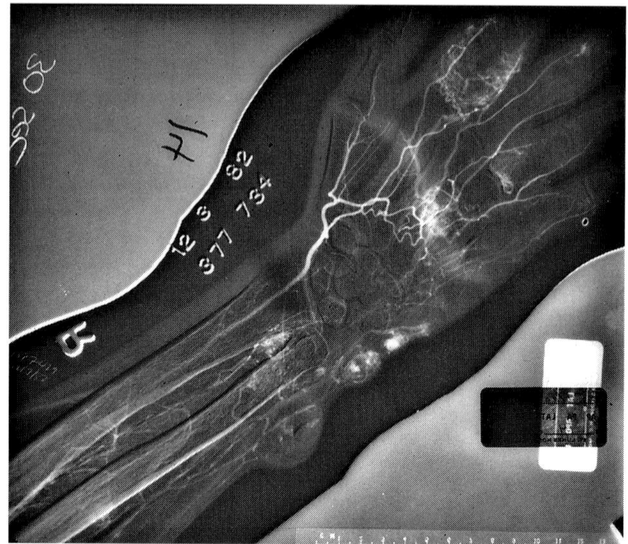

**FIGURE 23–22.** Radiograph of a patient with Maffucci syndrome and multiple spindle cell hemangiomas (some with phleboliths) on the lateral portion of the wrist and hand. Patient also has an enchondroma of the phalanx of the forefinger.

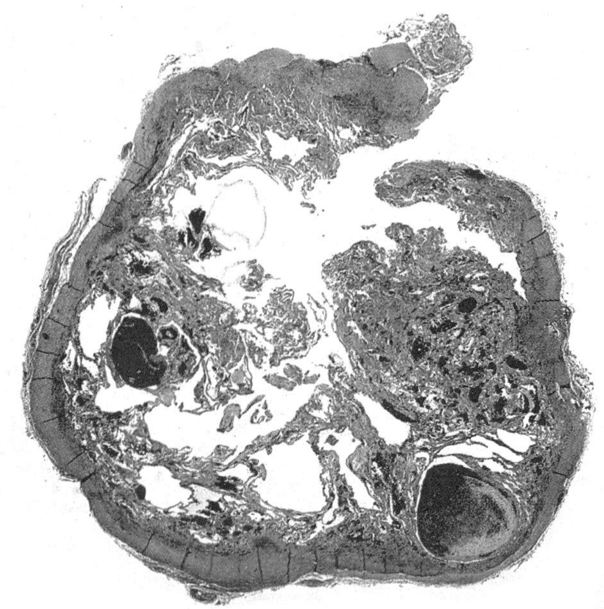

**FIGURE 23–24.** Subcutaneous spindle cell hemangioma with relative circumscription.

## Epithelioid Hemangioma (Angiolymphoid Hyperplasia with Eosinophilia, Histiocytoid Hemangioma)

Epithelioid hemangioma is an unusual but distinctive vascular tumor that was first described by Wells and Whimster[106] as *angiolymphoid hyperplasia with eosinophilia* and subsequently by others as *inflammatory angiomatous nodule, atypical or pseudopyogenic granuloma,*[95,96] and *histiocytoid hemangioma.*[104,105] The lesions reported in the Japanese literature as *Kimura's disease*[99,107–114] represent a different entity.

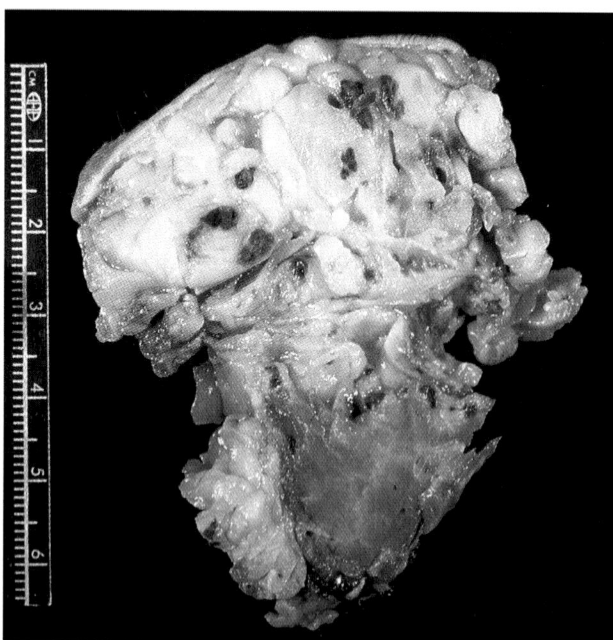

**FIGURE 23–23.** Gross specimen of a spindle cell hemangioma showing multiple lesions in the subcutis.

Epithelioid hemangiomas typically occur during early to mid adult life (age 20–40 years) and affect women more often than men. Most are situated superficially in the head and neck, particularly the region around the ear. As a result, they can be detected relatively early as small, dull red, pruritic plaques. Crusting, excoriation, bleeding, and coalescence of lesions are common secondary features. About half of the patients develop multiple lesions generally in the same area. Affected patients appear relatively well, although occasionally significant regional lymph node enlargement and eosinophilia of the peripheral blood accompany the lesions. These signs have suggested the possibility of an infectious agent, but to date none has been identified.

Typically, these tumors are circumscribed lesions of the subcutis or dermis (Figs. 23–30, 23–31), but occasionally they involve deep soft tissue and in rare instances involve or arise from vessels. Intravascular forms of this tumor not unexpectedly cause diagnostic problems for the pathologist; attention has been focused on this phenomenon by Rosai and Ackerman,[103] who described such lesions as *intravenous atypical vascular proliferation.*[103] Like many other hemangiomas, this lesion may have a vague lobular arrangement as a result of the clustering of small capil-

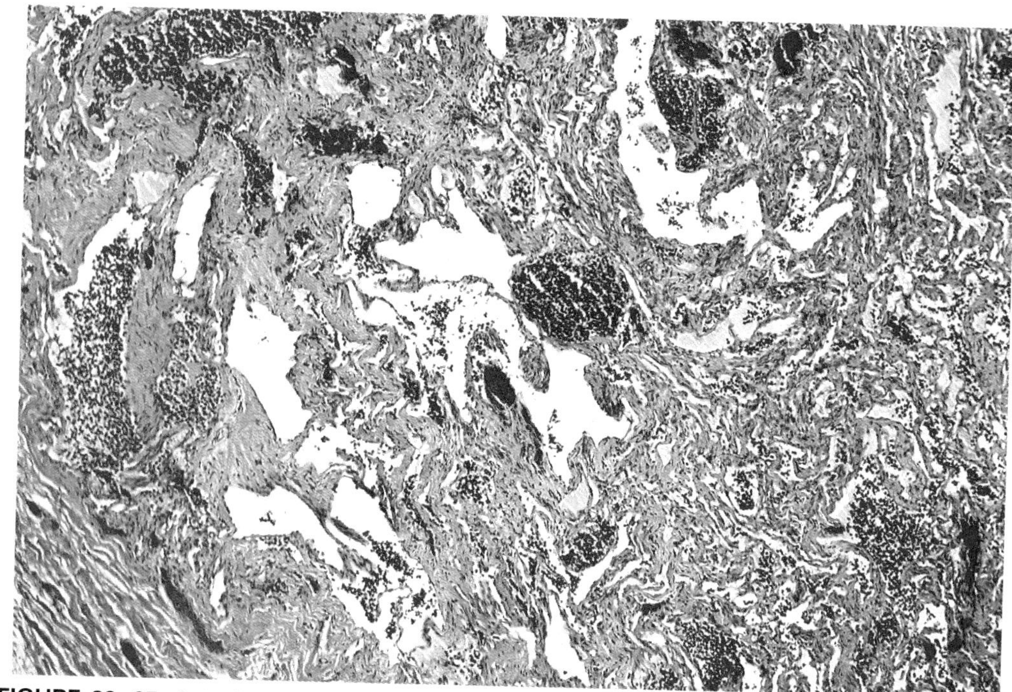

**FIGURE 23–25.** Spindle cell hemangioma with juxtaposition of the cellular and cavernous areas.

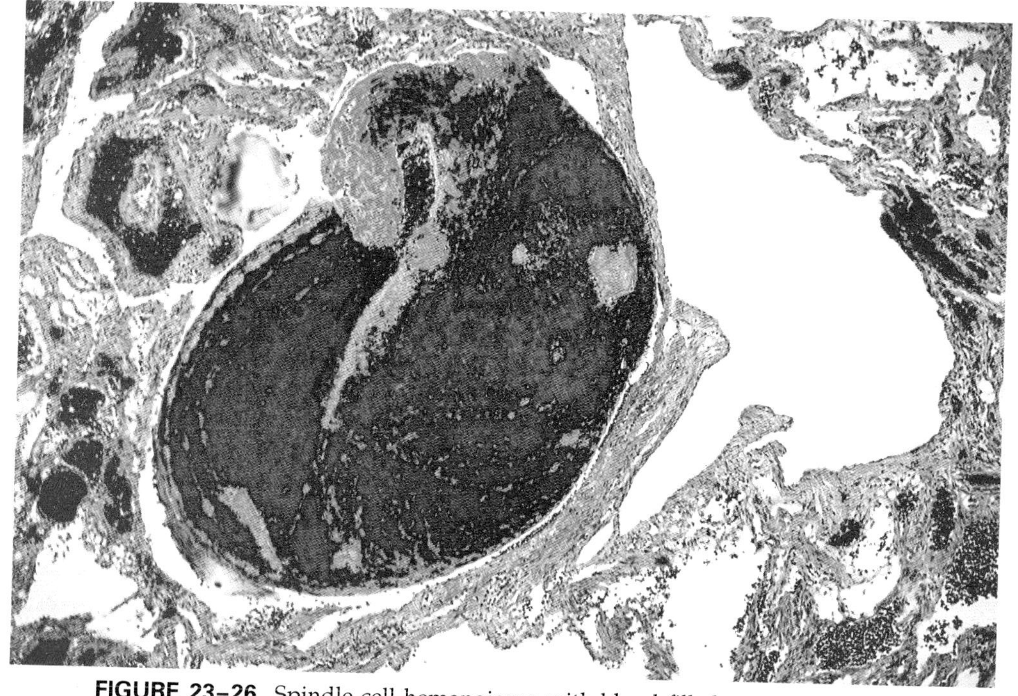

**FIGURE 23–26.** Spindle cell hemangioma with blood-filled cavernous spaces.

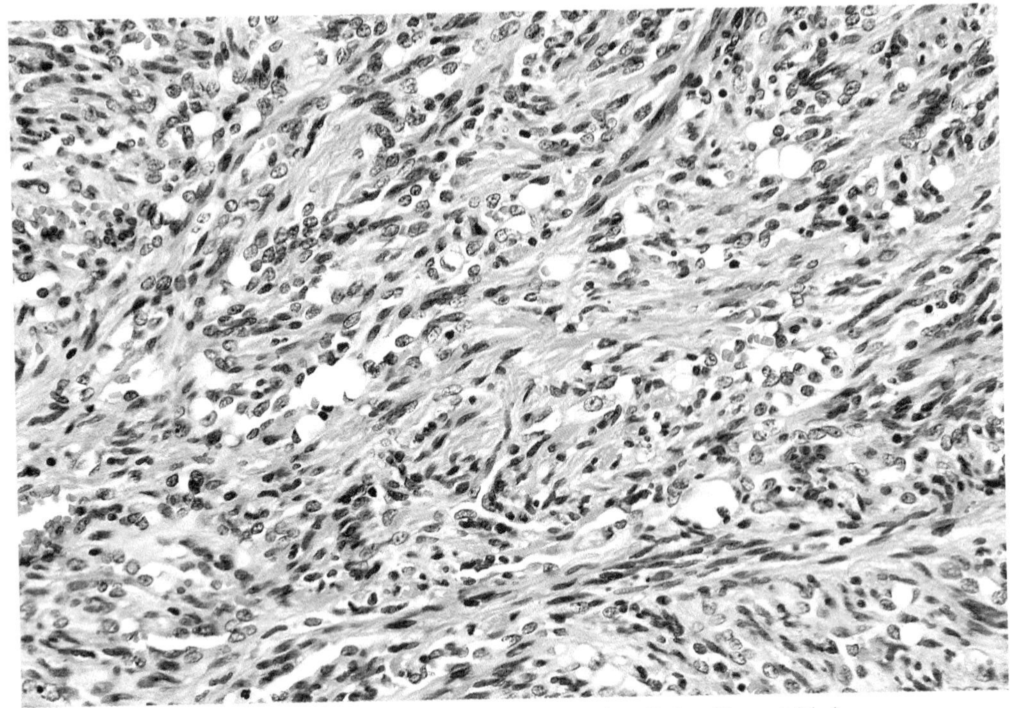

**FIGURE 23–27.** Spindle cell hemangioma with cellular (Kaposi-like) areas.

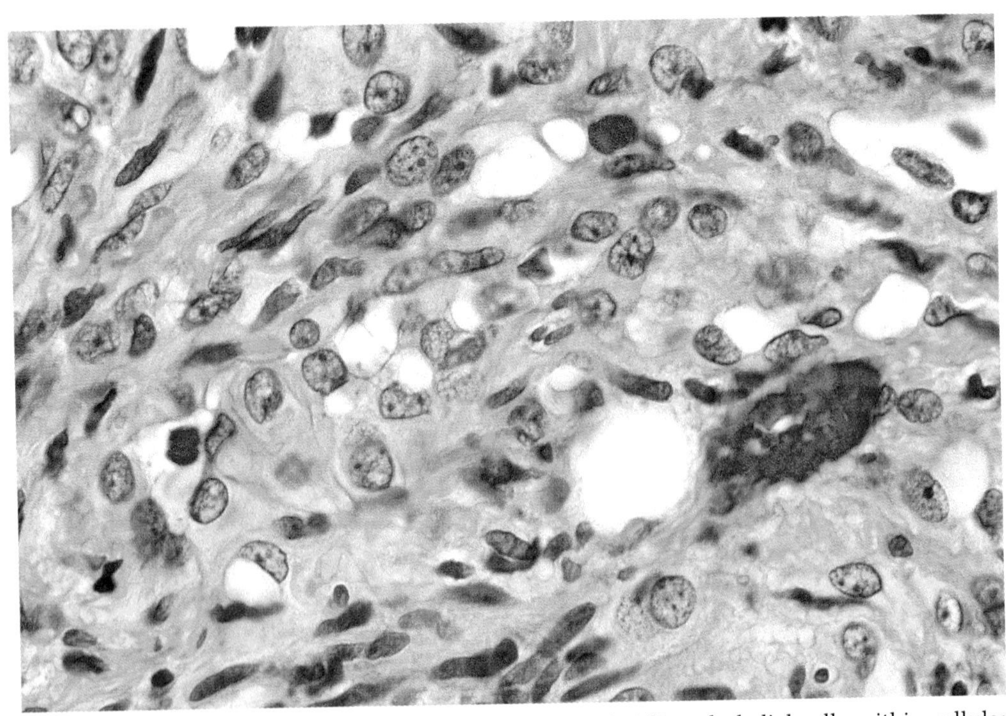

**FIGURE 23–28.** Spindle cell hemangioma with round "epithelioid" endothelial cells within cellular areas. Some show vacuolation.

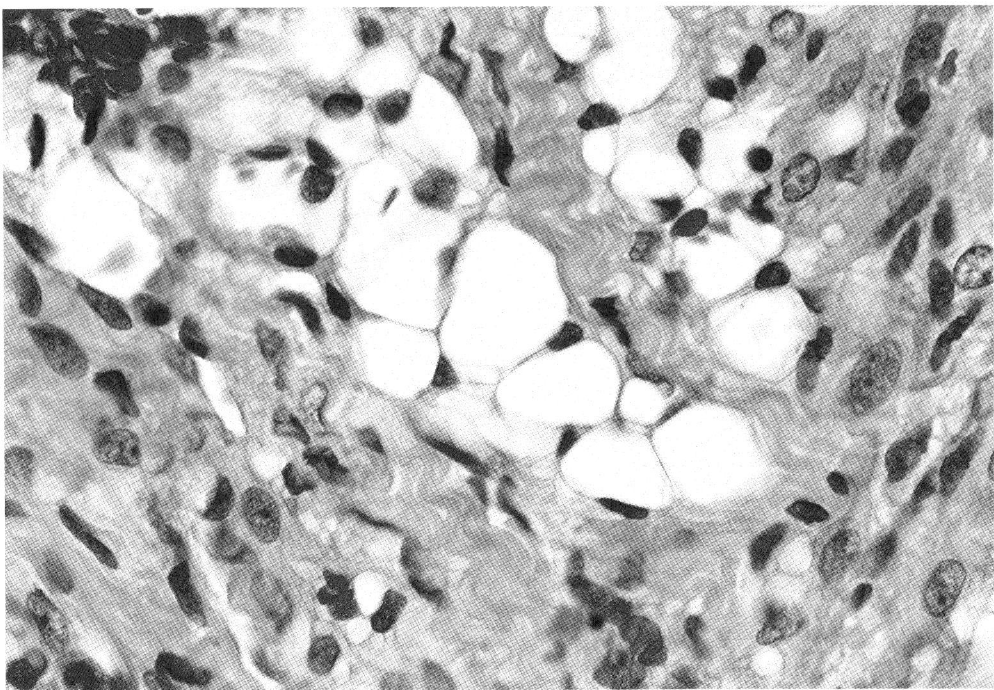

**FIGURE 23–29.** Spindle cell hemangioma with prominent vacuolation of endothelial cells. Such areas are frequently confused with fat.

lary-size vessels around a medium-size parent vessel (Fig. 23–32).

Many of the vessels are lined by distinct epithelioid endothelial cells (Figs. 23–33 to 23–36) with scalloped borders that protrude deeply into the lumen in a manner that has been likened to "tombstones." In small vessels the endothelium may assume a more conventional appearance. These epithelioid endothelial cells have rounded or lobated nuclei and abundant acidophilic cytoplasm containing occasional vacuoles that represent primitive vascular lumen formation. Although they have many of the ultrastructural features of endothelium, including micropinocytotic vesicles, antiluminal basal lamina, and Weibel-Palade bodies, they manifest certain modifications. Adjacent cells are often separated by rather large gaps and interdigitate only along their lateral basal borders by means of tight junctions. Organelles are more abundant in these cells and include increased numbers of mitochondria, smooth and rough endoplasmic reticulum, free ribosomes, and thin cytofilaments.

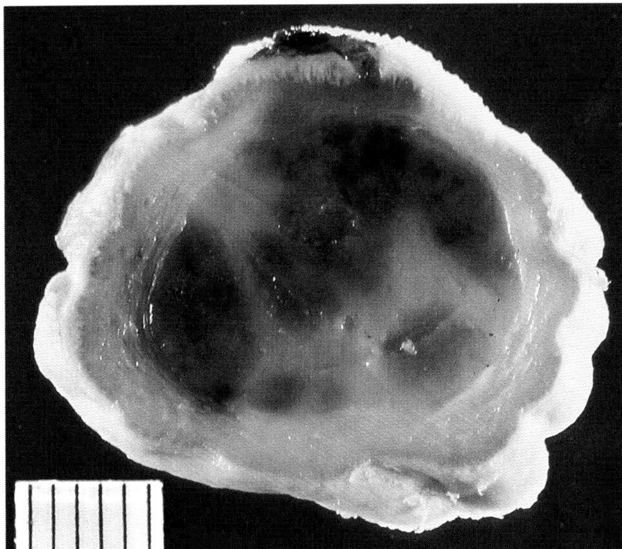

**FIGURE 23–30.** Gross appearance of a subcutaneous epithelioid hemangioma.

Histochemical reactions demonstrate increased hydrolytic and oxidative enzymes and decreased alkaline phosphatase compared to that of normal capillary endothelium. A mixture of inflammatory cells surrounds the vessels. Eosinophils are particularly characteristic of these tumors, but lymphocytes, mast cells, and plasma cells are also present. Lymphoid aggregates replete with germinal centers are occasionally present but are believed by some to be a feature of long-standing lesions or a peculiar host response.

Although about one-third of these lesions recur, virtually none has produced metastasis. One case reported by Reed and Terazakis[102] evidently gave rise to microscopic metastases in a regional lymph node, but this appears to be a unique event.[102] Rare lesions have been noted to regress spontaneously, but usu-

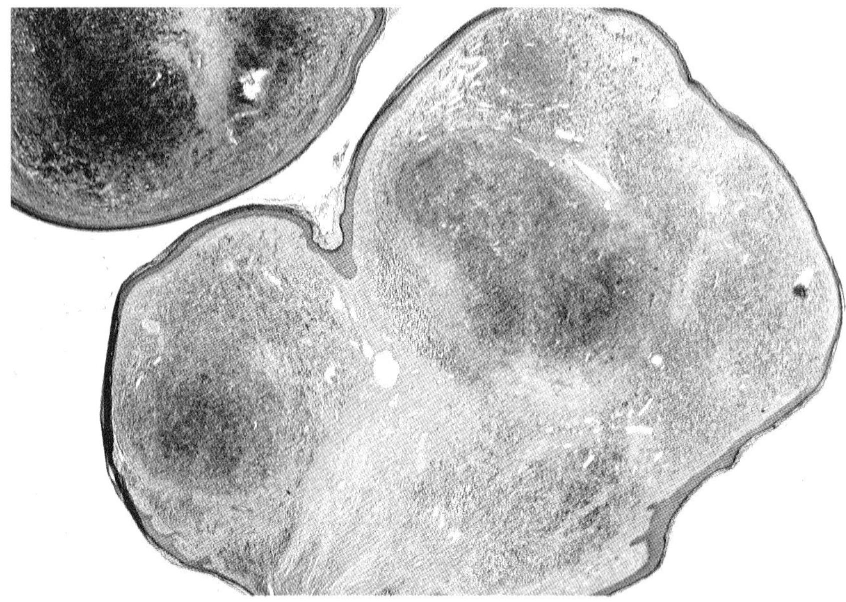

**FIGURE 23–31.** Low power view of an epithelioid hemangioma with nodules of vessels surrounded by a prominent lymphoid cuff.

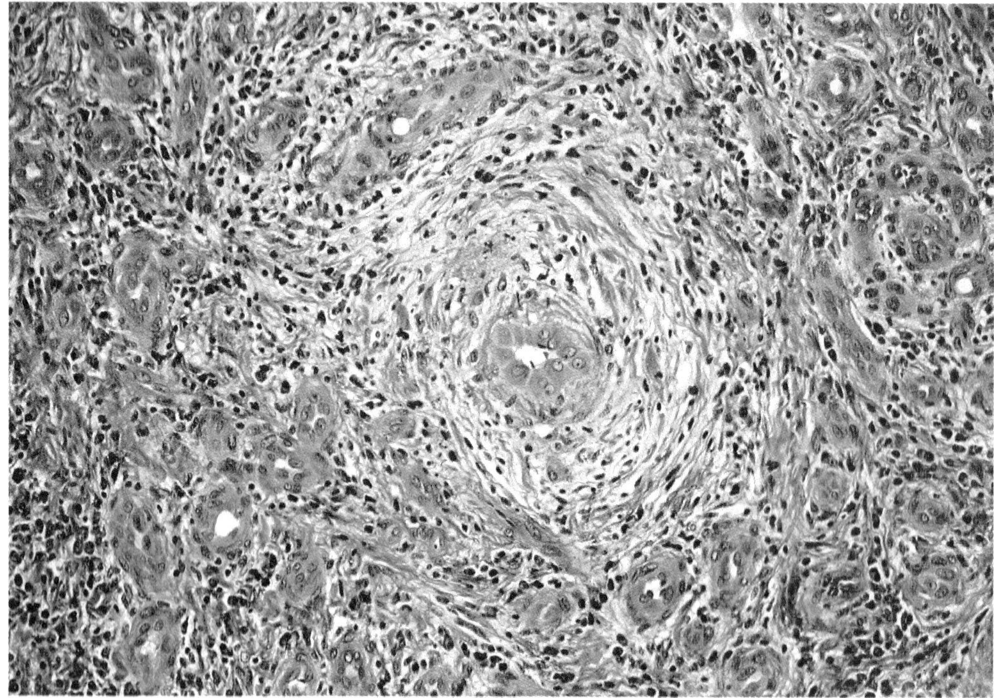

**FIGURE 23–32.** Epithelioid hemangioma with a central "parent" vessel surrounded by small vessels and dense inflammation.

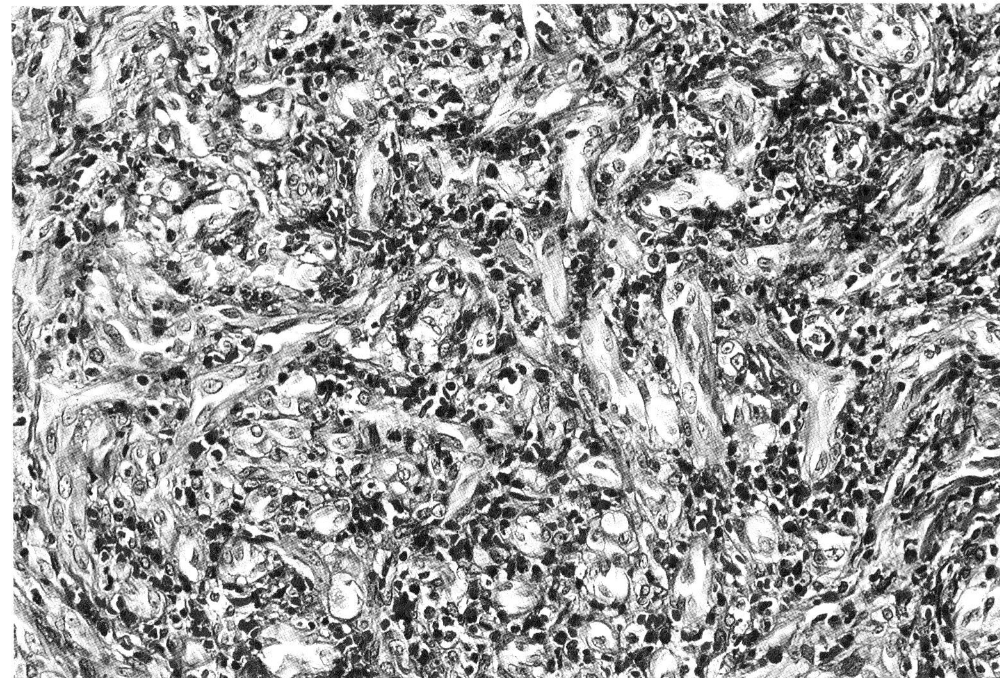

**FIGURE 23–33.** Epithelioid hemangioma. Vessels are lined by pale-staining cuboidal endothelial cells admixed with inflammatory elements, predominantly eosinophils.

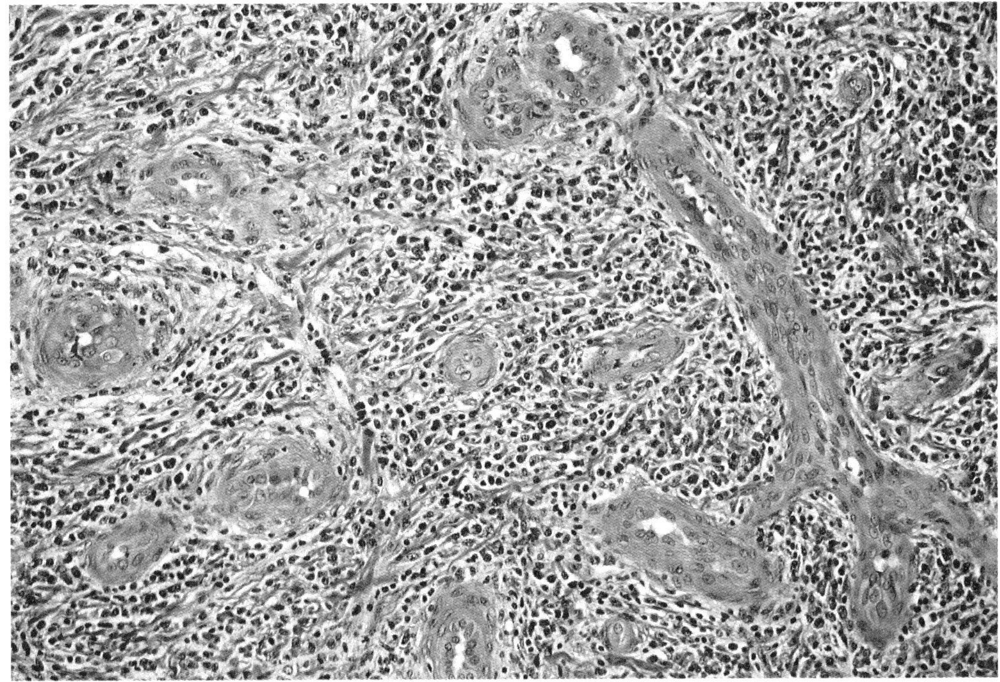

**FIGURE 23–34.** Epithelioid hemangioma in which some areas display more conventional-appearing endothelial cells interspersed with chronic inflammatory cells.

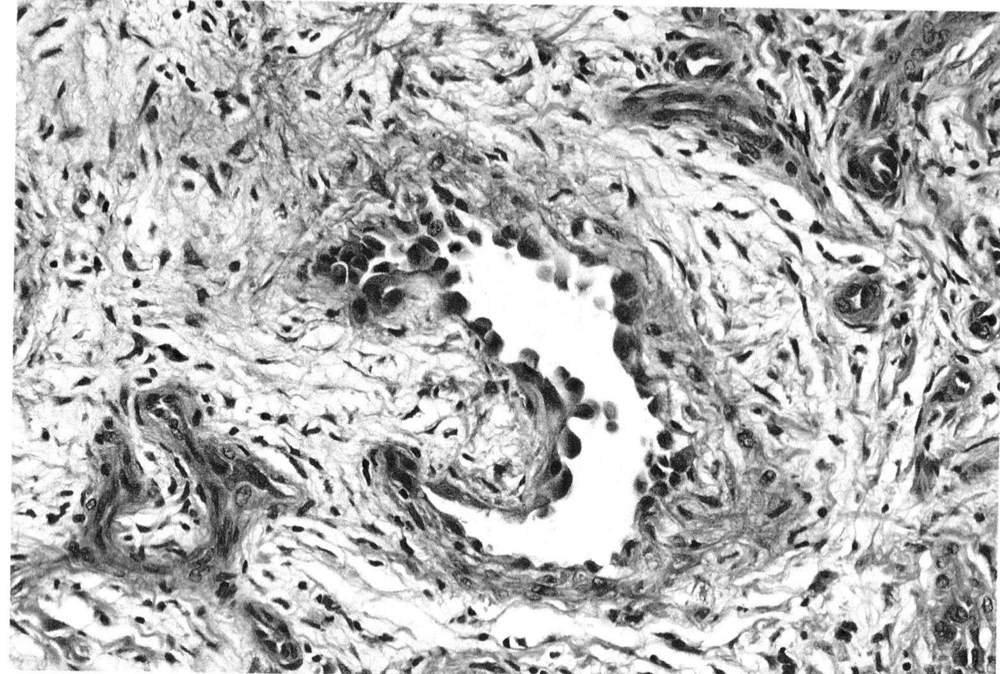

**FIGURE 23–35.** "Tombstone"-like arrangement of cells in large vessels of epithelioid hemangioma.

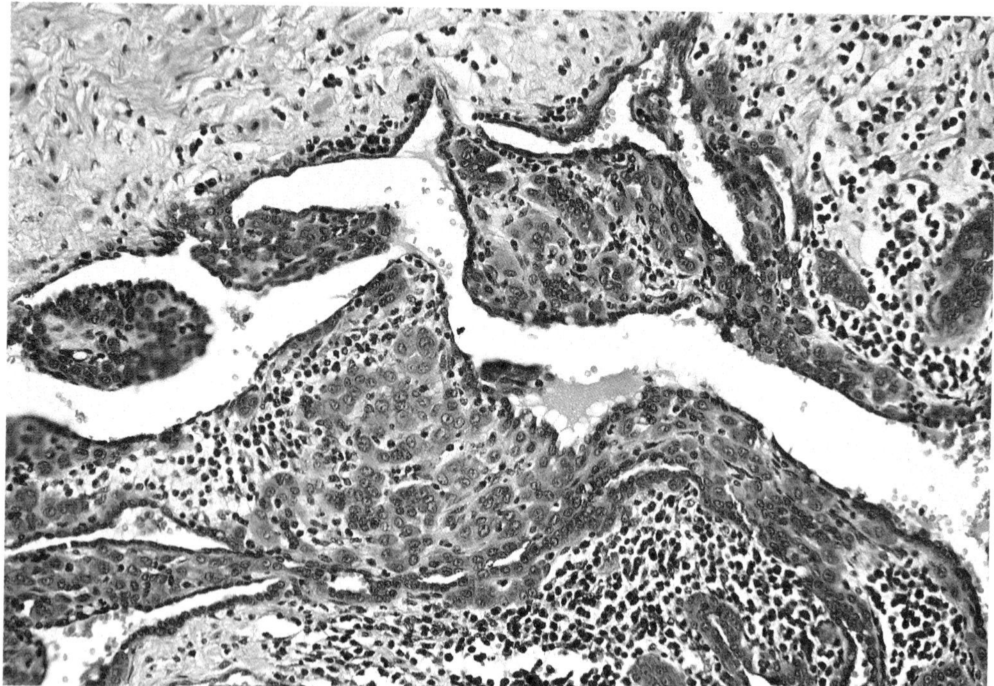

**FIGURE 23–36.** Epithelioid hemangioma involving the wall of a large vessel. This phenomenon should not be equated with malignancy.

ally surgical excision is required. About 80% of reported patients have responded at least partially to superficial radiotherapy,[99] but cryotherapy and injection of intralesional steroids have not met with success.[102]

Despite their benign nature, considerable controversy still exists as to the basic nature of these lesions; some authors consider them reactive and others neoplastic. We reviewed 96 epithelioid hemangiomas and were impressed that more than 60% were intimately associated with a large vessel that showed mural damage, rupture, or both.[97] These observations suggest that at least a significant number of soft tissue epithelioid hemangiomas are reactive lesions (Fig. 23–37) In this regard a rather impressive epithelioid hemangioma was reported to occur in a patient following a popliteal arteriovenous fistula.[100] Others have commented on the high incidence of arteriovenous shunts, particularly in deeply situated forms of epithelioid hemangioma. Although sharing many common histologic features and a benign clinical course, the lesions may be pathogenetically heterogeneous.

Many have speculated on the nature and significance of the epithelioid endothelial cell. In our opinion it seems to represent an altered functional state of endothelium, as it may be encountered in benign and malignant vascular tumors as well as in reactive vascular lesions. Rosai et al.,[104] noting the lobated nuclei, the decreased alkaline phosphatase, and the increased acid phosphatase compared with normal endothelium, referred to these cells as *histiocytoid.* The term *histiocytoid hemangioma,*[104] however, has been applied to a heterogeneous group of vascular lesions, including epithelioid hemangioma, hemangioendothelioma of bone, and epithelioid hemangioendothelioma (see Chapter 24), which vary considerably in presentation and behavior. For this reason, we have discouraged the use of "histiocytoid hemangioma" as a strict diagnostic term unless it is modified by some comment as to the level of malignancy of the lesions. It provides, however, an elegant concept for a group of lesions characterized by a peculiar epithelioid (or histiocytoid) endothelial cell.

### Kimura's Disease

First described by Kim in the Chinese literature and later by Kimura et al.[110] in the Japanese literature, Kimura's disease, a chronic inflammatory condition, appears to be endemic in the Asian population and occurs only infrequently in Westerners. Although formerly thought to be identical to epithelioid hemangioma (angiolymphoid hyperplasia), many data indi-

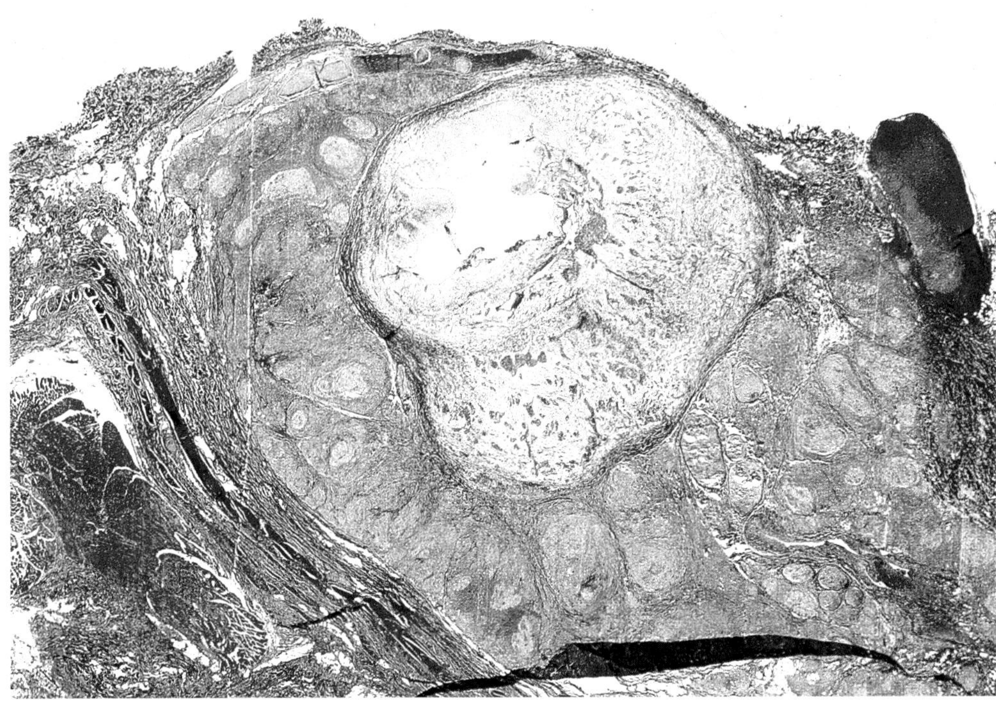

**FIGURE 23–37.** Changes of an epithelioid hemangioma arising from the walls of traumatized vessels. Note the prominent lymphocytic infiltrate around the lesions.

cate that they are two entirely unrelated lesions bearing only a few superficial histologic similarities.[107,108,111,114]

Kimura's disease presents as lymphadenopathy with or without an associated soft tissue mass. Peripheral eosinophilia is nearly always present. Increased serum immunoglobulin E (IgE), proteinuria, and nephrotic syndrome may also occur as part of the disease.[113,115] Lesions are most frequent in the subcutis of the head and neck area, although lesions have been noted in the groin, extremities, and chest wall. There is a striking male predilection in this disease. The lesions are characterized by dense lymphoid aggregates containing prominent germinal centers (Fig. 23–38). Within the germinal centers one occasionally identifies nuclear debris, polykaryocytes, and a delicate eosinophilic matrix. Immunohistochemical procedures reveal that IgE-bearing cells, corresponding to the distribution of dendritic reticulum cells, populate the germinal center. Thin-walled vessels, with the characteristics of postcapillary venules, reside adjacent to the germinal centers, occasionally dipping into the centers. Dense infiltrates of eosinophils adjacent to the lymphoid aggregates occasionally form "eosinophilic abscesses." During the late stages of the disease a dense hyaline fibrosis supervenes. The adherence of the mass to the surrounding structures often triggers alarm on the part of the surgeon regarding the possibility of malignancy. In affected lymph nodes there is exuberant follicular hyperplasia with preservation of the architecture. The changes in the germinal center are as described above for the soft tissue lesions.

The etiology of this condition is unknown, although the peripheral eosinophilia and elevated serum IgE suggest an immunologic reaction to an unknown stimulus. The lesions are benign, although recurrence may develop after surgical excision. There are no instances of malignancy supervening on these peculiar lymphoid proliferations.

Although Kimura's disease and angiolymphoid hyperplasia have in common a lymphoid infiltrate with eosinophils, there are rather striking differences. The vascular proliferation in Kimura's disease is relatively minor and is eclipsed by the inflammatory component. Moreover, the vessels in Kimura's disease are not lined by epithelioid endothelium but by more attenuated endothelial cells.

## Granulation Tissue-type Hemangioma (Pyogenic Granuloma)

The so-called pyogenic granuloma is a polypoid form of capillary hemangioma on the skin and mucosal surfaces. The inflammatory changes that often accompany these tumors may be so pronounced the lesions bear a striking resemblance to granulation tissue. In fact, most early pathologists considered these lesions

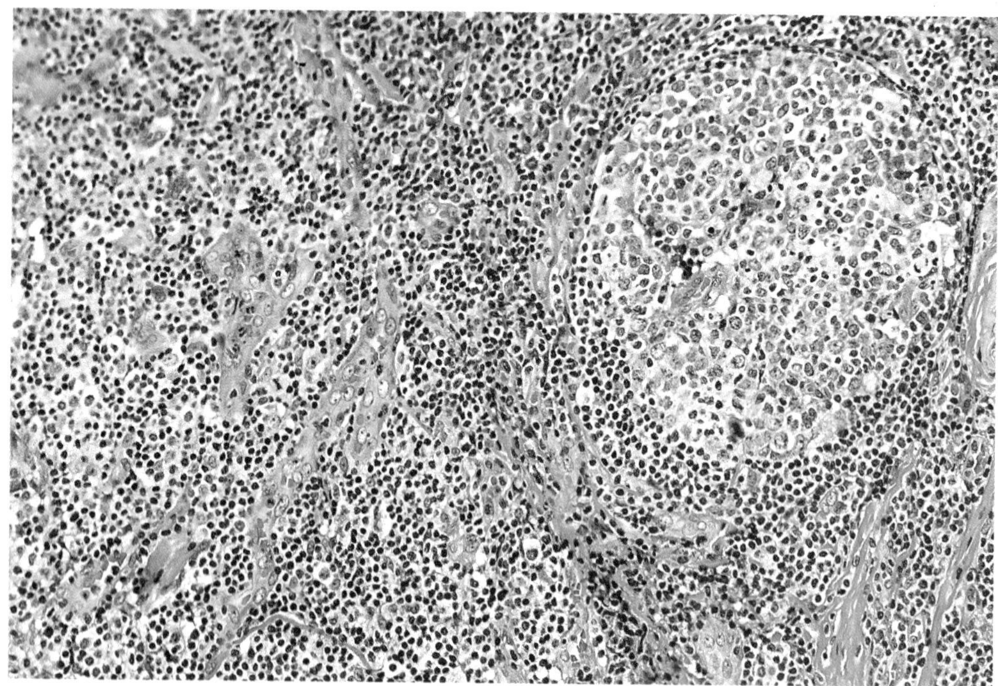

**FIGURE 23–38.** Kimura's disease. Lesion differs from epithelioid hemangioma in that the lymphoid component overshadows the minor vascular component.

to be infectious. Poncet and Dor, credited with the first description, believed these lesions were secondary to infection by *Botryomyces* organisms, whereas others implicated pyogenic bacteria, specifically staphylococci. Uncomplicated lesions, however, lack ulceration and inflammation and are similar to ordinary capillary hemangiomas except for their distinctive gross appearance and clinical symptoms.

These tumors may occur on either the skin or the mucosal surfaces, although the latter accounts for about 60% of all cases.[122] In the extensive review of 289 cases by Kerr,[122] the following were the most common sites, in descending order of frequency: gingiva (64 cases), finger (44 cases), lips (40 cases), face (28 cases), and tongue (20 cases). The genders are affected approximately equally, and the disease is evenly distributed over all decades. Approximately one-third develop following minor trauma. Multiple lesions may develop simultaneously, but this phenomenon almost always occurs in the cutaneous form rather than the mucosal form of the disease. There have been a few reports of disseminated (eruptive) forms of pyogenic granuloma,[119,121,128] with one following surgical removal of a solitary pyogenic granuloma. Disseminated pyogenic granulomas progress for a limited time and ultimately stabilize or regress. The mechanism for these initially alarming presentations is not clear, although some have suggested the release of angiogenic factors by the tumors. In the ordinary case the tumors develop rapidly and achieve their maximal size of several millimeters to a few centimeters within a few weeks or months. The well established lesion is a polypoid, friable, purple-red mass that bleeds easily and frequently ulcerates. Sessile forms of this tumor also occur, but they tend to be recurrent lesions.

The appearance of these lesions at low magnification immediately suggests the diagnosis because they are distinctly exophytic growths connected to the skin by stalks of varying diameter (Figs. 23–39 to 23–43) and occasionally are surrounded by a heaped-up collar of normal tissue. The adjacent epithelium is hyperkeratotic or acanthotic, but the epithelium overlying the lesion itself is flattened, atrophic, or ulcerated. The basic lesion is a lobular (cellular) hemangioma[124] set in a fibromyxoid matrix. Each lobule of the hemangioma is made up of a larger vessel, often with a muscular wall and surrounded by congeries of small capillaries. Most lesions, however, are altered by secondary inflammatory changes; as a result, they have been likened to granulation tissue. Both acute and chronic inflammatory cells are scattered throughout the lesion but, not unexpectedly, are most numerous at the surface. Secondary invading microorganisms are occasionally present in the superficial reaches of ulcerated lesions. Stromal edema may widely separate the capillary lumens, obscuring the lobular arrangement of the tumor (Fig. 23–42). Mitotic activity may be brisk in the endothelium and stromal fibroblasts when secondary changes such as edema and inflammation are present. In lesions that involute there is evidence to suggest they develop a progressive stromal and perivascular fibrosis. Rarely, the pyogenic granuloma may have areas in which the endothelium has an epithelioid appearance.

The clinical appearance of these lesions is quite characteristic and can serve as a useful diagnostic adjunct to the pathologist in difficult situations where a distinction between lesions, must be made (e.g., between a well differentiated angiosarcoma or an angiomatous form of Kaposi's sarcoma). In these situations it is useful to recall that the pyogenic

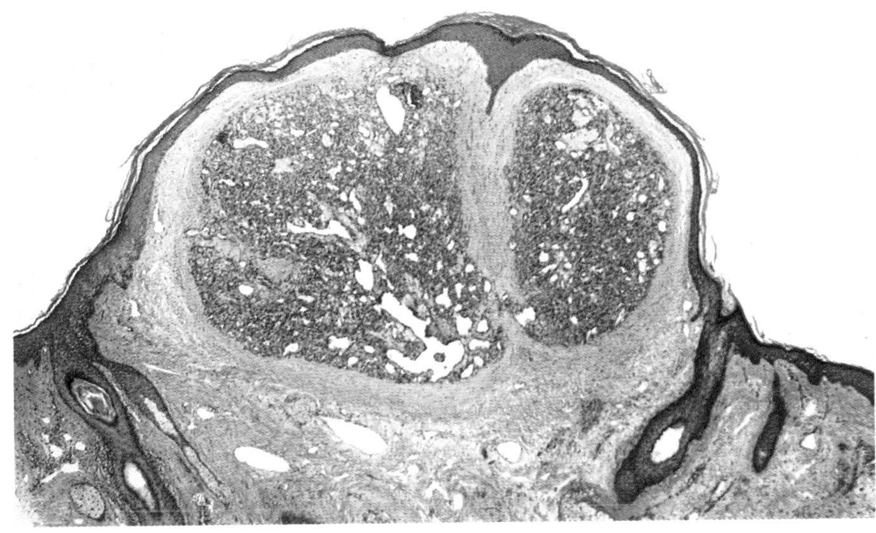

**FIGURE 23–39.** Granulation tissue-type hemangioma (pyogenic granuloma). Lesion is characterized by exophytic growth.

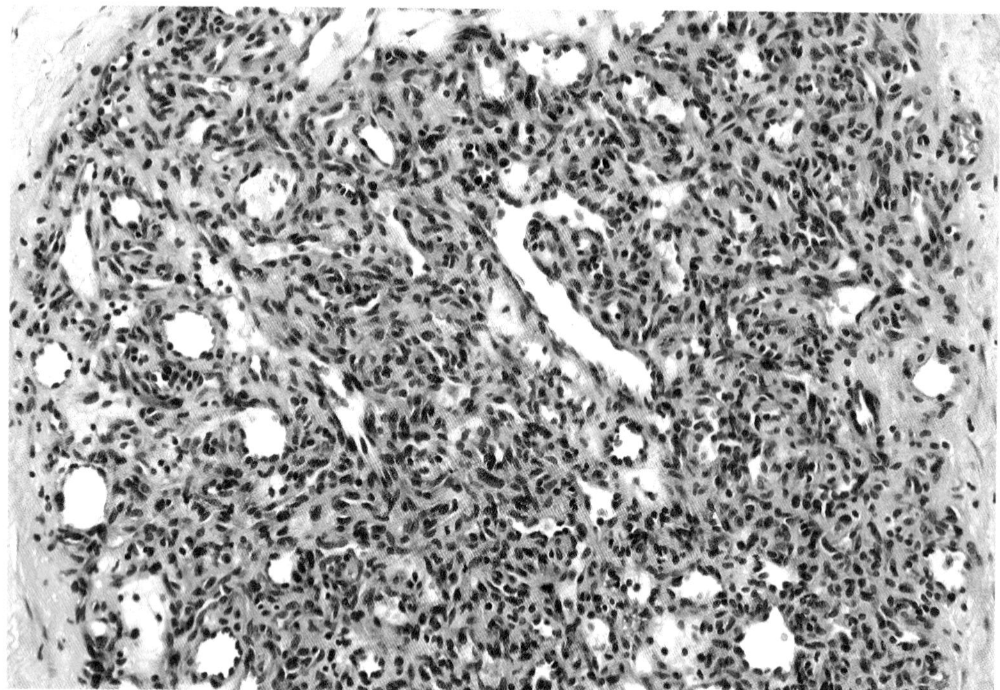

**FIGURE 23–40.** Lobular growth of vessels in a pyogenic granuloma.

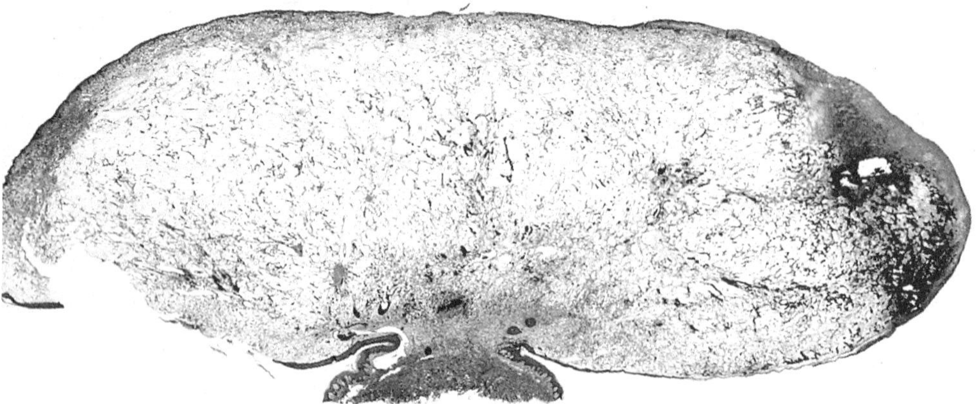

**FIGURE 23–41.** Pyogenic granuloma with ulceration of surface and marked stromal edema.

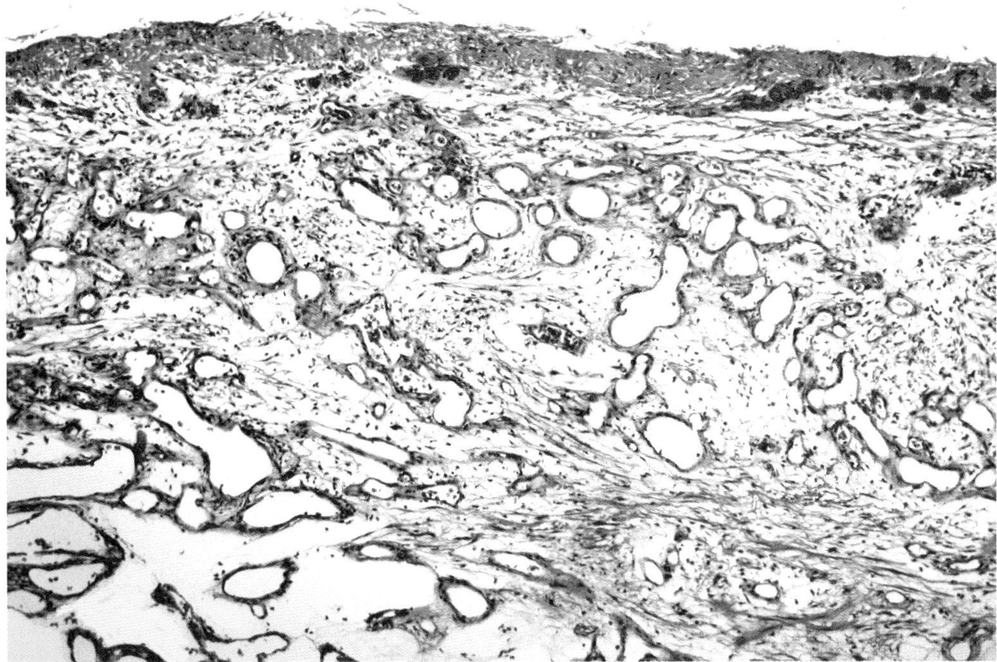

**FIGURE 23–42.** Stromal edema widely separating vessels of a pyogenic granuloma. (Same case as Fig. 23–41).

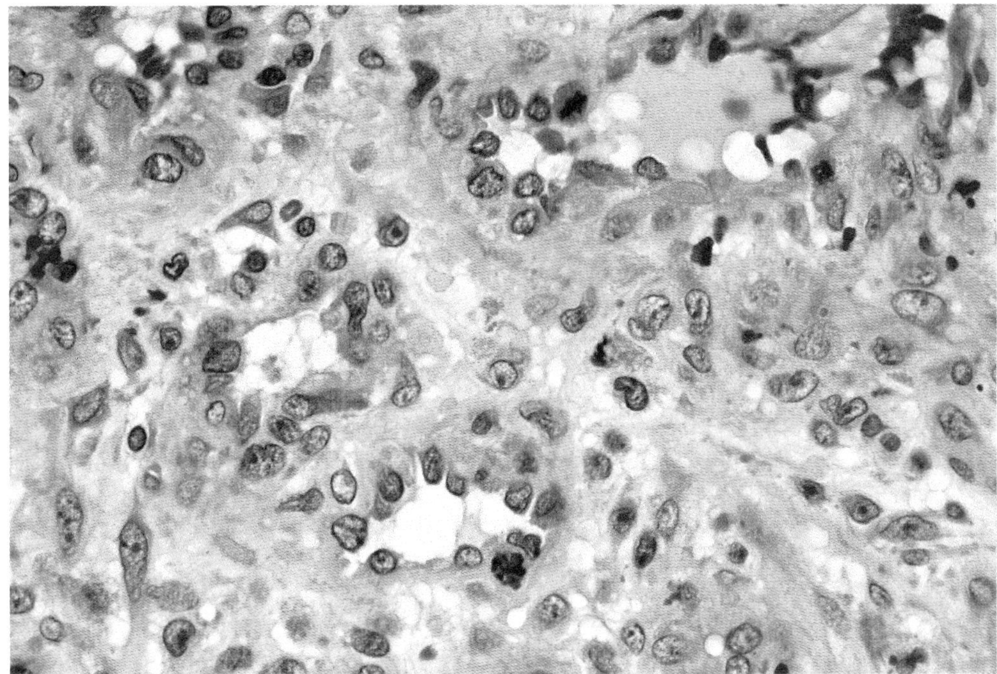

**FIGURE 23–43.** Mitotic activity in stromal and endothelial cells of a pyogenic granuloma.

granuloma is a more or less circumscribed lesion, often with a lobular arrangement, in contrast to the rambling, poorly confined nature of malignant vascular neoplasms. In particular, the manner in which even well differentiated angiosarcomas dissect through connective tissue and create irregular vascular spaces contrasts sharply with the pyogenic granuloma. Likewise, Kaposi's sarcoma is not well circumscribed and contains, in addition, at least focal cellular zones of spindled cells, which form the traditional slit-like vascular spaces. However, these diagnostic areas are often located in the central or deep areas of the tumor, whereas the well differentiated angiomatous component is seen peripherally or superficially. Thus in certain instances it is evident that a superficial biopsy of a vascular neoplasm may not be an adequate means to exclude malignancy.

Although the pyogenic granuloma is a benign lesion, 16% were noted to recur in one large series of tumors treated conservatively.[116] A significantly lower recurrence rate was noted in a series of 74 cases reported by Mills et al.[124] Recurrent disease may present as a solitary nodule or as multiple small satellite nodules around the site of the original lesion.[118,120,125,127,129] The phenomenon of *satellitosis* in this disease was analyzed by Warner and Wilson-Jones,[127] who found that most of these lesions occurred on the trunk, particularly the scapular area; and most had been incompletely excised initially. In contrast to the original tumors, the satellites are usually not pedunculated but, rather, are sessile and have an intact surface epithelium. In these respects they may grossly resemble ordinary hemangiomas. Although the rapid development of numerous satellites often causes considerable alarm on the part of the clinician, these lesions usually respond to reexcision and in some instances have even regressed spontaneously.

## Granuloma Gravidarum

Granuloma gravidarum is a specialized form of pyogenic granuloma that occurs on the gingival surface during pregnancy.[123] It is estimated that gingival changes occur in about 50% of pregnant women, but that only about 1% of this group develop localized tumors.[123] Typically, these lesions develop abruptly during the first trimester and arise from the interdental area of the gum. They are grossly and histologically indistinguishable from the ordinary form of pyogenic granuloma. They usually regress dramatically following parturition, although many persist as small mucosal nodules capable of renewed growth at the time of subsequent pregnancies. This unusual tumor has provided some of the most compelling evidence that the pyogenic granuloma lacks the degree of autonomous growth that characterizes most vascular tumors of adulthood. In fact, hormone sensitivity manifested by granuloma gravidarum has led some to conclude that the lesion should not be regarded as a true neoplasm but, rather, as exaggerated hyperplasia resulting from an altered physiologic state.

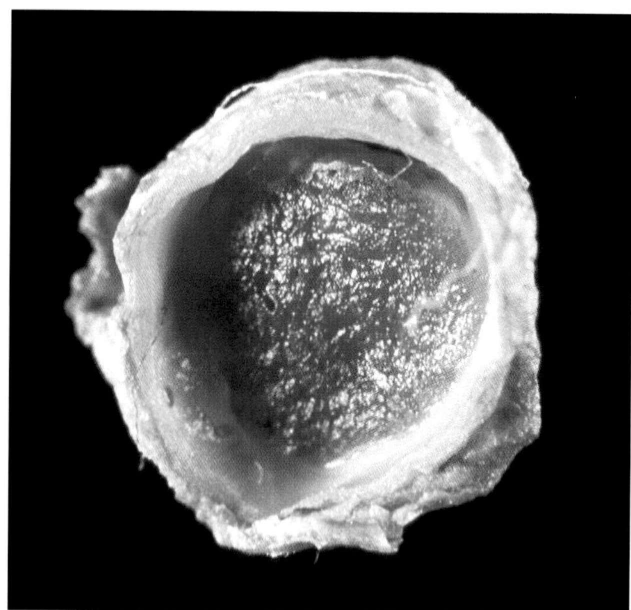

**FIGURE 23–44.** Gross specimen of the intravascular form of pyogenic granuloma.

## Intravenous Pyogenic Granuloma

An intravenous counterpart of pyogenic granuloma was recognized by Cooper et al.[117] This tumor is most common on the neck and upper extremity. It presents as a red-brown intravascular polyp that can be easily mistaken for an organizing thrombus (Figs. 23–44, 23–45). The tumor arises from the vein wall and protrudes deeply into the lumen but remains anchored to the wall by means of a narrow stalk containing the "feeder" vessels. The tumor is covered by a lining of endothelium, and the stroma often contains smooth muscle fibers, presumably remnants of the vein wall. Histologically, they are identical to uncomplicated pyogenic granulomas in that these tumors display no inflammatory or ulcerative change (Fig. 23–40). Like other pyogenic granulomas they are benign and display no tendency to spread in the bloodstream.

# DEEP HEMANGIOMAS OF MISCELLANEOUS SITES

Compared with cutaneous hemangiomas, those involving deep soft tissue structures are uncommon (Table 23–2), yet these tumors deserve special men-

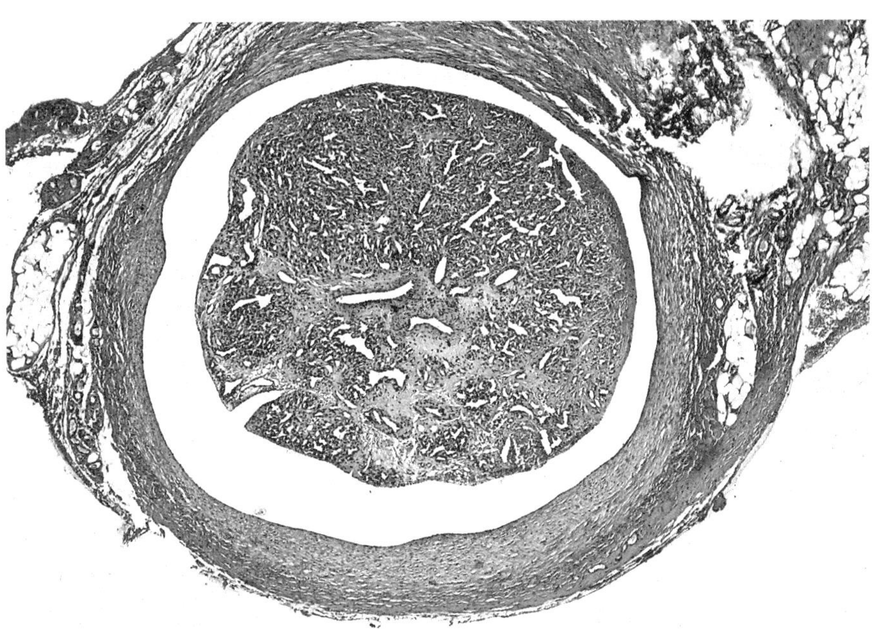

**FIGURE 23–45.** Intravascular pyogenic granuloma with preservation of the lobular arrangement of vessels.

tion because it is their unorthodox locations and different clinical presentations that create concern on the part of clinician and pathologist as to the possibility of malignancy.

## Intramuscular Hemangioma

The skeletal muscle hemangioma is probably the most common form of hemangioma of deep soft tissue, but it is nonetheless rare if one considers the spectrum of benign vascular neoplasms.[130–135] Watson and McCarthy[43] estimated that these lesions account for 0.8% of all benign vascular tumors, a figure that varies depending on the frequency with which incidental hemangiomas are excised at a given institution. Most intramuscular hemangiomas occur in young adults, with 80–90% manifesting before the age of 30 years.[130] The young age of affected patients and the long duration of symptoms in some cases raise the possibility that many of these lesions are congenital tumors that slowly give rise to symptoms during late childhood or early adult life. Unlike cutaneous hemangiomas, this form does not show a striking predilection for females and affects the genders in roughly equal numbers. Although any muscle can be affected, most intramuscular hemangiomas are located in the lower extremity, particularly the muscles of the thigh. In our experience at the Armed Forces Institute of Pathology (AFIP) there is some evidence that intramuscular hemangiomas of the capillary type have a greater predilection for the head and neck musculature and in this respect have a distribution similar to the juvenile form of capillary hemangiomas found in infants and young children.

Clinically, these lesions are more likely to pose diagnostic problems than superficial hemangiomas. They present simply as enlarging soft tissue masses with few signs or symptoms to belie their vascular nature. In particular, there is rarely any overlying discoloration of the skin, visible pulsation, or audible bruit. Radiography and arteriography are far more helpful for suggesting the diagnosis. Plain films may reveal phleboliths in addition to a soft tissue mass, and arteriography may demonstrate a highly vascular lesion with early venous runoff. Moreover, the vessels are oriented parallel to one another in a "striated" pattern.[130] This pattern, created by the orderly entry and proliferation of vessels between fascicles of muscle, is considered a helpful feature in support of the benignancy of the lesion. Pain is a frequent but not invariable symptom and is said to be more common with tumors involving long, narrow muscles where stretching of the muscle and nerve fibers by the tumor is more intense. Occasionally function is impaired or anatomic deformity occurs. Although a history of trauma is given in about one-fifth of cases, there is no indisputable evidence that the lesions are caused by trauma; it appears more likely that trauma merely aggravates the underlying tumor.

Intramuscular hemangiomas vary greatly in their gross and microscopic appearances, depending on whether they are of the capillary, cavernous, or mixed type. In many cases it is not possible to sharply classify these types because they are all part of the same histologic spectrum.

Intramuscular hemangiomas of the capillary type are most common and are most likely to be confused with a malignant tumor. Grossly, they may not ap-

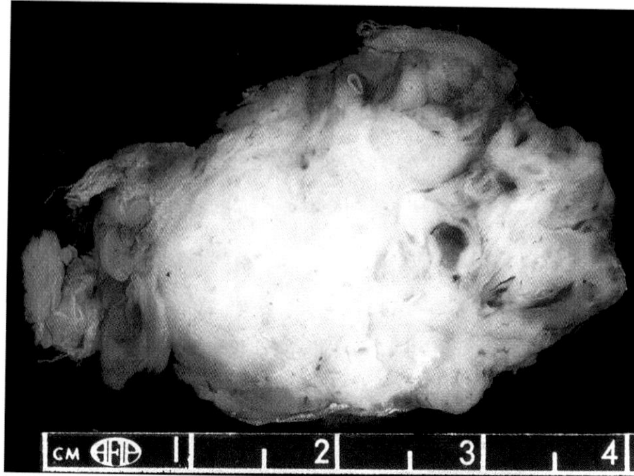


**FIGURE 23–46.** Gross appearance of an intramuscular hemangioma involving the medial thigh. Lesions often have a solid, nonhemorrhagic appearance.

pear especially vascular because they vary from tan to yellow or red (Fig. 23–46). They are composed of myriad small capillary-size vessels with plump nuclei that extend between individual muscle fibers (Figs. 23–47, 23–48, 23–49). Well developed lumen formation is apparent in most areas, although occasional tumors have a solidly cellular appearance similar to the early stage of the juvenile hemangioma. In occasional cases mitotic activity, intraluminal papillary tufting, and a proliferation of capillary vessels in perineural sheaths are present. Although seemingly disturbing features, none of these features is indicative of malignancy in these tumors.

On the other hand, the cavernous form of intramuscular hemangioma is easily recognized as a benign vascular tumor. Grossly, these lesions are blue-red masses composed of large vessels lined by bland, markedly attenuated endothelium, which seldom shows a significant degree of pleomorphism. The presence of adipose tissue in these tumors is common, and at times it may be so conspicuous as to suggest a diagnosis of lipoma. Many of the earlier tumors described as *infiltrating angiolipomas of muscle* or *benign mesenchymoma* may well be intramuscular hemangiomas with a striking fatty overgrowth.

The most important consideration in the differential diagnosis of these lesions is the distinction from an angiosarcoma of skeletal muscle. It should be recalled that angiosarcomas of deep soft tissue, specifically skeletal muscle, are rare (see Chapter 25); thus a vascular tumor of skeletal muscle is statistically more likely to be benign than malignant. Moreover, intramuscular hemangiomas do not develop the freely anastomosing sinusoidal pattern encountered in most well differentiated angiosarcomas, nor do they exhibit nuclear pleomorphism and hyperchromatism. As indicated earlier, some hemangiomas of skeletal muscle contain significant lipomatous components and therefore are occasionally confused with liposarcomas. Although well differentiated liposarcomas contain an in-

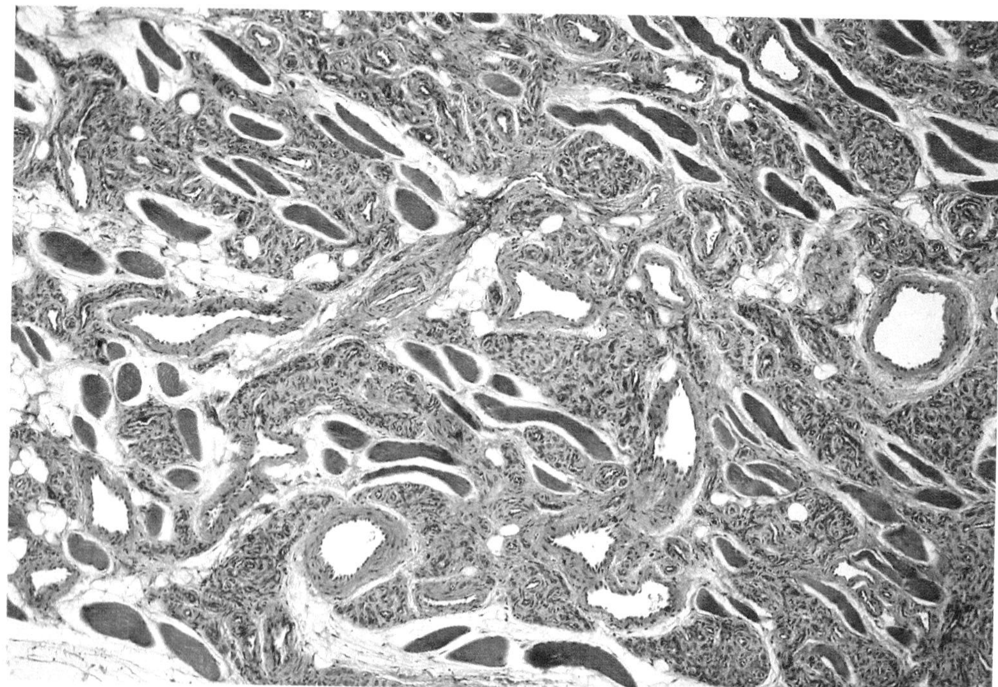

**FIGURE 23–47.** Intramuscular hemangioma with separation of muscle fibers by proliferating vessels. This pseudoinfiltrative pattern is often mistaken for evidence of malignancy.

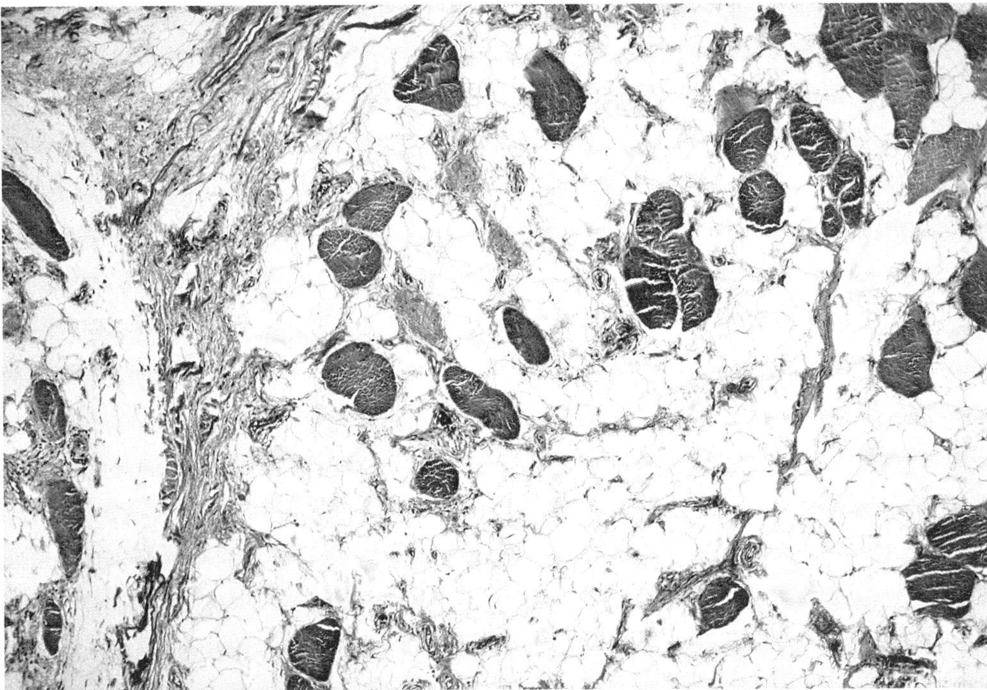

**FIGURE 23–48.** Intramuscular hemangioma with a significant admixture of fat. Such tumors have sometimes been classified as "angiolipomas" of muscle.

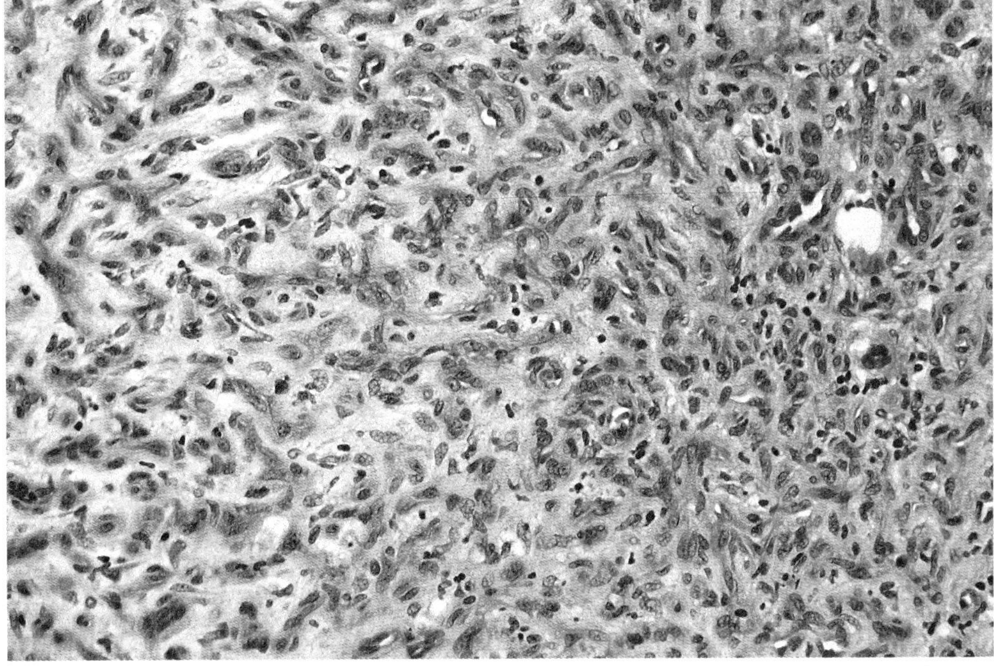

**FIGURE 23–49.** Small vessel (capillary) type of intramuscular hemangioma.

tricate vascular pattern, they rarely have the gaping vessels characteristic of hemangiomas, and they contain, in addition, lipoblasts. Finally, diffuse forms of hemangiomas (angiomatosis) involving skeletal muscle are histologically indistinguishable from intramuscular hemangiomas. The distinction of the two disorders must therefore be based on clinical parameters. In contrast to the intramuscular hemangioma, angiomatosis is usually a congenital or childhood lesion that involves an extensive body area, including muscle, skin, and bone. Intramuscular hemangiomas are best considered benign tumors with a small but definite risk of local recurrence attributable to the ease and adequacy of the initial excision. In our experience 18% of patients develop local recurrences, although other investigators have reported recurrences of more than 50%.[133] Metastases have not been recorded. Treatment is therefore best aimed at complete excision without resorting to radical surgery. Prior embolization of the tumor has been used as a means to facilitate surgical excision.[134]

## Synovial Hemangioma

Synovial hemangioma is a well recognized but rare entity. Theoretically, it can arise from any synovium-lined surface and therefore may be found along the course of tendons or in a joint space.[136–143] In the former location these lesions present in the same fashion as the common giant cell tumor, that is, as painless soft tissue swellings. The origin from synovium in these cases is only assumed because they may also involve superficial structures, and confinement by synovium is often not apparent. Thus the most characteristic form of synovial hemangioma is the intraarticular variety in which the tumor consists of a more or less discrete mass lined by a synovial membrane.[137,138,142] These tumors almost invariably involve the knee joint and classically present as recurrent episodes of pain, swelling, and joint effusion. The symptoms usually begin during childhood and persist several years before the time of diagnosis. In most instances a spongy compressible mass that decreases in size with elevation can be palpated over the joint. Plain films of the joint show nonspecific changes, including capsular thickening and vague soft tissue density and rarely erosion of bone or invasion of adjacent muscle. Arteriography is more diagnostic in that the pooling of blood over the mass suggests a vascular tumor. The tumor grows either as a discrete pedunculated lesion or as a diffuse process.

Histologically, the tumors are cavernous hemangiomas in which the vessels are separated by an edematous, myxoid, or focally hyalinized matrix occasionally containing inflammatory cells and siderophages (Fig. 23–50). The synovium overlying the tumor is sometimes thrown into villous projections, and its cells contain moderate to marked amounts of hemosiderin pigment (Figs. 23–50, 23–51). These synovial changes appear to be secondary phenomena but sometimes are so striking they raise the possibility of primary synovitis. Proper evaluation depends on the recognition that the underlying vessels are far too numerous and large for the area in question.

There is no general agreement concerning the pathogenesis of these lesions. It has been suggested by some that those lesions are not neoplasms but represent a reaction to trauma, although such a his-

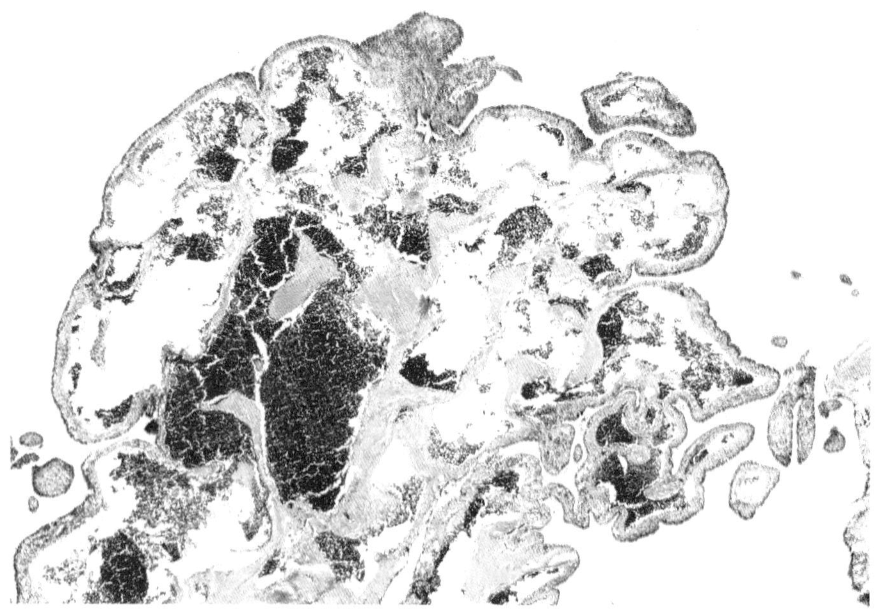

**FIGURE 23–50.** Synovial hemangioma depicting cavernous blood spaces located immediately subjacent to the synovial membrane.

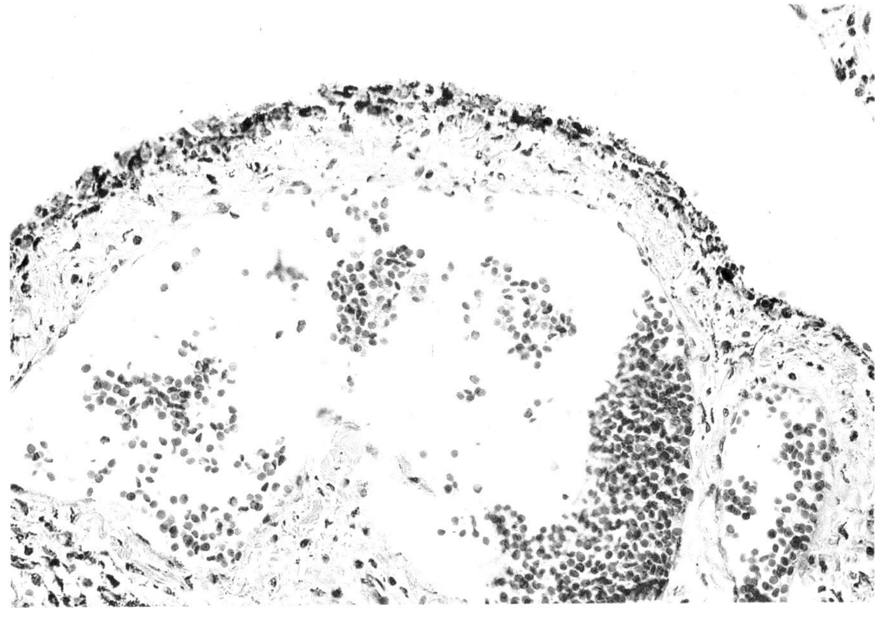

**FIGURE 23–51.** Synovial hemangioma. Pigmentation of synovial cells is a result of the presence of hemosiderin.

tory is given in only a small number of cases. On the other hand, the young age of most afflicted patients again raises the question as to whether these lesions represent congenital malformations or tumors, especially because occasional patients have been noted to have hemangiomas elsewhere.

Treatment of local or pedunculated tumors is relatively easy, consisting of simple extirpation. Diffuse lesions are more difficult to eradicate surgically, and small doses of radiation have sometimes been advocated.

### Hemangioma of Peripheral Nerves

Hemangiomas arising within the confines of the epineurium are rare. Of the few cases described in the literature several are probably unacceptable because they appear to involve nerve secondarily. Of the acceptable cases[144–148] there appears to be no characteristic age or anatomic distribution, although most occur in patients under the age of 40 years. Pain is a common symptom and may be accompanied by numbness and muscle wasting in the affected region. In one case symptoms of carpal tunnel syndrome were noted as a result of the location of the tumor in the median nerve. Involved nerves have included the trigeminal, ulnar, median, posterior tibial, and peroneal nerves. Histologically, most of the tumors have been cavernous hemangiomas with no histologic features suggesting malignancy.

Treatment of these benign tumors must be individualized. The benefits of total resection must be balanced against the morbidity of the procedure. Complete removal of an intraneural hemangioma has been accomplished by intrafascicular dissection using dissecting microscopy.[148] Such an approach offers complete removal with minimal morbidity.

## ANGIOMATOSIS (DIFFUSE HEMANGIOMA)

Angiomatosis is a rare, benign but clinically extensive vascular lesion of soft tissue that almost invariably becomes symptomatic during childhood.[149–153] These lesions probably begin during early intrauterine life when the limb buds form, grow proportionately with the fetus, and consequently affect large areas of the trunk or extremity (Fig. 23–52). We propose a com-

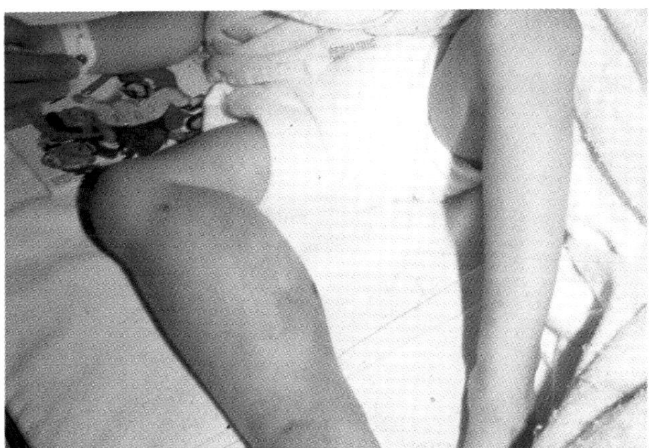

**FIGURE 23–52.** Child with angiomatosis affecting the entire lower leg.

bined clinicopathologic definition for this condition requiring that such lesions be histologically benign and affect a large segment of the body in a contiguous fashion.[153] Involvement may be of two types: either extensive vertical involvement of multiple tissue planes (e.g., subcutis, muscle, and bone) or extensive involvement of tissue of the same type (e.g., multiple muscles). More than half of patients present within the first two decades of life, usually with symptoms of diffuse persistent swelling sometimes associated with pain and discoloration. Only rarely is hypertrophy, gigantism, or clinical evidence of arteriovenous shunting present. On computed tomography (CT) scans the lesions appear as ill-defined nonhomogeneous masses that may resemble sarcoma except for the presence of serpiginous dense areas that correspond to thick-walled, tortuous vessels (Fig. 23–53). Because of the presence of large amounts of fat, these tumors often appear as predominantly fatty tumors (Fig. 23–54).

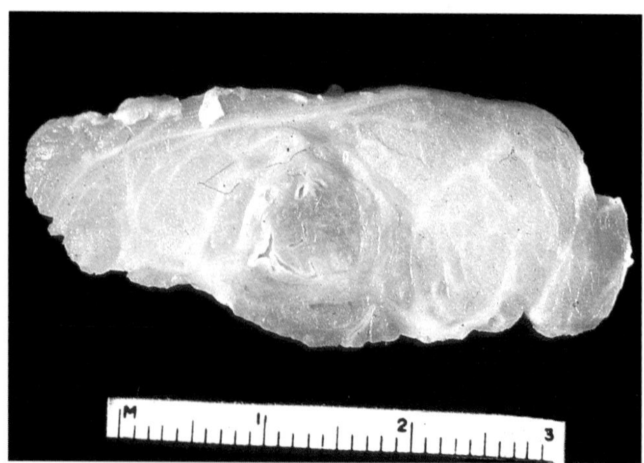

FIGURE 23–54. Cut section through a portion of angiomatosis. Pale appearance of muscle is typical and indicates replacement of fibers by vessels and fat.

Histologically, angiomatosis may assume one of two patterns. The first and more common pattern seen in most of the 50 cases we reviewed consisted of a melange of large venous, cavernous, and capillary-size vessels scattered haphazardly throughout soft tissue (Fig. 23–55). The venous vessels are remarkable for their irregular, thick walls that have occasional attenuations and herniations (Figs. 23–56, 23–57). A rather characteristic feature of these veins is the presence of small vessels clustered just adjacent to or in the wall of a large vein (Fig. 23–57). The second pattern, which occurs in a small number of cases, is virtually identical to that of a capillary hemangioma, except that the nodules of tumor diffusely infiltrate the surrounding soft tissue. The prominent amount of fat present in these lesions has led previous authors to use the term *infiltrating angiolipoma,* suggesting that angiomatosis is probably best regarded as a more generalized mesenchymal proliferation. One unique case, which featured a diffuse proliferation of glomus cells in addition to the vessels, offers some support to the foregoing idea.[153]

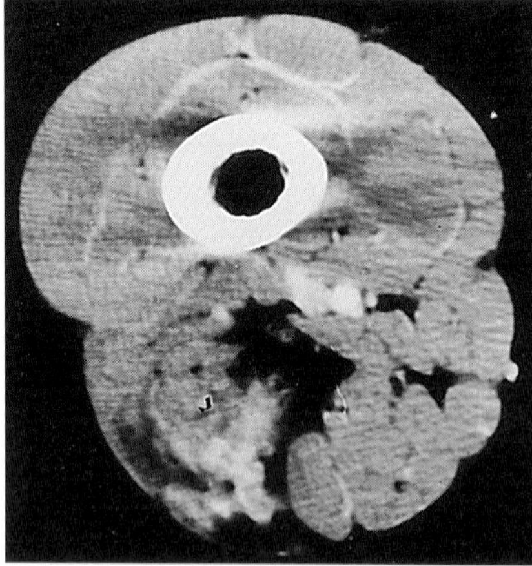

FIGURE 23–53. Computed tomography (CT) scan of angiomatosis illustrating diffuse nonhomogeneous regions in muscle. Serpiginous areas (arrow) represent tortuous vessels. (From Rao VK, Weiss SW. Angiomatosis of soft tissue: an analysis of the histologic features and clinical outcome in 51 cases. Am J Surg Pathol 16:764, 1992.)

In the study by Rao and Weiss,[153] nearly 90% of patients experienced recurrences, and 40% had more than one recurrence within a 5-year period. A somewhat lower recurrence rate was reported by Howat and Campbell.[152] This behavior contrasts with the recurrence rate of intramuscular hemangiomas, which is usually less than 50%. Although there has been speculation that recurrence rates may be higher in young children affected with this condition, it appears not to be true. There is no evidence that such lesions ever progress to frank malignancy, so the goal of therapy is to treat the lesions as conservatively as possible, balancing the need for complete surgical extirpation with the morbidity of the procedure.

Diagnosis of these unusual tumors may prove difficult. As indicated in the discussion of intramuscular hemangiomas, the distinction between angiomatosis and an intramuscular hemangioma is fundamentally based on clinical rather than pathologic criteria. However, we believe that the irregular venous channels with clustered small vessels in their walls are characteristic of angiomatosis and should certainly in small biopsy specimens prompt a dialogue with the clinician concerning the extent of the lesion.

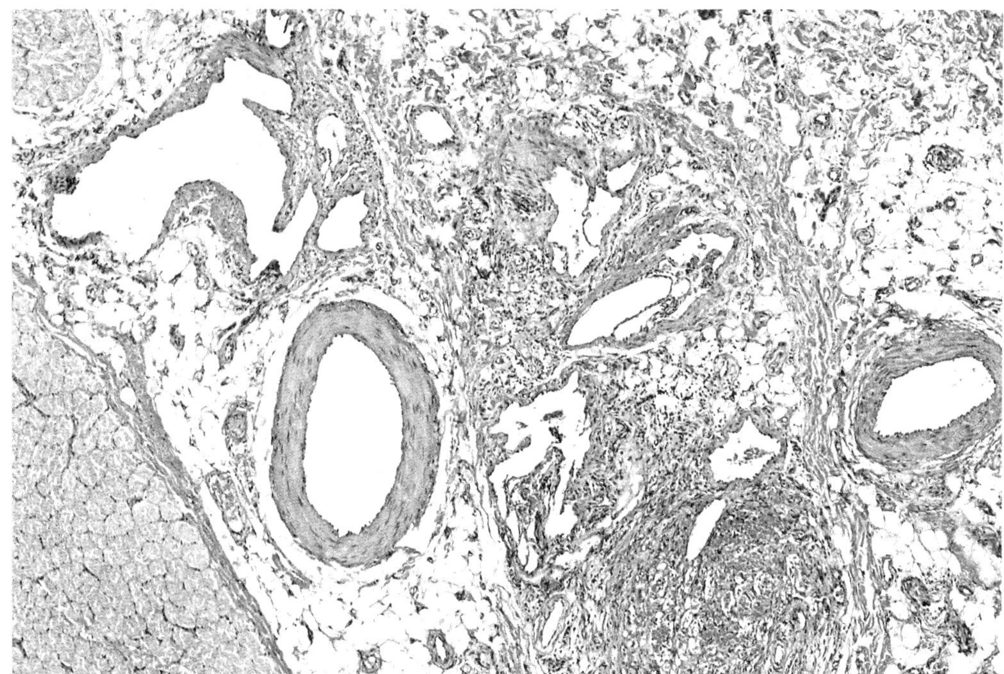

**FIGURE 23–55.** Angiomatosis with variously sized vessels involving muscle and fat.

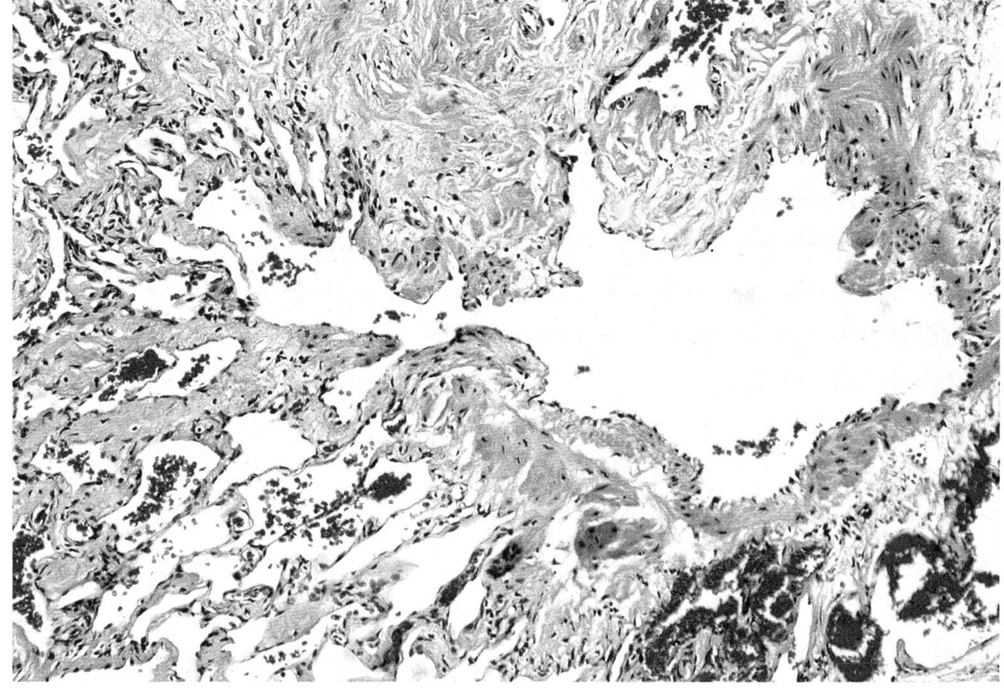

**FIGURE 23–56.** Angiomatosis with small vessels residing adjacent to and in the wall of a larger vessel.

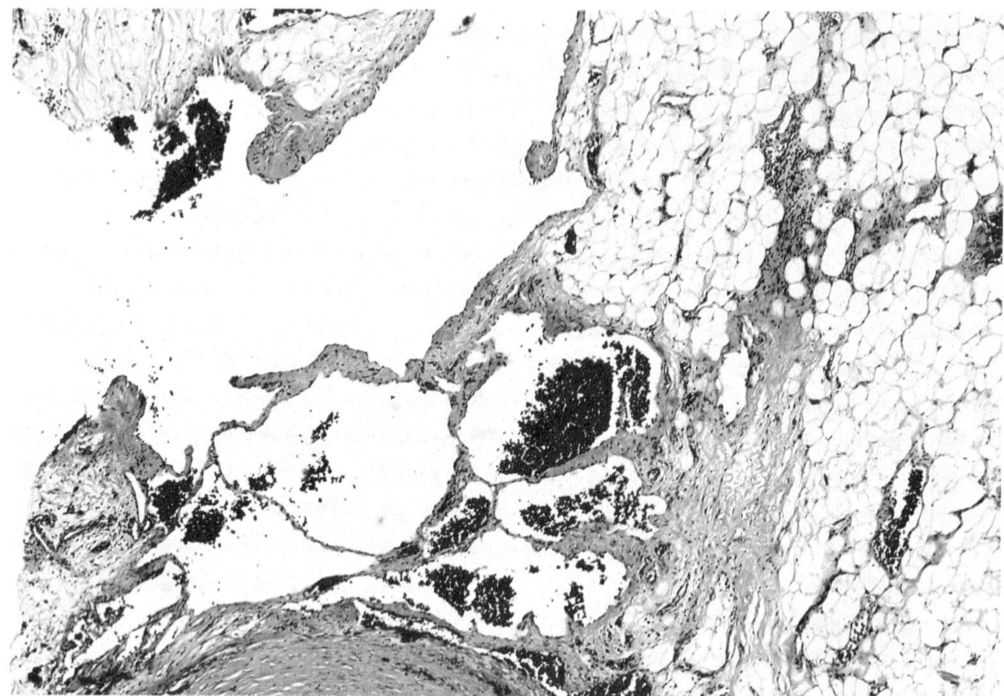

**FIGURE 23–57.** Venous vessel in angiomatosis illustrating irregular wall and herniations.

## VASCULAR ECTASIAS

Vascular ectasias are collectively a common group of lesions characterized by localized dilatation of preformed vessels.[154–160,163–167] Although most are cutaneous and share certain common histologic features, the clinical presentation and etiology are different. Thus in many instances a precise diagnosis depends on complete knowledge of the clinical history and gross appearance of the lesion in question. Of the many types of vascular ectasias, only the more significant ones are mentioned. The reader is referred to an excellent review of the subject for detailed discussions of the less common forms.[156]

### Nevus Flammeus (Nevus Telangiectaticus)

The most common form of ectasia is the *nevus flammeus,* or ordinary birthmark. These lesions are most common on the mid forehead, eyelids, and nape of the neck.[166,167] It has been estimated that about half of all infants have a nevus flammeus in the neck, which suggests a possible autosomal dominant mode of inheritance. Typically, the birthmark is a mottled macular lesion ranging in color from light pink to deep purple. Most are dull pink and are referred to as "salmon patches," or facetiously as "the affectionate peck of a stork." Most lesions eventually regress. Those on the forehead and eyelids are evanescent and disappear within the first year of life. Lesions on the nape of the neck fade more slowly, and their vestiges are documented in about 20% of the adult population.

The *port-wine stain* (*nevus vinosus*) is a specialized form of nevus flammeus. It differs from the latter in several respects; it grows proportionately with the child and demonstrates no tendency to fade. Although it begins as a smooth red to purple macular lesion on the face or extremity, it often acquires an elevated thickened surface that is more reminiscent of a true hemangioma. Some authors prefer to classify the port-wine stain and nevus flammeus as forms of hemangioma. Histologically, however, only dilatation of vessels in the mid and deep dermis is present, and in the early lesion even this change may not be pronounced. Comparison of port-wine stains with normal skin has not indicated any differences in immunostaining for factor VIII-associated protein, basement membrane protein, fibronectin, or various monoclonal antibodies specific for endothelium (e.g., PAL-E, ICAM-1, ELAM-1).[163] There does, however, appear to be a decrease in the number of perivascular nerves, suggesting that lack of neural control of the vascular bed results in their progressive dilatation.[165] Treatment of port-wine stains by laser therapy has been used.[158]

Aside from the cosmetic problems it poses, the port-wine stain may indicate the presence of more extensive vascular malformation. Port-wine stains of the face that occur in the distribution of the trigeminal nerve may be associated with ipsilateral vascular malformations of the leptomeninges and occasionally of the retina (*Sturge-Weber syndrome, encephalotrigeminal angiomatosis*). Seizures, hemiplegia, and mental retardation, which characterize the full-blown syndrome, are the result of cerebral atrophy induced by the meningeal malformation. *Klippel-Trenaunay syndrome* includes a port-wine stain associated with varicosities and hypertrophy (gigantism) of an extremity.[161,162] In most instances of this rare condition the lower extremity is affected, and the extensive varicosities and edema appear to be the result of agenesis of the deep venous structures. In a small number of patients there may be, in addition, a congenital arteriovenous fistula. It has been suggested that this subgroup be separately designated as *Parkes-Weber syndrome* because the problems with management are different.[161,162] In Parkes-Weber syndrome the major therapeutic thrust must be directed toward reducing or eliminating the arteriovenous fistula to prevent supervening congestive heart failure.

### Arterial Spiders

Arterial spiders (*nevus araneus*) represent another common form of ectasia, but unlike the nevus flammeus they are rarely found at birth. Instead, they represent acquired lesions associated with altered physiologic states (e.g., pregnancy, liver disease, hyperthyroidism); the lesions often regress with restoration of the normal state.[156] Grossly, they are characterized by a small central arteriole or "punctum" from which tiny radial vessels emanate. With application of pressure over the punctum the entire lesion blanches. With release of pressure the lesion reddens in a centrifugal direction. The vascular spider consists of a thick-walled arteriole, which dilates, branches as it approaches the surface epithelium, and eventually anastomoses with small capillaries of the dermis.

### Hereditary Hemorrhagic Telangiectasia (Osler-Weber-Rendu Disease)

Hereditary hemorrhagic-telangiectasia is characterized by vascular anomalies consisting of dilated capillaries and veins of the skin and mucosal membranes.[164] It is inherited as an autosomal dominant disease and commences with the development of numerous small red papules on the skin and mucosa, particularly in the region of the face, lips, oral mucosa, and tongue. Similar lesions may be found in the gastrointestinal, genitourinary, and pulmonary systems. The lesions usually appear during childhood, increase with age, and in the elderly may have an appearance similar to that of the vascular spider. In contrast to the spider, the lesions are prone to bleeding, so the course of the disease is marked by repeated bouts of hemorrhage. Treatment must be supportive because treatment of ectasias by such modalities as electrocoagulation can result in the formation of satellite lesions.

## REACTIVE VASCULAR PROLIFERATIONS

### Papillary Endothelial Hyperplasia (Vegetant Intravascular Hemangioendothelioma, Intravascular Angiomatosis)

Papillary endothelial hyperplasia is an exuberant, usually intravascular, endothelial proliferation that in many respects mimics an angiosarcoma.[168–178] It was first described by Masson, who designated it *vegetant intravascular hemangioendothelioma*.[174] He regarded it as a true neoplasm that displays degenerative changes including necrosis and thrombosis as it outgrows its blood supply. Henschen,[171] on the other hand, believed it was a primary endothelial proliferation occurring in response to inflammation and stasis in a vascular bed. His theory rested on the frequency with which this process occurred in vessels of inflamed hemorrhoids, urethral caruncles, and laryngeal polyps. Most evidence to date supports the contention that the lesion is an unusual form of organizing thrombus. Why only some thrombi display this form of organization is not clear.

Although this process may occur in virtually any vessel in the body, only those lesions that present as detectable masses are likely to come to the attention of the surgical pathologist. In our experience such lesions are most commonly located in veins on the head, neck, fingers, and trunk, where they appear as small, firm, superficial (deep dermis or subcutis) masses imparting a red to blue discoloration to the overlying skin (Fig. 23–58).[169] Usually a history of trauma is not elicited. Both the appearance and symptoms are nonspecific, so a biopsy is ultimately required to establish the identity of the lesion. In addition to its occurrence in a pure form in a dilated vessel, this lesion may be engrafted on a preexisting vascular lesion such as a hemangioma, pyogenic granuloma, or vascular malformation. In these cases the symptoms, appearance, and ultimate prognosis are related to the underlying lesion. In fact, most deeply situated papillary endothelial hyperplasias occur in intramuscular hemangiomas.

In its pure form the lesion is a small (average 2 cm), purple-red, multicystic mass containing clotted blood and surrounded by a fibrous pseudocapsule containing residual smooth muscle or elastic tissue of the preexisting vessel wall (Fig. 23–59). In vessels of small caliber that are markedly dilated, little or no muscle is demonstrable in the pseudocapsule. Rarely,

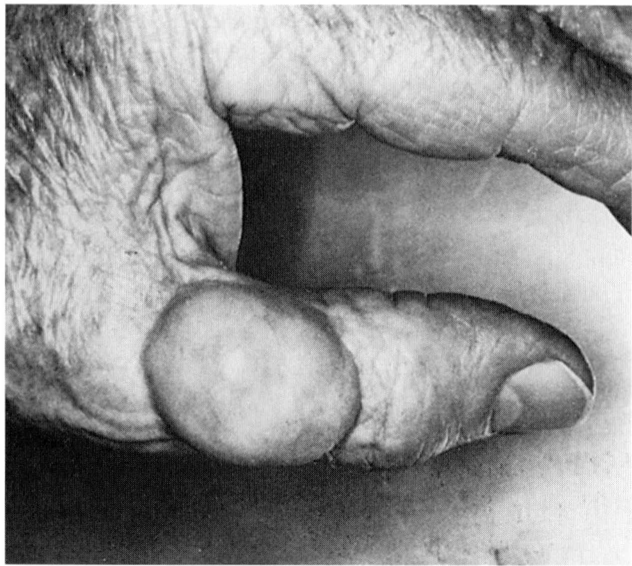

**FIGURE 23–58.** Papillary endothelial hyperplasia presenting as a localized nodule on the thumb.

rupture of the vessel of origin permits spilling over of the process into surrounding soft tissue, a phenomenon that should not be equated with malignancy. In our experience most of these lesions are intimately associated with thrombus material, lending support to the idea that they are unusual organizing thrombi. In the early lesion the ingrowth of endothelium along the contours of the thrombus partitions it into coarse papillae with fibrin cores (Fig. 23–60). In the well established or typical lesion, myriad small delicate papillae project into the lumen and closely simulate the tufting growth of the hemangiosarcoma. These papillae are composed of a single layer of endothelium surrounding a collagenized core. The endothelial cells appear plump or swollen but lack significant pleomorphism and mitotic figures. During the late stage, clumping and fusing of the papillae give rise to an anastomosing network of vessels embedded in a loose mesh-like stroma of connective tissue (Fig. 23–60D).

Ultrastructurally, the cells lining the papillae appear to be differentiated endothelial cells with numerous micropinocytotic vesicles at the luminal aspect, tight junctions along the lateral boundaries, and occasional intracytoplasmic Weibel-Palade bodies. Basal lamina invests the antiluminal surface of the cell. In addition, pericytes and undifferentiated cells can be identified on the antiluminal aspects of the endothelial cells.[172] The participation of several cell types is similar to the situation encountered in human granulation tissue and is further evidence of the reactive nature of this process.

The most significant aspect of this lesion is the regularity with which it is confused with an angiosarcoma. A helpful point in the differential diagnosis is its intravascular location, as angiosarcomas are almost never confined to a vascular lumen. As mentioned earlier, passive extension of this process into soft tissue may occur following vessel rupture. However, even in these cases the intravascular location of most of the lesion, coupled with the reactive changes in the vessel wall suggesting rupture, aid in the proper identification. On rare occasions papillary endothelial hyperplasia occurs extravascularly as a result of organization of a hematoma,[175] but this diagnosis should be made with caution. Apart from the usual intravascular location, papillary endothelial hyperplasia lacks

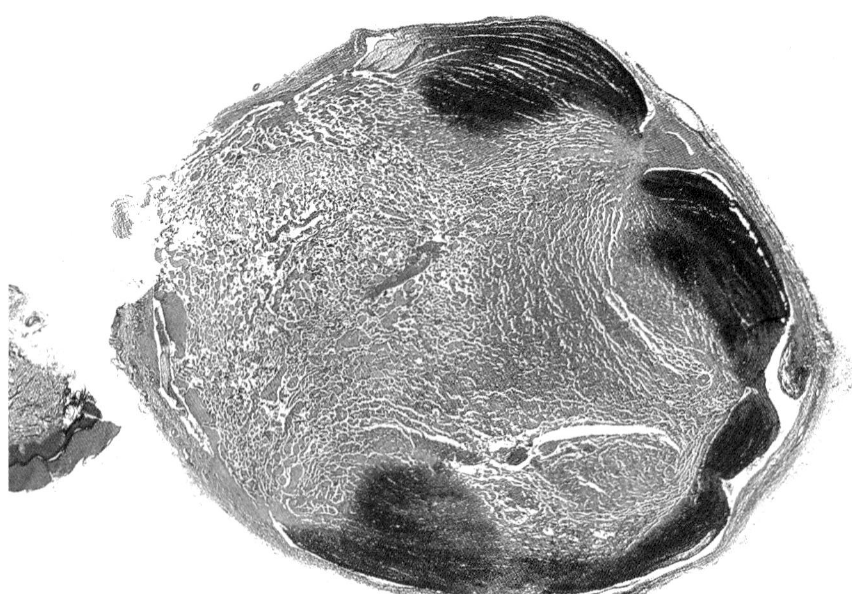

**FIGURE 23–59.** Organizing thrombus in a vessel showing early stages of papillary endothelial hyperplasia at the bottom of the picture.

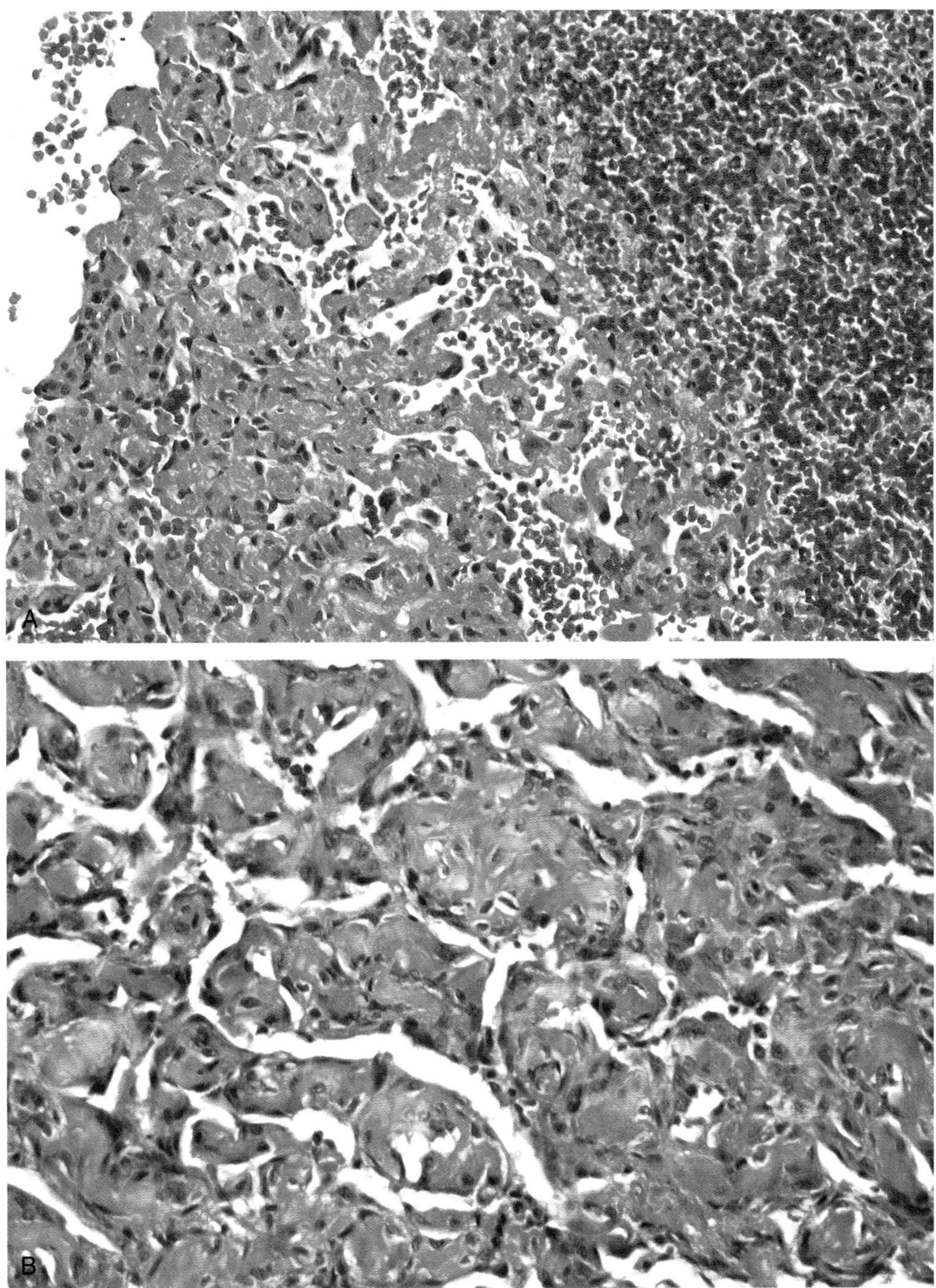


**FIGURE 23–60.** Stages of papillary endothelial hyperplasia. (**A**) Early stage is characterized by a thrombus with ingrowth of endothelial cells. Endothelium gradually subdivides the partially collagenized thrombus into coarse clumps (**B**) followed by papillae (**C**). (**D**) At the end-stage papillae fuse to form a loosely anastomotic "secondary" vascular pattern.

*Illustration continued on following page*

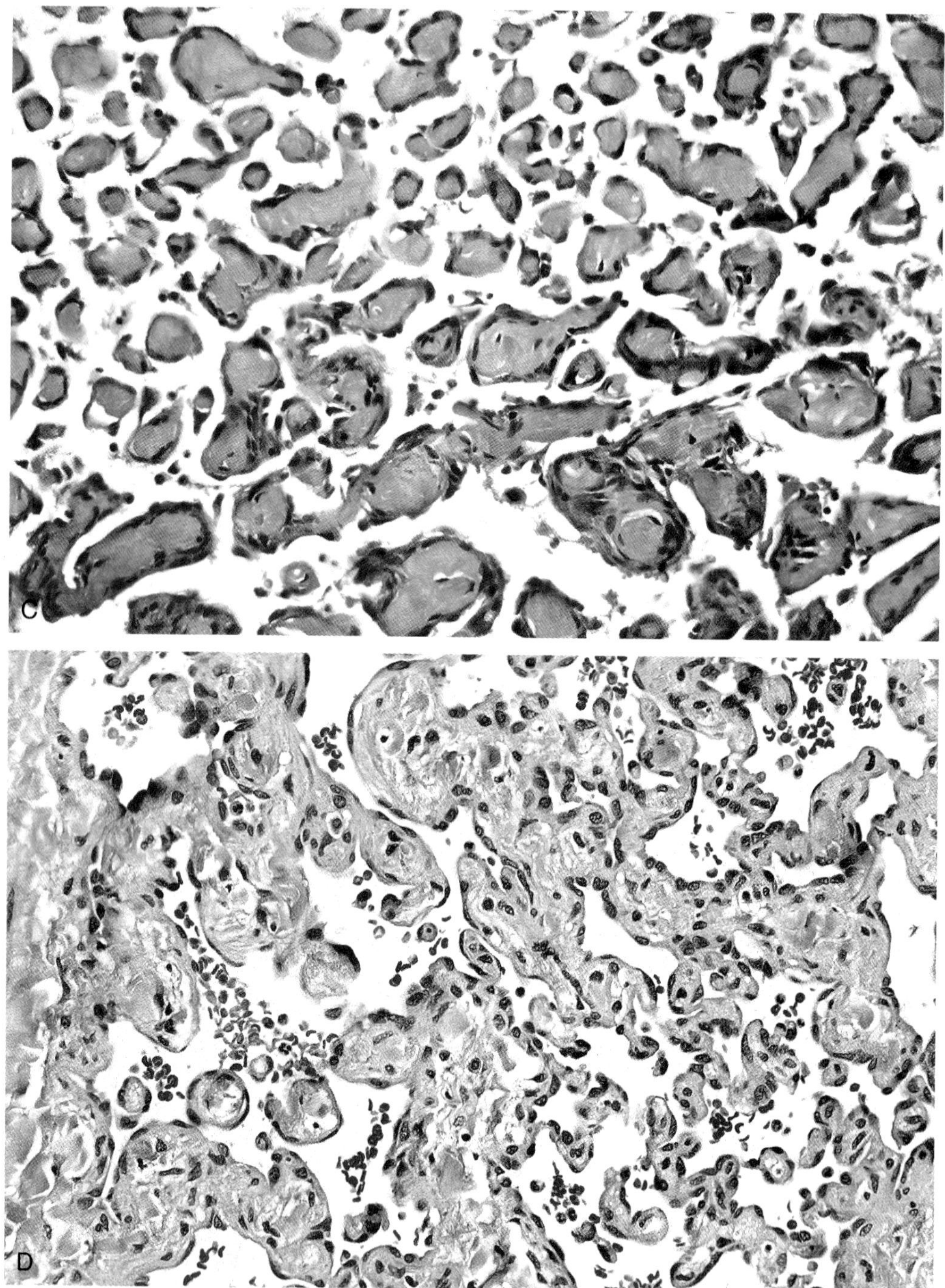


**FIGURE 23–60** *(Continued).*

the frank tissue necrosis, marked pleomorphism, and relatively high mitotic rate that characterize most angiosarcomas.

The prognosis of this lesion is excellent. Essentially all cases are cured by simple excision. Those that do recur are usually those that are superimposed on vascular tumors. The therapy in these cases should be dictated by the nature of the underlying lesions.

## Vascular Transformation of Lymph Nodes (Nodal Angiomatosis)

First described as *vascular transformation of lymph nodes*[179] and later as *nodal angiomatosis*,[178] this reactive change of lymph node occurs secondary to lymphatic or venous obstruction, or both, and has been observed particularly in axillary lymph nodes removed at the time of radical mastectomy for breast carcinoma.[177–180] The change may also occur in lymph nodes removed for a variety of other diagnostic or therapeutic reasons. Typically the change involves the subcapsular space and sinuses in either a segmental or diffuse fashion. In the most readily recognized case the small, ectatic, capillary-size vessels are well formed (Figs. 23–61, 23–62). Chan et al.[177] emphasized a greater range of changes in this condition than was previously appreciated. In extreme examples of vascular transformation the vessels may be closely packed and slightly attenuated so the resemblance to Kaposi's sarcoma is more than fleeting. Usually, however, there is maturation of the vessels toward the periphery of the lymph node such that ectatic capillaries are present immediately subjacent to the capsule. Extravasation of erythrocytes occurs; and in exceptional cases hyaline droplets, similar to those in Kaposi's sarcoma, are identified.

There are a number of features that serve to distinguish this lesion from Kaposi's sarcoma, including the overall preservation of lymph node architecture despite the expansion of the subcapsular and medullary sinuses, the peripheral maturation of the vessels, the lack of vessels arranged in distinct fascicles, and the presence of secondary sclerosis. However, the earliest stages of Kaposi's sarcoma of lymph nodes, as seen in the patient with acquired immunodeficiency syndrome (AIDS), may prove exceptionally difficult and at some times impossible to distinguish from vascular transformation of the lymph node.

## Glomeruloid Hemangioma

Glomeruloid hemangioma is a descriptive term coined by Chan et al.[181] for the reactive vascular proliferations that occur in *POEMS syndrome* (Takatsuki syndrome and Crowe-Fukase syndrome).[181–183,185] This syndrome is characterized by *p*olyneuropathy (peripheral neuropathy, papilledema), *o*rganomegaly (hepatosplenomegaly, lymphadenopathy), *e*ndocrinopathy

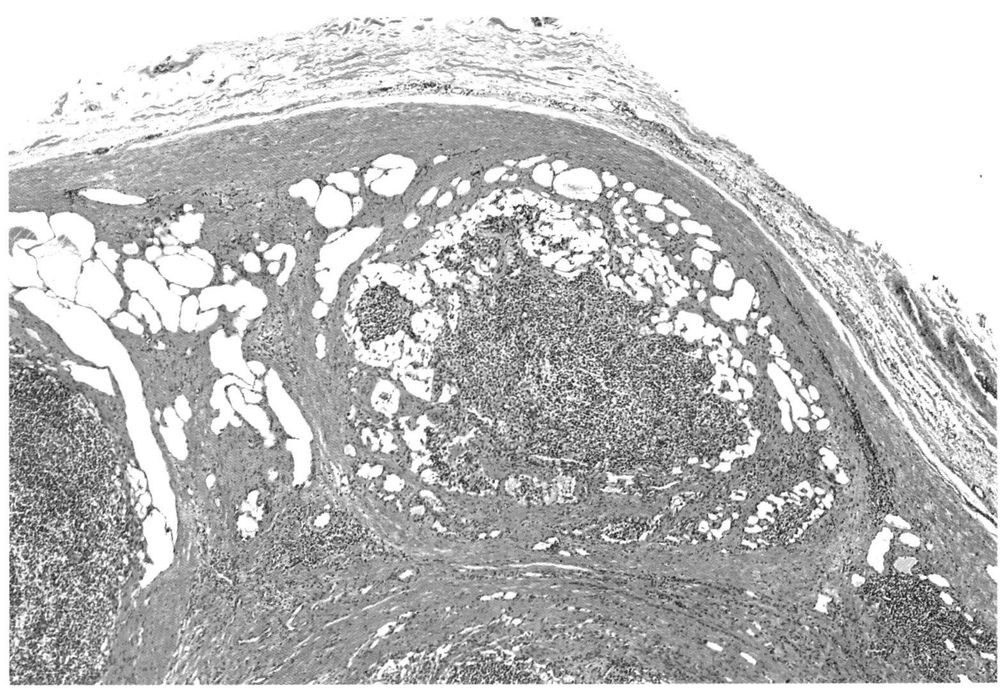

**FIGURE 23–61.** Vascular transformation in a lymph node (nodal angiomatosis). Vessels surround but preserve lymph follicles. Lymph node was removed as part of the regional lymph node dissection for carcinoma.

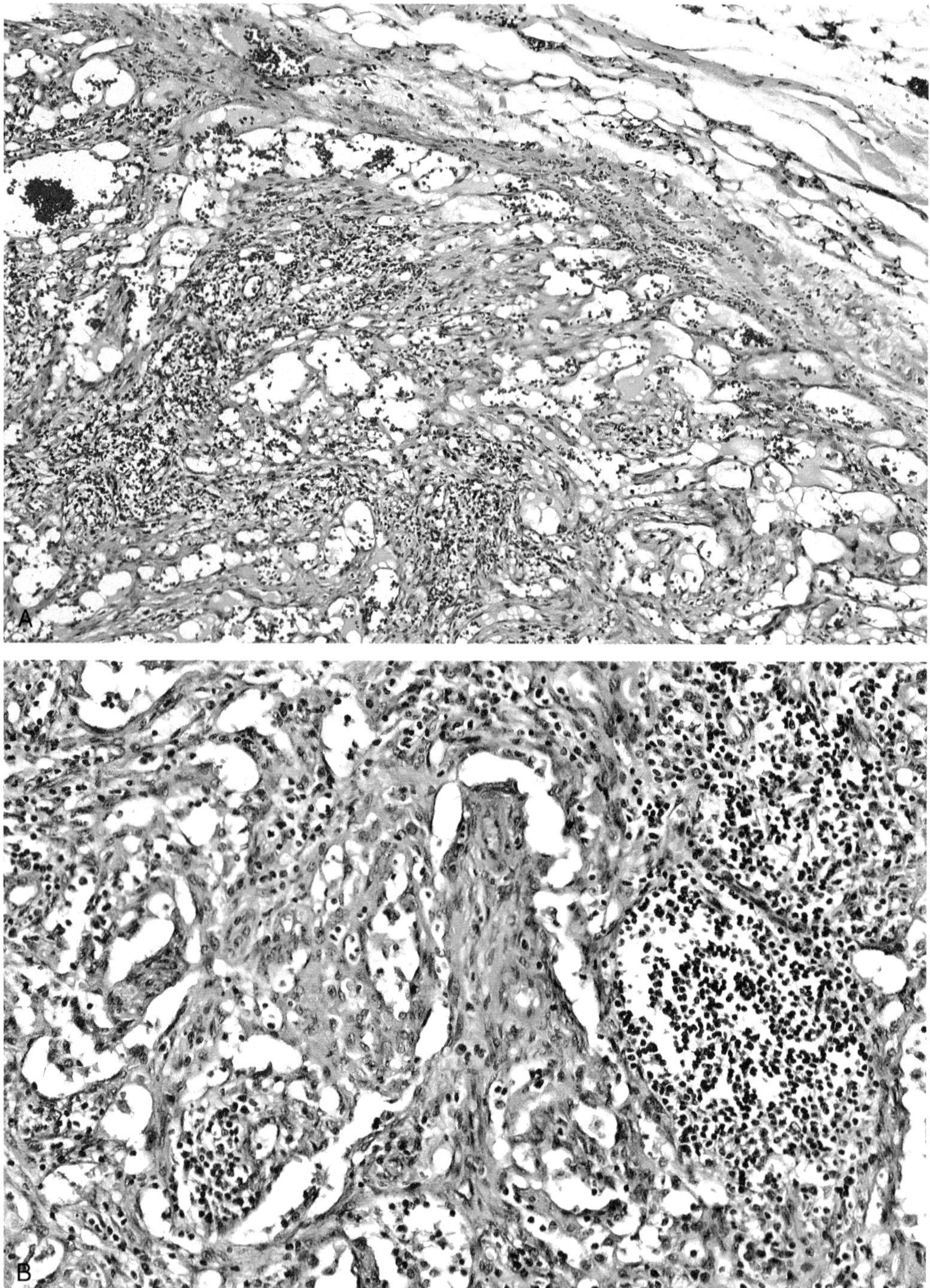


**FIGURE 23–62.** Vascular transformation of lymph node showing a subcapsular location (**A**) and prominent proliferation of vessels (**B**).

(amenorrhea, gynecomastia, impotence, adrenal insufficiency, hypothyroidism, glucose intolerance), *M*-protein (plasmacytosis, paraproteinemia, bone lesions), and *s*kin lesions (hyperpigmentation, hypertrichosis, angiomas); and in some instances it overlaps with multicentric Castleman's disease.[184]

The vascular lesions develop within the dermis underneath an intact, essentially normal epidermis. In the classic case, glomeruloid nests of capillaries lie in ectatic capillaries, creating a "vessel within a vessel" appearance (Figs. 23–63, 23–64). The intravascular capillaries are lined by normal-appearing endothelium and are filled with erythrocytes. A distinctive feature of the intravascular proliferation are the large round cells filled with eosinophilic globules corresponding to polytypic immunoglobulin (Fig. 23–65). Chan et al.[181] suggested that these cells, which reside principally outside the basal lamina, are closely related to endothelial cells rather than pericytes or smooth muscle cells. Their unusual appearance is probably induced by the presence of cytoplasmic immunoglobulin, which is derived from serum. In some cases of POEMS syndrome the vascular lesions are indistinguishable from an ordinary capillary hemangioma, and in other cases the lesions have features intermediate between a capillary hemangioma and the classic glomeruloid hemangioma, suggesting that they represent stages of the same process.

## Bacillary (Epithelioid) Angiomatosis

Bacillary (epithelioid) angiomatosis is a pseudoneoplastic vascular proliferation occurring almost exclusively in immunocompromised hosts.[186–194] It is caused by *Bartonella* (formerly *Rochalimaea*). *Bartonella* is a family of small gram-negative bacilli that includes a number of species pathogenic for humans: *B. henselae, B. qunitana, B. bacilliformis,* and *B. elizabethae. Bartonella henselae* and *quintana* have been shown to be the causative agents for bacillary angiomatosis and bacillary peliosis, as well as for *Bartonella* bacterial endocarditis and classic cat-scratch disease.[193,194]

Most cases of bacillary angiomatosis occur in men in the setting of AIDS. Bacillary angiomatosis usually presents as multiple pink, elevated skin lesions that may resemble a pyogenic granuloma. Usually their pink color distinguishes them from the dusky violaceous lesions of Kaposi's sarcoma. In some cases there are also liver, spleen, lymph node, bone, and soft tissue lesions.[186–189,192] In the classic case, bacillary angiomatosis consists of lobules of capillary-size vessels lined by plump (epithelioid) endothelium with clear cytoplasm (Fig. 23–66). Mild atypia and occasional mitotic figures may be present in the endothelial cells. Although the strikingly clear cytoplasm of the endothelial cells bears some similarity to the endothelial changes in epithelioid hemangioma, there is a neutrophilic infiltrate in the interstitium along with

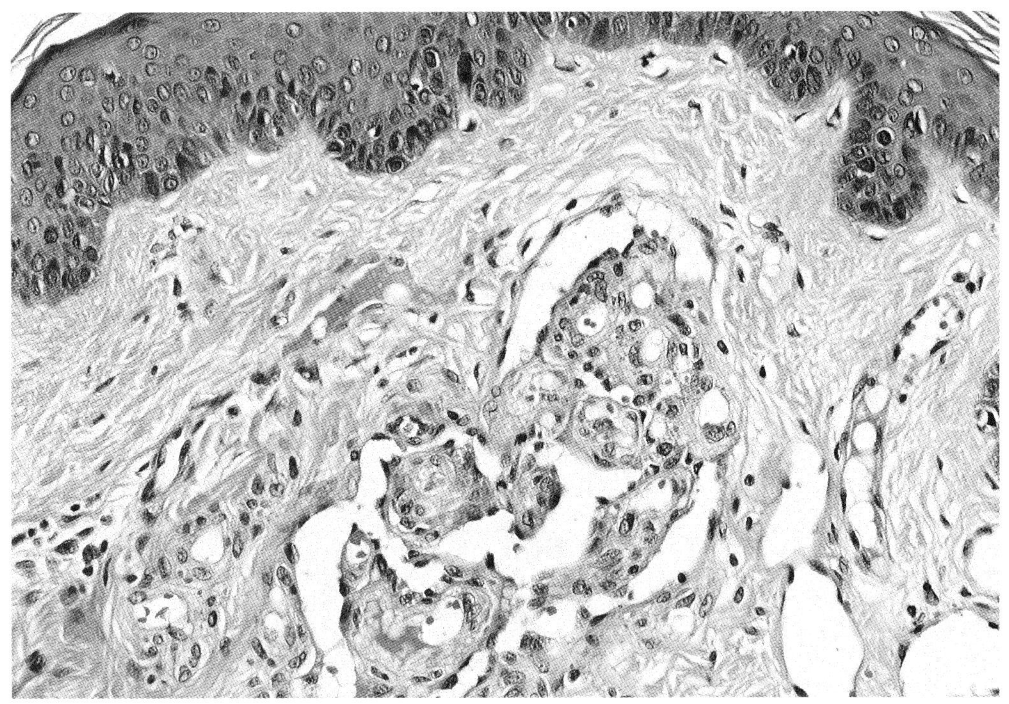

**FIGURE 23–63.** Glomeruloid hemangioma. (Case courtesy of Dr. C.D.M. Fletcher.)

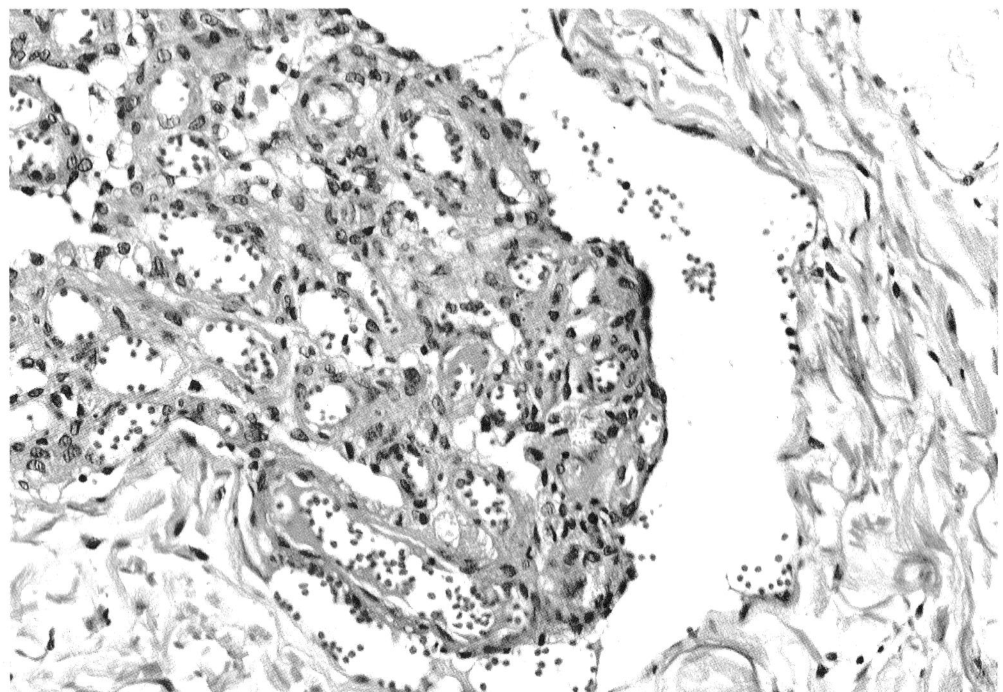

**FIGURE 23–64.** Glomeruloid hemangioma. (Case courtesy of Dr. C.D.M. Fletcher.)

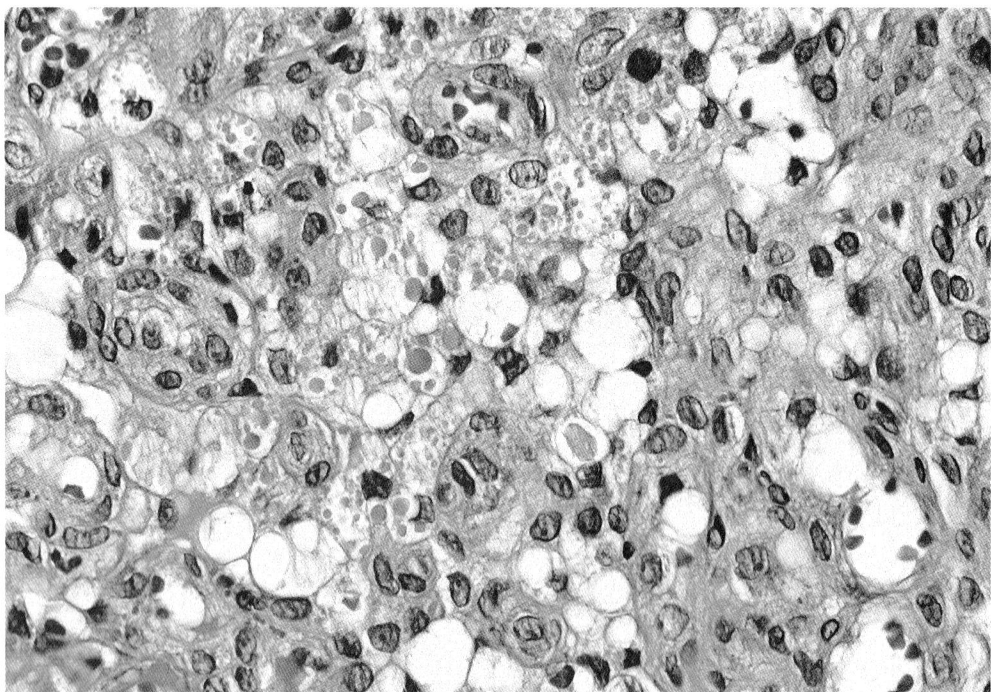

**FIGURE 23–65.** Hyaline droplets of immunoglobulin in a glomeruloid hemangioma. (Case courtesy of Dr. C.D.M. Fletcher.)

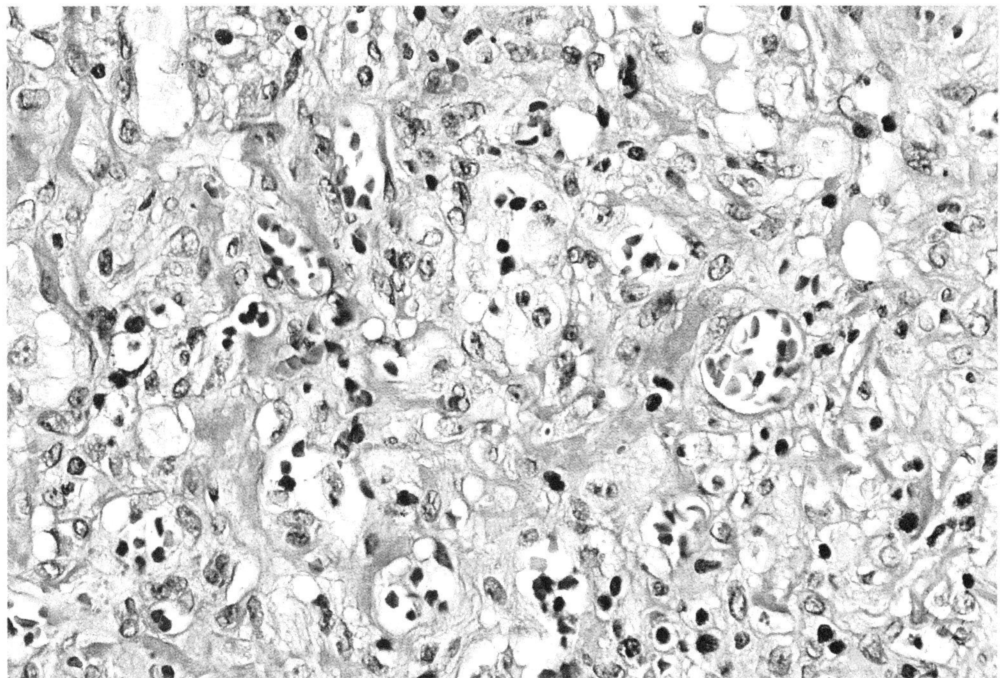

**FIGURE 23–66.** Bacillary angiomatosis showing endothelial cells with clear cytoplasm set in an inflammatory background.

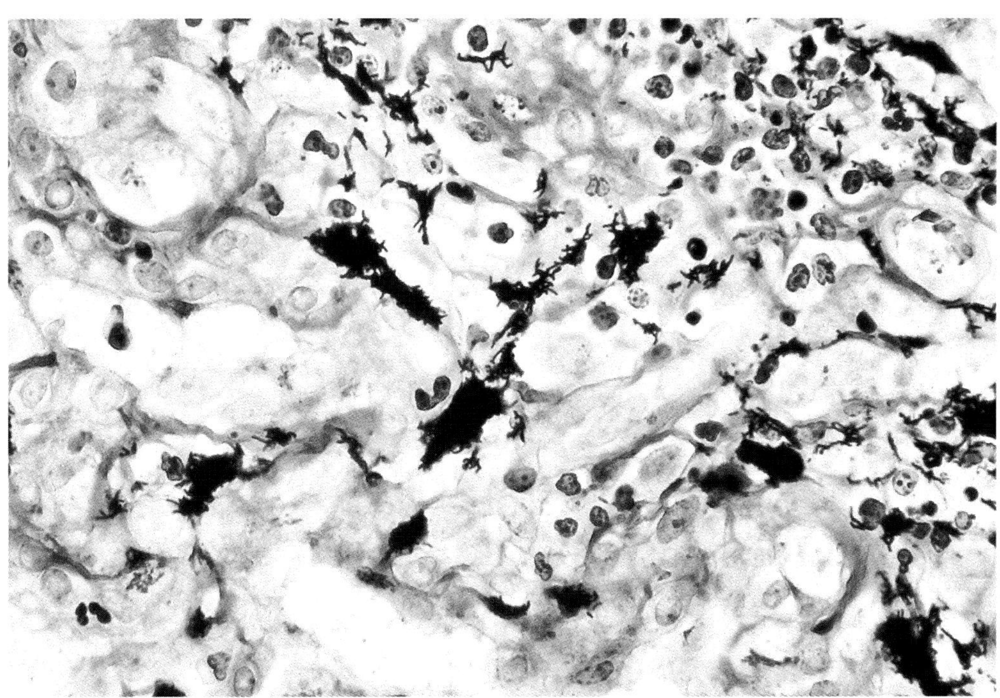

**FIGURE 23–67.** Warthin-Starry staining of bacillary angiomatosis showing numerous clumped rod-shaped organisms.

collections of pink coagulum containing clusters of the organisms that are easily identified with the Warthin-Starry stain (Fig. 23–67). Unfortunately, some bacillary angiomatosis does not display the foregoing distinctive changes and may be virtually indistinguishable from granulation tissue.[194] Obviously if the clinical setting suggests the diagnosis, one is obligated to rule out the diagnosis by means of special stains. On electron microscopy, the organisms appear as bacillary forms with a trilaminar cell wall. In the liver the organisms induce peliotic changes. Large numbers of organisms can be identified around the peliotic zones in the liver. Treatment of bacillary angiomatosis is effectively accomplished with erythromycin.

## REFERENCES


### General

1. Blei F, Walter J, Orlow SJ, Marchuk DA. Familial segregation of hemangiomas and vascular malformations as an autosomal dominant trait. Arch Dermatol 134:718, 1998.
2. Coffin CM, Dehner LP. Vascular tumors in children and adolescents: a clinicopathologic study of 228 tumors in 222 patients. Pathol Annu 1:97, 1993.
3. Enjolras O. Vascular tumors and vascular malformations: are we at the dawn of a better knowledge. Pediatr Dermatol 16: 238, 1994.
4. Enjolras O, Mulliken JB. Vascular tumors and vascular malformations. Adv Dermatol 13:375, 1998.
5. Enjolras O, Wassef M, Mazoyer E, et al. Infants with Kasabach Merritt syndrome do not have "true hemangiomas." J Pediatr 130:631, 1997.
6. Esterly NB. Cutaneous hemangiomas, vascular stains, and malformations, and associated syndromes. Curr Probl Dermatol 3:69, 1995.
7. Folkman J. Clinical application of research on angiogenesis. N Engl J Med 333:1757, 1995.
8. Johnson WC. Pathology of cutaneous vascular tumors. Int J Dermatol 15:239, 1976.
9. Madewell JE, Sweet DE. Tumors and tumorlike lesions in or about joints. In: Resnick D, Niwayama G (eds) Diagnosis of Bone and Joint Disorders, vol 3. WB Saunders, Philadelphia, 1981.
10. Mulliken JB, Glowacki J. Hemangiomas and vascular malformations in infants and children: a classification based on endothelial characteristics. Plast Reconstruct Surg 69:412, 1982.
11. North PE, Mizeracki JR, Thomas R, et al. Intramuscular "hemangiomas" are vascular malformations immunodistinctive from juvenile hemangiomas [abstract 61]. Mod Pathol 13:14A, 2000.
12. Powell J. Update on hemangiomas and vascular malformations. Curr Opin Pediatr 11:457, 1999.
13. Requena L, Sangueza OP. Cutaneous vascular anomalies. Part I. Hamartomas, malformations, and dilatations of preexisting vessels. Am Acad Dermatol 37:523, 1997.
14. Sarkar M, Mulliken JB, Koazakewich HP, et al. Thrombocytopenic coagulopathy (Kasabach-Merritt phenomenon) is associated with kaposiform hemangioendothelioma and not with common infantile hemangioma. Plast Reconstruct Surg 100: 1377, 1997.
15. Stout AP. Hemangioendothelioma: a tumor of blood vessels featuring vascular endothelial cells. Ann Surg 118:445, 1943.
16. Weiss SW. Vascular tumors: a deductive approach to diagnosis. Surg Pathol 2:185, 1989.

### Normal Structure and Function

17. Alberts B, Bray D, Lewis J, et al. Molecular Biology of the Cell, 3rd ed. Garland, New York, 1994, pp 1152–1154.
18. Arbiser JL. Angiogenesis: relevance for pathogenesis and treatment of dermatologic disease. Adv Dermatol 15:31, 1999.
19. Cines DB, Pollak ES, Buck CA, et al. Endothelial cells in physiology and in the pathophysiology of vascular disorders. Blood 91:3527, 1998.
20. Dejana E. Endothelial adherens junctions: implications in the control of vascular permeability and angiogenesis. J Clin Invest 98:1949, 1996.
21. Fajardo LF. The complexity of endothelial cells: a review. Am J Clin Pathol 92:241, 1989.
22. Hoyer LW. The factor VIII complex: structure and function. Blood 58:1, 1981.
23. Isner JM, Asahara T. Angiogenesis and vasculogenesis as therapeutic strategies for postnatal neovascularization. J Clin Invest 103:1231, 1999.
24. Majno G. Ultrastructure of the vascular membrane. In: Hamilton WF, Dow P (eds) Circulation, Handbook of Physiology, vol 3. American Physiological Society, Washington, DC, 1965.
25. Messmer K, Hammersen F (eds). Structure and Function of Endothelial Cells. Karger, Basel, 1983.
26. Thorgeirsson G, Robertson AL Jr. The vascular endothelium—pathobiologic significance [review]. Am J Pathol 93:801, 1978.
27. Turner RR, Beckstead JH, Warnke RA, et al. Endothelial cell phenotypic diversity. Am J Clin Pathol 87:569, 1987.
28. Wagner RC. Endothelial cell embryology and growth. In: Altura BM (ed) Advances in Microcirculation, vol 9. Karger, Basel, 1979.
29. Zetter BR. Endothelial heterogeneity: influence of vessel size, organ localization, and species specificity on the properties of cultured endothelial cells. In: Ryan U (ed) Endothelial Cells, vol 2. CRC Press, Boca Raton, FL, 1987.

### Hemangiomas (General)

30. Brizel HE, Raccuglia G. Giant hemangioma with thrombocytopenia: radioisotope demonstration of platelet sequestration. Blood 26:751, 1965.
31. Calonje E, Fletcher CDM. Sinusoidal hemangioma: a distinctive benign vascular neoplasm within the group of cavernous hemangiomas. Am J Surg Pathol 15:1130, 1991.
32. Chang J, Most D, Bresnick S, et al. Proliferative hemangiomas: an analysis of cytokine gene expression and angiogenesis. Plast Reconstruct Surg 103:1, 1999.
33. De Prost Y, Teillac D, Bodemer C, et al. Successful treatment of Kasabach-Merritt syndrome with pentoxifylline. J Am Acad Dermatol 25:854, 1991.
34. Edgerton MT, Hiebert JM. Vascular and lymphatic tumors in infancy, childhood, and adulthood: challenge of diagnosis and treatment. Curr Probl Cancer 7:1, 1978.
35. Ezekowitz RA, Mulliken JB, Folkman J. Interferon alpha-2a therapy for life-threatening hemangiomas of infancy. N Engl J Med 326:1456, 1992.
36. Hagood MF, Gathright JB. Hemangiomatosis of the skin and GI tract. Dis Colon Rectum 18:141, 1975.
37. Imperial R, Helwig EB. Verrucous hemangioma: a clinicopathologic study of 21 cases. Arch Dermatol 96:247, 1967.
38. Inceman S, Tangu Y. Chronic defibrination syndrome due to a giant hemangioma associated with microangiopathic hemolytic anemia. Am J Med 46:997, 1969.
39. Kasabach HH, Merritt KK. Capillary hemangioma with extensive purpura: report of a case. Am J Dis Child 59:1063, 1961.

40. Laberge-le Couteulx S, Jung HH, Labauge P, et al. Truncating mutations in CCM1 encoding KRIT1, cause hereditary cavernous angiomas. Nat Genet 23:189, 1999.
41. Laubauge P, Laberge S, Brunereau L, et al. Hereditary cerebral cavernous angiomas: clinical and genetic features in 57 French families. Lancet 352:1892, 1998.
42. Nichols GE, Gaffey MJ, Mills SE, et al. Lobular capillary hemangioma: an immunohistochemical study including steroid hormone receptor status. Am J Clin Pathol 97:77, 1992.
43. Watson WL, McCarthy WD. Blood and lymph vessel tumors. Surg Gynecol Obstet 71:569, 1940.
44. Weiss SW. Pedal hemangioma (venous malformation) occurring in Turner's syndrome: an additional manifestation of the syndrome. Hum Pathol 19:1015, 1988.
45. Wilson-Jones E. Malignant vascular tumors. Clin Exp Dermatol 1:287, 1976.

### Juvenile Hemangioma

46. Berard M, Sordello S, Ortega N, et al. Vascular endothelial growth factor confers a growth advantage in vitro and in vivo to stromal cells cultured from neonatal hemangioma. Am J Pathol 150:1315, 1997.
47. Bielenberg DR, Bucana CD, Sanchez R, et al. Progressive growth of infantile cutaneous hemangioma is directly correlated with hyperplasia and angiogenesis of adjacent epidermis and inversely correlated with expression of endogenous angiogenesis inhibitor, IFN-beta. Int J Oncol 14:401, 1999.
48. Bowers RE, Graham EA, Tomlinson KM. Spontaneous cure of strawberry nevi. Arch Dermatol 82:667, 1960.
49. Campbell JS. Congenital capillary hemangiomas of the parotid gland: a lesion characteristic of infancy. N Engl J Med 254:56, 1956.
50. Goldman RL, Perzik SL. Infantile hemangioma of the parotid gland: a clinicopathological study of 15 cases. Arch Otolaryngol 90:605, 1969.
51. Gonzalez-Crussi F, Hull MT, Grosfeld JL, et al. Congenital hemangioendothelioma: immunologic and ultrastructural studies. Lab Invest 38:387A, 1978.
52. Gonzalez-Crussi F, Reyes-Mugica M. Cellular hemangiomas (hemangioendotheliomas) in infants: light microscopic, immunohistochemical, and ultrastructural observations. Am J Surg Pathol 15:769, 1991.
53. Jang YC, Arumugam S, Ferguson M, et al. Changes in matrix composition during the growth and regression of human hemangiomas. J Surg Res 80:9, 1998.
54. Kraeling V, Razon MH, Boon UM. E-selectin is present in proliferating endothelial cells in human hemangiomas. Am J Pathol 145:1181, 1996.
55. Kumakiri M, Muramoto F, Tsukinaga T, et al. Crystalline lamellae in the endothelial cells of a type of hemangioma characterized by the proliferation of immature endothelial cells and pericytes. J Am Acad Dermatol 8:68, 1983.
56. Lister WA. The natural history of strawberry nevi. Lancet 1: 1429, 1938.
57. McFarland J. A congenital capillary angioma of the parotid gland: considerations of similar cases in the literature. Arch Pathol 9:820, 1930.
58. North PE, Waner M, Mizeracki A, Mihm MC. GLUT1: A newly discovered immunohistochemical marker for juvenile hemangiomas. Hum Pathol 31:11, 2000.
59. Pasyk KA, Grabb WC, Cherry GW. Cellular hemangioma: light and electron microscopic studies of two cases. Virchows Arch [Pathol Anat] 396:103, 1982.
60. Pasyk KA, Grabb WC, Cherry GW. Crystalloid inclusions in endothelial cells of cellular and capillary hemangiomas. Arch Dermatol 119:134, 1983.
61. Pasyk KA, Grabb WC, Cherry GW. Ultrastructure of mast cells in growing and involuting stages of hemangiomas. Hum Pathol 14:174, 1983.
62. Razon MJ, Kraling BM, Mulliken JB, Bischoff J. Increasing apoptosis coincides with onset of involution in infantile hemangioma. Microcirculation 5:189, 1998.
63. Takahashi K, Mulliken JB, Kozakewich HPW, et al. Cellular markers that distinguish the phases of hemangioma during infancy and childhood. J Clin Invest 93:2357, 1994.
64. Taxy JB, Gray SR. Cellular angiomas of infancy: an ultrastructucal study of two cases. Cancer 43:2322, 1979.
65. Verkarre V, Patey-Mariaud de Serre N, Vazeux R, et al. ICAM-3 and E-selectin endothelial cell expression diffentiate two phases of angiogenesis in infantile hemangiomas. J Cutan Pathol 26:17, 1999.
66. Walsh TS, Tompkins VN. Some observations on the strawberry nevus of infancy. Cancer 9:869, 1956.
67. Walter JW, Blei F, Anderson JL, et al. Genetic mapping of a novel familial form of infantile hemangioma. Am J Med Genet 82:77, 1999.
68. Wawro NM, Fredrickson RW, Tennant RW. Hemangioma of the parotid gland in the newborn and in infancy. Cancer 8: 595, 1955.
69. Yusunaga C, Sueshi K, Ohgami H, et al. Heterogeneous expression of endothelial cell markers in infantile hemangioendothelioma: immunohistochemical study of two solitary cases and one multiple one. Am J Clin Pathol 91:673, 1989.

### Acquired Tufted Angioma

70. Alessi E, Bertani E, Sala F. Acquired tufted hemangioma. Am J Dermatopathol 8:68, 1986.
71. Kumakiri M, Muramoto LF, Tsukinga I, et al. Crystalline lamellae in the endothelial cells of a type of hemangioma characterized by the proliferation of immature endothelial cells and pericytes-angioblastoma (Nakagawa). J Am Acad Dermatol 8:68, 1983.
72. Padilla RS, Orkin M, Rosai J. Acquired tufted angioma (progressive capillary hemangioma): a distinctive clinicopathologic entity related to lobular capillary hemangioma. Am J Dermatopathol 9:292, 1987.
73. Wilson-Jones E, Orkin M. Tufted angioma (angioblastoma): a benign progressive angioma, not to be confused with Kaposi's sarcoma or low-grade angiosarcoma. J Am Acad Dermatol 20: 214, 1989.

### Hobnail Hemangioma (Targetoid Hemosiderotic Hemangioma)

74. Guillou L, Calonje E, Speight P, et al. Hobnail hemangioma: a pseudomalignant vascular lesions with a reappraisal of targetoid hemosiderotic hemangioma. Am J Surg Pathol 23:97, 1999.
75. Mentzel TP, Partanen TA, Kutzner H. Hobnail hemangioma ("targetoid hemosiderotic hemangioma"): clinicopathologic and immunohistochemical analysis of 62 cases. J Cutan Pathol 26:279, 1999.
76. Rapini RP, Golitz LE. Targetoid hemosiderotic hemangioma. J Cutan Pathol 17:233, 1990.
77. Santa Cruz DJ, Aronberg J. Targetoid hemosiderotic hemangioma. J Am Acad Dermatol 19:550, 1988.
78. Vion B, Frenk E. Targetoid hemosiderotic hemangioma. Dermatology 184:300, 1992.

### Arteriovenous Hemangioma

79. Bluefarb SM, Adams LA. Arteriovenous malformation with angiodermatitis: stasis dermatitis simulating Kaposi's sarcoma. Arch Dermatol 96:176, 1967.
80. Earhart RN, Aeling JA, Nuss DD, et al. Pseudo-Kaposi's sarcoma: a patient with arteriovenous malformation and skin le-

sions simulating Kaposi's sarcoma. Arch Dermatol 110:907, 1974.
81. Lawton RL, Tidrick RT, Brintall ES. A clinicopathologic study of multiple congenital arteriovenous fistulae of the lower extremities. Angiology 8:161, 1957.
82. Strutton G, Weedon D. Acro-angiodermatitis: a simulant of Kaposi's sarcoma. Am J Dermatopathol 9:85, 1987.

## Spindle Cell Hemangioma

83. Battocchio S. Spindle cell hemangioendothelioma: further evidence against its proposed neoplastic nature. Histopathology 22:296, 1993.
84. Ding J, Hashimoto H, Imayama S, et al. Spindle cell hemangioendothelioma: probably a benign vascular lesion not a low-grade angiosarcoma: a clinocpathological, ultrastructural and immunohistochemical study. Virchows Arch A Pathol Anat Histopathol 420:77, 1992.
85. Fanburg JC, Meis-Kindblom JM, Rosenberg AE. Multiple enchondromas associated with spindle cell hemangioendothelioma: an overlooked variant of Maffucci's syndrome. Am J Surg Pathol 19:1029, 1995.
86. Fletcher CDM, Beham A, Schmid C. Spindle cell hemangioendothelioma: a clincopathological and immunohistochemical study indicative of a non neoplastic lesion. Histopathology 18: 291, 1991.
87. Hisaoka M, Koumo H, Aoki T, Hashimoto H. DNA flow cytometric and immunohistochemical analysis of proliferative activity in spindle cell hemangioendothelioma. Histopathology 27:451, 1995.
88. Imayama S, Murakamai Y, Hashimoto H, Hori Y. Spindle cell hemangioendothelioma exhibitis the ultrastructural features of a reactive vascular proliferation rather than of angiosarcoma. Am J Clin Pathol 97:279, 1992.
89. Murakami J, Sarker AB, Teramoto N, et al. Spindle cell hemangioendothelioma: a report of two cases. Acta Pathol Jpn 43:529, 1993.
90. Pellegrini AE, Drake RD, Qualman SJ. Spindle cell hemangioendotheioma: a neoplasm associated with Maffucci's syndrome. J Cutan Pathol 22:173, 1995.
91. Perkins P, Weiss SW. Spindle cell hemangioendothelioma: an analysis of 78 cases with reassessment of its pathogenesis and biologic behavior. Am J Surg Pathol 20:1196, 1996.
92. Scott GA, Rosai J. Spindle cell hemangioendothelioma. Am J Dermatopathol 10:281, 1988.
93. Weiss SW, Enzinger FM. Spindle cell hemangioendothelioma: a low grade angiosarcoma resembling a cavernous hemangioma and Kaposi's sarcoma. Am J Surg Pathol 10:521, 1986.

## Epithelioid Hemangioma

94. Castro C, Winkelmann RK. Angiolymphoid hyperplasia with eosinophilia in the skin. Cancer 34:1969, 1974.
95. Eady RAJ, Cowen T, Wilson-Jones E. Pseudopyogenic granuloma: the histopathogenesis in the light of ultrastructural studies. Br J Dermatol 95(Suppl):14, 1976.
96. Eady RAJ, Wilson-Jones E. Pseudopyogenic granuloma: enzyme histochemical and ultrastructural study. Hum Pathol 8: 653, 1977.
97. Fetsch JF, Weiss SW. Observations concerning the pathogenesis of epithelioid hemangioma (angiolymphoid hyperplasia). Mod Pathol 4:449, 1991.
98. Kindblom L-G, Fassina AS. Angiolymphoid hyperplasia with eosinophilia of the skin. Acta Pathol Microbiol Scand 89A:271, 1981.
99. Kitabatake T, Kurokawa H, Kurokawa S, et al. Radiotherapy for eosinophilic granuloma of the soft tissue (Kimura's disease). Strahlentherapie 144:407, 1972.
100. Moesner J, Pallesen R, Sorensen B. Angiolymphoid hyperplasia with eosinophilia (Kimura's disease): a case with dermal lesions in the knee and a popliteal arteriovenous fistula. Arch Dermatol 117:650, 1981.
101. Olsen TJ, Helwig EB. Angiolymphoid hyperplasia with eosinophilia: a clinicopathologic study of 116 patients. J Am Acad Dermatopathol 12:781, 1985.
102. Reed RJ, Terazakis N. Subcutaneous angioblastic lymphoid hyperplasia with eosinophilia (Kimura's disease). Cancer 29:489, 1972.
103. Rosai J, Ackerman LR. Intravenous atypical vascular proliferation: a cutaneous lesion simulating a malignant blood vessel tumor. Arch Dermatol 109:714, 1974.
104. Rosai J, Gold J, Landy R. The histiocytoid hemangiomas: a unifying concept embracing several previously described entities of skin, soft tissue, large vessels, bone, and heart. Hum Pathol 10:707, 1979.
105. Waldo E, Sidhu GS, Stahl R, et al. Histiocytoid hemangioma with features of angiolymphoid hyperplasia and Kaposi's sarcoma: a study by light microscopy, electron microscopy, and immunologic techniques. Am J Dermatopathol 5:525, 1983.
106. Wells GC, Whimster I. Subcutaneous angiolymphoid hyperplasia with eosinophilia. Br J Dermatol 81:1, 1969.

## Kimura's Disease

107. Chan JKC, Hui PK, Ng CS, et al. Epithelioid hemangioma (angiolymphoid hyperplasia with eosinophilia) and Kimura's disease in Chinese. Histopathology 15:557, 1989.
108. Googe PB, Harris NL, Mihm MC. Kimura's disease and angiolymphoid hyperplasia with eosinophils: two distinct histopathological entities. J Cutan Pathol 14:263, 1987.
109. Hui PK, Chan JKC, Ng CS, et al. Lymphadenopathy of Kimura's disease. Am J Surg Pathol 13:177, 1989.
110. Kimura T, Yoshimura S, Ishikawa E. Unusual granulation combined with hyperplastic change of lymphatic tissue. Trans Soc Pathol Jpn 37:179, 1948.
111. Kung ITM, Gibson JB, Bannatyne PM. Kimura's disease: a clinicopathological study of 21 cases and its distinction from angiolymphoid hyperplasia with eosinophilia. Pathology 16:39, 1984.
112. Kuo TT, Shih L-Y, Chan H-L. Kimura's disease: involvement of regional lymph nodes and distinction from angiolymphoid hyerplasia with eosinophilia. Am J Surg Pathol 12:843, 1988.
113. Quinibi WY, Al-Sibai MB, Akhtar M. Mesangioproliferative glomerulonephritis associated with Kimura's disease. Clin Nephrol 30:111, 1988.
114. Urabe A, Tsuneyoshi M, Enjoji M. Epithelioid hemangioma versus Kimura's disease: a comparative clinicopathologic study. Am J Surg Pathol 11:758, 1987.
115. Yamada A, Mitsuhashi K, Miyakawa Y, et al. Membranous glomerulonephritis associated with eosinophilic folliculitis of the skin (Kimura's disease): report of a case and review of the literature. Clin Nephrol 18:211, 1982.

## Granulation Tissue-type Hemangioma (Pyogenic Granuloma)

116. Bhaskar SN, Jacoway JR. Pyogenic granuloma: clinical features, incidence, histology, and result of treatment: report of 242 cases. J Oral Surg 24:391, 1966.
117. Cooper PH, McAllister HA, Helwig EB. Intravenous pyogenic granuloma: a study of 18 cases. Am J Surg Pathol 3:221, 1979.
118. Coskey RJ, Mehregan AH. Granuloma pyogenicum with multiple satellite recurrences. Arch Dermatol 96:71, 1967.
119. De Kaminsky AR, Otero AC, Kaminsky CA, et al. Multiple disseminated pyogenic granuloma. Br J Dermatol 98:461, 1978.
120. Grupper C, Pastel A. Pyogenic granuloma with multiple satellites. Bull Soc Fr Dermatol Syphilogr 76:496 1969.

121. Juhlin L, Sven-Olaf H, Ponten J, et al. Disseminated granuloma pyogenicum. Acta Dermatotvener (Stockh) 50:134, 1970.
122. Kerr DA. Granuloma pyogenicum. Oral Surg Oral Med Oral Pathol 4:158, 1951.
123. McDonald RH. Granuloma gravidarum. Am J Obstet Gynecol 72:1132, 1956.
124. Mills SE, Cooper PH, Fechner RE. Lobular capillary hemangioma: the underlying lesion of pyogenic granuloma. Am J Surg Pathol 4:471, 1980.
125. Nagashima N, Niizuma K. Multiple satellite granuloma telangiectaticum. Jpn J Dermatol 82:1, 1972.
126. Ulbright TM, Santa Cruz DI. Intravenous pyogenic granuloma: a case report with ultrastructural findings. Cancer 45:1646, 1980.
127. Warner J, Wilson-Jones E. Pyogenic granuloma recurring with multiple satellites: a report of 11 cases. Br J Dermatol 80:218, 1968.
128. Wilson BB, Greer KE, Cooper PH. Eruptive disseminated lobular capillary hemangioma (pyogenic granuloma). J Am Acad Dermatol 21:391, 1989.
129. Zaynoun ST, Juljulian HH, Kurban AK. Pyogenic granuloma with multiple satellites. Arch Dermatol 9:689, 1974.

### Intramuscular Hemangioma

130. Allen PW, Enzinger FM. Hemangiomas of skeletal muscle: an analysis of 89 cases. Cancer 29:8, 1972.
131. Angervall L, Nielsen JM, Stener B, et al. Concomitant arteriovenous vascular malformation in skeletal muscle. Cancer 44: 232, 1979.
132. Angervall L, Nilsson L, Stener B, et al. Angiographic, microangiographic, and histologic study of vascular malformation in striated muscle. Acta Radiol 7:65, 1968.
133. Beham A, Fletcher CDM. Intramuscular angioma: a clinicopathologic analysis of 74 cases. Histopathology 18:53, 1991.
134. Cohen AJ, Youkey JR, Clagett GP. Intramuscular hemangioma. JAMA 249:2680, 1983.
135. Godanich IF, Capanacci M. Vascular hamartomata and infantile angioectatic osteohyperplasia of the extremities. J Bone Joint Surg Am 44:815, 1962.

### Synovial Hemangioma

136. Bate TH. Hemangioma of the tendon sheath. J Bone Joint Surg Am 36:104, 1954.
137. Bennett GE, Cobey MC. Hemangioma of joints: report of five cases. Arch Surg 38:487, 1939.
138. Burman MS, Milgram JE. Hemangioma of tendon and tendon sheath. Surg Gynecol Obstet 50:397, 1930.
139. Cobey MC. Hemangioma of joints. Arch Surg 46:465, 1943.
140. Harkins HN. Hemangioma of a tendon sheath: report of a case with a study of 24 cases from the literature. Arch Surg 34:12, 1937.
141. Lichtenstein L. Tumors of synovial joints, bursae, and tendon sheath. Cancer 8:816, 1955.
142. Osgood RB. Tuberculosis of the knee joint: angioma of the knee joint. Surg Clin North Am 1:665, 1921.
143. Webster GV, Geschickter DF. Benign capillary hemangioma of digital flexor tendon sheath: case report. Ann Surg 122:444, 1945.

### Hemangioma of Peripheral Nerve

144. Kojima T, Ide Y, Marumo E, et al. Hemangioma of median nerve causing carpal tunnel syndrome. Hand 8:62, 1976.
145. Losli EJ. Intrinsic hemangiomas of the peripheral nerves. Arch Pathol 53:226, 1952.
146. Sato S. Uber das cavernose Angiom des peripherischen Nerven system. Arch Klin Chir 100:553, 1913.
147. Sommer R. Uber cavernose Angiome am peripheren Nervensystem. Dtsch Z Chir 173:65, 1922.
148. Wood MB. Intraneural hemangioma: report of a case. Plast Reconstr Surg 65:74, 1980.

### Angiomatosis (Diffuse Hemangioma)

149. Devaney K, Vinh TN, Sweet DE. Skeletal-extraskeletal angiomatosis: a clinicopathological study of fourteen patients and nosological considerations. J Bone Joint Surg Am 76:878, 1994.
150. Doederlein H. An unusually extensive hemangioma of diaphragm and of internal thoracic and abdominal wall as a cause of death in newborn. Zentralbl Allg Pathol 71:193, 1938.
151. Holden KR, Alexander F. Diffuse neonatal hemangiomatosis. Pediatrics 46:411, 1970.
152. Howat AJ, Campbell PE. Angiomatosis: a vascular malformation of infancy and childhood. Pathology 19:377, 1987.
153. Rao VK, Weiss SW. Angiomatosis of soft tissue: an analysis of the histologic features and clinical outcome in 51 cases. Am J Surg Pathol 16:764, 1992.

### Vascular Ectasias

154. Alderson MR. Spider naevi: their incidence in healthy school children. Arch Dis Child 38:286, 1963.
155. Barsky SH, Rosen S, Geer DE, et al. The nature and evolution of port wine stains: a computer-assisted study. J Invest Dermatol 74:154, 1980.
156. Bean WB. Vascular Spiders and Related Lesions of the Skin. Charles C Thomas, Springfield, IL, 1958.
157. Buecker JW, Ratz JL, Richfield DF. Histology of port-wine stain treated with carbon dioxide laser. J Am Acad Dermatol 10:14, 1984.
158. Finley JL, Arndt KA, Noe J, et al. Argon laser port-wine stain interaction. Arch Dermatol 120:613, 1984.
159. Finley JL, Clark RAF, Colvin RB, et al. Immunofluorescent staining with antibodies to factor VIII, fibronectin, and collagenous basement membrane protein in normal skin and port-wine stains. Arch Dermatol 118:971, 1982.
160. Finley JL, Noe JM, Arndt KA, et al. Port wine stains: morphologic variations and developmental lesions. Arch Dermatol 120:1453, 1984.
161. Letts RM. Orthopedic treatment of hemangiomatous hypertrophy of the lower extremity. J Bone Joint Surg Am 59:777, 1977.
162. Lindenauer SM. The Klippel-Trenaunay syndrome: varicosity, hypertrophy, and hemangioma with arteriovenous fistula. Ann Surg 162:303, 1965.
163. Neumann R, Leonhartsberger H, Knobler R, Hoenignsman H. Immunohistochemistry of port wine stains and normal skin with endothelium-specific antibodies PAL-E, anti-ICAM, anti-ELAM, and anti-factor VIIIrAG. Arch Dermatol 130:879, 1994.
164. Osler W. On a family form of recurring epistaxis associated with multiple telangiectases of the skin and mucous membranes. Bull Johns Hopkins Hosp 12:333, 1901.
165. Smoller B, Rosen S. Port-wine stains: a disease of altered neural modulation of blood vessels. Arch Dermatol 122:177, 1986.
166. Tan KL. Nevus flammeus of the nape, glabella, and eyelids. Clin Pediatr 11:112, 1972.
167. Wenzl JE, Burgert EO. The spider nevus in infancy and childhood. Pediatrics 33:227, 1964.

### Papillary Endothelial Hyperplasia

168. Barr RJ, Graham JH, Sherwin LA. Intravascular papillary endothelial hyperplasia: a benign lesion mimicking angiosarcoma. Arch Dermatol 114:723, 1978.
169. Clearkin KP, Enzinger FM. Intravascular papillary endothelial hyperplasia. Arch Pathol Lab Med 100:441, 1976.
170. Hashimoto H, Daimaru Y, Enjoji M. Intravascular papillary

edothelial hyperplasia: a clinicopathologic study of 91 cases. Am J Dermatopathol 5:539, 1983.
171. Henschen F. L'Endovasculite proliferante thrombopoietique dans la lesion vasculaire locale. Ann Anat Pathol (Paris) 9:113, 1932.
172. Kreutner A Jr, Smith RM, Trefny FA. Intravascular papillary endothelial hyperplasia: light and electron microscopic observations of a case. Cancer 42:2305, 1978.
173. Kuo T, Sayers P, Rosai J. Masson's "vegetant intravascular hemangioendothelioma": a lesion often mistaken for angiosarcoma. Cancer 38:1227, 1976.
174. Masson P. Hemangioendotheliome vegetant intravasculaire. Bull Soc Anat (Paris) 93:517, 1923.
175. Pins MR, Rosenthal DI, Springfield DS, et al. Florid extravascular papillary endothelial hyperplasia (Masson's pseudoangiosarcoma) presenting as a soft tissue sarcoma. Arch Pathol Lab Med 117:259, 1993.
176. Salyer WR, Salyer DC. Intravascular angiomatosis: development and distinction from angiosarcoma. Cancer 36:995, 1975.

### Vascular Transformation of Lymph Nodes

177. Chan JKC, Warnke RA, Dorfman R. Vascular transformation of sinuses in lymph nodes: a study of its morphological spectrum and distinction from Kaposi's sarcoma. Am J Surg Pathol 15:732, 1991.
178. Fayemi AO, Toker C. Nodal angiomatosis. Arch Pathol 99:170, 1975.
179. Haferkamp O, Rosenau W, Lennert K. Vascular transformation of lymph node sinuses due to venous obstruction. Arch Pathol 92:81, 1971.
180. Ostrowski ML, Siddiqui T, Barnes RE, et al. Vascular transformation of lymph node sinuses: a process displaying a spectrum of histologic features. Arch Pathol Lab Med 114:656, 1990.

### Glomeruloid Hemangioma

181. Chan JKC, Fletcher CDM, Hicklin GA, et al. Glomeruloid haemangioma: a distinctive cutaneous lesion of multicentric Castleman's disease associated with POEMS syndrome. Am J Surg Pathol 14:1036, 1990.
182. Ishikawa AO, Nihei Y, Ishikawa H. The skin changes of POEMS syndrome. Br J Dermatol 117:523, 1987.
183. Kanitakis J, Roger H, Soubrier M, et al. Cutaneous angiomas in POEMS syndrome: an ultrastructural and immunohistochemical study. Arch Dermatol 124:695, 1988.
184. Yang SG, Cho KH, Bang YJ, Kim CW. A case of glomeruloid hemangioma associated with multicentric Castleman's disese. Am J Dermatol 20:266, 1998.
185. Zak FG, Solomon A, Fellner MJ. Viscerocutaneous angiomatosis with dysproteinemia phagocytosis: its relationship to Kaposi's sarcoma and lymphoproliferative disorders. J Pathol 92: 594, 1966.

### Bacillary (Epithelioid) Angiomatosis

186. Baron AL, Steinbach LS, LeBoit PE, et al. Osteolytic lesions and bacillary angiomatosis in HIV infection: radiologic differentiation from AIDS-related Kaposi's sarcoma. Radiology 177: 77, 1990.
187. Chan JKC, Lewin KJ, Lombard CM, et al. Histopathology of bacillary angiomatosis of lymph node. Am J Surg Pathol 15: 430, 1991.
188. Cockerell CJ, Bergstresser PR, Myrie-Williams C, et al. Bacillary epithelioid angiomatosis occurring in an immunocompetent individual. Arch Dermatol 126:787, 1990.
189. LeBoit PE, Berger TG, Egbert BM, et al. Bacillary angiomatosis: the histopathology and differential diagnosis of a pseudoneoplastic infection in patients with human immunodeficiency virus disease. Am J Surg Pathol 13:909, 1989.
190. Reed JA, Brigati DJ, Flynn SD, et al. Immunocytochemical identification of Rochalimaea henselae in bacillary (epithelioid) angiomatosis, parenchymal bacillary peliosis, and persistent fever with bacteremia. Am J Surg Pathol 16:650, 1992.
191. Relman DA, Loutit JS, Schmidt TM, et al. The agent of bacillary angiomatosis: an approach to the identification of uncultured pathogens. N Engl J Med 323:1573, 1990.
192. Schnella RA, Greco MA. Bacillary angiomatosis presenting as a soft-tissue tumor without skin involvement. Hum Pathol 21: 567, 1990.
193. Spach DH, Koehler JF. Bartonella-associated infections. Infect Dis Clin North Am 12:137, 1998.
194. Wong R, Tappero J, Cockerell CJ. Bacillary angiomatosis and other Bartonella species infections. Semin Cutan Med Surg 16: 186, 1997.

# CHAPTER 24

# HEMANGIOENDOTHELIOMA: VASCULAR TUMORS OF INTERMEDIATE MALIGNANCY

The term *hemangioendothelioma* has become a useful designation for vascular tumors that have a biologic behavior intermediate between a hemangioma and a conventional angiosarcoma. Tumors included in this group have the ability to recur locally and have some ability to metastasize, but at a far reduced level compared to angiosarcoma. The risk of metastasis varies from tumor to tumor within this group. For example, the epithelioid hemangioendothelioma, the most aggressive member of this family, produces distant metastasis and death in a small but definite number of cases, whereas the retiform and Dabska-type hemangioendotheliomas, two closely related tumors, are rarely associated with regional lymph node metastasis. Whereas the spindle cell hemangioendothelioma (see Chapter 23) was previously considered in this group, it has been reclassified with the hemangiomas (i.e., spindle cell hemangioma) because it has no metastatic potential.

## EPITHELIOID HEMANGIOENDOTHELIOMA

The epithelioid hemangioendothelioma, an angiocentric vascular tumor, can occur at almost any age but rarely occurs during childhood[7,27,28]; it affects the sexes about equally. To date no predisposing factors have been identified; in particular, none of the 90 patients we have studied gave a history of ingesting oral contraceptives. The tumor develops as a solitary, slightly painful mass in either superficial or deep soft tissue, although in rare instances it occurs multifocally in a localized region of the body (Fig. 24–1). At least half of cases are closely associated with or arise from a vessel, usually a vein (Fig. 24–2). In some cases occlusion of the vessel accounts for more profound symptoms, such as edema or thrombophlebitis. Those tumors that arise from vessels usually have a variegated, white-red color and superficially resemble organizing thrombi, except that they are firmly attached to the surrounding soft tissue. Those that do not arise from vessels are white-gray and offer little hint of their vascular nature on gross inspection. Calcification is occasionally seen in large deeply situated tumors (Fig. 24–1).

### Microscopic Features

Lesions that arise from vessels have a characteristic appearance when seen at low power. They expand the vessel, usually preserving its architecture as they extend centrifugally from the lumen to the soft tissue (Figs. 24–3, 24–4). The lumen is filled with a combination of tumor, necrotic debris, and dense collagen. Unlike the epithelioid hemangioma (see Chapter 23), in which vascular differentiation proceeds through the formation of multicellular, canalized vascular channels, vascular differentiation in these tumors is more primitive and is expressed primarily at the cellular level. The tumors are composed of short strands or solid nests of rounded to slightly spindled endothelial cells (Figs. 24–5 to 24–9). Rarely are large, distinct vascular channels seen, except in the more peripheral portions of the tumor (Fig. 24–7). Instead, the tumor cells form small intracellular lumens, which are seen as clear spaces, or "vacuoles," that distort or "blister" the cell (Figs. 24–8, 24–9). Frequently confused with the mucin vacuoles of adenocarcinoma, these miniature lumens occasionally contain erythrocytes. The stroma varies from highly myxoid to hyaline. The myxoid areas are light blue on hematoxylin-eosin staining, and conventional histochemical treatment with aldehyde fuchsin pH 1.0 may reveal sulfated acid mucopolysaccharides. This

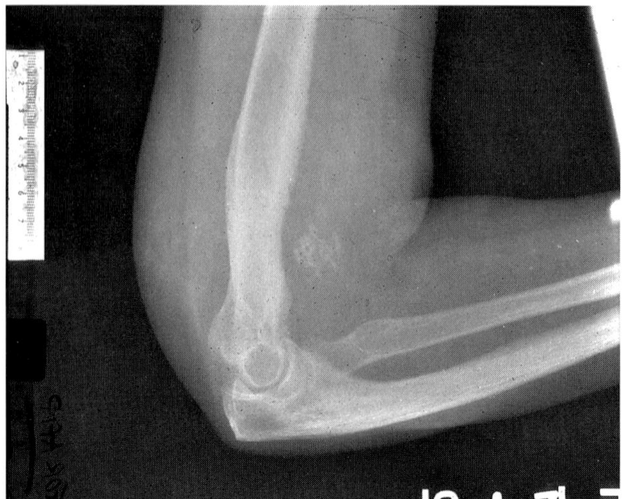

**FIGURE 24-1.** Plain film of arm showing an epithelioid hemangioendothelioma of the distal arm that has created erosion of bone. The mass is also partially calcified.

staining pattern should not be equated with cartilaginous differentiation; it simply reflects the tendency of some vascular tumors to produce sulfated acid mucins similar to the ground substance of vessel walls. Although occasional tumors do contain eosinophils and lymphocytes, rarely is this feature as pronounced as it is in the epithelioid hemangioma.

In most cases the tumors appear quite bland, and there is virtually no mitotic activity. In about one-fourth of cases the tumors contain areas with significant atypia, mitotic activity [more than 1 mitosis per 10 high power fields (HPF)], focal spindling of the cells, or necrosis (Figs. 24–10, 24–11, 24–12). Such features can be correlated with a more aggressive course, as discussed below. When metastases occur in this disease, they usually develop from tumors with these atypical features. Not unexpectedly, metastases also contain these features. In rare instances both primary and metastatic lesions appear bland cytologically.

## Differential Diagnosis

The differential diagnosis of this tumor includes metastatic carcinoma (or melanoma) and various sarcomas, which can assume an epithelioid appearance. In general, *carcinomas* and *melanomas* metastatic to soft tissue display far more nuclear atypia and mitotic activity than the epithelioid hemangioendothelioma and are rarely angiocentric. *Epithelioid angiosarcomas* are composed of solid sheets of highly atypical, mitotically active, epithelioid endothelial cells. Necrosis is common, and vascular differentiation is expressed primarily by the formation of irregular sinusoidal vascular channels. Occasional tumors have an architectural pattern (i.e., cords of epithelioid cells in a myxohyaline background) of an epithelioid hemangioendothelioma in some areas but solid sheets of epithelioid angiosarcoma in others. In our opinion these lesions should be regarded as conventional angiosarcomas, reserving the term epithelioid hemangioendothelioma for tumors that display the typical architectural pattern throughout.

*Epithelioid sarcoma* is perhaps the closest mimic of this tumor. Composed of nodules of rounded eosinophilic cells that surround cores of necrotic debris and collagen, epithelioid sarcoma develops primarily as a distal extremity lesion in young individuals. The polygonal cells usually blend and merge with the collagen in a close interplay between cell and stroma. In ambiguous cases, immunohistochemistry and electron microscopy may provide the most reliable clues for differentiation. With appropriate "cocktails" of monoclonal antibodies directed against a broad spectrum of cytokeratins, immunostaining is positive in virtually all carcinomas and epithelioid sarcomas. About one-fourth of epithelioid hemangioendotheliomas express cytokeratin,[9] but usually the staining is less intense and focal compared to epithelioid sarcoma. With optimal material, von Willebrand factor can be demonstrated in the cytoplasm of most epithelioid hemangioendotheliomas (Fig. 24–13). Accentuation of the staining is often noted around the cytoplasmic minilumens. The cells of epithelioid hemangioendothelioma express CD31 and CD34, and they bind *Ulex europaeus*. Reticulin staining highlights material

*Text continued on page 898*

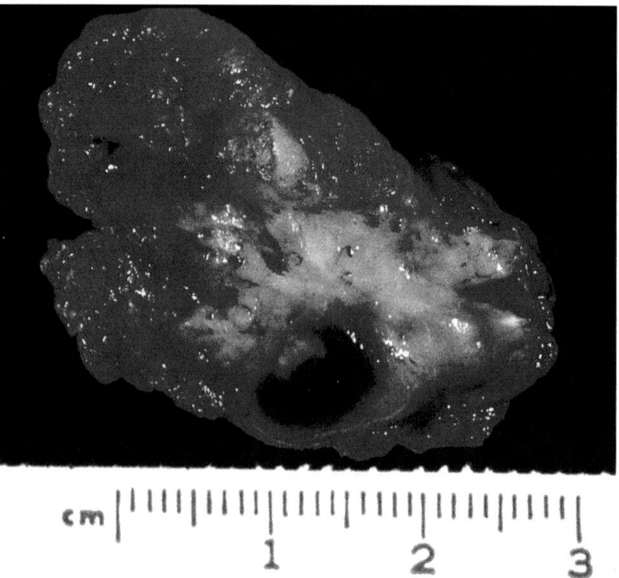


**FIGURE 24-2.** Gross specimen of epithelioid hemangioendothelioma. The tumor resembles an organizing thrombus in a small vein.

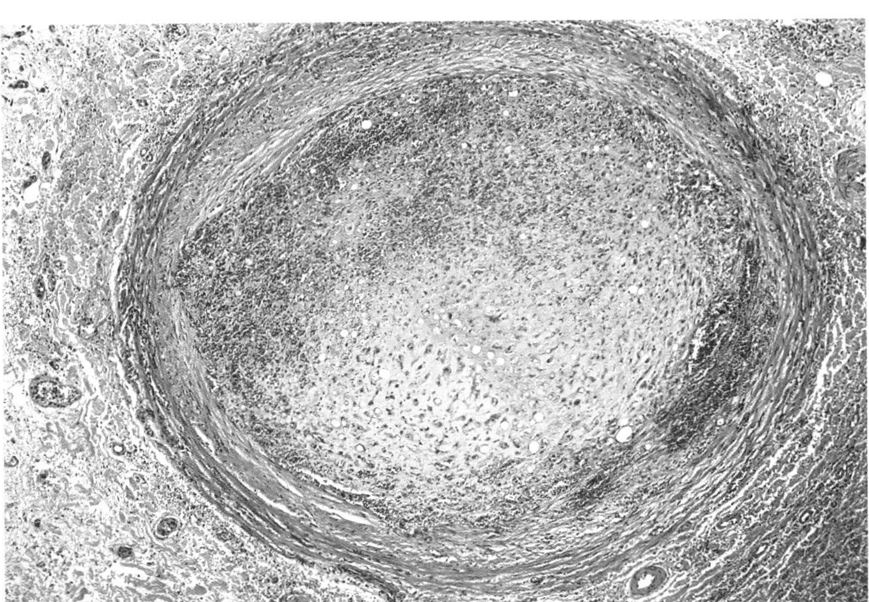

**FIGURE 24–3.** Epithelioid hemangioendothelioma.

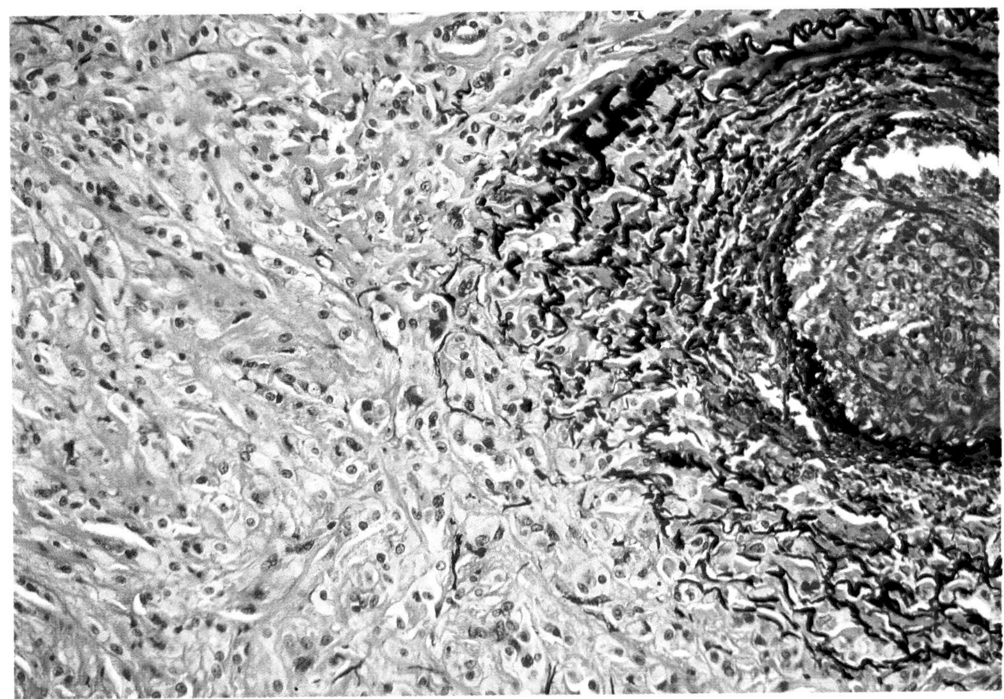

**FIGURE 24–4.** Epithelioid hemangioendothelioma arising in a small artery and extending centrifugally into soft tissue.

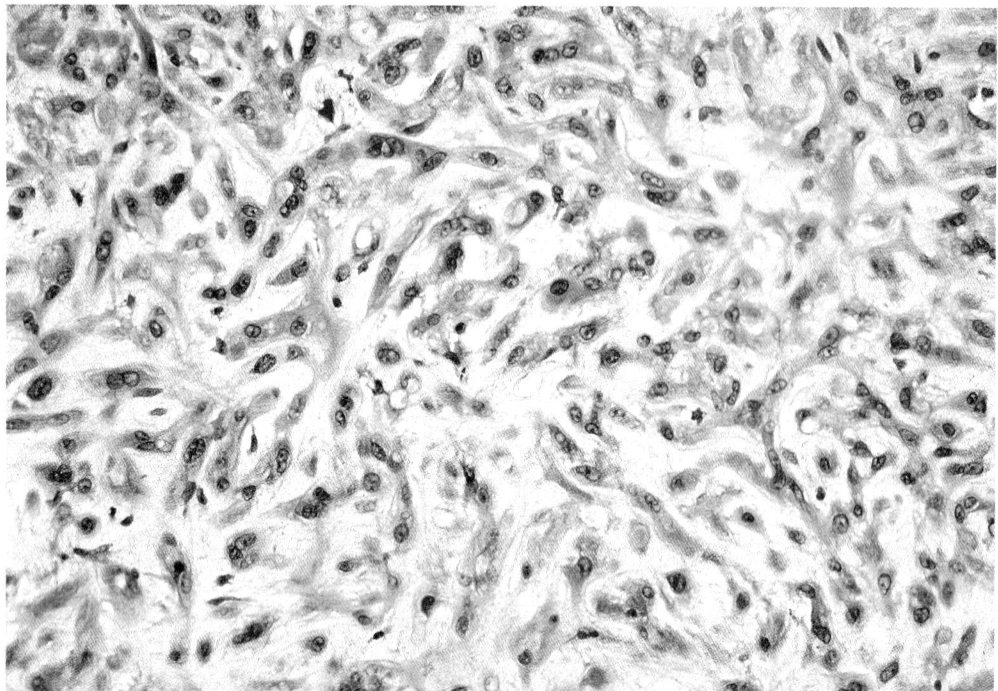

**FIGURE 24–5.** Epithelioid hemangioendothelioma composed of cords and chains of epithelioid endothelial cells in a myxoid background.

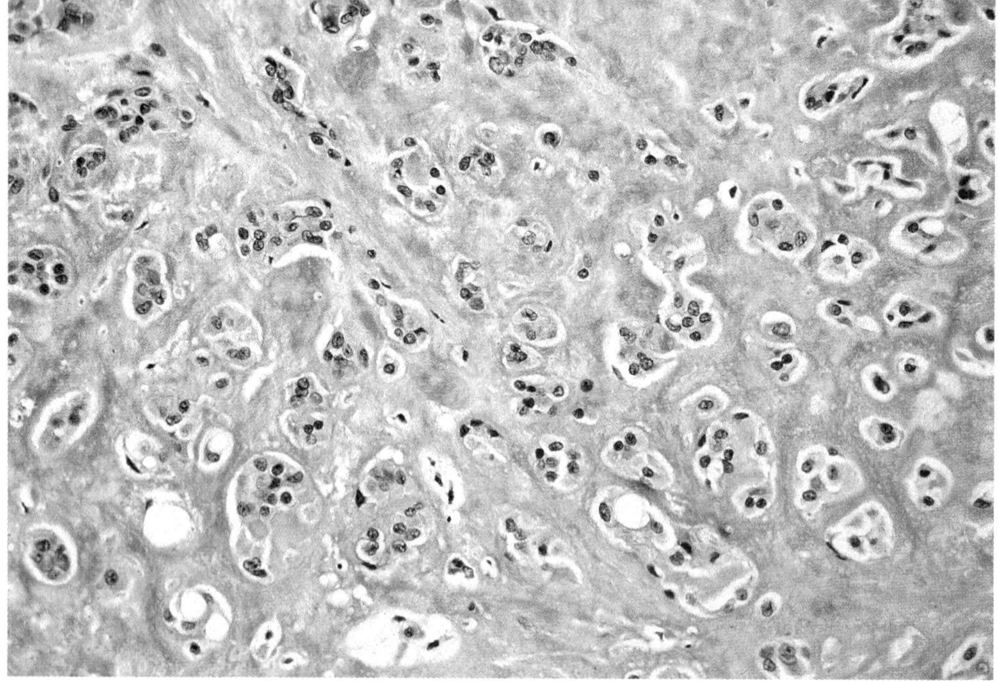

**FIGURE 24–6.** Epithelioid hemangioendothelioma with nests of cells in a hyalinized background.

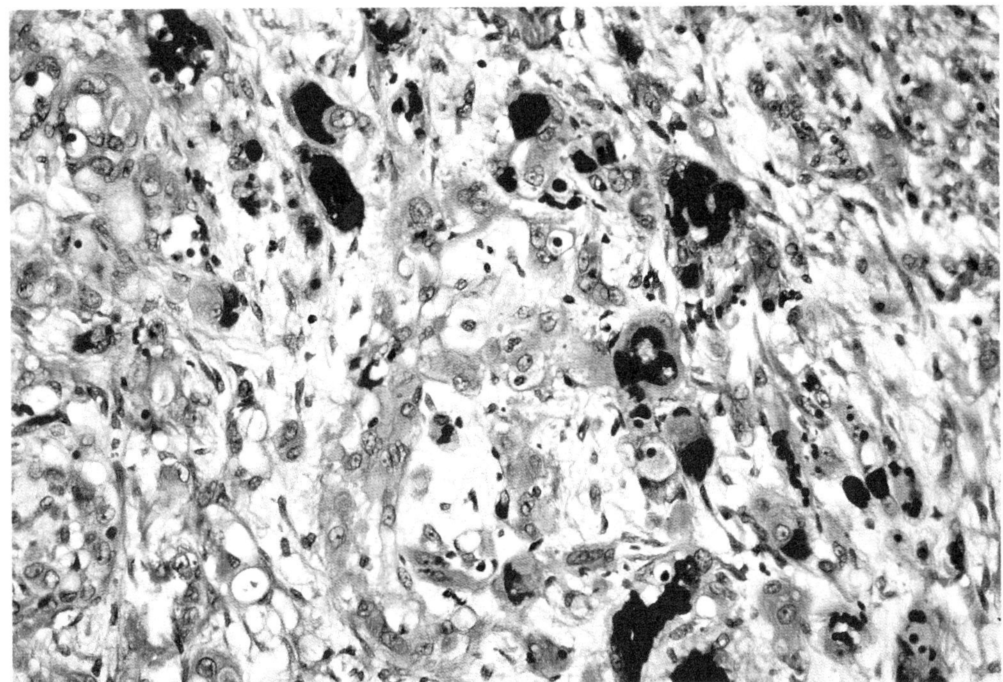

**FIGURE 24–7.** Peripheral areas of epithelioid hemangioendothelioma showing well formed capillary-size vessels.

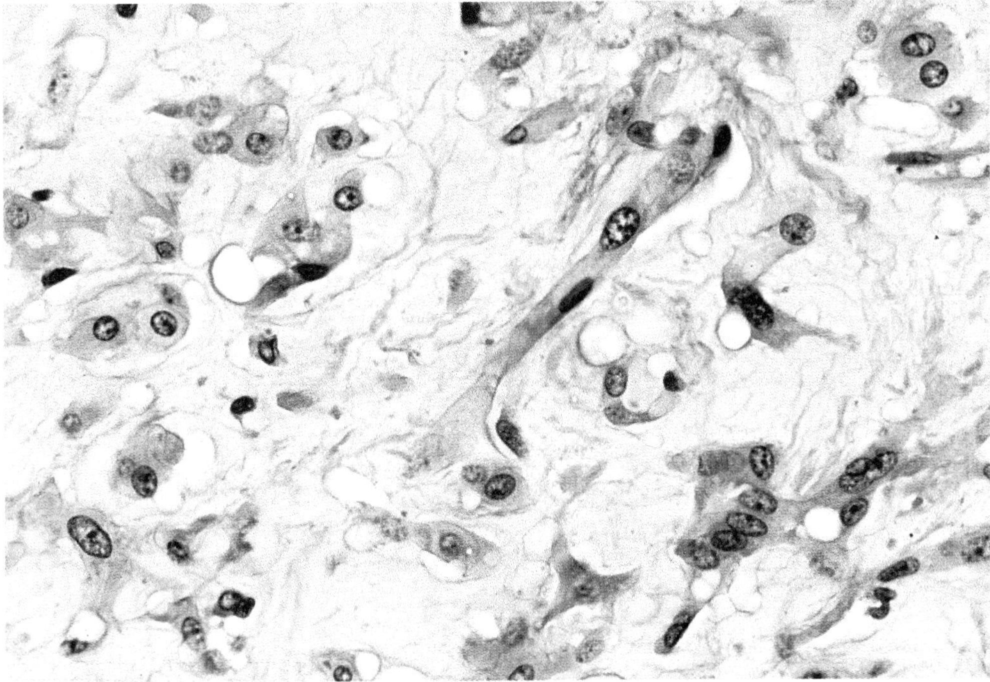

**FIGURE 24–8.** Cells of epithelioid hemangioendothelioma with characteristic intracytoplasmic vacuoles that "blister" the cell.

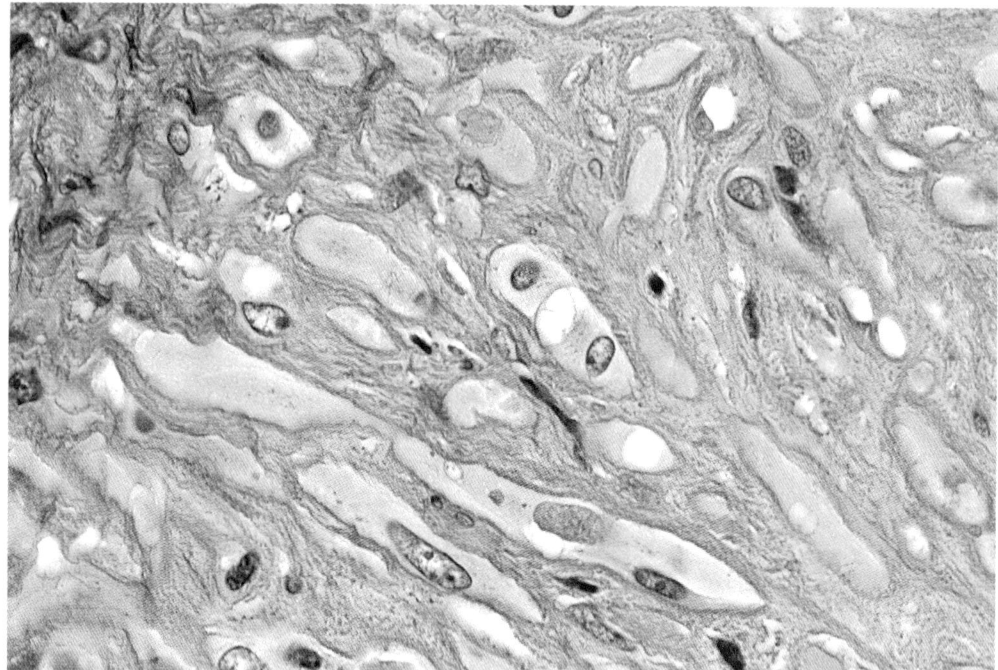

**FIGURE 24–9.** Epithelioid hemangioendothelioma with cytoplasmic vacuoles that "blister" the cell.

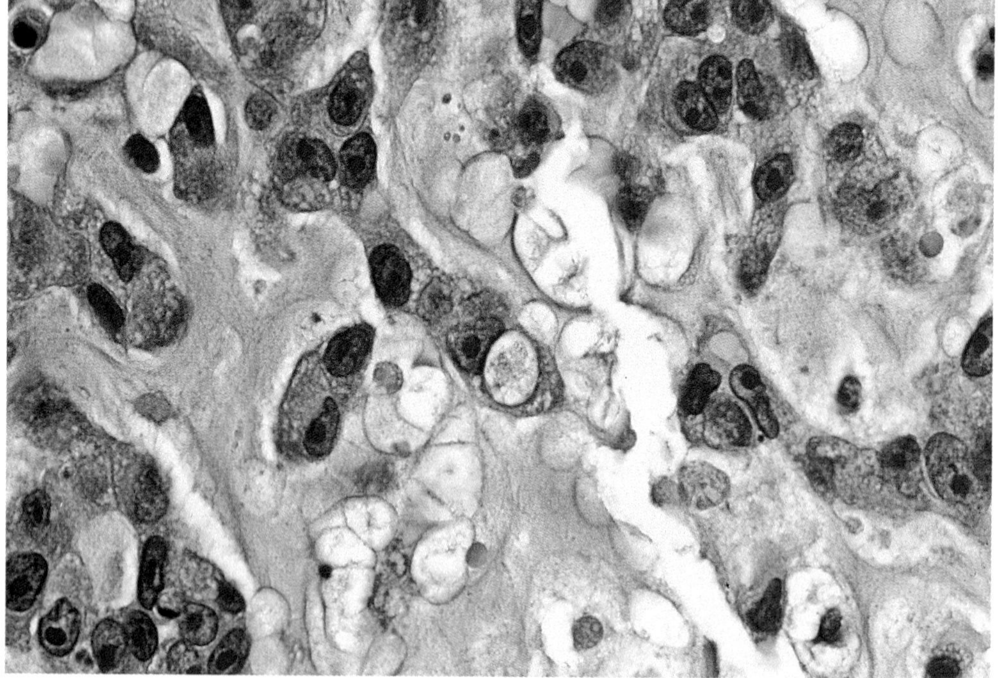

**FIGURE 24–10.** Malignant epithelioid hemangioendothelioma showing cells with marked atypia.

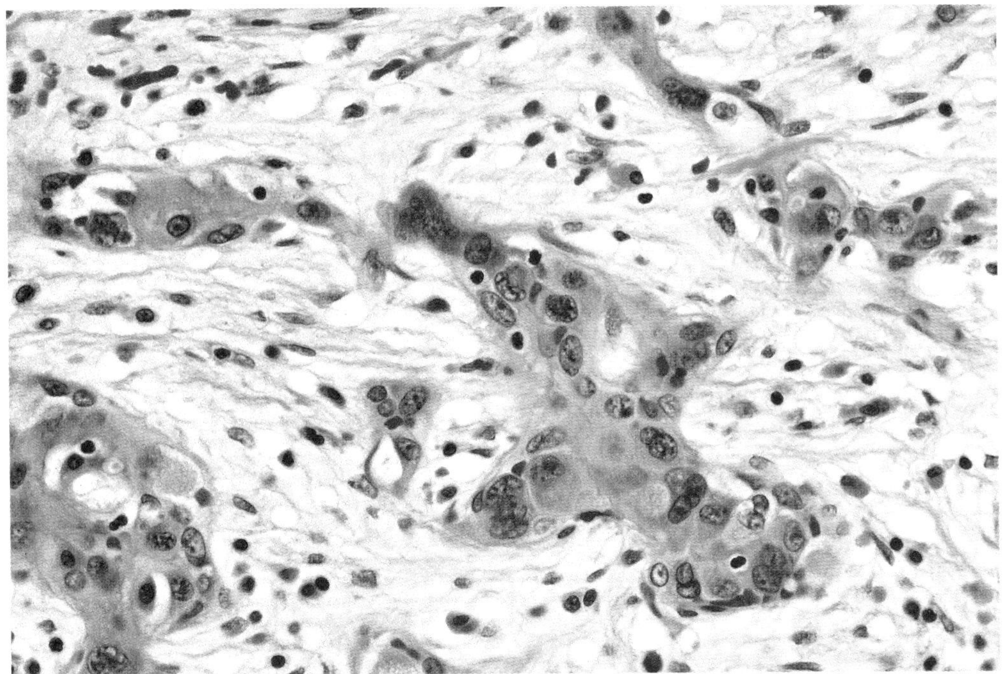

**FIGURE 24–11.** Malignant epithelioid hemangioendothelioma with cohesive nests of markedly atypical cells.

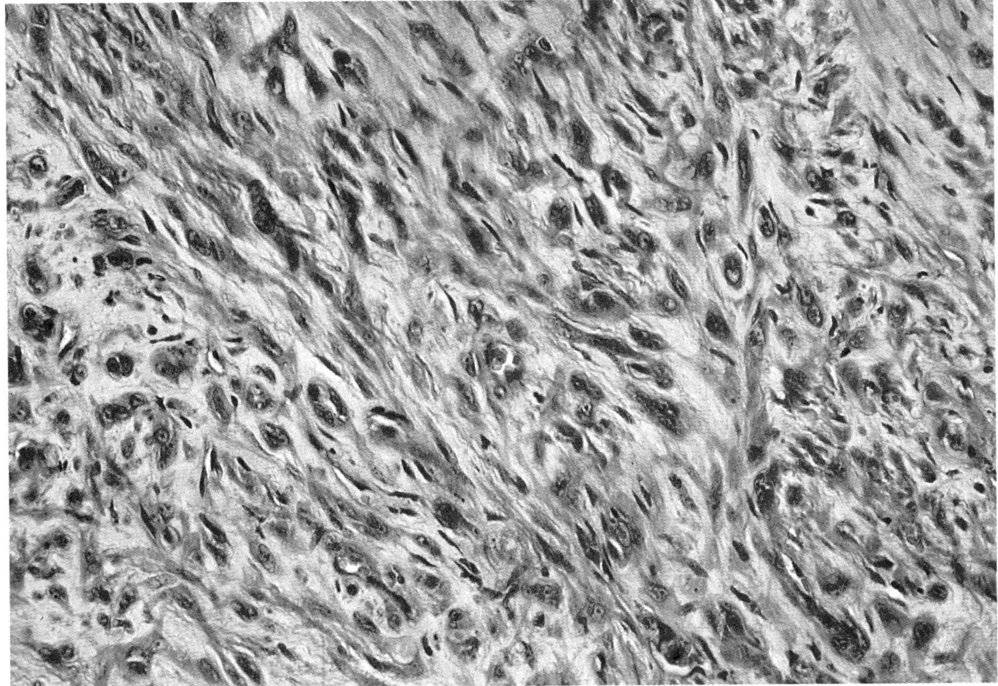

**FIGURE 24–12.** Marked spindling of cells in a malignant epithelioid hemangioendothelioma.

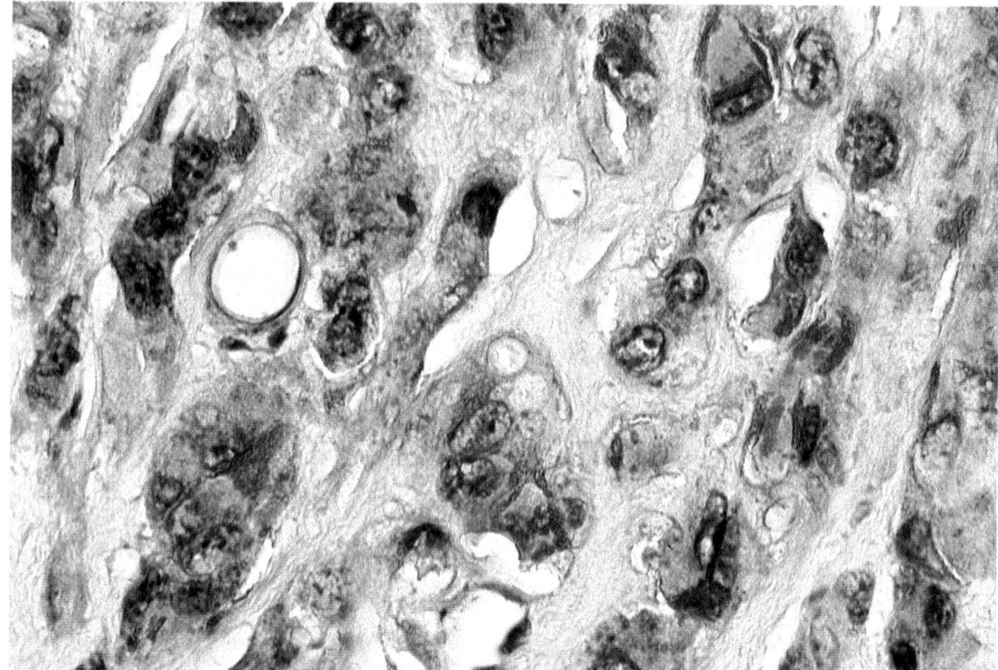

**FIGURE 24–13.** Positive von Willebrand factor (vWf: factor VIII-associated protein) immunostaining in an epithelioid hemangioendothelioma.

around individual cells and groups of cells comprising solid vascular channels (Fig. 24–7). By electron microscopy, the cells have the characteristics of endothelium, including well developed basal lamina, pinocytotic vesicles, and occasional Weibel-Palade bodies (Figs. 24–14, 24–15).[26,27] They differ from normal endothelium principally by the superabundance of intermediate filaments that crowd the cytoplasm.

## Behavior and Treatment

Although this tumor is capable of producing regional and distant metastasis, it does so far less frequently than conventional angiosarcoma. In our experience with 46 patients followed up for an average of 48 months, 6 (13%) developed a local recurrence, and 14 (31%) developed metastasis in regional lymph nodes, lung, liver, and bone (Table 24–1).[28] Fewer than half of the patients who developed metastases died of their disease, however. This is explained by the fact that half of all metastases are in regional lymph nodes, and excision of these structures may result in cure or at least long-term disease-free survival. Mentzel et al. have reported similar findings.[19]

Because the metastatic rate of epithelioid hemangioendotheliomas is higher than that for other members of the "hemangioendothelioma" family, some have suggested that these lesions be considered fully malignant sarcomas.[19] In our opinion this approach would prove to be a disservice for most patients with such soft tissue lesions who have an excellent long-term prognosis, which is quite different from those with conventional angiosarcomas. It must be emphasized, however, that for this designation to be mean-

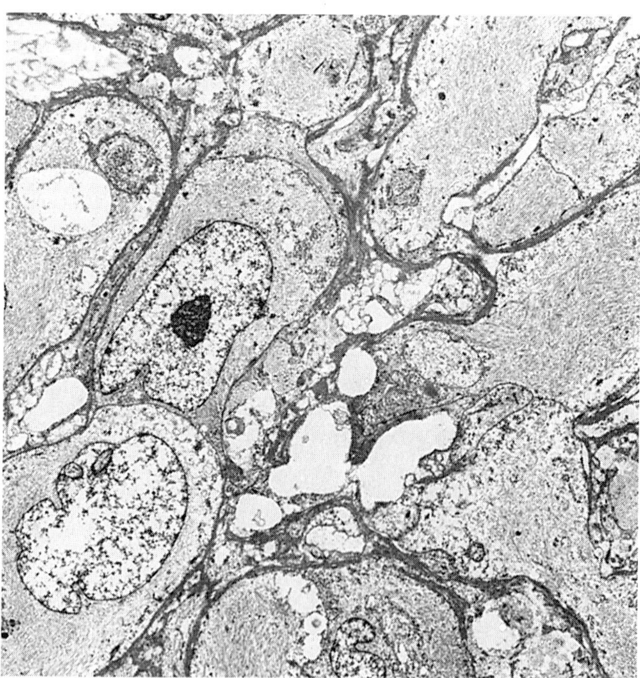

**FIGURE 24–14.** Electron micrograph of an epithelioid hemangioendothelioma showing complete investiture of cells with basal lamina, numerous intermediate filaments, and surface-oriented pinocytotic vesicles. (×2200)

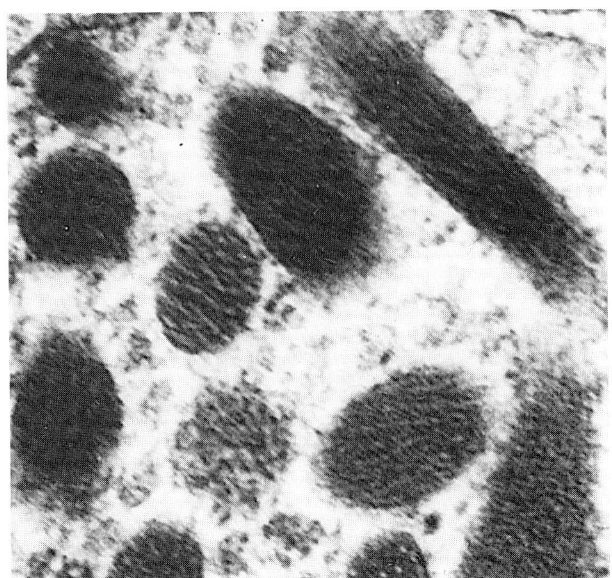

**FIGURE 24–15.** Weibel-Palade body in an epithelioid hemangioendothelioma. In longitudinal section the body has linear substructure; in cross section a dot matrix pattern is seen. (×75,200)

ingful the diagnosis should be restricted to lesions that demonstrate features of epithelioid hemangioendothelioma throughout. Lesions with solidly cellular zones of unequivocal angiosarcoma should be designated angiosarcoma and treated accordingly. Even so, about one-fourth of epithelioid hemangioendotheliomas display "atypical features," which we have defined as cellular atypia, mitotic activity (>1 mitosis per 10 HPF), necrosis, or extensive spindling. Compared to lesions lacking these features, they have a more aggressive course with a higher rate of metastasis and shorter interval between diagnosis and metastasis. Mentzel et al. have shown in a univariate analysis that similar features correlate with poor outcome.[19] For these reasons we have adopted the approach of identifying lesions with the above features as "atypical" or "malignant" epithelioid hemangioendotheliomas.

A small percentage of benign-appearing epithelioid hemangioendotheliomas metastasize and cause the death of the patient. In our experience this occurs in 10–15% of cases and seems to occur when the lesion acquires more atypical features over time. Because of the low grade nature of these tumors, complete and, ideally, wide local excision without adjuvant radiotherapy or chemotherapy is the treatment of choice. Histologically malignant forms are treated similarly to other sarcomas with at least radical local excision. Because the regional lymph nodes represent a common metastatic site, these structures should be evaluated as part of the treatment of this disease.

## Epithelioid Hemangioendotheliomas in Other Sites

Epithelioid hemangioendotheliomas occur in sites other than soft tissue.[1,2,4–6,8,10,11,13–15,17,18,21,22,24,25,29] In epithelial organs there is an even greater tendency for these tumors to be confused with carcinomas (Table 24–2). For example, in the lung they were initially believed to be an unusual form of intravascular bronchioloalveolar carcinoma[4,5] (Fig. 24–16) and in the liver a sclerosing form of cholangiocarcinoma. Their vascular nature has been confirmed in numerous reports. Identical tumors have also been reported in bone[15,25]; but in the older literature terms such as "angioglomoid tumor"[24] and "myxoid angioblastomatosis"[11,20] were used. They occur infrequently in the skin,[12,16,22] lymph nodes,[7,28,60] brain and meninges,[21] (Fig. 24–17) and peritoneum.[1] Although the basic features of the tumor are similar in the various organs, the clinical presentation and disease-related signs and symptoms differ. In the liver and lung the tumor occurs primarily in women and has a striking tendency to present in a multifocal fashion because of extensive growth along small vessels. The death rates from the disease in the lung and liver vary from 40% to 65%,[17,28] respectively, compared with a 13% death rate in soft tissues[28] (Table 24–1). Because of the indolent growth of these tumors, there has been considerable interest in performing liver transplantation in patients with this disease.[10,13,18] In a study by Marino et al.,[18] the projected 5-year survival rate of patients undergoing orthotopic liver transplantation was 76%, a figure that compares favorably with that for pa-

**TABLE 24–1** BEHAVIOR OF EPITHELIOID HEMANGIOENDOTHELIOMAS BY SITE

| | Soft Tissue | | Bone | Liver |
|---|---|---|---|---|
| **Behavior** | ***Weiss et al.[28] (46 Cases)*** | ***Mentzel et al.[19] (24 Cases)*** | ***Kleer et al.[16] (26 cases)*** | ***Makhlouf et al.[17] (60 cases)*** |
| Local recurrence | 6 (13%) | 3 (12%) | | |
| Metastasis | 14 (31%) | 5 (21%) | 8 (31%) | 37 (61%) |
| Mortality | 6 (13%) | 4 (18%) | 8 (31%) | 26 (43%) |

**TABLE 24–2** COMPARISON OF EPITHELIOID HEMANGIOENDOTHELIOMAS IN VARIOUS ORGANS

| Organ | Age | Gender | Multifocal | Angiocentricity |
|---|---|---|---|---|
| Soft tissue | 2nd to 9th decades | M = F | Rarely | One-half |
| Bone | 2nd to 8th decades | M = F | >50% | — |
| Lung | Median 40 years | F > M | Common | Intravascular spread common |
| Liver | Median 46 years | F > M | Common | Intravascular spread common |

M, males; F, females.

tients undergoing the procedure for nonmalignant disease.

## SPINDLE CELL HEMANGIOENDOTHELIOMA (SPINDLE CELL HEMANGIOMA)

Described in 1986 as a low-grade angiosarcoma with features of both cavernous hemangioma and Kaposi sarcoma,[31] spindle cell hemangioendothelioma was originally thought to have the ability to metastasize and was therefore considered within the spectrum of hemangioendothelioma. Extended follow-up in a large number of cases indicates that the lesion has no metastatic potential and that local recurrence may in fact represent contiguous growth along a vessel.[30] For these reasons the lesion is discussed in Chapter 23 as "spindle cell hemangioma."

## KAPOSIFORM HEMANGIOENDOTHELIOMA

The kaposiform hemangioendothelioma is a rare tumor that occurs nearly exclusively during the childhood and teenage years. It has features common to both capillary hemangioma and Kaposi sarcoma.[45] In the past these lesions have been reported anecdotally under a variety of names, including "kaposi-like infantile hemangioendothelioma,"[43] "hemangioma with Kaposi sarcoma-like features,"[40] and simply "hemangioendothelioma."[45] Although many were probably mistaken in the past for juvenile hemangiomas, there are compelling reasons for distinguishing between the two. The lesions occur in either superficial or deep soft tissue, although those in the latter sites, particularly the retroperitoneum, are associated with consumption coagulopathy and thrombocytopenia (Kasa-

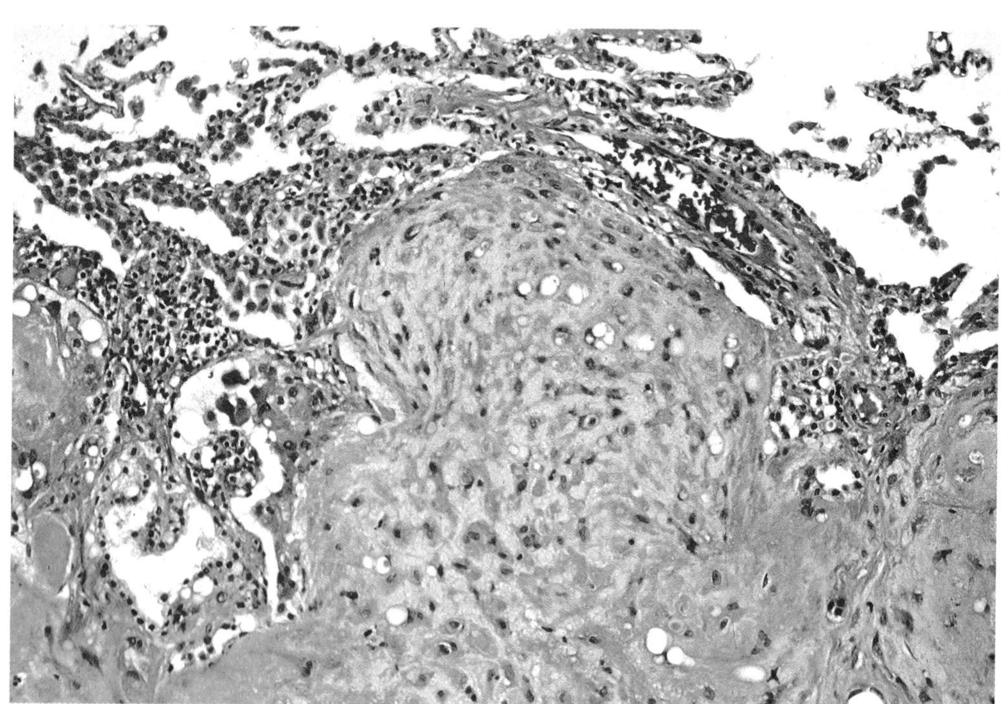

**FIGURE 24–16.** Epithelioid hemangioendothelioma of the lung (intravascular broncioloalveolar tumor).

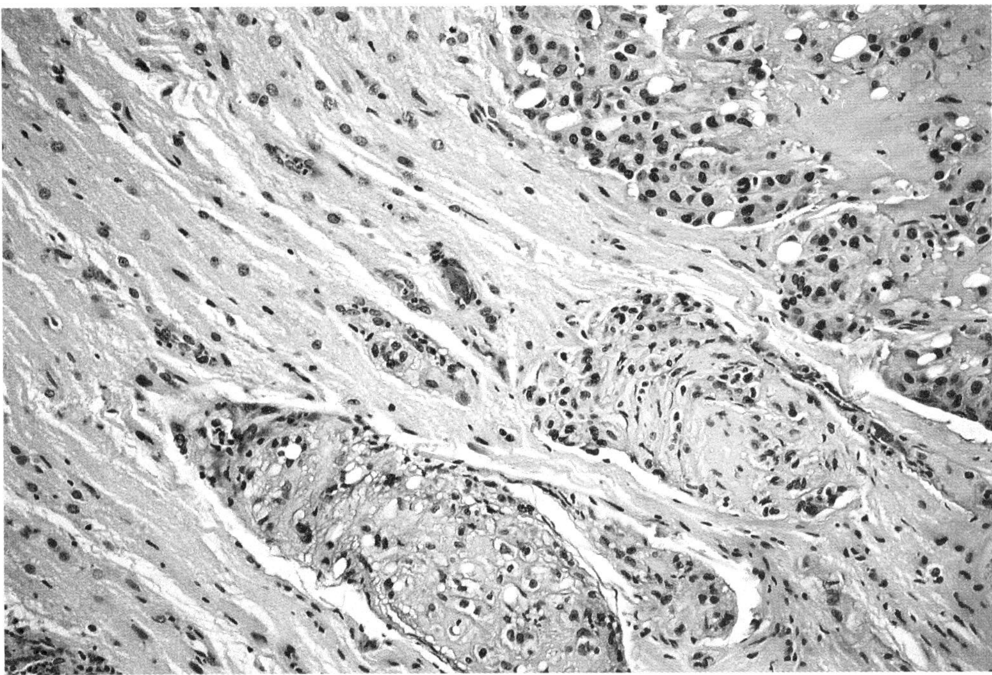

**FIGURE 24–17.** Epithelioid hemangioendothelioma of the meninges with brain involvement.

bach-Merritt syndrome). Interestingly, it now appears that most cases of Kasabach-Merritt syndrome occur with kaposiform hemangioendotheliomas and not with hemangiomas of the usual type as was previously assumed.[35,42] A small subset of cases is associated with lymphangiomatosis, which may either antedate the tumor or be discovered contemporaneously.[45] When these lesions occur on the skin they develop as an ill-defined violaceous plaque, in contrast to the polypoid red appearance of the typical juvenile hemangioma (Fig. 24–18). Those in deep soft tissue are composed of nodules that suggest both capillary hemangioma and Kaposi sarcoma. The ill-defined nodules contain a mixture of small, round, capillary-size vessels that blend with slit-like vessels (Figs. 24–19 to 24–24). Unlike the typical capillary hemangioma, which is made up of discrete lobules of small vessels, this tumor consists of irregular rambling nodules of tumor that infiltrate the soft tissues. In some cases the nodules contain glomeruloid nests of rounded or epithelioid endothelial cells with abundant eosinophilic cytoplasm containing fine granules of hemosiderin, hyaline globules, and cytoplasmic vacuoles, similar to those of the epithelioid hemangioendothelioma. Smaller amounts of hemosiderin and hyaline globules are also present in the spindled zones. Red blood cell fragments and microthrombi are identified between these cells and in the spindled endothelium. Atypia is usually minimal in these tumors, as are mitotic figures. In the tumors that have developed in the setting of lymphangiomatosis there is usually an abrupt transition between the two lesions (Fig. 24–25).

Immunohistochemically, these tumors have a profile suggesting lymphatic differentiation. They strongly express vascular endothelial growth factor receptor-3 (VEGFR-3), a sensitive marker of lymphatic differentiation[36] but only weakly von Willebrand factor (factor VIII-associated antigen). Most cells also express CD34 (Fig. 24–26). Large well-formed "feeder"

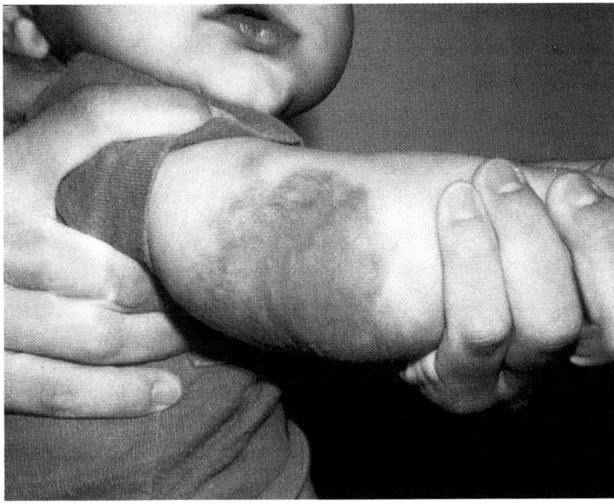

**FIGURE 24–18.** Kaposiform hemangioendothelioma with a violaceous plaque-like appearance on the arm of a child.

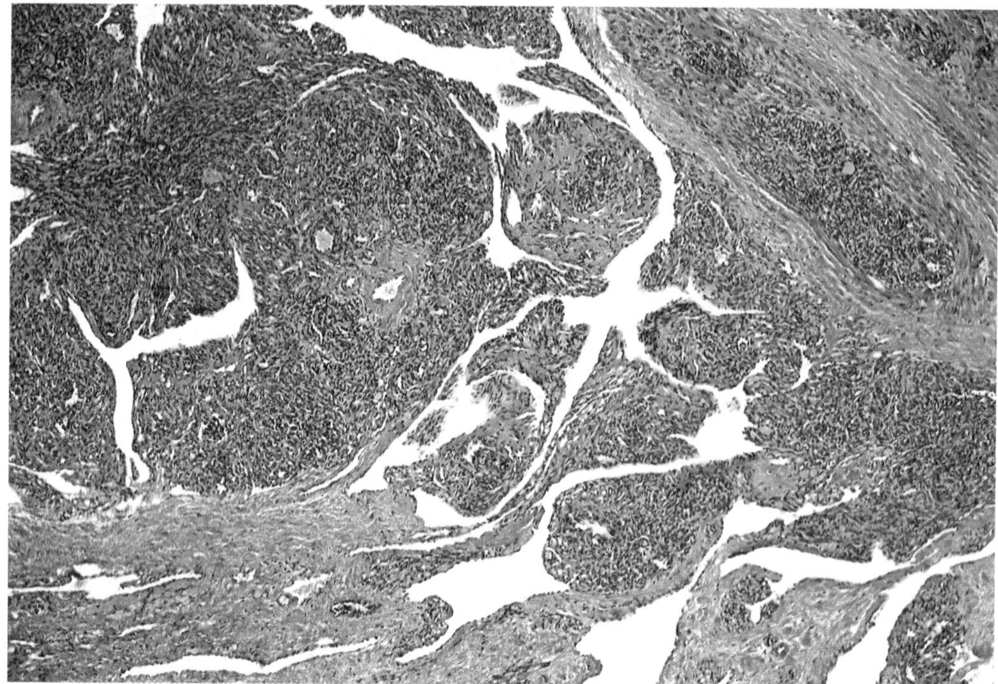

**FIGURE 24–19.** Kaposiform hemangioendothelioma with irregular nodules of tumor coursing through soft tissue.

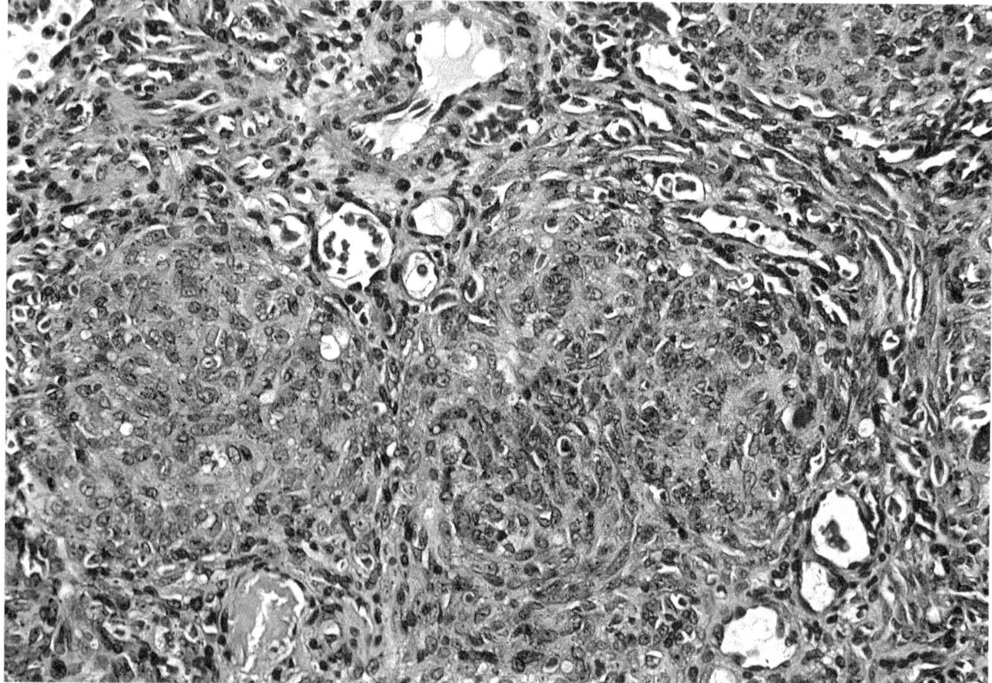

**FIGURE 24–20.** Kaposiform hemangioendothelioma with spindled zones merging with glomeruloid nests of rounded or epithelioid endothelial cells.

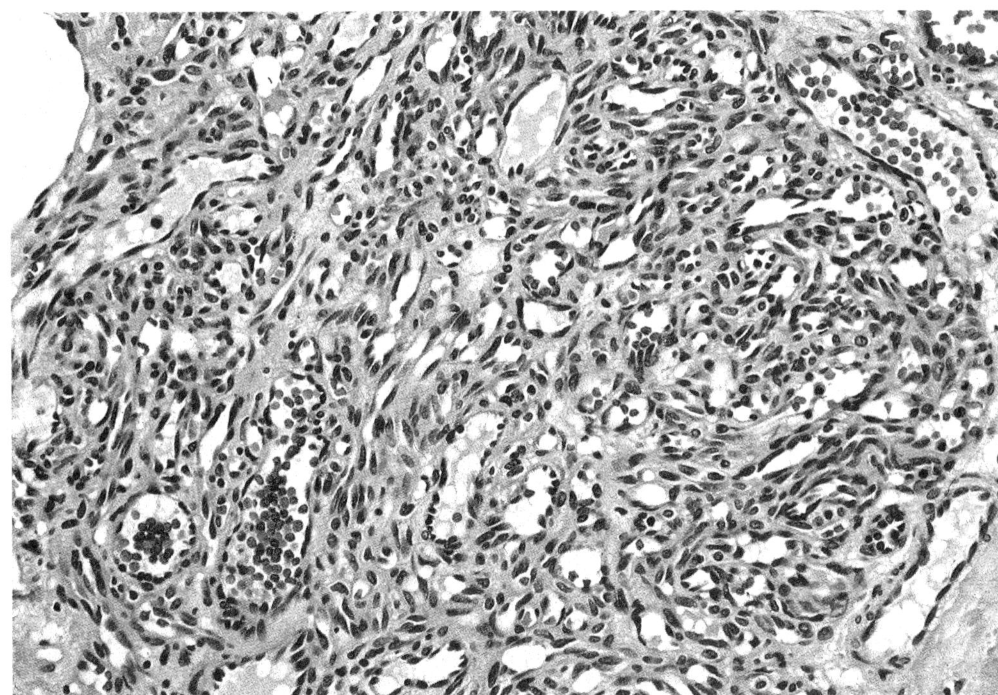

**FIGURE 24–21.** Capillary hemangioma-like areas in a kaposiform hemangioendothelioma.

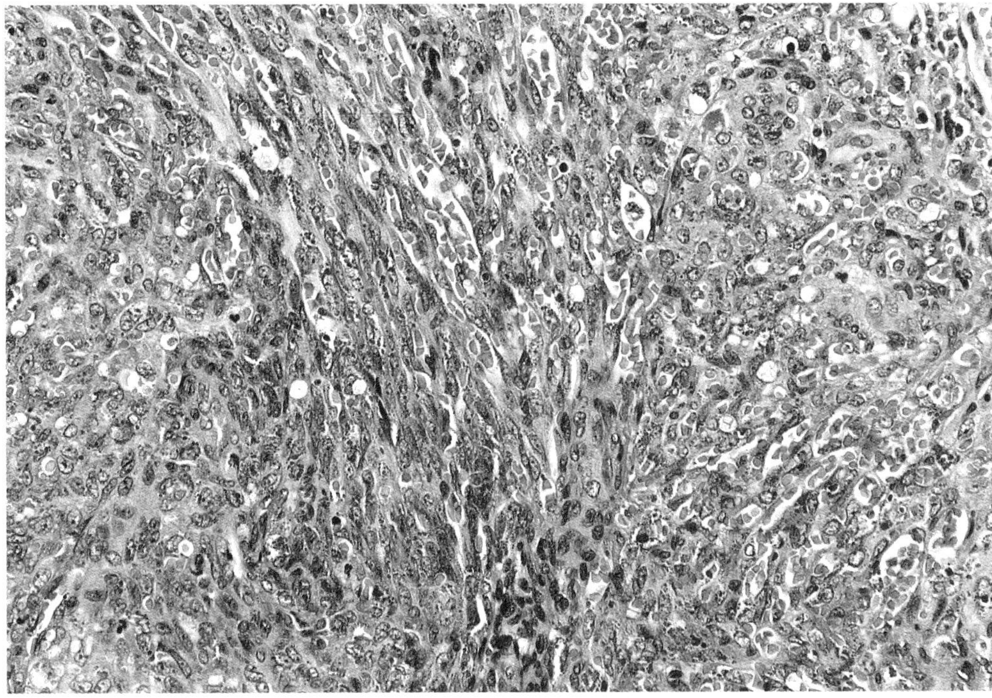

**FIGURE 24–22.** Kaposi-like areas in a kaposiform hemangioendothelioma.

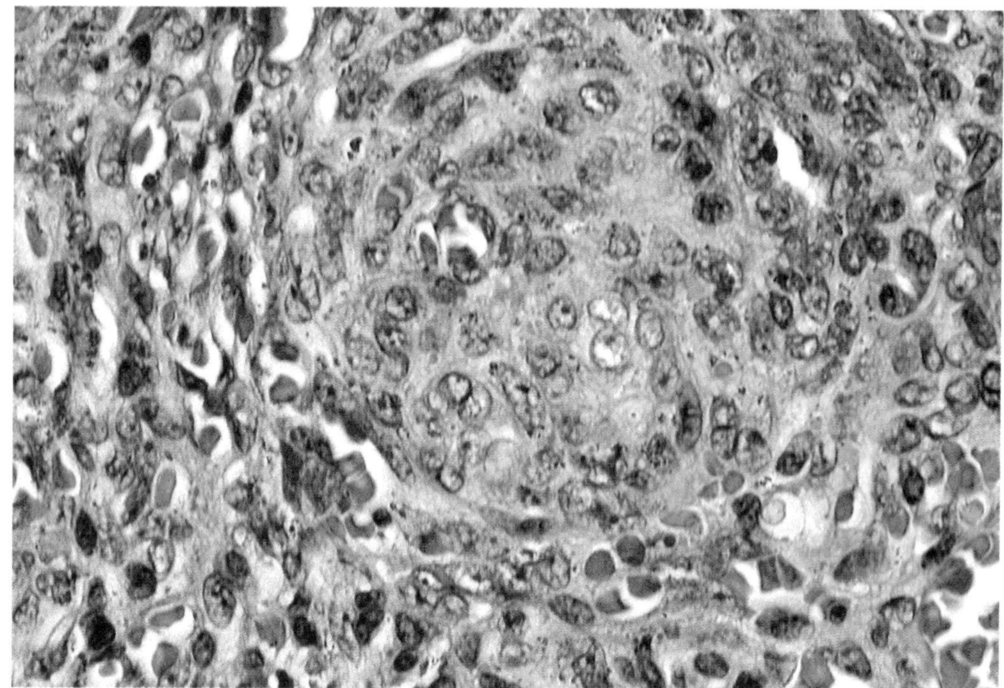

**FIGURE 24–23.** High power view of glomeruloid-like areas in a kaposiform hemangioendothelioma.

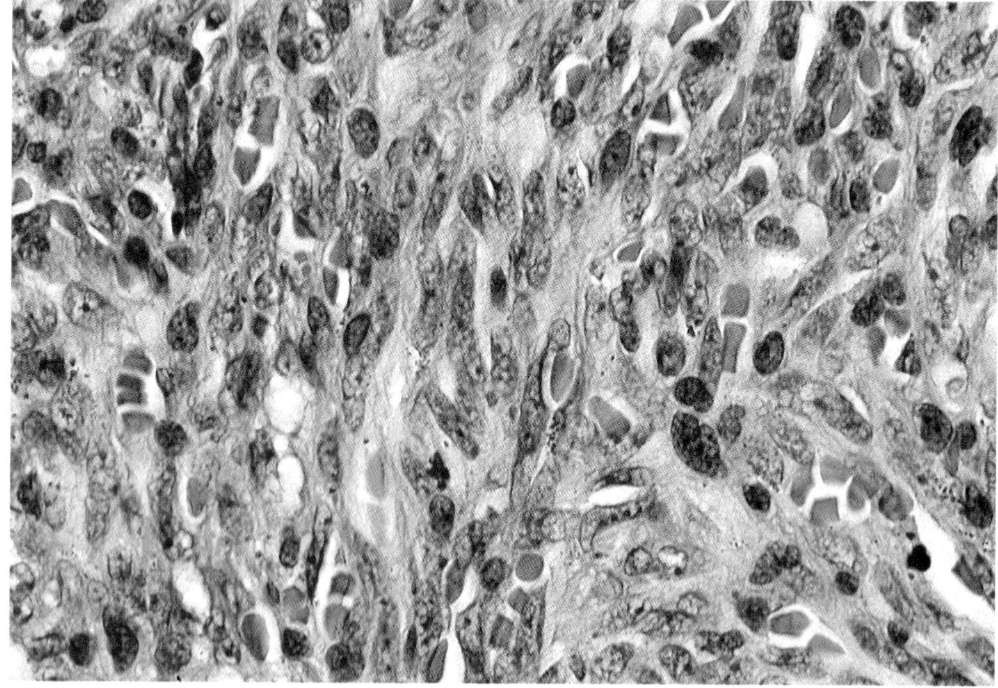

**FIGURE 24–24.** High power view of Kaposi-like areas in a kaposiform hemangioendothelioma.

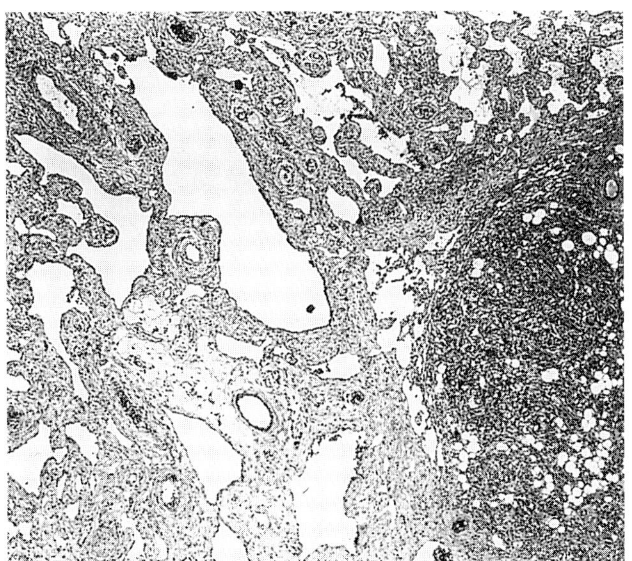

**FIGURE 24–25.** Kaposiform hemangioendothelioma associated with lymphangiomatosis. Lymphangioma is present on the left and the tumor nodule on the right. (×60)

vessels peripheral to the tumor nodules express conventional vascular endothelial markers. Ultrastructurally, the endothelial cells are arranged in cohesive nests with imperfect or partial lumen formation and are invested only partially with basal lamina (Fig. 24–27).

The behavior of this neoplasm is strongly influenced by its site, clinical extent, and the development of consumption coagulopathy. In contrast to juvenile hemangiomas, these lesions show no tendency to regress over time. Those located in the retroperitoneum and mediastinum are typically extensive, unresectable lesions associated with Kasabach-Merritt syndrome, which ultimately results in the death of the patient. More limited tumors in the superficial soft tissues are curable with wide local excision. To date none of these tumors has produced distant metastasis, although one case was marked by progressive local metastasis and involvement of regional lymph nodes.[38,45] Thus the challenge in these cases is not only to eradicate the tumor but also to support patients who have life-threatening hemorrhage from consumption coagulopathy. Some success has been reported using interferon-$\alpha$2A,[34] multimodality therapy,[33] and a chemotherapeutic regimen consisting of cyclophosphamide, vincristine, and actinomycin D.[37]

As implied, the two most important differential considerations in this disease are capillary (cellular) hemangioma of infancy and Kaposi sarcoma. Capillary hemangiomas are composed of distinct nodules of small capillary-size vessels. Although canalization can be imperfect during the early phase of growth, capillary hemangiomas do not display spindling of the cells, nor do they contain fragmented red blood cells and hemosiderin. Kaposi sarcoma is an excep-

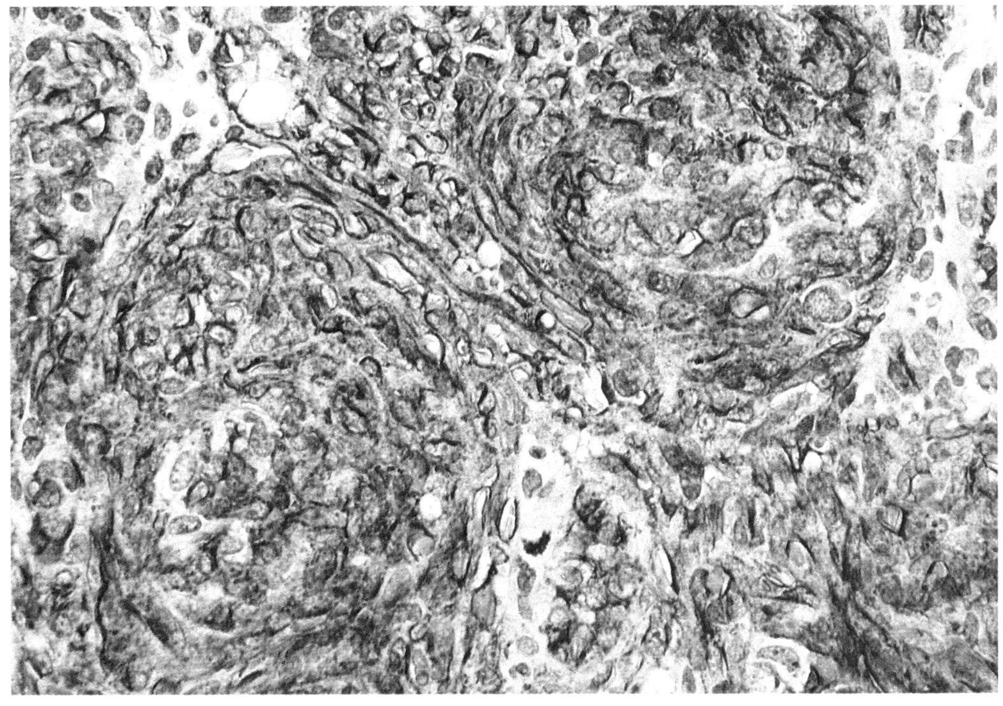

**FIGURE 24–26.** CD34 immunostaining of a kaposiform hemangioendothelioma.

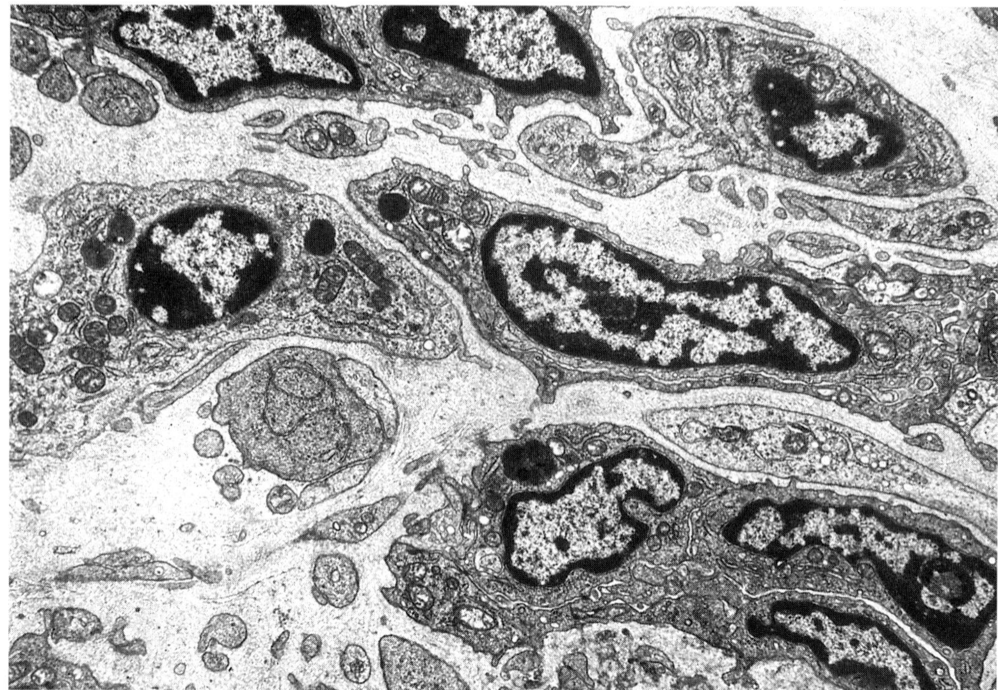

**FIGURE 24–27.** Electron micrograph of a kaposiform hemangioendothelioma illustrating primitive endothelial cells.

tionally rare tumor during childhood with the exception of lymphadenopathic forms, which have been described in Africa. It is characterized by uniform spindling of the cells and often a striking inflammatory infiltrate peripherally. Although clearly portions of kaposiform hemangioendothelioma may be indistinguishable from Kaposi sarcoma, the former shows much greater variation from area to area. HHV8 has not been associated with Kaposi form hemangioendothelioma thus far in contrast to Kaposi sarcoma. Acquired tufted hemangioma, occurring exclusively as a skin lesion usually in adults, bears an unmistakable similarity to kaposiform hemangioendothelioma and is most likely a closely related, if not identical, tumor occurring in adults without signs of consumption thrombocytopenia.

## HOBNAIL (DABSKA-RETIFORM) HEMANGIOENDOTHELIOMA

Hobnail hemangioendothelioma is a term we propose for two closely related tumors, the retiform hemangioendothelioma and Dabska-type hemangioendothelioma, both of which are characterized by a hobnail or cuboidal endothelial cell (Fig. 24–28). This cell is characterized by a high nuclear/cytoplasmic ratio and an apically placed, occasionally grooved nucleus that produces a surface bulge, accounting for the term "hobnail" or "matchstick." Hobnail endothelial cells vary in size and shape, from small lymphocytoid cells to larger cuboidal cells and in the extreme case tall columnar cells. Although the nature of this distinctive cell is not clear, it is often closely associated with lymphocytes and expresses VEGFR-3, which characterizes lymphatic endothelium, suggesting that both tumors are lymphatic neoplasms.[36] The two tumors have similar biologic behavior but display minor clinical and pathologic differences (Table 24–3). For purposes of clarity, the classic features of each is presented, but one must recognize that tumors with overlapping features occur and patients falling outside the normal age range for each tumor may be encountered.

Dabska-type hemangioendotheliomas were first described in 1969 in a small series of six patients.[48] All occurred in the skin or subcutis of infants and young children and were characterized by a distinctive small cuboidal or hobnail endothelial cell lining vascular spaces and forming intravascular glomeruloid papillations. Termed "endovascular papillary angioendothelioma," these rare tumors have never lent themselves to extensive studies. It has even been intimated that these lesions might not represent a distinct entity. More recently another low grade angiosarcoma, also characterized by hobnail endothelial cells but occurring in adults and forming long retiform vessels

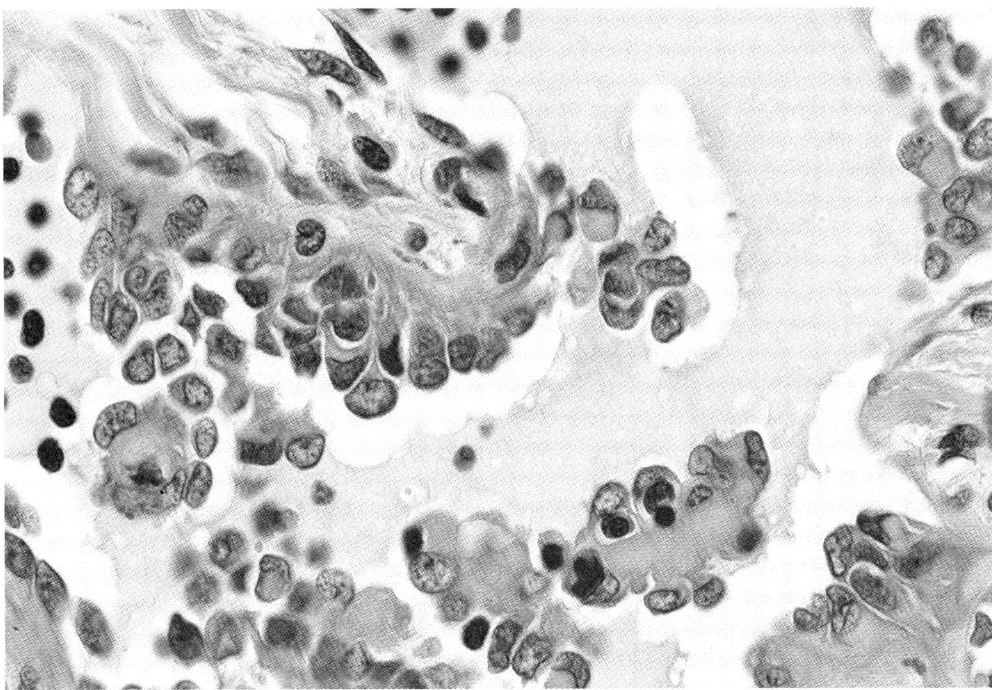

**FIGURE 24–28.** Hobnail, or "matchstick," endothelium, which characterizes the retiform and Dabska forms of hemangioendothelioma.

largely without intravascular papillations, has been described as "retiform hemangioendothelioma."[47]

## Clinical Features

Hobnail hemangioendothelimas may be seen in a broad age range, although lesions with classic features of the Dabska tumor typically occur in children, whereas retiform ones more commonly occur in adults (mean, fourth decade) (Table 24–3). Both, however, develop as ill-defined or plaque-like lesions of the skin and subcutaneous tissue sometimes associated with overlying violaceous discoloration. About one-half of cases occur in the distal portion of the extremity, but other sites may be affected. Rare cases of the Dabska type have been recorded in the spleen and in deep locations.[46,53]

## Microscopic Appearance

The Dabska type hemangioendothelioma is characterized by well formed vessels lined by cuboidal endothelium and featuring intraluminal growth of papillary endothelial structures (Figs. 24–29 to 24–33; Table 24–4). The vessels are often flanked by dense hyaline zones containing lymphocytes (Figs. 24–30 and 24–33). The papillations are lined by a hobnail endothelial cell with central hyaline cores (Fig. 24–31) composed of accumulated basement membrane material presumably synthesized by the tumor cells.[58] These structures have been compared to renal glomeruli. Intracytoplasmic vacuolation of the endothelium may be observed, a phenomenon seen in epithelioid vascular tumors. In some cases there is a close intermingling of endothelial cells with the intravascu-

**TABLE 24–3** COMPARISON OF DABSKA AND RETIFORM HEMANGIOENDOTHELIOMAS

| Parameter | Dabska | Retiform |
|---|---|---|
| Age | Children (25% adult) | Adults (15% child) |
| Location | Distal extremities (50%) | Distal extremities (50%) |
| Local recurrence | ~40% | ~60% |
| Lymph node metastasis | <10% | <10% |
| Distant metastasis | One case | None |
| Associations | Vascular/lymphatic malformation or tumor | Lymphedema, radiation |

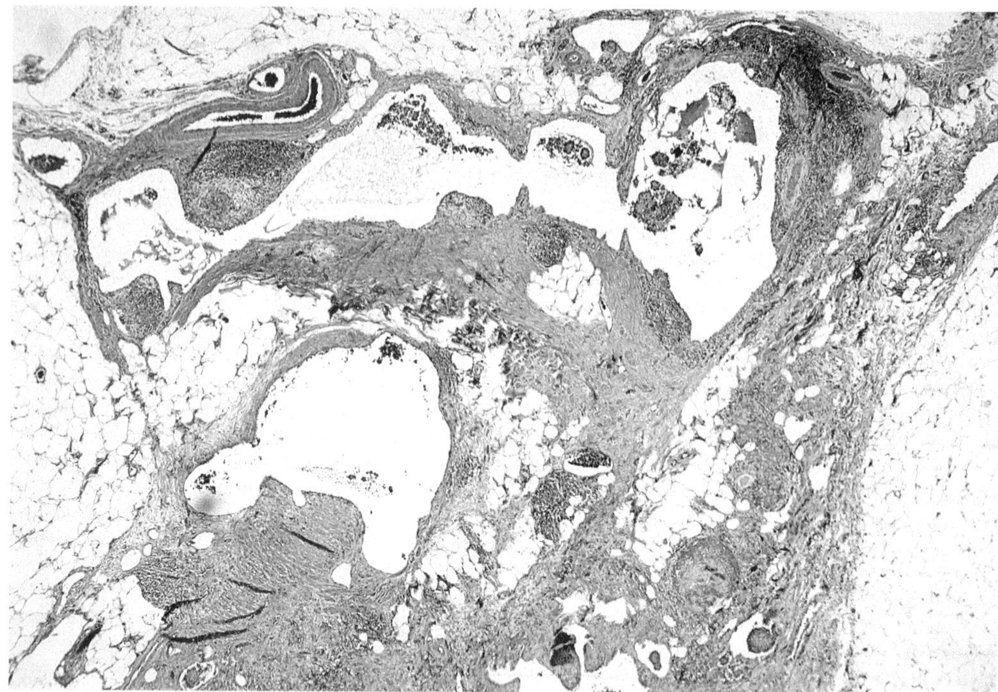

**FIGURE 24–29.** Dabska-type hobnail hemangioendothelioma with a lymphangiomatous background with intraluminal papillary growth.

lar lymphocytes, an observation that has led some to suggest that the tumor cells express some of the properties of the "high" endothelial cell of the postcapillary venule.[55] Although the intravascular papillations are admittedly the most spectacular part of the tumor, there is usually an underlying lesion, which may range from a lymphangioma to a more complex tumor with areas of hemangioma and lymphangioma (Fig. 24–29). Two cases in the literature have documented Dabska tumors arising in preexisting benign vascular tumors/malformations.[46,59]

The typical retiform hemangioendothelioma, on the other hand, consists of numerous elongated vessels, resembling the shape of the rete testis, that replace the dermis and extend into the subcutis (Table 24–4). These vessels are lined by a single layer of hobnail endothelial cells. (Figs. 24–34, 24–35). In the vicinity of the epidermal junction, the vessels may become ectatic such that the retiform pattern is lost. The vessels, often surrounded by hyaline sclerosis and lymphocytes, intercommunicate with one another; but dissection of the collagen planes by small groups of endothelial cells, as is seen in a conventional angiosarcoma, does not occur. Intraluminal papillary tufts of endothelial cells similar to the Dabska type hemangioendothelioma can be identified, but are usually infrequent (Fig. 24–36).

**TABLE 24–4** HISTOLOGIC COMPARISON OF DABSKA AND RETIFORM HEMANGIOENDOTHELIOMAS

| Feature | Dabska | Retiform |
|---|---|---|
| Hobnail endothelium | +++ | +++ |
| Lymphocytes | +++ | +++ |
| Perivascular hyalinization | +++ | +++ |
| Intravascular papillary tufts | +++ | + |
| Retiform vessels | − | +++ |
| Lymphangioma areas | ++ | − |

Although the foregoing descriptions seemingly depict two different lesions, one occasionally encounters hybrid tumors that defy precise classification. Such tumors may be made up of vessels lined by hobnail endothelium but not arranged in a retiform pattern and with only rare intraluminal papillations and no underlying vascular malformation. Such tumors underscore the need to create a designation that embraces all of the lesions under discussion.

### Immunohistochemical Findings

The immunohistochemistry of the Dabska and retiform lesions is remarkably similar. The neoplastic endothelial cells usually express factor von Willebrand

*Text continued on page 913*

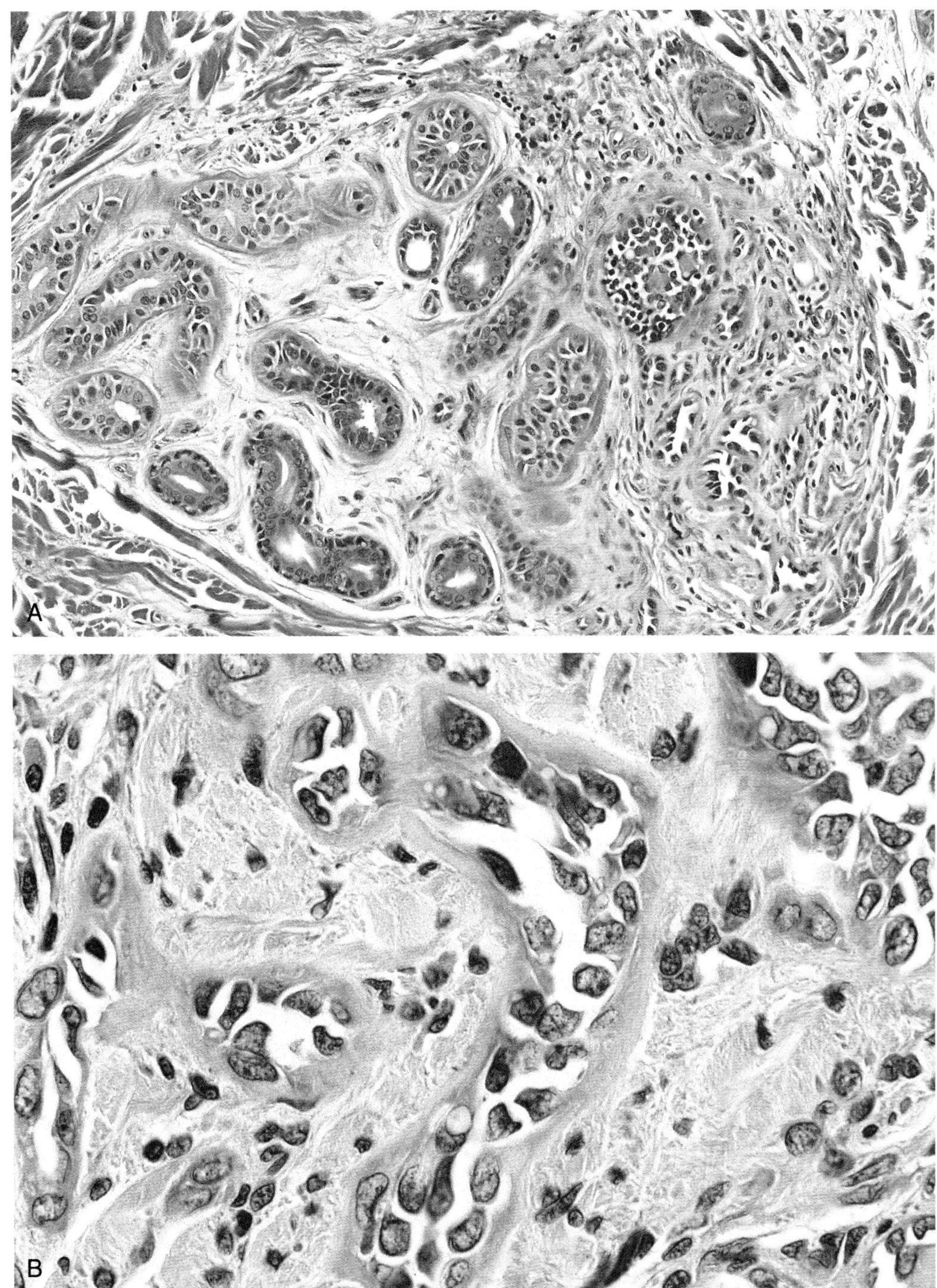


**FIGURE 24–30.** Dabska-type hemangioendothelioma with vessels lined by cuboidal-columnar endothelium (**A**) and surrounded by hyaline material (**B**).

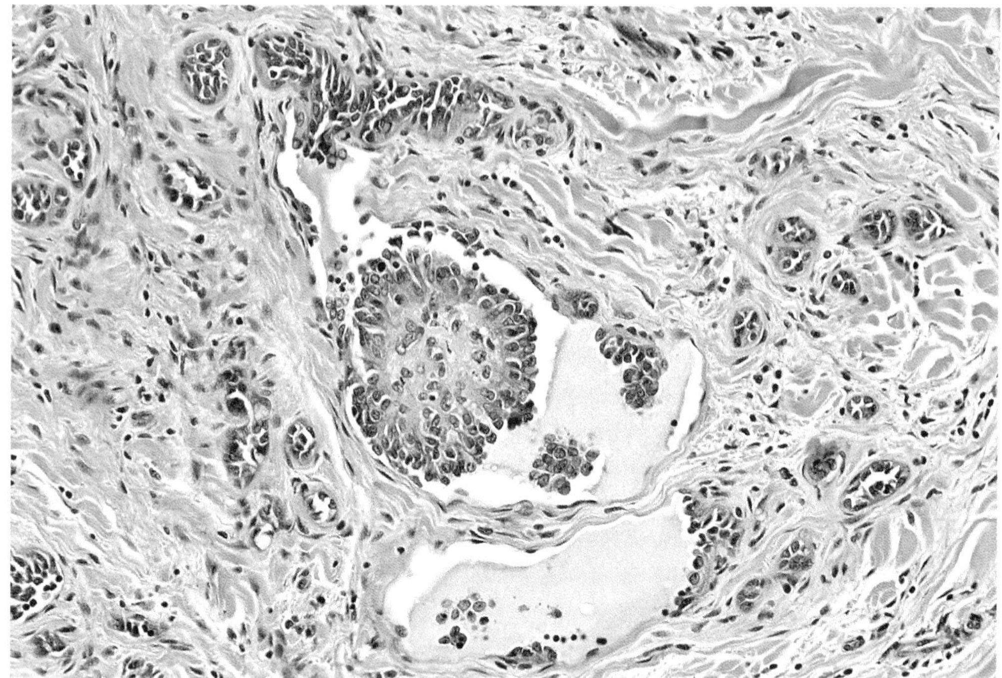

**FIGURE 24–31.** Intravascular papillations in a Dabska-type hemangioendothelioma.

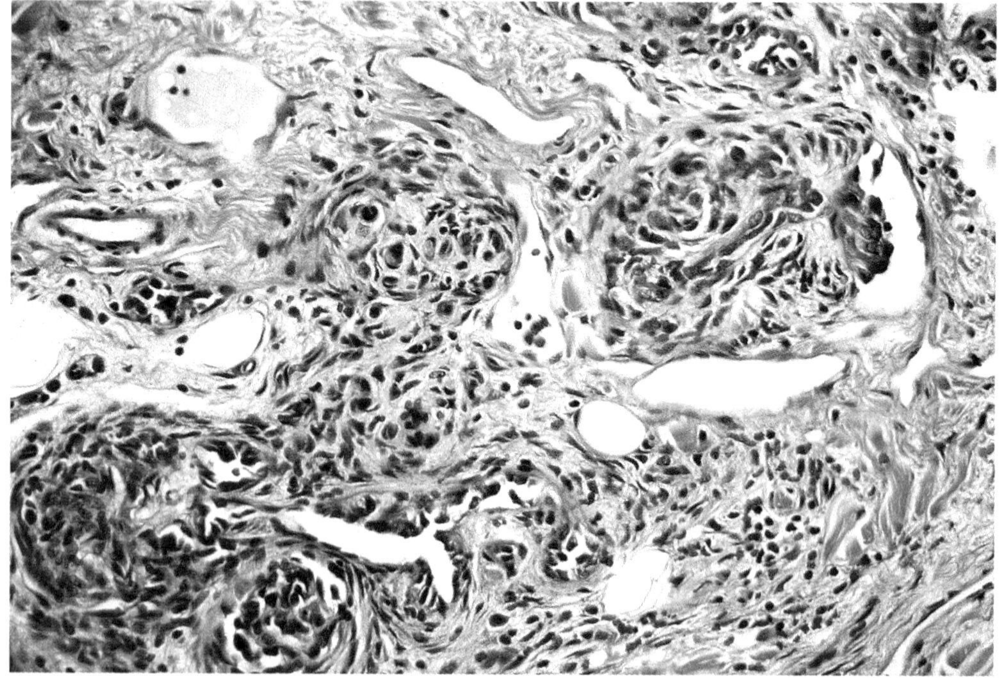

**FIGURE 24–32.** Solid areas of intravascular growth in a Dabska-type hemangioendothelioma.

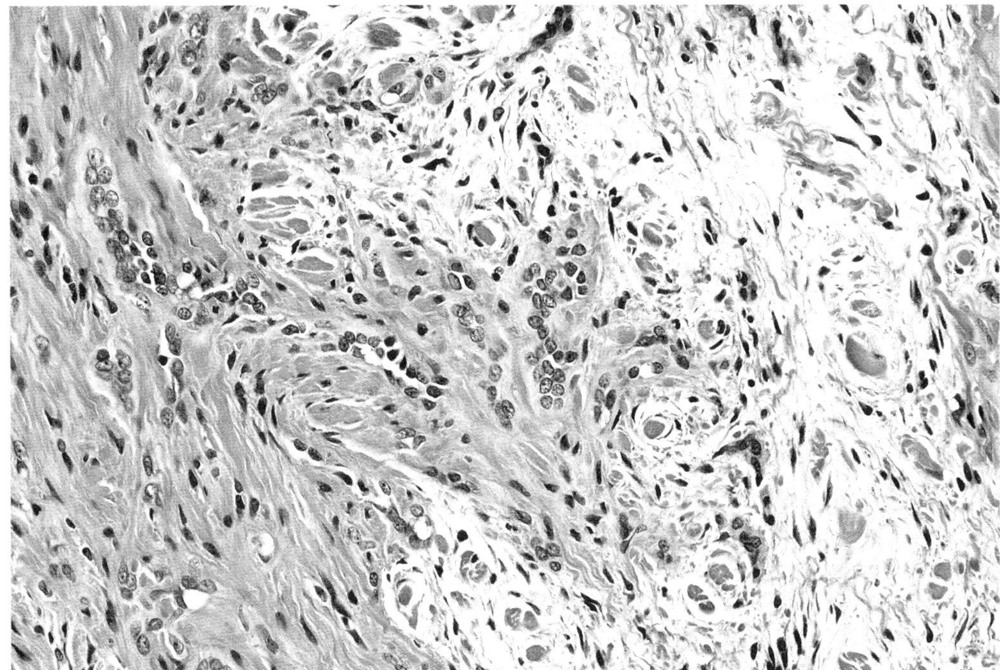

**FIGURE 24–33.** Dense hyaline sclerosis vessels in a Dabska tumor.

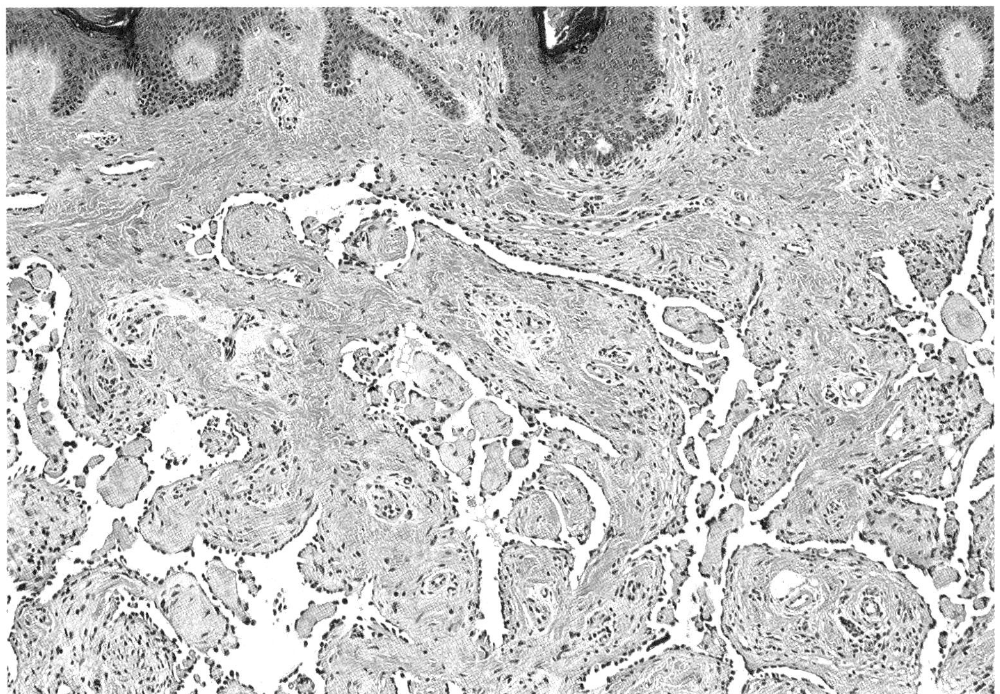

**FIGURE 24–34.** Retiform hemangioendothelioma involving the dermis.

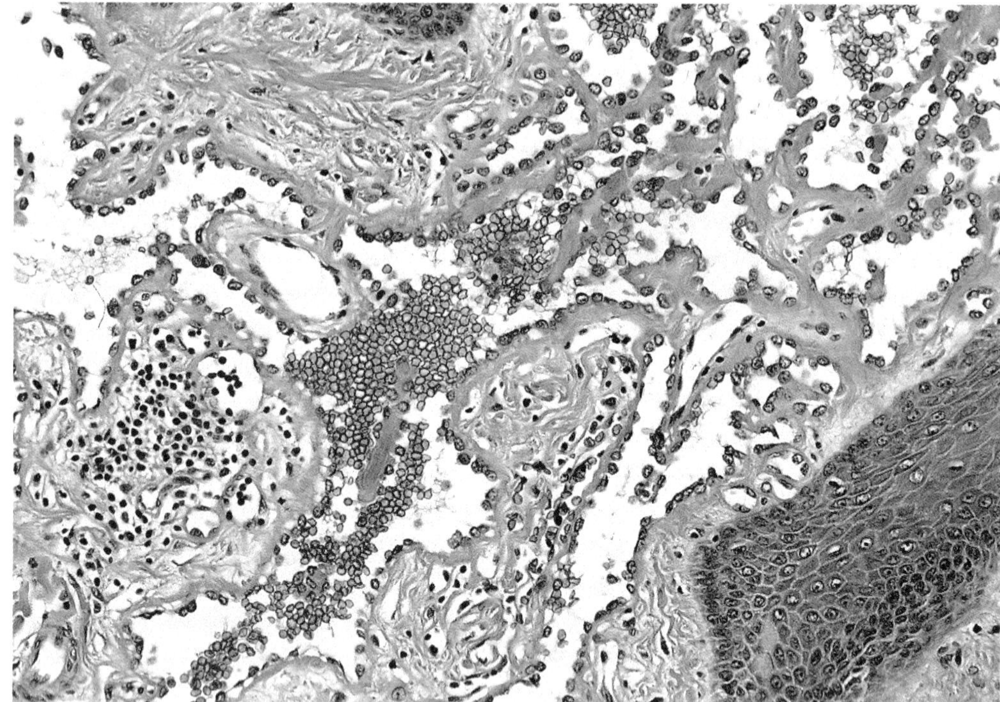

**FIGURE 24–35.** Retiform hemangioendothelioma with elongated vessels lined by cuboidal endothelium.

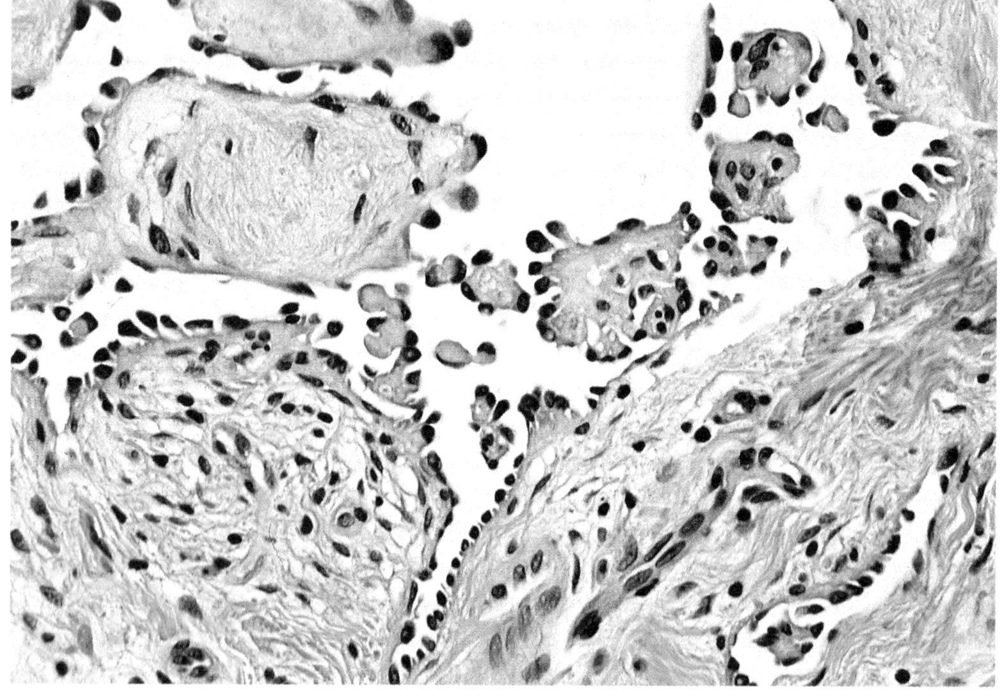

**FIGURE 24–36.** Retiform hemangioendothelioma with small intravascular papillations similar to a Dabska tumor.

factor, CD31, and CD34, although staining of the first two is usually significantly less intense than that of the last. In addition, these lesions strongly express VEGFR-3,[36,51] a receptor protein that appears to be a sensitive marker of lymphatic endothelium (Fig. 24–37). This staining profile, especially associated with the weak expression of factor VIII, is consistent with a tumor of lymphatic differentiation. For this reason Fanburg-Smith et al. suggested that the Dabska-type hemangioendothelioma be termed "papillary intralymphatic angioendothelioma" (PILA).[51] The lymphocytic infiltrate usually shows a mixture of B ($CD20^+$) and T ($CD3^+$) cells, although the intraluminal ones are predominantly T cells.[47]

### Discussion

Hobnail hemangioendotheliomas, regardless of whether they are of the Dabska or retiform type, appear to be low grade lesions with a capacity to extend to regional lymph nodes. Of the six patients reported by Dabska, two developed regional lymph node metastasis, and one eventually died of metastasis (as cited by Argani and Athanasian[46]). In the experience of Calonje et al. of retiform hemangioendotheliomas, nearly 60% of patients developed local recurrence and 1 of 14 patients developed a lymph node metastasis.[47] In our experience with 10 cases including both Dabska and retiform types, 4 developed local recurrences and 1 patient, with a tumor of an exclusively retiform pattern, developed a regional lymph node metastasis. In the series of Dabska-type hemangioendotheliomas reported by Fanburg-Smith et al. none of eight patients developed recurrence or metastasis during a median follow-up of 9 years.[51]

It should be emphasized that these data are based on tumors that fulfill a strict definition. Specifically, hobnail hemangioendotheliomas are composed of (hobnail) endothelium of low nuclear grade with an overall architectural pattern as described above. Intravascular tufts of atypical endothelium occur in angiosarcomas, but such lesions do not qualify as Dabska-type hemangioendotheliomas. There are also rare angiosarcomas characterized by high grade hobnail cells growing in solid sheets or as permeative vessels. These too should be designated angiosarcomas, rather than hobnail hemangioendotheliomas.

## POLYMORPHOUS HEMANGIOENDOTHELIOMA

Polymorphous hemangioendothelioma is a rare, presumably low grade, vascular tumor that to date has been reported primarily in lymph nodes[61] and only anecdotally in soft tissue.[61] It appears to affect adult men predominantly and is characterized by a variety of patterns in the same tumor and from tumor to tumor making it difficult to define a typical case histologically. These tumors may have angiomatous, spindled, solid, and retiform areas composed of cells

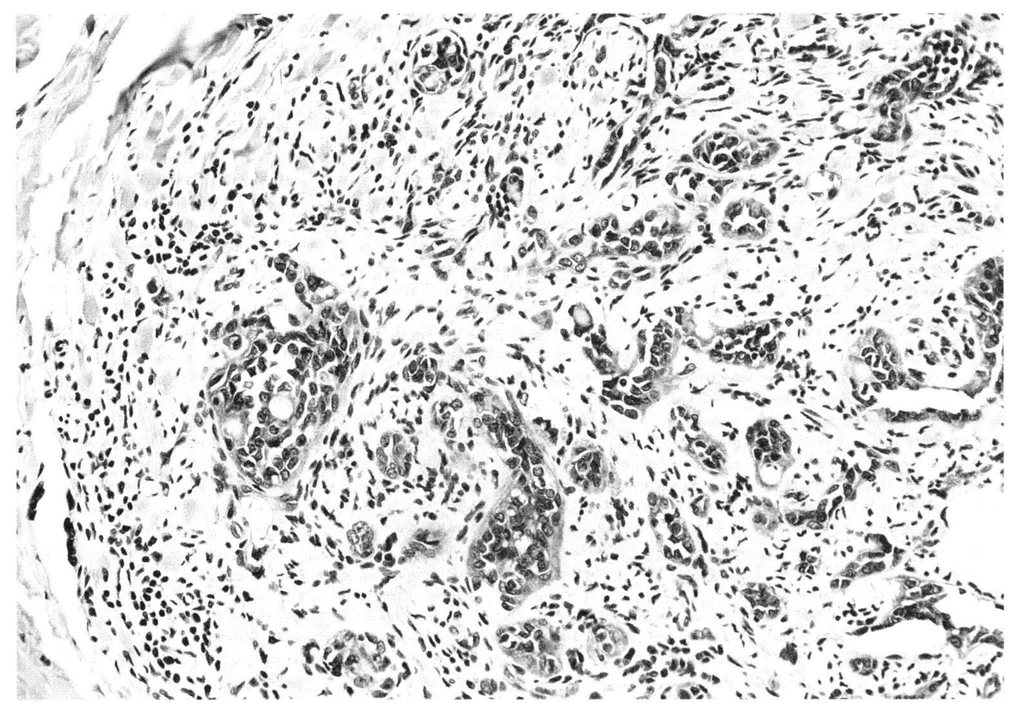

**FIGURE 24–37.** VEGFR-3 immunostaining in a Dabska tumor suggesting lymphatic differentiation.

of low nuclear grade that do not grow in a destructive or permeative pattern. In the two cases described by Nascimento et al., both had some areas containing hobnail endothelium. Although the designation "hemangioendothelioma" has been used for this group, only five of six reported cases have follow-up information. One of these patients developed metastatic disease within 4 years (cited by Nascimento et al.[62]), and two patients have only short-term follow-up. Until the lesions are fully characterized, these cases are perhaps best handled on an individual, and descriptive basis noting the predominant features and indicating the uncertainty of the long-term outlook.

## REFERENCES

### Epithelioid Hemangioendothelioma


1. Attanoos RL, Dallimore NS, Gibbs AR. Primary epithelioid hemangioendothelioma of the peritoneum: an unusual mimic of diffuse malignant mesothelioma. Histopathology 30:375, 1997.
2. Bhagavan BS, Dorfman HD, Murthy MSN, et al. Intravascular bronchioloalveolar tumor (IVBAT): a low-grade sclerosing epithelioid angiosarcoma of lung. Am J Surg Pathol 6:41, 1982.
3. Boudousquie AC, Lawce HJ, Sherman R, et al. Complex translocation (7;22) identified in an epithelioid hemangioendothelioma. Cancer Genet Cytogenet 92:116, 1996.
4. Corrin B, Manners B, Millard M, et al. Histogenesis of the so-called intravascular bronchiolo-alveolar tumor. J Pathol 128:163, 1979.
5. Dail DH, Liebow AA, Gmelich JT, et al. Intravascular, bronchiolar, and alveolar tumor of the lung (IVBAT): an analysis of twenty cases of a peculiar sclerosing endothelial tumor. Cancer 51:451, 1983.
6. Dean PJ, Haggitt RC, O'Hara CJ. Malignant epithelioid hemangioendothelioma of the liver in young women: relationship to oral contraceptive use. Am J Surg Pathol 9:695, 1985.
7. Ellis GL, Kratochvil FJ. Epithelioid hemangioendothelioma of the head and neck: a clinicopathologic report of twelve cases. Oral Surg Oral Med Oral Pathol 61:61, 1986.
8. Fukayama M, Nihei Z, Takizawa T, et al. Malignant epithelioid hemangioendothelioma of the liver spreading through the hepatic veins. Virchows Arch [Pathol Anat] 404:275, 1984.
9. Gray MH, Rosenberg AE, Dickersin GR, et al. Cytokeratin expression in epithelioid vascular neoplasms. Hum Pathol 21:212, 1990.
10. Hung CF, Jeng LB, Lee WC, et al. Liver transplantation for epithelioid hemangioendothelioma. Transplant Proc 30:3307, 1998.
11. Ishak KG, Sesterhenn IA, Goodman ZD, et al. Epithelioid hemangioendothelioma of the liver: a clinicopathologic and follow-up study of 32 cases. Hum Pathol 15:839, 1984.
12. Kato N, Tamura A, Okushiba M. Multiple cutaneous epithelioid hemangioendothelioma: a case with spindle cells. J Dermatol 25:453, 1998.
13. Kelleher MB, Iwatsuki S, Sheahan DG. Epithelioid hemangioendothelioma of the liver: clinicopathological correlation of 10 cases treated with orthotopic liver transplantation. Am J Surg Pathol 13:999, 1989.
14. Kiryu H, Hashimoto H, Hori Y. Ossifying epithelioid hemangioendothelioma. J Cutan Pathol 23:558, 1996.
15. Kitaichi M, Nagai S, Nishimura K, et al. Pulmonary epithelioid hemangioendothelioma in 21 patients including three with partial spontaneous regression. Eur Respir J 12:89; 1998.
16. Kleer CG, Unni KK, McLeod RA. Epithelioid hemangioendothelioma of bone. Am J Surg Pathol 20:1301, 1996.
17. Makhlouf HR, Ishak KG, Goodman ZD. Epithelioid hemangioendothelioma of the liver: a clinicopathologic study of 137 cases. Cancer 85:562, 1999.
18. Marino I, Todo S, Tzakis AG, et al. Treatment of hepatic epithelioid hemangioendothelioma with liver transplantation. Cancer 62:2079, 1988.
19. Mentzel T, Beham A, Calonje E, et al. Epithelioid hemangioendothelioma of skin and soft tissues: clinicopathologic and immunohistochemical study of 30 cases. Am J Surg Pathol 21:363, 1997.
20. Mirra JM, Kameda N. Myxoid angioblastomatosis of bones: a case report of a rare, multifocal entity with light, ultramicroscopic, and immunopathologic correlation. Am J Surg Pathol 9: 450, 1985.
21. Nora FE, Scheithauer BW. Primary epithelioid hemangioendothelioma of the brain. Am J Surg Pathol 20:707, 1996.
22. Quante M, Patel NK, Hill S, et al. Epithelioid hemangioendothelioma presenting in the skin: a clinicopathologic study of eight cases. Am J Dermatopathol 20:541, 1998.
23. Rosai J, Gold J, Landy R. The histiocytoid hemangiomas: a unifying concept embracing several previously described entities of skin, soft tissue, large vessels, bone, and heart. Hum Pathol 10:707, 1979.
24. Tang TT, Zuege RC, Babbitt DP, et al. Angioglomoid tumor of bone: a case report. J Bone Joint Surg Am 58:873, 1976.
25. Tsuneyoshi M, Dorfman HD, Bauer TW. Epithelioid hemangioendothelioma of bone: a clinicopathologic, ultrastructural, and immunohistochemical study. Am J Surg Pathol 10:754, 1986.
26. Vasquez M, Ordonez NG, English GW, Mackay B. Epithelioid hemangioendothelioma of soft tissue: report of a case with ultrastructural observations. Ultrastruct Pathol 22:73, 1998.
27. Weiss SW, Enzinger FM. Epithelioid hemangioendothelioma: a vascular tumor often mistaken for a carcinoma. Cancer 50:970, 1982.
28. Weiss SW, Ishak KG, Dail DH, et al. Epithelioid hemangioendothelioma and related lesions. Semin Diagn Pathol 3:259, 1986.
29. Weldon-Linne CM, Victor TA, Christ ML, et al. Angiogenic nature of the intravascular bronchioloalveolar tumor of the lung. Arch Pathol Lab Med 105:174, 1981.


### Spindle Cell Hemangioendothelioma


30. Perkins P, Weiss SW. Spindle cell hemangioendothelioma: a clinicopathologic study of 78 cases. Am J Surg Pathol 20:1196, 1996.
31. Weiss SW, Enzinger FM. Spindle cell hemangioendothelioma: a low-grade angiosarcoma resembling cavernous hemangioma and Kaposi's sarcoma. Am J Surg Pathol 10:521, 1986.


### Kaposiform Hemangioendothelioma


32. Beaubien ER, Ball NJ, Storwick GS. Kaposiform hemangioendothelioma: a locally aggressive vascular tumor. J Am Acad Dermatol 38:799, 1998.
33. Blei F, Karp N, Rofsky N, et al. Successful multimodal therapy for kaposiform hemangioendothelioma complicated by Kasabach-Merritt phenomenon: case report and review of the literature. Pediatr Hematol Oncol 15:295, 1998.
34. Deb G, Jenkner A, DeSio L, et al. Spindle cell (kaposiform) hemangioendothelioma with Kasabach-Merritt syndrome in an infant: successful treatment with alpha-2A interferon. Med Pediatr Oncol 28:358, 1997.
35. Enjolras O, Wassef M, Mazoyer E, et al. Infants with Kasabach-

Merritt syndrome do not have "true" hemangiomas. J Pediatr 130:631, 1997.
36. Folpe AL, Veikkola T, Valtola R, Weiss SW. Vascular endothelial growth factor receptor-3 (VEGFR-3): a marker of vascular tumors with presumed lymphatic differentiation, including Kaposi's sarcoma, kaposiform and Dabska-type hemangioendotheliomas, and a subset of angiosarcomas. Mod Pathol 13:180, 2000.
37. Hu B, Lachman R, Phillips J, et al. Kasabach-Merritt syndrome-associated kaposiform hemangioendothelioma successfully treated with cyclophosphamide, vincristine, and actinomycin D. J Pediatr Hematol Oncol 20:567, 1998.
38. Lai FM, Allen PW, Yuen PM, et al. Locally metastasizing vascular tumor: spindle cell, epithelioid, or unclassified hemangioendothelioma. Am J Clin Pathol 96:660, 1991.
39. Mentzel T, Massoleni G, Dei Tos AP, Fletcher CD. Kaposiform hemangioendothelioma in adults: clinicopathologic and immunohistochemical analysis of three cases. Am J Clin Pathol 108: 450, 1997.
40. Niedt GW, Greco MA, Wieczorek R, et al. Hemangioma with Kaposi's sarcoma-like features: report of 2 cases. Pediatr Pathol 9:567, 1989.
41. Pearl GS, Matthews WH. Congenital retroperitoneal hemangioendothelioma with Kasabach-Merritt syndrome. South Med J 72:239, 1979.
42. Sarkar M, Mulliken JB, Kozakewich HP, et al. Thrombocytopenic coagulopathy (Kasabach-Merritt phenomenon) is associated with kaposiform hemangioendothelioma and not with common infantile hemangioma. Plast Reconstruct Surg 100:1377, 1997.
43. Tsang WYW, Chang JKC. Kaposi-like infantile hemangioendothelioma: a distinctive vascular neoplasm of the retroperitoneum. Am J Surg Pathol 15:982, 1991.
44. Vin-Christian K, McCalmont TH, Frieden IJ. Kaposiform hemangioendothelioma: an aggressive, locally invasive vascular tumor that can mimic hemangioma of infancy. Arch Dermatol 133:1573, 1997.
45. Zukerberg LR, Nickoloff BJ, Weiss SW. Kaposiform hemangioendothelioma of infancy and childhood: an aggressive neoplasm associated with Kasabach-Merritt syndrome and lymphangiomatosis. Am J Surg Pathol 17:321, 1993.

### Hobnail (Dabska-Retiform) Hemangioendothelioma

46. Argani P, Athanasian E. Malignant endovascular papillary angioendothelioma (Dabska tumor) arising within a deep intramuscular hemangioma. Arch Pathol Lab Med 121:992, 1997.
47. Calonje E, Fletcher CDM, Wilson-Jones E, Rosai J. Retiform hemangioendothelioma: a distinctive form of low-grade angiosarcoma delineated in a series of 15 cases. Am J Surg Pathol 18: 115, 1994.
48. Dabska M. Malignant endovascular papillary angioendothelioma of the skin in childhood. Cancer 24:503, 1969.
49. Duke D, Dvorak A, Harris TJ, Cohen LM. Multiple retiform hemangioendotheliomas: a low grade angiosarcoma. Am J Dermatol 18:606, 1996.
50. Dulanto F, Armijo-Moreno M. Malignant endovascular papillary hemangioendothelioma of the skin. Acta Dermatovener (Stockh) 53:403, 1973.
51. Fanburg-Smith JC, Michal M, Partanen TA, et al. Papillary intralymphatic angioendothelioma (PILA): a report of twelve cases of a distinctive vascular tumor with phenotyic feature of lymphatic vessels. Am J Surg Pathol 23:1004, 1999.
52. Fukunaga M, Endo Y, Masui F, et al. Retiform hemangioendothelioma. Virchows Arch 428:301, 1996.
53. Katz JA, Mahoney DH, Shukla LW, et al. Endovascular papillary angioendothelioma in the spleen. Pediatr Pathol 8:185, 1988.
54. Magnin PH, Schroh RG, Barquin MA. Endovascular papillary angioendothelioma in children. Pediatr Dermatol 4:332, 1987.
55. Manivel JC, Wick MR, Swanson PE, et al. Endovascular papillary angioendothelioma of childhood: a vascular lesion possibly characterized by "high" endothelial cell differentiation. Hum Pathol 17:1240, 1986.
56. Miyachi Y, Imamura S. Very low-grade angiosarcoma. Dermatologica 162:206, 1981.
57. Morgan J, Robinson MJ, Rosen LB, et al. Malignant endovascular papillary angioendothelioma (Dabska tumor): a case report and review of the literature. Am J Dermatopathol 11:64, 1989.
58. Patterson K, Chandra RS. Malignant endovascular papillary angioendothelioma: a cutaneous borderline tumor. Arch Pathol Lab Med 109:671, 1985.
59. Quecedo E, Martinez-Escribano JA, Febrer I, et al. Dabska tumor developing within a preexisting vascular malformation. Am J Dermatopathol 18:303, 1996.
60. Sanz-Trelles A, Rodrigo-Fernandez I, Ayala-Carbonero A, Contreras-Rubio E. Retiform hemangioendothelioma: a new case in a child with diffuse endovascular papillary endothelial proliferation. J Cutan Pathol 24:440, 1997.

### Polymorphous Hemangioendothelioma

61. Chan JKC, Frizzera G, Fletcher DM, Rosai J. Primary vascular tumors of lymph nodes other than Kaposi's sarcoma: analysis of 39 cases and delineation of two new entitities. Am J Surg Pathol 16:335, 1992.
62. Nascimento AG, Keeney GL, Sciot R, Fletcher CD. Polymorphous hemangioendothelioma: a report of two cases one affecting extranodal soft tissues, and review of the literature. Am J Surg Pathol 21:1083, 1997.

# CHAPTER 25

# MALIGNANT VASCULAR TUMORS

## ANGIOSARCOMA

Angiosarcomas are malignant tumors that recapitulate many of the functional and morphologic features of normal endothelium. They may vary from highly differentiated tumors that resemble hemangiomas to those in which anaplasia makes them difficult to distinguish from carcinomas or melanomas. Consequently, the old literature is replete with terms such as hemangioendothelioma, lymphangioendothelioma, hemangioblastoma, lymphangiosarcoma, and hemangiosarcoma, attesting to the wide morphologic spectrum. It is not generally possible to determine whether these angiosarcomas display lymphatic or vascular differentiation, even though those arising in the setting of lymphedema have often been referred to as "lymphangiosarcomas" on the presumption that this impressive post hoc phenomenon indicated origin from lymphatics. For this reason the term "angiosarcoma" is used for all sarcomas showing endothelial differentiation regardless of whether the lesion is believed to be related to vascular or lymphatic endothelium. The ability to define specific differences between lymphatic and vascular endothelium by molecular and immunophenotypic methods may in time result in refinements of the classification of sarcomas,[23,32,39] however, and there already is some preliminary evidence that many angiosarcomas have a mixed phenotype.[6] In contrast to the term "angiosarcoma," the term "hemangioendothelioma" is used exclusively for vascular tumors of intermediate malignancy (see Chapter 24), thereby implying that the risk of metastatic disease is significantly lower than for angiosarcoma.

### Incidence

Angiosarcomas are collectively one of the rarest forms of soft tissue neoplasm. They account for a vanishingly small proportion of all vascular tumors, and they comprise less than 1% of all sarcomas as estimated by a 20-year study at the M.D. Anderson Hospital.[72] Although they may occur at any location in the body, they rarely arise from major vessels and have a decided predilection for skin and superficial soft tissue, a phenomenon that contrasts sharply with the deep location of most soft tissue sarcomas. These tumors rarely occur during childhood, but when they do they seem to occur in an epidemiologic pattern different from that of adults. For example, there is a greater tendency for them to develop in internal organs or with various disease states (e.g., Klippel-Trénaunay syndrome).[111] Analysis of 366 angiosarcomas reviewed at the Armed Forces Institute of Pathology (AFIP) during a 10-year period (Table 25–1) showed that one-third (121 cases) occurred in the skin, about one-fourth (89 cases) in soft tissue, and the remainder at other sites (e.g., breast, liver, bone, spleen).

The presentation and behavior of these tumors differs depending on location.[20–22] Hence angiosarcomas are more properly considered as several closely related tumors rather than as a single entity. We have divided them into several groups: cutaneous angiosarcoma of the usual type unassociated with lymphedema; cutaneous angiosarcoma associated with lymphedema (so-called lymphangiosarcoma); angiosarcoma of the breast; radiation-induced angiosarcoma; and angiosarcoma of deep soft tissue. There are also rare angiosarcomas that develop adjacent to foreign material,[58] in the vicinity of arteriovenous fistulas in renal transplant patients,[11,15,16,45,67] in other tumors,[61,62] or in association with rare genetic syndromes.[64,111] Although eclipsed in number by the other forms of angiosarcoma, these unusual associations suggest more than a fortuitous occurrence (see below).

**TABLE 25–1 ANATOMIC DISTRIBUTION OF ANGIOSARCOMAS: 1966–1976 (366 CASES)**

| Location | No. of Cases | % |
|---|---|---|
| Skin | 121 | 33 |
| Without lymphedema | 101 | |
| With lymphedema | 20 | |
| Soft tissue | 89 | 24 |
| Breast | 30 | 8 |
| Liver | 31 | 8 |
| Bone | 20 | 6 |
| Spleen | 16 | 4 |
| Heart and great vessels | 10 | 3 |
| Orbit | 10 | 3 |
| Pharynx/oral cavity | 13 | 4 |
| Other | 26 | 7 |
| *Total* | 366 | 100 |

Data are from the Armed Forces Institute of Pathology (AFIP).

## Etiologic Factors and Pathogenesis

Chronic lymphedema is the most widely recognized predisposing factor for angiosarcomas of skin and soft tissue, yet in our cases only about 10% of tumors have been associated with this condition (Table 25–1). Typically, lymphedema-associated angiosarcomas occur in women who have undergone radical mastectomy for breast carcinoma and have suffered chronic severe lymphedema for years. Chronic lymphedema occurring on a congenital,[86,89,95] idiopathic, traumatic, or infectious[85,91,95] basis also predisposes to angiosarcoma.

Several theories have been advanced to explain the association of lymphedema and angiosarcoma. Some have suggested that the growth and proliferation of obstructed lymphatics eventually fail to respond to normal control mechanisms. Others have subscribed to the idea that carcinogens in lymphatic fluid induce the neoplastic change. More recently it has been hypothesized that the lymphedematous extremity represents an "immunologically priviledged site"[92] (because of the loss of afferent lymphatic connections) and consequently is unable to perform immunologic surveillance of normally occurring mutant cell populations. This notion is supported by the observations that skin grafts survive for long periods when transferred to lymphedematous extremities.[92]

In the past it has been difficult to evaluate the role of radiation in the induction of angiosarcoma, as many patients who had undergone irradiation also had chronic lymphedema. There is now little doubt that there are bone fide postirradiation angiosarcomas.[112] Altogether, 5 of the 44 cases reported by Maddox and Evans,[41] 2 of the 44 reported by Sordillo et al.,[96] and a number of other small series and cases[13,17,77,120,122,127,128] attest to the fact that irradiation per se may lead to the development of angiosarcomas. To be considered radiation-induced, these tumors must be biopsy-proven angiosarcomas arising in the radiation field after an interval of several years; and they must not be associated with chronic lymphedema. More than half of the cases qualifying as postirradiation angiosarcomas have occurred following radiotherapy for another malignant tumor such as carcinoma of the cervix,[41] ovary,[13] endometrium,[87,120] or breast[17,116] and Hodgkin's disease.[122] Angiosarcomas that follow irradiation for genitourinary malignant tumors usually develop on the lower abdominal wall, whereas those following irradiation for breast carcinoma usually develop on the chest wall. The lumbar spinal area is often the site for those that arise after treatment of Hodgkin's disease.[122] The mean interval between irradiation and diagnosis has been approximately 12 years,[17,41] although longer intervals have been noted in patients who received low-dosage radiation for benign conditions such as eczema.[17]

A number of angiosarcomas have developed at the site of defunctionalized arteriovenous fistulas[5,11,14,16,33,45,67] in renal transplant patients. All of these patients were immunosuppressed, and it seems likely that the altered immune status plays a major role in tumorigenesis. However, it does not explain why these tumors, all angiosarcomas, occur in the immediate vicinity of the fistulas. Angiosarcomas also have been reported adjacent to foreign material introduced into the body iatrogenically or accidentally.[4,27,31,58,69] In an extensive review of the literature by Jennings et al.,[31] nine angiosarcomas associated with foreign material were identified. Common to all was a long latent period between the time of introduction of the foreign material and the development of the tumor. Although one case occurred within 3 years, the remainder appeared more than a decade later. A variety of solid materials were implicated, including shrapnel, steel, plastic and synthetic (usually Dacron) vascular graft material,[16,58,69,111] surgical sponges,[4,31] and bone wax.[31] The authors suggest that an exuberant host response in the form of a fibrous tissue capsule around the foreign material may represent an important intermediate step in the development of the sarcoma. We encountered an angiosarcoma in a long-standing gouty tophus, suggesting that urate deposits may function as the equivalent of foreign material.

Malignant change in a preexisting benign vascular tumor is probably an unusual event. Many cases attesting to this phenomenon probably represent errors in the original diagnosis. In one series of angiosarcomas, however, four occurred in preexisting benign lesions: three in port-wine stains and one in an irradiated lymphangioma.[111] Angiosarcomas have also been documented in benign and malignant nerve sheath tumors,[8,12,46,49,62] leiomyoma,[61] in the setting of neurofibromatosis,[111] Maffucci syndrome associated with spindle cell hemangioma,[111] bilateral retinoblastoma (Rb1 deletion),[19] Klippel-Trénaunay syndrome,[111] xeroderma pigmentosum,[36] as part of a malignant germ cell tumor,[65] and at the site of a herpes zoster lesion.[29] Finally, we have seen two cases of angiosarcoma complicating the course of Aicardi syndrome, an X-linked disorder associated with multiple congenital abnormalities including agenesis of the corpus callosum.[64] Both were high grade lesions in infants that grew rapidly over a few months. The gene associated with this syndrome has not been identified, and the putative mechanism for tumorigenesis is unknown.

Whereas there is strong circumstantial evidence linking human herpes virus 8 (HHV8) to Kaposi's sarcoma, there is no association with angiosarcoma.[35,37,38] Reports alleging findings to the contrary should be questioned.[44]

Unfortunately there is little information concerning the possible role of environmental carcinogens in the pathogenesis of soft tissue angiosarcomas. That such factors exist is suggested by the relatively strong evidence linking various substances to the induction of hepatic angiosarcomas (Kupffer cell sarcomas). About one-fourth of hepatic angiosarcomas[55] occur in patients who have received thorium dioxide (Thorotrast) for cerebral angiography, in vineyard workers exposed to $AsO_3$-containing insecticides, or in industrial workers exposed to vinyl chloride during the production of synthetic rubber.[3,42,55] A few cases have been recorded in patients receiving long-term androgenic anabolic steroids[21] and one in a patient taking estrogen.[28] Mutations of the K-*ras-2* gene have been detected in both sporadic and Thorotrast-induced hepatic angiosarcomas.[56]

Vascular endothelial growth factor (VEGF), an angiogenic cytokine, has become a recent focus in the study of tumor angiogenesis. This 45,000 dalton glycoprotein, normally produced by macrophages and stromal cells, stimulates growth and enhances permeability of endothelial cells. VEGF may also be produced by various tumors including some angiosarcomas, which express both VEGF and its receptors.[7,26] This observation implies that growth of angiosarcomas can occur by both autocrine and paracrine loops. Unfortunately, the ability to monitor treatment of angiosarcomas by serial VEGF serum concentrations has not proved practical.[24]

**TABLE 25-2 AGE DISTRIBUTION OF CUTANEOUS ANGIOSARCOMAS WITHOUT LYMPHEDEMA: 1966–1976 (101 CASES)**

| Age (Years) | No. of Cases | % |
|---|---|---|
| 0–11 | 11 | 11 |
| 11–20 | 9 | 9 |
| 21–30 | 6 | 6 |
| 31–40 | 5 | 5 |
| 41–50 | 18 | 18 |
| 51–60 | 10 | 10 |
| 61–70 | 17 | 17 |
| >70 | 22 | 22 |
| Unspecified | 3 | 2 |
| *Total* | 101 | 100 |

Data are from the AFIP.

**TABLE 25-3 GENDER DISTRIBUTION OF CUTANEOUS ANGIOSARCOMAS WITHOUT LYMPHEDEMA: 1966–1976 (101 CASES)**

| Gender | No. of Cases | % |
|---|---|---|
| Male | 62 | 62 |
| Female | 31 | 31 |
| Unknown | 8 | 7 |
| *Total* | 101 | 100 |

Data are from the AFIP.

## Cutaneous Angiosarcoma Not Associated with Lymphedema

Cutaneous angiosarcoma without lymphedema is the most common angiosarcoma. It primarily affects elderly persons (Tables 25-2, 25-3) and is usually located on the head and neck, particularly the area of the scalp (Table 25-4) and upper forehead. Because many patients with angiosarcomas are women with a full head of hair,[78] sun exposure as a tumorigenic agent is questionable. Clinically, the appearance of these lesions is variable. Most begin as ill-defined bruise-like areas with an indurated border; and for this reason they are apt to be considered benign. In a

**TABLE 25-4 ANATOMIC DISTRIBUTION OF CUTANEOUS ANGIOSARCOMAS WITHOUT LYMPHEDEMA: 1966–1976 (101 CASES)**

| Location | No. of Cases | % |
|---|---|---|
| Head and neck | 52 | 52 |
| Leg | 13 | 13 |
| Trunk | 13 | 13 |
| Arm | 8 | 8 |
| Generalized | 2 | 1 |
| Not specified | 13 | 13 |
| *Total* | 101 | 100 |

Data are from the AFIP.

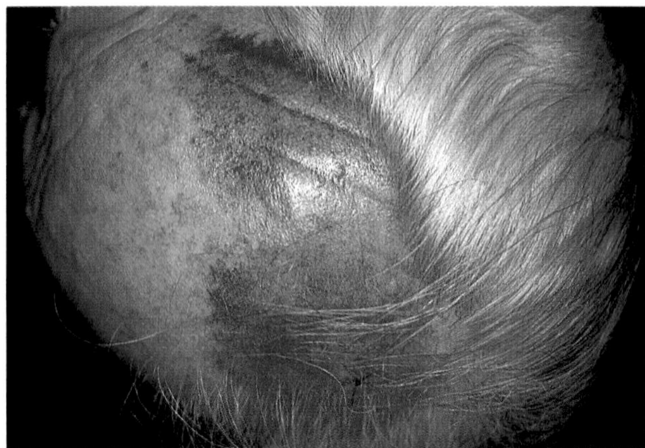

**FIGURE 25–1.** Angiosarcoma of the scalp in an elderly man. (Case courtesy of Dr. Vernon Sondak.)

small number of cases a diagnosis of facial edema is entertained. Large, advanced lesions are elevated, nodular, and occasionally ulcerated (Fig. 25–1). It is difficult to determine the extent of these lesions clinically. This fact, coupled with multifocality in about half of the cases, seriously complicates therapy and probably results in suboptimal initial therapy in a large number of cases. Preoperative mapping of angiosarcoma using grid-pattern biopsies or Moh's surgery has resulted in better delineation of tumor extent and treatment planning.[9]

Grossly, the tumors consist of ill-defined hemorrhagic areas (Fig. 25–2) that may flatten or ulcerate the overlying skin. Rarely, the epidermis displays verrucous hyperplasia.[74] On cut section the tumors are seen to have a microcystic or sponge-like quality due to the presence of blood-filled spaces. The tumors extensively involve the dermis and extend well beyond their apparent gross confines. In poorly differentiated, rapidly growing tumors, deep structures such as the subcutis and fascia may also be invaded. The periphery of the tumors contains a fringe of dilated lymphatic vessels surrounded by chronic inflammatory cells and usually small capillaries in which piling up and tufting of the endothelium suggests incipient malignant change.

Many cutaneous angiosarcomas are well to moderately differentiated lesions that form distinct vascular channels, albeit of irregular size and shape (Figs. 25–3 to 25–8). Such tumors at first may suggest poorly confined hemangiomas because of the numerous channels and the flattened innocuous appearance of the cells. Yet in contrast to true hemangiomas, the vascular channels seem to create their own tissue planes, dissecting through the dermal collagen (Fig. 25–6) and fascia or splitting apart groups of subcutaneous fat cells. Moreover, there is a tendency for the channels to communicate with each other, forming an anastomosing network of sinusoids (Figs. 25–4, 25–5). Although the cells resemble normal endothelium to some extent, they usually have larger, more chromatic nuclei and often pile up along the lumina, creating the papillations so typical of angiosarcomas (but which may also be seen in reactive vascular proliferations such as papillary endothelial hyperplasia).

A small number of cutaneous angiosarcomas are relatively high-grade tumors that are difficult to distinguish from carcinomas or high-grade fibrosarcomas (Fig. 25–7). These tumors may have occasional well-differentiated areas, as described earlier, that facilitate diagnosis. Others are composed exclusively of poorly differentiated areas. The cells in the poorly differenti-

*Text continued on page 925*

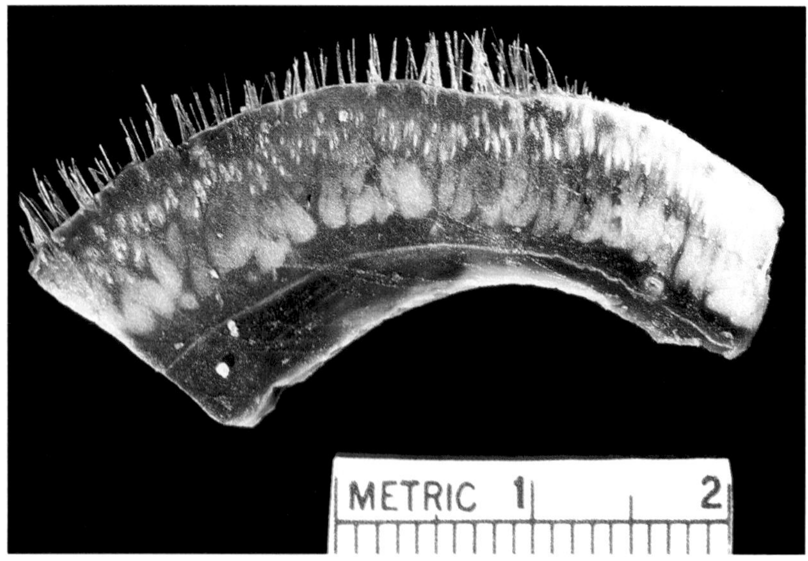


**FIGURE 25–2.** Angiosarcoma of the scalp. Hemorrhagic appearance frequently suggests a diagnosis of dissecting hemorrhage or hematoma.

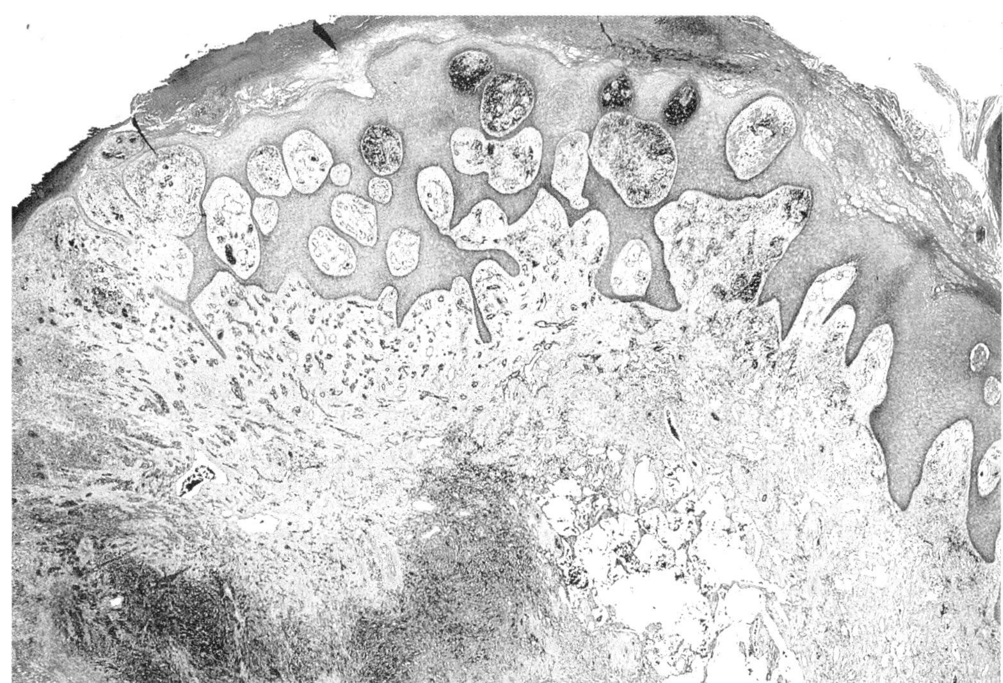

**FIGURE 25–3.** Cutaneous angiosarcoma composed of irregular vascular channels infiltrating the dermis. Some areas resemble a pyogenic granuloma.

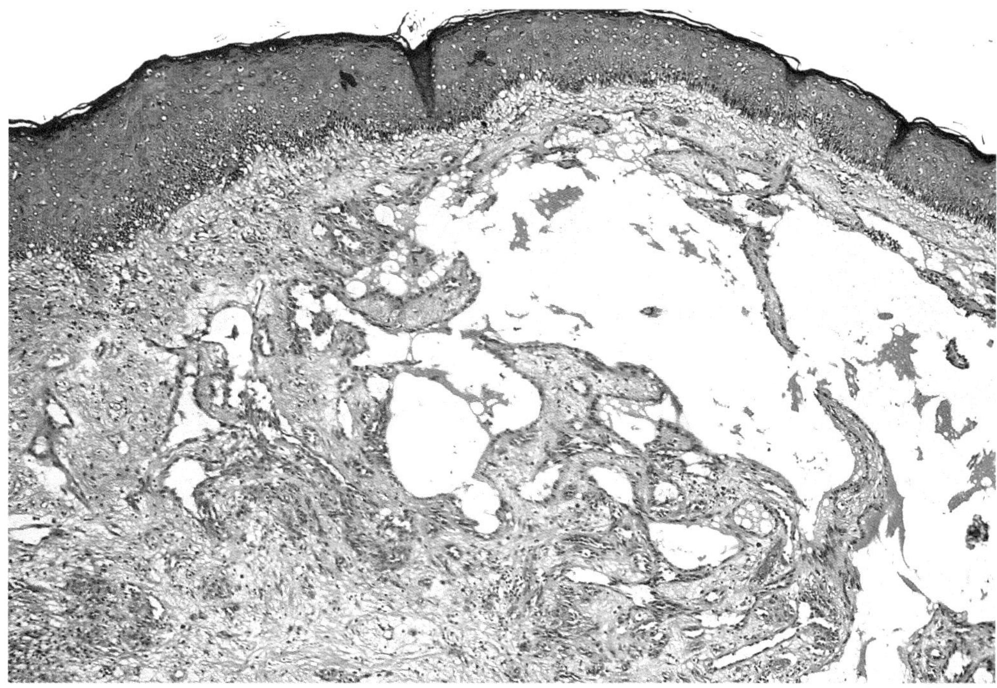

**FIGURE 25–4.** Cutaneous angiosarcoma with an irregular or sinusoidal pattern of vessels.

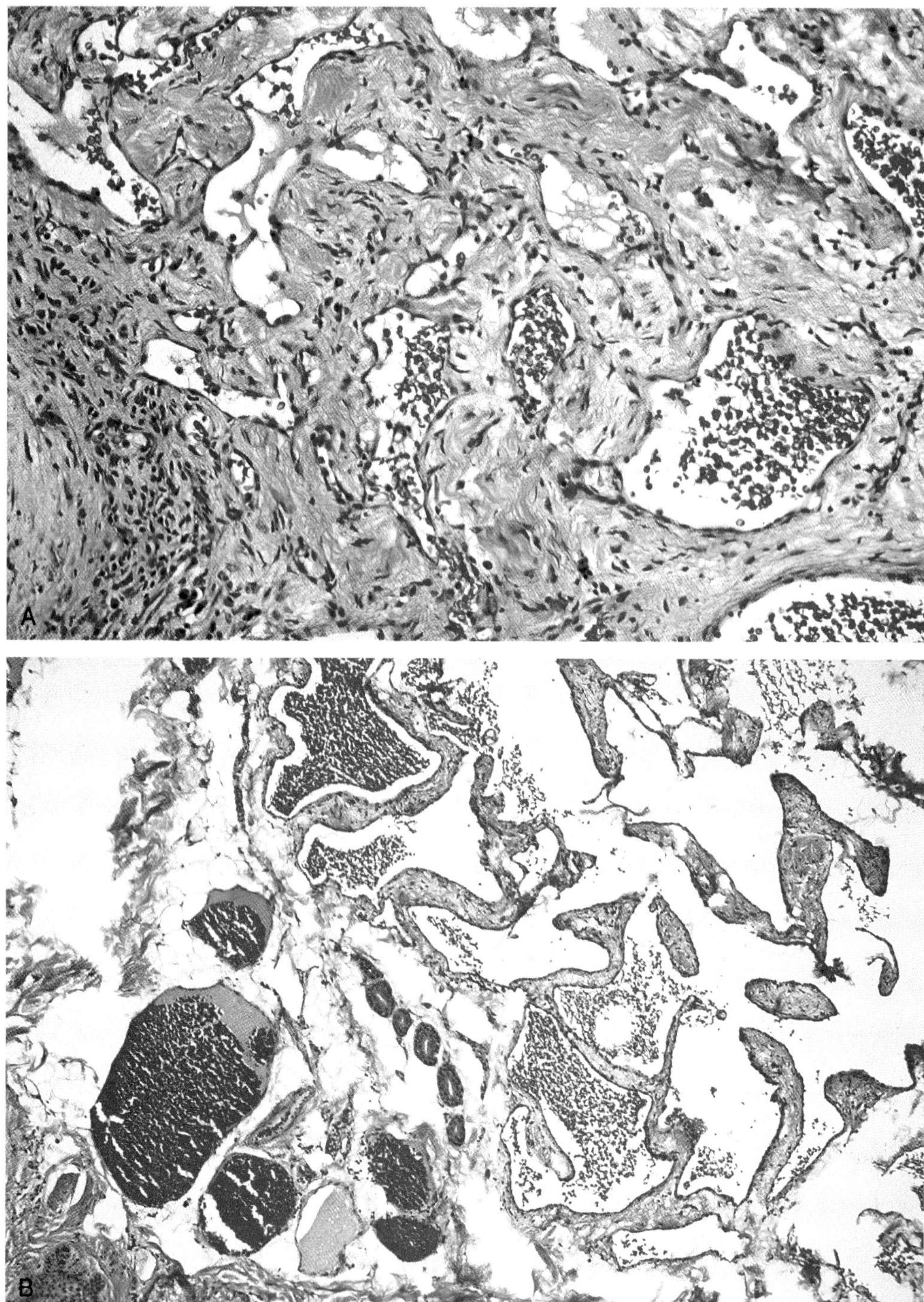

**FIGURE 25–5.** Varying patterns in cutaneous angiosarcomas. (**A**) Irregular ectatic vessels dissecting the dermis. (**B**) Large cavernous vascular spaces resembling a cavernous hemangioma.

*Illustration continued on opposite page*

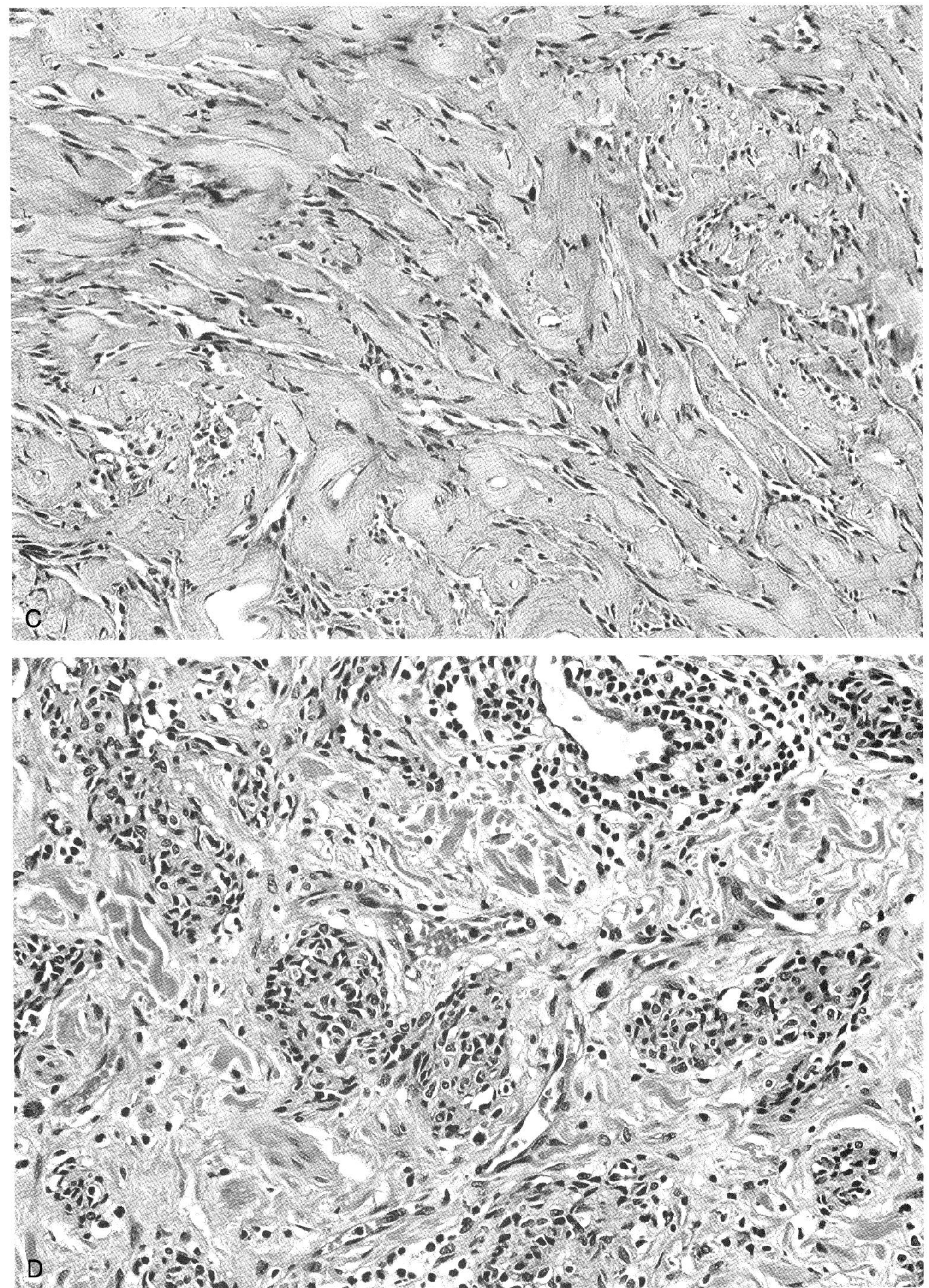


**FIGURE 25–5** *(Continued)*. (**C**) Slit-like vessels dissecting collagen. (**D**) Small clusters of slit-like vessels surrounded by chronic inflammatory cells.

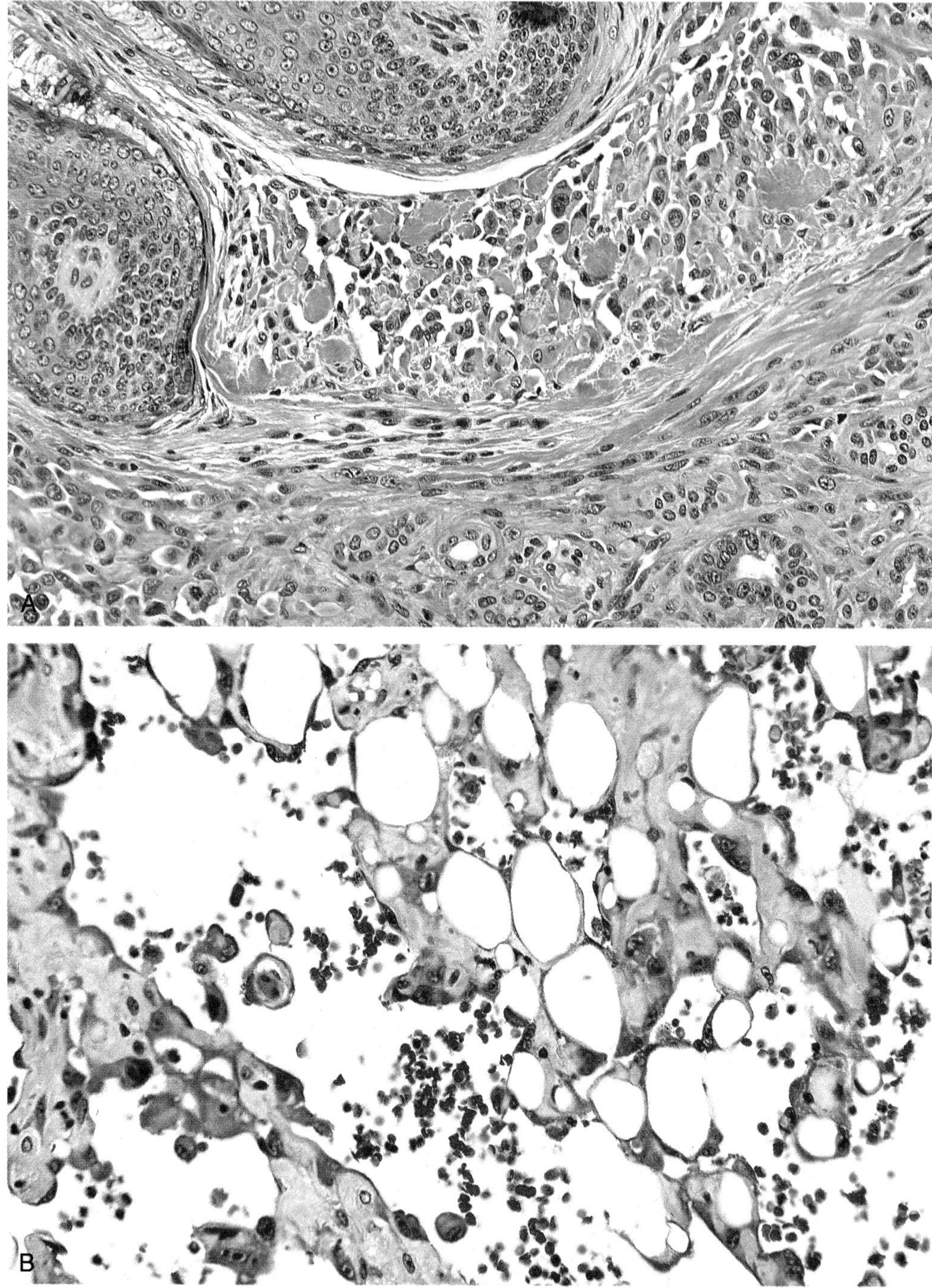

**FIGURE 25–6.** Infiltrative growth of an angiosarcoma around a hair shaft (**A**), within fat (**B**),

*Illustration continued on opposite page*

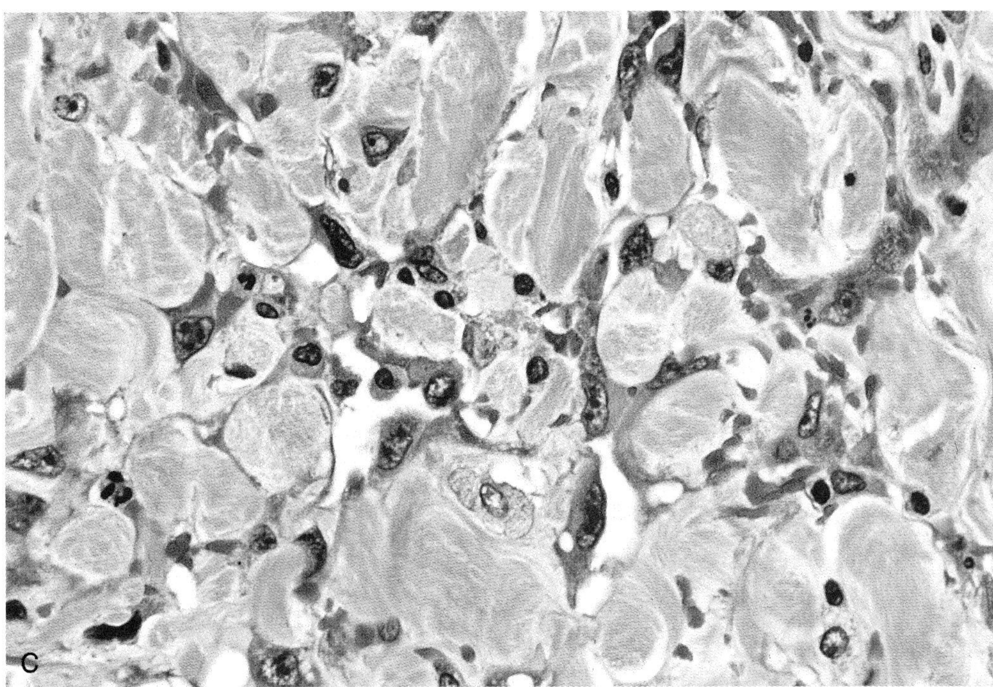


**FIGURE 25–6** *(Continued).* and between collagen bundles (**C**).

ated tumors may be pleomorphic and usually display prominent mitotic activity. A small number of angiosarcomas have a low grade appearance consisting of innocuous vessels infiltrating soft tissue and containing intraluminal papillations (Fig. 25–8). The diagnosis in these cases is based more on the pattern of growth than on the degree of cytologic atypia and mitotic activity.

### *Ultrastructural and Histochemical Findings*

The best-differentiated areas of these tumors have many of the features of normal endothelium, including a partial investiture of basal lamina along the antiluminal borders (Fig. 25–9), tight junctions between cells, pinocytotic vesicles, and occasional cytofilaments.[66,83] Weibel-Palade bodies, tubular structures found in normal endothelium, are present in a disappointingly small number of angiosarcomas[40,76,79,111] and, when present, are few in number. Poorly differentiated tumors, however, lack many and sometimes all of the foregoing features. However, in an ultrastructural study of 47 angiosarcomas, Mackay et al.[40] pointed out that poorly differentiated areas still display topographic features that suggest vascular differentiation, including a close relation between tumor cells and erythrocytes such that the latter lie between or sometimes within the cytoplasm of the former. Ramifying clefts between the cells suggest primitive or abortive vascular (luminal) differentiation. The authors did not note any ultrastructural differences between angiosarcomas arising in lymphedema and those that did not. Alkaline phosphatase, an enzyme found in vascular endothelium, has occasionally been identified.[81,83]

### *Immunohistochemical Findings*

Immunohistochemical confirmation of the diagnosis of angiosarcoma, even those that are poorly differentiated, can usually be accomplished using a panel of vascular markers. In recent years a number of new antibodies directed against various structural and protein products of endothelium has gradually replaced von Willebrand factor[30] in diagnostic importance. The latter, the most specific marker for endothelium, unfortunately lacks sensitivity in poorly differentiated vascular tumors, and the test may also be difficult to interpret because of a diffusion artifact. Use of CD34 and CD31, in our experience, identifies most angiosarcomas, including poorly differentiated ones, although there are a few caveats to be noted. CD34 (human hematopoietic progenitor cell antigen) is expressed by many angiosarcomas[54,57,63] and Kaposi's sarcoma, but it is also seen in some soft tissue tumors (e.g., epithelioid sarcoma) that may enter into the differential diagnosis of angiosarcoma.[14,57,68] CD31 (platelet-endothelial cell adhesion molecule), on the other hand, seems to be the more sensitive, more specific antigen for endothelial differentiation[53] (Fig. 25–10). In the context of soft tissue neoplasia, virtu-

*Text continued on page 930*

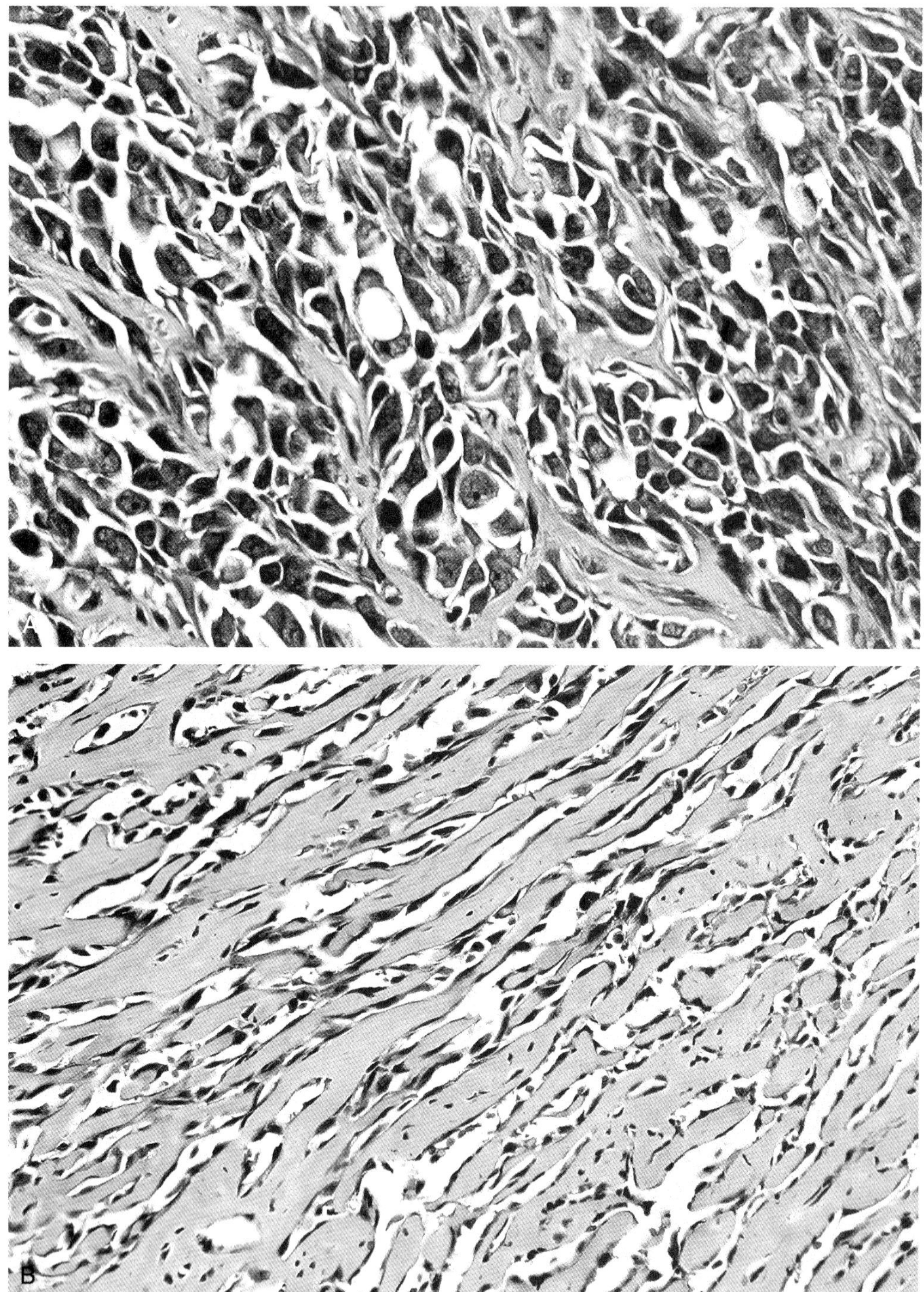


**FIGURE 25–7.** Variety of patterns in a high grade angiosarcoma, including a solid or medullary focus (**A**) and marked spindling of the cells (**B, C**).

*Illustration continued on opposite page*

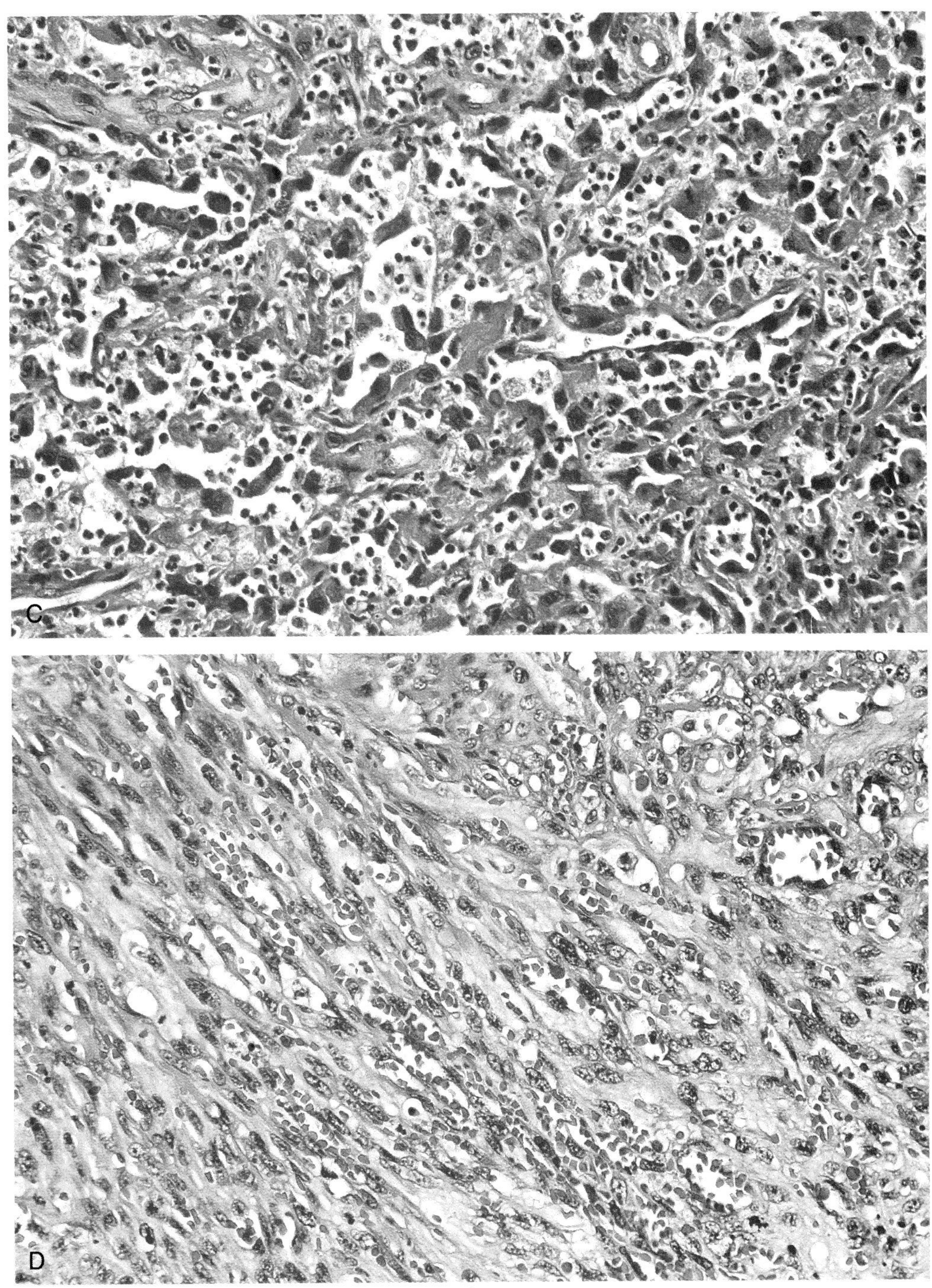


**FIGURE 25–7** *(Continued)*. (**D**) Highly pleomorphic tumor with rudimentary lumen formation.

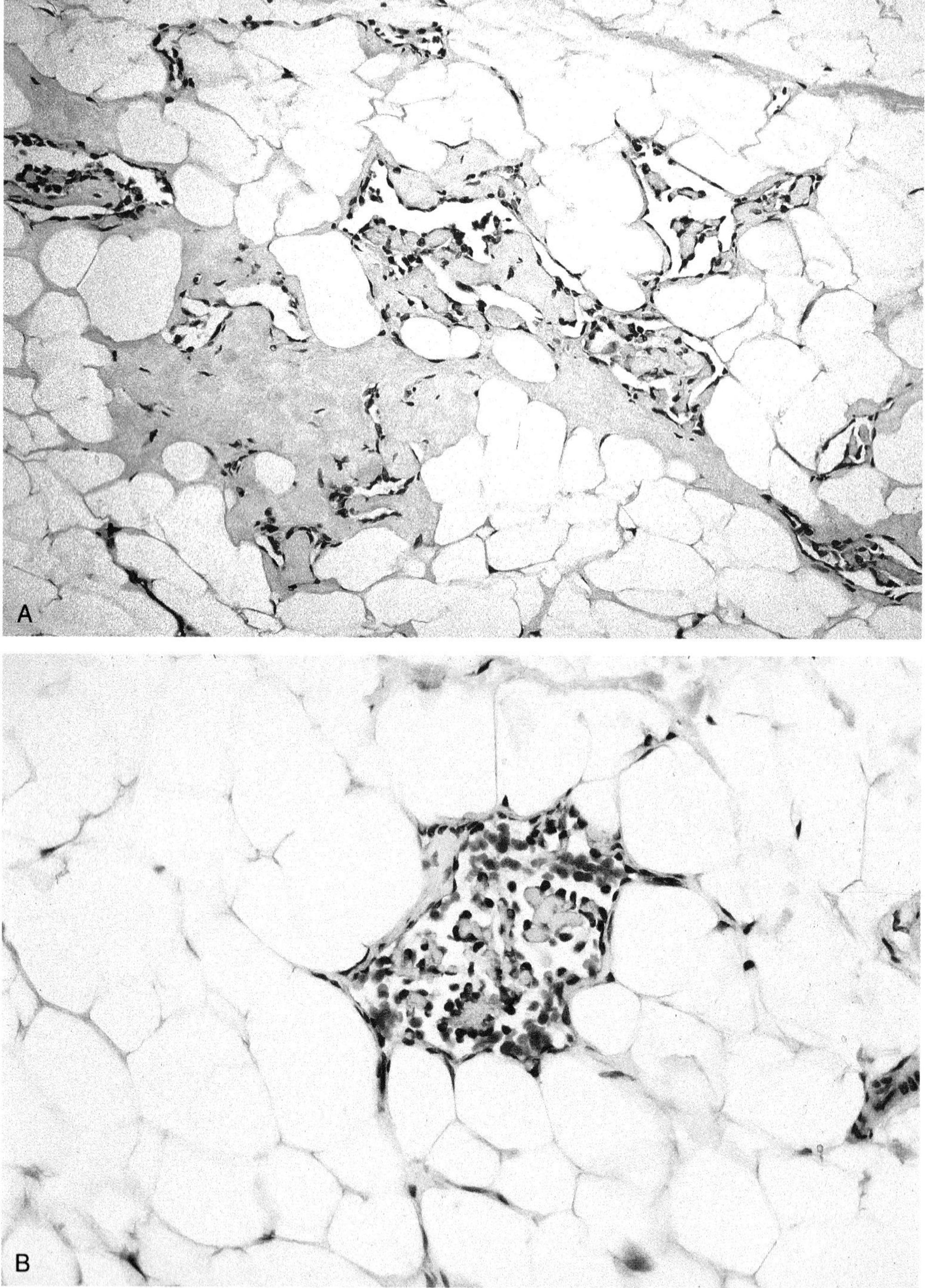


**FIGURE 25–8.** Low grade angiosarcoma with bland vessels dissecting fat (**A**), some with small intravascular papillations (**B**).

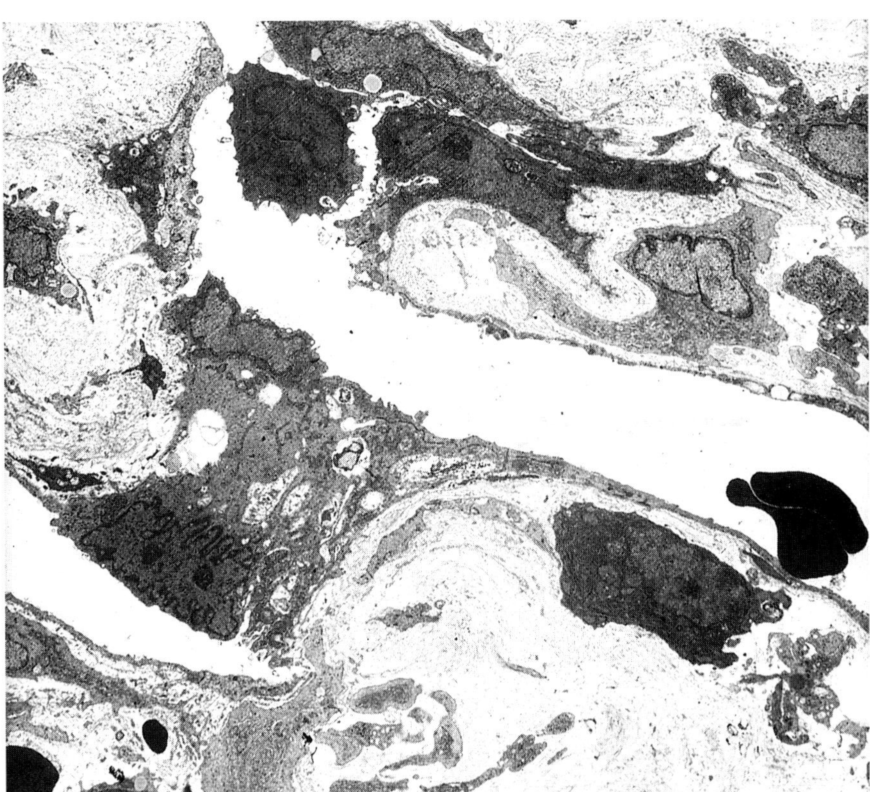

**FIGURE 25–9.** Electron micrograph of an angiosarcoma. An irregularly shaped blood vessel is lined by neoplastic endothelial cells with segments of basal lamina. Several perithelial cells and their processes are present outside the vessel wall (arrows). (Courtesy of Dr. Jerome B. Taxy.)

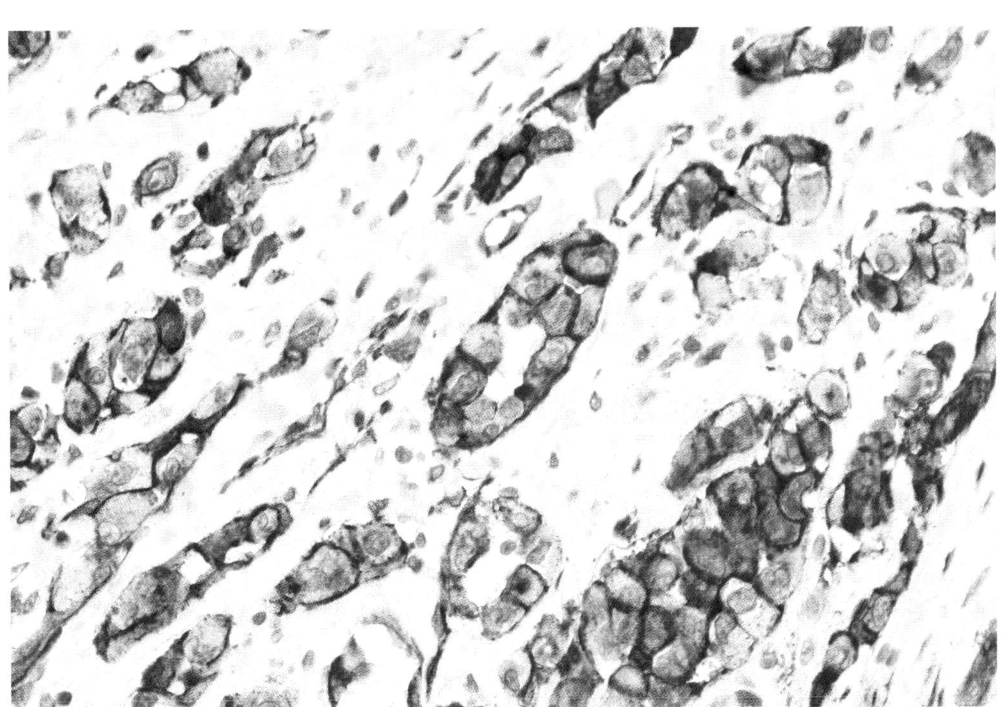

**FIGURE 25–10.** Immunostain for CD31 shows intense staining of most angiosarcoma cells.

ally all benign and malignant vascular tumors express this membrane protein, whereas more than 100 soft tissue tumors of nonvascular lineage do not.[18,52] The most prudent approach to the diagnosis of angiosarcomas, therefore, is to use immunohistochemical studies to rule out other diagnoses that may legitimately enter the differential diagnosis in a given case coupled with a panel of vascular markers (e.g., CD31, CD34) that, if positive, support the diagnosis of angiosarcoma.

A number of other substances have been employed to diagnose vascular tumors, but they are far less widely used than the foregoing. Nonimmunologic binding by *Ulex europaeus*, a plant lectin, to endothelium was formerly used as an adjunct with factor VIII-AG but is not specific, as it has been noted in other soft tissue tumors (e.g., synovial sarcoma, epithelioid sarcoma) and some carcinomas. Antibodies to thrombomodulin, an antagonist of factor VIII-AG, decorate most angiosarcomas but also react with various carcinomas, mesotheliomas, and trophoblastic tumors.[2,52,71] Although seldom required for diagnostic purposes, immunostains for laminin outline vascular channels by highlighting the basal lamina investing groups of neoplastic cells, and actin decorates pericytes occasionally present around neoplastic endothelium.[111]

A number of new biologic markers, which have not been extensively characterized in angiosarcomas, may prove useful for defining phenotypic differences among angiosarcomas. VEGFR-3, a sensitive lymphatic marker present in virtually all Kaposi's sarcomas, is present in about one-half of angiosarcomas[23] and co-localizes to the same cells that also express podoplanin, a 38-kDa membrane glycoprotein believed to be specific for lymphatic endothelium.[6] However, most angiosarcomas express podocalyxin as well as podoplanin, a substance that identifies vascular endothelium. Some have suggested that these findings support the hypothesis that most angiosarcomas display mixed lineage features. This of course makes the designation "angiosarcoma" all the more attractive.

### *Cytogenetic Findings*

Only a few angiosarcomas have been studied cytogenetically.[43,48,59] The chromosome number ranges from hypodiploid to hypertriploid. The most frequently abnormalities are gains in chromosomes 5, 8, and 20 and losses of chromosomes 7 and 22 and the Y chromosome.

### *Behavior and Treatment*

The prognosis of cutaneous angiosarcomas is poor,[78] partly because of the delay in seeking medical advice by patients, who are often elderly, and the tendency to underestimate and undertreat the tumors initially. In the largest series, 72 patients reported by Holden et al.,[79] only 12% survived 5 years or more, with one-half dying within 15 months of presentation. A comparably poor outlook was documented by Maddox and Evans[41] in their group of 17 patients, 16 of whom died of complications of the tumor. The series of 57 patients reported by Mark et al. documented a 5-year survival of 24%, although they included patients with organ-related angiosarcomas (e.g., heart, liver, breast).[80]

The most important factor for determining prognosis in many studies seems to be the size of the initial lesion. Tumors $<5$ cm in diameter have a significantly better prognosis than larger lesions.[41,79,80] Mark et al.[80] reported a 5-year survival of 32% for lesions $<5$ cm compared to 13% for those $>5$ cm. Grade has been correlated with outcome in some studies[41] but not in others.[78] Factors such as gender and location do not correlate with prognosis.[72] Death due to the disease results from local extension of the tumor or metastasis. Usually recurrences and metastases are noted within 2 years of diagnosis, although in the series of 12 cases reported by Haustein one patient died of extensive local disease without metastases.[76]

Sites affected by metastases are most commonly the cervical lymph nodes, followed by lung, liver, and spleen. Several long-term survivors of cutaneous angiosarcomas have been studied by Holden et al.,[79] who noted that they had all undergone radical radiotherapy, mostly wide-field electron beam therapy. Likewise, Mark et al. noted significantly improved survival in patients who underwent radiotherapy in addition to surgery.[80]

## Angiosarcoma Associated with Lymphedema

In 1949 Stewart and Treves[97] reported six patients who developed vascular sarcomas following radical mastectomy and axillary lymph node dissection for breast carcinoma. Although some of the patients had also undergone radiotherapy, the common denominator in each of the cases appeared to be the presence of chronic lymphedema, which usually supervened shortly after mastectomy. Since this original description, approximately 200 cases of vascular sarcomas complicating chronic lymphedema have been recorded. Not unexpectedly, most have occurred in women following mastectomy, although tumors have been documented on the abdominal wall following lymph node dissection for carcinoma of the penis[84] and the arm or leg affected by congenital,[86] idiopathic, or traumatic lymphedema. Other reports have noted the association of angiosarcoma with filarial lymphedema.[85–95] The pathogenesis of these unusual tumors is far from understood. It has been suggested that chronic lymphatic obstruction results in an abortive attempt at collateralization that eventually goes awry. Other explanations obviously must be considered, and localized defects in cellular immunity may play a role, as it has been noted that homografts transplanted to lymphedematous extremities survive far longer than those transplanted to the normal extremity of the same patient.[92] Moreover, it is possible that radiotherapy plays a secondary role in some cases by enhancing or aggravating the lymphedema.

### Clinical Findings

About 90% of all angiosarcomas associated with chronic lymphedema occur after mastectomy for breast carcinoma,[99] although the frequency of this complication has been estimated by Shirger[93] as only 0.45% of all women who survive 5 years after mastectomy. These patients are typically women in their seventh decade who have developed a significant degree of lymphedema, usually within a year of mastectomy. The tumors develop within 10 years of the original surgery, although the interval may be as short as 4 years or as long as 27 years. In rare instances the tumor has been reported in postmastectomy patients who have experienced little or no lymphedema. Whether some patients truly have no lymphedema must be questioned because minor degrees of lymphedema in obese patients could go undetected clinically.

When these tumors occur in congenital or idiopathic lymphedema, the affected patients are usually younger, the lymphedema is of longer duration, and any extremity may be affected. Most patients are in their fourth or fifth decade and have experienced lymphedema for 19–20 years. There has been one case of congenital lymphedema and angiosarcoma associated with Maffucci syndrome.[98]

Regardless of the clinical setting, the onset of cancer is heralded by the development of one or more polymorphic lesions superimposed on the brawny nonpitting edema of the affected extremity. Deeply situated lesions in the subcutis may impart only a mottled purple-red hue to the overlying skin, whereas the superficial lesion can be palpated as distinct nodules that coalesce to form large polypoid growths (Fig. 25–11). Ulceration, accompanied by a serosanguineous discharge, characterizes late lesions. Repeated healing and breakdown give rise to lesions of various stages that spread distally to the hands and feet or proximally to the chest wall or trunk in advanced cases of lymphangiosarcoma.

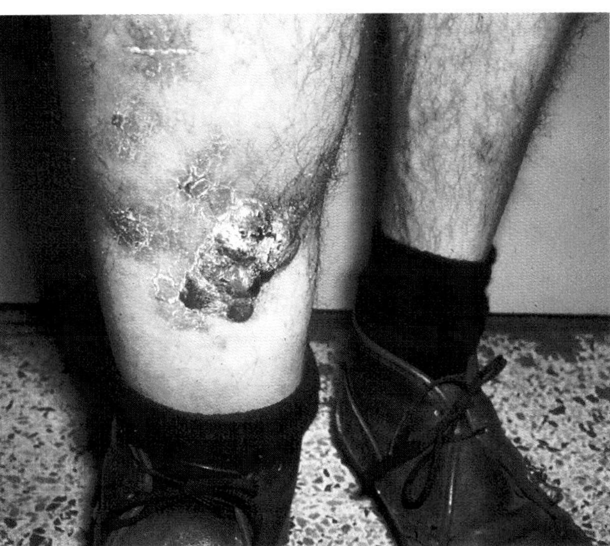

**FIGURE 25–11.** Angiosarcoma in a lymphedematous extremity.

### Microscopic Findings

Despite the fact that the term *lymphangiosarcoma* is commonly used, these lesions appear essentially identical to those of the head and neck described in the preceding sections. The hallmark of the lesion is the presence of small capillary-size vessels composed of obviously malignant cells that infiltrate soft tissue and skin. The lumens may be empty, filled with clear fluid, or engorged with erythrocytes, a finding that has made it difficult to classify these tumors as to blood vessel or lymphatic origin and has led to the suggestion that two lines of differentiation may be present. Lymphocytes are occasionally found around the neoplastic vessels, but because this feature is also seen in other angiosarcomas it does not provide sufficient evidence of lymphatic differentiation.

Perhaps the only feature that sets this tumor apart from the conventional angiosarcomas discussed in this chapter and provides some support for lymphatic differentiation is its association with areas of so-called lymphangiomatosis.[99] These changes appear to represent premalignant changes of small vessels, presumably lymphatics. The vessels become dilated and appear to form a diffuse ramifying network throughout the soft tissue (Fig. 25–12). They are lined by plump endothelial cells with hyperchromatic nuclei. These areas may merge imperceptibly with areas of frank angiosarcoma or may exist alone in patients who have not yet developed discrete clinical lesions.[87]

Therapy for this premalignant lesion is problematic. Such patients probably are at risk of developing angiosarcoma and deserve scrupulous follow-up care. It seems best to recommend therapy only for patients who have developed distinct clinical lesions.

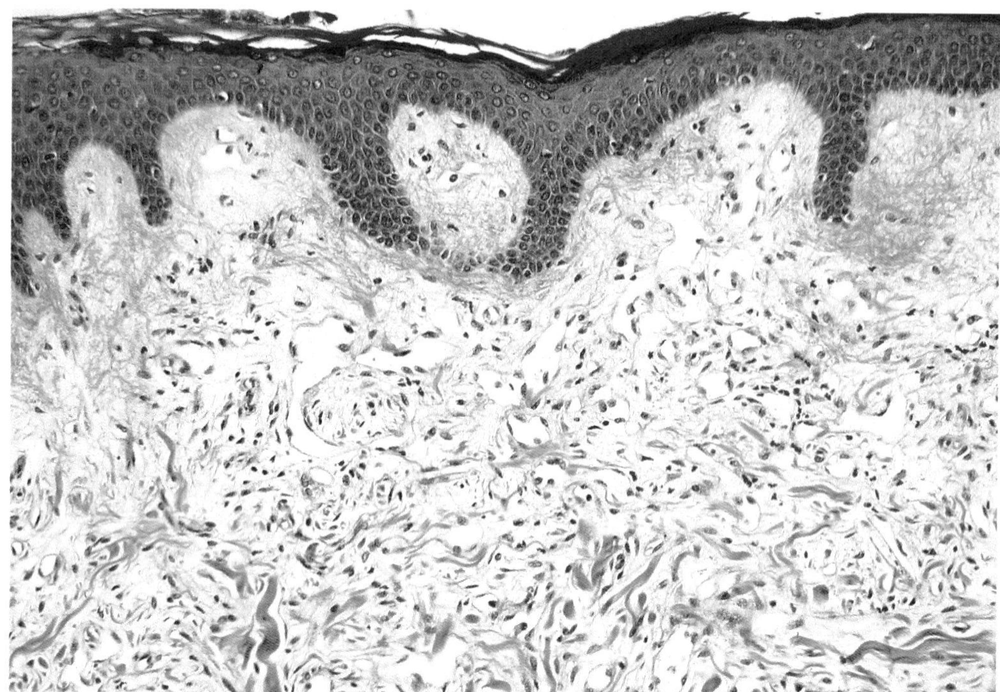

**FIGURE 25–12.** Diffuse proliferation of dermal lymphatic vessels (lymphangiomatosis) containing atypical endothelium. Lesion occurred in a patient a few years after mastectomy for breast carcinoma. Minimal lymphedema was present. Such changes have been considered "premalignant" and may herald the onset of frank angiosarcoma (lymphangiosarcoma). (×160)

### *Electron Microscopic Findings*

One of the most significant contributions of electron microscopy to the understanding of this disease has been to eradicate any lingering doubt concerning the possibility that these tumors represent carcinomas, specifically late recurrence of the original breast carcinoma.[88,94] Ultrastructurally, the best-differentiated areas of this tumor have features of capillary endothelial cells, including numerous pinocytotic vesicles, lateral desmosome-like attachments, and occasionally paranuclear filaments.[86,88] The cells are, furthermore, surrounded by basal lamina outside of which pericytes may be identified. Weibel-Palade bodies have also been identified.[88] There appear to be no differences ultrastructurally between the tumors that arise in lymphedema and those that do not,[40] although in one case reported by Kindblom et al.[88] the authors believed that some areas showed lymphatic as well as vascular differentiation. Although electron microscopy can document subtle degrees of endothelial differentiation not appreciated by light microscopy, poorly differentiated tumors understandably contain few ultrastructural features that would permit their recognition. In these areas, the cells resemble primitive mesenchymal cells containing abundant rough endoplasmic reticulum, glycogen, few intercellular attachments, and no luminal differentiation.[94]

### *Behavior and Treatment*

It is difficult to interpret survival data reliably because of the paucity of cases and the fact that early cases were treated suboptimally by modern standards. Woodward et al.[99] attempted a retrospective analysis of these tumors based on their experience at the Mayo Clinic and that reported in the literature. The mean (actuarial) survival time of patients with (lymph)angiosarcoma following mastectomy was 19 months, compared with 34 months for those developing the tumor outside this setting. The median survival time of patients with angiosarcoma and lymphedema in the experience of the Memorial Hospital is 31 months.[96] Only 6 of the 40 patients survived 5 years or longer. The salient point in both studies is that long-term survivors have usually been treated by initial radical ablative surgery, either limb disarticulation or hindquarter or forequarter amputation. Patients treated by less radical surgery or by irradiation run an unacceptably high risk of local recurrence. It is probable that "local recurrence" of this disease is an expression of extensive multifocal disease, a phenomenon that underscores the need to excise the lesions radically. Metastases to the lung, pleura, and chest wall are common and account for essentially all of the disease-related deaths.

## Angiosarcoma of the Breast

Angiosarcoma of the breast is a rare tumor, accounting for approximately 1 in 1700–2000 primary malignant tumors of the breast.[103,104] Despite its highly malignant nature, it may have a deceptively bland appearance, a phenomenon that has led to underdiagnosis in almost half of the reported cases. Unlike other angiosarcomas, this type occurs exclusively in women, usually during the third or fourth decade. Only occasional cases have been reported during the postmenopausal period. Several cases have been reported in pregnant women,[102,106,107] and at least one tumor rapidly enlarged with the onset of pregnancy.[103]

These lesions usually develop as rapidly growing masses that cause diffuse enlargement of the breast associated with blue-red discoloration of the skin (Fig. 25–13). Despite the appreciable size at the time of biopsy, the classic signs of ordinary mammary carcinoma, such as skin retraction, nipple discharge, and axillary node enlargement, are absent. The tumors are invariably located deep in the substance of the breast. They usually spread to involve the skin but seldom extend into the pectoral fascia. The tumors are ill-defined, hemorrhagic, spongy masses surrounded by a rim of vascular engorgement. The rim corresponds to a zone of well-differentiated but nonetheless neoplastic capillary-size vessels that can be compared with areas of a hemangioma except that their growth is more permeative. The main tumor mass shows the same changes that characterize other angiosarcomas. Likewise, metastasis may resemble the parent lesion or may show less differentiation. In one unusual case we reviewed, extramedullary hematopoiesis was present in the metastasis despite its absence in the original tumor.[106]

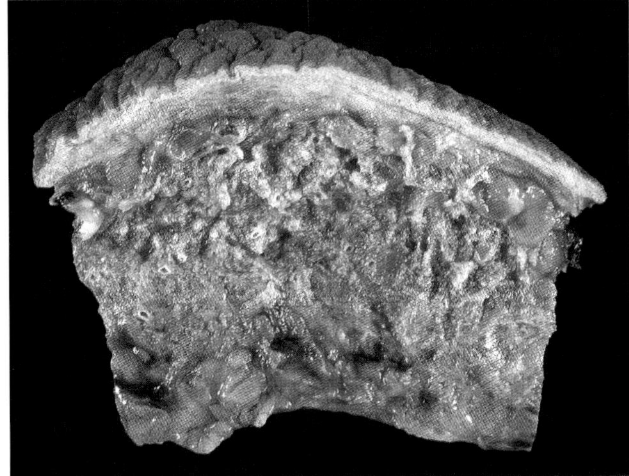

**FIGURE 25–13.** Angiosarcoma of the breast with a sponge-like quality.

### *Differential Diagnosis*

The differential diagnosis of this lesion lies principally in distinguishing it from *benign hemangioma* or *angiolipoma,* which on rare occasions involves the breast. In our experience angiosarcomas of the breast are ill-defined lesions that almost always contain cellular areas with atypia, mitotic activity, and necrosis. It is the presence of these features that ultimately distinguishes these tumors from hemangiomas. However, because some areas of an angiosarcoma can be well differentiated, it is advisable to totally embed small histologically benign or borderline lesions. Large lesions presenting the same diagnostic problem should be generously sampled. True hemangiomas or angiolipomas of the breast are usually sharply demarcated from normal breast tissue. The vessels of a hemangioma are regular in shape, whereas those of angiolipoma have typical microthrombi.

### *Behavior and Treatment*

Angiosarcomas are the most malignant of all breast tumors.[104] Of the approximately 50 patients reported in the literature, about 90% have died of the disease, usually within 2 years of diagnosis. Metastasis occurs relatively rapidly after diagnosis and most frequently involves the lungs, skin, and bone. In some instances massive bleeding from metastatic lesions appears to be the immediate cause of death.[101] In a study of 40 patients treated at two institutions, the survival rate was much better and could be correlated with the tumor grade. More than three-fourths of patients with grade I lesions were alive compared with fewer than one-fifth with grade III lesions.[100]

A similar trend was noted for 15 patients with breast angiosarcoma entered into the Connecticut Tumor Registry.[105] The best chance of survival is among patients who present shortly after the onset of symptoms with relatively small lesions and who undergo prompt mastectomy.[107] Less radical procedures almost always lead to local recurrence. Axillary lymph node dissection is not essential for management of this disease because metastasis to these structures, even in the face of large primary lesions, is rare. Adjuvant chemotherapy, particularly with dactinomycin, seems to be effective in some patients.

## Angiosarcoma of Soft Tissue

Angiosarcomas arising from and essentially restricted to deep soft tissue are uncommon. The estimate that one-fourth of angiosarcomas are of this type (Table 25–1) likely overestimates their frequency, as many are probably cutaneous angiosarcomas with deep extension. Even allowing for the difficulty of ascertain-

**TABLE 25-5 AGE DISTRIBUTION OF ANGIOSARCOMAS OF SOFT TISSUE: 1966–1976 (89 CASES)**

| Age (Years) | No. of Cases | % |
|---|---|---|
| 0–10 | 12 | 12 |
| 11–20 | 14 | 16 |
| 21–30 | 16 | 18 |
| 31–40 | 12 | 13 |
| 41–50 | 8 | 10 |
| 51–60 | 11 | 12 |
| >60 | 16 | 19 |
| *Total* | 89 | 100 |

Data are from the AFIP.

**TABLE 25-7 ANATOMIC DISTRIBUTION OF ANGIOSARCOMAS OF SOFT TISSUE: 1966–1976 (89 CASES)**

| Location | No. of Cases | % |
|---|---|---|
| Leg | 34 | 38 |
| Arm | 17 | 19 |
| Trunk | 22 | 25 |
| Head and neck | 13 | 15 |
| Unknown | 3 | 3 |
| *Total* | 89 | 100 |

Data are from the AFIP.

ing acceptable cases, it appears that these tumors do not display the relatively homogeneous clinical characteristics of other angiosarcomas. Rather, these tumors occur at any age and are evenly distributed throughout all decades (Tables 25–5, 25–6). About one-third develop in association with other conditions such as inherited diseases (neurofibromatosis, Klippel-Trénaunay syndrome, Maffucci syndrome), synthetic vascular grafts, and other neoplasms. Like the more common soft tissue sarcomas, this form of angiosarcoma has a propensity to occur on the extremities or in the abdominal cavity (Table 25–7), where it presents as a large, markedly hemorrhagic mass (Fig. 25–14). It is not unusual for these tumors to be confused with a chronic hematoma, even after biopsy of the tumor, if the biopsy material is limited or nonrepresentative. In the very young the large size of this tumor may result in hematologic abnormalities, such as thrombocytopenia, high-output cardiac failure from arteriovenous shunting, or even death due to massive exsanguination. Unlike angiosarcomas of the skin, deep angiosarcomas more commonly have an epithelioid appearance consisting of nests and clusters of round cells of high nuclear grade[108,110,111] (Figs. 25–15, 25–16). These so-called epithelioid angiosarcomas consist of sheets of highly atypical round cells with prominent nuclei, some of which contain intracytoplasmic lumens. In addition to factor VIII-AG, about one-third of cases also express cytokeratin,[25,108,111] a finding that may make distinction from a carcinoma problematic. The presence of CD31 therefore becomes an essential adjunctive stain.

**TABLE 25-6 GENDER DISTRIBUTION OF ANGIOSARCOMAS OF SOFT TISSUE: 1966–1976 (89 CASES)**

| Gender | No. of Cases | % |
|---|---|---|
| Male | 58 | 66 |
| Female | 28 | 32 |
| Unknown | 3 | 2 |
| *Total* | 89 | 100 |

Data are from the AFIP.

In one study, soft tissue angiosarcomas proved to be aggressive neoplasms.[111] Altogether, 53% of patients were dead of the disease within 1 year; another 31% had no evidence of disease at 46 months. Overall 20% of patients experienced local recurrences and 49% distant metastasis, most often to the lung followed by lymph node, bone, and soft tissue. The features statistically associated with poor outcome included older age, retroperitoneal location, large size, and high Ki67 values (>10%). In a smaller series of epithelioid angiosarcomas four of six patients died of the disease.[108]

## Radiation-induced Angiosarcoma

Although not a common postirradiation sarcoma, angiosarcomas have been documented following therapeutic irradiation for tumors of diverse types. In previous decades postirradiation angiosarcomas commonly presented as intraabdominal or abdominal wall masses following irradiation for carcinoma of the

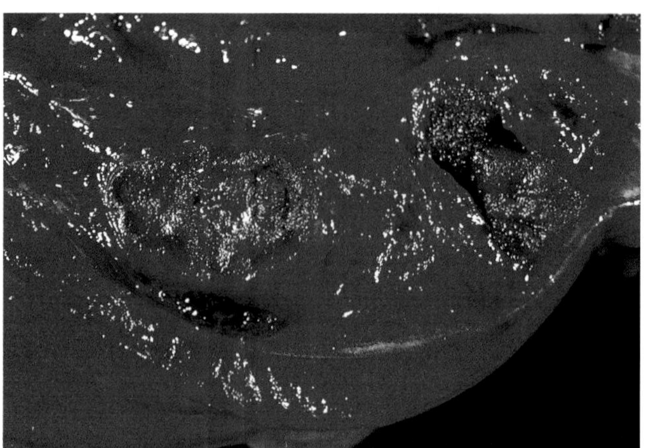

**FIGURE 25–14.** Angiosarcoma in deep soft tissue with prominent hemorrhage.

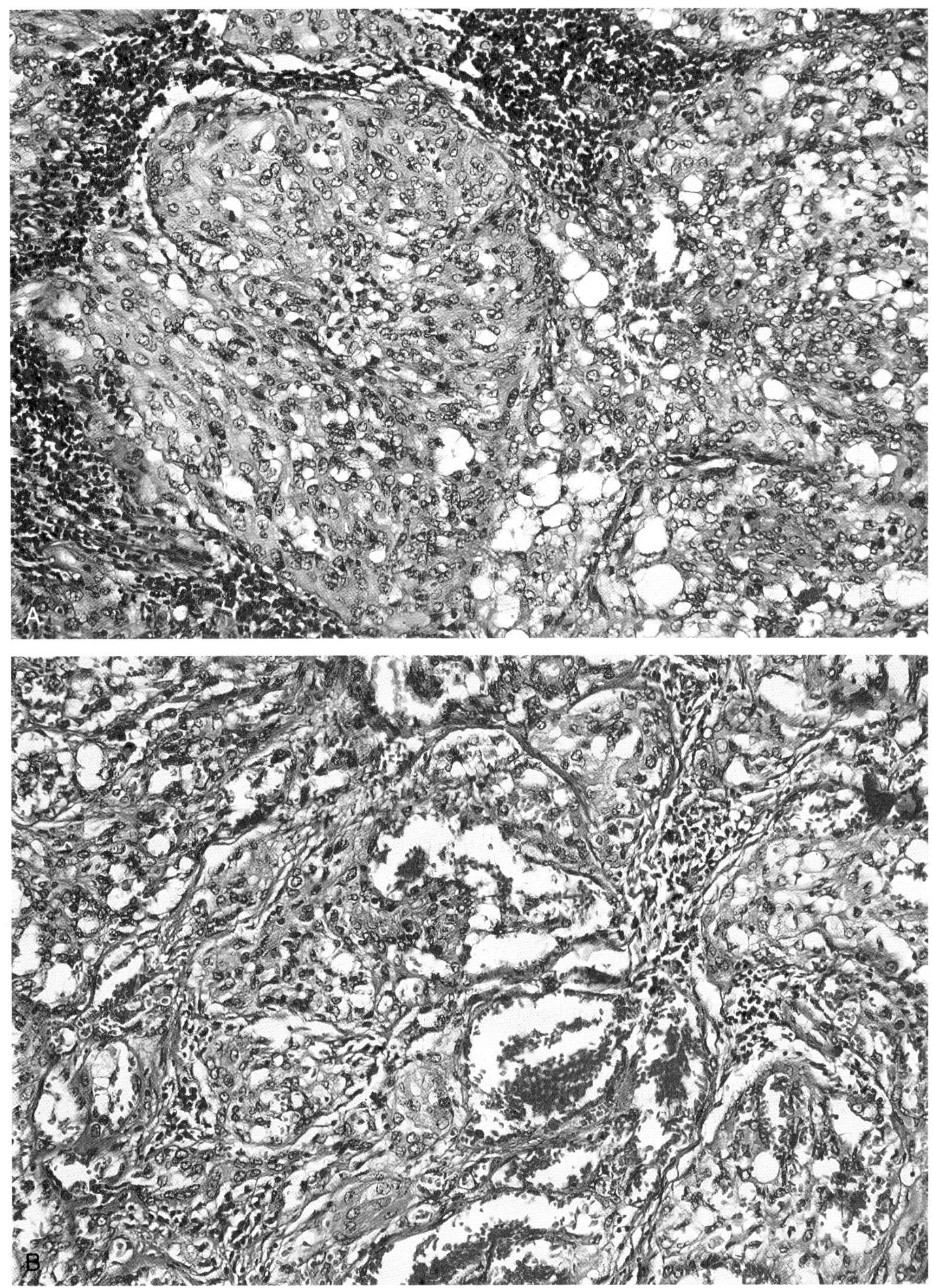


**FIGURE 25-15.** Angiosarcoma of deep soft tissue with a solid medullary pattern (**A**) with focal luminal differentiation (**B**).

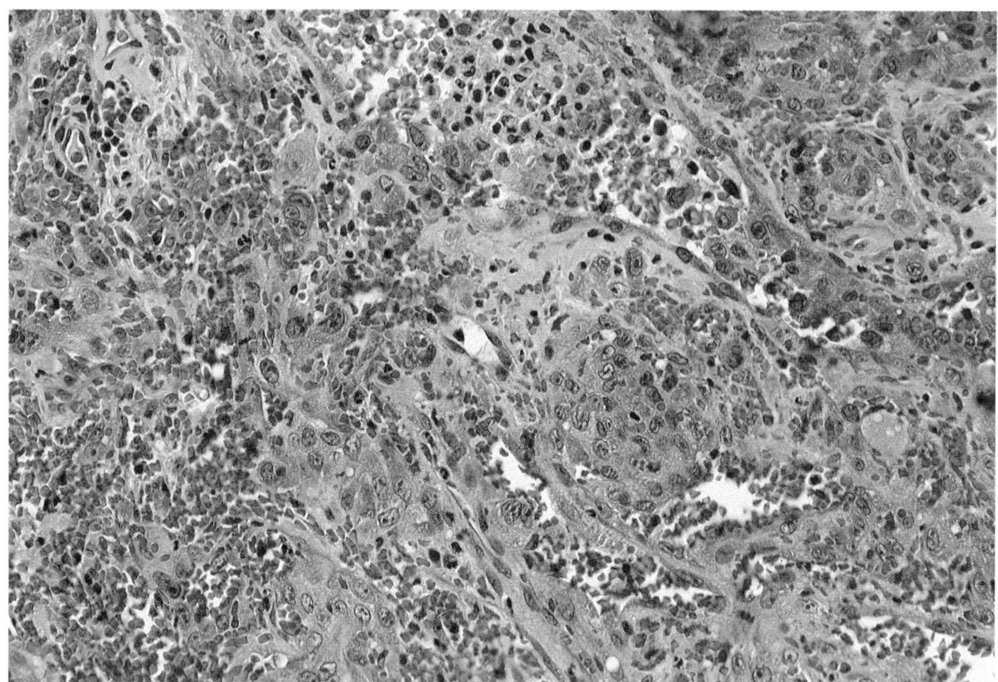

**FIGURE 25–16.** Epithelioid angiosarcoma of deep soft tissue.

cervix, ovary, or uterus, with a small number of cases occurring after irradiation for various other malignant or benign conditions.[75,77,127,128] During the last several years, however, the clinical profile seems to be changing. More than 50 angiosarcomas involving the skin or breast parenchyma have been reported in women who have had breast-sparing surgery and irradiation for mammary carcinoma often coupled with axillary lymph node dissection.[113–119,121,123–126] Based on a recent survey by the French Comprehensive Cancer Centers, 9 cases were identified from a cohort of 20,000 women treated conservatively for breast carcinoma.[117] These lesions occurred an average of 6 years after completion of therapy for the breast carcinoma, although many occurred after a latent period of less than 5 years. Most of these patients had not had lymphedema, suggesting that the significant commonality is irradiation. The onset of these lesions is heralded by ecchymoses or thickening of the skin with one or more elevated lesions (Fig. 25–17). Most are high grade lesions and have histologic features similar to those of other angiosarcomas. In the French experience all but one of the nine patients died of disease within 15 months of diagnosis. There are a few cases, such as the one reported by Moskaluk et al.,[118] that were low-grade or borderline vascular tumors that recurred repeatedly but did not metastasize. They seem to be the exception rather than the rule.

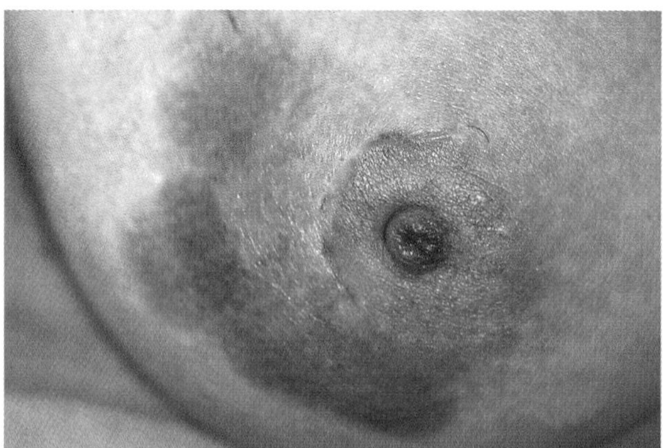

**FIGURE 25–17.** Cutaneous angiosarcoma of the breast after breast-conserving surgery and irradiation for carcinoma.

In addition to the foregoing lesions, there is a small number of "atypical vascular lesions" arising in this setting that do not fulfill the criteria of angiosarcoma and thus far have proved to be benign.[115] Four such cases were reported by Fineberg and Rosen,[115] and three were identified among the 20,000 cases reviewed by the French cancer centers.[117] These lesions usually present as small (<1 cm), solitary, elevated pink lesions that, unlike angiosarcoma, are not associated with any alterations or discoloration of the surrounding skin. They are circumscribed, intradermal nodules surrounded by a fibroblastic response; they consist of delicate vessels, possibly lymphatics, that ramify to a limited extent but do not extend into the subcutis (Fig. 25–18). The endothelium may protrude

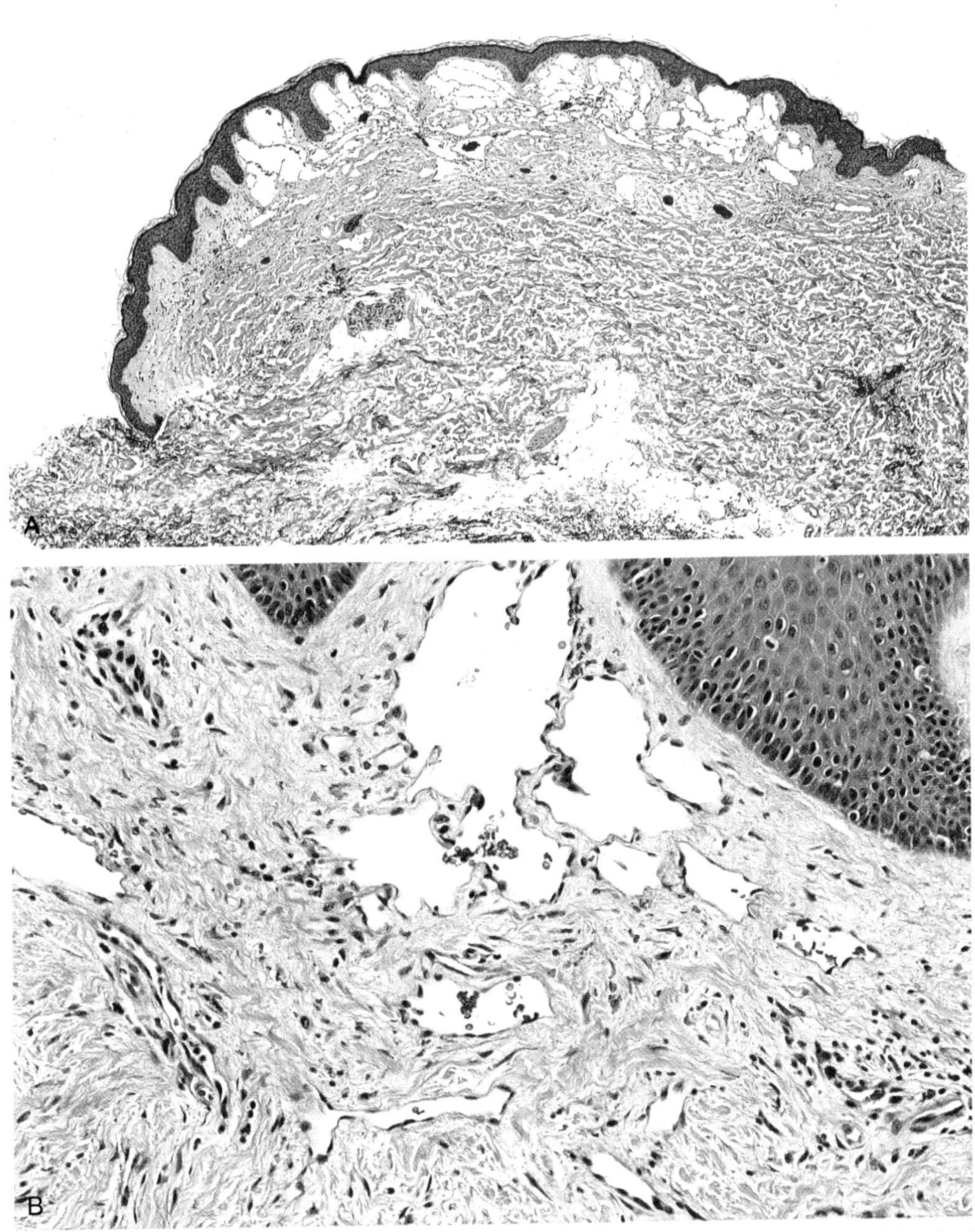


**FIGURE 25–18.** Atypical vascular lesion of the breast after breast-conserving surgery and irradiation for carcinoma. This lesion is a circumscribed dermal nodule (**A**) with minimal endothelial atypia but some anastomotic growth (**B**). Lesions of this type thus far have proved to be benign.

into the lumen, but it is typically one layer thick and of low nuclear grade. All four patients reported by Fineberg and Rosen were alive and well with follow-up periods as long as 10 years.[115] Although the number of cases is small and the amount of follow-up too limited to be dogmatic about these lesions, we are of the opinion that they are the result of radiation damage, rather than neoplastic or preneoplastic change.

## KAPOSI'S SARCOMA

In 1872 Kaposi[165] described five cases of an unusual tumor that principally affected the skin of the lower extremities in a multifocal, often symmetrical fashion. He considered the condition a round cell sarcoma that he termed "idiopathic multiple pigmented sarcoma of the skin." Since his description there have been dissenting opinions as to whether the lesions are hyperplasias or neoplasms. Studies analyzing Kaposi's sarcoma lesions for clonality by means of X-chromosome inactivation patterns have shown that the lesions can be monoclonal or polyclonal. In patients with multiple lesions, results have been contradictory. Some studies have illustrated clonality in separate lesions in the same patient,[183] suggesting that the disease is a disseminated monoclonal neoplasm, whereas others have found different inactivation patterns, suggesting a multifocal lesion arising from independently transformed cells.[153] Despite its precise position in the spectrum between neoplasia and hyperplasia,[138] there is general acceptance that Kaposi's sarcoma is a virus-associated if not virus-induced disease and that the course of the disease is strongly influenced by the immune status of the patient.

A number of potential causative viral agents have been considered in the past, including human immunodeficiency virus- (HIV-1), cytomegalovirus,[156] and papillomavirus.[160] The marked disparity of the disease in the various HIV risk groups and the failure to identify HIV in Kaposi's sarcoma cells rapidly cast doubt on the idea that HIV-1 was the causative agent.[130,131] In 1994 Chang and associates identified a virus in the Kaposi's sarcoma cells of a patient with acquired immunodeficiency syndrome (AIDS).[134] Termed Kaposi's sarcoma-associated herpes virus, it is most widely known as human herpes virus 8 (HHV8). It is the first human member of a group of viruses known as *Rhadinovirus*,[178] noteworthy because they rarely produce apparent disease in their normal host but become more virulent with transpecies infections. In addition to Kaposi's sarcoma, HHV8 has been associated with multifocal Castleman's disease and body cavity lymphomas.

At present there is strong circumstantial evidence that HHV8 is likely the causative agent of Kaposi's sarcoma.[199] This statement is supported by the following observations: (1) HHV8 infection as determined by antibodies to latency-associated nuclear antigen, a viral protein, parallels almost precisely the prevalence of Kaposi's sarcoma in AIDS risk groups and in various geographic areas of the world. The virus is present in most patients with Kaposi's sarcoma regardless of the clinical type, yet it is not present in the normal population to any significant degree. (2) There is a strong predictive value between detection of HHV8 genome in the blood of HIV-positive homosexual males and their subsequent development of Kaposi's sarcoma. (3) Virus can be identified in Kaposi's sarcoma cells.[133,141,158,161,169] (4) The genome of HHV8 contains homologues of cellular genes (e.g., v-*cyclin*) which can stimulate cell growth and angiogenesis.[175] (5) Introduction of HHV8 into human endothelial cells in vitro partially transforms the cells.[147] Infected cells exhibit prolongation of survival, acquisition of telomerase activity, and anchorage-independent growth.[142] Nonetheless, it has not yet been possible to demonstrate direct in vivo transmission from tumor to target cells or from human to human.

Despite all of the above evidence, it appears that the growth and maintenance of Kaposi's sarcoma may depend on a complex set of interactions.[151,154,177,189] For example, the product of the HIV-1 *TAT* gene is capable of stimulating the growth of Kaposi's sarcoma cells,[144,151] and HIV-infected T cells release a number of cytokines that also enhance tumor growth (paracrine effect). In addition, Kaposi's cells themselves produce a number of cytokines (e.g., VEGF) that through their receptors stimulate their own growth (autocrine effect).[172]

### Clinical Findings

Kaposi's sarcoma occurs in four principal clinical forms: chronic, lymphadenopathic, transplantation-associated, and AIDS-related.[135,170,174]

### Chronic Kaposi's Sarcoma

The chronic or classic form occurs primarily in men (90%) during late adult life (peak incidence sixth and seventh decades). The disease is prevalent in certain parts of the world including Poland, Russia, Italy, and the central equatorial region of Africa. In the latter region it accounts for up to 9% of all reported cancers.[132] It is rare in the United States, accounting for only 0.02% of all cancers. This form manifests a statistically significant association with a second malignant tumor or an altered immune state.[188] A study from Memorial Hospital indicates that about one-third of patients (34 of 92) with this form of Kaposi's sarcoma have or subsequently develop a second malignant tumor, and half of these neoplasms are of lymphoreticular origin, including leukemia, lymphoma, and multiple myeloma.[188] Kaposi's sarcoma may also be associated with pure red blood cell aplasia[185] and autoimmune hemolytic anemia.[185]

The disease commences with the development of multiple cutaneous lesions, usually on the distal portion of the lower extremity. Less commonly the lesions occur on the upper extremity and rarely in a visceral organ in the absence of cutaneous manifestations. The initial lesion is a blue-red nodule often accompanied by edema of the extremity. The latter sign has been interpreted by some as indicating deep soft tissue or lymphatic involvement by the tumor. The lesions slowly increase in size and number, spreading proximally and coalescing into plaques or polypoid growths that may resemble pyogenic granuloma. Occasional lesions even ulcerate. In some patients the early lesions regress; others evolve so that many stages of the disease are present at the same time. The course of the disease is characteristically prolonged.

### *Lymphadenopathic Kaposi's Sarcoma*

In contrast to the foregoing type, lymphadenopathic Kaposi's sarcoma occurs primarily in young African children who present with localized or generalized lymphadenopathy, with involvement of cervical, inguinal, and hilar lymph node chains and occasionally of ocular tissues and salivary gland. Skin lesions are usually sparse and, when they occur, develop more centrally than in the chronic form. The course of the disease is fulminant, which has been attributed to a tendency toward internal involvement.

### *Transplantation-associated Kaposi's Sarcoma*

The development of Kaposi's sarcoma in renal transplant patients is well established, although the incidence varies depending on the patient population, suggesting that genetic background influences the risk in the posttransplant setting as well. For example, in Western countries the incidence of posttransplantation Kaposi's sarcoma has been estimated at less than 1%, whereas in the Near East it approaches 4%. There are conflicting data as to whether the type of immunosuppression affects this risk.[182,193]

The disease develops several months to a few years after the transplant (average 16 months), and the extent of the disease can be correlated directly with the loss of cellular immunity as measured by the response to phytohemagglutinin (PHA), conconavalin A (Con A), pokeweed mitogen (PWM), and dinitrochlorobenzene (DNCB) skin testing. In a few instances of transplantation-associated Kaposi's sarcoma, the tumor occurred at a previous surgical site.[192]

The clinical course of this form of Kaposi's sarcoma depends on the stage of the disease and the ability to manipulate the immunosuppressive dosage successfully. In the experience cited by Qunibi et al.,[182] patients with disease restricted to the skin who could tolerate a 50% reduction in the immunosuppression dosage had a 100% response rate. Patients who develop organ or internal involvement succumb to their disease.

### *AIDS-related Kaposi's Sarcoma*

Caused by HIV-1, AIDS produces profound immunodeficiency and susceptibility to opportunistic infections and various tumors.[146] AIDS probably originated in Africa, where its epidemic proportions have been attributed to heterosexual transmission and to transmission via contaminated medical equipment (e.g., syringes).[181] In the United States most cases occur in the male homosexual population, although other risk groups, including intravenous drug users and hemophiliacs receiving factor VIII-enriched blood fractions, are also well recognized. Approximately 30% of patients with AIDS develop Kaposi's sarcoma, and in many instances diagnosis of the tumor leads to clinical recognition of the syndrome.[155] Kaposi's sarcoma, however, does not affect the known risk groups equally.[136] Roughly 40% of homosexual patients with AIDS have developed Kaposi's sarcoma compared with less than 5% in the other recognized risk groups. It has only rarely occurred in transfusion recipients.[197,315] As discussed above, the incidence of Kaposi's sarcoma in the AIDS population closely parallels the seropositivity for HHV8. It furthermore appears that in the homosexual male population in the United States the virus is probably transmitted sexually, as there is a strong correlation between seropositivity, the number of male sexual partners, and a history of sexually transmitted diseases.

In the AIDS syndrome, Kaposi's sarcoma develops in a young adult population (mean age 39 years). Initially the lesions are small, flat, pink patches (Fig. 25–19); they only later acquire the classic blue-violet papular appearance (Fig. 25–20). They occur in almost any location but have a predilection for lines of cleavage. Lesions on the tip of the nose have also been noted. Most patients present with multiple oral or cutaneous lesions and many with internal lesions.

## Microscopic Findings

There appears to be no fundamental difference in the appearance of Kaposi's sarcoma among the various clinical groups. In our experience, the early lesions of

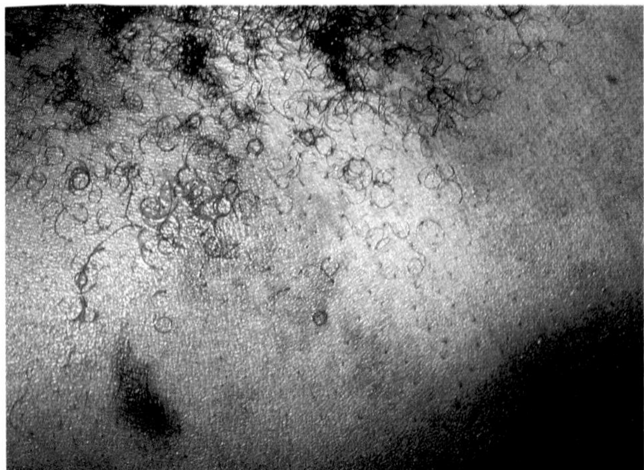

**FIGURE 25–19.** Early patch stage of Kaposi's sarcoma as seen in a patient with acquired immunodeficiency syndrome (AIDS). Lesion is flat and mottled. (Courtesy of Dr. Abe Macher.)

Kaposi's sarcoma are seen most commonly now in the AIDS patient, and the subtlety of changes in many cases presents an ongoing challenge to the surgical pathologist.

The earliest (*patch*) stage of Kaposi's sarcoma is a flat lesion characterized by proliferation of miniature vessels surrounding larger ectatic vessels. A slightly more advanced patch lesion displays, in addition, a loosely ramifying network of jagged vessels in the upper dermis (Figs. 25–21, 25–22). In some respects this stage resembles a well-differentiated angiosarcoma, except that the cells are so bland they closely resemble normal capillary or lymphatic endothelium. There is also a sparse infiltrate of lymphocytes and plasma cells surrounding the patch lesion. The histologic changes seen in patch lesions have also been noted in clinically normal areas of skin in patients who have Kaposi's sarcoma elsewhere. This observation underscores the diffuseness of the disease process.

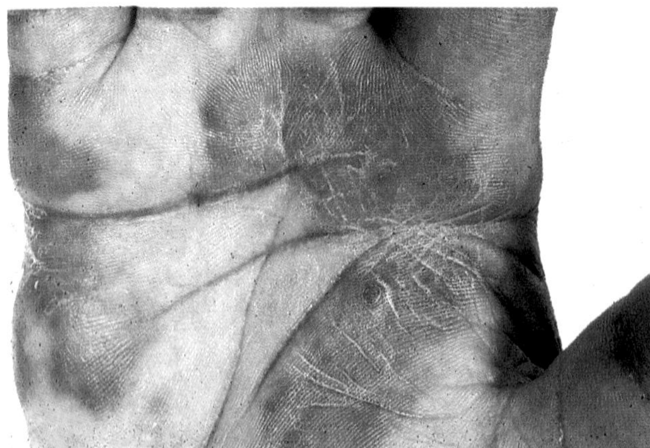

**FIGURE 25–20.** Advanced stage of Kaposi's sarcoma in an AIDS patient with a combination of patch, plaque, and nodular lesions. (Courtesy of Dr. Abe Macher.)

The more advanced (*plaque*) stage of the disease produces slight elevation of the skin; it is at this point that the vascular proliferation usually involves most of the dermis and may extend to the subcutis. A discernible but relatively bland spindle cell component, initially centered around the proliferating vascular channels, appears at this stage. In time the spindle cell foci coalesce and produce the classic nodular lesions of Kaposi's sarcoma. Diagnosis of the well established case is seldom difficult. Graceful arcs of spindle cells intersect one another in the manner of a well-differentiated fibrosarcoma (Figs. 25–23 to 25–26); but unlike fibrosarcoma, slit-like spaces containing erythrocytes separate the spindle cells and vascular channels (Fig. 25–24). In cross section these arcs of spindle cells are equally diagnostic by virtue of the sieve-like or honeycomb pattern they create. Inflammatory cells (lymphocytes and plasma cells), hemosiderin deposits, and dilated vessels are commonly seen at the periphery of nodular lesions (Fig. 25–23).[13] A characteristic, but probably not specific feature of the well established lesion is the presence of the hyaline globule. These periodic acid-Schiff (PAS)-positive, diastase-resistant spherules may be located both intracellularly and extracellularly[149] (Fig. 25–26). Some of the hyaline globules are effete erythrocytes, an idea that derives support from the finding of erythrocytes in phagolysosomes by ultrastructural analysis and by certain common histochemical features (positive for toluidine blue and endogenous peroxidase).[164]

Although the typical lesions of Kaposi's sarcoma are devoid of pleomorphism and a significant number of mitotic figures, histologically aggressive forms of Kaposi's sarcoma can be seen. They may result from progressive histologic dedifferentiation in otherwise typical cases. This phenomenon was observed in 5 of 14 autopsy cases reviewed by Cox and Helwig[139] and in two autopsy cases reported by Reed et al.[184] In our experience, poorly differentiated tumors may also arise ab initio and seem to be more common in cases of Kaposi's sarcoma originating in Africa. In these tumors the cells not only appear more pleomorphic but there may be a brisk level of mitotic activity. Kaposi's sarcoma, particularly in the setting of AIDS, may show transitional areas that appear more akin to angiosarcoma. These areas may contain large ectatic vascular spaces similar to a hemangioma or lymphangioma and in addition have papillary tufts lined by atypical endothelial cells (Fig. 25–25). The former feature was addressed in the literature, and such

*Text continued on page 945*

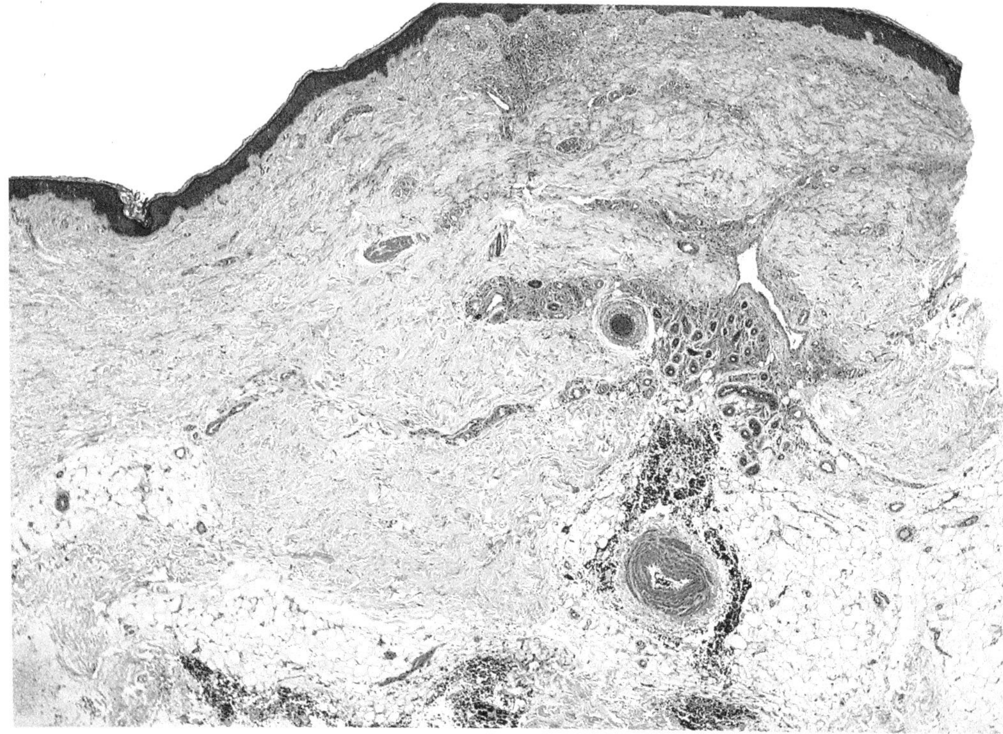

**FIGURE 25–21.** Early lesion of Kaposi's sarcoma in an AIDS patient. Lesions are flat or slightly elevated.

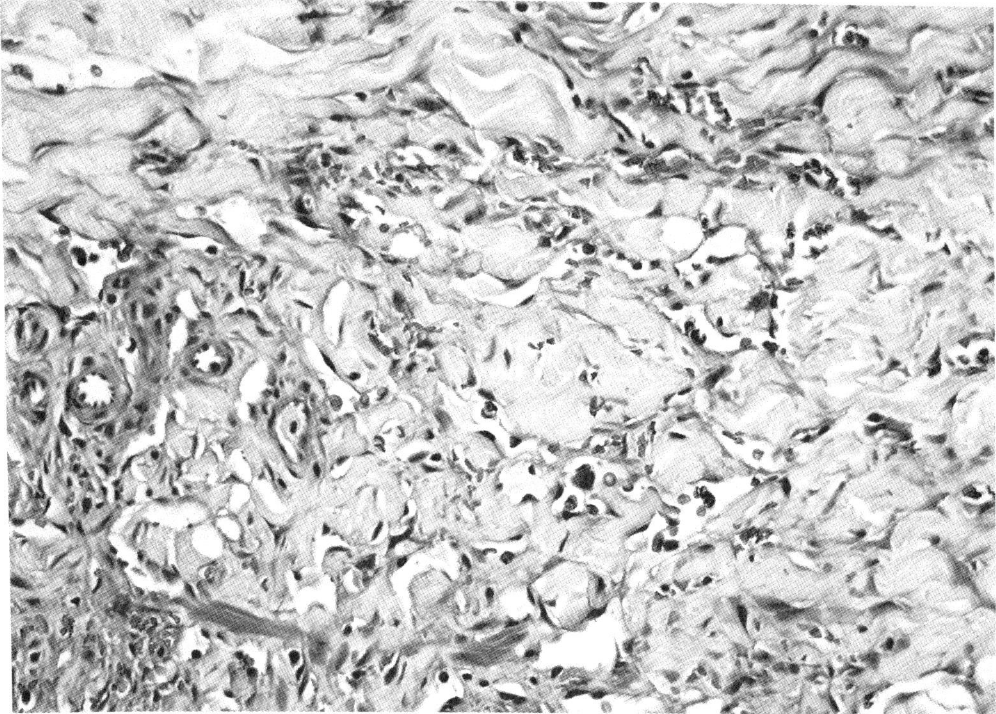

**FIGURE 25–22.** Early lesion of Kaposi's sarcoma illustrating irregular proliferation of miniature vessels in the dermis somewhat reminiscent of the pattern of an angiosarcoma.

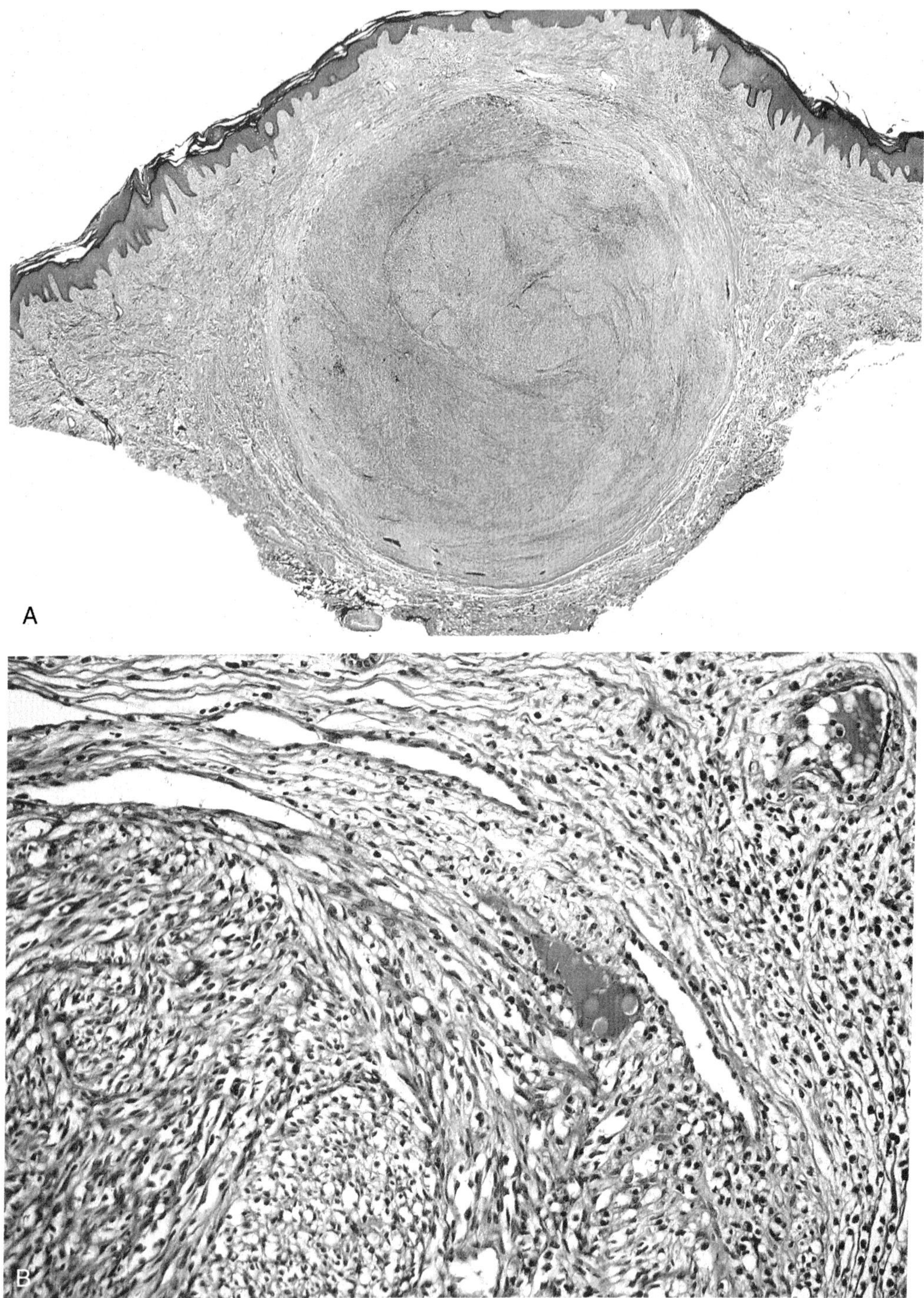

**FIGURE 25–23.** (**A**) Well established lesion of Kaposi's sarcoma. (**B**) Tumor nodule is circumscribed by lymphocytes and ectatic or crescentic vessels.

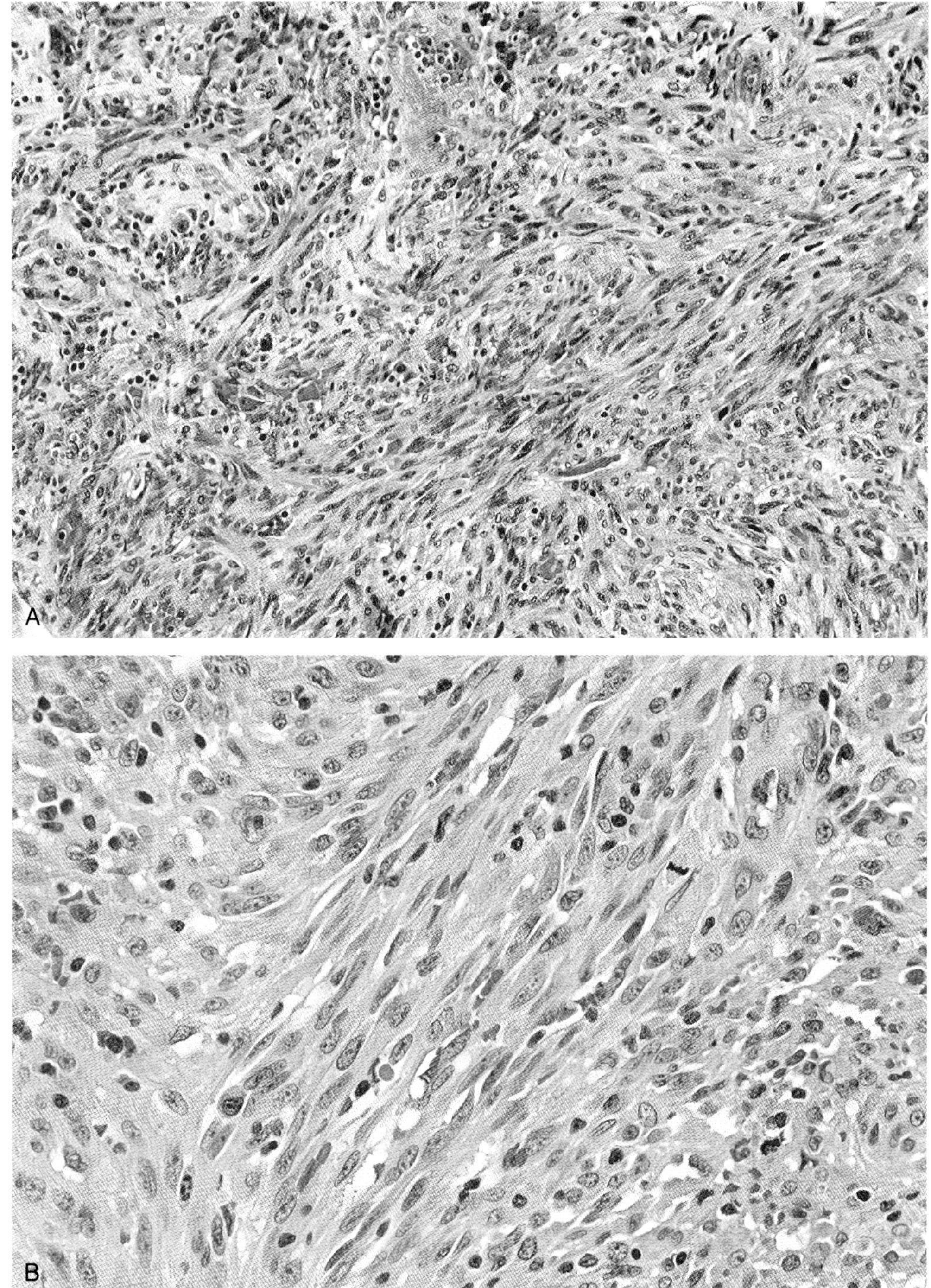

**FIGURE 25–24.** (**A**) Kaposi's sarcoma illustrating monomorphic spindle cells arranged in ill-defined fascicles. (**B**) Cells are separated by slit-like vessels containing erythrocytes.

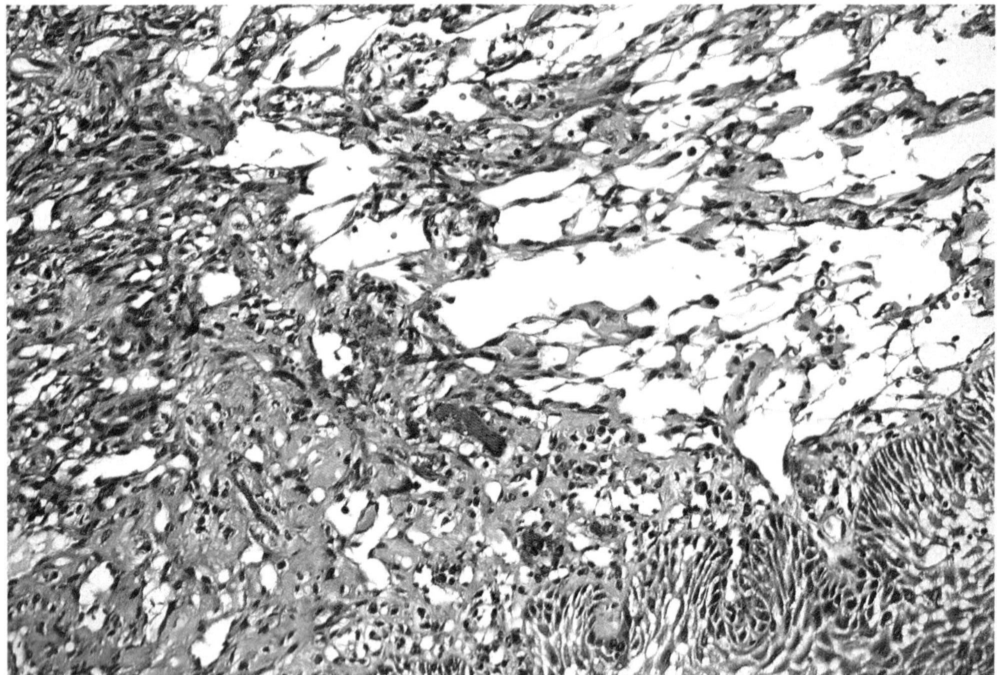

**FIGURE 25–25.** Kaposi's sarcoma with lymphangioma-like areas.

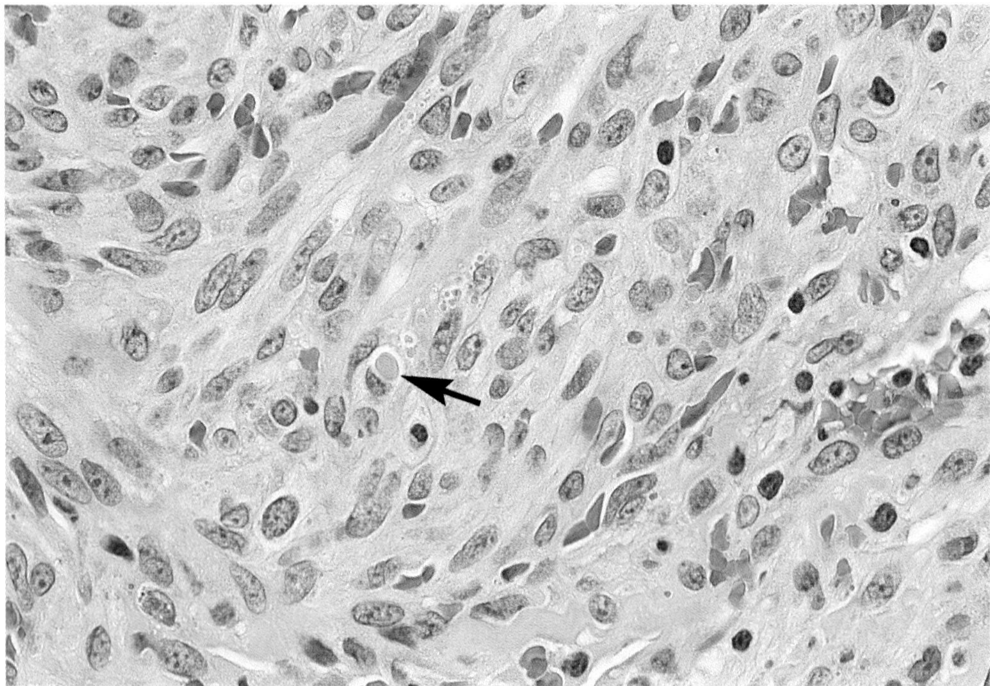

**FIGURE 25–26.** High-power view of Kaposi's sarcoma with hyaline globules. (H & E)

tumors were termed "lymphangioma-like Kaposi's sarcoma."[137,152]

Just as the early changes of Kaposi's sarcoma in the skin present a diagnostic challenge, so do early changes of this tumor in other organs (Fig. 25–27). A particularly common problem is the evaluation of lymph nodes in the AIDS patient. The earliest changes in lymph nodes may be represented by a mild angiectasia and proliferation of vessels in the subcapsular sinus. The interfollicular sinuses are gradually involved and expanded. The earliest stages may closely resemble the reactive lymph node condition known variously as nodal angiomatosis and vascular transformation of the subcapsular sinus, which occurs as a result of lymph node obstruction. Others have noted the similarity of these lymph nodes to Castleman's disease, when the proliferating vessels are centered around the follicles.[157,187] Accurate diagnosis of these histologically ambiguous lymph nodes should include complete sectioning of the block. This tactic often reveals more solidly cellular spindled foci, which confirm the diagnosis.[157] Well advanced cases of Kaposi's sarcoma involving lymph nodes do not present a problem of the same magnitude, as they exhibit partial or complete lymph node effacement by a monotonous spindle cell proliferation. Because patients with AIDS are prone to develop mycobacterial pseudotumors of the lymph node, special stains may be needed to distinguish these changes from Kaposi's sarcoma of the node.

## Special Studies

Immunohistochemical studies have contributed significantly to our understanding of the histogenesis of this tumor. In the past, variable reporting of factor VIII-AG in this tumor led to controversy concerning its endothelial nature. However, factor VIII-AG has proved to be highly variable in malignant vascular tumors, may be differentially expressed depending on the type of endothelium, and is subject to a great variety of interpretations because of a diffusion artifact. The use of numerous monoclonal antibodies directed against various structural substances in the endothelial cell has provided the opportunity to circumvent these problems. Several groups have provided support for the endothelial nature of Kaposi's sarcoma using a number of monoclonal antibodies, but their findings have led to apparently contradictory conclusions as to whether Kaposi's sarcoma is derived from vascular or lymphatic endothelium (Table 25–8). Rutgers et al.[186] concluded that the cells are more closely related to vascular endothelium because of immunostaining with three monoclonal antibodies (OKM5, anti-E92, HCl), which react with capillary but not lymphatic endothelium. Scully et al.[191] likewise

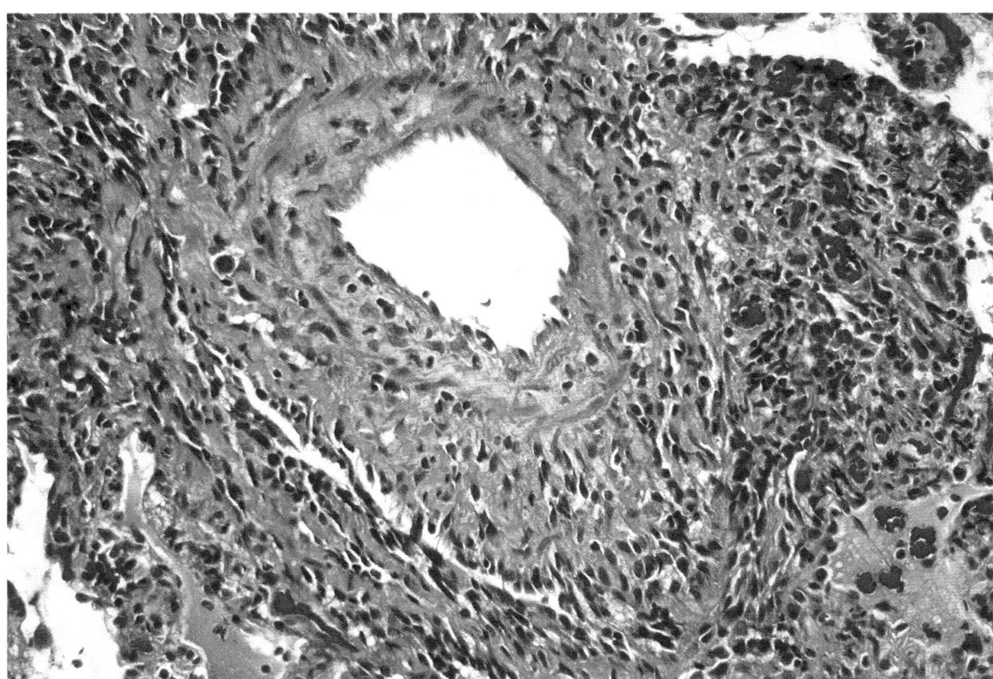

**FIGURE 25–27.** Kaposi's sarcoma involving lung. Note permeation of the septa and perivascular connective tissue.

**TABLE 25–8 HISTOCHEMICAL AND IMMUNOHISTOCHEMICAL STAINING OF KAPOSI'S SARCOMA**

| Factor | Normal Capillary | Normal Lymphatic | Kaposi's Sarcoma |
|---|---|---|---|
| Anti-factor VIII-AG[23] | + | +/− | −* |
| EN-4[162, 163] | + | + | + |
| PAL-E[162, 163] | + | − | − Early +/− late |
| OKM5[186] | + | − | +* |
| Anti-E92[186] | + | − | +* |
| HCl[186] | + | − | +* |
| HLA/DR/Ia[129] | + | − | −* |
| Alkaline phosphatase[129] | +++ | − | −* |
| 5-Nucleotidase[129] | + | +++ | +* |
| B721[190] | + | − | + |
| VEGFR-3[23, 32] | − | +++ | +++ |
| Podoplanin[6] | − | +++ | +++ |

*Spindle cells of tumor.

documented immunoreactivity in Kaposi's sarcoma cells utilizing an antibody (B721) that reacts with all vascular endothelium except for that of the renal glomerulus and sinusoids of the liver and spleen. Beckstead et al.,[129] on the other hand, argued for lymphatic endothelial differentiation because of the lack of HLA-DR/Ia and alkaline phosphatase and the intense 5-nucleotidase. Jones et al.[162,163] noted that the immunoreactivity of the tumor varies with the type or stage of the disease, with the early patch stage having the immunologic profile of a lymphatic tumor. These areas stain positively with a monoclonal antibody directed against all endothelium (EN-4) but do not stain with an antibody specific for vascular endothelium (PAL-E). More developed lesions, however, stain with EN-4 and are variable with PAL-E. Recently VEGFR-3, a relatively sensitive marker of lymphatic differentiation, has been identified in most Kaposi's sarcomas.[23,32,200] On balance, the weight of evidence supports lymphatic differentiation in this tumor.

## Ultrastructural Observations

Electron microscopy has traditionally supported the idea of endothelial differentiation in these tumors. In the early lesions slender endothelial cells with oval nuclei and small nucleoli line slit-like lumens (Fig. 25–28). Few intercellular junctions are noted, and focally gaps may be present between the cells. Fragmented basal lamina encircles the abluminal surface of the cells, and few if any pericytes are observed.[173] The latter observations seem to be more compatible with lymphatic than vascular differentiation. Advanced lesions not unexpectedly contain cells that have been variously described as "perithelial" or "fibroblastic," although immunohistochemical observations indicate that they are actually modified endothelial cells. Ultrastructurally, the spindled "perithelial" cells have lysosomes and ferritin and appear to be actively phagocytic.

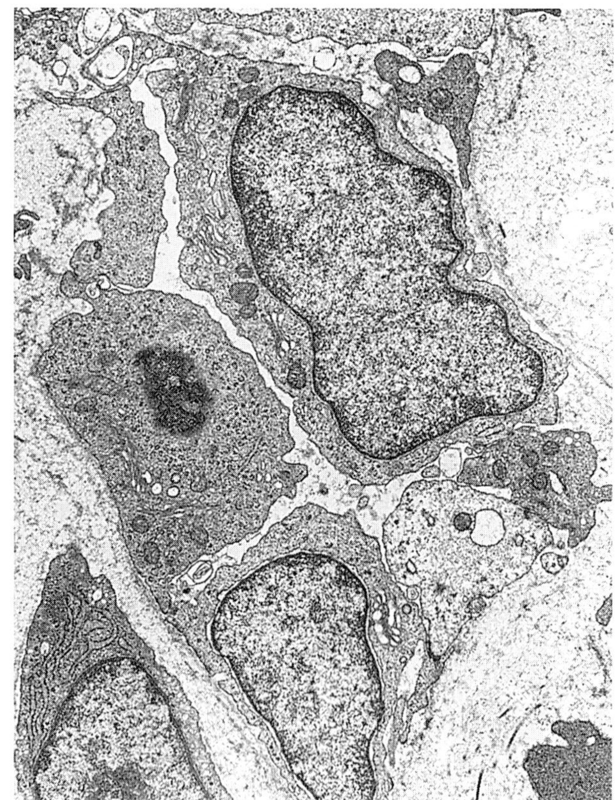

**FIGURE 25–28.** Electron micrograph of Kaposi's sarcoma. Cells exhibit endothelial characteristics and are surrounded by fragmented basal lamina. Pericytes are absent or greatly reduced. (×9000) (From McNutt NS, Fletcher V, Conant MA. Early lesions of Kaposi's sarcoma in homosexual men: an ultrastructural comparison with other vascular proliferations in the skin. Am J Pathol 111:62, 1983.)

### Differential Diagnosis

As indicated, recognition of the early changes of Kaposi's sarcoma, especially in the AIDS patient, remains one of the most difficult diagnostic problems. The irregular infiltrative pattern of the endothelial cells in early lesions is more helpful for the diagnosis than the degree of cytologic atypia, although the changes may be virtually indistinguishable from those in a well-differentiated angiosarcoma. An accurate clinical history becomes of paramount importance for establishing the diagnosis. The well advanced case may be confused with a fibrosarcoma. Features that distinguish a highly cellular form of Kaposi's sarcoma from a fibrosarcoma include the presence of ectatic vessels and inflammatory cells at the periphery of the lesions, the more curvilinear fascicles, and the presence of hyaline globules.

Arteriovenous malformations occasionally give rise to cutaneous lesions that clinically duplicate the picture of Kaposi's sarcoma. Such lesions have been termed "pseudo-Kaposi's sarcoma."[171] Histologically, these lesions consist of a proliferation of small capillary-size vessels occasionally surrounded by extravasated erythrocytes and hemosiderin. Frank spindling and formation of slit-like lumens are not seen. Arteriographic studies documenting the presence of an underlying arteriovenous malformation and the clinical findings of a bruit in the area of the lesions provide additional contrasting points.

The spindle cell hemangioendothelioma (see Chapter 24) is frequently confused with Kaposi's sarcoma. The presence of cavernous vessels and epithelioid endothelial cells (which are not seen in Kaposi's sarcoma) are the most reliable features for distinguishing the two tumors.

### Behavior and Treatment

The behavior of Kaposi's sarcoma is variable and is dependent on a number of interrelated factors, such as the immunologic competence of the host, the stage of the disease, and the presence or absence of opportunistic infections. In the chronic form of the disease, which occurs in more or less immunocompetent individuals who usually present with limited cutaneous disease, the disease-related mortality rate is 10–20%. Even in patients in this group who die of their disease, the duration of the disease is 8–10 years. An additional 25% of patients die of a second malignant tumor.[179]

Patients with AIDS who develop Kaposi's sarcoma have a far more aggressive course. The overall mortality rate of patients with Kaposi's sarcoma and AIDS is 41% during a relatively limited follow-up period; it is markedly influenced by the stage of the disease, the presence of opportunistic infections, and the presence of systemic symptoms. Eighty percent of patients who have avoided opportunistic infections are alive at 28 months compared with fewer than 20% who have an opportunistic infection.[166]

**TABLE 25–9 TRADITIONAL STAGING OF KAPOSI'S SARCOMA**

| | |
|---|---|
| Stage I: | Cutaneous, locally indolent |
| Stage II: | Cutaneous, locally aggressive, with or without regional lymph nodes |
| Stage III: | Generalized mucocutaneous or lymph node involvement, or both |
| Stage IV: | Visceral involvement |
| IVA: | No systemic signs or symptoms |
| IVB: | Systemic signs: 10% weight loss or fever over 100°F orally unrelated to an identifiable source of infection lasting more than 2 weeks |

Because of the relative paucity of Kaposi's sarcomas in the United States prior to the AIDS epidemic, there is relatively little reported experience with treatment of the disease. Surgery, formerly recommended, is no longer indicated other than for tissue diagnosis. The tendency toward multifocality, even with the chronic form of the disease, makes irradiation or chemotherapy (or both) the preferred therapy. The most common combination of drugs employs doxorubicin, bleomycin, and vincristine.[167] Interferon-$\alpha$ has also been shown to have efficacy against the tumors. To evaluate the efficacy of various drug combinations accurately, the AIDS Clinical Trials Group Oncology Committee has devised specific definitions of "clinical response" along with a staging system unique for AIDS-related Kaposi's sarcoma. This staging system replaces the traditional one (Table 25–9) and embraces a number of parameters including extent of tumor (T), status of the immune system (I), and severity of the illness (Table 25–10).[168]

## INTRAVASCULAR LYMPHOMATOSIS (ANGIOTROPIC LYMPHOMA)

Intravascular lymphomatosis, formerly called *proliferating angioendotheliomatosis,* is included in this chapter for historical interest only, as it has been conclusively identified as a lymphoma rather than an endothelial tumor. Originally described by Pfleger and Tappeiner, this unusual tumor was believed to represent diffuse neoplastic change of the endothelium throughout the body. Numerous recent reports attest to the fact that the tumor usually proves, in well studied cases, to be a lymphoma with a predilection for the intravascular spaces.[202–205,207]

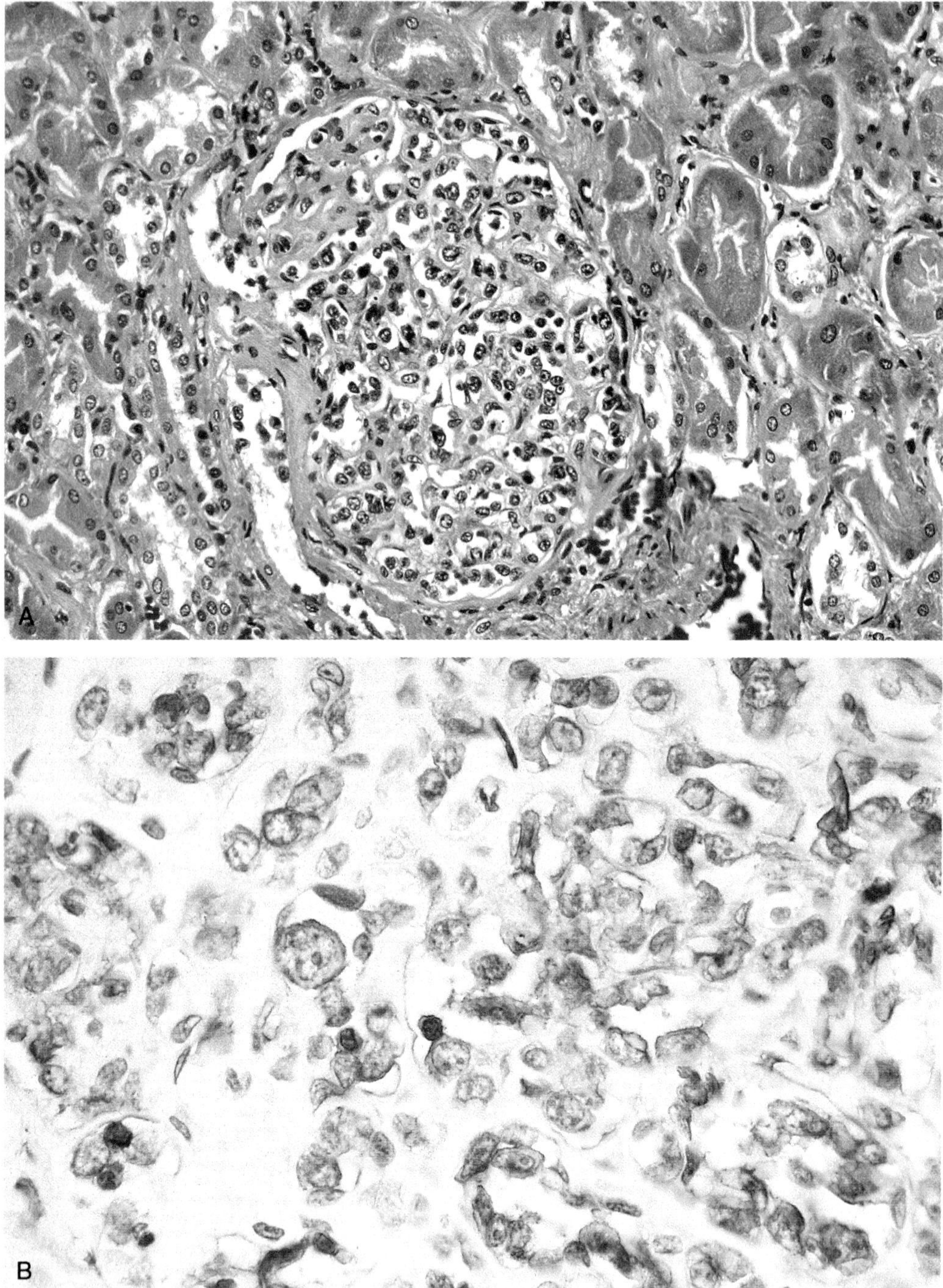

**FIGURE 25–29.** (**A**) Intravascular lymphomatosis (so-called proliferating angioendotheliomatosis) involving the renal glomerulus. (**B**) Cells are positive for leukocyte common antigen.

**TABLE 25–10 STAGING OF AIDS-RELATED KAPOSI'S SARCOMA**

| Parameter | Good Risk (0) (all of the following) | Poor Risk (1) (any of the following) |
|---|---|---|
| Tumor (T) | Confined to skin and/or lymph nodes and/or minimal oral disease* | Tumor-associated edema or ulceration; extensive oral KS; KS in nonnodal viscera |
| Immune system (I) | CD4 cells >200/μl | CD4 cells <200/μl |
| Systemic illness (S) | No history of OI or thrush; no "B" symptoms;† performance status >70 (Karnovsky) | History of OI and/or thrush; "B" symptoms; performance status <70; other HIV-related illness (e.g., lymphoma) |

Krown SE, Metroka C, Wernz JC. Kaposi's sarcoma in the acquired immune deficiency syndrome: a proposal for uniform evaluation, response, and staging criteria. J Clin Oncol 7:1201, 1989.

KS, Kaposi's sarcoma; OI, opportunistic infection; HIV, human immunodeficiency virus.

* Minimal oral disease is nonnodular KS confined to palate.

† B symptoms are unexplained fever, night sweats, >10% involuntary weight loss, or diarrhea persisting more than 2 weeks.

The disease occurs in adults and affects the genders equally. It begins with the development of multiple indurated erythematous nodules or plaques of the skin that bear a resemblance to erythema nodosum. Initially the general health of the patient is good, although occasionally fever and neurologic signs are present. Histologically, the small vessels of the dermis and subcutis are filled with plump mononuclear cells that occasionally appear to be in continuity with the endothelium (Fig. 25–29). The proliferating cells, accompanied by small fibrin thrombi, may virtually occlude small vessels. The cells have a high nucleocytoplasmic ratio, prominent nucleoli, and occasional mitotic figures. In patients dying of the disease, neoplastic cells are found in vessels throughout the body, and in some instances they infiltrate the parenchyma of organs. In the past the mistaken assumption that these tumors were derived from endothelium and not lymphocytes is partly explained by the fact that there is minimal involvement of bone marrow, lymph nodes, and spleen. Studies allegedly reporting factor VIII-AG or Weibel-Palade bodies[208] in the tumor probably sampled adjacent reactive endothelium rather than tumor. Immunohistochemical studies clearly demonstrate that the tumors have the immunologic profile of lymphomas[202,203,207,210]; most type as B cell lymphomas,[202,205,207] others as T cell lymphomas,[207] and still others as lymphomas of mixed phenotype.[203] It has been suggested that these unusual lymphomas have receptors that cause them to home selectively to endothelium.[206] Because of the differences in treatment protocols, it is particularly important that these lesions be distinguished from a true soft tissue sarcoma.

## REFERENCES

### General


1. Alles JU, Bosslet K. Immunocytochemistry of angiosarcomas: a study of 19 cases with especial emphasis on the applicability of endothelial cell specific markers to routinely prepared tissues. Am J Clin Pathol 89:463, 1988.
2. Appleton MA, Attonoos RL, Jasnai B. Thrombomodulin as a marker of vascular and lymphatic tumours. Histopathology 29:153, 1996.
3. Alrenga DP. Primary angiosarcoma of the liver: review article. Int Surg 60:198, 1975.
4. Ben-Ishak O, Kerner H, Brenner B, et al. Angiosarcoma of the colon developing in a capsule of a foreign body. Am J Clin Pathol 97:416, 1992.
5. Bessis D, Sotto A, Roubert P, Chabrier PE, et al. Endothelin-secreting angiosarcoma occurring at the site of an arteriovenous fistula for haemodialysis in a renal transplant receipient. Br J Dermatol 138:361, 1998.
6. Breiteneder-Geleff S, Soleiman A, Kowalski H. Angiosarcomas express mixed endothelial phenotypes of blood and lymphatic capillaries: podaplanin as a specific marker for lymphatic endothelium. Am J Pathol 154:385, 1999.
7. Brown LF, Tognazzi K, Dvorak HF, Harrist TJ. Strong expression of kinase insert domain-containing receptor, a vascular permeability factor/vascular endothelial growth factor receptor in AIDS-associated Kaposi's sarcoma and cutaneous angiosarcoma. Am J Pathol 148:1065, 1996.
8. Brown RW, Tornos C, Evans HL. Angiosarcoma arising from malignant schwannoma in a patient with neurofibromatosis. Cancer 70:1141, 1992.
9. Bullen R, Larson PO, Landeck AE, et al. Angiosarcoma of the head and neck managed by a combination of multiple biopsies to determine tumor margin and radiation therapy: report of three cases and review of the literature. Dermatol Surg 24:1105, 1998.
10. Burgdorf WHC, Mukai K, Rosai J. Immunohistochemical identification of factor VIII-related antigen in endothelial cells of cutaneous lesions of alleged vascular nature. Am J Clin Pathol 75:167, 1981.
11. Byers RJ, McMahon RFT, Freemont AJ, et al. Epithelioid angiosarcoma arising in an arteriovenous fistula. Histopathology 21:87, 1992.
12. Chaudhuri B, Ronan SG, Manaligod JR. Angiosarcoma arising in a plexiform neurofibroma. Cancer 46:605, 1980.
13. Chen KTK, Hoffman KD, Hendricks EJ. Angiosarcoma following therapeutic irradiation. Cancer 44:2044, 1979.
14. Cohen PR, Rapini RP, Farhood AI. Expression of the human hematopoietic progenitor cell antigen CD34 in vascular and spindle cell tumors. J Cutan Pathol 20:15, 1993.
15. Conlon PJ, Daly T, Doyle G, Carmody M. Angiosarcoma in the site of a ligated fistula in a renal transplant recipient. Nephrol Dial Transplant 8:259, 1993.

16. Dargent JL, Vermylen P, Abramowicz D, et al. Disseminated angiosarcoma presenting as a hemophagocytic syndrome in renal allograft recipient. Transplant Int 10:61, 1997.
17. Davies JD, Rees GJG, Mera SL. Angiosarcoma in irradiated postmastectomy chest wall. Histopathology 7:947, 1983.
18. DeYoung BR, Wick MR, Fitzgibbon JF, et al. CD31: an immunospecific marker for endothelial differentiation in human neoplasms. Appl Immunohistochem 1:97, 1993.
19. Dunkel IJ, Gerald WL, Rosenfield NS, et al. Outcome of patients with history of bilateral retinoblastoma treated for a second malignancy: the Memorial Sloan Kettering experience. Med Pediatr Oncol 30:59, 1998.
20. Eusebi V, Carcangiu ML, Dina R, et al. Keratin-positive epithelioid angiosarcoma of the thyroid: a report of four cases. Am J Surg Pathol 14:737, 1990.
21. Falk H, Thomas LB, Popper H, et al. Hepatic angiosarcoma associated with androgenic anabolic steroids. Lancet 2:1120, 1979.
22. Falk S, Krishnan J, Meis JM. Primary angiosarcoma of the spleen: a clinicopathologic study of 40 cases. Am J Surg Pathol 17:959, 1993.
23. Folpe AL, Veikkola T, Valtola R, Weiss SW. Vascular endothelial growth factor receptor-3 (VEGFR-3): a marker of vascular tumors with presumed lymphatic differentiation, including Kaposi's sarcoma, kaposiform and Dabska-type hemangioendotheliomas, and a subset of angiosarcomas. Mod Pathol 13: 180, 2000.
24. Fujimoto M, Kiyosawa T, Murata S, et al. Vascular endothelial growth factor in angiosarcoma. Anticancer Res 18:25, 1998.
25. Gray MH, Rosenberg AE, Dickersin GR, et al. Cytokeratin expression in epithelioid vascular neoplasms. Hum Pathol 21: 212, 1990.
26. Hashimoto M, Ohsawa A, Onhnishi A, et al. Expression of vascular endothelial growth factor and its receptor mRNA in angiosarcoma. Lab Invest 73:859, 1995.
27. Hayman J, Huygens H. Angiosarcoma developing around a foreign body. J Clin Pathol 36:515, 1983.
28. Hoch-Ligeti C. Angiosarcoma of liver associated with diethylstilbestrol. JAMA 240:1510, 1978.
29. Hudson CP, Hanno R, Callen JP. Cutaneous angiosarcoma in a site of healed herpes zoster. Int J Dermatol 23:404, 1984.
30. Jaffe EA. Endothelial cells and biology of factor VIII. N Engl J Med 296:377, 1977.
31. Jennings TA, Peterson L, Axiotis CA, et al. Angiosarcoma associated with foreign body material: a report of three cases. Cancer 62:2436, 1988.
32. Jussila L, Valtola R, Partanen TA, et al. Lymphatic endothelium and Kaposi's sarcoma spindle cells detected by antibodies against vascular endothelial growth factor receptor-3. Cancer Res 58:1599, 1998.
33. Keane MM, Carney DN. Angiosarcoma arising from a defunctionalized arteriovenous fistula. J Urol 149:364, 1993.
34. Kibe Y, Kishimoto S, Katoh N, et al. Angiosarcoma of the scalp associated with renal transplantation. Br J Dermatol 136: 752, 1997.
35. Lasota J, Miettinen M. Absence of Kaposi's sarcoma-associated virus (human herpesvirus-8) sequences in angiosarcoma. Virchows Arch 434:51, 1999.
36. Leake J, Sheehan MP, Rampling D, et al. Angiosarcoma complicating xeroderma pigmentosum. Histopathology 21:179, 1992.
37. Li N, Anderson WK, Bhawan J. Further confirmation of the association of human herpesvirus 8 with Kaposi's sarcoma. J Cutan Pathol 25:413, 1998.
38. Lin BT, Chen YY, Battifora H, Weiss LM. Absence of Kaposi's sarcoma-associated herpesvirus-like DNA sequences in malignant vascular tumors of the serous membranes. Mod Pathol 9: 1143, 1996.
39. Lymboussaki A, Partanene TA, Olofsson B, et al. Expression of the vascular endothelial growth factor C receptor VEGFR-3 in lymphatic endothelium of the skin and vascular tumors. Am J Pathol 153:395, 1998.
40. Mackay B, Ordoñez NG, Huang W-L. Ultrastructural and immunocytochemical observations on angiosarcomas. Ultrastruct Pathol 13:97, 1989.
41. Maddox JC, Evans HL. Angiosarcoma of skin and soft tissue: a study of 44 cases. Cancer 48:1907, 1981.
42. Makk L, Delorme F, Creech J, et al. Clinical and morphologic features of hepatic angiosarcoma in vinyl chloride workers. Cancer 37:149, 1976.
43. Mandahl N, Jin Y, Heim S, et al. Trisomy 5 and loss of the Y chromosome as the sole cytogenetic anomalies in a cavernous hemangioma/angiosarcoma. Genes Chromosomes Cancer 1: 315, 1990.
44. McDonagh DP, Liu J, Gaffey MJ, et al. Detection of Kaposi's sarcoma-associated herpesvirus-like DNA sequence in angiosarcoma. Am J Pathol 149:1363, 1996.
44a. McLaughlin ER, Brown LF, Weiss SW, et al. VEGF and its receptors are expressed in a pediatric angiosarcoma in a patient with Aicardi's syndrome. J Invest Dermatol 114:1209, 2000.
45. Medioni LD, Costes V, Leray H, et al. Angiosarcome sur fistule arterio-veineuse chez un transplante renal: une complication inhabituelle. Ann Pathol 16:200, 1996.
46. Meis JM, Kindblom L-G, Enzinger FM. Angiosarcoma arising in von Recklinghausen's disease (NF1): report of five additional cases. Mod Pathol 7:8A, 1994.
47. Millstein DI, Chik-Kwun T, Campbell EW. Angiosarcoma developing in a patient with neurofibromatosis (von Recklinghausen's disease). Cancer 47:950, 1981.
48. Molina A, Bangs CD, Donlon T. Angiosarcoma of the scalp with a complex hypotetraploid karyotype. Cancer Genet Cytogenet 41:268, 1989.
49. Morphopoulos GD, Banerjee SS, Ali HH, et al. Malignant peripheral nerve sheath tumour with vascular differentiation: a report of four cases. Histopathology 28:401, 1996.
50. Naka N, Ohsawa M, Tomita Y, et al. Prognostic factors in angiosarcoma: a multivariate analysis of 55 cases. J Surg Oncol 61:170, 1996.
51. Naka N, Tomita Y, Nakanishi H. Mutations of p53 tumor-suppressor in angiosarcoma. Int J Cancer 71:952, 1997.
52. Orchard GE, Zelger B, Jones EW, Jones RR. An immunocytochemical assessment of 19 cases of cutaneous angiosarcoma. Histopathology 28:235, 1996.
53. Parhams DV, Cordell JL, Micklem K, et al. JC70: a new monoclonal antibody that detects vascular endothelium associated antigen on routinely processed tissue sections. J Clin Pathol 43:752, 1990.
54. Poblet E, Gonzalez-Palacios F, Jimenez FJ. Different immunoreactivity of endothelial markers in well and poorly differentiated areas of angiosarcoma. Virchows Arch 428:217, 1996.
55. Popper H, Thomas LB, Telles NC, et al. Development of hepatic angiosarcoma in man induced by vinyl chloride, Thorotrast, and arsenic. Am J Pathol 92:349, 1978.
56. Przygodski RM, Finkelstein SD, Keohayong P, et al. Sporadic and Thorotrast-induced angiosarcoma of the liver manifest frequent and multiple point mutations in K-ras-2. Lab Invest 76: 153, 1997.
57. Ramani P, Bradley NJ, Fletcher CDM. QBEND/10, a new monoclonal antibody to endothelium: assessment of its diagnostic utility in paraffin sections. Histopathology 17:237, 1990.
58. Schneider T, Renney J, Hayman J. Angiosarcoma occurring

with chronic osteomyelitis and residual foreign material: case report of a late World War II wound complication. Aust N Z J Surg 67:578, 1997.

59. Schuborg C, Mertens F, Rydholm A, et al. Cytogenetic analysis of four angiosarcomas from deep and superficial soft tissue. Cancer Genet Cytogenet 100:52, 1998.
60. Swanson PE, Wick MR. Immunohistochemical evaluation of vascular neoplasms. Clin Dermatol 9:243, 1991.
61. Tallini G, Price FV, Carcangiu ML. Epithelioid angiosarcoma arising in uterine leiomyomas. Am J Clin Pathol 100:514, 1993.
62. Trassard M, LeDoussal V, Bui BN, Coindre JM. Angiosarcoma arising in a solitary schwannoma (neurilemoma) of the sciatic nerve. Am J Surg Pathol 20:1412, 1996.
63. Traweek ST, Kandalaft PL, Mehta P, et al. The human progenitor cell antigen (CD34) in vascular neoplasia. Am J Clin Pathol 96:25, 1991.
64. Tso CY, Sommer A, Hamoudi AB. Aicardi syndrome, metastatic angiosarcoma of the leg, and scalp lipoma. Am J Med Genet 45:594, 1993.
65. Ulbright TM, Clark SA, Einhorn LH. Angiosarcoma associated with germ cell tumors. Hum Pathol 16:268, 1985.
66. Waldo ED, Vuletin JC, Kaye GI. The ultrastructure of vascular tumors: additional observations and a review of the literature. Pathol Ann 12:278, 1977.
67. Wehrli BM, Janzen DL, Shokeir O, et al. Epithelioid angiosarcoma arising in a surgically constructed arteriovenous fistula: a rare complication of chronic immunosuppression in the setting of renal transplantation. Am J Surg Pathol 22:1154, 1998.
68. Weiss SW, Nickoloff BJ. CD-34 is expressed by a distinctive cell population in peripheral nerve, nerve sheath tumors, and related lesions. Am J Surg Pathol 17:1039, 1993.
69. Weiss WM, Riles TS, Gouge TH, et al. Angiosarcoma at the site of a Dacron vascular prosthesis: a case report and literature review. J Vasc Surg 14:87, 1991.
70. Wenig BM, Abbondanzo SL, Heffess CS. Epithelioid angiosarcoma of the adrenal glands: a clinicopathologic study of nine cases with a discussion of the implications of finding "epithelial-specific" markers. Am J Surg Pathol 18:62, 1994.
71. Yonezawa S, Maruyama I, Sakae K, et al. Thrombomodulin as a marker for vascular tumors: comparative study with factor VIII and Ulex europaeus I lectin. Am J Clin Pathol 88:405, 1987.

### Cutaneous Angiosarcoma

72. Bardwil JM, Mocega EE, Butler JJ, et al. Angiosarcomas of the head and neck region. Am J Surg 116:548, 1968.
73. Burgoon CF, Sodenberg M. Angiosarcoma. Arch Dermatol 99: 773, 1969.
74. Diaz-Cascajo C, Weyers W, Borghi S, Reichel M. Verrucous angiosarcoma of the skin: a distinct variant of cutaneous angiosarcoma. Histopathology 32:556, 1998.
75. Girard C, Johnson WC, Graham JH. Cutaneous angiosarcoma. Cancer 26:868, 1970.
76. Haustein UJ-F. Angiosarcoma of the face and scalp. Int J Dermatol 30:851, 1991.
77. Hodgkinson DJ, Soule EH, Woods JE. Cutaneous angiosarcoma of the head and neck. Cancer 44:1106, 1979.
78. Holden CA, Jones EW. Angiosarcoma of the face and scalp. J R Soc Med 78(Suppl 11):30, 1985.
79. Holden CA, Spittle MF, Jones EW. Angiosarcoma of the face and scalp: prognosis and treatment. Cancer 59:1046, 1987.
80. Mark RJ, Poen JC, Tran LM, et al. Angiosarcoma: a report of 67 patients and a review of the literature. Cancer 77:2400, 1996.
81. Newton JA, Apaull J, McGibbon DH, et al. Malignant angiosarcoma of the scalp: a case report with immunohistochemical studies. Br J Dermatol 112:97, 1985.
82. Reed RJ, Palomeque FE, Hairston MD III, et al. Lymphangiosarcomas of the scalp. Arch Dermatol 94:396, 1966.
83. Rosai J, Sumner HW, Kostianovsky M, et al. Angiosarcoma of the skin: a clinicopathologic and fine structural study. Hum Pathol 7:83, 1976.

### Angiosarcoma Associated with Lymphedema

84. Calnan J, Cowdell RH. Lymphangioendothelioma of the anterior abdominal wall: report of a case. Br J Surg 46:375, 1959.
85. Devi L, Bahuleyan CK. Lymphangiosarcoma of the lower extremity associated with chronic lymphedema of filarial origin. Ind J Cancer 14:176, 1977.
86. Dubin HU, Creehan EP, Headington JT. Lymphangiosarcoma and congenital lymphedema of the extremity. Arch Dermatol 110:608, 1974.
87. Jansey F, Szanto PB, Wright A. Postmastectomy lymphangiosarcoma in elephantiasis chirurgica: Stewart and Treves syndrome. Q Bull Northwest Univ Med School 31:301, 1957.
88. Kindblom L-G, Stenman G, Angervall L. Morphological and cytogenetic studies of angiosarcoma in Stewart-Treves syndrome. Virchows Arch [Pathol Anat Histopathol] 419:439, 1991.
89. Mackenzie DH. Lymphangiosarcoma arising in chronic congenital and idiopathic lymphoedema. J Clin Pathol 24:524, 1971.
90. Merrick T, Erlandson RA, Hajdu SI. Lymphangiosarcoma of a congenitally lymphedematous extremity. Arch Pathol 91:365, 1971.
91. Muller R, Hajdu SI, Brennan MF. Lymphangiosarcoma associated with chronic filarial lymphedema. Cancer 59:174, 1987.
92. Schreiber H, Barry FM, Russell WC, et al. Stewart-Treves syndrome: a lethal complication of postmastectomy lymphedema and regional immune deficiency. Arch Surg 114:82, 1979.
93. Shirger A. Postoperative lymphedema: etiologic and diagnostic factors. Med Clin North Am 46:1045, 1962.
94. Silverberg SG, Kay S, Koss LG. Postmastectomy lymphangiosarcoma: ultrastructural observations. Cancer 27:100, 1971.
95. Sordillo EM, Sordillo PP, Hajdu SI, et al. Lymphangiosarcoma after filarial infection. J Dermatol Surg Oncol 7:235, 1981.
96. Sordillo PP, Chapman R, Hajdu SI, et al. Lymphangiosarcoma. Cancer 48:1674, 1981.
97. Stewart FW, Treves N. Lymphangiosarcoma in postmastectomy lymphedema. Cancer 1:64, 1949.
98. Taswell HF, Soule EH, Coventry MB. Lymphangiosarcoma in chronic lymphedematous extremities: report of 13 cases and review of the literature. J Bone Joint Surg Am 44:277, 1962.
99. Woodward AH, Ivins JC, Soule EH. Lymphangiosarcoma arising in chronic lymphedematous extremities. Cancer 30:562, 1972.

### Angiosarcoma of Breast

100. Donnell RM, Rosen PP, Lieberman PH, et al. Angiosarcoma and other vascular tumors of the breast: pathologic analysis as a guide to prognosos. Am J Surg Pathol 5:629, 1981.
101. Kessler E, Kozenitsky IL. Haemangiosarcoma of breast. J Clin Pathol 24:530, 1971.
102. Khanna SK, Manchanda RL, Seigal RK, et al. Hemangioendothelioma (angiosarcoma) of the breast. Arch Surg 88:807, 1964.
103. McClanahan BJ, Hogg L. Angiosarcoma of the breast. Cancer 7:586, 1954.
104. McDivitt RW, Stewart FW, Berg JW. Tumors of the Breast. Atlas of Tumor Pathology, Fascicle 2, 2nd Series. Armed Forces Institute of Pathology, Washington, DC, 1966.

105. Merino MJ, Carter D, Berman M. Angiosarcoma of breast. Am J Surg Pathol 7:53, 1983.
106. Steingaszner LC, Enzinger FM, Taylor HB. Hemangiosarcoma of the breast. Cancer 18:352, 1965.
107. Tibbs D. Metastasizing hemangiomata: a case of malignant hemangioendoethelioma. Br J Surg 40:465, 1953.

### Angiosarcoma of Soft Tissue

108. Fletcher CDM, Beham A, Bekir S, et al. Epithelioid angiosarcoma of deep soft tissue: a distinctive tumor readily mistaken for an epithelial neoplasm. Am J Surg Pathol 15:915, 1991.
109. Lin BT, Colby T, Gown AM, et al. Malignant vascular tumors of the serous membranes mimicking mesothelioma: a report of 14 cases. Am J Surg Pathol 20:1431, 1996.
110. Maiorana A, Fante R, Fano RA, et al. Epithelioid angiosarcoma of the buttock: case report with immunohistochemical study on the expression of keratin polypeptides. Surg Pathol 4:325, 1991.
111. Meis-Kindblom JM, Kindblom LG. Angiosarcoma of soft tissue: a study of 80 cases. Am J Surg Pathol 22:683, 1998.

### Radiation-induced Angiosarcoma

112. Cafiero F, Gipponi M, Peressini A, et al. Radiation-associated angiosarcoma: diagnostic and therapeutic implications: two cases reports and review of the literature. Cancer 77:2496, 1996.
113. Cancellieri A, Eusebi V, Mambellin V, et al. Well-differentiated angiosarcoma of the skin following radiotherapy. Pathol Res Pract 187:301, 1991.
114. Edeiken S, Russo DP, Knecht J, et al. Angiosarcoma after tylectomy and radiation therapy for carcinoma of the breast. Cancer 70:644, 1992.
115. Fineberg S, Rosen PP. Cutaneous angiosarcoma and atypical vascular lesions of the skin and breast after radiation therapy for breast carcinoma. Am J Clin Pathol 102:757, 1994.
116. Givens SS, Ellerbroek NA, Butler JJ, et al. Angiosarcoma arising in an irradiated breast: a case report and review of the literature. Cancer 64:2214, 1989.
117. Marchal C, Weber B, de Lafontan B. Nine breast angiosarcomas after conservative treatment for breast carcinoma: a survey from French comprehensive cancer centers. Int J Radiat Oncol Biol Phys 44:113, 1999.
118. Moskaluk CA, Merino MJ, Danforth DN, et al. Low grade angiosarcoma of the skin of the breast: a complication of lumpectomy and radiation therapy for breast carcinoma. Hum Pathol 23:710, 1992.
119. Otis CN, Peschel R, McKhann C, et al. The rapid onset of cutaneous angiosarcoma after radiotherapy for breast cancer. Cancer 57:2130, 1986.
120. Paik HH, Komorowski R. Hemangiosarcoma of the abdominal wall following radiation therapy of endometrial carcinoma. Am J Clin Pathol 66:810, 1976.
121. Parham DM, Fisher C. Angiosarcomas of the breast developing post radiotherapy. Histopathology 31:189, 1997.
122. Richards PG, Bessell EM, Goolden AWG. Spinal extradural angiosarcoma occurring after treatment for Hodgkin's disease. Clin Oncol 9:165, 1983.
123. Rubin E, Maddox WA, Mazur MT. Cutaneous angiosarcoma of the breast 7 years after lumpectomy and radiation therapy. Radiology 174:258, 1990.
124. Sessions SC, Smenk RD. Cutaneous angiosarcoma of the breast after segmental mastectomy and radiation therapy. Arch Surg 127:1362, 1992.
125. Shaikh NA, Beaconsfield T, Walker M, et al. Postirradiation angiosarcoma of the breast: a case report. Eur J Surg Oncol 14: 449, 1988.
126. Stokkel MPM, Peterse HL. Angiosarcoma of the breast after lumpectomy and radiation therapy for adenocarcinoma. Cancer 69:1965, 1992.
127. Westerberg AH, Wiggers T, Henzen-Logmans SC, et al. Postirradiation angiosarcoma of the greater omentum. Eur J Surg Oncol 15:175, 1989.
128. Wovlov RB, Sato N, Azumi N, et al. Intraabdominal "angiosarcomatosis": report of two cases after pelvic irradiation. Cancer 67:2275, 1991.

### Kaposi's Sarcoma

129. Beckstead JH, Wood GS, Fletcher V. Evidence for the origin of Kaposi's sarcoma from lymphatic endothelium. Am J Pathol 119:294, 1985.
130. Beral V, Bull D, Darby S, et al. Risk of Kaposi's sarcoma and sexual practices associated with faecal contact in homosexual or bisexual men with AIDS. Lancet 339:632, 1992.
131. Bigga RJ, Melbye M, Kestems L, et al. Kaposi's sarcoma in Zaire is not associated with HTLV-III infection. N Engl J Med 311:1051, 1984.
132. Bluefarb SM. Kaposi's Sarcoma. Charles C Thomas, Springfield, IL, 1966.
133. Cathomas G, Stalder A, McGandy CE, Mihatsch MJ. Distribution of human herpesvirus 8 DNA in tumorous and nontumorous tissue of patients with acquired immunodeficiency syndrome with and without Kaposi's sarcoma. Mod Pathol 11: 415, 1998.
134. Chang Y, Cesarman E, Pessin MS, et al. Identification of herpesvirus-like DNA sequences in AIDS-associated Kaposi's sarcoma. Science 266:1865, 1994.
135. Chor PJ, Santa Cruz DJ. Kaposi's sarcoma: a clinicopathologic review and differential diagnosis. J Cutan Pathol 19:6, 1992.
136. Cohn DL, Judson FN. Absence of Kaposi's sarcoma in hemophiliacs with the acquired immunodeficiency syndrome. Ann Intern Med 101:401, 1984.
137. Cossu S, Satta R, Cottoni F, Massarelli G. Lymphangioma-like variant of Kaposi's sarcoma: clinicopathologic study of seven cases with review of the literature. Am J Dermatopathol 19:16, 1997.
138. Costa J, Rabson AS. Generalized Kaposi's sarcoma is not a neoplasm. Lancet 1:58, 1983.
139. Cox FH, Helwig EB. Kaposi's sarcoma. Cancer 12:289, 1959.
140. Dada MA, Chetty R, Biddolph SC, et al. The immunoexpression of bcl-2 and p53 in Kaposi's sarcoma. Histopathology 29: 159, 1996.
141. Dictor M, Rambech E, Way D, et al. Human herpesvirus 8 (Kaposi's sarcoma-associated herpesvirus) DNA in Kaposi's sarcoma lesions, AIDS Kaposi's sarcoma cell lines, endothelial Kaposi's sarcoma simulators, and the skin of immunosuppressed patients. Am J Pathol 148:2009, 1996.
142. Ecklung RE, Valatis J. Kaposi's sarcoma of lymph nodes. Arch Pathol 74:224, 1962.
143. Elford J, Tindall B, Sherkey T. Kaposi's sarcoma and insertive rimming [letter]. Lancet 339:938, 1992.
144. Ensoli B, Barillari G, Salahuddin SZ, et al. Tat protein of HIV-1 stimulates growth of cells derived from Kaposi's sarcoma: lesions of AIDS patients. Nature 345:84, 1990.
145. Ensoli B, Nakamura S, Salahuddin SZ, et al. AIDS-Kaposi's cells: long term culture with growth factor from retrovirus-infected $CD4^+$T cells. Science 242:430, 1988.
146. Fauci AS, Masur H, Gelmann EP, et al. The acquired immunodeficiency syndrome: an update. Ann Intern Med 102:800, 1985.
147. Flore O, Rafii S, Ely S, et al. Transformation of primary human endothelial cells by Kaposi's sarcoma-associated herpes virus. Nature 394:588, 1998.

148. Foreman KE, Wrone-Smith T, Boise LH, et al. Kaposi's sarcoma tumor cells preferentially express Bcl-xL. Am J Pathol 149:795, 1996.
149. Fukunaga M, Silverberg S. Hyaline globules in Kaposi's sarcoma: a light microscopic and immunohistochemical study. Mod Pathol 4:187, 1991.
150. Fukunaga M, Silverberg SG. Kaposi's sarcoma in patients with acquired immune deficiency syndrome: a flow cytometric DNA analysis of 26 lesions in 21 patients. Cancer 66:758, 1990.
151. Gallo RC. Some aspects of the pathogenesis of HIV-1-associated Kapsoi's sarcoma. Monogr Natl Cancer Inst 23:55, 1998.
152. Gange RW, Wilson-Jones E. Lymphangioma-like Kaposi's sarcoma: a report of 3 cases. Br J Dermatol 100:327, 1979.
153. Gill PS, Tsai YC, Rao AP, et al. Evidence for multiclonality in multicentric Kaposi's sarcoma. Proc Natl Acad Sci USA 95: 8257, 1998.
154. Giraldo G, Beth E, Buonaqurao FM. Kaposi's sarcoma: a natural model of interrelationships between viruses, immunologic responses, genetics, and oncogenesis. Antibiol Chemother 32:1, 1984.
155. Giraldo G, Beth E, Coeur P, et al. Kaposi's sarcoma: a new model in the search for viruses associated with human malignancies. J Natl Cancer Inst 49:1495, 1972.
156. Giraldo G, Beth E, Huang ES. Kaposi's sarcoma and its relationship to cytomegalovirus (CMV). III. CMV DNA and CMV early antigens in Kaposi's sarcoma. Int J Cancer 26:23, 1980.
157. Harris NL. Hypervascular follicular hyperplasia and Kaposi's sarcoma in patients at risk for AIDS. N Engl J Med 3120:462, 1984.
158. Herman PS, Shogreen LMR, White WL. The evaluation of human herpesvirus 8 (Kaposi's sarcoma-associated herpesvirus) in cutaneous lesions of Kaposi's sarcoma: a study of formalin-fixed paraffin-embedded tissue. Am J Dermatopathol 20: 7, 1998.
159. Hodak E, Hammel I, Feinmesser M, et al. Differential expression of p53 and Ki67 proteins in classic and iatrogenic Kaposi's sarcoma. Am J Dermatopathol 21:138, 1999.
160. Huang YQ, Li JJ, Rush MG, et al. HPV-16-related DNA sequences in Kaposi's sarcoma. Lancet 339:515, 1992.
161. Jin YT, Tsai ST, Yan JJ, et al. Detection of Kaposi's sarcoma-associated herpesvirus-like DNA sequence in vascular lesions: a reliable diagnostic marker for Kaposi's sarcoma. Am J Clin Pathol 105:360, 1996.
162. Jones RR, Jones EW. The histogenesis of Kaposi's sarcoma. Am J Dermatopathol 8:369, 1986.
163. Jones RR, Spaull J, Spry C, et al. The histogenesis of Kaposi's sarcoma in patients with and without AIDS. J Clin Pathol 39: 742, 1986.
164. Kao GF, Johnson FB, Sulica VI. The nature of the hyaline (eosinophilic) globules and vascular slits of Kaposi's sarcoma. Am J Dermatopathol 12:256, 1990.
165. Kaposi M. Idiopathisches multiples Pigmentsarkom der Haut. Arch Dermatol Syph 4:265, 1872.
166. Krigel RL. Prognostic factors in Kaposi's sarcoma. In: Friedman-Kien AE, Laubenstein LJ (eds) AIDS: The Epidemic of Kaposi's Sarcoma and Opportunistic Infections. Masson, New York, 1984.
167. Krown SE. Acquired immunodeficiency-associated Kaposi's sarcoma. Med Clin North Am 81:471, 1997.
168. Krown SE, Metroka C, Wernz JC. Kaposi's sarcoma in the acquired immune deficiency syndrome: a proposal for uniform evaluation, response, and staging criteria. J Clin Oncol 7:1201, 1989.
169. Li JJ, Huang YQ, Cockrell CJ, Friedman-Kien AE. Localization of human herpes-like virus type 8 in vascular endothelial cells and perivascular spindle shaped cells of Kaposi's sarcoma lesions by in situ hybridization. Am J Pathol 148:1741, 1996.
170. Lothe F. Kaposi's sarcoma. Acta Pathol Microbiol Scand 161:1, 1963.
171. Marshall ME, Hatfield ST, Hatfield DR. Arteriovenous malformation simulating Kaposi's sarcoma (pseudo Kaposi's sarcoma). Arch Dermatol 121:99, 1985.
172. Masood R, Cai J, Zheng T, et al. Vascular endothelial growth factor/vascular permeability factor is an autocrine growth factor for AIDS–Kaposi sarcoma. Proc Natl Acad Sci USA 94:979, 1997.
173. McNutt NS, Fletcher V, Conant MA. Early lesions of Kaposi's sarcoma in homosexual men: an ultrastructural comparison with other vascular proliferations in the skin. Am J Pathol 111: 62, 1983.
174. Mitsuyasu RT. Clinical variants and staging of Kaposi's sarcoma. Semin Oncol 14 (Suppl 3):13, 1987.
175. Moore PS, Chang Y. Kaposi's sarcoma-associated herpesvirus-encoded oncogenes and oncogenesis. J Natl Cancer Inst Mongr 23:65, 1998.
176. Murakami M, Sugita Y, Ishii N, et al. Detection and sequence diversity of Kaposi's sarcoma-associated herpesvirus (KHSV)/ human herpesvirus 8(HHV-8) DNA. Eur J Dermatol 9:13, 1999.
177. Nakamura S, Salahuddin SZ, Biberfeld P, et al. Kaposi's sarcoma cells: long-term culture with growth factor from retrovirus-infected CD4+T-cells. Science 242:426, 1988.
178. Neipel F, Albraecht J-C, Fleckenstein B. Human herpesvirus 8—the first human Rhadinovirus. Monogr Natl Cancer Inst 23:73, 1998.
179. O'Brien PH, Brasfield RD. Kaposi's sarcoma. Cancer 19:1497, 1966.
180. Pammer J, Plettenberg A, Weninger W, et al. CD40 antigen is expressed by endothelial cells and tumor cells in Kaposi's sarcoma. Am J Pathol 148:1387, 1996.
181. Pilot P, Taelman H, Minlangu KB, et al. Acquired immunodeficiency syndrome in a heterosexual population in Zaire. Lancet 2:65, 1984.
182. Qunibi WY, Barri Y, Alfurayh O, et al. Kaposi's sarcoma in renal transplant recipients: a report of 26 cases from a single institution. Transplant Proc 25:1402, 1993.
183. Rabkin CS, Janz S, Lash A. Monoclonal origin of multicentric Kaposi's sarcoma lesions. N Engl J Med 336:988, 1997.
184. Reed WB, Kamath HM, Weiss L. Kaposi sarcoma with emphasis on the internal manifestations. Arch Dermatol 110:115, 1974.
185. Reynolds WA, Winkelman RK, Soule EH. Kaposi's sarcoma: a clinicopathologic study with particular reference to its relationship to the reticuloendothelial system. Medicine 44:419, 1965.
186. Rutgers JL, Wieczorek R, Bonetti F, et al. The expression of endothelial cell surface antigens by AIDS-associated Kaposi's sarcoma. Am J Pathol 122:493, 1986.
187. Safai B, Johnson KG, Myskowski PL, et al. The natural history of Kaposi's sarcoma in the acquired immunodeficiency syndrome. Ann Intern Med 103:744, 1985.
188. Safai B, Mike V, Giraldo G, et al. Association of Kaposi's sarcoma with second primary malignancies: possible etiopathogenic implications. Cancer 45:1472, 1980.
189. Salahuddin SZ, Nakamura S, Bikerfeld P, et al. Angiogenic properties of Kaposi's sarcoma-derived cells after long term culture in vitro. Science 242:430, 1988.
190. Schwartz JL, Muhlbauer JE, Steiqbigel RT. Pre-Kaposi's sarcoma. J Am Acad Dermatol 11:377, 1984.
191. Scully PA, Steinman HK, Kennedy C, et al. AIDS-related Ka-

posi's sarcoma displays differential expression of endothelial surface antigens. Am J Pathol 130:244, 1988.
192. Shamroth JM, Ratanjee H, Kellen P, et al. Kaposi's sarcoma localized at the site of previous vascular surgery. Arch Dermatol 121:969, 1985.
193. Shmueli D, Sharpira Z, Yussim A, et al. The incidence of Kaposi's sarcoma in renal transplantation patients and its relation to immunosuppression. Transplant Proc 21:3209, 1989.
194. Silmonart T, Degraef C, Noel JC, et al. Overexpression of Bcl-2 in Kaposi's sarcoma-derived cells. J Invest Dermatol 111:349, 1998.
195. Velez-Garcia E, Robles-Cardona N, Fradera J. Kaposi's sarcoma in transfusion-associated AIDS. N Engl J Med 312:648, 1985.
196. Vogel J, Hinrichs SH, Reynolds RK, et al. The HIV tat gene induces dermal lesions resembling Kaposi's sarcoma in transgenic mice. Nature 335:606, 1988.
197. Volberding P. Therapy of Kaposi's sarcoma with interferon. In: Friedman-Kien AE, Laubenstein LJ (eds) AIDS: The Current Epidemic of Kaposi's Sarcoma and Opportunistic Infections. Masson, New York, 1984.
198. Weich HA, Salahuddin SZ, Gill P, et al. AIDS-associated Kaposi's sarcoma-derived cells in long-term culture express and synthesize smooth muscle alpha-actin. Am J Pathol 139:1251, 1991.
199. Weiss RA, Whitby D, Talbot S, et al. Human herpesvirus type 8 and Kaposi's sarcoma. Monogr Natl Cancer Inst 23:51, 1998.
200. Weninger W, Partanen TA, Breiteneder-Geleff S, et al. Expression of vascular endothelial growth factor receptor-3 and podoplanin suggests a lymphatic endothelial cell origin of Kaposi's sarcoma tumor cells. Lab Invest 79:243, 1999.

### Intravascular Lymphomatosis

201. Ansbacher L, Low N, Beck D, et al. Neoplastic angioendotheliosis, a clinicopathologic entity with multifocal presentation: case report. J Neurosurg 54:412, 1981.
202. Ansell J, Bhawan J, Cohen S, et al. Histiocytic lymphoma and malignant angioendotheliomatosis: one disease or two? Cancer 50:1506, 1982.
203. Bhawan J, Wolff SM, Ucci AA, et al. Malignant lymphoma and malignant angioendotheliomatosis: one disease. Cancer 55: 570, 1985.
204. Carroll TJ, Schelper RL, Goeken JA, et al. Neoplastic angioendotheliomatosis: immunopathologic and morphologic evidence for intravascular malignant lymphomatosis. Am J Clin Pathol 85:169, 1986.
205. Ferry JA, Harris NL, Picker LJ, et al. Intravascular lymphomatosis (malignant angioendotheliomatosis): a B-cell neoplasm expressing surface homing receptors. Mod Pathol 1:444, 1988.
206. Lin BT, Weiss LM, Battifora H. Intravascularly disseminated angiosarcoma: true neoplastic angioendotheliomatosis? Report of two cases. Am J Surg Pathol 21:1138, 1997.
207. Sheibani K, Battifora H, Winberg CD, et al. Further evidence that "malignant angioendotheliomatosis" is an angiotropic large-cell lymphoma. N Engl J Med 314:943, 1986.
208. Wick MR, Banks PM, McDonald TJ. Angioendotheliomatosis of the nose with fatal systemic dissemination. Cancer 48:2510, 1981.
209. Wick MR, Mills SE, Scheithauer BW, et al. Angioendotheliomatosis: an immunohistochemical reassessment. Lab Invest 52: 75A, 1985.
210. Wrotnowski U, Mills SE, Cooper PH. Malignant angioendotheliomatosis: an angiotropic lymphoma? Am J Clin Pathol 3:244, 1985.

# CHAPTER 26

# TUMORS OF LYMPH VESSELS

The lymphatic system, a diffuse network of endothelial channels, makes its appearance during the sixth week of human embryonic development. There is controversy as to whether it arises as an outgrowth from the venous system or differentiates *de novo* from adjacent mesenchyme Proponents of the first theory include Sabin, who demonstrated numerous connections between lymphatics and veins by means of injection techniques in a series of graded pig embryos. She concluded that the lymphatic system arose as buds from the venous system. Others maintain that these connections between veins and lymphatics occur only after the lymphatics have been laid down and the system differentiates from mesenchyme. In either event the lymphatic system develops in close association with the venous system and parallels the venous drainage of an organ. How these morphologic events translate into cellular events is not fully understood. It is known that vascular endothelial growth factor receptor-3 (VEGFR-3), a tyrosine kinase receptor, is important for lymphatic development.[9] Early in embryogenesis it is expressed by all endothelium but becomes restricted later during development to lymphatic endothelial cells (see Chapter 23).[4] Its ligand, VEGFC, is a potent lymphangiogenic factor that stimulates lymphatic endothelial proliferation and migration and lymphatic vessel enlargement. Identification of this receptor by immunohistochemistry has also proved useful for identifying tumors exhibiting lymphatic differentiation (see Chapter 24).[2]

In adults the lymphatics are an extensive unidirectional system of blunt-ending vessels that retrieve excess fluid from the interstitium, transport it to regional lymph nodes, and return it to the venous system by way of the thoracic duct. In addition, the lymphatics serve a special function in the absorption of protein and lipid from the liver and small intestine, respectively. These small vessels are nearly ubiquitous but are conspicuously absent in the brain, anterior chamber of the eye, and portions of organs served by an "open," or sinusoidal, blood system such as bone marrow and red pulp of spleen. The smallest lymphatic vessels approximate the size of the blood capillary and are made up of fragile endothelial channels situated in a background of reticulum fibers and ground substance. Larger collecting channels contain, in addition, valves, muscle fibers, and elastic tissue, although the latter two are never developed to the extent observed in veins.

At the level of light microscopy the small lymphatics closely resemble capillaries and sometimes are only tentatively identified by the nature of their contents. Fine structural analysis, however, has documented rather significant differences. Although the basic conformation of the endothelial cell of the lymphatic system is similar to that of the blood capillary, it is invested by neither a basement membrane nor pericytes, with the exception of large collecting lymphatic channels. The former finding is also borne out by immunohistochemical analysis. Whereas antibodies to type IV collagen and laminin demonstrate a linear pattern of immunoreactivity around vascular capillary endothelium, this pattern is lacking around lymphatic capillary endothelium.[1] Thus lymphatic endothelium is in direct contact with the interstitial space. This topographic relation is believed important for the expeditious recovery of fluid because a basement membrane serves as a partial diffusion barrier. In addition, there are thin "anchoring filaments" that terminate directly on the abluminal surface of the cell membrane and probably serve to maintain patency of the lymphatics during periods of increased interstitial pressure. The intercellular contacts between lymphatic endothelia are variable. Although tight junctions (zonula adherens), macula adherens, and desmosomes are present, there are many areas of simple overlapping of cells with no junctions.[3,7] This arrangement creates a "swinging door" effect so fluid can passively enter the lymphatic space during periods of increased interstitial pressure. Pinocytotic vesicles, thin cytofilaments, modest numbers of mitochondria, and endoplasmic reticulum, similar to those in capillaries, are also present in lymphatic cells. Further differences between vascular and lymphatic capillary endothelium have been demonstrated with the advent of numerous monoclonal antibodies directed against the structural components of endothelial cells.[5,8]

## LYMPHANGIOMAS

As with hemangiomas, it is often difficult to state whether lymphangiomas are true neoplasms, hamartomas, or lymphangiectasias. In actuality, this distinction is of little practical value because they are all benign lesions, and therapy is largely dictated by their location and clinical extent. Most regard lymphangiomas as malformations that arise from sequestrations of lymphatic tissue that fail to communicate normally with the lymphatic system (Fig. 26–1). These remnants may have some capacity to proliferate, but more importantly they accumulate vast amounts of fluid, which accounts for their cystic appearance. The fact that most lymphangiomas manifest clinically during childhood and develop in areas where the primitive lymph sacs occur (e.g., neck, axilla) provides presumptive evidence for this hypothesis. Some early workers such as Goetsch[26] considered these lesions to be true neoplasms capable of locally aggressive behavior, whereas others have suggested that they arise when inflammation causes fibrosis and obstruction of lymphatic channels. Although it is probable that some lymphangiomas are acquired lesions arising on an obstructive basis following surgery, irradiation, or infection in an affected part,[20,21,32] most seem to represent developmental lesions that appear relatively early in life.

Traditionally, lymphangiomas were divided into three groups.[6] The lymphangioma simplex, or capillary lymphangioma, is composed of small thin-walled lymphatics, whereas the cavernous lymphangioma consists of larger lymphatic channels with adventitial coats. The cystic lymphangioma, or cystic hygroma, is made up of large macroscopic lymphatic spaces that have investitures of collagen and smooth muscle. This classification has largely been replaced by the all-inclusive term "lymphangioma," as the distinction among some of these lesions was arbitrary and of little importance. In fact, many lymphangiomas have both cystic and cavernous components, which raises the possibility that the cystic lymphangioma is merely a long-standing cavernous lymphangioma in which the cavernous spaces have been converted to cystic spaces. Bill and Sumner[12] suggested that histologic differences are attributable to differences in anatomic location. Cystic lymphangiomas arise in areas such as the neck and axilla, where loose connective tissue allows expansion of the endothelium-lined channels; cavernous lymphangiomas develop in the mouth, lips, cheek, tongue, or other areas where dense connective tissue and muscle prevent expansion. We believe cystic and cavernous lymphangiomas are not sufficiently distinct to be treated separately. Differences between the two are mentioned as necessary.

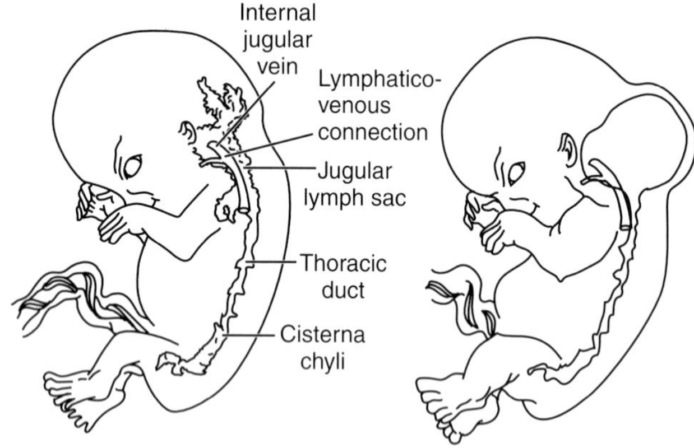


**FIGURE 26–1.** Proposed mechanism for formation of a lymphangioma. Lymphatic system in a normal fetus (**left**) with a patent connection between the jugular lymph sac and the internal jugular vein and a cystic hygroma from a failed lymphaticovenous connection (**right**). (Modified from Chervenak FA, Issacson G, Blakemore KJ. Fetal cystic hygroma: cause and natural history. N Engl J Med 309:822, 1983.)

### Clinical Findings

Compared with hemangiomas, lymphangiomas are relatively rare. Anderson,[11] reviewing 768 benign tumors at Babies Hospital in New York over a 15-year period, identified only 48 lymphangiomas; and Bill and Sumner[12] estimated that they accounted for 5 of 3000 admissions at Children's Orthopedic Hospital. Kindblom and Angervall[28] reported 100 lymphangiomas over a 5-year period at the Sahlgren Hospital. The gender incidence is roughly equal,[12,28] although a slight male predominance is often recorded. It is estimated that 50–65% of these tumors are present at birth, and as many as 90% manifest by the end of the second year of life.[10,12,14,16,22] In some series nearly one-third were documented during adult life.[28] Those that present during adult life are the superficial cutaneous lymphangiomas (lymphangioma circumscriptum),[20,23,32,37] some of which are acquired lymphangiectasias and intraabdominal lymphangiomas that present after long symptom-free intervals. Lymphangiomas affect almost any part of the body served by the lymphatic system but show a predilection for the head, neck, and axilla (Figs. 26–2, 26–3), sites that account for one-half to three-fourths of all lymphangiomas (Table 26–1). They also occur sporadically in various parenchymal organs including lung, gastrointestinal tract, spleen, liver, and bone. In the last three locations they occasionally signify the presence of diffuse or multifocal disease (see Lymphangiomatosis,

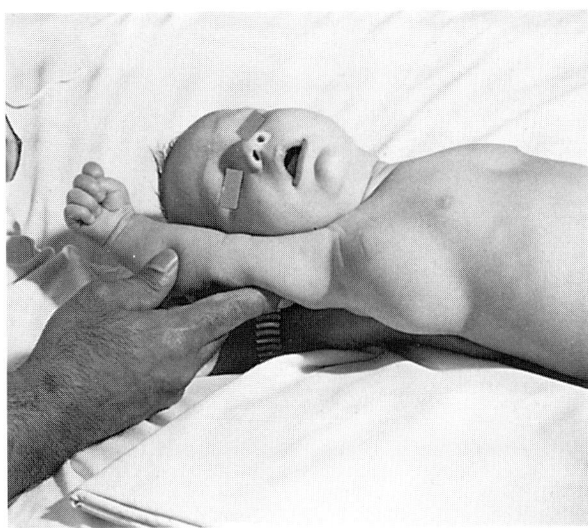

**FIGURE 26–2.** Lymphangioma (cystic hygroma) of the axilla.

**TABLE 26–1** ANATOMIC LOCATION OF LYMPHANGIOMAS (61 PATIENTS)

| Anatomic Location | No. |
|---|---|
| Head | 35 |
| Tongue | 8 |
| Check | 7 |
| Floor of the mouth | 7 |
| Parotid | 5 |
| Other | 8 |
| Neck | 25 |
| Trunk and extremities | 43 |
| Axilla | 15 |
| Pectoral | 10 |
| Arm | 6 |
| Scapula | 5 |
| Other | 7 |
| Internal | 6 |
| Mediastinum | 5 |
| Abdomen | 1 |

Modified from Bill AH, Sumner DS. A unified concept of lymphangioma and cystic hygroma. Surg Gynecol Obstet 120:79, 1965.
There are more than 61 tumors owing to the fact that large tumors were tabulated under several locations.

below). Lymphangiomas also occur in association with hemangiomas in Maffucci syndrome.[34]

The most common presentation of lymphangioma is that of a soft fluctuant mass that enlarges, remains static, or waxes and wanes during the period of clinical observation. In a few cases rapid enlargement can be related to an upper respiratory tract infection, which apparently causes obstruction in the lymphatics draining the tumor.

Lymphangioma (cystic hygroma) may also be detected in utero by ultrasonography. Such cases merit special comment, as they have been shown to be associated with hydrops fetalis and Turner syndrome, and they are associated with a high death rate[13,15] (Figs. 26–4, 26–5). Chervenak et al.[15] reported on 15 intrauterine cystic hygromas and found that 11 were associated with the cytogenetic abnormalities of Turner syndrome (45, X/O or 46,XO/46,XX). Of the 15 fetuses, 13 had severe hydrops, and none of the 15 ultimately survived. Thus it seems that defects in the lymphatic and vascular systems comprise part of Turner syndrome. The authors suggested that severe aberrations of the lymphatic system in this condition are incompatible with life; milder forms are compati-

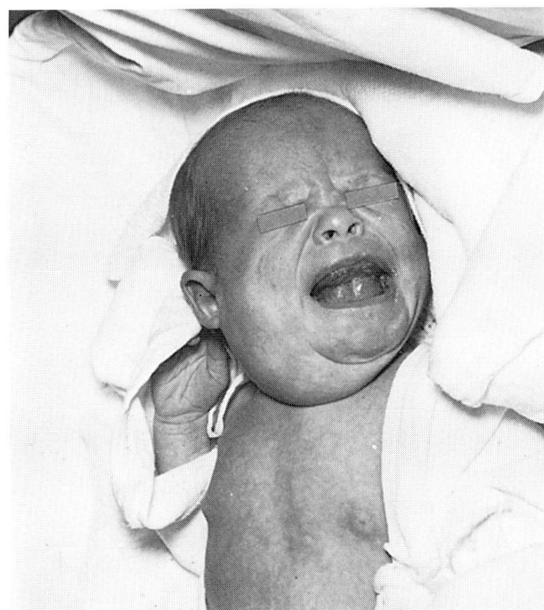

**FIGURE 26–3.** Lymphangioma (cystic hygroma) of the neck.

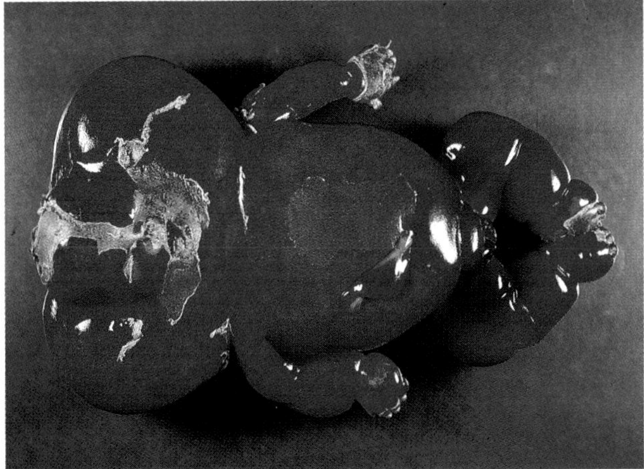

**FIGURE 26–4.** Abortus with Turner syndrome (XX/XO). A large cystic hygroma had been detected in utero by ultrasonography.

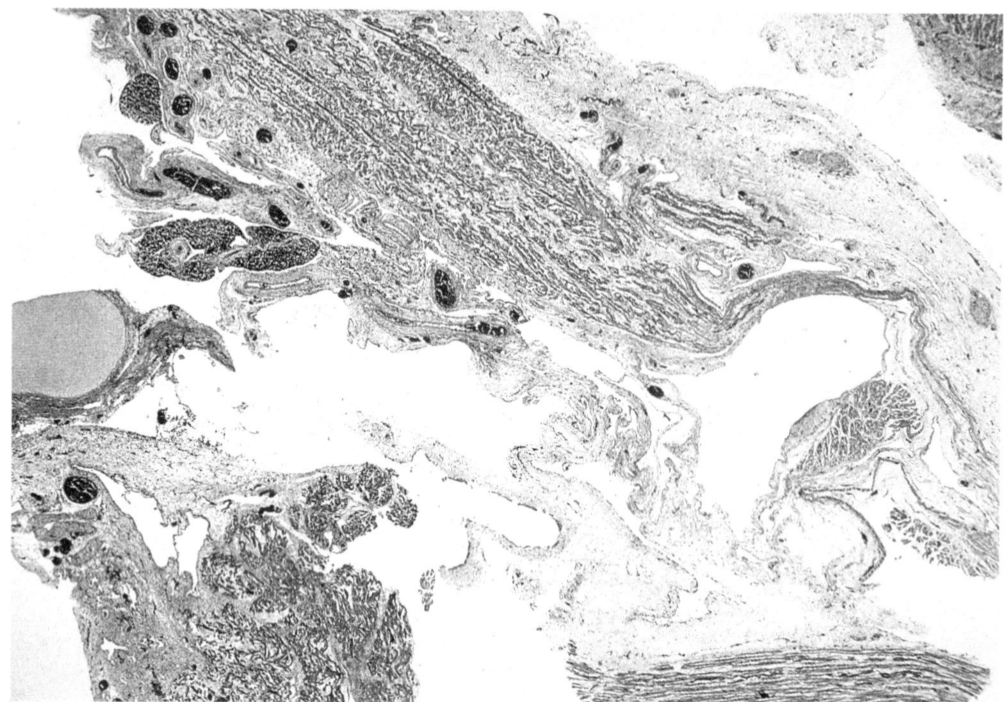

**FIGURE 26–5.** Section of a cystic hygroma from a fetus with Turner syndrome.

ble with survival but give rise to webbing of the neck and edema of the hands and feet, which characterize the Turner syndrome infantile phenotype (Fig. 26–6). Other syndromes may also be associated with fetal cystic hygroma, including Noonan syndrome, familial pterygium colli, fetal alcohol syndrome, and several chromosomal aneuploidies.[24] Because aneuploidic conditions may recur during subsequent pregnancies, cytogenetic analysis of fetuses born with cystic hygroma is indicated.

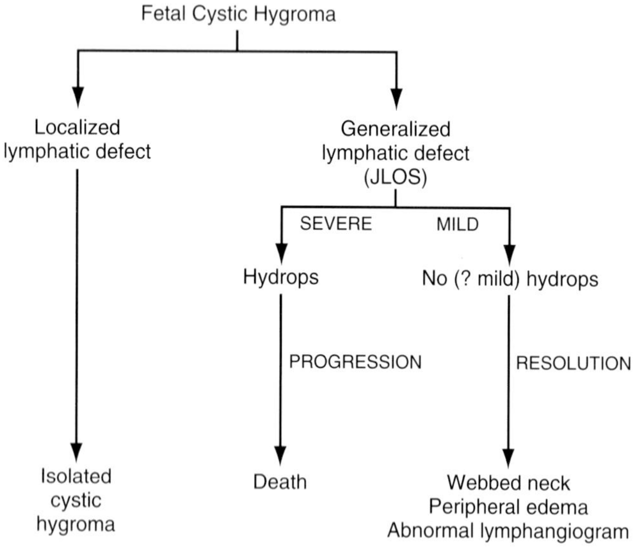

Fetal Cystic Hygroma

Localized lymphatic defect

Generalized lymphatic defect (JLOS)

SEVERE

MILD

Hydrops

No (? mild) hydrops

PROGRESSION

RESOLUTION

Isolated cystic hygroma

Death

Webbed neck
Peripheral edema
Abnormal lymphangiogram

**FIGURE 26–6.** Natural history of a fetal nuchal cystic hygroma. Generalized lymphatic defect results from the jugular lymphatic obstruction sequence. Depending on the severity of the obstruction, varying degrees of hydrops are noted. (Modified from Chervenak FA, Issacson G, Blakemore KJ. Fetal cystic hygroma: cause and natural history. N Engl J Med 309:822, 1983.)

## Lymphangiomas of the Head and Neck

Lymphangiomas are most common in the neck, where they typically lie in the supraclavicular fossa of the posterior cervical triangle or extend toward the crest of the shoulder. Less frequently they are located in the anterior cervical triangle just below the angle of the jaw. Tumors in this location are the ones most apt to present with significant airway or feeding problems.[18] About 10% of lymphangiomas of the neck extend into the mediastinum, illustrating the need for preoperative chest radiographs prior to planning a surgical approach. Grossly, these tumors are unicystic or multicystic masses that involve the superficial soft tissue and tend to bulge outward rather than extend inward (Fig. 26–3). Consequently, they usually do not compromise vital structures such as the trachea and esophagus unless they are large. In contrast to lymphangiomas of the neck, those involving the soft tissues of the lips, cheek, tongue, and mouth are usually of the cavernous type, frequently involve deep soft tissue structures, and cause functional impairment depending on their size.

## Intraabdominal Lymphangiomas

Intraabdominal tumors are rare (Fig. 26–7), as evidenced by the fact that Galifer et al.[25] tabulated only 139 cases from the English literature. Although 60% are present in patients under the age of 5 years, a significant percentage do not manifest until adult life.[16] The most common location is the mesentery, followed by the omentum, mesocolon, and retroperitoneum (Table 26–2). In addition to a palpable mass, patients with tumors in the first three locations often develop symptoms of an acute condition in the abdomen caused by the common complications of intestinal obstruction, volvulus, and infarction. In fact, a provisional diagnosis of acute appendicitis is frequently entertained because of the common occurrence of right lower quadrant pain. In contrast, retroperitoneal tumors produce few acute symptoms but ultimately are diagnosed by virtue of a large palpable mass causing displacement of one or more organs. Most arise in the lumbar area and cause displacement of the kidney, usually without urinary tract obstruction. Those arising in the superior portion of the retroperitoneum shift the pancreas and duodenum anteriorly.

In the past an abdominal lymphangioma was seldom diagnosed preoperatviely. The diagnosis can usually be suspected with a combination of radiologic studies.[29] Ultrasonography is useful for localizing and determining the cystic nature of the tumors. As seen by arteriography, the lesions are poorly vascularized; and in a few reported cases connections between lower extremity lymphatics and the tumors can be demonstrated with lymphography. On CT scans the tumors appear as multiple, homogeneous, nonenhancing areas with variable attenuation values, depending on whether the fluid is chylous or serous.

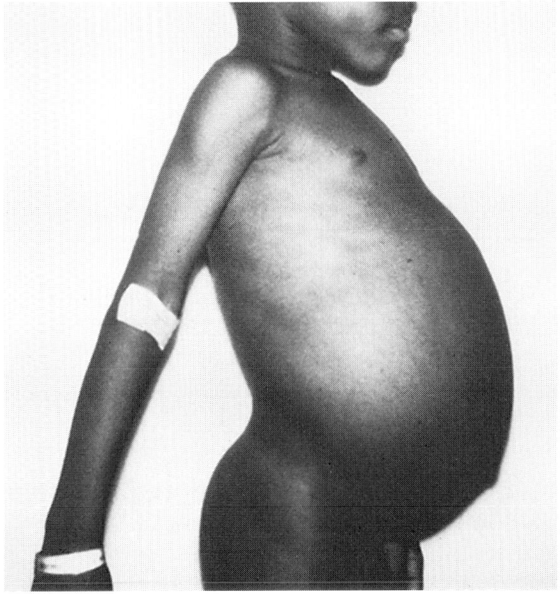

**FIGURE 26–7.** Large intraabdominal lymphangioma.

**TABLE 26–2** LOCATION OF 139 INTRAABDOMINAL LYMPHANGIOMAS

| Anatomic Location | No. of Cases | % |
|---|---|---|
| Mesentery | 96 | 69 |
| Jejunum | 25 | |
| Ileum | 44 | |
| Root of mesentery | 5 | |
| Not specified | 22 | |
| Omentum | 21 | 15 |
| Mesocolon | 15 | 11 |
| Retroperitoneum | 7 | 5 |
| *Total* | 139 | 100 |

Modified from Galifer RB, Pous JG, Juskiewenski S, et al. Intraabdominal cystic lymphangiomas in childhood. Prog Pediatr Surg 11:173, 1978.

## Cutaneous Lymphangiomas

Cutaneous lymphangiomas can be divided into superficial and deep forms.[21] The latter form is histologically and clinically identical to the usual cavernous lymphangioma and does not require additional elaboration (Fig. 26–8). The superficial intradermal form, sometimes referred to as *lymphangioma circumscriptum*,[21,32] has rather characteristic features. These lesions develop as multiple small vesicles or wart-like nodules that cover localized areas of skin (Fig. 26–9), although in some cases large areas of the body are affected. Histologically, dilated irregular lymphatic channels fill the papillary dermis and protrude into the epidermis, giving the impression of being "intraepidermal." The overlying epidermis is acanthotic and thrown into papillae. Generally, the lesions are asymptomatic unless they become irritated. They may arise de novo or be secondary to surgery or irradiation. In the latter setting some prefer to classify the lesions as "lymphangiectasis,"[20,21] although they are clinically and histologically indistinguishable from the *de novo* lesions.

Another form of cutaneous lymphangioma deserves special mention because of its mimicry of well differentiated angiosarcoma. The *acquired progressive lymphangioma (lymphangioendothelioma)* is a slowly growing cutaneous lymphangioma that occurs spontaneously in children and usually following surgery, irridiation, or minor forms of injury[17,26a,27,30,38] in adults (Figs. 26–10, 26–11, 26–12). Because of their association with irradiation some have also employed the term "benign lymphangiomatous papules following radiotherapy."[17] The two lesions, described as "atypical vascular lesions of the skin" by Fineberg and Rosen that

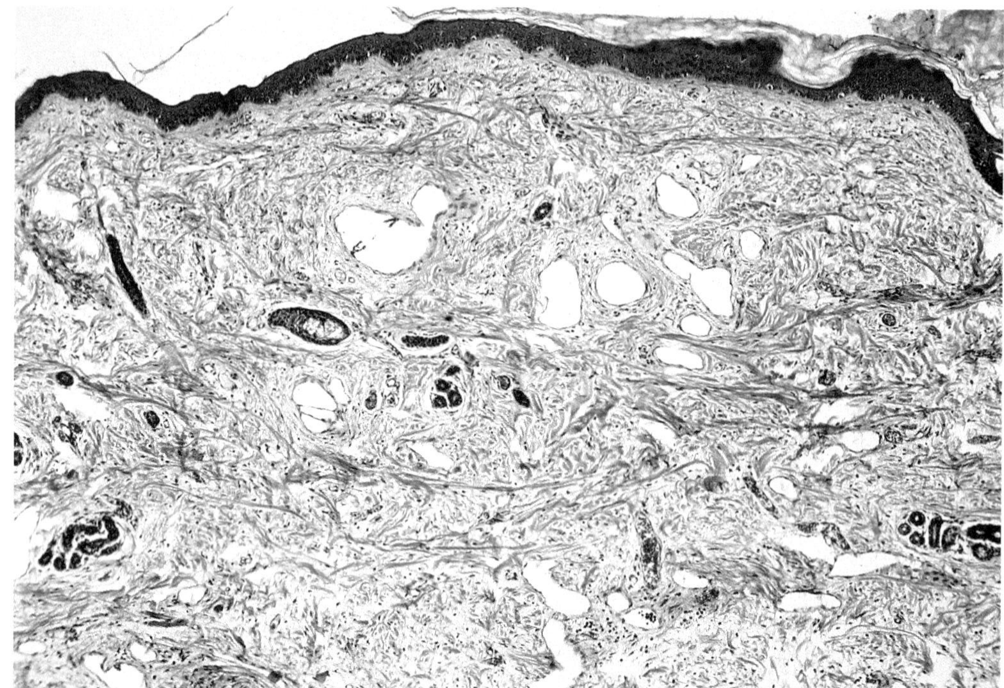

**FIGURE 26–8.** Cutaneous lymphangioma of the deep type. Dilated lymphatic channels extend over large areas of skin and involve superficial and deep dermis.

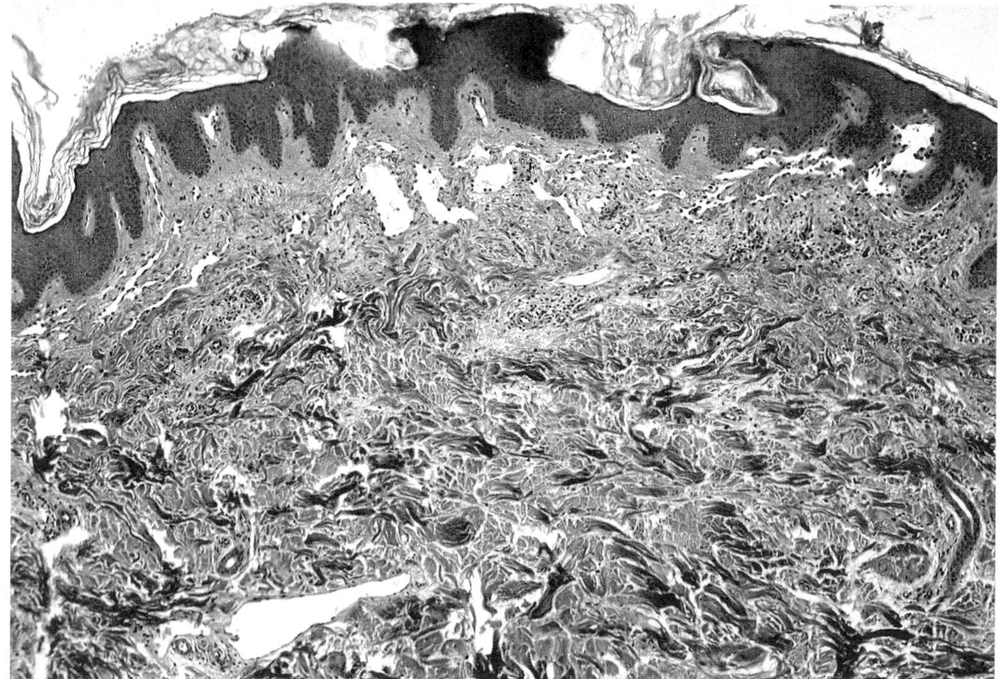

**FIGURE 26–9.** Cutaneous lymphangioma of superficial type (lymphangioma circumscriptum). Lymphatic vessels are localized and restricted to superficial dermis.

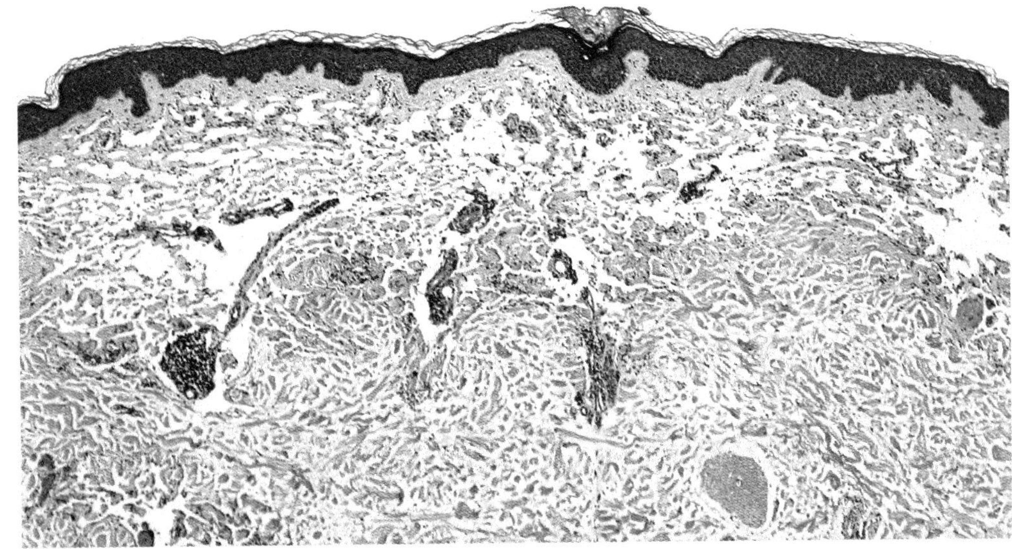

**FIGURE 26–10.** Acquired progressive lymphangioma with superficial proliferation of lymphatic vessels.

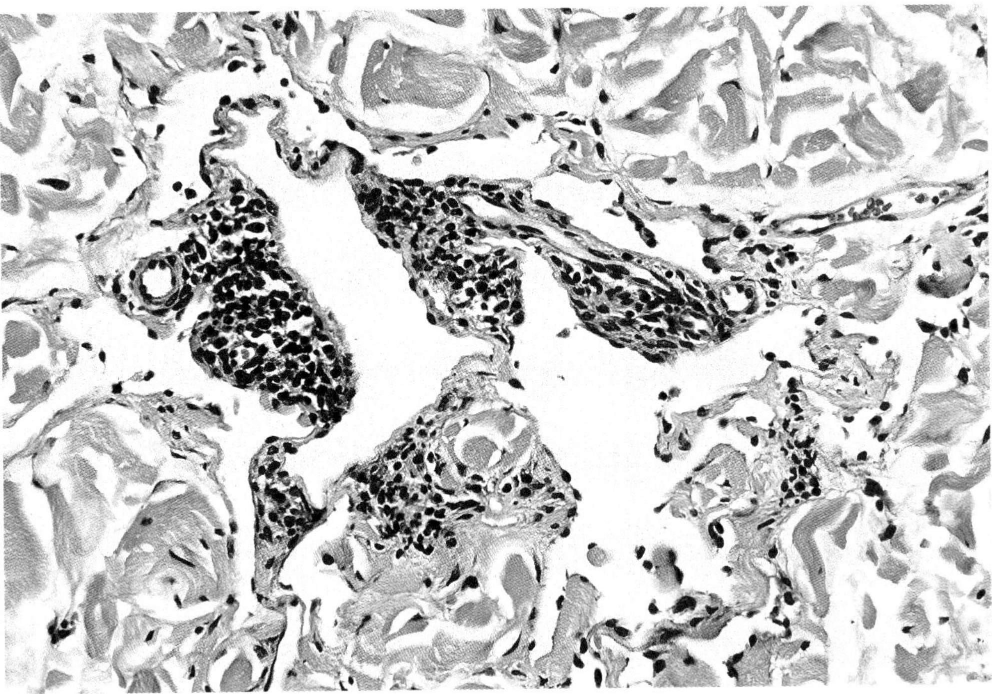

**FIGURE 26–11.** Acquired progressive lymphangioma with dissection of dermis by well differentiated lymphatic vessels.

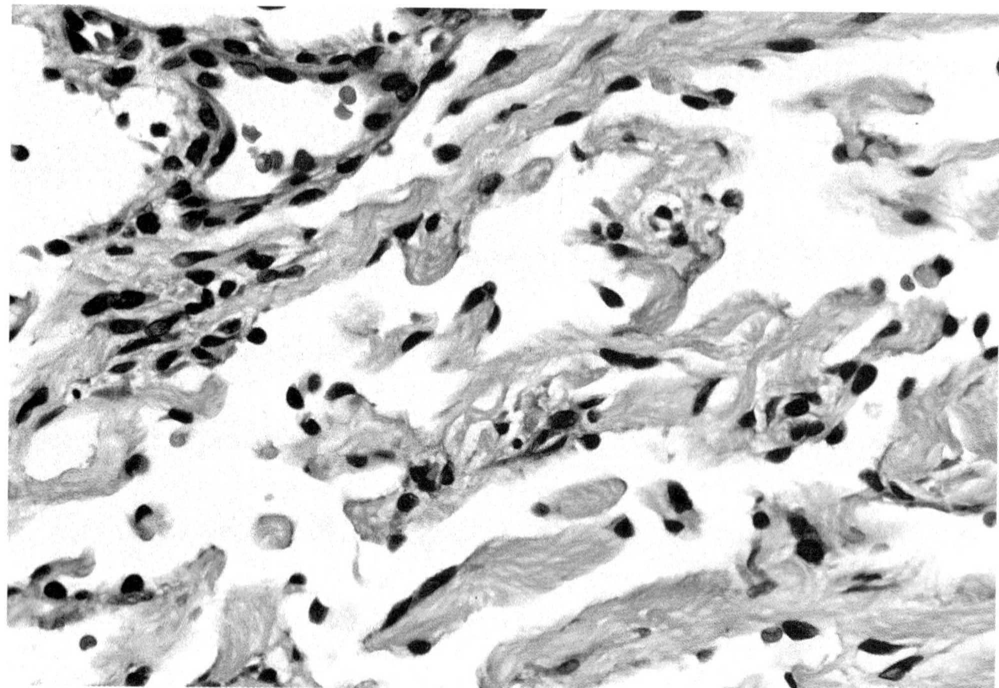

**FIGURE 26–12.** Acquired progressive lymphangioma with a single layer of endothelial cells without atypia.

occur after lumpectomy or irradiation may be closely related pathogenetically but are more limited in their growth.[19] Clinically, the lesion appears as one or more erythematous, white-tan or translucent vesicles. Those seen following irradiation occur after an interval of several months to years in the irradiated area. One of the most important clues to the diagnosis are the ectatic lymph vessels in the subpapillary region of the upper dermis that create the papular or vesicular appearance. The vessels ramify in the dermis and occasionally extend into the subcutis. The vessels, filled with clear fluid, are lined by attenuated endothelial cells that do not exhibit atypia, mitotic activity, or solid areas of growth. Lymphoid aggregates accompany the lymphatic channels. Follow-up of a limited number of cases has indicated a benign clinical course with no evidence of metastasis. In particular, three of the five patients reported following irradiation by Diaz-Cascajo et al. had follow-up of more than 3 years and were alive and well with neither recurrence nor metastasis.[17] In the series by Guillou and Fletcher, one of nine patients develolped a recurrence. Nonetheless, we believe this diagnosis of acquired progressive lymphangioma should be employed cautiously when dealing with postirradiation lesions in adults, as this situation is well recognized as a precursor to the development of angiosarcoma. In this setting it has been our approach to sample such lesions well, correlate the pathologic findings closely with the clinical features, and recommend close follow-up care.

## Gross and Microscopic Findings

Lymphangiomas vary from well circumscribed lesions made up of one or more large interconnecting cysts to ill-defined, sponge-like compressible lesions (Figs. 26–13 to 26–19) composed of microscopic cysts. The former are traditionally known as *cystic lymphan-*

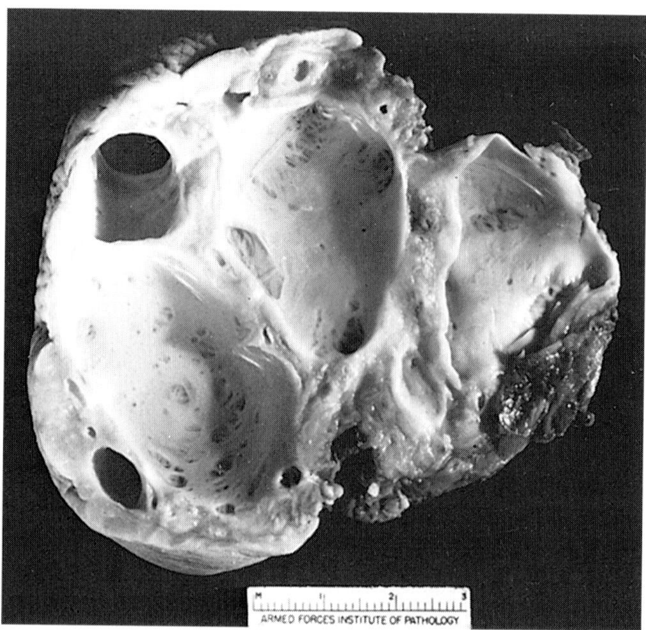


**FIGURE 26–13.** Cut section of a lymphangioma with thick-walled cysts of various size.

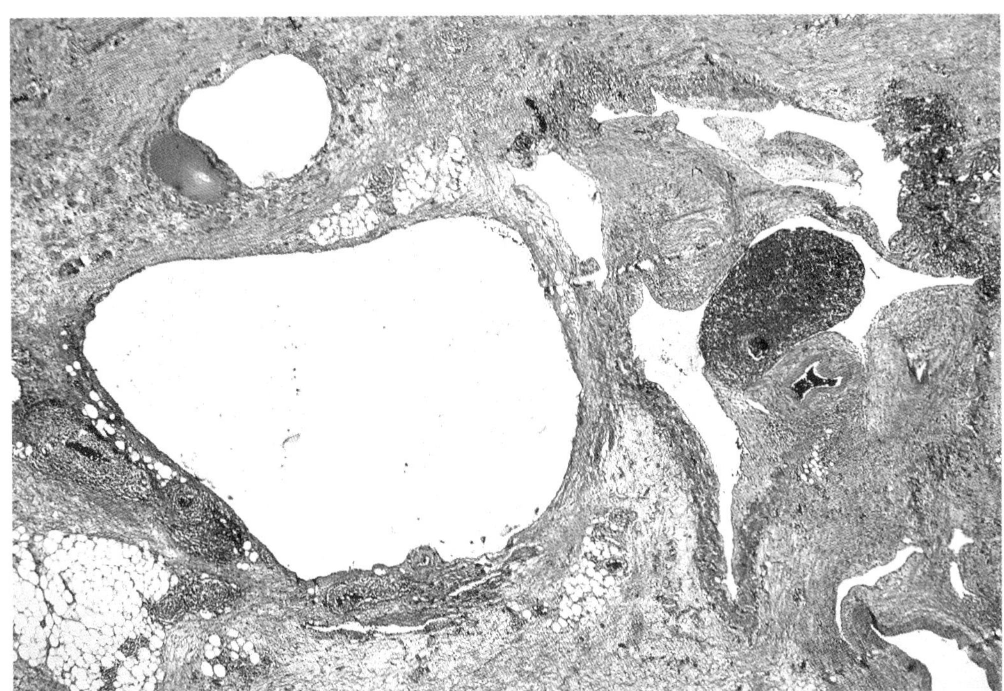

**FIGURE 26–14.** Low power view of lymphangioma.

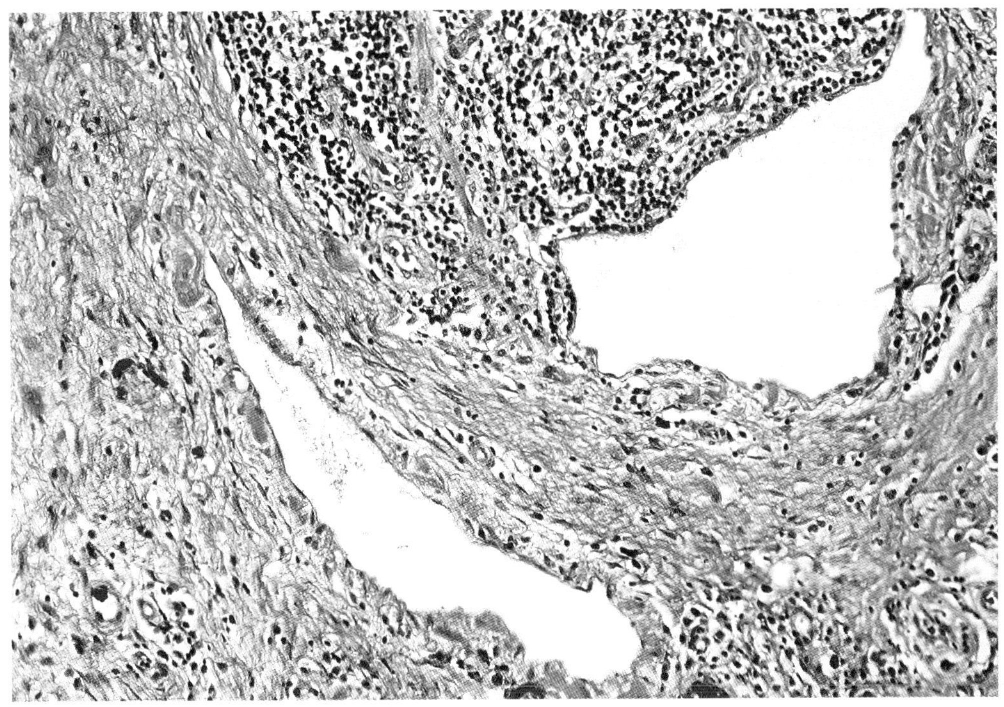

**FIGURE 26–15.** High power view of lymphangioma.

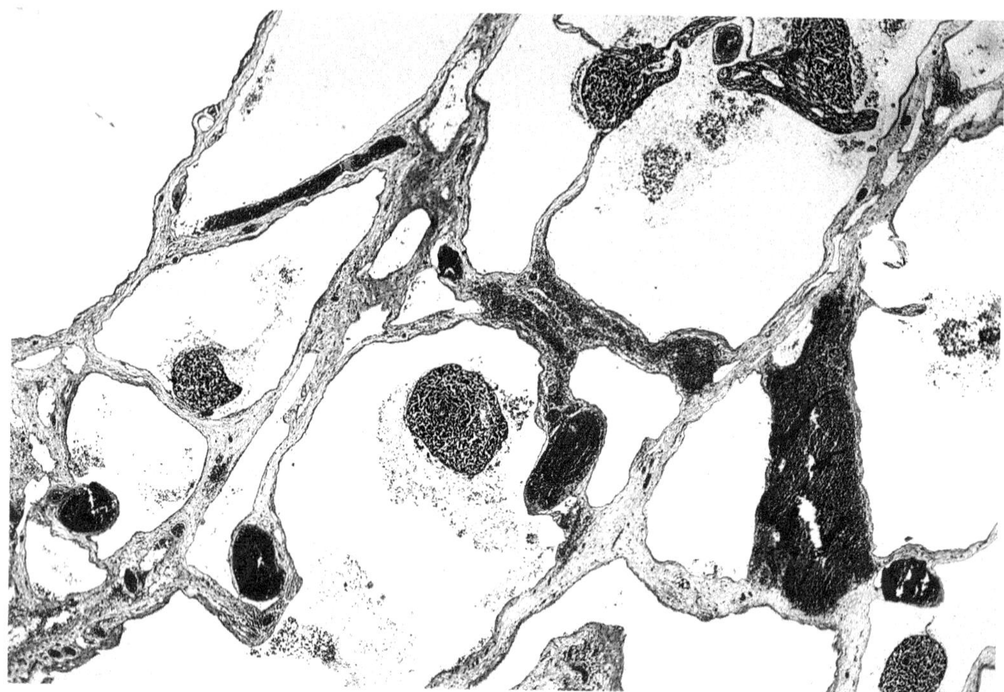

**FIGURE 26–16.** Lymphangioma containing dense lymphoid aggregates.

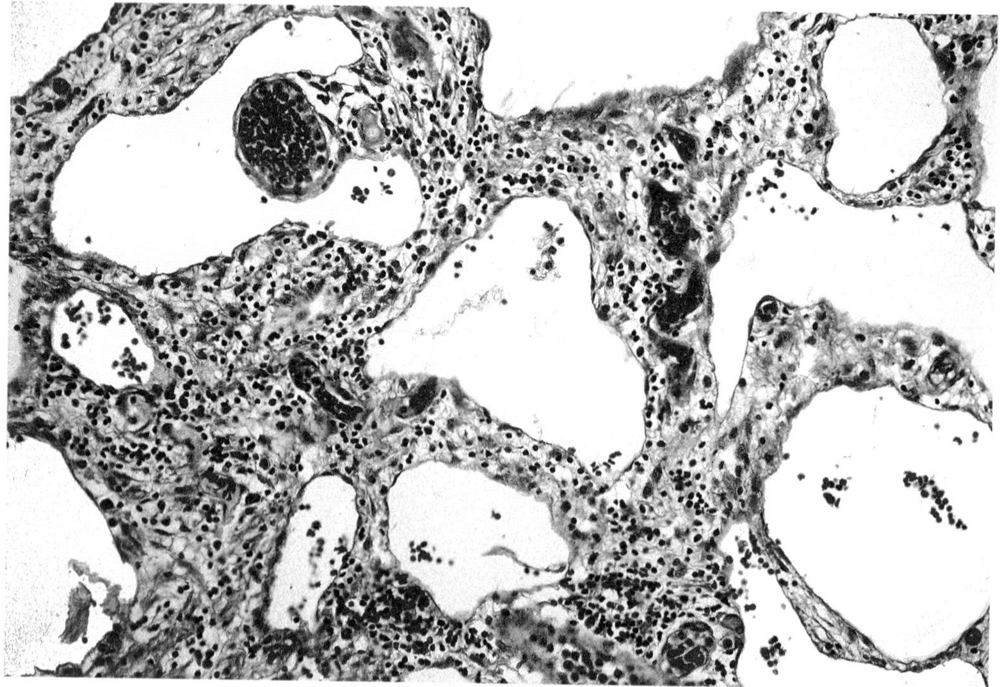

**FIGURE 26–17.** Lymphangioma with engorged vascular spaces.

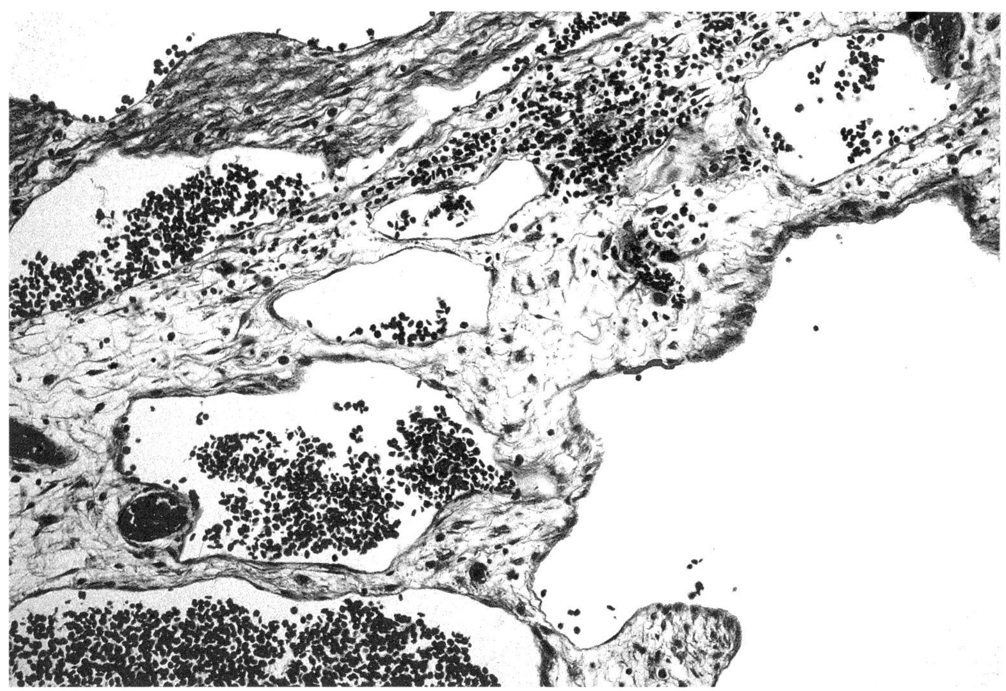

**FIGURE 26–18.** Lymphangioma with stromal hemorrhage.

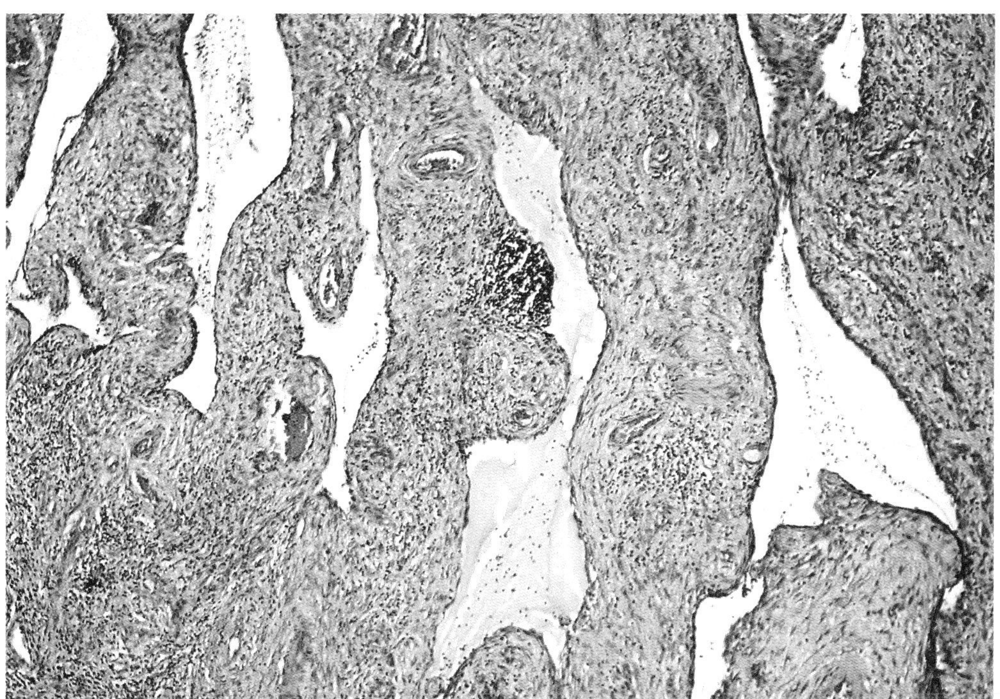

**FIGURE 26–19.** Inflamed intraabdominal lymphangioma.

*giomas (cystic hygroma)* and the latter as *cavernous lymphangiomas.* Tumors often combine features of the two, and their differences are offset by their overall similarities. Regardless of the size of the lymphatic spaces, both lesions are lined by attenuated endothelium resembling that in normal lymphatics. Small lymphatic spaces have only an inconspicuous adventitial coat surrounding them, whereas large lymphatic spaces have, in addition, fascicles of poorly developed smooth muscle. The lymphatic spaces classically are filled with proteinaceous fluid containing lymphocytes, although occasionally erythrocytes are present as well. The stroma is composed of a delicate meshwork of collagen punctuated by small lymphoid aggregates (Fig. 24–16). Occasionally the lymphoid aggregates become quite prominent, and such lesions have been descriptively termed "lymphangiolymphoma,"[28] an unfortunate choice of terms, as the lesions are not associated with, nor do they progress to, lymphomas. With repeated bouts of infection, the stroma of a lymphangioma becomes inflamed, edematous (Fig. 26–19), and ultimately fibrotic.

In most cases there is little difficulty establishing the correct diagnosis. However, lymphangiomas with secondary hemorrhage are sometimes confused with cavernous hemangiomas. Histologic features that favor the diagnosis of lymphangioma over hemangioma include the presence of lymphoid aggregates in the stroma and more irregular lumens with widely spaced nuclei. Because lymphatic endothelium may express factor VIII-associated antigen as well as CD31,[49] immunohistochemical procedures, with the possible exception of those for VEGFR-3,[2] are not especially reliable means of distinguishing hemangiomas from lymphangiomas. It has been our experience that if the diagnosis cannot be readily determined by routine hematoxylin and eosin-stained sections, ancillary studies usually do not contribute significant additional information.

It is more important to distinguish an intraabdominal lymphangioma from a cystic form of mesothelioma or microcystic adenoma of the pancreas. The cystic mesothelioma presents as a multicystic mass that affects a large area of peritoneum and requires repeated surgery for control (see Chapter 30). The clinical extent of the lesion is at variance with the lymphangioma, which usually involves a localized area of peritoneum. Cystic mesotheliomas are composed of gland-like spaces that show greater variation in size than the vascular spaces of the lymphangioma. Moreover, there is a transition from normal or reactive mesothelium to the glandular spaces of the mesothelioma. Out of context, however, the cells may look surprisingly similar. The cells of mesotheliomas have numerous microvilli, whereas those of lymphangiomas are smoothly contoured and resemble normal lymphatic endothelia. In ambiguous situations immunohistochemical procedures are easy, reliable means to make this distinction, as the cells of multicystic mesothelioma, like other mesothelial tumors but unlike lymphatic tumors, express cytokeratin and epithelial membrane antigen. Microcystic adenomas of the pancreas are composed of cystic spaces lined by cuboidal or low columnar, keratin-positive epithelium. The glandular spaces are more regular in shape than in lymphangioma and rest on a stroma containing a rich network of small blood capillaries, a feature usually not encountered in lymphangiomas.

## Behavior and Treatment

Although the lymphangioma is a benign lesion, it may cause significant morbidity because of its large size, critical location, or proclivity to become secondarily infected. Only rare cases are known to have regressed spontaneously, and eventually virtually all lesions require surgical treatment. The extent of the procedure should be dictated by the location and the desire to achieve a reasonable cosmetic result. For patients with lesions presenting early in life, the suggested time for surgery is between the ages of 18 and 24 months.[12] Usually cystic lymphangiomas are well circumscribed, are more amenable to complete excision, and are attended by a low rate of local recurrence. On the other hand, cavernous lymphangiomas in sites such as the tongue and palate have a tendency to insinuate themselves between muscle fibers, are difficult to excise, and are complicated by a high local recurrence rate[12]; in one series nerve palsies appeared in one-third of the patients.[18] A staged surgi-

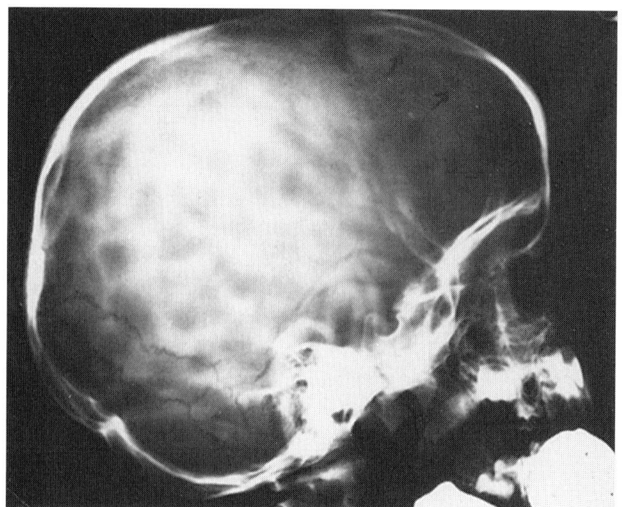

**FIGURE 26–20.** Male child with lymphangiomatosis affecting multiple bones and soft tissue sites. Multiple osteolytic lesions are present in the skull.

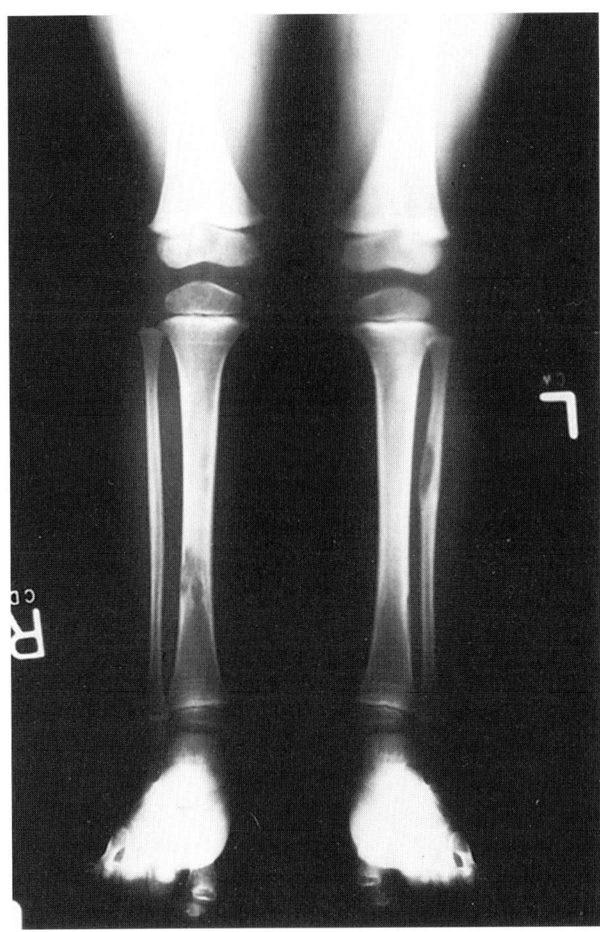


**FIGURE 26–21.** Lymphangiomatosis (same case as in Figure 26–18) with multiple, bilateral osteolytic lesions in long bones.

cal excision is often required to eradicate these tumors. Sclerosing agents and radiotherapy have been employed in the past but should not be used as alternatives to surgery. In fact, it should be emphasized that malignant transformation of previously irradiated lymphangiomas has been reported[23] (see Chapter 25).

## LYMPHANGIOMATOSIS

Lymphangioma affecting soft tissue or parenchymal organs in a diffuse or multifocal fashion is termed ***lymphangiomatosis***.[40,41,43,46–48,51] This rare disease can be conceptualized as the lymphatic counterpart of angiomatosis (see Chapter 23). It should be emphasized, however, that it is not always possible to distinguish angiomatosis from lymphangiomatosis clearly because overlap occurs between the two. By convention, the term lymphangiomatosis is reserved for lesions with predominantly, if not exclusively, lymphatic differentiation.

Like angiomatosis, this disease occurs principally in children and rarely manifests after age 20. Diagnosis of this condition at birth is uncommon because it seems that a latent period is required for these lesions to achieve sufficient size to become symptomatic. There is no gender predilection. The presenting symptoms are varied and depend on the site and extent of involvement. More than three-fourths of patients have multiple bone lesions. These well delimited osteolytic lesions with a variable degree of sclerosis (Figs. 26–20, 26–21, 26–22) are usually asymptomatic, are often discovered incidentally, and are frequently diagnosed as fibrous dysplasia or bone changes associated with hyperparathyroidism.[42] Acute symptoms more often relate to the presence of lymphangiomas in soft tissue, mediastinum, liver, spleen, or lung. The prognosis is determined by the extent of the disease.[49] Patients with liver, spleen, lung, and thoracic duct involvement usually have a poor prognosis,[49,50] as the lesions tend to be diffuse and are not amenable to surgical excision. On the other hand, patients with soft tissue involvement with or without skeletal involvement enjoy an excellent prognosis[44]

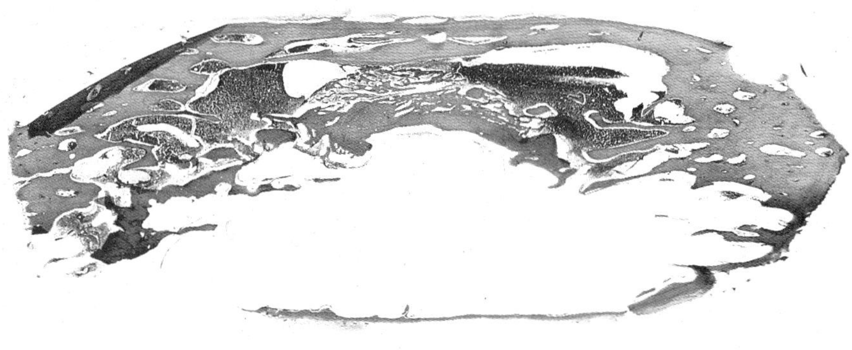

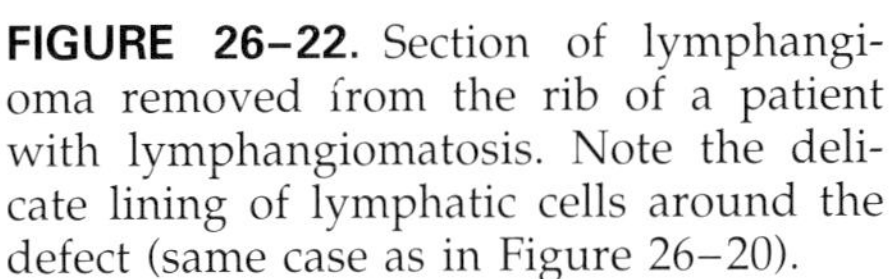
**FIGURE 26–22.** Section of lymphangioma removed from the rib of a patient with lymphangiomatosis. Note the delicate lining of lymphatic cells around the defect (same case as in Figure 26–20).

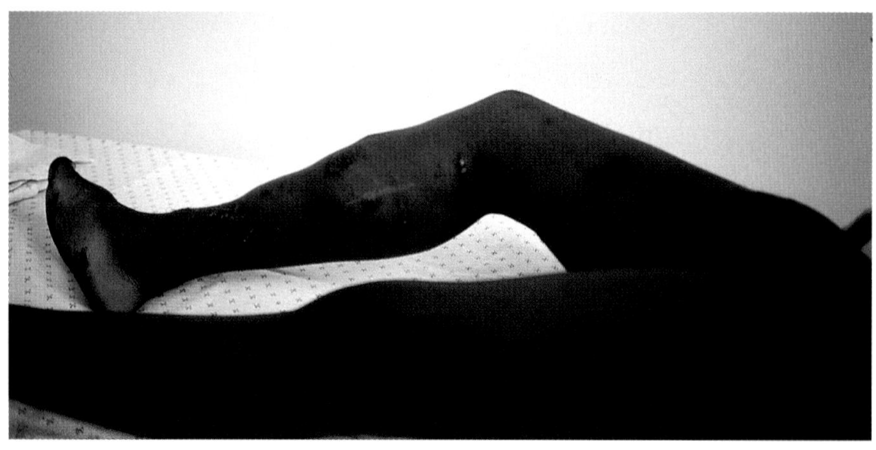

**FIGURE 26–23.** Lymphangiomatosis affecting one lower extremity.

because in most cases the bone lesions eventually stabilize and the soft tissue lesions respond to limited surgical resection. In contrast, patients with lesions in the vertebrae may develop cord compression and ultimately die of their disease.

Lymphangiomatosis affecting principally soft tissue and bone presents with fluctuant brawny swelling of an extremity that corresponds on the lymphangiogram to numerous interconnecting lymphatic channels (Fig. 26–23). The skin is thickened, and the soft tissue has a brown sponge-like quality due to the extensive replacement by proliferating lymphatic channels (Fig. 26–24). The proliferating vessels are lined by a single layer of flattened endothelium that ramifies in the soft tissue in a pattern analogous to a well differentiated angiosarcoma. Stromal hemosiderin deposits in the absence of active hemorrhage can be seen. Atypical features such as endothelial tufting, atypia, and mitotic activity of the lymphatic endothelium are not present. In these respects lymphangiomatosis is similar histologically to the deep portions of acquired progressive lymphangioma. The diagnosis of lymphangiomatosis may be difficult to establish when only bone biopsy is undertaken. To the unsuspecting pathologist the bland dilated lymph channels devoid of cells may appear so innocuous as to be overlooked altogether, and more emphasis may be placed on the surrounding bone resorption and atrophy. One or more vascular markers can be detected in the lymphatic endothelium, although CD31 seems to be the most sensitive.

The differential diagnosis of lymphangiomatosis includes angiomatosis, acquired progressive lymphangioma, and most importantly angiosarcoma. Although the infiltrative appearance at low power usually immediately suggests angiosarcoma, one is always struck by the apparent discordance between the infiltrative pattern, which suggests an aggressive process, and the relatively innocuous appearance of the lymphatic endothelia. Features such as endothelial redundancy and nuclear atypia, which are the hallmark of virtually all angiosarcomas, are absent in lymphangiomatosis and provide an important clue to the correct diagnosis. Angiomatosis is typically composed of vessels of varying size and mural complexity (see Chapter 23). Although some have a prominent capillary vascular component, the capillary vessels do not dissect and ramify throughout the soft tissue to the extent seen in lymphangiomatosis. The distinction between acquired progressive lymphangioma and lymphangiomatosis is more problematic. In our experience, portions of acquired progressive lymphangioma are virtually indistinguishable from lymphangiomatosis. Therefore one could conceptualize the acquired progressive lymphangioma in some cases as a limited or superficial form of lymphangiomatosis. The distinction between the two is therefore best made based on presentation and clinical extent, a situation analogous to the distinction between hemangioma and angiomatosis.

## LOCALIZED MASSIVE LYMPHEDEMA

Localized areas of massive lymphedema develop in morbidly obese individuals and frequently simulate a well differentiated liposarcoma.[52] The pathogenetic mechanism of this pseudoneoplastic condition appears to be localized lymphatic obstruction due to the weight of large dependent folds of fat. In some cases the condition is probably exacerbated by previous surgery that has interrupted lymphatics and contributes to obstruction. Patients with this condition usually weigh in excess of 300 pounds and develop lesions preferentially in the medial portion of the extremities. Clinically, the lesions are pendulous masses with a thickened hyperkeratotic or peau d'orange-like appearance of skin (Fig. 26–25). Radio-

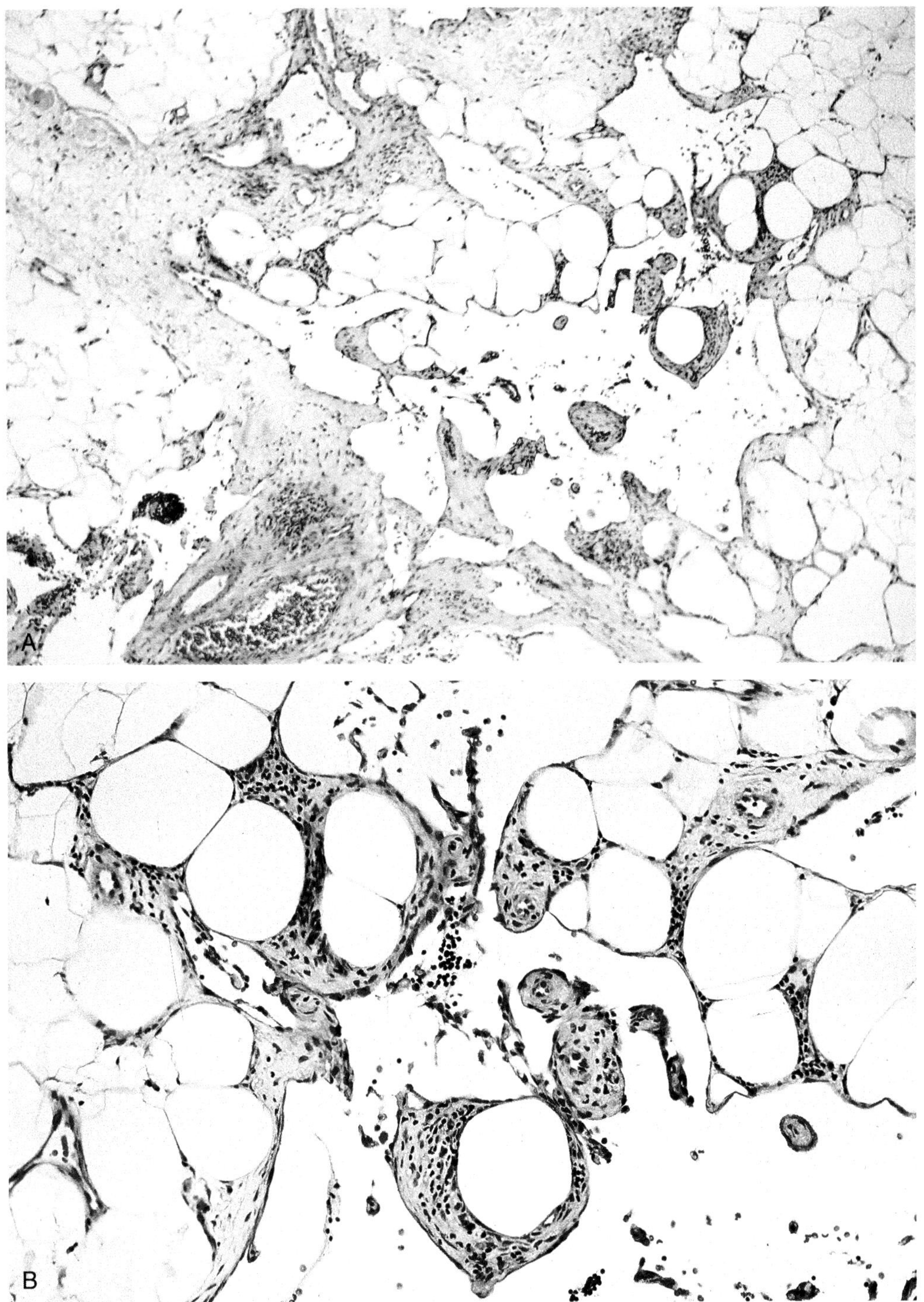


**FIGURE 26–24.** Persistently recurring lymphangiomatosis of the leg. Lymphatic channels diffusely involve soft tissue (**A**) and are composed of cells with little atypia (**B**).

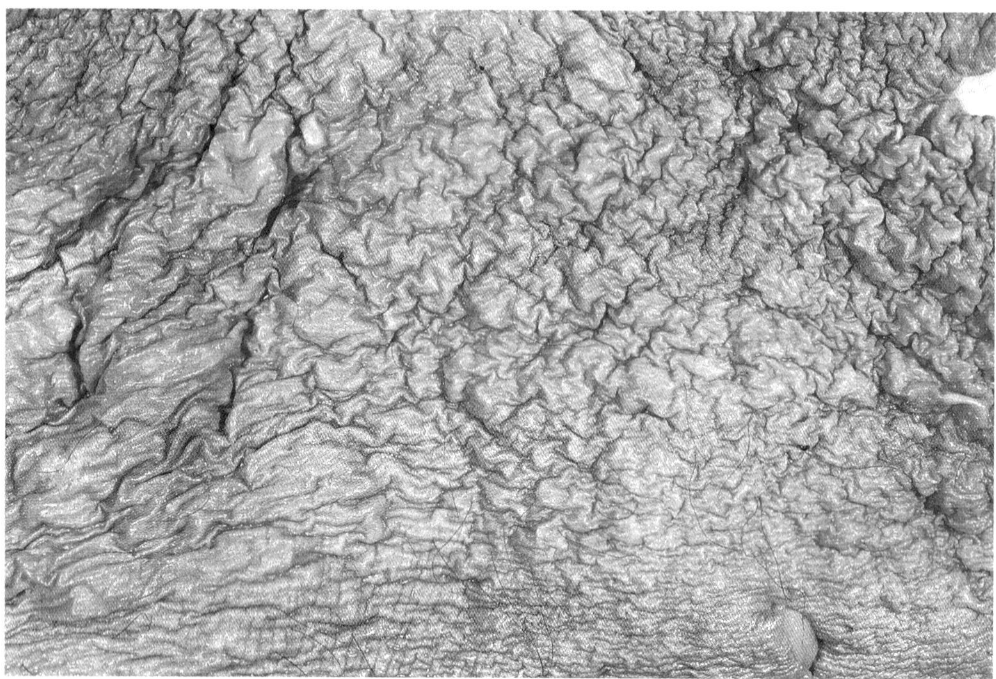

**FIGURE 26–25.** Localized massive lymphedema showing thickened pebble-like skin.

logically, the mass corresponds to expanded subcutaneous tissue with soft tissue "streaking" but without a discrete mass lesion. On cut section one is impressed by the amount of fibrous tissue traversing the fat and by the presence of cysts of various sizes that "weep" serous fluid (Fig. 26–26).

Histologically, the changes are those of chronic lymphedema. The overlying skin is thickened and occasionally hyperkeratotic (Fig. 26–27), whereas the underlying dermis is hyalinized and contains numerous small lymphatic channels surrounded by clusters of lymphocytes (Fig. 26–28). In the subcutis the interlobular septa are markedly expanded by edema fluid and mildly atypical fibroblasts such that the lobules of fat appear minimized. (Figs. 26–29, 26–30) At the interface of the septa and the residual fat one occasionally finds a fringe of reactive capillary-size vessels.

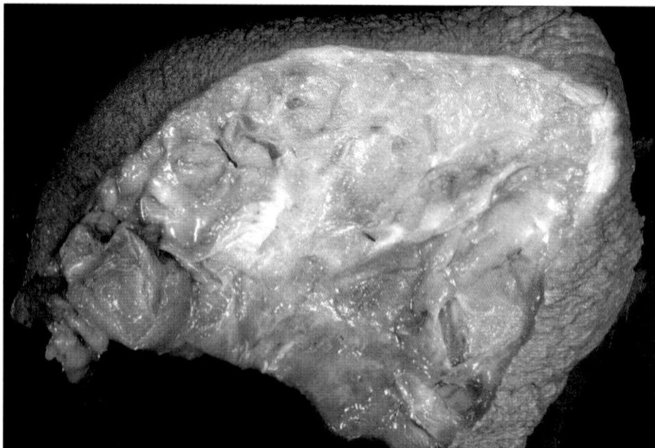

**FIGURE 26–26.** Localized massive lymphedema with multiple cysts of the subcutis and exaggerated fibrous trabeculae.

Although these lesions represent a reactive condition involving the lymphatic system, they are commonly confused with liposarcoma (see Chapter 17) because the expanded interlobular septa are misinterpreted as the fibrous bands of a sclerosing well differentiated liposarcoma. The salient observations when making this distinction are the overall preservation of the architecture of normal subcutaneous fat and the lack of significant atypia in the fibrous bands separating the fat. Because the underlying cause of the condition is morbid obesity, persistence or even recurrence of these lesions is to be expected following surgery. None has behaved in an aggressive manner.

## LYMPHANGIOSARCOMA

Traditionally, lymphangiosarcoma is defined as a vascular sarcoma arising in the setting of chronic lymphedema. Most occur in patients with postsurgical lymphedema, particularly as a result of radical mastectomy for breast carcinoma (**Stewart-Treves syndrome**), but they may develop in chronic lymphedema from almost any cause. Although the clinical setting suggests that these tumors arise from proliferating lymphatic endothelium, it is difficult to distin-

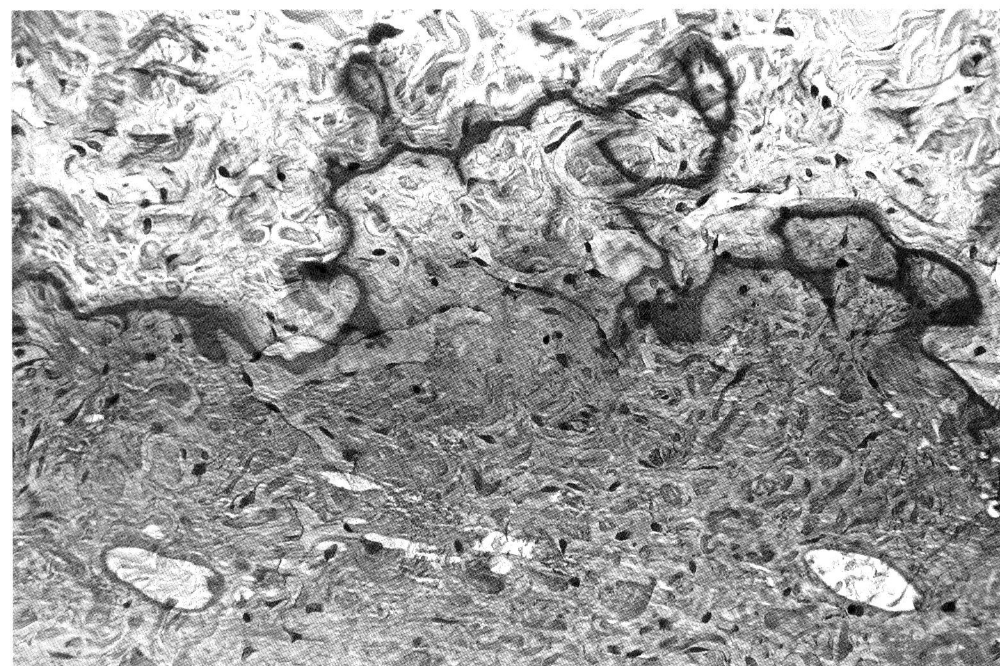

**FIGURE 26–27.** Thickened hyperkeratotic skin in localized massive lymphedema.

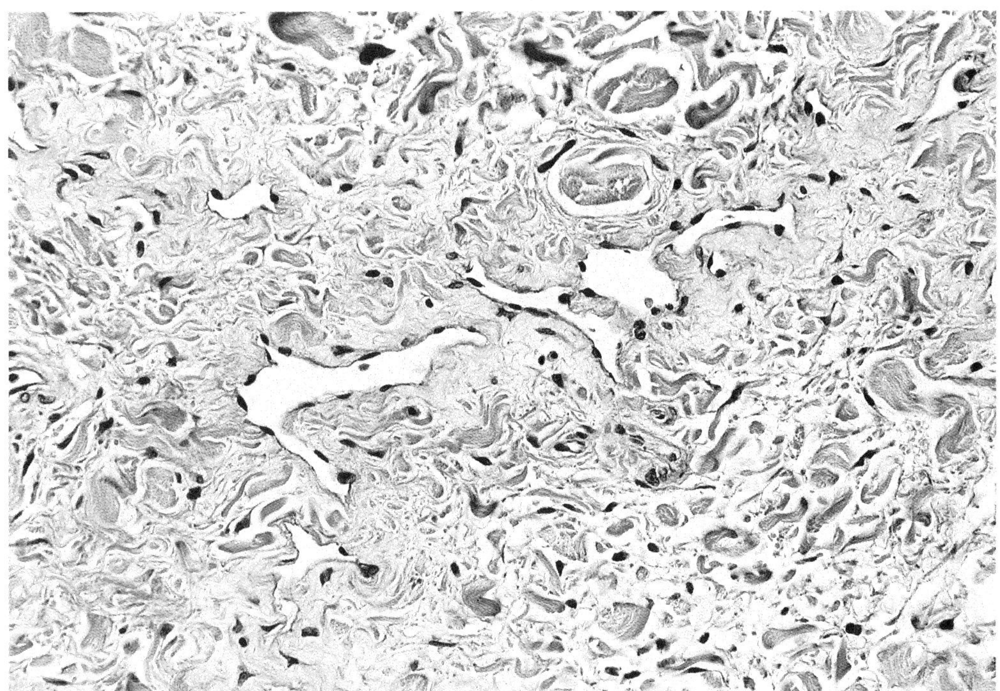

**FIGURE 26–28.** Irregular lymphatic channels in sclerotic dermis in localized massive lymphedema.

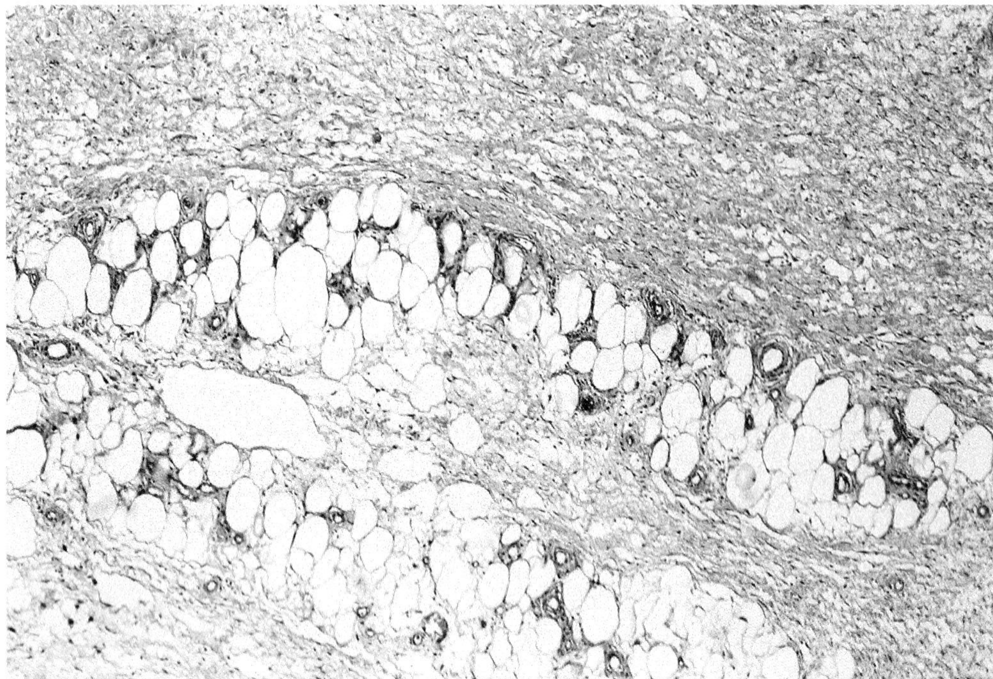

**FIGURE 26–29.** Widened fibrous trabeculae in the subcutis in massive localized lymphedema. Note fringe of capillaries of interface of fat and fibrous trabeculae.

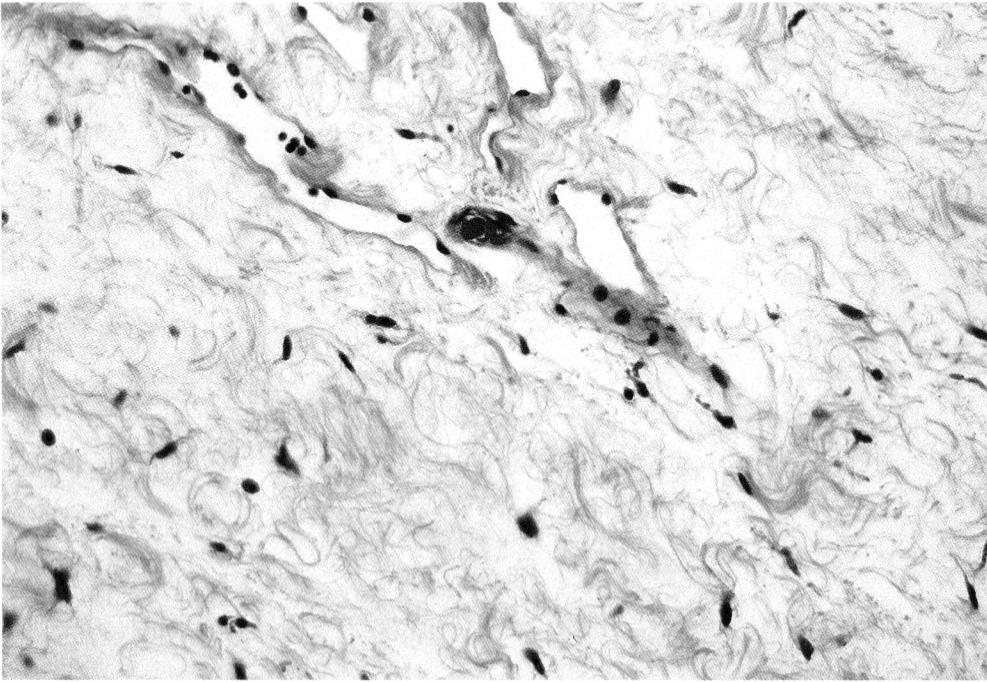

**FIGURE 26–30.** Mildly atypical fibroblasts in fibrous trabeculae within massive localized lymphedema.

guish them histologically from other forms of angiosarcoma. Hence they are discussed in Chapter 25.

## LYMPHANGIOMYOMA AND LYMPHANGIOMYOMATOSIS

Lymphangiomyomatosis is a rare disease characterized by proliferation of unusual, distinctive smooth muscle in the lymphatics and lymph nodes of the mediastinum, retroperitoneum, and often the pulmonary parenchyma.[81,88] These smooth muscle cells belong to the family of perivascular epithelioid cells (PEC) that co-express muscle and melanocytic[57,58,82] markers and that give rise to a number of neoplastic or quasineoplastic conditions including renal angiomyolipoma, sugar tumor of the lung and pancreas,[94] and clear-cell myomelanocytic tumor of the falciform ligament,[69] collectively termed PEComas.[58] Previously considered a multifocal malformation or hamartoma, lymphangiomyoma and lymphangiomyomatosis have variously been termed "intrathoracic angiomyomatous hyperplasia"[66] and "lymphangiopericytoma."[67] Localized lesions can be referred to as lymphangiomyoma, whereas extensive lesions involving large segments of the lymphatic chain with or without pulmonary involvement should be designated lymphangiomyomatosis.

### Clinical Findings

The disease occurs exclusively in women, usually during the reproductive years (mean age about 40 years). A significant number of patients have taken oral contraceptives; but in view of the common usage of these products, it is difficult to know the significance of this observation. A unique patient with pulmonary and abdominal lymphangiomyomatosis occurring in association with a solitary fibrous tumor of the lung, cavernous hemangioma of the liver, meningioma, papillary thyroid carcinoma, and parathyroid adenoma was recently reported by Cagnano et al.[60] Progressive dyspnea, the most common symptom, can be related to the almost constant presence of chylous pleural effusion or to pulmonary involvement, which occurs in about half of the patients.[64,93] Other symptoms include pneumothorax, hemoptysis, and rarely abdominal pain, chylous ascites,[73] and chyluria.[70,72]

Radiographic studies can be helpful for diagnosing this condition. Lymphography indicates obstruction in the major lymphatic ducts (Fig. 26–31A), ectatic lymph vessels distal to the obstruction, occasionally lymphatic-venous connections,[56] and general loss of lymph node architecture (Fig. 26–31B). Chest radiographs demonstrate changes highly characteristic of this condition (Fig. 26–32). In the fully developed

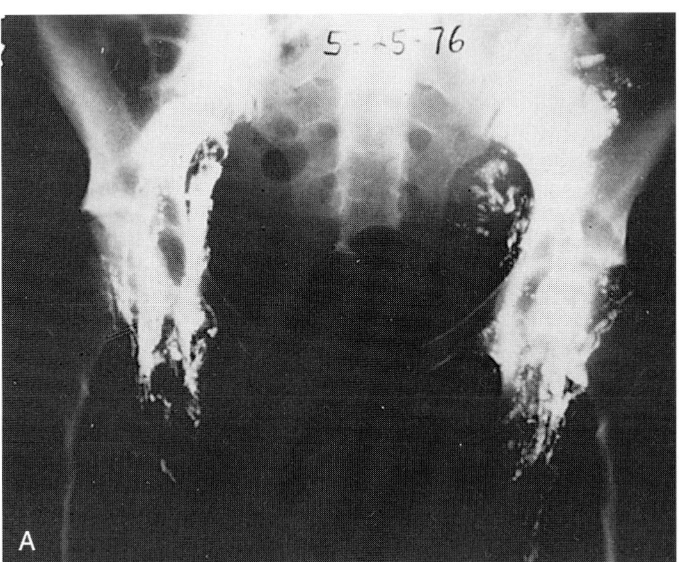


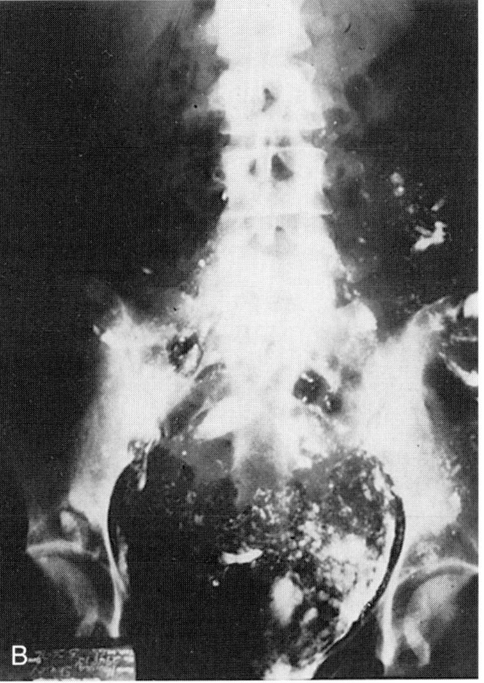


**FIGURE 26–31.** Lymphangiogram of a patient with lymphangiomyomatosis. (**A**) Initial film shows markedly dilated lymphatic vessels suggesting proximal obstruction. (**B**) Follow-up film (48 hours) shows amorphous collections of contrast material indicative of a loss of normal lymph node architecture. (Courtesy of Dr. Van Vliet, Grand Rapids, MI.)

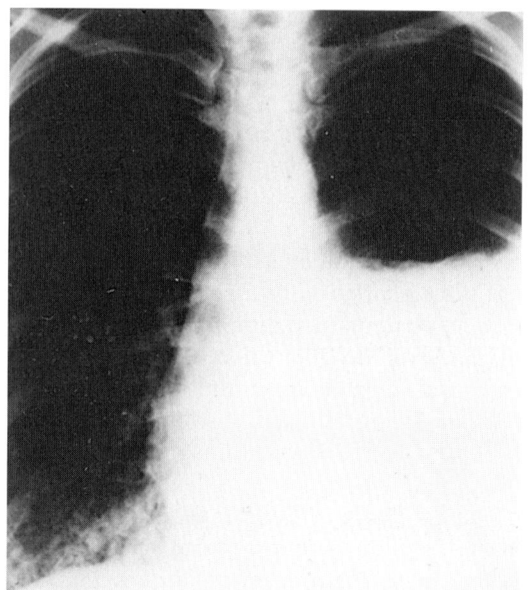

**FIGURE 26–32.** Chest radiograph in a patient with lymphangiomyomatosis. Lung volume is unaltered despite extensive interstitial disease. Massive (chylous) effusion is present on the left. (Courtesy of Dr. Van Vliet, Grand Rapids, MI.)

case a coarse reticular infiltrate with a bullous pattern is present throughout the lung. In contrast to chronic interstitial lung disease, the pulmonary volume is increased. Pulmonary function studies indicate airflow obstruction and markedly impaired gas exchange. The former defect results from poor communication of the emphysematous air spaces with the airways as a result of the proliferating muscle, whereas the latter defect is best explained by uneven ventilation or perfusion of the lung.[61]

## Gross Findings

At surgery these lesions are red to gray spongy masses that preferentially replace the thoracic duct and mediastinal lymph nodes (Fig. 26–33). Less often they involve the retroperitoneal lymph nodes only; and in particularly dramatic cases the entire lymphatic chain from neck to inguinal region is transformed into multiple confluent masses. Chylous effusion is encountered in most cases, and in some instances the pleural surfaces are noted to "weep" fluid, suggesting the presence of numerous abnormal communications between the lymphatics and the pleural surface. When the process affects the lungs as well, the organ has a honeycomb appearance with formation of numerous blebs or bullae.

## Microscopic Findings

The lymphangiomyoma has a remarkably uniform appearance. Smooth muscle cells are arranged in short fascicles around a ramifying network of endothelium-lined spaces (Figs. 26–34 to 26–37). The cells are plump with abundant grainy eosinophilic cytoplasm and nuclei devoid of pleomorphism and mi-

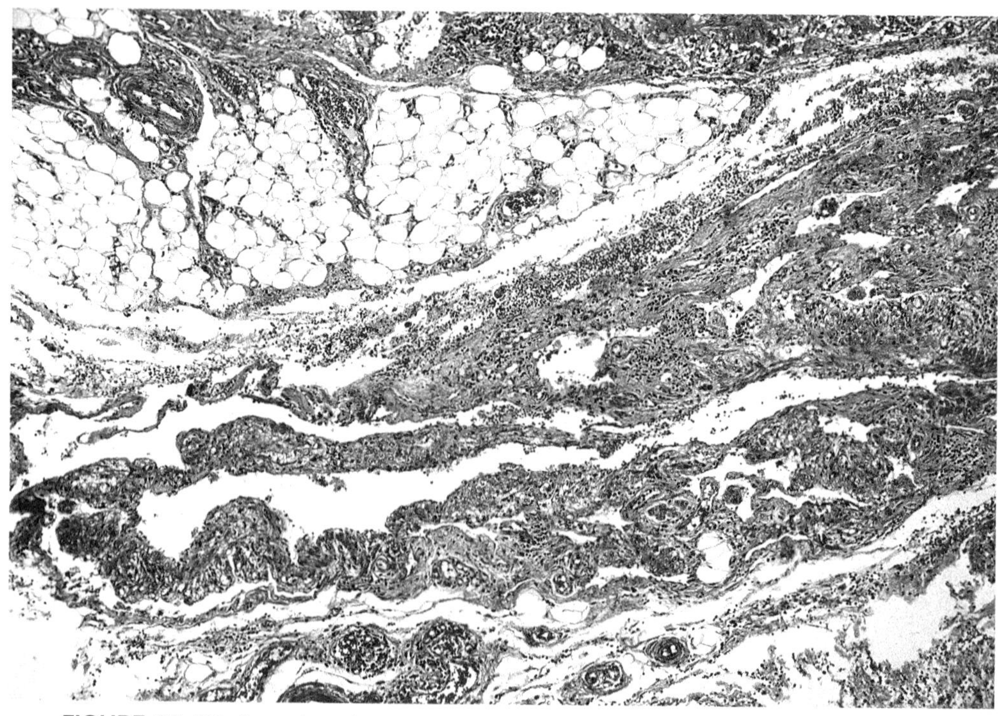

**FIGURE 26–33.** Lymphangiomyomatosis involving large lymphatic channels. (×25)

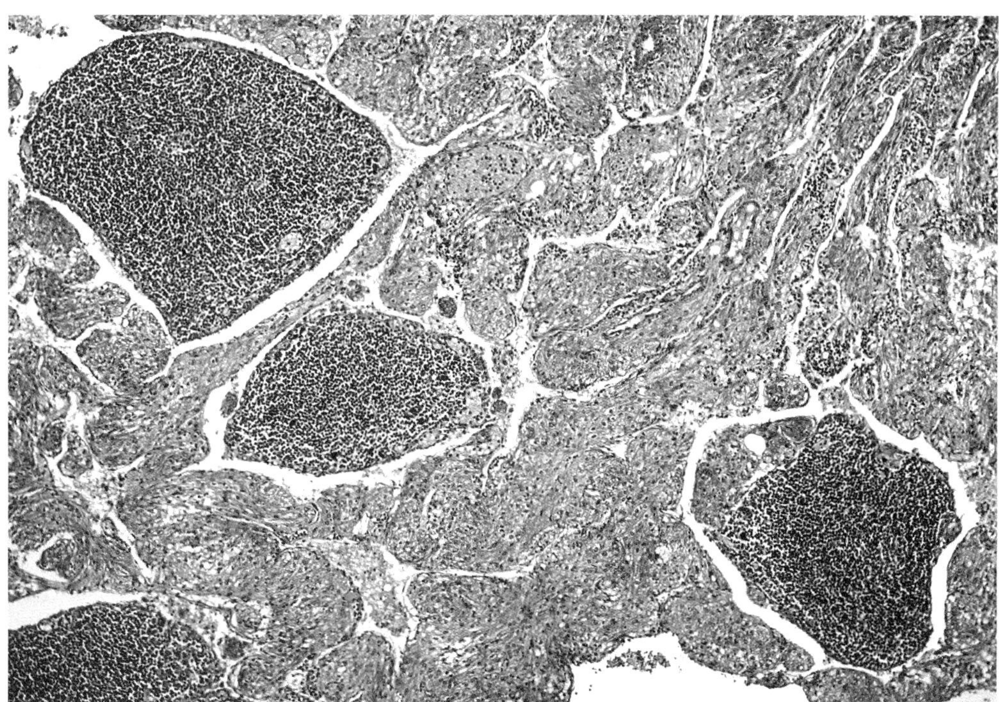

**FIGURE 26–34.** Lymphangiomyoma.

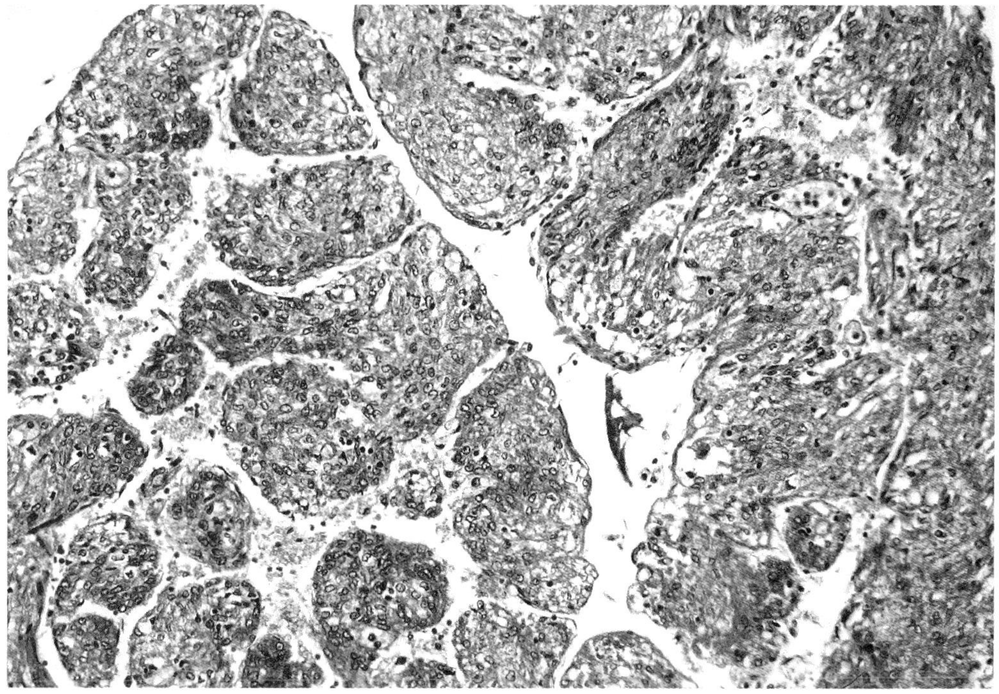

**FIGURE 26–35.** Lymphangiomyoma with the classic "pericytoma" pattern. (×150)

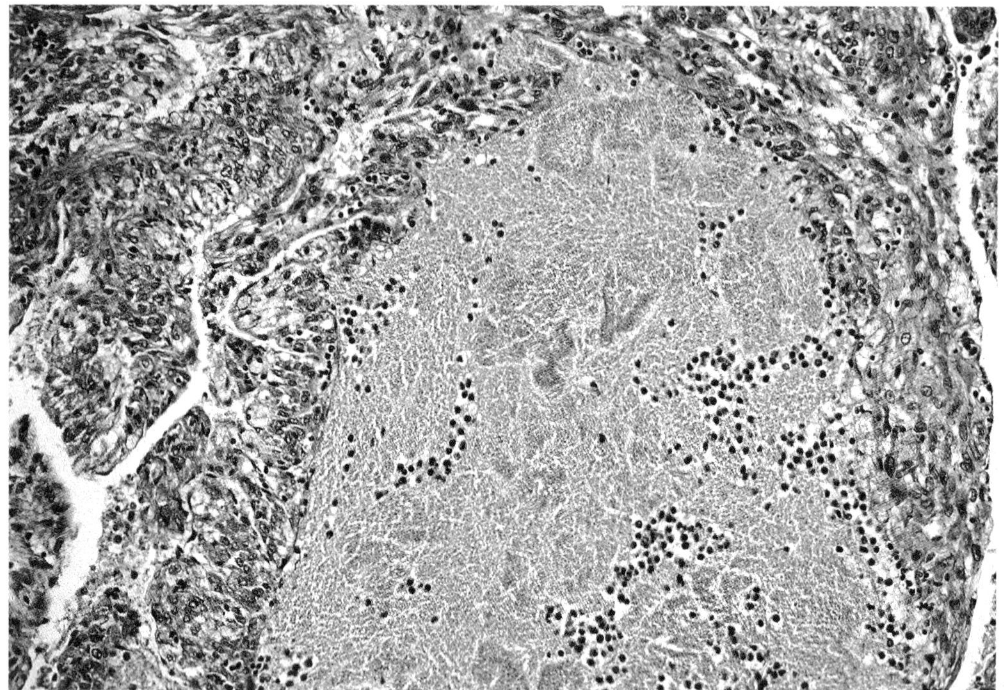

**FIGURE 26–36.** Lymphangiomyoma with lymph fluid in vascular spaces.

totic activity (Fig. 26–37). Occasionally, foci of lymphocytes are scattered between the muscle cells; in many instances they represent vestiges of preexisting lymph nodes. The vascular spaces are usually empty but are sometimes filled with eosinophilic material containing fat droplets and occasional lymphocytes.

In the lung the pathologic changes are extensive and severe (Figs. 26–38, 26–39). The primary lesion is a haphazard proliferation of smooth muscle cells that surround arterioles, venules, and lymphatics (Fig. 26–38B) and that diffusely thicken the alveolar septa. Secondary changes ensue, including bulla formation as a result of air trapping by obstructed bronchioles and hemorrhage and hemosiderin deposition as a result of venule destruction. Although the macroscopic appearance of honeycombing may initially suggest the diagnosis of end-stage interstitial fibrosis, the two lesions are quite different histologically. Lymphangiomyomatosis is characterized by an exclusive proliferation of smooth muscle cells that can be identified after applying a trichrome stain by their cytoplasmic fuchsinophilia (Fig. 26–38). The muscle proliferation that accompanies end-stage interstitial fibrosis (muscular cirrhosis) is less striking and is always associated with areas of fibrosis.

## Immunohistochemical Findings

The perivascular epithelioid cells that characterize lymphangiomyoma and its more extensive counterpart are characterized by co-expression of smooth muscle and melanocytic markers (Fig. 26–37B). These cells express actin (and less so desmin) along with a number of melanin-associated antigens such as gp100 (HMB45), melanoma-associated antigen recognized by T cells (MART-1), and microphthalmia transcription factor.[50,62,68] This unusual pattern of staining seems to reflect the presence of a melanin precursor substance that resides in the electron-dense, melanin-like granules that have been identifed in the cytoplasm of these cells. Because of the gender-restricted nature of this condition and the fact that hormonal manipulation seems to affect the growth of lesions in some cases, there has been a great deal of interest in identifying hormone receptor substances in these lesions by biochemical and immunohistochemical means. Some have reported nuclear estrogen or progesterone receptor protien[55,63,83] in these lesions seen with immununohistochemical procedures, whereas others have reported negative findings.[80] Measurements of receptor protein by biochemical methods have shown the levels to be minimally elevated.[87]

## Ultrastructural Findings

Several studies have confirmed the smooth muscle properties of the proliferating cells. The cells have numerous myofilaments with dense bodies.[54,73,84] Additional features of smooth muscle differentiation include plicated nuclei, pinocytotic vesicles on the cell

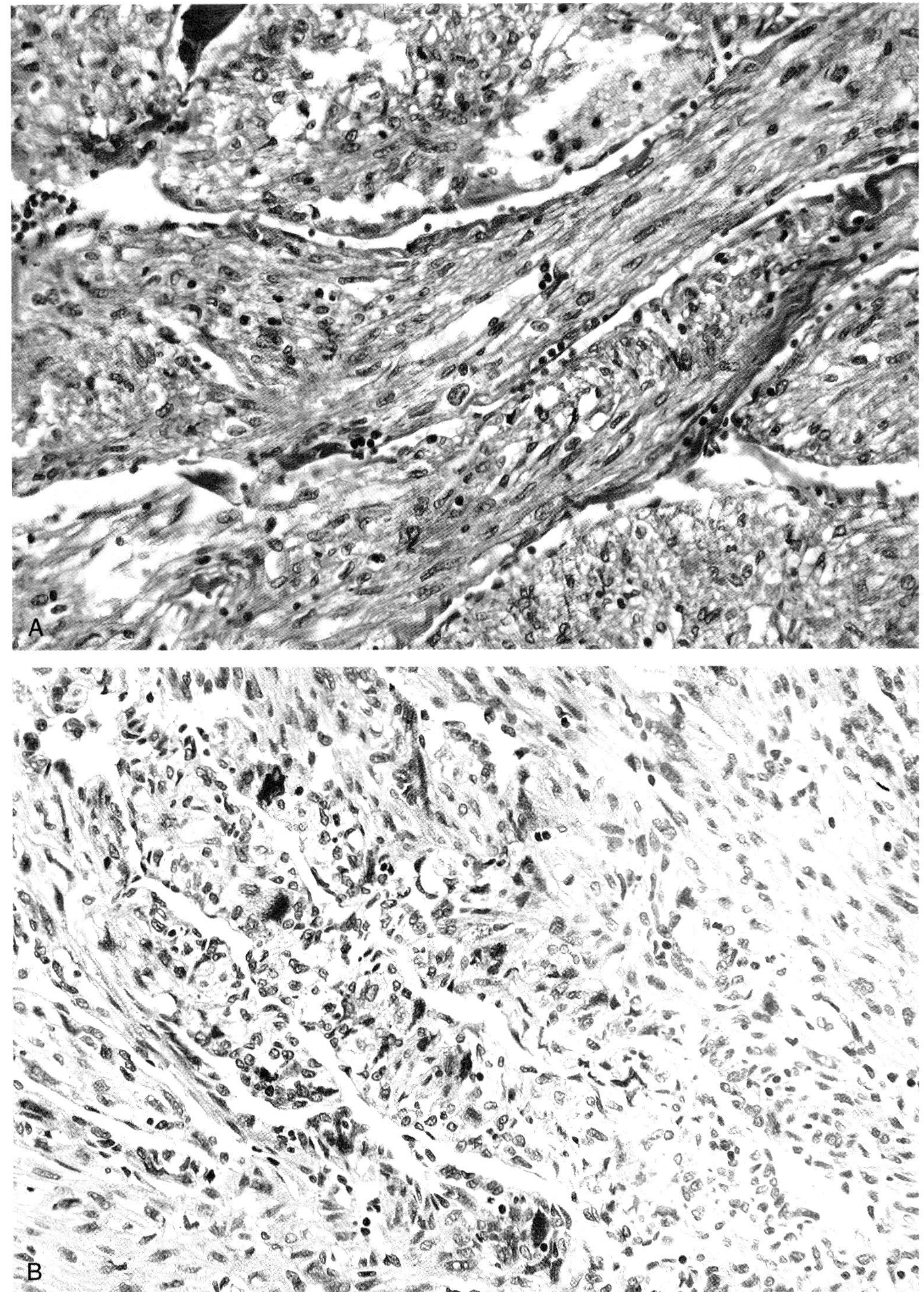


**FIGURE 26–37.** Lymphangiomyoma with distinctive partially vacuolated smooth muscle cells surrounding endothelium-lined spaces (**A**). These "perivascular epithelioid clear cells" co-express express smooth muscle and melanin markers. (**B**) This field shows focal positivity using HMB45 antibody.

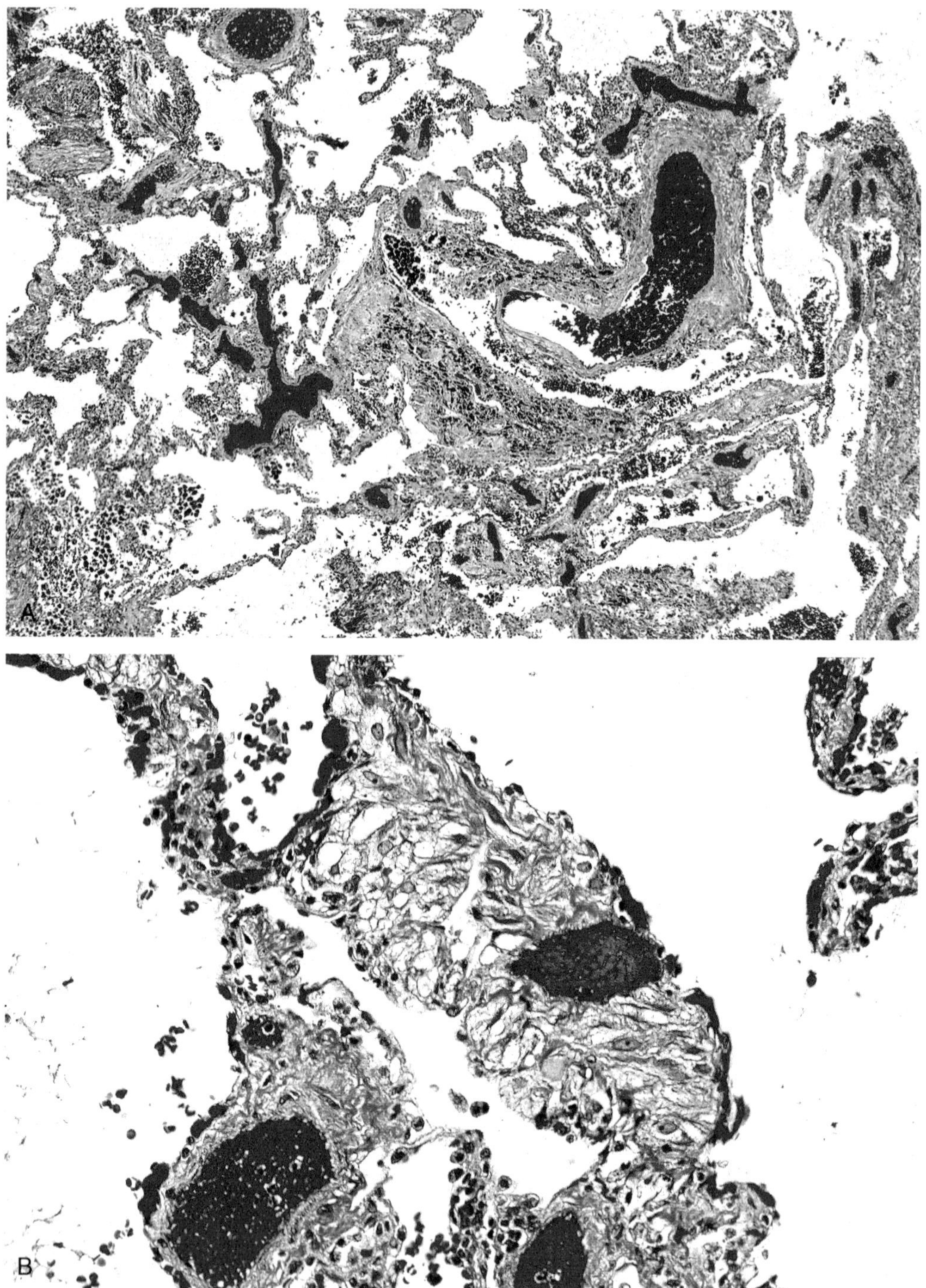


**FIGURE 26–38.** Lymphangiomyomatosis of the lung (**A**) with characteristic perivascular epithelioid cells (PEC) (**B**). (Trichrome stain)

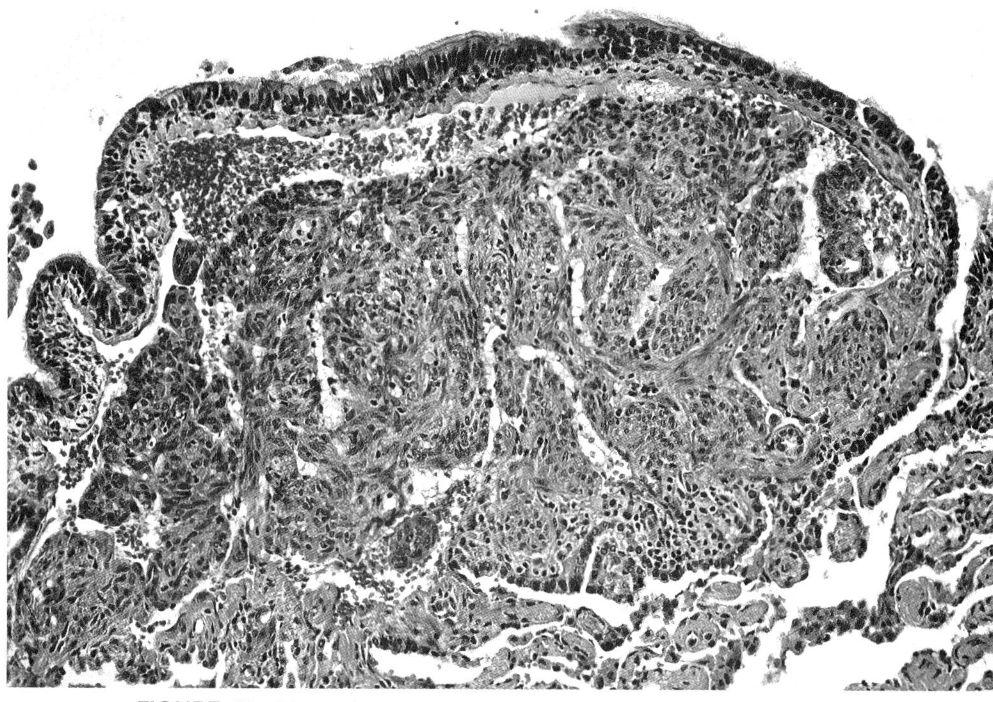

**FIGURE 26–39.** End-stage lung involved by lymphangiomyomatosis.

surface, and investiture by basal lamina. An unusual feature in these cells is the peculiar melanin-like, electron-dense granules containing a lamellar substructure[71] believed to be the source of the immunoreactivity for melanocytic markers. In one study of lung tissue, cells with the ultrastructural features of fibroblasts were identified in addition to typical smooth muscle cells. The authors suggested that the progenitor cell in the pulmonary lesion is an interstitial cell.[74] The cells lining the slit-like spaces resemble normal endothelia, but their discontinuous basal laminae and poorly formed intercellular attachments are more compatible with lymphatic than with vascular endothelium.[93]

## Differential Diagnosis

The full-blown case rarely presents diagnostic difficulty. Problems arise in limited forms of the disease when only one or two lymph nodes in the mediastinum or retroperitoneum are examined. Partial replacement of a lymph node might initially suggest the diagnosis of metastatic leiomyosarcoma (Fig. 26–40). The most helpful histologic feature is the consistent orientation of the smooth muscle cells around endothelial spaces. Leiomyosarcomas show no predictable or consistent polarization toward vessels, and except in extremely well differentiated cases they usually have more pleomorphism and mitotic activity. The presence of lipid droplets in the fluid bathing the smooth muscle cells in lymphangiomyomas is also suggestive of the diagnosis. Because the smooth muscle cells of lymphangiomyomatosis react with the HMB45 antibody but conventional smooth muscle cells do not, this antibody can be used to make this distinction as well.

Rarely, smooth muscle proliferations in the lung have features intermediate between those of lymphangiomyomatosis and of metastatic well differentiated leiomyosarcoma, or so-called benign metastasizing leiomyoma. One such case was reported by Banner et al.,[53] and we have reviewed a similar case. In our case, hundreds of microscopic smooth muscle nodules were present throughout the lung but bore no consistent relation to the lymphatics. They were composed of fusiform to spindled smooth muscle cells, only some of which had discernible linear striations. Follow-up information, indicating no apparent source for the tumor, strongly suggested primary smooth muscle proliferation. Such cases deserve the closest scrutiny and careful clinical evaluation to rule out pulmonary metastasis of a well-differentiated smooth muscle tumor of gynecologic, gastrointestinal, or retroperitoneal origin.

## Behavior and Treatment

The clinical course of patients with this disease is variable. Those with localized lesions may survive for long periods following surgical excision. Patients with

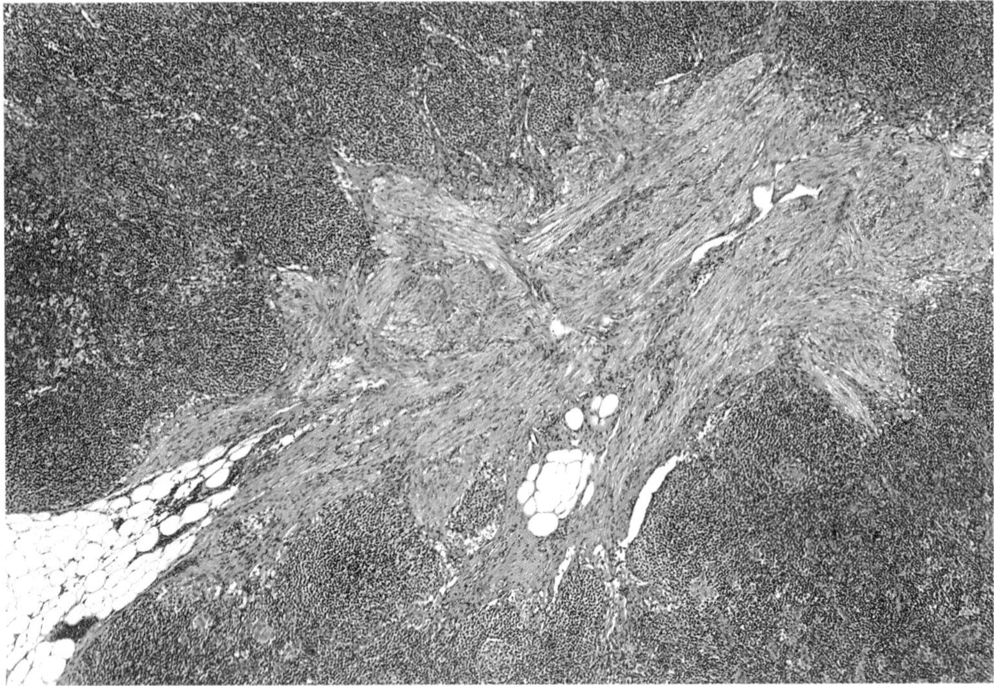

**FIGURE 26–40.** Lymph node partially involved by lymphangiomyomatosis.

pulmonary involvement usually experience progressive pulmonary insufficiency and die of the disease within 1–10 years of the diagnosis. Treatment of such patients is symptomatic. Obliteration of the pleural cavity by talc poudrage or instillation of nitrogen mustard prevents reaccumulation of chylous effusion,[76] and administration of medium-chain triglycerides reduces fluid and nutritional losses. Estrogen and progesterone receptor proteins have been detected in pulmonary or abdominal tissue in this disease.[59,78,87] Consequently, there has been a growing interest in treating these patients with ablative or manipulative hormonal therapy. The most favorable results have been reported in women treated with high doses of medroxyprogesterone, oophorectomy, or both. Little response has been noted following tamoxifen (an estrogen antagonist) or androgen therapy.[78,89] In one dramatic case reported by Svendsen et al.,[87] a patient treated with medroxyprogesterone and oophorectomy became appreciably worse when tamoxifen was added to her regimen and improved when it was discontinued.

## DISCUSSION

There is some lingering controversy as to whether lymphangiomyomatosis is part of the spectrum or a forme fruste of tuberous sclerosis. In support of their close relation is the fact that about 1% of patients with tuberous sclerosis have pulmonary changes similar if not identical to those of lymphangiomyomatosis.[86,91,92] Second, renal angiomyolipomas, considered one of the hallmarks of tuberous sclerosis and occurring in about 80% of patients, have been documented in about 15% of those with lymphangiomyomatosis.[79,90]

Those who doubt the relation of the two diseases have emphasized minor histologic and clinical differences. They state that the smooth muscle proliferation occurs preferentially around lymphatics in lymphangiomyomatosis but around vessels in tuberous sclerosis.[86] This, they believe, accounts for the high incidence of chylothorax in the former but not in the latter. Other differences include the fact that lymphangiomyomatosis is not an inherited disease as is tuberous sclerosis, is not associated with central nervous system lesions, and has never been documented in men.

Although the latter arguments seem to underscore significant differences between the two diseases, it should be emphasized that most cases of tuberous sclerosis are due to a spontaneous mutation and, therefore, it does not affect family members. Moreover, when pulmonary disease develops in tuberous sclerosis, more than three-fourths of the patients are female with minimal central nervous system symptoms.

It is our belief that overall the two diseases share more similarities than differences. In our experience there are indubitable cases of tuberous sclerosis in which the pulmonary and extrapulmonary lesions are identical to those of lymphangiomyomatosis (Figs. 26–32, 26–33). For these reasons we believe these diseases are two ends of a common spectrum.

## REFERENCES


### General

1. Barsky SH, Baker A, Siegel OP. Use of anti-basement membrane antibodies to distinguish blood vessel capillaries from lymphatic capillaries. Am J Surg Pathol 7:667, 1983.
2. Folpe AL, Veikkola T, Valtola R, Weiss SW. Vascular endothelial growth factor receptor-3 (VEGFR-3): a marker of vascular tumors with presumed lymphatic differentiation, including Kaposi's sarcoma, kaposiform and Dabska-type hemangioendotheliomas, and a subset of angiosarcomas. Mod Pathol 13:180, 2000.
3. Fraley EE, Weiss L. An electron microscopic study of lymphatic vessels in the penile skin of the rat. Am J Anat 109:85, 1961.
4. Kaipainen A, Korhonen J, Mustonen T, et al. Expression of the fms-like tyrosine kinase 4 gene becomes restricted to lymphatic endothelium during development. Proc Natl Acad Sci USA 92: 3566, 1995.
5. Knowles DM, Tolidjian B, Marboe C, et al. Monoclonal antihuman monocyte antibodies OKM1 and OKM5 possess distinctive tissue distributions including differential reactivity with vascular endothelium. J Immunol 132:2170, 1984.
6. Landing BH, Farber S. Tumors of the cardiovascular system. In: Atlas of Tumor Pathology. Armed Forces Institute of Pathology, Washington, DC, 1956.
7. Leak LV, Burke JF. Fine structure of the lymphatic capillary and the adjoining connective tissue area. Am J Anat 118:785, 1966.
8. Schlingemann RO, Dingjan GM, Emeis JJ, et al. Monoclonal antibody PAL-E specific for endothelium. Lab Invest 52:72, 1985.
9. Wilting J, Kurz H, Oh S-J, Christ B. Angiogenesis and lymphangiogenesis: analogous mechanisms and homologous growth factors. In: Little CD, Mironov V, Sage EH (ed) Vascular Morphogenesis: In Vivo, In Vitro, In Mente. Birkhauser, Boston, 1998.

### Lymphangiomas

10. Alqahtani A, Nguyen LT, Flageole H, et al. 25 years' experience with lymphangiomas in children. J Pediatr Surg 34:1164, 1999.
11. Anderson DH. Tumors of infancy and childhood. Cancer 4:890, 1951.
12. Bill AH, Sumner DS. A unified concept of lymphangioma and cystic hygroma. Surg Gynecol Obstet 120:79, 1965.
13. Byrne J, Blanc WA, Warburton D, et al. The significance of cystic hygroma in fetuses. Hum Pathol 15:61, 1984.
14. Castanon M, Margarit J, Carrasco R, et al. Long term follow up of nineteen cystic lymphangiomas treated with fibrin sealant. J Pediatr Surg 34:1276, 1999.
15. Chervenak FA, Isaacson G, Blakemore KJ. Fetal cystic hygroma: cause and natural history. N Engl J Med 309:822, 1983.
16. Chung JH, Suh YL, Park IA, et al. A pathologic study of abdominal lymphangiomas. J Korean Med Sci 14:257, 1999.
17. Diaz-Cascajo C, Borghi S, Weyers W, et al. Benign lymphangiomatous papules of the skin following radiotherapy: a report of five new cases and review of the literature. Histopathology 35:319, 1999.
18. Emery PJ, Bailey CM, Evans JNG. Cystic hygroma of the head and neck: a review of 37 cases. J Laryngol Otol 98:613, 1984.
19. Fineberg S, Rosen PP. Cutaneous angiosarcoma and atypical vascular lesions of the skin after radiation therapy for breast carcinoma. Am J Clin Pathol 102:757, 1994.
20. Fisher I, Orkin M. Acquired lymphangioma (lymphangiectasis). Arch Dermatol 101:230, 1970.
21. Flanagan BP, Helwig EB. Cutaneous lymphangioma. Arch Dermatol 113:24, 1977.
22. Fonkalsrud EW. Congenital malformations of the lymphatic system. Semin Pediatr Surg 3:62, 1994.
23. Fonkalsrud EW. Surgical management of congenital malformation of the lymphatic system. Am J Surg 28:152, 1974.
24. Fryns JP, Kleczkowska K, Vandenberghe F, et al. Cystic hygroma and hydrops fetalis in dup(11p) syndrome. Am J Med Genet 22:287, 1985.
25. Galifer RB, Pous JG, Juskiewenski S, et al. Intraabdominal cystic lymphangiomas in childhood. Prog Pediatr Surg 11:173, 1978.
26. Goetsch E. Hygroma colli cysticum and hygroma axillare: pathologic and clinical study and report of 12 cases. Arch Surg 36: 394, 1938.

26a. Guillou L, Fletcher CD. Benign lymphangioendothelioma (acquired progressive lymphangioma): a lesion not to be confused with well-differentiated angiosarcoma and patch stage Kaposi's sarcoma: clinicopathologic analysis of a series. Am J Surg Pathol 24:1047, 2000.

27. Kato H, Kadoya A. Acquired progressive lymphangioma occurring following femor arteriography. Clin Exp Dermatol 21:159, 1996.
28. Kindblom L-G, Angervall L. Tumors of lymph vessels. Contemp Issues Surg Pathol 18:163, 1991.
29. Koshy A, Tandon RK, Kapur BML, et al. Retroperitoneal lymphangioma. Am J Gastroenterol 69:485, 1978.
30. Meunier L, Barneon G, Meynadier J. Acquired progressive lymphangioma. Br J Dermatol 131:706, 1994.
31. Ngoc T, Ninh TX. Cystic hygroma in children: a report of 126 cases. J Pediatr Surg 9:191, 1974.
32. Peachy RO, Limm CC, Whimster IW. Lymphangioma of skin: a review of 65 cases. Br J Dermatol 83:519, 1970.
33. Prioleau PG, Santa Cruz DJ. Lymphangioma circumscripta following radical mastectomy and radiation therapy. Cancer 42: 1989, 1978.
34. Rosenquist GJ, Wolfe DC. Lymphangioma of bone. J Bone Joint Surg Am 34:158, 1968.
35. Singh S, Baboo M. Cystic lymphangioma in children: report of 32 cases including lesions at rare sites. Surgery 69:947, 1971.
36. Watson WL, McCarthy WD. Blood and lymph vessel tumors. Surg Gynecol Obstet 71:569, 1940.
37. Whimster IW. The pathology of lymphangioma circumscription. Br J Dermatol 10:35, 1974.
38. Wilson Jones E, Winkelmann RK, Zachary CB, Reda AM. Benign lymphangioendothelioma. J Am Acad Dermatol 23:229, 1990.
39. Witte MH, Witte CL. Lymphangiogenesis and lymphologic syndromes. Lymphology 19:21, 1986.

### Lymphangiomatosis

40. Asch MJ, Cohen AH, Moore TC. Hepatic and splenic lymphangiomatosis with skeletal involvement. Surgery 76:334, 1974.
41. Bell A, Simon BK. Chylothorax and lymphangiomas of bone: unusual manifestation of lymphatic disease. South Med J 71: 459, 1978.
42. Case records of the Massachusetts General Hospital. N Engl J Med 303:270, 1980.
43. Goldstein MR, Benchimol A, Cornell W, et al. Chylopericardium with multiple lymphangiomas of bone. N Engl J Med 280:1034, 1969.
44. Gomez CS, Calonje E, Ferrar DW, et al. Lymphangiomatosis of

the limbs: clinicopathologic analysis of a series with a good prognosis. Am J Surg Pathol 19:125, 1995.
45. Grunwald MH, Amichai B, Avinoach I. Acquired progressive lymphangioma. J Am Acad Dermatol 37:656, 1997.
46. Gutierrez RM, Spjut HJ. Skeletal angiomatosis: report of three cases and a review of the literature. Clin Orthop 85:82, 1972.
47. Harris R, Prandoni AS. Generalized primary lymphangiomas of bone: report of a case associated with congenital lymphedema of the forearm. Ann Intern Med 33:1302, 1950.
48. Najman E, Fabecic-Sabadi V, Temmer B. Lymphangioma in the inguinal region with cystic lymphangiomatosis of bone. J Pediatr 71:561, 1967.
49. Ramani P, Shah A. Lymphangiomatosis: histologic and immunohistochemical analysis of four cases. Am J Surg Pathol 17: 329, 1993.
50. Tazelaar HD, Kerr D, Yousem SA, et al. Diffuse pulmonary lymphangiomatosis. Hum Pathol 24:1313, 1993.
51. Tucker SM. Bilateral chylothorax with multiple osteolytic lesions: generalized abnormality of the lymphatic system. Proc R Soc Med 60:17, 1967.

### Localized Massive Lymphedema

52. Farshid G, Weiss SW. Massive localized lymphedema in the morbidly obese: a histologically distinct reactive lesions simulating liposarcoma. Am J Surg Pathol 22:1277, 1998.

### Lymphangiomyoma and Lymphangiomyomatosis

53. Banner AS, Carrington CB, Emory WB, et al. Efficacy of oophorectomy in lymphangioleiomyomatosis and benign metastasizing leiomyoma. N Engl J Med 305:204, 1981.
54. Basset F, Soler P, Marsac J, et al. Pulmonary lymphangiomyomatosis: three new cases studied with electron microscopy. Cancer 38:2357, 1976.
55. Berger U, Khaghani A, Pomerance A, et al. Pulmonary lymphangioleiomyomatosis and steroid receptors: an immunohistochemical study. Am J Clin Pathol 93:609, 1990.
56. Bhattacharyya AK, Balogh K. Retroperitoneal lymphangioleiomyomatosis: a 36-year benign course in a postmenopausal woman. Cancer 56:1144, 1985.
57. Bonetti F, Pea M, Martignoni G, et al. Cellular heterogeneity in lymphangiomyomatosis of the lung. Hum Pathol 22:727, 1991.
58. Bonetti F, Pea M, Martignoni G, et al. Clear cell (sugar) tumor of the lung is a lesion strictly related to angiomyolipoma: the concept of a family of lesions characterized by the presence of the perivascular epithelioid cells (PEC). Pathology 26:230, 1994.
59. Brentani MM, Carvalho RR, Saldiva PH, et al. Steroid receptors in pulmonary lymphangiomyomatosis. Chest 85:96, 1984.
60. Cagnano M, Benharroch D, Geffen DB. Pulmonary lymphangioleiomyomatosis: report of a case with associated multiple soft tissue tumors. Arch Pathol Lab Med 115:1257, 1991.
61. Carrington C, Cugell D, Gaensler E, et al. Lymphangioleiomyomatosis: physiologic-pathologic-radiologic correlations. Am Rev Respir Dis 116:977, 1977.
62. Chan JK, Tsang WY, Pan MY, et al. Lymphangiomyomatosis and angiomyolipoma: closely related entities characterized by hamartomatous proliferation of HMB-45 positive smooth muscle. Histopathology 22:445, 1993.
63. Colley MH, Geppert E, Franklin WA. Immunohistochemical detection of steroid receptors in a case of pulmonary lymphangioleiomyomatosis. Am J Surg Pathol 13:803, 1989.
64. Cornog JL, Enterline HT. Lymphangiomyoma: a benign lesion of chyliferous lymphatics synonymous with lymphangiopericytoma. Cancer 19:1909, 1966.
65. Corrin B, Liebow AA, Friedman PJ. Pulmonary lymphangiomyomatosis. Am J Pathol 79:348, 1975.
66. Eliasson AH, Phillips YY, Tenholder MF. Treatment of lymphangioleiomyomatosis: a meta-analysis. Chest 96:1352, 1989.
67. Enterline HT, Roberts B. Lymphangiopericytoma. Cancer 8:582, 1955.
68. Fetsch PA, Fetsch JF, Marincola FM, et al. Comparison of melanoma antigen recognized by T cells (MART-1) to HMB-45: additional evidence to support a common lineage for angiomyolipoma, lymphangiomyomatosis and clear cell sugar tumor. Mod Pathol 11:699, 1998.
69. Folpe AL, Goodman ZD, Ishak KG, Weiss SW. Clear cell myomelanocytic tumor of the falciform ligament/ligamentum teres in children and young adults: a novel member of the PEComa family of tumors. Am J Surg Pathol 24:1239, 2000.
70. Frack MD, Simon L, Dawson BH. The lymphangiomyomatosis syndrome. Cancer 22:428, 1968.
71. Fukuda Y, Kawamoto M, Yamamoto A, et al. Role of elastic fiber degradation in emphysema-like lesions of pulmonary lymphangiomyomatosis. Hum Pathol 21:1252, 1990.
72. Gray SR, Carrington CB, Cornog JL. Lymphangiomyomatosis: report of a case with ureteral involvement and chyluria. Cancer 35:490, 1975.
73. Joliat G, Stalder H, Kapanci Y. Lymphangiomyomatosis: a clinicoanatomical entity. Cancer 31:455, 1973.
74. Kane P, Lane B, Cordice J, et al. Ultrastructure of the proliferating cells in pulmonary lymphangiomyomatosis. Acta Pathol Lab Med 102:618, 1978.
75. Lack EE, Dolan MF, Finisio J, et al. Pulmonary and extrapulmonary lymphangioleiomyomatosis: report of a case with bilateral renal angiomyolipomas, multifocal lymphangioleiomyomatosis, and a glial polyp of the endocervix. Am J Surg Pathol 10: 650, 1986.
76. Lieberman J, Agliozzo CM. Intrapleural nitrogen mustard for treating chylous effusion of pulmonary lymphangioleiomyomatosis. Cancer 33:1505, 1974.
77. Matthews TJ, Hornall D, Sheppard MN. Comparison of the use of antibodies to alpha smooth muscle actin and desmin in pulmonary lymphangioleiomyomatosis. J Clin Pathol 46:479, 1993.
78. McCarty KS, Mossler JA, McLelland R, et al. Pulmonary lymphangiomyomatosis responsive to progesterone. N Engl J Med 303:1461, 1980.
79. Monteforte WJ, Kohnen PW. Angiomyolipomas in a case of lymphangiomyomatosis syndrome: relationship to tuberous sclerosis. Cancer 34:317, 1974.
80. Ohori NP, Yousem SA, Sonmez-Alpan E, et al. Estrogen and progesterone receptors in lymphangioleiomyomatosis, epithelioid hemangioendothelioma, and sclerosing hemangioma of the lung. Am J Clin Pathol 96:529, 1991.
81. Pachter MR, Lattes R. Mesenchymal tumors of the mediastinum. III. Tumors of lymph vascular origin. Cancer 16:108, 1963.
82. Peyrol S, Gindre D, Cordier AJF, et al. Characterization of the smooth muscle cell infiltrate and associated connective matrix of lymphangiomyomatosis: immunohistochemical and ultrastructural study of two cases. J Pathol 168:387, 1992.
83. Schiaffino E, Tavani E, Dellafiore L, et al. Pulmonary lymphangiomyomatosis: report of a case with immunohistochemical and ultrastructural findings. Appl Pathol 7:265, 1989.
84. Silverstein EF, Ellis K, Wolff M, et al. Pulmonary lymphangiomyomatosis. AJR 120:832, 1974.
85. Steffelaar JW, Nijkamp DA, Hilvering C. Pulmonary lymphangiomyomatosis: demonstration of smooth muscle antigens by immunofluorescent technique. Scand J Respir Dis 58:103, 1977.
86. Stovin PGI, Lum LC, Flower CDR, et al. The lungs in lymphangiomyomatosis and in tuberous sclerosis. Thorax 30:497, 1975.
87. Svendsen TL, Viskum K, Hansborg N, et al. Pulmonary lymphangioleiomyomatosis: a case of progesterone receptor posi-

tive lymphangioleiomyomatosis treated with medroxyprogesterone, oophorectomy, and tamoxifen. Br J Dis Chest 78:264, 1984.

88. Taylor JR, Ryu J, Colby TV, et al. Lymphangioleiomyomatosis: clinical course in 32 patients. N Engl J Med 323:1254, 1990.
89. Tomasian A, Greenberg MS, Rumerman H. Tamoxifen for lymphangioleiomyomatosis. N Engl J Med 306:745, 1982.
90. Vadas G, Pare JA, Thurlbeck MW. Pulmonary and lymph node myomatosis: review of literature and report of case. Can Med Assoc J 96:420, 1967.
91. Valensi QJ. Pulmonary lymphangiomyoma, a probable forme fruste of tuberous sclerosis: a case report and survey of the literature. Am Rev Respir Dis 108:1411, 1973.
92. Vejlens G. Specific pulmonary alterations in tuberous sclerosis. Acta Pathol Microbiol Scand 18:317, 1941.
93. Wolff M. Lymphangiomyoma: clinicopathological study and ultrastructural confirmation of its histogenesis. Cancer 31:988, 1973.
94. Zamboni G, Pea M, Martignoni G, et al. Clear cell "sugar" tumor of the pancreas: a novel member of the family of lesions characterized by the presence of perivascular epithelioid cells. Am J Surg Pathol 20:722, 1996.

# CHAPTER 27

# PERIVASCULAR TUMORS

Perivascular tumors are those that recapitulate the appearance of cells that support or invest blood vessels (i.e., glomus cells and pericytes). This perivascular group includes two relatively distinct tumors, the glomus tumor and the hemangiopericytoma.[75] The so-called solitary fibrous tumor is also included in this chapter because it bears a close similarity to the hemangiopericytoma. Although classic hemangiopericytomas and solitary fibrous tumors can usually be distinguished from one another, there are certainly intermediate or hybrid cases. It is possible that these lesions are part of a common family that will be clarified over time through cytogenetic and molecular studies.

## GLOMUS TUMOR

Glomus tumor is a distinctive neoplasm, the cells of which resemble the modified smooth muscle cells of the normal glomus body. It was originally considered a form of angiosarcoma until Masson[49] published his classic paper on the subject in 1924. His work was based on observations of three patients who had experienced strikingly similar symptoms. Each suffered paroxysms of lancinating pain in the upper extremity that abated abruptly after removal of the tumor. Masson compared the tumors to the normal glomus body and suggested that the lesion represented hyperplasia or overgrowth of this structure. It is now well accepted that the lesions are neoplastic and recapitulate the appearance of the modified smooth cells of the normal glomus body.

The normal glomus body is a specialized form of arteriovenous anastomosis that serves in thermal regulation. It is located in the stratum reticularis of the dermis and is most frequently encountered in the subungual region, the lateral areas of the digits, and the palm.[58] Glomus bodies are also identified in the precoccygeal soft tissue as one or more grouped structures (glomus coccygeum) varying in diameter from <1 to 4 mm. According to Popoff,[58] the structure does not develop until several months after birth and gradually undergoes atrophy during late adult life. Although it may be damaged in certain disease states, there is evidence that it may regenerate, probably as a result of differentiation of perivascular cells. The glomus body is made up of an afferent arteriole derived from the small arterioles supplying the dermis and branching into two or four preglomic arterioles (Figs. 27–1, 27–2, 27–3). These arterioles are endowed with the usual complement of muscle cells and an internal elastic lamina, but they blend gradually into a thick-walled segment with an irregular lumen known as the Sucquet-Hoyer canal. This region is the arteriovenous anastomosis proper. It is lined by plump cuboidal endothelial cells, which in turn are surrounded by longitudinal and circular muscle fibers but no elastic tissue. Scattered throughout the muscle fibers are the rounded, epithelioid "glomus" cells. These canals drain into a series of thin-walled collecting veins. The entire glomic complex is encompassed by lamellated collagenous tissue containing small nerves and vessels.

### Clinical Findings

Glomus tumors are uncommon, with an estimated incidence of 1.6% among the 500 consecutive soft tissue tumors reported from the Mayo Clinic.[67] The tumor is about equally common in both genders, although there is a striking female predominance (3:1) among patients with subungual lesions.[10,67,71] Most glomus tumors are diagnosed during adult life (20–40 years of age), although often symptoms have been present for several years before the diagnosis.[51,53] The lesions develop as small blue-red nodules that are usually located in the deep dermis or subcutis of the upper or lower extremity. The single most common site is the subungual region of the finger, but other common sites include the palm, wrist, forearm, and foot (Table 27–1). Glomus tumors probably also occur in the subcutaneous tissue near the tip of the spine, where they presumably arise from the glomus coccygeum (Fig. 27–4). However, many "incidental" glomus tumors arising in the region of the coccyx may well represent the normal glomus coccygeum[4,19] as

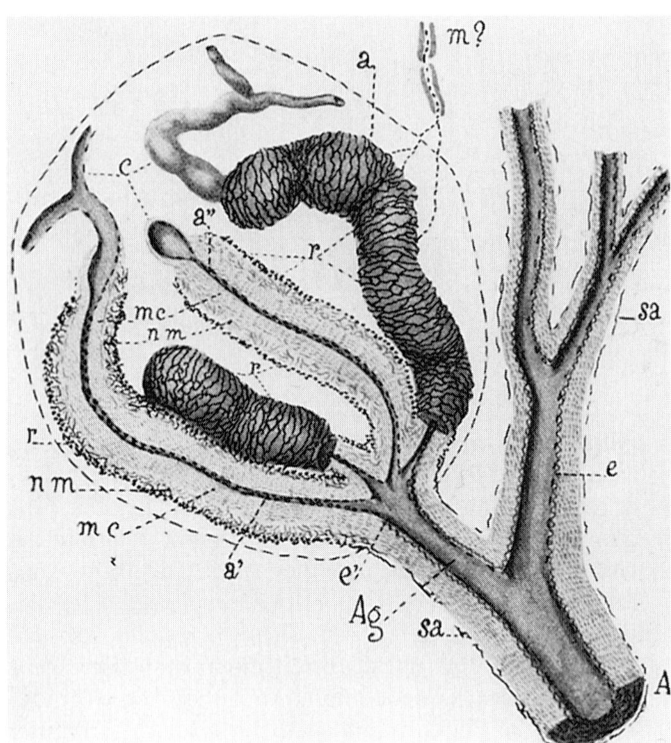


**FIGURE 27–1.** Normal glomus body according to Masson.[49] Afferent arteriole (**Ag**) gives rise to four preglomic arterioles, which blend with an irregular, thick-walled segment known as the Sucquet-Hoyer canal containing the arteriovenous anastomosis. It terminates in the collecting veins (**c**). (From Masson P. Le glomus neuromyoarterial des regions tactiles et ses tumeurs. Lyon Chir 21:257, 1924.)

this structure can reach several millimeters in diameter in the absence of clinical symptoms, suggesting a neoplasm.[24] These tumors also develop in sites where the normal glomus body may be sparse or even absent. Unusual locations have included the patella,[62] chest wall, bone,[11,44,46] stomach,[7,27,35,37,63,76] colon,[9] nerve,[16,43] eyelid, nose,[6] trachea,[40] and possibly mediastinum.[14] In our experience they have also occurred in the rectum, cervix, vagina, labia, and mesentery.

Most glomus tumors are solitary, although in two large studies the incidence of multiple lesions was estimated to be just under 10%.[25] There are several striking instances of patients with multiple lesions.[20,21,25,27,42,57] These reports indicate certain differences between the solitary and multiple forms of the disease. Multiple glomus tumors occur more often during childhood, are rarely subungual, and are less likely to be painful or symptomatic. Histologically, they are usually poorly circumscribed, occasionally plaque-like lesions that resemble cavernous hemangiomas[20] (see discussion of the glomangioma, below), in contrast to the ordinary glomus tumor, which is usually better circumscribed and more cellular. A few patients with multiple lesions have been known to have similarly affected family members or associated malformations.[45] Conant and Wiesenfeld[17] described nine affected members in one family which is compatible with an autosomal dominant mode of inheri-

**TABLE 27–1** ANATOMIC DISTRIBUTION OF GLOMUS TUMORS ACCORDING TO HISTOLOGIC SUBTYPE: AFIP, 506 CASES

| | Glomus Tumor | | Glomangioma | | Glomangiomyoma | |
|---|---|---|---|---|---|---|
| **Anatomic Location** | ***No. Cases*** | ***%*** | ***No. Cases*** | ***%*** | ***No. Cases*** | ***%*** |
| Upper extremities | 176 | 34 | 45 | 9 | 16 | 3 |
| Finger | 81 | | 9 | | 3 | |
| Lower extremities | 98 | 19 | 29 | 6 | 14 | 3 |
| Head and neck | 29 | 6 | 6 | 1 | 5 | 1 |
| Trunk | 24 | 5 | 8 | 2 | 0 | 0 |
| Other | 45 | 9 | 4 | 1 | 7 | 1 |
| *Total* | 372 | 73 | 92 | 19 | 42 | 8 |

AFIP, Armed Forces Institute of Pathology.

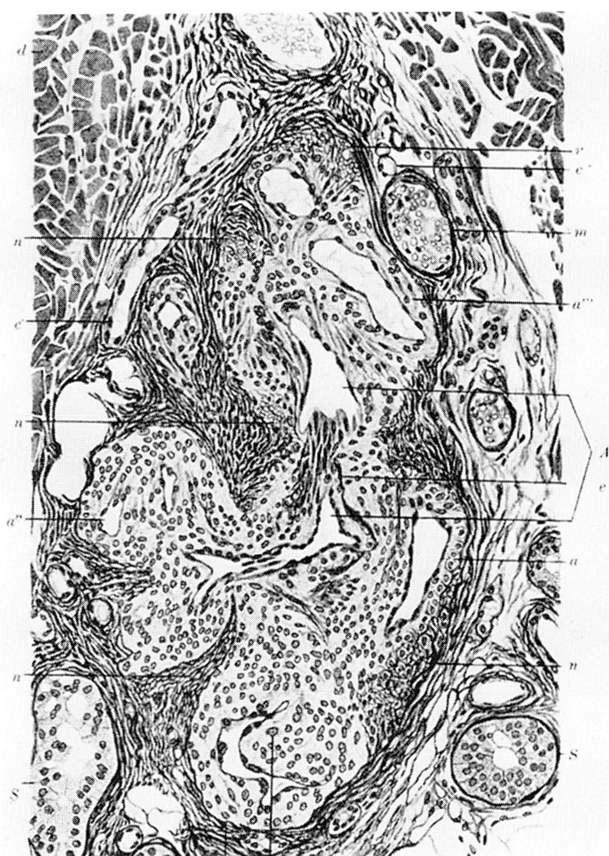

**FIGURE 27–2.** Histologic cross section through a glomus body according to Masson.[49] Glomic arterioles of Sucquet-Hoyer canal (**a**, **a″**, **a′ ″**,) contain glomus cells in their walls. Collecting veins are located at the periphery (**c**). Small nerves and collagen fibers encircle the glomus body. (From Masson P. Le glomus neuromyoarterial des regions tactiles et ses tumeurs. Lyon Chir 21:257, 1924.)

tance with incomplete penetrance. A gene for inherited glomangiomas has been localized to chromosome 1p21-22.[12] Glomus tumors have been noted in NF1.[57,64]

The symptoms produced by glomus tumors are characteristic and often well out of proportion to the size of the neoplasm. Paroxysms of pain radiating away from the lesion are the most common complaint. These episodes can be elicited by changes in temperature, particularly exposure to cold, and tactile stimulation of even minor degree. In some patients the pain is accompanied by additional signs of hypesthesia, muscle atrophy,[62] or osteoporosis of the affected part.[23,67] In unusual instances disturbances of autonomic function (e.g., Horner syndrome) have been reported.[49] Although the mechanism of pain production has not been fully elucidated, identification of nerve fibers containing immunoreactive substance P (a pain-associated vasoactive peptide) in glomus tumors suggests pain mediation through release of this substance.[41]

## Gross Findings

Grossly, the lesions are small blue-red nodules (usually <1 cm) that are immediately apparent on clinical examination. Subungual lesions may be more difficult to detect, and care should be taken to look for ridging of the nail or discoloration of the nail bed. Radiographs are helpful when they demonstrate a small scalloped osteolytic defect with a sclerotic border[28] in the terminal phalanx, as this finding is highly characteristic of a glomus tumor and epidermal inclusion cyst (Fig. 27–5). The more recent use of high-resolution MRI offers the promise of detecting extremely small soft tissue-based lesions.[36]

## Microscopic Findings

Glomus tumors have varying proportions of glomus cells, vascular structures, and smooth muscle tissue. According to the relative proportions, they have been divided into three groups: (1) glomus tumor proper; (2) glomangioma; and (3) glomangiomyoma. Although there is no significant difference in the age incidence in these three groups, the location of the tumors varies (Table 27–1). Glomus tumors are most common in the upper extremity and have a marked predilection for the finger, particularly the subungual region. Glomangiomas predominate on the hand and forearm and are usually the type encountered in patients with multiple or familial lesions. Glomangiomyomas are nearly equally divided between the upper and lower extremities.

The common form of ***glomus tumor*** accounts for about three-fourths of all cases in our material (Table 27–1). It is a well circumscribed lesion consisting of tight convolutes of capillary-sized vessels surrounded by collars of glomus cells set in a hyalinized or myxoid stroma (Fig. 27–6). Rarely, it appears as a poorly circumbscribed, diffuse lesion. Depending on the size of the nests of glomus cells, the tumor may have a highly vascular appearance reminiscent of a hemangiopericytoma or paraganglioma or a cellular appearance suggestive of an epithelial tumor[60] (Fig. 27–7). The glomus cell is quite distinctive, and its appearance is one of the most reliable means of distinguishing this tumor from others with similar growth patterns. The cell has a rounded, regular shape with a sharply punched-out rounded nucleus set off from the amphophilic or eosinophilic cytoplasm (Fig. 27–8). The outlines of the cells are not fully appreciated on routine hematoxylin-eosin-stained sections but can be accentuated with a periodic acid-Schiff (PAS) or toluidine blue stain on 1 $\mu$m sections. In these preparations a "chickenwire" network of matrix material is present between the cells.

Only rarely do glomus cells deviate from the fore-

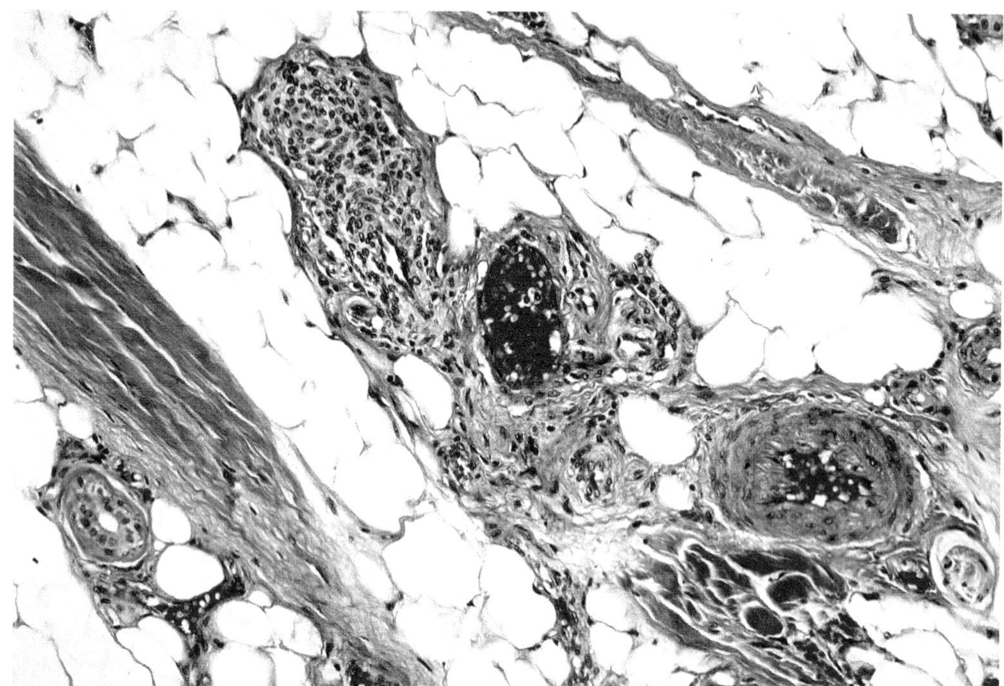

**FIGURE 27–3.** Normal glomus body from the foot. Arrows indicate the Sucquet-Hoyer canal with glomus cells.

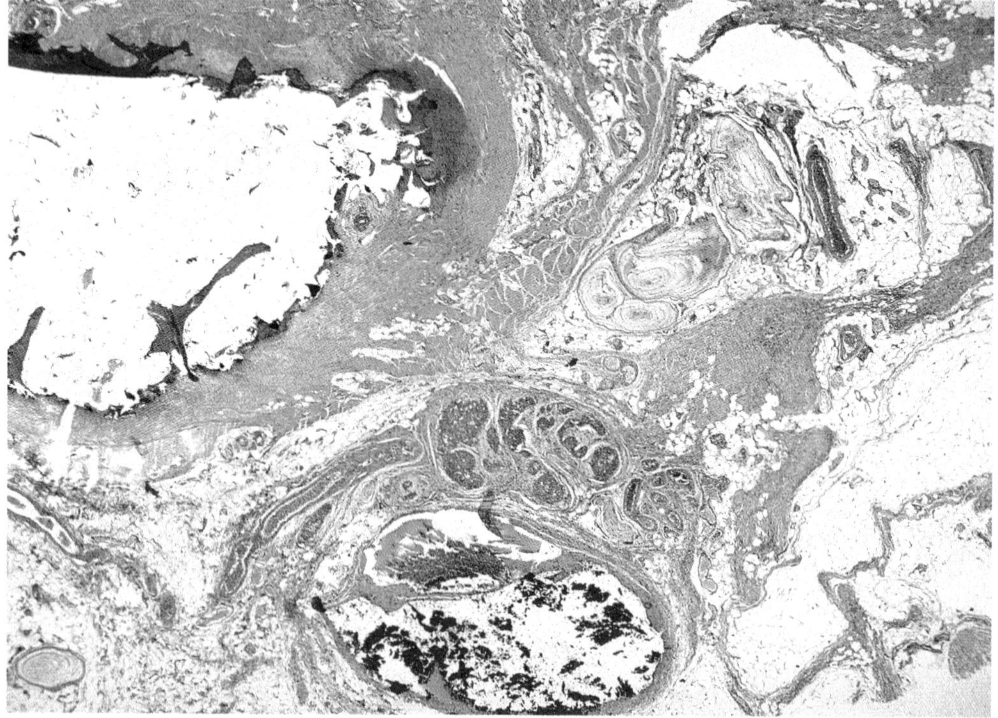

**FIGURE 27–4.** Glomus coccygeum located at the ventral tip of the coccyx.

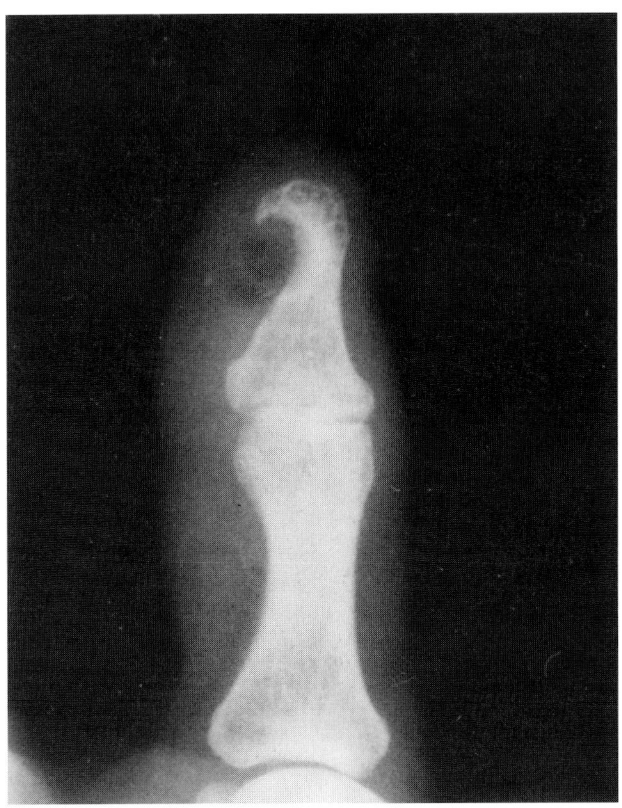

**FIGURE 27–5.** Postoperative radiograph showing a defect in the distal phalanx created by a subungual glomus tumor.

going description; but when they do, alterations in either the nucleus or the cytoplasm may be seen. Large hyperchromatic nuclei, probably representing a degenerative change analogous to that seen in some schwannomas, may replace the typical round, regular nuclei. If this change is present as an isolated finding in an otherwise typical glomus tumor, it should not be equated with malignancy. Such tumors are referred to as "symplastic glomus tumors" (see below). An even less common phenomenon is the acquisition of abundant granular, eosinophilic cytoplasm such that portions of the tumor appear "oncocytic"[66,69] (Fig. 27–9). Intravascular growth and signet-ring changes in the cells have been noted in a multifocal gastric glomus tumor.[27]

Although the cells are regarded as variants of smooth muscle cells, the cytoplasm is usually devoid of glycogen, and there is only minimal fuchsinophilia observed on staining with the Masson trichrome stain, two features that contrast with the staining reactions of conventional smooth muscle cells. Peripherally, the tumors have an ill-defined rim of collagen containing small nerves and vessels. This rim seldom serves as a complete or totally confining capsule, as isolated nests of glomus cells can be identified outside its boundaries and occasionally in the walls of small vessels surrounding the main tumor mass (Fig. 27–10). Vascular invasion is rarely seen in benign glomus tumors and does not appear to be predictive in and of itself of malignancy.

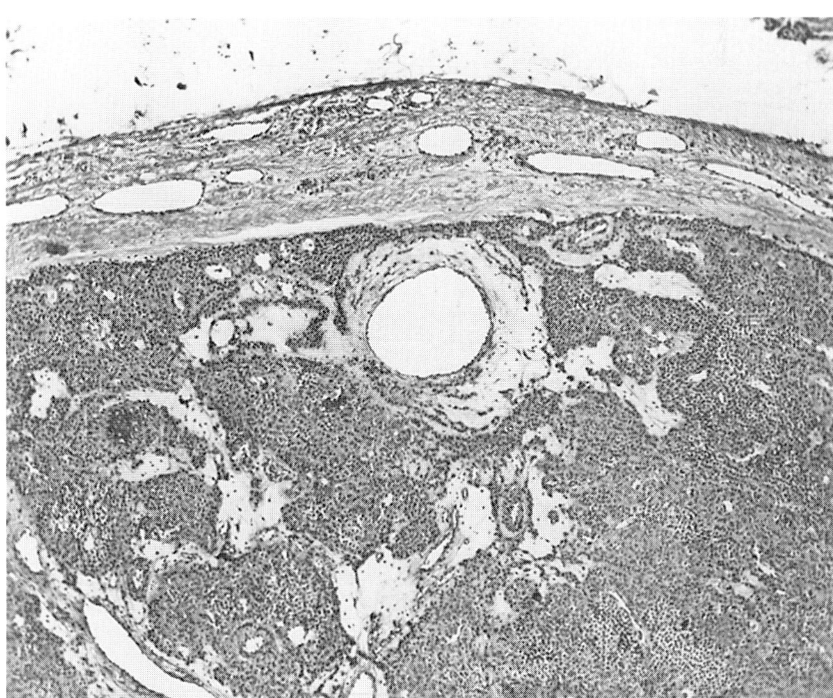

**FIGURE 27–6.** Common form of glomus tumor with a dense fibrous pseudocapsule surrounding solid sheets of cells. (×15)

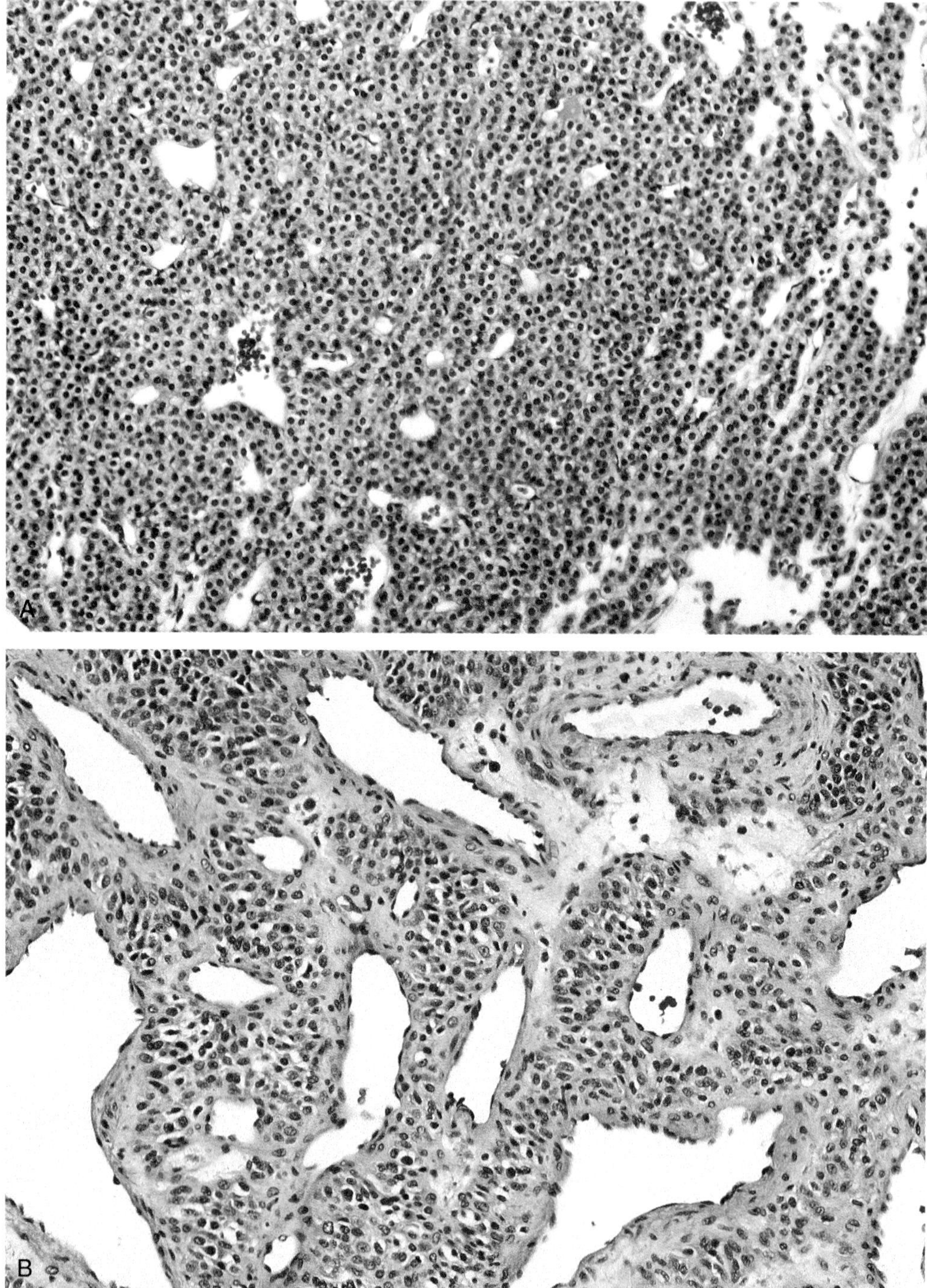


**FIGURE 27–7.** Variable patterns in glomus tumors. Most tumors are composed of solid sheets of cells interrupted by vessels of varying size (**A, B**).

*Illustration continued on opposite page*

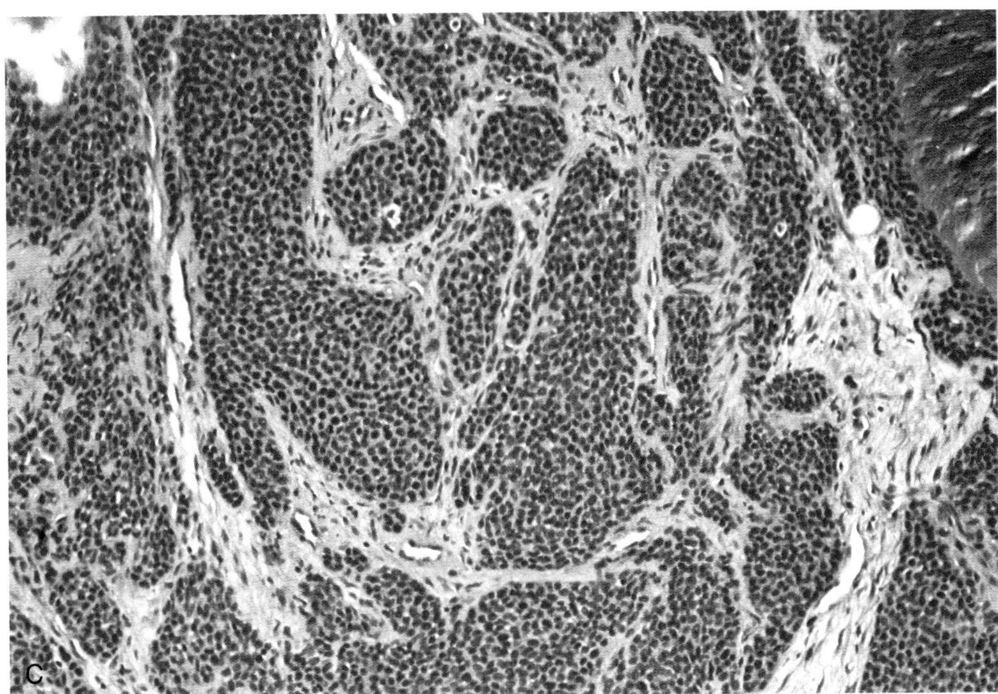


**FIGURE 27–7** *(Continued)*. Some areas have an organoid or epithelioid pattern of growth (**C**).

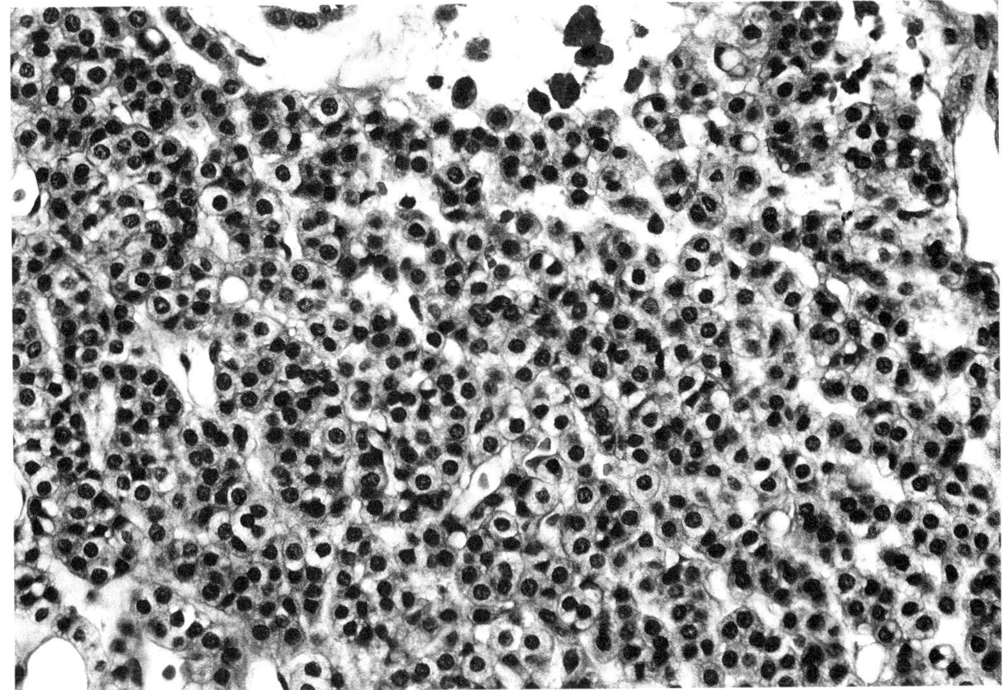

**FIGURE 27–8.** Glomus tumor with round cells exhibiting punched-out nuclei, pale cytoplasm, and a lacework of basement membrane material around the cells.

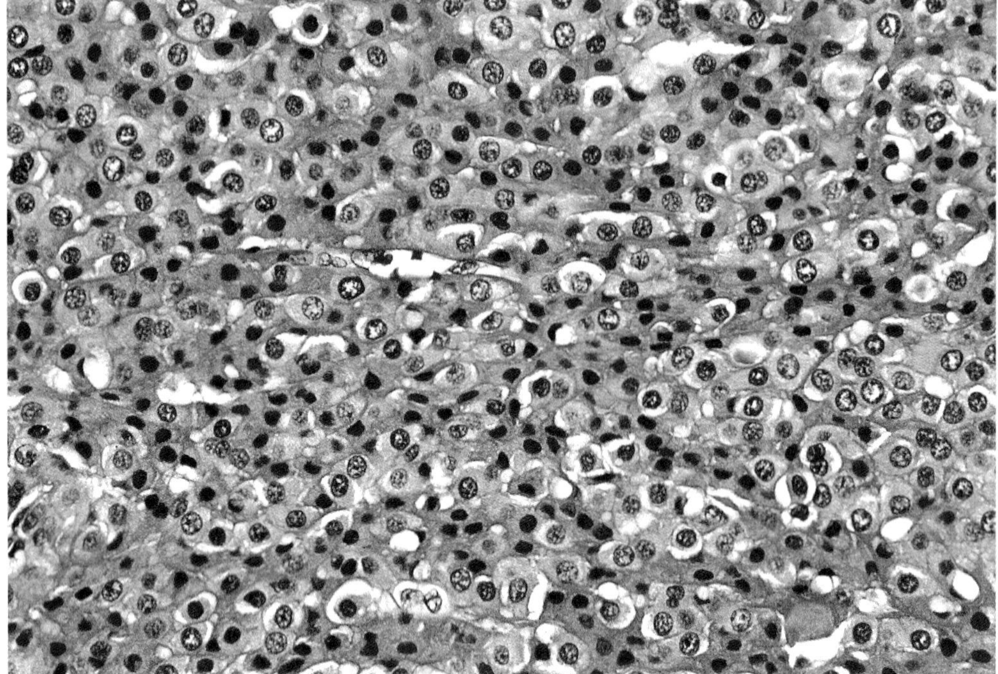

**FIGURE 27–9.** Oncocytic change in a glomus tumor.

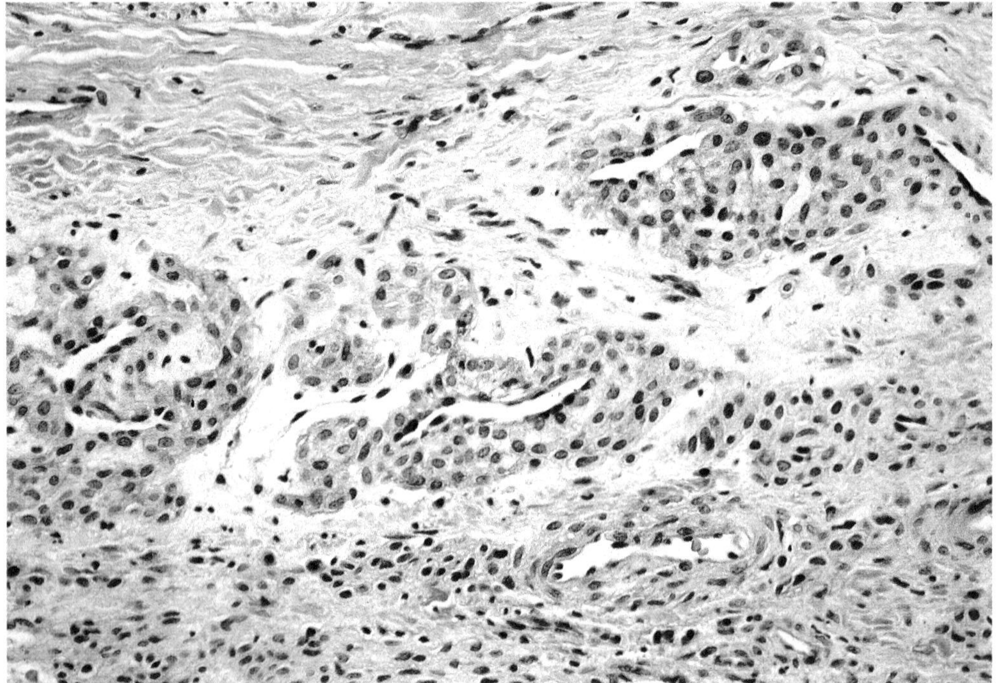

**FIGURE 27–10.** Proliferation of glomus cells in vessels at the periphery of a glomus tumor. This feature may be helpful for distinguishing solid glomus tumors from adnexal tumors.

In contrast to the common form of glomus tumor, ***glomangiomas*** are less well circumscribed and constitute only about one-fifth of cases. Grossly and microscopically, they resemble cavernous hemangiomas (Figs. 27–11, 27–12, 27–13). They are composed of gaping veins with small clusters of glomus cells in their walls. Secondary thrombosis and phlebolith formation may occur in these lesions just as they would in an ordinary hemangioma.

***Glomangiomyomas*** account for less than 10% of all glomus tumors and therefore are the least frequent type. Their overall pattern may be identical to that of the ordinary glomus tumor or the glomangioma. However, in contrast to the foregoing types, there is a gradual transition from glomus cells to elongated, mature smooth muscle cells.[78] This transition is most obvious in the region of large vessels, where the peripheral smooth muscle cells seem to blend with the tumor (Figs. 27–14, 27–15). The term ***glomangiopericytoma*** has been used recently for glomus tumors with prominent thin and thick-walled vessels and slight spindling of the glomus cells.[133] These tumors seem to be somewhat intermediate in appearance between glomangiomas and glomangiomyomas (Fig. 27–16).

Because glomus tumors are quite distinctive by virtue of their characteristic cells, location, and symptoms, errors in diagnosis are infrequent. Nonetheless, it has been our experience that highly cellular glomus tumors are occasionally mistaken for adnexal tumors or less frequently intradermal nevi. In the former instance, it is important to note the intimate relation of glomus cells around small vessels at the periphery of the tumor (Fig. 27–10) and the total lack of ductular differentiation or epithelial mucin production. Immunohistochemistry can reliably discriminate glomus tumors from solid forms of hidradenoma (the adnexal tumor most closely resembling a glomus tumor).[29] Virtually all hidradenomas contain immunoreactive keratin, whereas glomus tumors do not. In addition, hidradenomas frequently also express carcinoembryonic and epithelial membrane antigens, which are not encountered in glomus tumors. Likewise, S-100 protein is a reliable marker for distinguishing nevi from glomus tumors.[39] In the past, a reticulin stain was often used to discriminate glomus tumors from epithelial ones because the former displayed a delicate interstitial pattern of fiber deposition in contrast to the latter. This staining technique, which is often difficult to perform and interpret, has been largely replaced by immunohistochemistry. Although electron microscopy can serve as a diagnostic adjunct, it is seldom needed given the reliability of immunohistochemistry in most cases.

## Ultrastructural and Immunohistochemical Findings

The glomus cell is rounded or polygonal in shape and measures 8–12 $\mu$m with a rounded nucleus with

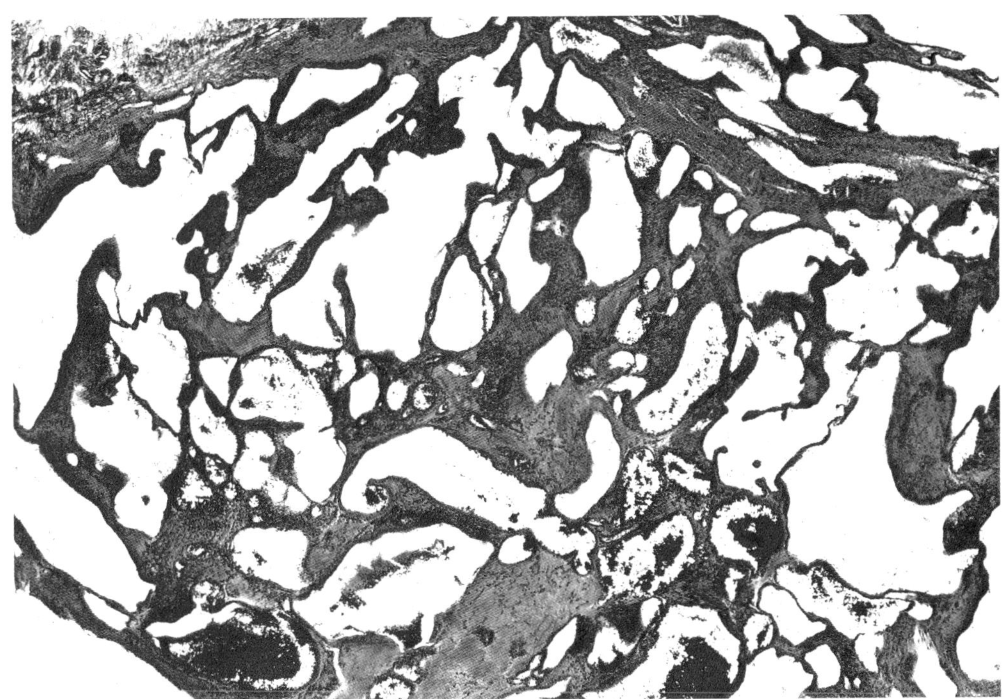

**FIGURE 27–11.** Partially collapsed glomangioma with dilated cavernous blood spaces.

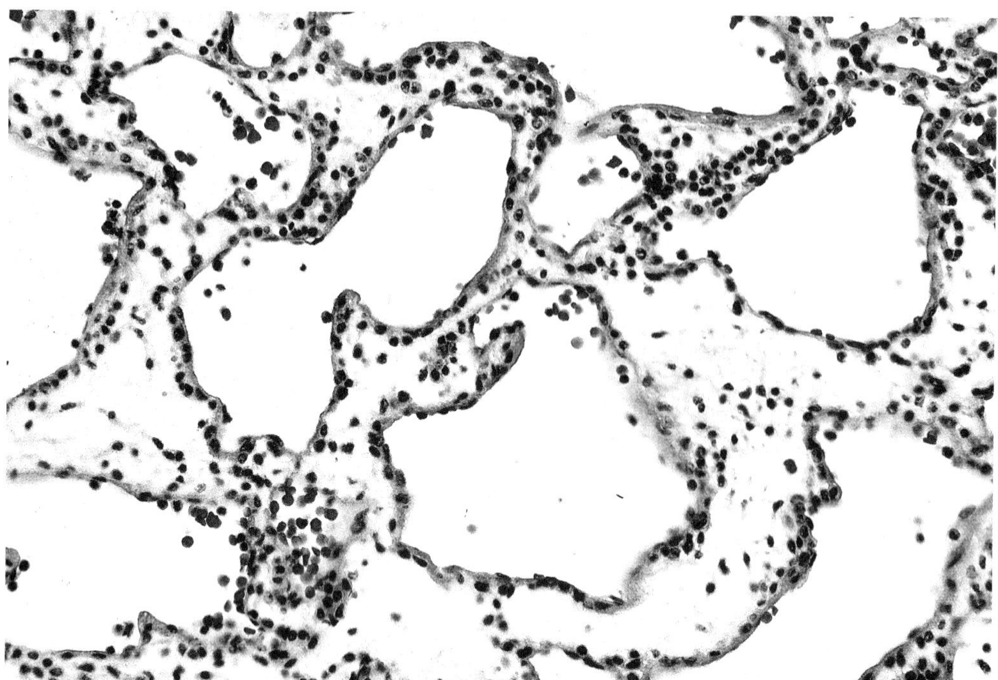

**FIGURE 27–12.** Glomangioma with cuffs of cells around dilated vessels.

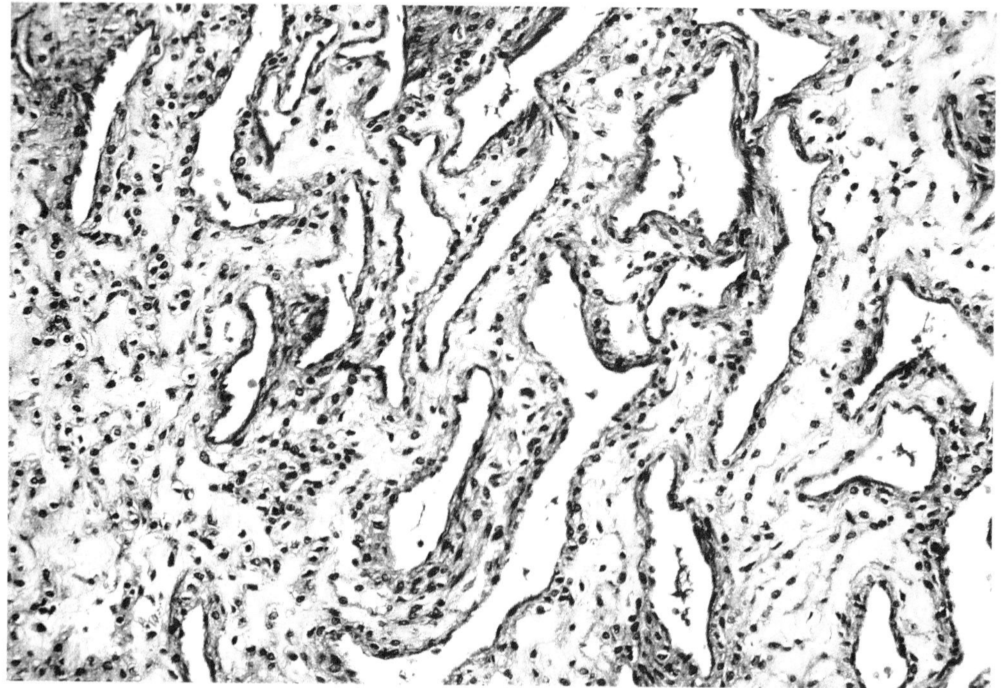

**FIGURE 27–13.** Glomangioma with marked hyalinization.

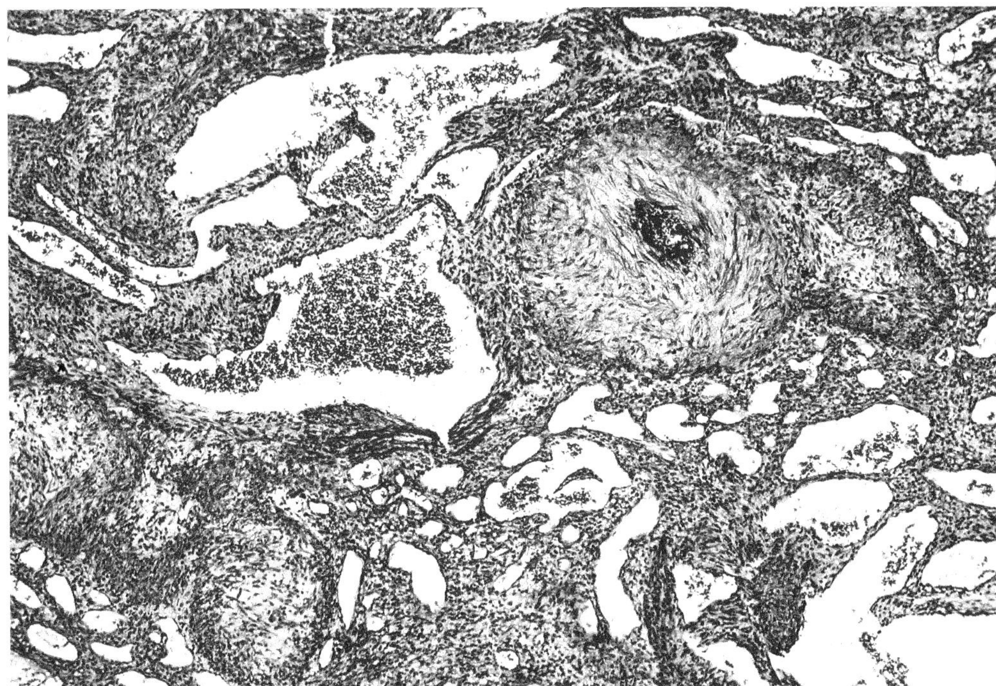

**FIGURE 27–14.** Glomangiomyoma. Note the blending of muscle in the vessels with tumor. (Masson trichrome stain)

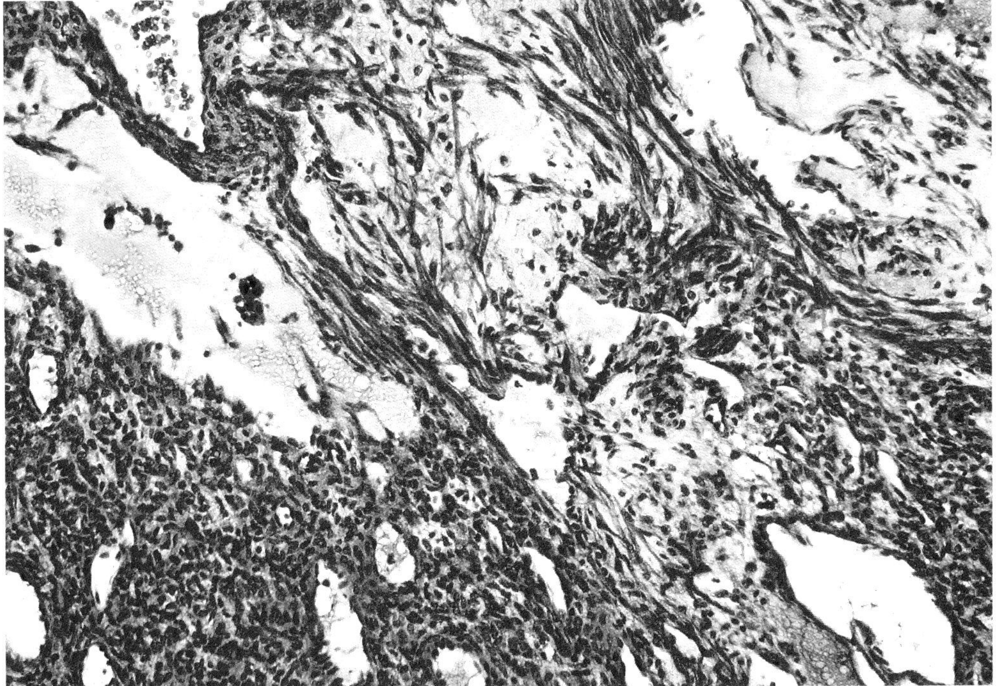

**FIGURE 27–15.** Glomangiomyoma. Glomus cells undergo transition to smooth muscle cells. (Masson trichrome stain)

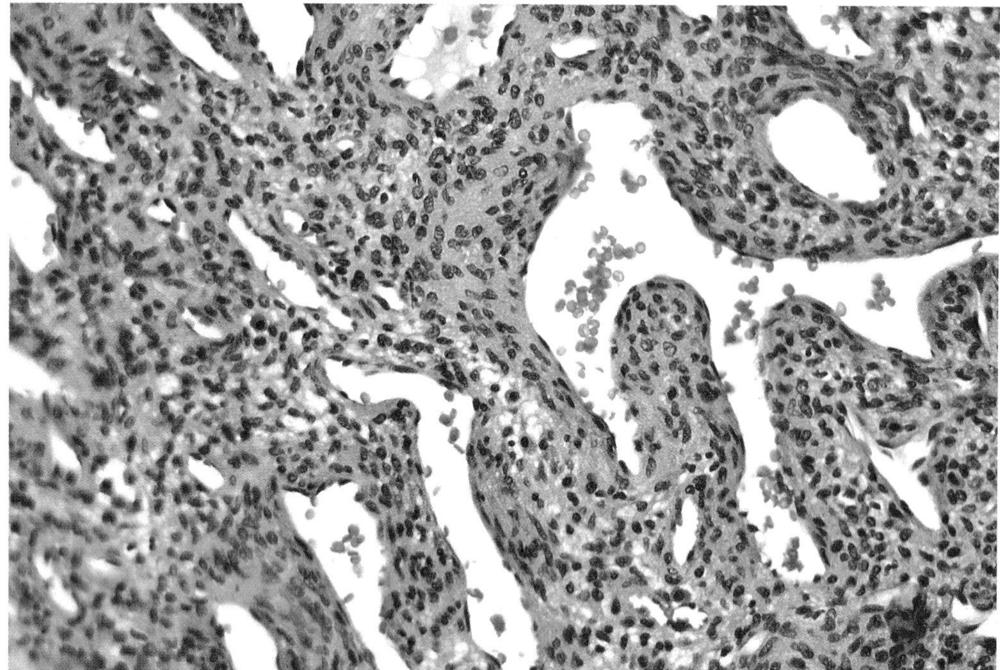

**FIGURE 27–16.** Glomus tumor that recurred with predominantly pericytic features: a so-called glomangiopericytoma.

occasional clefts and prominent nucleoli (Fig. 27–17). The cells are closely spaced and often interdigitate with each other along their short, knobby processes. Their surfaces are invested by a relatively thick basal lamina. The cytoplasm contains modest numbers of mitochondria and endoplasmic reticulum but is most notable for the bundles of thin (8 nm) actin-like filaments that fill the cytoplasm. The bundles are well oriented, have typical dense bodies, and occasionally terminate in dense attachment plaques on the cytoplasmic membrane.[73] In the glomus tumors with oncocytic features, not surprisingly the cytoplasm is filled with numerous mitochondria, making it more difficult to identify microfilaments.[69] Originally, glomus cells were thought to be pericytes on the basis of certain morphologic similarities noted in tissue culture.[52] However, as a result of determining the foregoing ultrastructural features the glomus tumor is generally considered more closely related to the smooth muscle cell. Certainly the quantity of myofilaments present in these cells exceeds that normally encountered in the pericyte, and the cell processes are less well developed than those of the latter cell. Vimentin and muscle actin isoforms can be identified in nearly all glomus tumors[15,18,28,56,58,59,65,191] (Fig. 27–18A). Desmin is much more variable, however, and has been reported in either no tumors[65] or in most of the tumors,[59,65] depending on the series. In concert with the ultrastructural features of the neoplasm, laminin and type IV collagen, two constituents of basal lamina, outline the cells or small groups of cells[27] (Fig. 27–18B). Nerve growth factor receptor and myelin-associated glycoprotein can be identified in some glomus tumors, although the meaning of this finding is not clear.[59]

### Behavior and Treatment

Most glomus tumors are benign and can be treated adequately by simple excision. Only 10% recur following conservative excision.[72] Infrequent local recurrences probably represent persistence of tumor following inadequate excision or infrequently a benign glomus tumor growing in a diffuse or infiltrative fashion[21,26,30,61] (see below).

## GLOMANGIOMATOSIS (DIFFUSE GLOMUS TUMOR)

Glomus tumors can present as diffusely infiltrating lesions similar to some vascular tumors and malformations. We refer to them as "glomangiomatosis" and conceptualize them as the glomoid counterpart of angiomatosis. Glomangiomatosis is rare, accounting for only 5% of glomus tumors with unusual or atypical features and a vanishingly smaller percent of all glomus tumors. This form of glomus tumor may be more prevalent among patients who present during childhood.[71] Other glomus tumors have been reported in the literature.[35,48,54,61,68] Typically such lesions are

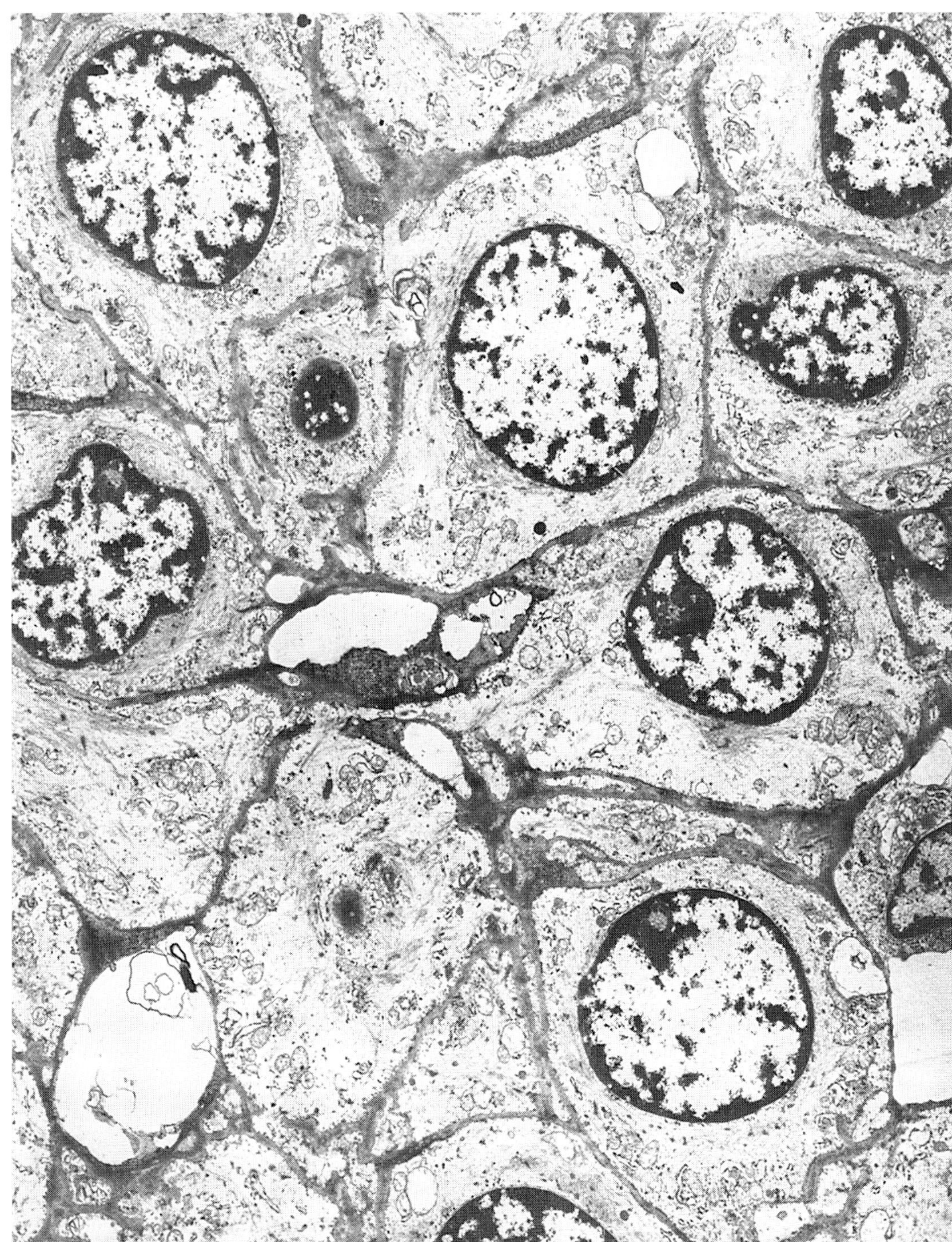

**FIGURE 27–17.** Electron micrograph of a glomus tumor. Cells are invested by dense basal lamina, have pinocytic vesicles along their surfaces, and contain cytoplasmic myofilaments with dense bodies. (Magnification reduced from ×5000) (Courtesy of the Department of Pathology, Veterans Administration Hospital, Hines, IL.)

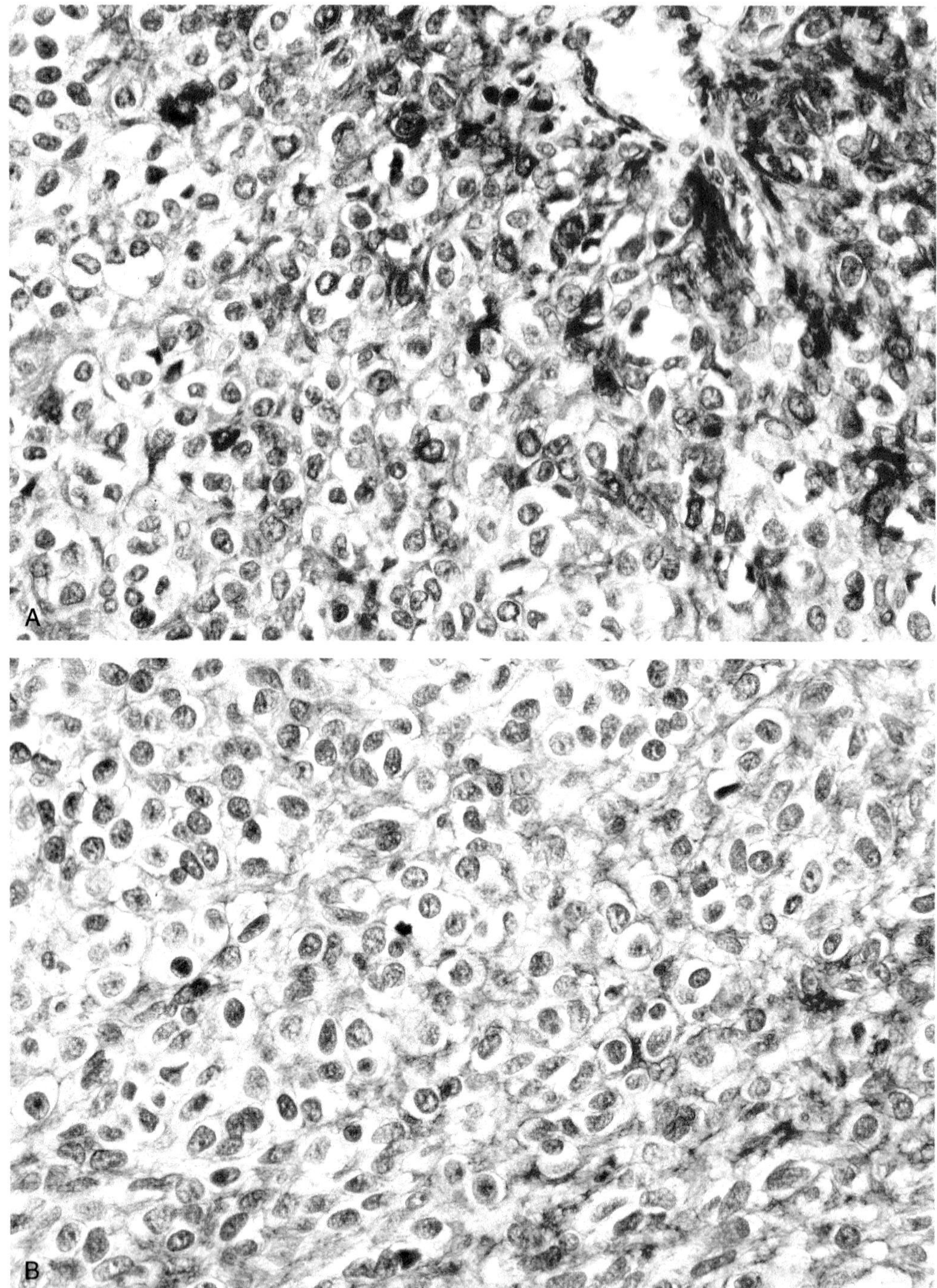


**FIGURE 27–18.** (**A**) Immunostains for actin reveal strong cytoplasmic positivity in glomus cells. (**B**) Immunostains for type IV collagen in a glomus tumor show intricate chicken-wire pattern between cells.

extensive, deep, and often pain-producing. Like angiomatosis, they consist of well formed vessels of varying size that grow in a diffuse or infiltrative fashion (Fig. 27–19). Mature fat sometimes accompanies the vessels. Clusters of glomus cells invest the vessels, particularly small vessels. There is no evidence that these lesions are malignant or undergo malignant transformation, but like angiomatosis they may be difficult to eradicate. In fact, we have seen one remarkable case in which microscopic residua of glomangiomatosis were associated with persistence of pain and required wide excision to alleviate symptoms. In general, the extent of excision is gauged by the symptomatic and cosmetic needs of the patient.

## ATYPICAL AND MALIGNANT GLOMUS TUMORS

Over the years the malignancy of glomus tumors has been more of a concept than a reality. Although several histologically malignant glomus tumors have been reported, biologic confirmation of malignancy in these cases was lacking[3,26,31–33,47,55,77] probably because many were superficial and therefore cured by therapy. A second compounding factor was the fact that the rare malignant glomus tumors that produced metastases lacked a benign glomus component, and so the accuracy of the diagnosis was questioned. The tumor reported by Lumley and Stansfeld that produced metastases is an example of this phenomenon.[48] Two other reports, one by Brathwaite and Poppiti[13] and a second by Watanabe et al.,[74] detailed two patients with malignant glomus tumors clearly arising in the setting of a benign glomus tumor. The first case, a mitotically active glomus tumor of the nose in a patient with multiple glomus tumors, produced disseminated disease documented at autopsy. The second case was a glomangiomyoma, which produced pulmonary metastases in 2 years.

Based on our experience we believe that a malignant glomus tumor can be diagnosed in the absence of a benign glomus component provided ancillary immunohistochemical data are available. In fact, only about one-half of malignant glomus tumors in our experience have a discernible benign component. The scheme in Table 27–2 is the one we propose for classifying glomus tumors with unusual features such as nuclear atypia and mitotic activity.

**TABLE 27–2 CLASSIFICATION OF GLOMUS TUMORS WITH ATYPICAL FEATURES**

| |
|---|
| Malignant Glomus Tumor |
| Marked atypia + mitotic activity (>5/50 HPF) *or* |
| Atypical mitotic figures *or* |
| Large size (>2 cm) + deep location |
| Glomus tumor of uncertain malignant potential |
| Superficial location + high mitotic activity (>5/50 HPF) *or* |
| Large size only *or* |
| Deep location only |
| Symplastic Glomus Tumor |
| Lacks criteria for malignant glomus tumor *and* |
| Marked nuclear atypia only |
| Glomangiomatosis |
| Lacks criteria for malignant glomus tumor or glomus tumor of uncertain malignant potential *and* |
| Diffuse growth resembling angiomatosis with prominent glomus component |

From Folpe AL, Fanburg-Smith JC, Miettinen M, Weiss SW. Atypical and malignant glomus tumors: analysis of 53 cases with a proposal for the reclassification of glomus tumors. Am J Surg Pathol 25:1, 2001.
HPF, high-power fields.

### Malignant Glomus Tumor

Malignant glomus tumors are defined as those that are (1) large ( > 2 cm) and deeply located; (2) have marked nuclear atypia and elevated mitotic rates [> 5 mitoses/50 high-power fields (HPF)]; or (3) display atypical mitotic figures. A compressed rim of benign glomus tumor surrounding the malignant areas is seen in about one-half of cases (Fig. 27–20). The malignant areas can assume one of two patterns (Figs. 27–21, 27–22). In the first, the tumor retains its architectural similarity to a benign glomus tumor and consists of sheets of round cells with a high nuclear/cytoplasmic ratio, high nuclear grade, and typical or atypical mitotic figures. At first glance these lesions resemble a round cell sarcoma such as Ewing's sarcoma (Fig. 27–22). In the second pattern, the malignant areas differ cytoarchitecturally from a glomus tumor and are composed of spindle or fusiform cells arranged in short fascicles reminiscent of a fibrosarcoma or leiomyosarcoma (Fig. 27–21). In the absence of a benign glomus component, the diagnosis of malignant glomus tumor nearly always presupposes the use of immunohistochemistry. Identification of cytoplasmic actin and the lattice-work of type IV collagen at least focally is highly suggestive of the diagnosis. Of the 21 glomus tumors meeting the criteria of malignancy detailed above, 38% developed metastases, providing support for the validity of the criteria.[22]

### Glomus Tumor of Uncertain Malignant Potential

Some glomus tumors fail to meet the minimum criteria of malignancy but display features that are clearly beyond the realm of an ordinary glomus tumor. We designate such lesions "glomus tumor of uncertain malignant potential." Most lesions falling into this category are superficial tumors with high mitotic activity and no significant nuclear atypia, or they are

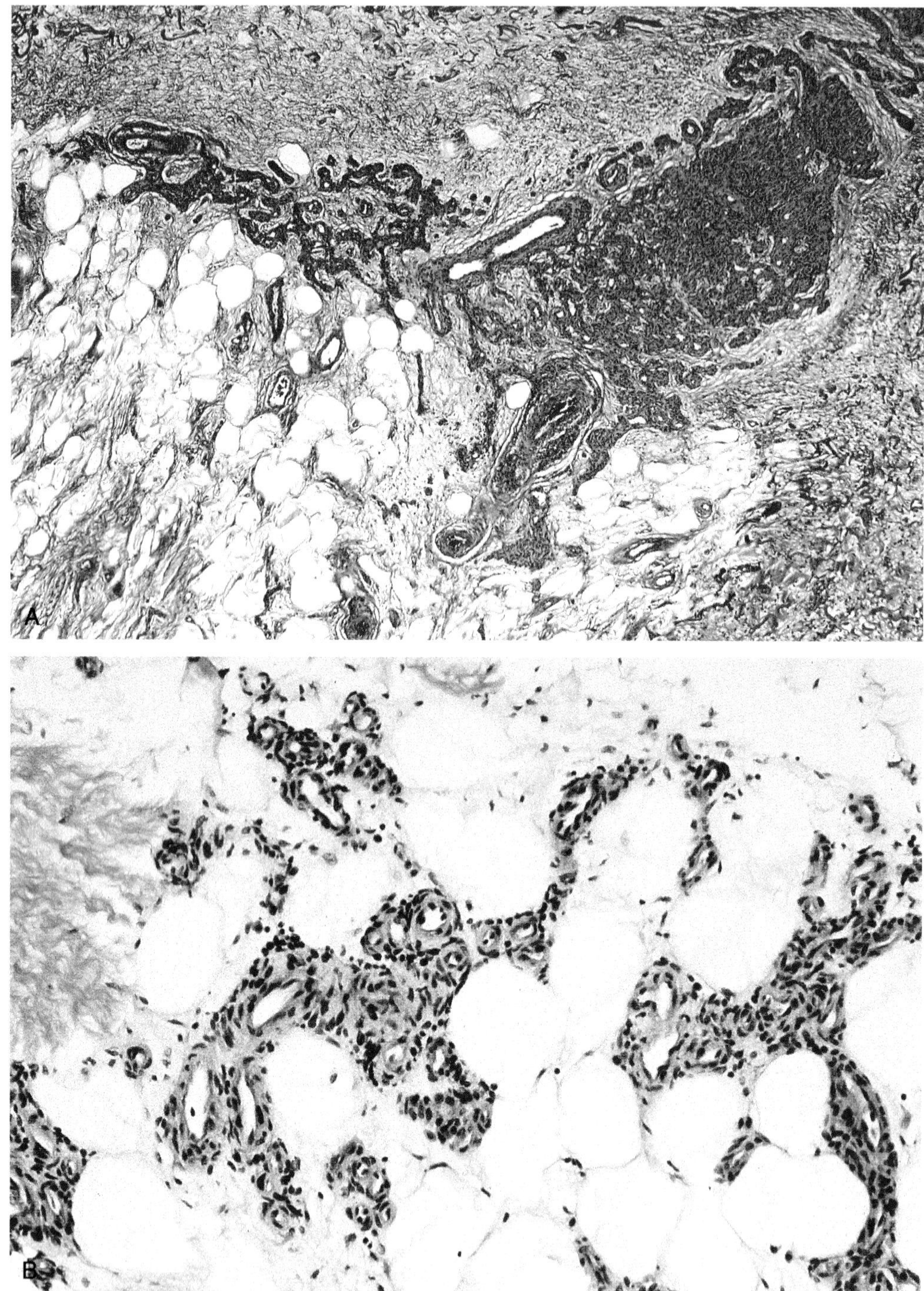


**FIGURE 27–19.** Diffuse glomus tumor (glomangiomatosis) with infiltrative growth of vessels (**A**), which are encircled by glomus cells (**B**).

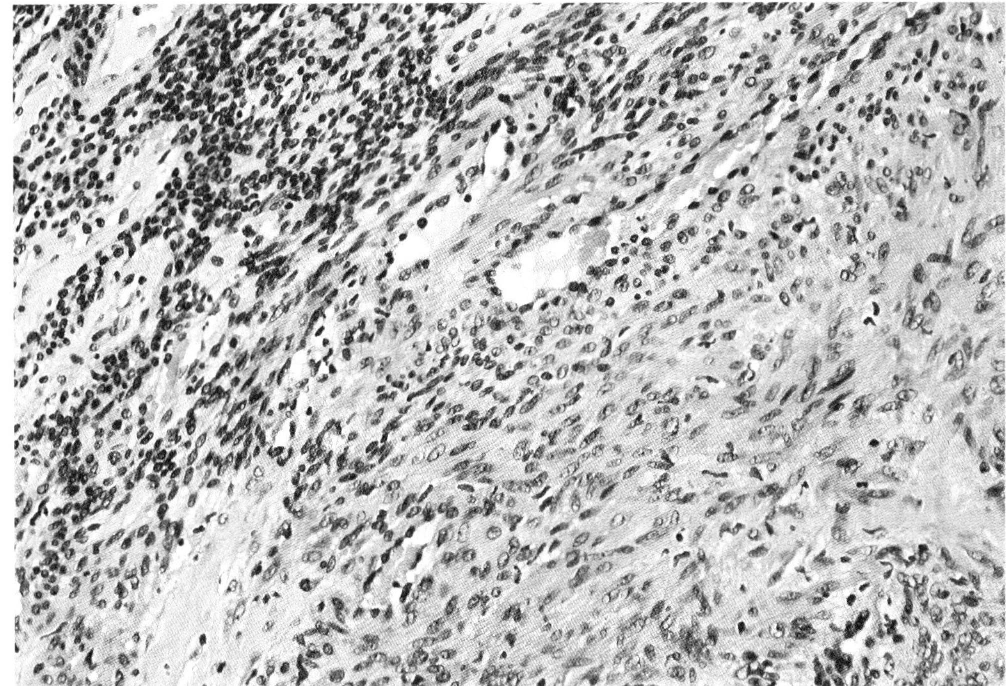

**FIGURE 27–20.** Malignant glomus tumor. There is a compressed rim of benign glomus tumor (upper right) next to a histologically malignant glomus tumor with a spindled pattern.

large or deep (Table 27–2). To date, the follow-up of glomus tumors of uncertain malignant potential has been uniformly good, but the number of cases is small and the follow-up relatively short. We believe that affixing the label "uncertain malignant potential" guarantees adequate follow-up for this problematic group of lesions.

### Symplastic Glomus Tumor

Glomus tumors that have marked nuclear atypia as their sole unusual feature can be labeled "symplastic glomus tumors" (Fig. 27–23). The marked nuclear atypia that characterizes tumors in this group appears to be a degenerative phenomenon that can be likened to symplastic change in leiomyomas. To date, symplastic glomus tumors have a benign course, similar to ordinary glomus tumors.

## HEMANGIOPERICYTOMA AND SOLITARY FIBROUS TUMOR FAMILY

Hemangiopericytoma was first described and named by Stout and Murray,[201–205] who postulated that it was composed mainly of pericytes, a cell first identified by Rouget in 1873[189] and further defined by Zimmerman in 1923.[226] This contractile, arborizing cell is arranged ubiquitously along capillaries and venules (Fig. 27–24). The multiple extensions of the cells encircle the vasculature, and there is evidence that they are the source of cells which can differentiate along osseous, fibroblastic, and adipogenic lines. Unfortunately, these cells do not have readily identifiable light microscopic and immunohistochemical features but are recognized ultrastructurally by their topographic relation to small vessels and their close association with basal lamina contiguous with that of the endothelium.

Over the years since Stout and Murray's description, the entity of hemangiopericytoma has been questioned. There are a number of inherent problems with this diagnosis. Apart from its topographic relation to a vessel, the pericyte lacks differentiating features at the light microscopic level that can be applied to recognition of a neoplastic counterpart.[113] Consequently, the diagnosis of hemangiopericytoma has traditionally rested principally on the presence of an architectural pattern, namely an elaborate branching pattern of small and large vessels.[114] This architectural pattern can be seen in a variety of other benign and malignant tumors and has led directly to the suggestion that the entity hemangiopericytoma may either not exist at all[118] or at best comprises a variant of other lesions. We subscribe to the view that there is a subset of lesions with a pericytic vascular pattern and that lack specific differentiation such that they cannot readily be classified as another tumor type.

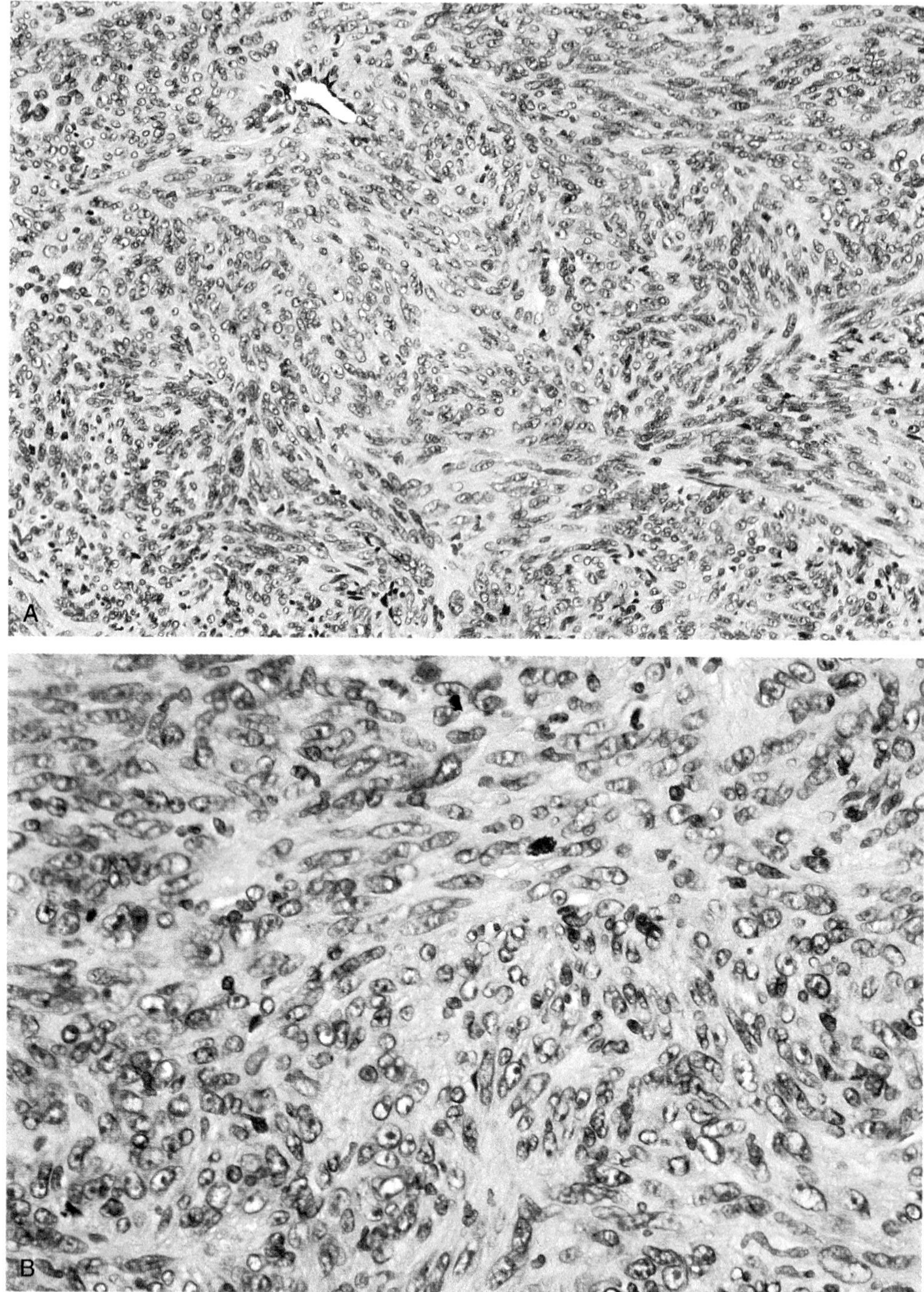


**FIGURE 27–21.** Malignant glomus tumor with a predominantly spindled pattern (**A**). Cells have myoid features with marked atypia and mitotic activity (**B**). Same case as in Figure 27–20.

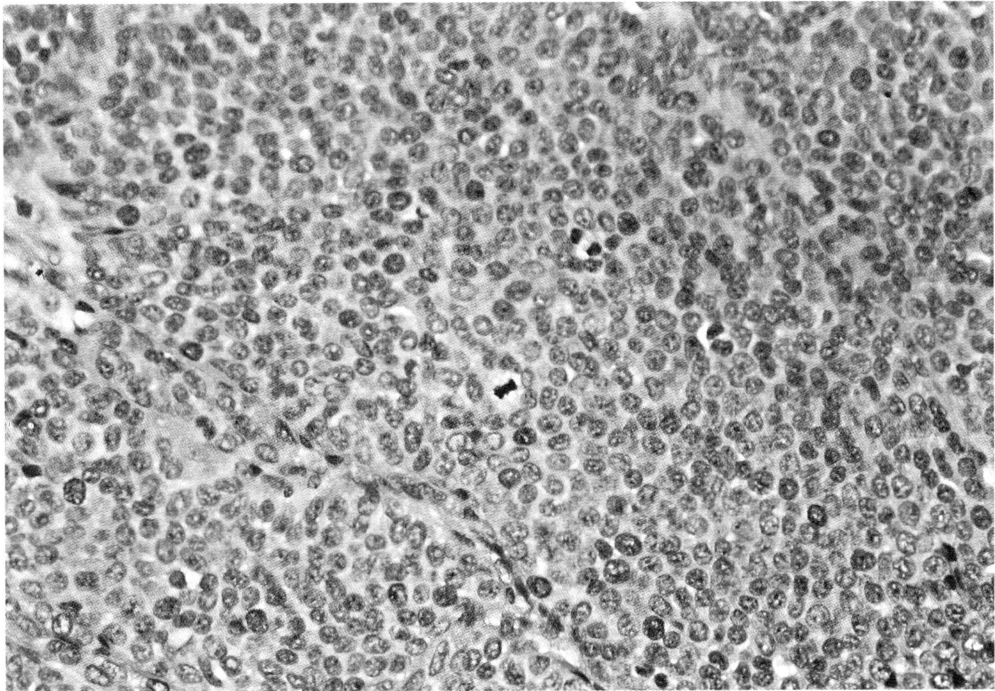

**FIGURE 27–22.** Malignant glomus tumor with the features of a predominantly round cell sarcoma. Such tumors may be confused with Ewing's sarcoma or lymphoma.

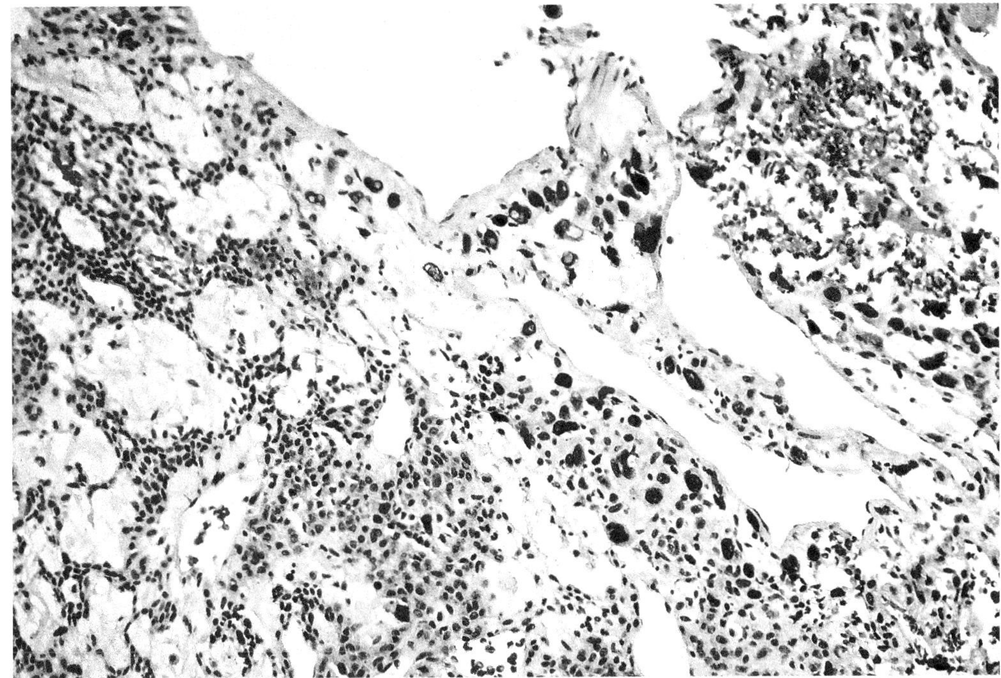

**FIGURE 27–23.** Glomus tumor with degenerative atypia ("symplastic glomus tumor").

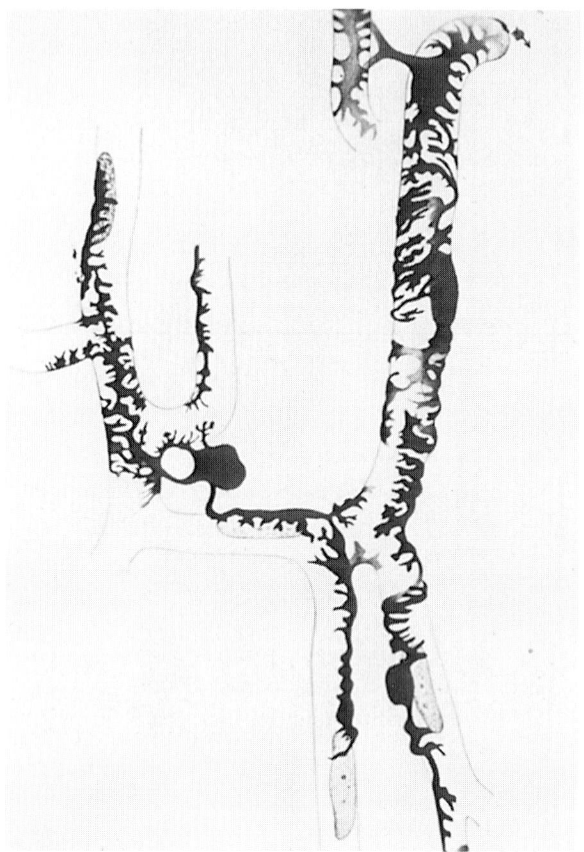

**FIGURE 27–24.** Pericytes, based on Zimmermann's original description of these cells. in 1923. Note the presence of multiple cytoplasmic processes. (From Zimmermann KW. Der feinere Bau der Blutkapillaren. Z Anat Entwicklungsgesch 68:29, 1923.)

For these lesions we use the term "hemangiopericytoma," recognizing that most of the cells comprising such lesions are not necessarily related to the normal pericyte.

It is strongly implied in the foregoing comments that efforts to exclude other diagnoses are undertaken before the "hemangiopericytoma" is diagnosed. For example, in a child myoid differentiation in a pericytic lesion suggests the diagnosis of myofibromatosis whereas keratin expression or glandular differentiation in a high grade round cell sarcoma with a pericytic pattern establishes the diagnosis of a synovial sarcoma. Even Stout apparently used this same general approach when he quipped, "it has been my general attitide in regard to hemangiopericytoma to reject it as a diagnosis if I can think of any other reasonable explanation for the tumor."[129]

The diagnosis of hemangiopericytoma has been further complicated by the current trend to draw close comparisons between the hemangiopericytoma and the so-called solitary fibrous tumor, a lesion that often displays a pericytic vascular pattern. The so1itary fibrous tumor was first described by Klemperer and Robin as a pleura-based lesion[152] and became known as "(localized) fibrous mesothelioma"[202] to distinguish it from the more aggressive diffuse epithelial mesotheliomas. The observations that both hemangiopericytoma and solitary fibrous tumors express the human progenitor antigen CD34 and can be associated with hypoglycemia forged an even closer link between the two. This has led to a prodigious number of reports describing solitary fibrous tumors in virtually every soft tissue site and many organs.* Although in some instances this trend has been the result of simply designating the "hemangiopericytoma" a "solitary fibrous tumor," unquestionably there are soft tissue lesions identical to pleural solitary fibrous tumors that previously passed unnoticed as unclassifiable mesenchymal tumors. Of course, the hope over the next several years is that molecular and cytogenetic studies will irrevocably link the two as a common entity, as occurred with Ewing's sarcoma and primitive neuroepithelial tumors, or dispel the idea altogether. To date, only a small number of hemangiopericytomas and solitary fibrous tumors have been studied cytogenetically, and in some of the reports it is difficult to judge the accuracy of the diagnosis.

We typically distinguish hemangiopericytomas and solitary fibrous tumors on the basis of general histopathologic features occasionally buttressed by immunohistochemistry (Table 27–3). One must, of course, recognize that in part those criteria presuppose ruling out specific differentiation in these tumors. Tumors with intermediate features or with roughly equal areas of hemangiopericytoma and solitary fibrous tumor are designated "hemangiopericytoma-solitary fibrous tumors" (see Fig. 27–47, below). We also seldom diagnose "malignant hemangiopericytoma," as most such lesions usually prove to be sarcomas of other types, notably synovial sarcoma. We reserve the diagnosis of malignant hemangiopericytoma for lesions in which areas of unequivocal benign hemangiopericytoma are present or when there is evidence that the lesion has evolved over time from a benign hemangiopericytoma into an overtly malignant one.

## HEMANGIOPERICYTOMA

Hemangiopericytoma is primarily a tumor of adult life (median age 45 years); it is rare in infants and children (Table 27–2). When it occurs during infancy or childhood, it differs in several aspects from its adult counterpart and therefore is discussed sepa-

---

*References [79,85,92,93,96,100,109,116,122–124,128,132,134,135,150,168,180,209,213,217,219,221,227].

**TABLE 27–3 COMPARISON OF HEMANGIOPERICYTOMA AND SOLITARY FIBROUS TUMOR**

| Parameter | Hemangiopericytoma | Solitary Fibrous Tumor |
|---|---|---|
| Location | Usually extremity | Usually body cavity, particularly pleura |
| Association with hypoglycemia | Yes | One-fourth[113] |
| Pericytic vascular pattern | +++ (Definitional) | Focal |
| Spindling | Typically not | Yes |
| Broad zones of hyalinization | Variable to focal | Typical |
| Histologic malignant forms | Small number | Small number |
| CD34 | Most positive | Virtually all positive |
| Cytogenetic abnormality | Abnormalities of 12q | Trisomy 21[102] |
| Comparative genomic hybridization | No gains/losses[163] | Frequent gains/losses[163] |

rately. The tumor occurs in the genders with equal frequency. Most patients with this tumor complain of a slowly enlarging painless mass that usually has reached a fairly large size by the time treatment is sought. The clinical duration varies; most hemangiopericytomas are present for several months or even years before removal. In one of our cases it had been present 30 years prior to surgery, and Stout and Cassel reported one that had been present 60 years.[204]

Tenderness and pain are infrequent and sometimes occur only during movement or exercise. Tumors in the pelvic fossa and the retroperitoneum may be associated with urinary retention, hydroureter, and hydronephrosis and rarely with constipation, abdominal distension, and vomiting. Except for one report of hemangiopericytomas in three members of one family, there is no evidence of increased familial incidence.[181] Other manifestations of the disease, caused by the rich vascularity of the hemangiopericytoma, are telangiectasia and elevated temperature of the overlying skin, unilateral varicose veins, and hemorrhoids sometimes associated with pulsation of the tumor and a distinct audible bruit. Because of these features some hemangiopericytomas have been clinically mistaken for vascular malformations or aneurysms.

*Hypoglycemia* has been noted in association with both hemangiopericytomas and solitary fibrous tumors,[85,86,178,179,188,195] most often those located in the pelvis and retropentoneum; it is mediated through production of insulin-like growth factors (IGFs) by the tumor. IGFs and insulin-like growth factor receptor (IGF-R) mRNA can be identified in tumor cells even in the absence of clinical hypoglycemia.[142,179] In patients with clinical hypoglycemia, symptoms abate with tumor removal. In addition, the IGFs stimulate proliferation of tumor cells through an autocrine loop that can be abolished when the receptors are inactivated. Hemangiopericytomas have been associated with ***oncogenic osteomalacia***,[181] although some display peculiar histologic features (see discussion of phosphaturic mesenchymal tumors, below).

## Anatomic Location

The tumor is most common in the lower extremity, especially the thigh, pelvic fossa, and retroperitoneum. Less frequently it affects the abdomen and upper extremity. Among the 106 cases in our series,[114] 37 were in the lower limb and 26 in the retroperitoneum and pelvis (Table 27–3). In the series reported by McMaster et al.,[159] the leading sites were the thigh and inguinal region, with about one-third occurring in these two locations. Most are deep-seated and are found in muscle tissue. Dermal and subcutaneous hemangiopericytomas are much less common, especially if one excludes those seen during infancy. We have also encountered two intravascular hemangiopericytoma-like tumors.

## Radiograph Findings

Features seen on radiography and computed tomography (CT) scans are not specific and consist of a well circumscribed, radiopaque soft tissue mass that often displaces neighboring structures such as the urinary bladder, colon, and ureter. Cystic changes are common, but calcification is rare and usually confined to large tumors of long duration. In fact, speckled calcification in small tumors makes one suspicious of a richly vascular synovial sarcoma, especially if the mass occurs in a young adult and is located near a large joint such as the knee.

Angiograms show a more characteristic picture; but they too are not sufficiently typical to permit an unequivocal diagnosis (Fig. 27–25). They show evidence of rapid circulation, indicated by a richly vascular mass with dilatation of the arteries and a diffuse capillary blush or opacification in the arterial phase (Fig. 27–21), a dense uniform tumor, and dilatation of the draining vessels in the vicinity of the tumor in the venous phase. Early visualization of veins, suggesting an arteriovenous shunt, is occasionally noted. Microangiographic studies of hemangiopericytomas have been carried out by Angervall et al.[81]

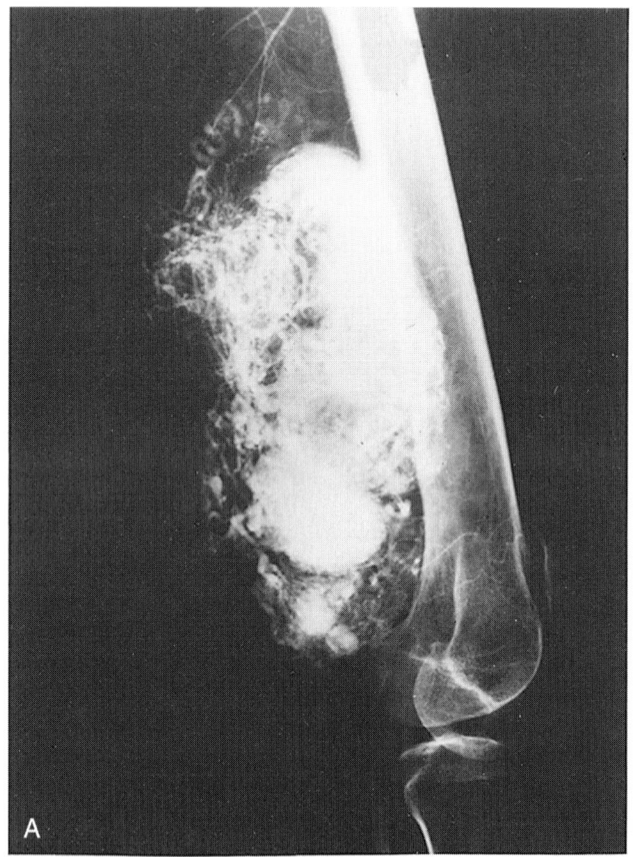


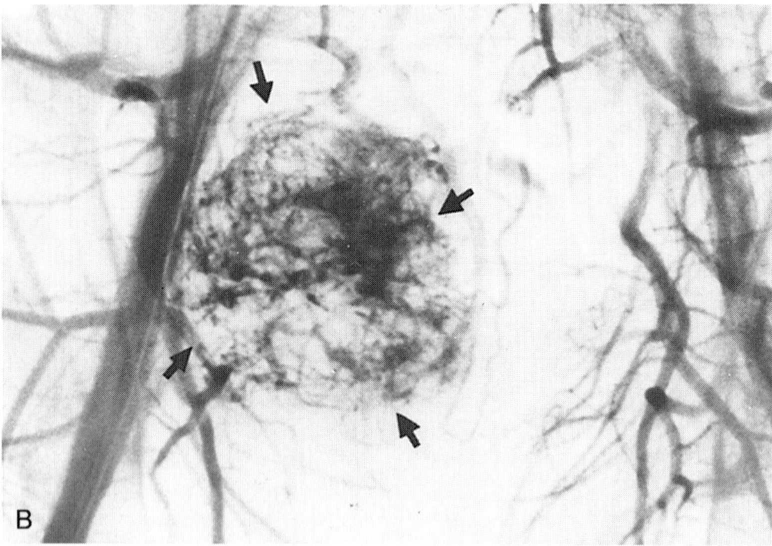


**FIGURE 27–25.** (**A**) Angiogram of a hemangiopericytoma in the left lower thigh shows capillary blush and tortuous veins draining the tumor. (**B**) Angiogram of a hemangiopericytoma in the pelvic fossa distinctly outlines the tumor (**arrows**). (From Enzinger FM, Smith BH. Hemangiopericytoma: an analysis of 106 cases. Hum Pathol 7:61, 1976.)

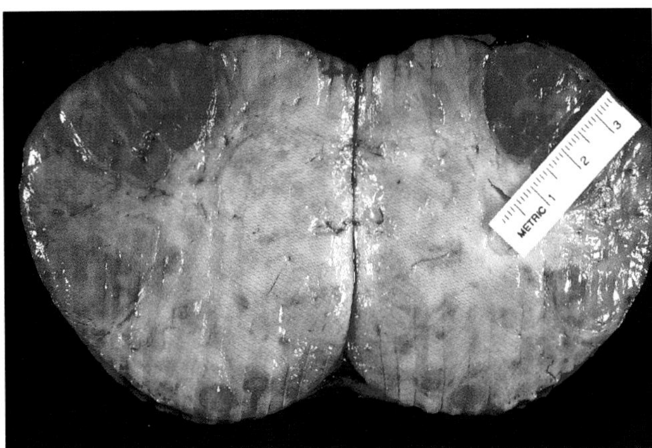


**FIGURE 27–26.** Gross specimen of a hemangiopericytoma.

## Gross Findings

Hemangiopericytoma usually presents as a solitary well circumscribed to fairly well circumscribed mass covered by a thin, richly vascular pseudocapsule. It averages 4–8 cm in diameter, but we have seen lesions as small as 1 cm and as large as 21 cm. There are also several reports in the literature of large hemangiopericytomas, including one that was 23 cm in greatest diameter.[125,165] On cut section the tumor is gray-white to red-brown, with a variable number of dilated vascular spaces and not infrequent areas of hemorrhage and cystic degeneration (Fig. 27–26) Necrosis is common in malignant forms of hemangiopericytoma.

## Microscopic Findings

For purposes of a definition, the diagnosis of a classic hemangiopericytoma depends on identification of the typical architectural vascular pattern in association with a population of relatively bland mesenchymal cells that display no discernible differentiation on light microscopy. Characteristically, the tumor consists of tightly packed round to fusiform cells with indistinct cytoplasmic borders that are arranged around an elaborate vasculature (Figs. 27–27 to 27–35). The vessels form a continuous ramifying vascular network that exhibits striking variation in caliber. As a rule, the dilated branching vessels divide and communicate with small or minute vessels that may be partly compressed and obscured by the surrounding cellular proliferation. Typically, the dividing sinusoidal vessels have a "staghorn," or "antler-like," configuration (Fig. 27–28). Commonly the vessels, particularly large ones, are invested with a thick coat of collagen that extends into the interstitium (Fig. 27–30). Broad zones of hyalinization are far less common in hemangiopericytomas than in solitary fibrous tumors.

*Text continued on page 1013*

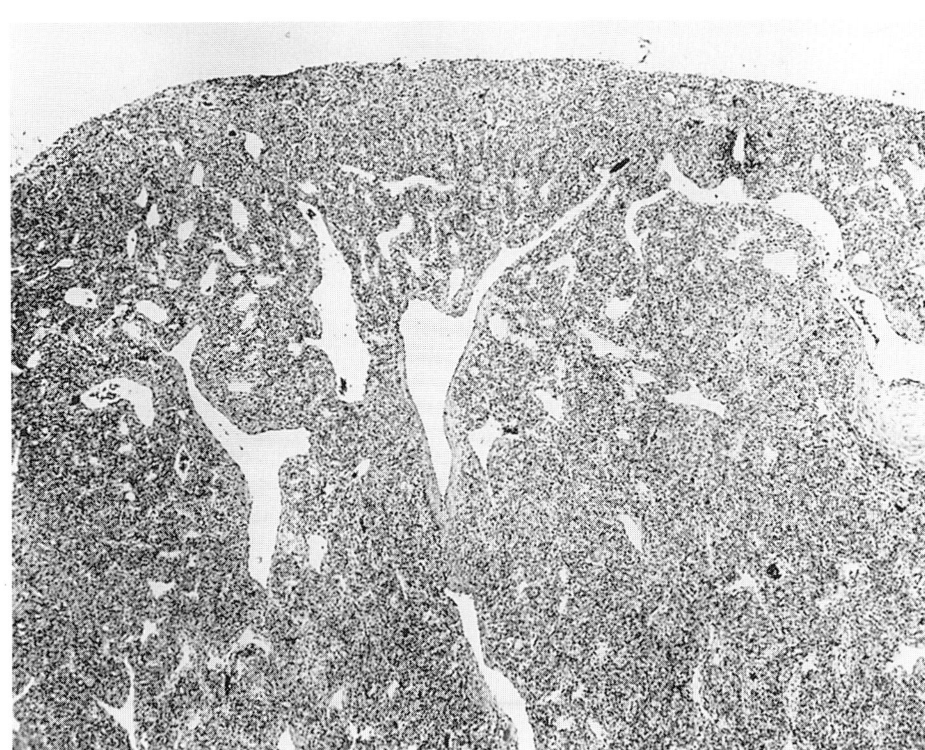

**FIGURE 27–27.** Hemangiopericytoma. Low-power view shows circumscription of the lesion and a characteristic vascular pattern consisting of anastomosing vessels of varying caliber. (×30)

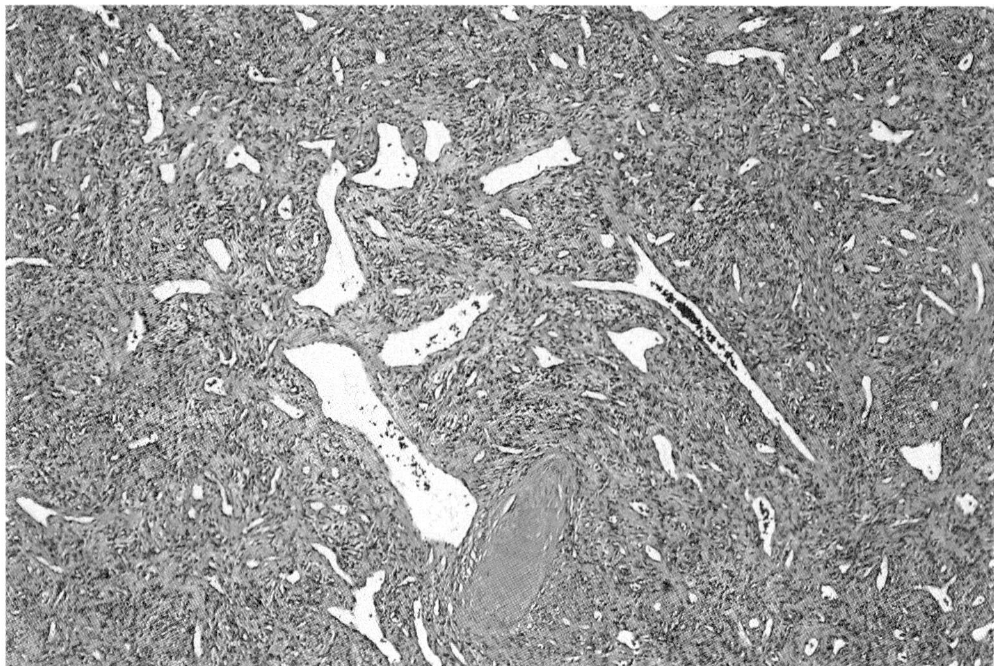

**FIGURE 27–28.** Hemangiopericytoma with a richly vascular pattern consisting of large and small vessels lined by a single layer of flattened endothelial cells.

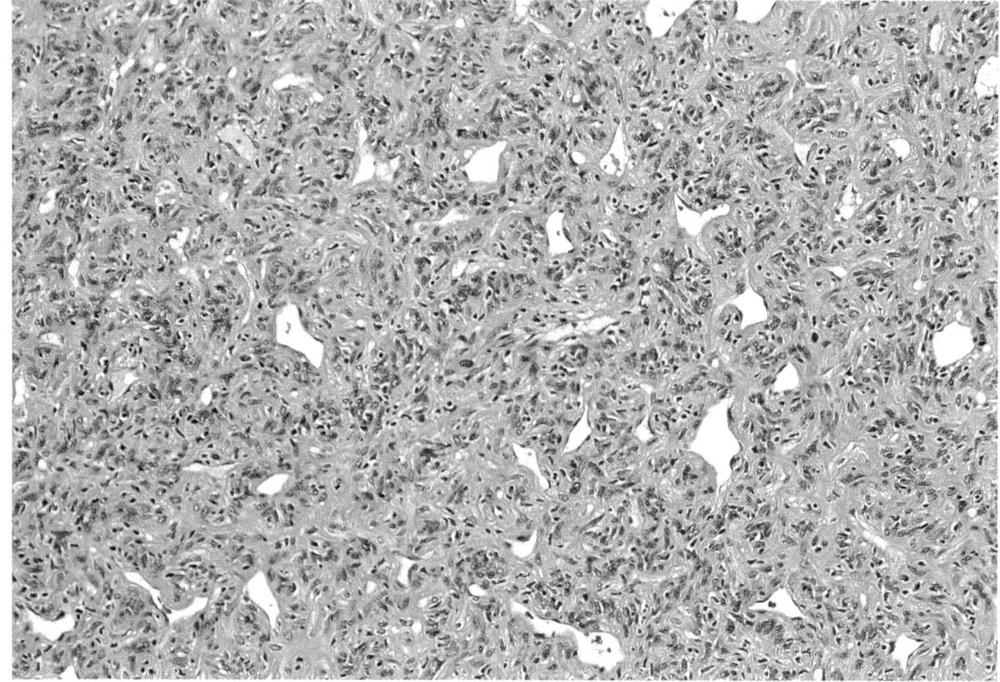

**FIGURE 27–29.** Hemangiopericytoma with predominantly small vessels.

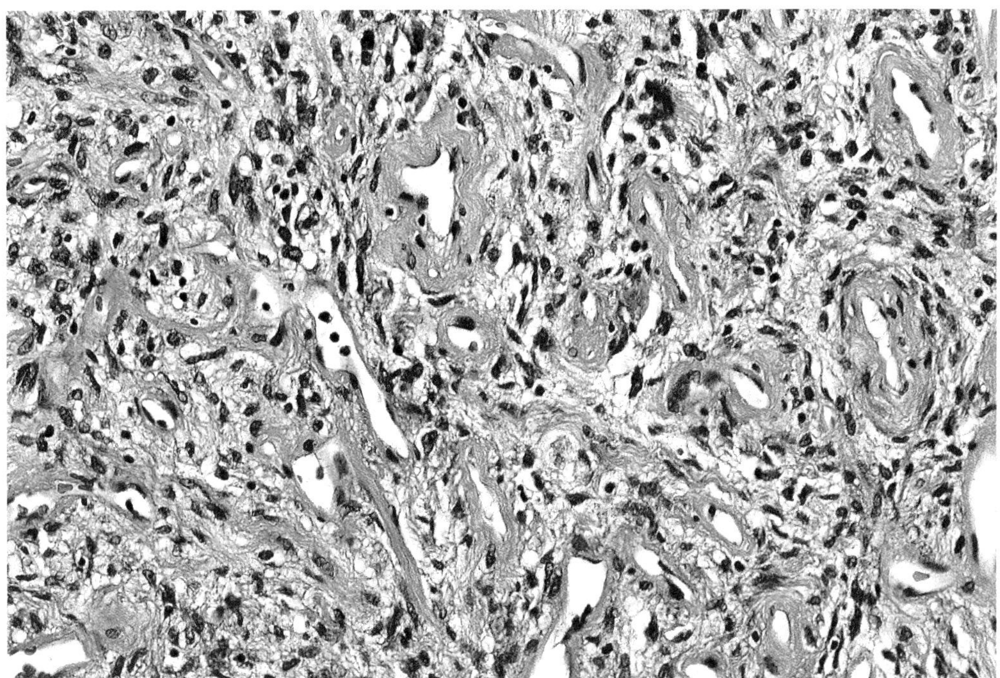

**FIGURE 27–30.** Hemangiopericytoma with perivascular hyalinization.

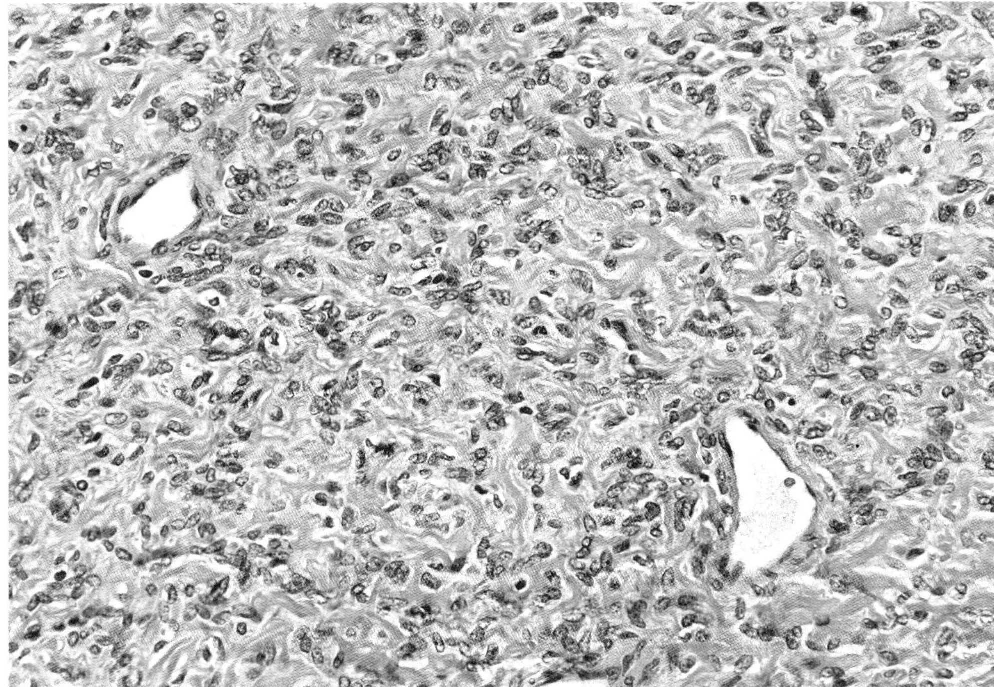

**FIGURE 27–31.** Hemangiopericytoma with interstitial hyalinization.

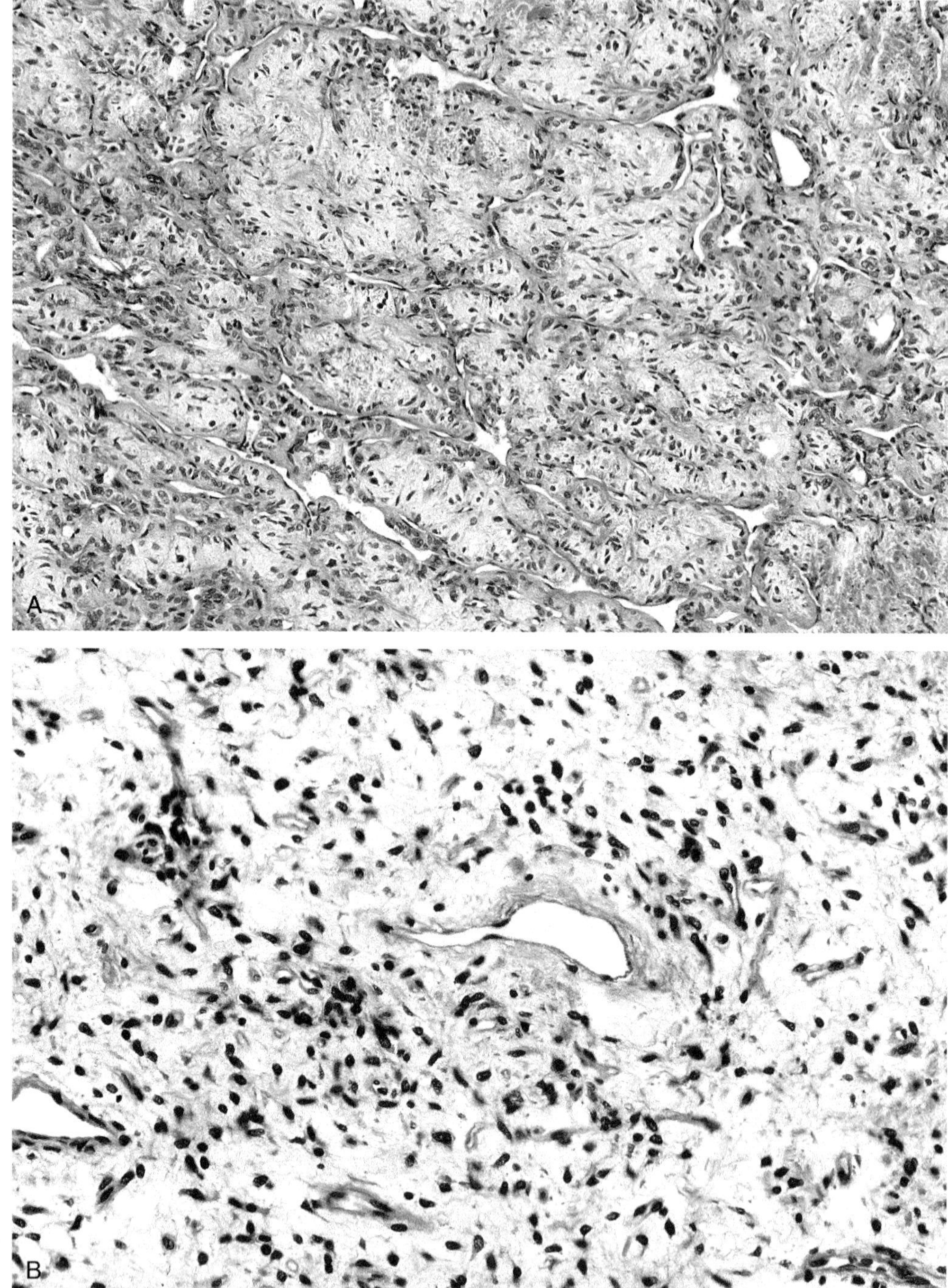


**FIGURE 27–32.** (**A**) Myoid change in a hemangiopericytoma. (**B**) At high power vessels are seen to be thicker and less elaborate than those in a myxoid liposarcoma.

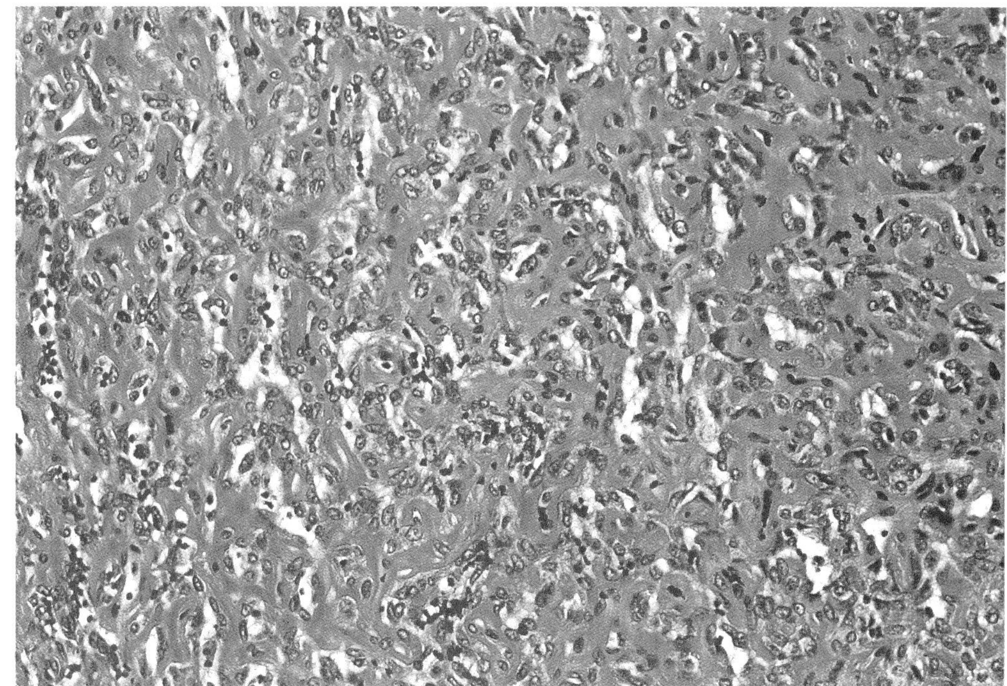

**FIGURE 27–33.** Pseudovascular pattern due to loss of cellular cohesion in a hemangiopericytoma.

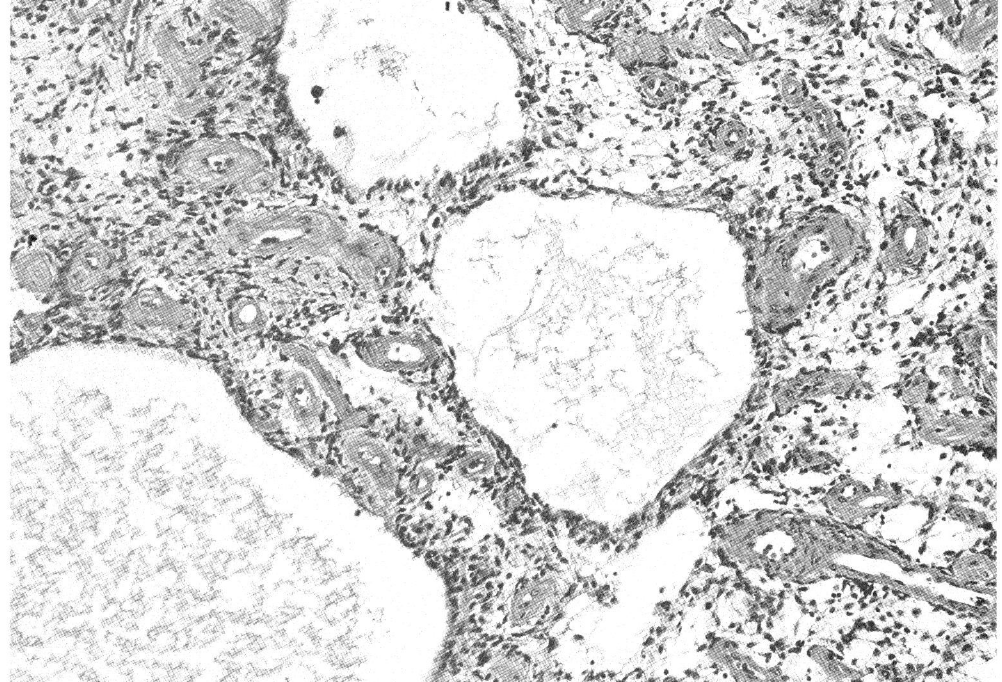

**FIGURE 27–34.** Cystic change in a hemangiopericytoma.

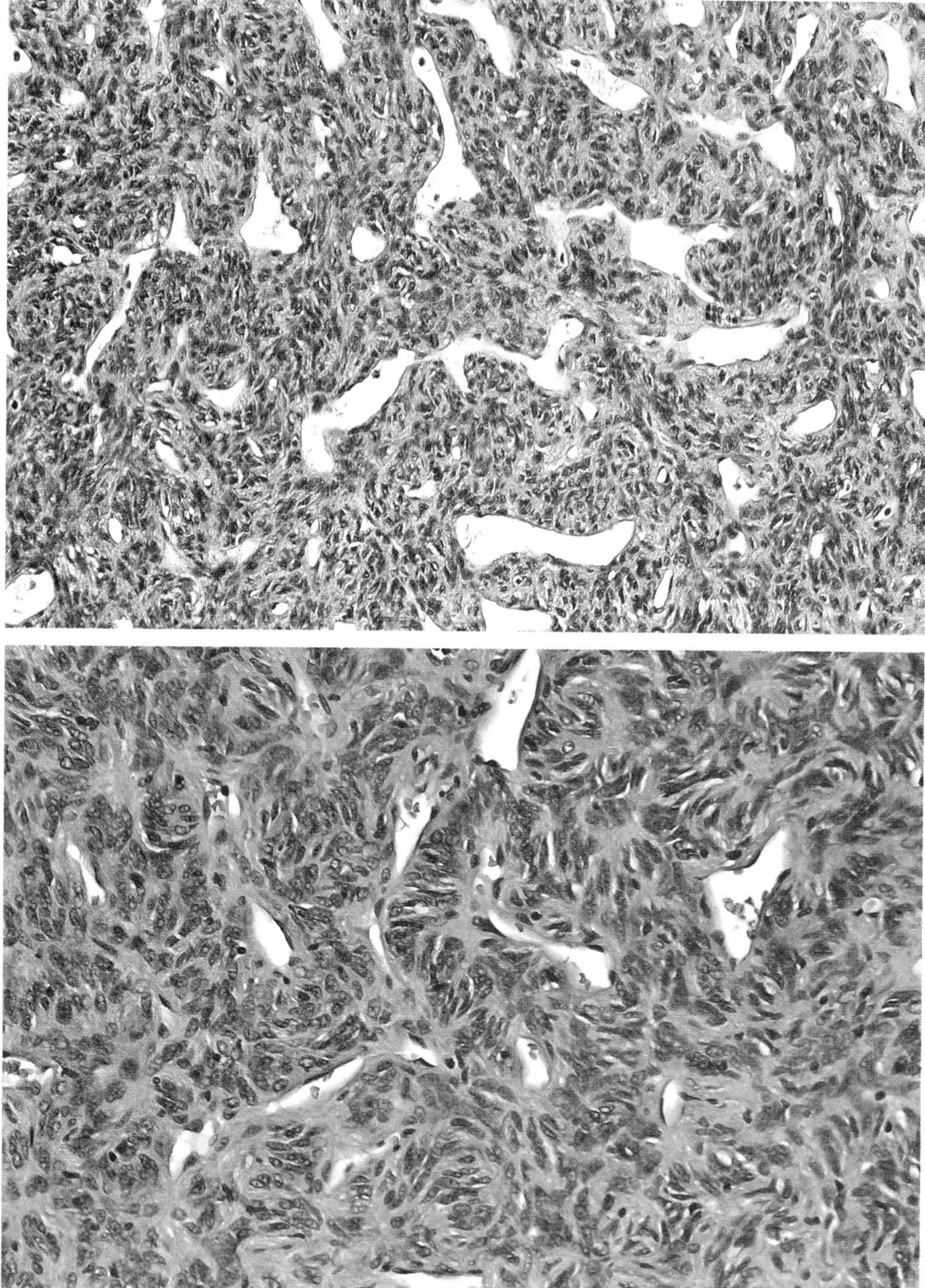

**FIGURE 27–35.** Cells in a hemangiopericytoma range from round/oval to slightly spindled.

In some hemangiopericytomas there are also focal spindle cell areas, but the spindle cells are never arranged in long bundles or fascicles as in the solitary fibrous tumor, fibrosarcoma, or synovial sarcoma. There are also solid cellular areas and sometimes focal palisading reminiscent of a neural tumor. Myxoid change is a common feature in the hemangiopericytoma (Fig. 27–32). When this change occurs throughout the lesion, there is a close similarity to myxoid liposarcoma. However, the presence of coarse-walled vessels and interstitial hyalinization and the absence of lipoblasts are important features that distinguish these hemangiopericytomas from myxoid liposarcomas.

A small subset of hemangiopericytomas contain a variable amount of fat as an integral part of the tumor.[94,120,213] These ***lipomatous hemangiopericytomas*** may be mistaken for well differentiated or dedifferentiated liposarcomas (see below). Unusual features that can confuse the histologic picture of hemangiopericytomas are the presence of pseudovascular spaces created by the loss of cellular cohesion (Fig. 27–33), cystic change (Fig. 27–34), and giant cells.

## Malignancy in Hemangiopericytomas

Malignancy in hemangiopericytomas has traditionally been a problematic area and which still requires further study. As indicated below, we employ a combination of mitotic activity, cellularity, hemorrhage, and necrosis to diagnose "malignant hemangiopericytoma" (see below), assuming there are areas of recognizable hemangiopericytoma with the classic vascular pattern of large vessels and hyalinization. We do not generally render the diagnosis "malignant hemangiopericytoma" for round cell sarcomas with a small-vessel pericytic pattern, as most of these lesions prove to be high grade sarcomas of various types, often round cell variants of synovial sarcoma.

## Immunohistochemical Findings

The cells of hemangiopericytomas usually contain vimentin as the sole intermediate filament, although rarely actin and desmin are present focally[162] even though light microscopic evidence of muscle differentiation may be absent. Most hemangiopericytomas express CD34 but usually in a smaller percentage of cases and to a lesser degree than solitary fibrous tumors[166] (Figs. 27–36, 27–37). Nonetheless, the presence of this antigen has served as an important adjunct in the diagnosis, particularly because is absent in some of the lesions (e.g., synovial sarcoma) considered in the differential diagnosis of hemangiopericytoma. Vascular antigens (von Willebrand factor and CD31) are absent in except in the endothelial cells lining the vascular spaces.

## Ultrastructural Findings

Numerous ultrastructural studies have been carried out, with most attempting to draw a close parallel between the cells of hemangiopericytomas and the normal pericyte.[88,154,166,172] Neoplastic cells were described as having rounded nuclei, an organelle-poor cytoplasm containing occasional arrays of microfilaments, cell processes, and poorly developed junctions. It has recently been pointed out that the cells comprising these tumors are fundamentally undifferentiated,[115] and it is only because of their topographic relation to blood vessels and their close association with periendothelial basement membrane that a relation to normal pericytes is inferred.[119] Moreover, mesenchymal cells that reside farther from the capillary may not display a close association with basement membrane.[88] Because of these issues, electron microscopy does not serve a primary diagnostic role for this disease and has essentially been replaced by a combination of histologic features and immunophenotypic analysis.

## Differential Diagnosis

Distinction of hemangiopericytoma from other neoplasms with prominent vascular patterns may cause considerable difficulty, but most hemangiopericytomas can be identified by their uniform cellular and vascular pattern and the dense reticulin meshwork that surrounds the individual tumor cells. Among the many tumors that mimic hemangiopericytoma, benign and malignant fibrous histiocytoma, synovial sarcoma, and mesenchymal chondrosarcoma are the most important. Careful sampling of the tumor reveals the correct diagnosis for most of these tumors.

***Fibrous histiocytoma***, particularly its deep subcutaneous form, usually displays a more prominent, more uniform spindle cell pattern than hemangiopericytoma, often with a distinct storiform arrangement of the tumor cells. There are, however, occasional examples of this tumor in which distinction may be exceedingly difficult. For unknown reasons most of these hybrid tumors seem to occur in the soft tissues of the orbit. A focal vascular pattern reminiscent of hemangiopericytoma is also seen in occasional malignant fibrous histiocytomas.

***Synovial sarcoma***, in about 10–20% of cases, exhibits a distinctive but focal hemangiopericytoma pattern. This pattern usually occurs in high grade round cell areas of the synovial sarcoma, and the caliber of the vascular channels does not have a broad range as

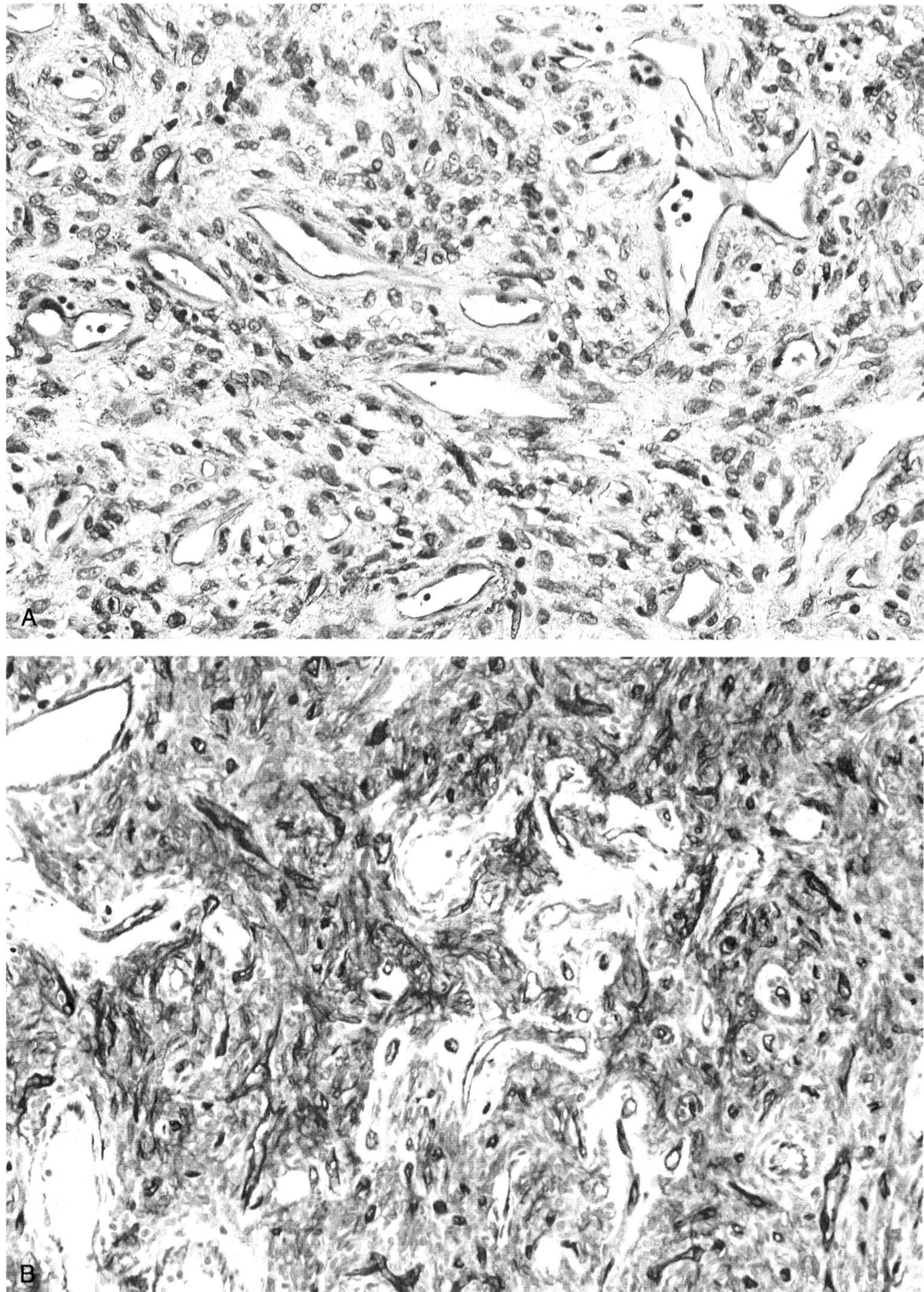


**FIGURE 27–36.** CD34 immunostain in hemangiopericytomas. Most tumors are positive, but staining may be relatively focal (**A**) or occasionally diffuse (**B**).

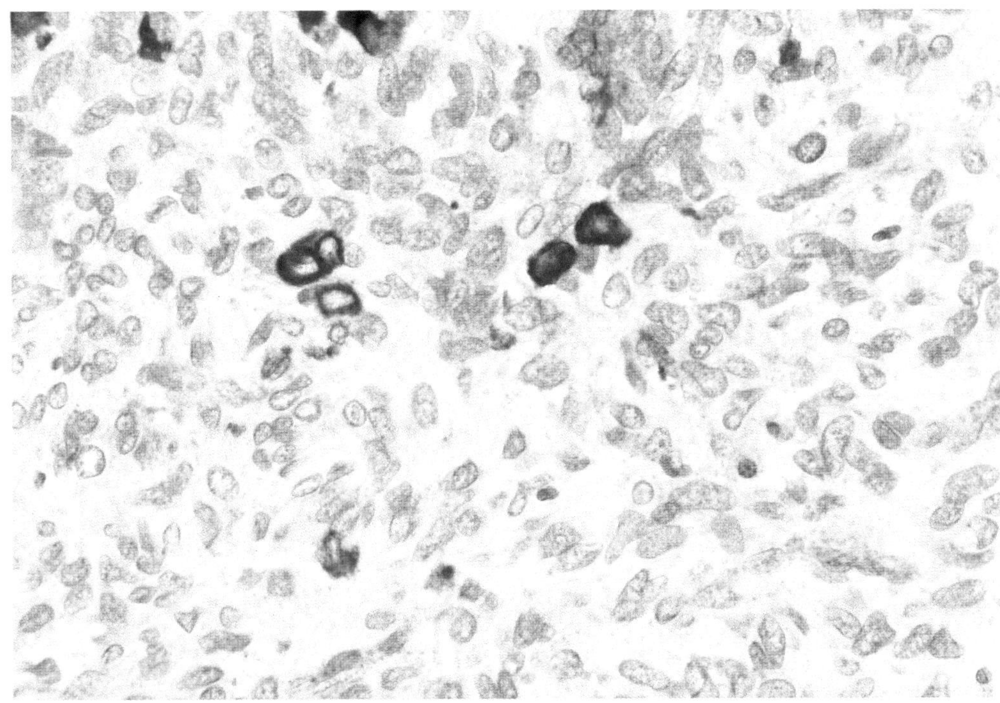

**FIGURE 27–37.** Rarely, tumor cells in hemangiopericytomas are desmin-positive.

is seen in hemangiopericytomas. Synovial sarcomas are almost always associated with distinct spindle cells and sometimes myxoid, hyalinized, and calcified areas, Moreover, the presence of a focal biphasic or glandular pattern or positive staining for immunoreactive cytokeratin permits an unequivocal diagnosis of synovial sarcoma. Clinical findings suggesting synovial sarcoma include a tumor that is painful, multinodular or multilobulated, and located near a large joint (especially the knee) in a patient 12–35 years of age (see Chapter 37).

*Mesenchymal chondrosarcoma* simulates the features of hemangiopericytoma in the closely packed small-cell areas but is readily recognizable by the presence of islands of well differentiated cartilage or, much less frequently, bone. Ill-defined foci of immature cartilage may also be present in the small-cell component (see Chapter 34).

*Juxtaglomerular tumors* that secrete renin and cause hypertension may also be misinterpreted as hemangiopericytomas,[126,178,187,215] especially those rare lesions that occur in extrarenal locations such as the retroperitoneum. In most of these neoplasms large epithelioid cells and thick-walled vessels are present, and some contain PAS-positive renin crystals.

## Cytogenetic and Molecular Analysis

Several balanced translocations have been observed in hemangiopericytomas, including t(12;19),[137,198] t(13;22),[155] and t(3:12).[157] The single most common abnormality are rearrangements of the long arm of chromosome 12, a site similar to those affected in lipomas and leiomyomas. Comparative genomic hybridization shows that hemangiopericytomas do not display any change in DNA copy numbers, unlike the solitary fibrous tumor.[163]

## Discussion

The difficulty of predicting the clinical behavior in hemangiopericytomas has been repeatedly stressed in the literature. Not surprisingly, the reported incidence of metastasis varies from approximately 10% to 60% depending on the diagnostic criteria and therapy. In the largest series of 106 hemangiopericytomas reported from the Armed Forces Institute of Pathology (AFIP), 17.2% of tumors metastasized,[114] although a recent study from the M.D. Anderson Cancer Hospital reported metastases in about 30% of patients, with a 5-year actuarial survival of 71%.[197] Significantly higher disease-free survival and lower local recurrence rates were associated with extremity lesions versus meningeal and retroperitoneal lesions.[197]

The criteria for malignancy vary from study to study. The criteria proposed by Enzinger and Smith identify overtly malignant or high grade lesions but fail to deal with low grade lesions. In their study, the large size of the lesion (>5 cm), an increased mitotic rate (≥4 mitoses/10 HPF), a high degree of cellularity, the presence of immature and pleomorphic tumor cells, and foci of hemorrhage and necrosis indicated a highly malignant course, significantly different from the other lesions (Fig. 27–38). McMaster et al.,[159] in a review of 60 cases from the Mayo Clinic, used similar but less stringent criteria for malignant behavior: either a slight degree of anaplasia and 1 mitosis/10 HPF or a moderate degree of cellular anaplasia and 1 mitosis/20 HPF. Most recently Middleton et al.[162] associated recurrence or metastasis with a trabecular pattern, necrosis, mitoses, vascular invasion, and cellular atypia. In our practice we identify lesions with the features reported by Enzinger and Smith as malignant, although we employ the term "low malignant potential" for lesions with lower levels of mitotic activity (1–3 mitoses/10 HPF) especially if they have any degree of atypia and cellularity.[114]

### Therapy

Complete local excision seems to be the primary treatment for tumors having a uniform histologic picture with no or minimal mitotic activity and without cellular pleomorphism or areas of necrosis or hemorrhage. Radical surgery, with or without adjunctive radiotherapy, is required for less well differentiated hemangiopericytomas. The ligation of afferent vessels or preoperative embolization has been advocated by some to shrink the tumor and minimize intraoperative hemorrhage. Reduction in the size of the tumor may also be accomplished by preoperative radiotherapy.

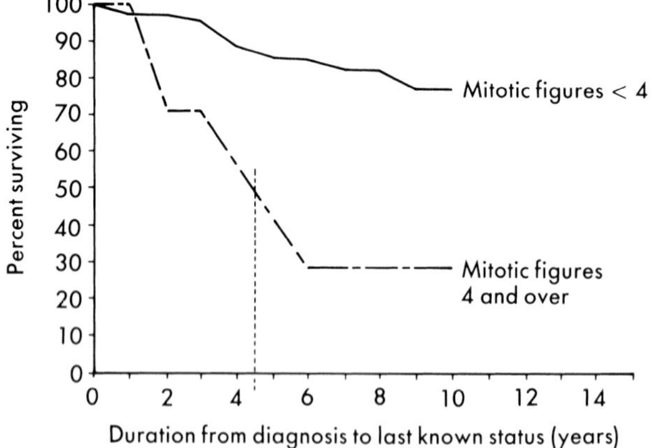


**FIGURE 27–38.** Actuarial survival rate of patients with hemangiopericytoma and relative survival based on the number of mitotic figures. Mitotic figures and necrosis are the two most important criteria when distinguishing benign from malignant hemangiopericytomas. (From Enzinger FM, Smith BH. Hemangiopericytoma: an analysis of 106 cases. Hum Pathol 7:61, 1976.)

## HEMANGIOPERICYTOMAS IN UNUSUAL SITES OR WITH UNUSUAL FEATURES

***Lipomatous hemangiopericytoma*** is a rare variant of hemangiopericytoma that contains a variable amount of mature fat as an integral part of the tumor[94,120,211] (Figs. 27–39, 27–40). These lesions have age and anatomic distibutions similar to those of conventional hemangiopericytomas. Microscopically, they consist of areas of histologically benign hemangiopericytoma admixed with microscopic or macroscopic areas of mature fat. In the typical case, about one-fourth to three-fourths of the tumor is mature fat. In some areas spindling of the pericytic areas creates a resemblance to a spindle cell lipoma. To date, all the lesions with follow-up information have behaved in a benign fashion, although a few have recurred. The principal significance of this variant is that it is easily mistaken for a well differentiated liposarcoma, particularly when only a small biopsy specimen is available. In these situations it is helpful to be apprised of the clinical features that suggest a relatively circumscribed, rather than an infiltrative, mass.

***Meningeal (cranial and intraspinal) hemangiopericytomas*** are indistinguishable from hemangiopericytomas at other sites and are no longer considered variants of meningioma.[104,144] Unlike conventional meningiomas, meningeal hemangiopericytomas lack S-100 protein and epithelial membrane antigen (EMA), and they do not display mutation in the NF2 locus on chromosome 22.[147,180] They have been shown to express vimentin as the sole intermediate filament. They occur at a younger age than meningiomas, grow more often along the sinuses, bleed profusely at operation, and have a tendency to recur. They may metastasize to extracranial sites.[127,218] Guthrie et al.,[130] in a review of 44 meningeal hemangiopericytomas, reported 5- and 15-year survival rates of 67% and 23%, respectively. Mena et al.,[160] in another large series, noted a recurrence rate of 60.6% and a metastatic rate of 23.4%.

***Hemangiopericytoma of the nasal passages and paranasal sinuses*** appears to be an entirely different histologic entity from hemangiopericytoma of soft tissue.[87,98,99,112,207] For that reason we believe the term hemangiopericytoma-like tumor of nasal passages is a better descriptor. Unlike conventional hemangiopericytomas, these lesions are composed predominantly of spindle cells arranged in short fascicles around an elaborate vasculature (Fig. 27–41). The vessels are not as elaborate or as hyalinized as those in conventional hemangiopericytomas. Mitotic activity is usually low or lacking altogether. Although typically having vimentin as the sole intermediate filament, a small sub-

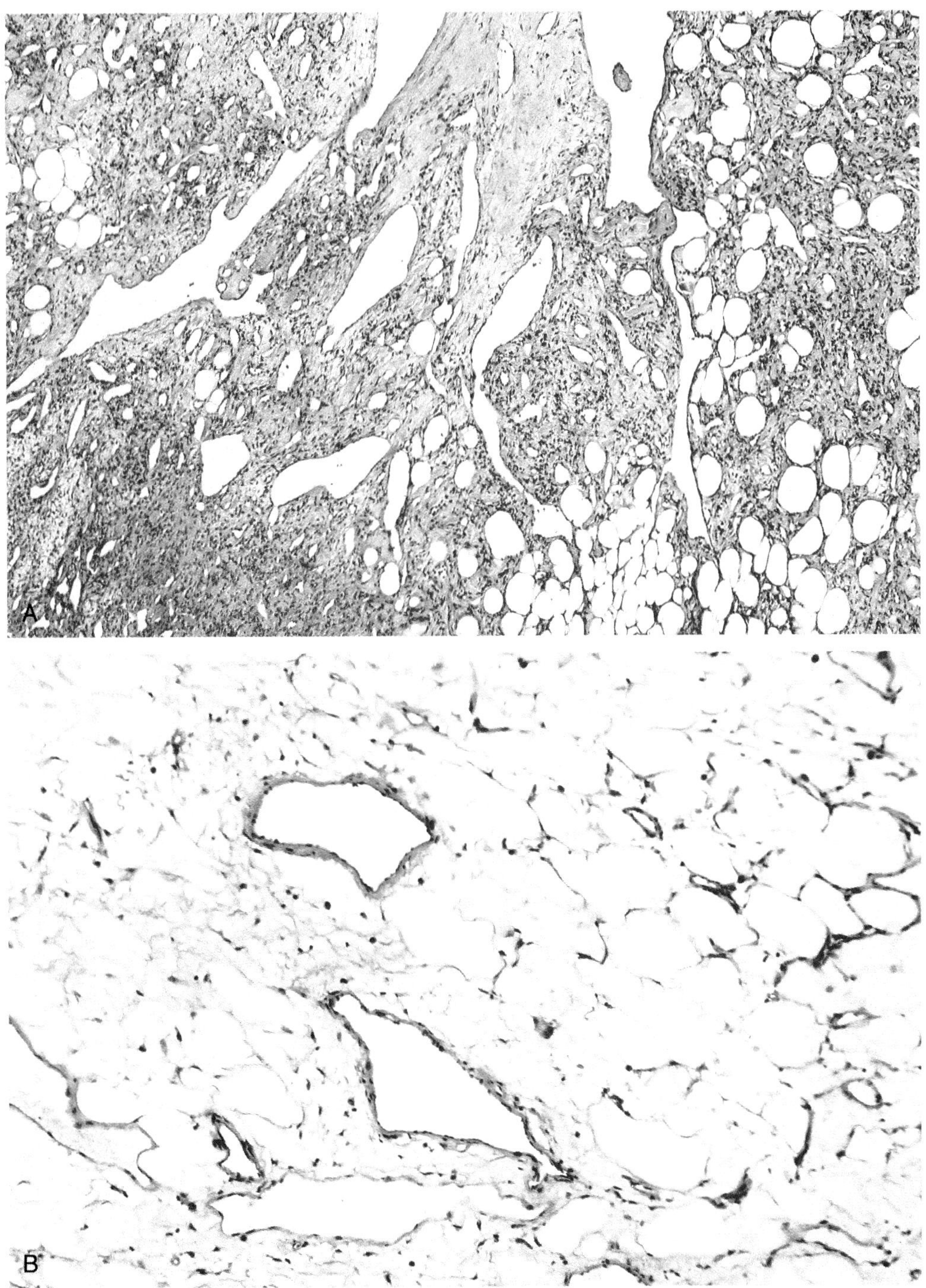

**FIGURE 27–39.** Lipomatous hemangiopericytoma, showing a range of appearances, from areas having only focal fat (**A**) to those that are predominantly fatty (**B**).

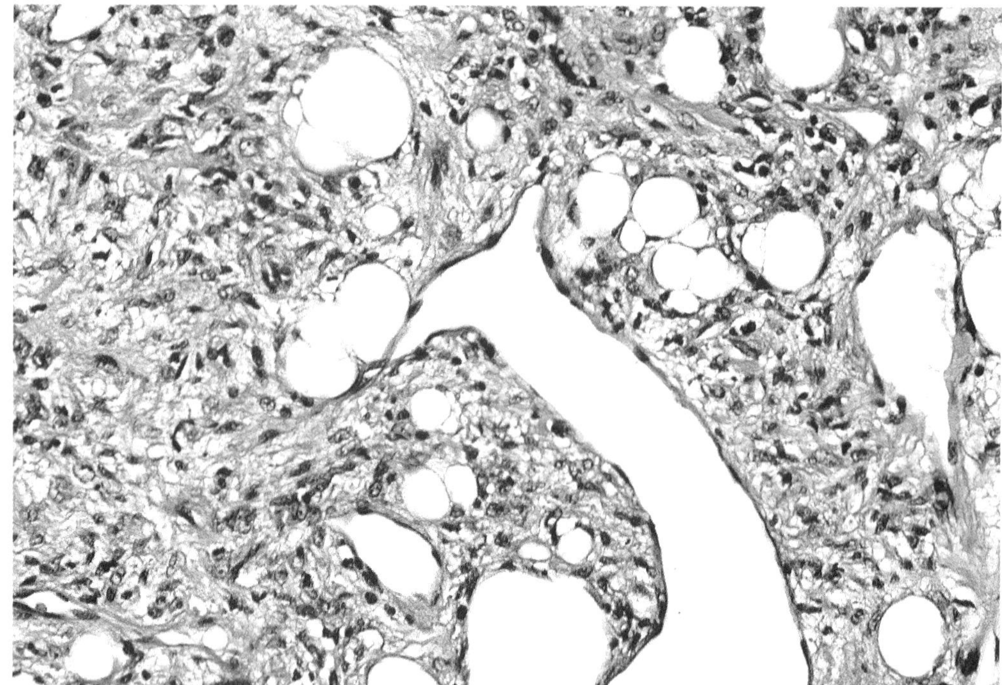

**FIGURE 27–40.** Lipomatous hemangiopericytoma.

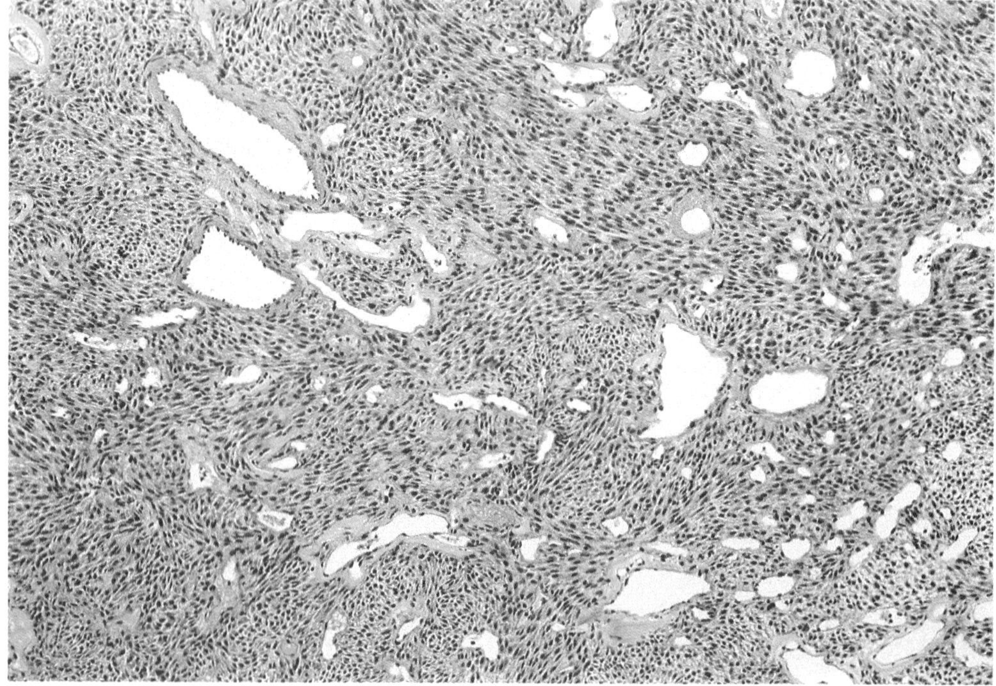

**FIGURE 27–41.** Hemangiopericytoma-like tumor of the nasal passage. Although the tumor has a pericytic vascular pattern, the cells tend to be plump fibroblastic cells arranged in short fascicles.

set contain immunoreactive actin and desmin. Most hemangiopericytomas at this site behave in a benign manner. For example, in the study of Abdel-Fattah et al.,[79] 44 cases were described as benign and six as malignant. In another series of nine cases,[110] four recurred but none metastasized.

***Myopericytomas***, an unusual group of superficial lesions with prominent vessels surrounded by concentrically arranged myoid cells that blend with similar stromal cells, have been reported by Grantner et al.[129] (Fig. 27–42). These lesions appear to be a hybrid between hemangiopericytomas and angiomyomas, but unlike hemangiopericytomas, they express both actin and desmin. Two of the five patients with follow-up information experienced recurrences.

***Orbital hemangiopericytomas*** are less common and are often difficult to distinguish from richly vascularized fibrous histiocytomas.[133,145,218] Croxatto and Font[101] reported a series of 30 cases with an 89% five-year survival rate.

***Hemangiopericytomas of miscellaneous sites.*** Although primary hemangiopericytomas have been documented in many organs including breast,[82,164,210] lung,[223] mediastinum, uterus, ovary, vagina,[194] and bone, it is prudent to remember that in many of these sites the diagnosis of hemangiopericytoma must be viewed with some degree of circumspection. For example, it is well recognized that endometrial stromal sarcomas of uterine, ovarian, or extra uterine origin and richly vascular renal cell carcinomas metastatic to bone or soft tissue run the risk of a mistaken diagnosis of hemangiopericytoma.

***Phosphaturic mesenchymal tumors*** are unusual lesions that produce osteomalacia presumably through secretion of a substance(s) that decreases renal tubular phosphate absorption. Although many bone and soft tissue tumors have been associated with oncogenic osteomalacia (e.g., osteosarcoma, chondroblastoma, chondromyxoid fibroma, malignant fibrous histiocytoma, giant cell tumor, hemangioma), there is a unique subgroup characterized by round to oval cells arranged in a pericytoma pattern and associated with lace-like calcification and giant cells.[177] Undoubtedly, some of these lesions have been reported as "hemangiopericytoma"; in our opinion they appear distinctive enough to warrant a separate designation (Fig. 27–43).

## INFANTILE HEMANGIOPERICYTOMA

Although the infantile hemangiopericytoma is usually described together with the adult hemangiopericytoma, it deserves separate consideration became of its different histologic picture and clinical behavior. Based on our cases, these lesions mostly occur in infants during the first year of life and, like juvenile hemangiomas, are mostly located in the subcutis and oral cavity. Tumors in older children and deep-seated

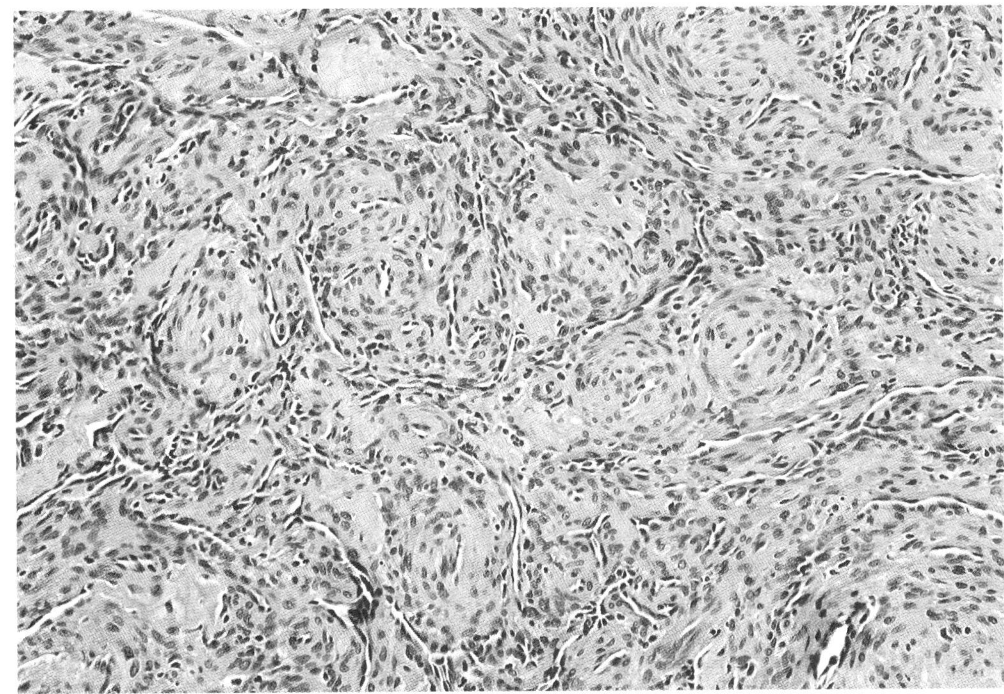

**FIGURE 27–42.** Myopericytoma. Muscle from the walls of small-caliber vessels spin off into the stroma of the lesion, giving it an appearance intermediate between a hemangiopericytoma and an angiomyoma.

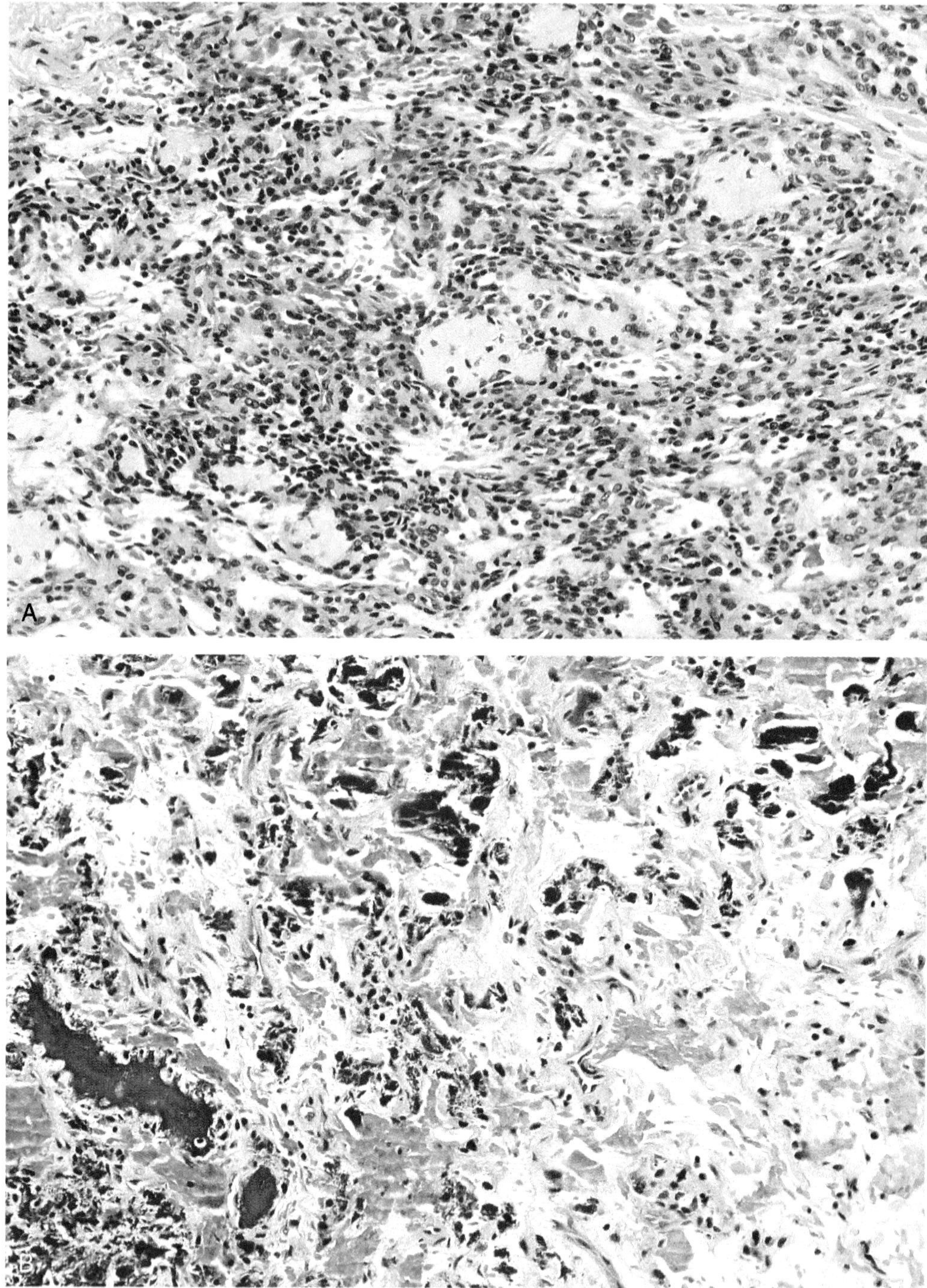

**FIGURE 27–43.** Phosphaturic mesenchymal tumor associated with osteomalacia. This distinctive subset of tumors are associated with oncogenic osteomalacia and consist of primitive mesencymal cells associated with a prominent vasculature (**A**) and calcification. (**B**) Some of these tumors have been labeled "hemangiopericytoma."

tumors in the muscle, mediastinum, and abdomen have also been described.[82,83,111,146,148] Alpers et al.[80] reported an infantile hemangiopericytoma of the tongue and sublingual region that was discovered at birth, grew in an infiltrative manner, and recurred rapidly after local excision. After 30 months the child was well with no evidence of further recurrence or metastasis. All lesions in our cases have been solitary, but there are rare accounts of patients with multiple lesions,[97,192] One was associated with Kasabach-Merritt syndrome.[97]

Microscopically, infantile hemangiopericytoma bears a close resemblance to the adult type, but many lesions, especially superficial ones, are multilobulated, often with distinct intravascular and perivascular satellite nodules outside the main tumor mass (Fig. 27–44A) and frequent endovascular growth (Fig. 27–44B). There is often increased mitotic activity and focal necrosis, features that indicate a poor prognosis for adult-type hemangiopericytomas but generally do not with the infantile form. Judging from our cases and the literature, most of these tumors tend to follow a benign clinical course; they are curable by local excision or may regress spontaneously.[95,97] In rare instances, however, there may be local infiltrative growth or recurrence and even metastasis.[146] Deep-seated lesions and those occurring in older children seem to pursue a more aggressive clinical course than superficial ones that appear during the first years of life.[80,83]

The hemangiopericytoma-like pattern found in the lobular or tufted hemangioma (a variant of lobular capillary hemangioma marked by dermal or subcutaneous capillary or vascular lobules), infantile myofibromatosis, and infantile fibrosarcoma must be distinguished from that of infantile hemangiopericytoma (see Chapters 11 and 23). Other benign and malignant neoplasms that may cause diagnostic difficulty include the juvenile hemangioma, glomus tumor, angiosarcoma, vascular forms of leiomyoma and leiomyosarcoma, stromal sarcoma, malignant peripheral nerve sheath tumor, mesothelioma, and liposarcoma.

## SOLITARY FIBROUS TUMOR

The solitary fibrous tumor was first described by Klemperer and Rabin in 1931 as a pleura-based lesion.[152] With the subsequent reports of Stout and Murray it became known as localized or solitary fibrous tumor of the pleura and peritoneum,[205] a term that served to distinguish it from the highly aggressive diffuse form of epithelial mesothelioma. With the appreciation that these lesions did not display mesothelial differentiation and occurred in diverse locations, "solitary fibrous tumor" has been rapidly embraced as the term of choice.[106,121–123,139,149,153,171,175,176,190,193,200,216,222] Although still best known as a pleural-based lesions, the solitary fibrous tumor has been reported in numerous sites including liver, orbit nasal passages, meninges, skin, respiratory tract, thyroid, and soft tissue.*

### Clinical Findings

Solitary fibrous tumors principally affect adults between the fourth and seventh decades of life (median 50 years). Most are located in the thoracic cavity where they are usually asymptomatic and are discovered incidentally on routine chest films or during workup of another abnormality.[107] Radiographically, serosal solitary fibrous tumors are rounded, sharply outlined, homogeneous densities or masses often on a pedicle that shifts with positional changes (Fig. 27–45). Sometimes the tumor is seen merely as an ovoid thickening of an interlobular fissure. Patients with large tumors report minor symptoms such as vague pleuritic pain, chronic cough, and shortness of breath. Arthritic pain and clubbing of the fingers (osteoarthropathy) occur in about 10% of patients.[113] Symptoms related to extrapleural solitary fibrous tumor are relatively nonspecific and relate simply to the presence of a mass usually in deep soft tissue. As indicated above, hemangiopericytoma/solitary fibrous tumors are associated with hypoglycemia in about 5% of cases due to secretion of insulin-like growth factors by the tumor.[121,143,158,169] Typical symptoms range from profuse sweating, headaches, and restlessness to disorientation, convulsions, and coma. One of our patients with hypoglycemia suffered four strokes within four consecutive days; another became manic, with psychotic manifestiations and a fasting blood glucose level as low as 18 mg/dl.

### Pathologic Findings

In its most common location the solitary fibrous tumor is an exophytic mass attached to the visceral or parietal pleura by means of a broad pedicle (Fig. 27–46). Less often the lesion grows from a serosal surface endophytically into the underlying organ (e.g., lung, liver)[150,223] and can present as a parenchymal lesion. It usually measures approximately 5–6 cm when first detected, although large lesions (20–30 cm) filling the hemithorax have been described. On cut section, regardless of the site of origin, the lesions are nodular, firm, gray-white masses occasionally with myxoid areas, hemorrhage, and necrosis.

In contrast to the classic hemangiopericytoma, the solitary fibrous tumor is composed principally of spindle cells, rather than round or fusiform cell (Fig.

*References [79,85,92,93,96,100,109,116,122–124,128,132,134,135,150,168,180,209,213,217,219,221,227].

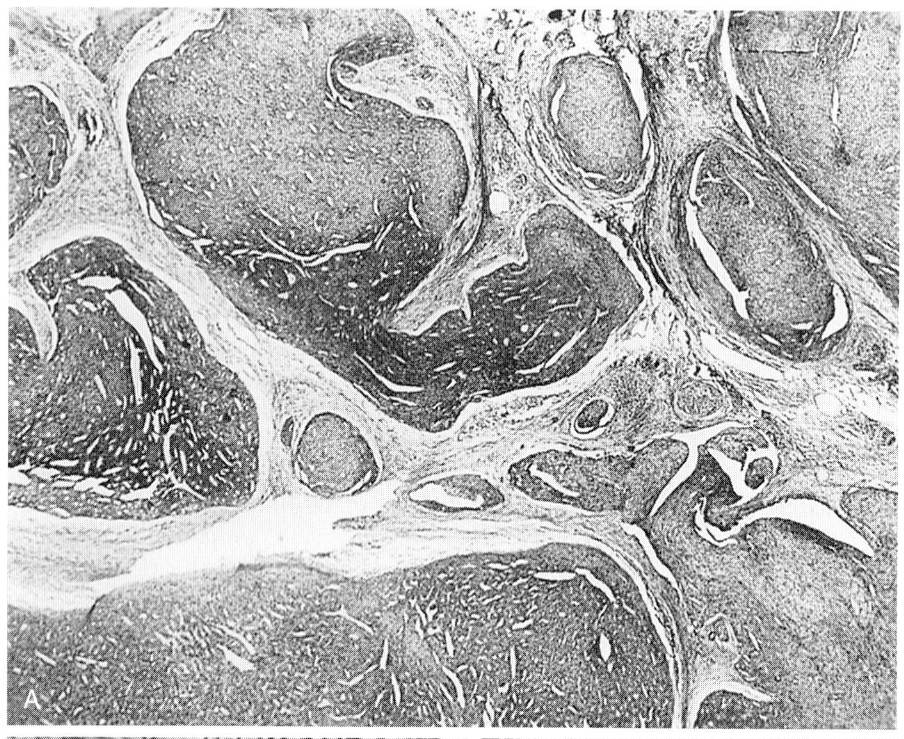


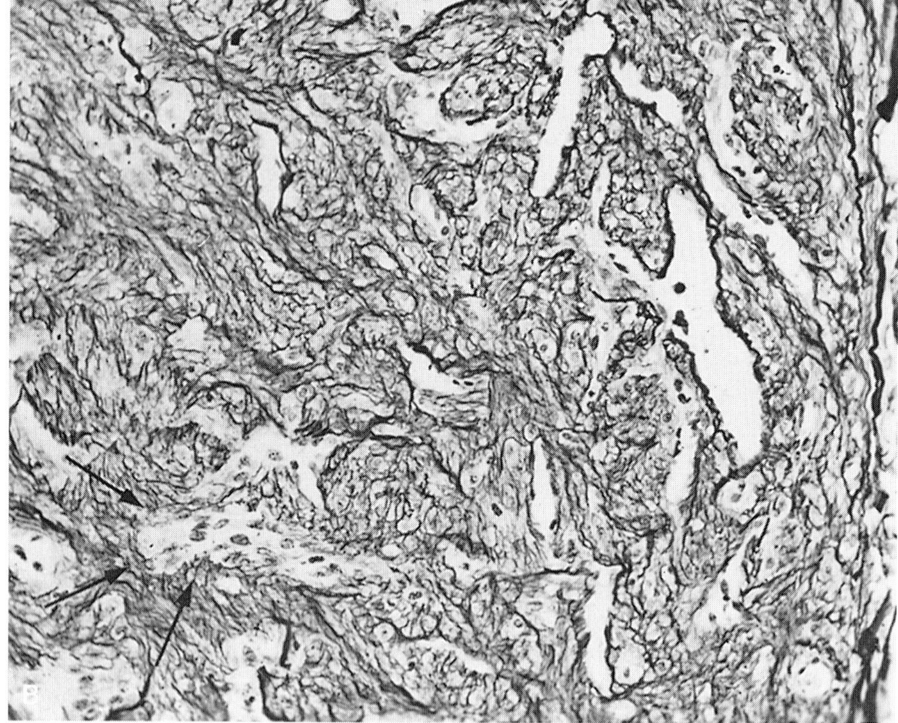


**FIGURE 27–44.** Infantile hemangiopericytoma with the typical multilobular arrangement of tumor cells (**A**) and intravascular endothelial proliferation (**B**) suggesting transition between hemangiopericytoma and hemangioma (arrows). (**A:** ×22, **B:** reticulin preparation, ×180) (From Enzinger FM, Smith BH. Hemangiopericytoma: an analysis of 106 cases. Hum Pathol 7:61, 1976.)

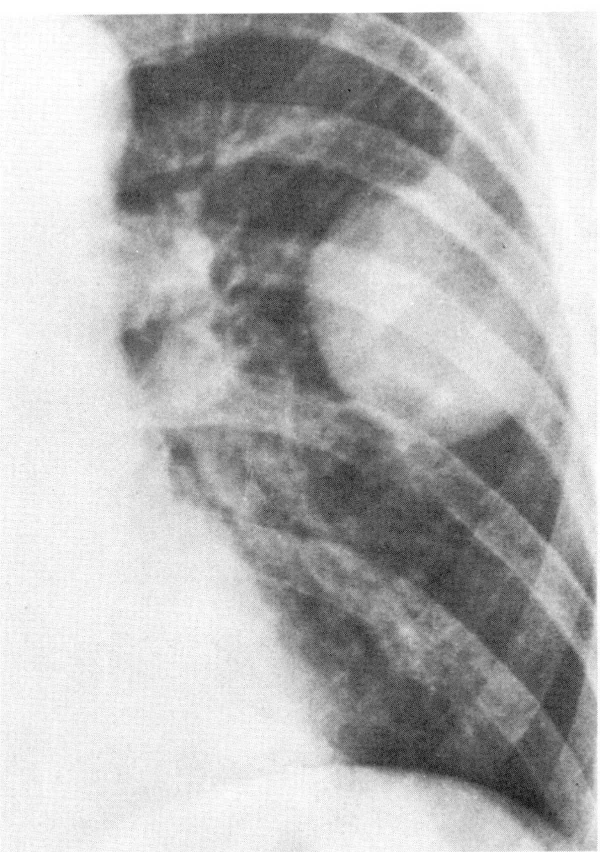

FIGURE 27-45. Radiograph of a solitary fibrous tumor of the pleura. Note the circumscribed mass in the left chest.

27-47). The arrangement of the cells varies from area to area in the same tumor (Figs. 27-48 to 27-53). In some zones the cells are arranged in short, ill-defined fascicles, whereas in others they are arranged randomly in what has been described as a "patternless pattern." A characteristic feature of the lesion that usually suggests the diagnosis even at low power are the relatively striking areas of hyalinization. In these areas the cells are usually arranged singly or in small parallel clusters next to dense collagen. Artifactual "cracks" develop between the cells and collagen or between groups of collagen fibers (Fig. 27-50). Myxoid change, as is seen in hemangiopericytomas, also develops in solitary fibrous tumors. The vascular pattern varies from narrow vascular clefts to gaping, branching vascular channels virtually indistinguishable from those of hemangiopericytoma. Usually, however, the degree of perivascular hyalinization is less striking.

Although the typical solitary fibrous tumor has little or no mitotic activity and only mild to moderate nuclear atypia, malignant forms occur, characterized by high cellularity, pleomorphism, and increased mitotic activity. Mitotic activity > 4 mitoses/10 HPF has been used to discriminate between benign and malignant forms at thoracic and extrathoracic sites.[117,217] Tumors judged to be malignant by their mitotic activity usually display a high level of cellularity, a distinct fascicular growth pattern similar to fibrosarcoma, and usually less interstitial collagen (Figs. 27-54, 27-55).

## Immunohistochemical and Ultrastructural Features

Virtually all solitary fibrous tumors of pleural and extrapleural origin consistently express CD34, variably express bcl-2,[123,139,165,213,218,225] and rarely express desmin[136] (Figs. 27-37, 27-52). Except for anecdotal cases[136] they lack cytokeratin and other mesothelial markers. This immunophenotype, buttressed by ultrastructural observations demonstrating myofibroblas-

*Text continued on page 1029*

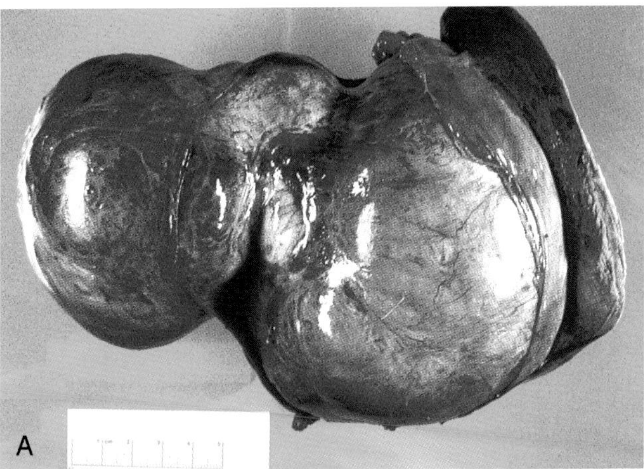

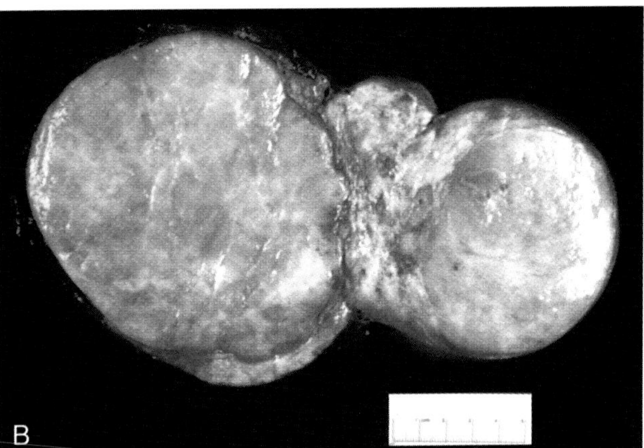

FIGURE 27-46. Solitary fibrous tumor growing as an exophytic mass from the surface of the liver (**A**). Cut section shows a dense white interior (**B**).

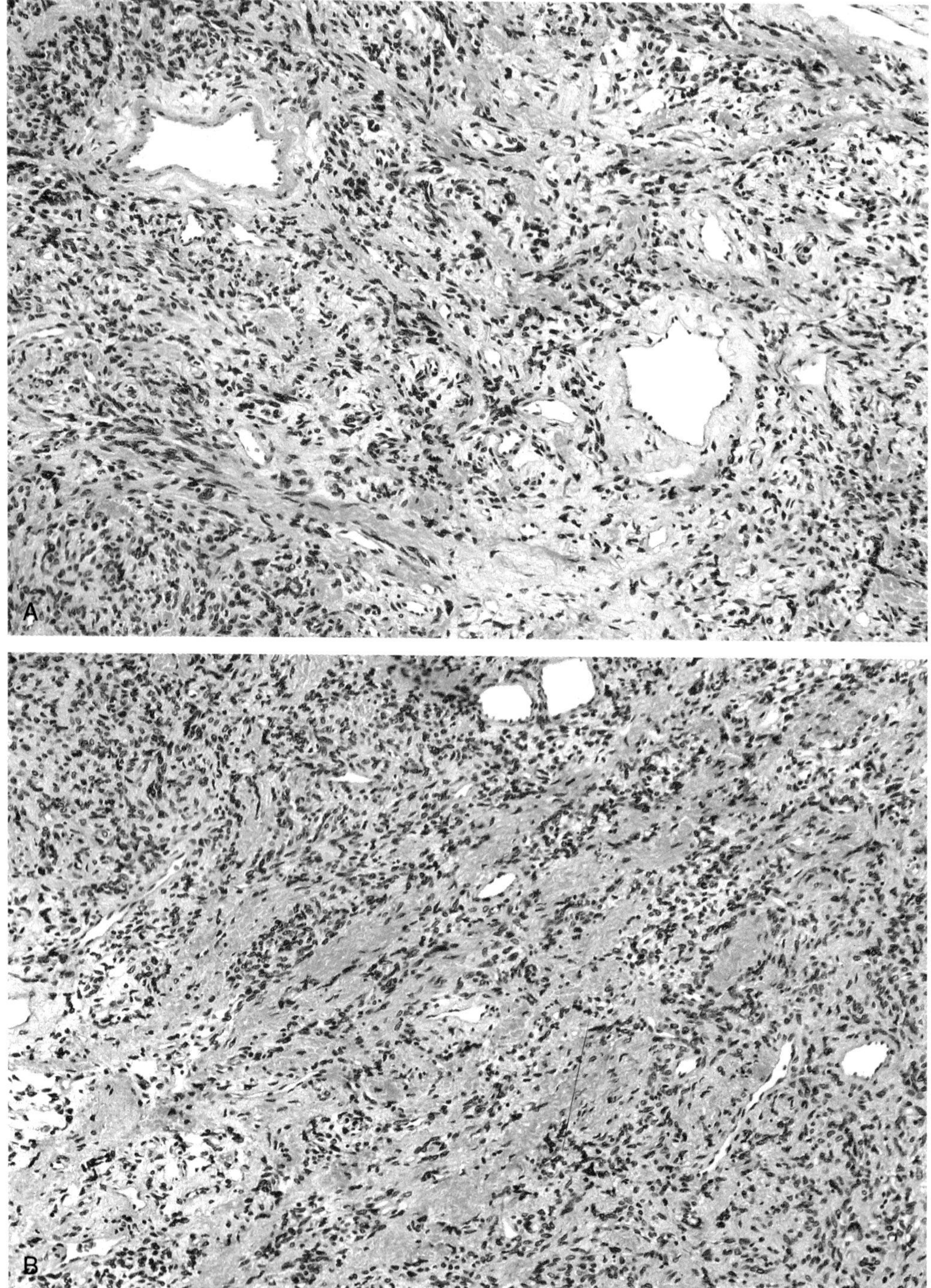

**FIGURE 27–47.** Tumor with features intermediate between a classic hemangiopericytoma and a classic solitary fibrous tumor. Tumor has a pericytic vascular pattern (**A**) but shows areas of interstitial hyalinization (**B**)

*Illustration continued on opposite page*

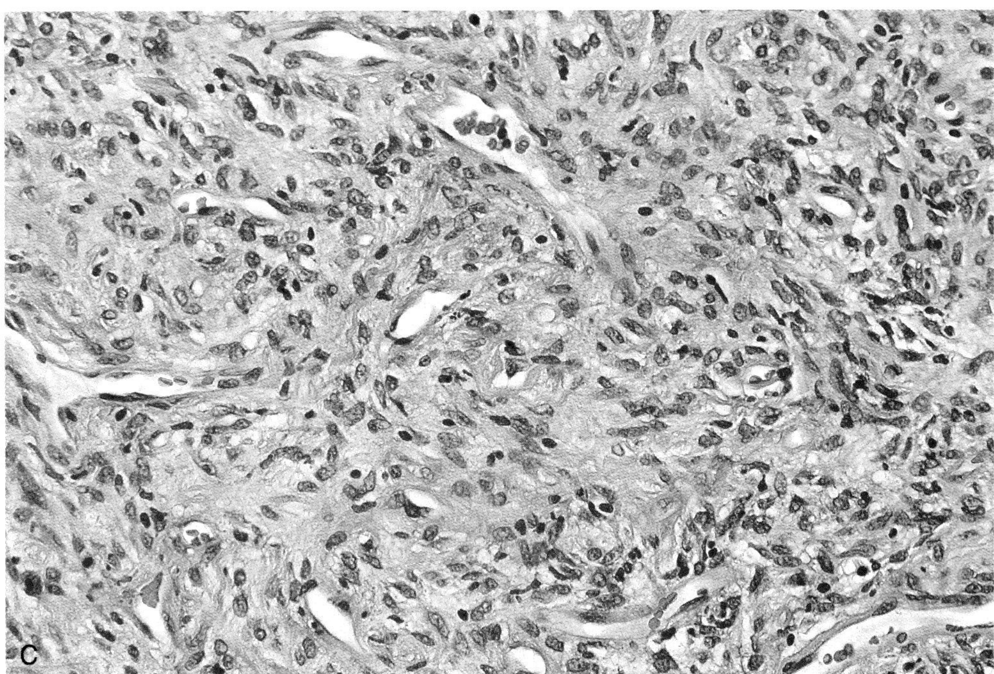

**FIGURE 27–47** *(Continued).* and more spindling of the tumor cells (**C**).

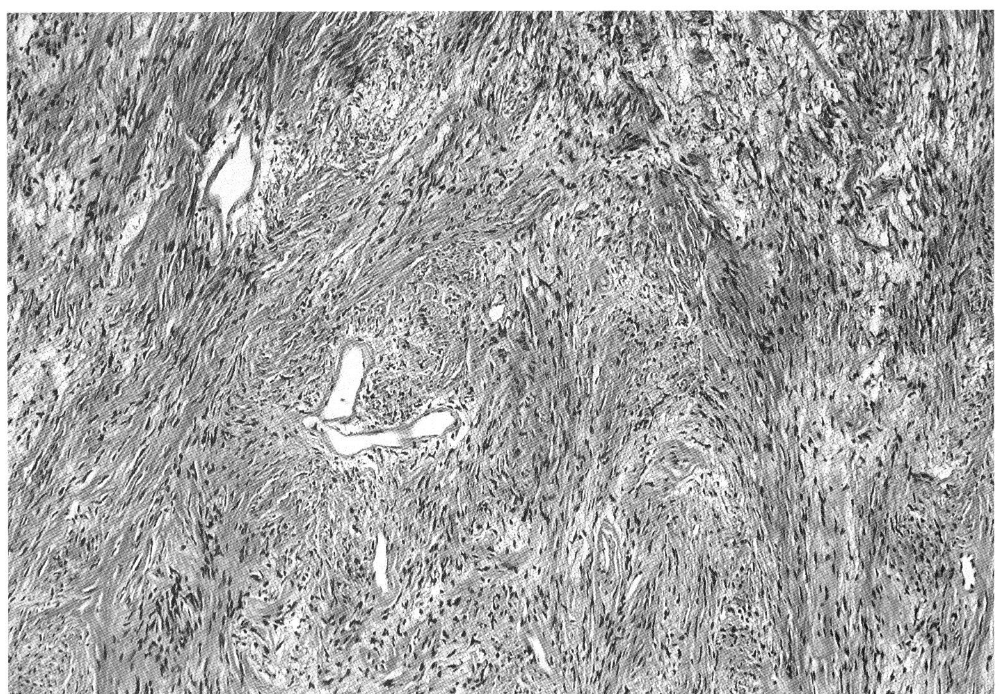

**FIGURE 27–48.** Solitary fibrous tumor with a heavily hyalinized area and focally prominent staghorn vessels.

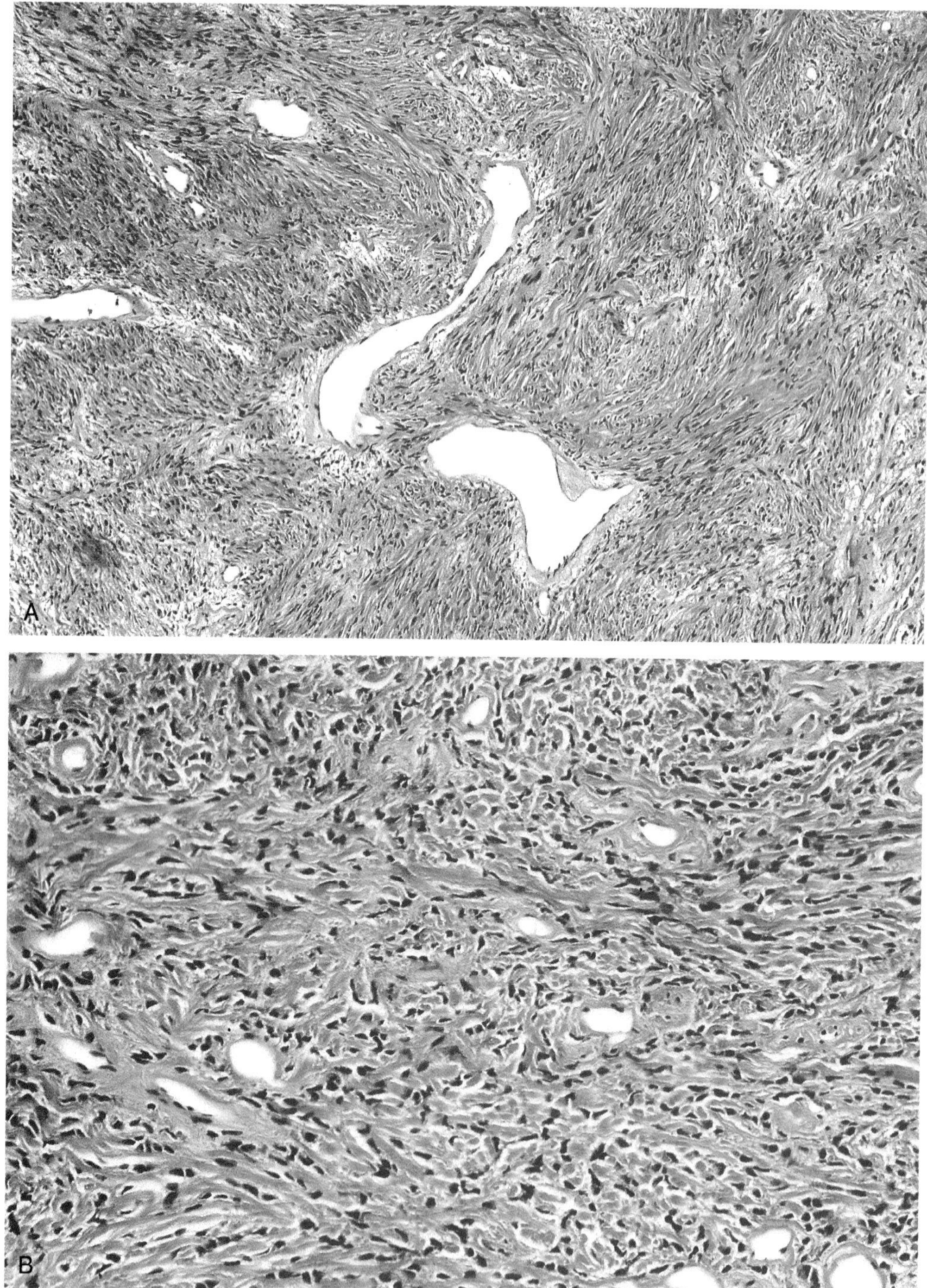


**FIGURE 27–49.** Solitary fibrous tumor showing a "pericytic" pattern (**A**) and "patternless pattern" (**B**) consisting of small fusiform cells randomly arranged between collagen bundles.

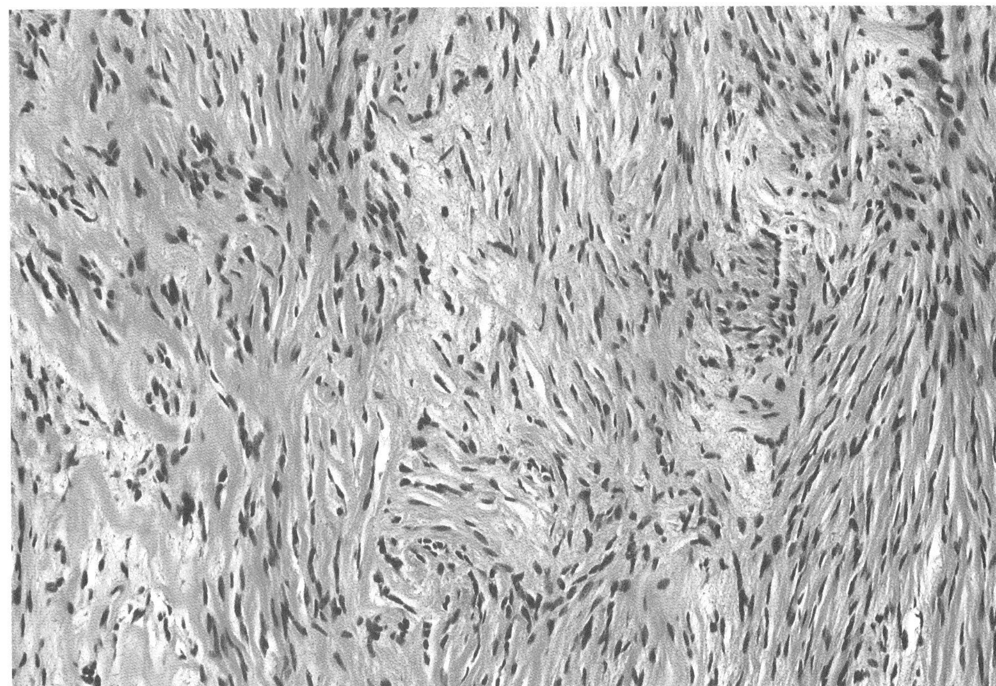

**FIGURE 27–50.** Solitary fibrous tumor with a characteristic cracking artifact between the cells and collagen.

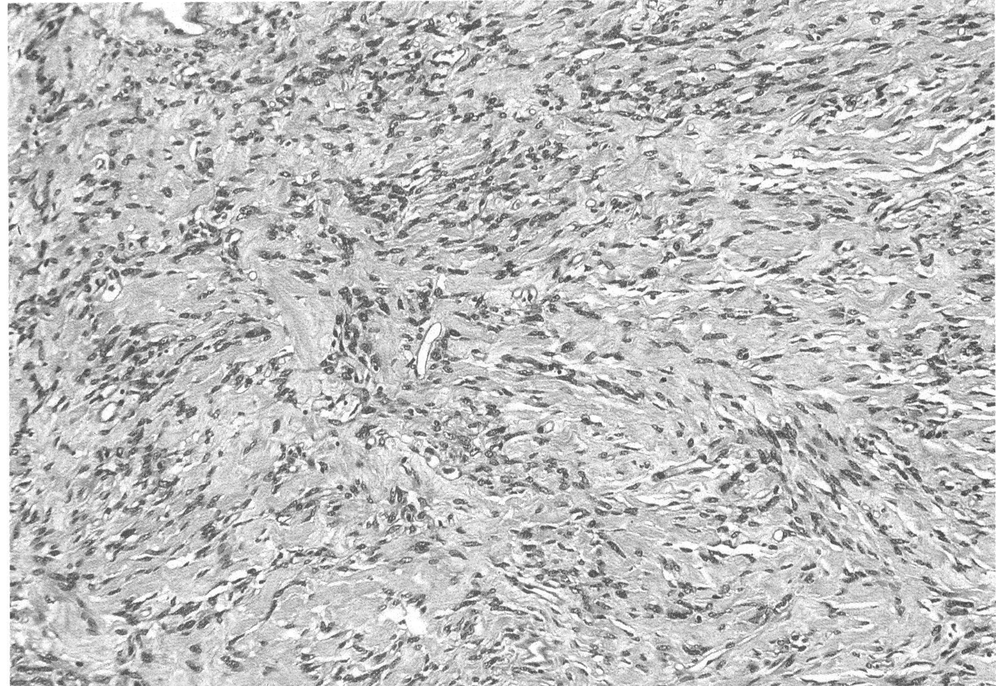

**FIGURE 27–51.** Solitary fibrous tumor with a staggered or grouped arrangement of cells in the collagen.

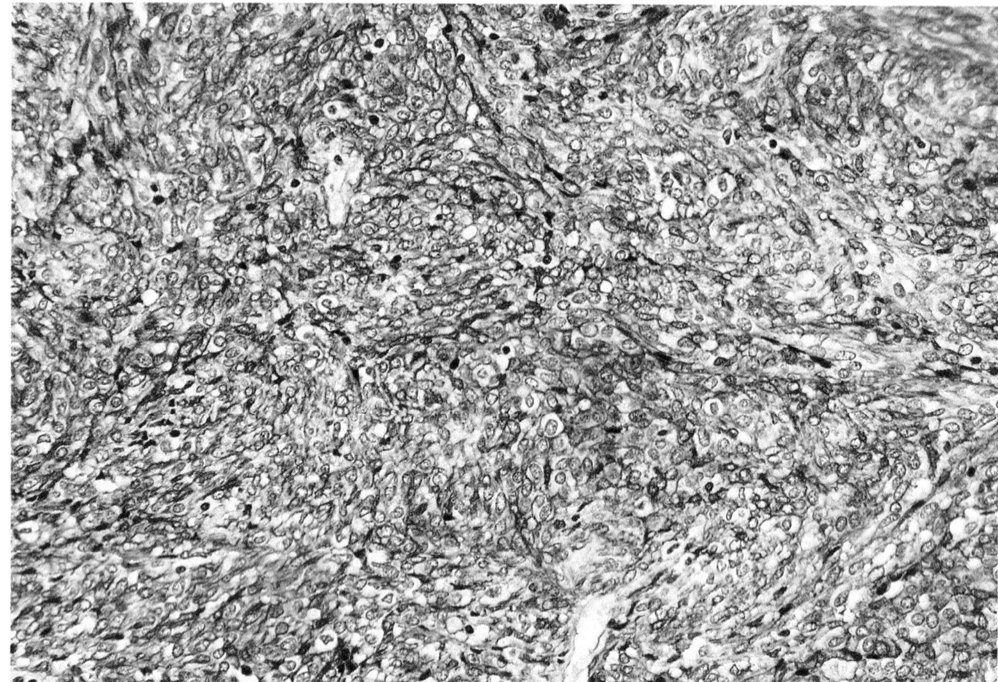

**FIGURE 27–52.** CD34 immunostain in a solitary fibrous tumor showing diffuse staining.

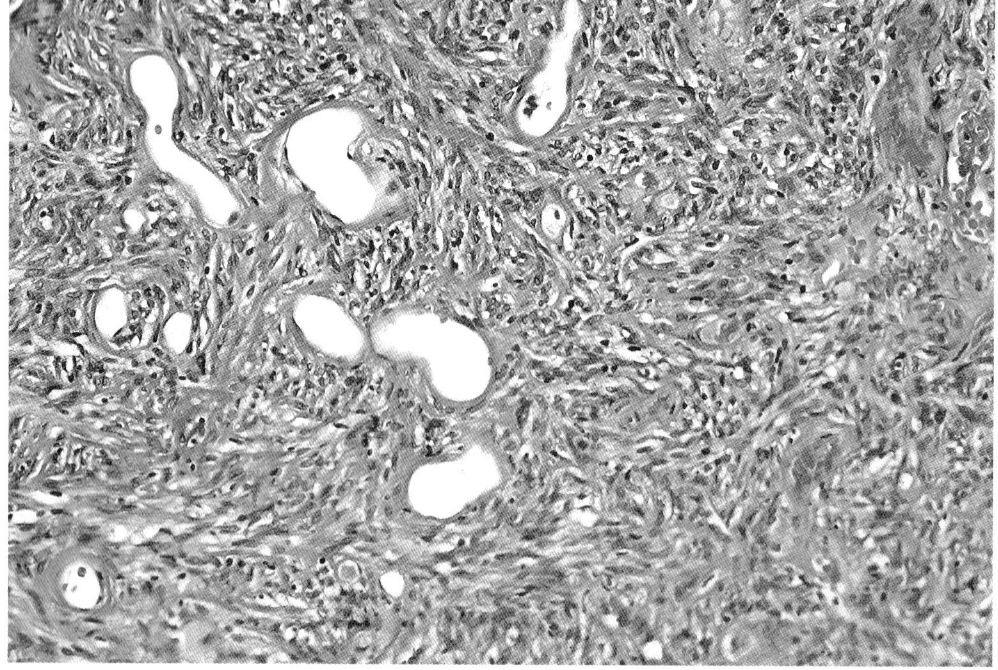

**FIGURE 27–53.** Solitary fibrous tumor with a hemangiopericytoma-like area.

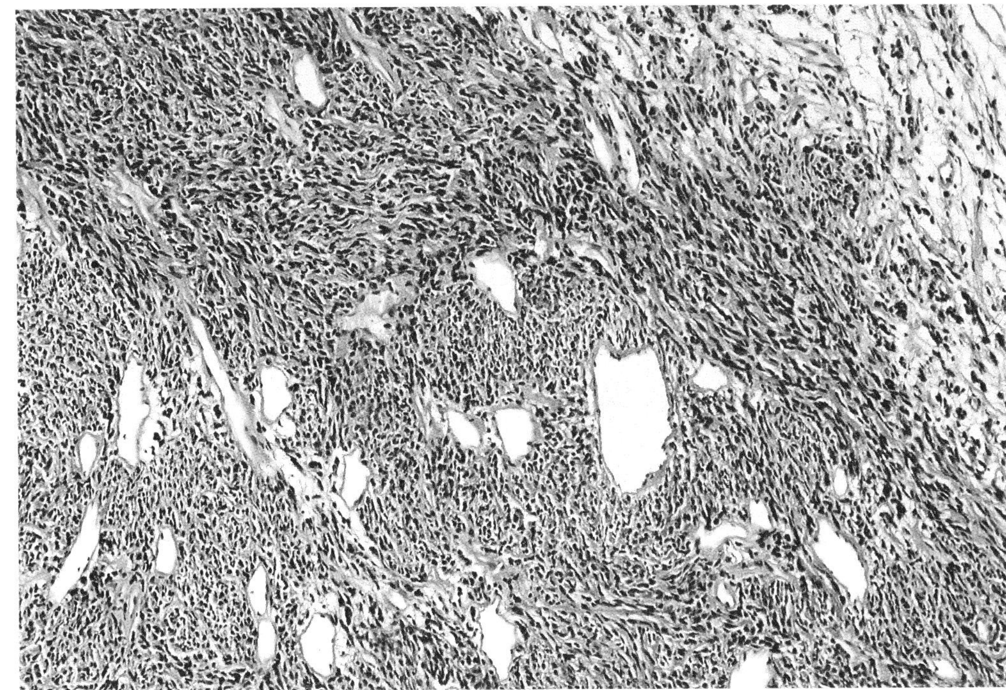

**FIGURE 27–54.** Malignant solitary fibrous tumor with heightened cellularity. Tumor also contained areas of histologically benign solitary fibrous tumor.

tic[91,136] and fibroblastic cells with rough endoplasmic reticulum, and occasional primitive junctions, has essentially debunked earlier views of mesothelial differentiation. Not only has the high sensitivity of CD34 for solitary fibrous tumors proved useful for distinguishing this tumor from desmoplastic mesothelioma,[123] it has resulted in a more accurate, consistent pattern of diagnosis, undoubtedly accounting for the large number of solitary fibrous tumors now diagnosed at extrathoracic sites.

## Clinical Behavior

Most solitary fibrous tumors behave in a benign fashion. In the most extensive series of thoracic solitary fibrous tumors reported from a single institution, two-thirds were judged benign on the basis of a number of histologic parameters.[117] All but two of the patients in this group were free of disease following simple excision or wedge resection of the lung. Malignant tumors had a more variable outcome. Approximately one-half of the patients were cured of their tumors following excision, whereas the remainder developed recurrences, metastases, or both (Table 27–4). Overall the metastatic rate of solitary fibrous tumors was 9% (16 of 169 with follow-up information). The features, which correlated statistically with malignancy, were increased cellularity, pleomorphism, increased mitotic activity (>4 mitoses/10 HPF), necrosis/hemorrhage, nonpedunculated growth, and an atypical location (e.g., parietal pleura, interlobar fissure, mediastinum, or endophytic growth into lung) (Table 27–5). It must be borne in mind that many of these features are co-dependent. For example, increased mitotic activity is nearly always accompanied by increased cellularity (Figs. 27–54, 27–55).

There is far less information concerning the behavior of extrathoracic solitary fibrous tumors. Of the slightly more than 100 cases reported in the literature, 5–10% have recurred, but metastases have been decidedly rare. Vallat-Decouvelaere et al. reported their experience from a large consultation service and indi-

**TABLE 27–4 CLINICAL BEHAVIOR OF INTRATHORACIC SOLITARY FIBROUS TUMORS**

| Histologic Diagnosis* | Recurrence (%) | Metastases (%) |
|---|---|---|
| Benign | 2 | 0 |
| Malignant† | 39 | 22 |

Data from England DM, Hochholzer L, McCarthy MJ. Localized benign and malignant fibrous tumors of the pleura: a clinicopathologic review of 223 cases. Am J Surg Pathol 13:640, 1989.

* There were 98 benign tumors with follow-up ranging from 1 to 317 months (median 57 months) and 71 malignant tumors with follow-up ranging from 2 to 372 months (median 31 months).

† Tumors were classified as malignant based on one or more of the following features in any portion of tumor: high cellularity with crowded overlapping nuclei, >4 mitoses/10 HPF, nuclear atypia, pleomorphic giant cells, and atypical mitoses.

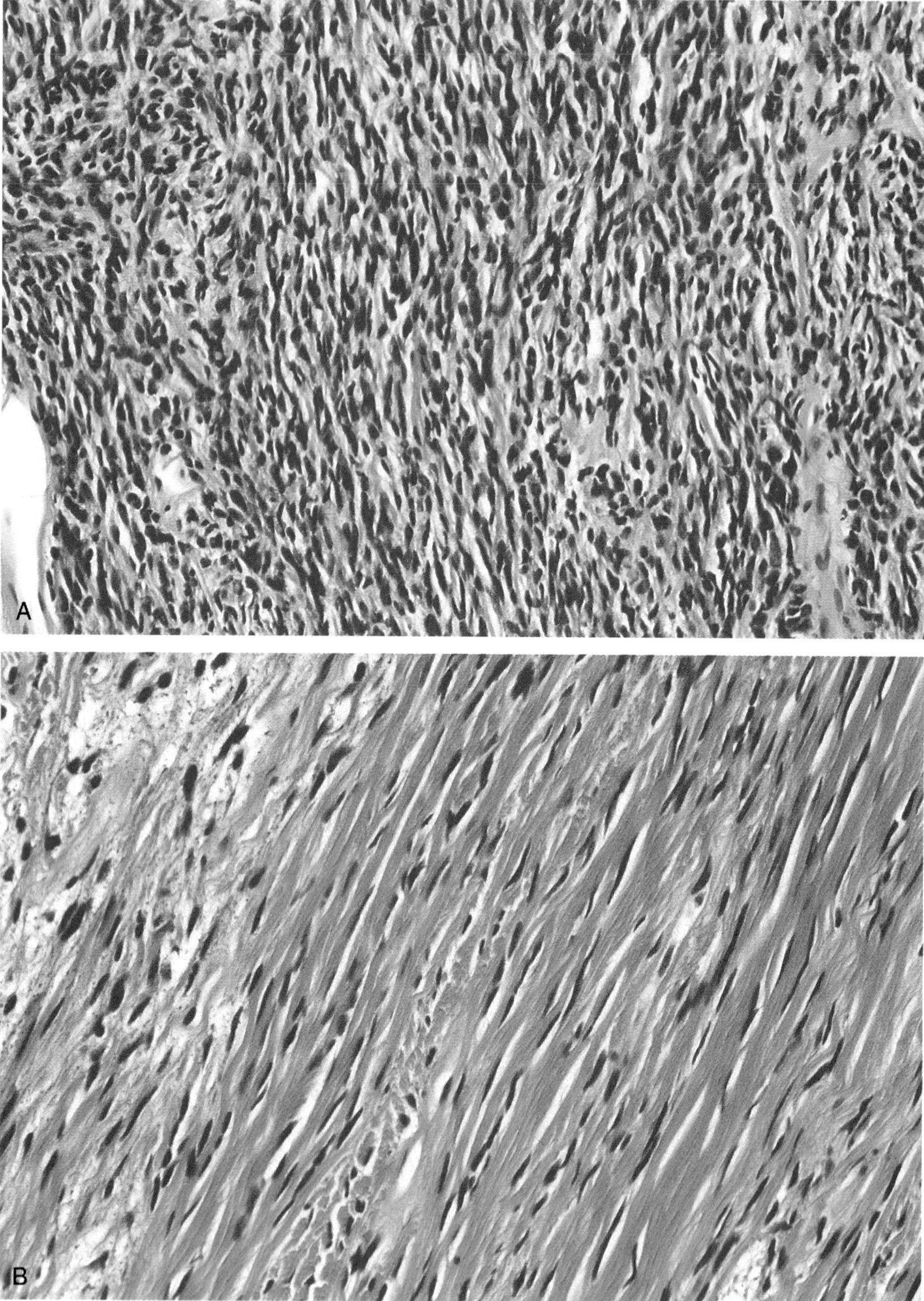


**FIGURE 27–55.** High-power view of a malignant solitary fibrous tumor with malignant areas (**A**). High-power view of benign areas for comparison (**B**). Same case as in Figure 27–54.

**TABLE 27–5 FEATURES ASSOCIATED WITH MALIGNANCY IN SOLITARY FIBROUS TUMORS**

| Thoracic[113] | Soft Tissue[213] |
|---|---|
| Histologic features | |
| Increased cellularity | Increased cellularity |
| Pleomorphism | Pleomorphism |
| Mitoses (>4/10 HPF) | Mitoses (>4/10 HPF) |
| Clinical/gross features | |
| Non pedunculated | |
| Atypical location (parietal pleura, parenchyma) | |
| Size >10 cm | |
| Necrosis/hemorrhage | |

cated that approximately 10% of extrathoracic solitary fibrous tumors have atypical features (cellularity, atypia, >4 mitoses/10 HPF, necrosis) or a history of local recurrence.[213] Eight of ten patients in this category developed local recurrences, and five died of distant metastasis. The authors suggested that the criteria employed, which were similar to those used for evaluating pleural lesions, identifies a more aggressive group and underscores the comparability of these lesions to their pleural counterpart.

## REFERENCES

### Glomus Tumor


1. Acebo E, Val-Vernal JF, Arce F. Giant intravenous glomus tumor. J Cutan Pathol 24:384, 1997.
2. Adair FE. Glomus tumor: a clinical study with a report of ten cases. Am J Surg 25:1, 1954.
3. Aiba M, Hirayama A, Kuramochi S. Glomangiosarcoma in a glomus tumor: an immunohistochemical and ultrastructural study. Cancer 61:1467, 1988.
4. Albrecht S, Zbieranowski I. Incidental glomus coccygeum: when a normal structure looks like a tumor. Am J Surg Pathol 14:922, 1990.
5. Anagostou CD, Papademetriou DG, Toumazani MN. Subcutaneous glomus tumors. Surg Gynecol Obstet 136:945, 1973.
6. Apfelberg DB, Teasler JL. Unusual locations and manifestations of glomus tumors (glomangiomas). Am J Surg 116:62, 1968.
7. Appleman HD, Helwig EB. Glomus tumors of the stomach. Cancer 23:203, 1969.
8. Bailey OT. The cutaneous glomus and its tumors: glomangiomas. Am J Pathol 11:915, 1935.
9. Barua R. Glomus tumor of the colon: first reported case. Dis Colon Rectum 31:138, 1988.
10. Beaton LI, Davis L. Glomus tumor: report of three cases: analysis of 271 recorded cases. Q Bull Northwest Univ Med School 15:245, 1941.
11. Bergstrand H. Multiple glomic tumors. Am J Cancer 29:470, 1937.
12. Boon LM, Brouillard P, Irrthum A, et al. A gene for inherited cutaneous venous anomalies ("glomangiomas") localizes to chromosome 1p21–22. Am J Hum Genet 65:125, 1999.
13. Brathwaite CD, Poppiti RJ. Malignant glomus tumor: a case report of widespread metastases in a patient with multiple glomus body hamartomas. Am J Surg Pathol 20:233, 1996.
14. Brindley GV. Glomus tumor of the mediastinum. J Thorac Surg 18:417, 1949.
15. Brooks JJ, Miettinen M, Virtanen I. Desmin immunoreactivity in glomus tumors. Am J Clin Pathol 87:292, 1987.
16. Calonje E, Fletcher CD. Cutaneous intraneural glomus tumor. Am J Dermatopathol 17:395, 1995.
17. Conant MA, Wiesenfeld SL. Multiple glomus tumors of the skin. Arch Dermatol 103:481, 1971.
18. Dervan PA, Tobbia IN, Casey M, et al. Glomus tumours: an immunohistochemical profile of 11 cases. Histopathology 14: 483, 1989.
19. Duncan L, Halverson J, DeSchryver-Kecskemeti K. Glomus tumor of the coccyx: a curable cause of coccygodynia. Arch Pathol Lab Med 115:78, 1991.
20. Eyster WH, Montgomery H. Multiple glomic tumors. Arch Dermatol Syph 62:893, 1950.
21. Faggioli GL, Bertoni F, Stella A, et al. Multifocal diffuse glomus tumor: a case report of glomangiomyoma and review of the literature. Int Angiol 7:281, 1988.
22. Folpe AL, Fanburg-Smith JC, Miettinen M, Weiss SW. Atypical and malignant glomus tumors: analysis of 53 cases with a proposal for the reclassification of glomus tumors. Am J Surg Pathol 25:1, 2001.
23. Freier DT, Lindenauer SM. Subcutaneous glomus tumor. Am J Surg 120:359, 1970.
24. Gatalica Z, Wang L, Lucio ET, Miettinen M. Glomus coccygeum in surgical pathology specimens: small troublemaker. Arch Pathol Lab Med 123:905, 1999.
25. Goodman TF, Abele DC. Multiple glomus tumors: a clinical and electron microscopic study. Arch Dermatol 103:11, 1971.
26. Gould EW, Manivel JC, Albores-Saavedra J, et al. Locally infiltrative glomus tumors and glomangiosarcomas: a clinical, ultrastructural, and immunohistochemical study. Cancer 65:310, 1990.
27. Haque S, Modlin IM, West AB. Multiple glomus tumors of the stomach with intravascular spread. Am J Surg Pathol 16:291, 1992.
28. Harris WR. Erosion of bone produced by glomus tumor. Can Med Assoc J 70:684, 1954.
29. Haupt HM, Stern JB, Berlin SJ. Immunohistochemistry in the differential diagnosis of nodular hidradenoma and glomus tumor. Am J Dermatopathol 14:310, 1992.
30. Hayes MM, Van der Westhuizen N, Holden GP. Aggressive glomus tumor of the nasal region: report of a case with multiple local recurrences. Arch Pathol Lab Med 117:649, 1993.
31. Hegyi L, Cormack GC, Grant JW. Histochemical investigation into the molecular mechanims of malignant transformation in a benign glomus tumour. J Clin Pathol 51:872, 1998.
32. Hirose T, Hasegawa T, Seki K, et al. Atypical glomus tumor in the mediastinum: a case report with immunohistochemical and ultrastructural studies. Ultrastruct Pathol 20:451, 1996.
33. Hiruta N, Kameda N, Tokudome T, et al. Malignant glomus tumor: a case report and review of the literature. Am J Surg Pathol 21:1096, 1997.
34. Ho KL, Pak MSY. Glomus tumor of the coccygeal region: case report. J Bone Joint Surg Am 62:141, 1980.
35. Hollingsworth JR, Ochsner JL. A multifocal diffuse glomus tumor. Am Surg 38:161, 1972.
36. Idy-Peretti I, Cermakova E, Dion E, et al. Subungual glomus tumor: diagnosis based on high-resolution MR images. AJR 159:1351, 1992.
37. Kanwar YS, Manaligod JR. Glomus tumor of the stomach: an ultrastructural study. Arch Pathol 99:392, 1975.

38. Kay S, Callahan WP, Murray MR, et al. Glomus tumors of the stomach. Cancer 4:726, 1951.
39. Kaye VM, Dehner LP. Cutaneous glomus tumor: a comparative immunohistochemical study with pseudoangiomatous intradermal melanocytic nevi. Am J Dermatopathol 13:2, 1991.
40. Kim YI, Kim JH, Sub JS, et al. Glomus tumor of the trachea: report of a case with ultrastructural observation. Cancer 15: 881, 1989.
41. Kishimoto S, Nagatani H, Miyashita A, et al. Immunohistochemical demonstration of substance P-containing nerve fibres in glomus tumours. Br J Dermatol 113:213, 1985.
42. Kiyosawa T, Umebayashi Y, Nakayama Y, Soeda S. Hereditary multiple glomus tumors involving the glans penis: a case report and review of the literature. Dermatol Surg 21:895, 1995.
43. Kline SC, Moore JR, deMente SH. Glomus tumor originating within a digital nerve. J Hand Surg 15:98, 1990.
44. Kobayashi Y, Kawaguchi T, Imoto K, et al. Intraosseous glomus tumor in the sacrum: a case report. Acta Pathol Jpn 40: 858, 1990.
45. Kohout E, Stout AP. The glomus tumor in children. Cancer 14: 555, 1961.
46. Lattes R, Bull DC. A case of glomus tumor with primary involvement of bone. Ann Surg 127:187, 1948.
47. Lopez-Rios F, Rodriguez-Peralto JL, Castano E, et al. Glomangiosarcoma of the lower limb: a case report with a literature review. J Cutan Pathol 24:571, 1997.
48. Lumley JSP, Stansfeld AG. Infiltrating glomus tumor of lower limb. BMJ 1:484, 1972.
49. Masson P. Le glomus neuromyoarterieal des regions tactiles et ses tumeurs. Lyon Chir 21:257, 1924.
50. Miettinen M, Lehto V-P, Virtanen I. Glomus tumor cells: evaluation of smooth muscle and endothelial cell properties. Virchows Arch [Cell Pathol] 43:139, 1983.
51. Mullis WF, Rosato FE, Rosato EF, et al. The glomus tumor. Surg Gynecol Obstet 135:705, 1972.
52. Murad J, Von Haam Z, Murthy MSN. The ultrastructure of hemangiopericytoma and a glomus tumor. Cancer 22:1239, 1968.
53. Murray MR, Stout AP. The glomus tumor: investigation of its distribution and behavior and the identity of its "epithelioid" cell. Am J Pathol 18:183, 1942.
54. Negri G, Schulte M, Mohr W. Glomus tumor with diffuse infiltration of the quadriceps muscle: a case report. Hum Pathol 28:750, 1997.
55. Noer H, Krogdahl A. Glomangiosarcoma of the lower extremity. Histopathology 18:365, 1991.
56. Nuovo MA, Grimes MM, Knowles DM. Glomus tumors: clinicopathologic and immunohistochemical analysis of forty cases. Surg Pathol 3:31, 1990.
57. Okada O, Demitsu T, Manabe M, Yoneda K. A case of multiple subungual glomus tumors associated with neurofibromatosis type 1. J Dermatol 26:535, 1999.
58. Popoff NW. The digital vascular system with reference to the state of the glomus in inflammation, arteriosclerotic gangrene, thromboangiitis obliterans, and supernumerary digits in man. Arch Pathol 18:295, 1934.
59. Porter PG, Bigler SA, McNutt M, et al. The immunophenotype of hemangiopericytoma and glomus tumors with special reference to muscle protein expression: an immunohistochemical study and review of the literature. Mod Pathol 4:46, 1991.
60. Pulitzer DR, Martin PC, Reed RJ. Epithelioid glomus tumor. Hum Pathol 26:1022, 1995.
61. Rao VK, Weiss SW. Angiomatosis of soft tissue: an analysis of the histologic features and clinical outcome in 51 cases. Am J Surg Pathol 16:764, 1992.
62. Riveros M, Pack GT. The glomus tumors: report of 20 cases. Ann Surg 133:394, 1951.
63. Salima H, Modlin IM, West AB. Multiple glomus tumors of the stomach with intravascular spread. Am J Surg Pathol 16: 291, 1992.
64. Sawada S, Honda M, Kamide R, Niimura M. Three cases of subungual glomus tumors with von Recklinghausen's neurofibromatosis. J Am Acad Dermatol 32:277, 1995.
65. Schürch W, Skalli O, Lagace R, et al. Intermediate filament proteins and actin isoforms as markers for soft tissue tumor differentiation and origin. III. Hemangiopericytomas and glomus tumors. Am J Pathol 136:771, 1990.
66. Shin DLH, Park SS, Lee JH, et al. Oncocytic glomus tumor of the trachea. Chest 98:1021, 1990.
67. Shugart RR, Soule EH, Johnson EW. Glomus tumor. Surg Gynecol Obstet 117:334, 1963.
68. Skelton HG, Smith KJ. Infiltrative glomus tumor arising from a benign glomus tumor: a distinctive immunohistochemical pattern in the infiltrative component. Am J Dermatopathol 21: 562, 1999.
69. Slater DN, Cotton DWK, Azzopardi JG. Oncocytic glomus tumour: a new variant. Histopathology 11:523, 1987.
70. Smyth M. Glomus cell tumors in the lower extremity: report of two cases. J Bone Joint Surg Am 53:157, 1971.
71. Stout AP. Tumors of the neuromyoarterial glomus. Am J Cancer 24:255, 1935.
72. Tsuneyoshi M, Enjoji M. Glomus tumor: a clinicopathologic and electron microscopic study. Cancer 50:1601, 1982.
73. Venkatachalam MA, Greally JG. Fine structure of glomus tumor: similarity of glomus cells to smooth muscle. Cancer 23: 1176, 1969.
74. Watanabe K, Sugino T, Saita A, et al. Glomangiosarcoma of the hip: report of a highly aggressive tumour with widespread distant metastases. Br J Dermatol 139:1097, 1998.
75. Weiss SW, Sobin LH. WHO Classification of Soft Tissue Tumours. Springer-Verlag, Berlin, 1994.
76. West AB, Buckley PJ. Mantle zone lymphoma in a gastric glomus tumor. Cancer 70:2246, 1992.
77. Wetherington RW, Lyle WG, Sangueza OP. Malignant glomus tumor of the thumb: a case report. J Hand Surg [Am] 22:1098, 1997.
78. Yang JS, Ko JW, Suh KS, Kim ST. Congenital multiple plaque like glomangiomyoma. Am J Dermatopathol 21:454, 1999.


### Hemangiopericytoma and Solitary Fibrous Tumor


79. Abdel-Fattah HM, Adams GL, Wick MR. Hemangiopericytoma of the maxillary sinus and skull base. Head Neck 12:77, 1990.
80. Alpers CE, Rosenau W, Finkbeiner WE, et al. Congenital (infantile) hemangiopericytoma of the tongue and the sublingual region. Am J Clin Pathol 81:377, 1984.
81. Angervall L, Kindblom LG, Nielsen JM, et al. Hemangiopericytoma: a clinicopathologic, angiographic and microangiographic study. Cancer 42:2412, 1978.
82. Arias-Stella J Jr, Rosen PP. Hemangiopericytoma of the breast. Mod Pathol 1:98, 1988.
83. Atkinson JB, Mahour GH, Isaacs H Jr, et al. Hemangiopericytoma in infants and children: a report of six patients. Am J Surg 148:372, 1984.
84. Aziza J, Mazerolles C, Selves J, et al. Comparison of the reactivities of monoclonal antibodies QBEND10 (CD34) and BNH9 in vascular tumors. Appl Immunohistochem 1:51, 1993.
85. Bainbridge TC, Singh RR, Mentzel T, Katenkamp D. Solitary fibrous tumor of urinary bladder: report of two cases. Hum Pathol 28:1204, 1997.
86. Baker DL, Oda D, Myall RW. Intraoral infantile hemangiopericytoma: literature review and addition of a case. Oral Surg Oral Med Oral Pathol 73:596, 1992.
87. Batsakis JG, Jacobs JB, Templeton AC. Hemangiopericytoma of

the nasal cavity: electron optic study and clinical correlations. J Laryngol Otol 97:361, 1983.
88. Battifora H. Hemangiopericytoma: ultrastructural study of five cases. Cancer 31:1418, 1973.
89. Benn JJ, Firth RG, Sonksen PH. Metabolic effect of an insulin-like factor causing hypoglycemia in a patient with haemangiopericytoma. Clin Endocrinol (Oxf) 32:769, 1990
90. Bommer G, Altenahr F, Kuhnau J Jr, et al. Ultrastructure of hemangiopericytoma associated with paraneoplastic hypoglycemia. Z Krebsforsch 85:231, 1976.
91. Briselli M, Mark EJ, Dickersin GR. Solitary fibrous tumor of the pleura: eight new cases and review of 360 cases in the literature. Cancer 47:2678, 1981.
92. Brunnemann RB, Ro JY, Ordonez NG, et al. Extrapleural solitary fibrous tumor: a clinicopathologic study of 24 cases. Mod Pathol 12:1034, 1999.
93. Carneiro SS, Scheithauer BW, Nascimento AG, et al. Solitary fibrous tumor of the meninges: a lesions distinct from fibrous meningioma: a clinicopathologic and immunohistochemical study. Am J Clin Pathol 106:217, 1996.
94. Ceballos KM, Munk PL, Masri BA, O'Connell JX. Lipomatous hemangiopericytoma: a morphologically distinct soft tissue tumor. Arch Pathol Lab Med 123:941, 1999.
95. Chen KT, Kassel SH, Medrano VA. Congenital hemangiopericytoma. J Surg Oncol 31:127, 1986.
96. Chilosi M, Facchetti F, Dei Tos AP, et al. Bcl-2 expression in pleural and extrapleural solitary fibrous tumours. J Pathol 181: 362, 1997.
97. Chung KC, Weiss SW, Kuzon WM. Multifocal congenital hemangiopericytomas associated with Kasabach-Merritt syndrome. Br J Plast Surg 48:240, 1995.
98. Compagno J. Hemangiopericytoma-like tumors of the nasal cavity: a comparison with hemangiopericytoma of soft tissues. Laryngoscope 88:460, 1978.
99. Compagno J, Hyams J. Hemangiopericytoma-like intranasal tumors: a clinicopathologic study of 23 cases. Am J Clin Pathol 66:672, 1976.
100. Cowper SE, Kilpatrick T, Proper S, Morgan MB. Solitary fibrous tumor of the skin. Am J Dermatopathol 21:213, 1999.
101. Croxatto JO, Font RL. Hemangiopericytoma of the orbit: a clinicopathologic study of 30 cases. Hum Pathol 13:199, 1982.
102. Dal Cin P, Sciot R, Fletcher CD, et al. Trisomy 21 in solitary fibrous tumor. Cancer Genet Cytogenet 86:58, 1996.
103. Dalton WT, Zolliker AS, McCaughey WT, et al. Localized primary tumors of the pleura: an analysis of 40 cases. Cancer 44: 1465, 1979.
104. D'Amore ESG, Manivel JG, Sung JH. Soft tissue and meningeal hemangiopericytomas: an immunohistochemical and ultrastructural study. Hum Pathol 21:414, 1990.
105. Dardick I, Hammar SP, Scheithauer BW. Ultrastructural spectrum of hemangiopericytoma: a comparative study of fetal, adult and neoplastic pericytes. Ultrastruct Pathol 13:111, 1989.
106. De Saint Aubain Somerhausen N, Rubin BP, Fletcher CD. Myxoid solitary fibrous tumor: a study of seven cases with emphasis on differential diagnosis. Mod Pathol 12:463, 1999.
107. Dictor M, Elner A, Andersson T, et al. Myofibromatosis-like hemangiopericytoma metastasizing as differentiated vascular smooth muscle and myosarcoma: myopericytes as a subset of "myofibroblasts." Am J Surg Pathol 16:1239, 1992.
108. Dingham RO. Hemangiopericytoma: report of two cases, one of congenital origin. Plast Reconstr Surg 21:399, 1958.
109. Dorfman DM, To K, Dickersin GR, et al. Solitary fibrous tumor of the orbit. Am J Surg Pathol 18:281, 1994.
110. Eichhorn JH, Dickersin GR, Bhan AK, et al. Sinonasal hemangiopericytoma: a reassessment with electron microscopy, immunohistochemistry, and long-term follow-up. Am J Surg Pathol 14:856, 1990.
111. Eimoto T. Ultrastructure of an infantile hemangiopericytoma. Cancer 40:2161, 1977.
112. Eneroth CM, Fluur E, Soderberg G, et al. Nasal hemangiopericytoma. Laryngoscope 80:17, 1970.
113. England DM, Hochholzer L, McCarthy MJ. Localized benign and malignant fibrous tumors of the pleura: a clinicopathologic review of 223 cases. Am J Surg Pathol 13:640, 1989.
114. Enzinger FM, Smith BH. Hemangiopericytoma: an analysis of 106 cases. Hum Pathol 7:61, 1976.
115. Erlandson RA, Woodruff JM. Role of electron microscopy in the evaluation of soft tissue neoplasms with emphasis on spindle cell and pleomorphic tumors. Hum Pathol 29:1372, 1998.
116. Ferreiro JA, Nascimento AG. Solitary fibrous tumour of the major salivary glands. Histopathology 28:261, 1996.
117. Fletcher CD, Dal Cin P, de Wever I, et al. Correlation between clinicopathologic features and karyotype in spindle cell sarcomas: a report of 130 cases from the CHAMP study group. Am J Pathol 154:1841, 1999.
118. Fletcher CDM. Hemangiopericytoma—a dying breed? Reappraison of an "entity" and its variant: a hypothesis. Curr Diagn Pathol 1:19, 1994.
119. Flint A, Weiss SW. CD-34 and keratin expression distinguishes solitary fibrous tumor (fibrous mesothelioma) of pleura from desmoplastic mesothelioma. Hum Pathol 265:428, 1995.
120. Folpe AL, Devaney K, Weiss SW. Lipomatous hemangiopericytoma: a rare variant of hemangiopericytoma that may be confused with liposarcoma. Am J Surg Pathol 23:1201, 1999.
121. Fukasawa Y, Takada A, Tateno M, et al. Solitary fibrous tumor of the pleura causing recurrent hypoglycemia by secretion of insulin-like growth factor II. Pathol Int 48:47, 1998.
122. Fukunaga M, Naganuma H, Nikaido T, et al. Extrapleural solitary fibrous tumor: a report of seven cases. Mod Pathol 10: 443, 1997.
123. Fukunaga M, Naganuma H, Ushigome S, et al. Malignant solitary fibrous tumour of the peritoneum. Histopathology 28: 463, 1996.
124. Gelb AB, Simmons ML, Weidner N. Solitary fibrous tumor involving the renal capsule. Am J Surg Pathol 20:1288, 1996.
125. Gensler S, Caplan LH, Laufman H. Giant benign hemangiopericytoma functioning as an arteriovenous shunt. JAMA 198: 203, 1966.
126. Gherardi G, Arya S, Hickler RB. Juxtaglomerular body tumor: a rare occult, but curable cause of lethal hypertension. Hum Pathol 5:236, 1974.
127. Goellner JR, Laws ER Jr, Soule EH, et al. Hemangiopericytoma of the meninges: Mayo Clinic experience. Am J Clin Pathol 70: 375, 1978.
128. Goodlad JR, Fletcher CDM. Solitary fibrous tumor at unusual sites: analysis of a series. Histopathology 19:515, 1991.
129. Grantner SR, Badizadegan K, Fletcher CD. Myofibromatosis in adults, glomangiopericytoma and myopericytoma: a spectrum of tumors showing perivascular myoid differentiation. Am J Surg Pathol 22:513, 1998.
130. Guthrie BL, Ebersold MJ, Scheithauer BW, et al. Meningeal hemangiopericytoma: histopathologic features, treatment, and long-term follow-up of 44 cases. Neurosurgery 25:514, 1989.
131. Hahn MJ, Dawson R, Esterly JA, et al. Hemangiopericytoma: an ultrastructural study. Cancer 31:255, 1973.
132. Hanau CA, Miettinenen M. Solitary fibrous tumor: histological and immunohistochemical spectrum of benign and malignant variants presenting at different sites. Hum Pathol 26:440, 1995.
133. Haney RF. Hemangiopericytoma of the orbit. Arch Ophthalmol 71:206, 1964.
134. Hasegawa T, Hirose T, Seki K, et al. Solitary fibrous tumor of the soft tissue: an immunohistochemical and ultrastructural study. Am J Clin Pathol 106:325, 1996.
135. Hasegawa T, Matsuno Y, Shimoda T, et al. Extrathoracic soli-

tary fibrous tumors: their histologic variability and potentially aggressive behavior. Hum Pathol 30:1464, 1999.
136. Hayes MM, Dietrich BE, Uys CJ. Congenital hemangiopericytomas of skin. Pediatr Dermatopathol 8:148, 1986.
137. Henn W, Wullich B, Thoennes M, et al. Recurrent t(12;19) (q13;q13.3) in intracranial and extracranial hemangiopericytoma. Cancer Genet Cytogenet 71:3009, 1993.
138. Herath SE, Stalboerger PG, Dahl RJ, et al. Cytogenetic studies of four hemangiopericytomas. Cancer Genet Cytogenet 72:137, 1994.
139. Hernandez FJ, Fernandez BB. Localized fibrous tumors of pleural: a light and electron microscopic study. Cancer 34: 1667, 1974.
140. Hiura M, Nogawa T, Nagai N, et al. Vaginal hemangiopericytoma: a light microscopic and ultrastructural study. Gynecol Oncol 21:376, 1985.
141. Hoeffel JC, Chardot C. Radiologic patterns of hemangiopericytoma of the leg. Am J Surg 123:591, 1972.
142. Hoog A, Sandberg Nordqvist AC, Hulting AL, et al. High molecular weight IGF-2 expression in a hemangiopericytoma associated with hypoglycaemia. APMIS 105:469, 1997.
143. Howard JW, Davis PL. Retroperitoneal hemangiopericytoma associated with hypoglycemia and masculinization. Del Med J 31:29, 1959.
144. Iwaki T, Fukui M, Takeshita I, et al. Hemangiopericytoma of the meninges: a clinicopathologic and immunohistochemical study. Clin Neuropathol 7:93, 1988.
145. Jakobiec FA, Howard GM, Jones IS, et al. Hemangiopericytoma of the orbit. Am J Ophthalmol 78:816, 1974.
146. Jenkins JJ III. Case 7, congenital malignant hemangiopericytoma. Pediatr Pathol 7:119, 1987.
147. Joseph JT, Lisle DK, Jacoby LB, et al. NF2 gene analysis distinguishes hemangiopericytoma from meningioma. Am J Pathol 147:1450, 1995.
148. Kauffman SL, Stout AP. Hemangiopericytoma in children. Cancer 13:695, 1960.
149. Kawai T, Mikata A, Torikata C, et al. Solitary (localized) pleural mesothelioma: a light and electron microscopic study. Am J Surg Pathol 2:365, 1978.
150. Kim H, Damjanov I. Localized fibrous mesothelioma of the liver: report of a giant tumor studied by light and electron microscopy. Cancer 52:1662, 1983.
151. Kishikawa M, Tsuda N, Fujii H. Ultrastructural study of hemangiopericytoma and hemangioendothelioma. J Electron Microsc 24:134, 1975.
152. Klemperer P, Rabin CB. Primary neoplasm of the pleura: a report of five cases. Arch Pathol 11:385, 1931.
153. Kottke-Marchant K, Hart WR, Broughan T. Localized fibrous tumor (localized fibrous mesothelioma) of the liver. Cancer 64: 1096, 1989.
154. Kuhn C III, Rosai J. Tumors arising from pericytes: ultrastructure and organ culture of a case. Arch Pathol 88:653, 1969.
155. Limon J, Rao U, Dal Cin P, et al. Translocation t(13;22) in hemangiopericytoma. Cancer Genet Cytogenet 21:309, 1986.
156. Lorigan JG, David CL, Evans HL, et al. The clinical and radiologic manifestations of hemangiopericytoma. AJR 153:345, 1989.
157. Mandahl N, Orndal C, Heim S, et al. Aberrations of chromosome segment 12q13-15 characterize a subgroup of hemangiopericytomas. Cancer 71:3009, 1993.
158. Masson EA, MacFarlane IA, Graham D, et al. Spontaneous hypoglycemia due to pleural fibroma: role of insulin like growth factors. Thorax 46:930, 1991.
159. McMaster MJ, Soule EH, Ivins JC. Hemangiopericytoma: a clinicopathologic study and long-term follow-up of 60 patients. Cancer 36:2232, 1975.
160. Mena H, Ribas JL, Pezeshkpour GH, et al. Hemangiopericytoma of the central nervous system: a review of 94 cases. Hum Pathol 22:84, 1991.
161. Mentzel T, Bainbridge TC, Katenkamp D. Solitary fibrous tumour: clinicopathologic, immunohistochemical, and ultrastructural analysis of 12 cases arising in soft tissues, nasal cavity and nasopharynx, urinary bladder, and prostate. Virchows Arch 430:445, 453, 1997.
162. Middleton LP, Duray PH, Merino MJ. The histological spectrum of hemangiopericytoma: application of immunohistiochemical analysis including proliferative markers to facilitate diagnosis and predict prognosis. Hum Pathol 29:636, 1998.
163. Miettinen MM, el-Rifai W, Sarlomo-Rikala M, et al. Tumor size-related DNA copy number changes occur in solitary fibrous tumors but not in hemangiopericytomas. Mod Pathol 10:1194, 1997.
164. Mittal KR, Gerald W, True LD. Hemangiopericytoma of the breast: report of a case with ultrastructural and immunohistochemical staining. Hum Pathol 17:1181, 1986.
165. Morris P, Stahl R, Liriano E, et al. Giant retroperitoneal pelvic hemangiopericytoma; J Cardiovasc Surg 32:778, 1991.
166. Murad TM, Von Haam E, Murthy MSN. Ultrastructure of a hemangiopericytoma and a glomus tumor. Cancer 22:1239, 1968.
167. Napi O, Ritter JH, Pettinato G, Wick MR. Hemangiopericytoma: histopathological pattern or clinicopathologic entity? Semin Diagn Pathol 12:221, 1995.
168. Nascimento AG. Solitary fibrous tumor: a ubiquitous neoplasm of mesenchymal differentiation. Adv Anat Pathol 3:338, 1996.
169. Nelson R, Bursan SO, Kiani R, et al. Hypoglycemic coma associated with benign pleural mesothelioma. J Thorac Cardiovasc Surg 69:306, 1975.
170. Nemes Z. Differentiation markers in hemangiopericytoma. Cancer 69:133, 1992.
171. Nielsen GP, O'Connell JX, Dickersin GR, Rosenberg AE. Solitary fibrous tumor of soft tissue: a report of 15 cases including 5 malignant examples with light microscopic and ultrastructural data. Mod Pathol 10:1028, 1997.
172. Nunnery EW, Kahn LB, Reddick RL, et al. Hemangiopericytoma: a light microscopic and ultrastructural study. Cancer 47: 906, 1981.
173. O'Brien P, Brasfield RD. Hemangiopericytoma. Cancer 18:249, 1965.
174. Ohmori H, Motoi M, Sato H, et al. Extrarenal renin-secreting tumor associated with hypertension. Acta Pathol Jpn 27:567, 1977.
175. Okike N, Bernatz PE, Woolner LB. Localized mesothelioma of the pleura: benign and malignant variants. J Thorac Cardiovasc Surg 75:363, 1978.
176. Osamura RY. Ultrastructure of a localized fibrous mesothelioma of the pleura: report of a case with histogenetic considerations. Cancer 39:139, 1977.
177. Park YK, Unni KK, Beabout JW, Hodgson SF. Oncogenic osteomalacia: a clinicopathologic study of 17 bone lesions. J Korean Med Sci 9:289, 1994.
178. Paullada JJ, Lisci-Gramilla A, Gonzales-Angulo A, et al. Hemangiopericytoma associated with hypoglycemia. Am J Med 44:990, 1968.
179. Pavelic K, Spaventi S, Gluncic V, et al. The expression and role of insulin-like growth factor II in malignant hemangiopericytomas. J Mol Med 77:865, 1999.
180. Perry A, Scheithauer BW, Nascimento AG. The immunophenotypic spectrum of meningeal hemangiopericytoma: a comparison with fibrous meningioma and solitary fibrous tumor of meninges. Am J Surg Pathol 21:1354, 1997.
181. Plukker JT, Koops HS, Molenaar I, et al. Malignant heman-

giopericytoma in three kindred members of one family. Cancer 61:841, 1988.

182. Porter PL, Bigler SA, McNutt M, et al. The immunophenotype of hemangiopericytomas and glomus tumors with special reference to muscle protein expression: an immunohistochemical study and review of the literature. Mod Pathol 4:46, 1991.
183. Ramsey HJ. Fine structure of hemangiopericytoma and hemangioendothelioma. Cancer 19:2005, 1966.
184. Rew DA, Allen JP. Late recurrence of an abdominal hemangiopericytoma. J R Soc Med 80:552, 1989.
185. Reynolds FC, Lansche WE. Hemangiopericytoma of the lower extremity. J Bone Joint Surg Am 40:921, 1958.
186. Rhodes RE Jr, Brown HA, Harrison EG Jr. Hemangiopericytoma of the nasal cavity: review of the literature and report of three cases. Arch Otolaryngol 79:505, 1964.
187. Robertson PW, Klidjian A, Harding LK, et al. Hypertension due to renin-secreting renal tumor. Am J Med 43:963, 1967.
188. Rose MG, Tallini G, Pollak J, Murren J. Malignant hypoglycemia associated with a large mesenchymal tumor: case report and review of the literature. Cancer J Sci Am 5:48, 1999.
189. Rouget C. Memoire sur le developpement, la structure, et proprietes physiologiques des capillaires sanguins et lymphatiques. Arch Physiol Norm Pathol 5:603, 1873.
190. Said JW, Nash G, Banks-Schlegel S, et al. Localized fibrous mesothelioma: an immunohistochemical and electron microscopic study. Hum Pathol 15:440, 1984.
191. Schurch W, Skalli O, Lagace R, et al. Intermediate filament proteins and actin isoforms as markers for soft tissue tumor differentiations and origin. III. Hemangiopericytomas and glomus tumors. Am J Pathol 136:771, 1990.
192. Seibert JJ. Multiple congenital hemangiopericytomas of the head and neck. Laryngoscope 88:1006, 1978.
193. Shabanah FH, Sayegh SF. Solitary (localized) pleural mesothelioma: report of two cases and review of the literature. Chest 60:558, 1971.
194. Silverberg SG, Willson MA, Board JA. Hemangiopericytoma of the uterus: an ultrastructural study. Am J Obstet Gynecol 110: 397, 1971.
195. Simon R, Greene RC. Perirenal hemangiopericytoma: a case associated with hypoglycemia. JAMA 189:155, 1964.
196. Smullens SN, Scotti D, Osterholm JL, et al. Preoperative embolization of retroperitoneal hemangiopericytomas as an aid in their removal. Cancer 50:1870, 1982.
197. Spitz FR, Bouvet M, Pisters PW, et al. Hemangiopericytoma: a 20 year single-institution experience. Ann Surg Oncol 5:350, 1998.
198. Sreekantaiah C, Bridge JA, Rao UN, et al. Clonal chromosomal abnormalities in hemangiopericytoma. Cancer Genet Cytogenet 54:173, 1991.
199. Staples JJ, Robinson RA, Wen BC, et al. Hemangiopericytoma: the role of radiotherapy. Int J Radiat Oncol Biol Phys 19:445, 1990.
200. Steinetz C, Clarke R, Jacobs GH, et al. Localized fibrous tumor of the pleura: correlation of histopathological, immunohistochemical, and ultrastructural features. Pathol Res Pract 186: 344, 1990.
201. Stout AP. Hemangiopericytoma: a study of 25 new cases. Cancer 2:1027, 1949.
202. Stout AP. Tumors featuring pericytes: glomus tumor and hemangiopericytoma. Lab Invest 5:217, 1956.
203. Stout AP, Cassel C. Hemangiopericytoma of omentum. Surgery 13:578, 1943.
204. Stout AP, Hamadi GM. Solitary (localized) mesothelioma of the pleura. Ann Surg 133:50, 1951.
205. Stout AP, Murray MR. Hemangiopericytoma: a vascular tumor featuring Zimmermann's pericytes. Ann Surg 116:26, 1942.
206. Stout AP, Murray MR. Localized pleural mesothelioma: investigation of its characteristics and histogenesis by the method of tissue culture. Arch Pathol 34:951, 1942.
207. Sugimoto T, Masuda T, Ucmura T, Tsuneyoshi M. Hemangiopericytoma-like intranasal tumor: a case report with an immunohistochemical study. Otolaryngol Head Neck Surg 113: 323, 1995.
208. Sullivan TJ, Wright JE, Wulc AE, et al. Haemangiopericytoma of the orbit. Aust NZ J Ophthalmol 20:325, 1992.
209. Suster S, Nascimento AG, Miettinen M, et al. Solitary fibrous tumors of soft tissues: a clinicopathologic and immunohistochemical study of 12 cases. Am J Surg Pathol 19:1257, 1995.
210. Tavassoli FA, Weiss S. Hemangiopericytoma of the breast. Am J Surg Pathol 5:745, 1981.
211. Theunissen PH, Ariens AT, Pannebakker MA, et al. Spatrezidiv eines Hamangioperizytoms mit lipomatoser Komponente. Pathologe 11:346, 1990.
212. Tulenko JF. Congenital hemangiopericytoma: case report. Plast Reconstr Surg 41:276, 1968.
213. Vallat-Decouvelaere AV, Dry SM, Fletcher CD. Atypical and malignant solitary fibrous tumors in extrathoracic locations: evidence of their comparability to intra-thoracic tumors. Am J Surg Pathol 22:1501, 1998.
214. Van de Rijn M, Lombard CM, Rouse RV. Expression of CD34 by solitary fibrous tumors of the pleura, mediastinum, and lung. Am J Surg Pathol 18:814, 1994.
215. Warshaw BL, Anand SK, Olsen DL, et al. Hypertension secondary to a renin-producing juxtaglomerular tumor. J Pediatr 94:247, 1979.
216. Westra WH, Gerald WL, Rosai JL. Solitary fibrous tumor: consistent CD34 immunoreactivity and occurrence in the orbit. Am J Surg Pathol 18:992, 1994.
217. Westra W, Grenko RT, Epstein J. Solitary fibrous tumor of the lower urinary tract: a report of five cases involving the seminal vesicles, urinary bladder, and prostate. Hum Pathol 31:63, 2000.
218. Winek RR, Scheithauer BW, Wick MR. Meningioma, meningeal hemangiopericytoma (angioblastic meningioma), peripheral hemangiopericytoma and acoustic schwannoma: a comparative immunohistochemical study. Am J Surg Pathol 13: 251, 1989.
219. Witkin GB, Rosai J. Solitary fibrous tumor of the mediastinum: a report of 14 cases. Am J Surg Pathol 13:547, 1989.
220. Witkin GB, Rosai J. Solitary fibrous tumor of the upper respiratory tract: a report of six cases. Am J Surg Pathol 15:842, 1991.
221. Yokoi T, Tsuzuki T, Yatabe Y, et al. Solitary fibrous tumour: significance of p53 and CD34 immunoreactivity in its malignant transformation. Histopathology 32:423, 1998.
222. Young RH, Clement PB, McCaughey WT. Solitary fibrous tumors ("fibrous mesotheliomas") of the peritoneum. Arch Pathol 114:493, 1990.
223. Yousem SA, Flynn SD. Intrapulmonary localized fibrous tumor: intraparenchymal so called localized fibrous mesothelioma. Am J Clin Pathol 89:365, 1988.
224. Yousem SA, Hochholzer L. Primary pulmonary hemangiopericytoma. Cancer 59:549, 1987.
225. Yu CCW, Hall PA, Fletcher CDM, et al. Haemangiopericytoma: the prognostic value of immunohistochemical staining with a monoclonal antibody to proliferating cell nuclear antigen (PCNA). Histopathology 19:29, 1991.
226. Zimmermann KW. Der feinere Bau der Blutkapillaren. Z Anat Entwicklungsgesch 68:29, 1923.
227. Zukerberg LR, Rosenberg AE, Randolph G, et al. Solitary fibrous tumor of the nasal cavity and paranasal sinuses. Am J Surg Pathol 15:126, 1991.

# CHAPTER 28

# BENIGN TUMORS AND TUMOR-LIKE LESIONS OF SYNOVIAL TISSUE

The synovial membrane forms the lining of joints, tendons, and bursae. In addition, its cells synthesize hyaluronate, a major component of synovial fluid, and facilitate the exchange of substances between blood and synovial fluid.[6] The synovial membrane varies considerably in appearance, depending on local mechanical factors and the nature of the underlying tissue. For instance, the synovial surface of joints subjected to high pressure is flat and acellular, whereas joints under less stress have a redundant surface lined by cells that resemble cuboidal or columnar epithelium.[35] Unlike epithelial lining cells, the synovial cells do not rest on a basal lamina but blend with the underlying stromal elements,[6] occasionally forming only an incomplete layer at the surface. Thus joint fluid and blood vessels may come in close contact with each other, a relation that probably enhances solute exchange between the two compartments.

Electron microscopically, the synovial membrane is composed of two cell types.[6,56] Type A cells are characterized by long filopodia that extend upward and form a ramifying network of overlapping processes devoid of junctional attachment.[6] In addition, they have a prominent Golgi apparatus, numerous vacuoles containing granular material, mitochondria, and pinocytotic vesicles. Under appropriate conditions these cells engage in phagocytosis. Type B cells are reminiscent of fibroblasts in their ultrastructural profile. They lack elaborate cytoplasmic processes and instead have a well developed rough endoplasmic reticulum. Although seemingly different, these cells probably represent functional modulations of the same cell because transitional forms are often seen.[56]

Synovial cells can also be characterized by means of monoclonal antibodies, although it is not yet possible to clearly relate a given antigenic phenotype with a given ultrastructural appearance. This is partly explained by the fact that when analyzed outside their normal milieu the cells may assume an altered appearance. It is also possible that a given antigenic phenotype is associated with a range of morphologic appearances. In any event, it appears that a significant proportion of cells lining the intimal surface of joints express antigens commonly associated with cells of the monocyte/macrophage series.[10,43,46] Synovial cells have provisionally been classified into three types by Burmester et al.[10] Type I cells are characterized by Ia antigens, Fc receptors, five monocyte differentiation antigens, and the property of phagocytosis. Type II cells have Ia antigens but no Fc receptors or monocyte differentiation antigens, and they are not phagocytic. Type III cells express fibroblastic but few monocytic antigens and unlike the first two cell types have the capacity to proliferate.

A number of benign tumors and tumor-like lesions arise from the synovium, such as chondroma of the tendon sheath, fibroma of the tendon sheath, synovial chondromatosis, and synovial hemangioma; yet only the giant cell tumor is considered prototypical. This tumor is the most common benign tumor of the tendon sheath and synovium and, moreover, is the only one that generally recapitulates the appearance of the normal synovial cell. It is occasionally referred to as "benign synovioma,"[68] an unfortunate term that connotes a benign form of synovial sarcoma. In actuality, giant cell tumors share few similarities with synovial sarcomas. In the localized form they occur principally on the digits and sometimes in an intraarticular location, sites where synovial sarcomas are rarely found. It is therefore preferable to consider giant cell tumors a distinct subset of synovium-based lesions and not as benign analogues of synovial sarcoma.

During the twentieth century, concepts concerning the pathogenesis of these lesions underwent constant revision. The earliest descriptions of the giant cell tumor of the tendon sheath indicate that it was considered a sarcoma until the classic description by Heurteux,[27] who suggested it was benign and proposed the term *myeloma of the tendon sheath.* Subsequent authors have emphasized the presence of foam cells and have consequently grouped these tumors with true xanthomas occurring in the setting of hyperlipidemia. Giant cell tumors, however, almost always arise in normolipemic persons and bear only a superficial similarity to tendinous xanthomas.

The most significant contribution to the understanding of giant cell tumors was made by Jaffe et al.,[30] who regarded the synovium of the tendon sheath, bursa, and joint as an anatomic unit that could give rise to a common family of lesions, including the giant cell tumor of the tendon sheath (nodular tenosynovitis), localized and diffuse forms of pigmented villonodular synovitis, and rare cases of extraarticular pigmented villonodular synovitis arising from bursae (pigmented villonodular bursitis or diffuse giant cell tumor of the tendon sheath). The differences in clinical extent and growth, they maintained, were influenced by the anatomic location. Lesions of the joints tended to expand inward and grow along the joint surface as the path of least resistance. Tumors of the tendon sheath, of necessity, grew outward, molded and confined by the shearing forces of the tendon. At present there has been no improvement of Jaffe et al.'s elegant unifying concept. On the other hand, their hypothesis that such lesions are reactive processes arising as a result of chronic inflammation is probably incorrect, as the preponderance of evidence indicates that they are neoplastic.

Although a number of terms have been applied in the literature, including fibrous histiocytoma of the synovium,[31] benign synovioma,[68] and nodular tenosynovitis,[5] we prefer the term *tenosynovial giant cell tumor* and divide the tumors into localized and diffuse forms, depending on their growth characteristics. The localized type primarily affects the digits and arises from the synovium of tendon sheaths or interphalangeal joints. The diffuse form occurs in areas adjacent to large weight-bearing joints such as the knee and ankle and in many instances represents extraarticular extension of pigmented villonodular synovitis. A small number of diffuse giant cell tumors have no intraarticular component and probably take origin from bursae associated with large joints. Pigmented villonodular synovitis restricted to the joint proper is not specifically discussed in this chapter; the reader is referred to several excellent works on the subject in the literature.[30,33]

## TENOSYNOVIAL GIANT CELL TUMOR, LOCALIZED TYPE (NODULAR TENOSYNOVITIS)

The localized form of giant cell tumor is characterized by a discrete proliferation of rounded synovial-like cells accompanied by a variable number of multinucleated giant cells, inflammatory cells, siderophages, and xanthoma cells. This tumor was first described by Chassaignac,[14] who referred to it as a "cancer of tendon sheath." It subsequently has been designated by other names, all of which serve to underscore the lack of agreement concerning its basic nature and line of differentiation.

### Clinical Findings

The giant cell tumor may occur at any age, but it is most common between 30 and 50 years. The gender ratio is skewed toward women.[31,39,63] The tumors occur predominantly on the hand, where they represent the most common neoplasm of that region[31] (Figs. 28–1, 28–2). Less common sites include the feet, ankles, and knees. In the experience of Ushijima et al.[63] (Table 28–1), 182 of 208 tumors occurred in the digits, most commonly in one of the fingers (158 cases); only 25 tumors were found in the larger joints, including the ankle/foot (10 cases), knee (8 cases), wrist (6 cases), and elbow (1 case). Finger lesions are typically located adjacent to the interphalangeal joint, although other sites may also be affected. Jaffe et al.[30] originally commented on the preference of these tumors to locate on the flexor surface, but subsequent workers have shown that the lesions may be more evenly distributed between flexor and extensor tendons.[25,31,63] They may even be found in a lateral or circumferential location.

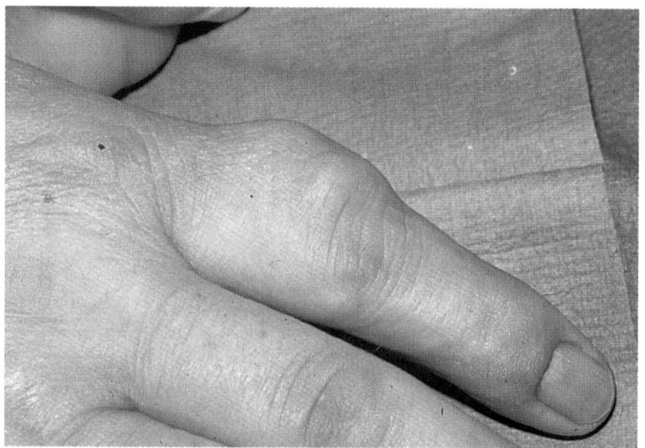

**FIGURE 28–1.** Localized giant cell tumor involving the proximal portion of the finger.

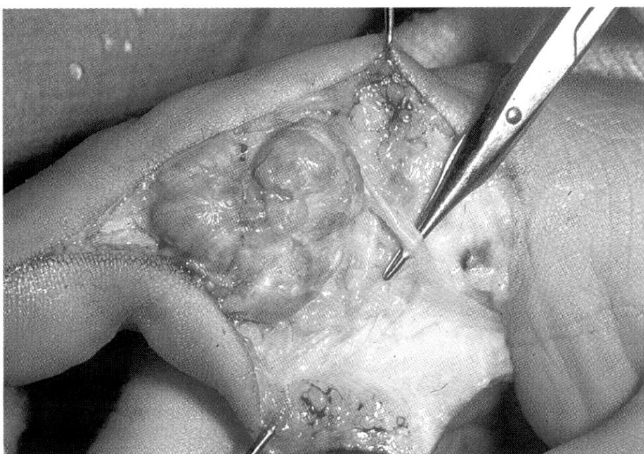

**FIGURE 28–2.** Localized giant cell tumor. Lobulated mass is present adjacent to the tendon (same case as in Figure 28–1).

The tumors develop gradually over a long time and often remain the same size for several years. On physical examination they are fixed to deep structures but are usually not attached to skin unless the lesion occurs in the distal portion of the fingers where skin is closely related to tendon. Serum cholesterol levels are normal. Antecedent trauma occurs in a variable number of patients, but its association with the lesions may be fortuitous. Radiographic studies usually document a circumscribed soft tissue mass in about half of the patients and occasionally various degenerative changes of the adjacent joint.[31] In only a small portion of patients, however, is there cortical erosion of bone.[32,38] According to Jones et al.,[31] erosion was observed in 10% of patients, but it was present in almost half of those reported by Fletcher and Horn.[22] Our experience parallels that of Jones et al., although obviously the incidence of bone changes is influenced by the selection of patients undergoing radiographic studies and by the location of the tumors. It has been suggested that giant cell tumors of the feet more frequently produce bone changes because the dense ligaments of that region are more likely to prevent outward growth of the tumor.[22] Invasion of adjacent bone is rare.[8]

**TABLE 28–1** ANATOMIC DISTRIBUTION OF GIANT CELL TUMOR OF THE TENDON SHEATH

| Location | No. of Cases |
|---|---|
| Digits | 183 |
| Fingers | 158 |
| Toes | 25 |
| Large joints | 25 |
| Ankle/foot | 10 |
| Knee | 8 |
| Wrist | 6 |
| Elbow | 1 |

Modified from Ushijima M, Hashimoto H, Tsuneyoshi M, et al. Giant cell tumor of the tendon sheath (nodular tenosynovitis): a study of 207 cases to compare the large joint group with the common digit group. Cancer 57:875, 1986.

## Gross Findings

Giant cell tumors are circumscribed lobulated masses that occasionally have shallow grooves along their deep surfaces created by the underlying tendons[68] (Figs. 28–3, 28–4). They are usually relatively small, ranging from 0.5 to 3.0–4.0 cm in diameter. Those on the feet are typically larger and more irregular in shape than those on the hands. On cut section the tumors have a mottled appearance: a pink-gray background flecked with yellow or brown, depending on the amount of lipid and hemosiderin. Tumors arising in the large joints are usually of greater size and more irregular in shape than tumors in the digits.[63]

## Microscopic Findings

In the experience of Wright,[68] who has studied the evolution of these tumors, the earliest lesion is a villous structure that projects into the synovial space of the tendon sheath. Limited space prevents continued growth into the cavity so ultimately the tumor grows outward in a cauliflower fashion and compresses synovium-lined clefts into its substance. At the stage at which most lesions are surgically excised, they are

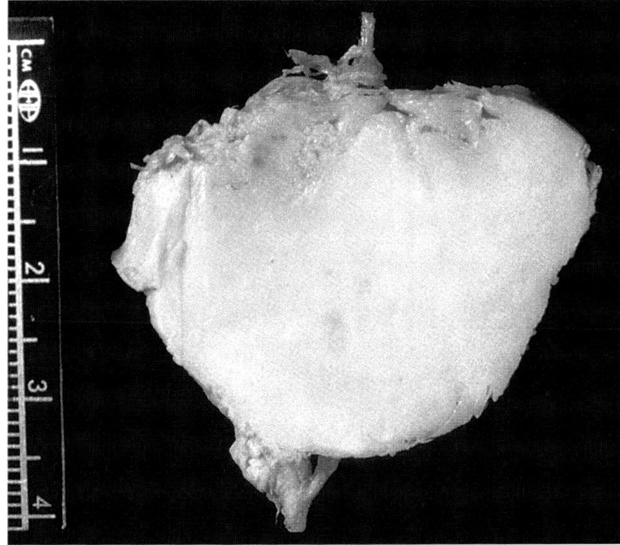


**FIGURE 28–3.** Gross appearance of giant cell tumor of the tendon sheath, localized type.

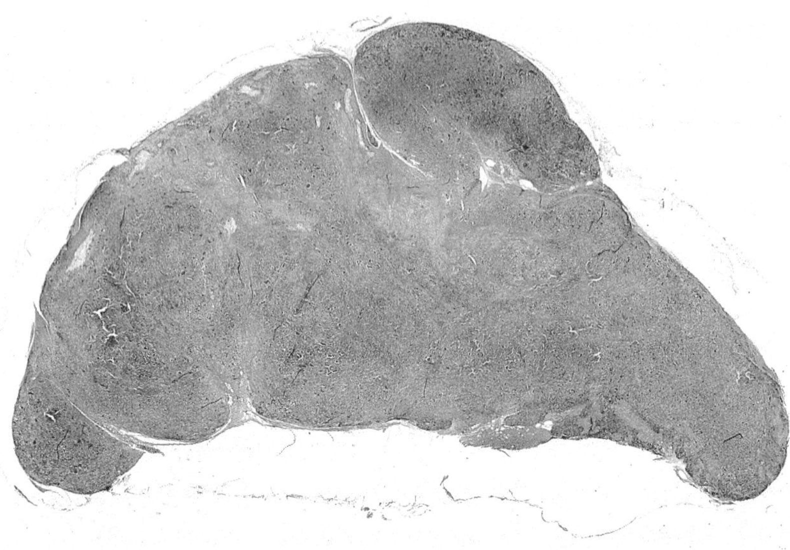

**FIGURE 28–4.** Localized giant cell tumor illustrating a late stage lesion. Deep synovial clefts are obliterated and replaced by fibrous bands that impart a vague lobular pattern to the tumor. Concave surface at the bottom is created by underlying tendon.

exophytic masses attached to the tendon sheath and have smooth but lobulated contours. They are partially invested by a dense collagenous capsule that penetrates the tumors, dividing them into vague nodules. The capsule is not totally confining, as isolated nests of tumor can be identified outside its bounds, especially at the deep margin where the tumor blends with the synovial membrane.

The appearance of the giant cell tumor varies depending on the proportion of mononuclear cells, giant cells, xanthoma cells, and the degree of collagenization (Figs. 28–5, 28–6, 28–7). Most tumors are moderately cellular and are composed of sheets of round or polygonal cells that blend with hypocellular collagenized zones in which the cells appear slightly spindled. Cleft-like spaces are occasionally present, particularly in lesions arising near large joints. Some probably represent synovium-lined spaces, whereas others are artificial spaces caused by shrinkage and loss of cellular cohesion. Multinucleated giant cells are scattered throughout the lesions. In the typical case they are relatively numerous but become sparse in highly cellular lesions, particularly recurrent ones (Fig. 28–8). These cells, which form by fusion of the more prevalent mononuclear cells, have a variable number of nuclei, ranging from as few as 3–4 to as many as 50–60. Xanthoma cells are also frequent, tend to be located geographically in these tumors, and often contain fine hemosiderin granules (Fig. 28–9). Cartilaginous and osseous metaplasia is a rare focal finding in these tumors.

The diagnosis of giant cell tumor per se is rarely difficult, but the evaluation of certain atypical features can be problematic. For instance, the presence of mitotic figures occasionally leads to a mistaken diagnosis of a malignant neoplasm. This feature occurs in more than half of the cases[68] and in our experience is a focal phenomenon in benign giant cell tumors. Rao and Vigorita[49] documented $\geq 3$ mitotic figures per 10 high-power fields (HPF) in more than 10% of their cases. Although it may indicate an actively growing lesion that is likely to recur, we have no evidence to suggest that such lesions metastasize (Figs. 28–10, 28–11). In about 1–5% of cases, tumor thrombi are observed in small veins draining these lesions (Fig. 28–12). Likewise, this feature does not correlate with the ability to produce metastasis based on preliminary follow-up information in our cases. In fact, because of the extreme rarity of metastasizing forms of giant cell tumor, it is justifiable to adopt a conservative approach when interpreting these atypical features.

## Differential Diagnosis

Occasionally, benign lesions located in the vicinity of the tendon sheath are confused with giant cell tumors, including foreign body granulomas, necrobiotic granulomas, tendinous xanthomas, and fibromas of the tendon sheath. *Granulomatous lesions,* however, are less localized and have a greater complement of inflammatory cells. *Necrobiotic granulomas* are characterized by cores of degenerating collagen rimmed by histiocytes and a prominent zone of proliferating capillaries. Giant cells are usually scarce or nonexistent. The distinction of giant cell tumor with a prominent xanthomatous component (Fig. 28–13) and *tendinous xanthoma* formerly represented a problem in differential diagnosis. As a result of the recognition and early treatment of hyperlipidemia, it is seldom a practical problem for the surgical pathologist today. In contrast to giant cell tumors, tendinous xanthomas that arise

*Text continued on page 1045*

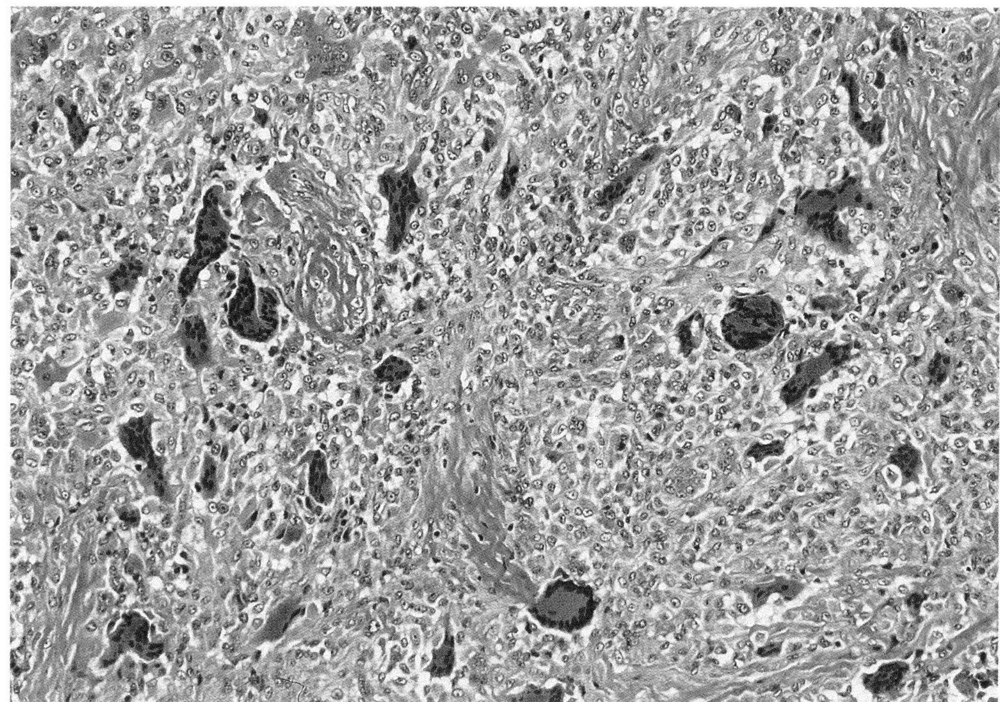

**FIGURE 28–5.** Localized form of giant cell tumor with a regular distribution of multinucleated giant cells admixed with round cells and collagen.

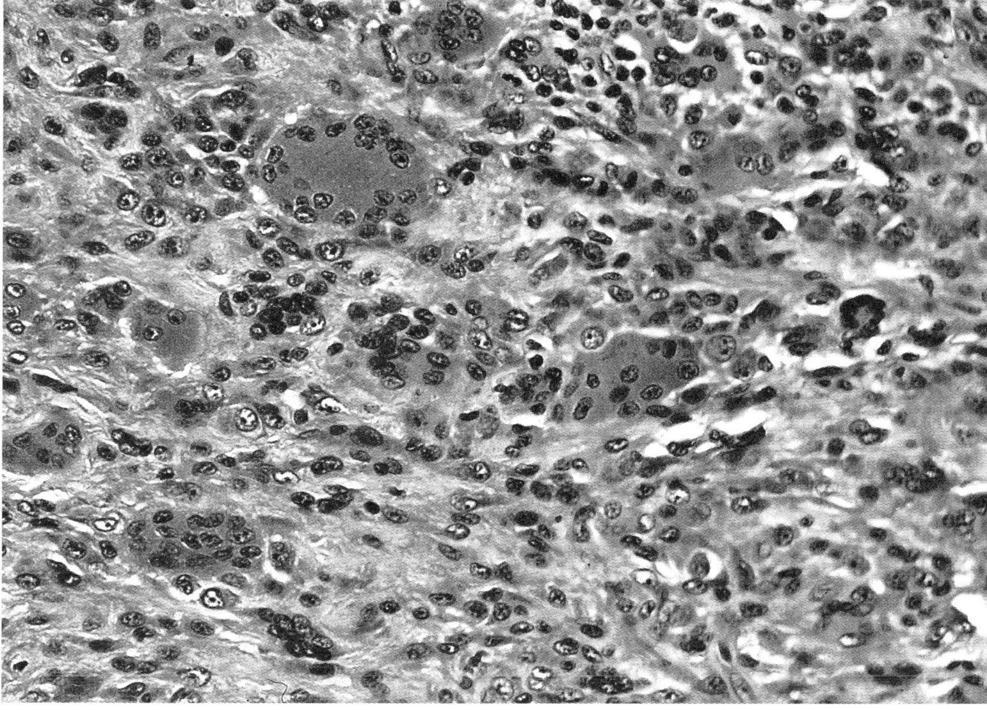

**FIGURE 28–6.** Giant cell-rich area of a localized form of giant cell tumor.

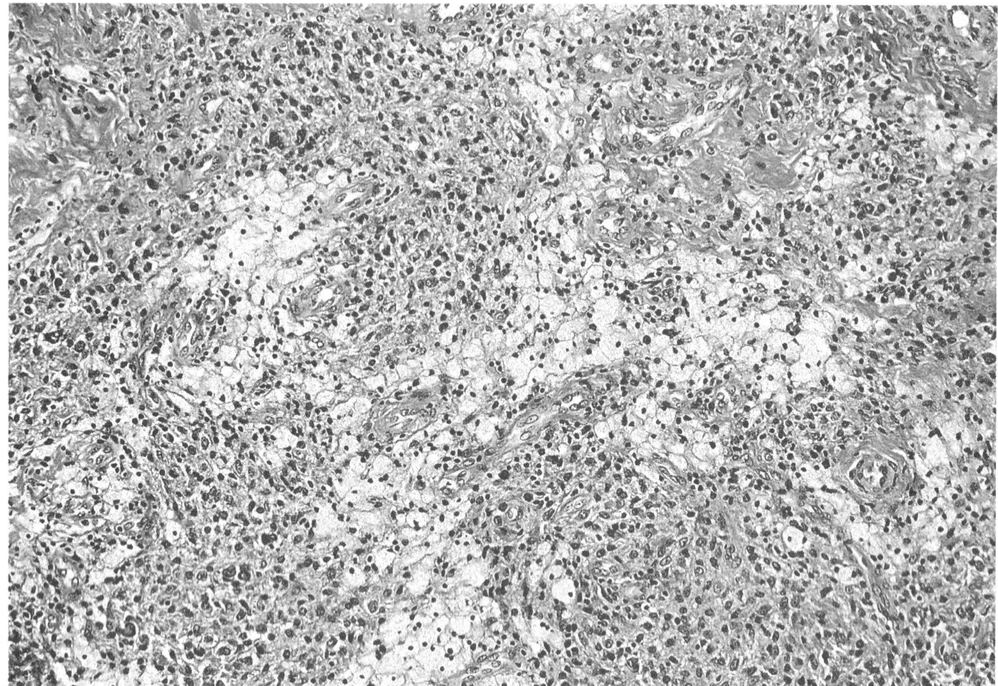

**FIGURE 28–7.** Localized form of giant cell tumor showing focal collections of xanthoma cells intermixed with round cells.

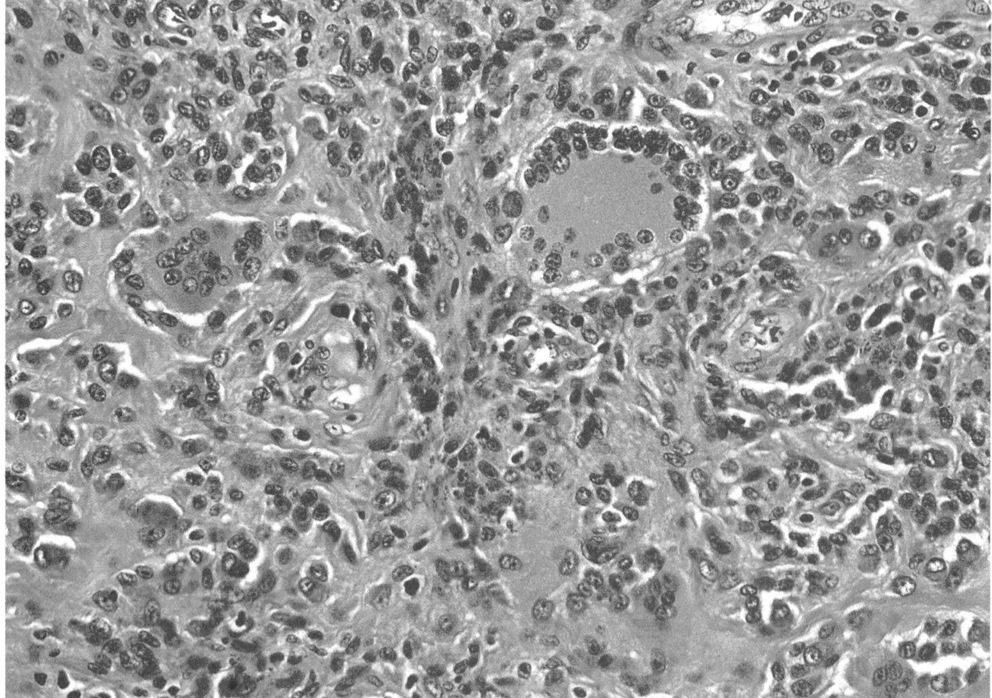

**FIGURE 28–8.** Rare giant cells admixed with round cells and areas of hemosiderin deposition in a giant cell-poor localized form of giant cell tumor.

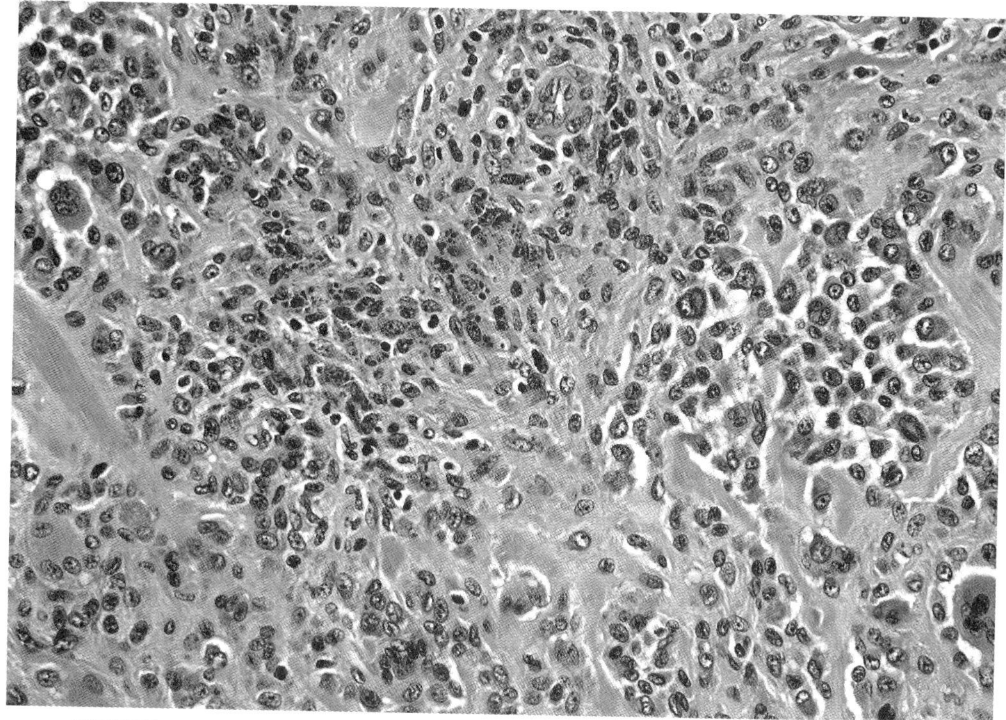

**FIGURE 28–9.** Abundant hemosiderin deposition in a localized giant cell tumor.

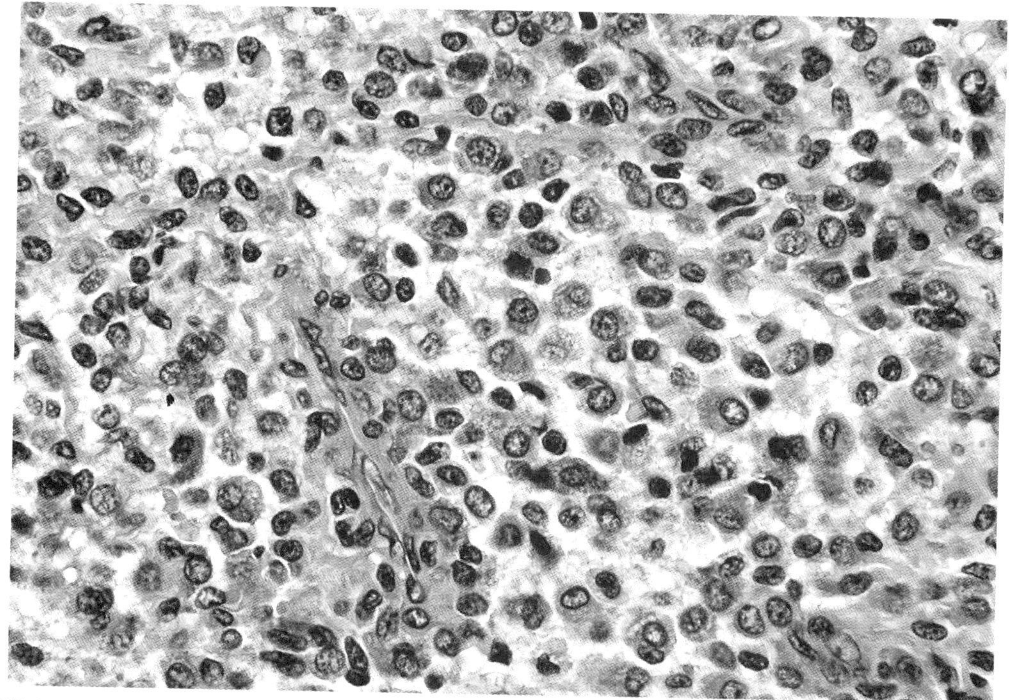

**FIGURE 28–10.** High-power view of round cells in a giant cell tumor with a paucity of giant cells. Some of the cells contain intracytoplasmic hemosiderin.

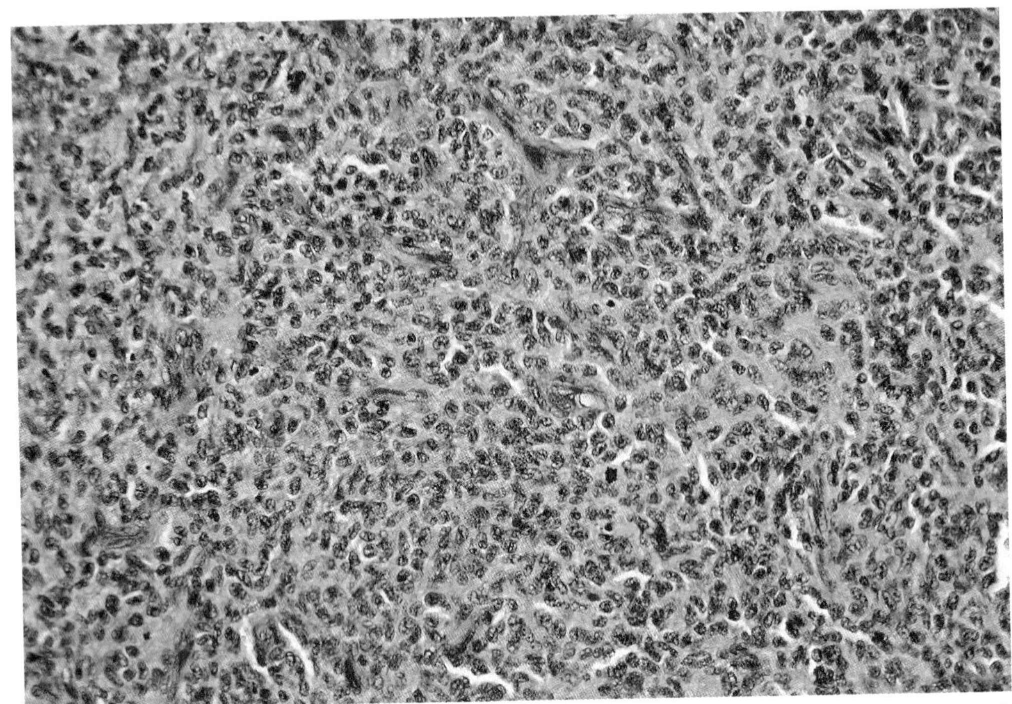

**FIGURE 28–11.** Cellular example of a localized form of giant cell tumor with a paucity of giant cells. Rare mitotic figures can be seen.

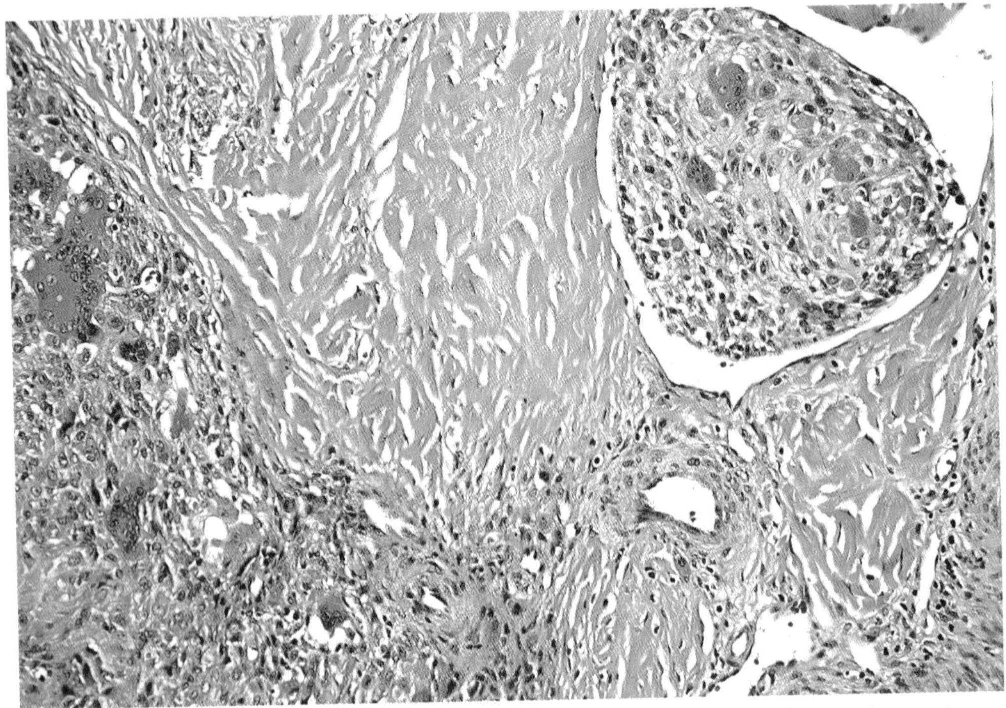

**FIGURE 28–12.** Focus of tumor in a vein in a localized giant cell tumor. This feature does not necessarily indicate malignancy.

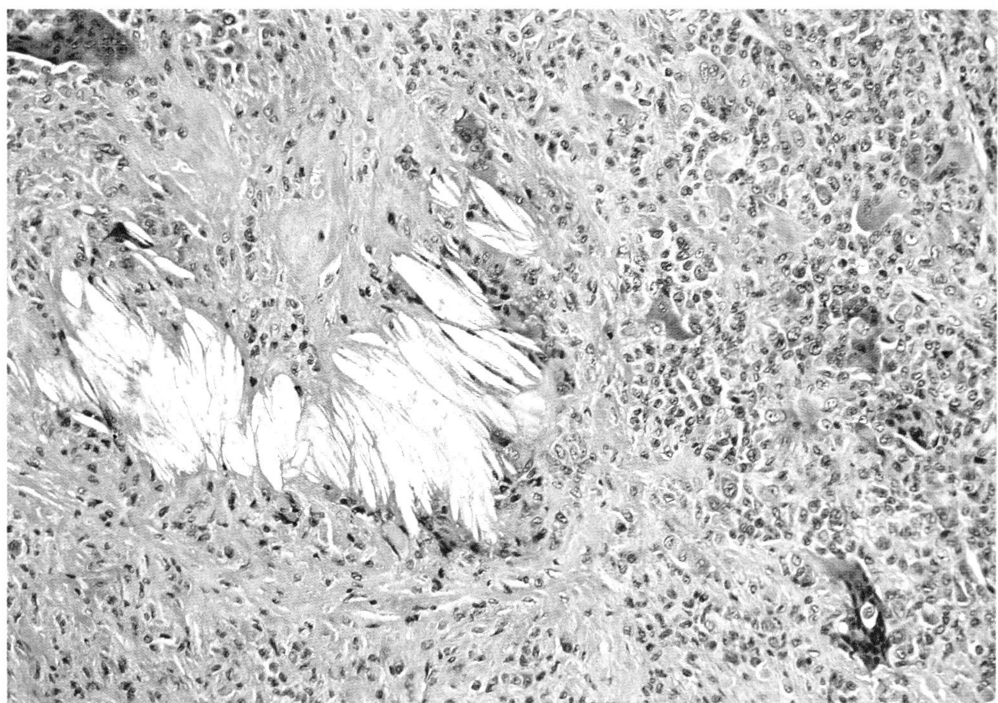

**FIGURE 28–13.** Cholesterol clefts in a localized giant cell tumor.

in the setting of hyperlipidemia are often multiple and occur in the tendon proper. Histologically, they consist almost exclusively of xanthoma cells, with only a few multinucleated giant cells and chronic inflammatory cells. "Cholesterol clefts" are characteristic of tendinous xanthomas but are usually absent in giant cell tumors. *Fibromas of the tendon sheath* bear some similarity to hyalinized forms of giant cell tumor (Fig. 28–14), and some believe that the former represents an end-stage of the latter.[36,53] In general, the cells of fibroma of the tendon sheath appear fibroblastic and are deposited in a more uniformly hyalinized stroma, although some lesions have focal features of giant cell tumors. Occasionally *epithelioid sarcomas* with numerous giant cells mimic a giant cell tumor. The relatively monomorphic population of cells and strong and diffuse expression of keratin distinguish it from giant cell tumor. Clefted areas of a giant cell tumor may also suggest the glandular component of a *biphasic synovial sarcoma,* but the cells lining the spaces are identical to those found in the solid portion of the tumor and lack epithelial features, as determined by immunohistochemistry.

## Ultrastructural and Immunohistochemical Findings

In most ultrastructural studies the cells of these lesions have been compared with normal synovium,[2,19] and the existence of both types of synovial cell has been used by some as support for a reactive process.[2] The predominant cell type has histiocyte-like features, with abundant electron-dense cytoplasm containing numerous ribosomes, a moderate number of mitochondria, and varying amounts of lysosomes.[63] These cells have a ruffled cell membrane, with pseudopodia and filopodia, and some show phagocytosis of erythrocytes or deposits of hemosiderin. A smaller proportion of cells are spindle-shaped fibroblast-like cells with well developed endoplasmic reticulum; rare cells have intracytoplasmic filaments with focal dense bodies, suggesting focal myofibroblastic differentiation.

Enzymatic and cell marker studies have supported the hypothesis that the cells are most closely related to monocytes and macrophages. They contain acid phosphatase, $\beta$-glucuronidase, and $\alpha$-naphthyl acetate esterase.[63,67]

Immunohistochemically, the mononuclear cells in giant cell tumors express CD68, HAM56, MAC387, and PG-M1[13,36,43,62] (Table 28–2). Some authors have taken this as evidence of monocyte/macrophage differentiation, whereas others have suggested a synovial origin,[13,43] given the similar immunophenotypic features of non-neoplastic synovium. A proportion of the mononuclear cells stain for factor XIIIa,[61] and rare cells also express actins.[36,43] About one-half of giant cell tumors contain occasional desmin-positive cells, the significance of which is unclear.[24] The multinucleated giant cells express CD68 and leukocyte common antigen, and several authors have suggested that

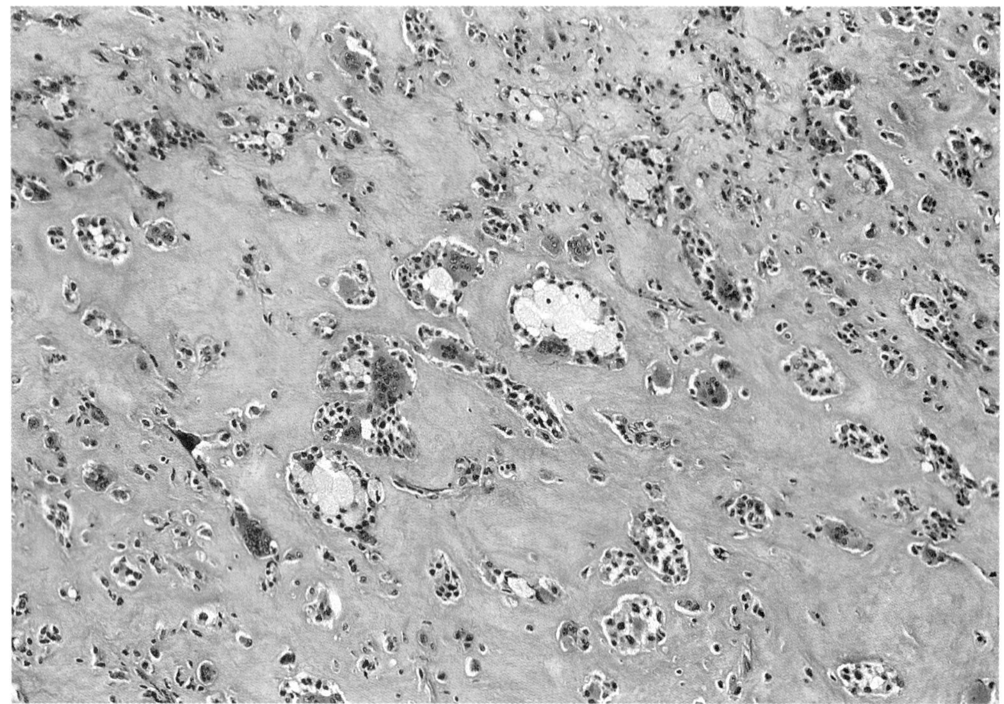

**FIGURE 28–14.** Localized giant cell tumor with extensive hyalinization bearing some resemblance to a fibroma of the tendon sheath.

these cells have features of osteoclasts based on the immunohistochemical expression of tartrate-resistant acid phosphatase, vitronectin receptor, calcitonin receptor, and parathyroid hormone-related peptide and receptor.[18,40,41,67] Only the mononuclear cells express Ki67 and proliferating cell nuclear antigen (PCNA), suggesting that they are the actively proliferating cells.[59,62,67]

## Cytogenetic Findings and DNA Ploidy

Several studies have reported clonal cytogenetic abnormalities in giant cell tumors of the tendon sheath (Table 28–3). Dal Cin et al.[17] found clonal abnormalities in five of six giant cell tumors, including three with t(1;2) (p11;q35–36), one with t(1;5)(p11;q22), and one with t(2;16)(q33;q24). More recently, Sciot et al.[58] found that rearrangements of 1p11–13 were the most frequent abnormality in both localized and diffuse forms of giant cell tumor. Other cytogenic aberrations, including abnormalities of 5q22 and 16q24, have also been described.[37,50] Mertens et al.[37] found cytogenetic aberrations in non-neoplastic synovial lesions, including hemorrhagic synovitis and rheumatoid synovitis. These cytogenetic data must be reconciled with molecular diagnostic studies indicating that

**TABLE 28–2** IMMUNOHISTOCHEMICAL FEATURES OF GIANT CELL TUMOR OF THE TENDON SHEATH AND REACTIVE SYNOVITIS

| | GCTTS | | Reactive Synovitis | |
|---|---|---|---|---|
| **Factor** | ***Mononuclear Cells*** | ***Giant Cells*** | ***Mononuclear Cells*** | ***Giant Cells*** |
| CD68 | + | + | + | + |
| MAC387 | + | − | + | − |
| HAM56 | + | − | + | − |
| LCA | +/− | + | − | + |
| S-100 protein | +/− | − | + | − |
| Keratins | − | − | − | − |
| Actins | + | − | − | − |
| Desmin | +/− | +/− | − | − |

Data are from Maluf et al.[36] and O'Connell et al.[43]
GCTTS, giant cell tumor of the tendon sheath.

**TABLE 28–3 CYTOGENETIC FINDINGS IN GIANT CELL TUMOR OF THE TENDON SHEATH**

| Study | Giant Cell Tumor Type | Cytogenetic Abnormality |
|---|---|---|
| Dal Cin et al.[17] | Localized | t(1;2)(p11;q35-36) |
| | Localized | t(1;2)(p11;q35-36) |
| | Localized | t(1;2)(p11;q35-36) |
| | Localized | t(1;5)(p11;q22) |
| | Localized | t(2;16)(q33;q24) |
| Ray et al.[50] | Localized | t(1,5;13)(p13;q35;q35;4), del (2)(q33), der (2)(pter-q31), t(5;14)(q13;q24), del (9)(p12), t (15q;22q) |
| Mertens et al.[37] | Localized | ins (5;1)(q31;p13p34) |
| Gonzalez-Campora et al.[26] | Diffuse | t(1;2)(pter-p22: :q24-pter), 5(1;14)(qter-p13: :q13-pter) |
| Rowlands et al.[51] | Diffuse | del (1)(q32q42), t5, t7, der (15)t (3;15)(q13;q24) |

these lesions are polyclonal, as seen by X chromosome inactivation analysis.[52,65]

DNA ploidy analysis of a small group of tenosynovial giant cell tumors indicates that diploid patterns are invariably present in the localized forms and in pigmented villonodular synovitis, whereas nearly half of diffuse tenosynovial giant cell tumors are aneuploid.[1] The latter group displays a higher proliferation index than the former two groups, a finding that may reflect rapid uncontrolled growth.

### Behavior and Treatment

Giant cell tumors are benign lesions that nonetheless have a capacity for local recurrence. In our experience it occurs in about 10–20% of cases, a rate roughly in accordance with that reported by others.[31,49,63] Recurrences seem to develop more often in highly cellular lesions with increased mitoses[68] and in patients who undergo simple enucleation, as microscopic residua are invariably left behind at the deep margin. Local excision with a small cuff of normal tissue is usually considered adequate therapy, even for lesions with increased cellularity and mitotic activity. Most are cured by this approach, and more extended surgery can always be planned at a later time for persistently recurring lesions.

### Discussion

Since the detailed description by Jaffe et al.[30] there has been much controversy as to whether giant cell tumors of the tendon sheath are a reactive or neoplastic process. Observation that trauma precedes about one-half of the cases, that some cases are multifocal,[9] and that similar lesions have been induced following intraarticular injections of blood in experimental animals[28,69] seem offset by cytogenetic studies indicating a clonal abnormality in these lesions, a finding that speaks strongly to a neoplastic process.[16,20] A neoplastic origin is also supported by the fact that this lesion is capable of a certain degree of autonomous growth, including local recurrence following surgical excision. Host factors may also affect the clinical behavior, as abnormalities of cellular immunity have been observed in some patients.[34] Finally, as discussed later in the chapter, rare giant cell tumors have given rise to metastatic disease.

## TENOSYNOVIAL GIANT CELL TUMOR, DIFFUSE TYPE (PROLIFERATIVE SYNOVITIS, FLORID SYNOVITIS, EXTRAARTICULAR PIGMENTED VILLONODULAR SYNOVITIS, PIGMENTED VILLONODULAR BURSITIS)

The diffuse tenosynovial giant cell tumor can be regarded as the soft tissue counterpart of pigmented villonodular synovitis of the joint space. In most instances the lesion probably represents extraarticular extension of a primary intraarticular process, a contention supported by the similarity in age, location, clinical presentation, and symptoms of the two processes. In rare instances this disease resides completely outside a joint, in which case its origin must be ascribed to the synovium of the bursa or tendon sheath.[1,18a,29,51,54] In their original description of villonodular synovitis, Jaffe et al. described four extraarticular cases (pigmented villonodular bursitis): two arising from the popliteal bursa, one from the bursa anserina, and one from the ankle bursa.[30] Additional cases have been reported in the thigh,[18a,47,48] groin (apparently arising from the iliopectineal bursa),[66] shoulder,[54] and knee.[51] Only 1 of 34 cases of pigmented villonodular synovitis reported by Atmore et al.[4] was located extraarticularly, and several of the cases reported by Arthaud[3] would probably also qualify as diffuse forms of giant cell tumor. In many instances it is difficult to define the origin of the tumor. Therefore we have employed the term *tenosynovial giant cell tumor of the diffuse type* when there is a poorly confined soft tissue mass with or without involvement of the adjacent joint.

Compared with the localized giant cell tumor, this form is uncommon and exhibits certain clinical differences. There is a tendency for these lesions to occur in young persons. About half of the cases are diagnosed prior to age 40 years, with a mean age similar to that for pigmented villonodular synovitis. Females are affected slightly more often than males. Typically, symptoms are of relatively long duration, often several years, and include pain and tenderness in the affected extremity. The additional presence of joint effusion, hemarthrosis, limitation of joint motion, and locking signify articular involvement in most cases. Its anatomic distribution parallels that of pigmented villonodular synovitis and includes the knee followed by the ankle and foot (Table 28–4). Uncommon locations are the finger, elbow, toe, and temporomandibular and sacroiliac areas. Radiographically, a soft tissue mass is usually evident and may be accompanied by osteoporosis, widening of the joint space, and cortical erosion of the adjacent bone (Fig. 28–15). Arteriography may suggest a neoplasm because of increased vascularity and early filling to the venous system.

At surgery the lesions are large, firm or sponge-like, multinodular masses. Color varies from white to yellow or brown, although usually staining with hemosiderin is less evident than in their articular counterparts, and they usually do not have grossly discernible villous patterns (Figs. 28–16, 28–17).

In contrast to localized giant cell tumors, this form is not surrounded by a mature collagenous capsule but instead grows in expansive sheets (Figs. 28–18, 28–19) interrupted by cleft-like or pseudoglandular spaces (Fig. 28–20). Many of the spaces represent residual synovial membrane, whereas others are probably artifactual. The predominant cell is round or polygonal (Fig. 28–21). Its cytoplasm may be clear or deeply brown when ladened with hemosiderin. Gradual transition between these cells, spindle cells, and xanthoma cells is common; and in some tumors the diagnosis of xanthoma is suggested. Multinucleated giant cells and chronic inflammatory cells are intermingled so the net effect is that of a highly polymorphic population of cells. In general, giant cells are less numerous than in localized tumors. In cellular areas the collagenous stroma is delicate and inconspicuous, whereas in hypocellular areas the stroma may be quite hyalinized.

These lesions usually present greater diagnostic problems than their localized counterparts. The pronounced cellularity, coupled with the clinical findings of an extensive, destructive mass is likely to lead to a diagnosis of malignancy. Particular problems arise in the early lesions, including a monomorphic popula-

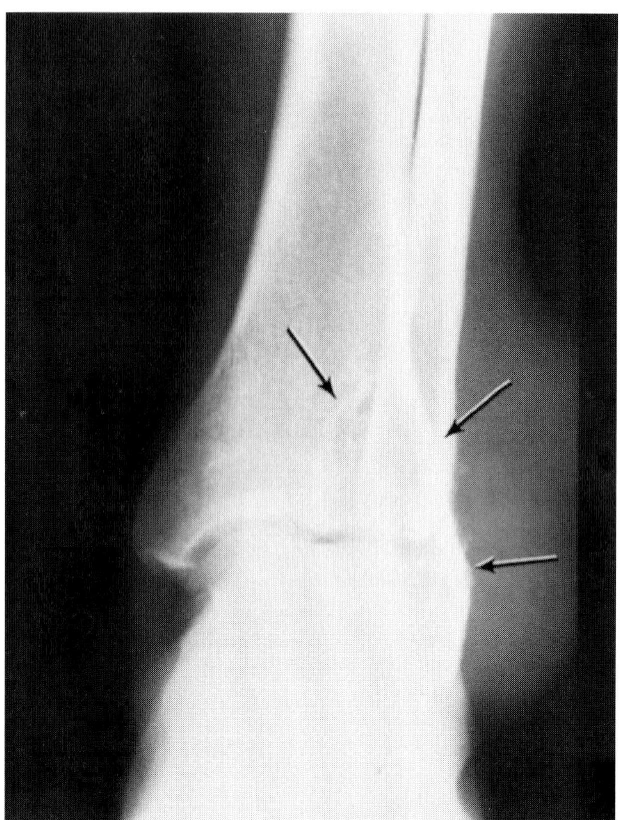

**FIGURE 28–15.** Radiograph of a diffuse form of giant cell tumor. Large soft tissue mass is present in the ankle region and has caused secondary destruction of the distal tibia and fibula (arrows). Minimal changes in the joint space suggest that the tumor arose in an extraarticular location.

**TABLE 28–4** ANATOMIC DISTRIBUTION OF DIFFUSE GIANT CELL TUMOR OF THE TENDON SHEATH (40 PATIENTS)

| Location | No. of Cases |
|---|---|
| Knee | 15 |
| Ankle and foot | 12 |
| Wrist | 5 |
| Finger | 3 |
| Elbow | 2 |
| Hip and sacroiliac region | 2 |
| Toe | 1 |
| *Total* | 40 |

Data are from the Armed Forces Institute of Pathology (AFIP).

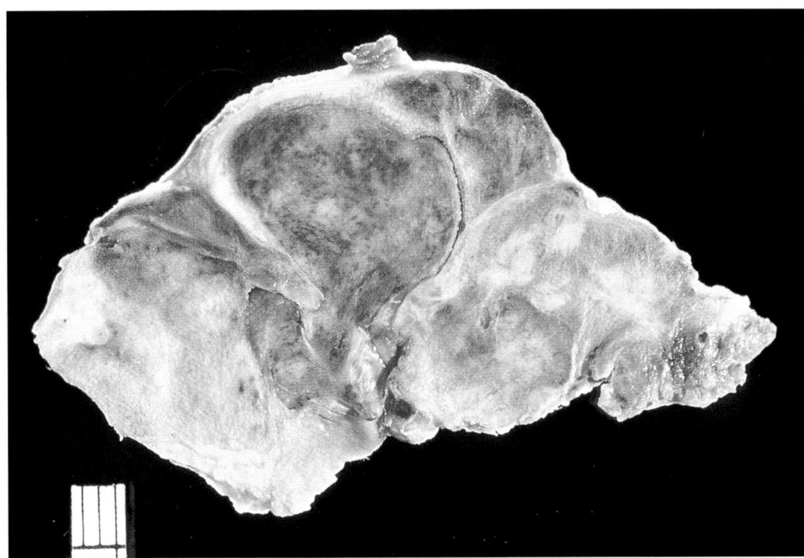

**FIGURE 28–16.** Diffuse form of giant cell tumor. The lesion has a multinodular appearance with variegated color. Shaggy villous projections, typical of pigmented villonodular synovitis, are not seen.

tion of round cells with a high nuclear to cytoplasmic ratio and a brisk mitotic rate (Figs. 28–22, 28–23). Focal necrosis may be present if torsion of a pedunculated tumor nodule has occurred. In such cases attention should be paid to the synovium-based location and to the apparent maturation of these tumor nodules at their periphery. In the peripheral zones the cells acquire a more prominent, slightly xanthomatous-appearing cytoplasm. Additional sections occasionally disclose focal giant cells, and iron staining may identify modest amounts of hemosiderin not discernible in routine sections. In more advanced lesions consisting of the classic polymorphic cellular population, other problems in differential diagnosis occur. For example, the pseudoglandular spaces are often misinterpreted as glandular spaces of a synovial sarcoma or the alveolar spaces of a rhabdomyosarcoma. The giant cell tumor shows great variation in type and arrangement of cells. Its geographic pattern of xanthomatous regions alternating with cellular hyalinized regions contrasts with the more uniform spindled appearance of most synovial sarcomas and the primitive round cells of childhood rhabdomyosarcomas. Diffuse giant cell tumors with prominent xanthomatous components must also be distinguished from inflammatory or xanthomatous forms of malignant fibrous histiocytoma. The latter, however, usually occur in the retroperitoneum and contain xanthomatous areas and spindled areas resembling the conventional forms of malignant fibrous histiocytoma. Moreover, most inflammatory forms of malignant fibrous histiocytoma have a predominantly acute inflammatory background, which contrasts with the modest number of chronic inflammatory cells that are present in giant cell tumors.

### Electron Microscopic and Immunohistochemical Features

The electron microscopic and immunohistochemical features of the diffuse type of giant cell tumor are similar to those found in the localized form. Similar to localized giant cell tumor, abnormalities of 1p have also been reported in their diffuse counterparts.[26,58] Rowlands et al.[51] reported a case with trisomy 5 and trisomy 7, similar to that described in cases of pigmented villonodular synovitis,[23,26,44,50] supporting a relation between these two lesions. Abdul-Karim et al.[1] found the proliferative index, as measured by flow cytometry, in the diffuse form of giant cell tumor to be significantly higher than that for the localized form of giant cell tumor or pigmented villonodular synovitis. Furthermore, an aneuploid DNA pattern was found in almost half of diffuse giant cell tumors, whereas all localized giant cell tumors and cases of pigmented villonodular synovitis were found to be diploid.

### Behavior and Treatment

Although much has been reported concerning the behavior and treatment of pigmented villonodular synovitis, there are few data concerning extraarticular forms of the disease. Preliminary follow-up information in our cases indicates that 40–50% of patients develop local recurrence. Recurrence rates for pigmented villonodular synovitis have been reported as 25% by Schwartz et al.[57], 46% by Byers et al.[11] and 33% in the recent series reported by de Saint Aubain Somerhausen and Fletcher.[18a] Recurrences can be correlated with a location in the knee and incomplete excision, with a cumulative probability of recurrence

*Text continued on page 1054*

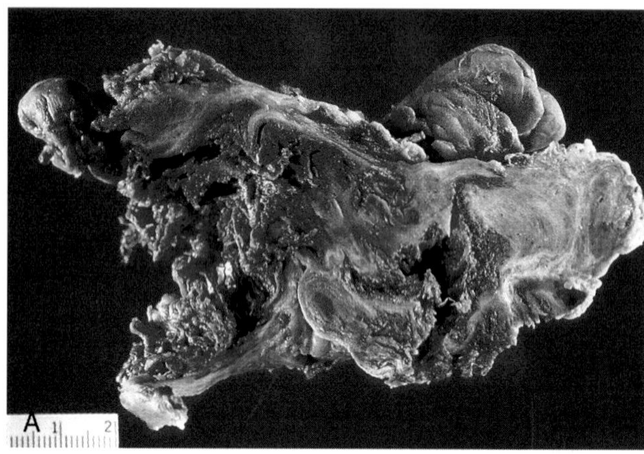

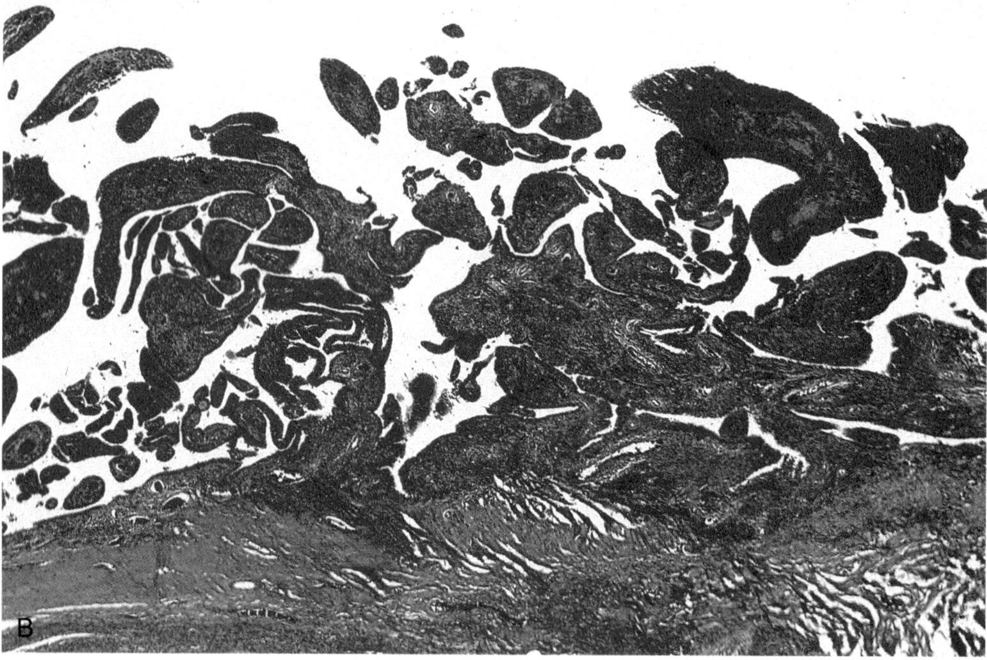

**FIGURE 28–17.** Intraarticular form of diffuse giant cell tumor (pigmented villonodular synovitis). Note the shaggy villous appearance in the gross (**A**) and microscopic (**B**) specimens.

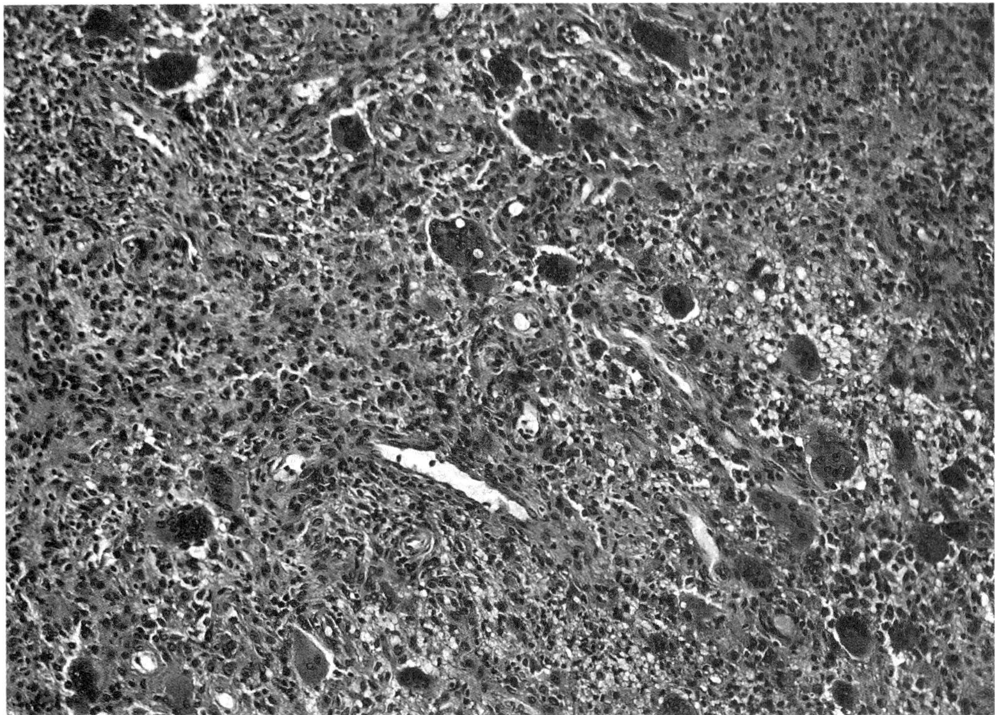

**FIGURE 28–18.** Diffuse form of giant cell tumor characterized by sheets of rounded synovial-like cells admixed with multinucleated giant cells and xanthoma cells with hemosiderin.

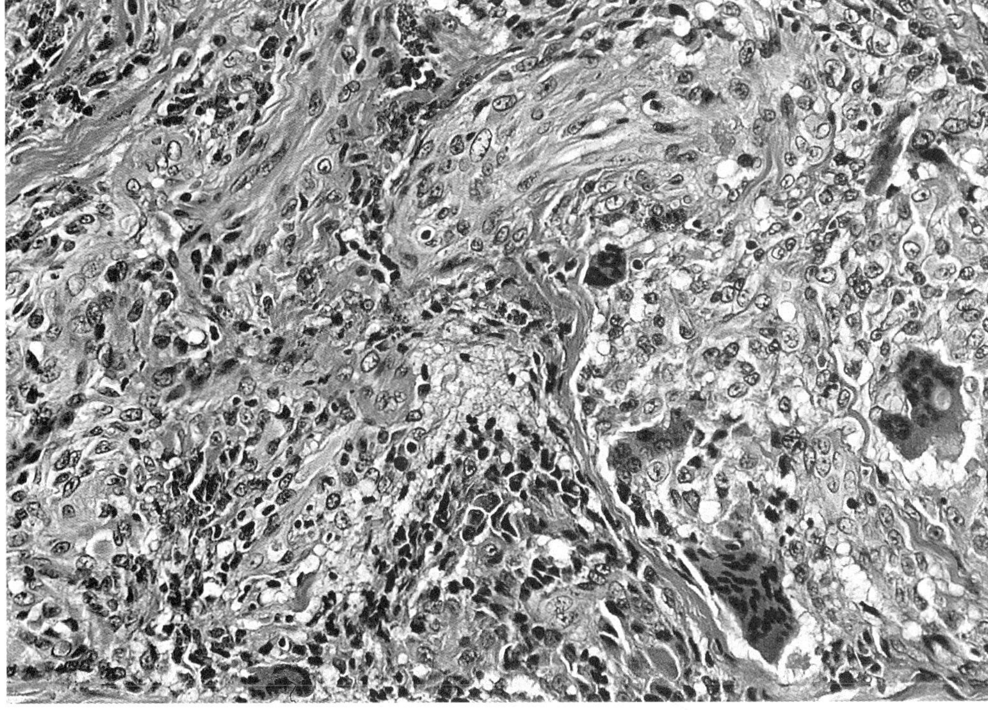

**FIGURE 28–19.** High-power view of diffuse type of giant cell tumor.

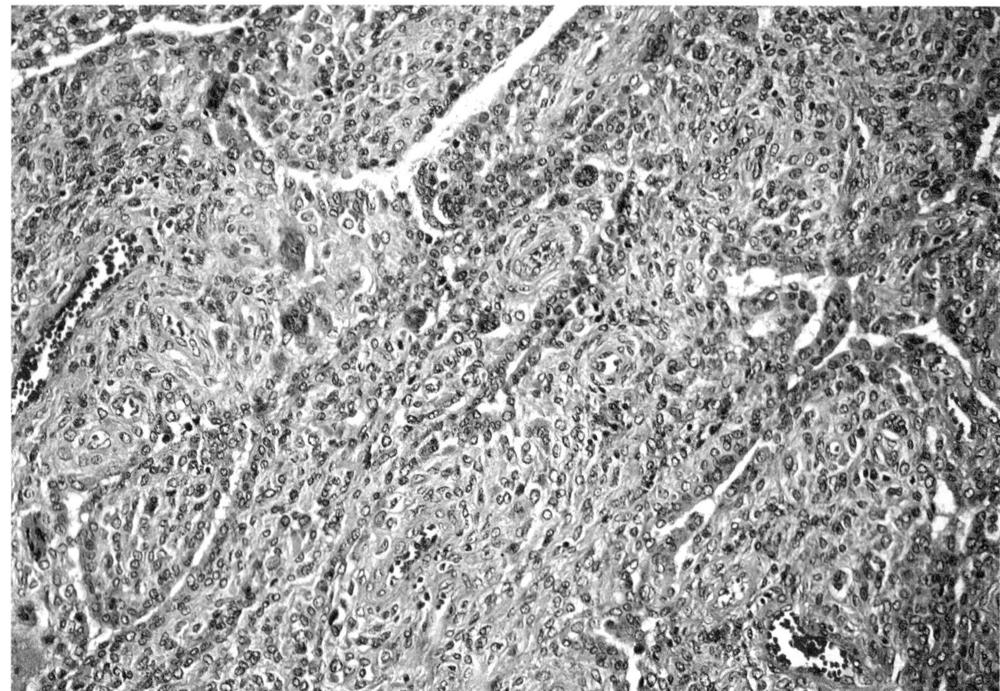

**FIGURE 28–20.** Pseudoglandular spaces in a diffuse giant cell tumor.

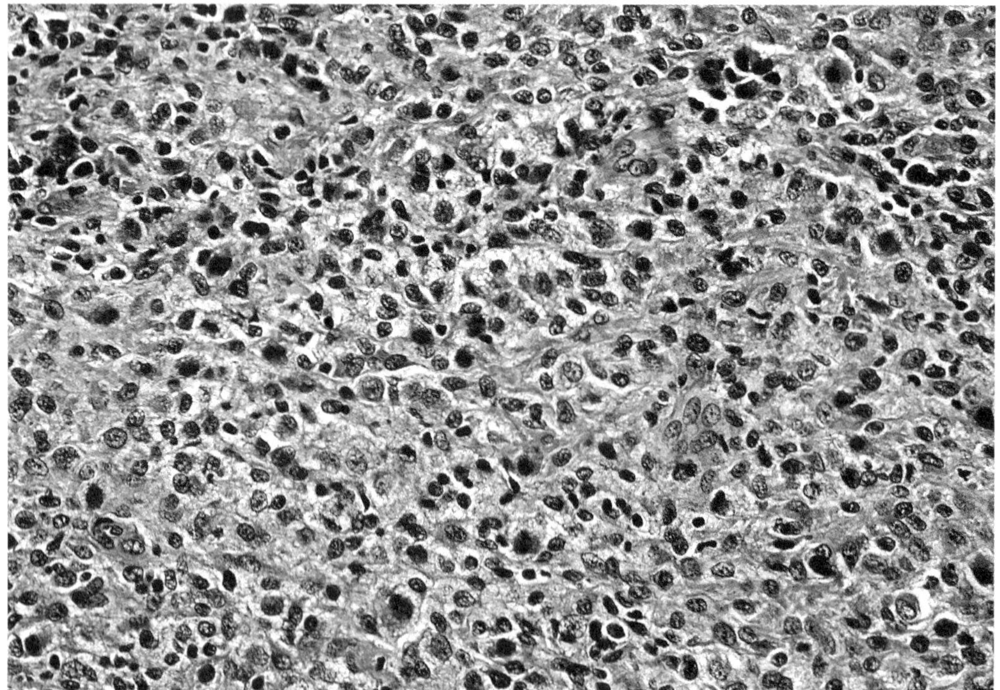

**FIGURE 28–21.** High-power view of monotonous round cells in a diffuse type of giant cell tumor.

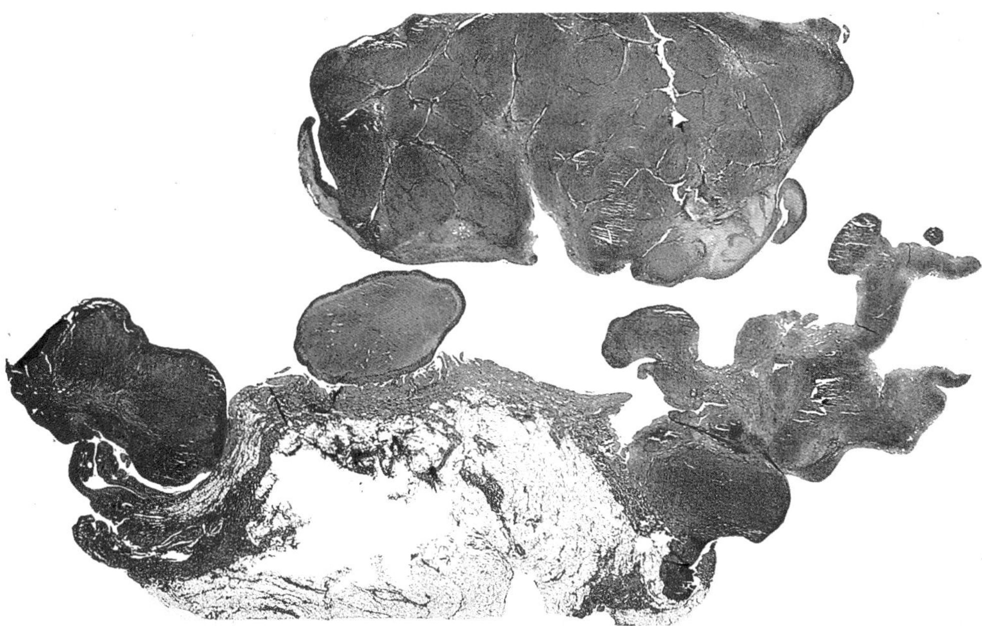

**FIGURE 28–22.** Early stage of a diffuse intraarticular giant cell tumor. Note necrosis of one of the nodules due to torsion of the tumor on its stalk.

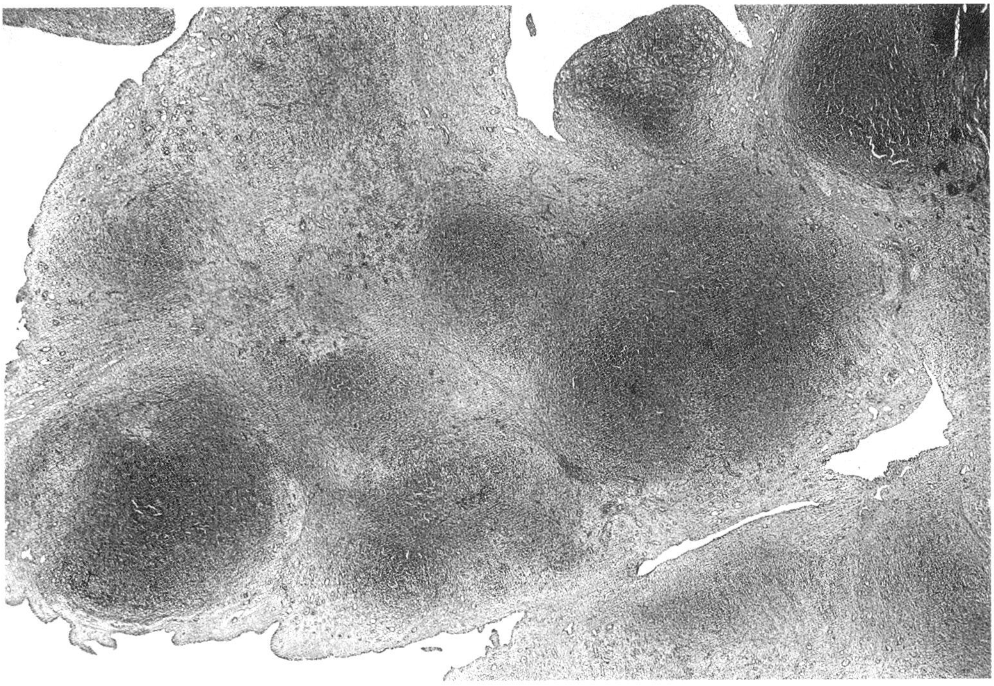

**FIGURE 28–23.** Early stage of a diffuse giant cell tumor (same case as Figure 28–22). The lesion has a distinctly nodular architecture.

of 15% at 5 years and 35% at 25 years,[57] however, morphologic features have not been found to be predictive of recurrence.[18a] We have also reported one diffuse recurrent giant cell tumor arising from the foot that metastasized to the lung after several years (Fig. 28–24). This case appears to be unique because metastases have not been observed in the collective experience of others.

Thus from a practical point of view, these lesions should be regarded as locally aggressive but nonmetastasizing lesions. Therapy should be based on a desire to remove the tumor as completely as possible without producing severe disability for the patient. Although wide excision or amputation is the best choice for local control of the disease, it implies significant morbidity, especially for lesions located adjacent to major joints. Less radical excision therefore is justified in these cases. Although radiotherapy has been endorsed for treatment of surgically unresectable villonodular synovitis,[45] there is no recorded experience concerning its use for this form of the disease.

## MALIGNANT GIANT CELL TUMOR OF THE TENDON SHEATH/PIGMENTED VILLONODULAR SYNOVITIS

Malignant giant cell tumors of the tendon sheath/pigmented villonodular synovitis comprise a rare group of tumors, the existence of which has been doubted by some and the diagnosis of which is difficult. The belief that the giant cell tumor is an inflammatory condition has led to the conclusion by some that malignant forms of this disease do not exist. Others have accepted any sarcoma that contains giant cells arising in the vicinity of a tendon as a "malignant giant cell tumor of the tendon sheath."[39] Consequently, malignant giant cell tumors of the tendon sheath as reported in the literature constitute a variety of lesions, including clear cell sarcoma, fibrosarcoma, epithelioid sarcoma, and malignant fibrous histiocytoma. Still others have implied that diffuse forms of the giant cell tumor, which behave in a locally aggressive fashion, should be considered malignant, although the morphologic appearance may remain unaltered during the course of the disease. Although each of these approaches has its validity, we have generally reserved the designation malignant giant cell tumor of the tendon sheath/pigmented villonodular synovitis for lesions in which a benign giant cell tumor or pigmented villonodular synovitis coexists with frankly malignant areas or when the original lesion was typical of a benign giant cell tumor or pigmented villonodular synovitis and the recurrence appeared malignant (Fig. 28–25). Defined in this fashion, true malignant giant cell tumors of the tendon sheath/pigmented villonodular synovitis comprise a rare group of tumors and are far outnumbered by benign lesions or even tumors with atypical features.

Carstens and Howell[12] were the first to report a malignant giant cell tumor. The original lesion was described as a giant cell tumor of the tendon sheath with atypical features that arose in the dorsum of the right foot. Following local excision, the lesion recurred repeatedly over many years and ultimately gave rise to numerous local metastases on the same extremity. Subsequently, Schajowicz described a case of pigmented villonodular synovitis of the knee that

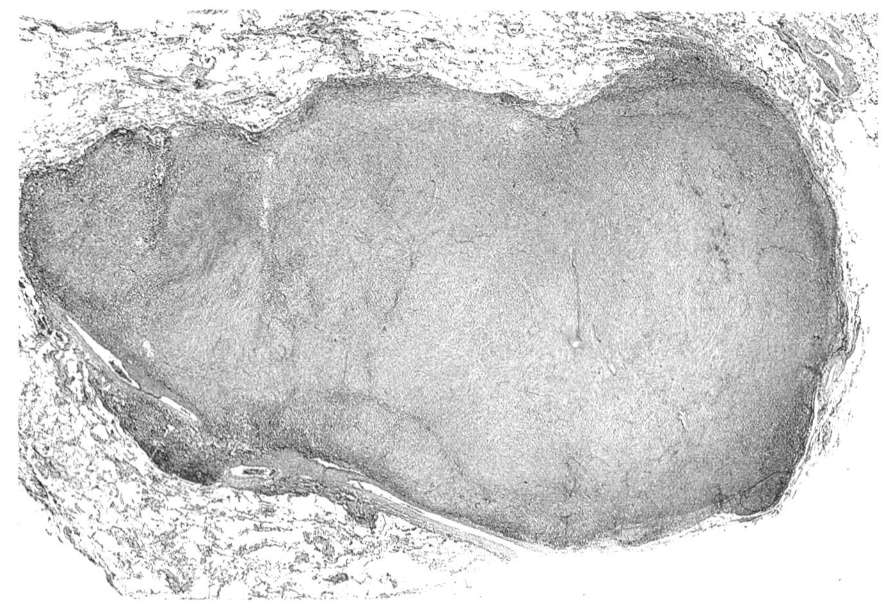

**FIGURE 28–24.** Pulmonary metastasis from a diffuse form of giant cell tumor of the foot.

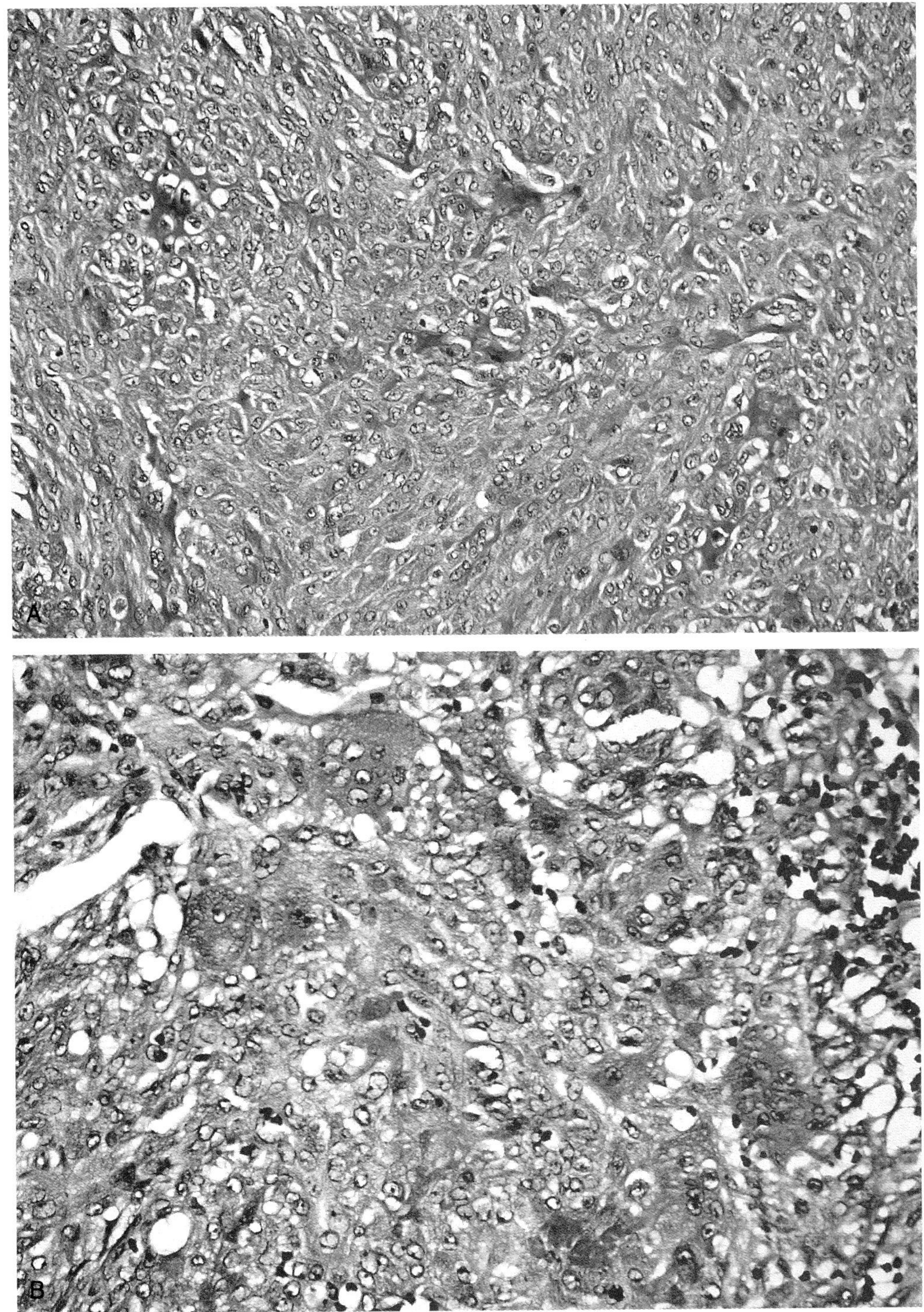


**FIGURE 28–25.** Low-power (**A**) and high-power (**B**) views of a malignant giant cell tumor of the tendon sheath. This tumor is characterized by sheets of large round cells devoid of intervening stroma.

**TABLE 28–5 CLINICAL FEATURES OF MALIGNANT GIANT CELL TUMOR OF THE TENDON SHEATH/PIGMENTED VILLONODULAR SYNOVITIS AND PIGMENTED VILLONODULAR SYNOVITIS**

| Parameter | PVNS | MPVNS |
|---|---|---|
| Age | 50% < 40 years | 12–79 years (peak: 6th decade) |
| Gender | Females > males | Females > males |
| Local recurrence (%) | 25–50 | 60–70 |
| Metastasis (%) | — | 60–70 |
| Died of tumor (%) | None | 40–50 |

Modified from Bertoni F, Unni KK, Beabout JW, et al. Malignant giant cell tumor of the tendon sheaths and joints (malignant pigmented villonodular synovitis). Am J Surg Pathol 21:153, 1997.
PVNS, pigmented villonodular synovitis; MPVNS, malignant pigmented villonodular synovitis.

recurred as a histologically malignant neoplasm and ultimately gave rise to pulmonary metastases.[55] There are several other documented cases of giant cell tumors of tendon sheath/pigmented villonodular synovitis that appeared histologically malignant following recurrence, some of which metastasized[1,15,18a,60] and others of which did not.[64]

Bertoni et al.[7] described three cases of typical pigmented villonodular synovitis that had histologic features of malignancy in recurrent lesions. No pathologic features were useful for predicting malignant transformation. In addition, they reported five cases of "malignant pigmented villonodular synovitis" that were primary (i.e., did not arise in previously documented pigmented villonodular synovitis) but had histologic features similar to those found in the cases of secondary malignant pigmented villonodular synovitis.

These tumors were characterized by nodules or sheets of oval to round cells with larger hyperchromatic nuclei and more prominent nucleoli than are found in typical cases of pigmented villonodular synovitis. Mitotic figures, including atypical mitoses, were seen, as was more extensive necrosis than is usually seen in pigmented villonodular synovitis. Furthermore, the zoning phenomenon seen in pigmented villonodular synovitis, in which the cells at the periphery of the nodules have smaller nuclei and more cytoplasm, was not found in the malignant cases (Table 28–5). In this series, four patients died with pulmonary or nodal metastases or owing to local extension into the pelvis or cranium; four patients were alive after wide aggressive surgical procedures. A similar case of "primary" malignant pigmented villonodular synovitis was reported by Nielsen and Kiaer.[42] It is still unclear whether these cases of "primary" malignant pigmented villonodular synovitis truly represent a malignant form of pigmented villonodular synovitis or are better interpreted as an intraarticular sarcoma with giant cells. Fanburg-Smith and Miettinen[21] reported 27 histologically malignant giant cell tumors of the tendon sheath, 6 of which were clinically malignant. The clinically malignant cases were characterized histologically by a diffuse infiltrative growth pattern, scant giant cells, nucleomegaly and macronucleoli, tumor cell dyscohesion, necrosis, and mitotic counts of more than 10 mitoses/10 HPF. Wide excision or amputation of true malignant forms of tenosynovial giant cell tumor/pigmented villonodular synovitis is indicated.

## MISCELLANEOUS CONDITIONS RESEMBLING DIFFUSE GIANT CELL TUMOR

Occasionally, reactive synovial lesions mimic the appearance of a diffuse giant cell tumor, particularly lesions of the intraarticular type (pigmented villonodular synovitis). Perhaps the most common condition that produces this picture is intraarticular hemorrhage. Long known to be associated with synovitis in hemophiliacs, intraarticular hemorrhage can give rise to hyperplastic changes of the synovium consisting of villous change and large deposits of hemosiderin.[75,76] However, only in the early stages of chronic hemarthrosis are the lesions reminiscent of pigmented villonodular synovitis. During the late stage the synovium is flattened and the subjacent tissue markedly fibrotic. A second, less well recognized condition is the synovitis associated with failed orthopedic prosthetic devices.[71–73,78,79] Collectively termed "detritic synovitis," these lesions are characterized by villous hyperplasia of the synovium (Fig. 28–26A). The subsynovial space is infiltrated with histiocytes, multinucleated giant cells, and a variable number of chronic inflammatory cells. The prosthetic material can be detected under polarized light as weakly birefringent intracellular or extracellular spicules (Fig. 28–26B). Usually it can also be stained with oil red O,

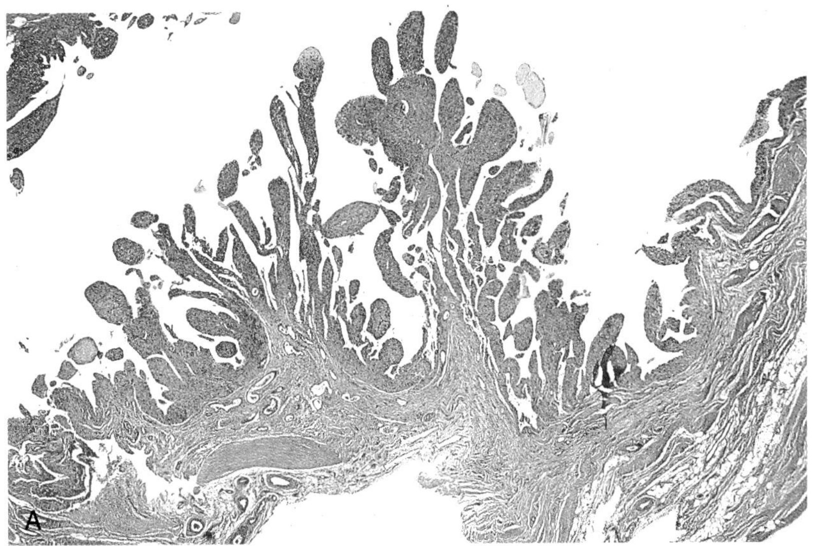

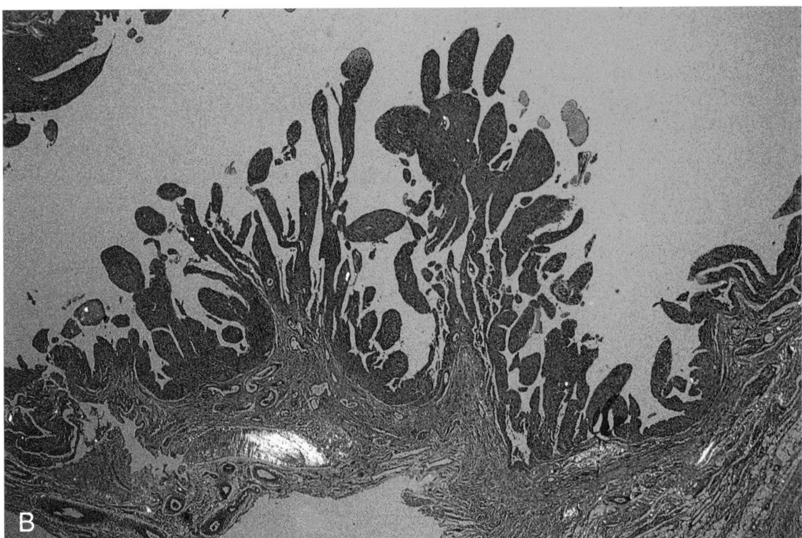

**FIGURE 28–26.** (**A**) Detritic synovitis showing villous configuration of the synovium. (**B**) Graft material is visible as birefringent particles in this partially polarized view.

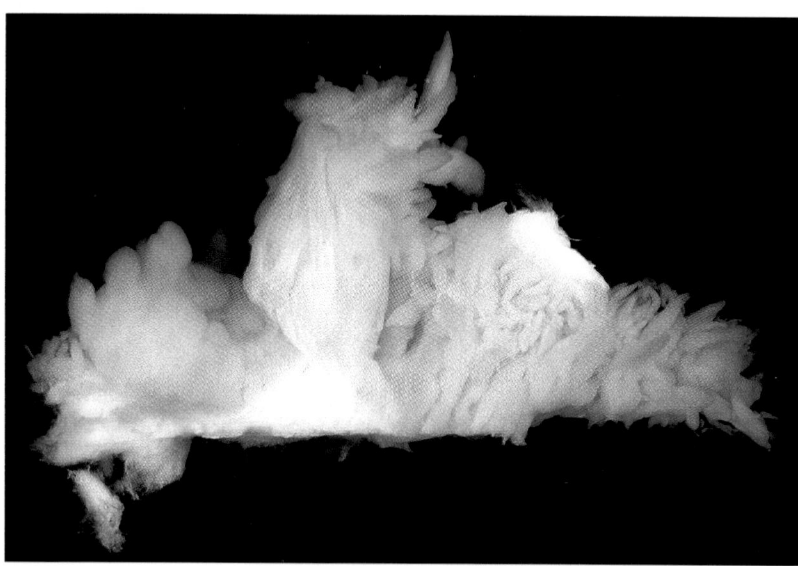

**FIGURE 28–27.** Gross appearance of synovium in a patient with α-mannosidase deficiency. Note that the synovium has delicate villous fronds.

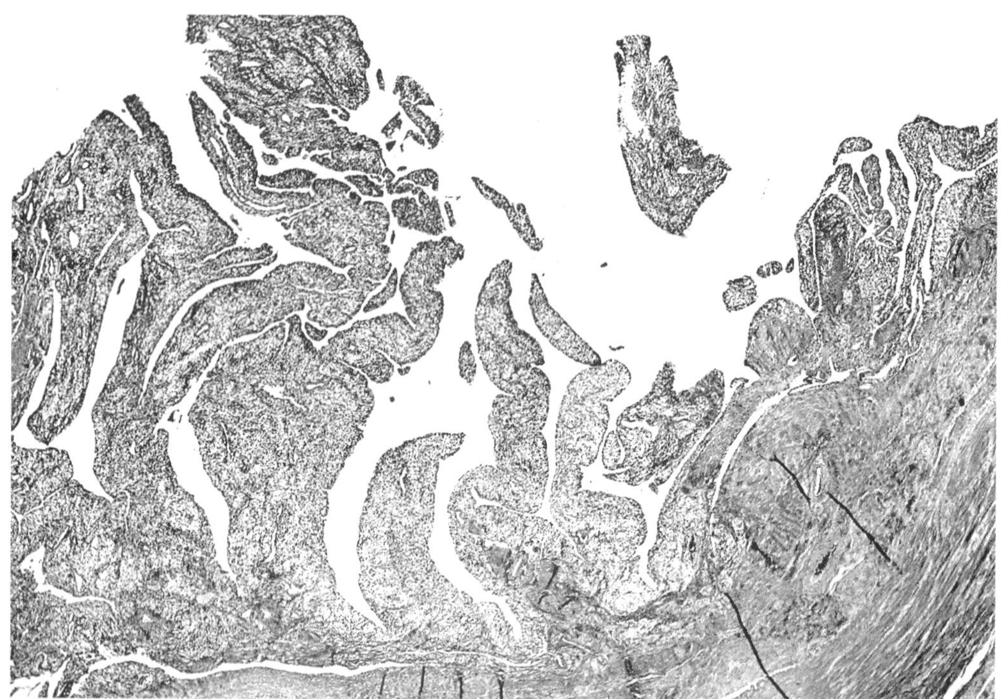

**FIGURE 28–28.** Synovitis due to α-mannosidase deficiency. At low power the lesion superficially resembles pigmented villonodular synovitis.

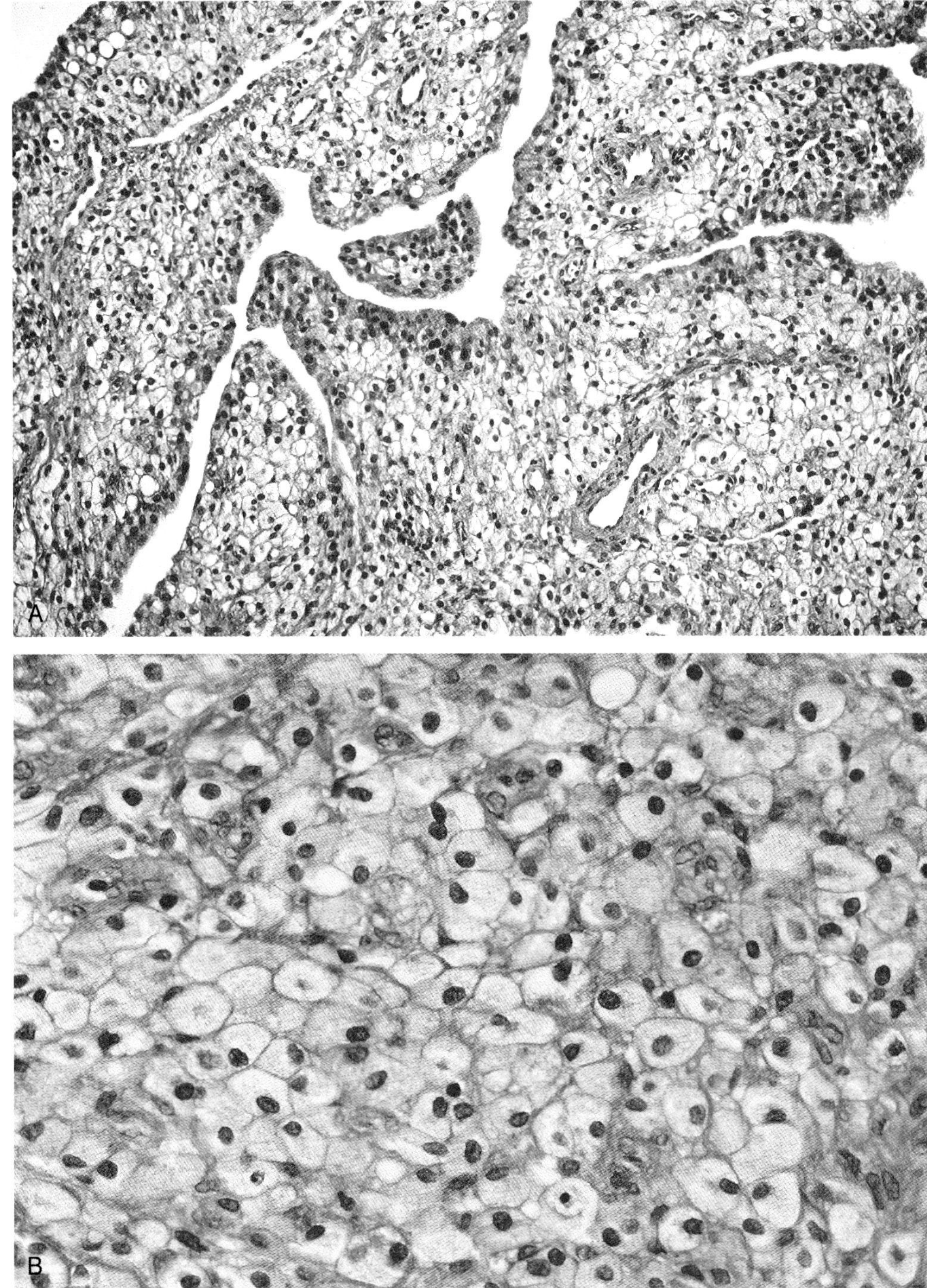

**FIGURE 28–29.** (**A**) Synovitis due to $\alpha$-mannosidase deficiency composed of synovial-lined papillary projections with centrally located vacuolated cells. (**B**) At high power the infiltrate consists of clear-appearing histiocytes containing PAS-positive, diastase-resistant bodies representing partially degraded oligosaccharides. (From Weiss SW, Kelly WD. Bilateral destructive synovitis associated with alpha-mannosidase deficiency. Am J Surg Pathol 7:487, 1983.)

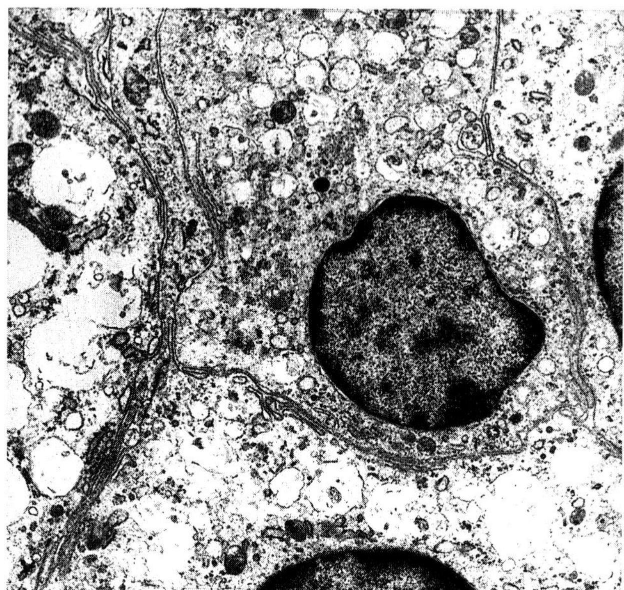

**FIGURE 28–30.** Electron micrograph of histiocytes from the synovium of a patient with α-mannosidase deficiency. Oligosaccharide is represented by granuloamorphous material in lysosomes. (From Weiss SW, Kelly WD. Bilateral destructive synovitis associated with alpha-mannosidase deficiency. Am J Surg Pathol 7:487, 1983.)

but it requires a long incubation period (up to 48 hours). These reactions can occur with polyethylene and silicone rubber devices and possibly also methylmethacrylate, which is used as a cement in metal prostheses. In addition, histiocytic reactions in the lymph nodes draining the regions of prosthetic devices have been reported.[70,74] Finally, we reviewed synovial tissue from a patient with α-mannosidase deficiency who developed bilateral destructive synovitis of the ankle region.[77] The hyperplastic villous-appearing synovium was infiltrated with clear-appearing histiocytes containing PAS-positive, diastase-resistant material representing partially degraded oligosaccharides in lysosomes (Figs. 28–27 to 28–30). Although definitive diagnosis requires an adequate clinical history with confirmatory biochemical data, the presence of a systemic disease was suspected because of the bilaterally symmetric distribution of the lesions, a distribution seldom encountered in pigmented villonodular synovitis.

## REFERENCES

### Giant Cell Tumor of Tendon Sheath

1. Abdul-Karim FW, El-Naggar A, Joyce MJ, et al. Diffuse and localized tenosynovial giant cell tumor and pigmented villonodular synovitis: a clinicopathologic and flow cytometric DNA analysis. Hum Pathol 23:729, 1992.
2. Alguacil-Garcia A, Unni KK, Goellner JR. Giant cell tumor of tendon sheath and pigmented villonodular synovitis: an ultrastructural study. Am J Clin Pathol 69:6, 1978.
3. Arthaud JB. Pigmented nodular synovitis: report of 11 lesions in nonarticular locations. Am J Clin Pathol 58:511, 1972.
4. Atmore WG, Dahlin DC, Ghormley RK. Pigmented villonodular synovitis: a clinical and pathologic study. Minn Med 39:196, 1956.
5. Baes H, Tanghe W. Nodular tenosynovitis. Dermatologica 149: 149, 1974.
6. Barland P, Novikoff AB, Hamerman D. Electron microscopy of the human synovial membrane. J Cell Biol 14:207, 1962.
7. Bertoni F, Unni KK, Beabout JW, et al. Malignant giant cell tumor of the tendon sheaths and joints (malignant pigmented villonodular synovitis). Am J Surg Pathol 21:153, 1997.
8. Booth KC, Campbell GS, Chase DR, et al. Giant cell tumor of tendon sheath with intraosseous invasion: a case report. J Hand Surg [Am] 20:1000, 1995.
9. Brown-Crosby E, Inglis A, Bullough PG. Multiple joint involvement with pigmented villonodular synovitis. Radiology 122:671, 1977.
10. Burmester GR, Dimitriu-Bona A, Waters SJ, et al. Identification of three major synovial lining cell populations by monoclonal antibodies directed to Ia antigens and antigens associated with monocytes/macrophages and fibroblasts. Scand J Immunol 17: 69, 1983.
11. Byers PD, Cotton RE, Deacon OW, et al. The diagnosis and treatment of pigmented villonodular synovitis. J Bone Joint Surg Br 50:290, 1968.
12. Carstens PHB, Howell RS. Malignant giant cell tumor of tendon sheath. Virchows Arch [Pathol Anat] 382:237, 1979.
13. Cavaliere A, Sidoni A, Bucciarelli E. Giant cell tumor of tendon sheath: immunohistochemical study of 20 cases. Tumori 83:841, 1997.
14. Chassaignac CME. Cancer de la gaine des tendons. Gaz Hosp Civ Milit 47:185, 1852.
15. Choong PF, Willen H, Nilbert M, et al. Pigmented villonodular synovitis: monoclonality in metastases: a case for neoplastic origin? Acta Orthop Scand 66:64, 1995.
16. Dal Cin P, Sciot R, De Snet L, et al. A new cytogenetic subgroup in tenosynovial giant cell tumors (nodular tenosynovitis) is characterized by involvement of 16q24. Cancer Genet Cytogenet 87:85, 1996.
17. Dal Cin P, Sciot R, Samson I, et al. Cytogenetic characterization of tenosynovial giant cell tumors (nodular tenosynovitis). Cancer Res 54:3986, 1994.
18. Darling JM, Goldring SR, Harada Y, et al. Multinucleated cells in pigmented villonodular synovitis and giant cell tumor of tendon sheath express features of osteoclasts. Am J Pathol 150: 1383, 1997.
18a. De Saint Aubain Somerhausen N, Fletcher CDM. Diffuse-type giant cell tumor: Clinicopathologic and immunohistochemical analysis of 50 cases with extraarticular disease. Am J Surg Pathol 24:479, 2000.
19. Eisenstein R. Giant cell tumor of tendon sheath. J Bone Joint Surg Am 50:476, 1968.
20. El-Naggar AK, Abdul-Karim FW. Tenosynovial giant cell tumors and other lesions traditionally considered to be reactive: further evidence for neoplastic etiology. Adv Anat Pathol 2:329, 1995.
21. Fanburg-Smith JC, Miettinen M. Malignant giant cell tumors of tendon sheath: histologic classification with clinical correlation. Clin Exp Pathol 46:16A, 1998.
22. Fletcher AG, Horn RC. Giant cell tumors of tendon sheath origin. Ann Surg 133:374, 1951.
23. Fletcher JA, Henkle C, Atkins L, et al. Trisomy 5 and trisomy 7 are nonrandom aberrations in pigmented villonodular synovi-

tis: confirmation of trisomy 7 in uncultured cells. Genes Chromosomes Cancer 4:264, 1992.

24. Folpe AL, Weiss SW, Fletcher CDM, et al. Tenosynovial giant cell tumors: evidence for a desmin-positive dendritic cell subpopulation. Mod Pathol 11:939, 1998.
25. Geweiler JA, Wilson JW. Diffuse biarticular pigmented villonodular synovitis. Radiology 93:845, 1969.
26. Gonzalez-Campora R, Salas Herrero E, Otal-Salaverri C, et al. Diffuse tenosynovial giant cell tumor of soft tissue: report of a case with cytologic and cytogenetic findings. Acta Cytol 39:770, 1995.
27. Heurteux MA. Myelome des gaines tendineuses. Arch Gen Med 167:40, 160, 1891.
28. Hoaglund FT. Experimental hemarthrosis. J Bone Joint Surg [Br] 49:285, 1967.
29. Horvath RR, Bostanche J, Altman MI. Diffuse type tenosynovial giant cell tumor of the ankle. J Am Podiatr Med Assoc 83:231, 1993.
30. Jaffe HL, Lichtenstein L, Sutro CJ. Pigmented villonodular synovitis, bursitis, and tenosynovitis: a discussion of the synovial and bursal equivalents of the tenosynovial lesions commonly denoted as xanthoma, xanthogranuloma, giant cell tumor, or myeloma of the tendon sheath, with some consideration of the tendon sheath lesion itself. Arch Pathol 31:731, 1941.
31. Jones FE, Soule EH, Coventry MB. Fibrous histiocytoma of synovium (giant cell tumor of tendon sheath, pigmented nodular synovitis). J Bone Joint Surg Am 51:76, 1969.
32. Karasick D, Karasick J. Giant cell tumor of tendon sheath: spectrum of radiologic findings. Skeletal Radiol 21:219, 1992.
33. Kindblom LG, Gunterberg B. Pigmented villonodular synovitis involving bone. J Bone Joint Surg Am 60:830, 1978.
34. Kinsella TD, Vasey F, Ashworth MA. Perturbations of humoral and cellular immunity in a patient with pigmented villonodular synovitis. Am J Med 58:444, 1975.
35. Lever JD, Ford EHR. Histological, histochemical, and electron microscopic observations on synovial membrane. Anat Rec 132: 525, 1958.
36. Maluf HM, DeYoung BR, Swanson PE, et al. Fibroma and giant cell tumor of tendon sheath: a comparative histological and immunohistological study. Mod Pathol 8:155, 1995.
37. Mertens FM, Örndahl C, Mandahl N, et al. Chromosome aberrations in tenosynovial giant cell tumors and nontumorous synovial tissue. Genes Chromosomes Cancer 6:212, 1993.
38. Moore JR, Weiland AJ, Curtis RM. Localized nodular tenosynovitis: experience with 115 cases. J Hand Surg [Am] 9:412, 1984.
39. Myers BW, Masi AT, Feigenbaum SL. Pigmented villonodular synovitis and tenosynovitis: a clinical epidemiologic study of 166 cases and literature review. Medicine 59:223, 1980.
40. Nakashima M, Ito M, Ohtsuru A, et al. Expression of parathyroid hormone (PTH)-related peptide (PTHrP) and PTH/PTHrP receptor in giant cell tumor of tendon sheath. J Pathol 180:80, 1996.
41. Neale SD, Kristelly R, Gundle R, et al. Giant cells in pigmented villonodular synovitis express an osteoclast phenotype. J Clin Pathol 50:605, 1997.
42. Nielsen AL, Kiaer T. Malignant giant cell tumor of synovium and locally destructive pigmented villonodular synovitis: ultrastructural and immunohistochemical study and review of the literature. Hum Pathol 20:765, 1989.
43. O'Connell JX, Fanburg JC, Rosenberg AE. Giant cell tumor of tendon sheath and pigmented villonodular synovitis: immunophenotype suggests a synovial cell origin. Hum Pathol 26:771, 1995.
44. Ohjimi Y, Iwasaki H, Ishituro M, et al. Short arm of chromosome 1 aberration recurrently found in pigmented villonodular synovitis. Cancer Genet Cytogenet 90:80, 1996.
45. O'Sullivan B, Cummings B, Catton C, et al. Outcome following radiation treatment for high-risk pigmented villonodular synovitis. Int J Radiat Oncol Biol Phys 32:777, 1995.
46. Palmer DG, Selvendran Y, Allen C, et al. Features of synovial membrane identified with monoclonal antibodies. Clin Exp Immunol 59:529, 1985.
47. Peterson LFA, Johnson EW Jr, Woolner LB. Extraarticular pigmented villonodular synovitis of the knee: report of a case. Am J Clin Pathol 30:158, 1958.
48. Probst FP. Extraarticular pigmented villonodular synovitis affecting bone: the role of angiography as an aid in its differentiation from similar bone-destroying conditions. Radiologe 13: 436, 1973.
49. Rao AS, Vigorita VJ. Pigmented villonodular synovitis (giant cell tumor of the tendon sheath and synovial membrane): a review of eighty-one cases. J Bone Joint Surg Am 66:76, 1984.
50. Ray RA, Morton CC, Lipinski KK, et al. Cytogenetic evidence of clonality in a case of pigmented villonodular synovitis. Cancer 67:121, 1991.
51. Rowlands CG, Roland B, Hwang WS, et al. Diffuse-variant tenosynovial giant cell tumor: a rare and aggressive lesion. Hum Pathol 25:423, 1994.
52. Sakkers RJ, de Jong D, van der Heul RO. X-chromosome inactivation in patients who have pigmented villonodular synovitis. J Bone Joint Surg Am 73:1532, 1991.
53. Satti MB. Tendon sheath tumours: a pathological study of the relationship between giant cell tumour and fibroma of tendon sheath. Histopathology 20:213, 1992.
54. Sawmiller CJ, Turowski GA, Sterling AT, et al. Extraarticular pigmented villondular synovitis of the shoulder: a case report. Clin Orthop 335:262, 1997.
55. Schajowicz F. Tumors and Tumor-like Lesions of Bone and Joints. Springer-Verlag, New York, 1981, p 521.
56. Schmidt D, Mackay B. Ultrastructure of human tendon sheath and synovium: implication for tumor histogenesis. Ultrastruct Pathol 3:269, 1982.
57. Schwartz HS, Unni KK, Pritchard DJ. Pigmented villonodular synovitis: a retrospective review of affected large joints. Clin Orthop 247:243, 1989.
58. Sciot R, Rosai J, Dal Cin P, et al. Analysis of 35 cases of localized and diffuse tenosynovial giant cell tumor: a report from the Chromosomes and Morphology (CHAMP) Study Group. Mod Pathol 12:576, 1999.
59. Seki K, Hirose T, Hasegawa T, et al. Giant cell tumor of tendon sheath: an immunohistochemical observation on the characteristics and the capacity of proliferation of tumor cells. Z Pathol 139:287, 1993.
60. Shinjo K, Miyake N, Takahashi Y. Malignant giant cell tumor of the tendon sheath: an autopsy report and review of the literature. Jpn J Clin Oncol 23:317, 1993.
61. Silverman JS, Knapik M. Fibroma of tendon sheath and tendosynovial giant cell tumors are rich in factor XIIIa dendrophages. J Histotechnol 19:45, 1996.
62. Tashiro H, Iwasaki H, Kikuchi M, et al. Giant cell tumors of tendon sheath: a single and multiple immunostaining analysis. Pathol Int 45:147, 1995.
63. Ushijima M, Hashimoto H, Tsuneyoshi M, et al. Giant cell tumor of the tendon sheath (nodular tenosynovitis): a study of 207 cases to compare the large joint group with the common digit group. Cancer 57:875, 1986.
64. Ushijima M, Hashimoto H, Tsuneyoshi M, et al. Malignant giant cell tumor of tendon sheath: a report of a case. Acta Pathol Jpn 35:699, 1985.
65. Vogrincic GS, O'Connell JX, Gilks CB. Giant cell tumor of tendon sheath is a polyclonal cellular proliferation. Hum Pathol 28:815, 1997.
66. Weisser JR, Robinson DW. Pigmented villonodular synovitis of

iliopectineal bursa: a case report. J Bone Joint Surg Am 33:988, 1951.

67. Wood GS, Beckstead JH, Medeiros LJ, et al. The cells of giant cell tumor of tendon sheaths resemble osteoclast. Am J Surg Pathol 12:444, 1988.
68. Wright CJE. Benign giant cell synovioma. Br J Surg 38:257, 1951.
69. Young JM, Hudacek AG. Experimental production of pigmented villonodular synovitis in dogs. Am J Pathol 30:799, 1954.

### Miscellaneous Conditions Resembling Diffuse Giant Cell Tumors

70. Albores-Saavedra J, Vuitch LF, Delgado R, et al. Sinus histiocytosis of pelvic lymph nodes after hip replacement: a histiocytic proliferation induced by cobalt-chromium and titanium. Am J Surg Pathol 18:83, 1994.
71. Christie AD, Weinberger KA, Dietrich M. Silicone lymphadenopathy and synovitis: complications of silicone elastomer finger joint prostheses. JAMA 237:1463, 1977.
72. Ewald FC, Sledge CB, Corson JM, et al. Giant cell synovitis associated with failed polyethylene patellar replacements. Clin Orthop 15:213, 1976.
73. Gordon M, Bullough PG. Synovial and osseous inflammation in failed silicone-rubber prostheses: a report of six cases. J Bone Joint Surg Am 64:574, 1982.
74. Gray MH, Talbert ML, Talbert WM, et al. Changes seen in lymph nodes draining sites of large joint prosthesis. Am J Surg Pathol 13:1050, 1989.
75. Rodnan GP, Brower TD, Hellstroma HR, et al. Post-mortem examination of an elderly severe hemophiliac, with observations on the pathologic findings in hemophilic joint disease. Arthritis Rheum 2:152, 1959.
76. Stein H, Duthie RB. Pathogenesis of chronic haemophilic arthropathy. J Bone Joint Surg Br 63:601, 1981.
77. Weiss SW, Kelly WD. Bilateral destructive synovitis associated with alpha-mannosidase deficiency. Am J Surg Pathol 7:487, 1983.
78. Worsing RA, Engber WD, Lange TA. Reactive synovitis from particulate Silastic. J Bone Joint Surg Am 64:581, 1982.
79. Yamashina M, Moatamed F. Periarticular reactions to microscopic erosion of silicone-polymer implants. Am J Surg Pathol 9:215, 1985.

# CHAPTER 29

# MESOTHELIOMA

Since Wagner et al.[241,243] demonstrated a high incidence of mesotheliomas among asbestos workers in the Cape Province of South Africa in 1960, mounting attention has been paid to this tumor, and numerous reports and reviews of mesothelioma have appeared in the medical literature. Mesothelioma is by no means a new disease, having been recognized as a distinctive clinicopathologic entity since the second half of the nineteenth century.[92,101] Sporadic reports of this neoplasm have been recorded in the literature under various synonyms, including endothelioma,[52] papillomatosis,[264] and carcinosarcoma.[26] Adami (1908)[1] is usually credited with coining the term *mesothelioma* and Klemperer and Rabin (1931)[120] with distinguishing and defining its epithelial and fibrous types.

The marked proliferation of reported cases in the medical literature is not only a reflection of widespread interest in the disease and its etiology and the evolution of more specific diagnostic criteria; it undoubtedly is also due to an actual increase in its rate of occurrence over the past decades.[37,127,226,244] Whitwell and Rawcliffe[253] identified only 12 cases during 1955–1963 but 38 cases during 1964–1970. Similarly, Newhouse and Thompson[151] encountered 10 cases prior to 1950 and 40 cases during 1951–1964. This steady increase in the number of newly observed cases parallels and follows the steep rise in the output and use of asbestos fibers in industrial countries during the first half of the twentieth century. Because there is a 20- to 40-year time lag between exposure to asbestos and development of the disease, this trend is likely to persist for several more years. The recent worldwide reduction in the industrial and commercial use of asbestos fibers is bound to cause the incidence of malignant mesothelioma to decrease, probably during the early twenty-first century.[37,127]

Mesothelioma is a tumor of adult life that mainly affects persons older than 50 years, and it is slightly more common in men than in women. It arises from the mesothelial cells of serosal surfaces and is about five times more common in the pleural cavity than in the peritoneal cavity. Not infrequently it involves both pleura and peritoneum as the result of direct extension through the diaphragm. It also occurs as a primary tumor in the pericardium[115,235] and tunica vaginalis testis,[22,80,109] but the incidence at those two sites accounts for less than 5% of all cases. Data as to incidence vary considerably, but the annual incidence of diffuse mesothelioma in the adult male population of the United States is estimated to be 7–13 per million.[218] Similarly, the reported incidence of asbestos exposure in patients with mesothelioma varies greatly, ranging from as little as 20% to as much as 99%.[20,262]

The prognosis differs slightly according to type. It is grave with the diffuse epithelial and biphasic types and even less favorable with the fibrous (sarcomatoid) type; nearly all patients with these tumors die of complications caused by the primary neoplasm within 12–18 months after diagnosis. Metastases do occur but usually at a late stage of the disease. There is still no effective mode of therapy, but multiagent chemotherapy and radiation therapy, in addition to surgery, seem to alleviate symptoms and prolong survival.

## HISTOLOGIC CLASSIFICATION

There are three principal forms of malignant mesothelioma: (1) epithelial; (2) fibrous (sarcomatoid); and (3) biphasic or mixed, with both epithelial and spindled features in close association. These three forms present almost exclusively as diffuse lesions, and so these terms are nearly synonymous with "diffuse mesothelioma," although there are infrequent but well documented tumors that develop as localized lesions.[65] Such lesions may represent an early form of what may develop into a diffuse disease. Epithelial and biphasic diffuse mesotheliomas display a wide range of growth patterns and cellular compositions, varying from well-differentiated tubulopapillary forms, which are readily recognizable, to poorly differentiated types consisting merely of solid nests and sheets of tumor cells that may be uniform in appearance or may have considerable cellular pleomor-

**TABLE 29–1 CLASSIFICATION OF MESOTHELIAL TUMORS**

| Tumor | Localized | Diffuse | Clinical Behavior |
|---|---|---|---|
| Adenomatoid tumor | Virtually always | | Benign |
| Well-differentiated papillary mesothelioma | Usually | Rarely | Benign/intermediate |
| Multicystic mesothelioma | Usually | Sometimes | Intermediate |
| Malignant mesothelioma | Rare | Virtually always | Malignant |

phism. Recognition of the fibrous or sarcomatoid type also may pose considerable diagnostic problems, often requiring immunohistochemical analysis.

There is only limited information as to the incidence and distribution of the various types. Among *diffuse mesotheliomas,* the epithelial type is by far the most common. For example, in the study by Leigh et al.[126] of 746 diffuse peritoneal mesotheliomas, 44% were of the epithelial type, 22% of the biphasic or mixed type, and 9% of the fibrous (sarcomatoid) type; in 25% there was no agreement among the reviewers as to the histologic type. Of 819 tumors reported by Hillerdal,[102] 50%, 34%, and 16% were of the epithelial, mixed, and fibrous types, respectively. Other studies have reported a similar distribution of the various types but with a substantial divergence in the incidence of the fibrous type.[245]

Less virulent forms of mesothelial tumors exist and include (1) the rare *well-differentiated papillary mesothelioma;* (2) *multicystic peritoneal mesothelioma,* a tumor frequently mistaken for lymphangioma; and (3) *benign mesothelioma of the genital tract,* a neoplasm often referred to as *adenomatoid tumor* to distinguish it from malignant diffuse mesotheliomas in the same locations. Commensurate with their excellent prognosis, the above lesions present with limited or localized disease and rarely are responsible for tumor-related death (Table 29–1).

## DIFFUSE MESOTHELIOMA

### Clinical Findings

The diffuse mesothelioma is mainly found in adults 45–75 years of age, regardless of whether it originates in the pleural, pericardial, or peritoneal cavity or the scrotum. Data as to the gender incidence vary considerably, but in most reviews, especially those with a large number of industrial workers, men outnumber women by a considerable margin.[2,7,8,140] Mesotheliomas in children are rare, but typical cases are present among our patients and are recorded in the literature.[3,11,87,117]

The clinical symptoms differ substantially and depend on the primary location of the neoplasm. *Diffuse pleural mesothelioma* usually manifests with chest pain, shortness of breath, and significant weight loss over a short period; it may also cause chronic cough, fever, and radiating pain in the shoulder or arm. Physical examination usually reveals decreased chest excursion, diminished or absent breath sounds, and in virtually all patients evidence of serous or hemorrhagic pleural effusion that accumulates rapidly and requires frequent aspiration. Pulmonary osteoarthropathy with arthritic pain and clubbing of the fingers or toes is encountered in 5–10% of cases, but it is much less common with diffuse mesothelioma than with solitary fibrous tumor of the pleura. Laboratory studies are not helpful in the diagnosis, although in some instances blood studies show leukocytosis and anemia, or there may be a thrombocytosis with thromboembolic episodes and pulmonary embolism.[148,193]

Patients with *diffuse peritoneal mesothelioma* usually give a history of nagging or burning abdominal or epigastric pain that is often more severe after meals. The pain is frequently accompanied by constipation, anorexia, nausea, or vomiting. Palpation of the abdomen discloses marked distension, increased density, and at times an ill-defined mass.[56,113] Ascites is often demonstrable[17,95]; it may be massive and frequently persists despite repeated paracenteses. Regional lymph nodes may be palpable and on biopsy are seen to contain metastatic deposits.[258] In some cases peritoneoscopy is helpful for the diagnosis.[33,143] Pericardial mesotheliomas tend to be associated with pericardial effusion, arrhythmia, or cardiac failure[235]; mesotheliomas of the tunica vaginalis are usually marked by a hydrocele or a scrotal mass.[80,109]

### Radiographic Findings

Radiographic and computed tomography (CT) examinations in patients with *diffuse pleural mesothelioma* show a rather distinct picture, but it rarely permits an unequivocal diagnosis (Fig. 29–1). The outstanding features are marked effusion, sometimes with compression of the adjacent lung and atelectasis, diffuse or irregular nodular thickening of the pleura or interlobular fissure, and not infrequently an intrathoracic mass. Less commonly widening or displacement of the mediastinum and a nodular infiltrate of the pulmonary parenchyma and pneumothorax secondary to invasion of the underlying visceral pleura and lung

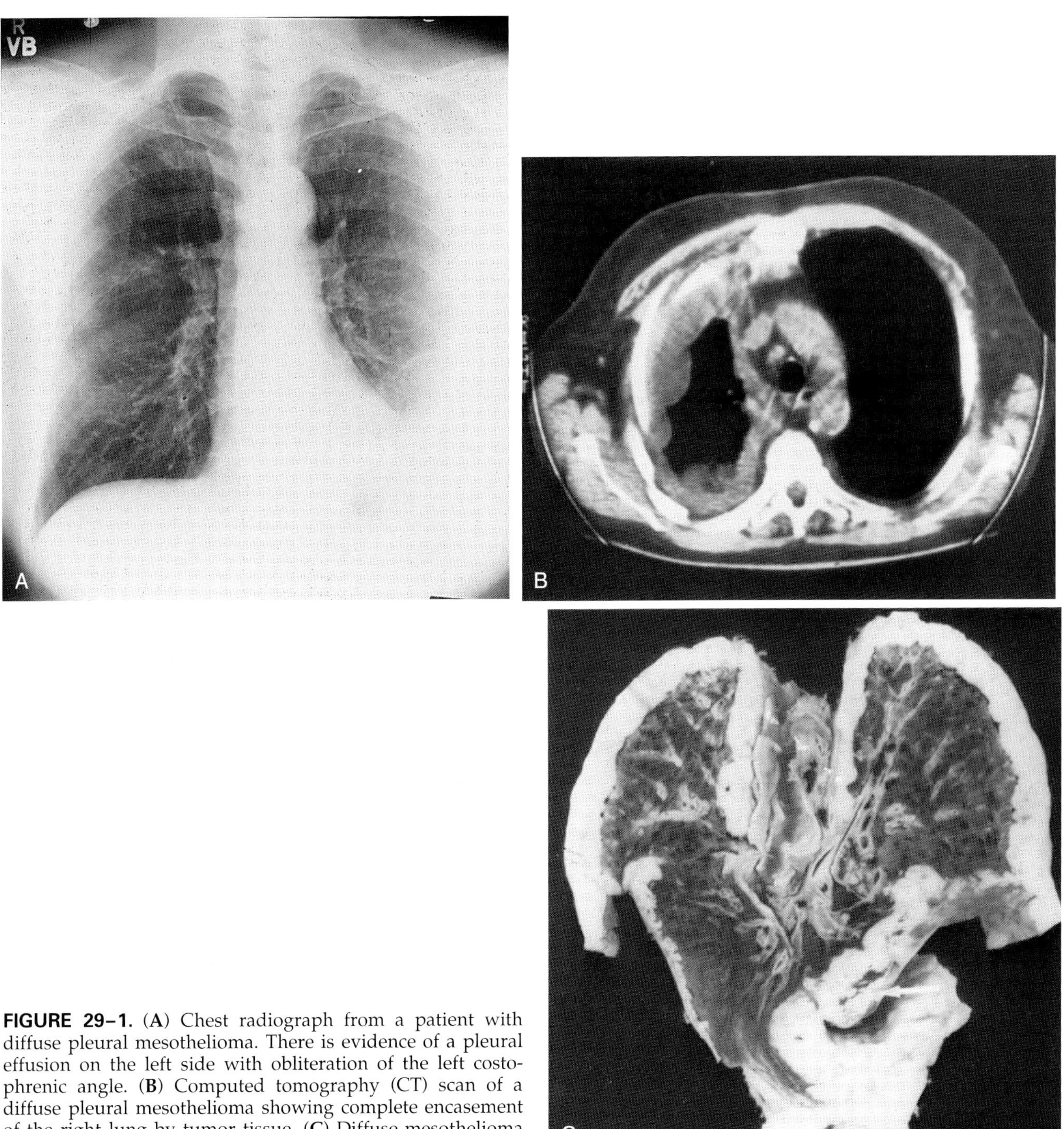


**FIGURE 29–1.** (**A**) Chest radiograph from a patient with diffuse pleural mesothelioma. There is evidence of a pleural effusion on the left side with obliteration of the left costophrenic angle. (**B**) Computed tomography (CT) scan of a diffuse pleural mesothelioma showing complete encasement of the right lung by tumor tissue. (**C**) Diffuse mesothelioma encasing and compressing both lungs of a 63-year-old man.

are present. Pulmonary fibrosis, however, is usually less severe than with asbestosis or carcinoma.[129]

Radiographic films and CT scans of *diffuse peritoneal mesothelioma* reveal thickening of the visceral and parietal peritoneum and omentum or multiple small nodules, often in association with ascites, signs of gastrointestinal tract dysfunction, and intestinal obstruction. There may also be pleural plaques in patients with asbestosis. Magnetic resonance imaging (MRI) may be superior to CT scans for demonstrating peritoneal masses, especially in the presence of ascites.[190,263] Both CT and MRI are critical for the preoperative evaluation of patients with diffuse mesothelioma to stage the lesion accurately and determine resectability.[172,226]

### Pleural and Ascitic Fluid

Pleural or ascitic fluid is viscous (owing to the high content of hyaluronic acid), amber-colored, or frankly hemorrhagic with demonstrable malignant cells in slightly more than half of the cases.[88] For example, in the series by Wanebo et al.,[246] pleural fluid was studied in 35 patients with diffuse mesotheliomas, but in only 15 were the cells recognized as malignant and in 5 as characteristic of mesothelioma. Markedly elevated levels of hyaluronic acid have been observed in a high percentage of cases, but they are also seen, although much less frequently, with carcinomas and sarcomas.

### Needle Biopsy

Needle biopsy guided by ultrasonography or CT scan is diagnostic in only a small percentage of cases, and thoracotomy and open biopsy may be necessary to establish the diagnosis. In many cases needle biopsy in combination with immunocytochemical and electron microscopic studies may permit a firm diagnosis of mesothelioma.[232]

### Mesothelioma and Asbestos Exposure

Although the association between pulmonary asbestosis and carcinoma was established during the early 1930s, the causal relation between asbestos exposure and mesothelioma was not recognized until 1960, when Wagner et al.[243] gave a detailed account of 47 diffuse mesotheliomas observed within a 5-year period in the asbestos regions of South Africa. In 1964 Selikoff et al.[206] reported on "asbestos exposure and neoplasia" in insulation workers of the New York area. Since publication of these reports, numerous studies carried out in England,[150,151,176] Scotland,[141] South Africa,[250] Canada,[138] the United States,[203] and other parts of the world have confirmed the observations of Wagner and colleagues and have demonstrated an increased incidence of mesothelioma not only among asbestos miners but also among industrial workers with a prolonged history of asbestos exposure.

Selikoff et al.,[207] in their classic study of 17,800 asbestos insulation workers, found that among 2271 consecutive deaths there were 175 mesotheliomas plus a large number of pulmonary carcinomas and carcinomas at other sites. In fact, in their series, cancer was responsible for 44% of all deaths, in contrast to the expected rate of 19%. Of the 175 cases of mesothelioma, 63 (36%) involved the pleura and 112 (64%) the peritoneum; most became apparent 25–40 years after the worker had started employment and been exposed to asbestos. This time lag between exposure and emergence of symptoms serves to explain not only the rarity of mesothelioma in young persons but also the surge in its incidence following a period in which the output and use of asbestos had risen markedly, especially in highly industrialized countries.

Exposure to asbestos is an occupational hazard not only in the mining and milling industries but also in the process of manufacturing, repairing, and installing (and removing) asbestos products such as thermal and electrical insulations, floor and ceiling tiles, automobile brake and clutch linings, cement tiles and pipes, and numerous other applications. Domestic exposure appears to be of lesser significance but has been observed in one or more relatives of asbestos workers and in persons and even animals living in the vicinity of asbestos mines and industries.

Multiple factors are important when determining the asbestos-related mesothelioma risk.[15] Asbestos fibers can be divided into two families: serpentine and amphibole (Table 29–2). Chrysotile is the main member of the serpentine family, whereas the amphibole family is composed of several members, including crocidolite, amosite, anthophyllite, tremolite, and actinolite. Several studies have showed a marked difference in the ability of these asbestos fiber types to induce mesothelioma. The highest risk is with expo-

**TABLE 29–2 CLASSIFICATION OF ASBESTOS FIBERS**

- Serpentines
  - Chrysotile (white asbestos)
- Amphiboles
  - Crocidolite (blue asbestos)
  - Amosite
  - Anthophyllite
  - Tremolite
  - Actinolite

sure to crocidolite, followed by amosite and tremolite. Chrysotile, the white asbestos found chiefly in Canada and Russia, accounts for more than 95% of the asbestos used commercially but rarely if ever causes mesothelioma.[15,121] Exposure to more than one type of fiber is common, however, and it has been suggested that the tumorigenicity of chrysotile is due to contamination with noncommercial amphiboles such as actinolite, tremolite, and anthophyllite.[47]

There are other properties of the type of asbestos fiber that determine mesothelioma risk. For example, the diameter of the fiber appears to be inversely related to mesothelioma risk, as fibers larger than 8 $\mu$m are much more likely to be associated with mesothelioma.[139,177] After inhalation, the fibrils are capable of passing into the pleural cavity. They may also be able to penetrate the bowel wall and migrate to the peritoneum, as suggested by animal experiments.[177,242] Occasionally they are carried to regional lymph nodes and other tissues such as the pancreas, liver, and kidney[122]; the curlier fibrils of chrysotile are less penetrating and are more readily removed by macrophages and lymphatics.[63] Finally, the greater biopersistence and ability to generate active oxygen radicals of crocidolite compared to other asbestos fiber types probably contribute to its greater tumorigenicity.[266]

Duration and intensity of exposure are also major factors when determining mesothelioma risk. Asbestos-related mesotheliomas characteristically have long latency periods. Lanphear and Buncher[123] found that 99% of patients with mesothelioma had a latent period of more than 15 years (median 32 years). Furthermore, there appears to be a direct relation between the intensity of exposure and cancer risk.

Most of the asbestos fibers in the body are too small to be visualized by light microscopy, but they are readily recognized in the lung as "asbestos bodies," asbestos fibers coated with acid mucopolysaccharides and hemosiderin granules. These segmented "nail-headed," golden-brown structures are difficult to distinguish from the ferruginous structures formed about a nonasbestos core, such as iron, talc, mica, carbon, and rutile. Assisting in the distinction of these fibers are the thin, transparent, usually straight central core of asbestos (Fig. 29–2), the refractile yellow core of talc and mica, and the black core of iron and rutile.[50] Examination by electron and scanning microscopy reveals that most ferruginous bodies have asbestos cores. Asbestos bodies are markedly increased in many construction workers and in patients with asbestosis or mesothelioma. The number of fibers seems to parallel the degree of exposure.[7,187]

More efficient ways of demonstrating and counting ferruginous bodies are examination of a lung juice smear[253] and particularly digestion of wet lung tissue with sodium hypochlorite and membrane filtration. Using the latter method, Smith and Naylor[213] found ferruginous bodies in 100% of consecutive autopsies, regardless of the cause of death. Likewise, Churg[47] found asbestos bodies in nearly all of the cases examined, but he noted a considerable increase in concentration in workers in certain asbestos-related occupa-

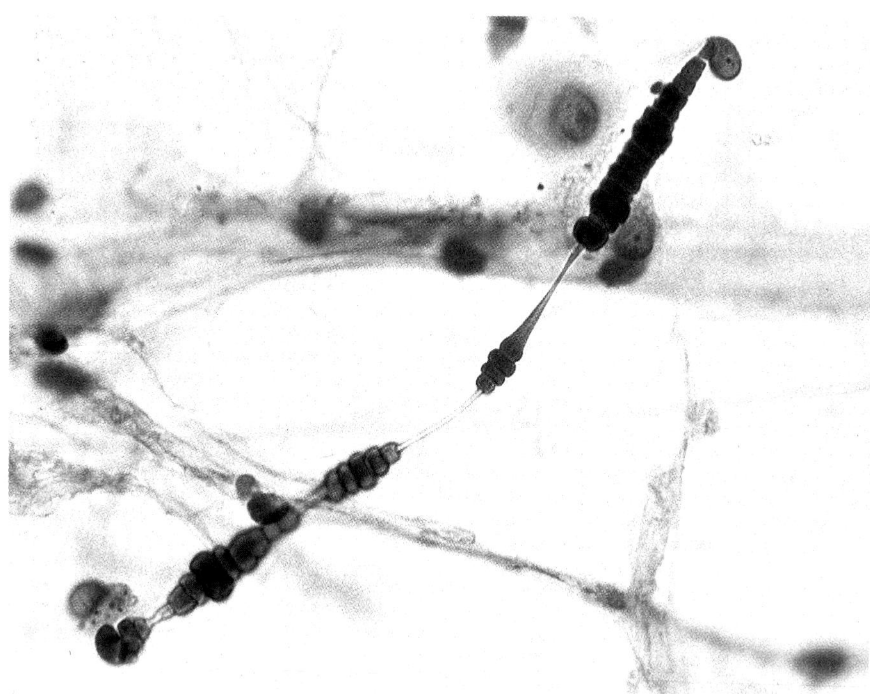

**FIGURE 29–2.** Ferruginous body with a thin, transparent, straight central core, consistent with an asbestos body.

tions and in patients with mesothelioma. Counts of asbestos fibers by electron microscopy are even more reliable than those with tissue digestion.[13] Electron diffraction patterns and especially energy-dispersive x-ray spectroscopy have been shown to be useful for the diagnosis and for distinguishing the various types of asbestos.[47,187]

Although measures have been taken in recent years to reduce asbestos exposure of industrial workers and the general population, it is likely—considering the long latent period of the disease—that the high incidence of mesothelioma will continue over the coming years. At particular risk are those who have been exposed to asbestos for several years, either as workers in the asbestos industry or by living in an asbestos-contaminated urban or industrial atmosphere. Also at risk are workers engaged in the demolition of buildings or refitting of ships containing asbestos packing around boilers and furnaces. With short or less intensive exposure, the incidence of mesothelioma is lower and the adverse effects are more delayed.[203] Smoking does not seem to enhance the risk of developing the disease.

Detailed descriptions of the prevalence of mesothelioma and the risk and environmental aspects of asbestos exposure were given in reviews by Kannerstein et al. in 1978,[114] Selikoff and Hammond in 1979,[207] and Craighead et al. in 1982, 1987, and 1989.[60–63] Although most mesotheliomas are related to asbestos exposure, other causes have also been proposed. Nonasbestos fibers, such as erionite, a naturally occurring mineral fiber found in central Turkey where it is used in the construction of houses, has been reported to be associated with a high prevalence of mesothelioma.[130,205] Pleural and peritoneal mesotheliomas have been associated with radiation exposure[93,208] and administration of thorium dioxide (Thorotrast).[219] Pleural mesotheliomas have been associated with chronic empyema[103] and peritoneal mesotheliomas with peritonitis.[184] Simian virus-40, a DNA papovavirus, has been linked with mesothelioma, as several studies have found simian virus-40-like sequences in both rodent[51] and human[173] mesotheliomas. Carbone et al.[41] found such sequences in 29 of 48 human mesotheliomas using the polymerase chain reaction, whereas Strickler et al. were unable to document these sequences in 50 mesotheliomas.[221] Similarly, Dhaene and colleagues were unable to detect nuclear expression of this viral oncoprotein in a large series of mesotheliomas.[77a] Finally, there have been several reports of mesothelioma arising in family members, although the relative roles of genetic and environmental influences are unclear.[70,97,166] Peterson et al. summarized the causes of non-asbestos-related mesothelioma.[175]

## Gross Findings

Initially the disease is characterized by numerous small nodules or plaques covering visceral and parietal serosal surfaces. At a later stage the individual nodules fuse and form a diffuse, sheet-like thickening that frequently encases and compresses the lungs or intestines and sometimes the liver and spleen (Figs. 29–1, 29–3). In the thoracic cavity the growth tends to be uniform but often is more pronounced in the serosal coverings of the lower lobe and diaphragm; in the peritoneum, involvement is usually more variable, and the diffuse or multinodular growth is often associated with large localized masses or a conglomerate of tumor nodules of variable size (Fig. 29–4). Massive involvement of the omentum is a common occurrence

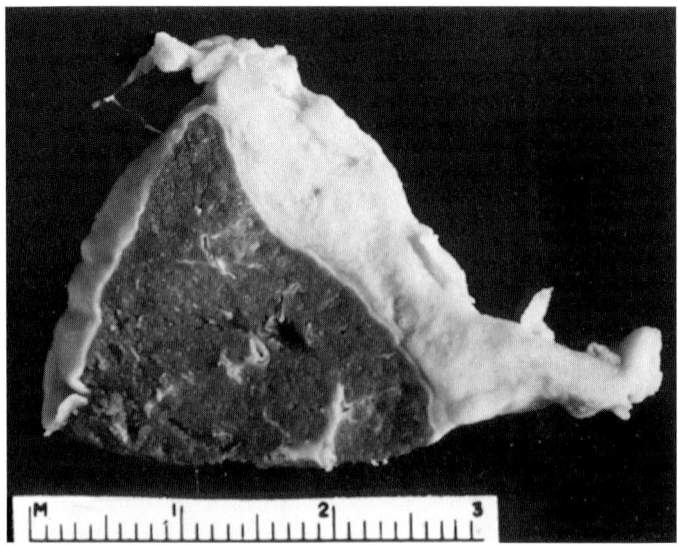


**FIGURE 29–3.** Diffuse epithelial mesothelioma of the serosal surface of the spleen in a 70-year-old woman. The tumor also encased the intestines and caused massive ascites.

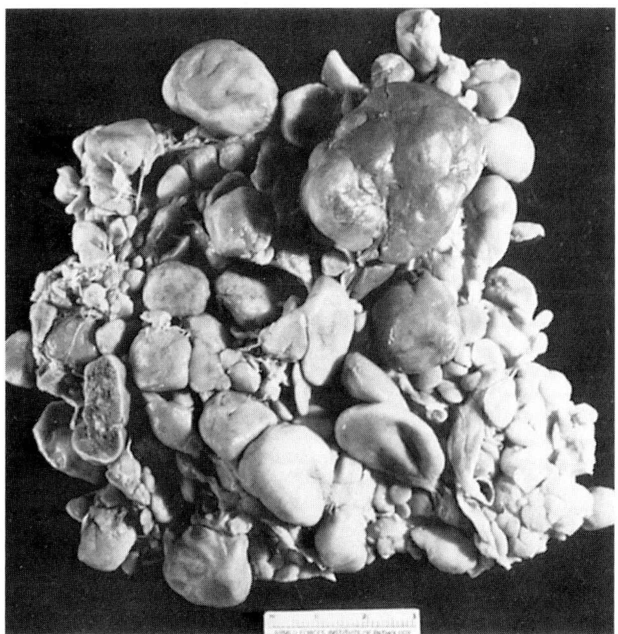

**FIGURE 29–4.** Peritoneal mesothelioma presenting as a conglomerate of variably sized tumor nodules.

that clinically may simulate the presence of a solitary localized neoplasm. The final stages of the disease are marked by massive encasement of the viscera with matting of the affected structures, commonly causing complete obliteration of the pleural or peritoneal cavity and severe, often fatal functional disturbances. In many cases the tumor tissue invades the adjacent lung or viscera, but in general invasion is more superficial than deep and is confined to the immediate subserosal tissues. Not infrequently the tumor extends through the chest or abdominal wall along a needle biopsy tract or a scar from a previous excision, a complication that must be given consideration when planning thoracoscopy, peritoneoscopy, or needle biopsy or when aspirating fluid for cytologic examination or to relieve symptoms. The excised tissue varies greatly in appearance and may be firm and rubbery or soft and gelatinous; on section it is generally gray-white and glistening, frequently with foci of hemorrhage or necrosis.

## Microscopic Findings

Although no two mesotheliomas are exactly alike and there is often a striking variation in different portions of the same neoplasm, most diffuse mesotheliomas are of the *epithelial type* and can be identified by their characteristic tubulopapillary pattern present at least focally. This pattern consists of papillary structures, branching tubules, and gland-like acinar and cystic spaces lined by rather uniform cuboidal or flattened epithelial-like cells with vesicular nuclei, one or two nucleoli, and abundant eosinophilic cytoplasm with distinct cytoplasmic borders (Figs. 29–5, 29–6). Mitotic figures are absent or rare in well-differentiated neoplasms, but they may be numerous in poorly differentiated ones. The surrounding matrix varies from myxoid to densely fibrous with or without hyalinization.

In addition to the typical tubulopapillary and tubuloglandular patterns, some tumors are composed of small uniform cells arranged in a delicate lace-like pattern, and others contain sheets of vacuolated cells vaguely reminiscent of liposarcoma (Fig. 29–7).[44a,211a] Others are marked by cleft-like structures or large, irregular, cystic spaces lined by a single layer of flattened epithelioid cells. In some of these cases fusion or rupture of the cystic spaces leads to the formation of large mucin-filled pools; in others the cystic structures are filled or replaced by multiple papillary projections with fibrous cores that bear a close resemblance to papillary carcinoma (Fig. 29–8).

There are also less well differentiated epithelial mesotheliomas in which the tubulopapillary pattern is largely inconspicuous or absent, and the tumor consists merely of small round or polygonal cells disposed in a linear or cord-like pattern or in clusters and solid nests and sheets (Figs. 29–9, 29–10). These tumors may resemble poorly differentiated carcinoma and therefore require ancillary immunohistochemical or electron microscopic studies (or both) for accurate diagnosis (discussed below). Associated with these changes is often a striking loss of cellular cohesion, with rounded or polygonal cells freely floating in the mucinous pools or dispersed in a loosely textured, myxoid stroma. This loss of cellular cohesion constitutes a frequent and useful feature in the differential diagnosis of mesothelioma. Calcospherites or psammoma bodies occur in approximately 5% of mesotheliomas, notably in those of the tubulopapillary type. Several unusual variants of epithelial mesothelioma have been described, including sporadic tumors that consist of nests of small hyperchromatic cells (*small-cell mesothelioma*),[135] pleomorphic variants, and those composed of cells with abundant glassy eosinophilic cytoplasm resembling a decidual reaction (*deciduoid mesothelioma*)[149] (Fig. 29–11). Although the latter variant was initially believed to have a predilection for arising in the peritoneum of young adult females without a history of asbestos exposure,[149,164c] subsequent reports have documented this tumor in the pleura of adults, some of whom had significant asbestos exposure.[164b,207a]

The second type, the *fibrous* or *sarcomatoid type* of diffuse mesothelioma, may be difficult to diagnose and is apt to be confused with fibrosarcoma, malignant fibrous histiocytoma, malignant hemangiopericy-

*Text continued on page 1075*

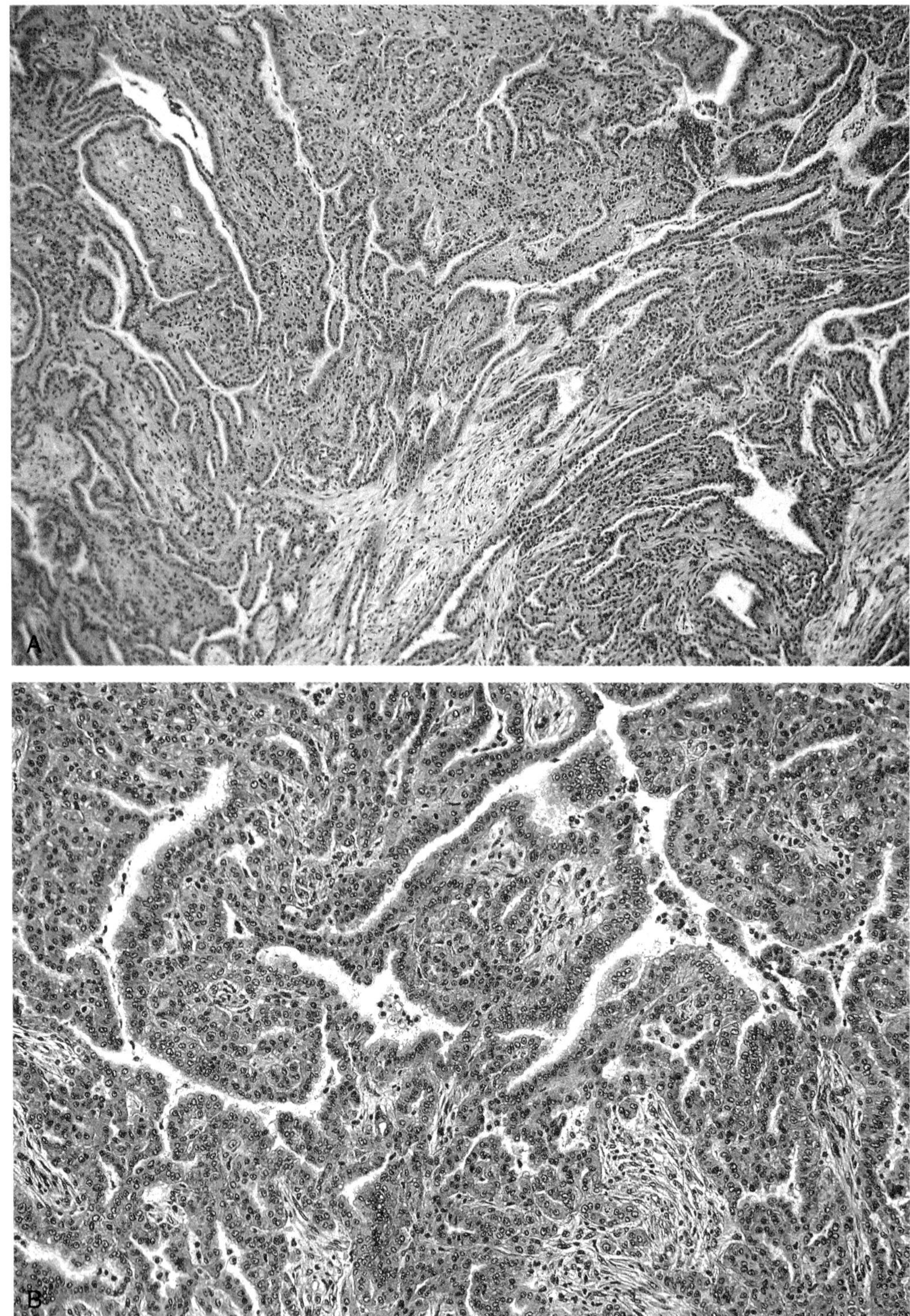


**FIGURE 29–5.** (**A**) Low-power view of a diffuse epithelial mesothelioma with a prominent tubulopapillary pattern. (**B**) Prominent tubulopapillary pattern composed of epithelioid cells with abundant eosinophilic cytoplasm in a diffuse epithelial mesothelioma.

*Illustration continued on opposite page*

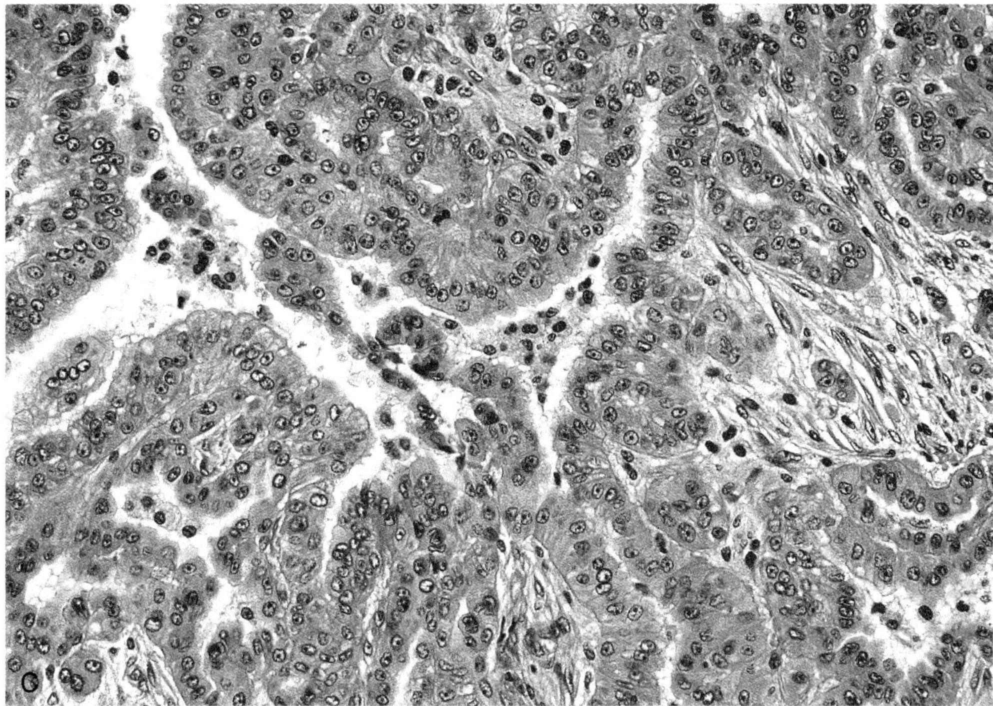

**FIGURE 29–5** *(Continued).* (**C**) Characteristic cytologic features of mesothelial cells in a diffuse epithelial mesothelioma with a prominent tubulopapillary pattern. The cells have vesicular nuclei with prominent nucleoli and abundant eosinophilic cytoplasm.

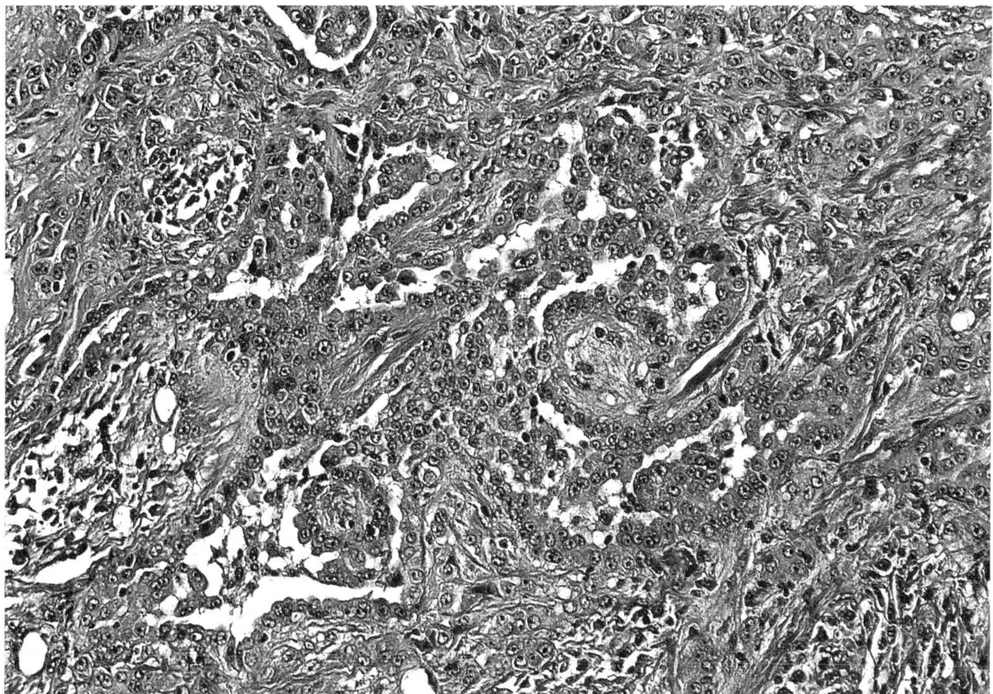

**FIGURE 29–6.** Papillary structures with fibrous cores are surrounded by malignant mesothelial cells.

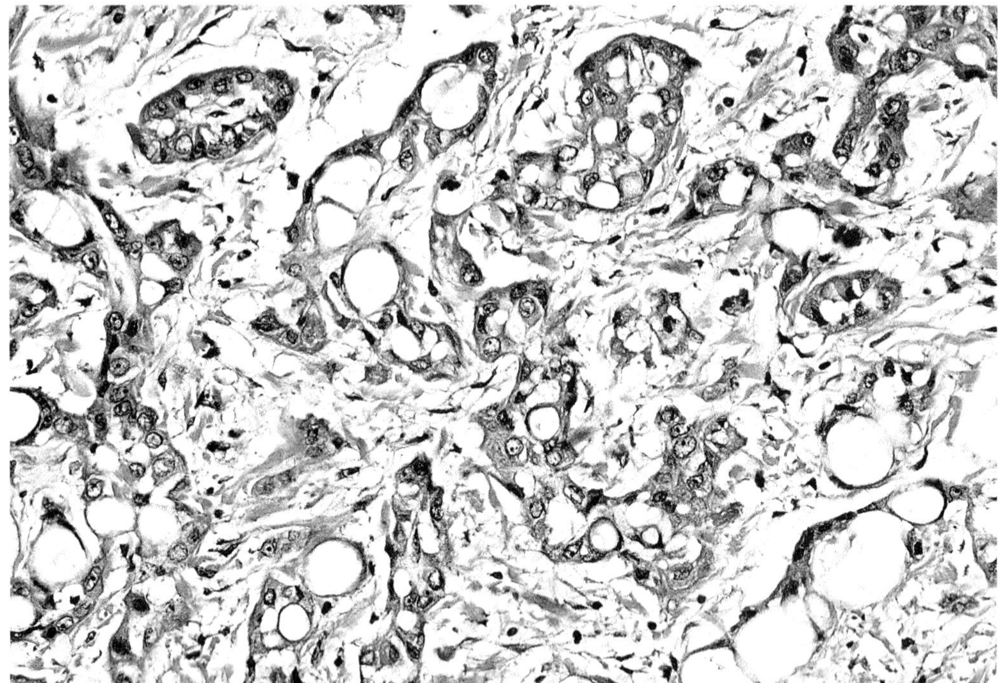

**FIGURE 29–7.** Diffuse epithelial mesothelioma with malignant cells arranged in a lace-like growth pattern reminiscent of that seen in adenomatoid tumors.

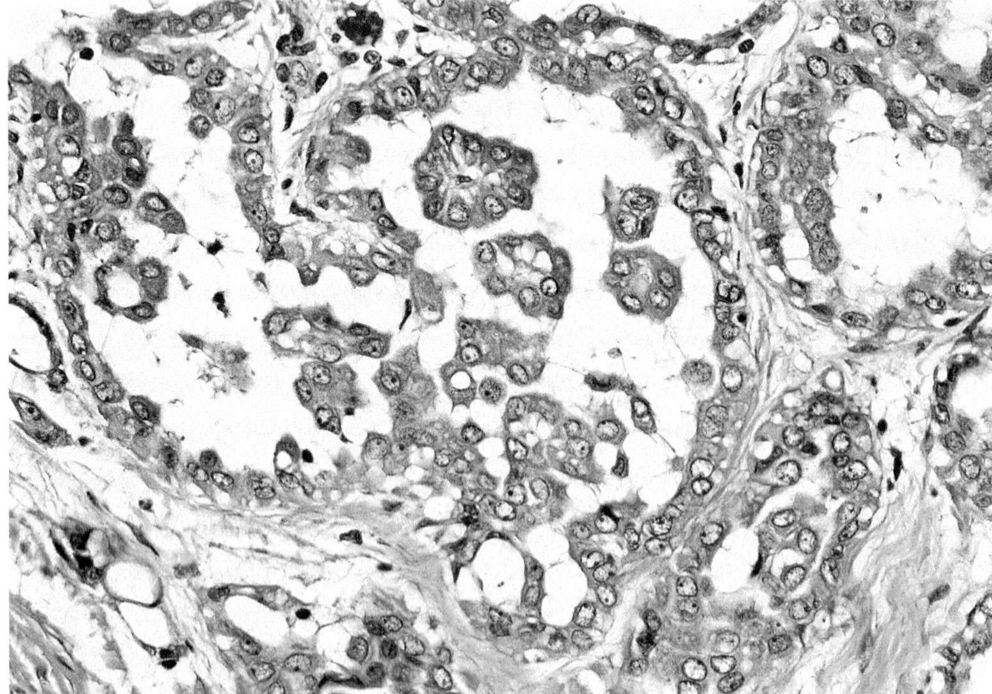

**FIGURE 29–8.** Multiple papillary projections with fibrous cores in a diffuse epithelial mesothelioma. These areas bear a close resemblance to papillary adenocarcinoma.

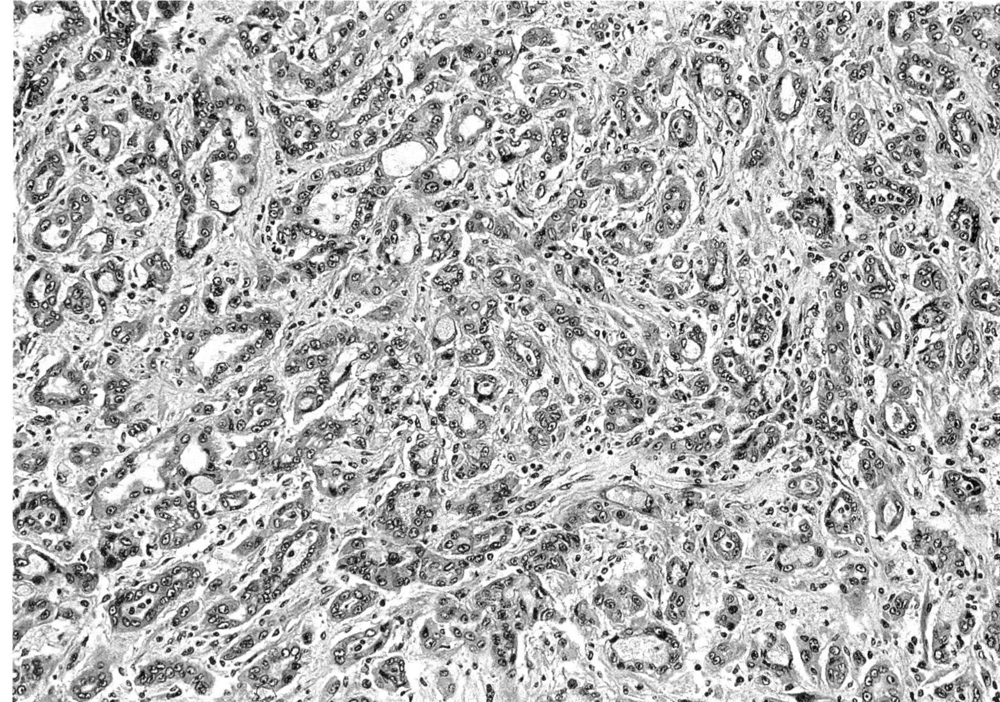

**FIGURE 29–9.** Diffuse epithelial mesothelioma composed predominantly of small tubules and cords.

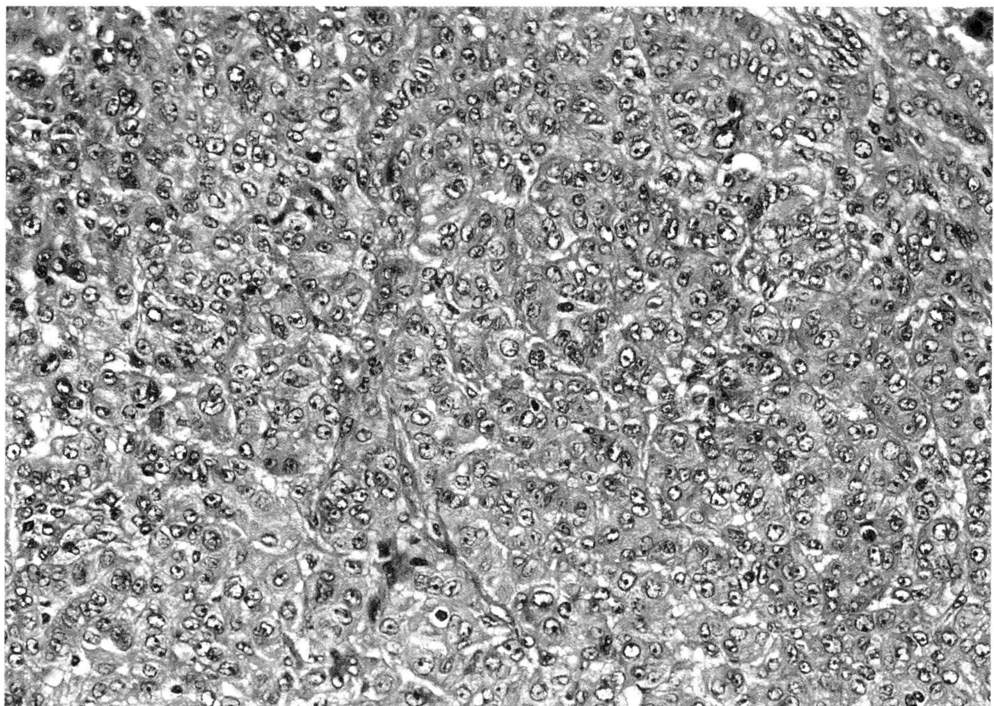

**FIGURE 29–10.** Solid sheet-like arrangement of malignant mesothelial cells with vesicular nuclei and macronucleoli.

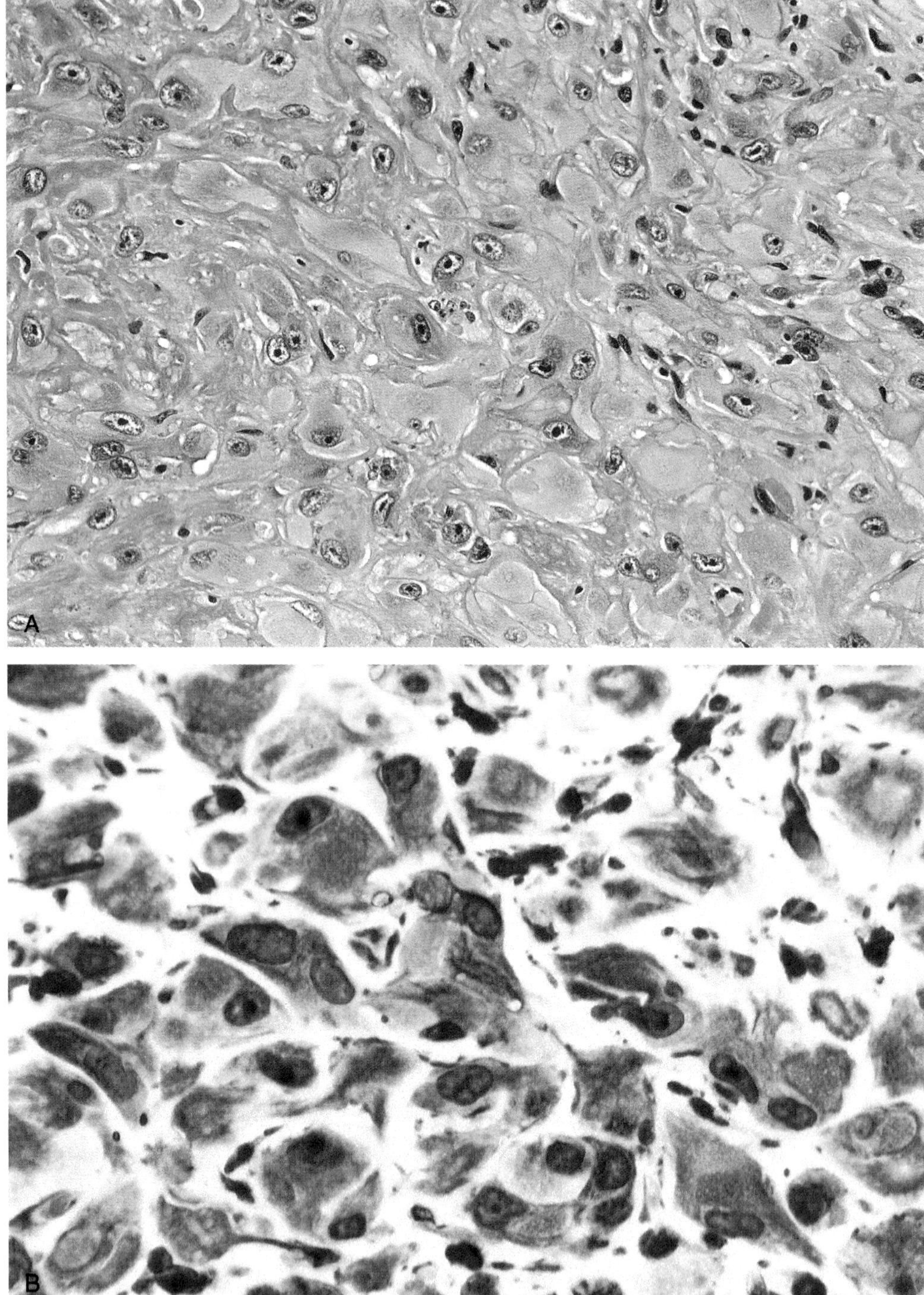

**FIGURE 29–11.** (**A**) Peritoneal deciduoid mesothelioma composed of cells with abundant glassy eosinophilic cytoplasm resembling a decidual reaction. (**B**) Diffuse cytokeratin immunoreactivity in a peritoneal deciduoid mesothelioma.

toma, or malignant solitary fibrous tumor (Fig. 29–12). As a rule, however, there are well oriented, spindle-shaped, fibroblast-like cells with nuclear hyperchromatism, pleomorphism, and occasional giant cells associated with areas of dense fibrosis, hyalinization, and necrosis. The presence of some of these fibrosing areas may cause confusion with a reactive fibrosing process (fibrous pleurisy); but as discussed below, the cellular atypia, increased mitotic activity, bland necrosis, and infiltrative growth are essential clues to the diagnosis.[134,137] There also may be a focal whorled, storiform, hemangiopericytoma-like or fibrosarcoma-like pattern. The term *desmoplastic diffuse mesothelioma* has been applied to richly collagenous tumors of this type (Fig. 29–13). Despite the extensive desmoplasia in these cases, the clinical course is that of a highly malignant neoplasm.[40,64,257] Osseous or cartilaginous metaplasia in some cases raises the question of chondrosarcoma or osteosarcoma[265] (Fig. 29–14). Rare tumors are composed of histiocytoid cells admixed with a dense polymorphous infiltrate composed of lymphocytes, plasma cells, eosinophils, and xanthoma cells.[99,118] Foci of epithelial differentiation are rare in the sarcomatoid type of diffuse mesothelioma and may be found only after careful scrutiny of multiple sections. In the absence of such areas, the diagnosis rests mainly on the presence of the diffuse and pleomorphic spindle cell pattern and the characteristic immunohistochemical and ultrastructural findings (discussed below).

The third type, the *mixed* or *biphasic type* of diffuse mesothelioma, consists of a mixture of epithelial and sarcomatous components that usually blend with one another such that transitional areas may be seen (Figs. 29–15, 29–16). Rarely in our experience do the two components abut one another in an abrupt fashion, as one sees in synovial sarcoma or carcinosarcomas of various organs. As in the diffuse fibrous type, osseous and cartilaginous differentiation occasionally occur.[265] Several investigators have noted the prevalence of the mixed type among patients with an occupational history of asbestos exposure.[139] Although there is some debate about the incidence of localized forms of epithelial and biphasic mesothelioma, there appears to be good documentation in a few cases.[65] Many alleged cases represent diffuse lesions that are inadequately staged, and others probably represent malignant forms of solitary fibrous tumor or biphasic tumors of other types (e.g., synovial sarcoma).

## Staining Characteristics

Special stains are helpful in the diagnosis of mesothelioma and particularly for differentiating this tumor from adenocarcinoma (Table 29–3). As in normal mesothelium, the occasional mucin droplets present in the tumor cells stain positively with alcian blue and colloidal iron (AMP) stains and lose their staining characteristics or stain less intensely after treating the sections with hyaluronidase. Unlike adenocarci-

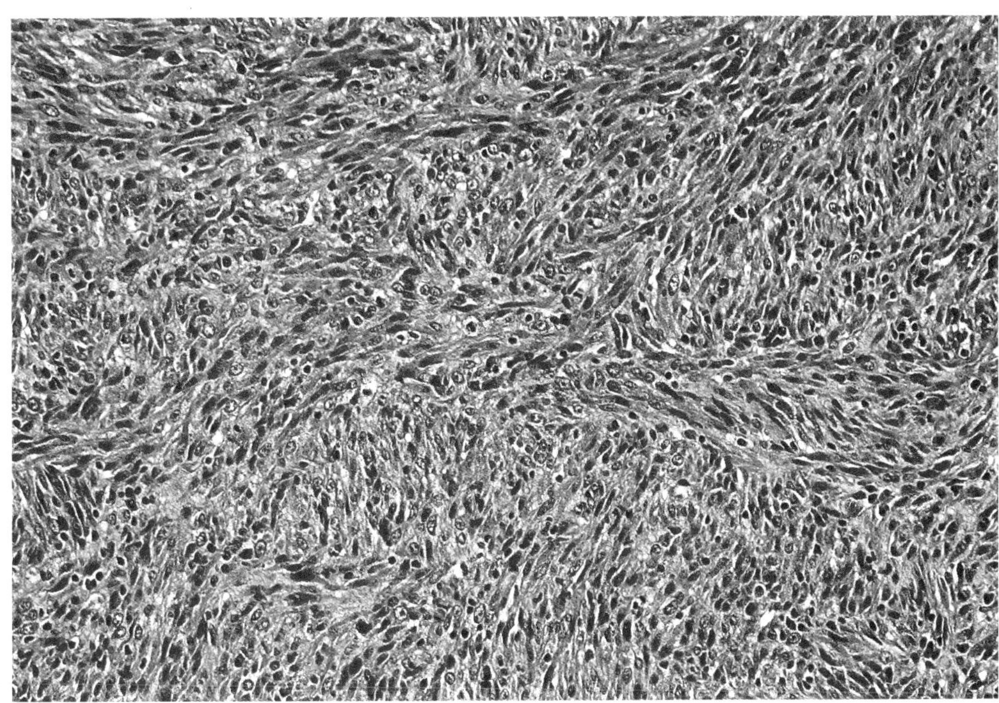

**FIGURE 29–12.** Fibrous (sarcomatoid) type of diffuse mesothelioma composed of spindle-shaped cells arranged in short fascicles.

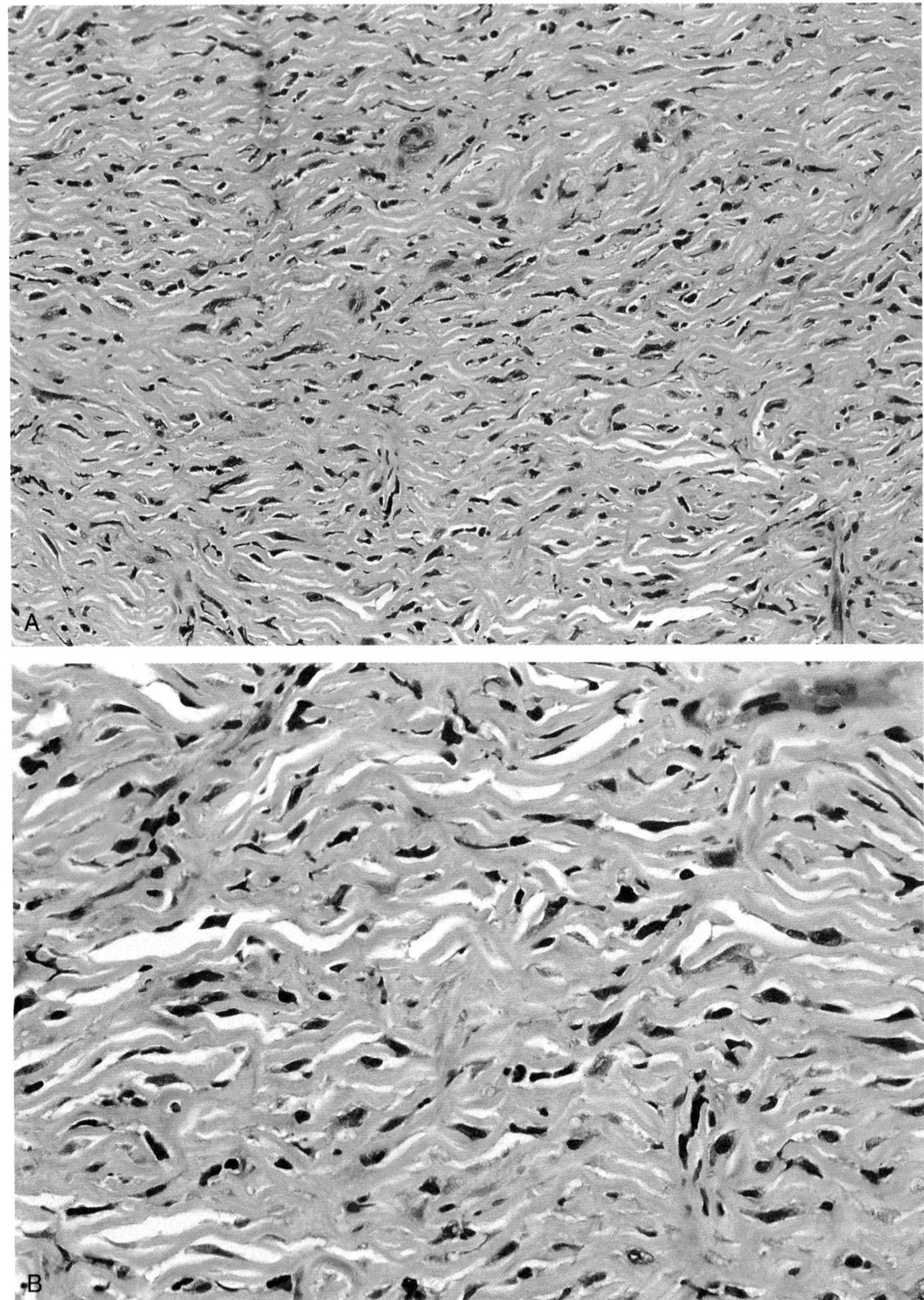


**FIGURE 29–13.** Low-power (**A**) and high-power (**B**) views of a desmoplastic diffuse mesothelioma. Such cases may be difficult to distinguish from pleural plaques.

*Illustration continued on opposite page*

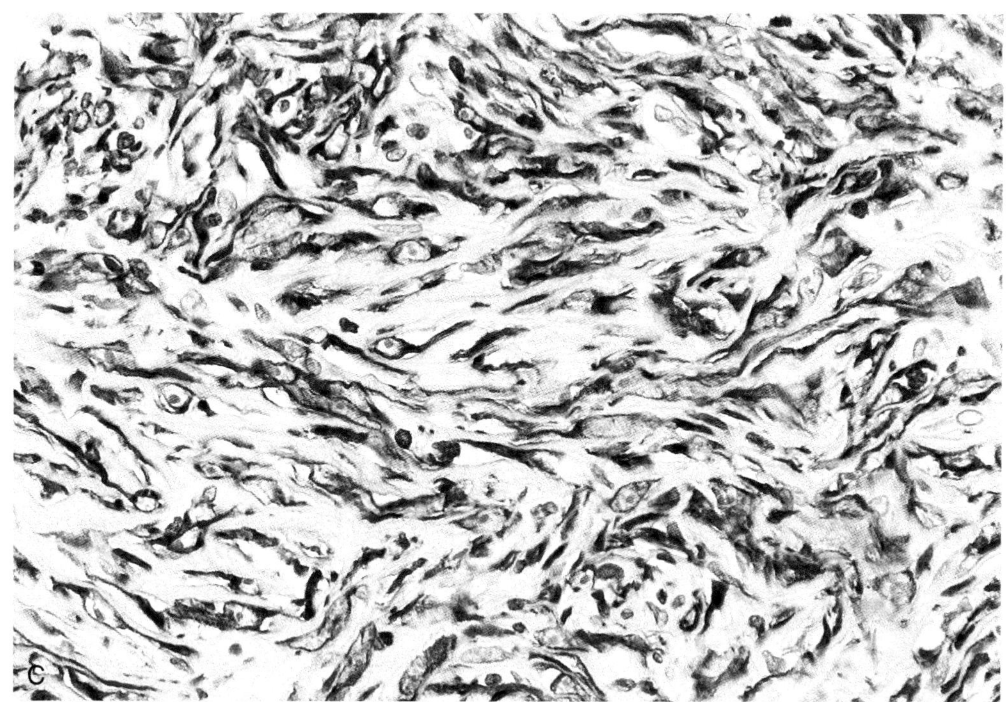

**FIGURE 29–13** *(Continued).* (**C**) Diffuse and strong immunoreactivity for low-molecular-weight cytokeratin (CAM5.2) in a desmoplastic diffuse mesothelioma.

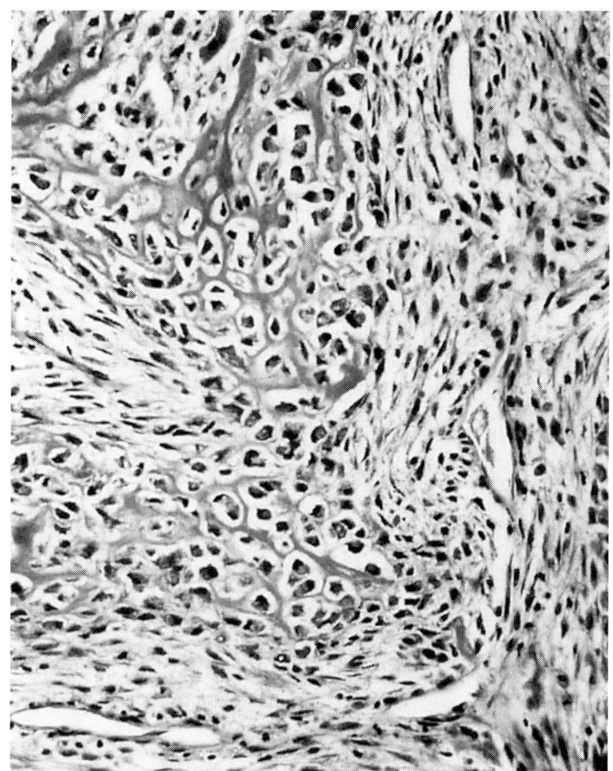

**FIGURE 29–14.** Malignant fibrous (sarcomatoid) mesothelioma with focal osteoid differentiation. (From Yousem SA, Hochholzer L. Malignant mesotheliomas with osseous and cartilaginous differentiation. Arch Pathol Lab Med 111:63, 1987.)

noma—and many synovial sarcomas—however, the mucin droplets do not stain with periodic acid-Schiff (PAS) after diastase digestion. Glycogen granules positive for PAS and sensitive to diastase digestion are present in the cytoplasm of many tumor cells, however.[28,84,212] Many of the intracellular droplets accept the mucicarmine stain and are metachromatic with toluidine blue and thionin preparations. Unfortunately, mucin droplets that stain positively for alcian blue (and negatively for PAS) are rare or entirely absent in at least half of the cases, especially in tumors that are less well differentiated.[186,189] The stromal mucin outside the tumor cells stains with alcian blue (pH 2.5) but is removed by hyaluronidase, a finding that mesothelioma shares with other sarcomas. However, acid mucin can be lost during processing in aqueous fixatives, and rare adenocarcinomas have alcian blue-positive stromal mucins.[128]

## Immunohistochemical Findings

Because of the lack of sensitivity and specificity of histochemical stains, immunostaining is indispensable for the diagnosis of mesothelioma. A specific marker for mesothelioma has not been found, and so a panel of antibodies is used to allow discrimination of mesothelioma from other neoplasms, particularly adenocarcinoma (Table 29–4). There have been numerous reviews on this subject, and various authors have

**TABLE 29-3 DIFFERENTIAL DIAGNOSIS OF MESOTHELIOMA AND ADENOCARCINOMA BASED ON INTRACELLULAR MUCIN***

| Stain | Malignant Epithelial Mesothelioma | Adenocarcinoma |
|---|---|---|
| PAS† | − | + |
| PAS-diastase | − | + |
| Alcian blue | + | + |
| Alcian blue-hyaluronidase | +/− | + |

* Including mucin in acinar spaces.
† Intracellular PAS-positive glycogen granules are present in many epithelial and biphasic mesotheliomas.

proposed antibody panels.[23,35,91,155,210,254] A number of antibodies may be useful for this differential diagnosis, including those to intermediate filaments, surface glycoproteins, myelomonocytic antigens, oncofetal antigens, and "antimesothelioma" antibodies, among others.[161]

### Intermediate Filaments

Almost all diffuse epithelial and biphasic mesotheliomas and most diffuse fibrous (sarcomatoid) mesotheliomas, stain for cytokeratins. As mesotheliomas become more sarcomatoid, they tend to express low-molecular-weight cytokeratins; hence CAM5.2 monoclonal antibodies are useful for recognizing the sarcomatoid variant. Because virtually all carcinomas are cytokeratin-positive, these stains are of little help in differentiating mesothelioma from adenocarcinoma.[59,104,111,165] Although both pulmonary adenocarcinomas and mesotheliomas express keratins 7, 8, 18, and 19, keratin 5 is frequently found in mesotheliomas but is usually absent in adenocarcinomas.[144] Clover et al.[57] found that an antibody to cytokeratin 5/6 stained all 23 epithelioid mesotheliomas but only 5 of 27 pulmonary adenocarcinomas using formalin-fixed paraffin-embedded tissues. Only 1 of 10 sarcomatoid mesotheliomas stained using this antibody. Similarly, Ordóñez[159] observed cytokeratin 5/6 reactivity in all 40 epithelial mesotheliomas but in none or 30 pulmonary adenocarcinomas. Although originally believed to be useful for distinguishing mesothelioma from pulmonary adenocarcinoma,[48] vimentin has been found to be expressed in as many as 50% of pulmonary adenocarcinomas,[73,107,156] thus limiting its utility in this differential diagnosis. There are also rare reports of mesotheliomas that express desmin.[105]

### Surface Glycoproteins

Cell surface glycoproteins have also been reported to be useful markers of mesothelioma. Epithelial membrane antigen stains most mesotheliomas with a prominent membranous pattern, whereas this marker stains the cytoplasm of pulmonary adenocarcinomas.[252] However, these patterns are not sufficiently consistent to be of diagnostic value.[127] SM-3 is a monoclonal antibody raised against the core protein of polymorphic epithelial mucin[36] and was initially believed to be useful in this differential diagnosis, as most pulmonary adenocarcinomas stained with this antibody, whereas staining was found to be rare in epithelial mesotheliomas.[214] Subsequent work by Ordónez found this antibody to be of no practical value.[157] The monoclonal antibodies B72.3 and Ber-EP4 are frequently used to distinguish mesothelioma from adenocarcinoma. B72.3 recognizes TAG-72 (tumor-associated glycoprotein), an antigen found in a wide variety of carcinomas but rarely found in meso-

**TABLE 29-4 DIFFERENTIAL DIAGNOSIS OF MESOTHELIOMA AND ADENOCARCINOMA BASED ON IMMUNOHISTOCHEMISTRY**

| Marker/Antibody | Malignant Mesothelioma | Adenocarcinoma |
|---|---|---|
| Vimentin | + | Up to 50% + |
| Cytokeratin | + | + |
| Epithelial membrane antigen | + (membranous) | + (cytoplasmic) |
| Carcinoembryonic antigen | − | + |
| Leu-M1 | − | + |
| Ber-EP4 | Up to 25% + | + |
| B72.3 | − | + |
| MOC-31 | − | + |
| Calretinin | + | − |
| Cytokeratin 5/6 | + | − |

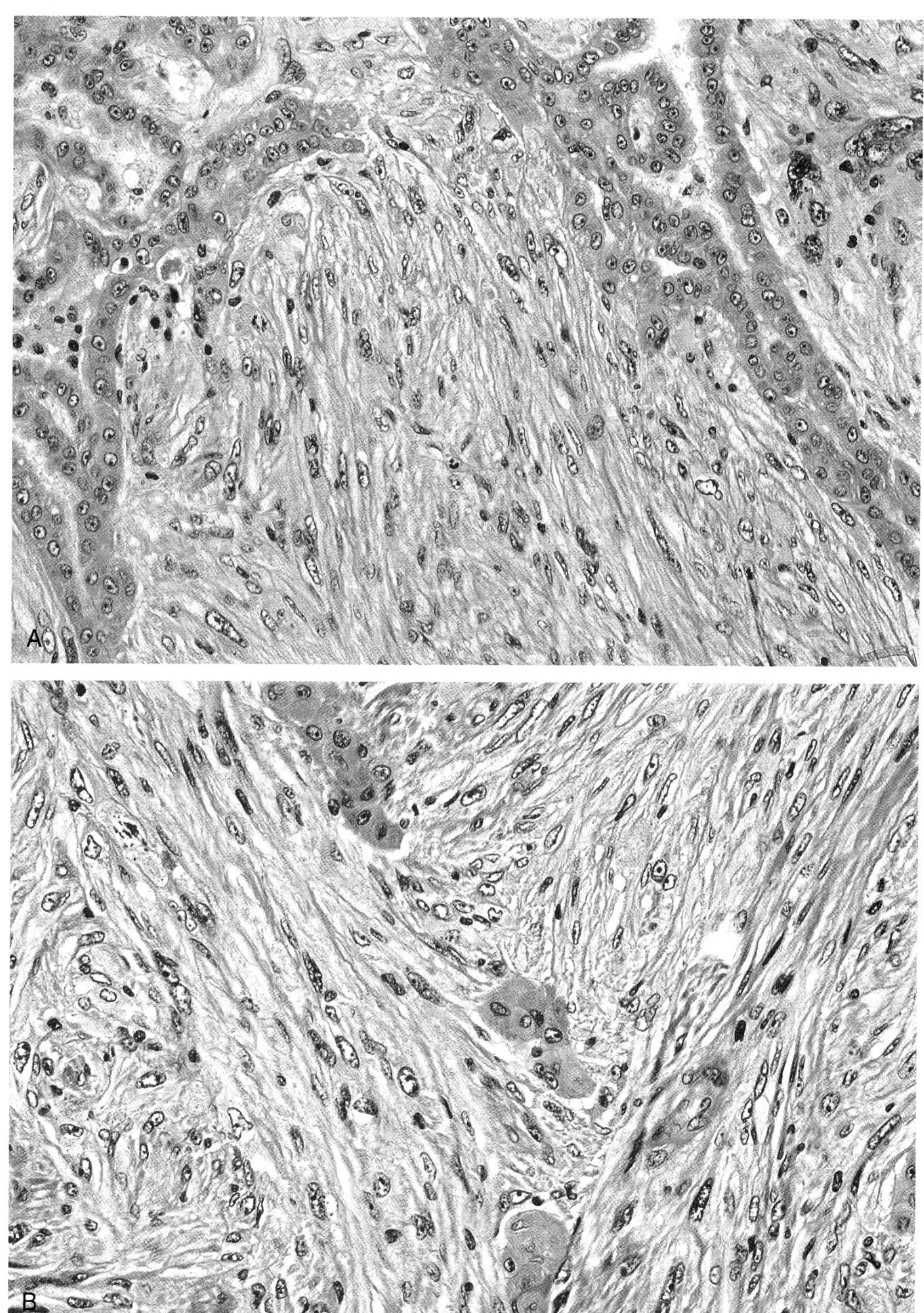

**FIGURE 29–15.** (**A**) Biphasic pleural mesothelioma. (**B**) High-power view of a biphasic pleural mesothelioma showing a gradual transition between epithelial and spindle-shaped cells.

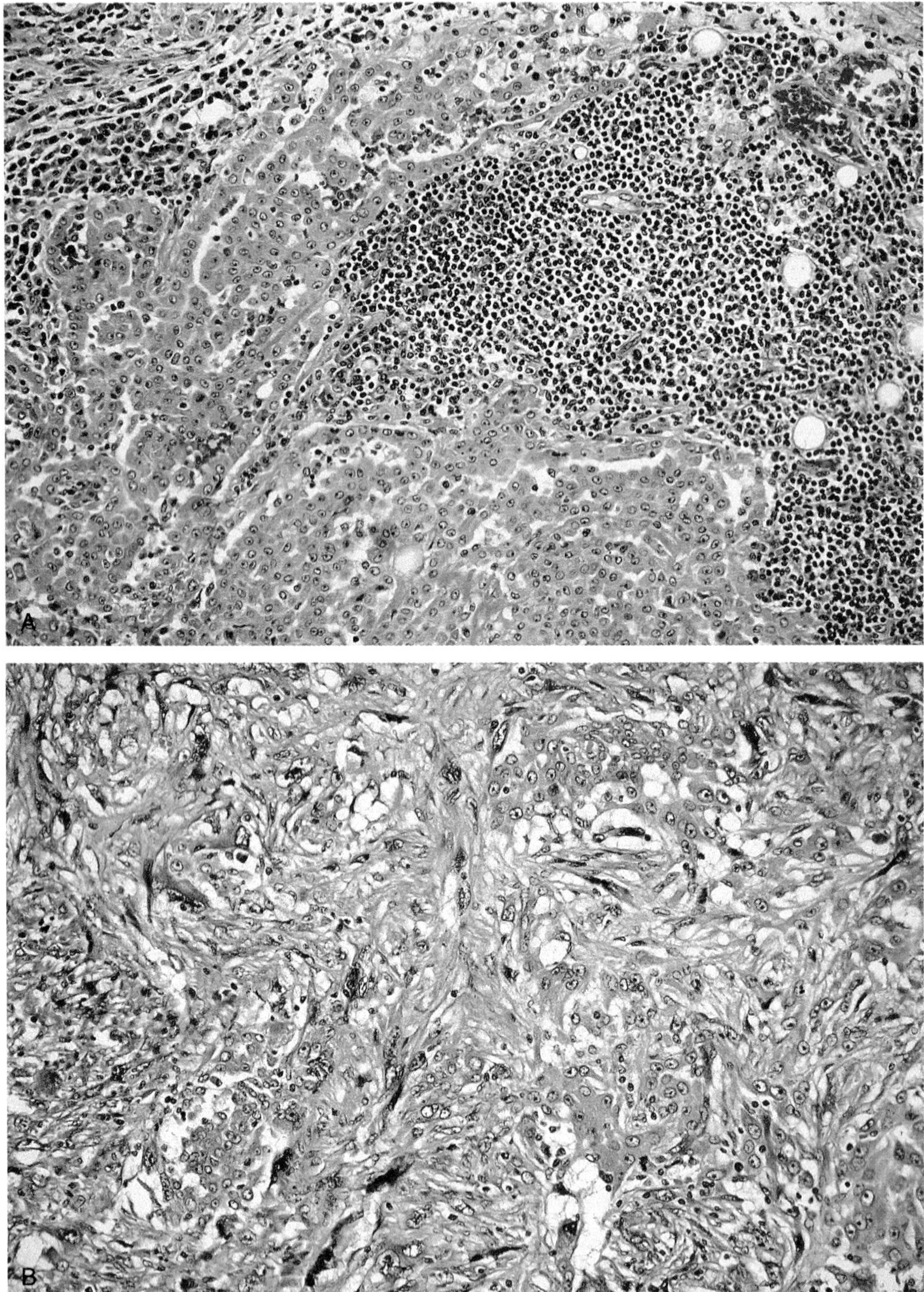


**FIGURE 29–16.** Unusual case of a diffuse pleural mesothelioma composed of roughly equal amounts of epithelial mesothelioma (**A**) and a high-grade malignant fibrous histiocytoma-like tumor. (**B**) Transitional area between epithelial mesothelioma and malignant fibrous histiocytoma-like area.

*Illustration continued on following page*

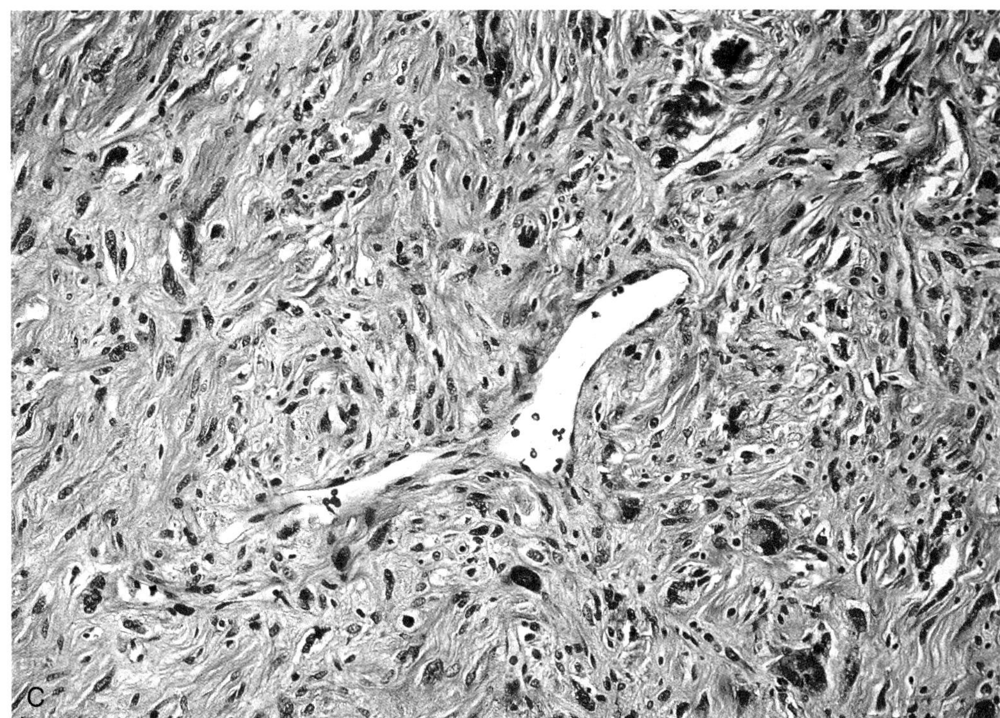


**FIGURE 29–16** *(Continued).* (**C**) High-power view of a malignant fibrous histiocytoma-like area in this unusual pleural mesothelioma.

theliomas.[108,236] Similarly, Ber-EP4 antibody recognizes a surface glycoprotein found in most adenocarcinomas but less commonly detected in mesotheliomas.[124,211] However, this antibody is not entirely specific, as it has been found to mark up to 26% of mesotheliomas.[90,160] Several other antibodies to surface glycoproteins have been evaluated in this context, including HEA 125,[240] 44-3A6,[157,217] and blood group-related antigens[110,116,152]; but none of these markers appears to offer any advantage over B72.3 or Ber-EP4.

## Myelomonocytic and Oncofetal Antigens

The antibody Leu-M1 (CD15) is commonly used in immunohistochemical panels devised to distinguish mesothelioma from adenocarcinoma. Leu-M1 is expressed in a variety of myeloproliferative disorders and various carcinomas, particularly pulmonary adenocarcinomas,[209,256] but it is rarely expressed in mesotheliomas. However, some report that only approximately 60% of pulmonary adenocarcinomas are stained by this antibody,[156,249] thereby limiting its utility.

Antibodies to the oncofetal antigen carcinoembryonic antigen (CEA) have long been used to distinguish pulmonary adenocarcinoma from mesothelioma. The early literature shows conflicting results, although it is likely these results can be attributed to the use of polyclonal antibodies and to differences in immunohistochemical techniques.[163] The studies using anti-CEA monoclonal antibodies have generally found a high frequency of staining in pulmonary adenocarcinomas, with rare staining in epithelial mesotheliomas.[72,255,259]

## "Antimesothelioma" and Miscellaneous Antibodies

Monoclonal antibodies generated against mesothelioma-associated antigens have been developed (Table 29–5). This long list of antibodies includes ME1,[153] HBME-1,[21,142,157] K1,[44] CD44-H,[4,16] anti-hyaluronate,[19]

**TABLE 29–5** PUTATIVE POSITIVE MARKERS OF MESOTHELIOMA

| Marker | Uses and Limitations |
|---|---|
| Calretinin | Moderate specificity, high sensitivity |
| Thrombomodulin | Moderate specificity, high sensitivity |
| Cytokeratin 5/6 | Moderate specificity, high sensitivity |
| CD44H | Moderate specificity and sensitivity |
| HBME-1 | Low specificity, high sensitivity |
| N-cadherin | Limited data |
| Hyaluronate receptor | Limited data |
| Wilms' tumor gene product | Limited data |

Modified from Attanoos RL, Gibbs AR. Pathology of malignant mesothelioma. Histopathology 30:403, 1997.

calretinin,[18,79,158] and the product of the Wilms' tumor gene.[32,168] None of these antibodies have complete specificity or sensitivity, although calretinin and cytokeratin 5/6 are emerging as particularly useful markers in this differential diagnosis (Fig. 29–17).

Finally, there is a long list of miscellaneous antigens that tend to be found much more commonly in pulmonary adenocarcinomas than in epithelial mesotheliomas, including thrombomodulin,[58,162] OV632,[75,81] E-cadherin,[125,174] MOC-31[45,161,194,215] and thyroid transcription factor-1 (TTF-1).[164a] Of these antibodies, MOC-31 and TTF-1 are particularly promising in that both appear to be present in almost all adenocarcinomas but are rarely expressed in mesotheliomas.

The immunohistochemical evaluation of mesotheliomas continues to be an area of intense research, and the search for a highly sensitive and specific anti-mesothelioma antibody will likely continue. At this point, most investigators advocate a broad panel of markers, most of which recognize pulmonary adenocarcinomas with high frequency, with relatively rare staining in mesotheliomas. Riera et al.[185] evaluated a large number of epithelial mesotheliomas and adenocarcinomas of various organs using a broad spectrum of antibodies with and without antigen retrieval techniques. Following statistical analysis, these authors found CEA and Ber-EP4 to have the best discriminatory value, followed by HBME-1, calretinin, and thrombomodulin. Others have proposed immunohistochemical panels, but the optimal panel has yet to be uniformly established.

## Ultrastructural Findings

Although mesotheliomas share some ultrastructural similarities with adenocarcinoma, they can be distinguished by the presence of abundant, long, slender, sometimes tortuous microvilli with a bush-like or shaggy appearance (Fig. 29–18).[167] The microvilli are found on the free surfaces of the tumor cells and in intracellular and intercellular lumens. The microvilli of adenocarcinoma are also located on the surface and inside cells but are generally much shorter, less numerous, and have a more club-like appearance[248] (Table 29–6). These differences are also readily discernible by scanning electron microscopy.[78,220,247] The characteristic appearance of numerous, long, slender, microvilli is lost in poorly differentiated neoplasms.[69,98,251] The cells of a mesothelioma are further marked by large nuclei with prominent nucleoli, a moderate number of mitochondria enveloped by rough endoplasmic reticulum, and frequently glycogen granules and bundles of intermediate filaments. There are smooth-surfaced intracellular vacuoles, but the Golgi apparatus and the associated smooth endoplasmic reticulum are rather inconspicuous. Suzuki et al.[229] observed rare lysosomes and osmiophilic lamellar structures in occasional tumor cells. Basal laminae

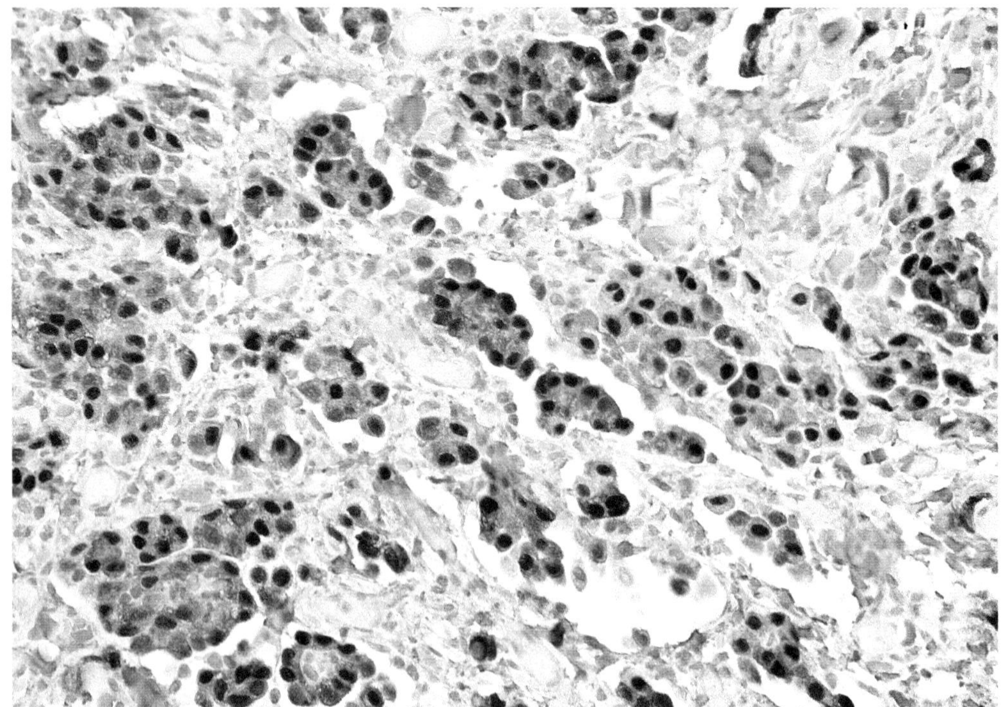

**FIGURE 29–17.** Diffuse immunoreactivity for calretinin in a diffuse epithelial mesothelioma of the pleura.

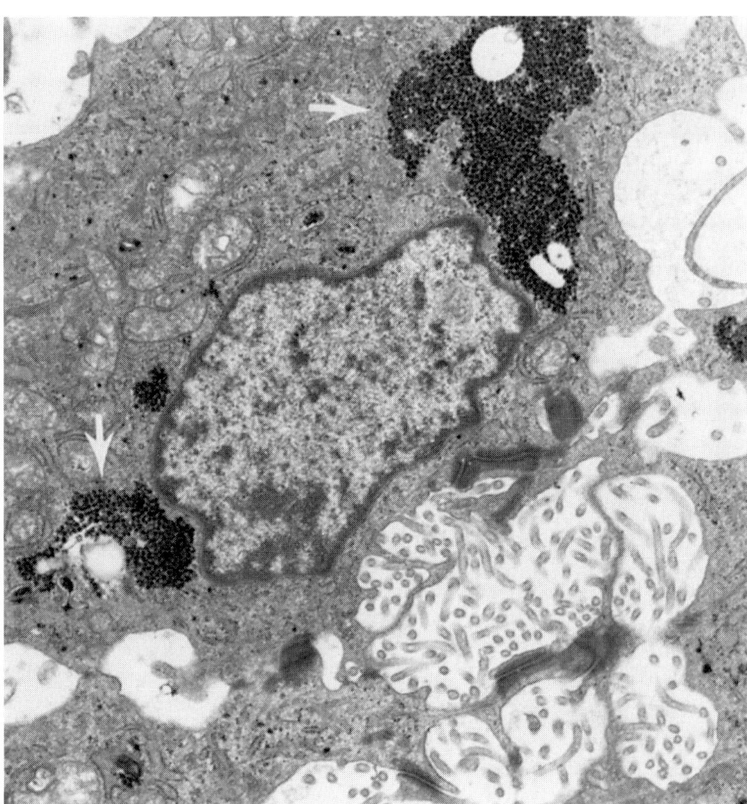

**FIGURE 29–18.** Electron microscopic view of a diffuse peritoneal mesothelioma in a 66-year-old woman. Note the intracellular and intercellular lumens with multiple slender microvilli and intracellular deposits of glycogen (arrows). (Courtesy Dr. Frederic I. Volini, West Suburban Hospital, Oak Park, IL.)

are present but are often interrupted or incomplete. There are also junctional structures or desmosomes between adjoining cells and intermediate filaments or tonofilaments often limited to the apical portion of the cell or arranged circumferentially around the nucleus. There are no ultrastructural differences between pleural and peritoneal mesotheliomas.[229]

Examination of the biphasic or mixed type of mesothelioma discloses a similar picture, but there are, in addition, fibroblast or myofibroblast-like cells with elongated nuclei and abundant rough endoplasmic reticulum and myofilaments with dense body formations and whorled aggregates of perinuclear intermediate filaments.[27] Forms transitional between the epithelial and spindle cells are not uncommon and can be recognized by the presence of intercellular microcavities with microvilli.[220] The latter feature has also been encountered in diffuse fibrous (sarcomatoid) mesotheliomas.

The extracellular spaces contain collagen fibers and colloidal iron-positive material, especially in close contact with the microvilli. None of the ultrastructural studies revealed asbestos fibers in the tumor cells, even in cases in which they were readily demonstrable in the surrounding pulmonary parenchyma.

## DNA Ploidy and Cytogenetic Findings

Numerous studies have evaluated the DNA content of mesotheliomas using flow cytometric techniques. Most malignant mesotheliomas are diploid, in contrast to adenocarcinomas, which are usually aneuploid.[38,82] For example, Burmer et al.[38] conducted a

**TABLE 29–6** DIFFERENTIAL DIAGNOSIS OF MESOTHELIOMA AND ADENOCARCINOMA BASED ON ULTRASTRUCTURAL FINDINGS

| Feature | Malignant Mesothelioma | Adenocarcinoma |
|---|---|---|
| Microvilli | Numerous, long, slender, "bushy" | Fewer, short, blunt, "club-like" |
| Desmosomes | ++ | + to ++ |
| Intermediate filaments | + to ++ | 0 to + |
| Basement membrane | ++ | ++ |
| Glycogen | ++ | 0 to + |

flow cytometric analysis of 46 mesotheliomas and found 65% to be diploid and 35% aneuploid. In a similar study, El-Naggar et al.[82] found 78% of malignant mesotheliomas to be diploid, whereas 88% of primary pulmonary adenocarcinomas were aneuploid. In contrast, several other studies have found aneuploidy in up to 60% of malignant mesotheliomas.[74,88,89,106] Whereas some have found aneuploidy to be an adverse prognostic factor,[74,106] others have not found the ploidy status to be of any prognostic significance.[71,179]

Most mesotheliomas harbor multiple cytogenetic abnormalities. The most frequent abnormalities involve partial loss of chromosome 1 (1p11-p22),[230,237] chromosome 3 (3p14-p25),[86,131,178,261] and chromosome 9 (9p).[25,42,119,261] Monosomy of chromosome 22[86] raises the possibility of involvement of the neurofibromatosis type 2 (NF2) tumor-suppressor gene in the pathogenesis of mesothelioma.[204]

## Differential Diagnosis

The differential diagnosis of diffuse mesothelioma depends on whether one is dealing with an epithelial, fibrous, or biphasic type. The differential diagnostic considerations for each of the types of diffuse mesothelioma are discussed below.

### *Epithelial Mesothelioma*

It is not always possible to distinguish well-differentiated epithelial mesothelial neoplasms from reactive mesothelial proliferations on the basis of a small biopsy specimen. In general, reactive or inflammatory mesothelial proliferations are limited to the serosal surfaces, where they may form small papillary structures, usually with gradual transitions between normal and hyperplastic mesothelium. These proliferations may arise in a variety of sites and settings. Rosai and Dehner[191] described proliferations of mesothelial-like cells in hernial sacs: They occurred in the inguinal region of children and followed hernial incarceration or some other mechanical injury. The lesions were marked by nodular proliferations of round or polygonal mesothelial cells associated with fibrin, hemosiderin, inflammatory cells, and a variable fibrovascular proliferation (Fig. 29–19). Similarly, nodular proliferations in the pericardium were described by Luthringer et al.[133] and in the lung by Chan et al.[43] These proliferations are composed of a mixed population of reactive mesothelial cells (cytokeratin-positive) and histiocytes ($CD68^{+}$), with the relative proportion of each depending on the clinical setting.[54,164]

Several features are useful for distinguishing mesothelioma from reactive mesothelial hyperplasia. Invasion into the underlying tissues is a useful indicator of mesothelioma but requires distinction from benign mesothelium, which may become entrapped in inflamed submesothelial connective tissue.[100] Entrapped benign mesothelial cells rarely extend deeper than the immediate subserosal fibrous layer, in contrast to mesothelioma, which shows more extensive and deeper invasion into the pleura, underlying chest wall, or lung, often accompanied by a desmoplastic stromal reaction. In addition, malignant mesothelial cells usually show more nuclear atypia and more prominent nucleoli than is seen in reactive mesothelial cells. The presence of necrotic mesothelial cells also favors a diagnosis of mesothelioma.[100] An excellent review of histologic features useful in separating benign and malignant mesothelial proliferations was provided by the US-Canadian Mesothelioma Reference Panel.[50a]

Immunohistochemical studies have found significant differences between reactive mesothelial proliferations and mesothelioma, but the extent of overlap of the two lesions makes it difficult to endorse these stains for making this important distinction in the individual case. Most epithelial mesotheliomas exhibit extensive, strong linear membrane staining using antibodies to epithelial membrane antigen, in contrast to the weak or undetectable staining seen in reactive mesothelial hyperplasia.[68,260] However, a negative reaction does not exclude mesothelioma. Several studies have found a significant difference in frequency of p53 immunoreactivity in reactive and malignant mesothelial proliferations.[39,136,146,182,202,238] For example, Cagle et al.[39] found 19 of 40 mesotheliomas to be p53-positive, whereas all 13 areas of reactive mesothelial hyperplasia or organizing pleuritis were negative. Because only about 50% of mesotheliomas stain for p53 protein, a negative stain would be relatively meaningless in the individual case. Antibodies to platelet-derived growth factor have also been found in up to one-half of mesotheliomas, whereas nonneoplastic mesothelium is usually weakly stained[12] or completely negative.[181] Some have also found a higher percentage of proliferating cells detected by antibodies to proliferating cell nuclear antigen (PCNA) in mesotheliomas than in nonneoplastic mesothelium,[181] but again there is considerable overlap between reactive and malignant proliferations.

Occasionally, collections of benign mesothelial cells are found in lymph nodes, mimicking metastatic mesothelioma. Although originally described in mediastinal lymph nodes,[34,199] benign mesothelial proliferations have also been described in abdominal lymph nodes found incidentally during staging procedures in patients with ovarian neoplasms.[53,55] In such cases there is also hyperplasia of peritoneal mesothelial cells, a common finding in patients with ovarian tumors.[53] In addition, collections of hyperplastic mesothelial cells have been reported in cervical and medi-

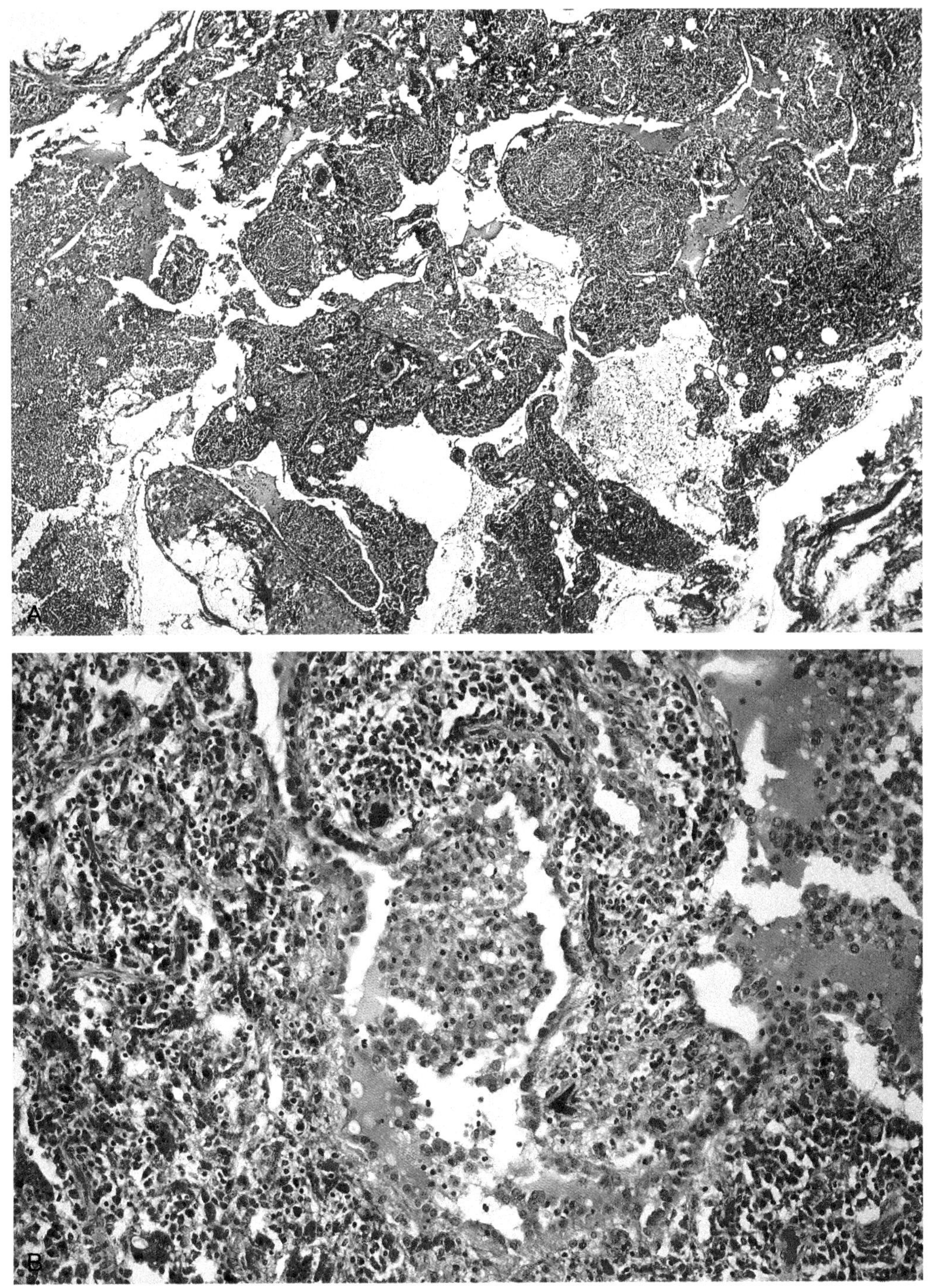

**FIGURE 29–19.** (**A**) Low-power view of reactive mesothelial hyperplasia in a hernial sac. (**B**) Reactive mesothelial proliferation admixed with chronic inflammatory cells and hemosiderin-laden macrophages.

*Illustration continued on following page*

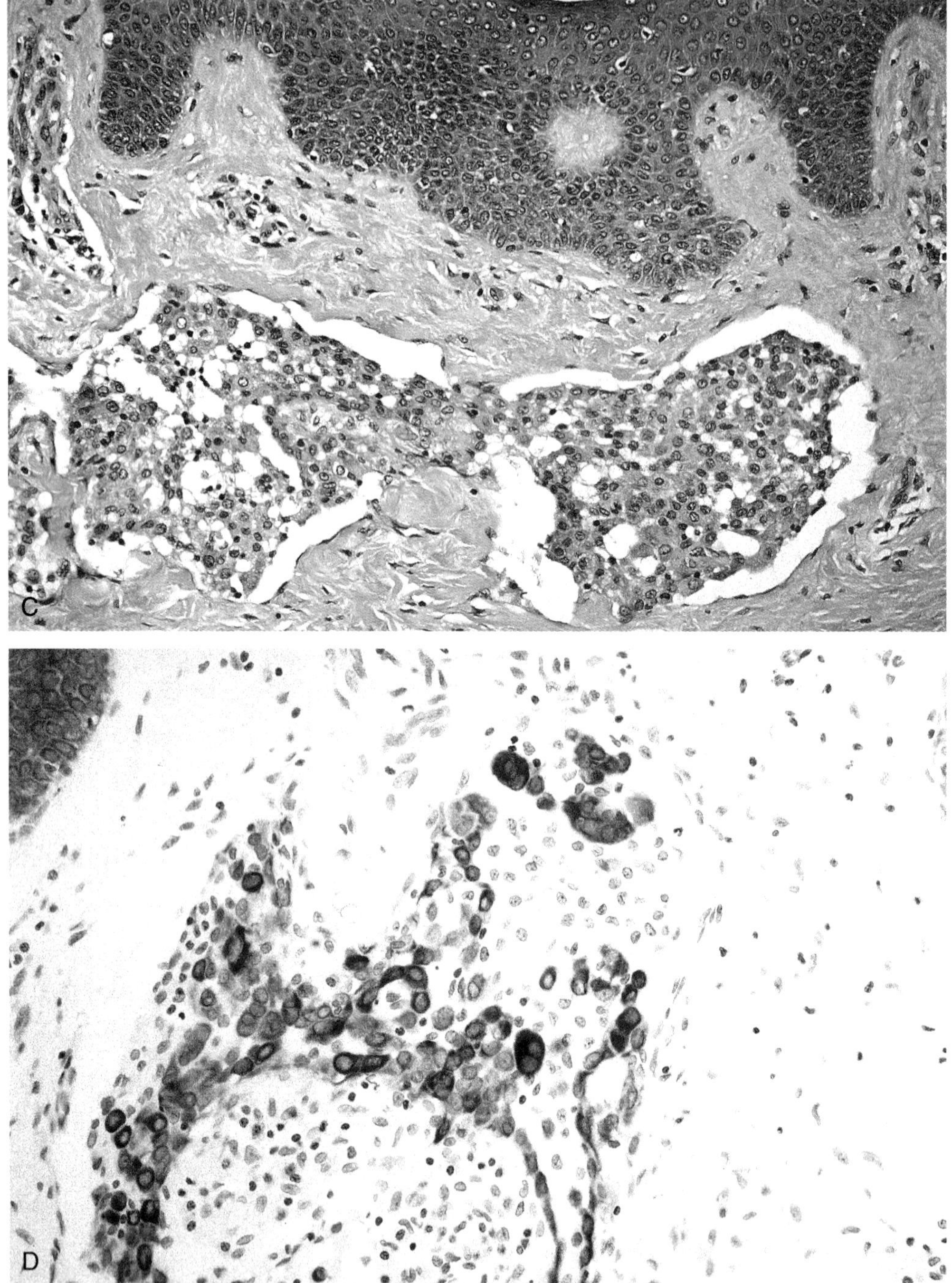


**FIGURE 29–19.** *(Continued).* (**C**) Benign-appearing mesothelial cells within dermal lymphatics in the same case as that depicted in **A** and **B.** This lesion is easily mistaken for metastatic carcinoma. (**D**) Strong cytokeratin immunoreactivity in mesothelial cells in dermal lymphatic channels. The surrounding endothelial cells do not stain for this marker.

astinal lymph nodes in patients with pleural or pericardial effusions,[10,96,169] presumably due to embolization via lymphatic channels.[222] Although metastatic mesothelioma in lymph nodes can occur in a sinusoidal distribution, features that suggest metastatic mesothelioma (rather than benign mesothelial proliferation) in lymph nodes include the identification of more than mild nuclear pleomorphism, tubulopapillary and alveolar patterns, and sclerosis.[238] Ultrastructural analysis may be useful for confirming the mesothelial nature of the cells in question.

Distinction of diffuse mesothelioma from adenocarcinoma and other primary or metastatic epithelial neoplasms is the most difficult diagnostic problem. Adenocarcinomas, particularly peripheral pulmonary adenocarcinomas, can show extensive pleural involvement and may be composed of large cells bearing a close resemblance to mesothelioma.[77] These tumors, however, arise invariably in the pulmonary parenchyma, a feature that may be evident on CT scans. Moreover, in contradistinction to mesothelioma, the intracellular mucin produced by many of these tumors stains well with PAS; in most instances the cells stain positively with anti-CEA, Leu-M1, and Ber-EP4. This also applies to metastases of occult carcinomas of the breast, ovary, and other visceral organs, which are usually multiple and involve both lungs. A detailed clinical history may prove helpful in some of these cases. In the peritoneal cavity distinguishing epithelial peritoneal mesothelioma from peritoneal and ovarian serous carcinomas may also be difficult (Fig. 29–20). Again, a battery of immunostains including B72.3, Ber-EP4, Leu-M1, calretinin, thrombomodulin, and cytokeratin 5/6 is useful for this distinction.[154] Tables 29–3, 29–4, and 29–6 provide guidelines for the histochemical, immunohistochemical, and ultrastructural differentiation of epithelial and mixed mesotheliomas from primary and metastatic adenocarcinomas.

### *Fibrous (Sarcomatoid) Mesothelioma*

The differential diagnosis of fibrous mesothelioma depends on the cellularity of the lesion. Hypocellular regions of desmoplastic mesothelioma may be difficult to distinguish from reactive fibrosis or pleural plaques, particularly in small biopsy specimens. Invasion of the subserosal connective tissues, chest wall, or lung parenchyma by neoplastic spindle cells is a highly sensitive, specific feature of desmoplastic malignant mesothelioma. In subtle cases, invasion of the underlying tissues may be highlighted by immunohistochemical stains for low-molecular-weight cytokeratins.[134] Because reactive submesothelial fibroblasts can be cytokeratin-positive, identification of staining in spindle cells in a thickened pleural lesion is of no diagnostic value. Bland necrosis characterized by necrotic foci accompanied by few if any inflammatory cells is a specific feature of desmoplastic malignant

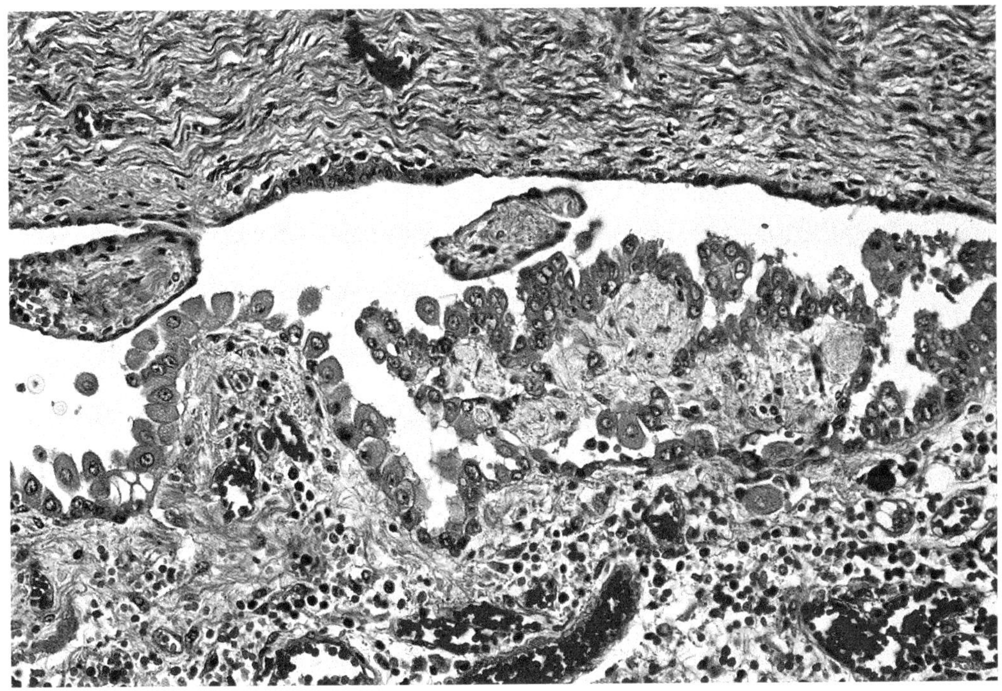

**FIGURE 29–20.** Diffuse epithelial mesothelioma attached to the surface of the ovary. Such tumors may be confused with ovarian or peritoneal serous adenocarcinoma.

mesothelioma, but it lacks sensitivity, as this feature is found in the minority of cases.[134] The presence of frankly sarcomatoid areas, characterized by spindle cells with marked hyperchromasia and nuclear pleomorphism, may also be useful for this distinction. Features useful for recognizing fibrous pleurisy include cellular zonation, with the more cellular areas oriented toward the luminal side of the pleura,[49] and a proliferation of capillaries oriented perpendicular to the pleural surface.[189] Data obtained from radiographic studies may also be of assistance. Mangano et al.[134] found no role for p53 immunohistochemistry in distinguishing these lesions.

More cellular examples of fibrous mesothelioma must be distinguished from benign and malignant variants of solitary fibrous tumor. Benign solitary fibrous tumors typically present as a pedunculated, well circumscribed mass composed of alternating hyper- and hypocellular zones with cytologically bland, patternless spindle cells deposited in a fibrous matrix. Immunohistochemically, the cells of solitary fibrous tumor uniformly express CD34 and rarely stain for cytokeratins. Malignant variants have a variable histologic appearance and may resemble a fibrosarcoma or malignant fibrous histiocytoma. Immunostaining for CD34 is less consistent in these lesions, but stains for cytokeratins are typically negative. One must also consider the possibility of a sarcoma that has metastasized to the pleura; the clinical history and radiographic data are most useful in this regard.

### Biphasic Mesothelioma

The differential diagnosis for biphasic mesothelioma is limited given the biphasic nature of this tumor. There is some resemblance to biphasic synovial sarcoma, but mesotheliomas are characterized by a mixture of epithelial and sarcomatous components that usually blend with one another such that transitional areas may be seen. Rarely in our experience do the two components abut one another in an abrupt fashion as one sees with synovial sarcoma or carcinosarcomas of various organs. Furthermore, it differs from most biphasic synovial sarcomas by the absence of intracellular PAS-positive mucin. In questionable cases, molecular genetic evaluation can be performed to detect the presence or absence of t(X;18), characteristic of synovial sarcoma.

## Prognosis and Therapy

The outlook is grave, and most patients with diffuse mesothelioma die of the disease within 1–2 years of diagnosis. Walz and Koch[245] reported a median survival of 13 months, with a 2-year survival rate of 29% and a 5-year rate of only 4%. Survival rates vary slightly according to tumor type, as most studies have found slightly longer survival for patients with diffuse epithelial mesothelioma compared to those with biphasic or sarcomatoid tumors.[30,67,76] Survival periods are equally short or even shorter for those with diffuse fibrous (sarcomatoid) mesothelioma with extensive desmoplasia. In fact, in the series reported by Cantin et al.[40] metastases occurred more frequently with desmoplastic than nondesmoplastic diffuse fibrous mesotheliomas. As the disease progresses, symptoms become increasingly severe, and many patients die of respiratory failure or intestinal obstruction. Additional complications are caused by extension of the tumor into neighboring tissues (e.g., lung, chest wall, diaphragm, intestinal wall, retroperitoneum) and by recurrence, sometimes along a needle tract of a previous aspiration or needle biopsy or the scar of a previous excision. Metastases do occur but at a relatively late stage of the disease. Kannerstein et al.[114] reported metastases in 18 of 50 autopsy cases. The most common sites of metastasis in their series were the regional lymph nodes, especially those in the mediastinum, abdomen, and supraclavicular region, and the liver, lungs, adrenal glands, and bone marrow. Sometimes lymph node metastases are the first manifestation of the disease. Blood-borne metastases are more commonly associated with fibrous (sarcomatoid) forms of diffuse mesothelioma than with any other microscopic type.[253] Other parameters reported to be adverse prognostic indicators include male gender,[67,218] advanced age,[9,193] poor performance status,[6,67] high white blood cell count,[67] advanced stage,[30,227] and high preoperative tumor volume[170] (Table 29–7).

As is evident from the survival rates, treatment is rarely effective, although remissions have been achieved. Single-modality therapy has not influenced survival, although palliation may be provided by surgery, chemotherapy, or radiation therapy alone. More recently, multimodality treatment with cytoreductive

**TABLE 29–7 REPORTED UNFAVORABLE PROGNOSTIC FACTORS FOR MALIGNANT PLEURAL MESOTHELIOMA**

| |
|---|
| Sarcomatoid type |
| High preoperative tumor volume |
| Poor performance status |
| Advanced age |
| Advanced stage |
| Male gender |
| High white blood cell count |
| Aneuploidy |

**TABLE 29–8 BRIGHAM STAGING SYSTEM FOR MALIGNANT PLEURAL MESOTHELIOMA**

| Stage | Definition |
|---|---|
| I | Confined to within capsule of parietal pleura: ipsilateral pleura, lung, pericardium, diaphragm, or chest wall disease limited to previous biopsy sites |
| II | Same as stage I plus positive intrathoracic lymph nodes |
| III | Local extension of disease into the chest wall or mediastinum, heart, or throughout the diaphragm or peritoneum; with or without extrathoracic or contralateral lymph node involvement |
| IV | Distant metastases |

Modified from Sugarbaker DJ, Strauss GM, Lynch TJ, et al. Node status has prognostic significance in the multimodality therapy of diffuse, malignant mesothelioma. J Clin Oncol 11:1172, 1993.

surgery (pleurectomy/decortication[183,196–198] or extrapleural pneumonectomy[197,224,225]) followed by chemotherapy and radiotherapy appears to prolong survival. Using extrapleural pneumonectomy followed by chemotherapy and radiotherapy, Sugarbaker et al.[223,224] reported a median survival of 21 months, with 2- and 5-year survival rates of 45% and 22%, respectively. Mitomycin C, cisplatin, doxorubicin, and cyclophosphamide appear to be the most active chemotherapic agents.[147,200,233] Because mesothelioma usually remains confined to the pleural or peritoneal cavities until late in its course (Table 29–8), intracavitary instillation of chemotherapeutic agents has been attempted with moderate success.[196,239]

The tendency for mesotheliomas to remain localized until late in their course and the relatively poor survival with conventional therapy has led to the unique opportunity to develop new therapies that might affect survival.[112] Mesothelioma cells secrete a variety of soluble factors, including transforming growth factor-$\beta$ (TGF$\beta$)[24,85] and interleukin-6 (IL-6),[201] which inhibit host immunity. Attempts to inhibit secretion of these soluble factors, thereby allowing the host immune system to eradicate the tumor, have been attempted in vitro[31] and in vivo,[14,29,46,94] in some cases as part of multimodality therapy.[171,216] Intrapleural photodynamic therapy has also been attempted,[231] although its success has been limited by significant morbidity.[132,234] Gene therapy is in its infancy, but trials are under way to test the efficacy of this mode of therapy in patients with mesothelioma.[5] This therapy is based on the use of a "suicide gene"; the gene encodes an enzyme, which produces a toxic metabolite that is transferred to tumor cells following administration of a nontoxic enzyme substrate.[83,145]

## WELL-DIFFERENTIATED PAPILLARY MESOTHELIOMA

The well-differentiated papillary mesothelioma, a rare mesothelial tumor, is sometimes referred to as *benign mesothelioma* or *papillary mesothelioma*.[267,268] The lesions are solitary[272] or multifocal[275,276] and are primarily located in the peritoneum, with a predilection for the omentum, mesentery, and pelvis; they may also arise from the spermatic cord and the surface of the testis. Rare cases have been described in the pericardium.[280] Many are incidental findings at surgical exploration or autopsy.[272,278]

Histologically, the lesion is characterized by a proliferation of uniform, cuboidal cells with centrally placed nuclei and inconspicuous nucleoli that line papillary structures (Figs. 29–21, 29–22). In some cases, the neoplastic cells form solid nests, tubules, or cords in the connective tissue stroma. Rarely, the features of papillary mesothelioma are associated with those of an adenomatoid tumor.[274] Multinucleated stromal giant cells with nucleoli arranged in a floret-like fashion may be present. Mitotic figures are absent or rare. The staining and electron microscopic features of the lining cells are typical of well-differentiated mesothelial cells.[271,277,282] As with malignant mesothelioma, negative staining of the cells with PAS after diastase digestion and the results of immunohistochemical studies, especially CEA and Leu-M1, help distinguish this lesion from surface papillary carcinoma.[272,279]

In our experience, localized, solitary tumors that have uniformly histologically benign features behave in a predictably benign fashion. Solitary tumors with slightly atypical cytologic features probably can also be expected to behave in a benign fashion if they are completely excised and are localized to one anatomic site.[272] Tumors that are widespread are much more likely to pursue a progressive clinical course and cannot be reliably regarded as benign neoplasms. Although there are reports of patients with widespread papillary mesotheliomas with histologically benign features that have behaved in a clinically benign fashion,[270] long-term follow-up is generally lacking in these cases.[281] Some of these lesions recur, often after many years, or progress to malignant mesothelioma with occasional distant metastases.[269] Furthermore, areas resembling well-differentiated papillary mesothelioma may be seen in diffuse malignant mesothelioma, albeit as a focal finding. The presence of ascites and clinical symptoms other than those attributable to torsion of a pedunculated tumor should raise the possibility of a malignancy. Unlike diffuse malignant mesothelioma, few have arisen in patients with a history of asbestos exposure.[270,273]

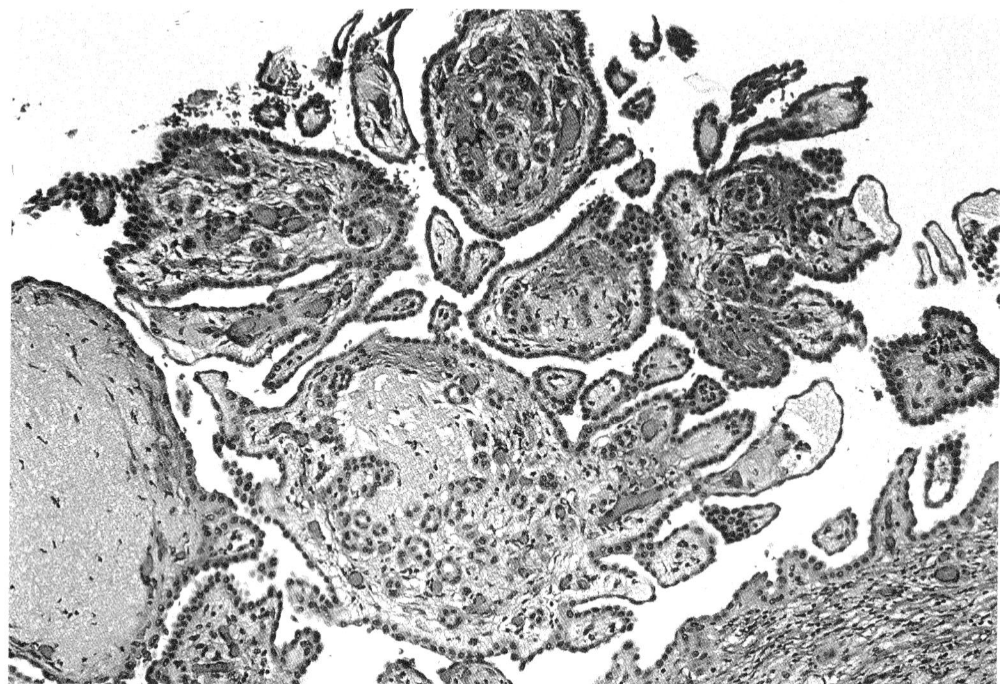

**FIGURE 29–21.** Low-power view of a well-differentiated papillary mesothelioma of the peritoneum. Papillary structures are lined by a single layer of cuboidal cells. Similar-appearing cells line tubules in the papillary cores.

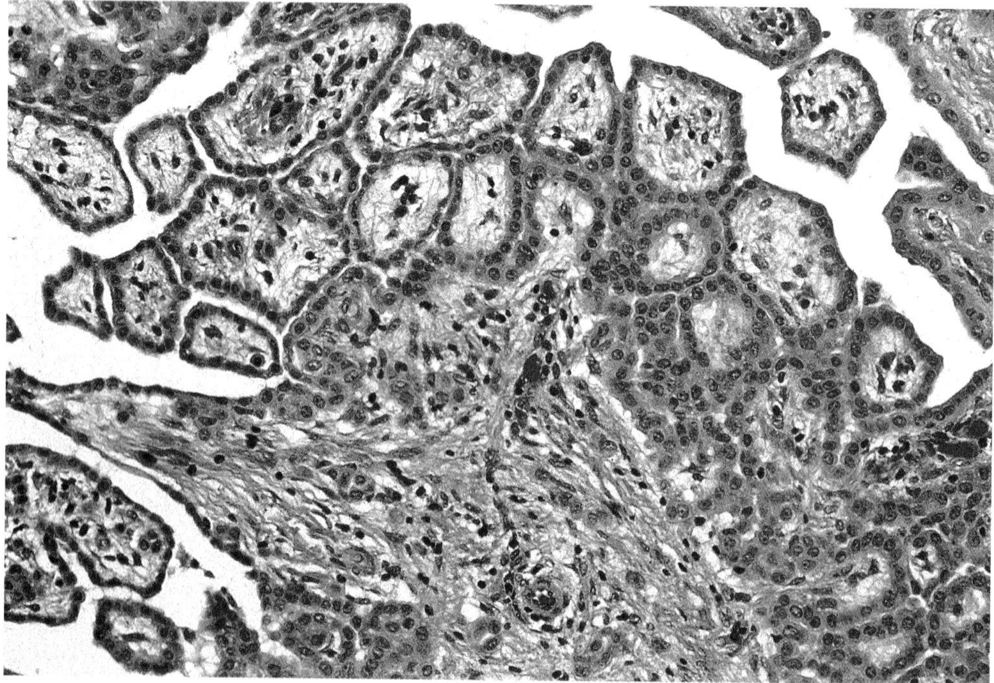

**FIGURE 29–22.** Cytologically bland mesothelial cells line papillary structures in a well-differentiated papillary mesothelioma of the peritoneum.

## MULTICYSTIC PERITONEAL MESOTHELIOMA

"Multicystic peritoneal mesothelioma" has been used to describe an unusual mesothelial lesion that deserves separate consideration because of its characteristic histologic picture and its benign behavior. In the past this lesion was often confused with cystic lymphangioma, mesenteric lymphatic cyst in basal cell nevus syndrome, or (despite its different clinical course) diffuse mesothelioma or even a disseminated form of mucin-producing adenocarcinoma. First described by Plaut[299] in 1928 as "loose cysts of the pelvis," this lesion has been referred to by a variety of names, including peritoneal inclusion cysts,[296] peritoneal cystosis,[290] benign cystic mesothelioma,[289,298,300] and multicystic mesothelial proliferation,[283] reflecting the controversial pathogenesis of this lesion.

Multicystic peritoneal mesothelioma occurs chiefly in adults, with a predilection for young and middle-aged women. It is usually noted because it produces vague lower abdominal pain or symptoms suggesting partial intestinal obstruction, such as distension, nausea, or vomiting. Rare patients present with an acute abdomen[305] or ascites.[295] The symptoms of the disease are relatively nonspecific, and a correct preoperative diagnosis is almost never rendered.

Exploratory laparotomy reveals a characteristic picture: Numerous thin-walled transparent cysts are unevenly distributed in the serosal and subserosal tissues of the parietal and visceral peritoneum of the abdomen and pelvis, often forming multicystic masses (Fig. 29–23). The lesions have a propensity to arise on the surface of the uterus, cul-de-sac, bladder, or rectum. The cysts measure a few millimeters in diameter to several centimeters and contain clear or blood-tinged fluid (Fig. 29–24). Occasionally, there are also multiple filamentous and string-like adhesions between the peritoneum, intestines, and viscera.[285,291]

Microscopic examination discloses one or more variously sized, round or irregularly shaped cystic space lined by a single layer of flattened or cuboidal mesothelial cells, sometimes displaying a brush border (Figs. 29–25, 29–26). Less commonly the cells are plump and protrude into the lumen in a hobnail or even papillary pattern. Focal squamous metaplasia is seen occasionally. The cystic spaces are separated by loose, edematous tissue often containing chronic inflammatory cells, fibrin deposits, and sometimes entrapped mesothelial cells resembling infiltrating carcinoma (so-called mural nodules) (Fig. 29–27). Transition between multicystic mesothelioma and adenomatoid tumor has been observed on several occasions[286,294] (Fig. 29–28). Unusual features include the presence of extracellular or intracellular hyaline globules[293] and calcifications.[288] The secreted material in the spaces stains positively with alcian blue and colloidal iron but negatively with PAS. Similarly staining material is found as a thin coating on the luminal surface of the tumor cells (Fig. 29–29) and rarely as small intracellular droplets.

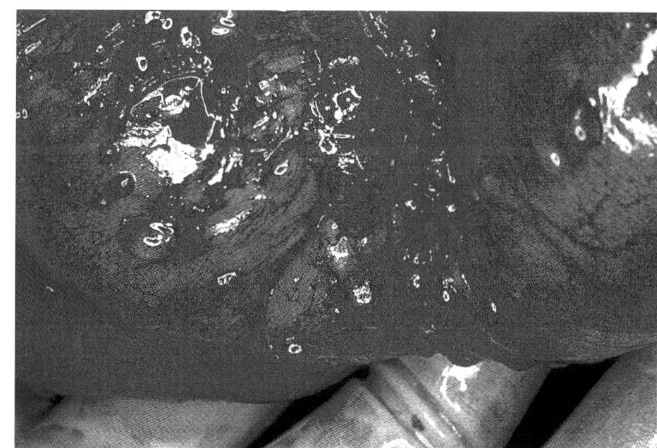

**FIGURE 29–23.** Multicystic mesothelioma diffusely involving the serosal surface of the intestine.

Like other forms of mesothelioma the lining cells are immunoreactive for cytokeratins and epithelial membrane antigen,[287,302,303] a feature that rules out cystic lymphangioma. Moreover, cystic lymphangioma occurs chiefly in male children and adolescents and microscopically is characterized by stromal aggregates of lymphocytes and an endothelial lining occasionally positive for factor VIII-related antigen and

*Text continued on page 1097*

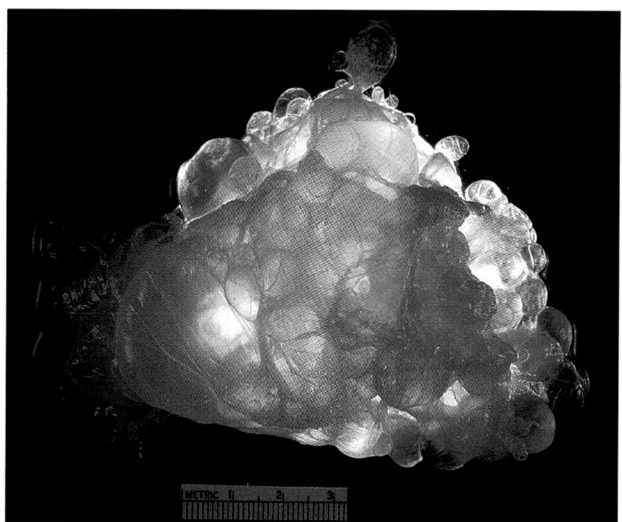


**FIGURE 29–24.** Multicystic peritoneal mesothelioma consisting of multiple transparent, fluid-filled cysts.

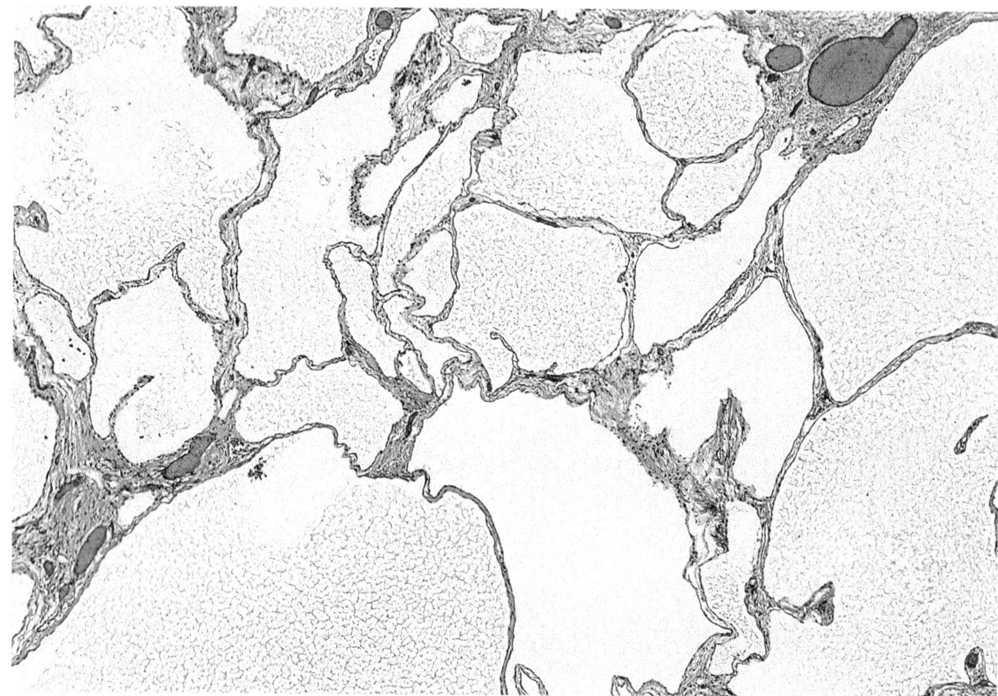

**FIGURE 29–25.** Multicystic mesothelioma composed of numerous mesothelial-lined cysts embedded in a delicate fibrovascular stroma.

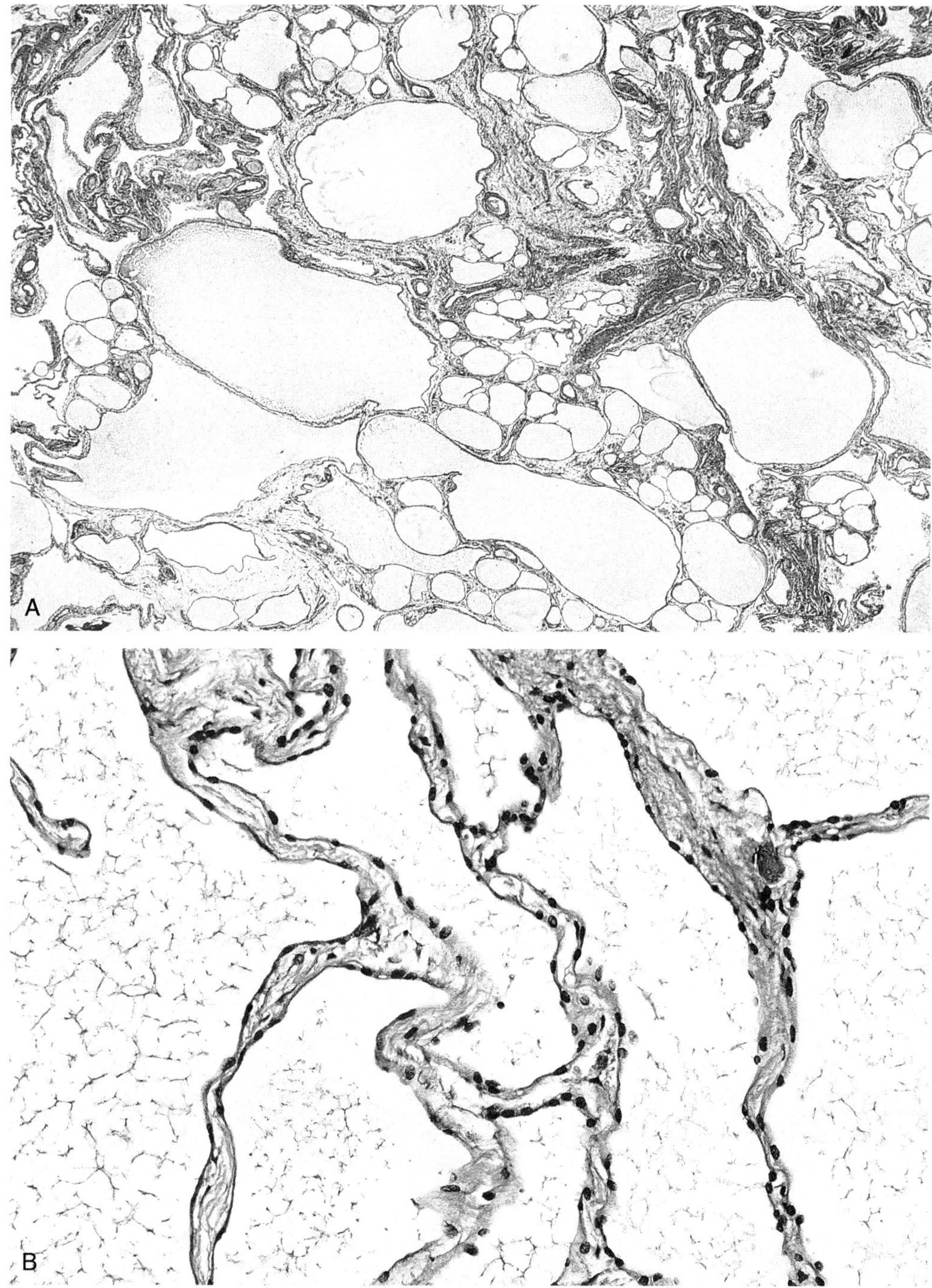


**FIGURE 29–26.** (**A**) Low-power view of a multicystic peritoneal mesothelioma mimicking a cystic lymphangioma. (**B**) Cysts are lined by cytologically bland flattened and cuboidal mesothelial cells.

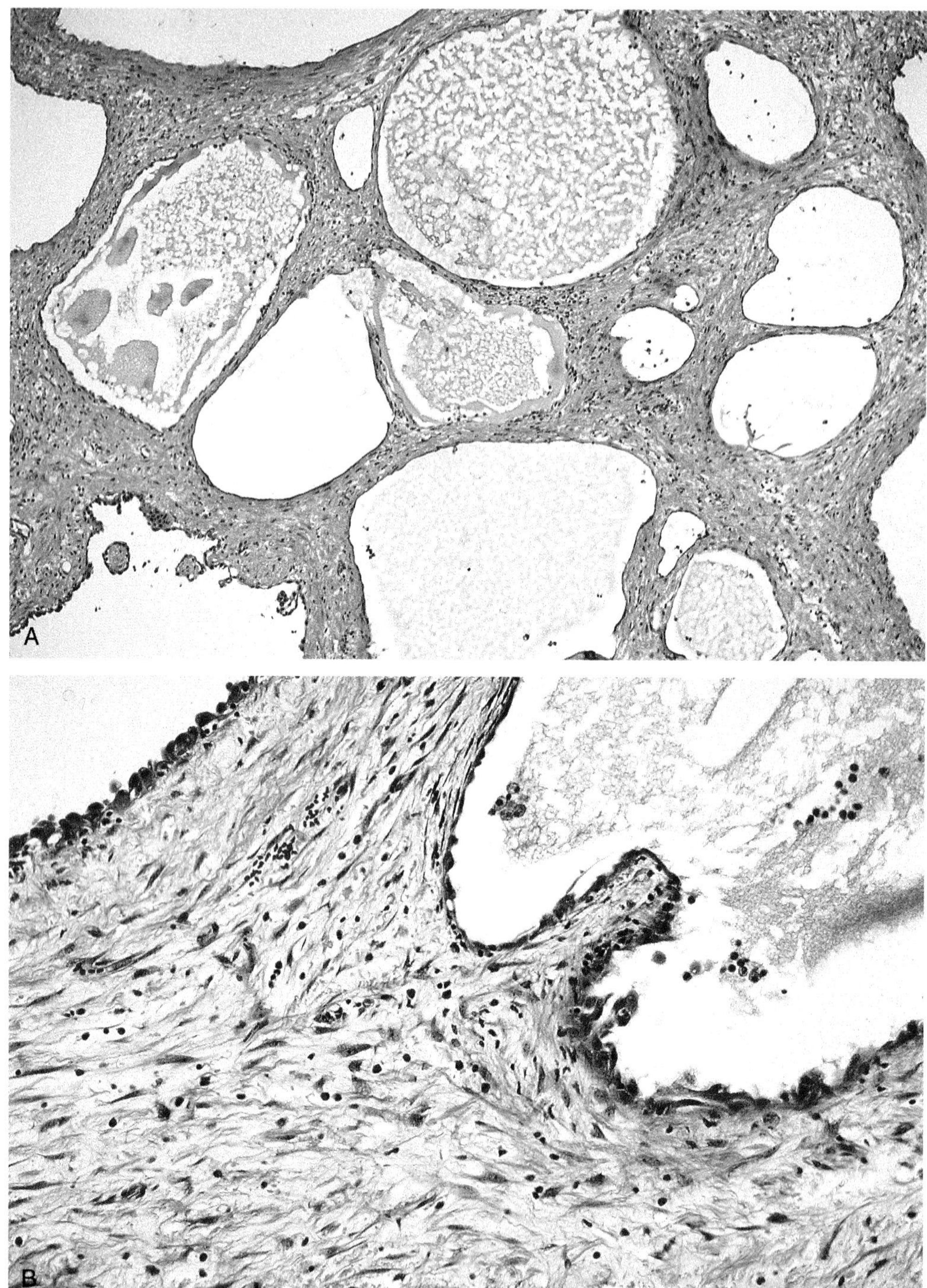


**FIGURE 29–27.** (**A**) Multicystic mesothelioma with secondary inflammatory changes. Rare cysts contain detached clumps of mesothelial cells. (**B**) Mesothelial spaces lie in an edematous, spindled stroma containing inflammatory cells.

*Illustration continued on opposite page*

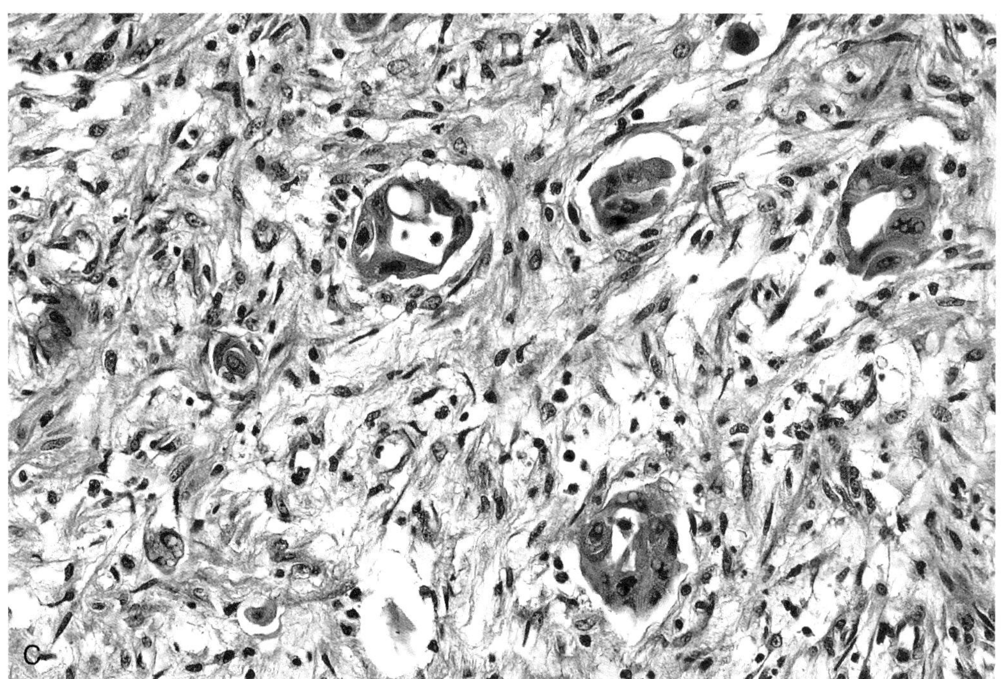

**FIGURE 29–27** *(Continued).* (**C**) Mesothelial cells entrapped in the wall of a multicystic mesothelioma closely mimicking infiltrating carcinoma.

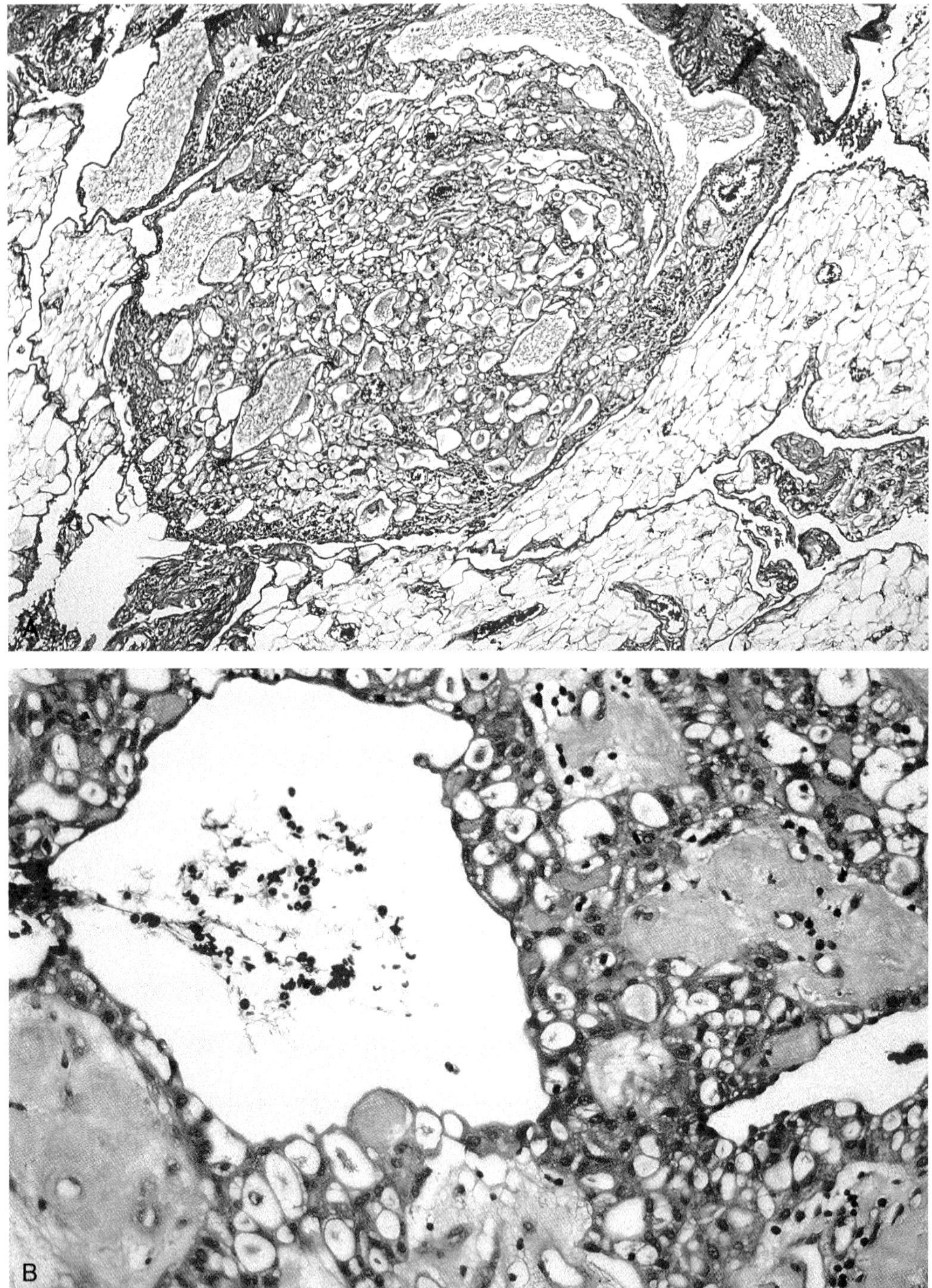

**FIGURE 29–28.** Low-power (**A**) and high-power (**B**) views of a multicystic mesothelioma with foci resembling adenomatoid tumor.

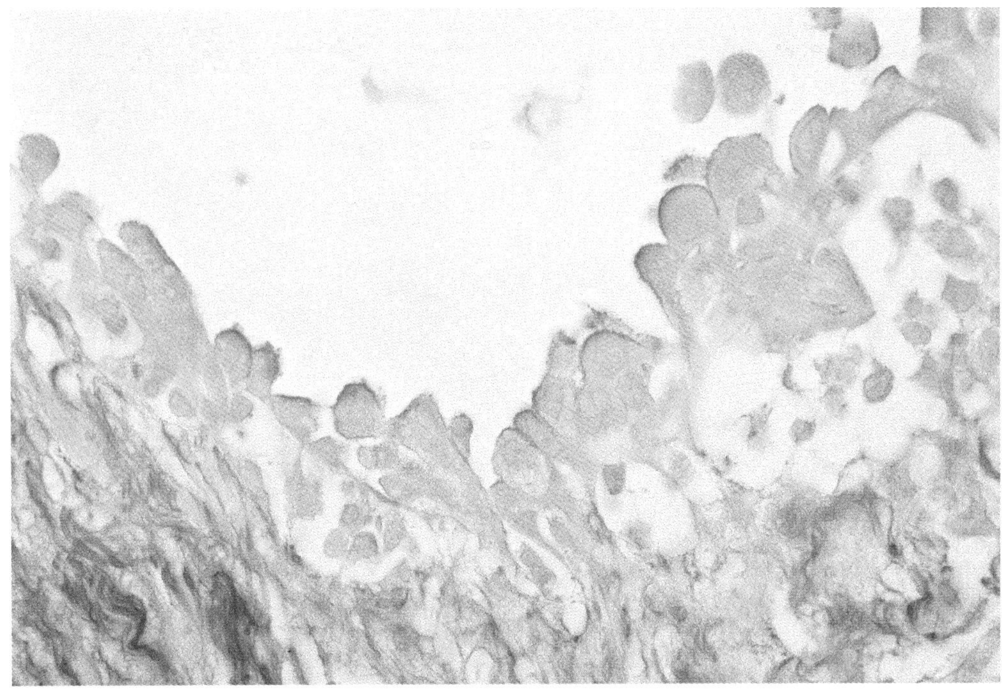

**FIGURE 29–29.** Colloidal iron stain showing a thin coating on the luminal surface of tumor cells in a multicystic mesothelioma.

negative for cytokeratins. A layer of smooth muscle tissue may surround the vascular structures. Other conditions that must be considered in the differential diagnosis are reactive mesothelial proliferations, well-differentiated papillary mesothelioma, ovarian and extraovarian papillary serous carcinomas, endometriosis, and microcystic adenoma of the pancreas (Fig. 29–30).

Electron microscopic studies reveal the ultrastructural characteristics of mesothelial cells,[297,301] especially slender microvilli on the luminal surfaces of the lining cells, well developed basal laminae, and tight desmosomal junctions (Fig. 29–31). There are also numerous intracytoplasmic filaments, ovoid mitochondria, and prominent rough endoplasmic reticulum (Fig. 29–32).

The clinical course is largely that of a benign lesion (Table 29–9). Among 25 patients with follow-up information reported by Weiss and Tavassoli,[305] 21 were alive, 2 died of other causes, and 2 died of the disease. The two patients who died were an infant who had a mixture of cystic and diffuse epithelial mesothelioma and a 47-year-old man who refused therapy and died 12 years after detection of the abdominal mass (Fig. 29–33).

The appropriate therapy seems to be total surgical excision for localized lesions and subtotal resection or debulking procedures for more extensive lesions.[305] Sometimes the large number of lesions and their small size preclude complete resection, with further spread and recurrence years after the initial excision. Rare cases have also been treated with sclerotherapy and transvaginal catheter drainage.[304]

The pathogenesis of this unusual lesion is not clear. The multiplicity of lesions, their spread and recurrence, and the reported transitions toward adenoma-

**TABLE 29–9** RELATION BETWEEN EXTENT OF MULTICYSTIC MESOTHELIOMA AT DIAGNOSIS AND CLINICAL OUTCOME

| Extent of Disease | No. of Patients | Alive | Died of Disease | Died of Other Causes | No Follow-up |
|---|---|---|---|---|---|
| Solitary | 6 | 3 | 1* | 0 | 2 |
| Localized | 15 | 7 | 0 | 8 | 0 |
| Diffuse | 16 | 11 | 1† | 2 | 2 |
| *Total* | 37 | 21 | 2 | 10 | 4 |

From Weiss SW, Tavassoli FA. Multicystic mesothelioma: an analysis of pathologic findings and biologic behavior in 37 cases. Am J Surg Pathol 12:737, 1988, with permission.

* Combined cystic/epithelial mesothelioma.

† Patient refused therapy.

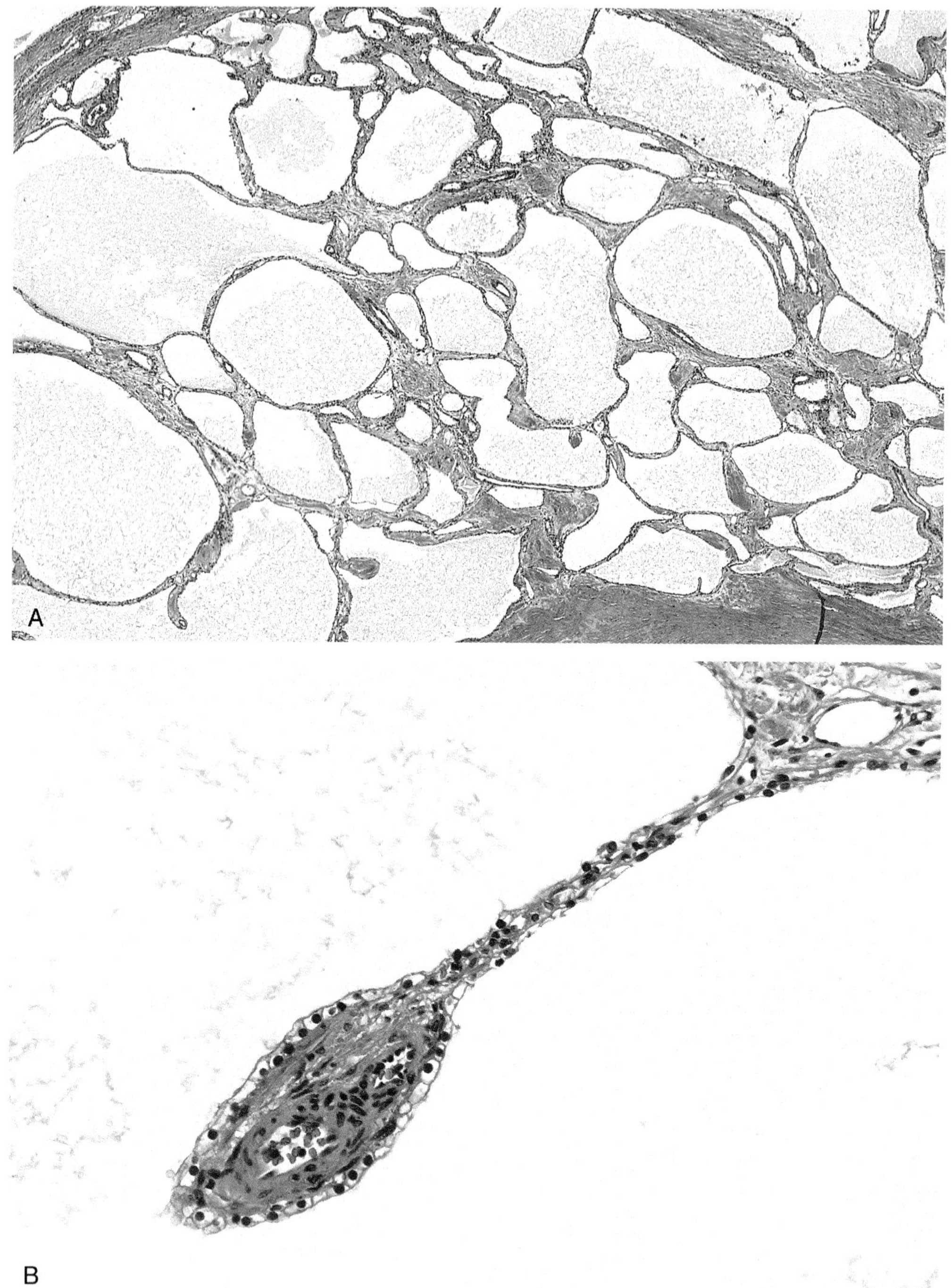


**FIGURE 29–30.** (**A**) Low-power view of a microcystic adenoma of the pancreas closely resembling multicystic mesothelioma. (**B**) Microcystic adenoma of the pancreas composed of cysts lined by cuboidal cells with vacuolated cytoplasm.

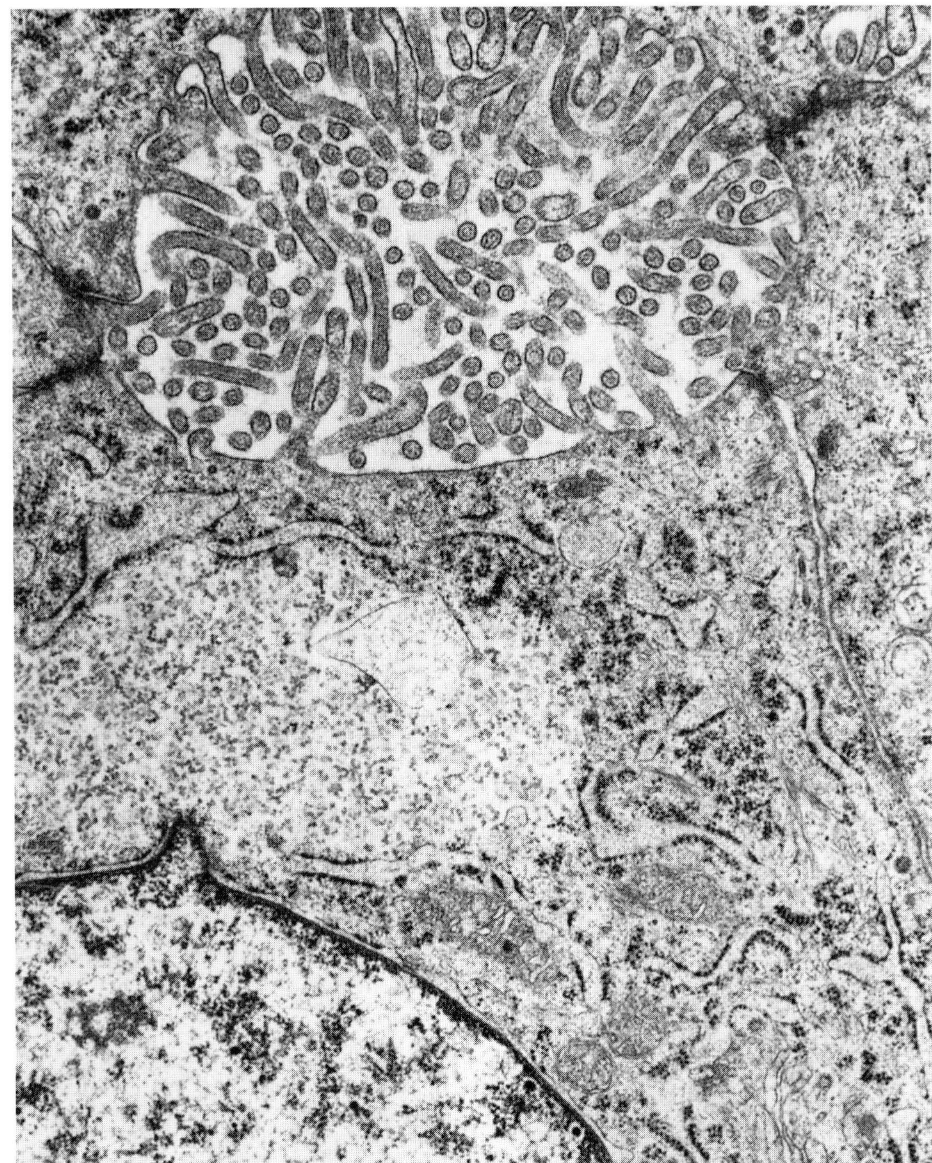

**FIGURE 29–31.** Electron microscopic view of a multicystic peritoneal mesothelioma showing intercellular space with numerous slender microvilli and deposits of intracellular glycogen. (From Mennemeyer R, Smith M. Multicystic, peritoneal mesothelioma: a report with electron microscopy of a case mimicking intraabdominal cystic hygroma (lymphangioma). Cancer 44:692, 1979.)

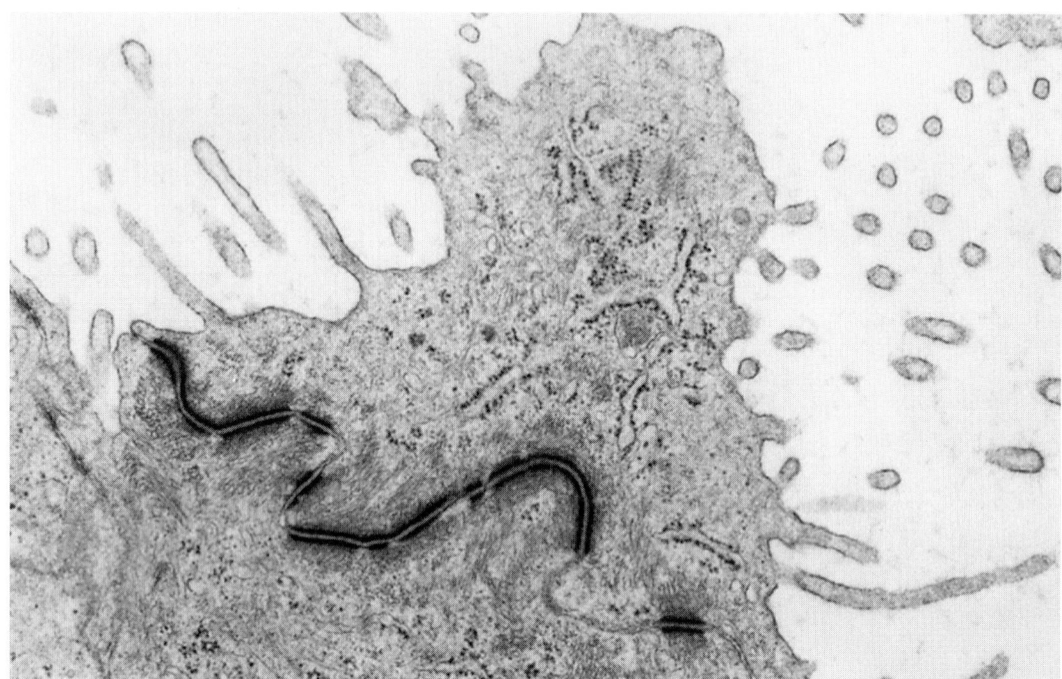

**FIGURE 29–32.** Electron microscopic view of a multicystic peritoneal mesothelioma with short microvilli, prominent tight desmosomal junctions, and converging microfilaments. (From Mennemeyer R, Smith M. Multicystic, peritoneal mesothelioma: a report with electron microscopy of a case mimicking intraabdominal cystic hygroma (lymphangioma). Cancer 44:692, 1979.)

toid tumor and rarely, with diffuse malignant mesothelioma support the contention that this is a neoplasm, even though 30–50% of patients have a history of abdominal surgery, pelvic inflammatory disease, or endometriosis.[296] The fact that this tumor is rare in the pleura[283] and is only occasionally associated with occupational asbestos exposure[284,292] suggests significant pathogenetic differences from the conventional form of diffuse malignant mesothelioma. Although diffuse epithelial mesothelioma presents at times as a multicystic growth, it usually can be identified by its less uniform gross appearance, its greater cellularity, and its cellular pleomorphism.

## ADENOMATOID TUMOR

Adenomatoid tumor is a clinically benign mesothelial neoplasm usually confined to the genital tract. It occurs in both genders; in men it most commonly is found in the epididymis (Fig. 29–34) but may also be

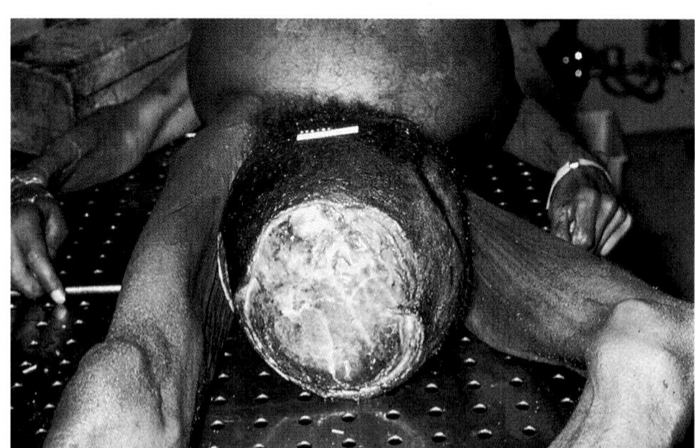

**FIGURE 29–33.** Multicystic peritoneal mesothelioma in a 47-year-old man. The patient refused therapy and died 12 years after initial detection of the tumor.

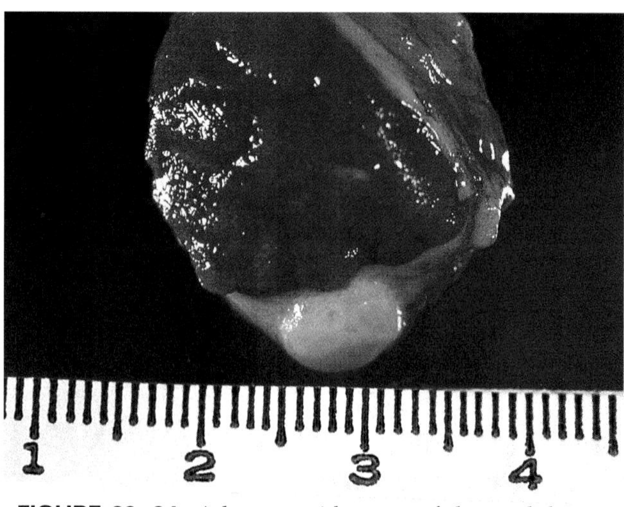


**FIGURE 29–34.** Adenomatoid tumor of the epididymis.

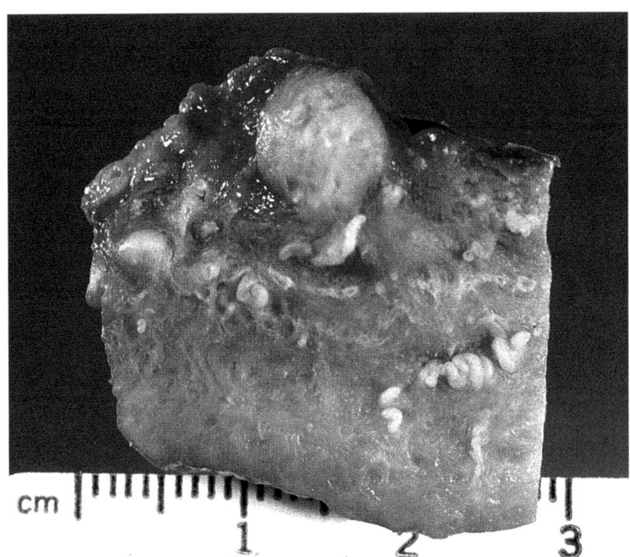


**FIGURE 29–35.** Adenomatoid tumor in the myometrium of a 44-year-old woman.

observed in the spermatic cord, testicular tunic, prostate, ejaculatory duct, and the parenchyma of the testis.[309,315,322] In women the lesion is most commonly seen in the uterus (Fig. 29–35) and fallopian tubes, but it may occur in the ovary.[311,320,329] Rarely, this lesion has been described in extragenital sites, including the small bowel mesentery,[308] omentum, retroperitoneum, adrenal gland,[321,328] pleura,[312] and heart.[318] Its mesothelial origin, first suggested by Masson et al. in 1942,[317] is now firmly established, but the earlier noncommittal term *adenomatoid tumor,* coined by Golden and Ash[310] in 1945, is still widely employed to distinguish this tumor from the rare papillary mesothelioma.

## Clinical Findings

In general, the tumor presents as a small indurated mass or swelling that is painless and nontender. It is usually an incidental finding at routine examination, surgery for some other cause (hysterectomy), or autopsy. It rarely occurs before the age of 20 years and is chiefly encountered in patients 30–60 years of age. The tumor is usually solitary, but multiple nodular lesions have been observed. A small number of these lesions in the scrotum are associated with hydroceles.

## Pathologic Findings

Gross examination reveals a firm mass generally less than 2 cm in greatest dimension. The mass is well circumscribed with a smooth, glistening, yellow-gray cut surface. On microscopic examination the tumor is seen to have a variable structural pattern ranging from irregularly arranged, dilated tubular channels and gland-like spaces lined by flattened or cuboidal cells to solid nests and strands of plump cells with abundant eosinophilic cytoplasm (Figs. 29–36,

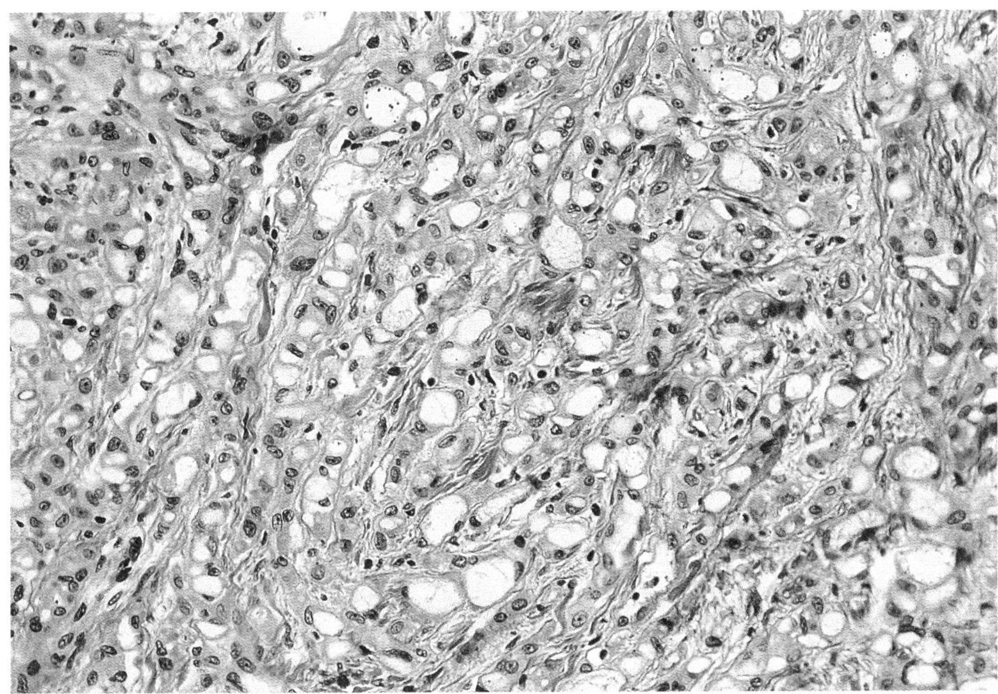

**FIGURE 29–36.** Benign mesothelioma of the genital tract (adenomatoid tumor) with a characteristic tubular pattern.

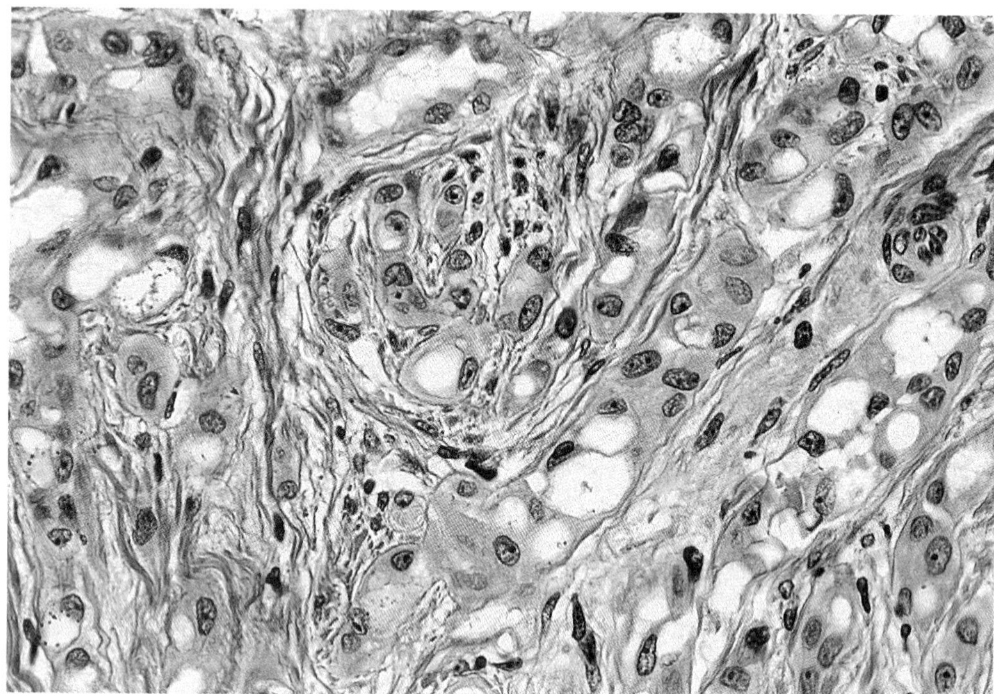

**FIGURE 29–37.** High-power view showing bland cytologic features of the mesothelial cells in an adenomatoid tumor.

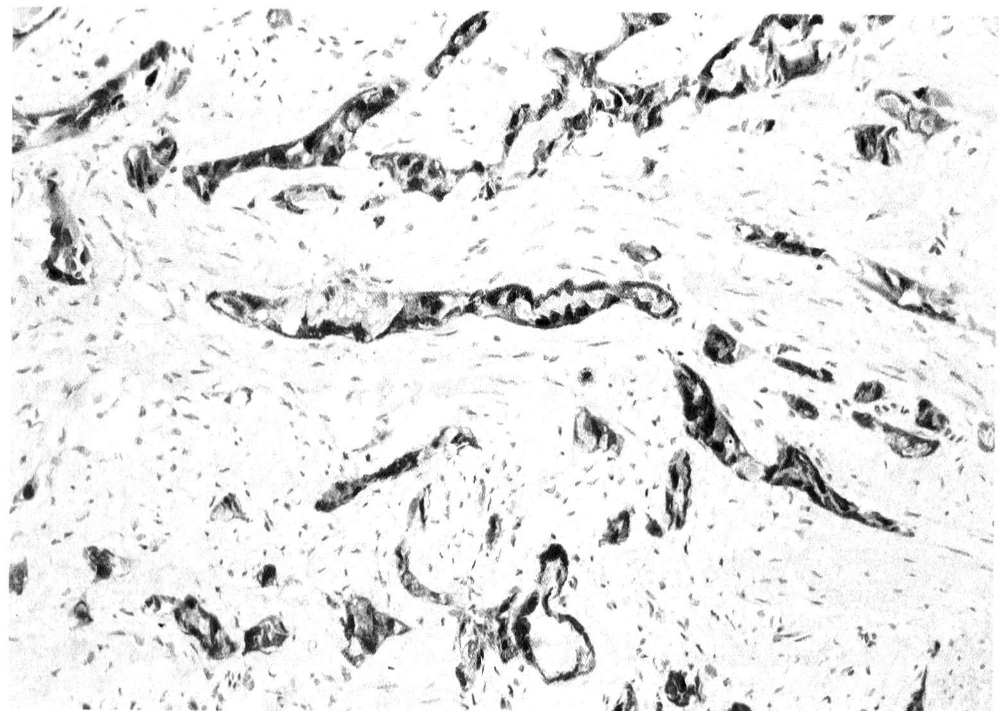

**FIGURE 29–38.** Diffuse calretinin immunoreactivity in an adenomatoid tumor of the fallopian tube.

29–37). As in other mesotheliomas, desquamated cells are often present in the dilated spaces. Lee et al.[313] distinguished canalicular, tubular, and plexiform patterns. The fibrous stroma may be sparse or abundant and may contain aggregates of lymphocytes. The smooth muscle component, which is present and even conspicuous in some cases, is likely residual. It has also been interpreted as an inherent part of the tumor and was cited as evidence for its origin in the müllerian duct. This theory of origin is not supported by several electron microscopic studies,[314,316,324,327] which revealed the characteristic features of mesothelial cells, including long, bushy microvilli on the luminal surfaces and intercellular spaces, irregular cytoplasmic protrusions, and desmosomes, often associated with tonofibrils. Like mesothelial cells at other sites, the cells stain positively for cytokeratins and do not stain for factor VIII-related antigen or CD31.[307,323,326] The latter stains are positive in histiocytoid (epithelioid) hemangioma of the testis, a tumor that must be distinguished from richly vascular variants of adenomatoid tumor.[306] Other markers of nonneoplastic and neoplastic mesothelial cells, including thrombomodulin and calretinin[325] (Fig. 29–38), have also been observed. Otis reported Ber-EP4 in 9 of 11 adenomatoid tumors[319] and cautioned that staining with this antibody does not exclude an adenomatoid tumor.

The tumor is benign, and local resection is adequate therapy. There are no reports of malignant transformation, although some diffuse malignant mesotheliomas have a prominent adenomatoid growth pattern.

## REFERENCES

### Diffuse Mesothelioma


1. Adami JG. Principles of Pathology. Lea & Febiger, Philadelphia, 1908.
2. Adams VI, Unni KK, Muhm JR, et al. Diffuse mesothelioma of pleura: diagnosis and survival in 92 cases. Cancer 58:1540, 1986.
3. Adrion A, Bosia S, Paoletti L, et al. Malignant peritoneal mesothelioma in a 17-year old boy with evidence of previous exposure to chrysotile and tremolite asbestos. Hum Pathol 25: 617, 1994.
4. Afify AM, Stern R, Jobes G, et al. Differential expression of CD44S and hyaluronic acid in malignant mesotheliomas, adenocarcinomas, and reactive mesothelial hyperplasias. Appl Immunohistochem 6:11, 1998.
5. Albelda SM. Gene therapy for lung cancer and mesothelioma. Chest 111:143, 1997.
6. Alberts AS, Falkson G, Goedhals L, et al. Malignant pleural mesothelioma: a disease unaffected by current therapeutic maneuvers. J Clin Oncol 6:527, 1988.
7. Antman KH. Clinical presentation and natural history of benign and malignant mesothelioma. Semin Oncol 8:313, 1981.
8. Antman KH. Natural history and epidemiology of malignant mesothelioma. Chest 103:737S, 1993.
9. Antman KH, Shemin R, Ryan L, et al. Malignant mesothelioma: prognostic variables in a registry of 180 patients, the Dana-Farber Cancer Institute and Brigham and Women's Hospital experience over two decades, 1965, 1988. J Clin Oncol 6: 147, 1988.
10. Argani P, Rosai J. Hyperplastic mesothelial cells in lymph nodes: report of six cases of a benign process that can simulate metastatic involvement by mesothelioma or carcinoma. Hum Pathol 29:339, 1998.
11. Armstrong GR, Raafat F, Ingram L, et al. Malignant peritoneal mesothelioma in childhood. Arch Pathol Lab Med 112:1159, 1988.
12. Ascoli V, Scalzo CC, Facciolo F, et al. Platelet-derived growth factor receptor immunoreactivity in mesothelioma and nonneoplastic mesothelial cells in serous effusions. Acta Cytol 39: 613, 1995.
13. Ashcroft T, Heppleston AG. The optical and EM determination of pulmonary asbestos fiber concentration and its relation to the human pathological reaction. J Clin Pathol 26:224, 1973.
14. Astoul P, Bertault Peres P, Durand A, et al. Pharmacokinetics of intrapleural recombinant interleukin-2 in immunotherapy for malignant pleural effusion. Cancer 73:308, 1994.
15. Attanoos RL, Gibbs AR. Pathology of malignant mesothelioma. Histopathology 30:403, 1997.
16. Attanoos RL, Webb R, Gibbs AR. CD44H expression in reactive mesothelium, pleural mesothelioma and pulmonary adenocarcinoma. Histopathology 30:260, 1997.
17. Averbach AM, Sugarbaker PH. Peritoneal mesothelioma: treatment approach based on natural history. Cancer Treat Res 81: 193, 1996.
18. Azam M, Linden MD, Amin MB. Calretinen and HBME-1 antibodies: a comparative immunohistochemical study. Mod Pathol 11:1003A, 1998.
19. Azumi N, Underhill CB, Kagan E, et al. A novel biotinylated probe specific for hyaluronate: its diagnostic value in diffuse malignant mesothelioma. Am J Surg Pathol 16:116, 1992.
20. Baas P, Schouwink H, Zoetmulder FAN. Malignant pleural mesothelioma. Ann Oncol 9:139, 1998.
21. Bateman AC, Al-Talib RK, Newman T, et al. Immunohistochemical phenotype of malignant mesothelioma: predictive value of CA125 and HBME-1 expression. Histopathology 30: 49, 1997.
22. Berti E, Schiaffino E, Minervini MS, et al. Primary malignant mesothelioma of the tunica vaginalis of the testis: immunohistochemistry and electron microscopy. Pathology 29:96, 1997.
23. Betta P-G, Andrion A, Donna A, et al. Malignant mesothelioma of the pleura: the reproducibility of the immunohistological diagnosis. Pathol Lab Pract 193:759, 1997.
24. Bielefeldt-Ohmann H, Fitzpatrick DR, Marzo AL, et al. Patho- and immunobiology of malignant mesothelioma: characterization of tumour infiltrating leukocytes and cytokine production in a murine model. Cancer Immunol Immunother 39:347, 1994.
25. Björkqvist A-M, Tammilehto L, Nordling S, et al. Comparison of DNA copy number changes in malignant mesothelioma, adenocarcinoma and large-cell anaplastic carcinoma of the lung. Br J Cancer 77:260, 1998.
26. Boehme M. Primates Sarcocarcinom der Pleura. Virchows Arch [Pathol Anat] 81:181, 1880.
27. Bolen JW, Hammar SP, McNutt MA. Reactive and neoplastic serosal tissue: a light microscopic, ultrastructural, and immunocytochemical study. Am J Surg Pathol 10:34, 1986.
28. Bollinger DJ, Wick MR, Dehner LP, et al. Peritoneal malignant mesothelioma versus serous papillary adenocarcinoma: a histochemical and immunohistochemical comparison. Am J Surg Pathol 13:659, 1989.
29. Boutin C, Nussbaum E, Monnet I, et al. Intrapleural treatment with recombinant gamma-interferon in early stage malignant pleural mesothelioma. Cancer 74:2460, 1994.
30. Boutin C, Rey F, Gouvernet J, et al. Thoracoscopy in pleural malignant mesothelioma: a prospective study of 188 consecutive patients. Cancer 72:394, 1993.

31. Bowman RV, Manning LS, Davis MR, et al. Chemosensitivity and cytokine sensitivity of malignant mesothelioma. Cancer Chemother Pharmacol 28:420, 1991.
32. Brainard JA, Goldblum JR. An immunohistochemical analysis of the Wilms' tumor gene product as a discriminator of peritoneal mesothelioma from primary peritoneal serous adenocarcinoma. Mod Pathol 11:582A, 1998.
33. Brenner J, Sordillo PP, Magill GB, et al. Malignant peritoneal mesothelioma: review of 25 patients. Am J Gastroenterol 75: 311, 1981.
34. Brooks JS, Livolsi VA, Pietra GG. Mesothelial cell inclusions in mediastinal lymph nodes mimicking metastatic carcinoma. Am J Clin Pathol 93:741, 1990.
35. Brown RW, Clark GM, Tandon AK, et al. Muliple marker immunohistochemical phenotypes distinguishing malignant pleural mesothelioma from pulmonary adenocarcinoma. Hum Pathol 24:347, 1993.
36. Burchell J, Gendler S, Taylor-Papadimitriou J, et al. Development and characterization of breast cancer reactive monoclonal antibodies directed against the core protein of the human milk mucin. Cancer Res 47:5476, 1987.
37. Burdorf A, Barendregt JJ, Swuste PHJJ, et al. Increasing incidence of mesothelioma in the future by professional exposure to asbestos in the past. Dutch J Med 141:1093, 1997.
38. Burmer GC, Rabinovitch PS, Kulander BG, et al. Flow cytometric analysis of malignant pleural mesotheliomas. Hum Pathol 20:777, 1989.
39. Cagle PT, Brown RW, Lebovitz RM. P53 immunostaining in the differentiation of reactive processes from malignancy in pleural biopsy specimens. Hum Pathol 25:443, 1994.
40. Cantin R, Al-Jabi M, McCaughey WT. Desmoplastic diffuse mesothelioma. Am J Surg Pathol 6:215, 1982.
41. Carbone M, Pass HI, Rizzo P, et al. Simian virus 40-like DNA sequences in human pleural mesothelioma. Oncogene 9:1781, 1994.
42. Center R, Lukeis R, Dietzch E, et al. Molecular deletion of 9p sequences in small cell lung cancer and malignant mesothelioma. Genes Chromosomes Cancer 7:47, 1993.
43. Chan JKC, Loo KT, Yau BKC, et al. Nodular histiocytic/mesothelial hyperplasia: a lesion potentially mistaken for a neoplasm in transbronchial biopsy. Am J Surg Pathol 21:658, 1997.
44. Chang K, Pai LH, Pass H, et al. Monoclonal antibody K1 reacts with epithelial mesothelioma but not with lung adenocarcinoma. Am J Surg Pathol 16:259, 1992.
44a. Chang HT, Yantiss RK, Nielsen GP, et al. Lipid-rich diffuse malignant mesothelioma: A case report. Hum Pathol 31:876, 2000.
45. Chen L-M, Lazcano O, Katzmann JA, et al. The role of conventional cytology, immunohistochemistry, and flow cytometric DNA ploidy in the evaluation of body cavity fluids: a prospective study of 52 patients. Am J Clin Pathol 109:712, 1998.
46. Christmas TI, Manning LS, Garlepp MJ, et al. Effect of interferon-alpha 2a on malignant mesothelioma. J Interferon Res 13:9, 1993.
47. Churg A. Fiber counting and analysis in the diagnosis of asbestos-related disease. Hum Pathol 13:381, 1982.
48. Churg A. Immunohistochemical staining for vimentin and keratin in malignant mesothelioma. Am J Surg Pathol 9:360, 1985.
49. Churg A, Green FHS. Pathology of Occupational Lung Disease, 2nd ed. Williams & Wilkins, Baltimore, 1998.
50. Churg A, Warnock ML, Green N. Analysis of the cores of ferruginous (asbestos) bodies from the general population. Lab Invest 40:31, 1975.
50a. Churg A, Colby TV, Cagle P, et al. The separation of benign and malignant mesothelial proliferations. Am J Surg Pathol 24: 1183, 2000.
51. Cicala C, Pompetti F, Carbone M. SV40 induces mesotheliomas in hamsters. Am J Pathol 142:1524, 1993.
52. Clarkson FA. Primary endothelioma of the pleura. Can Med Assoc J 4:192, 1914.
53. Clement PB, Young RH. Florid mesothelial hyperplasia associated with ovarian tumors: a potential source of error in tumor diagnosis and staging. Int J Gynecol Pathol 12:51, 1993.
54. Clement PB, Young RH. Histiocytic/mesothelial hyperlasia [letter]. Am J Surg Pathol 22:1036, 1998.
55. Clement PB, Young RH, Oliva E, et al. Hyperplastic mesothelial cells within abdominal lymph nodes: mimic of metastatic ovarian carcinoma and serous borderline tumor: a report of two cases associated with ovarian neoplasms. Mod Pathol 9: 879, 1996.
56. Clement PB, Young RH, Scully RE. Malignant mesotheliomas presenting as ovarian masses: a report of nine cases, including two primary ovarian mesotheliomas. Am J Surg Pathol 20: 1067, 1996.
57. Clover J, Oates J, Edwards C. Anti-cytokeratin 5/6: a positive marker for epithelioid mesothelioma. Histopathology 31:140, 1997.
58. Collins CL, Ordóñez NG, Schaefer R, et al. Thrombomodulin expression in malignant thrombomesothelioma and pulmonary adenocarcinoma. Am J Pathol 141:827, 1992.
59. Corson JM, Pinkus GS. Mesothelioma: profile of keratin proteins and carcinoembryonic antigen: an immunoperoxidase study of 20 cases and comparison with pulmonary adenocarcinoma. Am J Pathol 108:80, 1982.
60. Craighead JE. Current pathogenetic concepts of diffuse malignant mesothelioma. Hum Pathol 18:544, 1987.
61. Craighead JE. The epidemiology and pathogenesis of malignant mesothelioma. Chest 96:925, 1989.
62. Craighead JE, Abraham JL, Churg A, et al. The pathology of asbestos-associated diseases of the lung and pleural cavities: diagnostic criteria and proposed grading schema. Arch Pathol Lab Med 106:544, 1982.
63. Craighead JE, Mossman BT. The pathogenesis of asbestos-associated diseases. N Engl J Med 306:1446, 1982.
64. Crotty TB, Colby TV, Gay PC, et al. Desmoplastic malignant mesothelioma masquerading as sclerosing mediastinitis: a diagnostic dilemma. Hum Pathol 23:79, 1992.
65. Crotty TB, Myers JL, Katzenstein AA, et al. Localized malignant mesothelioma: a clinicopathologic and flow cytometric study. Am J Surg Pathol 18:357, 1994.
66. Crouch E, Churg A. Ferruginous bodies and the histologic evaluation of dust exposure. Am J Surg Pathol 8:109, 1984.
67. Curran D, Sahmoud T, Therasse P, et al. Prognostic factors in patients with pleural mesothelioma: the European Organization for Research and Treatment of Cancer experience. J Clin Oncol 16:145, 1998.
67a. Cury PM, Butcher DN, Fisher C, et al. Value of the mesothelium-associated antibodies thrombomodulin, cytokeratin 5/6, calretinin and CD44H in distinguishing epithelioid pleural mesothelioma from adenocarcinoma metastatic to the pleura. Mod Pathol 13:107, 2000.
68. Cury PM, Butcher DN, Corrin B, et al. The use of histological and immunohistochemical markers to distinguish pleural malignant mesothelioma and in situ mesothelioma from reactive mesothelial hyperplasia and reactive pleural fibrosis. J Pathol 189:251, 1999.
69. Dardick I, Al-Jabi M, McCaughey WTE, et al. Ultrastructure of poorly differentiated diffuse epithelial mesotheliomas. Ultrastruct Pathol 7:151, 1984.
70. Dawson A, Gibbs AR, Browne K, et al. Familial mesothelioma: details of 17 cases with histopathologic findings and mineral analysis. Cancer 70:1183, 1992.
71. Dazzi H, Thatcher N, Hasleton PS, et al. DNA analysis by

flow cytometry in malignant pleural mesothelioma: relationship to histology and survival. J Pathol 162:51, 1990.

72. Dejmek A, Hjerpe A. Carcinoembryonic antigen-like reactivity in malignant mesothelioma: a comparison between different commercially available antibodies. Cancer 73:464, 1994.
73. Dejmek A, Hjerpe A. Immunohistochemical reactivity in mesothelioma and adenocarcinoma: a stepwise logistic regression analysis. APMIS 102:255, 1994.
74. Dejmek A, Stromberg C, Wickstrom B, et al. Prognostic importance of the DNA ploidy pattern in malignant mesothelioma of the pleura. Anal Quant Cytol Histol 14:217, 1992.
75. Delahaye M, Hoogsteden HC, Van Der Kwast TH. Immunocytochemistry of malignant mesothelioma: OV632 as a marker of malignant mesothelioma. J Pathol 165:137, 1991.
76. De Pangher Manzini V, Brollo A, et al. Prognostic factors of malignant mesothelioma of the pleura. Cancer 72:410, 1993.
77. Dessy E, Pietra GG. Pseudomesotheliomatous carcinoma of lung: an immunohistochemical and ultrastructural study of three cases. Cancer 68:1747, 1991.

77a. Dhaene K, Verhulst A, van Marck E. SV40 large T-antigen and human pleural mesothelioma. Screening by polymerase chain reaction and tyramine-amplified immunohistochemistry. Virchows Arch 435:1, 1999.

78. Dionne PG, Wang NS. A scanning electron microscopic study of diffuse mesothelioma and some lung carcinomas. Cancer 40:707, 1977.
79. Doglioni C, Dei Tos AP, Laurino L, et al. Calretinen: a novel immunocytochemical marker for mesothelioma. Am J Surg Pathol 20:1037, 1996.
80. Eden CG, Bettochi C, Coker CB, et al. Malignant mesothelioma of the tunica vaginalis. J Urol 153:1053, 1995.
81. Edwards C, Oates J. OV632 and MOC-31 in the diagnosis of mesothelioma and adenocarcinoma: an assessment of their use in formalin fixed and paraffin wax embedded material. J Clin Pathol 48:626, 1995.
82. El-Naggar AK, Ordónez NG, Garnsey L, et al. Epithelioid pleural mesothelioma and pulmonary adenocarcinoma: a comparative DNA flow cytometric study. Hum Pathol 22:972, 1991.
83. Elshami AA, Kuchrczuk J, Zhang H, et al. Treatment of pleural mesothelioma in an immunocompetent rat model utilizing adenoviral transfer of HSV-thymidine kinase gene. Hum Gene Ther 7:141, 1996.
84. Fisher ER, Hellstrom HR. The periodic acid-Schiff reaction as an aid in the identification of mesothelioma. Cancer 13:837, 1960.
85. Fitzpatrick DR, Bielefeldt-Ohmann H, Hinbeck RP, et al. Transforming growth factor-$\beta$: antisense RNA-mediated inhibition affects anchorage-independent growth, tumorogenecity and tumour-infiltrating T-cells in malignant mesothelioma. Growth Factors 11:29, 1994.
86. Flejter WL, Li FP, Antman KH, et al. Recurring loss involving chromosomes 1, 3 and 22 in malignant mesothelioma: possible sites of tumor suppressor genes. Genes Chromosomes Cancer 1:148, 1989.
87. Fraire AE, Greenberg SD, Buffler P, et al. Mesothelioma of childhood. Cancer 62:838, 1988.
88. Friedman MT, Gentile P, Tarectecan A, et al. Malignant mesothelioma: immunohistochemistry and DNA ploidy analysis as methods to differentiate mesothelioma from benign reactive mesothelial cell proliferation and adenocarcinoma in pleural and peritoneal effusions. Arch Pathol Lab Med 120:959, 1996.
89. Frierson HF, Mills SE, Legier JF. Flow cytometric analysis of ploidy in immunohistochemically confirmed examples of malignant mesothelioma. Am J Clin Pathol 90:240, 1988.
90. Gaffey MJ, Mills SE, Swanson PE, et al. Immunoreactivity for BER-EP4 in adenocarcinomas, adenomatoid tumors, and malignant mesotheliomas. Am J Surg Pathol 16:593, 1992.
91. Garcia-Prats MD, Ballestin C, Sotelo T, et al. A comparative evaluation of immunohistochemical markers for the differential diagnosis of malignant pleural tumours. Histopathology 32:462, 1998.
92. Geschickter CF. Mesothelial tumors. Am J Cancer 26:378, 1936.
93. Gilks B, Hegedus C, Freeman H, et al. Malignant peritoneal mesothelioma after remote abdominal irradiation. Cancer 61: 2019, 1988.
94. Goey SH, Eggermont A, Punt CJ, et al. Intrapleural administration of interleukin-2 in mesotheliomas; a phase I-II study. Br J Cancer 72:1283, 1995.
95. Goldblum JR, Hart WR. Localized and diffuse mesotheliomas of the genital tract and peritoneum in women: a clinicopathological study of nineteen true mesothelial neoplasms, other than adenomatoid tumors, multicystic mesotheliomas and localized fibrous tumors. Am J Surg Pathol 19:1124, 1995.
96. Groisman GM, Amar M, Weiner P, et al. Mucicarminophilic histiocytosis (benign signet-ring cells) and hyperplastic mesothelial cells: two mimics of metastatic carcinoma within a single lymph node. Arch Pathol Lab Med 122:282, 1998.
97. Hammar SP, Bockus D, Remington F, et al. Familial mesothelioma: a report of two families. Hum Pathol 20:107, 1989.
98. Hammar SP, Bolen JW. Sarcomatoid pleural mesothelioma. Ultrastruct Pathol 9:337, 1985.
99. Henderson DW, Attwood HD, Constance TJ, et al. Lymphohistiocytoid mesothelioma: a rare lymphomatoid variant of sarcomatoid mesothelioma. Ultrastruct Pathol 12:367, 1988.
100. Henderson DW, Shilkin KB, Whitaker D. Reactive mesothelial hyperplasia vs. mesothelioma, including mesothelioma in situ: a brief review. Am J Clin Pathol 110:397, 1998.
101. Herzog F. Ein Fall von maligner Deckzellengeschwulst des Peritoneums. Zieglers 58:390, 1914.
102. Hillerdal G. Malignant mesothelioma 1982: review of 4710 published cases. Br J Dis Chest 77:321, 1983.
103. Hillerdal G, Berg J. Malignant mesothelioma secondary to chronic inflammation and old scars. Cancer 55:1968, 1985.
104. Holden J, Churg A. Immunohistochemical staining for keratin and carcinoembryonic antigen in the diagnosis of malignant mesothelioma. Am J Surg Pathol 8:277, 1984.
105. Hurliman NJ. Desmin and neural marker expression in mesothelial cells and mesotheliomas. Hum Pathol 25:753, 1994.
106. Isobe H, Sridhar KS, Doria R, et al. Prognostic significance of DNA aneuploidy in diffuse malignant mesothelioma. Cytometry 19:86, 1995.
107. Jasani B, Edwards RE, Thomas ND, et al. The use of vimentin antibodies in the diagnosis of malignant mesothelioma. Virchows Arch [Pathol Anat] 406:441, 1985.
108. Johnson VG, Schlom J, Paterson AJ, et al. Analysis of a human tumor-associated glycoprotein (TAG72) identified by monoclonal antibody B72.3. Cancer Res 46:850, 1986.
109. Jones MA, Young RH, Scully R. Malignant mesothelioma of the tunica vaginalis: a clinicopathologic analysis of 11 cases with review of the literature. Am J Surg Pathol 19:815, 1995.
110. Jordan D, Jagirdar J, Kaneko M. Blood group antigens, Lewis$^x$ and Lewis$^y$, in the diagnostic discrimination of malignant mesothelioma versus adenocarcinoma. Am J Pathol 135:931, 1989.
111. Kahn HJ, Thorner PS, Yeger H, et al. Distinct keratin patterns demonstrated by immunoperoxidase staining of adenocarcinomas, carcinoids, and mesotheliomas using polyclonal and monoclonal antikeratin antibodies. Am J Clin Pathol 86:566, 1986.
112. Kaiser LR. New therapies in the treatment of malignant pleural mesothelioma. Semin Thorac Cardiovasc Surg 9:383, 1997.
113. Kannerstein M, Churg J. Peritoneal mesothelioma. Hum Pathol 8:83, 1977.
114. Kannerstein M, Churg J, McCaughey WTF. Asbestos and mesothelioma: a review. Pathol Annu 13:81, 1978.

115. Kaul TK, Fields BL, Kahn DR. Primary malignant pericardial mesothelioma: a case report and review. J Cardiovasc Surg 35: 261, 1994.
116. Kawai T, Suzuki M, Torikata C, et al. Expression of blood group-related antigens and Helix pomatia agglutinin in malignant, pleural mesothelioma and pulmonary adenocarcinomas. Hum Pathol 22:118, 1991.
117. Kelsey A. Mesothelioma in childhood. Pediatr Hematol Oncol 11:461, 1994.
118. Khalidi HS, Battifora H. Lymphohistiocytoid mesothelioma: an immunohistochemical study. Mod Pathol 11:1036A, 1998.
119. Kivipensas P, Björkqvist A-M, Karhu R, et al. Gains and losses of DNA sequences in malignant mesothelioma by comparative genomic hybridization. Cancer Genet Cytogenet 89:7, 1996.
120. Klemperer P, Rabin CB. Primary neoplasms of the pleura: a report of five cases. Arch Pathol 11:385, 1931.
121. Landrigan PJ. Asbestos: still a carcinogen. N Engl J Med 338: 1618, 1998.
122. Langer AM, Selikoff IJ, Sastre A. Chrysotile asbestos in the lungs of persons in New York City. Arch Environ Health 22: 348, 1971.
123. Lanphear BP, Buncher CR. Latent period of malignant mesothelioma of occupational origin. Occup Med 7:718, 1992.
124. Latza U, Niedobitek G, Schwarting R, et al. Ber-EP4: new monoclonal antibody which distinguishes epithelia from mesothelia. J Clin Pathol 43:213, 1990.
125. Leers MPG, Aarts MMJ, Theunissen PHMH. E-cadherin and calretinin: a useful combination of immunohistochemical markers for differentiation between mesothelioma and metastatic adenocarcinoma. Histopathology 32:209, 1998.
126. Leigh J, Rogers AJ, Ferguson DA, et al. Lung asbestos fiber content and mesothelioma cell type, site, and survival. Cancer 68:135, 1991.
127. Leong AS-Y, Vernon-Roberts E. The immunohistochemistry of malignant mesothelioma. Pathol Annu 29:157, 1994.
128. Leong AS-YM, Stevens MW, Mukherjee TM. Malignant mesothelioma: cytologic diagnosis with histologic, immunohistochemical, and ultrastructural correlation. Semin Diagn Pathol 9:141, 1992.
129. Libshitz HI. Malignant pleural mesothelioma: the role of computed tomography. J Comput Tomogr 8:15, 1984.
130. Lilis R. Fibrous zeolites and endemic mesothelioma in Cappadocia, Turkey. J Occup Med 23:548, 1981.
131. Lu YY, Jhanwar SC, Cheng JQ, et al. Deletion mapping of the short arm of chromosome 3 in human malignant mesothelioma. Genes Chromosomes Cancer 9:76, 1994.
132. Luketich JD, Westkaemper J, Sommers KE, et al. Bronchoesophageal pleural fistula after photodynamic therapy for malignant mesothelioma. Ann Thorac Surg 62:283, 1996.
133. Luthringer DJ, Virmani R, Weiss SW, et al. A distinctive cardiovascular lesion resembling histiocytoid (epithelioid) hemangioma: evidence suggesting mesothelial participation. Am J Surg Pathol 14:993, 1990.
134. Mangano WE, Cagle PT, Churg A, et al. The diagnosis of desmoplastic malignant mesothelioma and its distinction from fibrous pleurisy: a histologic and immunohistochemical analysis of 31 cases including p53 immunostaining. Am J Clin Pathol 110:191, 1998.
135. Mayall FG, Gibbs AR. The histology and immunohistochemistry of small cell mesothelioma. Histopathology 20:47, 1992.
136. Mayall FG, Goddard H, Gibbs AR. P53 immunostaining in the distinction between benign and malignant mesothelial proliferations using formalin-fixed paraffin sections. J Pathol 168:377, 1992.
137. McCaughey WT, Colby TV, Battifora H, et al. Diagnosis of diffuse malignant mesothelioma: experience of a US/Canadian mesothelioma panel. Mod Pathol 4:342, 1991.
138. McDonald AD, Magner D, Eyssen G. Primary malignant mesothelial tumors in Canada, 1960–1968: a pathological review by the mesothelioma panel of the Canadian Tumor Reference Centre. Cancer 31:869, 1973.
139. McDonald JC, Armstrong B, Case B, et al. Mesothelioma and asbestos fiber type. Cancer 63:1544, 1989.
140. McDonald JC, McDonald AD. The epidemiology of mesothelioma in historical context. Eur Respir J 9:1932, 1996.
141. McEwen J, Finlayson A, Mair A, et al. Mesothelioma in Scotland. BMJ 4:575, 1970.
142. Miettinen M, Kovatich AJ. HBME-1: a monoclonal antibody useful in the differential diagnosis of mesothelioma, adenocarcinoma and soft-tissue and bone tumors. Appl Immunohistochem 3:115, 1995.
143. Moertel CG. Peritoneal mesothelioma. Gastroenterology 63:346, 1972.
144. Moll R, Dhouailly D, Sun TT. Expression of keratin-5 as a distinctive feature of epithelial and biphasic mesotheliomas: an immunohistochemical study using monoclonal antibodies AE14. Virchows Arch 58:129, 1989.
145. Moolten FL. Drug sensitivity ("suicide") genes for selective cancer therapy. Cancer Gene Ther 1:279, 1994.
146. Mullick SS, Green LK, Ramzy I, et al. P53 gene product in pleural effusions: practical use in distinguishing benign from malignant cells. Acta Cytol 40:855, 1996.
147. Nakano T, Chahinian AP, Shinjo M, et al. Cisplatin in combination with irinotecan in the treatment of patients with malignant pleural mesothelioma: a pilot phase II clinical trial and pharmacokinetic profile. Cancer 85:2375, 1999.
148. Nakano T, Fujii J, Tamura S. Thrombocytosis in patients with malignant pleural mesothelioma. Cancer 58:1699, 1986.
149. Nascimento AG, Keeney GL, Fletcher CDM. Deciduoid peritoneal mesothelioma: an unusual phenotype affecting young females. Am J Surg Pathol 18:439, 1994.
150. Newhouse ML, Berry G. Patterns of mortality in asbestos factory workers in London. Ann NY Acad Sci 330:53, 1979.
151. Newhouse ML, Thompson H. Mesothelioma of pleura and peritoneum following exposure to asbestos in the London area. Br J Ind Med 22:261, 1965.
152. Noguchi M, Nakajima T, Hirohashi S, et al. Immunohistochemical distinction of malignant mesothelioma from pulmonary adenocarcinoma with antisurfactant apoprotein, anti-Lewis[a], and anti-tn antibodies. Hum Pathol 20:53, 1989.
153. O'Hara CJ, Corson JM, Pinkus GS, et al. ME1: a monoclonal antibody that distinguishes epithelial-type malignant mesothelioma from pulmonary adenocarcinoma and extrapulmonary malignancies. Am J Pathol 136:421, 1990.
154. Ordónez NG. Role of immunohistochemistry in distinguishing epithelial peritoneal mesotheliomas from peritoneal and ovarian serous carcinomas. Am J Surg Pathol 22:1203, 1998.
155. Ordónez NG. The immunohistochemical diagnosis of epithelial mesothelioma. Hum Pathol 30:313, 1999.
156. Ordónez NG. The immunohistochemical diagnosis of mesothelioma: differentiation of mesothelioma and lung adenocarcinoma. Am J Surg Pathol 13:276, 1989.
157. Ordónez NG. The value of antibodies 44-3A6, SM3, HBME-1 and thrombomodulin in differentiating epithelial pleural mesothelioma from lung adenocarcinoma: a comparative study with other commonly used antibodies. Am J Surg Pathol 21:1399, 1997.
158. Ordónez NG. Value of calretinin immunostaining in differentiating epithelial mesothelioma from adenocarcinoma. Mod Pathol 11:929, 1998.
159. Ordónez NG. Value of cytokeratin 5/6 immunostaining in distinguishing epithelial mesothelioma of the pleura from lung adenocarcinoma. Am J Surg Pathol 22:1215, 1998.
160. Ordónez NG: Value of the Ber-EP4 antibody in differentiating

epithelial pleural mesothelioma from adenocarcinoma: the MD Anderson experience and a critical review of the literature. Am J Clin Pathol 109:85, 1998.

161. Ordónez NG. Value of the MOC-31 monoclonal antibody in differentiating epithelial pleural mesothelioma from lung adenocarcinoma. Hum Pathol 29:166, 1998.
162. Ordónez NG. Value of thrombomodulin immunostaining in the diagnosis of mesothelioma. Histopathology 31:25, 1997.
163. Ordónez NG, Mackay B. The roles of immunohistochemistry and electron microscopy in distinguishing epithelial mesothelioma of the pleura from adenocarcinoma. Adv Anat Pathol 3: 273, 1996.
164. Ordónez NG, Ro JY, Ayala AG. Lesions described as nodular mesothelial hyperplasia are primarily composed of histiocytes. Am J Surg Pathol 22:285, 1998.
164a. Ordónez NG. Value of thyroid transcript factor-1, E-cadherin, BG8, WT1, and CD44S immunostaining in distinguishing epithelial pleural mesothelioma from pulmonary and nonpulmonary adenocarcinoma. Am J Surg Pathol 24:598, 2000.
164b. Ordónez NG. Epithelial mesothelioma with deciduoid features. Report of four cases. Am J Surg Pathol 24:816, 2000.
164c. Orosz Z, Nagy P, Szentirmay Z, et al. Epithelial mesothelioma with deciduoid features. Virchows Arch 434:263, 1999.
165. Otis CN, Carter D, Cole S, et al. Immunohistochemical evaluation of pleural mesothelioma and pulmonary adenocarcinoma: a biinstitutional study of 47 cases. Am J Surg Pathol 11:445, 1987.
166. Otte KB, Sigstaard TI, Kjaerulff J. Malignant mesothelioma: clustering in the family producing asbestos cement in their home. Br J Ind Med 47:10, 1990.
167. Oury TD, Hammar SP, Roggli VL. Ultrastructural features of diffuse malignant mesotheliomas. Hum Pathol 29:1382, 1998.
168. Park S, Schalling M, Bernard A, et al. The Wilms tumour gene WT1 is expressed in murine mesoderm-derived tissues and mutated in a human mesothelioma. Nat Genet 4:415, 1993.
169. Parkash V, Vidwans M, Carter D. Benign mesothelial cells in mediastinal lymph nodes. Am J Surg Pathol 23:1264, 1999.
170. Pass HI, Temeck BK, Kranda K, et al. Preoperative tumor volume is associated with outcome in malignant pleural mesothelioma. J Thorac Cardiovasc Surg 115:310, 1998.
171. Pass HW, Temeck BK, Kranda K, et al. A phase II trial investigating primary immunochemotherapy for malignant pleural mesothelioma and the feasibility of adjuvant immunochemotherapy after maximal cytoreduction. Ann Surg Oncol 2:214, 1995.
172. Patz EF Jr, Shaffer K, Piwnica-Worms DR, et al. Malignant pleural mesothelioma: value of CT and MR imaging in predicting resectibility. AJR 159:961, 1992.
173. Pepper C, Jasani B, Navabi H, et al. Simian virus 40-large T antigen (SV4OLTAg) primer specific DNA amplification in human pleural mesothelioma tissue. Thorax 51:1074, 1996.
174. Peralta-Soler A, Knudsen KA, Jaurand MC, et al. The differential expression of N-cadherin and E-cadherin distinguishes pleural mesotheliomas from lung adenocarcinomas. Hum Pathol 26:1363, 1995.
175. Peterson JT, Greenberg SD, Buffler PA. Non-asbestos-related malignant mesothelioma: a review. Cancer 54:951, 1984.
176. Peto J, Hodgson JT, Matthews FE, et al. Continuing increase in mesothelioma mortality in Britain. Lancet 345:535, 1995.
177. Pooley FD, Clark N. Fiber dimensions and aspect ratio of crocidolite, chrysotile, and amosite particles detected in lung tissue specimens. Ann NY Acad Sci 330:711, 1979.
178. Popescu NC, Chahinian AP, DiPaolo JA. Non-random chromosome alterations in human malignant mesothelioma. Cancer Res 48:142, 1988.
179. Pyrhonen S, Laasonen A, Tammilheto L. Diploid predominance and prognostic significance of S-phase cells in malignant mesothelioma. Eur J Cancer 27:197, 1991.
180. Ramael M, Buysse C, Van den Bossche J, et al. Immunoreactivity for the $\beta$ chain of the platelet-derived growth factor receptor in malignant mesothelioma and non-neoplastic mesothelium. J Pathol 167:1, 1992.
181. Ramael M, Jacobs W, Weyler J, et al. Proliferation in malignant mesothelioma as determined by mitosis counts and immunoreactivity for proliferating cell nuclear antigen (PCNA). J Pathol 172:247, 1994.
182. Ramael M, Lemmens G, Eerdekens C, et al. Immunoreactivity for p53 protein in malignant mesothelioma and non-neoplastic mesothelium. J Pathol 168:371, 1992.
183. Rice TW, Adelstein DJ, Kirby TJ, et al. Aggressive multimodality therapy for malignant pleural mesothelioma. Ann Thorac Surg 58:24, 1994.
184. Riddell RH, Goodman MJ, Moossa AR. Peritoneal malignant mesothelioma in a patient with recurrent peritonitis. Cancer 48:134, 1981.
185. Riera JR, Astengo-Osuna C, Longmate JA, et al. The immunohistochemical diagnostic panel of epithelial mesothelioma: a re-evaluation after heat-induced epitope retrieval. Am J Surg Pathol 21:1409, 1997.
186. Roggli VL, Kolbeck J, Sanfilippo F. Pathology of human mesothelioma: etiology and diagnostic considerations. Pathol Annu 22:91, 1987.
187. Roggli VL, McGavran MH, Subach J, et al. Pulmonary asbestos counts and electron probe analysis of asbestos body cores in patients with mesothelioma: a study of 25 cases. Cancer 50: 2423, 1982.
188. Roggli VL, Pratt PC, Brody AR. Asbestos content of lung tissue in asbestos-associated diseases: a study of 110 cases. Br J Ind Med 43:18, 1986.
189. Roggli VL, Sanfilippo F, Shelburne JD. Mesothelioma. In: Roggli VL, Greenberg SD, Pratt PC (eds) Pathology of Asbestos--Associated Diseases, Little, Brown, Boston, 1992.
190. Ros PR, Yushok TJ, Buck JL, et al. Peritoneal mesothelioma: radiologic appearances correlated with histology. Acta Radiol 32:355, 1991.
191. Rosai J, Dehner LP. Nodular mesothelial hyperplasia in hernia sacs: a benign reactive condition simulating a neoplastic process. Cancer 35:165, 1975.
192. Rose RG, Palmer JD, Lougheed MN. Treatment of peritoneal mesothelioma with radioactive colloidal gold. Cancer 8:478, 1955.
193. Ruffie P, Feld R, Minkin S, et al. Diffuse malignant mesothelioma of the pleura in Ontario and Quebec: a retrospective study of 322 patients. J Clin Oncol 7:1157, 1989.
194. Ruitenbeek T, Gouw ASH, Poppema S. Immunocytology of body cavity fluids: MOC-31, a monoclonal antibody discriminating between mesothelial and epithelial cells. Arch Pathol Lab Med 118:265, 1994.
195. Rusch VW. Pleurectomy/decortication in the setting of multimodality treatment for diffuse malignant pleural mesothelioma. Semin Thorac Cardiovasc Surg 9:367, 1997.
196. Rusch VW, Niedzweicki D, Tao Y, et al. Intrapleural cisplatin and mitomycin for mesothelioma following pleurectomy: pharmacokinetic studies. J Clin Oncol 10:1001, 1992.
197. Rusch VW, Piantadosi S, Holmes EC. The role of extrapleural pneumonectomy in malignant pleural mesothelioma: a Lung Cancer Study Group trial. J Thorac Cardiovasc Surg 102:1, 1991.
198. Rusch VW, Saltz L, Venkatraman E, et al. A phase II trial of pleurectomy/decortication followed by intrapleural and systemic chemotherapy for malignant pleural mesothelioma. J Clin Oncol 12:1156, 1994.

199. Rutty GN, Lauder I. Mesothelial cell inclusions within mediastinal lymph nodes. Histopathology 25:483, 1994.
200. Samuels BL, Herndon JE, Harmon DC, et al. Dihydro-5-azacytidine and cisplatin in the treatment of malignant mesothelioma: a phase II study by the Cancer and Leukemia Group B. Cancer 982:1578, 1998.
201. Schmitter D, Lauber B, Fagg B, et al. Haemopoietic growth factors secreted by seven human pleural mesothelioma cell lines: interleukin-6 production as a common feature. Int J Cancer 51:296, 1992.
202. Segers K, Backhovens H, Singh SK, et al. Immunoreactivity for p53 and mdm2 and the detection of p53 mutations in human malignant mesothelioma. Virchous Arch 427:431, 1995.
203. Seidman H, Selikoff IJ, Hammond EC. Short-term asbestos work exposure and long-term observation. Ann NY Acad Sci 330:61, 1979.
204. Sekido Y, Pass HI, Bader S, et al. Neurofibromatosis type 2 gene is somatically mutated in mesothelioma but not in lung cancer. Cancer Res 55:1227, 1995.
205. Selcuk ZT, Coplu L, Kalyoncu AF, et al. Malignant pleural mesothelioma due to environmental mineral fibre in Turkey: analysis of 135 cases. Chest 102:790, 1992.
206. Selikoff IJ, Churg J, Hammond EC. Asbestos exposure and neoplasia. JAMA 188:22, 1964.
207. Selikoff IJ, Hammond EC. Health hazards of asbestos exposure. Ann NY Acad Sci 330:1, 1979.
207a. Shanks JH, Harris M, Banerjee SS, et al. Mesotheliomas with deciduoid morphology: A morphologic spectrum and a variant not confined to young females. Am J Surg Pathol 24:285, 2000.
208. Shannon VR, Besbitt JC, Libshitz HI. Malignant pleural mesothelioma after radiation therapy for breast cancer. Cancer 76: 437, 1995.
209. Sheibani K, Battifora H, Burke JS. Antigenetic phenotype of malignant mesotheliomas and pulmonary adenocarcinomas: an immunohistologic analysis demonstrating the value of Leu-M1 antigen. Am J Pathol 123:212, 1986.
210. Sheibani K, Esteban JM, Bailey A, et al. Immunopathologic and molecular studies as an aid to the diagnosis of malignant mesothelioma. Hum Pathol 23:107, 1992.
211. Sheibani K, Shin SS, Kezirian J, et al. Ber-EP4 antibody as a discriminant in the differential diagnosis of malignant mesothelioma versus adenocarcinoma. Am J Surg Pathol 15:779, 1991.
211a. Shimazaki H, Aida S, Iizuka Y, et al. Vacuolated cell mesothelioma of the pericardium resembling liposarcoma: A case report. Hum Pathol 31:767, 2000.
212. Silcocks PB, Herbert A, Wright DH. Evaluation of PAS-diastase and carcinoembryonic antigen staining in the differential diagnosis of malignant mesothelioma. J Pathol 149:133, 1986.
213. Smith MJ, Naylor B. A method for extracting ferruginous bodies from sputum and pulmonary tissue. Am J Clin Pathol 58: 250, 1972.
214. SooHoo WEJ, Ordónez NG. Expression of the core protein of polymorphic epithelial mucin as detected by SM-3 antibody in pulmonary adenocarcinoma and pleural malignant mesothelioma. Lab Invest 66:116A, 1992.
215. Sosolik RC, McGaughy VR, De Young BR. Anti-MOC 31: a potential addition to the pulmonary adenocarcinoma versus mesothelioma immunohistochemistry panel. Mod Pathol 10: 716, 1997.
216. Soulie P, Ruffie P, Trandafir L, et al. Combined systemic chemoimmunotherapy in advanced diffuse malignant mesothelioma: report of a phase I-II study of weekly cisplatin/interferon alpha-2a. J Clin Oncol 14:878, 1996.
217. Spagnolo DV, Whitaker D, Carrello S, et al. The use of monoclonal antibody 44-3A6 in cell blocks in the diagnosis of lung carcinoma, carcinomas metastatic to lung and pleura, and pleural malignant mesothelioma. Am J Clin Pathol 95:322, 1991.
218. Spirtas R, Beebe GW, Connelly RR, et al. Recent trends in mesothelioma incidence in the United States. Am J Ind Med 9: 397, 1986.
219. Stey C, Landolt-Weber U, Vetter W, et al. Malignant peritoneal mesothelioma after Thorotrast exposure. Am J Clin Oncol 18:313, 1995.
220. Stoebner B, Bernaudin JF, Nebut M, et al. Contribution of electron microscopy to the diagnosis of pleural mesothelioma. Ann NY Acad Sci 330:751, 1979.
221. Strickler HD, Goedert JJ, Fleming M, et al. Simian virus 40 and pleural mesothelioma in humans. Cancer Epidemiol Biomarkers Prev 5:473, 1996.
222. Suarez Vilela D, Izquierdo Garcia FM. Embolization of mesothelial cells in lymphatics: the route to mesothelial inclusions in lymph nodes? Histopathology 33:570, 1998.
223. Sugarbaker DJ. Diffuse malignant pleural mesothelioma: introduction. Semin Thorac Cardiovasc Surg 9:345, 1997.
224. Sugarbaker DJ, Garcia JP, Richards WG, et al. Extrapleural pneumonectomy in the multimodality therapy of malignant pleural mesothelioma: results in 120 consecutive patients. Ann Surg 224:228, 1996.
225. Sugarbaker DJ, Norberto JJ, Swanson SJ. Extrapleural pneumonectomy in the setting of multimodality therapy for diffuse malignant pleural mesothelioma. Semin Thorac Cardiovasc Surg 9:373, 1997.
226. Sugarbaker DJ, Norberto JJ, Swanson SJ. Surgical staging and work-up of patients with diffuse malignant pleural mesothelioma. Semin Thorac Cardiovasc Surg 9:356, 1997.
227. Sugarbaker DJ, Strauss GM, Lynch TJ, et al. Node status has prognostic significance in the multimodality therapy of diffuse, malignant mesothelioma. J Clin Oncol 11:1172, 1993.
228. Sussman J, Rosai J. Lymph node metastasis as the initial manifestation of malignant mesothelioma: report of six cases. Am J Surg Pathol 14:819, 1990.
229. Suzuki Y, Churg J, Kannerstein M. Ultrastructure of human malignant diffuse mesothelioma. Am J Pathol 85:241, 1976.
230. Taguchi T, Jhanwar S, Siegfried J, et al. Recurrent deletions of specific chromosomal sites in 1p, 3p, 6q, and 9p in human malignant mesothelioma. Cancer Res 53:4349, 1993.
231. Takita H, Dougherty TJ. Intracavitary photodynamic therapy for malignant pleural mesothelioma. Semin Surg Oncol 11:368, 1995.
232. Tao LC. Aspiration biopsy cytology of mesothelioma. Diagn Cytopathol 5:14, 1989.
233. Taub RN, Antman KH. Chemotherapy for malignant mesothelioma. Semin Thorac Cardiovasc Surg 9:361, 1997.
234. Teneck BK, Pass HI. Esophagal pleural fistula: a complication of photodynamic therapy. South Med J 88:271, 1995.
235. Thomason R, Schlegel W, Lucca M, et al. Primary malignant mesothelioma of the pericardium: case report and literature review. Tex Heart Inst J 21:170, 1994.
236. Thor A, Gorstein F, Ohuchi N, et al. Tumor-associated glycoprotein (TAG-72) in ovarian carcinomas defined by monoclonal antibody B72.3. J Natl Cancer Inst 76:995, 1986.
237. Tiainen M, Tammilehto L, Rautonen J, et al. Chromosomal abnormalities and their correlation with asbestos exposure and survival in patients with mesothelioma. Br J Cancer 60:618, 1989.
238. Tiniakaos DG, Healicon RM, Hair T, et al. P53 immunostaining as a marker of malignancy in cytologic preparations of body fluids. Acta Cytol 39:171, 1995.
239. Vlasveld LT, Gallee MP, Rodenhuis T, et al. Intraperitoneal chemotherapy for malignant peritoneal mesothelioma. Eur J Cancer 27:732, 1991.
240. Vortmeyer AO, Preuss J, Padberg B-C, et al. Immunocytochemical differential diagnosis of diffuse malignant pleural

mesotheliomas: a clinicomorphological study of 158 cases. Anticancer Res 11:889, 1991.
241. Wagner JC. Epidemiology of diffuse mesothelial tumors: evidence of an association from studies in South Africa and United Kingdom. Ann NY Acad Sci 132:575, 1965.
242. Wagner JC, Berry G, Timbrell V. Mesotheliomata in rats after inoculation with asbestos and other materials. Br J Cancer 28: 173, 1973.
243. Wagner JC, Sleggs AC, Marchand P. Diffuse pleural mesothelioma and asbestosis exposure in the Northwestern Cape Province. Br J Ind Med 17:260, 1960.
244. Walker AM, Laughlin JE, Friedlander ER, et al. Projections of asbestos related disease 1980–2009. J Occup Med 25:409, 1983.
245. Walz R, Koch HK. Malignant pleural mesothelioma: some aspects of epidemiology, differential diagnosis, and prognosis: histological and immunohistochemical evaluation and follow-up of mesotheliomas diagnosed from 1964 to January 1985. Pathol Res Pract 186:124, 1990.
246. Wanebo HJ, Martini N, Melamed MR, et al. Pleural mesothelioma. Cancer 38:2481, 1976.
247. Wang N. Electron microscopy in the diagnosis of pleural mesotheliomas. Cancer 31:1046, 1973.
248. Warhol MJ, Hickey WF, Corson JM. Malignant mesothelioma: ultrastructural distinction from adenocarcinoma. Am J Surg Pathol 6:307, 1982.
249. Warnock ML, Stoloff A, Thor A. Differentiation of adenocarcinoma of the lung from mesothelioma: periodic acid-Schiff, monoclonal antibodies B72.3 and Leu-M1. Am J Pathol 133:30, 1988.
250. Webster I. Mesotheliomatous tumors in South Africa: pathology and experimental pathology. Ann NY Acad Sci 132:623, 1965.
251. Weidner M. Malignant mesothelioma of peritoneum. Ultrastruct Pathol 15:515, 1991.
252. Weiss LM, Battifora H. The search for the optimal immunohistochemical panel for the diagnosis of malignant mesothelioma. Hum Pathol 24:345, 1993.
253. Whitwell F, Rawcliffe RM. Diffuse malignant pleural mesothelioma and asbestos exposure. Thorax 26:6, 1971.
254. Wick MR. Immunophenotyping of malignant mesothelioma. Am J Surg Pathol 21:1395, 1997.
255. Wick MR, Loy T, Mills ES, et al. Malignant epithelioid pleural mesothelioma versus peripheral pulmonary adenocarcinoma: a histochemical, ultrastructural, and immunohistologic study of 103 cases. Hum Pathol 21:759, 1990.
256. Wick MR, Mills SE, Swanson PE. Expression of "myelomonocytic" antigens in mesotheliomas and adenocarcinomas involving the serosal surfaces. Am J Clin Pathol 94:18, 1990.
257. Wilson GE, Hasleton PS, Chatterjee AK. Desmoplastic malignant mesothelioma: a review of 17 cases. J Clin Pathol 45:295, 1992.
258. Winslow DJ, Taylor HB. Malignant peritoneal mesotheliomas. Cancer 13:127, 1960.
259. Wirth PR, Legier J, Wright GL. Immunohistochemical evaluation of seven monoclonal antibodies for differentiation of pleural mesothelioma from lung adenocarcinoma. Cancer 67:655, 1991.
260. Wolanski K, Whitaker D, Shilkin KB, et al. The use of EMA and AgNOR testing in the differential diagnosis of mesothelioma from benign reactive mesotheliosis. Cancer 82:583, 1998.
261. Xiao S, Renshaw AA, Cibas EC, et al. Novel fluorescence in situ hybridization approaches in solid tumors: characterization of frozen specimens, touch preparations, and cytologic preparations. Am J Pathol 147:896, 1995.
262. Yates DH, Corrin B, Stidolph PN, et al. Malignant mesothelioma in south east England: clinicopathological experience of 272 cases. Thorax 52:507, 1997.
263. Yeh HC, Chahinian P. Ultrasonography and computed tomography of peritoneal mesothelioma. Radiology 135:705, 1980.
264. Yoshida T. Gleichzeitige Papillomatose der Pleura und des Peritoneums, zugleich ein Beitrag zur Frage des primaren Carcinoms der serosen Haute. Virchows Arch [Pathol Anat] 299: 363, 1937.
265. Yousem SA, Hochholzer L. Malignant mesotheliomas with osseous and cartilaginous differentiation. Arch Pathol Lab Med 111:62, 1987.
266. Zalma R, Bonneau L, Jaurand MC, et al. Formation of oxy-radicals by oxygen reduction arising from the surface activity of asbestos. Can J Med 65:2338, 1987.

### Well-Differentiated Papillary Mesothelioma

267. Addis BJ, Fox H. Papillary mesothelioma of ovary. Histopathology 7:387, 1983.
268. Barbera V, Rubino M. Papillary mesothelioma of the tunica vaginalis. Cancer 35:359, 1975.
269. Burrig KF, Pfitzer P, Hort W. Well-differentiated papillary mesothelioma of the peritoneum: a borderline mesothelioma. Virchows Arch [Pathol Anat] 417:1443, 1990.
270. Daya D, McCaughey WT. Well-differentiated papillary mesothelioma of the peritoneum: a clinicopathologic study of 22 cases. Cancer 65:292, 1990.
271. Goepel JR. Benign papillary mesothelioma of peritoneum: a histological, histochemical, and ultrastructural study of six cases. Histopathology 5:21, 1981.
272. Goldblum JR, Hart WR. Localized and diffuse mesotheliomas of the genital tract and peritoneum in women: a clinicopathological study of nineteen true mesothelial neoplasms, other than adenomatoid tumors, multicystic mesotheliomas, and localized fibrous tumors. Am J Surg Pathol 19:1124, 1995.
273. Grove A, Lidang-Jensen M, Donna A. Mesothelioma of the tunica vaginalis testis and hernial sacs. Virchows Arch [Pathol Anat] 415:283, 1989.
274. Hanrahan JB. A combined papillary mesothelioma and adenomatoid tumor of the omentum: report of a case. Cancer 16: 1497, 1963.
275. Hoekman K, Tognon G, Risse EK, et al. Well-differentiated papillary mesothelioma of the peritoneum: a separate entity. Eur J Cancer 32A:255, 1996.
276. Jatzko GR, Jester J. Simultaneous occurrence of a rectal carcinoma and a diffuse well-differentiated papillary mesothelioma of the peritoneum. Int J Colorectal Dis 12:326, 1997.
277. Lovell FA, Cranston PE. Well-differentiated papillary mesothelioma of the peritoneum. Am J Radiol 155:1245, 1990.
278. Mangal R, Taskin O, Franklin R. An incidental diagnosis of well-differentiated papillary mesothelioma in a woman operated on for recurrent endometriosis. Fertil Steril 63:196, 1995.
279. Mikuz G, Hopfel-Kreiner I. Papillary mesothelioma of the tunica vaginalis propria testis. Virchows Arch [Pathol Anat] 396: 231, 1982.
280. Sane AC, Roggli VL. Curative resection of a well-differentiated papillary mesothelioma of the pericardium. Arch Pathol Lab Med 119:266, 1995.
281. Swan N, Cottell DC, Sheahan K. Peritoneal mesotheliomas [letter]. Am J Surg Pathol 21:122, 1997.
282. Swerdlow M. Mesothelioma of the pelvic peritoneum resembling papillary cystadenocarcinoma of the ovary. Am J Obstet Gynecol 77:197, 1959.

### Multicystic Peritoneal Mesothelioma

283. Ball NJ, Urbanski SJ, Green FH, et al. Pleural multicystic mesothelial proliferation: the so-called multicystic mesothelioma. Am J Surg Pathol 14:375, 1990.
284. Blumberg NA, Murray JF. Multicystic peritoneal mesotheliomas: a case report. South Afr Med J 59:85, 1981.

285. Carpenter HA, Lancaster JR, Lee RA. Multilocular cysts of the peritoneum. Mayo Clin Proc 57:634, 1982.
286. Chan JKC, Fong MH. Composite multicystic mesothelioma and adenomatoid tumour of the uterus: different morphological manifestations of the same process? Histopathology 29:375, 1996.
287. Datta RV, Paty PB. Cystic mesothelioma of the peritoneum. Eur J Surg Oncol 23:461, 1997.
288. Hasan AK, Sinclair DJ. Case report: calcification in benign cystic peritoneal mesothelioma. Clin Radiol 48:66, 1993.
289. Hidvegi J, Schneider F, Rohonyi B, et al. Peritoneal benign cystic mesothelioma. Pathol Res Pract 187:103, 1991.
290. Jacobson E. Benign papillary mesothelial cystosis simulating serous cystadenocarcinoma of the ovary. Am J Obstet Gynecol 118:575, 1974.
291. Katsube Y, Mukai K, Silverberg SG. Cystic mesothelioma of the peritoneum: a report of five cases and review of the literature. Cancer 50:1615, 1982.
292. Kjellvold K, Nesland JM, Holm R, et al. Multicystic peritoneal mesothelioma. Pathol Res Pract 181:767, 1986.
293. Lamovec J, Sinkovec J. Multilocular peritoneal inclusion cysts (multicystic mesothelioma) with hyaline globules. Histopathology 28:466, 1996.
294. Livingston EG, Guis MS, Pearl ML, et al. Diffuse adenomatoid tumour of the uterus with a serosal papillary cystic component. Int J Gynecol Pathol 11:288, 1992.
295. McCullaghy M, Keen C, Dykes E. Cystic mesothelioma of the peritoneum: a rare cause of ascites in children. J Pediatr Surg 29:1205, 1994.
296. McFadden DE, Clement PB. Peritoneal inclusion cysts with mural mesothelial proliferation: a clinicopathologic analysis of six cases. Am J Surg Pathol 10:844, 1986.
297. Mennemeyer R, Smith M. Multicystic, peritoneal mesothelioma: a report with electron microscopy of a case mimicking intraabdominal cystic hygroma (lymphangioma). Cancer 44: 692, 1979.
298. Moore JH, Crum CP, Chandler JG, et al. Benign cystic mesothelioma. Cancer 45:2395, 1980.
299. Plaut A. Multiple peritoneal cysts and their histogenesis. Arch Pathol 5:754, 1928.
300. Schneider V, Partridge JR, Gutierrez F, et al. Benign cystic mesothelioma involving the female genital tract: report of four cases. Am J Obstet Gynecol 145:355, 1983.
301. Scucchi L, Mingazzini P, Di Stefano D, et al. Two cases of "multicystic peritoneal mesothelioma": description and critical review of the literature. Anticancer Res 14:715, 1994.
302. Sienkowski IK, Russell AJ, Dilly SA, et al. Peritoneal cystic mesothelioma: an electron microscopic and immunohistochemical study of two male patients. J Clin Pathol 39:440, 1986.
303. Takenouchi Y, Oda K, Takahara O, et al. Report of a case of benign cystic mesothelioma. Am J Gastroenterol 90:1165, 1995.
304. Van der Klooster JM, Lambers MD, van Bommel EF, et al. Successful catheter drainage of recurrent benign multicystic mesothelioma of the peritoneum. Neth J Med 50:246, 1997.
305. Weiss SW, Tavassoli FA. Multicystic mesothelioma: an analysis of pathologic findings and biologic behavior in 37 cases. Am J Surg Pathol 12:737, 1988.

### Adenomatoid Tumor

306. Banks ER, Mills SE. Histiocytoid (epithelioid) hemangioma of the testis: the so-called vascular variant of an "adenomatoid tumor." Am J Surg Pathol 14:584, 1990.
307. Barwick KW, Madri JA. An immunohistochemical study of adenomatoid tumors utilizing keratin and factor VIII antibodies: evidence for a mesothelial origin. Lab Invest 47:276, 1982.
308. Craig JR, Hart WR. Extragenital adenomatoid tumor: evidence for the mesothelial theory of origin. Cancer 43:1678, 1979.
309. Feuer A, Dewire DM, Foley WD. Ultrasonographic characteristics of testicular adenomatoid tumors. J Urol 155:174, 1996.
310. Golden A, Ash JE. Adenomatoid tumors of the genital tract. Am J Pathol 21:63, 1945.
311. Huang CC, Chang DY, Chen CK, et al. Adenomatoid tumor of the female genital tract. Int J Gynaecol Obstet 50:275, 1995.
312. Kaplan, MA, Tazelaar HD, Hayashi T, et al. Adenomatoid tumors of the pleura. Am J Surg Pathol 20:1219, 1996.
313. Lee MJ Jr, Dockerty MB, Thompson GJ, et al. Benign mesotheliomas (adenomatoid tumors) of genital tract. Surg Gynecol Obstet 91:221, 1950.
314. Mackay B, Bennington JL, Skoglund RW. The adenomatoid tumor: fine structural evidence for a mesothelial origin. Cancer 27:109, 1971.
315. Makarainen HP, Tammela TL, Karttunen TJ, et al. Intrascrotal adenomatoid tumors and their ultrasound findings. J Clin Ultrasound 21:33, 1993.
316. Marcus JB, Lynn JA. Ultrastructural comparison of an adenomatoid tumor, lymphangioma, hemangioma, and mesothelioma. Cancer 25:171, 1970.
317. Masson P, Riopelle JL, Simard LC. Le mesotheliome benin de la sphere genitale. Rev Can Biol 1:720, 1942.
318. Natarajan S, Luthringer DJ, Fishbein MC. Adenomatoid tumor of the heart: report of a case. Am J Surg Pathol 21:1378, 1997.
319. Otis CN. Uterine adenomatoid tumors: immunohistochemical characteristics with emphasis on Ber-EP4 immunoreactivity and distinction from adenocarcinoma. Int J Gynecol Pathol 15: 146, 1996.
320. Quigley JC, Hart WR. Adenomatoid tumors of the uterus. Am J Clin Pathol 76:627, 1981.
321. Raaf H, Grant L, Santoscoy C, et al. Adenomatoid tumors of the adrenal gland: a report of four new cases and a review of the literature. Mod Pathol 9:1046, 1996.
322. Racioppi M, d'Addessi A, di Pinto A, et al. Three consecutive cases of adenomatoid tumor of the epididymis: histological considerations and therapeutical implications: review of the literature. Arch Ital Urol Androl 68:115, 1996.
323. Said JW, Nash G, Lee M. Immunoperoxidase localization of keratin proteins, carcinoembryonic antigen, and factor VIII in adenomatoid tumors: evidence of mesothelial derivation. Hum Pathol 13:1106, 1982.
324. Salazar H, Kanbour A, Burgess F. Ultrastructure and observation on the histogenesis of mesotheliomas, adenomatoid tumors, of the female genital tract. Cancer 29:141, 1972.
325. Shintaku M, Sasaki M, Honda T. Thrombomodulin immunoreactivity in adenomatoid tumour of the uterus. Histopathology 28:375, 1996.
326. Stephenson TJ, Mills PM. Adenomatoid tumours: an immunohistochemical and ultrastructural appraisal of their histogenesis. J Pathol 148:327, 1986.
327. Taxy JB, Battifora H, Oyasu R. Adenomatoid tumors: a light-microscopic, histochemical, and ultrastructural study. Cancer 34:306, 1974.
328. Travis WD, Lack EE, Azumi N, et al. Adenomatoid tumor of the adrenal gland with ultrastructural and immunohistochemical demonstration of a mesothelial origin. Arch Pathol Lab Med 114:722, 1990.
329. Young RH, Silva EG, Scully RE. Ovarian and juxtaovarian adenomatoid tumors: a report of six cases. Int J Gynecol Pathol 10:364, 1991.

## CHAPTER 30

# BENIGN TUMORS OF PERIPHERAL NERVES

Benign tumors of peripheral nerves are relatively common lesions that differ from most soft tissue tumors in several important respects. Most soft tissue tumors arise from mesodermally derived tissue and display a range of features consonant with that lineage. Nerve sheath tumors arise from tissues considered to be of neuroectodermal or neural crest origin and display a range of features that mirror the various elements of the nerve (e.g., Schwann cell, perineurial cell). In rare instances they may even appear epithelioid (e.g., epithelioid schwannoma). Whereas most soft tissue tumors only seem to be encapsulated by virtue of the compression of surrounding tissues against their advancing border, the benign nerve sheath tumors arising in a nerve are completely surrounded by epi- or perineurium and therefore have a true capsule, a feature that may facilitate their enucleation. Finally, benign nerve sheath tumors represent the most important group of benign soft tissue lesions in which malignant transformation is an acknowledged phenomenon. Malignant peripheral nerve sheath tumors develop in preexisting neurofibromas in a subset of patients with neurofibromatosis 1, thereby providing an excellent model in which to study the molecular pathway of malignant transformaton.

This chapter discusses the two principal benign nerve sheath tumors—schwannoma (formerly neurilemoma) and neurofibroma, their variations, and associated syndromes. The schwannoma recapitulates in a more or less consistent fashion the appearance of the differentiated schwann cell, whereas the neurofibroma displays a spectrum of cell types ranging from schwann cell to fibroblast. Although the early literature often blurred or minimized the differences between schwannomas and neurofibromas, they are distinctive lesions that can be reproducibly distinguished from one another in most instances by their pattern of growth, cellular composition, associated syndromes, and cytogenetic alterations (Table 30–1). The perineurioma is a more recently recognized tumor that mirrors the normal perineurial cell, a barrier cell of the nerve sheath recognized by certain characteristic ultrastructural and immunophenotypic features. Several pseudotumorous lesions of nerve (e.g., traumatic neuroma, Morton's neuroma, nerve sheath ganglion) and two rare tumors, extracranial meningioma and pigmented neuroectodermal tumor of infancy, are also discussed in this chapter. The last two tumors are difficult to classify and are included because of their usually benign behavior and presumed neural crest lineage.

## EMBRYOGENESIS AND NORMAL ANATOMY

The peripheral nervous system can be defined as nervous tissue outside the brain and spinal cord. It is an extensive system which includes somatic and autonomic nerves, end-organ receptors, and supporting structures. It develops when axons lying close to one another grow out from the neural tube and are gradually invested with Schwann cells. Schwann cells arise from the neural crest, a group of cells that arise from and lie lateral to the neural tube and underneath the ectoderm of the developing embryo. The major peripheral nerve trunks form by fusion and division of segmental spinal nerves and, therefore, often contain mixtures of sensory, motor, and autonomic elements. Precise identification of these elements is not always possible solely on morphologic grounds. As the peripheral nerves form, the Schwann cells migrate peripherally from the spinal ganglia, orient themselves parallel to the axons, and encase them with their cytoplasm. In myelinated fibers only one axon segment is encased by one Schwann cell; and synthesis and spiraling of the schwannian plasma membrane around the axon create the myelin sheath. However, discontinuities of the myelin sheath exist at those points where adjacent Schwann cells meet but

**TABLE 30–1** COMPARISON OF SCHWANNOMA AND NEUROFIBROMA

| Parameter | Schwannoma | Neurofibroma |
|---|---|---|
| **Age** | 20–50 years | 20–40 years; younger in NF1 |
| **Common locations** | Head-neck; flexor portion of extremities; less often retroperitoneum and mediastinum | Cutaneous nerves; deep locations in NF1 |
| **Encapsulation** | Usually | Usually not |
| **Growth patterns** | Encapsulated tumor with Antoni A and B areas; plexiform type uncommon | Localized, diffuse and plexiform patterns |
| **Associated syndromes** | Most lesions sporadic; but some NF2, rarely NF1 | Most lesions sporadic; some NF1 |
| **S-100 protein immunostaining** | Strong and uniform | Variable staining of cells |
| **Malignant transformation** | Exceptionally rare | Rare in sporadic cases but occurs in 2–3% of NF1 patients |

where there is no lamination of the plasma membrane (nodes of Ranvier). In nonmyelinated nerves several axon segments are ensheathed by a common Schwann cell, but they are not enclosed beyond the initial stage of enfolding and therefore are invested with only a single or at most a few layers of schwannian plasma membrane. In humans the process of myelination commences during the eighteenth week of intrauterine life, is usually advanced by birth, and continues for several years postnatally.[2]

In the fully developed nerve a layer of connective tissue or epineurium surrounds the entire nerve trunk (Fig. 30–1). This structure varies in size depending of the location of the nerve, and it is composed of a mixture of collagen and elastic fibers along with mast cells. Several nerve fascicles lie within the confines of the epineurium, and each in turn is surrounded by a well defined sheath known as the perineurium. These small nerve fascicles anticipate the subsequent division of the nerve into smaller branches, and for this reason the terms *epineurium* and *perineurium* can be used interchangeably when referring to small nerves. The smallest connective tissue unit of the nerve is the endoneurium, an intricate network of collagen, blood vessels, and fibroblasts encircling individual nerve fibers.

Considerable emphasis has been placed on the nature of the perineurium.[13] The outer portion of the perineurium consists of layers of connective tissue, and the inner portion is represented by a multilayered, concentrically arranged sheath of flattened cells.[19] These cells, which are best defined by electron microscopy and immunohistochemistry, have been termed *perineurial fibroblasts, perineurial epithelium,*[19] or simply *perineurial cells.* They are continuous with the pia-arachnoid of the central nervous system and ap-

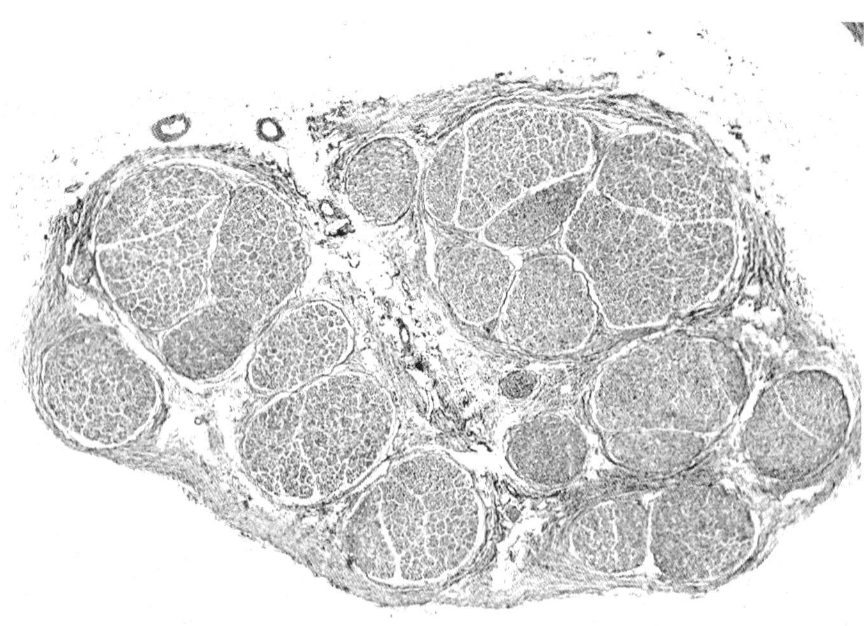

**FIGURE 30–1.** Normal sciatic nerve in cross section. The entire nerve is surrounded by epineurium, and smaller nerve fascicles are encompassed by perineurium.

pear to be important in maintaining a diffusion barrier for the peripheral nerve. It is not clear whether these cells are derived from Schwann cells, fibroblasts, or arachnoidal cells.[3,12] In contrast to Schwann cells, perineural cells express S-100 protein but not epithelial membrane antigen, an immunophenotypic profile identical to pia-arachnoid cells. Ultrastructurally, they form close junctions with each other and have basal lamina along the endoneurial and perineurial aspects of the cell,[19] features not encountered in the ordinary fibroblast and Schwann cell. The cytoplasm is rather poor in organelles except for the prominent, well aligned pinocytotic vesicles along their surface and occasional myofilaments. Peculiar acellular, collagen-rich, whorled structures known as *Renaut's bodies* are occasionally found directly underneath the perineurium. Their significance is unknown, but their frequency near joints has suggested a cushioning function.

Despite the undoubted importance of the investing connective tissue, the critical supporting element is the Schwann cell. It provides mechanical protection for the axon, produces and maintains the myelin sheath, and serves as a tube to guide regenerating nerve fibers. By light microscopy it is difficult to distinguish this cell from a fibroblast because their nuclei are similar. However, by electron microscopy a Schwann cell is easily identified by its intimate relation to its axons and by a continuous basal lamina that coats the surface of the cell facing the endoneurium. Current evidence suggests that the Schwann cell synthesizes this basal lamina[19] and is capable of synthesizing collagen precursors.[14] Except for occasional 10 nm fibrils, microtubules, and mitochondria, other cytoplasmic organelles are not especially prominent except during periods of increased metabolism (e.g., myelin synthesis).[15] Pi granules, flattened lamellations of osmiophilic material, are occasionally present in a perinuclear location, but their significance is unknown. In routine preparations it is difficult to distinguish the axon from the myelin sheath. This distinction, however, is easily accomplished with special stains. Silver stains selectively stain the axon (Fig. 30–2), whereas stains such as Luxol fast blue stain myelin. The variation in diameter of axon and myelin sheath can be appreciated with these stains. In general, moderate or heavily myelinated fibers correspond to sensory and motor fibers with fast conduction speeds, whereas lightly myelinated or unmyelinated fibers correspond to autonomic fibers with slower conduction speeds.[15] Ultrastructurally, the cytoplasm of the axon is characterized by numerous cytoplasmic filaments, slender mitochondria, and a longitudinally oriented endoplasmic reticulum. Nissl substance, a feature of the nerve cell body, is not present in the axoplasm. In addition, small vesicles

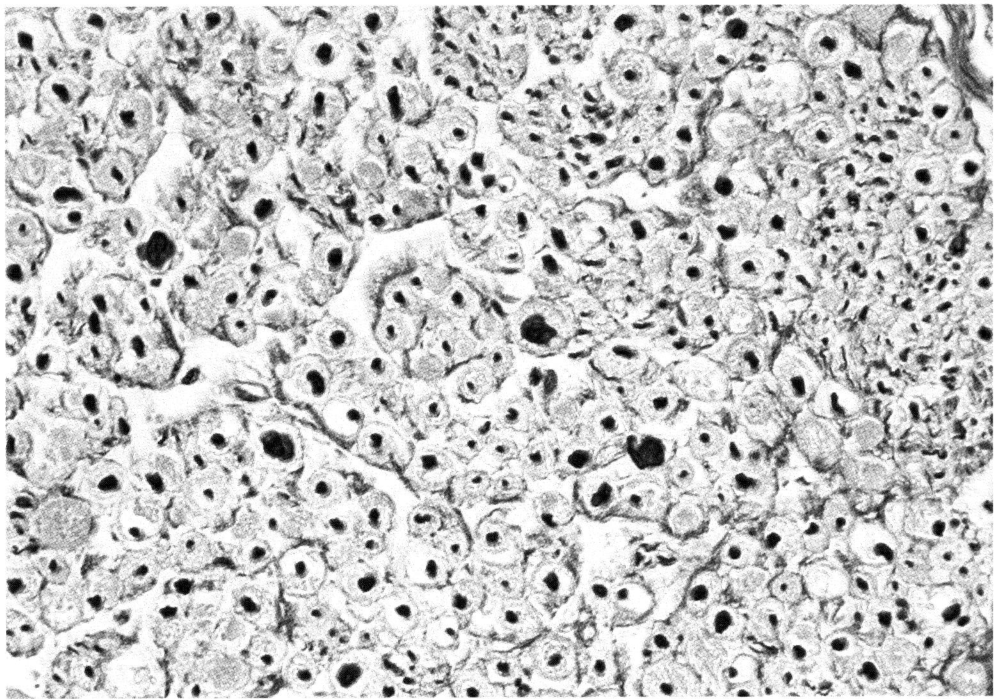

**FIGURE 30–2.** Normal peripheral nerve cut in cross section and stained with Bodian (silver) stain. Individual axons stain positively; surrounding myelin sheath does not stain. The thickness of axons and the myelin sheath varies and determines the conduction speed.

are observed occasionally; they may represent packets of neurotransmitter substance en route to the nerve terminal.

## TRAUMATIC (AMPUTATION) NEUROMA

Traumatic neuroma is an exuberant but nonneoplastic proliferation of a nerve occurring in response to injury or surgery. Under ideal circumstances the ends of a severed nerve reestablish continuity by an orderly growth of axons from proximal to distal stump through tubes of proliferating Schwann cells. However, if close apposition of the ends of nerve is not maintained or if there is no distal stump, a disorganized proliferation of the proximal nerve gives rise to a neuroma. Symptomatic neuromas are usually the result of surgery, notably amputation. Occasionally other surgical procedures such as cholecystectomy[25] have been incriminated in their pathogenesis. A rare form of traumatic neuroma is seen in rudimentary (supernumerary) digits that undergo autoamputation in utero. These lesions appear as raised nodules on the ulnar surface of the proximal fifth finger. They contain a disordered proliferation of nerves similar to a conventional traumatic neuroma (Fig. 30–3).[27]

Clinically, the neuroma presents as a firm nodule that is occasionally tender or painful. Strangulation of the proliferating nerve by scar tissue, local trauma, and infection have all been invoked as possible explanations of the pain. Grossly, the lesions are circumscribed, white-gray nodules seldom exceeding 5 cm in diameter; they are located in continuity with the proximal end of the injured or transected nerve. They consist of a haphazard proliferation of nerve fascicles, including axons with their investitures of myelin, Schwann cells, and fibroblasts. The fascicles are usually less well myelinated than the parent nerve and are embedded in a background of collagen (Fig. 30–4).

Traumatic neuromas are sometimes confused with palisaded encapsulated neuromas and neurofibromas. Participation of all elements of the nerve fascicles and identification of a damaged nerve distinguish a traumatic neuroma from neurofibroma. In areas where the fascicles are small and the matrix is poorly collagenized and highly myxoid, the similarity to neurofibroma may be striking (Fig. 30–5) and, therefore, may require identification of more subtle clues such as the characteristic collagen bundles of neurofibroma. Palisaded encapsulated neuromas arise exclusively in the skin, predominantly in women; they consist of a more circumscribed, orderly arrangement of nerve fascicles.

Treatment of traumatic neuromas is, in part, prophylactic. After traumatic nerve injury, an attempt should be made to reappose the ends of the severed nerve so regeneration of the proximal end proceeds down the distal trunk in an orderly fashion. Once a neuroma has formed, removal is indicated when it becomes symptomatic or when it must be distinguished from recurrent tumor in a patient who has had cancer-related surgery.[20] Simple excision of the lesion and reembedding the proximal nerve stump in an area away from the old scar constitute the conventional therapy.

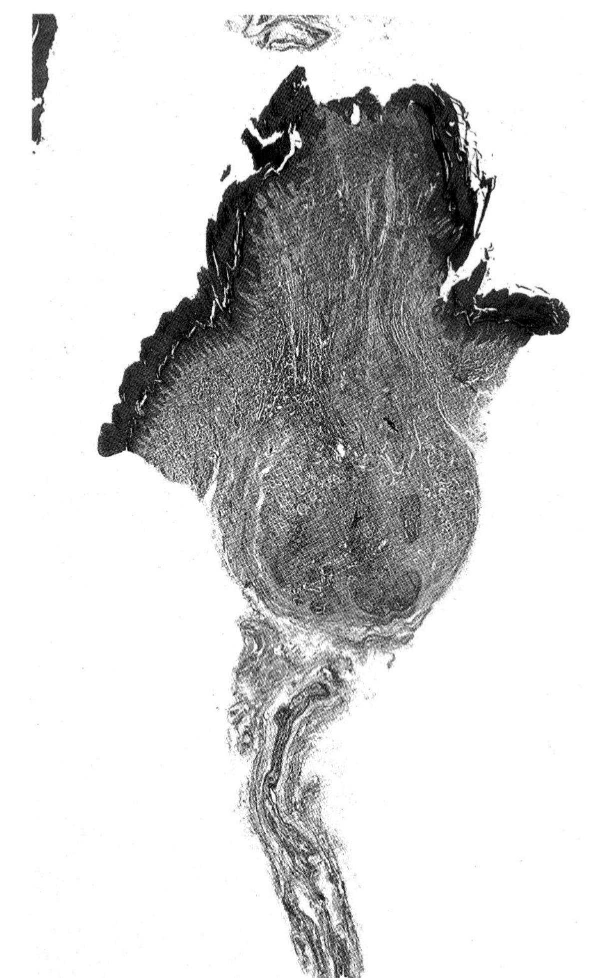

**FIGURE 30–3.** Rudimentary digit that underwent autoamputation in utero and showed areas of traumatic neuroma.

## MUCOSAL NEUROMA

Mucosal neuroma involves the mucosal surfaces of the lips, mouth, eyelids, and intestines in patients with type IIb multiple endocrine neoplasia (MEN-IIb), characterized by bilateral pheochromocytoma, C cell hyperplasia, medullary thyroid carcinoma, and parathyroid hyperplasia.[30] Because mucosal neuromas may represent an early manifestation of this life

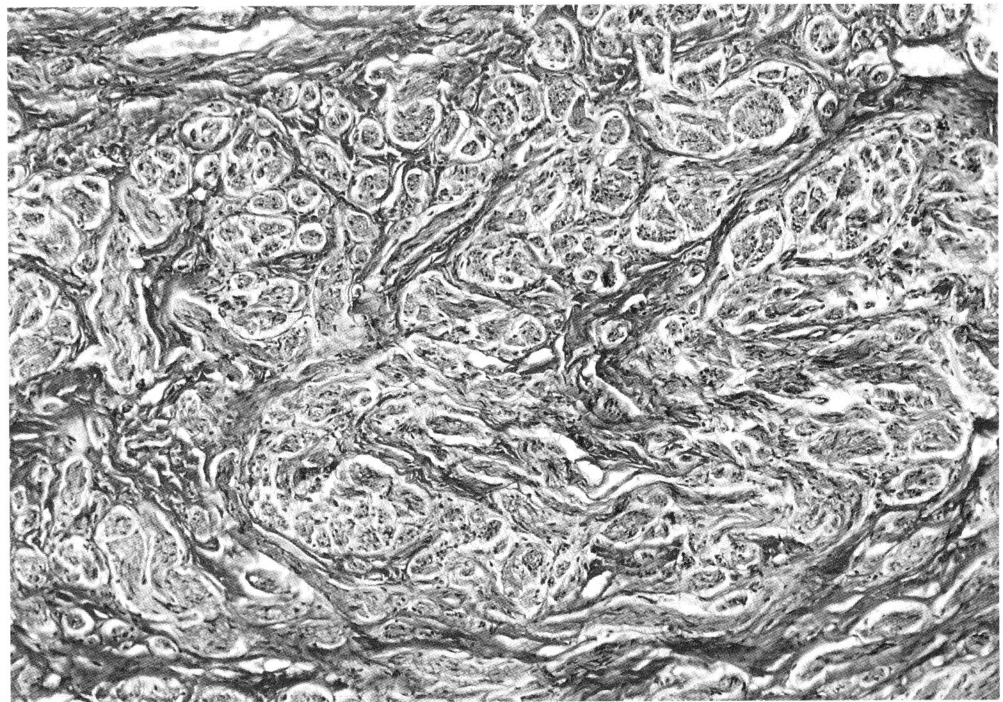

**FIGURE 30–4.** Traumatic neuroma composed of small proliferating fascicles of nerve enveloped in collagen.

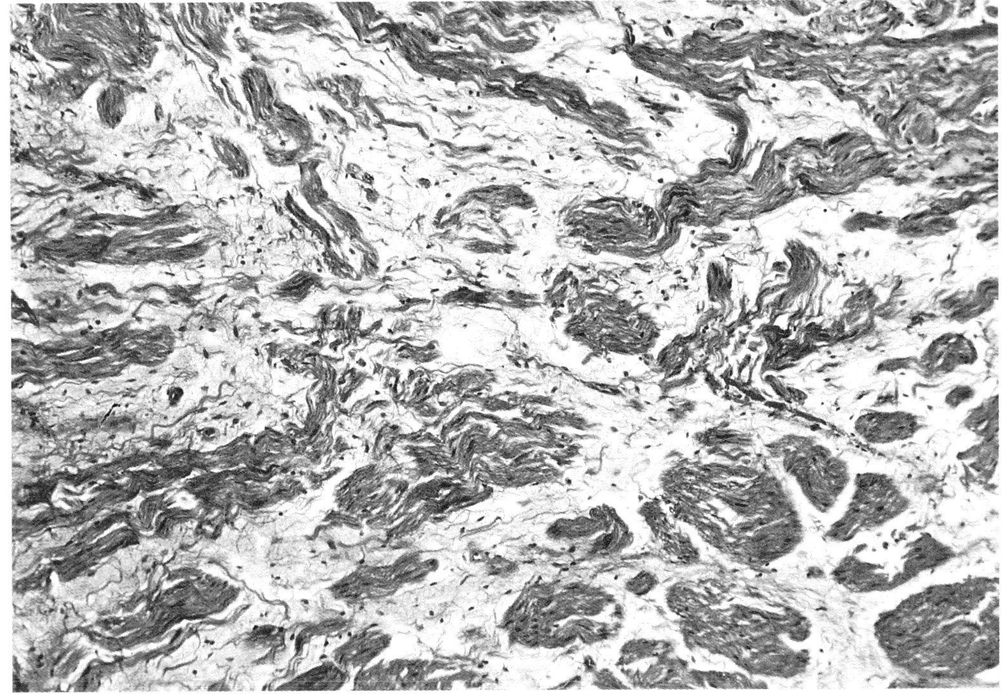

**FIGURE 30–5.** Myxoid areas in a traumatic neuroma resembling a neurofibroma.

threatening syndrome, recognition of these lesions is of more than academic interest. The lesions manifest during the first few decades of life and present as multiple nodules of varying size, which may result in diffuse enlargement of the affected area.

Histologically, the lesions are notable for the irregular, tortuous bundles of nerve with a prominent perineurium that lie scattered throughout the submucosa of the oral cavity (Fig. 30–6). The nerves and perineurium may be distinguished by a prominent degree of myxoid change. In the gastrointestinal tract both submucosal and myenteric plexus appear hyperplastic, with an increase in all elements of the plexus including schwann cells, neurons, and ganglion cells (Fig. 30–7).

## PACINIAN NEUROMA

Pacinian neuroma refers to localized hyperplasia or hypertrophy of the pacinian corpuscles, which occurs following trauma and commonly produces pain.[31,33,35] Typically it develops on the digits, where it produces a localized mass. Pacinian neuromas range in appearance from small nodules attached to the nerve by a slender stalk to one or more contiguous subepineural nodules (Fig. 30–8). Histologically, it consists of mature pacinian corpuscles that are increased in size or number (or both) and are often associated with degenerative changes and fibrosis of the adjacent nerve. The principal problem in the differential diagnosis is the distinction of these lesions from a normal pacinian body, which can achieve a size sufficient to be visualized macroscopically. For example, normal pacinian bodies can be identified in the abdominal cavity, where they are occasionally misinterpreted as tumor implants.[31] In pacinian neuromas the structures usually are larger than 1.5 mm in diameter. In general, a pacinian neuroma is diagnosed when the histologic features described above are associated with a discrete pain-producing mass. Pacinian neuromas should not be confused with "pacinian neurofibromas," a term used to describe a heterogeneous group of lesions that include neurofibroma, congenital nevi, and neurothekeoma.

## PALISADED ENCAPSULATED NEUROMA (SOLITARY CIRCUMSCRIBED NEUROMA)

Although the palisaded encapsulated neuroma was described more than two decades ago by Reed et al.,[42] its acceptance as a distinct entity was slow because of uncertainty as to its overlap with the common schwannoma. It has rather distinct clinical features, which in concert with its appearance warrant a separate term.[37,38,40,41] The palisaded encapsulated neuroma develops as a small asymptomatic nodule in the area of the face of adult patients and affects the genders equally. Affected patients do not display manifestations of neurofibromatosis 1 or MEN-IIb.

Histologically, it is composed of one or more circumscribed or encapsulated nodules that occupy the deep dermis and subcutaneous tissues (Fig. 30–9). In some cases the nodules form club-like extensions into the subcutaneous tissue.[39] They consist of a solid proliferation of Schwann cells and lack the variety of stromal changes (e.g., myxoid change, hyalinization) that may be encountered in schwannomas and neurofibromas (Fig. 30–10). Although superficially these neuromas may resemble schwannomas, particularly if minor degrees of nuclear palisading are noted, they differ by their presence of axons, best demonstrated with silver stains, that traverse the lesion in close association with the Schwann cells. Schwannomas may contain axons, but they are typically located peripherally immediately underneath the capsule. In most instances simple excision of these lesions has proved curative. In contrast to a traumatic neuroma these lesions are encapsulated, more uniform appearing, and unassociated with a damaged nerve.

## MORTON'S INTERDIGITAL NEUROMA (LOCALIZED INTERDIGITAL NEURITIS, MORTON'S TOE, MORTON'S METATARSALGIA)

Morton's interdigital neuroma is not a true tumor but, rather, a fibrosing process of the plantar digital nerve that results in paroxysmal pain in the sole of the foot, usually between the heads of the third and fourth metatarsals and less often between the second and third.[43–48] The pain typically commences with exercise, is alleviated by rest, and may radiate into the toes or leg. In some cases a small area of point tenderness can be defined, although generally no mass can be palpated. The condition is almost always unilateral. Because women are affected more often than men, the wearing of ill-fitting high-heeled shoes has been incriminated in the pathogenesis of this condition. Lesions histologically similar to Morton's neuroma are sometimes seen adjacent to nerves in the hand, where they are undoubtedly related to chronic occupational or recreational injury.

At surgery the characteristic lesion is a firm fusiform enlargement of the plantar digital nerve at its bifurcation point. In advanced cases the nerve may be firmly attached to the adjacent bursa and soft tissue.

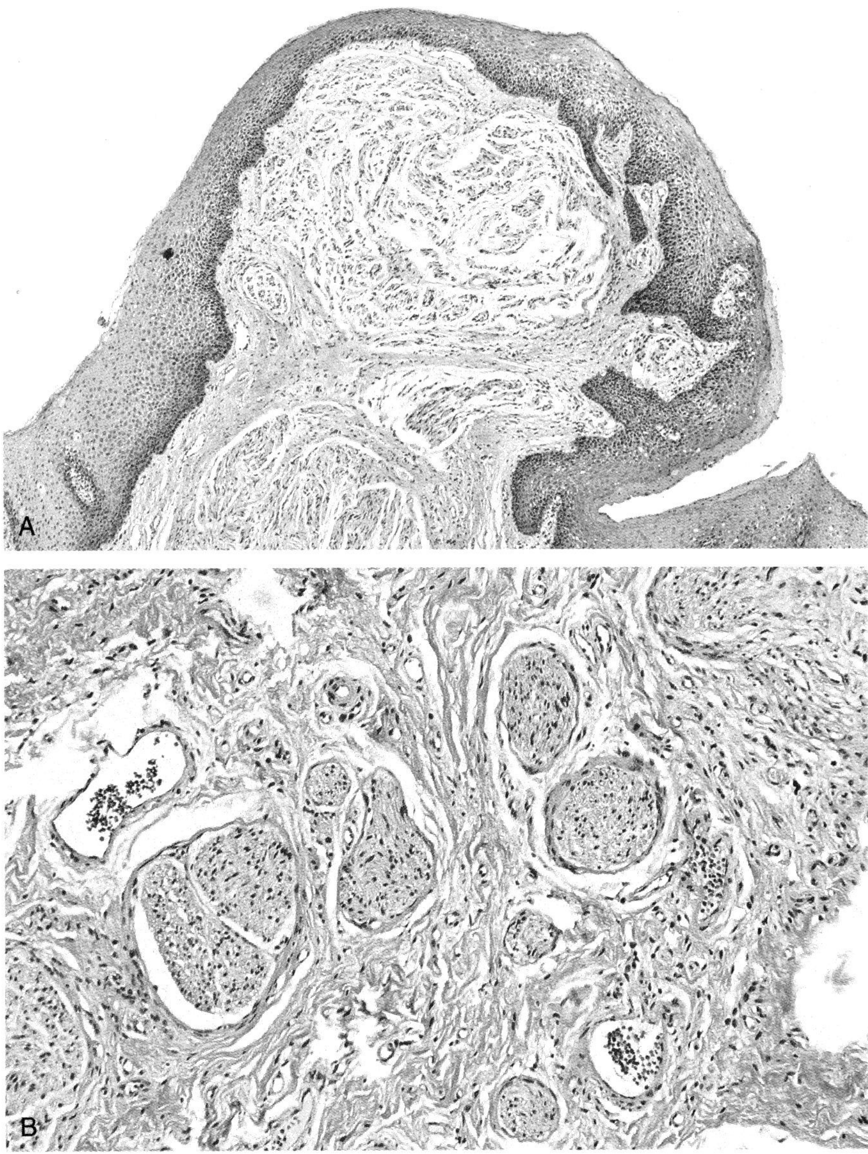


**FIGURE 30–6.** Mucosal neuroma from a patient with multiple endocrine neoplasia type IIb (**A**). Irregular, convoluted nerves with prominent perineurium and focal myxoid change lie in submucosal tissue (**B**).

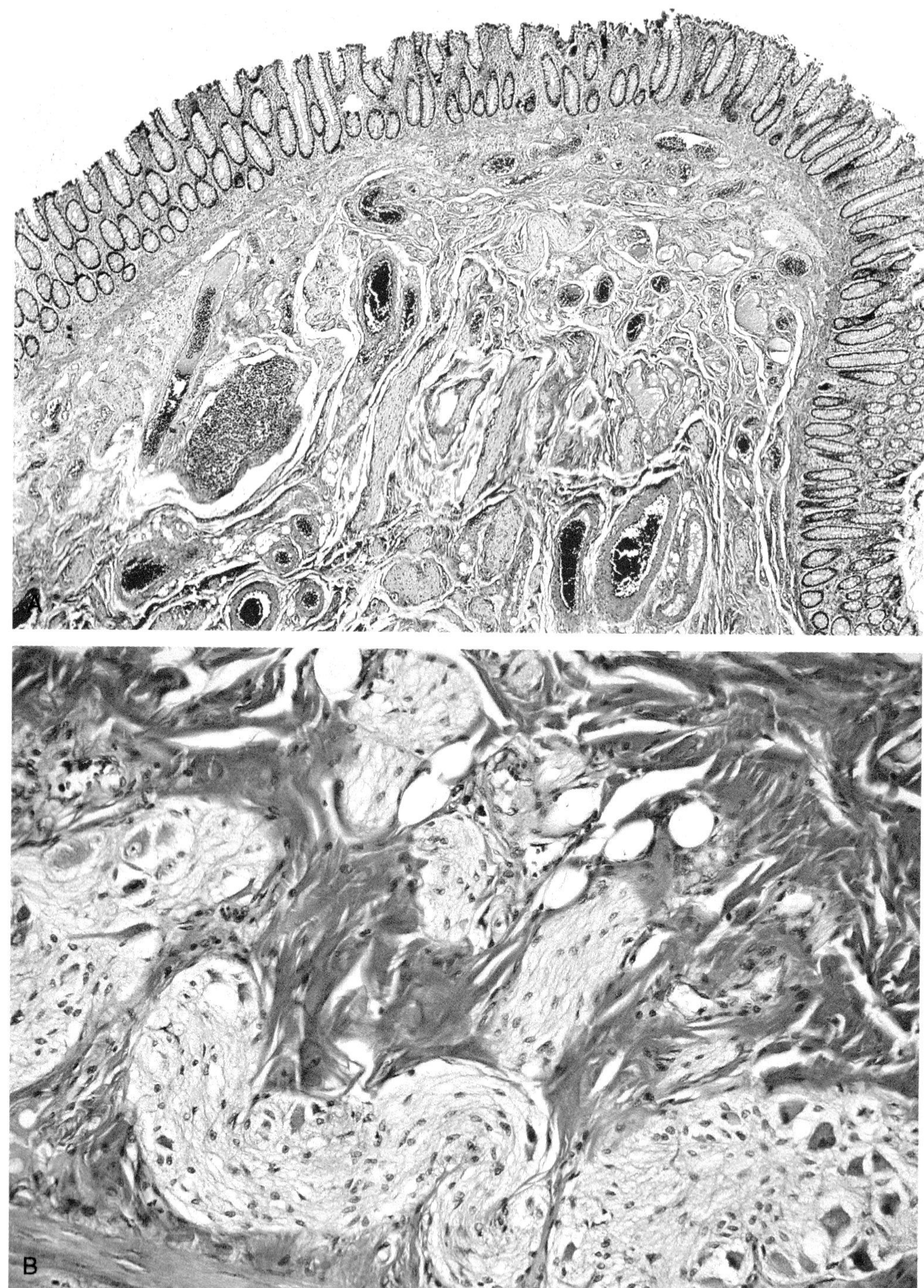


**FIGURE 30–7.** Gangioneuromatosis of the gastrointestinal tract in a patient with MEN-IIb (**A**). Autonomic nerves in the muscle wall are increased in size and number (**B**).

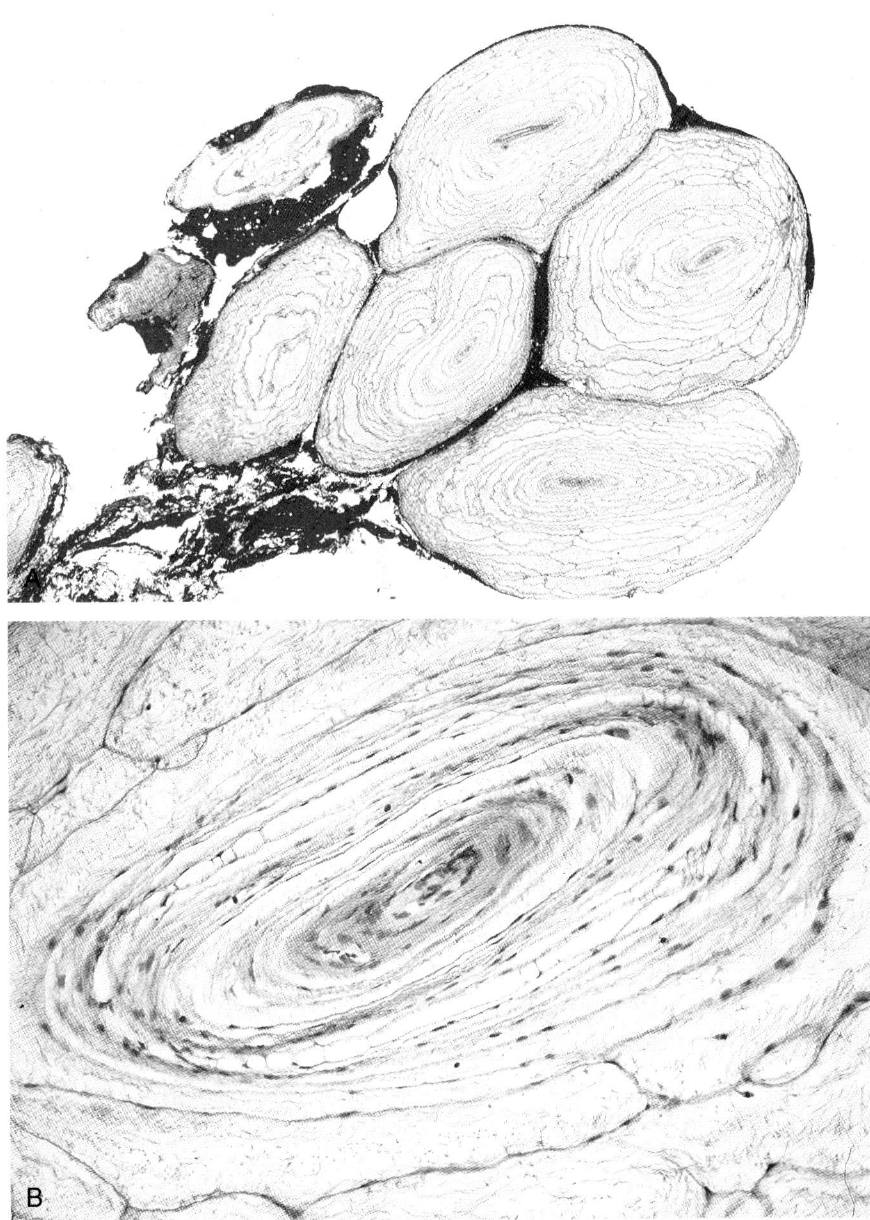

**FIGURE 30–8.** Pacinian neuroma (**A**). High power view (**B**).

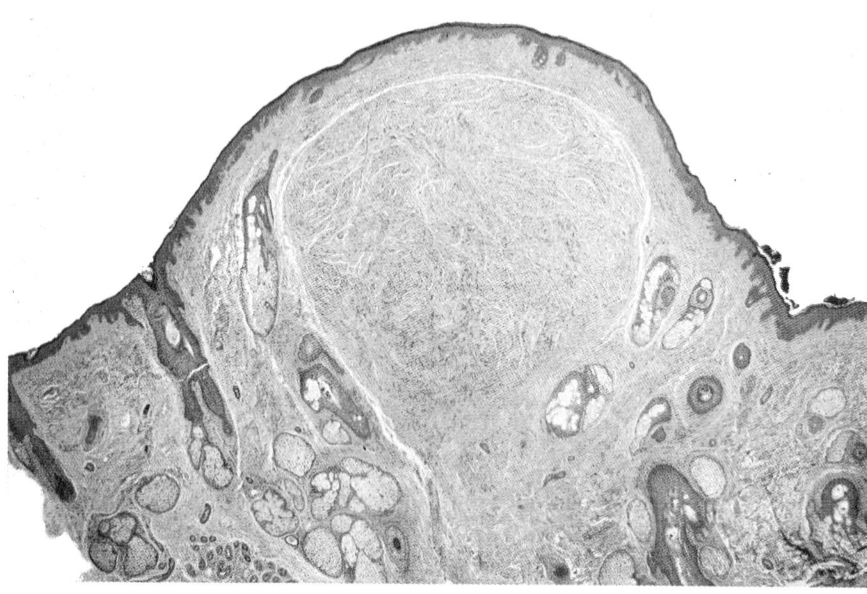

**FIGURE 30–9.** Palisaded encapsulated neuroma.

Although grossly the lesion resembles a traumatic neuroma or neurofibroma, it is different histologically. Proliferative changes characterize traumatic neuromas, whereas degenerative changes are the hallmark of Morton's neuroma. Edema and fibrosis occur in the nerve (Fig. 30–11A). Hyalinization of endoneurial vessels is also present in some cases (Fig. 30–11B). Elastic fibers are diminished in the center of the lesions but are increased at its periphery, where they have a bilaminar appearance similar to the elastic fibers in an elastofibroma.[45] As the lesion progresses, the fibrosis becomes marked and envelops the epineurium and perineurium in a concentric fashion and may even extend into the surrounding tissue. Pathogenetically, the changes have been explained by compression of the neurovascular bundles by the adjacent metatarsal heads. Whether the injury is primarily neural or is mediated via vascular ischemia is not resolved. Although conservative measures such as wearing of orthopedic footwear have been used, the most successful therapy consists in removing the affected nerve segment.

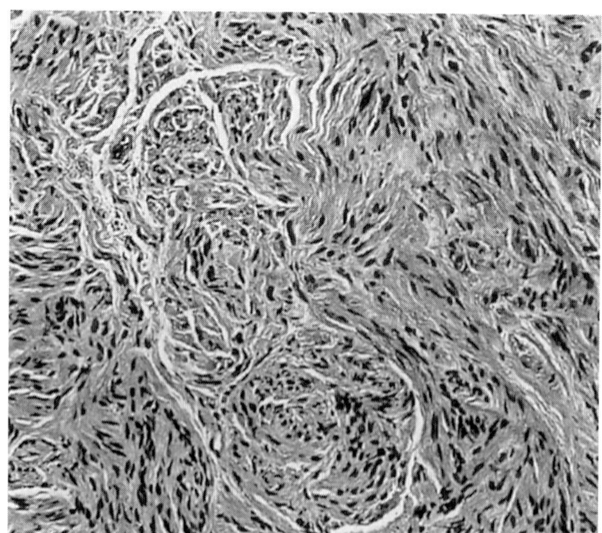

**FIGURE 30–10.** Palisaded encapsulated neuroma with irregular bundles of nerves containing both nerve and nerve sheath cells.

## GANGLIONEUROMA

Because of the overlap between ganglioneuroma and primitive neuroblastic tumors, ganglioneuroma is discussed in Chapter 32.

## NERVE SHEATH GANGLION

Rarely ganglia occur in intraneural locations.[49–51] Such lesions present as tender masses with pain or numbness in the distribution of the affected nerve. Most of these lesions are located in the external popliteal nerve[49] at the head of the fibula, which suggests that a particular type of injury or irritation leads to their development. The nerve exhibits localized swelling that corresponds to myxoid change with secondary cyst formation. In some cases, however, the unlined cysts dominate the histologic picture and cause marked displacement of the nerve fascicles toward one side of the sheath (Fig. 30–12). This lesion, like its soft tissue counterpart, represents a degenerative process rather than a neoplasm. The myxoid zones in these lesions have unfortunately led to some confusion with the so-called nerve sheath myxoma or neurothekeoma. This entity is a true neoplasm probably

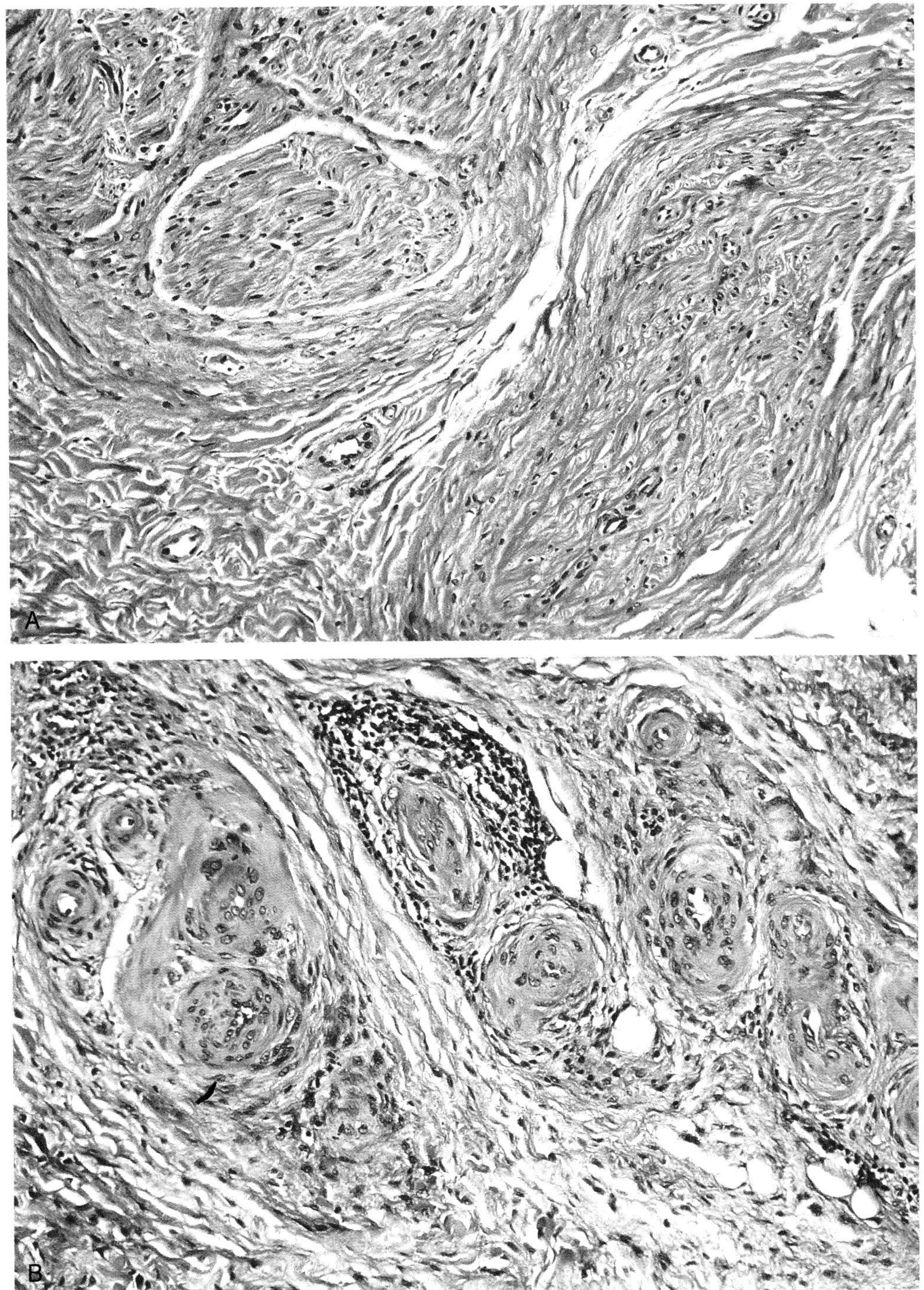

**FIGURE 30–11.** Morton's neuroma. Dense perineural (**A**) and perivascular (**B**) fibrosis characterize the lesion.

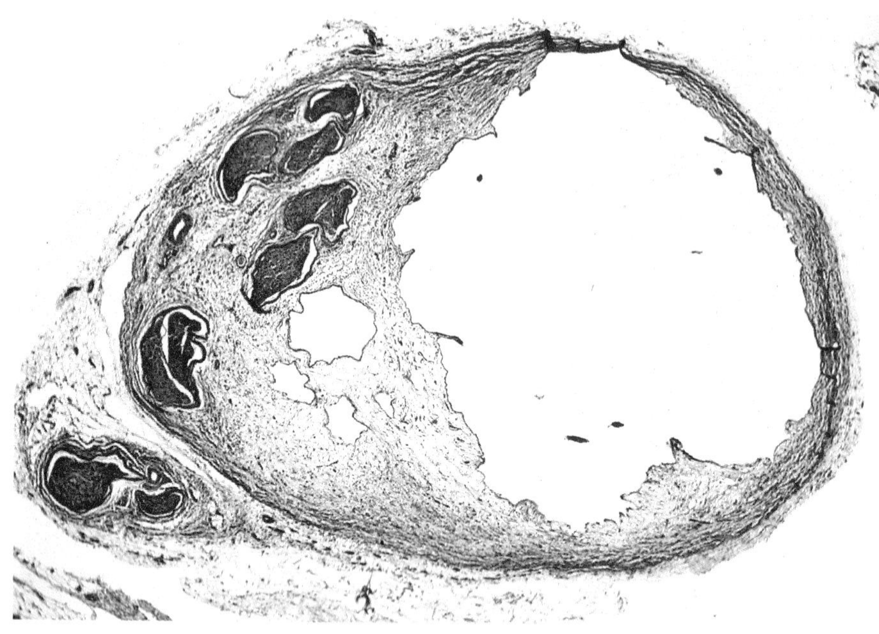

**FIGURE 30–12.** Ganglion of nerve sheath. Connective tissue of the nerve undergoes myxoid change and cystification.

of Schwann cell origin and is quite distinct from nerve sheath ganglion (see discussion of neurothekeoma, below). Therapy of a nerve sheath ganglion consists of local excision, although decompression is acceptable if the integrity of the nerve is threatened.

## NEUROMUSCULAR HAMARTOMA (NEUROMUSCULAR CHORISTOMA; BENIGN TRITON TUMOR)

Tumors composed of skeletal muscle and neural elements are collectively referred to as *Triton tumors* in accord with an early hypothesis concerning their histogenesis (see Chapter 31), The best recognized of these mosaic tumors is the malignant peripheral nerve sheath tumor with rhabdomyoblastic differentiation (malignant Triton tumor), although combinations such as rhabdomyosarcoma with ganglion cells (ectomesenchymoma) also occur. Benign lesions composed of neural and skeletal muscle differentiation are rare and are represented principally by the neuromuscular hamartoma or choristoma and the neurofibroma with a rhabdomyomatous component. "Benign Triton tumor" is often used loosely to refer to neuromuscular hamartomas, although it is technically incorrect if these are hamartomas or choristomas that occur when primitive mesenchyme of developing limb buds is included in the nerve sheath. Karyotypic analysis in one case was normal, supporting a hamartomatous process.[59]

Of the fewer than 20 cases reviewed from the literature, all occurred in young children and developed as masses in various large nerve trunks, particularly the brachial and sciatic.[52–60] The case described by O'Connell and Rosenberg[57] presented as multiple lesions outside the nerve. Because of their strategic locations, neurologic symptoms are prominent. The tumors are multinodular masses subdivided by fibrous bands into smaller nodules or fascicles. Each fascicle is composed of highly differentiated skeletal muscle fibers that vary in size but are often larger than normal. Intimately associated with the skeletal muscle and sharing the same perimysial sheath are both small myelinated and nonmyelinated nerves (Fig. 30–13). Smooth muscle is rarely present.[59] At times the fibrous component surrounding the lesions is so dense and cellular it suggests the diagnosis of fibromatosis replacing muscle and nerve. Follow-up information in our cases and those in the literature supports their benignity. Even incomplete excision has resulted in amelioration of symptoms and progressive decrease in size. Therefore, after a correct diagnosis treatment should be conservative and aimed primarily at maintaining the integrity of the nerve.

## NEUROFIBROMA

Neurofibromas may assume one of three growth patterns: localized, diffuse, or plexiform. The localized form is seen most commonly as a superficial, solitary tumor in normal individuals. Diffuse and plexiform neurofibromas have a close association with neurofibromatosis 1 (NF1), the latter being nearly pathognomonic of the disease. They are, therefore, discussed in that context later.

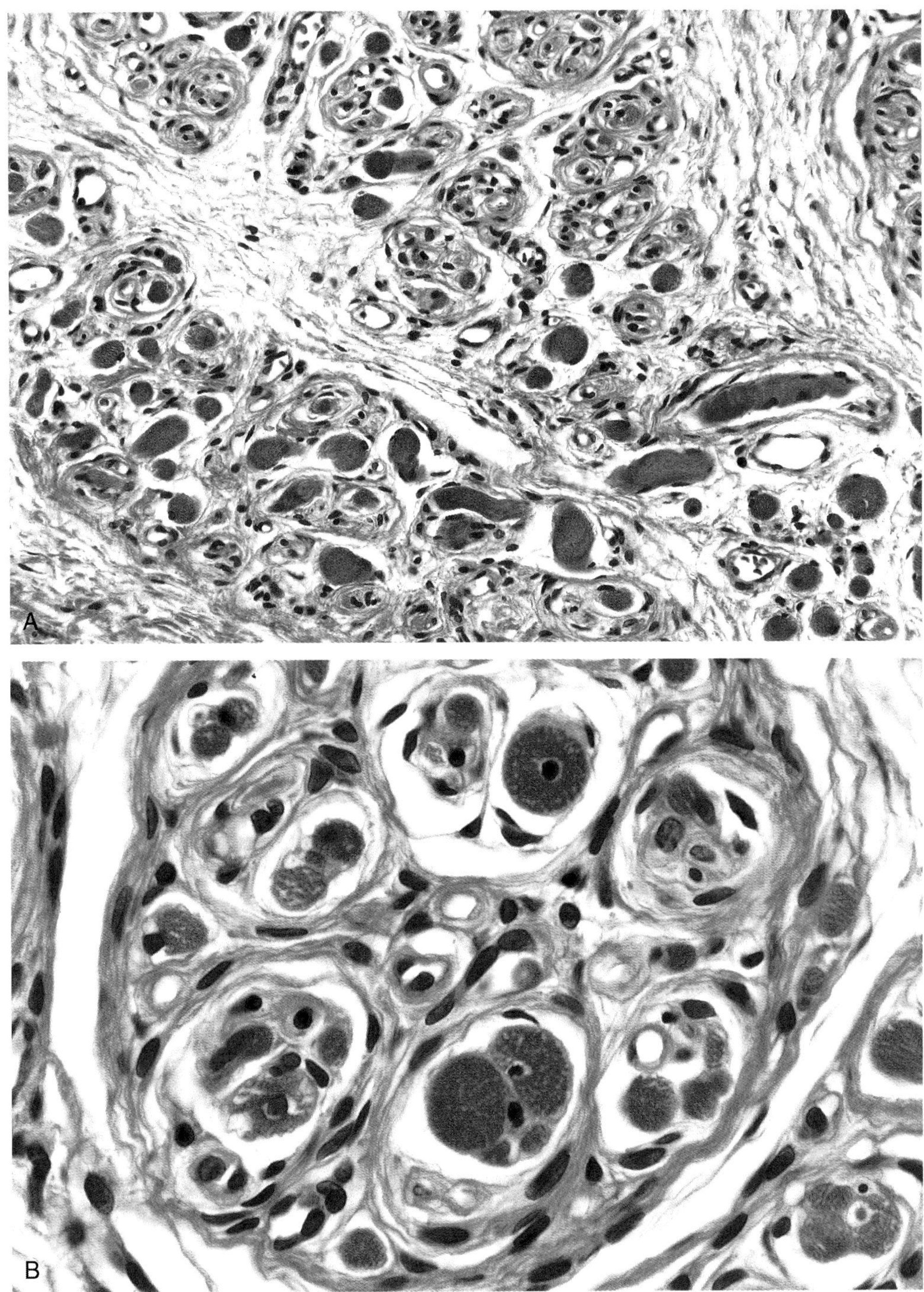


**FIGURE 30–13.** Neuromuscular hamartoma composed of short bundles of mature nerve and muscle (**A**). High power view of neuromuscular hamartoma (**B**).

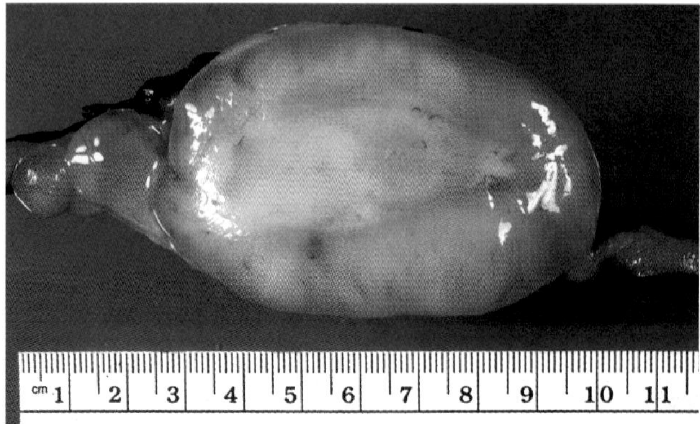


**FIGURE 30–14.** Gross specimen of neurofibroma arising as fusiform expansion of nerve. (Case courtesy of Dr. Steve Bonsib.)

## Localized (Sporadic) Neurofibroma

Localized neurofibromas occur most often as sporadic lesions in patients who do not have NF1. Their exact incidence is unknown because of the difficulty in excluding the diagnosis of NF1 in some persons such as the young, in whom the initial presentation of the disease may be a solitary neurofibroma, or patients who have no affected family members. Despite these problems, it appears that sporadic neurofibromas outnumber those occurring in NF1. In the series by Geschickter[128] about 90% of neurofibromas were of the solitary or sporadic type, and the remainder were found in the setting of NF1.

### Clinical Findings

Localized sporadic neurofibromas, like their inherited counterparts, affect the genders equally. Most develop in persons between the ages of 20 and 30 years.[128] Because most are superficial lesions of the dermis or subcutis, they are found evenly distributed over the body surface. They grow slowly as painless nodules and produce few symptoms. Grossly they are glistening tan-white tumors that lack the secondary degenerative changes common to schwannomas. If they arise in major nerves, they expand the structure in a fusiform fashion, and normal nerve can be seen entering and exiting from the mass (Fig. 30–14). If such a lesion remains confined by the epineurium, it has a true capsule. More commonly these tumors arise in small nerves and readily extend into soft tissue. Such tumors appear circumscribed but are nonencapsulated.

### Microscopic Findings

Histologically, the neurofibroma varies, depending on its content of cells, mucin, and collagen (Figs. 30–15 to 30–19). In its most characteristic form the neurofibroma contains interlacing bundles of elongated cells with wavy, dark-staining nuclei. The cells are intimately associated with wire-like strands of collagen that have been likened to "shredded carrots." Small to moderate amounts of mucoid material separate the cells and collagen. The stroma of the tumor is dotted

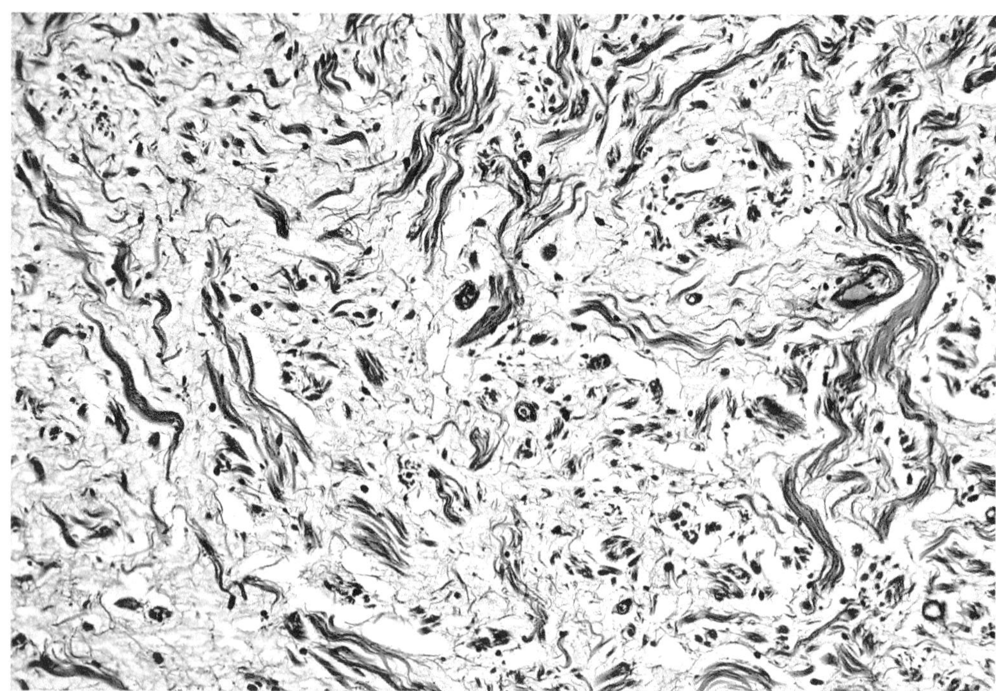

**FIGURE 30–15.** Neurofibroma with a myxoid matrix containing neoplastic cells and ropey collagen bundles.

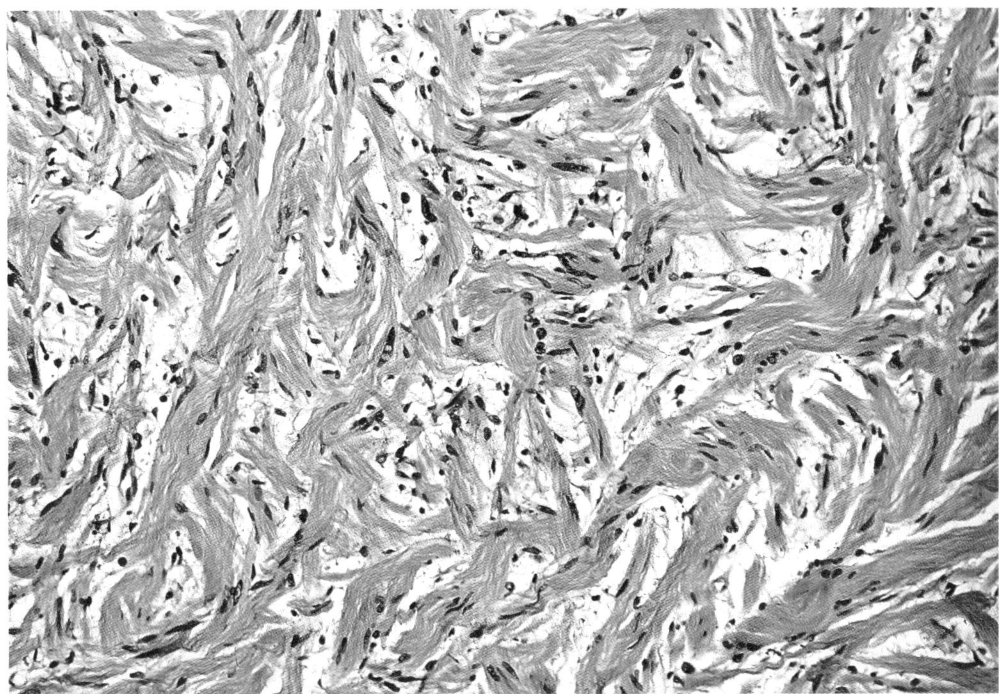

**FIGURE 30–16.** Neurofibroma with dense collagen bundles.

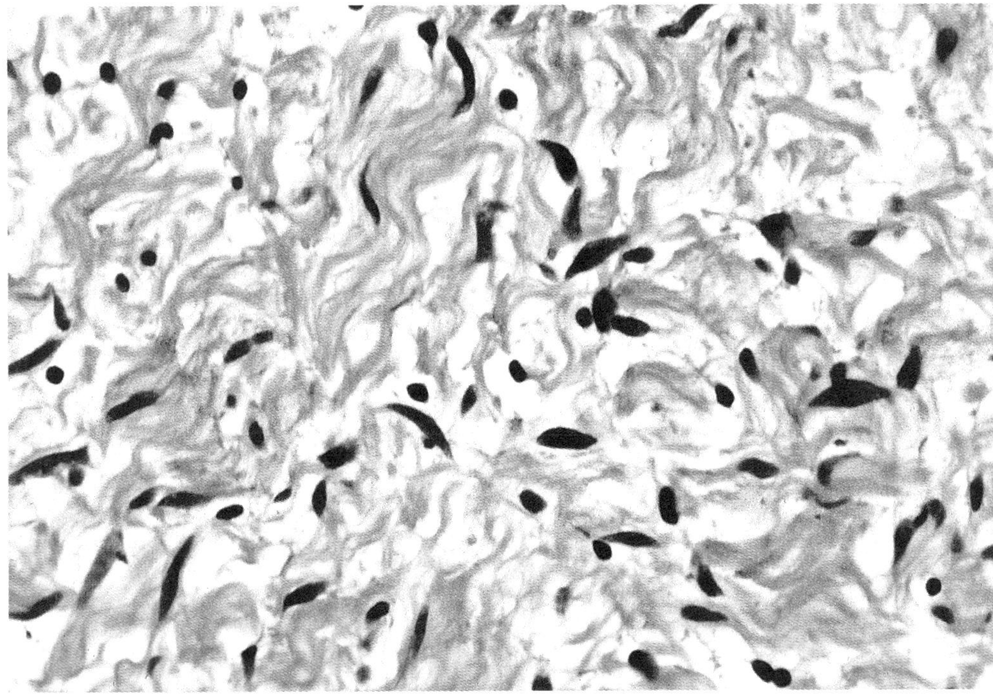

**FIGURE 30–17.** Neurofibroma with Schwann cells of an irregular shape, mononuclear cells, and occasional mast cells.

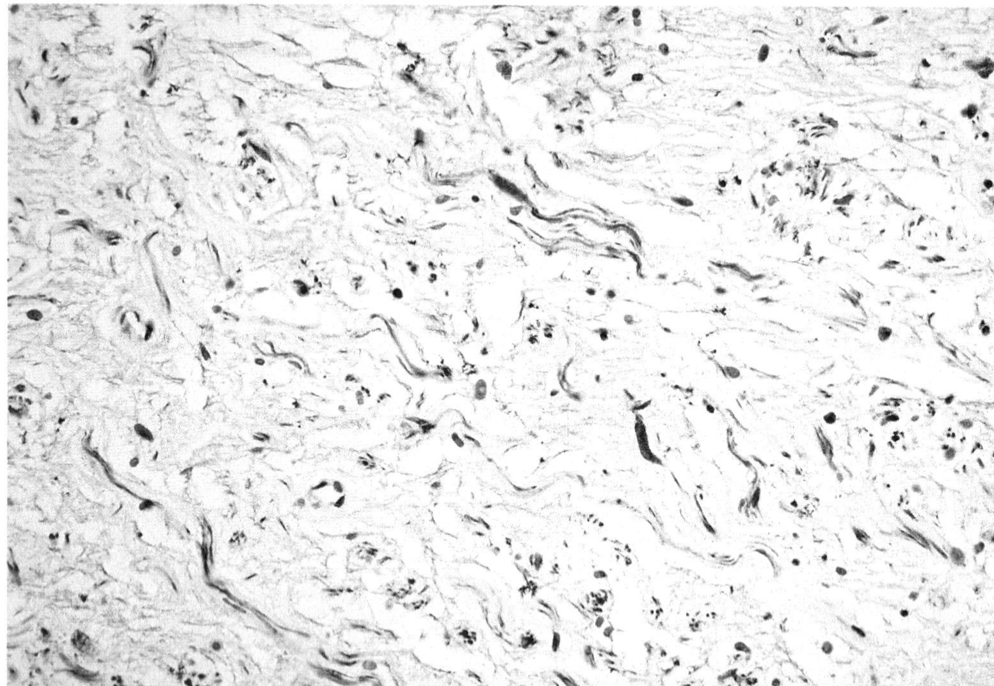

**FIGURE 30–18.** S-100 protein immunostain of a neurofibroma illustating that not all cells in the lesion express the antigen.

with occasional mast cells, lymphocytes, and rarely xanthoma cells. Less frequently the neurofibroma is highly cellular and consists of Schwann cells set in a uniform collagen matrix devoid of mucosubstances (Fig. 30–16). The cells may be arranged in short fascicles, whorls, or even a storiform pattern. In certain respects these cellular neurofibromas resemble Antoni A areas of a schwannoma. Unlike schwannoma, they are not encapsulated and lack a clear partition into two zones. Moreover, small neurites can usually be demonstrated throughout these tumors. Least commonly these tumors are highly myxoid and easily confused with myxomas; this form of neurofibroma usually occurs on the extremities. These hypocellular neoplasms contain pools of acid mucopolysaccharide with widely spaced Schwann cells. In contrast to the cells of myxoma, neurofibroma cells usually have a greater degree of orientation. The vascularity is also more prominent; and with careful searching features of specific differentiation (e.g., Wagner-Meissner bodies) may be found. Rare variations in neurofibromas are epithelioid change of the schwann cells (Fig. 30–19) and skeletal muscle.[58,62] We encountered one extraordinary case containing benign glands and a rare rosette. S-100 protein can be identified in these tumors but stains only a subset of cells in keeping with the observation that neurofibromas often contain a varied population of cells (Fig. 30–18).

Although solitary neurofibromas are not associated with the same incidence of malignant change as their inherited counterparts, the exact risk is unknown. It is probably extraordinarily small. Simple excision of these tumors is considered adequate therapy.

## NEUROFIBROMATOSIS

Neurofibromatosis, also named *von Recklinghausen's disease* for the man who described the disease in 1882, was formerly considered a single disease but is now known to be two clinically and genetically distinct diseases.[72,73,83,89,97,131] The more common disease, formerly known as the peripheral form of neurofibromatosis, is designated *neurofibromatosis 1*, whereas the less common disease, formerly known as the central form, is designated *neurofibromatosis 2 (bilateral acoustic neurofibromatosis)*.

A common genetic disease, NF1 affects 1 in every 2500 to 3000 live births,[65] and it accounts for one admission out of 3100 at the Mayo Clinic.[66] It is inherited as an autosomal dominant trait with a high rate of penetrance. Because only half of the patients with this disease have affected family members, the disease in the remaining patients represents new mutations. The mutation rate, estimated at $10^{-4}$ per gamete per generation, is among the highest for a dominantly inherited trait. About 80% of new mutations are of paternal origin.

NF1 is associated with deletions, insertions, or mutations in the NF1 gene, a tumor suppressor gene located in the pericentromeric region of chromosome

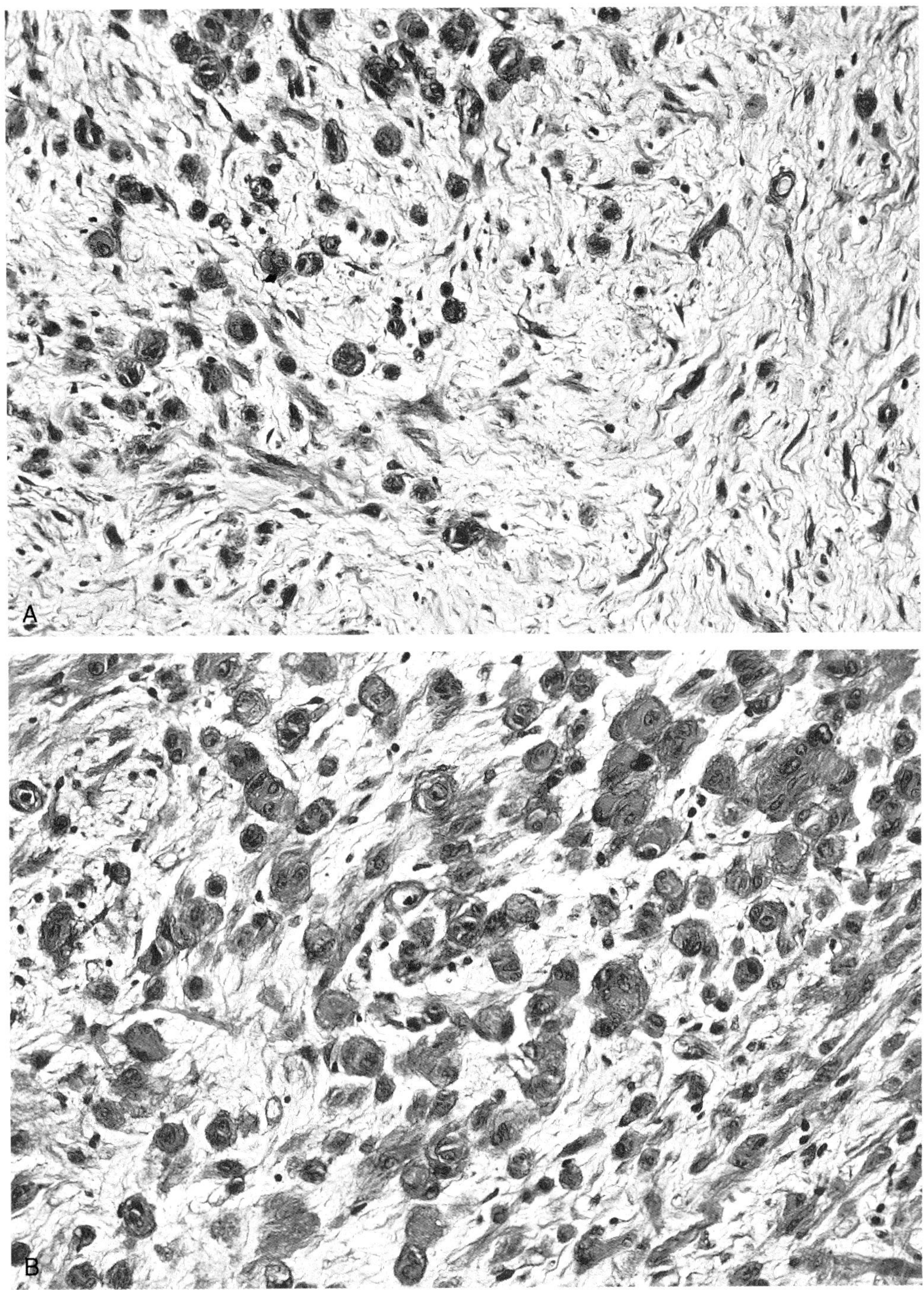


**FIGURE 30–19.** Epithelioid neurofibroma arising in a nerve in a patient with neurofibromatosis 1 (NF1) (**A**) shows transition between epithelioid areas and those with appearance of conventional neurofibroma. High power view of epithelioid areas (**B**).

17.[63] Spanning a distance of 300 kb and containing within it three additional genes, it is one of the largest human genes identified to date. It encodes a protein known as neurofibromin, which has been localized to various portions of the cells[99] including the microtubular system. It is ubiquitously distributed in all tissues. Although the function of neurofibromin is not fully defined, it is homologous to the family of GAP proteins (guanosine triphosphatose activating protein), which are believed to be important in the control of cell growth through their downregulation of the *ras* gene. Given the protean manifestations of this disease, which range from malignant tumors to developmental and cognitive defects, neurofibromin probably has a role far more encompassing than we currently understand.

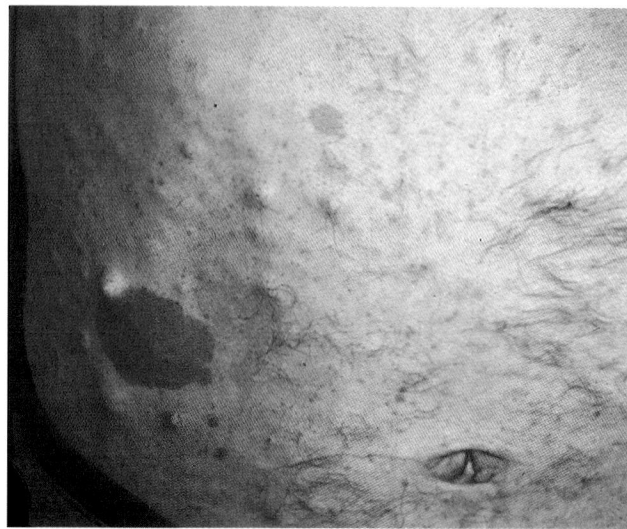

**FIGURE 30–20.** Café au lait spot. These pigmented lesions usually herald the onset of NF1. They are usually multiple, occur on unexposed surfaces, and typically are several centimeters in diameter.

## Clinical Findings

Clinically, there are a number of cardinal signs and symptoms of the disease, two or more of which must be present (Table 30–2) to establish the diagnosis. It should be emphasized that the severity of the disease varies widely from patient to patient and from family to family. To date it has not been possible to predict a clinical phenotype from the genetic mutation. That, coupled with the fact that there are more than 200 mutations for NF1 (none of which predominates), explains in large part why population-based screening for the gene is not done.

In the typical patient, NF1 becomes evident within the first few years of life when café au lait spots develop. These pigmented macular lesions resemble freckles, especially during the early stage when they are small. Typically they become much larger and darker with age and occur mainly on unexposed surfaces of the body (Fig. 30–20). One of the most characteristic locations for these spots is the axilla (axillary freckle sign). Pathologically, they are characterized by an increase in melanin pigment in the basal layer of the epidermis. The pigment may be present in the form of giant melanosomes (macromelanosomes), a feature that has been used as a means of histologically distinguishing them from other pigmented lesions[78] (e.g., freckle, lesions of Albright's disease). However, it has been emphasized that the giant granules are not invariably found[104]; their presence may be a function of the age of the lesion. In adults only lesions larger than 1.5 cm are considered café au lait spots for purposes of diagnosis.[69] Because the number of café au lait spots increases with age and more than 90% of patients with neurofibromatosis have these lesions, their number serves as a useful guideline when making the diagnosis. Not only do these lesions herald the onset of the disease, but in older patients they often give some indication as to the form and severity of the disease.[69] For instance, patients with few café au lait spots tend to have either (1) late onset of palpable neurofibromas, (2) localization of neurofibromas to one segment of the body, or (3) NF2.

Neurofibromas, the hallmark of the disease, make their appearance during childhood or adolescence after the café au lait spots. The time course varies greatly: Some tumors emerge at birth, and others appear during late adult life (Fig. 30–21). They may be found in virtually any location and in unusual instances may be restricted to one area of the body (segmental neurofibromatosis).[88] Unusual symptoms have been related to the presence of these tumors in

**TABLE 30–2** DIAGNOSTIC CRITERIA FOR NEUROFIBROMATOSIS 1

*Neurofibromatosis 1 is diagnosed in an individual with two or more of the following signs or factors.*

- Six or more café au lait macules: >5 mm in greatest diameter in prepubertal individuals; >15 mm in greatest diameter in postpubertal individuals
- Two or more neurofibromas of any type or one plexiform neurofibroma
- Freckling in the axillary or inguinal region
- Optic glioma
- Two or more Lisch nodules (iris hamartomas)
- A distinctive osseous lesion such as sphenoid dysplasia or thinning of long bone cortex with or without pseudoarthrosis
- First-degree relative (parent, sibling, offspring) with neurofibromatosis 1 by the above criteria

From National Institutes of Health.[90]

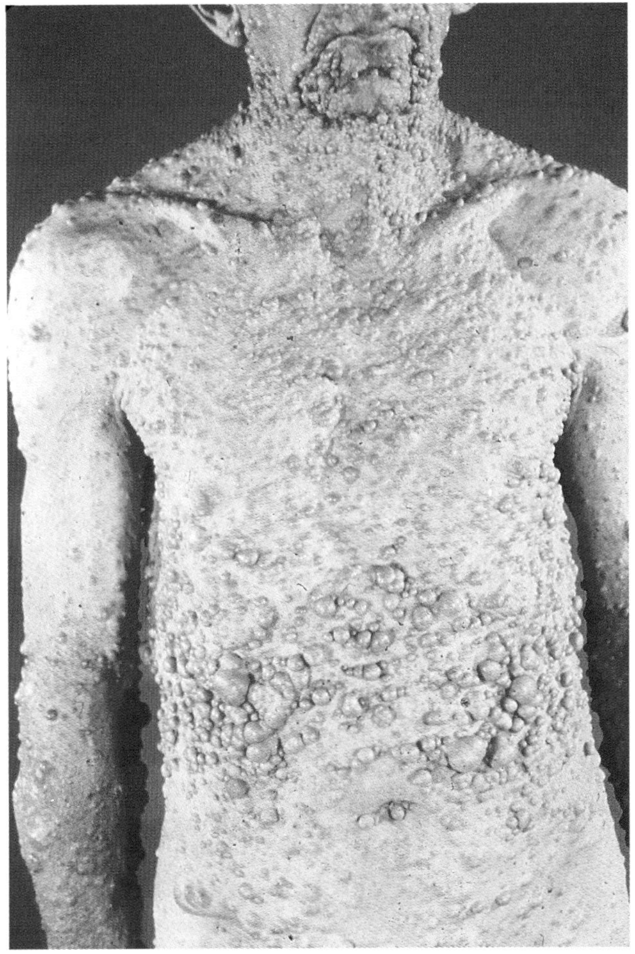

**FIGURE 30–21.** Male patient with neurofibromatosis of long duration.

various organs, including the gastrointestinal tract,[76] appendix,[87] larynx,[92] blood vessels,[73,101,102] and heart.[95] The tumors are usually slowly growing lesions. Acceleration of their growth rate has been noted during pregnancy and at puberty. Sudden increase in the size of one lesion should always raise the question of malignant change.

In addition to peripheral neurofibromas, patients with NF1 may also develop central nervous system tumors, including optic nerve glioma, astrocytoma, and a variety of heterotopias. Vestibular schwannoma, the hallmark of NF2, is virtually never encountered in NF1. Unusual "bright lesions" may be detected by T2-weighted magnetic resonance imaging (MRI) in the brain of up to 50% of children with NF1, although the precise nature and significance of these lesions is unknown.

Pigmented hamartomas of the iris (Lisch nodules)[98] may also be found. These asymptomatic lesions are not present in normal individuals or in those with NF2 (Figs. 30–22, 30–23). Although they cannot be correlated with other specific manifestations of NF1, they are helpful for establishing the diagnosis.

Skeletal abnormalities occur in almost 40% of patients with this disease.[66,69,109] They include erosive defects secondary to impingement by soft tissue tumors and primary defects, such as scalloping of the vertebra, congenital bowing of long bones with pseudoarthrosis, unilateral orbital malformations, and cystic osteolytic lesions. In the past the intraosseous cystic lesions were believed to be skeletal neurofibromas, but most of these lesions have a histologic appearance similar to that of a nonossifying fibroma or fibrous cortical defect. They are characterized by fascicles of fibroblasts arranged in short intersecting fascicles (sometimes in a storiform pattern) and punctuated with occasional giant cells.

Gynecomastia may develop in young men with neurofibromatosis. Histologically, it does not have the appearance of true gynecomastia and thus has been termed *pseudogynecomastia*. The breast stroma is hyalinized and contains small nerve fibers and fibroblasts, some of which are multinucleated. In addition to these well recognized signs and symptoms, the disease may also be associated with diverse symptoms not clearly referable to the presence of tumors. They include disorders of growth, sexual maturation and mentation,[69] and abnormalities of the lung.[85,100,107] Certain tumors, including schwannoma,[168] pheochro-

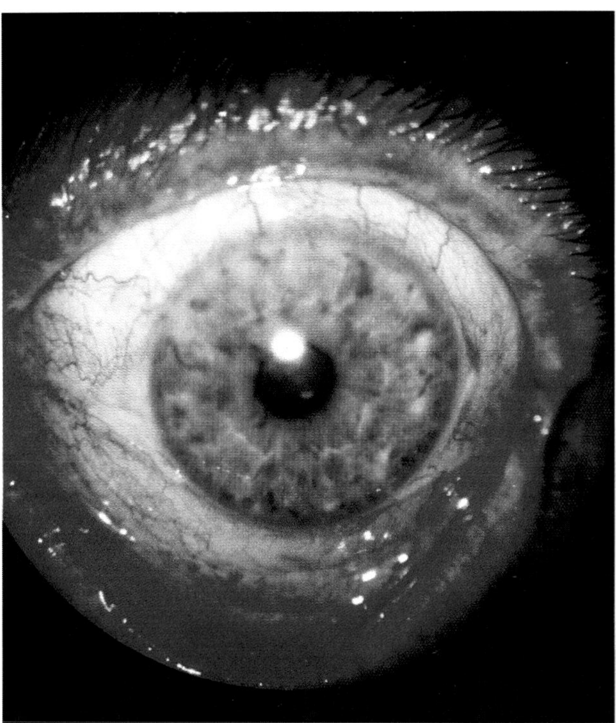

**FIGURE 30–22.** Lisch nodule in a patient with NF1. Pigmented areas are seen as brown areas in the iris.

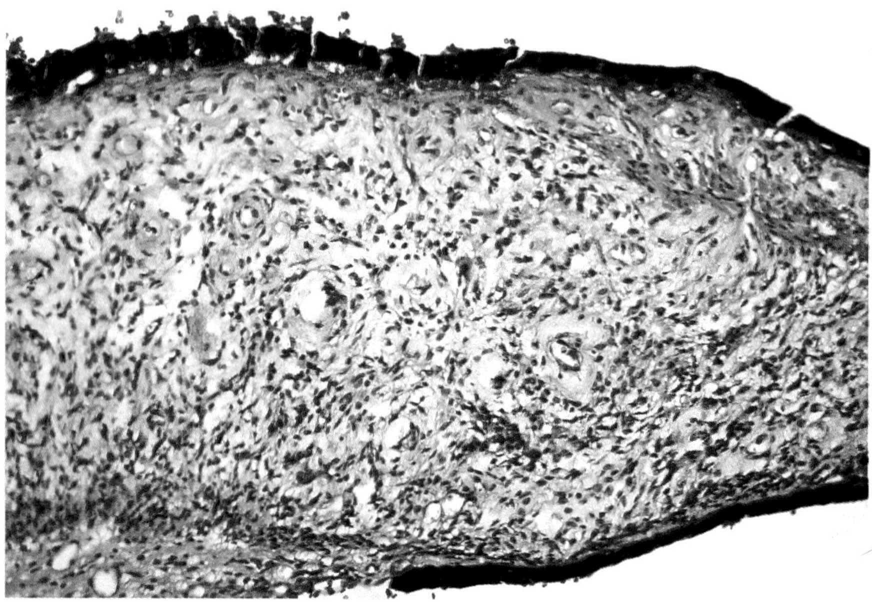

**FIGURE 30–23.** Lisch nodule showing collections of pigment in the iris.

mocytoma,[69] ganglioneuroma, nephroblastoma,[106] gastrointestinal stromal tumor, and leukemia,[71,86] have been reported with this disease.

## Variants of NF1

In addition to classic NF1, there appear to be variant forms in which the features are atypical or incomplete[67] (Table 30–3) They include (1) *segmental NF* manifesting as neurofibromas in a segmental distribution, possibly due to somatic mosaicism of NF1 mutations; (2) *gastrointestinal NF;* (3) *familial spinal NF;* and (4) *familial café au lait spots.*

**TABLE 30–3 NEUROFIBROMATOSIS AND VARIANTS**

"Classic" neurofibromatosis 1 (NF1)
Whole gene deletion phenotype NF1
Alternate forms of NF1 (incomplete/atypical features)
- Mixed NF
- Localized NF
  - Segmental NF
  - Gastrointestinal NF
  - Familial spinal NF
  - Familial café au lait spots
- Related forms of NF1 (conditions with additional features)
  - NF/Noonan syndrome
  - Watson syndrome

"Classic" neurofibromatosis 2 (bilateral vestibular schwannomas)
Schwannomatosis

Modified from Carey JC, Viskochil DH. Neurofibromatosis type 1: a model condition for the study of the molecular basis of variable expressivity in human disorders. Am J Med Genet 89:7, 1999.

## Pathological Findings

Several types of neurofibroma occur with this disease. They are distinguished on the basis of their gross and microscopic appearances.

### *Localized Neurofibroma*

Localized neurofibroma is the most common type encountered, but it is histologically the least characteristic because essentially identical lesions occur on a sporadic basis. These tumors are typically located in the dermis and subcutis but may be located in deep soft tissue as well. The tumors are larger than solitary neurofibromas. Large pendulous tumors of the skin are often alluded to as *fibroma molluscum.*

Histologically, these tumors are no different from solitary neurofibromas and embrace a spectrum from highly cellular to highly myxoid tumors. Malignant degeneration may occur but is more common in deeply situated lesions. The presence of mitotic activity is required to document malignant change because nuclear pleomorphism is seen in benign lesions.

### *Plexiform Neurofibroma*

Plexiform neurofibroma is virtually pathognomonic of this disease, provided the definition of a plexiform neurofibroma is stringent (Figs. 30–24 to 30–27). Plexiform neurofibromas essentially always develop during early childhood, often before the cutaneous neurofibromas have fully developed. Those plexiform neurofibromas involving an entire extremity give rise

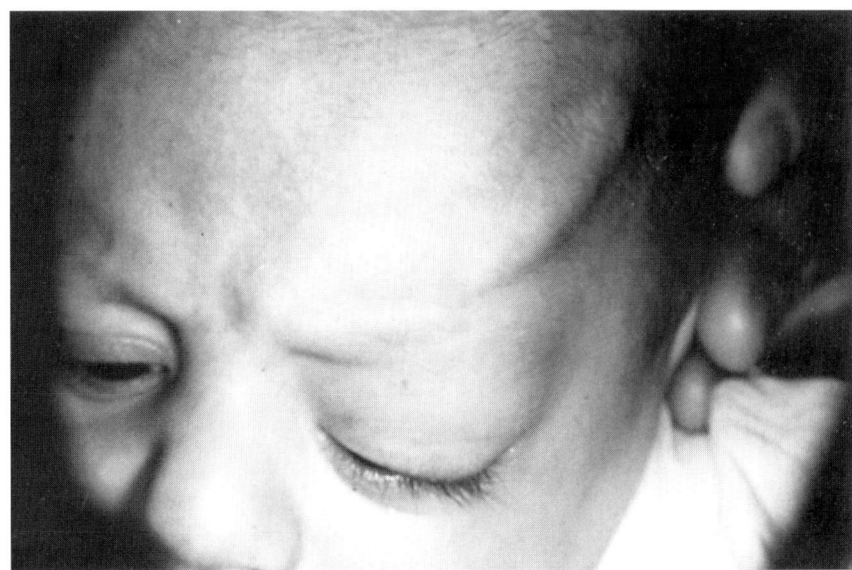

**FIGURE 30–24.** Plexiform neurofibroma in the subcutis of the scalp and involving the upper eyelid. Note the irregular, tortuous contour of the tumor. Lesions of this type are virtually pathognomonic of NF1.

to the condition known as *elephantiasis neuromatosa,* in which the extremity is enlarged (Fig. 30–28). The overlying skin is loose, redundant, and hyperpigmented, and the underlying bone may be hypertrophied, a phenomenon probably related to the increased vascular supply to the limb. Macroscopically,

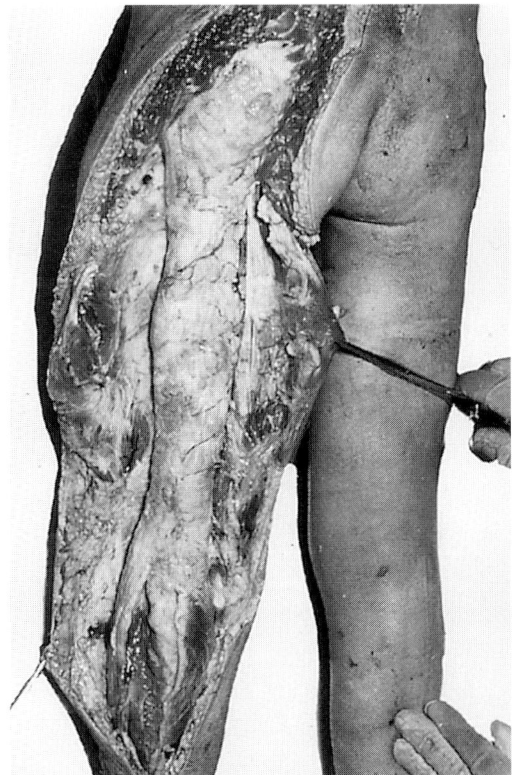

**FIGURE 30–25.** Plexiform neurofibroma of the lower extremity in a patient with NF1.

plexiform neurofibromas are large lesions that affect large segments of a nerve, distorting it and contorting it into a "bag of worms" (Fig. 30–26). Smaller lesions, which simply have a plexiform pattern when viewed microscopically rather than macroscopically, should not be interpreted as plexiform neurofibromas for purposes of establishing the diagnosis of NF1.

Microscopically, the lesion consists of a tortuous mass of expanded nerve branches, which are seen cut in various planes of section (Figs. 30–29 to 30–31). In the early stages the nerves may simply have an increase in the endoneurial matrix material, resulting in wide separation of the small nerve fascicles (Fig. 30–30). With continued growth the cells spill out of the nerves into soft tissue, creating a diffuse backdrop of neurofibromatous tissue (Fig. 30–31) such that NF1 lesions can have both plexiform and diffuse areas. Plexiform neurofibromas, like localized neurofibromas, may display nuclear atypia. Because these lesions are at greatest risk to undergo malignant transformation, care should be paid to lesions displaying

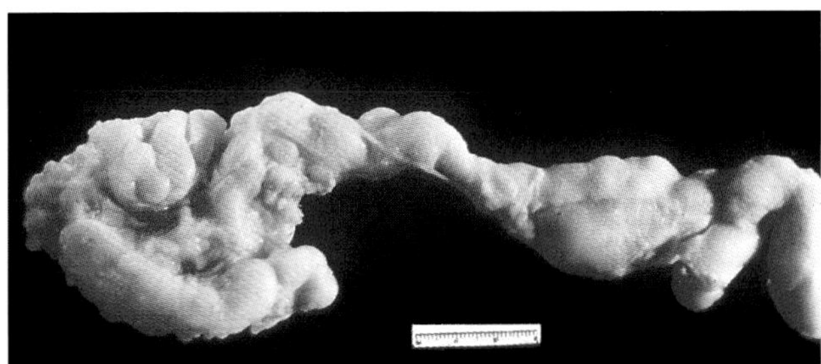

**FIGURE 30–26.** Gross appearance of a plexiform neurofibroma. The nerve is converted to a thick convoluted mass, which has been likened to a "bag of worms."

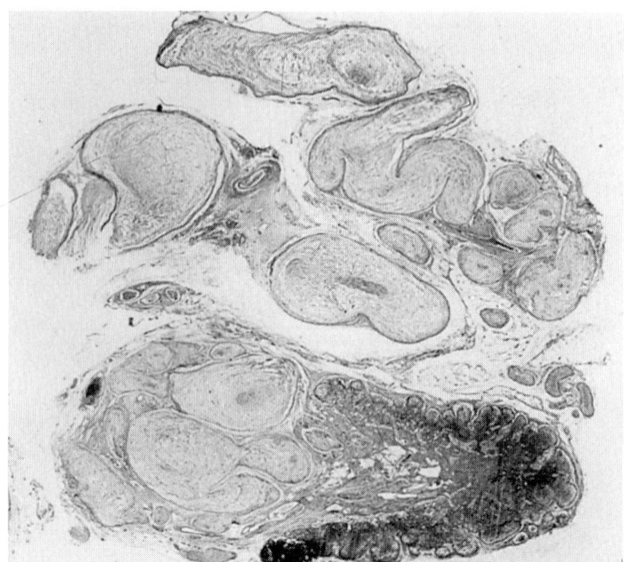

**FIGURE 30–27.** Plexiform neurofibroma involving nerve and extending into the hilum of a lymph node. Apparent lymph node involvement does not indicate malignancy but simply reflects the diffuseness of the process. (×5)

heightened cellularity and atypia. The sequence of histologic changes and the inherent problems are discussed later.

Electron microscopy of these lesions has documented the participation of several cell types.[68,82,174] The predominant cell is the Schwann cell, which is surrounded by basal lamina (Fig. 30–32). These cells may invest small axons, spiral around themselves, or lie singly in the matrix. A significant number of fibroblasts are also present, which are distinguished from Schwann cells by their prominent endoplasmic reticulum and their lack of basal lamina. It has been suggested that these lesions are really hamartomas because of the polymorphic population of cells. Although the early lesions have many of the features of a hyperplastic process, the advanced lesions manifest a capacity of autonomous growth and malignant transformation, characteristics of a true neoplasm.

### *Diffuse Neurofibroma*

Diffuse neurofibroma is an uncommon but distinctive form that occurs principally in children and young adults. Some have termed these lesions *paraneurofibroma*[5] to indicate the extension of the tumor beyond the confines of the perineurium. It is not yet clear how often this tumor is associated with neurofibromatosis. In our consultation experience, about 10% of patients with this lesion also have neurofibromatosis.

Clinically, this tumor is most common in the head and neck region and presents as a plaque-like elevation of the skin. On cut section, the entire subcutis between superficial fascia and dermis is thickened by firm, grayish tissue (Fig. 30–33). As its name implies, this form of neurofibroma is ill-defined and spreads extensively along connective tissue septa and between fat cells. Despite its infiltrative growth, it does not destroy but, rather, envelops the normal structures it encompasses in much the same fashion as dermatofibrosarcoma protuberans (Fig. 30–34). It differs from the conventional neurofibroma in that it has a uniform matrix of fine fibrillary collagen. The Schwann cells, which lie suspended in the matrix, are usually less elongated than those of conventional neurofibromas and have short fusiform or even round contours (Figs. 30–35, 30–36). The tumor contains clusters of Meissner body-like structures, a characteristic feature of this lesion that serves to distinguish it from the superficial aspect of dermatofibrosarcoma protuberans

*Text continued on page 1137*

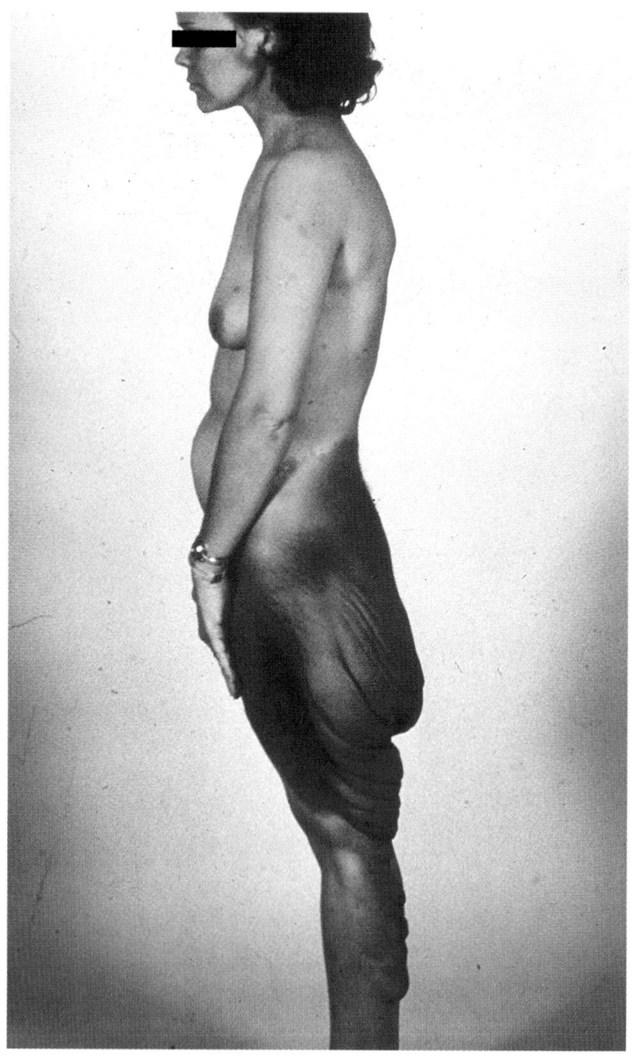

**FIGURE 30–28.** Patient with NF1 and a large neurofibroma of leg resulting in elephantiasis neuromatosa.

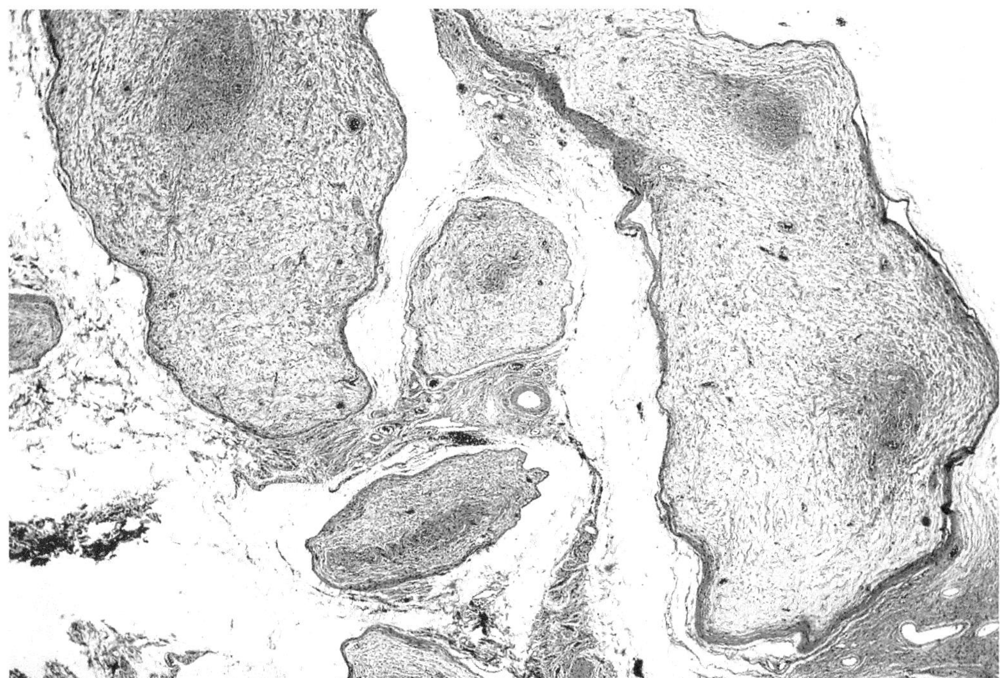

**FIGURE 30–29.** Plexiform neurofibroma with tortuous enlargement of the nerves.

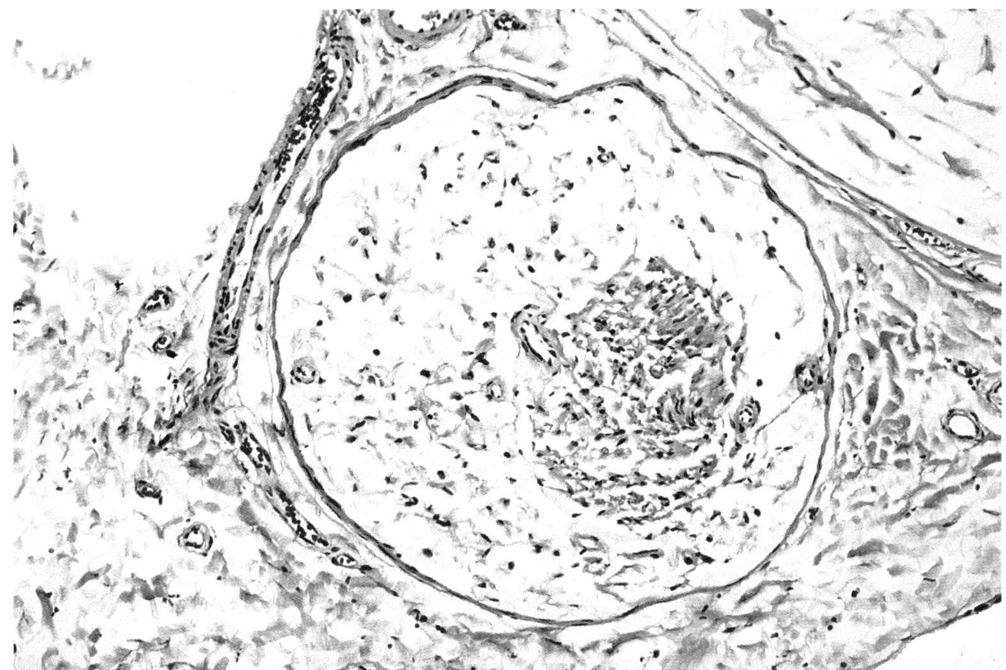

**FIGURE 30–30.** Plexiform neurofibroma with expansion of the endoneurium by myxoid ground substance.

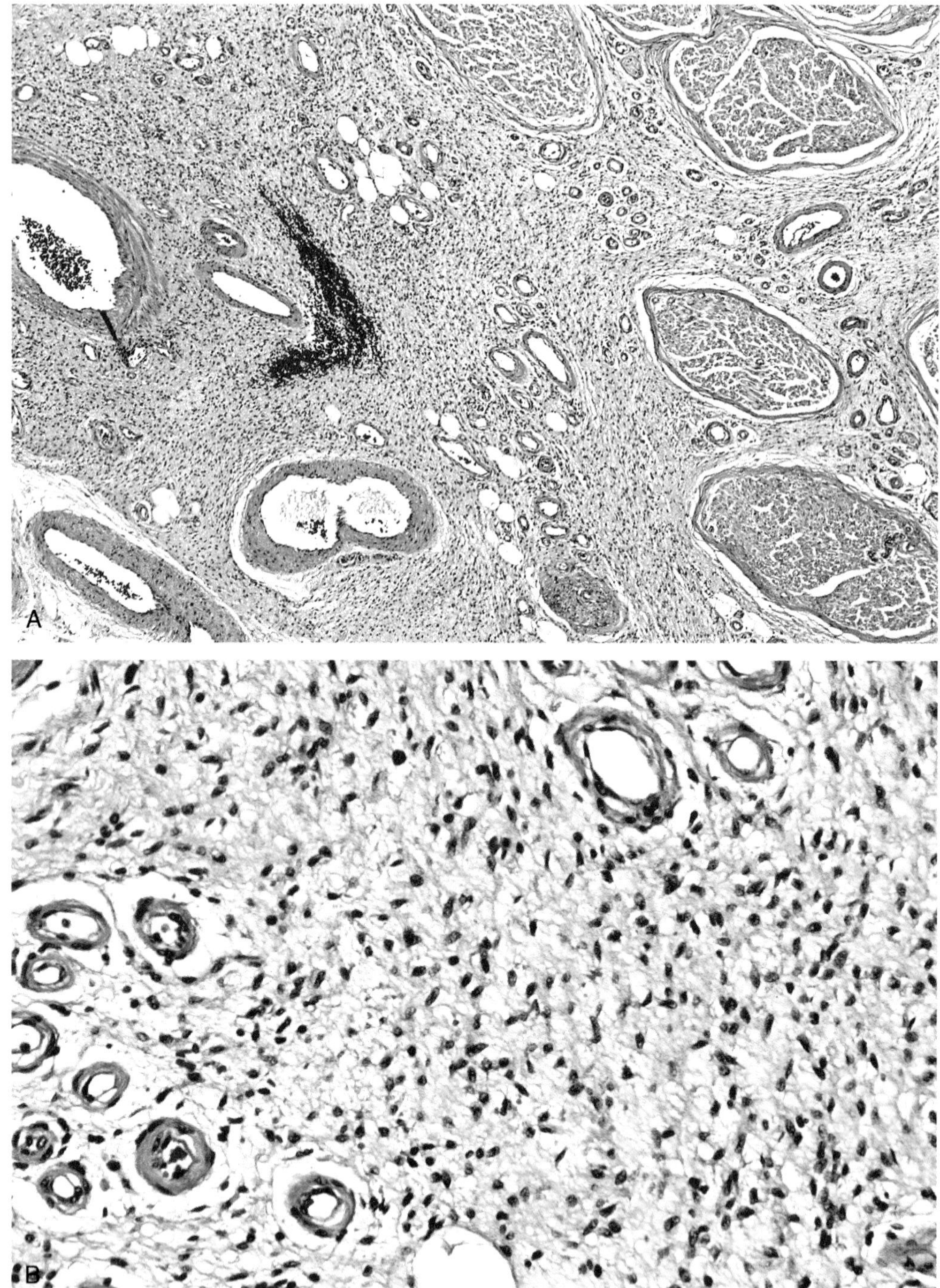

**FIGURE 30–31.** (**A, B**) Portion of a plexiform neurofibroma illustrating the lesion spilling out into soft tissue. These areas may resemble areas of diffuse neurofibroma.

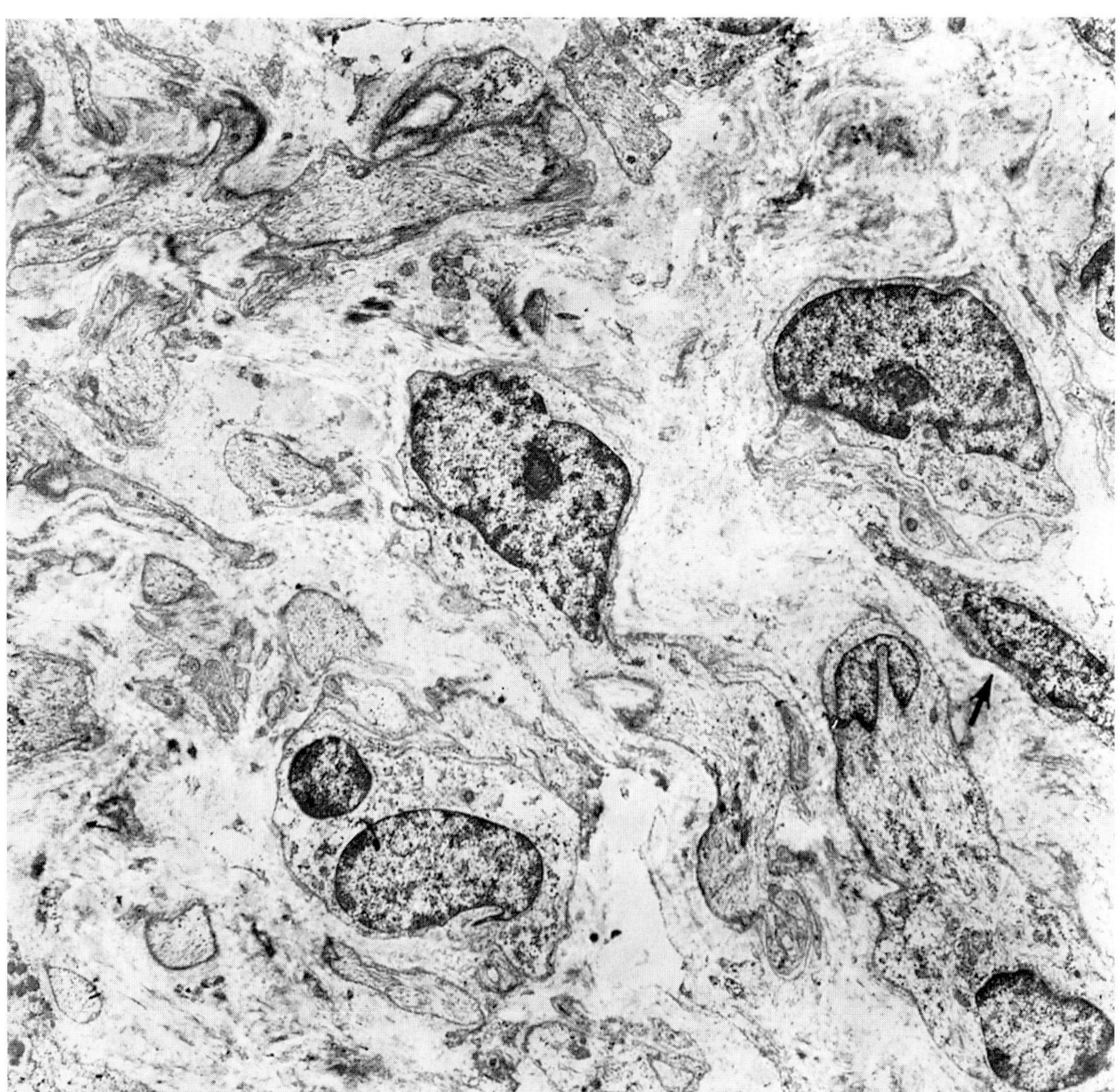

**FIGURE 30–32.** Electron micrograph of a neurofibroma with predominantly Schwann cells and occasional fibroblasts (arrow). (×5775)

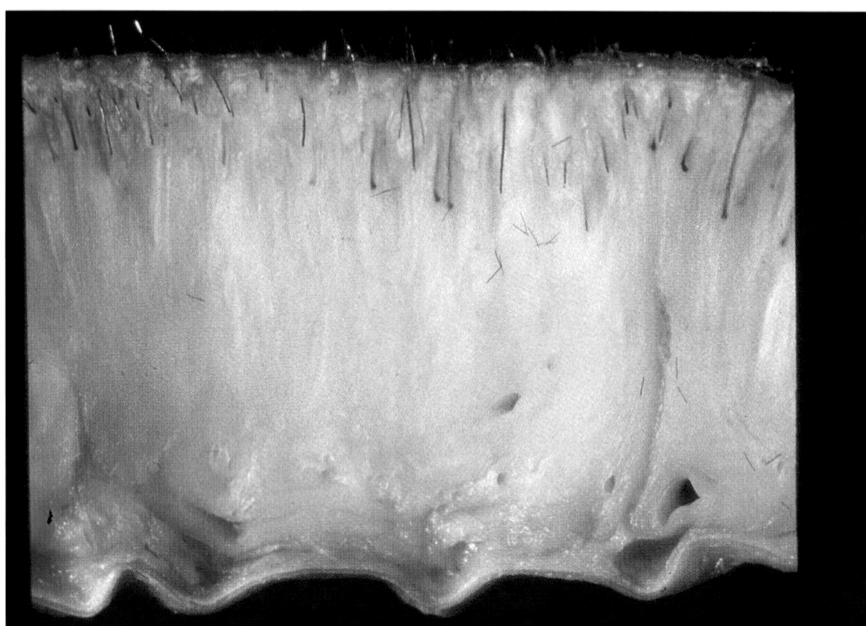

**FIGURE 30–33.** Diffuse neurofibroma presenting as an ill-defined expansion of the subcutaneous region of the scalp.

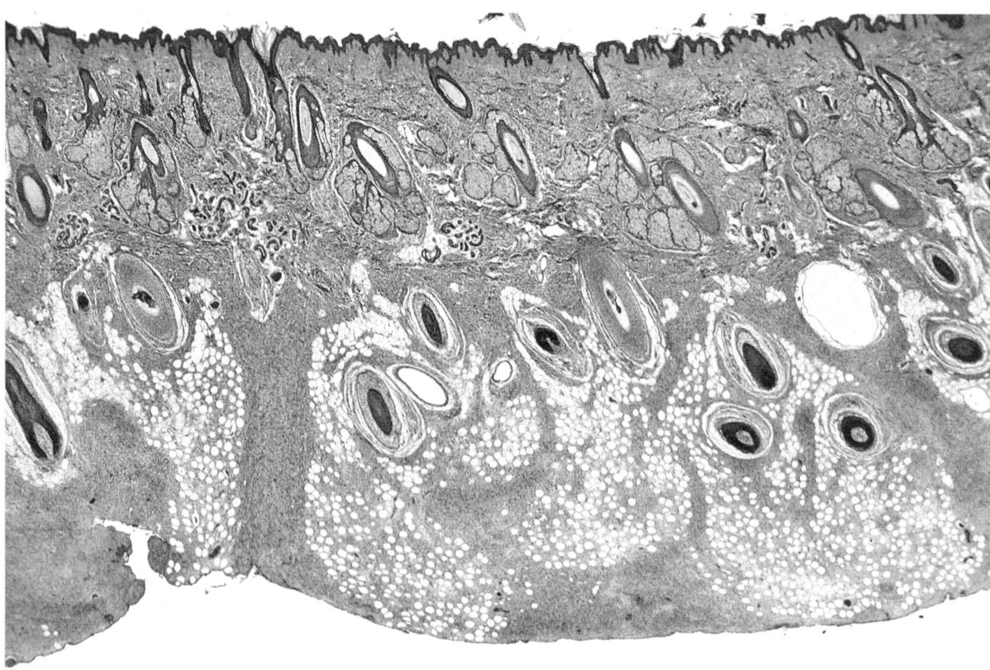

**FIGURE 30–34.** Diffuse neurofibroma with extensive permeation of subcutaneous tissue similar to a dermatofibrosarcoma protuberans.

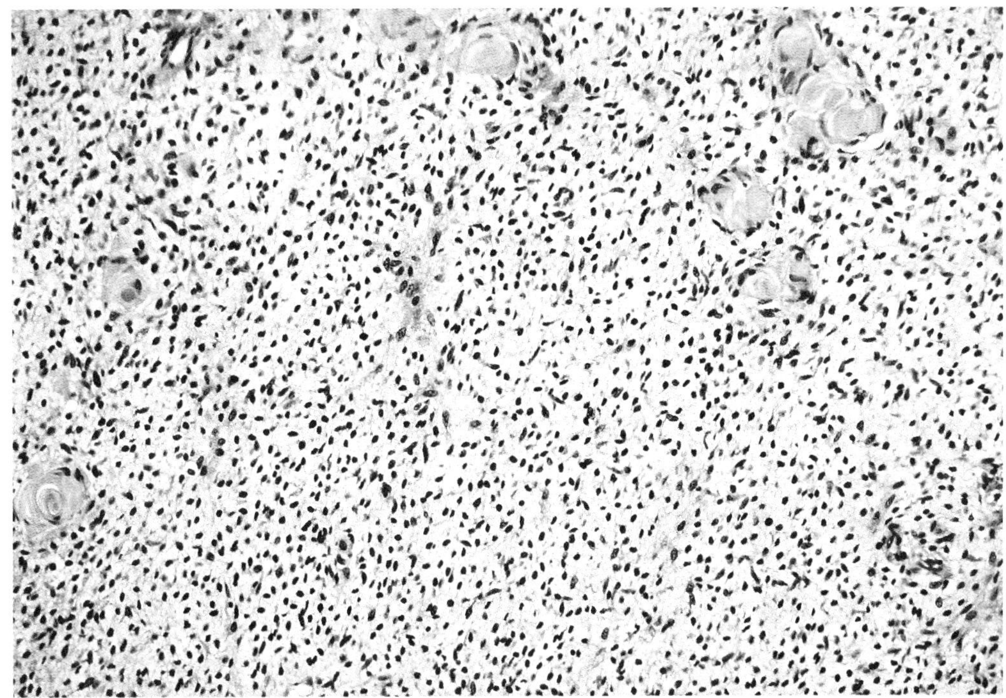

**FIGURE 30–35.** Diffuse neurofibroma showing the fine fibrillary collagenous background punctuated with Wagner-Meissner bodies.

(Fig. 30–37). Some diffuse neurofibromas consist of a rather complex arrangement of several mesenchymal elements in addition to the neurofibromatous tissue (Fig. 30–38). These tumors, which seem to be more common in neurofibromatosis, consist of neurofibromatous tissue admixed with mature fat or large ectatic vessels. The latter structures at times are so striking they eclipse the neural component and can result in the erroneous impression of exuberant granulation tissue. Rarely, nuclear palisading is present in diffuse neurofibromas.

### Pigmented Neurofibroma

Neurofibromas containing melanin-bearing pigmented cells are rare,[113] comprising fewer than 1% of all neurofibromas referred to the Armed Forces Institute of Pathology (AFIP) in consultation.[64,70] Most occur in patients with NF1 and are of the diffuse type, although some have features of both diffuse and plexiform types (Fig. 30–39). The pigment is not usually appreciated on gross examination and requires histologic examination. The pigmented cells, which are dendritic or epithelioid in shape, are dispersed throughout the tumors but have a tendency to cluster and localize toward the superficial portions of the lesion (Fig. 30–40). They express both S-100 protein and melanin markers in contrast to the surrounding nonpigmented cells, which express S-100 protein only. Because of the diffuse pattern of growth these lesions may recur, but metastasis has not been recorded.

These lesions should be distinguished from pigmented forms of dermatofibrosarcoma protuberans (Bednar tumor), a tumor that in the past was sometimes referred to as a "storiform pigmented neurofibroma." The uniform fibroblastic cells, repetitive storiform pattern, and lack of S-100 protein immunoreactivity usually make this distinction apparent. The distinction between congenital pigmented nevi with neuroid features and pigmented neurofibroma is less clear-cut. The lack of a junctional or superficial nevoid component supports the diagnosis of a pigmented neurofibroma over that of a congenital neuroid nevus.

## Malignant Change in Neurofibromas

In a small percentage of NF1 patients a malignant peripheral nerve sheath tumor (MPNST) emerges from a preexisting neurofibroma, usually a deep-seated plexiform lesion (Figs. 30–41, 30–42). Although the genetic events underlying this transformation are not completely understood, it appears that inactivation of the *CDKN2A* (also known as *INK4A*) gene, which encodes two proteins (p16 and p19) important for cell cycle regulation, is a significant event.[80,81,91] By immunohistochemistry p16 can be demonstrated in neurofibromas but is lacking in

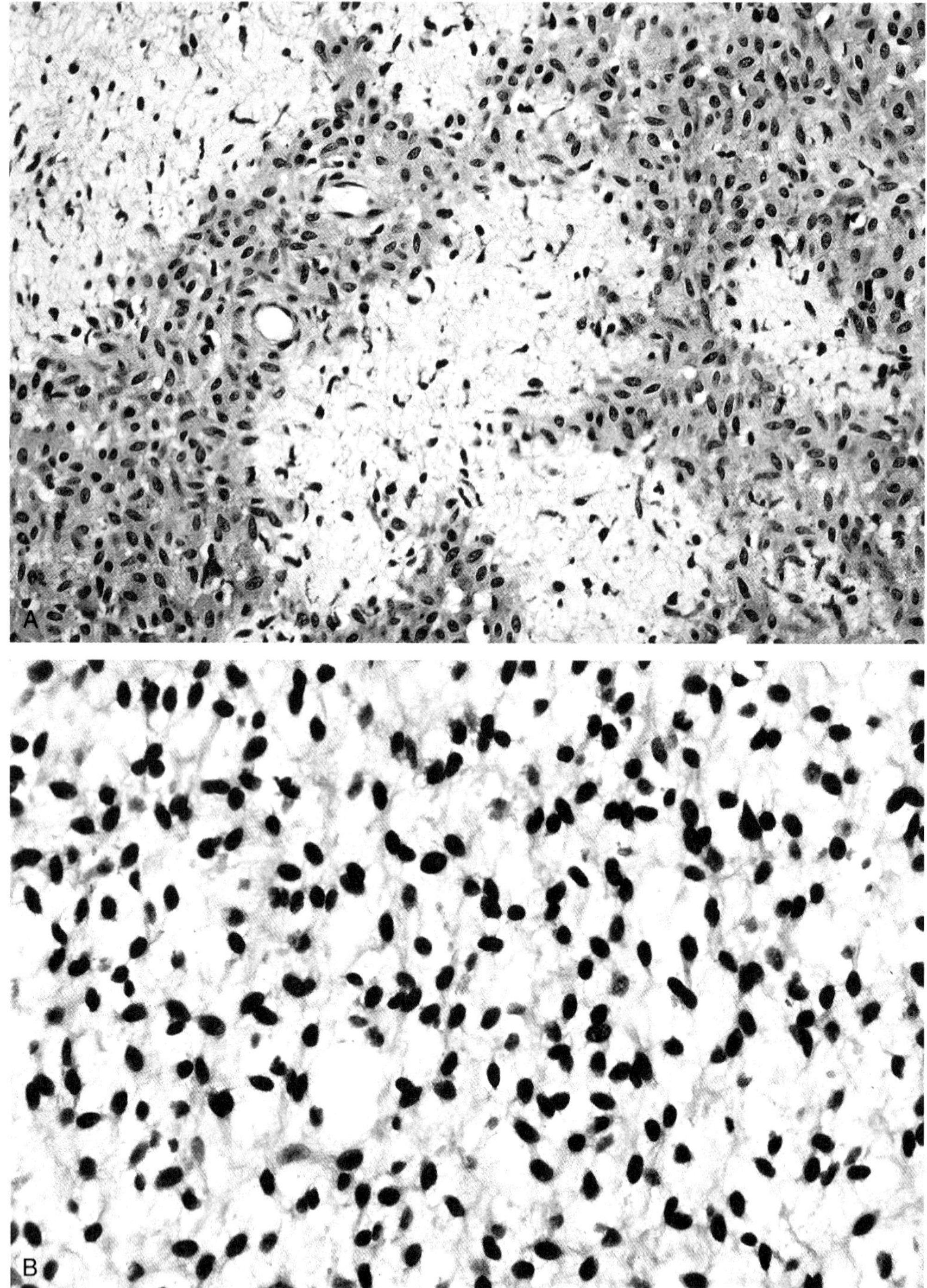

**FIGURE 30–36.** Diffuse neurofibroma with characteristic short fusiform or rounded Schwann cells. Shown at medium (**A**) and high power (**B**).

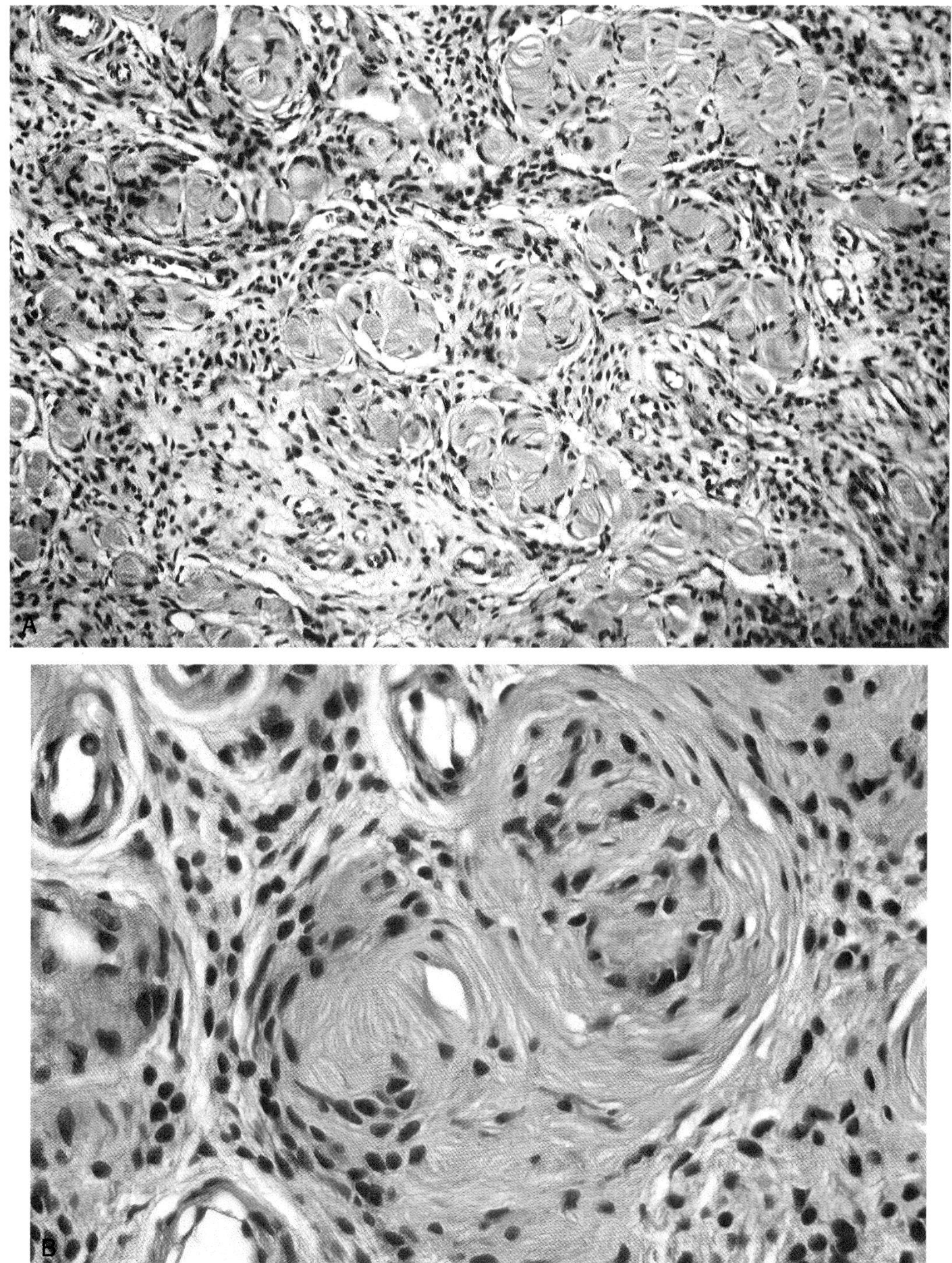

**FIGURE 30–37.** Wagner-Meissner bodies in a diffuse neurofibroma at medium (**A**) and high (**B**) power.

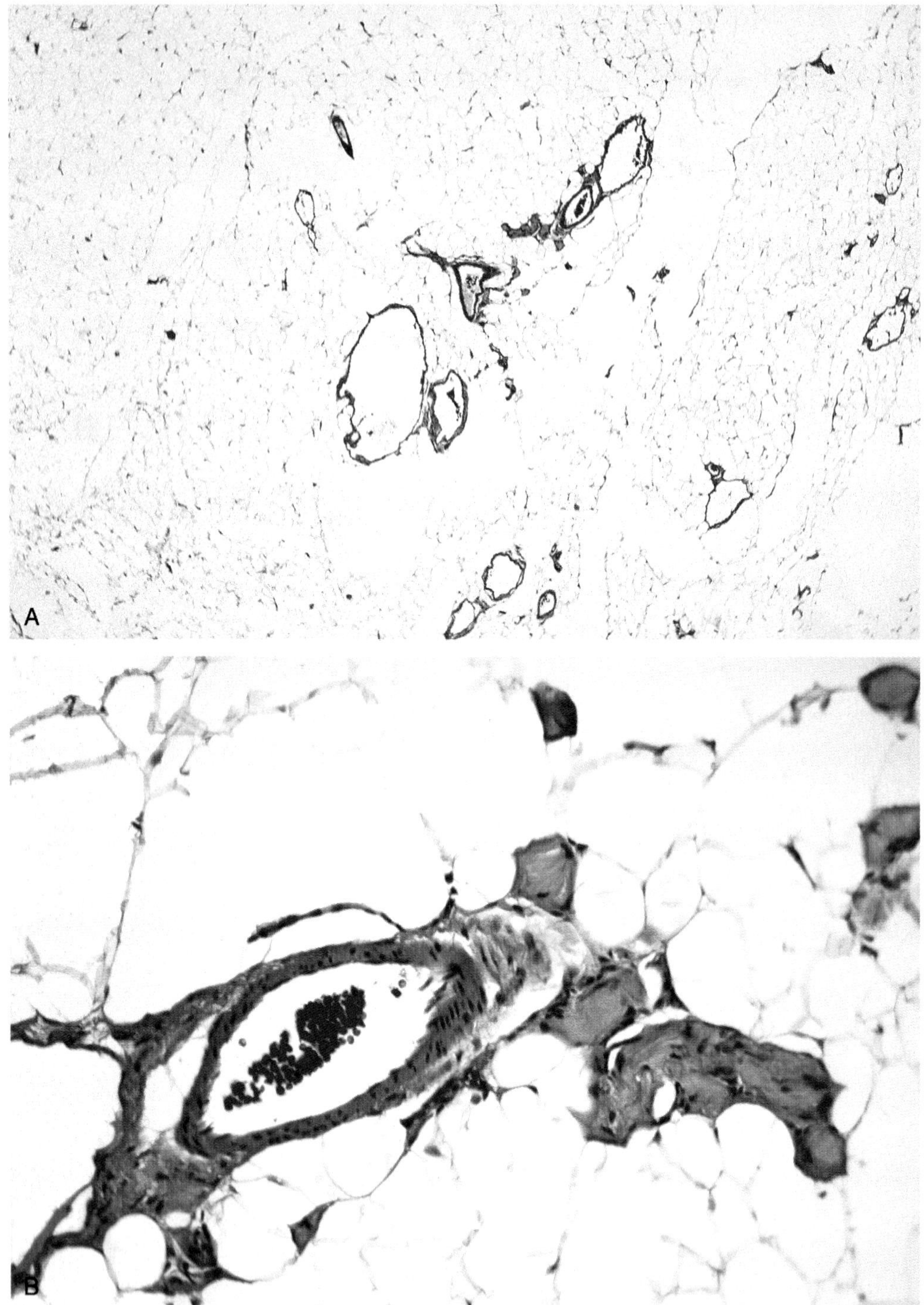

**FIGURE 30–38.** (**A**) Diffuse neurofibroma with extensive fatty overgrowth. (**B**) Wagner-Meissner bodies in the fat identify the neural nature of the lesion.

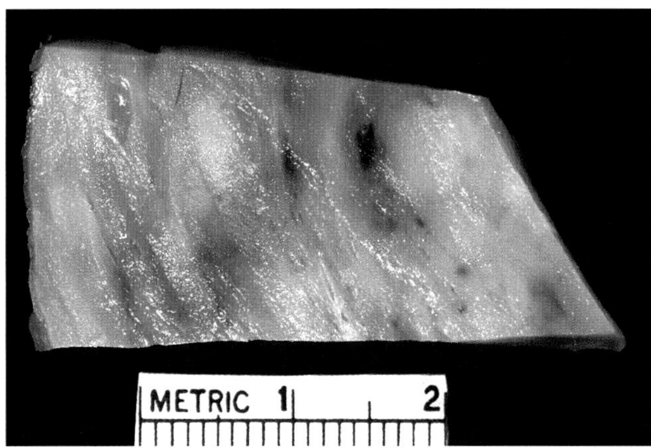


**FIGURE 30–39.** Pigmented neurofibroma developing in a neurofibroma of the diffuse type.

MPNSTs. Although immunostaining for one or more protein markers such as p16 may prove to have diagnostic utility, the distinction between neurofibromas and low grade MPNSTs is still made by light microscopy.

The histologic demarcation between a neurofibroma with atypical histologic features and a low grade MPNST is difficult because, in effect, these lesions represent a histologic continuum (Figs. 30–43 to 30–46). Furthermore, in neurofibromas that have undergone malignant transformation, it is commonplace to have neurofibroma with a range of atypical features adjacent to areas of frank MPNST. To date there has been no large study correlating the number and degree of atypical features in neurofibromas with either outcome or with molecular alterations. A small study with short-term follow-up by Lin et al.[84] suggested that cellularity, atypia, and low levels of mitotic activity were still associated with good outcome. We agree with others[7] that the mere presence of mitotic figures in an otherwise innocuous neurofibroma is not sufficient for a diagnosis of malignancy, but it should be pointed out that mitotic activity and cellularity seem to co-vary; it is unusual to encounter a mitotically activity neurofibroma without some increase in cellularity. The following paragraphs represent our general approach to this problem, and Table 30–4 details the criteria and terms we and others employ.[7] In the final analysis, although labels are convenient, borderline neurofibromatous lesions require careful sampling, dialogue with the clinician, and potentially complete removal depending on the clinical setting.

*Neurofibroma* is the term we use for conventional neurofibromas and those with nuclear atypia only (Fig. 30–43). The latter, as an isolated focal or diffuse change, is common in neurofibromas and does not correlate with malignancy. Although some use the term "atypical neurofibroma" for such lesions, we prefer not to use a term that could be miscontrued as reflecting concern about malignancy.

*Neurofibroma with atypical features* is the term we use for neurofibromas that have any combination of atypical features that fall short of the minimum criteria

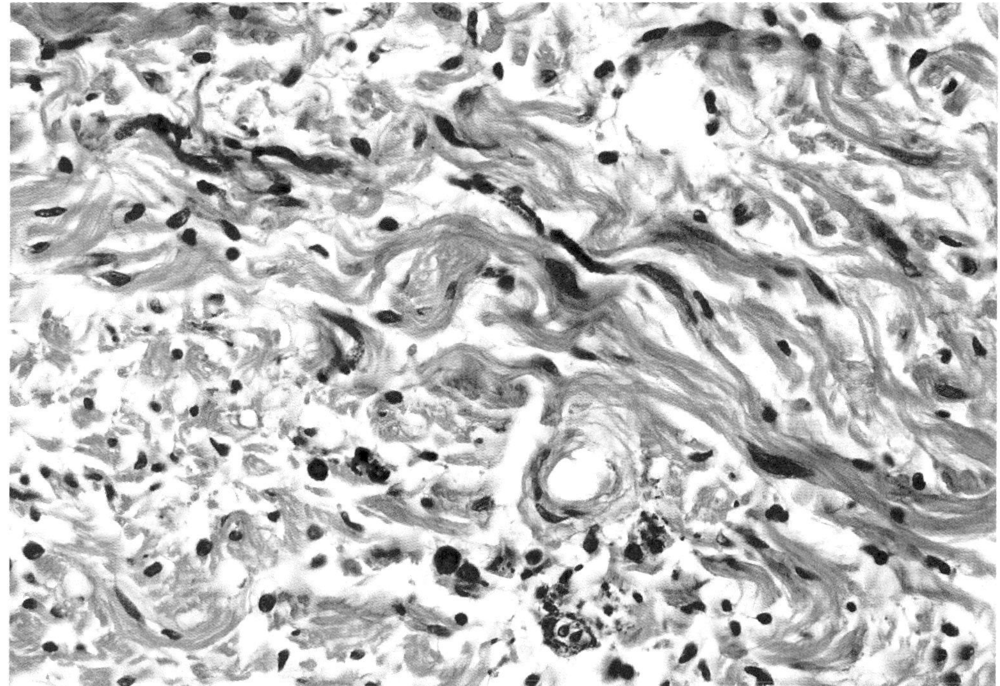

**FIGURE 30–40.** Pigmented neurofibroma. Melanin pigment is present in irregularly shaped Schwann cells.

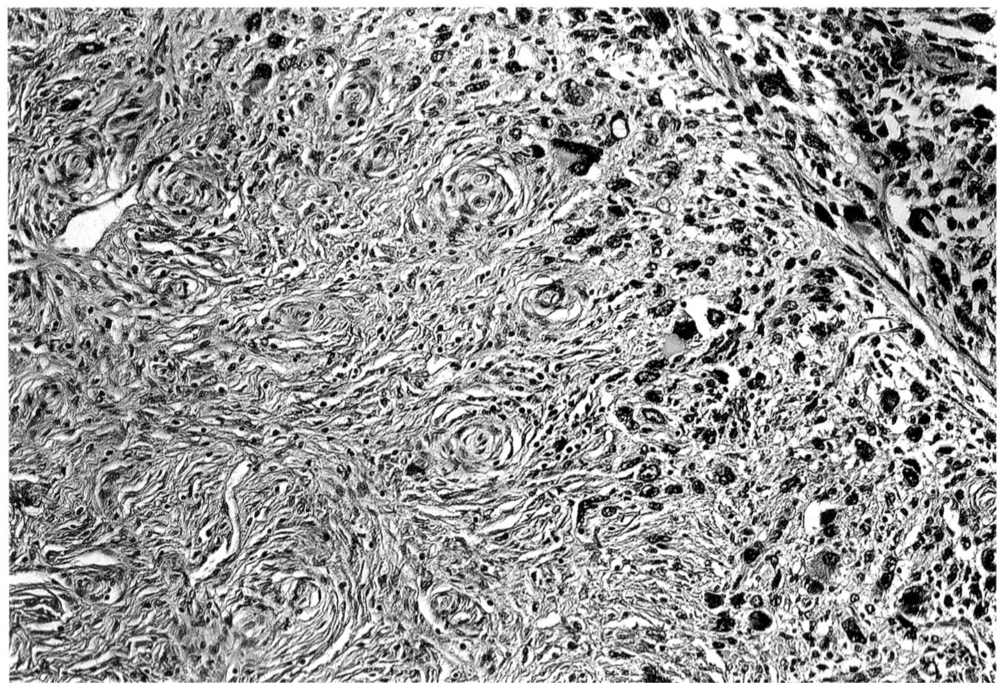

**FIGURE 30–41.** Neurofibroma with malignant transformation (right).

for a diagnosis of low grade MPNST (Fig. 30–44). This category excludes lesions characterized by nuclear atypia only.

*Low grade MPNST arising in neurofibroma* is the term used when there is generalized nuclear atypia, increased cellularity, and usually low levels of mitotic activity (Figs. 30–45, 30–46). Nuclear atypia consists of nuclear enlargement and hyperchromatism. Some suggest that nuclear enlargement should be at least three times the size of a normal schwann cell nucleus.[7] If mitotic activity is not present, we diagnosis a low grade MPNST if the cellularity is marked (consisting of nearly back-to-back cells forming sheets or fascicles).

## Discussion

Unlike solitary neurofibromas, those encountered in neurofibromatosis may cause significant morbidity. The large number of lesions usually makes surgical therapy impossible. Therefore surgery has traditionally been reserved for lesions that are large, painful, or located in strategic areas where continued expansion would compromise organ function. Even after

**TABLE 30–4** NEUROFIBROMAS WITH ATYPICAL AND MALIGNANT FEATURES

| Features | | | Diagnostic Terms | |
|---|---|---|---|---|
| ***Nuclear Atypia**** | ***Cellularity*** | ***Mitoses*** | ***Scheithauer et al.*** | ***Weiss-Goldblum*** |
| Usually focal; occasionally diffuse | — | — | Atypical neurofibroma | Neurofibroma |
| Absent | + | Absent | Cellular neurofibroma | Neurofibroma |
| Absent | + | + | Cellular neurofibroma | Neurofibroma with atypical features |
| Diffuse | + | — | Low grade MPNST | Low grade MPNST if cellularity is extreme with back-to-back cells or fascicles; otherwise neurofibroma with atypia features |
| Diffuse | + | + | Low grade MPNST | Low grade MPNST |

MPNST, malignant peripheral nerve sheath tumor.

* Nuclear atypia is nuclear enlargement and hyperchromatism. Scheithauer et al. used nuclear enlargement of at least three times the normal Schwann cell for a diagnosis of malignancy.

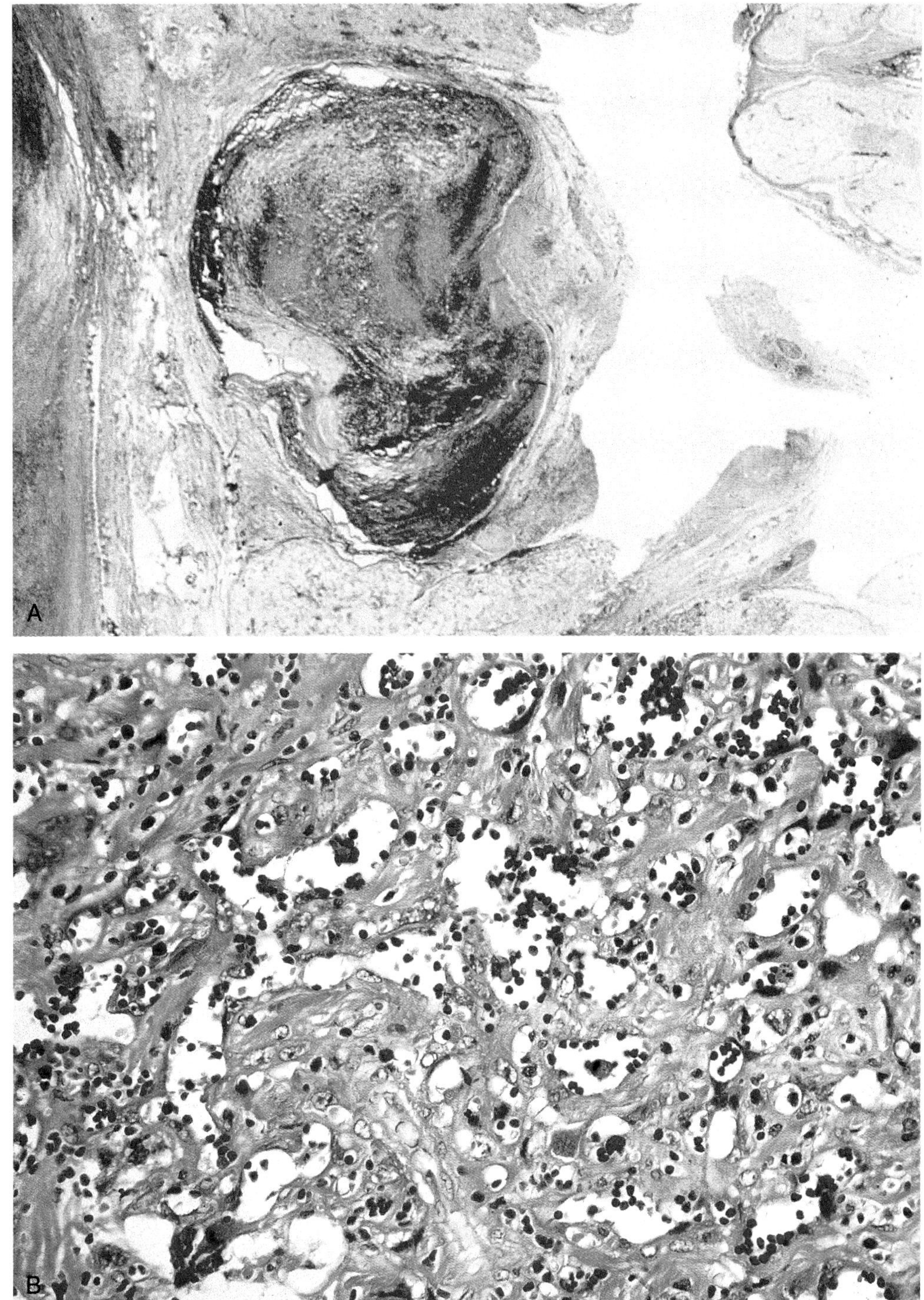


**FIGURE 30–42.** (**A**) Plexiform neurofibroma with an area of angiosarcoma (hemorrhagic zone). The tumor was an epithelioid angiosarcoma. (**B**) This pattern of malignant transformation is rare and is discussed in Chapter 32.

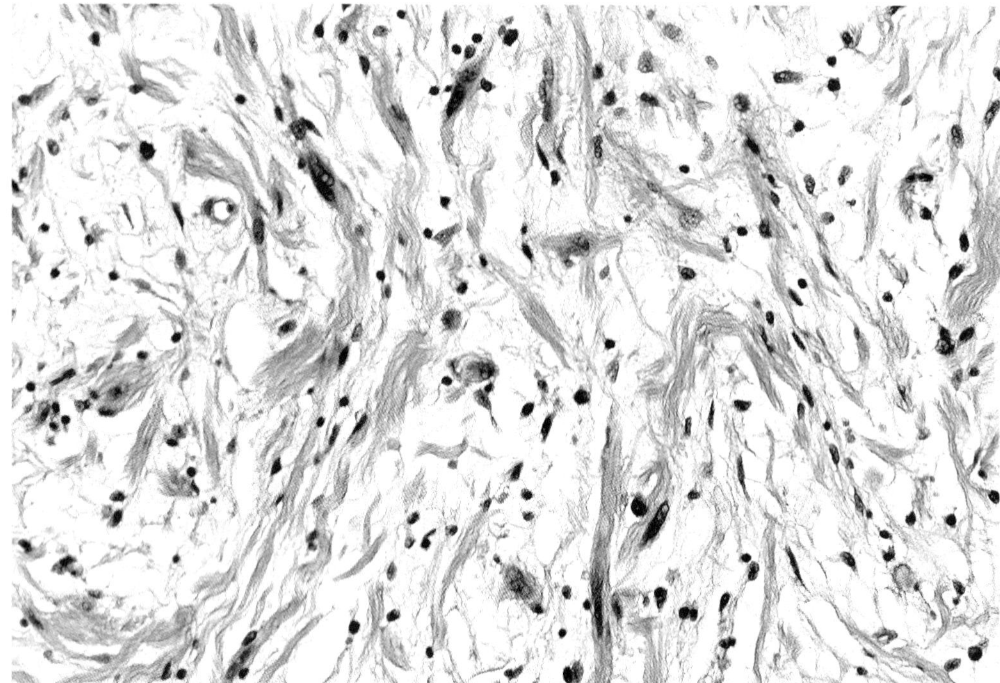

**FIGURE 30–43.** Neurofibroma with nuclear atypia of occasional cells without increased cellularity or mitotic activity.

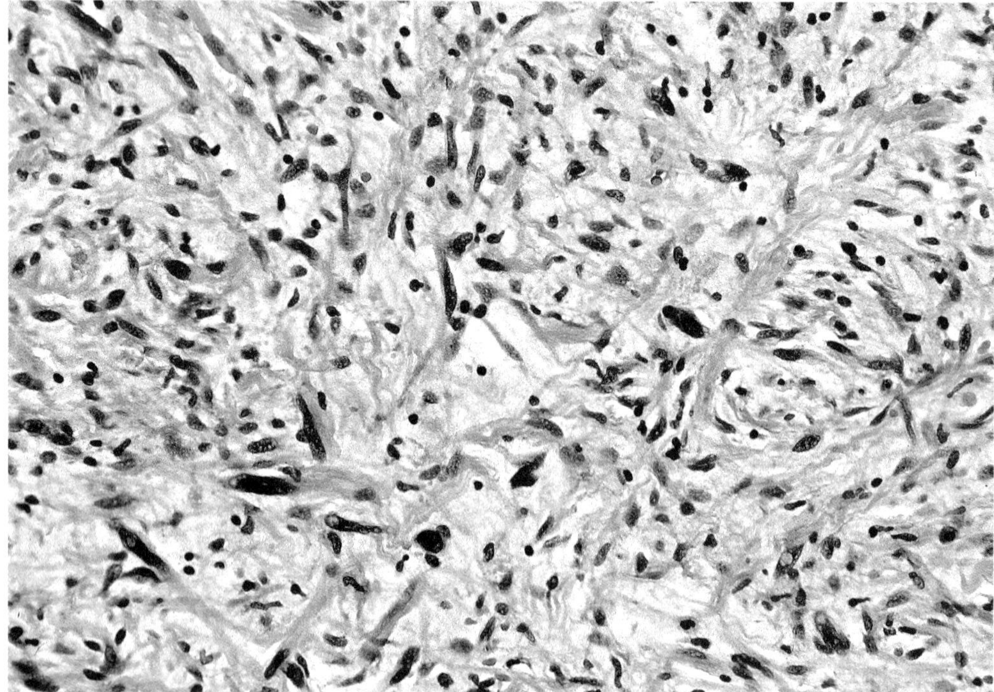

**FIGURE 30–44.** Neurofibroma with moderate cellularity and nuclear atypia. We use the designation neurofibroma with atypical features for changes of this type. This change was adjacent to areas of frank sarcoma.

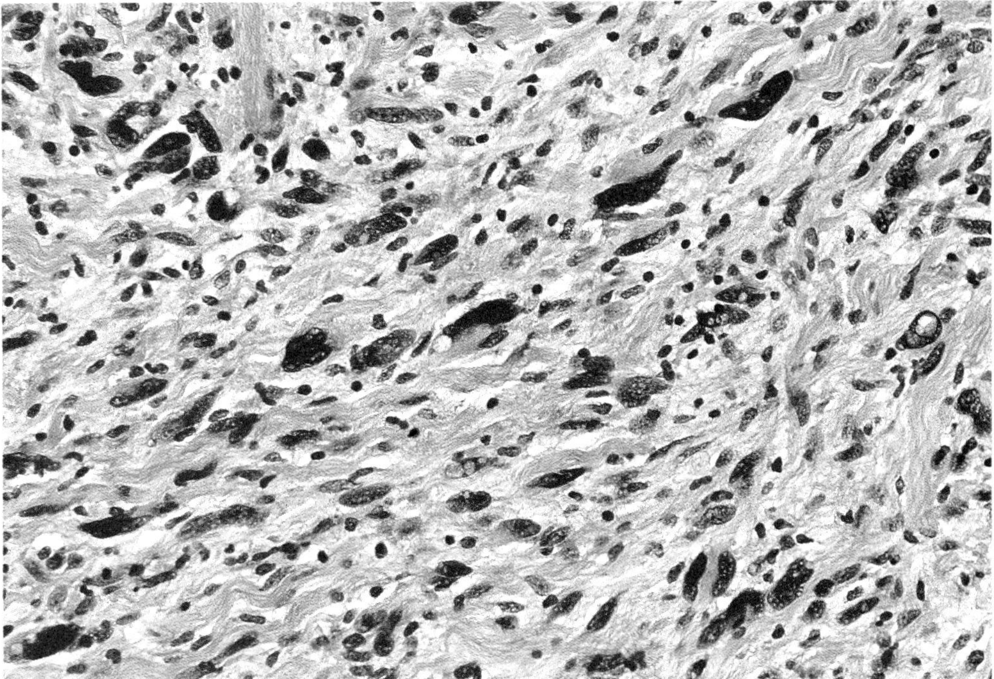

**FIGURE 30–45.** Low grade malignant peripheral nerve sheath tumor arising in a neurofibroma. This "neurofibromatous" lesion is characterized by marked cellularity such that cells are nearly back-to-back. The nuclear atypia is marked and generalized.

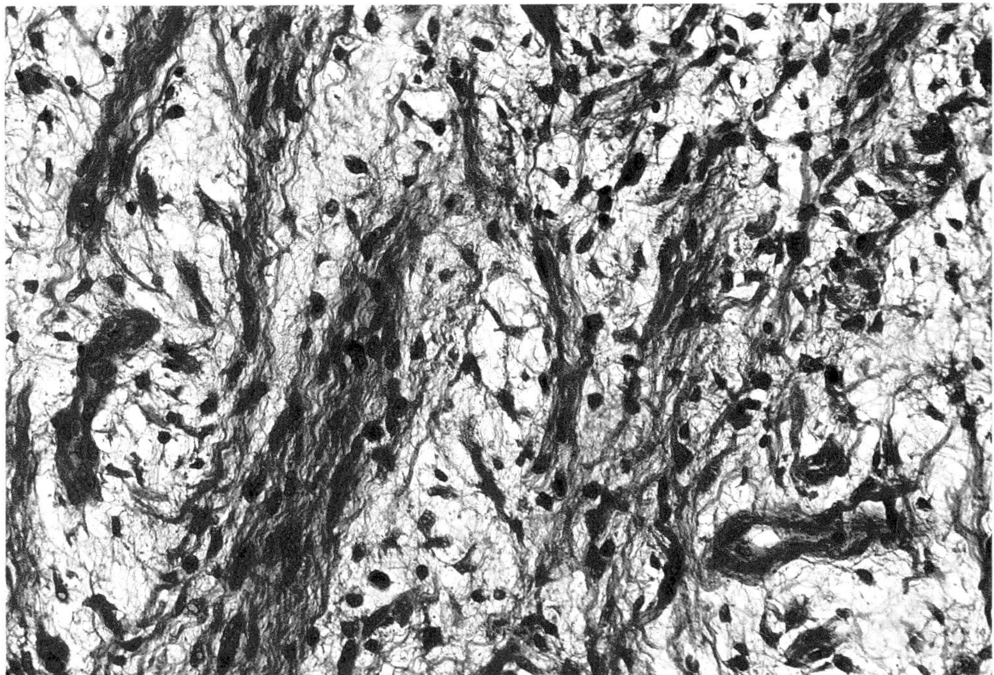

**FIGURE 30–46.** Low grade malignant peripheral nerve sheath tumor arising in a neurofibroma. There is generalized marked atypia and increased cellularity such that the cells appear arranged in small fascicles. Low levels of mitotic activity were identified in the lesion.

attempted complete excision of these lesions, clinical recurrences occasionally develop, a phenomenon related to the ill-defined nature of the tumors.

A problem of more importance is that of malignant transformation. The exact incidence is difficult to determine and has been estimated at 2–29% of patients with the disease.[65,69,77,93,103] The often-quoted frequency of 13%[77] is too high an estimate in our opinion because it is based on ascertainment of cases reported in the literature. The true incidence is probably closer to the lower figure of 2%.[69] This estimate is reinforced by the follow-up study of a nationwide cohort of 212 Danish patients with neurofibromatosis.[105] Of the 212 patients, 9 developed a sarcoma of nerve or soft tissue origin, and 16 developed a glioma. Most malignant tumors occurred in the proband group (84 patients), who, by definition, required hospitalization and were probably more severely affected by the disorder. The authors suggest that the natural history of neurofibromatosis may be more accurately reflected by the largest group of patients, relatives of the probands (128 patients) who did not require hospitalization and whose prognosis may have been better than previously thought. Both groups, however, had decreased survival rate after 40 years when compared with the general population.

In our experience, the patients at greatest risk to develop sarcomas are those who have had neurofibromatosis for many years.[74] More than three-fourths of patients with neurofibromatosis and MPNST have had the disease 10 years or longer. Only rarely do sarcomas complicate the course of patients who have had the disease less than 5 years. Typically, patients developing sarcomas present with rapid enlargement or pain in a preexisting neurofibroma. Both symptoms, especially the former, should always lead to biopsy. Unfortunately, the prognosis for patients developing an MPNST in this setting is poor (see Chapter 32).

## SCHWANNOMA (NEURILEMOMA)

Schwannoma is an encapsulated nerve sheath tumor consisting of two components: a highly ordered cellular component (Antoni A area) and a loose myxoid component (Antoni B area). The presence of encapsulation and the two types of Antoni areas plus uniformly intense immunostaining for S-100 protein[9] distinguish schwannoma from neurofibroma.

### Clinical Findings

Schwannomas occur at all ages but are most common in persons between the ages of 20 and 50 years.[128] They affect the genders in roughly equal numbers. The tumors have a predilection for the head, neck, and flexor surfaces of the upper and lower extremities.[168] Consequently, the spinal roots and the cervical, sympathetic, vagus, peroneal, and ulnar nerves are most commonly affected. Deeply situated tumors predominate in the posterior mediastinum and the retroperitoneum. Schwannomas are usually solitary sporadic lesions. In a population-based study of schwannomas, about 90% were sporadic, 3% occurred in patients with NF2, 2% in those with schwannomatosis, and 5% in association with multiple meningiomas in patients with or without NF2.[111] Rarely schwannomas occur as part of NF1.[138] Most schwannomas, whether sporadic or inherited, display inactivation mutations of the NF2 gene (see below).

Schwannoma is a slowly growing tumor that is usually present several years before diagnosis. When it involves small nerves, it is freely movable except for a single point of attachment. In large nerves the tumor is movable except along the long axis of the nerve where the attachment restricts mobility.

Pain and neurologic symptoms are uncommon unless the tumor becomes large. In some instances the patient is vaguely aware that the tumor waxes and wanes in size,[168] a phenomenon that might be related to fluctuations in the amount of cystic change in the lesion. Of particular significance is the posterior mediastinal schwannoma, which often originates from or extends into the vertebral canal. Such lesions, termed dumbbell tumors,[61] pose difficult management problems because patients may develop profound neurologic difficulties.

### Gross Findings

Because these tumors arise in nerve sheaths, they are surrounded by a true capsule consisting of the epineurium. Depending on the size of the involved nerve, the appearance of the tumor varies. Tumors of small nerves may resemble neurofibromas by virtue of their fusiform shape, and they often eclipse or obliterate the nerve of origin. In large nerves the tumors present as eccentric masses over which the nerve fibers are splayed.

On cut section these tumors have a pink, white, or yellow appearance and usually measure less than 5 cm (Figs. 30–47, 30–48). Tumors in the retroperitoneum and mediastinum may be considerably larger. As a result, these tumors are more likely to manifest secondary degenerative changes such as cystification and calcification (see discussion of the ancient schwannoma, below).

### Microscopic Findings

Most schwannomas are uninodular masses surrounded by a fibrous capsules consisting of epineu-

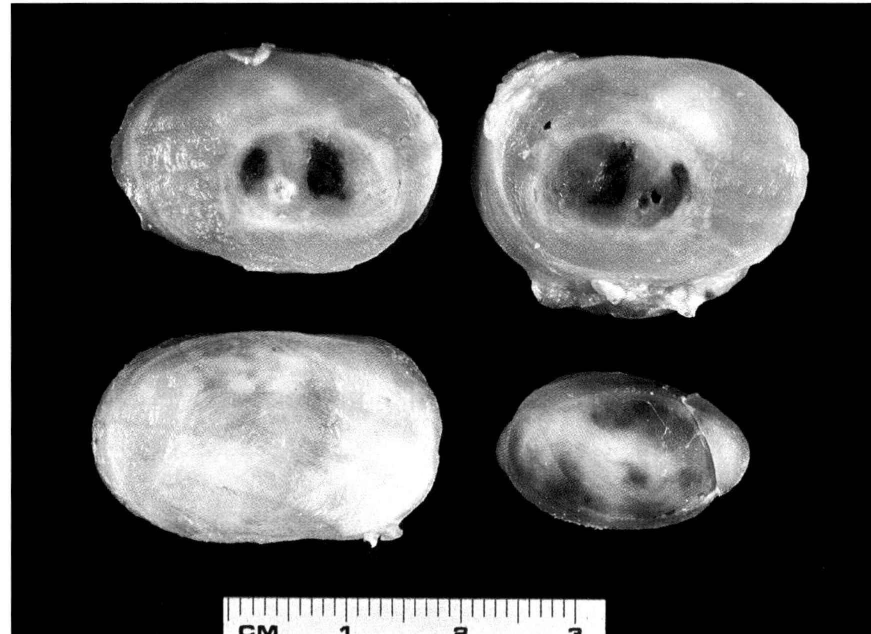


**FIGURE 30–47.** Multiple transverse sections through a schwannoma. Tumors are well circumscribed and colony display foci of hemorrhage and cyst formation.

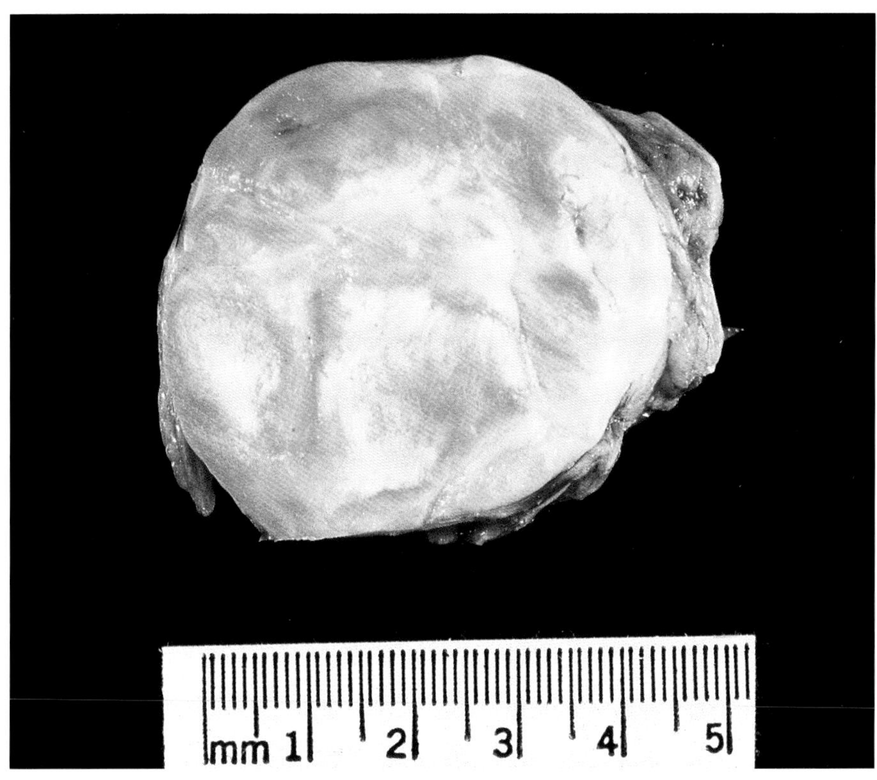


**FIGURE 30–48.** Mottled yellow-white appearance of a presacral schwannoma.

rium and residual nerve fibers (Fig. 30–49). Neurites are generally not demonstrable in the substance of the tumor. In rare cases the schwannoma arises intradermally or, as mentioned above, manifest as a plexiform or multinodular growth similar to a plexiform neurofibroma.

The hallmark of a schwannoma is the pattern of alternating Antoni A and B areas (Figs. 30–50 to 30–60). The relative amounts of these two components vary, and they may blend imperceptibly or change abruptly. Antoni A areas are composed of compact spindle cells that usually have twisted nuclei, indistinct cytoplasmic borders, and occasionally clear intranuclear vacuoles. They are arranged in short bundles or interlacing fascicles (Figs. 30–51, 30–52, 30–53). In highly differentiated Antoni A areas there may be nuclear palisading, whorling of the cells (similar to meningioma), and Verocay bodies, formed by two compact rows of well aligned nuclei separated by fibrillary cell processes (Fig. 30–51). Mitotic figures are occasionally present but can usually be dismissed if the lesion otherwise has all the hallmarks of schwannoma. S-100 protein, an acidic protein common to supporting cells of the central and peripheral nervous system, can be demonstrated in schwannomas,[8,9] particularly in the Antoni A areas.

Antoni B areas are far less orderly and less cellular. The spindle or oval cells are arranged haphazardly in the loosely textured matrix, which is punctuated by microcystic change, inflammatory cells, and delicate collagen fibers (Figs. 30–54 to 30–57). The large, irregularly spaced vessels, which are characteristic of schwannomas, become most conspicuous in the hypocellular Antoni B areas (Figs. 30–58, 30–59). Their gaping tortuous lumens are often filled with thrombus material in various stages of organization, and their walls are thickened by dense fibrosis. Glands and benign epithelial structures may occur in schwannoma (Fig. 30–61).[127] Judging from the number and type of glands, this seems to represent true epithelial differentiation in the tumor rather than entrapment or induced proliferation of normal structures.[115,125] On occasion, schwannomas develop cystic spaces lined by Schwann cells that assume a round or epithelioid appearance. This change may be confused with true epithelial differentiation (Fig. 30–62). Such tumors have been referred to as pseudoglandular schwannomas.[119] Rarely, schwannomas contain a significant population of small lymphocyte-like Schwann cells arranged around collagen nodules forming giant rosettes (Figs. 30–63, 30–64) or around vessels forming perivascular rosettes.[129]

## Ultrastructural and Immunohistochemical Findings

Electron microscopy has provided some of the best evidence in support of the separate natures of schwannomas and neurofibromas. In contrast to the neurofibroma, which contains a mixture of cell types,

*Text continued on page 1160*

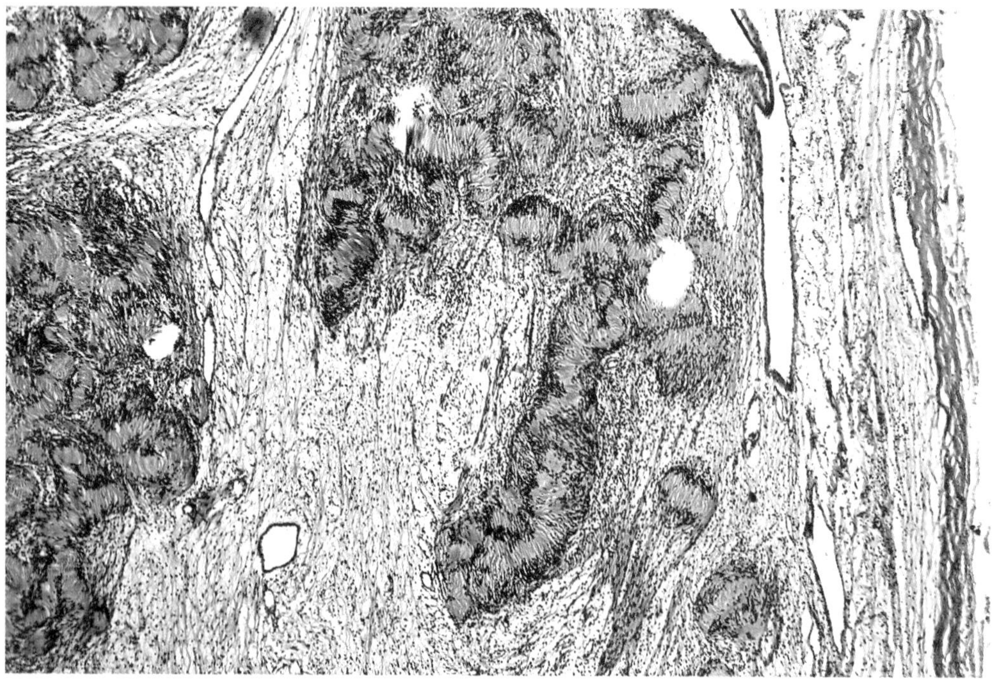

**FIGURE 30–49.** Schwannoma with a discrete confining capsule.

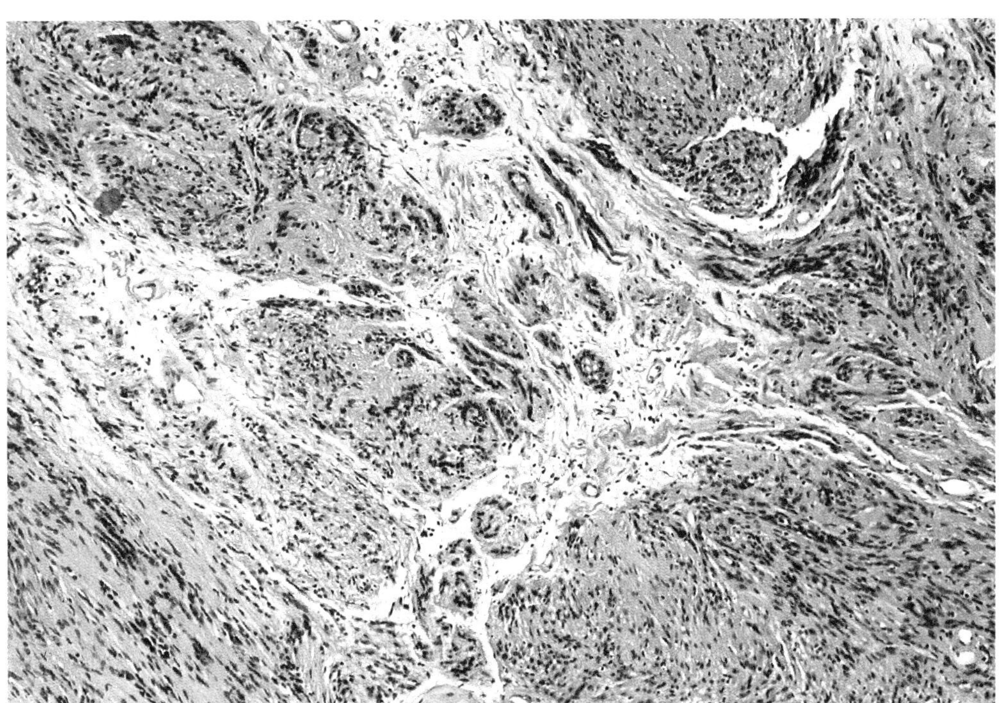

**FIGURE 30–50.** Schwannoma with alternating Antoni A and B areas.

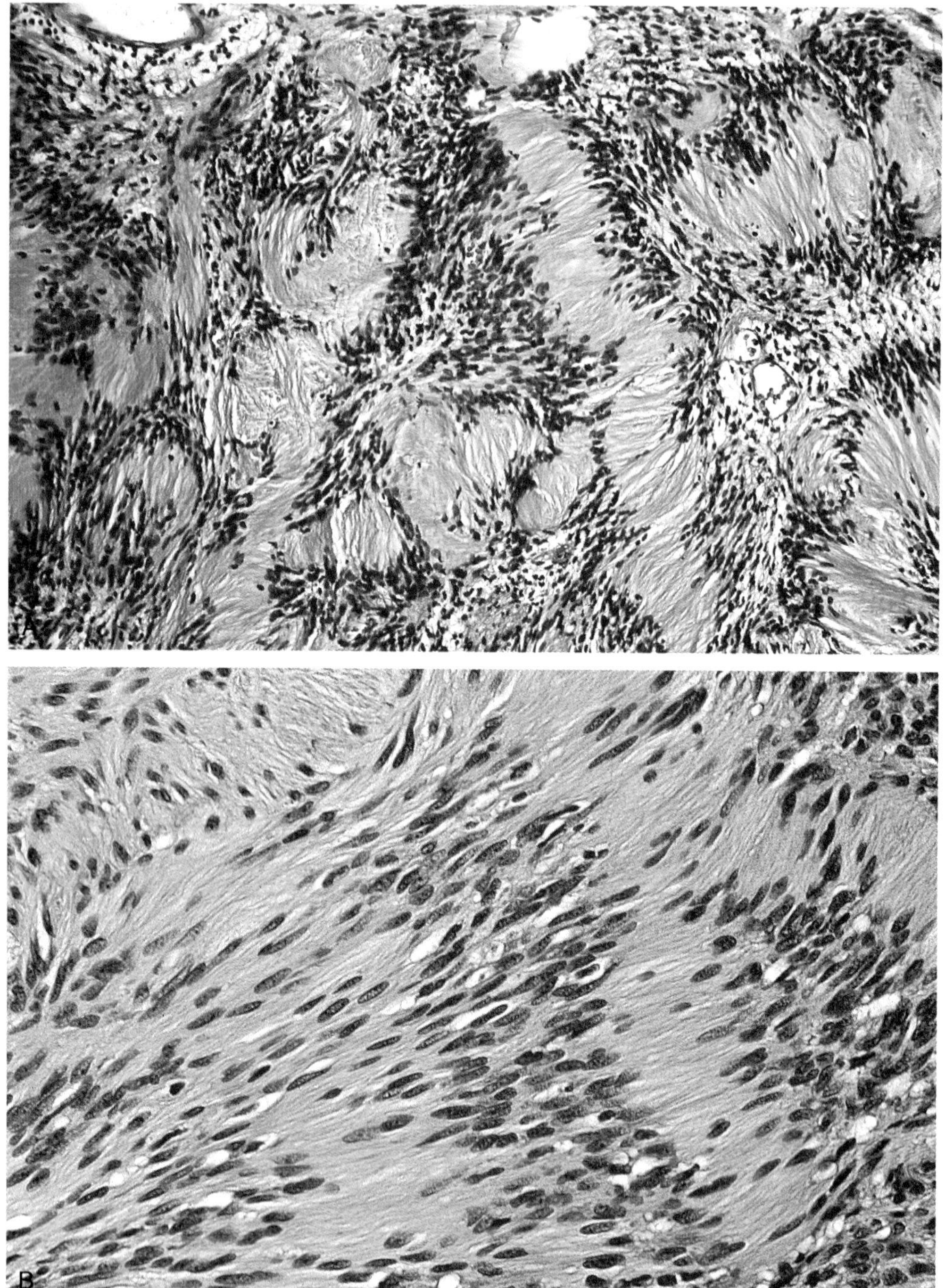

**FIGURE 30–51.** (**A**) Antoni A areas illustrating nuclear palisading with Verocay bodies. (**B**) High power view shows nuclear palisading.

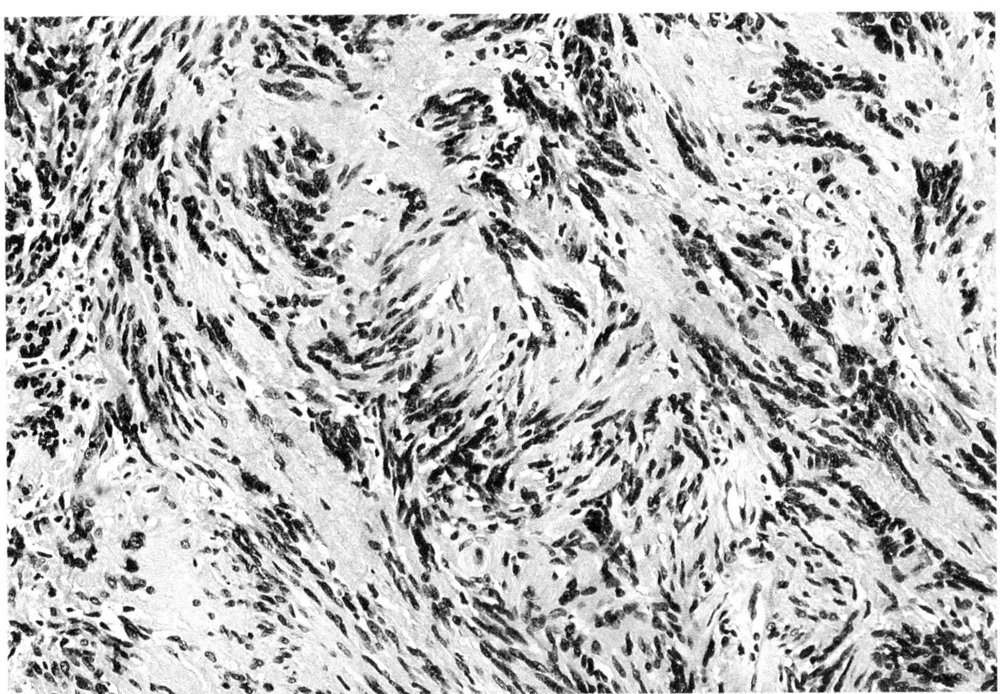

**FIGURE 30–52.** Antoni A areas with short fascicles and focal nuclear palisading.

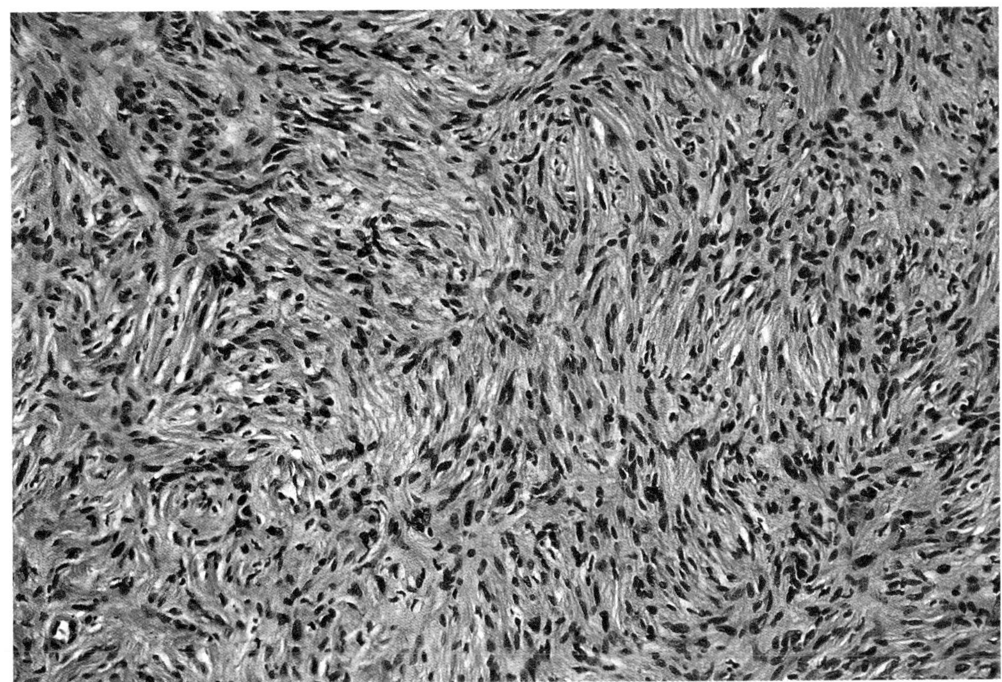

**FIGURE 30–53.** Antoni A areas with ill-defined fascicles without nuclear palisading.

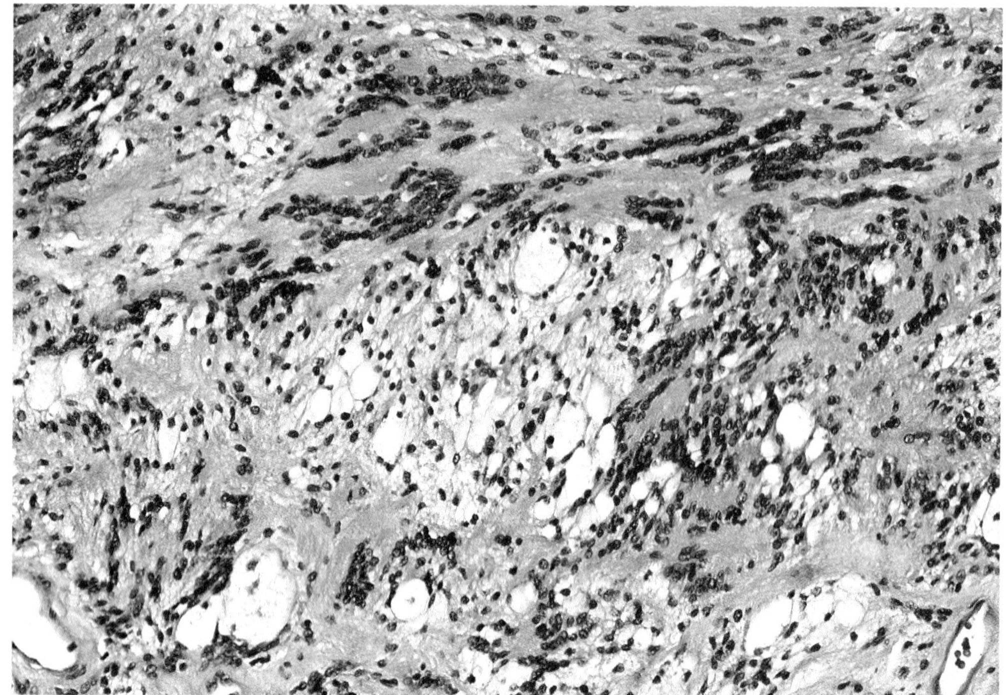

**FIGURE 30–54.** Transition between Antoni A areas and loosely textured Antoni B areas (center).

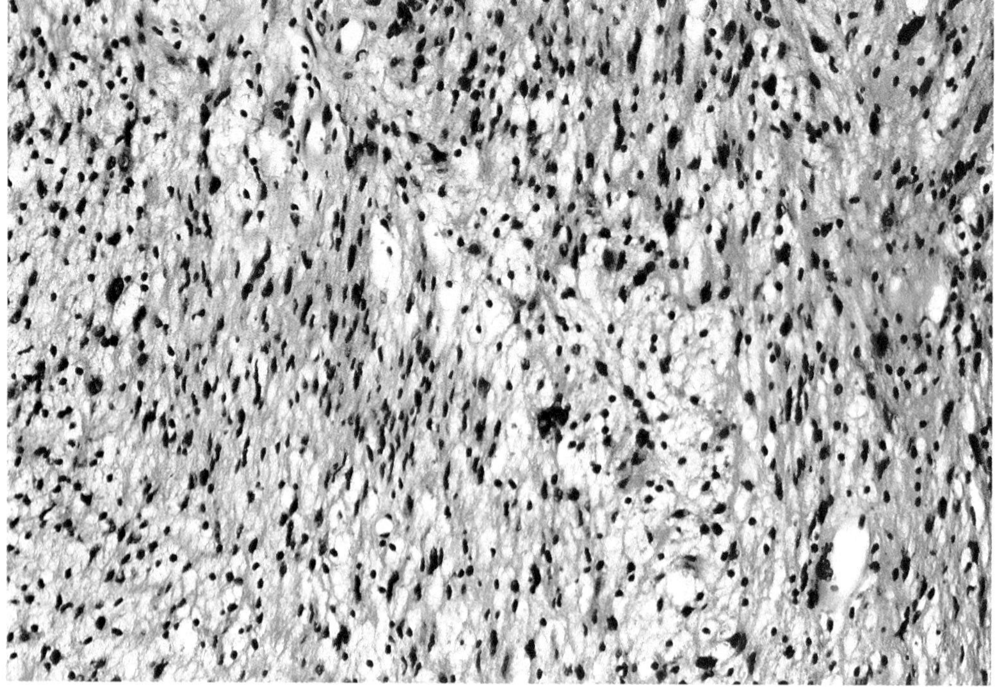

**FIGURE 30–55.** Antoni B areas in a schwannoma.

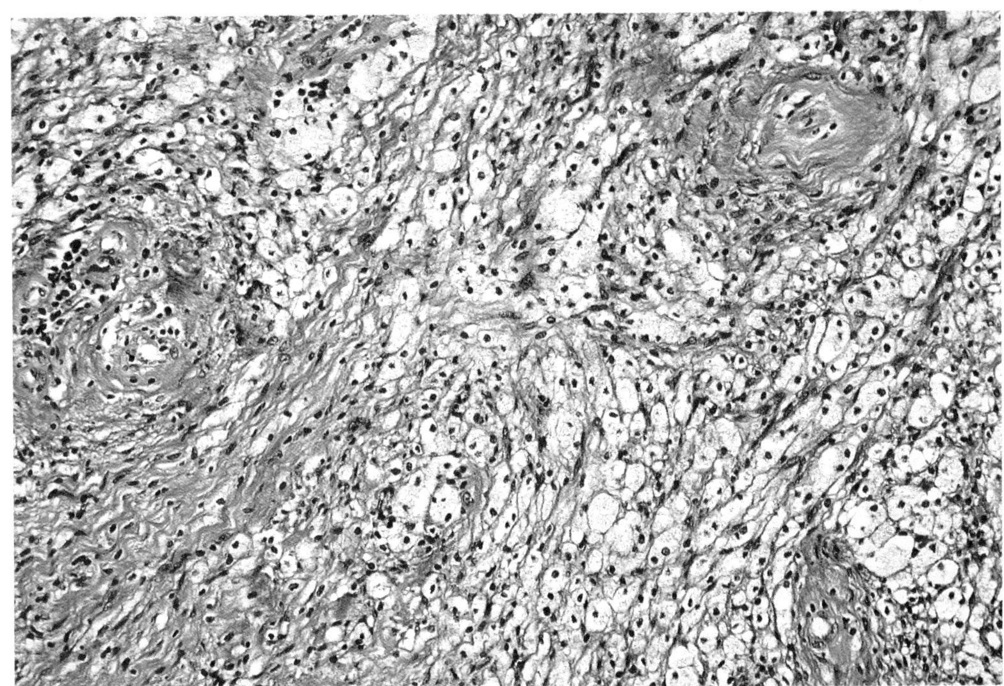

**FIGURE 30–56.** Antoni B areas with xanthomatous change.

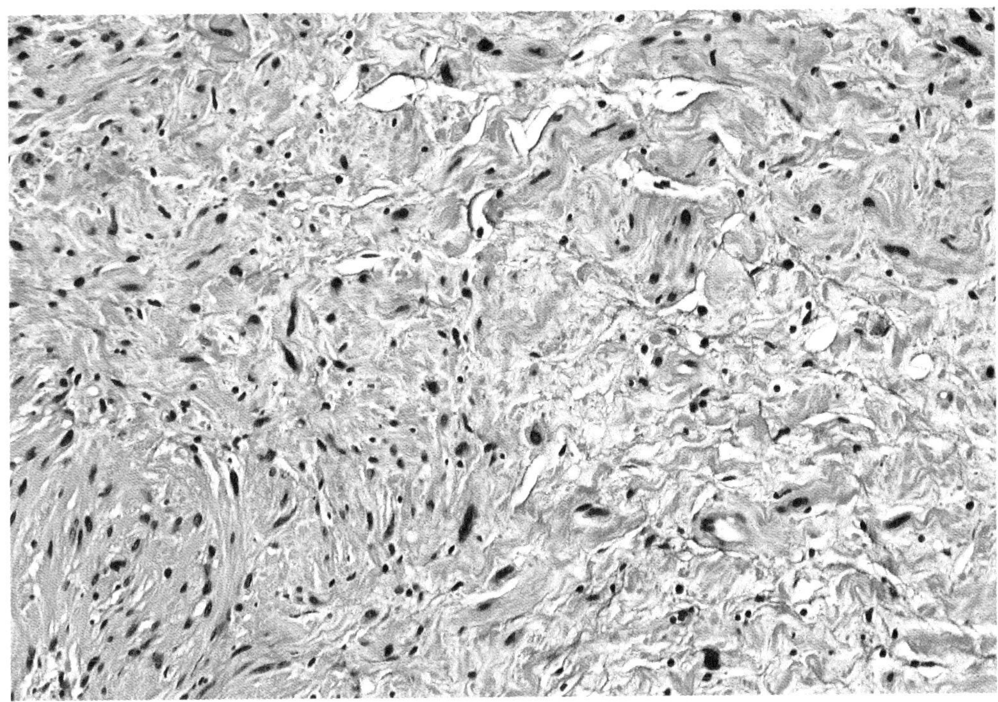

**FIGURE 30–57.** Antoni B areas with hyalinization.

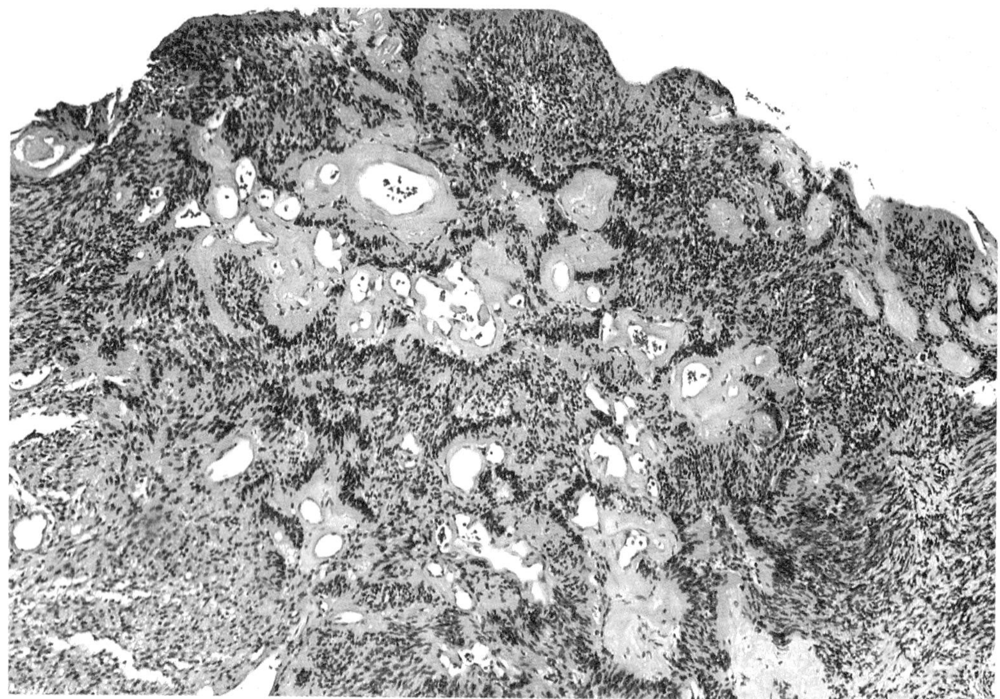

**FIGURE 30–58.** Ectatic irregularly shaped vessels with surrounding hyalinization are a common feature of schwannomas.

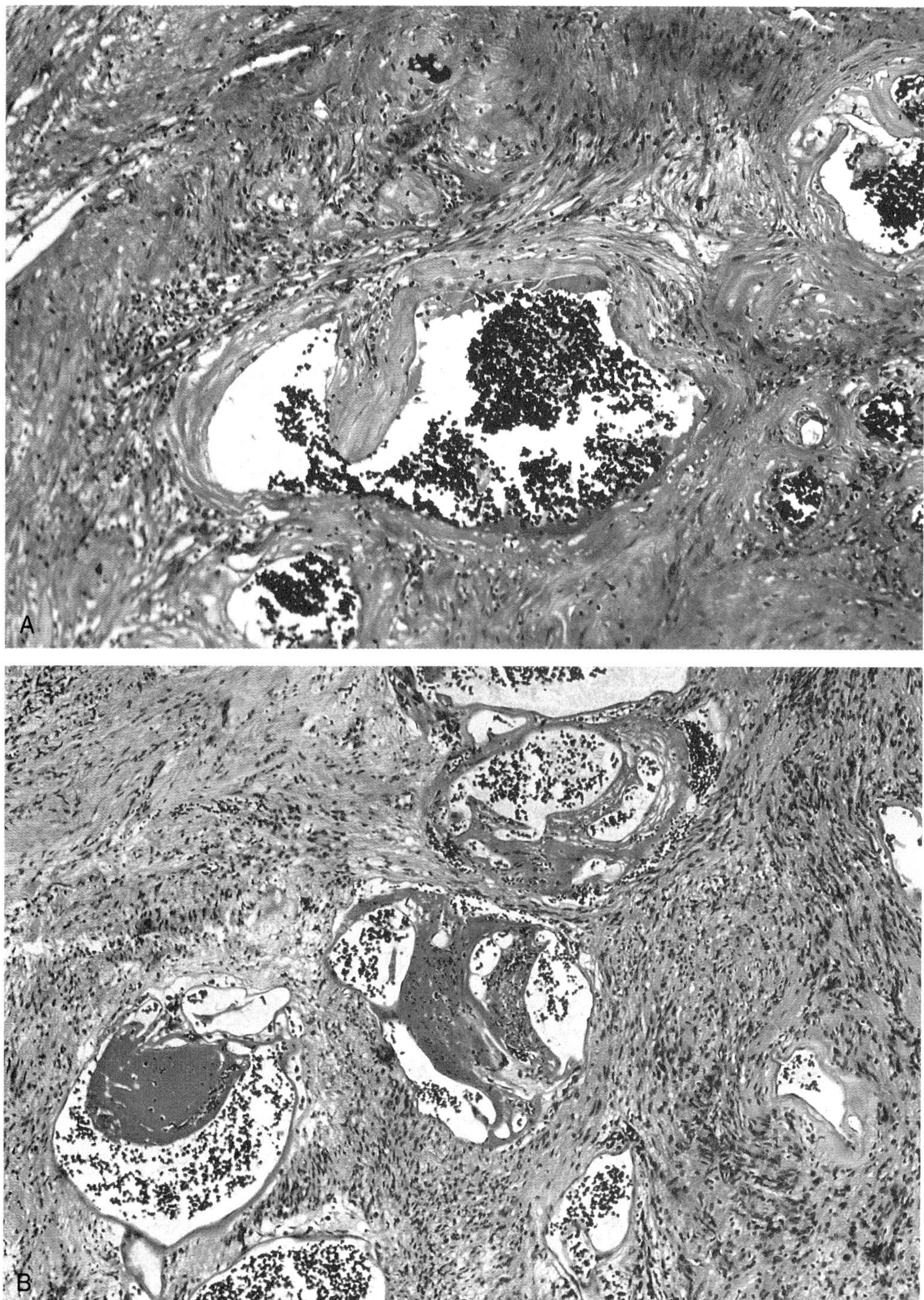


**FIGURE 30–59.** Hyalinized (**A**) and partially thrombosed (**B**) vessels in a schwannoma.

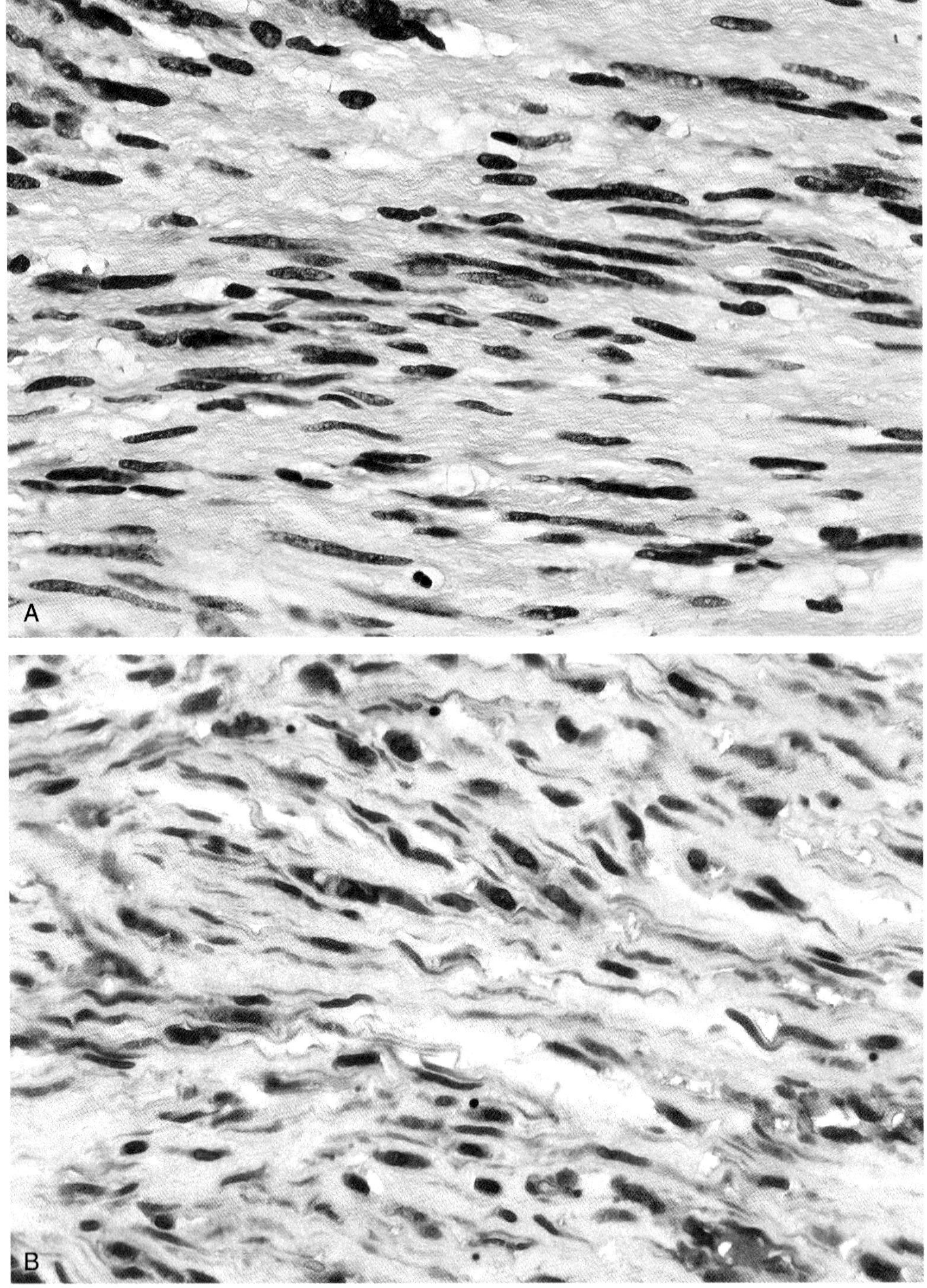


**FIGURE 30–60.** Differentiated Schwann cells (**A**) expressing S-100 protein (**B**) in a schwannoma.

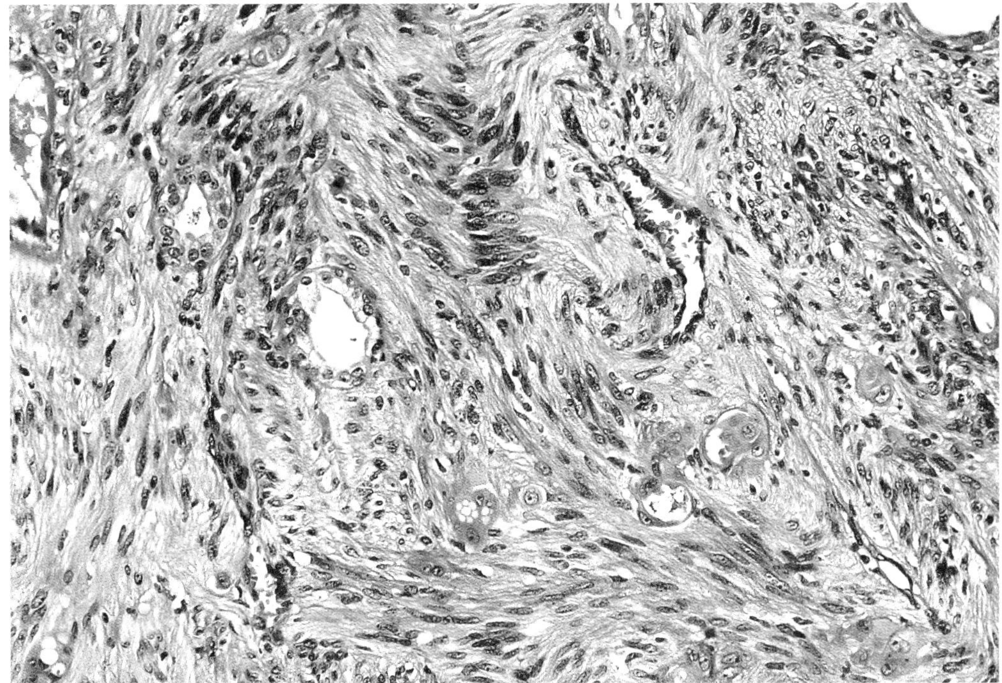

**FIGURE 30–61.** Schwannoma with benign glands and squamous islands.

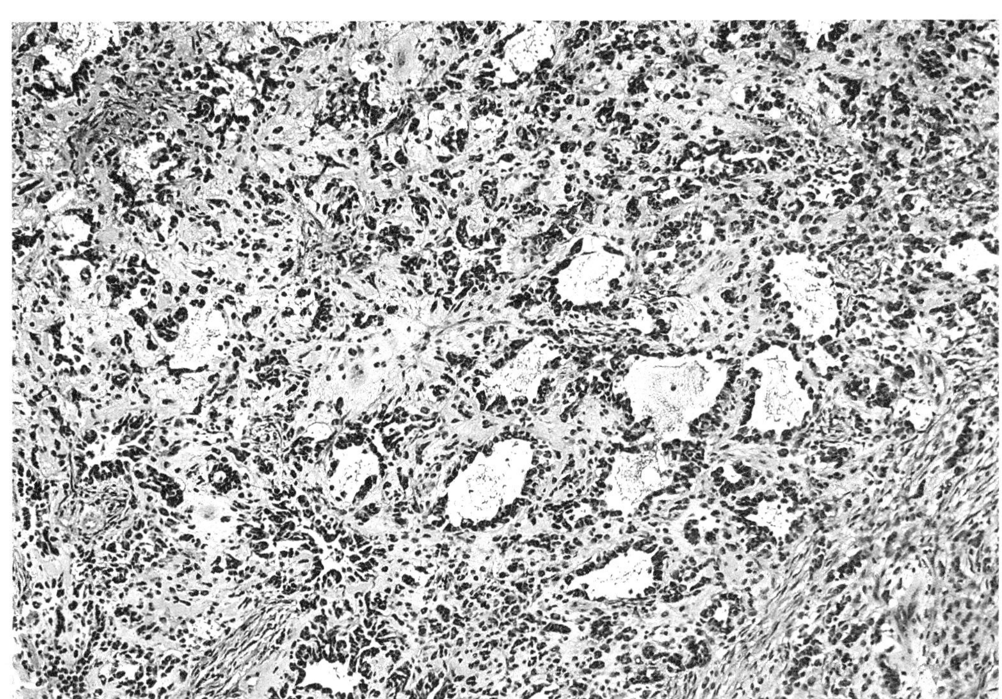

**FIGURE 30–62.** Schwannoma with cystic spaces resembling glands or dilated lymphatics (a so-called pseudoglandular schwannoma).

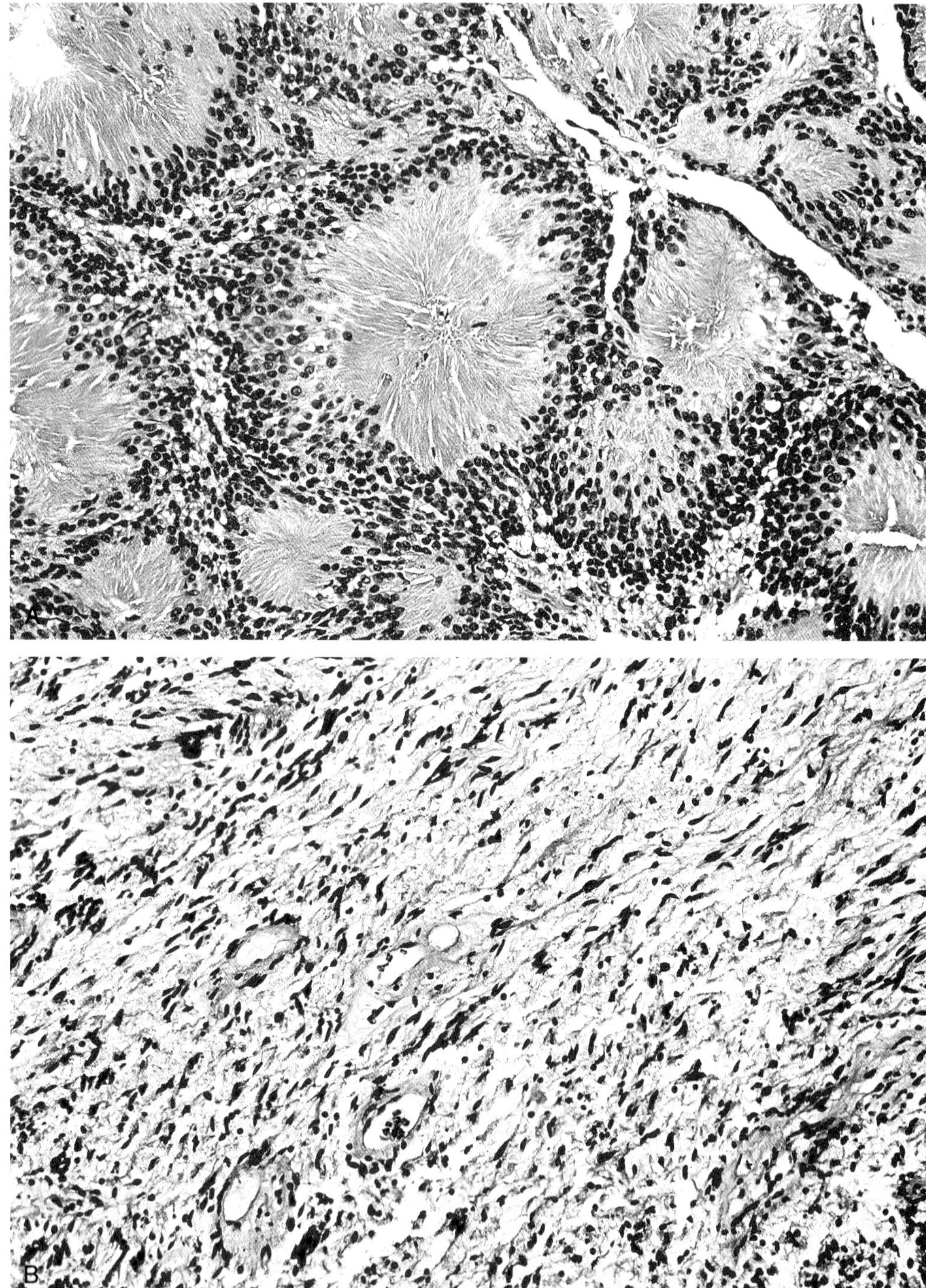


**FIGURE 30–63.** Neuroblastoma-like schwannoma composed of rounded Schwann cells forming rosettes (**A**). Other areas had a more conventional appearance (**B**).

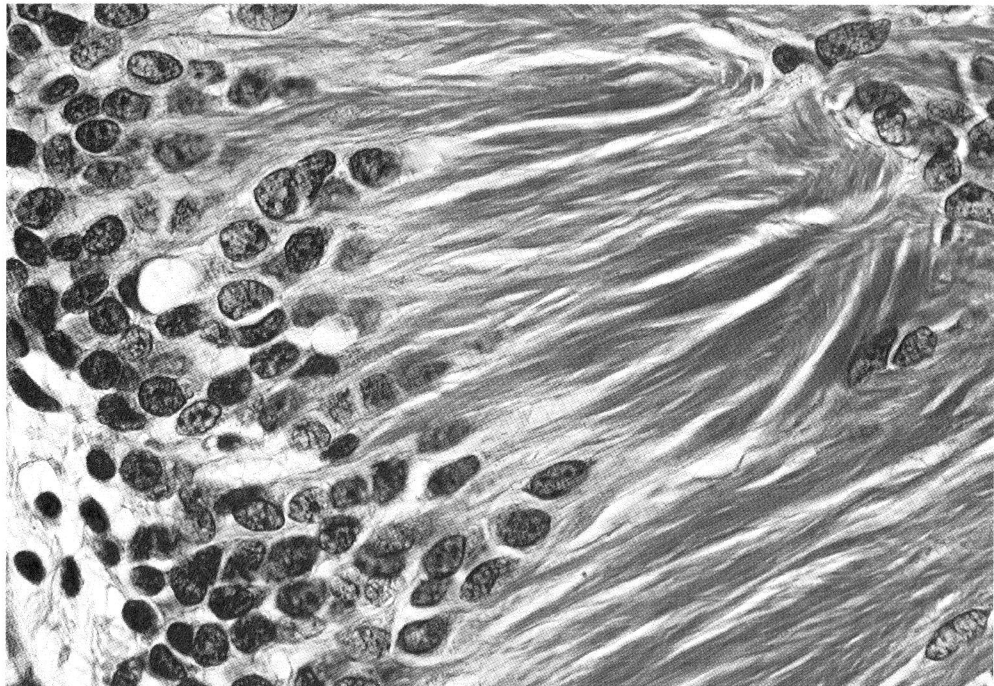

**FIGURE 30–64.** Giant rosette in a schwannoma formed by the radial arrangement of Schwann cells around a collagen core. (Masson trichrome stain)

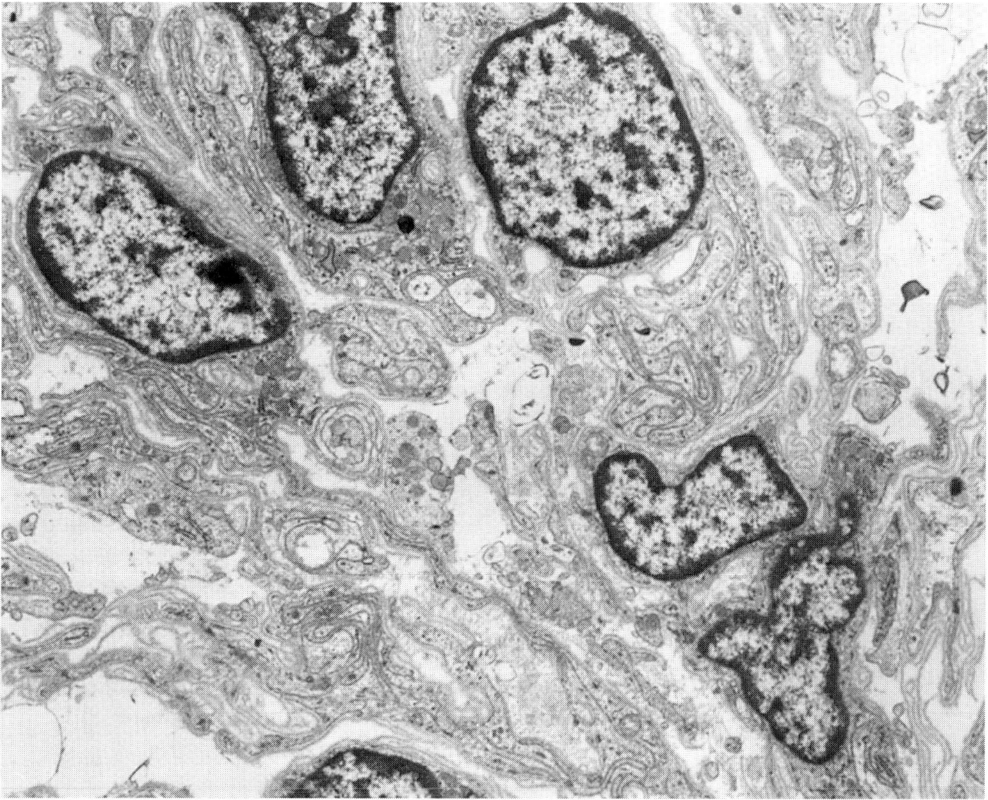

**FIGURE 30–65.** Electron micrograph of a schwannoma. Cells give off long cytoplasmic processes, which lie in layers adjacent to the cell body and are invested by well formed continuous basal lamina. (From Taxy JB, Battifora H. In: Trump B, Jones RT (eds) Diagnostic Electron Microscopy. Wiley, New York, 1980.)

the schwannoma consists almost exclusively of Schwann cells.[10,82] These cells have attenuated cell processes that emanate from the cell body and lie in undulating layers adjacent to the cell body.[82,123,159,174] Basal lamina consisting of electron-dense material (measuring approximately 50 nm) coats the surface of the Schwann cell and lies in redundant stacks between the cells along with typical and long-spacing collagen (Fig. 30–65). The cytoplasm of the Schwann cell contains a flattened, occasionally invaginated nucleus, microfibrils, occasional lysosomes, and scattered mitochondria. In Antoni B areas the Schwann cells have increased numbers of lysosomes and myelin figures with only a fragmented basal lamina, suggesting that these are degenerated Antoni A areas.

In concert with ultrastructural observations, most cells in schwannomas have the antigenic phenotype of Schwann cells. S-100 protein is strongly expressed by most cells in a schwannoma, in contrast to the cells of neurofibromas, which variably express the antigen. Leu-7 and occasionally glial fibrillary acidic protein are present in these tumors. Although the expression of S-100 protein is somewhat diminished in the Antoni B areas, immunostaining for this protein is so consistent and of such intensity that it serves as an important diagnostic tool. In our experience it is most valuable for diagnosing a severely degenerated schwannoma in which the amount of myxoid change or fibrosis obscures the neoplastic nature of the lesion altogether. It usually also distinguishes deeply situated schwannomas from well differentiated leiomyosarcomas. This important differential point is especially difficult in biopsy material from large intraabdominal or retroperitoneal masses. The difficulty can be further compounded by the fact that schwannomas and leiomyosarcomas can display equivalent degrees of nuclear palisading. Whereas S-100 protein immunostaining is nearly always observed in schwannomas, it is seldom observed in leiomyosarcomas in our experience. Additional helpful stains include the Masson trichrome stain to document the presence or absence of longitudinal striations.

## Discussion

Schwannomas behave in a benign fashion. In Stout's series of 50 cases[168] none recurred after simple or even incomplete excision. Malignant change is rare[134,153,158] and from a practical point of view can be discounted. Among the well over 1000 schwannomas we have seen, there has been only one instance of true malignant transformation. In that case the original tumor had the features of a classic schwannoma, whereas the recurrent tumor, 8 years later, had areas of malignancy. The patient later succumbed to metastatic disease. Woodruff et al. presented nine acceptable cases,[179] including two of their own, in a comprehensive review of the literature. Others have subsequently been reported.[150] As a group, these tumors occur in adults without NF1 but with a longstanding mass. Unlike neurofibromas, in which supervening malignancy resembles a spindle cell sarcoma, malignancy in schwannomas usually has an epithelioid appearance. Areas of a conventional schwannoma are identified alongside confluent expanses of large, round, atypical eosinophilic cells (Fig. 30–66C,D).[117] McMenamin and Fletcher have noted microscopic collections of these epithelioid cells in schwannomas and suggested that they represent an early stage of malignant transformation (Fig. 30–66A,B).[150]

## Schwannoma with Degenerative Change (Ancient Schwannoma)

Ancient schwannomas are those displaying marked nuclear atypia on a degenerative basis.[110,120] They are usually large tumors of long duration, and a significant number are located in deep structures such as the retroperitoneum.[120] Degenerative changes include cyst formation, calcification, hemorrhage, and hyalinization (Figs. 30–67 to 30–72). The tumor itself is usually infiltrated by large numbers of siderophages and histiocytes. One of the most treacherous aspects of this tumor is the degree of nuclear atypia encountered. The Schwann cell nuclei are large, hyperchromatic, and often multilobed but lack mitotic figures (Figs. 30–68, 30–71). These tumors behave as ordinary schwannomas; therefore the nuclear atypia can be regarded as a purely degenerative change.

## Cellular Schwannoma

First described in 1969 by Harkin and Reed[5] and later by Woodruff et al.,[177] the cellular schwannoma has become a well recognized variant of the schwannoma,[118,126,147,176] that because of its cellularity, mitotic activity, and occasional presence of bone destruction is diagnosed as malignant in more than one-fourth of cases.[171] In our opinion and others,[7] most of the lesions reported as plexiform MPNSTs of infancy and childhood[151] and congenital neural hamartoma (fascicular schwannoma) are cellular schwannomas. Defined as a schwannoma composed predominantly or exclusively of Antoni A areas that lack Verocay bodies, cellular schwannoma occurs in a similar age group as classic schwannoma but tends to develop more often in deep structures such as the posterior mediastinum and retroperitoneum. Only about one-fourth develop in the deep soft tissues of the extremities. It may present as a palpable asymptomatic mass noted ra-

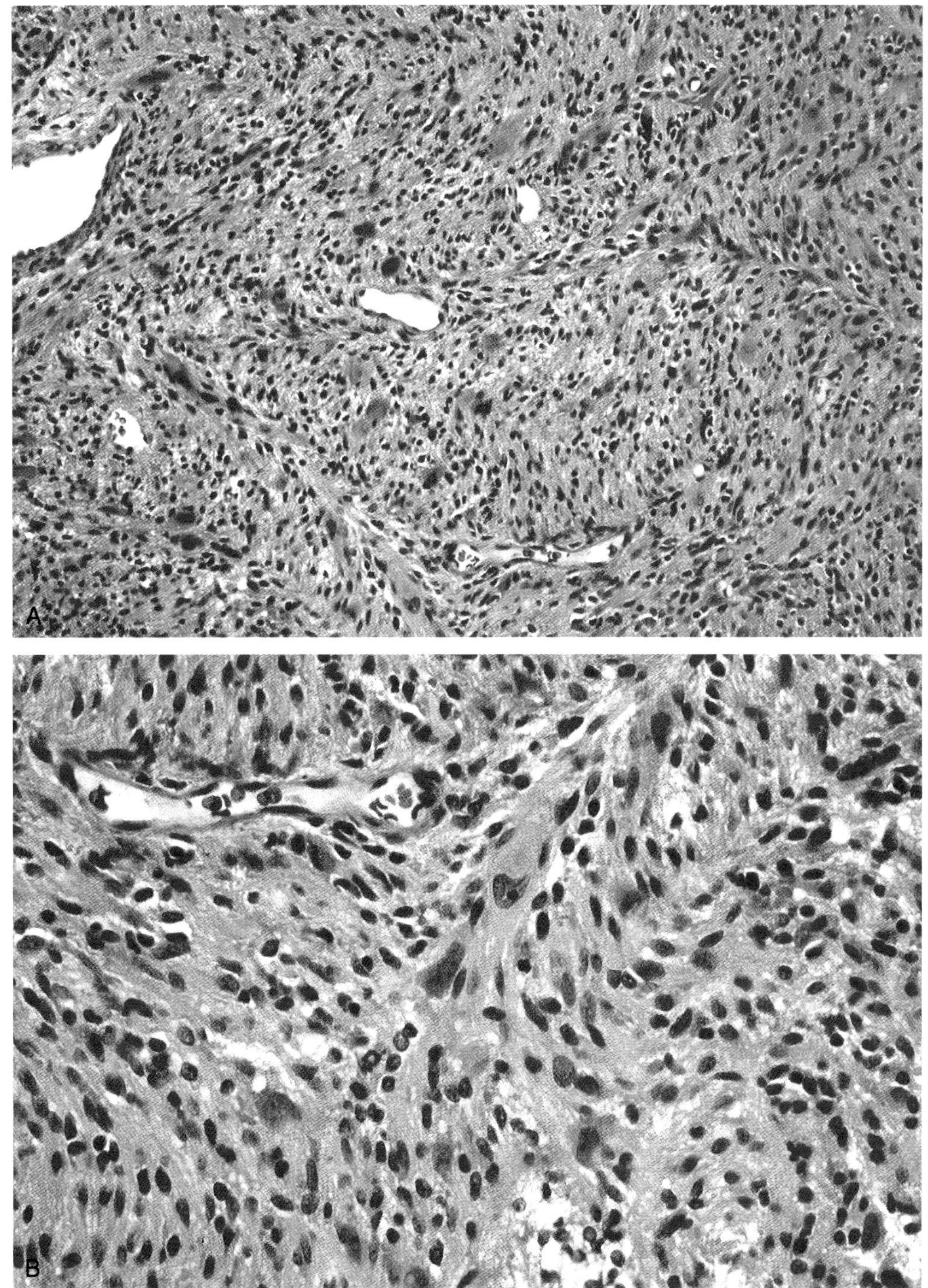


**FIGURE 30–66.** Schwannoma with scattered atypical (**A, B**) cells and frank malignant change (**C, D**).

*Illustration continued on following page*

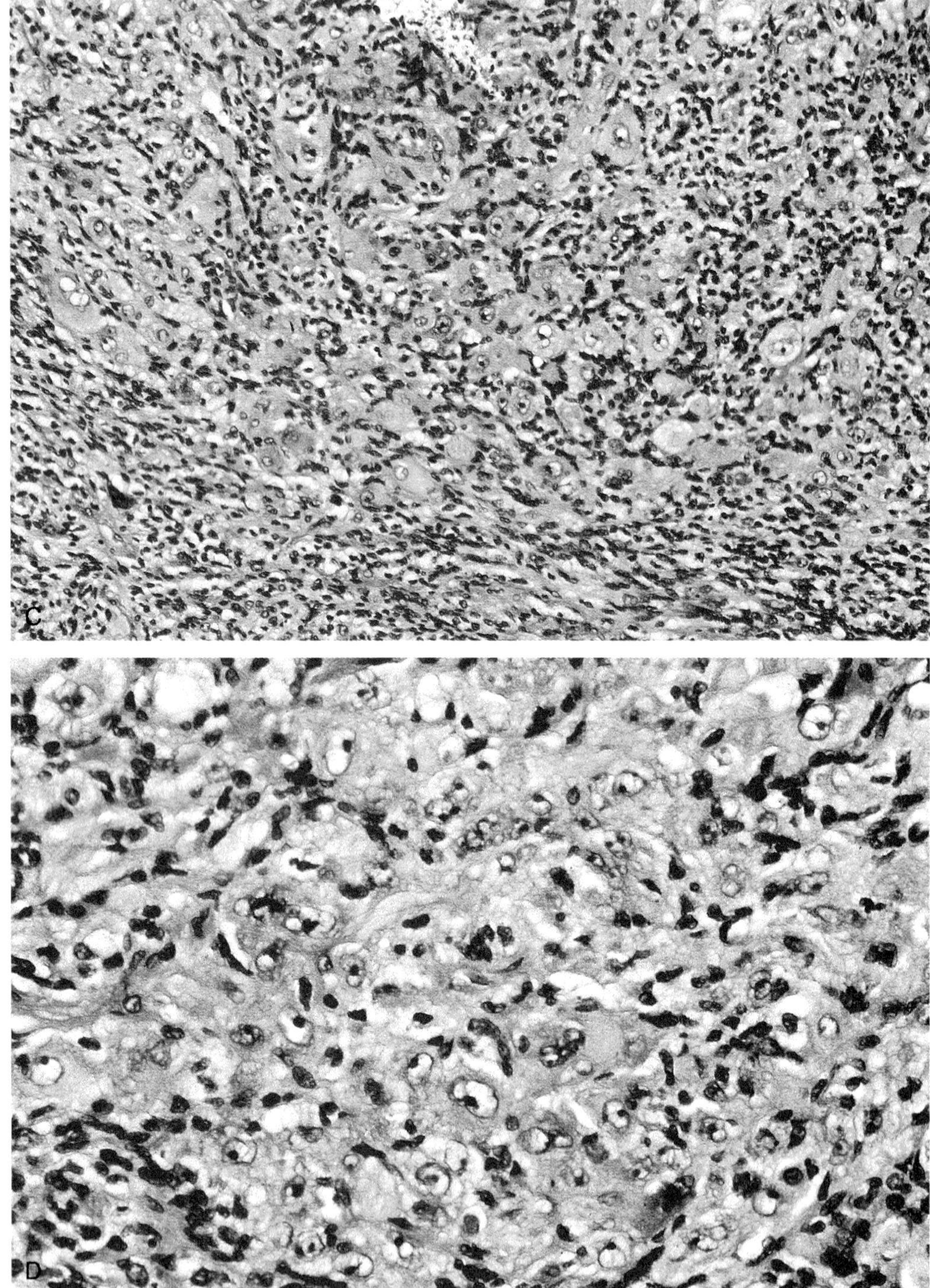

**FIGURE 30–66** *(Continued).* Scattered atypical cells within otherwise benign schwannoma (**A, B**) have been described as the "precursor" lesion to frank malignancy which is diagnosed by confluent areas of obviously malignant cells (**C, D**).

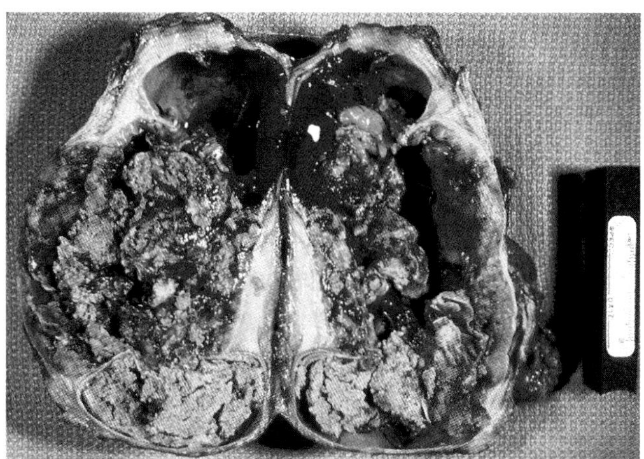

**FIGURE 30–67.** Gross specimen of a schwannoma of the retroperitoneum with extensive degenerative changes (ancient schwannoma). Tumors are characterized by areas of old and new hemorrhage, cyst formation, and calcification.

diographically or as a mass producing neurologic symptoms. Like classic schwannomas, the lesions appear circumscribed, if not encapsulated, and occasionally are multinodular or plexiform. Usually homogeneously tan in color, they commonly have hemorrhage but seldom display cystic degeneration[7] (Fig. 30–73). Underneath their capsule they may contain lymphoid aggregates. Antoni A areas dominate the histologic picture but small amounts of Antoni B may be present, usually not exceeding 10% of the lesion.[7] In addition to short intersecting fascicles and whorls of Schwann cells, the Antoni A areas may display long, sweeping fascicles of Schwann cells sometimes arranged in a herringbone fashion (Figs. 30–74, 30–75). The presence of this pattern often suggests the diagnosis of fibrosarcoma or leiomyosarcoma to those unfamiliar with cellular schwannomas. Mitotic activity may be observed but usually is low [<4 mitoses per 10 high power fields (HPF)].[176] Focal areas of necrosis are seen in up to 10% of cases. The cells fringing the necrotic zones, however, are differentiated Schwann cells and lack the hyperchromatism and anaplasia so typical of those surrounding areas of zonal necrosis in MPNSTs. Like classic schwannomas, the cellular schwannoma displays diffuse, strong immunoreactivity for S-100 protein. Most cellular schwannomas are diploid with a low S-phase fraction (6–7%).[118]

Important factors that suggest a benign diagnosis include cellularity that is disproportionately high compared with the levels of mitoses and atypia, sharp circumscription if not encapsulation, perivascular hyalinization, occasionally focal Antoni B areas, and invariably strong, diffuse immunoreactivity for S-100 protein. Staining for S-100 protein is an invaluable adjunct for this diagnosis, particularly if one is dealing with material obtained by small-needle biopsies of large retroperitoneal or mediastinal masses. In fact, we rarely diagnose malignancy based on needle biopsies of differentiated spindle cell tumors if staining for S-100 protein is strongly positive because of the possibility of a cellular schwannoma.

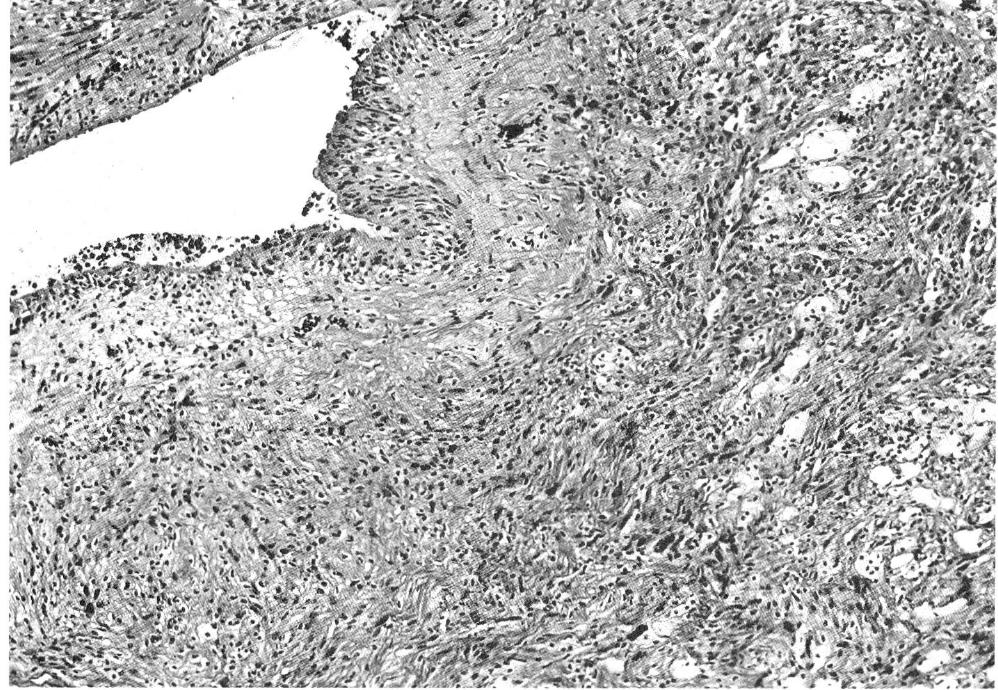

**FIGURE 30–68.** Ancient schwannoma with cyst formation and interstitial hyalinization.

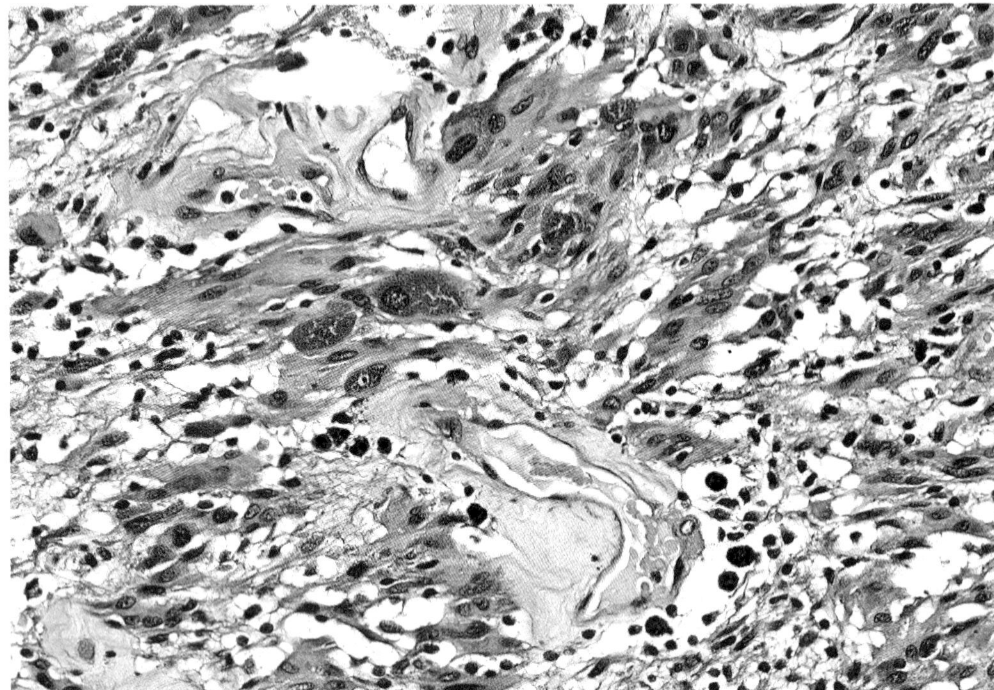

**FIGURE 30–69.** Ancient schwannoma with degenerative atypia and perivascular hyalinization. Note the lipofuscin-like pigment in the Schwann cells.

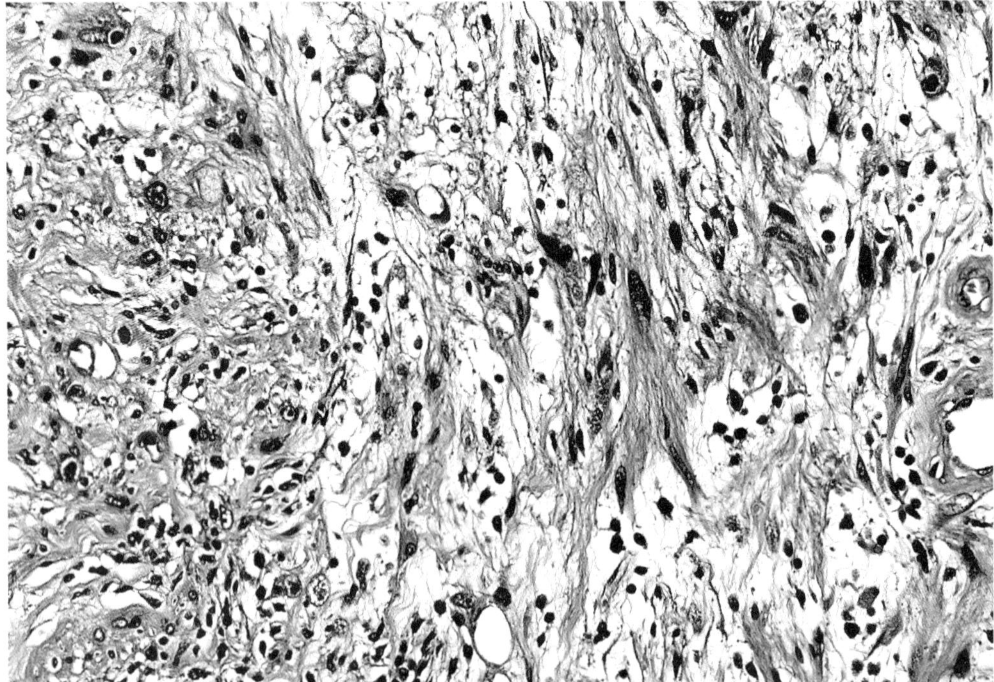

**FIGURE 30–70.** Ancient schwannoma.

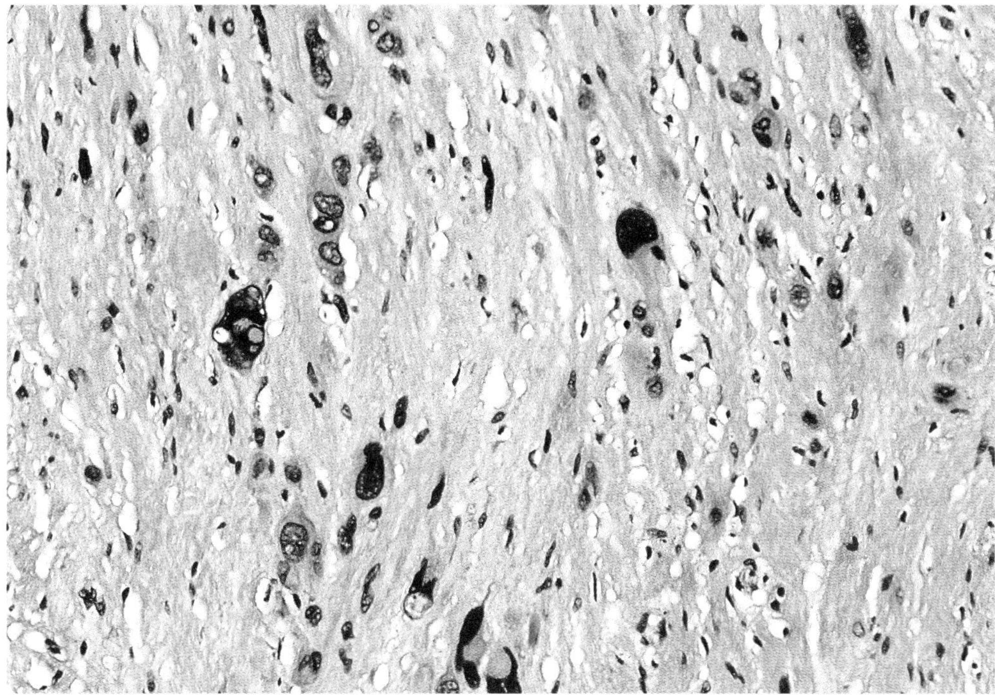

**FIGURE 30–71.** Ancient schwannoma with extensive hyalinization.

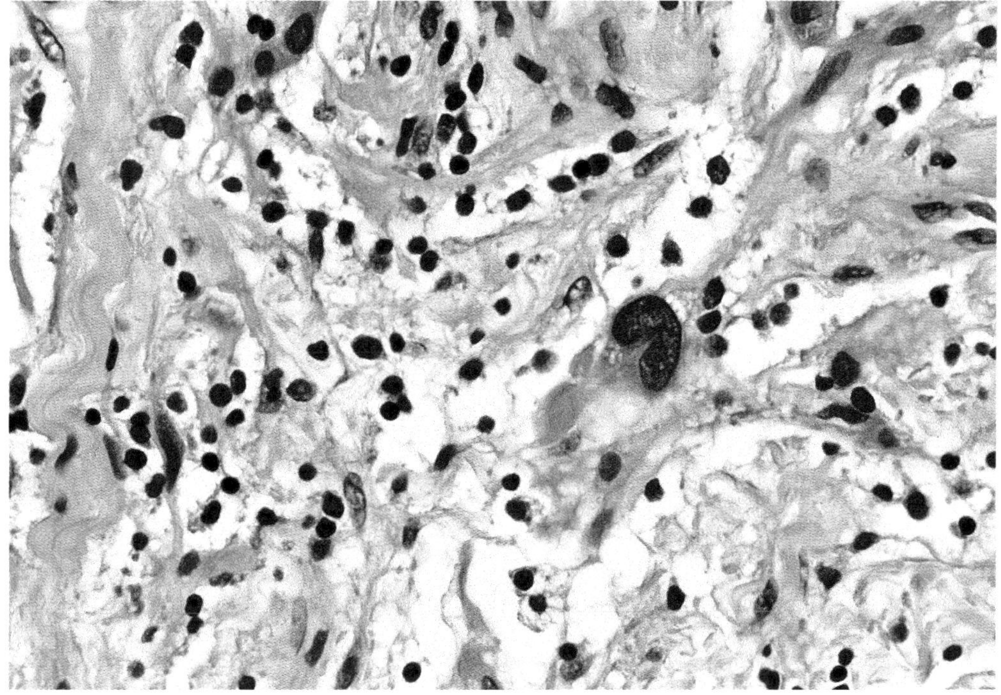

**FIGURE 30–72.** Degenerative atypia in an ancient schwannoma.

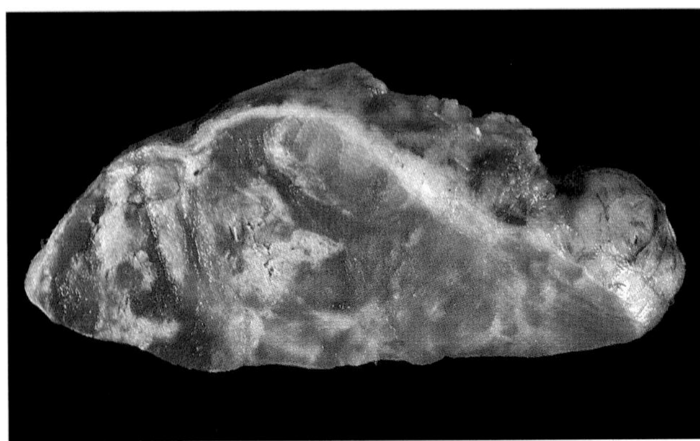

**FIGURE 30–73.** Cellular schwannoma with a characteristic tawny yellow color.

Although initial skepticism was expressed about the biologic behavior of cellular schwannomas, with some suggesting that it was in fact a low grade MPNST, several large studies with extended follow-up information[118,125,147,176] have reaffirmed the initial findings of Woodruff et al. More than 100 cases have been reported, with nearly one-third having follow-up periods of more than 5 years. Fewer than 5% of patients have developed recurrences, and none has developed metastatic disease. In most of the cases reported by White et al.,[176] treatment was conservative and consisted of surgical excision only. That these truly represent variants of schwannoma is indicated not only by histologic but also by ultrastructural and cytogenetic similarities.[147]

## Plexiform Schwannoma

About 5% of schwannomas grow in a plexiform or multinodular pattern,[178] which may or may not be apparent macroscopically (Figs. 30–76, 30–77, 30–78). Unlike plexiform neurofibromas, which are considered nearly pathognomonic of NF1, the association of plexiform schwannomas with NF1 or NF2 is considerably weaker.[178] Of the approximately 50 cases reported in the literature, there have been only a few cases associated with NF1[125,137,142] or NF2.[136,160,173] Plexiform schwannomas usually occur in the skin and infrequently in deep sites. Like classic schwannoma, they are encapsulated but as a group tend to be more cellular. It is important to be aware of this fact, as there is a risk of misinterpreting a lesion as a sarcoma arising in a plexiform neurofibroma. Attention to the fact that the lesion does not have a level of atypia commensurate with the mitotic activity, lacks geographic necrosis, and displays strong S-100 protein staining provides good support for benignancy in such cases.

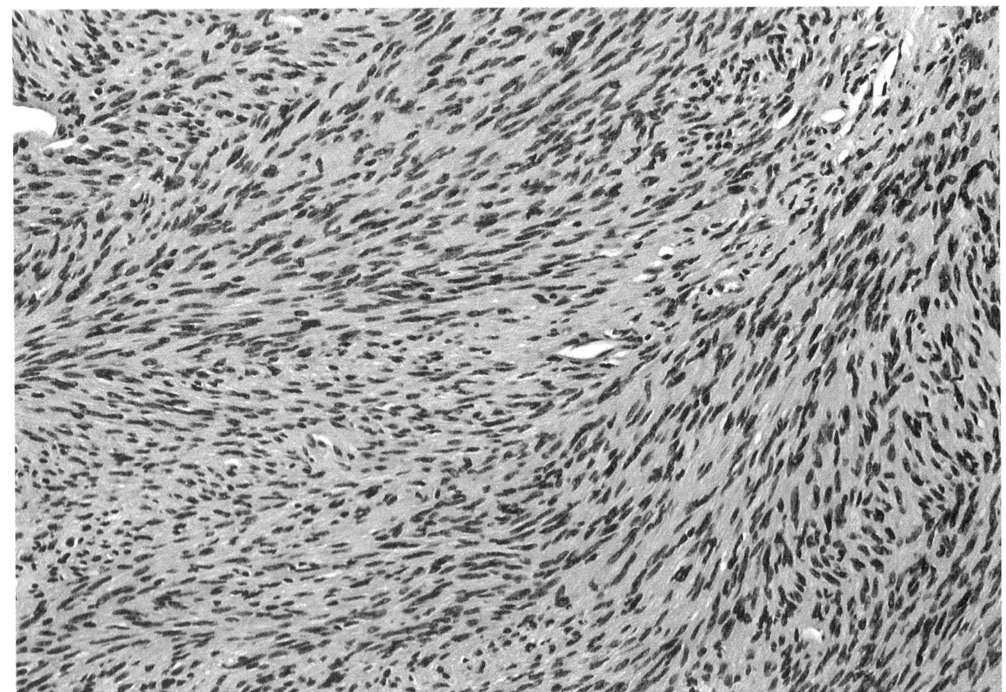

**FIGURE 30–74.** Cellular schwannoma with long fascicles of Schwann cells without Antoni B areas or Verocay bodies.

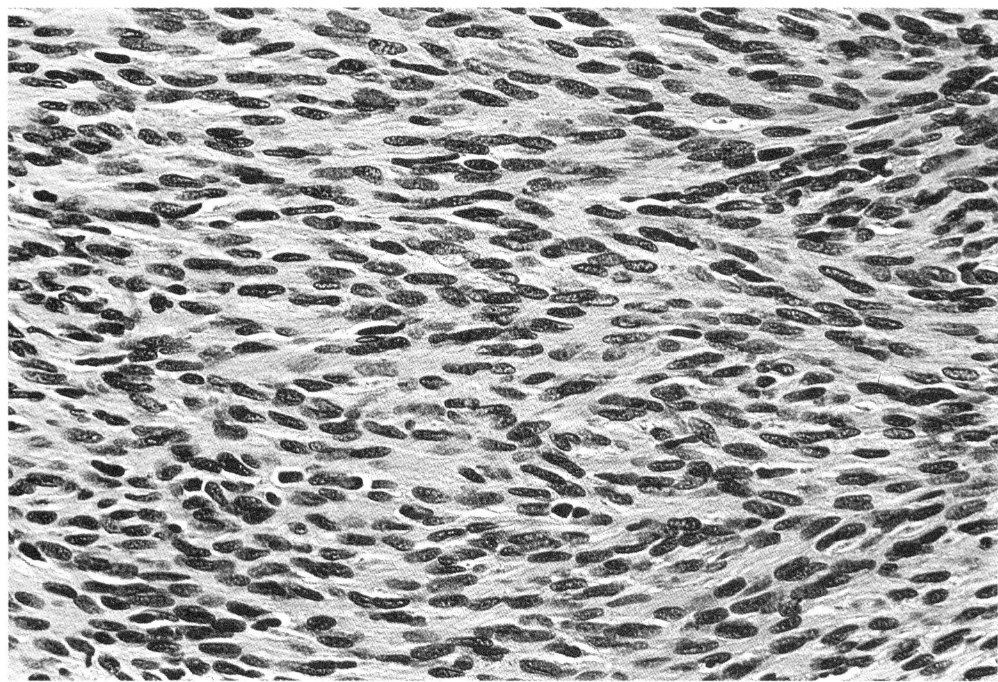

**FIGURE 30–75.** Cellular schwannoma consisting of differentiated Schwann cells without mitotic activity.

### Epithelioid Schwannoma

Schwannomas consisting predominantly or exclusively of epithelioid Schwann cells have been described by Kindblom et al.[144] Like conventional schwannoma they develop as a circumscribed or encapsulated mass in the superficial soft tissues.[144,165] The tumor is composed of small rounded schwann cells arranged singly, in small aggregates, or in cords within a collagenous or partially myxoid stroma (Fig. 30–79). Areas of conventional schwannoma may be seen in some tumors. The epithelioid schwann cells are small and rounded with sharp cytoplasmic borders and occasionally intranuclear cytoplasmic (pseudo) inclusions. Although occasional atypical cells are seen, they seem to represent a degenerative change, as these tumors virtually always lack mitotic figures and have low proliferative activity as measured by Ki67 immunostaining.[144] The cells may be associated with dense collagen cores forming irregular collagen rosettes similar to those seen in the neuroblastoma-like schwannoma. Immunohistochemistry, electron microscopy, or both are helpful, if not essential, for establishing the diagnosis. Virtually all cells strongly express S-100 protein (Fig. 30–80A); immunostains for type IV collagen outlines a latticework of basement membrane material around individual cells and groups of cells (Fig. 30–80B). The combination of these two stains is highly suggestive of the diagnosis as few tumors co-express these two antigens to this degree. Electron microscopy shows that the cells resemble differentiated Schwann cells. Of the few cases reported, the behavior has been uniformly benign.

The differential diagnosis of these lesions includes notably epithelioid forms of MPNST. Although the two bear some similarity, epithelioid forms of MPNST should be diagnosed only when the constitutent cells are cytologically malignant. Most have large nuclei with prominent macronuclei reminiscent of malignant melanoma.

## NEUROFIBROMATOSIS 2 (BILATERAL ACOUSTIC NEUROFIBROMATOSIS)

Neurofibromatosis 2 is a far rarer disease than NF1, affecting 1 in 50,000 persons. Like NF1, this disease is inherited as an autosomal dominant trait with a high rate of penetrance (95%). The NF2 gene is a tumor suppressor gene located on chromosome 22, which encodes a 595 amino acid member of the moesin-ezrine-radixin cytoskeleton-associated proteins. Variously known as "merlin" or "schwannomin," the protein localizes to the motile portions (e.g., ruffled borders) of the cell. Most cases of NF2 are associated with inactivating mutations of the allele, resulting in absence of the gene product merlin (see below) in the tumors.[132,133,140,141,145,146,154,166,170,172,175] Curiously, a significant but small number of cases of NF2 and sporadic schwannomas have either no NF2 inactivation or in-

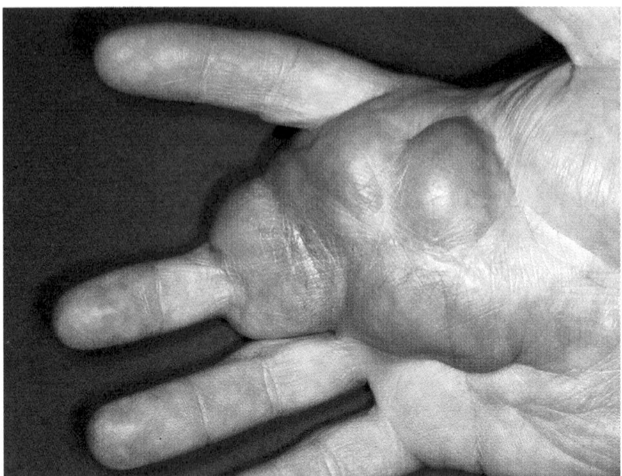

**FIGURE 30–76.** Plexiform schwannoma.

activation of only one allele. The mechanism of oncogenesis in these cases is less clear; it has been suggested that they have undetectable mutations[166] or alternative pathways of merlin inactivation.[143]

The onset of NF2 is usually during adolescence or early adult life, with the development of tinnitus or hearing loss due to the presence of bilateral acoustic schwannomas, which usually affect the vestibular portion of the VIII nerve (Table 30–5). Café au lait spots and neurofibromas are rare or absent in this form of neurofibromatosis. In addition to acoustic schwannomas, other central nervous system tumors occur commonly, including schwannomas of other cranial nerves, meningioma, ependymoma, and glioma. Approximately one-half to two-thirds of patients with NF2 also develop cutaneous schwannomas, but it appears that patients with multiple schwannomas in the absence of bilateral acoustic schwannomas, so-called schwannomatosis, have a disease different from NF2 (see schwannomatosis).

Histologically, the schwannomas occurring in NF2 are fundamentally no different from those that occur sporadically. Although there does not appear to be any malignant transformation of NF2-related schwannomas, the patients nonetheless experience significant morbidity and mortality from this disorder. Because of the critical location of many of these tumors in the cranium or spinal cord, patients may succumb to the space-occupying effects of their tumors.

**TABLE 30–5 DIAGNOSTIC CRITERIA FOR NEUROFIBROMATOSIS 2**

**Definite NF2**
- Bilateral vestibular schwannoma (VS) *or*
- Family history of NF2 (first degree relative) *plus*
  - Unilateral VS at age <30 years or
  - Any two of the following: meningioma, glioma, schwannoma, juvenile posterior subcapsular lelenticular opacities/juvenile cortical cataract

**Presumptive or probable NF2**
- Unilateral VS at age <30 *plus* at least one of following: meningioma, glioma, schwannoma, or juvenile posterior subcapsular lenticular opacities/juvenile cortical cateract *or*
- Multiple meningiomas (two or more) plus (1) unilateral vestibular schwannomas at age <30 years *or* (2) one of the following: glioma, schwannoma, or juvenile posterior subcapsular lenticular opacities/juvenile cortical cataract

From Gutman MD, Aylsworth A, Carley J, et al. The diagnostic evaluation and multidisciplinary management of neurofibromatosis 1 and neurofibromatosis 2. JAMA 278:51, 1997.

## SCHWANNOMATOSIS

The entity of multiple schwannomas, or "schwannomatosis,"[148] has been variously considered an attenuated form of NF2 or a completely different disease.[116,157,163,164] As a result of standardization of criteria for the diagnosis of NF2 complemented by better imaging techniques to detect acoustic nerve tumors and buttressed by genetic testing, it has been possible to identify a distinct group of patients with multiple schwannomas of peripheral, cranial nerves, or spinal nerves who never develop bilateral acoustic schwannomas and who rarely have affected family members.[139,163] Such patients are now regarded as having a separate disorder, designated "schwannomatosis" (Table 30–6).

Clinically, this disease affects men and women equally. They present with multiple, often painful schwannomas involving skin or soft tissue. In some patients the schwannomas have a striking segmental distribution. Although some develop schwannomas related to cranial or spinal nerves they do not de-

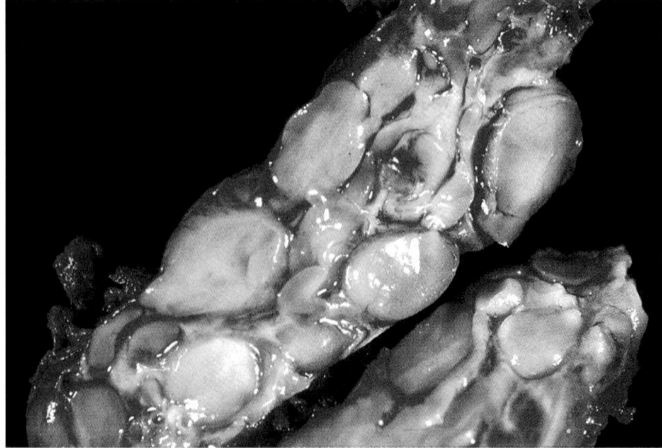

**FIGURE 30–77.** Gross specimen of a plexiform schwannoma illustrating a multinodular pattern of growth.

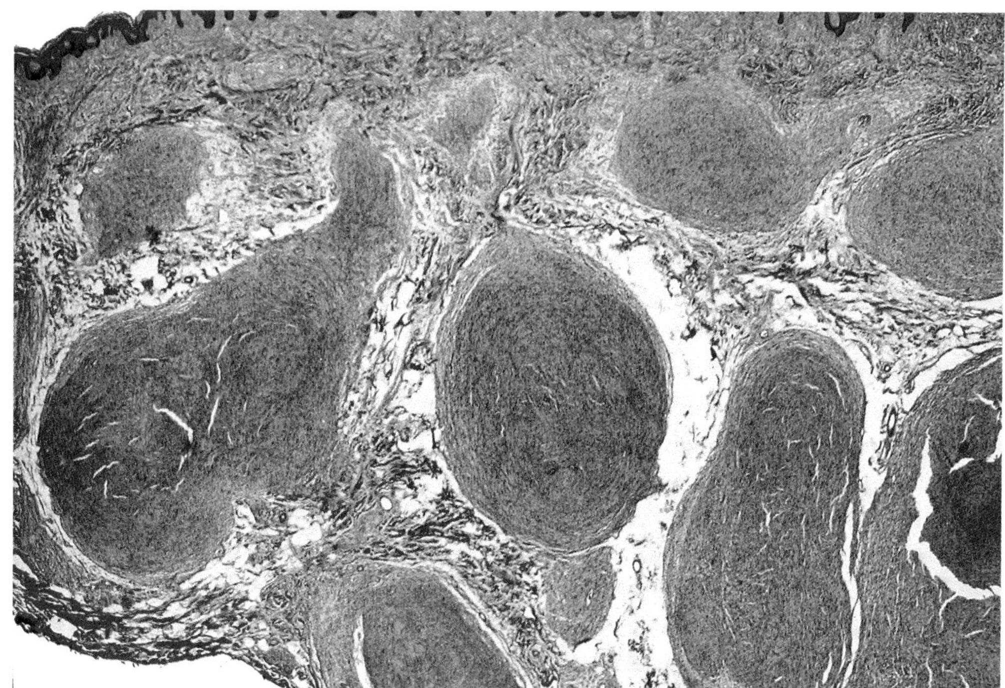

**FIGURE 30–78.** Plexiform schwannoma involving the dermis.

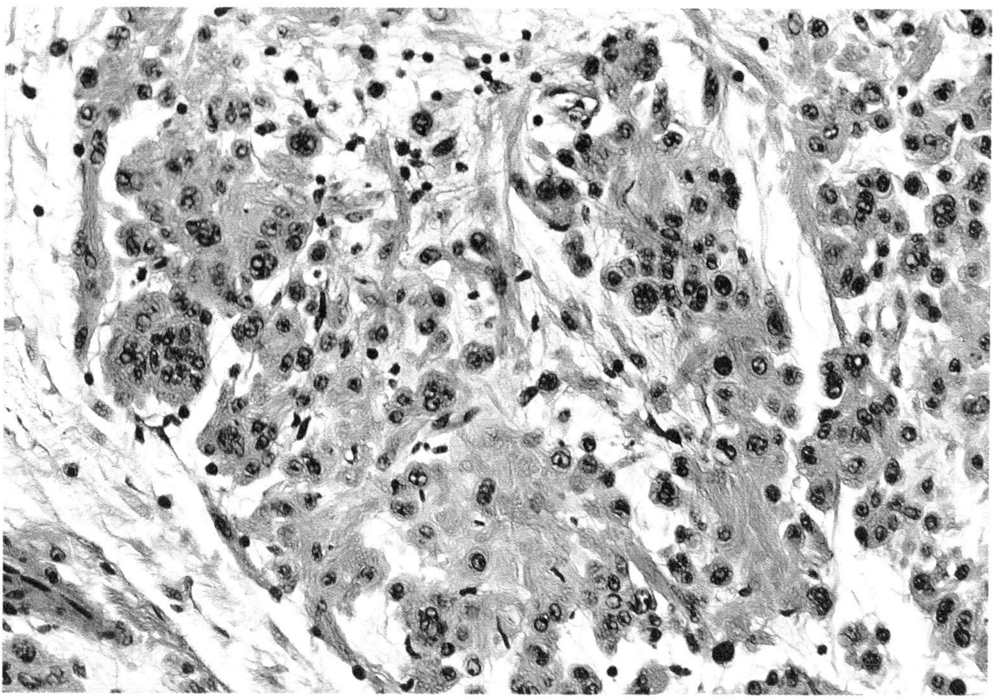

**FIGURE 30–79.** Epithelioid schwannoma. Note the cohesive nests of bland epithelioid cells.

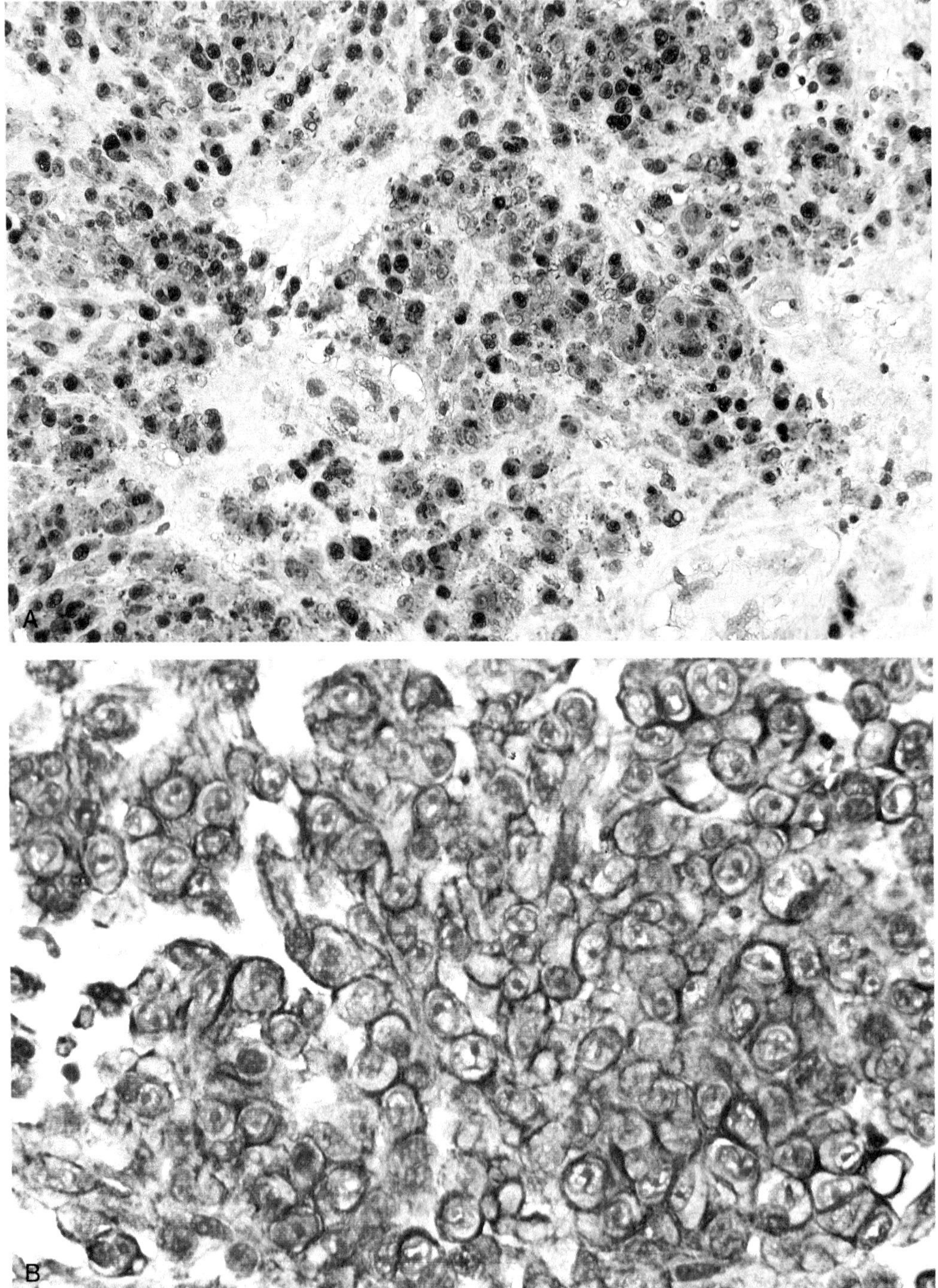


**FIGURE 30–80.** Epithelioid schwannoma with S-100 protein (**A**) and intricate pattern of type IV collagen immunoreactivity (**B**). The latter is reflective of basal lamina material surrounding the cells.

**TABLE 30–6 DIAGNOSTIC CRITERIA FOR SCHWANNOMATOSIS**

**Definite schwannomatosis**
- Two or more pathologically proven schwannomas *plus*
- Lack of radiographic evidence of vestibular nerve tumor at age >18 years

**Presumptive or probable schwannomatosis**
- Two or more pathological proven schwannomas without symptoms of VIII nerve dysfunction at age >30 years *or*
- Two or more pathologically proven schwannomas in an anatomically limited distribution (single limb or segment of the spine) without symptoms of VIII nerve dysfunction at any age.

From Jacoby LB, Jones D, Davis K, et al. Molecular analysis of the NF2 tumor-suppressor gene in schwannomatosis. Am J Hum Genet 61:1293, 1997.

velop the various other forms of central nervous system tumors seen in NF2, such as astrocytoma, ependymoma, and meningioma.

By molecular analysis, nearly all patients have NF2 mutations in their tumors but not in normal tissues, indicating that they have somatic rather than germ cell line mutations of this allele.[139] Some of these patients appear to be somatic mosaics, thereby accounting for the segmental distribution of the tumor. Of interest is the fact that in some patients each of the tumors harbors different NF2 mutations, leading to speculation that a second gene may be involved in this disease. The effect of such a gene would be to render the NF2 locus more suspectible to mutational damage such that a variety of somatic NF2 mutations might evolve.

## MELANOTIC SCHWANNOMA

A rare form of pigmented neural tumor commonly arising from the sympathetic nervous system was described in 1932 by Millar[189] as *malignant melanotic tumor of ganglion cells,* discussed under the term *melanocytic schwannoma* by Fu et al.,[183] and recently redesignated *psammomatous melanotic schwannoma* by Carney,[180] who noted its association with Carney syndrome. Based on our experience and that in the literature, the lesion is a distinctive neoplasm of adult life that differs significantly from classic schwannoma despite the similarity in names.[180–190] The tumor arises commonly from the spinal or autonomic nerves near the midline. However, a number of cases have been reported in the stomach and in bone and soft tissues. Unusual sites include the heart, bronchus, liver, and skin.[180] More than half of patients with the tumor have evidence of *Carney syndrome,* which includes *myxomas* of the heart, skin, and breast, *spotty pigmentation* due to lentigenes, blue nevus, and the distinctive epithelioid blue nevus,[181] *endocrine overactivity* manifested by Cushing's disease (pigmented nodular adrenal disease), acromegaly (pituitary adenoma), or sexual precocity (Sertoli cell tumor). The tumor typically develops at an earlier age (average 22.5 years) in patients with Carney syndrome than in those without the syndrome (average 33.2 years).[180] About 20% of patients with melanotic schwannomas have multiple tumors, and in such patients there is an even higher probability that other manifestations of Carney's complex will be present.[180] The symptoms related specifically to the tumor depend on its location and rate of growth, but most commonly they are pain and neurologic symptoms in the affected part. Most striking is a case reported by Fu et al.,[183] in which the patient lost sympathetic nerve function in the ipsilateral lower extremity. In one of our cases, a well encapsulated lesion of the mediastinum, the patient was symptom-free, and the lesion was detected on a routine chest radiograph.

The tumors are usually circumscribed or encapsulated and vary from black-brown to gray-blue. It is often difficult to make out cellular detail in these tumors because of the heavy pigment deposits. Usually there are at least focal areas with little or no pigment, so the character of the cells can be evaluated. The cells vary in shape from polygonal to spindled and blend gradually from one to another (Figs. 30–81, 30–82). This feature, coupled with the ill-defined borders of the cytoplasm, often imparts a syncytial quality to the tumors that is somewhat reminiscent of a schwannoma. Likewise, the nuclei may display clear intranuclear cytoplasmic (pseudo) inclusions characteristic of schwann cells. Nuclear chromatism may be marked, and the nucleoli are often prominent. Occasionally there is vague palisading or formation of whorled structures such that the tumor resembles a schwannoma or neurofibroma. Ganglion cell differentiation has not been observed in our material, although in the original case attenuated cytoplasmic processes led Millar[189] to conclude that the tumor cells were ganglionic. Psammoma bodies are present in most cases in our experience. Carney reported them in all of his cases but noted that extensive sampling was necessary to document them in some.[180]

The melanin pigment may be coarsely clumped or finely granular and varies from area to area. Tinctorially it is similar to dermal melanin and stains positively with the Fontana stain and negatively for iron and periodic acid-Schiff (PAS). In this respect it differs from the faint and focal pigment seen in conventional schwannomas, which is neural melanin. On immunohistochemical studies, these tumors strongly express S-100 protein and a melanoma-associated antigen (HMB-45). Ultrastructurally there is a spectrum of maturation, including premelanosomes and mela-

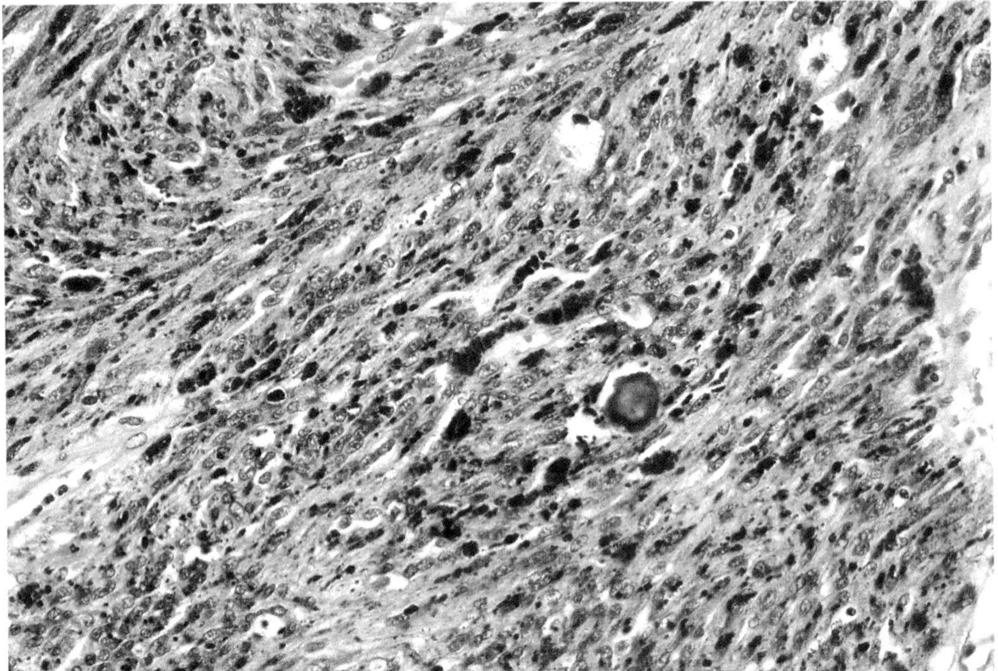

**FIGURE 30–81.** Melanotic schwannoma with heavy melanin deposits and a psammoma body.

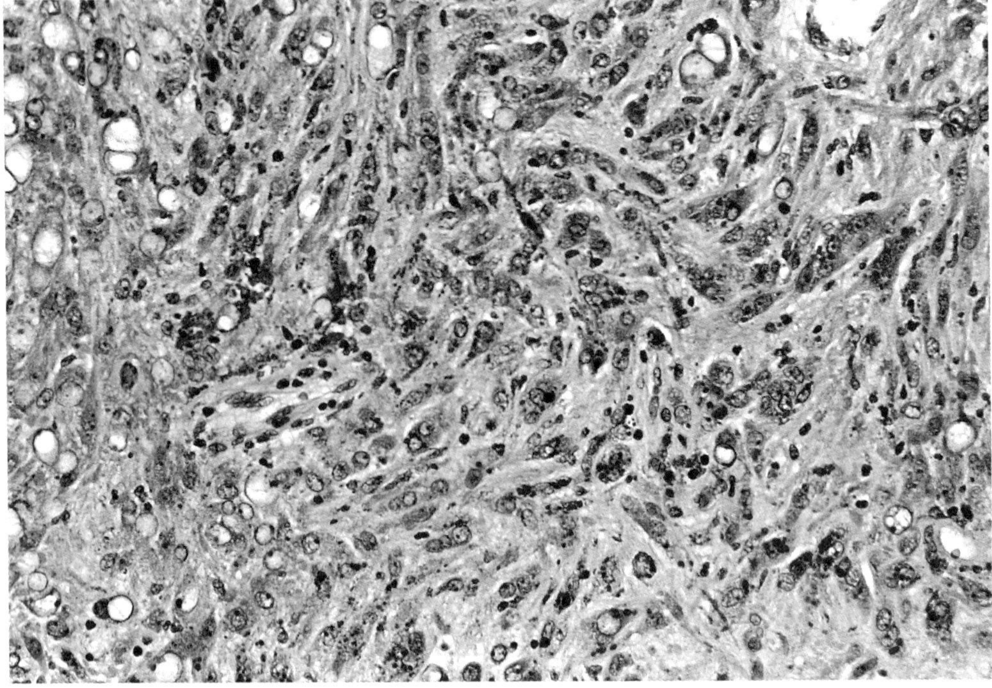

**FIGURE 30–82.** Melanotic schwannoma with a less pigmented area.

nosomes, which leads one to conclude that the pigment is synthesized by the tumor cell. Except for the presence of melanosomes, the cells resemble Schwann cells with elaborate cytoplasmic processes that interdigitate or spiral in the manner of mesaxons.

The biologic behavior of these tumors is difficult to predict, and metastases can occur in the absence of overt malignant features. Neither tumor size nor ploidy predicts malignant behavior. In the past it was thought that most of these lesions had a benign, indolent course. Metastases, for example, were reported in only 13% of patients with melanotic schwannomas and Carney syndrome.[180] A review of approximately 60 cases in the literature has disclosed metastasis in 26%.[190] Furthermore, only 53% of patients followed for more than 5 years were disease-free, suggesting that long-term follow up is required to fully judge metastatic risk. Although all may be potentially malignant, we have designated those with significant mitotic activity as malignant melanotic schwannomas. When metastases develop they too abound with melanin pigment.

The usual problem in differential diagnosis is distinguishing this tumor from a metastatic malignant melanoma. Primary melanotic schwannomas usually do not have the degree of nuclear atypia or mitotic activity expected in a metastatic melanoma. The peculiar syncytial quality of the cells and particularly the psammomatous calicification are important features of melanotic schwannoma that metastatic melanomas lack.

## PERINEURIOMA

Perineurioma is a rare soft tissue tumor composed of cells resembling those of the normal perineurium.[191,195,197,202,204] It was first described in 1978 by Lazarus and Trombetta[201] on the basis of ultrastructural findings. Although several cases were published after that early description,[191,192,203,211] the tumor has been slow to gain wide recognition and acceptance because of the lack of clear-cut criteria for diagnosis. Tumors that have been identified as perineuriomas have had varying histologic appearances and considerable overlap with neurofibroma, indicating that it is not possible to recognize these tumors consistently on the basis of light microscopy alone. Rather, it requires light microscopy with ultrastructural or immunohistochemical confirmation.[195] There are two distinct forms of perineurioma: the intraneural perineurioma and the extraneural or soft tissue perineurioma.

### Intraneural Perineurioma

Intraneural perineurioma is a rare condition that has recently been shown to be an intraneural clonal proliferation of perineurial cells. Many lesions formerly diagnosed as "localized hypertrophic neuropathy" are probably examples of intraneural perineurioma. The lesions usually develop in a nerve in the upper extremity of a young individual. Characteristic signs and symptoms include muscle weakness, denervation changes seen by electromyography, and in extreme cases muscle atrophy. The affected nerve displays a fusiform expansion extending several centimeters in length (Fig. 30–83). On cross section the entire nerve is expanded by the formation of tiny "onion bulbs" consisting of concentric layers of perineurial cells ensheathing a central axon and schwann cell (Fig. 30–84). The perineurial cells occasionally spin off the sheath and communicate with adjacent ones. Because of the highly organized nature of these lesion, the usual impression is that of a reactive or reparative process. However, with immunostains for epithelial membrane antigen (EMA) and S-100 protein, the striking preponderance of perineurial cells becomes readily apparent. Immunostains for EMA highlight the ensheathing perineural cells, leaving the central portion of the "onion bulb" devoid of staining. With S-100 protein or neurofilament protein immunostains, highlighting schwann cells and axons respectively, a reverse staining pattern is noted (Fig. 30–85).

The question of whether the intraneural perineurioma is a true neoplasm or an unusual reactive process has been debated and is reflected in the variety of terms employed for this lesion. The best evidence to date suggests that they are indeed neoplastic. These lesions are associated with significant proliferative activity [as reflected by MIB-1 and proliferating cell nuclear antigen (PCNA) immunoreactivity] and clonal alterations of chromosome 22.[194]

The behavior of intraneural perineurioma has been uniformly benign, with neither recurrences nor metastases reported. Nonetheless, there are no standard guidelines for the treatment of this condition. MRI has been successful in determining the extent of nerve involvement,[206] but because complete resection with nerve grafting does not completely restore function[199] this option should be carefully weighed against the degree of nerve compromise.

### Soft Tissue (Extraneural) Perineurioma

Soft tissue perineuriomas, although more common than their intraneural counterpart, are still relatively rare.[197,205,207,210] They occur in adults, and none has been associated with either NF1 or NF2. They have been associated with alternations of chromosome 22 but not the NF2 locus per se.[197,200] Of the reported cases they appear to occur primarily in the superficial soft tissues particularly of the hand. Only rare exam-

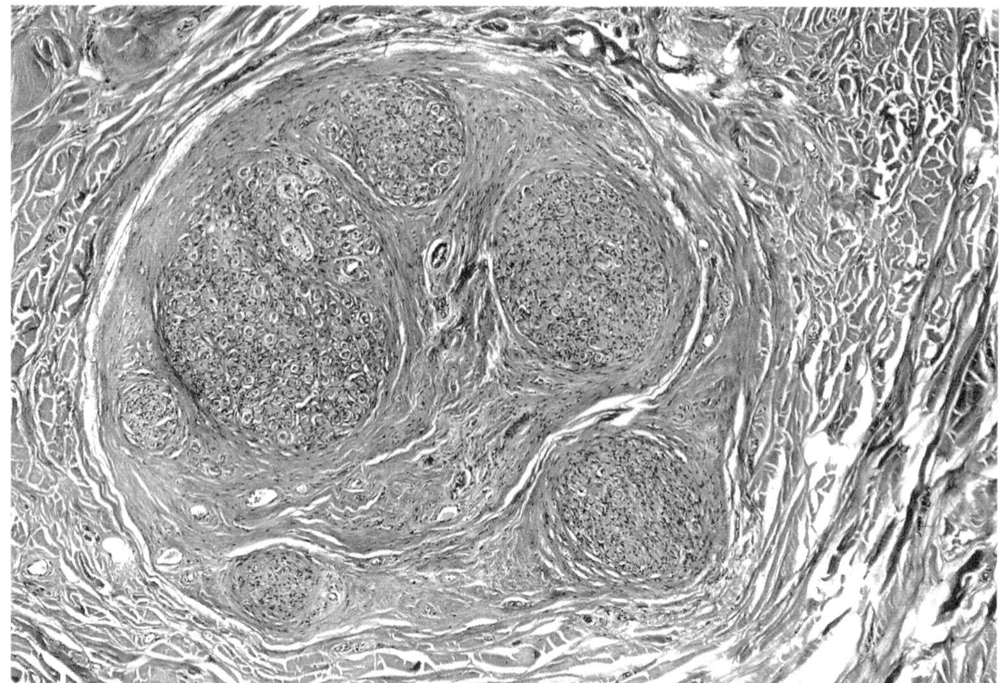

**FIGURE 30–83.** Intraneural perineurioma.

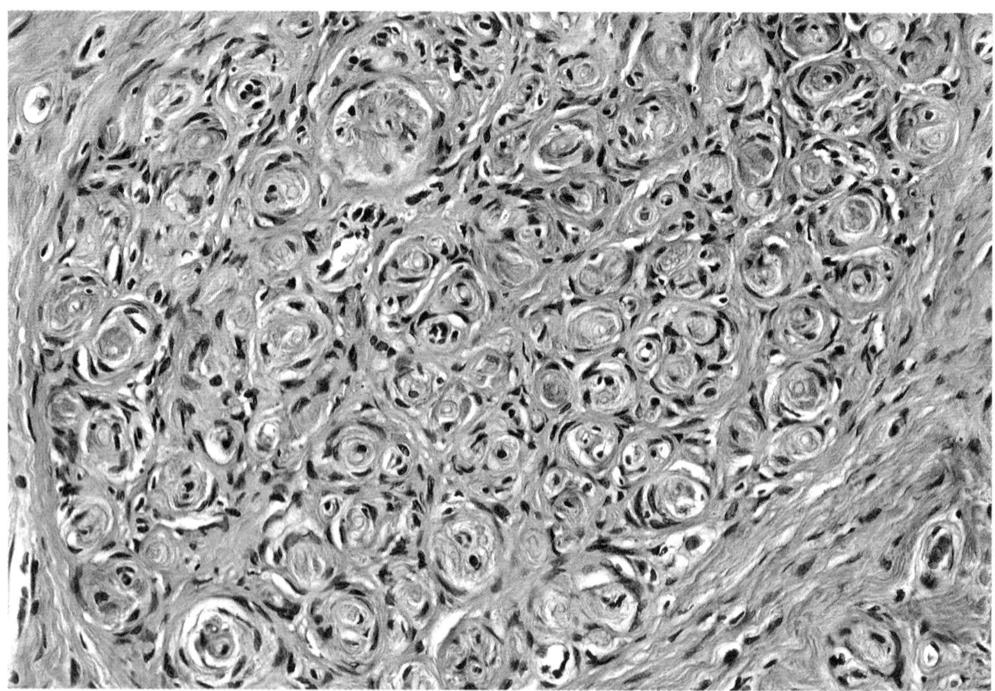

**FIGURE 30–84.** Intraneural perineurioma with "onion bulb" expansion of the nerve sheath.

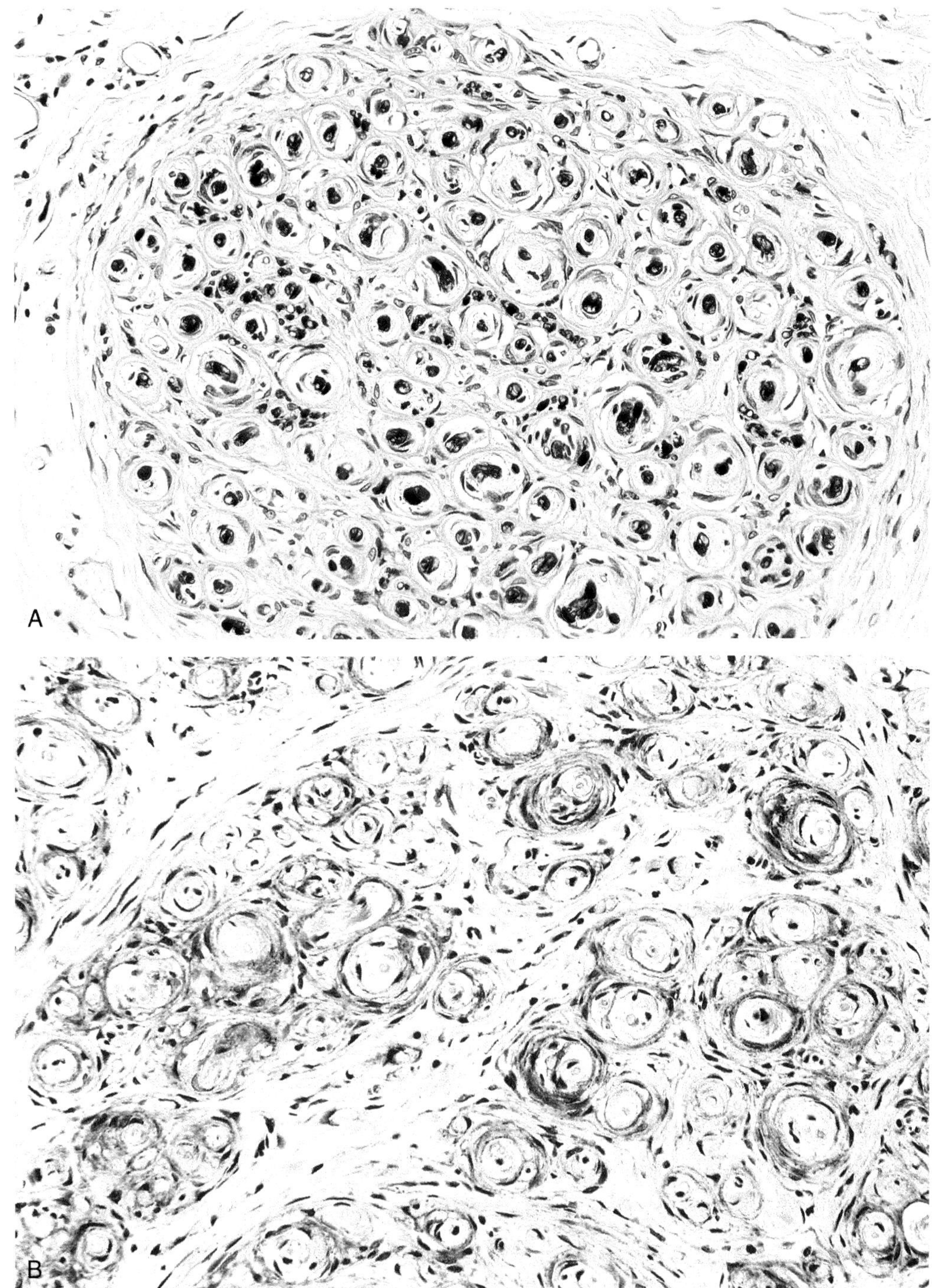


**FIGURE 30–85.** Intraneural perineurioma. S-100 protein immunostain decorates Schwann cells but not perineurial cells (**A**). Epithelial membrane antigen (EMA) immunostain shows reverse pattern with positively staining perineurial component and no staining of Schwann cells (**B**).

ples have been reported in deep sites such as the abdominal cavity.

The lesions are circumscribed white masses ranging in size from 1 cm to nearly 20 cm. The most common appearance of a soft tissue perineurioma is a spindle cell lesion composed of slender fibroblast-like cells arranged in a vague fascicular or storiform pattern or sometimes forming whorls (Fig. 30–86). The lesions vary greatly in their cellularity. Cellular lesions with little stroma and a storiform pattern closely resemble dermatofibrosarcoma protuberans or benign fibrous hitiocytoma. In lesions with a prominent myxoid stroma, the perineurial cells are widely separated with their myriad processes appearing as delicate, hair-like extensions (Fig. 30–87). In highly collagenized perineuriomas the slender processes may appear to ramify within or dissect through the matrix. Ossification occurs rarely.[204]

An unusual variant of soft tissue perineurioma has been described by Fetsch and Miettinen as *sclerosing perineurioma*.[196] These lesions occurred primarily in young men and affect the hand exclusively. Unlike the foregoing forms of perineurioma the cells in these lesions range from spindled to distinctly rounded and are arranged in cords, trabeculae, and chains. In addition to EMA immunoreactivity, nearly half of the lesions also expressed smooth muscle or muscle-specific actin. The differential diagnosis includes a variety of epithelioid lesions (e.g., epithelioid hemangioendothelioma, adnexal tumors) and fibrosing lesions (fibroma of the tendon sheath, calcifying fibrous pseudotumor, fibrosing tenosynovial giant cell tumor). Because it is a recently recognized tumor, it is likely that many perineuriomas were previously diagnosed as fibrous histiocytoma, dermatofibrosarcoma protuberans, neurofibroma, or meningioma. Although it is occasionally possible to suspect the diagnosis of a perineurioma when distinct whorls are present in a tumor or when a presumed "neurofibroma" fails to stain for S-100 protein, the diagnosis must be confirmed with immunohistochemistry. NF2 deletions have been observed in this tumor.[205]

Definitionally, all benign perineuriomas are EMA-positive and S-100 protein-negative (Fig. 30–88). Because EMA staining in perineuriomas is membranous, it may be difficult to appreciate if the cell processes are widely separated. Consequently high power examination of the tumor may be necessary. Type IV collagen and laminin, two components of the basement memberane, also decorate the abundant basal lamina elaborated by the perineurial cell. This finding, however, is not specific for perineurial tumors and is seen in a variety of other soft tissue lesions, particularly conventional schwannomas. Electron microscopic identification may be used in lieu of immunohistochemistry, although we seldom find it necessary. The attributes of perineurial cells include slender, nontapered processes containing large num-

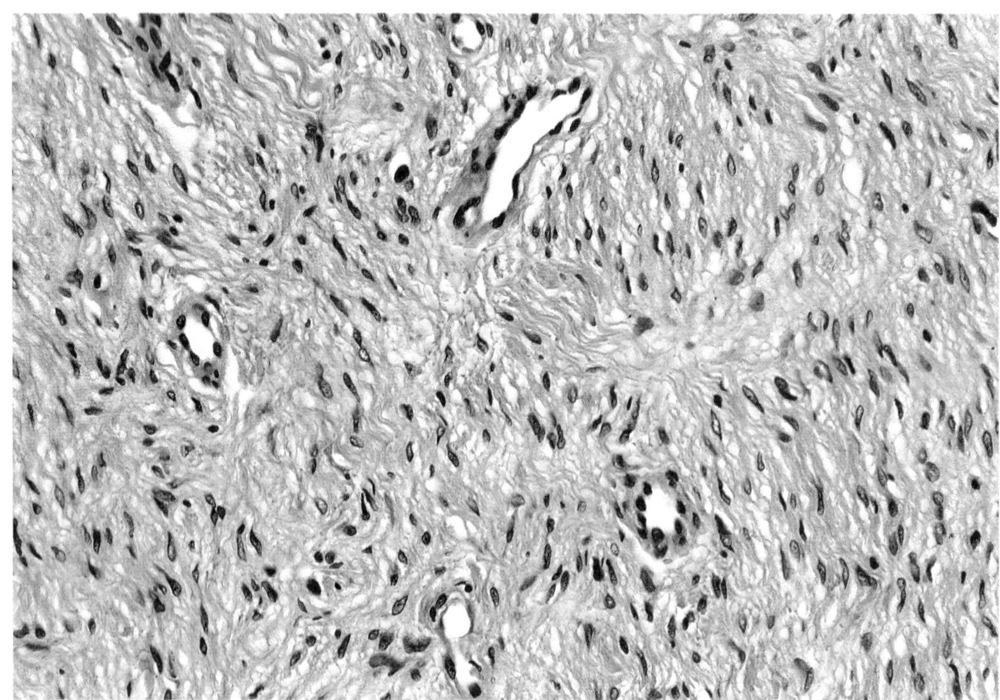

**FIGURE 30–86.** Extraneural (soft tissue) perineurioma with slender perineurial cells arranged in short fascicles.

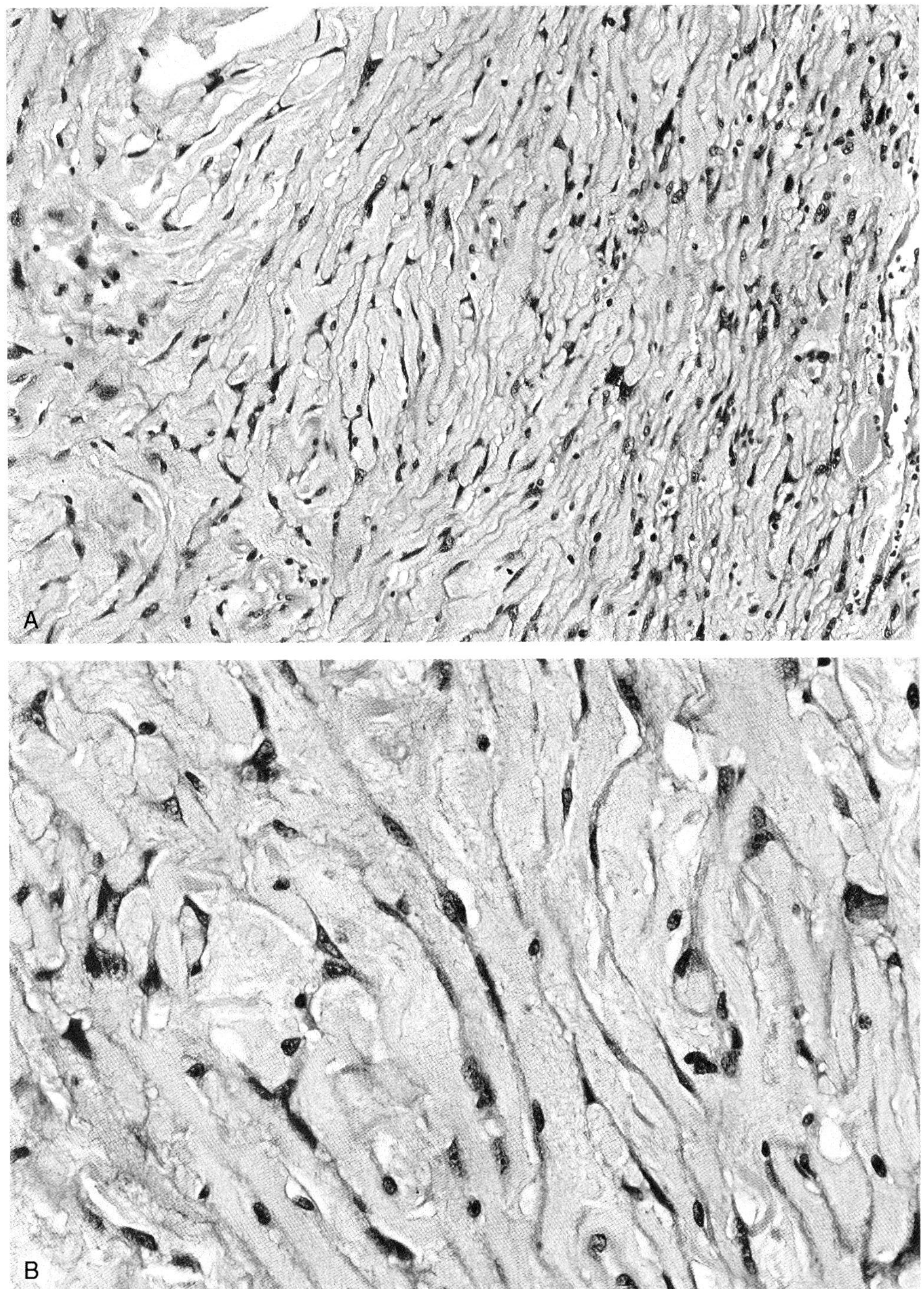


**FIGURE 30–87.** (**A**) Extraneural (soft tissue) perineurioma with cytologic atypia. (**B**) High power view illustrating slender cell processes. The tumor behaved in an aggressive fashion.

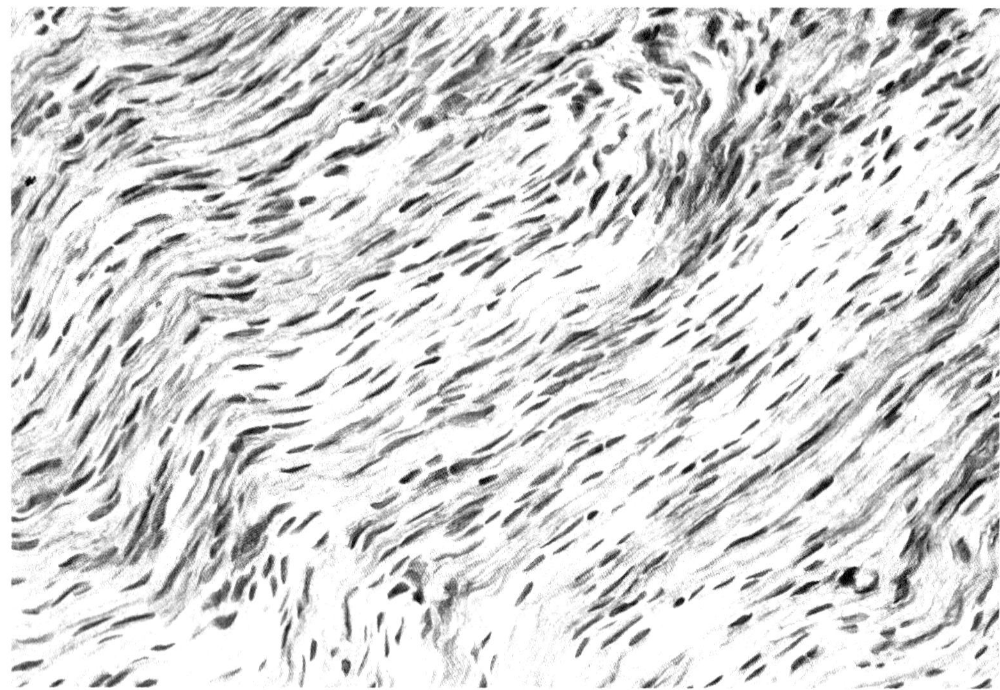

**FIGURE 30–88.** EMA immunostaining of a perineurioma.

bers of pinocytotic vesicles and partial investment with basal lamina (Figs. 30–89, 30–90). Ribosome lamellar complexes were described in one perineurioma by Dhimes et al.[193]

All the perineuriomas reported have had an excellent course without recurrence or metastasis. Conservative excision is considered adequate therapy.

### Malignant Perineurioma

By convention, the term perineurioma is used to refer to lesions with histologically benign or, at most, minimally atypical features. Hirose et al. demonstrated that a small subset of otherwise typical malignant peripheral nerve sheath tumors (<5%) display perineurial features.[198] Until these lesions are studied more extensively these lesions are diagnosed as "perineurial malignant peripheral nerve sheath tumor," or "malignant peripheral nerve sheath tumor with perineurial differentiation," rather than as "malignant perineurioma."

## GRANULAR CELL TUMOR

The granular cell tumor is a benign neural tumor characterized by large granular-appearing eosinophilic cells.[212–229,231–248,251–256,259–269,272–282] Although originally considered a muscle tumor by Abrikossoff[212] in 1926, its close association with nerve and immunohistochemical characteristics firmly identify it as a neural lesion, but it is sufficiently distinctive to be separated from neurofibroma and schwannoma. Older terms for this tumor are *granular cell myoblastoma,*[215] *granular cell neuroma, granular cell neurofibroma,* and *granular cell schwannoma.*[232] Reactive granular lesions consisting of collections of granular-appearing histiocytes at sites of trauma comprise a separate, unrelated entity[270] (see Chapter 13).

Granular cell tumors are fairly common; for example, Vance and Hudson[280] found one case among 346 surgical specimens. The granular cell tumor generally occurs as a small, poorly circumscribed nodule that may be solitary or multiple and always pursues a benign clinical course. Malignant granular cell tumor is a well established but rare entity, with fewer than 100 reported cases. It is discussed separately below.

Granular cell tumors occur in patients of any age but are most common in those in the fourth, fifth, and sixth decades of life; they are rare in children.[258] It is about twice as common in women as in men. In some but not all reviews, African American patients outnumber Whites by a considerable margin.[236] In one series, for example, two-thirds of the patients were African American. As a rule, the lesion manifests as a solitary painless nodule located in the dermis or subcutis and less frequently in the submucosa, smooth muscle, or striated muscle (Fig. 30–91). It is also found in the internal organs, particularly the larynx, bronchus, stomach, and bile duct. Usually the nodule is smaller than 3 cm and has been noted for less than 6 months.

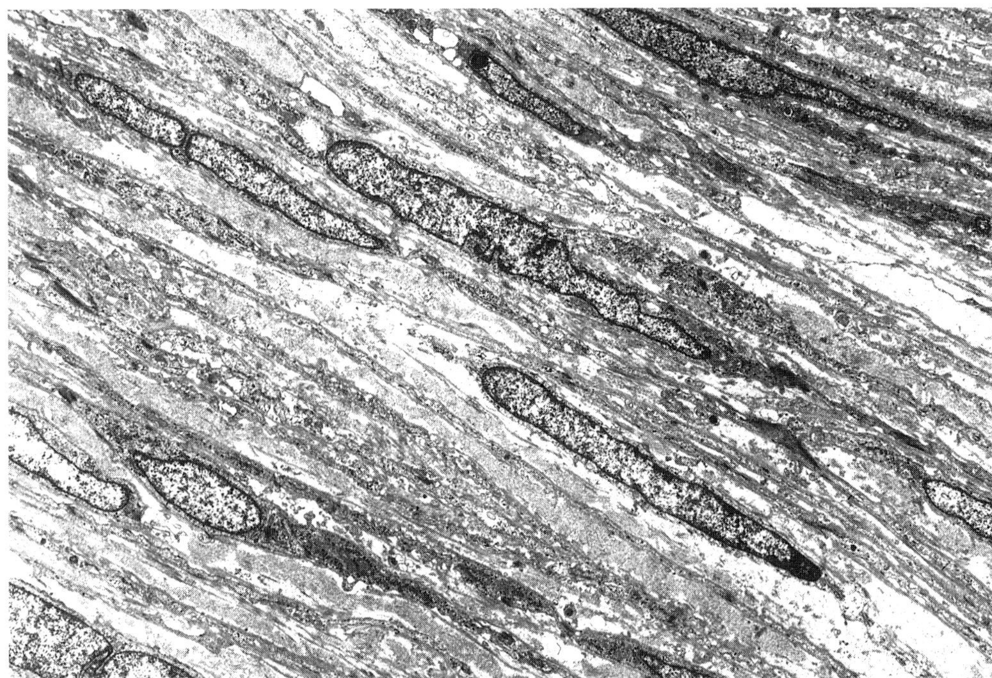

**FIGURE 30–89.** Electron micrograph of a perineurioma showing slender elongated cells invested with basal lamina.

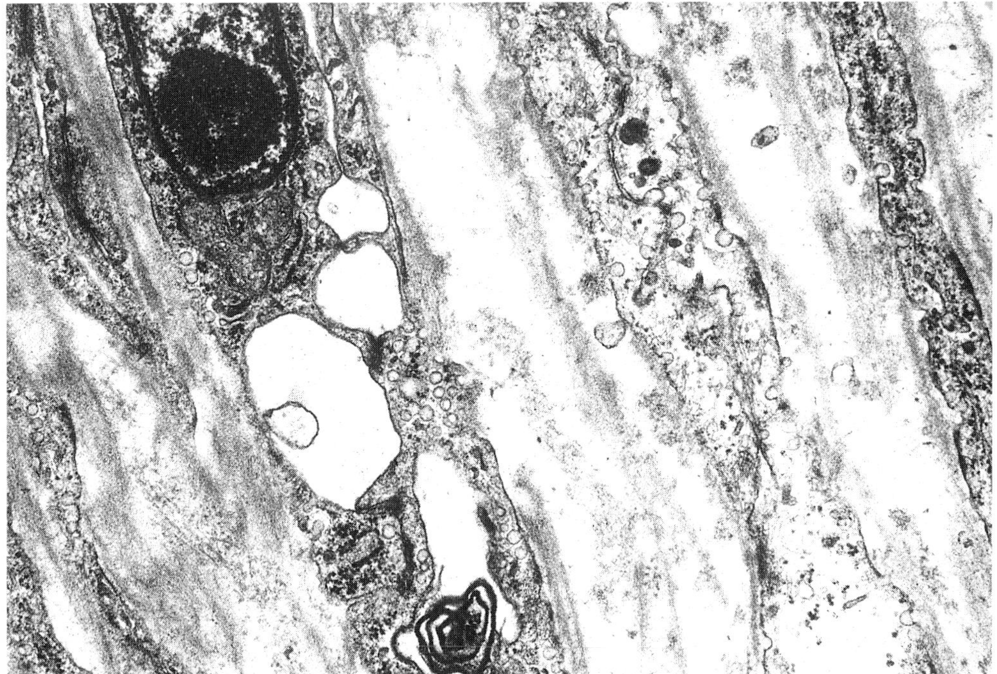

**FIGURE 30–90.** Electron micrograph of a perineurioma. A process of the perineurial cell is invested in basal lamina and has surface-oriented pinocytotic vesicles.

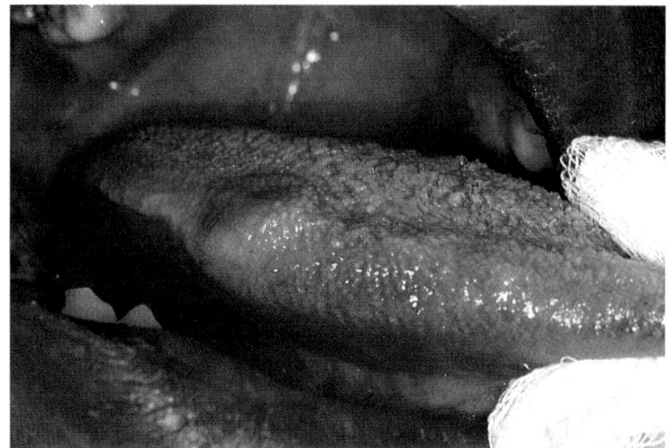

**FIGURE 30–91.** Granular cell tumor of the tongue.

Approximately 10–15% of patients with a granular cell tumor have lesions at multiple sites, frequently involving the subcutis, submucosa, and one or more visceral structures. The number of lesions varies greatly from patient to patient, but as many as 50 nodules have been counted in some cases. Multiple lesions may appear synchronously or over a period of many years. Increased familial incidence is extremely uncommon, but it has been reported.[220,254] There is no record in the literature or in our cases of multiple (or solitary) granular cell tumors occurring in a patient with the stigmata of neurofibromatosis.

## Pathologic Findings

Granular cell tumors tend to be poorly circumscribed; consequently, the tumor is usually removed together with portions of the adjacent adipose tissue or muscle. In most cases the nodule measures less than 3 cm in diameter, and on cut section it is characteristically pale yellow-tan or yellow-gray. About two-thirds of the nodules are located in the dermal, subcutaneous, or submucosal tissues. Some are associated with marked acanthosis or pseudoepitheliomatous hyperplasia of the overlying squamous epithelium, a striking feature that has repeatedly caused this process to be mistaken for squamous cell carcinoma (Fig. 30–92).[240] Another important, histogenetically significant feature is the close association between granular cells and peripheral nerves. Frequently the granular cells encompass small nerves or replace them almost entirely and are recognizable only by the residual neurites that can be demonstrated with the Bodian method or similar silver preparations (Fig. 30–93). At times clusters of granular cells are also surrounded by circumferentially arranged spindle cells in the manner of perineurium.

The cells of granular cell tumor are rounded, polygonal, or slightly spindled in character, with nuclei ranging from small and dark to large with vesicular chromatin (Figs. 30–94 to 30–97). Mild to moderate amounts of nuclear atypia may be seen but in and of itself is not indicative of malignancy (Fig. 30–96). The eosinophilic cytoplasm is fine to coarsely granular. The granules, representing phagolysosomes are strongly PAS-positive, disastase-resistant (Fig. 30–97). Smaller cells containing coarse particles that are strongly PAS-positive are interspersed between the granular cells (interstitial cells, angulate body cells).

The growth pattern varies; the cells tend to be disposed in ribbons or nests divided by slender fibrous connective tissue septa or in large sheets with no particular cellular arrangement. Older lesions frequently exhibit marked desmoplasia, and some of these can be identified only by the presence of a few scattered nests of granular cells in a dense mass of collagen.

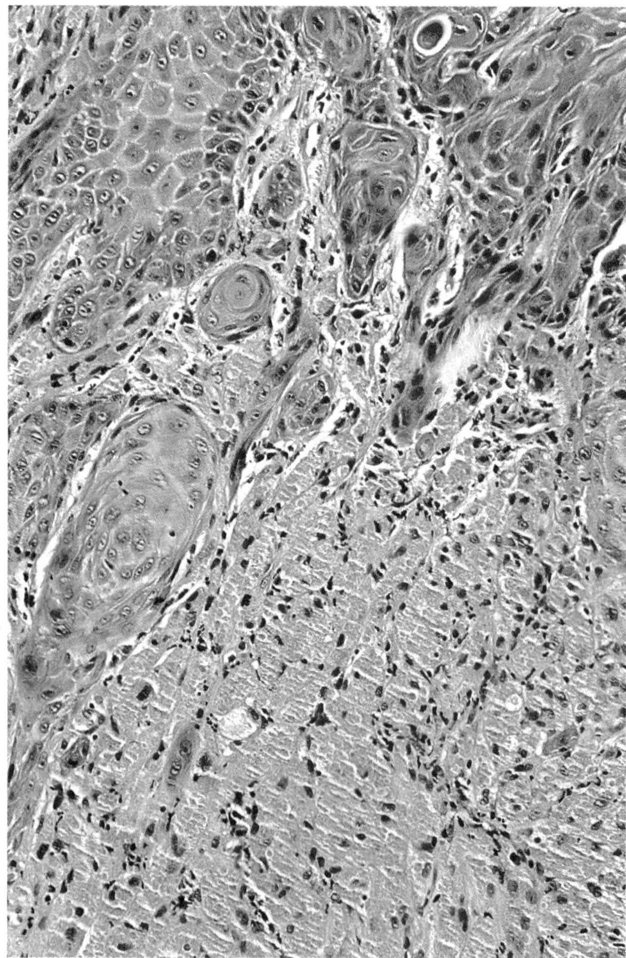

**FIGURE 30–92.** Granular cell tumor with pseudoepitheliomatous hyperplasia of the overlying skin.

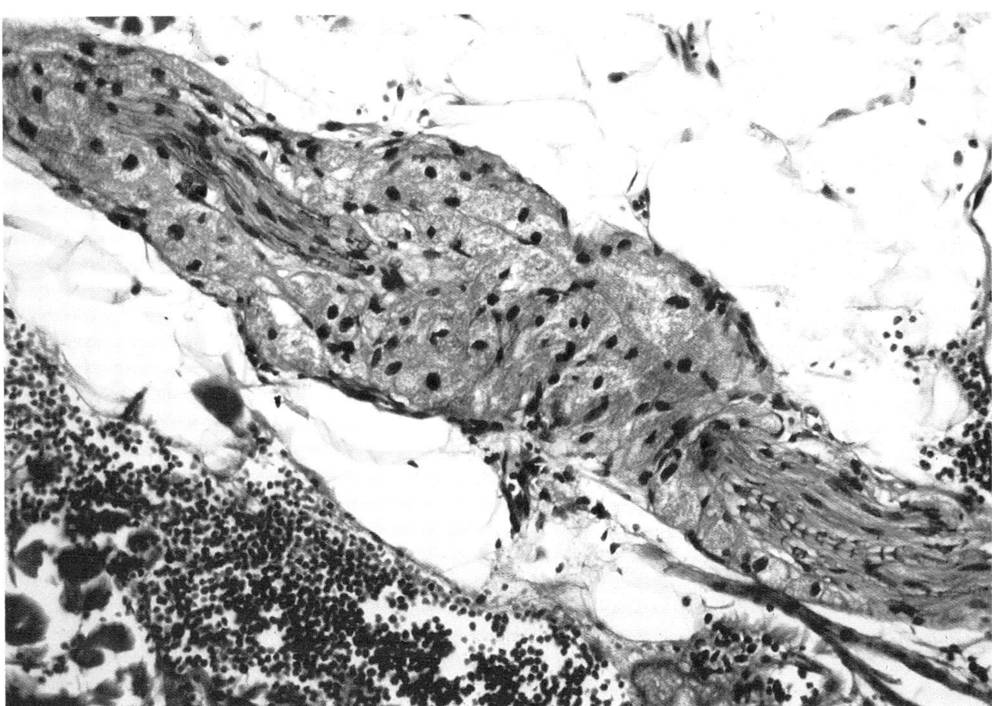

**FIGURE 30–93.** Granular cell tumor involving a small nerve.

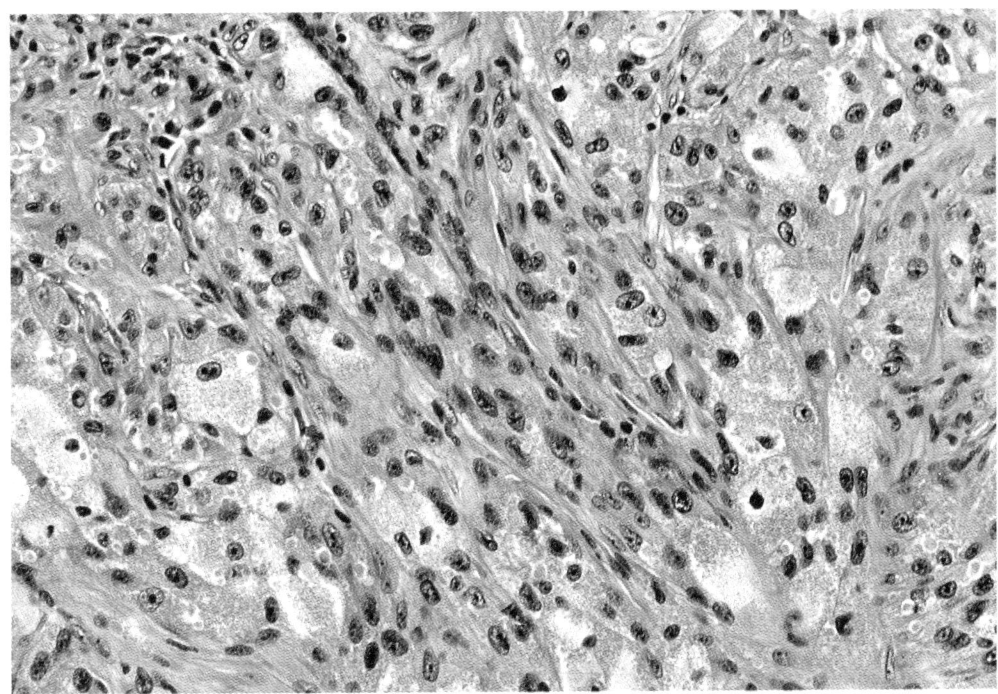

**FIGURE 30–94.** Granular cell tumor with spindled and rounded tumor cells.

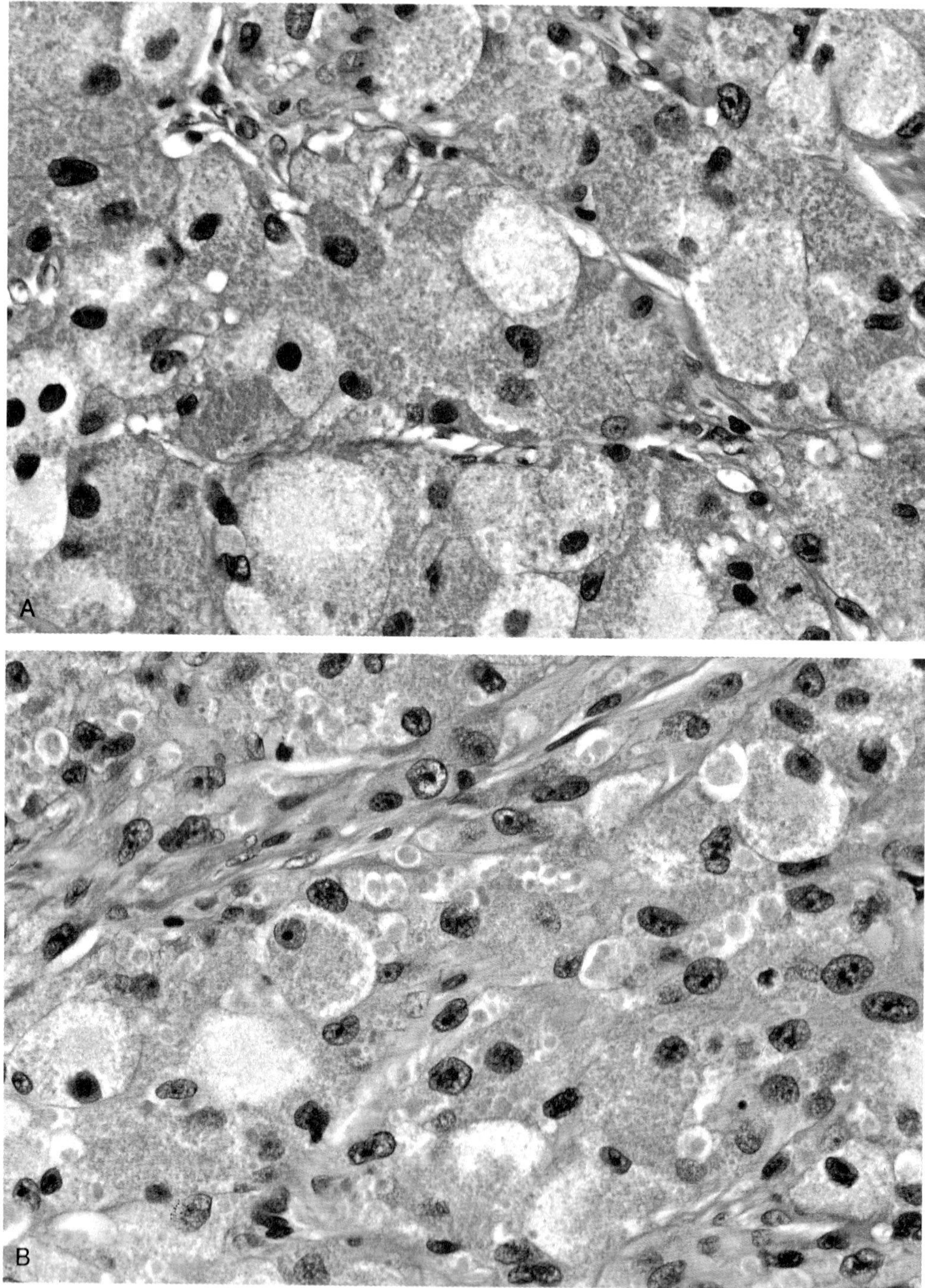


**FIGURE 30–95.** Granular cell tumor with a range of nuclear appearances. Some nuclei are small and dark (**A**), and others are larger with a vesicular nuclear chromatin pattern (**B**).

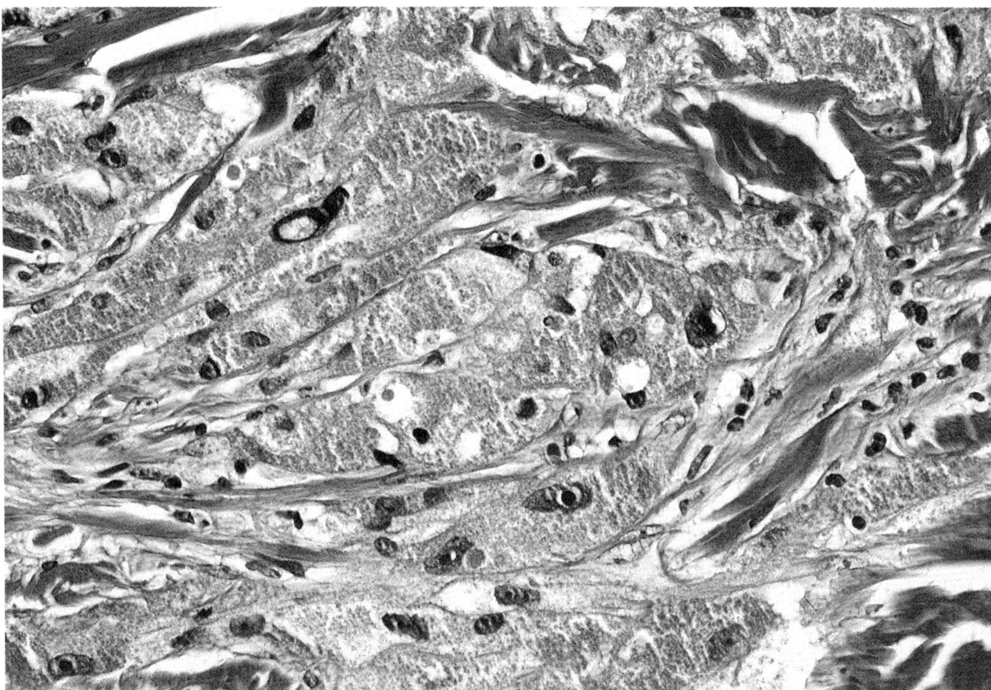

**FIGURE 30–96.** Benign granular cell tumor with atypical cells. This change does not per se indicate malignancy.

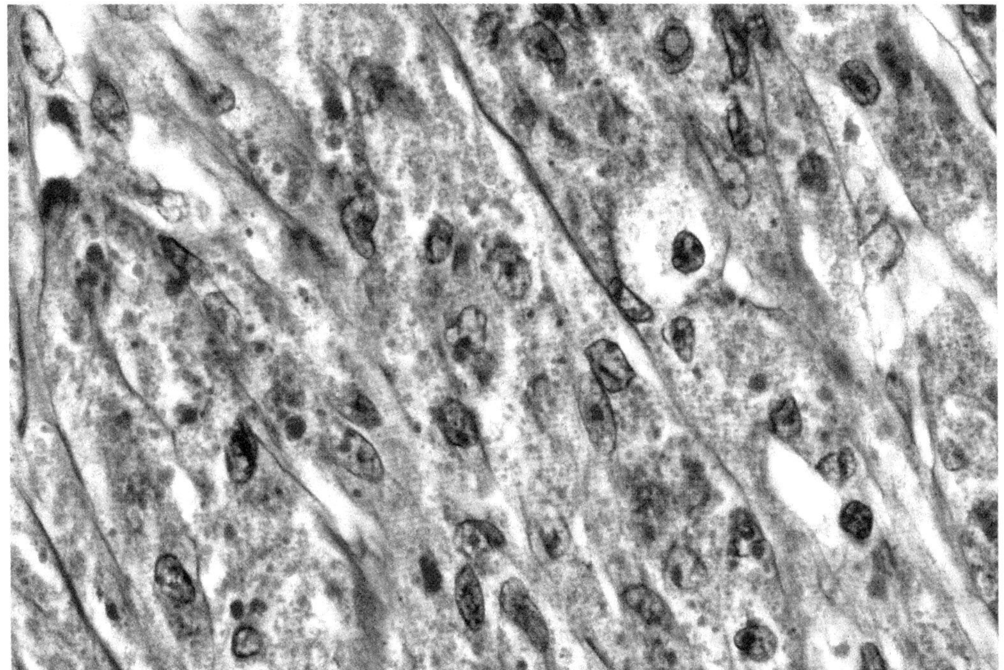

**FIGURE 30–97.** Periodic acid-Schiff (PAS)-positive diastase-resistant bodies in a granular cell tumor.

Less frequently the granular cells involve or replace the musculature; they grow along the muscle fibers or even seem to extend within the sarcolemmal sheath. They may also be found in smooth muscle tissue, in fibrous tissue such as tendons, fascia, or ligaments, and rarely in small lymphoid aggregates or even lymph nodes, a feature that should not be confused with lymph node metastasis (Fig. 30–98).

Unlike the cells of most benign and malignant muscle tumors, the granular cells do not contain glycogen. There are several detailed accounts of the various histochemical staining reactions in the early literature.[213,216,218,271,282]

Immunohistochemical investigation reveals positive staining for S-100 protein (Fig. 30–99), neuron-specific enolase, laminin, and various myelin proteins. Because the characteristic granules are lysosomal in nature, it is not surprising that granular cell tumors are also strongly positive for the panmacrophage antigen CD68 (Kp1).[230,245] The cells do not react with antibodies for neurofilament proteins or glial fibrillary acidic protein (GFAP).[253,255,270] According to Nathrath and Remberger,[256] the interstitial cells stain for myelin protein.

Ultrastructurally, the granular cell tumor shows a highly characteristic picture that has been well described in the literature. Typically the intracellular granules consist of membrane-bound, presumably autophagic vacuoles that contain cellular debris, including mitochondria, myelin figures, fragmented rough endoplasmic reticulum, and, according to some authors, myelinated and nonmyelinated axon-like structures (Figs. 30–100, 30–101). There are also small interstitial cells with angulated bodies containing packets of parallel microtubules (Fig. 30–102), microfilaments, and lipid material as well as cells with multiple cytoplasmic processes, partly surrounded by incomplete basal laminae.

## Differential Diagnosis

A number of benign mesenchymal tumors have a granular appearance. Differentiation from other benign neoplasms should not be difficult. The coarsely granular cytoplasm and the absence of cross-striations and glycogen distinguish the benign granular cell tumor from rhabdomyoma; the absence of lipid droplets distinguishes it from hibernoma and fibroxanthoma. Awareness of the frequent association of dermal granular cell tumor and marked acanthosis of the overlying squamous epithelium prevents a mistaken diagnosis of squamous cell carcinoma.

Finally, reactive changes that occur in association with surgical trauma or other types of injury may simulate a benign granular cell tumor. The granular cells in these lesions tend to be associated with inflammatory elements and areas of necrosis, and they stain more intensely with the alcian blue stain and PAS preparation (see Chapter 13). This tumor also lacks the ribbon-like or nest-like cellular orientation of granular cell tumors. Sobel and Churg,[270,271] who gave a detailed account of this lesion, found

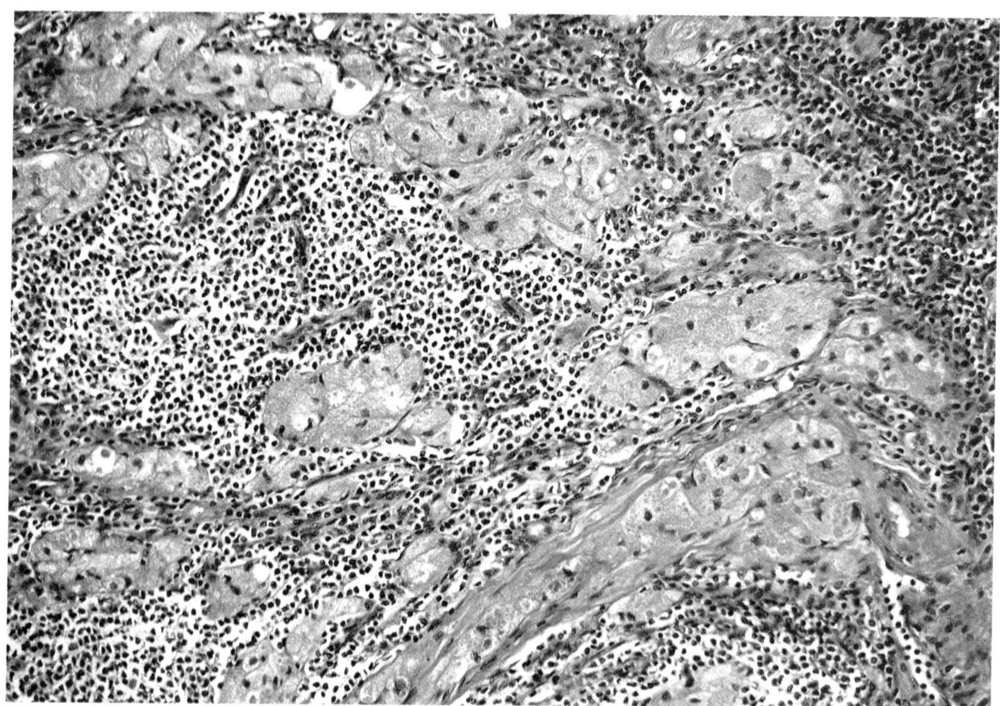

**FIGURE 30–98.** Granular cell tumor involving a lymph node.

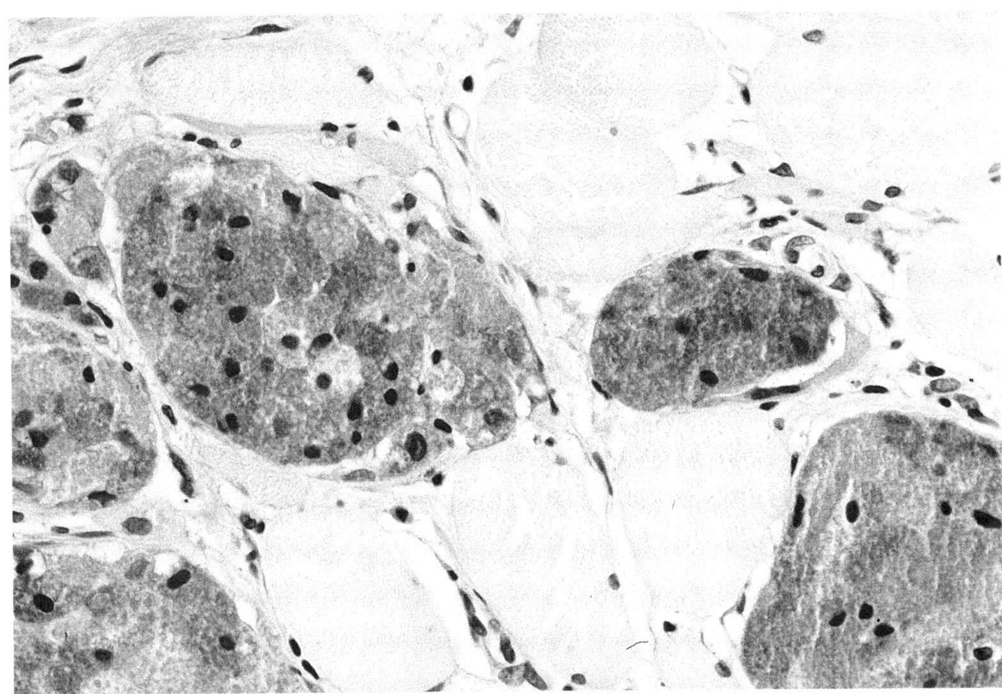

**FIGURE 30–99.** S-100 protein immunoreactivity in a granular cell tumor.

several such lesions in scars from cesarean sections. A massive granular reaction to epoxy polymer may also occur near prosthetic joint replacements (see Chapter 13).

## Discussion

Early accounts uniformly regarded the granular cell tumor as one with muscle differentiation. This view gradually changed with the observation that nerves and neuromas occasionally display granular changes. In addition, electron microscopy and immunohistochemistry showed that the granular cell tumor had schwannian features. The tumors stain positively for S-100 protein, myelin proteins (PO and P2), and myelin-associated glycoproteins, suggesting that the granules are myelin or myelin breakdown products[253,268] as was originally suggested by Fisher and Wechsler.[232] The angular bodies in the interstitial cells are not marked by antibodies to S-100 protein, but they are positive on staining with antibodies to myelin protein.[253] Excluding the malignant tumors, recurrence is rare. Of 92 cases reported by Strong et al.,[274] 6 recurred, one of them after 10 years. Hence local surgical excision is curative in nearly all cases.

## Malignant Granular Cell Tumor

Malignant granular tumors constitute fewer than 2% of all granular cell tumors. Ravich et al.[263] are usually credited with the first account of this entity. It occurred in the wall of the urinary bladder of a 31-year-old woman who died of metastatic disease 17 months after the tumor was removed surgically and diagnosed as a malignant granular cell tumor. Since their report, about 80 additional cases have been described,[214,240,278,279] including the largest series of 46 reported by Fanburg-Smith et al.[229]

In most respects malignant tumors are similar to benign ones except they are rarely encountered during childhood and tend to be, on average, larger than their benign counterpart. A history of long clinical duration and recent rapid growth has been observed in some cases, suggesting the possibility of malignant transformation from a preexisting benign granular cell tumor, analogous to the malignant transformation of neurofibromas.

Although in the earlier literature a variety of malignant soft tissue tumors were labeled malignant granular cell tumors (e.g., granular cell leiomyosarcoma), this diagnosis should be restricted to neoplasms that are histologically similar to benign granular cell tumors but that have a constellation of histologic features that portend an increased risk for metastasis.[229] Such features include necrosis, spindling, vesicular nuclei with prominent nucleoli, increased mitotic activity (>2 mitoses/10 HPF), high nucleocytoplasmic ratio, and pleomorphism. Tumors with three or more of these features are considered malignant and have an approximately 40% risk of causing death (Figs.

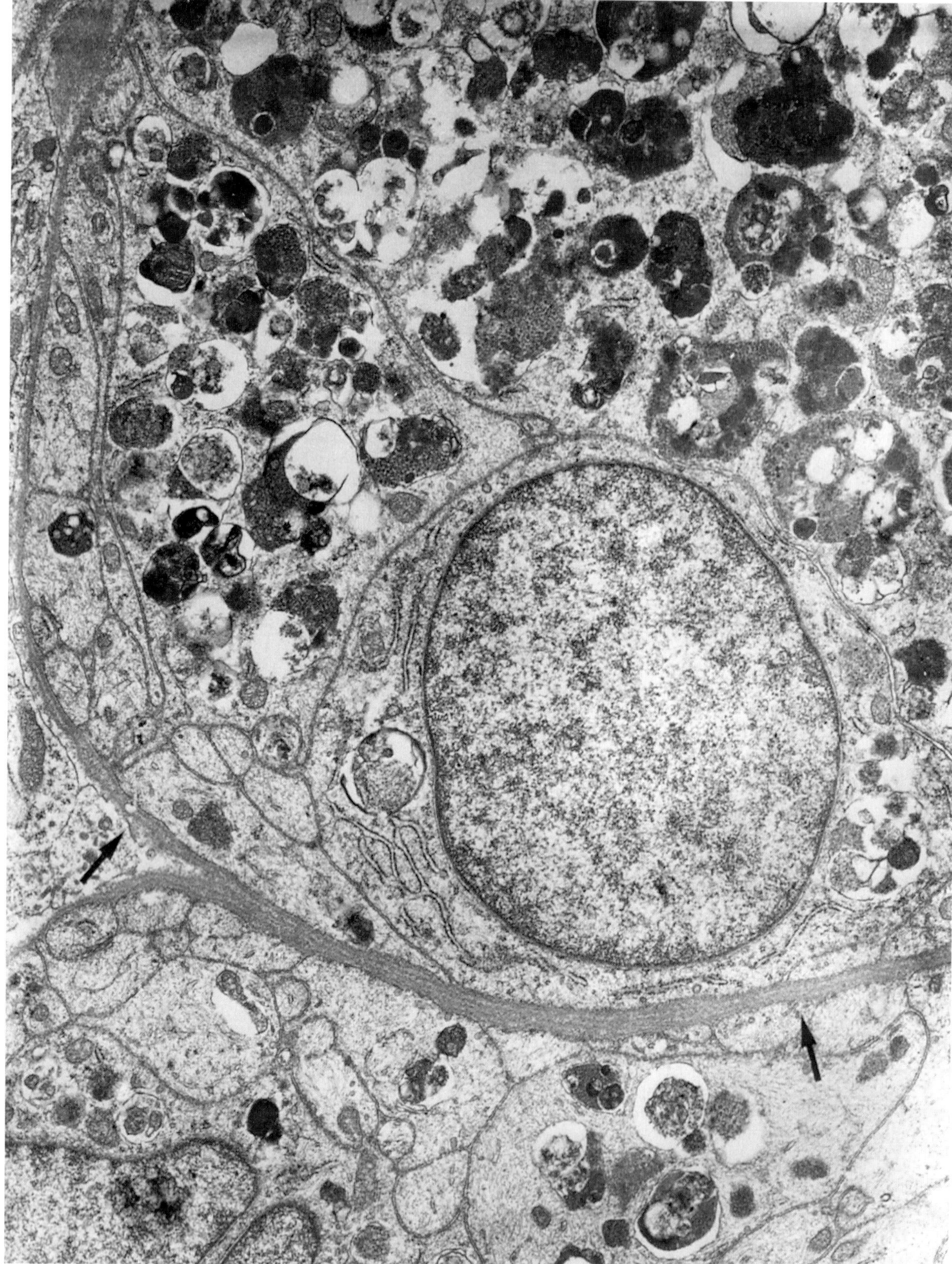

**FIGURE 30–100.** Ultrastructure of granular cell tumor. Large autophagic granules in the cytoplasm of the tumor cell are surrounded by a distinct basal lamina (arrows). (Courtesy of Dr. Zelma Molnar, Veterans Administration Hospital, Hines, IL.)

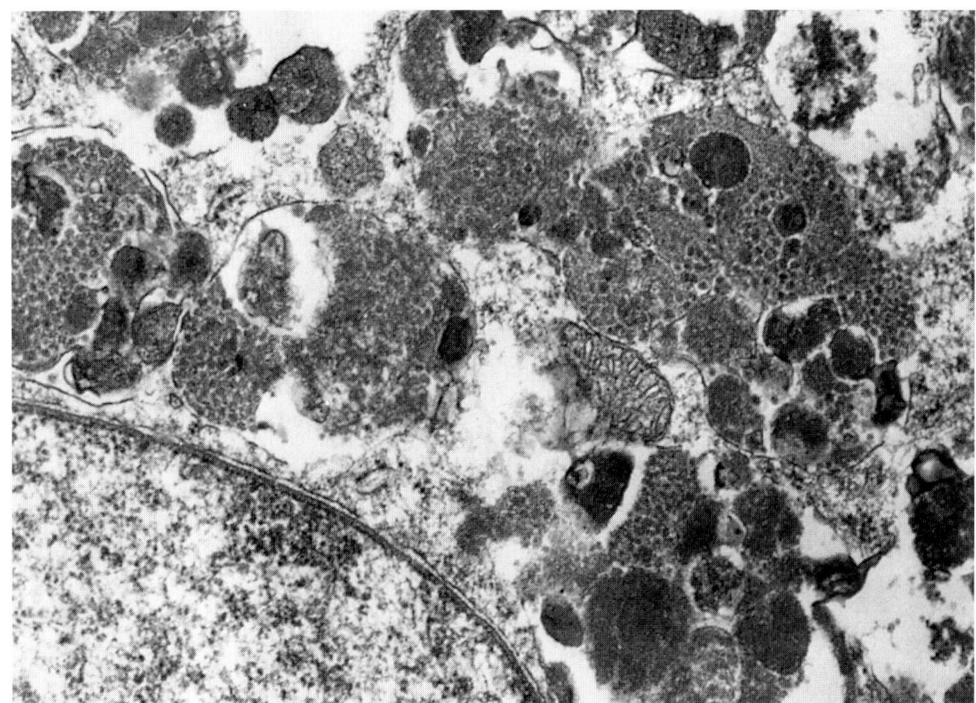

**FIGURE 30–101.** Large vacuoles containing finely granular structures and small masses of electron-dense material.

30–103, 30–104). Tumors with fewer than three features (termed "atypical granular cell tumor") have an excellent outcome with no metastases. This system provides a systematic approach to identifying lesions with a signficant risk of metastasis. When employing this system we usually require that features such as spindling and atypia be prominent in the tumor and not simply a focal change.

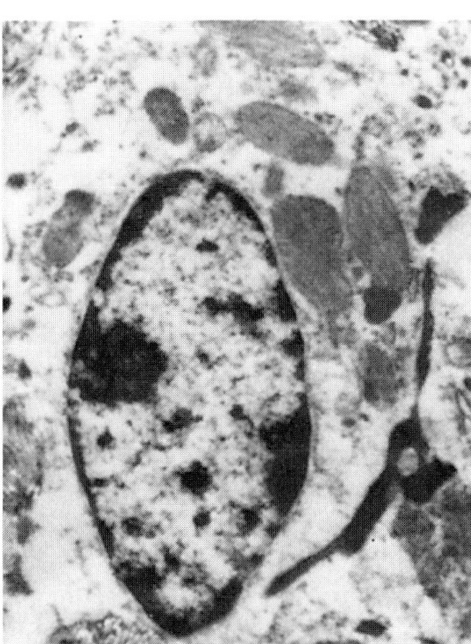

**FIGURE 30–102.** Angulated bodies in interstitial cell of a granular cell tumor. (×7800)

Frankly malignant granular cell tumors should be distinguished from other malignant tumors that display granular cytoplasm from time to time, such as leiomyosarcoma, malignant fibrous histiocytoma, and angiosarcoma.[249,250,257] It is useful to keep in mind that granular cell tumors, even malignant ones, usually originate in superficial soft tissues, and their granularity tends to be a diffuse, uniform change as contrasted with the focal granularity in other malignant lesions.

Typically the malignant form of granular cell tumor recurs before it metastasizes, usually within less than 1 year. Metastasis occurs through the lymphatics and bloodstream; and lymph node metastases and metastases to the lung, liver, and bone are common. The interval between excising the primary tumor and the appearance of metastasis is variable, but in most cases it takes several years before the metastatic lesions become apparent.

## CONGENITAL (GINGIVAL) GRANULAR CELL TUMOR

The term *congenital (gingival) granular cell tumor* and its synonyms *congenital epulis, congenital granular cell myoblastoma,* and *granular cell fibroblastoma* have been applied to a variant of the granular cell tumor that is indistinguishable in its structure and staining characteristics from this tumor but differs by its exclusive

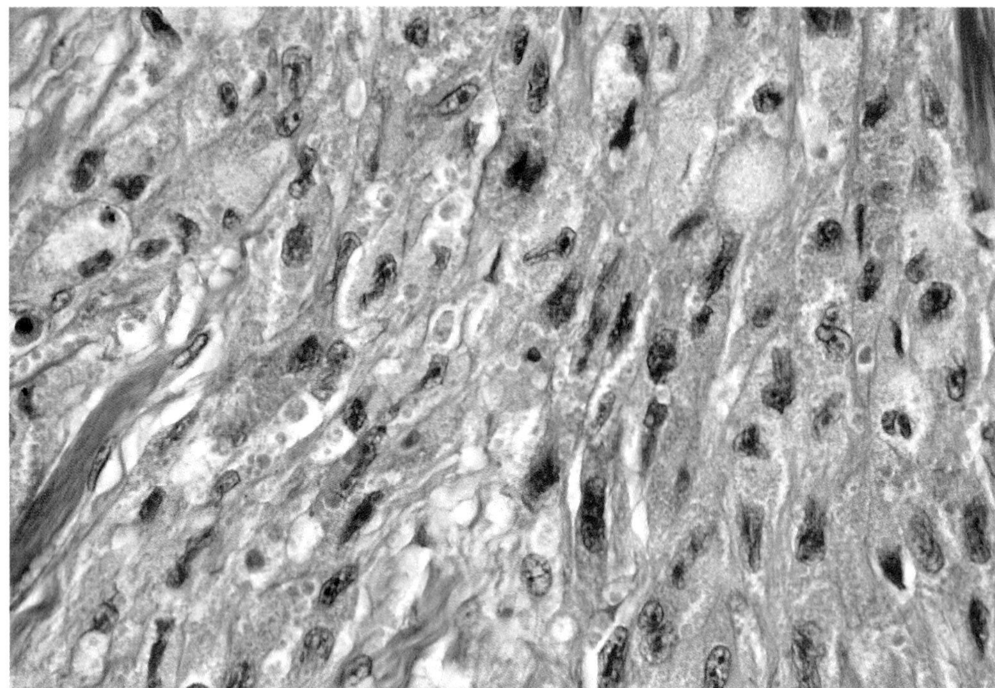

**FIGURE 30–103.** Malignant granular cell tumor with nuclear atypia, spindling, and prominent nucleoli.

occurrence in infants at or immediately after birth and by its characteristic location in the labial aspect of the dental ridge, with a predilection for the upper jaw.[283–295] It also differs from adult granular cell tumors by its prominent vascularity, the presence of scattered remnants of odontogenic epithelium, and the strong phosphatase activity of the tumor cells (Fig. 30–105). Moreover, it lacks interstitial cells with angulate bodies and does not show immunostaining for laminin or S-100 protein.[262,286,290] About 10% of these lesions are multiple, and approximately 90% afflict girls.[283,289,295] Characteristically, the condition manifests as a protruding, round or ovoid nodule covered by a smooth mucosal surface and firmly attached to the gum by a broad base or infrequently by a pedicle. Ulceration of the mucosa is uncommon, and microscopically there is no evidence of pseudoepitheliomatous hyperplasia of the overlying squamous epithelium.[289] Like other forms of granular cell tumor, the nodules are small, averaging 1–2 cm in greatest diameter.

There is usually no further growth after birth and no tendency toward local recurrence. In fact, even without therapy, most congenital granular cell tumors cease to grow or regress spontaneously. In Cussen and MacMahon's case,[284] for instance, the lesion almost completely disappeared after 4 months and could no longer be detected after 3 years. Lack et al.[284] reported that lesions treated later in the neonatal period were smaller and exhibited some evidence of involution. There is no record of a malignant counterpart of this tumor. The exact nature of this condition is still not clear, and there is little support for an origin from odontogenic epithelial cells.

## NEUROTHEKEOMA (NERVE SHEATH MYXOMA)

In 1969 Harkin and Reed[5] described an unusual myxoid tumor of probable nerve sheath origin under the term *myxoma of nerve sheath.*[305] Its distinctive appearance led them to distinguish it provisionally from variants of neurofibroma. Later, Gallager and Helwig[302] reported 53 similar cases under the name *neurothekeoma* to stress its nerve sheath origin, and others utilized the term *bizarre cutaneous neurofibroma,*[303] dermal nerve sheath myxoma.[296,297] Some tumors, mistakenly called *pacinian neurofibromas,* are also neurothekeomas.

They usually arise during childhood and early adult life and have a predilection for the upper portion of the body, such as the head, neck, and shoulder. Mucous membranes are rarely involved. They are situated in the dermis and subcutis and in an exceptional instance occur in deep soft tissue.

Histologically, the tumor is divided into distinct lobules by fibrous connective tissue (Figs. 30–106, 30–107). Each lobule consists of a myxoid matrix composed of either hyaluronic acid[302] or sulfated acid mucins (Figs. 30–108, 30–109).[302] Usually the cells dis-

*Text continued on page 1193*

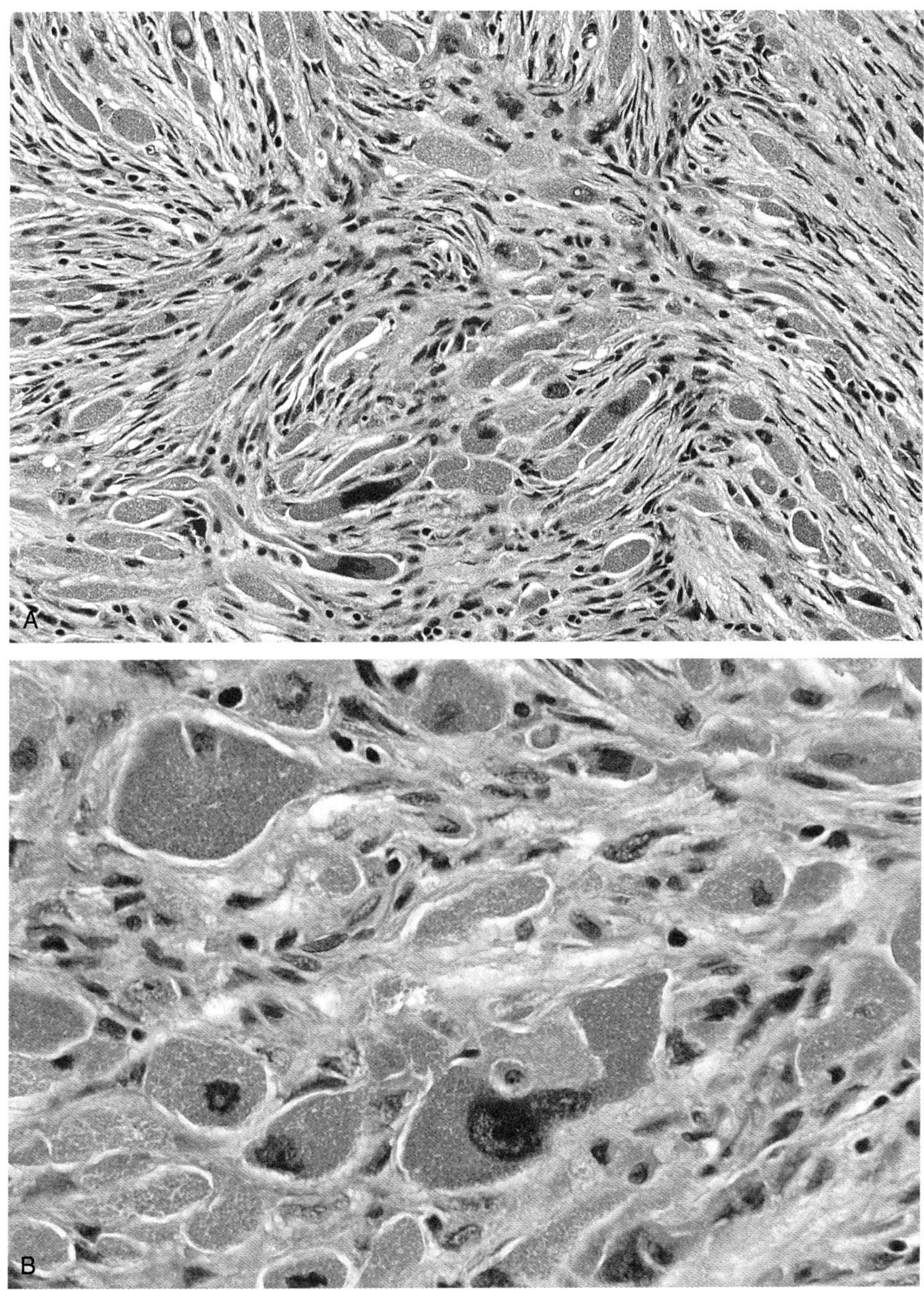

**FIGURE 30–104.** (**A, B**) Malignant granular cell minor illustrating profound nuclear atypia, prominent nucleoli, and spindling. Mitotic figures were also identified.

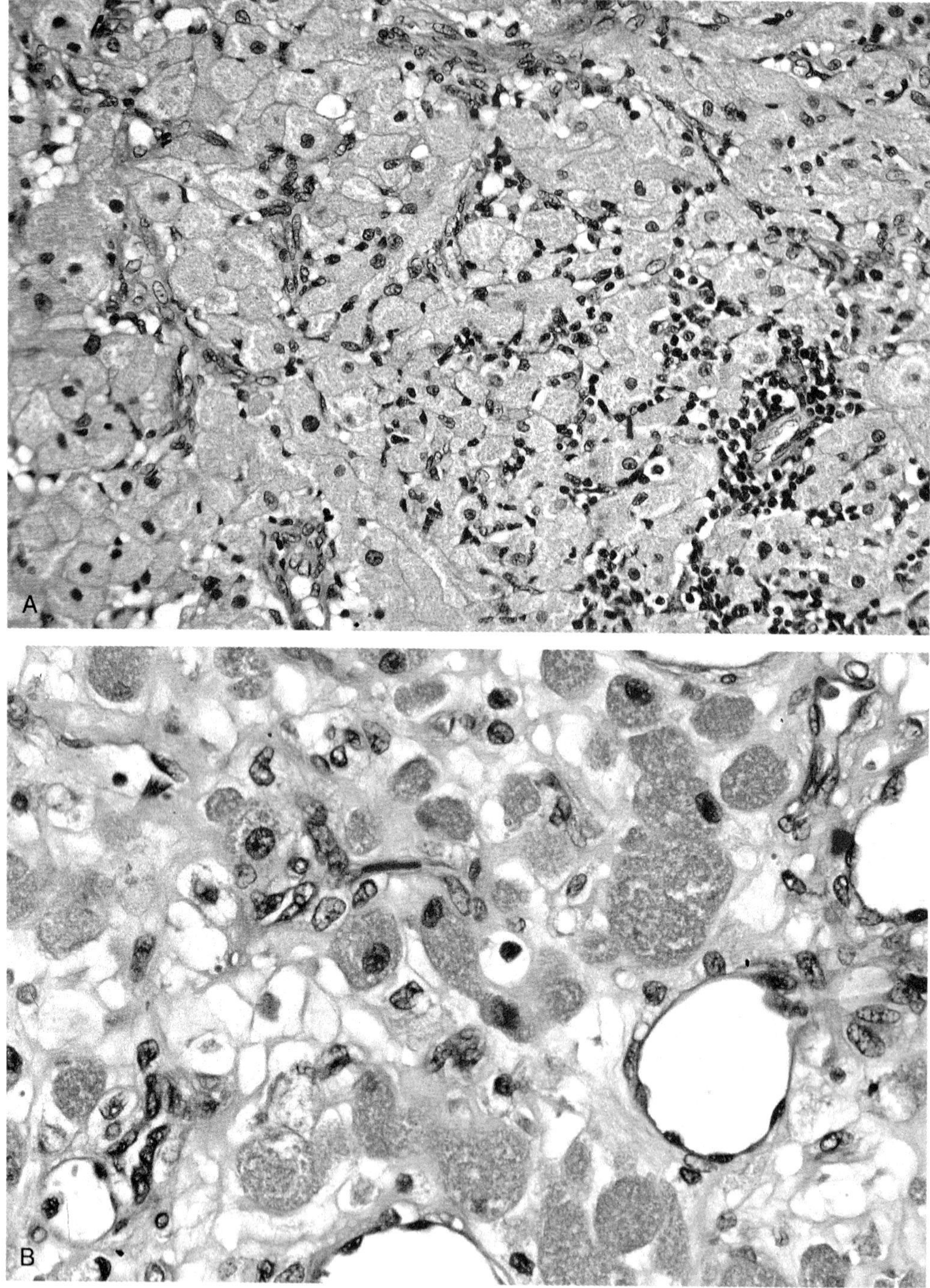

**FIGURE 30–105.** (**A, B**) Congenital granular cell tumor.

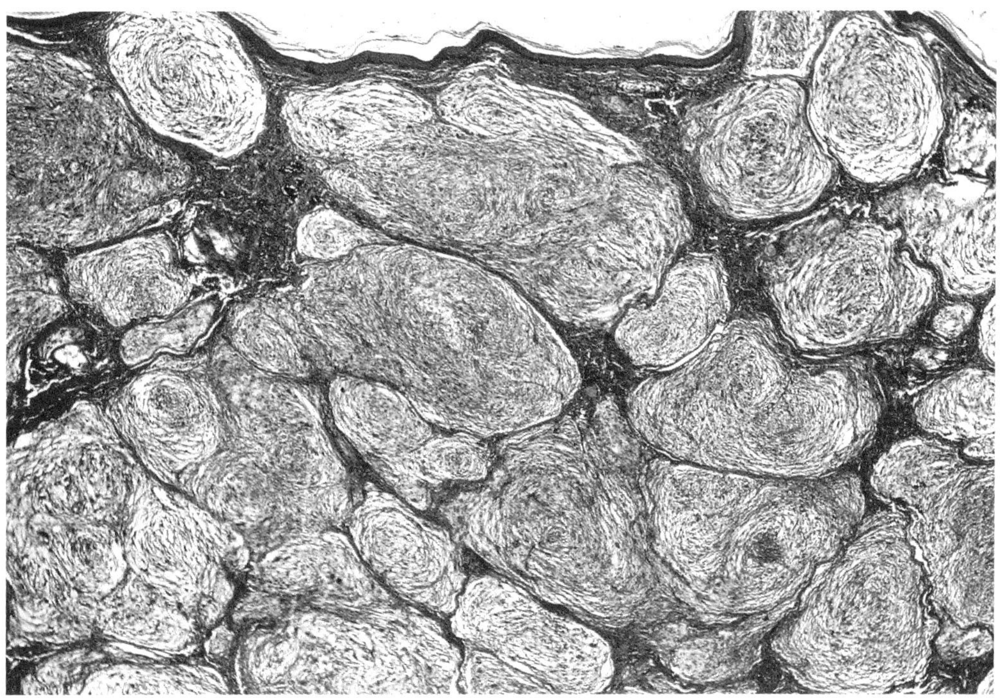

**FIGURE 30–106.** Neurothekeoma involving the dermis. Not the prominent septae.

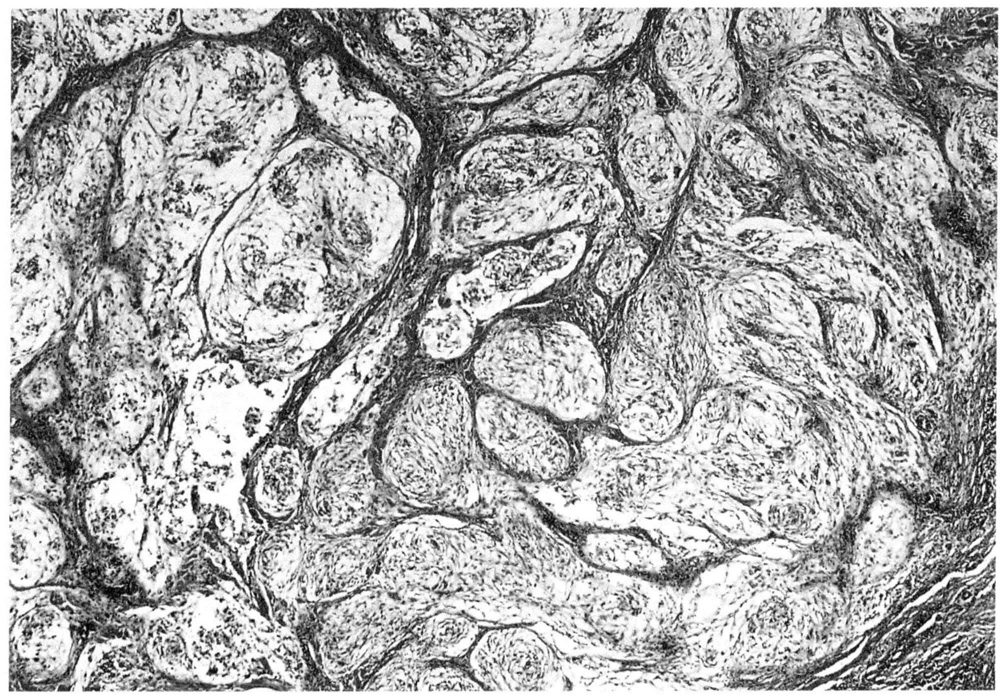

**FIGURE 30–107.** Neurothekeoma.

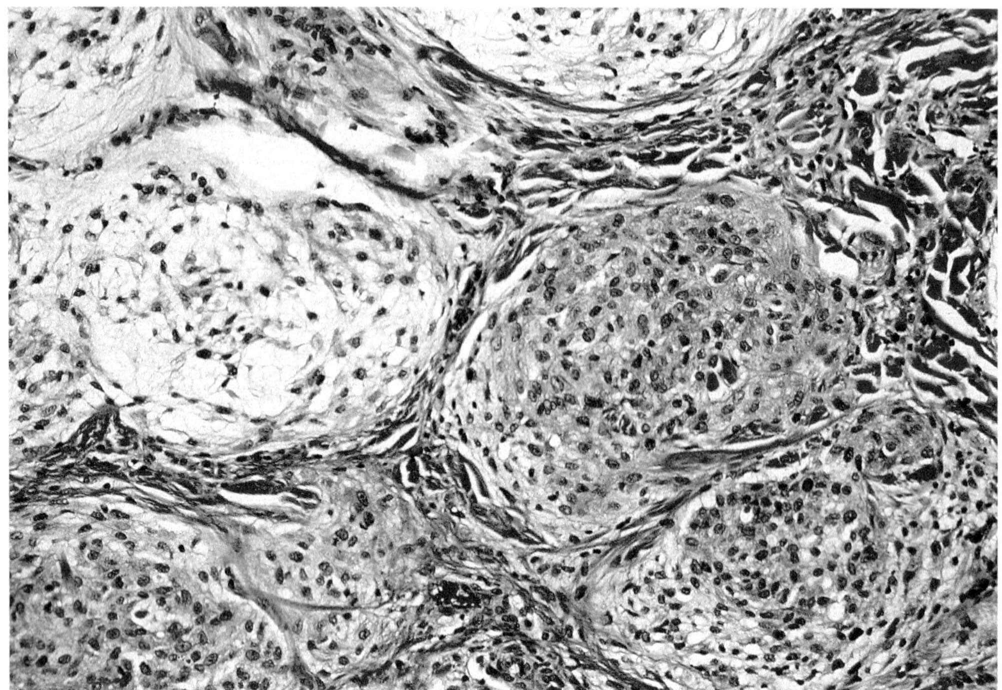

**FIGURE 30–108.** Myxoid and cellular nodules in a neurothekeoma.

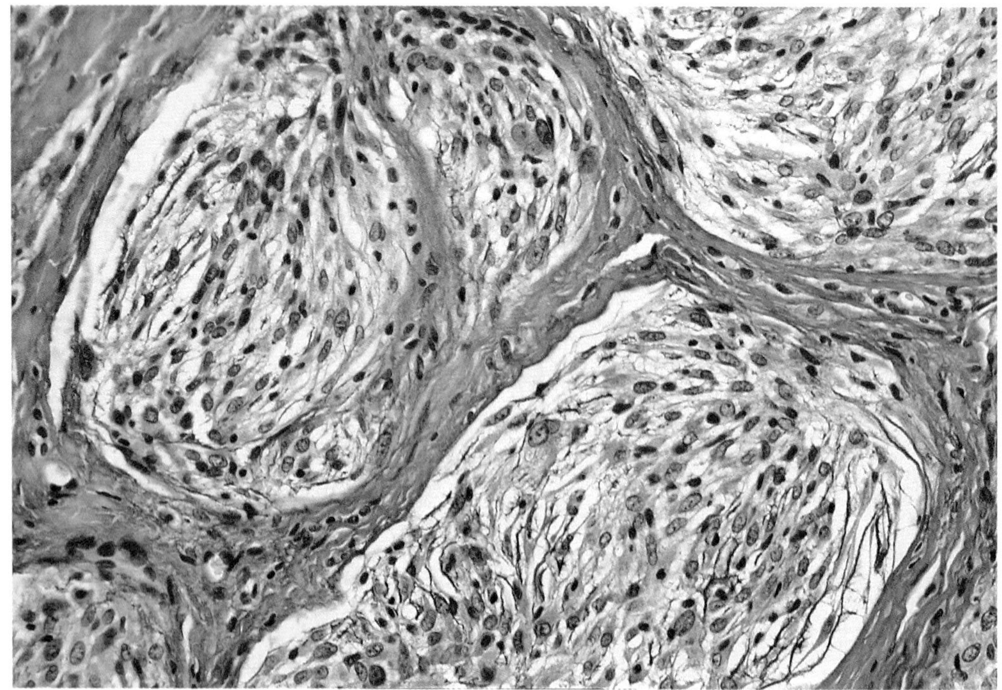

**FIGURE 30–109.** Cellular nodules in a neurothekeoma.

play little pleomorphism and few mitotic figures. Benign giant cells are occasionally present in the lobules, and rarely neurites are identified among the tumor cells. Although most tumors are quite myxoid, some tumors are more cellular, with marked nuclear atypia, mitoses, extension into fat or skeletal muscle, or vascular invasion (Fig. 30–110). Known as *cellular neurothekeoma*[299,301] or *cellular neurothekeoma with atypical features*,[300] they may be mistaken for sarcoma to those unfamiliar with the basic architectural pattern of the tumor. The most helpful clues to the recognition of cellular neurothekeomas with atypical features are the superficial dermal location and the distinctive septate architecture.

Neurothekeoma is usually regarded as a variant of a nerve sheath tumor because of its overall histologic similarity to a neurofibroma and its infrequent origin from a nerve. Some have questioned this concept, however, and have suggested that there may be two different lesions or subtypes included under this term.[299,301] The observation that S-100 protein is usually easily demonstrated in highly myxoid neurothekeomas but not in the more cellular forms has been used as evidence that the two lesions are different entities (Fig. 30–111). We doubt that this is the case. Overall cellular neurothekeomas are similar in appearance to the more myxoid one; furthermore, PGP9.5, a broad neural marker, has been identified in both.[306]

The differential diagnosis of this unusual tumor includes notably focal mucinosis, myxoid malignant fibrous histiocytoma, and myxoid neurofibroma. Focal mucinosis does not display the degree of circumscription, lobulation, or cellularity seen in neurothekeoma. Myxoid malignant fibrous histiocytomas are poorly circumscribed, more pleomorphic lesions with a more elaborate and organized vasculature and no septations. Moreover, most develop as large, deeply situated tumors in adults in contrast to neurothekeoma, which occurs principally in the superficial soft tissues of young individuals. Distinction of this tumor from neurofibroma is more of an academic point, as they are probably related. In general, the multinodularity and the whorled arrangement of the cells of neurothekeoma contrasts with most neurofibromas. Rarely the tumor recurs.

## EXTRACRANIAL MENINGIOMA

Extracranial meningiomas are rare tumors that occur in the skin or soft tissue of the scalp or along the vertebral axis.[307,308] By definition they are not associated with an underlying meningioma of the neuraxis, and extracranial extension of an intracranial tumor should always be considered before accepting a meningioma in soft tissue or skin as a primary tumor. Although true extracranial meningiomas probably arise from ectopic arachnoid lining cells, their precise

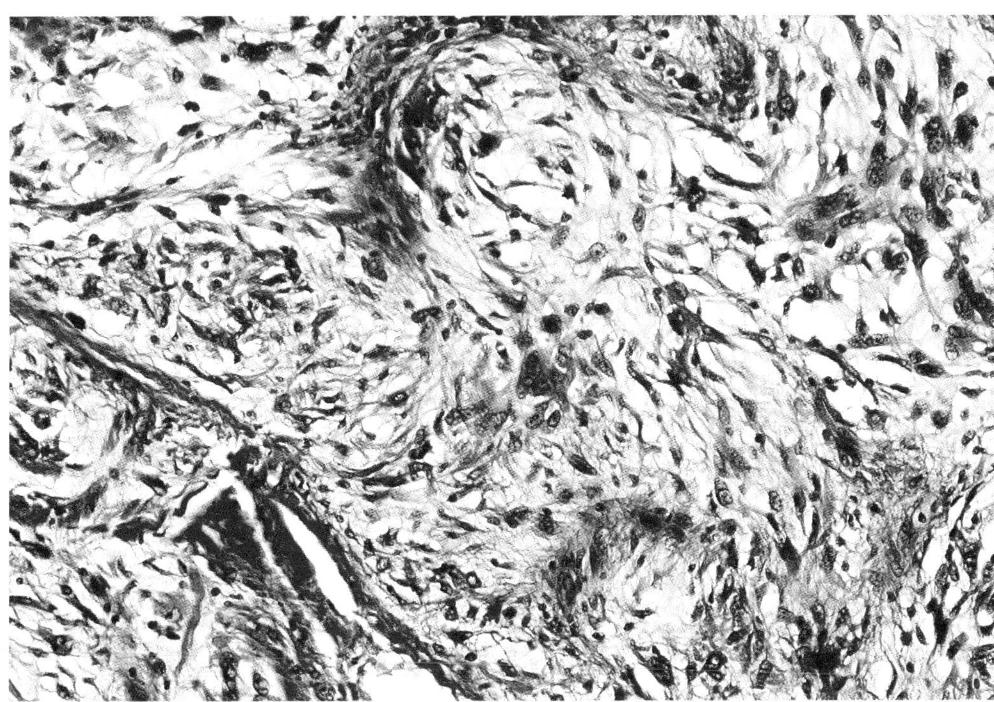

**FIGURE 30–110.** Nuclear atypia in a neurothekeoma, a feature not associated with aggressive behavior.

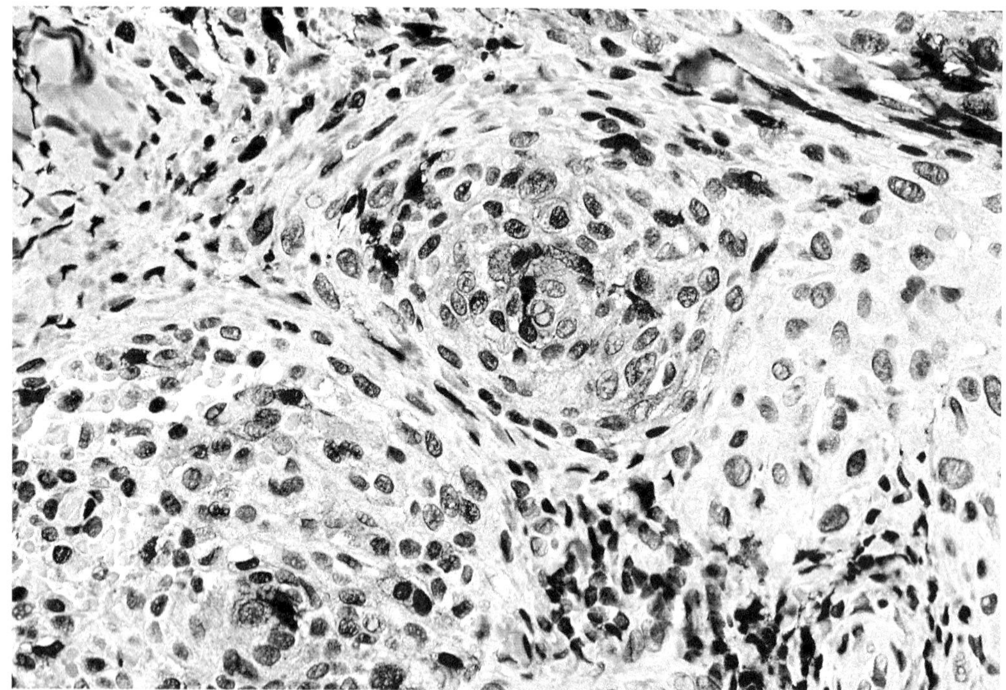

**FIGURE 30–111.** S-100 protein immunoreactivity in a neurothekeoma.

presentation and localization suggest at least two pathogenetic mechanisms.[307]

One form of extracranial meningioma, termed type I by Lopez et al.,[307] arises in the skin of the scalp, forehead, and paravertebral areas and as a result may be mistaken clinically for cutaneous lesions, including epidermal inclusion cyst, skin tag, and nevus. The pathogenesis is probably similar to that of meningocele and is believed to be the result of abnormalities of neural tube closure with relocation of meningeal tissue in the surrounding skin and subcutis (Fig. 30–112). This proposal explains the congenital nature of the type I tumor and its distribution, which coincides with that of meningocele. The similarity of this tumor to meningocele is heightened by its histologic appearance. Although some consist of solid, isolated nests of meningothelial cells in the skin, others may contain a rudimentary stalk or cystic cavity (Fig. 30–113). Such lesions occupy an intermediate position in the spectrum between meningocele and extracranial meningioma and have been named *meningeal hamartomas*. The type I meningioma is benign, although persistence of a connection with the central nervous system can lead to postoperative meningitis or neurologic deficits.

The second form of extracranial meningioma (type II) (Fig. 30–114) may occur at any age, but adults are usually affected. These tumors are situated in the vicinity of the sensory organs (eye, ear, nose) or along the paths of the cranial and spinal nerves. Symptoms associated with the tumor are related to its size, location, and growth rate. Histologically, these lesions are indistinguishable from the ordinary intracranial meningioma. The solid nests of meningothelial cells are arranged in sheets or whorls and occasionally are punctuated by psammoma bodies (Fig. 30–115). In addition to surgical removal, appropriate studies to exclude an intracranial component are recommended for these more deeply situated tumors.

## GLIAL HETEROTOPIAS

Like ectopic meningeal rests, ectopic deposits of glial tissue occur occasionally on the scalp and rarely in other soft tissue sites.[310–312] Over the years they have been called a variety of names, including nasal glioma, glial hamartoma, and heterotopic glial tissue.[309] The common presentation of a glial heterotopia is that of a polypoid mass at the root of the nose or to one side of the bridge of the nose in an infant, which grows commensurately with the infant. In most cases the lesions lack a communication with the brain; in the few that do communicate with the brain, the connection occurs through the cribriform plate such that rhinorrhea may be an accompanying symptom. Histologically, the lesions consist of mats of mature glial tissue which, in addition to astrocytes, may

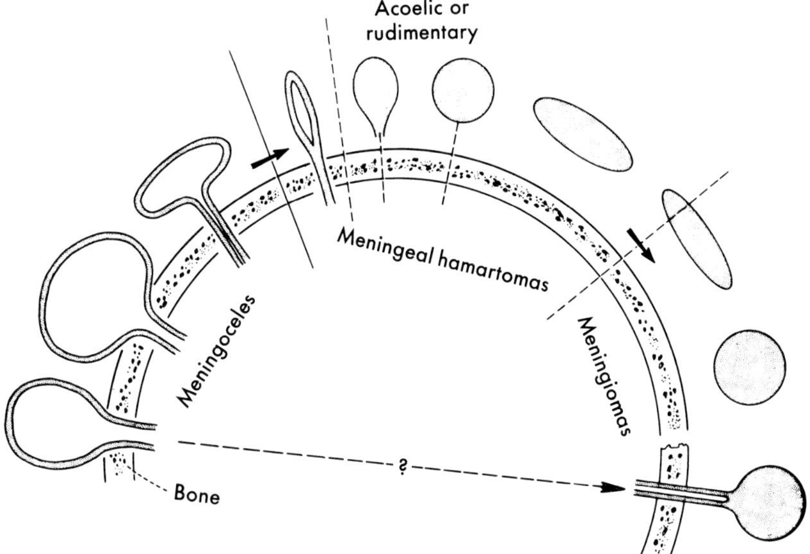


**FIGURE 30–112.** Histogenesis of cutaneous meningiomas. Note the possible relations between meningoceles, meningeal hamartomas, and type I extracranial meningiomas. The first retain their connections with the central nervous system and are predominantly cystic, whereas the last two lose the connections and are solid. (From Lopez DA, Silvers DN, Helwig EB. Cutaneous meningiomas: a clinicopathologic study. Cancer 34:728, 1974.)

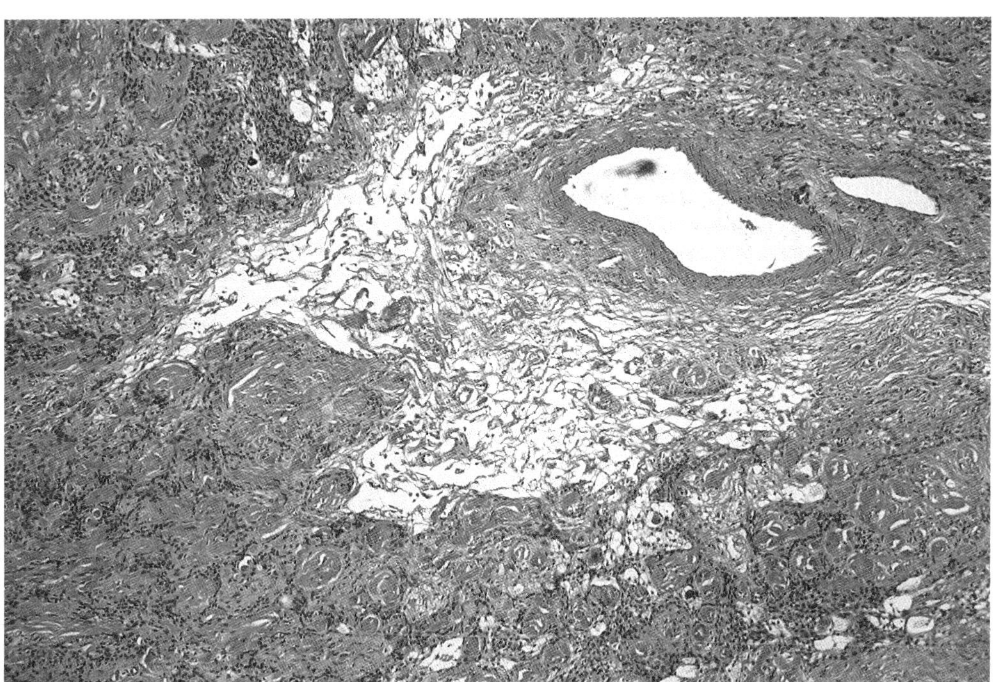

**FIGURE 30–113.** Type I ectopic meningioma from a child. Note the partially cystic central area.

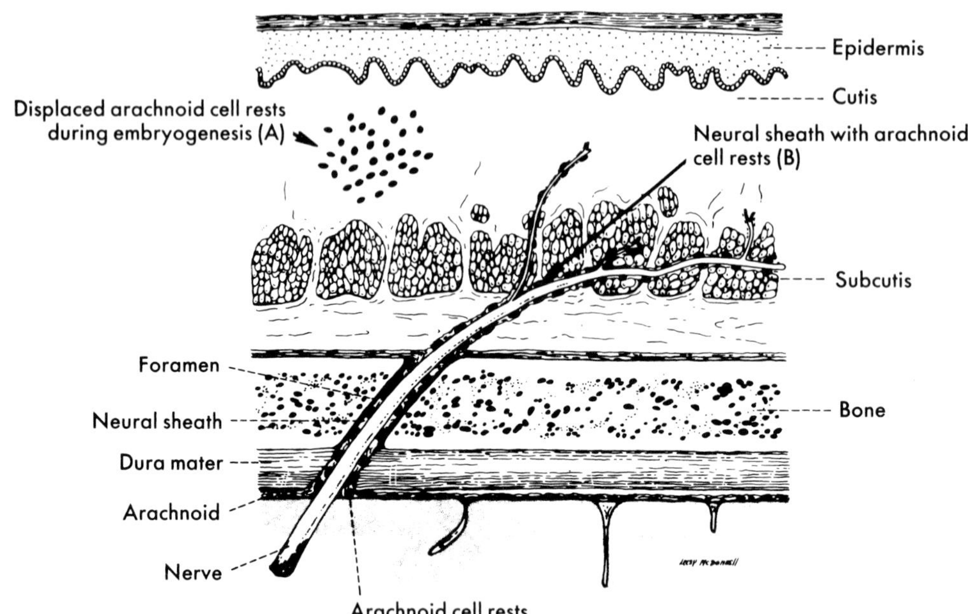


**FIGURE 30–114.** Primary cutaneous meningiomas. There are two possible origins of primary cutaneous meningiomas. (**A**) Type I may result from abnormalities of neural tube closure with resultant ectopic arachnoid cell rests. (**B**) Type II, which occurs in adults and follows the distribution of the sensory organs and nerves, probably is derived from arachnoid rests in nerve sheaths. (From Lopez DA, Silvers DN, Helwig EB. Cutaneous meningiomas: a clinicopathologic study. Cancer 34: 728, 1974.)

also contain neurons (Fig. 30–116). Although most glial heterotopias may be viewed as variants of encephalocele, in which the communication with the brain is lost, we have encountered two glial heterotopias on the chest wall of adults, suggesting that other pathogenetic mechanisms allow the development of these unusual lesions.

## MELANOTIC NEUROECTODERMAL TUMOR OF INFANCY (RETINAL ANLAGE TUMOR, MELANOTIC PROGONOMA)

First described in 1918 by Krompecher, the melanotic neuroectodermal tumor of infancy, a rare tumor of disputed histogenesis, has been referred to as *congenital melanocarcinoma, melanotic adamantinoma, retinal anlage tumor, melanotic progonoma,* and *pigmented epulis of infancy.*[313–336] Although most current studies support a neural crest origin of this tumor, there is little evidence that the tumor specifically represents retinal anlage. Therefore we prefer the less fanciful term *melanotic neuroectodermal tumor of infancy.*

### Clinical Findings

The tumor usually develops during the first year of life and presents as a protruding mass in the upper or lower jaw. The skin or mucosa is tightly stretched over the lesion, but it is rarely if ever ulcerated. Radiographically, the tumor is a cystic radiolucent lesion with a capacity for local destruction and displacement of the developing teeth (Fig. 30–117). Patients with this tumor in unusual sites such as the anterior fontanelle, epididymis,[318,319,336] mediastinum,[329] and brain,[334] develop symptoms referable to those sites. The few cases reported in the uterus[329] and shoulder[328] and those in adults[327] should be disregarded because they represent different lesions altogether. We have encountered one of these tumors in the soft tissues of the extremity, and it has also been reported in long bone.

### Gross and Microscopic Findings

Grossly, the tumor ranges in color from slate gray to blue-black, depending on the amount of melanin pigment. It is composed of irregular alveolar spaces lined by cuboidal cells containing varying amounts of melanin pigment (Fig. 30–118). In addition, small, round, less well differentiated cells resembling those of neuroblastoma lie in the alveolar space or as isolated nests in a fibrous stroma. Neurofibrillary material, resembling glial tissue, may be seen in association with these cells in the spaces. In two exceptional cases, glial tissue was found outside the epithelial islands. One case was a tumor arising in the brain in which the entire stroma was glial,[334] and the second was a tumor arising in a glial heterotopia of the oropharynx.[325]

The cuboidal cells have the electron microscopic features of epithelial and melanocytic cells.[316] They are bounded by basal laminae and elaborately interdigitate laterally with neighboring cells, forming desmosomes. Both mature and immature melanosomes

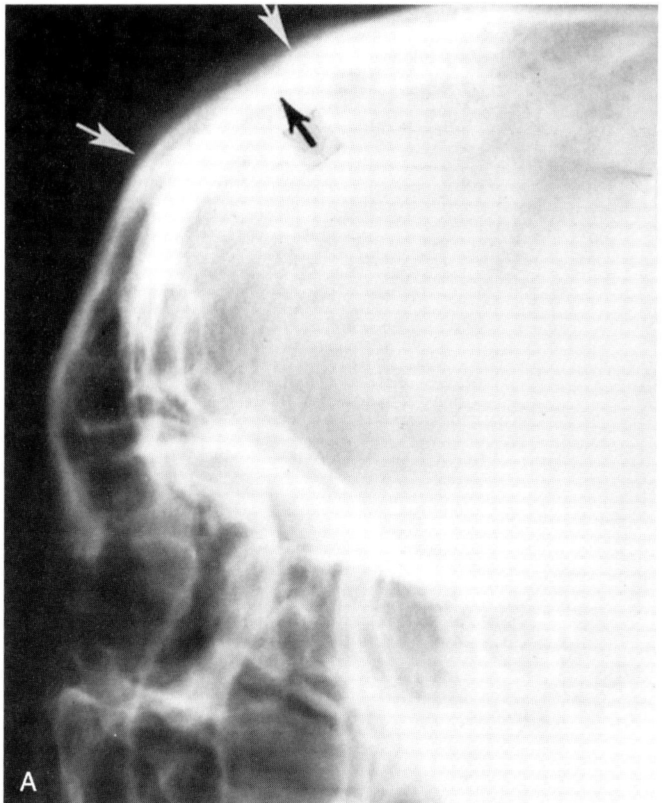


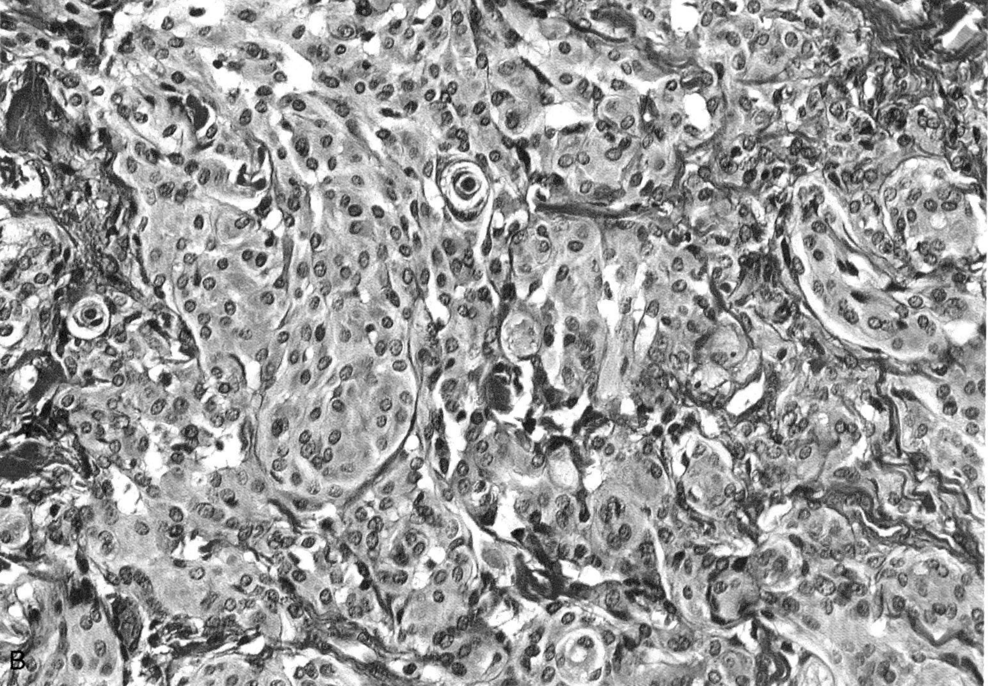


**FIGURE 30–115.** Primary cutaneous meningioma of the frontal area of the scalp. (**A**) Radiograph demonstrates extracranial location of frontal mass. The outer table of the skull is partly eroded (between the white arrows) whereas the inner table is intact (black arrow). (**B**) Tumor consists of whorls of plump epithelioid cells indistinguishable from cells of the intracranial form of meningioma.

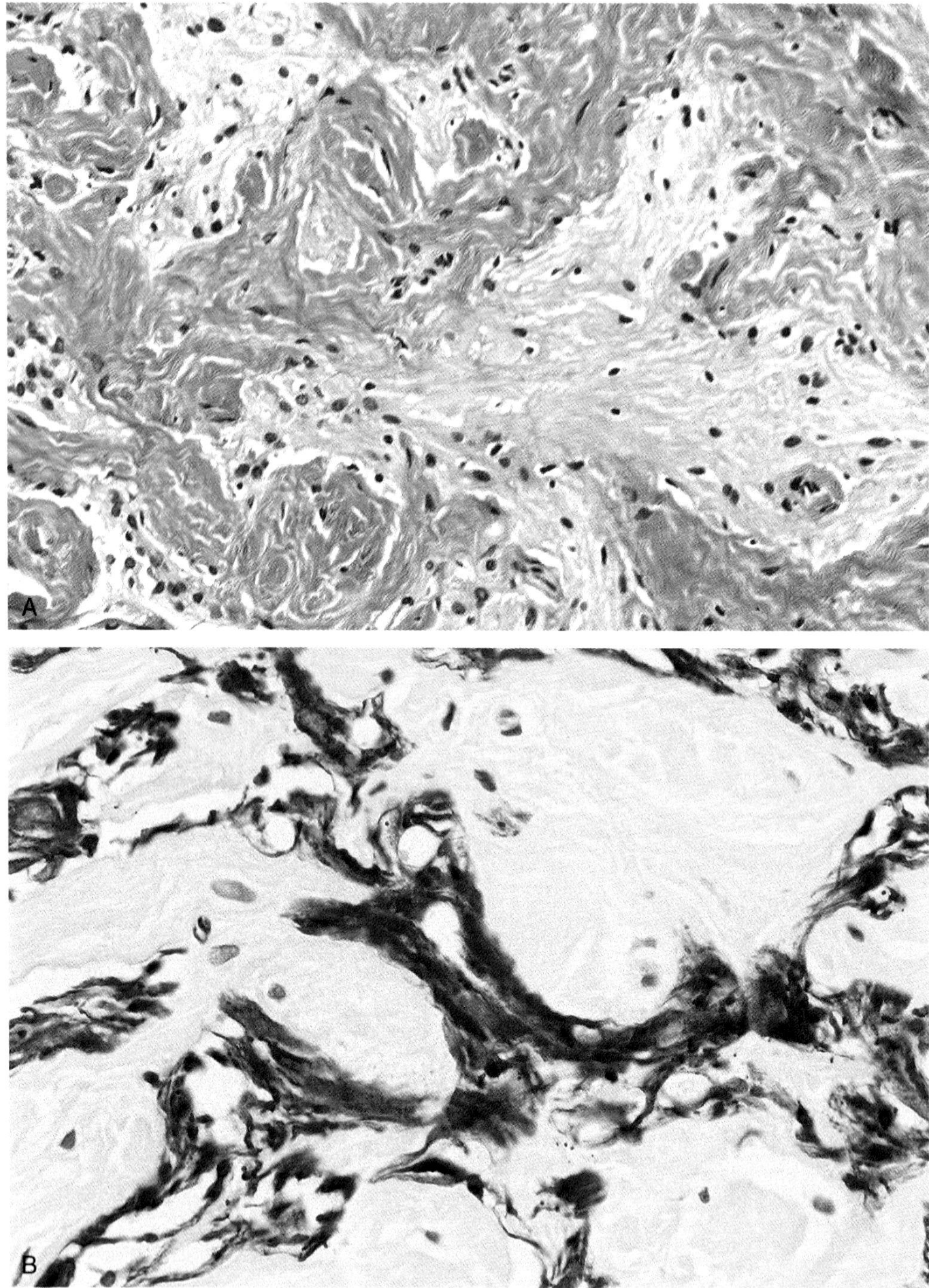


**FIGURE 30–116.** (**A**) Glial heterotopia with lightly staining glial tissue interspersed between collagen (dark areas). (**B**) Immunostaining for glial fibrillary acidic protein highlights glial tissue against the negatively staining backdrop of collagen.

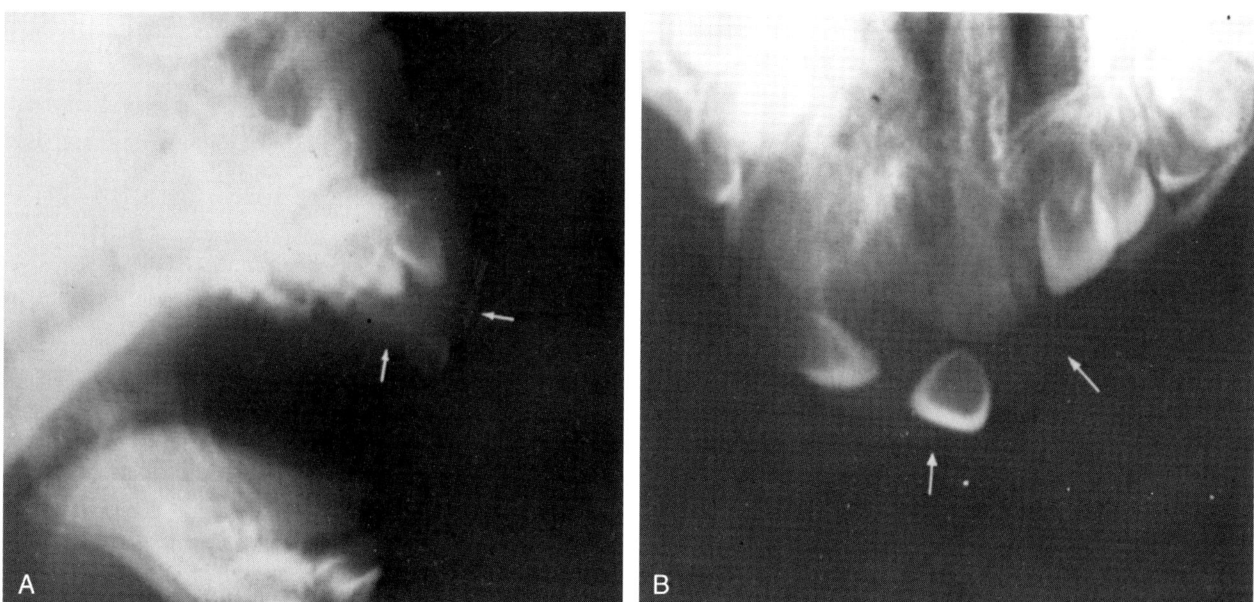


**FIGURE 30–117.** Radiograph of pigmented neuroectodermal tumor of infancy (retinal anlage tumor) in the maxilla. Tumor is represented by vaguely outlined soft tissue mass (arrows) with destruction of the maxilla (**A**) and displacement of teeth (**B**).

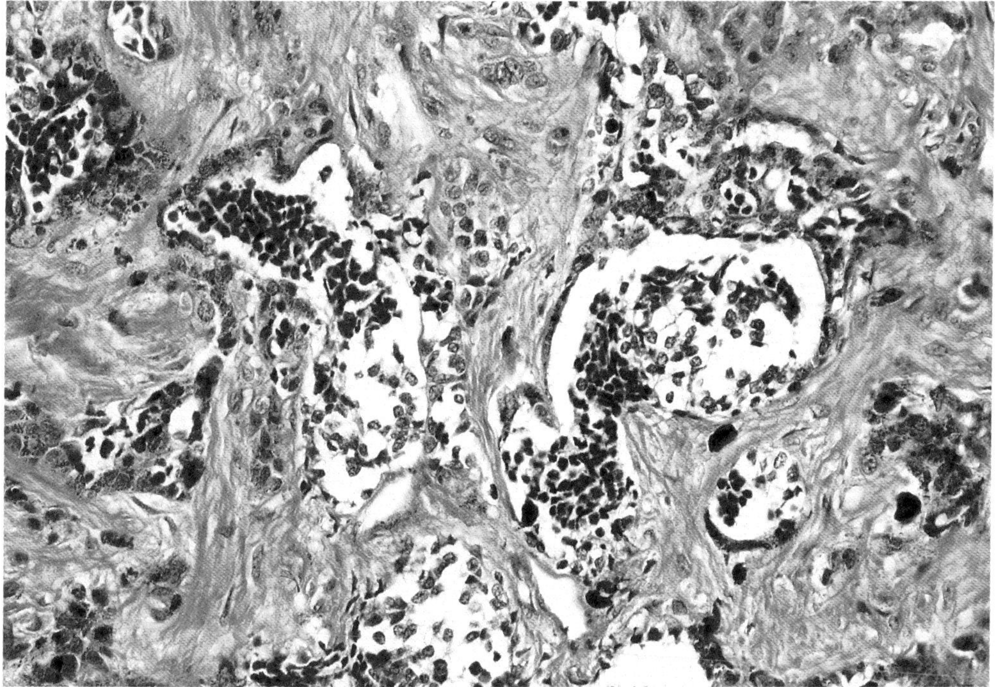

**FIGURE 30–118.** Pigmented neuroectodermal tumor of infancy with flattened pigmented epithelial cells lining alveolar spaces. Immature, nonpigmented rounded cells lie clumped in the spaces. (×160)

similar to those of melanocytes and melanoma cells are present in the cytoplasm. Functionally they share certain properties of the melanocyte in that melanization of these cells may be increased by agents that induce similar changes in melanocytes of animals.[316] Immunohistochemically, the cuboidal cells express cytokeratin and a melanoma-associated antigen (HMB-45). Neuron-specific enolase, Leu-7, and synaptophysin are variably present in the epithelial cells and the small neuroblastic element.

The round, less well differentiated cells contain few organelles but are believed to be neuroblastic by virtue of their elongated cell processes, dense-core vesicles,[316] and intracytoplasmic neurofilamentous material.[316,320] Their association with glial-like areas and, in one case, with ganglioneuromatous areas[316] provides further support for this contention.

## Discussion

Traditionally, this tumor was considered benign, but in a large series from the AFIP nearly half of those with follow-up information recurred, and 5–10% of cases reported in the literature have produced metastasis.[316,322,326] One case, a stillborn, was noted to have multiple metastases at delivery.[326] A second case, a tumor of the epididymis, produced micrometastases in regional lymph nodes[322]; and two others metastasized as primitive neuroblastic tumors devoid of melanin.[316,322] Although metastasis is a relatively uncommon event, attempts to eradicate the tumor at the time of initial surgery are endorsed. Unfortunately it has not been possible to predict recurrence or metastasis in this disease by conventional parameters or by utilization of more sophisticated techniques such as flow cytometery.

The histogenesis of this tumor has been controversial. The concepts of a congenital melanoma and an odontogenic tumor are now obsolete for various reasons. The former does not account for the primitive neuroblastic component, and the latter does not take into consideration tumors at sites where there are no odontogenic rests. To date the most appealing theory is that the tumor is derived from neural crest.[314,316] This concept allows latitude in the distribution of the lesions, accounts for the presence of pigmented and neuroblastic elements, and explains the rare tumor associated with increased levels of vanillylmandelic acid.[314,316] It does not seem necessary to compare this tumor specifically with the developing retina; in fact, the embryologic evidence against this possibility has been extensively summarized.[314] It seems more probable that this tumor merely reflects a primitive stage or degree of differentiation common to many types of pigmented neuroepithelium.

## REFERENCES

### General


1. Angevine JB. The nervous tissue. In: Bloom M, Fawcett D (eds) A Textbook of Histology. Chapman & Hall, New York, 1994, pp 309–364.
2. Asbury AK, Johnson PC. Pathology of peripheral nerve. In: Major Problems in Pathology, vol 9. WB Saunders, Philadelphia, 1978.
3. Erlandson RA. The enigmatic perineural cell and its participation in tumors and in tumor-like entities. Ultrastruct Pathol 15: 335, 1991.
4. Feany MB, Anthony DC, Fletcher CD. Nerve sheath tumours with hybrid features of neurofibroma and schwannoma: a conceptual challenge. Histopathology 32:404, 1998.
5. Harkin JC, Reed RJ. Tumors of the peripheral nervous system. In: Atlas of Tumor Pathology, 2nd series, Fascicle 3. Armed Forces Institute of Pathology, Washington, DC, 1969.
6. Ortiz-Hidalgo C, Weller RO. Peripheral nervous system. In: Sternberg SS (ed) Histology for Pathologists. Raven Press, New York, 1992.
7. Scheithauer BW, Woodruff JM, Erlandson RA. Tumors of the peripheral nervous system. In: Atlas of Tumor Pathology. American Registry of Pathology, Washington, DC, 1999.
8. Steffansson K, Wollmann R, Jerkovic M. S-100 protein in soft tissue tumors derived from Schwann cells and melanocytes. Am J Pathol 106:261, 1982.
9. Weiss SW, Langloss JM, Enzinger FM. The role of the S-100 protein in the diagnosis of soft tissue tumors with particular reference to benign and malignant Schwann cell tumors. Lab Invest 49:299, 1983.
10. Woodruff JM. Pathology of major peripheral nerve sheath neoplasms. In: Weiss SW, Brooks JJ (eds) Soft Tissue Tumors. Williams & Wilkins, Baltimore, 1996.
11. Woodruff JM. Tumors and tumorlike conditions of the peripheral nerve. In: Ninfo V, Chung EB, Cavazzana AO (eds) Tumors and Tumorlike Lesions of Soft Tissue. Churchill Livingstone, New York, 1991.


### Embryogenesis and Normal Anatomy


12. Bunge MB, Wood PM, Tynan LB, et al. Perineurium originates from fibroblasts: demonstration in vitro with a retroviral marker. Science 243:229, 1989.
13. Burkel WE. The histological fine structure of perineurium Anat Rec 158:177, 1967.
14. Church RL, Tanzer M, Pfeiffer SE. Collagen and procollagen production by a clonal line of Schwann cells. Proc Natl Acad Sci USA 70:1943, 1973.
15. Elvin LG. The structure and composition of motor, sensory, and autonomic nerves and nerve fibers. In: Bourne GH (ed) The Structure and Function of Nervous Tissue. Structure I, vol 1. Academic, San Diego, 1968, p 325.
16. Nathaniel EJH, Pease DC. Collagen and basement membrane formation by Schwann cells during nerve regeneration. J Ultrastruct Res 9:550, 1963.
17. Ochoa J, Mair WGP. The normal sural nerve in man. I. Ultrastructure and numbers of fibers and cells. Acta Neuropathol (Berl) 13:197, 1969.
18. Ochoa J, Mair WGP. The normal sural nerve in man. II. Changes in axons and Schwann cells due to aging. Acts Neuropathol (Berl) 13:217, 1969.
19. Shantha TK, Bourne GH. The perineural epithelium—a new concept. In: Bourne GH (ed) The Structure and Function of Nervous Tissue. Structure I, vol 1. Academic, New York, 1968, p 379.

### Traumatic (Amputation) Neuroma

20. Boldrey F. Amputation neuroma in nerves implanted in bone. Ann Surg 118:1052, 1943.
21. Cieslak AK, Stout AP. Traumatic and amputation neuromas. Arch Surg 53:646, 1946.
22. Das Gupta TW, Brasfield RD. Amputation neuromas in cancer patients. NY J Med 69:2129, 1969.
23. Haymaker W. The pathology of peripheral nerve injuries. Milit Surg 102:448, 1948.
24. Huber CC, Lewis LD. Amputation neuroma: their development and prevention. Arch Surg 1:85, 1920.
25. Hume RH, Buxton RW. Post cholecystectomy amputation neuroma. Am Surg 20:698, 1954.
26. Lassmann H, Ammerer HP. Schwann cells and perineurium in neuroma: some morphological aspects. Virchows Arch [Cell Pathol] 15:313, 1974.
27. Shapiro L, Juhlin E, Brownstein MH. Rudimentary polydactyly: an amputation neuroma. Arch Dermatol 108:223, 1973.
28. Snyder CC, Knowles RP. Traumatic neuromas. J Bone Joint Surg Am 47:641, 1965.

### Mucosal Neuroma

29. Carney JA, Hayles AB. Alimentary tract manifestations of multiple endocrine neoplasia, type 2b. Mayo Clin Proc 52:543, 1977.
30. Williams ED, Pollack DJ. Multiple mucosal neuromata with endocrine tumors: a syndrome allied to von Recklinghausen's disease. J Pathol 91:71, 1966.

### Pacinian Neuroma

31. Dembinski AS, Jones JW. Intra-abdominal pacinian neuroma: a rare lesions in an unusual location. Histopathology 19:89, 1991.
32. Fletcher CDM, Theaker JM. Digital pacinian neuroma: a distinctive hyperplastic lesion. Histopathology 15:249, 1989.
33. Fraitag S, Sherardi R, Wechsler J. Hyperplastic pacinian corpuscles: an uncommonly encountered lesion of the hand. J Cutan Pathol 21:457, 1994.
34. Hart WR, Thompson NW, Hildreth DH, et al. Hyperplastic pacinian corpuscles: a cause of digital pain. Surgery 70:730, 1971.
35. Rhode CM, Jennings WD Jr. Pacinian corpuscle neuroma of digital nerves. South Med J 68:86, 1975.
36. Schuler FA III, Adamson JE. Pacinian neuroma: an unusual cause of finger pain. Plast Reconstr Surg 62:576, 1978.

### Palisaded Encapsulated Neuroma

37. Albrecht S, Kahn HJK, From L. Palisaded encapsulated neuroma: an immunohistochemical study. Mod Pathol 2:403, 1989.
38. Argenyi ZB, Cooper PH, Santa Cruz D. Plexiform and other unusual variants of palisaded encapsulated neuroma. J Cutan Pathol 20:34, 1993.
39. Argenyi ZB, Santa Cruz D, Bromley C. Comparative light-microscopic and immunohistochemical study of traumatic and palisaded encapsulated neuromas of the skin. Am J Dermatopathol 14:505, 1992.
40. Dakin MC, Leppard B, Theaker JM. The palisaded encapsulated neuroma (solitary circumscribed neuroma). Histopathology 20:405, 1992.
41. Fletcher CDM. Solitary circumscribed neuroma of the skin (so-called palisaded, encapsulated neuroma): a clinicopathologic and immunohistochemical study. Am J Surg Pathol 13:574, 1989.
42. Reed RJ, Fine RM, Meltzer HD. Palisaded encapsulated neuromas of the skin. Arch Dermatol 106:865, 1972.

### Morton's Interdigital Neuroma

43. Bennett GL, Graham CE, Mauldin DM. Morton's interdigital neuroma: a comprehensive treatment protocol. J Foot Ankle Surg 16:760, 1995.
44. Lassmann G, Lassmann H, Stockinger L. Morton's metatarsalgia: light and electron microscopic observations and their relations to entrapment neuropathies. Virchows Arch [Pathol Anat] 370:307, 1976.
45. Reed RJ, Bliss BO. Morton's neuroma: regressive and productive intermetatarsal elastofibrositis. Arch Pathol 95:123, 1973.
46. Scotti TM. The lesion of Morton's metatarsalgia (Morton's toe). Arch Pathol 63:91, 1957.
47. Wu KK. Morton's interdigital neuroma: a clinical review of its etiology treatment and results. J Foot Ankle Surg 35:112, 1996.
48. Young G, Lindsey J. Etiology of symptomatic recurrent interdigital neuromas. J Am Podiatr Med Assoc 83:255, 1993.

### Nerve Sheath Ganglion

49. Barrett R, Cramer F. Tumors of the peripheral nerves and so-called ganglia of the peroneal nerve. Clin Orthop 27:135, 1963.
50. Cobb CA III, Moiel RN. Ganglion of the peroneal nerve: report of two cases. J Neurosurg 41:255, 1974.
51. Guardjian ES, Larsen RD, Lindner DW. Intraneural cyst of the peroneal and ulnar nerves: report of two cases. J Neurosurg 23:76, 1965.

### Neuromuscular Hamartoma (Neuromuscular Choristoma; Benign Triton Tumor)

52. Awasthi D, Kline DG, Beckman EN. Neuromuscular hamartoma (benign Triton tumor) of the brachial plexus. J Neurosurg 75:795, 1991.
53. Bonneau R, Brochu P. Neuromuscular choristoma: a clinicopathologic study of two cases. Am J Surg Pathol 7:521, 1983.
54. Louhimo I, Rapola J. Intraneural muscular hamartoma: report of two cases in small children. J Pediatr Surg 7:696, 1972.
55. Markel SF, Enzinger FM. Neuromuscular hamartoma: a benign "Triton tumor" composed of mature neural and striated muscle elements. Cancer 49:140, 1982.
56. Mitchell A, Scheithauer BW, Ostertag H, et al. Neuromuscular hamartoma. Am J Clin Pathol 103:460, 1995.
57. O'Connell JX, Rosenberg AE. Multiple cutaneous neuromuscular choristomas: report of a case and a review of the literature. Am J Surg Pathol 14:93, 1990.
58. Orlandi E. Sopra un caso di rhabdomioma del nervo ischiatico. Arch Sci Med (Torino) 19:113, 1895.
59. Van Dorpe JV, Sciot R, De Vos R, et al. Neuromuscular choristoma (hamartoma) with smooth and striated muscle component: case report with immunohistochemical and ultrastructural analysis. Am J Surg Pathol 21:1090, 1997.
60. Zwick DL, Livingston K, Clapp L. Intracranial nerve rhabdomyoma/choristoma in a child: a case report and discussion of possible histogenesis. Hum Pathol 20:390, 1989.

### Neurofibroma and NF1

61. Akwari OE, Payne WAS, Onofrio BM, et al. Dumbbell neurogenic tumors of the mediastinum. Mayo Clin Proc 53:353, 1978.
62. Azzopardi JG, Eusebi V, Tison V, et al. Neurofibroma with rhabdomyomatous differentiation: benign "Triton" tumor of the vagina. Histopathology 7:561, 1983.
63. Barker D, Wright E, Nguyen L, et al. Gene for von Recklinghausen neurofibromatosis is in the pericentromeric region of chromosome 17. Science 236:1100, 1987.
64. Bird CC, Wills RA. The histogenesis of pigmented neurofibromas. J Pathol 976:631, 1969.

65. Brasfield RD, Das Gupta TK. Von Recklinghausen's disease: a clinicopathological study. Ann Surg 175:86, 1972.
66. Canale DJ, Bebin J. Von Recklinghausen disease of the nervous system. In: Vinken PJ, Bruyn GW (ed) Handbook of Clinical Neurology, vol 14, American Elsevier, New York, 1972, p 132.
67. Carey JC, Viskochil DH. Neurofibromatosis type 1: a model condition for the study of the molecular basis of variable expressivity in human disorders. Am J Med Genet 89:7, 1999.
68. Chino F, Tsuruhara T. Electron microscopic study of von Recklinghausen's disease. Jpn J Med Sci 21:249, 1968.
69. Crowe FW, Schull WJ, Neel JV. A Clinical, Pathological, and Genetic Study of Multiple Neurofibromatosis. Charles C Thomas, Springfield, IL, 1956.
70. Fetsch JF, Michal M, Miettinen M. Pigmented (melanotic) neurofibroma: a clinicopathologic and immunohistochemical analysis of 19 lesions from 17 patients. Am J Surg Pathol 24:331, 2000.
71. Fraumeni JF. Neurofibromatosis and childhood leukemia. BMJ 4:489, 1971.
72. Friedman JM. Epidemiology of neurofibromatosis type 1. Am J Med Genet 89:1, 1999.
73. Greene J, Fitzwater J, Burgess J. Arterial lesions associated with neurofibromatosis. Am J Clin Pathol 62:481, 1974.
74. Guccion JG, Enzinger FM. Malignant schwannoma associated with von Recklinghausen's neurofibromatosis. Virchows Arch [Pathol Anat] 383:43, 1979.
75. Gutman D, Aylsworth A, Carley J, et al. The diagnostic evaluation and multindisciplinary management of neurofibromatosis I and neurofibromatosis 2. JAMA 278:51, 1997.
76. Hochberg FH, DaSilva AB, Galdabini J, et al. Gastrointestinal involvement in von Recklinghausen's neurofibromatosis. Neurology 24:1144, 1974.
77. Hosoi K. Multiple neurofibromatosis (von Recklinghausen's disease) with special reference to malignant transformation. Arch Surg 22:258, 1931.
78. Jimbow K, Szabo G, Fitzpatrick TB. Ultrastructure of giant pigmented granules (macromelanosomes) in the cutaneous pigmented macules of neurofibromatosis. J Invest Dermatol 61: 300, 1973.
79. Korf BR. Plexiform neurofibromas. Am J Med Genet 89:31, 1999.
80. Kourea HP, Cordon-Cardo C, Dudas M, et al. Expression of $p27^{kip}$ and other cell cycle regulators in malignant peripheral nerve sheath tumors and neurofibromas. Am J Pathol 155: 1885, 1999.
81. Kourea HP, Orlow I, Scheithauer BW, et al. Deletions of the INK4A gene occur in malignant peripheral nerve sheath tumors but not in neurofibromas. Am J Pathol 155:1855, 1999.
82. Lassmann H, Jurecka W, Lassmann W, et al. Different types of benign nerve sheath tumors: light microscopy, electron microscopy, and autoradiography. Virchows Arch [Pathol Anat] 375: 197, 1977.
83. Lichtenstein BW. Neurofibromatosis (von Recklinghausen's disease of nervous system): analysis of a total pathologic picture. Arch Neurol Psychiatry 62:822, 1949.
84. Lin BT, Weiss LM, Medeiros LJ. Neurofibroma and cellular neurofibroma with atypia: a report of 14 tumors. Am J Surg Pathol 21:1443, 1997.
85. Massaro D, Katz S, Mathews MJ, et al. Von Recklinghausen's neurofibromatosis associated with cystic lung disease. Am J Med 38:233, 1965.
86. McEvoy MW, Mann JR. Neurofibromatosis with leukemia. BMJ 3:641, 1971.
87. Merck C, Kindblom LG. Neurofibromatosis of the appendix in von Recklinghausen's disease. Acta Pathol Microbiol Scand 83A:623, 1975.
88. Miller RM, Sparkes RS. Segmental neurofibromatosis. Arch Dermatol 113:837, 1977.
89. Mulvihill JJ, Parry DM, Sherman JL, et al. Neurofibromatosis 1 (Recklinghausen disease) and neurofibromatosis 2 (bilateral acoustic neurofibromatosis). Ann Intern Med 113:39, 1990.
90. National Institutes of Health. Neurofibromatosis: National Institutes of Health Consensus Development Conference Statement, vol 6(12). US Department of Health and Human Services, Bethesda, July 13–15, 1987, pp 1–9.
91. Nielsen GP, Stemmer-Rachamimov AO, Ino Y, et al. Malignant transformation of neurofibromas in neurofibromatosis 1 is associated with CDKN2A/p16 inactivation. Am J Pathol 155: 1879, 1999.
92. Pleasure J, Geller SA. Neurofibromatosis in infancy presenting with congenital stridor. Am J Dis Child 113:390, 1967.
93. Preston FW, Walsh WS, Clarke TS. Cutaneous neurofibromatosis (von Recklinghausen's disease). Arch Surg 64:13, 1952.
94. Prieto VG, McNutt NS, Lugo J, Reed JA. Differential expression of the intermediate filament peripherin in cutaneous neural lesions and neurotized melanocytic nevi. Am J Surg Pathol 21:1450, 1997.
95. Pung S, Hirsch EF. Plexiform neurofibromatosis of the heart and neck. Arch Pathol 59:341, 1955.
96. Rao UN, Sonmez-Alpan E, Michalopoulos GK. Hepatocyte growth factor and c-MET in benign and malignant peripheral nerve sheath tumors. Hum Pathol 28:1066, 1997.
97. Rasmussen SA, Friedman JM. NF1 gene and neurofibromatosis 1. Am J Epidemiol 151:33, 2000.
98. Riccardi VM. Von Recklinghausen neurofibromatosis. N Engl J Med 305:1617, 1981.
99. Roudebush M, Slabe T, Sundaram V, et al. Neurofibromin colocalizes with mitochondria in cultured cell. Exp Cell Res 23:161, 1997.
100. Sagel SS, Forrest JV. Interstitial lung disease in neurofibromatosis. South Med J 68:647, 1975.
101. Salyer WR, Salyer DC. The vascular lesions of neurofibromatosis. Angiology 25:510, 1974.
102. Schorn D, Griessel PJ, Ziady F. Neurofibromatosis with renovascular hypertension. S Afr Med J 48:1537, 1974.
103. Scott OLS. Disease of the skin. In: Sorsby A (ed) Clinical Genetics. Butterworth, London, 1953, p 580.
104. Silvers DN, Greenwood RS, Helwig EG. Café-au-lait spots without giant pigment granules: occurrence in suspected neurofibromatosis. Arch Dermatol 110:87, 1974.
105. Sorensen SA, Mulvihill JJ, Nielsen A. Long-term follow-up of von Recklinghausen neurofibromatosis: survival and malignant neoplasms. N Engl J Med 314:1010, 1986.
106. Stay EJ, Vawter G. The relationship between nephroblastoma and neurofibromatosis (von Recklinghausen's disease). Cancer 39:2550, 1977.
107. Webb WR, Goodman PC. Fibrosing alveolitis in patients with neurofibromatosis. Radiology 122:289, 1977.
108. Weiss B, Bollag G, Shannon K. Hyperactive Ras as a therapeutic target in neurofibromatosis type 1. Am J Med Genet 89:14, 1999.
109. Zorab P, Edwards H. Spinal deformity in neurofibromatosis. Lancet 2:823, 1972.

### Schwannoma, NF2, and Schwannomatosis

110. Ackerman LV, Taylor FH. Neurogenous tumors within the thorax. Cancer 4:669, 1951.
111. Antiheimo J, Sankila R, Carpen O, et al. Population based analysis of sporadic and type 2 neurofibromatosis-associated meningiomas and schwannomas. Neurology 54:71, 2000.
112. Argeny Z, Goodenberger ME, Strauss JS. Congenital neural hamartoma ("fascicular schwannoma"): a light microscopic, immunohistochemical and ultrastructural study. Am J Dermatopathol 12:283, 1990.

113. Bird CC, Willis RA. The histogenesis of pigmented neurofibromas. J Pathol 97:631, 1969.
114. Brandes WW. A malignant neurinoma (schwannoma) with epithelial elements. Arch Pathol 16:649, 1933.
115. Brooks JJ, Draffen RM. Benign glandular schwannoma. Arch Pathol Lab Med 116:192, 1992.
116. Buenger KM, Porter NC, Dozier SE, et al. Localized multiple neurilemomas of the lower extremity. Cutis 51:36, 1993.
117. Carstens H, Schrodt G. Malignant transformation of a benign encapsulated neurilemoma. Am J Clin Pathol 51:144, 1969.
118. Casadei GP, Scheithauer BW, Hirose T, et al. Cellular schwannoma: a clinicopathologic DNA flow cytometric and prolifration marker study of 71 cases. Cancer 75:1109, 1995.
119. Chan JK, Fok KO. Pseudoglandular schwannoma. Histopathology 29:481, 1996.
120. Dahl I. Ancient neurilemoma (schwannoma). Acta Pathol Microbiol Scand 85A:812, 1977.
121. Das Gupta TK, Brasfield RD, Strong EW, et al. Benign solitary schwannomas (neurilemomas). Cancer 24:355, 1979.
122. Denecke K. Uber zwei Falle von metastasierenden Neurinomen des Magendarmkanals. Beitr Path Anat 89:242, 1932.
123. Fisher ER, Vuzevski VD. Cytogenesis of schwannoma (neurilemoma), neurofibroma, dermatofibroma, and dermatofibrosarcoma as revealed by electron microscopy. Am J Clin Pathol 49: 141, 1968.
124. Fittipaldi C. Contributo allo studio dei neurinomi. Riv Patol Nerve Ment 39:521, 1932.
125. Fletcher CDM, Davies SE. Benign plexiform (multinodular) schwannoma: a rare tumor unassociated with neurofibromatosis. Histopathology 19:971, 1986.
126. Fletcher CDM, Davies SE, McKee PH. Cellular schwannoma: a distinct pseudosarcomatous entity. Histopathology 11:21, 1987.
127. Fletcher CDM, Madziwa D, Heyderman E, et al. Benign dermal schwannoma with glandular elements—true heterology or a local "organizer" effect? Clin Exp Dermatol 11:475, 1986.
128. Geschickter CF. Tumors of the peripheral nerves. Am J Cancer 25:377, 1935.
129. Goldblum JR, Beals TF, Weiss SW. Neuroblastoma-like neurilemoma. Am J Surg Pathol 18:266, 1994.
130. Gulcke N. Zur Klinik des Neurinomas. Arch Klin Chir 142: 478, 1926.
131. Gutmann DH, Aylsworth A, Carey JC, et al. The diagnostic evalution and multidisciplinary management of neurofibromatosis 1 and neurofibromatosis 2. JAMA 278:71, 1997.
132. Gutmann DH, Geist RT, Xu H, et al. Defects in neurofibromatosis 2 protein function can arise at multiple levels. Hum Mol Genet 7:335, 1998.
133. Gutmann DH, Giordano MJ, Fishback AS, Guha A. Loss of merlin expression in sporadic menilngiomas, ependymomas and schwannomas. Neurology 49:267, 1997.
134. Hanada M, Tanaka T, Kanayama S, et al. Malignant transformation of intrathoracic ancient neurilemoma in a patient without Von Recklinghausen's disease. Acta Pathol Jpn 32:527, 1982.
135. Hasegawa SL, Mentzel T, Fletcher CD. Schwannomas of the sinonasal tract and nasopharynx. Mod Pathol 10:777, 1997.
136. Ishida T, Kuroda M, Motoi T, et al. Phenotypic diversity of neurofibromatosis 2: association with plexiform schwannoma. Histopathology 32:264, 1998.
137. Iwashita T, Enjoji M. Plexiform neurilemoma: a clincopathologic and immunohistochemical analysis of 23 tumors from 20 patients. Virchows Arch [Pathol Anat] 422:305, 1986.
138. Izumi AK, Rosato FE, Wood MG. Von Recklinghausen's disease associated with multiple neurilemomas. Arch Dermatol 104:172, 1971.
139. Jacoby LB, Jones D, Davis K, et al. Molecular analysis of the NF2 tumor-suppressor gene in schwannomatosis. Am J Hum Genet 61:1291, 1997.
140. Jacoby LB, MacCollin B, Barone R, et al. Frequency and distribution of NF2 mutations in schwannomas. Genes Chromosomes Cancer 17:45, 1996.
141. Jacoby LB, Pulaski K, Rouleau GA, et al. Clonal analysis of human meningiomas and schwannomas. Cancer Res 50:6783, 1990.
142. Kao GF, Laskin WB, Olsen TG. Solitary cutaneous plexiform neurilemoma (schwannoma): a clinicopathologic, immunohistochemical, and ultrastructural study of 11 cases. Mod Pathol 2:20, 1989.
143. Kimura Y, Koga H, Araki N, et al. The involvement of calpain-dependent proteolyisis of the tumor suppressor NF2 (merlin) in schwannomas and meningiomas. Nat Med 4:915, 1998.
144. Kindblom LG, Meis-Kindblom JM, Havel G, Busch C. Benign epithelioid schwannoma. Am J Surg Pathol 22:762, 1998.
145. Kluwe L, Mautner VF. A missense mutation in the NF2 gene results in moderate and mild clinical phenotypes of neurofibromatosis type 2. Hum Genet 97:224, 1996.
146. Lekanne Deprez RH, Bianchi AB, Groen NA, et al. NF2 gene transcript mutations in sporadic meningiomas and vestibular schwannomas. Am J Hum Genet 54:1022, 1994.
147. Lodding L, Kindblom L-G, Angervall L, et al. Cellular schwannoma: a clinicopathologic study of 29 cases. Virchows Arch [Pathol Anat] 416:237, 1990.
148. MacCollin M, Woodfin W, Kronn D, Short MP. Schwannomatosis: a clinical and pathologic study. Neurology 46:1072, 1996.
149. Mandybur TI. Melanotic nerve sheath tumors. J Neurosurg 41: 187, 1974.
150. McMenamin ME, Fletcher CDM. Epithelioid malignant change in benign schwannomas [abstract 54]. Mod Pathol 13:13A, 2000.
151. Meis-Kindblom JM, Enzinger FM. Plexiform malignant peripheral nerve sheath tumor of infancy and childhood. Am J Surg Pathol 18:479, 1994.
152. Murray MR, Stout AP. Schwann cells versus fibroblasts as the origin of the specific nerve sheath tumor. Am J Pathol 16:41, 1940.
153. Nayler SJ, Leiman G, Omar T, Cooper K. Malignant transformation in a schwannoma. Histopathology 29:189, 1996.
154. Parry DM, MacCollin MM, Kaiser-Kupfer MI, et al. Germ-line mutations in the neurofibromatosis 2 gene correlations with disease severity and retinal abnormalities. Am J Hum Genet 59:529, 1996.
155. Prichard RW, Custer RP. Pacinian neurofibroma. Cancer 5:297, 1952.
156. Prose PH, Gherardo GJ, Coblenz A. Pacinian neurofibroma. AMA Arch Dermatol 76:65, 1957.
157. Purcell SM, Dixon SL. Schwannomatosis: an unusual variant of neurofibromatosis or a distinct clinical entity? Arch Dermatol 125:390, 1989.
158. Rasbridge SA, Browse NL, Tighe JR, et al. Malignant nerve sheath tumor arising in a benign ancient schwannoma. Histopathology 14:525, 1989.
159. Razzuk MA, Urschel HC, Martin JA, et al. Electron microscopical observations on mediastinal neurilemoma, neurofibroma, and ganglioneuroma. Ann Thorac Surg 15:73, 1973.
160. Reith JD, Goldblum JR. Multiple cutaneous plexiform schwannomas: report of a case and review of the literature with particular reference to the association with types 1 and 2 neurofibromatosis and schwannomatosis. Arch Pathol Lab Med 120:399, 1996.
161. Saxen E. Tumours of tactile end-organs. Acta Pathol Microbiol Scand 25:66, 1948.

162. Schochet SS Jr, Barret DA II. Neurofibroma with aberrant tactile corpuscles. Acta Neuropathol (Berl) 28:161, 1974.
163. Seppala MT, Sainio MA, Haltia MJ, et al. Multiple schwannomas: schwannomatosis or neurofibromatosis 2. J Neurosurg 89: 36, 1998.
164. Shishiba T, Niimura M, Ohtsuka F, Tsuru N. Multiple cutaneous neurilemomas as a skin manifestation of neurilemomatosis. J Am Acad Dermatol 10:744, 1984.
165. Smith K, Mezebish D, Williams JP, et al. Cutaneous epithelioid schwannomas: a rare variant of benign peripheral nerve sheath tumor. J Cutan Pathol 25:50, 1998.
166. Stemmer AO, Xu L, Gonzalez-Agosti C, et al. Universal absence of merlin but not other ERM family members in schwannomas. Am J Pathol 151:1649, 1997.
167. Stenman G, Kindblom LG, Johansson M, et al. Clonal chromosome abnomalities and in vitro growth characteristics of classical and cellular schwannomas. Cancer Genet Cytogenet 57:121, 1991.
168. Stout AP. The peripheral manifestations of specific nerve sheath tumor (neurilemoma). Am J Cancer 24:751, 1935.
169. Sun CN, White HJ. An electron microscopic study of a schwannoma with special reference to banded structures and peculiar membranous multiple-chambered spheroids. J Pathol 114:13, 1974.
170. Takeshima H, Nishi T, Yamamoto K, et al. Loss of merlin-p85 protein complex in NF2 related tumors. Int J Oncol 12:1073, 1998.
171. Trassard M, LeDoussal V, Bui BN, Coindre JM. Angiosarcoma arising in a solitary schwannoma (neurilemoma) of the sciatic nerve. Am J Surg Pathol 20:1412, 1996.
172. Trofatter JA, MacCollin MM, Rutter JL, et al. A novel neurofibromatosis 2 tumor suppressor. Cell 72:791, 1993.
173. Val-Bernal JF, Figols J, Vazquez-Barquero A. Cutaneous plexiform schwannoma associated with neurofibromatosis type 2. Cancer 76:1181, 1995.
174. Waggener JD. Ultrastructure of benign peripheral nerve sheath tumors. Cancer 19:699, 1966.
175. Welling DB, Guida M, Goll F, et al. Mutational spectrum in the neurofibromatosis type 2 gene in sporadic and familial schwannomas. Hum Genet 98:189, 1996.
176. White W, Shiu MH, Rosenblum MK, et al. Cellular schwannoma: a clinicopathologic study of 57 patients and 58 tumors. Cancer 66:1266, 1990.
177. Woodruff JM, Godwin TA, Erlandson RA, et al. Cellular schwannoma: a variety of schwannoma sometimes mistaken for a malignant tumor. Am J Surg Pathol 5:733, 1981.
178. Woodruff JM, Marshall ML, Godwin TA, et al. Plexiform (multinodular) schwannoma: a tumor simulating the plexiform neurofibroma. Am J Surg Pathol 7:691, 1983.
179. Woodruff JM, Selig AM, Crowlely K, Allen PW. Schwannoma with malignant transformation: a rare distinctive peripheral nerve tumor. Am J Surg Pathol 18:882, 1994.

### Melanotic Schwannoma

180. Carney JA. Psammomatous melanotic schwannoma: a distinctive heritable tumor with special associations including cardiac myxoma and the Cushing syndrome. Am J Surg Pathol 14:206, 1990.
181. Carney JA, Ferreiro JA. The epithelioid blue nevus: a multicentric familial tumor with important associations, including cardiac myxoma and psammomatous melanotic schwannoma. Am J Surg Pathol 20:259, 1996.
182. Font RL, Truong LD. Melanotic schwannoma of soft tissues: electron microscopic observations and review of the literature. Am J Surg Pathol 8:129, 1984.
183. Fu YS, Kaye GI, Lattes R. Primary malignant melanocytic tumors of the sympathetic ganglia with an ultrastructural study of one. Cancer 36:2029, 1975.
184. Killeen RM, Davy CL, Bauserman SC. Melanocytic schwannoma. Cancer 62:174, 1988.
185. Krausz T, Azzopardi JG, Pearse E. Malignant melanoma of the sympathetic chain: with consideration of pigmented nerve sheath tumors. Histopathology 8:881, 1984.
186. Leger F, Vital C, Rivel J, et al. Psammomatous melanotic schwannoma of a spinal nerve root: relationship the Carney complex. Pathol Res Pract 192:1142, 1996.
187. Lowman RM, LiVolsi VA. Pigmented (melanotic) schwannomas of the spinal canal. Cancer 46:391, 1980.
188. Mennenmeyer RP, Hammar SP, Tytus JS, et al. Melanotic schwannomas: clinical and ultrastructural studies of three cases with evidence of intracellular melanin synthesis. Am J Surg Pathol 3:3, 1979.
189. Millar WG. A malignant melanotic tumor of ganglion cells arising from thoracic sympathetic ganglion. J Pathol Bacteriol 35:351, 1932.
190. Vallat-Decouvelacre AV, Wassef M, Lot G, et al. Spinal melanoticc schwannoma: a tumour with poor prognosis. Histopathology 35:558, 1999.

### Perineurioma

191. Ariza A, Bilbao JM, Rosai J. Immunohistochemical detection of epithelial membrane antigen in normal perineurial cells and perineurioma. Am J Surg Pathol 12:678, 1988.
192. Carneiro F, Brandao O, Correia AC, et al. Spindle cell tumor of the breast. Ultrastruct Pathol 15:335, 1991.
193. Dhimes P, Martizez-Gonzalez MA, Carabias E, Perez-Espejo G. Ultrastructural study of a perineurioma with ribosome-lamella complexes. Ultrastruct Pathol 20:167, 1996.
194. Emory TS, Scheithauer BW, Horose T, et al. Intraneural perineurioma: a clonal neoplasm associated with abnormalities of chromosome 22. Am J Clin Pathol 103:696, 1995.
195. Erlandson RA. The enigmatic perineurial cell and its participation in tumors and in tumorlike entities. Ultrastruct Pathol 15: 335, 1991.
196. Fetsch JF, Miettinen M. Sclerosing perineurioma: a clinicopathologic study of 19 cases of a distinctive soft tissue lesion with a predilection for the fingers and palms of young adults. Am J Surg Pathol 21:1433, 1997.
197. Giannini C, Scheithauer BW, Jenkins RB, et al. Soft tissue perineurioma: evidence for an abnormality of chromosome 22, criteria for diagnosis, and review of the literature. Am J Surg Pathol 21:164, 1997.
198. Hirose T, Scheithauer BW, Sano T. Perineurial malignant peripheral nerve sheath tumor (MPNST): a clinicopathologic, immunohistochemical and ultrastructural study of seven cases. Am J Surg Pathol 22:1369, 1998.
199. Jazayeri MA, Robinson JH, Legolvan DP. Intraneural perineurioma involving the median nerve. Plast Reconstr Surg 105: 2089, 2000.
200. Lasota J, Wozniak A, Debiec-Rychter M. Loss of chromosome 22q and lack of NF2 mutations in perineuriomas [abstract 46]. Mod Pathol 13:11a, 2000.
201. Lazarus SS, Trombetta LD. Ultrastructural identification of a benign perineurial cell tumor. Cancer 41:1823, 1978.
202. Mentzel T, Dei Tos AP, Fletcher CD. Perineurioma (storiform perineural fibroma): clinicopathologic analysis of four cases. Histopathology 25:261, 1994.
203. Ohno T, Park P, Akai M, et al. Ultrastructural study of a perineurioma. Ultrastruct Pathol 5:495, 1988.
204. Rank JP, Rostad SW. Perineurioma with ossification: a case report with immunohistochemical and ultrastructural studies. Arch Pathol Lab Med 122:366, 1998.
205. Sciot R, Cin PD, Hagemeijer A, et al. Cutaneous sclerosing

perineurioma with cryptic NF2 gene deletion. Am J Surg Pathol 23:849, 1999.

206. Simmons Z, Mahadeen ZI, Kothari MJ, et al. Localized hypertrophic neuropathy: magnetic resonance imaging findings and long term follow up. Muscle Nerve 22:28, 1999.
207. Smith K, Skelton H. Cutaneous fibrous perineuroma. J Cutan Pathol 25:333, 1998.
208. Theaker JM, Fletcher CDM. Epithelial membrane antigen expression by the perineurial cell: further studies of peripheral nerve lesions. Histopathology 14:581, 1989.
209. Theaker JM, Gatter KC, Puddle J. Epithelial membrane antigen expression by the perineurium of peripheral nerve and in peripheral nerve tumors. Histopathology 13:171, 1987.
210. Tsang WYW, Chan JKC, Chow LTC, et al. Perineurioma: an uncommon soft tissue neoplasm distinct from localized hypertrophic neuropathy and neurofibroma. Am J Surg Pathol 16: 756, 1992.
211. Weidenheim KM, Campbell WG. Perineurial cell tumor: immunohistochemical and ultrastructural characterization: relationship to other peripheral nerve tumors with a review of the literature. Virchows Arch [Pathol Anat] 408:375, 1986.

### Granular Cell Tumor

212. Abrikossoff A. Ueber Myome ausgehened von der quergestreiften willkuerlichen Muskulatur. Virchows Arch [Pathol Anat] 260:215, 1926.
213. Alkek DS, Johnson WC, Graham JH. Granular cell myoblastoma, a histological and enzymatic study. Arch Dermatol 98: 543, 1968.
214. Al-Sarraf M, Loud A, Vaitkevicius V. Malignant granular cell tumor. Arch Pathol 91:550, 1971.
215. Aparicio SR, Lumsden CE. Light- and electron-microscopic studies on the granular cell myoblastoma of the tongue. J Pathol 97:339, 1969.
216. Armin A, Connelly EM, Rowden G. An immunoperoxidase investigation of S-100 protein in granular cell myoblastomas: evidence for Schwann cell derivation. Am J Clin Pathol 79:37, 1983.
217. Ashburn LL, Rodger RC. Myoblastomas, neural origin: report of six cases, one with multiple tumors. Am J Clin Pathol 22: 440, 1952.
218. Bangle R. A morphologic and histochemical study of granular cell myoblastoma. Cancer 5:950, 1952.
219. Bangle R Jr. An early granular cell myoblastoma confined within a small peripheral myelinated nerve. Cancer 6:790, 1953.
220. Baraf CS, Bender B. Multiple cutaneous granular cell myoblastoma. Arch Dermatol 89:243, 1964.
221. Buley ID, Gatter KC, Kelly PMA, et al. Granular cell tumours revisited: an immunohistological and ultrastructural study. Histopathology 12:263, 1988.
222. Bussany-Caspari W, Hammar CH. Zur Malignitaet der sogenannten Myoblastenmyome. Zentralbl Allg Pathol 98:401, 1958.
223. Cadotte M. Malignant granular cell myoblastoma. Cancer 33: 1417, 1974.
224. Carstens PH. Ultrastructure of granular cell myoblastoma. Acta Pathol Microbiol Scand 78:685, 1970.
225. Christ ML, Ozzello L. Myogenous origin of a granular cell tumor of the urinary bladder. Am J Clin Pathol 56:736, 1971.
226. Compagno J, Hyams VJ, Ste-Marie P. Benign granular cell tumors of the larynx: a review of the 36 cases with clinicopathologic data. Ann Otol Rhinol Laryngol 84:308, 1975.
227. Donhuijsen K, Samtleben W, Leder LD, et al. Malignant granular cell tumor. J Cancer Res Clin Oncol 95:93, 1979.
228. Dunnington JH. Granular cell myoblastoma of the orbit. Arch Ophthalmol 40:14, 1948.
229. Fanburg-Smith JC, Meis-Kindblom JM, Fante R, Kindblom LG. Malignant granular cell tumor of soft tissue: diagnostic criteria and clinicopathologic correlation Am J Surg Pathol 22:779, 1998.
230. Filie AC, Lage JM, Azumi N. Immunoreactivity of S-100 protein, alpha-1 antitrypsin, and CD68 in adult and congenital granular cell tumors. Mod Pathol 9:888, 1996.
231. Finkel G, Lane B. Granular cell variant of neurofibromatosis: ultrastructure of benign and malignant tumors. Hum Pathol 13:959, 1982.
232. Fisher ER, Wechsler H. Granular cell myoblastoma—a misnomer: EM and histochemical evidence concerning its Schwann cell derivation and nature (granular cell schwannoma). Cancer 15:936, 1962.
233. Fust JA, Custer RP. Granular cell "myoblastoma" and granular cell neurofibromas: separation of the neurogenous tumors from the myoblastoma group. Am J Pathol 24:674, 1948.
234. Fust JA, Custer RP. On the neurogenesis of so-called granular cell myoblastoma. Am J Clin Pathol 19:522, 1949.
235. Gamboa L. Malignant granular cell myoblastoma. Arch Pathol 60:663, 1955.
236. Garancis JC, Komorowski RA, Kuzma JF. Granular cell myoblastoma. Cancer 25:542, 1970.
237. Goodman MD, Cooper PH. Granular cell tumor (myoblastoma) of the stomach; case report with ultrastructural findings and review of the literature. Am J Dig Dis 17:1117, 1972.
238. Harrer WV, Patchefsky AS. Malignant granular cell myoblastoma of the posterior mediastinum. Chest 61:95, 1972.
239. Hunter DT, Dewar JP. Malignant granular cell myoblastoma: report of a case and review of the literature. Am Surg 26:554, 1960.
240. Jardines L, Cheung L, LiVolsi V, et al. Malignant granular cell tumors: report of a case and review of the literature. Surgery 116:49, 1900.
241. Kindblom LG, Olsson KM. Malignant granular cell tumor: a clinico-pathologic and ultrastructural study of a case. Pathol Res Pract 172:384, 1981.
242. Klemperer P. Myoblastoma of the striated muscle. Am J Cancer 20:324, 1934.
243. Krieg AF. Malignant granular cell myoblastoma: a case report. Arch Pathol 74:251, 1962.
244. Kubacz GJ. Malignant granular cell myoblastoma: report of a case. Aust N Z J Surg 40:291, 1971.
245. Kurtin PJ, Bonin DM. Immunohistochemical demonstration of the lysosome associated glycoprotein CD68 (KP1) in granular cell tumors and schwannomas. Hum Pathol 25:1172, 1994.
246. Lack EE, Worsham GF, Callihan MD, et al. Granular cell tumor: a clinicopathologic study of 110 patients. J Surg Oncol 13:301, 1980.
247. Mackenzie DH. Malignant granular cell myoblastoma. J Clin Pathol 20:739, 1967.
248. Madhavan M, Aurora AL, Sen SB. Malignant granular cell myoblastoma. Indian J Cancer 11:360, 1974.
249. McWilliam LJ, Harris M. Granular cell angiosarcoma of the skin: histology, electron microscopy, and immunohistochemistry of a newly recognized tumor. Histopathology 9:1205, 1985.
250. Mentzel T, Wadden C, Fletcher CD. Granular cell change in smooth muscle tumours of skin and soft tissue. Histopathology 24:223, 1994.
251. Miettinen M, Lehtonen E, Lehtola H, et al. Histogenesis of granular cell tumour: an immunological and ultrastructural study. J Pathol 142:221, 1984.
252. Moscovic EA, Azar HA. Multiple granular cell tumors ("myoblastomas"): case report with electron microscopic observations and review of the literature. Cancer 20:2032, 1967.
253. Mukai M. Immunohistochemical localization of S-100 protein and peripheral nerve myelin proteins (P2 protein and PO protein) in granular cell tumors. Am J Pathol 112:139, 1983.

254. Murray DE, Seaman E, Ultzinger W. Granular cell myoblastomas in successive generations. J Surg Oncol 1:193, 1969.
255. Nakazato Y, Ishizeki J, Takahashi K, et al. Immunohistochemical localization of S-100 protein in granular cell myoblastoma. Cancer 49:1624, 1982.
256. Nathrath WBJ, Remberger K. Immunohistochemical study of granular cell tumours: demonstration of neuron specific enolase, S-100 protein, laminin, and alpha-1-antichymotrypsin. Virchows Arch A Pathol Anat Histopathol 408:421, 1986.
257. Nistal M, Paniagua R, Pizazo ML, et al. Granular changes in vascular leiomyosarcoma. Virchows Arch [Pathol Anat] 386: 239, 1980.
258. Papageorgiou S, Litt JZ, Pomeranz JR. Multiple granular cell myoblastomas in children. Arch Dermatol 96:168, 1967.
259. Pearse AGE. The histogenesis of granular cell myoblastoma. J Pathol Bacteriol 62:351, 1950.
260. Propst A, Weiser G. Das granulare Neuron Feyrters. Wien Klin Wochenschr 83:31, 1971.
261. Rao TV, Puri R, Reddy GNN. Intracranial trigeminal nerve granular cell myoblastoma: case report. J Neurosurg 59:706, 1983.
262. Ratzenhofer M. Granulaere falsche Neurome (sog. Myoblastenmyome) und sekundaere Wucherung de Deckepithels. Virchows Arch [Pathol Anat] 320:138, 1951.
263. Ravich A, Stout AP, Ravich RA. Malignant granular cell myoblastoma involving the urinary bladder. Ann Surg 121: 361, 1945.
264. Robertson AJ, McIntosh W, Lamont P, et al. Malignant granular cell tumor (myoblastoma) of the vulva: report of a case and review of the literature. Histopathology 5:69, 1981.
265. Ross RC, Miller TR, Foote FW. Malignant granular cell myoblastoma. Cancer 5:112, 1952.
266. Save-Soderbergh I. Basal lamina in granular cell tumors. Hum Pathol 6:637, 1975.
267. Seo IS, Azarelli B, Warner TF, et al. Multiple visceral and cutaneous granular cell tumors: ultrastructural and immunocytochemical evidence of Schwann cell origin. Cancer 53:2104, 1984.
268. Smolle J, Konrad K, Kerl H. Granular cell minors contain myelin-associated glycoprotein: an immunohistochemical study using Leu-7 monoclonal antibody. Virchows Arch A Pathol Anat Histopathol 406:1, 1985.
269. Sobel HJ. Granular cell myoblastoma: an electron-microscopic and cytochemical study illustrating the genesis of granules and aging of myoblastoma cells. Am J Pathol 65:59, 1971.
270. Sobel HJ, Arvin E, Marquet E, et al. Reactive granular cell in sites of trauma. Am J Clin Pathol 61:223, 1974.
271. Sobel HJ, Churg J. Granular cells and granular cell lesions. Arch Pathol 77:132, 1974.
272. Sobel HJ, Schwarz R, Marquet E. Light and electron microscopic study of the origin of granular cell myoblastoma. J Pathol 109:101, 1973.
273. Steffelaar JW, Nap M, van Haelst UJGM. Malignant granular cell tumor: report of a case with special reference to carcinoembryonic antigen. Am J Surg Pathol 6:665, 1982.
274. Strong EW, McDivitt RW, Brasfield RD. Granular cell myoblastoma. Cancer 25:415, 1970.
275. Svejda J, Horn V. Disseminated granular-cell pseudotumor: so-called metastasizing granular cell myoblastoma. J Pathol Bacteriol 76:343, 1958.
276. Toto PD, Restarski J. Histogenesis of the granular-cell myoblastoma. Oral Surg Oral Med Oral Pathol 24:384, 1967.
277. Tsuneyoshi M, Enjoji M. Granular cell tumor: a clinicopathological study of 48 cases. Fukuoka Acta Med 69:495, 1978.
278. Tyagi SP, Khan MH, Tyagi N. Malignant granular cell tumor. Indian J Cancer 15:77, 1978.
279. Usui M, Ishii S, Yamawaki S, et al. Malignant granular cell tumor of the radial nerve: an autopsy observation with electron microscopic and tissue culture studies. Cancer 39:1547, 1977.
280. Vance S, Hudson R. Granular cell myoblastoma. Am J Clin Pathol 52:208, 1969.
281. Weiser G. Granularzelltumor (Granulares Neuron Feyrter) und Schwannsche Phagen: electronenoptische Untersuchung von 3 Faellen. Virchows Arch [Pathol Anat] 380:49, 1978.
282. Whitten JB. The fine structure of an intraoral granular-cell myoblastoma. Oral Surg Oral Med Oral Pathol 26:202, 1968.


### Congenital (Gingival) Granular Cell Tumor


283. Bhaskar SN, Akamine R. Congenital epulis (congenital granular cell fibroblastoma). J Oral Surg 8:517, 1955.
284. Cussen LJ, MacMahon RA. Congenital granular cell myoblastoma. J Pediatr Surg 10:249, 1975.
285. Fuhr AH, Krogh PHJ. Congenital epulis of the newborn: centennial review of the literature and a report of a case. J Oral Surg 30:30, 1972.
286. Ganley CJ, El Attar AM. Congenital myoblastoma of the newborn. Oral Surg Oral Med Oral Pathol 20:645, 1965.
287. Henefer EP, Abaza NA, Anderson SP. Congenital granular cell epulis: report of a case. Oral Surg Oral Med Oral Pathol 47: 515, 1979.
288. Koppang HS. Congenital gingival granular-cell myoblastoma. Oral Surg Oral Med Oral Pathol 34:98, 1972.
289. Lack E, Crawford BE, Worsham GF, et al. Gingival granular cell tumors of the newborn (congenital "epulis"): a clinical and pathologic study of 21 patients. Am J Surg Pathol 5:37, 1981.
290. Lack EE, Perez-Atayde AR, McGill TJ, et al. Gingival granular cell tumor of the newborn (congenital "epulis"): ultrastructural observations relating to histogenesis. Hum Pathol 13:686, 1982.
291. Lifshitz MS, Flotte TJ, Greco MA. Congenital granular cell epulis: immunohistochemical and ultrastructural observations. Cancer 53:1845, 1984.
292. Matthews JB, Mason GI. Oral granular cell myoblastoma: an immunohistochemical study. J Oral Pathol 11:343, 1982.
293. Slootweg P, de Wilde P, Vooijs P, et al. Oral granular cell lesions: an immunohistochemical study with emphasis on intermediate-sized filament proteins. Virchows Arch [Pathol Anat] 402:35, 1983.
294. Tucker JC, Rusnock EJ, Azumi N. Gingival granular cell tumors of the newborn: an ultrastructural and immunohistochemical study. Arch Pathol Lab Med 114:895, 1990.
295. Volkmann J. Myoblastenmyom: eine stelene angeborene Oberkiefergeschwulst bei einem Neugeborenen. Zentralbl Chir 56: 2982, 1929.


### Neurothekeoma (Nerve Sheath Myxoma)


296. Angervall L, Kindblom L, Haglid K. Dermal nerve sheath myxoma. Cancer 53:1752, 1984.
297. Aronson PJ, Fretzin DF, Potter BS. Neurothekeoma of Gallager and Helwig (dermal nerve sheath myxoma variant): report of a case with electron microscopic and immunohistochemical studies. J Cutan Pathol 12:506, 1985.
298. Barnhill RL, Dickersin GR, Nickeleit V, et al. Studies on the cellular origin of neurothekeoma: clinical, light microscopic, immunohistochemical, and ultrastructural observations. J Am Acad Dermatol 25:80, 1991.
299. Barnhill RL, Mihm MC Jr. Cellular neurothekeoma: a distinctive variant of neurothekeoma mimicking nevomelanocytic tumors. Am J Surg Pathol 14:113, 1990.
300. Busam KJ, Mentzel T, Colpaert C, et al. Atypical or worrisome features in cellular neurothekeoma: a study of 10 cases. Am J Surg Pathol 22:1067, 1998.
301. Calonje E, Wilson-Jones E, Smith NP, et al. Cellular "neurothekeoma": an epithelioid variant of pilar leiomyoma? Mor-

phological and immunohistochemical analysis of a series. Histopathology 20:397, 1992.
302. Gallager RL, Helwig EB. Neurothekeoma: a benign cutaneous tumor of nerve sheath origin. Am J Clin Pathol 74:759, 1980.
303. King D, Barr R. Bizarre cutaneous neurofibromas. J Cutan Pathol 7:21, 1980.
304. MacDonald DM, Wilson-Jones E. Pacinian neurofibroma. Histopathology 1:247, 1977.
305. Pulitzer DR, Reed RJ. Nerve sheath myxoma. Am J Dermatopathol 7:409, 1985.
306. Wang AR, May D, Bourne P, Scott G. PGP: a marker for cellular neurothekeoma. Am J Surg Pathol 23:1401, 1999.

### Extracranial Meningioma

307. Lopez DA, Silvers DN, Helwig EB. Cutaneous meningiomas: a clinicopathologic study. Cancer 34:728, 1974.
308. Theaker JM, Fleming KA. Meningioma of the scalp: a case report with immunohistochemical features. J Cutan Pathol 14: 49, 1987.

### Glial Heterotopias

309. Orkin M, Fisher I. Heterotopic brain tissue (heterotopic neural rest). Arch Dermatol 94:699, 1966.
310. Rios JJ, Diaz-Cano SL, Rivera-Hueto F, et al. Cutaneous ganglion cell choristoma. J Cutan Pathol 18:469, 1991.
311. Shepherd NA, Coates PJ, Brown AA. Soft tissue giomatosis—heterotopic glial tissue in the subcutis: a case report. Histopathology 11:655, 1987.
312. Skelton HG, Smith KJ. Glial heterotopia in the subcutaneous tissue overlying T-12. J Cutan Pathol 26:523, 1999.

### Melanotic Neuroectodermal Tumor of Infancy

313. Allen M, Harrison W, Jahrsdoerfer R. Retinal anlage tumors. Am J Clin Pathol 51:309, 1969.
314. Borello ED, Gorlin RJ. Melanotic neuroectodermal tumor of infancy: a neoplasm of neural crest origin. Cancer 19:196, 1966.
315. Cutler LS, Chaudhry AP, Topazian R. Melanotic neuroectodermal tumor of infancy: an ultrastructural, literature review, and reevaluation. Cancer 48:257, 1981.
316. Dehner LP, Sibley RK, Sauk JJ, et al. Malignant melanotic neuroectodermal tumor of infancy: a clinical, pathologic, ultrastructural, and tissue culture study. Cancer 43:1389, 1979.
317. Dooling EC, Chi JEG, Gilles FH. Melanotic neuroectodermal tumor of infancy: its histological similarities to fetal pineal gland. Cancer 39:1535, 1977.
318. Duckworth R, Seward GR. Amelanotic ameloblastic odontoma. Oral Surg Oral Med Oral Pathol 19:73, 1965.
319. Eaton WL, Ferguson JP. A retinoblastic teratoma of the epididymis. Cancer 9:718, 1956.
320. Frank GL, Koten HE. Melanotic hamartoma ("retinal anlage tumor") of the epididymis. J Pathol Bacteriol 93:549, 1967.
321. Hayward AF, Fickling BW, Lucas RB. An electron microscope study of a pigmented tumor of the jaw of infants. Br J Cancer 23:702, 1969.
322. Johnson RE, Scheithauer BW, Dahlin DC. Melanotic neuroectodermal tumor of infancy. Cancer 52:661, 1983.
323. Kapadia SH, Frisman DM, Hitchcock CL, et al. Melanotic neuroectodermal tumor of infancy. Am J Surg Pathol 17:566, 1993.
324. Koudstall J, Oldhoff J, Panders AK, et al. Melanotic neuroectodermal tumor of infancy. Cancer 22:151, 1968.
325. Lee SC, Henry MM, Gonzalez-Crussi F. Simultaneous occurrence of melanotic neuroectodermal tumor and brain heterotopia in the oropharynx. Cancer 38:249, 1976.
326. Lindahl F. Malignant melanotic progonoma: one case. Acta Pathol Microbiol Scand 78A:532, 1970.
327. Lurie HI. Congenital melanocarcinoma, melanocytic adamantinoma, retinal anlage tumor, progonoma, and pigmented epulis of infancy: summary and review of the literature and report of the first case in an adult. Cancer 14:1090, 1961.
328. Lurie HI, Isaacson C. A melanotic progonoma in the scapula. Cancer 14:1088, 1961.
329. Misugi K, Okajima H, Newton WA, et al. Mediastinal origin of a melanotic progonoma or retinal anlage tumor: ultrastructural evidence for neural crest origin. Cancer 18:477, 1965.
330. Navas Palacios JJ. Malignant melanotic neuroectodermal tumor: light and electron microscopic study. Cancer 46:529, 1980.
331. Pettinato G, Manivel C, d'Amore ESG, et al. Melanotic neuroectodermal tumor of infancy: an immunohistochemical study. Histopathology 12:425, 1988.
332. Schulz DM. A malignant melanotic neoplasm of the uterus resembling the retinal anlage tumor. Am J Clin Pathol 28:524, 1957.
333. Stirling RW, Powell G, Fletcher CDM. Pigmented neuroectodermal tumor of infancy: an immunohistochemical study. Histopathology 12:425, 1988.
334. Stowens D, Lin TH. Melanotic progonoma of the brain. Hum Pathol 5:105, 1974.
335. William AO. Melanotic ameloblastoma ("progonoma") of infancy showing osteogenesis. J Pathol Bacteriol 93:545, 1967.
336. Zone RM. Retinal analage tumor of the epididymis: a case report. J Urol 103:106, 1970.

# CHAPTER 31

# MALIGNANT TUMORS OF THE PERIPHERAL NERVES

Malignant tumors arising from peripheral nerves or displaying differentiation along the lines of the various elements of the nerve sheath (e.g., Schwann cell, perineural cell, fibroblast) are collectively referred to as malignant peripheral nerve sheath tumors (MPNSTs). This term replaces a number of earlier terms including ***malignant schwannoma, neurofibrosarcoma,*** and ***neurogenic sarcoma.*** Because MPNSTs recapitulate the appearance of various cells of the nerve sheath, they range in appearance from tumors that resemble a neurofibroma to those indistinguishable from a fibrosarcoma. Rarely, tumors arising from nerves or neurofibromas display aberrant lines of differentiation. For example, angiosarcomas may arise in nerves or in preexisting neurofibromas. By convention these tumors are not considered MPNSTs but are classified according to their aberrant line of differentiation. Although primitive neuroectodermal tumors also arise from peripheral nerves, they are considered along with neuroblastic tumors and Ewing's sarcoma in Chapter 32.

The diagnosis of MPNSTs has traditionally been one of the most difficult and elusive among soft tissue diseases because of the lack of standardized diagnostic criteria. Although there is general agreement that if a sarcoma arises from a peripheral nerve or a neurofibroma it can usually be considered an MPNST, there has been less agreement over the years as to the diagnostic criteria for tumors occurring outside these settings. As a result, the incidence of this sarcoma has varied in the literature. In 1931 Stewart and Copeland,[108] reporting their experience from Memorial Hospital in New York, maintained that "neurogenic sarcomas" comprise most of the fibrosarcomas of soft tissue and that most occurred in patients without neurofibromatosis. Likewise, Geschickter,[37] in a review of cases from the Johns Hopkins Hospital, concluded that the tumor was among the most common of all soft tissue sarcomas. Both studies reflect a liberal diagnostic approach and willingness to accept many spindled collagen-producing sarcomas as neural, especially if they occur in certain locations or produce characteristic symptoms. On the other hand, Stout[110] proposed a stricter definition of the tumor. In his opinion, these tumors could not be distinguished from fibrosarcomas on histologic grounds, and their diagnosis rested on the documented origin from nerve or neurofibroma or association with von Recklinghausen's disease. The rarity of the tumor in Stout's experience and its high association with neurofibromatosis reflect in large part his stringent criteria.

A sarcoma is assumed to be a MPNST if one of three criteria can be met: (1) the tumor arises from a peripheral nerve, (2) it arises from a preexisting benign nerve sheath tumor, usually a neurofibroma; or (3) the tumor displays a constellation of histologic features that are seen in tumors arising in the foregoing situations and are generally accepted as reflecting schwann cell differentiation by light microscopy. These features include the (1) dense and hypodense fascicles alternating in a "marble-like" pattern consisting of (2) asymmetrically tapered spindled cells with irregular buckled nuclei or (3) immunohistochemical or electron microscopic evidence of schwann cell differentiation in the context of a fibrosarcomatous-appearing tumor. In addition, there are features that are less specific but frequently occur in schwann cell tumors, including nuclear palisading, whorled structures that vaguely suggests large tactoid structures, peculiar "hyperplastic" perivascular change, and occasionally heterologous elements (e.g., cartilage, bone, skeletal muscle). Obviously, these criteria allow inclusion of only MPNSTs that are reasonably well differentiated or have not yet obscured their site of origin. Nonetheless, this approach offers an acceptable degree of diagnostic reproducibility and eliminates the potpourri of spindle cell tumors that have been diagnosed as MPNSTs in the past.

## CLINICAL FINDINGS

The MPNSTs account for approximately 5–10% of all soft tissue sarcomas, about one-fourth to one-half occur with neurofibromatosis 1 (NF1).[31,53,128] Obviously the diagnostic criteria and type of pathologic material affect these figures, as illustrated by the fact that the association with NF1 varies from about one-fourth[37] to more than two-thirds in the literature. In large series in which there has been consistency in histologic diagnoses, the percents of patients with MPNSTs having and not having NF1 is roughly equal.[53] Patients with NF1 are clearly at increased risk to develop these tumors, although earlier estimates that patients with NF1 had a risk as high as 13% of developing an MPNST are gross overestimates according to current studies. About 3–5% of patients with NF1 develop MPNSTs[106] (see Chapter 30). Patients with NF1 develop sarcomas usually after a relatively long latent period (10–20 years[45]), and in some cases the MPNSTs are multiple.[105] MPNST in childhood is recognized, but infrequent.[9,15,24]

The exact mechanism of malignant transformation or tumor progression in NF1 is not fully understood, but it seems to involve a multistep process in which genes other than the NF1 gene also participate (see below). Aside from the foregoing genetic predilection to develop MPNSTs, little is known about the pathogenesis of these tumors in humans. About 10–20% of cases occur as a result of therapeutic or occupational irradiation after a latent period of more than 15 years.[30,31,34,63,128] These tumors do not differ significantly from other MPNSTs.

Experimentally, these tumors can be induced in laboratory animals by transplacental injection of ethylnitrosourea[62] or administration of methylcholanthrene.[99] As a result of these studies, it has been suggested that a search for chemical carcinogens in the environment might prove fruitful.

The MPNST is typically a disease of adult life, as most tumors occur in patients 20–50 years of age.[5,19–21,31,45,106] Patients with NF1 develop these tumors at an earlier age, however. The average age at the time of diagnosis for patients with NF1 was 29 and 36 years in the Mayo Clinic[31] and Memorial Sloan Kettering[53] studies, respectively, compared with 40 and 44 years, respectively, for patients without the disease. Our experience indicates an average age of 32 years for both groups but a wider age range among patients without NF1.[45] The gender ratio of patients with MPNST varies, depending on patient selection. Men predominate in studies that report a high percentage of patients with NF1 as a result of the bias toward men in this disease.[20,31,45,128] In studies of sporadic cases of MPNST, the gender ratio is roughly equal to or slightly biased toward women.[20,38] These observations parallel our experience. Eighty percent of patients with NF1 and MPNST are men,[45] whereas only 56% of patients with sporadic MPNST are men.[45]

Like other sarcomas, these lesions present as enlarging masses that are usually noted several months before diagnosis. Pain is variable but seems to be more prevalent in those with NF1. In fact, pain or sudden enlargement of a preexisting mass in this setting should lead to immediate biopsy to exclude the possibility of malignant transformation of a neurofibroma. Fluorodeoxyglucose positron emission tomography (FDG PET), which allows visualization of glucose metabolism by cells, has been reasonably successful in identifying malignant change in plexiform neurofibromas,[33] although it has a small false-positive rate. MPNSTs that arise from major nerves typically give rise to a striking constellation of sensory and motor symptoms, including projected pain, paresthesias, and weakness. The symptoms rarely antedate the detection of a mass.

Most MPNSTs arise in association with major nerve trunks, including the sciatic nerve, brachial plexus, and sacral plexus. Consequently, the most common anatomic sites include the proximal portions of the upper and lower extremities and the trunk. Comparatively few arise in the head and neck, a feature that contrasts with the distribution of the schwannoma.

## GROSS FINDINGS

In its classic form, an MPNST arises as a large fusiform or eccentric mass in a major nerve (Fig. 31–1). Thickening of the nerve proximally and distally to the main mass usually indicates spread of the neoplasm along the epineurium and perineurium. In NF1 patients MPNSTs may develop in a preexisting neurofibroma (Fig. 31–2). Most of these lesions are deeply situated; only rare ones arise from superficial neurofibromas. Regardless of the clinical setting, the gross appearance of the MPNST is essentially similar to that of other soft tissue sarcoma. It is usually large, averaging more than 5 cm in diameter, and has a fleshy, opaque, white-tan surface marked by areas of secondary hemorrhage and necrosis. This appearance contrasts with the white mucoid appearance of the typical neurofibroma.

## MICROSCOPIC FINDINGS

Most MPNSTs resemble fibrosarcomas in their overall organization (Figs. 31–3 to 31–6) with certain modifications. Classically, the cells recapitulate the features of the normal Schwann cell. Unlike the symmetrically spindled cells of fibrosarcoma, they have markedly irregular contours. In profile the nuclei are wavy,

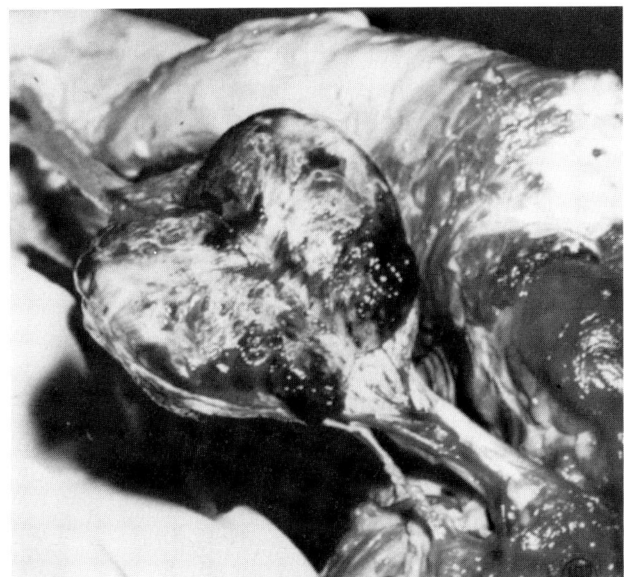

**FIGURE 31–1.** Malignant peripheral nerve sheath tumor (MPNST) arising as a large fusiform mass from the sciatic nerve. Cut section of tumor shows prominent hemorrhage and necrosis.

buckled, or comma-shaped, whereas when viewed en face they are asymmetrically oval (Fig. 31–7). The cytoplasm is lightly stained and usually indistinct. The cells can range from spindled in shape to fusiform or even rounded such that the lesion can mimic a fibrosarcoma or even a round cell sarcoma (Fig. 31–8).

The cells are arranged in sweeping fascicles, but there is greater variation in organization than in the fibrosarcoma. Densely cellular fascicles alternate with hypocellular, myxoid zones (Fig. 31–6), which swirl and interdigitate with one another creating a marble-like effect (Fig. 31–3). Others display a peculiar nodular, curlicue, or whorled arrangement of spindled cells (Figs. 31–9, 31–10) crudely suggesting tactoid differentiation. Nuclear palisading may be present, but in our cases it has occurred in fewer than 10% of all MPNSTs and, when present, is usually of a focal nature (Fig. 31–11).

There are several other subtle features that are quite characteristic of MPNSTs. Because they are not completely specific, they must be evaluated in the context of the foregoing discussion before a given tumor is termed an MPNST. These features include hyaline bands (Fig. 31–12) and nodules, which in cross section can be likened to giant rosettes (Fig. 31–12B), extensive perineural and intraneural spread of tumor (Fig. 31–13), and a peculiar proliferation of tumor in the subendothelial zones of vessels so the neoplastic cells appear to herniate into the lumen (Fig. 31–14). Small vessels may also proliferate in the walls of or around large vessels (Fig. 31–14B). Likewise, heterotopic elements, present in about 10–15% of MPNSTs, seem to be more common in MPNSTs than in other sarcomas.[22,24] Their presence may initially suggest the diagnosis in a tumor that otherwise resembles fibrosarcoma.

Mature islands of cartilage and bone are the most

*Text continued on page 1225*

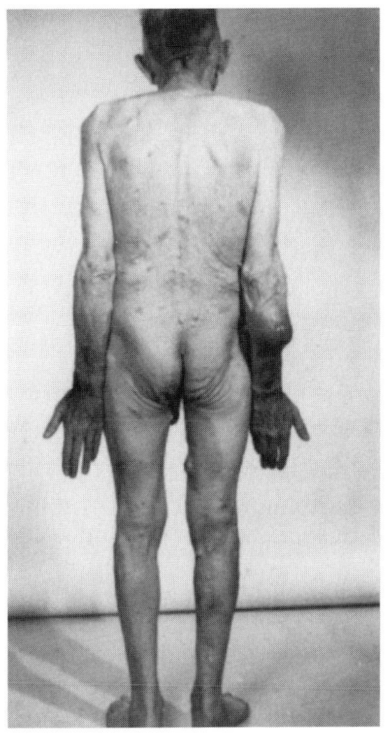

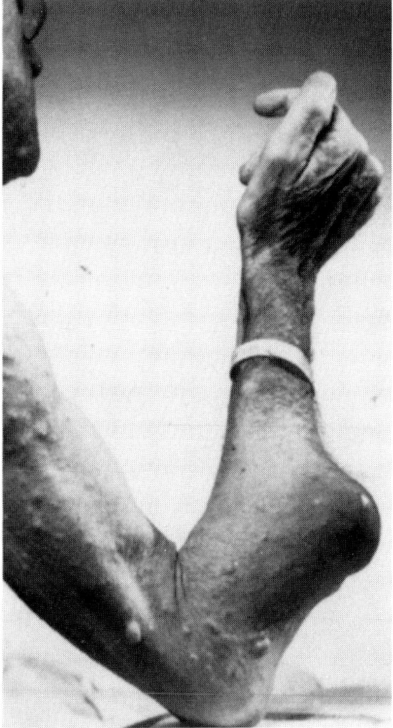

**FIGURE 31–2.** MPNST of the arm in a patient with long-standing neurofibromatosis.

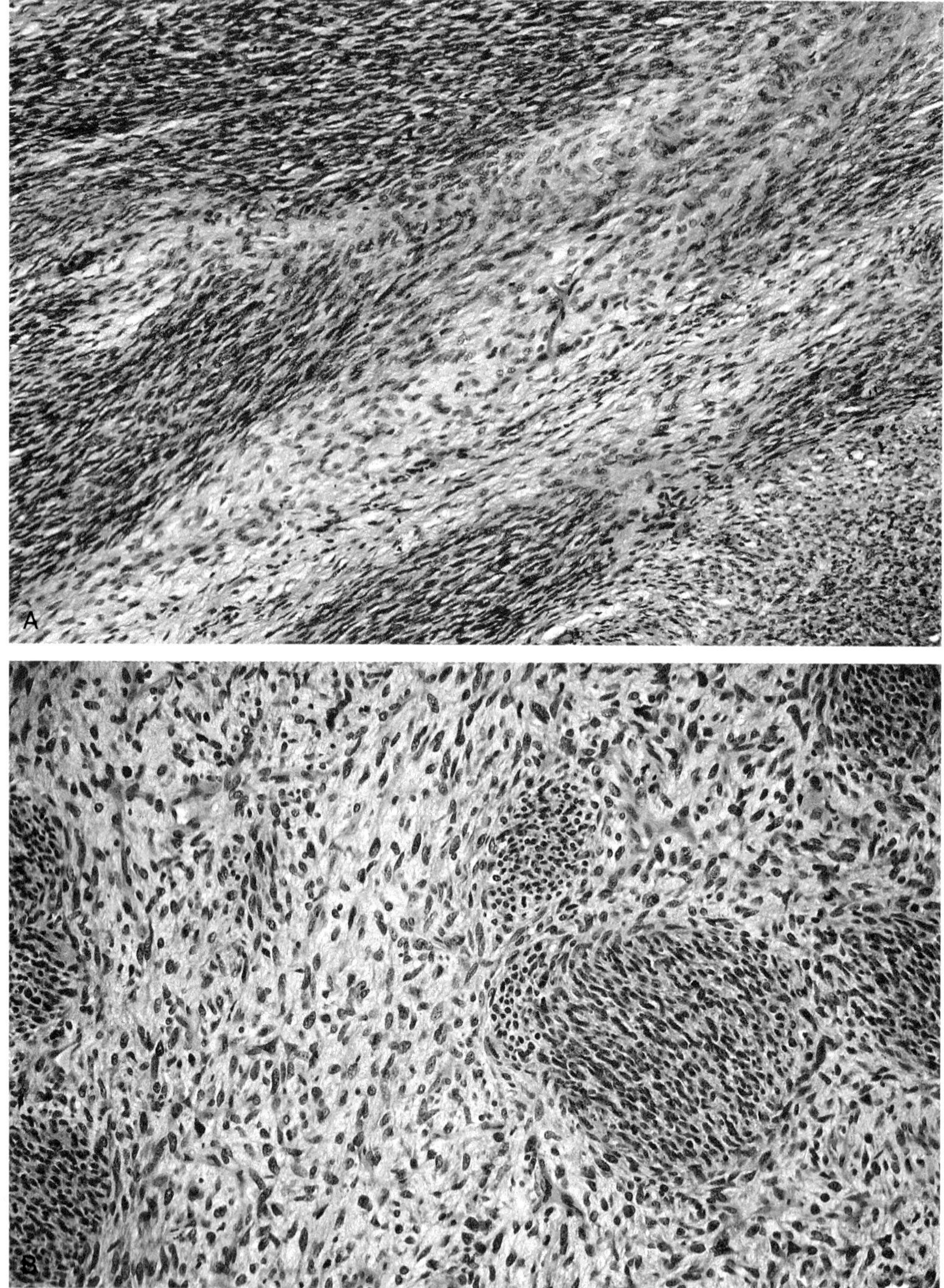

**FIGURE 31–3.** (**A, B**) Typical appearance of an MPNST with densely cellular areas alternating with less cellular ones, creating a marbleized appearance.

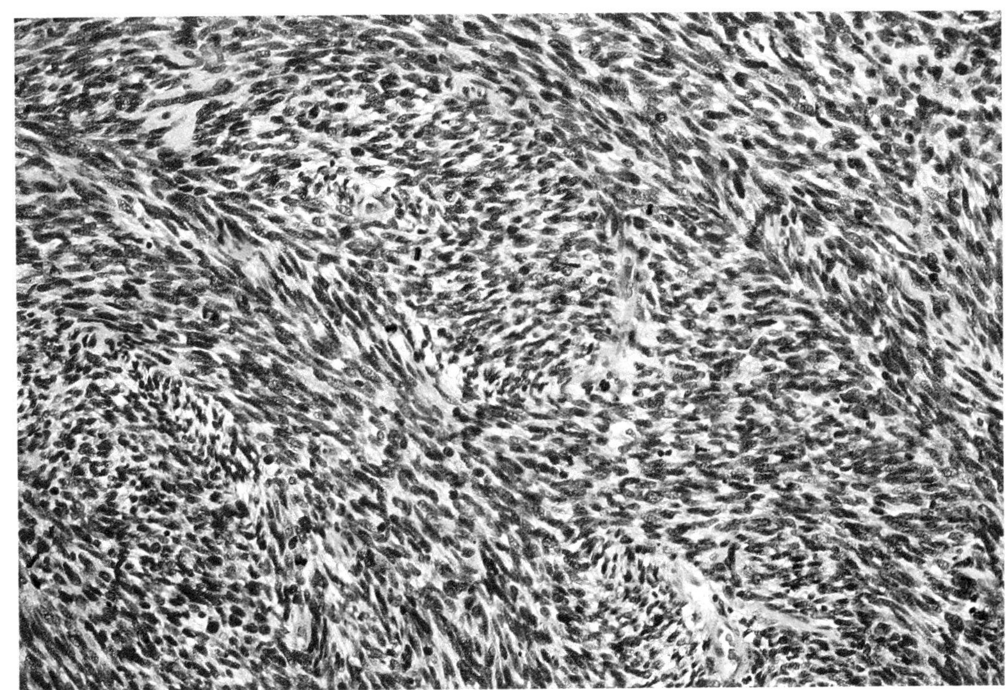

**FIGURE 31–4.** MPNST consisting exclusively of dense fascicles of spindled cells, similar to a fibrosarcoma.

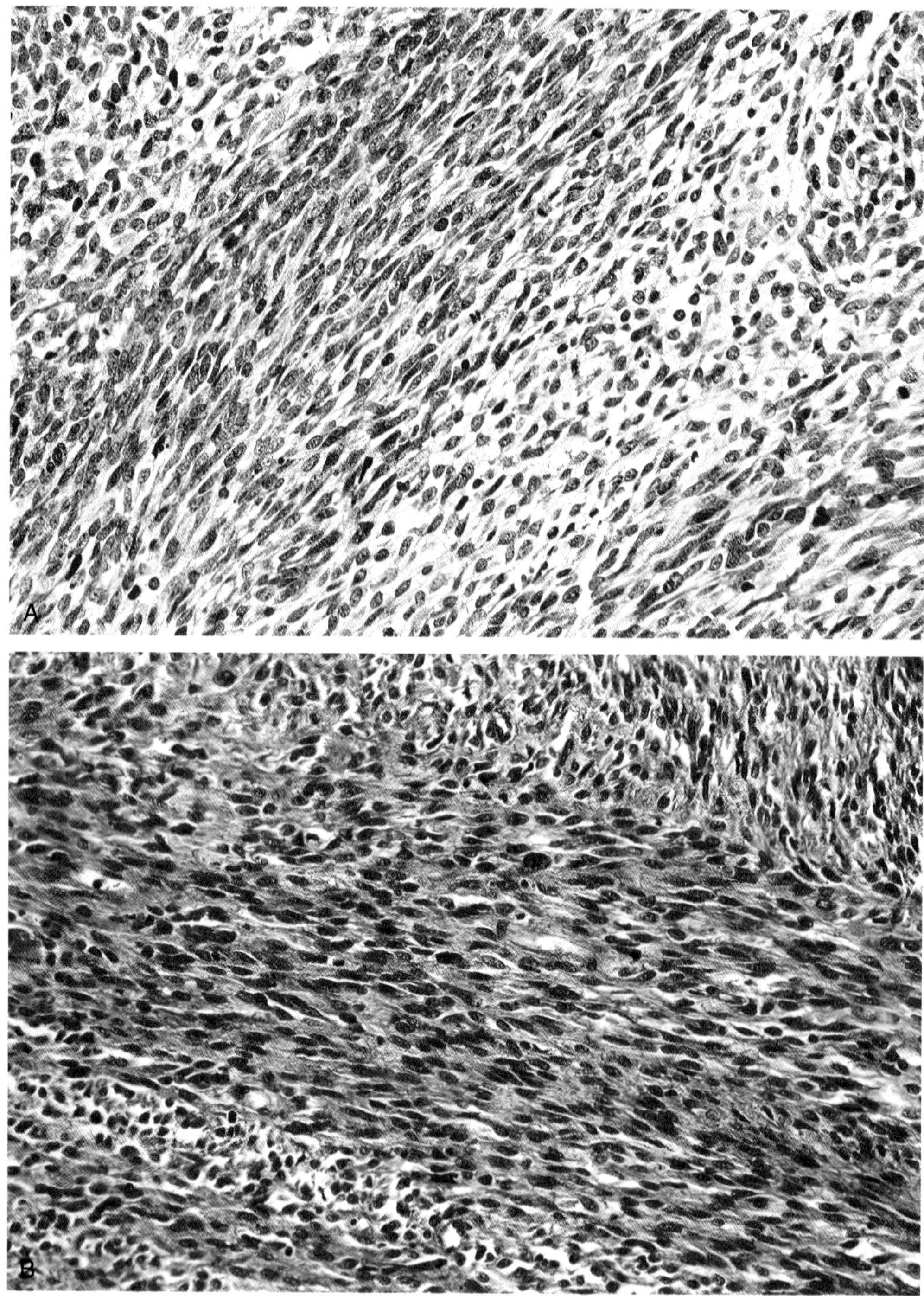

**FIGURE 31–5.** (**A, B**) Cellular fascicles of an MPNST.

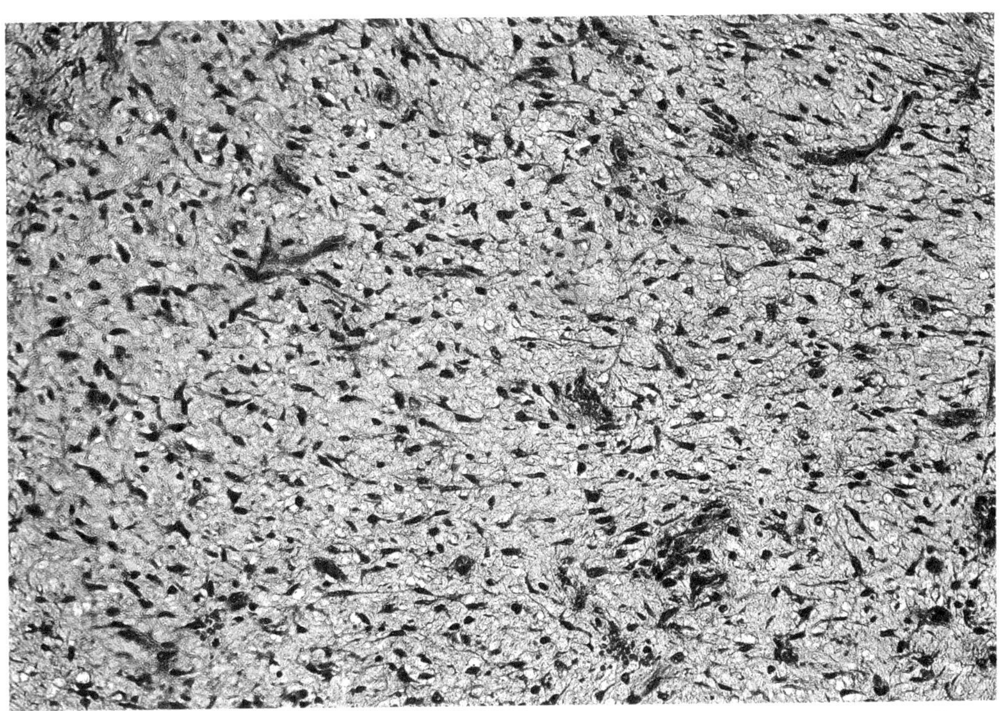

**FIGURE 31–6.** Myxoid area in an MPNST showing randomly arranged Schwann cells.

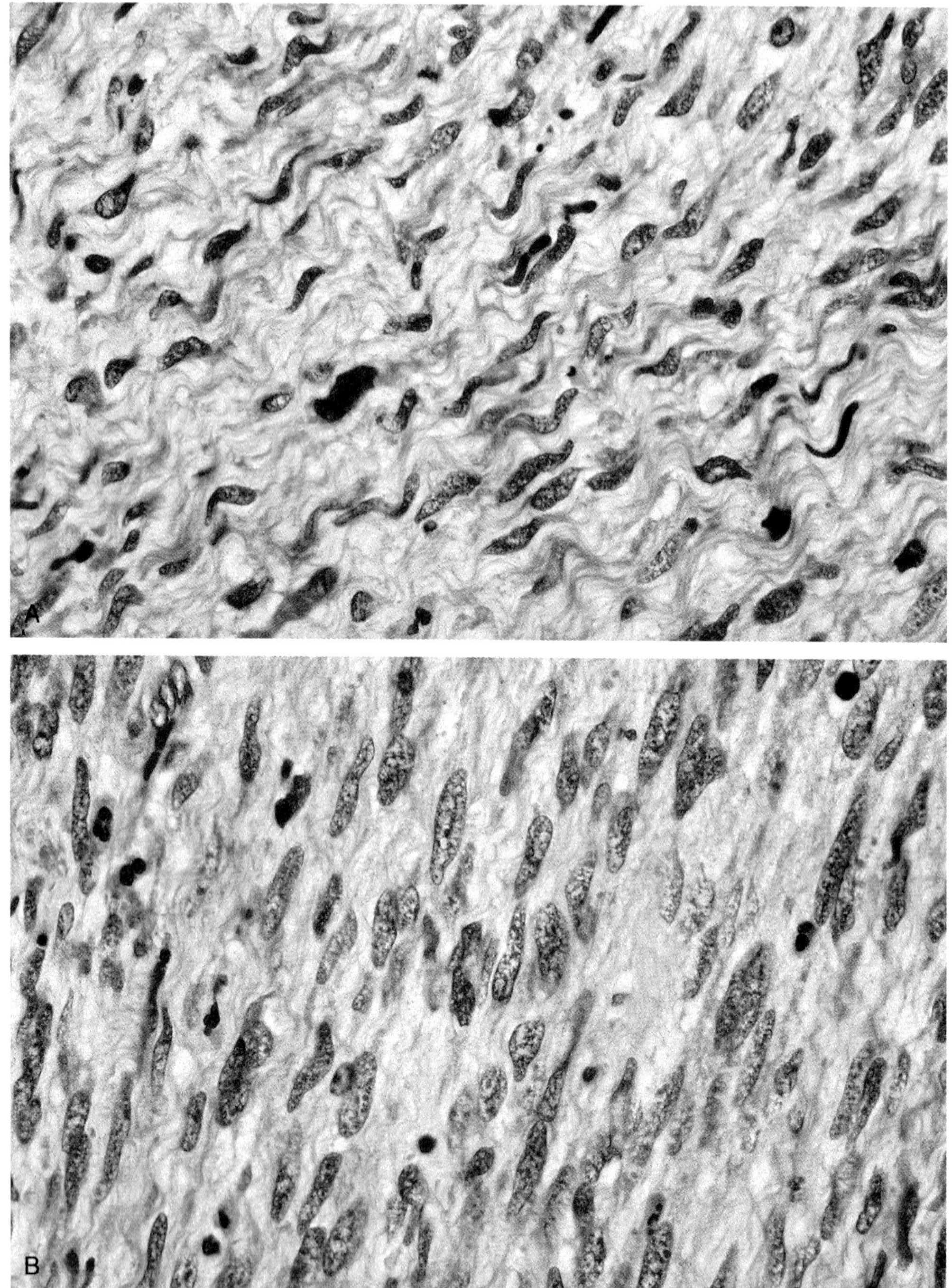


**FIGURE 31–7.** Cells in an MPNST with well differentiated areas (**A**) in which cells have an irregular, buckled shape characteristic of Schwann cells to less differentiated areas (**B**).

*Illustration continued on following page*

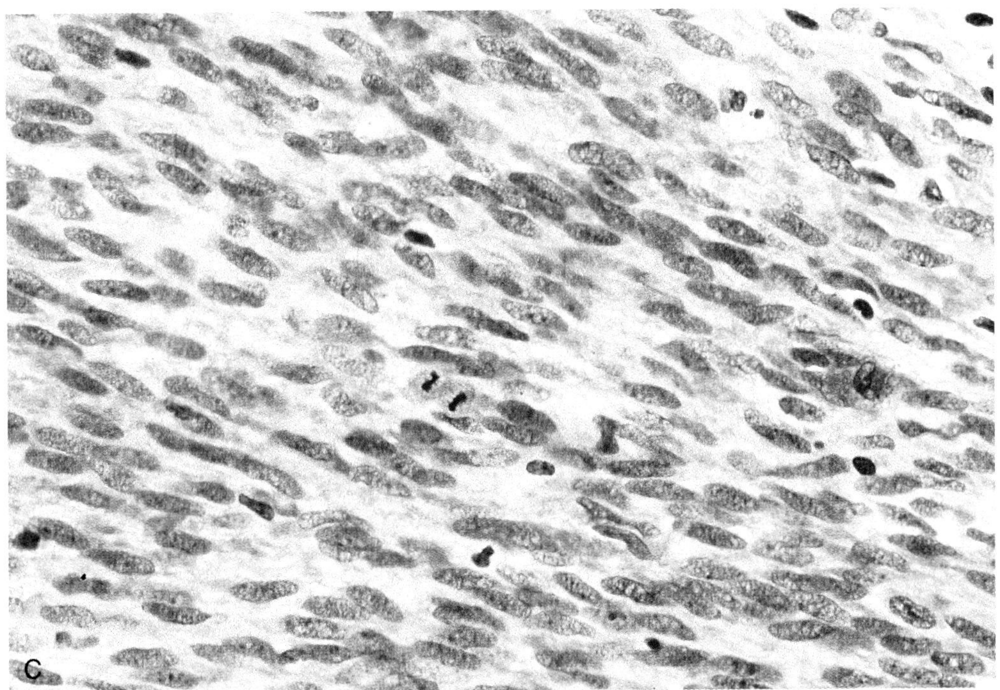


**FIGURE 31–7** *(Continued).* (**C**) S-100 protein immunostain shows focal weak staining of cells in an MPNST.

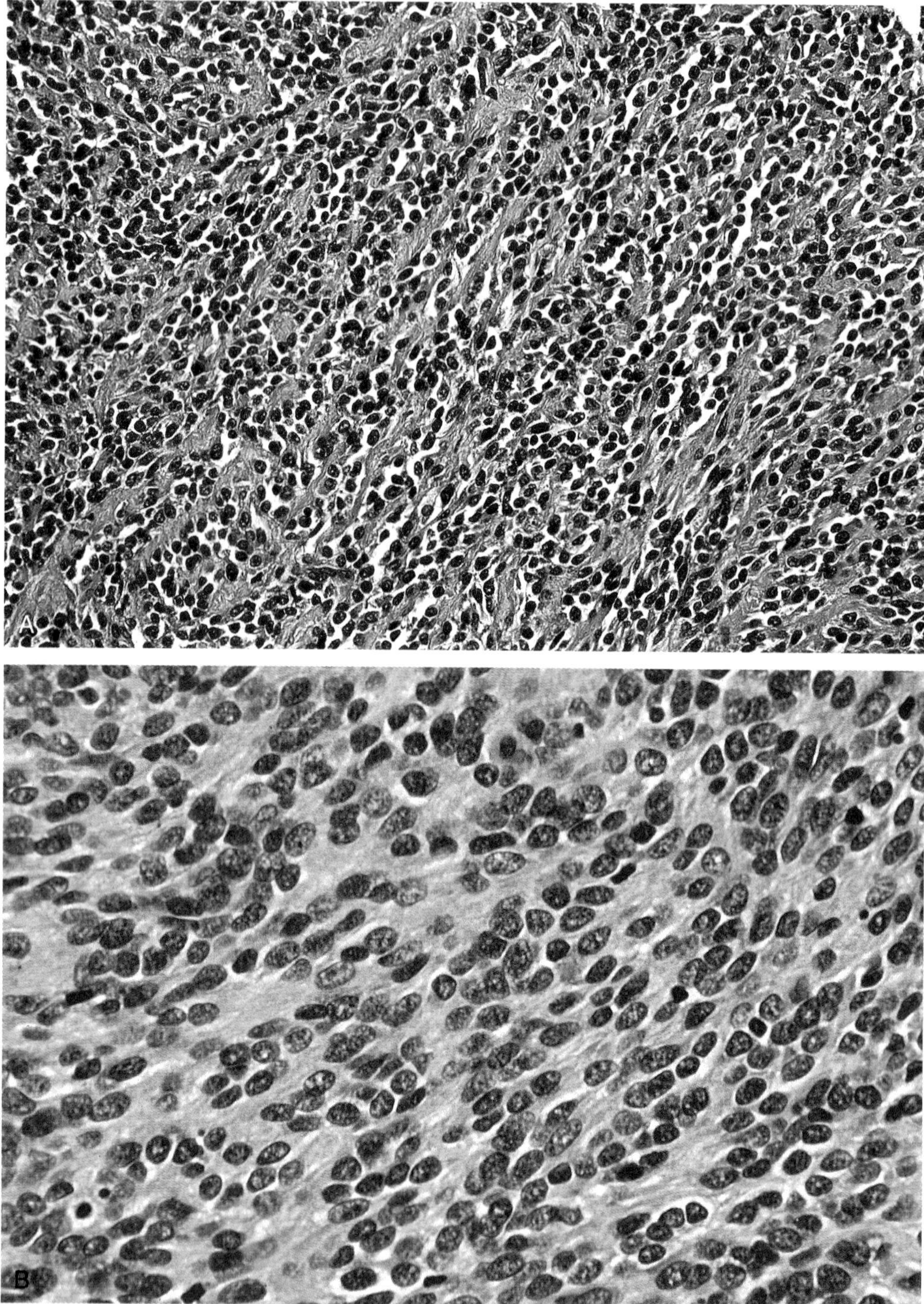

**FIGURE 31–8.** MPNST with areas composed of rounded (**A**) or short fusiform (**B**) cells. (**B**) Vague palisading of nuclei can be seen.

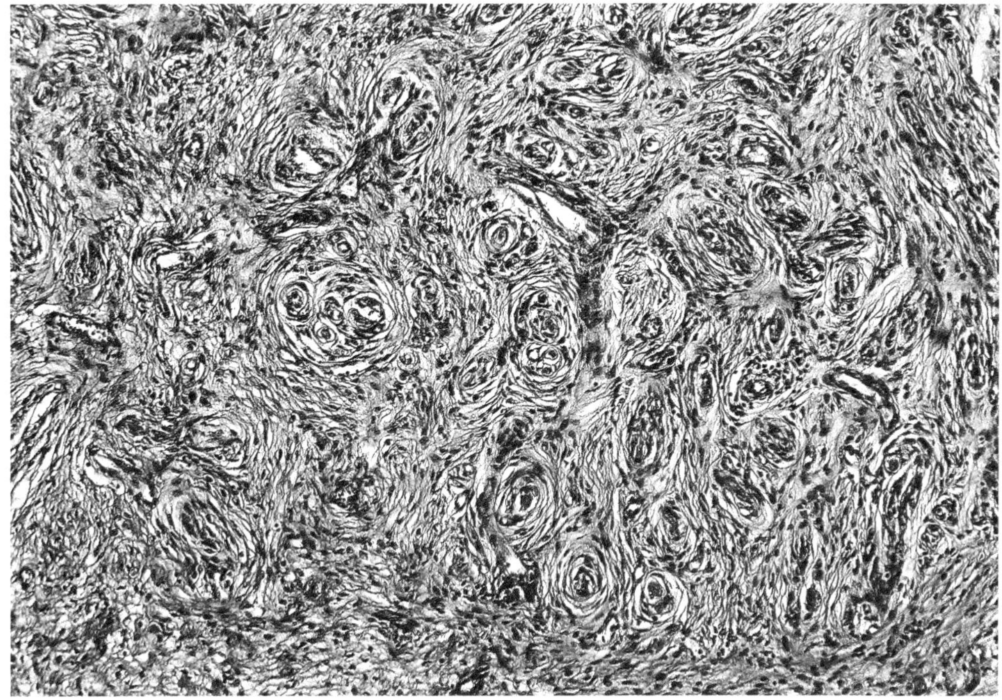

**FIGURE 31–9.** Low grade MPNST with a curlicue arrangement of cells.

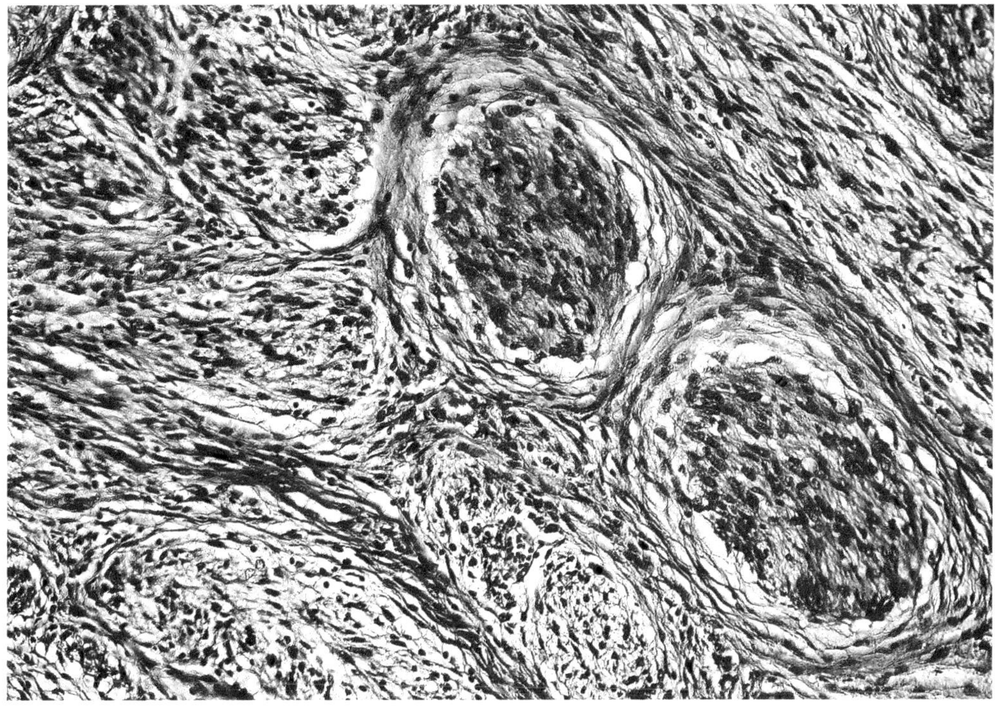

**FIGURE 31–10.** Whorled structures in an MPNST.

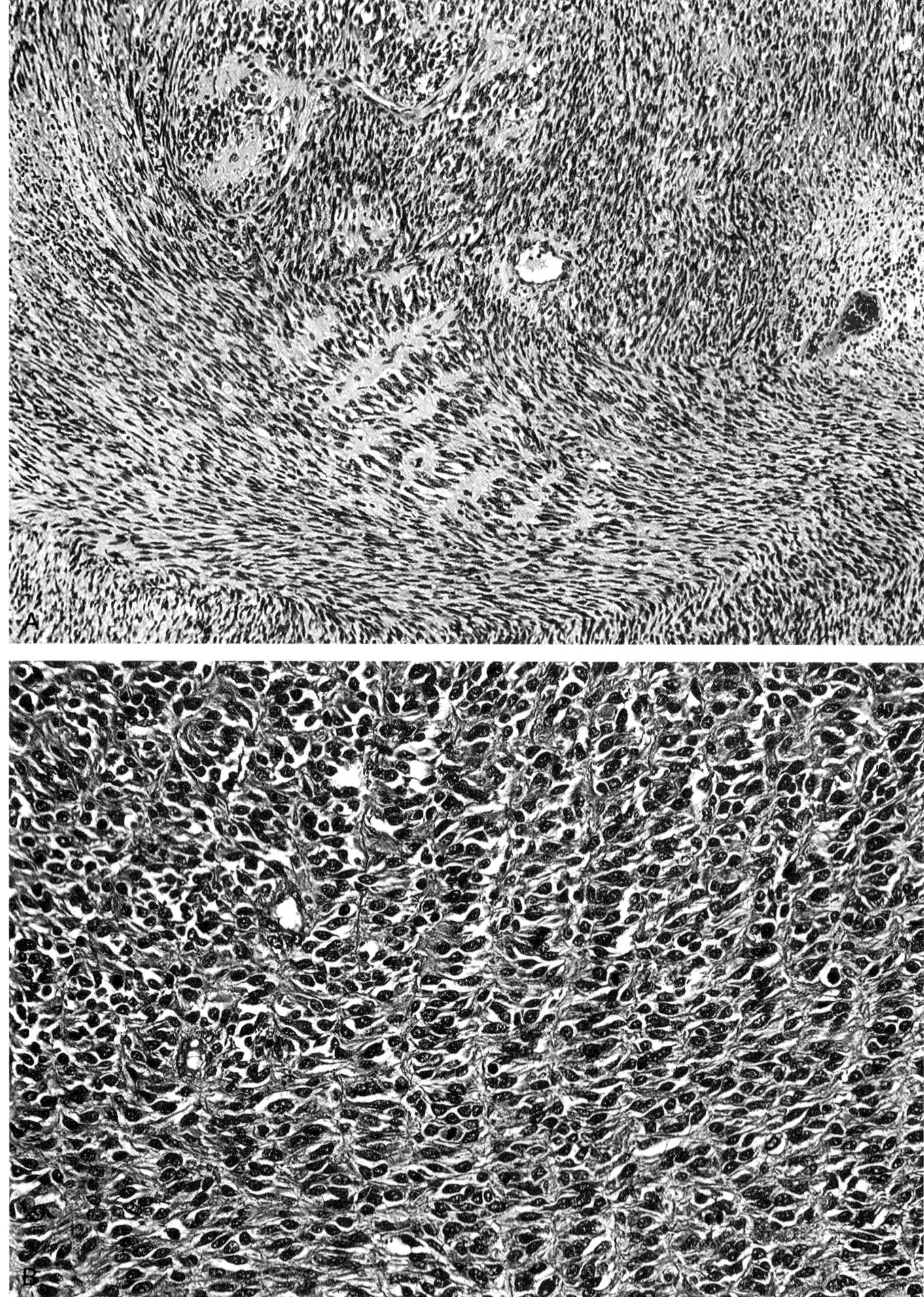

**FIGURE 31–11.** (**A, B**) Nuclear palisading is an uncommon feature in an MPNST. It may also be seen in schwannomas and some leiomyosarcomas.

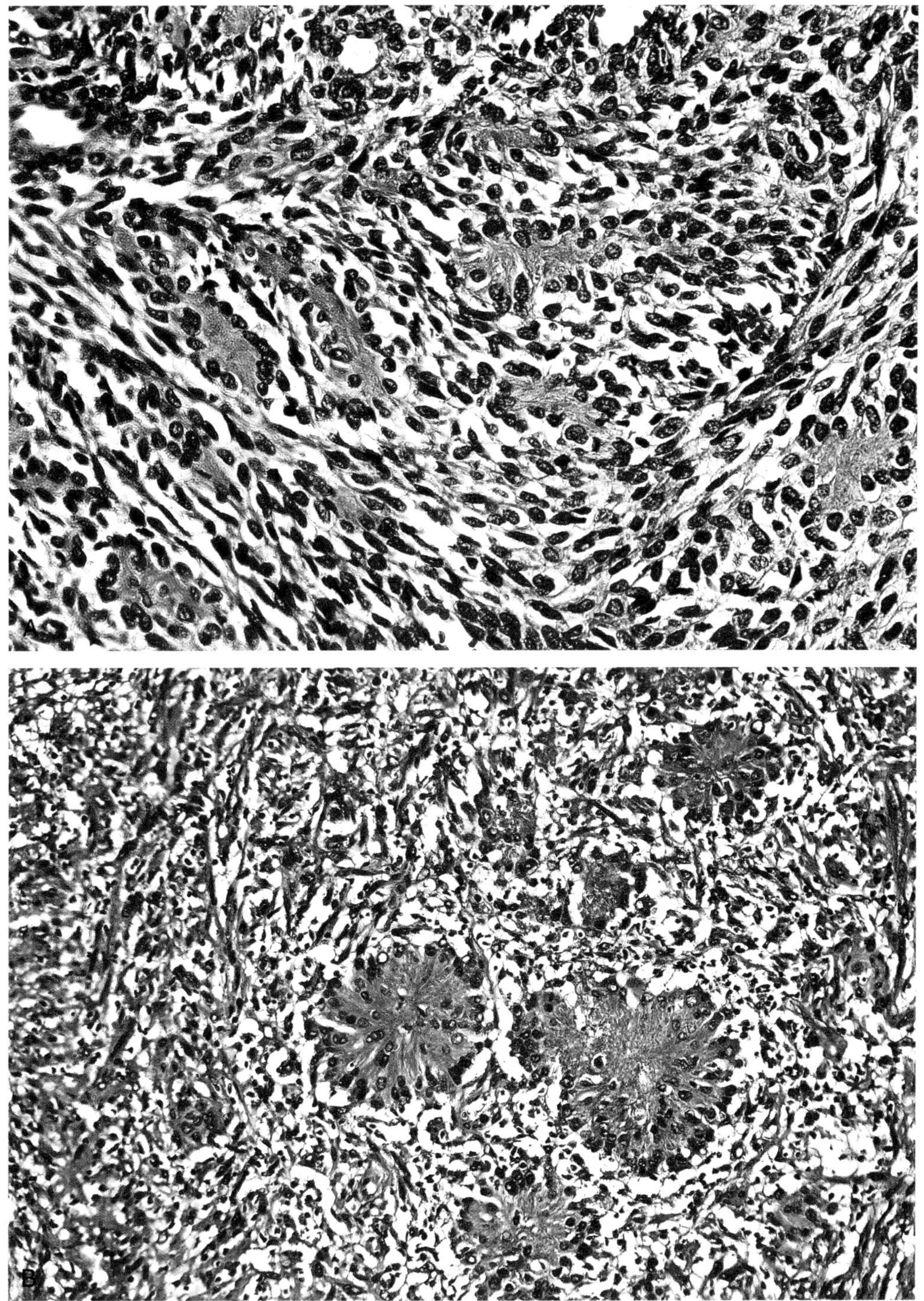

**FIGURE 31–12.** Hyalinized cords (**A**) and nodules (**B**) are uncommon but distinctive features of MPNSTs.

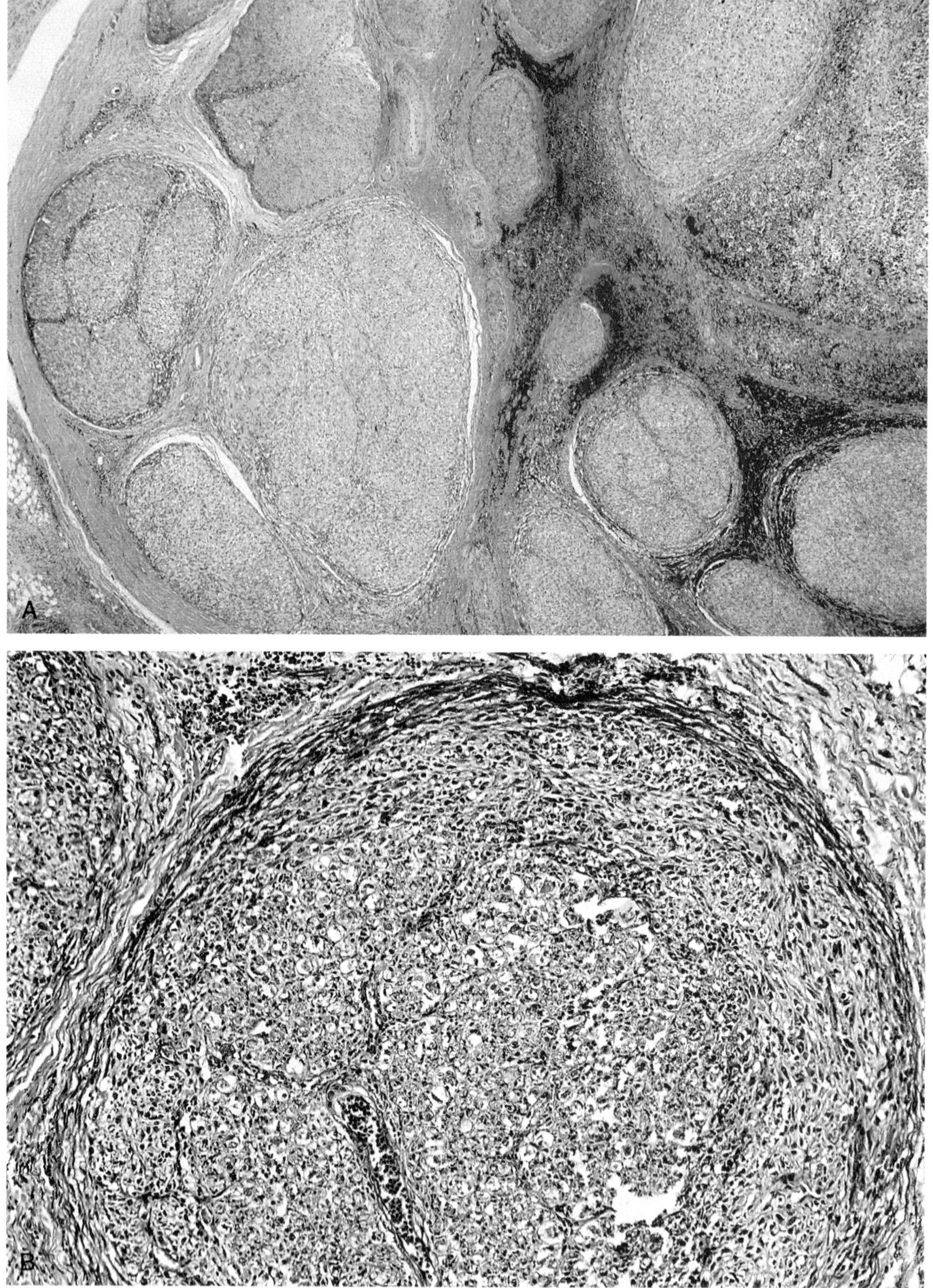

**FIGURE 31–13.** (**A**) Replacement of a peripheral nerve by an MPNST. (**B**) High power view showing insinuation of a tumor between the nerve fascicles.

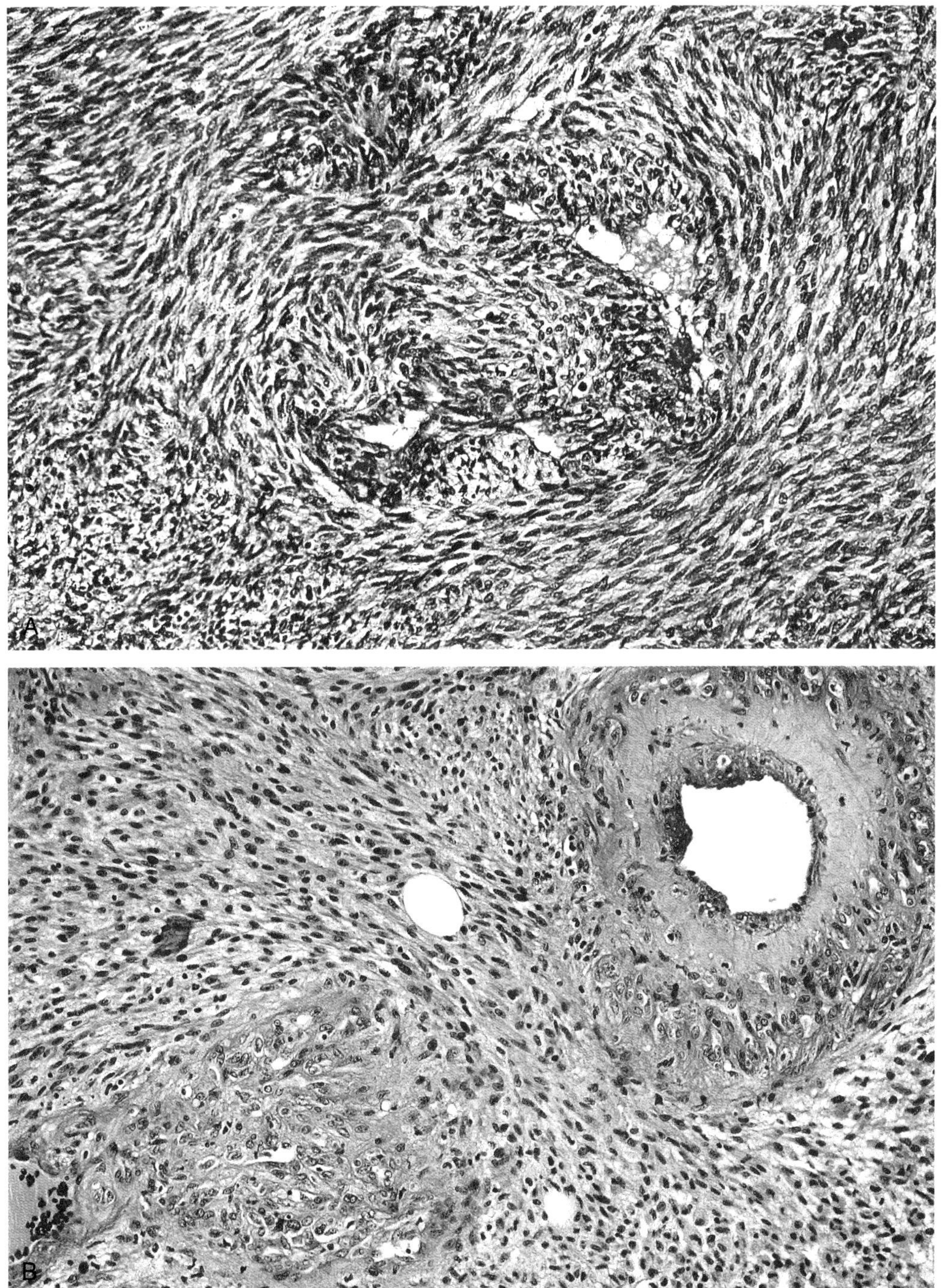

**FIGURE 31–14.** Peculiar changes around small vessels in MPNST. In **A** the tumor appears to herniate into lumens of vessels, whereas in **B** there is a small proliferation of small vessels in the walls of large vessels in MPNSTs.

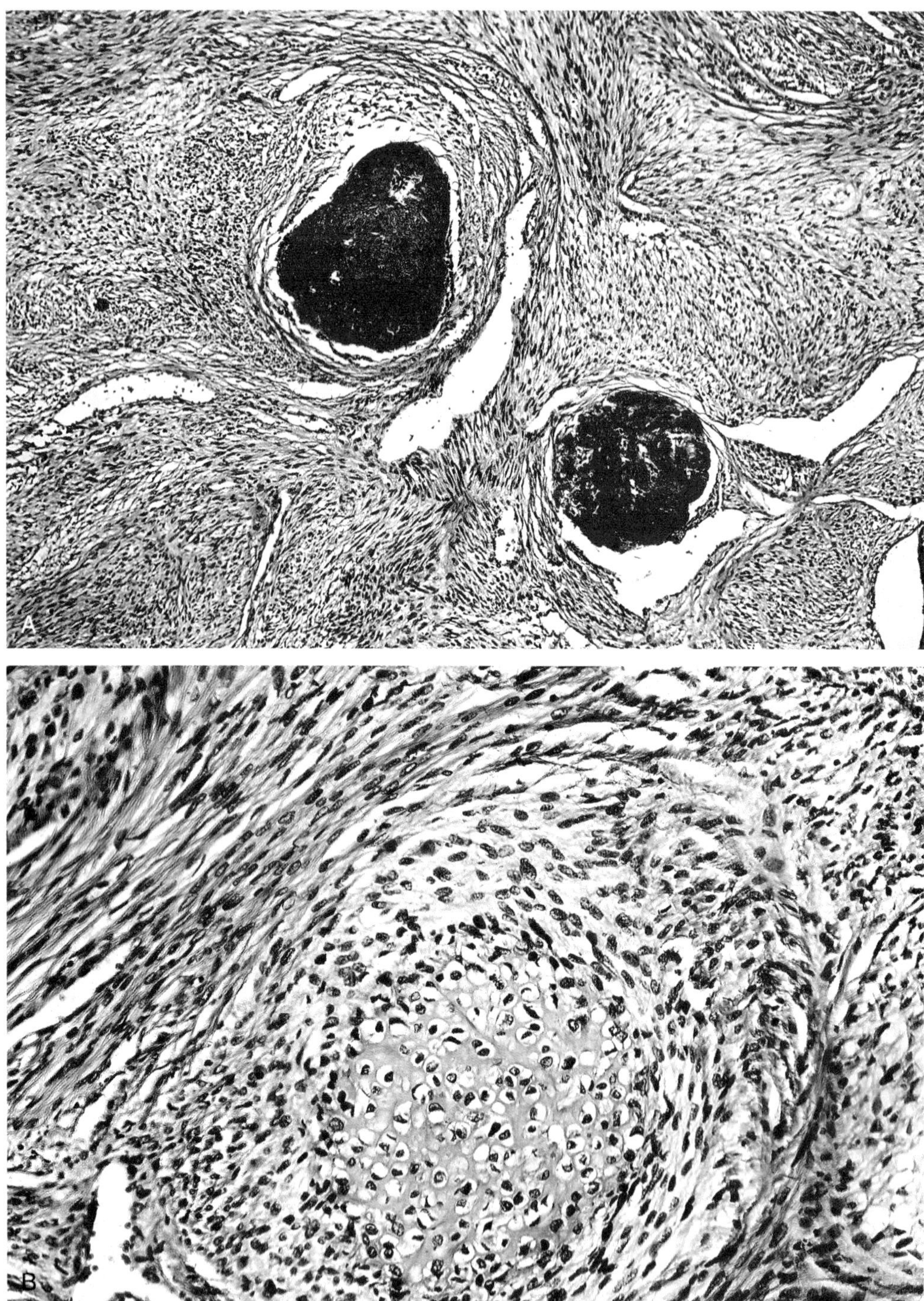

**FIGURE 31–15.** Heterologous elements with a malignant peripheral nerve sheath tumor are most often bone (**A**) and cartilage (**B**).

common elements (Fig. 31–15), whereas skeletal muscle and mucin-secreting glands are rare. In addition, we have seen one MPNST with squamous differentiation; and one MPNST reported in the literature arising in von Recklinghausen's disease showed foci of liposarcoma, although the illustrations are not entirely convincing.[20] These unusual MPNSTs seem to occur more often in NF1 and have been referred to in the past as *malignant mesenchymomas of nerve sheath*.[47] Because they are composed predominantly of recognizable schwannian elements, we still consider them variants of MPNST.

Although most MPNSTs conform to this description, a small percentage appear quite different. Some of these tumors closely resemble neurofibromas except they manifest a greater degree of cellularity, pleomorphism, and mitotic activity. These MPNSTs are typically found in the setting of von Recklinghausen's disease and have sometimes been termed *malignant neurofibromas*. If the lesion fulfills the criteria of malignancy as detailed in Chapter 30, we refer to it as a *low grade malignant peripheral nerve sheath tumor arising in a neurofibroma*. At the opposite end of the spectrum are anaplastic MPNSTs, which may be difficult to distinguish from other pleomorphic sarcomas (Fig. 31–16). They contain sheets of plump, spindled and giant cells intermixed with areas of hemorrhage and necrosis. These pleomorphic tumors have been documented more often in the setting of von Recklinghausen's disease. To some extent this may indicate the general reluctance to diagnosis an anaplastic MPNST outside the setting of NF1. Diagnosis of these tumors depends on identifying areas of typical MPNST. Infrequently, MPNSTs contain areas of primitive neuroepithelial differentiation consisting of cords or nests of small round cells[1] and in extraordinary cases even rosettes (Fig. 31–17). Primitive neuroepithelial differentiation appears to be a more common feature of MPNSTs in children.[81]

## IMMUNOHISTOCHEMICAL FINDINGS

A number of antigens are useful for identifying nerve sheath differentiation, including S-100 protein, Leu-7, PGP9.5, and myelin basic protein. Other antigens have also been studied in these tumors.[44,55] S-100 protein, the most widely used antigen for neural differentiation, can be identified in 50–90% of MPNSTs, although typically the staining is focal and limited to a small number of cells[75,90,123,126] (Fig. 31–7C). Because it is rare to encounter an MPNST with strong, diffuse immunoreactivity for S-100 protein, such a staining pattern always suggests reconsideration of various benign diagnoses, notably cellular schwannoma. Leu-7 and myelin basic protein are found in about 50% and 40% of MPNSTs, respectively.[126] None of these markers is specific for neural differentiation, so some have suggested using a panel of antibodies.[126] We generally use S-100 protein coupled with a number of other

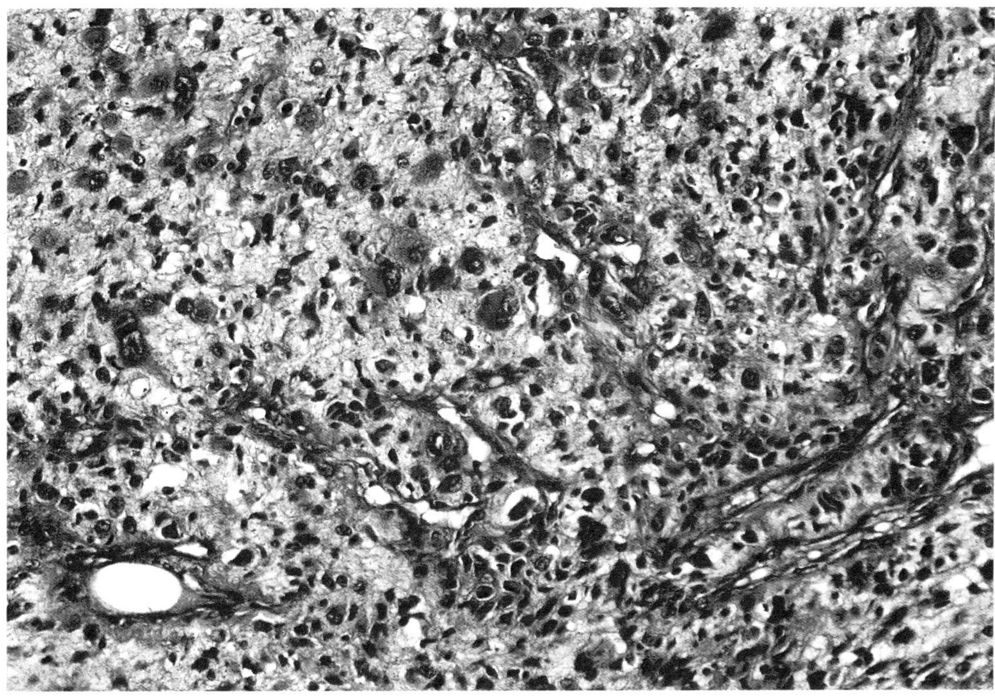

**FIGURE 31–16.** Pleomorphic areas in an MPNST.

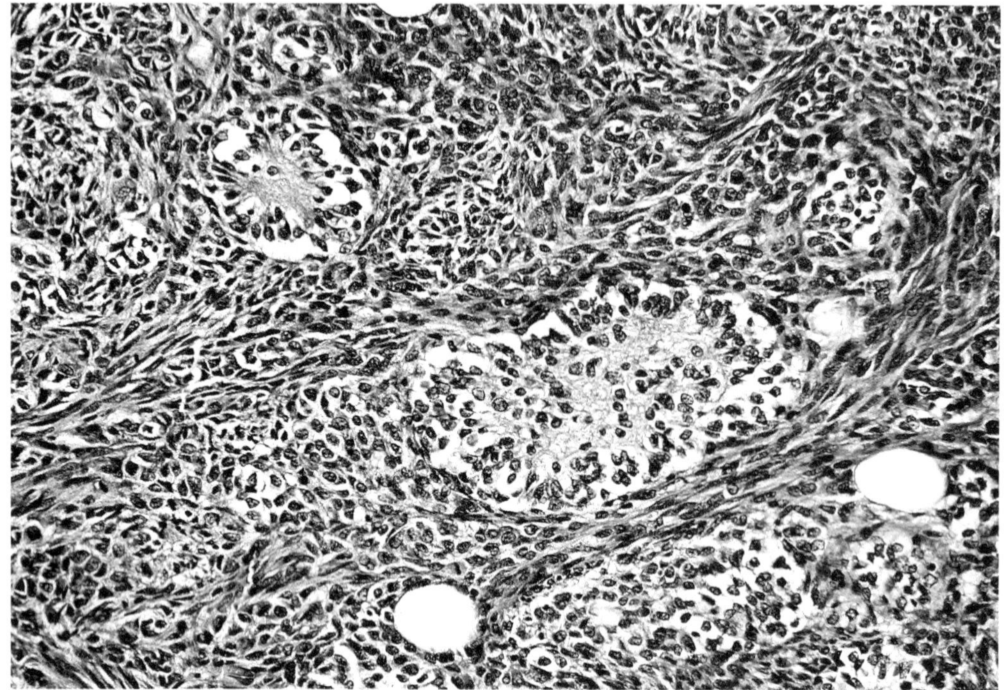

**FIGURE 31–17.** Primitive neuroectodermal differentiation in the form of a rosette in an MPNST.

antigens (e.g., keratin) that can rule out other diagnostic possibilities such as monophasic synovial sarcoma (see Chapter 8). p53 immunoreactivity is also detected in more than half of MPNSTs, in contrast to its usual absence in neurofibromas.[46,60,76]

## ELECTRON MICROSCOPIC FINDINGS

The MPNSTs are characterized by many of the same features as benign nerve sheath tumors. Most significantly, the spindled or polygonal cells give off nontapered branching cytoplasmic processes that extend for appreciable distances from the cell body and contain microtubules and neurofilaments (Fig. 31–18). The processes usually lie close to one another and form junctional complexes.[78] In well differentiated MPNSTs, the cells and processes are coated with basal lamina,[12,13,32,50,78] and occasional wisps of cytoplasm curl around themselves in the manner of mesaxon formation.[78] In less well differentiated MPNSTs, the cell processes are broader,[32] and the basal laminae are poorly developed or incomplete.[32,78] The matrix contains collagen in various forms (e.g., typical, long spacing, and broad amianthoid fibers)[92] and wisps and scrolls of basal lamina. One unique MPNST contained annulate lamellae.[41] These ultrastructural features are most compatible with schwannian differentiation. However, there is some evidence that fibroblast-like cells may participate in MPNSTs associated with von Recklinghausen's disease,[12] just as they participate in benign neurofibromas. Nonetheless, it should be recalled that the perineurial fibroblast and Schwann cell are closely related and may represent structural modulations of the same cell determined by their locations in the nerve sheath.[17]

## DIFFERENTIAL DIAGNOSIS

Most MPNSTs are easily diagnosed as malignant tumors, and the major challenge resides in distinguishing them from other sarcomas such as fibrosarcoma, monophasic synovial sarcoma, and leiomyosarcoma. As implied previously, fibrosarcoma and synovial sarcoma have a more uniform fascicular pattern, contain symmetric fusiform cells resembling fibroblasts, and obviously lack features of neural differentiation. Monophasic synovial sarcoma often contains densely hyalinized or calcified areas (or both) in combination with areas suggesting rudimentary epithelial differentiation in the form of clusters of round cells with clear cytoplasm.

Immunostaining for cytokeratin and S-100 protein also aids in the differential diagnosis. Immunoreactive cytokeratin can be detected in a significant number of monophasic synovial sarcomas but is absent except in the malignant peripheral nerve sheath tumor with glands (see p. 1233). Whereas S-100 protein is identi-

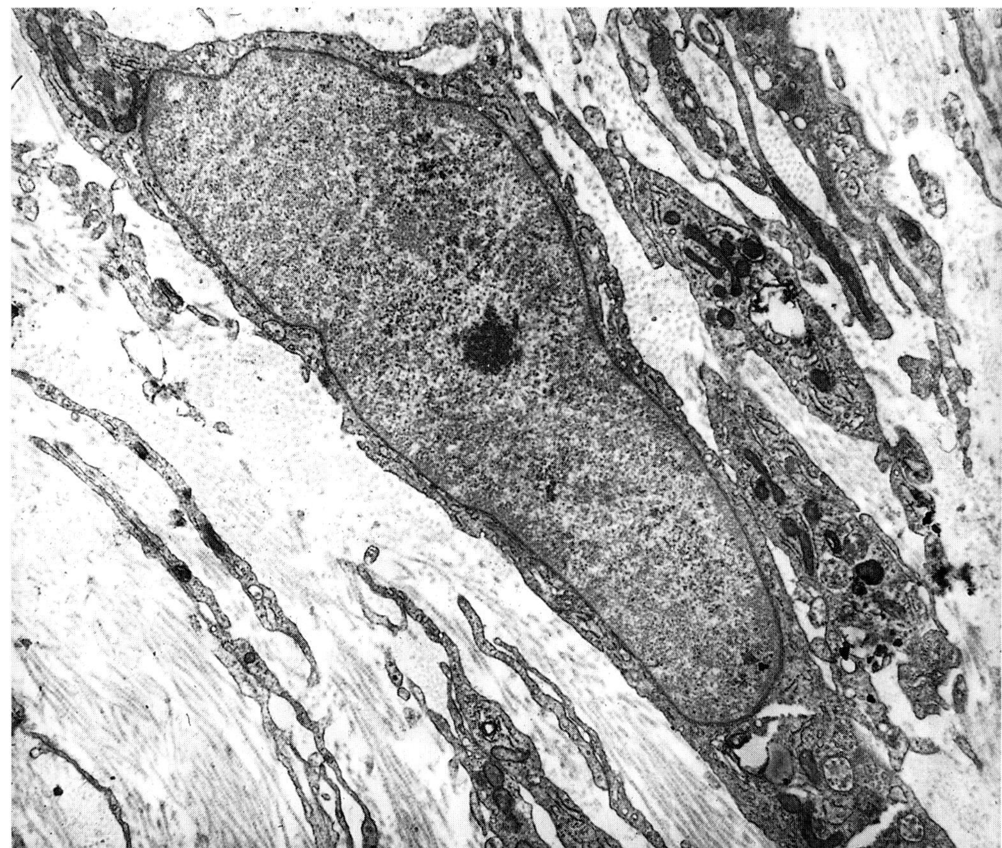

**FIGURE 31–18.** Electron micrograph of an MPNST illustrating an asymmetrically tapered cell with cell processes of adjacent cells lying parallel to it.

fied in up to 30% of synovial sarcomas, it is present in 50–90% of MPNSTs.[21,75,90,123,126] Typically the staining is focal, and the number of immunoreactive cells is small compared with neurofibroma and schwannoma, reflecting either a loss of differentiation or a shift from a Schwann cell (S-100 protein-positive) to a perineural cell (S-100 protein-negative) population. Myelin basic protein has been identified in about half of MPNSTs,[126] but there are far fewer data concerning the specificity of immunostaining for this antigen in mesenchymal tumors. Neuron-specific enolase and neurofilament proteins have also been identified in MPNSTs, where their presence has been interpreted as evidence that these tumors occasionally display neuronal differentiation.[75]

Leiomyosarcoma can usually be distinguished from MPNST without undue difficulty. Its cells have distinct eosinophilic cytoplasm, centrally placed blunt-ended nuclei, and occasional juxtanuclear vacuoles. In ambiguous situations special stains are helpful, as the cytoplasm of leiomyosarcoma is fuchsinophilic with longitudinal striations (Masson trichrome stain) and contains at least moderate amounts of glycogen [periodic acid-Schiff (PAS) preparation]. The cytoplasm of MPNSTs is usually less fuchsinophilic (with no longitudinal striations) and contains little or no glycogen. An important diagnostic problem is the distinction of neurofibromas with one or more unusual features from a MPNST. This occurs typically with "borderline" neurofibromatous lesions of von Recklinghausen's disease. A diagnosis of malignancy depends on the findings of enhanced cellularity, diffuse atypia, and usually at least a low level of mitotic activity. This problem is discussed in greater detail in Chapter 30. In rare instances, one encounters a typical neurofibroma in which small foci may appear malignant by virtue of the foregoing criteria. We have interpreted such lesions as *neurofibroma with focal malignant change* and recommend conservative excision if the focus constitutes a small portion of the entire neurofibroma and the focus appears totally removed by the excision. Preliminary follow-up in these cases supports this conservative approach to management.

The criterion of mitotic activity paradoxically

does not apply to schwannomas. Schwannoma displaying mitotic activity pursues a benign course, and rarely has this tumor been known to undergo malignant degeneration. Thus when material from a small biopsy specimen is evaluated, it is hazardous to attempt to distinguish a cellular schwannoma from a MPNST solely on the basis of mitotic activity. In this situation, a larger sample of the mass is necessary to determine if the tumor in question has an Antoni A and B pattern, perivascular hyalinization, encapsulation, or other typical features of a schwannoma.

## MOLECULAR AND CYTOGENETICS

The development of MPNST from neurofibroma appears to be a multistep process in which a number of genes participate, leading to gain in function of some and a loss of function of others. Patients with NF1 have germline inactivation of NF1. However, there has been uncertainty as to whether neurofibromas arise when there is inactivation of one or both NF1 alleles. Evidence suggests that both alleles are inactivated in neurofibromas[101] and MPNSTs,[84] and that schwann cells derived from NF1-deleted (neurofibromin-deficient) animals acquire increased proliferative capacity and angioinvasive properties.[58,59] The progression of a neurofibroma to an MPNST is associated with a number of additional chromosomal alterations.[3,80,86,103] The most common alterations are genomic gains involving 17q, 7p, 5p, 8q, and 12q. Less common alterations are genomic losses of 9p, 13q, and 1p. Notably, 9p includes the *CDKN2* gene, a cyclin-dependent kinase inhibitor that is inactivated in more than 50% of MPNSTs but not in neurofibromas.[64,65] This gene produces two protein products, p16 and p19. The former negatively regulates cell cycling through the *Rb* pathway, whereas the latter negatively regulates cycling through the p53 pathway. Thus inactivation of this gene favors increased proliferation. That *p53* is ultimately affected in MPNST is suggested by finding immunostaining for p53 in a large number of MPNSTs but not in neurofibromas.[46,60,76]

## CLINICAL BEHAVIOR

Most MPNSTs are high grade sarcomas, with a high likelihood of producing local recurrence and distant metastasis. Although the prognosis reported in the early literature for this disease was often dismal, the survival reported from large cancer referral centers in which patients have undergone sophisticated radiologic imaging and extensive surgery often coupled with adjuvant radiation or chemotherapy has improved. Based on three large studies from the Mayo Clinic and Memorial Sloan-Kettering Cancer Hospital,[53,63,128] the local recurrence rate varies from 40% to 65% and the metastatic rate from 40% to 68% (Table 31–1). The 5-year survival based on a study of 134 patients with tumors from all sites was 52%,[128] although lower survival rates (15%) are recorded when the lesions occur at sites for which it is difficult to achieve good margins (e.g., retroperitoneum, thoracic cavity).[53,63] There appear to be a number of prognostic variables in this disease, including the size of the lesion, location, stage, grade, status of surgical margins, necrosis, and use of adjuvant radiation (Table 31–2). In a multivariate analysis the status of surgical margins and a history of irradiation emerge as independent prognostic variables. Thus patients who have positive surgical margins or who have radiation-induced sarcomas have a worse prognosis than the group as a whole.

In the past a large body of literature indicated that tumors associated with NF1 have a particularly poor prognosis compared with those occurring on a sporadic basis. This was not surprising because of the tendency of tumors in NF1 to be large, central, and deep. More recent large studies have not confirmed this finding, however.[53,120] In a large series from Memorial Hospital in which the authors compared tumors of roughly comparable size and location (buttock and leg) in patients with and without NF1, there was no significant difference in behavior. Approximately 40% of patients in both groups developed local recurrence, and it could be correlated with the type of surgery and the presence of positive margins.[53,120] Sixty-five percent of patients in both groups developed distant metastasis with a comparable inter-

**TABLE 31–1** CLINICAL BEHAVIOR OF MALIGNANT PERIPHERAL NERVE SHEATH TUMORS BY SITE[53,63,128]

| Location | No. of Cases | Recurrence (%) | Metastasis (%) | 5-Year Survival (%) |
|---|---|---|---|---|
| All sites | 134 | 43 | 40 | 52 |
| Lower extremity/buttock | 43 | 40 | 63 | 39 |
| Paraspinal | 25 | 65 | 68 | 16 |

**TABLE 31–2 CORRELATION BETWEEN PROGNOSTIC VARIABLES AND SURVIVAL IN MALIGNANT PERIPHERAL NERVE SHEATH TUMORS**

| Prognostic Factor | 5-Year Survival (%) | Univariate Analysis ($p$) | Multivariate Analysis ($p$) |
|---|---|---|---|
| Size (cm) | | | |
| <5 | 70 | <0.0001 | 0.24 |
| 5.1–10.0 | 57 | | |
| 10.1–15 | 43 | | |
| >15 | | | |
| Location | | | |
| Nonextremity | 43 | 0.0064 | 0.20 |
| Extremity | 70 | | |
| History of NF1 | | | |
| Yes | 36 | 0.0074 | 0.075 |
| No | 57 | | |
| History of XRT | | | |
| Yes | | 0.0004 | **0.023** |
| No | 58 | | |
| Stage | | | |
| 1 | 65 | 0.0340 | |
| 2 | 60 | | |
| 3 | 46 | | |
| Grade | | | |
| 1 | 65 | 0.0074 | 0.39 |
| 2 | 61 | | |
| 3 | 35 | | |
| 4 | 55 | | |
| Surgical margin | | | |
| Positive | 22 | 0.0030 | **0.0044** |
| Negative | 67 | | |
| Close | 43 | | |
| Unknown | 37 | | |
| Use of IORT/BT | | | |
| Yes | 72 | 0.039 | 0.32 |
| No | 50 | | |
| Necrosis | | | |
| Yes | 37 | 37 | |
| No | 62 | 0.0099 | |

NF1, neurofibromatosis 1; XRT, x-irradiation; IORT/BT, intraoperative radiotherapy/brachytherapy.
The $p$ values in boldface represent statistically significant parameters.
From Wong WW, Hirose T, Scheithauer BW, et al. Malignant peripheral nerve sheath tumor: analysis of treatment outcome. Int J Radiol Oncol Biol Phys 42:351, 1998.

val between surgery and metastasis (14–18 months).[53] The overall 5-year survival rate in the experience of Wanebo et al. was 43.7%, with factors such as the age of the patient, size and location of tumor, and margins most influential for outcome.[120] Likewise, the most recent study by Wong et al. based on Mayo Clinic experience could not confirm that NF1 by itself was an independent variable for prognosis.[128]

The most common metastatic site for MPNST is the lung, followed by bone and pleura. Fewer than 10% of patients with metastasis developed regional node deposits, indicating that routine lymph node dissections do not play an important role in the treatment of this disease. This also emphasizes the fact that metastatic spindle cell lesions with Schwann cell-like features are apt to be metastatic desmoplastic or neurotropic melanomas or some other spindle cell tumor mimicking MPNST. One should also be aware of the propensity of this tumor to spread for considerable distances along the nerve sheath, and there are reports of tumors entering the subarachnoid space of the spinal cord via this route.[108] Therefore it is wise to obtain a frozen section of the nerve margins to assess the adequacy of the excision. In the experience of most, regional lymph node metastasis is uncommon,[38,108] consequently, lymph node dissections do not play a role in the primary surgical therapy of this disease. However, in our experience, lymph node metastasis may be seen in the presence of widely metastatic disease.

Although MPNST does not occur often in the pediatric age group, it appears to have a course roughly comparable to adult. Meis et al., in a retrospective review based on consultation material, noted metastasis in 50% of patients at 2 years.[81] A report from a large cancer center, however, reported 41% survival at 10 years and related the prognosis closely to whether the patient underwent radical surgery. Survival at 10 years was 80% for patients who had undergone radical surgery compared to only 14% for those who did not.[10]

## MALIGNANT PERIPHERAL NERVE SHEATH TUMOR WITH RHABDOMYOBLASTIC DIFFERENTIATION (MALIGNANT TRITON TUMOR)

In the broadest sense, a Triton tumor is any neoplasm with both neural and skeletal muscle differentiation; included are the neuromuscular hamartoma (benign Triton tumor),[43,93,95] medulloblastoma with rhabdomyosarcoma,[134] rhabdomyosarcoma with ganglion cells (ectomesenchymoma), and MPNST with rhabdomyosarcoma.[7,22,91,130] The term ***malignant Triton tumor*** is usually applied only to the MPNST with rhabdomyosarcoma because it is the most widely recognized of the foregoing entities.[49,91,114,127] This composite neoplasm was first described in 1938 by Masson and Martin,[74] who suggested that the neural elements in the tumor induced differentiation of skeletal muscle in much the same fashion as normal nerve was believed to induce the regeneration of skeletal muscle in the Triton salamander. As a result, these tumors were eventually accorded the name of the amphibian.

A review of all reported cases of Triton tumors in the literature attests to their relative rarity and their tendency to occur in NF1.[132] Slightly more than half of the reported cases in the literature have occurred in conjunction with von Recklinghausen's disease.[7,29] However, our experience suggests the tumor may occur outside the setting of NF1 more often than is generally appreciated. Low estimates of sporadic cases seem to result from errors in diagnosis, as evidenced by the fact that most cases are referred to us with a diagnosis of fibrosarcoma or rhabdomyosarcoma, depending on the prominence of the muscle component. Because most reported cases occur in patients with von Recklinghausen's disease, affected individuals are usually young (average age 35 years). The tumors are widely distributed, but most occur on the head, neck, and trunk. Like other MPNSTs, symptoms are related to a progressively enlarging mass that may give rise to neurologic symptoms. The 5-year survival based on a literature review by Brooks et al. was 12%.[7]

The hallmark of this tumor is the presence of rhabdomyoblasts scattered throughout a stroma indistinguishable from an ordinary MPNST (Figs. 31–19, 31–20). The number of rhabdomyoblasts varies greatly from tumor to tumor and even from area to area in the same tumor. They are usually relatively mature, and their abundant eosinophilic cytoplasm contrasts sharply with the pale-staining cytoplasm of the schwann cells. Cross-striations can be identified but, as in rhabdomyosarcomas, are more readily identified in cells with elongated tapered cytoplasm. Both desmin and nuclear regulatory proteins (MyoD1 and myogenin) can be demonstrated in the rhabdomyoblasts (Fig. 31–20B), although the latter tends to be present in only the most mature elements (see Chapter 22).

The histogenesis of these unusual tumors has occasioned much discussion. Although Masson believed that one cell line induced the other, it seems just as likely that both cell lines originate from less well differentiated neural crest cells. Normally the neural crest contributes to the formation of mesenchyme in certain vertebrates and ultimately forms portions of branchial cartilage, connective tissue, and muscle in the facial region.[124] Thus these tumors recapitulate both the schwannian and the mesenchymal potentiality of the neural crest.

## MALIGNANT PERIPHERAL NERVE SHEATH TUMOR WITH GLANDS (GLANDULAR MALIGNANT SCHWANNOMA)

In 1892 Garre[36] reported a patient with von Recklinghausen's disease and an MPNST of the sciatic nerve. Scattered throughout the schwannian background of the tumor were numerous well differentiated glands. Since that time, slightly more than 20 additional tumors have been reported, probably making it among the rarest of MPNSTs with aberrant differentiation.[14,18,26,35,87,104] Almost all of these tumors have occurred in patients with von Recklinghausen's disease, a fact that easily accounts for the young median age (about 30 years)[127] of affected patients. The tumors usually arise from major nerves, including the sciatic, median, brachial plexus, and spinal nerves.

Characteristically, they have a spindle cell background indistinguishable from ordinary MPNSTs and may contain other heterotopic elements such as muscle, cartilage, and bone. The glands are usually few in number and are made up of well differentiated, nonciliated cuboidal or columnar cells with clear cyto-

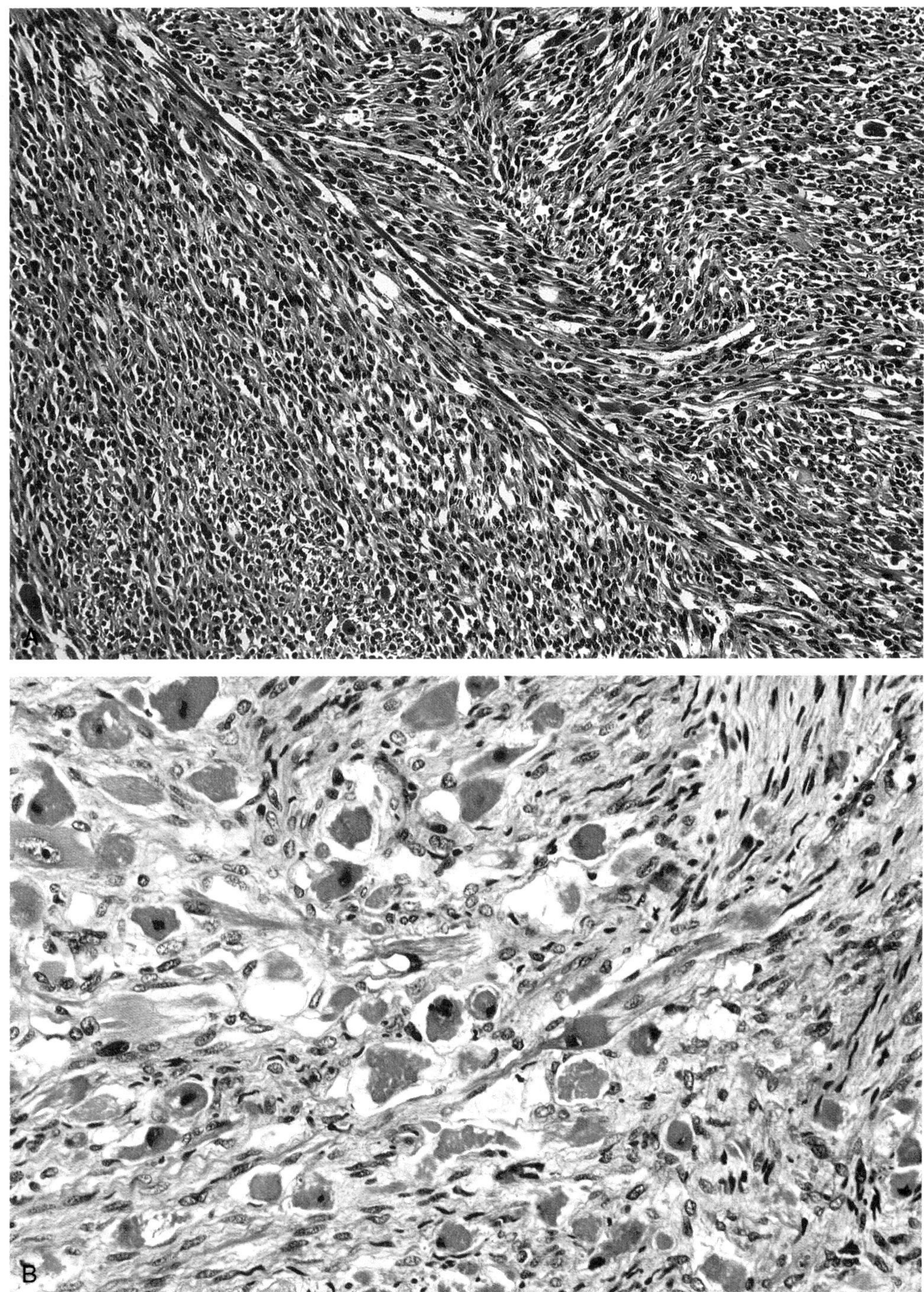

**FIGURE 31–19.** (**A**) Malignant peripheral nerve sheath tumor with rhabdomyoblastic differentiation (malignant Triton tumor). (**B**) Rounded or elongated large rhabdomyoblasts are scattered throughout the tumor.

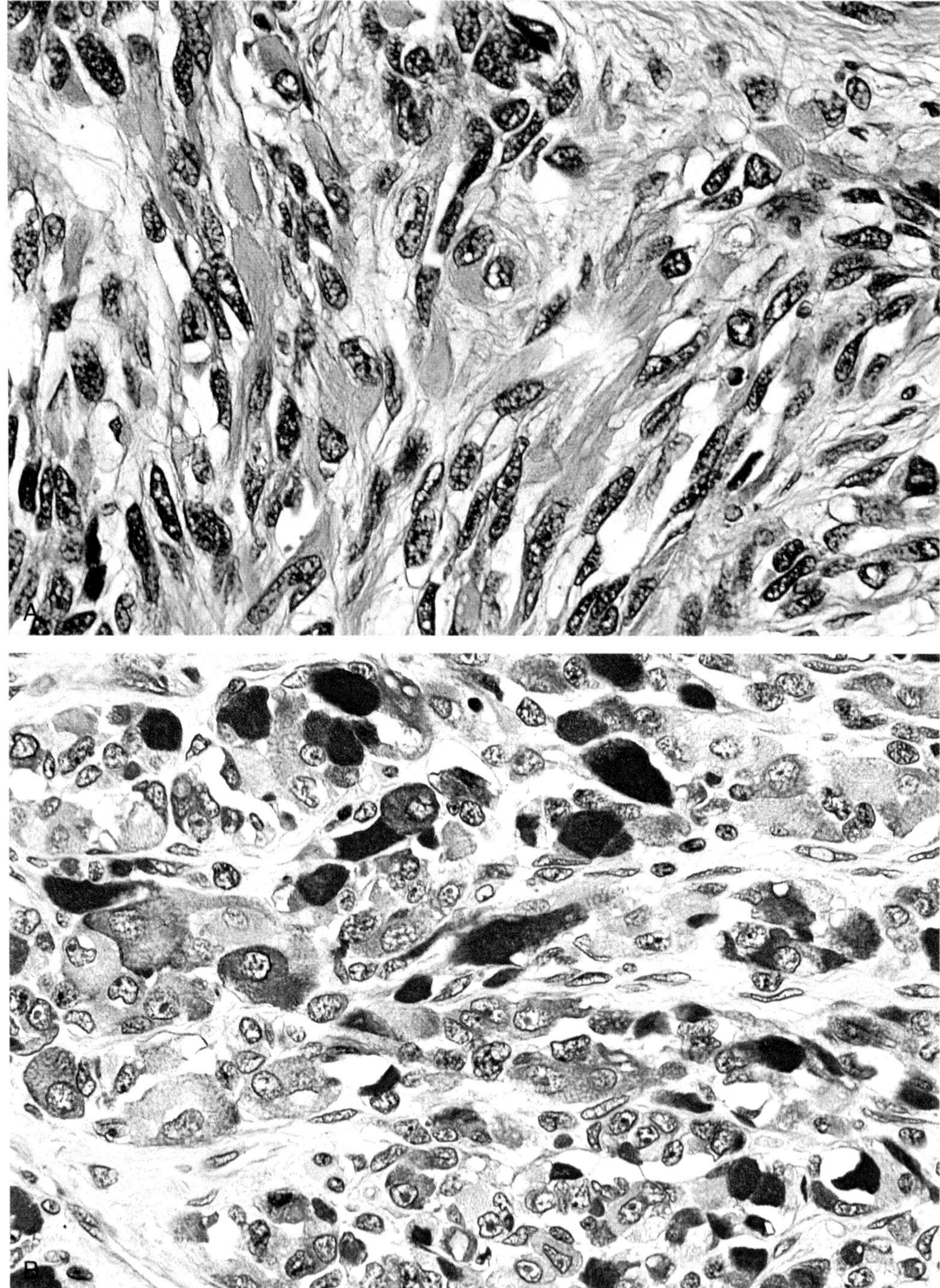

**FIGURE 31–20.** Rhabdomyoblasts in an MPNST (**A**) showing desmin immunoreactivity (**B**).

plasm and occasional goblet cells (Figs. 31–21, 31–22, 31–23). Intracellular and extracellular mucin, which are histochemically identical to conventional epithelial mucins, can be demonstrated in the glands (Fig. 31–22). We have even encountered one that contained squamous islands in addition to glands (Fig. 31–23). By electron microscopy, the glands are seen to have features of intestinal epithelium and have numerous well oriented microvilli with core rootlets.[117] Some of the cells in the glands are argyrophilic and contain dense-core granules,[122] others have documented ependymal differentiation.[26] Somatostatin immunoreactivity was noted in the glands of one glandular schwannoma.[122] Rarely the glands appear histologically malignant.

It may be difficult to distinguish these tumors from biphasic synovial sarcomas because the glandular elements may be virtually identical. It is principally the spindled element that distinguishes them, although obviously the presence of goblet cells or neuroendocrine differentiation favors the diagnosis of a glandular MPNST. In synovial sarcomas the spindled element resembles a conventional fibrosarcoma and may secondarily hyalinized or calcified. Subtle degrees of epithelial differentiation may also be evident in the spindled stroma of the synovial sarcoma. This feature is not present in glandular MPNSTs because the epithelial elements invariably arise rather abruptly from the stroma. The immunologic phenotype of synovial sarcoma and glandular MPNST differs. The former often contains keratin-positive cells in the spindled zones (and occasionally S-100 protein-positive ones), whereas the latter displays only focal S-100 protein positivity. The addition of other neural antigens such as nerve growth factor receptor (NGFR) and PGP9.5 may improve the sensitivity and specificity of the diagnosis.[128]

Although the glandular elements set this tumor apart as a peculiar histologic variant, they serve essentially no role in grading the tumor or predicting its biologic behavior. Tumors with a highly malignant schwannian component may be expected to do poorly regardless of the degree of differentiation of the glands. Most tumors reported in the literature seem to fall into this category. On the other hand, tumors with a low grade schwannian element may do extremely well, as illustrated by the fact that the two patients with tumors of this type reported by Woodruff and Christensen[131] are alive and well. It should be noted in passing, however, that certain rare (benign) schwannomas with glandular elements should be clearly distinguished from glandular MPNSTs. Usually they are superficial lesions with glands that resemble adnexal structures, leading some to question whether they are entrapped elements.

The source of the epithelial elements in these tumors has remained controversial. Some authors have suggested that they arise from heterotopic ependymal cells located in the peripheral nerve,[21,37] and some claim to have documented ependymal features. The

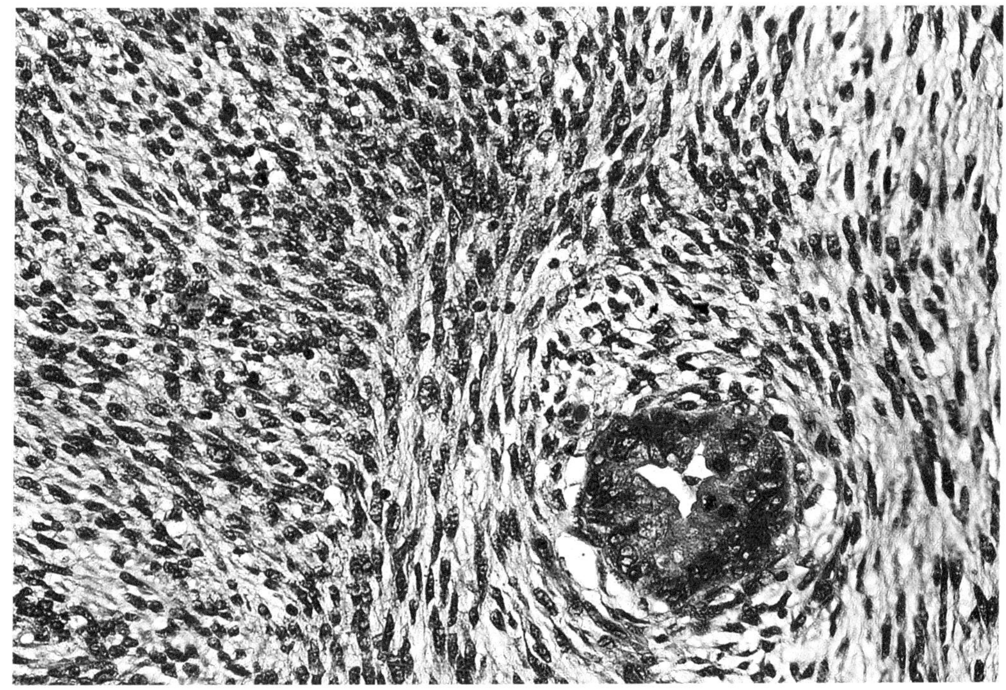

**FIGURE 31–21.** MPNST with glandular differentiation. Glands in this case appeared malignant.

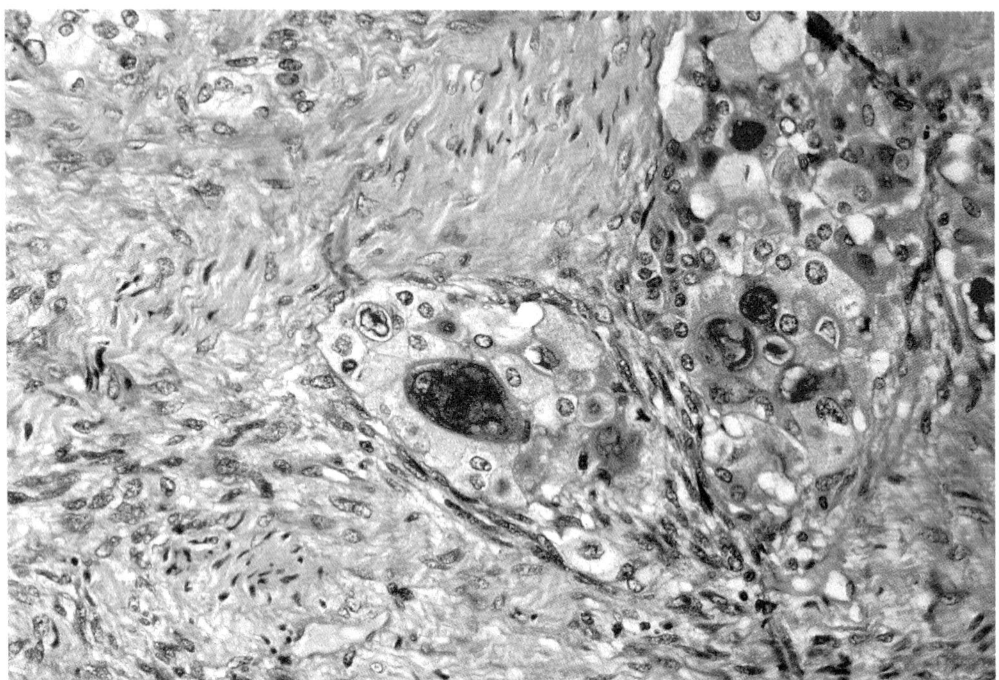

**FIGURE 31–22.** Glands in an MPNST containing carminophilic mucin.

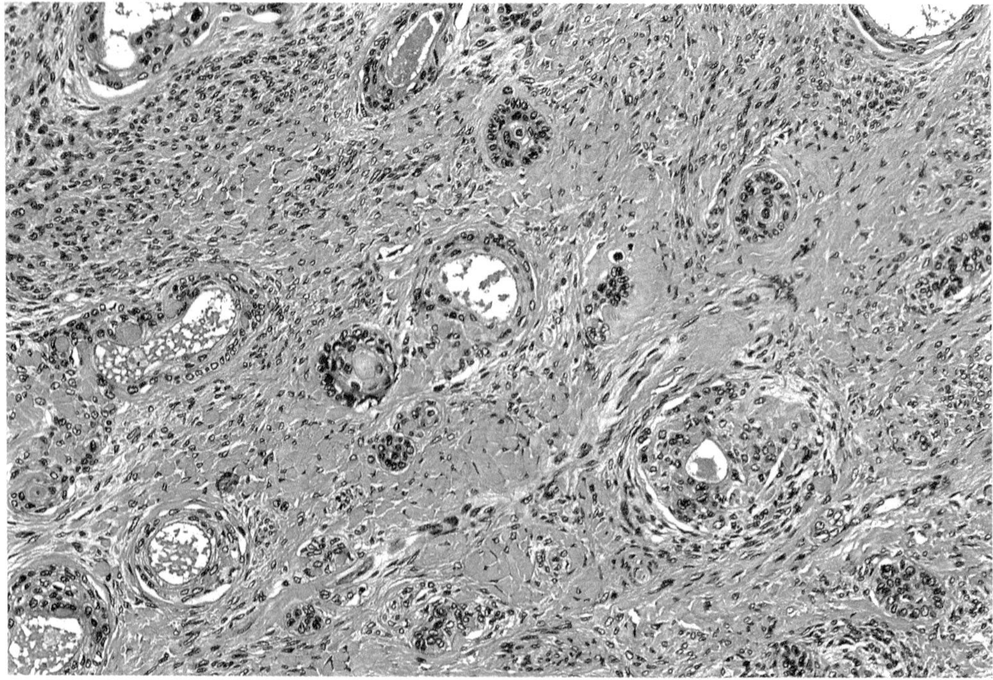

**FIGURE 31–23.** MPNST with glands and squamous islands.

presence of goblet cells in these glands, the degree of mucin production, and the consistent absence of blepharoplasts argue against this interpretation. A more tenable suggestion is that the Schwann cell or a less committed precursor differentiates along epithelial and schwannian lines.

## MALIGNANT PERIPHERAL NERVE SHEATH TUMOR WITH ANGIOSARCOMA

Slightly more than 20 angiosarcomas arising in nerve sheath tumors have been reported, making these tumors largely curiosities.[6,8,11,82,85,89] Most have developed in patients with NF1 and not surprisingly, therefore, were associated with either plexiform neurofibroma, MPNST, or both. Anecdotal reports attest to the fact that angiosarcoma may also occur in benign schwannomas,[82] normal nerves,[85] and sporadic MPNSTs.[89] Because of the strong association with NF1, these tumors usually occur in young individuals. They are indistinguishable from MPNSTs and have conventional-appearing angiosarcomas that may be microscopic or macroscopic in size. The prognosis is poor, and most of the patients have succumbed to the disease.

## EPITHELIOID MALIGNANT PERIPHERAL NERVE SHEATH TUMOR (EPITHELIOID MALIGNANT SCHWANNOMA)

Epithelioid MPNST is an unusual form of MPNST that closely resembles carcinoma or melanoma by virtue of the fact that the tumor is composed predominantly or exclusively of schwann cells with a polygonal epithelioid appearance.[2,16,67,70,77,112] Although we estimated that 5% or fewer MPNSTs belong to this group, this estimate may be far too generous. In fact, for many years the exact nature of this unusual group of tumors was questioned, as indicated by Stewart and Copeland: "We have observed tumors of deeper nerve trunks which looked like certain nonpigmented melanomas yet did not run the clinical course of melanoma. Are those melanomas or neurosarcomas?"[108]

There is convincing evidence that these tumors do represent nerve sheath tumors rather than melanomas or metastatic carcinomas. First, the tumors follow a distribution similar to that of the ordinary MPNST, with most occurring in patients 20–50 years of age. In our experience with 26 cases, the median age was 36 years; men were affected slightly more often than women. Most of the tumors reported in the literature originated in major nerves, including the sciatic, tibial, peroneal, facial, antebrachial cutaneous, and digital nerves. In our experience, 8 of 10 deeply situated epithelioid MPNSTs originated from a major nerve, including the sciatic nerve (three cases) and the brachial plexus, femoral, radial, and median nerves (one case each). It is the cases in which origin from a nerve or neurofibroma cannot be documented that pose the most challenging and sometimes unresolvable problems in diagnosis. Although this form of MPNST may occur in NF1, it seems to occur less frequently than in ordinary MPNSTs. Lodding et al.[70] encountered one case in their series of 16, whereas none of our 26 patients had the disease.[67]

Histologically, the tumor is variable. In our cases the most characteristic appearance is that of short cords of large epithelioid cells arranged in a vague nodular pattern (Figs. 31–24 to 31–27). The cells in these tumors usually have large, round nuclei with prominent melanoma-like nuleoli (Fig. 31–26). The tumors may appear densely cellular or myxoid (Fig. 31–26B), depending on the accumulation of acid mucin between the cords, and there is often subtle blending of the epithelioid areas with spindled areas resembling the conventional MPNST (Fig. 31–28). However, it is our belief that the term *epithelioid MPNST* should be reserved for tumors in which the predominant pattern is epithelioid. Although the combination of all of these features is usually sufficient to make the correct diagnosis, many tumors lack this distinctive appearance. In fact, most tumors reported in the literature have resembled melanomas or carcinomas and have consisted simply of small nests of epithelioid cells admixed with a spindled component.

There are a number of rather unusual forms of epithelioid MPNST that deserve comment. Some contain a predominance of clear cells, and others are made up of rhabdoid cells with a prominent glassy eosinophilic perinuclear zone corresponding ultrastructurally to the presence of whorls of intermediate filaments (Fig. 31–27). Still other tumors consist of sheets of rounded pleomorphic cells suggestive of a pleomorphic carcinoma (Fig. 31–29).

Consequently, the diagnosis has largely depended on an established origin from a nerve. In the absence of this feature, the diagnosis is sometimes suspected by a delicate "mesenchymal" pattern of collagenization and a transition to spindled "schwannian" areas (Fig. 31–28). Unlike many melanomas, neither melanin pigment nor glycogen can be demonstrated in the cytoplasm of these tumors. In one unique case we reviewed, the diagnosis of "malignant epithelioid schwannoma" was established by virtue of the presence of true rosettes in a tumor that otherwise resembled melanoma (Fig. 31–17). It should be emphasized that a clear-cut distinction from melanoma or carcinoma is not always possible on routine sections, a

*Text continued on page 1240*

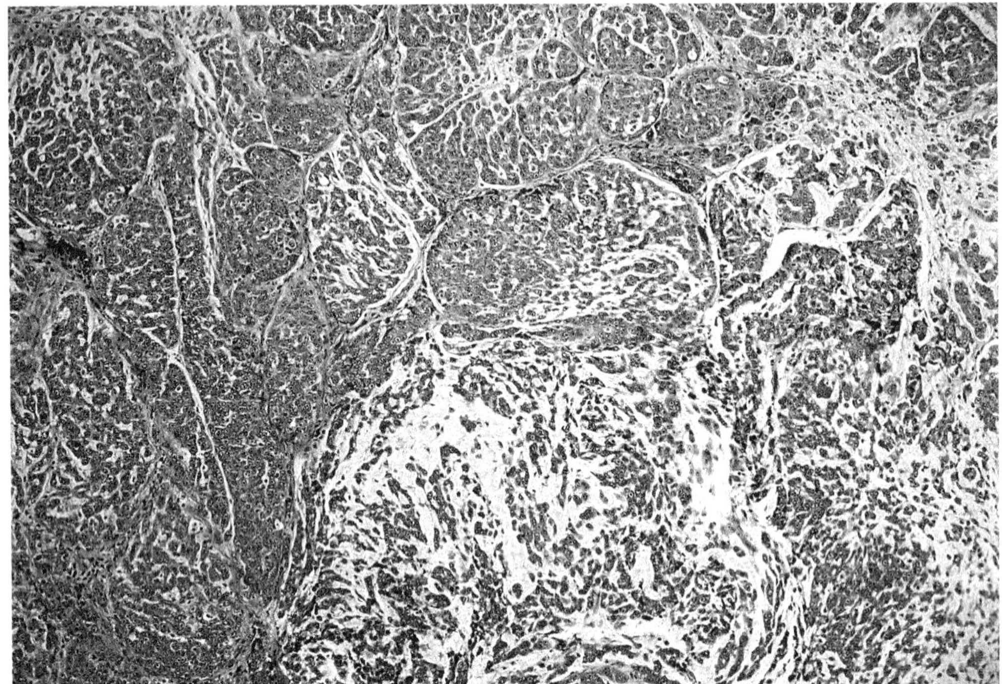

**FIGURE 31–24.** Epithelioid malignant peripheral nerve sheath tumor showing vague nodular growth. The tumor varies from slightly myxoid to cellular.

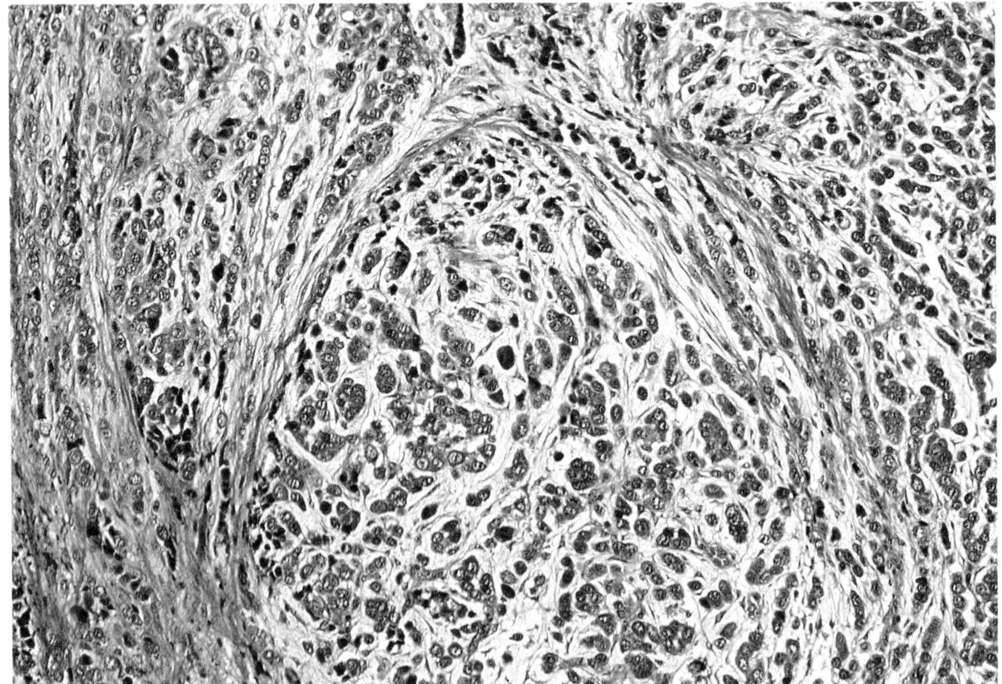

**FIGURE 31–25.** Epithelioid MPNST cords of epithelioid cells.

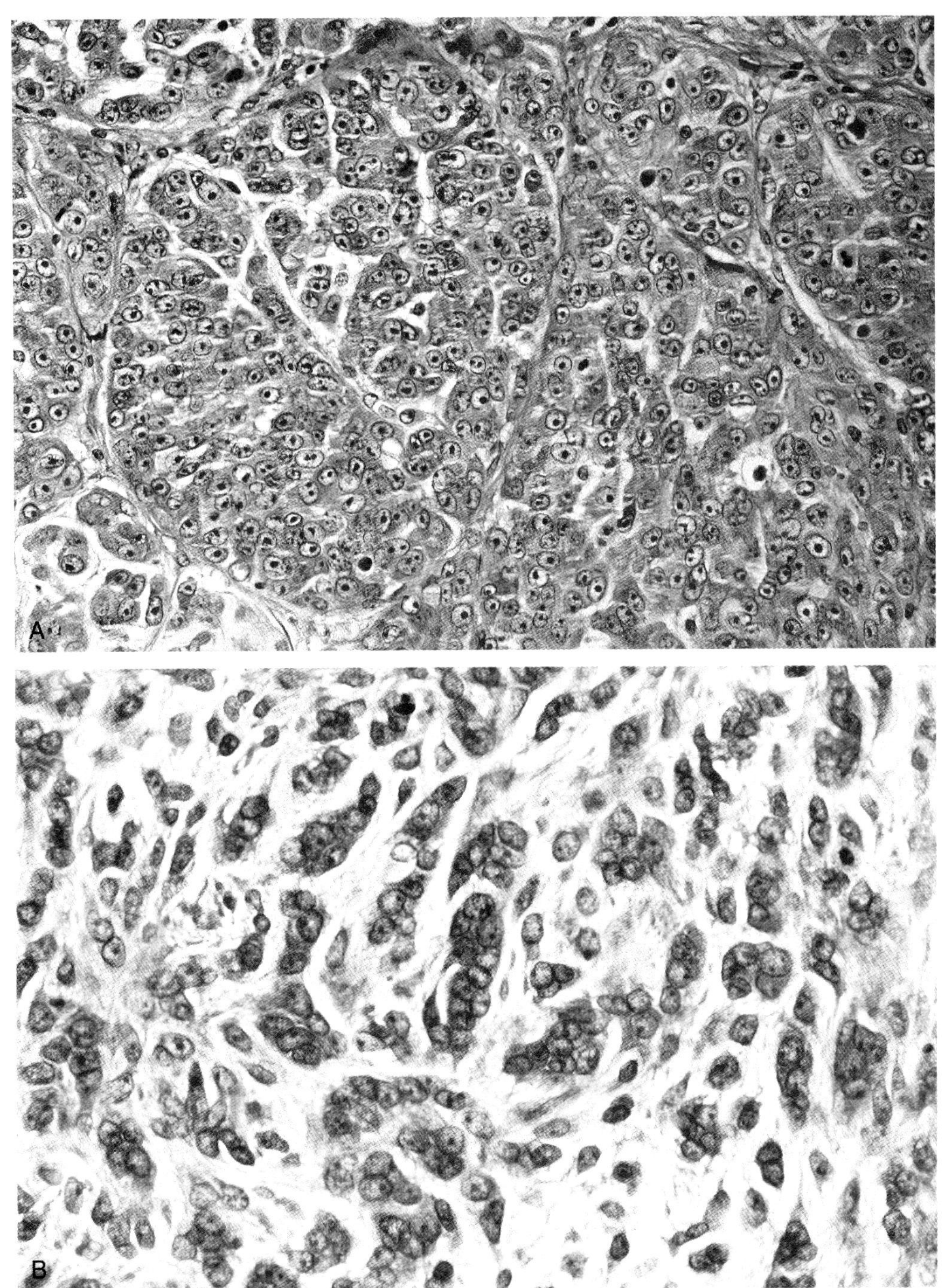

**FIGURE 31–26.** Epithelioid malignant peripheral nerve sheath tumor showing the polygonal shape of cells and prominent nucleoli (**A**). In some areas groups of cells are seperated by myxoid stroma (**B**).

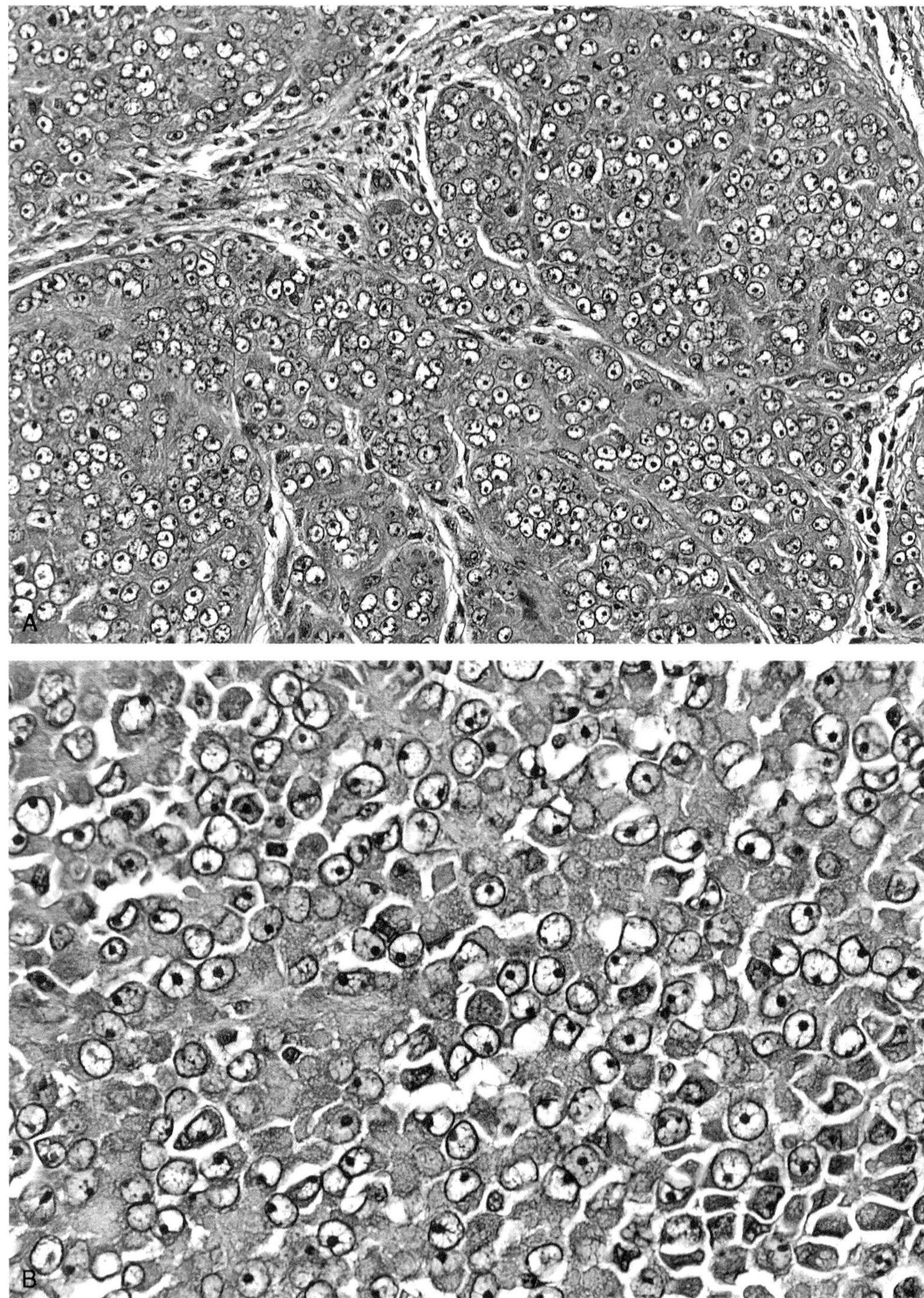


**FIGURE 31–27.** (**A**) Epithelioid malignant peripheral nerve sheath tumor with rhabdoid cells. (**B**) High power view of rhabdoid cells shows a glassy perinuclear zone.

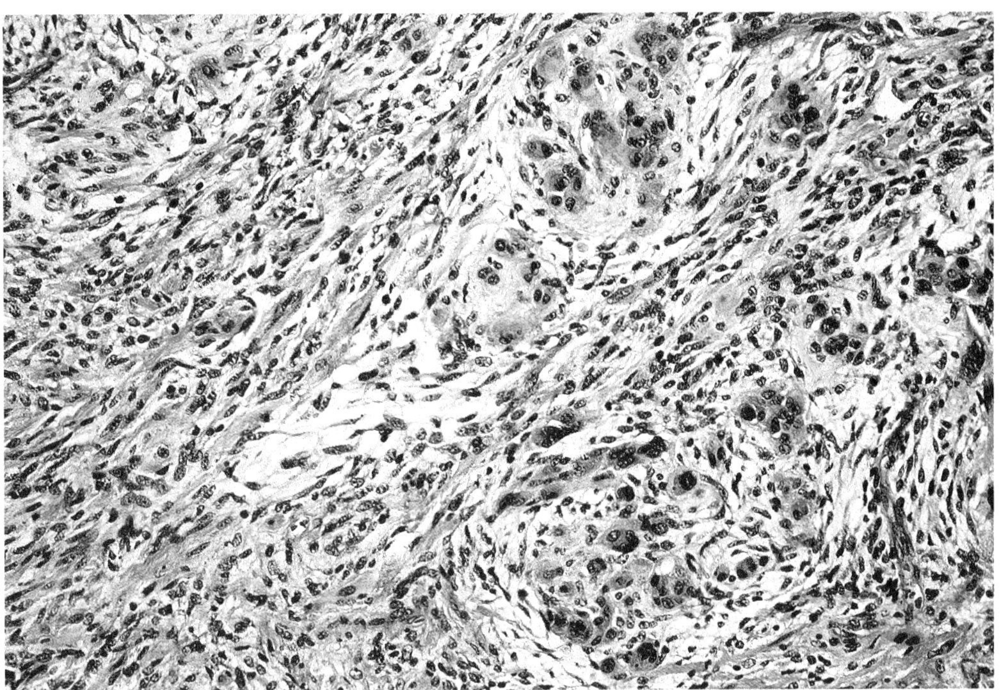

**FIGURE 31–28.** MPNST with focal epithelioid differentiation.

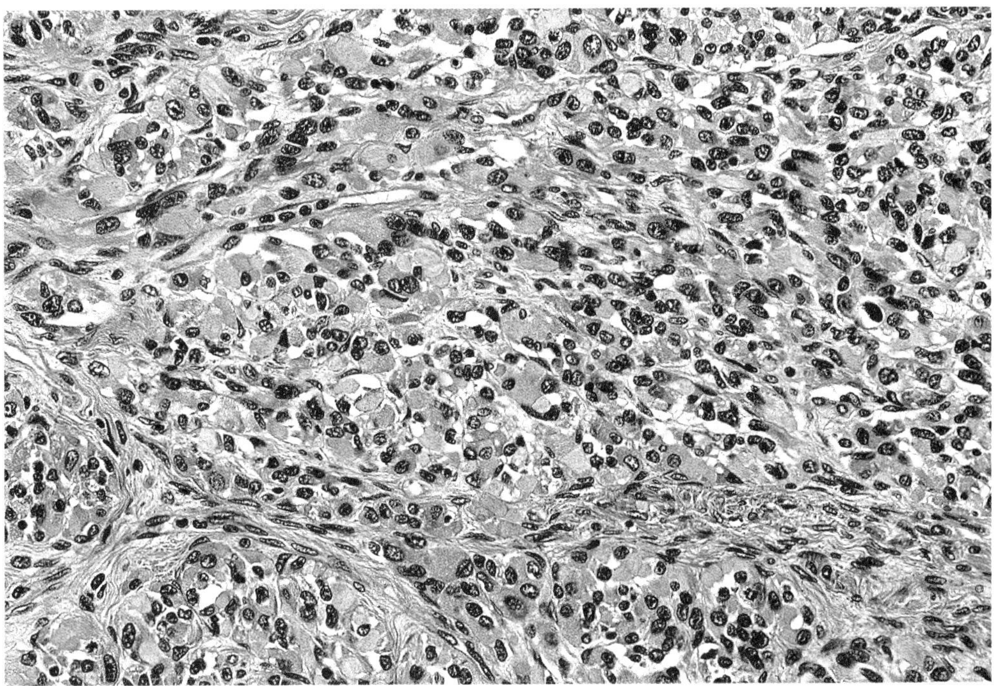

**FIGURE 31–29.** Epithelioid MPNST composed of pleomorphic epithelioid cells.

dilemma compounded by the fact that occasionally metastatic spindled melanomas are virtually indistinguishable from MPNST.

In our experience, about 80% of these tumors are strongly and diffusely positive for S-100 protein, a pattern of immunoreactivity that contrasts with conventional MPNST[67] (Fig. 31–30). They do not express melanoma-associated antigen, and only rarely is keratin present. Therefore the presence of either keratin or melanin-related antigens in a malignant epithelioid tumor argues against the diagnosis of epithelioid MPNST. Type IV collagen can be identified readily between individual cells and groups of cells with immunohistochemical procedures; regrettably, the pattern of basal lamina deposition does not help distinguish this tumor from melanoma, which also shares considerable overlap.[67]

The ultrastructural features of epithelioid MPNST vary as a function of differentiation. Whereas it is possible to identify interlocking cell processes invested with basal lamina and displaying cell junctions, these features are not invariably present.

Despite the limited number of reported cases, there is no doubt that they are fully malignant tumors and should be treated accordingly. At least half of the patients reported in the literature developed distant metastases, usually in the lung. In our experience with 10 patients with tumors in deep soft tissue, 3 developed metastatic disease.[67] Because of the melanoma-like appearance of these tumors, the question has been raised as to whether they commonly spread to regional lymph nodes. Lodding et al. noted lymph node metastasis in 3 of their 14 cases,[70] but we had no instances of lymph node metastasis in 16 cases.[67] Until additional cases adequately address the question, it seems prudent at least to evaluate these tumors clinically before deciding on definitive therapy.

## SUPERFICIAL EPITHELIOID MPNST

A significant number of epithelioid MPNSTs occur in the superficial soft tissues. Until recently, such tumors were unrecognized probably because they were diagnosed as other forms of malignancy. In our recent study of epithelioid MPNSTs, more than half of the tumors occurred in the dermis or subcutaneous tissue. Unlike deep lesions, they were not multinodular but, rather, uninodular masses circumscribed by the capsule of a preexisting nerve or neurofibroma. In the nodule the cells are arranged in small groups or cohesive nests somewhat reminiscent of those in a nevus. The cells typically mold to one another with little or no intervening stroma, although the nests are separated by a fibrous or myxoid stroma. The cells, however, display the same prominence of nucleoli and mitotic activity as those in soft tissue. Like their deep counterparts, S-100 protein can usually be identified. The behavior of this group of lesions is quite good, probably because of their superficial location,

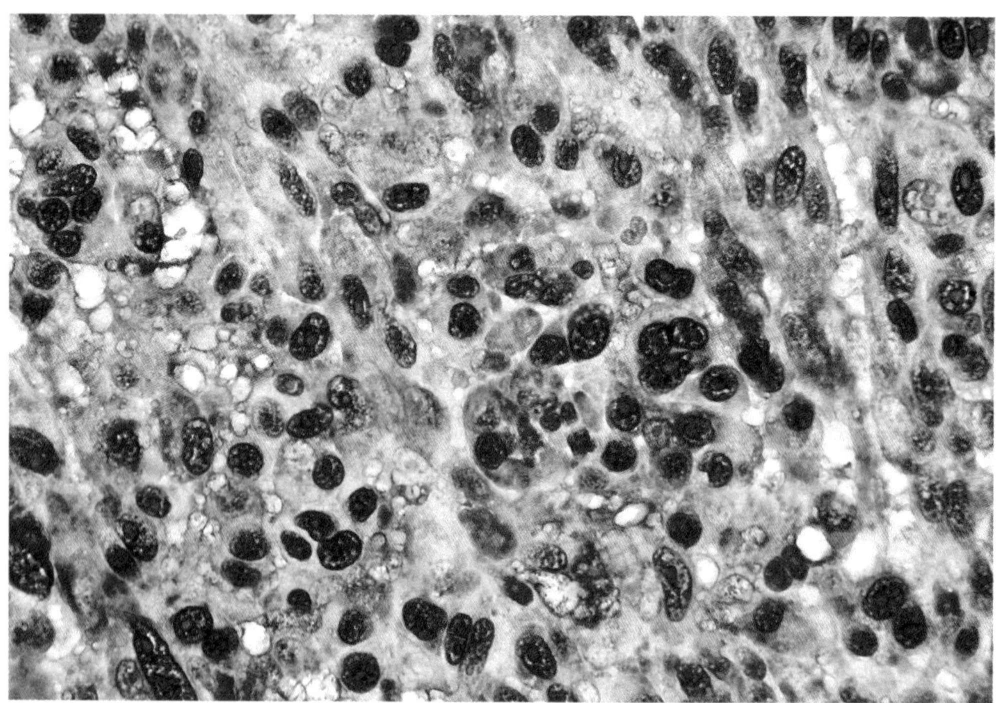

**FIGURE 31–30.** S-100 protein immunostaining in an epithelioid MPNST.

sharp circumscription, and small size. In this group only 1 of 16 patients in our review developed metastasis to the lung. This tumor should be distinguished from epithelioid schwannoma, a benign nerve sheath tumor that does not have the atypia or mitotic activity of epithelioid MPNSTs.

## CLEAR CELL SARCOMA (MALIGNANT MELANOMA OF SOFT PARTS)

Described in 1968 by Enzinger,[148] clear cell sarcoma has become a well accepted clinicopathologic entity.[135–149,151–158,160,163–166,168–173] Although it produces melanin,[137,139,147,163,170] it differs from the conventional melanoma in several important respects. It is a deeply situated tumor that is nearly always intimately associated with tendons or aponeuroses. It lacks junctional changes and rarely even involves epidermis. Cytogenetic analysis of a small number of clear cell sarcomas indicates that in most there is a translocation of chromosomes 12 and 22, an alteration not encountered in malignant melanoma.[140,141,164,166,168,173] Although the term *malignant melanoma of soft parts* is used as a synonym for this tumor, it is important that this lesion not be loosely considered a malignant melanoma but, rather, a unique lesion.

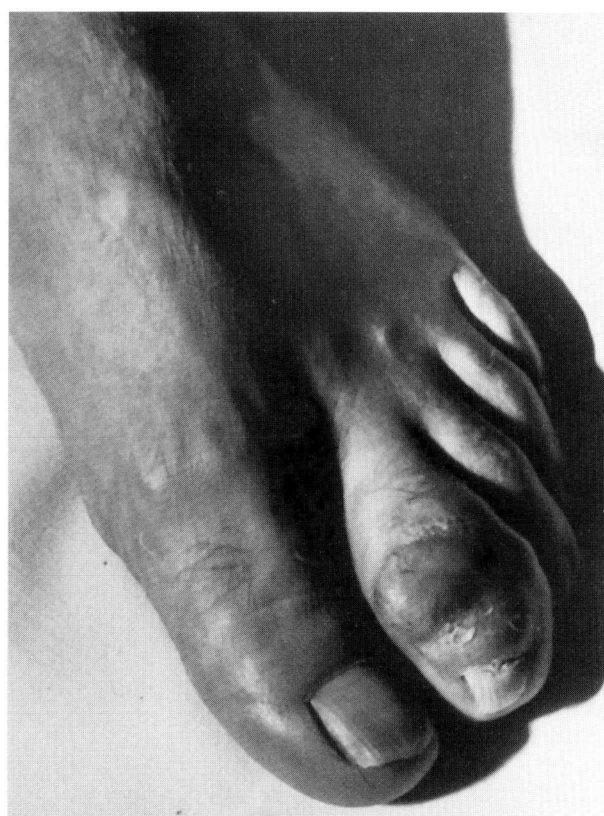

**FIGURE 31–31.** Clear cell sarcoma of the second toe.

### Clinical Findings

Clear cell sarcoma mainly affects young adults between the ages of 20 and 40 years, but in rare instances it occurs in the very young and the very old. The age range in our series of 141 patients[143] was 7–83 years (median 27 years). Women were affected more commonly than men. The principal sites of the neoplasm are the extremities, especially the region of the foot and ankle; 63 (43%) of our 141 cases originated in this general region (Fig. 31–31). Next in frequency are the knee, thigh, and hand, where another 51 (36%) of the cases occurred. The head and neck region and the trunk are only rarely involved (Table 31–3). Clear cell sarcoma is usually deep-seated and, like epithelioid sarcoma, is often intimately bound to tendons or aponeuroses. The overlying skin tends to be uninvolved, although many of the large tumors extend into the subcutis and lower dermis.

At the time of diagnosis, the tumor presents as a slowly enlarging mass causing tenderness or pain in about half of the cases. At the time of operation the duration of symptoms varies substantially, averaging 2 years but ranging from a few weeks to 20 years. In fact, clear cell sarcomas that have been present for 5 years or more not uncommon. A history of trauma or injury to the site of the tumor is given by slightly fewer than half of the patients. Calcification is occasionally noted radiologically in addition to a soft tissue mass.

### Pathologic Findings

Macroscopically, the tumor consists of a circumscribed, lobulated or multinodular gray-white mass. Frequently the mass is attached to tendons or aponeuroses, but there is no connection with the overly-

**TABLE 31–3** ANATOMIC DISTRIBUTION OF 141 CLEAR CELL SARCOMAS

| Location | No. of Patients | Percent |
|---|---|---|
| Head and neck | 1 | 0.8 |
| Trunk | 3 | 2.1 |
| Upper extremity | 31 | 22.0 |
| Lower extremity (foot 28; knee 21; heel 15; ankle 11) | 106 | 75.1 |
| *Total* | **141** | **100.0** |

Data are from Montgomery et al.[160]

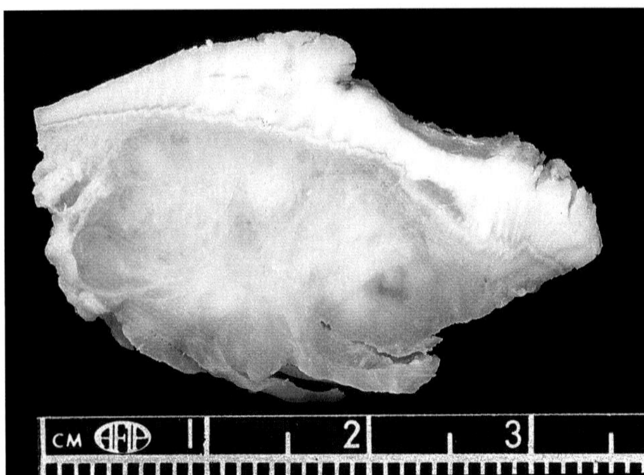


**FIGURE 31–32.** Clear cell sarcoma diffusely infiltrating a tendon (top) and skeletal muscle (bottom).

ing skin (Figs. 31–32, 31–33). The tumor ranges in size from 1 cm to more than 10 cm; most are 2–6 cm. The cut surface may be distorted by focal hemorrhage, necrosis, or cystic change. Foci of dark brown or black pigmentation occur in a small number of cases (Fig. 31–33).

Microscopic examination discloses a rather uniform pattern composed of compact nests or fascicles of rounded or fusiform cells with a clear cytoplasm bordered and defined by a delicate framework of fibrocollagenous tissue, which is often contiguous with adjacent tendons or aponeuroses (Figs. 31–34 to 31–41). The individual cells have a fairly regular appearance, but they vary somewhat from tumor to tumor. In most instances they have round to ovoid vesicular nuclei with prominent basophilic nucleoli and clear or pale-staining cytoplasm (Fig. 31–42A). They are associated with occasional multinucleated giant cells with 10–15 peripherally placed nuclei similar to those of the surrounding mononuclear tumor cells (Fig. 31–38). Less commonly the cells have a finely stippled eosinophilic cytoplasm and resemble those of a fibrosarcoma. Sometimes clear cells and eosinophilic cells coexist in different portions of the same neoplasm with focal transitions. It should also be noted that when degenerative changes occur in a tumor the cells may appear small and condensed and shrink from the dense fibrous scaffolding (Fig. 31–40). This combination of changes can result in the mistaken diagnosis of alveolar rhabdomyosarcoma or some other type of round cell tumor. Rarely, especially in recurrent and metastatic neoplasms, the cells may become more pleomorphic with features suggesting diagnoses such as carcinoma or melanoma (Fig. 31–41). Mitotic figures tend to be rare and usually number fewer than 2 or 3 mitoses/10 high power fields (HPF). Occasionally myxoid stroma is prominent, leading to consideration of other myxoid sarcomas. The clear cell appearance is a result of the presence of large amounts of intracellular glycogen. Reticulin preparations accentuate the nest-like pattern and clearly outline the collagenous framework that separates the cellular aggregates. In some tumors, the nest-like pattern is absent or inconspicuous. Intracellular melanin is rarely seen with hematoxylin-eosin stain but can be detected in more than half of cases with histochemical stains for melanin. It is also noteworthy that in some instances melanin is absent in the primary tumor but is abundant in the metastasis, and that many clear cell sarcomas contain hemosiderin that may stain positively with Fontana's stain or Warthin-Starry preparation (Fig. 31–43). In cases of doubt, an iron preparation is necessary to distinguish melanin from hemosiderin.

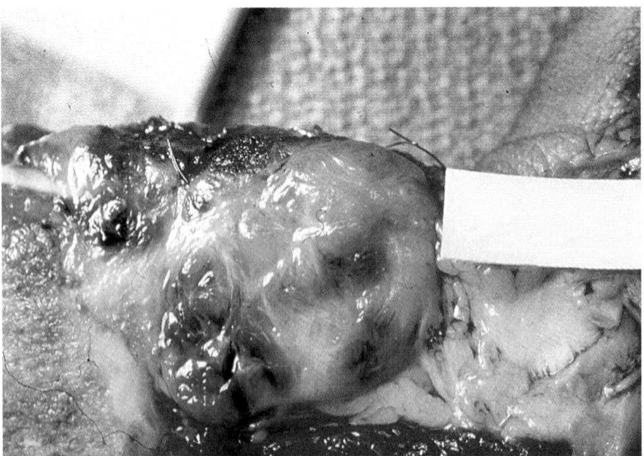

**FIGURE 31–33.** Clear cell sarcoma showing pigmented areas.

Immunohistochemically, the cells of nearly all cases express S-100 protein (Fig. 31–44). Most also express antigens associated with melanin synthesis (HMB-45, melan-A, Mel-CAM, microphthalmia transcription factor) reflective of melanin synthesis. Neuron-specific enolase, Leu-7, and LN3 have also been noted in these lesions. Ultrastructurally, the tumor consists of oval or fusiform cells with rounded nuclei, evenly dispersed chromatin at the nuclear membrane, and a large, centrally placed, single nucleolus. The cytoplasm contains multiple, rounded and swollen mitochondria, membrane-bound vesicles, and ribosomes and polyribosomes in varying numbers. There are also aggregates of rough endoplasmic reticulum, scanty amounts of glycogen, and occasional lipid droplets. Mononuclear and multinuclear cells display similar ultrastructural characteristics. Melanosomes in varying stages of development are present in most cases. Some show dense pigmentation, and others exhibit the typical lamellar, striated, or "barrel-stave"

*Text continued on page 1248*

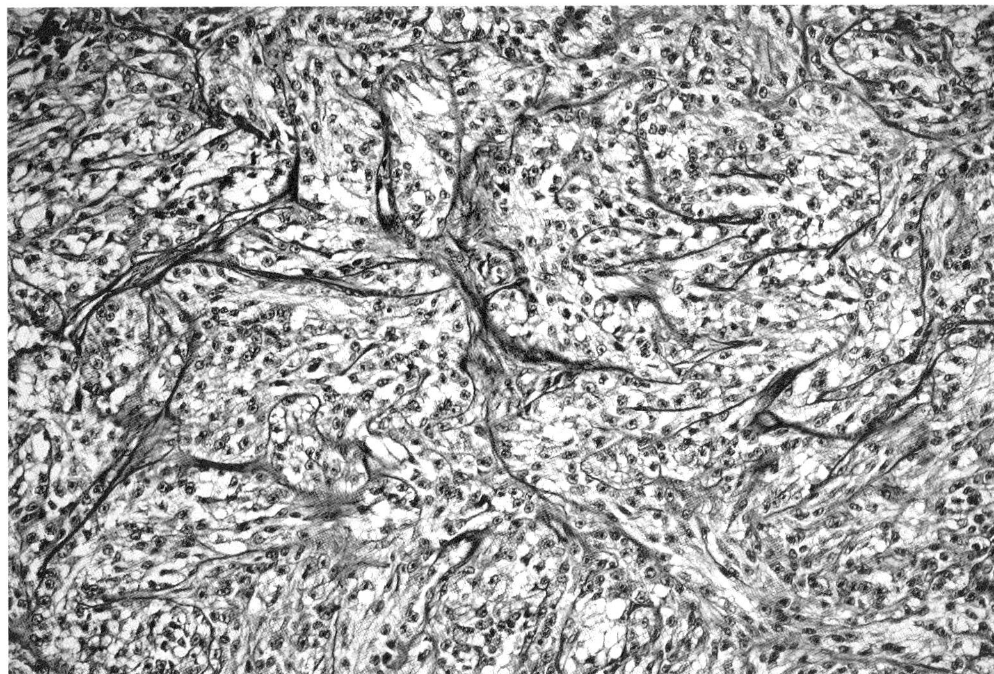

**FIGURE 31–34.** Clear cell sarcoma. Fibrous tissue septa divide the tumor into well defined nests and groups of pale-staining tumor cells.

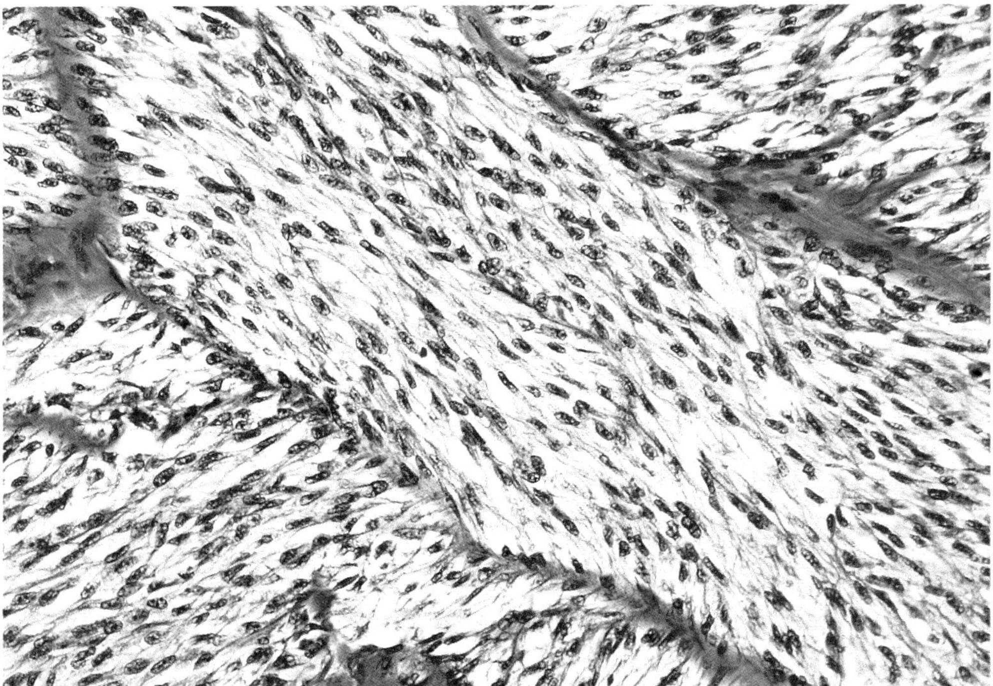

**FIGURE 31–35.** Clear cell sarcoma showing arrangement of the pale-staining tumor cells in short fascicles separated by dense fibrous septa.

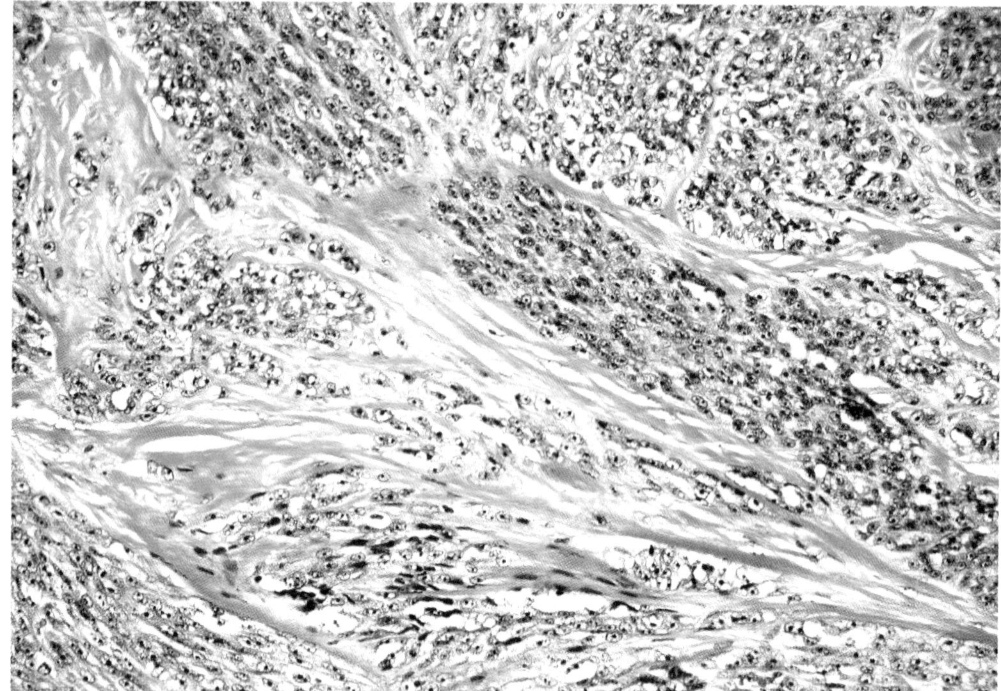

**FIGURE 31–36.** Clear cell sarcoma subdivided by dense fibrous bands.

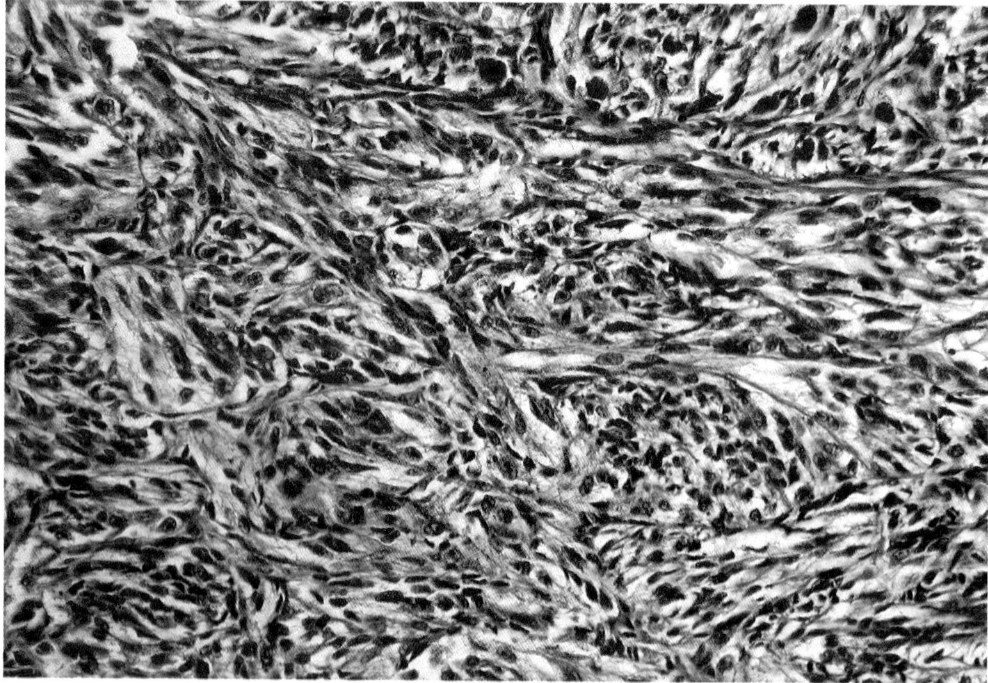

**FIGURE 31–37.** Clear cell sarcoma with cytoplasmic melanin pigment.

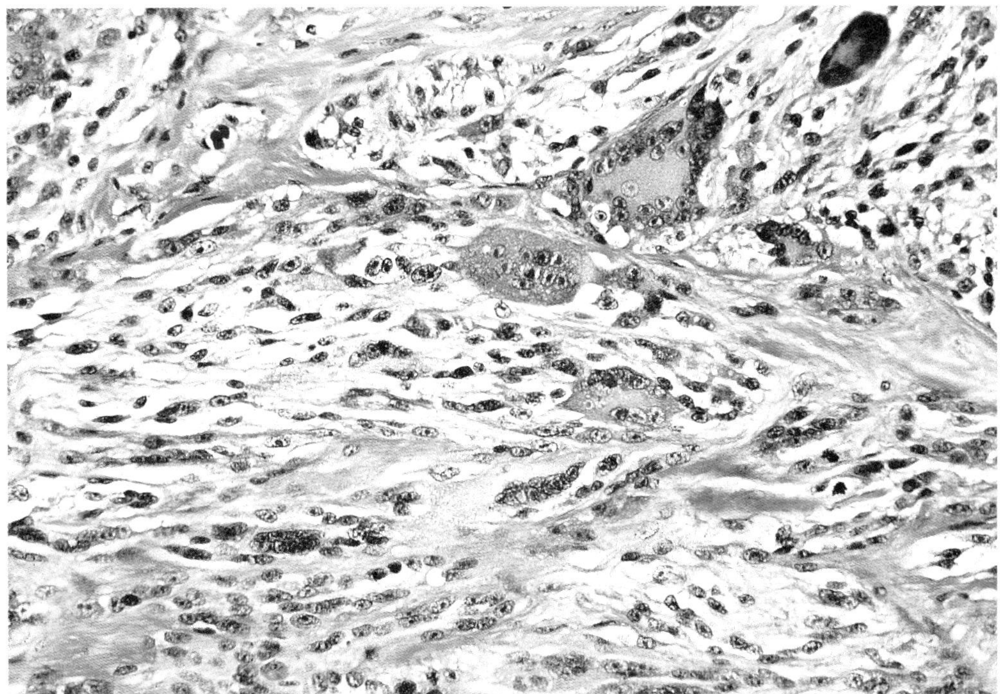

**FIGURE 31–38.** Clear cell sarcoma with scattered multinucleated giant cells. The giant cells have a wreath of peripherally placed nuclei of uniform size and shape.

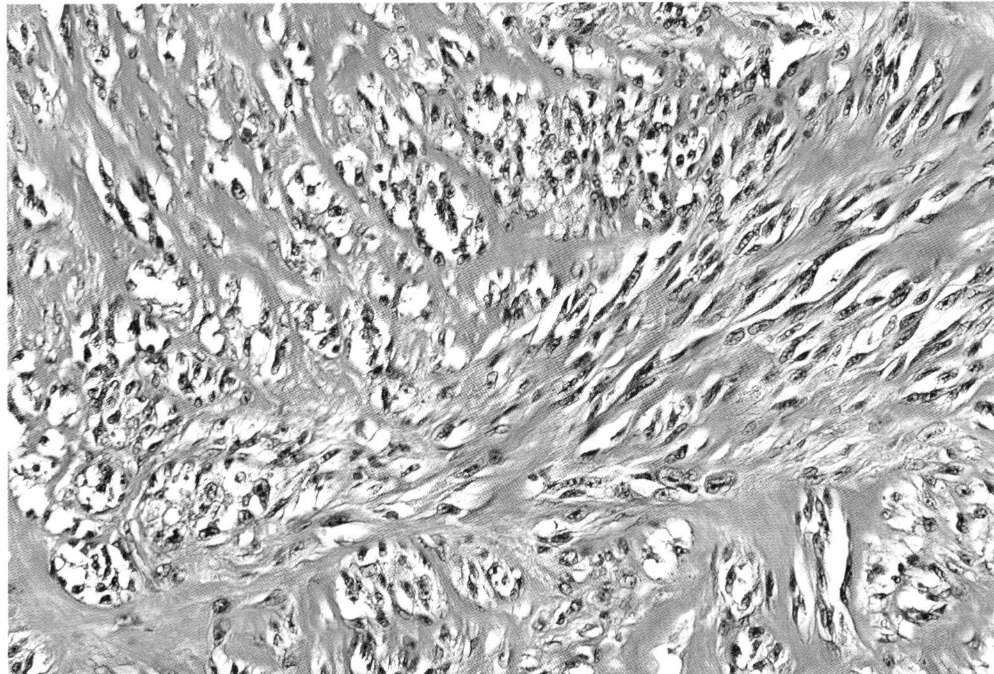

**FIGURE 31–39.** Clear cell sarcoma with areas of dense hyalinization.

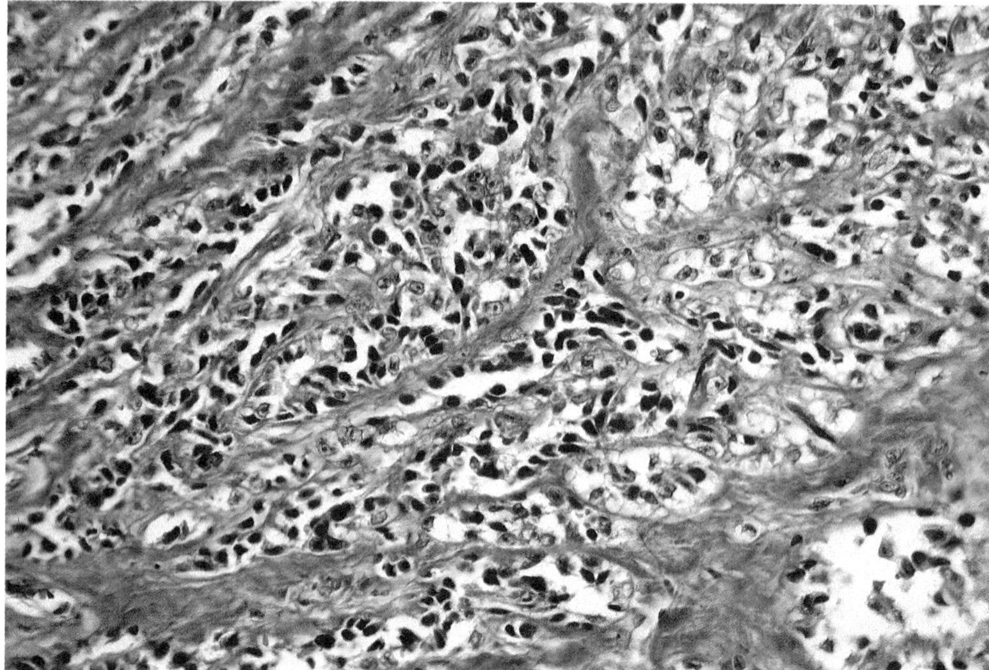

**FIGURE 31–40.** Clear cell sarcoma with degeneration. Cells can acquire a "small cell" appearance that is misleading.

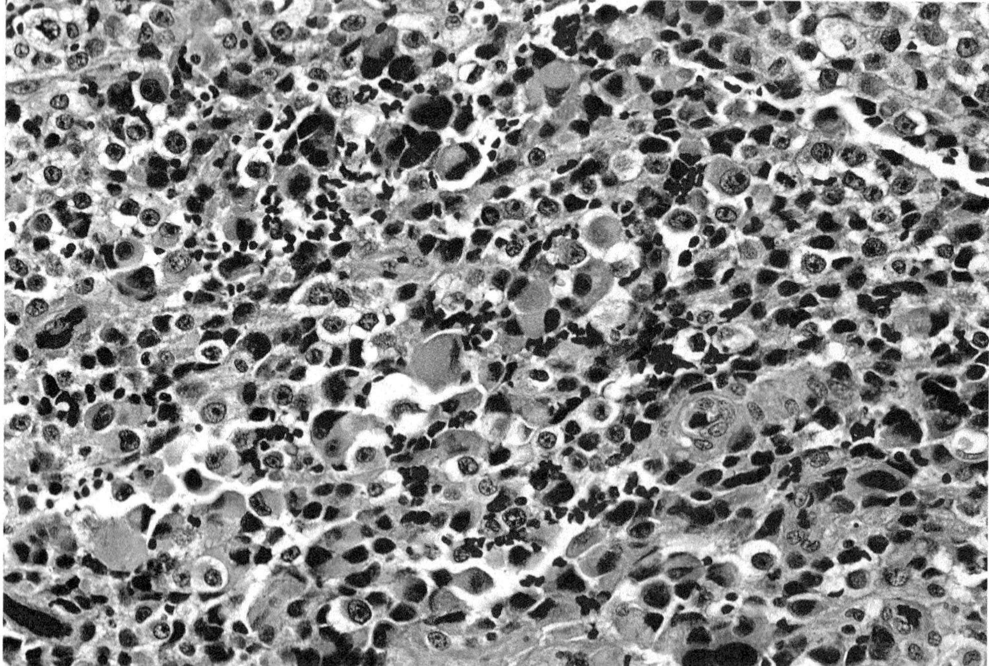

**FIGURE 31–41.** Metastatic clear cell sarcoma with marked pleomorphism and essentially no spindling. Metastasic deposits of this type resemble carcinoma or melanoma.

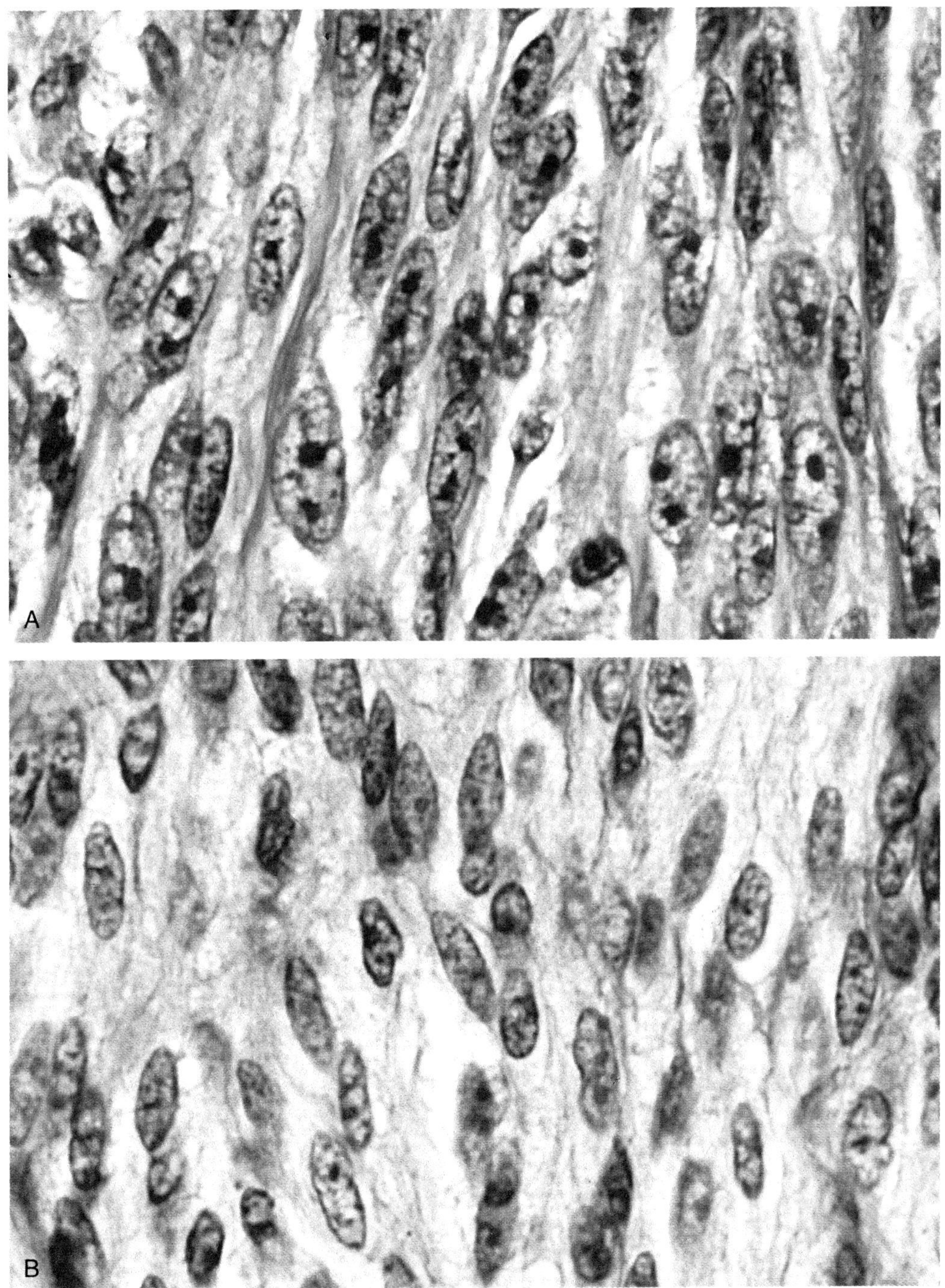


**FIGURE 31–42.** Comparison of cytologic features of clear cell sarcoma and a cellular blue nevus at the same magnification. (**A**) Clear cell sarcoma has prominent vesicular nuclei with a large single nucleolus. (**B**) Cellular blue nevus cells are smaller with a less vesicular nuclear chromatin pattern and small pinpoint nuclei.

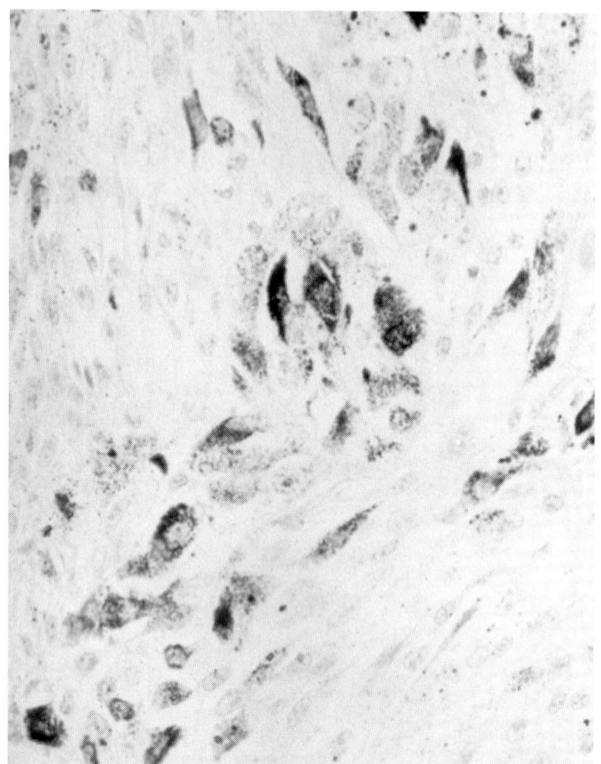

**FIGURE 31–43.** Clear cell sarcoma. Fontana's stain reveals melanin pigment in some of the tumor cells. (Fontana stain; ×400)

internal structure of premelanosomes (Fig. 31–45). Basal laminae surround groups of closely apposed neoplastic cells. Collagen fibers are abundant in the extracellular spaces. Benson et al.[138] also described occasional cells with stubby or finger-like dendritic processes, a few of which contained longitudinally aligned filaments.

## Differential Diagnosis

Although several of the tumors in our series and the literature were initially diagnosed as synovial sarcoma and a relation between the tumors was claimed in the literature (tendosynovial sarcoma), a reliable microscopic distinction of the tumors is feasible if attention is paid to the absence of a biphasic cellular pattern and intracellular mucin and, in more than half of cases, to the presence of intracellular melanin. Tsuneyoshi et al.[172] distinguished between "synovial" and "melanotic" types of clear cell sarcoma, a rather arbitrary and subjective division that is not possible in our opinion.

Differentiation from fibrosarcoma may be more problematic, particularly in those that lack the clear cell appearance of the tumor cells and consist of spindle-shaped cells with eosinophilic cytoplasm and smaller, less prominent nucleoli. In these cases, special stains may help in arriving at a reliable diagnosis, as the cells of fibrosarcoma are not arranged in dis-

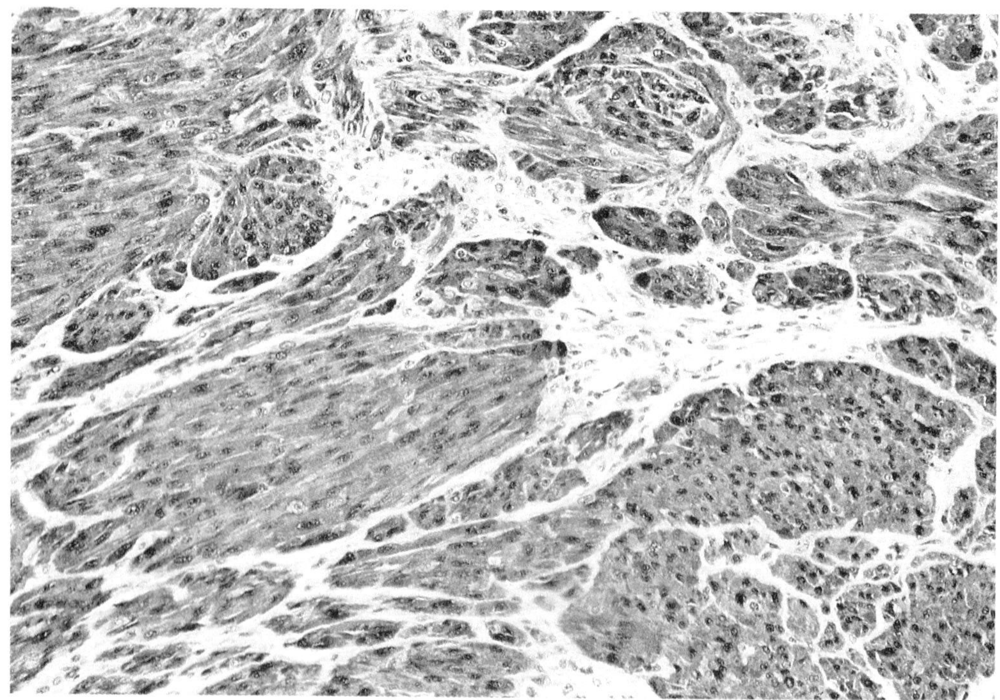

**FIGURE 31–44.** Strong S-100 protein immunostaining in a clear cell sarcoma.

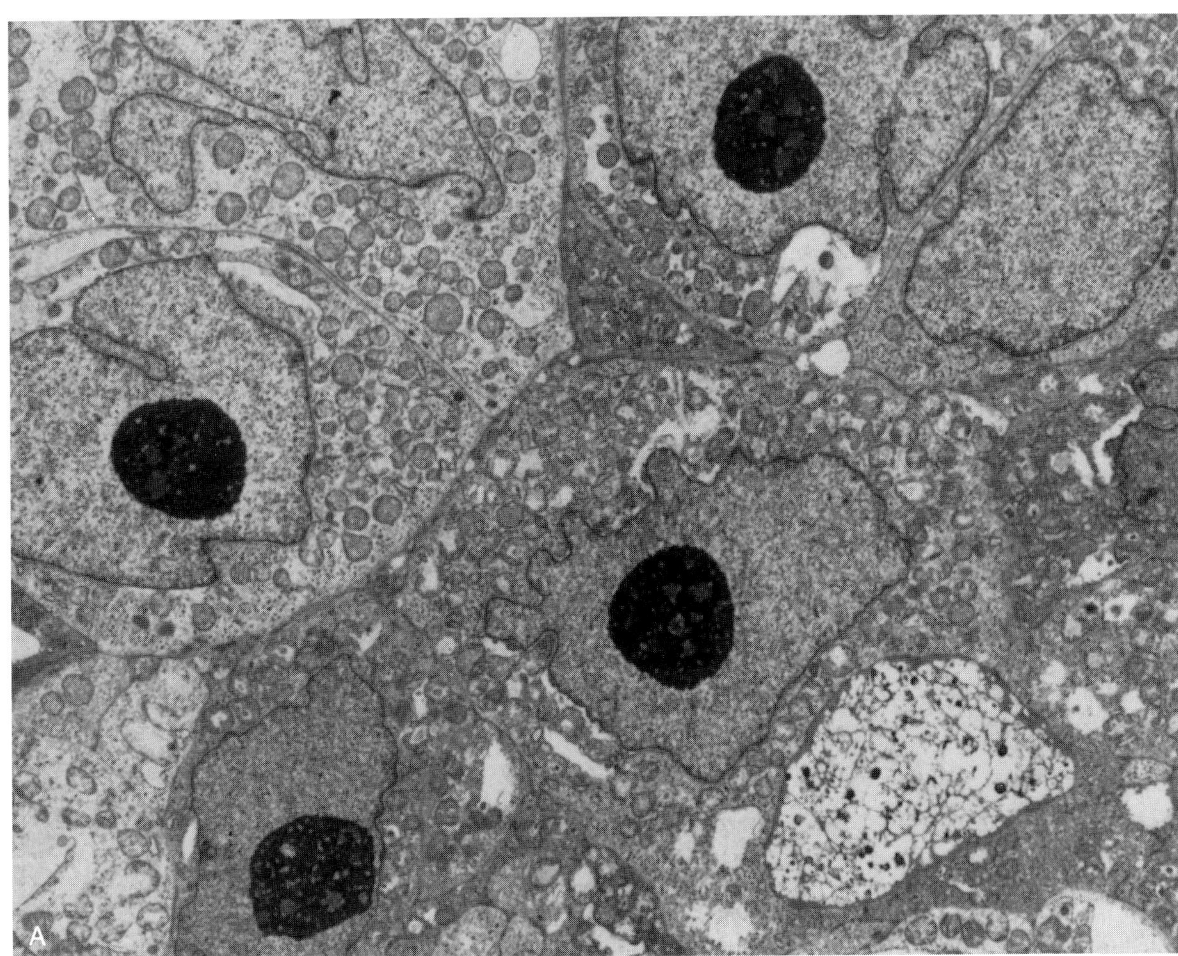


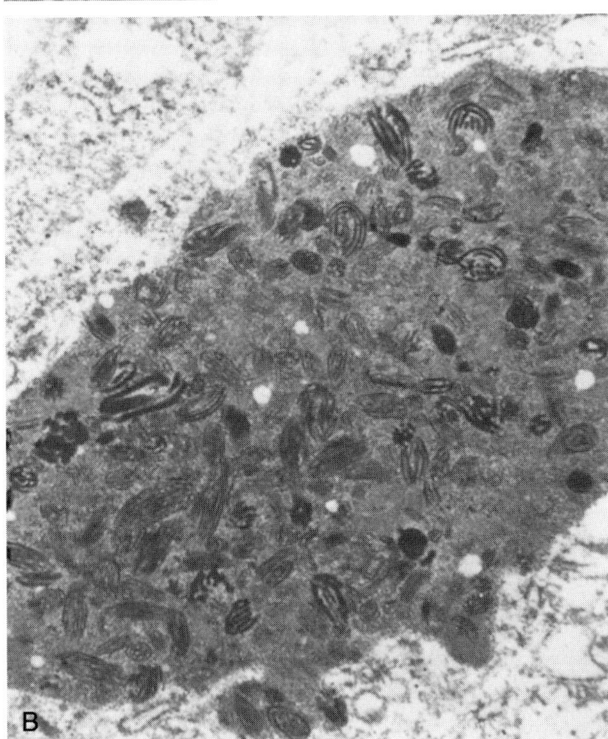


**FIGURE 31–45.** (**A**) Clear cell sarcoma (malignant melanoma of soft parts) showing tumor cells with irregular nuclear profiles, strikingly prominent nucleoli, and numerous mitochondria (×4600) (From Benson JD, Kraemer BB, Mackay B. Malignant melanoma of soft parts: an ultrastructural study of four cases. Ultrastruct Pathol 8:57, 1985.) (**B**) Melanosomes with typical lamellar or "barrel-stave" internal structure in a clear cell sarcoma. (×40,500)

tinct cellular aggregates, lack immunoreactivity for S-100 protein, and are devoid of glycogen. Distinction from an epithelioid form of MPNST and a spindle cell melanoma may be much more difficult and in fact is impossible in rare cases. The MPNST, however, is often associated with a large peripheral nerve or with manifestations of neurofibromatosis; moreover, its cells rarely contain glycogen, have dense hyperchromatic nuclei, and display more prominent mitotic activity. MPNSTs with melanin formation do exist, but they are rare in our experience. As a rule, desmoplastic or spindle cell malignant melanoma,[186] a more common condition, involves the dermis and is associated with pigmentation or junctional changes in the overlying or adjacent skin. Its cells also have prominent nucleoli, infrequent mitotic figures, and intracellular glycogen. The exhibit positive immunostaining for S-100 proteins; but they are rarely as pale-staining or as uniform as those of clear cell sarcoma. The prominent nucleoli and the more fusiform appearance of the tumor cells also assist in the differentiation from metastatic renal cell carcinoma. Owing to the fact that cellular blue nevus can occur at a similar age, and in similar locations, and have certain common histologic features including clear spindled cells associated with giant cells, distinction from clear cell sarcoma can be problematic. Fundamentally, the cells of a clear cell sarcoma are larger, with a vesicular nuclear chromatin pattern and prominent nucleoli. In cellular blue nevi the small cells typically have pinpoint nucleoli (Fig. 31–42).

## Clinical Course and Behavior

Even in cases treated by seemingly adequate therapy, the prognosis is poor, and many patients develop recurrences and metastases. In the large Armed Forces Institute of Pathology (AFIP) experience based on consultation material,[143] 54% were alive and 46% had died. Of the 53 patients who had died, 50 died of metastatic disease and 3 from unrelated causes. In 24 of the 50 cases the tumor recurred locally before metastasis. Of the living patients, 34 were well without recurrence or metastasis, 21 with one or more recurrences, and 7 with metastatic disease. However, patients with multiple recurrences[154,156] spanning two to three decades before the metastases appear have been recorded. A study from The Netherlands of 30 patients reported a 5-year survival of 54% and of 65% in patients with localized diseases.[144] Patients who developed local recurrence or regional lymph node metastases eventually developed distant metastasis as well, indicating a clear need for controlling the local disease. Prognostic factors in this disease include tumor size[160,167] and necrosis.[167] Other factors such as age, location, depth, or proliferation index have been found to be independent prognostic factors. The most common sites of metastasis are the lung, lymph nodes, and bone.[116,128] Because of the frequency of regional lymph node metastases, the question of prophylactic lymph node dissection has been raised. Although there is no answer to this question at present, there may be a role for sentinel lymph node biopsy in this disease as is currently carried out for breast carcinoma and malignant melanoma.[144] The fact that some tumors have recurred or metastasized 10 years or more after the initial tumor indicates that long-term follow-up is necessary before one can safely assume that the patient has been cured.

## Discussion

There seems to be no doubt that clear cell sarcoma is a neuroectodermal tumor bearing some histologic similarity to cellular blue nevus in terms of its lack of epidermal involvement, its architectural pattern, and to some extent its cytologic features. Although sometimes referred to as "deep melanoma of soft parts," clear cell sarcoma should be considered distinct from cutaneous malignant melanoma. In more than three-fourths of cases the clear cell sarcoma has a unique translocation t(12;22)(q13;q12) that has never been identified in malignant melanoma. This translocation fuses the *ATF-1* gene on chromosome 12 with the *EWS* gene on chromosome 22, *ATF-1* is a transcription factor, the effect of which may be similar in nature to that of the Ewing's sarcoma/primitive neuroectodermal tumor (EWS-PNET) translocation. Clear cell sarcoma has also been reported to have increased copies of chromosomes 7 and 8 in addition to abnormalities of chromosome 22. In contrast, the gene for cutaneous melanoma has been localized to 1p.

# NEUROTROPIC-DESMOPLASTIC MELANOMAS

Neurotropic-desmoplastic melanomas are a distinctive subset of melanomas that display varying degrees of desmoplasia and neurotropism.[174,176–181,183–191] Although we refer to them as a common entity, they are often divided into desmoplastic or neurotropic forms in the dermatologic literature. The reason for even considering these lesions in this chapter is that we have found they are frequently mistaken for benign and malignant nerve sheath tumors as well as reactive fibroblastic proliferations. These lesions were first described in the seminal paper by Conley et al.[177] as desmoplastic melanoma. Noting that these lesions occurred commonly in the head and neck region, these authors were impressed by the remarkable desmoplastic properties of the tumors. Reed and Leonard[185]

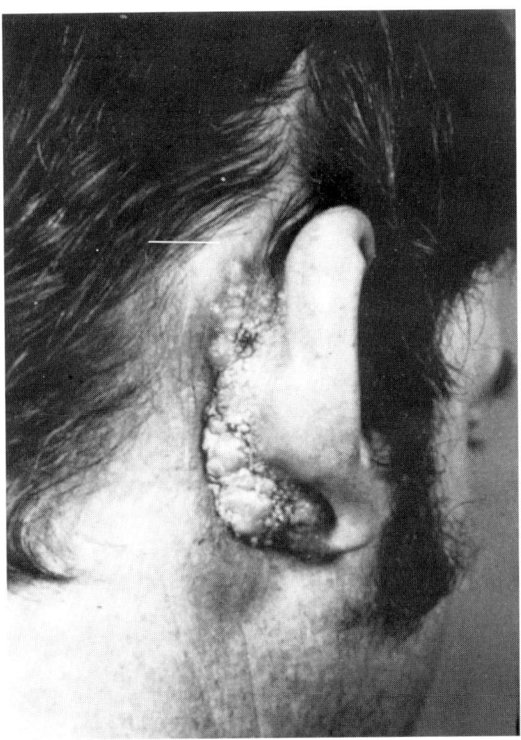

**FIGURE 31–46.** Neurotropic melanoma. Tumor arose in the posterior auricular region and produced a wart-like nonpigmented mass. Lesion recurred several times in the same region before metastasizing to the paraspinal area.

later described a subset of desmoplastic melanomas as "neurotropic melanoma" and commented on their tendency to migrate toward and spread along nerves. In fact, both features may be seen to a varying degree in a given case. The term *neurotropic melanoma* is not used for conventional melanomas that simply display focal neurotropism. Most of these lesions probably originate from melanocytes of the epidermis, whereas only a small fraction arise *de novo* from the dermal structures. The size, appearance, and degree of melanocytic atypia in the precursor lesion are variable. It is not uncommon, in our experience, that a precursor lesion is overlooked entirely and that progression or recurrence of the lesion is assumed to be a primary soft tissue neoplasm.

About three-fourths of neurotropic melanomas occur on the head and neck, usually in adult patients (Fig. 31–46). Cases in children have been recognized, and unusual sites such as the vulva may be affected. The most common precursor lesion is lentigo maligna melanoma, but these tumors may also arise in superficial spreading and acral lentiginous melanomas (see Fig. 31–49). Apart from the precursor lesion, the main tumor mass is firm and scar-like in consistency (Figs. 31–47, 31–48) and is made up of spindled or slightly oval cells that form short packet-like fascicles, vaguely reminiscent of carcinoma, that infiltrate the connective tissue (Figs. 31–49, 31–50, 31–51). In some cases, collections of tumor cells with Schwann cell features, in a rudimentary fashion, recapitulate the appearance of small nerves. Fine or dense collagen fibrils surround the cells. In other areas the cells lose their cohesion with one another and infiltrate singly. These areas are often collections of tumor cells that can be identified in the endoneurium and perineurium of normal nerves (Fig. 31–52) and are believed to be one of the reasons for the high rate of local recurrence of this lesion following conservative excision. Occasionally this perineural growth is flagged by an associated lymphocytic response, which is helpful for identifying tumor (Fig. 31–52B). In recurrent tumors the cells acquire a more epithelial appearance and usually have more pleomorphism so they look distinctly carcinomatous. Axons can be demonstrated in the tumor, but melanin pigment is absent, although it can be identified in the precursor lesion.

Ultrastructurally, the cells in a neurotropic melanoma do not contain melanosomes or premelanosomes but express schwann cell features to a variable degree.[179,187] Most desmoplastic-neurotropic melanomas exhibit positive immunostaining for S-100 protein, although it can be quite focal.[184] In these preparations the long attenuated shape of these schwannian cells is easily appreciated (Fig. 31–53). Immunostains for gp100 (HMB45) are almost always negative, but microphthalmia transcription factor, a nuclear regulatory protein in melanin-producing cells, is present in nearly one-half of desmoplastic melanomas.[182] We have not encountered microphthalmia transcription factor in MPNSTs, so this antigen will probably play an increasingly important role in distinguishing the

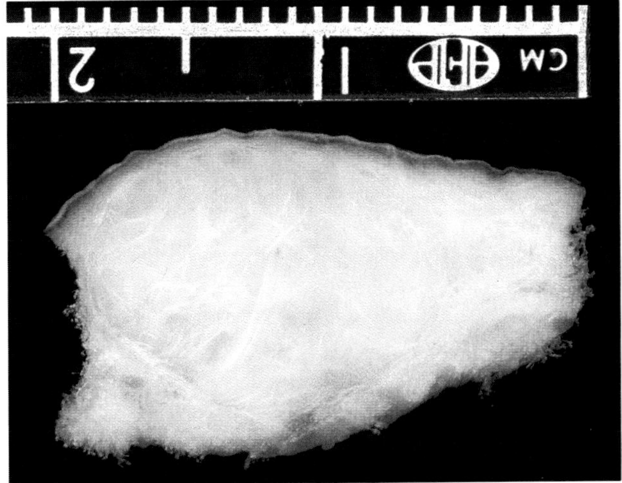

**FIGURE 31–47.** Neurotropic melanoma. Note the ill-defined scar-like quality of this dermal tumor.

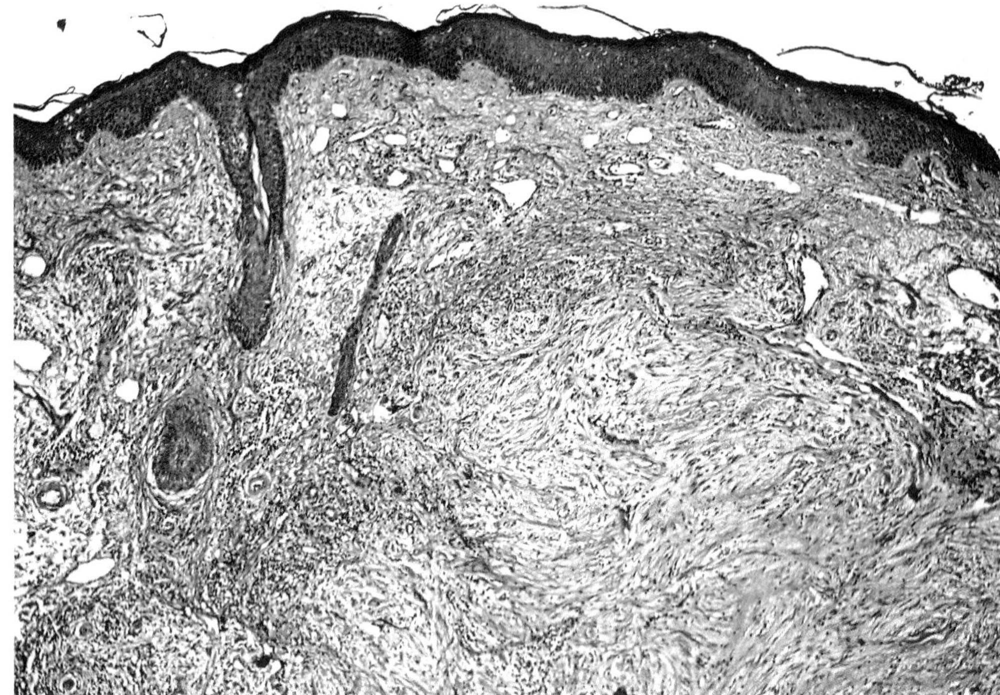

**FIGURE 31–48.** Neurotropic melanoma. This highly desmoplastic tumor was present in the mid and deep dermis. No epidermal lesion was present in the sections studied.

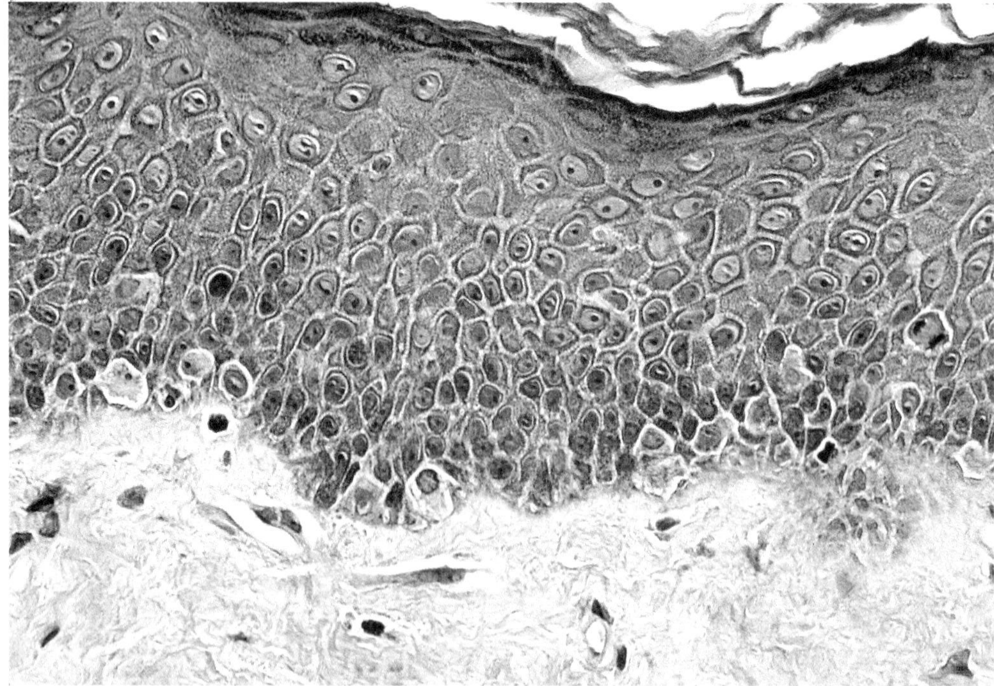

**FIGURE 31–49.** Neurotropic melanoma showing minimal melanocytic dysplasia at the surface of the lesion.

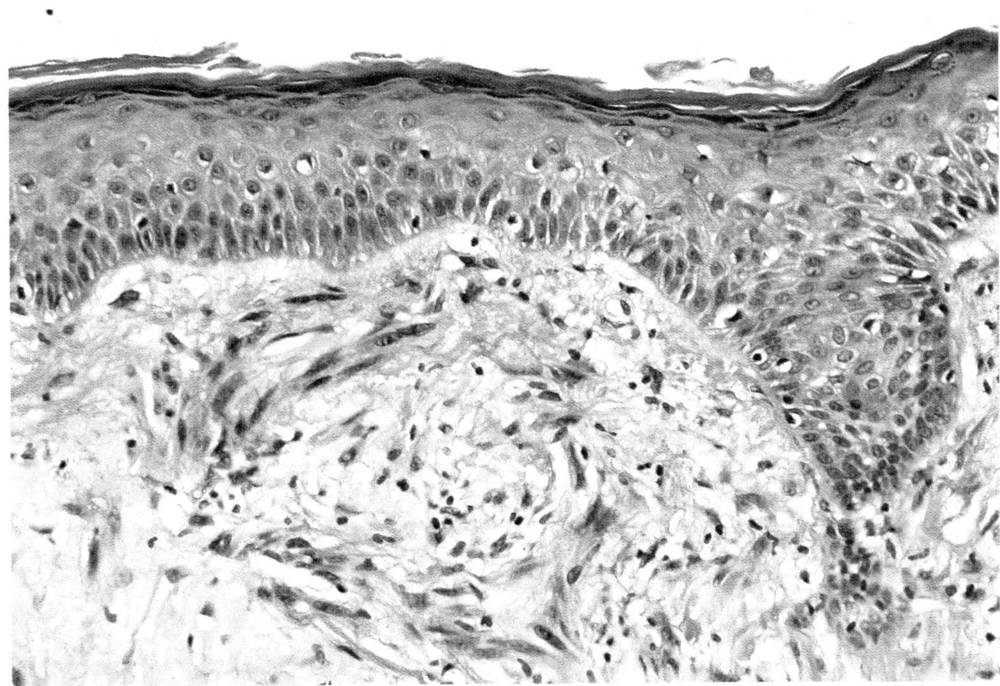

**FIGURE 31–50.** Neurotropic melanoma with subtle spindle cell proliferation in the superficial dermis.

MPNST from this form of melanoma. Although the presence of S-100 protein immunostaining is usually reliable for distinguishing desmoplastic melanoma from various reactive fibroblastic proliferations, there have been rare instances of S-100 immunoreactivity noted in scars and fibromatosis. Therefore it is always important to make an independent assessment of the nature of the positive-staining cells.

These lesions are fully malignant tumors. Most present as Clark's level IV or V lesions. Of the collected cases in the literature, about one-third of patients died of their tumors. Local recurrence occurs in about half of patients and can be predicted by excision with margins of less than 1 cm, head and neck location, level V invasion, and tumor thickness of more than 4 mm. Common metastatic sites are the regional lymph nodes and lung. It should be noted that occasionally conventional melanomas display neurotropic or schwann cell features in a metastatic site.[178,179] Thus a lymph node with metastatic tumor reminiscent of a MPNST could be either a conventional or neurotropic melanoma but rarely an MPNST (Fig. 31–29).

## EXTRASPINAL (SOFT TISSUE) EPENDYMOMA

Soft tissue ependymomas are rare tumors that occur in subcutaneous locations dorsal to the sacrum and coccyx or in deep soft tissue anterior to the sacrum and posterior to the rectum.[192–203] Many that occur in the latter location represent ependymomas of the cauda equina that have extended through the sacral foramina to present as presacral masses.[203] Those situated dorsally to the sacrum represent the more significant group in terms of soft tissue tumors; consequently, this discussion is restricted to this group. Pathogenetically, the dorsal coccygeal ependymoma may arise from normal remnants of the neural tube (coccygeal medullary vestige) or from abnormal remnants resulting from embryologic malformations. The latter contention is supported by the fact that a significant proportion of patients with this tumor[193] have developmental abnormalities such as spina bifida.

Characteristically, these tumors present as longstanding masses that are often diagnosed preoperatively as pilonidal cysts, teratomas, or sweat gland tumors. Although a few have prove to be extensive at the time of initial surgery,[193] most are encapsulated and easily separated from the fascia overlying the sacrum and coccyx. Grossly, they are myxoid multilobulated masses with focal areas of hemorrhage and necrosis (Fig. 31–54). Most resemble the ependymomas arising from the cauda equina and are of the "myxopapillary type." Cuboidal or columnar cells are arranged on fibrovascular stalks in a papillary configuration (Fig. 31–55), Secondary perivascular degenerative changes result in the peculiar myxoid and hyalinized appearance that characterizes the myxopapillary ependymoma. In cases where the degeneration

*Text continued on page 1259*

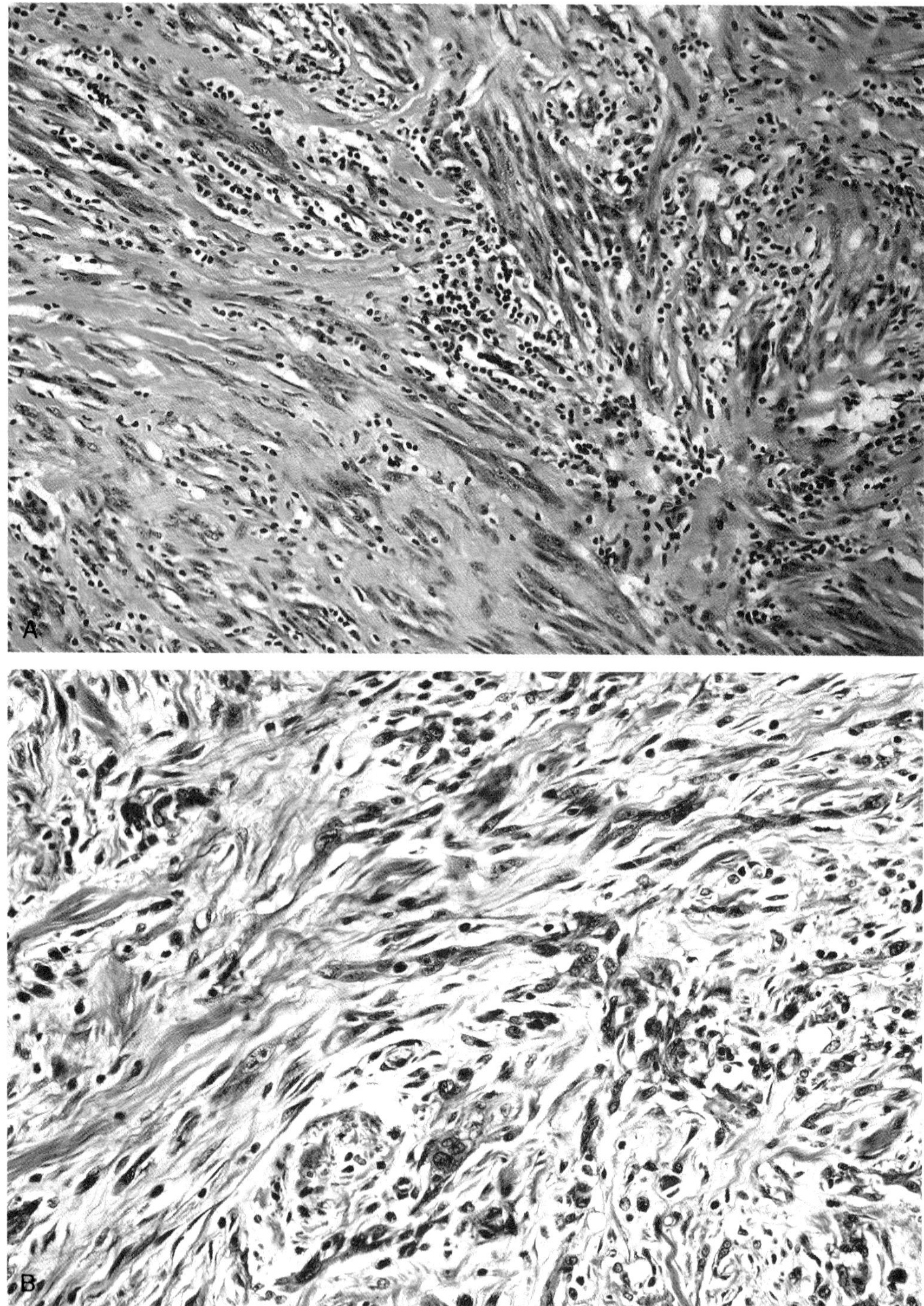


**FIGURE 31–51.** Various patterns in a neurotropic melanoma. Obvious areas of malignancy (**A**) have atypical cells arranged in short packets or fascicles. In other areas the spindled cells are arranged in slender packets or cords (**B**).

*Illustration continued on opposite page*

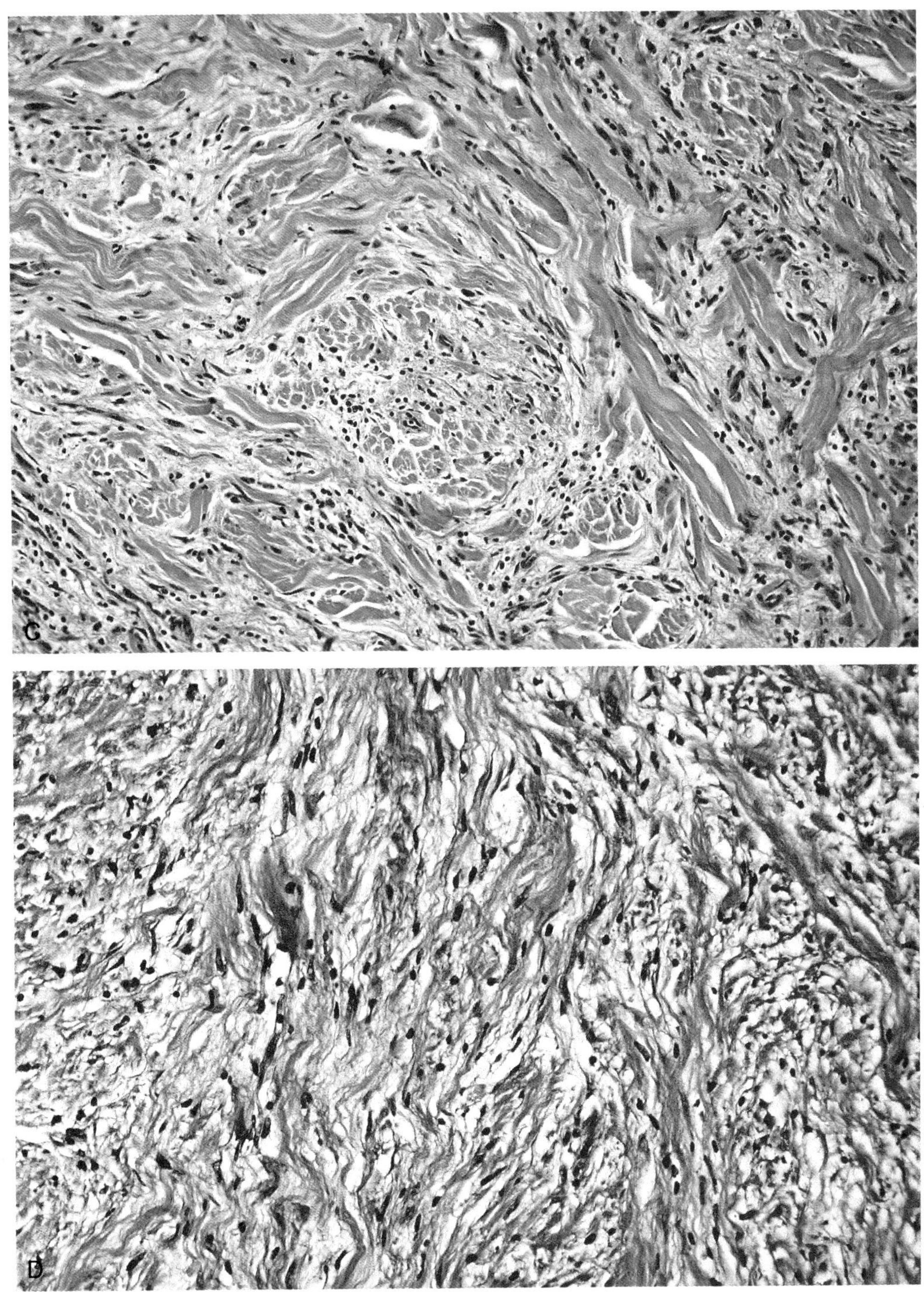

**FIGURE 31–51** *(Continued)*. Desmoplasia can be marked with thick bands of collagen (**C**). Areas with delicate collagen and widely separated neoplastic cells resemble neurofibroma (**D**).

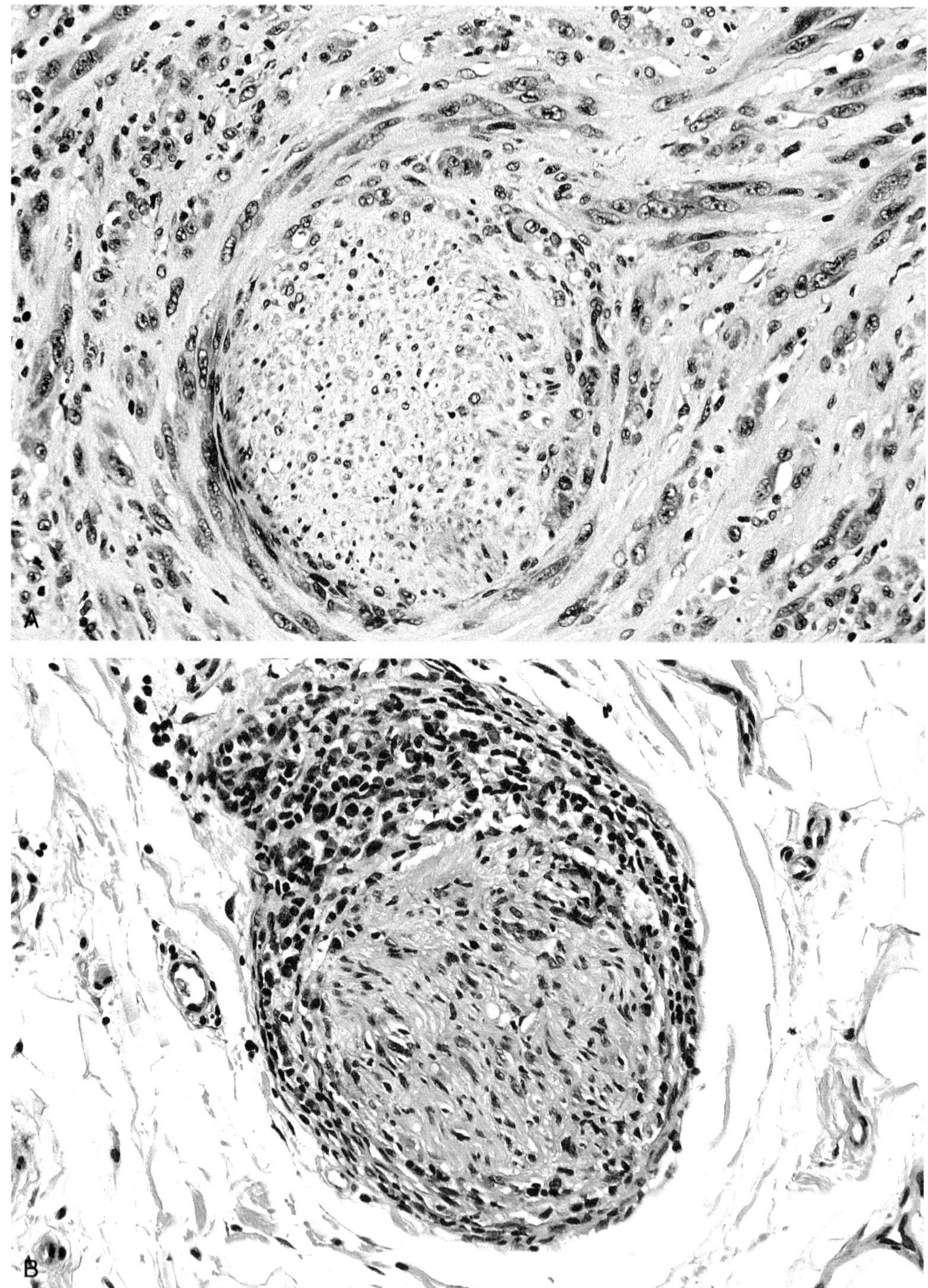

**FIGURE 31–52.** Neurotropic melanoma showing targeting of tumor cells around a nerve (neurotropism) (**A**). Occasionally perineural deposits are associated with lymphocytic response, a subtle clue that the lesion may be a melanoma rather than a malignant Schwann cell tumor (**B**).

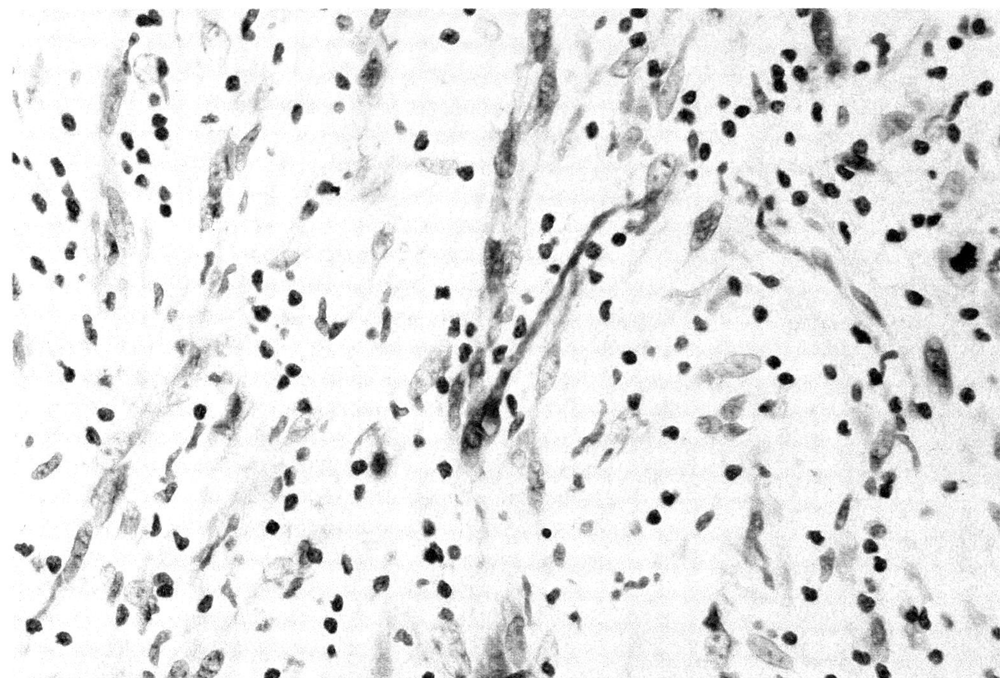

**FIGURE 31–53.** Immunostaining of neurotropic melanoma for S-100 protein, illustrating elongated schwannian cells.

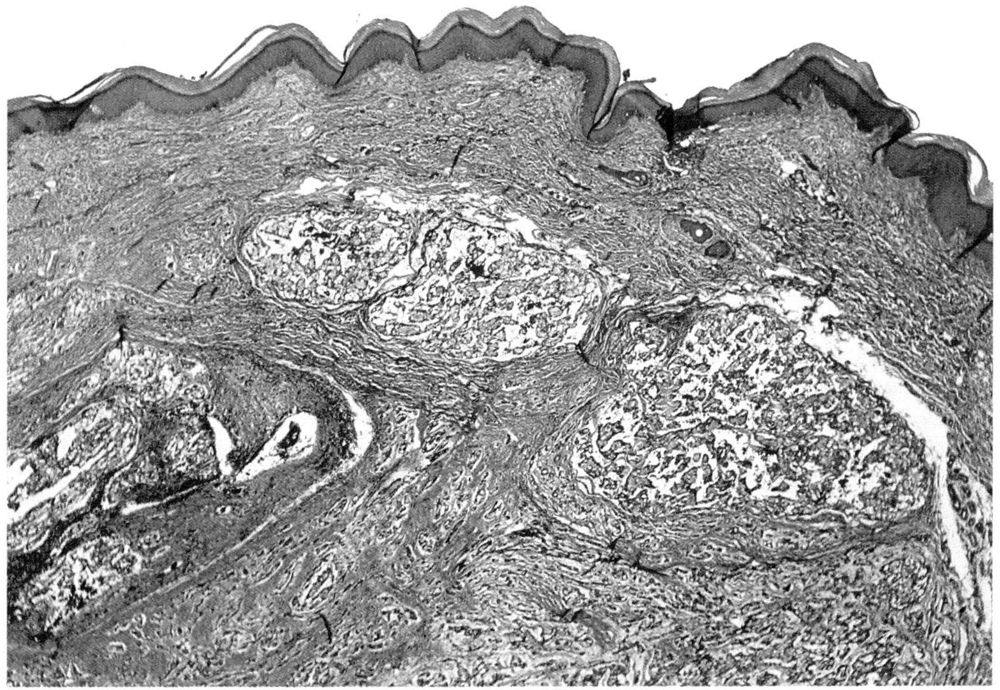

**FIGURE 31–54.** Extraspinal ependymoma presenting in a dorsococcygeal location.

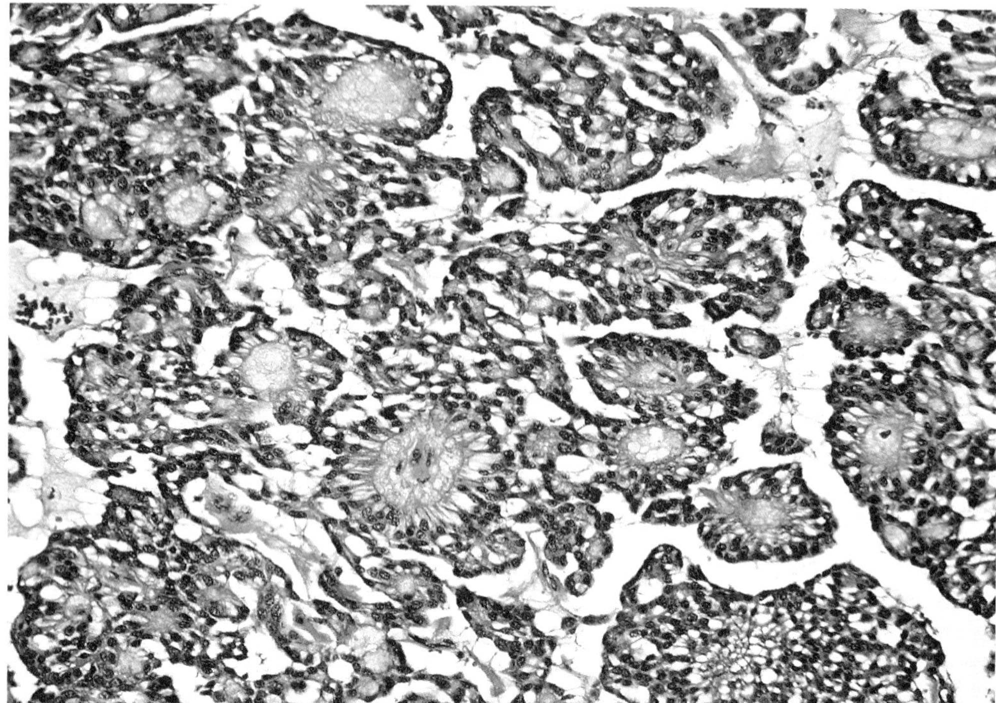

**FIGURE 31–55.** Extraspinal ependymoma. Tumor resembles a myxopapillary ependymoma of the cauda equina and contains perivascular pseudorosettes and papillary structures.

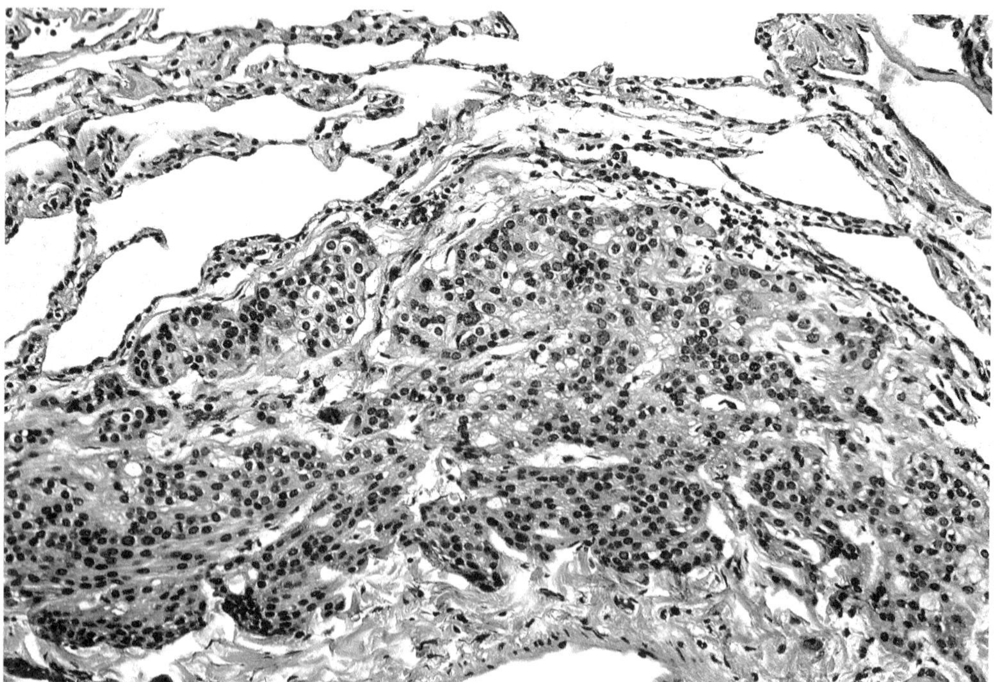

**FIGURE 31–56.** Extraspinal ependymoma metastatic to lung. Nests of tumor may mimic the pattern of carcinoma or carcinoid tumor.

is not marked, the tumor may resemble the more cellular papillary ependymoma of the brain. The cells are usually wall differentiated with apically polarized nuclei. Occasionally blepharoplasts are demonstrated by means of special stains (phosphotungstic acid-hematoxylin stain). Carminophilic intracytoplasmic mucin is not present in these cells despite its presence in the closely related "choroid plexus papilloma."[203] Ultrastructurally these cells have many of the features of normal ependymal cells. They contain microvilli and lateral desmosomes at their apical surfaces, whereas elaborate interdigitations of the plasma membrane and underlying basement membrane material characterize the basal surfaces. Parallel arrays of fine filaments and occasional microtubules are found in the cytoplasm.

Although ependymomas are, in general, low grade neoplasms and usually pose only problems in control of local disease, dorsal coccygeal ependymomas have a greater propensity to metastasize than their intraspinal counterparts. This has been ascribed to their easier accessibility to lymphatic channels and to the longer survival time associated with these tumors. Thus of 11 primary dorsal coccygeal ependymomas, 3 metastasized either to regional (inguinal) nodes or the lung. Metastasis to the lung may be mistaken for a carcinoid tumor (Fig. 31–56). Distant metastasis is a late event, usually occuring 10 years or more after diagnosis of the primary tumor. Adequate treatment of these tumors consists in wide local excision with irradiation for residual or inoperable disease. The protracted course of this disease underscores the need for extended follow-up care and even resection of isolated metastases if and when they appear.

## REFERENCES

### Malignant Peripheral Nerve Sheath Tumor


1. Abe S, Imamura T, Partk P, et al. Small round-cell type of malignant peripheral nerve sheath tumor. Mod Pathol 11:747, 1998.
2. Alvira MM, Mandybur TI, Menefee MG. Light microscopic and ultrastructural observations of a metastasizing malignant epithelioid schwannoma. Cancer 38:1977, 1976.
3. Berner J-M, Sorlie T, Mertens F, et al. Chromosome band 9p21 is frequently altered in malignant peripheral nerve sheath tumors: studies of CDKN2A and other genes in the pRB pathway. Genes Chromosomes Cancer 26:151, 1999.
4. Biggs FJ. Neurosarcoma of the median nerve. Med J Aust 1:687, 1935.
5. Bojsen-Moller M, Myrhe-Jensen O. A consecutive series of 30 malignant schwannomas: survival in relation to clinicopathological parameters and treatment. Acta Pathol Microbiol Scand 92A:147, 1984.
6. Bricklin AS, Rushton HW. Angiosarcoma of venous origin arising in radial nerve. Cancer 39:1556, 1977.
7. Brooks JS, Freeman M, Enterline HT. Malignant "Triton" tumors: natural history and immunohistochemistry of nine new cases with literature review. Cancer 55:2543, 1985.
8. Brown RW, Tornos C, Evans HI. Angiosarcoma arising from malignant schwannoma in a patient with neurofibromatosis. Cancer 70:1141, 1992.
9. Carli M, Morgan M, Bisogno G, et al. Malignant peripheral nerve sheath tumors in childhood (MPNST): a combined experience of the Italian and German co-operative studies: SIOP XXVII meeting. Med Pediatr Oncol 25:243, 1995.
10. Casanova M, Ferrari A, Spreafico F, et al. Malignant peripheral nerve sheath tumors in children: a single-institution twenty-year experience. J Pediatr Hematol Oncol 21:509, 1999.
11. Chaudhuri B, Ronan SG, Manaligod JR. Angiosarcoma arising in a plexiform nerofibroma: a case report. Cancer 46:605, 1980.
12. Chitale AR, Dickerson GR. Electron microscopy in the diagnosis of malignant schwannomas: a report of six cases. Cancer 51:1448, 1983.
13. Chiu HF, Troster M. Ultrastructure of malignant schwannomas. Lab Invest 40A:246, 1979.
14. Christensen WN, Strong EW, Bains MS, Woodruff JM. Neuroendocrine differentiation in the glandular peripheral nerve sheath tumor: pathologic distinction form the biphasic synovial sarcoma with glands. Am J Surg Pathol 12:417, 1988.
15. Coffin CM, Dehner LP. Peripheral neurogenic tumors of the soft tissues of children and adolescents: a clinicopathologic study of 139 cases. Pediatr Pathol 9:387, 1989.
16. Cohn I. Epithelial neoplasms of peripheral and cranial nerves: report of three cases: review of the literature. Arch Surg 17:117, 1928.
17. Conley K, Rubinstein LJ, Spence AM. Studies on experimental malignant nerve sheath tumors maintained in tissue and organ culture systems II. Electron microscopy observations. Acta Neuropathol (Berl) 34:293, 1976.
18. Cross PA, Clarke NW. Malignant nerve sheath tumor with epithelial elements. Histopathology 12:547, 1988.
19. D'Agostino AN, Soule EH, Miller RH. Primary malignant neoplasm of nerves (malignant neurilemomas) in patients without manifestations of multiple neurofibromatosis (von Recklinghausen's disease). Cancer 16:1003, 1963.
20. D'Agostino AN, Soule EH, Miller RH. Sarcomas of the peripheral nerves and somatic soft tissues associated with multiple neurofibromatosis (von Recklinghausen's disease). Cancer 16:1015, 1963.
21. Daimaru Y, Hashimoto H, Enjoji M. Malignant peripheral nerve-sheath tumors (malignant schwannomas): an immunohistochemical study of 29 cases. Am J Surg Pathol 9:434, 1985.
22. Daimaru Y, Hashimoto H, Enjoji M. Malignant "Triton" tumors: a clinicopathologic and immunohistochemical study of nine cases. Hum Pathol 15:768, 1984.
23. Das Gupta TK, Brasfield RD. Solitary malignant schwannoma. Ann Surg 171:419, 1970.
24. De Cou JM, Rao BN, Parham DM, et al. Malignant peripheral nerve sheath tumors: the St. Jude Children's Research Hospital experience. Ann Surg Oncol 2:524, 1995.
25. Denlinger RH, Koestner A, Wechsler W. Indication of neurogenic tumors in C3HeB/FEJ mice by nitrosourea derivatives. Int J Cancer 13:559, 1974.
26. DeSchryver K, Santa Cruz DJ. So-called glandular schwannoma: ependymal differentiation in a case. Ultrastruct Pathol 6:167, 1984.
27. DiCarlo EF, Woodruff JM, Bansal M, et al. The purely epithelioid peripheral nerve sheath tumor. Am J Surg Pathol 10:478, 1986.
28. Doorn PF, Molenaar WM, Buter J, et al. Malignant peripheral nerve sheath tumors in patients with and without neurofibromatosis. Eur J Surg Oncol 21:78, 1995.
29. Ducatman BS, Scheithauer BW. Malignant peripheral nerve

sheath tumor with divergent differentiation. Cancer 54:1049, 1984.
30. Ducatman BS, Scheithauer BW. Port-irradiation neurofibrosarcoma. Cancer 51:1028, 1983.
31. Ducatman BS, Scheithauer BW, Piepgras DG. Malignant peripheral nerve sheath tumors: a clinicopathologic study of 120 cases. Cancer 57:2006, 1986.
32. Erlandson RA, Woodruff JM. Peripheral nerve sheath tumors: an electron microscopic study of 43 cases. Cancer 49:273, 1982.
33. Ferner RE, Lucas JD, O'Doherty MJ, et al. Evaluation of fluorodeoxyglucose postiron emisssion tomography (FDG PET) in the detection of malignant peripheral nerve sheath tumours arising from within plexiform neurofibromas in neurofibromatosis 1. J Neurol Neurosurg Psychiatry 68:353, 2000.
34. Foley KM, Woodruff JM, Ellis F, Posner JB. Radiation-induced malignant and atypical MPNST. Ann Neurol 7:311, 1980.
35. Foraker AG. Glandlike elements in a peripheral neurosarcoma. Cancer 1:286, 1948.
36. Garre C. Uber sekundare Maligne Neurome. Beitr Z Chir Z 9:465, 1892.
37. Geschickter CF. Tumors of the peripheral nerves. Am J Cancer 25:377, 1935.
38. Ghosh BC, Ghosh L, Huvos AG, et al. Malignant schwannoma: a clinicopathologic study. Cancer 31:184, 1973.
39. Giannestras NJ, Bronson JL. Malignant schwannoma of the medial plantar branch of the posterior tibial nerve (unassociated with von Recklinghausen's disease). J Bone Joint Surg Am 57:701, 1975.
40. Goldman RL, Jones SE, Heusinkveld RS. Combination chemotherapy of metastatic malignant schwannoma with vincristine, Adriamycin, cyclophosphamide, and imidazole carboxamide: a case report. Cancer 39:1955, 1977.
41. Goodlad JR, Fletcher CDM. Malignant peripheral nerve sheath tumour with annulate lamellae mimicking pleomorphic malignant fibrous histiocytoma. J Pathol 164:23, 1991.
42. Gore I. Primary malignant tumors of nerves: a report of eight cases. Cancer 2:278, 1951.
43. Gratia. Une curieuse anomalie anatomique constituee par la presence de tissu musculaire strie dans la substance du nerf pneumogastrique. Ann Med Vet 33:649, 1884.
44. Gray MH, Rosenberg AE, Dickersin GR, et al. Glial fibrillary acidic protein and keratin expression by benign and malignant nerve sheath tumors. Hum Pathol 20:1089, 1989.
45. Guccion JG, Enzinger FM. Malignant schwannoma associated with von Recklinghausen's neurofibromatosis. Virchows Arch [Pathol Anat] 383:43, 1979.
46. Halling KC, Scheithauer BW, Halling AC, et al. p53 expression in neurofibroma and malignant peripheral nerve sheath tumor: an immunohistochemical study of sporadic and NF-1 associated tumors. Am J Clin Pathol 106:282, 1996.
47. Harkin JC, Reed RJ. Tumors of the peripheral nervous system. In: Atlas of Tumor Pathology, 2nd series, fascicle 3. Armed Forces Institute of Pathology, Washington, DC, 1969.
48. Hedeman LA, Lewinsky BS, Lochridge GK, et al. Primary malignant schawannoma of the gasserian ganglion: report of two cases. J Neurosurg 48:279, 1978.
49. Heffner DK, Gnepp DR. Sinonasal fibrosarcomas, malignant schwannomas, and "Triton" tumors: a clinicopathologic study of 67 cases. Cancer 70:1089, 1992.
50. Herrera GA, deMoraes HP. Neurogenic sarcomas in patients with neurofibromatosis (von Recklinghausen's disease): light, electron microscopy and immunohistochemistry study. Virchows Arch [Pathol Anat] 403:361, 1984.
51. Hirose T, Maeda T, Furuya K. Malignant peripheral nerve sheath tumor of the pancreas with perineural cell differentiation. Ultrastruct Pathol 22:227, 1998.
52. Hirose T, Scheithauer BW, Sano T. Perineural malignant peripheral nerve sheath tumor (MPNST): a clinicopathologic, immunohistochemical, and ultrastructural study of seven cases. Am J Surg Pathol 22:1368, 1998.
53. Hruban RH, Shiu MH, Senie RT, et al. Malignant peripheral nerve sheath tumors of the buttock and lower extremity. Cancer 66:1253, 1990.
54. Janwar SC, Chen Q, Li FP, et al. Cytogenetic analysis of soft tissue sarcomas: recurrent chromosome abnormalities in malignant peripheral nerve sheath tumors (MPNST). Cancer Genet Cytogenet 78:138, 1994.
55. Johnson K, Glick AD, Davis BW. Immunohistochemical evaluation of Leu-7, myelin basic protein, S-100 protein, glial fibrillary acidic protein, and LN3 immunoreactivity in nerve sheath tumors and sarcomas. Arch Pathol Lab Med 112:155, 1988.
56. Karcioglu Z, Somren A, Mathes SJ. Ectomesenchymoma: a malignant tumor of migratory neural crest (ectomesenchyme) remnants showing ganglionic, schwannian, melanocytic, and rhabdomyoblastic differentiation. Cancer 39:2486, 1977.
57. Katz LD, Creech JL, Makk L. Giant retroperitoneal sarcoma of nerve sheath origin. South Med J 67:349, 1974.
58. Kim HA, Ling B, Ratner N. NF1 deficient mouse Schwann cells are angiogenic and invasive and can be induced to hyperproliferate: reversion of some phenotypes by an inhibitor of farnesyl protein transferase. Mol Cell Biol 17:862, 1997.
59. Kim HA, Rosenbaum T, Marchionni MA, et al. Schwann cells from neurofibromin-deficient mice exhibit activation of p21-ras, inhibition of cell proliferation, and morphological changes. Oncogene 11:325, 1995.
60. Kindblom LG, Ahlden M, Meis-Kindblom JM, Stenman G. Immunohistochemical and molecular analysis of p53, MDM2, proliferating cell nuclear antigen and Ki67 in benign and malignant peripheral nerve sheath tumors. Virchows Arch 427:19, 1995.
61. King R, Busam K, Rosai J. Metastatic malignant melanoma resembling malignant peripheral nerve sheath tumor: report of 16 cases. Am J Surg Pathol 23:1499, 1999.
62. Koestner A, Swenberg JA, Wechslar W. Transplacental production of ethylnitrosourea of neoplasms of the nervous system in Sprague-Dawley rats. Am J Pathol 63:37, 1971.
63. Kourea HP, Bilsky MH, Leung DH, et al. Subdiaphragmatic and intrathoracic paraspinal malignant peripheral nerve sheath tumors: a clinicopathologic study of 25 patients and 26 tumors. Am J Cancer 82:2191, 1998.
64. Kourea HP, Cordon-Cardo C, Dudas M, et al. Expression of $p27^{kip}$ and other cell cycle regulators in malignant peripheral nerve sheath tumors and neurofibromas. Am J Pathol 155: 1885, 1999.
65. Kourea HP, Orlow I, Scheithauer BW, et al. Deletions of the INK4A gene occur in malignant peripheral nerve sheath tumors but not in neurofibromas. Am J Pathol 155:1855, 1999.
66. Krumerman MS, Stingle W. Synchronous malignant glandular schwannomas in congenital neurofibromatosis. Cancer 41:2444, 1978.
67. Laskin WB, Weiss SW, Bratthauer GL. Epithelioid variant of malignant peripheral nerve sheath tumor (malignant epithelioid schwannoma). Am J Surg Pathol 15:1136, 1991.
68. Laurian N, Zohar Y. Malignant neurilemoma of parotid gland. J Laryngol Otol 84:1267, 1970.
69. Legius E, Marchuk DA, Collins FS, et al. Somatic deletion of the neurofibromatosis type I gene in a neurofibrosarcoma supports a tumor suppressor gene hypothesis. Nat Genet 3:122, 1993.
70. Lodding P, Kindblom LG, Angervall L. Epithelioid malignant schwannoma: a study of 14 cases. Virchows Arch [Pathol Anat] 409:433, 1986.
71. Maeda T, Furuya K, Kiyasu Y, Kawasaki H. Malignant periph-

eral nerve sheath tumor of the pancreas with perineurial cell differentiation. Ultrastruct Pathol 22:227, 1998.
72. Mannarino E, Watts JW. Malignant tumors arising from peripheral nerves. J Int Coll Surg 37:550, 1962.
73. Maseritz IH. Neurogenic sarcoma. J Bone Joint Surg Am 24:586, 1942.
74. Masson P, Martin JF. Rhabdomyomes des nerfs. Bull Assoc Fr Etud Cancer 27:751, 1938.
75. Matsunou H, Shimoda T, Kakimoto S, et al. Histopathologic and immunohistochemical study of malignant tumors of peripheral nerve sheath (malignant schwannoma). Cancer 56:2269, 1985.
76. McCarron KF, Goldblum JR. Plexiform neurofibroma with and without associated malignant peripheral nerve sheath tumor: a clinicopathologic and immunohistochemical analysis of 54 cases. Mod Pathol 11:612, 1998.
77. McCormick LJ, Hazard JB, Dickson JA. Malignant epithelioid neurilemoma (schwannoma). Cancer 7:725, 1954.
78. McKay B, Osborne BM. The contribution of electron microscopy to the diagnosis of tumors. Pathol Annu 8:359, 1978.
79. McKeen EA, Bodurtha J, Meadows AT, et al. Rhabdomyosarcoma complicating multiple neurofibromatosis. J Pediatr 93:992, 1978.
80. Mechtersheimer G, Otano-Joos M, Ohl S, et al. Analysis of chromosomal imbalances in sporadic and NF-1 associated peripheral nerve sheath tumors by comparatie genomic hybridization. Genes Chromosomes Cancer 25:362, 1999.
81. Meis JM, Enzinger FM, Martz KL, et al. Malignant peripheral nerve sheath tumors (malignant schwannoma) in children. Am J Surg Pathol 16:694, 1992.
82. Meis JM, Kindblom LG, Enzinger FM. Angiosarcoma arising in peripheral nerve sheath tumors: report of 5 additional cases. Lab Invest 70:80A, 1994.
83. Mennemeyer RP, Hallman KO, Hammar SP, et al. Melanotic schwannoma: clinical and ultrastructural studies of three cases with evidence of intracellular melanin synthesis. Am J Surg Pathol 3:3, 1979.
84. Menon AG, Anderson KM, Riccardi VM, et al. Chromosome 17p deletions and p53 gene mutations associated with the formation of malignant neurofibrosarcomas in von Recklinghausen's neurofibromatosis. Proc Natl Acad Sci USA 87:5435, 1990.
85. Mentzel T, Katenkamp D. Intraneural angiosarcoma and angiosarcoma arising in benign and malignant peripheral nerve sheath tumours: clinicopathological and immunohistochemical analysis of four cases. Histopathology 35:114, 1999.
86. Mertens F, Rydholm A, Bauer HF, et al. Cytogenetic findings in malignant peripheral nerve sheath tumors. Int J Cancer 61:793, 1995.
87. Michel SL. Epithelial elements in a malignant neurogenic tumor of the tibial nerve. Am J Surg 113:404, 1967.
88. Miracco C, Montesco MC, Santopietro R, et al. Proliferative activity, angiogenesis and necrosis in peripheral nerve sheath tumors: a quantitatiaave evaluation for prognosis. Mod Pathol 9:1108, 1996.
89. Morphopoulos GD, Banerjee SS, Ali HH, et al. Malignant peripheral nerve sheath tumor with vascular differentiation: a report of four cases. Histopathology 28:401, 1996.
90. Nakajima T, Watanaba S, Soto Y, et al. An immunoperoxidase study of S-100 protein distribution in normal and neoplastic tissues. Am J Surg Pathol 6:715, 1982.
91. Ordóñez NG, Tornos C. Malignant peripheral nerve sheath tumor of the pleura with epithelial and rhabdomyoblastic differentiation: report of a case clinically simulating mesothelioma. Am J Surg Pathol 21:1515, 1997.
92. Orenstein JM. Amianthoid fibers in synovial sarcoma and a malignant schwannoma. Ultrastruct Pathol 4:163, 1983.
93. Orlandi E. Rhabdomyoma del nervo ischiatico. Arch Sci Med (Torino) 19:113, 1895.
94. Payne RA. Metaplasia in a nerve sheath sarcoma in von Recklinghausen's disease. Br J Surg 47:688, 1960.
95. Raney B, Schnaufer L, Ziegler M. Treatment of children with neurogenic sarcoma: experience at the Children's Hospital of Philadelphia 1958–1984. Cancer 59:1, 1987.
96. Rao SB, Dinakar I. Neurofibroma of sciatic nerve. Indian J Cancer 7:226, 1970.
97. Rao UN, Sonmez-Alpan E, Michalopoulos GK. Hepatocyte growth factor and c-MET in benign and malignant peripheral nerve sheath tumors. Hum Pathol 28:1066, 1997.
98. Reynolds JE, Fletcher JA, Lytle CH, et al. Molecular characterization of a 17q11.2 translocation in a malignant schwannoma cell line. Hum Genet 90:450, 1992.
99. Rigdon RH. Neurogenic tumors produced by methylcholanthrene in the white Pekin duck. Cancer 8:906, 1955.
100. Rubinstein LJ, Conley FK, Herman MM. Studies on experimental malignant nerve sheath tumors maintained in tissue and organ culture systems. I. Light microscopy observations. Acta Neuropathol (Berl) 34:277, 1976.
101. Sawada S, Florell S, Purandare SM, et al. Identification of NF1 mutations in both alleles of a dermal neurofibroma. Nat Genet 14:110, 1996.
102. Schaldenbrand JD, Appelman HD. Solitary stromal gastrointestinal tumors in von Recklinghausen's disease with minimal smooth muscle differentiation. Hum Pathol 15:229, 1994.
103. Schmidt H, Wuerl P, Taubert H, et al. Genomic imbalances of 7p and 17q in malignant peripheral nerve sheath tumors are clinically relevant. Genes Chromosomes Cancer 25:205, 1999.
104. Smith TA, Machen SK, Fisher C, Goldblum JR. Usefulness of cytokeratin subsets for distinguishing monophasic synovial sarcoma from malignant peripheral nerve sheath tumor. Am J Clin Pathol 112:641, 1999.
105. Sordillo PP, Helson L, Hajdu SI, et al. Malignant schwannoma: clinical characteristics, surgery, and response to therapy. Cancer 47:2503, 1981.
106. Sorensen SA, Mulvihill JJ, Nielsen A. Long-term follow-up of von Recklinghausen neurofibromatosis. N Engl J Med 305:1617, 1981.
107. Spence AM, Rubenstein LJ, Conley FK, et al. Studies on experimental malignant nerve sheath tumors maintained in tissue and organ culture systems. III. Melanin pigment and melanogenesis in experimental neurogenic tumors, a reappraisal of the histogenesis of pigmented nerve sheath tumors. Acta Neuropathol (Berl) 35:27, 1976.
108. Stewart TW, Copeland MM. Neurogenic sarcoma. Am J Cancer 15:1235, 1931.
109. Storm FK, Eilber FR, Mirra J, et al. Neurofibrosarcoma. Cancer 45:126, 1980.
110. Stout AP. The malignant tumors of the peripheral nerves. Am J Cancer 25:1, 1935.
111. Strauss BL, Gutman DDH, Dehner LP, et al. Molecular analysis of malignant triton tumors. Hum Pathol 30:984, 1999.
112. Taxy JB, Battifora HB. Epithelioid schwannoma: diagnosis by electron microscopy. Ultrastruct Pathol 2:19, 1981.
113. Trassard M, LeDoussal V, Bui BN, Coindere JM. Angiosarcoma arising in a solitary schwannoma (neurilemoma) of the sciatic nerve. Am J Surg Pathol 20:1412, 1996.
114. Travis JA, Sandberg AA, Neff JR, Bridge JA. Cytogenetic findings in malignant Triton tumor. Genes Chromosomes Cancer 9:1, 1994.
115. Trojanowski JQ, Kleinman GM, Proppe KH. Malignant tumors of nerve sheath origin. Cancer 46:1202, 1980.
116. Tsuneyoshi M, Enjoji M. Primary malignant peripheral nerve tumors (malignant schwannomas): a clinicopathologic and electron microscopic study. Acta Pathol Jpn 29:363, 1979.

117. Uri AK, Witzleben CL, Raney RB. Electron microscopy of glandular schwannoma. Cancer 53:493, 1984.
118. Vauthey JN, Woodruff JM, Brennan MF. Extremity malignant peripheral nerve sheath tumors (neurogenic sarcomas): a 10 year experience. Ann Surg Oncol 2:126, 1995.
119. Vieta JO, Pack GT. Malignant neurilemomas of peripheral nerves. Am J Surg 82:416, 1951.
120. Wanebo JE, Malik JM, Vandenberg SR, et al. Malignant peripheral nerve sheath tumors: a clinicopathologic study of 28 cases. Cancer 71:1247, 1993.
121. Wang AR, Weiss SW, Reed JA, Scott G. PGP9.5 and N-CAM are sensitive markers for malignant peripheral nerve sheath tumors (PMNSTs). Mod Pathol 13:16A, 2000.
122. Warner TFCS, Louie R, Hafez GR, et al. Malignant nerve sheath tumor containing endocrine cells. Am J Surg Pathol 7:583, 1983.
123. Weiss SW, Langloss JM, Enzinger FM. The role of S-100 protein in the diagnosis of soft tissue tumors with particular reference to benign and malignant Schwann cell tumors. Lab Invest 49:299, 1983.
124. Weston JA. The migration and differentiation of neural crest cells. Adv Morphogen 8:41, 1970.
125. White HR. Survival in malignant schwannoma: an 18-year study. Cancer 27:720, 1971.
126. Wick MR, Swanson PE, Scheithauer BW, et al. Malignant peripheral nerve sheath tumor: an immunohistochemical study of 62 cases. Am J Clin Pathol 87:425, 1987.
127. Wong SY, Teh M, Tan YO, et al. Malignant glandular Triton tumor. Cancer 67:1076, 1991.
128. Wong WW, Hirose T, Scheithauer BW, et al. Malignant peripheral nerve sheath tumor: analysis of treatment outcome. Int J Radiat Oncol Biol Phys 42:351, 1998.
129. Woodruff JM. Peripheral nerve tumors showing glandular differentiation (glandular schwannoma). Cancer 37:2399, 1976.
130. Woodruff JM, Chernik NL, Smith MC, et al. Peripheral nerve tumors with rhabdomyosarcomatous differentiation (malignant "Triton" tumors). Cancer 32:426, 1973.
131. Woodruff JM, Christensen WN. Glandular peripheral nerve sheath tumors. Cancer 72:3618, 1993.
132. Woodruff JM, Perino G. Non-germ cell or teratomatous malignant tumors showing rhabdomyoblastic differentiation with emphasis on the malignant Triton tumor. Semin Diagn Surg Pathol 11:69, 1994.
133. Wuerker RB, Kirkpatrick JB. Neuronal microtubules, neurofilaments, and microfilaments. Int Rev Cytol 33:45, 1972.
134. Zimmerman LE, Font RL, Andersen SR. Rhabdomyosarcomatous differentiation in malignant intraocular medulloepitheliomas. Cancer 30:817, 1972.

### Clear Cell Sarcoma (Malignant Melanoma of Soft Parts)

135. Angervall L, Stener B. Clear cell sarcoma of tendons: a study of four cases. Acta Pathol Microbiol Scand 77:589, 1969.
136. Aue G, Hedges LK, Schwartz HS, et al. Clear cell sarcoma or malignant melanoma of soft parts: molecular analysis of microsatellite instability with clinical correlations. Cancer Genet Cytogenet 105:24, 1998.
137. Bearman RM, Noe J, Kempson R. Clear cell sarcoma with melanin pigment. Cancer 36:977, 1975.
138. Benson JD, Kraemer BB, Mackay B. Malignant melanoma of soft parts: an ultrastructural study of four cases. Ultrastruct Pathol 8:57, 1985.
139. Boudreaux D, Waisman J. Clear cell sarcoma with melanogenesis. Cancer 41:1387, 1978.
140. Bridge JA, Borek DA, Neff JR, et al. Choromosomal abnormalities in clear cell sarcoma: implication for histogenesis. Am J Clin Pathol 93:26, 1990.
141. Bridge JA, Sreekantaiah C, Neff JR, et al. Cytogenetic findings in clear cell sarcoma of tendons and aponeuroses: malignant melanoma of soft parts. Cancer Genet Cytogenet 52:101, 1991.
142. Carpenter WM, Tsaknis PJ, Konzelman JL, et al. Clear cell sarcoma of tendons and aponeuroses. Oral Surg Oral Med Oral Pathol 45:580, 1978.
143. Chung EB, Enzinger FM. Malignant melanoma of soft parts: a reassessment of clear cell sarcoma. Am J Surg Pathol 7:405, 1983.
144. Deenik W, Mooi WJ, Rutgers EJ, et al. Clear cell sarcoma (malignant melanoma) of soft parts: a clinicopathologic study of 30 cases. Cancer 86:969, 1999.
145. Dutra FR. Clear cell sarcoma of tendons and aponeuroses: three additional cases. Cancer 25:942, 1970.
146. Eckhardt JJ, Pritchard DL, Soule EH. Clear cell sarcoma: a clinicopathologic study of 27 cases. Cancer 52:1482, 1983.
147. Ekfors TO, Rantakokko V. Clear cell sarcoma of tendons and aponeuroses: malignant melanoma of soft tissue: report of four cases. Pathol Res Pract 165:422, 1979.
148. Enzinger FM. Clear cell sarcoma of tendons and aponeuroses: an analysis of 21 cases. Cancer 18:1163, 1968.
149. Epstein AL, Martin AO, Kempson R. Use of a newly established human cell line (SU-CCS-1) to demonstrate the relationship of clear cell sarcoma to malignant melanoma. Cancer Res 44:1265, 1984.
150. Hernandez EJ. Malignant blue nevus: a light and electron microscopic study. Arch Dermatol 107:741, 1973.
151. Hirata K. Clear cell sarcoma arising from the right plantar aponeurosis. Orthop Surg (Tokyo) 20:1326, 1969.
152. Hoffman GJ, Carter D. Clear cell sarcoma of tendons and aponeuroses with melanin. Arch Pathol 95:22, 1973.
153. Kindblom LG, Lodding P, Angervall L. Clear cell sarcoma of tendons and aponeuroses: an immunohistochemical and electron microscopic analysis indicating neural crest origin. Virchows Arch [Pathol Anat] 401:109, 1983.
154. Kubo T. Clear cell sarcoma of patellar tendon studied by electron microscopy. Cancer 24:948, 1969.
155. Lucas DR, Nascimento AG, Sim FH. Clear cell sarcoma of soft tissues: Mayo Clinic experience with 35 cases. Am J Surg Pathol 16:1197, 1992.
156. Mackenzie DH. Clear cell sarcoma of tendon and aponeuroses with melanin production. J Pathol 114:231, 1974.
157. Mackenzie DH. Two types of soft tissue sarcoma of uncertain histogenesis. Br J Cancer 25:458, 1971.
158. Mechtersheimer G, Tilgen W, Klar E, et al. Clear cell sarcoma of tendons and aponeuroses: case presentation with special reference to immunohistochemical findings. Hum Pathol 20:914, 1989.
159. Merkow LP, Burt RC, Hayeslip DW, et al. A cellular and malignant blue nevus: a light and electron microscopic study. Cancer 24:888, 1969.
160. Montgomery EA, Meis JM, Ramos AG, et al. Clear cell sarcoma of tendons and aponeurosis: a clinicopathologic study of 58 cases with analysis of prognostic factors. Int J Surg Pathol 1:59, 1993.
161. Mrozek K, Karakousis CP, Perez-Mesa C, et al. Translocation t(12;22)(q13;q12.2-12.3) in a clear cell sarcoma of tendons and aponeuroses. Genes Chromosomes Cancer 6:249, 1993.
162. Parker JB, Marcus PB, Martin JH. Spinal melanotic clear cell sarcoma: a light and electron microscopic study. Cancer 46: 718, 1980.
163. Raynor AC, Vargas-Crotes F, Alexander RW, et al. Clear cell sarcoma with melanin pigment: a possible soft tissue variant of malignant melanoma: case report. J Bone Joint Surg Am 61:276, 1979.
164. Reeves BR, Fletcher CD, Gusterson BA. Translocation t(12;22)(q12;q13) is a nonrandom rearrangement in clear cell sarcoma. Cancer Genet Cytogenet 64:101, 1992.

165. Rodriguez HA, Ackerman LV. Cellular blue nevus: clinicopathological study of 45 cases. Cancer 21:393, 1968.
166. Rodriquez E, Sreekantaiah C, Reuter VE, et al. t(12;22)(q13;q13) and trisomy 8 are nonrandom aberrations in clear cell sarcoma. Cancer Genet Cytogenet 64:107, 1992.
167. Sara AS, Evans HL, Benjamin RS. Malignant melanoma of soft parts (clear cell sarcoma): a study of 17 cases with emphasis on prognostic factors. Cancer 15:367, 1990.
168. Stenman G, Kindblom LG, Angervall L. Reciprocal translocation t(12;22)(q13;q13) in clear cell sarcoma of tendons and aponeuroses. Genes Chromosomes Cancer 4:122, 1992.
169. Swanson PE, Wick MR. Clear cell sarcoma: an immunohistochemical analysis of six cases and comparison with other epithelioid neoplasms of soft tissue. Arch Pathol Lab Med 113:55, 1989.
170. Toe TK, Saw D. Clear cell sarcoma with melanin: report of two cases. Cancer 41:235, 1978.
171. Travis JA, Bridge JA. Significance of both numerical and structural chromosomal abnormalities in clear cell sarcoma. Cancer Genet Cytogenet 64:104, 1992.
172. Tsuneyoshi M, Enjoji M, Kubo T. Clear cell sarcoma of tendons and aponeuroses: a comparative study of 13 cases with provisional subgrouping into the melanotic and synovial types. Cancer 42:243, 1978.
173. Zucman J, Delattre O, Desmaze C, et al. EWS and aTF-gene fusion induced by t(12;22) translocation in malignant melanoma of soft parts. Nat Genet 4:341, 1993.

### Neurotropic (Desmoplastic) Melanoma

174. Ackerman AB, Godomski J. Neurotropic malignant melanoma and other neurotropic neoplasms in the skin. Am J Dermatopathol 6(Suppl):63, 1984.
175. Barr RJ, Morales RV, Graham JH. Desmoplastic nevus: a distinct histologic variant of mixed spindle cell and epithelioid cell nevus. Cancer 46:557, 1980.
176. Bruijm JA, Mihm MC, Barnhill RL. Desmoplastic melanoma. Histopathology 20:197, 1992.
177. Conley J, Lattes R, Orr W. Desmoplastic malignant melanoma: a rare variant of spindle cell melanoma. Cancer 28:914, 1971.
178. Dabbs DJ, Bolen JW. Superficial spreading malignant melanoma with neurosarcomatous metastasis. Am J Clin Pathol 82:109, 1984.
179. DiMaio SM, Mackay B, Smith JL, et al. Neurosarcomatous transformation in malignant melanoma: an ultrastructural study. Cancer 50:2345, 1982.
180. Egbert B, Kempson R, Sagebiel R. Desmoplastic malignant melanoma: a clinicopathologic study of 25 cases. Cancer 62: 2033, 1988.
181. Jain S, Allen PW. Desmoplastic malignant melanoma and its variants. Am J Surg Pathol 13:358, 1989.
182. Koch MB, Arbiser AK, Weiss SW, et al. Melanoma cell adhesion molecule (Mel-CAM) and microphthalmia transcription factor (MiTF) expression distinguish desmoplastic/sarcomatoid melanoma (DM) from morphological mimics [abstract 357]. Mod Pathol 13:63, 2000
183. Labrecque P, Hu C, Winkelman RK. On the nature of desmoplastic melanoma. Cancer 38:1025, 1976.
184. Longacre TA, Egbert BM, Rouse RV. Desmoplastic and spindle cell malignant melanoma: an immunohistochemical study. Am J Surg Pathol 20:1489, 1996.
185. Reed PJ, Leonard DD. Neurotropic melanoma: a variant of desmoplastic melanoma. Am J Surg Pathol 3:301, 1979.
186. Reiman HM, Goellner JR, Woods JE, et al. Desmoplastic melanoma of the head and neck. Cancer 60:2269, 1987.
187. Smithers BM, McLeod GR, Little JH. Desmoplastic neural transforming and neurotropic melanoma: a review of 45 cases. Aust N Z J Surg 60:967, 1990.
188. Valensi Q. Desmoplastic malignant melanoma: a light and electron microscopic study of two cases. Cancer 43:1148, 1979.
189. Warner TFCS, Hafez GR, Buchler DA. Neurotropic melanoma of the vulva. Cancer 49:999, 1982.
190. Warner TFCS, Hafez GR, Finch RE, et al. Schwann cell features in neurotropic melanoma. J Cutan Pathol 8:177, 1981.
191. Warner TFCS, Lloyd RV, Hafez GR, et al. Immunocytochemistry of neurotropic melanoma. Cancer 53:254, 1984.

### Extraspinal (Soft Tissue) Ependymoma

192. Adson AW, Moersch FP, Kernohan JW. Neurogenic tumors arising from the sacrum. Arch Neurol Psychiatry 41:535, 1939.
193. Anderson MS. Myxopapillary ependymomas presenting in the soft tissues over the sacrococcygeal region. Cancer 19:585, 1966.
194. Brindley GV. Sacral and presacral tumors. Ann Surg 121:721, 1945.
195. Heath MH. Presacral ependymoma: case report and review of the literature. Am J Clin Pathol 39:161, 1963.
196. Hendren TH, Hardin CA. Extradural metastatic ependymoma. Surgery 54:880, 1963.
197. Jackman RJ, Clark PL, Smith ND. Retrorectal tumors. JAMA 145:956, 1951.
198. Kernohan JW, Fletcher-Kernohan HA. Ependymomas: a study of 109 cases. Assoc Res Nerv Dis 16:182, 1937.
199. Lovelady SB, Dockerty MB. Extragenital pelvic tumors in women. Am J Obstet Gynecol 58:215, 1949.
200. Mallory FB. Three gliomata of ependymal origin: two in the fourth ventricle, one subcutaneous over the coccyx. J Med Res 8:1, 1902.
201. Ross ST. Sacral and presacral tumors. Am J Surg 76:687, 1948.
202. Vagaiwala MR, Robinson JS, Galicich JH, et al. Metastasizing extradural ependymoma of the sacrococcygeal area: case report and review of the literature. Cancer 44:326, 1979.
203. Wolff M, Santiago H, Duby MM. Delayed distant metastasis from a subcutaneous sacrococcygeal ependymoma: case report with tissue culture, ultrastructural observations, and review of the literature. Cancer 30:1046, 1972.

# CHAPTER 32

# PRIMITIVE NEUROECTODERMAL TUMORS AND RELATED LESIONS

Neuroblastoma and the related tumors ganglioneuroblastoma and ganglioneuroma are derived from primordial neural crest cells that migrate from the mantle layer of the developing spinal cord and populate the primordia of the sympathetic ganglia and adrenal medulla. Cytogenetic and molecular genetic data have contributed to our understanding of this group of tumors and have been incorporated along with multiple other parameters into management decisions and prognostication for these patients. Although there are histologic similarities, extraskeletal Ewing's sarcoma and peripheral neuroepithelioma are clearly distinct from neuroblastoma. A number of lines of evidence suggest that extraskeletal Ewing's sarcoma and peripheral neuroepithelioma are closely related tumors, the former representing a less differentiated form of the latter. For the purposes of this chapter, these tumors are referred to as the Ewing's sarcoma/primitive neuroectodermal tumor (ES/PNET) family of tumors.

## NEUROBLASTOMA AND GANGLIONEUROBLASTOMA

Neuroblastoma, ganglioneuroblastoma, and ganglioneuroma can be conceptualized as three maturational manifestations of a common neoplasm. Neuroblastoma, the least differentiated, resembles the fetal adrenal medulla and is made up of primitive neuroblasts. Ganglioneuroblastoma (differentiating neuroblastoma) has primitive neuroblasts along with maturing ganglion cells; the number and arrangement of the cells vary so the tumor assumes a wide range of appearances and is associated with a wide range of biologic behavior. Ganglioneuroma, a fully differentiated tumor, is characterized by a mixture of mature Schwann cells and ganglion cells. Neuroblastoma and ganglioneuroblastoma are discussed together because both are considered malignant. In contrast, pure ganglioneuromas are benign tumors requiring only conservative therapy and so are considered separately.

### Etiologic and Genetic Factors

Most neuroblastomas occur on a sporadic basis, but in a small number of patients there appears to be a genetic predisposition that follows an autosomal dominant pattern of inheritance.[80,82] There are rare reports of patients with neuroblastoma with a constitutional deletion or rearrangement of the distal short arm of chromosome 1 as the sole abnormality, suggesting the presence of a tumor-suppressor gene at this locus.[15,83,118] The tumor tends to be less common in African Americans than Whites; and in certain parts of the world, notably the Burkitt's lymphoma belt in Africa, it is practically nonexistent.[87] In situ neuroblastomas, small microscopic foci of neuroblastoma confined to the adrenal and discovered incidentally at autopsy, are rather common (1 in 200 infants dying of other causes), in dramatic contrast with the low incidence of clinical neuroblastoma.

A number of cytogenetic abnormalities have been identified in neuroblastomas, although the exact manner in which they are etiologically linked to the tumor is not fully understood.[11] The most common abnormality is a deletion or rearrangement of the short arm of chromosome 1,[13,55] a finding present in up to 70% of neuroblastomas.[21] The common region of loss is between 1p36.2 and 1p36.3,[22,149] suggesting loss or inactivation of a gene or genes critical to the development and progression of this tumor. A number of candidate tumor-suppressor genes have been mapped to this locus, including the zinc finger gene *HKR3*.[89] Several groups have also identified a potential second tumor-suppressor locus proximal to 1p36, and deletions in this locus are associated with N-*myc* (also referred to as *MYCN*) amplification (described below).[23,124,136] Some authors have found random involvement of the maternal and paternal alleles of 1p in tumors with loss of heterozygosity of this locus,[32] whereas others have found preferential loss of the maternal allele, suggesting the process of genomic imprinting.[24]

Other cytogenetic abnormalities have been found with lower frequency in neuroblastomas, including abnormalities of 14q,[52,135] 11q,[132] and 9p.[137] Gain of 17q has also been found in some cases and has been associated with more aggressive clinical behavior.[19,21,112]

Extrachromosomal double-minute chromatin bodies and homogeneously staining regions, representing sites of N-*myc* amplified sequences, are additional common findings. N-*myc* amplification occurs in approximately 20–25% of neuroblastomas and is strongly predictive of poor outcome, independent of stage or age.[18,125,126] Because the N-*myc* copy number in a given tumor is relatively constant with respect to time,[14] N-*myc* amplification appears to be an intrinsic property of a given tumor and probably occurs as an early event following alterations of 1p.[15]

More recently, attention has been focused on abnormalities in the nerve growth factor/nerve growth factor receptor pathway. Neurotrophic ligands such as nerve growth factor, brain-derived neurotrophic factor, and neurotrophin 3 bind to tyrosine kinase receptors known as TRK-A, TRK-B, and TRK-C, respectively, and induce differentiation in sympathetic neurons.[62,74] As discussed below, high TRK-A expression has been correlated with favorable clinical stage and outcome and is inversely related to N-*myc* amplification.[101] Brodeur et al.[11] postulated that failure to maintain an intact nerve growth factor/receptor pathway results in neuroblasts that remain in a relatively undifferentiated state, making them vulnerable to subsequent mutational events such as 1p loss and N-*myc* amplification. This pathway also appears to be important in the regression or differentiation of these tumors in some patients.[15]

There are fewer data regarding TRK-B and TRK-C, although expression of full-length TRK-B has been associated with N-*myc* amplification.[103] In contrast, high expression of TRK-C has been found in patients with lower-stage tumors[152] and is usually not expressed in N-*myc* amplified tumors.

## Clinical Findings

Neuroblastoma is the third most common malignant tumor and the most common extracranial solid tumor in children; it occurs at a rate of about 1 per 10,000 live births.[6] At most large children's centers it accounts for 10–12% of all malignant tumors, preceded in frequency by leukemias and brain tumors.[39] It develops at a relatively younger patient age than rhabdomyosarcomas and ES/PNETs. About one-fourth of neuroblastomas are congenital, some of which are detected prenatally owing to the widespread use of ultrasonography.[68,123] In general, the tumors diagnosed prenatally are found in the adrenal gland, are often cystic, are of a favorable clinical stage, have favorable biologic features (lack of N-*myc* amplification), and have an excellent prognosis.[1] Half are diagnosed by the age of 2 years and 90% by the age of 5 years; only sporadic cases are seen during adolescence or adult life.[35,122] The peak age at the time of presentation is about 18 months. In most large series there is a slight male predominance documented as 1.22:1.00 by Kinnear-Wilson and Draper[73] and 1.26:1.00 by DeLorimier et al.[39] The distribution of neuroblastomas and ganglioneuroblastomas generally follows the distribution of the sympathetic ganglia; hence they are found in a paramidline position at any point between the base of the skull and the pelvis, in addition to the adrenal medulla and organ of Zuckerkandl. Some cases possibly also arise from the dorsal root ganglia. This location would explain those dumbbell-shaped neuroblastomas in which significant enlargement of the intervertebral foramen occurs.[129] In the experience reported by DeLorimier et al.[39] based on the California Tumor Registry, 134 of 212 tumors occurred in the retroperitoneum, 33 in the mediastinum, 5 in the cervical region, and 6 in the sacral region. About half of all retroperitoneal tumors arise in the adrenal, although the difficulty determining the origin of large tumors must be acknowledged.

The constellation of symptoms varies depending on the age of the patient, location of the mass, and presence or absence of associated clinical syndromes. Usually patients with neuroblastomas appear wasted and chronically ill and manifest a variety of nonspecific signs and symptoms such as fever, weight loss, gastrointestinal tract disturbances including watery diarrhea,[121] and anemia. In half of the patients, a nodular fixed mass extending across the midline can be palpated on physical examination. So protean are the manifestations that half of neuroblastomas are misdiagnosed initially, and a significant number of patients are diagnosed as having rheumatic fever because of the frequent occurrence of fever and joint pain.[27] About one-third of neonates with neuroblastoma present with blue-red cutaneous metastases, which have been likened to blueberries (blueberry muffin baby).[45] Although hypertension is neither as common nor as severe as with pheochromocytomas, about one-fifth of the patients have this symptom, which remits with tumor removal.[148] A relatively rare presentation of neuroblastoma usually associated with a good prognosis is the "myoclonus-opsoclonus" syndrome. Characterized by rapid, alternating eye movements and myoclonic movements of the extremities, this symptom complex disappears following tumor eradication, suggesting that it is due to a circulating antitumor factor that cross-reacts with cerebellar cells.[113] Other neuroblastomas have been associated with myasthenia gravis,[119] Cushing syndrome,[38] von Recklinghausen's disease,[81] fetal hydantoin syndrome,[111] Hirschsprung's disease,[88] oncocytoid renal cell carcinoma,[96] and neurodevelopmental anomalies including focal cortical dysplasia.[8]

## Radiographic Findings

Retroperitoneal neuroblastomas cause anterior, lateral, and downward displacement of the kidney, usually without hydronephrosis or calyceal distortion. Calcification, a characteristic finding, occurs in about half of the tumors.[41] Typically the calcification consists of finely stippled densities in the central portion of the tumor, although peripheral linear densities may also be seen. Metastatic lesions commonly occur in bone and result in osteolytic lesions that display a peculiar predilection for the skull, femur, and humerus; occasionally they are bilaterally symmetric in their distribution. Radiolabeled metaiodobenzylguanidine (MIBG) is incorporated into catecholamine-secreting cells and has been used to detect bone and soft tissue involvement by neuroblastoma.[53,147]

According to the International Neuroblastoma Staging System (INSS),[16,17] extensive radiographic studies are required to define the extent of disease and identify metastatic foci. Computed tomography (CT), magnetic resonance imaging (MRI), and MIBG scans are used to evaluate the primary tumor, whereas bone radiography and scintigraphy, abdominal CT scans or MRI, chest radiography (with or without chest CT scans or MRI), in addition to bilateral posterior iliac crest bone marrow aspirates and biopsies, are required to determine the presence or absence of metastatic disease.

## Laboratory Findings

About 80–90% of patients with neuroblastoma have elevated levels of catecholamines (norepinephrine, epinephrine) and their metabolites [vanillylmandelic acid (VMA), homovanillic acid (HVA), and 3-methoxy-4-hydroxyphenylglycol (MHPG)] in their urine (Fig. 32–1).[27] This may reflect increased production or diminished storage of these substances by the tumor. Measurement of these substances has proved useful for the diagnosis and for monitoring the course of the disease during therapy. Persistent elevation following surgery suggests significant residual disease, and the metabolite levels are sometimes elevated before a recurrence is clinically evident. The VMA/HVA ratio has been reported to be of prognostic significance, as ratios of 1.5 or more are associated with an improved prognosis.[44] Neuropeptide Y, a biologically active polypeptide that co-localizes with catecholamines, is found in high levels in the serum of patients with neuroblastomas compared with the levels in those with ganglioneuroblastoma or ganglioneuroma. It is released during surgical manipulation of tumors, decreases following tumor removal, and reappears with recrudescence of disease, suggesting that it too may prove useful for monitoring the disease.[76,77]

Serum ferritin can be detected in the serum of patients with active disease and is also used as a prognostic indicator. This iron-binding protein, presumably synthesized by the tumor, is capable of coating the surface of T lymphocytes and is responsible for E rosette inhibition, a phenomenon observed in patients with advanced neuroblastoma.[60] The presence of elevated serum neuron-specific enolase[143] and lactate dehydrogenase[130] has also been correlated with survival rates of patients with neuroblastoma.

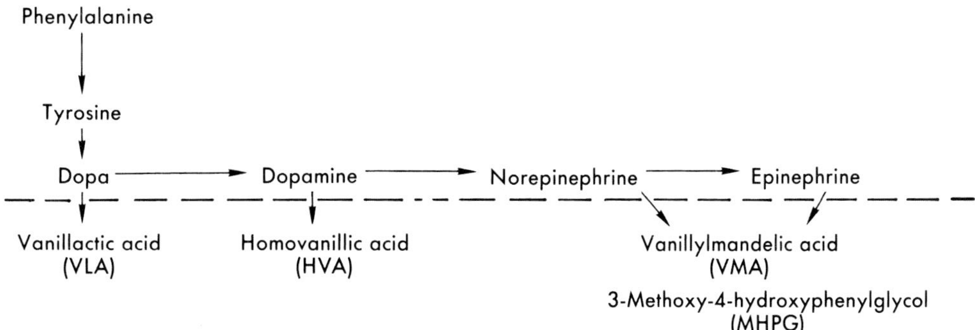


**FIGURE 32–1.** Metabolic pathway showing enzymatic conversion of phenylalanine to epinephrine. Catabolites below the dotted line are those that may be present in the urine of patients with neuroblastoma.

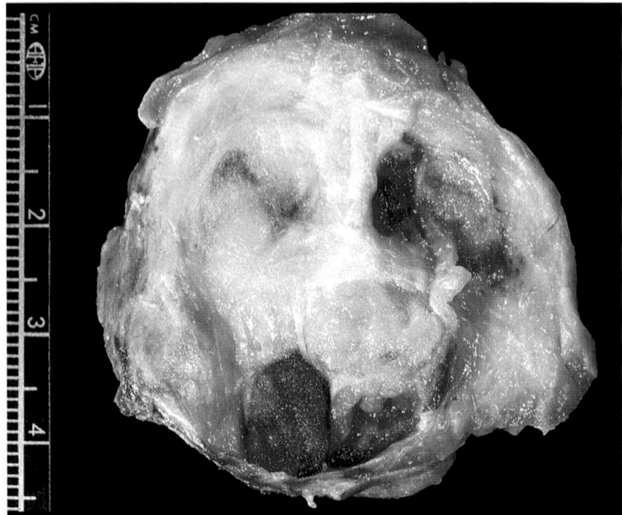

**FIGURE 32–2.** Ganglioneuroblastoma. Hemorrhagic areas corresponded to neuroblastoma, whereas the remainder of the tumor was ganglioneuroma.

## Gross Findings

Neuroblastomas are lobulated masses averaging 6–8 cm in diameter; they are intimately related to the adrenal gland or sympathetic chain. At surgery they often appear to have delicate membranous capsules that are easily ruptured to yield the soft, fleshy, gray, partially hemorrhagic tumor. Tumors composed of large expanses of differentiated ganglioneuroma associated with neuroblastomatous foci (nodular ganglioneuroblastoma) have gray hemorrhagic nodules set in a firm white-gray tumor mass (Fig. 32–2).[3]

## Microscopic Findings

The nomenclature of neuroblastomas has undergone significant revision. Old classification schemes utilizing terms such as "ganglioneuroblastoma" without further modification ignore the vast range of behavior that can be encountered with tumors that have both neuroblastic and ganglionic elements. The recently devised International Neuroblastoma Pathology Classification (INPC) has similarities to the systems proposed by Shimada et al.[128] and Joshi et al.[69–71] and is an age-linked classification dependent on the degree of neuroblastic differentiation, cellular turnover index, and the presence or absence of Schwannian stromal development. Equivalent terms in old classification systems are indicated in Table 32–1 and depicted in Fig. 32–3.

### *Neuroblastoma*

The term "neuroblastoma" refers to a tumor that is composed mostly of neuroblasts, which may display a variable degree of ganglionic differentiation (see below). These tumors are further subdivided into undifferentiated, poorly differentiated, and differentiating forms, depending on the percentage of cells showing

**TABLE 32–1** NOMENCLATURE OF NEUROBLASTOMA

| INPC System | Shimada System | Joshi System | Conventional System |
|---|---|---|---|
| Neuroblastoma (Schwannian stroma-poor) | | Neuroblastoma | |
| Undifferentiated type | Stroma-poor, undifferentiated histology | Undifferentiated type | Neuroblastoma |
| Poorly differentiated type | Stroma-poor, undifferentiated histology | Poorly differentiated type | Neuroblastoma |
| Differentiating type | Stoma-poor, differentiated histology | Differentiating type | Ganglioneuroblastoma |
| | | Ganglioneuroblastoma | |
| Ganglioneuroblastoma, nodular (Composite Schwannian stroma/rich stroma-dominant and stroma-poor) | Stroma-rich, nodular type | Nodular type | Composite ganglioneuroblastoma |
| Ganglioneuroblastoma, intermixed (Schwannian stroma-rich) | Stroma-rich, intermixed type | Intermixed type | Composite ganglioneuroblastoma |
| Ganglioneuroma (Schwannian stroma-dominant) | | | |
| Maturing | Stroma-rich, well-differentiated | Borderline type | Ganglioneuroblastoma |
| Mature | Ganglioneuroma | Ganglioneuroma | Ganglioneuroma |

INPC, International Neuroblastoma Pathology Committee.

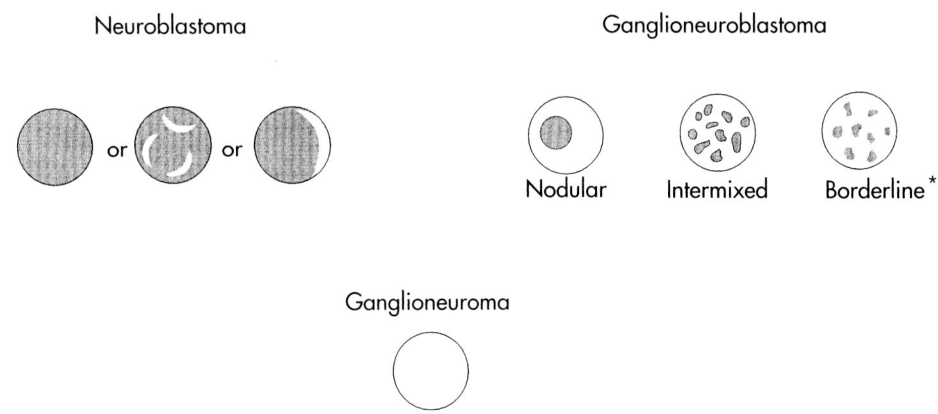


**FIGURE 32–3.** Terminology of neuroblastic tumors. Shaded areas represent the neuroblastomatous component. *Equivalent to maturing ganglioneuroma in INPC system. Unshaded areas are the ganglioneuromatous component. (Modified from Joshi VV, Cantor AB, Altshuler G, et al. Age-linked prognostic categorization based on a new histologic grading systems of neuroblastomas: a clinicopathologic study of 211 cases from the Pediatric Oncology Group. Cancer 69:2199, 1992.)

ganglionic differentiation. Undifferentiated forms display no ganglionic differentiation, whereas the other two forms display less than or more than 5% differentiating cells, respectively. Unlike ganglioneuroblastomas, Schwannian stromal development comprises less than 50% of the neoplasm.

The most primitive neuroblastomas resemble the anlage of the developing sympathetic nervous system and adrenal medulla (Fig. 32–4). They are composed of sheets of small round cells that are divided into small lobules by delicate fibrovascular stroma (Figs. 32–5, 32–6). The cells, which are almost devoid of cytoplasm, have round to polygonal deeply staining nuclei similar to those of lymphocytes (Fig. 32–7). Out of context, poorly differentiated neuroblastoma may be mistaken for round cell sarcomas (e.g., ES/PNETs), lymphoma, or nucleated erythrocytes of erythroblastosis fetalis (Fig. 32–8), especially if cellular preservation is poor and the cells are artifactually crushed. Diagnosis of poorly differentiated neuroblastoma is sometimes suggested by the presence of calcification or morula-like clusters of cells that represent the earliest form of rosette formation or by ancillary immunohistochemical or ultrastructural studies documenting neuroblastic features (discussed below). With progressive differentiation, the neuroblasts acquire attenuated cytoplasmic processes (neurites) (Fig. 32–9), which are polarized toward a central point to form a rosette with a solid central core (Homer Wright rosette) (Fig. 32–10). In addition, the stroma contains mats of neuropil, which are tangled networks of cell processes. In the most differentiated neuroblastomas, some of the cells show partial or even complete ganglionic differentiation (Fig. 32–11). Ganglionic differentiation is heralded by enlargement of the cells with acquisition of a discernible rim of eosinophilic cytoplasm. Binucleation occurs, and the nuclear chromatin pattern is distinctly vesicular.

### Ganglioneuroblastoma

Ganglioneuroblastomas are tumors in which a portion of the lesion has the appearance of a neuroblastoma as described above and contains, in addition, a partial ganglioneuromatous stroma (see Ganglioneuroma, below). The exact amount and arrangement of this stroma further determines the subclassification of the ganglioneuroblastoma. Nodular ganglioneuroblastomas contain gross nodules of neuroblastoma abutting large expanses of ganglioneuroma (Figs. 32–12, 32–13). This form of ganglioneuroblastoma was previously referred to as "ganglioneuroblastoma with focal complete differentiation" by Beckwith and Martin[5] and as "composite neuroblastoma" by Stout.[198] The second, or intermixed, form of ganglioneuroblastoma consists of microscopic nests of neuroblastoma situated in a ganglioneuromatous stroma (Fig. 32–14). The nests of neuroblasts appear discrete but unencapsulated. According to the INPC, the subtype described as "stroma-rich, well-differentiated" ganglioneuroblastoma in the original Shimada classification and the "borderline-type" ganglioneuroblastoma in the Joshi system is now referred to as "ganglioneuroma, maturing subtype" (Figs. 32–15, 32–16, 32–17).

## Immunohistochemical Findings

A number of neuroectodermal antigens can be identified in neuroblastomas, although generally the extent and intensity are functions of the level of differentiation.[4,150] Neuron-specific enolase is probably the most sensitive but also the least specific marker for neuro-

*Text continued on page 1274*

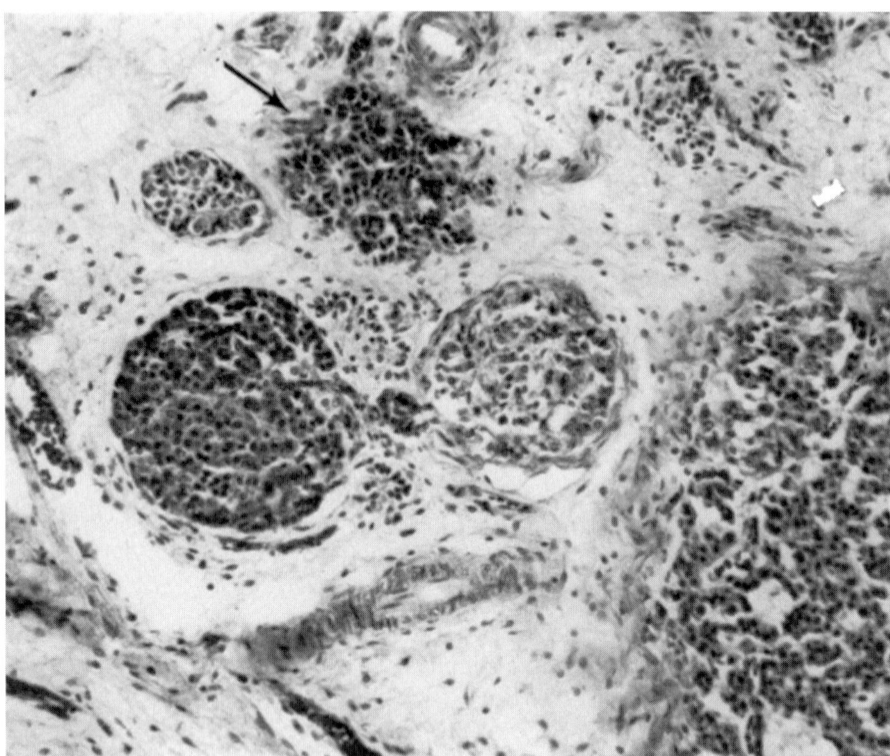

**FIGURE 32–4.** Clusters of primitive neuroblasts (arrow) from the periadrenal area in a developing fetus.

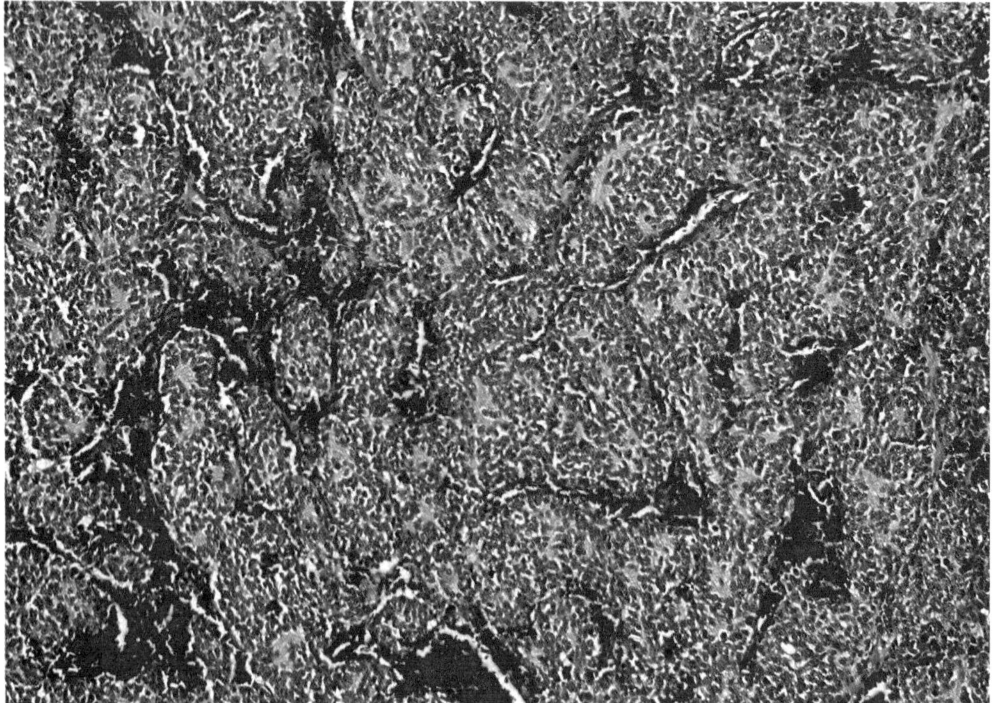

**FIGURE 32–5.** Poorly differentiated neuroblastoma with hemorrhagic fibrovascular septa that divide the tumor into small lobules.

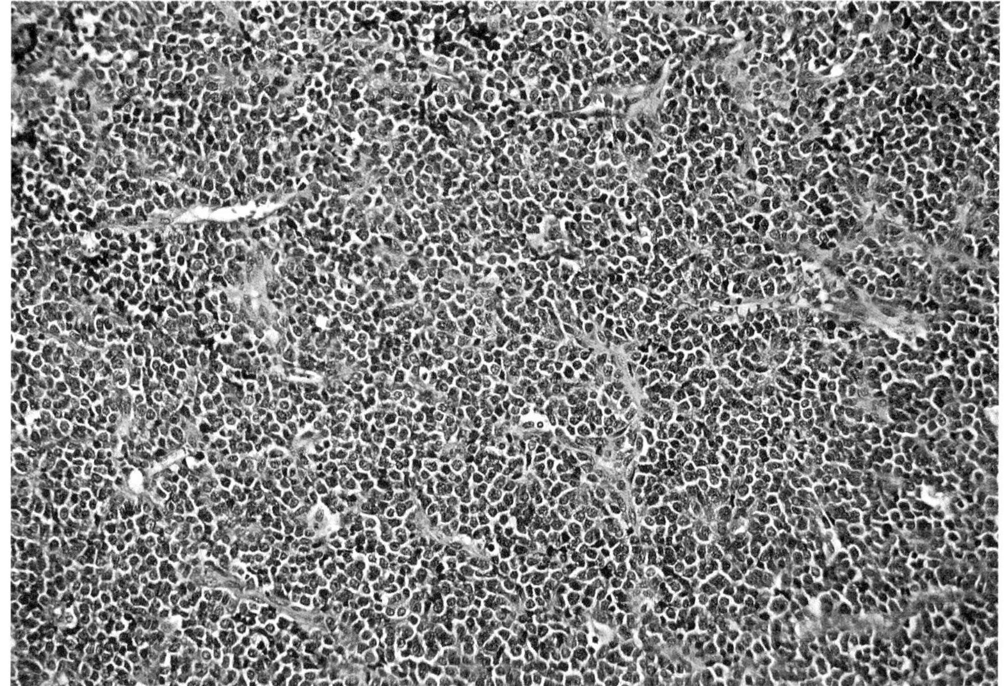

**FIGURE 32–6.** Poorly differentiated neuroblastoma composed of monotonous sheets of cells with little cytoplasm divided by fibrovascular septa.

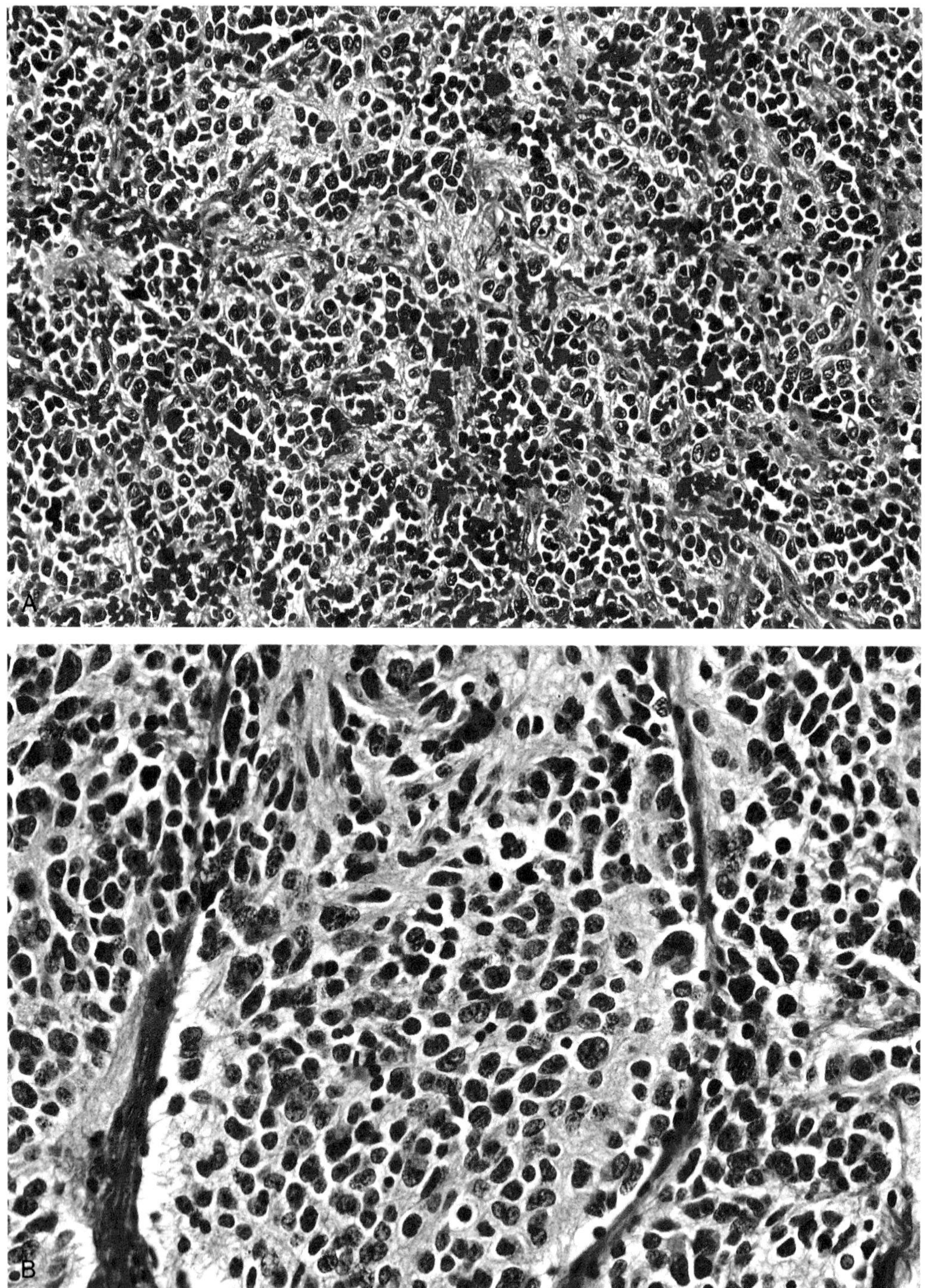

**FIGURE 32–7.** Low-power (**A**) and high-power (**B**) views of a poorly differentiated neuroblastoma composed of a sheet-like proliferation of monotonous small round cells with little cytoplasm.

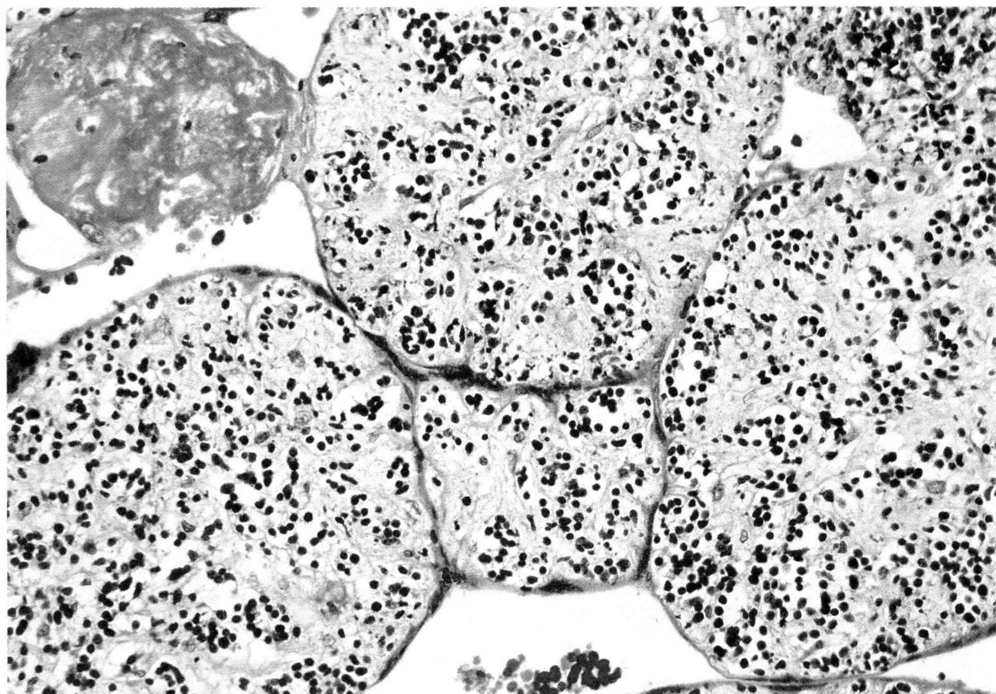

**FIGURE 32–8.** Congenital neuroblastoma involving the placenta. Tumor cells resemble nucleated erythrocytes and may be misinterpreted as evidence of erythroblastosis fetalis.

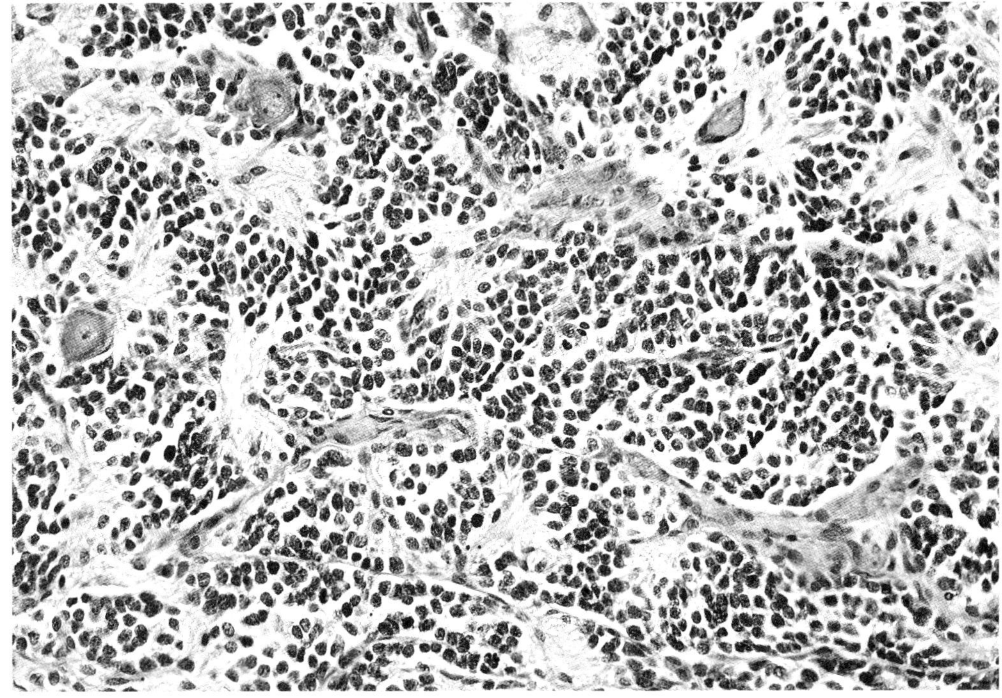

**FIGURE 32–9.** Poorly differentiated neuroblastoma. In this area of the tumor the neuroblasts have attenuated cytoplasmic processes that are polarized toward a central point to form Homer Wright rosettes.

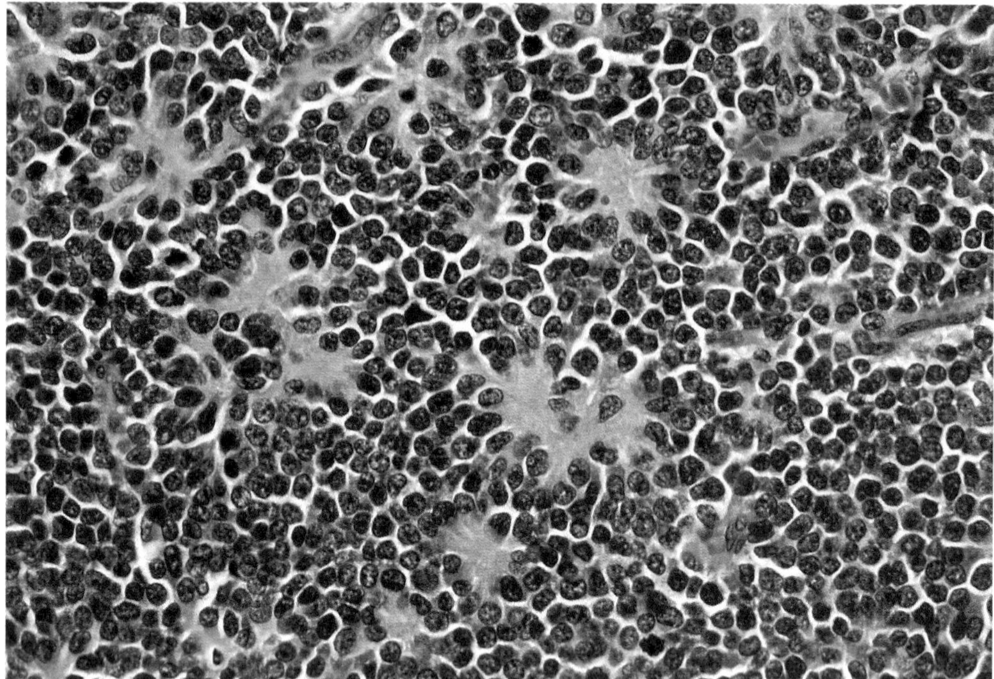

**FIGURE 32–10.** Homer Wright rosettes in a poorly differentiated neuroblastoma.

blastomas. It can be identified at least focally in even poorly differentiated tumors and is identified with increasing intensity in differentiating tumors, ganglioneuroblastomas, and ganglioneuromas. Because it is present in a variety of other small round cell tumors such as ES/PNETs and rhabdomyosarcomas, it cannot be used alone for the differential diagnosis. Neurofilament protein, the intermediate filament characteristic of neuronal cells, can be identified in many neuroblastomas, although the immunoreactivity appears to depend greatly on the degree of differentiation and method of fixation.[100,109] S-100 protein is strongly expressed in the ganglioneuromatous portions of these tumors. In addition, Shimada et al.[127] found that some neuroblastomas show S-100 protein immunoreactivity in elongated spindle-shaped cells in the supportive stroma surrounding nests of tumor cells. These cells may represent precursor cells capable of producing a differentiated neuromatous stroma,[10] and several studies have found a favorable prognostic influence of S-100 protein staining in these tumors.[2,58,127] Other markers that have proved useful for diagnosing neuroblastoma include protein gene product 9.5, chromogranin, vasoactive intestinal peptide, and synaptophysin.[25,59,108] All are best demonstrated in the more differentiated tumors. Glial fibrillary acidic protein and myelin basic protein are usually not identified in neuroblastomas unless they contain more differentiated foci.[99] Although immunoreactivity for enzymes of catecholamine synthesis (tyrosine hydroxylase, dopamine decarboxylase) can be detected in neuroblastomas, it tends to be weak. Preliminary reports have described immunolocalization of $\beta$-integrins,[48] transforming growth factor-$\beta$ (TGF$\beta$),[95] neural cell adhesion molecule (NCAM)[99] and microtubule-associated protein in these tumors.

A monoclonal antibody (NB-84) raised to neuroblastoma cells that recognizes a 57-kDa unknown antigen has been reported to be a sensitive marker of neuroblastomas.[141] Although this antibody is highly sensitive for recognizing neuroblastic tumors,[50,97] it lacks complete specificity, as up to 20% of ES/PNETs are marked by this antibody. The absence of the *MIC2* gene product in neuroblastoma is useful for distinguishing these tumors from ES/PNETs.

## Ultrastructural Findings

Ultrastructurally, neuroblastomas exhibit a wide range of cytologic differentiation.[120,140] The least differentiated cells may be difficult to distinguish from primitive cells in other types of tumors because they have scant rims of cytoplasm, few organelles other than free ribosomes, and small numbers of heterogeneous granules measuring about 50 nm. More differentiated cells can be clearly recognized as neural by virtue of attenuated cytoplasmic processes containing fine neurofilaments (8–12 nm) and microtubules (24–26 nm). Dense-core neurosecretory granules, presumably representing the site of conversion of dopamine to nor-

*Text continued on page 1279*

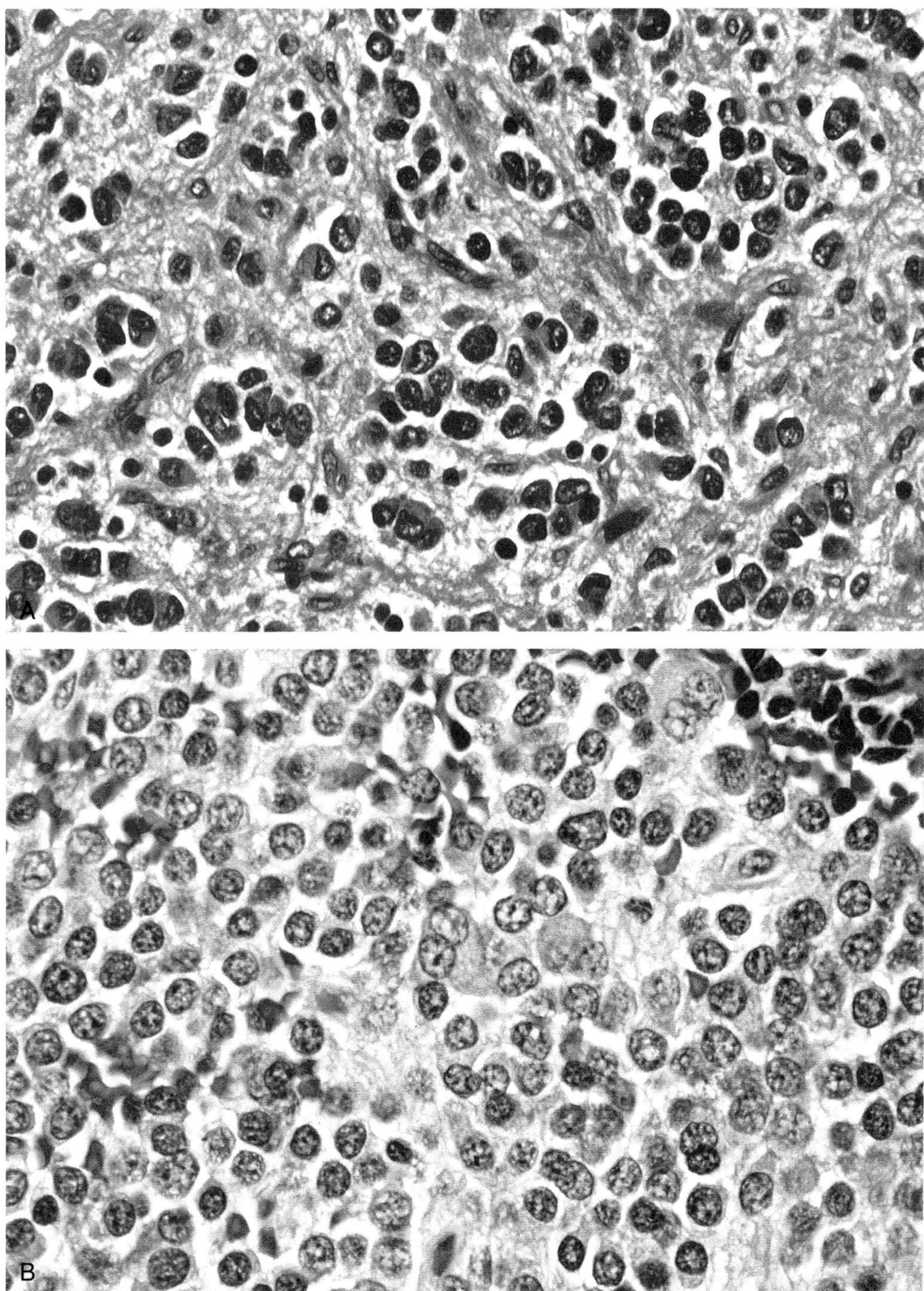


**FIGURE 32–11.** (**A**) Neuroblastoma composed predominantly of small round cells with little cytoplasm. Rare cells have a discernible rim of eosinophilic cytoplasm suggesting incipient ganglionic differentiation. (**B**) Neuroblastoma with focal ganglionic differentiation. A binucleated cell is apparent in the center of this photomicrograph.

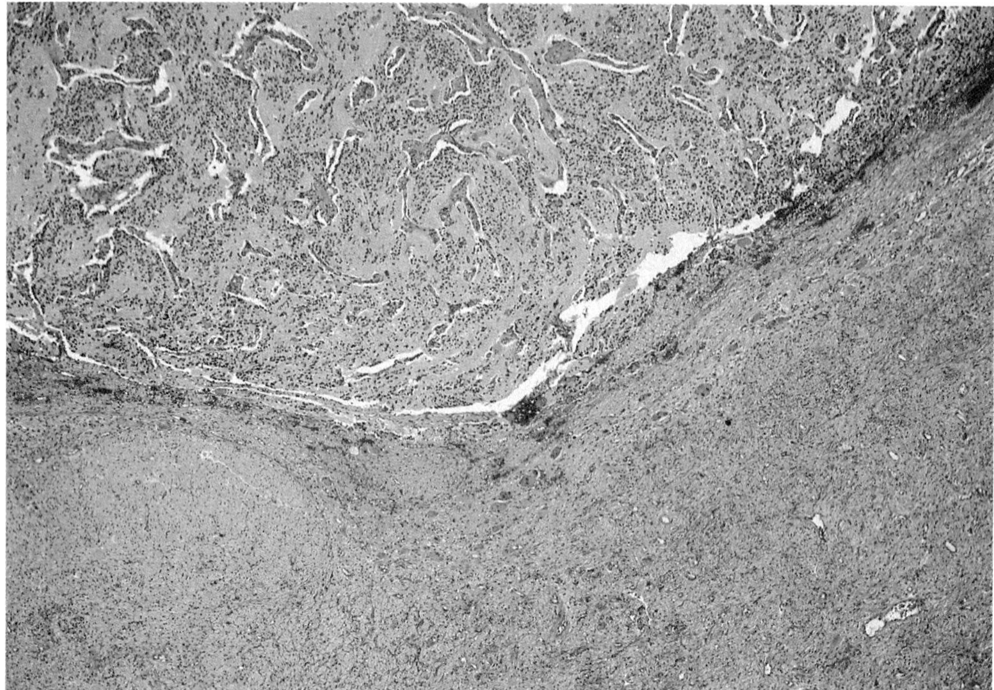

**FIGURE 32–12.** Low-power view of nodular ganglioneuroblastoma. Areas with neuroblastic differentiation are sharply circumscribed and separated from ganglioneuromatous zones.

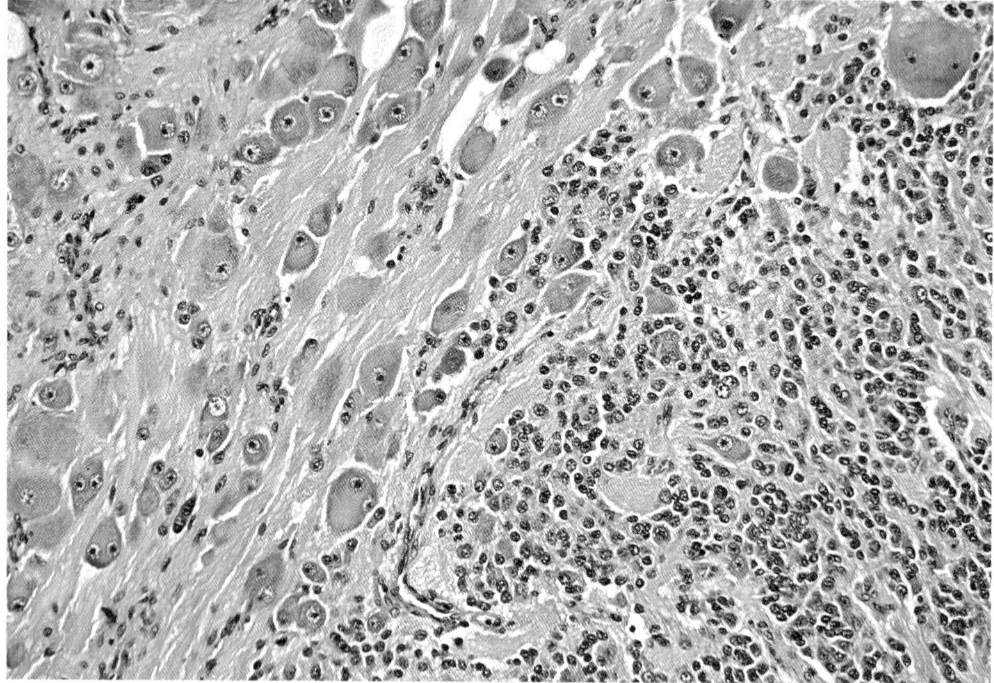

**FIGURE 32–13.** Nodular ganglioneuroblastoma. Areas of ganglioneuroma abruptly give way to areas of neuroblastoma.

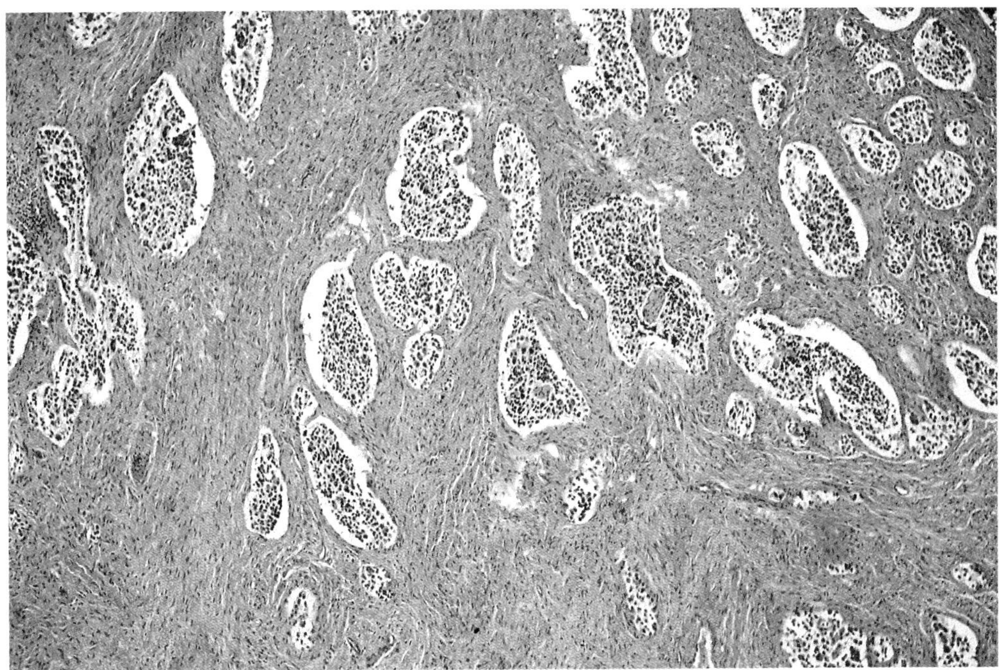

**FIGURE 32–14.** Ganglioneuroblastoma with patchy nodules of immature neuroblasts set in a mature ganglioneuromatous stroma.

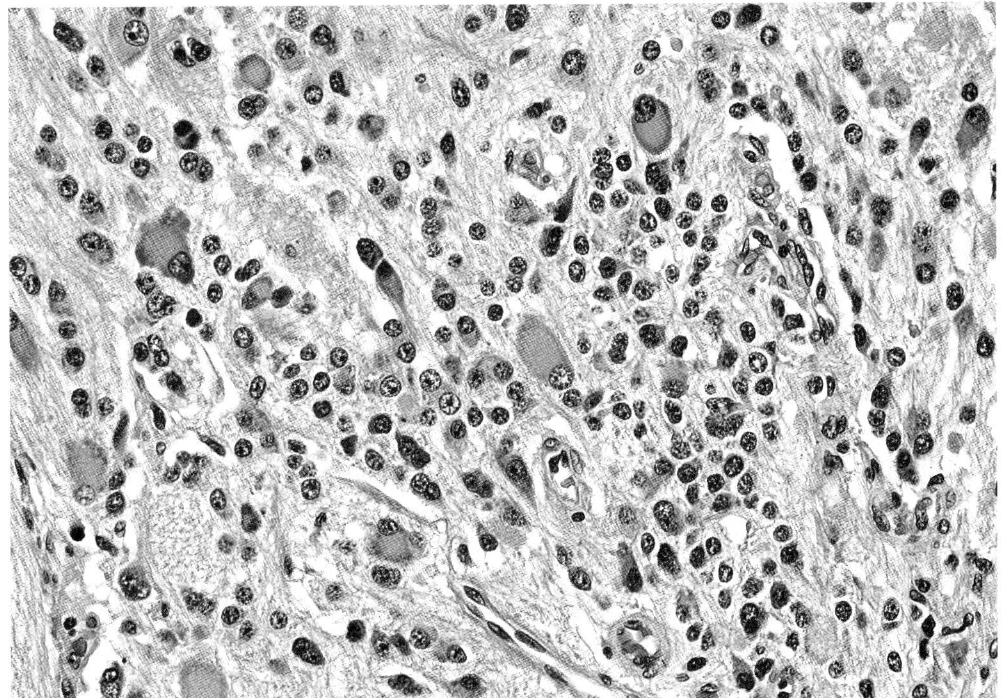

**FIGURE 32–15.** Ganglioneuroblastoma composed of an intimate admixture of neuroblasts and ganglion cells deposited in a fibrillary stroma.

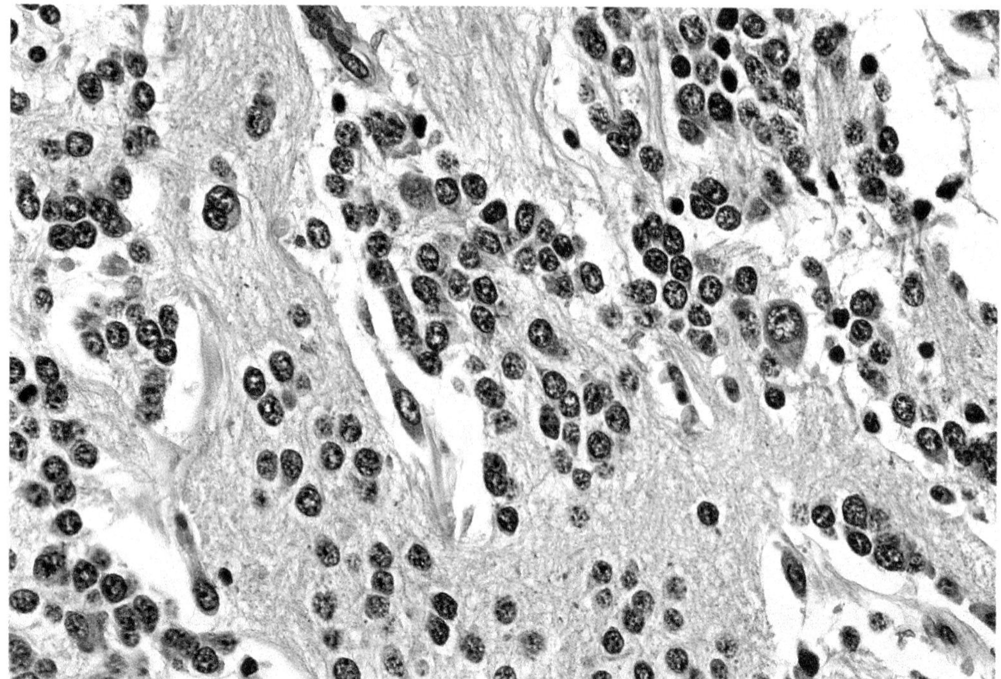

**FIGURE 32–16.** Ganglioneuroblastoma. This area is composed predominantly of neuroblasts in a fibrillary stroma. Rare binucleated forms and cells with obvious ganglionic differentiation are present.

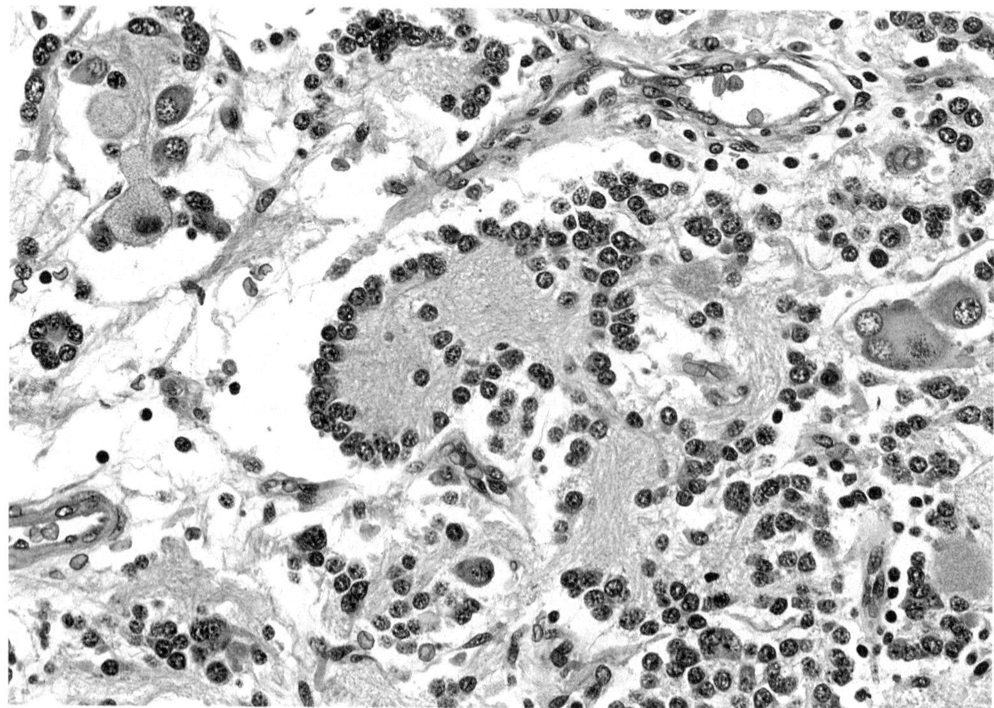

**FIGURE 32–17.** Homer Wright rosettes in a ganglioneuroblastoma.

epinephrine, vary in numbers. Although they typically occur in small clusters in the elongated cell processes, they may also be found in the cell body. The granules, measuring approximately 100 nm in diameter, contain central dense cores surrounded by clear halos and delicate outer membranes. Occasionally clear vesicles are also noted. The significance of the latter structures is not certain, although they may contain acetylcholine or may be exhausted sites of catecholamine stores. Ganglionic differentiation in these tumors is accompanied by an increase in the cytoplasm, with concomitant increases in mitochondria, ribosomes, polysomes, and perinuclear Golgi apparatus. Small dense-core granules are found randomly throughout the cytoplasm (Fig. 32–18). In addition, large heterogeneous granules containing myelin figures are present in significant numbers and are believed to represent sites for storage of degraded catecholamines. Ganglioneuromatous areas contain, in addition to mature ganglion cells, a proliferation of Schwann cells characterized by long tapered cytoplasmic processes invested with basal lamina.

## Differential Diagnosis

The young age of the patient, the location along the sympathetic chain, and elevated urinary catecholamines establish the diagnosis of neuroblastoma in most cases. Evaluation of needle biopsy specimens of poorly differentiated nonfunctioning tumors, however, may present diagnostic problems. The usual problem is the distinction of neuroblastoma from rhabdomyosarcoma or ES/PNETs, but fortunately immunohistochemical and electron microscopic studies have greatly improved the accuracy of the light microscopic diagnosis.

The clinical presentations of neuroblastoma and rhabdomyosarcoma may be similar. Both occur in young persons, often in intraabdominal locations. Rhabdomyosarcomas usually show more variability

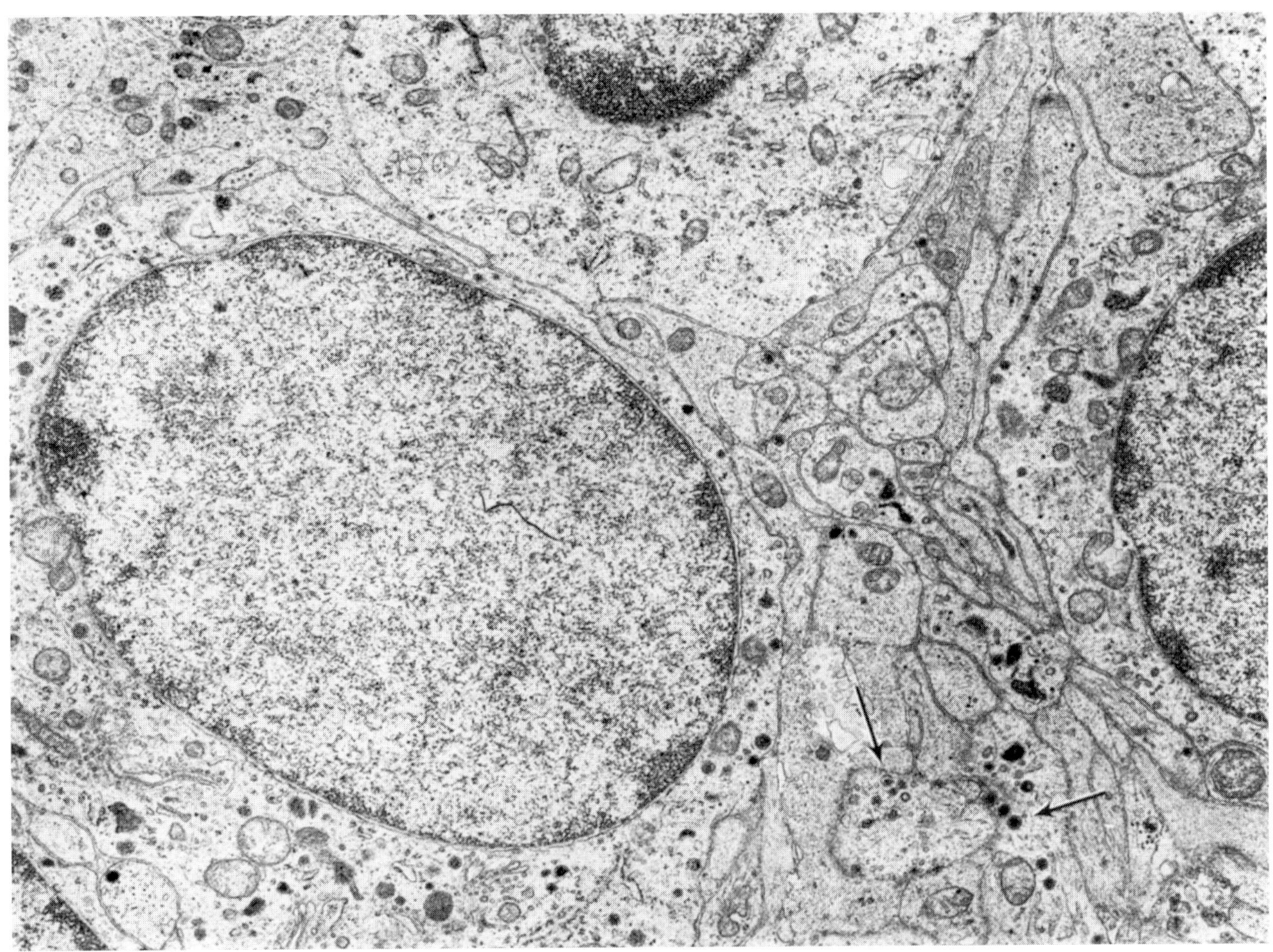

**FIGURE 32–18.** Electron micrograph of a neuroblastoma. Cells have numerous intertwining processes containing dense-core granules (arrows). Occasional dense-core granules are also present in the cell body. (Courtesy Dr. Tim Triche, National Cancer Institute, Bethesda, MD.)

in the size and shape of cells and nuclei. The cytoplasm is usually more abundant, more sharply outlined, and endowed with an eosinophilic hue. Careful search for differentiated areas reveals typical strap cells and tadpole cells. Differentiated rhabdomyoblasts have both thin (8 nm) and thick (12 nm) myofilaments and occasionally Z-band material ultrastructurally. Moreover, most rhabdomyosarcomas have moderate amounts of cytoplasmic glycogen, in contrast to neuroblastoma. The immunohistochemical detection of myogenic antigens, including actin, desmin, MyoD1, and myogenin, is extremely useful for confirming the diagnosis.

Although patients with ES/PNETs usually are relatively older than those with neuroblastoma, we have found that the two tumors can be difficult to distinguish by light microscopy alone, particularly when cellular preservation is not optimal. In well preserved specimens, extraskeletal Ewing's sarcomas have more regular nuclei, more finely stippled chromatin patterns, and cytoplasm filled with glycogen. Usually the cells are arranged in sheets and lobules. The similarity between neuroblastoma and peripheral neuroepithelioma may be striking, given the presence of Homer Wright rosettes in both tumors. However, neuroblastomas usually have a more fibrillary background, often have foci of calcification, and show evidence of ganglionic differentiation in many cases. Although the product of the *MIC2* gene (CD99) can be detected immunohistochemically in almost all cases of ES/PNET and in other round cell tumors with low frequency, neuroblastomas have not been found to express this antigen. Thus membranous immunoreactivity for this antigen virtually excludes neuroblastoma as a diagnostic consideration.

**TABLE 32–2 TWO-YEAR SURVIVAL RATES FOR NEUROBLASTOMA BY PROGNOSTIC FACTOR**

| Factor | No. of Patients | Survival (%) |
|---|---|---|
| Overall | 124 | 60 |
| Age | | |
| <2 years | 73 | 77 |
| 2 + years | 51 | 38 |
| Neuron-specific enolase | | |
| Normal (1–100 ng/ml) | 60 | 76 |
| Abnormal (>100 ng/ml) | 23 | 17 |
| Ferritin | | |
| Normal (0–150 ng/ml) | 64 | 83 |
| Abnormal (>150 ng/ml) | 39 | 19 |
| E rosette inhibition | | |
| Normal (0–15%) | 56 | 60 |
| Abnormal (>15%) | 27 | 54 |
| VMA/HVA ratio | | |
| High (>1) | 28 | 84 |
| Low (<1) | 22 | 44 |
| Stage | | |
| I | 15 | 100 |
| II | 27 | 82 |
| III | 18 | 42 |
| IV | 51 | 30 |
| IV-S | 13 | 100 |
| Pathology (Shimada system) | | |
| Favorable type | 52 | 94 |
| Unfavorable type | 36 | 39 |

From Evans AE, Angio GJ, Propert K, et al. Prognostic factors in neuroblastoma. Cancer 59:1853, 1987.
VMA/HVA, vanillylmandelic acid/homovanillic acid.

## Behavior and Treatment

Despite recent therapeutic advances, the survival rates of patients with neuroblastoma have remained relatively unchanged over the past two decades, a finding that contrasts with the prognosis of other childhood sarcomas. Survival rates depend on a number of partially interrelated factors (Tables 32–2, 32–3), including age at diagnosis, clinical stage, histologic type, extent of S-100 protein staining, presence of N-*myc* amplification, DNA ploidy, presence of 1p and other cytogenetic abnormalities, degree of TRK-A expression, and certain laboratory findings (e.g., serum ferritin, neuron-specific enolase, lactate dehydrogenase).

Age and clinical stage, independent variables, are the two most important prognostic factors. Children less than 1 year of age at diagnosis have a far better prognosis than children who are diagnosed after 1 year of age.[20,34,44,46] Likewise, patients with localized neuroblastoma have an excellent prognosis. The staging system used for neuroblastoma has evolved over the past 25 years. The system proposed by Evans et al.[46] in 1971 was adopted by the Children's Cancer Group and was the first to gain wide acceptance.[79] The surgicopathologic staging system proposed by Hayes et al.[61] and modified by the Pediatric Oncology Group[105] gained popularity during the 1980s. In 1993 the International Neuroblastoma Staging System

**TABLE 32–3 FAVORABLE PROGNOSTIC FACTORS FOR NEUROBLASTOMA**

- Young age (<1 year)
- Favorable histologic type
- Low stage (1, 2, 4S)
- No N-*myc* amplification
- Hyperdiploid or near-triploid DNA content
- No allelic loss of 1p
- High expression of TRK-A
- Normal serum ferritin, neuron-specific enolase, and lactate dehydrogenase
- High urinary VMA/HVA ratio

(INSS) was established[16] with elements borrowed from the staging systems of both Evans et al. and the Pediatric Oncology Group (Table 32–4). Patients with stage 1 or 2 disease have a significantly longer survival than do patients with stage 3 or 4 disease. The location of the tumor, although important, is closely related to the stage of the disease. For instance, cervical, thoracic, and pelvic tumors have better prognoses than retroperitoneal and adrenal tumors but usually are detected at an earlier clinical stage.

A notable exception to the trend of decreasing survival rate with increasing clinical disease is a special group of stage 4 lesions designated 4S. These tumors otherwise would be stage 1 or 2, but there is also remote disease confined to the liver, skin, or bone marrow, without radiographic evidence of bone metastases. Despite their tumor dissemination, these patients have a paradoxically favorable prognosis and a high rate of spontaneous tumor regression.[46] Van Noesel et al.[146] reported on 119 patients with stage 4S neuroblastoma and found that 33 (28%) died, usually as a complication of hepatomegaly with renal failure, respiratory failure, or both. All but one of the patients who died was diagnosed during the first 4 weeks of life. In addition, progression to stage 4 disease and death were strongly related to N-*myc* amplification. Hachitanda and Hata[57] found that most patients with stage 4S disease were less than 1 year of age, had favorable histology, and had an excellent outcome, although there was a subgroup with a poor prognosis who had unfavorable histopathologic and biologic features. Thus a thorough histologic evaluation and N-*myc* amplification are necessary to predict the outcome for this subgroup of patients.[72]

**TABLE 32–4 INTERNATIONAL NEUROBLASTOMA STAGING SYSTEM**

| Stage | Definition |
|---|---|
| 1 | Localized tumor confined to the area of origin; complete gross resection, with or without microscopic residual disease; representative ipsilateral lymph nodes negative for tumor |
| 2A | Localized tumor with incomplete gross excision; representative ipsilateral nonadherent lymph nodes negative for tumor |
| 2B | Localized tumor with or without complete gross excision, with ipsilateral nonadherent lymph nodes positive for tumor<br>Enlarged contralateral lymph nodes negative for tumor |
| 3 | Unresectable unilateral tumor infiltrating across the midline, with or without regional lymph node involvement; *or* localized unilateral tumor with contralateral regional lymph node involvement; *or* midline tumor with bilateral extension by infiltration or by lymph node involvement |
| 4 | Any primary tumor with dissemination to distant lymph nodes, bone, bone marrow, liver, skin, and/or other organs except as defined for stage 4S |
| 4S | Localized primary tumor (as defined for stage 1, 2A, or 2B), with dissemination limited to skin, liver, and/or bone marrow |

Modified from Brodeur GM, Pritchard J, Berthold F, et al. Revisions in the international criteria for neuroblastoma diagnosis, staging and response to treatment. J Clin Oncol 11:1466, 1993.

The reason for the excellent prognosis in patients with stage 4S disease is not completely understood.[92] Some authors have conceptualized stage 4S as multiple primary tumors rather than metastases[37]; others have hypothesized that stage 4S is a premalignant condition in which the final mutogenic event has not yet occurred.[75] In this respect, stage 4S could be considered comparable to in situ adrenal neuroblastoma, which regresses in most instances. Pritchard and Hickman[114] suggested that a developmental time switch for apoptosis is the most likely mechanism for spontaneous regression of neuroblastoma. Thus massive apoptosis of tumor cells, possibly through mediation by activated caspase 3,[77a] may be important in tumor regression,[66,67] whereas inhibition of apoptosis by the Bcl-2 oncoprotein might be associated with tumor progression and resistance to therapy.[26,63]

In the past it has been difficult to correlate the degree of differentiation with the outcome because, as indicated previously, terms such as "ganglioneuroblastoma" encompassed a broad range of tumors.[94] In 1984 Shimada and associates[128] proposed a new histologic system that has generally replaced earlier systems for purposes of predicting the clinical course (Table 32–5). It divides neuroblastomas into those that have a differentiated stroma (stroma-rich) and those that do not (stroma-poor). The latter group, composed of pure neuroblastomas and some ganglioneuroblastomas, is further subdivided by the age of the patient, the degree of cellular maturation, and nuclear pathologic characteristics (mitosis-karyorrhexis index) into favorable and unfavorable subtypes.

The Shimada system appears to accurately identify two groups of patients (unfavorable stroma-poor, nodular stroma-rich) with a notably poor prognosis.[31] This is a more complex system than earlier ones and introduces an entirely new nomenclature, with which pathologists are less familiar. The Joshi system,[69–71] detailed above, blends the basic observations of the Shimada system with more traditional terms. The more recent studies of the International Neuroblastoma Pathology Committee[129a,129b] have shown the prognostic importance of histologic subtype using their proposed classification scheme.

**TABLE 32–5 HISTOLOGIC TYPE OF NEUROBLASTOMA AND ITS EFFECT ON 2-YEAR SURVIVAL RATES**

| Stromal Character | Survival (%) |
|---|---|
| Stroma-rich | |
| Favorable histology | |
| Well-differentiated type | 100 |
| Intermixed type | 92 |
| Unfavorable histology | |
| Nodular type | 18 |
| Stroma-poor | |
| Favorable histology | 84 |
| Age <18 months; MKI <200/5000 | |
| Age 18–60 months; MKI <100/5000 and differentiating | |
| Unfavorable histology | 4.5 |
| Age <18 months; MKI >200/5000 | |
| Age 18–60 months; MKI >100/5000 or undifferentiated | |
| Age >5 years | |

Modified from Shimada H, Chatten J, Newton WA Jr, et al. Histopathologic prognostic factors in neuroblastic tumors: definition of subtypes of ganglioneuroblastoma and an age-linked classification of neuroblastoma. J Natl Cancer Inst 73:405, 1984.
MKI, mitotic-karyorrhectic index.

Numerous studies have attested to the importance of N-*myc* amplification to the prognosis of neuroblastoma.[11,18,126,144,145] Consequently, it is mandatory that a small aliquot of tissue be obtained and frozen at the time of surgery from every suspected neuroblastoma. Approximately 20–25% of patients with neuroblastoma have N-*myc* amplification.[104,131] Up to 30% of patients with advanced-stage disease have N-*myc* amplification, whereas fewer than 5% of patients with low-stage disease have this feature (Table 32–6). There are relatively few cases in the literature of patients with low-stage disease and N-*myc* amplification, although there are several reports of patients with these features who have had prolonged survival.[47,79] On the other hand, patients with 4S disease and N-*myc* amplification have an aggressive clinical course.[57,146]

The presence or absence of N-*myc* amplification is closely linked to other biologic variables. Tumor cell ploidy seems to provide data complementary to N-*myc* amplification. Near-diploid or tetraploid levels of DNA are associated with advanced-stage disease, N-*myc* amplification, poor response to therapy, and a less favorable outcome.[85,86] In contrast, hyperdiploidy is associated with lower-stage disease, better response to therapy, and a good prognosis.

There is also a strong correlation between N-*myc* amplification and allelic loss of chromosome 1p.[23,51] In the study by Caron et al.,[23] there was 100% three-year event-free survival for patients with stage 1, 2, or 4S disease without allelic loss of chromosome 1p compared to 34% three-year event-free survival among those with such loss. These authors found that loss of chromosome 1p was the most powerful prognostic factor by multivariate analysis, but it has not been established if allelic loss of 1p and N-*myc* amplification are independent prognostic variables.[54,90,91] Brown et al.[19] found gain of 17q to be an important independent prognostic variable that is strongly linked to 1p deletion, N-*myc* amplification, advanced tumor stage, and older patient age.

There is an inverse relation between N-*myc* amplification and the level of TRK-A expression.[101,102,138] Nakagawara et al.[102] found a strong correlation between TRK-A expression and favorable tumor stage, younger patient age, normal N-*myc* copy number, and a favorable prognosis. A high level of TRK-A expression was associated with an 86% five-year cumulative survival, compared to 14% for those with a low level of TRK-A expression. Similar results have been reported by others.[9,33,134]

Based on N-*myc* amplification, DNA ploidy, allelic loss of 1p, and TRK-A expression, three genetically distinct groups of neuroblastoma emerge (Table 32–7).[11] Hyperdiploid or near-triploid tumors virtually never show N-*myc* amplification, rarely show allelic loss of 1p, and have high TRK-A expression. These patients are usually younger than 1 year of age, generally have favorable-stage disease, and have an excellent prognosis. Most infants whose neuroblastomas are detected by screening studies fall into this category.[110,133,142] A second group of tumors have near-diploid or near-tetraploid DNA content, lack N-*myc* amplification, show allelic loss of 1p in 25–50% of cases, and usually have low TRK-A expression. These patients are more likely to be older than 1 year of age, have advanced-stage disease, and have an intermediate prognosis. Patients with near-diploid or near-tetraploid tumors with N-*myc* amplification virtually always have allelic loss of 1p and low or absent TRK-A expression. These patients are almost always older

**TABLE 32–6 CORRELATION AMONG N-*myc* AMPLIFICATION, STAGE, AND SURVIVAL**

| Stage at Diagnosis | N-*myc* Amplification (%) | 3-Year Survival (%) |
|---|---|---|
| 1, 2 | <5 | 90 |
| 4S | 5–10 | 80 |
| 3, 4 | 30–35 | 30 |
| *Total* | 25–30 | 50 |

Modified from Brodeur GM, Maris JM, Yamashiro BJ, et al. Biology and genetics of human neuroblastomas. J Pediatr Hematol Oncol 19:93, 1997.

**TABLE 32–7 CLINICAL AND GENETIC TYPES OF NEUROBLASTOMA**

| Feature | Type 1 | Type 2 | Type 3 |
|---|---|---|---|
| DNA ploidy | Hyperdiploid or near-triploid | Near-diploid or near-tetraploid | Near-diploid or near-tetraploid |
| N-*myc* | Normal | Normal | Amplified |
| 1p Allelic loss | <5% | 25–50% | 80–90% |
| *TRK-A* expression | High | Low | Low or absent |
| Age | <1 year | >1 year | >1 year |
| Stage | 1, 2, or 4S | 3 or 4 | 3 or 4 |
| 3-Year survival | 95% | 25–50% | <5% |

Modified from Brodeur GM, Maris JM, Yamashiro BJ, et al. Biology and genetics of human neuroblastomas. J Pediatr Hematol Oncol 19:93, 1997.

than 1 year of age, have advanced-stage disease, and have a poor response to treatment with a rapidly progressive course.[15]

A number of other genes have also been implicated as having a prognostic impact on neuroblastoma, including other tumor-suppressor genes (e.g., *DCC*),[116] genes related to the multidrug resistance phenotype (*MDR*1, *MRP*),[30,39,40,107] genes related to invasion and metastasis (including CD44[49,84] and membrane-type matrix metalloproteinases[121]), other proto-oncogenes (including H-*ras*),[139] and telomerase activity.[64,87a] Elevated serum ferritin, neuron-specific enolase, lactate dehydrogenase, and the urinary VMA/HVA ratio also correlate with survival rates but not with the same level of statistical significance as the preceding factors.[44]

At the time of diagnosis about two-thirds of patients harbor metastatic disease, a finding that emphasizes the need for thorough clinical evaluation before instituting therapy. Metastatic disease is most common in bone, lymph nodes, liver, and skin. Although the presence of metastasis does not necessarily portend death from disease, bone metastasis accompanied by overt radiologic changes is a notable exception. This pattern of metastasis almost always signifies a fatal outcome.

A small number of tumors (1–2%) undergo spontaneous regression or maturation (Fig. 32–19), most of-

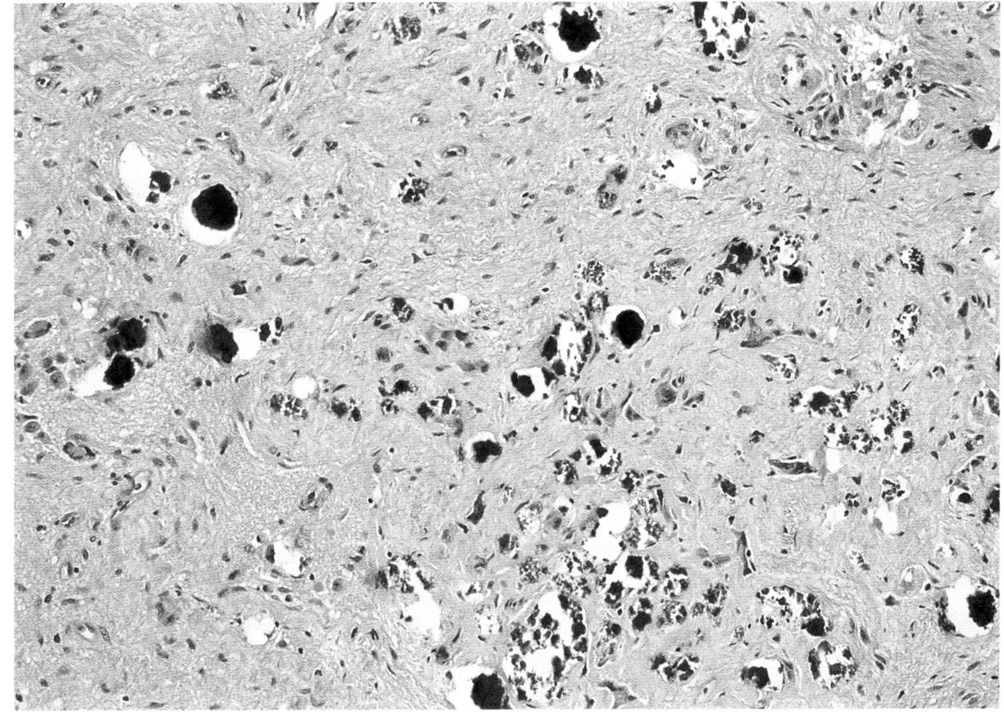

**FIGURE 32–19.** Zone of maturation in a neuroblastoma following therapy. There is extensive calcification of the neuromatous stroma, which is devoid of primitive neuroblasts.

ten in children under 1 year of age.[151] It is generally believed that most clinical cures of neuroblastoma, particularly in patients with stage 4S disease, represent tumor regression rather than maturation,[45] although tumor maturation is well documented in the literature.[42,56] In many recent cases the question has been raised as to whether therapy induced the maturation. Early cases, such as the one described by Cushing and Wolback,[36] leave little doubt that it represents a natural sequence of events in rare cases. In this instance the patient received no therapy apart from administration of Coley's toxin following biopsy. Histologically, hypocellular zones with amorphic or plump degenerating cells may be seen in tumors undergoing regression, as these changes have been described in resected tumors from untreated patients who were identified by a mass screening program.[65]

Management of patients with neuroblastoma is determined by the risk for recurrent disease based on age, stage, and selected biologic features, resulting in low, intermediate, and high risk groups.[27,28] Low-risk patients are generally managed with surgery alone, even if the tumor has unfavorable biologic prognostic factors or residual microscopic disease remains after surgery.[29,93,105,106,111a] The treatment of patients with 4S disease should be individualized. Because of the risk of respiratory failure secondary to hepatomegaly in patients with 4S disease who are less than 4 weeks of age, chemotherapy or irradiation prior to surgery has been recommended.[146] For patients with 4S disease who are more than 4 weeks of age, biologic markers can place the patients in low and high risk groups. Low risk 4S patients can be treated with surgery alone, whereas adjuvant therapy has been recommended for patients with 4S disease who have unfavorable biologic markers.[146]

Intermediate risk patients generally require chemotherapy and second-look surgery.[27] Multiagent regimens including cyclophosphamide, ifosfamide, doxorubicin, etoposide, and cisplatin have been found to be the most effective.[12] Patients with high risk disease are generally treated with postoperative dose-intensive chemotherapy, which has improved the complete and partial response rates but has not had a significant impact on ultimate survival. Autologous bone marrow[115] and peripheral blood stem cell transplantation[43] have also been used in this setting. To remove tumor from autologous marrow intended for transplantation, magnetic microspheres targeted with monoclonal antibodies against the tumor have been employed.[117] Minimal residual tumor can be detected by flow cytometric analysis[78] or the reverse transcriptase-polymerase chain reaction (RT-PCR)[98] and may serve as an additional component of surveillance for neuroblastoma patients.

## Ganglioneuroma

Ganglioneuromas are fully differentiated tumors that contain no immature elements. They are rare compared with other benign neural tumors, such as neurilemoma and neurofibroma, but they outnumber neuroblastomas along the sympathetic axis by about 3:1 according to Stout's estimate.[198] In our experience, ganglioneuromas differ significantly in terms of age distribution and location compared with neuroblastomas. Most ganglioneuromas are diagnosed in patients older than 10 years and are most often located in the posterior mediastinum, followed by the retroperitoneum (Table 32–8). Only a minor proportion occur in the adrenal proper.[157,159] The differences in distribution of neuroblastomas and ganglioneuromas support the idea that most ganglioneuromas develop de novo rather than by way of maturation in a preexisting neuroblastoma.

Ganglioneuromas may also be found at other sites, including the skin,[153,170,176] retro- or parapharynx,[190,199] and gastrointestinal tract.[168,197] In the gastrointestinal tract, polypoid ganglioneuromas have been reported in association with Cowden syndrome,[158,181] tuberous sclerosis,[165] familial polyposis coli,[187,188] and juvenile polyposis.[184,189] Ganglioneuromatous polyposis has been described in patients with type 1 neurofibromatosis,[164,169,196] and multiple endocrine neoplasia type IIb (MEN-IIb).[175]

Clinically, ganglioneuromas present as large masses in the retroperitoneum or mediastinum; they are usu-

**TABLE 32–8 AGE AND ANATOMIC DISTRIBUTIONS OF GANGLIONEUROMA: 1970–1980 (88 CASES)**

| Parameter | No. of Cases |
|---|---|
| Age (years) | |
| 0–4 | 5 |
| 5–9 | 9 |
| 10–19 | 23 |
| 20–29 | 22 |
| 30–39 | 12 |
| 40–49 | 4 |
| 50–59 | 6 |
| 60–69 | 4 |
| >69 | 3 |
| Location | |
| Mediastinal | 34 |
| Retroperitoneal | 27 |
| Adrenal | 19 |
| Pelvic | 5 |
| Cervical | 2 |
| Parapharyngeal | 1 |

Data are from the Armed Forces Institute of Pathology (AFIP).

ally of longer duration than neuroblastomas. Most patients have normal levels of urinary catecholamine metabolites, although there is an increased incidence of elevated values in patients with extremely large tumors.[182] Extreme elevations should prompt careful evaluation for occult neuroblastomatous foci. On radiographic examination, about one-third are seen to have intralesional calcification.[178,195] Ultrasonographic studies reveal a hypoechoic lesion that is typically hypovascular. The tumor has low attenuation on CT scans and low signal intensity on T1-weighted images and high signal intensity on T2-weighted images.[177,191] Clinically, patients may present with sweating, hypertension, virilization,[173] and diarrhea.[185] Diarrheal symptoms in patients with these tumors have been related to the presence of vasoactive intestinal peptide, which can be localized to the cytoplasm of the ganglion cell by means of immunoperoxidase techniques.[155,179,193,194]

Grossly, the ganglioneuroma is a well circumscribed tumor with a fibrous capsule. On cut section it is gray to yellow and sometimes displays a trabecular or whorled pattern similar to that of leiomyoma (Fig. 32–20). Histologically, it has a uniform appearance throughout. The background consists of bundles of longitudinal and transversely oriented Schwann cells that crisscross each other in an irregular fashion (Figs. 32–21, 32–22). Rarely, fat is present in the stroma. Scattered throughout the schwannian backdrop are relatively mature ganglion cells (Figs. 32–23 to 32–26). Although they may occur in an isolated fashion, usually they are found in small clusters or nests. In general, they are not fully mature and lack satellite cells and Nissl bodies. Typically, their voluminous cytoplasm is bright pink and contains one to three nuclei, which may exhibit a mild to moderate degree of atypia. Pigment is sometimes present in the ganglion cells and is believed to represent catecholamine products that undergo autooxidation to a melanin-like substance (neuromelanin).[187] Although the pigment has tinctorial properties of dermal melanin (Fontana-positive), ultrastructurally it does not have the regular subunit structure but consists instead of large lysosomal structures with myelin figures.[186] There are now a number of reports in the literature of composite tumors composed of ganglioneuroma and pheochromocytoma,[180] some of which have arisen in patients with type 1 neurofibromatosis[162] or MEN-II.[156,183]

Biologically, ganglioneuromas are benign tumors. Of the 146 tumors studied by Stout,[198] none metastasized. However, it should be pointed out that rarely an apparent "metastatic" focus of ganglioneuroma is encountered in a lymph node adjacent to the main tumor mass or at a more distant site (Fig. 32–27).[161,171,174] It is assumed that these lesions represent neuroblastomas in which the metastasis and the primary tumor matured. Rare ganglioneuromas undergo malignant transformation.[154,163,166,167,172,192] Some have been in de novo ganglioneuromas and others in ganglioneuromas arising as a result of maturation in a neuroblastoma. Malignant transformation of a ganglioneuroma in a human immunodeficiency virus (HIV)-positive patient has been reported.[160] Most commonly, the malignant component resembles a malignant peripheral nerve sheath tumor (Fig. 32–28).

*Text continued on page 1289*

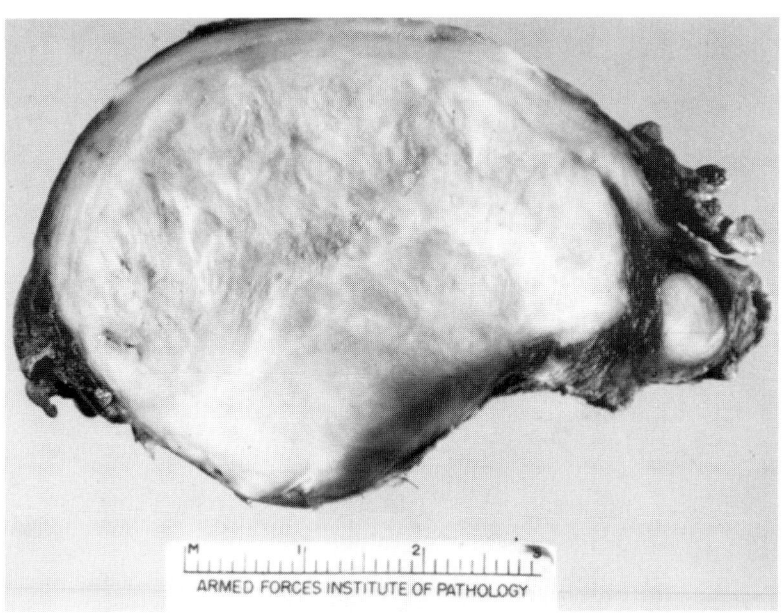


**FIGURE 32–20.** White whorled gross appearance of a ganglioneuroma.

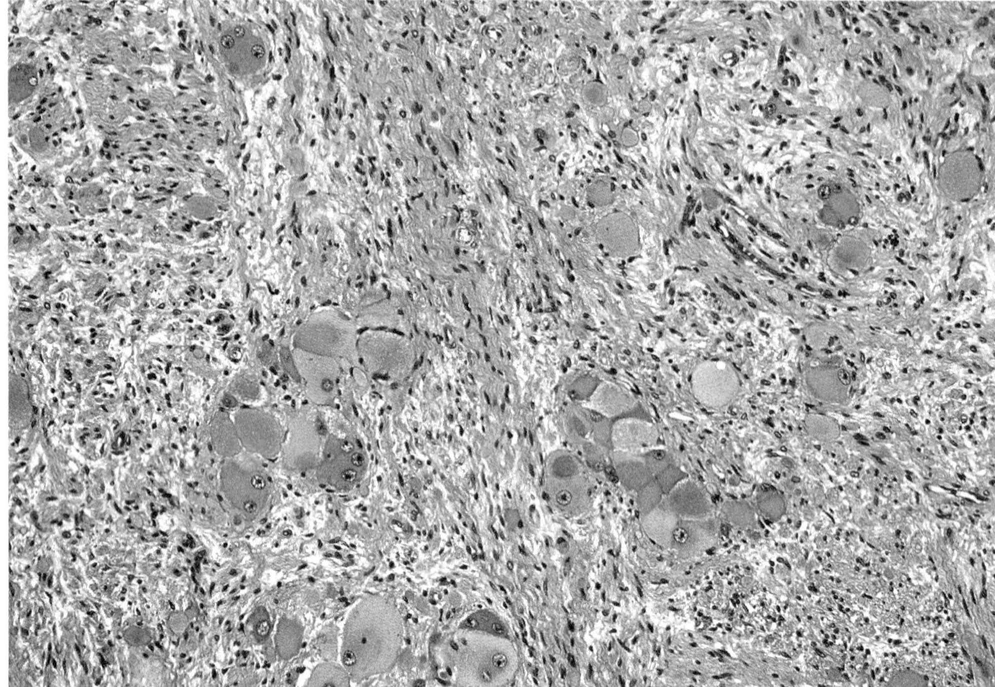

**FIGURE 32–21.** Ganglioneuroma composed of clusters of ganglion cells deposited in a neuromatous stroma.

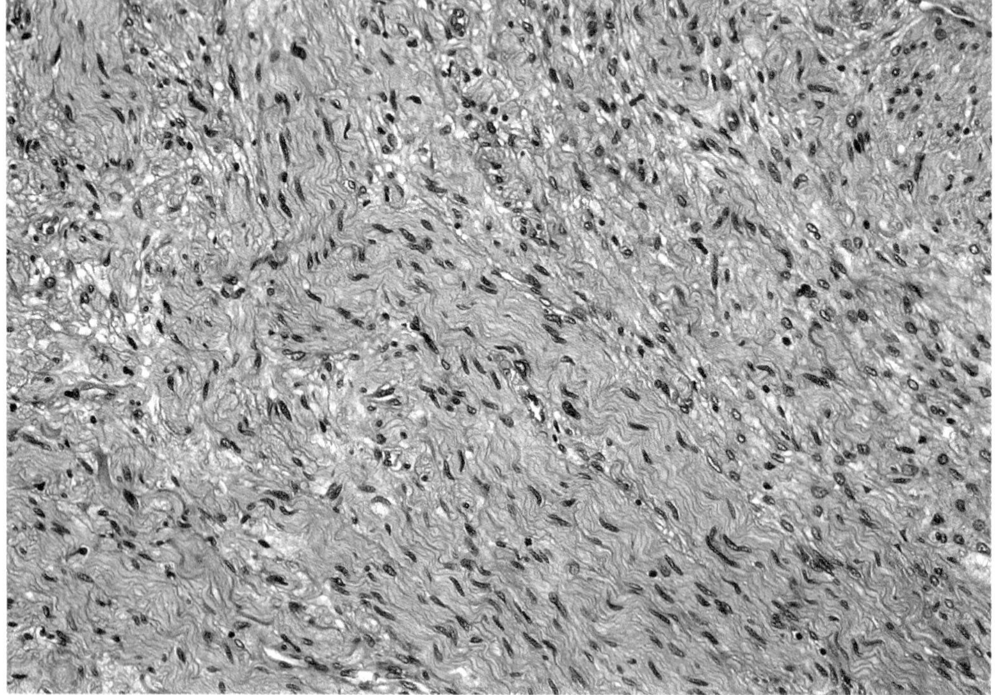

**FIGURE 32–22.** Neuromatous stroma devoid of ganglion cells in a ganglioneuroma.

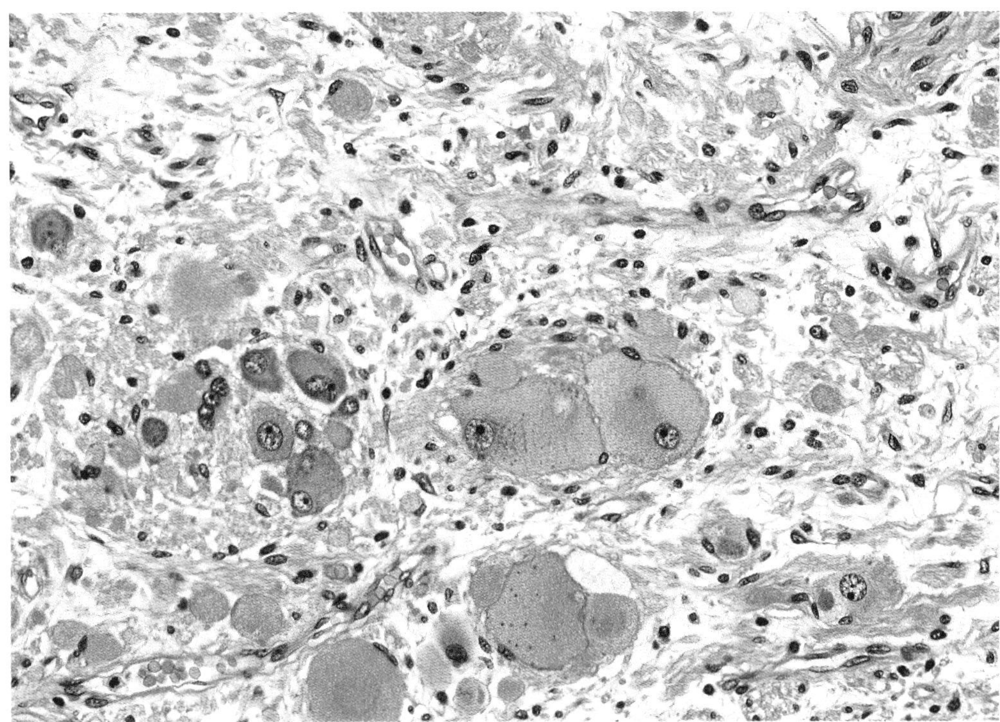

**FIGURE 32–23.** Ganglioneuroma with clusters of variably sized ganglion cells.

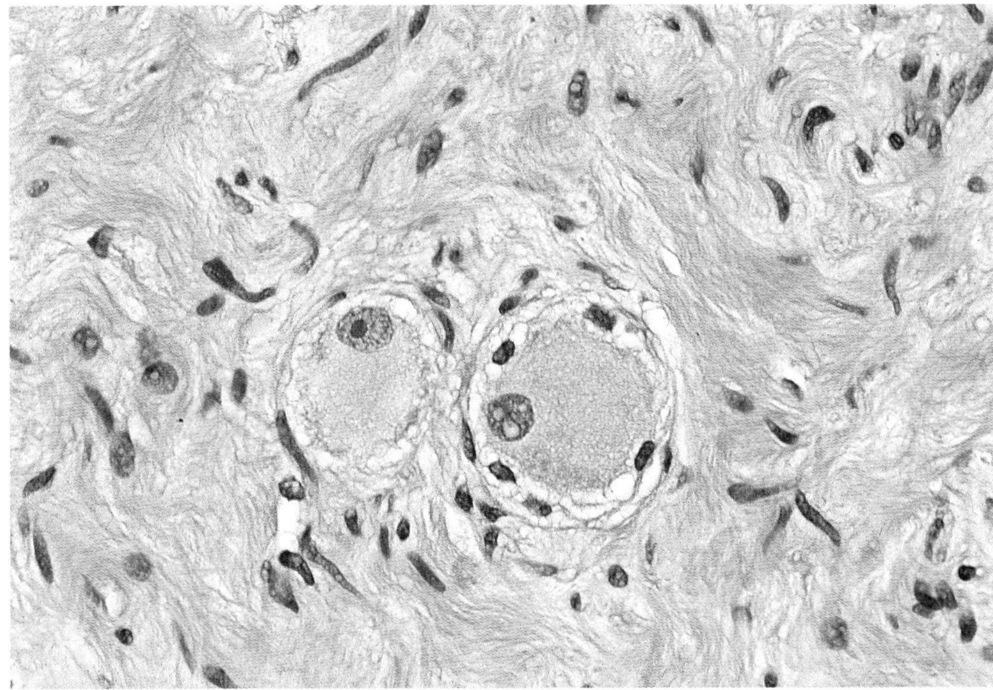

**FIGURE 32–24.** Mature ganglion cells with satellite cells in a ganglioneuroma.

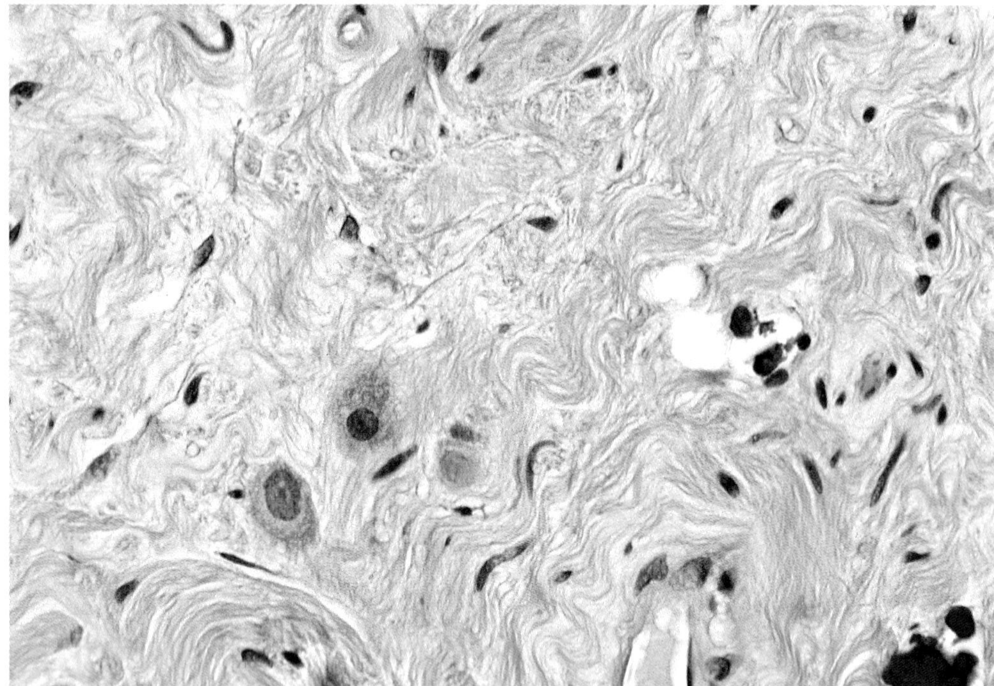

**FIGURE 32–25.** Ganglion cells from a ganglioneuroma having less Nissl substance and fewer satellite cells than their normal counterparts. Focal calcification is seen.

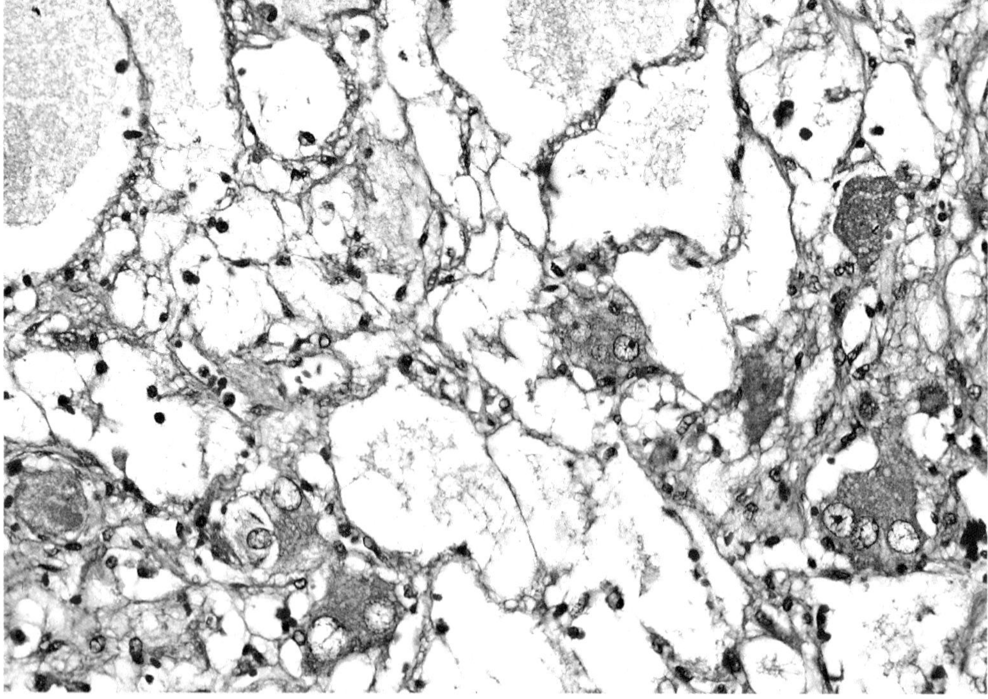

**FIGURE 32–26.** Cystic change in a ganglioneuroma obscuring the basic architecture of this lesion. Obvious ganglion cells can still be identified.

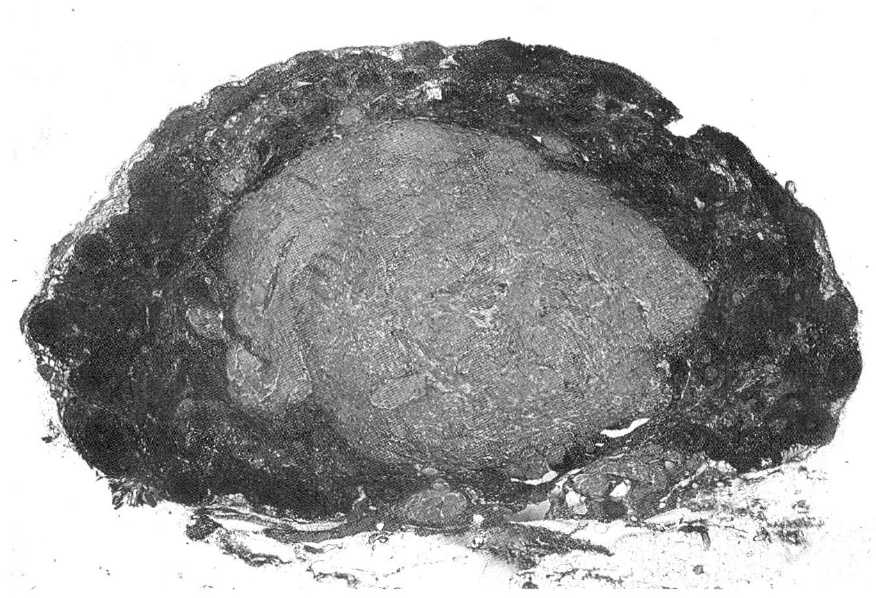

**FIGURE 32–27.** Apparent metastatic focus of a ganglioneuroma in a lymph node probably representing maturation of a neuroblastoma.

## GANGLION CELL CHORISTOMA

Collections of mature ganglion cells in the skin as an isolated, incidental finding have been termed "ganglion cell choristomas."[201–203] Rios et al.[203] reported such a tumor in a 14-year-old child. It consisted of a poorly circumscribed collection of mature ganglion cells in the dermis. The tumor was not associated with elevated levels of urinary VMA secretion, nor was the patient known to have a neuroblastoma. Lee et al.[201] described a slightly different dermal lesion containing a superficial ganglionic component associated with a deep dermal neuromatous component. Traumatic pharyngeal neuromas arising adjacent to autonomic ganglia may contain ganglion cells and thus may superficially resemble a ganglioneuroma.[200]

## EXTRASKELETAL EWING'S SARCOMA/PRIMITIVE NEUROECTODERMAL TUMOR FAMILY

There has been a remarkable evolution in the concepts regarding the histogenesis and relation of skeletal and extraskeletal Ewing's sarcoma and peripheral neuroepithelioma (also sometimes referred to as peripheral or adult neuroblastoma or, more commonly, primitive neuroectodermal tumor). In 1918, Arthur Purdy Stout[338] reported the case of a 42-year-old man with an ulnar nerve tumor composed of undifferentiated round cells that formed rosettes. Three years later James Ewing[250] reported a round cell neoplasm in the radius of a 14-year-old girl, calling it a "diffuse endothelioma of bone" and proposing an endothelial derivation. Over the next decades, there was much debate regarding the histogenesis of this neoplasm.[229,230,337,352] Some authors challenged its very existence as a distinct entity,[352] whereas others believed the tumor was derived from Oberling's bone marrow reticular cell.[337] It was not until 1975 that Angervall and Enzinger[207] described the first Ewing's sarcomas arising in soft tissue (extraskeletal ES). Subsequent reports confirmed the clinical and pathologic features of extraskeletal ES.[259,314,332]

At about the same time, Seemayer et al.[320] described peripheral neuroectodermal tumors (PNETs) that were unrelated to structures of the peripheral or sympathetic nervous system; subsequently Jaffe et al.[271] reported similar tumors in bone. In 1979 Askin et al.[211] described the "malignant small-cell tumor of the thoracopulmonary region" (Askin tumor) as having histologic features similar to those of PNETs but with a unique clinicopathologic profile. With the advent of immunohistochemical, cytogenetic, and molecular genetic techniques, it became apparent that the aforementioned lesions have overlapping features, supporting a common histogenesis.[239]

Identification of a common cytogenetic abnormality, t(11;22)(q24;q12), in Ewing's sarcoma[213] and PNET[350] has been used as a strong argument to support the hypothesis that these two neoplasms are histogenetically related. Since these early reports, numerous additional studies have found this translocation or variants involving 22q12, the site of the Ewing's sarcoma (*EWS*) gene, in 90–95% of Ewing's sarcoma and PNET.[253,345] As discussed below, identification of the novel fusion transcript that results from this translocation lends support to this relation. The two tumors

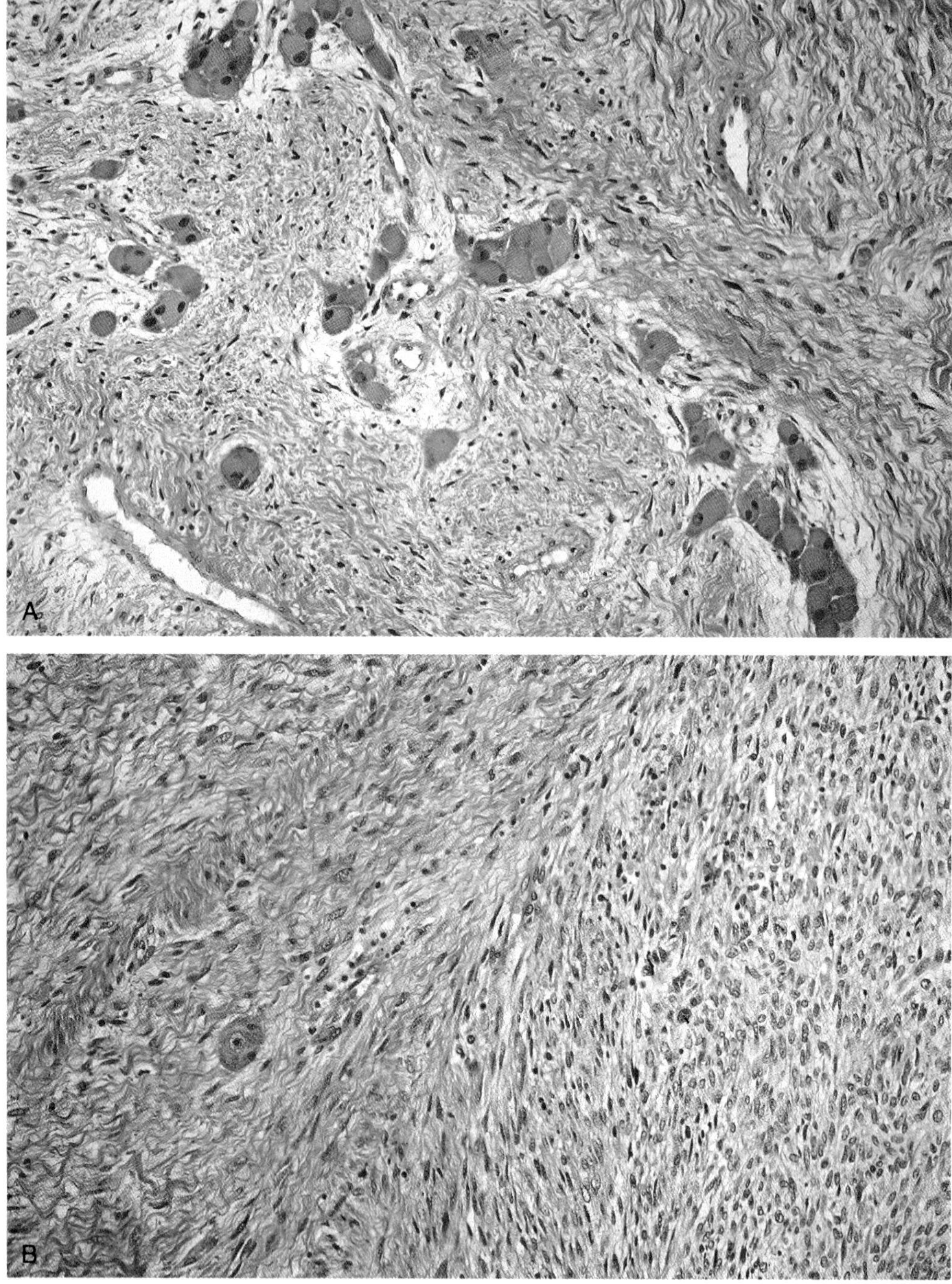


**FIGURE 32–28.** Rare example of malignant transformation of a ganglioneuroma to a malignant peripheral nerve sheath tumor. (**A**) Ganglioneuromatous portion of the tumor. (**B**) Interface between a ganglioneuroma and a malignant peripheral nerve sheath tumor.

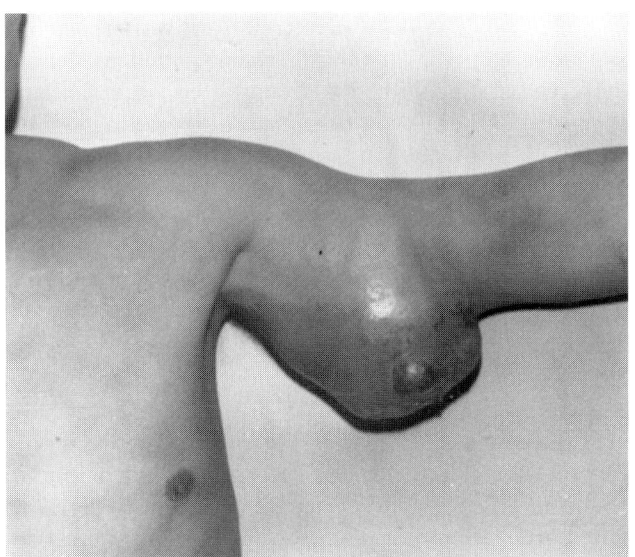

**FIGURE 32–29.** Primitive neuroectodermal tumor (peripheral neuroepithelioma) of the upper arm.

also share a consistent pattern of proto-oncogene expression (c-*myc*, c-*myb*, c-*src*, c-*mil*/*raf*),[217,334] which is distinct from that found in neuroblastomas; they also have the same cholinergic neurotransmitter enzymes and neural-associated glycolipid profile.[224] Finally, as many as 95% of Ewing's sarcomas and PNETs have been found to express the product of the *MIC2* gene,[335] further establishing a link between these tumors.

It is clear that there is a spectrum of clinical and pathologic features in this group of tumors. The discussion below elaborates on this spectrum for tumors arising in extraskeletal locations.

## Clinical Features

Most patients with ES/PNETs are adolescents or young adults, the majority of whom are less than 30 years of age.[239] Although the mean age for PNET is similar to that of extraskeletal ES, there tends to be a broader age range for the former, with a significant number of patients over the age of 40 years.[225,265,267,282,290,318] In contrast, patients with extraskeletal ES are rarely over age 40.[243,324] Both tumors are slightly more common in males than in females. African Americans rarely seem to be affected by this group of tumors.[255]

PNET most commonly arises in the extremities (Fig. 32–29). Studies reporting a high incidence of lesions in the paravertebral areas, especially in close relation to the vertebral foramina, possibly have included neuroblastomas. In our experience, the most common anatomic sites are the upper thigh and buttock followed by the upper arm and shoulder. Tumors that are intimately attached to a major nerve may give rise to signs and symptoms related to diminished neurologic function. There is no increased tendency for these tumors to occur in patients with von Recklinghausen's disease.

The principal sites of extraskeletal ES are the paravertebral region and chest wall, generally in close association with the vertebrae or the ribs (Fig. 32–30). These tumors may also arise in the soft tissues of the lower extremities and rarely in the pelvic and hip regions, the retroperitoneum, and the upper extremities.[207,259] Unusually they have been described in the lung,[223,344] uterus,[327] ovary,[276] urinary bladder,[216] myocardium,[228] parotid gland,[238] and kidney.[218,256,291,311,323]

In general, the tumor presents as a rapidly growing, deeply located mass measuring 5–10 cm in greatest diameter. Superficially located cases do occur but are rare.[215,266,321] The tumor is painful in about one-third of cases. If peripheral nerves or the spinal cord are involved, there may be progressive sensory or motor disturbances. As with other round cell sarcomas, the preoperative duration of symptoms is usually less than 1 year. Unlike neuroblastoma, catecholamine levels are within normal limits.[219]

## Pathologic Findings

The gross appearance of the tumor varies. In general, it is multilobulated, soft, and friable; it rarely exceeds 10 cm in greatest diameter. Its cut surface has a gray-yellow or gray-tan appearance, often with large areas of necrosis, cyst formation, or hemorrhage. Despite the extensive necrosis, calcification is rare.

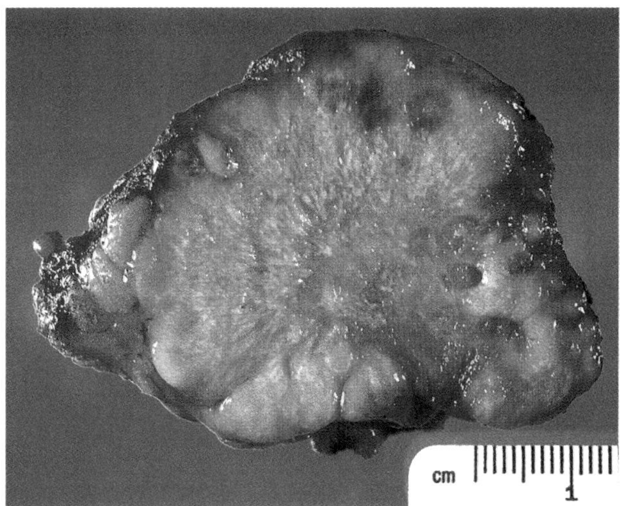


**FIGURE 32–30.** Gross photograph of a primitive neuroectodermal tumor from the chest wall of a 10-year-old boy. Foci of necrosis are apparent.

There is a spectrum of histologic change in this family of tumors, but criteria distinguishing Ewing's sarcoma, so-called atypical Ewing's sarcoma (large cell variant), and PNET are varied, as discussed below (Table 32–9). Because these lesions comprise a spectrum of histogenetically related tumors, the precise criteria for designating a tumor an extraskeletal ES, atypical Ewing's sarcoma or PNET are less critical.

The typical case of extraskeletal ES is marked by a solidly packed, lobular round cell pattern of striking uniformity (Figs. 32–31, 32–32). The individual cells have a round or ovoid nucleus measuring about 10–15 $\mu$m in diameter, with a distinct nuclear membrane, fine powdery chromatin, and one or two minute nucleoli. There are no multinucleated giant cells. The cytoplasm is ill-defined, scanty, and pale staining; and in many cases it is irregularly vacuolated as a result of intracellular deposits of glycogen (Figs. 32–33, 32–34). Intracellular glycogen is present in most cases, but the amount varies from tumor to tumor and sometimes in different portions of the same neoplasm. In addition, glycogen droplets may compress and indent the nucleus (Fig. 32–35). The number of mitotic figures varies, and in many cases the paucity of mitotic figures contrasts with the immature appearance of the tumor cells.[207]

Although the tumor is richly vascular, the thin-walled vessels are compressed and obscured by the closely packed tumor cells; the rich vascularity is often discernible only in areas of degeneration and necrosis (Fig. 32–36). In fact, the association of distinct vascular structures with degenerated or necrotic "ghost" cells is a common striking feature that has been described as the "filigree" pattern of Ewing's sarcoma (Fig. 32–37).[277] Aside from the prominent vascularity, there is occasionally a pseudovascular or pseudoalveolar pattern caused by small fluid-filled pools or spaces amid the solidly arranged tumor cells (Fig. 32–38), a feature occasionally misinterpreted as angiosarcoma or alveolar rhabdomyosarcoma by those unfamiliar with this secondary change. Presumably, this pattern was responsible for Ewing's initial designation of the tumor as a "diffuse endothelioma."[250]

In some cases the cells show increased nuclear size or cellular atypism. They have been described in the literature as "small cell" (lymphocytoid), "large cell," or "atypical" Ewing's sarcoma (Fig. 32–39).[297,299]

The typical PNET is composed of sheets or lobules of small round cells containing darkly staining, round or oval nuclei (Fig. 32–40). The cytoplasm is indistinct except in areas where the cells are more mature and the elongated hair-like cytoplasmic extensions coalesce to form rosettes (Fig. 32–41). Most of the rosettes are similar to those seen in neuroblastomas and contain a central solid core of neurofibrillary material (Homer Wright rosette). Rarely, the rosettes resemble those of retinoblastoma and contain a central lumen or vesicle (Flexner-Wintersteiner rosette). Some tumors are composed of cords or trabeculae of small round cells. These areas bear a resemblance to a carcinoid tumor or a small-cell undifferentiated carcinoma, although histogenetically they are properly compared with primitive neuroepithelium. About 10–20% of PNETs display spindled areas that resemble a primitive fibrosarcoma or malignant schwannoma (Fig. 32–42). There are also rare tumors with glial, ependymal, cartilaginous, or epithelial differentiation.[264]

## Ultrastructural Features

Similar to the spectrum of histologic findings, there is also an ultrastructural spectrum of neural differentiation in the ES/PNET family (Table 32–10). Extraskeletal ES has primitive undifferentiated cells with uniform round or ovoid nuclei, a smooth nuclear envelope, and finely granular chromatin with one or

*Text continued on page 1299*

**TABLE 32–9 SPECTRUM OF LIGHT MICROSCOPIC FEATURES ACROSS THE ES/PNET FAMILY OF TUMORS**

| Feature | Classic Ewing's sarcoma | Atypical Ewing's sarcoma | PNET |
|---|---|---|---|
| Cell shape | Uniform, round | Irregular | Irregular |
| Chromatin | Fine | Coarse | Coarse |
| Nucleoli | Pinpoint | More prominent | Prominent |
| Glycogen | Abundant | Moderate | Scant |
| Rosettes | Absent | Absent | Present |

Modified from Navarro S, Cavazanna AO, Llombart-Bosch A, et al. Comparison of Ewing's sarcoma of bone and peripheral neuroepithelioma: an immunocytochemical and ultrastructural analysis of two primitive neuroectodermal neoplasms. Arch Pathol Lab Med 118:608, 1994.

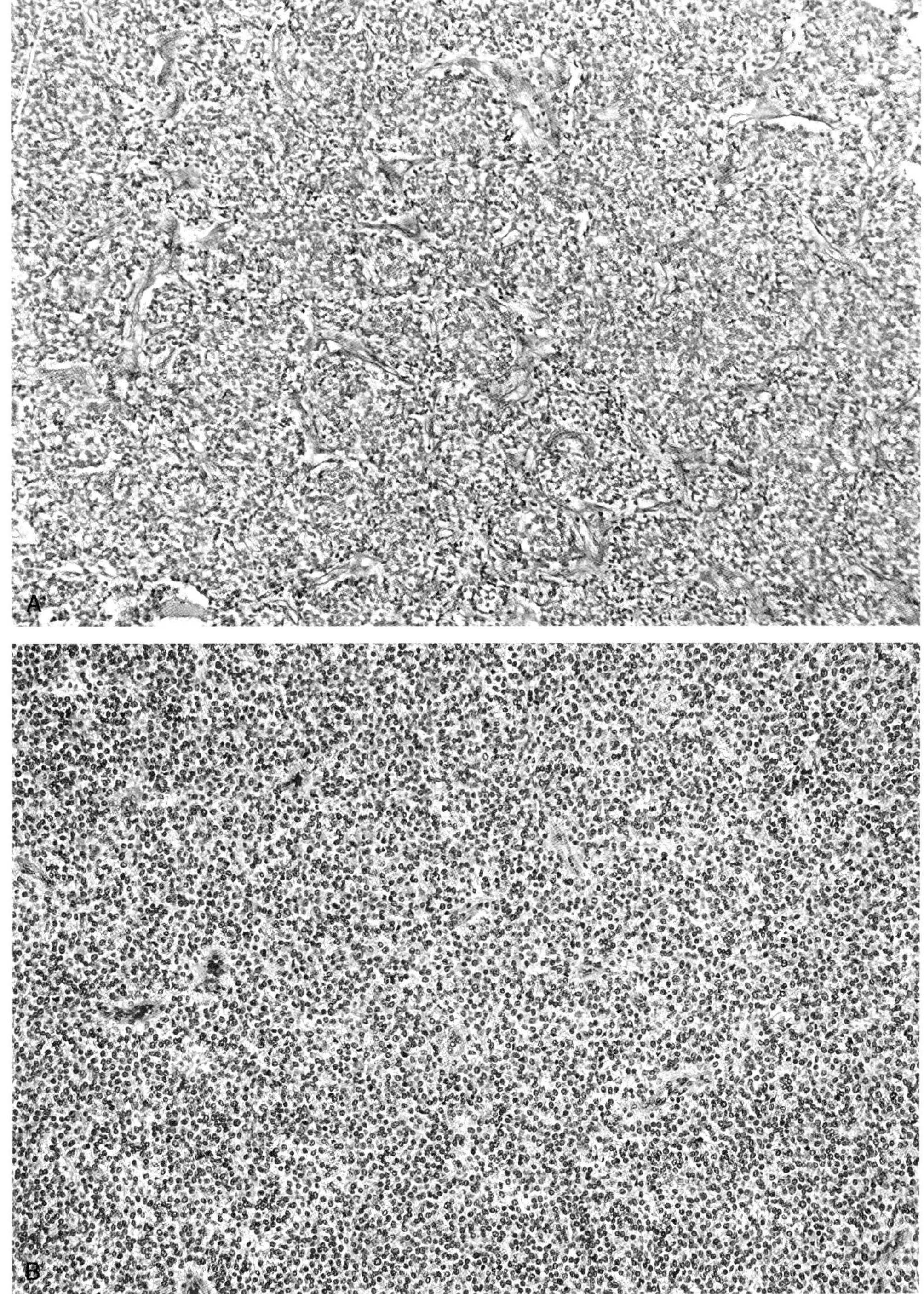

**FIGURE 32–31.** (**A**) Low-power view of extraskeletal Ewing's sarcoma characterized by a lobular round cell pattern of striking uniformity. (**B**) Typical low-power view of the monotonous appearance of this tumor.

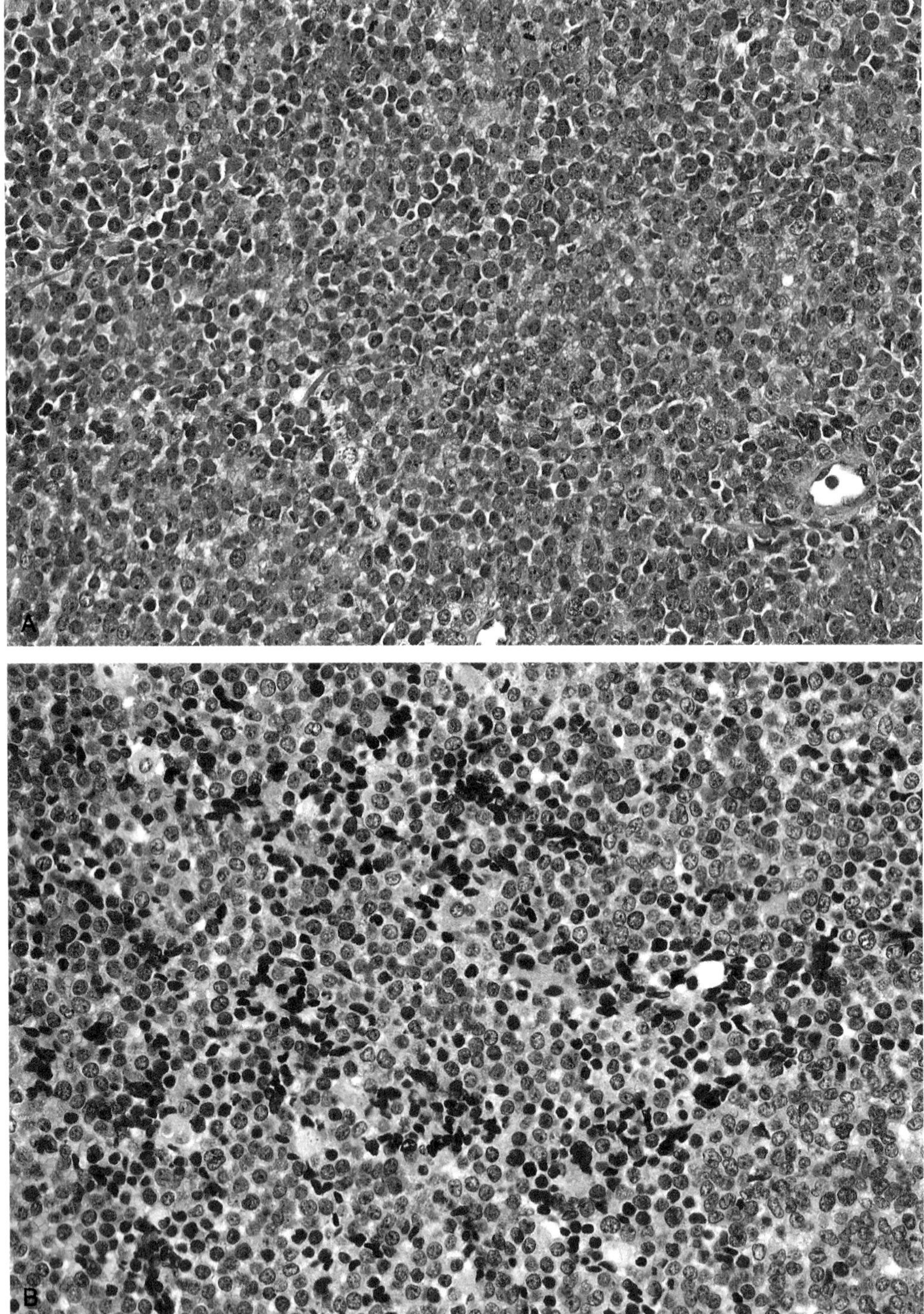

**FIGURE 32–32.** (**A**) Extraskeletal Ewing's sarcoma composed of a monotonous proliferation of round cells. Homer Wright rosettes are not seen. (**B**) Admixture of small round cells with crushed darker-staining cells.

*Illustration continued on opposite page*

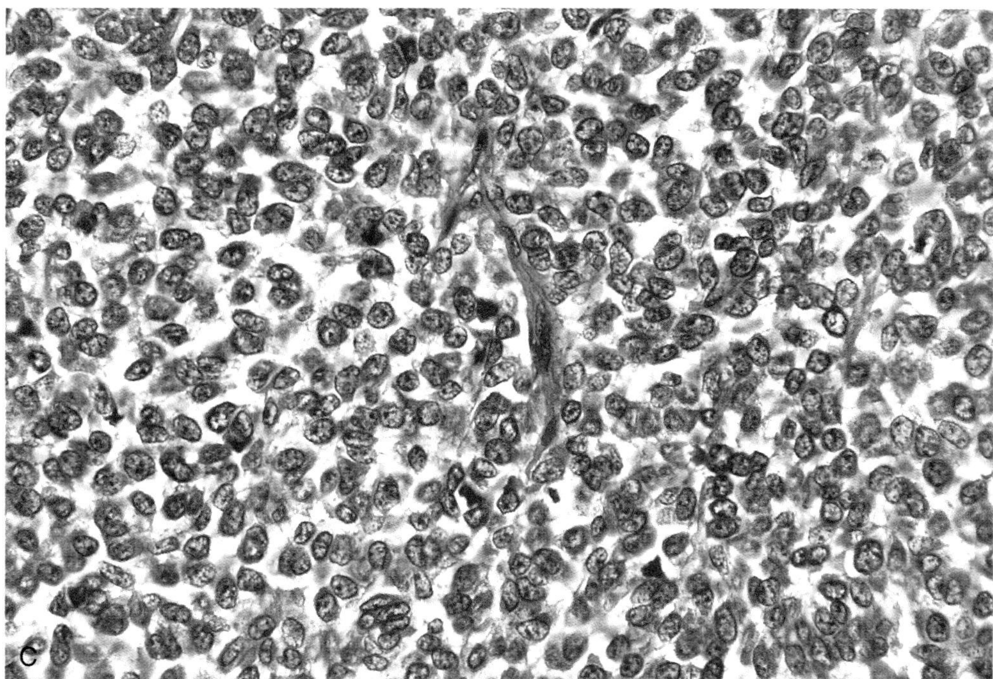

**FIGURE 32–32** *(Continued).* (**C**) High-power view of round cell proliferation in an extraskeletal Ewing's sarcoma.

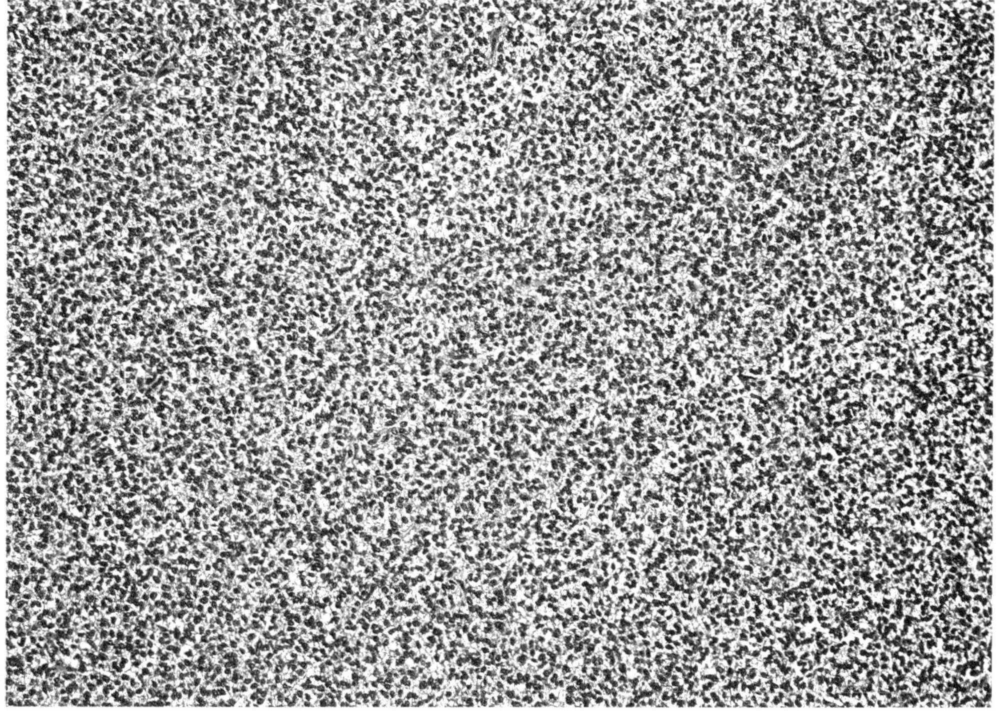

**FIGURE 32–33.** Low-power view of extraskeletal Ewing's sarcoma composed of cells with abundant cleared-out cytoplasm secondary to glycogen deposition.

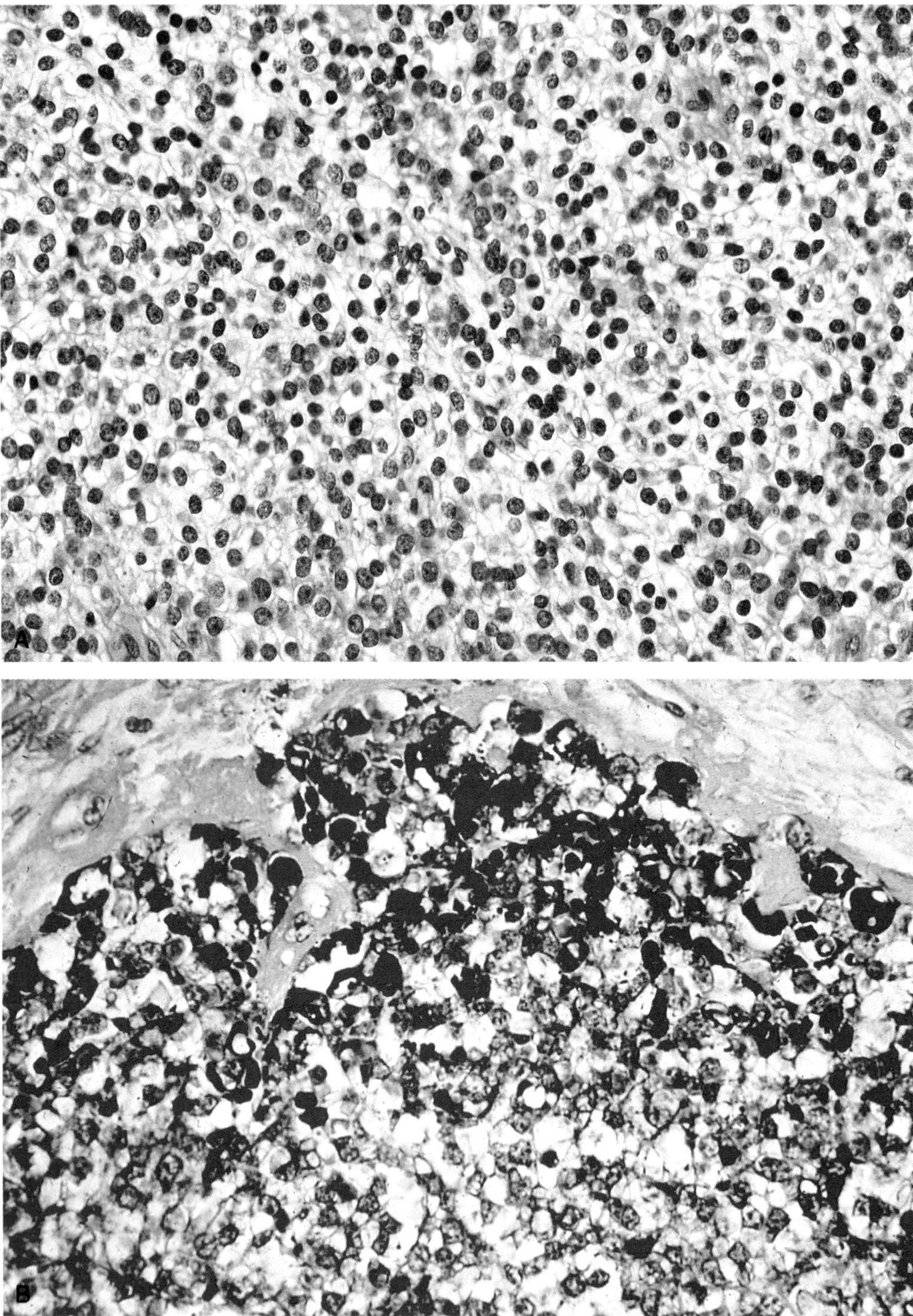

**FIGURE 32–34.** (**A**) Cells with abundant cleared-out cytoplasm and clearly defined cell borders in extraskeletal Ewing's sarcoma. (**B**) Extraskeletal Ewing's sarcoma. PAS preparation reveals intracellular glycogen, especially in the peripheral portion of the tumor.

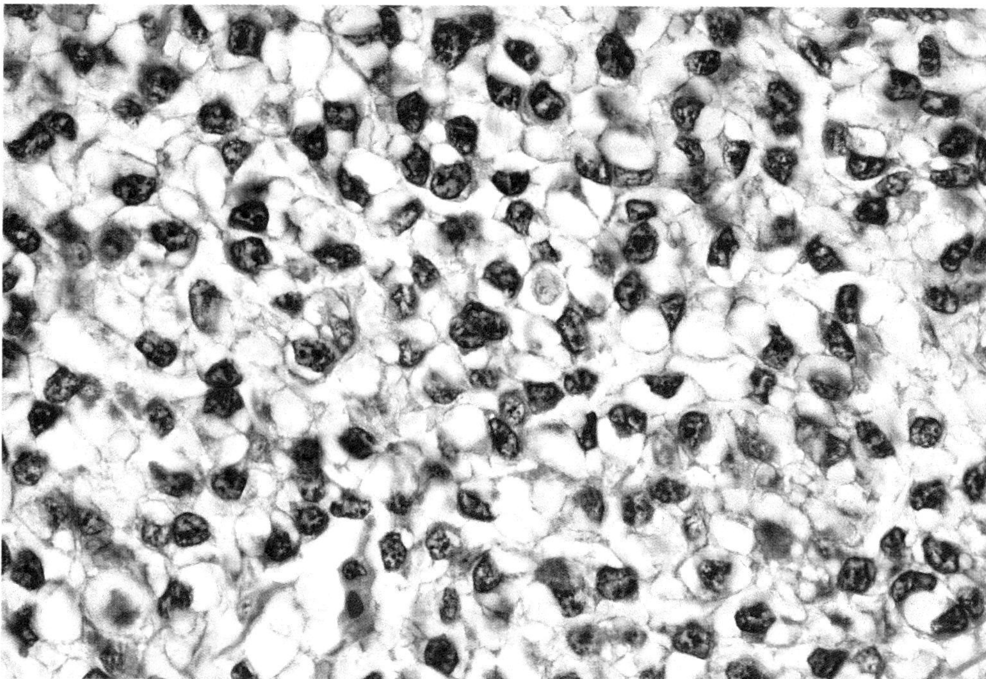

**FIGURE 32–35.** Extraskeletal Ewing's sarcoma. Cytoplasmic vacuoles secondary to the deposition of intracellular glycogen often indent the nuclei.

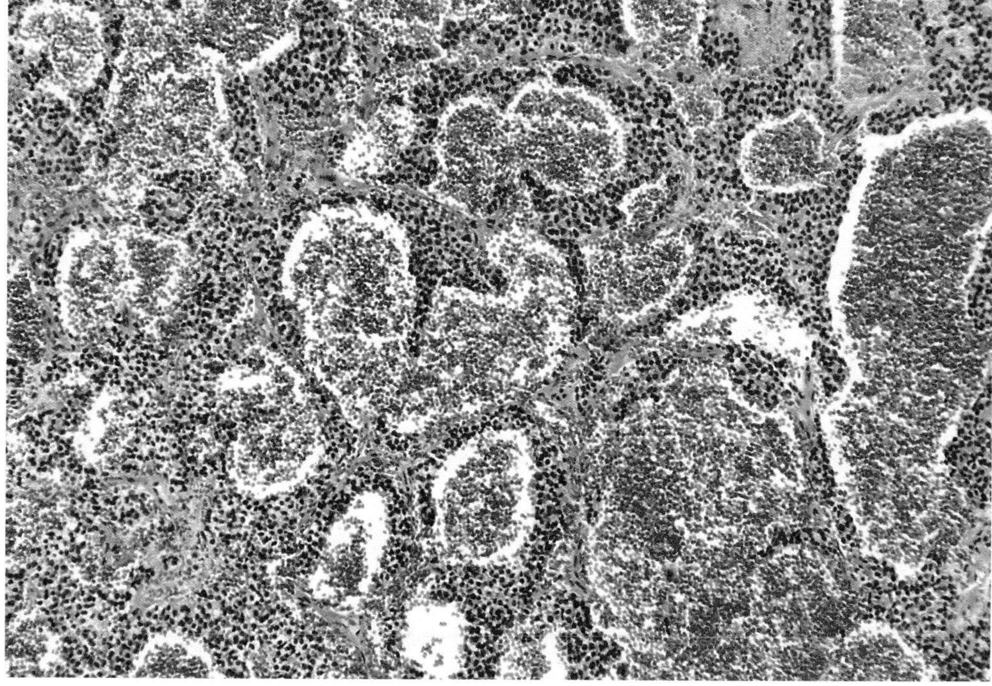

**FIGURE 32–36.** Hemorrhagic zone in extraskeletal Ewing's sarcoma resembling a vascular neoplasm.

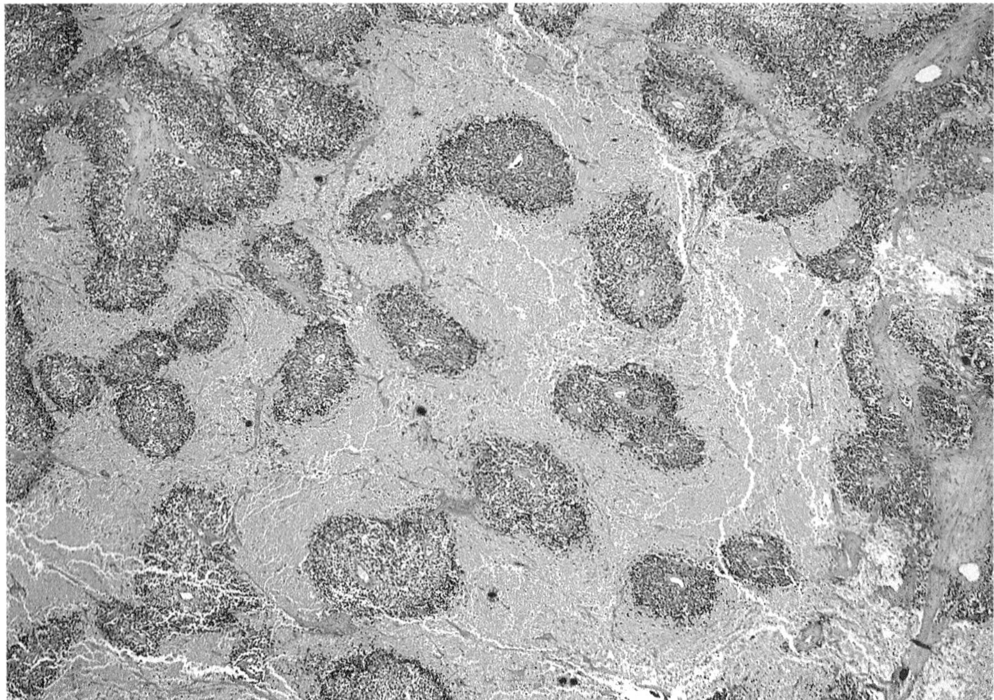

**FIGURE 32–37.** Extensive zones of necrosis in extraskeletal Ewing's sarcoma. There is maintenance of the tumor cells around blood vessels.

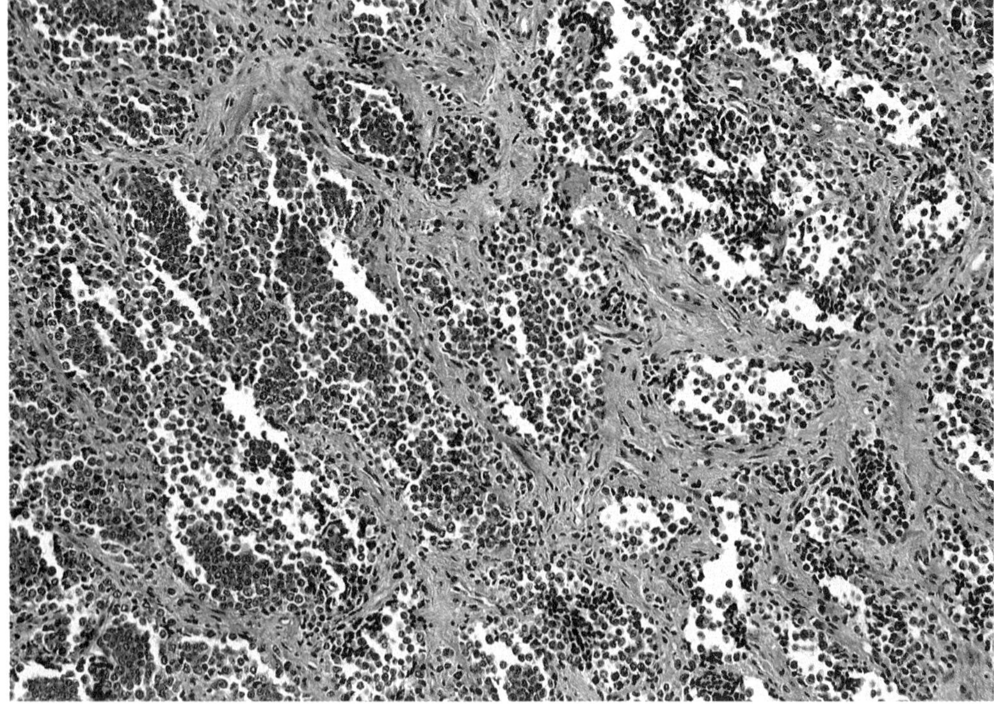

**FIGURE 32–38.** Pseudoalveolar pattern in an extraskeletal Ewing's sarcoma superficially resembling an alveolar rhabdomyosarcoma.

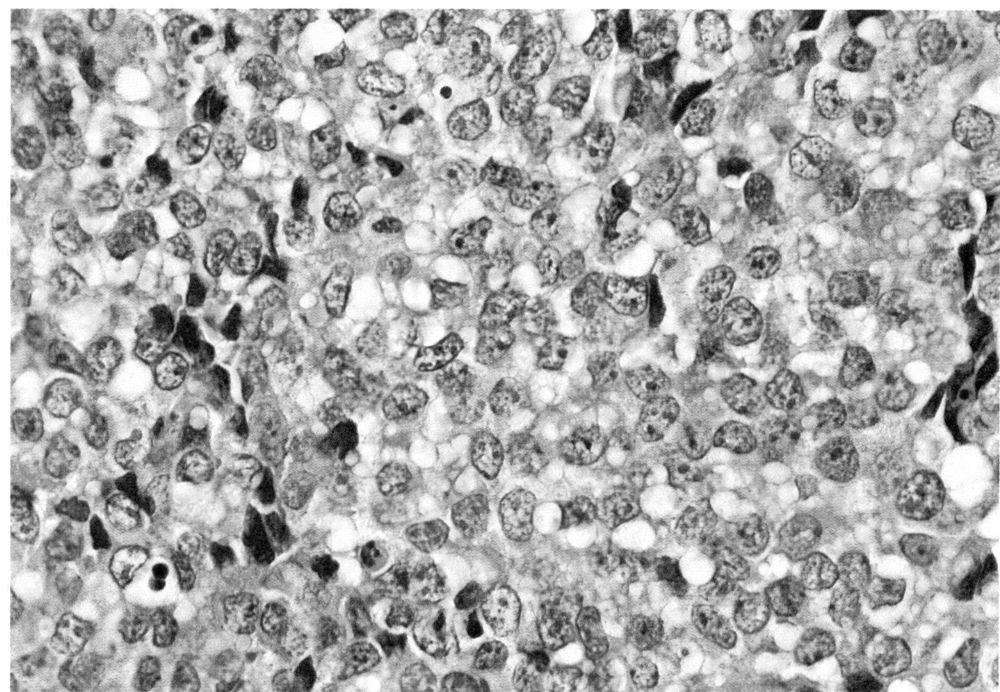

**FIGURE 32–39.** High-power view of large cells in an extraskeletal Ewing's sarcoma. The cells have vesicular chromatin and prominent nucleoli. Such tumors have been described as atypical or large-cell variants of Ewing's sarcoma.

two small nucleoli (Fig. 32–43).[279,298,299] Characteristically, the cytoplasm contains few organelles, including a small number of mitochondria, a poorly developed Golgi complex, and abundant glycogen, sometimes containing small lipid droplets. There are also free ribosomes, inconspicuous rough endoplasmic reticulum, occasional membrane-bound dense bodies (presumably lysosomes), and bundles of intermediate nonspecific filaments. The cells are closely apposed and are joined by infrequent, rudimentary cell junctions. Bundles of myofilaments, Weibel-Palade bodies, and distinct basal laminae are absent.[249,351]

On the other end of the spectrum, the typical PNET is characterized by the presence of elongated cell processes that interdigitate with each other and contain small dense-core granules (neurosecretory granules) that measure 50–100 nm and occasionally contain microtubules.[220,346] The processes are most highly developed in the center of the rosette and in the neurofibrillary areas, where they form a tangled mass. They are also noted in areas that display little neurofibrillary differentiation by light microscopy.

## Immunohistochemical Findings

For many years, a diagnosis of ES/PNET was essentially an immunohistochemical diagnosis of exclusion. More recently, numerous data have been published regarding the product of the *MIC2* gene (HBA71 antigen, glycoprotein p30/32, or CD99) in this group of tumors, confirming the high sensitivity of this marker

**TABLE 32–10** SPECTRUM OF ULTRASTRUCTURAL FEATURES ACROSS THE ES/PNET FAMILY OF TUMORS

| Feature | Classic Ewing's sarcoma | Atypical Ewing's sarcoma | PNET |
|---|---|---|---|
| Organelles | Scarce | Moderate | Abundant |
| Dense-core granules | Absent | Rare | Abundant |
| Neurotubules | Absent | Rare | Abundant |
| Neuritic processes | Absent | Rare | Abundant |

Modified from Navarro S, Cavazanna AO, Llombart-Bosch A, et al. Comparison of Ewing's sarcoma of bone and peripheral neuroepithelioma: an immunocytochemical and ultrastructural analysis of two primitive neuroectodermal neoplasms. Arch Pathol Lab Med 118:608, 1994.

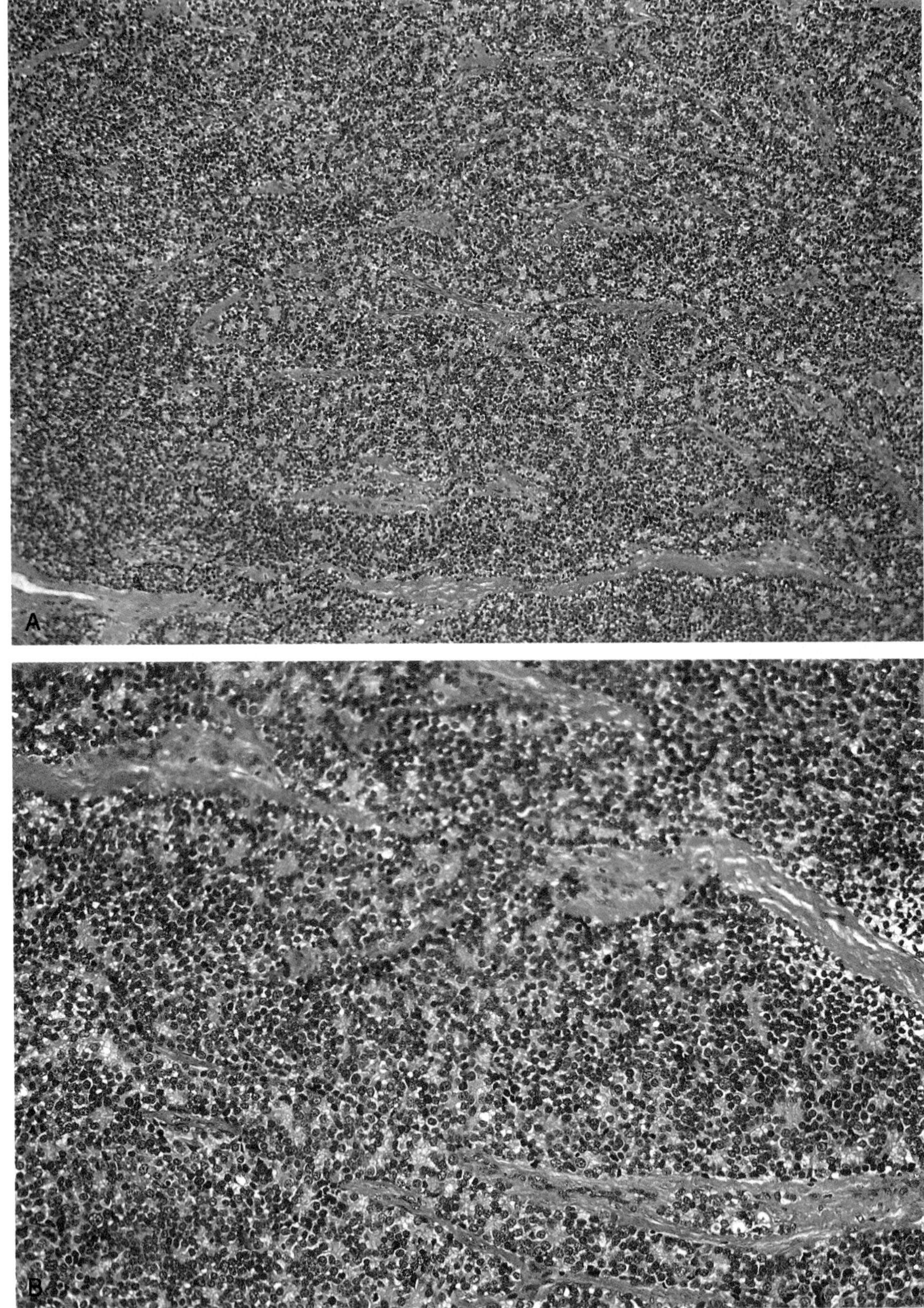

**FIGURE 32–40.** (**A, B**) Primitive neuroectodermal tumor (peripheral neuroepithelioma) with distinctive lobular architecture and numerous Homer Wright rosettes apparent at low magnification.

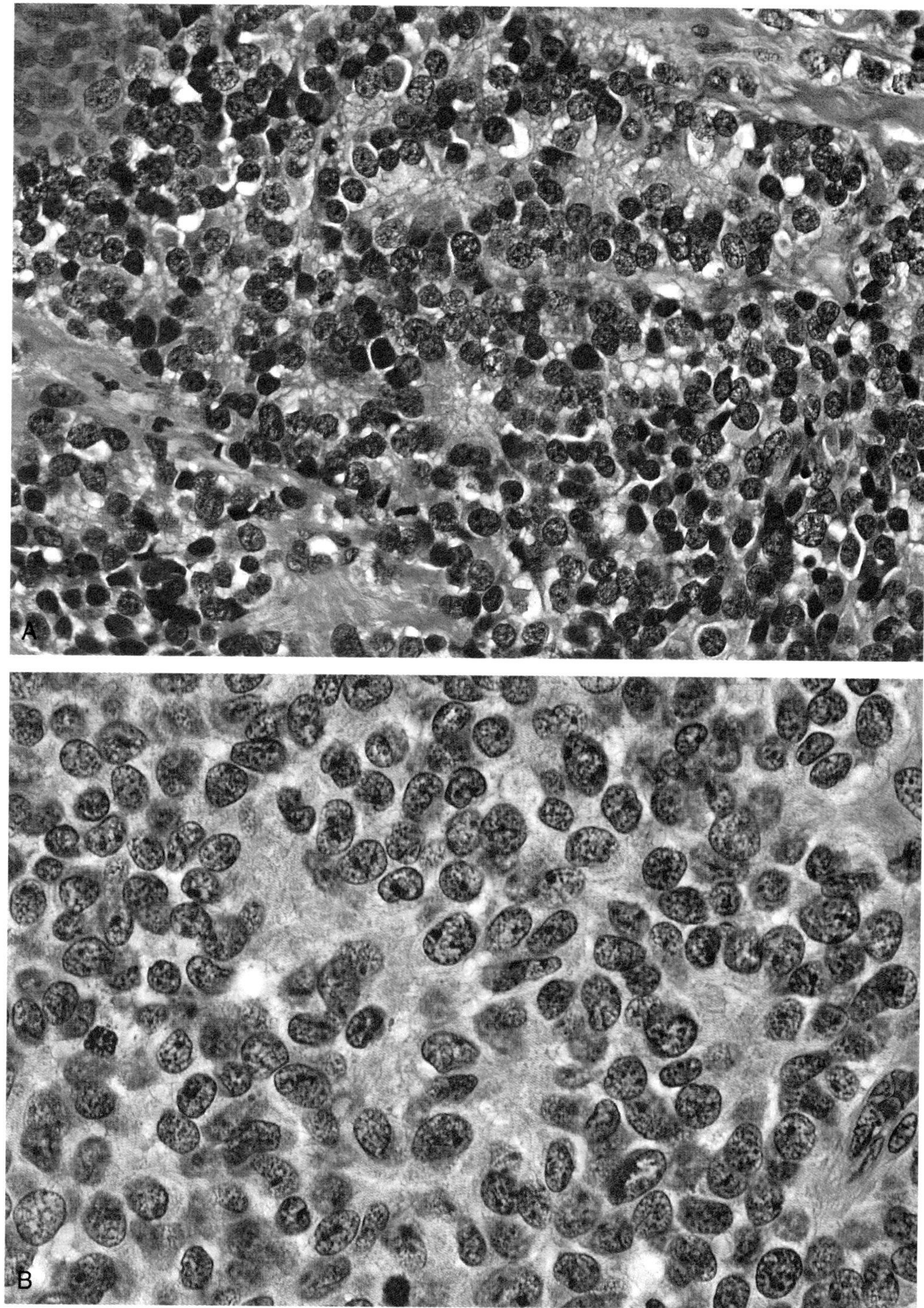

**FIGURE 32–41.** (A, B) Primitive neuroectodermal tumor (peripheral neuroepithelioma). Large cells with vesicular nuclei and prominent nucleoli surround a central fibrillary core (Homer Wright rosettes).

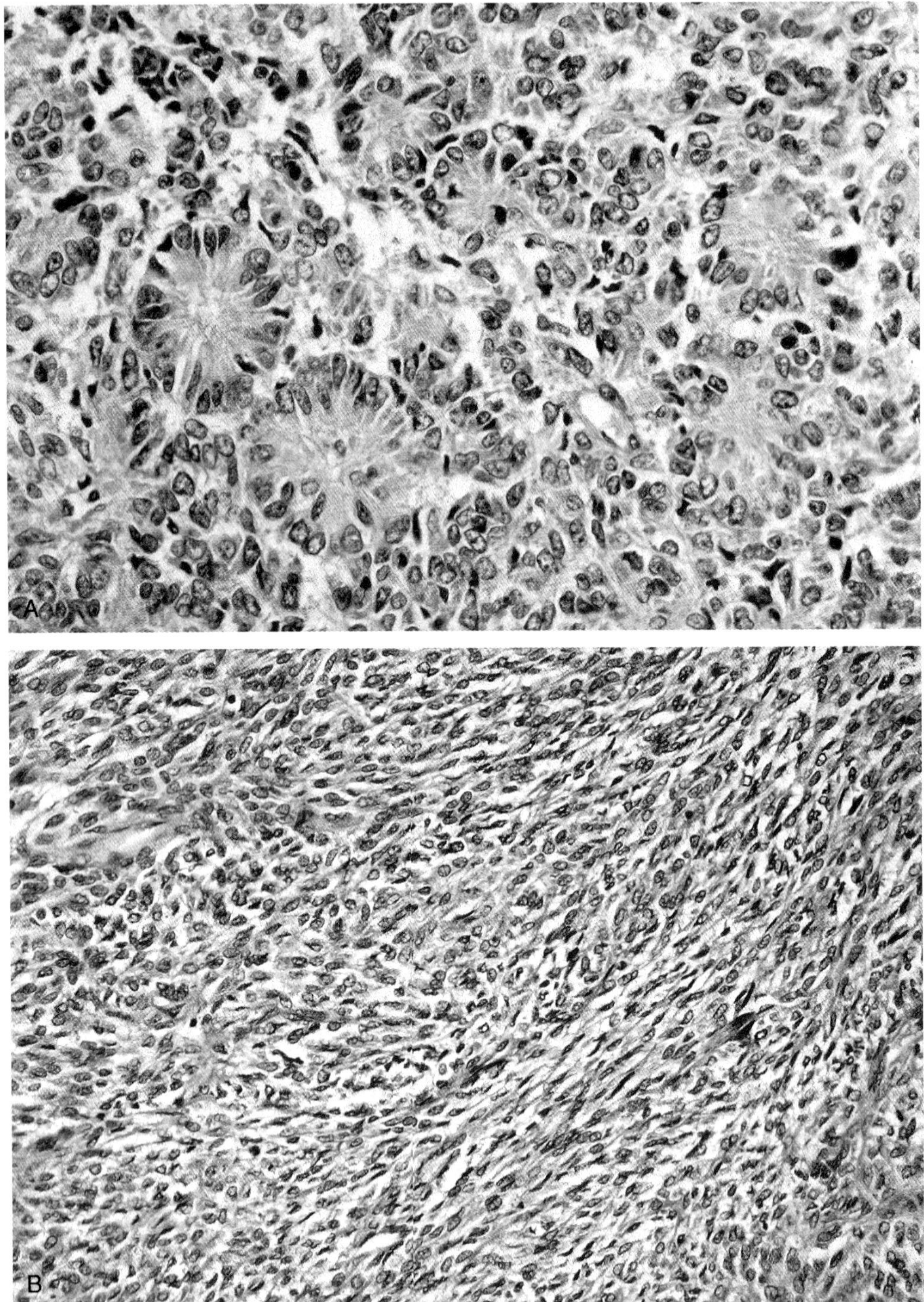


**FIGURE 32–42.** Primitive neuroectodermal tumor (peripheral neuroepithelioma) with round cell areas containing rosettes (**A**) and spindled areas (**B**) coexisting in the same tumor.

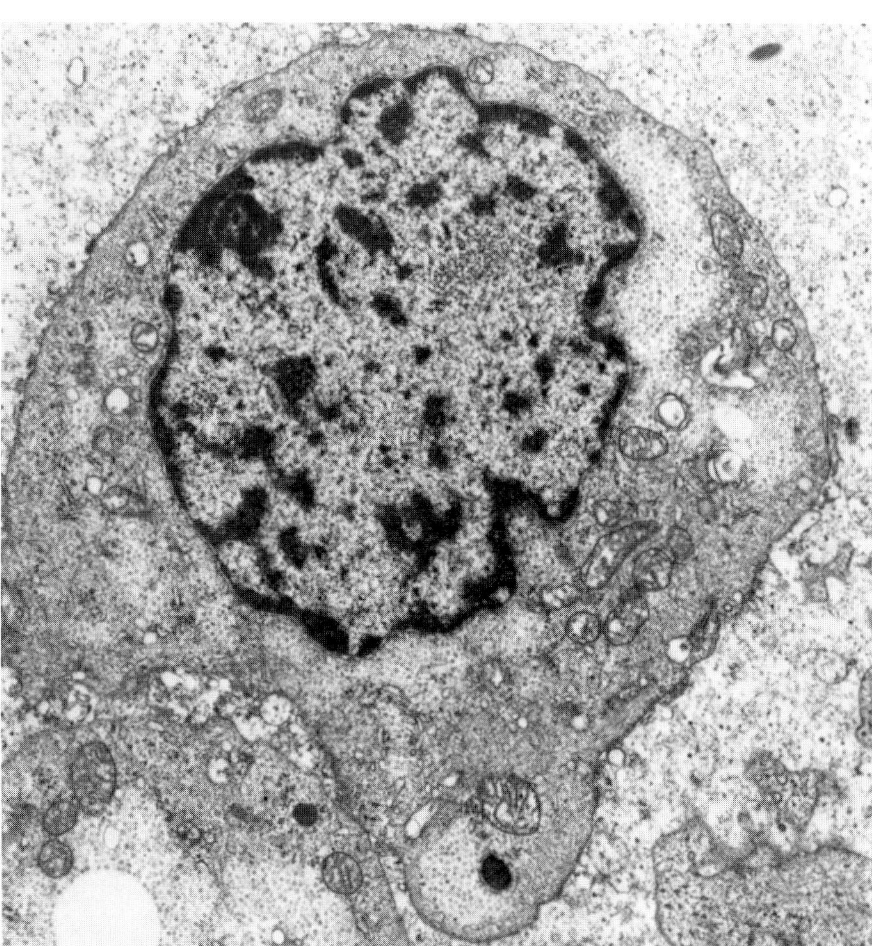

**FIGURE 32–43.** Electron microscopic view of a tumor in the extraskeletal Ewing's sarcoma/primitive neuroectodermal tumor family. This cell has a prominent nucleus with marginated chromatin, few organelles, and abundant glycogen.

for the ES/PNET family (Fig. 32–44).[206,251,308,312,348] The *MIC2* gene is a pseudoautosomal gene located on the short arms of the sex chromosomes,[261] and its product is a membranous glycoprotein that can be detected immunohistochemically using a variety of antibodies, including 12E7 and O13. Although initially believed to be highly specific, it is apparent that virtually all other round cell tumors in the differential diagnosis, on rare occasion, show membranous immunoreactivity for the *MIC2* gene product, including lymphomas, particularly T-lymphoblastic lymphoma[313] and precursor B-lymphoblastic lymphoma,[305] Merkel cell carcinoma,[309,331] small-cell carcinoma,[287] rhabdomyosarcoma,[268] small-cell osteosarcoma,[244] desmoplastic small round cell tumor,[257] and mesenchymal chondrosarcoma (Table 32–11).[262] Notably, childhood neuroblastomas have not been reported to stain for this antigen. Thus although immunostains for CD99 are highly sensitive for recognizing the ES/PNET family of tumors, this marker should be used as part of a panel of immunostains, given the lack of complete specificity.

Many ES/PNETs also stain for myriad neural markers, including neuron-specific enolase, Leu-7, S-100 protein, synaptophysin, and PGP 9.5.[222,283,286,322] Although PNETs tend to express one or more of these neural markers with greater frequency than ex-

**TABLE 32–11 FREQUENCY OF CD99 IMMUNOREACTIVITY IN ES/PNET FAMILY AND OTHER SMALL ROUND CELL TUMORS**

| Diagnosis | Positive (%) |
|---|---|
| ES/PNET | 95 |
| T-lymphoblastic lymphoma | 92 |
| Poorly differentiated synovial sarcoma | 50 |
| Small cell osteosarcoma | 23 |
| Rhabdomyosarcoma | 21 |
| Desmoplastic small round cell tumor | 16 |
| Small-cell carcinoma | 9 |
| Merkel cell carcinoma | 9 |
| Neuroblastoma | 0 |

Data are from Scotlandi et al.[319] and Stevenson et al.[335]

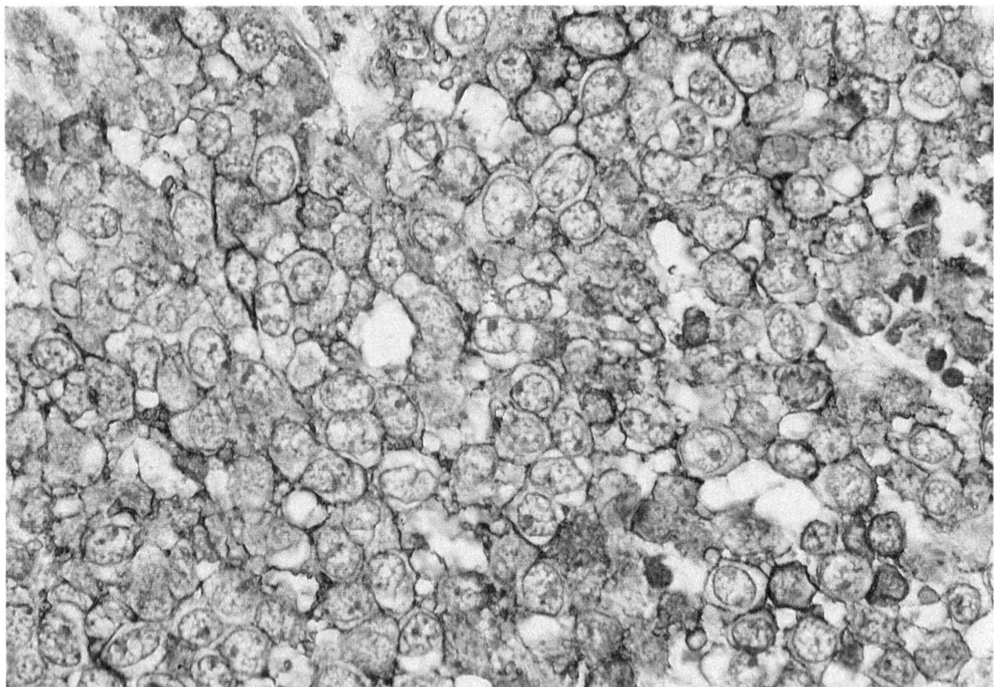

**FIGURE 32–44.** Strong membranous CD99 immunoreactivity in an extraskeletal Ewing's sarcoma/primitive neuroectodermal tumor.

traskeletal ES, there is significant overlap. It must be kept in mind that in many of the reported studies the immunohistochemical expression of neural markers is used as one of the criteria to differentiate cases of extraskeletal ES from PNET. Shanfeld et al.[322] found that the degree of immunohistochemical expression of neural markers in tumors that lack light microscopic evidence of neural differentiation was not predictive of clinical behavior. In addition, the degree of expression of these antigens has not been found to be related to the specific *EWS* gene fusion type.[205] Up to 20% of tumors have focal immunoreactivity for low-molecular-weight cytokeratins,[262a,284,302] although these tumors do not express cytokeratins 7 or 19, a useful finding for distinguishing them from poorly differentiated synovial sarcoma.[288] Desmin has been described in two PNETs that had rosettes (seen on light microscopy) and neural features (seen by electron microscopy) but had no ultrastructural evidence of muscle differentiation.[306] In addition, there are several reports of "biphenotypic small-cell sarcomas" with both neuroectodermal and muscle differentiation.[235,330]

## Cytogenetic Findings

Approximately 90–95% of ES/PNETs are characterized by rearrangements of the *EWS* gene on 22q12 and *ETS*-related oncogenes, most commonly *FLI1* on 11q24 (Table 32–12).[241,242] Less commonly, the *EWS* gene is fused with other *ETS*-related genes, including *ERG* on 21q22,[243,328] *ETV1* on 7p22,[272,326] *E1AF* on 17q12,[274] or *FEV* on 2q33[310] (Fig. 32–45). The translocation breakpoints are restricted to introns 7–10 of the *EWS* gene and introns 3–9 of the *ETS*-related genes,[354] with the most common fusion being between exon 7 of *EWS* and exons 5 or 6 of *FLI1*.[236,353] These translocations result in a novel chimeric gene that encodes for a chimeric transcript and protein, the function of which is largely unknown; however, *EWS/FLI1* antagonists have been found to inhibit growth of tumor cells in vitro.[280,339,342] Given the limitations of traditional cytogenetic techniques for detecting these translocations,[226,245] the ability to detect fusion transcripts by molecular genetic techniques (fluorescence in situ hybridization[260,293,294] and RT-PCR[247,248,329]) using fixed, paraffin-embedded tissues[204,281,319] has greatly facilitated the diagnosis of these tumors. Although highly sensitive and specific for the ES/PNET

**TABLE 32–12** TUMORS REPORTED TO HAVE t(11;22)(q24;q12)

| |
|---|
| Skeletal and extraskeletal Ewing's sarcoma |
| Primitive neuroectodermal tumor |
| Malignant small-cell tumor of thoracopulmonary region (Askin's tumor) |
| Olfactory neuroblastoma |
| Small-cell osteosarcoma |
| Mesenchymal chondrosarcoma |

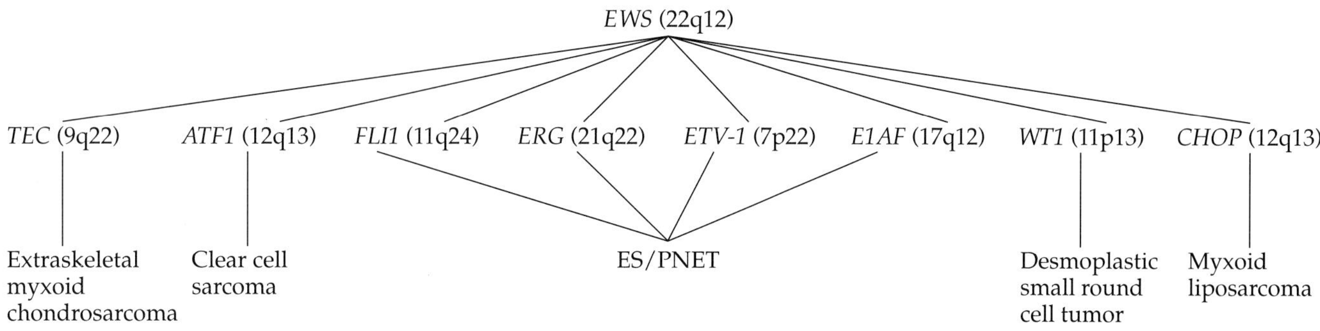


**FIGURE 32–45.** Critical role of the *EWS* gene (22q12) in the molecular genesis of sarcomas.

family of tumors, Thorner et al.[341] reported four tumors with this fusion transcript that lacked morphologic and immunohistochemical features typical of this group of tumors. Furthermore, there are several reports of biphenotypic sarcomas with both myogenic and neural differentiation with the *EWS/FLI1* fusion transcript.[235,330]

Secondary cytogenetic abnormalities that occur in this group of tumors have been described, including trisomy 8,[210,295] trisomy 12,[292] and t(1;16).[246,333] These cytogenetic abnormalities lack sufficient sensitivity and specificity for diagnostic purposes.

## Differential Diagnosis

Although a histogenetic relation between PNET and extraskeletal ES has been clearly established, the issue as to whether there is any clinical significance in differentiating between these lesions has yet to be resolved. Part of the difficulty lies in the variability of criteria for classifying lesions as either extraskeletal ES or PNET.[225,265,269,282] Whereas some studies require histologic evidence of rosette formation for a diagnosis of PNET, others require immunohistochemical evidence of neural differentiation, with or without rosettes. For example, in the study by Schmidt et al.,[318] a tumor was designated a PNET if it had Homer Wright rosettes on light microscopy or co-expressed two or more neural markers by immunohistochemistry. Using such criteria, the authors found that patients with PNET had a more aggressive clinical course than those with extraskeletal ES. Using identical criteria, however, others were unable to distinguish significant clinical differences between these tumors.[307,325] In the past, we diagnosed PNET if the tumor showed well-defined rosettes of the Homer Wright or Flexner-Wintersteiner type, if there were two or more positive neural markers, or if there was ultrastructural evidence of neural differentiation. Such arbitrary designations may become obsolete if future prospective studies fail to reveal significant clinical differences between these entities. Currently, we prefer to classify these tumors as members of the ES/PNET family, followed by a comment as to the presence or absence of light microscopic, immunohistochemical (Table 32–13), or ultrastructural features supporting neural differentiation.

Neuroblastoma enters the differential diagnosis because of the young age of some patients, the frequent paravertebral location of the tumor, and the presence of rosette-like structures of the Homer Wright type in some of the tumors. The average age of patients with ES/PNET is older than that of patients with neuroblastoma by a significant margin. Furthermore, patients with neuroblastoma often have elevated urinary catecholamine metabolite levels, a feature not found

**TABLE 32–13** IMMUNOHISTOCHEMICAL ANALYSIS OF ROUND CELL TUMORS

| Tumor | CD99 | NB-84 | NSE | S-100 | Desmin | Myogenin/ MyoD1 | CK | LCA |
|---|---|---|---|---|---|---|---|---|
| ES/PNET | ● | ◗ | ◗ | ◗ | — | — | ◗ | — |
| Rhabdomyosarcoma | ◗ | ◗ | ◗ | ◗ | ● | ● | ◗ | — |
| Neuroblastoma | — | ● | ● | ◗ | — | — | — | — |
| Desmoplastic small round cell tumor | ◗ | ◗ | ● | ◗ | ● | — | ● | — |
| Mesenchymal chondrosarcoma | ● | — | ● | ◗ | — | — | ◗ | — |
| Lymphoblastic lymphoma | ● | — | — | — | — | — | — | ● |

CK, cytokeratin; LCA, leukocyte common antigen; ● = usually positive; ◗ = rarely positive.

in patients with ES/PNET. The presence of mats of neuropil and ganglionic differentiation are usually features of primary or metastatic neuroblastoma, although focal ganglionic differentiation has rarely been described in ES/PNETs.[278,289] Intracellular glycogen is rare in neuroblastomas and may be discernible only by electron microscopy. Also, in contrast to neuroblastomas, the necrotic areas in ES/PNETs rarely undergo calcification.[343] Expression of CD99, as previously mentioned, all but excludes neuroblastoma as a diagnostic consideration. Although the monoclonal antibody NB84 is a highly sensitive marker of neuroblastoma, it is found in up to 20% of ES/PNETs. Finally, neuroblastoma is characterized by a consistent cytogenetic abnormality (deletion of the short arm of chromosome 1) and lacks the t(11;22) found in the ES/PNET family of tumors (Table 32–14).

Alveolar rhabdomyosarcoma may display similar densely packed cellular areas, especially at its periphery, but in general its nuclei contain more chromatin and tend to be more irregular in outline. When multiple sections are examined, the solid round cell areas are nearly always associated with areas showing loss of cellular cohesion and a distinct alveolar pattern, multinucleated giant cells with marginally placed nuclei, and in about 20–30% of cases eosinophilic cells characteristic of rhabdomyoblasts with or without cross-striations. Furthermore, most rhabdomyosarcomas show positive immunostaining for muscle markers, including myogenin and MyoD1, although desmin is rarely detected in ES/PNETs. It must also be kept in mind that some rhabdomyosarcomas exhibit membranous staining for CD99. Detection of t(2;13)(q35;q14) characteristic of alveolar rhabdomyosarcoma by cytogenetic or molecular genetic techniques is useful for distinguishing alveolar rhabdomyosarcoma from ES/PNET.[248]

Malignant (non-Hodgkin's) lymphoma is often suspected because of the undifferentiated appearance of the tumor cells. This diagnosis can be ruled out in most cases if attention is paid to the lobular arrangement and monotonous uniformity of the nuclei in ES/PNETs, the presence of stainable intracellular glycogen, and the lack of reticulin fibrils in the tumor lobules. The presence or absence of lymph node involvement may be significant, as lymph node metastasis of ES/PNET is rare. Furthermore, malignant lymphomas almost always express leukocyte common antigen. Because CD99 is found in most T cell lymphoblastic lymphomas[313,348] and rare lymphoblastic lymphomas do not express leukocyte common antigen,[231,305] a panel of antibodies that include T and B cell markers (e.g., CD20 and CD79a) are useful for avoiding an erroneous diagnosis.

Metastatic pulmonary small-cell carcinoma and cutaneous neuroendocrine carcinoma (Merkel cell carcinoma) must be considered in the differential diagnosis, particularly when the tumor occurs in patients older than 45 years and is located superficially. In general, metastatic pulmonary small-cell carcinoma can be ruled out if a thorough clinical history and radiographic studies fail to reveal pulmonary involvement. The cells of Merkel cell carcinoma have large, closely packed nuclei and little cytoplasm, and they are frequently arranged in a trabecular pattern. This tumor is chiefly located in the dermis or subcutis, and two-thirds occur in patients over 60 years of age. Although cutaneous ES/PNETs exist,[266] they generally occur in much younger patients, with a peak incidence during the second decade of life. Immunohistochemically, virtually all Merkel cell carcinomas have a characteristic globular or punctate pattern of staining with CAM5.2. Furthermore, almost all of these tumors stain for cytokeratin 20,[227] a marker generally

**TABLE 32–14** CYTOGENETIC FINDINGS IN ROUND CELL TUMORS

| Tumor | Cytogenetics | Genes |
|---|---|---|
| ES/PNET | t(11;22)(q24;q12) | *FLI1/EWS* |
| | t(21;22)(q22;q12) | *ERG/EWS* |
| | t(7;22)(p22;q12) | *ETV1/EWS* |
| | t(17;22)(q12;q12) | *E1AF/EWS* |
| | t(2;22)(q33;q12) | *FEV/EWS* |
| Alveolar rhabdomyosarcoma | t(2;13)(q35;q14) | *PAX3/FKHR* |
| | t(1;13)(p36;q14) | *PAX7/FKHR* |
| Neuroblastoma | $1p^-$ | |
| Desmoplastic small round cell tumor | t(11;22)(p13;q12) | *WT1/EWS* |
| Round cell liposarcoma | t(12;16)(q13;p11) | *CHOP/FUS* |
| | t(12;22)(q13;q12) | *CHOP/EWS* |
| Poorly differentiated synovial sarcoma | t(X;18)(p11;q11) | *SSX1 or SSX2/SYT* |

absent in metastatic small-cell carcinomas and ES/PNETs. Finally, most pulmonary small-cell carcinomas and Merkel cell carcinomas are negative for CD99.[287,309]

Mesenchymal chondrosarcoma is a rare neoplasm that typically occurs in young adults, with an extraosseous location in approximately 20% of cases.[296] Histologically, the neoplasm is characterized by a biphasic appearance of small nests or nodules of well differentiated cartilage intimately admixed with undifferentiated round cells, often arranged around a hemangiopericytoma-like vascular pattern. Although the biphasic appearance is characteristic, it may not be seen on a small biopsy specimen, making distinction from ES/PNETs difficult. Immunohistochemically, mesenchymal chondrosarcoma usually expresses neural markers such as neuron-specific enolase and S-100 protein. The diffuse membranous expression of CD99[262] and identification of the t(11;22) translocation[316] in this tumor raise the possibility that mesenchymal chondrosarcoma is part of the ES/PNET family of tumors.

Small-cell osteosarcoma typically occurs in young patients and is composed of cells similar to those seen in ES/PNETs. The diagnosis can be made only if osteoid is identified, but osteoid may be only focally present in the tumor and is often not identified in small biopsy specimens. Most tumors express neural markers, including neuron-specific enolase and Leu-7,[301] and some express cytokeratins, actins,[244] and rarely CD99.[335] One small-cell osteosarcoma with a t(11;22) translocation has been reported.[300]

Poorly differentiated synovial sarcoma is composed of small round cells often arranged around a hemangiopericytoma-like vasculature. However, unless one sees other areas of biphasic or monophasic synovial sarcoma, this lesion may be difficult to distinguish from malignant hemangiopericytoma or ES/PNETs. Because only approximately 50% of poorly differentiated synovial sarcomas express cytokeratins[254] and some show membranous CD99 immunoreactivity,[240,254] the immunohistochemical distinction of poorly differentiated synovial sarcoma from ES/PNET is difficult in some cases. We have found cytokeratin subsets useful in this regard, as 60–70% of poorly differentiated synovial sarcomas stain for cytokeratins 7 and 19, whereas ES/PNETs rarely if ever express these antigens.[288] Finally, detection of t(X;18) by conventional cytogenetics or the resultant SSX1/SYT or SSX2/SYT fusion transcript by molecular genetic techniques may serve as a diagnostic aid in these cases as well.[347]

The desmoplastic small round cell tumor typically presents in young adults, usually men, as a large intraabdominal mass with multiple peritoneal implants.[257,258] Rare examples of this tumor have also been described in the pleura, central nervous system, and peripheral soft tissues.[257] Histologically, it is composed of sharply outlined islands of tumor cells separated by a desmoplastic stroma containing myofibroblasts and prominent vascularity. The tumor nests often show peripheral palisading and central necrosis. The individual tumor cells are relatively uniform, small, and round to oval with hyperchromatic nuclei, inconspicuous nucleoli, and scanty cytoplasm. Immunohistochemically, these lesions have a polyphenotypic profile, with co-expression of cytokeratin, vimentin, desmin, and neuron-specific enolase. The pattern of desmin immunoreactivity is unique, with a characteristic perinuclear dot-like pattern of staining. Most cases studied thus far have been negative for CD99, although up to 20% in the series by Gerald et al. showed membranous CD99 immunoreactivity.[257] This tumor also has a unique cytogenetic abnormality: t(11;22)(p13;q12).[317] The breakpoint on chromosome 22 is the same as that seen in the ES/PNET family of tumors, but the locus on chromosome 11 involves the Wilms' tumor gene (*WT1*). The resultant *EWS/WT1* fusion transcript can be detected using RT-PCR.[237] Intraabdominal desmoplastic small round cell tumors[303] and unusual tumors with phenotypic features of both the desmoplastic small round cell tumor and ES/PNET[275] have been found to harbor the *EWS/FLI1* fusion transcript. However, the *EWS/WT1* fusion transcript has been found only in desmoplastic small round cell tumors.

## Clinical Behavior and Therapy

Until the introduction of modern therapy, the outlook for patients with an ES/PNET was bleak, and only a small percentage of patients with this tumor survived. For instance, in the series of extraskeletal ESs reported by Angervall and Enzinger in 1975,[207] 22 of the 35 patients with follow-up information died of metastatic disease, most commonly to the lung and skeleton. Similarly, many of the larger studies of PNET suggested that these tumors are highly aggressive neoplasms that rapidly give rise to metastatic disease and death. Jurgens et al.[273] cited a survival rate of approximately 50% at 3 years, whereas Kushner et al.[282] found that only 25% of patients with tumors >5 cm were alive at 24 months. Marina et al.[290] reported a 10.8-month disease control interval, a period significantly shorter than that of classic osseous Ewing's sarcoma. Although several studies suggest that patients with a PNET have a worse prognosis than those with extraskeletal ES,[233,265,285,286,290,318] others have not found this to be the case.[307,325,340] The data on this subject are difficult to interpret given the differences in diagnostic criteria for classifying tumors as extraskeletal ES or PNET.

Parham et al.[307] studied 63 ES/PNETs from patients who were treated uniformly to determine the prognostic significance of neuroectodermal differentiation. Tumors were classified as PNET if they showed rosettes or immunohistochemical expression of at least two neural markers (or both). Using another classification scheme, tumors were classified as PNET if they showed rosettes or immunohistochemical expression of at least four neural markers (or both). Finally, using a third classification scheme, tumors that showed ultrastructural evidence of neural differentiation were classified as PNETs. Using any of the above classification schemes, the authors were unable to show any significant difference in clinical outcome for patients with or without neuroectodermal differentiation. Future prospective studies using uniform diagnostic criteria to evaluate large numbers of patients who are uniformly treated should shed light on this unresolved issue.

The prognosis for patients with ES/PNETs has steadily improved, as most patients with localized tumors are now cured by surgery, radiation therapy/multiagent chemotherapy, or both.[349] Preoperative chemotherapy using vincristine, doxorubicin, and cyclophosphamide (and more recently ifosfamide and etoposide)[208,232,263] have allowed more conservative surgical procedures with better postsurgical function. The role of surgery in the treatment of this disease is controversial. While some have found the extent of surgical excision to be of prognostic significance,[204a,304] others have found this not to be the case.[315] The role of bone marrow transplantation in high risk patients has yet to be resolved.[212,336] Minimal residual disease can be detected in peripheral blood by RT-PCR.[252]

Key prognostic factors that adversely influence the outcome of the disease are the presence of metastatic disease at the time of initial diagnosis, large tumor size, extensive necrosis (filigree pattern), central axis tumors, and poor response to initial chemotherapy.[209,214,221,270] More recently, several studies have found that the type of *EWS/FLI1* fusion transcript may be prognostically relevant,[236,353] as patients with type 1 *EWS/FLI1* fusion transcripts appear to have longer disease-free survival than those with other fusion transcript types. De Alava et al. found that patients with type 1 fusion transcripts have tumors with lower proliferative rates, and they generally respond better to chemotherapy than those with other types of fusion transcript.[234] However, Ginsburg et al. found no significant clinical differences between those tumors with *EWS/FLI1* or *EWS/ERG* fusion transcripts. An excellent review of the molecular biology of the ES/PNET family was provided by de Alava and Gerald.[237a]

## OLFACTORY NEUROBLASTOMA (ESTHESIONEUROBLASTOMA)

Described in 1924 by Berger and Luc,[359] the olfactory neuroblastoma is a specialized form of neuroectodermal tumor arising in the superior turbinate, cribriform plate, and upper one-third of the nasal cavity.[368,380,385] Its origin has been debated and has been variously attributed to the neuroectodermal cells of the olfactory placode, sympathetic fibers (ganglionic loci of the nervus terminalis) in the anterior portion of the nasal cavity, the sphenopalatine ganglion, and the organ of Jacobson. Its location high in the nasal vault, however, and the fact that the tumor cells have ultrastructural features of olfactory nerve cells favor origin from the olfactory placode.[358,371,386,390,395]

### Clinical Features

Most patients with this tumor are adults, with a peak incidence during the fifth and sixth decades of life.[361,371] Unlike neuroblastomas, these tumors rarely arise during early childhood.[384] Men and women are equally affected. For localized lesions, the most common presentation is unilateral nasal obstruction and epistaxis, followed less frequently by lacrimation, rhinorrhea, and anosmia. Extensive lesions involving the sinuses are accompanied by frontal headache and diplopia. There are several reports of patients presenting with the syndrome of inappropriate antidiuretic hormone secretion.[355,369] Radiographically, spotty calcification may be detected in the tumor, although the specific bone changes depend on the extent of the tumor. MRI and CT scans are useful for delineating the anatomic extent of the tumor and determining resectability.[378,389]

### Gross and Microscopic Findings

Grossly, the lesions are fleshy, gray polypoid masses that may have areas of hemorrhage and necrosis. Histologically, there is a spectrum of pathologic features, with some tumors closely resembling childhood neuroblastoma and others resembling paragangliomas.[371,386] Some tumors are composed of small round cells with hyperchromatic nuclei and scanty cytoplasm. True rosettes with a central lumen (Flexner or olfactory rosettes) and pseudorosettes containing a core of neurofibrillary material (Homer Wright rosettes) can be found. Such tumors span a spectrum from those with few mitotic figures, minimal nuclear pleomorphism, prominent fibrillary matrix, and an absence of necrosis to those with numerous mitotic figures, marked nuclear pleomorphism, minimal or absent fibrillary matrix, and extensive areas of necrosis.[372] Other tumors are composed of nodules of medium-sized polygonal cells with uniform ovoid nuclei, inconspicuous nucleoli, and relatively abundant, slightly eosinophilic, granular cytoplasm, reminiscent of the cells seen in paragangliomas (Figs. 32–46, 32–47).[371] According to Hirose et al.,[371] most olfactory neuroblastomas have characteristics of both classic neuroblastoma and paraganglioma. A prominent glomeruloid capillary network is often seen in the stroma.[370] Focal ganglionic differentiation is occasionally present.[363,371,386]

## Immunohistochemical and Ultrastructural Findings

Immunohistochemically, virtually all tumors express one or more markers of neuronal or neuroendocrine differentiation, including synaptophysin, neuron-specific enolase, neurofilament protein, and chromogranin.[357,396] Synaptophysin and chromogranin tend to be expressed more frequently by paraganglioma-like tumors (Fig. 32–48), whereas neurofilament protein is more commonly expressed by tumors that closely resemble neuroblastoma.[371] A fine network of cells that are positive for S-100 protein and vimentin surround the neuroblasts in a diagnostically distinctive fashion,[364,371,388] bringing to mind the sustentacular network that is positive for S-100 protein in paragangliomas. Tumors with Flexner type (olfactory) rosettes stain for cytokeratin and epithelial membrane antigen,[358,394] but even tumors without such epithelial structures can exhibit focal cytokeratin immunoreactivity.[371] This is in contrast to the diffuse cytokeratin staining typical of neuroendocrine carcinomas. Unlike the ES/PNET family of tumors, olfactory neuroblastoma does not express CD99.[356,365,383]

Ultrastructurally, the cells have features of primitive neuroblasts, including dense-core (neurosecretory) granules and cell processes containing microtubules.[376,377,381] There are often numerous pleomorphic mitochondria and extensive paranuclear Golgi complexes. Sustentacular-like cells, with long, slender processes that encompass individual or groups of tumor cells, may be seen.[371]

## DNA Ploidy Status and Cytogenetic Findings

Almost 75% of olfactory neuroblastomas are aneuploid or polyploid, although the ploidy status does not appear to correlate with clinical behavior.[371] Relatively few olfactory neuroblastomas have been evaluated cytogenetically; several have shown complex cytogenetic aberrations.[374,393] The t(11;22)(q24;q12) characteristic of the ES/PNET family of tumors has been detected in some tumors diagnosed as olfactory neuroblastoma,[362,393] but recent studies have been unable to detect the *EWS/FLI1* fusion transcript in pri-

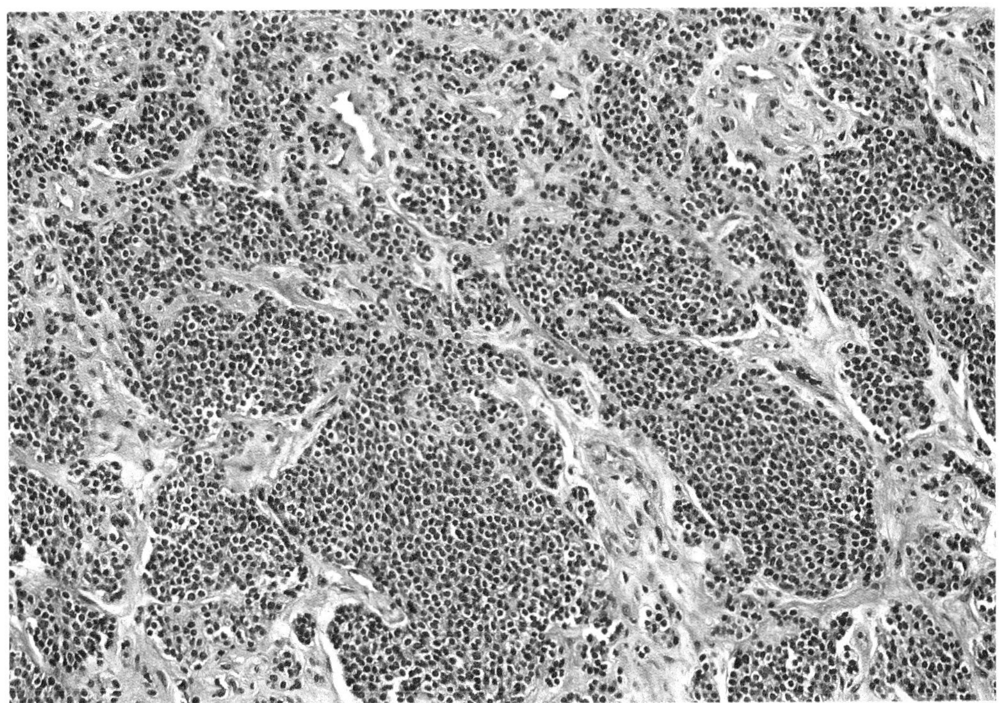

**FIGURE 32–46.** Low-power view of an olfactory neuroblastoma composed of nests of uniform ovoid cells in a fibrovascular stroma.

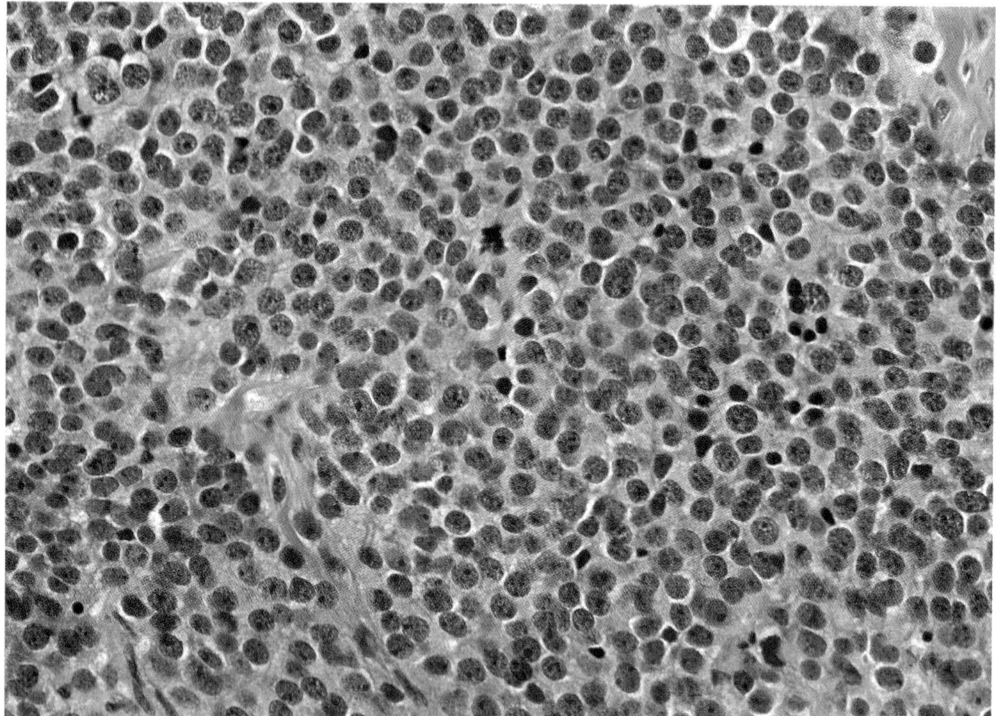

**FIGURE 32–47.** Olfactory neuroblastoma composed of uniform ovoid cells with powdery chromatin, small nucleoli, and eosinophilic granular cytoplasm.

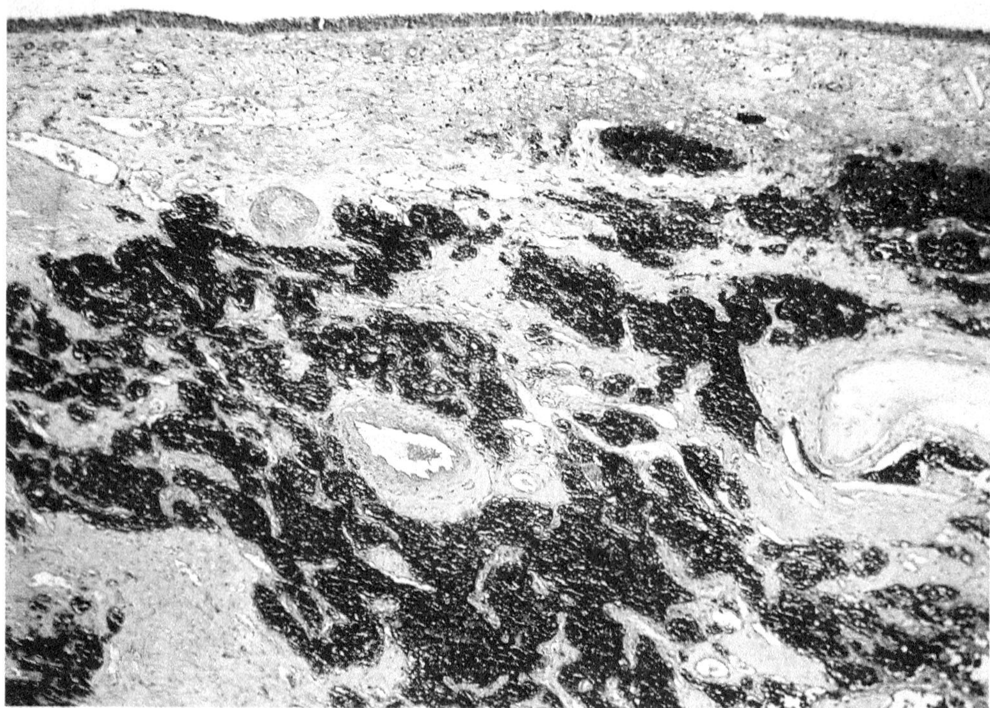

**FIGURE 32–48.** Diffuse synaptophysin immunoreactivity in an olfactory neuroblastoma.

mary olfactory neuroblastomas using either fluorescence in situ hybridization or RT-PCR.[356,377,379]

## Therapy and Prognosis

The initial management of an olfactory neuroblastoma usually involves multimodality therapy. This strategy has allowed improved survival, although late recurrences and metastases are still common. In more recent series, 5-year survival rates have ranged from 69%[382] to 78%.[366,367] Treatment and survival are strongly dependent on stage. The most widely used staging system was proposed by Kadish et al.[375] Stage A patients, with tumors limited to the nasal cavity, have a crude 5-year survival rate of 90.0%.[368] Stage B patients, with tumors involving the nasal cavity and one or more paranasal sinuses, have a 70.9% survival rate.[368] Stage C patients, with disease extending beyond the nasal cavity and sinuses, have a 46.7% survival rate.[368] Because of the frequency of endocranial invasion, a combined otolaryngologic and neurosurgical approach with bicoronal incision and frontal lobe exposure is often required.[361] Numerous studies have validated the added survival advantage of radiation therapy, chemotherapy, or both.[360,373,391,397]

Mills and Frierson[380] and others have pointed out that even the Kadish staging system is not fully predictive of survival rates. In their experience with 21 olfactory neuroblastomas, completeness of the surgical excision was the only feature that correlated with prognosis. Furthermore, no histologic features could be correlated significantly with survival rates. On the other hand, Hirose et al.[371] found that the development of metastatic disease was closely linked to histologic subtype. None of the four patients with paraganglioma-like tumors developed metastatic disease, compared to four of five patients with neuroblastoma-like tumors, and 7 of 13 patients whose tumors had combined features of paraganglioma and neuroblastoma. Strong S-100 protein staining of sustentacular-like cells and a low Ki-67 labeling index were also associated with prolonged survival. Several studies have reported relatively frequent immunohistochemical staining for P53 in these tumors.[371,387] Papadaki et al. found no evidence of *p53* gene mutations in 14 olfactory neuroblastomas,[387] but *p53* wild-type hyperexpression detected immunohistochemically was associated with an increased risk of local recurrence.

## REFERENCES

### Neuroblastoma and Ganglioneuroblastoma


1. Acharya S, Jayabose S, Cogan SJ, et al. Prenatally diagnosed neuroblastoma. Cancer 80:304, 1997.
2. Ambros IM, Zellner A, Roald B, et al. Role of ploidy, chromosome 1p, and Schwann cells in the maturation of neuroblastoma. N Engl J Med 334:1505, 1996.
3. Askin FB, Perlman EJ. Neuroblastoma and peripheral neuroectodermal tumors. Am J Clin Pathol 109(Suppl 1):S23, 1998.
4. Becker H, Wirnsberger G, Ziervogel K, et al. Immunohistochemical markers in (ganglio)neuroblastomas. Acta Histochem Suppl 38:107, 1990.
5. Beckwith JB, Martin RF. Observations on the histopathology of neuroblastoma. J Pediatr Surg 3:106, 1968.
6. Beckwith JB, Perrin EV. In situ neuroblastomas: a contribution to the natural history of neural crest tumors. Am J Pathol 43: 1089, 1963.
7. Biegel JA, White PS, Marshall HN, et al. Constitutional 1p36 deletion in a child with neuroblastoma. Am J Hum Genet 52: 176, 1993.
8. Blatt J, Hamilton RL. Neurodevelopmental anomalies in children with neuroblastoma. Cancer 82:1603, 1998.
9. Borrello MG, Bongarzone I, Pierotti MA, et al. TRK and RET proto-oncogene expression in human neuroblastoma specimens: high-frequency of trk expression in nonadvanced stages. Int J Cancer 54:540, 1993.
10. Brodeur GM. Schwann cells are antineuroblastoma agents. N Engl J Med 334:1537, 1996.
11. Brodeur GM, Azar C, Brother M, et al. Neuroblastoma: effect of genetic factors on prognosis and treatment. Cancer 70:1685, 1992.
12. Brodeur GM, Castleberry RP. Neuroblastoma In: Pizzo PA, Poplack DG (eds) Principles and Practice of Pediatric Oncology. Lippincott, Philadelphia, 1997, p 761.
13. Brodeur GM, Green AA, Hayes FA, et al. Cytogenetic features of human neuroblastomas and cell lines. Cancer Res 41:4678, 1981.
14. Brodeur GM, Hayes RA, Green AA, et al. Consistent N-myc copy number in simultaneous or consecutive neuroblastoma samples for sixty individual patients. Cancer Res 47:4248, 1987.
15. Brodeur GM, Maris JM, Yamashiro BJ, et al. Biology and genetics of human neuroblastomas. J Pediatr Hematol Oncol 19: 93, 1997.
16. Brodeur GM, Pritchard J, Berthold F, et al. Revisions in the international criteria for neuroblastoma diagnosis, staging and response to treatment. J Clin Oncol 11:1466, 1993.
17. Brodeur GM, Seeger RC, Barrett A, et al. International criteria for diagnosis, staging, and response to treatment in patients with neuroblastoma. J Clin Oncol 6:1874, 1988.
18. Brodeur GM, Seeger RC, Schwab M, et al. Amplification of N-myc in untreated human neuroblastomas correlates with advanced disease stage. Science 224:1121, 1984.
19. Brown N, Cotterill S, Lastowska M, et al. Gain of chromosome on 17q and adverse outcome in patients with neuroblastoma. N Engl J Med 340:1954, 1999.
20. Carlsen NLT, Christensen IJ, Schroeder H, et al. Prognostic factors in neuroblastomas treated in Denmark from 1943 to 1980: a statistical estimate of prognosis based on 253 cases. Cancer 58:2726, 1986.
21. Caron H. Allelic loss of chromosome 1 and additional chromosome 17 material are both unfavourable prognostic markers in neuroblastoma. Med Pediatr Oncol 24:215, 1995.
22. Caron H, Peter M, van Sluis P, et al. Evidence for two tumour suppressor loci on chromosomal band 1p35-36 involved in neuroblastoma: one probably imprinted, another associated with N-myc amplifications. Hum Mol Genet 4:535, 1995.
23. Caron H, van Sluis P, de Kraker J, et al. Allelic loss of chromosome 1p as a predictor of unfavorable outcome in patients with neuroblastoma. N Engl J Med 334:225, 1996.
24. Caron H, van Sluis P, van Hoeve M, et al. Allelic loss of chromosome 1p36 in neuroblastoma is of preferential maternal

origin and correlates with N-myc amplification. Nat Genet 4: 187, 1993.
25. Carter RL, Al-Sam SZ, Corbett RP, et al. A comparative study of immunohistochemical staining for neuron-specific enolase, protein gene product 9.5 and S-100 protein in neuroblastoma, Ewing's sarcoma and other round cell tumours in children. Histopathology 16:461, 1990.
26. Castle VP, Heidelberger KP, Bromberg J, et al. Expression of the apoptosis-suppressing protein Bcl-2 in neuroblastoma is associated with unfavourable histology and N-myc amplification. Am J Pathol 143:1543, 1993.
27. Castleberry RP. Biology and treatment of neuroblastoma. Pediatr Oncol 44:919, 1997.
28. Castleberry RP, Pritchard J, Ambros P, et al. The International Neuroblastoma Risk Groups (INRG): a preliminary report. Eur J Cancer 33:2113, 1997.
29. Castleberry RP, Shuster JJ, Altshuler G, et al. Infants with neuroblastoma and regional lymph node metastases have a favorable outlook after limited postoperative chemotherapy: a Pediatric Oncology Group study. J Clin Oncol 10:1299, 1992.
30. Chan HSL, Haddad G, Thorner PS, et al. P-glycoprotein expression as a predictor of the outcome of therapy for neuroblastoma. N Engl J Med 325:1608, 1991.
31. Chatten J, Shimada H, Sather HN, et al. Prognostic value of histopathology in advanced neuroblastoma: a report from the Children's Cancer Study Group. Hum Pathol 19:1187, 1988.
32. Cheng JM, Hiemstra JL, Schneider SS, et al. Preferential amplification of the paternal allele of the N-myc gene in human neuroblastomas. Nat Genet 4:191, 1993.
33. Cogner P, Barbany G, Dominici C, et al. Coexpression of messenger RNA for TRK proto-oncogene and low affinity nerve growth factor receptor in neuroblastoma with favorable prognosis. Cancer Res 53:2044, 1993.
34. Coldman AJ, Fryer CJH, Elwood JM, et al. Neuroblastoma: influence of age at diagnosis, stage, tumor site, and sex on prognosis. Cancer 46:1896, 1980.
35. Cowan JM, Dayal Y, Schwaitzberg S, et al. Cytogenetic and immunohistochemical analysis of an adult anaplastic neuroblastoma. Am J Surg Pathol 21:957, 1997.
36. Cushing H, Wolback SB. Transformation of malignant paravertebral sympathoblastoma into benign ganglioneuroma. Am J Pathol 3:203, 1927.
37. D'Angio GJ, Lyster KM, Urunay G. Neuroblastoma: stage IV-S: a special entity? Memorial Sloan-Kettering Cancer Center Bull 2:61, 1971.
38. Dehner LP. Pediatric Surgical Pathology. Mosby, St. Louis, 1975.
39. DeLorimier AA, Bragg KU, Linden G. Neuroblastoma in childhood. Am J Dis Child 118:441, 1969.
40. Dhooge CRM, De Moerloose BMJ, Benoit YCN, et al. Expression of the MDR1 gene product P-glycoprotein in childhood neuroblastoma. Cancer 80:1250, 1997.
41. Duckett JW, Koop CE. Neuroblastoma. Urol Clin North Am 4: 285, 1977.
42. Dyke PC, Mulkey DA. Maturation of ganglioneuroblastoma to ganglioneuroma. Cancer 20:1343, 1967.
43. Eguchi H, Takaue Y, Kawano Y, et al. Peripheral blood stem cell autografts for the treatment of children over 1 year old with stage IV neuroblastoma: a long-term follow-up. Bone Marrow Transplant 21:1011, 1998.
44. Evans AE, Angio GJ, Propert K, et al. Prognostic factors in neuroblastoma. Cancer 59:1853, 1987.
45. Evans AE, Chatten J, D'Angio GJ, et al. A review of 17 IV-S neuroblastoma patients at the Children's Hospital of Philadelphia. Cancer 45:833, 1980.
46. Evans AE, D'Angio GJ, Randolph JA. A proposed staging for children with neuroblastoma: Children's Cancer Study Group A. Cancer 27:374, 1971.
47. Fabbretti G, Valenti C, Loda M, et al. N-myc gene amplification/expression in localized stroma-rich neuroblastoma (ganglioneuroblastoma). Hum Pathol 24:294, 1993.
48. Favrot MC, Combaret V, Goillot E, et al. Expression of integrin receptors on 45 clinical neuroblastoma specimens. Int J Cancer 49:347, 1991.
49. Favrot MC, Combaret V, Lasset C. CD44—a new prognostic marker for neuroblastoma. N Engl J Med 329:1965, 1993.
50. Folpe AL, Patterson K, Gown AM. Antineuroblastoma antibody NB-84 also identifies a significant subset of other small blue round cell tumors. Appl Immunohistochem 5:239, 1997.
51. Fong CT, Dracopoli NC, White PS, et al. Loss of heterozygosity for chromosome 1p in human neuroblastomas: correlation with N-myc amplification. Proc Natl Acad Sci USA 86:3753, 1989.
52. Fong CT, White PS, Peterson K, et al. Loss of heterozygosity for chromosomes 1 or 14 defines subsets of advanced neuroblastomas. Cancer Res 52:1780, 1992.
53. Geatti O, Shapiro B, Sisson JC, et al. Iodine-131 metaiodobenzylguanadine scintigraphy for the location of neuroblastoma: preliminary experience in ten cases. J Nucl Med 26:736, 1985.
54. Gehring M, Berthold F, Edler L, et al. The 1p deletion is not a reliable marker for the prognosis of patients with neuroblastoma. Cancer Res 55:5366, 1995.
55. Gilbert F, Feder M, Balaban G, et al. Human neuroblastomas and abnormalities of chromosome 1 and 17. Cancer Res 44: 5444, 1984.
56. Griffin ME, Bolande RP. Familial neuroblastoma with regression and maturation to ganglioneurofibroma. Pediatrics 43:377, 1969.
57. Hachitanda Y, Hata J-I. Stage IVS neuroblastoma: a clinical, histological, and biological analysis of 45 cases. Hum Pathol 27:1135, 1996.
58. Hachitanda Y, Tsuneyoshi M. Neuroblastoma with a distinct organoid pattern: a clinicopathologic, immunohistochemical and ultrastructural study. Hum Pathol 25:67, 1994.
59. Hachitanda Y, Tsuneyoshi M, Enjoji M. Expression of pan-neuroendocrine proteins in 53 neuroblastic tumors. Arch Pathol Lab Med 113:381, 1989.
60. Hann HWL, Evans AE, Cohen IJ, et al. Biologic differences between neuroblastoma stages IV-S and IV: measurement of serum ferritin and E-rosette inhibition in 30 children. N Engl J Med 305:425, 1981.
61. Hayes FA, Green A, Hustu HO, et al. Surgicopathologic staging of neuroblastoma: prognostic significance of regional lymph node metastases. J Pediatr 102:59, 1983.
62. Hempstead GL, Martin-Zanca D, Kaplan DR, et al. High-affinity NGF binding requires coexpression of the trk proto-oncogene and the low-affinity NGF receptor. Nature 350:678, 1991.
63. Hickman JA. Apoptosis induced by anticancer drugs. Cancer Metastasis Rev 11:121, 1992.
64. Hiyama E, Hiyama K, Yokoyama T, et al. Correlating telomerase activity levels with human neuroblastoma outcomes. Nat Med 1:249, 1995.
65. Ijiri R, Tanaka Y, Kato K, et al. Clinicopathologic study of mass-screened neuroblastoma with special emphasis on untreated observed cases. A possible histologic clue to tumor regression. Am J Surg Pathol 24:807, 2000.
66. Ikeda H, Hirato J, Akami M, et al. Bcl-2 oncoprotein expression and apoptosis in neuroblastoma. J Pediatr Surg 30:805, 1995.
67. Ikeda H, Hirato J, Akami M, et al. Massive apoptosis detected by in-situ DNA nick end labeling in neuroblastoma. Am J Surg Pathol 20:649, 1996.

68. Jennings RW, LaQuaglia MP, Leong K, et al. Fetal neuroblastoma: prenatal diagnosis and natural history. J Pediatr Surg 28:1168, 1993.
69. Joshi VV, Cantor AB, Altshuler G, et al. Age-linked prognostic categorization based on a new histologic grading system of neuroblastomas: a clinicopathologic study of 211 cases from the Pediatric Oncology Group. Cancer 69:2199, 1992.
70. Joshi VV, Cantor AB, Altshuler G, et al. Recommendations for modification of terminology of neuroblastic tumors and prognostic significance of Shimada classification: a clinicopathologic study of 213 cases from the Pediatric Oncology Group. Cancer 69:2183, 1992.
71. Joshi VV, Silverman JF, Altshuler G, et al. Systematization of primary histopathologic and fine-needle aspiration cytology feature and description of unusual histopathologic features of neuroblastic tumors: a report from the Pediatric Oncology Group. Hum Pathol 24:493, 1993.
72. Katzenstein HM, Bowman LC, Brodeur GM, et al. Prognostic significance of age, MYCN oncogene amplification, tumor cell ploidy, and histology in 110 infants with stage D(S) neuroblastoma: The Pediatric Oncology Group experience—A Pediatric Oncology Group study. J Clin Oncol 16:2007, 1998.
73. Kinnear-Wilson LM, Draper GJ. Neuroblastoma, its natural history and prognosis: a study of 487 cases. BMJ 3:301, 1974.
74. Klein R, Jing S, Nanduri V, et al. The trk proto-oncogene encodes a receptor for nerve growth factor. Cell 65:189, 1991.
75. Knudson AG Jr, Meadows AT. Regression of neuroblastoma IV-S: a genetic hypothesis. N Engl J Med 302:1254, 1980.
76. Kogner P, Björk O, Theodorsson E. Neuropeptide Y as a marker in pediatric neuroblastoma. Med Pediatr Oncol 21:217, 1993.
77. Kogner P, Björk O, Theodorsson E. Neuropeptide Y in neuroblastoma: increased concentration in metastasis, release during surgery, and characterization of plasma and tumor extracts. Med Pediatr Oncol 21:317, 1993.
77a. Koizumi H, Ohkawa I, Tsukahara T, et al. Apoptosis in favourable neuroblastomas is not dependent on Fas (CD95/APO-1) expression but on activated caspase 3 (CPP32). J Pathol 189:410, 1999.
78. Komada Y, Zhang X-L, Zhou Y-W, et al. Flow cytometric analysis of peripheral blood and bone marrow for tumor cells in patients with neuroblastoma. Cancer 82:591, 1998.
79. Kushner BH, Cheung N-KV, LaQuaglia MP, et al. International Neuroblastoma Staging System stage 1 neuroblastoma: a prospective study and literature review. J Clin Oncol 14:2174, 1996.
80. Kushner BH, Gilbert F, Helson L. Familial neuroblastoma: case reports, literature review, and etiologic considerations. Cancer 57:1887, 1986.
81. Kushner BH, Hajdu SI, Helson L. Synchronous neuroblastoma and von Recklinghausen's disease: a review of the literature. J Clin Oncol 3:117, 1985.
82. Kushner BH, Helson L. Monozygotic siblings discordant for neuroblastoma: etiologic implications. J Pediatr 107:405, 1985.
83. Laureys G, Speleman F, Opdenakker G, et al. Constitutional translocation t(1;17)(p36;q12-21) in a patient with neuroblastoma. Genes Chromosomes Cancer 2:252, 1990.
84. Leone A, Seeger RC, Hong CM, et al. Evidence for nm23 RNA overexpression, DNA amplification and mutation in aggressive childhood neuroblastomas. Oncogene 8:855, 1993.
85. Look AT, Hayes FA, Nitschke R, et al. Cellular DNA content as a predictor of response to chemotherapy in infants with unresectable neuroblastoma. N Engl J Med 311:231, 1984.
86. Look AT, Hayes FA, Shuster JJ, et al. Clinical relevance of tumor cell ploidy and N-myc gene amplification in childhood neuroblastoma: a Pediatric Oncology Group study. J Clin Oncol 9:581, 1991.
87. Lopez-Ibor B, Schwartz AD. Neuroblastoma. Pediatr Clin North Am 32:755, 1985.
87a. Maitra A, Yashima K, Rathi A, et al. The RNA component of telomerase as a marker of biologic potential and clinical outcome in childhood neuroblastic tumors. Cancer 85:741, 1999.
88. Maris JM, Chatten J, Meadows AT, et al. Familial neuroblastoma: a three generation pedigree and further association with Hirschsprung disease. Med Pediatr Oncol 28:1, 1997.
89. Maris JM, Jensen SJ, Sulman EP, et al. Cloning, chromosomal localization, and physical mapping and genomic characterization of HKR3. Genomics 35:289, 1996.
90. Maris JM, White PS, Beltinger CP, et al. Significance of chromosome 1p loss of heterozygosity in neuroblastoma. Cancer Res 55:4664, 1995.
91. Martinsson T, Shoberg P-M, Hedborg F, et al. Deletion of chromosome 1p loci and microsatellite instability in neuroblastomas analyzed with a short-tandem repeat polymorphisms. Cancer Res 55:5681, 1995.
92. Matthay KK. Stage IV S neuroblastoma: what makes it special? J Clin Oncol 16:2003, 1998.
93. Matthay KK, Sather HN, Seeger RC, et al. Excellent prognosis of stage II neuroblastoma is independent of residual disease and radiation therapy. J Clin Oncol 7:236, 1989.
94. Mauakinen J. Microscopic patterns as a guide to prognosis of neuroblastomas in childhood. Cancer 29:1637, 1972.
95. McCune BK, Patterson K, Chandra RS, et al. Expression of transforming growth factor-beta isoforms in small round cell tumors of childhood: an immunohistochemical study. Am J Pathol 142:49, 1993.
96. Medeiros LJ, Palmedo G, Krigman HR, et al. Oncocytoid renal cell carcinoma after neuroblastoma: a report of four cases of a distinct clinicopathologic entity. Am J Surg Pathol 23:772, 1999.
97. Miettinen M, Chatten J, Paetau A, et al. Monoclonal antibody NB84 in the differential diagnosis of neuroblastoma and other small round cell tumors. Am J Surg Pathol 22:327, 1998.
98. Miyajima Y, Kato K, Numata S, et al. Detection of neuroblastoma cells in bone marrow and peripheral blood at diagnosis by the reverse transcriptase-polymerase chain reaction for tyrosine hydroxylase mRNA. Cancer 75:2757, 1995.
99. Molenaar WM, deLeiji L, Trojanowski JQ. Neuroectodermal tumors of the peripheral and central nervous system share neuroendocrine N-CAM-related antigens with small cell lung carcinoma. Acta Neuropathol (Berl) 83:46, 1991.
100. Mukai M, Torikata C, Iri H, et al. Expression of neurofilament triplet proteins in human neural tumors: an immunohistochemical study of paraganglioma, ganglioneuroma, ganglioneuroblastoma, and neuroblastoma. Am J Pathol 122:28, 1986.
101. Nakagawara A, Arima M, Azar CG, et al. Inverse relationship between trk expression and N-myc amplification in human neuroblastomas. Cancer Res 52:1364, 1992.
102. Nakagawara A, Arima-Nakagawara M, Scavarda NJ, et al. Association between high levels of expression of the TRK gene and favorable outcome in human neuroblastoma. N Engl J Med 328:847, 1993.
103. Nakagawara A, Azar CG, Scavarda NJ, et al. Expression and function of TRK-B and BDNF in human neuroblastomas. Mol Cell Biol 14:759, 1994.
104. Nisen PD, Waber PG, Rich MA, et al. N-myc oncogene RNA expression in neuroblastoma. J Natl Cancer Inst 80:1633, 1988.
105. Nitschke R, Smith EI, Altshuler G, et al. Treatment of grossly unresectable localized neuroblastoma: a Pediatric Oncology Group study. J Clin Oncol 9:1181, 1991.
106. Nitschke R, Smith EI, Shochat S, et al. Localized neuroblas-

toma treated by surgery: a Pediatric Oncology Group study. J Clin Oncol 6:1271, 1988.
107. Norris MD, Bordow SB, Marshall GM, et al. Expression of the gene for multidrug-resistance-associated protein and outcome in patients with neuroblastoma. N Engl J Med 334:231, 1996.
108. Oppendal BR, Brandtzaeg P, Kemshead JT. Immunohistochemical differentiation of neuroblastomas from other round cell neoplasms of childhood using panel of mono- and polyclonal antibodies. Histopathology 11:351, 1987.
109. Osborn M, Dirk T, Kaser H, et al. Immunohistochemical localization of neurofilaments and neuron specific enolase in 29 cases of neuroblastoma. Am J Pathol 122:433, 1986.
110. Parker I. Newborn screening for neuroblastoma. Curr Opin Pediatr 9:70, 1997.
111. Pendergrass TW. Fetal hydantoin syndrome in neuroblastoma. Lancet 2:2150, 1976.
111a. Perez CA, Matthay KK, Atkinson JB, et al. Biologic variables in the outcomes of stages I and II neuroblastoma treated with surgery as primary therapy: A Children's Cancer Group Study. J Clin Oncol 18:18, 2000.
112. Plantaz D, Mohapatra G, Matthay KK, et al. Gain of chromosome 17 is the most frequent abnormality detected in neuroblastoma by comparative genomic hybridization. Am J Pathol 150:81, 1997.
113. Pranzatelli MR. The neurobiology of the opsoclonus-myoclonus syndrome. Clin Neuropharmacol 15:186, 1992.
114. Pritchard J, Hickman JA. Why does stage 4s neuroblastoma regress spontaneously? Lancet 344:869, 1994.
115. Pritchard J, McElwain TJ, Graham-Pole J. High-dose melphalan with antologous marrow for treatment of advanced neuroblastoma. Br J Cancer 45:86, 1982.
116. Reyes-Mugica M, Lin P, Yokota J, et al. Status of deleted in colorectal cancer gene expression correlates with neuroblastoma metastasis. Lab Invest 78:669, 1998.
117. Reynolds CP, Seeger RC, Vo DD, et al. Model system for removing neuroblastoma cells from bone marrow monoclonal antibodies and magnetic immunobeads. Cancer Res 46:5882, 1986.
118. Roberts T, Chernova A, Cowell JK. Molecular characterization of the 1p22 breakpoint region spanning the constitutional translocation breakpoint in a neuroblastoma patient with a t(1; 10)(p22;q21). Cancer Genet Cytogenet 100:10, 1998.
119. Robinson MJ, Howard RN. Neuroblastoma, presenting as myasthenia gravis in a child aged 3 years. Pediatrics 43:111, 1969.
120. Romansky SG, Crocker DW, Shaw KNF. Ultrastructural studies on neuroblastoma. Cancer 42:2392, 1978.
121. Sakakibara M, Koizumi S, Saikawa Y, et al. Membrane-type matrix metalloproteinase-1 expression and activation of gelatinase A as prognostic markers in advanced pediatric neuroblastoma. Cancer 85:231, 1999.
122. Salter JE, Gibson D, Ordonez NG, et al. Neuroblastoma of the anterior mediastinum in a 80-year-old woman. Ultrastruct Pathol 19:305, 1995.
123. Saylors RL III, Cohn SL, Morgan ER, et al. Prenatal detection of neuroblastoma by fetal ultrasonography. Am J Pediatr Hematol Oncol 16:356, 1994.
124. Schleiermacher G, Peter M, Michon J, et al. Two distinct deleted regions on the short arm of chromosome 1 in neuroblastoma. Genes Chromosomes Cancer 10:275, 1994.
125. Seeger RC, Brodeur GM, Sather H. Association of multiple copies of the N-myc oncogene with rapid progression of neuroblastoma. N Engl J Med 313:111, 1985.
126. Seeger RC, Wada R, Brodeur GM, et al. Expression of N-myc by neuroblastomas with one or multiple copies of the oncogene. Prog Clin Biol Res 271:41, 1988.
127. Shimada H, Aoyama C, Chiba T, et al. Prognostic subgroups for undifferentiated neuroblastoma: immunohistochemical study with anti-S-100 protein antibody. Hum Pathol 16:471, 1985.
128. Shimada H, Chatten J, Newton WA Jr, et al. Histopathologic prognostic factors in neuroblastic tumors: definition of subtypes of ganglioneuroblastoma and an age-linked classification of neuroblastoma. J Natl Cancer Inst 73:405, 1984.
129. Shimada Y, Sato K, Abe E. Congenital dumbbell neuroblastoma. Spine 20:1295, 1995.
129a. Shimada H, Ambros IM, Dehner LP, et al. The International Neuroblastoma Pathology Classification (the Shimada System). Cancer 86:364, 1999.
129b. Shimada H, Ambros IM, Dehner LP, et al. Terminology and morphologic criteria of neuroblastic tumors. Recommendations by the International Neuroblastoma Pathology Committee. Cancer 86:349, 1999.
130. Shuster JJ, McWilliams NB, Castleberry R, et al. Serum lactate dehydrogenase in childhood neuroblastoma: a Pediatric Oncology Group recursive partitioning study. Am J Clin Oncol 15: 295, 1992.
131. Slavc I, Ellenbogen R, Jung W-H, et al. myc Gene amplification and expression in primary human neuroblastoma. Cancer Res 50:1459, 1990.
132. Srivatsan ES, Ying KL, Seeger RC. Deletion of chromosome 11 and of 14q sequences in neuroblastoma. Genes Chromosomes Cancer 7:32, 1993.
133. Steve J, Parker L, Roy P, et al. Is neuroblastoma screening evaluation needed and feasible? Br J Cancer 71:1125, 1995.
134. Suzuki T, Bodenmann E, Shimada H, et al. Lack of high-affinity nerve growth factor receptors in aggressive neuroblastomas. J Natl Cancer Inst 85:377, 1993.
135. Takayama H, Suzuki T, Mugishima H, et al. Deletion mapping of chromosome 14q and 1p in human neuroblastoma. Oncogene 7:1185, 1992.
136. Takeda O, Homma C, Maseki N, et al. There may be two tumor suppressor genes on chromosome arm 1p closely associated with biologically distinct subtypes of neuroblastoma. Genes Chromosomes Cancer 10:30, 1994.
137. Takita J, Hayashi Y, Yokota J. Loss of heterozygosity in neuroblastomas—an overview. Eur J Cancer 33:1971, 1997.
138. Tanaka T, Hiyama E, Sugimoto T, et al. trkA Gene expression in neuroblastoma: the clinical significance of an immunohistochemical study. Cancer 76:1086, 1995.
139. Tanaka T, Slamon DJ, Shimada H, et al. A significant association of Ha-RAS p21 in neuroblastoma cells with patient prognosis. Cancer 68:1296, 1991.
140. Taxy JB. Electron microscopy in the diagnosis of neuroblastoma. Arch Pathol Lab Med 104:355, 1980.
141. Thomas JO, Nijjar J, Turley H, et al. NB84: a new monoclonal antibody for the recognition of neuroblastoma in routinely processed material. J Pathol 163:69, 1991.
142. Treuner J, Schilling FH. Neuroblastoma mass screening: the arguments for and against. Eur J Cancer 31A:565, 1995.
143. Tsuchida Y, Honna T, Iwanaka T, et al. Serial determination of serum neuron-specific enolase in patients with neuroblastoma and other pediatric tumors. J Pediatr Surg 22:419, 1987.
144. Tsuda H, Shimosato Y, Upton MP, et al. Retrospective study on amplification of N-myc and c-myc genes in pediatric solid tumors and its association with prognosis and tumor differentiation. Lab Invest 59:321, 1988.
145. Tsuda T, Obara M, Hirano H, et al. Analysis of N-myc amplification in relation to disease stage and histologic types in human neuroblastomas. Cancer 60:820, 1987.
146. Van Noesel MM, Hahlan K, Hakvoort-Cammel SGAJ, et al. Neuroblastoma 4S: a heterogeneous disease with variable risk factors and treatment strategies. Cancer 80:834, 1997.

147. Voute PA, Hoefnagel CA, Marcuse HR, et al. Detection of neuroblastoma with $^{131}$I-meta-iodobenzylguanadine. Prog Clin Biol Res 175:389, 1985.
148. Weinblatt ME, Heisel MA, Siegel SE. Hypertension in children with neurogenic tumors. Pediatrics 71:947, 1983.
149. White PS, Maris JM, Beltinger C, et al. A region of consistent deletion in neuroblastoma maps within 1p36.2-.3. Proc Natl Acad Sci USA 92:5520, 1995.
150. Wirnsberger GH, Becker H, Ziervogel K, et al. Diagnostic immunohistochemistry of neuroblastic tumors. Am J Surg Pathol 16:49, 1992.
151. Yamamoto K, Hanada R, Kikuchi A, et al. Spontaneous regression of localized neuroblastoma detected by mass screening. J Clin Oncol 16:1265, 1998.
152. Yamashiro DJ, Nakagawara A, Ikegaki N, et al. Expression of TRK-C in favorable human neuroblastomas. Oncogene 12:37, 1996.

### Ganglioneuroma

153. Argenyi ZB. Cutaneous neural heterotopias and related tumors relevant for the dermatopathologist. Semin Diagn Pathol 13:60, 1996.
154. Banks E, Yum M, Brodhecker C, et al. A malignant peripheral nerve sheath tumor in association with paratesticular ganglioneuroma. Cancer 64:1738, 1989.
155. Bjellerup P, Theodorsson E, Cogner P. Somatostatin and vasoactive intestinal peptide (VIP) in neuroblastoma and ganglioneuroma: chromatographic characterization and release during surgery. Eur J Cancer 31A:481, 1995.
156. Brady S, Lechan RM, Schwaitzberg SD, et al. Composite pheochromocytoma/ganglioneuroma of the adrenal gland associated with multiple endocrine neoplasia type 2A: case report with immunohistochemical analysis. Am J Surg Pathol 21:102, 1997.
157. Braslis KG, Jones A. Ganglioneuroma of the adrenal medulla. Aust NZ J Surg 67:816, 1997.
158. Carney JA, Go VLW, Sizemore GW, et al. Alimentary tract ganglioneuromatosis—a major component of the syndrome of multiple endocrine neoplasia, type 2B. N Engl J Med 295:1287, 1976.
159. Celik V, Unal G, Ozgultekin R, et al. Adrenal ganglioneuroma. Br J Surg 83:263, 1996.
160. Chandrasoma P, Shibata D, Radin R, et al. Malignant peripheral nerve sheath tumor arising in an adrenal ganglioneuroma in an adult male homosexual. Cancer 57:2022, 1986.
161. Chen GH, He JN. Malignant ganglioneuroma of adrenals with metastasis to liver and spleen. Chin Med J 993:261, 1986.
162. Chetty R, Duhig JD. Bilateral pheochromocytoma-ganglioneuroma of the adrenal in type 1 neurofibromatosis. Am J Surg Pathol 17:837, 1993.
163. Damiani S, Manetto V, Carrillo G, et al. Malignant peripheral nerve sheath tumor arising in a "de novo" ganglioneuroma: a case report. Tumori 77:90, 1991.
164. D'Amore ES, Manivel JC, Pettinato G, et al. Intestinal ganglioneuromatosis: mucosal and transmural types: a clinicopathologic and immunohistochemical study of six cases. Hum Pathol 22:276, 1991.
165. Devoede G, Lemieux B, Massé S, et al. Colonic hamartomas in tuberous sclerosis. Gastroenterology 94:182, 1988.
166. Drago G, Pasquier B, Pasquier D, et al. Malignant peripheral nerve sheath tumor arising in a "de novo" ganglioneuroma: a case report and review of the literature. Med Pediatr Oncol 28: 216, 1997.
167. Fletcher CDM, Fernando IN, Braimbridge MV, et al. Malignant nerve sheath tumor arising in a ganglioneuroma. Histopathology 12:445, 1988.
168. Freeman BD, Zuckerman GR, Callery MP. Duodenal ganglioneuroma: a rare cause of upper GI hemorrhage. Am J Gastroenterol 91:262, 1996.
169. Fuller CE, Williams GT. Gastrointestinal manifestations of type 1 neurofibromatosis (von Recklinghausen's disease). Histopathology 19:1, 1991.
170. Gambini C, Rongioletti F. Primary congenital cutaneous ganglioneuroma. J Am Acad Dermatol 35:353, 1996.
171. Garvin JH, Lack EE, Berenberg W, et al. Ganglioneuroma presenting with differentiated skeletal metastases: report of a case. Cancer 54:357, 1984.
172. Ghali VS, Gold JE, Vincent RA, et al. Malignant peripheral nerve sheath tumor arising spontaneously from retroperitoneal ganglioneuroma: a case report, review of the literature, and immunohistochemical study. Hum Pathol 23:72, 1992.
173. Godlewski G, Nguyen Trong AH, Tang J, et al. Virilizing adrenal ganglioneuroma containing Leydig cells. Acta Chir Belg 93:181, 1993.
174. Goldman RL, Winterling AN, Winterling CC. Maturation of tumors of sympathetic nervous system: report of long-term survival in two patients, one with disseminated osseous metastases, and review of cases from the literature. Cancer 18: 1510, 1965.
175. Haggitt RC, Reid BJ. Hereditary gastrointestinal polyposis syndromes. Am J Surg Pathol 10:871, 1986.
176. Hammond RR, Walton JC. Cutaneous ganglioneuromas: a case report and review of the literature. Hum Pathol 27:735, 1996.
177. Ichikawa T, Ohtomo K, Araki T, et al. Ganglioneuroma: computed tomography and magnetic resonance features. Br J Radiol 69:114, 1996.
178. Johnson GL, Hruban RH, Marshall FF, et al. Primary adrenal ganglioneuroma: CT finding in four patients. AJR 169:169, 1997.
179. Kimura N, Yamamoto H, Okamoto H, et al. Multiple hormone gene expression in ganglioneuroblastoma with watery diarrhea, hypokalemia, and achlorhydria syndrome. Cancer 71: 2841, 1993.
180. Lamovec J, Frković-Grazio S, Bracko M. Nonsporadic cases and unusual morphological features in pheochromocytoma and paraganglioma. Arch Pathol Lab Med 122:63, 1988.
181. Lashner BA, Riddell RH, Wynans CS. Ganglioneuromatosis of the colon and extensive glycogenic acanthosis in Cowden's disease. Dig Dis Sci 31:213, 1986.
182. Lucas K, Gula NG, Knisely AS, et al. Catecholamine metabolites in ganglioneuroma. Med Pediatr Oncol 22:240, 1994.
183. Matias-Guiu X, Garrastazu MT. Composite phaeochromocytoma-ganglioneuroblastoma in a patient with multiple endocrine neoplasia type IIA. Histopathology 32:281, 1998.
184. Mendelsohn G, Diamond MP. Familial ganglioneuromatous polyposis of the large bowel: report of a family with associated juvenile polyposis. Am J Surg Pathol 8:515, 1984.
185. Mendelsohn G, Eggleston JC, Olson JL, et al. Vasoactive intestinal peptide and its relationship to ganglion cell differentiation in neuroblastic tumors. Lab Invest 41:144, 1979.
186. Mullins JD. A pigmented differentiating neuroblastoma: a light and ultrastructural study. Cancer 46:522, 1980.
187. O'Dowd GM, Gaffney EF. Pigmented ganglioneuroblastoma: a tumour cell "storage disease"? Histopathology 22:591, 1993.
188. Perkins JT, Blackstone MO, Riddell RH. Adenomatous polyposis coli and multiple endocrine neoplasia type 2B. Cancer 55: 375, 1985.
189. Pham BN, Villaneuva RP. Ganglioneuromatous proliferation associated with juvenile polyposis coli. Arch Pathol Lab Med 113:91, 1989.
190. Preidler KW, Ranner G, Szolar D, et al. Retropharyngeal ganglioneuroma: ultrasound, CT and MRI findings in a 57-year-old patient. Eur J Radiol 19:108, 1995.
191. Radin R, David CL, Goldfarb H, et al. Adrenal and extra-

adrenal retroperitoneal ganglioneuroma: imaging findings in 13 adults. Radiology 202:703, 1997.
192. Ricci A, Parham DM, Woodruff JM, et al. Malignant peripheral nerve sheath tumors arising from ganglioneuromas. Am J Surg Pathol 8:19, 1984.
193. Schmid KW, Dockhorn-Dworniczak B, Fahrenkamp A, et al. Chromogranin A, secretogranin II and vasoactive intestinal peptide in phaeochromocytomas and ganglioneuromas. Histopathology 22:527, 1993.
194. Schulman DI, McClenathan DT, Harmel RP, et al. Ganglioneuromatosis involving the small intestine and pancreas of a child and causing hypersecretion of vasoactive intestinal polypeptide. J Pediatr Gastroenterol Nutr 22:212, 1996.
195. Schulman H, Laufer L, Barki Y, et al. Ganglioneuroma: an "incidentaloma" of childhood. Eur Radiol 8:582, 1998.
196. Shekitka KM, Sobin LH. Ganglioneuromas of the gastrointestinal tract: relation to von Recklinghausen disease and other multiple tumor syndromes. Am J Surg Pathol 18:250, 1994.
197. Srinivasan R, Mayle JE. Polypoid ganglioneuroma of colon. Dig Dis Sci 43:908, 1998.
198. Stout AP. Ganglioneuroma of the sympathetic nervous system. Surg Gynecol Obstet 84:101, 1947.
199. Walsh C, Anderhuber W, Preidler K, et al. Retro- and parapharyngeal ganglioneuroma. J Laryngol Otol 110:87, 1996.

### Ganglion Cell Tumors

200. Daneshvar A. Pharyngeal traumatic neuromas and traumatic neuromas with mature ganglion cells (pseudoganglioneuromas). Am J Surg Pathol 14:565, 1990.
201. Lee JY, Martinez AJ, Abell E. Ganglioneuromatous tumor of the skin: a combined heterotopia of ganglion cells and hamartomatous neuroma: report of a case. J Cutan Pathol 15:58, 1988.
202. Radice F, Gianotti R. Cutaneous ganglion cell tumor of the skin: case report and review of the literature. Am J Dermatopathol 15:488, 1993.
203. Rios JJ, Diaz-Cano SJ, Rivera-Hueto F, et al. Cutaneous ganglion cell choristoma: report of a case. J Cutan Pathol 18:469, 1991.

### Extraskeletal Ewing's Sarcoma/Primitive Neuroectodermal Tumor Family

204. Adams V, Hany MA, Schmid M, et al. Detection of t(11;22)(q24;q12) translocation breakpoint in paraffin-embedded tissue of the Ewing's sarcoma family by nested reverse transcription-polymerase chain reaction. Diagn Mol Pathol 5:107, 1996.
204a. Ahmad R, Mayol BR, Davis M, et al. Extraskeletal Ewing's sarcoma. Cancer 85:725, 1999.
205. Amann G, Zoubek A, Salzer-Kuntschik M, et al. Relation of neuroglial marker expression and EWS gene fusion types in MIC2/CD99-positive tumors of the Ewing family. Hum Pathol 30:1058, 1999.
206. Ambros IM, Ambros PF, Strehl S, et al. MIC2 is a specific marker for Ewing's sarcoma and peripheral primitive neuroectodermal tumors: evidence of a common histogenesis of Ewing's sarcoma and peripheral primitive neuroectodermal tumors from MIC2 expression and specific chromosomal aberration. Cancer 67:1886, 1991.
207. Angervall L, Enzinger FM. Extraskeletal neoplasm resembling Ewing's sarcoma. Cancer 36:240, 1975.
208. Antman K, Crowley J, Balcerzak SP, et al. A Southwest Oncology Group and Cancer and Leukemia Group B Phase II Study of doxorubicin, dacarbazine, iphosfamide and mesna in adults with advanced osteosarcoma, Ewing's sarcoma and rhabdomyosarcoma. Cancer 82:1288, 1998.
209. Arai Y, Kun LE, Brooks MT, et al. Ewing's sarcoma: local tumor control and patterns of failure following limited-volume radiation therapy. Int J Radiat Oncol Biol Phys 21:1501, 1991.
210. Armengol G, Tarkkanen M, Virolainen M, et al. Recurrent gains of 1q8 and 12 in the Ewing family of tumours by comparative genomic hybridization. Br J Cancer 75:1403, 1997.
211. Askin FB, Rosai J, Sibley RK, et al. Malignant small cell tumor of the thoracopulmonary region in childhood. Cancer 43:2438, 1979.
212. Atra A, Whelan JS, Calvagna V, et al. High-dose busulphan/melphalan with autologous stem cell rescue in Ewing's sarcoma. Bone Marrow Transplant 20:843, 1997.
213. Aurias A, Rimbaut C, Buffe D, et al. Chromosomal translocation in Ewing's sarcoma. N Engl J Med 309:496, 1983.
214. Baldini EH, Demetri GD, Fletcher CDM, et al. Adults with Ewing's sarcoma/primitive neuroectodermal tumor. Adverse effect of older age and primary extraosseous disease on outcome. Ann Surg 230:79, 1999.
215. Banerjee SS, Agbamu DA, Eyden BP, et al. Clinicopathological characteristics of peripheral primitive neuroectodermal tumour of skin and subcutaneous tissue. Histopathology 31:355, 1997.
216. Banerjee SS, Eyden BP, McVey RJ, et al. Primary peripheral primitive neuroectodermal tumour of the urinary bladder. Histopathology 30:486, 1997.
217. Batsakis JD, El-Naggar AK. Ewing's sarcoma and primitive neuroectodermal tumors: cytogenetic synosures seeking a common histogenesis. Adv Anat Pathol 4:207, 1997.
218. Benesch M, Urban C. Is primitive neuroectodermal tumor of the kidney a distinct entity? Cancer 82:1414, 1998.
219. Berthold F, Kracht J, Lampert F, et al. Ultrastructural, biochemical, and cell culture studies of a presumed extraskeletal Ewing's sarcoma with special reference to differential diagnosis from neuroblastoma. J Cancer Res Clin Oncol 103:293, 1982.
220. Bolen JW, Thorning D. Peripheral neuroepithelioma: a light and electron microscopic study. Cancer 46:2456, 1980.
221. Cangir A, Vietti TJ, Gehan EA, et al. Ewing's sarcoma metastatic at diagnosis: results and comparisons of two Intergroup Ewing Sarcoma Studies. Cancer 66:887, 1990.
222. Carter RL, Al-Sam SZ, Corbett RP, et al. A comparative study of immunohistochemical staining for neuron-specific enolase, protein gene product 9.5, and S-100 protein in neuroblastoma, Ewing's sarcoma, and other round cell tumours in children. Histopathology 16:461, 1990.
223. Catalan RL, Murphy T. Primary primitive neuroectodermal tumor of the lung. AJR 169:1201, 1997.
224. Cavazzana AO, Magnani JL, Ross RA, et al. Ewing's sarcoma is an undifferentiated neuroectodermal tumor. Prog Clin Biol Res 271:487, 1988.
225. Cavazzana AO, Ninfo B, Roberts J, et al. Peripheral neuroepithelioma: a light microscopic immunocytochemical, and ultrastructural study. Mod Pathol 5:71, 1992.
226. Chan JKC. Molecular analysis of primitive neuroectodermal tumors: a new model for the study of solid tumors showing specific chromosomal translocations. Adv Anat Pathol 1:87, 1994.
227. Chan JKC, Suster S, Wenig BM, et al. Cytokeratin 20 immunoreactivity distinguishes Merkel cell (primary cutaneous neuroendocrine) carcinomas and salivary gland small cell carcinomas from small cell carcinomas of various sites. Am J Surg Pathol 21:226, 1997.
228. Charney DA, Charney JM, Ghali BS, et al. Primitive neuroectodermal tumor of the myocardium: a case report, review of the literature, immunohistochemical, and ultrastructural study. Hum Pathol 27:1365, 1996.
229. Colville HC, Willis RA. Neuroblastoma metastases in bones, with a criticism of Ewing's endothelioma. Am J Pathol 9:421, 1933.

230. Connor CL. A further consideration of Ewing's sarcoma. Am J Cancer 22:41, 1934.
231. Cossman J, Chused TM, Fisher RI, et al. Diversity of immunologic phenotypes of lymphoblastic lymphoma. Cancer Res 43: 4486, 1993.
232. Craft AW, Cotterill SJ, Bullimore JA, et al. Long-term results from the first UKCCSG Ewing's tumour study (ET-1): United Kingdom Children's Cancer Study Group (UKCCSG) and the Medical Research Council of Bone Sarcoma Working Party. Eur J Cancer 33:1061, 1997.
233. Daugaard S, Kamby C, Sunde LM, et al. Ewing's sarcoma: a retrospective study of histological and immunohistochemical factors and their relation to prognosis. Virchows Arch 414:243, 1989.
234. De Alava E, Antonescu C, Panizo A, et al. Why do Ewing's sarcomas with EWS-FLI-1 type 1 transcripts behave better? Mod Pathol 11:981A, 1998.
235. De Alava E, Dolores Lovano M, Sola I, et al. Molecular features in a biphenotypic small cell sarcoma with neuroectodermal and muscle differentiation. Hum Pathol 29:181, 1998.
236. De Alava E, Kawai A, Healey JH, et al. EWS-FLI-1 fusion transcript structure is an independent determinant of prognosis in Ewing's sarcoma. J Clin Oncol 16:1248, 1998.
237. De Alava E, Ladanyi M, Rosai J, et al. Detection of chimeric transcripts in desmoplastic small round cell tumor and related developmental tumors by reverse transcriptase-polymerase chain reaction. Am J Pathol 147:1584, 1995.
237a. De Alava E, Gerald WL. Molecular biology of the Ewing's sarcoma/primitive neuroectodermal tumor family. J Clin Oncol 18:204, 2000.
238. Deb RA, Desai SB, Amonkar PP, et al. Primary primitive neuroectodermal tumour of the parotid gland. Histopathology 33: 375, 1998.
239. Dehner LP. Primitive neuroectodermal tumor and Ewing's sarcoma. Am J Surg Pathol 17:1, 1993.
240. Dei Tos AP, Wadden C, Calonje E, et al. Immunohistochemical demonstration of glycoprotein p30/32$^{MIC2}$ (CD99) in synovial sarcoma: a potential cause of diagnostic confusion. Appl Immunohistochem 3:168, 1995.
241. Delattre O, Zucman J, Melot T, et al. The Ewing family of tumors: a subgroup of small-round-cell tumors defined by specific chimeric transcripts. N Engl J Med 331:294, 1994.
242. Delattre O, Zucman J, Plougastel B, et al. Gene fusion with an ETS-binding domain caused by chromosome translocation in human tumors. Nature 359:162, 1992.
243. Desmaze C, Brizard F, Turc-Carel C, et al. Multiple chromosomal mechanisms generate an EWS/FLI-1 or an EWS/ERG fusion gene in Ewing tumors. Cancer Genet Cytogenet 97:12: 1997.
244. Devaney K, Vinh TN, Sweet DE. Small cell osteosarcoma of bone: an immunohistochemical study with differential diagnostic considerations. Hum Pathol 24:1211, 1993.
245. Douglass EC. Chromosomal rearrangements in Ewing's sarcoma and peripheral neuroectodermal tumor (PNET). Semin Dev Biol 1:393, 1990.
246. Douglass EC, Rowe ST, Valentine M, et al. A second nonrandom translocation, der(16)t(1;16)(q21;q13), in Ewing's sarcoma and peripheral neuroectodermal tumor. Cytogenet Cell Genet 53:87, 1990.
247. Downing JR, Head DR, Parham DM, et al. Detection of the (11;22)(q24;q12) translocation of Ewing's sarcoma and peripheral neuroectodermal tumor by reverse transcription polymerase chain reaction. Am J Pathol 143:1294, 1993.
248. Downing JR, Khandekar A, Shurtleff SA, et al. Multiplex RT-PCR assay for the differential diagnosis of alveolar rhabdomyosarcoma and Ewing's sarcoma. Am J Pathol 146:622, 1995.
249. Erlandson A. Ultrastructural distinction between rhabdomyosarcoma and other undifferentiated "sarcomas." Ultrastruct Pathol 11:83, 1987.
250. Ewing J. Diffuse endothelioma of bone. Proc NY Pathol Soc 21:17, 1921.
251. Fellinger EJ, Garin-Chesa P, Glasser DB, et al. Comparison of cell surface antigen HBA71 (p30/32MIC2), neuron specific enolase, and vimentin in the immunohistochemical analysis of Ewing's sarcoma of bone. Am J Surg Pathol 16:746, 1992.
252. Fidelia-Lambert MN, Zhuang Z, Tsokos M. Sensitive detection of rare Ewing's sarcoma cells in peripheral blood by reverse transcriptase polymerase chain reaction. Hum Pathol 30:78, 1999.
253. Fletcher JA. Cytogenetic observations in malignant soft tissue tumors. Adv Pathol Lab Med 4:235, 1991.
254. Folpe AL, Schmidt RA, Chapman D, et al. Poorly differentiated synovial sarcoma: immunohistochemical distinction from primitive neuroectodermal tumors and high-grade malignant peripheral nerve sheath tumors. Am J Surg Pathol 22:673, 1998.
255. Fraumeni JF Jr, Glass AG. Rarity of Ewing's sarcoma among U.S. Negro children. Lancet 1:366, 1979.
256. Furman J, Murphy WM, Jelsma PF, et al. Primary primitive neuroectodermal tumor of kidney: case report and review of the literature. Am J Clin Pathol 106:339, 1996.
257. Gerald W, Ladanyi M, de Alava E, et al. Clinical, pathologic and molecular spectrum of desmoplastic small round cell tumor based on review of 109 cases. J Clin Oncol 16:3028, 1998.
258. Gerald WL, Rosai J. Desmoplastic small cell tumor with divergent differentiation. Pediatr Pathol 9:177, 1989.
259. Gillespie JJ, Roth LM, Wills ER, et al. Extraskeletal Ewing's sarcoma: histologic and ultrastructural observations in three cases. Am J Surg Pathol 3:99, 1979.
260. Ginsberg JP, de Alava E, Ladanyi M, et al. EWS-FLI1 and EWS-ERG gene fusions are associated with similar clinical phenotypes in Ewing's sarcoma. J Clin Oncol 17:1809, 1999.
261. Goodfellow PJ, Darling SM, Thomas NS, et al. A pseudoautosomal gene in man. Science 234:740, 1986.
262. Granter SR, Renshaw AA, Fletcher CDM, et al. CD99 reactivity in mesenchymal chondrosarcoma. Hum Pathol 27:1273, 1996.
262a. Gu M, Antonescu CR, Guiter G, et al. Cytokeratin immunoreactivity in Ewing's sarcoma. Prevalence in 50 cases confirmed by molecular diagnostic studies. Am J Surg Pathol 24:410, 2000.
263. Gururangan S, Marina NM, Luo X, et al. Treatment of children with peripheral primitive neuroectodermal tumor or extraosseous Ewing's tumor with Ewing's-directed therapy. J Pediatr Hematol Oncol 20:55, 1998.
264. Hachitanda Y, Tsuneyoshi M, Enjoji M, et al. Congenital primitive neuroectodermal tumor with epithelial and glial differentiation: an ultrastructural and immunohistochemical study. Arch Pathol Lab Med 114:101, 1990.
265. Hartman KR, Triche TJ, Kinsella TJ, et al. Prognostic value of histopathology in Ewing's sarcoma: long-term follow-up of distal extremity primary tumors. Cancer 67:163, 1991.
266. Hasegawa SL, Davison JM, Rutten A, et al. Primary cutaneous Ewing's sarcoma: immunophenotypic and molecular cytogenetic evaluation of five cases. Am J Surg Pathol 22:310, 1998.
267. Hashimoto H, Tsuneyoshi M, Daimaru Y, et al. Extraskeletal Ewing's sarcoma: a clinicopathologic and electron microscopic analysis of 8 cases. Acta Pathol Jpn 35:1087, 1985.
268. Hess E, Cohen C, DeRose PB, et al. Nonspecificity of p30/32$^{MIC2}$ immunolocalization with the O13 monoclonal antibody in the diagnosis of Ewing's sarcoma: application of an algorithmic immunohistochemical analysis. Appl Immunohistochem 5:94, 1997.
269. Hijazi Y, Tsokos M, Steinberg S, et al. Neuroectodermal differ-

entiation does not play a role in the prognosis of Ewing's sarcoma versus primitive neuroectodermal tumor. Mod Pathol 9:21A, 1995.

270. Horowitz ME, Malawer MM, Woo SY, et al. Ewing's sarcoma family of tumors Ewing's sarcoma of bone and soft tissue and the peripheral primitive neuroectodermal tumors. In: Pizzo PA, Poplack DG (eds) Principles and Practice of Pediatric Oncology, 3rd ed. Lippincott-Raven, Philadelphia, 1997, p 831.
271. Jaffe R, Santamaria M, Yunis EJ, et al. The neuroectodermal tumor of bone. Am J Surg Pathol 8:885, 1984.
272. Jeon I-S, Davis JN, Braun BS, et al. A variant Ewing's sarcoma translocation (7;22) fuses the EWS gene to the ETS gene ETV-1. Oncogene 10:1229, 1995.
273. Jurgens H, Bier V, Harms D, et al. Malignant peripheral neuroectodermal tumors: a retrospective analysis of 42 patients. Cancer 61:349, 1988.
274. Kaneko Y, Yoshida K, Handa M, et al. Fusion of the ETS-family gene E1AF to EWS by t(17;22)(q12;q12) chromosome translocation in an undifferentiated sarcoma of infancy. Genes Chromosomes Cancer 15:115, 1996.
275. Katz RL, Quezado M, Senderowicz AM, et al. An intra-abdominal small round cell neoplasm with features of primitive neuroectodermal and desmoplastic round cell tumor and a EWS/FLI-1 fusion transcript. Hum Pathol 28:502, 1997.
276. Kawauchi S, Fukuda T, Miyamoto S, et al. Peripheral primitive neuroectodermal tumor of the ovary confirmed by CD99 immunostaining, karyotypic analysis, and RT-PCR for EWS/FLI-1 chimeric mRNA. Am J Surg Pathol 22:1417, 1998.
277. Kissane JM, Askin FB, Foukes M, et al. Ewing's sarcoma of bone: clinicopathologic aspects of 303 cases from the Intergroup Ewing's sarcoma study. Hum Pathol 14:773, 1983.
278. Kobayashi S, Kurose A, Miki H, et al. Peripheral primitive neuroectodermal tumor similar to ganglioneuroblastoma. Clin Exp Pathol 46:36A, 1998.
279. Komiya S, Irie K, Sasaguri Y, et al. An ultrastructural study of extraskeletal Ewing's sarcoma. Acta Pathol Jpn 34:445, 1984.
280. Kovar H, Aryee DN, Jug G, et al. EWS/FLI-1 antagonists induce growth inhibition of Ewing tumor cells in vitro. Cell Growth Differ 7:429, 1996.
281. Kumar S, Pack S, Kumar D, et al. Detection of EWS-FLI-1 fusion in Ewing's sarcoma/peripheral primitive neuroectodermal tumor by fluorescence in situ hybridization using formalin-fixed paraffin-embedded tissue. Hum Pathol 30:324, 1999.
282. Kushner BH, Hajdu SI, Gulati SC, et al. Extracranial primitive neuroectodermal tumors: the Memorial Sloan-Kettering Cancer Center experience. Cancer 67:1825, 1991.
283. Ladanyi M, Heinemann FS, Huvos AG, et al. Neural differentiation in small round cell tumors of bone and soft tissue with the translocation t(11;22)(q24;q12): an immunohistochemical study of 11 cases. Hum Pathol 21:1245, 1990.
284. Ladanyi M, Lewis R, Gari-Chesa P, et al. EWS rearrangement in Ewing's sarcoma and peripheral neuroectodermal tumor: molecular detection and correlation with cytogenetic analysis and MIC2 expression. Diagn Mol Pathol 2:141, 1993.
285. Llombart-Bosch A, Lacombe MJ, Peydro-Olaya A, et al. Malignant peripheral neuroectodermal tumors of bone other than Askin's neoplasm: characterization of fourteen new cases with immunohistochemistry and electron microscopy. Virchows Arch 412:421, 1988.
286. Llombart-Bosch A, Terrier-Lacombe MJ, Peydro-Olaya A, et al. Peripheral neuroectodermal sarcoma of soft tissue (peripheral neuroepithelioma): a pathologic study of ten cases with differential diagnosis regarding other small, round-cell sarcomas. Hum Pathol 20:273, 1989.
287. Lumadue JA, Askin FB, Perlman EJ. MIC-2 analysis of small cell carcinoma. Am J Clin Pathol 102:692, 1994.
288. Machen SK, Gautam R, Fisher C, et al. The utility of cytokeratin subsets in poorly differentiated synovial sarcoma versus peripheral primitive neuroectodermal tumor. Histopathology 33:501, 1998.
289. Maeda G, Masui F, Yokoyama R, et al. Ganglion cells in Ewing's sarcoma following chemotherapy: a case report. Pathol Int 48:475, 1998.
290. Marina NM, Etchbanas E, Parham DM, et al. Peripheral primitive neuroectodermal tumor (peripheral neuroepithelioma) in children: a review of the St. Jude experience and controversies of diagnosis and management. Cancer 64:1952, 1989.
291. Marley DF, Liapis H, Humphrey DA, et al. Primitive neuroectodermal tumor of the kidney—another enigma: a pathologic, immunohistochemical and molecular diagnostic study. Am J Surg Pathol 21:354, 1997.
292. Maurici D, Perez-Atayde A, Grier HE, et al. Frequency and implications of chromosome 8 and 12 gains in Ewing's sarcoma. Cancer Genet Cytogenet 100:1106, 1998.
293. McManus AP, Gusterson BA, Pinkerton CR, et al. Diagnosis of Ewing's sarcoma and related tumours by fluorescence in-situ hybridization detection of chromosome 22q12 translocations on tumour touch imprints. J Pathol 176:137, 1995.
294. Monforte-Munoz H, Lopez-Terrada D, Affendie H, et al. Documentation of EWS gene rearrangements by fluorescence in-situ hybridization (FISH) in frozen sections of Ewing's sarcoma-peripheral primitive neuroectodermal tumor. Am J Surg Pathol 23:309, 1999.
295. Mugneret F, Lizard S, Aurias A, et al. Chromosomes in Ewing's sarcoma. II. Nonrandom additional changes, trisomy 8, and der (16)t(1;16). Cancer Genet Cytogenet 32:239, 1988.
296. Nakashima Y, Unni KK, Shives TS, et al. Mesenchymal chondrosarcoma of bone and soft tissue: a review of 111 cases. Cancer 57:2444, 1986.
297. Nascimento AG, Unni KK, Pritchard DJ, et al. A clinicopathologic study of 20 cases of large-cell (atypical) Ewing's sarcoma of bone. Am J Surg Pathol 4:29, 1980.
298. Navarro S, Cavazzana AO, Llombart-Bosch A, et al. Comparison of Ewing's sarcoma of bone and peripheral neuroepithelioma: an immunocytochemical and ultrastructural analysis of two primitive neuroectodermal neoplasms. Arch Pathol Lab Med 118:608, 1994.
299. Navas-Palacios JJ, Aparicio-Duque R, Valdes MD. On the histogenesis of Ewing's sarcoma: an ultrastructural, immunohistochemical, and cytochemical study. Cancer 53:1882, 1984.
300. Noguera R, Navarro S, Triche TJ. Translocation t(11;22) in small cell osteosarcoma. Cancer Genet Cytogenet 45:121, 1990.
301. O'Connell JX, Manghan DC, Mankin HJ, et al. Small cell osteosarcoma: an immunohistochemical and flow cytometric study. Mod Pathol 6:9A, 1993.
302. O'Neil-Smith K, Wittenberg KH, Efird JT, et al. Ewing's sarcoma and peripheral primitive neuroectodermal tumor: a proposal for a standardized classification scheme based on morphologic, immunohistochemical and clinical features. Mod Pathol 9:36A, 1996.
303. Ordi J, de Alava E, Torne A, et al. Intraabdominal desmoplastic small round cell tumor with EWS/ERG fusion transcript. Am J Surg Pathol 22:1026, 1998.
304. Ozaki T, Hillmann A, Hoffmann C, et al. Significance of surgical margin on the prognosis of patients with Ewing's sarcoma: a report from the Cooperative Ewing's Sarcoma Study. Cancer 78:892, 1996.
305. Ozdemirli M, Fanburg-Smith JC, Hartmann B-P, et al. Precursor B-lymphoblastic lymphoma presenting as a solitary bone tumor and mimicking Ewing's sarcoma: a report of four cases and review of the literature. Am J Surg Pathol 22:795, 1998.
306. Parham DM, Dias P, Kelly DR, et al. Desmin positivity in primitive neuroectodermal tumors of childhood. Am J Surg Pathol 6:43, 1992.

307. Parham DM, Hijazi Y, Steinberg SM, et al. Neuroectodermal differentiation in Ewing's sarcoma family of tumors does not predict tumor behavior. Hum Pathol 30:911, 1999.
308. Perlman EJ, Dickman BS, Askin FB, et al. Ewing sarcoma: routine diagnostic utilization of MIC 2 analysis: a Pediatric Oncology Group/Children's Cancer Group Intergroup study. Hum Pathol 25:304, 1994.
309. Perlman EJ, Lumadue JA, Hawkins AL, et al. Primary cutaneous neuroendocrine tumors: diagnostic use of cytogenetic and MIC2 analysis. Cancer Genet Cytogenet 82:30, 1995.
310. Peter M, Couturier J, Pacquement H, et al. A new member of ETS family fused to EWS in Ewing tumors. Oncogene 14:1159, 1997.
311. Quezado M, Benjamin DR, Tsokos M. EWS/FLI-1 fusion transcripts in three peripheral primitive neuroectodermal tumors of the kidney. Hum Pathol 28:767, 1997.
312. Ramani P, Rampling D, Link M. Immunocytochemical study of 12E7 in small round cell tumors of childhood: an assessment of its sensitivity and specificity. Histopathology 23:557, 1993.
313. Riopel M, Dickman PS, Link MP, et al. MIC2 analysis in pediatric lymphomas and leukemias. Hum Pathol 25:396, 1994.
314. Rud NP, Reiman HM, Pritchard DJ, et al. Extraosseous Ewing's sarcoma: a study of 42 cases. Cancer 64:1548, 1989.
315. Sailer SL, Harmon DC, Mankin HJ, et al. Ewing's sarcoma: surgical resection as a prognostic factor. Int J Radiat Oncol Biol Phys 15:43, 1988.
316. Sainati L, Scapinello A, Montaldi A, et al. A mesenchymal chondrosarcoma of a child with the reciprocal translocation (11;22)(q24;q12). Cancer Genet Cytogenet 71:144, 1993.
317. Sawyer JR, Tryka AF, Lewis JM. A novel reciprocal chromosome translocation t(11;22)(p13;q12) in an intraabdominal desmoplastic small round-cell tumor. Am J Surg Pathol 16:411, 1992.
318. Schmidt D, Herrmann C, Jurgens H, et al. Malignant peripheral neuroectodermal tumor and its necessary distinction from Ewing's sarcoma: a report from the Kiel Pediatric Tumor Registry. Cancer 68:2251, 1991.
319. Scotlandi K, Serra M, Manara MC, et al. Immunostaining of the p30/32$^{MIC2}$ antigen and molecular detection of EWS rearrangements for the diagnosis of Ewing's sarcoma and peripheral neuroectodermal tumor. Hum Pathol 27:408, 1996.
320. Seemayer TA, Thelmo WL, Boland R, et al. Peripheral neuroectodermal tumors. Perspect Pediatr Pathol 2:151, 1975.
321. Sexton CW, White WL. Primary cutaneous Ewing's family sarcoma: report of a case with immunostaining for glycoprotein p30/32$^{MIC2}$. Am J Dermatopathol 18:601, 1996.
322. Shanfeld RL, Edelman J, Willis JE, et al. Immunohistochemical analysis of neural markers in peripheral primitive neuroectodermal tumors (pPNET) without light microscopic evidence of neural differentiation. Appl Immunohistochem 5:78, 1997.
323. Sheaff M, McManus A, Scheimberg I, et al. Primitive neuroectodermal tumor of the kidney confirmed by fluorescence in-situ hybridization. Am J Surg Pathol 21:461, 1997.
324. Shimada H, Newton WA Jr, Soule EH, et al. Pathologic features of extraosseous Ewing's sarcoma: a report from the Intergroup Rhabdomyosarcoma Study. Hum Pathol 19:442, 1988.
325. Siebenrock KA, Nascimento AG, Rock MG. Comparison of soft tissue Ewing's sarcoma and peripheral neuroectodermal tumor. Clin Orthop 329:288, 1996.
326. Smith LM, Adams RH, Brothman AR, et al. Peripheral primitive neuroectodermal tumor presenting with diffuse cutaneous involvement and 7;22 translocation. Med Pediatr Oncol 30:357, 1998.
327. Sorensen JB, Schultze HR, Madsen DL, et al. Primitive neuroectodermal tumor (PNET) of the uterine cavity. Eur J Obstet Gynecol Reprod Biol 76:181, 1998.
328. Sorensen PHB, Lessnick SL, Lopez-Terrada D, et al. A second Ewing's sarcoma translocation, t(21;22), fuses the EWS gene to another ETS-family transcription factor, ERG. Nat Genet 6:146, 1994.
329. Sorensen PHB, Liu XF, Delattre O, et al. Reverse transcriptase PCR amplification of EWS-FLI-1 fusion transcripts as a diagnostic test for peripheral primitive neuroectodermal tumors of childhood. Diagn Mol Pathol 2:147, 1993.
330. Sorensen PHB, Shimada H, Liu XF, et al. Biphenotypic sarcomas with myogenic and neural differentiation express the Ewing's sarcoma EWS/FLI-1 fusion gene. Cancer Res 55:1385, 1995.
331. Soslow RA, Wallace M, Goris J, et al. MIC2 gene expression in cutaneous neuroendocrine carcinoma (Merkel cell carcinoma). Appl Immunohistochem 4:235, 1996.
332. Soule EH, Newton W Jr, Moon TE, et al. Extraskeletal Ewing's sarcoma: a preliminary review of 26 cases encountered in the Intergroup Rhabdomyosarcoma Study. Cancer 42:259, 1978.
333. Stark B, Mor C, Jeison M, et al. Additional chromosomal 1q aberrations and der(16) t(1;16), correlation to the phenotypic expression and clinical behavior of the Ewing family of tumors. J Neurooncol 31:3, 1997.
334. Stephenson CF, Bridge JA, Sandberg AA. Cytogenetic and pathologic aspects of Ewing's sarcoma and neuroectodermal tumors. Hum Pathol 23:1270, 1993.
335. Stevenson AJ, Chatten J, Bertoni F, et al. CD99 (p30/32$^{MIC2}$) neuroectodermal/Ewing's sarcoma antigen as an immunohistochemical marker: review of more than 600 tumors and the literature experience. Appl Immunohistochem 2:231, 1994.
336. Stewart DA, Gyonyor E, Paterson AH, et al. High-dose melphalan ± total body irradiation and autologous hematopoietic stem cell rescue for adult patients with Ewing's sarcoma or peripheral neuroectodermal tumor. Bone Marrow Transplant 18:315, 1996.
337. Stout AP. A discussion of the pathology and histogenesis of Ewing's tumor of bone marrow. AJR 50:334, 1943.
338. Stout AP. Tumor of the ulnar nerve. Proc NY Pathol Soc 18:2, 1918.
339. Tanaka K, Iwakuma T, Harimaya K, et al. EWS-FLI-1 antisense oligodioxynucleotide inhibits proliferation of human Ewing's sarcoma and primitive neuroectodermal tumor cells. J Clin Invest 99:239, 1997.
340. Terrier P, Henry-Amar M, Triche TJ, et al. Neuro-ectodermal differentiation of Ewing's sarcoma of bone associated with an unfavourable prognosis? Eur J Cancer 31A:307, 1995.
341. Thorner P, Squire J, Chilton-MacNeill S, et al. Is the EWS/FLI-1 fusion transcript specific for Ewing's sarcoma and peripheral primitive neuroectodermal tumor? A report of four cases showing this transcript in a wider range of tumor types. Am J Pathol 148:1125, 1996.
342. Toretsky JA, Connell Y, Neckers L, et al. Inhibition of EWS-FLI-1 fusion protein with antisense oligodioxynucleotides. J Neurooncol 31:9, 1997.
343. Triche TJ, Ross WE. Glycogen-containing neuroblastoma with clinical and histopathological features of Ewing's sarcoma. Cancer 41:1425, 1978.
344. Tsuji S, Hisaoka M, Morimitsu Y, et al. Peripheral primitive neuroectodermal tumour of the lung: report of two cases. Histopathology 33:369, 1998.
345. Turc-Carel C, Aurias A, Mugneret F, et al. Chromosomes in Ewing's sarcoma. I. An evaluation of 85 cases and remarkable consistency of t(11;22)(q24;q12). Cancer Genet Cytogenet 32: 229, 1988.
346. Ushigome S, Shimoda T, Takaki K, et al. Immunocytochemical and ultrastructural studies of the histogenesis of Ewing's sarcoma and putatively related tumors. Cancer 64:52, 1989.
347. Van de Rijn M, Barr FG, Xiong QB, et al. Poorly differentiated

synovial sarcoma: an analysis of clinical, pathologic and molecular genetic features. Am J Surg Pathol 23:106, 1999.
348. Weidner N, Tjoe J. Immunohistochemical profile of monoclonal antibody O13: antibody that recognizes glycoprotein p30/32[MIC2] and is useful in diagnosing Ewing's sarcoma and peripheral neuroepithelioma. Am J Surg Pathol 18:486, 1994.
349. Wexler LH, DeLaney TF, Tsokos M, et al. Ifosfamide and etoposide plus vincristine, doxorubicin and cyclophosphamide for newly diagnosed Ewing's sarcoma family of tumors. Cancer 78:901, 1996.
350. Whang-Peng J, Triche TJ, Knutsen T, et al. Chromosome translocation in peripheral neuroepithelioma. N Engl J Med 311: 584, 1984.
351. Wigger HJ, Salazar GH, Blanc WA. Extraskeletal Ewing's sarcoma: an ultrastructural study. Arch Pathol 101:446, 1977.
352. Willis RA. Metastatic neuroblastoma in bone presenting the Ewing's syndrome, with a discussion of "Ewing's sarcoma." Am J Pathol 16:317, 1940.
353. Zoubek A, Dockhorn-Dworniczak B, Delattre O, et al. Does expression of different EWS chimeric transcripts define clinically distinct risk groups of Ewing tumor patients? J Clin Oncol 14:1245, 1996.
354. Zucman J, Melot T, Desmaze C, et al. Combinatorial generation of variable fusion proteins in the Ewing family of tumors. EMBO J 12:4481, 1993.

### Olfactory Neuroblastoma

355. Al Ahwal M, Jaj N, Nabholtz JM, et al. Olfactory neuroblastoma: report of a case associated with inappropriate antidiuretic hormone secretion. J Otolaryngol 23:437, 1994.
356. Argani P, Perez-Ordonez B, Xiao H, et al. Olfactory neuroblastoma is not related to the Ewing family of tumors: absence of EWS/FLI-1 gene fusion and MIC2 expression. Am J Surg Pathol 22:391, 1998.
357. Axe S, Kuhajada FP. Esthesioneuroblastoma: intermediate filaments, neuroendocrine and tissue-specific antigens. Am J Clin Pathol 88:139, 1987.
358. Banerjee AK, Sharma BS, Vashista RK, et al. Intracranial olfactory neuroblastoma: evidence for olfactory epithelial origin. J Clin Pathol 45:299, 1992.
359. Berger L, Luc R. L'esthesioneuroepitheliome olfactif. Bull Assoc Fr Etude Cancer 13:410, 1924.
360. Bhattacharyya N, Thornton AF, Joseph MP, et al. Successful treatment of esthesioneuroblastoma and neuroendocrine carcinoma with combined chemotherapy and proton radiation: results in 9 cases. Arch Otolaryngol Head Neck Surg 123:34, 1997.
361. Broich G, Pagliari A, Ottaviani F. Esthesioneuroblastoma: a general review of the cases published since the discovery of the tumour in 1924. Anticancer Res 17:2683, 1997.
362. Cavazzana AO, Navarro S, Noguera R, et al. Olfactory neuroblastoma is not a neuroblastoma but is related to primitive neuroectodermal tumor (PNET). Prog Clin Biol Res 271:463, 1988.
363. Chan JKC, Lau WH, Yuen RWS. Ganglioneuroblastic transformation of olfactory neuroblastoma. Histopathology 14:425, 1989.
364. Choi HS, Anderson PJ. Immunohistochemical diagnosis of olfactory neuroblastoma. J Neuropathol Exp Neurol 44:18, 1985.
365. Devaney K, Wenig BM, Abbondanzo SL. Olfactory neuroblastoma and other round cell lesions of the sinonasal region. Mod Pathol 9:658, 1996.
366. Dulguerov P, Calcaterra T. Esthesioneuroblastoma: the UCLA experience 1970–1990. Laryngoscope 102:843, 1992.
367. Eden BV, Debo RF, Larner JM, et al. Esthesioneuroblastoma: long term outcome and patterns of failure—the University of Virginia experience. Cancer 73:2556, 1994.
368. Elkon D, Hightower SI, Lim ML, et al. Esthesioneuroblastoma. Cancer 44:1087, 1979.
369. Ferlito A, Rinaldo A, Devaney KO. Syndrome of inappropriate antidiuretic hormone secretion associated with head neck cancers: review of the literature. Ann Otol Rhinol Laryngol 107: 878, 1997.
370. Gaudin PB, Rosai J. Florid vascular proliferation associated with neural and neuroendocrine neoplasms: a diagnostic clue and potential pitfall. Am J Surg Pathol 19:642, 1995.
371. Hirose T, Scheithaeuer BW, Lopes MB, et al. Olfactory neuroblastoma: an immunohistochemical, ultrastructural, and flow cytometric study. Cancer 76:4, 1995.
372. Hyams VJ, Batsakis JG, Micjaels LE. Tumors of the upper respiratory tract. In: Atlas of Tumor Pathology, 2nd Series, Fascicle 25. Armed Forces Institute of Pathology, Washington, DC, 1988, p 240.
373. Irish J, Dasgupta R, Freeman J, et al. Outcome and analysis of the surgical management of esthesioneuroblastoma. J Otolaryngol 26:1, 1997.
374. Jin Y, Mertens F, Artheden K, et al. Karyotypic features of malignant tumors of the nasal cavity and paranasal sinuses. Int J Cancer 60:637, 1995.
375. Kadish S, Goodman M, Wang CC. Olfactory neuroblastoma: a clinical analysis of 17 cases. Cancer 37:1571, 1976.
376. Kahn LB. Esthesioneuroblastoma: a light and electron microscopic study. Hum Pathol 5:364, 1974.
377. Kumar S, Perlman E, Pack S, et al. Absence of EWS/FLI1 fusion in olfactory neuroblastomas indicates these tumors do not belong to the Ewing's sarcoma family. Hum Pathol 30: 1356, 1999.
378. Li C, Yousem DM, Hayden RE, et al. Olfactory neuroblastoma: MR evaluation. Am J Neuroradiol 14:1167, 1993.
379. Mezzelani A, Tornielli S, Minoletti F, et al. Esthesioneuroblastoma is not a member of the primitive peripheral neuroectodermal tumour-Ewing's group. Br J Cancer 81:586, 1999.
380. Mills SE, Frierson HF. Olfactory neuroblastoma: a clinicopathologic study of 21 cases. Am J Surg Pathol 9:317, 1985.
381. Min K-W. Usefulness of electron microscopy in the diagnosis of "small" round cell tumors of the sinonasal region. Ultrastruct Pathol 19:347, 1995.
382. Morita A, Ebersold MJ, Olsen KD, et al. Esthesioneuroblastoma: prognosis and treatment. Neurosurgery 32:706, 1993.
383. Nelson RS, Perlman EJ, Askin FB. Is esthesioneuroblastoma a peripheral neuroectodermal tumor? Hum Pathol 26:639, 1995.
384. Nguyen QA, Villablanca JG, Siegel SE, et al. Esthesioneuroblastoma in the pediatric age-group: the role of chemotherapy and autologous bone marrow transplantation. Int J Pediatr Otorhinolaryngol 37:45, 1996.
385. Oberman HA, Rice DH. Olfactory neuroblastoma: a clinicopathologic study. Cancer 38:2494, 1976.
386. Ordóñez NG, MacKay B. Neuroendocrine tumors of the nasal cavity. Pathol Annu 28:77, 1993.
387. Papadaki H, Kounelis S, Kapadia SB, et al. Relationship of p53 gene alterations with tumor progression and recurrence in olfactory neuroblastoma. Am J Surg Pathol 20:715, 1996.
388. Schmidt JL, Zarbo RJ, Clark JL. Olfactory neuroblastoma: clinicopathologic and immunohistochemical characterization of four representative cases. Laryngoscope 100:1052, 1990.
389. Schuster JJ, Phillips CD, Levine PA. MR of esthesioneuroblastoma (olfactory neuroblastoma) and appearance after craniofacial resection. Am J Neuroradiol 15:1169, 1994.
390. Silva EG, Butler JJ, Mackay B, et al. Neuroblastomas and neuroendocrine carcinomas of the nasal cavity: a proposed new classification. Cancer 50:2388, 1982.
391. Slevin NJ, Irwin CJ, Banerjee SS, et al. Olfactory neural tumors: the role of external beam radiotherapy. J Laryngol Otol 110:1012, 1996.

392. Sorensen PHB, Wu JK, Berean KW, et al. Olfactory neuroblastoma is a peripheral neuroectodermal tumor related to Ewing's sarcoma. Proc Natl Acad Sci USA 93:1038, 1996.
393. Szymas J, Wolf G, Kowalczyk D, et al. Olfactory neuroblastoma: detection of genomic imbalances by comparative genomic hybridization. Acta Neurochir (Wien) 139:839, 1997.
394. Takahashi H, Ohara S, Yamada M, et al. Esthesioneuroepithelioma: a tumor of true olfactory epithelium origin: an ultrastructural and immunohistochemical study. Acta Neuropathol (Berl) 75:147, 1987.
395. Taxy JB, Bharani NK, Mills SE, et al. The spectrum of olfactory neural tumors: a light-microscopic immunohistochemical and ultrastructural analysis. Am J Surg Pathol 10:687, 1986.
396. Trojanowski JQ, Lee V, Pillsbury N, et al. Neuronal origin of human esthesioneuroblastoma demonstrated with antineurofilament monoclonal antibodies. N Engl J Med 307:159, 1982.
397. Zappia JJ, Carroll WR, Wolf GT, et al. Olfactory neuroblastoma: the results of modern treatment approaches at the University of Michigan. Head Neck 15:190, 1993.

# CHAPTER 33

# PARAGANGLIOMA

The paraganglia are widely dispersed collections of specialized neural crest cells that arise in association with the segmental or collateral autonomic ganglia throughout the body. This system includes the adrenal medulla, chemoreceptors (i.e., carotid and aortic bodies), vagal body, and small groups of cells associated with the thoracic, intraabdominal, and retroperitoneal ganglia. Although the paraganglia are closely related structures, the present trend is to regard them as a large group of embryologically similar structures that manifest certain anatomic differences and functional specializations. For example, the adrenal medulla is a neuroendocrine organ that secretes large amounts of epinephrine and norepinephrine; its cells are chromaffin-positive, and tumors arising from this organ are often functionally active. On the other hand, the carotid and aortic bodies are chemoreceptors specialized to detect changes in the blood pH and oxygen tension. Although catecholamine storage can be documented in their chief cells by sensitive fluorometric techniques, their cells are usually chromaffin-negative, and tumors arising from these structures are usually nonfunctional.

According to Glenner and Grimley,[15] the extraadrenal paraganglion system can be divided into several anatomic groups (Figs. 33–1, 33–2). The *branchiomeric paraganglia* arise in association with arterial vessels and cranial nerves of the head and neck region, including the jugulotympanic, intercarotid (carotid body), subclavian, laryngeal, coronary, aorticopulmonary, and orbital paraganglia. Their cells are generally chromaffin-negative and are arranged in small cohesive nests (zellballen). The carotid body tumor and glomus jugulare tumor epitomize the neoplasms arising from branchiomeric paraganglia.

The *intravagal paraganglia* are located in the perineurium of the vagus nerve, usually at the level of the jugular or nodose ganglion. The tumors arising from these structures are histologically and cytochemically indistinguishable from those arising in the branchiomeric paraganglia. In fact, those arising from the jugular ganglion and invading the temporal bone may be difficult to distinguish from glomus jugulare tumors.

*Aorticosympathetic paraganglia* arise in association with the sympathetic nervous system, particularly at the bifurcation of the aorta (Figs. 33–2, 33–3, 33–4). They may also be found along the courses of the iliac and femoral vessels and in the thorax. Tumors arising from these structures vary in chromaffinicity, functional activity, and histologic appearance. Some resemble branchiomeric paragangliomas, whereas others may be virtually indistinguishable from adrenal pheochromocytomas.

The nomenclature of paragangliomas is confusing, and before the work of Glenner and Grimley[15] it was poorly standardized. Early authors classified paragangliomas according to the chromaffin reaction (i.e., chromaffin and nonchromaffin paragangliomas) on the assumption that catecholamine-secreting tumors such as pheochromocytomas would be chromaffin-positive and nonfunctional tumors chromaffin-negative. The chromaffin reaction is an unreliable procedure that does not always correspond to functional activity and is not specific for catecholamines. Moreover, nonfunctional tumors such as carotid body paragangliomas synthesize and store small amounts of catecholamine, further underscoring the fact that the chromaffin reaction is at best only a crude means of classifying this group of tumors. The most rational approach is that paragangliomas be named according to their anatomic site and further modified depending on whether functional activity is documented clinically. Thus the common nonfunctioning carotid body tumor would be designated "carotid body paraganglioma, nonfunctional." This nomenclature is used herein.

## CAROTID BODY PARAGANGLIOMA (CHEMODECTOMA, NONCHROMAFFIN PARAGANGLIOMA)

The normal carotid body lies on the posterior aspect of the bifurcation of the common carotid artery, usually buried in the adventitia of the vessel.[6] It is a

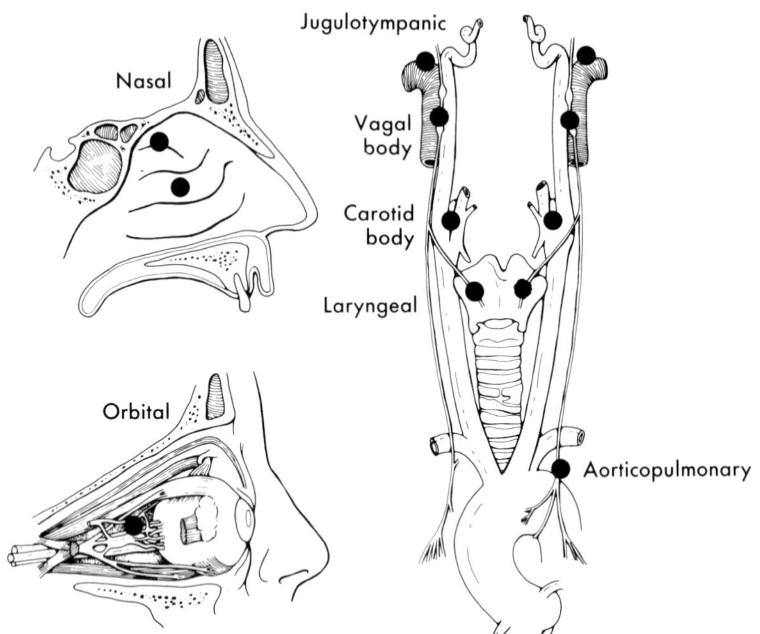


**FIGURE 33–1.** Distribution of branchiomeric paraganglia. (Modified from Lack EE, Cubilla AL, Woodruff JM, et al. Paragangliomas of the head and neck region: a clinical study of 69 patients. Cancer 39:397, 1977.)

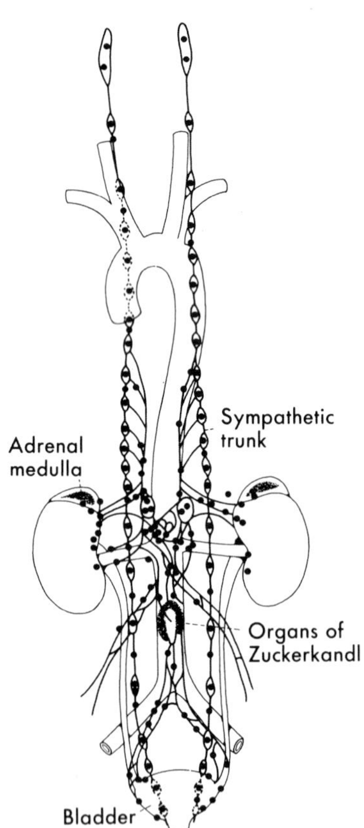


**FIGURE 33–2.** Distribution of aorticosympathetic paraganglia. [Modified from Glenner CG, Grimley PM. Tumors of the extraadrenal paraganglion system (including chemoreceptors). In: Atlas of Tumor Pathology, Fascicle 9, 2nd Series. Armed Forces Institute of Pathology, Washington, DC, 1974.]

specialized chemoreceptor that monitors changes in the arterial oxygen tension and pH of the blood and, in turn, influences in a reflex fashion the rate and depth of respiration and to a lesser extent the heart rate. It is among the largest of the paraganglia and can usually be identified during routine autopsy as a small red body approximately the size of a rice grain. It may assume a size of several millimeters in persons with chronic lung disease or those subjected to the chronic hypoxemia of high altitudes as a result of compensatory hyperplasia.

The carotid body receives its blood supply from the common or external carotid and its innervation primarily from sensory (afferent) fibers of the glossopharyngeal (IX) nerve, with lesser contributions from the vagus (X) nerve and superior cervical ganglion of the sympathetic nervous system. The organ is made up of round or polygonal cells (chief cells) surrounded by delicate sustentacular cells, an arrangement that creates the nest-like (zellballen) appearance. The chief cells have small dense-core granules measuring 100–200 nm, which are the sites of norepinephrine storage as confirmed by the formalin vapor-induced fluorescence of the cells (see Special Staining and Other Procedures, below).

The exact function of the chief cells is unclear, although it seems likely that they influence the level of activity of the autonomic nerves in the organ. The sustentacular cells are modified Schwann cells that appear to conduct nerves to their synaptic terminations on the chief cells. Although the chief cells and

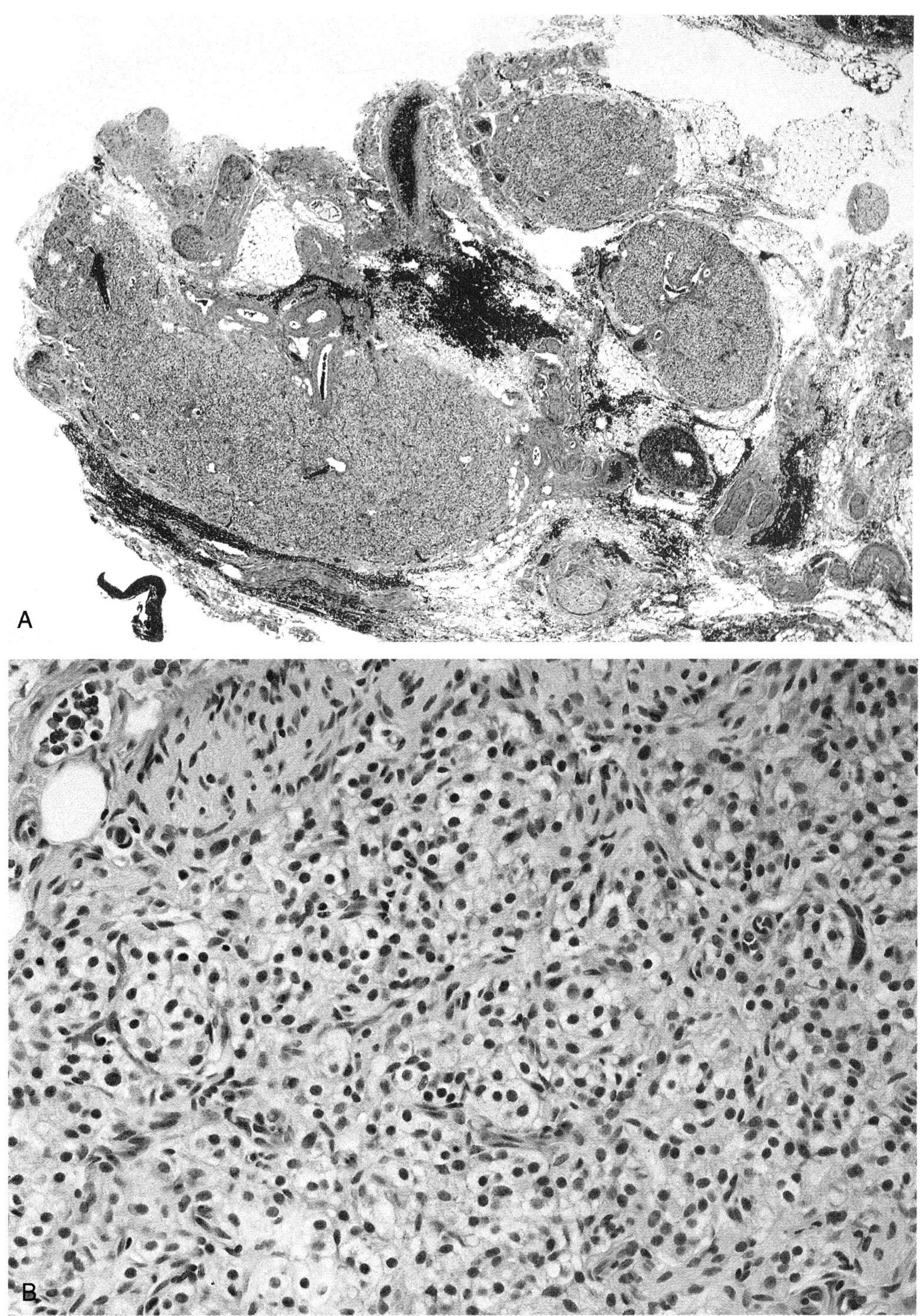


**FIGURE 33–3.** (**A, B**) Organ of Zuckerkandl removed at autopsy from a child.

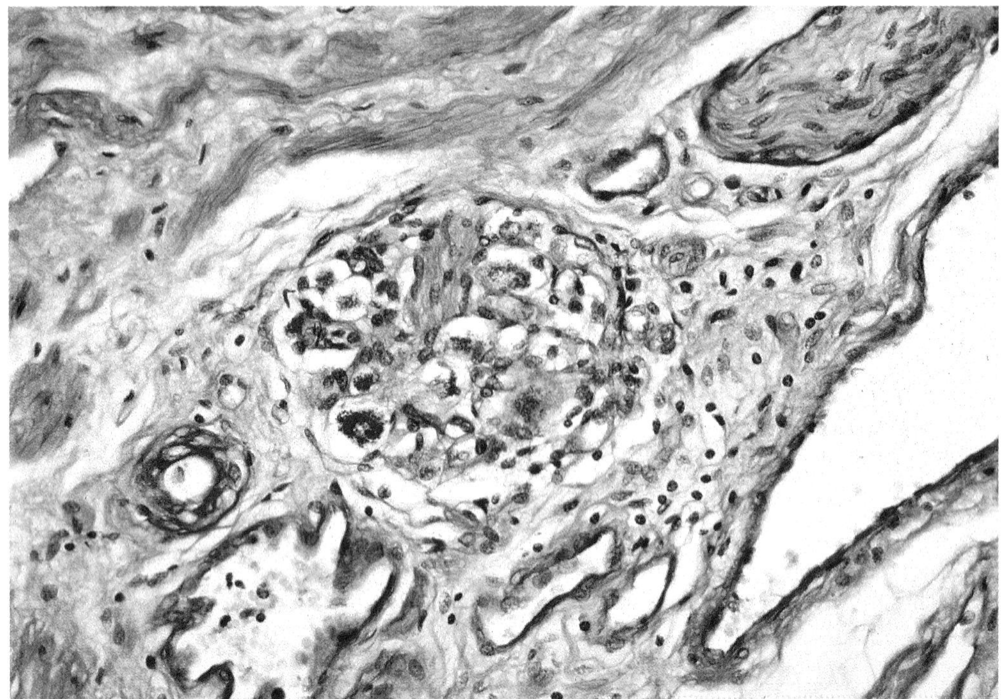

**FIGURE 33–4.** Normal paraganglion located in association with a small autonomic nerve in the retroperitoneum. Pigment, probably lipochrome, is present in some of the paraganglion cells.

sustentacular cells are believed to be of neural crest origin, the supporting structures of the body are presumably of mesenchymal origin.

The carotid body tumor is the most common of the extraadrenal paragangliomas. In the review of the literature by Saldana et al.[53] and in the experience of Memorial Hospital reported by Lack et al.,[31] about 60% of all head and neck paragangliomas arise from the carotid body. The overall incidence of these tumors, however, is low, calculated to be 0.012% of the surgical specimens at Memorial Hospital.[30] The tumor is considerably more common in areas of high altitude such as Peru, Mexico, and Colorado. In fact, Saldana et al.[53] observed that it is nearly 10 times more frequent in high altitude areas in Peru than in sea level locales, suggesting that prolonged hyperplasia of the organ may eventually progress to neoplasia. Men are affected about as often as women in most series, except those reported at high altitudes, where women predominate.[53] Usually the tumor occurs in patients between the ages of 40 and 60 years, although occasional cases in children have been reported.[51,56]

The most common sign is a painless, slowly enlarging mass located in the upper portion of the neck below the angle of the jaw (Fig. 33–5). The tumor is usually movable from side to side but not in a vertical direction. A bruit may be audible over the tumor, and pressure on the tumor may cause an increase in the heart rate (carotid sinus syndrome). Large tumors encroaching on nearby structures cause a variety of associated symptoms. Lesions impinging on the hypopharynx cause hoarseness, whereas involvement of the vagus or sympathetic nerve results in vocal cord paralysis or Horner syndrome. Rarely, carotid body

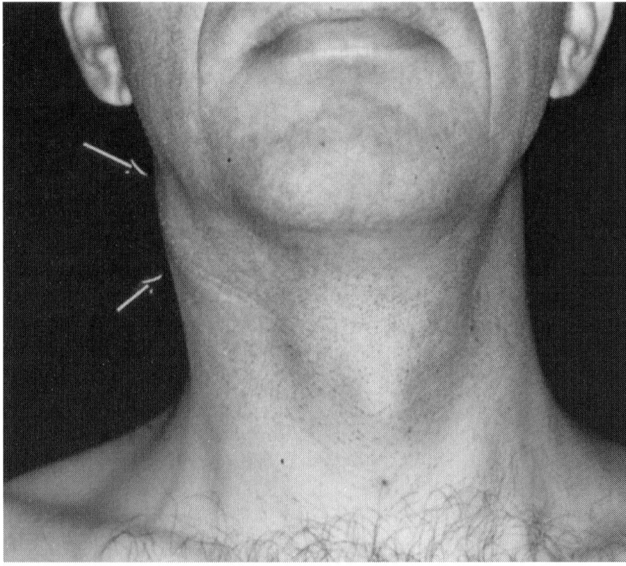

**FIGURE 33–5.** Patient with a carotid body paraganglioma of the right cervical region (arrows). (Courtesy Dr. Thomas J. Whelan, Honolulu, HI.)

tumors are functional[10,14,20] resulting in clinical hypertension. In the past, the level of accurate preoperative diagnosis was extremely low, and these tumors were often confused with tuberculous lymphadenitis, branchial cleft cyst, metastatic carcinoma, carotid artery aneurysm, schwannoma, or lymphoma. Selective arteriography has led to more preoperative diagnoses.[34,35] Typically, these studies indicate enlarged, tortuous carotid vessels with widening and lateral displacement of the bifurcation point (Fig. 33–6). They are also useful for documenting the extent of the lesion. Contralateral carotid angiography is necessary in some patients to exclude bilateral tumors or to document the amount of collateral cerebral blood flow should ligation of the carotid vessels be necessary during surgery.

## Familial and Multifocal Tumors

Paragangliomas have a tendency to occur multifocally. Approximately 7% of carotid body tumors are bilateral,[17] although seldom do both tumors come to clinical attention simultaneously.[46] Approximately 10% of carotid body tumors are familial.[17,58] In the study by Grufferman et al.[17] familial tumors were identified in 88 of 923 patients with carotid body tumors. Of these 88 patients, 31.4% had bilateral tumors compared to 4.4% of patients with sporadic carotid body tumors. A similar frequency of bilateral familial paragangliomas has been reported by others.[12,39,61] Most familial paragangliomas arise in the carotid bodies, and these patients tend to be younger than those with sporadic tumors and have a more even gender distribution. In addition, patients with familial paragangliomas more often have multifocal tumors, most commonly involving the carotid body and glomus jugulare. Evaluation of numerous kindreds suggests that familial cases are inherited with an autosomal dominant pattern of inheritance with incomplete penetrance.[49,50] However, van der Mey et al.[62] noted that children of female carriers never developed these tumors, whereas offspring of male carriers had a 50% risk, suggesting the process of genomic imprinting.[22,23]

Linkage analysis performed in kindreds with familial paragangliomas has revealed evidence of linkage to 11q22.3-q23.2,[2,3,42,64] the site of the *PGL1* tumor-suppressor gene,[63] although there appears to be some genetic heterogeneity, as some cases show linkage to 11q13.[36,37] Genetic counseling based on DNA linkage analysis has detected presymptomatic tumors in some patients.[5,48]

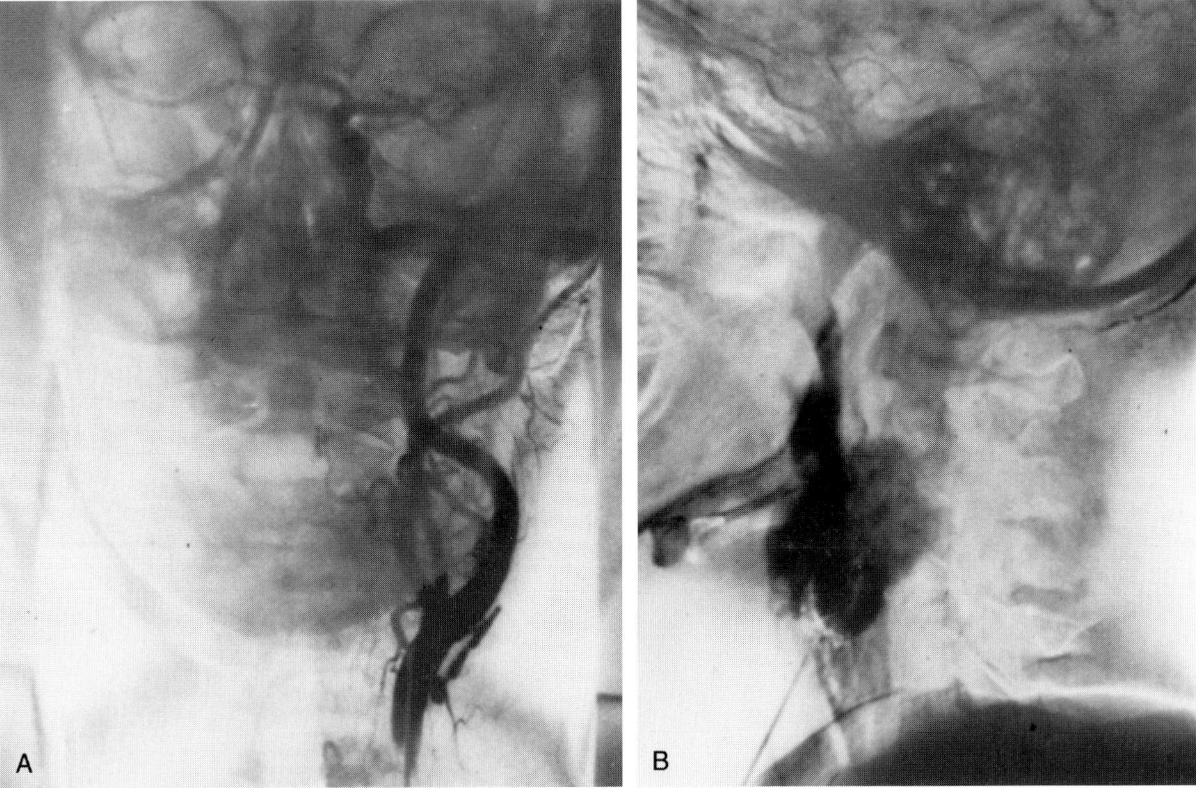


**FIGURE 33–6.** (**A**) Carotid angiography demonstrates widening and lateral displacement of the carotid bifurcation point caused by a carotid body tumor. (**B**) Tumor blush is evident during a later phase of the study.

Rare paragangliomas have been reported in patients with von Hippel-Lindau disease. The tumors in these cases have been found in the carotid body,[24,67] glomus jugulare,[8] mediastinum,[4] retroperitoneum,[8] and sella.[54] Although it is clear that familial paragangliomas not associated with von Hippel-Lindau disease do not have mutations in the von Hippel-Lindau gene located on chromosome 3p,[7,57] too few cases of von Hippel-Lindau- associated paragangliomas have been reported to determine the frequency of mutations at 3p. Sporadic paragangliomas have been associated with mutations of 3p21.[65]

## Gross and Microscopic Findings

Carotid body tumors typically lie in the bifurcation of the common carotid artery (Fig. 33–7A) and may be only partially attached to the vessel or may completely encase it. The intimacy of this relationship is a major factor in determining the surgical resectability of a given tumor. Most carotid body tumors have a lobular, beefy red to brown appearance and measure a few centimeters in diameter (Fig. 33–7B). Hemorrhage and fibrosis are seen in some cases. The tumor is surrounded by a thin or incomplete capsule of connective tissue that is periodically penetrated by fine nerve branches. In the central portion of the neoplasm, the round or polygonal epithelioid cells are arranged in small nests (zellballen) around an elaborate vasculature that can be clearly outlined with a reticulin preparation (Fig. 33–8). In contrast to the normal gland, the zellballen of the carotid body tumor are larger and more irregular in shape, and the cells comprising the tumor are usually larger and more atypical than normal chief cells. Their centrally located nuclei have finely clumped chromatin, and the cytoplasm has either an amphophilic or granular eosinophilic appearance (Fig. 33–9). The cytoplasm of one cell occasionally envelops that of an adjacent cell, a phenomenon termed "cell embracing." Frequently, shrinkage or retraction of the cells away from the tiny vessels results in loss of the classic zellballen pattern. In these regions the cells seem to be arranged in short ribbons or cords similar to those in a carcinoid tumor, in pseudoglands as in an adenocarcinoma, or in pseudorosettes as in a neuroblastic tumor. Paragangliomas with these patterns are often misdiagnosed, a fact that emphasizes the need for special staining procedures. In addition to the specific staining procedures for paragangliomas discussed below, staining for glycogen and mucin is occasionally useful because the stains are negative in paragangliomas and often positive in carcinomas. Another peculiar but frequent artifact of the carotid body tumor is the foamy or vacuolar cytoplasmic change of the chief cell (Fig. 33–10). The cytoplasm contains one or more clear vacuoles that indent the small pyknotic nucleus in the same fashion that fat droplets displace or indent the nucleus of the lipoblast. It is possible to distinguish these cells from true lipoblasts by their close association with other cells having the conventional features of chief cells. Markedly sclerotic carotid body tumors have little or no nesting pattern, and small aggregates of cells lie isolated in the collagenized matrix (Fig. 33–11). Spindling of the chief cell occurs in a small number of cases. This change, descriptively termed "sarcomatoid" by Lack et al.,[30,31] does not appear to affect the prognosis adversely. Occasionally, carotid

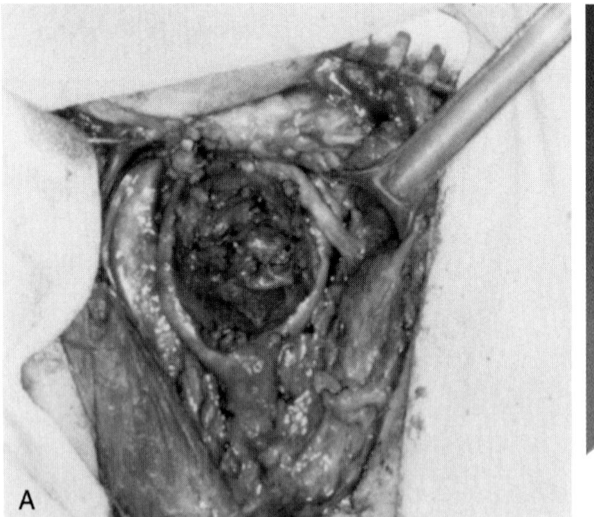


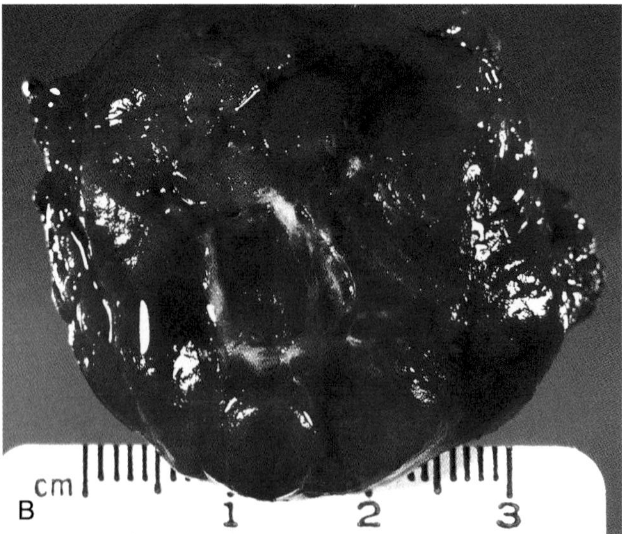


**FIGURE 33–7.** (**A**) Carotid body tumor located at the bifurcation of the internal and external carotid arteries. (**B**) Cut section of a carotid body tumor. (**A:** Courtesy Dr. Thomas J. Whelan, Honolulu, HI.)

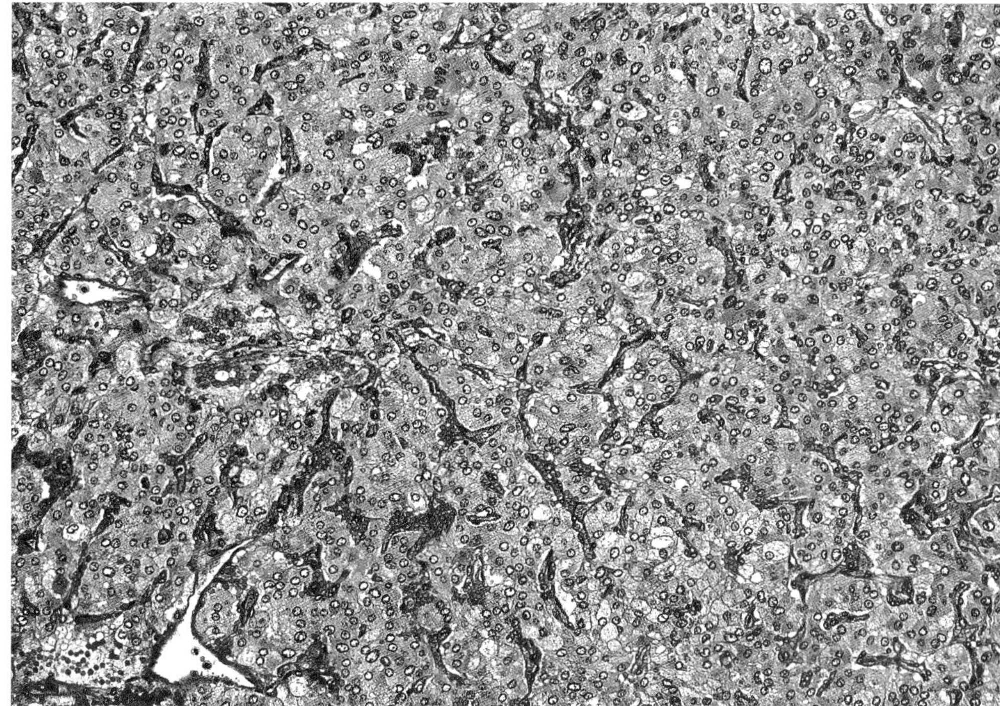

**FIGURE 33–8.** Medium-power view of a carotid body paraganglioma with a zellballen pattern.

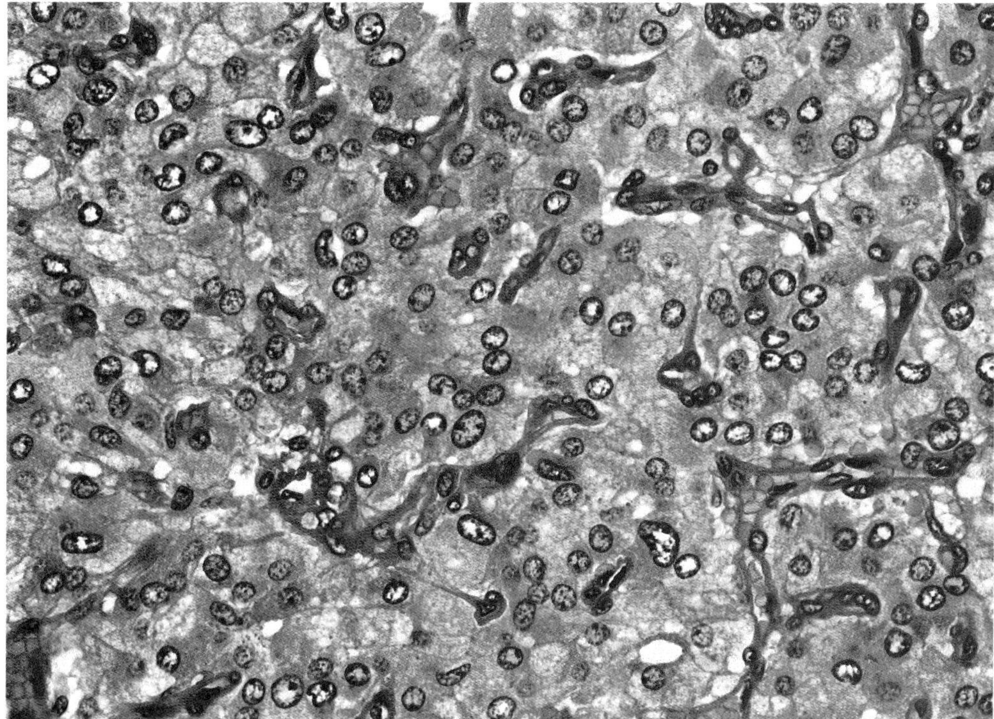

**FIGURE 33–9.** High-power view of a carotid body paraganglioma composed of nests of uniform round cells surrounding a delicate vasculature.

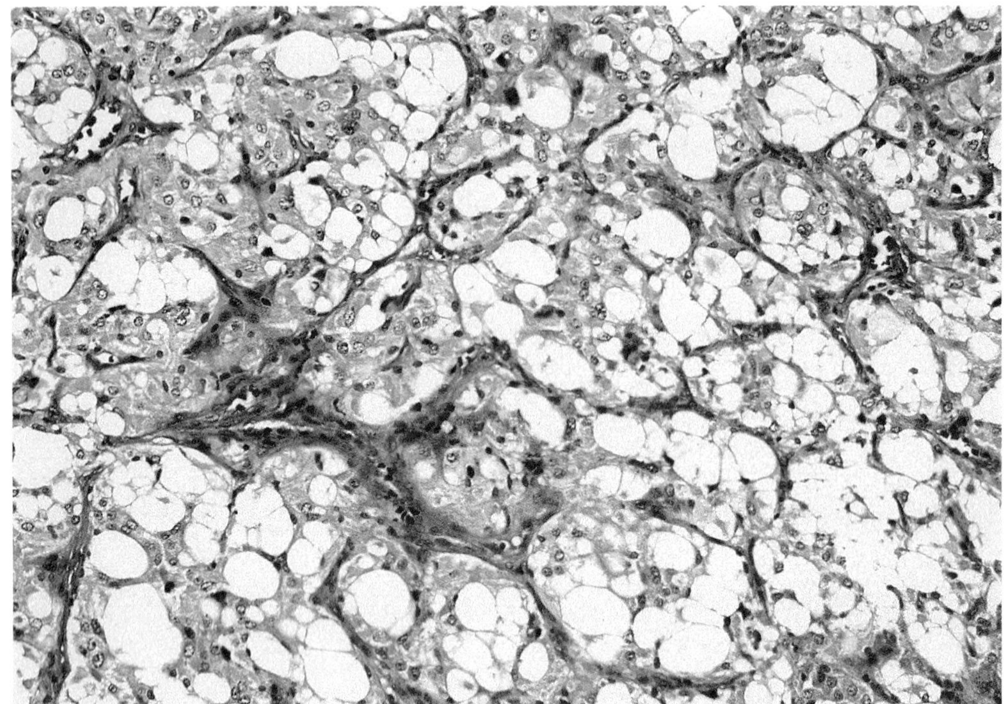

**FIGURE 33–10.** Vacuolated cells in a carotid body paraganglioma, some of which resemble lipoblasts.

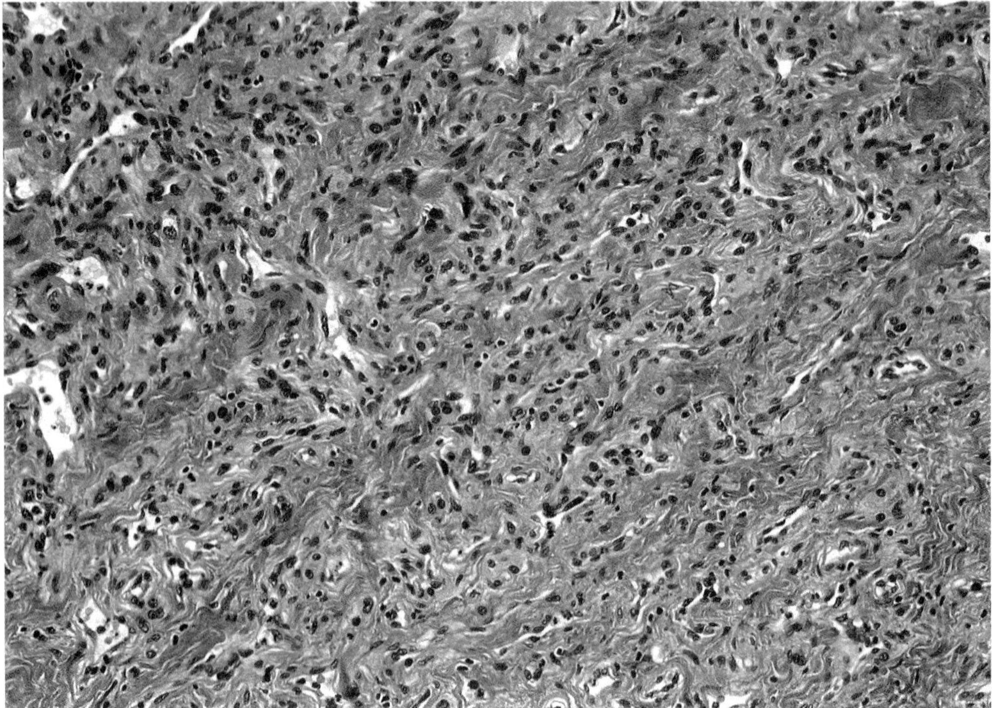

**FIGURE 33–11.** Hyalinized carotid body paraganglioma with isolated neoplastic cells surrounded by dense fibrous stroma.

body tumors are mistaken for vascular tumors (Fig. 33–12), specifically hemangiopericytomas, if the vessels become ectatic and compress the intervening chief cells (Figs. 33–13, 33–14).

## Malignant Carotid Body Tumors

It is usually difficult to recognize the potentially metastasizing carotid body tumor because many are virtually devoid of "malignant" features. A few, however, have atypical features that we believe warrant a diagnosis of malignancy. These tumors are characterized by extremely large zellballen, which blend into broad sheets made up of pleomorphic cells with mitotic figures (Fig. 33–15). Focal necrosis is usually present in the zellballen, and vascular invasion may also be documented. Tumors with these features are uncommon, so an outright diagnosis of malignancy is infrequent. It should be emphasized that nuclear pleomorphism and giant cell formation may be seen in benign carotid body tumors (Figs. 33–16, 33–17) and should not be regarded as evidence sufficient to declare the lesion malignant.

## Special Staining and Other Procedures

In the past the chromaffin reaction, based on the observation that chromic acid oxidizes catecholamines (i.e., norepinephrine, epinephrine) and indoleamines (i.e., serotonin) to a brown polymer, was used to identify tissue containing catecholamines. As indicated by Glenner and Grimley,[15] it is an insensitive, nonspecific, capricious method for demonstrating catecholamines. It is usually invalidated by prior formalin fixation, excessive washing, or dehydration of the tissue; and it fails to detect small amounts of catecholamine. Moreover, it does not invariably identify tissues that presumably have large amounts of this substance, possibly because of anoxic loss of the biogenic amine, low concentration of the substance in a given cell, or differences in the protein envelope surrounding the compound. Although both the normal carotid body and carotid body paraganglioma contain small amounts of catecholamines, the chromaffin reaction is not sensitive enough to detect these quantities. Consequently, with few exceptions, carotid body tumors are chromaffin-negative.

A more sensitive, reliable technique is formaldehyde-induced fluorescence of these compounds. When exposed to vaporous formaldehyde, catecholamines form a green fluorescent dicyclic compound, whereas serotonin forms a yellow compound. This method may be used with fresh or frozen tissue and usually can identify catecholamines successfully in carotid body tumors.

Because catecholamines can reduce silver salts, the modified Grimelius stain (2% silver nitrate) for argyrophil granules[28] can be used to diagnose carotid

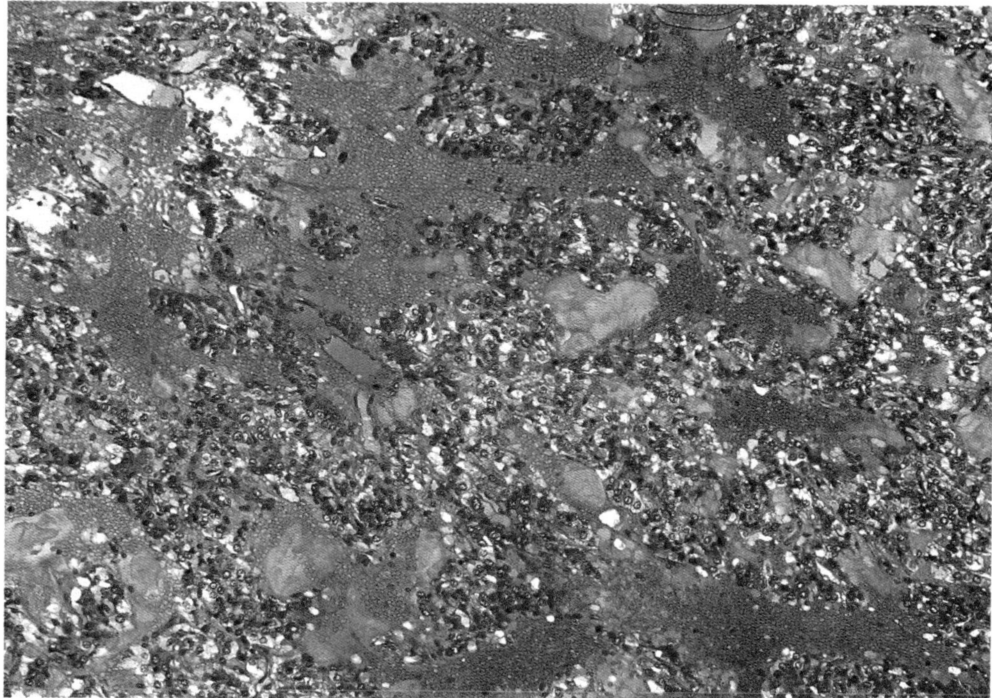

**FIGURE 33–12.** Carotid body paraganglioma with marked congestion of vessels simulating a vascular neoplasm.

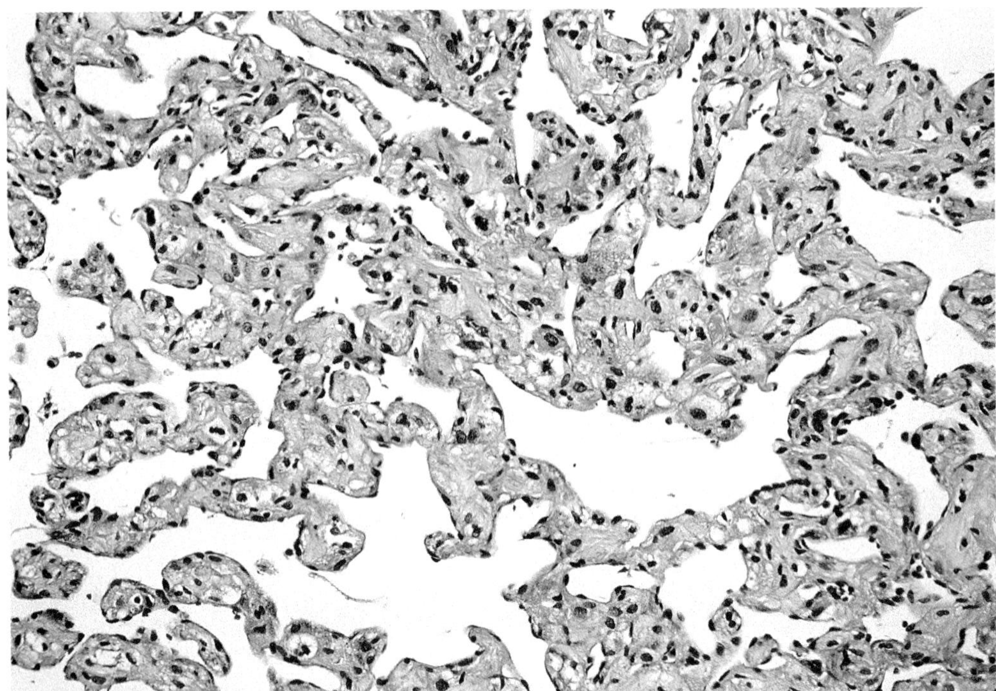

**FIGURE 33–13.** Paraganglioma with ectatic vasculature simulating the appearance of a hemangiopericytoma.

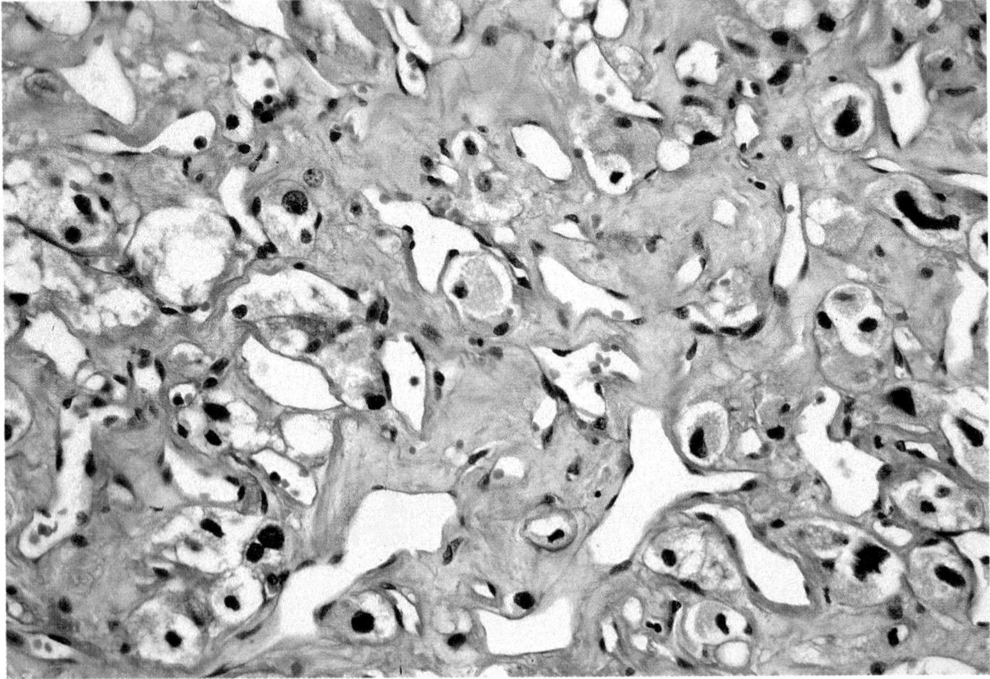

**FIGURE 33–14.** High-power view of a hyalinized carotid body paraganglioma with a hemangiopericytoma-like vasculature.

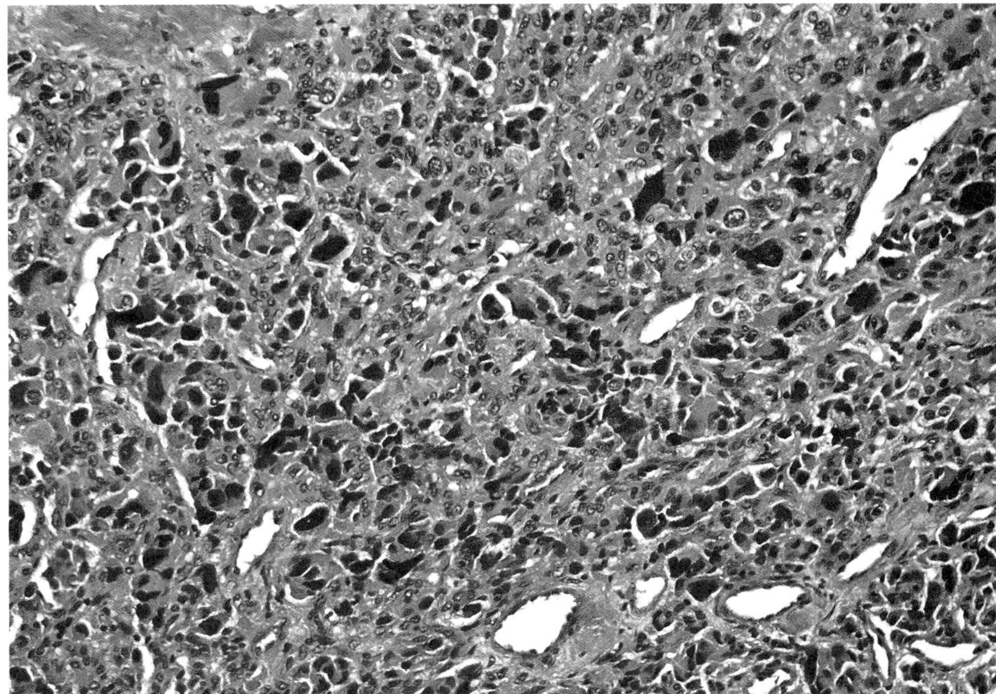

**FIGURE 33–15.** Malignant carotid body tumor composed of broad sheets of pleomorphic cells with rare mitotic figures.

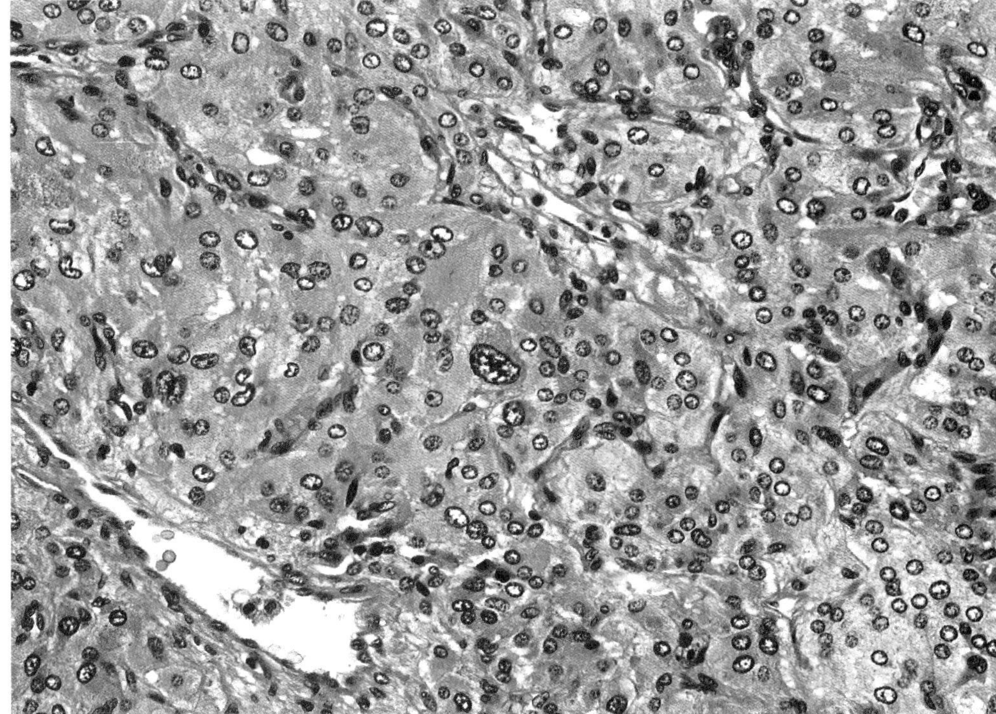

**FIGURE 33–16.** Rare atypical cell found in an otherwise typical carotid body paraganglioma.

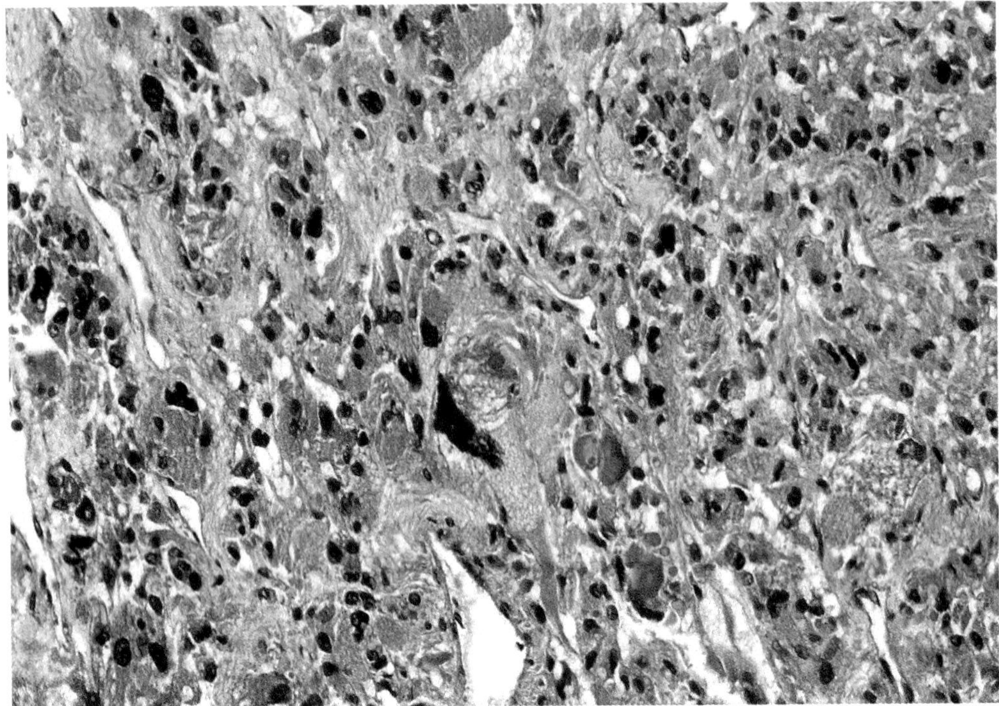

**FIGURE 33–17.** Carotid body paraganglioma containing scattered atypical cells with smudgy nuclear chromatin.

body tumors (Fig. 33–18). This procedure is by no means as specific as the fluorescence technique described earlier, but it offers the advantage that it can be performed on paraffin-embedded tissue. Caution must be exercised when interpreting these stains because degenerating cells are argyrophilic, as are other neural crest tumors. Fontana's stain for argentaffin granules is usually negative in carotid body tumors. False-positive reactions may occur as a result of lipochrome pigment in sustentacular cells.

## Immunohistochemical Findings

With optimally fixed material, neuron-specific enolase, synaptophysin, neurofilament protein, and chromogranin (Fig. 33–19) can be demonstrated in the chief cells of most, if not all, branchiomeric paragangliomas.[25,29,32,55] In addition, the delicate sustentacular network can be elegantly demonstrated using antibodies to S-100 protein (Fig. 33–20), and in a few instances these same cells co-express glial fibrillary acidic protein. A variety of other polypeptides can also be demonstrated in chief cells,[9,27,47] but the immunologic profile seems to vary slightly, depending on the type of paraganglioma. For example, 10 of 11 carotid body tumors expressed multiple peptide hormones in the experience reported by Warren et al.[66] They included various combinations of the following: serotonin, leu-enkephalin, gastrin, substance P, vasoactive intestinal peptide, somatostatin, bombesin, melanocyte-stimulating hormone, and adrenocorticotropic hormone (ACTH). Only a few tumors of the glomus tympanicum expressed these hormones, and none were detected in glomus jugulare tumors. The incidence of neuropeptide hormones in paragangliomas collated from all sites is detailed in Table 33–1.

**TABLE 33–1 IMMUNOHISTOCHEMICAL FINDINGS IN PARAGANGLIOMAS**

| Substance | % Positive ($n$ = 99) |
|---|---|
| Neuron-specific enolase | 100 |
| Leu-enkephalin | 76 |
| Met-enkephalin | 75 |
| Somatostatin | 67 |
| Pancreatic polypeptide | 51 |
| Vasoactive intestinal peptide | 43 |
| Substance P | 31 |
| Adrenocorticotropic hormone | 28 |
| Calcitonin | 23 |
| Bombesin | 15 |
| Neurotensin | 12 |

From Linnoila RI, Lack EE, Steinberg SM, et al. Decreased expression of neuropeptides in malignant paragangliomas: an immunohistochemical study. Hum Pathol 19:47, 1988.

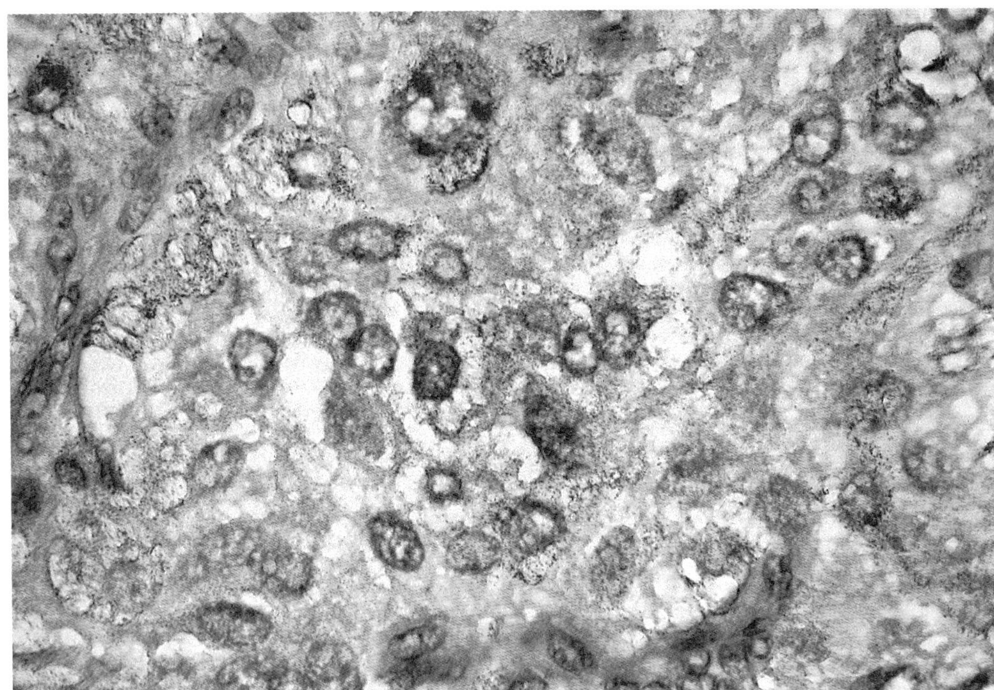

**FIGURE 33–18.** Delicate intracytoplasmic argyrophilic granules in a paraganglioma. (Grimelius stain)

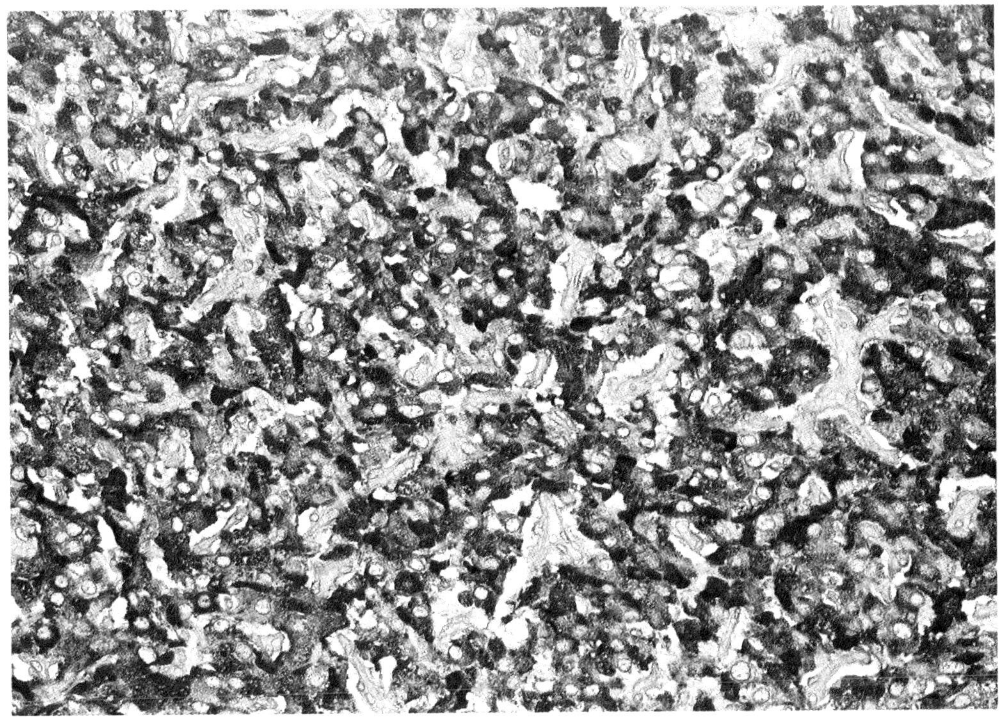

**FIGURE 33–19.** Diffuse immunostaining for chromogranin A in a carotid body paraganglioma.

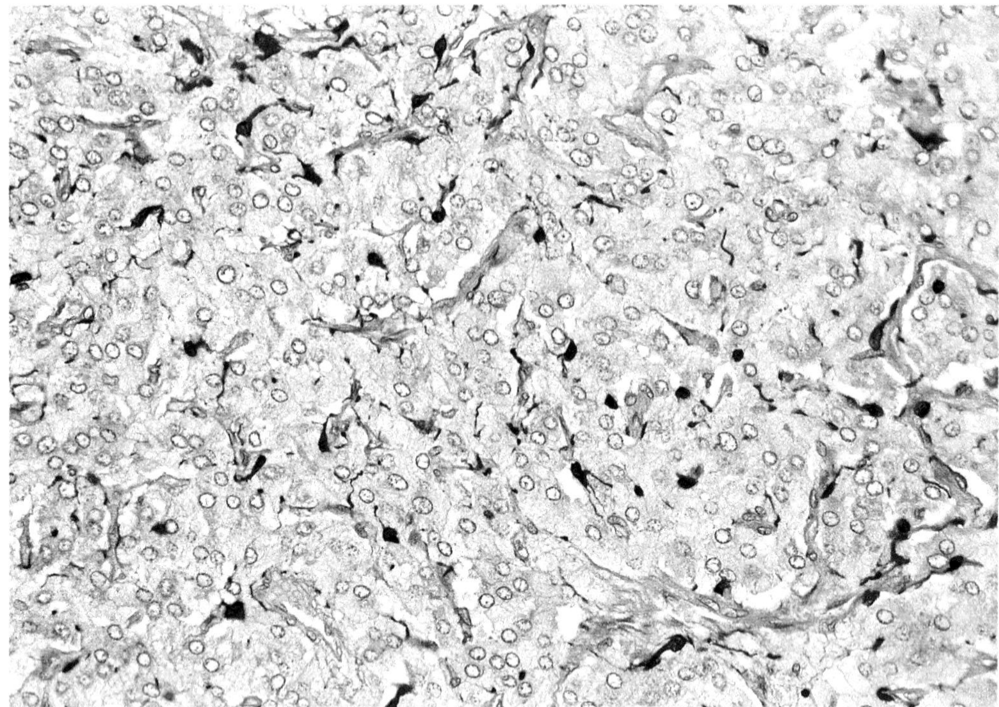

**FIGURE 33–20.** Paraganglioma with a delicate sustentacular network outlined by the immunostain for S-100 protein.

### Ultrastructural Findings

Electron microscopic studies have been performed by a number of investigators, and their results are similar.[1,16] The predominant cell, which resembles the normal chief cell, is round or polyhedral and closely interdigitates with other cells by means of intercellular junctions. The number of ribosomes and mitochondria vary from cell to cell, so the density of the cytoplasm ranges from "dark" to "light." The hallmark of the cell is the presence of small dense-core granules measuring 100–200 nm in diameter (Fig. 33–21); they represent sites of catecholamine storage and in rare sections can be demonstrated to arise from the Golgi apparatus.[1] Sustentacular cells, which have elongated cell processes, are usually not demonstrable in carotid body tumors,[1,30] although Min found their identification diagnostically useful for distinguishing paraganglioma from other neuroendocrine tumors.[43] In the few cases where they were present, they were markedly reduced in number.[16] Their relative rarity provides additional support for the contention that these carotid body lesions are true neoplasms and not hyperplasias. The number of nerve fibers is markedly reduced, and if present they do not bear the normal relation to chief cells.

### Behavior and Treatment

Most carotid body tumors are benign and are cured if total excision can be accomplished at the time of the initial surgery. A small number of patients develop metastases. Patients who develop local tumor recurrence or who have untreated tumors of long duration seem to be at greatest risk for this complication. The incidence of metastasis is estimated at 6–9%.[30,46] Gaylis and Mieny[13] reported an incidence of 30% which they claimed was the result of extended follow-up information. The incidence of malignancy, reported as 50% from an early study at the Mayo Clinic, was based on an evaluation of histologic features alone and was not borne out by subsequent follow-up information.[21]

About half of the metastases appear in regional lymph nodes, and the remainder occur at distant sites, particularly lung and bone. Typically, there is a long interval between the time of diagnosis and the appearance of metastasis. The patient reported by Gustilo et al.[19] developed a metastasis in the pelvis 35 years after resection of the primary tumor. Thus extended follow-up care is advisable.

Technologic advances in vascular surgery and anesthesia now make it possible to resect more carotid

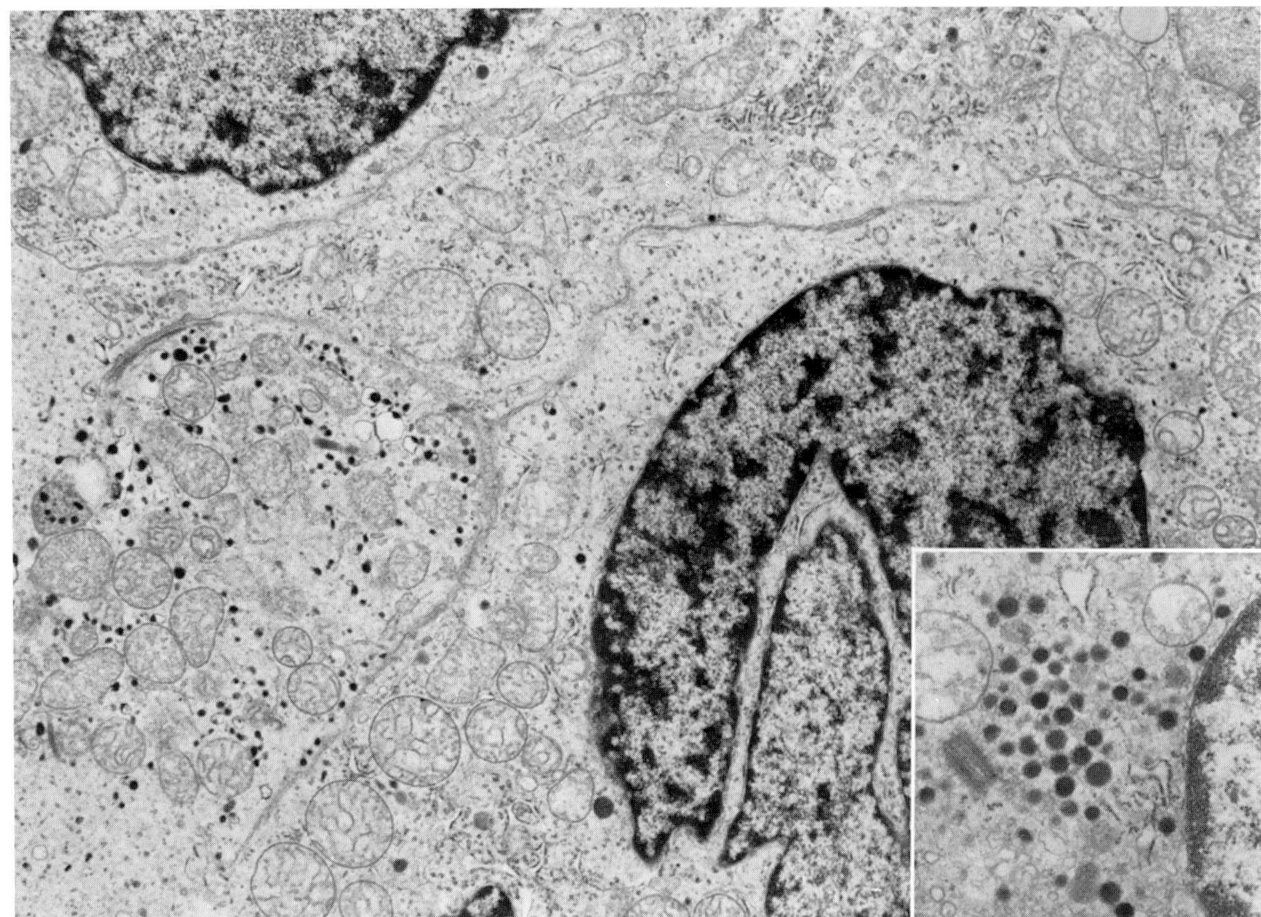

**FIGURE 33–21.** Electron micrograph of a paraganglioma illustrating closely apposed cells characterized by small dense-core granules **(inset)**. (From Taxy JB, Battifora H. The electron microscope in the diagnosis of soft tissue tumors. In: Trump B, Jones RT (eds) Diagnostic Electron Microscopy. Wiley, New York, 1980.)

body tumors with fewer complications than previously.[33] Bilateral carotid arteriography is advisable before surgery, to document the extent of the lesion, determine the presence of a contralateral lesion, and assess the degree of collateral cerebral blood flow should ligation of the carotid artery become necessary. Functional activity should be excluded by means of preoperative catecholamine levels. Patients with functional tumors should be premedicated in the same fashion as patients with adrenal pheochromocytomas.[40]

Localized lesions are easily removed by subadventitial dissection of the carotid artery with preservation of the entire system. More extensive lesions that wrap themselves around the vessel may require resection of the vessel with grafting.[11,38] Selection of patients for the latter procedure is usually based on several factors, including patient age, degree of histologic aggressiveness, and whether basic functions such as swallowing or breathing are compromised. The most common complication of surgery is damage to cranial nerves.[41,46] A small number of patients with bilateral tumors develop postoperative baroreceptor failure and hypertension secondary to bilateral loss of carotid sinus function.[45,52] Extensive intraoperative blood loss can be significantly reduced by preoperative tumor embolization.[35,59] Radiotherapy has been advocated for unresectable lesions and for metastases.[18,26,44,60]

## JUGULOTYMPANIC PARAGANGLIOMA (GLOMUS JUGULARE TUMOR)

Paragangliomas involving the temporal bone and specifically the middle ear take their origin from the paraganglia that follow the auricular branch of the vagus nerve or the tympanic branch of the glossopharyngeal nerve or those related to the bulb of the jugular vein. Although it is conventional to refer to these tumors collectively as glomus jugulare tumors, some prefer to designate the tumors involving the middle ear as glomus tympanicum and to reserve the term glomus jugulare for those that grow upward from the jugular bulb[76,83,89] given the differences in surgical approaches. In some cases, particularly those of long duration, it is difficult to define the origin of the tumor.

Paraganglioma is the most common neoplasm of the middle ear, and those in the temporal bone represent the second most common type of extraadrenal paraganglioma. Most occur in women, and the peak incidence is during the fifth decade. The manner of presentation depends on the rate of growth and the location. Those that arise in the temporal bone usually extend laterally, eventually presenting as a mass in the middle ear or the external auditory canal. In such patients the initial symptoms develop early and include dizziness, pulsating tinnitus, and conductive hearing loss. Usually after several years, discoloration of the tympanic membrane or a friable hemorrhagic mass in the auditory canal appears. Often an aural polyp, cholesteatoma, or vascular tumor is erroneously diagnosed.[86] Tumors of the jugular bulb, in contrast, grow upward, enlarging the jugular foramen and producing characteristic crescentic erosions of the bone crest between the jugular vein and carotid artery radiographically.[91,92] Although these tumors also involve the middle ear, they often, in addition, extend to the base of the brain, causing palsies of the cranial nerves in almost 40% of patients.[68,90] Additional studies utilizing computed tomography (CT), magnetic resonance imaging (MRI), and angiography are useful for determining the size and extent of the lesion, possible synchronous lesions, and the extent of intracranial extension and for assessing the relation of the tumor to major vessels.[69,88]

The incidence of overt functional activity is estimated at 1% in jugulotympanic paragangliomas.[89] One particularly striking case was reported in which the patient experienced cyclic changes in blood pressure at 10- to 17-minute intervals associated with increased norepinephrine levels.[90] Several other jugulotympanic paragangliomas have given rise to hypertensive crises during intraoperative manipulation.[72,91] Jackson et al.[82] reported an increased incidence of perioperative gastrointestinal complications, including cholecystitis and pancreatitis, possibly related to the production of cholecystokinin.

Histologically, these tumors are virtually identical to carotid body tumors. They are usually arranged in a zellballen configuration, although the zellballen are smaller and less uniform than those of the carotid body tumor (Figs. 33–22, 33–23). They are usually highly vascular tumors, a feature that has often led to the mistaken diagnosis of hemangioma when biopsy specimens of these tumors are obtained from the external auditory canal. Typically, the tumors are chromaffin-negative, although argyrophilic granules can be demonstrated by means of the Grimelius stain, and catecholamine storage can be documented using formalin-induced fluorescence.

Ultrastructurally, the tumors are composed of chief cells with small dense-core granules, occasional microtubules, and cilia. One report has described rhomboid crystals with a periodicity of 6–9 nm and delimited by a single membrane. Sustentacular cells are scarce.[78] The immunohistochemical findings are similar to those of carotid body tumors with minor differences.

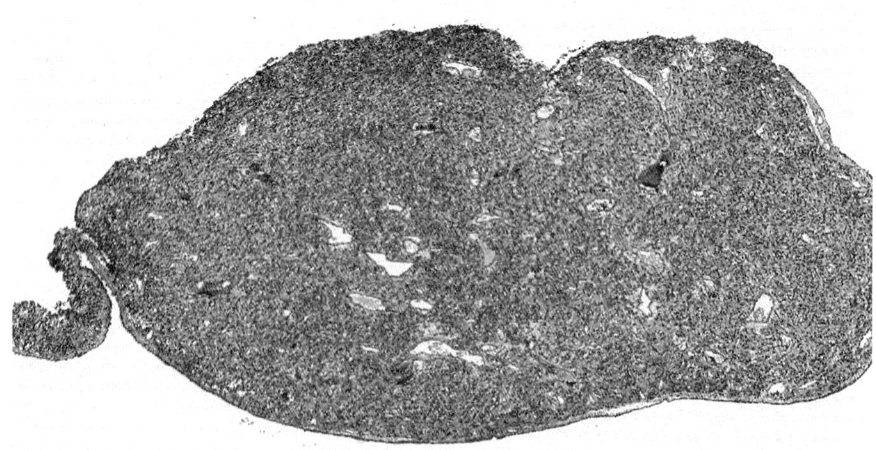

**FIGURE 33–22.** Low-power view of a jugulotympanic paraganglioma.

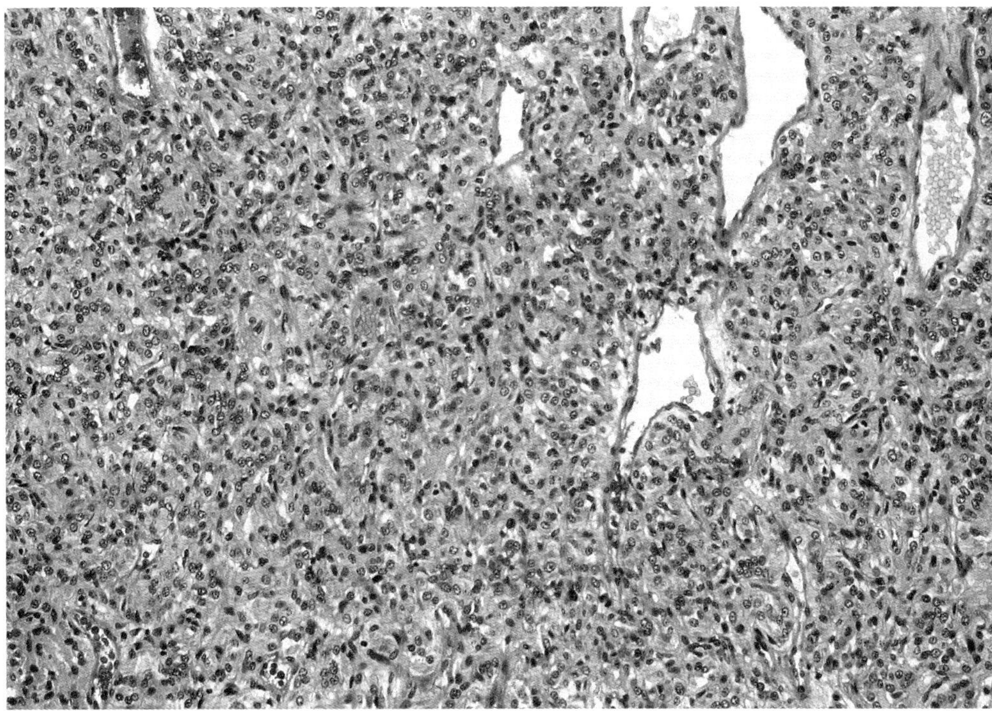

**FIGURE 33–23.** Jugulotympanic paraganglioma with the characteristic zellballen arrangement of cells similar to that seen in carotid body tumors.

The behavior and treatment of jugulotympanic paragangliomas can be most accurately assessed by clinical stage. The Fisch classification[87] combines glomus typanicum and jugulare tumors (Table 33–2), whereas the Glascock/Jackson[77] classification systems separate these two groups, given the differences in surgical approach depending on site (Tables 33–3, 33–4).[91] For patients with surgically curable tumors, the type of operation performed is in turn dependent on tumor site, tumor size, and the relation of the tumor to major vessels.[80]

Type I glomus typanicum tumors are generally treated with a transcanal tympanotomy, whereas a postauricular approach is generally used for type II, III, and IV glomus typanicum tumors.[83] Preoperative embolization is usually performed to reduce intraop-

**TABLE 33–2** FISCH CLASSIFICATION FOR PARAGANGLIOMAS OF THE GLOMUS TYPANICUM AND GLOMUS JUGULARE

| Type | Criteria |
|---|---|
| A | Tumor limited to the middle ear cleft (typanicum) |
| B | Tumor limited to the tympanomastoid area with no bone destruction in the infralabyrinthine compartment of the temporal bone |
| C | Tumor involving the infralabyrinthine compartment of the temporal bone |
| C1 | Jugular foramen and jugular bulb involvement |
| C2 | Vertical portion of carotid canal |
| C3 | Horizontal portion of carotid canal |
| $D_1$ | Tumor with intracranial extension <2 cm in diameter |
| $D_2$ | Tumor with intracranial extension >2 cm in diameter |

From Oldring D, Fisch U. Glomus tumors of the temporal region: surgical therapy. Am J Otol 1:7, 1979.

**TABLE 33–3** GLASCOCK/JACKSON CLASSIFICATION FOR PARAGANGLIOMAS OF THE GLOMUS TYPANICUM

| Type | Criteria |
|---|---|
| I | Small mass limited to the promontory |
| II | Tumor completely filling the middle ear space |
| III | Tumor filling the middle ear and extending into the mastoid |
| IV | Tumor filling the middle ear, extending into the mastoid or through the tympanic membrane to fill the external auditory canal; may also extend anteriorly to the internal carotid artery |

From Jackson CG. Skull base surgery. Am J Otol 3:161, 1981.

**TABLE 33–4 GLASCOCK/JACKSON CLASSIFICATION OF PARAGANGLIOMAS OF THE GLOMUS JUGULARE**

| Type | Criteria |
|---|---|
| I | Small tumor involving the jugular bulb, middle ear, and mastoid |
| II | Tumor extending into the internal auditory canal (± intracranial extension) |
| III | Tumor extending into the petrous apex (± intracranial extension) |
| IV | Tumor extending beyond the petrous apex into the clivus or infratemporal fossa (± intracranial extension) |

From Jackson CG. Skull base surgery. Am J Otol 3:161, 1981.

erative blood loss.[85] Incompletely excised tumors may be treated with postoperative radiation therapy.[73]

Type I and II glomus jugulare tumors are generally treated via a skull base approach,[76] whereas type III and IV tumors often require an infratemporal fossa approach.[74,91] Injury to cranial nerves is the most common postoperative complication.[81]

The clinical course of paragangliomas arising in these locations is usually benign, although some patients develop metastatic disease. In the study by Brown,[71] 138 of the 150 patients with low stage tumors were alive without disease at 10 years. In contrast, 14 of 81 patients with higher stage disease died as a direct result of their tumor. In only 2 of 231 patients did metastasis develop, one to the lung and one to the liver. This rate is slightly lower than the 4% rate reported by Borsanyi[70] derived from 200 cases reported in the literature. Fuller et al.,[75] who analyzed 73 cases from the Mayo Clinic, found no metastasis; a similar experience was reported by Cole[72] with 20 glomus jugulare tumors. Johnstone et al.[84] reviewed 20 jugulare typanic paragangliomas that produced metastasis and found that the common metastatic sites were lung (nine cases), vertebra or bone (six cases), and liver (four cases). Only 3 of the 20 tumors produced metastasis in regional lymph nodes.

## VAGAL PARAGANGLIOMA (VAGAL BODY TUMOR)

The first vagal body tumor was described by Stout in 1935; since that time approximately 200 additional cases have been reported in the English literature, making it the third most common paraganglioma of the head and neck after carotid body and glomus jugulare tumors.[96,97,102] These tumors arise from small dispersed collections of paraganglia that follow the cervical course of the vagus nerve, particularly at the level of the jugular and nodose ganglia. These paraganglia usually lie just underneath the perineurium but occasionally are embedded in the substance of the nerve. Consequently, vagal body tumors develop as high cervical masses between the mastoid process and the angle of the jaw in the parapharyngeal space. The close relation with the nerves at the base of the brain results in neurologic symptoms, including weakness of the tongue, vocal cord paralysis, hoarseness, and in some cases Horner syndrome.[94,100] Rarely are these tumors functional.[101] Like glomus jugulare tumors, these lesions are more frequent in women than in men, and in about 10–15% of cases multiple tumors have been noted.[99] They can be clearly distinguished from carotid body tumors arteriographically because they usually lie above the carotid bifurcation, causing anterior displacement of the vessels without widening of the bifurcation point. At surgery the tumor is usually wrapped around the nerve, although occasionally the nerve fibers are splayed over the tumor, presumably in cases where the lesion arises from intravagal paraganglia.[93]

Histologically, vagal body paragangliomas are similar to carotid body tumors, except they are often traversed by dense fibrous bands representing the residual vagal perineurium (Fig. 33–24). Ultrastructurally, the tumors contain chief cells that show a gradation in cytoplasmic density similar to the light and dark cells of the carotid body. They contain dense-core neurosecretory granules, some of which have a more elongated, or "pleomorphic," appearance than those of the carotid body tumor.[98] Sustentacular cells and synaptic endings on chief cells have been found in some cases[95] but not in others.[99]

Approximately 10–20% of vagal body tumors metastasize, most commonly to regional lymph nodes, although distant metastasis to lung and bone also occur.[93,103] Local infiltration of the internal carotid artery[93,94] and extension into the cranial vault represent significant problems in disease control. Surgical resection is the treatment of choice, although it is usually not possible to excise these lesions without sacrificing the vagus nerve.

## MEDIASTINAL PARAGANGLIOMA (AORTIC BODY TUMOR, MEDIASTINAL AORTICOSYMPATHETIC PARAGANGLIOMA)

Mediastinal paragangliomas arise from paraganglia associated with the pulmonary artery and aortic arch or from the segmental paraganglia associated with the sympathetic chain. The former tumors are located

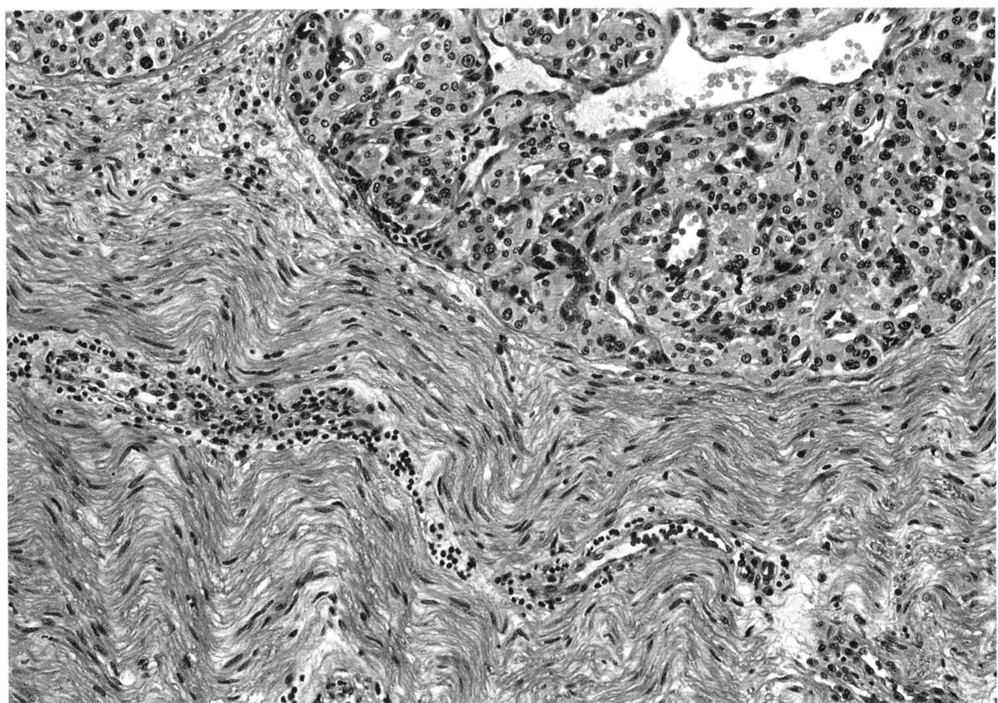

**FIGURE 33–24.** Vagal body paraganglioma embedded in the vagal nerve.

in the anterior mediastinum and are termed "aortic body tumors," whereas the latter are located in the posterior mediastinum and are the mediastinal equivalent of retroperitoneal (extraadrenal) paragangliomas.

Aortic body paragangliomas can originate at any site where the aortic body chemoreceptor has been identified: (1) anterolateral to the aortic arch; (2) lateral to the innominate artery; (3) at the angle of the ductus arteriosus and descending aorta; and (4) to the upper right of the main pulmonary artery.[15] Most reported cases have occurred in persons over age 40 years, and they affect the genders equally. They may be associated with paragangliomas at other sites.[108,113]

Clinically, although many of these tumors are found incidentally in asymptomatic patients, a significant number of patients present with symptoms related to catecholamine secretion, including headache, hypertension, and sweating.[107] Radiographically, the tumors are highly vascular masses of the anterior or superior mediastinum that are fed by vessels from the subclavian, internal mammary, or intercostal arteries, with early drainage into the superior vena cava.[109,111] Histologically, they are identical to the tumors of the carotid body.[104–106]

Although formerly regarded as relatively benign lesions, Olson and Salyer[114] emphasized the rather aggressive course of the anterior mediastinal paraganglioma. Although only about 10% of patients develop metastasis, most eventually die of the disease. Of the 41 cases reported in the literature and reviewed by Olson and Salyer,[114] only 19 patients were alive and well without evidence of disease. Of the remainder, 14 had either inoperable disease or died as a result of the tumor. Three were alive with residual mediastinal tumor, four had tumor documented incidentally at autopsy, one was lost to follow-up, and one had multiple tumors. In a review of the literature of anterior and middle mediastinal paragangliomas, Lamy et al.[112] found a high rate of local recurrence (56%) and documented metastasis in 21 of 79 (27%) reported cases. Optimum therapy is complete surgical excision, using cardiopulmonary bypass if necessary.[109,112] When complete excision cannot be accomplished, the prognosis is guarded, as slow progression and death from tumor may ensue.

Posterior mediastinal paragangliomas are far less common than the foregoing type.[110] In contrast, they occur in younger persons (average age 29 years) and in about half of cases are associated with symptoms referable to functional activity by the tumor. In the remainder of the patients, the mass, which is usually located in the costovertebral sulcus at the level of the fifth to seventh ribs, is discovered incidentally at the time of chest radiography.

The tumors are related to the sympathetic chain, and for this reason they can be considered histogenetically and embryologically similar to the extraadrenal paragangliomas of the retroperitoneum. They may combine features of classic carotid body tumor or adrenal pheochromocytoma. The histologic features of the retroperitoneal paraganglioma, discussed in the following section, are equally applicable to this tumor.

In the study by Moran et al.,[113] 12 of 16 mediastinal paragangliomas were located in the posterior mediastinum. Two patients in this series developed metastatic disease, both with posterior mediastinal paragangliomas. Complete surgical excision is the preferred treatment and is usually accomplished more readily than with paragangliomas in the anterior mediastinum.

## RETROPERITONEAL PARAGANGLIOMA

Approximately 10–20% of paragangliomas of the retroperitoneum arise outside the adrenal from paraganglia that lie along the aortic axis in close association with the sympathetic chain. The largest collection of paraganglia includes the organs of Zuckerlandl (Figs. 33–3, 33–4), paired structures overlying the aorta at the level of the inferior mesenteric artery. These structures are prominent during early infancy but gradually regress after 12–18 months of age, leaving behind only small microscopic residua. Although they are believed to serve chemoreceptor functions in animals, their physiologic role in humans is not understood. Most extraadrenal paragangliomas arise from this organ, whereas a smaller number are derived from the paraganglia lying at other points along the aortic or iliac vessels.

Retroperitoneal paragangliomas occur at a relatively earlier age than those of the head and neck. Most occur in persons 30–45 years of age, although the malignant forms may have an even younger median age.[121,145] Men and women are affected in approximately equal numbers in most series. Occasionally these tumors are multiple, or they may be associated with paragangliomas of other sites[141] or with other tumors such as gastric stromal tumors and pulmonary chondromas as a component of Carney's triad.[115,116,119,120,122]

Back pain and a palpable mass are the two most common presenting symptoms. About 10% of patients present initially with metastatic disease, and about 20% of these tumors are discovered incidentally at the time of autopsy. Symptoms related to production of norepinephrine occur in 25–60% of patients with these tumors. Such patients develop chronic or intermittent hypertension, headaches, and palpitations. In contrast, functional adrenal paragangliomas (pheochromocytomas) may be associated with increased serum levels of epinephrine and norepinephrine, and the exact constellation of symptoms depends on the relative amounts of each. Hypertension predominates in norepinephrine-secreting tumors, whereas hypotension, hypovolemia, palpitations, and tachyarrhythmias are hallmarks of those producing large amounts of epinephrine.[131,151] The difference in secretory patterns is believed to be related to the presence of methyltransferase in some adrenal pheochromocytomas (which converts norepinephrine to epinephrine) and its absence in extraadrenal paragangliomas. Rare retroperitoneal tumors induce hypertension by compressing renal vessels, resulting in renal ischemia.[144]

Extraadrenal paragangliomas are rarely diagnosed preoperatively unless the lesion is functional. In the latter instance, the diagnosis can be established by measuring total urinary catecholamines, and the lesions can be localized by means of angiography. Scintigraphic localization of both adrenal and extraadrenal lesions has been accomplished by means of iodine 131($^{131}$I) metaiodobenzylguanidine (MIBG), a structural analogue of norepinephrine.[139,156] It is concentrated in adrenergic tissue by the same mechanism as that of a neurotransmitter and has allowed visualization of paragangliomas as small as 0.2 g.[152] Localization of these tumors has also been accomplished using the radiolabeled somatostatin analogue octreotide.[128,154] CT scans and MRI are also highly sensitive for detecting small tumors.[129,149]

### Gross and Microscopic Findings

These tumors are partially encapsulated brown masses that usually measure several centimeters in diameter (Fig. 33–25). Hemorrhage is a common finding. Histologically, retroperitoneal paragangliomas may resemble a branchiomeric paraganglioma or adrenal pheochromocytoma, or they may combine features of both. Most, however, are similar to the adrenal pheochromocytoma.

They are composed of small polygonal or slightly spindled cells with an amphophilic or eosinophilic cytoplasm. The cells are arranged in short, irregular anastomosing sheets around a delicate vasculature (Figs. 33–26, 33–27). The cell outlines are often indistinct so the sheets have a syncytial quality. Eosinophilic globules may be identified in the cytoplasm of the cells and vary in size from a few micrometers to the size of a nucleus. These structures seem to represent remnants of dense-core granules, and their presence has been correlated with benignancy (see below). Rare tumors are composed of cells with a melanin-like cytoplasmic pigment (neuromelanin).[134,143] Hemorrhage in these nests of cells is not infrequent (Fig. 33–28). Although few retroperitoneal paragangliomas resemble carotid body tumors in their entirety, it is

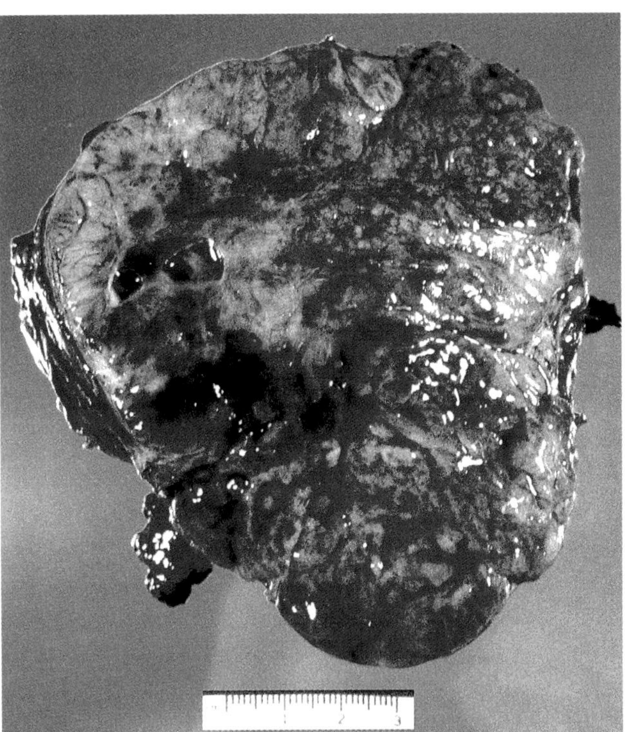

**FIGURE 33–25.** Gross appearance of a retroperitoneal paraganglioma with brown cut surface and focal hemorrhage.

often possible to find occasional areas in these lesions where the cells are round and grow in small nests. A few retroperitoneal paragangliomas are highly pleomorphic lesions made up of spindled or angular cells with deeply eosinophilic cytoplasm and large hyperchromatic nuclei. Such tumors grow in extremely large sheets and often lack the organization of the usual paraganglioma (Fig. 33–29).

On initial inspection these pleomorphic tumors are worrisome and may be mistaken for carcinomas, except that little mitotic activity accompanies the pleomorphic changes. In rare instances, areas of ganglioneuroma are encountered in retroperitoneal paragangliomas (Fig. 33–30). Chromaffin reactions are positive in about two-thirds of retroperitoneal paragangliomas, according to Brantigan and Katase,[117] although not all such tumors are functional (Fig. 33–31). Argyrophilic granules were demonstrated in all the retroperitoneal paragangliomas reported by Lack et al.[133]

## Criteria of Malignancy

The criteria of malignancy for paragangliomas have been controversial. In the opinion of some, the only definite criterion of malignancy is metastatic disease. Linnoila et al.[136] analyzed various features in clinically benign and malignant paragangliomas and concluded that extraadrenal location, coarse nodularity, confluent necrosis, and absence of hyaline globules may be predictive of malignancy (Table 33–5). Altogether, 71% of malignant tumors had two or three of these features, whereas 89% of benign tumors had one or none. The same authors suggested that decreased expression of a variety of neuropeptides may also correlate with malignancy and may therefore serve as an adjunctive means of identifying aggressive behavior. Benign lesions typically express five or more neuropeptides and malignant lesions only two.[137] Clarke et al.[121] found extraadrenal location, male gender, young age, tumor weight, and Ki-67 labeling index to be predictive of malignancy (Table 33–6). Several other studies have found a positive correlation between high proliferative index as measured with the MIB-1 antibody and malignant clinical behavior.[117a,143a] The relative value of flow cytometry has been studied in regard to the evaluation of malignancy in these tumors.[126,147] Although tumors that have metastasized are more often aneuploid or tetraploid than those that have not, there is significant

**TABLE 33–5** HISTOLOGIC FEATURES OF CLINICALLY BENIGN AND MALIGNANT SYMPATHOADRENAL PARAGANGLIOMAS

| Histologic Feature | Malignant ($n$ = 64) | Benign ($n$ = 64) | $p$ |
|---|---|---|---|
| Zellballen pattern (%) | 44 | 30 | NS |
| Trabecular pattern (%) | 21 | 30 | NS |
| Mixed patterns (%) | 33 | 38 | NS |
| Diffuse (sold pattern) (%) | 0 | 3 | NS |
| Confluent tumor necrosis (%) | 32 | 6 | 0.0023 |
| Mitotic rate (mean/30 HPF) | 3 | 1 | NS |
| Hyaline globules (%) | 32 | 59 | 0.013 |
| Extensive local/vascular invasion (%) | 32 | 11 | 0.022 |

Modified from Linnoila RI, Keiser HR, Steinberg SM, et al. Histopathology of benign versus malignant sympathoadrenal paragangliomas: clinicopathologic study of 120 cases including unusual histologic features. Hum Pathol 21:1168, 1990.
NS, not significant; HPF, high-power fields.

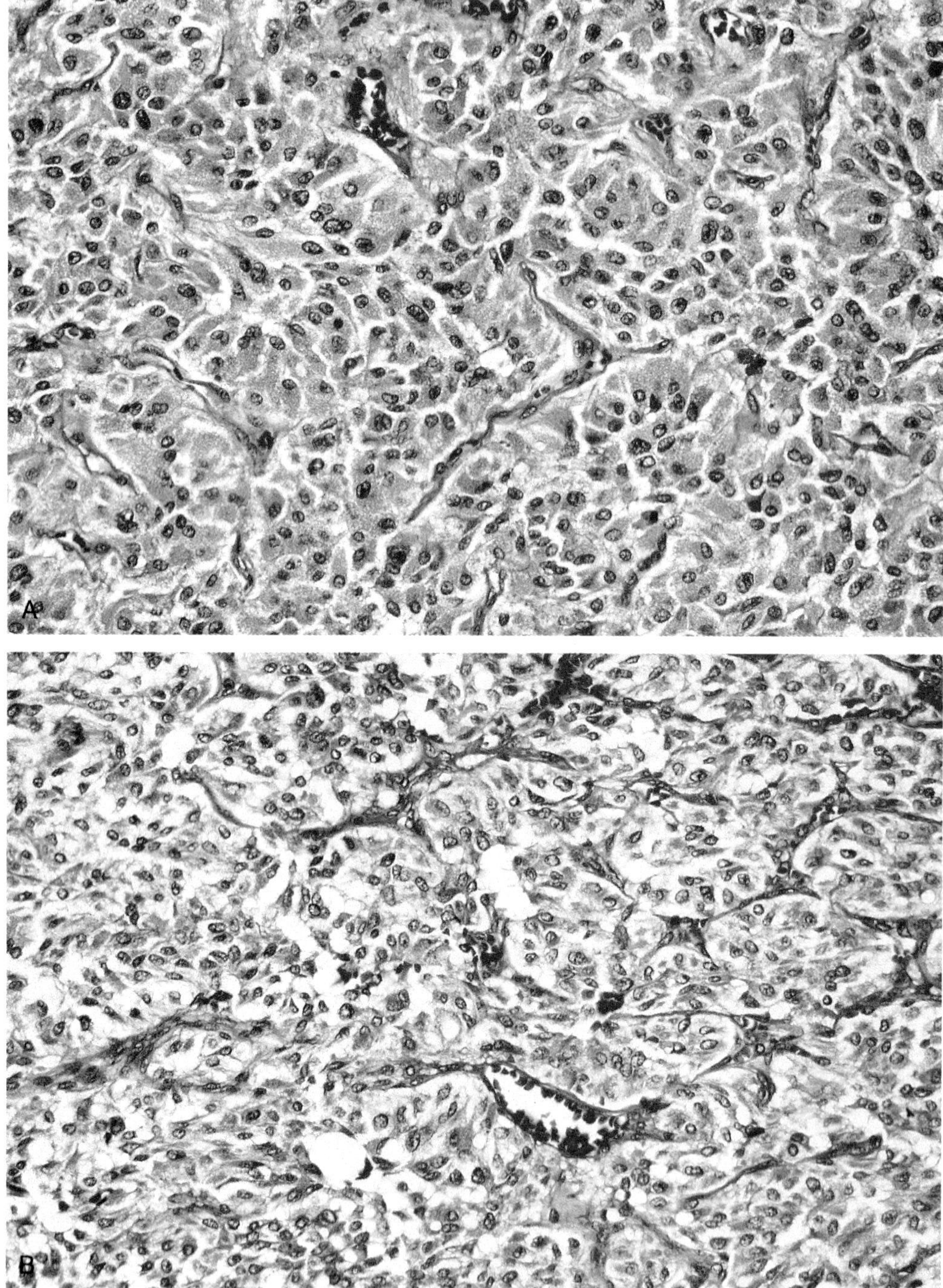

**FIGURE 33–26.** (**A**) Extraadrenal paraganglioma with sheet-like growth of cells in one area. (**B**) In other areas cells have lost cohesion, with formation of clear spaces.

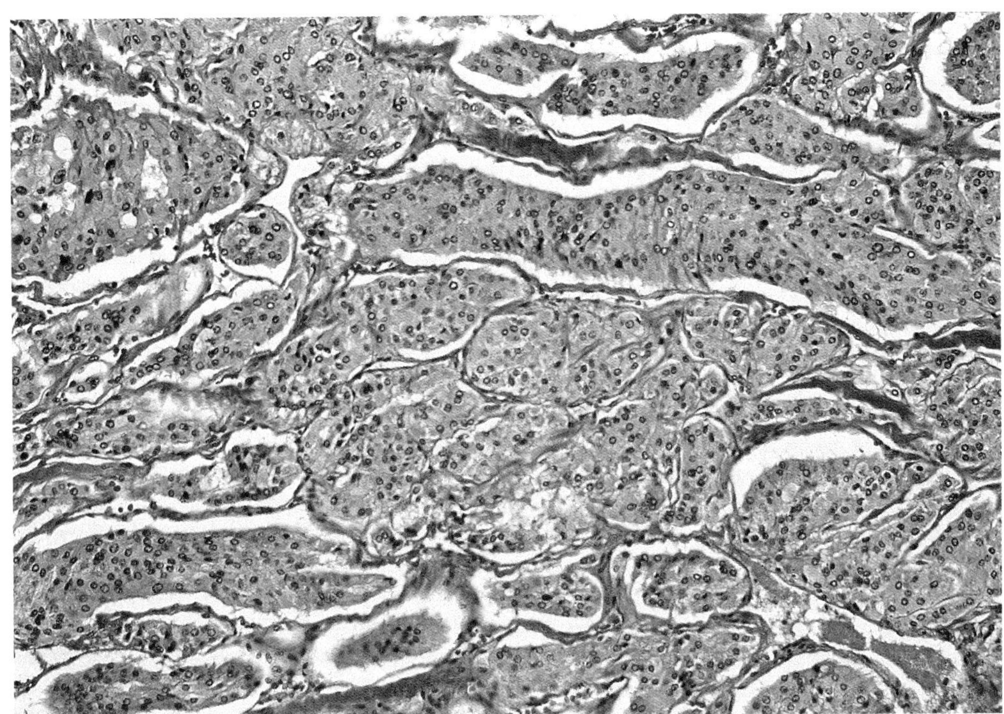

**FIGURE 33–27.** Carcinoid-like pattern in a retroperitoneal paraganglioma.

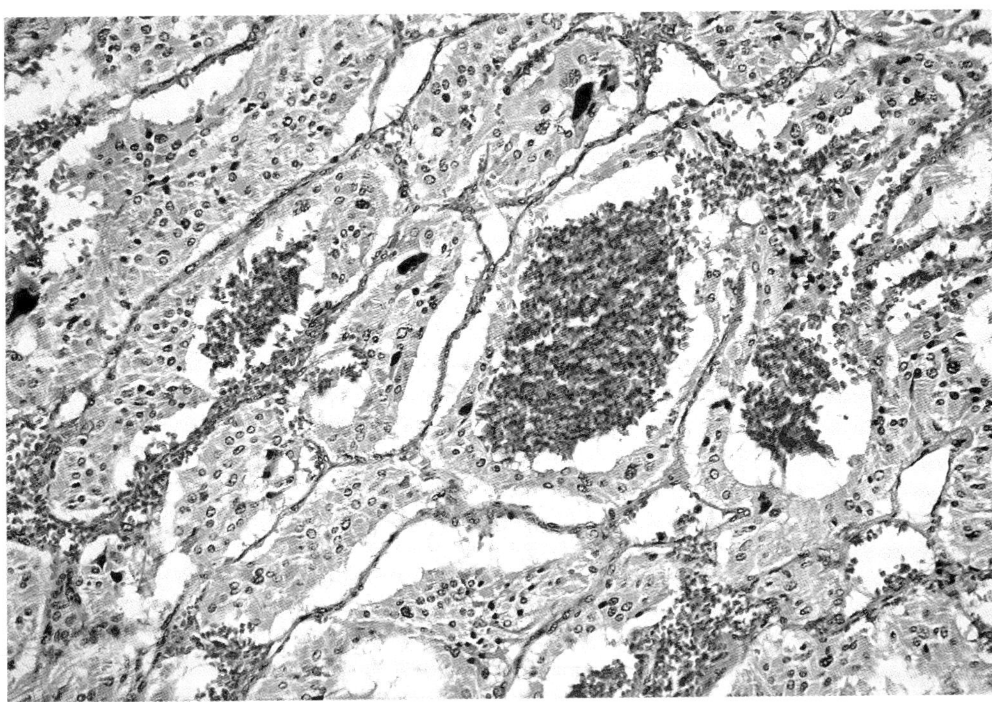

**FIGURE 33–28.** Paraganglioma with cystic hemorrhage.

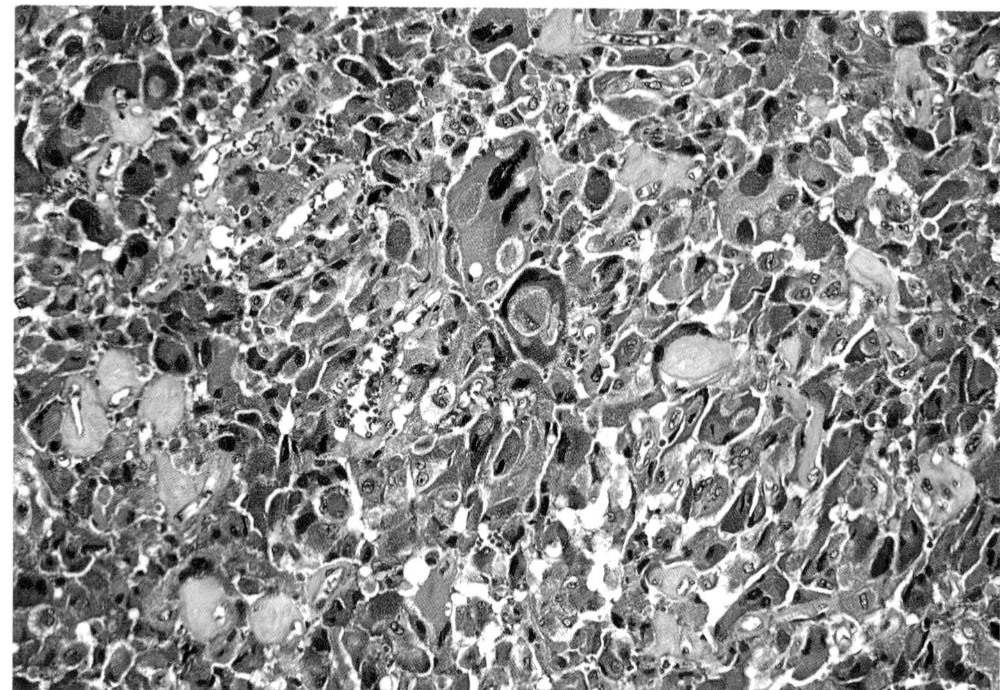

**FIGURE 33–29.** Pleomorphic form of a retroperitoneal paraganglioma. Cells are large and angular and have a deeply staining cytoplasm. Cell embracing, a general feature of paragangliomas, is evident in this tumor.

overlap of these two groups such that ploidy analysis is not particularly helpful in the individual case (Table 33–7).[117a] Analogous to the situation with neuroblastoma, the extent of S-100 protein staining of sustentacular cells has also been found to be of prognostic significance.[142,155]

## Immunohistochemical Findings

The immunologic profile of this form of paraganglioma is similar to that of the branchiomeric forms in that neuron-specific enolase, neurofilament protein, synaptophysin, and chromogranin can be identified in chief cells, which in turn are surrounded by a sustentacular network of cells that stain positively for S-100 protein.[118,124] Leu-enkephalin, an opiate-like pentapeptide that comprises part of the $\beta$-endorphin molecule, can be identified in many adrenal and extraadrenal paragangliomas.[123] This finding is to be expected in view of the fact that this pentapeptide is produced by normal and hyperplastic adrenal medullary cells. Insulin-like growth factor II, a polypeptide of 67 amino acids that is homologous to the $\beta$-chain of proinsulin, has been identified in adrenal tissues, the carotid body, and paraganglia and can also be localized to most chief cells in adrenal and extraadrenal paragangliomas.[135,153] Its significance is unclear, but it is known to have a mitogenic influence on fibroblasts and can enhance differentiation in myoblasts and neuroblastoma cell lines. A variety of neuropeptides

**TABLE 33–6 CLINICAL AND PATHOLOGIC FEATURES OF CLINICALLY BENIGN AND MALIGNANT SYMPATHOADRENAL PARAGANGLIOMAS**

| Parameter | Malignant ($n$ = 10) | Benign ($n$ = 23) | $p$ |
|---|---|---|---|
| Male gender (%) | 90 | 44 | 0.08 |
| Mean age (years) | 38 | 49 | 0.05 |
| Neurofibromatosis (%) | 0 | 100 | 0.04 |
| Tumor weight, mean (g) | 481 | 124 | 0.05 |
| Ki-67 index, mean (%) | 5 | 1 | 0.0009 |
| Extraadrenal site (%) | 40 | 9 | 0.03 |

Modified from Clarke MR, Weyant RJ, Watson CG, et al. Prognostic markers in pheochromocytoma. Hum Pathol 28:522, 1998.

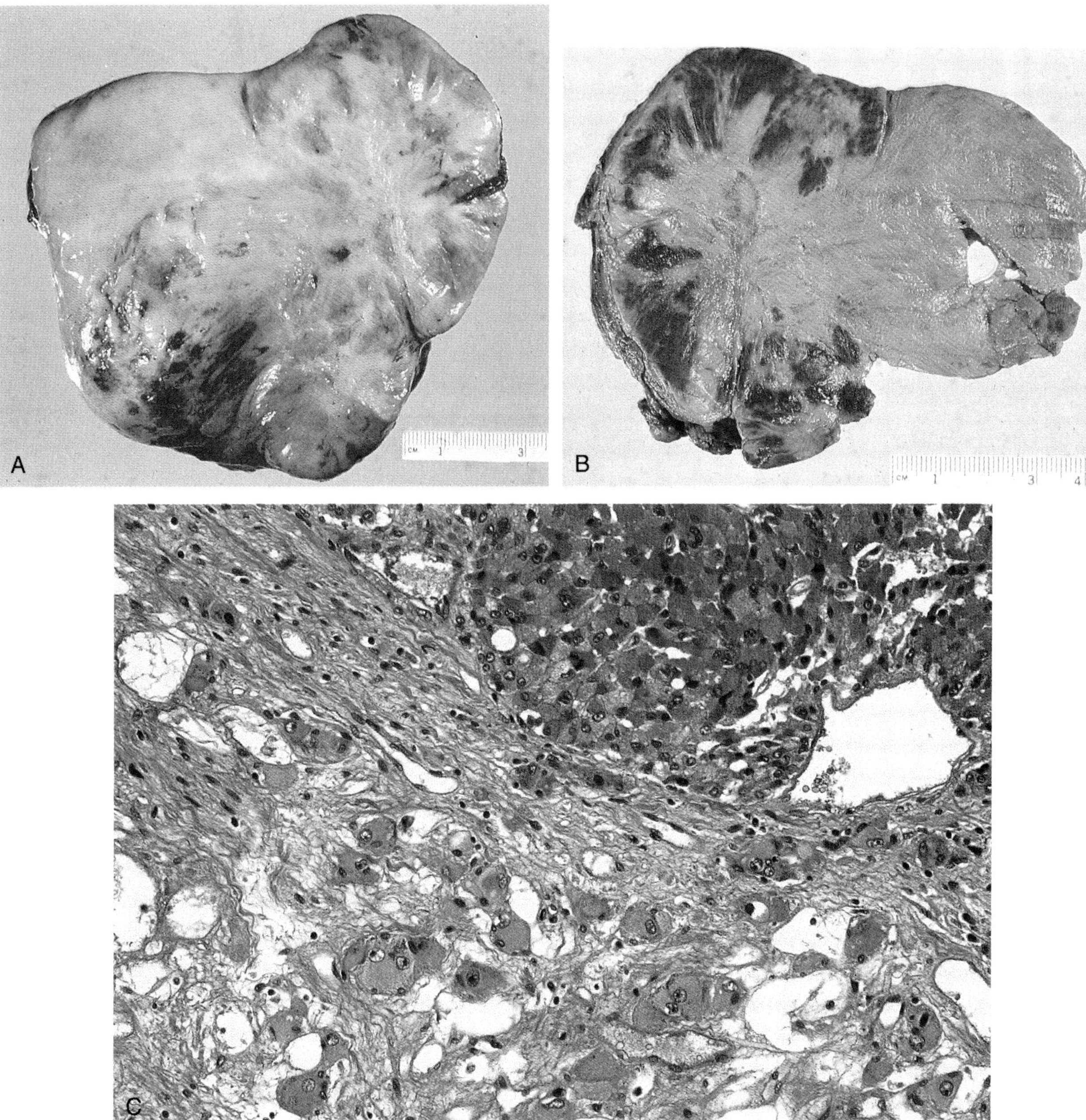

**FIGURE 33–30.** (**A**) Gross appearance of a retroperitoneal paraganglioma mixed with a ganglioneuroma. Most of the tumor was composed of ganglioneuromatous elements (white areas) with a lesser component of paraganglioma (brown areas). (**B**) Chromaffin reaction accentuates the paragangliomatous portions of this tumor. (**C**) Histologic appearance of a mixed retroperitoneal paraganglioma with ganglioneuromatous elements characterized by prominent ganglion cells.

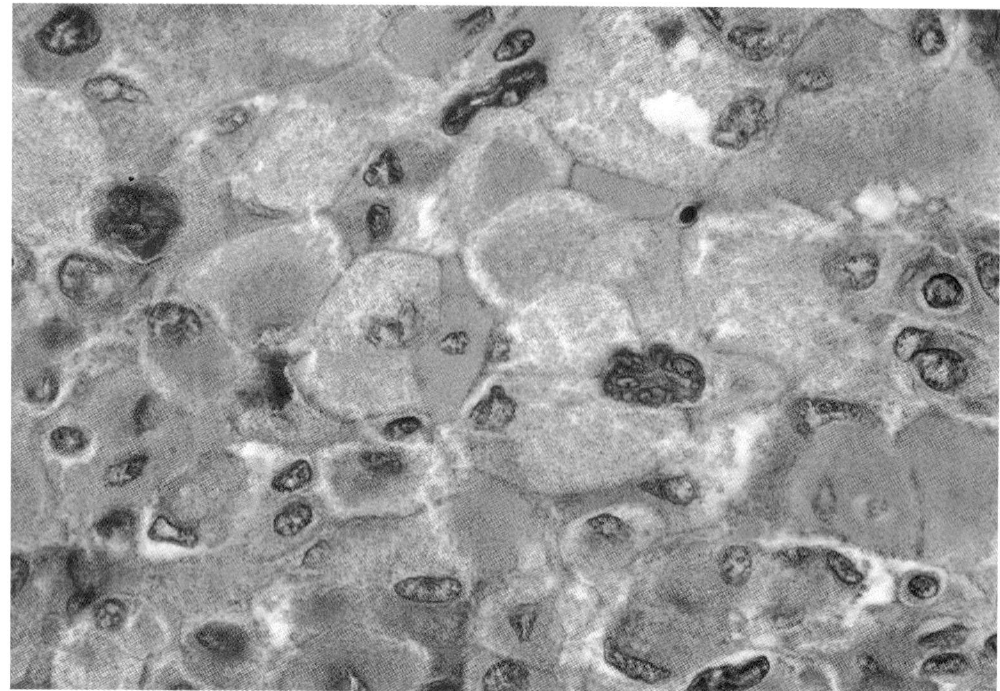

**FIGURE 33–31.** Chromaffin-positive granules in the cells of a retroperitoneal paraganglioma.

can be localized to the chief cells (detailed in Table 33–1).[137]

## Behavior and Treatment

Early reports in the literature consistently indicated that extraadrenal paragangliomas had a more aggressive course than those in the adrenal.[125,133,140,151] A study based on experience from Memorial Hospital offers evidence to the contrary.[150] Approximately 50% of both adrenal and extraadrenal tumors were malignant, as evidenced by metastatic disease or locally aggressive behavior. The 5-year survival rate was 77% for patients with adrenal tumors and 82% for those with extraadrenal tumors, figures that are not significantly different. When patients with malignant tumors were compared by site, there was still no statistical difference in disease-free survival rates.

Clarke et al.[121] studied 66 pheochromocytomas and retroperitoneal paragangliomas, 10 of which metastasized. Of the 10 tumors that metastasized, 4 were extraadrenal.

There is little correlation between the functional activity of the tumor and the degree of malignancy. Dissemination of this tumor occurs both lymphatically and hematogenously, and the most common sites of metastasis are the regional lymph nodes, bone, liver, and lung.[146]

If a retroperitoneal paraganglioma is suspected clinically, appropriate steps to document functional activity should be undertaken before surgery. Premedication of patients with $\beta$-adrenergic blocking agents is mandatory to avert intraoperative hypertensive crises or tachyarrhythmias during surgical manipulation of the tumor. Surgery should be aimed at complete removal, as adjunctive therapies including radiother-

**TABLE 33–7** DNA PLOIDY PATTERN BY FLOW CYTOMETRY IN PATIENTS WITH EXTRAADRENAL PARAGANGLIOMAS

| Ploidy Pattern | Benign | Malignant | Total |
|---|---|---|---|
| DNA diploid | 20 | 0 | 20 |
| DNA aneuploid | 4 | 1 | 5 |
| DNA tetraploid | 5 | 2 | 7 |
| *Total* | 29 | 3 | 32 |

Modified from Pang LC, Tsao KC. Flow cytometric DNA analysis for the determination of malignant potential in adrenal and extraadrenal pheochromocytomas or paragangliomas. Arch Pathol Lab Med 117:1142, 1993.

apy, chemotherapy,[130,148] and treatment with MIBG[138] can only be considered palliative. Because of the excellent localization of these tumors by modern radiographic techniques, some have advocated laparoscopic surgery as an alternative to laparotomy.[149] It has been suggested that serum neuropeptide Y levels are a reliable, sensitive means of following patients, as levels of this substance can be correlated with tumor recurrence.[127,132]

## MISCELLANEOUS PARAGANGLIOMAS

Paragangliomas may arise in numerous locations other than those already mentioned, including the nasopharynx,[196] larynx,[174,175,203] orbit,[159,214] gallbladder,[193] duodenum,[166] kidney,[190] thyroid,[182,191] bladder,[200,204] prostate,[165,170,207] lung,[208] pancreas,[176] and heart.[180,181] Although it has been claimed that they may also arise in the extremities from paraganglia that follow the arterial vessels, systematic microscopic search by Karnauchow[188] of 38 autopsy cases failed to reveal acceptable structures. Moreover, some cases reported as paragangliomas of the extremity seem in reality to be alveolar soft part sarcomas. In our opinion, paraganglioma of the extremity should be diagnosed with great reserve and only after alternative diagnoses such as carcinoma, melanoma, and alveolar soft part sarcoma have been excluded by appropriate staining procedures, clinical history taking, and electron microscopic studies.

### Nasopharyngeal Paraganglioma

Most paragangliomas involving the nasopharynx arise from adjacent structures, such as the glomus jugulare and vagal body, and extend secondarily into this region.[164] Primary nasopharyngeal tumors arising from submucosal paraganglia are rare, and this diagnosis is an exclusionary one. These tumors are pulsatile blue masses arising high in the nasopharynx. They produce symptoms of dysphonia, dysphagia, nasal obstruction, and epistaxis.[196] Their appearance is similar to that of the carotid body tumor.

### Laryngeal Paraganglioma

Laryngeal paragangliomas arise from the paired paraganglia situated in the soft tissue of the larynx. The superior pair are located at the level of the superior margin of the thyroid cartilage, whereas the inferior pair are located at the border of the thyroid and cricoid cartilage. Aberrant locations near the upper tracheal rings have also been identified. Most laryngeal paragangliomas occur in women, mainly during the fourth to sixth decades of life.[174] Almost all arise above the level of the vocal cords and involve the ipsilateral aryepiglottic fold. Affected patients usually develop hoarseness, dysphagia, and dyspnea. These tumors are histologically similar to other branchiomeric paragangliomas. The relative malignancy of these tumors has been disputed.[175,199] Barnes et al.[162] maintained that almost all are benign, with fewer than 2% exhibiting aggressive behavior. The high incidence of metastasis, reported as 25% in a review of the literature by Gallivan et al.,[178] is most likely the result of misdiagnosis of laryngeal carcinomas or atypical carcinoids.

### Orbital Paraganglioma

Orbital paragangliomas are rare tumors that are presumed to arise from the paraganglia associated with the ciliary ganglion. They produce symptoms of visual loss and throbbing pain and deficits of one or more cranial nerves. Unfortunately, many orbital paragangliomas reported in the past are, in fact, alveolar soft part sarcomas that have been misdiagnosed. Excluding 13 of the 29 reported cases, Archer et al.[159] found that the 16 acceptable orbital paragangliomas occurred at a wide range of ages (3–68 years) with an equal gender distribution. Nearly 40% of those treated with exenteration recurred, but none of the tumors to date has produced metastatic disease.

### Gangliocytic Paraganglioma

Described in 1962 by Taylor and Helwig,[213] gangliocytic paraganglioma is an unusual tumor that combines features of paraganglioma, carcinoid, and ganglioneuroma. It almost always occurs in the second portion of the duodenum,[172,177] although rarely the third portion of the duodenum is involved. Recently, a single case with typical histology was described in the appendix.[216] The tumor predominantly affects men and makes its appearance during adult life with the onset of gastrointestinal tract bleeding. Most can be demonstrated on upper gastrointestinal tract series as pedunculated or sessile lesions that arise in the submucosa and deform the overlying mucosa.

Histologically, the tumors are distinctive. They are composed of epithelioid areas that may appear indistinguishable from conventional paraganglioma (Figs. 33–32, 33–33) or may have a ribbon-like or trabecular arrangement similar to that of carcinoid (Fig. 33–34). The epithelioid areas are surrounded by a delicate network of Schwann cells and nerve axons (Fig. 33–35). Scattered among the epithelioid areas are variably differentiated ganglion cells. Although most do not appear fully differentiated, they can be easily recognized by their abundant cytoplasm, vesicular nuclei, and faint cytoplasmic basophilia. A prominent neuromatous stroma is seen in some gangliocytic

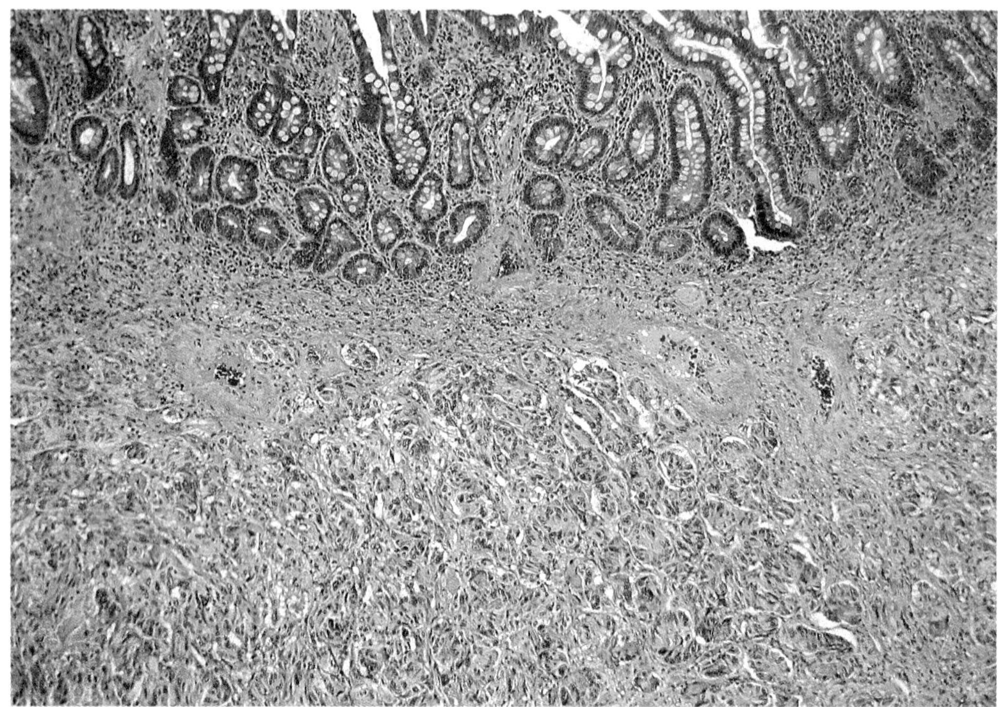

**FIGURE 33–32.** Low-power view of a gangliocytic paraganglioma.

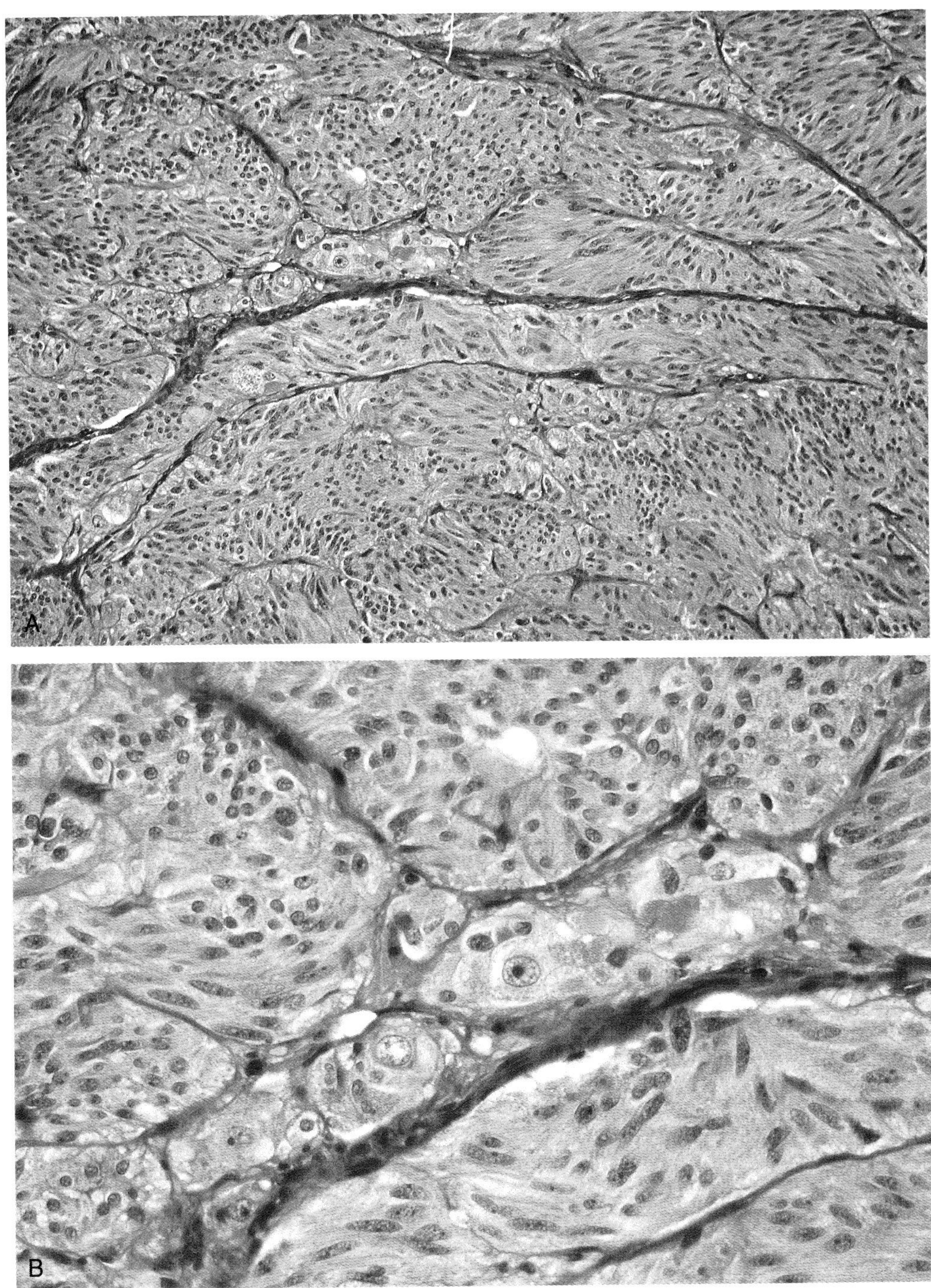


**FIGURE 33–33.** (**A**) Gangliocytic paraganglioma with a typical low-power appearance. (**B**) Focal differentiating ganglion cells are seen in epithelioid areas.

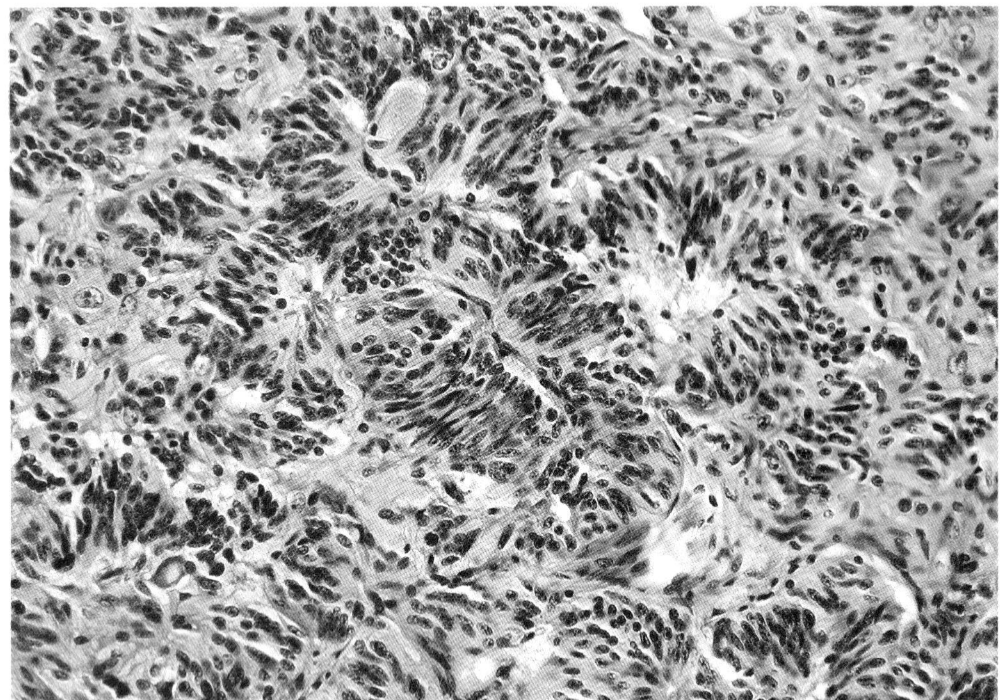

**FIGURE 33–34.** Carcinoid-like area in a gangliocytic paraganglioma.

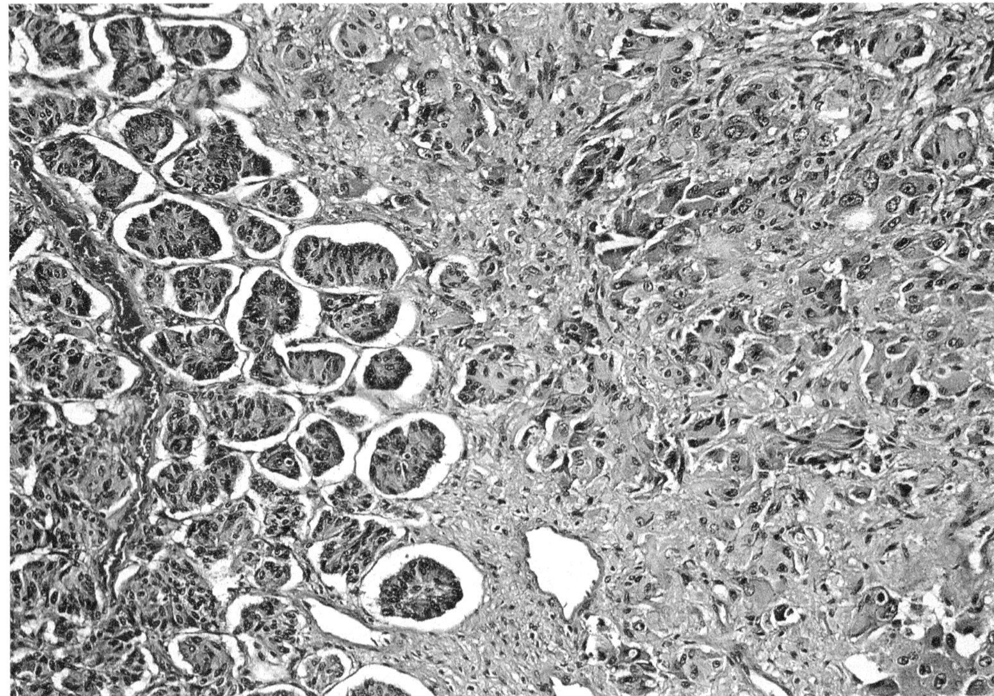

**FIGURE 33–35.** Gangliocytic paraganglioma consisting of an admixture of carcinoid-like areas and ganglion cells.

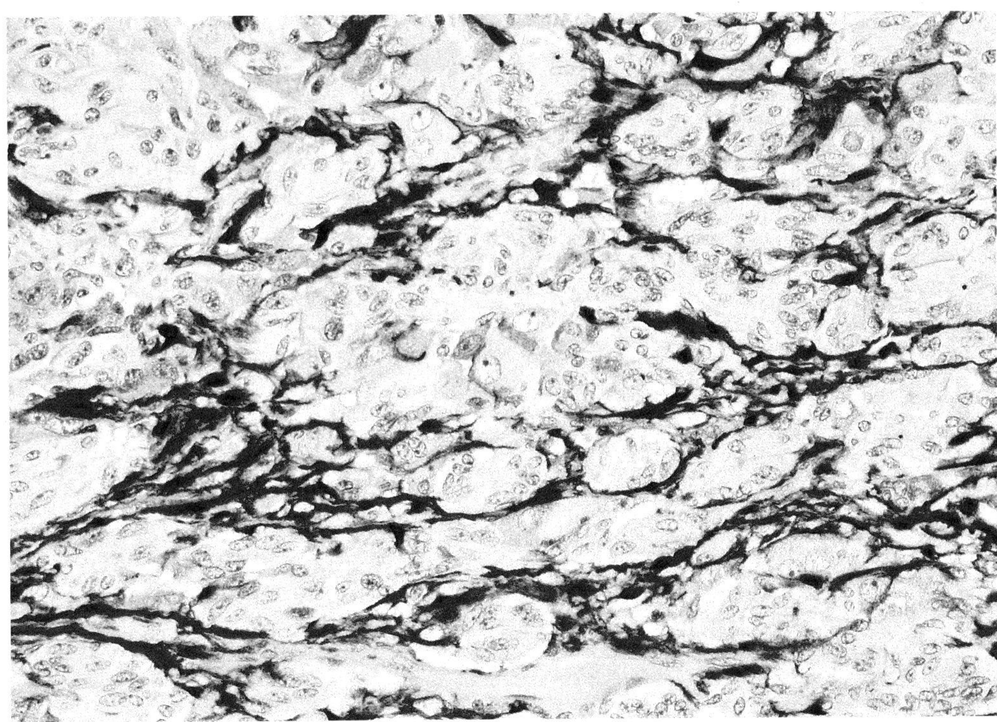

**FIGURE 33–36.** S-100 protein-positive sustentacular network surrounding epithelioid nests in a gangliocytic paraganglioma.

paragangliomas, so portions of the tumor out of context resemble ganglioneuroma.

A variety of antigens can be identified in the epithelioid cells of these tumors, including neuron-specific enolase,[179,206] insulin,[202] glucagon,[202] leu-enkephalin,[201] pancreatic polypeptide,[215] somatostatin,[215] vasoactive intestinal peptide,[202] and serotonin.[202] Chromogranin has been identified in carcinoid-like areas of these tumors.[194,215] The ganglion cells express neuron-specific enolase, synaptophysin, and neurofilament protein, whereas S-100 protein is easily demonstrable in the sustentacular network surrounding the epithelioid cells (Fig. 33–36). It has been postulated that this tumor arises from the primordium of the pancreas, which undergoes hyperplasia and recapitulates, in an exaggerated fashion, the endodermal-neuroectodermal complexes of van Campenout, which normally occur in the duodenum. As pointed out by Scheithauer et al.,[206] about half of the paragangliomas of the cauda equina also show ganglionic differentiation, so it does not seem necessary to specifically impute van Campenout complexes in the pathogenesis of this type of paraganglioma. Almost all tumors have proved to be benign, with only rare reports of lymph node metastases.[161,171,183,215] Hence simple excision to prevent recurrent gastrointestinal hemorrhage is usually adequate therapy.

## Paraganglioma of the Cauda Equina

Paraganglioma of the cauda equina has been recognized only recently as a distinct entity, with fewer than 80 cases having been reported in the literature.[160] Early cases were probably misdiagnosed as ependymomas or carcinomas. Men are affected slightly more often than women, and the tumor occurs most frequently in patients 50–60 years of age. Most present with "cauda equina syndrome," which includes lower back pain, weakness of the extremity, or urinary or fecal incontinence. Extreme elevations in cerebrospinal fluid protein can be documented in a significant proportion of cases.[209] The tumors are extramedullary, intradural masses that may or may not be attached to the cauda equina. The tumors resemble other paragangliomas in all respects, although in almost one-half of tumors, ganglionic differentiation may be seen.[209] The chief cells contain neuron-specific enolase, neurofilament protein, synaptophysin, and chromogranin, as well as other peptides including somatostatin and ACTH.[195] Unlike paragangliomas from other sites, cauda equina tumors often express cytokeratins[169,184,189,198] (Fig. 33–37), which correlates with the ultrastructural finding of cytoplasmic intermediate filaments, in addition to dense-core neurosecretory granules.[167,212] Thus the precise relation between these

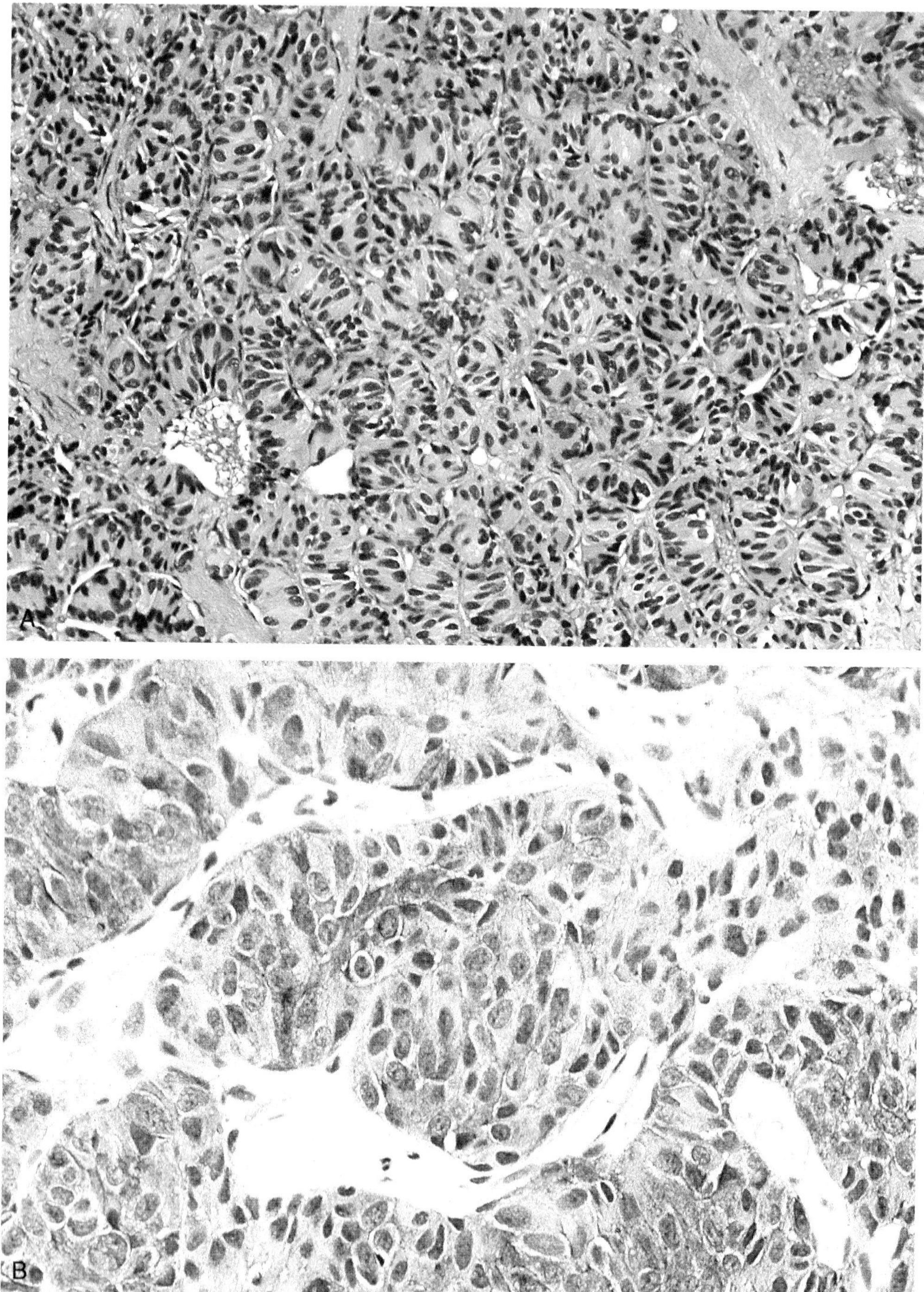


**FIGURE 33–37.** (**A**) Typical histologic appearance of a paraganglioma of the cauda equina. The same tumor was diffusely immunoreactive for synaptophysin (**B**) and cytokeratin (**C**).

*Illustration continued on opposite page*

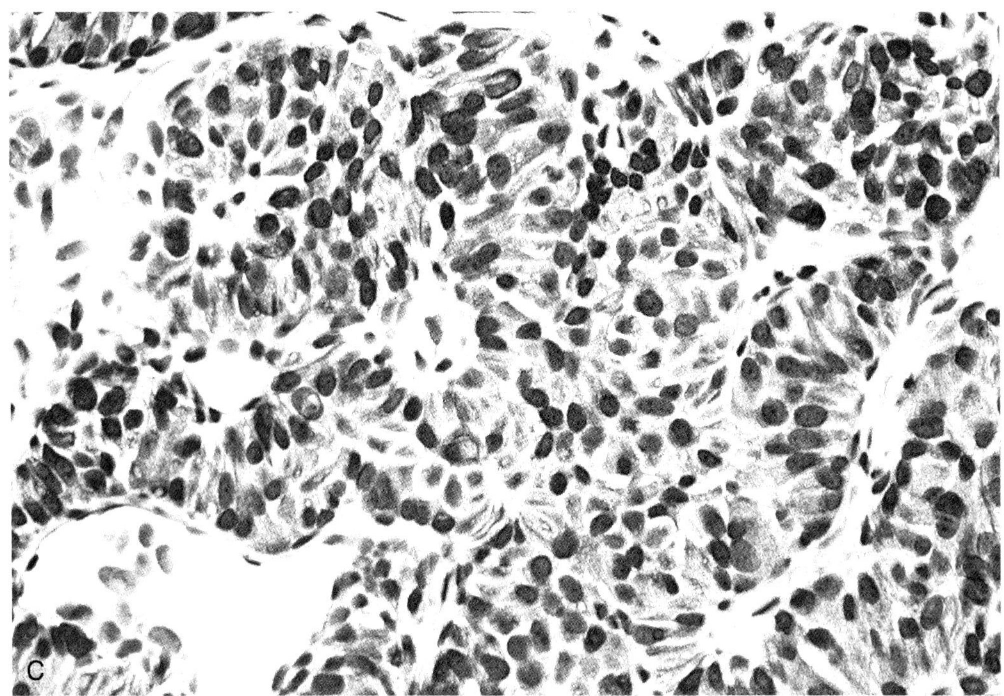


**FIGURE 33–37** *(Continued).*

tumors and paragangliomas from other sites is somewhat obscure. Although most are benign, their location may complicate complete surgical excision, leading to local recurrence in about 10% of patients.[157,163,173,209] There are rare reports of intracranial and intraspinal metastasis.[205,211] Radiotherapy has been recommended for unencapsulated or incompletely excised tumors.[160]

## Cardiac Paraganglioma

Cardiac paraganglioma is one of the rarest forms of paraganglioma, with fewer than 40 cases reported in the literature.[158,168,180,185,187,197] Most have occurred in women at an average age of 45 years. The tumor arises primarily on the left atrium or in the interventricular groove at the aortic root and commonly gives rise to hypertensive symptoms. The lesions are histologically and immunohistochemically similar to other forms of paraganglioma. Treatment of these inaccessible tumors usually requires resection of the posterior atrial wall with coronary artery bypass.[186,192] Although most are clinically benign, rare tumors have given rise to distant metastasis.

## REFERENCES

### Carotid Body Paraganglioma

1. Alpert LI, Bochetto JF Jr. Carotid body tumor: ultrastructural observations. Cancer 34:564, 1974.
2. Baysal BE, van Schothorst EM, Farr JE, et al. A high-resolution STS, AST, a gene-based physical map of the hereditary paraganglioma region on chromosome 11q23. Genomics 44:214, 1997.
3. Baysal BE, van Schothorst EM, Farr JE, et al. Repositioning the hereditary paraganglioma critical region on chromosome band 11q23. Hum Genet 104:219, 1999.
4. Bender BU, Altehofer C, Januszewicz A, et al. Functioning thoracic paraganglioma: association with von Hippel-Lindau syndrome. J Clin Endocrinol Metab 82:3356, 1997.
5. Bikhazi PH, Roeder E, Attaie A, et al. Familial paragangliomas: the emerging impact of molecular genetics on evaluation and management. Am J Otol 20:639, 1999.
6. Biscoe TJ. Carotid body: structure and function. Physiol Rev 51:437, 1971.
7. Chew SL, Lavender P, Jain A, et al. Absence of mutations in the MEN2A region of the RET proto-oncogene in non-MEN2A phaeochromocytomas. Clin Endocrinol (Orf) 42:17, 1995.
8. Choyke PL, Glenn GM, McClellan MW, et al. von Hippel-Lindau disease: genetic, clinical and imaging features. Radiology 194:629, 1995.
9. Fried G, Wikstrom LM, Hoog A, et al. Multiple neuropeptide immunoreactivities in a renin-producing human paraganglioma. Cancer 74:142, 1994.
10. Fries JG, Chamberlin JA. Extraadrenal pheochromocytoma: literature review and report of a cervical pheochromocytoma. Surgery 63:268, 1968.
11. Fruhwirth J, Koch G, Hauser H, et al. Paragangliomas of the carotid bifurcation: oncological aspects of vascular surgery. Eur J Surg Oncol 22:88, 1996.
12. Gardner T, Dalsing M, Weisberger E, et al. Carotid body tumors, inheritance, and a high incidence of associated cervical paragangliomas. Am J Surg 172:196, 1996.
13. Gaylis H, Mieny CJ. The incidence of malignancy in carotid body tumors. Br J Surg 64:885, 1977.
14. Glenner GG, Crout JR, Roberts WC. A functional carotid-

body-like tumor secreting levarterenol. Arch Pathol 73:230, 1962.

15. Glenner GG, Grimley PM. Tumors of the extraadrenal paraganglion system (including chemoreceptors). In: Atlas of Tumor Pathology, Fascicle 9, 2nd Series. Armed Forces Institute of Pathology, Washington, DC, 1974.
16. Grimley PM, Glenner GC. Histology and ultrastructure of carotid body paragangliomas: comparison with the normal gland. Cancer 20:1473, 1967.
17. Grufferman S, Gillman MW, Pasternak LR, et al. Familial carotid body tumors: case report and epidemiological review. Cancer 46:2116, 1982.
18. Guedea F, Mendenhall WM, Parsons JT, et al. Radiotherapy for chemodectoma of the carotid body and ganglion nodosum. Head Neck 13:509, 1991.
19. Gustilo RB, Lober PH, Salovich EL. Chemodectoma metastasizing to bone: case report. J Bone Joint Surg Am 47:155, 1965.
20. Hamberger CA, Hamberger CB, Wersall J, et al. Malignant catecholamine-producing tumor of the carotid body. Acta Pathol Microbiol Scand [A] 69:489, 1967.
21. Harrington SW, Claggett OT, Dockerty MB. Tumors of the carotid body: clinical and pathologic considerations of 20 tumours affecting 19 patients (1 bilateral). Ann Surg 114:820, 1941.
22. Heutink P, van der Mey AG, Sandkuijl LA, et al. A gene subject to genomic imprinting and responsible for hereditary paragangliomas maps to chromosome 11q23-qter. Hum Mol Genet 1:7, 1992.
23. Heutink P, van Schothorst EM, van der Mey AG, et al. Further localization of the gene for hereditary paragangliomas and evidence for linkage in unrelated families. Eur J Hum Genet 2:148, 1994.
24. Hull MT, Roth LM, Glover JL, et al. Metastatic carotid body paraganglioma in von Hippel-Lindau disease. Arch Pathol Lab Med 106:235, 1982.
25. Johnson TL, Zarbo RJ, Lloyd RV, et al. Paragangliomas of the head and neck: immunohistochemical neuroendocrine and intermediate filament typing. Mod Pathol 1:216, 1988.
26. Kawai A, Healey JH, Wilson SC, et al. Carotid body paraganglioma metastatic to bone: report of two cases. Skeletal Radiol 27:103, 1998.
27. Kitahara M, Mori T, Seki H, et al. Malignant paraganglioma presenting as Cushing syndrome with virilism in childhood: production of cortisol, androgens, and adrenocorticotrophic hormone by the tumor. Cancer 72:3340, 1993.
28. Kliewer CE, Cochran AJ. A review of the histology, ultrastructure, immunohistology, and molecular biology of extraadrenal paragangliomas. Arch Pathol Lab Med 113:1209, 1989.
29. Kliewer KE, Wen DR, Cancilla PA, et al. Paragangliomas: assessment of prognosis by histologic, immunohistochemical and ultrastructural techniques. Hum Pathol 20:29, 1989.
30. Lack EE, Cubilla AL, Woodruff JM. Paragangliomas of the head and neck region: a pathologic study of tumors from 70 patients. Hum Pathol 10:199, 1979.
31. Lack EE, Cubilla AL, Woodruff JM, et al. Paragangliomas of the head and neck region: a clinical study of 69 patients. Cancer 39:397, 1977.
32. Lam KY, Chan ACL. Paragangliomas: a comparative, clinical, histologic, and immunohistochemical study. Int J Surg Pathol 1:111, 1993.
33. LaMuraglia GM, Fabian RL, Brewster DC, et al. The current surgical management of carotid body paragangliomas. J Vasc Surg 15:1038, 1992.
34. Leonetti JP, Donzelli JJ, Littooy FN, et al. Perioperative strategies in the management of carotid body tumors. Otolaryngol Head Neck Surg 117:111, 1997.
35. Liapis C, Gougoulakis A, Karydakis V, et al. Changing trends in management of carotid body tumors. Am Surg 61:989, 1995.
36. Mariman EC, van Beersum SE, Cremers CW, et al. Analysis of a second family with hereditary nonchromaffin paragangliomas locates the underlying gene at the proximal region of chromosome 11q. Hum Genet 91:357, 1993.
37. Mariman EC, van Beersum SE, Cremers CW, et al. Fine mapping of putatively imprinted gene for familial nonchromaffin paragangliomas to chromosome 11q13.1: evidence for genetic heterogeneity. Hum Genet 95:56, 1995.
38. Matticari S, Credi G, Pratesi C, et al. Diagnosis and surgical treatment of carotid body tumors. J Cardiovasc Surg 86:233, 1995.
39. McCaffrey TV, Meyer FB, Michels VV, et al. Familial paragangliomas of the head and neck. Arch Otolaryngol Head Neck Surg 120:1211, 1994.
40. McGuirt WF, Harker LA. Carotid body tumors. Arch Otolaryngol 101:58, 1975.
41. McPherson GAD, Halliday AW, Mansfield AO. Carotid body tumours and other cervical paragangliomas: diagnosis and management in 25 patients. Br J Surg 76:33, 1989.
42. Milunsky J, DeStefano AL, Huang XL. Familial paragangliomas: linkage to chromosome 11q23 and clinical implications. Am J Med Genet 72:66, 1997.
43. Min KW. Diagnostic usefulness of sustentacular cells in paragangliomas: immunocytochemical and ultrastructural investigation. Ultrastruct Pathol 22:369, 1998.
44. Mitchell DC, Clyne CAC. Chemodectoma of the neck: the response to radiotherapy. Br J Surg 72:903, 1985.
45. Netterville JL, Reilly KM, Robertson D, et al. Bilateral carotid body tumors: etiology and management of physiological changes resulting from bilateral excision. Laryngoscope (in press).
46. Netterville JL, Reilly KM, Robertson D, et al. Carotid body tumors: a review of 30 patients with 46 tumors. Laryngoscope 105:115, 1995.
47. Omura M, Sato T, Cho R, et al. A patient with malignant paraganglioma that simultaneously produces adrenocorticotropic hormone and interleukin-6. Cancer 74:1634, 1994.
48. Oosterwijk JC, Jansen JC, van Schothorst EM, et al. First experiences with genetic counseling based on predictive DNA diagnosis in hereditary glomus tumours (paragangliomas). J Med Genet 33:379, 1996.
49. Parkin J. Familial multiple glomus tumors and pheochromocytomas. Ann Otolaryngol 90:60, 1981.
50. Pereira D, Hunter K. Familial multicentric nonchromaffin paragangliomas. Clin Oncol 6:273, 1980.
51. Perel Y, Schlumberger M, Marguerite G, et al. Pheochromocytoma and paraganglioma in children: a report of 24 cases of the French Society of Pediatric Oncology. Pediatr Hematol Oncol 14:413, 1997.
52. Robertson DI, Hollister AS, Biaggioni I, et al. The hypertension of baroreflex failure. N Engl J Med 329:1449, 1993.
53. Saldana MJ, Salem LE, Travezan R. High altitude hypoxia and chemodectomas. Hum Pathol 4:251, 1973.
54. Scheithauer BW, Parameswaran A, Burdick B. Intrasellar paraganglioma: report of a case in a sibship of von Hippel-Lindau disease. Neurosurgery 38:395, 1996.
55. Schmid KW, Schröder S, Dockhorn-Dworniczak B, et al. Immunohistochemical demonstration of chromogranin A, chromogranin B, and secretogranin II in extra-adrenal paragangliomas. Mod Pathol 7:347, 1994.
56. Shamblin WR, ReMine WH, Sheps SG, et al. Carotid body tumor (chemodectoma): clinicopathologic analysis of 90 cases. Am J Pathol 122:732, 1971.
57. Skoldberg F, Grimelius L, Woodward ER, et al. A family with hereditary extra-adrenal paragangliomas without evidence for mutations in the von Hippel-Lindau disease or RET genes. Clin Endocrinol (Oxf) 48:11, 1998.

58. Sobol SM, Dailey JC. Familial multiple cervical paragangliomas: report of a kindred and review of the literature. Otolaryngol Head Neck Surg 102:382, 1992.
59. Tikkakoski T, Luotonen J, Leinonen S, et al. Preoperative embolization in the management of neck paragangliomas. Laryngoscope 107:821, 1997.
60. Valdagni R, Amichitti M. Radiation therapy of carotid body tumors. Am J Clin Oncol 13:45, 1990.
61. Van Baars F, van den Broek P, Cremers C, et al. Familial nonchromaffinic paragangliomas (glomus tumors): clinical aspects. Laryngoscope 91:988, 1981.
62. Van der Mey AGL, Maaswinkel-Mooy PD, Cornelisse CJ, et al. Genomic imprinting in hereditary glomus tumors: evidence for a new genetic theory. Lancet 2:1291, 1989.
63. Van Schothorst EM, Beekman M, Torremans P, et al. Paragangliomas of the head and neck region show complete loss of heterozygosity at 11q22-q23 in chief cells and the flow-sorted DNA aneuploid fraction. Hum Pathol 29:1045, 1998.
64. Van Schothorst EM, Jansen JC, Bardoel AF, et al. Confinement of PGL, an imprinted gene causing hereditary paragangliomas, II-cM interval on 11q22-q23 and exclusion of DRD2 and NCM as candidate genes. Eur J Hum Genet 4:267, 1996.
65. Vargas MP, Zhuang Z, Wang C, et al. Loss of heterozygosity on the short arm of chromosomes 1 and 3 in sporadic pheochromocytoma and extra-adrenal paraganglioma. Hum Pathol 28:411, 1997.
66. Warren WH, Lee I, Gould VE, et al. Paragangliomas of the head and neck: ultrastructural and immunohistochemical analysis. Ultrastruct Pathol 8:333, 1985.
67. Zanelli M, van der Walt JD. Carotid body paraganglioma in von Hippel-Lindau disease: a rare association. Histopathology 29:178, 1996.


### Jugulotympanic Paraganglioma


68. Alshaikhly A, Hamid AM, Azadeh B. Glomus tympanicum chemodectoma: unusual radiological findings. J Laryngol Otol 108:607, 1994.
69. Amand VK, Leonetti JP, Al-Mefty O. Neurovascular considerations in surgery of glomus tumors with intracranial extensions. Laryngoscope 103:722, 1993.
70. Borsanyi SJ. Glomus jugulare tumors. Laryngoscope 72:1336, 1962.
71. Brown JS. Glomus jugulare tumors revisited: a ten-year statistical follow-up of 231 cases. Laryngoscope 95:284, 1985.
72. Cole JM. Glomus jugulare tumors of the temporal bone: radiation of glomus tumor of the temporal bone. Laryngoscope 89: 1623, 1979.
73. De Jong AL, Coker NJ, Jenkins HA, et al. Radiation therapy in the management of paragangliomas of the temporal bone. Am J Otol 16:283, 1995.
74. Fisch U. Infratemporal fossa approach for glomus tumors of the temporal bone. Ann Otol Rhinol Laryngol 91:474, 1982.
75. Fuller AM, Brown HA, Harrison EG Jr, et al. Chemodectomas of the glomus jugulare. Laryngoscope 77:218, 1967.
76. Glascock ME, Harris PF, Newsome G. Glomus tumors: diagnosis and treatment. Laryngoscope 84:2006, 1974.
77. Glascock ME, Jackson CG, Dickens JRE, et al. Glomus jugulare tumors of the temporal bone: surgical management of glomus tumors. Laryngoscope 89:1640, 1979.
78. Horvath KK, Ormos J, Ribari O. Crystals in a jugulotympanic paraganglioma. Ultrastruct Pathol 10:257, 1986.
79. Jackson CG. Skull base surgery. Am J Otol 3:161, 1981.
80. Jackson CG, Cueva RA, Thedinger BA, et al. Conservation surgery for glomus jugulare tumors: the value of early diagnosis. Laryngoscope 100:1031, 1990.
81. Jackson CG, Cueva RA, Thedinger BA, et al. Cranial nerve preservation in lesions of the jugular fossa. Otolaryngol Head Neck Surg 105:687, 1991.
82. Jackson CG, Gulya AJ, Knox GW, et al. A paraneoplastic syndrome associated with glomus tumors of the skull base: early observations. Otolaryngol Head Neck Surg 100:583, 1989.
83. Jackson CG, Welling DB, Chironais P, et al. Glomus tympanicum tumors: contemporary concepts in conservation surgery. Laryngoscope 99:875, 1989.
84. Johnstone PA, Foss RD, Desilets DJ. Malignant jugulotympanic paraganglioma. Arch Pathol Lab Med 114:976, 1990.
85. Murphy TP, Brackmann DE. Effects of preoperative embolization on glomus jugulare tumors. Laryngoscope 99:1244, 1989.
86. Negerian CA, McKenna MJ, Nadol JB Jr. Non-paraganglioma jugular foramen lesions mascarading as glomus jugulare tumors. Am J Otol 16:94, 1995.
87. Oldring D, Fisch U. Glomus tumors of the temporal region: surgical therapy. Am J Otol 1:7, 1979.
88. Rodgers GK, Applegate L, de la Cruz A. Magnetic resonance angiography: analysis of vascular lesions of the temporal bone and skull base. Am J Otol 14:56, 1993.
89. Schwaber MK. Diagnosis and management of catecholamine secreting tumors: glomus tumors. Laryngoscope 54:1008, 1984.
90. Spector GJ, Sobel S, Thawley SE, et al. Glomus jugulare tumors of the temporal bone: patterns of invasion in the temporal bone. Laryngoscope 89:1628, 1979.
91. Stewart KL. Paragangliomas of the temporal bone. Am J Otolaryngol 14:219, 1993.
92. Wright JW Jr, Wright JW III, Hicks GW. Glomus jugulare tumors of the temporal bone: radiologic appearance of glomus tumors. Laryngoscope 89:1620, 1975.


### Vagal Paraganglioma


93. Biller HF, Lawson W, Som P, et al. Glomus vagal tumors. Ann Otol Rhinol Laryngol 98:21, 1989.
94. Borba LAB, Al-Mefty O. Intravagal paragangliomas: report of four cases. Neurosurgery 38:569, 1996.
95. Chaudhry AP, Haar JG, Kous A, et al. A nonfunctioning paraganglioma of vagus nerve. Cancer 43:1689, 1979.
96. Davidson J, Gullane P. Glomus vagale tumors. Otolaryngol Head Neck Surg 99:66, 1988.
97. Gulya AJ. The glomus tumor and its biology. Laryngoscope 103(Suppl):7, 1993.
98. Heinrich MC, Harris AE, Bell WR. Metastatic intravagal paraganglioma: case report and review of the literature. Am J Med 78:1017, 1985.
99. Kahn LB. Vagal body tumor (nonchromaffin paraganglioma, chemodectoma, and carotid-body-like tumor) with cervical node metastasis and familial association: ultrastructural study and review. Cancer 38:2367, 1976.
100. Leonetti JP, Brackmann DE. Glomus vagale tumor: the significance of early vocal cord paralysis. Otolaryngol Head Neck Surg 100:533, 1989.
101. Tannir NM, Cortas N, Allam C. A functioning catecholamine-secreting vagal body tumor: a case report and review of the literature. Cancer 52:932, 1983.
102. Urquhart AC, Johnson JT, Myers EN, et al. Glomus vagal: paraganglioma of the vagus nerve. Laryngoscope 104:440, 1994.
103. Walsh RM, Leen EJ, Gleeson MJ, et al. Malignant vagal paraganglioma. J Laryngol Otol 111:883, 1997.


### Mediastinal Paraganglioma


104. Assaf HM, al-Momen AA, Martin JG. Aorticopulmonary paraganglioma: a case report with immunohistochemical studies and literature review. Arch Pathol Lab Med 116:1085, 1992.
105. Bird DJ, Seiler MW. Aorticopulmonary paraganglioma (aortic body tumor): report of a case. Ultrastruct Pathol 15:475, 1991.

106. Castanon J, Gil-Aguado M, de la Llana R, et al. Aortopulmonary paraganglioma, a rare aortic tumor: a case report. J Thorac Cardiovasc Surg 106:1232, 1993.
107. Gallivan MVE, Chun B, Rowden G, et al. Intrathoracic paravertebral malignant paraganglioma. Arch Pathol Lab Med 104:4, 1980.
108. Herrera MF, van Heerden JA, Puga FJ, et al. Mediastinal paraganglioma: a surgical experience. Ann Thorac Surg 56:109, 1993.
109. Kern JA, Milbrandt TA, Rolf S, et al. Resection of multiple mediastinal paragangliomas with cardiopulmonary bypass. Ann Thorac Surg 64:1824, 1997.
110. Lack EE, Stillinger RA, Colvin DB, et al. Aortico-pulmonary paraganglioma: report of a case with ultrastructural study and review of the literature. Cancer 43:269, 1979.
111. Lacquet LK. Aortopulmonary paraganglioma, a rare tumor. J Thorac Cardiovasc Surg 109:398, 1995.
112. Lamy AL, Fordet GJ, Luoma A, et al. Anterior and middle mediastinum paraganglioma: complete resection is the treatment of choice. Ann Thorac Surg 57:249, 1994.
113. Moran CA, Suster S, Fishback N, et al. Mediastinal paragangliomas: a clinicopathologic and immunohistochemical study of 16 cases. Cancer 72:2358, 1993.
114. Olson JL, Salyer WR. Mediastinal paragangliomas (aortic body tumor): a report of four cases and a review of the literature. Cancer 41:2405, 1978.

### Retroperitoneal Paraganglioma

115. Acha T, Picazo B, Garcia-Martin FJ, et al. Carney's triad: apropos of a new case. Med Pediatr Oncol 22:216, 1994.
116. Argos MD, Ruiz A, Sanchez F, et al. Gastric leiomyoblastoma associated with extraadrenal paraganglioma and pulmonary chondroma: a new case of Carney's triad. J Pediatr Surg 28: 1545, 1993.
117. Brantigan CO, Katase RY. Clinical and pathologic features of paraganglioma of the organ of Zuckerkandl. Surgery 65:898, 1969.
117a. Brown HM, Komorowski RA, Wilson SD, et al. Predicting metastasis of pheochromocytomas using DNA flow cytometry and immunohistochemical markers of cell proliferation. Cancer 86:1583, 1999.
118. Capella C, Riva C, Cornaggia M, et al. Histopathology, cytology, and cytochemistry of pheochromocytomas and paragangliomas including chemodectomas. Pathol Res Pract 183:176, 1988.
119. Carney JA. The triad of gastric epithelioid leiomyosarcoma, pulmonary chondroma, and functioning extraadrenal paraganglioma: a five year review. Medicine 62:159, 1983.
120. Carney JA, Sheps SG, Go VLW, et al. The triad of gastric leiomyosarcoma, functioning extraadrenal paraganglioma, and pulmonary chondroma. N Engl J Med 296:1517, 1977.
121. Clarke MR, Weyant RJ, Watson CG, et al. Prognostic markers in pheochromocytoma. Hum Pathol 28:522, 1998.
122. De Jong E, Mulder W, Nooitgedacht E, et al. Carney's triad. Eur J Surg Oncol 24:147, 1998.
123. DeLellis RA, Tischler AS, Lee AK, et al. Leu-enkephalin-like immunoreactivity in proliferative lesions of the human adrenal medulla and extraadrenal paraganglia. Am J Surg Pathol 7:29, 1983.
124. Fraga M, Garcia-Caballero T, Antunez J, et al. A comparative immunohistochemical study of pheochromocytomas and paragangliomas. Histol Histopathol 8:429, 1993.
125. Glenn F, Gray GF. Functional tumors of the organ of Zuckerkandl. Ann Surg 183:578, 1976.
126. Gonzales-Campora R, Diaz Cano S, Lerma-Puertas E, et al. Paragangliomas: static cytometric studies of nuclear DNA patterns. Cancer 71:820, 1993.
127. Hellman LJ, Cohen PS, Averbuch SD, et al. Neuropeptide Y distinguishes benign from malignant pheochromocytoma. J Clin Oncol 7:720, 1989.
128. Hurst RD, Modlin IM. Use of radiolabeled somatostatin analogs in the identification and treatment of somatostatin receptor-bearing tumors. Digestion 54(Suppl 1):88, 1993.
129. Jalil ND, Pattou FN, Combemale F, et al. Effectiveness and limits of preoperative, imaging studies for the localization of pheochromocytomas and paragangliomas; a review, of 282 cases. French Association of Surgery (AFC), and the French Association of Endocrine Surgeons (AFCEN). Eur J Surg 164: 23, 1998.
130. Kimura S, Iwai M, Fukuda T, et al. Combination chemotherapy for malignant paraganglioma. Int Med 36:35, 1997.
131. Kimura N, Miura Y, Nagatsu I, et al. Catecholamine synthesizing enzymes in 70 cases of functioning and non-functioning phaeochromocytoma and extra-adrenal paraganglioma. Virchows Arch [Pathol Anat Histopathol] 421:25, 1992.
132. Kuvshinoff BW, Nussbaum MS, Richards AI, et al. Neuropeptide Y secretion from a malignant extraadrenal retroperitoneal paraganglioma. Cancer 70:2350, 1992.
133. Lack EE, Cubilla AL, Woodruff JM, et al. Extraadrenal paragangliomas of the retroperitoneum. a clinicopathologic study of 12 tumors. Am J Surg Pathol 4:109, 1980.
134. Lack EE, Kim H, Reed K. Pigmented ("black") extraadrenal paraganglioma. Am J Surg Pathol 22:265, 1998.
135. Li SL, Goko H, Xu ZD, et al. Expression of insulin-like growth factor (IGF)-II in human prostrate, breast, bladder and paraganglioma tumors. Cell Tissue Res 291:469, 1998.
136. Linnoila RI, Keiser HR, Steinberg SM, et al. Histopathology of benign versus malignant sympathoadrenal paragangliomas: clinicopathologic study of 120 cases including unusual histologic features. Hum Pathol 21:1168, 1990.
137. Linnoila RI, Lack EE, Steinberg SM, et al. Decreased expression of neuropeptides in malignant paragangliomas: an immunohistochemical study. Hum Pathol 19:47, 1988.
138. Loh KC, Fitzgerald PA, Matthay KK, et al. The treatment of malignant pheochromocytoma with iodine-131 metaiodobenzylguanidine: a comprehensive review of 116 reported patients. J Endocrinol Invest 20:648, 1997.
139. Maurea S, Cuocolo A, Reynolds JC, et al. Iodine-131-metaiodobenzylguanidine scintigraphy in preoperative and postoperative evaluation of paragangliomas: comparison with CT and MRI. J Nucl Med 34:173, 1993.
140. Melicow MM. One hundred cases of pheochromocytoma (107 tumors) at the Columbia-Presbyterian Medical Center 1926–1976: a clinicopathologic analysis. Cancer 40:1987, 1977.
141. Mena J, Bowen JC, Hollier LH. Metachronous bilaternal nonfunctional intercarotid paraganglioma (carotid body tumor) and functional retroperitoneal paraganglioma: report of a case and review of the literature. Surgery 114:107, 1993.
142. Montresor E, Iacono C, Nifosi F, et al. Retroperitoneal paragangliomas: role of immunohistochemistry in the diagnosis of malignancy and in assessment of prognosis. Eur J Surg 160: 547, 1994.
143. Moran CA, Albores-Saavedra J, Wenig BM, et al. Pigmented extraadrenal paragangliomas: a clinicopathologic and immunohistochemical study of five cases. Cancer 79:398, 1997.
143a. Nagura S, Katoh R, Kawaoi A, et al. Immunohistochemical estimations of growth activity to predict biological behavior of pheochromocytomas. Mod Pathol 12:1107, 1999.
144. Nakano S, Kigoshi T, Uchida K, et al. Hypertension and unilateral renal ischemia (Page kidney) due to compression of a retroperitoneal paraganglioma. Am J Nephrol 16:91, 1996.
145. Olson JR, Abell MR. Nonfunctional nonchromaffin paragangliomas of the retroperitoneum. Cancer 23:1358, 1969.
146. O'Riordain DS, Young WF Jr, Grant CS, et al. Clinical spec-

trum and outcome of functional extraadrenal paraganglioma. World J Surg 20:916, 1996.

147. Pang LC, Tsao KC. Flow cytometric DNA analysis for the determination of malignant potential in adrenal and extraadrenal pheochromocytomas or paragangliomas. Arch Pathol Lab Med 117:1142, 1993.
148. Patel SR, Winchester DJ, Benjamin RS. A 15-year experience with chemotherapy of patients with paraganglioma. Cancer 76:1476, 1995.
149. Pattou FN, Combemale FP, Poirette JF, et al. Questionability of the benefits of routine laparotomy as the surgical approach for pheochromocytomas and abdominal paragangliomas. Surgery 120:1006, 1996.
150. Pommier RF, Vetto JT, Billingsly K, et al. Comparison of adrenal and extraadrenal pheochromocytomas. Surgery 114:1160, 1993.
151. Scott HW Jr, Oates JA, Nies AS, et al. Pheochromocytoma: recent diagnosis and management. Ann Surg 183:587, 1976.
152. Sisson JC, Frager MS, Valk TW, et al. Scintigraphic localization of pheochromocytoma. N Engl J Med 305:12, 1981.
153. Suzuki T, Watanabe K, Sugino T, et al. Immunocytochemical demonstration of IGF-II immunoreactivity in human phaeochromocytoma and extraadrenal paraganglioma. J Pathol 167: 199, 1992.
154. Tenenbaum F, Lumbroso J, Schlumberger M, et al. Comparison of radiolabeled octreotide and metaiodobenzylguanidine (MIBG) scintigraphy in malignant pheochromocytoma. J Nucl Med 36:1, 1995.
155. Unger P, Hoffman K, Pertsemlidis D, et al. S-100 protein-positive sustentacular cells in malignant and locally aggressive adrenal pheochromocytomas. Arch Pathol Lab Med 115:484, 1991.
156. Van Gils AP, van Erkel AR, Falk TH, et al. Magnetic resonance imaging or metaiodobenzylguanidine scintigraphy for the demonstration of paragangliomas? Correlations and disparities. Eur J Nucl Med 21:239, 1994.

### Miscellaneous Paragangliomas

157. Aggarwal S, Deck JH, Kucharczyk W. Neuroendocrine tumor (paraganglioma) of the cauda equina: MRI and pathologic findings. Am J Neuroradiol 14:1003, 1993.
158. Araust DJ, Banner NR, Canton AM, et al. Location, localization, and surgical treatment of cardiac pheochromocytoma. Am J Cardiol 69:283, 1992.
159. Archer KF, Hurwitz JJ, Balogh JM, et al. Orbital nonchromaffin paraganglioma: a case report and review of the literature. Ophthalmology 96:1659, 1989.
160. Bak J, Olsson Y, Grimelius L, et al. Paraganglioma of the cauda equina: a case report and review of the literature. APMIS 104:234, 1996.
161. Barbareschi M, Frigo B, Aldovini E, et al. Case report: duodenal gangliocytic paraganglioma. Virchows Arch 416:81, 1989.
162. Barnes L, Ferlito A, Wenig BM. Laryngeal paragangliomas: a review and report of a single case. J Laryngol Otol 111:197, 1997.
163. Batra V, Trivedi C. Paraganglioma of the cauda equina. JAPI (J Assoc Physician's India) 40:750, 1992.
164. Batsakis JG. Paragangliomas of the head and neck. In: Tumors of the Head and Neck. Williams & Wilkins, Baltimore, 1979.
165. Boyle M, Gaffney EF, Thurston A. Paraganglioma of the prostatic urethra: a report of three cases and a review of the literature. Br J Urol 77:445, 1996.
166. Buetow PC, Levine MS, Buck JL, et al. Duodenal gangliocytic paraganglioma: CT MR imaging and US findings. Radiology 204:745, 1997.
167. Cabello A, Ricoy JR. Paraganglioma of the cauda equina. Cancer 52.751, 1983.
168. Casanova J, Maura CS, Torres JP, et al. Intrapericardial paraganglioma. Eur J Cardiothorac Surg 10:287, 1996.
169. Chetty R, Pillay P, Jaichand V. Cytokeratin expression in adrenal phaaeochromocytomas and extra-adrenal paragangliomas. J Clin Pathol 51:477, 1998.
170. Denford A, Vaughan M, Mayall F. Paraganglioma as an unusual mimic of carcinoma in the prostate. Br J Urol 80:677, 1997.
171. Dookhan DB, Miettinen M, Finkel G, et al. Recurrent duodenal gangliocytic paraganglioma with lymph node metastasis. Histopathology 22:399, 1993.
172. Evans JD, Wilson PG, Barber PC, et al. Duodenal gangliocytic paraganglioma presenting as an ampullary tumor. Int J Pancreatol 20:131, 1996.
173. Faro SH, Turtz AR, Koenigsberg RA, et al. Paraganglioma of the cauda equina with associated intramedullary cyst: MR findings. Am J Neuroradiol 18:1588, 1997.
174. Ferlito A, Barnes L, Wenig BM. Identification, classification, treatment and prognosis of laryngeal paraganglioma: review of the literature and eight new cases. Ann Otol Rhinol Laryngol 103:525, 1994.
175. Ferlito A, Milroy CM, Wenig BM, et al. Laryngeal paraganglioma versus atypical carcinoid tumor. Ann Otol Rhinol Laryngol 104:78, 1995.
176. Fujino Y, Nagata Y, Ogino K, et al. Nonfunctional paraganglioma of the pancreas: report of a case. Surg Today 28:209, 1998.
177. Furihata M, Sonobe H, Iwata J, et al. Immunohistochemical characterization of a case of duodenal gangliocytic paraganglioma. Pathol Int 46:610, 1996.
178. Gallivan MVE, Chun B, Rowden G, et al. Laryngeal paraganglioma: a case report with ultrastructural analysis and literature review. Am J Surg Pathol 3:85, 1979.
179. Hamid QA, Bishop AE, Rode J, et al. Duodenal gangliocytic paraganglioma: a study of 10 cases with immunocytochemical neuroendocrine markers. Hum Pathol 17:1151, 1986.
180. Hamilton BH, Francis IR, Gross BH, et al. Intrapericardial paragangliomas (pheochromocytomas): imaging features. AJR 168:109, 1997.
181. Heufelder AE, Hofbauer LC. Greetings from below the aortic arch: the paradigm of cardiac paraganglioma. J Clin Endocrinol Metab 81:891, 1996.
182. Hughes JH, El-Mofty S, Sessions D, et al. Primary intra thyroidal paraganglioma with metachronous carotid body tumor: report of a case and review of the literature. Pathol Res Pract 193:791, 1997.
183. Inai K, Kobuke T, Yonehara S, et al. Duodenal gangliocytic paraganglioma with lymph node metastasis in a 17-year old boy. Cancer 63:2540, 1989.
184. Ironside JW, Royds JA, Taylor CD, et al. Paraganglioma of the cauda equina; a histological, ultrastructural and immunocytochemical study of two cases with review of the literature. J Pathol 145:195, 1985.
185. Jebara VA, Uva MS, Farge A, et al. Cardiac pheochromocytomas. Ann Thorac Surg 53:356, 1992.
186. Jeevanandam C, Oz MC, Shapiro B, et al. Surgical management of cardiac pheochromocytoma: resection versus transplantation. Ann Surg 221:415, 1995.
187. Johnson TL, Shapiro B, Beierwaltes WH, et al. Cardiac paragangliomas: a clinicopathologic and immunohistochemical study of four cases. Am J Surg Pathol 9:827, 1985.
188. Karnauchow PN. Investigation into the occurrence of paraganglia in lower limbs. Lab Invest 6:368, 1957.
189. Labrousse F, Leboutet MJ, Petit B, et al. Cytokeratin expression in paragangliomas of the cauda equina. Clin Neuropathol 18:208, 1999.
190. Lagace R, Tremblany M. Non-chromaffin paraganglioma of

kidney with distant metastasis. Can Med Assoc J 99:1095, 1968.

191. LaGuette J, Matias-Guiu X, Rosai J. Thyroid paraganglioma: a clinicopathologic and immunohistochemical study of three cases. Am J Surg Pathol 21:748, 1997.
192. Lewis IH, Yousif D, Mullis SL, et al. Management of cardiac pheochromocytoma. J Cardiothorac Vasc Anesth 8:223, 1994.
193. Miller TA, Webber TR, Appleman HD. Paraganglioma of the gallbladder. Arch Surg 15:631, 1972.
194. Min KW. Gangliocytic paraganglioma of the duodenum: report of a case with immunocytochemical and ultrastructural investigation. Ultrastruct Pathol 21:587, 1997.
195. Moran CA, Rush W, Mena H. Primary spinal paragangliomas: a clinicopathological and immunohistochemical study of 30 cases. Histopathology 31:167, 1997.
196. Nguyen QA, Gibbs PM, Rice DH. Malignant nasal paraganglioma: a case report and review of the literature. Otolaryngol Head Neck Surg 113:157, 1995.
197. Orr LA, Pettigrew RI, Churchwell AL, et al. Gadolinium utilization in the MR evaluation of cardiac paraganglioma. Clin Imaging 21:404, 1997.
198. Orrell JM, Hales SA. Paragangliomas of the cauda equina have a distinctive cytokeratin immunophenotype. Histopathology 21:479, 1992.
199. Ozunlu A, Dundar A, Satar B, et al. Laryngeal paraganglioma: a review and report of a single case. J Laryngol Otol 110:519, 1996.
200. Papadimitriou JC, Drachenberg CB. Giant mitochondria with paracrystalline inclusions in paraganglioma of the urinary bladder: correlation with mitochondrial abnormalities in paragangliomas of other sites. Ultrastruct Pathol 18:559, 1994.
201. Perrone T. Duodenal gangliocytic paraganglioma and carcinoid. Am J Surg Pathol 10:147, 1986.
202. Perrone T, Sibley RK, Rosai J. Duodenal gangliocytic paraganglioma: an immunohistochemical and ultrastructural study and a hypothesis concerning its origin. Am J Surg Pathol 9:31, 1985.
203. Peterson KL, Fu YS, Calcaterra T. Subglottic paraganglioma. Head Neck 19:54, 1997.
204. Rhaman SI, Matthews LK, Shaikh H, et al. Primary paraganglioma of the bladder in 14-year-old boy. Br J Urol 75:682, 1995.
205. Roche PH, Figarella-Branger D, Regis J, et al. Cauda equina paraganglioma with subsequent intracranial and intraspinal metastases. Acta Neurochir (Wien) 138:475, 1996.
206. Scheithauer BW, Nora FE, LeChago J, et al. Duodenal gangliocytic paraganglioma: clinicopathologic and immunocytochemical study of 11 cases. Am J Clin Pathol 86:559, 1986.
207. Shapiro B, Gonzalez E, Weissman A, et al. Malignant paraganglioma of the prostate: case report, depiction by meta-iodobenzylguanidine scintigraphy and review of the literature. Q J Nucl Med 41:36, 1997.
208. Skodt V, Jacobsen GK, Helsted M. Primary paraganglioma of the lung: report of two cases and review of the literature. APMIS 103:597, 1995.
209. Sonnenland PRL, Scheithauer BW, LeChago J, et al. Paraganglioma of the cauda equina region: clinicopathologic study of 31 cases with special reference to immunocytology and ultrastructure. Cancer 58:1720, 1986.
210. Steel TR, Botterill P, Sheehy JP. Paraganglioma of the cauda equina with associated syringomyelia: case report. Surg Neurol 42:489, 1994.
211. Strommer KN, Brandner S, Sarioglu AC, et al. Symptomatic cerebellar metastasis and late local recurrence of a cauda equina paraganglioma: case report. J Neurosurg 83:166, 1995.
212. Taxy JB. Paraganglioma of the cauda equina: report of a rare tumor. Cancer 51:1904, 1983.
213. Taylor HB, Helwig EB. Benign nonchromaffin paragangliomas of the duodenum. Virchows Arch [Pathol Anat] 335:356, 1962.
214. Thacker WC, Duckworth JK. Chemodectoma of the orbit. Cancer 23:1233, 1969.
215. Tomic S, Warner T. Pancreatic somatostatin-secreting gangliocytic paraganglioma with lymph node metastasis. Am J Gastroenterol 91:607, 1996.
216. Van Eeden S, Offerhaus GJA, Peterse HL, et al. Gangliocytic paraganglioma of the appendix. Histopathology 36:47, 2000.

# CHAPTER 34

# CARTILAGINOUS SOFT TISSUE TUMORS

Benign extraosseous cartilaginous lesions are uncommon and usually present as tumor-like masses. Although still unclear as to whether most are neoplastic or metaplastic in origin, some have been shown to be clonal, suggesting a neoplastic process. In the past we rather arbitrarily employed the term *soft part* or *extraskeletal chondroma* for small well defined solitary nodules of hyaline cartilage that are unattached to bone and occur primarily in the distal extremities, especially the fingers and hand. We have used the same designation for the rare chondroma-like lesions that occur in the gastrointestinal and respiratory tracts. These lesions, however, must be distinguished from the cartilaginous rests of branchial origin that are usually found in the soft tissues of the lateral neck in infants and small children[25] and from the metaplastic cartilage encountered in some benign lipomatous (chondrolipoma) and fibromatous (calcifying aponeurotic fibroma) neoplasms; they must also be distinguished from multiple cartilaginous nodules in the synovium (synovial chondromatosis) and from the cartilage in myositis ossificans and its variants.

Malignant cartilaginous tumors also occur as primary soft tissue neoplasms, but they are much less common than primary chondrosarcomas of bone. There are chiefly two distinctive types: *myxoid chondrosarcoma* and *mesenchymal chondrosarcoma*. There are sporadic reports of other morphologic types of extraskeletal chondrosarcoma, but these entities are in need of further definition.[81]

*Well differentiated extraosseous chondrosarcomas* resembling hyaline cartilage are rare. In fact, if such a tumor is encountered in soft tissue, it is more likely an extension or metastasis of a bone tumor than a primary soft tissue neoplasm. Well differentiated chondrosarcomas do arise from the synovium, however, sometimes secondary to synovial chondromatosis,[18,20,32,34,44] and from the periosteum (periosteal chondrosarcoma).[31] They also appear following radiation therapy or injection of radioactive material, usually after a latent period of many years. For example, Ghalib et al.[66] recorded a chondrosarcoma of the larynx that appeared 40 years after a course of irradiation for hyperthyroidism, and Schajowicz et al.[105] reported a chondrosarcoma of the axilla secondary to injection of Thorotrast for the diagnosis of hemangioma. Rare instances of chondrosarcoma also occur in the respiratory tract, especially the nasal passages, larynx, trachea, and bronchi. They are found in the heart and great vessels, especially the pulmonary artery. Chondrosarcomas of the urinary bladder and uterus are most likely malignant mixed mesodermal tumors or carcinosarcomas that have differentiated along two or more cell lines but have been sampled inadequately. Equally rare are chondrosarcomas of the mammary gland. Most display an epithelial or fibroadenomatous component, and many show transitions toward liposarcoma or osteosarcoma.

## EXTRASKELETAL CHONDROMA

Extraskeletal chondroma, a benign cartilaginous tumor that occurs predominantly in the hands and feet, has a benign clinical course. Its variable histologic appearance not infrequently leads to a mistaken diagnosis of chondrosarcoma. Much of the literature regarding this entity consists of case reports and small series, although there are two comprehensive reports of this entity, including the Mayo Clinic report of 70 tumors[11] and 104 cases from the files of the Armed Forces Institute of Pathology (AFIP).[10]

### Clinical Findings

The tumor occurs primarily in the soft tissues of the hands and feet, usually with no connection to the underlying bone. Its predominant single site is the fingers, where more than 80% of extraskeletal chondromas are found. Less frequent sites include the hands, toes, feet, and trunk; rare cases have been described in the dura,[9,40] larynx,[17,23,27] pharynx,[43] oral cavity,[7,42] and skin.[1] Extraskeletal chondroma usually manifests as a slowly enlarging nodule or mass that seldom causes pain or tenderness; the tumor mainly affects adults 30–60 years of age and is rare in children.[24,35] It is often associated with tendons, tendon sheaths, or joint capsules[4]; unlike periosteal chondroma,[28,30] it is located outside the periosteum. Nearly all of the tumors are solitary, although Dellon et al.[15] described bilateral chondromas in the right index and left ring fingers of a patient with renal failure. In addition, Humphreys et al.[21] described an unusual case of multiple cutaneous chondromas of the face in a patient whose brother and nephew were similarly affected, suggesting an autosomal dominant mode of inheritance. In general, however, multiple chondroid lesions are more likely forms of synovial chondromatosis. The association of pulmonary chondroma, gastric epithelioid stromal tumor, and extraadrenal paraganglioma is known as *Carney's triad.*

Radiographically, the lesion is well demarcated and does not involve bone, although some tumors cause compression deformities or bone erosion. Discrete, irregular, ring-like or curvilinear calcifications are often demonstrable[46] (Fig. 34–1). Computed tomography (CT) and magnetic resonance imaging (MRI) are useful for determining the exact site of the tumor and its relation to the adjacent bone.[14,82]

## Pathologic Findings

Excised chondromas are usually well demarcated, have rounded or ovoid configurations, and are firm on palpation. Occasional chondromas are soft or friable with focal cystic change. Nearly all are small, seldom exceeding 3 cm in greatest diameter. They

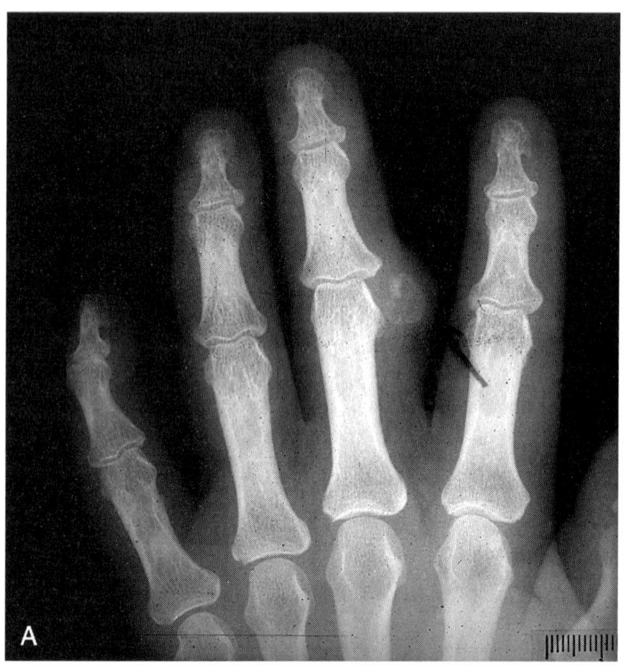
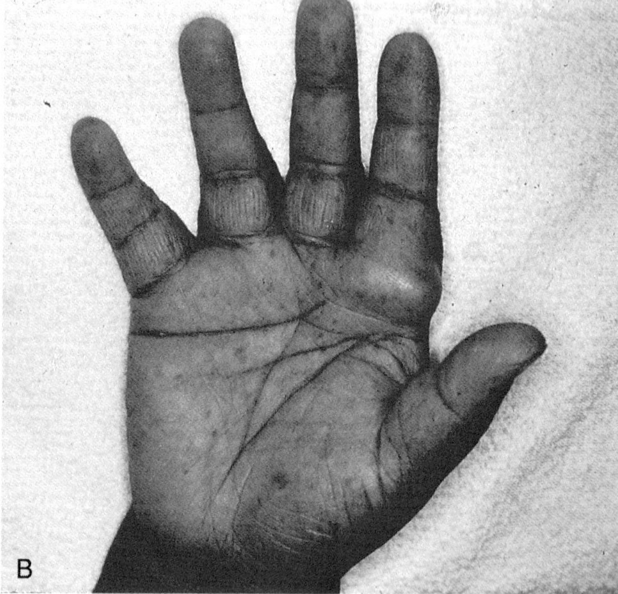
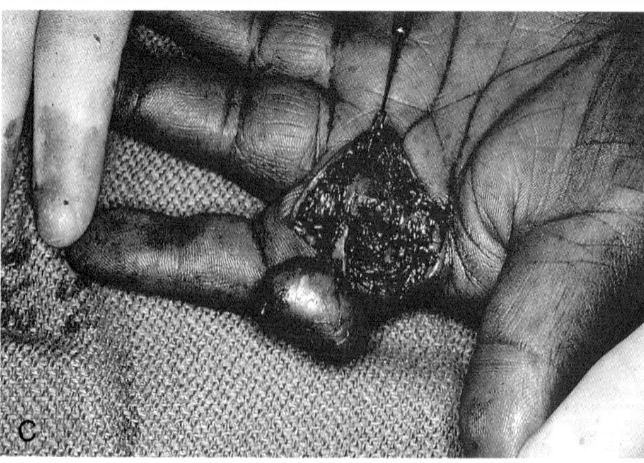

**FIGURE 34–1.** Chondroma of soft parts. (**A**) Radiograph of the left third finger showing a small soft tissue mass with foci of calcification. (**B**) Chondroma of soft parts at the base of the right second finger. (**C**) Intraoperative specimen of enucleated chondroma of soft parts shown in (**B**).

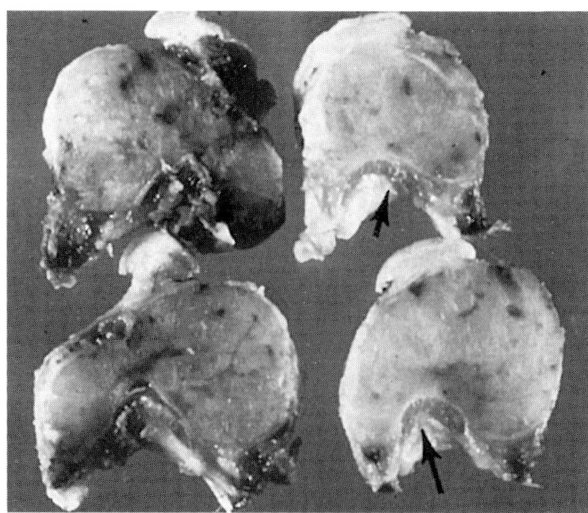

**FIGURE 34–2.** Cross sections of a chondroma of soft parts removed from the second toe of a 62-year-old woman. The tumor is well circumscribed and is firmly attached to a tendon (arrows). (From Chung EB, Enzinger FM. Benign chondromas of soft parts. Cancer 41:1414, 1978.)

may be attached to the tendon or tendon sheath (Fig. 34–2). Microscopically, they vary considerably in appearance. About two-thirds consist of mature or fairly mature hyaline cartilage arranged in a more or less distinct lobular pattern with sharp borders (Fig. 34–3). Some of these tumors are altered by focal fibrosis (*fibrochondroma*) or ossification (*osteochondroma*)[36]; others show myxoid change (*myxochondroma*), sometimes together with focal hemorrhage. About one-third display focal or diffuse calcification, usually a late feature that may completely obscure the cartilaginous nature of the tumor and may mimic tumoral calcinosis. The calcified material is granular, floccular, or crystalline and often outlines the contours of the chondrocytes in a lace-like pattern (Figs. 34–4, 34–5, 34–6). Calcification tends to be more pronounced in the center than at the periphery of the tumor lobule. It is often accompanied by cellular degeneration and necrosis, which accounts for the softened gross appearance of some of these tumors. As noted by Del Rosario et al.,[16] some tumors have cells with periodic acid-Schiff (PAS)-positive, diastase-resistant intracytoplasmic hyaline globules, which may represent a glycoproteinaceous secretory product.

A striking feature that occurs in about 15% of the tumors is a focal granuloma-like proliferation of epithelioid and multinucleated giant cells somewhat reminiscent of a fibroxanthoma or a giant cell tumor[45] (Figs. 34–7, 34–8). This proliferation is most conspicuous at the tumor margin and along the interlobular vascular channels. There are also rare extraskeletal chondromas in which the presence of plump immature-appearing cells on a myxoid background simulates a chondrosarcoma (Fig. 34–9). In general, however, these tumors can be recognized as chondromas by the presence of more mature, less cellular cartilaginous areas at the periphery. There are also several reports of extraskeletal chondromas that exhibit chondroblastic features and multinucleated giant cells.[22,45]

Like normal chondrocytes, the cells of the extraskeletal chondroma are positive for vimentin and S-100 protein.[45] The electron microscopic picture reveals chondrocytes with large indented nuclei, abundant rough endoplasmic reticulum, and occasional membrane-bound vacuoles. Short microvillous processes, or filopodia, extend from the cytoplasmic surfaces into the surrounding intercellular matrix (Fig. 34–10). In calcified cases the latter contains variously sized aggregates of hydroxyapatite crystals.

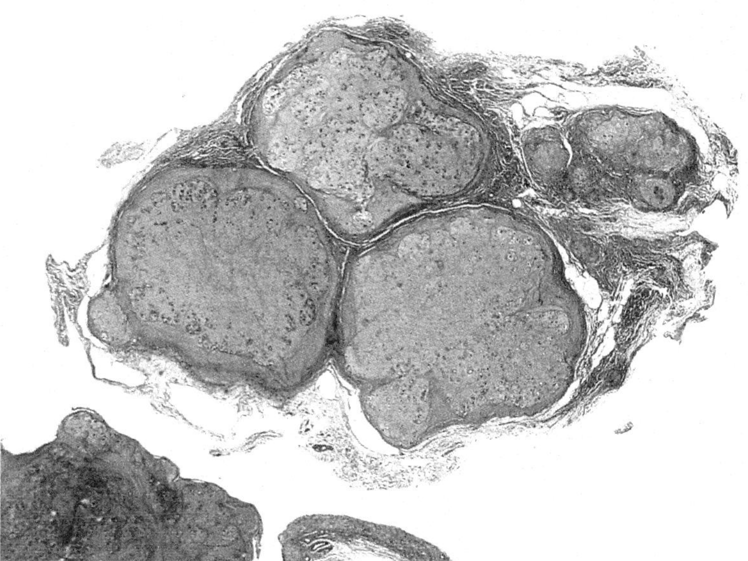

**FIGURE 34–3.** Cross section of a chondroma of soft parts showing circumscription and a multinodular growth pattern.

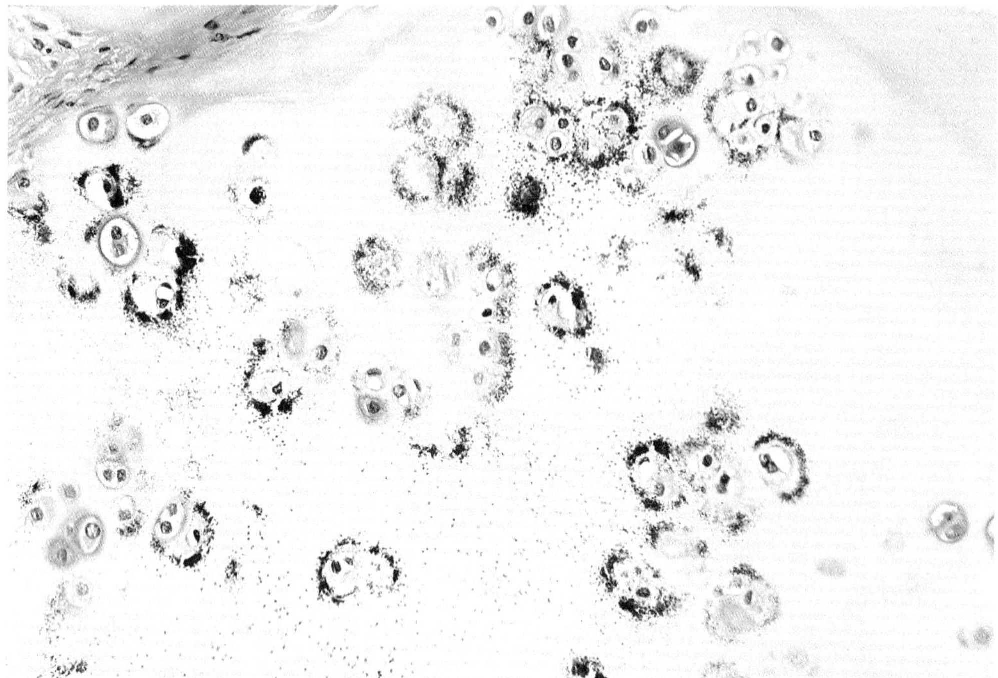

**FIGURE 34–4.** Chondroma of soft parts consisting of mature hyaline cartilage with nests of benign-appearing cells in lacunae.

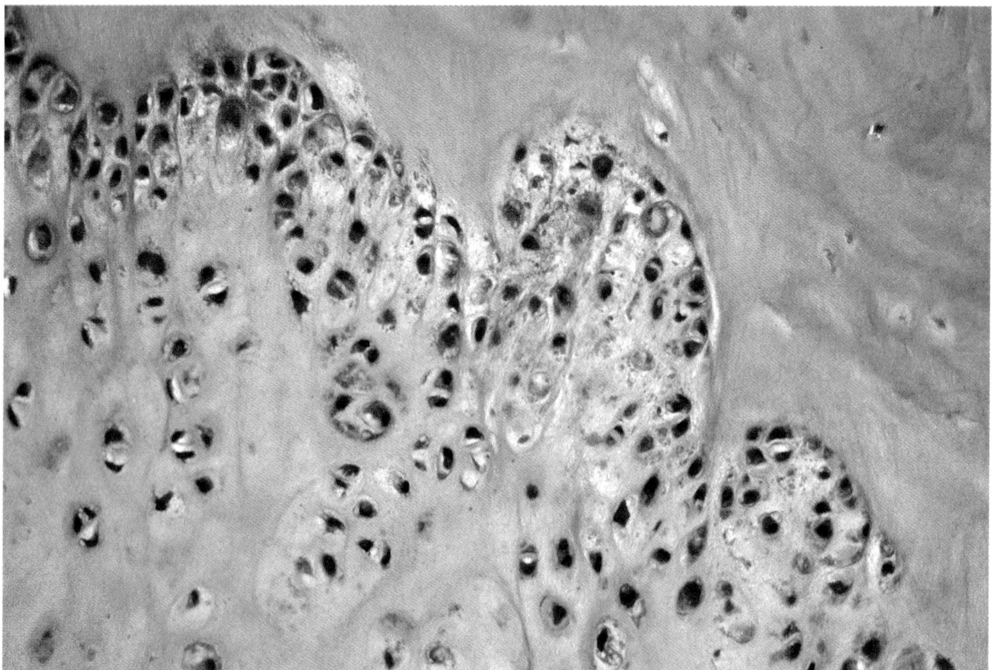

**FIGURE 34–5.** Chondroma of soft parts with a hypercellular zone at the periphery of a lobule.

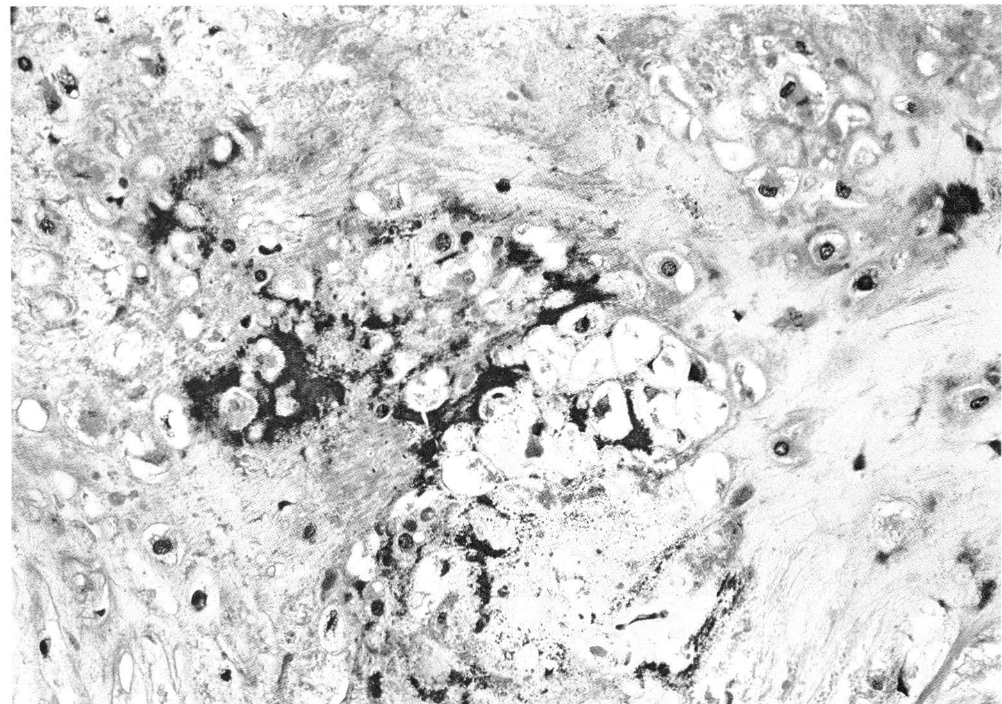

**FIGURE 34–6.** Calcified chondroma of soft parts. Calcium deposits surround and partly replace the cartilage cells.

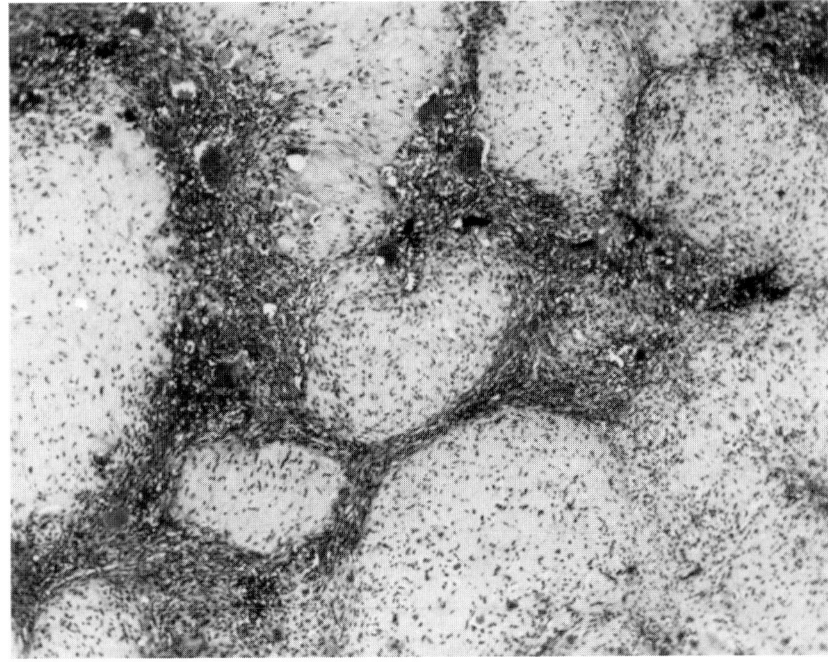

**FIGURE 34–7.** Chondroma of soft parts altered by a granuloma-like proliferation of epithelioid and multinucleated giant cells.

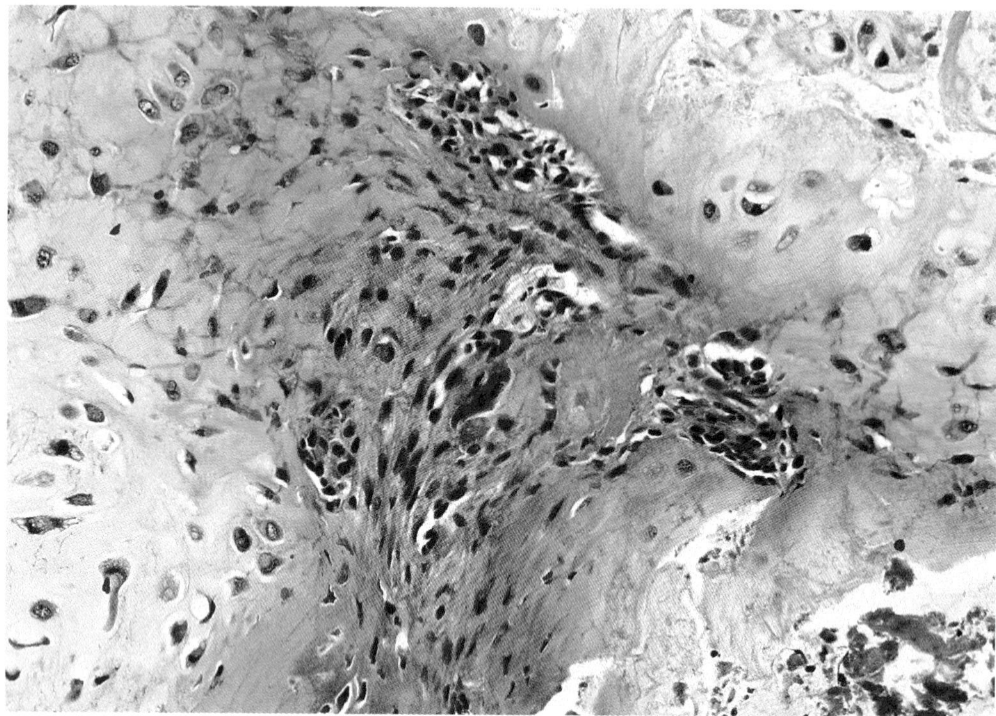

**FIGURE 34–8.** High-power view of interlobular septa in a chondroma of soft parts. Rare multinucleated giant cells are seen.

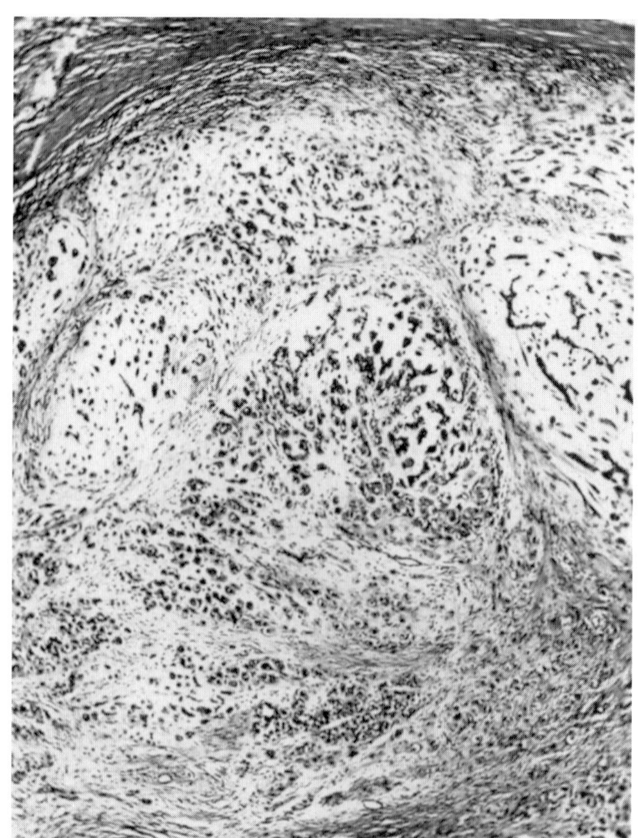

**FIGURE 34–9.** Chondroma of soft parts consisting of immature-appearing cells in a myxoid matrix reminiscent of an extraskeletal myxoid chondrosarcoma.

The cytogenetic data on soft tissue chondromas are limited. Clonal chromosomal abnormalities have been identified in some cases,[8,29] including monosomy 6 and rearrangement of chromosome 11.[12]

## Differential Diagnosis

Distinction from other benign lesions should not be difficult. *Calcifying aponeurotic fibroma* is characterized by short bar-like foci of cartilaginous metaplasia in a dense, poorly circumscribed fibromatous background. It occurs in the hand rather than in the distal portion of the digits and almost always affects patients younger than 25 years. *Tumoral calcinosis* may mimic a heavily calcified chondroma, but it lacks cartilage and usually shows a distinct histiocytic response to the calcified material. *Giant cell tumors* have more uniform cellular patterns and rarely have metaplastic cartilage or bone. Radiography usually allows distinction from *periosteal* or *juxtacortical chondroma,* a small well circumscribed tumor located underneath the periosteum that causes erosion of the underlying cortex with "ledges" or "buttresses" at the margin of the tumor[5] and from *subungual osteochondroma,*[2,3] a lesion that has cartilage overlying well developed bone.

*Synovial chondromatosis* differs from extraskeletal chondroma by its occurrence in large joints, such as

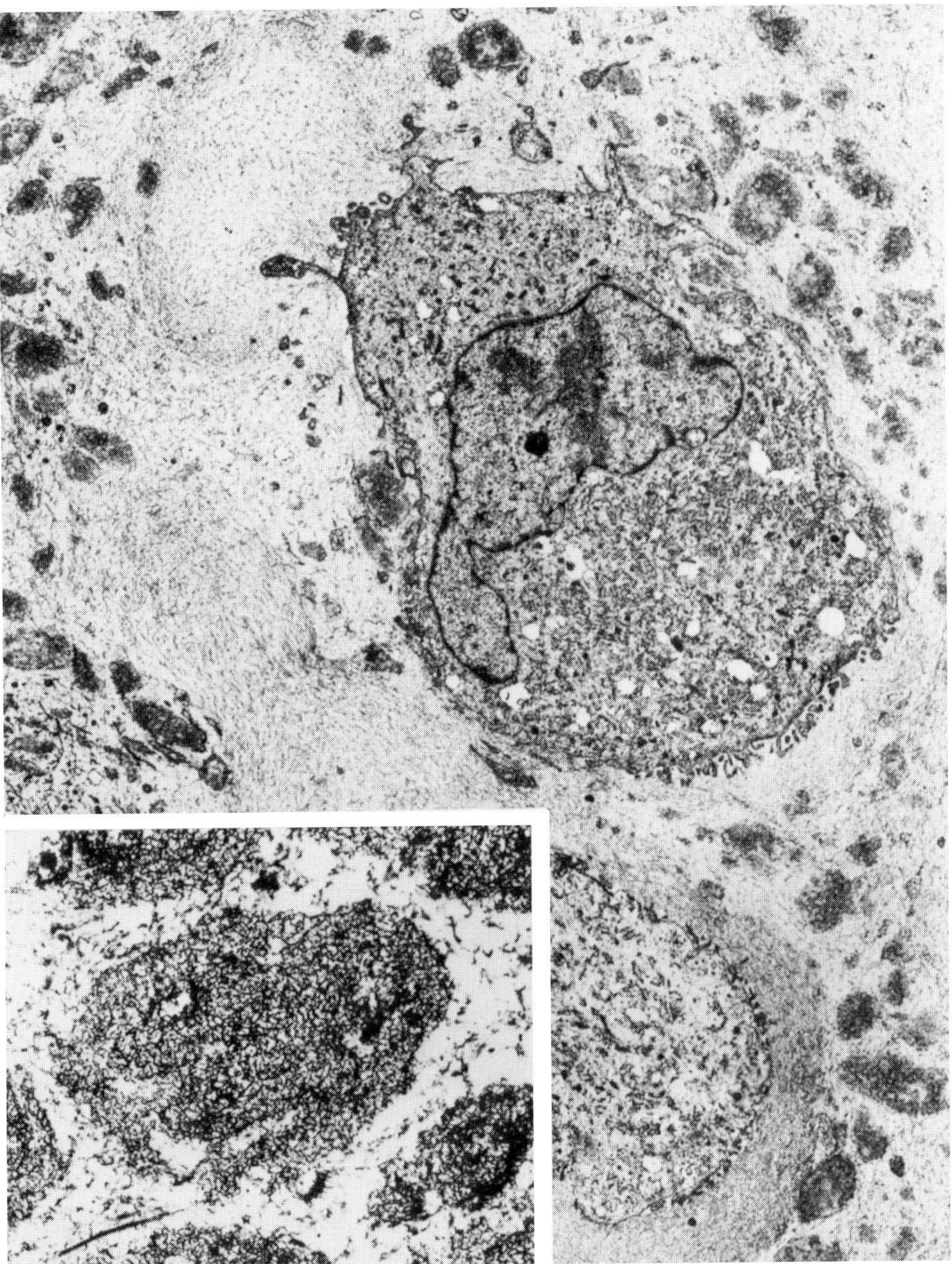

**FIGURE 34–10.** Electron micrograph of a calcified chondroma of soft parts showing loosely spaced cartilage cells with abundant rough endoplasmic reticulum, free ribosomes, and short irregular microvillous processes surrounded by aggregates of calcium crystals. (**Inset**) Aggregates of hydroxyapatite crystals under high magnification. (From Chung EB, Enzinger FM. Benign chondromas of soft parts. Cancer 41: 1414, 1978.)

the knee, hip, elbow, or shoulder joint[19,33,37,38] and the formation of numerous, small, metaplastic cartilaginous or osteocartilaginous nodules of varying size attached to the synovial membrane of the joint, tendon sheath, or lining of the adjacent extraarticular bursa (Figs. 34–11, 34–12, 34–13). Rarely it occurs in the surrounding soft tissues (extraarticular synovial chondromatosis).[39,41] These synovial nodules often become detached and are found as loose bodies in the joint space. Some are hypercellular with clustering of tumor cells and increased mitotic activity. Most become calcified or ossified and can be readily demonstrated by routine radiography as multiple, small, discrete radiopaque bodies (loose bodies or joint mice).

*Nonmineralized "loose bodies"* are demonstrable on arthrograms, CT scans, or MRI as multiple filling defects outlined by contrast material.[26] Bone scintigraphy also shows intense radionuclide uptake in the nodules.[82] As in soft part chondromas, hypercellularity, binucleate cells, and nuclear atypia are compatible with a benign clinical course.

Rare instances of *chondrosarcoma* arising in synovial chondromatosis have been reported.[6,13] *Periosteal chondrosarcoma* must also be included in the differential diagnosis.[31]

Drawing a sharp line between *myxoid chondrosarcoma* and the *myxoid variant of chondroma* may be difficult, especially with those rare tumors that exhibit a moderate degree of cellular pleomorphism. Usually, however, the cartilage cells of chondromas are better differentiated, especially in the peripheral portion of the tumor; they tend to be less cellular and smaller; and as a rule they occur in the soft tissues of the hands and feet, unusual locations for myxoid chondrosarcoma.

### Discussion

Although some of the chondroblastic or myxoid forms of extraskeletal chondroma cause concern because of their atypical cellular features, there is no evidence that these tumors behave differently from the well differentiated forms composed of adult-type hyaline cartilage. We have seen a few tumors that recurred locally, but all were treated effectively by reexcising the tumor. It is noteworthy that we have never encountered transformation of extraskeletal chondroma to chondrosarcoma, although this is by no means rare with chondroid lesions of bone. Local excision is the preferred mode of therapy.

## EXTRASKELETAL MYXOID CHONDROSARCOMA

The extraskeletal myxoid chondrosarcoma bears a superficial resemblance to myxoid liposarcoma, but its distinctive structure and staining characteristics identify it as a separate entity and establish its chondroblastic origin. The tumor is relatively rare: Tsuneyoshi et al.[115] noted an incidence of 2.3% among 603 soft tissue sarcomas.

Extraskeletal myxoid chondrosarcoma has also been reported as "chordoid sarcoma"[88] and by Hajdu et al.[72] as *tendosynovial sarcoma,* a term coined for a group of neoplasms that have a close association with tendosynovial structures, including synovial sarcoma, epithelioid sarcoma, clear-cell sarcoma, and extraskeletal myxoid chondrosarcoma. Myxoid chondrosarcoma occurs primarily in the deep tissues of the extremities, especially the musculature. Because a morphologically identical tumor also occurs in bone,

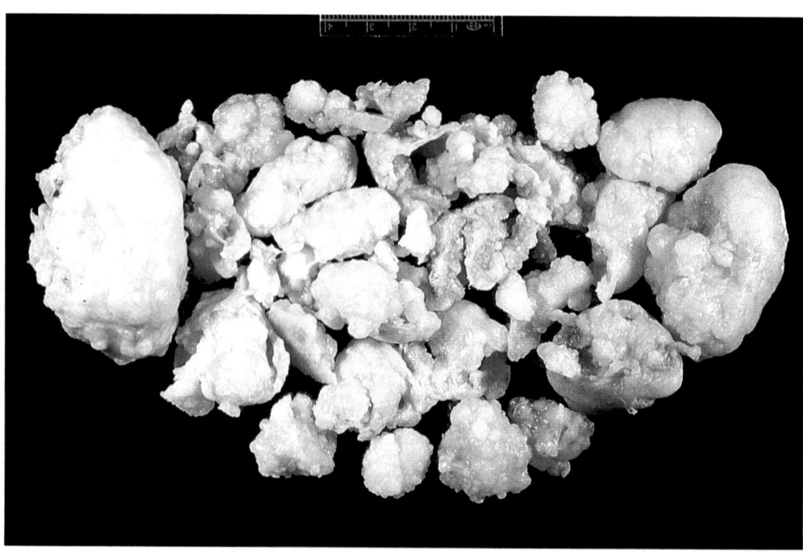

**FIGURE 34–11.** Conglomerate of variably sized nodules of synovial chondromatosis.

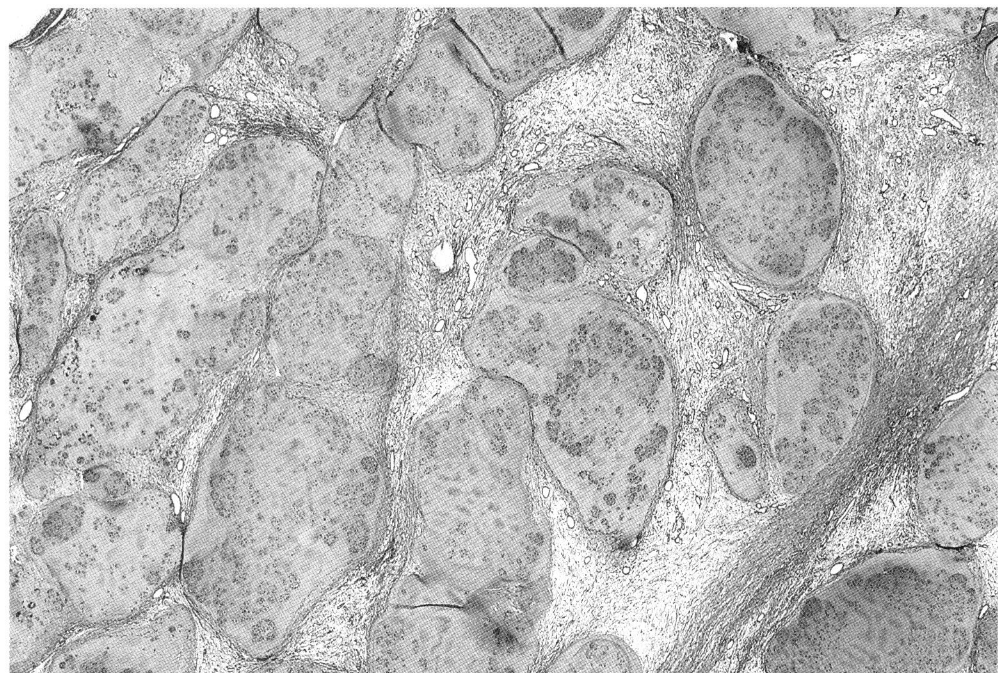

**FIGURE 34–12.** Synovial chondromatosis of the left knee.

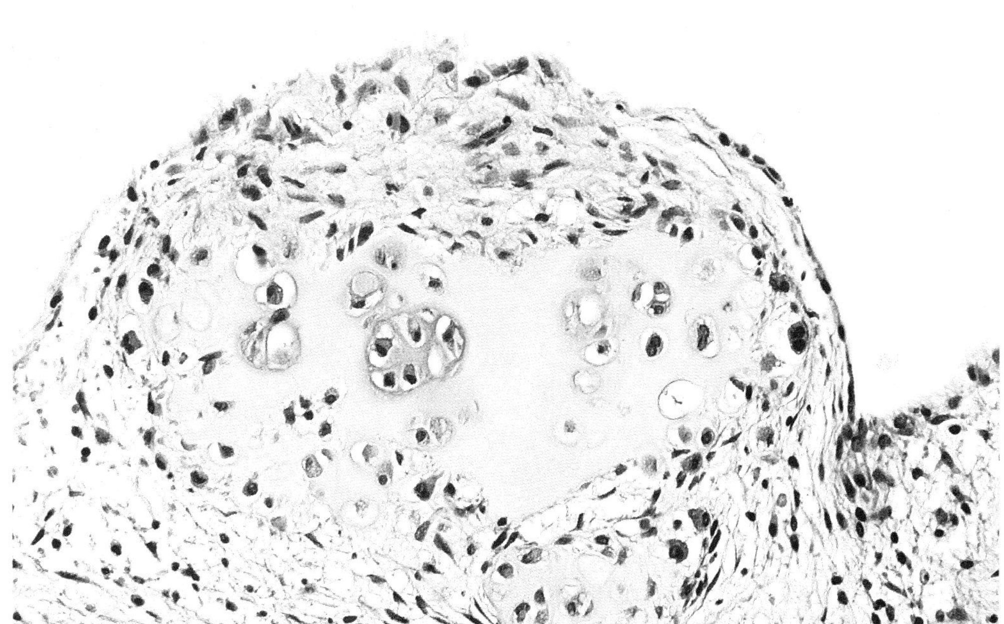

**FIGURE 34–13.** High-power view of synovial chondromatosis with a nodule of metaplastic cartilage underneath the synovium.

radiographic examination, CT scan, or MRI may be necessary to establish its soft tissue origin. It is a relatively slow-growing tumor but has a propensity for local recurrence and eventually pulmonary metastasis, sometimes years after the initial diagnosis.

## Clinical Findings

The tumor most commonly afflicts patients older than 35 years, and only a few cases have been encountered in children and adolescents.[70,71] Most series have found a peak incidence during the fifth or sixth decades of life.[59,92] Men are affected about twice as often as women. The clinical signs and symptoms are nonspecific. Most patients present with a slowly growing, deep-seated mass that causes pain and tenderness in approximately one-third of cases. Complications such as ulceration and hemorrhage may be encountered with large tumors. The duration of symptoms varies considerably, ranging from a few weeks to several years. Some patients have a history of trauma prior to discovery of the tumor, but as with other sarcomas the significance of this finding remains uncertain and is probably coincidental.

More than two-thirds of the tumors occur in the extremities, especially the thigh and popliteal fossa, similar to myxoid liposarcoma.[47,92,102] Most are deep-seated, although occasional tumors are confined to the subcutis; the latter may be difficult to distinguish from myxoid forms of chondroma. There are also accounts of synovial and pleural myxoid chondrosarcomas.[69,81] Rare tumors have been described in unusual locations including the mediastinum,[111] retroperitoneum,[64] abdomen,[78] and fingers.[47] Radiography, CT scans, and MRI show a soft tissue mass with no distinctive radiologic features that would set the tumor apart from other types of soft tissue sarcoma.[65,86,121]

## Pathologic Findings

Macroscopically, the neoplasm occurs as a soft to firm, ovoid, lobulated to nodular mass that is generally well circumscribed, often with a distinct fibrous capsule. On section, it has a gelatinous, gray to tan-brown surface, its color largely dependent on the amount of hemorrhage, a frequent feature of the tumor (Fig. 34–14). Occasionally hemorrhage is so prominent the tumor is mistaken for a hematoma.[58] Despite the distinct multinodular pattern, there is no evidence of multicentric origin.

The size of the tumor varies from a few centimeters to 15 cm or more; most, however, are 4–7 cm in greatest diameter at the time of excision. Meis-Kindblom et al.[92] reported a size range from 1.1 to 25.0 cm and a median tumor size of 7 cm.

Microscopically, a characteristic multinodular pattern is clearly evident (Fig. 34–15). The individual tumor nodules consist of round or slightly elongated cells of uniform shape and size separated by variable amounts of mucoid material (Figs. 34–16 to 34–20). The individual cells have small hyperchromatic nuclei

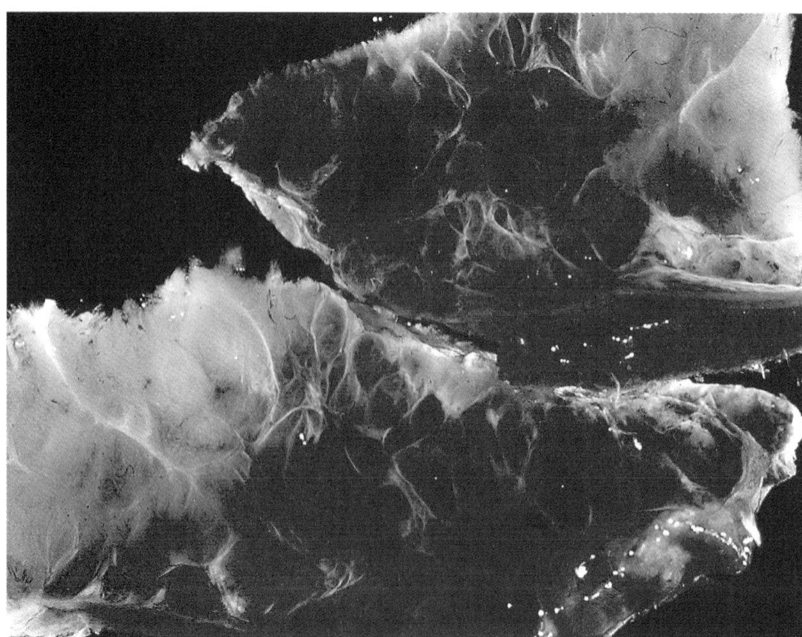

**FIGURE 34–14.** Gross appearance of an extraskeletal myxoid chondrosarcoma with a characteristic gelatinous appearance and a multinodular growth pattern. The dark appearance of some of the nodules is the result of hemorrhage.

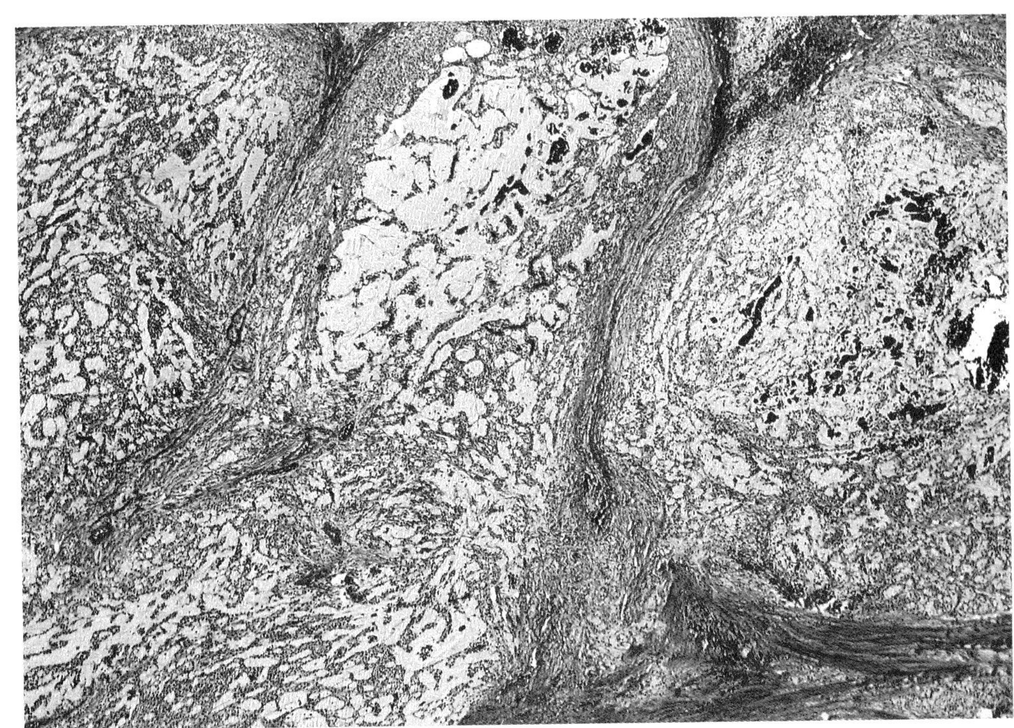

**FIGURE 34–15.** Low-power view of an extraskeletal myxoid chondrosarcoma with a characteristic nodular arrangement.

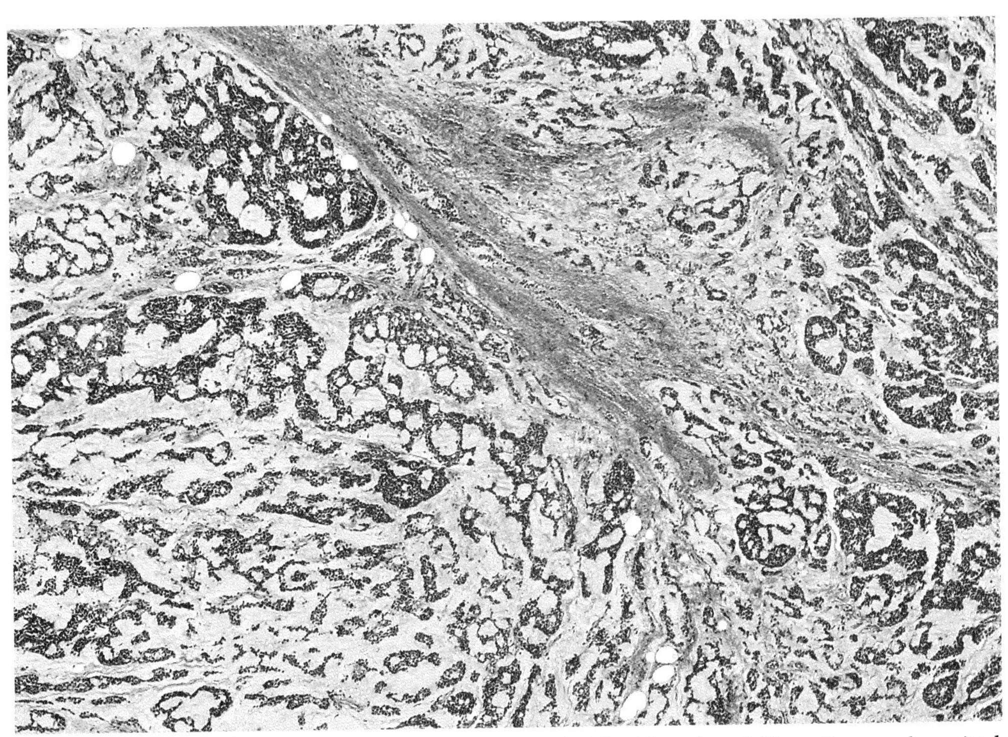

**FIGURE 34–16.** Extraskeletal myxoid chondrosarcoma. Cords of eosinophilic cells are deposited in an abundant myxoid stroma.

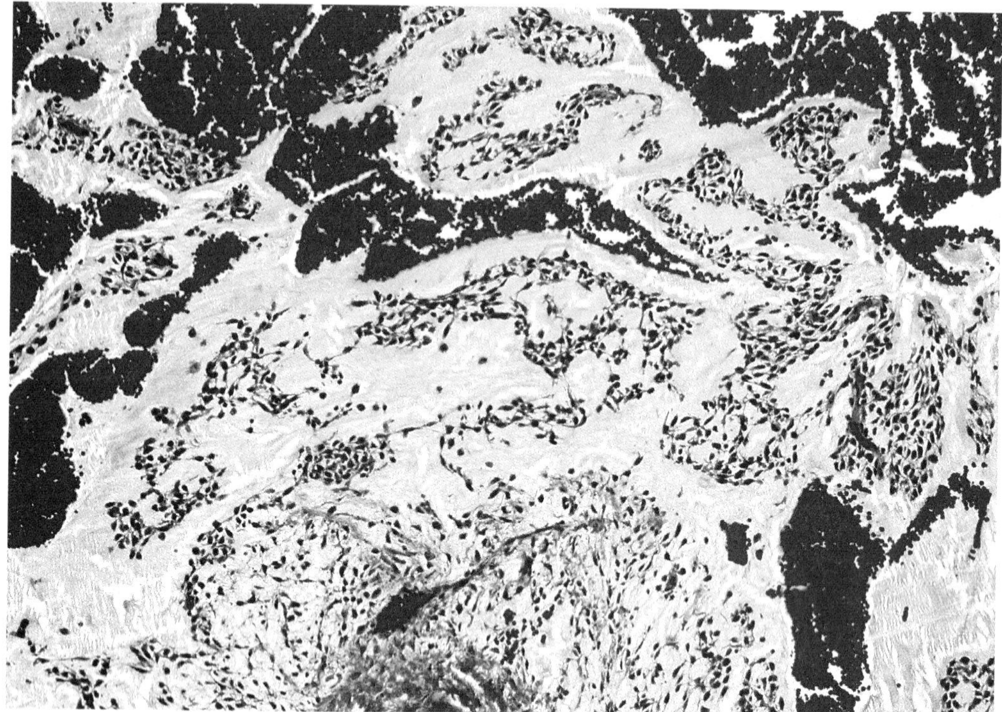

**FIGURE 34–17.** Characteristic alignment of tumor cells in strands and cords separated by large amounts of mucoid material in an extraskeletal myxoid chondrosarcoma. Note the areas of hemorrhage, a characteristic feature of this tumor.

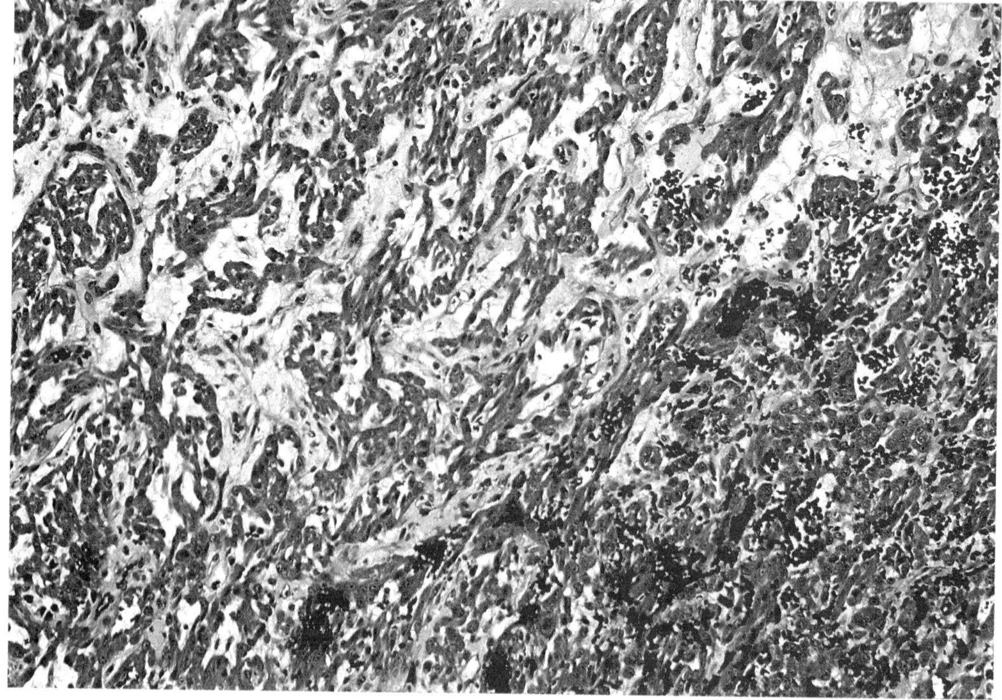

**FIGURE 34–18.** Extraskeletal myxoid chondrosarcoma. Cords of spindle-shaped cells with deeply eosinophilic cytoplasm are separated by mucoid material.

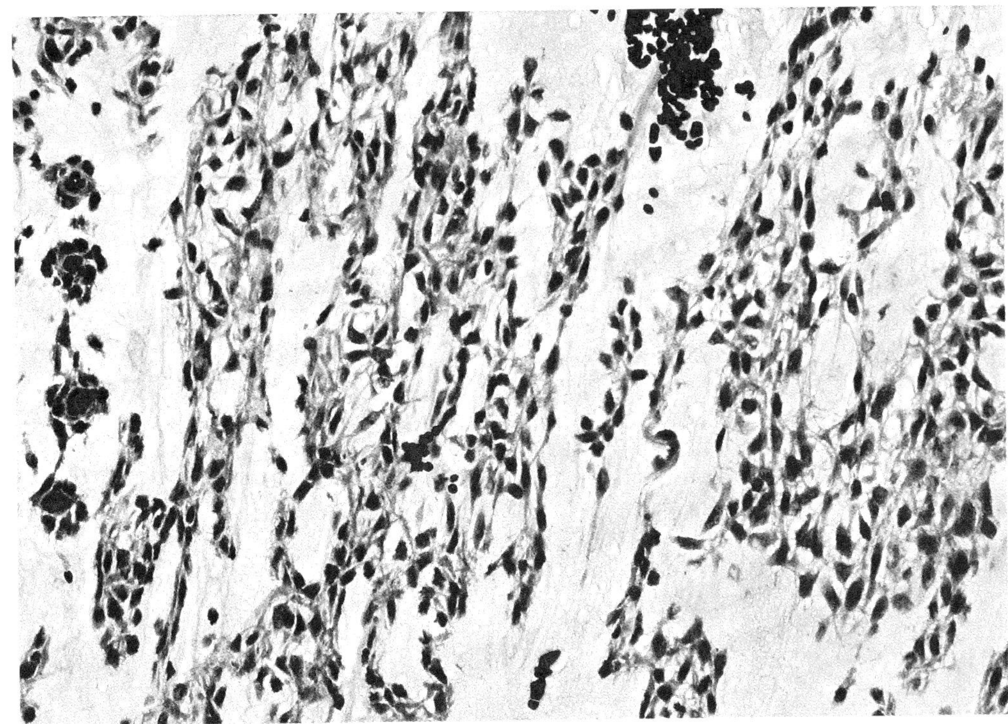

**FIGURE 34–19.** Extraskeletal myxoid chondrosarcoma with strands of small eosinophilic cells widely separated by mucoid material.

and a narrow rim of deeply eosinophilic cytoplasm, features characteristic of chondroblasts (Fig. 34–21). Occasional cells are vacuolated. Unlike chondrosarcoma of bone, differentiated cartilage cells with distinct lacunae are rare; but on careful and prolonged search of multiple sections they are detected in about one-third of the tumors. Mitotic figures are rare in typical cases but may be numerous in less well differentiated and more cellular forms of the tumor.[118]

Characteristically, the individual cells are arranged in short anastomosing cords, strands, or pseudoacini, often creating a lace-like appearance. Less frequently the cellular elements are disposed in small loosely textured whorls or aggregates, reminiscent of an epithelial neoplasm. Rarely, cellular foci composed of fibroblastic/myofibroblastic spindle-shaped cells are present.[47] Indeed, if these features prevail throughout the tumor, a definitive diagnosis of chondrosarcoma may not be possible. Although most extraskeletal myxoid chondrosarcomas are highly myxoid tumors, a distinct subset are hypercellular with less myxoid stroma between the neoplastic cells; they are composed of large cells with vesicular nuclei and prominent nucleoli (Fig. 34–22). These tumors are best diagnosed by identifying typical less cellular areas of extraskeletal myxoid chondrosarcoma or by cytogenetics (discussed below). Some tumors are composed of a cellular proliferation of relatively small round cells closely resembling extraskeletal Ewing's sarcoma/primitive neuroectodermal tumor (Fig. 34–23). Even more rarely, typical extraskeletal myxoid chondrosarcomas are associated with or progress to a high grade sarcoma resembling malignant fibrous histiocytoma (dedifferentiated extraskeletal myxoid chondrosarcoma).[101]

In the more typical tumors, the extracellular mucinous material is abundant and consists largely of chondroitin 4-sulfate, chondroitin 6-sulfate, and keratan sulfate.[62] It stains deeply with the colloidal iron stain and the alcian blue preparation; unlike other richly mucinous soft tissue tumors (with the exception of myxochondroma and chordoma), the staining reaction is not inhibited by pretreating the sections with hyaluronidase. The mucinous matrix also stains with the mucicarmine stain, metachromatically with toluidine blue, and a deep purple with the aldehyde-fuchsin preparation at pH 1.7. The intensity of mucin staining depends on the pH of the staining solution.[48,80] Kindblom and Angervall,[81] using the critical electrolyte method designed by Scott and Dorling,[107] demonstrated that alcian blue stained the matrix with a magnesium chloride concentration up to 0.55 M compared with a concentration of only 0.1 M for myxoid liposarcoma and intramuscular myxoma. As in normal cartilage cells, intracellular PAS-positive and diastase-sensitive material (glycogen) is another

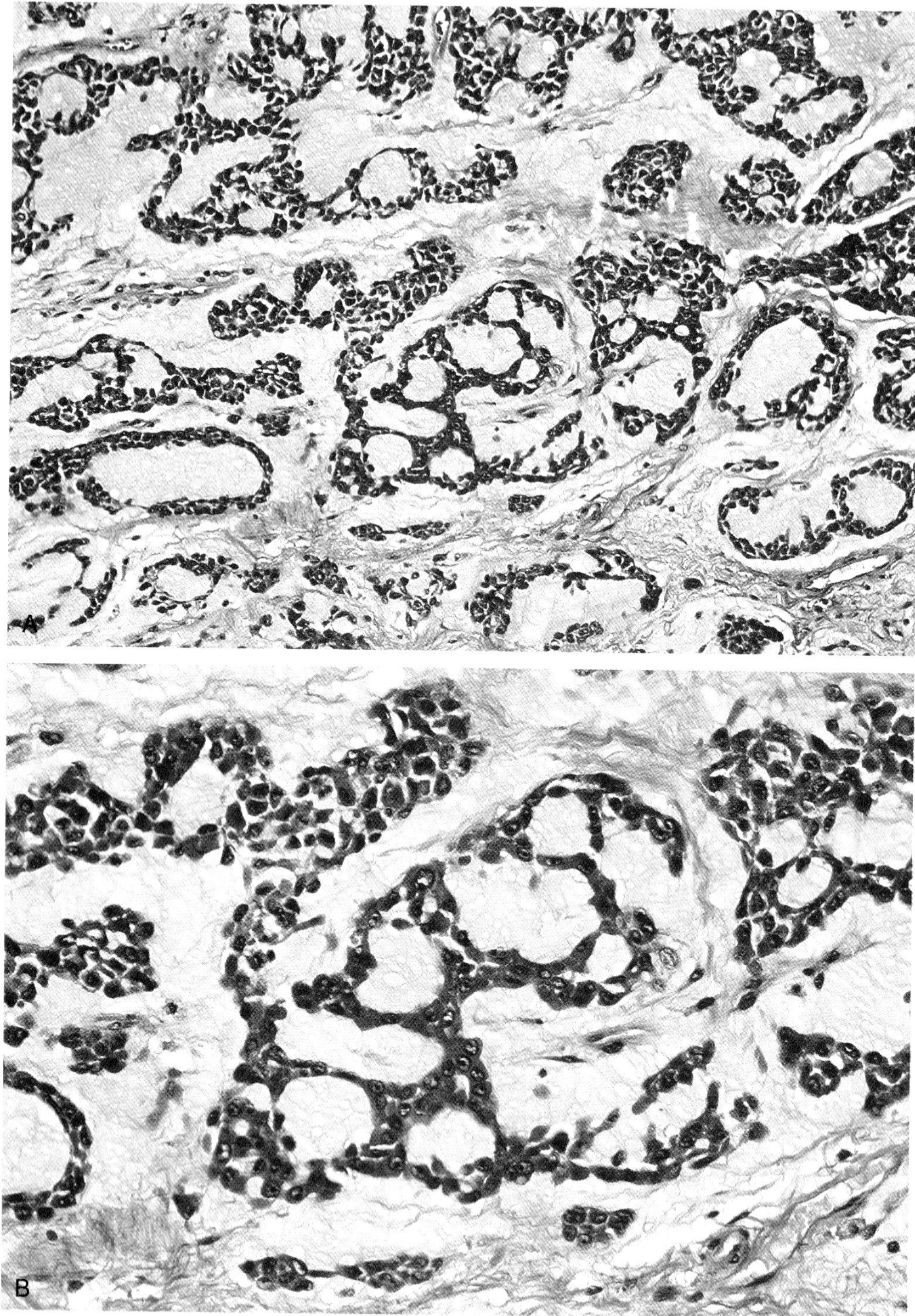


**FIGURE 34–20.** (**A**) Extraskeletal myxoid chondrosarcoma composed of cells arranged in a pseudoacinar pattern. (**B**) High-power view of densely eosinophilic epithelioid cells arranged in pseudoacini.

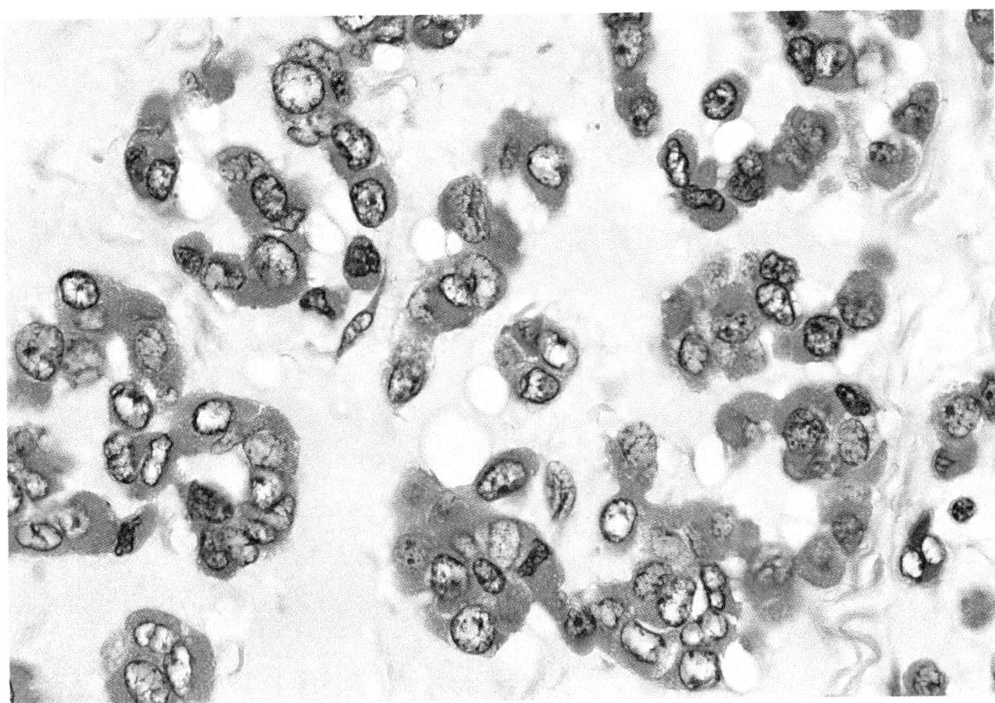

**FIGURE 34–21.** High-power view of chondroblasts in an extraskeletal myxoid chondrosarcoma. The cells are surrounded by a rim of deeply eosinophilic cytoplasm.

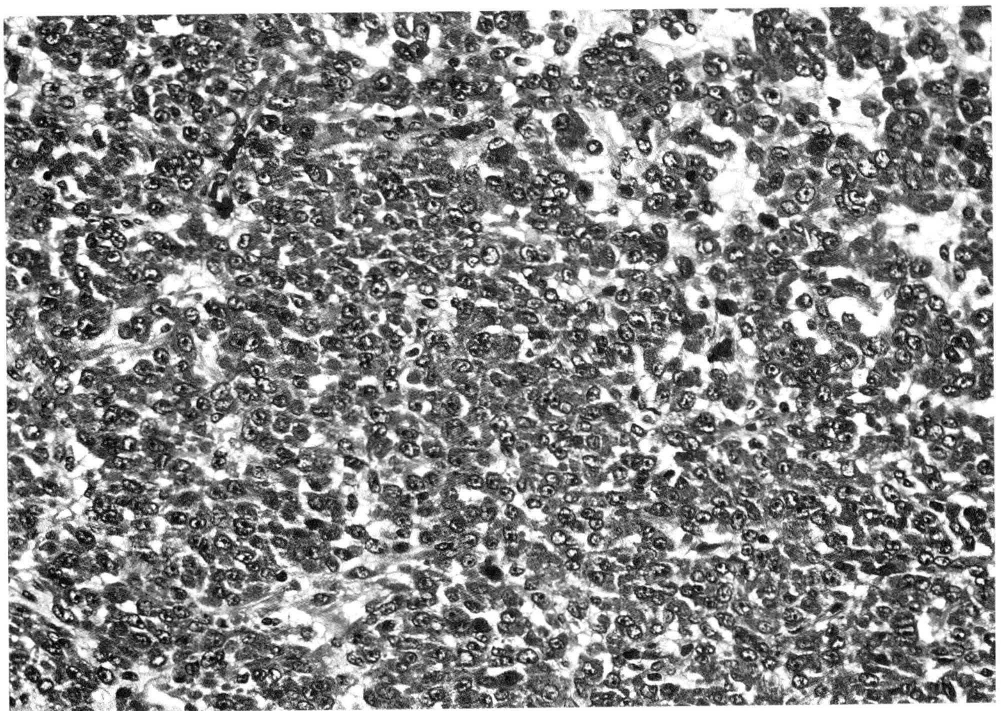

**FIGURE 34–22.** Cellular variant of an extraskeletal myxoid chondrosarcoma composed of large cells with vesicular nuclei and deeply eosinophilic cytoplasm. Other areas of typical myxoid chondrosarcoma were present in this tumor.

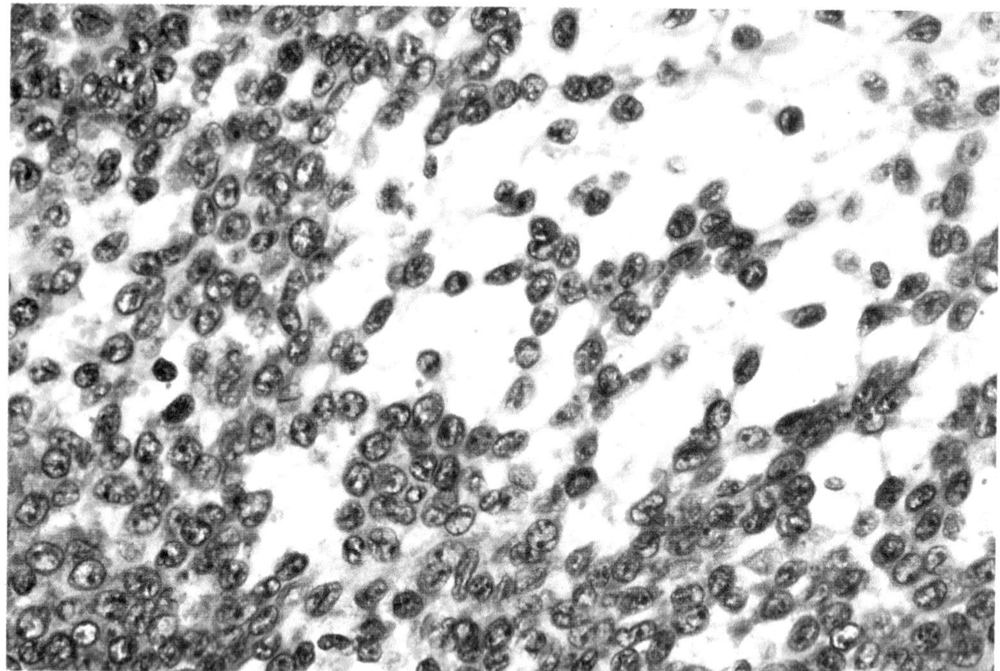

**FIGURE 34–23.** Cellular variant of extraskeletal myxoid chondrosarcoma composed of small round cells mimicking an extraskeletal Ewing's sarcoma/primitive neuroectodermal tumor.

typical feature of the tumor. Secondary changes such as fibrosis and hemorrhage are common, but calcification or bone formation is rare.

## Immunohistochemical Findings

The cells of myxoid chondrosarcoma stain strongly for vimentin, and S-100 protein immunoreactivity has been reported in many cases.[47,71] More recently, Dei Tos et al.[56] found that only 7 of 39 (17.8%) myxoid chondrosarcomas stained for this antigen. Given that most of the lesions in the differential diagnosis stain for S-100 protein, these authors argued that the absence of S-100 protein is diagnostically useful for recognizing myxoid chondrosarcoma. We have found that slightly fewer than one-half of extraskeletal myxoid chondrosarcomas stain for S-100 protein, often with rather focal and weak immunoreactivity. As with many other types of sarcoma, rare cases show focal immunoreactivity for cytokeratins.[46,92,95] Some authors have found evidence of neuroendocrine differentiation in rare examples of this tumor, as evidenced by staining for neuron-specific enolase, chromogranin, or synaptophysin[51,92] and identification of dense-core granules on ultrastructural examination.[72a,116]

## Ultrastructural Findings

The tumor is composed of fusiform spindle-shaped or ovoid cells with round, often indented or clefted nuclei, distinct nucleoli, and abundant cytoplasm with a well developed Golgi complex, glycogen granules, microfilaments, and a prominent rough endoplasmic reticulum containing granular amorphous material[58,89,92,98] (Fig. 34–24). Densely packed bundles or parallel arrays of microtubules may also be present, a feature that has been observed in myxoid chondrosarcomas of bone and other neoplasms as well.[55,87,112,120] The cellular surfaces are slightly scalloped, and there are finger-like cytoplasmic projections (Fig. 34–25), but these features are less well pronounced than in normally developing chondroblasts.[119] There are also intracytoplasmic inclusions of matrix material and macular or desmosomal intercellular attachments without tonofilaments. The extracellular spaces contain copious amounts of an amorphous, granular or finely fibrillary matrix and a varying number of collagen fibers.[91,92,99]

## Cytogenetic Findings

Extraskeletal myxoid chondrosarcoma is characterized by a balanced translocation: t(9;22)(q22;q12).[67,73,74,106,110,117] The breakpoint involves the *EWS* gene on chromosome 22q12[68] and the *CHN* (or *TEC*) gene on 9q22,[52] resulting in the formation of a chimeric gene that activates the transcription of target genes involved in cell proliferation.[84] The *EWS/CHN* fusion transcript has been detected in approximately 65% of cases.[49,50] Brody et al.[50] did not detect this

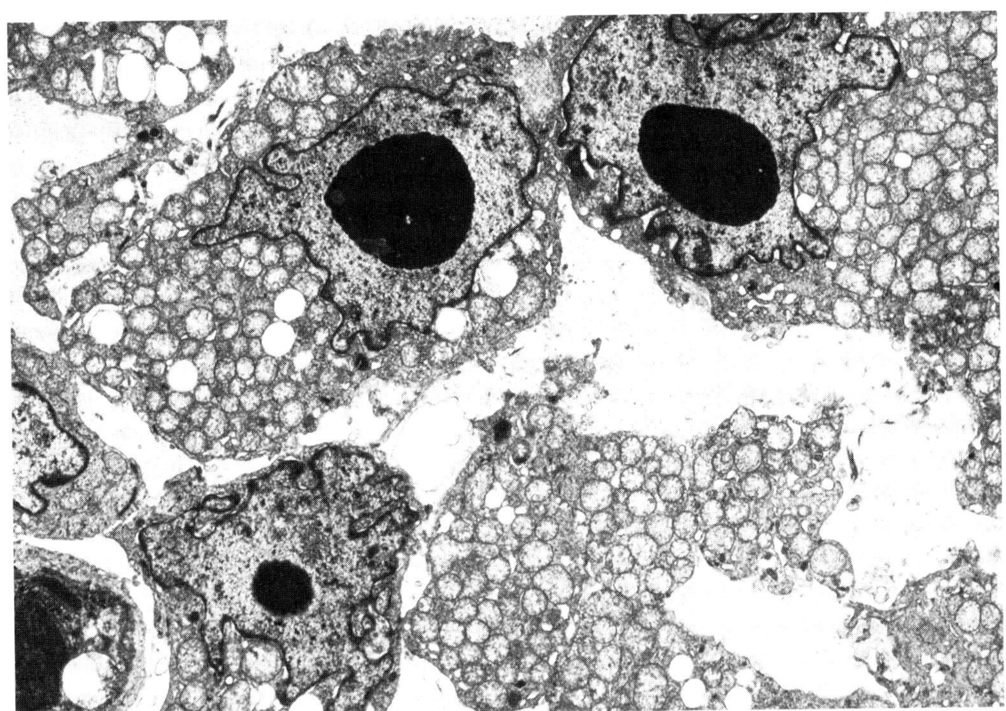

**FIGURE 34–24.** Electron micrograph of an extraskeletal myxoid chondrosarcoma with numerous mitochondria in chondroblasts.

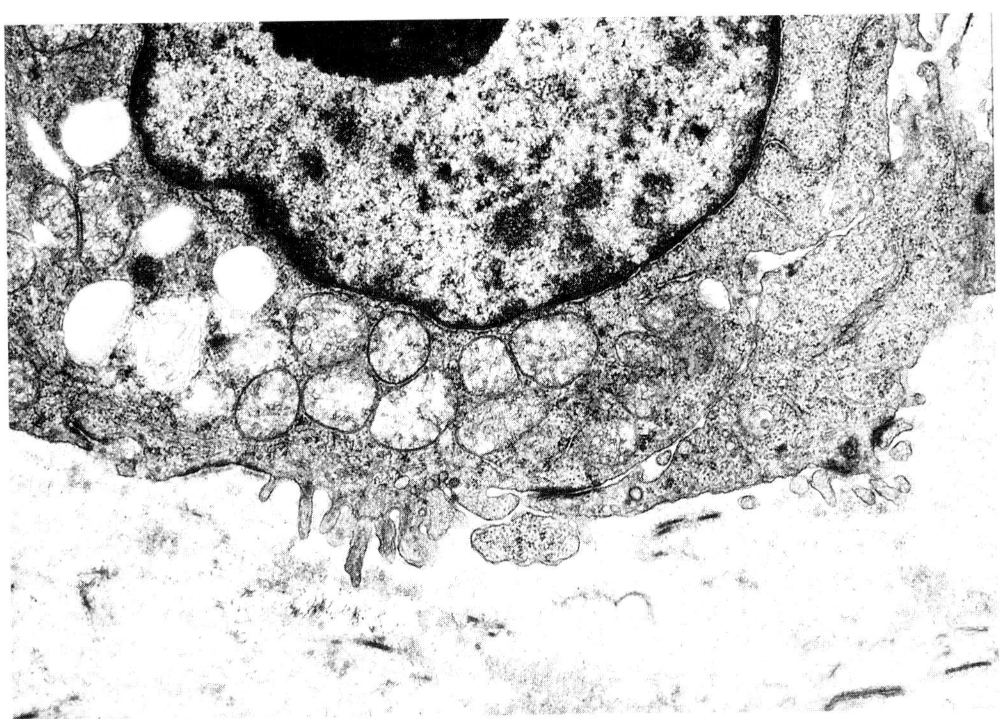

**FIGURE 34–25.** Electron micrograph of an extraskeletal myxoid chondrosarcoma with the finger-like cytoplasmic projections characteristic of this tumor.

**TABLE 34–1 LIGHT MICROSCOPIC FEATURES OF EXTRASKELETAL MYXOID CHONDROSARCOMA AND DIFFERENTIAL DIAGNOSTIC CONSIDERATIONS**

| Diagnosis | Cellularity | Vascularity | Pleomorphism | Matrix |
|---|---|---|---|---|
| Myxoma | 1+ | 1+ | 0 | HA |
| Myxoid liposarcoma | 1+ | 3+ (fine) | 1+ | HA |
| Myxoid MFH | 1+ to 2+ | 3+ (coarse) | 2+ to 3+ | HA |
| Myxoid chondrosarcoma | 1+ (cords) | 1+ | 1+ | CS |

MFH, malignant fibrous histiocytoma; HA, hyaluronic acid; CS, chondroitin sulfate.

fusion transcript in four skeletal myxoid chondrosarcomas, suggesting that this lesion is pathogenetically distinct from its extraskeletal counterpart. Less often, this tumor is characterized by a t(9;17) (q22;q11) exhibiting fusion between *RBP56* (also known as *TAF2N*) on 17q11 with the *CHN* gene.[49a,95a,108a]

## Differential Diagnosis

Among the various types of chondroid tumor, the "cartilage tumors in soft tissue" described by Lichtenstein and Goldman[85] bear some resemblance to myxoid chondrosarcoma. They differ, however, by their exclusive occurrence in the hand, their comparatively small size, and their benign behavior. They show a close similarity to the myxoid variant of soft part chondroma. *Chondromyxoid fibroma* rarely occurs as a periosteal tumor or in soft tissue as secondary tissue implantations.[83,100] It can be recognized by its greater degree of cellular pleomorphism and condensation of the tumor cells underneath a narrow, richly vascularized fibrous band that borders the individual tumor nodules. In addition, there may be multinucleated giant cells and foci of calcification or ossification, features rarely seen in myxoid chondrosarcomas.

*Juxtacortical (parosteal) chondrosarcomas* lack the myxoid component and show a broad attachment to the perichondrium or periosteum of the involved bone, sometimes with invasion of the underlying cortex and cortical irregularities on radiographs.[90,104] *Chordoma,* especially its myxoid form, enters the differential diagnosis, but this diagnosis is unlikely if the tumor occurs outside its usual location in the sacrococcygeal region, the base of the skull, or the cervical spine. Extraskeletal myxoid chondrosarcoma shows no radiographic evidence of bone involvement and lacks multivacuolated, physaliphorous tumor cells. Immunohistochemically, chordoma co-expresses S-100 protein and markers of epithelial differentiation (epithelial membrane antigen and cytokeratins, particularly cytokeratins 8 and 19).[94,95] Ultrastructurally, the cells show peculiar multilayered structures composed of rough endoplasmic reticulum and mitochondria in close juxtaposition.

Myxoma and myxoid liposarcoma must also be considered in the differential diagnosis (Table 34–1). *Myxoma* displays a similar paucity of vascular structures, but it is less cellular, as the cytologically bland cells are separated by abundant myxoid stroma. *Myxoid liposarcoma,* on the other hand, displays a striking plexiform vascular pattern and contains typical lipoblasts, especially at the margin of the tumor lobules. S-100 protein is found in approximately 40% of myxoid liposarcomas[57] and does not help distinguish this tumor from extraskeletal myxoid chondrosarcoma. Both myxoma and myxoid liposarcoma can be clearly distinguished from myxoid chondrosarcoma by the absence of stainable mucin after treating the sections with hyaluronidase (Table 34–2).

Still another problem is the distinction of extraskeletal myxoid chondrosarcoma from benign and malignant *mixed tumors of salivary gland origin (pleomorphic adenoma)* and *sweat gland origin (chondroid syringoma).* Although most of these tumors are more superficially located than chondrosarcoma, rare tumors arise in the deep subcutaneous or subfascial soft tissues.[79,93] These tumors display a curious modulation between epithelioid and spindled areas. Although the immunophenotype of deeply situated myoepithelial lesions is incompletely defined, we reserve this diagnosis for lesions that clearly express epithelial and myoepithelial markers, including cytokeratin, S-100 protein, glial fibrillary acidic protein, and calponin.[60,63,79]

**TABLE 34–2 CRITICAL ELECTROLYTE CONCENTRATION OF MYXOID SOFT TISSUE TUMORS**

| Tumor | Critical Electrolyte Conc. |
|---|---|
| Intramuscular myxoma | 0.1 |
| Myxoid liposarcoma | 0.1 |
| Myxoid malignant fibrous histiocytoma | 0.2 |
| Botryoid rhabdomyosarcoma | 0.2 |
| Myxoid chondrosarcoma | 0.5 |

From Kindblom LG, Angervall L. Histochemical characterization of mucosubstances in bone and soft tissue tumors. Cancer 36:985, 1975.

The rare *parachordoma* must also be distinguished from myxoid chondrosarcoma, given its usually benign clinical behavior.[53,77,103,108] Microscopically, it is typically lobulated and contains nests of vacuolated cells deposited in a myxoid matrix, resembling the physaliphorous cells of chordoma. The tumor cells contain intracytoplasmic glycogen, and the stromal mucoid material is rich in hyaluronic acid, which stains positively with alcian blue stain and is sensitive to predigestion with hyaluronidase. Although there are relatively few immunohistochemical studies of parachordoma (Table 34–3), this tumor typically coexpresses S-100 protein and epithelial markers (keratin and epithelial membrane antigen).[61,63] Ultrastructurally, parachordoma exhibits incomplete epithelial differentiation with primitive desmosome-like cell junctions, fragmented internal lamina, and microvillous cytoplasmic projections. Intermediate filaments are usually abundant and may be arranged in bundles.[61]

There are few data regarding cytogenetic abnormalities in parachordoma, although Tihy et al.[114] reported a case with structural rearrangements involving chromosomes 2 and 4 as well as loss of chromosomes 9, 10, 20, and 22. Folpe et al.[63] described a case with trisomy 15 and monosomies of chromosomes 1, 16, and 17.

*Myxopapillary ependymoma* can be distinguished by its perivascular growth, positivity for glial fibrillary acidic protein, and the presence of glial-type microfilaments.[109]

## Discussion

Although the clinical behavior of myxoid chondrosarcoma varies considerably from case to case, it is in general a relatively slow-growing tumor that recurs and eventually metastasizes in most cases. Of the 31 patients in the series by Enzinger and Shiraki,[59] 20 were alive at last follow-up, but six of these patients developed recurrence and two developed metastasis. Four died of metastatic disease and seven of unrelated causes. In the more recent study by Meis-Kindblom et al.[92] local recurrences and metastasis developed in 48% and 16% of patients, respectively. Estimated 5-, 10-, and 15-year survival rates were 90%, 70%, and 60%, respectively. Similarly, the 10-year survival rate in the study from the Mayo Clinic was 78%.[96]

Late recurrence and metastasis are common. In the series from the AFIP[59] one patient developed a recurrence 18 years after the initial excision; in another case pulmonary metastasis became evident 10 years after surgical removal of the tumor and 4 years after removal of a regional lymph node metastasis. Tanaka and Asao[113] observed recurrence 30 years after initial presentation. In the series of Saleh et al.,[102] 3 of the 10 patients with metastasis were alive at 13, 14, and 16 years after the initial therapy. The most frequent metastatic sites are the lung, soft tissues, and lymph nodes.

Radical local excision with or without adjunctive radiotherapy seems to be the treatment of choice. Good results with high-dose irradiation (6000 cGy) have been reported,[75] but chemotherapy has not been found to be efficacious.[97]

Several reports have suggested that tumor cellularity predicts prognosis,[54,59,62,96] whereas Meis-Kindblom et al.[92] found that cellularity was not prognostically significant. Other studies have also been unable to correlate histologic features with clinical outcome.[49,76,102] Several clinical parameters have been found to be of prognostic significance, including increasing patient age, large tumor size, and proximal tumor location.[92] There seems to be little doubt as to the chondroblastic origin of myxoid chondrosarcoma; the close histologic resemblance of the tumor cells to chondroblasts, the typical staining characteristics, and the presence of occasional foci of more mature and readily identifiable cartilage cells clearly support this concept.

**TABLE 34–3 IMMUNOHISTOCHEMICAL FEATURES OF EXTRASKELETAL MYXOID CHONDROSARCOMA AND DIFFERENTIAL DIAGNOSTIC CONSIDERATIONS**

| Tumor | CAM5.2 | CK7 | CK19 | EMA | S-100 | CEA | Actin |
|---|---|---|---|---|---|---|---|
| Myxoid chondrosarcoma | − | − | − | − | +/− | − | − |
| Parachordoma | + | − | − | + | + | − | − |
| Chordoma | + | +/− | + | + | + | + | − |
| Myxoid liposarcoma | − | − | − | − | +/− | − | − |
| Mixed tumor | + | N/A | N/A | +/− | + | − | +/− |

CAM5.2, cell adhesion molecule; EMA, epithelial membrane antigen; CEA, carcinoembryonic antigen; N/A, not available.

# EXTRASKELETAL MESENCHYMAL CHONDROSARCOMA

First described as a distinct entity by Lichtenstein and Bernstein in 1959,[140] extraskeletal mesenchymal chondrosarcoma is a cartilaginous tumor of characteristic bimorphic appearance composed of sheets of primitive mesenchymal cells and interspersed islands of well differentiated cartilaginous tissue.[126,127,151] Because of the latter, extraskeletal mesenchymal chondrosarcoma has traditionally been considered a variant of chondrosarcoma, although emerging cytogenetic data have raised the alternative idea that these lesions may be closely related to extraskeletal Ewing's sarcoma/primitive neuroectodermal tumor (ES/PNET) (see below). Until more evidence is available, we have continued to classify this tumor as a variant of chondrosarcoma. Because of its prominent vascular pattern, several cases reported in the earlier literature were initially interpreted as hemangiopericytoma with cartilaginous differentiation.[148] Mesenchymal chondrosarcoma is a rare tumor that is two to three times more common in bone than in soft tissue.[136,147] Unlike myxoid chondrosarcoma, it is a rapidly growing tumor with a high incidence of metastasis.

## Clinical Findings

This neoplasm differs from other forms of chondrosarcoma by its preponderance in young adults 15–35 years of age and its slightly more frequent occurrence in females than in males. The tumor may also occur in young children.[125,138] Louvet et al.[142] pointed out a relation between the age of the patient and the location of the tumor: Patients with neural and muscular forms of the disease are considerably younger (mean age 23.5 years) than those with mesenchymal chondrosarcomas arising from the musculature (mean age 43.9 years). The principal anatomic sites of extraskeletal mesenchymal chondrosarcoma are the region of the head and neck, particularly the orbit, the cranial and spinal dura mater, and the occipital portion of the neck, followed by the lower extremities, especially the thigh[135,136,147] (Table 34–4). Rare tumors have also been described in the pleura,[143] retroperitoneum,[133] cerebellum,[144] and labia majus.[141] In comparison, mesenchymal chondrosarcomas of bone arise chiefly in the jaws and ribs.[147,157,159]

Orbital lesions tend to produce exophthalmos, orbital pain, blurring of vision, and headaches[123,137,139,154]; intracranial and intraspinal tumors are accompanied by vomiting, headaches, and various motor and sensory defects.[124,149,152] Tumors in the extremities usually manifest as painless, slowly enlarging masses situated in the musculature. We have reviewed cases in which a metastasis from a primary mesenchymal chondrosarcoma of bone mimicked a soft tissue tumor. Therefore a bone survey is essential, particularly when the tumor occurs in an unusual location. In most cases radiography reveals a well defined soft tissue mass, often with irregular radiopaque stipplings, arcs, flecks, or streaks as the result of focal calcification or bone formation in cartilaginous areas[153] (Fig. 34–26). CT scans, MRI, and angiography are helpful for outlining the tumor prior to surgical therapy.

**TABLE 34–4 ANATOMIC DISTRIBUTION OF 51 EXTRASKELETAL MESENCHYMAL CHONDROSARCOMAS**

| Anatomic Location | No. of Patients | % |
|---|---|---|
| Upper extremities | 6 | 12 |
| Lower extremities | 18 | 35 |
| Orbit | 5 | 10 |
| Trunk | 8 | 16 |
| Dura/meninges | 11 | 21 |
| Head and neck | 3 | 6 |
| *Total* | 51 | 100 |

Data are from Guccion et al.,[135] Huvos et al.,[136] and Nakashima et al.[147]

## Pathologic Findings

Grossly, mesenchymal chondrosarcoma presents as a multilobulated circumscribed mass that shows considerable variation in size. In the series by Guccion et al.[135] the smallest tumor was 2.5 cm in greatest diameter and the largest 37 cm. Cut sections show a mixture of fleshy soft gray-white tissue and scattered foci of irregularly sized cartilage and bone. At times there are also small areas of hemorrhage and necrosis, but hemorrhage is much less prominent than in myxoid chondrosarcoma.

Microscopically, mesenchymal chondrosarcoma exhibits a characteristic bimorphic pattern composed of sheets of undifferentiated round, oval, or spindle-shaped cells and small, usually well defined islets or nodules of well differentiated, benign-appearing cartilaginous tissue, frequently with central calcification and ossification (Figs. 34–27, 34–28, 34–29). The undifferentiated cells have ovoid or elongated hyperchromatic nuclei and scanty, poorly outlined cytoplasm; they are arranged in small aggregates or in a hemangiopericytoma-like pattern about sinusoidal vascular channels lined by a single layer of endothelium (Figs. 34–30, 34–31). Solid cellular and richly vascular patterns may be present in different portions of the same neoplasm. The cartilaginous foci are usually well defined, but there are also poorly circum-

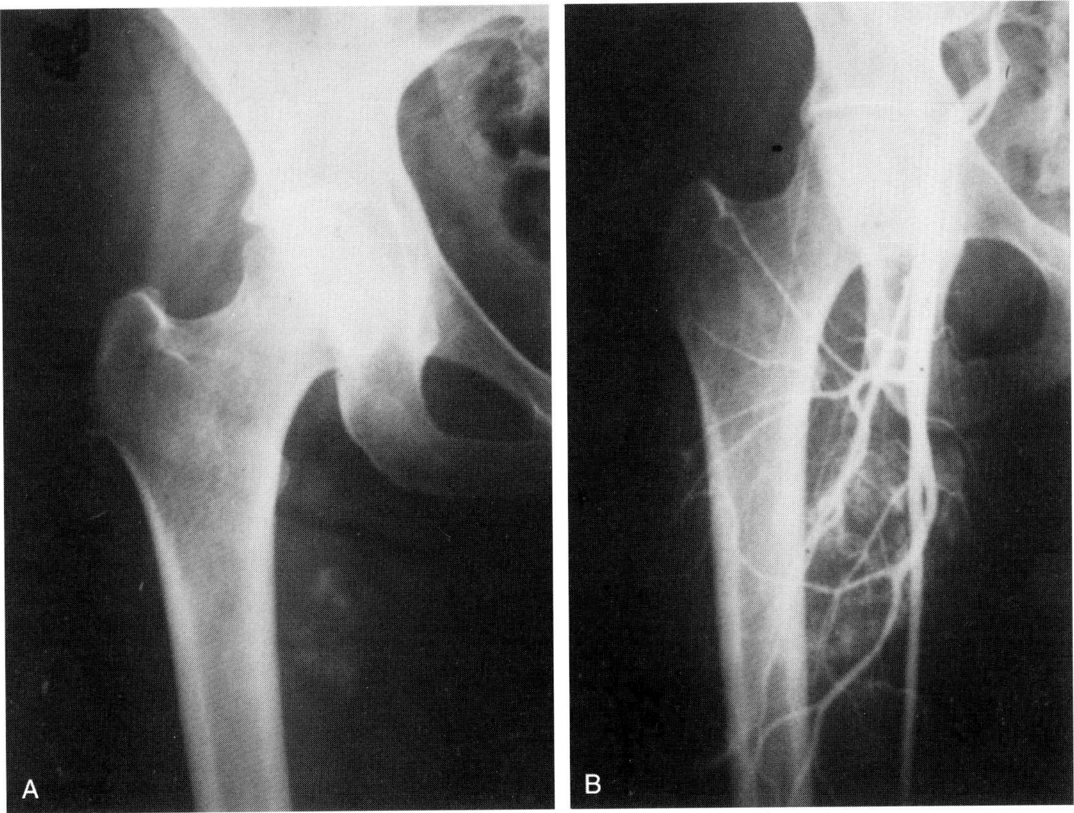


**FIGURE 34–26.** Extraskeletal mesenchymal chondrosarcoma of the right thigh. (**A**) Radiograph of a soft tissue mass with focal calcification. (**B**) Angiogram demonstrates the rich vascularity of the tumor.

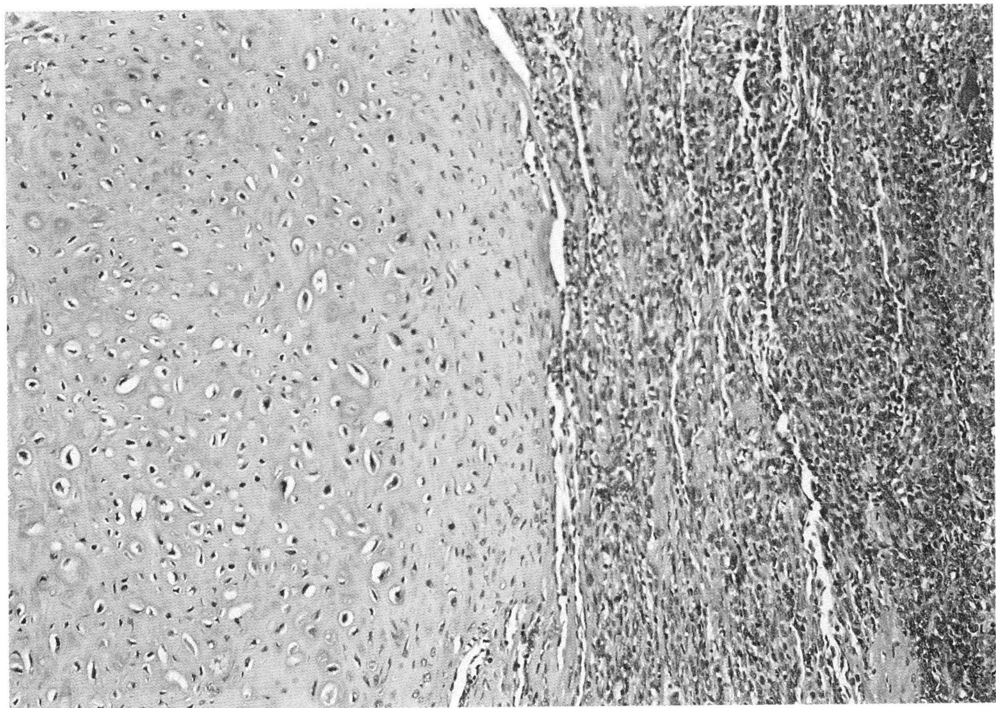

**FIGURE 34–27.** Low-power view of a mesenchymal chondrosarcoma with the characteristic bimorphic picture: islands of well-differentiated cartilage surrounded by sheets of small, undifferentiated tumor cells.

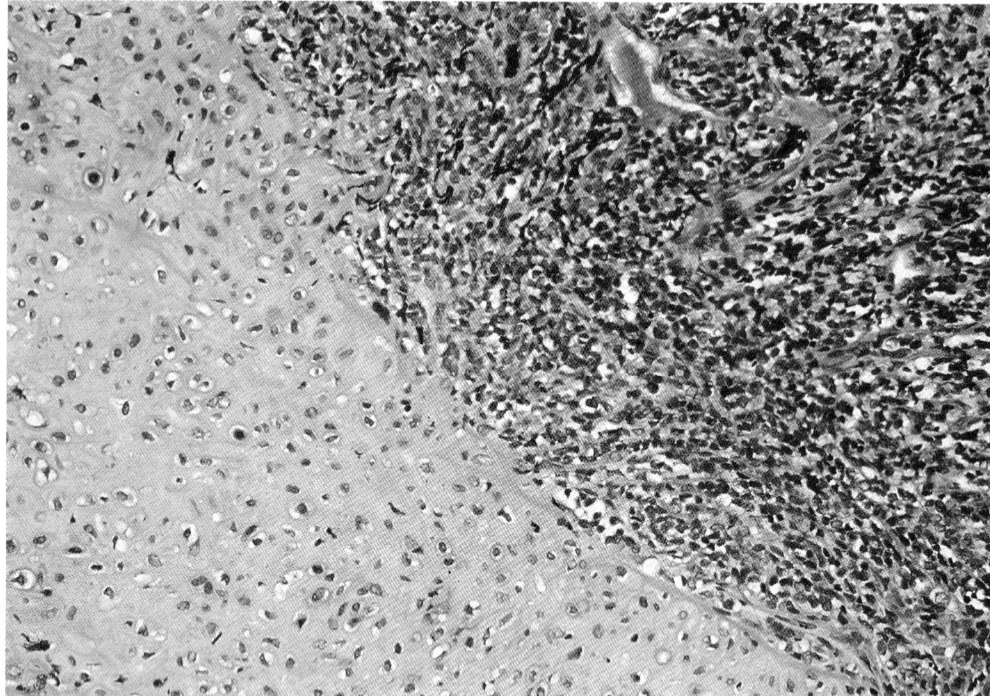

**FIGURE 34–28.** Sharp demarcation between small, undifferentiated tumor cells and well-differentiated cartilage in a mesenchymal chondrosarcoma.

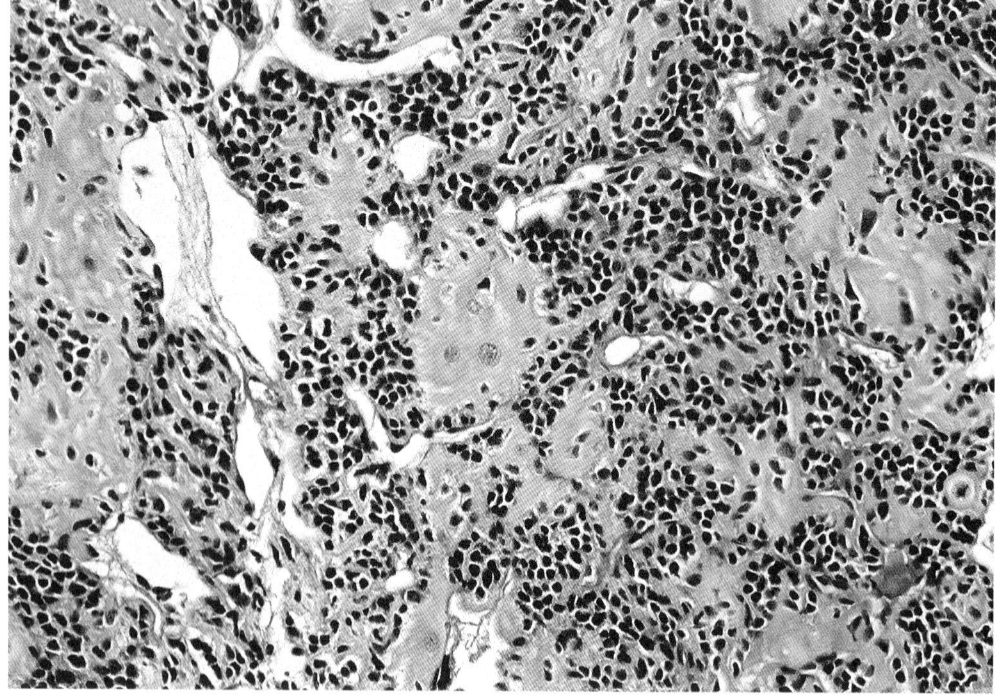

**FIGURE 34–29.** Extraskeletal mesenchymal chondrosarcoma with an intimate admixture of islands of cartilaginous tissue and small round cells.

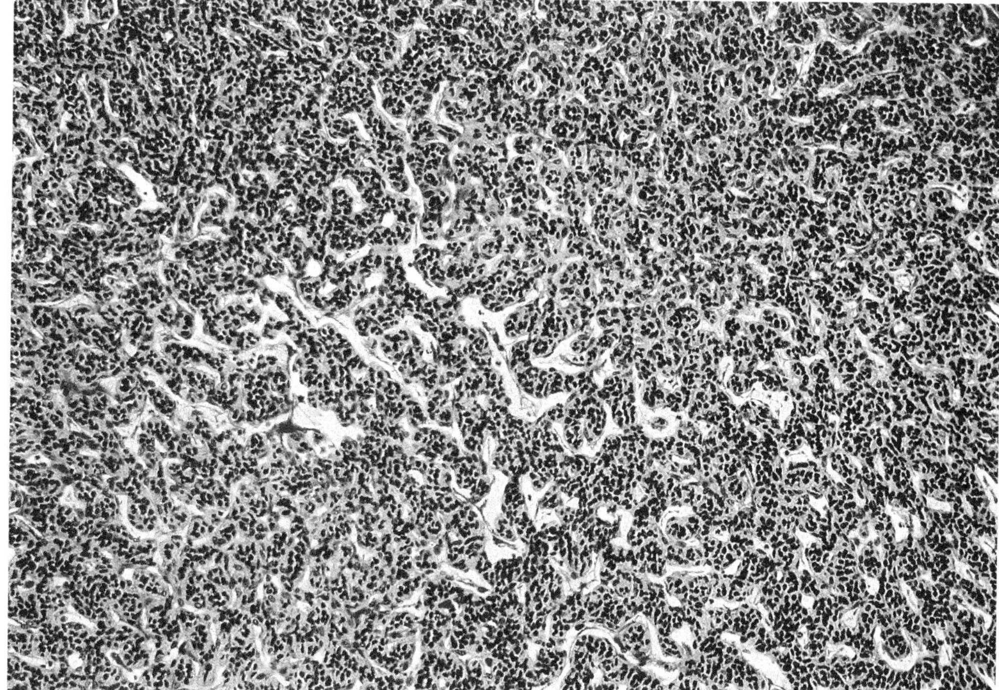

**FIGURE 34–30.** Small round cells surround a prominent hemangiopericytoma-like vasculature in an extraskeletal mesenchymal chondrosarcoma.

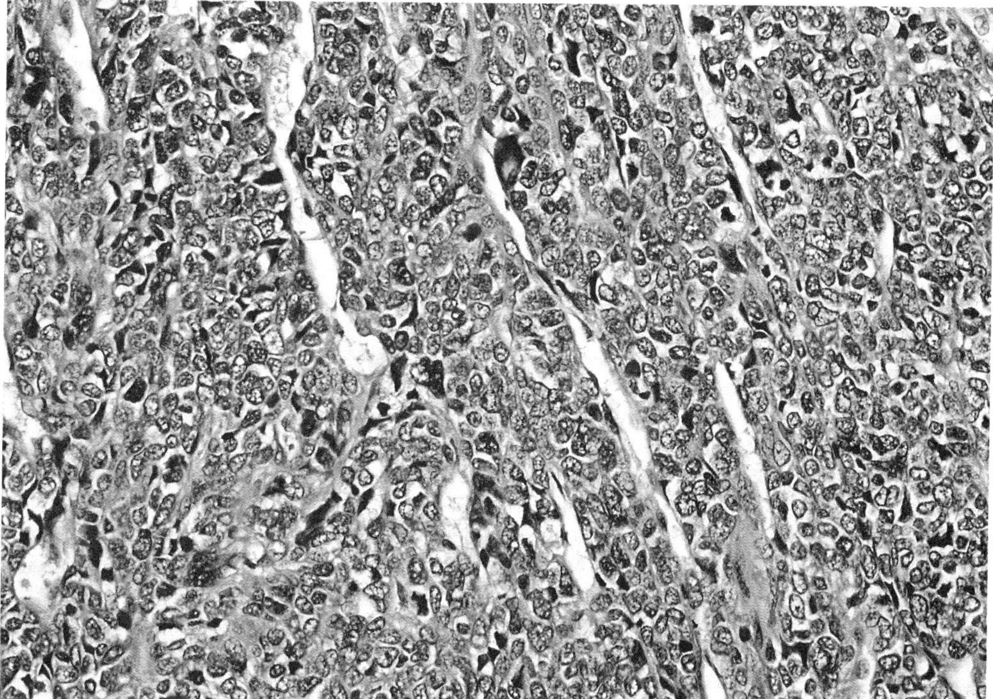

**FIGURE 34–31.** High-power view of small round cells surrounding hemangiopericytoma-like vessels in an extraskeletal mesenchymal chondrosarcoma.

scribed cartilaginous areas that blend with the undifferentiated tumor cells. Spindle cell areas, with or without collagen formation, are present in some cases but are rarely a prominent feature of the tumor. The staining characteristics of the cartilaginous areas are indistinguishable from those of other forms of chondrosarcoma.

Immunohistochemically, the cartilaginous portion of the tumor typically shows strong S-100 protein positivity, whereas only isolated cells in the undifferentiated areas stain for this antigen.[155,158] Moreover, as in other round cell tumors, the undifferentiated cells may stain for neuron-specific enolase and Leu-7. Stains for desmin, actin, cytokeratin, and epithelial membrane antigen are typically negative.

In the absence of the cartilaginous foci, the undifferentiated areas may closely resemble other round cell sarcomas, particularly ES/PNETs. Although early reports on the product of the *MIC2* gene (CD99) indicated that the undifferentiated areas of extraskeletal mesenchymal chondrosarcoma were negative for this antigen,[122,128,160] a subsequent report by Granter et al.[134] found that all 11 of their cases showed strong membranous immunoreactivity for CD99 in these undifferentiated areas. In addition, 8 of 11 cases showed weak staining in the well differentiated chondroid areas. The divergent results may be due to the use of different antibodies and different antigen retrieval techniques. Nevertheless, immunostaining for CD99 does not allow distinction of extraskeletal mesenchymal chondrosarcoma from ES/PNETs.

## Ultrastructural Findings

The cells in well differentiated cartilaginous areas have irregular round to stellate or scalloped configurations with short cytoplasmic processes, large ovoid nuclei, abundant rough endoplasmic reticulum with focal sac-like dilatations, a well developed Golgi apparatus, and variable amounts of glycogen.[129,146] The extracellular spaces contain filamentous, finely granular material. In contrast, the undifferentiated, round, ovoid, or polygonal cells have large nuclei, prominent nucleoli and inconspicuous cytoplasm with few organelles. The cellular elements are closely packed with cohesive cell membranes and desmosomes but without cytoplasmic projections. Fibroblast-like cells with increased rough endoplasmic reticulum and occasional desmosome-like junctions may also be present in the tumor. Basal laminae are confined to the interspersed endothelial cells and pericytes.[131]

## Cytogenetic Findings

There are relatively few cytogenetic studies of well characterized examples of mesenchymal chondrosarcoma. Most of these tumors have been shown to harbor complex cytogenetic alterations.[130,145,156] Sainati et al.[150] identified one case of osseous mesenchymal chondrosarcoma with t(11;22)(q24;q12), which is typical of the ES/PNET family of tumors, raising the possibility that this tumor may also be histogenetically related to the aforementioned group of tumors.

## Differential Diagnosis

Although typical mesenchymal chondrosarcomas pose no particular diagnostic problem, recognition of this tumor may be difficult with small biopsy or needle biopsy specimens that demonstrate only one of the two tissue elements. In particular, tumors without the cartilaginous element may be mistaken for ES/PNET, malignant hemangiopericytoma, or poorly differentiated synovial sarcoma with a prominent hemangiopericytoma-like pattern. Although we have observed well differentiated cartilage in one case of benign hemangiopericytoma, it is a rare finding; and as a rule the presence of cartilage excludes a diagnosis of hemangiopericytoma. Metaplastic cartilage may also occur in poorly differentiated synovial sarcoma, but it is much less common than foci of calcification or bone. Careful search for a biphasic pattern or epithelial differentiation with antibodies against cytokeratin or epithelial membrane antigen is indicated in difficult cases.

Distinction from differentiated forms of extraskeletal chondrosarcoma may also cause some diagnostic difficulty. These rare tumors, however, always display a more uniform pattern and lack the contrasting differentiated and undifferentiated areas.

## Discussion

Mesenchymal chondrosarcoma is a fully malignant tumor that pursues a rapid clinical course and metastasizes in a high percentage of cases.[135] Nakashima et al.[147] reported 5- and 10-year survival rates of 54.6% and 27.3%, respectively. Earlier studies by Huvos et al.[136] and Dahlin and Henderson[127] revealed similar 10-year survival rates.

The principal metastatic site is the lung. Lymph node metastasis is less common than with myxoid chondrosarcoma. Several of our patients had a protracted clinical course and late metastases, but there seems to be no reliable prognostic relation to the patient's age or degree of cellular differentiation. Combined radical surgery and chemotherapy or radiotherapy appears to be the treatment of choice.

Although presumed to be closely related to chondrosarcoma, the presence of t(11;22)(q24;q12) in one mesenchymal chondrosarcoma and the frequent expression of the *MIC2* gene product raises the possibility of a closer relation to the ES/PNET tumor family. Goji et al.[132] identified focal chondrocytic differentiation in a ES/PNET cell line with t(11;22), supporting this hypothesis.

## REFERENCES

### Extraskeletal Chondroma


1. Ando K, Goto Y, Hirabayashi N, et al. Cutaneous cartilaginous tumor. Dermatol Surg 21:339, 1995.
2. Apfelberg DB, Druker D, Maser MR, et al. Subungual osteochondroma: differential diagnosis and treatment. Arch Dermatol 115:472, 1979.
3. Ayala F, Lembo G, Montesano M. A rare tumor: subungual chondroma: report of a case. Dermatologica 167:339, 1983.
4. Bansal M, Goldman AB, DiCarlo EF, et al. Soft tissue chondromas: diagnosis and differential diagnosis. Skeletal Radiol 22: 309, 1993.
5. Bauer TW, Dorfman HD, Latham JT. Periosteal chondroma. Am J Surg Pathol 6:631, 1982.
6. Bertoni F, Unni KK, Beabout JW, et al. Chondrosarcomas of the synovium. Cancer 67:155, 1991.
7. Blum MR, Danford M, Speight PM. Soft tissue chondroma of the cheek. J Orol Pathol Med 22:334, 1993.
8. Bridge JA, Bhatia PS, Anderson JR, et al. Biologic and clinical significance of cytogenetic and molecular cytogenetic abnormalities in benign and malignant cartilaginous lesions. Cancer Genet Cytogenet 69:79, 1993.
9. Brownlee RD, Sevick RJ, Rewcastle NB, et al. Intracranial chondroma. Am J Neuroradiol 18:889, 1997.
10. Chung EB, Enzinger FM. Benign chondromas of soft parts. Cancer 41:1414, 1978.
11. Dahlin C, Salvador H. Cartilaginous tumors of the soft tissues of the hands and feet. Mayo Clin Proc 49:721, 1974.
12. Dal Cin P, Qi H, Sciot R, et al. Involvement of chromosomes 6 and 11 in a soft tissue chondroma. Cancer Genet Cytogenet 93:177, 1997.
13. Davis RI, Hamilton A, Biggart JD. Primary synovial chondromatosis: a clinicopathologic review and assessment of malignant potential. Hum Pathol 29:683, 1998.
14. De Beuckeleer LH, De Schepper AM, Ramon F, et al. Magnetic resonance imaging of cartilaginous tumors: a retrospective study of 79 patients. Eur J Radiol 21:34, 1995.
15. Dellon A, Weiss SW, Mitch WE. Bilateral extraosseous chondromas of the hand in a patient with chronic renal failure. Am Soc Surg Hand 3:139, 1978.
16. Del Rosario AD, Bui HX, Singh J, et al. Intracytoplasmic eosinophilic hyaline globules in cartilaginous neoplasms: a surgical, pathological, ultrastructural, and electron probe x-ray microanalytic study. Hum Pathol 25:1283, 1994.
17. Devaney KO, Ferlito A, Silver CE. Cartilaginous tumors of the larynx. Ann Otol Rhinol Laryngol 104:251, 1995.
18. Dunn EJ, McGavran M, Nelson P, et al. Synovial chondrosarcoma: report of a case. J Bone Joint Surg Am 56:811, 1974.
19. Gilbert SR, Lachiewicz PF. Primary synovial osteochondromatosis of the hip: report of two cases with long-term follow-up after synovectomy and a review of the literature. Am J Orthop 26:555, 1997.
20. Hermann G, Klein MJ, Abdelwahab IF, et al. Synovial chondrosarcoma arising in synovial chondromatosis of the right hip. Skeletal Radiol 26:366, 1997.
21. Humphreys TR, Herzberg AJ, Elenitsas R, et al. Familial occurrence of multiple cutaneous chondromas. Am J Dermatopathol 16:56, 1994.
22. Isayama T, Iwasaki H, Kikuchi M. Chondroblastoma-like extraskeletal chondroma. Clin Orthop 268:214, 1991.
23. Johnson DB, McGrath F, Ryan MJ. Laryngeal chondroma: an unusual cause of upper airway obstruction. Clin Radiol 50:412, 1995.
24. Kamysz JW, Zawin JK, Gonzalez-Crussi F. Soft tissue chondroma of the neck: a case report and review of the literature. Pediatr Radiol 26:145, 1996.
25. Karlin CA, De Smet AA, Neff J, et al. The variable manifestations of extraarticular synovial chondromatosis. AJR 137:731, 1981.
26. Kramer J, Recht M, Deely DM, et al. MR appearance of idiopathic synovial osteochondromatosis. J Comp Assist Tomogr 17:772, 1993.
27. Lewis JE, Olsen KD, Inwards CY. Cartilaginous tumors of the larynx: clinicopathologic review of 47 cases. Ann Otol Rhinol Laryngol 106:94, 1997.
28. Mandahl N, Heim S, Arheden K, et al. Chromosomal rearrangements in chondromatous tumors. Cancer 65:242, 1990.
29. Mandahl N, Willen H, Rydholm A, et al. Rearrangement of band q13 on both chromosomes 12 in a periosteal chondroma. Genes Chromosomes Cancer 6:121, 1993.
30. Nguyen TP, Burk DL Jr. Musculoskeletal case of the day: periosteal (juxtacortical) chondroma. AJR 165:203, 1995.
31. Nojima T, Unni KK, McLeod RA, et al. Periosteal chondroma and periosteal chondrosarcoma. Am J Surg Pathol 9:661, 1985.
32. Ontell F, Greenspan A. Chondrosarcoma complicating synovial chondromatosis: findings with magnetic resonance imaging. Can Assoc Radiol J 45:318, 1994.
33. Ozaki J, Tomita Y, Nakagawa Y, et al. Synovial chondromatosis of the acromioclavicular joint: a case report. Arch Orthop Trauma Surg 112:152, 1993.
34. Perry BE, McQueen DA, Lin JJ. Synovial chondromatosis with malignant degeneration to chondrosarcoma. J Bone Joint Surg Am 70:1259, 1987.
35. Pollock L, Malone M, Shaw DG. Childhood soft tissue chondroma: a case report. Pediatr Pathol Lab Med 15:437, 1995.
36. Reith JD, Bauer TW, Joyce MJ. Paraarticular osteochondroma of the knee: a report of 2 cases and review of the literature. Clin Orthop 334:225, 1997.
37. Rogachefsky RA, Zlatkin MB, Greene TL. Synovial chondromatosis of the distal radioulnar joint: a case report. J Hand Surg [Am] 22:1093, 1997.
38. Ruth RM, Groves RJ. Synovial osteochondromatosis of the elbow presenting with ulnar nerve neuropathy. Am J Orthop 25: 843, 1996.
39. Sviland L, Malcolm AJ. Synovial chondromatosis presenting as painless soft tissue mass: a report of 19 cases. Histopathology 27:275, 1995.
40. Takano M, Oka H, Kawano N, et al. Dural chondroma with fat tissue. Acta Neurochir (Wien) 139:690, 1997.
41. Tibrewal SB, Iossifidis A. Extra-articular synovial chondromatosis of the ankle. J Bone Joint Surg Br 77:659, 1995.
42. Tosios K, Laskaris G, Eveson J, et al. Benign cartilaginous tumor of the gingiva: a case report. Int J Oral Maxillofac Surg 22:231, 1993.
43. Wang BH, Guan XL, Xiao LF, et al. Soft tissue chondroma of the parapharyngeal space: a case report. J Laryngol Otol 112: 294, 1998.
44. Wuisman PI, Noorda RJ, Jutte PC. Chondrosarcomas secondary to synovial chondromatosis: report of two cases and review of the literature. Arch Orthop Trauma Surg 116:307, 1997.
45. Yamada T, Irisa T, Nakano S, et al. Extraskeletal chondroma with chondroblastic and granuloma-like elements. Clin Orthop 315:257, 1995.

46. Zlatkin MB, Lander PH, Begin LR, et al. Soft tissue chondromas. AJR 144:1263, 1985.

### Extraskeletal Myxoid Chondrosarcoma

47. Abramovici LA, Steiner GC, Bonar F. Myxoid chondrosarcoma of soft tissue and bone: a retrospective study of 11 cases. Hum Pathol 26:1215, 1995.
48. Angervall L, Enerback L, Knutson H. Chondrosarcoma of soft tissue origin. Cancer 32:507, 1973.
49. Antonescu CR, Argani P, Erlandson RA, et al. Skeletal and extraskeletal myxoid chondrosarcoma: a clinicopathologic, ultrastructural and molecular comparative study. Mod Pathol 12: 18A, 1998.
49a. Bjerkehagen B, Dietrich C, Reed W, et al. Extraskeletal myxoid chondrosarcoma: multimodal diagnosis and identification of a new cytogenetic subgroup characterized by t(9;17)(q22; q11). Virch Arch 435:524, 1999.
50. Brody RI, Ueda T, Hamelin A, et al. Molecular analysis of the fusion of EWS to an orphan nuclear receptor gene in extraskeletal myxoid chondrosarcoma. Am J Pathol 150:1049, 1997.
51. Chieng DC, Erlandson RA, Antonescu C, et al. Neuroendocrine differentiation in adult soft tissue sarcomas with features of extraskeletal myxoid chondosarcoma: report of seven cases. Mod Pathol 12:23A, 1998.
52. Clark J, Benjamin H, Gill S, et al. Fusion of the EWS gene to CHN, a member of the steroid/thyroid receptor gene superfamily, in a human myxoid chondrosarcoma. Oncogene 12:229, 1996.
53. Dabska M. Parachordoma: a new clinicopathologic entity. Cancer 40:1586, 1977.
54. Dardick I, Lagace R, Carlier MT, et al. Chordoid sarcoma (extraskeletal myxoid chondrosarcoma): a light and electron microscopic study. Virchows Arch [Pathol Anat] 399:61, 1983.
55. DeBlois G, Wang S, Kay S. Microtubular aggregates within rough endoplasmic reticulum: an unusual ultrastructural feature of extraskeletal myxoid chondrosarcoma. Hum Pathol 17: 469, 1986.
56. Dei Tos AP, Wadden C, Fletcher CDM. Extraskeletal myxoid chondrosarcoma: an immunohistochemical reappraisal of 39 cases. Appl Immunohistochem 5:73, 1997.
57. Dei Tos AP, Wadden C, Fletcher CDM. S-100 protein staining and liposarcoma: its diagnostic utility in the high grade myxoid (round cell) variant. Appl Immunohistochem 4:95, 1996.
58. Elizalde JM, Ereno C, Florencio MR, et al. Extraskeletal myxoid chondrosarcoma: a clinicopathologic and immunohistochemical study of two cases. Tumori 79:283, 1993.
59. Enzinger FM, Shiraki M. Extraskeletal myxoid chondrosarcoma: an analysis of 34 cases. Hum Pathol 3:421, 1972.
60. Ferreiro JA, Nascimento AG. Hyaline-cell rich chondroid syringoma: a tumor mimicking malignancy. Am J Surg Pathol 19:912, 1995.
61. Fisher C, Miettinen M. Parachordoma: a clinicopathologic and immunohistochemical study of four cases of an unusual soft tissue neoplasm. Ann Diagn Pathol 1:3, 1997.
62. Fletcher CD, Powell G, McKee PH. Extraskeletal myxoid chondrosarcoma: a histochemical and immunohistochemical study. Histopathology 10:499, 1986.
63. Folpe AL, Agoff SN, Willis J, et al. Parachordoma is immunohistochemically and cytogenetically distinct from axial chordoma and extraskeletal myxoid chondrosarcoma. Am J Surg Pathol 23:1059, 1999.
64. Fukuda T, Ishikawa H, Ohnishi V, et al. Extraskeletal myxoid chondrosarcoma arising from the retroperitoneum. Am J Clin Pathol 85:514, 1986.
65. Gebhardt MC, Parekh SG, Rosenberg AE, et al. Extraskeletal myxoid chondrosarcoma of the knee. Skeletal Radiol 28:354, 1999.
66. Ghalib SH, Warner ED, DeGowin EL. Laryngeal chondrosarcoma after thyroid irradiation. JAMA 210:1762, 1969.
67. Gibas Z, Miettinen M, Limon J, et al. Cytogenetic and immunohistochemical profile of myxoid chondrosarcoma. Am J Clin Pathol 103:20, 1995.
68. Gill S, McManus AP, Crew AJ, et al. Fusion of the EWS gene to a DNA segment from 9q22-31 in a human myxoid chondrosarcoma. Genes Chromosomes Cancer 12:307, 1995.
69. Goetz SP, Robinson RA, Landas SK. Extraskeletal myxoid chondrosarcoma of the pleura: report of a case clinically simulating mesothelioma. Am J Clin Pathol 97:498, 1992.
70. Greenspan A, Unni KK, Blake L, et al. Extraskeletal myxoid chondrosarcoma: an unusual tumour in a 6-year old boy. Can Assoc Radiol J 45:62, 1994.
71. Hachitanda Y, Tsuneyoshi M, Daimaru Y, et al. Extraskeletal myxoid chondrosarcoma in young children. Cancer 61:2521, 1988.
72. Hajdu SI, Shiu MH, Fortner JG. Tendosynovial sarcoma: a clinicopathologic study of 136 cases. Cancer 39:1201, 1977.
72a. Harris M, Coyne J, Tariq M, et al. Extraskeletal myxoid chondrosarcoma with neuroendocrine differentiation: A pathologic, cytogenetic, and molecular study of a case with a novel translocation t(9;17)(q22;q11.2). Am J Surg Pathol 24:1020, 2000.
73. Hinrichs SH, Jaramillo MA, Gumerlock PH, et al. Myxoid chondrosarcoma with a translocation involving chromosomes 9 and 22. Cancer Genet Cytogenet 14:219, 1985.
74. Hirabayashi Y, Ishida T, Yoshida MA, et al. Translocation (9; 22)(q22;q12): a recurrent chromosome abnormality in extraskeletal myxoid chondrosarcoma. Cancer Genet Cytogenet 81: 33, 1995.
75. Hitchon H, Nobler MP, Wohl M, et al. The radiotherapeutic management of chordoid sarcoma. Am J Clin Oncol 13:208, 1990.
76. Janbhekar NA, Baraniya J, Baruah R, et al. Extraskeletal myxoid chondrosarcoma: clinicopathologic, histochemical, and immunohistochemical study of 10 cases. Int J Surg Pathol 5:77, 1997.
77. Karabela-Bouropolou V, Skourtas C, Liapi-Avgei G, et al. Parachordoma: a case report of a very rare soft tissue tumor. Pathol Res Pract 192:972, 1996.
78. Karabinis VD, Arnold TE, Hameed M, et al. Myxoid chondrosarcoma of the abdominal aorta. Int Surg 78:59, 1993.
79. Kilpatrick SE, Hitchcock MG, Kraus MD, et al. Mixed tumors and myoepitheliomas of soft tissue: a clinicopathologic study of 19 cases with a unifying concept. Am J Surg Pathol 21:13, 1997.
80. Kindblom LG, Angervall L. Histochemical characterization of mucosubstances in bone and soft tissue tumors. Cancer 36:985, 1975.
81. Kindblom LG, Angervall L. Myxoid chondrosarcoma of the synovial tissue: a clinicopathologic, histochemical, and ultrastructural analysis. Cancer 52:1886, 1983.
82. Kransdorf MJ, Meis JM. Extraskeletal osseous and cartilaginous tumors of the extremities. Radiographics 13:853, 1993.
83. Kyriakos M. Soft tissue implantation of chondromyxoid fibroma. Am J Surg Pathol 3:363, 1979.
84. Labelle Y, Bussieres J, Courjal F, et al. The EWS/TEC fusion protein encoded by the t(9;22) chromosomal translocation in human chondrosarcomas is a highly potent transcriptional activator. Oncogene 18:3303, 1999.
85. Lichtenstein L, Goldman RL. Cartilage tumors in soft tissues, particularly in the hand and foot. Cancer 17:1203, 1964.
86. Lin WY, Wang SJ, Yeh SH. Radionuclide imaging in extraskeletal myxoid chondrosarcoma. Clin Nucl Med 20:524, 1995.
87. Mackay B, Ayala AG. Intracisternal tubules in human melanoma cells. Ultrastruct Pathol 1:1, 1980.

88. Martin RF, Melnick PJ, Warner NE, et al. Chordoid sarcoma. Am J Clin Pathol 59:623, 1973.
89. Martinez-Tello FJ, Navas-Palacios JJ. Ultrastructural study of conventional chondrosarcomas and myxoid and mesenchymal chondrosarcomas. Virchows Arch [Pathol Anat] 396:197, 1982.
90. Matsumoto K, Hukuda S, Ishizawa M, et al. Parosteal (juxtacortical) chondrosarcoma of the humerus associated with regional lymph node metastasis: a case report. Clin Orthop 290: 168, 1993.
91. Mehio AR, Ferenczy A. Extraskeletal myxoid chondrosarcoma with "chordoid" features (chordoid sarcoma). Am J Clin Pathol 70:700, 1978.
92. Meis-Kindblom JM, Bergh P, Gunterberg B, et al. Extraskeletal myxoid chondrosarcoma: a reappraisal of its morphologic spectrum and prognostic factors based on 117 cases. Am J Surg Pathol 23:636, 1999.
93. Michal M, Miettinen M. Myoepitheliomas of the skin and soft tissues: report of 12 cases. Virchows Arch 434:393, 1999.
94. Naka T, Iwamoto Y, Shinohara N, et al. Cytokeratin subtyping in chordomas and the fetal notochord: an immunohistochemical analysis of aberrant expression. Mod Pathol 10:545, 1997.
95. O'Hara BJ, Paetau A, Miettinen M. Keratin subsets and monoclonal antibody HBME-1 in chordoma: immunohistochemical differential diagnosis between tumors simulating chordoma. Hum Pathol 29:119, 1998.
95a. Panagopoulos I, Mencinger M, Dietrich CV, et al. Fusion of the RBP56 and CHN genes in extraskeletal myxoid chondrosarcomas with translocation t(9;17)(q22;q11). Oncogene 18: 7594, 1999.
96. Oliveira AM, Sebo TJ, McGrory JE, et al. Extraskeletal myxoid chondrosarcoma: A clinicopathologic, immunohistochemical, and ploidy analysis of 23 cases. Mod Pathol 13:900, 2000.
97. Patel SR, Burgess MA, Papadopoulos NE, et al. Extraskeletal myxoid chondrosarcoma: long-term experience with chemotherapy. Am J Clin Oncol 18:161, 1995.
98. Payne C, Dardick I, Mackay B. Extraskeletal myxoid chondrosarcoma with intracisternal microtubules. Ultrastruct Pathol 18:257, 1994.
99. Povysil C, Matejovsky Z. A comparative ultrastructural study of chondrosarcoma, chordoid sarcoma, chordoma, and chordoma periphericum. Pathol Res Pract 179:546, 1985.
100. Rahimi A, Beabout JW, Ivins JC, et al. Chondromyxoid fibroma: a clinicopathologic study of 76 cases. Cancer 30:726, 1972.
101. Ramesh K, Gahukamble L, Sarma NH, et al. Extraskeletal myxoid chondrosarcoma with dedifferentiation. Histopathology 27:381, 1995.
102. Saleh G, Evans HL, Ro JY, et al. Extraskeletal myxoid chondrosarcoma: a clinicopathologic study of ten patients with long-term follow-up. Cancer 70:2827, 1992.
103. Sangueza OP, White CR. Parachordoma. Am J Dermatopathol 16:185, 1994.
104. Schajowicz F. Juxtacortical chondrosarcoma. J Bone Joint Surg Br 59:473, 1977.
105. Schajowicz F, Defilippi-Novoa CA, Firpo CA. Thorotrast-induced chondrosarcoma of the axilla. AJR 100:931, 1967.
106. Sciot R, Dal Cin P, Fletcher C, et al. t(9;22)(q22-31;q11-12) is a consistent marker of extraskeletal myxoid chondrosarcoma: evaluation of three cases. Mod Pathol 8:765, 1995.
107. Scott JE, Dorling J. Differential staining of acid glucosaminoglycans (mucopolysaccharides) by alcian blue in salt solutions. Histochemie 5:221, 1965.
108. Shin HJC, Mackay B, Ichinose H, et al. Parachordoma. Ultrastruct Pathol 18:249, 1994.
108a. Sjogren H, Meis-Kindblom J, Kindblom L-G, et al. Fusion of the EWS–related TAF2N to TEC in extraskeletal myxoid chondrosarcoma. Cancer Res 59:5064, 1999.
109. Specht C, Smith TW, De Girolami U, et al. Myxopapillary ependymoma of the filum terminale. Cancer 58:310, 1986.
110. Stenman G, Andersson H, Mandahl M, et al. Translocation t(9; 22)(q22;q12) is a primary cytogenetic abnormality in extraskeletal myxoid chondrosarcoma. Int J Cancer 62:398, 1995.
111. Suster S, Moran CA. Malignant cartilaginous tumors of the mediastinum: clinicopathological study of six cases presenting as extraskeletal soft tissue masses. Hum Pathol 28:588, 1997.
112. Suzuki T, Kaneko H, Kojima K, et al. Extraskeletal myxoid chondrosarcoma characterized by microtubular aggregates in the rough endoplasmic reticulum and tubuline immunoreactivity. J Pathol 156:51, 1988.
113. Tanaka N, Asao T. Chordoid sarcoma of the soft tissue of the nape of the neck: a case with a 20-year follow-up. Virchows Arch [Pathol Anat] 379:261, 1978.
114. Tihy F, Scott P, Russo P, et al. Cytogenetic analysis of a parachordoma. Cancer Genet Cytogenet 105:14, 1998.
115. Tsuneyoshi M, Enjoji M, Iwasaki H, et al. Extraskeletal myxoid chondrosarcoma: a clinicopathologic and electron microscopic study. Acta Pathol Jpn 31:439, 1981.
116. Tucker JA, King JAC, Vollmer RT, et al. Evidence for neuroendocrine differentiation in extraskeletal myxoid chondrosarcoma. Clin Exp Pathol 46:68A, 1998.
117. Turc-Carel C, Dal Cin P, Rao U, et al. Recurrent breakpoints at 9q31 and 22q12.2 in extraskeletal myxoid chondrosarcoma. Cancer Genet Cytogenet 30:145, 1988.
118. Ueda Y, Okada Y, Nakanishi I. Cellular variant of extraskeletal myxoid chondrosarcoma of abdominal wall: a case report with comparative immunohistochemical study on cartilaginous collagenous proteins in various myxoid mesenchymal tumors. J Cancer Res Oncol 118:147, 1992.
119. Weiss SW. Ultrastructure of the so-called "chordoid sarcoma": evidence supporting cartilaginous differentiation. Cancer 37: 300, 1976.
120. Wetzel WJ, Reuhl KR. Microtubular aggregates in the rough endoplasmic reticulum of a myxoid chondrosarcoma. Ultrastruct Pathol 1:519, 1980
121. Whitten CG, el-Khoury GY, Benda JA, et al. Case report 829: intramuscular myxoid chondrosarcoma. Skeletal Radiol 23:153, 1994.

### Extraskeletal Mesenchymal Chondrosarcoma

122. Ambros IM, Ambros PF, Strehl S, et al. MIC2 is a specific marker for Ewing's sarcoma and peripheral primitive neuroectodermal tumors. Cancer 67:1886, 1991.
123. Bagchi M, Husain N, Goel MM, et al. Extraskeletal mesenchymal chondrosarcoma of the orbit. Cancer 72:2224, 1993.
124. Cho BK, Chi JG, Wang KC, et al. Intracranial mesenchymal chondrosarcoma: a case report and literature review. Childs Nerv Syst 9:295, 1993.
125. Crawford JG, Oda D, Egbert M, et al. Mesenchymal chondrosarcoma of the maxilla in a child. J Oral Maxillofac Surg 53: 938, 1995.
126. Dabska M, Huvos AG. Mesenchymal chondrosarcoma in the young. Virchows Arch [Pathol Anat] 399:89, 1983.
127. Dahlin DC, Henderson ED. Mesenchymal chondrosarcoma: further observations on a new entity. Cancer 15:410, 1962.
128. Devaney K, Abbondanzo SL, Shekitka KM, et al. MIC2 detection in tumors of bone and adjacent soft tissue. Clin Orthop 310:176, 1995.
129. Dickersin GR, Rosenberg AE. The ultrastructure of small-cell osteosarcoma, with a review of the light microscopy and differential diagnosis. Hum Pathol 22:267, 1991.
130. Dobin SM, Donner LR, Speights VO Jr. Mesenchymal chondrosarcoma: a cytogenetic, immunohistochemical and ultrastructural study. Cancer Genet Cytogenet 83:56, 1995.
131. Fu YS, Kay S. A comparative ultrastructural study of mesen-

chymal chondrosarcoma and myxoid chondrosarcoma. Cancer 33:1531, 1974.

132. Goji J, Sano K, Nakamura H, et al. Chondrocytic differentiation of peripheral neuroectodermal tumor cell line in nude mouse xenograph. Cancer Res 52:421, 1992.
133. Gonzalez-Campora R, Otal Salaverri C, Gomez-Pascual A, et al. Mesenchymal chondrosarcoma of the retroperitoneum: report of a case diagnosed by fine needle aspiration biopsy with immunohistochemical and electron microscopic demonstration of S-100 protein in undifferentiated cells. Acta Cytol 39:1237, 1995.
134. Granter SR, Renshaw AA, Fletcher CD, et al. CD99 reactivity in mesenchymal chondrosarcoma. Hum Pathol 27:1273, 1996.
135. Guccion JG, Font RL, Enzinger FM, et al. Extraskeletal mesenchymal chondrosarcoma. Arch Pathol 95:336, 1973.
136. Huvos AG, Rosen G, Dabska M, et al. Mesenchymal chondrosarcoma: a clinicopathologic analysis of 35 patients with emphasis on treatment. Cancer 51:1230, 1983.
137. Jacobs JL, Merriam JC, Chadburn A, et al. Mesenchymal chondrosarcoma of the orbit: report of three new cases and review of the literature. Cancer 73:399, 1994.
138. Kruse R, Simon RG, Stanton R, et al. Mesenchymal chondrosarcoma of the cervical spine in a child. Am J Orthop 26:279, 1997.
139. Lauer SA, Friedland S, Goodrich JT, et al. Mesenchymal chondrosarcoma with secondary orbital invasion. Ophthal Plast Reconstr Surg 11:182, 1995.
140. Lichtenstein L, Bernstein D. Unusual benign and malignant chondroid tumors of bone: a survey of some mesenchymal cartilage tumors and malignant chondroblastic tumors including a few multicentric ones and chondromyxoid fibromas. Cancer 12:1142, 1959.
141. Lin J, Yip KM, Maffulli N, et al. Extraskeletal mesenchymal chondrosarcoma of the labium majus. Gynecol Oncol 60:492, 1996.
142. Louvet C, de Gramont A, Krulik M, et al. Extraskeletal mesenchymal chondrosarcoma: case report and review of the literature. J Clin Oncol 3:858, 1985.
143. Luppi G, Cesinaro AM, Zaboli A, et al. Mesenchymal chondrosarcoma of the pleura. Eur Respir J 9:840, 1996.
144. Malik SN, Farmer PM, Hajdu SI, et al. Mesenchymal chondrosarcoma of the cerebellum. Ann Clin Lab Sci 26:496, 1996.
145. Mandahl N, Heim S, Arheden K, et al. Chromosomal rearrangements in chondromatous tumors. Cancer 65:242, 1990.
146. Mawad JK, Mackay B, Raymond AK, et al. Electron microscopy in the diagnosis of small round cell tumors of bone. Ultrastruct Pathol 18:263, 1994.
147. Nakashima Y, Unni KK, Shives TC, et al. Mesenchymal chondrosarcoma of bone and soft tissue: a review of 111 cases. Cancer 57:2444, 1986.
148. Reeh MJ. Hemangiopericytoma with cartilaginous differentiation involving orbit. Arch Ophthalmol 75:82, 1966.
149. Rushing EJ, Armonda RA, Ansari Q, et al. Mesenchymal chondrosarcoma: a clinicopathologic and flow cytometric study of 13 cases presenting in the central nervous system. Cancer 77: 1884, 1996.
150. Sainati L, Scapinello A, Montaldi A, et al. A mesenchymal chondrosarcoma of a child with the reciprocal translocation (11;22)(q24;q12). Cancer Genet Cytogenet 71:144, 1993.
151. Salvador AH, Beabout JW, Dahlin DC. Mesenchymal chondrosarcoma: observations on 30 new cases. Cancer 28:605, 1971.
152. Scheithauer BW, Rubinstein LJ. Meningeal mesenchymal chondrosarcoma: report of 8 cases with review of the literature. Cancer 42:2744, 1978.
153. Shapeero LG, Vanel D, Couanet D, et al. Extraskeletal mesenchymal chondrosarcoma. Radiology 186:819, 1993.
154. Shinaver CN, Mafee MF, Choi KH. MRI of mesenchymal chondrosarcoma of the orbit: case report and review of the literature. Neuroradiology 39:296, 1997.
155. Swanson PE, Lillemoe TJ, Manivel JC, et al. Mesenchymal chondrosarcoma: an immunohistochemical study. Arch Pathol Lab Med 114:943, 1990.
156. Szymanska J, Tarkkanen M, Wiklund T, et al. Cytogenetic study of extraskeletal mesenchymal chondrosarcoma: a case report. Cancer Genet Cytogenet 86:170, 1996.
157. Takahashi K, Sato K, Kanazawa H, et al. Mesenchymal chondrosarcoma of the jaw: report of a case and review of 41 cases in the literature. Head Neck 15:459, 1993.
158. Ushigome S, Takakuwa T, Shinagawa T, et al. Ultrastructure of cartilaginous tumors and S-100 protein in the tumors: with reference to the histogenesis of chondroblastoma, chondromyxoid fibroma, and mesenchymal chondrosarcoma. Acta Pathol Jpn 34:1285, 1984.
159. Vencio EF, Reeve CM, Unni KK, et al. Mesenchymal chondrosarcoma of the jaw bones: clinicopathologic study of 19 cases. Cancer 82:2350, 1998.
160. Weidner N, Tjoe J. Immunohistochemical profile of monoclonal antibody O13: antibody that recognizes glycoprotein p30/ $32^{MIC2}$ and is useful in diagnosing Ewing's sarcoma and peripheral neuroepithelioma. Am J Surg Pathol 18:486, 1994.

# CHAPTER 35

# OSSEOUS SOFT TISSUE TUMORS

We are principally concerned in this chapter with the following extraskeletal bone-forming lesions: (1) myositis ossificans and related nonneoplastic, heterotopic ossifications, (2) fibrodysplasia (myositis) ossificans progressiva, and (3) extraskeletal osteosarcoma.

*Myositis ossificans,* by far the most common of the lesions, is a localized, self-limiting ossifying process that follows mechanical trauma in most cases. Identical lesions also occur in persons with no apparent history of preceding injury, and in some of these cases an infectious process has been claimed as a possible cause or initiating factor. Whereas most of these lesions originate in muscle tissue, morphologically similar proliferations also arise in the subcutis, tendons, fasciae, and periosteum. Depending on their location, these heterotopic ossifications have been variously classified as *panniculitis ossificans, fasciitis ossificans, florid reactive periostitis,* and *fibroosseous pseudotumor of digits.*

Not further discussed in this chapter are other rare heterotopic ossifications that occur after various kinds of soft tissue injury. Such lesions have been described in surgical scars, particularly those of the abdomen,[24,25,41] in burns,[19] and in association with dislocations of the elbow and other joints and total hip arthroplasty.[3] They have also been observed in patients with tetanus,[5,39] in hemophiliacs, in paraplegics secondary to traumatic spinal injury,[14,42] following pharmacologically induced paralysis,[2] and in patients with spina bifida, myelomeningocele, syringomyelia, cerebral palsy, or poliomyelitis, probably induced by passive movement or forced exercise.[8,13,15] Repeated minor soft tissue trauma is also the cause of the "drill bone" or "shooter bone" in the deltoid and pectoralis muscles, the "rider bone" in the adductor muscles of the thigh, and the "shoemaker's bone" in the rectus muscle of the lower abdominal wall—all lesions that are rarely encountered today but have been repeatedly described in the earlier literature.

In addition to these more deeply seated lesions, localized bone formations in the dermis and subcutis are not particularly rare. They may be solitary or multiple, and they occur spontaneously or in connection with a variety of neoplastic (e.g., linear basal cell nevus, basal cell carcinoma, chondrosyringoma, calcifying epithelioma) and nonneoplastic (e.g., scars, acne, puncture wounds, injections, organizing hematomas, pseudohypoparathyroidism, dermatomyositis) processes. Many of these lesions have been reported as *osteoma cutis,* but they too seem to be products of metaplasia rather than neoplasia.[4,12,33]

*Fibrodysplasia ossificans progressiva (myositis ossificans progressiva)* is a heritable disorder in which massive crippling ossification occurs following diffuse fibroblastic proliferation in muscle and associated soft tissues, especially those of the back, shoulder, and neck. The process has its onset during early childhood and follows a relentless clinical course with total disability in its later stages. Although microscopically the early phase of the lesion may be confused with fibromatosis, it can be definitively identified radiographically in nearly all cases by the presence of microdactylia and other malformations of the hands and feet.

*Extraskeletal osteosarcoma,* the only true neoplasm discussed in this chapter, is a highly malignant tumor that afflicts a much older age group than osteosarcoma of bone. Occasionally it occurs in radiation-damaged tissues. With vanishingly rare exceptions, there is no convincing evidence that it ever occurs as a malignant transformation of heterotopic ossification, including myositis ossificans.

## NONNEOPLASTIC HETEROTOPIC OSSIFICATIONS

### Myositis Ossificans

Myositis ossificans is a benign ossifying process that is generally solitary and well circumscribed. It is found most commonly in the musculature, but it may also occur in other tissues, especially in tendons[34] and subcutaneous fat.[27] The latter lesions are sometimes referred to as *panniculitis ossificans* or *fasciitis ossificans*. Distinguishing between traumatic and nontraumatic forms of myositis ossificans seems to serve little purpose, as both forms are morphologically identical and are most likely secondary to some kind of injury.

Despite countless reports of this lesion in the literature, myositis ossificans still causes considerable difficulties in diagnosis. This is particularly true of the early stage of the disease, in which the immature and highly cellular portions of the lesions are often confused with those of extraskeletal osteosarcoma. In fact, there are several reports of cases in which the lesion was initially diagnosed incorrectly and the patient was treated by unnecessarily radical surgery. Late stage myositis ossificans, consisting almost entirely of mature lamellar bone, is sometimes misinterpreted as an osteoma.

As Ackerman[1] and others have pointed out, the term *myositis ossificans* is a misnomer because the lesion is not necessarily confined to the musculature, is devoid of bone in its early proliferative phase, and lacks a significant degree of inflammation. If inflammation occurs, it is usually minimal and is mostly evident in the tissues surrounding the lesion. For these reasons myositis ossificans and related processes have also been discussed under the designations "pseudomalignant osseous tumors of soft tissues"[7] and "extraosseous localized, nonneoplastic bone and cartilage formation."[1] Although undoubtedly these terms are more accurate and less confining, they are more cumbersome and so far have not been widely accepted in the literature. For this reason the conventional term *myositis ossificans* is retained for this chapter.

### Clinical Findings

The initial complaint, noted within hours or days after injury, is pain or tenderness, followed by a diffuse, doughy soft tissue swelling. Later, usually during the second or third week after onset, the swelling becomes more circumscribed and indurated and gradually changes into a mass that is distinctly outlined and firm to stony on palpation. The mass averages 3–6 cm in greatest diameter, but lesions measuring as large as 15 cm have been observed.

The condition chiefly affects young, vigorous, athletically active adolescents and adults, predominantly males, but it may also be found in older persons and females. For unknown reasons myositis ossificans is rare in small children,[9,16,20] and most ossifying soft tissue lesions in this age group are examples of fibrodysplasia ossificans progressiva. In about 80% of cases the lesion involves the limbs; the favored sites in the lower extremity are the quadriceps muscle and the gluteus muscle and in the upper extremity the flexor muscles, especially the brachialis muscle. Trauma-induced lesions have also been described in the head and neck, particularly in the masseter and sternocleidomastoid muscles.[28,37,43] Wasman et al.[40] described a myositis ossificans-like lesion arising in the median nerve. Deep-seated lesions may involve both muscle and underlying periosteum.

Some myositis ossificans-like lesions are confined to the subcutaneous fat (*panniculitis ossificans*). These lesions prevail in the upper extremity and, unlike the intramuscular lesions, predominate in women rather than men. Rarely, similar lesions arise in the mesentery, typically in middle-aged to elderly men following abdominal surgery. Such lesions show a tendency to recur.[41]

Laboratory findings in myositis ossificans are largely normal. There are no significant changes in serum calcium or phosphorus levels, but sometimes the erythrocyte sedimentation rate, white blood cell count, and alkaline phosphatase levels are slightly elevated; these changes return to normal after the lesion is removed.

### Radiographic Findings

At the initial stage, radiographs show merely a slight increase in soft tissue density. Calcification is rarely seen before the end of the third week after injury and initially presents as rather faint, irregular, floccular radiopacities, sometimes described as the "dotted veil" pattern of myositis ossificans. As the lesion progresses and becomes increasingly calcified, it presents as a well outlined soft tissue mass that is most densely calcified at its periphery. Calcification becomes clearly apparent radiographically 4–6 weeks after the onset of the lesion; it proceeds from the periphery toward the center of the process, but even in late lesions the central core tends to remain uncalcified (Figs. 35–1, 35–2). The presence of a distinct radiolucent cleft between the lesion and the underlying bone helps distinguish myositis ossificans from osteochondroma.[30] Angiograms reveal a diffuse blush and fine neovascularity during the early phase of the process.[44] The appearance of myositis ossificans on computed tomography (CT) and magnetic resonance imaging (MRI) has been described in detail by Kransdorf et al.[21,22] among others.[11,36]

### Pathologic Findings

Grossly, most of the lesions measure 3–6 cm in greatest diameter. They tend to be well circumscribed and cut with a gritty sensation; they are white, soft, and rather gelatinous (or hemorrhagic) in the center and yellow-gray with a rough granular surface at the periphery (Fig. 35–3).

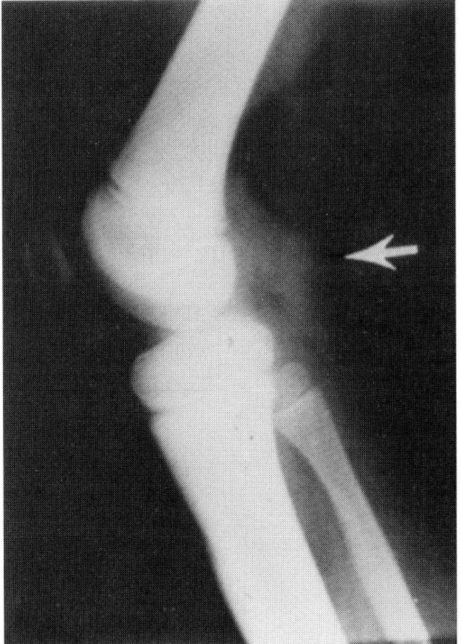
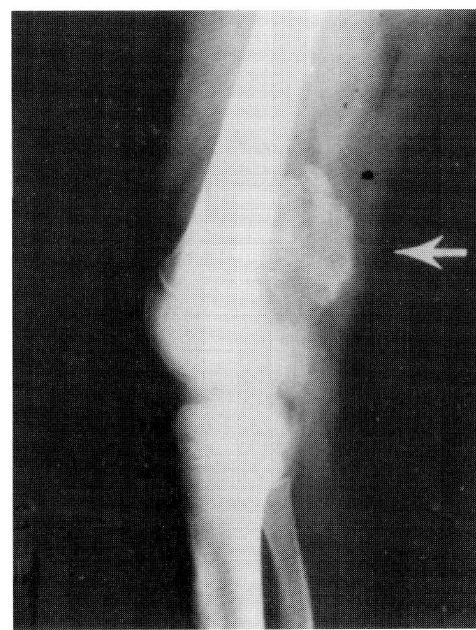

**FIGURE 35–1.** Myositis ossificans of the popliteal fossa showing evidence of progressive ossification within a 22-day period.

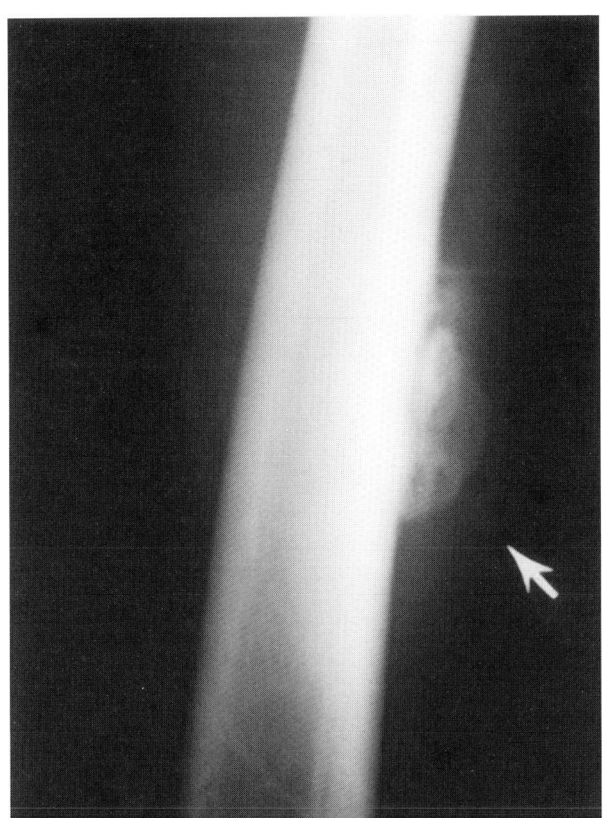

**FIGURE 35–2.** Radiograph of myositis ossificans (arrow) of the upper thigh. The lesion had been present for 5 weeks.

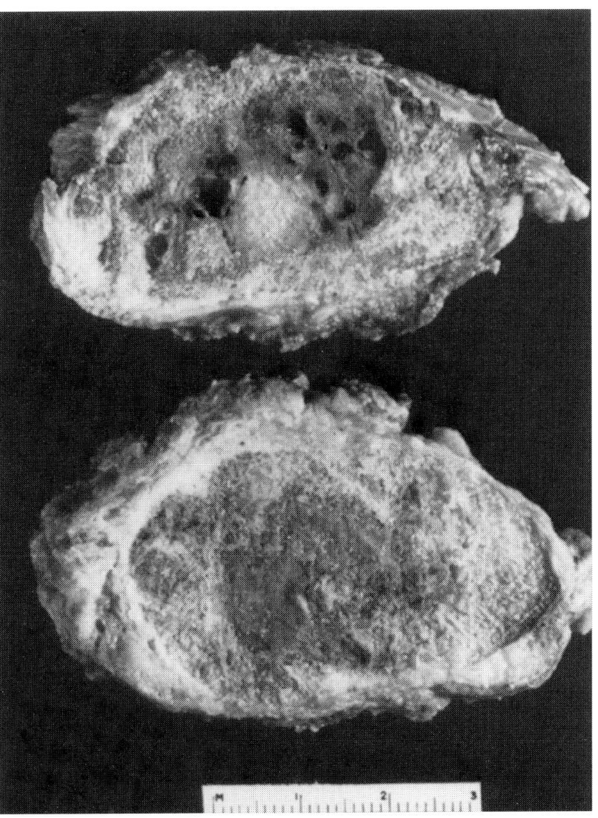

**FIGURE 35–3.** Gross picture of myositis ossificans showing a hemorrhagic center surrounded by a broad zone of ossification and small amounts of residual muscle tissue.

Myositis ossificans is generally characterized by the presence of a distinct zonal pattern that reflects different degrees of cellular maturation, a pattern that is most conspicuous in lesions of 3 weeks' or more duration (Figs. 35–4, 35–5, 35–6). In these cases the innermost portion of the lesion is composed of immature, loosely textured, often richly vascular fibroblastic tissue bearing a close resemblance to nodular fasciitis or granulation tissue (Fig. 35–7). The constituent fibroblasts and myofibroblasts display a mild degree of cellular pleomorphism and rather prominent mitotic activity. They are intermingled with a varying number of macrophages, chronic inflammatory cells, fibrinous material, and not infrequently multinucleated giant cells. In addition, there may be prominent endothelial proliferation, focal hemorrhage, fibrin, and entrapped atrophic or necrotic muscle fibers.

Bordering these areas is an intermediate zone in which the cells become condensed into ill-defined trabeculae consisting of a mixture of fibroblasts, osteoblasts, and varying amounts of osteoid separated by thin-walled, ectatic vascular channels (Figs. 35–8, 35–9, 35–10). Farther toward the periphery the osteoid increasingly undergoes calcification and evolves into mature lamellar bone (Fig. 35–11). Not infrequently islets of immature or mature cartilage are present and precede bone formation. Characteristically, bone formation is most prominent at the margin of the lesion, often with rimming of the osteoid by a monolayer of osteoblasts showing little variation in size and shape. The bone is separated from the surrounding muscle tissue by a zone of loose, myxoid, or compressed fibrous tissue. The surrounding muscle often shows atrophic changes, sometimes together with a mild inflammatory infiltrate and focal sarcolemmal proliferation. In some lesions, particularly those arising in the subcutaneous fat (*panniculitis ossificans*), the zonal pattern is absent or inconspicuous. Older lesions consist only of mature lamellar bone together with interspersed fat cells, fibrous tissue, and thin-walled vascular spaces indistinguishable from osteoma. Ultrastructurally, myositis ossificans consists of fibroblasts and myofibroblasts with focally condensed myofilaments, macrophages, and preosteoblasts and osteoblasts with numerous mitochondria and prominent rough endoplasmic reticulum.[32]

### Malignant Transformation of Myositis Ossificans

We have seen no convincing cases of malignant transformation of myositis ossificans, but there are several accounts in the literature in which transformation of myositis ossificans into extraskeletal osteosarcoma is claimed.[17,18,31,35] In most of these cases, the presence of myositis ossificans is poorly documented, and in only a few is the diagnosis based on biopsy. In some of the reported cases, long duration and dedifferentiation of a well differentiated osteosarcoma may have simulated an origin in myositis ossificans.

### Differential Diagnosis

It is of paramount importance to distinguish this lesion from extraskeletal osteosarcoma (Table 35–1). This is best accomplished on the basis of the charac-

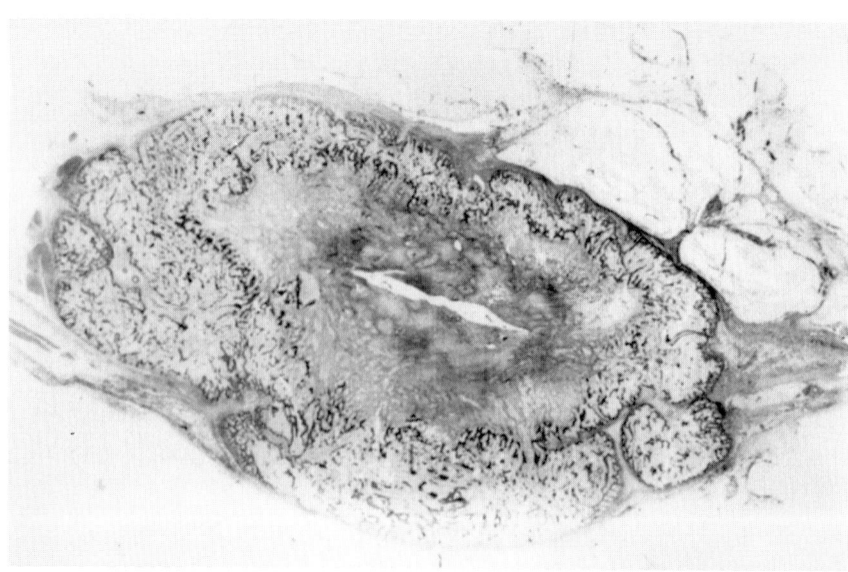

**FIGURE 35–4.** Cross section of myositis ossificans showing the typical zoning phenomenon: a fibroblastic center and a broad zone of ossification at the periphery.

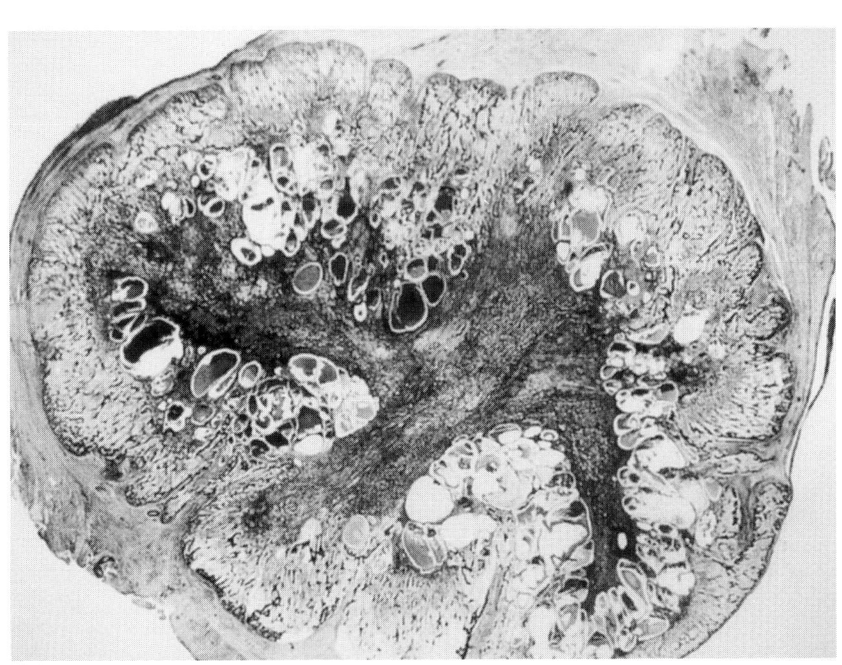

**FIGURE 35–5.** Myositis ossificans with features similar to those seen in Figure 35–4; but in addition there are dilated vessels and focal hemorrhage in the more central portion of the lesion.

teristic zoning phenomenon of myositis ossificans, that is, the presence of immature cellular areas in the center and more mature, ossifying areas with osteoblastic rimming at the periphery. In sharp contrast, osteosarcoma displays a more disorderly growth of hyperchromatic and often pleomorphic cells with lace-like rather than trabecular osteoid formation and sometimes a "reverse zoning effect" (i.e., osteoid or bone formation in the interior and older portion of the lesion and immature spindle cell formation at its margin). Moreover, unlike myositis ossificans, extraskeletal osteosarcoma shows a greater degree of cellular atypia, no subsidence of growth at the periphery, and infiltration of neighboring tissues in a destructive manner. Mitotic figures are present in the immature portions of myositis ossificans and osteosarcoma, but several clearly atypical or tripolar forms point toward malignancy. Confusion of myositis ossificans with osteosarcoma is most likely with small biopsy specimens obtained during the initial proliferative phase or obtained from the cellular center of an early lesion. The differential diagnosis may also be a problem in cases in which the lesion lacks the characteristic zoning phenomenon and grows in an irregular multifocal or multilobulated fashion, as in most cases of fibroosseous pseudotumor involving the distal portions of the fingers or toes (discussed below). Because extraskeletal osteosarcomas occur rarely in young persons,

**TABLE 35–1** DIFFERENTIAL DIAGNOSTIC FEATURES OF MYOSITIS OSSIFICANS, FIBROOSSEOUS PSEUDOTUMOR OF THE DIGITS, AND EXTRASKELETAL OSTEOSARCOMA

| Lesion | Peak Age | Site | Zoning | Pleomorphism | Atypical Mitoses |
|---|---|---|---|---|---|
| Myositis ossificans | 2nd–3rd Decades | Muscles of lower or upper extremities | Immature central areas, mature lamellar bone at periphery | Absent to mild | Absent |
| Fibroosseous pseudotumor | 2nd–3rd Decades | Digits | Usually absent | Absent to mild | Absent |
| Extraskeletal osteosarcoma | 6th–7th Decades | Muscles of lower or upper extremities | If present, has central osteoid or bone and atypical spindled cells at periphery | Moderate to severe | Present |

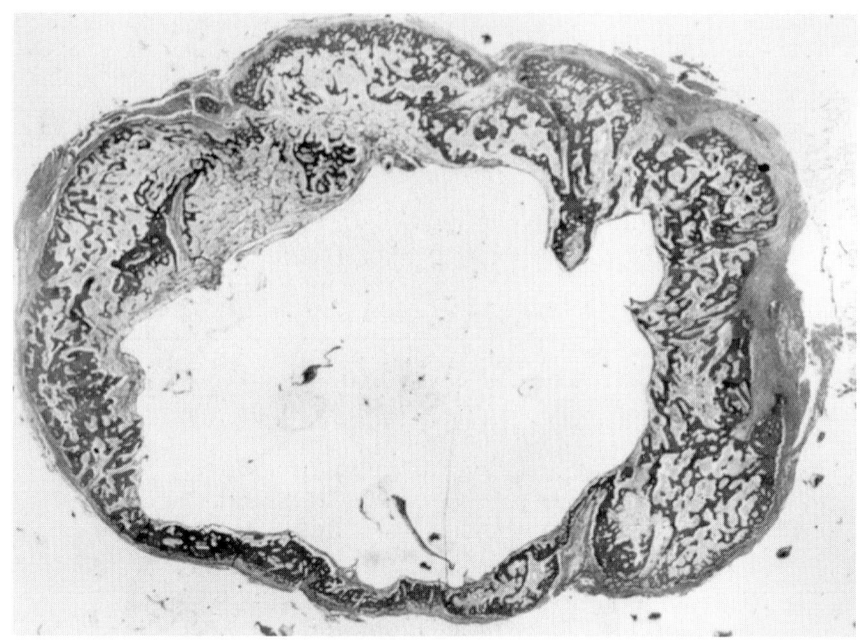

**FIGURE 35-6.** Late form of myositis ossificans with a central fluid-filled space surrounded by mature bone and dense fibrous tissue.

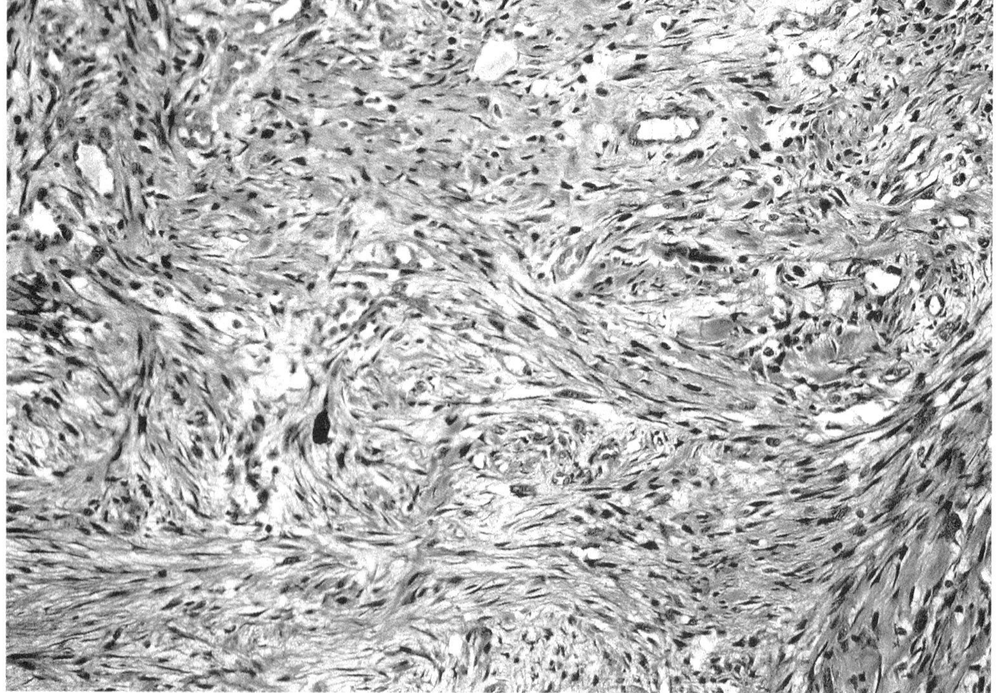

**FIGURE 35-7.** Central portion of myositis ossificans showing fibroblastic/myofibroblastic proliferation closely resembling nodular fasciitis.

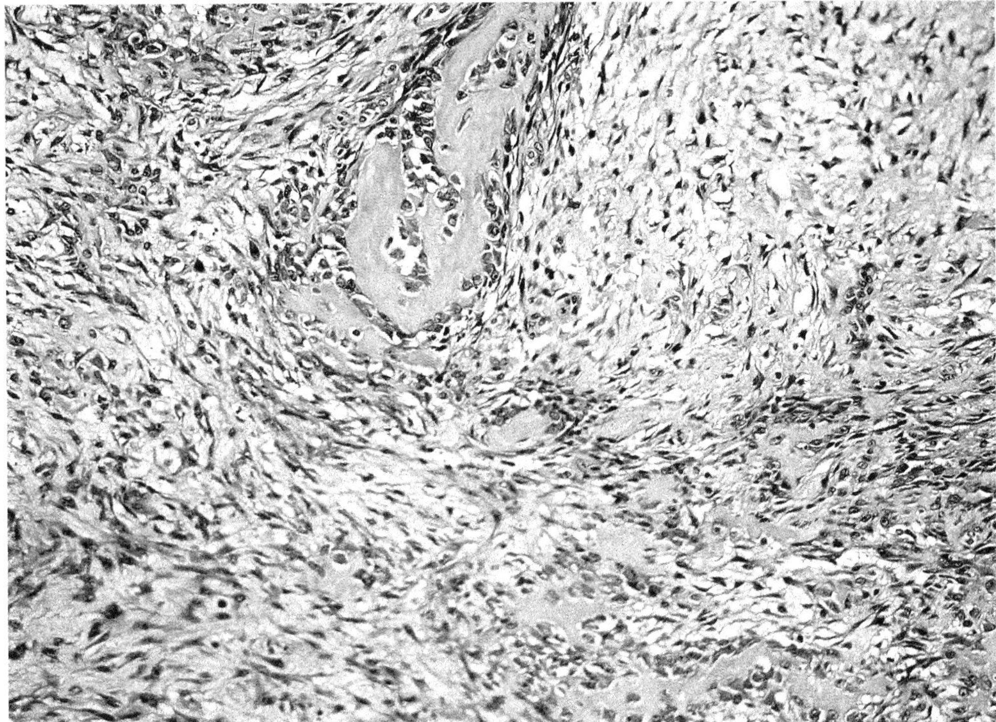

**FIGURE 35–8.** Intermediate portion of myositis ossificans with transition from proliferating spindle-shaped cells to trabeculae of osteoid lined by plump osteoblasts.

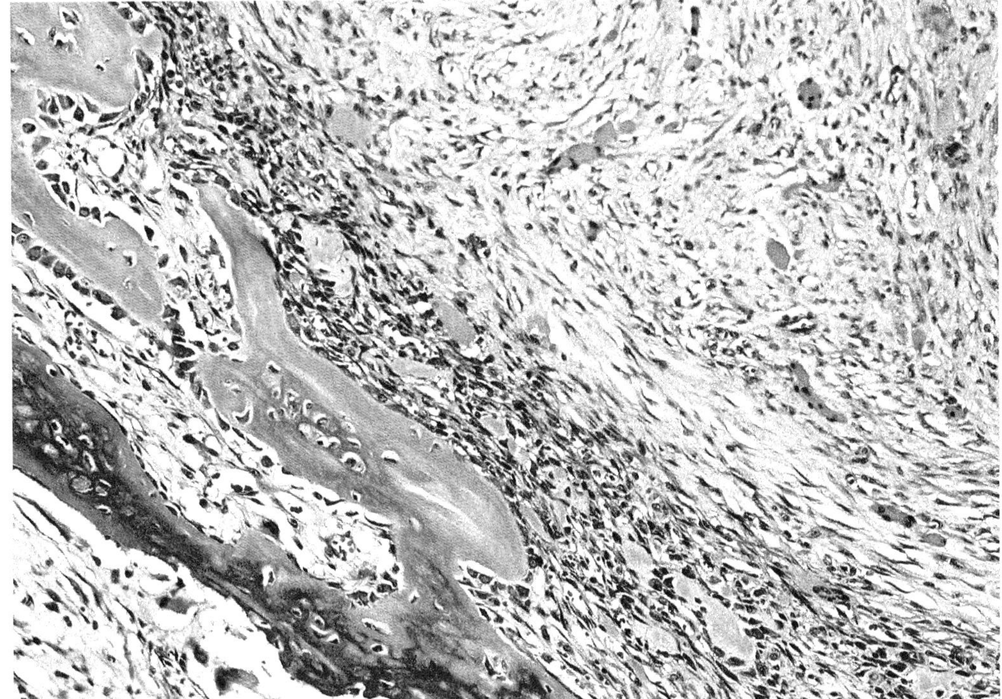

**FIGURE 35–9.** Osteoblast-lined osteoid adjacent to spindle cell proliferation resembling nodular fasciitis in a case of myositis ossificans.

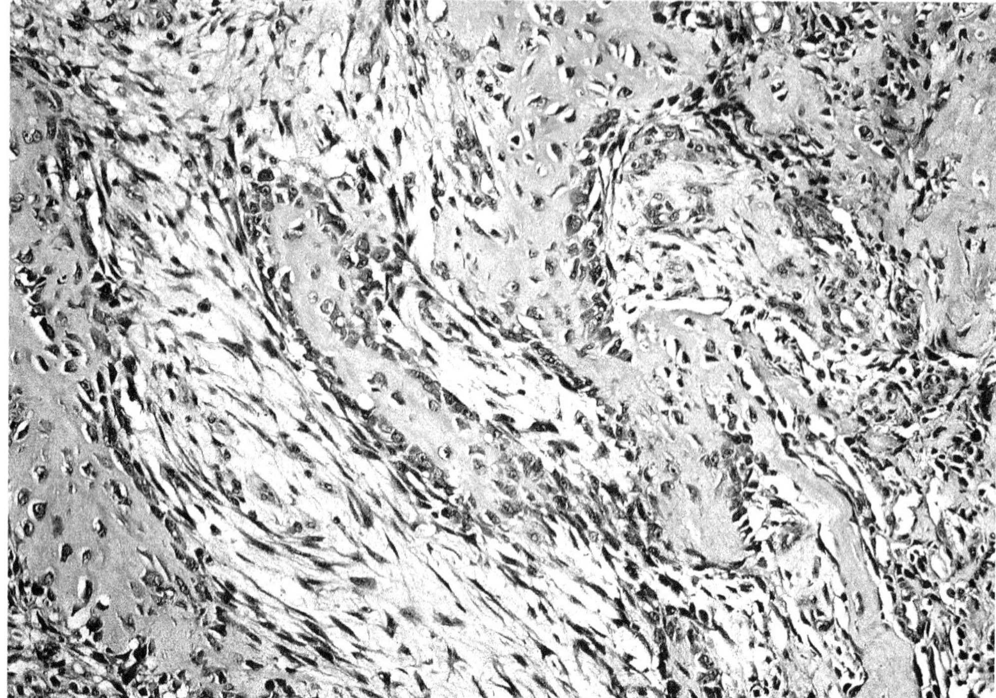

**FIGURE 35–10.** Myositis ossificans. Numerous osteoblasts are seen lining osteoid, surrounded by a cytologically bland proliferation of spindle-shaped cells.

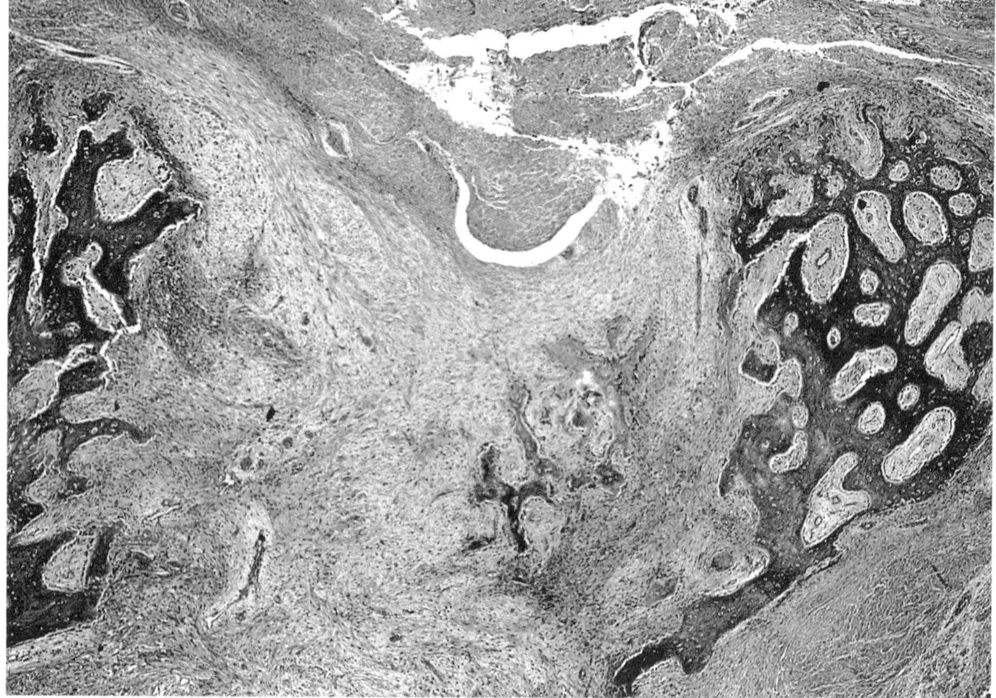

**FIGURE 35–11.** Low magnification view of a peripheral portion of myositis ossificans displaying a zone of osteoid trabeculae rimmed by osteoblasts, underneath which is a proliferation of spindle-shaped cells.

consideration of the age of the patient may help reach a correct diagnosis.[38]

Rarely, a soft tissue metastasis of a silent osteoblastic carcinoma can masquerade as myositis ossificans. Benign lesions also may be confused with myositis ossificans, including purely reactive lesions such as nodular fasciitis, proliferative myositis, posttraumatic periostitis, and exuberant fracture callus. Proliferative myositis rarely contains minute foci of osteoid or bone, but characteristically this feature is associated with a diffuse proliferation of plump fibroblasts resembling ganglion cells. Posttraumatic periostitis manifests as an ossified mass that is attached to bone with a broad base. Exuberant callus is usually associated with a discernible fracture line on standard radiographs.

### *Pathogenesis*

Although there is general agreement that myositis ossificans is a nonprogressive benign process without neoplastic potential, its pathogenesis is still poorly understood. In cases with a definite history of traumatic injury it can be assumed that the process commences with tissue necrosis or hemorrhage, or both, followed by exuberant reparative fibroblastic and vascular proliferation, eventually leading to progressive ossification. The exact environmental or humoral conditions underlying the ossifying process are unclear. Detachment and intramuscular implantation of periosteal cells are not necessary prerequisites for the ossification because this ossifying process also takes place in the subcutis and at other sites that are a considerable distance from bone. Similarly, the occurrence of ectopic ossifications in paraplegics and patients with tetanus may be explained by trauma resulting from passive exercise rather than disturbed neurotrophic factors. The source of the osteoblasts remains an enigma. They may be transformed fibroblasts, or they may be derived from primitive perivascular mesenchymal cells secondary to injury and necrosis of muscle and other tissues.[6]

A satisfactory explanation of the so-called nontraumatic cases of myositis ossificans is even more problematic.[10,26] It is likely that in most of these cases minor injury such as a spontaneous muscle tear or a similar disruptive lesion associated with heavy manual labor, weight lifting, or some other strenuous exercise or activity has been overlooked or forgotten; yet it is difficult to exclude the possibility that some of these cases are caused or initiated by an infectious process. Lagier and Cox[23] reported a patient who had had an antiinfluenza vaccination 15 days before the onset of the lesion. A similar infectious origin has been considered for the related fibroosseous pseudotumor of the digits.[45]

### *Discussion*

Because myositis ossificans is a benign, self-limiting process, the prognosis is excellent, and there is no need for further therapy once the diagnosis of myositis ossificans has been established by biopsy or local excision. However, if only a biopsy was done or if the lesion was partly excised at an early phase of its growth, it may continue to grow for a limited period; in these cases repeated radiographic examinations should be obtained during the follow-up period to document the maturation of the lesion and the absence of destructive growth. Spontaneous regression of myositis ossificans has also been observed.[29]

## Fibroosseous Pseudotumor of the Digits

Fibroosseous pseudotumor of the digits, a heterotopic ossification closely related to myositis ossificans, occurs in the subcutaneous tissue of the digits.[48] It has been previously described under various names, including *florid reactive periostitis of the tubular bones of hands and feet,*[50,59] *pseudomalignant osseous tumor of the soft tissues,*[55] and *parosteal fasciitis.*[52] This lesion appears to be closely related to bizarre parosteal osteochondromatous proliferation (Nora's lesion) and acquired osteochondroma.[47] Clinically, this process presents as a painful, localized, fusiform, often erythematous swelling in the soft tissues of the fingers, especially the region of the proximal phalanx[48] (Fig. 35–12) and less commonly, the toes.[46,49,57,58] It predominantly affects young adults and, unlike myositis ossificans, is more common in women.

Radiographically, it is usually an ill-defined soft tissue mass with focal calcification that lacks the typical zoning pattern of myositis ossificans.[21,22] There may be thickening of the adjacent periosteum, and rare cases erode adjacent bone.[56,60] Histologically, the lesion closely resembles myositis ossificans but lacks its orderly zonal pattern; it consists merely of an irregular, often nodular mixture of loosely arranged fibroblasts, a prominent myxoid matrix, and deposits of osteoid rimmed by uniform osteoblasts[48] (Figs. 35–13 to 35–16). Multinucleated giant cells may be seen, and in some cases there is a mild lymphoplasmacytic infiltrate. Immunohistochemically, the spindle-shaped cells express vimentin and actin,[58] suggesting myofibroblastic differentiation.

The major differential diagnosis is with extraskeletal osteosarcoma. The latter lesion typically occurs in older patients and rarely involves the digits. Furthermore, extraskeletal osteosarcoma is characterized by more pleomorphic hyperchromatic cells and atypical mitotic figures. Bizarre parosteal osteochondromatous proliferation (Nora's lesion), similar to fibrooseous pseudotumor, predominantly involves the short tubu-

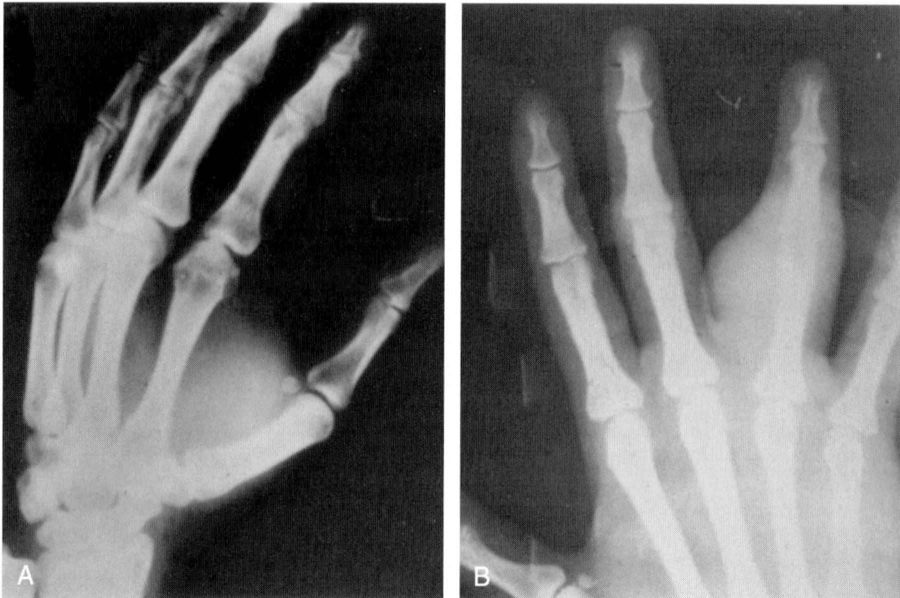


**FIGURE 35–12.** Radiographs of fibroosseous pseudotumor of the thenar eminence (**A**) and the right ring finger (**B**).

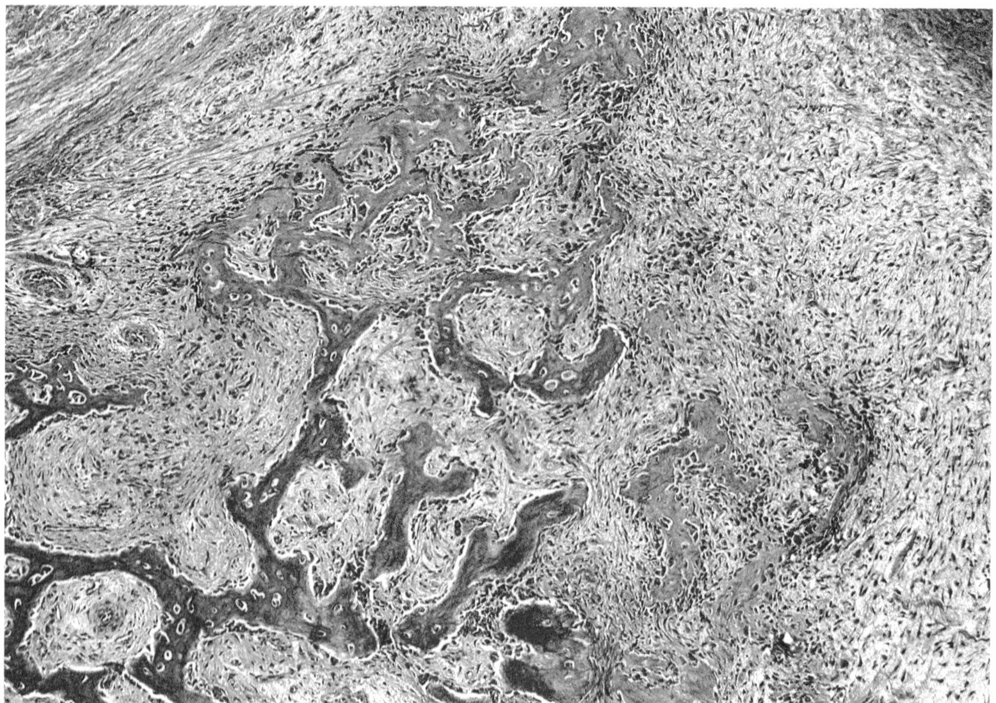

**FIGURE 35–13.** Fibroosseous pseudotumor of the right index finger showing a peripheral zone of proliferating spindle cells and a central zone of osteoid.

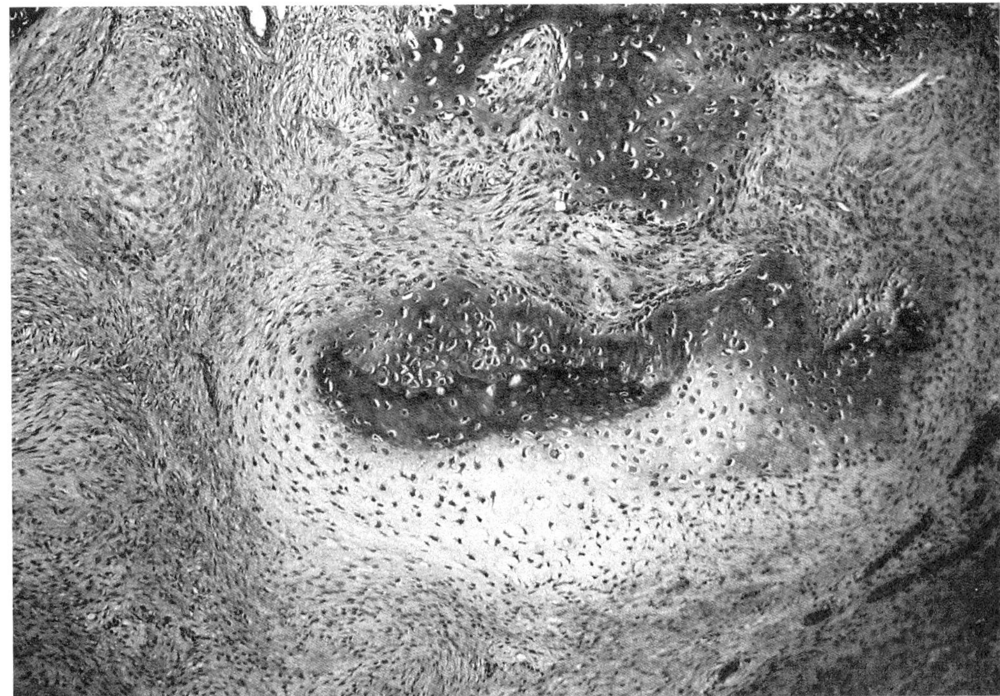

**FIGURE 35–14.** Fibroosseous pseudotumor with osteoblast-rimmed osteoid material and a surrounding chondroid zone.

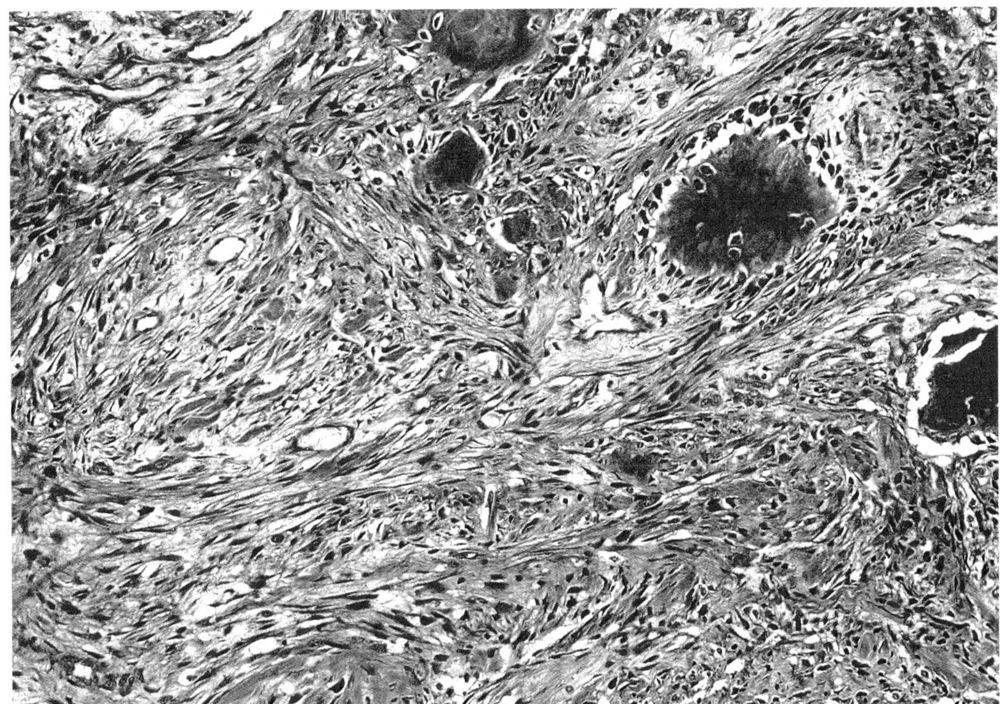

**FIGURE 35–15.** High magnification view of fibroosseous pseudotumor with proliferation of spindle-shaped cells adjacent to trabeculae of osteoid resembling myositis ossificans.

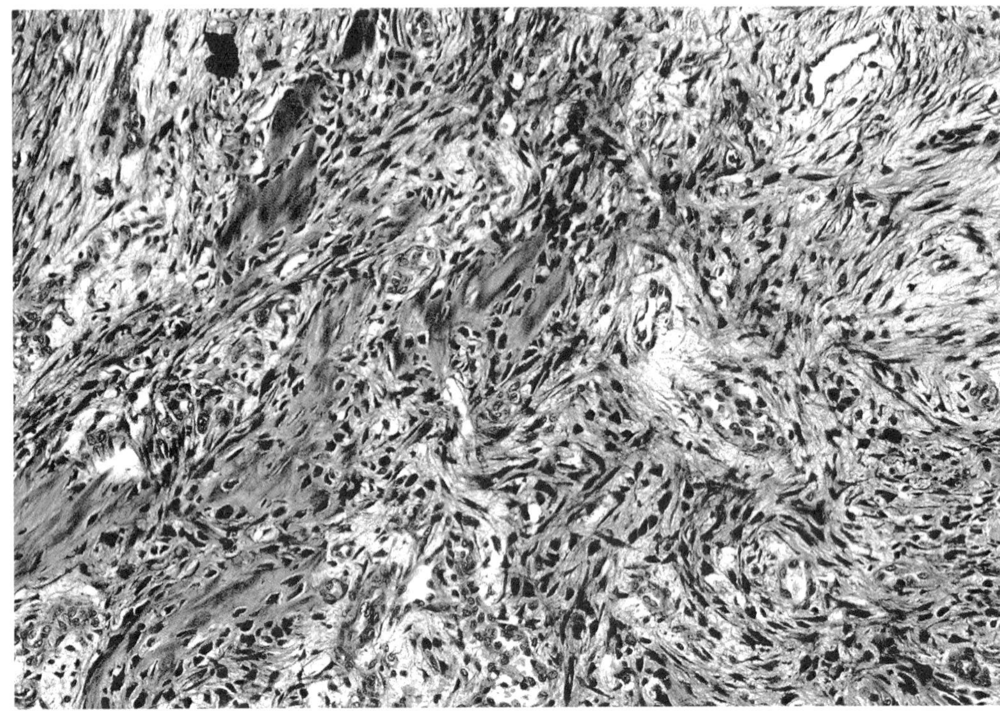

**FIGURE 35–16.** Fibroosseous pseudotumor with an admixture of proliferating cytologically bland spindle-shaped cells and osteoid.

lar bones of the hands and feet of young adults.[51,53,54] Given the overlapping clinical and histologic features, it has been proposed that this lesion most likely represents an intermediate step between fibroosseous pseudotumor of the digits and acquired osteochondroma (Turret exostosis).[47] Nora's lesion presents as a well delineated mass attached to the bone surface. Histologically, a zonal architecture is apparent at low magnification with central or basally located new bone surrounded by a peripheral cap of cartilage. The cartilage often shows foci of hypercellularity with binucleated cells which may result in a misinterpretation of malignancy if the entire clinical and radiographic picture is not considered.

As with the conventional form of myositis ossificans, the exact pathogenetic mechanism of this process is not clear. In the series by Dupree and Enzinger[48], a history of trauma was given in only 9 of 21 patients. Similarly, Spjut and Dorfman reported a history of trauma in 5 of 12 cases.[59] Some have postulated that an infectious process serves as the nidus for this lesion based on the elevated white blood cell counts and increased streptolysin O titers in some patients.[45] Most are cured by complete excision, and local recurrences are generally related to inadequate excision. Of the seven cases with follow-up information in the series from the Armed Forces Institute of Pathology (AFIP), only one patient developed a local recurrence.[48] Spjut and Dorfman reported local recurrence in only 1 of 10 patients.[59]

## FIBRODYSPLASIA (MYOSITIS) OSSIFICANS PROGRESSIVA

Fibrodysplasia (myositis) ossificans progressiva is a rare, slowly progressive hereditary disease that principally affects children under the age of 10 years. It is characterized by progressive fibroblastic proliferation and subsequent calcification and ossification of subcutaneous fat, muscles, tendons, aponeuroses, and ligaments. The disorder is often associated with symmetric malformations of the digits, especially microdactyly or adactyly of the thumbs and great toes, which precede onset of the fibroblastic proliferations and calcifications. Its prevalence in children, diffuse or multinodular soft tissue involvement, progressive clinical course, and increased familial incidence distinguish it from localized myositis ossificans. Sporadic cases have been described in the literature since the seventeenth century.

### Clinical Findings

The disease has its onset primarily between birth and 6 years of age, although in rare instances it arises in older children and even in young adults.[66] Males and females are about equally affected, and there is no predilection for any particular race.[97] As in localized myositis ossificans, the lesion presents as a painful, doughy soft tissue swelling that most commonly begins in the upper paraspinal muscles and spreads from the axial to the appendicular skeleton, typically from cranial to caudal and from the proximal to the distal extremities[91] (Fig. 35–17). This typical progression may be modified by injury, immunization, or surgery.[84] The preosseous lesion is a highly vascular fibroblastic proliferation that is histologically similar to that seen in the infantile forms of fibromatosis.[81,82] During the later stages the fibroblastic proliferation is replaced by endochondral ossification with mature lamellar bone having bone marrow elements that may involve an entire muscle from origin to insertion.[82] This causes progressive muscle stiffening, immobilization, and contraction deformities, leading to severe changes in posture and gait as well as increasing difficulties in respiration.[83] In fact, patients with fibrodysplasia ossificans progressiva are much more likely to suffer a catastrophic fall resulting in traumatic brain injury, intracranial hemorrhage, or death than are those without this disease.[75] Involvement of the masseter muscle may impair normal mastication and result in severe weight loss. Many patients die during early adult life from respiratory failure or pneumonia.[97]

Malformation or the absence of one or more digits is an almost constant finding that helps distinguish this disease from infantile forms of fibromatosis. The malformations are usually present at birth or appear soon thereafter; in the earliest stage they are best identified radiographically (Fig. 35–18); they consist mainly of bilateral shortening of the fingers (microdactyly), absence of both thumbs and great toes (adactyly), or digital deviations, particularly valgus position of the great toe (bilateral hallux valgus). Frequently other digits are also involved.[95] Connor and Evans,[68] in a review of 34 affected patients, reported hallux valgus in 79%, short first metacarpals in 59%, and deviation (clinodactyly) of the fifth fingers in 42%. In 29 of the 34 cases the skeletal alterations were present at birth. Sometimes the significance of these osseous malformations is not immediately recognized,

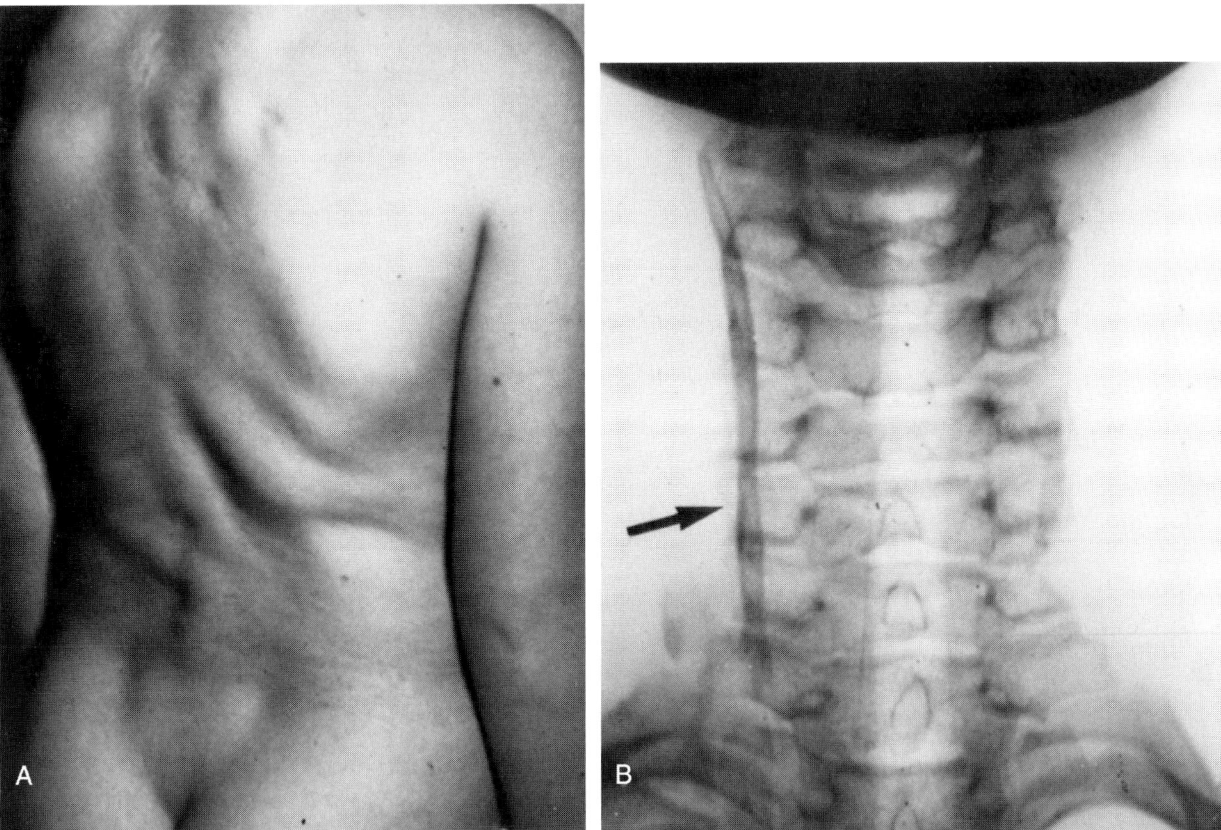

**FIGURE 35–17.** (**A**) Fibrodysplasia (myositis) ossificans progressiva involving the back of a child with ill-defined, indurated nodules caused by focal fibroblastic proliferation and ossification of the musculature. (**B**) Radiograph of linear ossification of paraspinal muscles (arrow). (Courtesy of Prof. Dr. Günther Möbius, Schwerin.)

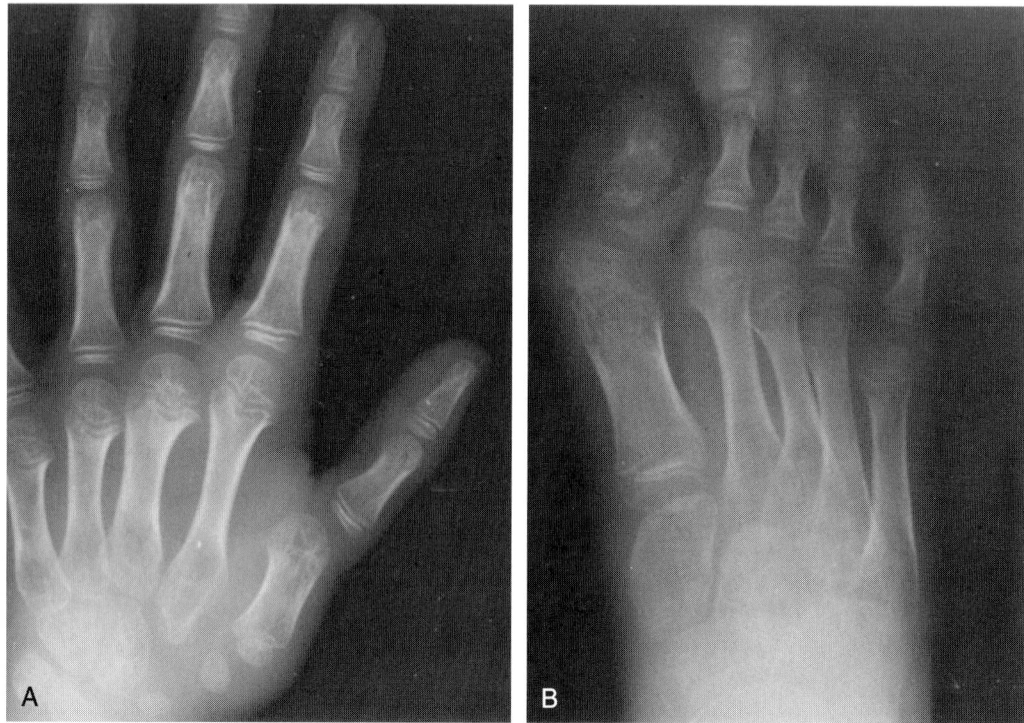


**FIGURE 35–18.** Fibrodysplasia (myositis) ossificans progressiva. (**A**) Radiograph shows shortening and deviation of the thumb. (**B**) Radiograph shows malformation of the great toe, a relatively common radiographic finding in this disease.

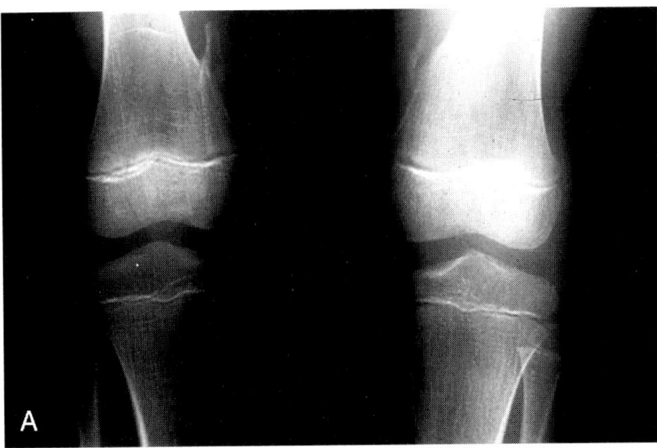


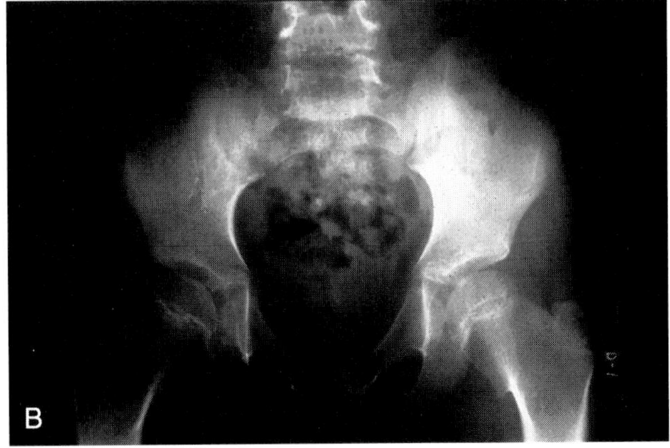


**FIGURE 35–19.** (**A**) Radiograph of both knees of a 7-year-old boy with fibrodysplasia (myositis) ossificans progressiva. Ossification is demonstrated along the medial femoral condyles bilaterally as well as the medial left tibial metaphysis along sites of ligamentous insertions producing pseudoexostoses. (**B**) Radiograph of the pelvis of the same patient showing bilateral broad short femoral necks and small pseudoexostoses along the medial femoral metaphyses.

and surgical correction is attempted, precipitating ectopic ossification. Additional radiographic changes, which appear at a later stage of the disease, consist of bony bridges in muscles and tendons; contractures and ankylosis of the shoulder, elbow, spine, and other joints[61,70,94]; exostosis of the tibia and other bones; metaphyseal widening of long bones[88]; and osteoporosis (Fig. 35–19). CT scans and MRI may help demonstrate early changes of the disease[65] (Fig. 35–20); bone scans reveal increased tracer uptake at the sites of ossification.[76] Deformity of the ears, absence of teeth, deafness, and sexual infantilism may also be part of the clinical picture.[92] Laboratory findings are generally unremarkable, except for elevated alkaline phosphatase levels. Basic fibroblast growth factor, a potent stimulator of angiogenesis, has been found to be significantly elevated in the urine in patients with acute flareups of fibrodysplasia ossificans progressiva.[79] Although the human leukocyte antigen HLA-B27 is common in patients with disorders of heterotopic bone formation,[86] this antigen has not been found with increased prevalence in patients with fibrodysplasia ossificans progressiva.[64]

## Pathologic Findings

There are essentially two stages of the disease. The first consists of nodular swelling of muscle and subcutis caused by interstitial edema, perivascular lymphocytic inflammation, and a loose proliferation of fibroblasts, usually in the endomysium and perimysium[74] (Fig. 35–21). During the second stage, collagen is laid down between the fibroblasts, followed by variable muscular atrophy, calcification, ossification of the collagenized fibrous tissue, and formation of mature bone and cartilage. Unlike localized myositis ossificans, the ossification occurs in the center of the nodules. The nodules often interconnect, leading eventually to the formation of bony bridges that replace muscles, tendons, and ligaments. Histochemical and ultrastructural studies show active fibroblasts with prominent endoplasmic reticulum, collagen fibers of normal periodicity, and increased mucosubstances.[87] Gannon et al.[73] found that the cells in the early preosseous fibroblastic stage are immunoreactive for bone morphogenetic protein 2/4 (discussed below), whereas the cells of infantile fibromatosis do not stain for this antigen.

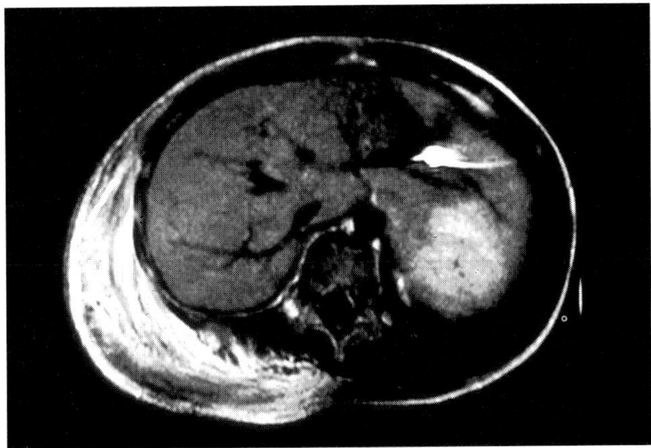

**FIGURE 35–20.** Fibrodysplasia (myositis) ossificans progressiva. Magnetic resonance image of the same patient depicted in Figure 35–19 reveals a large soft tissue mass that extended along the deep and superficial muscles of the back from the lower neck to the lower thoracic spine.

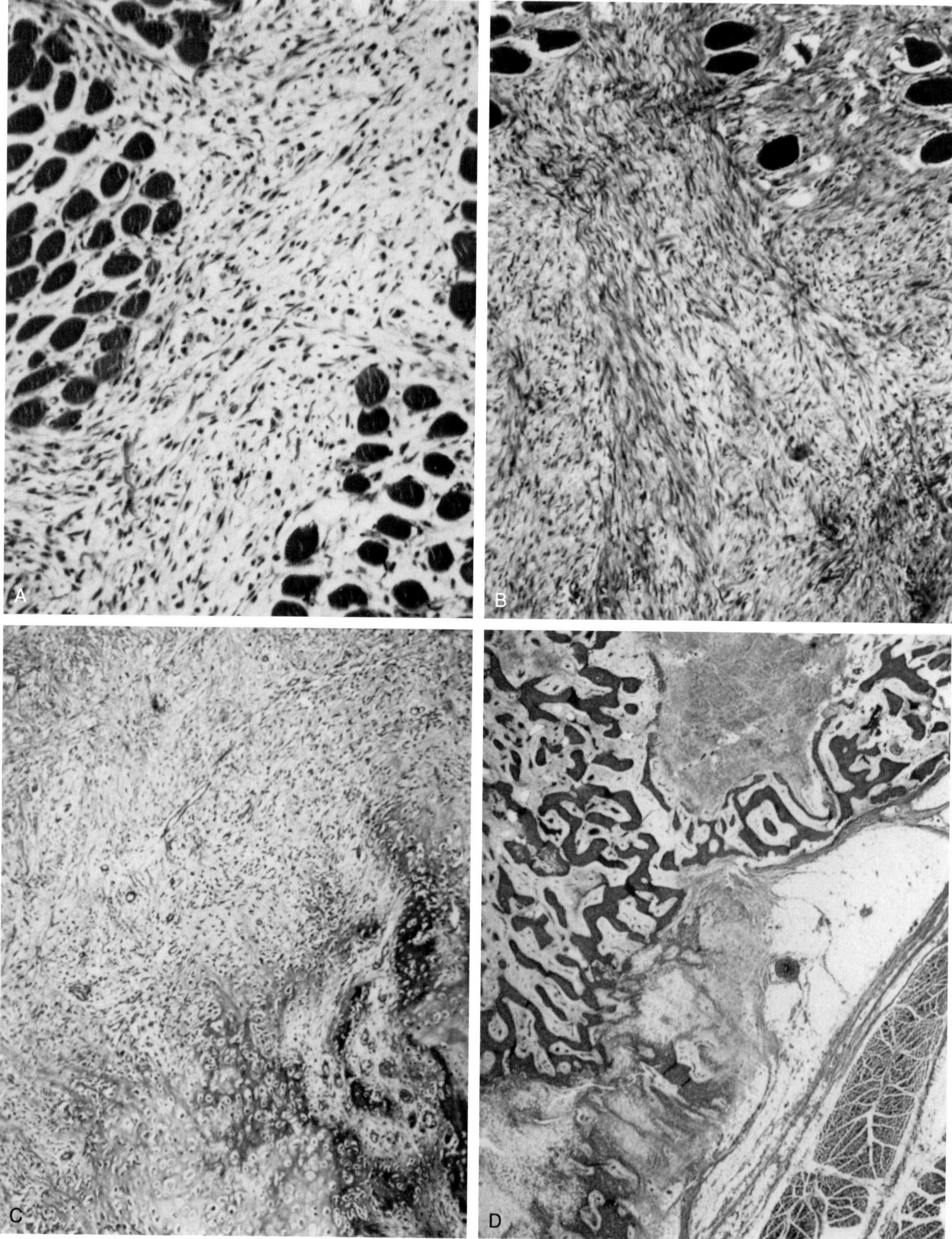


**FIGURE 35–21.** Fibrodysplasia (myositis) ossificans progressiva of the scapular region in a 7-year-old girl. (**A, B**) Edema and ill-defined, loosely textured fibroblastic proliferation of muscle that superficially resembles infantile fibromatosis, proliferative myositis, or nodular fasciitis. (**C, D**) Irregular ossification of the fibroblastic tissue lacking the zoning phenomenon of localized myositis ossificans.

### Genetic Aspects of Fibrodysplasia Ossificans Progressiva

A rare disease, fibrodysplasia ossificans progressiva is inherited in an autosomal dominant pattern,[71] and most cases appear to be due to new mutations, probably related to the low reproductive fitness of afflicted individuals.[80,100] In addition, there is variable expression of this disorder, as some patients have a milder form of the disease.[69,78] Janoff et al.[77] reported this disease in two half-sisters with the same unaffected mother and different unaffected fathers, suggesting that the mother has a mutant gene in numerous ova but that the mutant gene is present in few or no somatic cells (gonadal mosaicism).[71]

The gene or genes that are mutated in fibrodysplasia ossificans progressiva are unknown. Genetic linkage studies are difficult given that most cases appear to arise from new mutations. The underlying biochemical process has been elucidated by Shafritz et al.[96] and others[67,85] by the finding of overexpression of bone morphogenetic protein 4 (BMP4) in the cells of the early fibroproliferative lesion in patients with this disease. This gene is a member of the transforming growth factor $\beta$ gene superfamily[99] and has been mapped to chromosome 14q22-q23.[98] The BMP genes have the ability to induce the complete cellular program of endochondral bone formation and likely play a critical role in the pathogenesis of this disease. However, Xu and Shore[100] were unable to identify any mutations in the *BMP4* gene suggesting an abnormality of a regulatory gene.

### Prognosis and Therapy

The outlook is poor, and usually the disease proves fatal within a period of 10–15 years, frequently as the result of severe respiratory insufficiency caused by progressive immobilization of the thorax. Biopsy and trauma may lead to the development of new lesions and should be avoided. Dietary measures, steroids,[72] and agents binding minerals or blocking calcification (EDTA and EHDP) have been tried with disappointing results. High does of intravenous disodium etidronate may be helpful for decreasing pain, swelling, and acute flareups of this disease,[62,89] but excessive use can result in ricket-like osseous abnormalities.[90] Isotretinoin, a retinoid capable of inhibiting differentiation of mesenchymal cells into cartilage and bone, has not been found to be an effective mode of therapy.[103]

The differential diagnosis includes the battered child syndrome,[102] ectopic bone formation with multiple congenital anomalies,[93] pseudohypoparathyroidism,[63] and dermatomyositis with multiple calcifications.[101] The latter entity is also associated with shortening of the metacarpal and metatarsal bones, exostoses, and multiple subcutaneous ossifications.[68] Finally, as mentioned earlier, the initial noncalcified fibrous proliferation of fibrodysplasia ossificans progressiva may be mistaken for a juvenile form of fibromatosis.

## EXTRASKELETAL OSTEOSARCOMA

Compared with osteosarcoma of bone, extraskeletal osteosarcoma is rare, accounting for approximately 1–2% of all soft tissue sarcomas.[150] It may be defined as a malignant mesenchymal neoplasm that produces osteoid, bone, or chondroid material. It is located in the soft tissues without attachment to the skeleton, as determined by radiographic examination or inspection during the operative procedure. Included in our material and among the reported cases are also a number of osteosarcomas of soft tissues that developed several years after radiotherapy for carcinoma or some other malignant epithelial or mesenchymal neoplasm.[123]

Excluded from this chapter are osteosarcomas arising in the breast,[149] urinary bladder,[160] prostate,[144] and other visceral organs[113,135] because in many of these tumors there is a participating epithelial component suggesting carcinosarcoma. We have also excluded malignant mesenchymomas, a rather nebulous entity that exhibits by definition two or more well defined malignant mesenchymal components.

There are few reliable data in the literature as to the incidence of extraskeletal osteosarcoma. Allan and Soule[104] encountered 26 cases among 2100 soft tissue sarcomas, an incidence of 1.24%. Lorentzon et al.,[136] in a study of the Swedish Cancer Registry, found four extraskeletal osteosarcomas (1.65%) among 242 osteosarcomas of bone. They calculated an annual incidence of two to three cases per million population.

### Clinical Findings

Although osteosarcomas of bone occur chiefly during the first two decades of life, extraskeletal osteosarcomas are rarely encountered in patients under 40 years of age. In a series of 40 extraskeletal osteosarcomas reported from the Mayo Clinic,[133] the mean age was 50.7 years (range 23–81 years), and in a series of 25 cases from Denmark, Jensen et al.[128] reported a mean age of 67 years (range 35–82 years). A similar age incidence was reported by Fine and Stout[124] and others.[145] The data as to the gender incidence vary, and both male and female predominance has been reported. Lee et al.[133] found a male/female ratio of 1.9:1.0.

There are no specific signs or symptoms. Generally the tumor presents as a progressively enlarging soft tissue mass that is painful in about one-third of patients. Large and late examples of the tumor may ulcerate through the skin but usually only after biopsy or some other surgical procedure. The duration of symptoms varies from a few weeks to many years, although most present within 6–8 months following the initiation of symptoms.[128,133]

Among the various anatomic sites, the muscles of the thigh are most commonly affected; the large muscles of the pelvic and shoulder girdles and retroperitoneum are other relatively common sites (Table 35–2). Most of the tumors are deep-seated and fixed to the underlying tissues, but occasional lesions are freely movable and are confined to the subcutis or even the dermis.[107,114] There are also reports of extraskeletal osteosarcomas arising in unusual locations including the larynx,[115] tongue,[137] mediastinum,[116] spermatic cord,[108] penis,[106,147] and central nervous system.[142] The laboratory findings show no specific abnormalities. Alkaline phosphatase is usually normal with localized disease, but it is elevated in the presence of metastases. With conventional radiographs, CT scan, and MRI, extraskeletal osteosarcoma manifests as a soft tissue mass with spotty to massive calcifications and no evidence of bone involvement[140,141,155] (Figs. 35–22, 35–23, 35–24A).

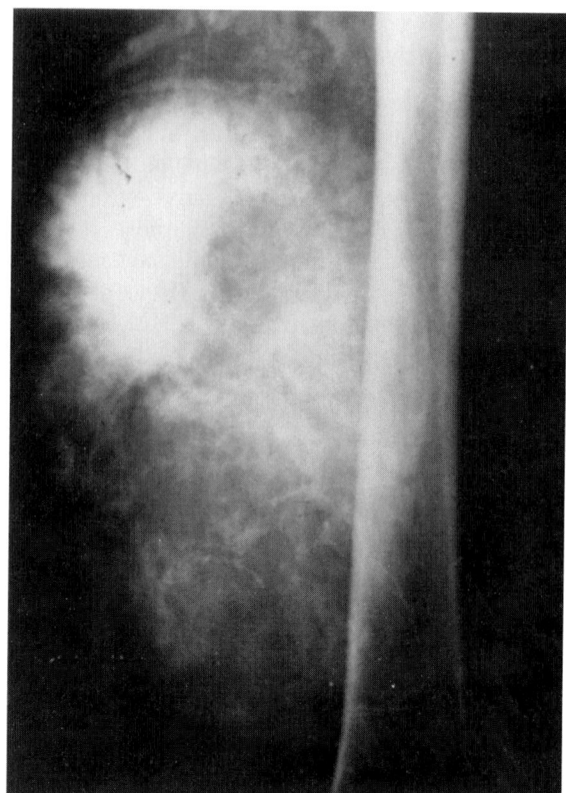

**FIGURE 35–22.** Radiograph of extraskeletal osteosarcoma of the mid-thigh demonstrating a soft tissue mass with extensive ossification. (From Chung EB, Enzinger FM. Extraskeletal osteosarcoma. Cancer 60:1132, 1987.)

## Pathogenesis

Mechanical injury has been considered to be a causative agent,[136] but as with other neoplasms the etiologic significance of trauma is difficult to assess. Preceding trauma has been reported in 12.5%[114] to 23.0%[133] of patients. There are also reports of osteosarcoma arising at the sites of a previous injection[132] and fracture.[110] Extraskeletal osteosarcomas arising in myositis ossificans are rare and most of these reports are poorly documented.[126,127] Eckardt et al.[120] observed an osteosarcoma of the thigh in a 32-year-old-man that developed in a heterotopic ossification of dermatomyositis 28 years after onset of the disease. Unlike osteosarcoma of bone, the tumor has not been reported in siblings, but Mirra et al.[139] reported a unique case of an extraskeletal osteosarcoma that arose in the mother of a daughter who had previously died of skeletal osteosarcoma.

**TABLE 35–2** ANATOMIC DISTRIBUTION OF 153 EXTRASKELETAL OSTEOSARCOMAS

| Anatomic Location | No. of Patients | % |
|---|---|---|
| Lower extremity | 82 | 53 |
| Thigh | 56 | |
| Other | 26 | |
| Upper extremity | 30 | 20 |
| Trunk | 18 | 12 |
| Retroperitoneum | 17 | 11 |
| Head and neck | 5 | 3 |
| Other | 1 | 1 |
| *Total* | 153 | 100 |

Data are from references 114, 128, and 133.

## Radiation-Induced Extraskeletal Osteosarcoma

Since Martland[138] described the development of osteogenic sarcoma in patients engaged in the manufacture of luminous watch dials, numerous cases of osseous and extraosseous postradiation osteosarcomas have been reported in the literature.[131,134] Most of the extraosseous osteosarcomas occurred in patients who underwent radiation therapy for a malignant neoplasm such as a mammary carcinoma,[149] uterine and ovarian carcinoma,[105] seminoma,[112] Wilms' tumor,[109] Hodgkin's disease, neuroblastoma,[154] astrocytoma,[154] or retinoblastoma.[130] In most instances the tumor became apparent 4 years or more after radiotherapy.

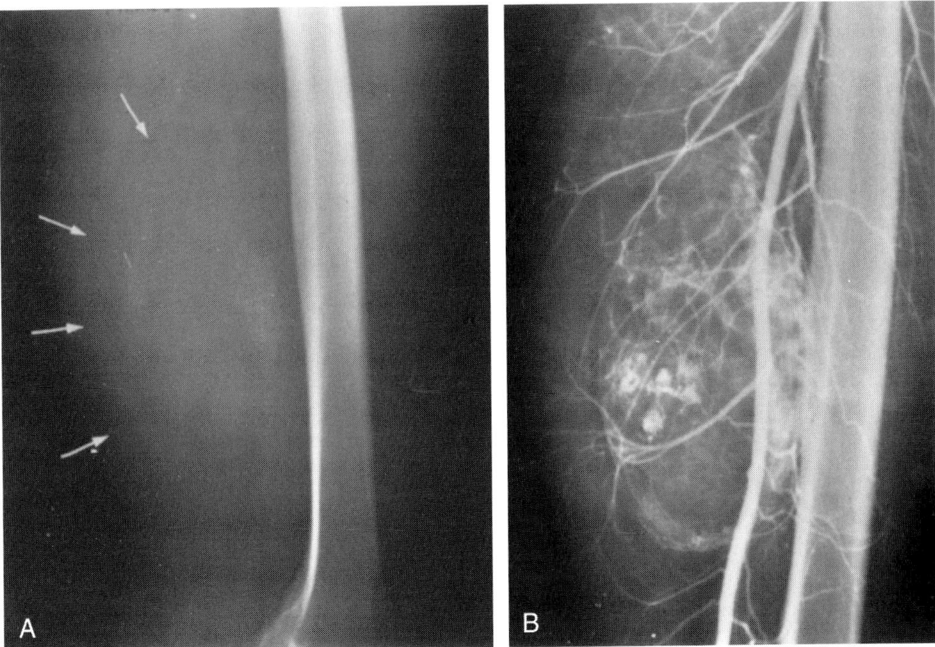


**FIGURE 35–23.** (**A**) Radiograph of extraskeletal osteosarcoma shows a soft tissue mass with areas of ossification (arrows). (**B**) There is a moderate degree of vascularization in the angiogram with focal neovascularity and stretching and displacement of arteries.

Assessment of these cases is facilitated by the presence of chronic radiodermatitis in the skin overlying the tumor or radiation change in the surrounding muscle tissue.[131] As with extraskeletal chondrosarcomas, there are also sporadic cases that developed following diagnostic procedures with radioactive thorium dioxide (Thorotrast). One of these, an extraskeletal osteosarcoma of the mandibular region in a 51-year-old man, appeared 30 years after a Thorotrast angiogram of the carotid artery.[125]

## Pathologic Findings

Macroscopically, there is little that would permit a reliable diagnosis. The tumor varies in its gross appearance from a well circumscribed mass with a distinct pseudocapsule to an infiltrating tumor without discernible borders. Frequently, it is firm to stony on palpation. Less often it presents as a soft or multicystic mass. On section it usually displays a granular white surface with yellow flecks and multiple foci of necrosis and hemorrhage. Most of the tumors measure 5–10 cm when excised (Fig. 35–24B).

Microscopically, extraskeletal osteosarcomas have in common the presence of neoplastic osteoid and bone, not infrequently together with neoplastic cartilage. There is a striking variation in the relative prominence of this material and the associated osteoblastic and fibroblastic elements. Extraskeletal osteosarcomas, like osteosarcomas of bone, range from tumors that resemble fibrosarcoma or malignant fibrous histiocytoma (*fibroblastic osteosarcoma*) to extremely cellular tumors with an irregular round or spindle cell pattern with considerable pleomorphism and mitotic activity (*osteoblastic osteosarcoma*). Usually the osteoid is deposited in a fine, ramifying, lace-like or coarsely trabecular pattern, occasionally showing transitions toward sheaths of osteoid or mature-appearing bone (Figs. 35–25, 35–26, 35–27) Unlike in myositis ossificans where the most mature portion is located at the periphery, there is often a "reverse zoning phenomenon" (i.e., central deposition of osteoid material and atypical spindle cell proliferation at the periphery). Atypical cartilage of variable cellularity, with or without myxoid areas or focal bone formation, is present in many cases (Fig. 35–28), but it rarely becomes a dominating feature (*chondroblastic osteosarcoma*). There is also a varying number of benign and malignant multinucleated giant cells of the osteoclastic type that are often associated with hemorrhage (*osteoclastic* or *giant cell osteosarcoma*) (Fig. 35–29). The vascular pattern varies substantially. Occasional lesions with markedly dilated vascular spaces resemble a vascular tumor (*telangiectatic osteosarcoma*)[118,139] (Fig. 35–30). Well differentiated forms resembling parosteal osteosarcoma, and tumors with a small-cell pattern (*small-cell osteosarcoma*) have also been described[107,159] (Fig. 35–31). Metastatic lesions closely resemble their primary neoplasms.

Like many other mesenchymal tumors, extraskeletal

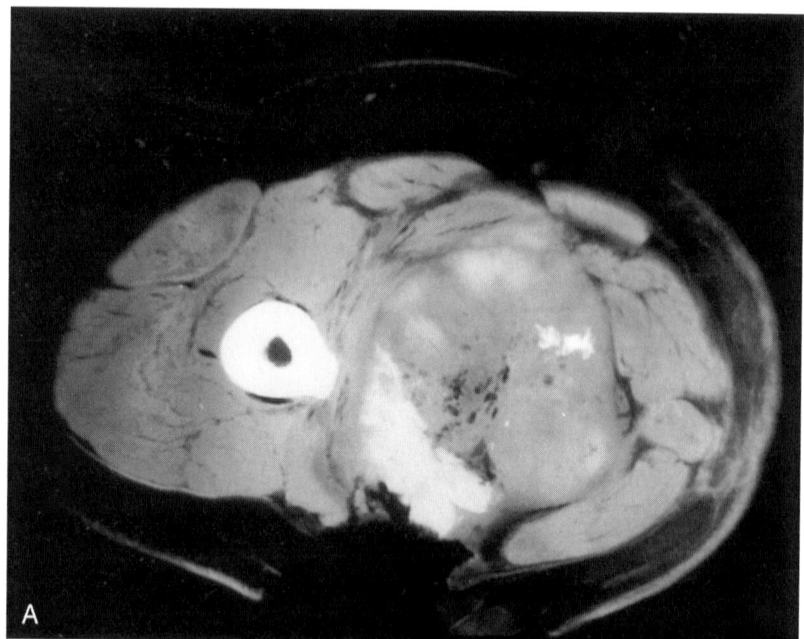


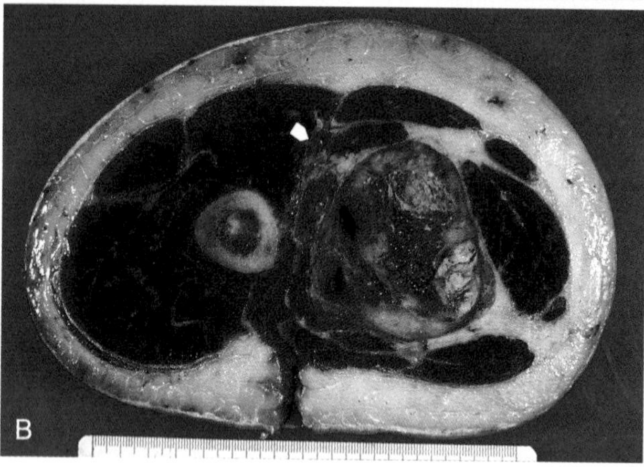


**FIGURE 35–24.** Computed tomography scan (**A**) and cross-section of extraskeletal osteosarcoma of the thigh (**B**). Note the circumscription of the tumor, areas of hemorrhage, and the absence of bone involvement.

osteosarcomas stain positively for vimentin. More recently, monoclonal antibodies to osteocalcin and osteonectin have been utilized to recognize skeletal and extraskeletal osteosarcoma.[111,121,122,148,151] Fanburg-Smith et al.[122] found that an antibody to osteocalcin was 82% sensitive for extraskeletal osteosarcoma neoplastic cells, with immunostaining of neoplastic cells away from bone in 91% of cases and in 75% for bony tumor matrix. They reported 100% specificity for osteoblasts, as this antigen was nonreactive in all nonbone cells. However, an antibody to osteonectin was not specific for osteoblasts. Focal positivity for desmin, actin, S-100 protein, and cytokeratins has been reported in some cases.[128]

## Ultrastructural Findings

There are only a few studies of the ultrastructural features of extraskeletal osteosarcoma, but all indicate that they are indistinguishable from those found in primary osteosarcoma of bone.[129,146] Characteristically, the tumor cells vary considerably in appearance. They have irregularly shaped, large nuclei with crenated or indented nuclear membranes. There is a prominent endoplasmic reticulum that ranges from narrow tubular to markedly dilated structures, often enveloping mitochondria and having a finely granular content. There are also scattered free ribosomes, a well developed Golgi complex, varying amounts of filamentous material, and occasional lysosomes and lipid inclusions. Pinocytotic vesicles and desmosomes or tight junctions are absent or rare. Rao et al.[145] described, in addition, a cell with "interdigitating short processes, abundant filaments, and scarce endoplasmic reticulum." Occasionally there are multinucleated osteoclast-like giant cells with numerous mitochondria and multiple cellular processes.[156,157] The extracellular spaces contain a feltwork of interlacing collagen fi-

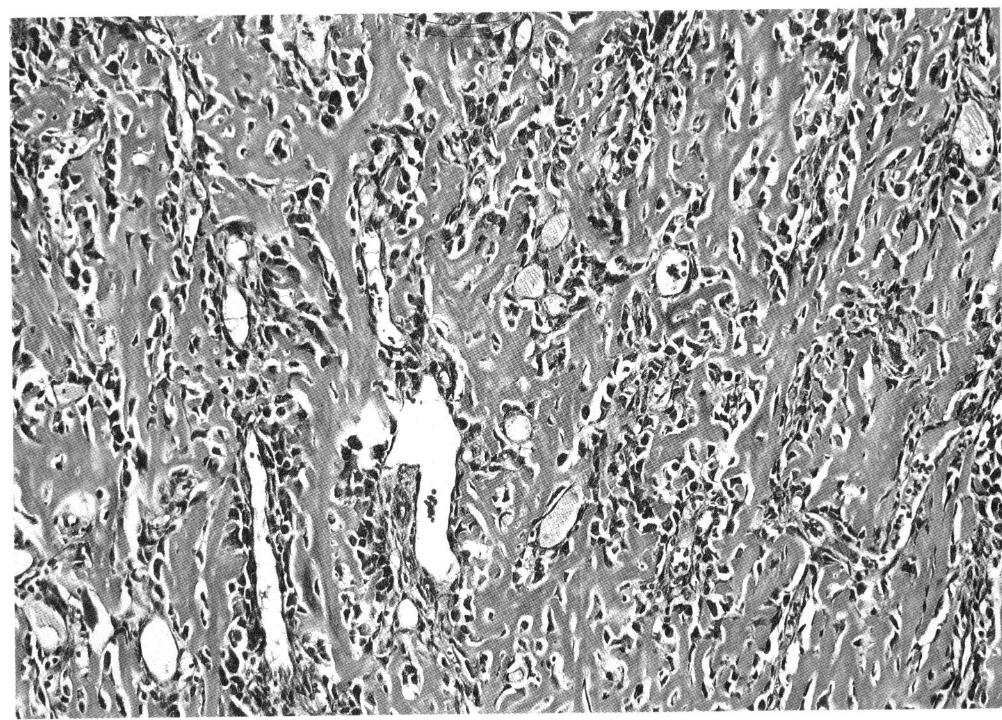

**FIGURE 35–25.** Extraskeletal osteosarcoma with large hyperchromatic cells separated by hyalinized collagen and osteoid.

bers, sometimes with scattered delicate electron-dense particles and deposits of needle-shaped, crystalline hydroxyapatite.

## Differential Diagnosis

It is not always easy to distinguish extraskeletal osteosarcoma from other benign and malignant bone- and cartilage-forming soft tissue lesions. The differentiation from myositis ossificans and other reactive reparative processes has already been discussed (Table 35–1). Among malignant tumors, metaplastic bone is infrequently found in synovial sarcoma, epithelioid sarcoma, malignant fibrous histiocytoma, liposarcoma, malignant melanoma, and other mesenchymal or epithelial neoplasms. In most of these neoplasms osteoid or bone is confined to a small portion of the tumor and is relatively well differentiated without the disorderly pattern and cellular pleomorphism of osteosarcoma. For some of them, however, it is exceedingly difficult to reach a definitive diagnosis and to exclude osteosarcoma. In fact, at times the only distinguishing feature between extraskeletal osteosarcoma and malignant fibrous histiocytoma with metaplastic bone are the relatively small amounts of neoplastic osteoid and bone in the latter tumor. According to Dorfman and Bhagavan,[117] the presence of the osseous and chondroid elements in the fibrous septa and pseudocapsule favor malignant fibrous histiocytoma. Bane et al.[107] believed that the production of any neoplastic osteoid or bone in a malignant fibrohistiocytic tumor, no matter how focal, warrants a diagnosis of osteosarcoma. Thus the distinction between malignant fibrous histiocytomas with bone and extraskeletal osteosarcomas is sometimes arbitrary, residing with the definitional criteria of the author.

Parosteal osteosarcoma may also make its appearance as a bulky lobulated densely ossified extraosseous mass focally indistinguishable from an extraskeletal osteosarcoma. In most cases this relatively low grade tumor can be positively identified by its greater overall differentiation, its broad attachment to a thickened cortical bone, and its tendency to encircle the shaft of the bone and cause cortical erosion.[119,152] Differential diagnostic considerations must also include periosteal osteogenic sarcoma,[153] a more aggressive and less well differentiated osteoblastic tumor that is often marked by a prominent chondroblastic component, and the rare "high grade surface osteosarcoma."[158]

## Prognosis

The outlook is grave, and most patients with this tumor succumb to metastatic growth within 2–3 years after the initial diagnosis. In the series by Bane

*Text continued on page 1414*

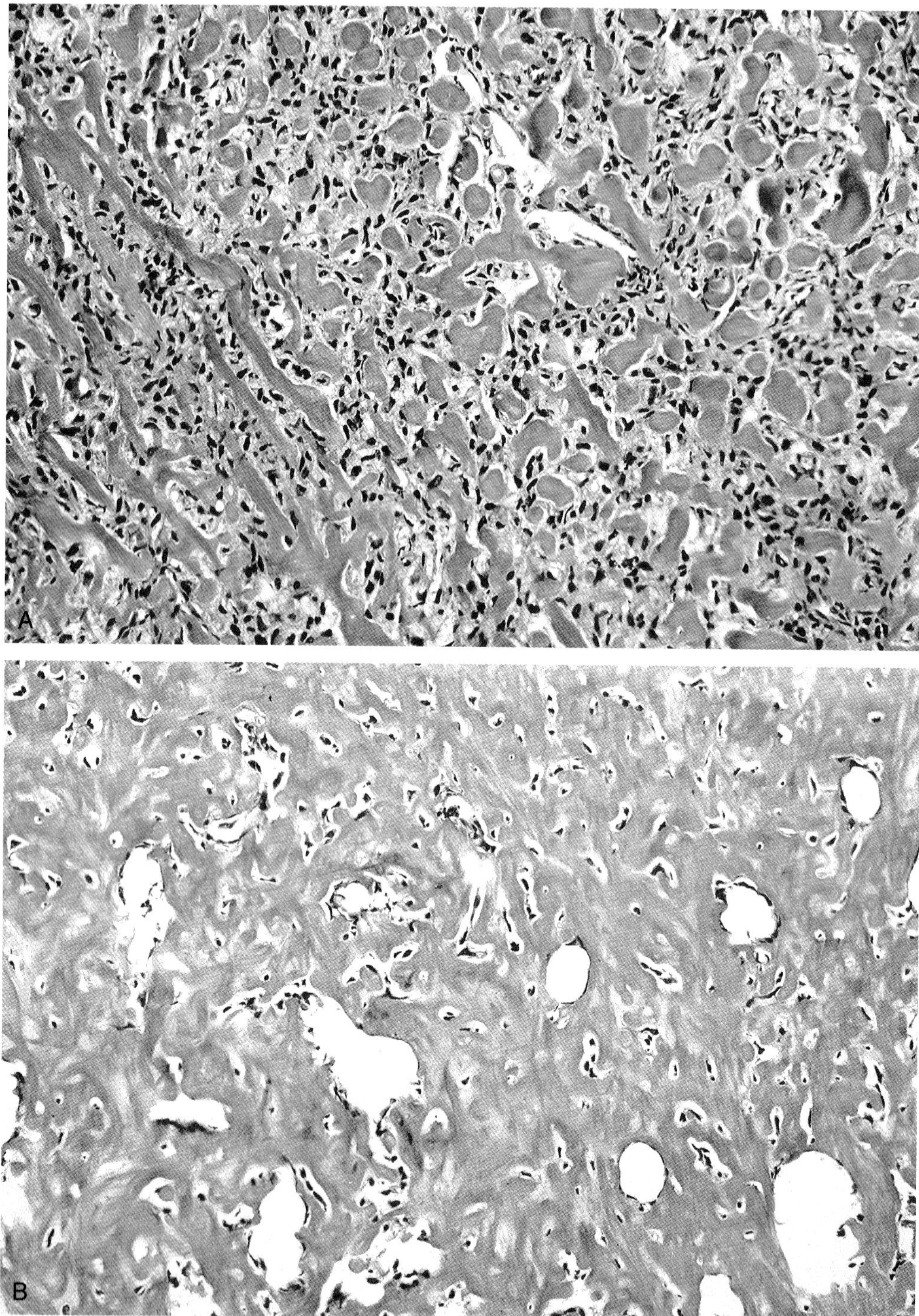


**FIGURE 35–26.** Extraskeletal osteosarcoma of the retroperitoneum. (**A**) Malignant cells are compressed by osteoid material. (**B**) In this portion of the tumor there is a broad expanse of osteoid with relatively few malignant cells.

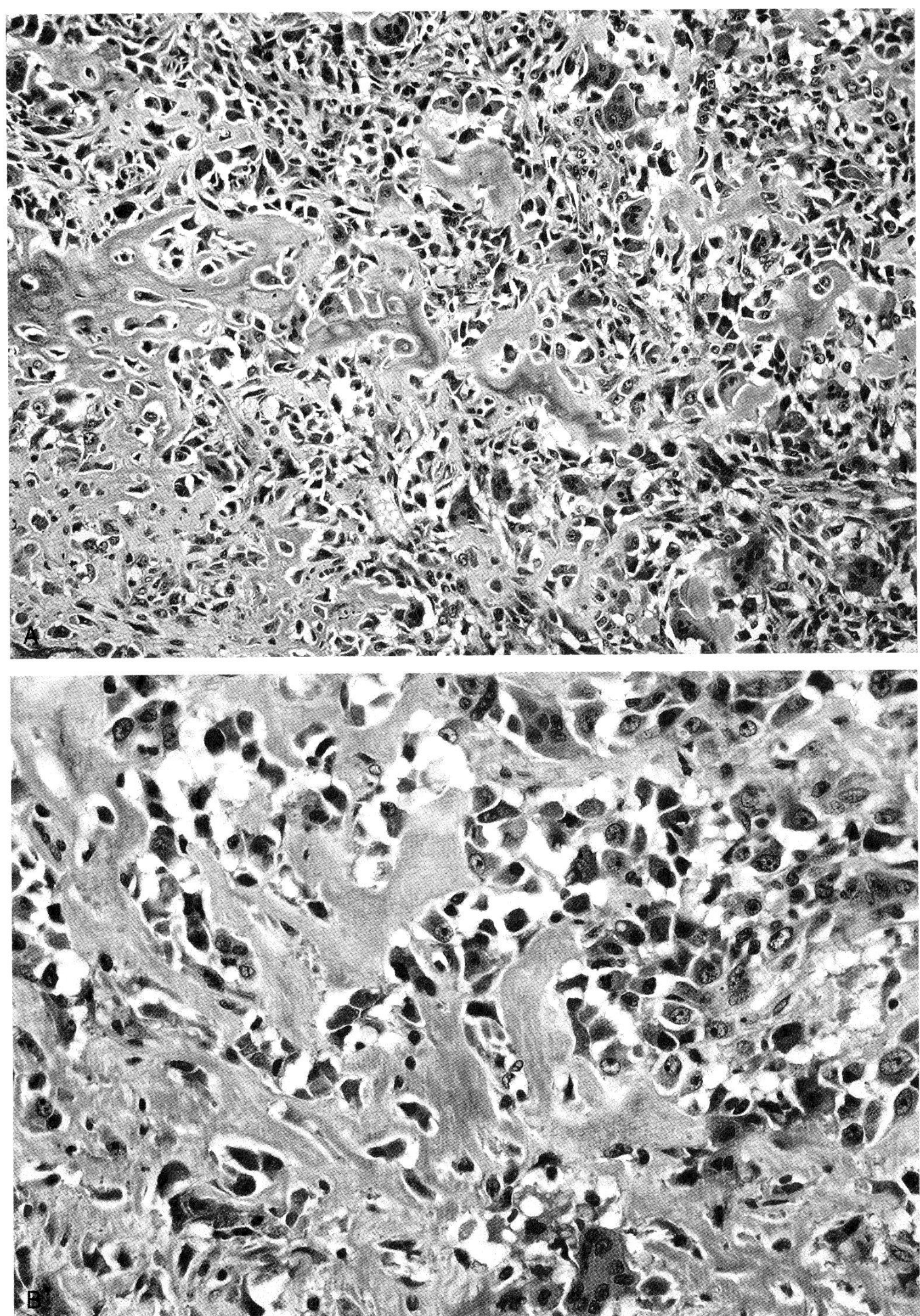


**FIGURE 35–27.** (**A**) Extraskeletal osteosarcoma of the thigh. Bands of osteoid material are seen between pleomorphic spindle-shaped and epithelioid cells. (**B**) High magnification view of malignant cells depositing osteoid in an extraskeletal osteosarcoma.

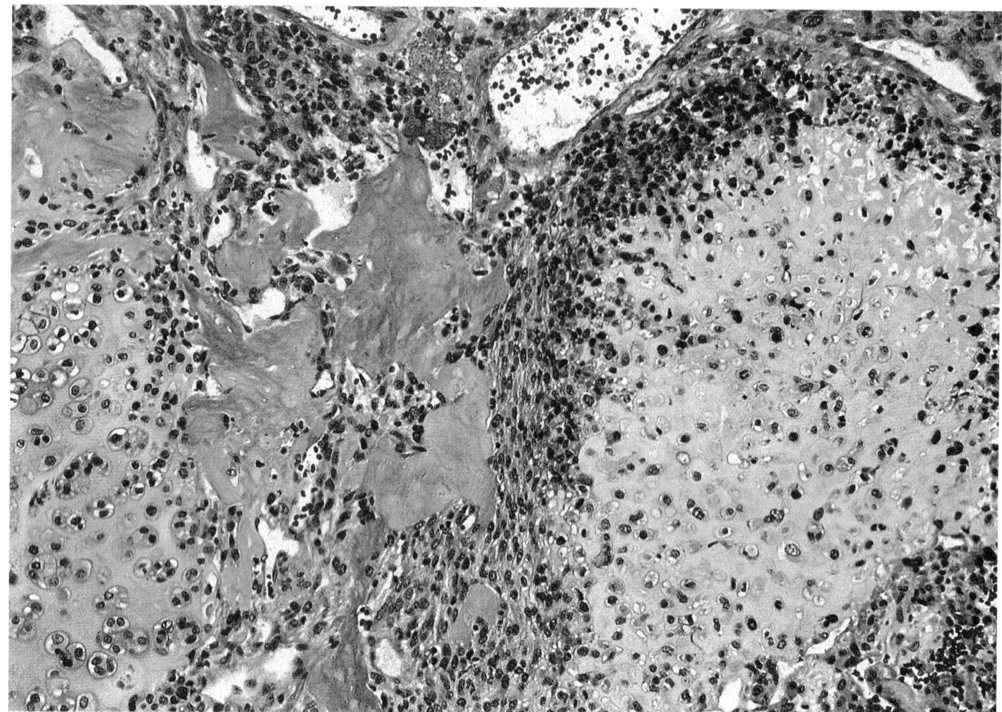

**FIGURE 35–28.** Osteoblastic osteosarcoma with chondroblastic and osteoblastic areas adjacent to one another.

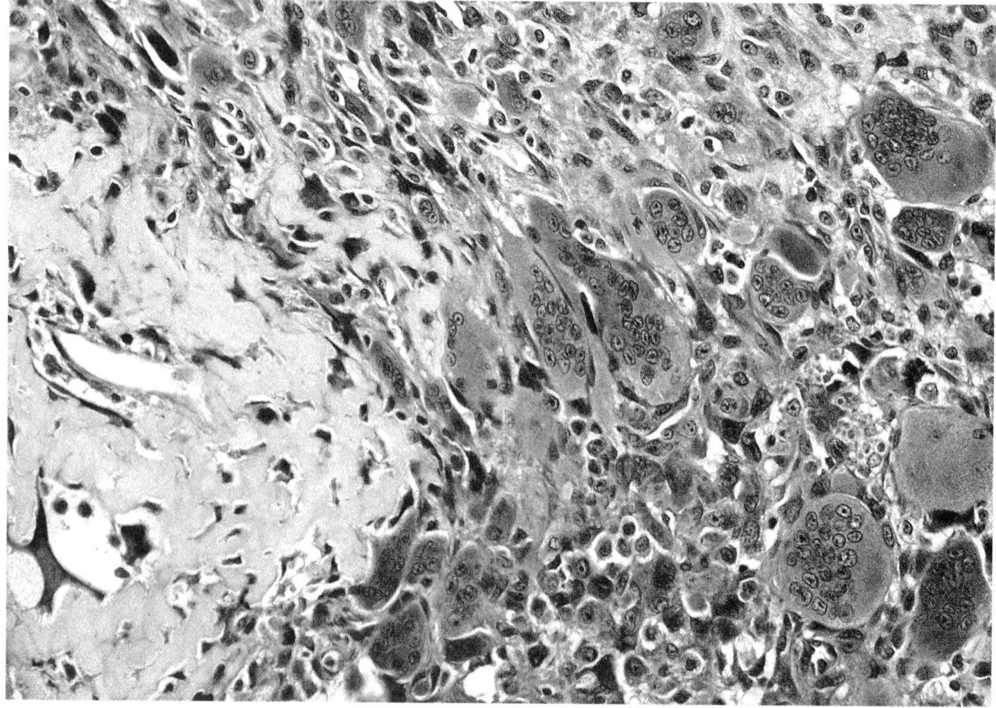

**FIGURE 35–29.** Osteoclast-like giant cells in an extraskeletal osteosarcoma.

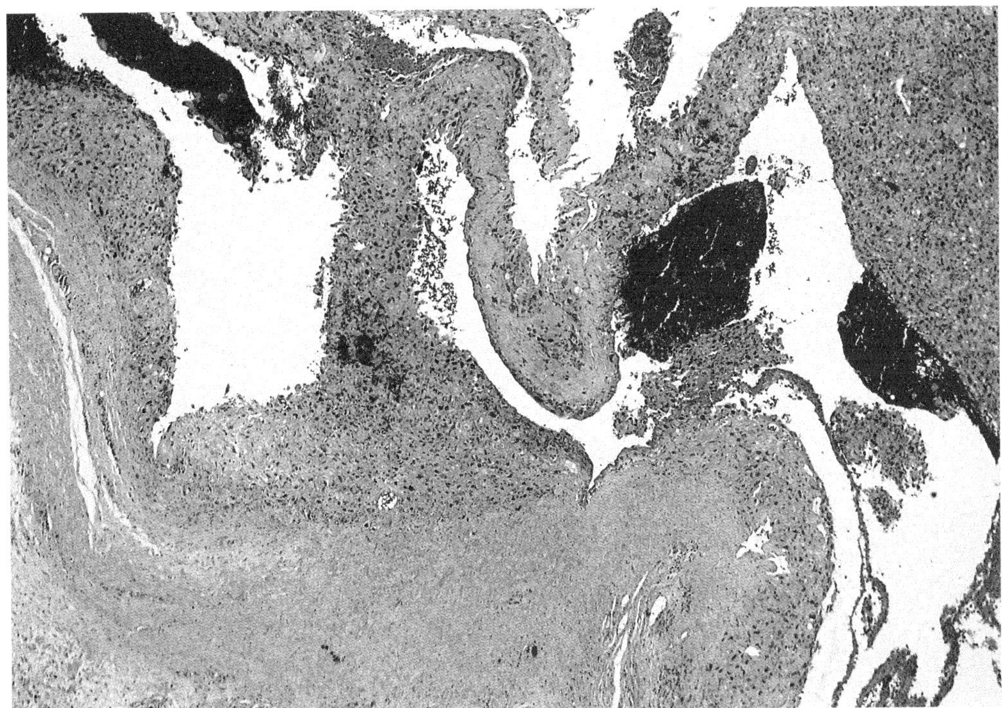

**FIGURE 35–30.** Telangiectatic extraskeletal osteosarcoma with markedly dilated blood-filled spaces lined by pleomorphic tumor cells.

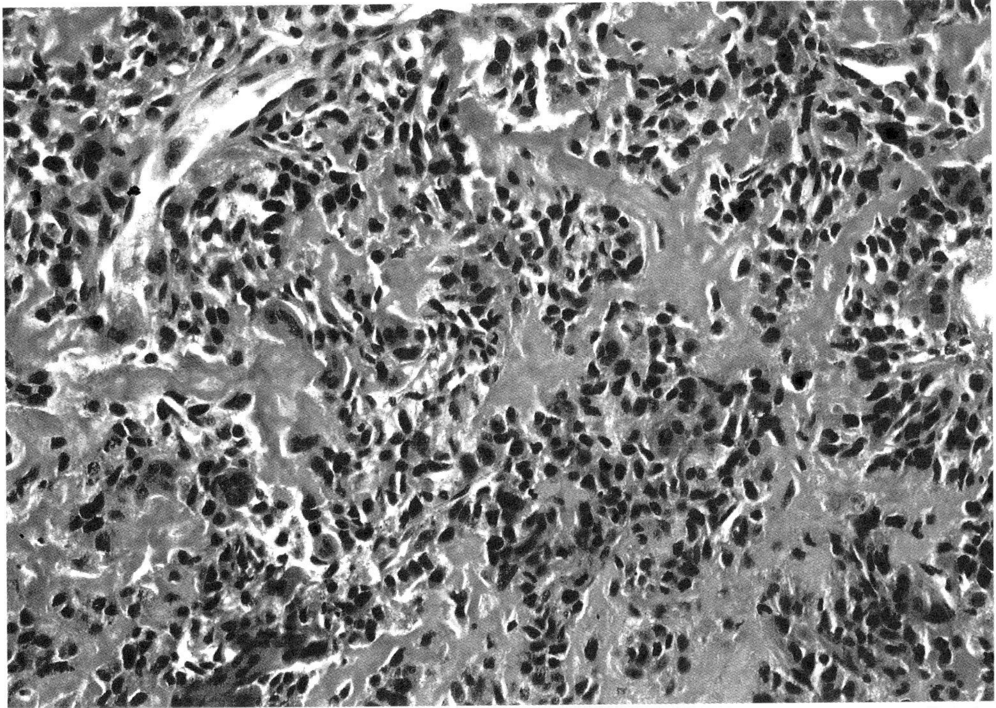

**FIGURE 35–31.** Extraskeletal osteosarcoma composed predominantly of small round cells adjacent to bands of osteoid.

et al.,[107] 13 (50%) of 26 tumors recurred locally and 16 (61.5%) metastasized; five patients had distant metastases at presentation. Similarly, Lee et al.[133] reported local recurrences and distant metastases in 45% and 65% of patients, respectively, with 33 of 40 patients (83%) dying of tumor during the follow-up period. The lungs constitute the most common metastatic site, followed by the liver, bones, regional lymph nodes, and soft tissue. Despite the dismal prognosis, combination therapy with radical surgery (possibly limb-sparing segmental resection as an alternative to amputation), radiotherapy, and sequential preoperative or postoperative chemotherapy[143] should be carried out in the hope of improving survival.

Tumor size, histologic subtype, and proliferation index have been proposed as prognostic variables. Bane et al.[107] found that a tumor size of 5 cm or more was an unfavorable prognostic indicator, although tumor size was not found to be of prognostic significance in several other reports.[128,133] Chung and Enzinger[114] found that patients with the fibroblastic type of extraskeletal osteosarcoma had a slightly better prognosis than those with other histologic subtypes, whereas Lee et al.[133] reported that patients with the chondroblastic type fared slightly better. Others were unable to correlate the histologic subtype with prognosis.[107,128] The Ki-67 proliferation index was correlated with survival in the study by Jensen et al.,[128] with significantly longer survival in patients with tumors with Ki-67 indices less than 24%.

## REFERENCES

### Myositis Ossificans and Related Lesions


1. Ackerman LV. Extra-osseous localized non-neoplastic bone and cartilage formation (so-called myositis ossificans): clinical and pathological confusion with malignant neoplasms. J Bone Joint Surg Am 40:279, 1958.
2. Ackman JB, Rosenthal DI. Generalized periarticular myositis ossificans as a complication of pharmacologically induced paralysis. Skeletal Radio l 24:395, 1995.
3. Akrengart L. Periarticular heterotopic ossification after total hip arthroplasty: risk factors and consequences. Clin Orthop 263:49, 1991.
4. Alling CC, Martinez MG, Ballard JB, et al. Osteoma cutis. J Oral Surg 32:195, 1974.
5. Asa DK, Bertorini TE, Pinals RS. Myositis ossificans circumscripta: a complication of tetanus. Am J Med Sci 292:40, 1986.
6. Chalmers J, Gray DH, Rush J. Observations on the induction of bone in soft tissues. J Bone Joint Surg Br 57:36, 1975.
7. Chaplin DM, Harrison MHM. Pseudomalignant osseous tumor of soft tissue: report of two cases. J Bone Joint Surg Br 54:334, 1972.
8. Costello FV, Brown A. Myositis ossificans complicating anterior poliomyelitis. J Bone Joint Surg Br 33:594, 1951.
9. Cushner FD, Morwessel RM. Myositis ossificans in children. Orthopedics 18:287, 1995.
10. Dahl I, Angervall L. Pseudosarcomatous proliferative lesions of soft tissue with or without bone formation. Acta Pathol Microbiol Scand 85A:577, 1977.
11. De Smet AA, Norris MA, Fisher DR. Magnetic resonance imaging of myositis ossificans: analysis of seven cases. Skeletal Radiol 21:503, 1992.
12. Fawcett HA. Hereditary osteoma cutis. J R Soc Med 76:697, 1983.
13. Freiberg JA. Para-articular calcification and ossification following acute anterior poliomyelitis in an adult. J Bone Joint Surg Am 34:339, 1952.
14. Hardy AG, Dickson JW. Pathological ossification in traumatic paraplegia. J Bone Joint Surg Br 45:76, 1963.
15. Hess WE. Myositis ossificans occurring in poliomyelitis. Arch Neurol Psychiatry 66:606, 1951.
16. Howard CB, Porat S, Bar-Oon E, et al. Traumatic myositis ossificans of the quadriceps in infants. J Pediatr Orthop 7:80, 1998.
17. Huvos AG. The spontaneous transformation of benign into malignant soft tissue tumors (with emphasis on extraskeletal osseous, lipomatous, and schwannian lesions). Am J Surg Pathol (Suppl) 9:7, 1985.
18. Järvi OH, Kvist HTA, Vainio PV. Extraskeletal retroperitoneal osteosarcoma probably arising from myositis ossificans. Acta Pathol Microbiol Scand 74:11, 1968.
19. Johnson MK, Lawrence JF. Metaplastic bone formation (myositis ossificans) in the soft tissues of the hand. J Bone Joint Surg Am 57:999, 1975.
20. Jouve JL, Cottalorda J, Bollini G, et al. Myositis ossificans: report of seven cases in children. J Pediatr Orthop 6:33, 1997.
21. Kransdorf MJ, Meis JM. Extraskeletal osseous and cartilaginous tumors of the extremities. Radiographics 13:853, 1993.
22. Kransdorf MJ, Meis JM, Jelinek JS. Myositis ossificans: MR appearance with radiologic-pathologic correlation. AJR 157:1243, 1991.
23. Lagier R, Cox JN. Pseudomalignant myositis ossificans. Hum Pathol 6:653, 1975.
24. Lehrman A, Pratt JH, Parkhill EM. Heterotopic bone in laparotomy scars. Am J Surg 104:591, 1962.
25. Marteinsson B, Musgrove J. Heterotopic bone formation in abdominal incisions. Am J Surg 130:23, 1975.
26. Merchan EC, Sanchez-Herrera S, Valdazo GA, et al. Circumscribed myositis ossificans: report of nine cases without history of injury. Acta Orthop Belg 59:273, 1993.
27. Miller LF, O'Neill C. Myositis ossificans in paraplegics. J Bone Joint Surg Am 31:283, 1949.
28. Myoken Y, Sugata T, Tanaka S. Traumatic myositis ossificans of the temporal and masseter muscle. Br J Oral Maxillofac Surg 36:76, 1998.
29. Nisolle JF, Delaunois L, Trigaux JP. Myositis ossificans of the chest wall. Eur Respir J 9:178, 1996.
30. Norman A, Dorfman HD. Juxtacortical circumscribed myositis ossificans: evolution and radiographic features. Radiology 96:301, 1970.
31. Pack GT, Braund RR. Development of sarcoma in myositis ossificans. JAMA 119:776, 1942.
32. Povysil C, Matejovsky Z. Ultrastructural evidence of myofibroblasts in pseudomalignant myositis ossificans. Virchows Arch [Pathol Anat] 381:189, 1979.
33. Roth SI, Stowell RE, Helwig EB. Cutaneous ossification: report of 120 cases and review of the literature. Arch Pathol 76:44, 1963.
34. Rothberg AS. Tendinitis ossificans traumatica. Am J Surg 58:285, 1942.
35. Shanoff LB, Spira M, Hardy S. Myositis ossificans: evolution to osteogenic sarcoma. Am J Surg 113:537, 1967.
36. Shirkhoda A, Armin AR, Bis KG, et al. MR imaging of myositis ossificans: variable patterns at different stages. J Magn Res Imaging 5:287, 1995.
37. Steiner M, Gould AR, Cushner GM, et al. Myositis ossificans

traumatica of the masseter muscle: review of the literature and report of two additional cases. Oral Surg Oral Med Oral Pathol Oral Radiol Endod 84:703, 1997.
38. Sumiyoshi K, Tsuneyoshi M, Enjoji M. Myositis ossiificans: a clinicopathologic study of 21 cases. Acta Pathol Jpn 35:1109, 1985.
39. Tompkins GS, Lachiewicz PF. Myositis ossificans after tetanus: treatment aided by quantitative technetium Tc 99m pyrophosphate radionuclide imaging. J South Orthop Assoc 4:239, 1995.
40. Wasman JK, Willis J, Makley J, et al. Myositis ossificans-like lesion of nerve. Histopathology 30:75, 1997.
41. Wilson JD, Montague CJ, Salcuni P, et al. Heterotopic mesenteric ossification ('intraabdominal myositis ossificans'): report of five cases. Am J Surg Pathol 23:1464, 1999.
42. Wittenberg RH, Peschke U, Botel U. Heterotopic ossification after spinal cord injury: epidemiology and risk factors. J Bone Joint Surg Br 74:215, 1992.
43. Woolgar JA, Beirne JC, Triantafyllou A. Myositis ossificans traumatica of sternocleiomastoid muscle presenting as cervical lymph-node metastasis. Int J Oral Maxillofac Surg 24:170, 1995.
44. Yagmai I. Myositis ossificans: diagnostic value of arteriography. AJR 128:811, 1977.

### Fibroosseous Pseudotumor of the Digits

45. Angervall L, Stener B, Stener I, et al. Pseudomalignant osseous tumor of soft tissue. J Bone Joint Surg Br 51:654, 1969.
46. Chan KW, Khoo US, Ho CM. Fibroosseous pseudotumor of the digits: report of a case with immunohistochemical and ultrastructural studies. Pathology 25:193, 1993.
47. Dorfman HD, Czerniak B. Reactive and metabolic conditions simulating neoplasms of bone. In: Bone Tumors. Mosby, St. Louis, 1998, p 1143.
48. Dupree WB, Enzinger FM. Fibroosseous pseudotumor of the digits. Cancer 58:2103, 1986.
49. Horie Y, Morimura T. Fibro-osseous pseudotumor of the digits arising in the subungual region: a rare benign lesion simulating extraskeletal osteosarcoma. Pathol Int 45:536, 1995.
50. Landsman JC, Shall JF, Seitz WH, et al. Florid reactive periostitis of the digits. Orthop Rev 19:831, 1990.
51. Lindeque BG, Simson IW, Fourie PA. Bizarre parosteal osteochondromatous proliferation of a phalanx. Arch Orthop Trauma Surg 110:58, 1990.
52. McCarthy EF, Ireland DCR, Sprague BL, et al. Parosteal (nodular) fasciitis of the hand. J Bone Joint Surg Am 58:714, 1976.
53. Meneses MF, Unni KK, Swee RG. Bizarre parosteal osteochondromatous proliferation of bone (Nora's lesion). Am J Surg Pathol 17:691, 1993.
54. Nora FE, Dahlin DC, Beabout JW. Bizarre parosteal osteochondromatous proliferations of the hands and feet. Am J Surg Pathol 7:245, 1983.
55. Patel MR, Desai SS. Pseudomalignant osseous tumor of soft-tissue: a case report and review of literature. J Hand Surg [Am] 11:66, 1986.
56. Prevel CD, Hanel DP. Fibro-osseous pseudotumor of the distal phalanx. Ann Plast Surg 36:321, 1996.
57. Schutte HE, van der Heul RO. Pseudomalignant, nonneoplastic osseous soft-tissue tumors of hands and foot. Radiology 176:149, 1990.
58. Sleater J, Mullins D, Chun K, et al. Fibro-osseous pseudotumor of the digit: a comparison to myositis ossificans by light microscopy and immunohistochemical methods. J Cutan Pathol 23:373, 1995.
59. Spjut HJ, Dorfman HD. Florid reactive periostitis of the tubular bones of the hands and feet: a benign lesion which may simulate osteosarcoma. Am J Surg Pathol 5:423, 1981.
60. Tang JB, Gu YQ, Xia RG, et al. Fibro-osseous pseudotumor that may be mistaken for a malignant tumor in the hand: a case report and review of the literature. J Hand Surg [Am] 21:714, 1996.

### Fibrodysplasia (Myositis) Ossificans Progressiva

61. Baysal T, Elmali N, Kutlu R, et al. The Stoneman: myositis (fibrodysplasia) ossificans progressiva. Eur Radiol 8:479, 1998.
62. Brantus J-F, Meunier PJ. Effects of intravenous etidronate and oral corticosteroids in fibrodysplasia ossificans progressiva. Clin Orthop 346:117, 1998.
63. Bronsky D, Kushner DS, Dubin A, et al. Idiopathic hypoparathyroidism and pseudohypoparathyroidism: case report and review of the literature. Medicine 27:317, 1958.
64. Calvert GT, Shore EM. Human leukocyte antigen B27 allele is not correlated with fibrodysplasia ossificans progressiva. Clin Orthop 346:66, 1998.
65. Caron KH, DiPietro MA, Aisen AM, et al. MR imaging of early fibrodysplasia ossificans progressiva. J Comput Assist Tomogr 14:318, 1990.
66. Cohen RB, Hahn GV, Tabas JA, et al. The natural history of heterotopic ossification in patients who have fibrodysplasia ossificans progressiva: a study of forty-four patients. J Bone Joint Surg Am 75:215, 1993.
67. Connor JM. Fibrodysplasia ossificans progressiva-lessons from rare maladies. N Engl J Med 335:591, 1996.
68. Connor JM, Evans DAP. Fibrodysplasia ossificans progressiva: the clinical features and natural history of 34 patients. J Bone Joint Surg Am 64:76, 1982.
69. Connor JM, Skirton H, Lunt PW. A three-generation family with fibrodysplasia ossificans progressiva. J Med Genet 30:687, 1993.
70. Connor JM, Smith R. The cervical spine in fibrodysplasia ossificans progressiva. Br J Radiol 55:492, 1982.
71. Delatycki M, Rogers JG. The genetics of fibrodysplasia ossificans progressiva. Clin Orthop 346:15, 1998.
72. Dixon TF, Mulligan L, Nassim R, et al. Myositis ossificans progressiva: report of a case in which ACTH and cortisone failed to prevent reossification after excision of ectopic bone. J Bone Joint Surg Br 36:445, 1954.
73. Gannon FH, Kaplan FS, Olmsted E, et al. Bone morphogenetic protein 2/4 in early fibromatous lesions in fibrodysplasia ossificans progressiva. Hum Pathol 28:339, 1997.
74. Gannon FH, Valentine BA, Shore EM, et al. Acute lymphocytic infiltation in an extremely early lesion of fibrodysplasia ossificans progressiva. Clin Orthop 346:19, 1998.
75. Glaser DL, Rocke DN, Kaplan FS. Catastrophic falls in patients who have fibrodysplasia ossificans progressiva. Clin Orthop 346:110, 1998.
76. Gulaldi NC, Elahi N, Sasani J, et al. Tc-99m MDP scanning in a patient with extensive fibrodysplasia ossificans progressiva. Clin Nucl Med 20:188, 1995.
77. Janoff HB, Muenke M, Johnson LO, et al. Fibrodysplasia ossificans progressiva in two half—sisters: evidence for maternal mosaicism. Am J Med Genet 61:320, 1996.
78. Janoff HB, Tabas JA, Shore EM, et al. Mild expression of fibrodysplasia ossificans progressiva: a report of 3 cases. J Rheumatol 22:976, 1995.
79. Kaplan F, Sawyer J, Connors S, et al. Urinary basic fibroblast growth factor: a biochemical marker for preosseous fibroproliferative lesions in patients with fibrodysplasia ossificans progressiva. Clin Orthop 346:59, 1998.
80. Kaplan FS, McCluskey W, Hahn G, et al. Genetic transmission of fibrodysplasia ossificans progressiva: report of a family. J Bone Joint Surg Am 75:1214, 1993.
81. Kaplan FS, Strear CM, Zasloff MA. Radiographic and scintigraphic features of modeling and remodeling in the hetero-

topic skeleton of patients who have fibrodysplasia ossificans progressiva. Clin Orthop 304:238, 1994.

82. Kaplan FS, Tabas JA, Gannon FH, et al. The histopathology of fibrodysplasia ossificans progressiva: an endochondral process. J Bone Joint Surg Am 75:220, 1993.
83. Kussmaul WG, Esmail AN, Sagar Y, et al. Pulmonary and cardiac function in advanced fibrodysplasia ossificans progressiva. Clin Orthop 346:104, 1998.
84. Lanchoney TF, Cohen RB, Rocke DM, et al. Permanent heterotopic ossification at the injection site after diphtheria-tetanus-pertussus immunizations in children who have fibrodysplasia ossificans progressiva. J Pediatr 126:762, 1995.
85. Lanchoney TF, Olmsted EA, Shore EM, et al. Characterization of bone morphogenetic protein 4 receptor in fibrodysplasia ossificans progressiva. Clin Orthop 346:38, 1998.
86. Lopez de Castro JA. Structure, function, and disease association of HLA-B27. Curr Opin Rheumatol 6:371, 1994.
87. Maxwell WA, Spicer SS, Miller RL, et al. Histochemical and ultrastructural studies in fibrodysplasia ossificans progressiva (myositis ossificans progressiva). Am J Pathol 87:483, 1977.
88. O'Reilly M, Renton P. Metaphyseal abnormalities in fibrodysplasia ossificans progressiva. Br J Radiol 66:112, 1993.
89. Oz BB, Boneh A. Myositis fibrodysplasia ossificans progressiva: a 10-year follow-up on a patient treated with etidronate disodium. Acta Paediatr 83:1332, 1994.
90. Pazzaglia U, Beluffie G, Ravelli A, et al. Chronic intoxication by ethane-1-hydroxy-1, 1 disphosphonate EHDP in a child with myositis ossificans progressiva. Pediatr Radiol 23:439, 1993.
91. Rocke DM, Zasloff M, Peeper J, et al. Age- and joint-specific risk of initial heterotopic ossification in patients who have fibrodysplasia ossificans progressiva. Clin Orthop 301:243, 1994.
92. Rogers JG, Geho WB. Fibrodysplasia ossificans progressiva: a survey of 42 cases. J Bone Joint Surg Am 61:909, 1979.
93. Rosborough D. Ectopic bone formation associated with multiple anomalies. J Bone Joint Surg Br 48:499, 1966.
94. Sawyer JR, Klimkiewicz JJ, Iannotti JP, et al. Mechanism for superior subluxation of the glenohumeral joint in fibrodysplasia ossificans progressiva. Clin Orthop 346:130, 1998.
95. Schroeder HW, Zasloff M. The hand and foot malformations in fibrodysplasia ossificans progressiva. Johns Hopkins Med J 147:73, 1980.
96. Shafritz AB, Shore EM, Gannon FH, et al. Overexpression of an osteogenic morphogen in fibrodysplasia ossificans progressiva. N Engl J Med 355:555, 1996.
97. Smith R. Fibrodysplasia (myositis) ossificans progressiva: clinical lessons from a rare disease period. Clin Orthop 346:7, 1998.
98. Van den Wijngaard A, Weghuis DO, Boersma CJC, et al. Fine mapping of human bone morphogenetic protein-4 gene (BMP4) to chromosome 14q22-q23 by in situ hybridisation. Genomics 27:559, 1995.
99. Wozney JM, Rosen V. Bone morphogenetic protein and bone morphogenetic protein gene family in bone formation and repair. Clin Orthop 346:26, 1998.
100. Xu M, Shore EM. Mutational screening of the bone morphogenetic protein 4 gene in a family with fibrodysplasia ossificans progressiva. Clin Orthop 346:53, 1998.
101. Young JW. Case report 314: diagnosis: juvenile dermatomyositis with changes of the hallux typical of fibrodysplasia (myositis) ossificans progressiva. Skeletal Radiol 13:318, 1985.
102. Youssef L, Schmidt TL. Battered child syndrome simulating myositis. J Pediatr Orthop 3:392, 1983.
103. Zasloff MA, Rocke DM, Crofford LJ, et al. Treatment of patients who have fibrodysplasia ossificans progressiva with isotretinoin. Clin Orthop 346:121, 1998.

### Extraskeletal Osteosarcoma

104. Allan CJ, Soule EH. Osteogenic sarcoma of the somatic soft tissues: clinicopathologic study of 26 cases and review of the literature. Cancer 27:1121, 1971.
105. Ascenzi A, Casagrande A, Ribotta G. On radiation-induced extraskeletal osteosarcoma: report of a case. Tumori 66:261, 1980.
106. Bacetic D, Knezevic M, Stogsic Z, et al. Primary extraskeletal osteosarcoma of the penis with a malignant fibrous histiocytoma-like component. Histopathology 33:184, 1998.
107. Bane BL, Evans HL, Ro JY, et al. Extraskeletal osteosarcoma: a clinicopathologic review of 26 cases. Cancer 65:2726, 1990.
108. Beiswanger JC, Woodruff RD, Savage PD, et al. Primary osteosarcoma of the spermatic cord with synchronous bilateral renal cell carcinoma. Urology 49:957, 1997.
109. Belasco JB, Meadoves AC. Extraskeletal osteogenic sarcoma after treatment of Wilms' tumors. Cancer 50:1894, 1982.
110. Berry MP, Jenkin RD, Fornasier VL, et al. Osteosarcoma at the site of previous fracture: a case report. J Bone Joint Sug Am 62:1216, 1980.
111. Bosse A, Vollmer E, Bocker W, et al. The impact of osteonectin for differential diagnosis of bone tumors. Pathol Res Pract 186: 651, 1990.
112. Boyer CW, Navin JJ. Extraskeletal osteogenic sarcoma: a late complication of radiation therapy. Cancer 18:628, 1965.
113. Burke AP, Virmani R. Osteosarcomas of the heart. Am J Surg Pathol 15:289, 1991.
114. Chung EB, Enzinger FM. Extraskeletal osteosarcoma. Cancer 60:1132, 1987.
115. Dahm LJ, Schaefer SD, Carder HM, et al. Osteosarcoma of the soft tissue of the larynx: report of a case with light and electron microscopic studies. Cancer 42:2343, 1978.
116. De Nictolis M, Goteri G, Brancorsini D, et al. Extraskeletal osteosarcoma of the mediastinum associated with long-term patient survival: a case report. Anticancer Res 15:275, 1995.
117. Dorfman HD, Bhagavan BS. Malignant fibrous histiocytoma of soft tissue with metaplastic bone and cartilage formation. Skeletal Radiol 8:45, 1982.
118. Dubec JJ, Munk PL, O'Connell JX, et al. Soft tissue osteosarcoma with telangiectatic features: MR imaging findings in two cases. Skeletal Radiol 26:732, 1997.
119. Dwinnell LA, Dahlin DC, Ghormley RK. Parosteal (juxtacortical) osteogenic sarcoma. J Bone Joint Surg Am 36:732, 1954.
120. Eckardt JJ, Ivins JC, Perry HO, et al. Osteosarcoma arising in heterotopic ossification of dermatomyositis: case report and review of the literature. Cancer 48:1256, 1981.
121. Fanburg JC, Rosenberg AE, Weaver DL, et al. Osteocalcin and osteonectin immunoreactivity in the diagnosis of osteosarcoma. Am J Clin Pathol 108:464, 1997.
122. Fanburg-Smith JC, Bratthauer GL, Miettinen M. Osteocalcin and osteonectin immunoreactivity in extraskeletal osteosarcoma: a study of 28 cases. Hum Pathol 30:32, 1999.
123. Fang Z, Yokoyama R, Mukai K, et al. Extraskeletal osteosarcoma: a clinicopathologic study of four cases. Jpn J Clin Oncol 25:55, 1995.
124. Fine G, Stout AP. Osteogenic sarcoma of the extraskeletal soft tissues. Cancer 9:1027, 1956.
125. Hasson J, Hartman KS, Milikow E, et al. Thorotrast-induced extraskeletal osteosarcoma of the cervical region: report of a case. Cancer 36:1827, 1975.
126. Huvos AG. Osteogenic sarcoma of bones and soft tissues in older persons: a clinicopathologic analysis of 117 patients older than 60 years. Cancer 57:1442, 1986.
127. Järvi OH, Kvist HTA, Vainio PV. Extraskeletal retroperitoneal osteosarcoma probably arising from myositis ossificans. Acta Pathol Microbiol Scand 74:11, 1968.
128. Jensen ML, Schumacher B, Myhre Jensen O, et al. Extraskeletal

osteosarcomas: a clinicopathologic study of 25 cases. Am J Surg Pathol 22:588, 1998.

129. Katenkamp D, Stiller D, Waldmann G. Ultrastructural cytology of human osteosarcoma cells. Virchows Arch [Pathol Anat] 381:49, 1978.
130. Kauffman SL, Stout AP. Extraskeletal osteogenic sarcomas and chondrosarcomas in children. Cancer 16:432, 1963.
131. Laskin WB, Silverman TA, Enzinger FM. Postradiation soft tissue sarcomas: an analysis of 52 cases. Cancer 62:2330, 1988.
132. Lee JH, Griffiths WJ, Bottomley RH. Extraosseous osteogenic sarcoma following an intramuscular injection. Cancer 40:3097, 1977.
133. Lee JSY, Fetsch JF, Wasdhal DA, et al. A review of 40 patients with extraskeletal osteosarcoma. Cancer 76:2253, 1995.
134. Logue JP, Cairnduff F. Radiation induced extraskeletal osteosarcoma. Br J Radiol 64:171, 1991.
135. Loos JH, El-Naggar AK, Ro JY, et al. Primary osteosarcoma of the lung: report of two cases and review of the literature. J Thorac Cardiovasc Surg 100:867, 1990.
136. Lorentzon R, Larsson SE, Boquist L. Extra-osseous osteosarcoma: a clinical and histopathological study of four cases. J Bone Joint Surg Br 61:205, 1979.
137. Loyzaga JM, Fernandez Machin P, Sala J. Osteogenic sarcoma of the tongue: case report and review of the literature. Pathol Res Pract 192:75, 1996.
138. Martland HS. Occupational poisoning in manufacture of luminal watch dials. JAMA 92:466, 1929.
139. Mirra JM, Fain JS, Ward WG, et al. Extraskeletal telangiectatic osteosarcoma. Cancer 71:3014, 1993.
140. Moser RP Jr. Musculoskeletal case of the day: extraskeletal osteosarcoma of the thigh. AJR 162:1463, 1994.
141. Murphey MD, Robbin MR, McRae JA, et al. The many faces of osteosarcoma. Radiographics 17:1205, 1997.
142. Ohara M, Hayashi K, Shinohara C, et al. Primary osteosarcoma of the cerebrum with immunohistochemical and ultrastructural studies: report of a case. Acta Neuropathol (Berl) 88:384, 1994.
143. Patel SR, Benjamin RS. Primary extraskeletal osteosarcoma: experience with chemotherapy. J Natl Cancer Inst 87:1331, 1995.
144. Rachman R, Di Massa EV. Pelvic extraskeletal osteosarcoma associated with prostatic adenocarcinoma. Am J Clin Pathol 44:556, 1965.
145. Rao U, Cheng A, Didolkar MS. Extraosseous osteogenic sarcoma: clinicopathologic study of eight cases and review of literature. Cancer 41:1488, 1978.
146. Reddick RL, Michelitch HJ, Levine AM, et al. Osteogenic sarcoma: a study of the ultrastructure. Cancer 45:64, 1980.
147. Sacker AR, Oyama KK, Kessler S. Primary osteosarcoma of the penis. Am J Dermatopathol 16:285, 1994.
148. Serra M, Morini M, Scotlandi K, et al. Evaluation of osteonectin as a diagnostic marker of osteogenic bone tumors. Hum Pathol 23:1326, 1992.
149. Silver SA, Tavassoli FA. Primary osteogenic sarcoma of the breast: a clinicopathologic analysis of 50 cases. Am J Surg Pathol 22:925, 1998.
150. Sordillo PP, Hajdu SI, Magill GB, et al. Extraosseous osteogenic sarcoma: a review of 48 patients. Cancer 51:727, 1983.
151. Takada J, Ishii S, Ohta T, et al. Usefulness of a novel monoclonal antibody against human osteocalcin in immunohistochemical diagnosis. Virchows Arch A Pathol Anat Histopathol 420:507, 1992.
152. Unni KK, Dahlin DC, Beabout JW, et al. Parosteal osteogenic sarcoma. Cancer 37:2644, 1976.
153. Unni KK, Dahlin DC, Beabout JW, et al. Periosteal osteogenic sarcoma. Cancer 37:2476, 1976.
154. Varela-Duran J, Dehner LP. Postirradiation osteosarcoma in childhood: a clinicopathologic study of three cases and review of the literature. Am J Pediatr Hematol Oncol 2:263, 1980.
155. Varma DG, Ayala AG, Guo SQ, et al. MRI of extraskeletal osteosarcoma. J Comput Assist Tomogr 17:414, 1993.
156. Waxman M, Vuletin JC, Saxe BI, et al. Extraskeletal osteosarcoma: light and electron microscopic study. Mt Sinai J Med 48:322, 1981.
157. Williams AH, Schwinn CP, Parker JW. The ultrastructure of osteosarcoma: a review of 20 cases. Cancer 37:1293, 1976.
158. Wold LE, Unni KK, Beabout JW, et al. High-grade surface osteosarcomas. Am J Surg Pathol 8:181, 1984.
159. Yi ES, Shmookler BM, Malaver MM, et al. Well-differentiated extraskeletal osteosarcoma: a soft-tissue homologue of parosteal osteosarcoma. Arch Pathol Lab Med 115:906, 1991.
160. Young RH, Rosenberg AE. Osteosarcoma of the urinary bladder: report of a case and review of the literature. Cancer 59:174, 1987.

# CHAPTER 36

# BENIGN SOFT TISSUE TUMORS AND PSEUDOTUMORS OF MISCELLANEOUS TYPE

This chapter discusses a heterogeneous group of benign tumors or pseudotumors in which the line of differentiation is in question. Many of the lesions are characterized by abundant myxoid stroma (intramuscular myxoma, juxtaarticular myxoma, cutaneous myxoma, aggressive angiomyxoma, and ganglion, among others); there is evidence that the cells in these lesions are fibroblastic or have some features of myofibroblasts. Other lesions discussed in this chapter, particularly ossifying fibromyxoid tumor and parachordoma, are pathologic curiosities in which the differentiation (and in the case of parachordoma, its very existence) has been disputed since their initial descriptions. Nevertheless, these entities are characterized by clinical and pathologic features that make them unique, despite uncertainties as to their differentiation.

## TUMORAL CALCINOSIS

Tumoral calcinosis is a distinct clinical and histologic entity that is characterized by tumor-like periarticular deposits of calcium that are found foremost in the regions of the hip, shoulder, and elbow. The disorder occurs predominantly in otherwise healthy children, adolescents, and young adults, is more often multiple than solitary, and not infrequently affects two or more siblings of the same family. Unlike similar calcifications associated with renal insufficiency, hypervitaminosis D, and milk-alkali syndrome, there are no demonstrable abnormalities in calcium metabolism.

The term *tumoral calcinosis* was coined by Inclan in 1943,[15] but this condition was recognized as an entity much earlier. In 1899, Duret observed this process in siblings: a 17-year-old girl and her younger brother who had multiple calcifications in the neighborhood of the hip and elbow joint.[10] Later, in 1935, Teutschlaender gave a detailed account of another typical case, an 11-year-old girl with multiple lesions in the shoulder and elbow regions which had their onset at age 2 years. He thought that this process was secondary to fat necrosis and used the term "lipid calcinosis."[41–43] Since these descriptions, almost 250 acceptable examples of this growth have been reported under various names, including calcifying bursitis,[7] calcifying collagenolysis,[46] and Kikuyu bursa.[23] In New Guinea the natives aptly refer to it as "hip stones."[5,31]

### Clinical Findings

The principal manifestation of the disease is the presence of a large, firm, subcutaneous calcified mass that is asymptomatic and slowly growing, often gradually enlarging over many years; it is usually located in the vicinity of a large joint, especially the trochanteric and gluteal regions of the hip, the lateral portion of the shoulder, and the posterior elbow (Table 36–1). It is less frequent in the hands, feet, and knees. The lesion is firmly attached to the underlying fascia, muscle, or tendon and may infiltrate these structures, but it is unrelated to bone. Approximately two-thirds of patients have multiple lesions, some of which are bilateral and symmetric. The mass is usually asymptomatic and only rarely causes discomfort, tenderness, or pain. The underlying joints are unaffected, and with few exceptions patients with tumoral calcinosis are in good health. In fact, small and more deep-seated lesions are frequently overlooked and are often incidental findings during examination for some other

**TABLE 36–1 ANATOMIC LOCATIONS OF 105 CASES OF TUMORAL CALCINOSIS**

| Site | No. of Cases | % |
|---|---|---|
| Hips | 33 | 31 |
| Buttocks | 27 | 26 |
| Upper extremities | 16 | 15 |
| Lower extremities | 12 | 11 |
| Spine/sacrum | 7 | 7 |
| Miscellaneous | 10 | 10 |
| *Total* | 105 | 100 |

Modified from Pakasa NM, Kalengayi RM. Tumoral calcinosis: a clinicopathological study of 111 cases with emphasis on the earliest changes. Histopathology 31:18, 1997.

cause. Large lesions, measuring 20 cm or more in diameter, are not particularly rare.[33] Association with calcifying skin lesions, dental abnormalities, and angioid retinal streaks has been reported.[1,11,13,37]

Tumoral calcinosis typically has its onset during the first and second decades of life; it is rare in patients older than 50 years. Overall, males and females are about equally affected. In the series of Pakasa and Kalengayi,[33] males predominated over females at a ratio of 1.5:1.0 in patients who developed the disease during the first two decades of life; during adulthood, women were affected about twice as often. Approximately two-thirds of cases involve Blacks, predominantly African and African Americans.[17,28,33] About half affect siblings, and in some instances several generations of the same family are involved.[27,32,37] Complications of the disease are rare. Occasionally there is ulceration of the overlying skin with secondary infection, fistula formation, and discharge of a yellow-white chalky fluid.[33] There is no association with scleroderma or other collagen vascular diseases.

Laboratory examinations show no evidence of increased calcium levels, but in many patients there is slight to moderate hyperphosphatemia.[38,49] Calcitriol (1,25-dihydroxyvitamin $D_3$) may also be elevated, but serum alkaline phosphatase and uric acid levels are normal.

## Radiologic Findings

Examination with radiography or computed tomography (CT) reveals a subcutaneous conglomerate of multiple, rounded opacities separated by radiolucent lines (fibrous septa) imparting a "chicken wire" pattern of lucencies[39] with distinct fluid levels in some of the nodules[12] (Figs. 36–1, 36–2). There are no associated bony abnormalities; despite the large amounts of calcium in the lesion, there is no evidence of osteoporosis in the skeleton as in patients with renal insufficiency and secondary hyperparathyroidism. Scintigraphic examination is useful, especially for identifying multiple lesions and assessing therapy.[6] For instance, all seven patients reported by Balachandran et al.[3] had abnormal scintigrams with increased tracer concentration.

## Pathologic Findings

Study of the gross specimen discloses a firm, rubbery mass that is unencapsulated, extends into the adjacent muscles and tendons, and is usually 5–15 cm in greatest diameter. On sectioning, the mass consists of a framework of dense fibrous tissue containing spaces filled with yellow-gray, pasty, calcareous material or chalky, milky liquid that is easily washed out, resulting in irregular cystic cavities (Fig. 36–3). Chemical analysis of the intra- and extracellular calcified material reveals hydroxyapatite.[37]

Microscopically, active and inactive phases of the disease can be distinguished, often together in the same lesion (Figs. 36–4, 36–5). Slavin et. al.[37] proposed a three-stage classification scheme to describe these lesions, spanning from cellular lesions devoid of calcification to cellular cystic lesions with calcification, and finally hypocellular calcified lesions. In the active (cellular) phase, a central mass of amorphous or granular calcified material is bordered by a florid proliferation of mono- or multinuclear macrophages, osteoclast-like giant cells, fibroblasts, and chronic inflammatory elements. Pakasa and Kalengayi[33] described fibrohistiocytic nodules during the early proliferative phase characterized by fibroblast-like cells, foamy histiocytes, occasional mononuclear macrophages, and hemosiderin-laden macrophages. During the inactive phase there is merely calcified material surrounded by dense fibrous material extending into the adjacent tissues or a cystic space surrounded by calcium deposits. Sometimes the calcified material forms small psammoma body-like masses with concentric layering of calcium (calcospherites) that bear a superficial resemblance to ova of parasites (Fig. 36–6). Examination with electron microscopy reveals histiocytes with and without lipid inclusions, needle-shaped hydroxyapatite crystals, crystalline aggregates with a dense central core, and laminated calcospherites.[14,19] Hydroxyapatite crystals and noncrystalline calcific deposits arise primarily in intracytoplasmic membrane-bound vesicles and mitochondria.

## Differential Diagnosis

Morphologically, identical periarticular lesions may be encountered in patients with chronic renal disease and secondary hyperparathyroidism,[25,26,34] but most

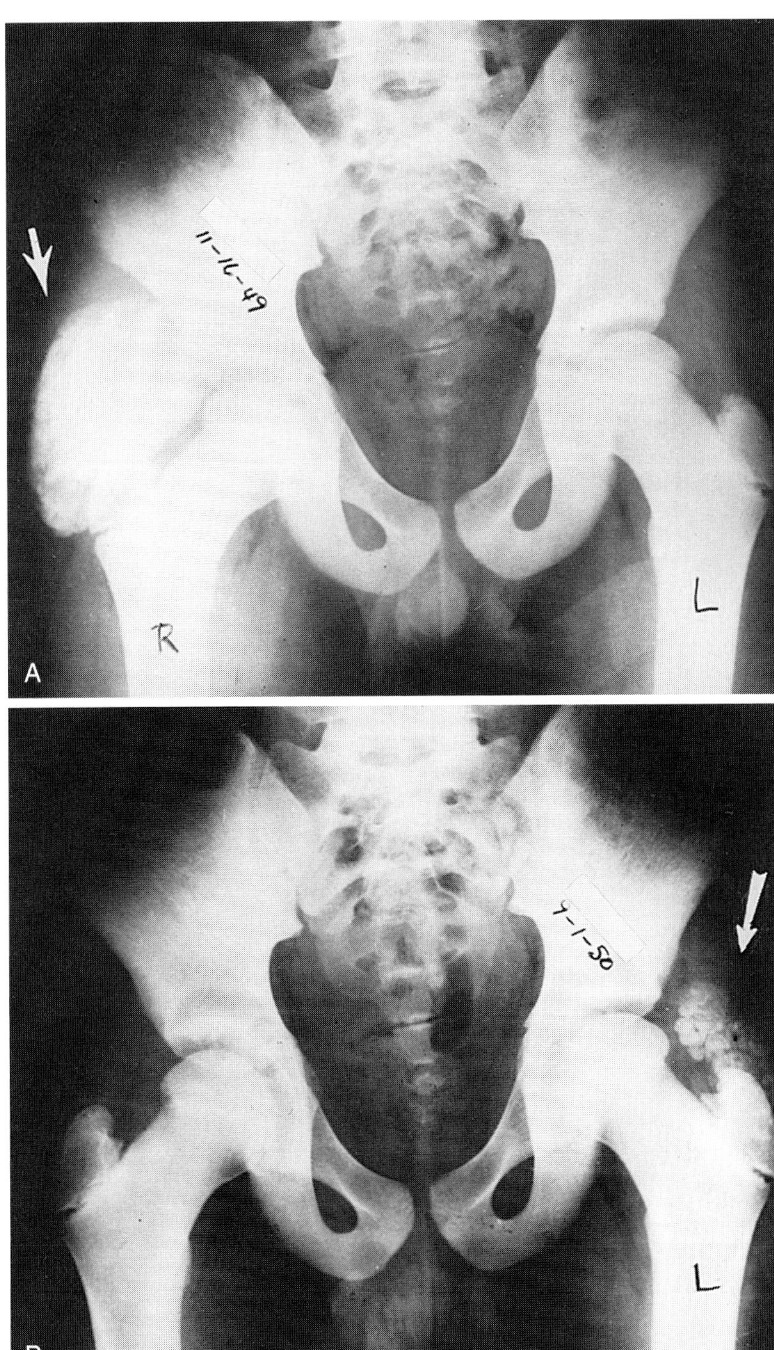


**FIGURE 36–1.** Radiograph of tumoral calcinosis involving the soft tissues of both hips (arrows). Nine months after the calcified mass in the right hip (**A**) was removed, a second mass developed in the left hip (**B**).

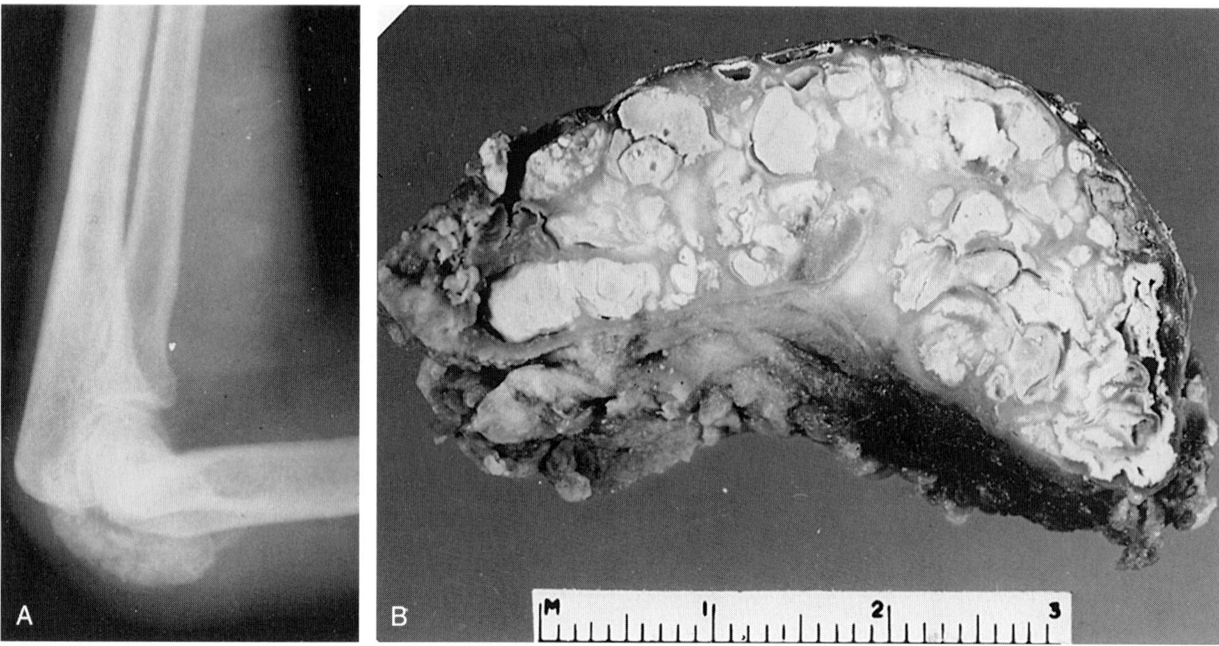


**FIGURE 36–2.** Tumoral calcinosis in the right elbow region of an 18-year-old man. (**A**) Radiograph shows calcified mass in the elbow region. (**B**) Cross section of tumor revealing a conglomerate of calcified masses surrounded by dense collagenous tissue.

patients with these lesions are older than those with tumoral calcinosis, have additional calcifications in visceral organs such as the kidney, lung, heart, and stomach, and have abnormally low calcium levels. There are also tumoral calcinosis-like lesions and vascular calcifications associated with hyperphosphatemia in patients with end-stage renal disease undergoing hemodialysis.[2,26] Similar calcifying soft tissue lesions, but associated with hypercalcemia, occur in patients with hypervitaminosis D,[4] hyperparathyroidism, and milk-alkali syndrome (Burnett syndrome),[36] a rare condition associated with prolonged antacid therapy for peptic ulcer, and in patients with excessive osteolysis and mobilization of calcium in destructive neoplastic and infectious lesions of bone.[16] In all of these lesions a detailed clinical history and laboratory data aid in reaching a reliable diagnosis (Table 36–2).

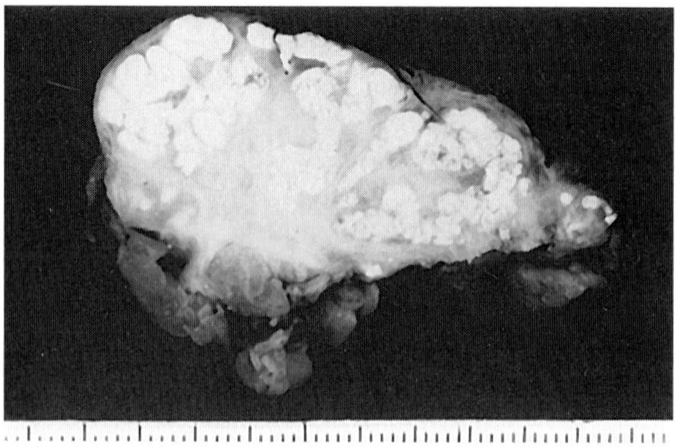

**FIGURE 36–3.** Cross section of tumoral calcinosis of the right thigh showing multilocular calcification of densely collagenous tissue.

Calcinosis universalis and calcinosis circumscripta likewise are located in the skin and subcutis and are associated with normal serum calcium and phosphorus levels. Calcinosis universalis forms multiple nodules or plaques that occur mainly in children and are associated in about half of the cases with manifestations of scleroderma or dermatomyositis. It may ultimately lead to limited mobility, contractures, and ankylosis. Calcinosis circumscripta, on the other hand, chiefly affects middle-aged women and most commonly involves the hand and wrist, including tendon sheaths. It is associated in a large percentage of cases

**TABLE 36–2** TUMOR-LIKE CALCIFIC LESIONS IN SOFT TISSUE

- Tumoral calcinosis
- Chronic renal failure with secondary hyperparathyroidism
- Milk-alkali syndrome
- Hypervitaminosis D
- Bone destruction secondary to infection/neoplasm

Modified from McGregor DH, Mowry M, Cherian R, et al. Nonfamilial tumoral calcinosis associated with chronic renal failure and secondary hyperparathyroidism: report of two cases with clinicopathological, immunohistochemical, and electron microscopic findings. Hum Pathol 26:607, 1995.

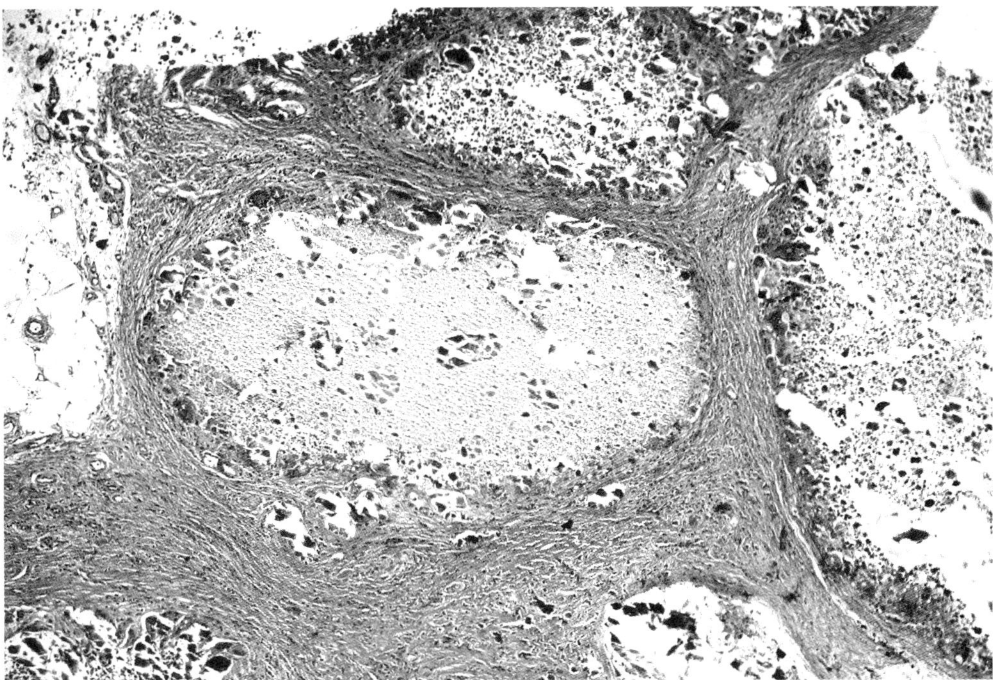

**FIGURE 36–4.** Tumoral calcinosis. Amorphous calcified material bordered by a florid proliferation of macrophages and multinucleated, osteoclast-like giant cells. The nodules are separated by bands of dense fibrous tissue.

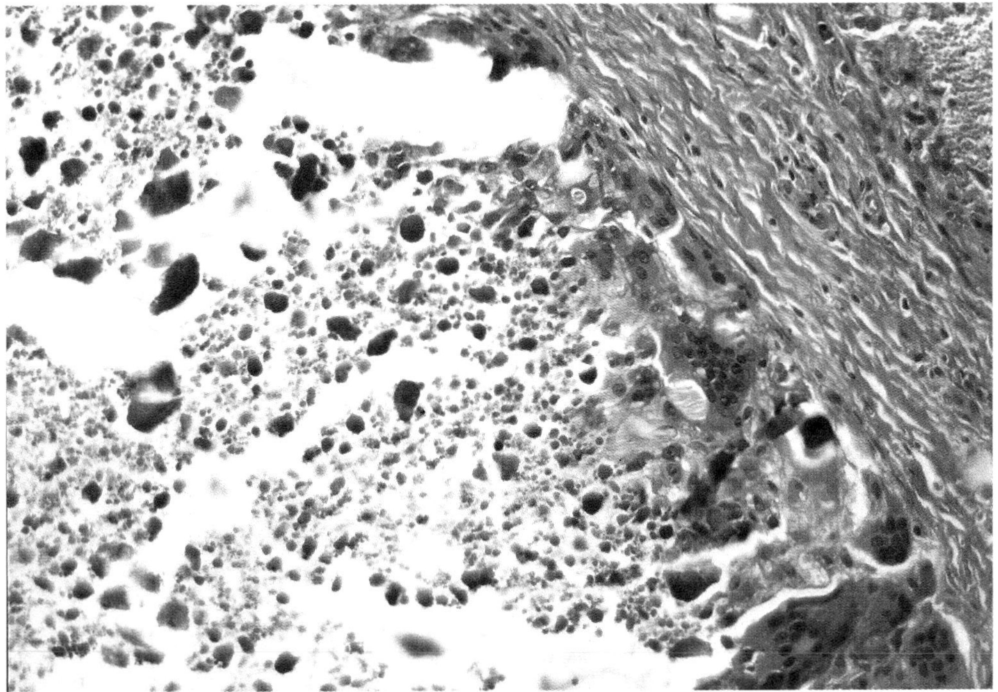

**FIGURE 36–5.** Tumoral calcinosis with a characteristic mixture of calcified material, histiocytes, and multinucleated giant cells.

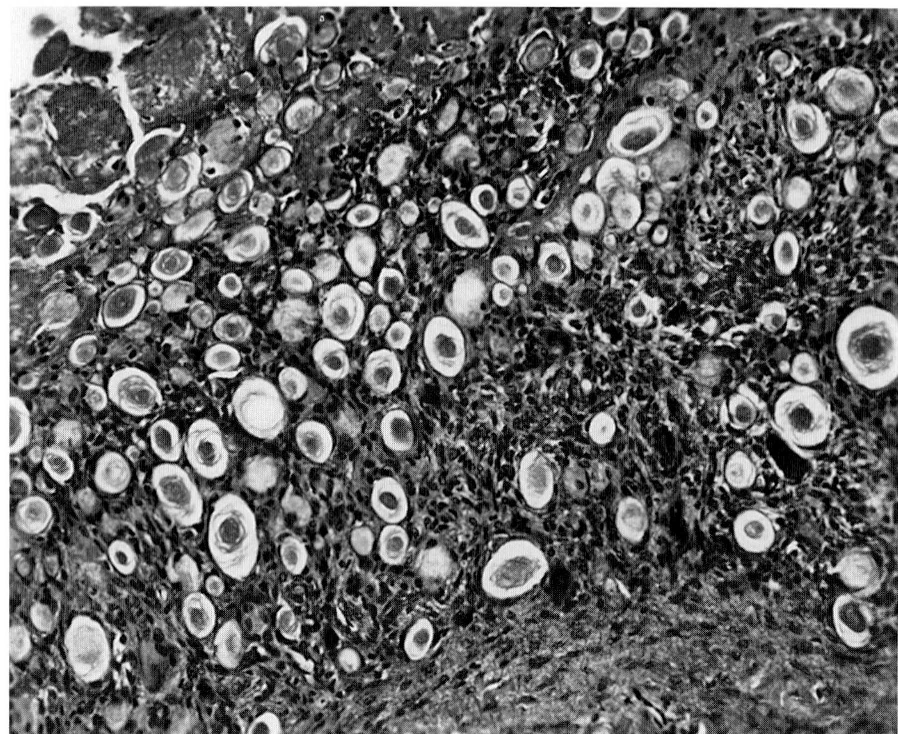

**FIGURE 36–6.** Variant of tumoral calcinosis with numerous calcospherites simulating a parasitic infection.

with Raynaud's disease or scleroderma, sclerodactyly, or polymyositis.[18] In one such case secondary infection led to severe, fatal amyloidosis.[48] The CREST syndrome is a related condition involving *c*alcinosis cutis, *R*aynaud's phenomenon, *e*sophageal hypomotility, *s*clerodactyly, and *t*elangiectasis.

There are also dystrophic calcifications, as in calcareous tendinitis, that show an identical microscopic picture but are smaller and develop in damaged tissue secondary to minor injury, ischemic necrosis, or a necrotizing infectious process.[35] Calcifications of tendons and ligaments have also been reported in patients undergoing long-term therapy with etretinate, a synthetic vitamin A derivative prescribed for acne, psoriasis, and various keratinization disorders.[9] Other forms of calcification, such as those of the scrotal skin, are not uncommon, but the exact cause is still not clear.[45]

## Discussion

Tumoral calcinosis is an inborn error in calcium metabolism that is inherited according to a dominant or recessive pattern.[21,37] Laboratory studies reveal normal calcium levels, but in many cases there is elevation of serum phosphorus levels, probably the result of increased tubular reabsorption or reduced renal excretion of phosphorus. Calcitriol (1,25-dihydroxyvitamin $D_3$) levels are also increased in some patients.[22,29] Slavin et al.[37] described a family in which 7 of 13 siblings developed tumoral calcinosis. All seven had hyperphosphatemia and normocalcemia. One had increased phosphorus levels prior to the onset of the calcification, but in the remaining six siblings without calcifications, phosphorus levels were normal. Trauma is rarely reported by patients with tumoral calcinosis,[8] but minor repeated trauma and tissue injury seem to play a role in the calcifying process; it probably serves as a trigger mechanism that leads to a chain of events, beginning with hemorrhage, fat necrosis, fibrosis, and collagenization and ending with collagenolysis and ultimately massive calcification. Several authors have proposed that the pressure of sleeping on the hard ground may explain the principal sites of calcification in African Blacks.[24,47]

## Prognosis

The treatment of choice is surgical removal of the lesion as early as possible, when the lesion is still small and amenable to total resection.[44] Incomplete excision may lead to recurrence, secondary infection, or abscess formation. Treatment with radiation or cortisone is largely ineffective.[20] Calcium deprivation and $PO_4$-binding antacids have been effectively employed as an alternative mode of therapy.[30] Others, however, report no response to a low phosphorus diet and oral aluminum hydroxide gel.[40]

## INTRAMUSCULAR MYXOMA

A number of benign mesenchymal lesions are characterized by abundant myxoid matrix, a small number of inconspicuous stellate-shaped or spindle-shaped cells, and a poorly developed vascular pattern. Most seem to be composed of modified fibroblasts that produce excessive amounts of glycosaminoglycans rich in hyaluronic acid and little collagen.[50] Chief among them is the intramuscular myxoma, a relatively uncommon benign mesenchymal lesion that is of particular importance because it is almost always cured by local excision yet is easily mistaken for a myxoid sarcoma.

### Clinical Findings

Intramuscular myxoma is a tumor of adult life that occurs primarily in patients 40–70 years of age.[54,59,60] In our experience it is rare in young adults and virtually nonexistent in children and adolescents. About two-thirds of the patients are women.[58,64] There is no evidence of increased familial incidence.

The clinical manifestations are nonspecific, and it is difficult to diagnose the tumor before biopsy and microscopic examination. In most patients the sole presenting sign is a painless, palpable mass that is firm, slightly movable, and often fluctuant. Pain or tenderness is present in fewer than one-fourth of patients.[54] As one would expect, pain and occasional numbness, paresthesia, and muscle weakness distal to the lesion are mostly associated with tumors of large size. Because of the relative lack of symptoms, most of the tumors are present for several months or years before they are excised. The rate of growth varies, however, and there is no close relation between size and clinical duration. A history of trauma is given in fewer than one-fourth of the cases. There is also nothing in the clinical history that indicates the tumor is etiologically related to thyroid dysfunction, as in myxedema.

By far the most frequent sites of the tumor are the large muscles of the thigh, shoulder, buttocks, and upper arm (Fig. 36–7). Rare lesions also have been reported in the head and neck.[66,69] The exact location in the musculature varies: Some tumors are completely surrounded by muscle tissue, and others are firmly attached on one side to muscle fascia. There are also myxomas of identical appearance that seem to arise from the periosteum, subchondral epiphysis, and joint capsule. Angiographic examination reveals a poorly vascularized soft tissue mass surrounded by well vascularized muscle tissue.[60] Magnetic resonance imaging reveals a well-defined tumor exhibiting low signal intensity relative to skeletal muscle on T1-weighted images and a hyperintense appearance relative to muscle on T2-weighted images.[52,61,68]

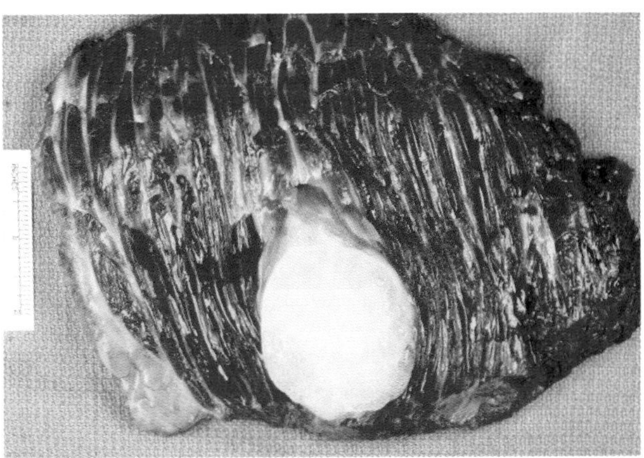

**FIGURE 36–7.** Intramuscular myxoma showing a uniform yellowish white cut surface. The tumor characteristically appears well circumscribed.

### Multiple Intramuscular Myxomas and Fibrous Dysplasia

Although most intramuscular myxomas are solitary, there are occasional patients in whom two or more myxomas are present, usually in the same region of the body. Microscopically, these tumors are in no way different from the solitary intramuscular myxomas. Nearly all are associated with monostotic or rarely polyostotic fibrous dysplasia of bone, generally in the same anatomic region where the myxomas are located[51,56,63,71] (Fig. 36–8). In this setting, females are affected significantly more commonly than males. Often there is a long interval between the appearances of the two processes. In most cases the fibrous dysplasia is noted during the growth period, whereas the multiple myxomas, like their solitary forms, become apparent many years later during adult life.[72] Rarely, multiple intramuscular myxomas are detected before the osseous lesions.[53] If specifically sought, radiologically evident bone abnormalities are seen in many patients with intramuscular myxomas.[64] In the case of Mazabraud et al.,[63] an osteosarcoma developed in a patient with fibrous dysplasia and multiple myxomas.

### Pathologic Findings

The gross appearance is characteristic and changes little from case to case. Most tumors are ovoid or globular and have a glistening gray-white or white appearance, depending on the relative amounts of collagen and myxoid material (Fig. 36–9). They consist of a mass of stringy gelatinous material with occasional small fluid-filled, cyst-like spaces, and they are covered by bundles of skeletal muscle or fascial tissue (Fig. 36–10). Although on gross examination

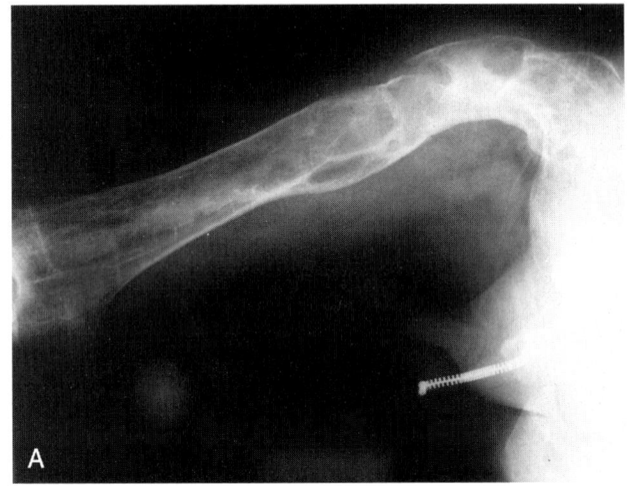


**FIGURE 36–8.** Patient with multiple intramuscular myxomas and fibrous dysplasia. (**A**) Characteristic radiographic features of fibrous dysplasia involving the humerus show a shepherd's crook deformity. (**B**) Histologic appearance of fibrous dysplasia. An intramuscular myxoma was found in the soft tissues adjacent to the humerus.

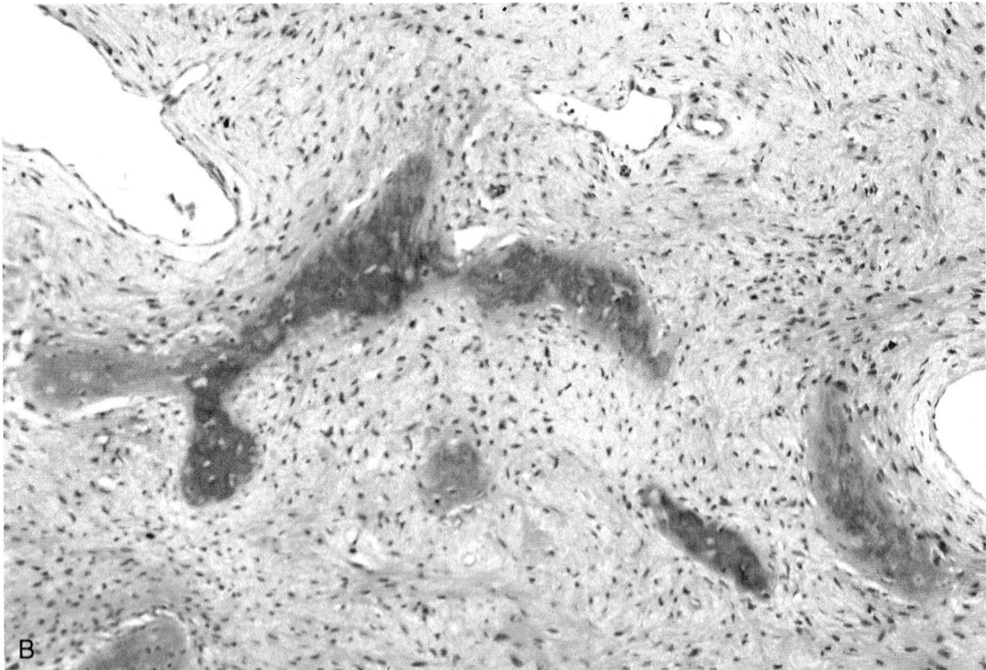

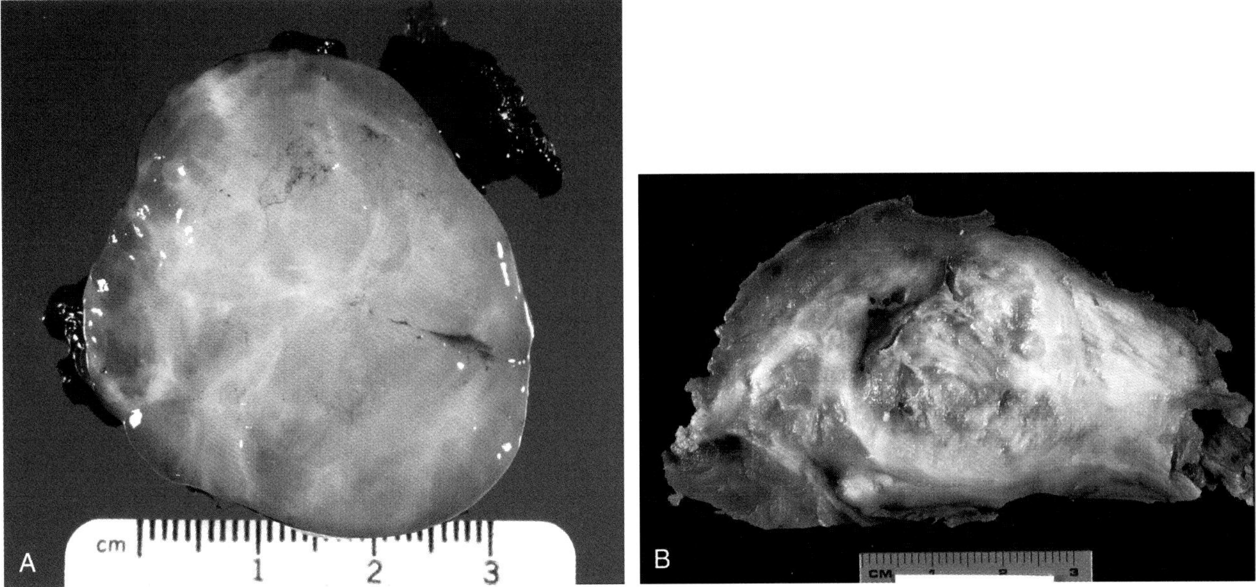


**FIGURE 36–9.** Gross appearances of intramuscular myxoma. (**A**) The tumor has a mucoid, gelatinous cut surface with thin fibrous septa. (**B**) Fibrous-appearing intramuscular myxoma.

most of the tumors appear to be well circumscribed, many infiltrate the adjacent musculature or are surrounded by edematous muscle tissue, which may serve as a cleavage plane for the surgeon. The size varies greatly. Most measure 5–10 cm in greatest diameter, but some lesions are 20 cm or larger.

On histologic examination the tumor varies little in its appearance and is composed of relatively small numbers of inconspicuous cells, abundant mucoid material, and a loose meshwork of reticulin fibers (Figs. 36–11, 36–12, 36–13). Characteristically, mature collagen fibers and vascular structures are sparse, a feature that has also been demonstrated by microangiography.[60] Fluid-filled cystic spaces are seen occasionally (Figs. 36–14, 36–15), but they are rarely a prominent feature.[67] The constituent cells have small, hyperchromatic, pyknotic-appearing nuclei and scanty cytoplasm that sometimes extends along the reticulin fibers with multiple processes, giving the cell a stellate appearance (Figs. 36–16, 36–17). There is little cellular pleomorphism, and there are no multinucleated giant cells. In some cases there are also scattered macrophages with small intracellular droplets of lipid material (Fig. 36–18). The small size of these droplets and the absence of nuclear deformation or scalloping afford their distinction from lipoblasts (Fig. 36–19). At the periphery, where the tumor merges with the surrounding muscle, fat cells and atrophic muscle fibers are occasionally scattered in the mucoid substance. These residual muscle fibers can be misinterpreted as evidence of rhabdomyoblastic differentiation, resulting in a misdiagnosis of rhabdomyosarcoma.

Some intramuscular myxomas show focal areas of hypercellularity and hypervascularity, which may cause further confusion with a sarcoma (Fig. 36–20). In the study by Nielsen et al.,[65] 38 of 51 cases of intramuscular myxoma (76%) had hypercellular zones that occupied 10–80% of the tumor. However, even in these hypercellular zones, the cells lack nuclear atypia, and there is a paucity of mitotic figures and an absence of necrosis. Areas of more typical hypocellular intramuscular myxoma allow their definitive recognition.

Immunohistochemically, the cells stain positively for vimentin; unlike lipoblasts, they do not stain for S-100 protein.[58,62] Rare cells may also stain for actin.[66] Cells and reticulin fibers are suspended in large amounts of mucoid material that stains positively with alcian blue, mucicarmine, and colloidal iron stains. The mucoid material is depolymerized by prior treatment of the sections with hyaluronidase.[60]

Ultrastructural examination discloses predominantly fibroblast- and myofibroblast-like cells with prominent rough endoplasmic reticulum, microfilamentous material, a prominent Golgi complex, and pinocytotic and secretory vesicles, together with a mixture of amorphous and granular material and collagen fibers in the extracellular spaces (Fig. 36–21A). There are also macrophage-like cells with small lipid droplets or secretory vacuoles and multiple cytoplasmic processes[55,58] (Fig. 36–21B).

*Text continued on page 1435*

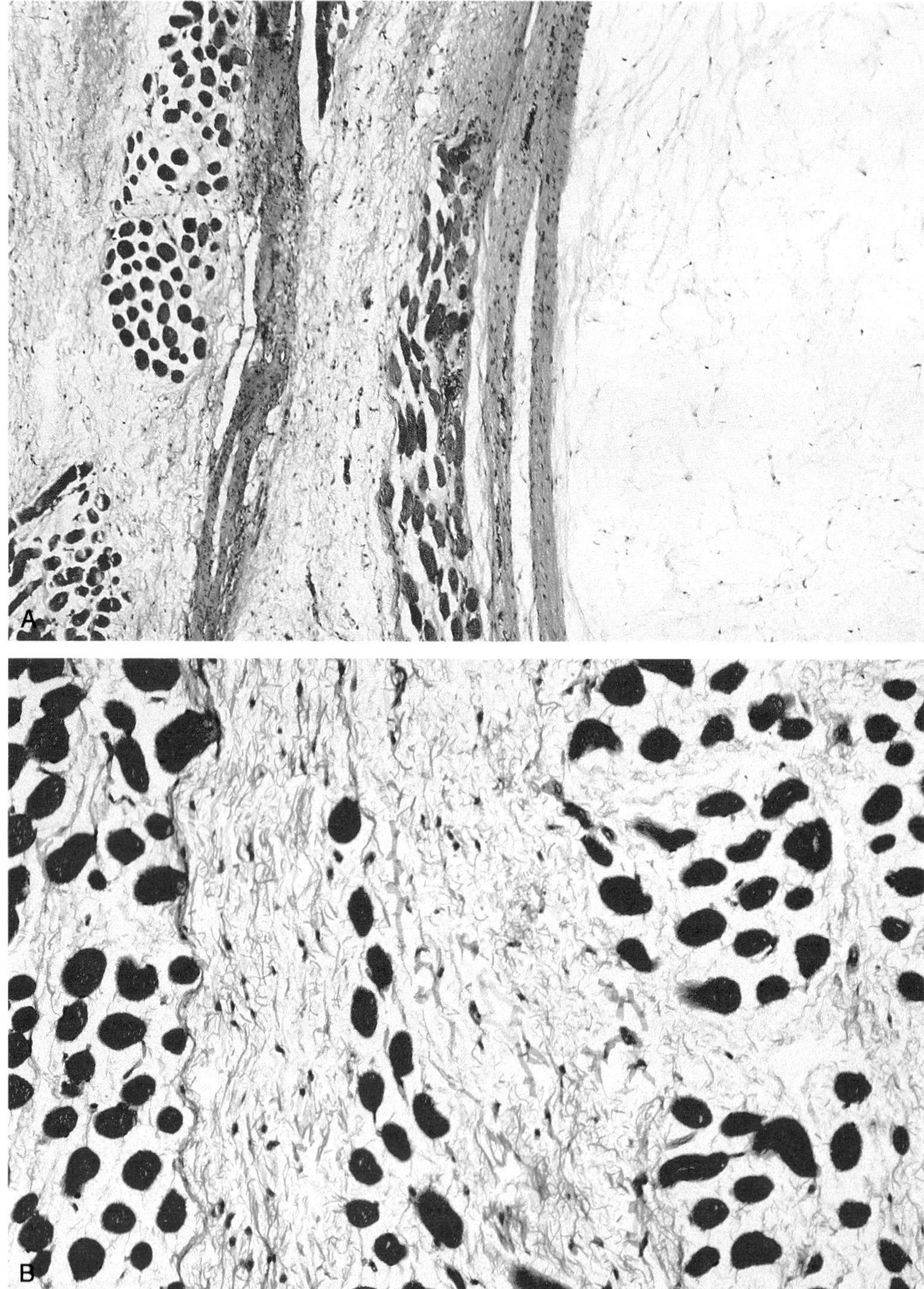


**FIGURE 36–10.** Intramuscular myxoma. Although grossly well circumscribed, the tumor infiltrates the surrounding skeletal muscle (**A**). Higher magnification appearance of the peripheral portion of an intramuscular myxoma with atrophy of the surrounding skeletal muscle (**B**).

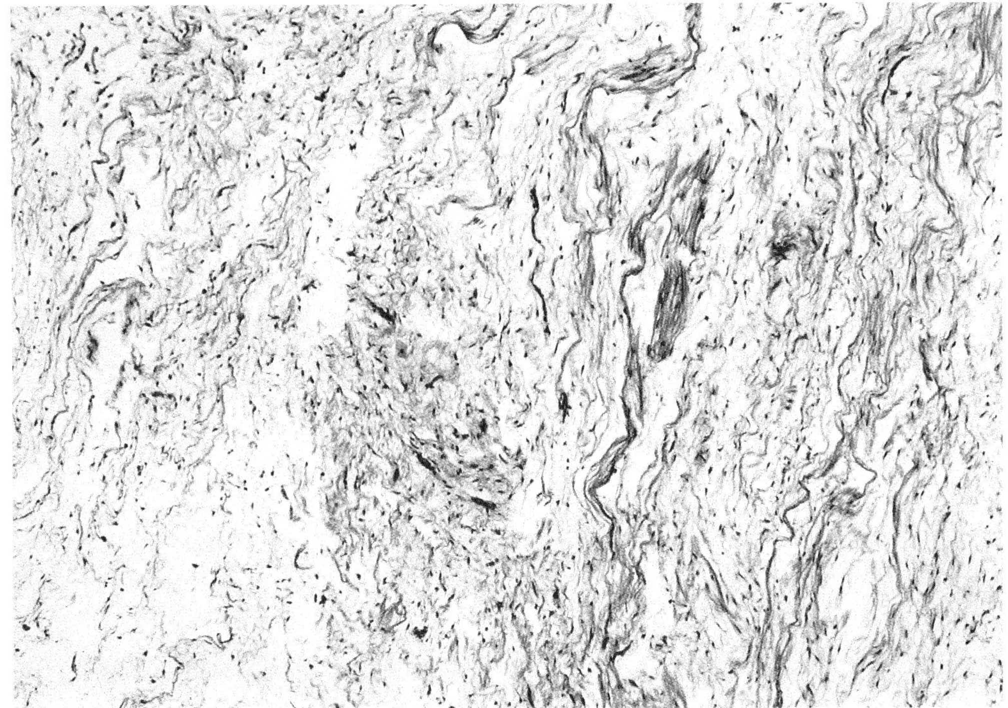

**FIGURE 36–11.** Low magnification appearance of intramuscular myxoma characterized by a paucity of cells, abundance of mucoid material, and almost complete absence of vascular structures.

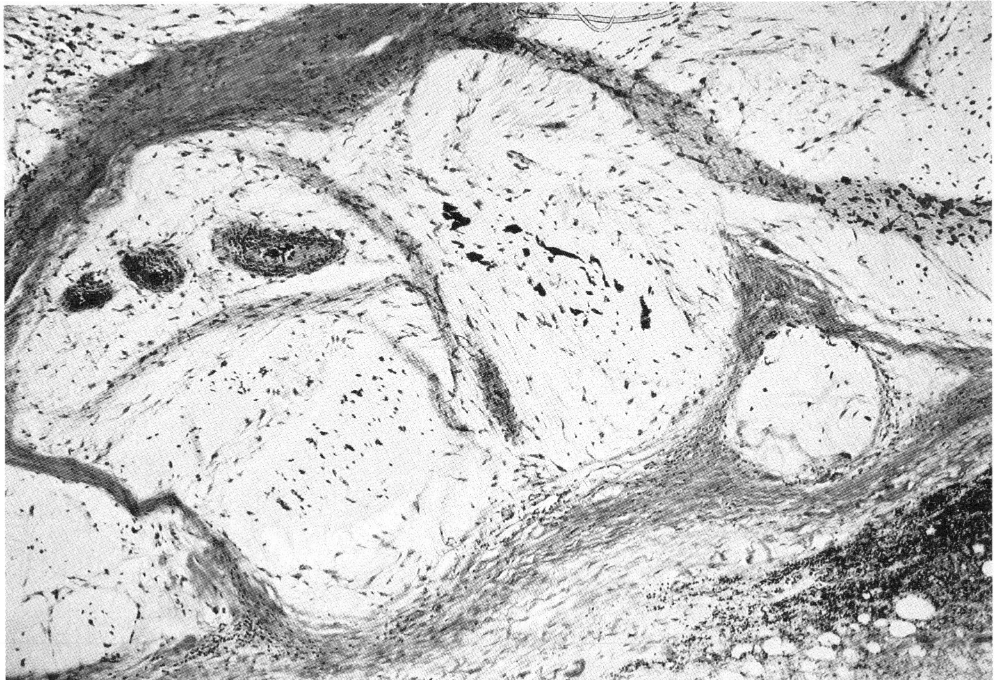

**FIGURE 36–12.** Intramuscular myxoma. Intersecting fibrous septa give the tumor a multilobular appearance.

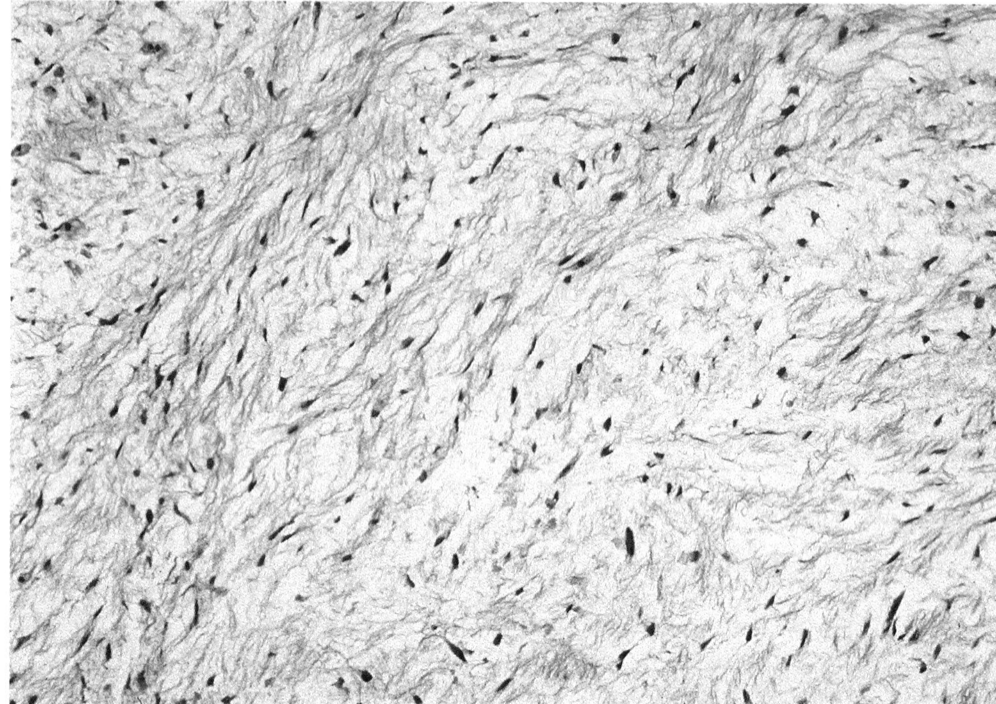

**FIGURE 36–13.** Intramuscular myxoma. The tumor cells are widely separated by abundant mucoid material and generally do not touch one another.

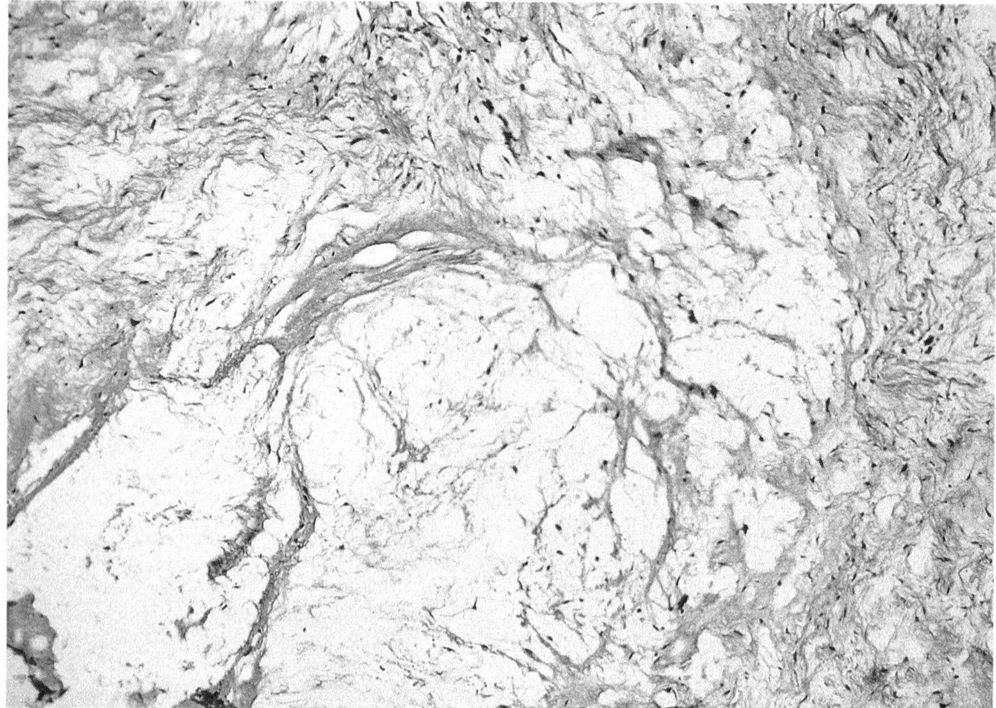

**FIGURE 36–14.** Intramuscular myxoma with prominent fluid-filled cystic spaces.

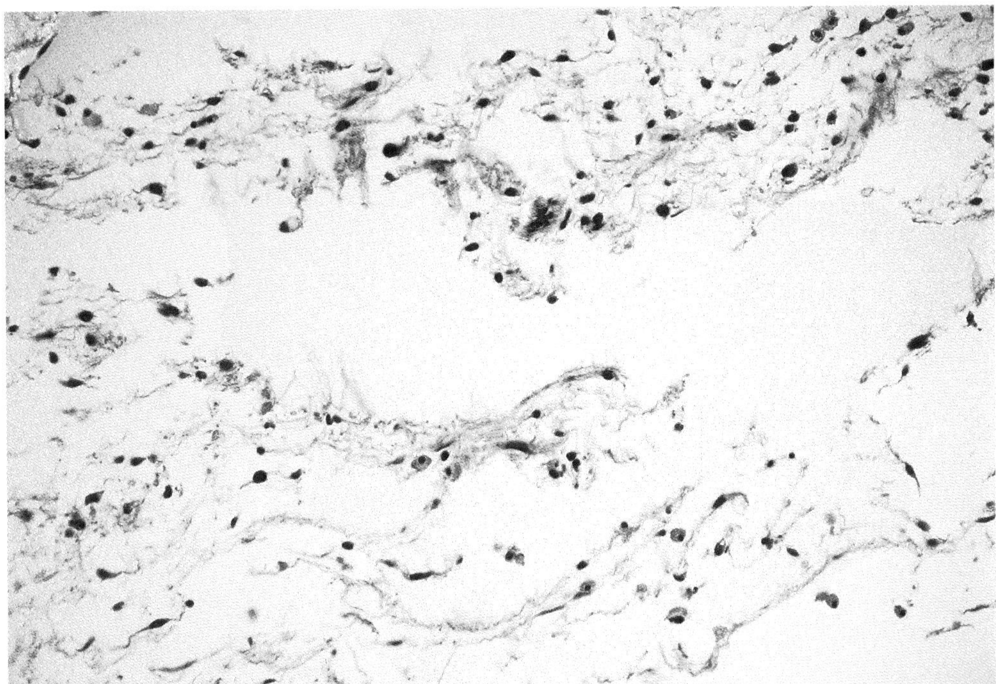

**FIGURE 36–15.** Cystic area in an intramuscular myxoma.

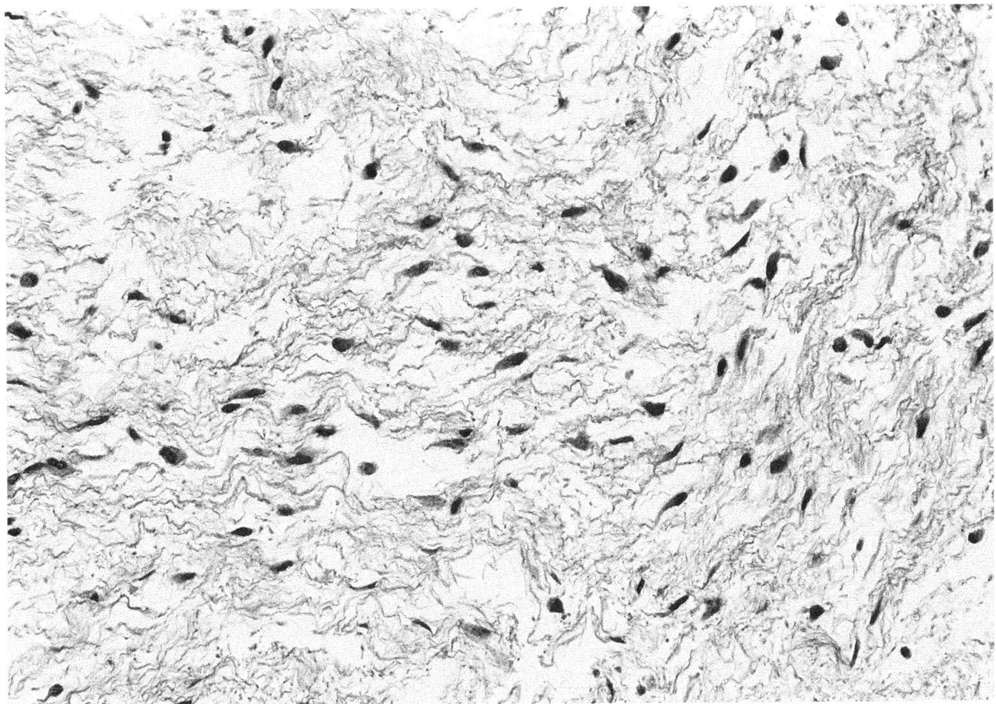

**FIGURE 36–16.** Intramuscular myxoma. The tumor is composed of cytologically bland spindled and stellate-shaped cells that are widely separated by myxoid stroma.

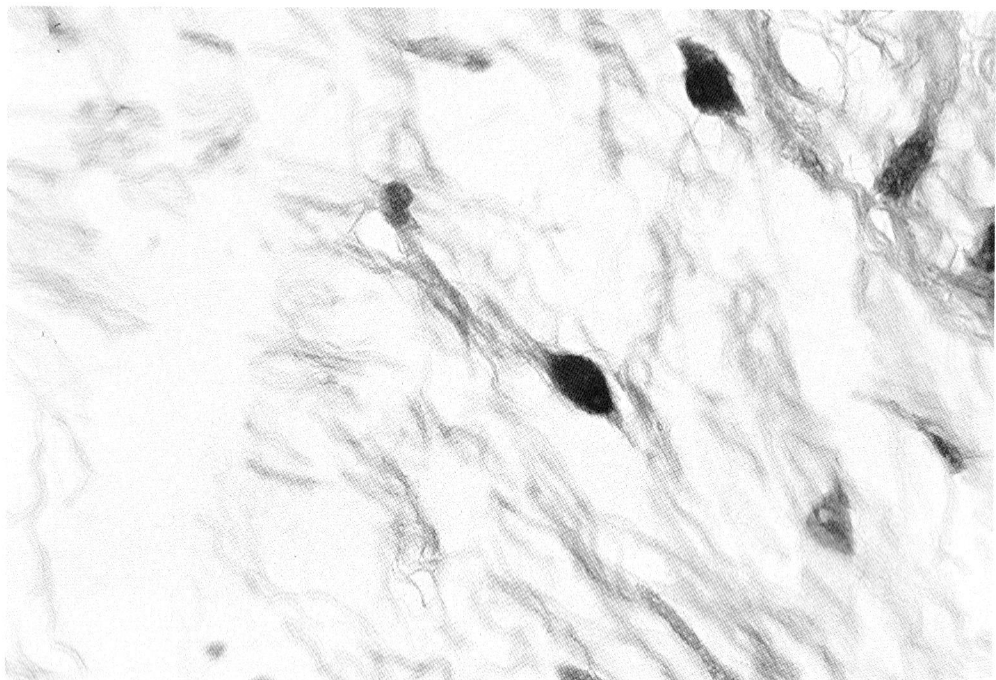

**FIGURE 36–17.** High magnification appearance of pyknotic cells with tapered cytoplasm in an intramuscular myxoma.

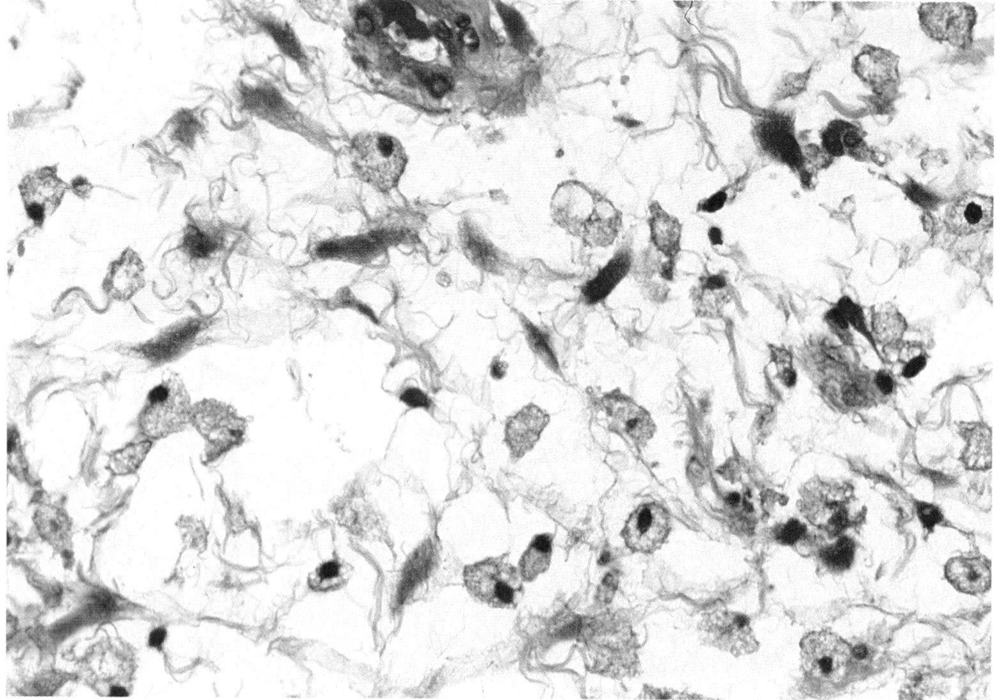

**FIGURE 36–18.** Intramuscular myxoma with collection of macrophages with small intracellular droplets of lipid material.

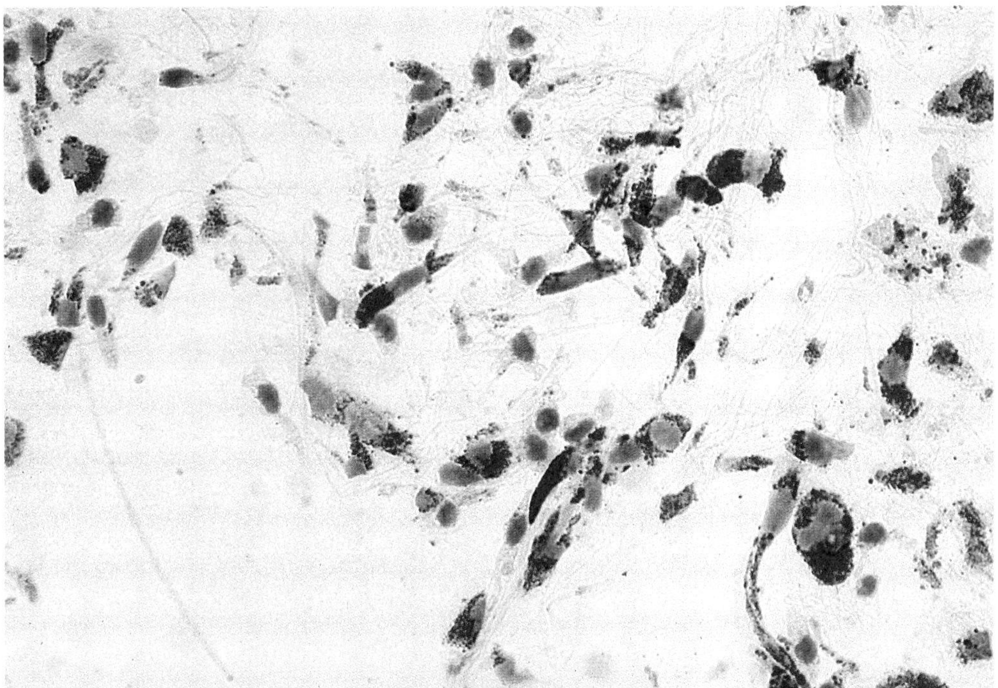

**FIGURE 36–19.** Frozen section of intramuscular myxoma with granular oil red O-positive intracellular lipid material mimicking a liposarcoma.

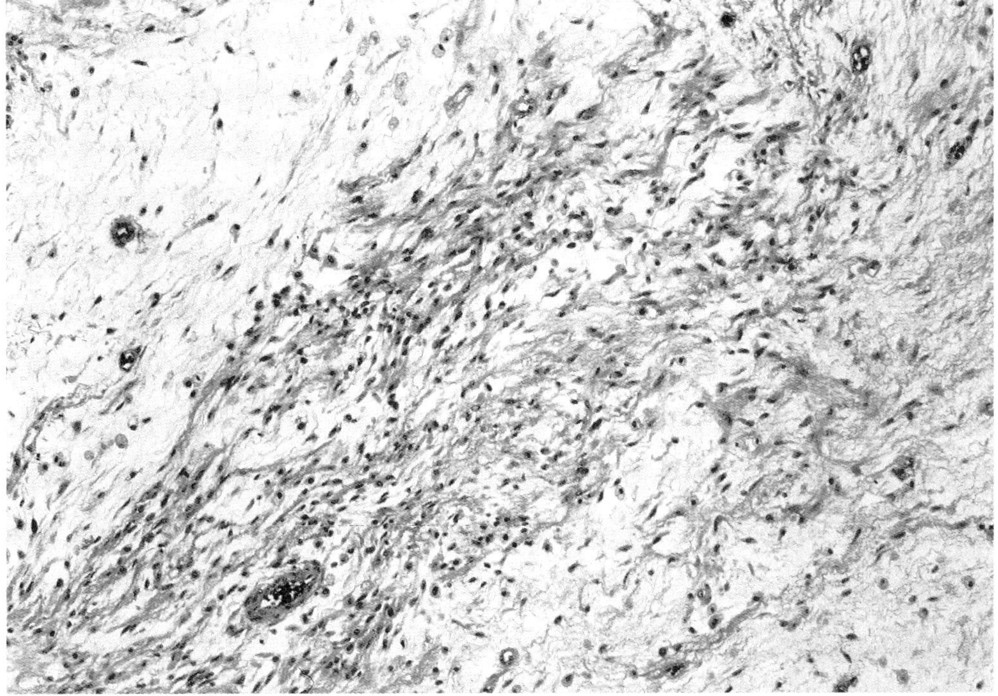

**FIGURE 36–20.** Hypercellular focus in an otherwise typical intramuscular myxoma.

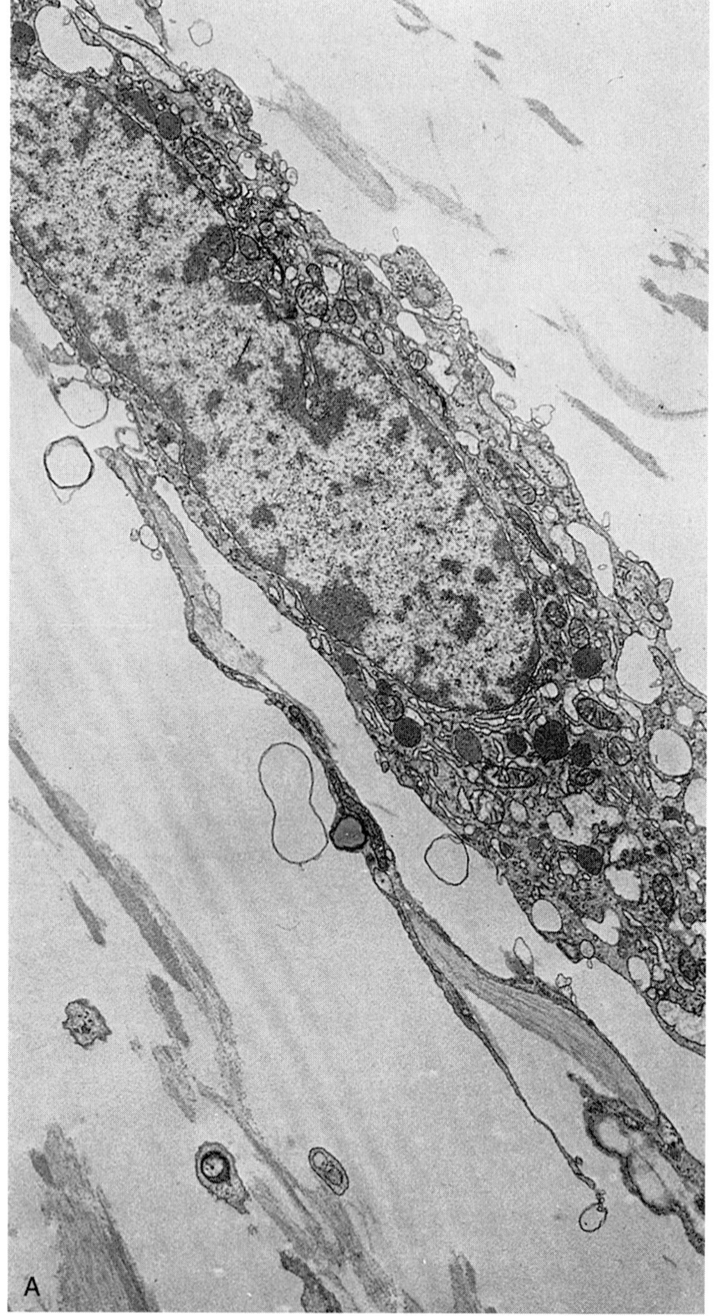


**FIGURE 36–21.** (**A**) Electron microscopy of an intramuscular myxoma with fibroblast-like cells; note the prominent rough endoplasmic reticulum and collagen fibers in the extracellular spaces. (**B**) Electron microscopy of an intramuscular myxoma. Macrophage-like cells with multiple membrane-bound lipid droplets. (**A, B:** Courtesy of Veterans Administration Hospital, Ann Arbor, MI.)

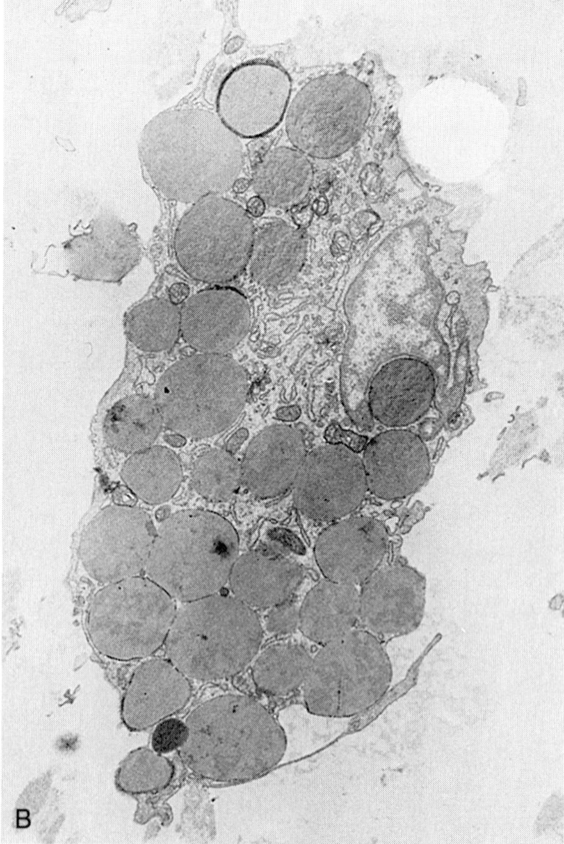

**TABLE 36–3 DIFFERENTIAL DIAGNOSIS OF INTRAMUSCULAR MYXOMA**

| Tumor Type | Pleomorphism | Vascularity | Matrix |
|---|---|---|---|
| Intramuscular myxoma | — | Inconspicuous | Hyaluronic acid |
| Myxoid liposarcoma | + | Fine, plexiform | Hyaluronic acid |
| Myxoid chondrosarcoma | + | Irregular | Chondroitin sulfate |
| Myxoid MFH | +++ | Coarse, curvilinear | Hyaluronic acid |

MFH, malignant fibrous histiocytoma.

### Differential Diagnosis

Numerous benign and malignant myxoid neoplasms are apt to be confused with intramuscular myxoma (Table 36–3). At times the tumor is difficult to distinguish from myxolipoma, myxoid neurofibroma, neurothekeoma, myxochondroma, and nodular fasciitis, conditions discussed in previous chapters. More importantly, intramuscular myxoma may be confused with richly myxoid malignant tumors. *Myxofibrosarcoma (low-grade myxoid malignant fibrous histiocytoma)*, similar to intramuscular myxoma, predominantly affects adults and may arise either in superficial or deep soft tissues. At the low end of the spectrum, myxofibrosarcoma is a hypocellular neoplasm composed of spindle-shaped cells deposited in an abundant myxoid stroma. However, the cells always demonstrate a greater degree of nuclear hyperchromasia and cytologic atypia than those of intramuscular myxoma. Many of these neoplasms also have prominent curvilinear blood vessels, often with perivascular tumoral condensation. *Myxoid liposarcoma* is characterized by a regular plexiform vasculature with spindle-shaped or stellate cells with mild cytologic atypia deposited in a myxoid stroma. In addition, the identification of cells with adipocytic differentiation, including well-formed lipoblasts, is useful for this distinction. *Extraskeletal myxoid chondrosarcoma* is composed of nests and cords of cells with densely eosinophilic cytoplasm deposited in a chondroitin sulfate-rich stroma. Although blood vessels are often not conspicuous, these lesions frequently show areas of hemorrhage and hemosiderin deposition. Immunostaining for S-100 protein, when positive, is useful for recognizing this entity, although fewer than one half of all cases stain for this antigen. Finally, *low-grade fibromyxoid sarcoma* is a rare neoplasm that also occurs in the deep soft tissues of adults. Histologically, this tumor is composed of cytologically uniform spindle-shaped cells deposited in a variably collagenous and myxoid matrix, often with a swirling arrangement of tumor cells around thin-walled capillaries.

### Discussion

Despite their frequently large size and prominent myxoid appearance, intramuscular myxomas are benign and rarely recur locally.[57,59] In a series by Nielsen et al.,[65] none of the 32 patients for whom follow-up information was available developed a local recurrence, including those with hypercellular lesions. In the series reported by Ireland et al.,[59] 2 of 39 intramuscular myxomas recurred, which were described as "cellular" and "moderately cellular." They were successfully treated by reexcision.

The lack of progressive growth, the paucity of vascular structures, and the apparent immutability of the tumor cells make it highly unlikely that myxoma, as Stout[70] had suggested, is a tumor of primitive mesenchyme. Instead, it seems much more likely that this tumor and similar benign myxomatous lesions in the corium and subcutis arise from modified fibroblasts that produce excessive amounts of glycosaminoglycans, which in turn, as has been shown experimentally, inhibit the polymerization of normal collagen. There is no convincing evidence that trauma is an important factor in the genesis of intramuscular myxoma. The occasional association with fibrous dysplasia, however, suggests an underlying localized error in tissue metabolism.

## JUXTAARTICULAR MYXOMA

Juxtaarticular myxoma is marked by the accumulation of mucinous material in the vicinity of the large joints, most commonly the knee but occasionally near the shoulder, elbow, hip, or ankle (Table 36–4). It almost always arises in adults, particularly men, with a predilection for the third through fifth decades of

**TABLE 36–4 ANATOMIC LOCATION OF 65 JUXTAARTICULAR MYXOMAS**

| Site | No. of Cases | % |
|---|---|---|
| Knee | 57 | 88.0 |
| Shoulder | 3 | 4.5 |
| Elbow | 3 | 4.5 |
| Hip | 1 | 1.5 |
| Ankle | 1 | 1.5 |
| *Total* | 65 | 100.0 |

Modified from Meis JM, Enzinger FM. Juxtaarticular myxoma: a clinical and pathological study of 65 cases. Hum Pathol 23:639, 1992.

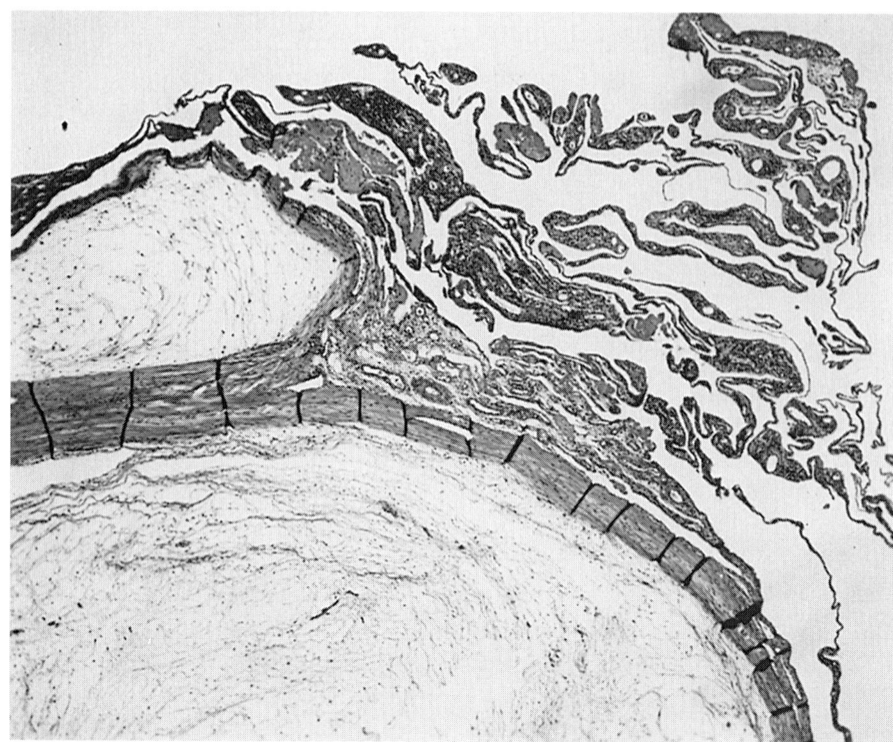

**FIGURE 36–22.** Juxtaarticular myxoma with a dense fibrous capsule and attached synovial villi.

life. The growth typically presents as a swelling or mass that is sometimes rapidly enlarging and is not infrequently associated with pain or tenderness.[77,79] These lesions may be associated with antecedent trauma and can arise adjacent to a joint with osteoarthritis. Some lesions are discovered incidentally during total knee or hip arthroplasty.[79,80] When in the region of the knee, it is frequently found together with meniscal and parameniscal cysts, small myxoma-like masses embedded in the lateral or medial semilunar cartilage.[73,74,76] The radiologic features are similar to those found with intramuscular myxoma.[75,78]

Grossly, most lesions are 2–6 cm, but some are as large as 12 cm at the time of excision.[79] They typically have a mucoid cystic or multicystic appearance on cut section.

Histologically, juxtaarticular myxoma closely resembles intramuscular myxoma and is composed of scattered small, spindle-shaped or stellate-shaped fibroblast-like cells deposited in a richly myxoid matrix that often contains variously sized thin- or thick-walled cystic spaces (Fig. 36–22). Occasionally, there are hypercellular areas with slight cellular pleomorphism, features that may arouse suspicion of a low-grade myxoid sarcoma. The process involves not only the periarticular soft tissues and the overlying cutaneous fat, but also the joint capsule, tendons, and rarely skeletal muscle. Some lesions have areas of hemorrhage and hemosiderin deposition with scattered chronic inflammation and reactive fibroblastic proliferation.

Juxtaarticular myxoma is benign but is apt to recur after incomplete excision. In the series by Meis and Enzinger,[79] recurrences appeared in 10 of the 29 patients for whom follow-up information was available, including one lesion that recurred four times.

The cause if this condition is not clear, but it may represent an exuberant reactive fibroblastic proliferation with overproduction of mucin. Sciot et al. described a case with clonal chromosomal changes, including trisomy 7 and a translocation between chromosomes 8 and 22.[81]

## MYXOMA OF THE JAW

Although myxoma of the jaw is primarily a bone tumor, it occasionally manifests in the soft tissues as a myxomatous swelling or mass overlying a radiographically demonstrable osteolytic defect of the mandible or maxilla.[86,90,91] It may also displace and destroy teeth, extend into the adjacent maxillary sinus,[87] and involve the soft tissues of the face.[89] It chiefly affects young adults, with a predilection for females; it is slightly more frequent in the mandible than in the maxilla.[95] Rare lesions have been described in infants and children.[82,84]

Microscopically, myxomas of the jaw are poorly circumscribed myxoma-like masses that differ from other myxomatous lesions merely by a slightly greater degree of cellularity and cellular pleomorphism and a higher rate of mitosis. Rare lesions also have epithelial inclusions presumed to be of odontogenic origin.[93] The cells are immunoreactive with antibodies against vimentin and S-100 protein but not desmin or cytokeratin.[92] Similar to normal odontogenic epithelium, the epithelial inclusions stain for cytokeratin 19.[93] Electron microscopic examination reveals the presence of fibroblasts and myofibroblasts.[88,94] Surgical removal of the growth is often difficult, and the lesion is apt to recur, especially when it is treated by curettage rather than excision.[85] More cellular forms may be difficult to distinguish from fibrous dysplasia and ossifying fibroma.[83]

## CUTANEOUS MYXOMA (SUPERFICIAL ANGIOMYXOMA)

*Cutaneous myxoma,* also known as *superficial angiomyxoma,* was first described by Allen et al.[96] in 1988 and was more fully characterized by Calonje et al.[98] in 1999. This lesion should be distinguished from the other cutaneous myxoid lesions with which it may be confused because it has a propensity for local recurrence.

Cutaneous myxoma arises slightly more commonly in males, predominantly middle-aged adults, although rare congenital examples have been described.[97,98] There is a predilection for the trunk, lower extremities, and head and neck; some arise in the genital region of both males and females.[99] Histologically identical lesions have been described in Carney's complex, particularly those that are multiple and arise in the eyelids and external ear.[106,114] Clinically, most appear as polypoid or papulonodular cutaneous lesions which may be confused with a cyst, skin tag, or neurofibroma.[98]

As seen by light microscopy, this lesion has a lobular or multinodular appearance at low magnification (Figs. 36–23, 36–24); most are poorly circumscribed with extension into the underlying subcutaneous tissue and rarely skeletal muscle. A sparse proliferation of spindle- and stellate-shaped cells are deposited in an extensive myxoid stroma that is sensitive to hyaluronidase digestion (Figs. 36–25, 36–26). The cells have indistinct cell borders and oval nuclei with inconspicuous nucleoli; mitotic figures are rare. Binucleated or multinucleated cells may be seen, as are scattered cells with intranuclear cytoplasmic pseudoinclusions. There is often a prominent vasculature that is focally arborizing, reminiscent of that seen in myxoid liposarcomas (Fig. 36–27). A mixed inflammatory infiltrate is common, particularly stromal neutrophils, a feature unique to this tumor when compared to other cutaneous myxoid lesions.[98] Up to

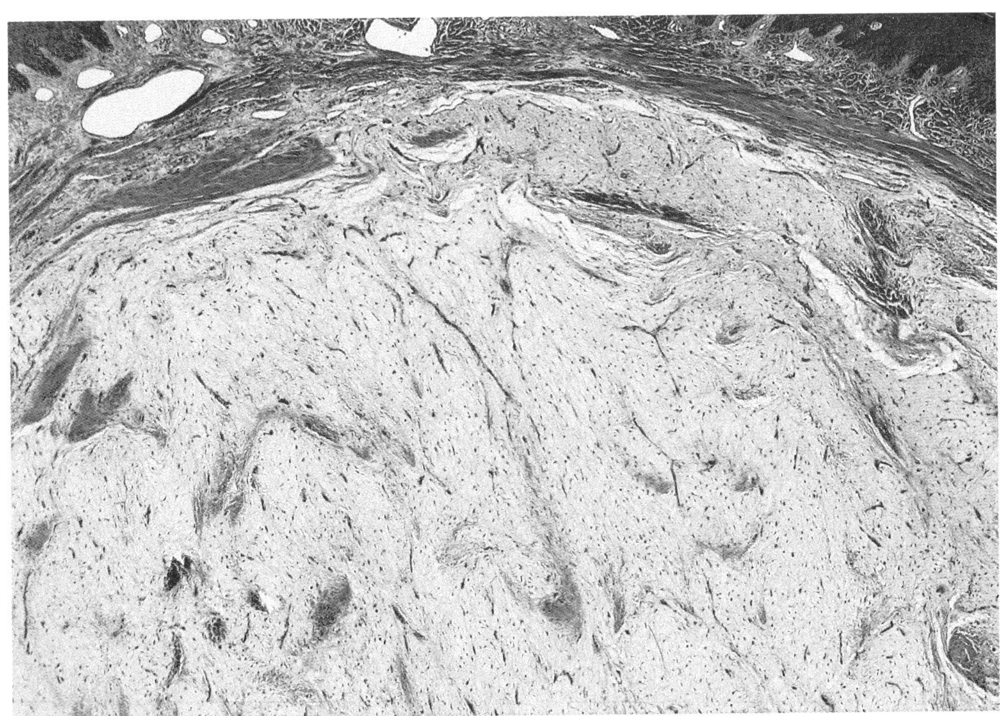

**FIGURE 36–23.** Cutaneous myxoma (superficial angiomyxoma). At low magnification, the tumor is hypocellular with prominent myxoid stroma; it appears fairly well circumscribed at its superficial aspect.

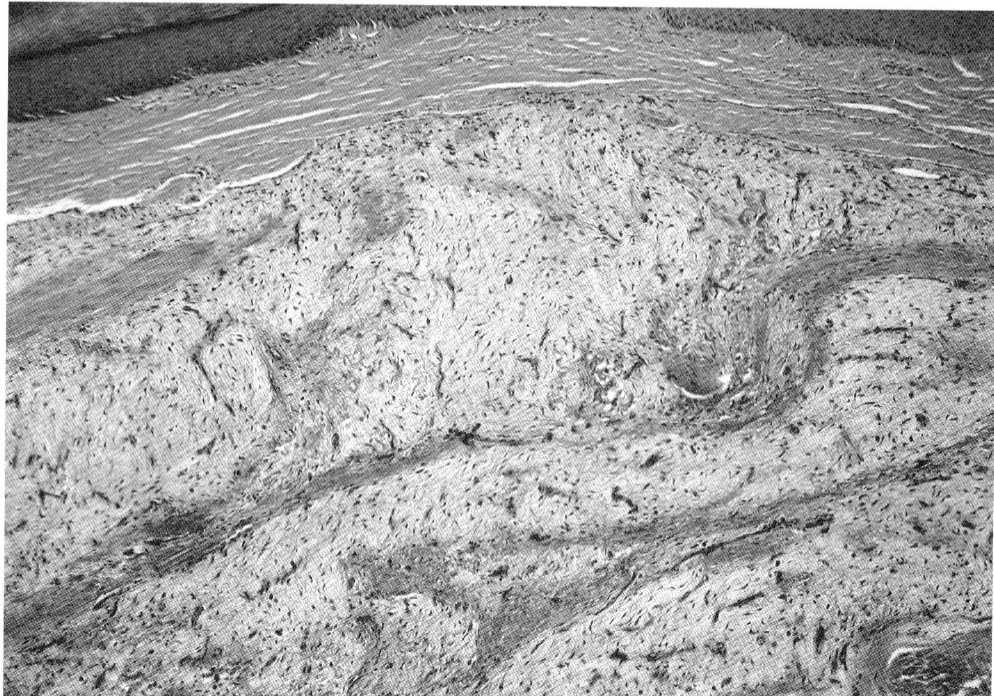

**FIGURE 36–24.** Multilobular appearance of a cutaneous myxoma.

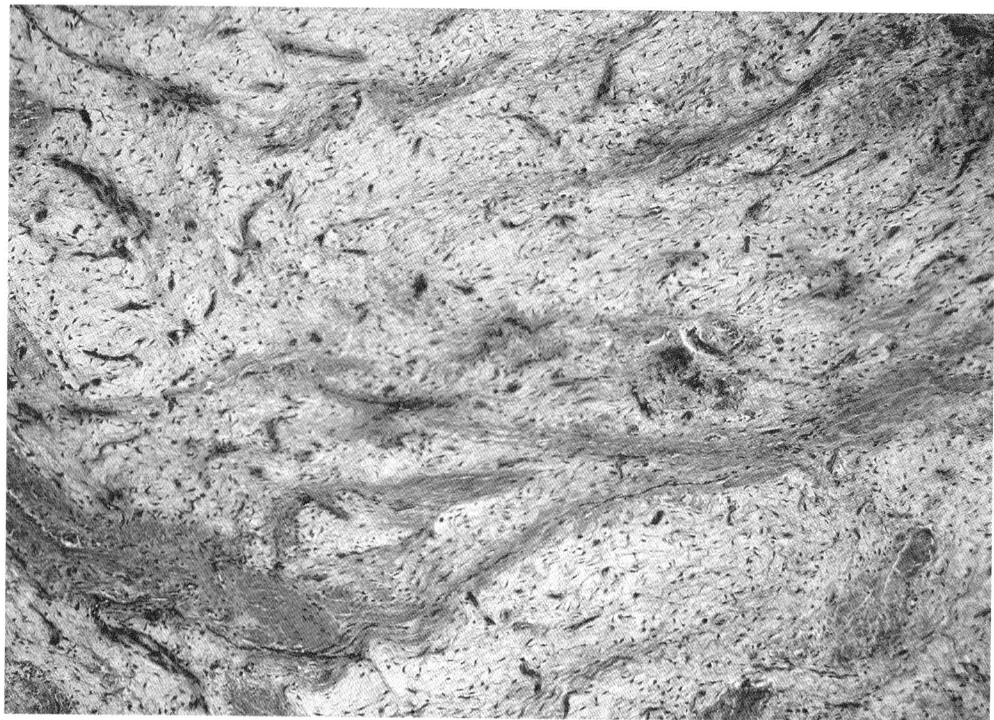

**FIGURE 36–25.** Cutaneous myxoma. Fibrous septa subdivide the tumor into ill-defined lobules.

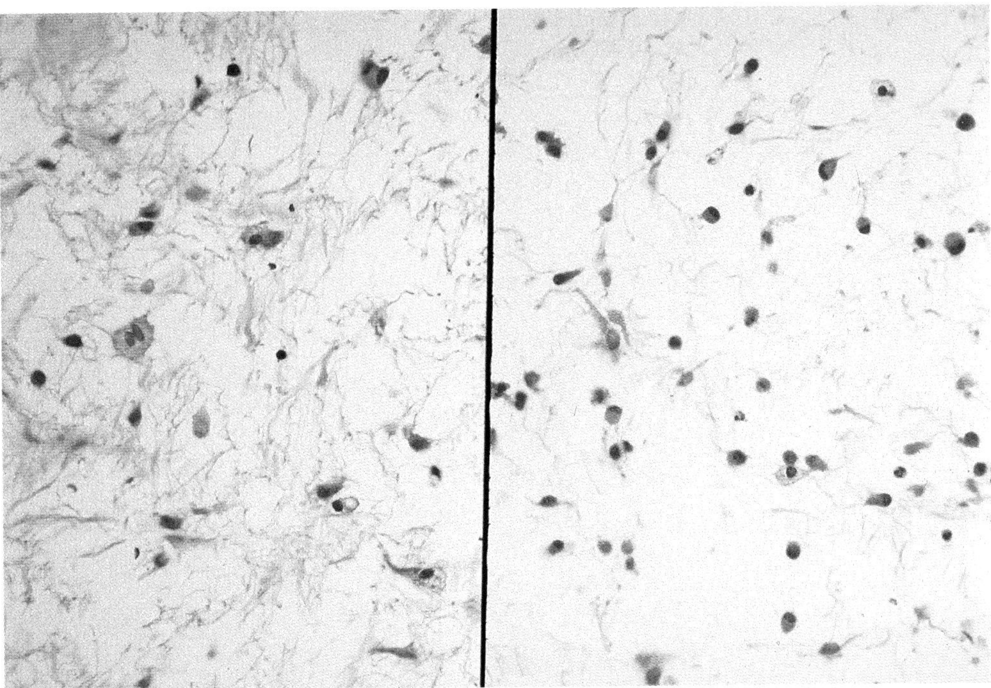

**FIGURE 36–26.** Cutaneous myxoma stained with alcian blue stain without (**left**) and with (**right**) pretreatment with hyaluronidase.

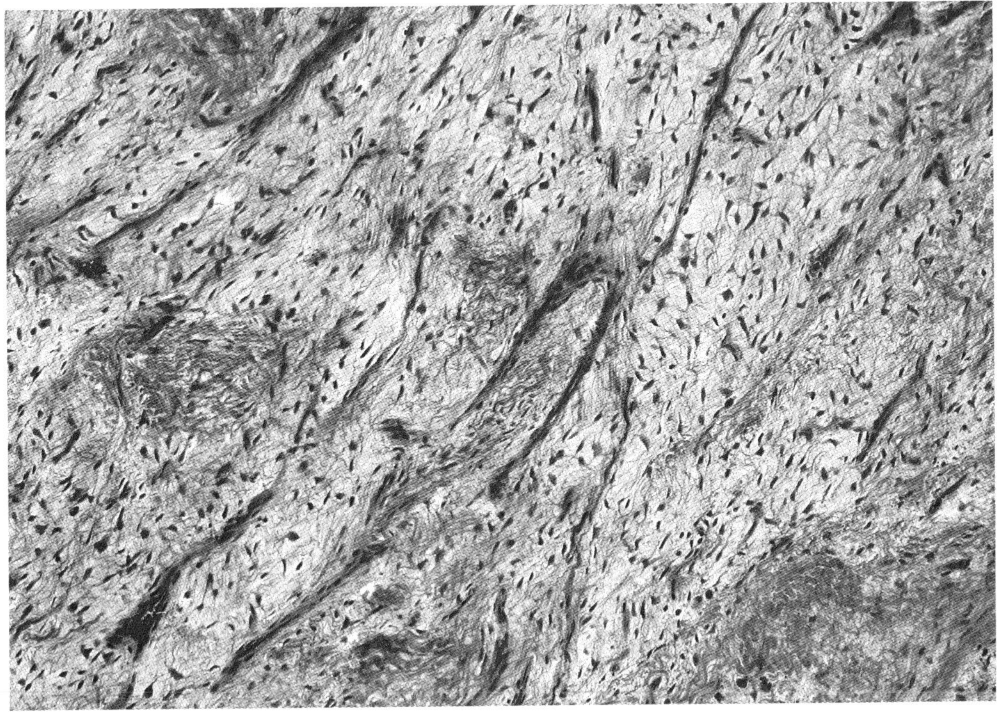

**FIGURE 36–27.** Cutaneous myxoma. A prominent arborizing vasculature is present, mimicking that found in myxoid liposarcoma.

one-third of these tumors have epithelial structures consisting of basaloid buds, epithelial strands, or epidermoid (keratin-filled) cysts, possibly as a result of entrapment of adnexal structures by the neoplasm[96,98] (Figs. 36–28, 36–29, 36–30).

Immunohistochemically, the tumor cells consistently express vimentin but do not stain for cytokeratins or S-100 protein.[98] Rare cells stain for smooth muscle actin, possibly representing focal myofibroblastic differentiation.[100]

The differential diagnosis of cutaneous myxoma is extensive and includes aggressive angiomyxoma, focal cutaneous mucinosis, cutaneous myxoid cyst, dermal nerve sheath myxoma (neurothekeoma), myxoid neurofibroma, myxoid liposarcoma, and myxofibrosarcoma.

Some cutaneous myxomas arise in the genital region[99] and so may be confused with *aggressive angiomyxoma*. The latter lesion, however, tends to be larger, involves deeper structures, and has a vascular pattern that differs from that of cutaneous myxoma. *Focal cutaneous mucinosis* lacks the lobular architecture, stromal neutrophils, and epithelial structures found in cutaneous myxoma. The distinction between these two entities is of clinical importance, as the former does not recur locally. *Cutaneous myxoid cyst* is easily distinguished given its almost exclusive location on the fingers. *Neurothekeoma* has a more pronounced lobular growth pattern and is characterized by plumper cells that are invariably positive for S-100 protein. *Myxoid neurofibroma* is composed of cells with wavy or buckled nuclei that are also S-100 protein-positive.

*Myxoid liposarcoma* is usually more deeply located and larger than cutaneous myxoma, and it is characterized by a plexiform vasculature with scattered lipoblasts. *Myxofibrosarcoma* has a greater degree of nuclear atypia and hyperchromasia as well as curvilinear vessels often lined by hyperchromatic tumor cells.

Cutaneous myxoma has a propensity for local recurrence if incompletely excised. In the series by Allen et al.,[96] 8 of 20 (40%) tumors recurred, including five of eight tumors with epithelial components. Calonje et al.[98] reported a recurrence rate of 30%, including one case that recurred three times. In the latter series, recurrences developed a median of 12 months following initial excision, particularly those that were incompletely excised. No cutaneous myxoma has been reported to metastasize.

## CUTANEOUS AND CARDIAC MYXOMAS, SPOTTY PIGMENTATION, AND ENDOCRINE OVERACTIVITY (CARNEY'S COMPLEX)

The triad of cutaneous and cardiac myxomas, spotty pigmentation, and endocrine overactivity, first described by Carney et al.[104] in 1985, principally affects young adults and consists of cutaneous and cardiac myxomas (Fig. 36–31), spotty pigmentation, and endocrine overactivity. The disorder is familial and is transmitted as an autosomal dominant trait.[106] Evidence has suggested involvement of chromosomes

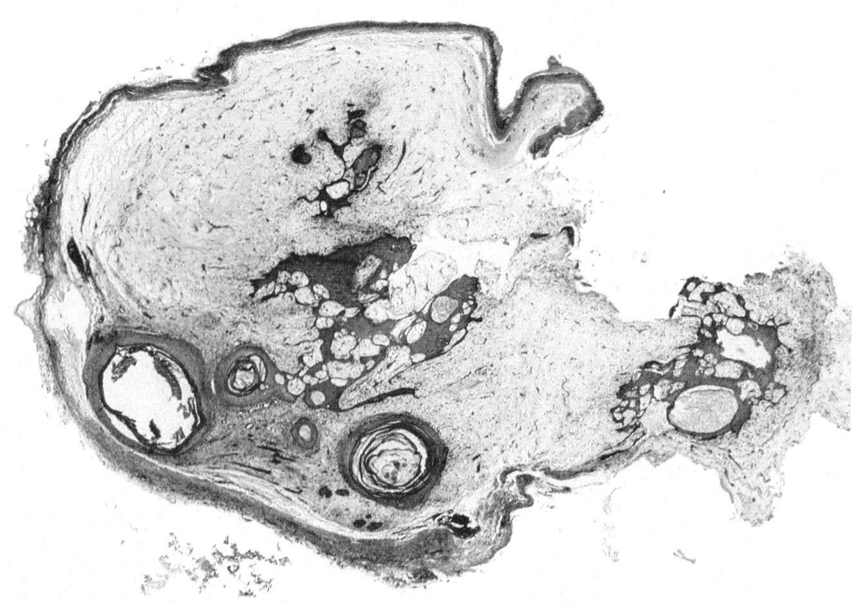

**FIGURE 36–28.** Cutaneous myxoma in a patient with Carney's complex. Note the adnexal structures surrounded by myxoid matrix.

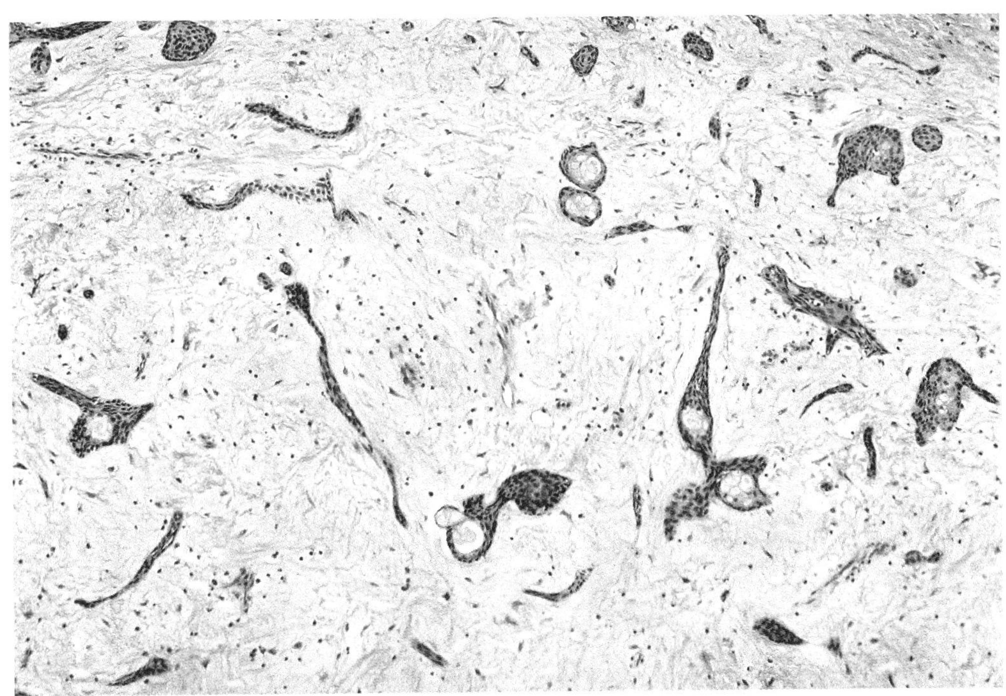

**FIGURE 36–29.** Cutaneous myxoma in a patient with Carney's complex. Numerous epithelial strands are found in the substance of the neoplasm.

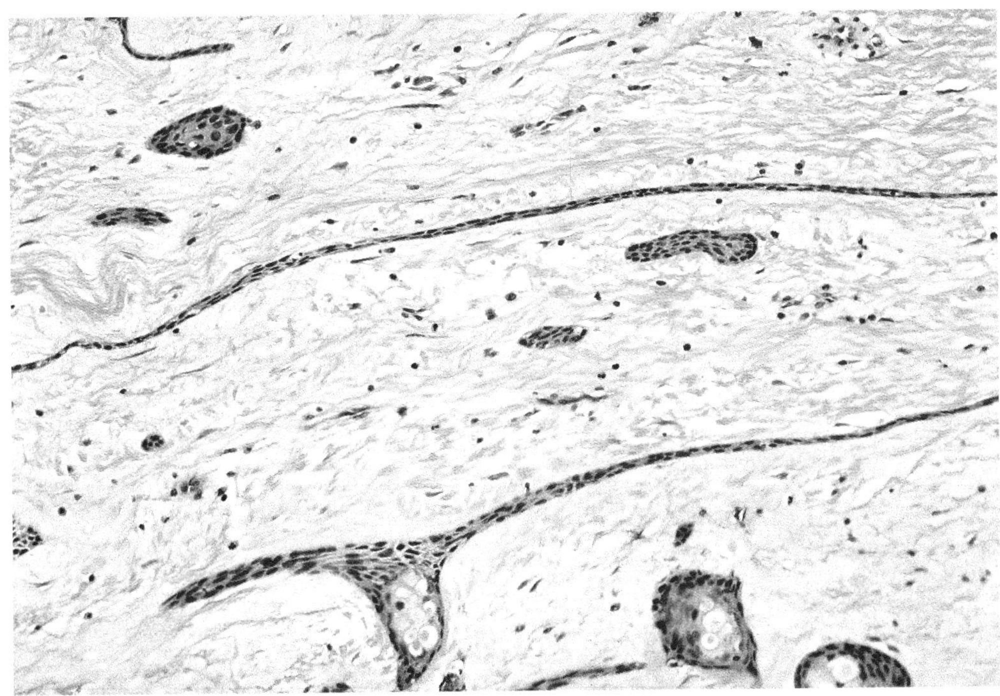

**FIGURE 36–30.** High magnification view of elongated epithelial strands which appear to be compressed by the surrounding neoplasm in a cutaneous myxoma in a patient with Carney's complex.

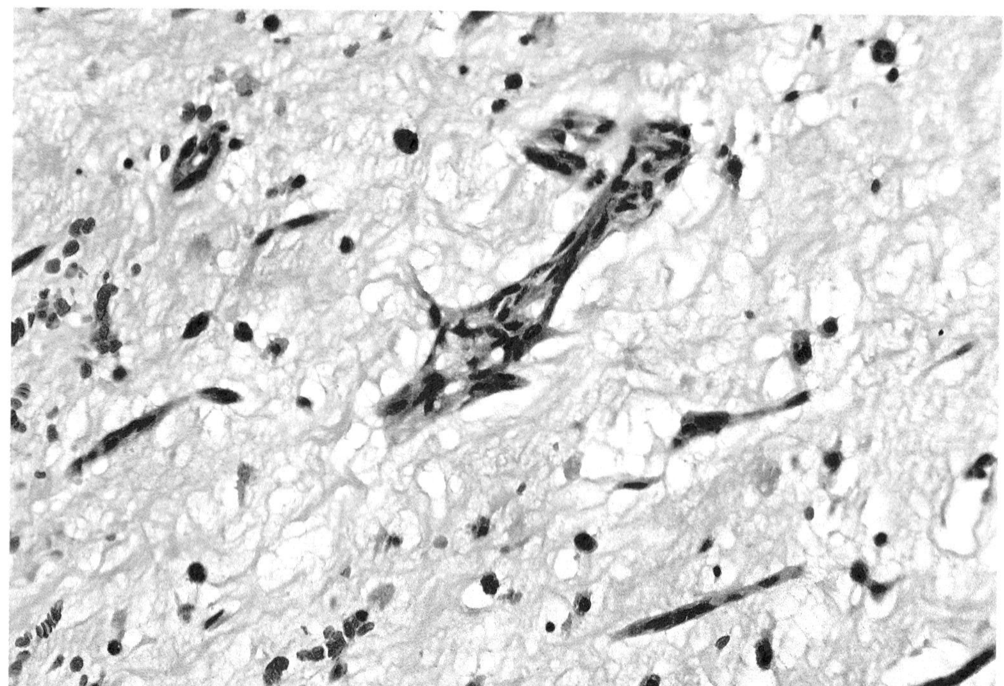

**FIGURE 36–31.** Cardiac myxoma in a patient with Carney's complex.

2p15-16[121,123,125] and 17q2,[109] although not all patients have abnormalities at these loci, suggesting genetic heterogeneity.[116,118]

The cutaneous myxomas have a predilection for the eyelids and range from small sessile papules to large pedunculated, finger-like masses; they are multiple in most cases and are characterized by an appearance during early adulthood (mean age 18 years).[105] The lesions are found in the dermis or subcutaneous tissue, are usually sharply circumscribed, and are characterized by cytologically bland spindled and stellate-shaped cells deposited in an abundant myxoid stroma with a prominent capillary vasculature, identical to sporadic cutaneous myxomas discussed in the previous section. They are often associated with a basaloid proliferation of the surface epithelium, which may cause misclassification of some of these lesions as basal cell carcinoma or trichofolliculoma.[114] More recently, Ferreiro and Carney reported the association of myxomas of the external ear with Carney's complex.[114] Of the 152 patients with this complex known to these authors, 22 (14%) had myxomas of the external ear. Furthermore, 22 of 26 patients (85%) with ear myxomas were found to have Carney's complex. Multifocal myxoid fibroadenomas and myxomatosis of the breast are also occasional components of this complex.[108]

The most serious components of the syndrome are psammomatous melanotic schwannoma[102] (see Chapter 30) and cardiac myxoma.[101,124] Cardiac myxomas, regardless of their association with this syndrome, may be associated with peripheral tumor emboli,[113,115] and up to 24% of all patients with cardiac myxomas die of its complications.[112]

The spotty skin pigmentation includes lentigines that predominantly affect the face, particularly the vermilion border of the lips,[111] and blue nevi, including epithelioid blue nevi.[103,107] Endocrine overactivity may be due to the presence of primary pigmented nodular adrenocortical disease resulting in Cushing's syndrome,[117,120] pituitary adenoma resulting in acromegaly, or sexual precocity associated with testicular lesions, particularly large-cell calcifying Sertoli's cell tumor.[110,119] Thyroid gland abnormalities ranging from follicular hyperplasia to cystic carcinoma have been associated with Carney's complex.[122]

## CUTANEOUS MYXOID CYST

Cutaneous myxoid cyst, which has received relatively little attention in the literature, is characterized by a soft, dome-shaped nodule located in the corium of the distal and dorsal portions of the fingers and infrequently the toes close to the nail. With the exception of small children, it occurs at virtually any age and is about twice as common in women as in men.[126] In general, the nodule is small, slow-growing and rarely exceeds 2 cm in greatest diameter.[127–129] Typically it consists of a small number of spindle- and stellate-shaped fibroblasts producing small amounts of gly-

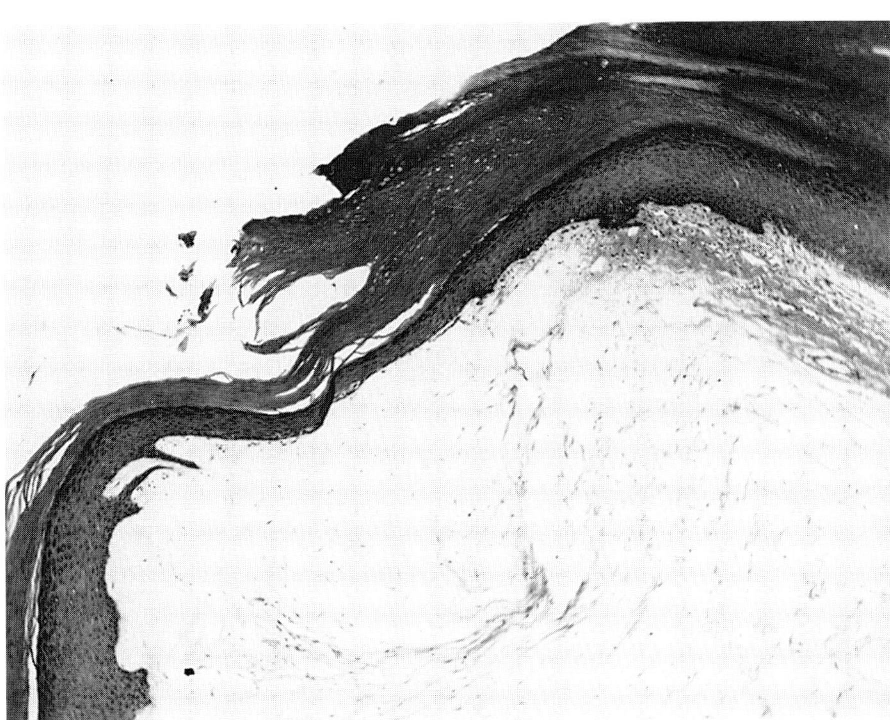

**FIGURE 36–32.** Cutaneous myxoid cyst of the index finger in the region of the nail bed.

cosaminoglycans (mucopolysaccharides) at the expense of collagen (Fig. 36–32). Many contain small fluid-filled cavities, but few of these cavities are bordered by collagenous walls as in ganglia. Not infrequently the nodules are covered by wart-like verrucous skin and are associated with grooving or other dystrophic changes of the nail and Heberden's nodes. Radiologic examination frequently reveals osteoarthritis in the adjacent terminal joint. Treatment may be difficult. Recurrence after incision and drainage and even excision is a common event, and some reviewers recommend wide excision with full-thickness skin grafting.[127] Others report good results with multiple injections of topical steroids (triamcinolone acetonide).[129] A morphologically similar giant fibromyxoid growth was described in association with a meningomyelocele scar and compound nevi.[130]

## FOCAL CUTANEOUS MUCINOSIS AND MYXEDEMA

Although originally believed to be synonymous with cutaneous myxoma,[137] *focal cutaneous mucinosis* is an asymptomatic localized accumulation of hypocellular mucinous material with scattered small spindle-shaped cells predominantly in the dermis of the face, trunk, and oral region of adult patients[131,144,146] (Figs. 36–33, 36–34). Unlike cutaneous myxoma, it lacks a distinct lobular or multinodular architecture, and it has few blood vessels and lacks stromal neutrophils.[98] Preexisting dermal collagen bundles are retained and separated by abundant myxoid stroma. It is curable by local excision and does not locally recur.

*Localized myxedema* is histologically indistinguishable from focal cutaneous mucinosis, but it is clinically marked by a large, discrete, often bilateral, nonpitting nodule or plaque in the pretibial region and less commonly in the dorsal aspects of the ankle and foot, often with hyperpigmentation of the overlying skin. Characteristically, it affects patients who have hyperthyroidism or have been cured of hyperthyroidism but continue to show exophthalmos (Graves' ophthalmopathy), probably because of blocking thyroid-stimulating hormone (TSH) receptor autoantibodies.[134–136,141,143]

The term *scleromyxedema* or *papular mucinosis* has been used to describe a nodular accumulation of mucinous material and proliferating fibroblasts in the dermis causing a "cobblestone" appearance of the skin. This process has been associated with a variety of conditions, including human immunodeficiency virus (HIV) infection,[133,142] dermatomyositis,[139] systemic lupus erythematosus,[138,140] mycosis fungoides[145] and abnormal serum gamma globulin.[132,147]

## GANGLION

Ganglion is by far the most common and best known of the more superficially located myxoid lesions. It occurs as a unilocular or multilocular cystic or myx-

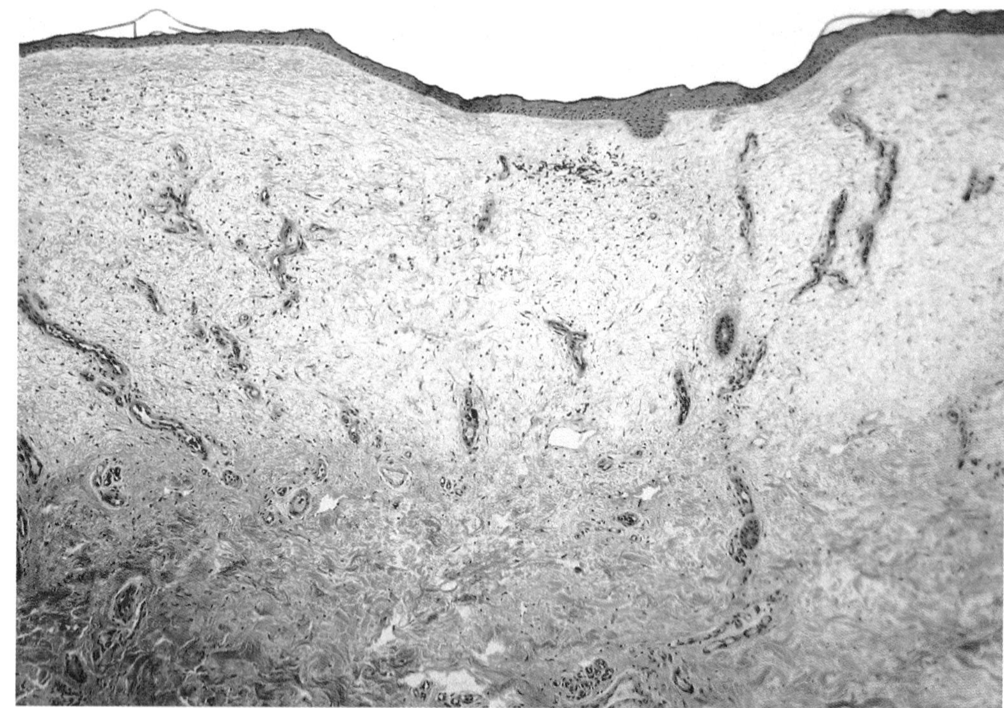

**FIGURE 36–33.** Focal cutaneous mucinosis. There is a localized accumulation of hypocellular mucinous material with scattered small spindle-shaped cells in the dermis.

oid mass on the dorsal surface of the wrist in young persons, especially women, generally 25–45 years of age. Less often it is found on the volar surface of the wrist or fingers and the dorsum of the foot and toes.[148,151–154,157,158] In about half of the cases the condition is associated with tenderness or mild pain and causes interference of function. In Carp and Stout's series,[150] a history of trauma was given by about half of the patients.

Ganglia usually measure 1.5–2.5 cm in diameter. They are frequently attached to the joint capsule and tendon sheaths and probably are due to excessive mucin production by fibroblasts rather than disintegration of preformed fibrous structures. There is no communication between the ganglion and the joint space. Some of these lesions are easily confused with myxomas, especially during the initial myxoid stage of development. Most, however, are readily recognized by their location and the presence of multiple thick-walled cystic spaces of variable size in association with myxoid areas. Focal myxoid change is noted in the earliest stage (Fig. 36–35). Subsequently, microscopic cysts develop and coalesce into larger ones until finally the lesion assumes its typical form of a dominant cyst (Fig. 36–36). Sarpyener et al.[155] described multiple ganglia of the hands, wrists, feet, and ankles in a 4-year-old mentally retarded boy with bilateral ptosis of the eyelids. Ganglion-like lesions may also arise in the subperiosteal region or bone.[149,156] Intraneural ganglion-like lesions (nerve sheath ganglion) and neurothekeoma are discussed and illustrated in Chapter 30.

## AGGRESSIVE ANGIOMYXOMA

The term *aggressive angiomyxoma* was coined by Steeper and Rosai in 1983 for a morphologically distinctive, slow-growing myxoid neoplasm that occurs chiefly in the genital, perineal, and pelvic regions of adult women.[178] Despite its bland histologic features, it has a propensity for local recurrence.

### Clinical and Radiologic Findings

The neoplasm predominantly affects reproductive-age females with a peak incidence during the third decade of life. The female/male ratio is more than 6:1,[166] but this tumor has been increasingly recognized as arising in the inguinal region, along the spermatic cord, or in the scrotum or pelvic cavity of men.[159,163,170,179] In women, the vulvar region is the most common site of involvement and may be initially misdiagnosed clinically as a Bartholin's cyst, periurethral cyst, or hernia.[168] Although slowly growing, these lesions aggressively infiltrate the perivaginal and perirectal soft tissues.

The radiologic features of this tumor have been well described.[161,162] Magnetic resonance imaging

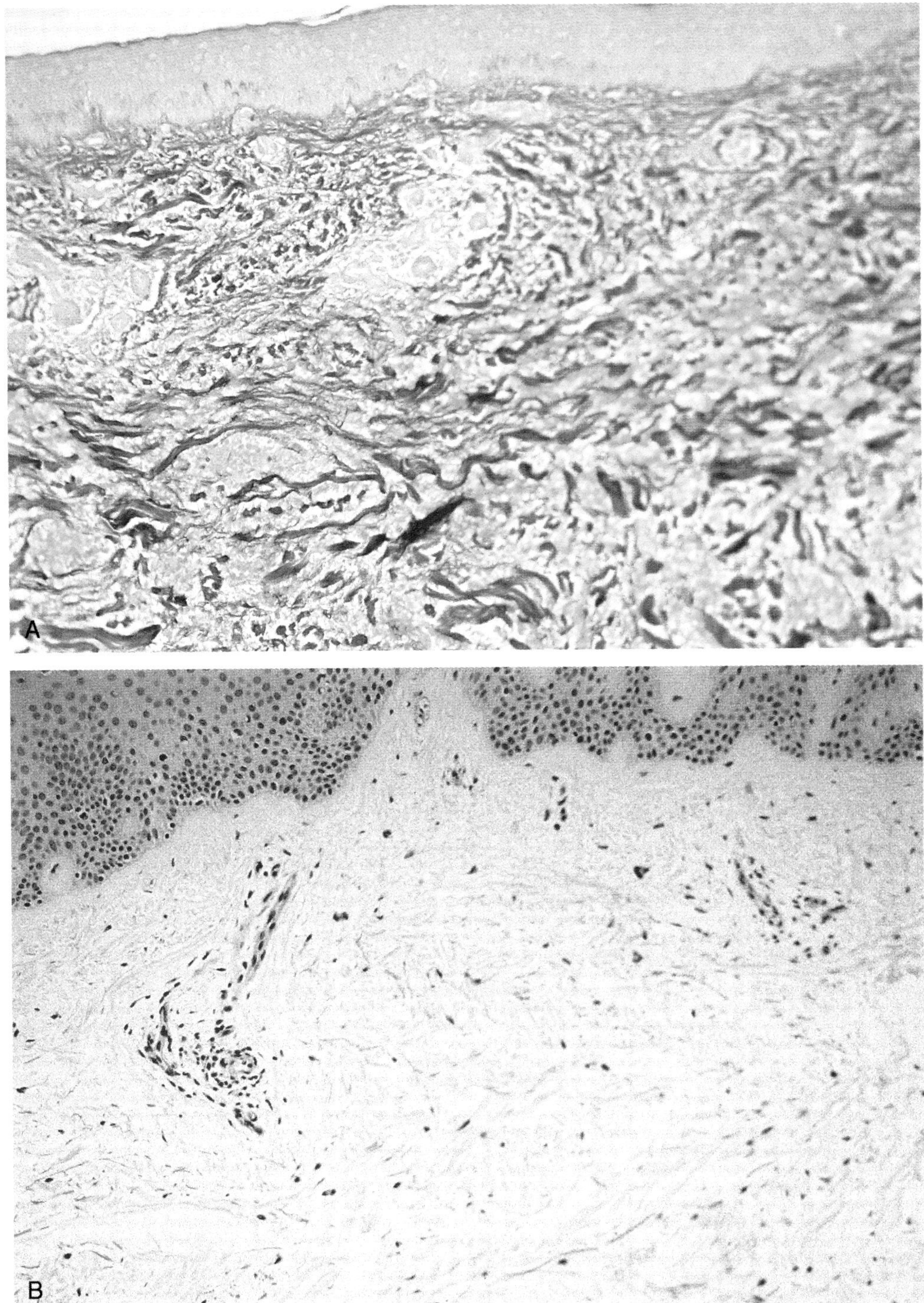


**FIGURE 36–34.** Focal cutaneous mucinosis stained with alcian blue stain without (**A**) and with (**B**) pretreatment with hyaluronidase.

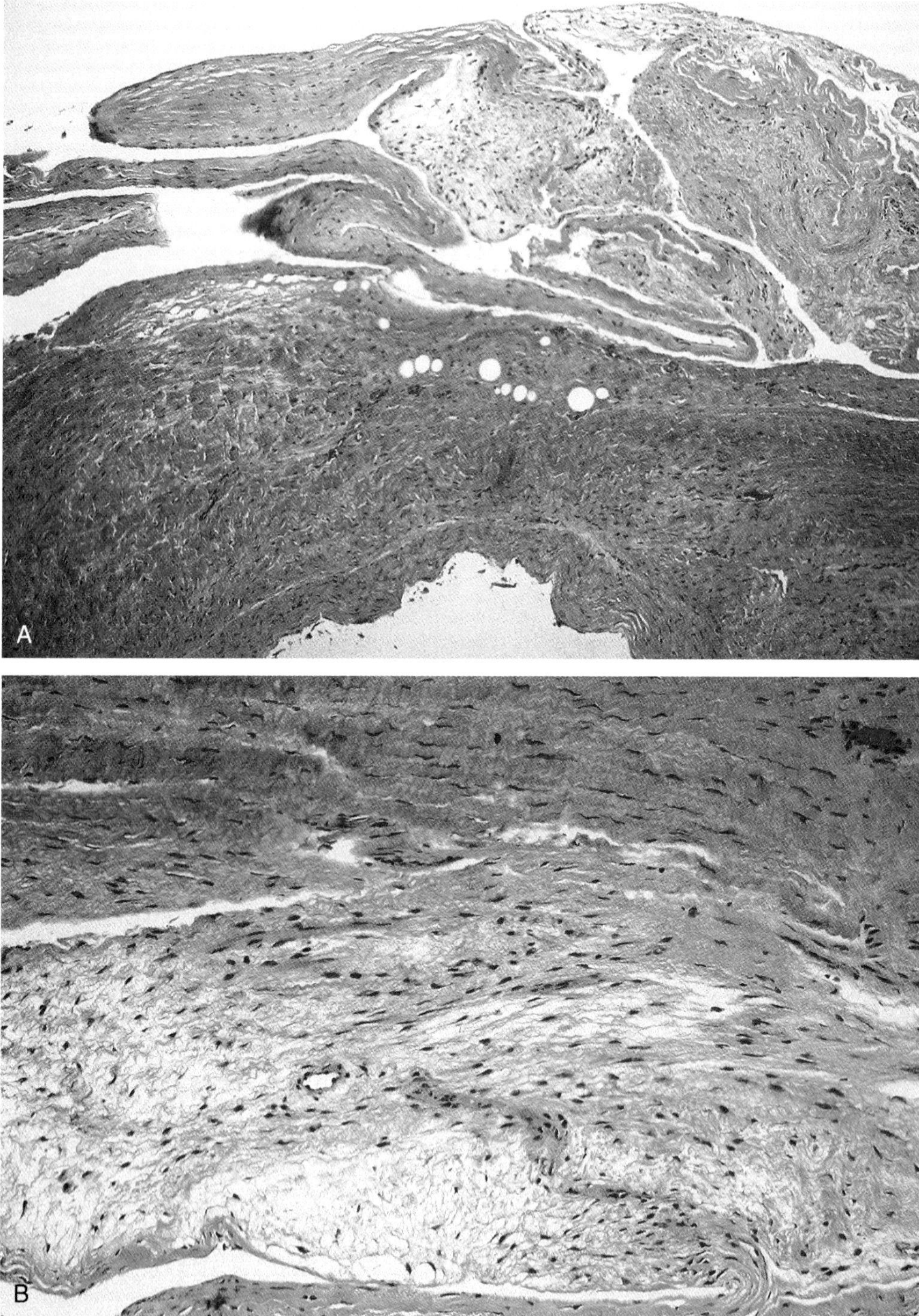


**FIGURE 36–35.** (**A**) Low magnification view of a ganglion with an irregular thick-walled cystic space and focal myxoid change in the surrounding matrix. (**B**) High magnification view of focal myxoid change with bland spindle-shaped cells in a ganglion.

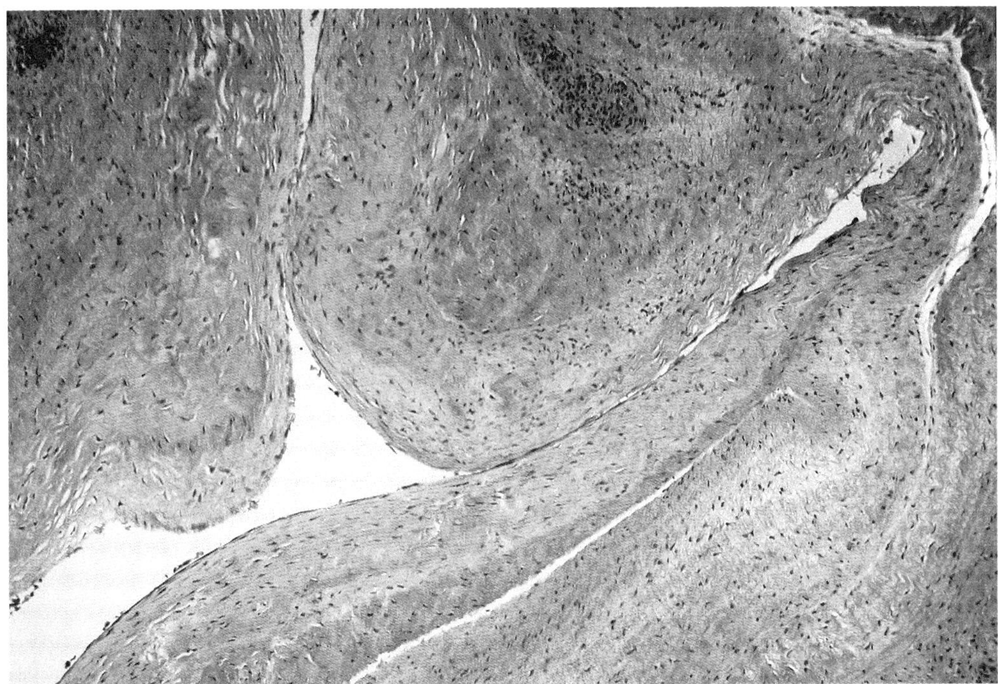

**FIGURE 36–36.** Ganglion. Dominant cyst with prominent myxoid change in the surrounding soft tissue.

(MRI) reveals a mass with high signal intensity on T2-weighted images with translevator extension and growth around perineal structures.[164,175]

## Pathologic Findings

Grossly, angiomyxomas are soft, partly circumscribed, or polypoid; on cross section they have a gelatinous appearance and range in size from a few centimeters to 20 cm or more. Steeper and Rosai reported an angiomyxoma of the pelvis and retroperitoneum in a 34-year-old woman that measured 60 × 20 cm in greatest diameter.[178] In the series by Fetsch et al.[166] 23 of 27 tumors were 10 cm or larger. Most have a lobulated appearance. Although some areas of the tumor may be sharply marginated, others show adherence or infiltration into the surrounding soft tissues.

Microscopically, the tumor is composed of widely scattered spindle- and stellate-shaped cells with ill-defined cytoplasm and variably sized, thin- or thick-walled vascular channels in a myxoid stroma that is rich in collagen fibers and, like other richly myxoid tumors, often contains foci of hemorrhage (Figs. 36–37 to 36–40). Although the cellularity is usually low and uniform throughout the tumor, some lesions have focal areas of increased cellularity, particularly around large vessels and at the periphery of the tumor.[166,168] The cells have small round to oval hyperchromatic nuclei with small centrally located nucleoli (Fig. 36–41). Mitotic figures are rare or absent and are not atypical. The stroma is characterized by prominent myxoid change with fine collagen fibrils, often with areas of erythrocyte extravasation. A characteristic feature of this tumor is the presence of variably sized vessels that range from small thin-walled capillaries to large vessels with secondary changes including perivascular hyalinization and medial hypertrophy (Fig. 36–42). Mast cells are often prominent, and some tumors have perivascular lymphoid aggregates. Small bundles of spindle-shaped cells with eosinophilic cytoplasm may be present, frequently adjacent to blood vessels.[168] These cells have more conventional features of smooth muscle cells, with cigar-shaped nuclei and perinuclear vacuoles. As noted by Granter et al.,[168] occasional aggressive angiomyxomas have features overlapping those seen in angiomyofibroblastomas, including epithelioid cells arranged in cords around blood vessels and multinucleated cells, suggesting that these two lesions are on a morphologic spectrum.

## Immunohistochemical and Electron Microscopic Findings

Immunohistochemically, the cells of aggressive angiomyxoma show diffuse staining for vimentin. Although earlier reports of this entity noted an absence of desmin staining,[159] more recent studies have shown

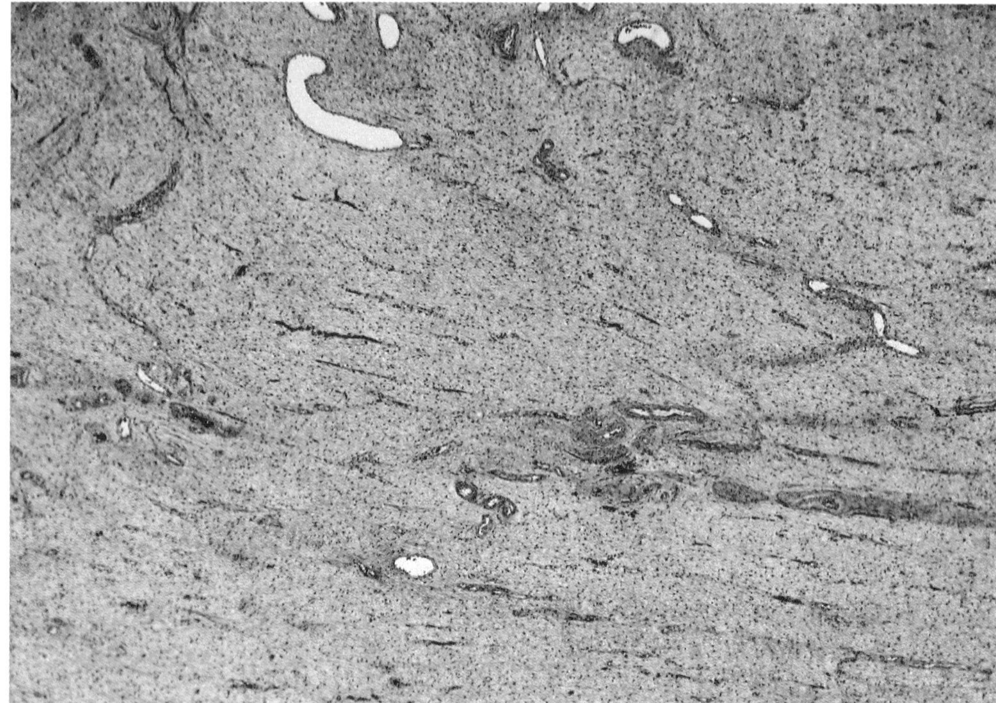

**FIGURE 36–37.** Aggressive angiomyxoma. The tumor is hypocellular and has prominent thin- and thick-walled vascular channels surrounded by a myxoid stroma.

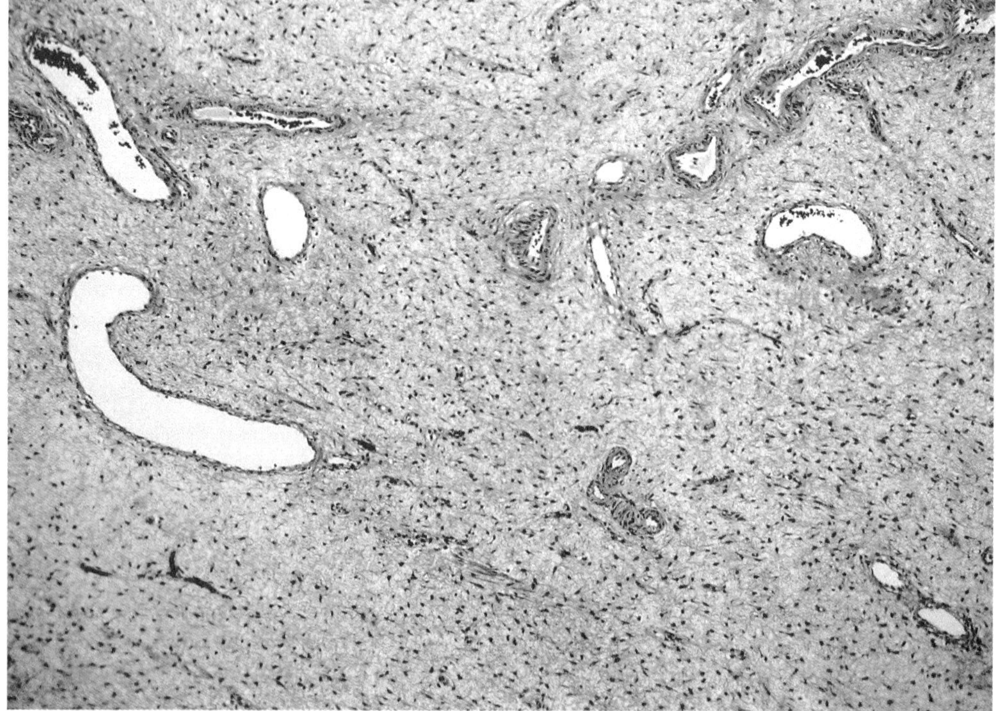

**FIGURE 36–38.** Aggressive angiomyxoma. Spindle-shaped cells are evenly distributed in a myxoid stroma. Prominent vessels are apparent.

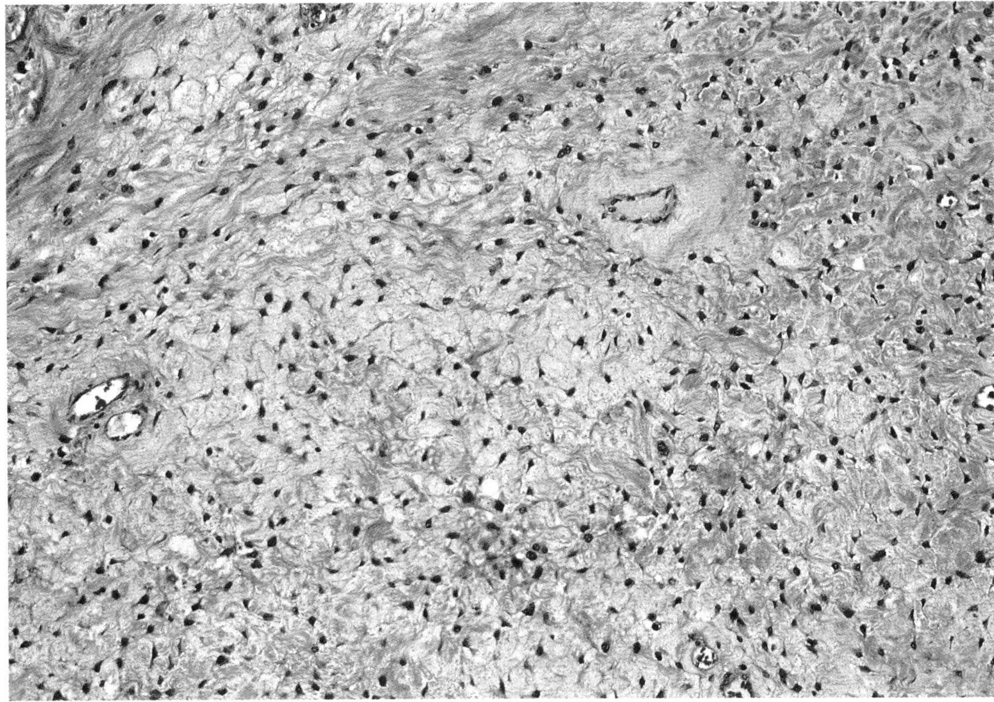

**FIGURE 36–39.** Aggressive angiomyxoma. Cytologically bland spindled and stellate-shaped cells are evenly distributed in a myxoid stroma.

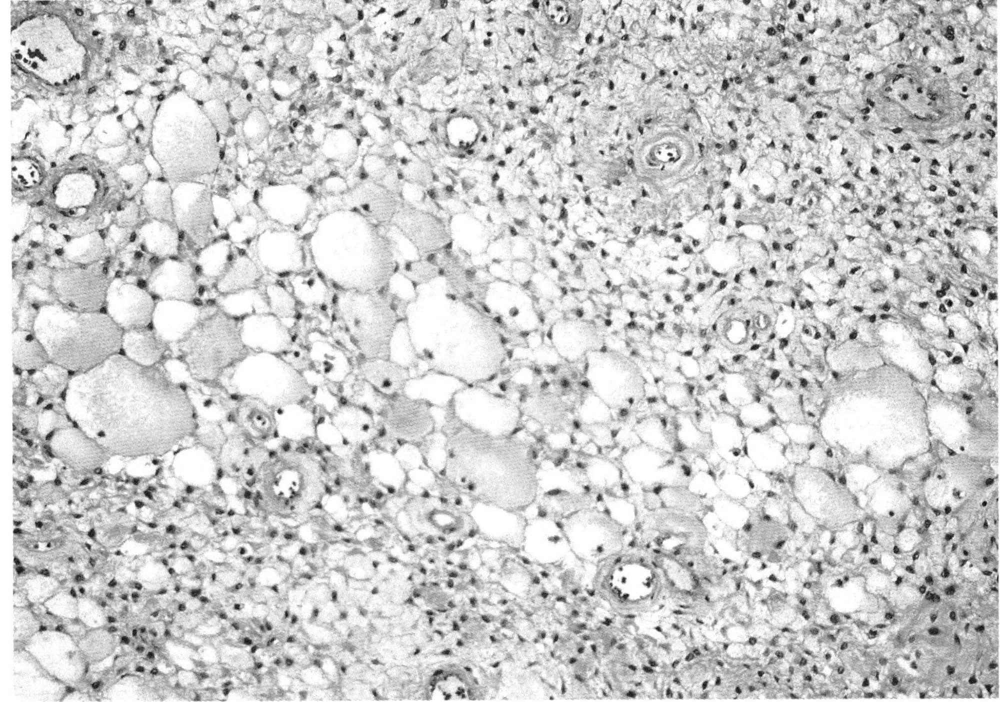

**FIGURE 36–40.** Microcystic change in an aggressive angiomyxoma.

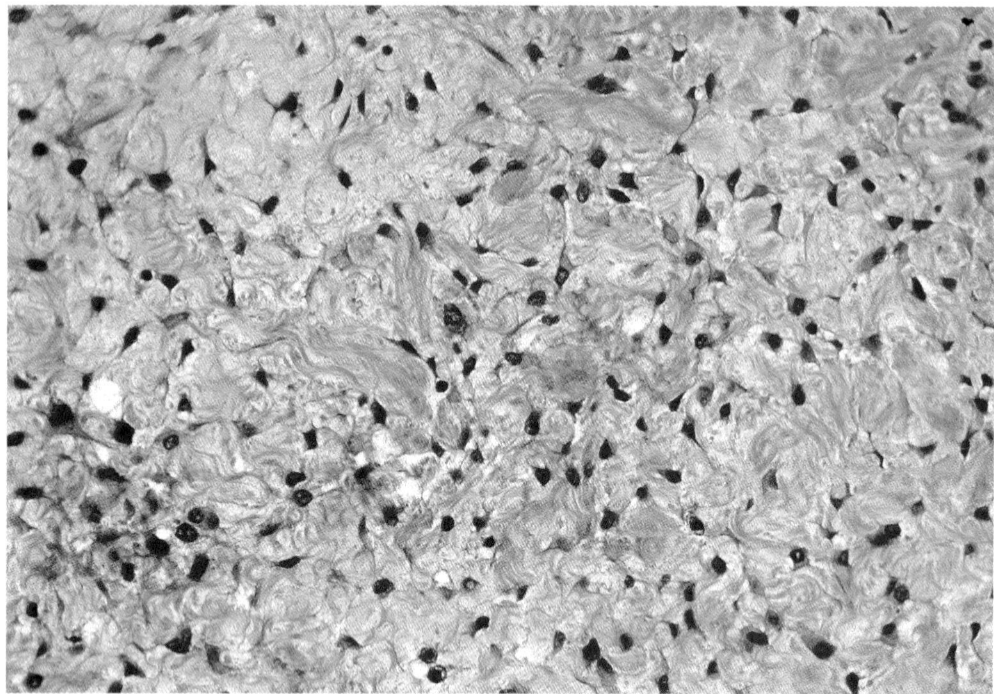

**FIGURE 36–41.** High magnification view of bland spindled and stellate-shaped cells in an aggressive angiomyxoma.

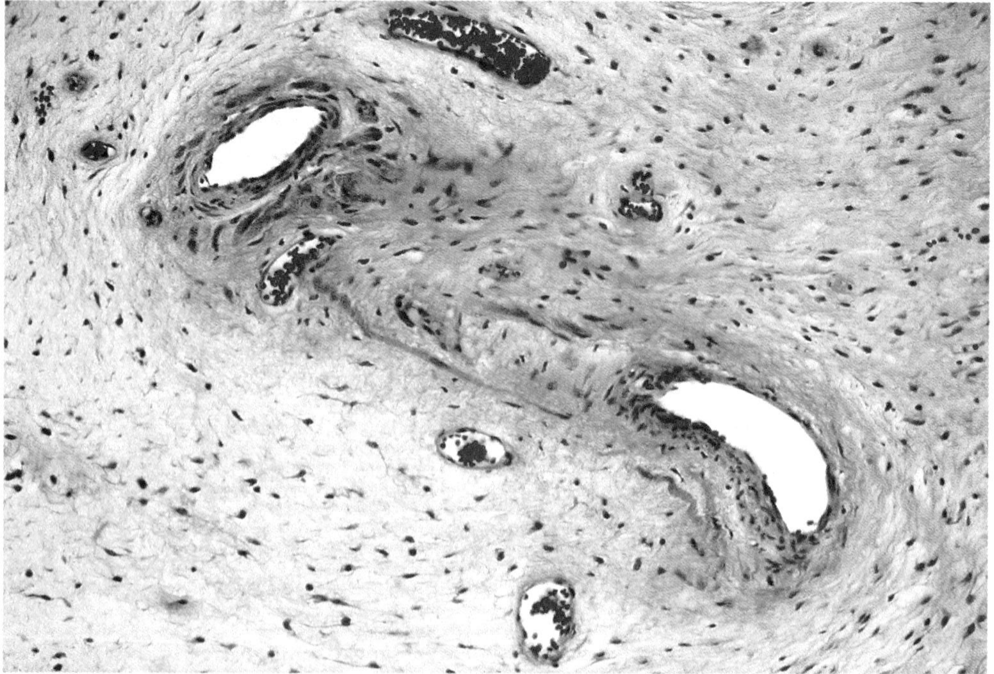

**FIGURE 36–42.** Characteristic thin- and thick-walled vascular channels in an aggressive angiomyxoma.

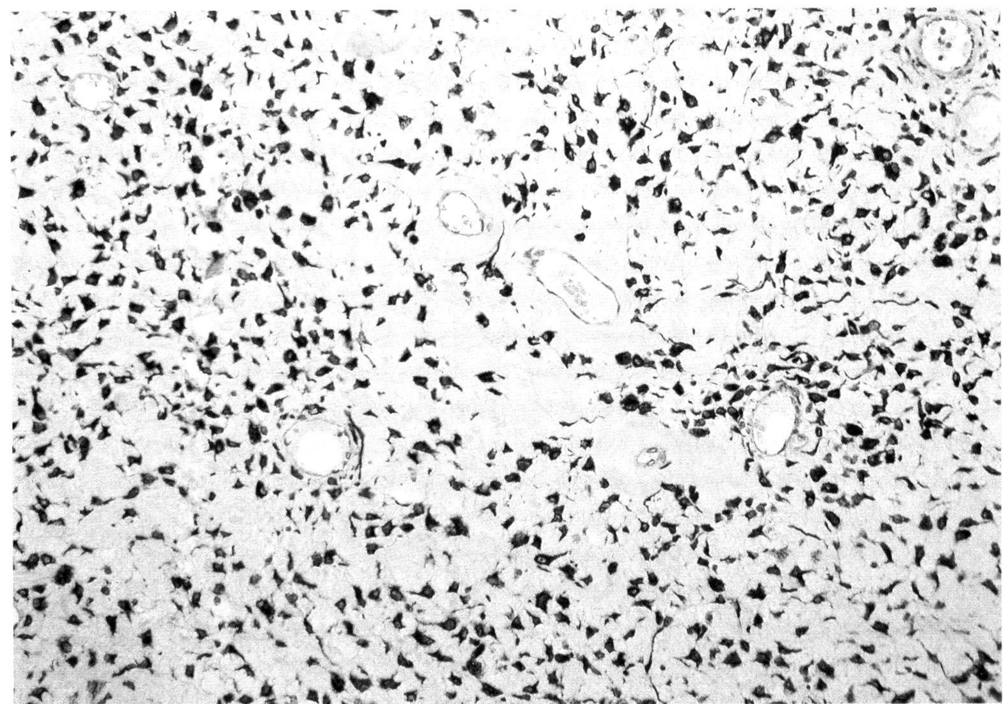

**FIGURE 36–43.** Diffuse desmin immunoreactivity in an aggressive angiomyxoma.

that most cases stain either focally or diffusely (Fig. 36–43) for this antigen[166,168] (Table 36–5). Immunostains for muscle-specific actin and smooth muscle actin are also positive in most cases, whereas S-100 protein and cytokeratins are not expressed by the neoplastic cells.[160,174] A variable proportion of cells in some aggressive angiomyxomas also express CD-34[166,176] and Factor XIIIa.[176] Both estrogen and progesterone receptors have been detected suggesting a hormonal role in the development or growth of these lesions.[165,166,169] Electron microscopic examination shows fibroblast-like[159] or myofibroblast-like cells,[177] often with delicate cytoplasmic processes extending into the surrounding myxoid matrix, which consists of a mixture of finely granular material and scattered collagen fibers.

## Differential Diagnosis

Aggressive angiomyxoma must be differentiated from other benign myxoid neoplasms given its propensity for local recurrence. *Angiomyofibroblastoma,* originally described by Fletcher et al. in 1992,[167] is a neoplasm that arises in the subcutaneous tissues of the vulva, vagina, and rarely the scrotum. Most are small and well circumscribed, and they are composed of plump epithelioid cells arranged in a striking perivascular distribution. Binucleated and multinucleated cells are commonly seen. The lesion rarely assumes a myxoid appearance as is found in aggressive angiomyxoma, and there are typically numerous thin-walled vessels with perivascular hyalinization.[174] As previously stated, aggressive angiomyxoma and angiomyofibro-

**TABLE 36–5** IMMUNOHISTOCHEMICAL DATA IN SERIES OF AGGRESSIVE ANGIOMYXOMAS

| Marker | Fetsch et al.[166] | Granter et al.[168] | Total (%) |
|---|---|---|---|
| Desmin | 22/22 | 13/14 | 35/36 (97) |
| Smooth muscle actin | 19/20 | 10/11 | 29/31 (94) |
| Muscle-specific actin | 16/19 | 11/12 | 27/31 (87) |
| CD-34 | 8/16 | — | 8/16 (50) |
| Estrogen receptor | 13/14 | — | 13/14 (93) |
| Progesterone receptor | 9/10 | — | 9/10 (90) |
| S-100 protein | 0/20 | 0/14 | 0/34 (0) |

blastoma have overlapping histologic and immunohistochemical features. However, the distinction between these two entities is of clinical importance, as aggressive angiomyxoma has a much higher risk of recurrence than angiomyofibroblastoma, a lesion that is usually cured following simple excision (Table 36–6).

Aggressive angiomyxoma also shares histologic features with *myxomas of the intramuscular and juxtaarticular types,* but these tumors arise in different anatomic sites and are generally less cellular, less vascular, and have more abundant stromal mucin than the aggressive angiomyxoma.

*Cutaneous myxoma* is a relatively rare neoplasm that typically involves the dermis or subcutaneous tissue (or both) and rarely arises in the vulvar or perineal region.[166] This lesion is characteristically lobular or multinodular and is composed of a sparsely cellular proliferation of stellate and spindle-shaped cells deposited in an abundant myxoid matrix. It has variable vascularity but lacks thick-walled large vessels as are seen in the aggressive angiomyxoma, and the neoplastic cells do not express desmin.

*Myxoid neurofibroma* may also closely resemble aggressive angiomyxoma but is composed of cells with wavy or buckled nuclei, occasionally with the formation of Wagner-Meissner bodies, and diffuse immunoreactivity for S-100 protein. These lesions also lack the characteristic vascularity of aggressive angiomyxoma.

*Myxoid leiomyoma,* a tumor that may reach a large size and is frequently found in the pelvic region, differs from aggressive angiomyxoma by its less prominent vascular pattern and the presence of widely scattered smooth muscle cells in a myxoid matrix. The tumor cells are larger and have more abundant eosinophilic cytoplasm than those of aggressive angiomyxoma, and they tend to be arranged in small packets or loose fascicles.

*Pelvic fibromatosis* primarily affects women between the ages of 20 and 35 years. Like aggressive angiomyxoma, pelvic fibromatosis is an infiltrative process and often entraps surrounding soft tissue structures; it is composed of more elongated spindle-shaped cells separated by abundant collagen and arranged in sweeping fascicles. Some pelvic fibromatoses have striking myxoid change, but areas of more typical fibromatosis are invariably present. Although these lesions have a uniform distribution of small to medium-size vessels, they lack the large caliber thick-walled vessels characteristic of aggressive angiomyxoma.

Because aggressive angiomyxoma may become extremely large and has a tendency to infiltrate the surrounding soft tissues, a low-grade myxoid sarcoma is not infrequently considered. *Myxoid liposarcoma* arises only rarely in the pelvic region and can be distinguished by its characteristic fine plexiform vasculature and the identification of scattered lipoblasts. *Myxofibrosarcoma (low-grade myxoid malignant fibrous histiocytoma)* is distinguished from aggressive angiomyxoma by the presence of cells with more obvious cytologic atypia and hyperchromasia and its characteristic curvilinear vascular pattern.

## Discussion

Aggressive angiomyxoma tends to recur in a high percentage of cases (Fig. 36–44), but there is no evidence that it is capable of metastasis. Steeper and Rosai reported five cases with more than 12 months follow-up, four of which recurred locally, one as late as 14 years after local excision.[178] Begin et al.[159] described six cases with follow-up data, all of which recurred within 9–84 months after excision. A 36% rate of local recurrence was reported by both Fetsch et al.[166] and Granter et al.[168] in more recently published series. Neither size nor cellularity correlate with the risk of local recurrence. Because many of these tumors have infiltrative borders, complete excision is often difficult and likely accounts for the high rate of local recurrence.

Clonal cytogenetic aberrations have been reported in some aggressive angiomyxomas, including a pericentric inversion of 12p11.2,[171] loss of an X chromosome,[173] and a translocation involving 12q14-15.[172] A low Ki-67 index is in keeping with its characteristic

**TABLE 36–6 DIFFERENTIAL DIAGNOSTIC FEATURES OF AGGRESSIVE ANGIOMYXOMA AND ANGIOMYOFIBROBLASTOMA**

| Feature | Aggressive Angiomyxoma | Angiomyofibroblastoma |
|---|---|---|
| Gross appearance | Poorly circumscribed, infiltrative | Circumscribed |
| Size | Large (many ≥10 cm) | Most ≤3 cm |
| Cellularity | Uniform | Perivascular hypercellularity |
| Cell shape | Spindled | Epithelioid |
| Vasculature | Variably sized, thick-walled | Numerous, thin-walled, often perivascular hyalinization |
| Multinucleation | Absent | Present |
| Recurrence | 50% | Rare |

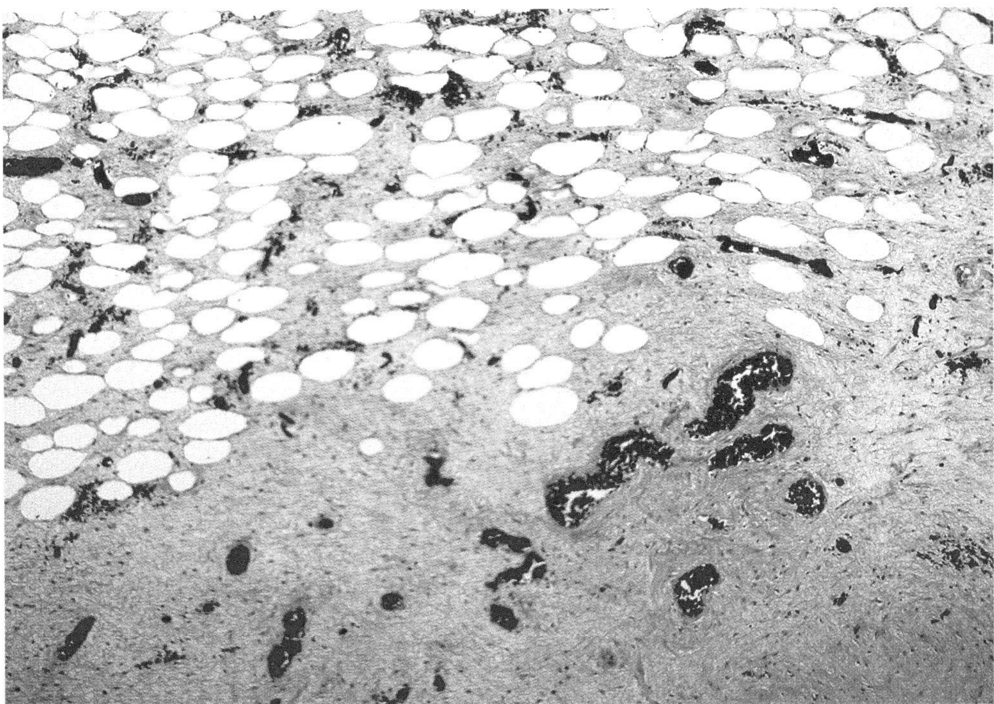

**FIGURE 36–44.** Infiltration of surrounding adipose tissue in an aggressive angiomyxoma. This pattern of infiltration likely accounts for the high rate of local recurrence of this tumor.

slow growth.[166] Although the line of differentiation has been debated since its initial description, most report features of myofibroblastic differentiation by either immunohistochemistry or ultrastructural analysis. Tumors with composite features of aggressive angiomyxoma and angiomyofibroblastoma raise the possibility that these two lesions are related and possibly derived from a primitive mesenchymal cell normally found in the lower female genital tract that has the capability of myofibroblastic differentiation. In our experience these two lesions are reasonably distinctive such that they can be reliably distinguished in virtually all cases.

## OSSIFYING FIBROMYXOID TUMOR OF SOFT TISSUE

The ossifying fibromyxoid tumor of soft tissue, first described in 1989,[183] is a rare tumor of uncertain differentiation that most commonly arises in the extremities and virtually always acts in a clinically benign fashion. It almost exclusively affects adults, with only rare examples having been documented in young children.[181] Men are affected more commonly than women. Most patients present with a small, painless, well defined, often lobulated subcutaneous mass that involves the extremities in approximately 70% of cases (Table 36–7). Less commonly involved sites include the trunk, head and neck, mediastinum, and retroperitoneum.[188,192,193] Radiographic studies usually reveal a well circumscribed mass with an incomplete ring of peripheral calcification and scattered calcifications in the substance of the neoplasm[190] (Fig. 36–45).

**TABLE 36–7** ANATOMIC LOCATION OF 59 CASES OF OSSIFYING FIBROMYXOID TUMOR

| Site | No. of Cases |
|---|---|
| Upper extremity | 20 (34%) |
| Shoulder/upper arm | 10 |
| Elbow/forearm | 4 |
| Hands/fingers | 6 |
| Lower extremity | 20 (34%) |
| Buttock/thigh | 11 |
| Knee/lower leg | 4 |
| Foot | 5 |
| Trunk | 11 (19%) |
| Chest wall | 9 |
| Abdomen | 1 |
| Flank | 1 |
| Head and neck | 8 (13%) |
| *Total* | 59 (100%) |

Modified from Enzinger FM, Weiss SW, Liang CY. Ossifying fibromyxoid tumor of soft parts: a clinicopathological analysis of 59 cases. Am J Surg Pathol 13:817, 1989.

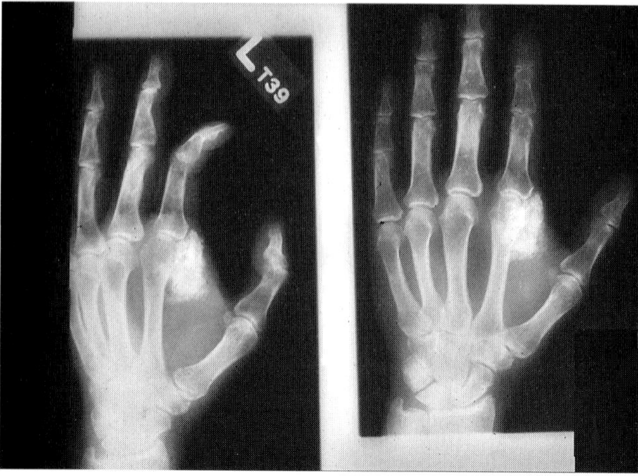


**FIGURE 36–45.** Typical radiographic appearance of ossifying fibromyxoid tumor of soft tissue. The tumor is well circumscribed and has extensive calcification.

## Pathologic Findings

Grossly, most tumors are well circumscribed, spherical, and lobulated or multinodular, typically covered by a thick fibrous pseudocapsule (Figs. 36–46, 36–47). Most measure 3–5 cm, but occasional lesions are 15 cm or larger. On cut section, the tumor is tan-white and often has a gritty texture.

Microscopically, most are located in the subcutaneous tissue, but some are attached to tendons, fascia, or involve the underlying skeletal muscle. The tumor is composed of uniform round, ovoid, or spindle-shaped cells arranged in nests and cords and deposited in a variably myxoid and collagenous stroma[182,186] (Figs. 36–48 to 36–52). In approximately 80% of cases there is an incomplete shell of lamellar bone found at the periphery of the nodules, either within or immediately underneath a dense fibrous pseudocapsule and sometimes extending into the substance of the tumor (Fig. 36–53). Despite extensive sampling, up to 20% of cases are nonossifying.[184]

The constituent cells, which vary little in size and shape, are characterized by pale-staining vesicular nuclei with minute nucleoli and small amounts of eosinophilic cytoplasm (Fig. 36–54). The cells may be deposited in a variety of patterns, including cords, nests, or sheets; or they may be randomly distributed in a fibromyxoid matrix. Some are predominantly myxoid and composed of alcian blue-positive, hyaluronidase-sensitive acid mucopolysaccharides, occasionally forming microcysts.[197] Other tumors are predominantly collagenous, sometimes with a gradual transition between densely hyalinized collagen and osteoid. Small foci of calcification and metaplastic cartilage may also be seen in the tumor nodules. Most have a rich vasculature, with many vessels exhibiting perivascular hyalinization and others subintimal fibrin deposition or thrombosis.

Rare ossifying fibromyxoid tumors have areas of hypercellularity, increased mitotic activity, or both. Others show extensive osteoid deposition in the central portion of the tumor. These rare cases have been referred to as "atypical" or "malignant" variants of ossifying fibromyxoid tumor[185] (Figs. 36–55, 36–56).

## Immunohistochemical and Ultrastructural Findings

Immunohistochemically, the cells are positive for vimentin and express S-100 protein in about 70% of

*Text continued on page 1461*

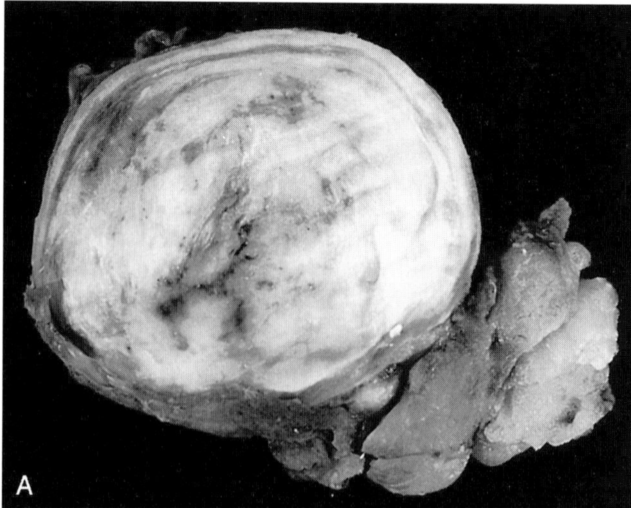


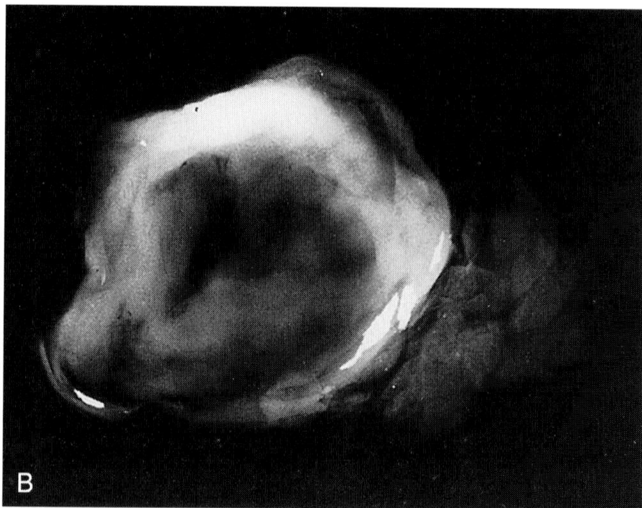


**FIGURE 36–46.** Ossifying fibromyxoid tumor with a well circumscribed mass covered by a pseudocapsule (**A**). Radiographic examination reveals multiple areas of calcification, particularly in the capsular region of the tumor (**B**).

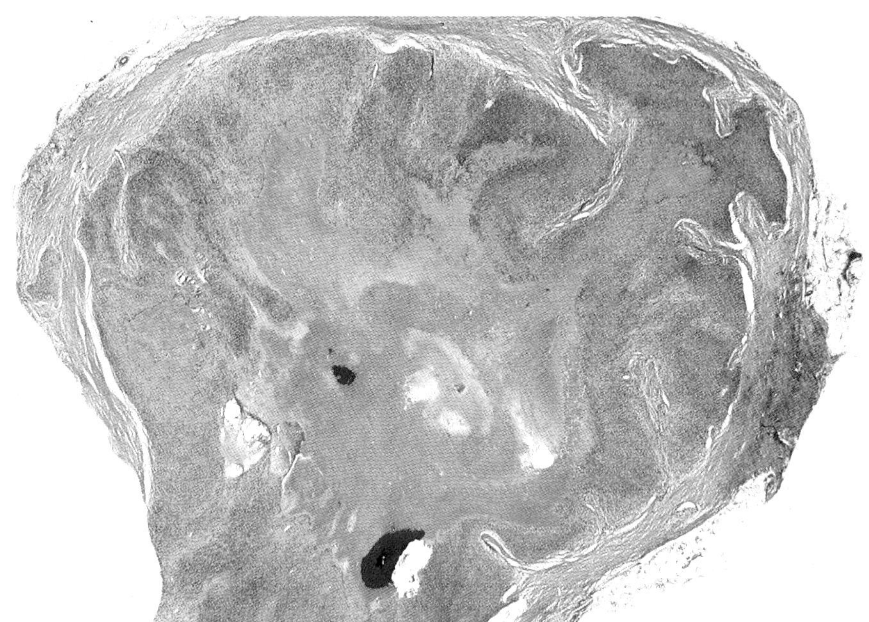

**FIGURE 36–47.** Ossifying fibromyxoid tumor of soft tissue. A pseudocapsule almost completely surrounds the neoplasm.

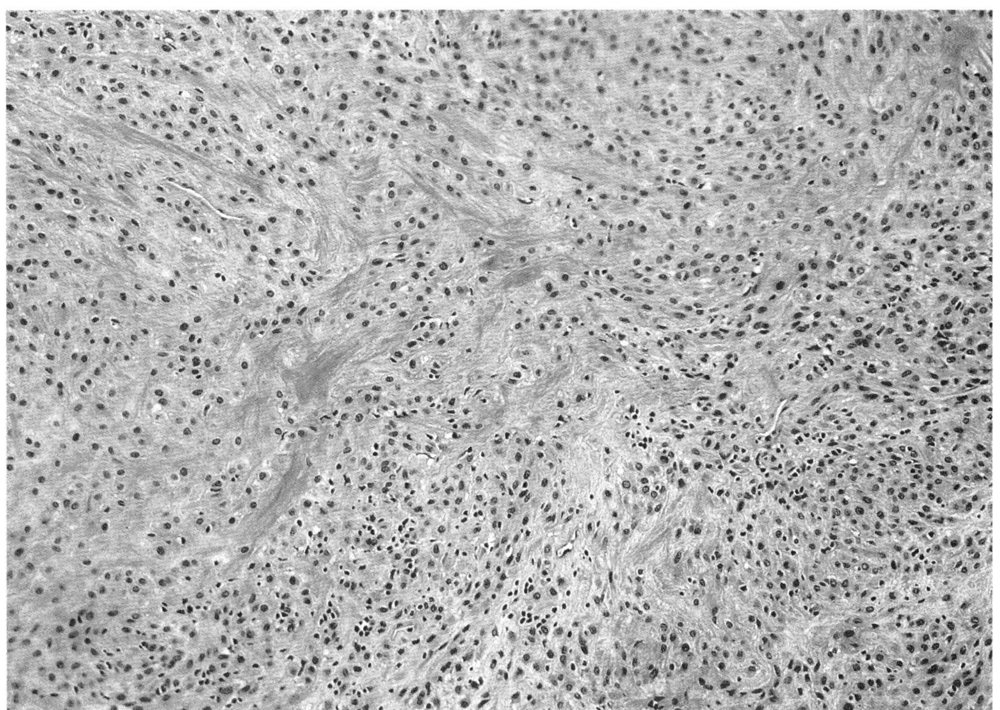

**FIGURE 36–48.** Low magnification appearance of an ossifying fibromyxoid tumor. The cells are arranged in a variety of patterns and deposited in a variably hyalinized and myxoid matrix.

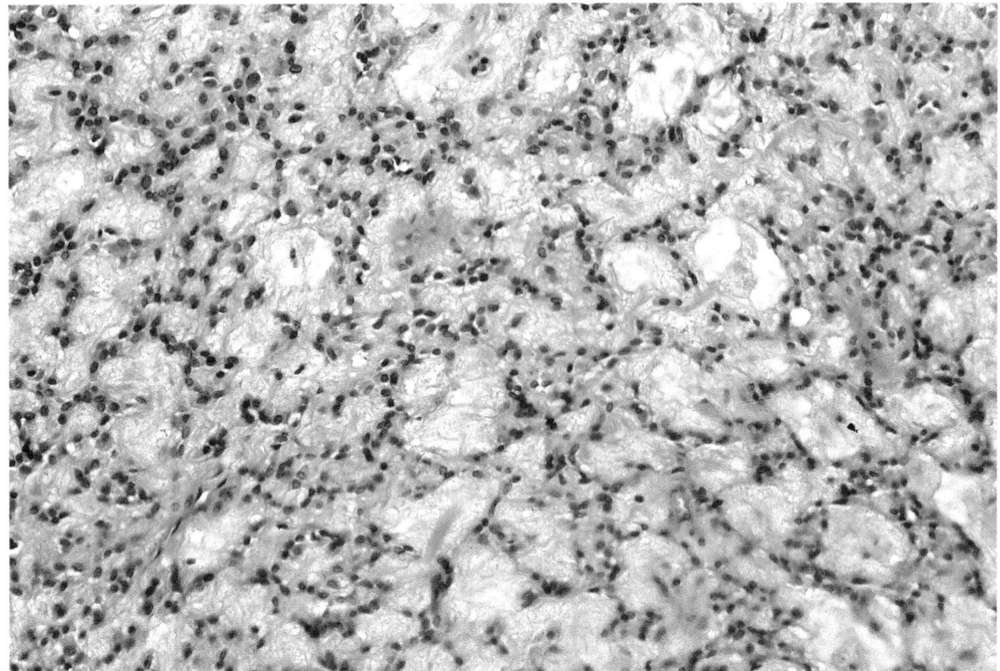

**FIGURE 36–49.** Ossifying fibromyxoid tumor. Cords of small tumor cells are suspended in a myxoid matrix.

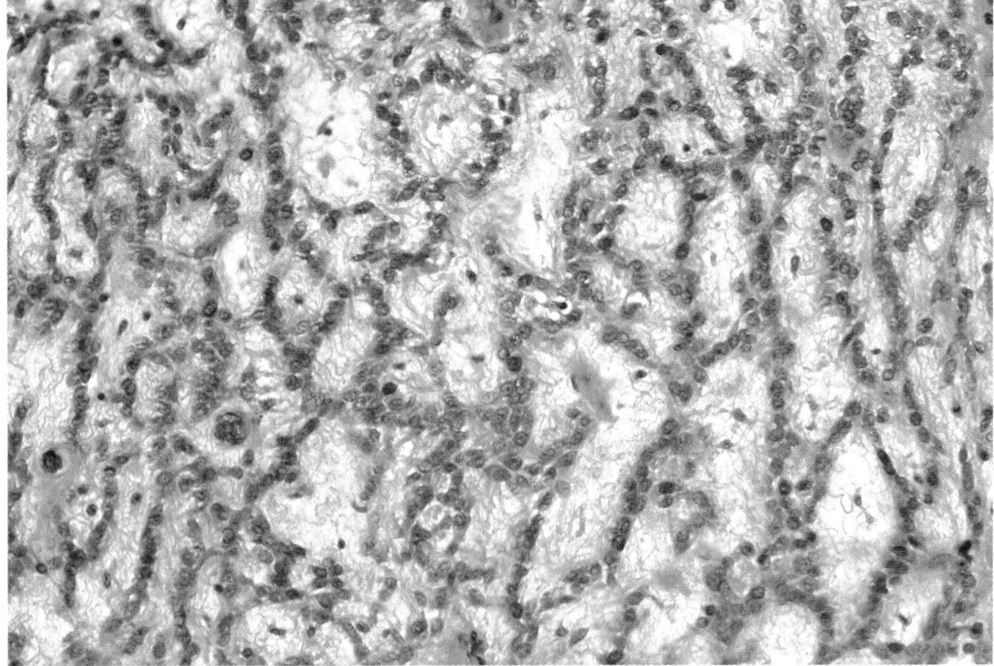

**FIGURE 36–50.** Thin cords of epithelioid tumor cells in an ossifying fibromyxoid tumor.

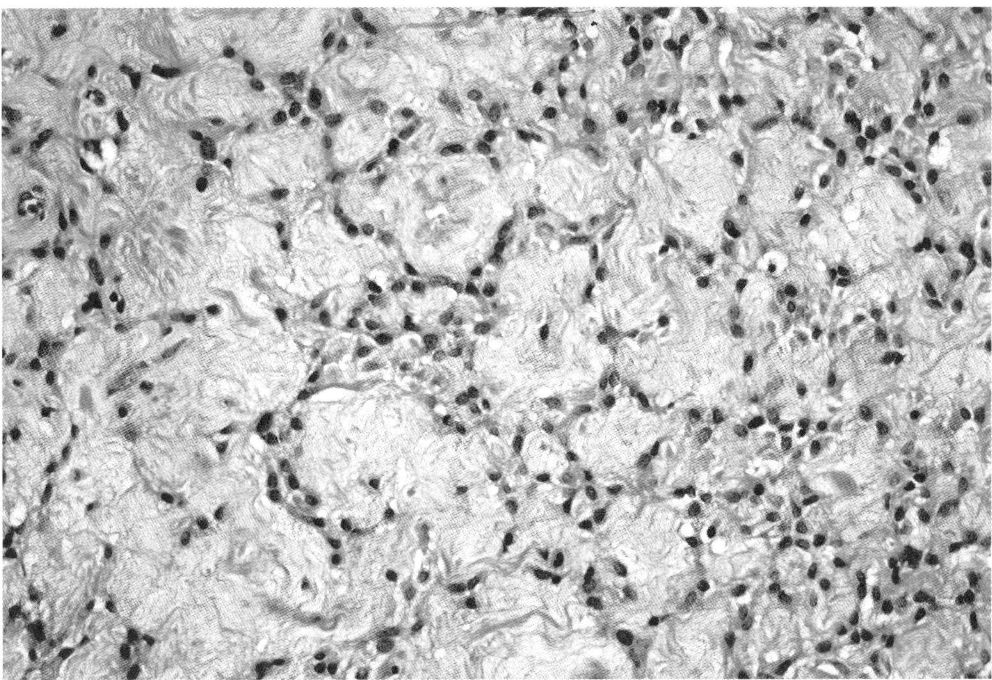

**FIGURE 36–51.** Less cellular zone in an ossifying fibromyxoid tumor.

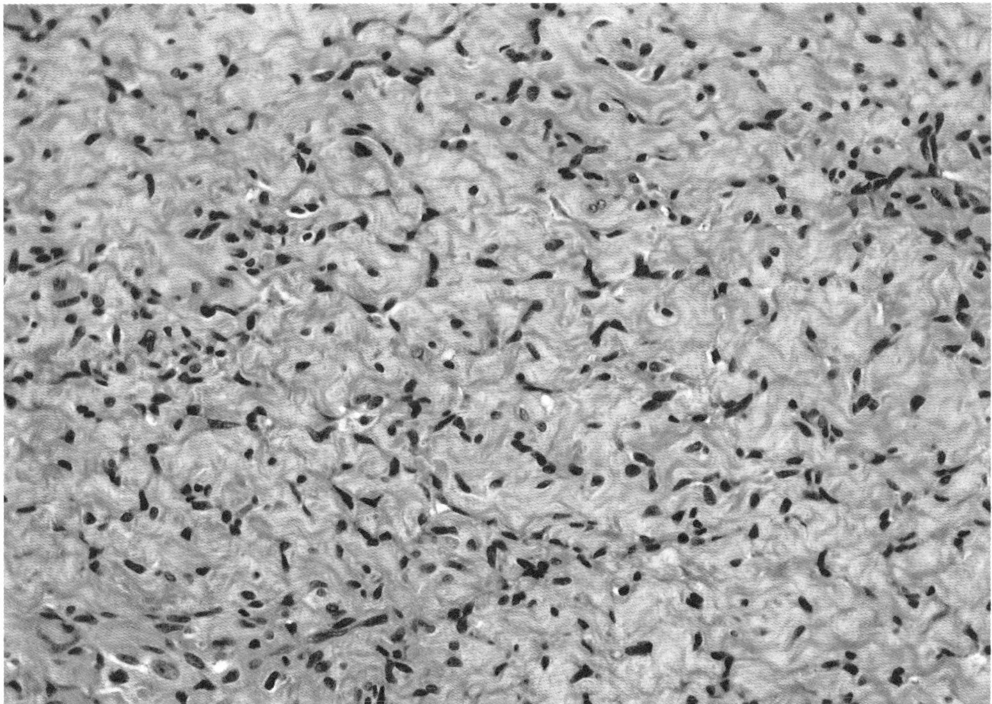

**FIGURE 36–52.** Fibrous zone in an ossifying fibromyxoid tumor, with compression of cords of tumor cells.

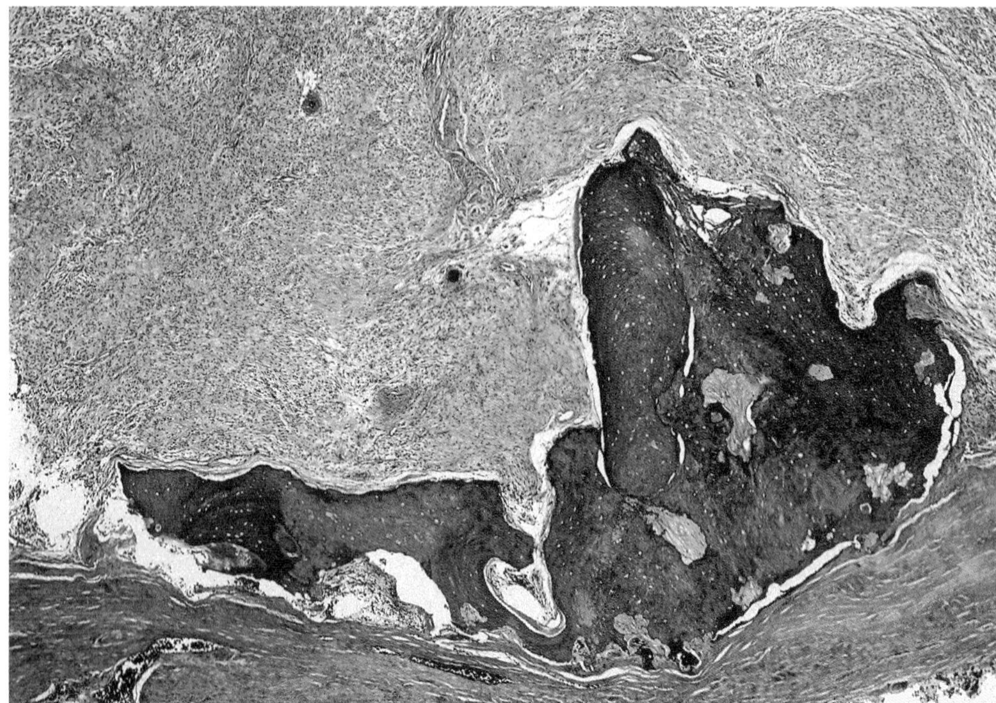

**FIGURE 36–53.** Ossifying fibromyxoid tumor with an incomplete rim of lamellar bone.

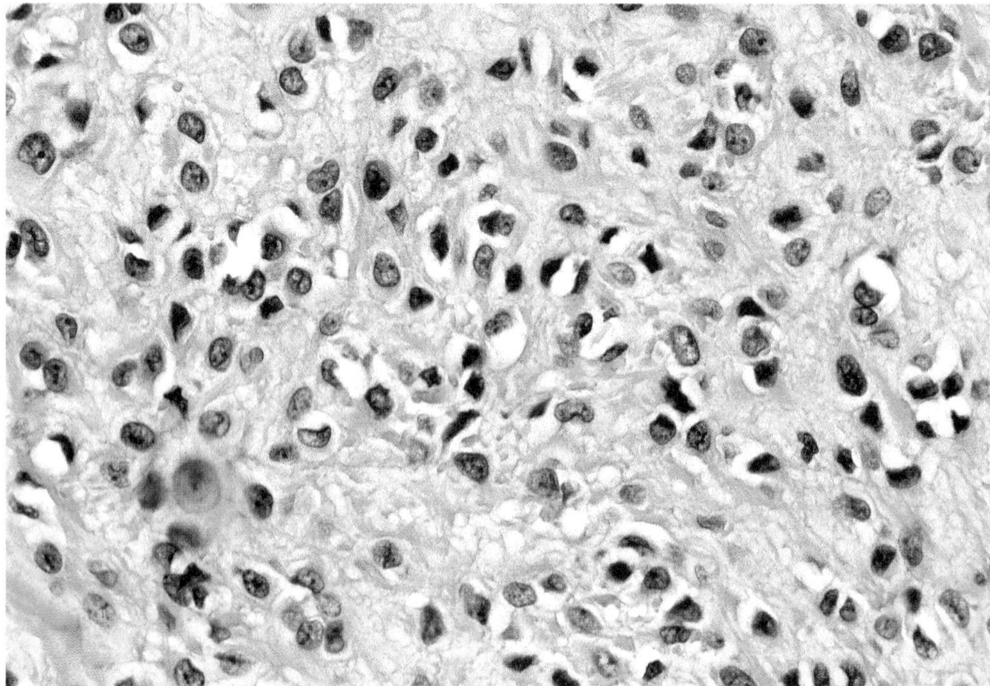

**FIGURE 36–54.** High magnification view of bland epithelioid cells with vacuolated or eosinophilic cytoplasm in an ossifying fibromyxoid tumor.

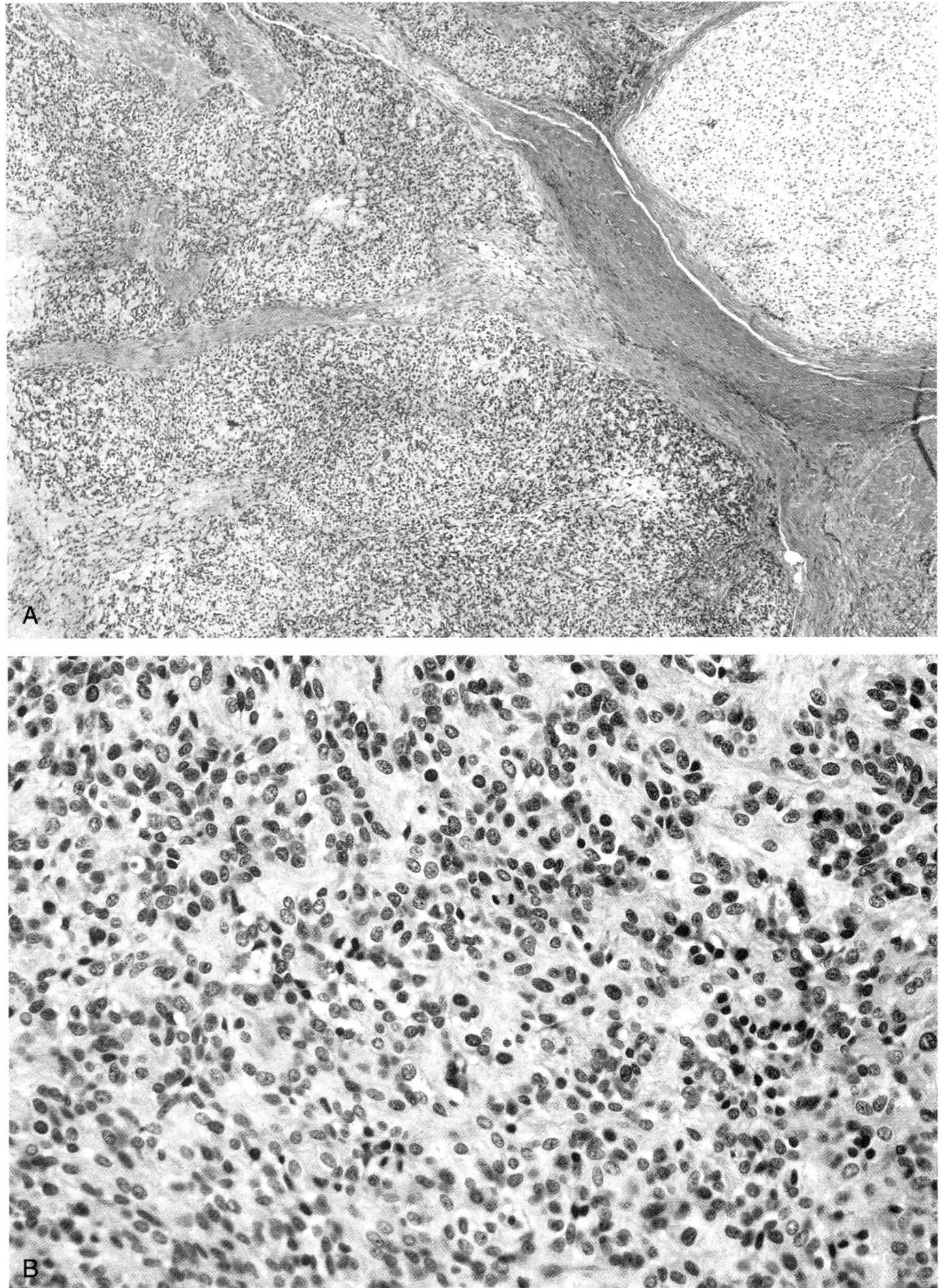


**FIGURE 36–55.** (**A**) Low magnification view of an ossifying fibromyxoid tumor with a characteristic multilobular appearance. Some of the lobules are strikingly cellular, a feature that raises concern for malignancy. (**B**) High magnification view of a cellular focus in an "atypical" ossifying fibromyxoid tumor.

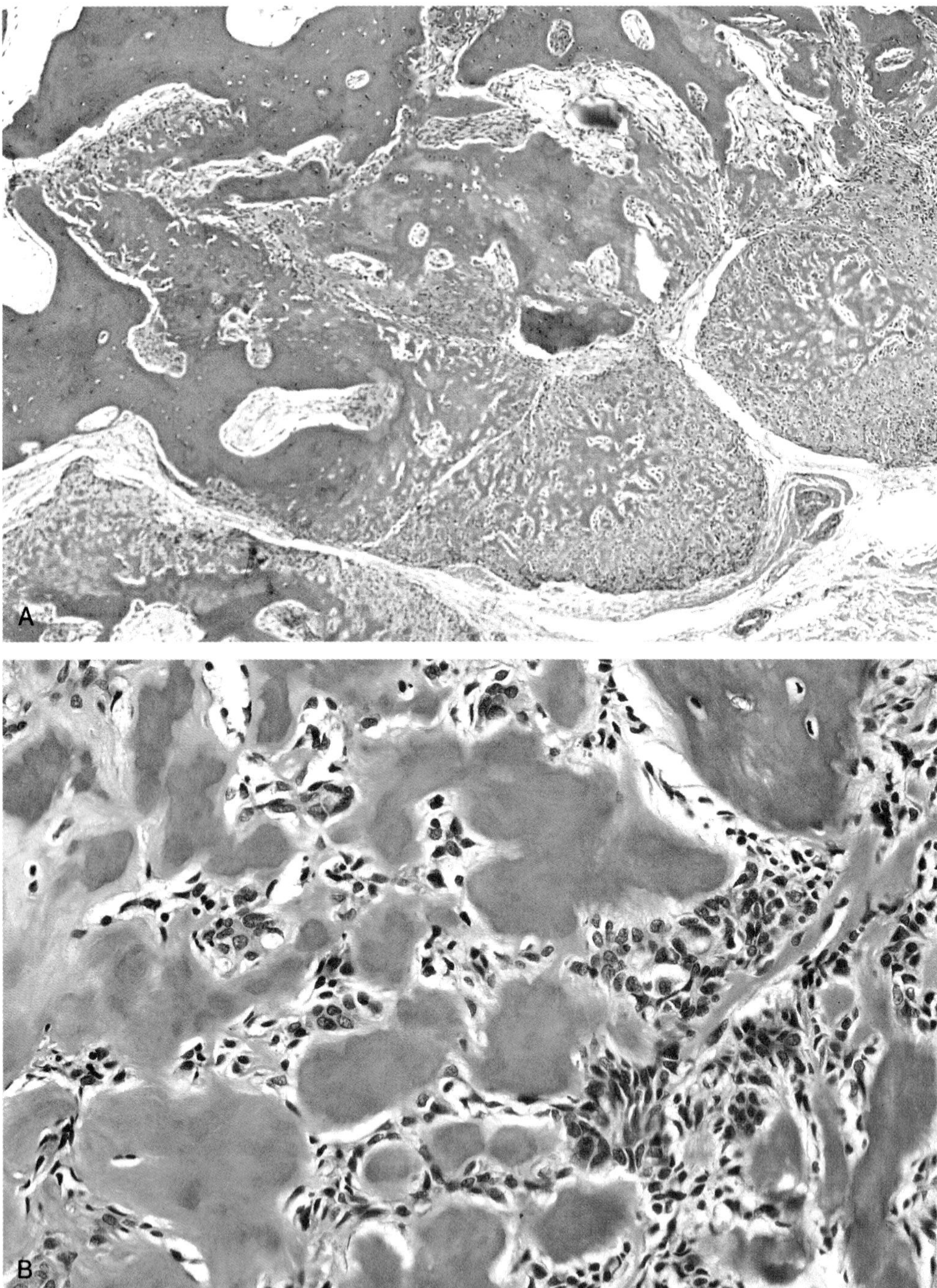


**FIGURE 36–56.** (**A**) Recurrent lesion in a 50-year-old man who had a typical ossifying fibromyxoid tumor resected 2 years earlier. (**B**) This lesion was more cellular than this patient's original tumor and showed areas reminiscent of a low-grade osteosarcoma with formation of abundant osteoid.

cases (Fig. 36–57), but immunoreactivity for the latter tends to be less intense than in schwannoma.[187,191] The cells may also express Leu-7, neuron-specific enolase, and glial fibrillary acidic protein. Some stain focally for desmin or smooth muscle actin,[195] but they do not express cytokeratins.[189]

Electron microscopy reveals the cells to have abundant intracytoplasmic intermediate filaments often in a perinuclear whorl, short fragments of thick external lamina, and complex sometimes interdigitating cell processes (Fig. 36–58).[180] Ribosome-lamellar complexes have also been described.[184]

## Differential Diagnosis

The differential diagnosis includes benign and malignant epithelioid nerve sheath tumors (epithelioid neurofibroma, epithelioid schwannoma, epithelioid malignant peripheral nerve sheath tumor), chondroid syringoma (cutaneous mixed tumor), myxoid chondrosarcoma, and epithelioid smooth muscle tumors.

The ossifying fibromyxoid tumor has many features in common with *nerve sheath tumors;* as discussed below, there is some evidence to support neural differentiation of the tumor cells. However, ossifying fibromyxoid tumor has not been documented to arise from a peripheral nerve, and the architectural and cytologic features are not typical of either epithelioid neurofibroma or epithelioid schwannoma. The cells also lack the cytologic atypia characteristic of epithelioid malignant peripheral nerve sheath tumors.

The absence of epithelial markers in the ossifying fibromyxoid tumor helps exclude *chondroid syringoma* as a diagnostic consideration. The lobulated architecture and arrangement of the neoplastic cells into cord-like structures bears some resemblance to *myxoid chondrosarcoma,* but the stroma of ossifying fibromyxoid tumor varies between myxoid and collagenous and the neoplastic cells have less eosinophilic cytoplasm than those of myxoid chondrosarcoma. Histochemically, periodic acid-Schiff (PAS) staining usually reveals abundant intracytoplasmic glycogen in the cells of myxoid chondrosarcoma, a feature lacking in ossifying fibromyxoid tumors. The ultrastructural characteristics of the two tumors are also quite distinctive. *Epithelioid smooth muscle tumors* usually express myoid antigens and lack S-100 protein, and they exhibit ultrastructural evidence of myoid differentiation.

## Discussion

The clinical behavior of the ossifying fibromyxoid tumor varies. Most of the reported tumors have followed a benign clinical course, but almost one-third recur locally. In the original report by Enzinger et al.,[183] 11 of 41 patients (27%) in whom follow-up information was available experienced one or more recurrences. In addition, one patient with three recurrences developed a similar tumor in the contralateral thigh that was presumed to be a metastasis. The patient committed suicide shortly after discovery of the

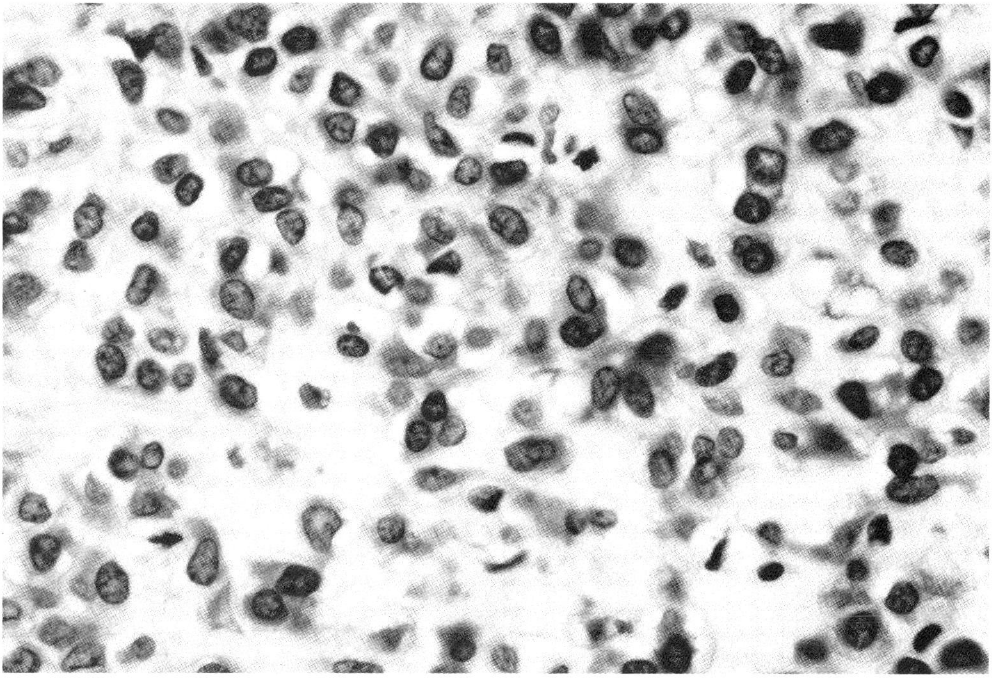

**FIGURE 36–57.** Ossifying fibromyxoid tumor with strong S-100 protein immunoreactivity.

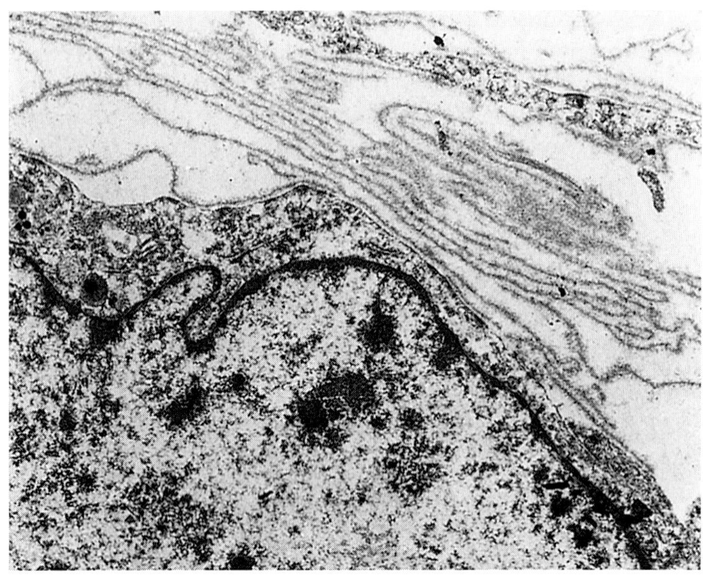

**FIGURE 36–58.** Electron micrograph of an ossifying fibromyxoid tumor with reduplication and scroll formation of external laminae, suggesting a tumor with neural differentiation. (From Enzinger FM, Weiss SW, Liang CY. Ossifying fibromyxoid tumor of soft parts: a clinicopathological analysis of 59 cases. Am J Surg Pathol 13:817, 1989.)

contralateral lesion. One additional patient developed a recurrence that histologically progressed to a well differentiated osteosarcoma. Yoshida et al.[196] observed a tumor of this type in a 54-year-old man that had its onset in the right thigh and over a period of 10 years involved the upper arm and neck with invasion of the mediastinum and vertebrae. In 1995, Kilpatrick et al.[185] reported six "atypical" and "malignant" ossifying fibromyxoid tumors. All of the tumors in this report had histologic features of malignancy, including areas of increased cellularity, increased mitotic activity, or deposition of centrally placed osteoid. Although meaningful follow-up was not available in four of these cases, one patient, a 68-year-old man with a 9 cm deep soft tissue mass adjacent to the greater trochanter, developed a local recurrence and histologically proven pulmonary metastases. Complete surgical incision is the therapy of choice to reduce the risk of local recurrence and the potential for histologic progression to a more aggressive lesion.[194]

The line of differentiation of this tumor has been disputed since its initial description, with cartilaginous, myoepithelial, osteogenic, and myoid origins suggested. The preponderance of evidence is more suggestive of peripheral nerve sheath differentiation. The encapsulation and the immunohistochemical expression of neural antigens including S-100 protein, Leu-7, neuron-specific enolase, and glial fibrillary acidic protein (GFAP) are in keeping with this theory. Furthermore, the ultrastructural features suggest schwannian differentiation, albeit incomplete, prompting some to suggest that this lesion could be regarded as a low-grade malignant peripheral nerve sheath tumor.[184] The fact that malignant forms of this tumor have displayed clear-cut osteosarcomatous areas has led to an opposing view that they represent an unusual bone or cartilage-producing tumor.

## PARACHORDOMA

Parachordoma is a rare tumor of characteristic histologic appearance and uncertain histogenesis. It was first described by Laskowski in 1951 as "chordoma periphericum."[211] In 1977, Dabska coined the term "parachordoma" in what still remains the largest series (10 cases) reported in the literature.[199] Since that time, fewer than 50 cases have been described, mostly in the form of case reports or small series.[203,206–209,220] Relatively few cases have been studied by immunohistochemistry or cytogenetics, and distinction of parachordoma from chordoma and extraskeletal myxoid chondrosarcoma can be problematic. Distinction among these entities is of clinical importance, however, as there are significant differences in therapy and prognosis.

### Clinical Findings

The tumor affects patients of all ages although there is a peak incidence in the second through fourth decades of life. Males are affected slightly more commonly than females. Most arise in the deep soft tissues of the extremities, usually in the muscles of the thigh, calf, upper arm or forearm.

### Pathologic Findings

Grossly, the parachordoma forms a nodular mass ranging in size from 1 to 12 cm in greatest dimension;

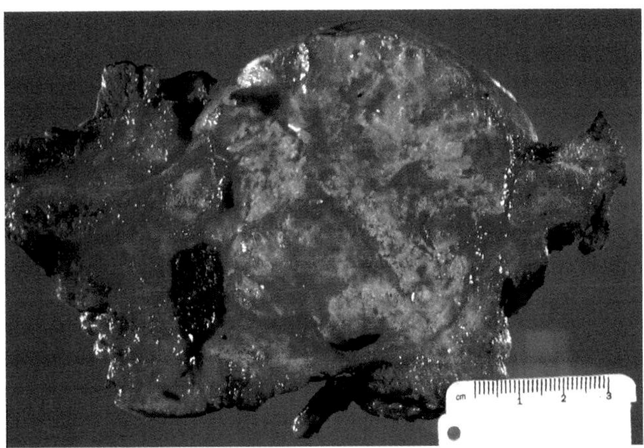

**FIGURE 36–59.** Gross appearance of a parachordoma arising in the chest wall of a 55-year-old man.

most are 3–7 cm (Fig. 36–59). Microscopically, it consists of small nests of pale-staining cells resembling the cells of the notochord. The tumor is composed predominantly of round eosinophilic cells arranged in cords, chains, or pseudoacini reminiscent of myxoid chondrosarcoma (Figs. 36–60 to 36–63). Not uncommonly the cells show a transition to spindle-shaped cells (Fig. 36–64) or small, round glomoid cells[205] (Fig. 36–65). All lesions have a population of cells with vacuolated cytoplasm resembling physaliferous cells found in chordomas (Figs. 36–66, 36–67). There is usually only a mild degree of nuclear atypia, and mitotic figures are rare, usually with fewer than one mitotic figure per 20 high power fields (HPF). The cells are deposited in a matrix that varies from myxoid to hyaline (Fig. 36–68) and contains a high concentration of hyaluronic acid, as evidenced by reduction of alcian blue staining after hyaluronidase predigestion.[205] Although grossly well circumscribed, there are frequently small nests of cells that are separate from the main tumor and trail off into the surrounding soft tissue structures, sometimes evoking a desmoplastic stromal response (Fig. 36–69).

## Immunohistochemical and Electron Microscopic Findings

By immunohistochemistry, the cells characteristically co-express cytokeratins (Fig. 36–70), including cytokeratins 8/18, epithelial membrane antigen, S-100 protein, Leu-7, and vimentin.[203,205,216] In addition, type IV collagen surrounds groups of cells in a nest-like fashion.[205] Immunostains for CD-34, actin, glial fibrillary acidic protein, and calponin are typically negative. Electron microscopy reveals the cells to have evidence of incomplete epithelial differentiation, with primitive cell junctions, fragmented basal lamina, and microvillous projections.[198,203,219,221]

*Text continued on page 1469*

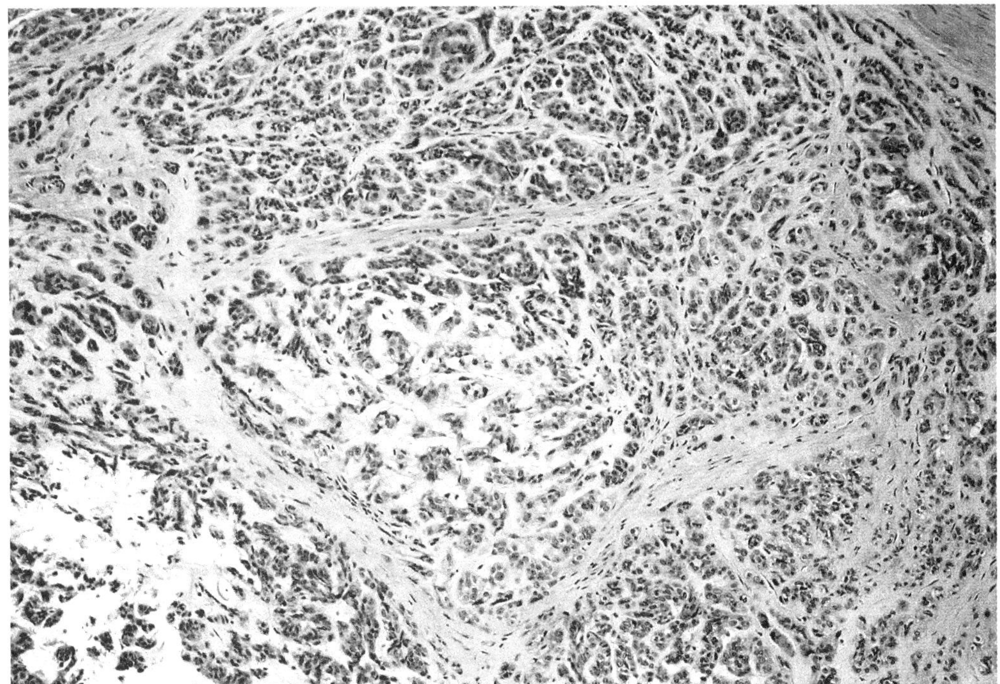

**FIGURE 36–60.** Parachordoma showing multinodular masses of epithelioid to spindle cells, with a variably myxochondroid matrix.

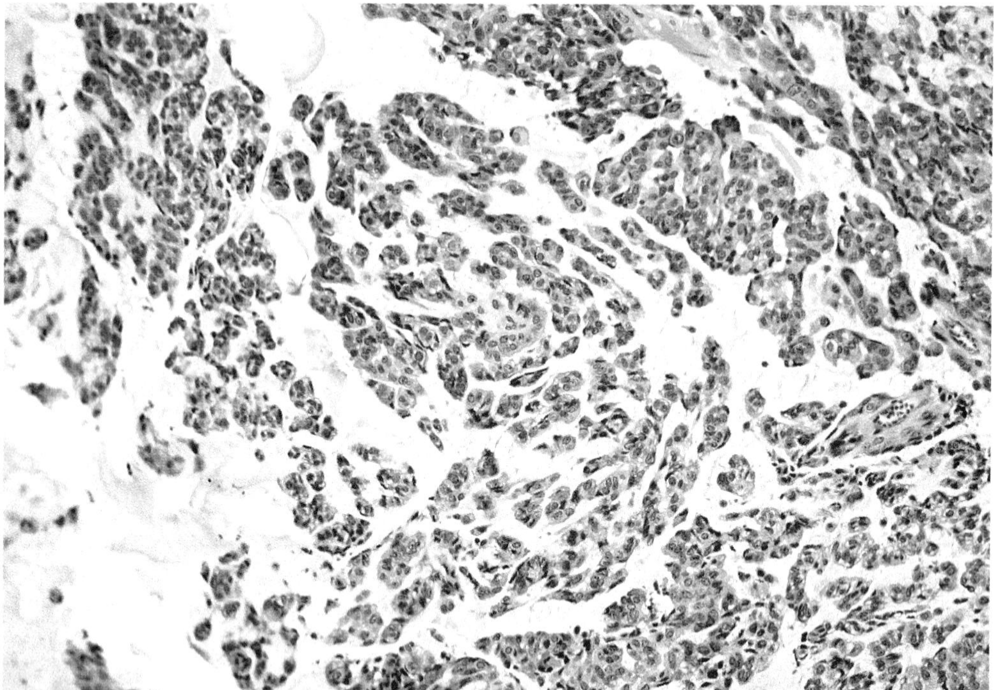

**FIGURE 36–61.** Parachordoma. Nests of epithelioid cells are suspended in a myxoid matrix.

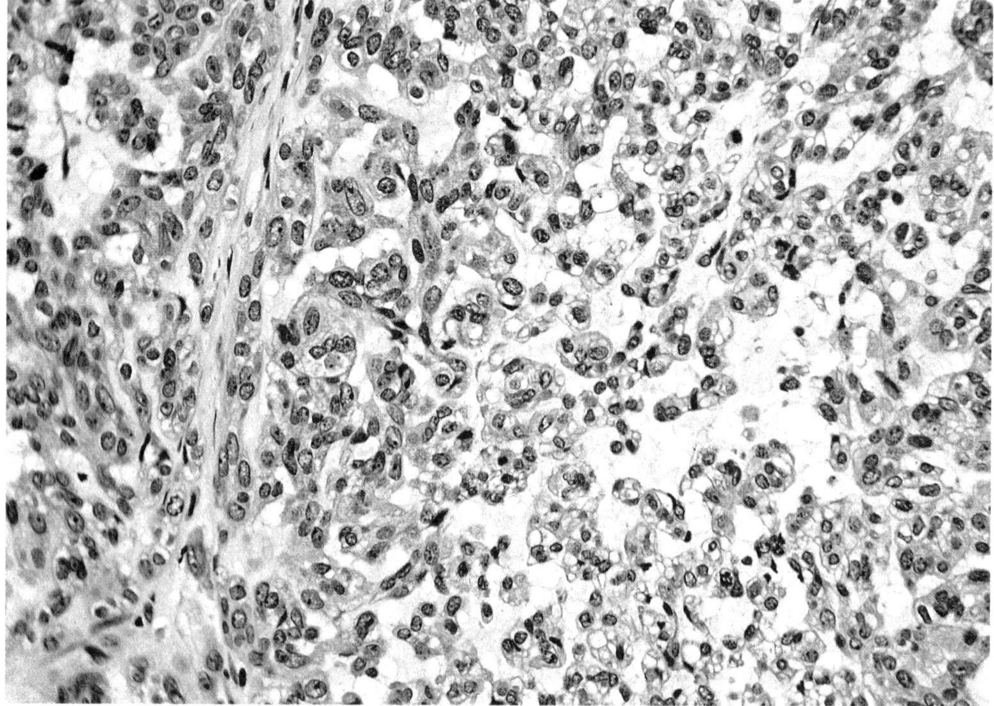

**FIGURE 36–62.** Parachordoma. Nests and cords of epithelioid to spindle-shaped cells are deposited in a myxochondroid matrix.

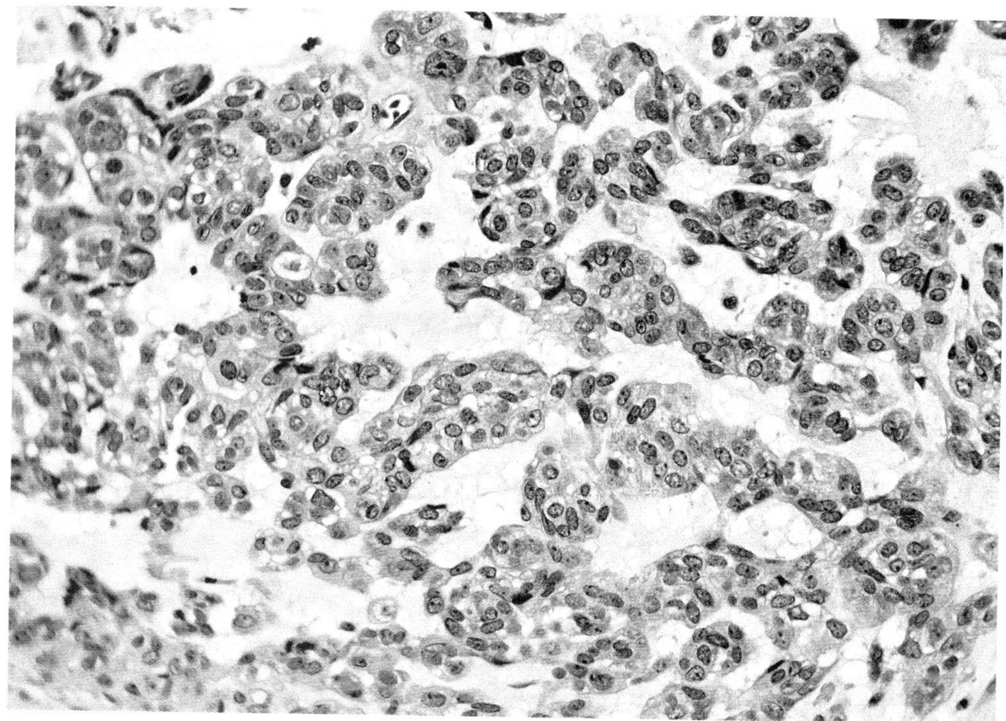

**FIGURE 36–63.** Nests of uniform-appearing epithelioid cells suspended in a myxochondroid matrix in a parachordoma.

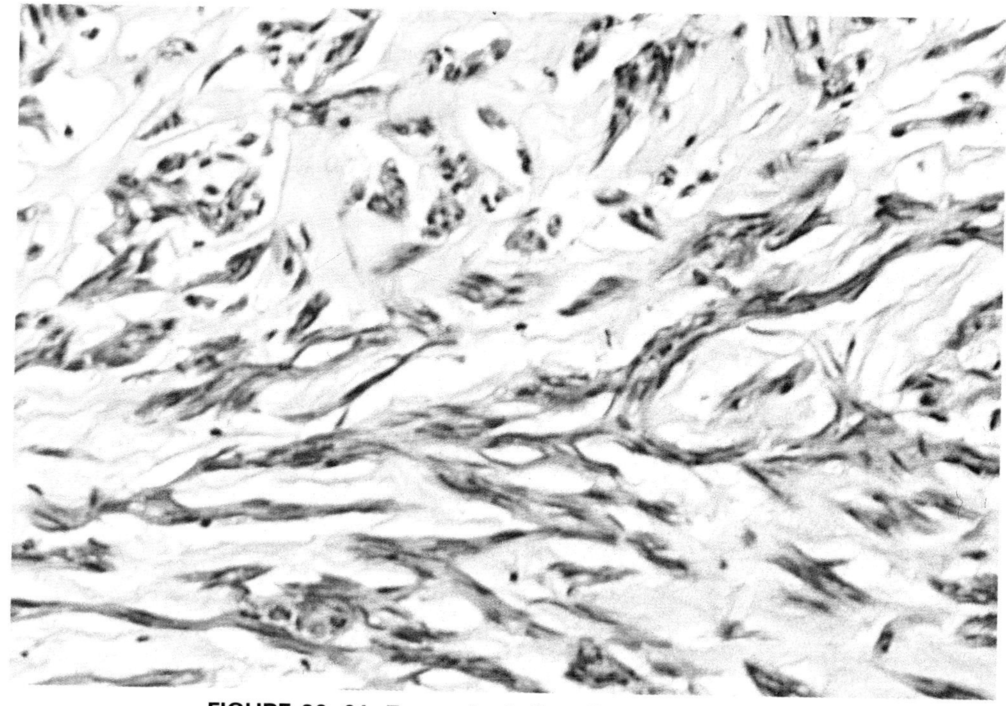

**FIGURE 36–64.** Focus of spindle cells in parachordoma.

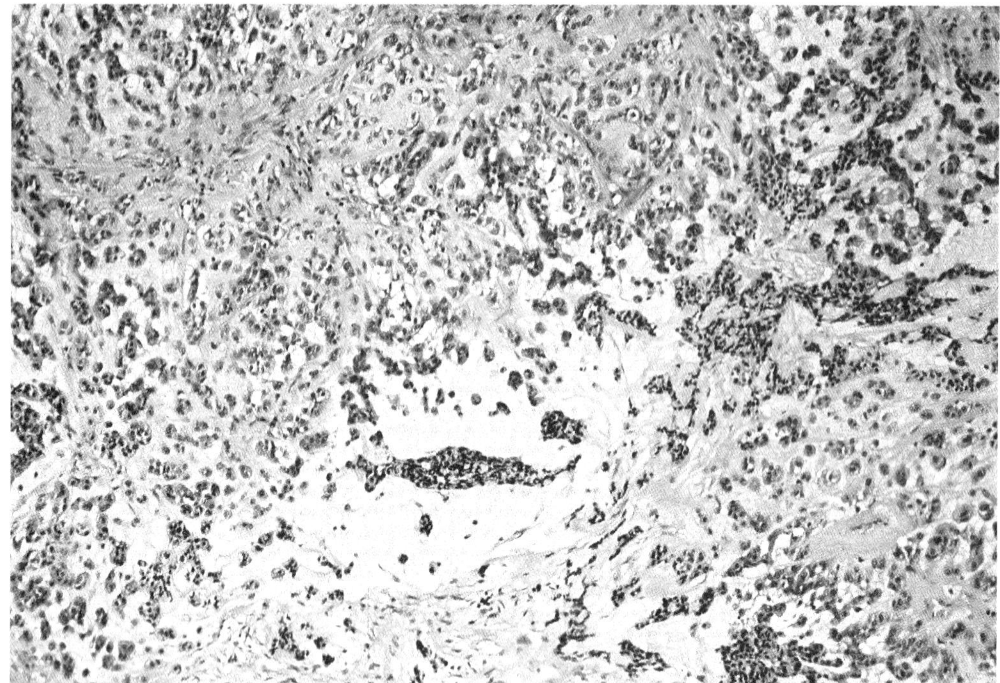

**FIGURE 36–65.** Transition from large epithelioid cells to small glomoid cells in a parachordoma.

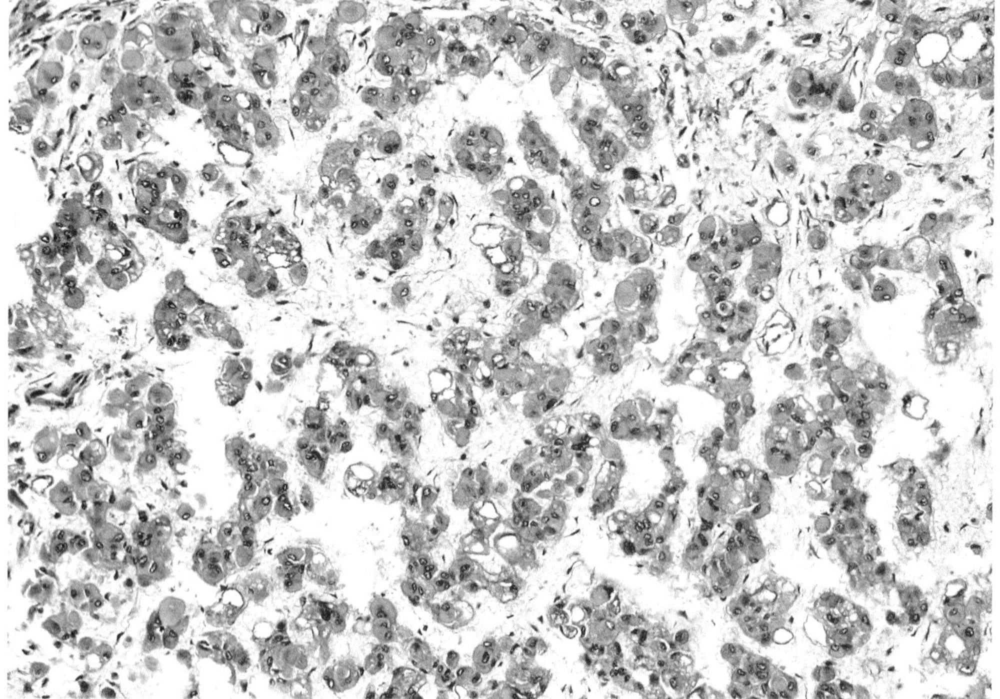

**FIGURE 36–66.** Chordoma-like area in a parachordoma. Nests of large cells with abundant eosinophilic and vacuolated cytoplasm are suspended in a myxochondroid matrix.

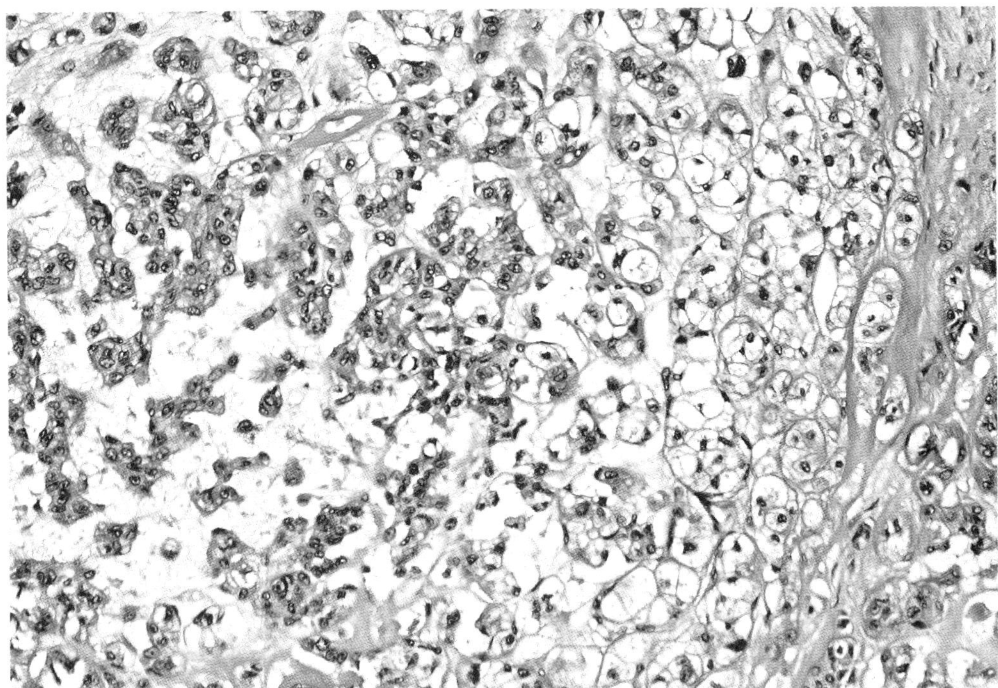

**FIGURE 36–67.** Parachordoma. Transition from eosinophilic cells to cells with clear, vacuolated cytoplasm.

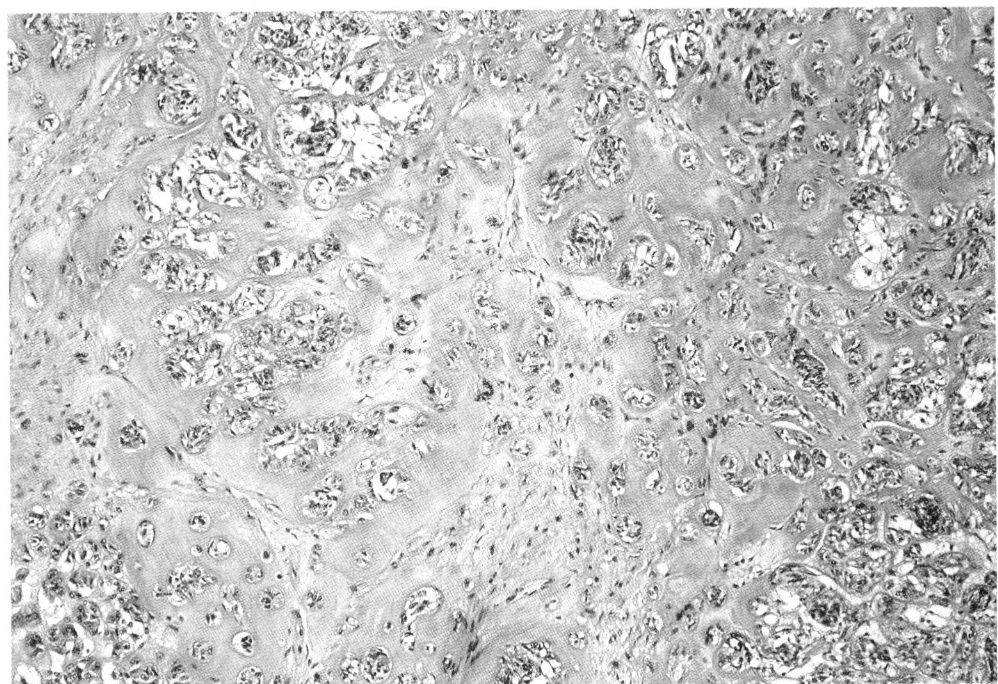

**FIGURE 36–68.** Parachordoma with a densely hyalinized matrix.

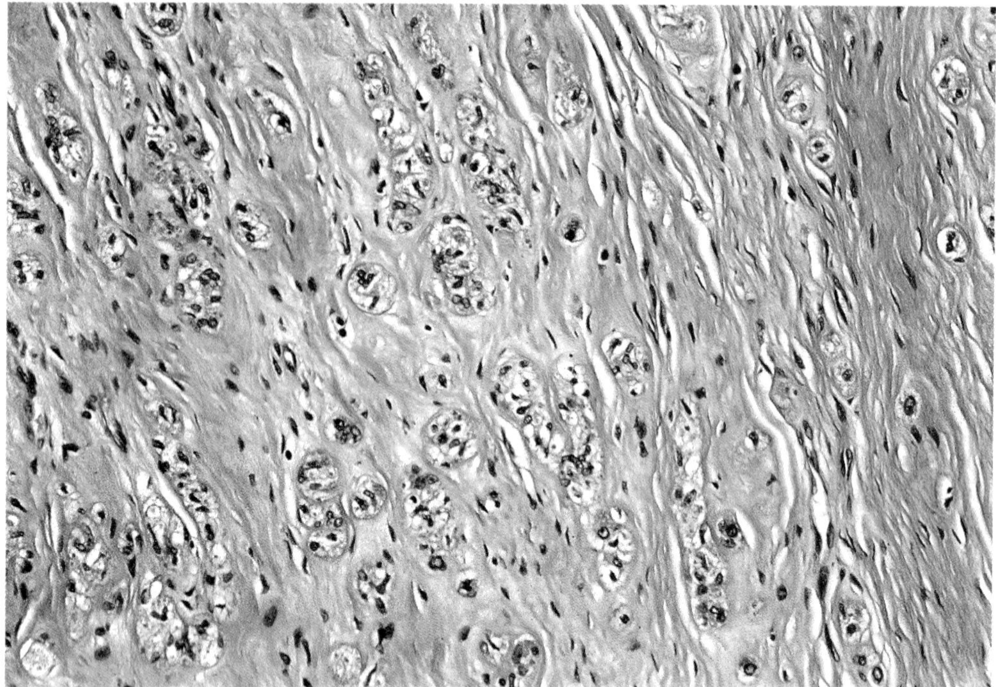

**FIGURE 36–69.** Periphery of a parachordoma with infiltrating small nests and single cells in a desmoplastic background.

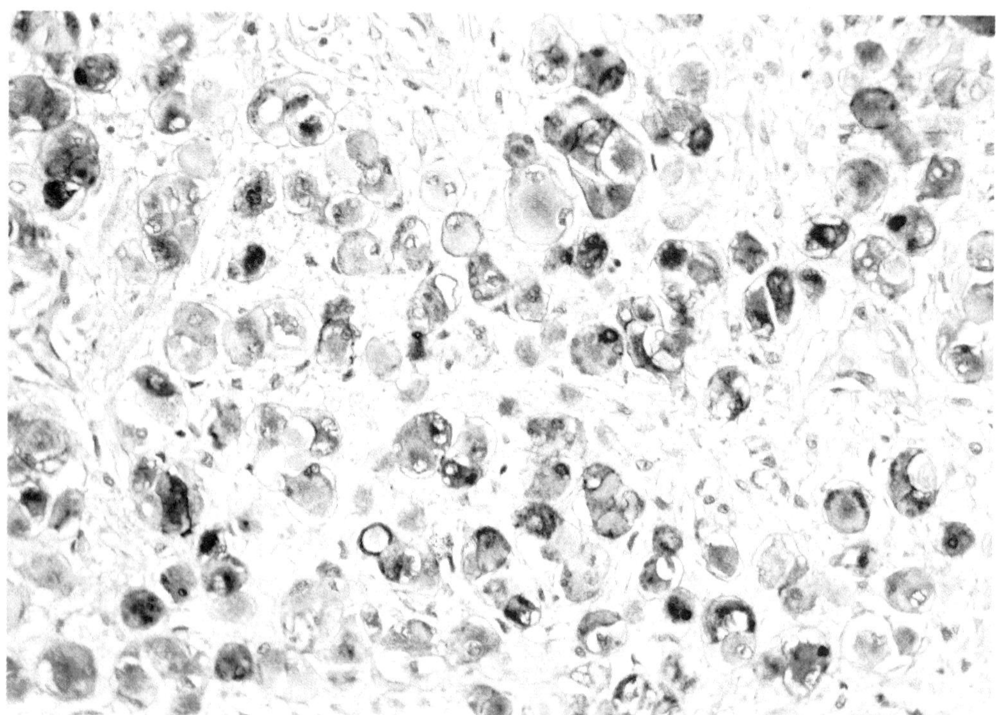

**FIGURE 36–70.** Parachordoma with strong immunoreactivity for high-molecular-weight cytokeratin.

## Cytogenetic Findings

Few parachordomas have been studied by cytogenetics. In a series of seven parachordomas reported by Folpe et al.,[205] one patient had multiple cytogenetic aberrations including trisomy 15 and monosomies of chromosomes 1, 16, and 17. Tihy et al.[222] reported a parachordoma with small der2 (2)5(2;4),del(3q) and loss of chromosomes 9, 19, 20, and 22. Limon et al.[213] reported a tumor with a complex karyotype, although this tumor may represent an ossifying fibromyxoid tumor.[205]

## Differential Diagnosis

Parachordoma has many features overlapping with those in *chordoma,* and, in fact, many consider this tumor to be the peripheral counterpart of axial chordoma.[199] Both are characterized by round cells with vacuolated cytoplasm (physalipherous-like) arranged in nests and cords. Unlike the chordoma, parachordoma shows a blending of these vacuolated epithelioid cells with spindle-shaped cells and small glomoid cells. In contrast to chordoma, the matrix of parachordoma is abolished by hyaluronidase predigestion. There is also significant immunophenotypic overlap between these lesions as both are characterized by expression of low-molecular-weight cytokeratins, epithelial membrane antigen, S-100 protein, and vimentin (Table 36–8). Chordomas express cytokeratins 1/10 and 19, both of which are absent in parachordomas.[203,205,215,218] Furthermore, type IV collagen is only rarely and focally expressed in chordoma, in contrast to the nest-like arrangement around groups of cells in the parachordoma.[205,212]

Distinction from *extraskeletal myxoid chondrosarcoma* may also be difficult. The spindled and glomoid components seen in parachordoma are not typical of this lesion. The stromal mucin in extraskeletal myxoid chondrosarcomas is hyaluronidase-resistant, unlike that found in parachordoma. Ultrastructurally, the cells of the extraskeletal myxoid chondrosarcoma lack evidence of epithelial differentiation; rather, they are characterized by abundant rough endoplasmic reticulum and dilated cisternae containing microtubular aggregates.[200] Immunohistochemically, extraskeletal myxoid chondrosarcoma only rarely shows focal cytokeratin positivity, and less than one-half are S-100 protein-positive[201] (Table 36–8). Finally, extraskeletal myxoid chondrosarcoma is characterized by a t(9;22), which appears to be specific for this lesion.

Some authors have suggested that parachordoma is a deep soft tissue variant of *myoepithelioma,*[210] but in our opinion they are different tumors. Most true myoepithelial tumors arise in the subcutaneous tissue, have well defined epithelial components, and show evidence of myoepithelial differentiation by immunohistochemistry. There is little ultrastructural or immunohistochemical support for myoepithelial differentiation in parachordoma, as the latter usually does not express myoid markers (including smooth muscle actin and calponin) or GFAP.[205] Although Kilpatrick et al. argued that previously reported parachordomas most likely fall into the category of mixed tumor/myoepithelioma,[204,210] O'Connell and Berean[217] suggested just the opposite—that some tumors reported as mixed tumor/myoepithelioma may be parachordomas.

## Discussion

Parachordoma is an indolent neoplasm but has the potential for local recurrence, possibly related to the small tumor nodules that are often present outside the main mass.[205] According to the review of the literature by Folpe et al.,[205] local recurrences have been reported in 6 of 24 cases with follow-up information, although in most instances there is no comment as to the completeness of surgical excision.[207,208] Some of these recurrences appeared many years after the initial excision. For example, Dabska reported a local recurrence 19 years after the initial therapy.[199] Rare examples of this tumor have been reported to metastasize. Limon et al.[213] reported metastasis of a tumor that originated on the palm to an axillary lymph node after 7 years. However, the authenticity of this case as a true parachordoma has been questioned.[205] Miettinen et al.[214] reported a 67-year-old woman with a popliteal mass who developed widespread pulmonary metastasis and death at 12 months. The latter tumor was unusual in that it had a high mitotic rate

**TABLE 36–8** IMMUNOHISTOCHEMICAL FEATURES OF LESIONS IN THE DIFFERENTIAL DIAGNOSIS OF PARACHORDOMA

| Tumor Type | S-100 | EMA | Cam5.2 | CK 7 | CK 19 | CK 1/10 | CEA |
|---|---|---|---|---|---|---|---|
| Parachordoma | + | + | + | − | − | − | − |
| Chordoma | + | + | + | +/− | + | + | + |
| Extraskeletal myxoid chondrosarcoma | +/− | − | − | − | − | − | − |

and areas of necrosis. Wide local excision is the treatment of choice.

The line of differentation of this tumor remains a subject of intense debate; as previously mentioned, some have doubted its very existence.[204] We believe there is sufficient evidence to support the concept of parachordoma as a distinctive clinicopathologic entity characterized by an indolent clinical course. An excellent review of this controversial subject was provided by Fisher.[202]

## AMYLOID TUMOR (AMYLOIDOMA)

Although systemic amyloid deposition is much more common than localized deposits, the latter have been reported in virtually every anatomic site. Such deposits may arise in association with immunocytic dyscrasias, including multiple myeloma and plasmacytoid lymphoma; but they may also be associated with long-term hemodialysis and a variety of chronic infectious or inflammatory diseases (tuberculosis, osteomyelitis, rheumatoid arthritis).[228] There are also localized deposits of amyloid that occur with no clinical evidence of immunocytic dyscrasia or any other coexisting or preexisting disease; these lesions are rare and are found mainly in the soft tissues[233,241] or as solitary or multiple nodules in the respiratory,[224,230] urinary,[223,229,231] and gastrointestinal tracts.[225,240,249] There are also reports of localized amyloid tumors in the region of the head and neck,[244,246] including the orbit,[236] breast,[235,242] mediastinum,[237] heart,[248] liver,[251] bone,[226,238,239] nervous system,[234] and skin, where they are usually much smaller and occur as multiple macules or papules in the upper dermis.[232]

Grossly, the tumor consists of a lobulated nodule or mass with a white-yellow or pink-yellow waxy surface. Microscopic examination discloses amorphous faintly eosinophilic material that is PAS-positive and metachromatic with the crystal violet stain. The deposits are typically surrounded by histiocytes and multinucleated giant cells associated with a variable lymphoplasmacytic infiltrate. The plasma cells usually show no evidence of immaturity or cellular atypia (Figs. 36–71, 36–72). In most cases the interspersed vessel walls are diffusely thickened by amyloid deposits. Rare lesions also show prominent areas of metaplastic bone or cartilage.[243,252] Elastic stains help distinguish the tumor from elastofibroma, and the absence of a fibroblastic proliferation distinguishes it from tumoral calcinosis. In addition, the deposited amyloid stains positively with the Congo red preparation, showing an "apple-green" birefringence under polarized light (Fig. 36–73). The Congo red affinity is abolished by prior treatment of the sections with potassium permanganate in most reactive or inflammatory forms of the disease characterized by amyloid A protein (AA).[246,250] The subtypes of amyloid can be further differentiated by immunohistochemical demonstration of the kappa and lambda light chains in

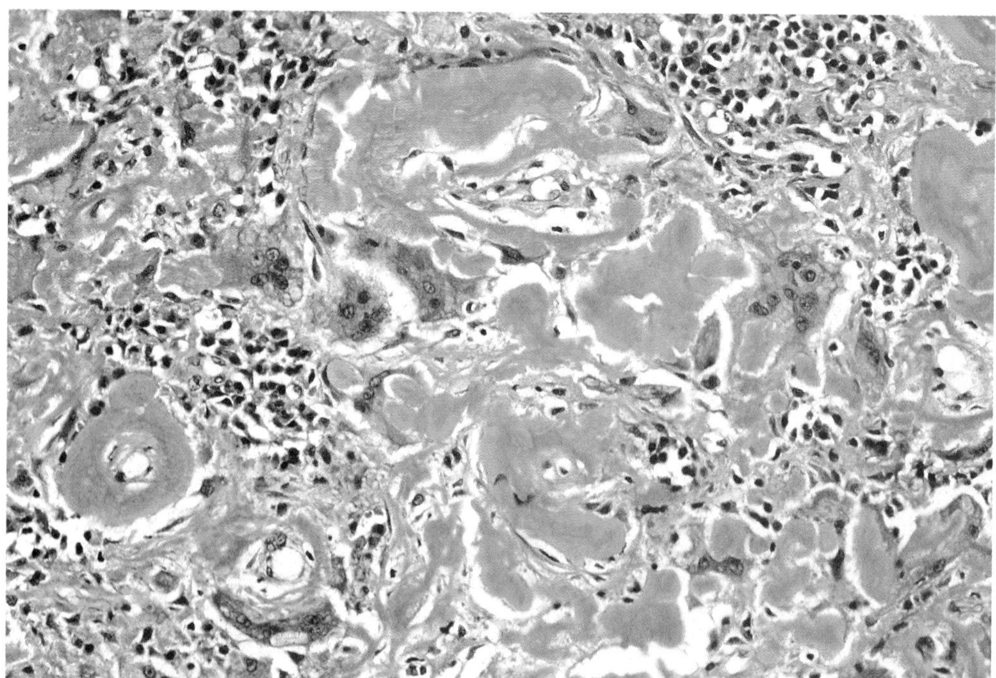

**FIGURE 36–71.** Amyloid tumor with amorphous deposits of amyloid associated with foreign body-type giant cells and plasma cells.

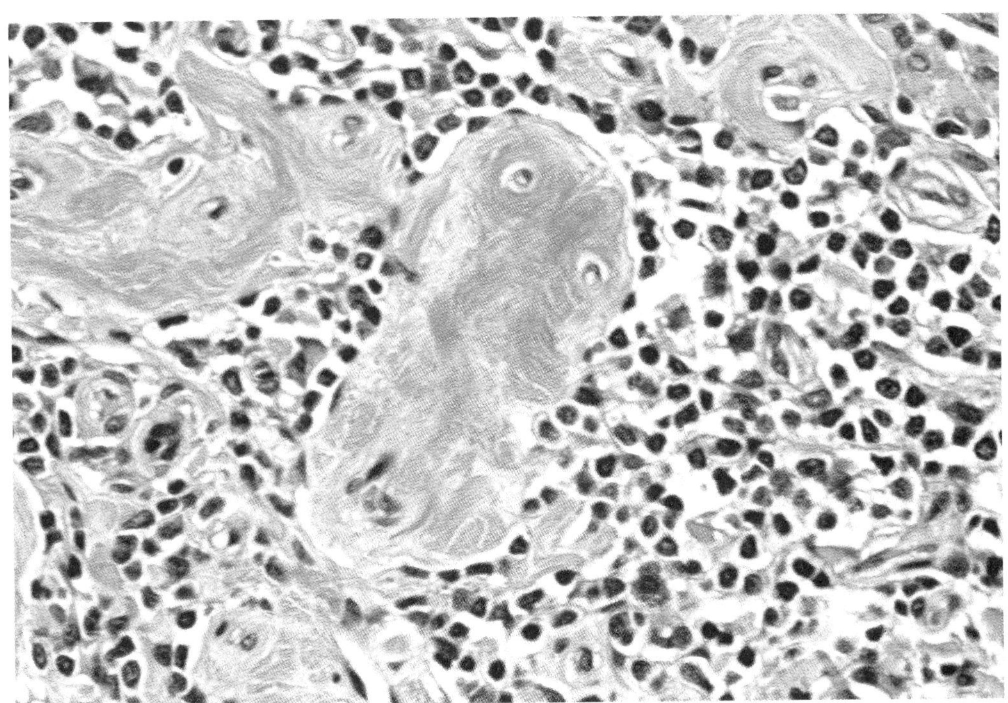

**FIGURE 36–72.** High magnification of amyloid tumor with prominent plasma cell infiltrates surrounding deposits of amyloid.

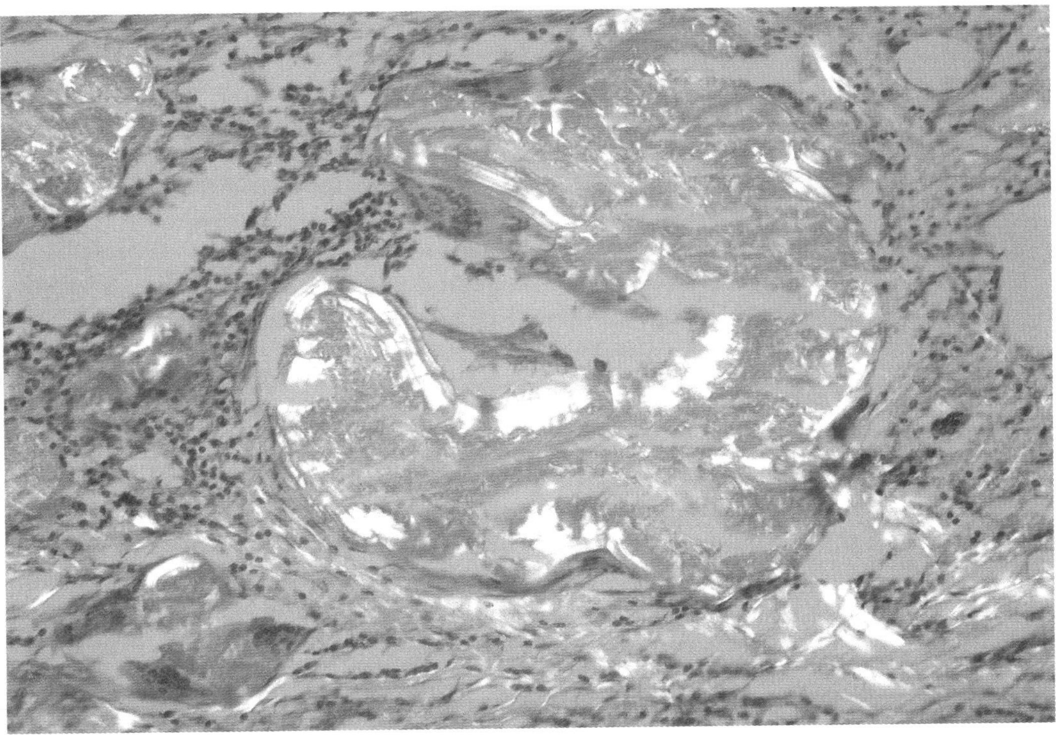

**FIGURE 36–73.** Apple-green birefringence under polarized light in an amyloid tumor.

AL amyloid, amyloid A protein in AA amyloid, and $\beta_2$-microglobulin in hemodialysis-associated amyloid.[227] Electron microscopy shows that the amyloid consists of fine, straight, nonbranching fibrils that measure 70–100 nm in diameter.

Early reports often provided no information as to the type of amyloid comprising the tumor-like mass. More recent reports have described deposits of both the AA[233,235] and AL[238,247] types with few reports of $\beta_2$-microglobulin amyloid.[245] Laeng et al.[234] detected monoclonal rearrangements of the heavy-chain immunoglobulin gene in amyloidomas of the nervous system, providing strong support for the concept that at least some of these lesions are composed of AL-producing B-cell clones capable of terminal differentiation. Of the 14 soft tissue amyloidomas reported by Krishnan et al.,[233] 10 were associated with plasmacytoid lymphoma (nine cases) or myeloma (one case). In their review of the literature of amyloidoma of bone, Pambuccian et al.[238] found all lesions to be composed of AL amyloid, with many patients progressing to generalized disease.

## PLEOMORPHIC HYALINIZING ANGIECTATIC TUMOR OF SOFT PARTS

Initially described in a series of 14 cases by Smith et al.,[257] pleomorphic hyalinizing angiectatic tumor of soft parts (PHAT) is a rare yet distinctive low-grade neoplasm that differs in several respects from schwannomas and conventional malignant fibrous histiocytomas. Since its initial description, few additional cases of PHAT have been reported in the literature,[253–256] and it is likely that this neoplasm continues to be mistaken for the above entities, among others. Accurate recognition of this neoplasm is of clinical importance given its propensity for local recurrence.

### Clinical Findings

PHAT characteristically arises in adults as a slowly enlarging mass that is often present for several years before coming to clinical attention. In most cases the clinical impression is that of a hematoma, a benign neoplasm, or even Kaposi's sarcoma. Males and females are affected equally. The single most common site of the tumor is the subcutaneous tissue of the lower extremities. In the original series of 14 cases described by Smith et al.,[257] 11 tumors arose in the subcutaneous tissue, including 8 in the lower extremities and 1 each in the buttock, chest wall, and arm. However, three tumors arose in skeletal muscle, one each in the shoulder, thigh, and chest wall. The tumor ranges in size from 2 to 8 cm in greatest dimension, with most being in the range of 4–6 cm.

### Pathologic Findings

Grossly, most tumors have a lobulated appearance with a cut surface that varies in color from white-tan to maroon (Fig. 36–74). Rare lesions have a prominent cystic component, and others show conspicuous myxoid change. The tumors are not encapsulated; although some have fairly well demarcated borders, most show diffusely infiltrative margins with trapping of normal tissues at the tumor periphery.

Microscopically, the most striking feature at low magnification is the presence of clusters of thin-walled ectatic blood vessels scattered throughout the lesion. The vessels range in size from small to macroscopic, and they tend to be distributed in small clusters (Figs. 36–75, 36–76). Typically the ectatic vessels are lined by endothelium with a thick subjacent rim of amorphous eosinophilic material that is often surrounded by lamellated collagen. Some vessels show organizing intraluminal thrombi with papillary endothelial hyperplasia. Hyaline material emanates from the vessels and extends into the stroma of the neoplasm, trapping neoplastic cells. The constituent cells are plump, spindled, and rounded with pleomorphic nuclei arranged in sheets or occasionally in fascicles reminiscent of fibrosarcoma (Fig. 36–77). In general, the cells resemble those seen in pleomorphic malignant fibrous histiocytoma and have hyperchromatic,

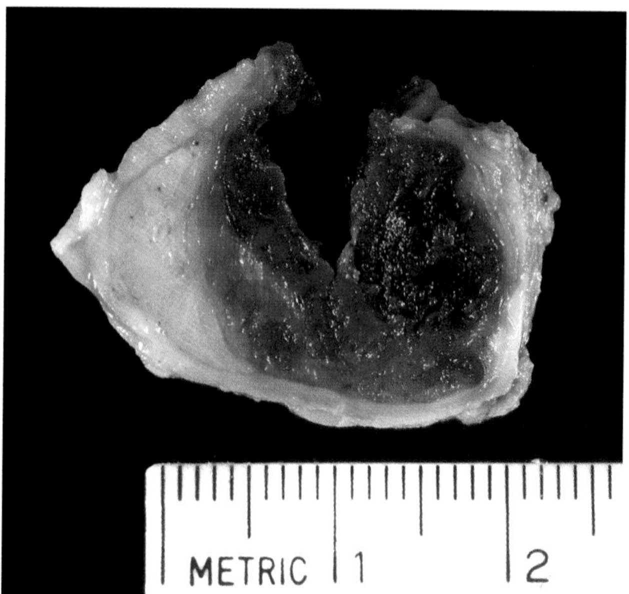


**FIGURE 36–74.** Pleomorphic hyalinizing angiectatic tumor. Gross specimen with a hemorrhagic appearance.

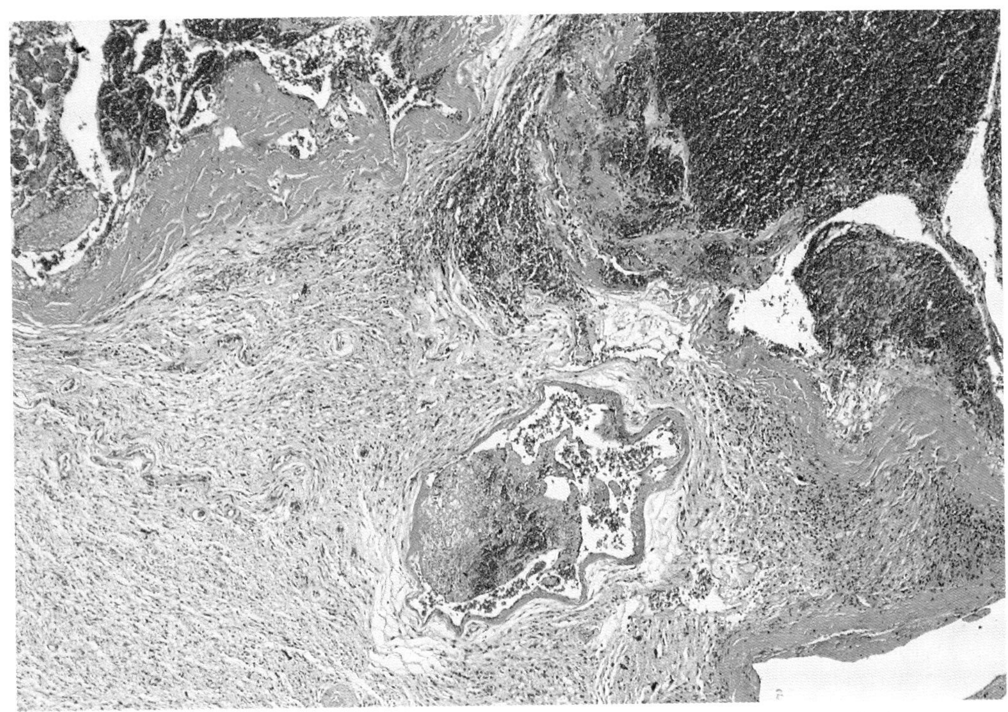

**FIGURE 36–75.** Pleomorphic hyalinizing angiectatic tumor with clusters of thin-walled ectatic vessels, a characteristic feature of this tumor.

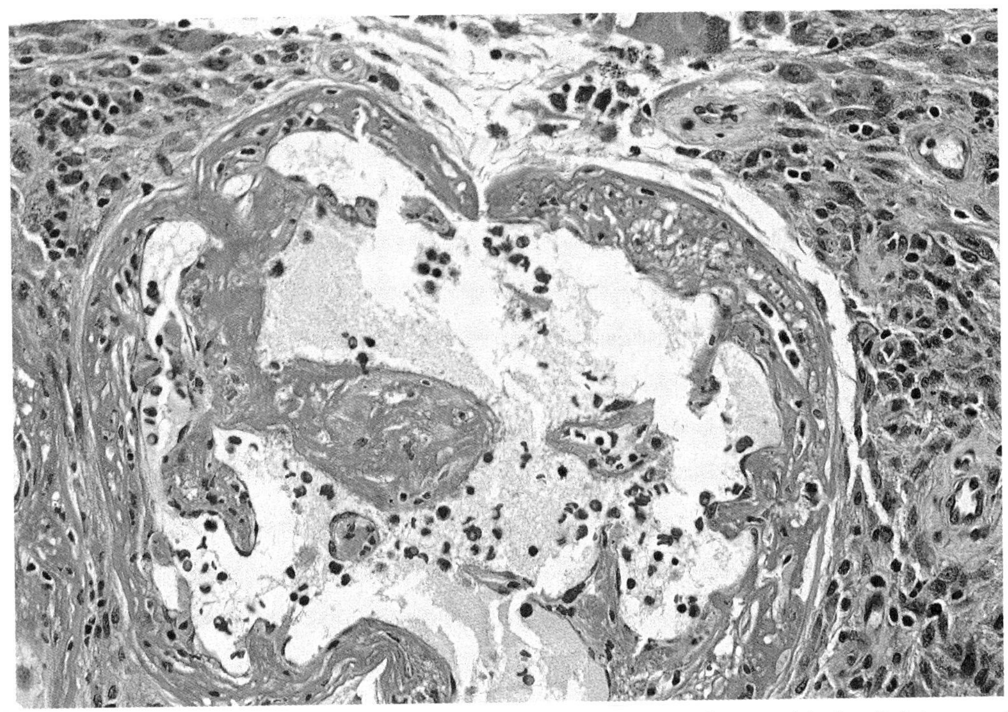

**FIGURE 36–76.** Characteristic high power view of a vessel in a pleomorphic hyalinizing angiectatic tumor.

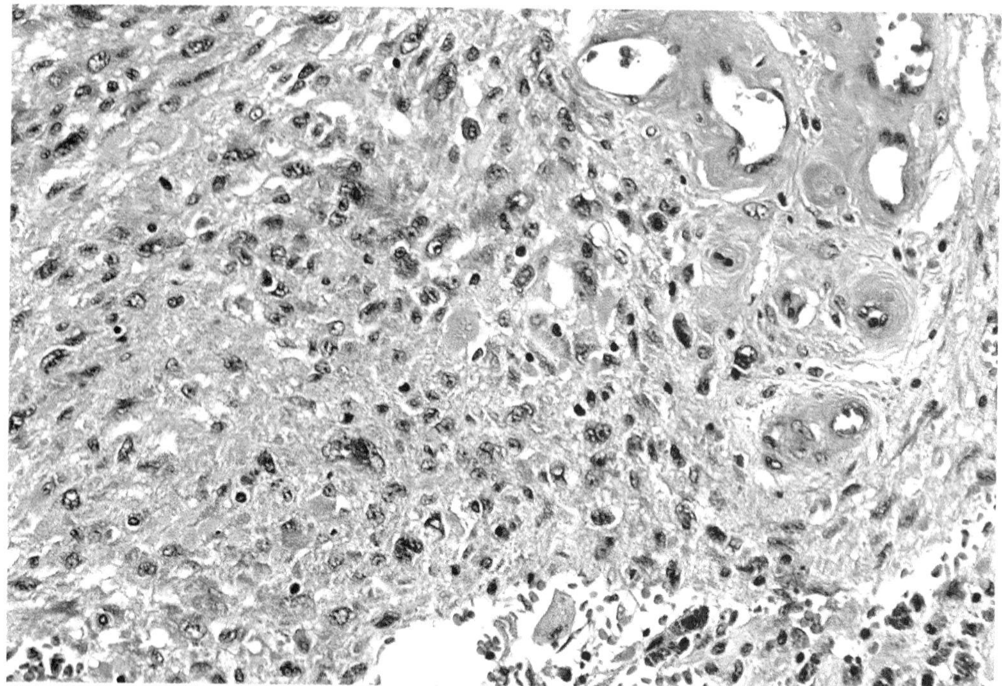

**FIGURE 36–77.** Pleomorphic nuclei in a pleomorphic hyalinizing angiectatic tumor. Despite the marked nuclear pleomorphism, mitotic figures are scarce.

pleomorphic nuclei lacking discernible cytoplasmic differentiation.[257] Not uncommonly, intranuclear cytoplasmic inclusions are prominent (Fig. 36–78). Despite the striking degree of nuclear pleomorphism, mitotic figures are scarce (usually <1 mitosis/50 HPF). Occasional tumor cells, particularly those adjacent to ectatic vessels, contain intracytoplasmic hemosiderin. The tumors have a variable inflammatory infiltrate, most prominently mast cells, although in some lesions lymphocytes, plasma cells, and eosinophils are conspicuous. Foci of psammomatous calcification are occasionally present.

Immunohistochemistry shows that the neoplastic cells do not stain for S-100 protein, thereby helping to exclude schwannoma as a diagnostic consideration. The cells consistently express vimentin, and most also stain for CD-34. Immunoreactivity for Factor XIIIa may be present,[255,256] but the tumors generally do not express actin, desmin, cytokeratin, epithelial membrane antigen, factor VIII-related antigen, or CD-31. Groisman et al.[255] reported immunoreactivity for vascular endothelial growth factor (VEGF), a secreted protein implicated in tumor-associated angiogenesis, in both tumoral and endothelial cells.

Few PHATs have been evaluated by electron microscopy. The neoplastic cells lack specific evidence of differentiation and generally contain large numbers of cytoplasmic filaments which have been confirmed to represent vimentin filaments by immunoelectron microscopy.[257]

## Differential Diagnosis

PHAT bears a striking resemblance to *schwannoma,* although several light microscopic and immunohistochemical features allow their distinction. Unlike schwannoma, PHAT is not encapsulated and usually grows in an infiltrative manner. It lacks distinct Antoni A and B zones and does not express S-100 protein.

The tumor also resembles *psammomatous melanotic schwannoma,* as psammomatous calcifications are sometimes found in PHAT and intranuclear inclusions raise the possibility of a neural neoplasm. Unlike psammomatous melanotic schwannoma, which co-expresses S-100 protein and HMB45, PHAT lacks these antigens.

The pronounced nuclear pleomorphism in the absence of specific features of differentiation also raises the possibility of *malignant fibrous histiocytoma.* Despite the striking cellularity in many PHATs, this tumor lacks significant mitotic activity. In addition, intranuclear cytoplasmic inclusions are not a feature of malignant fibrous histiciocytoma, nor is expression of CD-34.

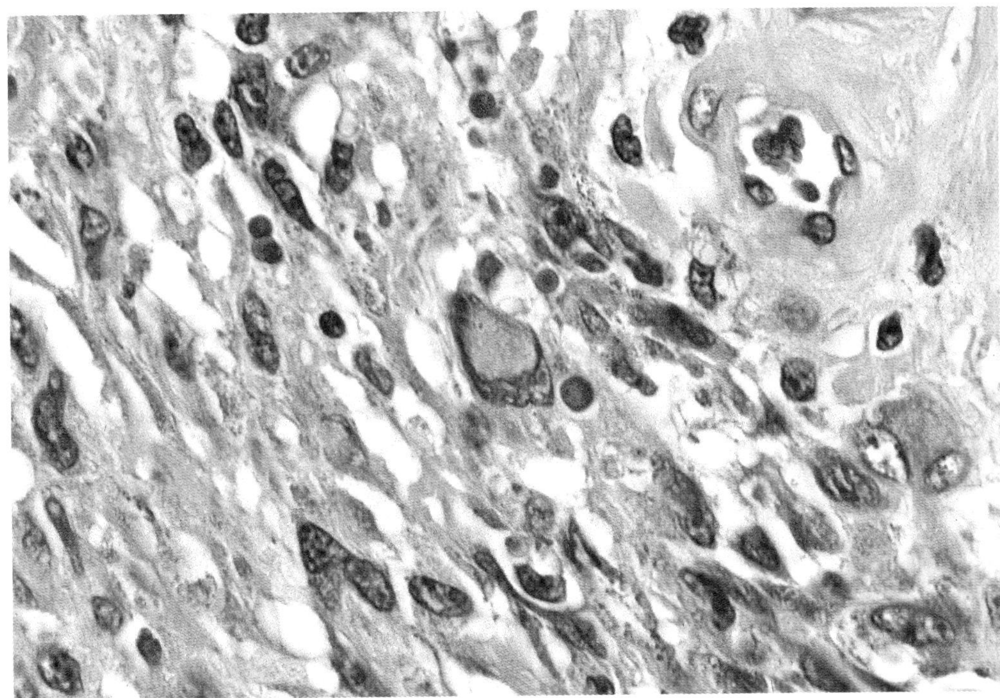

**FIGURE 36–78.** Pleomorphic hyalinizing angiectatic tumor with tumor cells that have prominent intranuclear cytoplasmic inclusions.

## Discussion

The clinical behavior of PHAT is characterized by local recurrence; metastases have not been documented. In the original study by Smith et al.,[257] follow-information available for eight patients revealed that four (50%) developed local recurrence, including one patient with an aggressive recurrence necessitating amputation and another who suffered multiple recurrences over a 25-year period. Wide local excision is recommended as the best therapeutic approach whenever possible.

Because of the paucity of reports of this neoplasm, its true nature has yet to be elucidated. The absence of S-100 protein immunoreactivity essentially negates the possibility that it is an unusual neural neoplasm. Some have suggested that PHAT is related to solitary fibrous tumor and giant cell angiofibroma given the overlapping histologic and immunohistochemical features,[253,254] but the expression of CD-34 in PHAT seems to be a less consistent finding than in these other neoplasms.

The most striking histologic feature of PHAT is the hyalinizing angiectatic vasculature. This may reflect, in part, the slow growth of the tumor, as suggested by the low Ki-67 index and S-phase fraction.[253,257] It has also been suggested that deposition of hyaline material leads to progressive vascular obliteration and tumoral hypoxia, which in turn promotes vascular endothelial growth factor production by the neoplastic cells, resulting in active angiogenesis.[255]

## REFERENCES

### Tumoral Calcinosis


1. Abraham Z, Rozner I, Rozenbaum M. Tumoral calcinosis: report of a case and brief review of the literature. J Dermatol 23: 545, 1996.
2. Apostolou T, Tziamalis M, Christodoulidou C, et al. Regression of massive tumoral calcinosis of the ischium in a dialysis patient after treatment with reduced calcium dialysate and i.v. administration. Clin Nephrol 50:247, 1998.
3. Balachandran S, Abbud Y, Prince MJ, et al. Tumoral calcinosis: scintigraphic studies of an affected family. Br J Radiol 53:960, 1980.
4. Bauer JM, Freyberg RH. Vitamin D intoxication with metastatic calcification. JAMA 130:1208, 1946.
5. Berg D. Tumoral calcinosis. Br J Surg 59:570, 1972.
6. Boskey AL, Vigorita VJ, Spencer O, et al. Chemical, microscopic, and ultrastructural characterization of the mineral deposits in tumoral calcinosis. Clin Orthop 178:258, 1983.
7. Carnett J. The calcareous deposits of so-called calcifying subacromial bursitis. Surg Gynecol Obstet 41:404, 1925.
8. Chen WS, Eng HL. Tumoral calcinosis after thumb tip injury: case report. J Trauma 38:952, 1995.
9. DiGiovanna JJ, Helfgott RK, Gerber LH, et al. Extraspinal tendon and ligament calcification associated with long-term therapy with etretinate. N Engl J Med 315:1177, 1986.
10. Duret MH. Tumeurs multiples et singulieres des bourses ser-

euses (endotheliomes peut etre d'origine parasitaire). Bull Mem Soc Anat (Paris) 74:725, 1899.

11. Gall G, Metzker A, Garlick J, et al. Head and neck manifestations of tumoral calcinosis. Oral Surg Oral Med Oral Pathol 77:158, 1994.
12. Geirnaerdt MJ, Kroon HM, van der Heul RO, et al. Tumoral calcinosis. Skeletal Radiol 24:148, 1995.
13. Ghanchi F, Ramsay A, Coupland S, et al. Ocular tumoral calcinosis: a clinicopathologic study. Arch Ophthalmol 114:341, 1996.
14. Hatori M, Oomamiuda K, Kokubun S. Hydroxyapatite crystals in tumoral calcinosis: a case report. Tohoku J Exp Med 180: 359, 1996.
15. Inclan A. Tumoral calcinosis. JAMA 121:490, 1943.
16. Irnell L, Werner I, Grimelius L. Soft tissue calcification in hyperparathyroidism. Acta Med Scand 187:145, 1970.
17. Jain SP. Tumoral calcinosis in Somalia and Ethiopia: a report of twenty-one cases and brief review of literature. East Afr Med J 66:476, 1989.
18. Katayama I, Higashi K, Mukai H, et al. Tumoral calcinosis in scleroderma. J Dermatol 16:82, 1989.
19. Kindblom LG, Gunterberg B. Tumoral calcinosis: an ultrastructural analysis and consideration of pathogenesis. APMIS 96: 368, 1988.
20. Lafferty FW, Reynolds ES, Pearson OH. Tumoral calcinosis: a metabolic disease of obscure etiology. Am J Med 38:105, 1965.
21. Lyles KW, Burkes EJ, Ellis GJ, et al. Genetic transmission of tumoral calcinosis: autosomal dominant with variable clinical expressivity. J Clin Endocrinol Metabol 60:1093, 1985.
22. Lyles KW, Halsey DL, Friedman NE, et al. Correlation of serum concentrations of 1,25-dihydroxyvitamin D, phosphorus, and parathyroid hormone in tumoral calcinosis. J Clin Endocrinol Metabol 67:88, 1988.
23. Maathuis JB, Koten JW. Kikuyu-bursa and tumoral calcinosis. Trop Geogr Med 21:389, 1969.
24. McClatschie S, Bremner AD. Tumoral calcinosis: an unrecognized disease. BMJ 1:153, 1969.
25. McGregor D, Burn J, Lynn K, et al. Rapid resolution of tumoral calcinosis after renal transplantation. Clin Nephrol 51: 54, 1999.
26. McGregor DH, Mowry M, Cherian R, et al. Nonfamilial tumoral calcinosis associated with chronic renal failure and secondary hyperparathyroidism: report of two cases with clinicopathological, immunohistochemical, and electron microscopic findings. Hum Pathol 26:607, 1995.
27. McGuinness FE. Hyperphosphataemic tumoral calcinosis in Bedouin Arabs: clinical and radiological features. Clin Radiol 50:259, 1995.
28. McKee PH, Llomba NG, Hutt MSR. Tumoral calcinosis: a pathological study of 56 cases. Br J Dermatol 107:669, 1982.
29. Mitnick PD, Goldfarb S, Slatopolsky E, et al. Calcium and phosphate metabolism in tumoral calcinosis. Ann Intern Med 92:482, 1980.
30. Mozzaffarian G, Lafferty FW, Pearson OH. Treatment of tumoral calcinosis with phosphorus deprivation. Ann Intern Med 77:741, 1972.
31. Murthy DP. Tumoral calcinosis: a study of cases from Papua, New Guinea. J Trop Med Hyg 93:403, 1990.
32. Narchi H. Hyperostosis with hyperphasphatemia: evidence of familial occurrence and association with tumoral calcinosis. Pediatrics 99:745, 1997.
33. Pakasa NM, Kalengayi RM. Tumoral calcinosis: a clinicopathological study of 111 cases with emphasis on the earliest changes. Histopathology 31:18, 1997.
34. Pecovnik-Balon B, Kramberger S. Tumoral calcinosis in patients on hemodialysis: case report and review of the literature. Am J Nephrol 17:93, 1997.
35. Pedersen HE, Key JA. Pathology of calcareous tendinitis and subdeltoid bursitis. Arch Surg 62:50, 1951.
36. Randall RE Jr, Strauss MB, McNeely WF. The milk-alkali syndrome. Arch Intern Med 107:163, 1961.
37. Slavin RE, Wen J, Kumar D, et al. Familial tumoral calcinosis: a clinical, histopathologic, and ultrastructural study with an analysis of its calcifying process and pathogenesis. Am J Surg Pathol 17:788, 1993.
38. Smack D, Norton SA, Fitzpatrick JE. Proposal for a pathogenesis-based classification of tumoral calcinosis. Int J Dermatol 35: 265, 1996.
39. Steinbach LS, Johnston JO, Tepper EF, et al. Tumoral calcinosis: radiologic-pathologic correlation. Skeletal Radiol 24:573, 1995.
40. Steinherz R, Chesney RW, Eisenstein B, et al. Elevated serum calcitriol concentrations do not fall in response to hyperphosphatemia in familial tumoral calcinosis. Am J Dis Child 139: 816, 1985.
41. Teutschlaender O. Die symmetrisch for schreitende Lipocalcinogranulomatose (Hygromatosis lipocalcinogranulomatosa progrediens) und andere Schleimbeutelveranderungen (sog "Bursitis calcarea" und Lipoma arborescens). Zieglers Beitr 103:499, 1939.
42. Teutschlaender O. Lipid Calcinosis (Lipoid Kalkgicht). Zieglers Beitr 110:402, 1947.
43. Teutschlaender O. Zur Kenntnis der progressiven Lipocalcinogranulomatose der Muskulatur. Virchows Arch [Pathol Anat] 295:424, 1935.
44. Tezelman S, Siperstein AE, Duh QY, et al. Tumoral calcinosis: controversies in the etiology and alternatives in the treatment. Arch Surg 128:737, 1993.
45. Theuvenet WJ, Nolthenius-Puylaert T, Giedrpcy JZL, et al. Massive deformation of the scrotal wall by idiopathic calcinosis of the scrotum. Plast Reconstr Surg 74:539, 1984.
46. Thomson JEM, Tanner FJ. Tumoral calcinosis. J Bone Joint Surg Am 31:132, 1949.
47. Thomson JG. Calcifying collagenolysis (tumoural calcinosis). Br J Radiol 39:526, 1966.
48. Wheeler CE, Curtis AC, Cawley EP, et al. Soft tissue calcification with special reference to its occurrence in the "collagen diseases." Ann Intern Med 36:1050, 1952.
49. Wilber JF, Slatopolsky E. Hyperphosphatemia and tumoral calcinosis. Ann Intern Med 68:1044, 1968.

### Intramuscular Myxoma

50. Allen PW. Myxoma is not a single entity: a review of the concept of myxoma. Ann Diagn Pathol 4:99, 2000.
51. Cabral CE, Guedes P, Fonseca T, et al. Polyostotic fibrous dysplasia associated with intramuscular myxomas: Mazabraud's syndrome. Skeletal Radiol 27:278, 1998.
52. Caraway NP, Staerkel GA, Fanning CV, et al. Diagnosing intramuscular myxoma by fine needle aspiration: a multi-disciplinary approach. Diagn Cytopathol 11:255, 1994.
53. Court-Payen M, Ingemann Jensen L, Bjerregaard B, et al. Intramuscular myxoma and fibrous dysplasia of bone: Mazabraud's syndrome; a case report. Acta Radiol 38:368, 1997.
54. Enzinger FM. Intramuscular myxoma. Am J Clin Pathol 43: 104, 1965.
55. Feldman P. A comparative study including ultrastructure of intramuscular myxoma and myxoid liposarcoma. Cancer 43: 512, 1979.
56. Fujii K, Inoue M, Araki Y, et al. Multiple intramuscular myxomas associated with polyostotic fibrous dysplasia. Eur J Radiol 22:152, 1996.
57. Gober GA, Nicholas RW. Case report 800: intramuscular myxoma. Skeletal Radiol 22:452, 1993.
58. Hashimoto H, Tsuneyoshi M, Daimaru Y, et al. Intramuscular

myxoma: a clinicopathologic, immunohistochemical, and electron microscopic study. Cancer 58:740, 1986.
59. Ireland DC, Soule EH, Ivins JC. Myxoma of somatic soft tissues: a report of 58 patients, 3 with multiple tumors and fibrous dysplasia of bone. Mayo Clin Proc 48:401, 1973.
60. Kindblom LG, Stener B, Angervall L. Intramuscular myxoma. Cancer 34:1737, 1974.
61. Kransdorf MJ, Moser RP Jr, Jelinek JS, et al. Intramuscular myxoma: MR features. J Comput Assist Tomogr 13:836, 1989.
62. Lombardi T, Lock C, Samson J, et al. S-100, alpha-smooth muscle actin and cytokeratin 19 immunohistochemistry in odontogenic and soft tissue myxomas. J Clin Pathol 48:759, 1995.
63. Mazabraud A, Semat P, Roze R. A propos de l'association de fibromyxomes des tissus mous a la dysplasie fibreuse des os. Presse Med 75:2223, 1967.
64. Miettinen M, Hockerstedt K, Reitamo J, et al. Intramuscular myxoma: a clinicopathologic study of 23 cases. Am J Clin Pathol 84:265, 1985.
65. Nielsen GP, O'Connell JX, Rosenberg AE. Intramuscular myxoma: a clinicopathologic study of 51 cases with emphasis on hypercellular and hypervascular variants. Am J Surg Pathol 22:122, 1998.
66. Orlandi A, Bianchi L, Marino B, et al. Intramuscular myxoma of the face: an unusual localization; a clinicopathological study. Dermatol Surg 21:251, 1995.
67. Pettersson H, Hudson TM, Springfield DS, et al. Cystic intramuscular myxoma: report of a case. Acta Radiol Diagn (Stockh) 26:425, 1985.
68. Schwartz HS, Walker R. Recognizable magnetic resonance imaging characteristics of intramuscular myxoma. Orthopedics 20:431, 1997.
69. Serrat A, Verrier A, Espeso A, et al. Intramuscular myxoma of the temporalis muscle. J Oral Maxillofac Surg 56:1206, 1998.
70. Stout AP. Myxoma, the tumor of primitive mesenchyme. Ann Surg 127:706, 1948.
71. Szendroi M, Rahoty P, Antal I, et al. Fibrous dysplasia associated with intramuscular myxoma (Mazabraud's syndrome): a long-term follow-up of three cases. J Cancer Res Clin Oncol 124:401, 1998.
72. Wirth WA, Leavitt D, Enzinger FM. Multiple intramuscular myxomas: another extraskeletal manifestation of fibrous dysplasia. Cancer 27:1167, 1971.

### Juxtaarticular Myxoma

73. Becton JL, Young HH. Cysts of semilunar cartilage of the knee. Arch Surg 90:708, 1965.
74. Bennett GE, Shaw MB. Cysts of the semilunar cartilages. Arch Surg 33:92, 1936.
75. Daluiski A, Seeger LL, Doberneck SA, et al. A case of juxta-articular myxoma of the knee. Skeletal Radiol 24:389, 1995.
76. Gallo GA, Sryan RS. Cysts of the semilunar cartilages of the knee. Am J Surg 116:65, 1968.
77. Ghormley RK, Dockerty MB. Cystic myxomatous tumors about the knee: their relation to cysts of the menisci. J Bone Joint Surg [Am] 25:306, 1943.
78. King DG, Saifuddin A, Preston HV, et al. Magnetic resonance imaging of juxta-articular myxoma. Skeletal Radiol 24:145, 1995.
79. Meis JM, Enzinger FM. Juxtaarticular myxoma: a clinical and pathological study of 65 cases. Hum Pathol 23:639, 1992.
80. Noble J, Hamblen DL. The pathology of the degenerate meniscus lesion. J Bone Joint Surg Br 57:180, 1975.
81. Sciot R, Dal Cin P, Samson I, et al. Clonal chromosomal changes in juxta-articular myxoma. Virchows Arch 434:177, 1999.

### Myxoma of the Jaws

82. Ang HK, Ramani P, Michaels L. Myxoma of the maxillary antrum in children. Histopathology 23:361, 1993.
83. Balough G, Inovay J. Recurrent mandibular myxoma: report of a case. J Oral Surg 30:121, 1972.
84. Caleffi E, Toschi S, Bocchi A. Myxoma of the maxilla: surgical treatment of an unusual case in a child. Plast Reconstruct Surg 93:1274, 1994.
85. Deron PB, Nikolovski N, Den Hollander JC. Myxoma of the maxilla: a case with extremely aggressive biologic behavior. Head Neck 18:495, 1996.
86. Ghosh BC, Huvos AG, Gerold FP, et al. Myxoma of the jaw bones. Cancer 31:237, 1973.
87. Greenfield SD, Friedman O. Myxoma of maxillary sinus. NY State J Med 51:1319, 1951.
88. Hasleton PS, Simpson W, Craig RDP. Myxoma of the mandible: a fibroblastic tumor. Oral Surg Oral Med Oral Pathol 46:396, 1978.
89. Kaffe I, Naor H, Buchner A. Clinical and radiological features of odontogenic myxoma of the jaws. Dentomaxillofac Radiol 26:299, 1997.
90. Kangur T, Dahlin D, Tulington E. Myxomatous tumors of the jaws. J Oral Surg 33:523, 1975.
91. Kawai T, Murakami S, Kishino M, et al. MR images of a maxillary myxoma. AJR 167:1343, 1996.
92. Lombardi T, Kuffer R, Bernard JP, et al. Immunohistochemical staining for vimentin filaments and S-100 protein in myxoma of the jaws. J Oral Pathol 17:175, 1988.
93. Lombardi T, Lock C, Samson J, et al. S100, alpha-smooth muscle actin and cytokeratin 19 immunohistochemistry in odontogenic and soft tissue myxomas. J Clin Pathol 48:759, 1995.
94. Moshiri S, Oda D, Worthington P, et al. Odontogenic myxoma: histochemical and ultrastructural study. J Oral Pathol Med 21:401, 1992.
95. Slootweg PJ, Wittkampf AR. Myxoma of the jaws: an analysis of 15 cases. J Maxillofac Surg 14:46, 1986.

### Cutaneous Myxoma (Superficial Angiomyxoma)

96. Allen PW, Dymock RB, McCormac LB. Superficial angiomyxomas with and without epithelial components: report of 30 tumors in 28 patients. Am J Surg Pathol 12:519, 1988.
97. Bedlow AJ, Sampson SA, Holden CA. Congenital superficial angiomyxoma. Clin Exp Dermatol 22:237, 1997.
98. Calonje E, Guerin D, McCormick D, et al. Superficial angiomyxoma: clinicopathologic analysis of a series of distinctive but poorly recognized tumors with tendency for recurrence. Am J Surg Pathol 23:910, 1999.
99. Fetsch JF, Laskin WB, Tavassoli FA. Superficial angiomyxoma (cutaneous myxoma): a clinicopathologic study of 17 cases arising in the genital region. Int J Gynecol Pathol 16:325, 1997.
100. Wilk M, Schmoeckel C, Kaiser HW, et al. Cutaneous angiomyxoma: a benign neoplasm distinct from cutaneous focal mucinosis. J Am Acad Dermatol 33:352, 1995.

### Carney's Complex

101. Basson CT, MacRae CA, Korf B, et al. Genetic heterogeneity of familial atrial myxoma syndromes (Carney's complex). Am J Cardiol 79:994, 1997.
102. Carney JA. Psammomatous melanotic schwannoma: a distinctive, heritable tumor with special associations, including cardiac myxoma and the Cushing syndrome. Am J Surg Pathol 14:206, 1990.
103. Carney JA, Ferreiro JA. The epithelioid blue nevus: a multicentric familial tumor with important associations, including cardiac myxoma and psammomatous melanotic schwannoma. Am J Surg Pathol 20:259, 1996.
104. Carney JA, Gordon H, Carpenter PC, et al. The complex of

myxomas, spotty pigmentation, and endocrine overactivity. Medicine 64:270, 1985.

105. Carney JA, Headington JT, Su WPD. Cutaneous myxomas: a major component of the complex of myxomas, spotty pigmentation, and endocrine overactivity. Arch Dermatol 122:790, 1986.
106. Carney JA, Hruska LS, Beauchamp GD, et al. Dominant inheritance of the complex of myxomas, spotty pigmentation, and endocrine overactivity. Mayo Clin Proc 61:165, 1986.
107. Carney JA, Stratakis CA. Epithelioid blue nevus and psammomatous melanotic schwannoma: the unusual pigmented skin tumors of the Carney's complex. Semin Diagn Pathol 15:216, 1998.
108. Carney JA, Toorkey BC. Myxoid fibroadenoma and allied conditions (myxomatosis) of the breast: a heritable disorder with special associations including cardiac and cutaneous myxomas. Am J Surg Pathol 15:713, 1991.
109. Casey M, Mah C, Merliss AD, et al. Identification of a novel genetic locus for familial cardiac myxomas and Carney's complex. Circulation 98:2560, 1998.
110. Chang B, Borer JG, Tan PE, et al. Large-cell calcifying sertoli cell tumor of the testis: case report and review of the literature. Urology 52:520, 1998.
111. Chrousos GP, Stratakis CA. Carney's complex and the familial lentiginosis syndromes: linked to inherited neoplasias and developmental disorders, and genetic loci. J Intern Med 243:573, 1998.
112. Cook CA, Lund BA, Carney JA. Mucocutaneous pigmented spots and oral myxomas: the oral manifestations of the complex of myxomas, spotty pigmentation and endocrine activity. Oral Surg Oral Med Oral Pathol 63:175, 1987.
113. Feldman AR, Keeling JH. Cutaneous manifestations of atrial myxoma. J Am Acad Dermatol 21:1080, 1989.
114. Ferreiro JA, Carney JA. Myxomas of the external ear and their significance. Am J Surg Pathol 18:274, 1994.
115. Gardner SS, Solomon AR. Cutaneous and cardiac myxomas: an important association. Semin Dermatol 10:148, 1991.
116. Irvine AD, Armstrong DK, Bingham EA, et al. Evidence for a second genetic locus in Carney's complex. Br J Dermatol 139: 572, 1998.
117. Kirschner LS, Taymans SE, Stratakis CA. Characterization of the adrenal gland pathology of Carney's complex, and molecular genetics of the disease. Endocr Res 24:863, 1998.
118. Milunsky J, Huang XL, Baldwin CT, et al. Evidence for genetic heterogeneity of the Carney's complex (familial atrial myxoma syndromes). Cancer Genet Cytogenet 106:173, 1998.
119. Noszian IM, Balon R, Eitelberger FG, et al. Bilateral testicular large-cell calcifying Sertoli's cell tumor and recurrent cardiac myxoma in a patient with Carney's complex. Pediatr Radiol 25:S236, 1995.
120. Stratakis CA, Carney JA, Kirschner LS, et al. Synaptophysin immunoreactivity in primary pigmented nodular adrenocortical disease: neuroendocrine properties of tumors associated with Carney's complex. J Clin Endocrinal Metab 84:1122, 1999.
121. Stratakis CA, Carney JA, Lin JP, et al. Carney's complex, a familial multiple neoplasia and lentiginosis syndrome: analysis of 11 kindreds and linkage to the short arm of chromosome 2. J Clin Invest 97:699, 1996.
122. Stratakis CA, Courcoutsakis NA, Abati A, et al. Thyroid gland abnormalities in patients with the syndrome of spotty skin pigmentation, myxomas, endocrine overactivity, and schwannomas. J Clin Endocrinol Metab 82:2037, 1997.
123. Stratakis CA, Jenkins RB, Pras E, et al. Cytogenetic and microsatellite alterations in tumors from patients with the syndrome of myxomas, spotty skin pigmentation, and endocrine overactivity (Carney's complex). J Clin Endocrinol Metab 81:3607, 1996.
124. Tatebe S, Ohzeki H, Miyamura H, et al. Carney's complex in association with right atrial myxoma. Ann Thorac Surg 58:561, 1994.
125. Taymans SE, Kirschner LS, Giatzakis C, et al. Radiation hybrid mapping of chromosomal region 2p15-p16: integration of expressed and polymorphic sequences maps at the Carney's complex (CNC) and Doyne honeycomb retinal dystrophy (DHRD) loci. Genomics 56:344, 1999.


### Cutaneous Myxoid Cyst


126. Arner O, Lindholm A, Romanus R. Mucous cysts of fingers. Acta Chir Scand 111:314, 1956.
127. Constant E, Royer JR, Pollard RJ, et al. Mucous cysts of the fingers. Plast Reconstr Surg 43:241, 1969.
128. Gross RE. Recurring myxomatous, cutaneous cysts of the fingers and toes. Surg Gynecol Obstet 65:289, 1937.
129. Johnson WC, Graham JH, Helwig EB. Cutaneous myxoid cyst. JAMA 191:15, 1965.
130. McCalmont CS, White WL, Jorizzo JL. Giant fibromyxoid tumor of the adventitial dermis: forme fruste of trichodiscoma. Am J Dermatopathol 13:403, 1991.


### Focal Cutaneous Mucinosis and Myxedema


131. Buchner A, Merrell PW, Leider AS, et al. Oral focal mucinosis. Int J Oral Maxillofac Surg 19:337, 1990.
132. Clark BJ, Mowat A, Fallowfield ME, et al. Papular mucinosis: is the inflammatory cell infiltrate neoplastic? The presence of a monotypic plasma cell population demonstrated by in situ hybridization. Br J Dermatol 135:467, 1996.
133. Dapaire-Duclos F, Renuy F, Dandurand M, et al. Papular mucinosis with rapid spontaneous regression in an HIV-infected patient. Eur J Dermatol 8:353, 1998.
134. Gimlette TMD. Pretibial myxoedema. BMJ 5195:348, 1960.
135. Howsden SM, Herndon JH Jr, Freeman RG. Lichen myxedematosus. Arch Dermatol 111:1325, 1975.
136. Ishizawa T, Sugiki H, Anzai S, et al. Pretibial myxedema with Graves' disease: a case report and review of the Japanese literature. J Dermatol 25:264, 1998.
137. Johnson WC, Helwig EB. Cutaneous focal mucinosis: a clinicopathological and histochemical study. Arch Dermatol 93:13, 1966.
138. Kand N, Tsuchida T, Watanabe T, et al. Cutaneous lupus mucinosis: a review of our cases and the possible pathogenesis. J Cutan Pathol 24:553, 1997.
139. Kaufmann R, Greiner D, Schmidt P, et al. Dermatomyositis presenting as plaque-like mucinosis. Br J Dermatol 138:889, 1998.
140. Maruyama M, Miyauchi S, Hashimoto K. Massive cutaneous mucinosis associated with systemic lupus erythematosus. Br J Dermatol 137:450, 1997.
141. Omohundro C, Dijkstra JW, Camisa C, et al. Early onset pretibial myxedema in the absence of ophthalmopathy: a morphologic evolution. Cutis 58:211, 1996.
142. Rongioletti F, Ghigliotti G, De Marchi R, et al. Cutaneous mucinoses and HIV infection. Br J Dermatol 139:1077, 1998.
143. Shishido M, Kuroda K, Tsukifuji R, et al. A case of pretibial myxedema associated with Graves' disease: an immunohistochemical study of serum-derived hyaluronan-associated protein. J Dermatol 22:948, 1995.
144. Soda G, Baiocchini A, Bosco D, et al. Oral focal mucinosis of the tongue. Pathol Oncol Res 4:304, 1998.
145. Vazquez-Doval FJ, Sola MA. Mucinosis of the mammary areolae and mycosis fungoides. Clin Exp Dermatol 21:374, 1996.
146. Wilk M, Schmoeckel C. Cutaneous focal mucinosis: a histopathological and immunohistochemical analysis of 11 cases. J Cutan Pathol 21:446, 1994.

147. Wu MT, Chang CH, Yu HS, et al. Scleromyxoedema with prominent linear eruption and polyclonal gammopathy. Clin Exp Dermatol 22:110, 1997.

### Ganglion

148. Barnes WE, Larsen RD, Posch JL. Review of the ganglia of the hand or wrist with analysis of surgical treatment. Plast Reconstr Surg 34:570, 1964.
149. Bauer TW, Dorfman HD. Intraosseous ganglion: a clinicopathologic study of 11 cases. Am J Surg Pathol 6:207, 1982.
150. Carp L, Stout AP. A study of ganglion: with especial reference to treatment. Surg Gynecol Obstet 47:460, 1928.
151. Englert HM. Die ganglioplastischen Tumoren oder Gangliome der Hand. Chirurg 44:35, 1973.
152. McEvedy V. Simple ganglia. Br J Surg 49:585, 1961.
153. Oertel YC, Beckner ME, Engler WF. Cytologic diagnosis and ultrastructure of fine-needle aspirates of ganglion cysts. Arch Pathol Lab Med 110:938, 1986.
154. Salyer WR, Salyer DC. Myxoma-like features of organizing thrombi in arteries and veins. Arch Pathol 99:307, 1975.
155. Sarpyener MA, Ozcurumez O, Seyhan F. Multiple ganglions of tendon sheaths. J Bone Joint Surg Am 50:985, 1968.
156. Sime FH, Dahlin DC. Ganglion cysts of bone. Mayo Clin Proc 46:484, 1971.
157. Soren A. Pathogenesis, clinic and treatment of ganglion. Arch Orthop Trauma Surg 99:247, 1982.
158. Zachariae L, Vibe-Hansen H. Ganglia recurrence rate elucidated by a follow-up of 347 operated cases. Acta Chir Scand 139:625, 1973.

### Aggressive Angiomyxoma

159. Begin LR, Clement PB, Kirk ME, et al. Aggressive angiomyxoma of pelvic soft parts: a clinicopathologic study of nine cases. Hum Pathol 16:621, 1985.
160. Bigotti G, Coli A, Gasbarri A, et al. Angiomyofibroblastoma and aggressive angiomyxoma: two benign mesenchymal neoplasms of the female genital tract: an immunohistochemical study. Pathol Res Pract 195:39, 1999.
161. Catalano O. Case report: aggressive angiomyxoma of the pelvic soft tissues; US and CT findings. Clin Radiol 53:782, 1998.
162. Chien AJ, Freeby JA, Win DT, et al. Aggressive angiomyxoma of the female pelvis: sonographic, CT and MR findings. AJR 171:530, 1998.
163. Clatch RJ, Drake WK, Gonzalez JG. Aggressive angiomyxoma in men: a report of two cases associated with inguinal hernias. Arch Pathol Lab Med 117:911, 1993.
164. Davani N, Chablani BN, Saba PR. Aggressive angiomyxoma of pelvic soft tissues: MR imaging appearance. AJR 170:1113, 1998.
165. De Salvia D, Fais GF, Lauri F, et al. Aggressive angiomyxoma of the vulva: expression of estroprogestinic receptors and follow-up. Clin Exp Obstet Gynecol 25:141, 1998.
166. Fetsch JF, Laskin WB, Lefkowitz M, et al. Aggressive angiomyxoma: a clinicopathologic study of 29 female patients. Cancer 78:79, 1996.
167. Fletcher CD, Tsang WY, Fisher C, et al. Angiomyofibroblastoma of the vulva: a benign neoplasm distinct from aggressive angiomyxoma. Am J Surg Pathol 16:373, 1992.
168. Granter SR, Nucci MR, Fletcher CDM. Aggressive angiomyxoma: reappraisal of its relationship with angiomyfibroblastoma in a series of 16 cases. Histopathology 30:3, 1997.
169. Htwe M, Deppisch LM, Saint-Julien JS. Hormone-dependent aggressive angiomyxoma of the vulva. Obstet Gynecol 86:697, 1995.
170. Iezzoni JC, Fechner RE, Wong LE, et al. Aggressive angiomyxoma in males: a report of four cases. Am J Clin Pathol 104:391, 1995.
171. Kazmierczak B, Dal Cin P, Wanschura S, et al. Cloning and molecular characterization of part of a new gene fused to HMGIC in mesenchymal tumors. Am J Pathol 152:431, 1998.
172. Kazmierczak B, Wanschura S, Meyer-Bolte K, et al. Cytogenetic and molecular analysis of an aggressive angiomyxoma. Am J Pathol 147:580, 1995.
173. Kenny-Moynihan MB, Hagen J, Richman B, et al. Loss of an X-chromosome in aggressive angiomyxoma of female soft parts: a case report. Cancer Genet Cytogenet 89:61, 1996.
174. Ockner DM, Sayadi H, Swanson PE, et al. Genital angiomyofibroblastoma: comparison with aggressive angiomyxoma and other myxoid neoplasms of skin and soft tissue. Am J Clin Pathol 107:36, 1997.
175. Outwater EK, Marchetto BE, Wagner BJ, et al. Aggressive angiomyxoma: findings on CT and MR imaging. AJR 172:435, 1999.
176. Silverman JS, Albukerk J, Tamsen A. Comparison of angiomyofibroblastoma and aggressive angiomyxoma in both sexes: four cases composed of bimodal CD 34 and factor XIIIa positive dendritic cell subsets. Pathol Res Pract 193:673, 1997.
177. Skalova A, Michal M, Husek K, et al. Aggressive angiomyxoma of the pelvicoperineal region. Am J Dermatopathol 15:446, 1993.
178. Steeper TA, Rosai J. Aggressive angiomyxoma of the female pelvis and perineum: report of nine cases of a distinctive type of gynecologic soft-tissue neoplasm. Am J Surg Pathol 7:463, 1983.
179. Tsang WY, Chan JK, Fisher C, et al. Aggressive angiomyxoma: a report of four cases occurring in men. Am J Surg Pathol 16:1059, 1992.

### Ossifying Fibromyxoid Tumor of Soft Tissue

180. Donner LR. Ossifying fibromyxoid tumor of soft parts: evidence supporting Schwann cell origin. Hum Pathol 23:200, 1992.
181. Ekfors TO, Kulju T, Aaltonen M, et al. Ossifying fibromyxoid tumour of soft parts: report of four cases including one mediastinal and infantile. APMIS 106:1124, 1998.
182. Enzinger FM. Critical commentary. Pathol Res Pract 189:605, 1993.
183. Enzinger FM, Weiss SW, Liang CY. Ossifying fibromyxoid tumor of soft parts: a clinicopathological analysis of 59 cases. Am J Surg Pathol 13:817, 1989.
184. Fisher C, Hedges M, Weiss SW. Ossifying fibromyxoid tumor of soft parts with stromal cyst formation and ribosome-lamella complexes. Ultrastruct Pathol 18:593, 1994.
185. Kilpatrick SE, Ward WG, Mozes M, et al. Atypical and malignant variants of ossifying fibromyxoid tumor: clinicopathologic analysis of six cases. Am J Surg Pathol 19:1039, 1995.
186. Kyriakos M. Ossifying fibromyxoid tumor: something new to mull over. Am J Clin Pathol 95:107, 1991.
187. Miettinen M. Ossifying fibromyxoid tumor of soft parts: additional observations on a distinctive soft tissue tumor. Am J Clin Pathol 95:142, 1991.
188. Motoyama T, Ogose A, Watanabe H. Ossifying fibromyxoid tumor of the retroperitoneum. Pathol Int 46:79, 1996.
189. Nakayama F, Kuwahara T. Ossifying fibromyxoid tumor of soft parts of the back. J Cutan Pathol 23:385, 1996.
190. Schaffler G, Raith J, Ranner G, et al. Radiographic appearance of an ossifying fibromyxoid tumor of soft parts. Skeletal Radiol 26:615, 1997.
191. Schofield JB, Krausz T, Stamp GWH, et al. Ossifying fibromyxoid tumour of soft parts: immunohistochemical and ultrastructural analysis. Histopathology 22:101, 1993.
192. Thompson J, Castillo M, Reddick RL, et al. Nasopharyngeal nonossifying variant of ossifying fibromyxoid tumor: CT and MR findings. Am J Neuroradiol 16:1132, 1995.

193. Williams SB, Ellis GL, Mies JM, et al. Ossifying fibromyxoid tumour (of soft parts) of the head and neck: a clinicopathological and immunohistochemical study of nine cases. J Laryngol Otol 107:75, 1993.
194. Williamson MER, Dallimore N. A new bony lump for general surgeons: ossifying fibromyxoid tumour of soft parts. Eur J Surg 160:53, 1994.
195. Yang P, Hirose T, Hasegawa T, et al. Ossifying fibromyxoid tumor of soft parts: a morphological and immunohistochemical study. Pathol Int 44:448, 1994.
196. Yoshida H, Minamizaki T, Yumoto T, et al. Ossifying fibromyxoid tumor of soft parts. Acta Pathol Jpn 41:480, 1991.
197. Zamecnik M, Michel M, Simpson RH, et al. Ossifying fibromyxoid tumor of soft parts: a report of 17 cases with emphasis on unusual histological features. Ann Diagn Pathol 1:73, 1997.

### Parachordoma

198. Carstens PH. Chordoid tumor: a light, electron microscopic and immunohistochemical study. Ultrastruct Pathol 19:291, 1995.
199. Dabska M. Parachordoma: a new clinicopathologic entity. Cancer 40:1586, 1977.
200. De Blois D, Wang S, Kay S. Microtubular aggregates within endoplasmic reticulum: an unusual ultrastructural feature of extraskeletal myxoid chondrosarcoma. Hum Pathol 17:469, 1996.
201. Dei Tos AP, Wadden C, Fletcher CDM. Extraskeletal myxoid chondrosarcoma: an immunohistochemical reappraisal of 39 case. Appl Immunohistochem 5:73, 1997.
202. Fisher C. Parachordoma exists: but what is it? Adv Anat Pathol 7:141, 2000.
203. Fisher C, Miettinen M. Parachordoma: a clinicopathologic and immunohistochemical study of four cases of an unusual soft tissue neoplasm. Ann Diagn Pathol 1:3, 1997.
204. Fletcher CDM, Kilpatrick SE. Parachordomas [letter]. 21:1120, 1997.
205. Folpe AL, Agoff SN, Willis J, et al. Parachordoma is immunohistochemically and cytogenetically distinct from axial chordoma and extraskeletal myxoid chondrosarcoma. Am J Surg Pathol 23:1059, 1999.
206. Hirowaka M, Manabe T, Sugihara K. Parachordoma of the buttock: an immunohistochemical case study and review. Jpn J Clin Oncol 24:336, 1994.
207. Imlay SP, Argenyi ZD, Stone MS, et al. Cutaneous parachordoma: a light microscopic and immunohistochemical report of two cases and review of the literature. J Cutan Pathol 25:279, 1998.
208. Ishida T, Oda H, Oka T, et al. Parachordoma: an ultrastructural and immunohistochemical study. Virchows Arch [Pathol Anat] 422:239, 1993.
209. Karabela-Bouropoulou V, Skourtas C, Liapi-Avgeri G, et al. Parachordoma: a case report of a very rare soft tissue tumor. Pathol Res Pract 192:972, 1996.
210. Kilpatrick SE, Hitchcock MG, Kraus MD, et al. Mixed tumors and myoepetheliomas of soft tissue: a clinicopathologic study of 19 cases with a unifying concept. Am J Surg Pathol 21:13, 1997.
211. Laskowski J. Zarys onkologii. In: Kolodziejska H (ed) Pathology of Tumors. PZWL, Warsaw, 1995, pp 91–99.
212. Leong ASY, Vinyuvat S, Suthipintawong C, et al. Patterns of basal lamina immunostaining in soft-tissue and bony tumors. Appl Immunohistochem 5:1, 1997.
213. Limon J, Babinska M, Denis A, et al. Parachordoma: a rare sarcoma with clonal chromosomal changes. Cancer Genet Cytogenet 102:78, 1998.
214. Miettinen M, Karaharju E, Jarvinen H. Chordoma with a massive spindle-cell sarcomatous transformation: a light- and electron-microscopic and immunohistochemical study. Am J Surg Pathol 11:563, 1987.
215. Naka T, Iwamoto Y, Shinohara N, et al. Cytokeratin subtyping in chordomas and the fetal notochord: an immunohistochemical analysis of aberrant expression. Mod Pathol 10:545, 1997.
216. Niezavitowski A, Limon J, Wasilewska A, et al. Parachordoma: a clinicopathologic, immunohistochemical, electron microscopic, flow cytometric, and cytogenetic study. Gen Diagn Pathol 141:49, 1995.
217. O'Connell JX, Berean KW. Parachordomas [letter]. Am J Surg Pathol 21:1120, 1997.
218. O'Hara BJ, Paetau A, Miettinen M. Keratin subsets and monoclonal antibody HBME-1 in chordoma: immunohistochemical differential diagnosis between tumors simulating chordoma. Hum Pathol 29:119, 1998.
219. Povysil C, Matejovsky Z. A comparative ultrastructural study of chondrosarcoma, chordoid sarcoma, chordoma, and chordoma pheriphericum. Pathol Res Pract 179:546, 1985.
220. Sangueza OP, White CR. Parachordoma. Am J Dermatopathol 16:185, 1994.
221. Shin HJ, Mackay B, Ichinose H, et al. Parachordoma. Ultrastruct Pathol 18:249, 1994.
222. Tihy F, Scott P, Russo P, et al. Cytogenetic analysis of a parachordoma. Cancer Genet Cytogenet 105:14, 1998.

### Amyloid Tumor

223. Bhagwandeen BS, Taylor S. Primary localized amyloidoma of the bladder with a monoclonal plasma cell infiltrate. Pathology 20:67, 1988.
224. Chen KTK. Amyloidosis presenting in the respiratory tract. Pathol Annu 1:253, 1989.
225. Deans GT, Hale RJ, McMahon RF, et al. Amyloid tumor of the colon. J Clin Pathol 48:592, 1995.
226. Dee CH, Missirian RJ, Chernoff IJ. Primary amyloidoma of the spine: a case report and review of the literature. Spine 23:497, 1998.
227. Feiner HD. Pathology of dysproteinemia: light chain amyloidosis, non-amyloid immunoglobulin deposition disease, cryoglobulinemia syndromes, and macroglobulinemia of Waldenstriauom. Hum Pathol 19:1255, 1988.
228. Glenner GG. Amyloid deposits and amyloidosis: the $\beta$-fibrilloses. N Engl J Med 302:1283, 1980.
229. Hamidi AK, Liepnieks JJ, Bihrle R, et al. Local synthesis of amyloid fibril precursor in AL amyloidosis of the urinary tract. Amyloid 5:49, 1998.
230. Ihling C, Weirich G, Gaa A, et al. Amyloid tumors of the lung: an immunocytoma? Pathol Res Pract 192:446, 1996.
231. Khan SM, Birch PJ, Bass PS, et al. Localized amyloidosis of the lower genitourinary tract: a clinicopathologic and immunohistochemical study of nine cases. Histopathology 21:143, 1992.
232. Kibbi AG, Rubeiz NG, Zaynon ST, et al. Primary localized cutaneous amyloidosis. Int J Dermatol 31:95, 1992.
233. Krishnan J, Chu WS, Elrod JP, et al. Tumoral presentation of amyloidosis (amyloidomas) in soft tissue: a report of 14 cases. Am J Clin Pathol 100:135, 1993.
234. Laeng RH, Aftermatt HJ, Scheithauer BW, et al. Amyloidomas of the nervous system: a monoclonal B-cell disorder with monotypic amyloid light chain gamma amyloid production. Cancer 82:362, 1998.
235. Luo JH, Rotterdam H. Primary amyloid tumor of the breast: a case report and review of the literature. Mod Pathol 10:735, 1997.
236. Massry GG, Harrison W, Hornblass A. Clinical and computer tomographic characteristics of amyloid tumor of the lacrimal gland. Ophthalmology 103:1233, 1996.

237. Ossnoss KZ, Harrell DD. Isolated mediastinal mass in primary amyloidosis. Chest 78:786, 1980.
238. Pambuccian SE, Horyd ID, Cawte T, et al. Amyloidoma of bone: a plasma cell/plasmacytoid neoplasm; report of three cases and review of the literature. Am J Surg Pathol 21:179, 1997.
239. Porchet F, Sonntag VK, Vrodos N. Cervical amyloidoma of C2: case report and review of the literature. Spine 23:133, 1998.
240. Senapati A, Fletcher C, Bultitude MI, et al. Amyloid tumor of the rectum. J R Soc Med 88:48, 1995.
241. Sidoni A, Alberti PF, Bravi S, et al. Amyloid tumours in the soft tissues of the legs: case report and review of the literature. Virchows Arch 432:563, 1998.
242. Silverman JF, Dabbs DJ, Norris HT, et al. Localized primary (AL) amyloid tumor of the breast: cytologic, histologic, immunohistochemical, and ultrastructural observations. Am J Surg Pathol 10:539, 1986.
243. Symonds DA, Eichelberger MF, Sager GL. Calcifying amyloidoma of the breast. South Med J 88:1169, 1995.
244. Thompson LDR, Derringer GA, Wenig BM. Amyloidosis of the larynx: a clinicopathologic study of 11 cases. Mod Pathol 13:528, 2000.
245. Tomm Y, Htwe M, Chandra R, et al. Bilateral beta 2-microglobulin amyloidomas of the buttocks in a long-term hemodialysis patient. Arch Pathol Lab Med 118:651, 1994.
246. Van Rijswijk MH, Van Heusdan CW. The potassium permanganate method: a reliable method for differentiating amyloid AA from other forms of amyloid in routine laboratory practice. Am J Pathol 97:43, 1979.
247. Vavrina J, Muller W, Gebbers JO. Recurrent amyloid tumor of the parotid gland. Eur Arch Otorhinolaryngol 252:53, 1995.
248. Warner KJ, Blackwell GG, Herrera GA, et al. Cardiac amyloidoma with IgM-kappa gammopathy. Arch Pathol Lab Med 118:1148, 1994.
249. Watanabe T, Kato K, Sugitani M, et al. A case of solitary amyloidosis localized within the transverse colon presenting as a submucosal tumor. Gastrointest Endosc 49:644, 1999.
250. Weiss SW. Tumoral amyloidosis of soft tissue (amyloidoma): new approaches to an old problem. Am J Clin Pathol 100:91, 1993.
251. Yamamoto T, Maeda N, Kawasaki H. Hepatic failure in a case of multiple myeloma-associated amyloidosis (kappa-AL). J Gastroenterol 30:393, 1995.
252. Yokoo H, Nakazato Y. Primary localized amyloid tumor of the breast with osseous metaplasia. Pathol Int 48:545, 1998.


### Pleomorphic Hyalinizing Angiectatic Tumor of Soft Parts


253. Fukunaga M, Ushigome S. Pleomorphic hyalinizing angiectatic tumor of soft parts. Pathol Int 47:784, 1997.
254. Gallo C, Murer B, Roncaroli F. Pleomorphic hyalinizing angiectatic soft-tissue tumor: description of a case. Pathologica 89:531, 1997.
255. Groisman GM, Bejar J, Amar M, et al. Pleomorphic hyalinizing angiectatic tumor of soft parts: immunohistochemical study including the expression of vascular endothelial growth factor. Arch Pathol Lab Med 124:423, 2000.
256. Silverman JS, Dana MM. Pleomorphic hyalinizing angiectatic tumor of soft parts: immunohistochemical case study shows cellular composition by $CD34^+$ fibroblasts and $XIIIa^+$ dendrophages. J Cutan Pathol 24:377, 1997.
257. Smith MEF, Fisher C, Weiss SW. Pleomorphic hyalinizing angiectatic tumor of soft parts: a low-grade neoplasm resembling neurilemoma. Am J Surg Pathol 20:21, 1996.

# CHAPTER 37

# MALIGNANT SOFT TISSUE TUMORS OF UNCERTAIN TYPE

The neoplasms described in this chapter are a heterogeneous group of tumors that are considered to be of uncertain histogenesis because they have no precise normal tissue counterpart. Each is characterized by its own distinctive clinical and pathologic features. These tumors are grouped together in this chapter simply for convenience.

## SYNOVIAL SARCOMA

Synovial sarcoma is a clinically and morphologically well defined entity that has been described extensively in the literature. It occurs primarily in the para-articular regions of the extremities, usually in close association with tendon sheaths, bursae, and joint capsules. Despite its name, it is uncommon in joint cavities and is encountered in areas with no apparent relation to synovial structures, such as the parapharyngeal region, abdominal wall, pleura, and heart.

Its microscopic resemblance to developing synovium was suggested early in the literature, but its origin from preformed synovial tissues has never been substantiated. Indeed, there are such significant immunophenotypic and ultrastructural differences between synovial sarcoma and normal synovium that most regard the label "synovial sarcoma" a fanciful designation that has its roots in the descriptive works of the earlier literature. Smith,[119] for example, used the term *synovioma,* whereas Lejars and Rubens-Duval,[67] preferred the term *synovial endothelioma.* It should be noted in passing that the term *tendosynovial sarcoma,* coined by Hajdu et al.,[42,117] is not restricted to synovial sarcoma but embraces a collection of sarcomas including epithelioid sarcoma, clear cell sarcoma, and extraskeletal myxoid chondrosarcoma. For this reason it has no diagnostic purpose, although it has some conceptual value in the opinion of some. Although synovial sarcoma continues to be the term of choice, some have suggested that it be replaced by the term "carcinosarcoma" of soft tissue, a term that more accurately captures the essence of this lesion.

The reported data on the frequency of this tumor vary. Pack and Ariel[99] observed an incidence of 8.4% among all malignant tumors of somatic soft tissues studied at Memorial Hospital. In other studies, the reported incidence has ranged from as low as 5.6%[130] to as high 10%[7] among all soft tissue sarcomas. In the material from the Armed Forces Institute of Pathology (AFIP), synovial sarcoma is the fourth most common type of sarcoma after malignant fibrous histiocytoma, liposarcoma, and rhabdomyosarcoma.

The criteria for the histologic diagnosis vary among institutions, but several basic and closely interrelated types are recognized: the classic *biphasic type,* with distinct epithelial and spindle cell components in varying proportions; the *monophasic fibrous type,* a fibrosarcoma-like spindle cell tumor with no demonstrable epithelial component; and at the other extreme of the morphologic spectrum the *monophasic epithelial type.* The biphasic and monophasic fibrous types are about equally common, although definitive recognition of the latter type requires immunohistochemical demonstration of epithelial differentiation or the characteristic cytogenetic or molecular genetic alteration found in this tumor. Theoretically, a pure monophasic epithelial synovial sarcoma exists but is impossible to identify without cytogenetic data. In practice, predominantly epithelial forms of synovial sarcoma are diagnosed by recognizing small fibrosarcomatous foci, having cytogenetic data, or both. Synovial sarcoma may also present as a poorly differentiated round cell sarcoma often arranged in a pericytomatous pattern.

## Clinical Findings

### *Age and Gender Incidence*

Synovial sarcoma is most prevalent in adolescents and young adults 15–40 years of age. In the series by Cadman et al.[7] the median age at the time of operation was 31.3 years, with 83.6% of the patients being between 10 and 50 years. The tumor may arise in children 10 years of age or younger, and there are several reports in the literature of this tumor arising in newborns.[27,100,112] Males are affected more often than females, with an average male/female ratio of 1.2:1.0. There does not appear to be a predilection for any particular race.

### *Clinical Complaints*

The most typical presentation is that of a palpable, deep-seated swelling or mass associated with pain or tenderness in slightly more than half of cases. Less frequently, pain or tenderness is the only manifestation of the disease. There may be minor limitation of motion, but severe functional disturbance or weight loss is seldom encountered; when it does occur, it is nearly always associated with poorly differentiated, large tumors of long duration. The mechanism for the common symptoms of pain and tenderness is unknown, but there is no evidence that an inflammatory process ever precedes the onset of the tumor. Other clinical complaints are rare and are related to the location of the tumor. Patients with synovial sarcomas in the hypopharynx, for instance, often suffer from difficulty swallowing and breathing and not infrequently have alteration or loss of voice.[20] Primary or secondary involvement of nerves may cause projected pain, numbness, and paresthesia.

The preoperative duration of symptoms varies considerably. Generally, the tumor grows slowly and insidiously, often giving a false impression as to the degree of malignancy, delaying diagnosis and therapy. In most cases the duration is 2–4 years, but there are also cases in which a slow-growing mass or pain at the tumor site has been noted for as long as 20 years prior to operation. Not infrequently these cases are wrongly diagnosed initially as arthritis, synovitis, or bursitis.

### *Trauma*

Although most patients with synovial sarcoma fail to give a definitive history of antecedent trauma, there are patients with such a history in our cases and in the literature; most had sustained a minor or major injury during athletic or recreational activities. The interval between the episode of trauma and onset of the tumor varies considerably, ranging from a few weeks to as long as 40 years. For example, Vincent[141] described a 60-year-old man who had suffered an injury of the right hip at age 20 years and 40 years later developed a synovial sarcoma in the same location. In some cases trauma may be merely a coincidence related to the predominance of synovial sarcomas in the extremities, as suggested by reports of patients who suffered injury *after* the presence of a mass had been noted.[44] There are rare reports of synovial sarcoma arising in the field of previous therapeutic irradiation[88,136] and one of a tumor associated with a metal implant used for hip replacement surgery.[65]

### *Anatomic Location*

Synovial sarcomas occur predominantly in the extremities, where they tend to arise in the vicinity of large joints, especially the knee region (Table 37–1). They are intimately related to tendons, tendon sheaths, and bursal structures, usually just beyond the confines of the joint capsule; less frequently they are attached to fascial structures, ligaments, aponeuroses, and interosseous membranes. They are rare in joint cavities; according to our material and most reviews, intraarticular synovial sarcomas account for fewer than 5% of all cases.[51,80]

**TABLE 37–1** SYNOVIAL SARCOMA AFIP, 345 CASES

| Anatomic Location | No. of Cases |
|---|---|
| Head-neck | 31 (9.0%) |
| Neck | 12 |
| Pharynx | 7 |
| Larynx | 7 |
| Other | 5 |
| Trunk | 28 (8.1%) |
| Chest | 10 |
| Abdominal wall | 9 |
| Other | 9 |
| Upper extremities | 80 (23.2%) |
| Forearm-wrist | 24 |
| Shoulder | 22 |
| Elbow-upper arm | 20 |
| Hand | 14 |
| Lower extremities | 206 (59.7%) |
| Thigh-knee | 102 |
| Foot | 45 |
| Lower leg-ankle | 33 |
| Hip-groin | 22 |
| Other | 4 |
| *Total* | 345 (100.0%) |

AFIP, Armed Forces Institute of Pathology.

In most series, 85–95% of all synovial sarcomas arise in the extremities, with a predilection for the lower extremities. In the lower extremities, most arise in the vicinity of the knee, with fewer arising in the foot, lower leg-ankle region, and hip-groin. Tumors arising in the upper extremities, which account for approximately 15% of all cases, are fairly evenly distributed between the forearm-wrist region, shoulder, elbow-upper arm region, and hand.

Following the extremities, the head and neck region is the second most common site of synovial sarcoma, accounting for up to 10% of all cases.[2,30] Most of these tumors seem to originate in the paravertebral connective tissue spaces and manifest as solitary retropharyngeal or parapharyngeal masses near the carotid bifurcation. Additional cases in this general area have been reported in the soft palate,[78] tongue,[49] parotid gland,[40] and tonsil.[24] Because of the unusual location, synovial sarcomas in this region are often misdiagnosed.

About 5–10% of synovial sarcomas arise in the trunk, including the chest wall[36] and abdominal wall.[28,75] Like synovial sarcomas at other sites, these neoplasms are usually deep-seated. Fetsch and Meis,[28] who reviewed 27 cases culled from the AFIP material, noted a large number of cystic tumors among their cases. The age and gender incidence of these tumors and their behavior corresponds to that of synovial sarcomas at other sites.

Synovial sarcoma has been described at virtually every anatomic site including the skin,[33] heart,[43,53,93] lung,[57,105,145] pleura,[37] prostate,[52] kidney,[60] central nervous system,[61] bone,[12] esophagus,[3] and peripheral nerve.[94,126] With tumors arising in these unusual sites, definitive recognition becomes more difficult, but some of these cases have been amply confirmed by molecular genetic techniques.[48]

## Radiographic Findings

Radiographic studies may be helpful for suggesting a clinical or preoperative diagnosis of synovial sarcoma, largely because of the presence of calcification. Most synovial sarcomas present on x-ray films as round or oval, more or less lobulated swellings or masses of moderate density, usually located in close proximity to a large joint. The underlying bone tends to be uninvolved, but in about 15–20% of the cases, there is a periosteal reaction, superficial bone erosion, or invasion. Massive bone destruction, which is rare, is mostly caused by poorly differentiated synovial sarcomas of long duration and large size.[55,106] In the series by Strickland and Mackenzie,[123] 18 of 65 cases showed some alteration of bone, mostly pressure atrophy and periosteal proliferation.

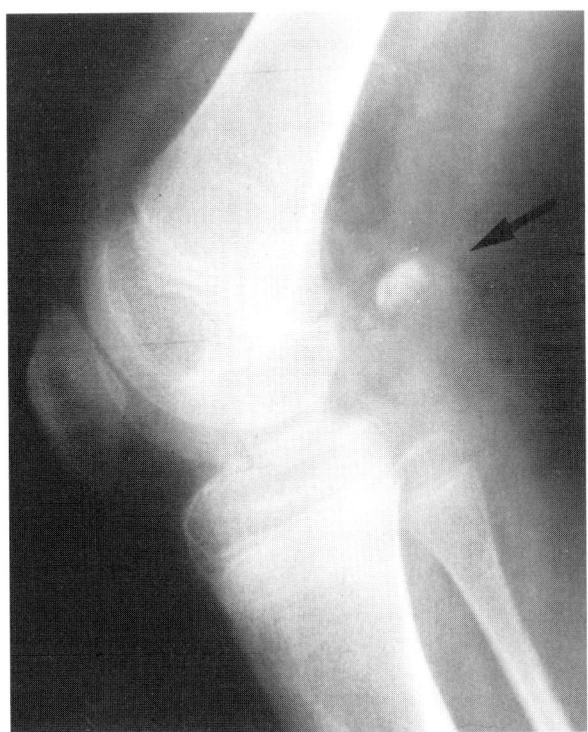

**FIGURE 37–1.** Radiograph of a synovial sarcoma originating in the popliteal fossa. Note the focal calcification in the tumor (arrow), a feature that is present in about 20% of these cases.

The most striking radiologic characteristic, found in 15–20% of synovial sarcomas, is the presence of multiple small, spotty radiopacities caused by focal calcification and, less frequently, bone formation.[79,111] In most instances these changes consist merely of fine stippling, but in some cases large portions of the tumor are marked or even outlined by radiopaque masses (Figs. 37–1, 37–2, 37–3). Confusion with other tumors is possible, but radiopacities are not observed in most other forms of sarcoma with the exception of extraosseous osteosarcoma, a tumor that tends to segregate in an older group of individuals.

Computed tomography (CT) and magnetic resonance imaging (MRI) have become valuable tools for determining the site of origin and extent of the lesion. Like conventional radiographs, they show a paraarticular heterogeneous septated mass, often with associated calcification or bone erosion, but they do not provide a specific or diagnostic picture.[47]

## Gross Findings

The gross appearance varies depending on the rate of growth and the location of the tumor. Slow-growing lesions tend to be sharply circumscribed, round, or

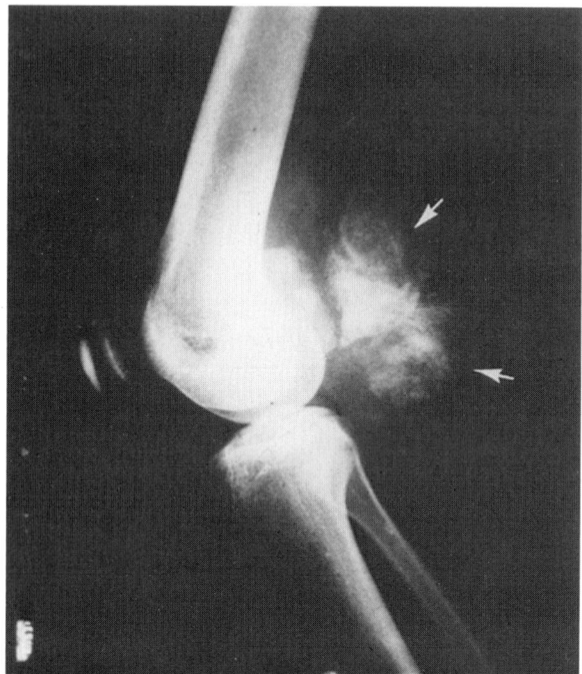

**FIGURE 37-2.** Massive calcification and ossification in a synovial sarcoma of the popliteal fossa (arrows). In general, tumors with extensive calcification carry a better prognosis than those without.

multilobular; as a result of compression of adjacent tissues by the expansively growing tumor, they are completely or partially invested by a smooth, glistening pseudocapsule (Fig. 37-4). Cyst formation may be prominent, and occasional lesions present as multicystic masses (Fig. 37-5). Most of the tumors are firmly attached to surrounding tendons, tendon sheaths, or the exterior wall of the joint capsule; not infrequently portions of these structures adhere to the gross specimen (Fig. 37-6). On palpation they are either soft or firm, depending on their collagen content. On section they are yellow to gray-white. They may attain a size of 15 cm or more, but in the average case they measure 3-5 cm in greatest diameter. As already mentioned, calcification is common but rarely a discernible gross feature. Less well differentiated and more rapidly growing synovial sarcomas tend to be poorly circumscribed and commonly exhibit a rather variegated and often friable or shaggy appearance, frequently with multiple areas of hemorrhage, necrosis, and cyst formation. Markedly hemorrhagic tumors have been confused with angiosarcomas or even organizing hematomas.

## Microscopic Findings

Unlike most other types of sarcoma, the tumor is composed of two morphologically different types of cells that form a characteristic biphasic pattern: *epithelial cells,* resembling those of carcinoma, and fibrosarcoma-like *spindle cells,* sometimes incorrectly designated as *stromal cells.* Transitional forms between epithelial and spindle cells suggest a close relation, which is also supported by tissue culture, ultrastructural, immunohistochemical, and molecular genetic findings. Depending on the relative prominence of the two cellular elements and the degree of differentiation, synovial sarcomas form a continuous morphologic spectrum and can be broadly classified into the (1) *biphasic type,* with distinct epithelial and spindle cell components in varying proportions; (2) *monophasic fibrous type;* (3) rare *monophasic epithelial type;* and (4) *poorly differentiated (round cell) type.*

### *Biphasic Synovial Sarcoma*

The classic synovial sarcoma—the biphasic type—is generally readily recognizable by the coexistence of

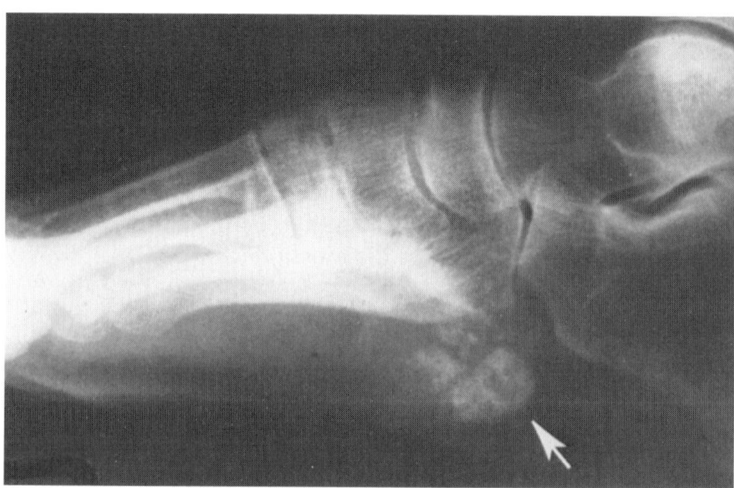

**FIGURE 37-3.** Radiograph of a synovial sarcoma of the planta pedis showing extensive calcification of the tumor (arrow).

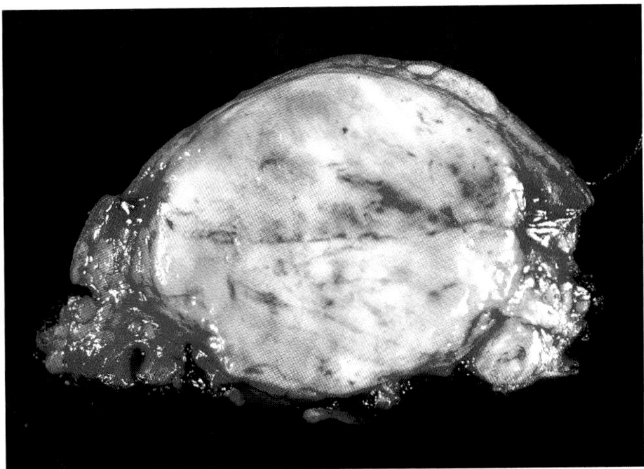

**FIGURE 37–4.** Photomicrograph of a high-grade monophasic fibrous synovial sarcoma. The tumor has a fleshy gray-tan appearance with focal hemorrhage.

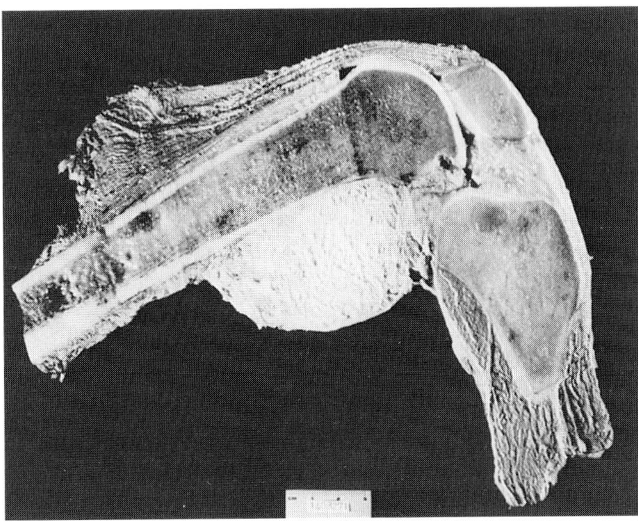

**FIGURE 37–6.** Synovial sarcoma of the lower thigh and popliteal region, the most common single location of this neoplasm.

morphologically different but histogenetically related epithelial cells and fibroblast-like spindle cells (Figs. 37–7, 37–8, 37–9). The epithelial cells are characterized by large, round or oval, vesicular nuclei and abundant pale-staining cytoplasm with distinctly outlined cellular borders. The cells are cuboidal to tall and columnar; they are disposed in solid cords, nests, or glandular structures that contain granular or homogeneous eosinophilic secretions (Figs. 37–10, 37–11). The glandular spaces lined by epithelial cells must be distinguished from cleft-like artifacts that are the result of tissue shrinkage. Outpouchings of the cyst-like spaces into the surrounding uninvolved tissue may wrongly suggest on origin within a bursa, particularly because some of these spaces are lined by a single layer of epithelial cells bearing a resemblance to normal synovium.

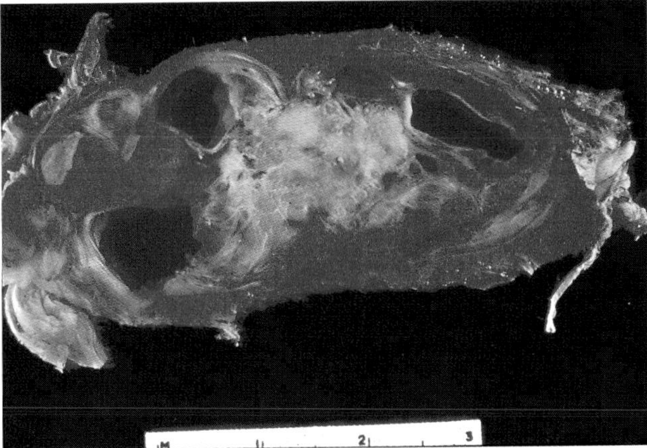

**FIGURE 37–5.** Multicystic synovial sarcoma of the knee region.

Not infrequently cuboidal or flattened epithelial cells also cover small villous or papillary structures often with spindle cells rather than connective tissue in the papillary core. A diagnosis of squamous cell carcinoma is also suggested by focal squamous metaplasia, including the occasional formation of squamous pearls and keratohyalin granules.

The surrounding spindle cell or fibrous component consists mostly of well oriented, rather plump, spindle-shaped cells of uniform appearance with small amounts of indistinct cytoplasm and oval dark-staining nuclei. Generally the cells form solid, compact sheets that are virtually indistinguishable from fibrosarcoma (Figs. 37–12, 37–13), except perhaps for the absence of long sweeping fascicles or a herringbone pattern, a more irregular nodular arrangement, and fewer mitotic figures. Mitotic figures in synovial sarcoma occur in both epithelial and spindle-shaped cells, but as a rule only the poorly differentiated forms of the tumor exhibit more than two mitotic figures per high power field (HPF). Occasionally there is nuclear palisading (Fig. 37–14); but in contrast to leiomyosarcomas and malignant peripheral nerve sheath tumors, this feature is typically confined to a small portion of the tumor.

Commonly, the cellular portions of synovial sarcoma alternate with less cellular areas displaying hyalinization, myxoid change, or calcification. The collagen in the hyalinized zones may be diffusely distributed or form narrow bands or plaque-like masses sometimes associated with a markedly thickened basement membrane separating epithelial and spindle cell elements (Fig. 37–15). The myxoid areas are generally less conspicuous and tend to occupy

*Text continued on page 1494*

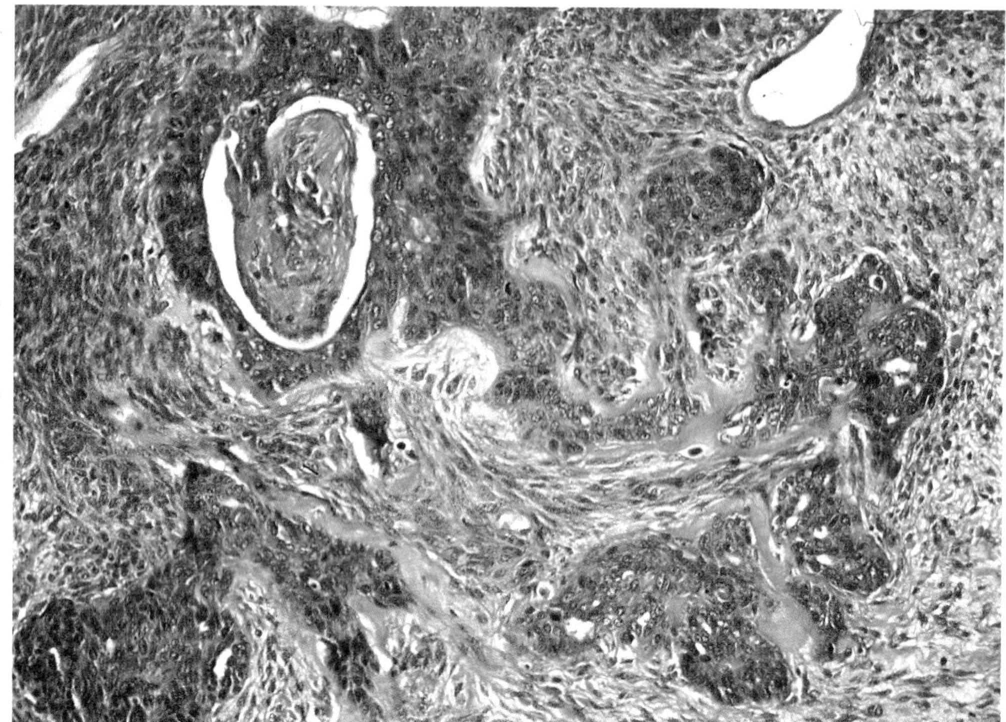

**FIGURE 37–7.** Biphasic synovial sarcoma showing close apposition of epithelial structures with malignant spindle cells.

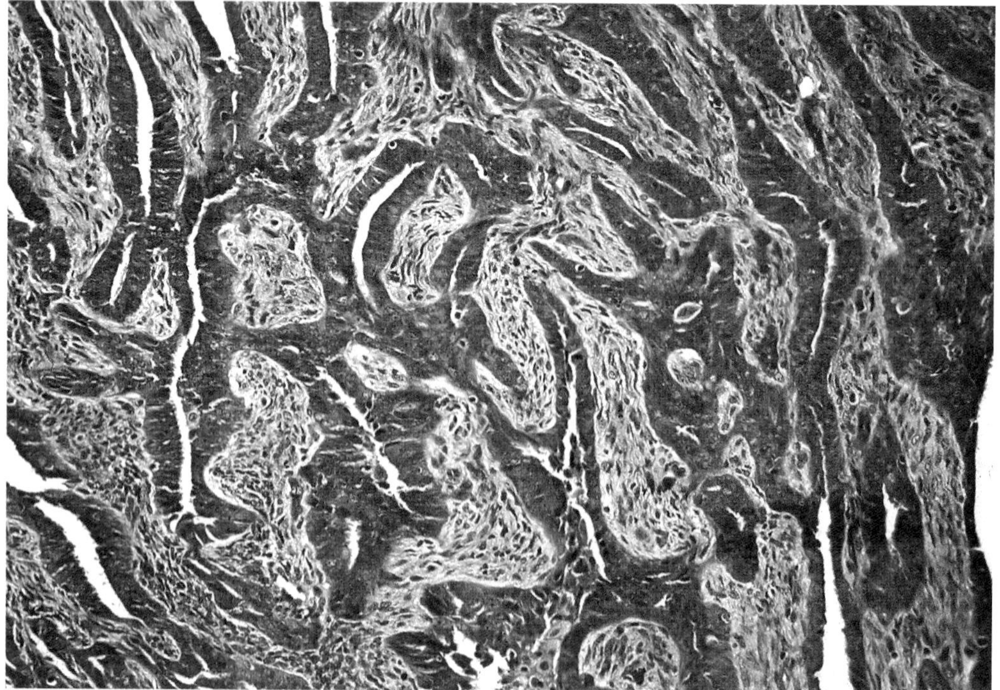

**FIGURE 37–8.** Typical biphasic synovial sarcoma with columnar epithelial cells surrounded by spindle cell elements.

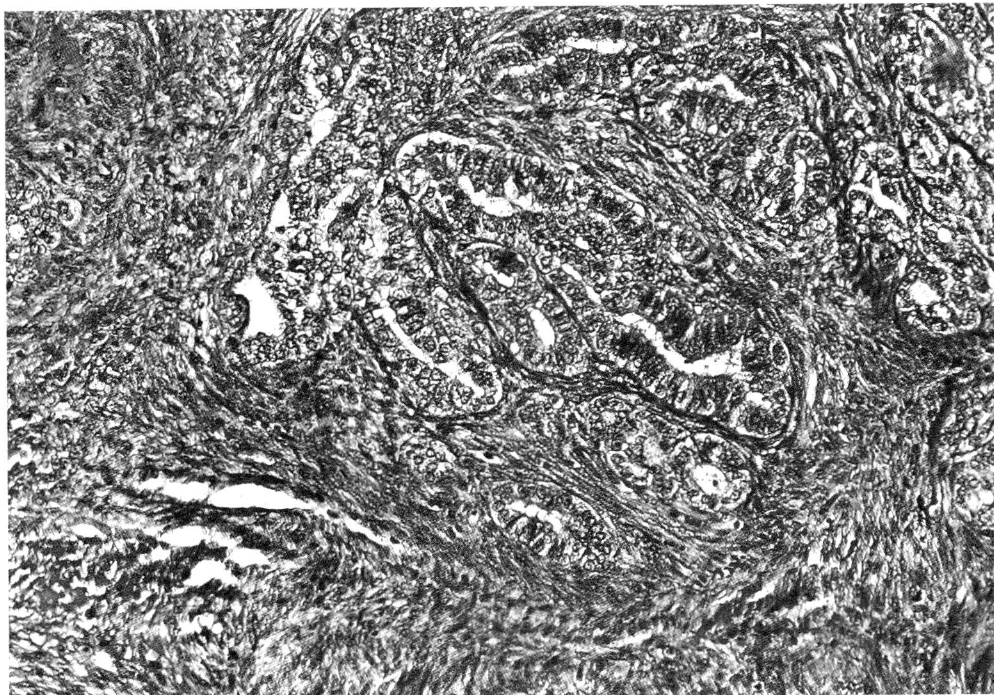

**FIGURE 37–9.** Biphasic synovial sarcoma with glandular epithelial structures adjacent to a malignant spindle cell component.

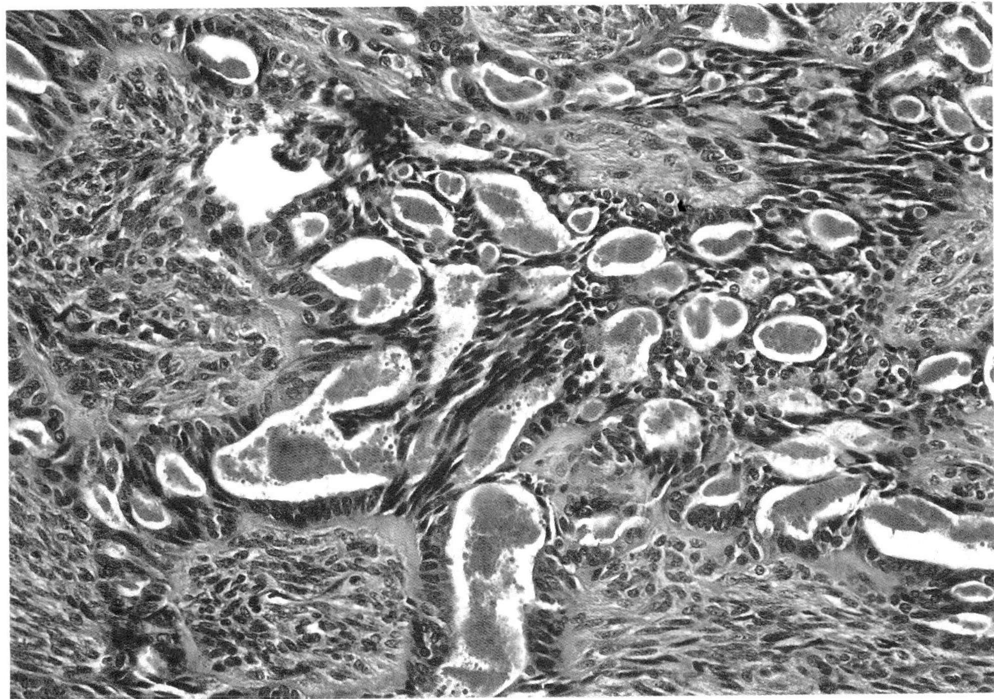

**FIGURE 37–10.** Biphasic synovial sarcoma. The epithelial structures have intraluminal eosinophilic secretions.

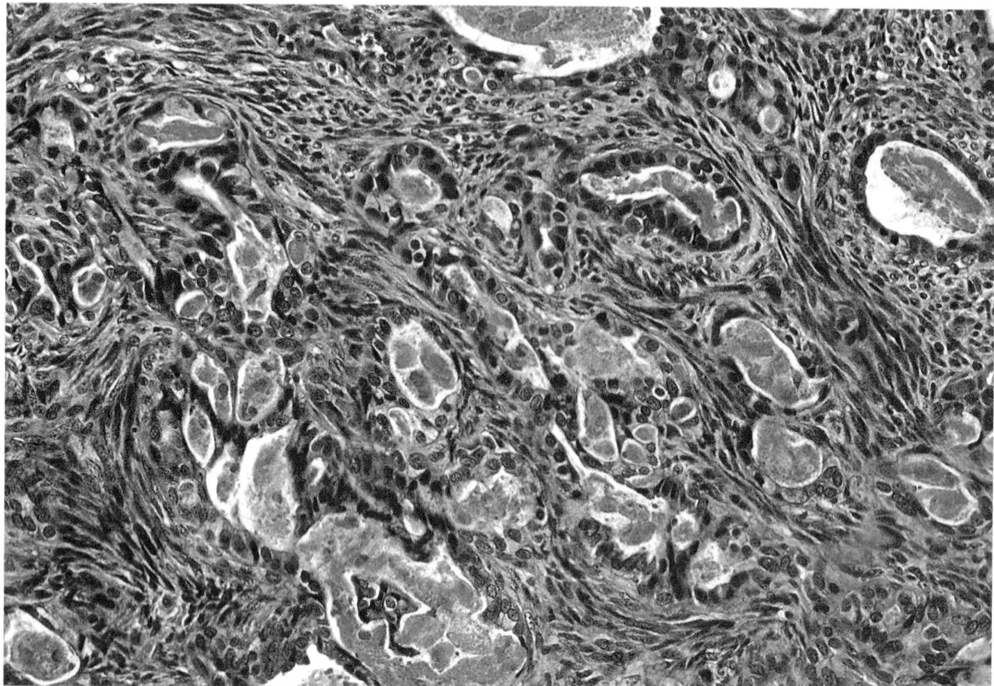

**FIGURE 37–11.** Biphasic synovial sarcoma with prominent intraluminal eosinophilic secretions in epithelial elements.

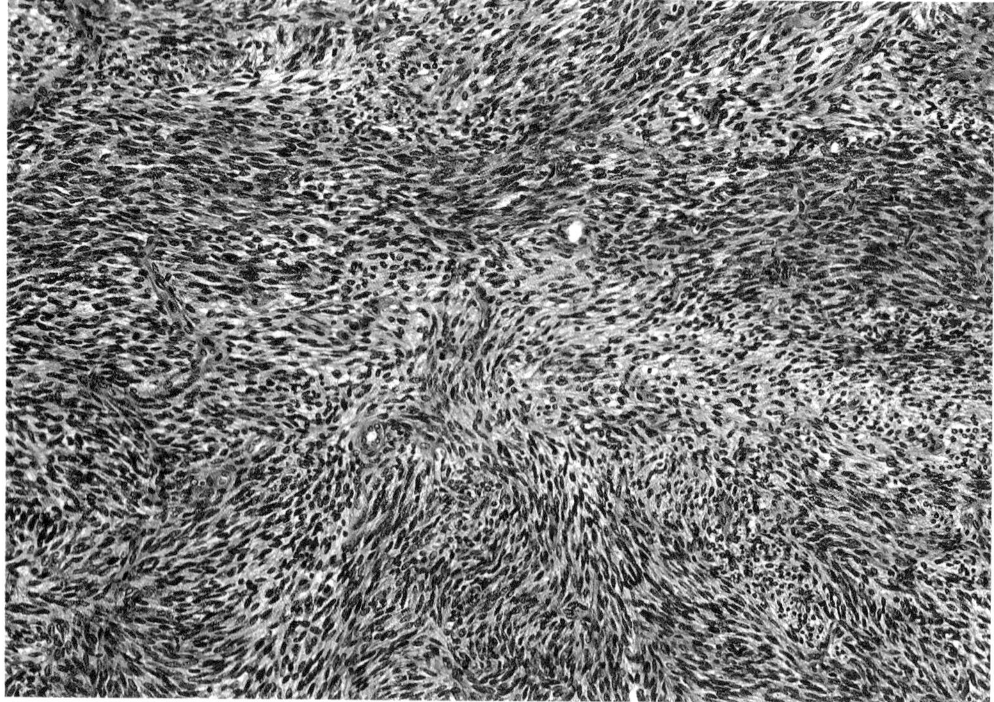

**FIGURE 37–12.** Fibrosarcoma-like area in a synovial sarcoma. Note the alternating darkly staining and lightly staining regions, imparting a marbled appearance.

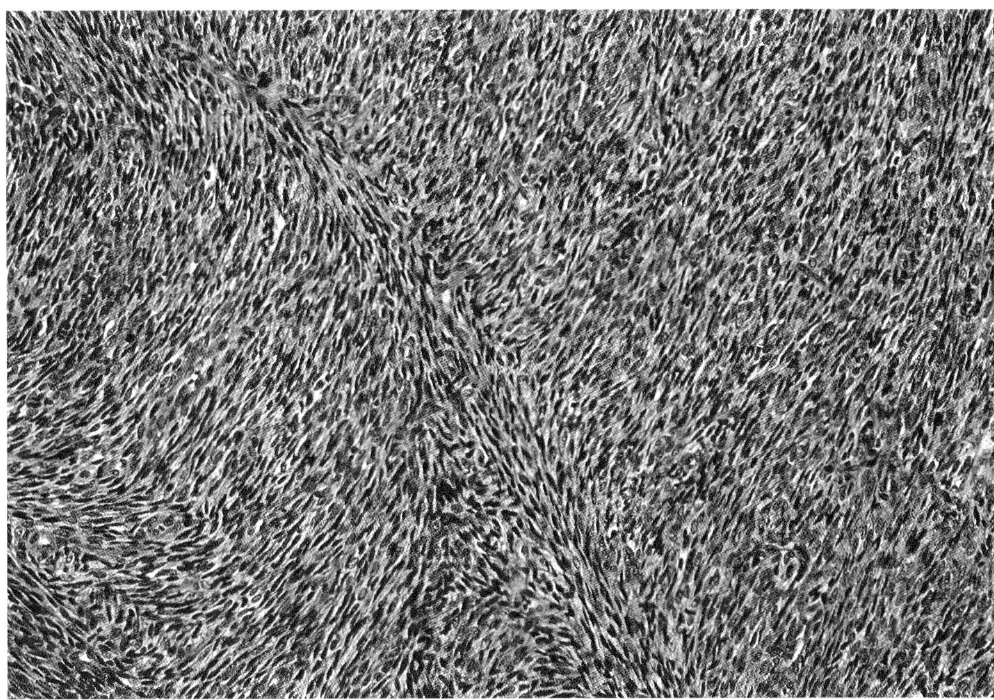

**FIGURE 37–13.** Fibrosarcoma-like area in a synovial sarcoma. The spindle cells are arranged in distinct fascicles.

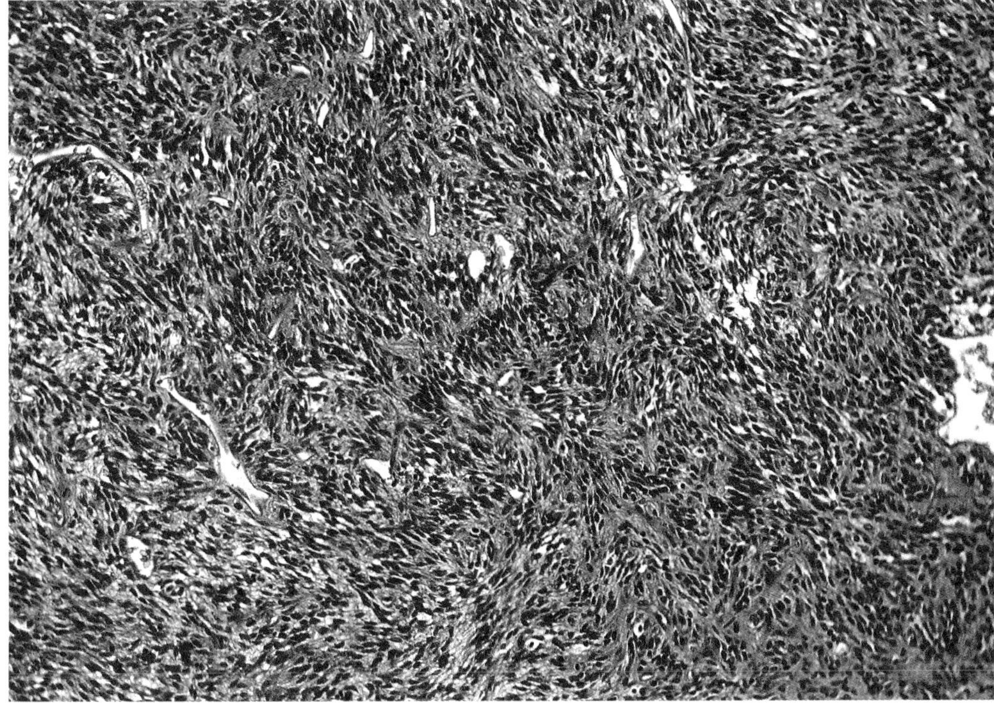

**FIGURE 37–14.** Synovial sarcoma with focal nuclear palisading reminiscent of a neural tumor.

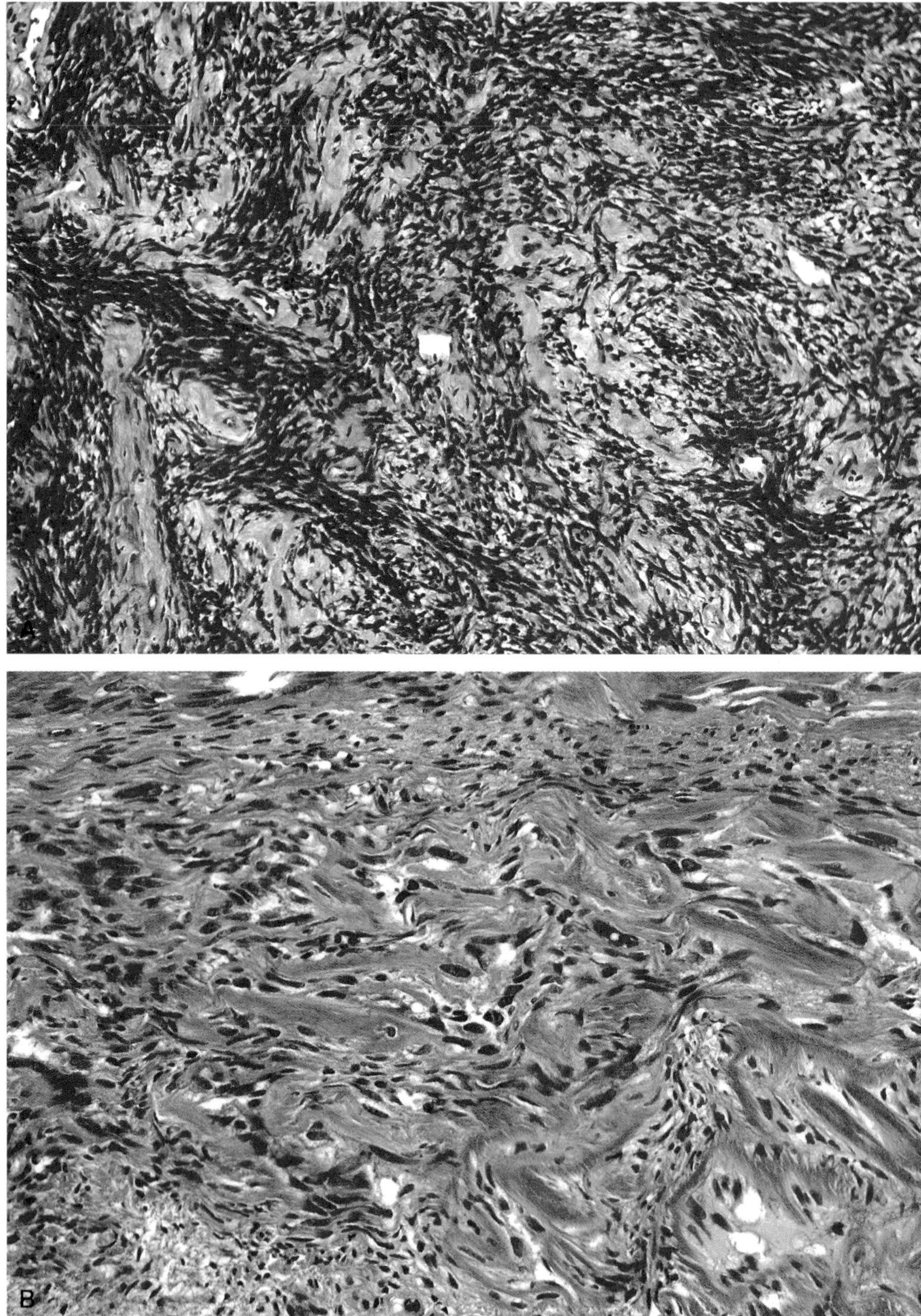


**FIGURE 37–15.** (**A**) Monophasic synovial sarcoma with prominent perivascular hyalinization. (**B**) Thick collagen bands separate malignant spindle cells in a monophasic synovial sarcoma. This pattern of hyalinization is characteristic of this tumor.

*Illustration continued on opposite page*

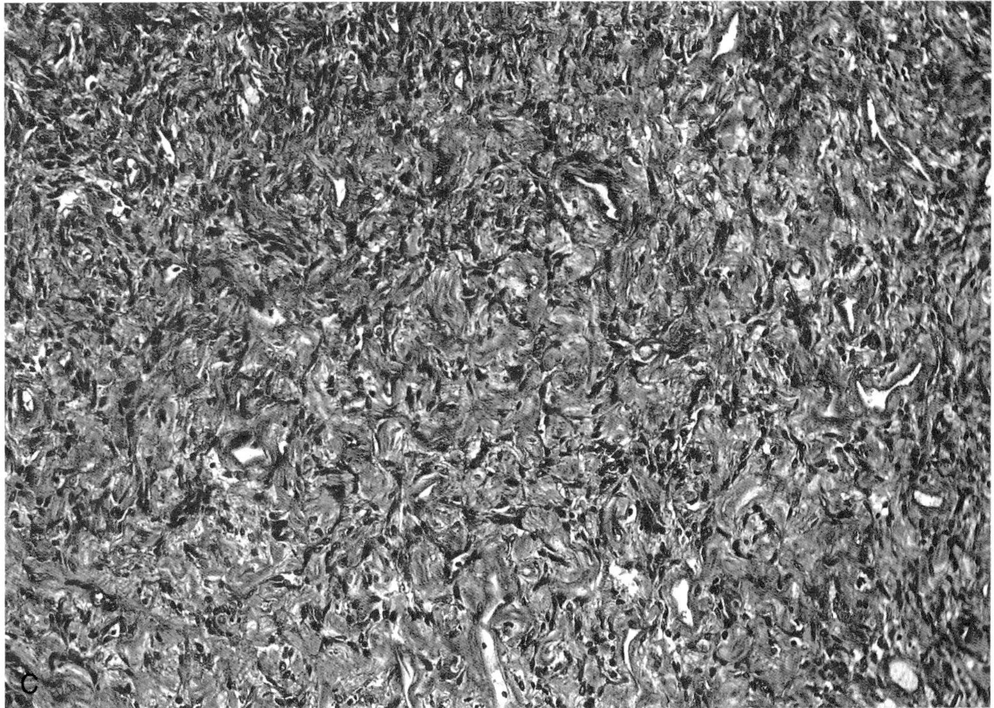

**FIGURE 37–15** *(Continued).* (**C**) Extensive hyalinization in a synovial sarcoma with compression of neoplastic cells.

only a small, ill-defined portion of the tumor, although some cases are predominantly myxoid[63,89] (Fig. 37–16).

Calcification with or without ossification is another diagnostically important and characteristic feature that is present to a varying degree in about 20% of synovial sarcomas. It may be inconspicuous and consist merely of a few small irregularly distributed spherical concretions, or it may be extensive and occupy a large portion of the neoplasm[86,139] (Fig. 37–17). In general, calcification is preceded by hyalinization and is more pronounced at the periphery of the tumor than at its center. Rarely, chondroid changes are present, nearly always together with focal calcification and ossification.

Mast cells are yet another typical feature of synovial sarcoma; they show no particular arrangement but are more numerous in the spindle cell than in the epithelial portions of the neoplasm. Inflammatory elements and multinucleated giant cells are rare.

The degree of vascularity varies. In some cases it is a dominant feature, and there are numerous dilated vascular spaces resembling hemangiopericytoma (Fig. 37–18); in others there are merely a few scattered vascular structures. Secondary changes such as hemorrhage are most prominent in poorly differentiated tumors. Scattered lipid macrophages, siderophages, multinucleated giant cells, and deposits of cholesterol may be present but are much less conspicuous in synovial sarcomas than in synovitis (Fig. 37–19).

### *Monophasic Fibrous Synovial Sarcoma*

The monophasic fibrous form of synovial sarcoma is a relatively common neoplasm, the existence of which has been confirmed by positive immunostaining of some or most of the spindle cells for epithelial antigens, by ultrastructural features such as occasional intercellular spaces with filopodia,[31] and by identical cytogenetic and molecular genetic abnormalities found in the biphasic type (discussed below). Because this type is closely related to the biphasic type and merely represents one extreme of its morphologic spectrum, the discussed morphologic parameters of the spindle cell portion of the biphasic type, such as cellular appearance, hyalinization, myxoid change, mast cell infiltrate, hemangiopericytomatous vasculature, and focal calcification, apply equally to the monophasic fibrous type.

In some cases, an obvious epithelial component can be identified by extensive sampling. Even in those cases without obvious epithelial differentiation, however, many monophasic fibrous synovial sarcomas have foci in which the cells have a more epithelioid appearance and appear to be more cohesive than the surrounding spindle-shaped cells. The cells in these foci have more eosinophilic cytoplasm but otherwise have the same nuclear features as the surrounding spindle-shaped cells. Such areas often have immunohistochemical evidence of epithelial differentiation (Fig. 37–20).

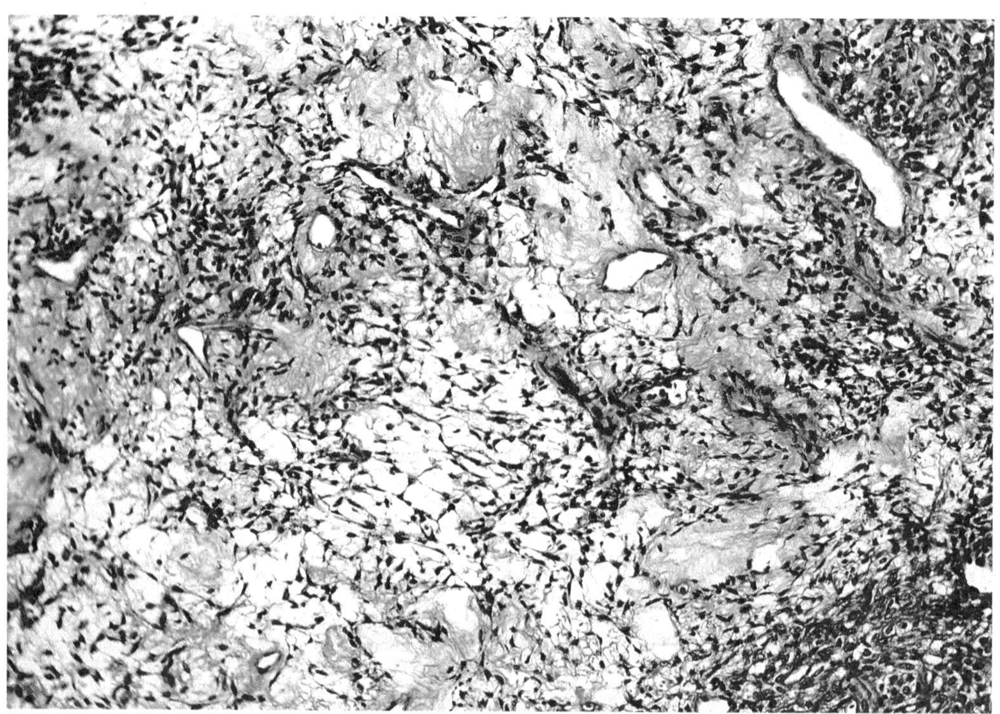

**FIGURE 37–16.** Prominent myxoid change in synovial sarcoma.

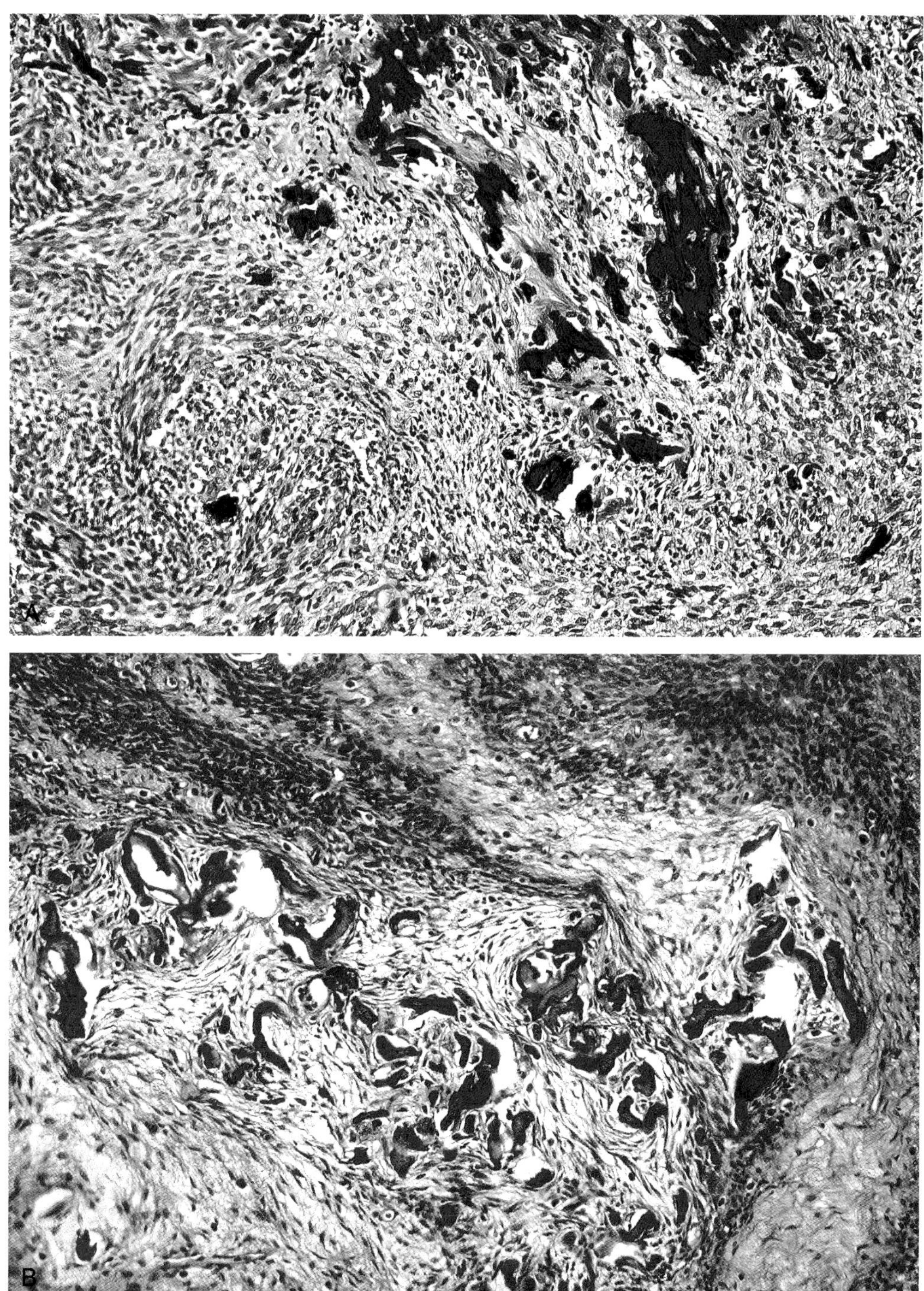


**FIGURE 37–17.** (**A**) Calcification in a synovial sarcoma, a common feature of this neoplasm. (**B**) Note the focus of calcification in this small monophasic fibrous synovial sarcoma of the foot.

*Illustration continued on following page*

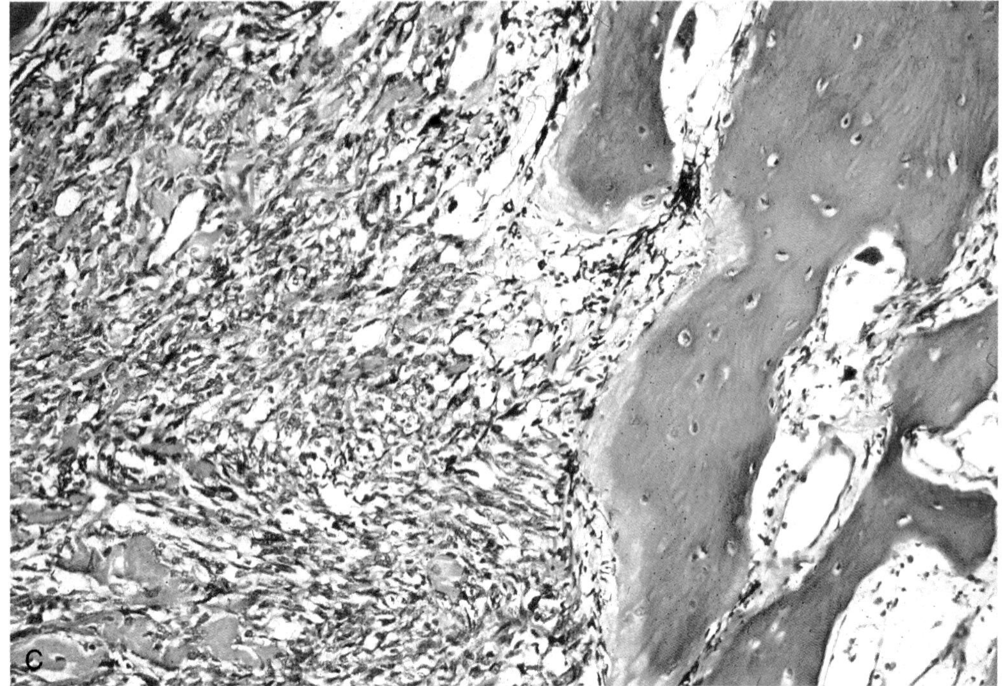


**FIGURE 37–17** *(Continued).* (**C**) Monophasic fibrous type of synovial sarcoma with osseous metaplasia.

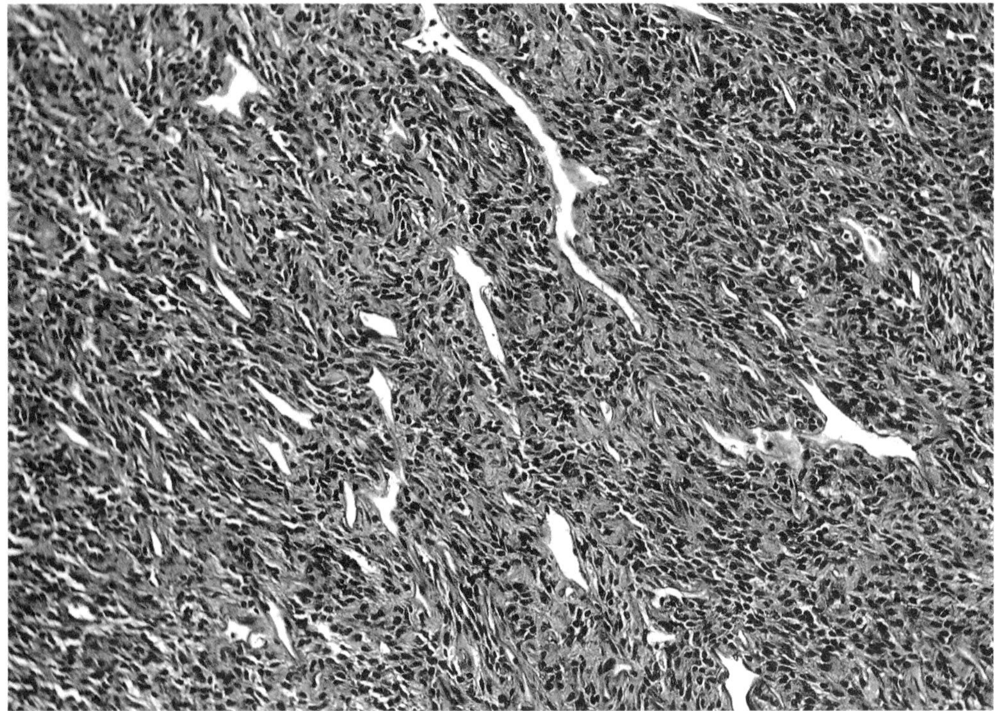

**FIGURE 37–18.** Prominent hemangiopericytomatous vasculature in a synovial sarcoma.

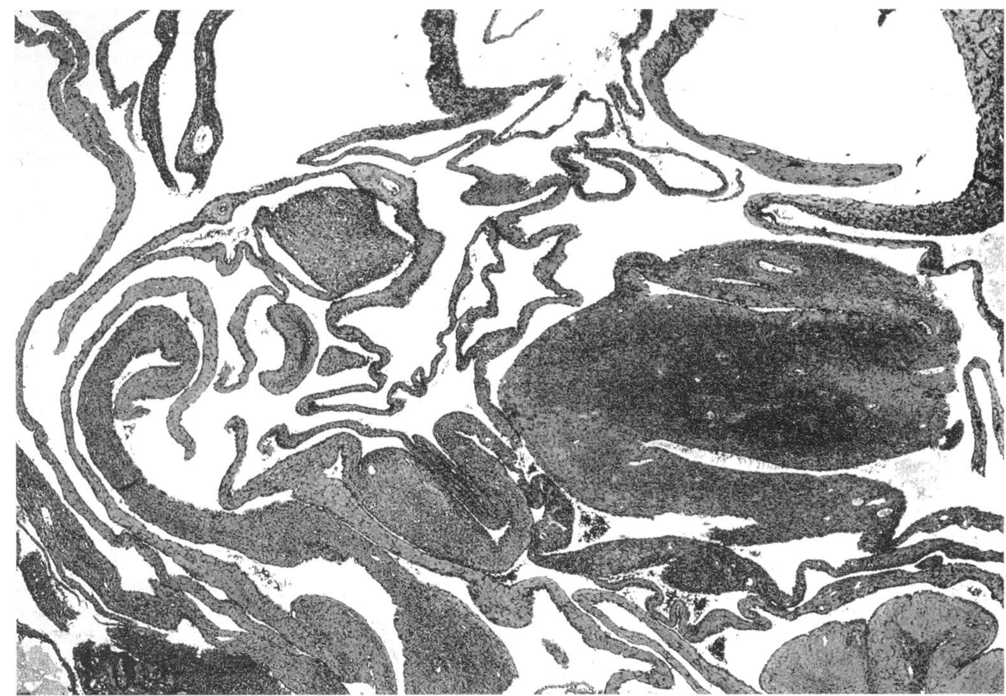

**FIGURE 37–19.** Cystic synovial sarcoma. Malignant spindle cells are seen in the thickened fibrous septa.

### *Monophasic Epithelial Synovial Sarcoma*

What has been said about the diagnosis of the monophasic fibrous type of synovial sarcoma applies also to the monophasic epithelial synovial sarcoma, a rarely recognized neoplasm. In our experience it is often difficult to render this diagnosis with any degree of certainty. In fact, it might be argued that this variant exists only conceptually as a means of validating the entire (epithelial) biphasic spectrum of synovial sarcoma. However, with the ability to analyze tumors for the characteristic translocation and fusion transcript, it is now feasible to diagnose monophasic epithelial synovial sarcoma in epithelial tumors that otherwise would be misdiagnosed as other benign or malignant epithelial neoplasms.[127] The most important differential considerations are metastatic carcinoma, melanoma, and adnexal tumors. However, other epithelioid mesenchymal tumors should also be considered including epithelioid sarcoma and epithelioid malignant peripheral nerve sheath tumor. We have encountered several likely tumors of this type, but all of these had minute foci of spindle cell differentiation and, strictly speaking, were biphasic synovial sarcomas with an exceptionally prominent epithelial pattern (Figs. 37–21, 37–22, 37–23). Farris and Reed[26] and Majeste and Beckman[76] described lesions of this histologic type as "monophasic glandular synovial sarcoma and carcinoma of the soft tissues" and as "synovial sarcoma with an overwhelming epithelial component," respectively. The latter tumor also displayed a distinct spindle cell pattern in a small portion of the tumor. Obviously, as with the monophasic fibrous type, other features must be weighed when making this diagnosis, such as the age of the patient, the location of the tumor, and the presence of mast cells, calcifications, and periodic acid-Schiff (PAS)-positive eosinophilic amorphous material in the glands. Cytogenetic or molecular genetic data would be most useful for confirming the diagnosis of this rare tumor. It must be emphasized that neither the large size of a tumor nor its long duration and staining characteristics entirely rule out metastatic carcinoma.

### *Poorly Differentiated Synovial Sarcoma*

The poorly differentiated synovial sarcoma can be thought of as a form of tumor progression that can be superimposed on any of the other synovial sarcoma subtypes. Recognition of this subtype of synovial sarcoma is of practical importance not only because it poses a special problem in diagnosis but also because it behaves more aggressively and metastasizes in a significantly larger percentage of cases.[73,135] The incidence of the poorly differentiated type among synovial sarcomas is difficult to estimate, but in the study by Machen et al.,[73] 21 of 34 (62%) synovial sarcomas had poorly differentiated foci, in some cases accounting for up to 90% of the neoplasm.

Histologically, poorly differentiated synovial sarcoma may have three patterns[81]: a large cell or epithelioid pattern composed of variably sized rounded nuclei with prominent nucleoli (Fig. 37–24), a small-cell

*Text continued on page 1502*

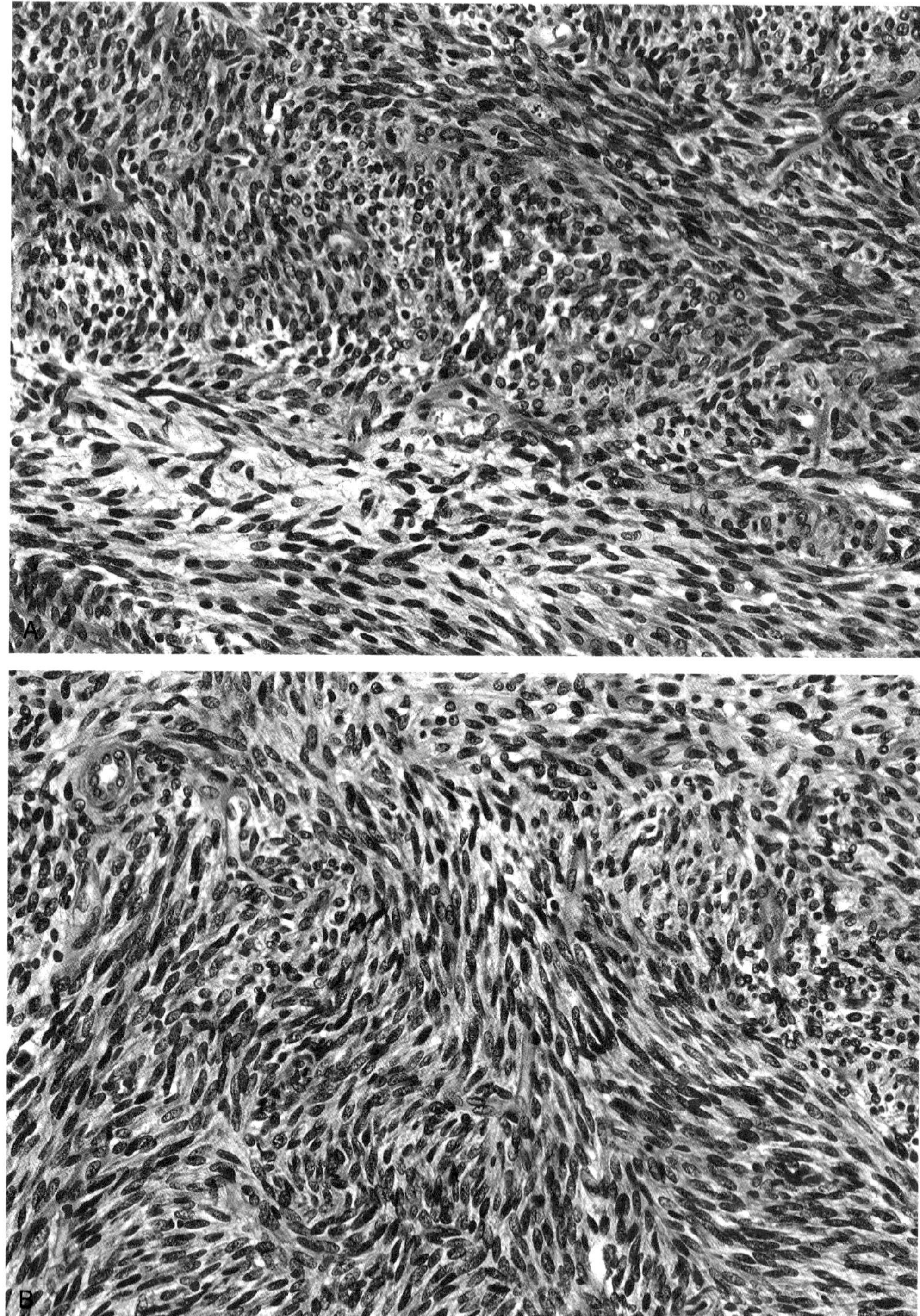


**FIGURE 37–20.** (**A**) High magnification view of a monophasic fibrous synovial sarcoma. The malignant spindle cells are relatively uniform with respect to one another. (**B**) Uniform spindle cells in a monophasic fibrous synovial sarcoma.

*Illustration continued on opposite page*

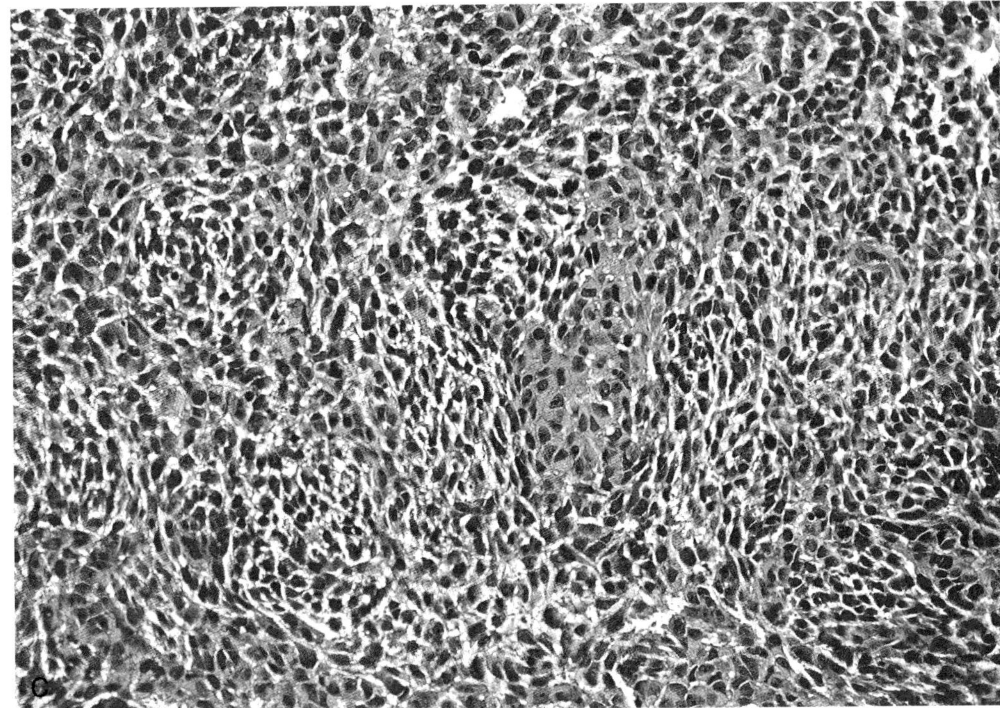

**FIGURE 37–20** *(Continued).* (**C**) Epithelioid area in a monophasic fibrous synovial sarcoma. A small group of cells have increased amounts of eosinophilic cytoplasm and appear more cohesive.

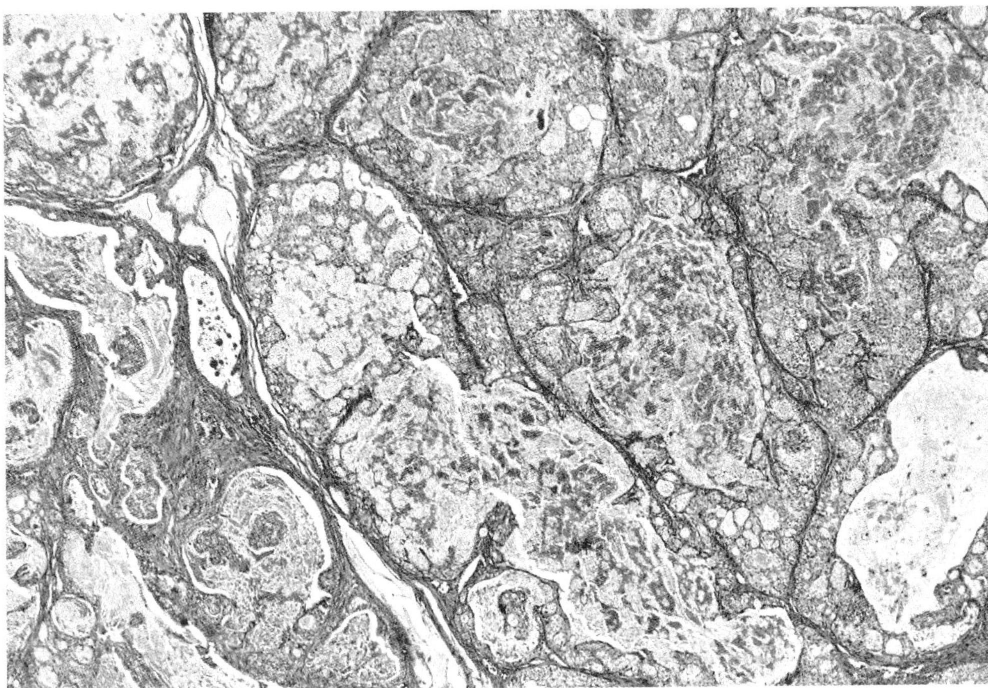

**FIGURE 37–21.** Monophasic epithelial-type synovial sarcoma. A cribriform glandular pattern was prominent throughout this neoplasm.

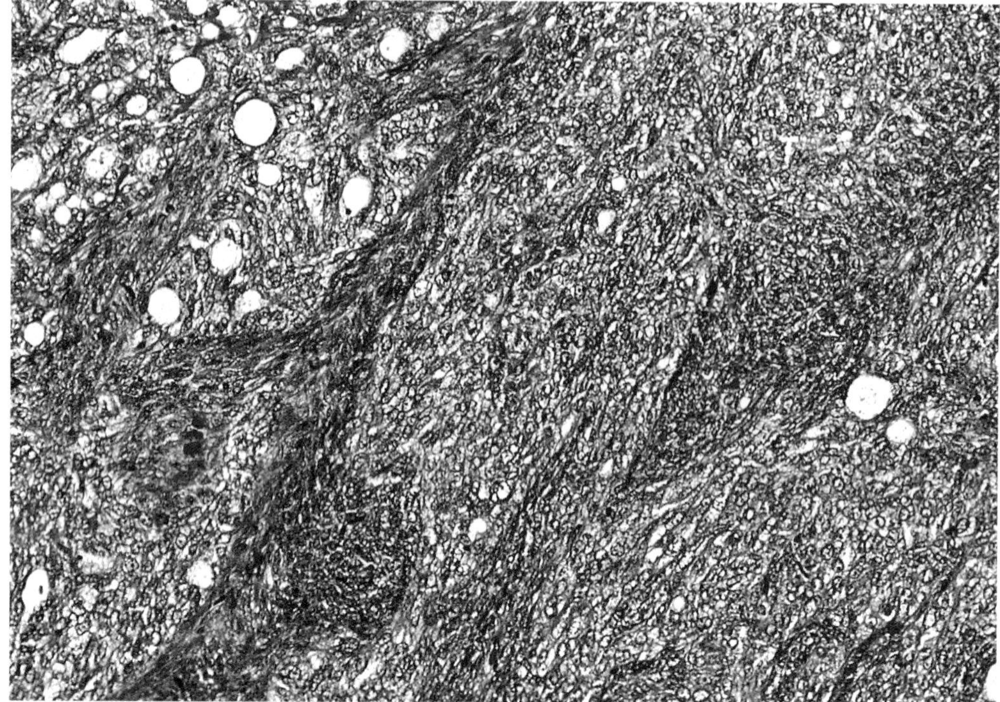

**FIGURE 37–22.** Predominantly epithelial-type synovial sarcoma. Small areas with a well developed spindle cell pattern are present.

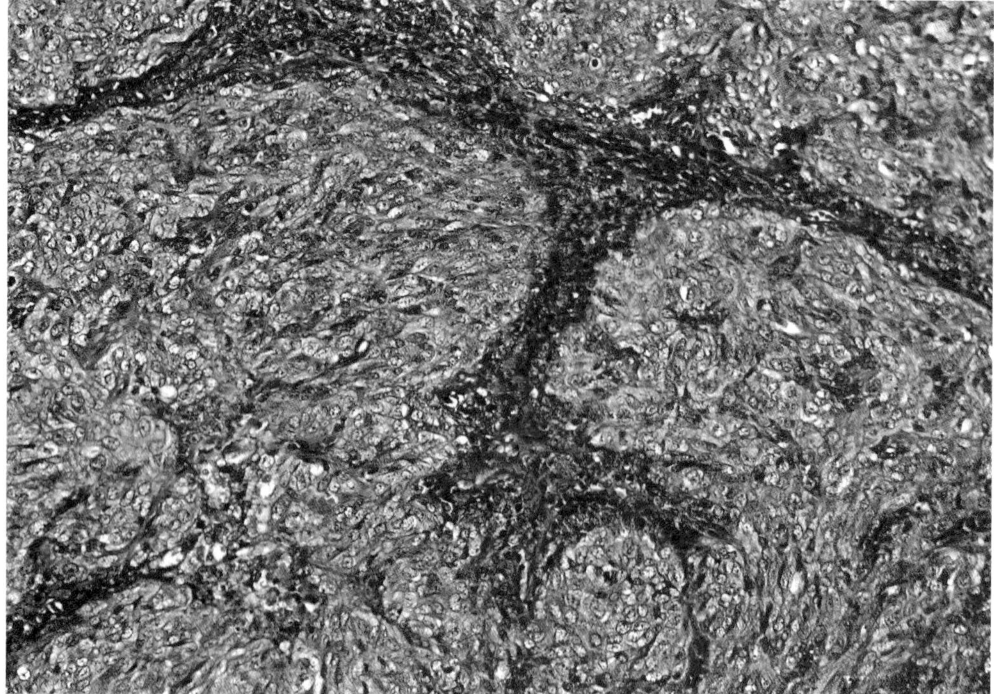

**FIGURE 37–23.** Predominantly epithelial-type synovial sarcoma. Most of this tumor was composed of sheets of cohesive epithelioid cells with only small foci of spindle cell differentiation.

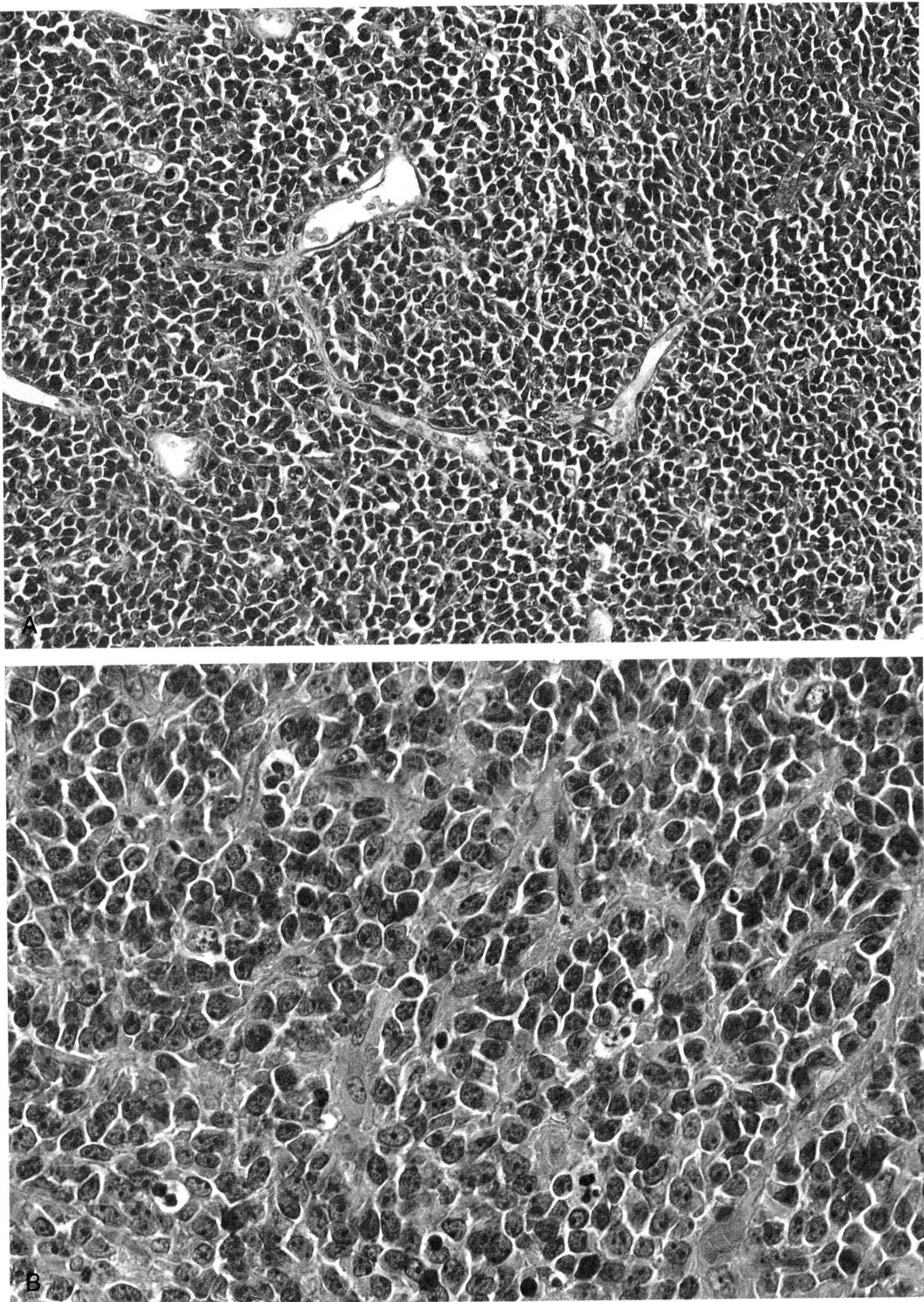

**FIGURE 37–24.** Poorly differentiated area of a synovial sarcoma. (**A**) Low magnification view with a prominent hemangiopericytomatous vasculature. (**B**) Note the cytologic features of round cells in poorly differentiated synovial sarcoma.

pattern with nuclear features similar to other small round cell tumors, and a high grade spindle cell pattern composed of spindle-shaped cells with high grade nuclear features and a high mitotic rate (Fig. 37–25) often accompanied by necrosis. Such tumors often have a richly vascular pattern with dilated thin-walled vascular spaces resembling those of malignant hemangiopericytoma. In fact, it appears that a high percentage of sarcomas interpreted as malignant hemangiopericytomas are actually examples of poorly differentiated synovial sarcoma. Occasionally, cells with intracytoplasmic hyaline inclusions imparting a rhabdoid morphology may be found in poorly differentiated areas.[73] Distinguishing this tumor from other round cell sarcomas such as extraskeletal Ewing's sarcoma/primitive neuroectodermal tumor (PNET) may be exceedingly difficult and often requires ancillary immunohistochemical or molecular genetic techniques.[35,135]

### *Special Staining Procedures*

Two distinctive types of mucinous material are present in synovial sarcomas. Secretions in the epithelial cells, intracellular clefts, and pseudoglandular spaces stain positively with the PAS, colloidal iron, alcian blue, and mucicarmine stains. The staining characteristics of the mucinous secretions remain unaltered after treatment of the secretions with diastase and hyaluronidase, but in general and in distinction to adenocarcinomas, the mucinous material is more conspicuous in the intracellular clefts and pseudoglandular spaces than in the secreting epithelial cells. Buonassisi and Ozzello[6] identified the mucinous material as chondroitin sulfate B and heparin-related glycosaminoglycans using tissue cultures. Nakamura et al.[92] analyzed six synovial sarcomas and found—in addition to hyaluronic acid, chondroitin sulfate, and heparatin sulfate—sialic acid in the epithelial elements. Sialic acid was absent in the spindle cell areas. In contrast to mesothelioma, granular intracellular glycogen that stains positively for PAS is never a striking feature of synovial sarcoma.

The second type of mucinous material, stromal or mesenchymal mucin, which is elaborated by the spindle cells, also stains positively for colloidal iron and alcian blue stains, but it is weakly carminophilic and stains negatively with the PAS preparation. It is present in the interstices of the spindle cell or fibrosarcoma-like areas and the loosely textured myxoid portions of the tumor. This material is rich in hyaluronic acid and, like other mesenchymal mucins, is completely removed by prior treatment of the secretions with hyaluronidase. PAS and alcian blue preparations—as well as various metachromatic stains and naphthol AS-D chloroacetate esterase—are also useful for identifying the mast cell infiltrate.

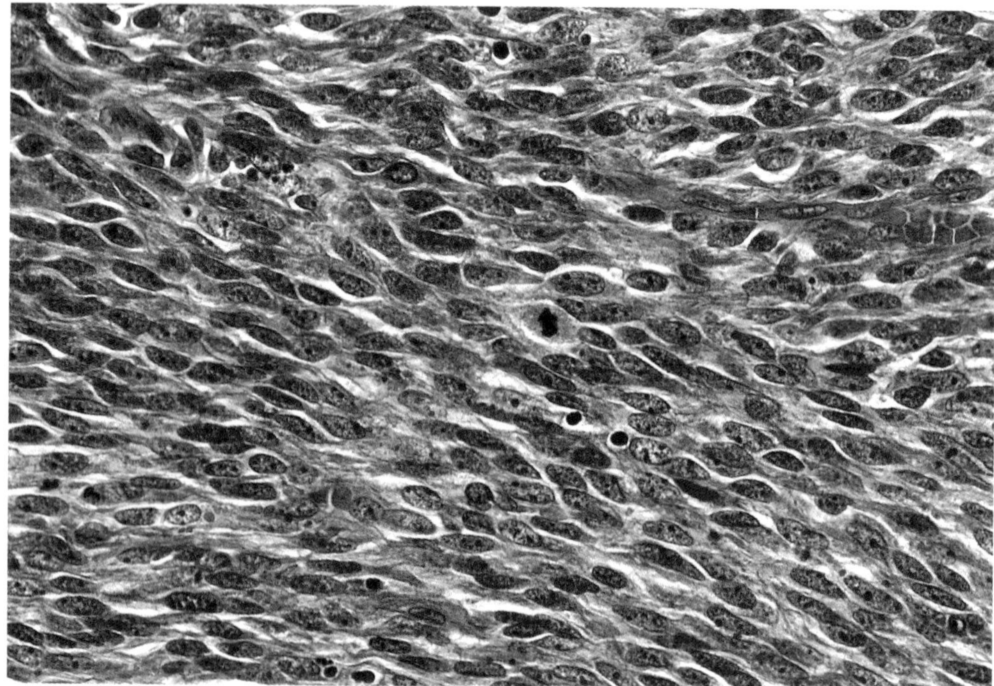

**FIGURE 37–25.** Poorly differentiated synovial sarcoma composed of spindle cells with high-grade nuclear features.

### *Immunohistochemical Findings*

Most synovial sarcomas display immunoreactivity for cytokeratins and epithelial membrane antigen[1,13,14,98,110] (Fig. 37–26). In an immunohistochemical study of 100 synovial sarcomas by Guillou et al.,[41] focal positivity for epithelial membrane antigen and cytokeratin was found in 97% and 69% of cases, respectively. In this study, only 1 of 100 cases was negative for both of these epithelial markers. In our experience and that reported in the literature,[54,70] approximately 90% of all synovial sarcomas are cytokeratin-positive. In general, the intensity of staining is more pronounced in the epithelial cell component than the spindle cell component. In some lesions of the monophasic fibrous type, only a few isolated cells express these antigens, making it necessary to stain and examine multiple sections from different portions of the tumor[39,84] (Fig. 37–27). Poorly differentiated variants usually, but not always, express these epithelial markers. In the study by Folpe et al.,[35] all nine poorly differentiated synovial sarcomas stained for epithelial membrane antigen, whereas only 30% and 50% stained for low- and high-molecular-weight cytokeratins, respectively. Similarly, van de Rijn et al.[135] found staining for epithelial membrane antigen and cytokeratin in 95% and 42% of poorly differentiated synovial sarcomas, respectively. In contrast to other spindle cell sarcomas, the cells of synovial sarcomas express cytokeratins 7 and 19.[45,83,121] Because some synovial sarcomas stain for epithelial membrane antigen but not cytokeratin, and vice versa, both markers should be used in an attempt to demonstrate epithelial differentiation in these tumors.[30]

Although not emphasized until recently, up to 30% of synovial sarcomas show focal immunoreactivity for S-100 protein.[29,41,121] Most of these S-100 protein-positive synovial sarcomas co-express epithelial markers, but the occasional synovial sarcoma may express S-100 protein in the absence of epithelial markers, thereby causing confusion with malignant peripheral nerve sheath tumors. In such cases the detection of cytokeratins 7 and 19 may be useful for recognizing monophasic fibrous synovial sarcomas.[121]

CD99, the product of the *MIC2* gene, can be immunohistochemically detected in the cytoplasm or membrane of cells in 60–70% of synovial sarcomas.[21,103] In addition, bcl-2 protein has been reported in 75–100% of synovial sarcomas, typically in a strong and diffuse fashion.[46,101,124,140] Unlike many other spindle cell tumors, synovial sarcoma is virtually always negative for CD34.[124,137]

### *Ultrastructural Findings*

The biphasic tumors are composed of epithelial and spindle cells with transitional forms between the two

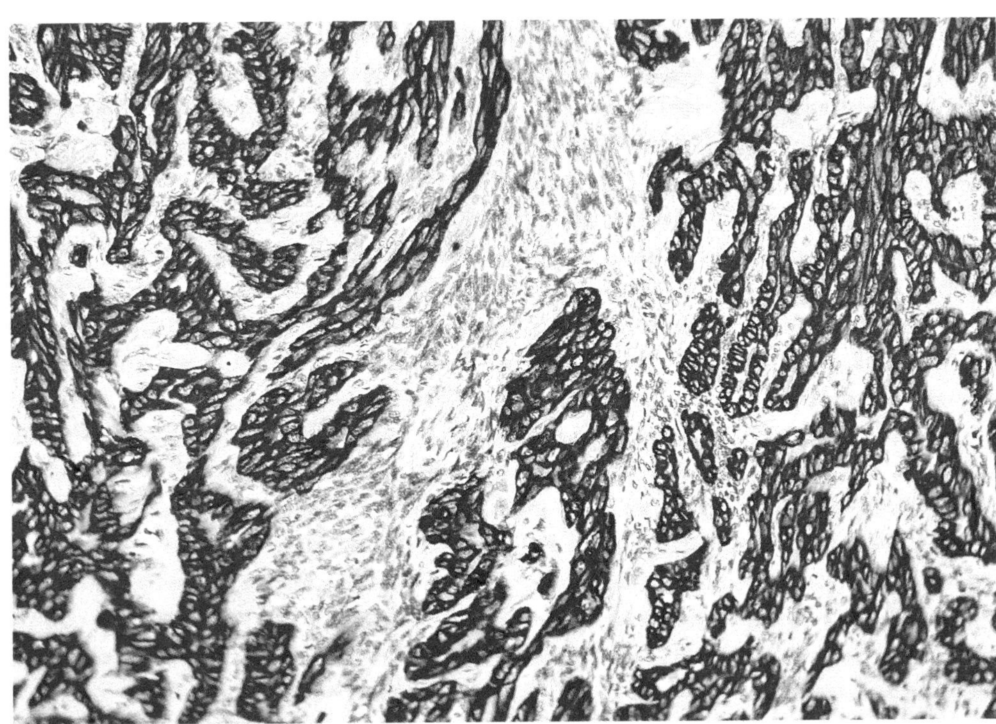

**FIGURE 37–26.** High molecular weight cytokeratin immunoreactivity highlights the epithelial elements in this biphasic synovial sarcoma.

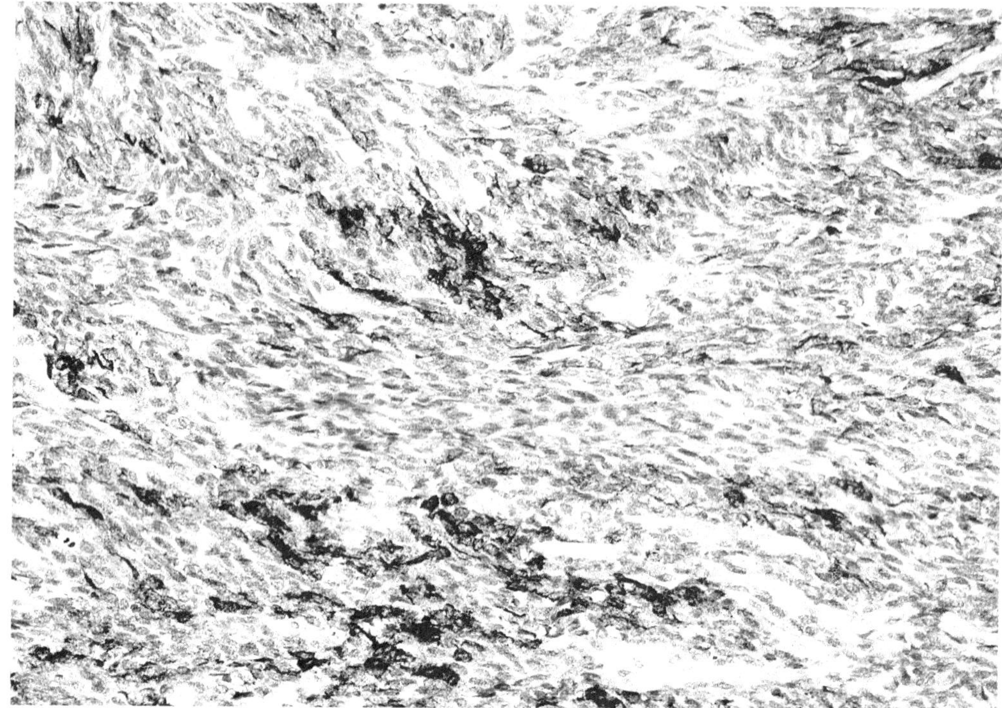

**FIGURE 37–27.** Focal immunoreactivity for cytokeratin 7 in this monophasic fibrous synovial sarcoma.

cell types. The epithelial cells have sharply defined ovoid nuclei with narrow, dense rims of chromatin and abundant cytoplasm containing mitochondria, a prominent Golgi complex, rare paranuclear aggregates of intermediate filaments, lysosomes, and smooth and rough endoplasmic reticulum, sometimes arranged in stacked arrays. On rare occasions tonofilaments are found in the epithelial cells, especially in the areas of squamous metaplasia. Frequently, the epithelial cells are disposed in clusters or gland-like structures, with microvilli or villous filopodia on the surfaces facing the intercellular or pseudoglandular spaces. Many of the spaces contain electron-dense mucinous material. In contrast to the cells of normal synovium, the epithelial cells are interconnected by junctional complexes, zonulae adherens, or desmosome-like structures. The fibroblast-like spindle cells have irregularly outlined nuclei, marginated chromatin, and small nucleoli. The cytoplasm contains mitochondria and a prominent Golgi apparatus, but there is less cytoplasm and a less well developed rough endoplasmic reticulum than that of typical fibroblasts. A continuous basal lamina, a structure that is absent in normal synovium, often separates the epithelial clusters and gland-like structures from the surrounding spindle-shaped cells[16,69,87,102] (Fig. 37–28).

The ultrastructural features of the monophasic fibrous type are indistinguishable from those of the spindle cell areas of the biphasic type. There are, however, identifying features of early epithelial differentiation, such as intercellular or cleft-like spaces of varying size bordered by multiple microvilli, as well as poorly developed junctions or desmosome-like structures. In addition, there are occasional cell clusters similar to those seen in the biphasic type. There is no distinct basal lamina, but there are occasional fragments of basal lamina or condensed ground substance at the cell surfaces.[22,62] Tsuneyoshi et al.[130] described the presence of membrane-bound secretory granules and tabulated bodies containing filamentous structures.

### *Cytogenetic and Molecular Genetic Findings*

A consistent, specific translocation, most commonly a balanced reciprocal translocation, t(X;18)(p11.2;q11.2), is found in more than 90% of all synovial sarcoma subtypes.[18,68,131,132] This translocation involves the *SYT* gene on chromosome 18 and either the *SSX1* or *SSX2* gene on the *X* chromosome.[11,15,17,116] The *SYT/SSX* fusion messenger RNA can be detected by reverse transcriptase-polymerase chain reaction (RT-PCR)[34] or fluoresence in situ hybridization (FISH)[72,115] using frozen or paraffin-embedded tissue.[4,66,91,129,143,146] These techniques are particularly useful for monophasic fibrous and poorly differentiated synovial sarcomas which may be difficult to distinguish from other spindle cell and round cell sarcomas, respectively. Although this translocation has been described in rare

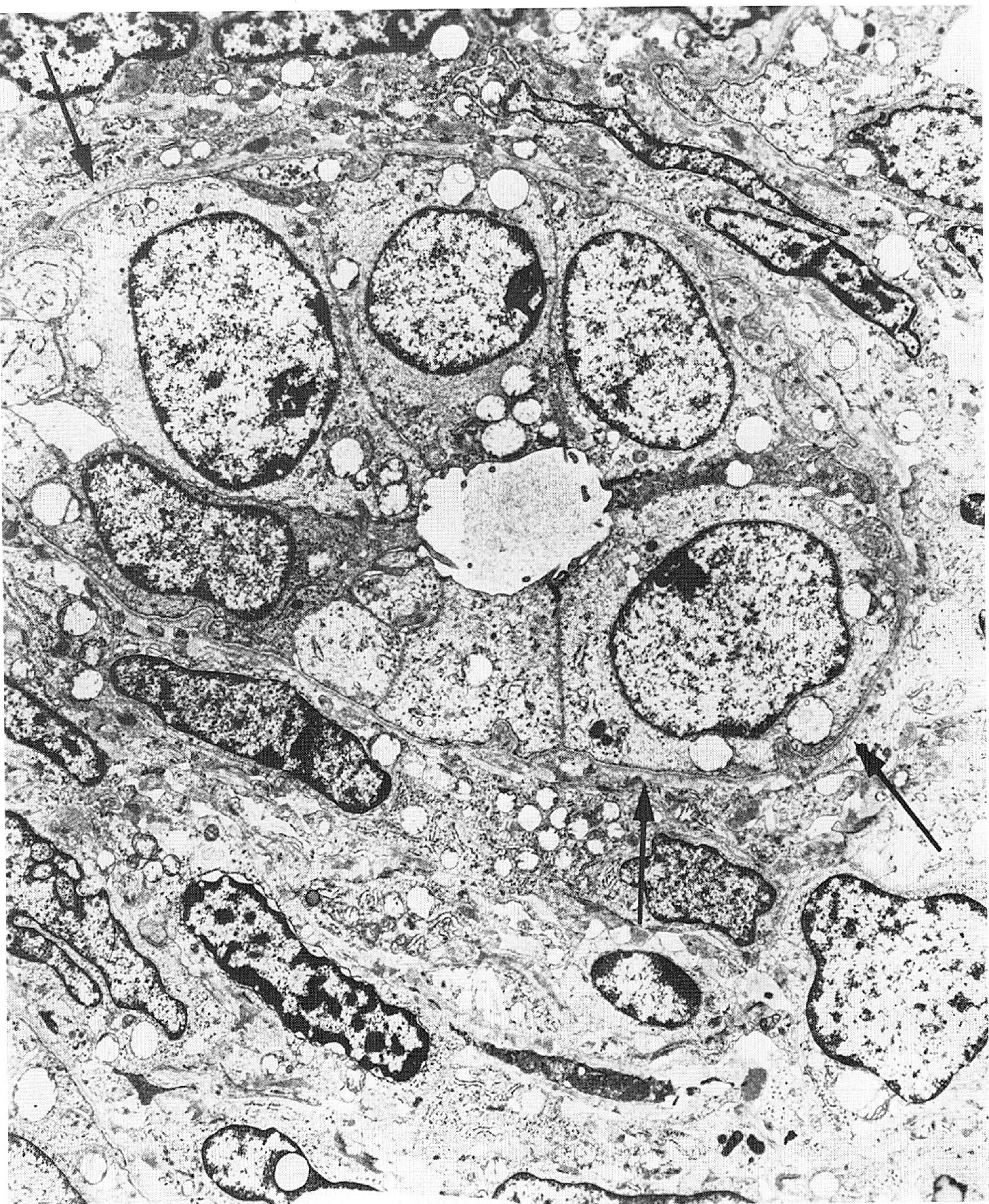

**FIGURE 37–28.** Electron micrograph of a biphasic synovial sarcoma showing short microvilli in the small pseudoglandular space and separation of the epithelial and fibroblast-like spindle cell elements by a distinct basal lamina (arrows). (Courtesy of Dr. R.F. Armstrong, Victoria Hospital, London, Canada.)

fibrosarcomas[77] and malignant fibrous histiocytomas,[68] such reports likely represent misdiagnosed synovial sarcomas, as this translocation has yet to be convincingly demonstrated in any other tumor type.[134]

Although there is disagreement,[15,34,115] some have found a correlation between the histologic subtype of synovial sarcoma and the breakpoint site.[19,59,104] Involvement of the *SSX2* gene has been associated with the monophasic fibrous synovial sarcoma, although almost half of this variant involved *SSX1*.[59] Kawai et al.[59] found a significantly longer metastasis-free survival period in those patients with localized tumors involving the *SSX2* gene, although the biologic explanation for this observation remains unclear. Several studies have shown the *SYT-SSX1* fusion transcript to be associated with a higher Ki-67 index and higher mitotic rate than the *SYT-SSX2* fusion transcript, suggesting that fusion type is related to proliferative activity.[50,93a]

## Differential Diagnosis

Distinguishing synovial sarcoma from other neoplasms may be difficult, and in many instances a reliable diagnosis is not possible without immunohistochemical examination. The differential diagnosis depends on the subtype of synovial sarcoma, as discussed below.

### *Differential Diagnosis of Biphasic Synovial Sarcoma*

In general, biphasic synovial sarcoma causes few problems with the diagnosis, especially if the tumor is located in the extremities near a large joint and occurs in a young adult. However, when the tumor arises in an unusual site, *carcinosarcoma, glandular malignant peripheral nerve sheath tumor* (MPNST) and *malignant mesothelioma* enter the differential diagnosis. In carcinosarcomas of any site, the glandular element usually shows a significantly greater degree of nuclear pleomorphism than the epithelial component seen in biphasic synovial sarcoma. Similarly, the spindle cell component of carcinosarcomas is usually more cytologically atypical. Glandular MPNST, a rare neoplasm, usually can be recognized by the presence of intestinal-type epithelium with goblet cells, the occasional association with rhabdomyosarcomatous elements (Triton tumor), and the occurrence in patients with manifestations of neurofibromatosis type 1.[10,142]

Rare synovial sarcomas have been described in the pleura and peritoneum and thus may cause confusion with malignant mesothelioma. However, the latter tumor typically presents in older patients, often male, usually with a history of significant asbestos exposure. Furthermore, malignant mesotheliomas involve the pleura or peritoneum diffusely and only rarely present as a localized mass. Histologically, malignant mesotheliomas with spindled and epithelial areas usually show a gradual transition between these two areas. Synovial sarcomas, on the other hand, have a sharp abutment of gland with stroma. Additional histologic, histochemical, and immunohistochemical differences between these tumors usually allow their distinction. Finally, identification of a t(X;18) or *SYT-SSX* fusion transcript would confirm a diagnosis of synovial sarcoma in extremely difficult cases.

### *Differential Diagnosis of Monophasic Fibrous Synovial Sarcoma*

The monophasic fibrous synovial sarcoma may resemble a number of other spindle cell neoplasms including fibrosarcoma, leiomyosarcoma, MPNST, hemangiopericytoma, and spindle cell carcinoma. Often an immunohistochemical panel is necessary to recognize this variant, and in difficult cases cytogenetic or molecular genetic techniques can confirm the diagnosis. This tumor can be distinguished from *fibrosarcoma* by its frequent location near large joints, its irregular and often multilobular growth pattern, the plump appearance of the nuclei, and the focal whorled arrangement of the spindle cells. In general, mitotic figures are less common than in fibrosarcomas. Additional factors that suggest a synovial sarcoma are the presence of mast cells, foci of calcification, the presence of a hemangiopericytomatous vasculature, and most importantly the demonstration of cytokeratin or epithelial membrane antigen in the neoplastic cells. It is likely that many so-called fibrosarcomas reported in the older literature are actually monophasic fibrous synovial sarcomas.

Some monophasic fibrous synovial sarcomas contain spindle cells with more eosinophilic cytoplasm, reminiscent of *leiomyosarcoma.* However, leiomyosarcomas typically have cells arranged in better defined fasicles that intersect at right angles to each other. The nuclei are blunt-ended, often with a paranuclear vacuole, and the cytoplasm is more densely eosinophilic. Although some leiomyosarcomas express cytokeratins, particularly cytokeratins 8 and 18, virtually all of these tumors stain strongly for smooth muscle actin, and many others express muscle-specific actin or desmin. The absence of bcl-2 protein in leiomyosarcoma may also be useful for this distinction.[124]

The *malignant peripheral nerve sheath tumor* may bear a close resemblance to the monophasic fibrous type of synovial sarcoma. Obvious origin from a nerve suggests a diagnosis of MPNST, although rare examples of synovial sarcoma have also been described as arising in nerves.[94] Synovial sarcomas do not arise from preexisting neurofibromas or in patients with neurofibromatosis type 1. Both MPNST and monophasic synovial sarcoma may have alternating areas of hyper-

and hypocellularity, imparting a marbled appearance at low magnification. Neuroid-type whorls and perivascular or subintimal involvement of blood vessels by the neoplastic cells suggest a diagnosis of MPNST.[30]

Cytologically, the cells of MPNSTs are often wavy or buckled and appear to have been pinched at one end with bulbous protrusion of the opposite end of the nucleus. Immunohistochemically, approximately two-thirds of MPNSTs stain focally for S-100 protein. Because S-100 protein has been found in up to 30% of synovial sarcomas,[41] this marker alone cannot distinguish between these two neoplasms. Similarly, although up to 90% of synovial sarcomas express epithelial markers, rare MPNSTs express either cytokeratin or epithelial membrane antigen. In this context, cytokeratins 7 and 19 may be useful in that virtually all synovial sarcomas express cytokeratin 7, cytokeratin 19, or both, whereas both of these antigens are rarely expressed in MPNSTs.[121] Electron microscopy often shows schwannian differentiation in MPNSTs, although it is less well developed in poorly differentiated tumors and appears to be related to the degree of S-100 protein immunoreactivity.[32]

Many synovial sarcomas exhibit a prominent hemangiopericytomatous vascular pattern, which can result in an erroneous diagnosis of *hemangiopericytoma*. The latter tumor is rare and by definition the diagnosis is one of exclusion. Typically, this vascular pattern is present as a focal phenomenon in synovial sarcomas, whereas by definition, hemangiopericytomas have this vasculature throughout the entire neoplasm, including myxoid and hyalinized zones. In addition, the hemangiopericytoma lacks immunohistochemical evidence of epithelial differentiation and expresses CD-34 in up to 80% of cases, a marker typically absent in synovial sarcomas.

#### Differential Diagnosis of Monophasic Epithelial Synovial Sarcoma

Distinction of purely epithelial forms of synovial sarcoma from *adnexal* or *metastatic carcinoma* is virtually impossible in the absence of a focal biphasic pattern. Fortunately, most of these tumors, when carefully sampled, have focal spindle cell areas that are sufficiently characteristic to allow a specific diagnosis.

#### Differential Diagnosis of Poorly Differentiated Synovial Sarcoma

In most instances, poorly differentiated synovial sarcoma resembles a number of other small round cell neoplasms including extraskeletal Ewing's sarcoma/primitive neuroectodermal tumor (ES/PNET), neuroblastoma, rhabdomyosarcoma, malignant hemangiopericytoma, mesenchymal chondrosarcoma, and lymphoma. A diagnosis of poorly differentiated synovial sarcoma is made simpler if one can identify a lower grade component that is typical of either monophasic or biphasic synovial sarcoma. In the absence of such a component, or if only a small amount of tissue composed entirely of round cells is available, distinction from the aforementioned entities invariably requires ancillary techniques for diagnosis.

Although CD99 is a highly sensitive marker of the ES/PNET family of tumors,[122] this antigen may also be found in synovial sarcomas including poorly differentiated variants.[21] Furthermore, epithelial markers may be absent in poorly differentiated synovial sarcomas and focally present in ES/PNET.[114] Machen et al.[74] found cytokeratins 7 and 19 useful for this distinction in that most poorly differentiated synovial sarcomas, including those that lack cytokeratins AE1/AE3 and epithelial membrane antigen, express cytokeratin 7, cytokeratin 19, or both, whereas these antigens are typically absent in the ES/PNET family of tumors. Identification of the *EWS/FLI-1* or *SYT/SSX* fusion transcript is most useful for confirming diagnoses of ES/PNET and poorly differentiated synovial sarcoma, respectively.

*Neuroblastoma* arises from structures of the sympathetic nervous system during early childhood, characteristically has Homer Wright rosettes, and lacks expression of both CD99 and epithelial markers. *Rhabdomyosarcoma* can be excluded by the absence of desmin, myogenin, or MyoD1; appropriate T and B cell markers help exclude *lymphoma*. Distinction from *malignant hemangiopericytoma* may be exceedingly difficult given that some poorly differentiated synovial sarcomas lack immunohistochemical evidence of epithelial differentiation. In such cases, detection of the *SYT/SSX* fusion transcript can confirm a diagnosis of poorly differentiated synovial sarcoma.

Some poorly differentiated synovial sarcomas are composed of large epithelioid cells, sometimes accompanied by cells with rhabdoid features. Such tumors may be difficult to distinguish from *metastatic carcinoma, epithelioid sarcoma,* and *malignant extrarenal rhabdoid tumor*. Recognition of a lower grade area more typical of synovial sarcoma is the most useful way to distinguish these neoplasms. In the absence of such foci, a broad immunohistochemical panel coupled with ultrastructural and molecular genetic data can usually resolve this dilemma.

### Discussion

#### Recurrence and Metastasis

Although traditionally considered to be a high grade malignancy, advancements in therapy have lowered the incidence of recurrence and metastasis with improved long-term survival. As one would expect, the prognosis is poorest in cases treated merely by local excision with inadequate margins and without any adjunctive therapy. In these cases recurrence rates as high as 70% and 83%[2,82] are reported. With more adequate surgical excision or with adjunctive radiotherapy the recurrence rate has been reported to be significantly lower (less than 40%). In most cases the recurrent growth manifests within the first 2 years after initial therapy, although this is not true in all instances. For example, Sutro[125] observed a synovial sarcoma that recurred at 35 years. In addition, patients with more than one recurrence are not rare, and we have observed cases with four, five, and even six recurrences over a period of several years.

Metastatic lesions develop in about half of cases, most commonly to the lung, followed by the lymph nodes and the bone marrow. In our series,[73] all patients who developed metastatic disease had involvement of one or both lungs; similarly, in the series of Ryan et al.[109] the lung was affected in 94% of cases and the lymph nodes in 10%.

There are numerous accounts of late metastasis and long periods of survival after metastasis. Thunold and Bang[128] observed a woman who had a calcified synovial sarcoma removed at age 14 years and developed lung metastasis 26 years later. On the other hand, there are rare instances in which pulmonary metastasis is already present at the time of or prior to the initial diagnosis. Microscopically, the metastatic lesions are largely similar to the primary neoplasm, but metastases of biphasic tumors often exhibit a more prominent spindle cell pattern than the primary lesion, a lesser degree of cellular differentation, and increased mitotic activity. Care should be exercised when interpreting pulmonary metastasis of any spindle cell sarcoma to avoid interpreting entrapped alveolar spaces as evidence of biphasic differentiation.

### *Prognosis*

Reported 5-year survival rates for synovial sarcoma range from 36% to 76%[90] and up to 82% in heavily calcified tumors[139] (Table 37–2). Reported 10-year survival rates range from 20%[95] to 63%.[90] The differences in the 5- and 10-year survival rates reflect the relatively high incidence of late metastases. Numerous clinical and microscopic factors have been reported to influence the length of survival (Table 37–3). Major clinical factors associated with a more favorable clinical outcome include young age of the patient (15 years or younger),[23,64,96] tumor size smaller than 5 cm,[5,73,118] distal extremity location,[96] and low tumor stage.[71]

A wide array of histologic features have been reported to be of prognostic significance, but there is often disagreement among studies. There is still no agreement as to the prognostic significance of the microscopic subtype. Whereas some have found biphasic synovial sarcomas to behave in a more indolent fashion than monophasic tumors,[8,62] others have not found this to be so.[23,25] In most of these studies, the authors categorize the tumors as biphasic or monophasic fibrous or epithelial types. It is difficult to compare the results of these studies, however, because of great differences in the criteria used to distinguish the synovial sarcoma subtypes. In the study by Machen et al.[73] the amount of each tumor composed of spindled and epithelial areas was evaluated semiquantitatively and was not found to be of prognostic significance.

Two histologic patterns of synovial sarcoma have special clinical significance. Extensively calcified synovial sarcomas appear to have a better long-term prognosis. In a series of extensively calcified synovial sarcomas by Varela-Duran and Enzinger,[139] local recurrence and pulmonary metastases were detected in 32% and 29% of patients, respectively. In our own study of extremity synovial sarcomas,[73] 24% of cases had areas of calcification ranging from 5% to 20% of the tumors, but we did not find that the presence or extent of calcification had an impact on clinical be-

**TABLE 37–2 SYNOVIAL SARCOMA: REPORTED 5-YEAR SURVIVAL RATES**

| Study | Year | % |
|---|---|---|
| Varela-Duran and Enzinger[139]* | 1982 | 82 |
| Tsuneyoshi et al.[130] | 1983 | 51 |
| Golouh et al.[39] | 1990 | 64 |
| Schmidt et al.[112]** | 1991 | 63 |
| Oda et al.[96] | 1993 | 54 |
| Bergh et al.[5] | 1999 | 60 |

* Heavily calcified synovial sarcomas.
** Synovial sarcomas of children and adolescents (7-year survival rates).

**TABLE 37–3 FAVORABLE AND UNFAVORABLE PROGNOSTIC FACTORS BY MULTIVARIATE ANALYSIS FOR SYNOVIAL SARCOMA**

Low risk for metastasis
- Patient age <25 years
- Tumor size <5 cm
- Absence of poorly differentiated areas

High risk for metastasis
- Patient age >40 years
- Tumor size ≥5 cm
- Poorly differentiated areas

Modified from Bergh P, Meis-Kindblom JM, Gherlinzoni F, et al. Synovial sarcoma: identification of low and high risk groups. Cancer 85:2596, 1999.

havior. On the other hand, it is clear that tumors with poorly differentiated areas generally behave more aggressively and metastasize in a higher percentage of cases than those without such areas.[5,135] In our own study the risk of an adverse outcome was significantly greater when 20% or more of the tumor was composed of poorly differentiated areas.[73] Thus, thorough sampling of these tumors is required to determine the presence and extent of poorly differentiated areas. Other histologic features reported to have an adverse prognostic impact include the presence of rhabdoid cells,[96] extensive tumor necrosis,[107] high mitotic index (>10 mitoses/10HPF),[73,118] and high nuclear grade.[73,96] Aneuploidy,[23] high proliferating cell nuclear antigen (PCNA) score[71,95] and increased apoptotic index[59a] have also been reported to be adverse prognostic indicators, but it is not clear whether these techniques are more predictive than the mitotic index alone. In addition, *p53* mutations[113] and the co-expression of hepatocyte growth factor and its receptor (c-MET)[97] have been associated with a poor prognosis. It has also been suggested that synovial sarcoma patients with the *SYT/SSX2* fusion transcript are more likely to have a longer disease-free survival than those with the *SYT/SSX1* fusion transcript.[59]

### Therapy

Local control of synovial sarcoma is clearly related to the adequacy of initial surgical excision. Simple local excision without ancillary therapy is incapable of checking the growth and spread of the tumor, and most reviewers recommend extensive surgery as the therapy of choice, including radical local excision, often with removal of an entire muscle or muscle group, and amputation, depending mainly on the size of the tumor and its location. Because radical local excision is often impossible with tumors situated near a large joint—the favored location of synovial sarcoma—adjunctive radiotherapy in addition to local excision of the tumor is favored over amputation.[90,118,144] In the study by Mullen and Zagars of 85 patients with localized synovial sarcoma treated with conservative surgery and radiotherapy,[90] 5-, 10-, and 15-year survival rates of 76%, 63%, and 57%, respectively, were reported.

More recently, trials have evaluated the possible beneficial role of adjunctive chemotherapy with adriamycin,[90] cisplatin and doxorubicin,[56] and particularly ifosfamide.[108] There is some suggestion that these agents improve disease-free and overall survivals. Additionally, surgical metastasectomy, particularly wedge or segmental resection of solitary or multiple pulmonary metastases,[9,133,138] may also improve long-term survival.

### Line of Differentiation

There is still considerable debate as to the exact line of differentiation of this neoplasm. This uncertainty is also reflected in the new edition of the World Health Organization Soft Tissue Classification in which synovial sarcoma is placed among the "miscellaneous soft tissue tumors." The cells of the synovial sarcoma differ in several aspects from normal synovium, and synovial sarcoma is not known to arise from a benign synovial lesion such as villonodular synovitis or giant cell tumor of the tendon sheath.

In the past, most discussion centered on whether synovial sarcomas arose from preformed synovium. The largely outdated concept that sarcomas arise from mature, preformed tissue has given way to a discussion as to whether these tumors have cellular features that resemble normal synovium. As previously mentioned, synovial sarcomas rarely arise in joint cavities, and these tumors may arise in locations in which normal synovial structures are rare or nonexistent, including the lung, heart, and abdominal wall. Furthermore, there are significant immunohistochemical and ultrastructural differences between the cells of synovial sarcoma and those of the synovial lining. For example, nonneoplastic synovial cells react only with vimentin and do not express epithelial markers, nor do they show ultrastructural evidence of epithelial differentiation.[38,85] Moreover, fibroblastic (type B) synoviocytes characteristically express the vascular cell adhesion molecule (VCAM-1) and the enzyme uridine diphosphoglucose dehydrogenase, neither of which is detectable in the spindle cells of the monophasic synovial sarcoma.[120] In fact, on the strength of these findings, some reviewers believe that the term synovial sarcoma should be abandoned and the term *connective tissue carcinosarcoma* or *soft tissue carcinoma* used instead.[16,38,85] The term synovial sarcoma is so well established in the literature, however, there seems little reason to alter it at present until there is a consensus as to the appropriate choice of alternate terms.

## ALVEOLAR SOFT PART SARCOMA

Alveolar soft part sarcoma is a clinically and morphologically distinct soft tissue sarcoma that was first defined and named by Christopherson et al. in 1952.[151] Before their report, typical cases had been described under various designations including malignant myoblastoma,[166] angioendothelioma,[173] and even liposarcoma.[158] Since 1952 numerous examples of these tumors have been reported and have been studied immunohistochemically and electron microscopically; but there is still uncertainty as to their exact nature. Alveolar soft part sarcomas are uniformly malignant; there is no benign counterpart of the tumor.

Alveolar soft part sarcoma is an uncommon neoplasm; its frequency among our cases is estimated at 0.5–1.0% of all soft tissue sarcomas. It is even less common in other series. Ekfors et al.[156] for example, found only one alveolar soft part sarcoma among 246 malignant soft tissue tumors in Finland, an incidence of 0.4%.

## Clinical Findings

This tumor occurs principally in adolescents and young adults and is most frequently encountered in patients 15–35 years of age[174,175] (Table 37–4). Female patients outnumber males, especially among patients under 25 years of age.[193] Infants and children are affected less frequently. There are two main locations of the tumor. When it occurs in adults, it is seen predominantly in the lower extremities, especially the anterior portion of the thigh. For example, in a study of 102 alveolar soft part sarcomas by Lieberman et al.,[174] 39.5% involved the soft tissues of the buttock or thigh. The tumor has also been described in a variety of unusual locations including the female genital tract,[183,191,198] mediastinum,[160] and lung.[205] When the tumor affects infants and children, it is often located in the region of the head and neck, especially the orbit and tongue; tumors in the head and neck tend to be smaller, probably because of earlier detection[167,178,180,203] (Table 37–5).

Alveolar soft part sarcoma usually presents as a slowly growing, painless mass that almost never causes functional impairment. Because of the relative lack of symptoms it is easily overlooked; in a number of cases metastasis to the lung or brain is the first manifestation of the disease.[176,190,196] Headache, nausea, and visual changes are often associated with cerebral metastasis. As a rule, the tumor is richly vascular, causing pulsation or a distinctly audible bruit in some instances. Massive hemorrhage is often encountered during surgical removal. In rare instances there is erosion or destruction of the underlying bone.[177] Hypervascularity with prominent draining veins and prolonged capillary staining are usually demonstrable with angiography and CT scans. On MRI, the tumor typically demonstrates high signal intensity on both T2- and T1-weighted images.[168,206]

**TABLE 37–4 AGE DISTRIBUTION OF 102 ALVEOLAR SOFT PART SARCOMAS**

| Age (Years) | No. of Patients | % |
|---|---|---|
| 0–9 | 12 | 12 |
| 10–19 | 17 | 17 |
| 20–29 | 42 | 41 |
| ≥30 | 31 | 30 |
| *Total* | 102 | 100 |

Modified from Lieberman PH, Brennan MF, Kimmel M, et al. Alveolar soft-part sarcoma: a clinicopathologic study of half a century. Cancer 63:1, 1989.

**TABLE 37–5 ANATOMIC DISTRIBUTION OF 102 ALVEOLAR SOFT PART SARCOMAS**

| Location | No. of Patients | % |
|---|---|---|
| Buttock/thigh | 40 | 39.5 |
| Leg/popliteal | 17 | 16.6 |
| Chest wall/trunk | 13 | 12.9 |
| Forearm | 10 | 9.7 |
| Arm | 8 | 8.5 |
| Back/neck | 6 | 6.4 |
| Tongue | 4 | 3.2 |
| Retroperitoneum | 4 | 3.2 |
| *Total* | 102 | 100.0 |

Modified from Lieberman PH, Brennan MF, Kimmel M, et al. Alveolar soft-part sarcoma: a clinicopathologic study of half a century. Cancer 63:1, 1989.

## Pathologic Findings

The gross specimen tends to be poorly circumscribed, soft, and friable; on section it consists of yellow-white to gray-red tissue, often with large areas of necrosis and hemorrhage. Frequently the tumor is surrounded by numerous tortuous vessels of large caliber.

The microscopic picture varies little from tumor to tumor, and the uniformity of the microscopic picture is a constant and typical feature of the lesion. Characteristically, dense fibrous trabeculae of varying thickness divide the tumor into compact groups or compartments of irregular size that in turn are subdivided into sharply defined nests or aggregates of tumor cells (Figs. 37–29, 37–30). These cellular aggregates are separated from one another by thin-walled, sinusoidal vascular channels lined by a single layer of flattened endothelial cells. In most instances the cellular aggregates exhibit central degeneration, necrosis, and loss of cohesion resulting in a pseudoalveolar pattern (Fig. 37–31). This pattern should not be confused with the more irregular alveolar pattern of alveolar rhabdomyosarcoma. Less frequently, the nest-like pattern is inconspicuous or absent entirely, and the tumor is merely composed of uniform sheets of large granular cells with few or no discernible vascular channels (Fig. 37–32). This more solid, or compact type of alveolar soft part sarcoma occurs mainly in infants and children and is often associated with a more favorable prognosis.

The individual cells are large, rounded, or more

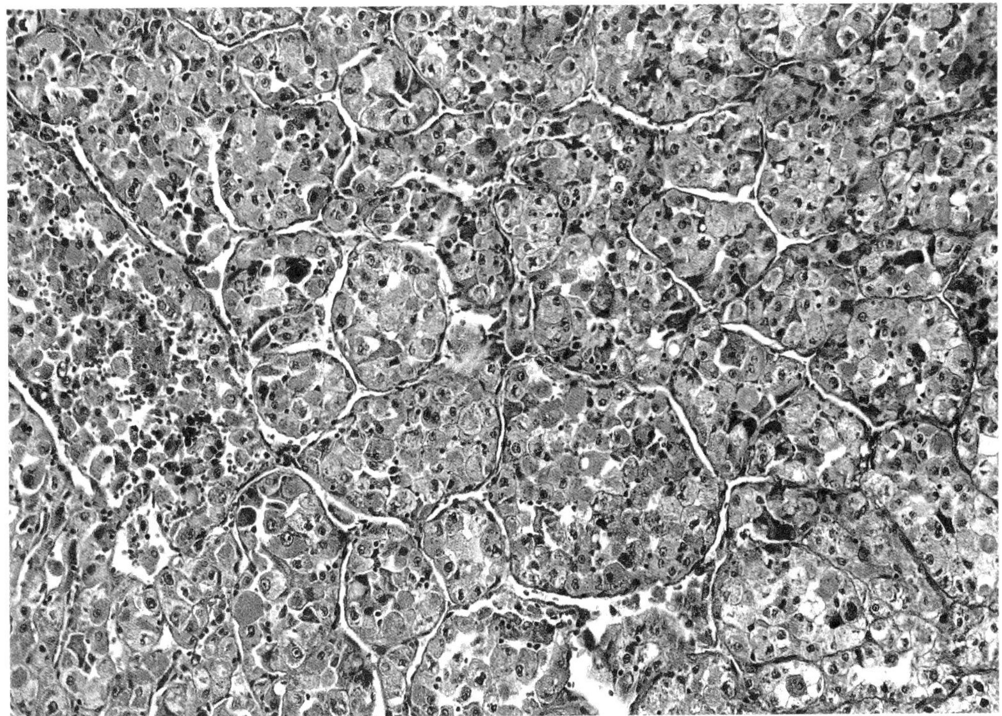

**FIGURE 37–29.** Alveolar soft part sarcoma with a typical organoid arrangement of tumor cells.

often polygonal and display little variation in size and shape. They have distinct cell borders and one or more vesicular nuclei with small nucleoli and abundant granular, eosinophilic, and sometimes vacuolated cytoplasm. Mitotic figures are scarce. Rare pleomorphic tumors have been reported in the literature[157] (Fig. 37–33).

At the margin of the tumor there are usually numerous dilated veins, probably the result of multiple arteriovenous shunts in the neoplasm similar to hemangiopericytoma and paraganglioma. Vascular invasion is a constant, striking finding that explains the tendency of the tumor to develop metastasis at an early stage of the disease (Fig. 37–34).

Histochemical stains are useful for establishing the diagnosis in that PAS preparation reveals varying amounts of intracellular glycogen and characteristically PAS-positive, diastase-resistant rhomboid or rod-shaped crystals (Fig. 37–35). Masson[179] in 1959 was the first to describe and depict these crystals as a diagnostic feature of alveolar soft part sarcoma; Shipkey et al. in 1964[202] were the first to examine them by electron microscopy. According to our material, the typical crystalline material is present in at least 80% of the tumors; in the remainder there are merely PAS-positive granules, probably precursors of the crystals. The crystals are a feature of both primary and metastatic alveolar soft part sarcomas.

## Immunohistochemical Findings

Numerous immunohistochemical studies have attempted to elucidate the histogenesis of this unusual tumor, often resulting in contradictory results.[161,162,169,182,187,197] The cells of alveolar soft part sarcomas generally do not stain with antibodies against cytokeratin, epithelial membrane antigen, neurofilaments, glial fibrillary acidic protein, serotonin, or synaptophysin; but they occasionally express S-100 protein and neuron-specific enolase.[174,194] The reports in regard to staining for muscle markers differ somewhat (Table 37–6), but most investigators have reported immunoreactivity for vimentin, muscle-specific actin, or desmin in the tumor cells.[165,182] Other myogenic markers including Z-protein, myosin, and $\beta$-enolase have been found in rare alveolar soft part sarcomas.[152,174,180]

In 1991 Rosai et al.[199] detected the myogenic nuclear regulatory protein MyoD1 by immunohistochemistry, and it was confirmed by Western blot analysis. In contrast, Cullinane et al.[154] were unable to detect MyoD1 by Northern blot analysis. Using paraffin-embedded samples, Wang et al.[209] were unable to detect nuclear expression of MyoD1 in 12 alveolar soft part sarcomas, although there was considerable granular cytoplasmic immunoreactivity. In addition, all cases were negative for myogenin, another myo-

*Text continued on page 1517*

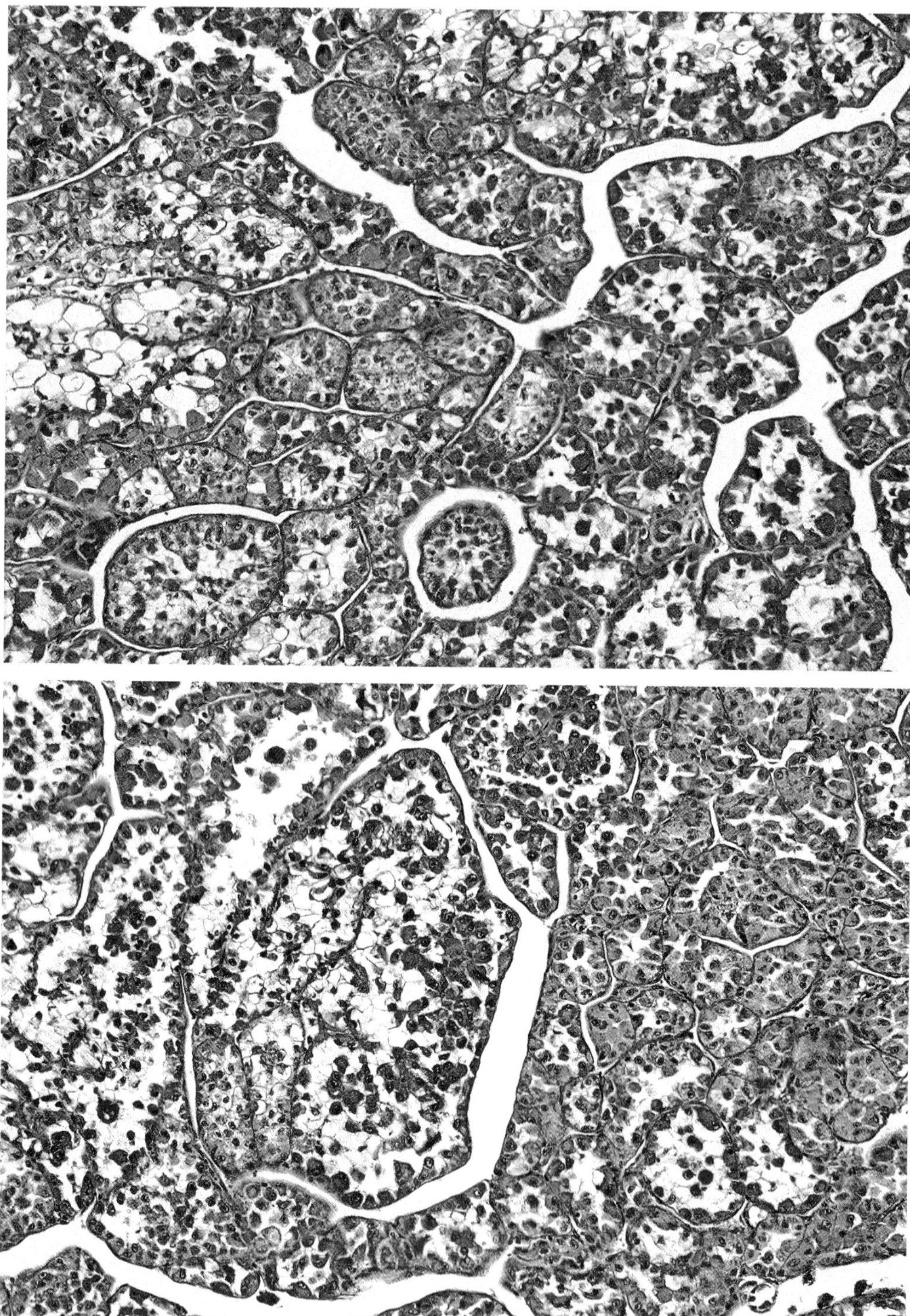

**FIGURE 37–30.** Alveolar soft part sarcoma with nests of large tumor cells with central loss of cellular cohesion resulting in a pseudoalveolar pattern. The cell nests are separated by thin-walled, sinusoidal vascular spaces.

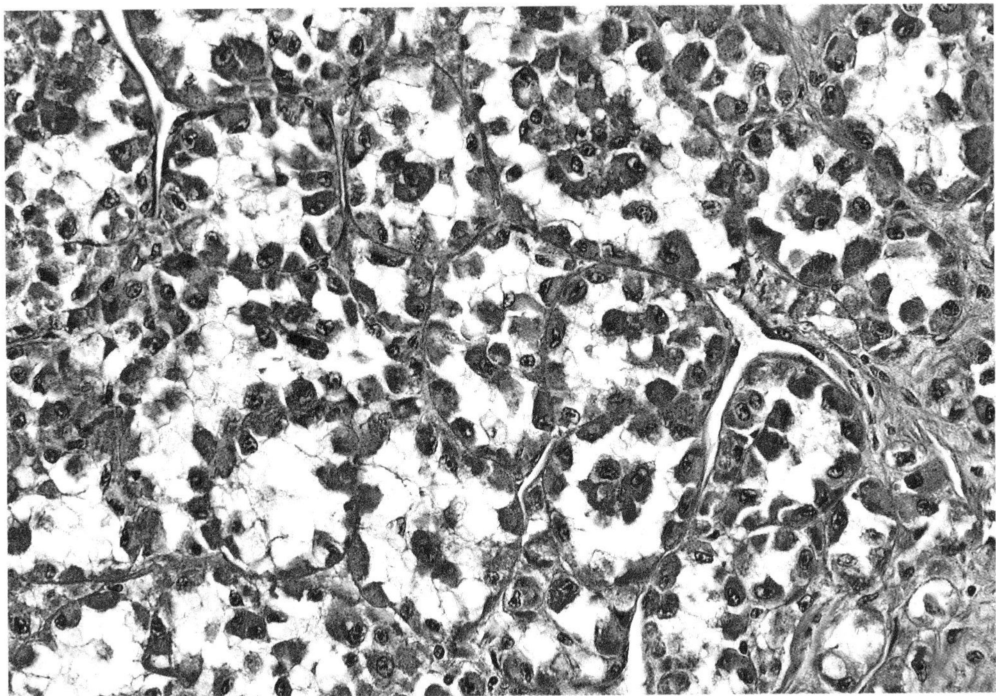

**FIGURE 37–31.** Prominent pseudoalveolar growth pattern in an alveolar soft part sarcoma.

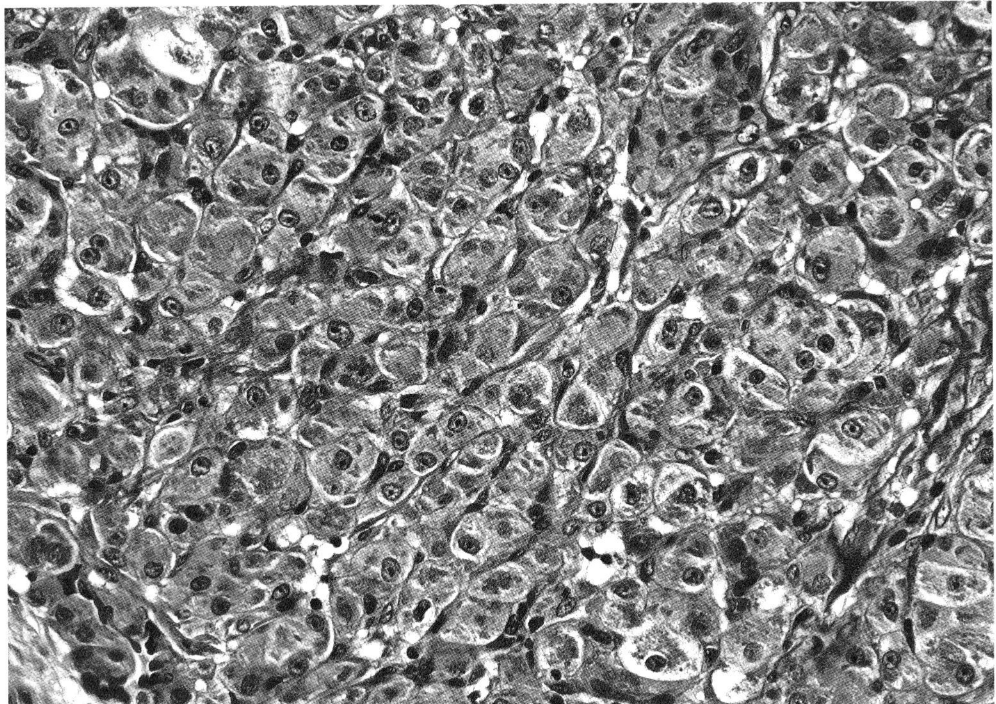

**FIGURE 37–32.** Alveolar soft part sarcoma without the clustering or nest-like arrangement of tumor cells. This variant occurs mainly in children and often carries a more favorable prognosis.

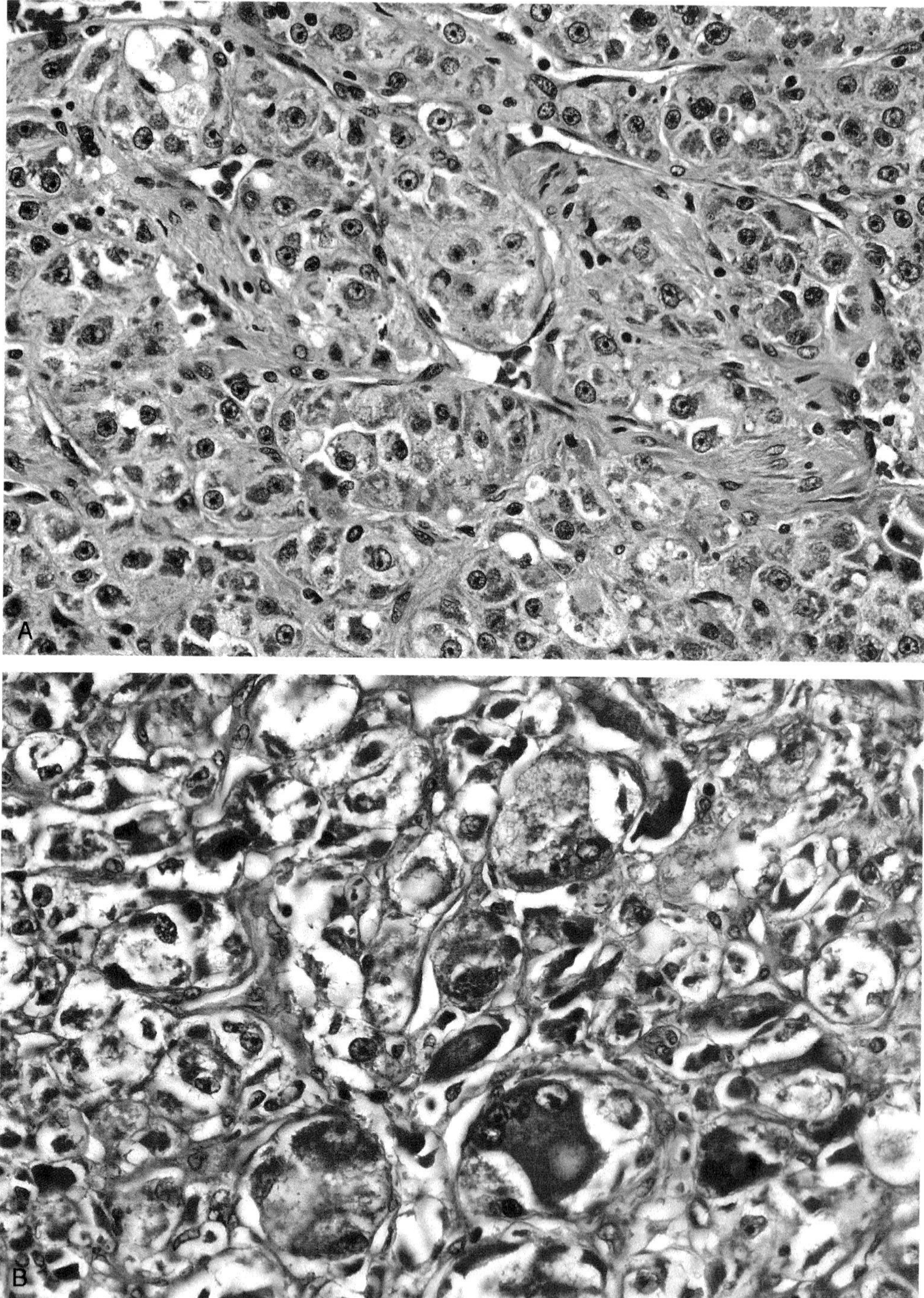


**FIGURE 37–33.** Range of cytologic atypia in alveolar soft part sarcomas. (**A**) This is the typical cytologic appearance of alveolar soft part sarcoma, with relatively uniform nuclei and prominent nucleoli. (**B**) Scattered atypical cells in an alveolar soft part sarcoma.

*Illustration continued on opposite page*

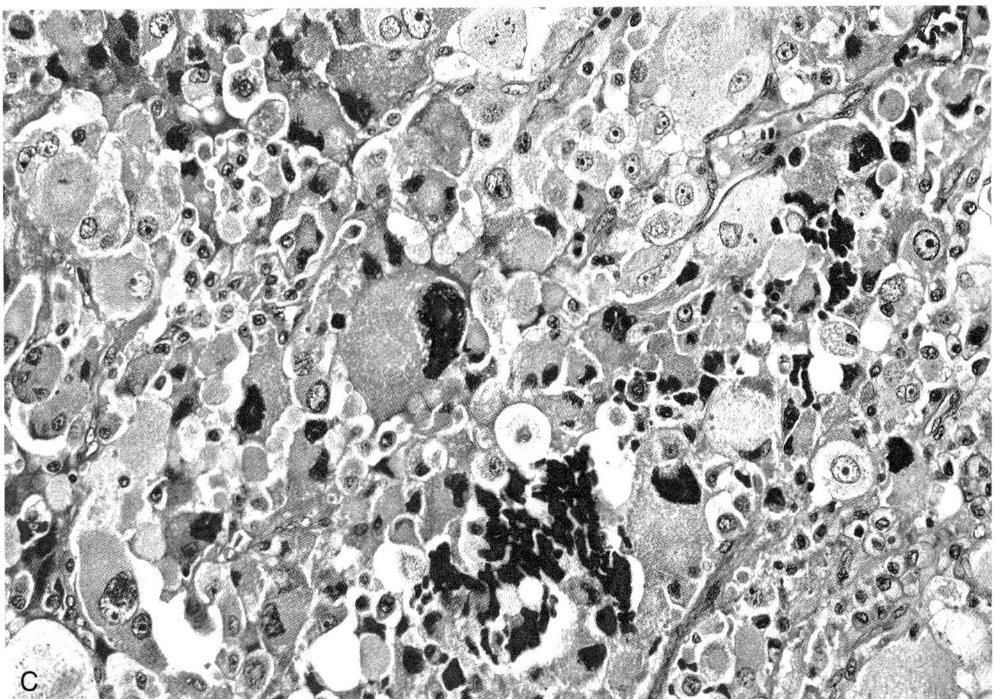


**FIGURE 37–33** *(Continued).* (**C**) Marked cytologic atypia in an alveolar soft part sarcoma.

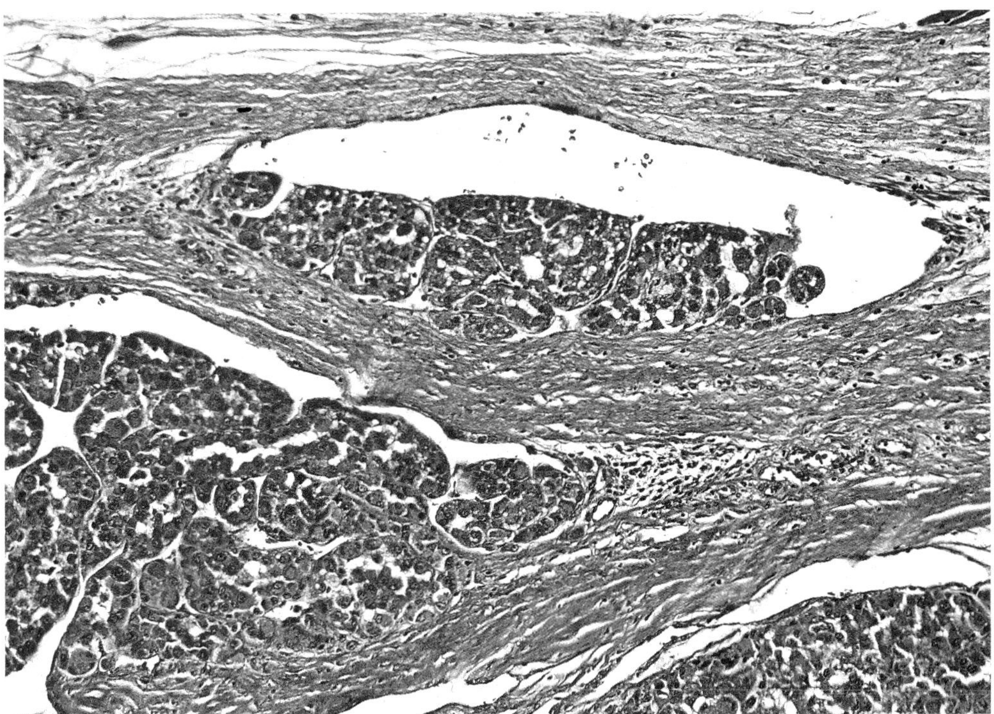

**FIGURE 37–34.** Dilated peripheral vein with tumor invasion.

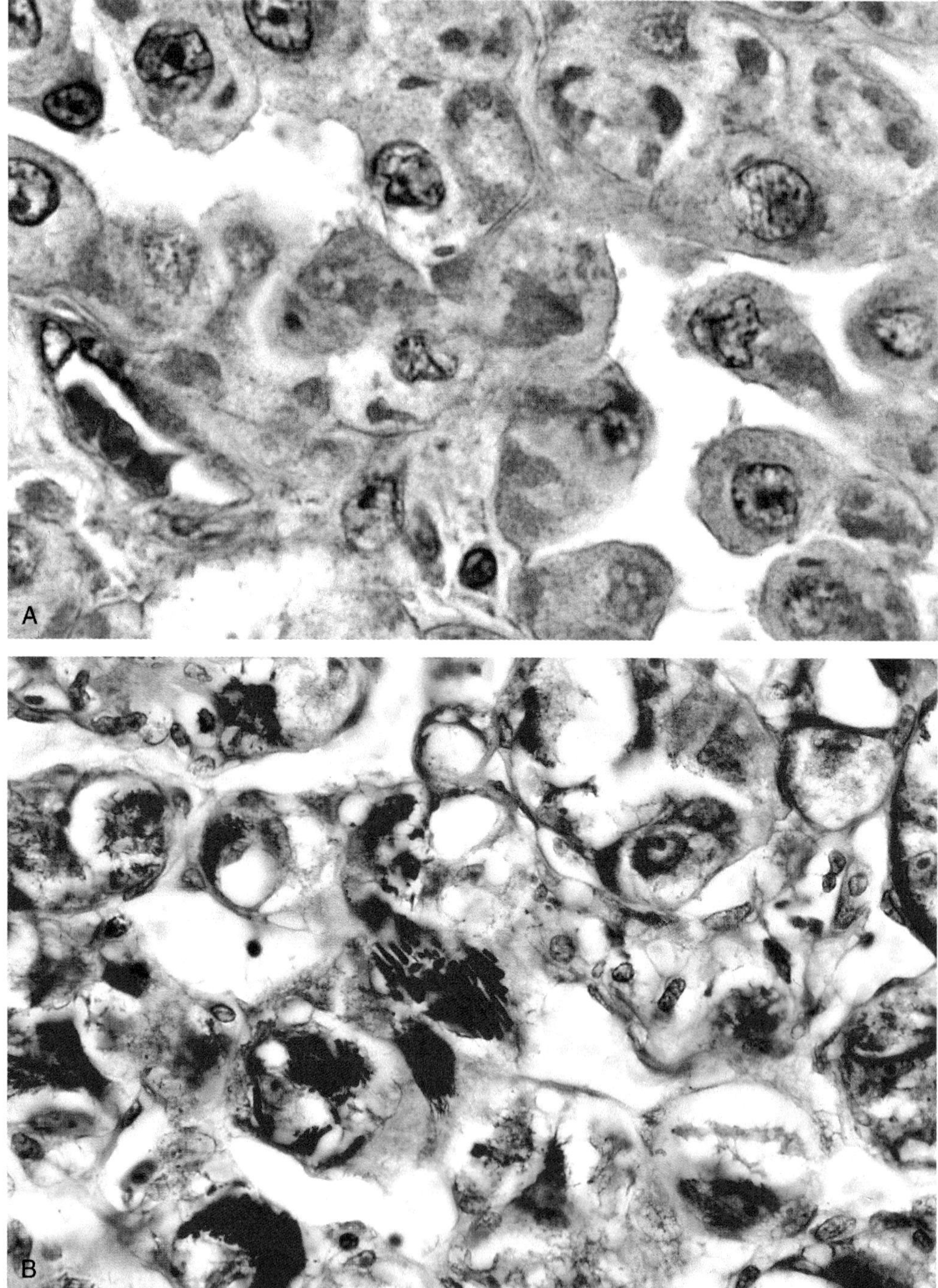


**FIGURE 37–35.** (**A**) High magnification view of an alveolar soft part sarcoma. There is focal condensation of eosinophilic cytoplasm. (**B**) Periodic acid-Schiff (PAS) staining with diastase reveals varying amounts of intracellular crystalline material.

*Illustration continued on opposite page*

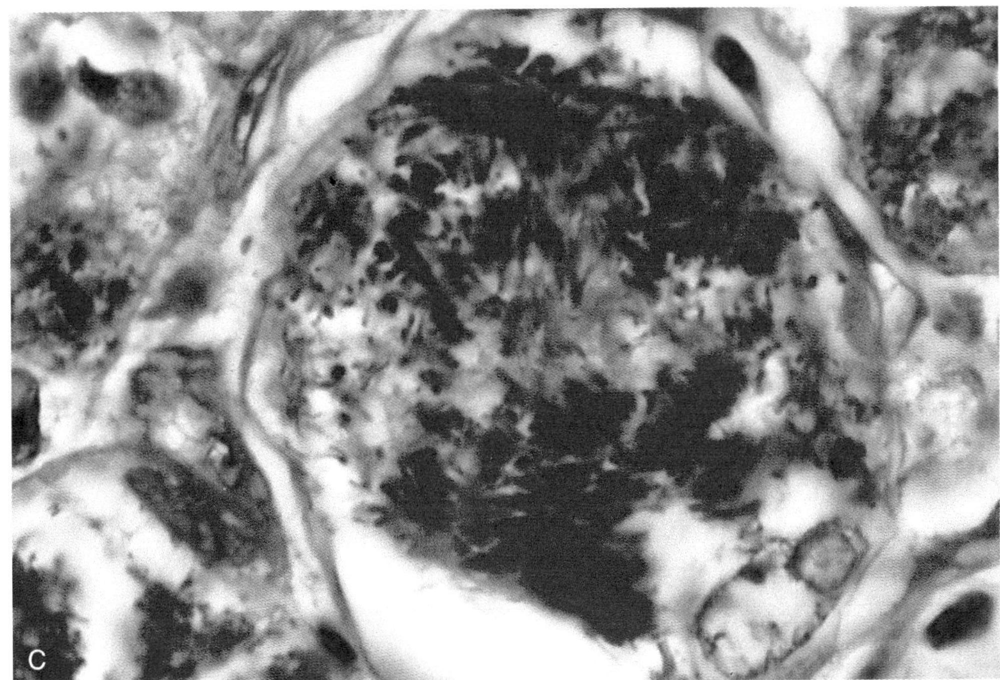

**FIGURE 37–35** *(Continued).* (**C**) High magnification view of crystalline material, diagnostic of alveolar soft part sarcoma.

genic nuclear regulatory protein. Similar results were recently reported by Gomez et al.[163]

## Electron Microscopic Findings

Electron microscopy shows the cells to contain numerous mitochondria, a prominent smooth endoplasmic reticulum, glycogen, and a well developed Golgi apparatus. Characteristically, there are also rhomboid, rod-shaped, or spicular crystals with a regular lattice pattern and sparse electron-dense secretory granules (Fig. 37–36). Both crystals and dense granules are membrane-bound and consist of crystallized and uncrystallized filaments 6 nm in diameter, suggesting transitions between the two structures. The filaments are arranged in a parallel fashion with

**TABLE 37–6** IMMUNOHISTOCHEMICAL DATA ON MUSCLE DIFFERENTIATION IN ALVEOLAR SOFT PART SARCOMAS

| Study | Year | Myoglobin | MSA | SMA | Desmin | MyoD1/Myogenin |
|---|---|---|---|---|---|---|
| Auerbach and Brooks[147] | 1987 | 0/12 | ND | ND | 0/9 | ND |
| Coira et al.[152] | 1991 | 1/1 | 1/1 | 1/1 | 1/1 | ND |
| Cullinane et al.[154] | 1992 | ND | 0/1 | ND | 0/1 | 0/1 |
| Foshini et al.[161] | 1988 | 0/2 | ND | 0/2 | 0/2 | ND |
| Hirose et al.[165] | 1990 | ND | 3/5 | 4/5 | 3/5 | ND |
| Lieberman et al.[174] | 1989 | ND | 0/14 | ND | 5/14 | ND |
| Miettinen and Ekfors[182] | 1990 | ND | 4/7 | ND | 3/7 | ND |
| Mukai et al.[187] | 1989 | 0/3 | 3/3 | ND | 3/3 | ND |
| Ordóñez et al.[194] | 1989 | ND | 2/14 | ND | 6/14 | ND |
| Persson et al.[197] | 1988 | 0/10 | 6/10 | ND | 8/10 | ND |
| Rosai et al.[199] | 1991 | 0/1 | 1/1 | 1/1 | 1/1 | 1/1 |
| Wang et al.[209] | 1996 | 0/11 | 0/11 | 0/11 | 6/11 | 0/11 |
| Gomez et al.[163] | 1999 | ND | 0/19 | ND | 0/19 | 0/19 |
| *Total* | | 1/40 (2.5%) | 20/86 (23%) | 6/20 (30%) | 36/97 (37%) | 1/32 (3%) |

Modified from Foschini MP, Eusebi V. Alveolar soft-part sarcoma: a new type of rhabdomyosarcoma? Semin Diagn Pathol 11:58, 1994.
MSA, muscle-specific actin; SMA, smooth-muscle actin; ND, not done.

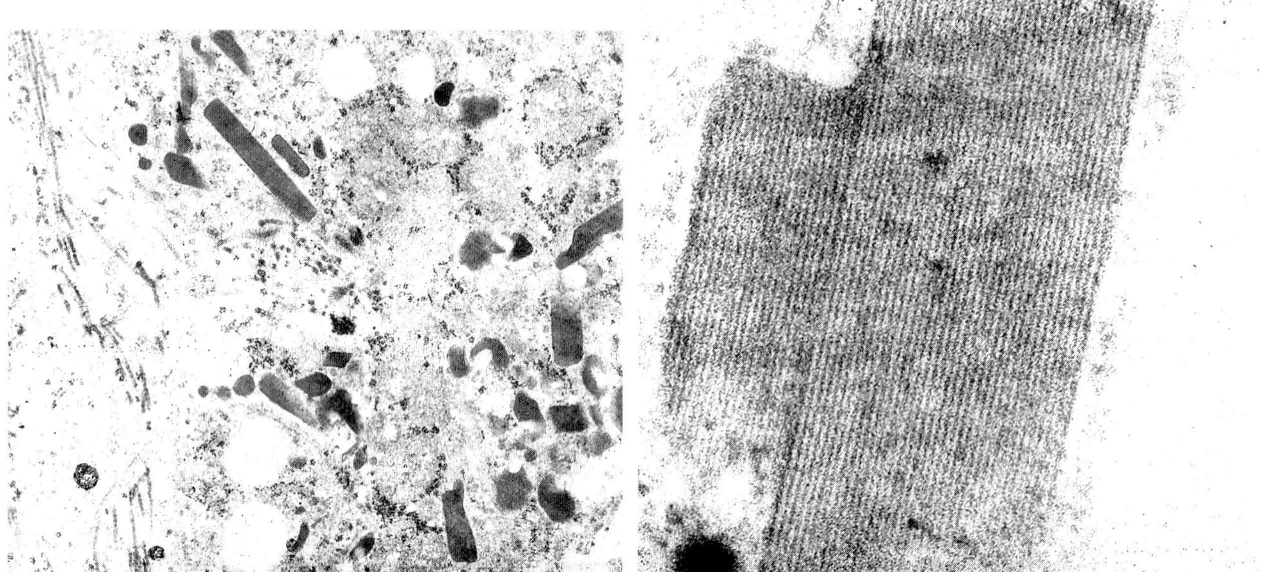

**FIGURE 37–36.** Electron micrographs depicting intracellular crystalline structures in an alveolar soft part sarcoma.

a periodicity of 10 nm.[186] The large polygonal cells are separated from the intervening vascular channels by a basal lamina, occasional circumferentially arranged spindle-shaped cells, and collagen fibers. Rare desmosomes or hemidesmosomes are present between the individual cells and between cells and surrounding basal laminae.[170] There is no evidence of smooth muscle or striated muscle differentiation,[181,188] but Mukai et al.[185] using digital image analysis of the crystalline material demonstrated structural similarities to actin filaments. More recently, tubular aggregates probably representing complex extensions or invaginations of cell membranes have been identified,[189,192] as have marked mitochondrial abnormalities.[149]

Several cytogenetic aberrations have been reported in alveolar soft part sarcomas. Craver et al.[153] described a case with trisomy 8, and there are several reports of abnormalities involving 17q25.[164,200,207] Analysis by comparative genomic hybridization has revealed gains at 1q, 8q, 12q, and 16p.[172]

## Differential Diagnosis

The differential diagnosis chiefly includes metastatic *renal cell carcinoma, paraganglioma,* and *granular cell tumor* (Table 37–7). Alveolar rhabdomyosarcoma is sometimes confused with alveolar soft part sarcoma but more because of the similarity in name than in the microscopic picture.

*Renal cell carcinoma,* primary or metastatic, often bears a striking resemblance to alveolar soft part sarcoma (Fig. 37–37), but in most cases it can be distinguished by the absence of the characteristic PAS-positive crystalline material. The pale-staining cytoplasm of its cells and the fat content of renal cell carcinoma are less reliable features because each may be encountered in degenerated forms of alveolar soft part sarcoma (Fig. 37–38). Immunoreactivity for epithelial membrane antigen is useful for confirming a diagnosis of renal cell carcinoma, as this antigen is absent in alveolar soft part sarcoma. Glycogen is present in

**TABLE 37–7** DIFFERENTIAL DIAGNOSTIC FEATURES OF ALVEOLAR SOFT PART SARCOMA

| Lesion | Glycogen | Crystals | Immunohistochemistry |
|---|---|---|---|
| Alveolar soft part sarcoma | + | + | Variable muscle markers |
| Renal cell carcinoma | + | – | Epithelial membrane antigen |
| Paraganglioma | – | – | Neuroendocrine markers (synaptophysin, chromogranin); S-100 protein in sustentacular cells |
| Granular cell tumor | – | – | S-100 protein |

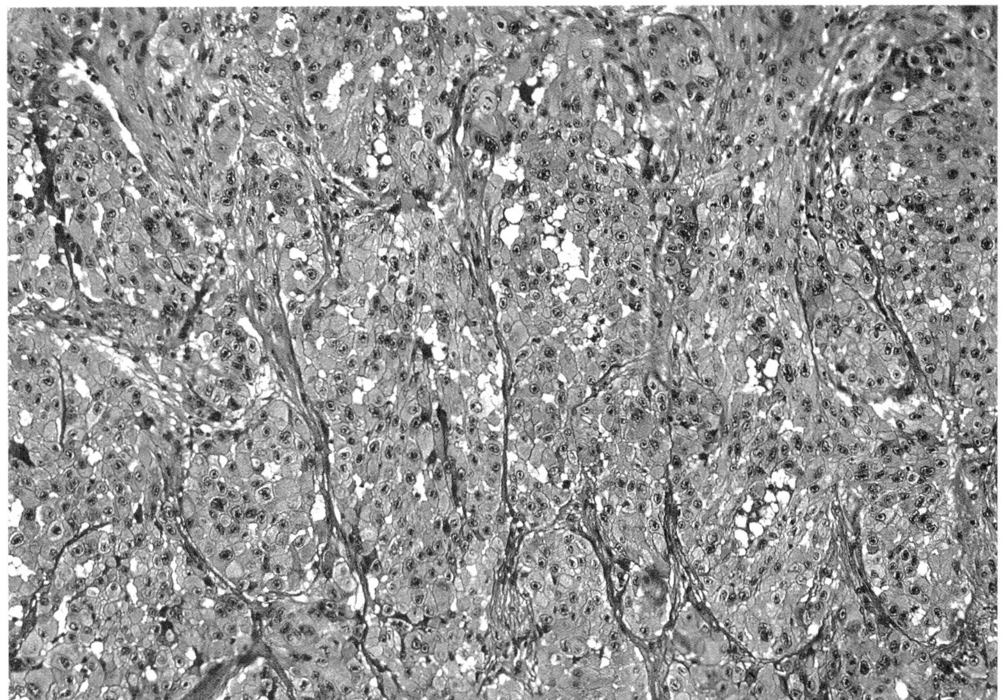

**FIGURE 37–37.** Metastatic renal cell carcinoma simulating an alveolar soft part sarcoma.

both tumors, but it is absent in *granular cell tumor* and *paraganglioma*. It is also noteworthy that the cells of granular cell tumor are less well defined, have a distinctly granular cytoplasm, and show strongly positive immunostaining for S-100 protein; moreover, they do not display the rich vascular pattern of alveolar soft part sarcoma.

The clinical features are also of value in the differential diagnosis. Primary renal cell carcinomas are usually demonstrable radiographically in the retroperitoneum. Renal cell carcinoma, paraganglioma, and malignant granular cell tumor chiefly affect patients over 40 years of age; they are rare in patients younger than 25 years. Moreover, as mentioned elsewhere, there is no record that a "bona fide" paraganglioma has ever occurred in the extremities.

## Discussion

Despite numerous immunohistochemical and electron microscopic studies, the exact nature and tissue type of alveolar soft part sarcoma remains uncertain. Over the years, several concepts concerning the nature of this tumor have been entertained. A variant of paraganglioma was first proposed by Smetana and Scott,[204] who emphasized the morphologic resemblance of alveolar soft part sarcoma to paraganglioma and favored a chemoreceptor origin. They stressed the close ultrastructural resemblance between alveolar soft part sarcomas and carotid body tumors, including the presence of chief cells, peripheral spindle-shaped cells, and electron-dense secretory-like granules. Strong evidence against this concept, however, is not only the abundance of glycogen and PAS-positive, diastase-resistant crystalline material in the tumor cells but also that the cells of alveolar soft part sarcomas are not argyrophilic with Grimelius stain, do not stain with antibodies to neurofilaments, chromogranin, synaptophysin, serotonin, and met-enkephalin, and contain no intracellular catecholamines as indicated by the complete absence of formaldehyde vapor-induced fluorescence in the tumor cells.[156,184] Furthermore, alveolar soft part sarcomas differ in several clinical aspects from paragangliomas. They prevail in patients younger than 30 years, involve chiefly the extremities, and behave in a malignant manner with frequent metastasis to lung, brain, and bone. There is also some question as to the existence of paraganglionic structures in the muscles of the extremities. We have never encountered paraganglia or related structures in the soft tissues of the limbs, nor were they detected by Karnauchow and Magner,[171] who carried out a systematic search for such structures in the thigh.

Skeletal muscle differentiation has been suggested by many over the years, but a number of studies have also detracted from this concept. Fisher and Reidbord[159] first suggested the possibility of skeletal

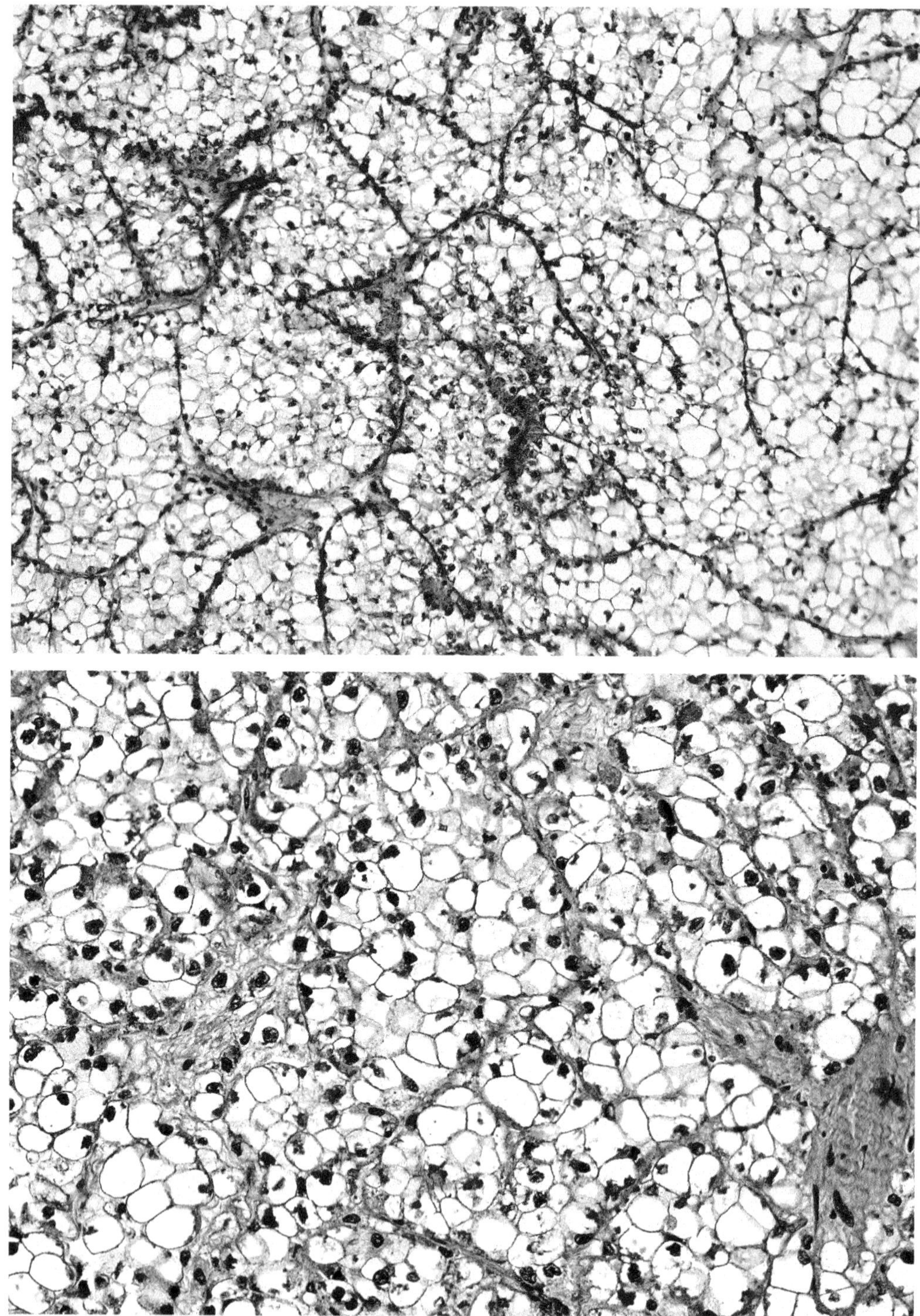

**FIGURE 37–38.** Alveolar soft part sarcoma simulating a renal cell carcinoma of clear cell type. The cytoplasmic clearing likely represents a degenerative feature of this tumor.

muscle differentiation on the basis of the resemblance of the membrane-bound crystals to those in nemaline myopathy and rhabdomyoma. This concept was strengthened by immunohistochemical studies that demonstrated the potential of the tumor cells to express desmin and muscle-specific actin. Others, however, were unable to confirm these results or, finding only a few desmin-positive cells, questioned their significance.[147,174] Although the initial detection of MyoD1 in a case of alveolar soft part sarcoma reported by Rosai et al.[199] seemed to lend support to the concept of skeletal muscle differentiation, others have been unable to duplicate this finding.[154,163,209] On balance, there is no convincing evidence that alveolar soft part sarcomas exhibit skeletal muscle differentiation using more sophisticated techniques.

Still another concept of the histogenesis was offered by DeSchryver-Kecskemeti et al.,[155] who contended that the cytoplasmic granules of alveolar soft part sarcomas are similar to the renin granules of juxtaglomerular tumors and proposed the name "angioreninoma." There is, however, no sign of hyperreninism (e.g., hypertension, hypokalemia, aldosteronism) in patients with alveolar soft part sarcoma; according to Mukai et al.,[184] immunostaining for renin is negative and plasma renin levels are normal. Moreover, similar PAS-positive crystals have been observed in a human muscle spindle[150] and in a variety of tumors, including rhabdomyoma, islet cell tumor, paraganglioma, schwannoma, and Warthin's tumor.

### Clinical Behavior and Therapy

The ultimate prognosis is poor despite the relatively slow growth of the tumor. Lieberman et al.,[174] in a study of 91 cases with follow-up information, reported a 77% survival rate at 2 years, 60% at 5 years, and 38% at 10 years in patients who presented without metastasis. Only 15% of the patients were alive after 20 years. Auerbach and Brooks[147] reported an overall 5-year survival rate of 67%. Metastases tend to occur early in the course of the disease, and there are many reports of patients who present with pulmonary or brain metastasis. On the other hand, metastasis may also be delayed for many years; Lillehei et al.[176] reported a patient who developed brain metastases 33 years after the initial presentation, emphasizing the need for long-term follow-up.

The most important prognostic parameters appear to be age at diagnosis, tumor size, and the presence of metastasis at presentation.[162,174,195] In the study by Lieberman et al.[174] there was an increased risk of metastasis at presentation with increasing age, as only 17% of patients who presented during the first decade of life had metastatic disease compared to 32% in patients older than 30 years of age. Improved prognosis in children may in part be related to the location of the tumor, its small size, and its better resectability.[157] In addition, patients who present with metastatic disease tend to have primary tumors that are larger than those in patients who do not have metastasis at presentation.[174] Although the development of metastatic disease clearly worsens the prognosis,[174] resection of solitary brain metastases may be of prognostic benefit.[148,208] The principal metastatic sites are the lungs, followed by the brain and skeleton. Metastasis to lymph nodes are infrequent.

Treatment is not particularly promising, and the relatively slow growth of the tumor must be considered when one is assessing the effect of therapy. Most reviewers recommend radical surgical excision of primary and metastatic lesions combined with radiotherapy or chemotherapy (or both). There is no consensus as to the effect of chemotherapy; according to Lieberman et al.,[174] there is little difference in survival rates between patients treated by postoperative irradiation or chemotherapy, although Sherman et al.[201] reported improved local control with adjuvant radiotherapy in patients without metastatic disease at presentation.

## EPITHELIOID SARCOMA

The term *epithelioid sarcoma* has been applied to a morphologically distinctive neoplasm that is likely to be confused with a variety of benign and malignant conditions, especially a granulomatous process, a synovial sarcoma, and an ulcerating squamous cell carcinoma. The tumor mainly afflicts young adults; its principal sites are the fingers, hands, and forearms. In fact, epithelioid sarcoma is the most common soft tissue sarcoma in the hand and wrist, followed by alveolar rhabdomyosarcoma and synovial sarcoma. It is not surprising, therefore, that earlier tumors were described as synovial sarcoma,[211] sarcoma aponeuroticum,[220] and large cell sarcoma of the tendon sheath.[213]

### Clinical Findings

Epithelioid sarcoma is most prevalent in adolescents and young adults 10–35 years of age (median age 26 years).[216,224] It is rare in children and older persons,[238,240] but no age group is exempt. Male patients outnumber females by about 2:1.[216,257] The racial distribution is similar to that in the overall population. As mentioned, the tumor has a propensity to occur in the finger, hand, and forearm, followed in frequency by the knee and lower leg, especially the pretibial region, the buttocks and thigh, the shoulder and arm, and the ankle, foot, and toe (Table 37–8). It is rare in the trunk and head and neck region[242,244,276] with the exception of the scalp. Other unusual sites include the penis[222,236,253] and vulva.[235,241]

**TABLE 37-8 ANATOMIC DISTRIBUTION OF 215 EPITHELIOID SARCOMAS**

| Location | No. of Patients | % |
|---|---|---|
| Hand/fingers | 65 | 30 |
| Forearm/wrist | 37 | 17 |
| Knee/lower leg | 31 | 15 |
| Buttock/thigh | 22 | 10 |
| Shoulder/arm | 20 | 9 |
| Ankle/foot/toes | 19 | 9 |
| Trunk | 12 | 6 |
| Head and neck | 9 | 4 |
| *Total* | 215 | 100.0 |

From Chase DR, Enzinger FM. Epithelioid sarcoma: diagnosis, prognostic indicators, and treatment. Am J Surg Pathol 9:241, 1985.

The tumor occurs in both the subcutis and deeper tissues. When located in the subcutis, it usually presents as a firm nodule that may be solitary or multiple, has a callus-like consistency, and is often described as a "woody hard knot" or "firm lump" that is slow-growing and painless. Nodules situated in the dermis are often elevated above the skin surface and frequently become ulcerated weeks or months after they are first noted. Such lesions are often erroneously diagnosed as an "indurated ulcer," "draining abscess," or "infected wart" that fails to heal despite intensive therapy (Figs. 37–39, 37–40, 37–41). Deep-seated lesions are usually firmly attached to tendons, tendon sheaths, or fascial structures; they tend to be larger and less well defined and manifest as areas of induration or as multinodular lumpy masses, sometimes moving slightly with motion of the extremity (Fig. 37–42). Pain or tenderness is rarely a prominent symptom, with the exception of the tumors that encroach on large nerves. The size of the tumor varies substantially and ranges from a few millimeters to 15 cm or more. Most of the tumors, however, measure 3–6 cm in diameter. Because many lesions are multinodular, determination of their exact size is often impossible.

Radiographic examination typically reveals a soft tissue mass with an occasional speckled pattern of calcification. Cortical thinning and erosion of underlying bone may be present, but invasion and destruction of adjacent bone are rare. MRI is useful for revealing the anatomic extent of the tumor.[260]

## Pathologic Findings

Gross inspection usually shows the presence of one or more nodules measuring 0.5–5.0 cm in greatest diameter. Deep-seated tumors, attached to tendons or fascia, tend to be larger and present as firm, multinodular masses with irregular outlines. The cut surface has a glistening gray-white or gray-tan mottled surface with focal yellow or brown areas caused by focal necrosis or hemorrhage.

The principal microscopic characteristics are the distinct nodular arrangement of the tumor cells, their tendency to undergo central degeneration and necrosis, and their epithelioid appearance and cytoplasmic eosinophilia. The nodular pattern, probably the most conspicuous single feature of epithelioid sarcoma, varies somewhat. In some tumors the nodules are well circumscribed; in others they are less well defined and are often compacted into irregular multinodular masses (Figs. 37–43, 37–44, 37–45). Multiple nodules are less common in tissue obtained at the initial operation than in recurrent tumors. In rare cases the presence of multiple small superficial satellite nodules near the operative site may mimic a skin disease.[234] Necrosis of the tumor nodules is a common finding (Fig. 37–46); it is most prominent in the center of the nodules and at times is associated with hemorrhage and cystic change. Fusion of several necrotizing nodules results in a "geographic" lesion with scalloped margins (Fig. 37–47). When the tumor spreads within a fascia or aponeurosis, it forms fes-

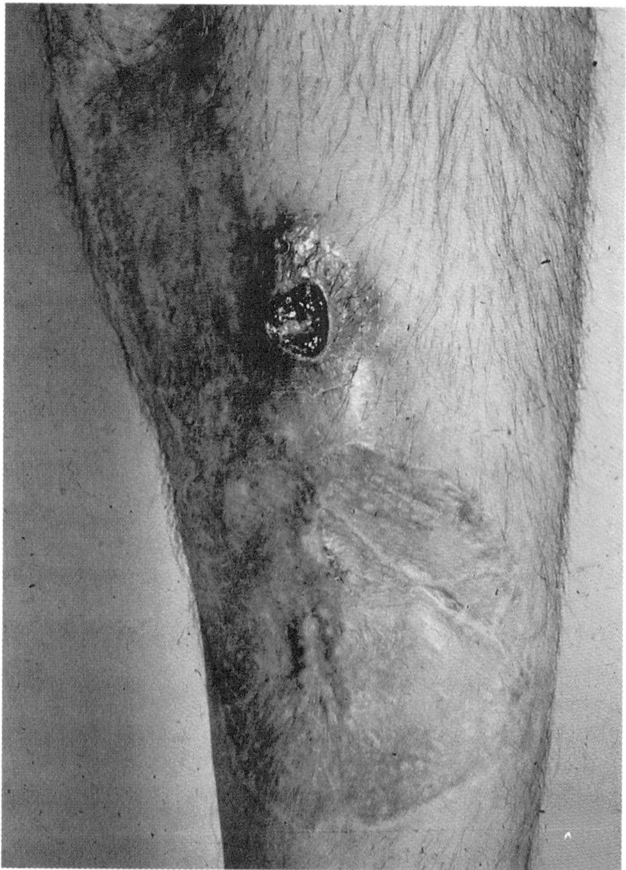

**FIGURE 37–39.** Recurrent ulcerating epithelioid sarcoma of the anterior tibial region in a 21-year-old man.

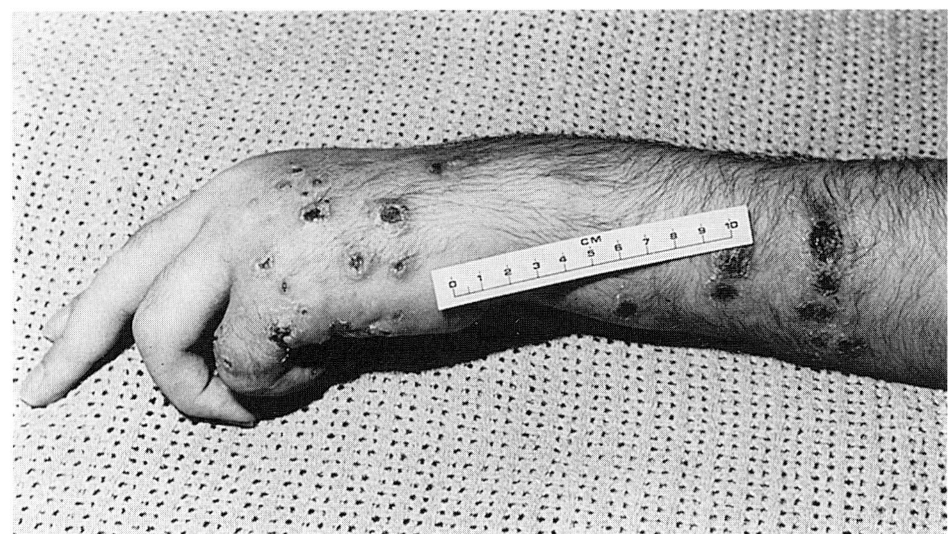


**FIGURE 37–40.** Recurrent epithelioid sarcoma of the hand and forearm with multiple, ulcerated (punched-out) satellite lesions of the skin. (From Heenan P, Quirk CJ, Papadimitriou JM. Epithelioid sarcoma: a diagnostic problem. Am J Dermatopathol 8:95, 1986.)

toon-like or garland-like bands punctuated by areas of necrosis. Not infrequently the tumor grows along the neurovascular bundle and invests large vessels or nerves. Vascular invasion takes place, but in our experience it is rarely a prominent feature of the tumor.

Lesions located or extending into the dermis often ulcerate through the skin and may simulate an ulcerating squamous cell carcinoma, especially because of the pronounced epithelioid appearance and eosinophilia of the tumor cells. This process occurs mainly in areas with small amounts of subcutaneous fat such as the fingers and the prepatellar and pretibial regions.

The constituent cellular elements range from large ovoid or polygonal cells with deeply eosinophilic cytoplasm (suggesting a rhabdomyosarcoma or malignant rhabdoid tumor) to plump spindle-shaped cells (reminiscent of a fibrosarcoma or malignant fibrous histiocytoma) (Figs. 37–48, 37–49, 37–50). In some of the latter tumors the spindle cell pattern predominates and obscures the characteristic epithelioid features and nodularity (Figs. 37–51, 37–52). The "fibroma-like variant of epithelioid sarcoma" reported by Mirra et al.[251] is presumably of this type. In general, cellular pleomorphism is minimal. Usually, epithelioid and spindle-shaped cells merge imperceptibly, and there is never the distinct biphasic or pseudoglandular pattern as in synovial sarcomas (Fig.

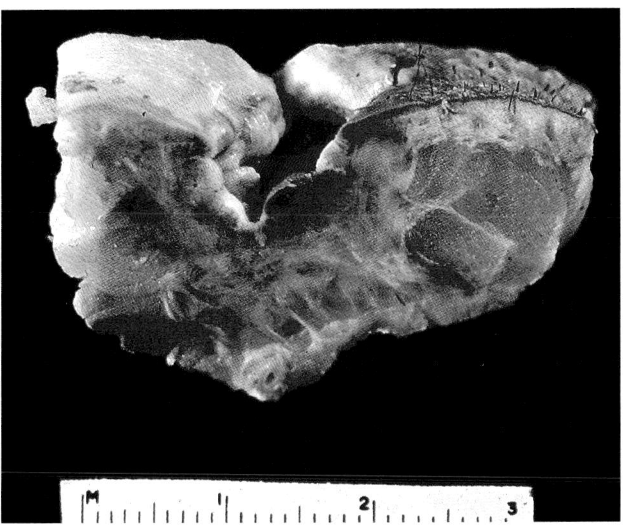

**FIGURE 37–41.** Ulcerating epithelioid sarcoma of the hand with indurated margins.

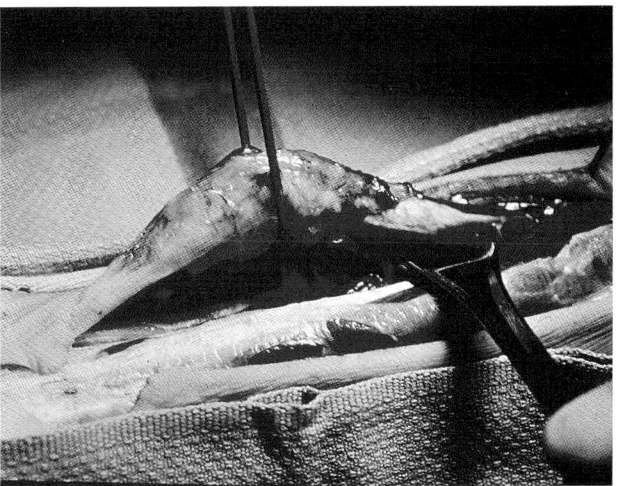

**FIGURE 37–42.** Epithelioid sarcoma of the wrist infiltrating the tendon of the flexor carpi ulnaris in a 28-year-old man. (From Enzinger FM. Epithelioid sarcoma: a sarcoma simulating a granuloma or a carcinoma. Cancer 26:1029, 1970.)

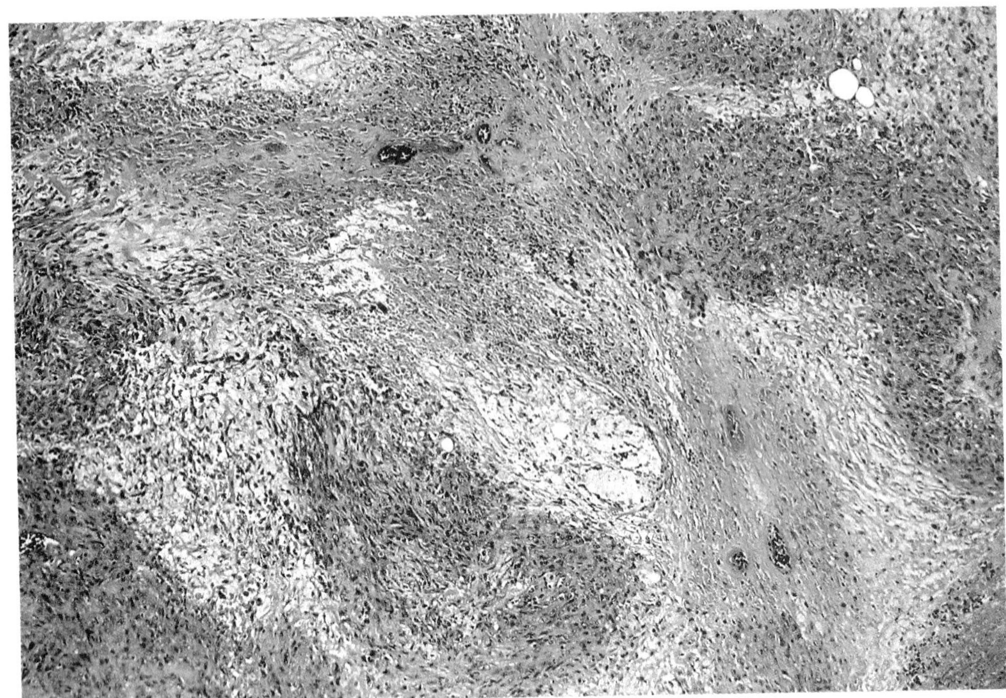

**FIGURE 37–43.** Typical low magnification appearance of an epithelioid sarcoma with a pseudogranulomatous pattern.

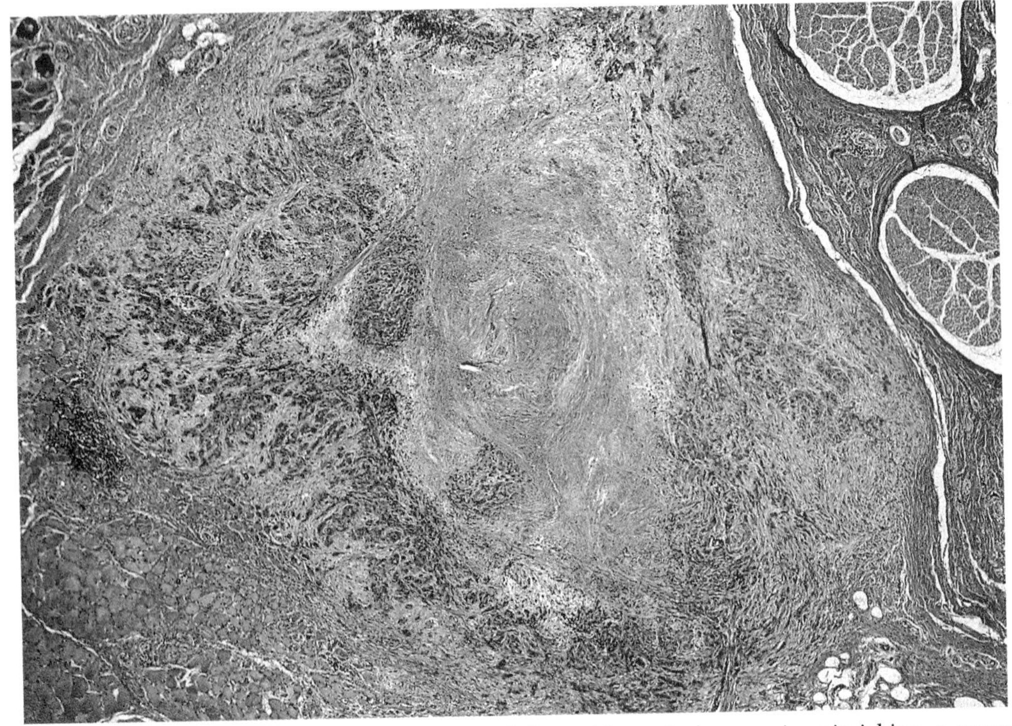

**FIGURE 37–44.** Epithelioid sarcoma. Note the nodules with central necrosis mimicking a necrotizing granulomatous process.

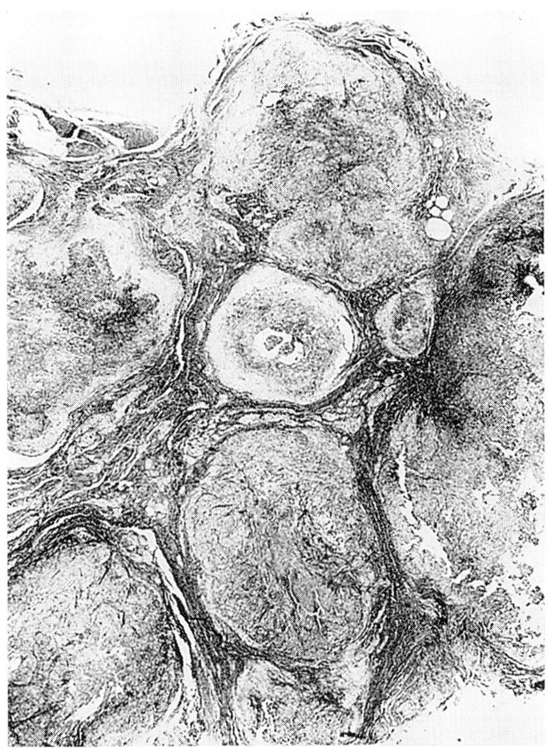

**FIGURE 37-45.** Epithelioid sarcoma with a conglomerate of tumor nodules with central necrosis. (From Enzinger FM. Epithelioid sarcoma: a sarcoma simulating a granuloma or a carcinoma. Cancer 26:1029, 1970.)

37-53). In some tumors the loss of cellular cohesion and secondary hemorrhage may closely simulate an angiosarcoma; in others the presence of intracellular lipid droplets suggests the incipient lumen formation of endothelial cells seen in epithelioid hemangioendotheliomas. Intercellular deposition of dense hyalinized collagen is common and, together with the eosinophilic cytoplasm, contributes to the deeply eosinophilic appearance of the tumor. Calcification and bone formation are found in 10-20% of cases, but cartilaginous metaplasia is rare[218] (Fig. 37-54). Aggregates of chronic inflammatory cells along the peripheral margin of the tumor nodules are present in most cases and may mimic a chronic inflammatory process (Fig. 37-55).

Special staining techniques contribute little to the diagnosis. The cytoplasm stains a deep red-brown with the Masson trichrome stain. There is no stainable intracellular mucin, but alcian blue-positive and hyaluronidase-sensitive mesenchymal mucin is often found in the surrounding matrix. There may also be some intracellular glycogen.

## Immunohistochemical Findings

Most epithelioid sarcomas stain for both low- and high-molecular weight cytokeratins (Fig. 37-56), epi-

*Text continued on page 1532*

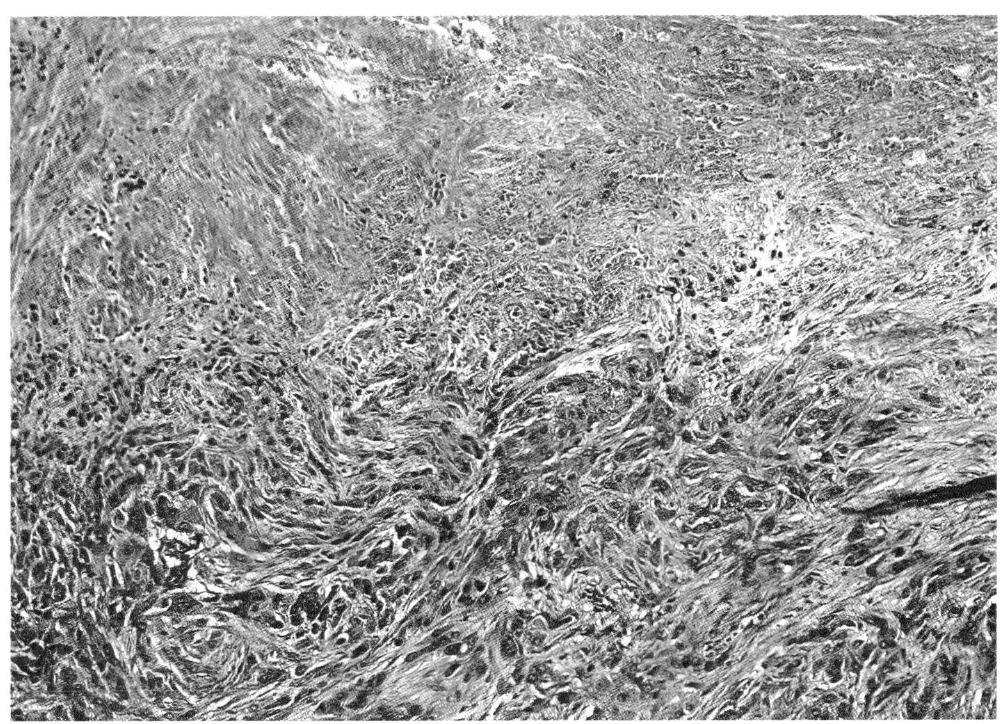

**FIGURE 37-46.** Epithelioid sarcoma with central necrosis of the tumor nodule.

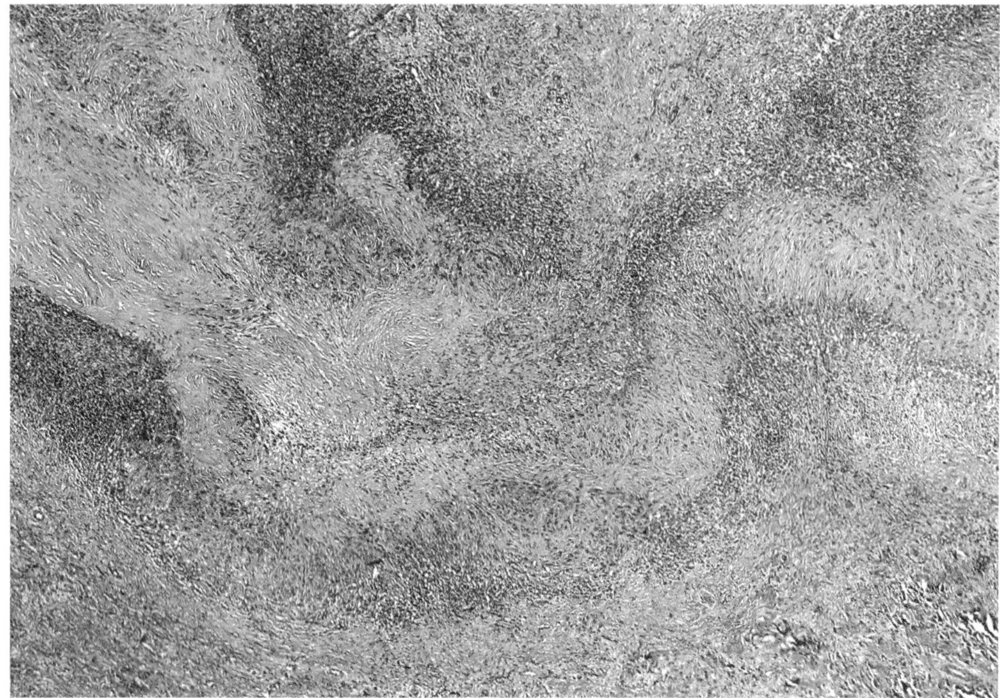

**FIGURE 37–47.** Epithelioid sarcoma. Fusion of several necrotizing nodules results in areas of geographic necrosis with scalloped margins.

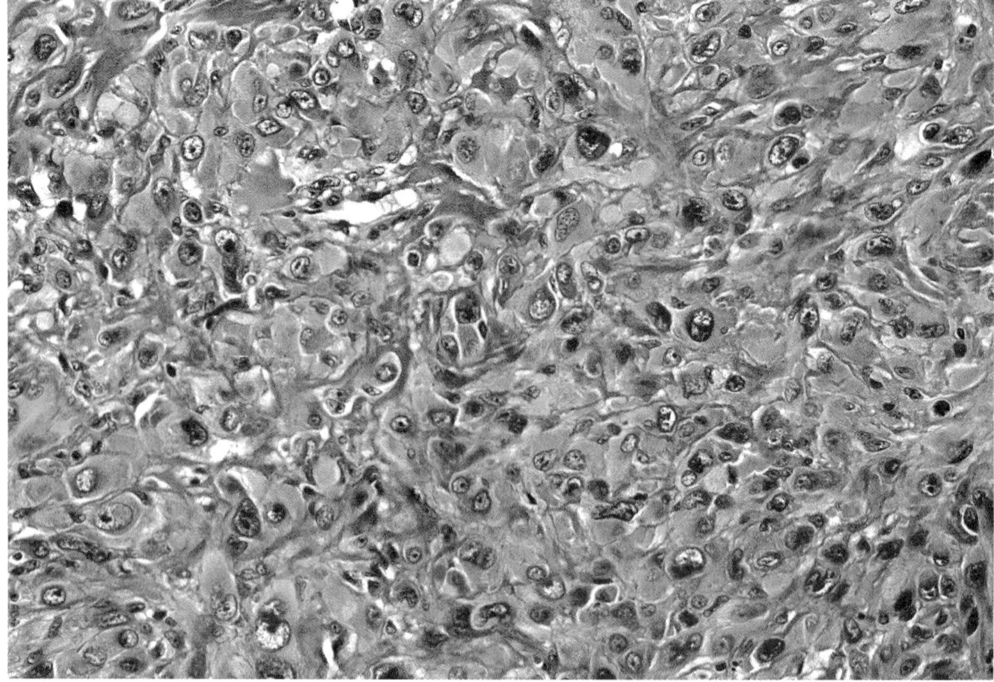

**FIGURE 37–48.** Cytologic features of malignant epithelioid cells in an epithelioid sarcoma.

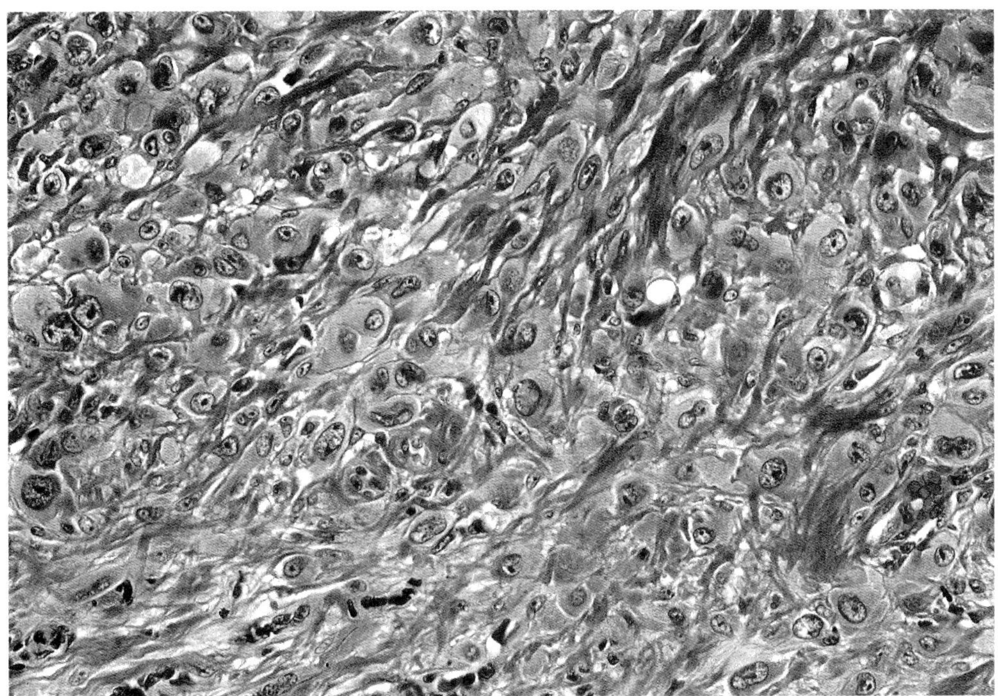

**FIGURE 37–49.** Close interplay between collagen and malignant epithelioid cells with densely eosinophilic cytoplasm in an epithelioid sarcoma.

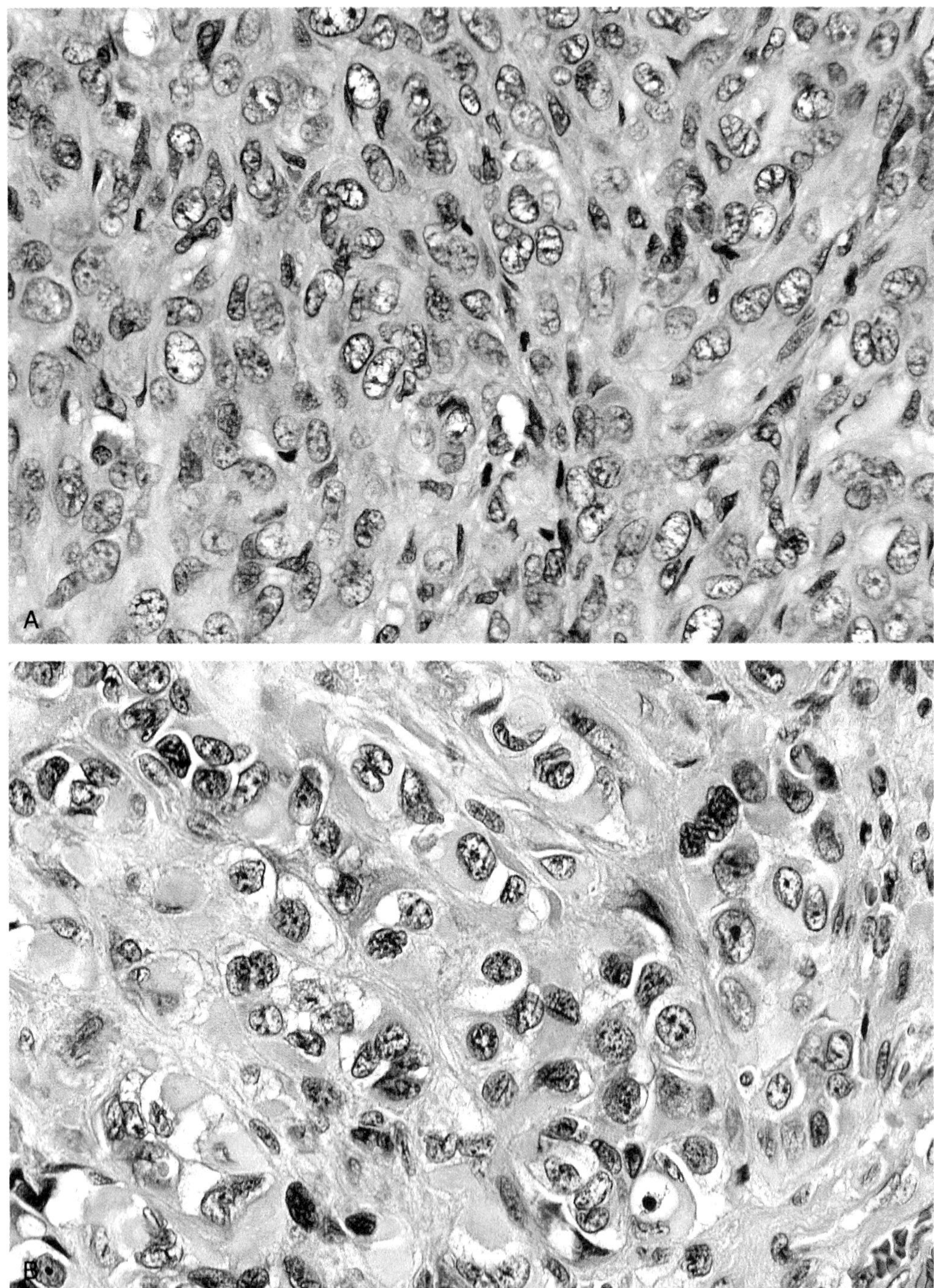


**FIGURE 37–50.** (**A, B**) Cytologic appearance of malignant epithelioid cells in epithelioid sarcoma. Most of the tumor cells have abundant deeply eosinophilic cytoplasm.

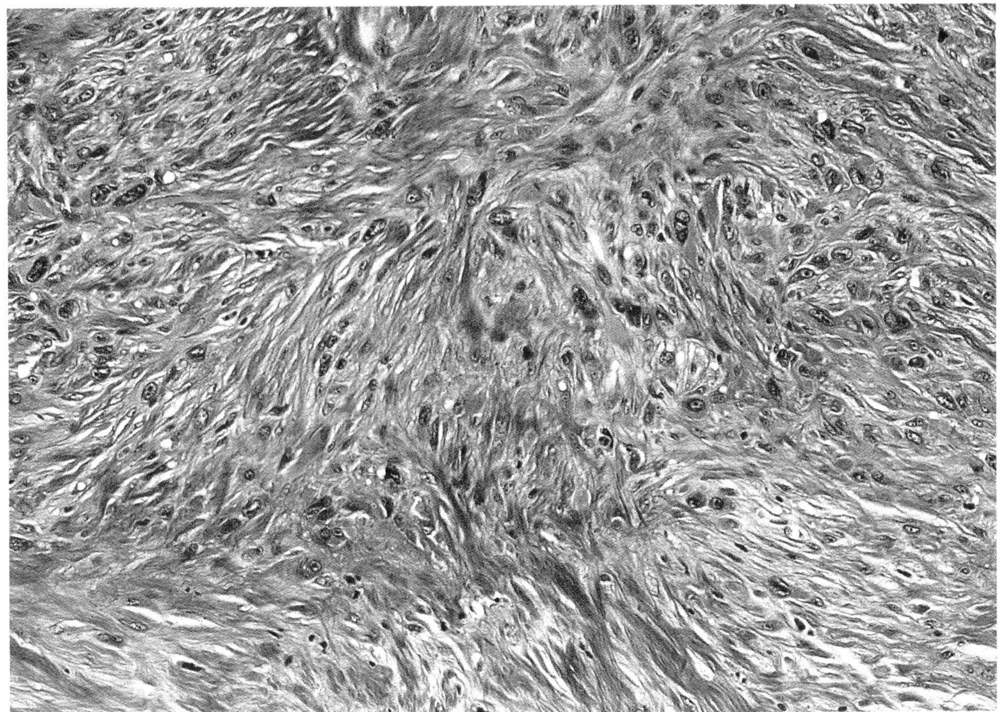

**FIGURE 37–51.** Epithelioid sarcoma with a predominantly spindle cell pattern.

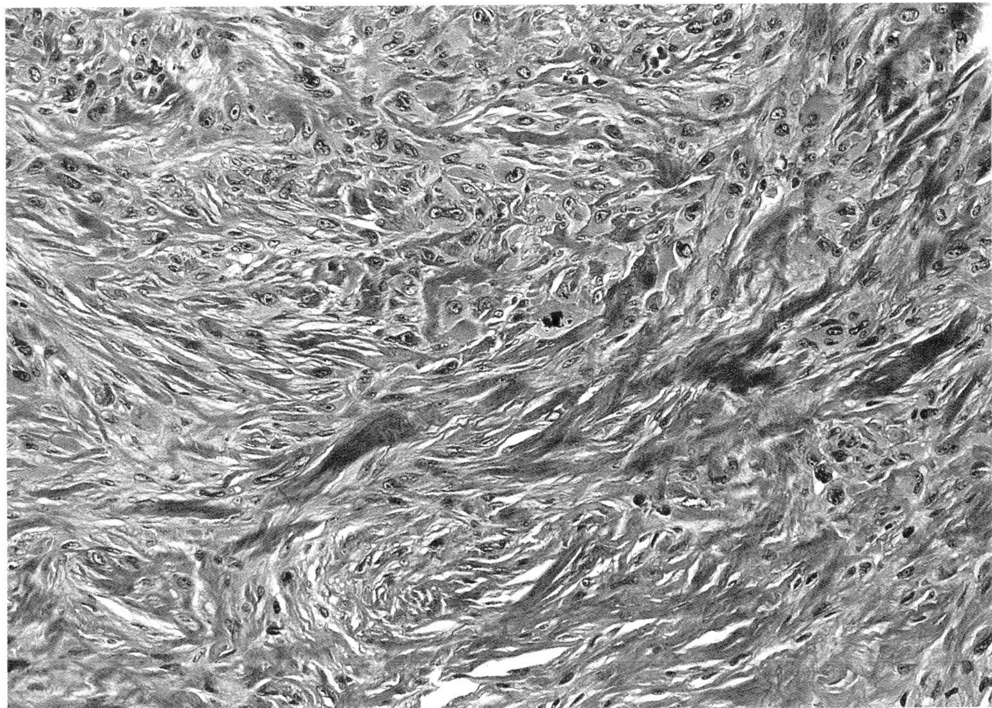

**FIGURE 37–52.** Interplay between dense collagen bundles and malignant spindle cells in an epithelioid sarcoma.

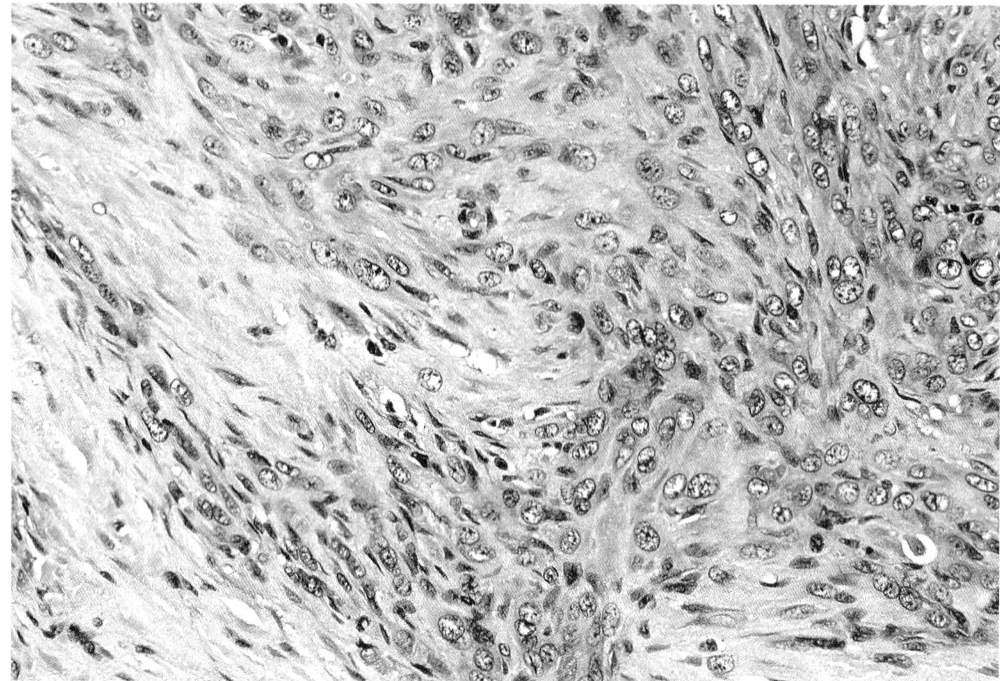

**FIGURE 37–53.** Transition from epithelioid to spindle cells and interdigitating collagen bundles in an epithelioid sarcoma.

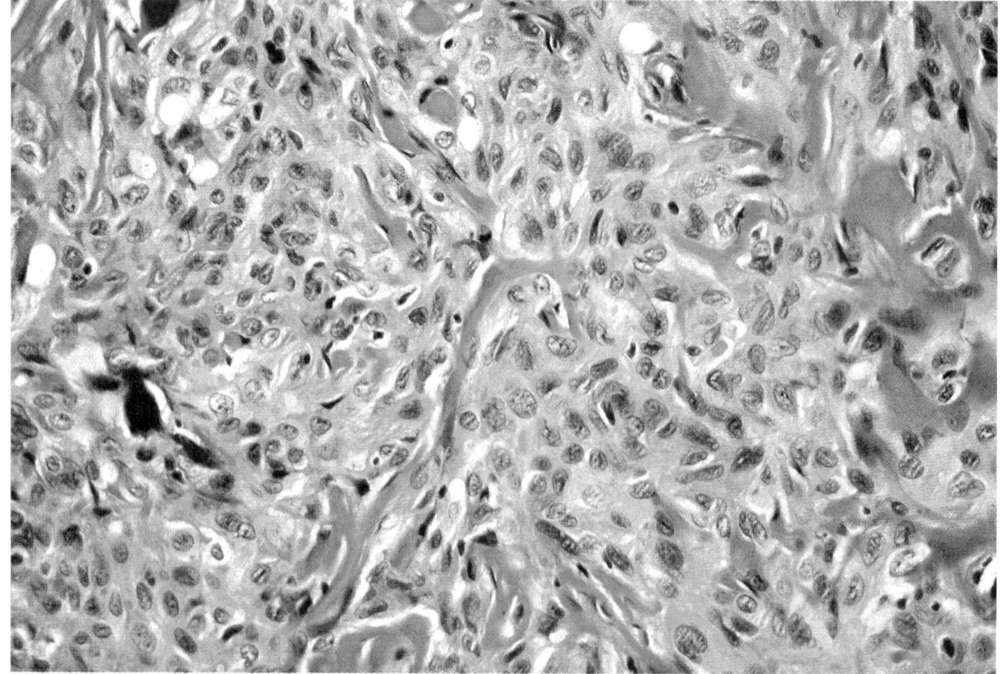

**FIGURE 37–54.** Focal calcifications in an epithelioid sarcoma, an unusual feature of this neoplasm.

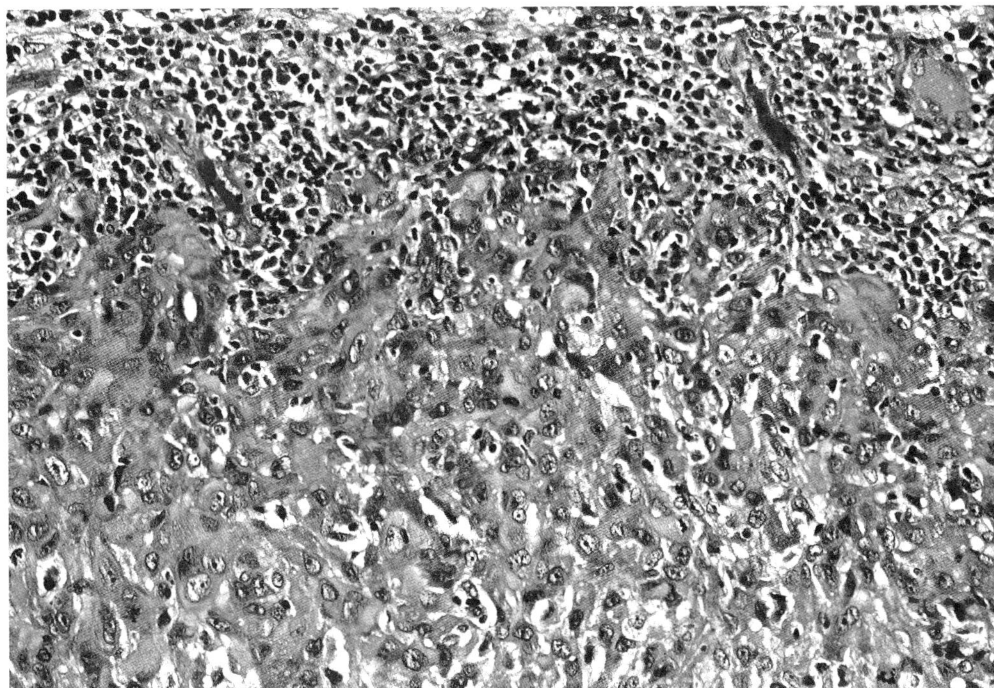

**FIGURE 37–55.** Aggregates of chronic inflammatory cells along the peripheral margin of a tumor nodule in an epithelioid sarcoma.

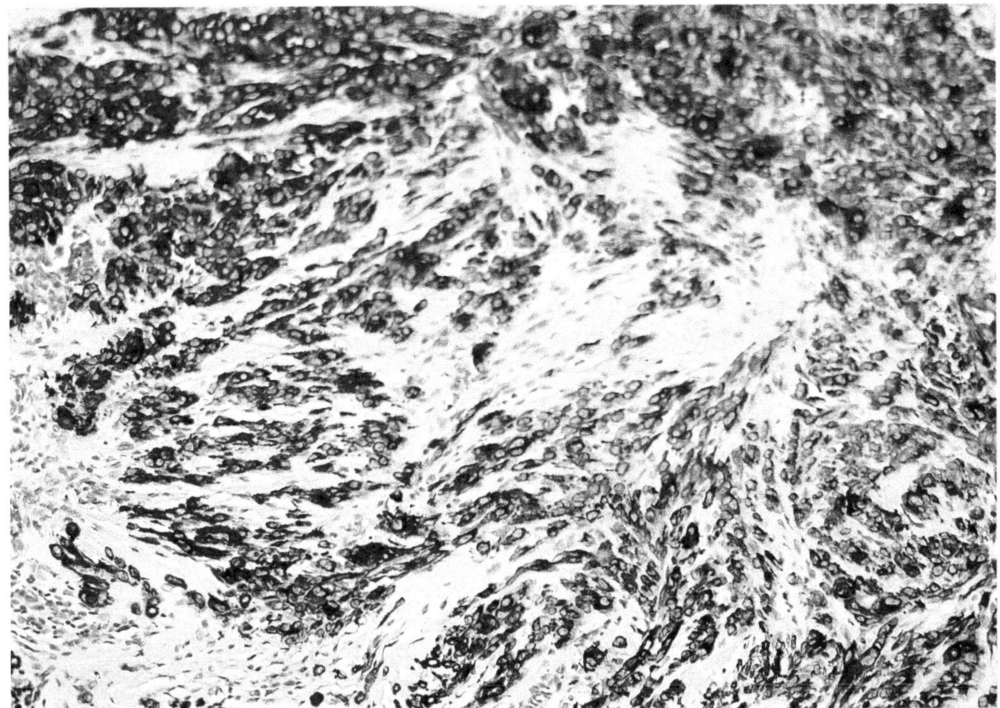

**FIGURE 37–56.** Strong cytokeratin immunoreactivity typical of epithelioid sarcoma.

thelial membrane antigen, and vimentin.[217,221,226,255] The degree of immunoreactivity, however, varies considerably from tumor to tumor and in different portions of the same neoplasm. Usually the presence of cytokeratin is more pronounced in epithelioid areas than in spindled areas. In addition, up to 60–70% of cases stain for CD-34,[248,274] a finding that may be useful in epithelioid sarcomas that do not stain for vimentin[210] (Fig. 37–57). Antibodies directed against S-100 protein, neurofilament protein, carcinoembryonic antigen, factor VIII-related antigen, and CD-31 are typically negative.

## Ultrastructural Findings

Most investigators report polygonal and spindle-shaped cells with ovoid, indented nuclei containing small amounts of marginally placed chromatin. The cytoplasm contains arrays of rough endoplasmic reticulum, a prominent Golgi apparatus, free ribosomes, and occasional mitochondria, lysosomes, and droplets of osmiophilic material. Intermediate filaments are a common, often striking feature. They may be arranged longitudinally as in myofibroblasts, but they more often form paranuclear masses or whorls, a feature that probably accounts for the voluminous cytoplasm and the striking epithelioid (and often rhabdoid) appearance of the tumor cells[239,246,250] (Fig. 37–58). There are occasionally interdigitating cellular processes with maculae adherens or intercellular desmosome-like junctions and small intercellular cystic or cleft-like spaces surrounded by filopodia. As in synovial sarcomas there may be light and dark tumor cells; but unlike this tumor's glandular structures, intracellular cystic spaces and basal laminae are absent in the epithelioid sarcoma.[249,252,273]

## Cytogenetic Findings

Cytogenetic data for epithelioid sarcomas are relatively limited. Cordoba et al.[219] described a case with a t(8;22)(q22;q11), and Quezado et al.[259] described allelic loss on 22q in six of ten informative cases. The 22q site is the location of the NF2 tumor suppressor gene, and abnormalities of this gene predispose to the hereditary tumor neurofibromatosis type 2 syndrome.[272] Interestingly, Rose et al.[261] described an epithelioid sarcoma arising in a patient with neurofibromatosis type 2. Other cytogenetic abnormalities described in this tumor include gains at 11q, 1q, 6p and 9q[244a] and aberrations of 18q[238] and 8q.[267]

## Differential Diagnosis

The frequency with which the tumor is mistaken for a benign process is chiefly a result of its deceptively harmless appearance during the initial stage of the disease. Small superficially located tumors with a

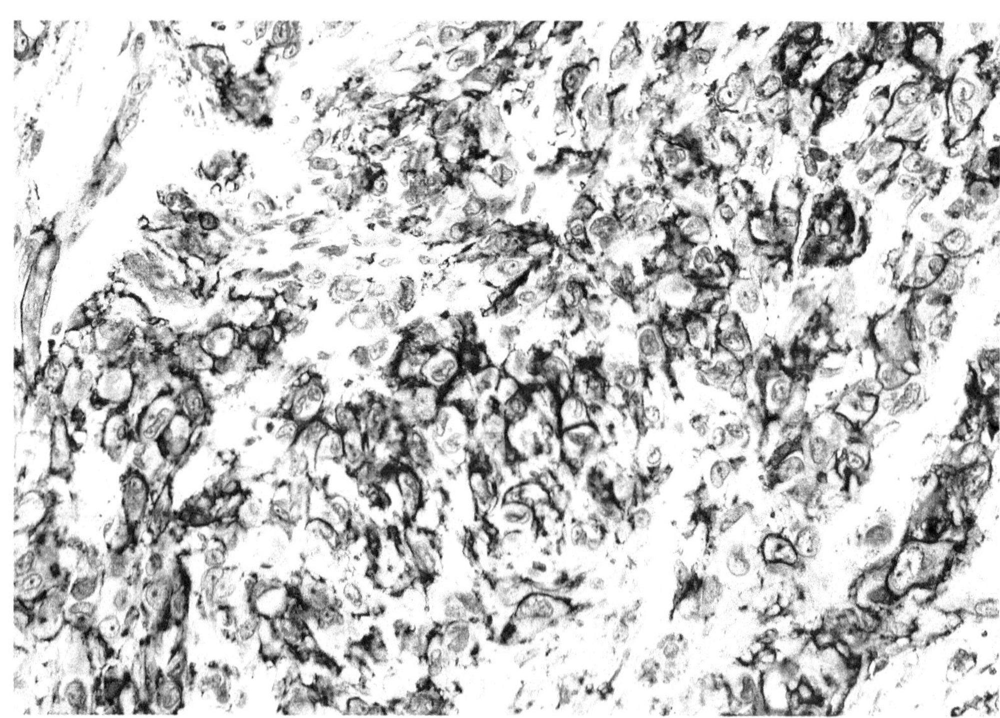

**FIGURE 37–57.** Membranous immunoreactivity for CD34 in an epithelioid sarcoma. This antigen is found in up to 70% of cases.

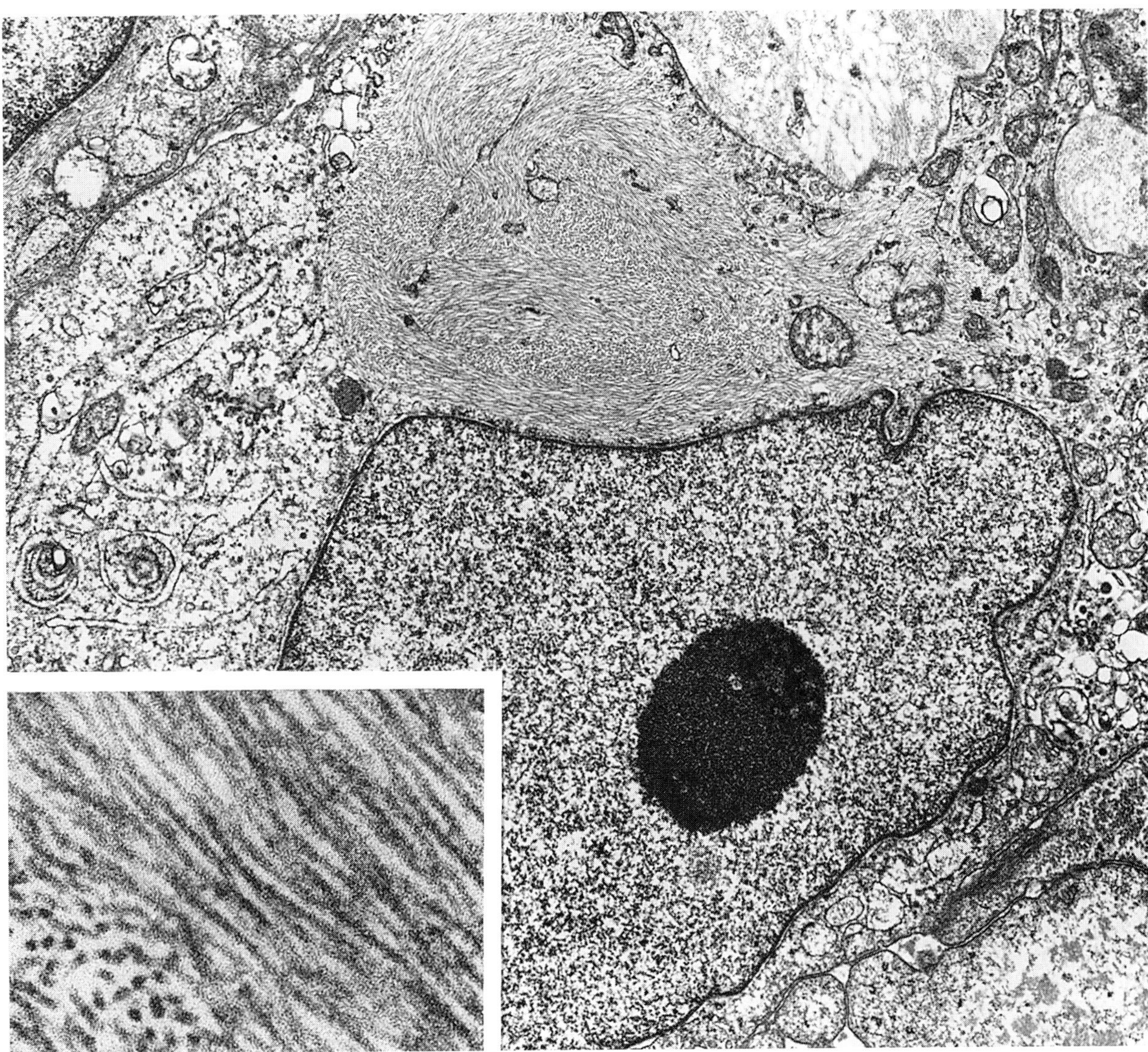

**FIGURE 37–58.** Ultrastructure of an epithelioid sarcoma showing polygonal cells with a paranuclear mass of intermediate filaments. (**Inset**) High-power view of intracytoplasmic bundles of intermediate filaments ranging in diameter from 7 to 12 nm. (From Mukai M, Torikata C, Iri H, et al. Cellular differentiation of epithelioid sarcoma: an electron-microscopic, enzyme histochemical, and immunohistochemical study. Am J Pathol 119:44, 1985.)

nodular or multinodular pattern are likely to be mistaken for an inflammatory process, particularly a *necrotizing infectious granuloma, necrobiosis lipoidica, granuloma annulare,* or *rheumatoid nodule.* In contrast to the latter processes, the individual cells in the epithelioid sarcoma tend to be more sharply defined, are larger and more eosinophilic, and stain positively for cytokeratins and epithelial membrane antigen. The epithelioid features, nodularity, and immunostaining for cytokeratin also aid in differentiating epithelioid sarcoma from nodular fasciitis, fibrous histiocytoma, and fibromatosis.

Epithelioid sarcoma may also be mistaken for a wide array of epithelioid-appearing malignant soft tissue neoplasms (Fig. 37–59). The cytologic features of the constituent cells are reminiscent of those seen in both *epithelioid malignant peripheral nerve sheath tumor* (MPNST) and *melanoma.* Unlike epithelioid sarcoma, epithelioid MPNST tends to stain strongly for S-100 protein[243] and virtually never expresses cytokeratins, although epithelial membrane antigen may be rarely detected.[271] Similarly, malignant melanoma virtually always expresses S-100 protein, and many lesions also stain for HMB-45.

This lesion also has overlapping features with those found in *epithelioid angiosarcoma.* Histologically, both

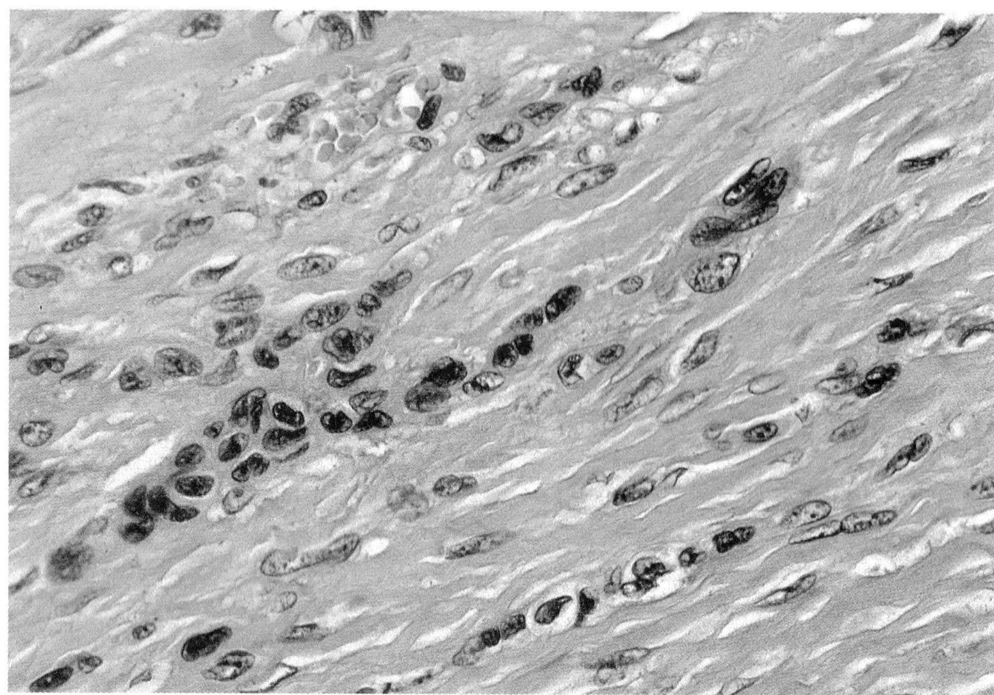

**FIGURE 37–59.** Peripheral portion of an epithelioid sarcoma with cording of epithelioid cells mimicking invasive lobular carcinoma of the breast.

are composed of large epithelioid cells, and both often have cells with cytoplasmic vacuoles. Furthermore, epithelioid sarcoma may have a hemorrhagic pseudoangiosarcomatous pattern.[231] Confusion between these two entities is compounded by the fact that epithelioid angiosarcomas not uncommonly express cytokeratins,[228,247] and both may stain for CD-34. The absence of specific endothelial markers such as factor VIII-related antigen and CD-31 in epithelioid sarcoma allows their distinction.[266,275]

In some cases distinction from *synovial sarcoma* is difficult. It can be successfully accomplished in most cases, however, if attention is paid to the persistent absence of a biphasic pattern, pseudoglandular structures, intracellular mucin, and the larger size and prominent eosinophilia of the tumor cells in epithelioid sarcoma. Moreover, dermal involvement and ulceration are much more common with epithelioid sarcoma than with synovial sarcoma. In some cases the location of the tumor suggests the correct diagnosis. Epithelioid sarcomas are most common in the fingers and the hand, and synovial sarcomas prevail in the vicinity of the knee and other large joints. Immunohistochemically, cytokeratin 7 is expressed in most synovial sarcomas but is rare in epithelioid sarcomas.[233,248] Furthermore, synovial sarcomas rarely express CD-34.

Some epithelioid sarcomas are difficult to distinguish from ulcerating *squamous cell carcinoma*. However, epithelioid sarcoma lacks keratin pearls and dyskeratosis in the adjacent epithelium.

## "Proximal-type" Epithelioid Sarcoma

In 1997 Guillou et al.[231] described a "proximal-type" epithelioid sarcoma characterized by its propensity to arise in axial locations and its more aggressive behavior and histologically by a predominance of large epithelioid cells with marked cytologic atypia, frequently with intracytoplasmic hyaline inclusions, imparting a rhabdoid appearance to the tumor cells (Figs. 37–60, 37–61, 37–62). They were described as having an immunophenotype similar to that of classic epithelioid sarcoma, although some stained focally for desmin and smooth muscle actin.[231,278] As described, these tumors have many features overlapping those of malignant extrarenal rhabdoid tumors (discussed below). Although Guillou et al.[231] argued that a number of tumors reported as malignant extrarenal rhabdoid tumor arising in proximal locations represent this unusual form of epithelioid sarcoma, we are not yet convinced that the "proximal-type" epithelioid sarcoma represents a distinct clinicopathologic entity. In fact, we believe it more likely represents a variant of malignant extrarenal rhabdoid tumor. In either case it should not be confused with the classic form of epithelioid sarcoma. As yet, there are no cytogenetic data reported for this form of epithelioid sarcoma.

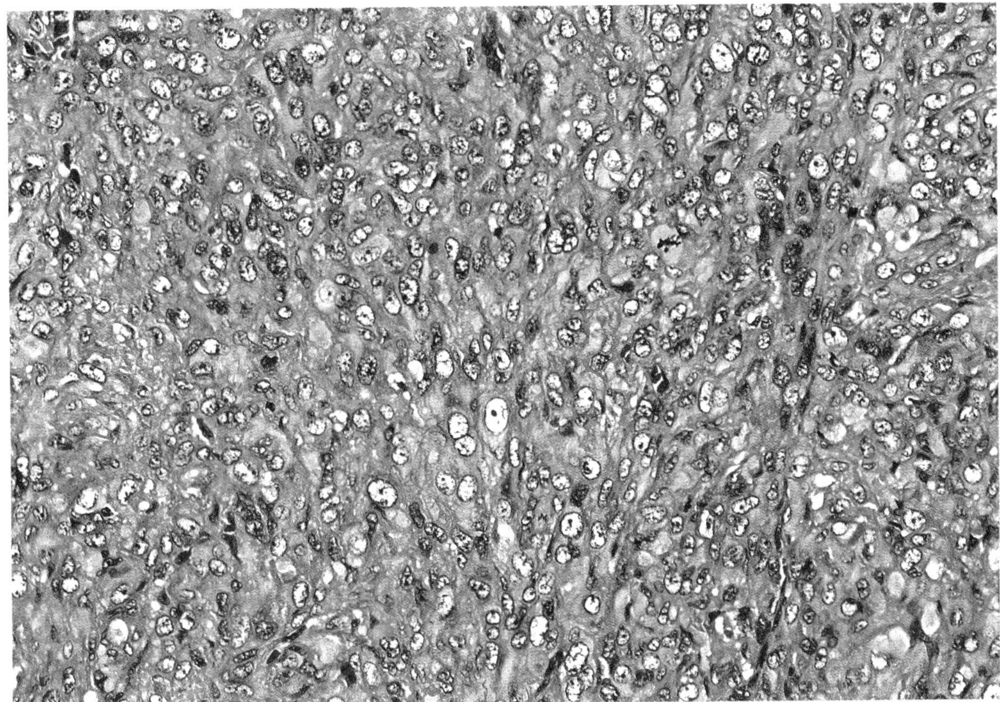

**FIGURE 37–60.** "Proximal-type" epithelioid sarcoma composed of sheets of large epithelioid cells with marked cytologic atypia.

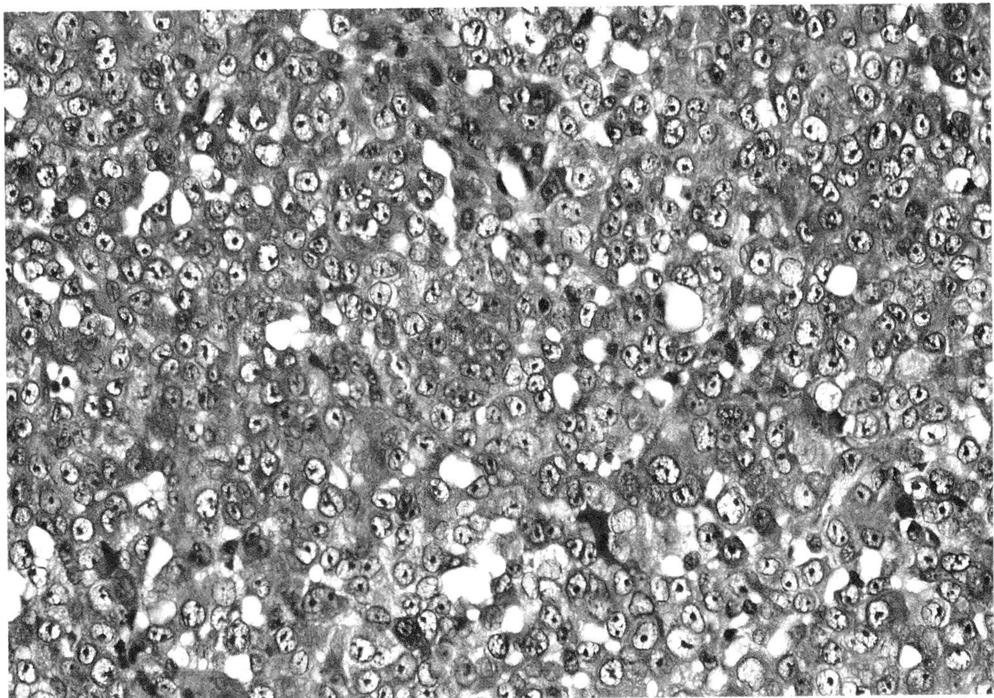

**FIGURE 37–61.** Sheets of large epithelioid cells with macronucleoli in a "proximal-type" epithelioid sarcoma.

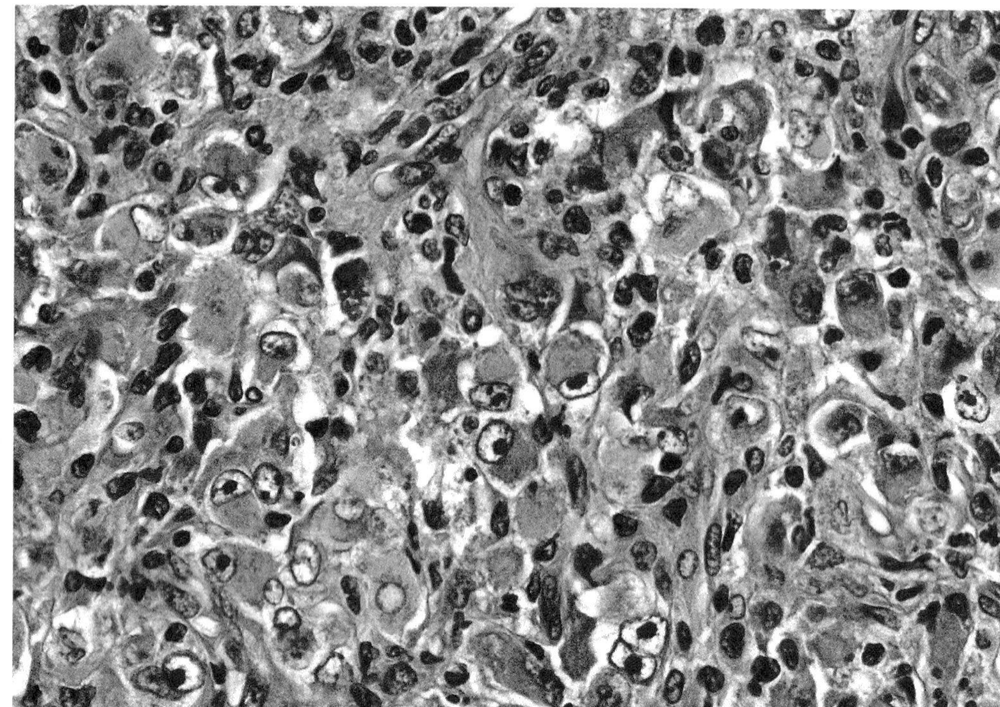

**FIGURE 37–62.** "Proximal-type" epithelioid sarcoma composed of large epithelioid cells with marked cytologic atypia and intracytoplasmic hyaline inclusions, imparting a rhabdoid appearance.

Interestingly, some examples of classic epithelioid sarcoma have aberrations of 22q similar to those described for malignant extrarenal rhabdoid tumor.

## Clinical Course and Therapy

Epithelioid sarcoma has a high risk for local recurrence and metastasis and requires long-term follow-up, given that recurrence or metastasis may occur many years after the initial diagnosis. In the study from the AFIP published in 1985,[216] follow-up data, available in 202 patients, showed recurrence and metastatic rates of 77% and 45%, respectively; 32% of patients died as a direct result of their tumor. The most common sites of metastasis were regional lymph nodes (34%) and the lung (51%) and less frequently the skin, central nervous system, and soft tissue (Table 37–9). The scalp was the site of metastasis in 22% of the cases. The interval between the initial surgical procedure and the first recurrence averaged 1 year 6 months in the fatal cases and 2 years 1 month in the nonfatal cases; the time to metastasis averaged 4 years 1 month in the fatal cases versus 3 years 4 months in the nonfatal cases.

Multiple recurrences, often as the result of marginal resection, are a characteristic feature of the tumor. One of the patients reported by Chase and Enzinger was treated for recurrent tumor growth in the left pretibial region on 11 occasions during a 16-year period.[216] Another patient had 20 surgical procedures for recurrent growth within a period of 10 years. The recurrent tumor generally presents as confluent nodules in the dermis or along tendons and fascial structures at or near the original tumor site. As previously mentioned, there are also cases where the skin adjacent and proximal to the tumor is studded with small, crater-like ulcerated nodules or plaques, a striking picture unlike that of any other recurrent soft tissue sarcoma.[234] In fact, the tendency for this tumor to track along an extremity some distance from the

**TABLE 37–9** SITE OF METASTATIC DISEASE IN 83 METASTASIZING EPITHELIOID SARCOMAS

| Location | No. of Cases | % |
|---|---|---|
| Lung | 42 | 51 |
| Lymph nodes | 28 | 34 |
| Scalp | 18 | 22 |
| Bone | 11 | 13 |
| Brain | 11 | 13 |
| Liver | 10 | 12 |
| Pleura | 9 | 11 |

Modified from Chase DR, Enzinger FM. Epithelioid sarcoma: diagnosis, prognostic indicators, and treatment. Am J Surg Pathol 9:241, 1985.

original scar suggests local "metastasis," rather than local "recurrence" in the strict sense of the word. Recurrence generally develops within the first year after diagnosis, but recurrence may be late; in one of the cases reported by Chase and Enzinger[216] it became apparent 25 years after the primary tumor was removed by local excision.

Intravascular growth and lymph node involvement are ominous features: in one series, for instance, six of eight patients with intravenous extension of the tumor or lymph node involvement developed pulmonary metastases. Conversely, 9 of 10 patients without these features were alive 2 to more than 13 years after diagnosis.[263] Metastasis may occur early in the course of disease and may even manifest before detection of the primary tumor,[270] or it may occur many years following the initial diagnosis. For example, one patient in the study from the AFIP developed metastatic disease 19 years after the initial diagnosis.[216] Prognosis therefore should be rendered with considerable caution, even if the patient appears to be well and free of tumor 5 years after the initial diagnosis.

Prognosis depends on various factors, including the gender of the patient, the site, size, and depth of the tumor, the number of mitotic figures, the presence or absence of hemorrhage, necrosis, and vascular invasion, and the adequacy of the initial excision (Table 37–10). In the series by Chase and Enzinger,[216] the survival rate for females was 78% compared to 64% for males. The improved outcome in females was even more pronounced in the series of Bos et al.,[215] who reported a 5-year survival rate of 80% in females compared to 40% in males.

Tumor site also appears to be prognostically important in that tumors arising in the distal extremities have a more favorable prognosis than those in the trunk and proximal portion of the limbs.[216] Large tumor size is also associated with a more aggressive clinical course.[225,232] For example, in the series by Evans and Baer,[225] six of seven patients with tumors 5 cm or larger developed metastasis, compared to only two of ten patients with smaller tumors.

**TABLE 37–10** REPORTED ADVERSE PROGNOSTIC FEATURES FOR EPITHELIOID SARCOMA

| |
|---|
| Male gender |
| Non-distal extremity tumors |
| Large tumor size (≥5 cm) |
| Increased tumor depth |
| High mitotic index |
| Hemorrhage |
| Necrosis |
| Vascular invasion |
| Inadequate initial excision |

Flow cytometric DNA analysis has revealed inconsistent results.[223,237,254] In the study from the Mayo Clinic,[232] 13 of 23 tumors were diploid, 6 were aneuploid, and 4 were tetraploid. Neither DNA content nor S-phase fraction correlated with clinical behavior.

Accurate assessment and comparison of the efficacy of treatment is difficult, especially if the cases are derived from multiple sources, as in the AFIP material. It is clearly evident, however, that the initial therapy (marginal resection) was inadequate in many cases and that a more aggressive surgical approach is required to prevent recurrent growth.[232,262,269] Adequate treatment requires early radical local excision or amputation if the primary tumor is situated in the fingers or toes. Amputation should also be considered as treatment for recurrent growth but does not seem to offer any benefit to patients with distant metastasis.[277] Regional lymph node dissection should be included among the therapeutic modalities because lymph node metastasis is a fairly common occurrence in epithelioid sarcoma. In all cases surgical treatment should be combined with radiotherapy and multiagent chemotherapy over a prolonged period, similar to the chemotherapy given for other adult-type sarcomas. Shimm and Suit[265] reported local control and a low rate of recurrence with preoperative or postoperative radiation therapy and resection.

## Discussion

There is still no consensus as to the exact nature and cell type of epithelioid sarcoma. Not surprisingly, a synovial origin is often suggested in view of the intimate association of the tumor with tendons and aponeuroses, the mixture of epithelioid and spindle-shaped cell elements, and the presence of mucinous material in the surrounding ground substance. It is further supported by the immunostaining for cytokeratin,[245] the ultrastructural demonstration of light and dark cells and microvilli in some of the cases, and the reported occurrence of a morphologically distinct epithelioid and synovial sarcoma that presented at two locations in the same knee.[264] There are, however, a number of contrasting features: the predominant location of epithelioid sarcoma in the hand, the persistent absence of pseudoglandular structures and intracellular mucin droplets, the lack of basal laminae ultrastructurally, and distinctive cytogenetic alterations. Over the past years it has also been suggested that epithelioid sarcoma is a tumor of primitive mesenchymal cells with fibroblastic and histiocytic differentiation,[229,268] a primitive mesenchymal tumor with differentiation along histiocytic and synovial lines,[214] a fibrosarcoma,[227] a tumor of myofibroblasts altered by massive production of intermediate filaments,[212,256] a malignant giant cell tumor of the tendon sheath,[226] and a tumor related to nodular tenosynovitis and arising from synovioblastic mesenchyme.[249]

Trauma to the site of the tumor may be a contributing factor and has been reported in a large number of cases. In the series by Chase and Enzinger,[216] for example, unsolicited reports of antecedent trauma were given in 20% of cases. Prat et al.[257] reported a history of trauma in 6 of 22 patients, including one case in which an epithelioid sarcoma of the hand developed following exposure to plutonium. Another case, reported by Bloustein et al.,[214] originated in the scar tissue of a cesarean section. Puissegur-Lupo et al.[258] observed an epithelioid sarcoma that arose in scar tissue 17 months after traumatic amputation of three fingers of the right hand.

## DESMOPLASTIC SMALL ROUND CELL TUMOR

Desmoplastic small round cell tumor (DSRCT) is a relatively uncommon entity that typically involves the abdominal or pelvic peritoneum (or both) of young males and pursues an aggressive clinical course. The lesion is characterized by a proliferation of small round cells deposited in an abundant desmoplastic stroma, and it is characterized immunohistochemically by multiphenotypic differentiation. This lesion has had a variety of names, including undifferentiated malignant epithelial tumor involving serosal surfaces of the scrotum and abdomen in young males,[328] desmoplastic small-cell tumor with divergent differentiation,[305] intraabdominal desmoplastic small round cell tumor,[291,306,320] malignant small-cell epithelial tumor of the peritoneum co-expressing mesenchymal-type intermediate filaments,[322] intraabdominal neuroectodermal tumor of childhood with divergent differentiation,[333] and desmoplastic small-cell tumor with multiphenotypic differentiation.[301] Given the fact that this lesion may arise in an extraabdominal location and may also arise in adult patients, desmoplastic small round cell tumor is now the most commonly used name for this neoplasm.

### Clinical Findings

Most patients with this tumor are 15–35 years of age, although patients as young as 5 years[285] and as old as the seventh and eighth decades of life[299,335] have been reported. In a study of 109 patients with this tumor by Gerald et al.,[303] the patients ranged in age from 6 to 49 years (mean 22 years). Males far outnumber females at a ratio of approximately 4:1.[303,318]

**TABLE 37–11 ANATOMIC DISTRIBUTION OF 109 CASES OF DESMOPLASTIC SMALL ROUND CELL TUMOR**

| Location | No. of Patients | % |
|---|---|---|
| Abdominal cavity | 103 | 94 |
| Thoracic region | 4 | 4 |
| Posterior cranial fossa | 1 | 1 |
| Hand | 1 | 1 |
| *Total* | 109 | 100 |

From Gerald WL, Ladanyi M, de Alava E, et al. Clinical, pathologic, and molecular spectrum of tumors associated with t(11;22) (p13;q12): desmoplastic small round-cell tumor and its variants. J Clin Oncol 16:3028, 1998.

Most present with a large abdominal and/or pelvic mass with extensive peritoneal involvement, usually without an identifiable visceral site of origin (Table 37–11). The most common complaint is abdominal distension, often associated with pain and constipation. Other signs and symptoms are intestinal or ureteral obstruction, ascites, difficulty with urination, and impotence.[289,300] Although most tumors arise in the aforementioned sites, this tumor has also been described in the paratesticular region,[292,296,309] ovary,[336] pleura,[286,323] parotid gland,[335] hand,[279] and central nervous system.[330] Ordóñez reported a 10-year-old boy who presented with a mass in the liver and bilateral lung metastasis without ascites or other evidence of peritoneal involvement.[318]

### Pathologic Findings

Grossly, the tumor forms a solid, large multilobulated mass that is white or gray-white on cross section, sometimes distorted by cystic change and areas of necrosis. Microscopically, most tumors are composed of sharply demarcated nests of varying size with small round or oval cells embedded in a hypervascular desmoplastic stroma (Figs. 37–63, 37–64, 37–65). Large tumor cell nests often have central necrosis (Fig. 37–66). The tumor cells appear undifferentiated and have small hyperchromatic nuclei with inconspicuous nucleoli and scant amounts of eosinophilic cytoplasm (Fig. 37–67). In most cases the nuclei are relatively uniform, but some tumors show focal areas with increased nuclear atypia, and rare tumors are composed predominantly of markedly atypical cells.[318] The cells may be arranged in a variety of patterns including large nests with central necrosis, tubular-like structures, trabeculae separated by fibrovascular septa reminiscent of a "zellballen" pattern, and cords of single cells similar to lobular carcinoma of the breast[295,318] (Fig. 37–68). Typically, the cellular aggregates are surrounded and separated by abun-

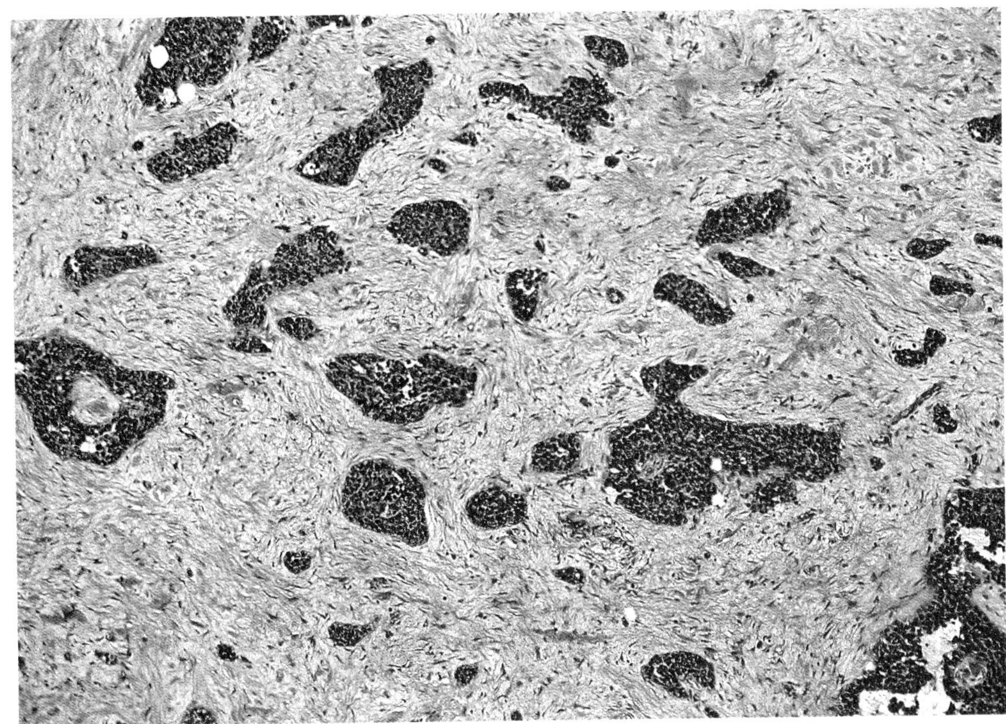

**FIGURE 37–63.** Desmoplastic small round cell tumor. Nests of undifferentiated tumor cells are surrounded by abundant fibrous stroma.

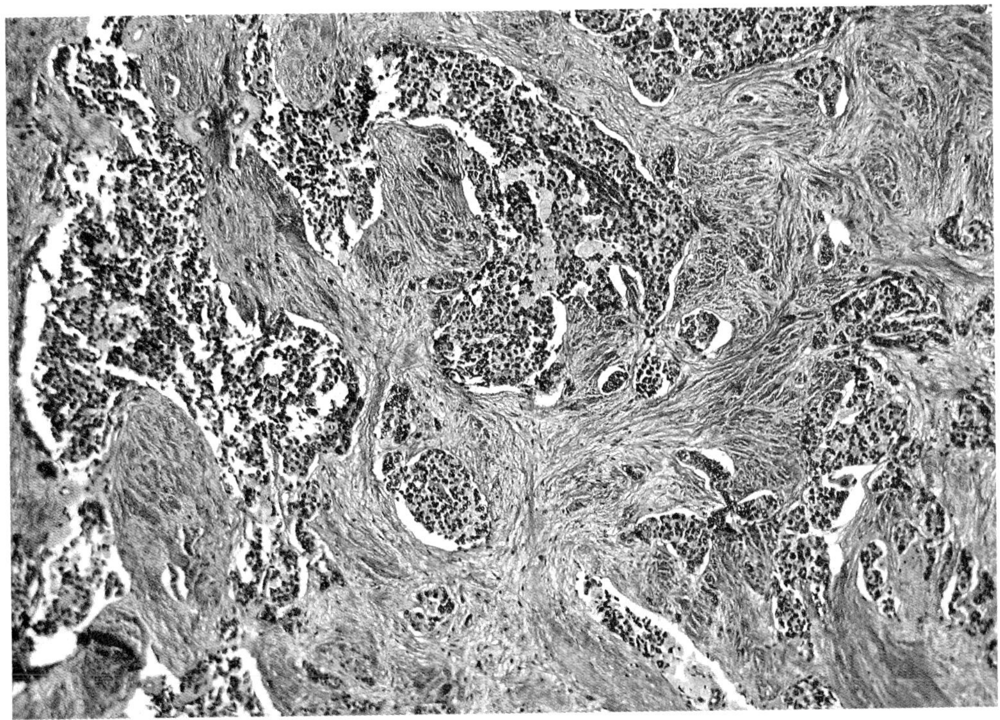

**FIGURE 37–64.** Nests of undifferentiated tumor cells are separated by a dense fibrous stroma in this desmoplastic small round cell tumor.

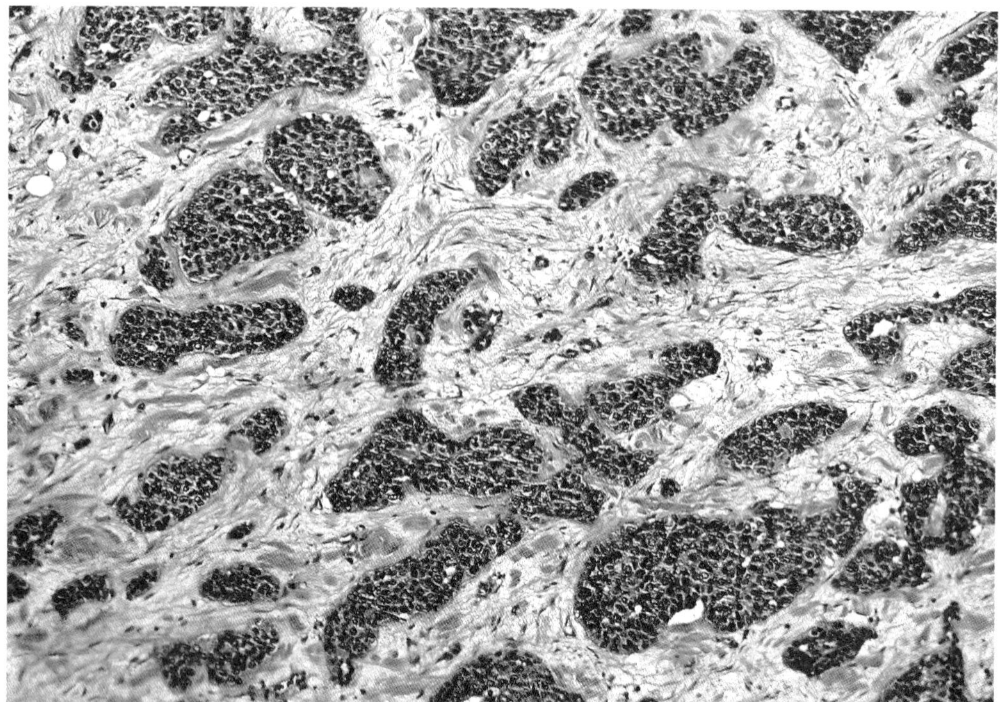

**FIGURE 37–65.** Prominent desmoplastic stroma surrounds varying sized nests of tumor cells in a desmoplastic small round cell tumor.

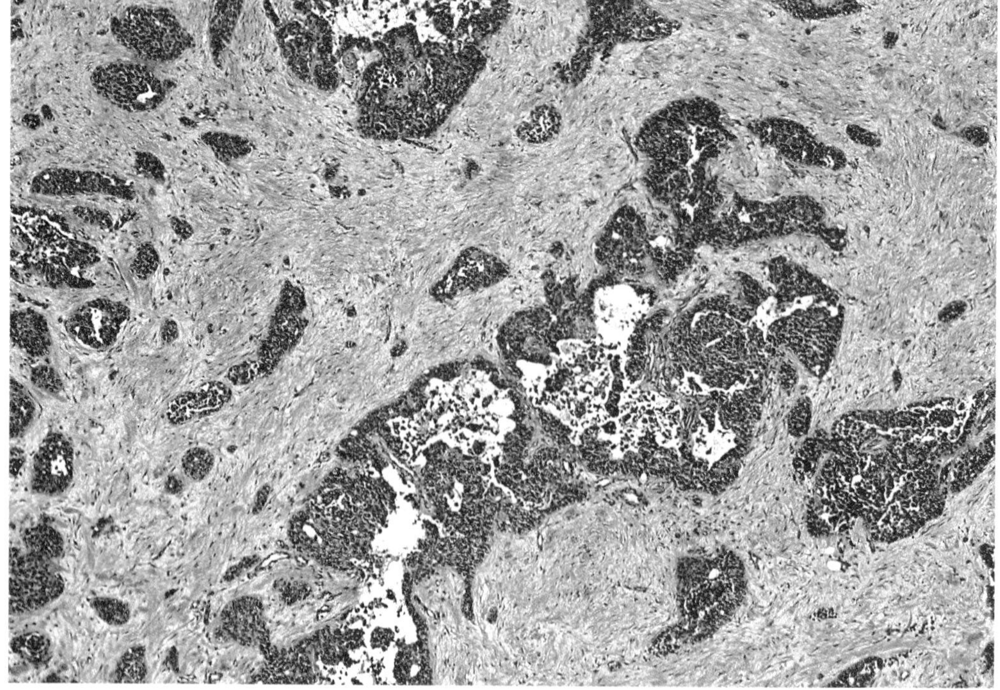

**FIGURE 37–66.** Desmoplastic small round cell tumor. Larger tumor nests show central necrosis.

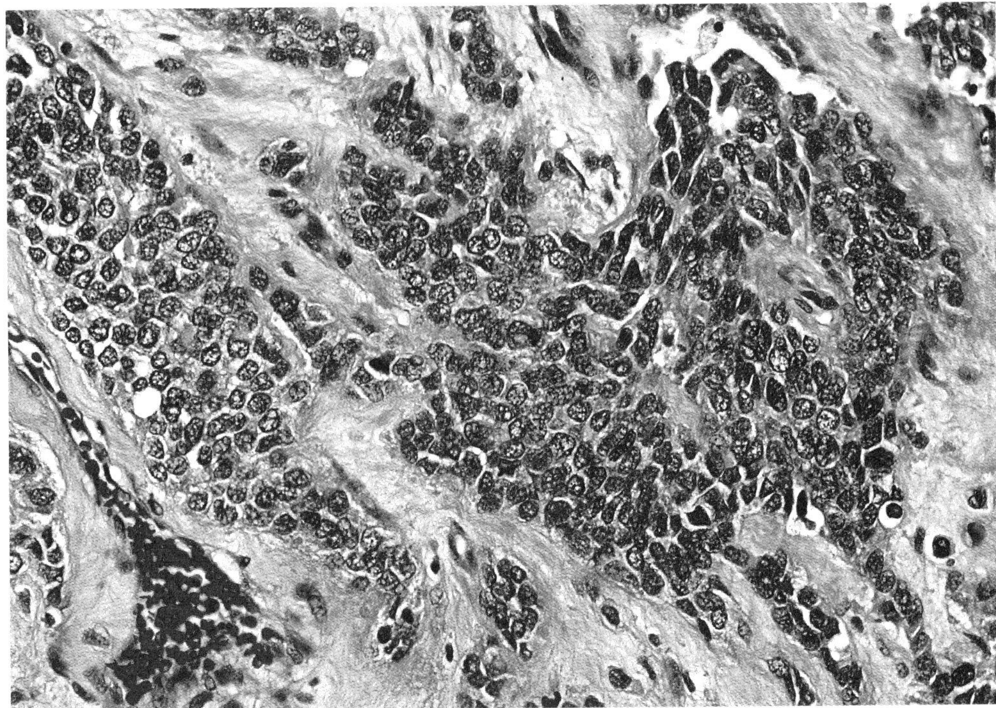

**FIGURE 37–67.** Desmoplastic small round cell tumor. The tumor cells appear undifferentiated and have small hyperchromatic nuclei with inconspicuous nucleoli.

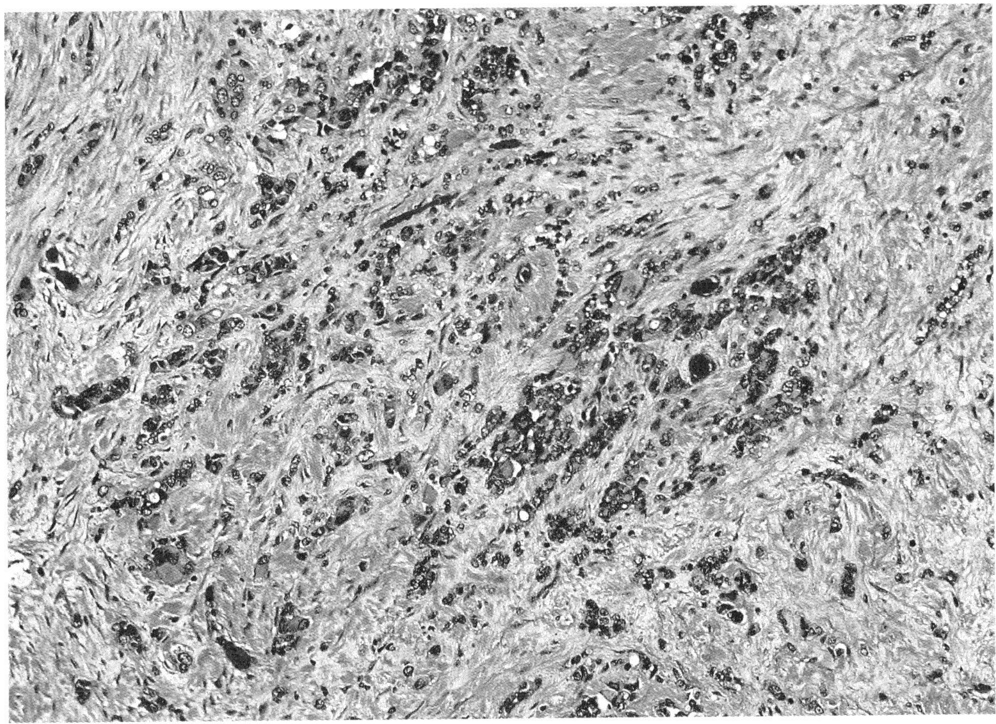

**FIGURE 37–68.** Desmoplastic small round cell tumor. Cords of cells are surrounded by a dense fibrous stroma mimicking lobular carcinoma of the breast.

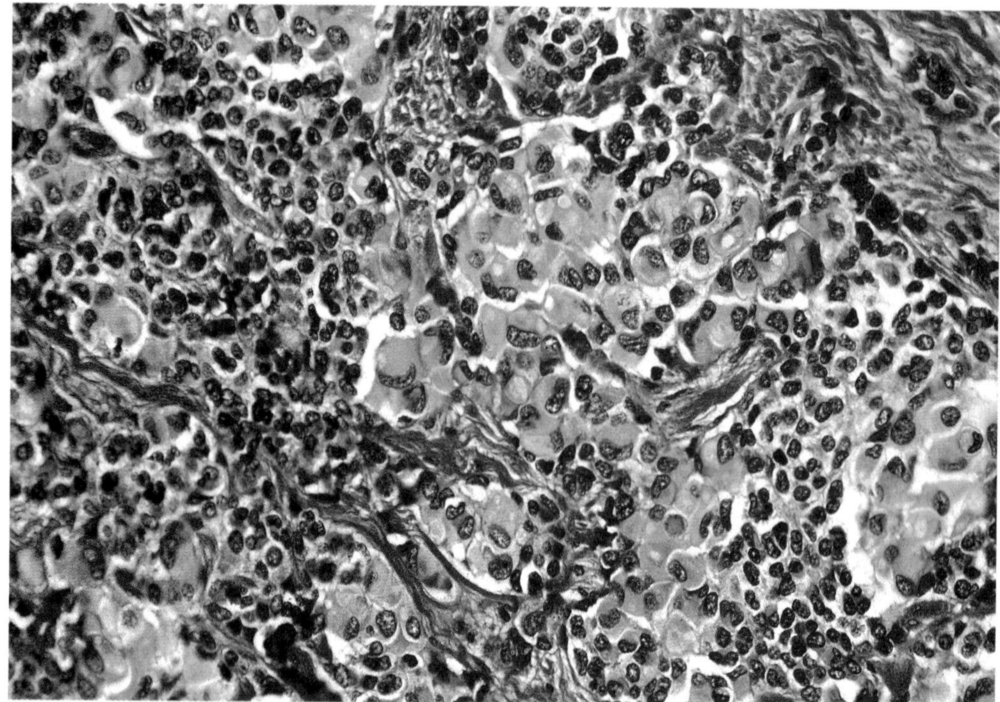

**FIGURE 37–69.** Focus of cells with a rhabdoid appearance in a desmoplastic small round cell tumor.

dant fibrous connective tissue with only a scattering of spindle-shaped fibroblasts and myofibroblasts. Occasionally, the tumor cells have more abundant cleared-out or vacuolated cytoplasm or a signet ring-like appearance. A relatively common finding is the presence of rhabdoid-like foci in which the tumor cells have paranuclear intracytoplasmic hyaline inclusions composed of aggregates of intermediate filaments[303] (Fig. 37–69). Other rare features include Homer Wright-like rosettes, papillary areas, zones that resemble traditional cell carcinoma,[245,318] and areas composed predominantly of cells with a spindled morphology. In the recent study by Ordóñez[318] two-thirds of the tumors had the classic histologic features of DSRCT, whereas one-third had atypical histologic features.

## Immunohistochemical Findings

The tumor is characterized by a polyphenotypic profile with expression of epithelial, mesenchymal, and neural markers (Table 37–12). Virtually all tumors stain for epithelial markers, including cytokeratins and epithelial membrane antigen. In a study by Gerald et al.[303] cytokeratins and epithelial membrane antigen were expressed in 86% and 93% of cases, respectively. Occasionally immunostains for cytokeratin reveal a dot-like pattern of cytoplasmic immunoreactivity. Stains for cytokeratin 20 (positive in Merkel cell carcinoma) and cytokeratins 5/6 (positive in malignant mesothelioma) are negative in DSRCT,[319] although epithelial markers including MOC-31 and Ber-EP4 are commonly expressed.

Virtually all DSRCTs stain for vimentin,[280,319] but perhaps the most useful diagnostic marker is desmin. Up to 90% of cases stain for this antigen, typically

**TABLE 37–12** SUMMARY OF IMMUNOHISTOCHEMICAL DATA ON DESMOPLASTIC SMALL ROUND CELL TUMORS REPORTED IN THE LITERATURE

| Marker | No. of Positive Cases | % |
|---|---|---|
| Cytokeratin | 97/107 | 91 |
| Desmin | 107/117 | 91 |
| EMA | 64/73 | 88 |
| Vimentin | 87/103 | 84 |
| NSE | 88/107 | 82 |
| Synaptophysin | 11/43 | 26 |
| S-100 protein | 13/74 | 18 |
| Neurofilament protein | 6/50 | 12 |
| CD99 | 4/33 | 12 |
| Chromogranin | 7/64 | 11 |

Modified from Ordóñez NG. Desmoplastic small round cell tumor. II. An ultrastructural and immunohistochemical study with emphasis on new immunohistochemical markers. Am J Surg Pathol 22:1314, 1998.

with a perinuclear dot-like pattern, a unique pattern of desmin immunoreactivity peculiar to DSRCT (Fig. 37–70). Although often taken as evidence of myogenic differentiation, immunostains for nuclear myogenic regulatory proteins including MyoD1 and myogenin are negative; rare lesions express muscle-specific or smooth muscle actin.[313,319]

A variety of neural antigens have been detected in DSRCTs, most commonly neuron-specific enolase and Leu-7, having been reported in 82% and 49% of cases, respectively.[319] However, immunoreactivity for more specific markers of neuroendocrine differentiation including synaptophysin and chromogranin are rare in this tumor.[283,319]

CD99 and NB-84 are markers that have been more recently utilized in the differential diagnosis of small round cell neoplasms. Although CD99 is a highly sensitive marker for the ES/PNET family, it is not completely specific and has been detected in many other round cell neoplasms, including up to one-third of DSRCTs.[319] Similarly, although NB-84 is a sensitive marker of neuroblastoma, it has been reported in other tumors, including up to 50% of DSRCTs.[298,316]

A high-molecular-weight glycoprotein, CA-125 is often present in mucinous carcinomas of the ovary and adenocarcinomas of the uterine cervix and endometrium.[315] It has also been found to be expressed by the tumor cells in DSRCTs.[319] Interestingly, some patients with DSRCTs have elevated serum levels of CA-125,[321] which may return to normal levels following aggressive treatment.[297,336]

### Ultrastructural Findings

The most striking ultrastructural feature of this tumor is the intracellular whorls and packets of microfilaments that are usually located near the nucleus, often compressing the nucleus or pushing it toward the periphery. There are a moderate number of mitochondria, free ribosomes, and small lakes of glycogen. Dense-core granules are infrequently found.[294,334] The cells are closely apposed with occasional filopodia, tight cell junctions, or small desmosomes with tonofilaments. Sometimes the cell clusters are partly enveloped by a basal lamina.[319] Z-band material and thick or thin filaments suggesting myogenic differentiation are not seen.

### Cytogenetic and Molecular Genetic Findings

The identification of a unique cytogenetic abnormality t(11;22)(p13;q12) in this tumor has helped to establish the DSRCT as a distinct clinicopathologic entity.[287,304,325,326] The breakpoints involve the *EWS* gene on 22q12 and the Wilms' tumor gene (*WT1*) on 11p13.[302,312] *WT1* is a tumor suppressor gene that encodes a zinc-finger-type transcription factor that nor-

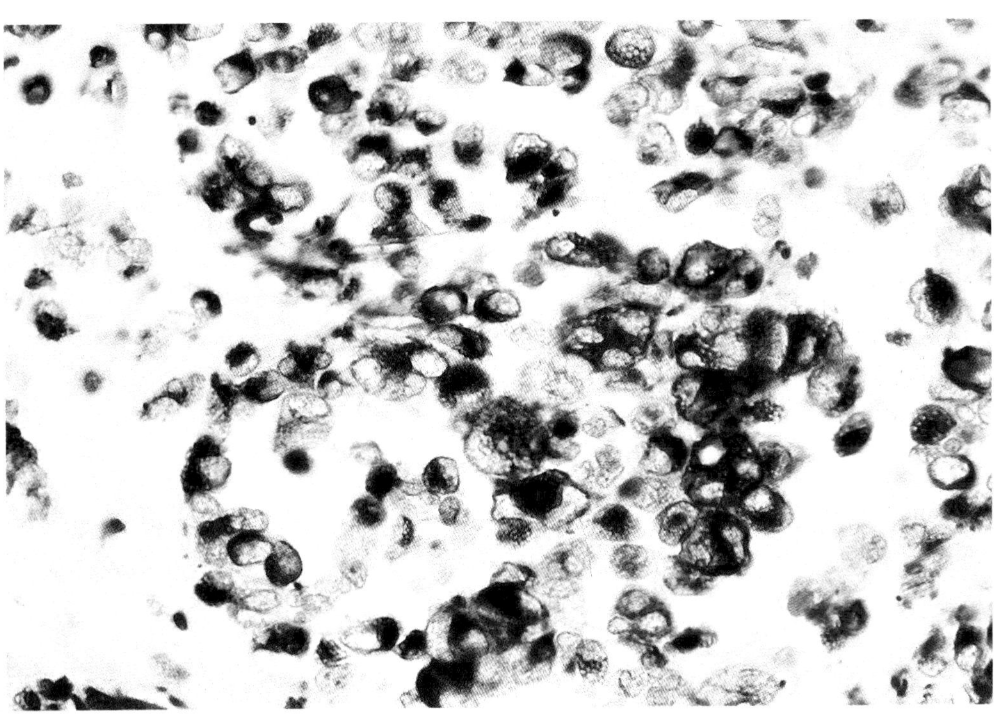

**FIGURE 37–70.** Typical perinuclear dot-like pattern of desmin immunoreactivity peculiar to desmoplastic small round cell tumors.

mally represses promoters that control expression of growth factors such as platelet-derived growth factor (PDGFA).[302,307,314] The fusion protein appears to induce expression of PDGFA, a potent mitogen and chemoattractant for fibroblasts and endothelial cells, thus serving as a potential link between the unique translocation and histologic characteristics of this tumor.[314]

The fusion transcript can be detected by molecular genetic techniques including the reverse transcriptase-polymerase chain reaction (RT-PCR)[282,288,293] and fluorescence in situ hybridization.[324] Most commonly, this fusion involves exon 7 of *EWS* and exon 8 of *WT1;* rare variant fusions have been described.[281,329] Although the *EWS-WT1* fusion product has been described only in DSRCTs, (Table 37–13) rare tumors have been reported to have the fusion products characteristically identified in the ES/PNET family, including *EWS-ERG*[317] and *EWS-FLI1*.[310] Newer polyclonal anti-WT1 antibodies have been developed that detect the WT1 protein in DSRCTs,[284,290,307a] a marker which will likely facilitate this diagnosis in the absence of tissue for molecular genetic analysis.

## Differential Diagnosis

The DSRCT must be differentiated from other small round cell tumors including extraskeletal ES/PNET, rhabdomyosarcoma, neuroblastoma, lymphoma, poorly differentiated carcinoma, small-cell carcinoma, Merkel cell carcinoma, and malignant mesothelioma. When arising in the typical clinicopathologic setting, DSRCTs can be easily distinguished from these other entities, although ancillary techniques including immunohistochemistry and molecular genetics are invariably required. The immunohistochemical expression of epithelial, mesenchymal, and neural antigens, particularly the dot-like pattern of desmin staining, are useful for arriving at a diagnosis. Procuring frozen tissue for molecular genetic analysis to identify the *EWS-WT1* fusion transcript is valuable, particularly in lesions with an atypical immunophenotype.[331] Given the immunophenotypic features that overlap with those of many of the aforementioned tumors, a panel of immunostains is generally required.

The differential diagnosis of DSRCT continues to broaden as its pathologic profile has expanded. Thus a variety of neoplasms including sarcomatoid carcinoma, spindle cell sarcomas of various types, metastatic adenocarcinoma, and malignant extrarenal rhabdoid tumor may occasionally be entertained as diagnostic considerations. As above, a combination of immunohistochemical and molecular genetic analysis should allow for this distinction.

**TABLE 37–13 SENSITIVITY AND SPECIFICITY OF THE *EWS-WT1* FUSION TRANSCRIPT FOR DESMOPLASTIC SMALL ROUND CELL TUMORS**

| Diagnosis | *EWS-WT1*-Positive | % |
|---|---|---|
| DSRCT | 11/12 | 92 |
| Primitive neuroectodermal tumor family | 0/8 | 0 |
| Wilms' tumor | 0/17 | 0 |
| Alveolar rhabdomyosarcoma | 0/13 | 0 |
| Nonalveolar rhabdomyosarcoma | 0/9 | 0 |

Modified from de Alava E, Ladanyi M, Rosai J, et al. Detection of chimeric transcripts in desmoplastic small round cell tumor and related developmental tumors by reverse transcriptase polymerase chain reaction: a specific diagnostic assay. Am J Pathol 147:1584, 1995.
DSRCT, desmoplastic small round cell tumors.

## Clinical Behavior

The DSRCT is a highly aggressive neoplasm with an extremely poor prognosis. In the series reported by Ordóñez et al. in 1993,[320] 16 of 22 patients died of the disease within 8–50 months after the initial therapy. In a follow-up study published in 1998,[318] 25 of 35 patients for whom follow-up information was available died of widespread metastasis, and the remainder were alive with disease. In a study from the Memorial Sloan Kettering Cancer Center,[327] 13 of 32 patients treated with an extensive debulking procedure (>90% of tumor removed) followed by systemic chemotherapy remained progression-free, although three of these patients died from toxicity related to treatment. Although the prognosis remains dismal, improved survival is correlated with a complete or good response to multimodality therapy, including extensive surgical debulking.[311] Complete excision is often impossible because of the irregular outline of the tumor and the presence of multiple implants in the peritoneum.

## Discussion

The exact nature of this tumor is still uncertain. Some have speculated that the DSRCT is derived from mesothelial or submesothelial cells, given the predominant location of this tumor in mesothelial cell-lined cavities and the immunohistochemical expression of both epithelial and mesenchymal antigens. The cells of the DSRCT invariably express desmin, as do normal mesothelial cells, submesothelial mesenchymal cells,[332] and some malignant mesotheliomas.[308] However, there are a number of immunohistochemical differences between the DSRCT and mesothelioma such as the expression of MOC-31, Ber-EP4, and Leu-M1 in DSRCTs (usually absent in malignant mesotheliomas) and the absence of cytokeratins 5/6 and thrombomodulin (usually present in malignant mesotheliomas).[319] Furthermore, there is no ultrastructural evidence of mesothelial differentiation in DSRCTs; as previously noted, rare tumors arise in locations not lined by mesothelial cells.

## MALIGNANT EXTRARENAL RHABDOID TUMOR

Malignant rhabdoid tumor of the kidney, initially described in 1978 and thought to be a "rhabdomyosarcomatoid variant of Wilms' tumor," has subsequently been defined as a distinct clinicopathologic entity different from Wilms' tumor.[353,383,389] Most tumors that arise in the kidney occur in children less than 1 year of age and have an aggressive clinical course: The majority of patients die of widespread metastatic disease within a short time from the initial diagnosis.

Subsequently, tumors with a histologic appearance similar to that of tumors arising in the kidney have been described in virtually every extrarenal anatomic site including the skin,[347] soft tissues,[384] urogenital tract,[356,365] gastrointestinal tract,[367,375,392] liver,[351] thymus,[363] and most prominently the central nervous system,[344,376,377] among others. It is often difficult to determine from the descriptions of these tumors whether they represent "pure" extrarenal rhabdoid tumors composed exclusively of cells with a rhabdoid morphology or they represent focal rhabdoid areas within a "parent" neoplasm of recognizable phenotype.[391] We believe therefore that the term "extrarenal rhabdoid tumor" as it pertains to soft tissue should used for tumors with a predominant rhabdoid morphology and in which no other clear line of differentiation can be documented. In this regard, it should be noted that carcinomas of various types may have rhabdoid features, including transitional cell carcinoma of the bladder,[354,361] colorectal adenocarcinoma,[346,386] renal cell carcinoma,[352a,388] Merkel cell carcinoma,[364] collecting duct carcinoma,[388] and vulvar carcinoma.[360] In addition, rhabdoid features have been described in other types of neoplasms such as melanomas,[340,341,345,362] mesotheliomas,[368] meningiomas,[374] lymphomas,[388] and sarcomas of various types (endometrial stromal sarcoma,[369] rhabdomyosarcoma,[359] leiomyosarcoma,[364] synovial sarcoma,[366] myxoid chondrosarcoma,[385] and desmoplastic small round cell tumor[303]). Clinically, extrarenal rhabdoid tumors occur over a much broader age range than those found in the kidney, although these lesions are far more common in children, occasionally arising as congenital lesions. Like their renal counterparts, extrarenal rhabdoid tumors are generally characterized by an aggressive clinical behavior, as fewer than 50% of patients survive more than 5 years regardless of the type of therapy employed.[391]

### Pathologic Findings

Extrarenal rhabdoid tumor is characterized by a population of large polygonal cells with eccentric nuclei, vesicular chromatin, prominent nucleoli, and abundant cytoplasm containing acidophilic and PAS-positive hyaline inclusions or globules (Figs. 37–71, 37–72, 37–73). As described below, the inclusions correlate ultrastructurally to a paranuclear intracellular mass composed of compact bundles or whorls of intermediate filaments 10 nm in length[353] (Figs. 37–74, 37–75, 37–76). Some benign tumors, including pleomorphic adenomas and myoepitheliomas of the salivary glands, have intracytoplasmic hyaline inclusions,[349,352] but these tumors lack the nuclear cytologic atypia to designate them as having a rhabdoid morphology. Evaluation of multiple sections may be required to determine if the rhabdoid cells are a component of a "composite" extrarenal rhabdoid tumor with a recognizable neoplastic phenotype (Fig. 37–77). In addition, ancillary techniques such as immunohistochemistry, electron microscopy, and molecular genetic analysis is often necessary to recognize such a "parent" neoplasm, particularly if the rhabdoid cells comprise a substantial portion of the tumor.

### Immunohistochemical and Ultrastructural Findings

A variety of antigens may be detected in the cells of "pure" extrarenal rhabdoid tumor including epithelial (Fig. 37–78), mesenchymal, and neural antigens.[348,373,391] Although this polyphenotypic immunohistochemical profile is also characteristic of DSRCT, histologic and molecular genetic differences allow distinction between these tumors.

Ultrastructurally, rhabdoid cells are characterized by paranuclear aggregates or whorls of intermediate filaments 10 nm in size. Additionally, the cytoplasm contains a moderate amount of dilated rough endoplasmic reticulum, few mitochondria, lysosomes, lipid droplets, and free ribosomes.[384,385]

### Cytogenetic Findings

Relatively limited cytogenetic data are available, but renal rhabdoid tumors may have aberrations of chromosomes 11 (at 11p15) and 22 (at 22q11).[357,358,370,379,381] Schofield et al.[380] reported loss of heterozygosity on 22q in 80% of renal rhabdoid tumors, suggesting the presence of a tumor suppressor gene at this locus.

Of the extrarenal rhabdoid tumors, those arising in

*Text continued on page 1550*

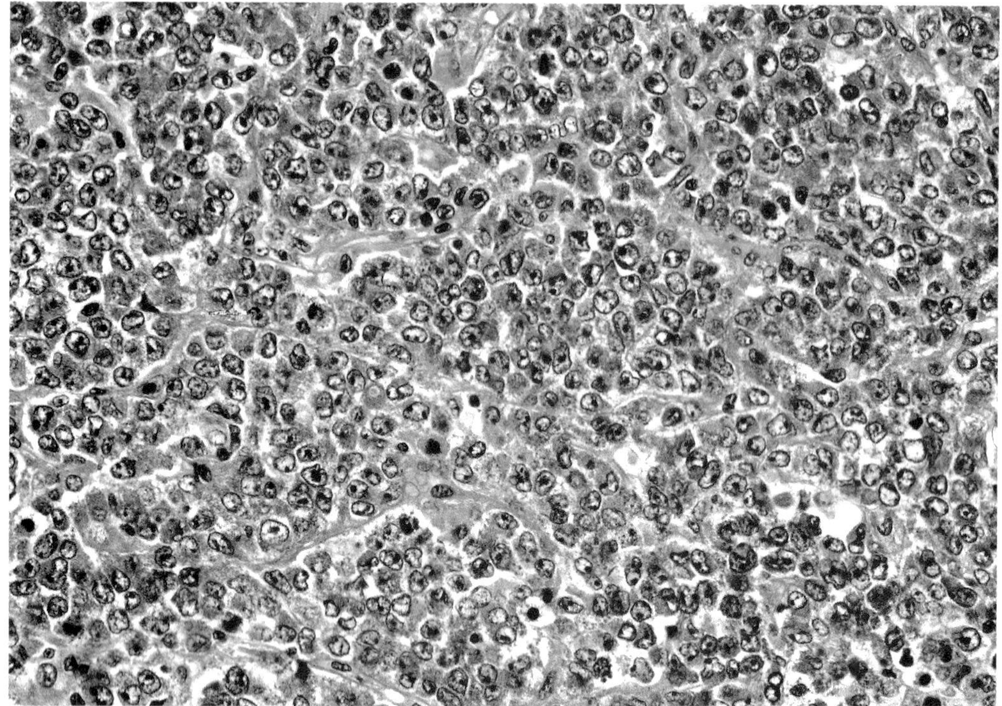

**FIGURE 37–71.** Malignant extrarenal rhabdoid tumor composed of nests of large epithelioid cells.

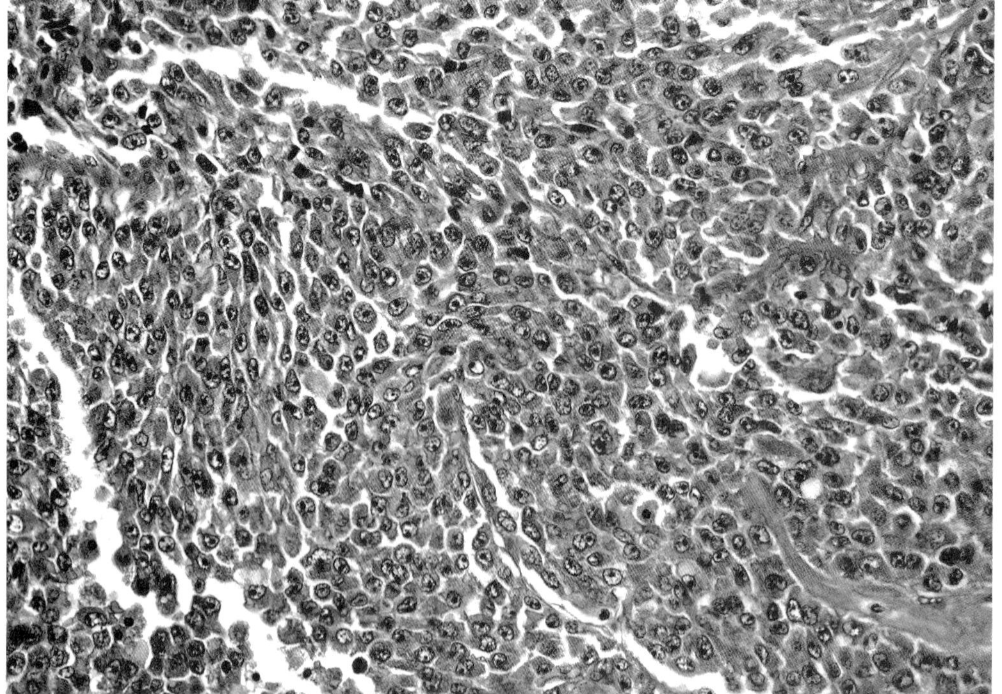

**FIGURE 37–72.** Sheets of large epithelioid cells with abundant eosinophilic cytoplasm in a malignant extrarenal rhabdoid tumor.

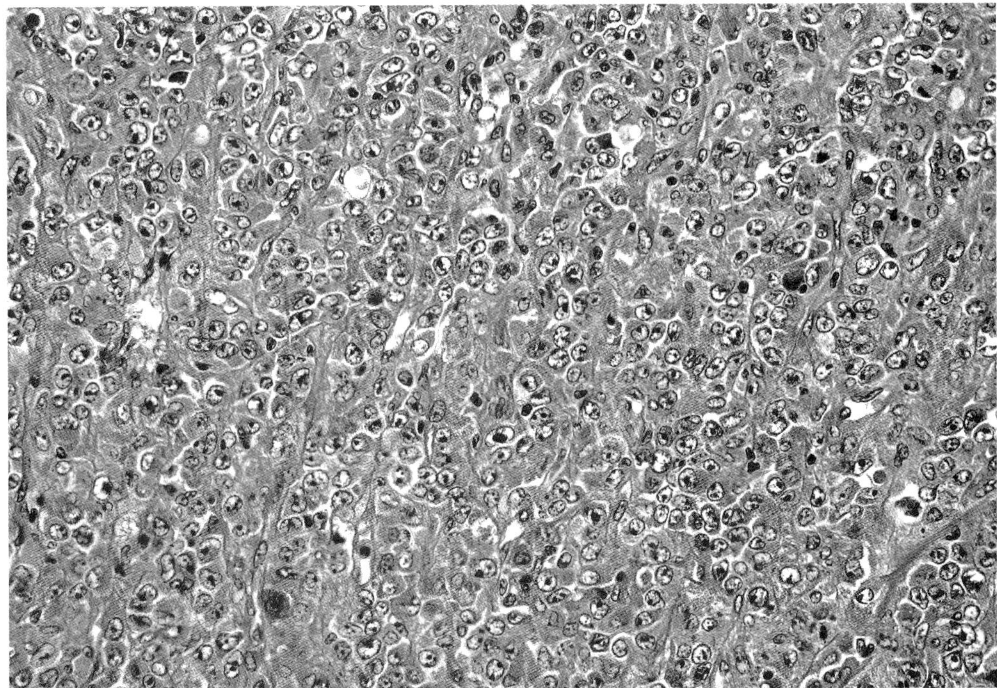

**FIGURE 37–73.** Malignant extrarenal rhabdoid tumor with a sheet of uniform large epithelioid cells having macronucleoli and abundant eosinophilic cytoplasm.

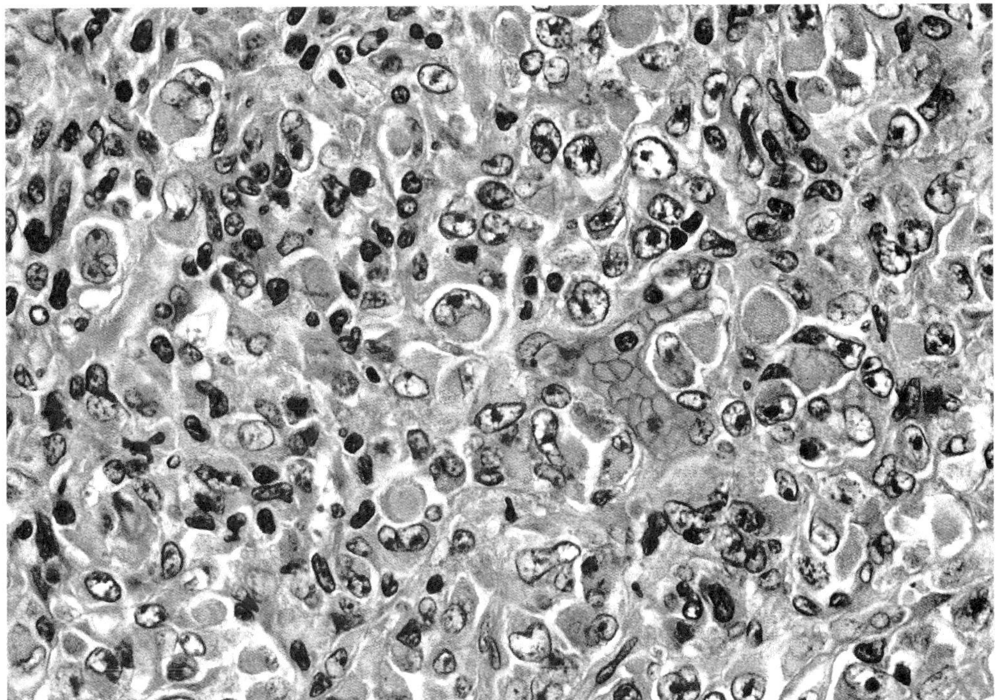

**FIGURE 37–74.** Malignant extrarenal rhabdoid tumor. The tumor cells have eccentric nuclei with macronucleoli.

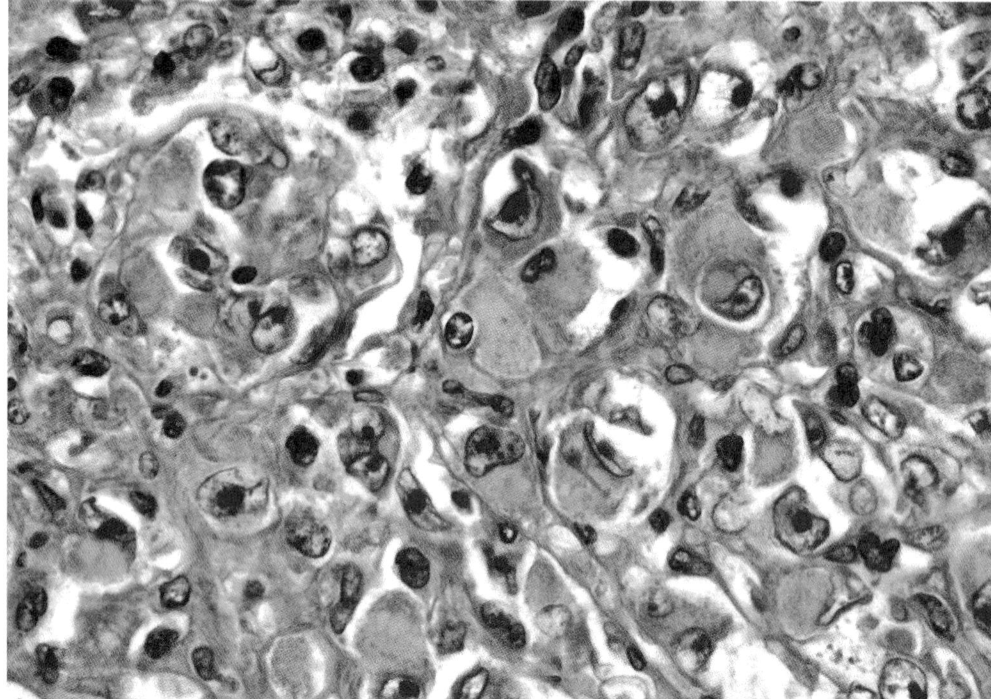

**FIGURE 37–75.** High magnification view of paranuclear intracytoplasmic hyaline inclusions in a malignant extrarenal rhabdoid tumor.

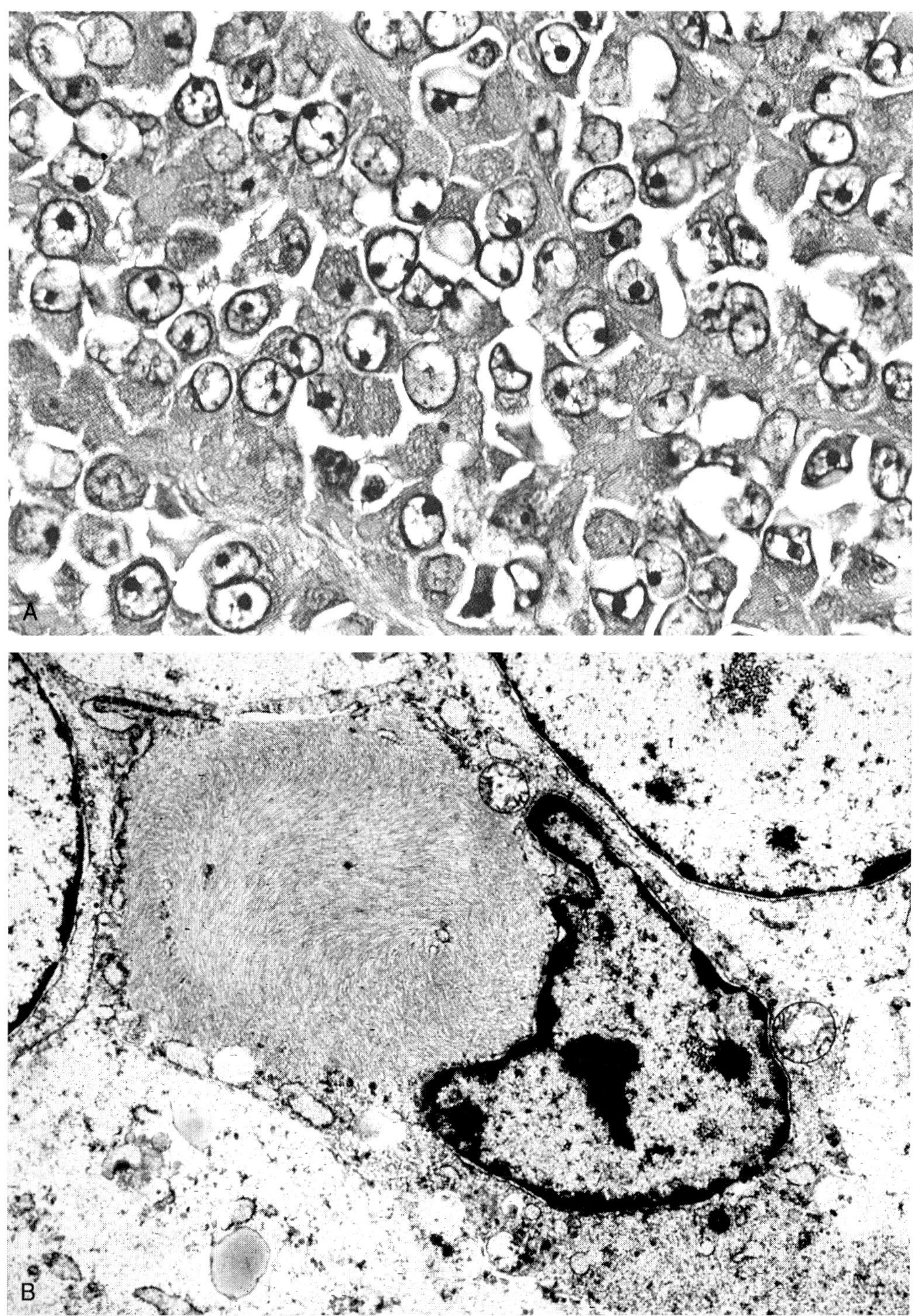


**FIGURE 37–76.** Malignant extrarenal rhabdoid tumor. (**A**) Cells with rhabdoid morphology. (**B**) Ultrastructural correlate, with a paranuclear whorl of intermediate filaments.

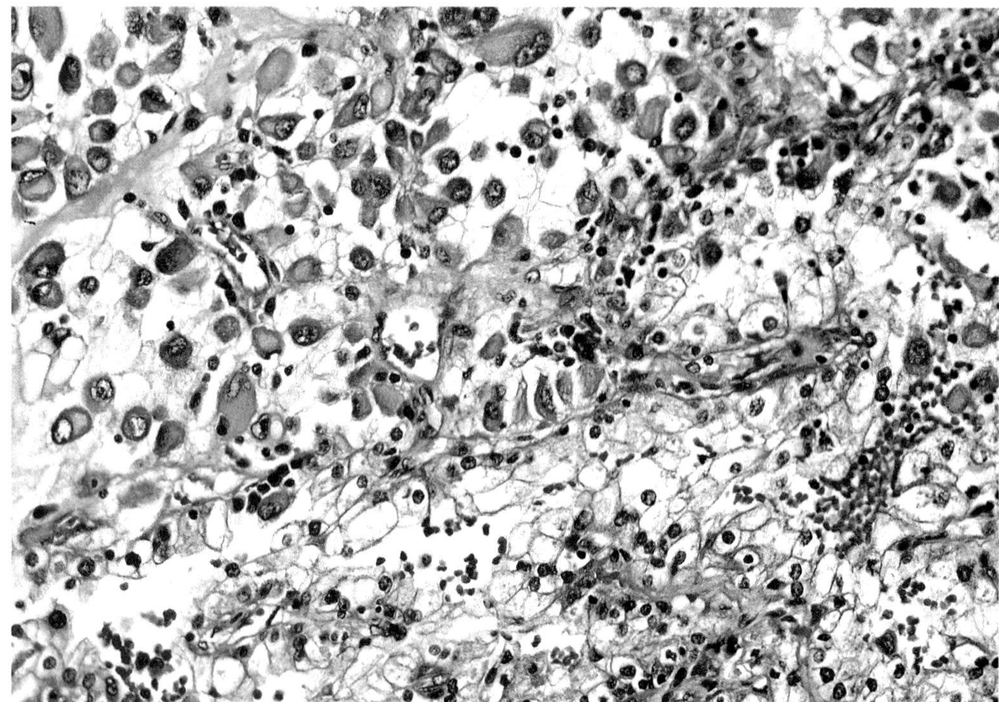

**FIGURE 37–77.** "Composite" extrarenal rhabdoid tumor with a typical clear cell renal cell carcinoma appearance at the bottom and cells with rhabdoid features near the top.

the central nervous system are the best characterized cytogenetically. Tumors in this location consistently demonstrate monosomy 22 with or without partial deletion of the remaining chromosome 22.[338,343,355] For example, in a study by Burger et al.,[344] seven of eight rhabdoid tumors of the central nervous system were found to have monosomy 22 by fluorescence in situ hybridization. More recently, extrarenal rhabdoid tumors outside of the central nervous system have also been found to harbor abnormalities of chromosome 22[337,339,373,378,382] (22q11–12), although this appears to be a less consistent finding than those found in the central nervous system. The *hSNF5/INII* gene has been reported to be mutated in rhabdoid tumors and remains a candidate gene important for the development of this unusual tumor.[339,371,387]

### Discussion

Because of the definitional issues regarding the malignant rhabdoid tumor of soft tissue, it is difficult to cite meaningful studies from the literature. It has been proposed that the rhabdoid phenotype represents a "final common pathway" for the evolution of many tumors to a higher-grade, more clinically aggressive neoplasm[372,391] analogous to the tumor progression seen with dedifferentiated sarcomas[342,350] and sarcomatoid carcinomas.[390] We believe there is ample evidence to support the existence of malignant extrarenal rhabdoid tumor as a clinicopathologic entity, rather than simply a pattern of tumor progression, analogous to the situation with malignant fibrous histiocytoma.

## MALIGNANT MESENCHYMOMA

The term malignant mesenchymoma has been applied to a large array of tumors utilizing a variety of diagnostic criteria. The evolution of the term and its various uses are discussed below. At present, this term serves little diagnostic use and should probably be abandoned altogether for the approach detailed below. From a historic point of view, Stout[397] coined this term for nonepithelial malignant tumors "showing two or more unrelated, differentiated tissue types in addition to the fibrosarcomatous element." He applied the term to a wide variety of neoplasms; after his initial report of 8 cases in 1948 he collected 355 cases by 1959.[395] Others, however, used this term in an entirely different setting. For example, Symmers and Nangle[398] and Ewing and Harrison[394] employed it for a group of myxoid liposarcomas because of their lipoblastic, myxoid, and vascular components. Thomas and Kothare[399] applied it to a poorly differentiated sarcoma with "tissue similar to embryonal mesenchyme."

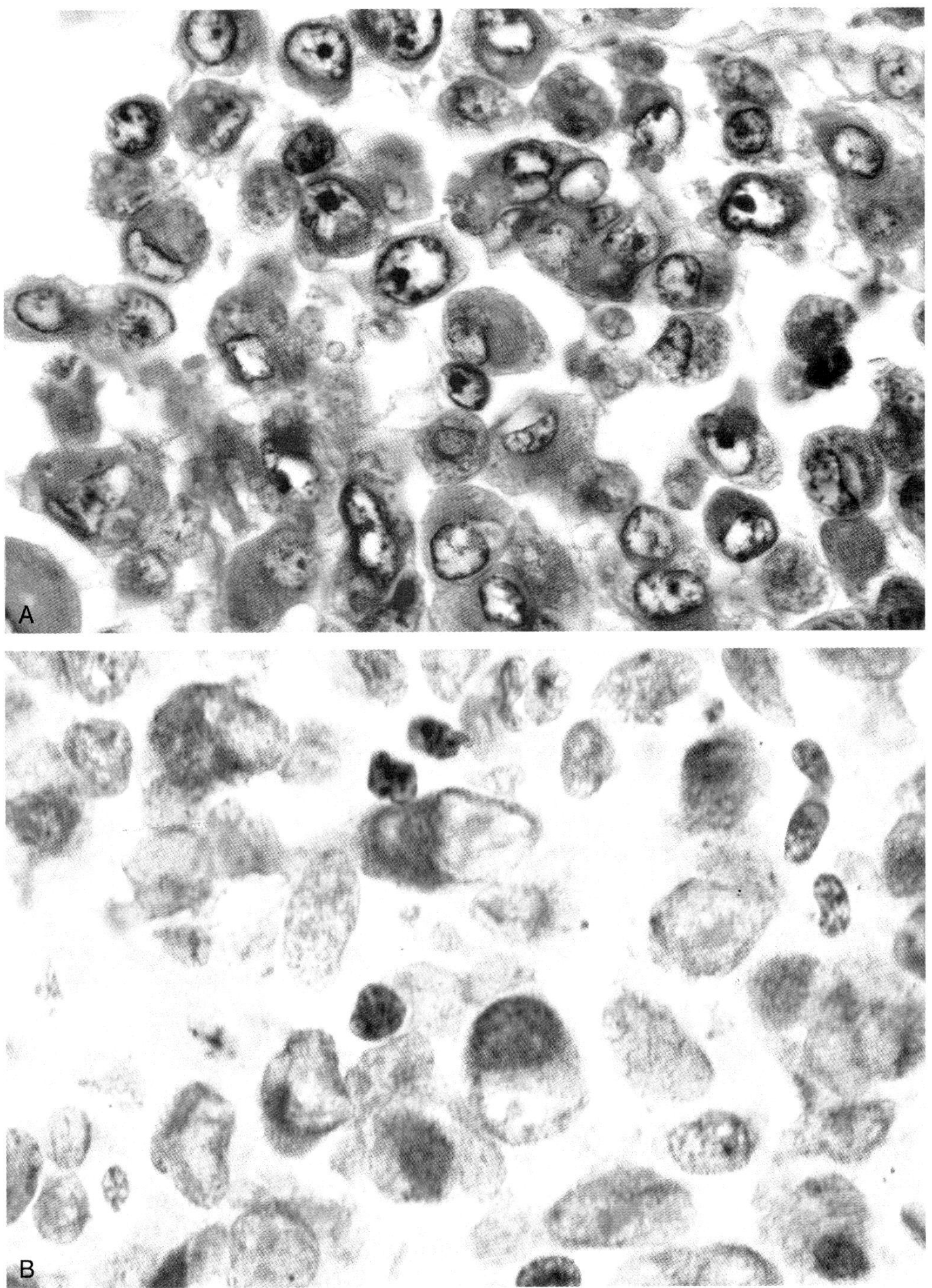

**FIGURE 37–78.** Malignant extrarenal rhabdoid tumor. (**A**) High magnification view of rhabdoid cells. (**B**) Paranuclear immunoreactivity for Cam5.2 in rhabdoid cells.

In 1991 Newman and Fletcher[396] attempted to refine the criteria for this diagnosis by excluding a variety of morphologic patterns that were judged to show no specific differentiation, such as fibrosarcoma, hemangiopericytoma, myxofibrosarcoma, and pleomorphic malignant fibrous histiocytoma. In addition, although the authors attempted to exclude "dedifferentiated" sarcomas, it appears as if some of these cases and some reported by Brady et al.[393] are actually dedifferentiated liposarcomas with a minor well differentiated liposarcomatous element.

There remain several neoplasms that qualify as malignant mesenchymoma but are frequently treated (rather arbitrarily) as distinct and separate entities. For example, malignant peripheral nerve sheath tumors may contain areas of rhabdomyosarcoma (malignant Triton tumor), yet these lesions have never been categorized as "malignant mesenchymoma." Likewise, osseous and cartilagenous differentiation has been accepted as a component of some well differentiated liposarcomas. Thus there seem to be as many exceptions to the rules as there are rules themselves for the diagnosis of malignant mesenchymoma.

For all of these reasons, we believe the label "malignant mesenchymoma" is best deleted from classification schemes. Sarcomas displaying two or more lines of differentiation are best diagnosed by identifying the lines of differentiation, their approximate amounts, and the grade of the most aggressive component. To continue to use the term "malignant mesenchymoma" unites a diverse group of lesions while eclipsing far more important issues of histologic grade. The suggestion that "malignant mesenchymoma" behaves less aggressively than the level of differentiation suggests is based on six cases, four of which had less than 5 years of follow-up.[396]

## INFLAMMATORY MYXOHYALINE TUMOR OF THE DISTAL EXTREMITIES WITH VIROCYTE OR REED-STERNBERG-LIKE CELLS

In 1997 Montgomery et al.[403] first reported 49 cases of a previously undescribed tumor of the distal extremities with unusual histologic features often prompting a misdiagnosis of an inflammatory or infectious process. Because of the presence of scattered bizarre cells with vesicular nuclei and macronucleoli and a prominent inflammatory background, the authors coined the term *inflammatory myxohyaline tumor of distal extremities with virocyte or Reed-Sternberg-like cells.* In this initial report, local recurrences occurred in almost one-fourth of the patients, although none developed metastatic disease. Subsequently, Meis-Kindblom and Kindblom[400] reported a series including one patient with biopsy-proven metastasis and used the term "acral myxoinflammatory fibroblastic sarcoma" to describe their cases. It is clear that the two terms refer to identical lesions even though minor differences were noted in the latter paper.

### Clinical Findings

Although the age range is broad, most patients with this tumor are in the fourth and fifth decades of life.[400–403] Males and females are affected equally, and most patients present with a slowly growing, painless, ill-defined mass of the distal extremities. The upper extremities are affected more commonly than the lower extremities with the single most common site being the soft tissues of the fingers and hand, although some lesions arise in the lower arm and wrist. On the lower extremities, these tumors may arise in the toes, feet, ankles, and lower legs (Table 37–14). In our experience, rare lesions also arise on the trunk. Some patients report mild pain and decreased mobility of the affected site, and occasionally there is a history of antecedent trauma. Clinically, the lesion is often thought to represent a ganglion cyst or some form of tenosynovitis.

### Pathologic Findings

Grossly, the tumor is typically multinodular and poorly circumscribed, and it is often removed piecemeal by the surgeon (Fig. 37–79). Gelatinous-appearing areas are conspicuous in the lesions with extensive myxoid change. The tumors range in size from 1 to 8 cm (mean 3–4 cm).

Histologically, at low magnification the tumor is multinodular and poorly circumscribed and frequently involves surrounding tendon sheaths and the synovium of adjacent joints (Fig. 37–80). Most arise

**TABLE 37–14 ANATOMIC DISTRIBUTION OF 95 INFLAMMATORY MYXOHYALINE TUMORS OF THE DISTAL EXTREMITIES**

| Anatomic Site | No. of Cases |
|---|---|
| Upper extremities | 65 (68%) |
| Fingers/hands | 53 |
| Wrist/lower arm | 10 |
| Miscellaneous | 2 |
| Lower extremities | 30 (32%) |
| Toes/feet | 16 |
| Ankles/lower leg | 13 |
| Miscellaneous | 1 |

Data are from references 400 and 402.

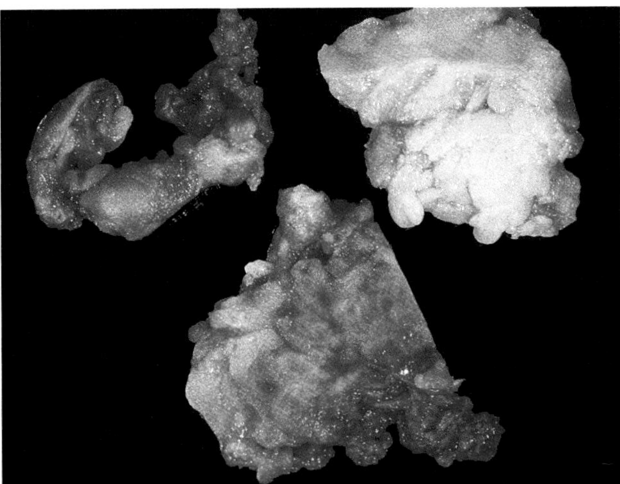

**FIGURE 37–79.** Gross specimen of an inflammatory myxohyaline tumor showing multinodular focally gelatinous mass. (From Montgomery EA, Devaney KO, Giordano TJ, et al. Inflammatory myxohyaline tumor of distal extremities with virocyte or Reed-Sternberg-like cells: a distinctive lesion with features simulating inflammatory conditions, Hodgkin's disease, and various sarcomas. Mod Pathol 11: 384, 1998.)

in the subcutaneous tissue, but some involve the dermis and others focally infiltrate skeletal muscle. Destruction or invasion of underlying bony structures has not been reported.

The most striking feature at low magnification is that of a dense inflammatory infiltrate merging with myxoid or hyaline zones (Figs. 37–81, 37–82). In most cases, leukocytes and plasma cells predominate, although neutrophils and eosinophils are conspicuous in some tumors (Fig. 37–83). Germinal centers are occasionally encountered. The amount of myxoid and hyalinized stroma varies from case to case. Some tumors are composed predominantly of hypocellular myxoid zones (Fig. 37–84), whereas in other tumors there may be only focal myxoid change. Hyaline zones contain a sparse mixture of inflammatory and neoplastic cells and often resemble the hyalinized zones of inflammatory myofibroblastic tumor (Fig. 37–85). Hemosiderin deposition may be conspicuous.

Examination of more cellular zones reveals bizarre atypical cells deposited in a hyalinized or myxoid stroma and allows for recognition of this lesion as a neoplastic process. These atypical cells range in shape from plump spindled cells to histiocytoid or epithelioid cells (Fig. 37–86). The spindled cells have a moderate degree of nuclear atypia, whereas the larger epithelioid cells often have large vesicular nuclei with macronucleoli and prominent eosinophilic cytoplasm, imparting a close similarity to virocytes or Reed-Sternberg cells (Figs. 37–87, 37–88) Despite the marked degree of nuclear atypia, there is a paucity of mitotic figures, typically with fewer than 2 mitoses/50 HPF. Ganglion-like cells resembling those seen in

*Text continued on page 1559*

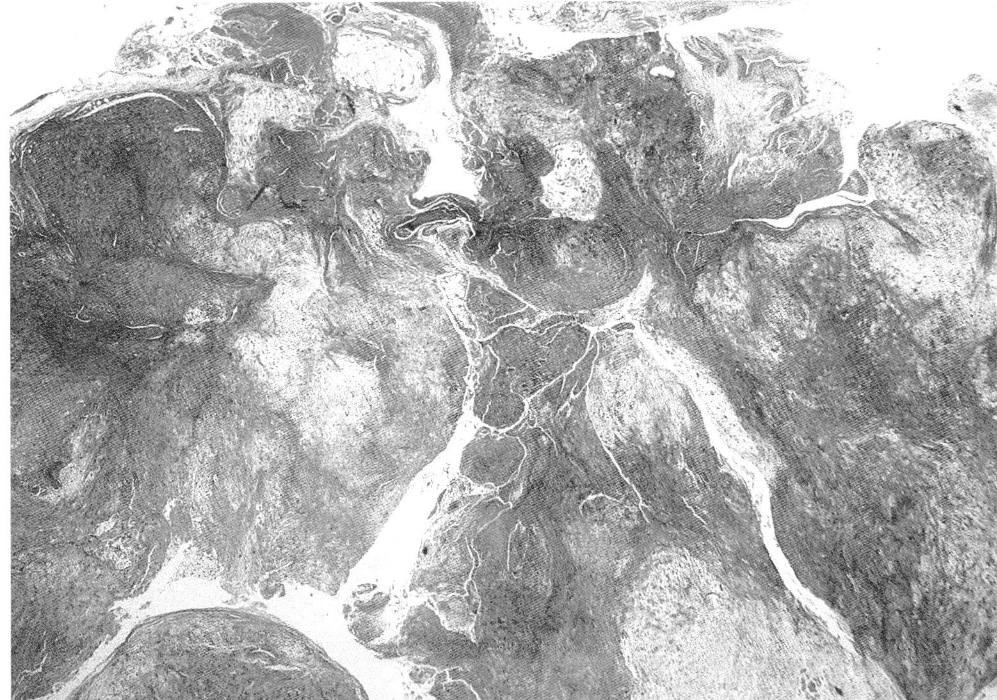

**FIGURE 37–80.** Low power view of inflammatory myxohyaline tumor illustrating a mixture of myxoid, hyaline, and inflammatory zones.

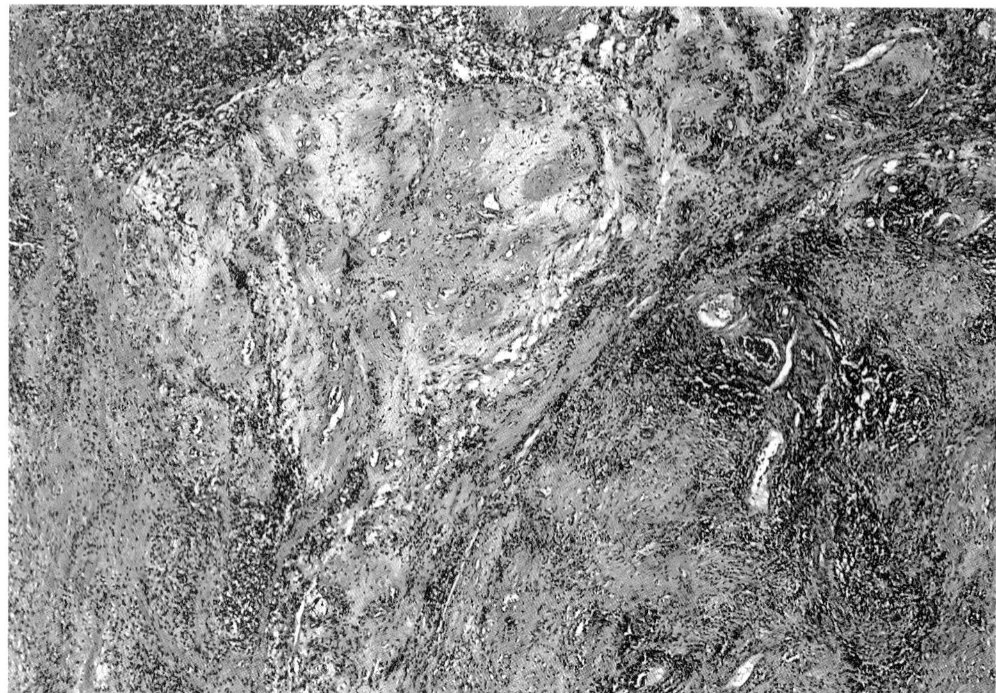

**FIGURE 37–81.** Admixture of myxoid, hyaline, and inflammatory zones in an inflammatory myxohyaline tumor.

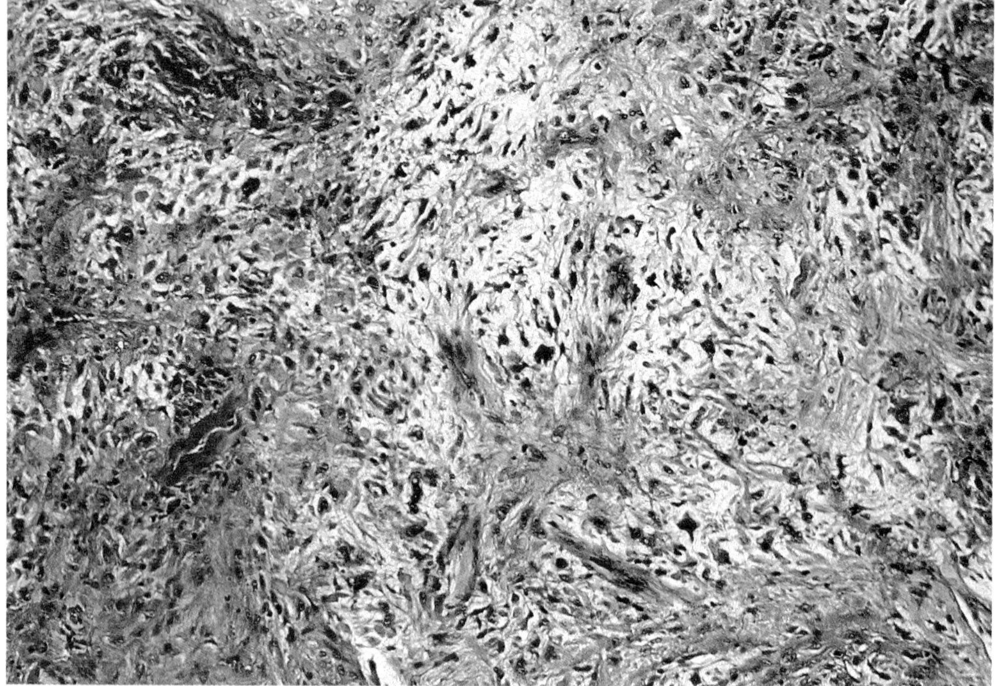

**FIGURE 37–82.** Inflammatory myxohyaline tumor. Note the transition between myxoid and hyaline zones.

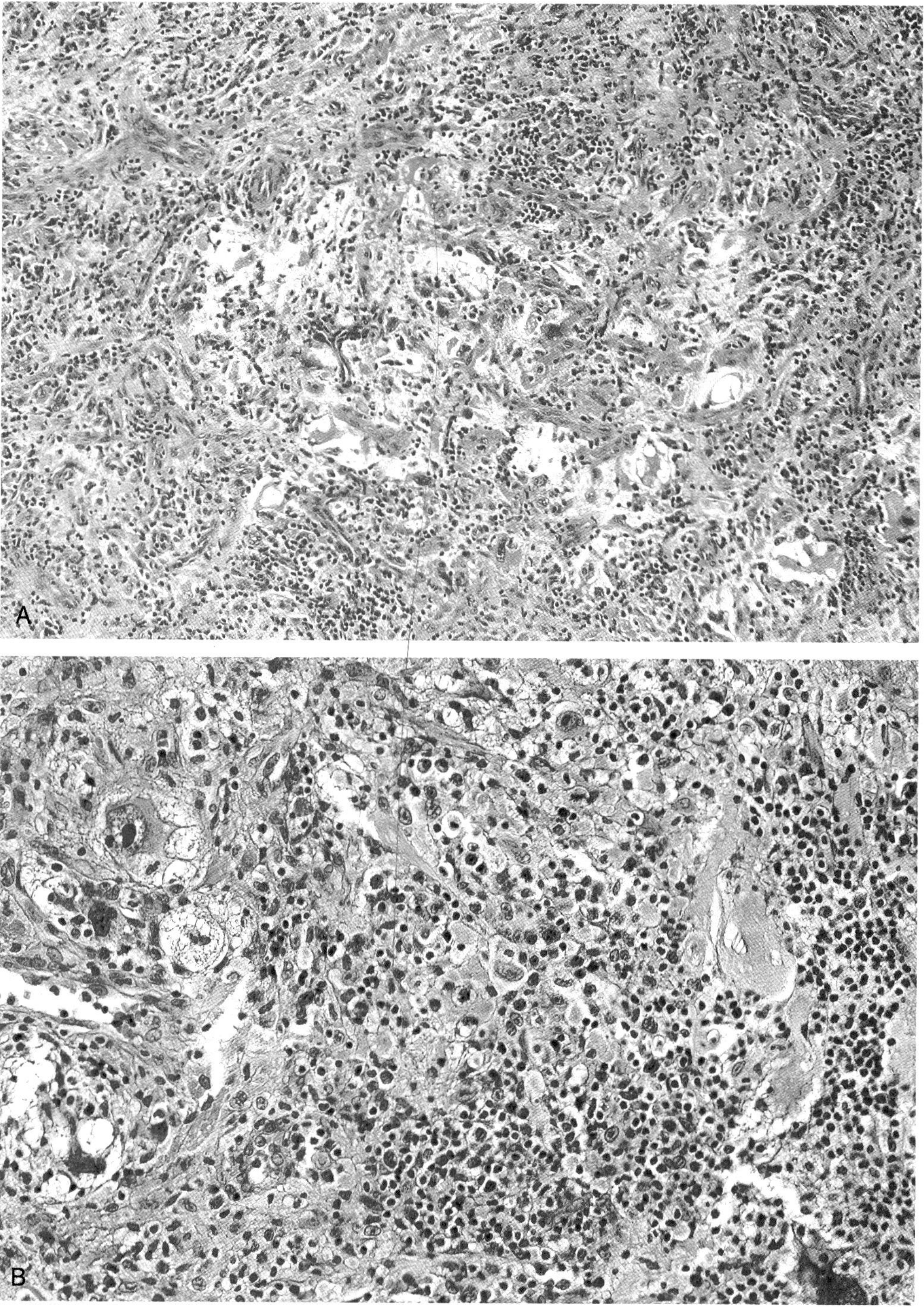

**FIGURE 37–83.** (**A, B**) Inflammatory myxohyaline tumor with prominent inflammatory zones.

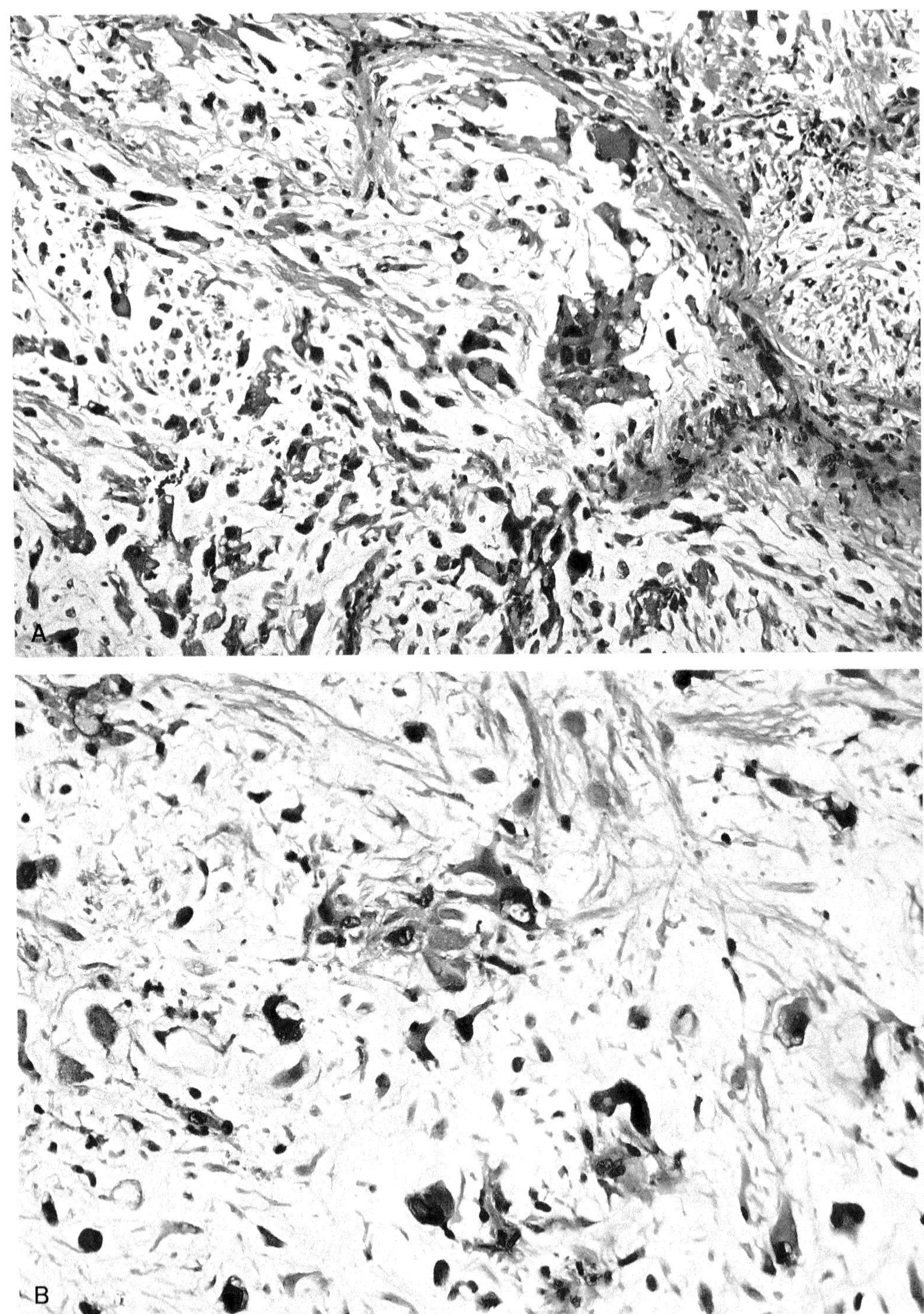


**FIGURE 37–84.** Myxoid zones in inflammatory myxohyaline tumor. Cells with smudgy nuclei are prominent.

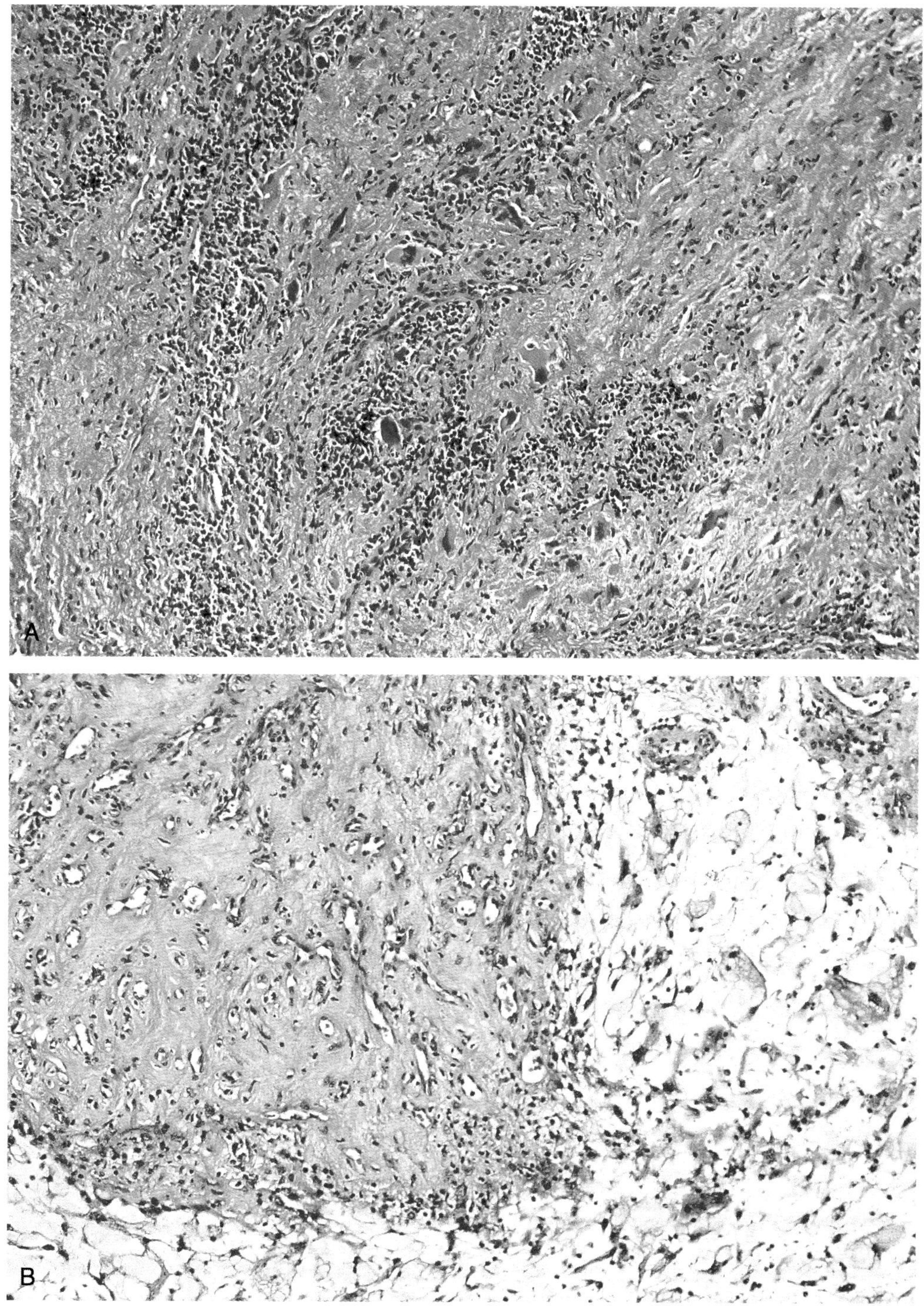


**FIGURE 37–85.** Inflammatory myxohyaline tumor. (**A**) Hyaline area with prominent inflammatory component. (**B**) Sharp transition between myxoid and hyaline zones.

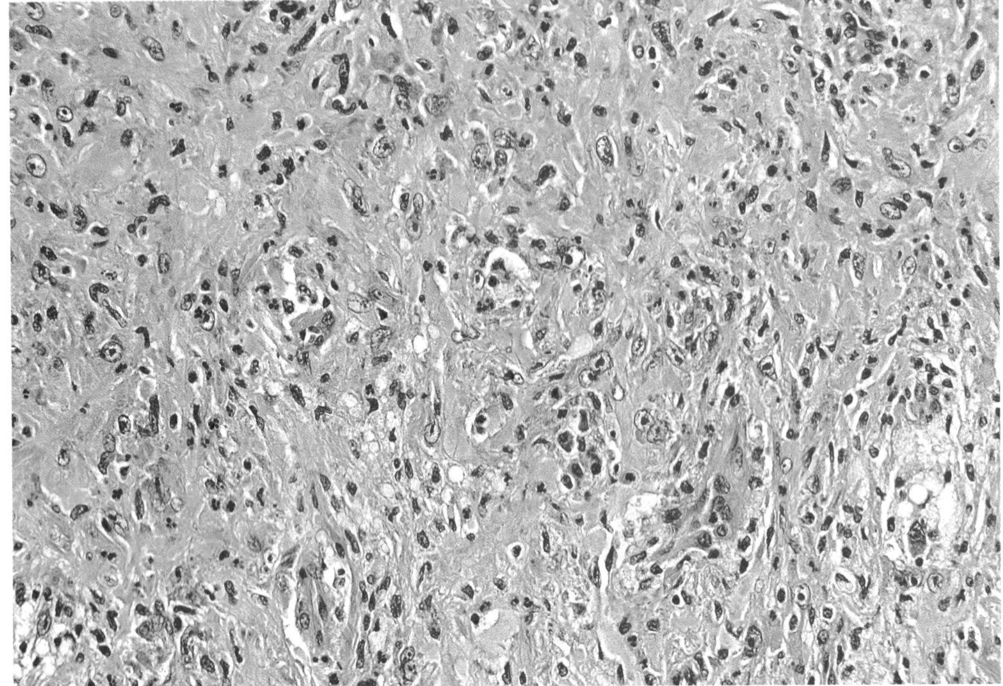

**FIGURE 37–86.** Inflammatory myxohyaline tumor. Neoplastic cells range from spindled to epithelioid.

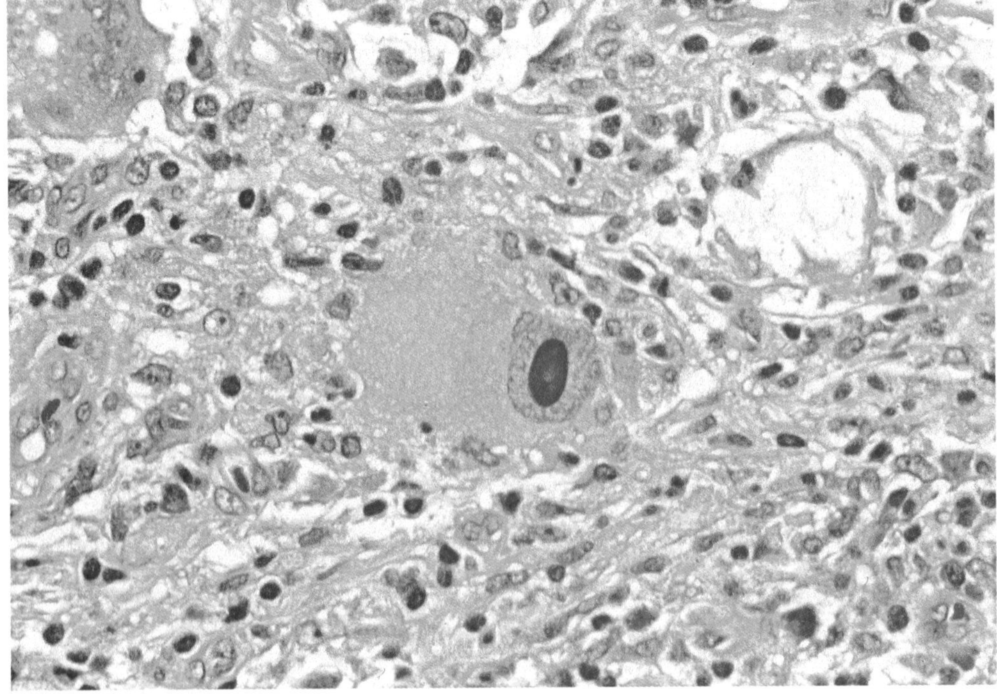

**FIGURE 37–87.** Enlarged tumor cell with a large eosinophilic nucleolus resembling a virocyte in an inflammatory myxohyaline tumor.

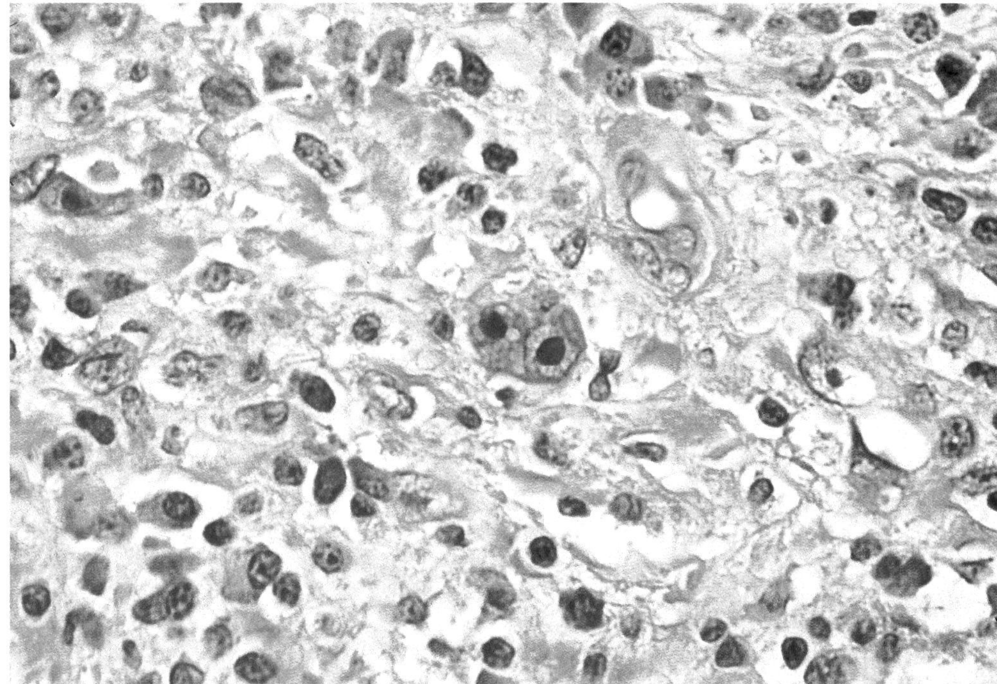

**FIGURE 37–88.** Inflammatory myxohyaline tumor with cells resembling Reed-Sternberg cells.

proliferative fasciitis may be widely scattered throughout the neoplasm or form small nodular collections. Some bizarre cells have multivacuolated cytoplasm resembling lipoblasts (Fig. 37–89) and others appear to engulf inflammatory cells. Multinucleated giant cells including Touton-type giant cells are occasionally encountered (Fig. 37–90). In addition, there is often an intermingling of round mononuclear cells with bland nuclear features and small amounts of amphophilic cytoplasm. Necrosis is present in occasional cases.

## Immunohistochemical Findings

The mononuclear and larger bizarre cells consistently stain for vimentin, with variable immunoreactivity for CD-68, CD-34, and smooth muscle actin[400] (Table 37–15). Immunostains for S-100 protein, HMB-45, desmin, epithelial membrane antigen, leukocyte common antigen, CD-15 (Leu-M1), and CD-30 (Ki-1) are typically negative. Rare cases show focal immunoreactivity for cytokeratins. The lymphocytic infiltrate is predominantly composed of T cells with a smaller component of B cells.

## Electron Microscopic Findings

The bizarre neoplastic cells characteristically have a single, often clefted nucleus with one or more large nucleoli and occasional intranuclear cytoplasmic inclusions.[400] There are abundant rough endoplasmic reticulum and mitochondria, as well as densely packed perinuclear whorls of intermediate filaments, although actin-type and thin filaments are not seen. Small lipid droplets, glycogen, and scattered lysosomes may also be seen in the cytoplasm.

## Differential Diagnosis

Because of the wide array of appearances of this tumor, the differential diagnosis in part depends on the

**TABLE 37–15** IMMUNOHISTOCHEMICAL DATA ON INFLAMMATORY MYXOHYALINE TUMORS OF THE DISTAL EXTREMITIES

| Marker | No. of Cases Stained |
|---|---|
| Vimentin | 35/35 (100%) |
| CD-68 | 23/35 (66%) |
| CD-34 | 7/25 (28%) |
| Cytokeratin | 4/38 (11%) |
| Smooth muscle actin | 2/33 (6%) |
| CD-15 | 0/5 |
| CD-30 | 0/12 |
| EMA | 0/28 |
| S-100 protein | 0/44 |
| Desmin | 0/6 |

Data are from references 400 and 402.

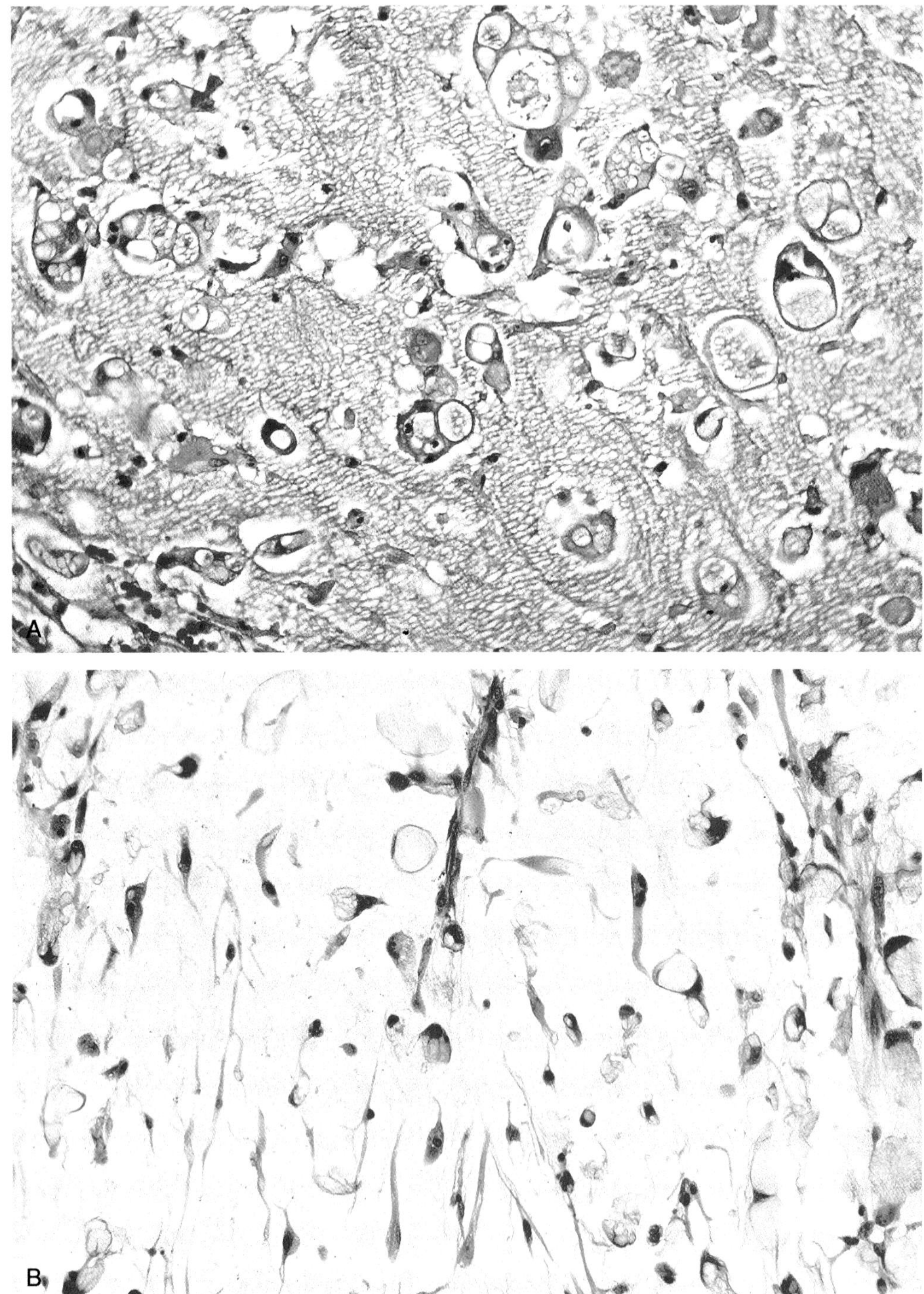


**FIGURE 37–89.** Myxoid zones in an inflammatory myxohyaline tumor. (**A**) Bizarre cells are distended with stromal mucin. (**B**) Pseudolipoblasts are prominent in this tumor.

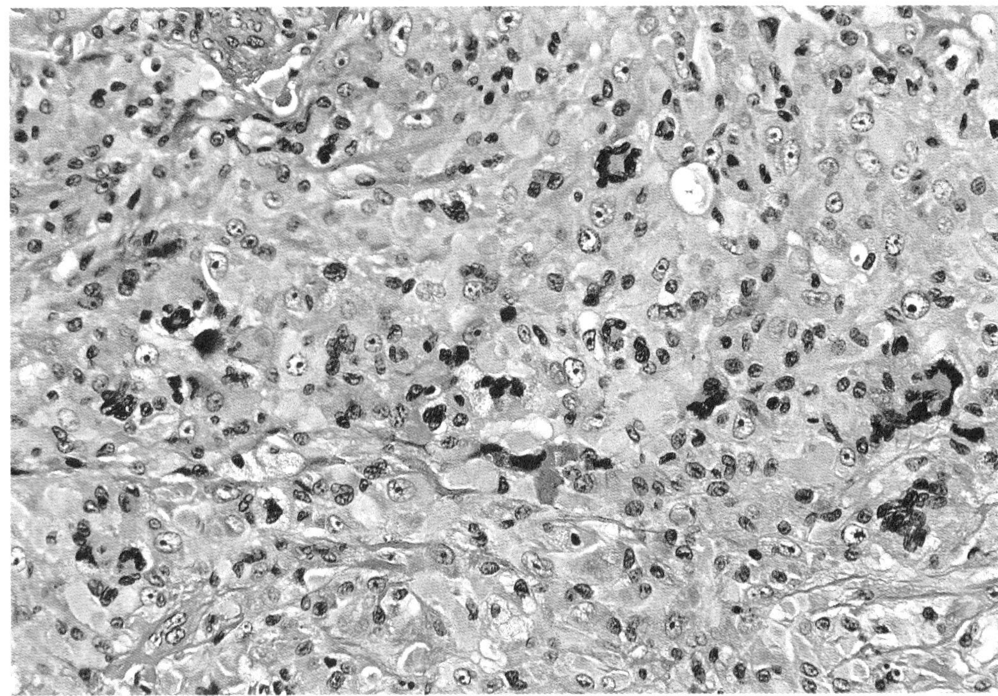

**FIGURE 37–90.** Scattered multinucleated giant cells in a cellular zone of inflammatory myxohyaline tumor.

cellularity of the lesion and the relative amount of myxoid and hyaline stroma. An infectious or inflammatory process is often considered, given the prominent inflammatory background, cells with virocyte-like nuclei, and necrosis. Special stains for microbial organisms are invariably negative, as are immunohistochemical stains for cytomegalovirus. Montgomery et al.[402] analyzed 10 cases by the PCR for the presence of Epstein-Barr virus (EBV). Although four patients were found to harbor EBV, the level of amplification was compatible with latent, rather than active, viral infection.

*Giant cell tumor of the tendon sheath* is often a diagnostic consideration given the location of the tumor, the prominent inflammatory component, and the presence of Touton-like giant cells and hemosiderin. Recognition of the large bizarre cells, which are widely scattered in some cases, is critical for distinguishing these lesions. This tumor also has histologic features that overlap with those found in *inflammatory myofibroblastic tumor* and *inflammatory fibrosarcoma,* although the cells of inflammatory myxohyaline tumor are more bizarre than those seen in the latter and lack the well developed immunohistochemical and ultrastructural features of myofibroblasts. Moreover, the acral location of the inflammatory myxohyaline tumor is not characteristic of either inflammatory myofibroblastic tumor or inflammatory fibrosarcoma, both of which are most commonly found in the abdomen or thorax.

Myriad benign and malignant myxoid lesions also enter the differential diagnosis for lesions with prominent myxoid stroma. The inflammatory myxohyaline tumor can be distinguished from benign myxoid lesions by recognizing large bizarre cells that would not be found in any benign myxoid soft tissue neoplasm. Distinction from *myxoid malignant fibrous histiocytoma* is the most difficult aspect of the differential diagnosis, although both tumors have enough distinguishing characteristics to support the contention that they are distinct entities. Focal areas of high-grade pleomorphic storiform malignant fibrous histiocytoma are often seen in myxoid malignant fibrous histiocytomas, whereas such high-grade areas would not be found in inflammatory myxohyaline tumors. Additional differences include the alternating myxoid and hyalinized zones, a more striking inflammatory infiltrate, the presence of virocyte-like cells, and the acral location typical of inflammatory myxohyaline tumor.

The presence of Reed-Sternberg-like cells also suggests the possibility of *Hodgkin's disease* in some cases. Immunohistochemically, the large atypical cells lack expression of CD-15 and CD-30 as one would expect to find in the Reed-Sternberg cells of Hodgkin's disease.

**TABLE 37–16 CLINICAL BEHAVIOR OF INFLAMMATORY MYXOHYALINE TUMORS OF THE DISTAL EXTREMITIES**

| Study | No. of Cases With Follow-up | Follow-up Interval (Median) | Local Recurrence | Metastasis |
|---|---|---|---|---|
| Meis-Kindblom et al.[400] | 36 | 6 months to 45 years (5 years) | 24/36 (67%) | 2/36 (6%) |
| Montgomery et al.[402] | 27 | 6 months to 10 years (53 months) | 6/27 (22%) | 0/27 (0%) |

## Discussion

In the original series of 51 cases reported by Montgomery et al.,[402] follow-up information was obtained in 27 patients with a median follow-up period of 53 months. Of these 27 patients, 6 (22%) developed at least one local recurrence 15 months to 10 years after the initial excision, but none developed metastatic disease. In the subsequent study of 44 cases by Meis-Kindblom and Kindblom,[400] follow-up information obtained in 36 patients revealed a local recurrence rate of 67%, including eight patients who had two local recurrences and five who had at least three local recurrences. The rather striking difference in recurrence rates between these studies probably reflects a difference in the referral base. The cases reported from the AFIP[400] were largely ascertained retrospectively, and many were not originally diagnosed as sarcoma, whereas those reported by Montgomery et al.[402] were ascertained prospectively and all were diagnosed as low-grade sarcomas and treated more aggressively. One patient reported by Meis-Kindblom and Kindblom[400] developed a histologically documented inguinal lymph node metastasis 1.5 years after the initial excision. A second patient developed suspected pulmonary metastases 2 years after the first local recurrence and 5 years after the initial presentation, although the metastases were not documented histologically (Table 37–16). At this point, wide local excision without adjuvant therapy appears to be adequate treatment for this tumor.

## REFERENCES

### Synovial Sarcoma

1. Abenoza P, Manivel JC, Swanson PE, et al. Synovial sarcoma: ultrastructural study and immunohistochemical analysis by a combined peroxidase-antiperoxidase/avidin-biotin-peroxidase complex procedure. Hum Pathol 17:1107, 1986.
2. Amble FR, Olsen KD, Nascimento AG, et al. Head and neck synovial cell sarcoma. Otolaryngol Head Neck Surg 107:631, 1992.
3. Anton-Pacheco J, Kano I, Cuadros J, et al. Synovial sarcoma of the esophagus. J Pediatr Surg 31:1703, 1996.
4. Argani P, Zakowski MF, Klimstra DS, et al. Detection of the SYT-SSX chimeric RNA of synovial sarcoma in paraffin embedded tissue and its application in problematic cases. Mod Pathol 11:65, 1998.
5. Bergh P, Meis-Kindblom JM, Gherlinzoni F, et al. Synovial sarcoma: identification of low and high risk groups. Cancer 85:2596, 1999.
6. Buonassisi V, Ozzello L. Sulfated mucopolysaccharide reproduction by synovial sarcoma cells in vivo and in tissue culture. Cancer Res 33:874, 1973.
7. Cadman NL, Soule EH, Kelly PJ. Synovial sarcoma: an analysis of 134 tumors. Cancer 18:613, 1965.
8. Cagle LA, Mirra JM, Storm FK, et al. Histologic features relating to prognosis in synovial sarcoma. Cancer 59:1810, 1987.
9. Choong PFM, Pritchard DJ, Sim FH, et al. Long-term survival in high grade soft tissue sarcoma: prognostic factors in synovial sarcoma. Int J Oncol 7:161, 1995.
10. Christensen WN, Strong EW, Bains MS, et al. Neuroendocrine differentiation in the glandular peripheral nerve sheath tumor. Am J Surg Pathol 12:417, 1988.
11. Clark J, Rocques PJ, Crew AJ, et al. Identification of novel genes, SYT and SSX involved in the t(X;18)(p11.2;q11.2) translocation found in human synovial sarcoma. Nat Genet 7:502, 1994.
12. Cohen IJ, Issakov J, Avigad S, et al. Synovial sarcoma of bone delineated by spectral karyotyping. Lancet 350:1679, 1997.
13. Corson JM, Weiss LM, Banks-Schlegel SP, et al. Keratin proteins and carcinoembryonic antigen in synovial sarcomas: an immunohistochemical study of 24 cases. Hum Pathol 15:615, 1984.
14. Corson JM, Weiss LM, Banks-Schlegel SP, et al. Keratin proteins in synovial sarcoma. Am J Surg Pathol 7:107, 1983.
15. Crew AJ, Clark J, Fisher C, et al. Fusion of SYT to two genes, SSX1 and SSX2 encoding protein with homology to the Krappel-associated box in human synovial sarcoma. EMBO J 14: 2333, 1995.
16. Dardick I, Ramjohn S, Thomas MJ, et al. Synovial sarcoma: interrelationship of the biphasic and monophasic subtypes. Pathol Res Pract 187:871, 1991.
17. De Leeuw B, Balemans M, Olde Weghuis D, et al. Identification of two alternative fusion genes, SYT-SSX1 and SYT-SSX2, in t(X;18)(p11.2;q11.2)-positive synovial sarcomas. Hum Mol Genet 4:1097, 1995.
18. De Leeuw B, Berger W, Sinke RJ, et al. Identification of a yeast artificial chromosome (YAC) spanning the synovial sarcoma-specific t(x;18)(p11.2;q11.2) breakpoint. Genes Chromosomes Cancer 6:182, 1993.
19. De Leeuw B, Suijkerbuijk RF, Olde Weghuis D, et al. Distinct Xp11.2 breakpoint regions in synovial sarcoma revealed by metaphase and interphase FISH: relationship to histologic subtypes. Cancer Genet Cytogenet 73:89, 1994.
20. Dei Tos AP, Dal Cin P, Sciot R, et al. Synovial sarcoma of the larynx and hypopharynx. Ann Otol Rhinol Laryngol 107:1080, 1998.
21. Dei Tos AP, Wadden C, Calonje E, et al. Immunohistochemical demonstration of glycoprotein p30/32mic2 (CD99) in synovial sarcoma: a potential cause of diagnostic confusion. Appl Immunohistochem 3:168, 1995.

22. Dickersin GR. Synovial sarcoma: a review and update, with emphasis on the ultrastructural characterization of the nonglandular component. Ultrastruct Pathol 15:379, 1991.
23. El-Naggar AK, Ayala AG, Abdul-Karim FW, et al. Synovial sarcoma: a DNA flow cytometric study. Cancer 65:2295, 1990.
24. Engelhardt J, Leafstedt SW. Synovial sarcoma of tonsil and tongue base. South Med J 76:243, 1983.
25. Evans HL. Synovial sarcoma: a study of 23 biphasic and 17 probable monophasic examples. Pathol Annu 15:309, 1980.
26. Farris KB, Reed RJ. Monophasic, glandular, synovial sarcomas and carcinomas of the soft tissues. Arch Pathol Lab Med 106: 129, 1982.
27. Ferrari A, Casanova M, Massimino M, et al. Synovial sarcoma: report of a series of 25 consecutive children from a single institution. Med Pediatr Oncol 32:32, 1999.
28. Fetsch JF, Meis JM. Synovial sarcoma of the abdominal wall. Cancer 72:469, 1993.
29. Fischer C, Schofield J. S-100 protein positive synovial sarcoma. Histopathology 19:375, 1991.
30. Fisher C. Synovial sarcoma. Ann Diagn Pathol 2:401, 1998.
31. Fisher C. Synovial sarcoma: ultrastructural and immunohistochemical features of epithelial differentiation in monophasic and biphasic tumors. Hum Pathol 17:996, 1986.
32. Fisher C, Carter RL, Ramachandra S, et al. Peripheral nerve sheath differentiation in soft tissue sarcomas: an ultrastructural and immunohistochemical study. Histopathology 20:115, 1992.
33. Flieder DB, Moran CA. Primary cutaneous synovial sarcoma: a case report. Am J Dermatopathol 20:509, 1998.
34. Fligman I, Lonardo F, Jhanwar SC, et al. Molecular diagnosis of synovial sarcoma and characterization of a variant SYT-SSX2 fusion transcript. Am J Pathol 147:1592, 1995.
35. Folpe AL, Schmidt RA, Chapman D, et al. Poorly differentiated synovial sarcoma: immunohistochemical distinction from primitive neuroectodermal tumors and high-grade malignant peripheral nerve sheath tumors. Am J Surg Pathol 22:673, 1998.
36. Fujimoto K, Hashimoto S, Abe T, et al. Synovial sarcoma arising from the chest wall: MR imaging findings. Radiat Med 15: 411, 1997.
37. Gaertner E, Zeren EH, Fleming MV, et al. Biphasic synovial sarcomas arising in the pleural cavity: a clinicopathologic study of five cases. Am J Surg Pathol 20:36, 1996.
38. Ghadially FN. Is synovial sarcoma a carcinosarcoma of connective tissue? Ultrastruct Pathol 11:147, 1987.
39. Golouh R, Vuzevski V, Bracko M, et al. Synovial sarcoma: a clinicopathologic study of 36 cases. J Surg Oncol 45:20, 1990.
40. Grayson W, Nayler SJ, Jena GP. Synovial sarcoma of the parotid gland: a case report with clinicopathologic analysis and review of the literature. South Afr J Surg 36:32, 1998.
41. Guillou L, Wadden C, Kraus MD, et al. S-100 protein reactivity in synovial sarcomas: a potentially frequent diagnostic pitfall; immunhistochemical analysis of 100 cases. Appl Immunohistochem 4:167, 1996.
42. Hajdu SI, Shiu MH, Fortner JG. Tendosynovial sarcoma: a clinicopathological study of 136 cases. Cancer 39:1201, 1977.
43. Hall TC, Jensen DA, Lohse JR, et al. Synovial sarcoma with t(X:18) chromosomal translocation, cardiac involvement, and peripheral embolus. Med Pediatr Oncol 32:141, 1999.
44. Hamperl H. Malignes Synovialom und Trauma. Zentralbl Chir 94:889, 1969.
45. Hazelbag HM, Mooi WJ, Fleuren GJ, et al. Chain-specific keratin specific profile of epithelioid soft-tissue sarcoma: an immunohistochemical study on synovial sarcoma and epithelioid sarcoma. Appl Immunohistochem 4:176, 1996.
46. Hirakawa N, Naka T, Yamamoto I, et al. Overexpression of bcl-2 protein in synovial sarcoma: a comparative study of other soft tissue spindle cell sarcomas and an additional analysis by fluorescence in situ hybridization. Hum Pathol 27:1060, 1996.
47. Hirsch RJ, Yousem DM, Loevner LA, et al. Synovial sarcomas of the head and neck: MR findings. AJR 169:1185, 1997.
48. Hisaoka M, Hashimoto H, Iwamasa T. Primary synovial sarcoma of the lung: report of two cases confirmed by molecular detection of SYT-SSX fusion gene transcripts. Histopathology 34:205, 1999.
49. Holtz F, Magielski JF. Synovial sarcomas of the tongue base: the seventh reported case. Arch Otolaryngol 111:271, 1985.
50. Inagaki H, Nagasaka T, Otsuka T, et al. Association of SYT-SSX fusion types with proliferative activity in prognosis in synovial sarcoma. Mod Pathol 13:482, 2000.
51. Ishida T, Iijima T, Moriyama S, et al. Intra-articular calcifying synovial sarcoma mimicking synovial chondromatosis. Skeletal Radiol 25:766, 1996.
52. Iwasaki H, Ishiguro M, Ohjimi Y, et al. Synovial sarcoma of the prostate with t(X;18)(p11.2;q11.2). Am J Surg Pathol 23:220, 1999.
53. Iyengar V. Lineberger AS, Kerman S, et al. Synovial sarcoma of the heart: correlation with cytogenetic findings. Arch Pathol Lab Med 119:1080, 1995.
54. Jorgensen LJ, Lyon H, Myhre-Jensen O, et al. Synovial sarcoma: an immunohistochemical study of the epithelioid component. APMIS 102:191, 1994.
55. Kaakaji Y, Valle DE, McCarthy KE, et al. Case 4: synovial sarcoma. AJR 171:868, 1998.
56. Kampe CE, Rosen G, Eilber F, et al. Synovial sarcoma: a study of intensive chemotherapy in 14 patients with localized disease. Cancer 72:2161, 1993.
57. Kaplan MA, Goodman MB, Satish J, et al. Primary pulmonary sarcoma with morphologic features of monophasic synovial sarcoma and chromosome translocation t(X;18). Am J Clin Pathol 105:195, 1996.
58. Katenkamp D, Stiller D. Synovial sarcoma of the abdominal wall: light microscopic, histochemical and electron microscopic investigations. Virchows Arch [Pathol Anat] 388:349, 1980.
59. Kawai A, Woodruff J, Healey JH, et al. SYT-SSX gene fusion as a determinant of morphology and prognosis in synovial sarcoma. N Engl J Med 338:153, 1998.
59a. Kawauchi S, Fukuda T, Oda Y, et al. Prognostic significance of apoptosis in synovial sarcoma: Correlation with clinicopathologic parameters, cell proliferative activity, and expression of apoptosis-related proteins. Mod Pathol 13:755, 2000.
60. Kim D-H, Sohn JH, Lee MC, et al. Primary synovial sarcoma of the kidney. Am J Surg Pathol 24:1097, 2000.
61. Kleinschmidt-DeMasters BK, Mierau GW, Sze CJ, et al. Unusual dural and skull-based mesenchymal neoplasms: a report of four cases. Hum Pathol 29:240, 1998.
62. Krall RA, Kostianovsky M, Patchefsky AS. Synovial sarcoma: a clinical, pathological, and ultrastructural study of 26 cases supporting the recognition of a monophasic variant. Am J Surg Pathol 5:137, 1981.
63. Krane JF, Bertoni F, Fletcher CDM. Myxoid synovial sarcoma: an underappreciated morphologic subset. Mod Pathol 12:456, 1999.
64. Ladenstein R, Truener J, Koscielniak E, et al. Synovial sarcoma of childhood and adolescence: report of the German CWS-81 study. Cancer 71:3647, 1993.
65. Lamovec J, Zidar A, Cucek-Plenicar M. Synovial sarcoma associated with total hip replacement. A case report. J Bone Joint Surg Am 70:1558, 1988.
66. Lasota J, Jasinski M, Debiec-Rychter M, et al. Detection of the SYT-SSX fusion transcripts in formaldehyde-fixed, paraffin embedded tissue: a reverse transcription polymerase chain reaction amplification assay useful in the diagnosis of synovial sarcoma. Mod Pathol 11:626, 1998.

67. Lejars F, Rubens-Duval H. Les sarcomes primitifs des synoviales articulaires. Rev Chir (Paris) 41:751, 1910.
68. Limon J, Dal Cin P, Sandberg AA. Translocations involving the X chromsome in solid tumors: presentation of two sarcomas with t(X;18)(q13;p11). Cancer Genet Cytogenet 23:87, 1986.
69. Lombardi L, Rilke F. Ultrastructural similarities and differences of synovial sarcoma, epithelioid sarcoma and clear cell sarcoma of tendons and aponeuroses. Ultrastruct Pathol 6:209, 1984.
70. Lopes JM, Bjerkehagen B, Holm R, et al. Immunohistochemical profile of synovial sarcoma with emphasis on the epithelial-type differentiation: a study of 49 primary tumours, recurrences and metastasis. Pathol Res Pract 190:168, 1994.
71. Lopes JM, Hannisdal E, Bjerkehagen B, et al. Synovial sarcoma: evaluation of prognosis with emphasis on the study of DNA ploidy and proliferation (PCNA and Ki-67) markers. Anal Cell Pathol 16:45, 1998.
72. Lu Y-J, Birdsall S, Summersgill B, et al. Dual colour flourescence in situ hybridization to paraffin-embedded samples to deduce the presence of the der(X)t(X;18)(p11.2;q11.2) an involvement of either the SSX1 or SSX2 gene: a diagnostic and prognostic aid for synovial sarcoma. J Pathol 187:490, 1999.
73. Machen SK, Easley KA, Goldblum JR. Synovial sarcoma of the extremities: a clinicopathologic study of 34 cases, including semi-quantitative analysis of spindled, epithelial and poorly differentiatad areas. Am J Surg Pathol 23:268, 1999.
74. Machen SK, Fisher C, Gautam RS, et al. Utility of cytokeratin subsets for distinguishing poorly differentiated synovial sarcoma from peripheral primitive neuroectodermal tumour. Histopathology 33:501, 1998.
75. Machinami R, Kashima T. Synovial sarcoma of the abdominal wall. J Pathol 182:A25, 1997.
76. Majeste RM, Beckman EN. Synovial sarcoma with an overwhelming epithelial component. Cancer 61:2527, 1988.
77. Mandahl N, Heim S, Arheden K, et al. Multiple karyotypic rearrangements, including t(X;18) (p11;q11), in a fibrosarcoma. Cancer Genet Cytogenet 30:323, 1998.
78. Massarelli G, Tanda F, Salis B. Synovial sarcoma of the soft palate: report of a case. Hum Pathol 9:341, 1978.
79. Maxwell JR, Yao L, Eckardt JJ, et al. Case report 878: densely calcifying synovial sarcoma of the hip metastatic to the lungs. Skeletal Radiol 23:673, 1994.
80. McKinney CD, Mills SE, Fechner RF. Intraarticular synovial sarcoma. Am J Surg Pathol 16:1017, 1992.
81. Meis-Kindblom JM, Stenman G, Kindblom L-C. Differential diagnosis of small round cell tumors. Semin Diagn Pathol 13: 213, 1996.
82. Menendez LR, Brien E, Brien WW. Synovial sarcoma: a clinicopathalogic study. Orthop Rev 21:465, 1992.
83. Miettinen M. Keratin subsets in spindle cell sarcomas: keratins are widespread but synovial sarcoma contains a distinct keratin polypeptide pattern and desmoplakins. Am J Pathol 135: 505, 1991.
84. Miettinen M, Lehto VP, Virtanen I. Monophasic synovial sarcoma of spindle-cell type: epithelial differentiation as revealed by ultrastructural features, content of prekeratin and binding of peanut agglutinin. Virchows Arch [Cell Pathol] 44:187, 1983.
85. Miettinen M, Virtanen I. Synovial sarcoma—a misnomer. Am J Pathol 117:18, 1984.
86. Milchgrub S, Ghandur-Mnaymneh L, Dorfman HD, et al. Synovial sarcoma with extensive osteoid and bone formation. Am J Surg Pathol 17:357, 1993.
87. Mirra JM, Wang S, Bhuta S. Synovial sarcoma with squamous differentiation of its mesenchymal glandular elements: a case report with light-microscopic, ultramicroscopic and immunologic correlation. Am J Surg Pathol 8:791, 1984.
88. Mischler NE. Synovial sarcoma of the neck associated with previous head and neck radiation therapy. Arch Otolaryngol 104:482, 1978.
89. Moffatt EJ, Lieu K, Layfield LJ. Demonstration of myxoid change in fine-needle aspiration of synovial sarcoma: a case report. Diagn Cytopathol 18:188, 1998.
90. Mullen JR, Zagars GK. Synovial sarcoma outcome following conservation surgery and radiotherapy. Radiother Oncol 33:23, 1994.
91. Nagao K, Ito H, Yoshida H. Chromosomal translocation t(X; 18) in human synovial sarcomas analyzed by fluorescence in situ hybridization using paraffin embedded tissue. Am J Pathol 148:601, 1996.
92. Nakamura T, Nakata K, Hata S, et al. Histochemical characterization of mucosubstances in synovial sarcoma. Am J Surg Pathol 8:429, 1984.
93. Nicholson AG, Rigby M, Lincoln C, et al. Synovial sarcoma of the heart. Histopathology 30:349, 1997.
93a. Nilsson G, Skytting B, Xie Y, et al. The SYT-SSX1 variant of synovial sarcoma is associated with a high rate of tumor cell proliferation and poor clinical outcome. Cancer Res 59:3180, 1999.
94. O'Connell JX, Browne WL, Gropper PT, et al. Intraneural biphasic synovial sarcoma: an alternative "glandular" tumor of peripheral nerve. Mod Pathol 9:738, 1996.
95. Oda Y, Hashimoto H, Takeshita S, et al. The prognostic value of immunohistochemical staining for proliferating cell nuclear antigen in synovial sarcoma. Cancer 72:478, 1993.
96. Oda Y, Hashimoto H, Tsuneyoshi M, et al. Survival in synovial sarcoma: a multivariate study of prognostic factors with special emphasis on the comparison between early death and long-term survival. Am J Surg Pathol 17:35, 1993.
97. Oda Y, Sakamoto A, Saito T, et al. Expression of hepatocyte growth factor (HGF)/scatter factor and its receptor c-MET correlates with poor prognosis in synovial sarcoma. Hum Pathol 31:185, 2000.
98. Ordóñez NG, Mahfouz SM, Mackay B. Synovial sarcoma: an immunohistochemical and ultrastructural study. Hum Pathol 21:733, 1990.
99. Pack GT, Ariel IM. Synovial sarcoma (malignant synovioma): a report of 60 cases. Surgery 28:1047, 1950.
100. Pappo AS, Fontanesi J, Luo X, et al. Synovial sarcoma in children and adolescents: the St. Jude Children's Research Hospital Experience. J Clin Oncol 12:2360, 1994.
101. Pilotti S, Mezzelani A, Azzarelli A, et al. Bcl-2 expression in synovial sarcoma. J Pathol 184:337, 1998.
102. Povysil C. Synovial sarcoma with squamous metaplasia. Ultrastruct Pathol 7:207, 1984.
103. Renshaw AA. O13 (CD99) in spindle cell tumors: reactivity with hemangiopericytoma, solitary fibrous tumor, synovial sarcoma and meningioma but rarely with sarcomatoid mesothelioma. Appl Immunohistochem 3:250, 1995.
104. Renwick PJ, Reeves BR, Dal Cin P, et al. Two categories of synovial sarcoma defined by divergent chromosome translocation breakpoints in Xp11.2, with implications for the histologic sub-classification of synovial sarcoma. Cytogenet Cell Genet 70:58, 1995.
105. Roberts CA, Seemeyer TA, Neff JR, et al. Translocation (X;18) in primary synovial sarcoma of the lung. Cancer Genet Cytogenet 88:49, 1996.
106. Robinson DL, Destian S, Hinton DR. Synovial sarcoma of the neck: radiographic findings with a review of the literature. Am J Otolaryngol 15:46, 1994.
107. Rooser B, Willen H, Huguson A, et al. Prognostic factors in synovial sarcoma. Cancer 63:2182, 1989.
108. Rosen G, Forscher C, Lowenbraun S, et al. Synovial sarcoma: uniform response of metastases to high dose of ifosfamide. Cancer 73:2506, 1994.

109. Ryan JR, Baker LH, Benjamin RS. The natural history of metastatic synovial sarcoma: experience of the Southwest Oncology Group. Clin Orthop 164:257, 1982.
110. Salisbury JR, Isaacson PG. Synovial sarcoma: an immunohistochemical study. J Pathol 147:49, 1985.
111. Sanchez Reyes JM, Alcaraz Mexia M, Quinones Tapia D, et al. Extensively calcified synovial sarcoma. Skeletal Radiol 26:671, 1997.
112. Schmidt D, Thum P, Harms D, et al. Synovial sarcoma in children and adolescents: a report from the Kiel Pediatric Tumor Registry. Cancer 67:1667, 1991.
113. Schneider-Stock R, Onnasch D, Haeckel C, et al. Prognostic significance of p53 gene mutations and p53 protein expression in synovial sarcomas. Virchows Arch 435:407, 1999.
114. Shanfeld RL, Edelman J, Willis JE, et al. Immunohistochemical analysis of neural markers in peripheral primitive neuroectodermal tumors (pPNET) without light microscopic evidence of neural differentiation. Appl Immunohistochem 5:78, 1997.
115. Shipley J, Crew J, Birdsall S, et al. Interphase fluorescence in situ hybridization and reverse transcription polymerase chain reaction as a diagnostic aid for synovial sarcoma. Am J Pathol 148:559, 1996.
116. Shipley JM, Clark J, Crew AJ, et al. The t(X;18)(p11.2;q11.2) translocation found in human synovial sarcomas involves two distinct loci on the X chromosome. Oncogene 9:1447, 1994.
117. Shiu MH, McCormack PM, Hajdu SI, et al. Surgical treatment of tendosynovial sarcoma. Cancer 43:889, 1979.
118. Singer S, Baldini EH, Demetri GD, et al. Synovial sarcoma: prognostic significance of tumor size, margin of resection, and mitotic activity for survival. J Clin Oncol 14:1201, 1996.
119. Smith LW. Synoviomata. Am J Pathol 3:355, 1927.
120. Smith MEF, Fisher C, Wilkinson LS, et al. Synovial sarcoma lacks synovial differentiation. Histopathology 26:279, 1995.
121. Smith TA, Machen SK, Fisher C, et al. Utility of cytokeratin subsets in distinguishing monophasic synovial sarcoma from malignant peripheral nerve sheath tumor. Am J Clin Pathol 112:641, 1999.
122. Stevenson AJ, Chatten J, Bertoni F, et al. CD99 (p30/32 MIC2) neuroectodermal/Ewing's sarcoma antigen as an immunohistochemical marker: a review of more than 600 tumors and the literature experience. Appl Immunohistochem 2:231, 1994.
123. Strickland B, Mackenzie DH. Bone involvement in synovial sarcoma. J Fac Radiologists (Lond) 10:64, 1959.
124. Suster S, Fisher C, Moran CA. Expression of bcl2 oncoprotein in benign and malignant spindle cell tumors of soft tissue, skin, serosal surfaces and gastrointestinal tract. Am J Surg Pathol 22:863, 1998.
125. Sutro CJ. Synovial sarcoma of the soft parts in the first toe: recurrence after 35 years' interval. Bull Hosp Joint Dis 37:105, 1976.
126. Tacconi L, Thom M, Thomas DG. Primary monophasic synovial sarcoma of the brachial plexus: report of a case and review of the literature. Clin Neurol Neurosurg 98:249, 1996.
127. Tajima K, Fuyama S, Yamaguchi H, et al. Pure monophasic, epithelial synovial sarcoma without a spindle cell component. Histopathology 34:78, 1999.
128. Thunold J, Bang G. Synovial sarcoma: a case report. Acta Orthop Scand 47:231, 1976.
129. Tsuji S, Hisaoka M, Morimitsu Y, et al. Detection of SYT-SSX fusion transcripts in synovial sarcoma by reverse transcription-polymerase chain reaction using archival paraffin embedded tissues. Am J Pathol 153:1807, 1998.
130. Tsuneyoshi M, Yokoyama K, Enjoji M. Synovial sarcoma: a clinicopathologic and ultrastructural study of 42 cases. Acta Pathol Jpn 33:23, 1983.
131. Turc-Carel C, Dal Cin P, Limon J, et al. Involvement of chromosome X in primary cytogenetic change in human neoplasia: nonrandom translocation in synovial sarcoma. Proc Natl Acad Sci USA 84:1981, 1987.
132. Turc-Carel C, Dal Cin P, Limon J, et al. Translocation X;18 in synovial sarcoma. Cancer Genet Cytogenet 23:9, 1986.
133. Ueda T, Uchida A, Kodama K, et al. Aggressive pulmonary metastasectomy for soft tissue sarcoma. Cancer 72:1919, 1993.
134. Van de Rijn M, Barr FG, Collins MH, et al. Absence of SYT-SSX fusion products in soft tissue tumors other than synovial sarcoma. Am J Clin Pathol 112:43, 1999.
135. Van de Rijn M, Barr FG, Xiong Q-B, et al. Poorly differentiated synovial sarcoma: an analysis of clinical, pathologic, and molecular genetic features. Am J Surg Pathol 23:106, 1999.
136. Van de Rijn M, Barr FG, Xiong Q-B, et al. Radiation-associated synovial sarcoma. Hum Pathol 28:1325, 1997.
137. Van de Rijn M, Rouse RV. CD34: a review. Appl Immunohistochem 2:71, 1994.
138. Vangeel AM, Pastorino U, Jauch KW, et al. Surgical treatment of lung metastases: the European organization for research and treatment of cancers—soft tissue and bone sarcoma group study of 255 patients. Cancer 77:675, 1996.
139. Varela-Duran J, Enzinger FM. Calcifying synovial sarcoma. Cancer 50:345, 1982.
140. Viguer JM, Jimenez-Heffernan JA, Vicandi B, et al. Cytologic features of synovial sarcoma with emphasis on the monophasic fibrous variant: a morphologic and immunocytochemical analysis of bcl-2 protein expression. Cancer 84:50, 1998.
141. Vincent RG. Malignant synovioma. Ann Surg 152:777, 1960.
142. Woodruff JM, Christensen WN. Glandular peripheral nerve sheath tumors. Cancer 72:3618, 1993.
143. Yang P, Hirose T, Hasegawa T, et al. Dual-colour fluorescence in situ hybridization analysis of synovial sarcoma. J Pathol 184:7, 1998.
144. Yokoyama K, Shinohara N, Kondo M, et al. Prognostic factors in synovial sarcoma: a clinicopathologic study of 18 cases. Jpn J Clin Oncol 25:131, 1995.
145. Zeren H, Moran CA, Suster S, et al. Primary pulmonary sarcomas with features of monophasic synovial sarcoma: a clinicopathological, immunohistochemical, and ultrastructural study of 25 cases. Hum Pathol 26:474, 1995.
146. Zilmer M, Harris CP, Steiner DS, et al. Use of non-breakpoint DNA probes to detect the t(X;18) in interphase cells from synovial sarcoma: implications for detection of diagnostic tumor translocations. Am J Pathol 152:1171, 1998.

### Alveolar Soft Part Sarcoma

147. Auerbach HE, Brooks JJ. Alveolar soft part sarcoma: a clinicopathologic and immunohistochemical study. Cancer 60:66, 1987.
148. Bindal RK, Sawaya RE, Leavens ME, et al. Sarcoma metastatic to the brain: results of surgical treatment. Neurosurgery 35: 185, 1994.
149. Cardinalli IA, Selig MK, Dickersin GR. Alveolar soft-part sarcoma with unusual mitochondrial findings: a case report. Ultrastruct Pathol 22:321, 1998.
150. Carstens HB. Membrane-bound cytoplasmic crystals, similar to those in alveolar soft part sarcoma, in a human muscle spindle. Ultrastruct Pathol 14:423, 1990.
151. Christopherson WM, Foote FW Jr, Stewart FW. Alveolar soft-part sarcoma: structurally characteristic tumors of uncertain histogenesis. Cancer 5:100, 1952.
152. Coira BM, Sachdev R, Moscovic E. Skeletal muscle markers in alveolar soft part sarcoma. Am J Clin Pathol 94:799, 1991.
153. Craver RD, Heinrich SD, Correa H, et al. Trisomy 8 in alveolar soft part sarcoma. Cancer Genet Cytogenet 81:94, 1995.
154. Cullinane C, Thorner PS, Greenberg ML, et al. Molecular genetic, cytogenetic and immunohistochemical characterization

of alveolar soft part sarcoma: implication for cell origin. Cancer 70:2444, 1992.

155. DeSchryver-Kecskemeti K, Kraus FT, Engleman BA. Alveolar soft-part sarcoma: a malignant angioreninoma: histochemical, immunocytochemical, and electron-microscopic study of four cases. Am J Surg Pathol 6:5, 1982.
156. Ekfors TO, Kalimo H, Rantakokko V, et al. Alveolar soft part sarcoma: a report of two cases with some histochemical and ultrastructural observations. Cancer 43:1672, 1979.
157. Evans HL. Alveolar soft-part sarcoma: a study of 13 typical examples and one with a histologically atypical component. Cancer 55:912, 1985.
158. Fender FA. Liposarcoma: report of a case with intracranial metastasis. Am J Pathol 9:909, 1933.
159. Fisher ER, Reidbord H. Electron microscopic evidence suggesting myogenous derivation of the so-called alveolar soft part sarcoma. Cancer 27:150, 1971.
160. Flieder DB, Moran CA, Suster S. Primary alveolar soft-part sarcoma of the mediastinum: a clinicopathologic and immunohistochemical study of two cases. Histopathology 31:469, 1997.
161. Foschini MP, Ceccarelli C, Eusebi V, et al. Alveolar soft part sarcoma: immunological evidence of rhabdomyoblastic differentation. Histopathology 13:101, 1988.
162. Foschini MP, Eusebi V. Alveolar soft-part sarcoma: a new type of rhabdomyosarcoma? Semin Diagn Pathol 11:58, 1994.
163. Gomez JA, Amin MB, Ro JY, et al. Immunohistochemical profile of myogenin and MyoD1 does not support skeletal muscle lineage in alveolar soft part sarcoma: a study of 19 tumors. Arch Pathol Lab Med 123:503, 1999.
164. Heimann P, Devalck C, Debusscher C, et al. Alveolar soft-part sarcoma: further evidence by FISH for the involvement of chromosome band 17q25. Genes Chromosomes Cancer 23:194, 1998.
165. Hirose T, Kudo E, Hasegawa T, et al. Cytoskeletal properties of alveolar soft part sarcoma. Hum Pathol 21:204, 1990.
166. Horn RC, Stout AP. Granular cell myoblastoma. Surg Gynecol Obstet 76:315, 1943.
167. Hunter BC, Devaney KO, Ferlito A, et al. Alveolar soft part sarcoma of the head and neck region. Ann Otol Rhinol Laryngol 107:810, 1998.
168. Iwamoto Y, Morimoto N, Chuman H, et al. The role of MR imaging in the diagnosis of alveolar soft part sarcoma: a report of 10 cases. Skeletal Radiol 24:267, 1995.
169. Jong R, Kandel R, Fornasier V, et al. Alveolar soft part sarcoma: review of nine cases including two cases with unusual histology. Histopathology 32:63, 1998.
170. Kamei T, Ishihara Y, Takahashi M, et al. An ultrastructural and histochemical study of alveolar soft part sarcoma with special reference to the nature of the crystals. Acta Pathol Jpn 34:435, 1984.
171. Karnauchow N, Magner D. The histogenesis of alveolar soft part sarcoma. J Pathol Bacteriol 89:169, 1963.
172. Kiuru-Kuhlefelt S, El-Rifai W, Sarlomo-Rikala M, et al. DNA copy number changes in alveolar soft part sarcoma: a comparative genomic hybridization study. Mod Pathol 11:227, 1998.
173. Kolodny A. Angioendothelioma of bone. Arch Surg 12:854, 1926.
174. Lieberman PH, Brennan MF, Kimmel M, et al. Alveolar soft-part sarcoma: a clinicopathologic study of half a century. Cancer 63:1, 1989.
175. Lieberman PH, Foote FW, Stewart FW, et al. Alveolar soft part sarcoma. JAMA 198:1047, 1966.
176. Lillehei KO, Kleinschmidt-DeMasters B, Mitchell DH, et al. Alveolar soft part sarcoma: an unusually long interval between presentation and brain metastasis. Hum Pathol 24:1030, 1993.
177. Lorigan JG, O'Keeffe FN, Evans HL, et al. The radiologic manifestations of alveolar soft-part sarcoma. AJR 153:335, 1989.
178. Marker P, Jensen ML, Siemssen SJ. Alveolar soft-part sarcoma of the oral cavity: report of a case and review of the literature. J Oral Maxillofac Surg 53:1203, 1995.
179. Masson P. Tumeurs Humaines: Histologie, Diagnostics et Techniques, 2nd ed. Librairie Maloine, Paris, 1959.
180. Matsuno Y, Mukai K, Itabashi M, et al. Alveolar soft part sarcoma: a clinicopathologic and immunohistochemical study of 12 cases. Acta Pathol Jpn 40:199, 1990.
181. Menesce LP, Eyden BP, Edmondson D, et al. Immunophenotype and ultrastructure of alveolar soft part sarcoma. J Submicrosc Cytol Pathol 25:377, 1993.
182. Miettinen M, Ekfors T. Alveolar soft part sarcoma: immunohistochemical evidence of muscle cell differentiation. Am J Clin Pathol 93:32, 1990.
183. Morimitsu Y, Tanaka H, Owanaga F, et al. Alveolar soft part sarcoma of the uterine cervix. Acta Pathol Jpn 43:204, 1993.
184. Mukai M, Iri H, Nakajima T, et al. Alveolar soft-part sarcoma: a review of the histogenesis and further studies based on electron microscopy, immunohistochemistry, and biochemistry. Am J Surg Pathol 7:679, 1983.
185. Mukai M, Torikata C, Iri H, et al. Alveolar soft part sarcoma: an elaboration of a three dimensional configuration of the crystalloids by digital image processing. Am J Pathol 116:398, 1984.
186. Mukai M, Torikata C, Iri H. Alveolar soft part sarcoma: an electron microscopic study especially of uncrystallized granules using a tannic acid containing fixative. Ultrastruct Pathol 14:41, 1990.
187. Mukai M, Torikata C, Shimoda T, et al. Alveolar soft part sarcoma: assessment of immunohistochemical demonstration of desmin using paraffin sections and frozen sections. Virchows Arch [Pathol Anat] 414:503, 1989.
188. Nakano H. Alveolar soft part sarcoma: histogenesis. Anticancer Res 18:4207, 1998.
189. Nakano H, Park P, Ohno T. Ultrastructural studies of tubules, analogous to skeletal cell T-tubules in alveolar soft part sarcoma. J Orthop Sci 3:143, 1998.
190. Nakashima Y, Kotoura Y, Kasakura K, et al. Alveolar soft-part sarcoma: a report of 10 cases. Clin Orthop 294:259, 1993.
191. Nielsen GP, Oliva E, Young RH, et al. Alveolar soft-part sarcoma of the female genital tract: a report of nine cases and review of the literature. Int J Gynecol Pathol 14:283, 1995.
192. Ohno T, Park P, Higaki S, et al. Smooth tubular aggregates associated with plasmalemmal invaginations in alveolar soft part sarcoma. Ultrastruct Pathol 18:383, 1994.
193. Ordóñez NG. Alvolar soft part sarcoma: a review and update. Adv Anat Pathol 6:125, 1999.
194. Ordóñez NG, Ro JY, Mackay B. Alveolar soft part sarcoma: an ultrastructural and immunocytochemical investigation of its histogenesis. Cancer 63:1721, 1989.
195. Pappo AS, Parham DM, Cain A, et al. Alveolar soft part sarcoma in children and adolescents: clinical features and outcome of 11 patients. Med Pediatr Oncol 26:81, 1996.
196. Perry JR, Bilbao JM. Metastatic alveolar soft part sarcoma presenting as a dural-based cerebral mass. Neurosurgery 34:168, 1994.
197. Persson S, Willems JS, Kindblom LG, et al. Alveolar soft part sarcoma: an immunohistochemical, cytologic, and electron-microscopic study and a quantitative DNA analysis. Virchows Arch [Pathol Anat] 412:499, 1988.
198. Radig K, Buhtz P, Roessner A. Alveolar soft part sarcoma of the uterine corpus: report of two cases and review of the literature. Pathol Res Pract 194:59, 1998.
199. Rosai J, Dias P, Parham DM, et al. MyoD1 protein expression

in alveolar soft part sarcoma as confirmatory evidence of its skeletal muscle nature. Am J Surg Pathol 15:974, 1991.
200. Sciot R, Dal Cin P, De Vos R, et al. Alveolar soft-part sarcoma: evidence for its myogenic origin and for the involvement of 17q25. Histopathology 23:439, 1993.
201. Sherman N, Vavilala M, Pollock R, et al. Radiation therapy for alveolar soft-part sarcoma. Med Pediatr Oncol 22:380, 1994.
202. Shipkey FH, Lieberman PH, Foote FW, et al. Ultrastructure of alveolar soft part sarcoma. Cancer 17:821, 1964.
203. Simmons WB, Haggerty HS, Ngan B, et al. Alveolar soft part sarcoma of the head and neck: a disease of children and young adults. Int J Pediatr Otorhinolaryngol 17:139, 1989.
204. Smetana HF, Scott WF. Soft tissue tumors of peculiar character and uncertain origin (malignant tumors of nonchromaffin paraganglia). Milit Surg 109:330, 1951.
205. Sonobe H, Ro JY, Mackay B, et al. Primary pulmonary alveolar soft-part sarcoma: report of a case. Int J Surg Pathol 2:57, 1994.
206. Temple HT, Scully SP, O'Keefe RJ, et al. Clinical presentation of alveolar soft part sarcoma. Clin Orthop 300:213, 1994.
207. Van Echten J, van den Berg E, van Baarlen J, et al. An important role for chromsome 17, band q25, in the histogenesis of alveolar soft part sarcoma. Cancer Genet Cytogenet 82:57, 1995.
208. Wang CH, Lee N, Lee LS. Successful treatment for solitary brain metastasis from alveolar soft part sarcoma. J Neurooncol 25:161, 1995.
209. Wang NP, Bacchi CE, Jiang JJ, et al. Does alveolar soft-part sarcoma exhibit skeletal muscle differentiation? An immnunocytochemical and biochemical study of myogenic regulatory protein expression. Mod Pathol 9:496, 1996.

### Epithelioid Sarcoma

210. Arber DA, Kandalaft PL, Mehta P, et al. Vimentin negative epithelioid sarcoma: the value of immunohistochemical panel that includes CD-34. Am J Surg Pathol 17:302, 1993.
211. Berger L. Synovial sarcomas in serous bursae and tendon sheaths. Am J Cancer 34:501, 1938.
212. Blewitt RW, Aparicio SGR, Bird CC. Epithelioid sarcoma, a tumour of myofibroblasts. Histopathology 7:573, 1983.
213. Bliss BO, Reed RJ. Large cell sarcomas of tendon sheath. Am J Clin Pathol 49:776, 1968.
214. Bloustein PA, Silverberg SG, Waddell WR. Epithelioid sarcoma: case report with ultrastructural review, histogenetic discussion, and chemotherapeutic data. Cancer 38:2390, 1976.
215. Bos GD, Pritchard DJ, Reiman HM, et al. Epithelioid sarcoma: an analysis of fifty-one cases. J Bone Joint Surg Am 70:862, 1998.
216. Chase DR, Enzinger FM. Epithelioid sarcoma: diagnosis, prognostic indicators, and treatment. Am J Surg Pathol 9:241, 1985.
217. Chase DR, Enzinger FM, Weiss SW, et al. Keratin in epithelioid sarcoma: an immunohistochemical study. Am J Surg Pathol 8:435, 1984.
218. Chetty R, Slavin JL. Epithelioid sarcoma with extensive chondroid differentiation. Histopathology 24:400, 1994.
219. Cordoba JC, Parham DM, Meyer WH, et al. A new cytogenetic finding in a epithelioid sarcoma, t(8;22)(q22;q11). Cancer Genet Cytogenet 72:151, 1994.
220. Dabska M, Koszarowski T. Clinical and pathologic study of aponeurotic (epithelioid) sarcoma. Pathol Annul 17:129, 1982.
221. Daimaru Y, Hashimoto H, Tsuneyoshi M, et al. Epithelial profile of epithelioid sarcoma: an immunohistochemical analysis of eight cases. Cancer 59:134, 1987.
222. Dominguez C, Broseta E, Alonso C, et al. Epithelioid sarcoma of penis simulating Peyronie's disease. Br J Urol 72:975, 1993.
223. El-Naggar AK, Garcia GM. Epithelioid sarcoma: flow cytometric study of DNA content and regional DNA heterogeneity. Cancer 69:1721, 1992.
224. Enzinger FM. Epithelioid sarcoma: a sarcoma simulating a granuloma or a carcinoma. Cancer 26:1029, 1970.
225. Evans HL, Baer SC. Epithelioid sarcoma: a clinicopathologic and prognostic study of 26 cases. Semin Diagn Pathol 10:286, 1993.
226. Fisher C. Epithelioid sarcoma: the spectrum of ultrastructural differentiation in seven immunohistochemically defined cases. Hum Pathol 19:265, 1988.
227. Fisher ER, Horvat B. The fibrocytic derivation of the so-called epithelioid sarcoma. Cancer 30:1074, 1972.
228. Fletcher CDM, Beham A, Bekir S, et al. Epithelioid angiosarcoma of deep soft tissue: a distinctive tumor readily mistaken for an epithelioid neoplasm. Am J Surg Pathol 15:915, 1991.
229. Frable WJ, Kay S, Lawrence W, et al. Epithelioid sarcoma: an electron microscopic study. Arch Pathol 95:8, 1973.
230. Gross E, Rao BN, Pappo A, et al. Epithelioid sarcoma in children. J Pediatr Surg 31:1663, 1996.
231. Guillou L, Wadden C, Coindre J-M, et al. "Proximal-type" epithelioid sarcoma, a distinctive aggressive neoplasm showing rhabdoid features: clinicopathologic, immunohistochemical, and ultrastructural study of a series. Am J Surg Pathol 21: 130, 1997.
232. Halling AC, Wollan PC, Pritchard DJ, et al. Epithelioid sarcoma: a clinicopathologic review of 55 cases. Mayo Clin Proc 71:636, 1996.
233. Hazelbag HM, Mooi WJ, Fleuren GJ, et al. Gene-specific keratin profile of epithelioid soft-tissue sarcomas: an immunohistochemical study on synovial sarcoma and epithelioid sarcoma. Appl Immunohistochem 4:176, 1996.
234. Heenan PJ, Quirk CJ, Papadimitriou JM. Epithelioid sarcoma: a diagnostic problem. Am J Dermatopathol 8:95, 1986.
235. Hernandez-Ortiz MJ, Valenzuela-Ruiz P, Gonzalez-Estecha A, et al. Fine needle aspiration cytology of primary epithelioid sarcoma of the vulva: a case report. Acta Cytol 39:100, 1995.
236. Huang DJ, Stanisic TH, Hansen KK. Epithelioid sarcoma of the penis. J Urol 147:1370, 1992.
237. Ishida T, Oka T, Matsushita H, et al. Epithelioid sarcoma: an electron-microscopic, immunohistochemical, and DNA flow cytometric analysis. Virchows Arch [Pathol Anat] 421:401, 1992.
238. Iwasaki H, Ohjimi Y, Ishiguro M, et al. Epithelioid sarcoma with an 18q aberration. Cancer Genet Cytogenet 91:46, 1996.
239. Kanai T, Irisawa R, Kusama H, et al. Ultrastructural observation of epithelioid sarcoma. J Dermatol 20:691, 1993.
240. Kodet R, Smelhaus V, Newton WA Jr, et al. Epithelioid sarcoma in childhood: an immunohistochemical, electron microscopic and clinicopathologic study of 11 cases under 15 years of age and review of the literature. Pediatr Pathol 14:433, 1994.
241. Konefka T, Senkus E, Emerich J, et al. Epithelioid sarcoma of the Bartholin's gland primarily diagnosed as vulvar carcinoma. Gynecol Oncol 54:393, 1994.
242. Kuhel WI, Monihan N, Shanahan EM, et al. Epithelioid sarcoma of the neck: a rare tumor mimicking metastatic carcinoma from an unknown primary. Otolaryngol Head Neck Surg 117:S210, 1997.
243. Laskin WB, Weiss SW, Bratthauer GL. Epithelioid variant of malignant peripheral nerve sheath tumor (malignant epithelioid schwannoma). Am J Surg Pathol 15:1136, 1991.
244. Leroy X, Delobelle A, Lefebvre JL, et al. Epithelioid sarcoma of the tongue. J Clin Pathol 50:869, 1997.
244a. Lushnikova T, Knuutila S, Miettinen M. DNA copy number changes in epithelioid sarcoma and its variants: A comparative genomic hybridization study. Mod Pathol 13:1092, 2000.
245. Manivel JC, Wick MR, Dehner LP, et al. Epithelioid sarcoma: an immunohistochemical study. Am J Clin Pathol 87:319, 1987.

246. Meis JM, Mackay B, Ordóñez NG. Epithelioid sarcoma: an immunohistochemical and ultrastructural study. Surg Pathol 1: 13, 1988.
247. Meis-Kindblom JM, Kindblom LG. Angiosarcoma of soft tissue: a study of cases. Am J Surg Pathol 22:683, 1998.
248. Miettinen M, Fanburg-Smith JC, Virolainen M, et al. Epithelioid sarcoma: an immunohistochemical analysis of 112 classical and variant cases and a discussion of the differential diagnosis. Hum Pathol 30:934, 1999.
249. Miettinen M, Lehto VP, Vartio T, et al. Epithelioid sarcoma: ultrastructural and immunohistologic features suggesting synovial origin. Arch Pathol Lab Med 106:620, 1982.
250. Mills SE, Fechner RE, Bruns DE, et al. Intermediate filaments in eosinophilic cells of epithelioid sarcoma: a light microscopic, ultrastructural, and electrophoretic study. Am J Surg Pathol 5:199, 1981.
251. Mirra JM, Kessler S, Bhuta S, et al. The fibroma-like variant of epithelioid sarcoma: a fibrohistiocytic/myoid cell lesion often confused with benign and malignant spindle cell tumors. Cancer 69:1382, 1992.
252. Mukai M, Torikata C, Iri H, et al. Cellular differentiation of epithelioid sarcoma: an electron-microscopic, enzyme-histochemical, and immunohistochemical study. Am J Pathol 119: 44, 1985.
253. Ormsby AH, Liou LS, Oriba HA, et al. Epithelioid sarcoma of the penis: report of an unusual case and review of the literature. Ann Diagn Pathol 4:88, 2000.
254. Pastel-Levy C, Bell DA, Rosenberg AE, et al. DNA flow cytometry of epithelioid sarcoma. Cancer 70:2823, 1992.
255. Persson S, Kindblom LG, Angerval L. Epithelioid sarcoma: an electron-microscopic and immunohistochemical study. Appl Pathol 6:1, 1988.
256. Pisa R, Novelli P, Bonetti F. Epithelioid sarcoma: a tumor of myofibroblasts, or not. Histopathology 8:353, 1984.
257. Prat J, Woodruff JM, Marcove RC. Epithelioid sarcoma: an analysis of 22 cases indicating the prognostic significance of vascular invasion and regional lymph node metastasis. Cancer 41:1472, 1978.
258. Puissegur-Lupo ML, Perret WJ, Millikan LE. Epithelioid sarcoma: report of a case. Arch Dermatol 121:394, 1985.
259. Quezado MM, Middleton LP, Bryant B, et al. Allelic loss on chromosome 22q in epithelioid sarcomas. Hum Pathol 29:604, 1998.
260. Romero JA, Kim EE, Moral IS. MR characteristics of epithelioid sarcoma. J Comp Assist Tomogr 18:929, 1994.
261. Rose DSC, Fisher C, Smith MEF. Epithelioid sarcoma arising in a patient with neurofibromatosis type 2. Histopathology 25: 379, 1994.
262. Ross HM, Lewis JJ, Woodruff JM, et al. Epithelioid sarcoma: clinical behavior and prognostic factors of survival. Ann Surg Oncol 4:491, 1997.
263. Santiago H, Feinerman LK, Lattes R. Epithelioid sarcoma: a clinical and pathological study of nine cases. Hum Pathol 3: 133, 1972.
264. Schiffman R. Epithelioid sarcoma and synovial sarcoma in the same knee. Cancer 45:158, 1980.
265. Shimm DS, Suit HD. Radiation therapy of epithelioid sarcoma. Cancer 52:1022, 1983.
266. Smith MEF, Brown JI, Fisher C. Epithelioid sarcoma: presence of vascular-endothelial cadherin and lack of epithelial cadherin. Histopathology 33:425, 1998.
267. Sonobe H, Ohtsuki Y, Sugimoto T, et al. Involvement of 8q, 22q, and monosomy 21 in an epithelioid sarcoma. Cancer Genet Cytogenet 96:178, 1997.
268. Soule EH, Enriquez P. Atypical fibrous histiocytoma, malignant histiocytoma, and epithelioid sarcoma: a comparative study of 65 tumors. Cancer 30:128, 1972.
269. Steinberg BD, Gelberman RH, Mankin HJ, et al. Epithelioid sarcoma in the upper extremity. J Bone Joint Surg Am 74:28, 1992.
270. Sugarbaker PH, Auda S, Webber BL. Early distant metastases from epithelioid sarcoma of the hand. Cancer 48:852, 1981.
271. Swanson PE, Dehner LP, Sirgi KE, et al. Cytokeratin immunoreactivity in malignant tumors of bone and soft tissue: a reappraisal of cytokeratin as a reliable marker in diagnostic immunohistochemistry. Appl Immunohistochem 2:103, 1994.
272. Trofatter JA, MacCollin MM, Rutter JL, et al. A novel Moesin-, Ezrin-, Radixin-like gene is a candidate for the neurofibromatosis 2 tumor suppressor. Cell 72:791, 1993.
273. Tsuneyoshi M, Enjoji M, Shinohara N. Epithelioid sarcoma: a clinicopathologic and electron microscopic study. Acta Pathol Jpn 30:411, 1980.
274. Van de Rijn M, Rouse RV. CD-34: a review. Appl Immunohistochem 2:71, 1994.
275. Von Hochstetter AR, Meyer VE, Grant JW, et al. Epithelioid sarcoma mimicking angiosarcoma: the value of immunohistochemistry in the differential diagnosis. Virchows Arch A Pathol Anat 418:271, 1991.
276. White VA, Heathcote JG, Hurwitz JJ, et al. Epithelioid sarcoma of the orbit. Ophthalmology 101:1680, 1994.
277. Whitworth PW, Pollock RE, Mansfield PF, et al. Extremity epithelioid sarcoma: amputation vs local resection. Arch Surg 126:1485, 1991.
278. Zidar A. "Proximal type" epithelioid sarcoma: report of seven cases. Clin Exp Pathol 46:77A, 1998.


### Desmoplastic Small Round Cell Tumor


279. Adsay V, Cheng J, Athanasian E, et al. Primary desmoplastic small cell tumor of soft tissues and bone of the hand. Am J Surg Pathol 23:1408, 1999.
280. Amato RJ, Ellerhorst JA, Ayala AG. Intraabdominal desmoplastic small cell tumor: report and discussion of five cases. Cancer 78:845, 1996.
281. Antonescu CR, Gerald WL, Magid MS, et al. Molecular variants of the EWS-WT1 gene fusion in desmoplastic small round cell tumor. Diagn Mol Pathol 7:24, 1998.
282. Argatoff LH, O'Connell JX, Mathers JA, et al. Detection of the EWS/WT1 gene fusion by reverse transcriptase-polymerase chain reaction and the diagnosis of intra-abdominal desmoplastic small round tumor. Am J Surg Pathol 20:406, 1996.
283. Asano T, Fukuda Y, Fukunaga Y, et al. Intra-abdominal desmoplastic small cell tumor in an adolescent suggesting a neurogenic origin. Acta Pathol Jpn 43:275, 1993.
284. Barnoud R, Sabourin J-C, Pasquier D, et al. Immunohistochemical expression of WT1 by desmoplastic small round cell tumor: a comparative study with other small round cell tumors. Am J Surg Pathol 24:830, 2000.
285. Basade MM, Vege DS, Nair CN, et al. Intra-abdominal desmoplastic small round cell tumor in children: a clinicopathologic study. Pediatr Hematol Oncol 13:95, 1996.
286. Bian Y, Jorden AG, Rupp M, et al. Effusion cytology of desmoplastic small round cell tumor of the pleura: a case report. Acta Cytol 37:77, 1993.
287. Biegel JA, Conard K, Brooks JJ. Translocation (11;22)(p13;q12): primary change in intraabdominal desmoplastic small round cell tumor. Genes Chromosomes Cancer 7:119, 1993.
288. Brodie SG, Stocker SJ, Wardlaw JC, et al. EWS and WT-1 gene fusion in desmoplastic small round cell tumor of the abdomen. Hum Pathol 26:1370, 1995.
289. Carroll JC, Klauber GT, Kretschmar CS, et al. Urological aspects of intra-abdominal desmoplastic small round cell tumor of childhood: a preliminary report. J Urol 151:172, 1994.
290. Charles AK, Moore IE, Berry PJ. Immunohistochemical detec-

tion of the Wilms' tumour gene WT1 in desmoplastic small round cell tumours. Histopathology 30:312, 1997.

291. Cheung NYA, Khoo US, Chart KW. Intraabdominal desmoplastic small round-cell tumour. Histopathology 20:531, 1989.
292. Cummings OW, Ulbright TM, Young RH, et al. Desmoplastic small round cell tumors of the paratesticular region: a report of six cases. Am J Surg Pathol 21:219, 1997.
293. De Alava E, Ladanyi M, Rosai J, et al. Detection of chimeric transcripts in desmoplastic small round cell tumor and related developmental tumors by reverse transcriptase polymerase chain reaction: a specific diagnostic assay. Am J Pathol 147: 1584, 1995.
294. Devaney K. Intra-abdominal desmoplastic small round cell tumor of the peritoneum in a young man. Ultrastruct Pathol 18: 389, 1994.
295. Dorsey BV, Benjamin LE, Rauscher F, et al. Intra-abdominal desmoplastic small round-cell tumor: expansion of the pathologic profile. Mod Pathol 9:703, 1996.
296. Farhat F, Culine S, Lhomme C, et al. Desmoplastic small round cell tumors: results of a four-drug chemotherapy regimen in five adult patients. Cancer 77:1363, 1996.
297. Fizazi K, Farhat F, Theodore C, et al. Ca125 and neuron-specific enolase (NSE) as tumour markers for intra-abdominal desmoplastic small round-cell tumours. Br J Cancer 75:76, 1997.
298. Folpe AL, Patterson K, Gown AM. Antineuroblastoma antibody NB-84 also identifies a significant subset of other small blue round cell tumors. Appl Immunohistochem 5:239, 1997.
299. Fukunaga M, Endo Y, Takaki K, et al. Postmenopausal intra-abdominal desmoplastic small cell tumor. Pathol Int 46:281, 1996.
300. Furman J, Murphy WM, Wajsman Z, et al. Urogenital involvement by desmoplastic small round-cell tumor. J Urol 158:1506, 1997.
301. Gerald W, Rosai J. Desmoplastic small cell tumor with multiple-phenotypic differentiation. Zentralbl Pathol 139:141, 1993.
302. Gerald W, Rosai J, Ladanyi M. Characterization of the genomic breakpoint and chimeric transcripts in the EWS-WT1 gene fusion of desmoplastic small round cell tumor. Proc Natl Acad Sci USA 92:1028, 1995.
303. Gerald WL, Ladanyi M, de Alava E, et al. Clinical, pathologic, and molecular spectrum of tumors associated with t(11; 22)(p13;q12): desmoplastic small round-cell tumor and its variants. J Clin Oncol 16:3028, 1998.
304. Gerald WL, Ladanyi M, de Alava E, et al. Desmoplastic small round-cell tumor: a recently recognized tumor type associated with a unique gene fusion. Adv Anat Pathol 2:341, 1995.
305. Gerald WL, Rosai J. Desmoplastic small cell tumor with divergent differentiation. Pediatr Pathol 9:177, 1989.
306. Gerald WL, Miller HK, Battifora H, et al. Intraabdominal desmoplastic small round-cell tumor: report of 19 cases of a distinctive type of high-grade polyphenotypic malignancy affecting young individuals. Am J Surg Pathol 15:499, 1991.
307. Haber DA, Buckler AJ. WT1: a novel tumor suppressor gene inactivated in Wilms' tumor. New Biol 4:97, 1992.
307a. Hill DA, Pfeifer JD, Marley EF, et al. WT1 staining reliably differentiates desmoplastic small round cell tumor from Ewing sarcoma/primitive neuroectodermal tumor. Am J Clin Pathol 114:345, 2000.
308. Hurlimann J. Desmin and neural marker expression in mesothelial cells and mesotheliomas. Hum Pathol 25:753, 1994.
309. Kawano N, Inayama Y, Nagashima Y, et al. Desmoplastic small round-cell tumor of the paratesticular region: report of an adult case with demonstration of EWS and WT1 gene fusion using paraffin-embedded tissue. Mod Pathol 12:729, 1999.
310. Katz RL, Quezado M, Senderowicz AM, et al. An intra-abdominal small round cell neoplasm with features of primitive neuroectodermal and desmoplastic round cell tumor and a EWS/FLI-1 fusion transcript. Hum Pathol 28:502, 1997.
311. Kushner BH, LaQuaglia MP, Wollner N, et al. Desmoplastic small round-cell tumor: prolonged progression-free survival with aggressive multi-modality therapy. J Clin Oncol 14:1526, 1996.
312. Ladanyi M, Gerald W. Fusion of the EWS and WT1 genes in the desmoplastic small round cell tumor. Cancer Res 54:2837, 1994.
313. Lamovec J. Intra-abdominal desmoplastic small round-cell tumour with expression of muscle specific actin. Histopathology 24:577, 1994.
314. Lee SB, Kolquist KA, Nichols K, et al. EWS-WT1 translocation product induces PDGFA in desmoplastic small round-cell tumor. Nat Genet 17:309, 1997.
315. Loy TS, Quesenberry JT, Sharp SC. Distribution of CA125 in adenocarcinomas: an immunohistochemical study of 481 cases. Am J Clin Pathol 98:175, 1992.
316. Miettinen M, Chatten J, Paetau A, et al. Monoclonal antibody NB84 in the differential diagnosis of neuroblastoma and other small round cell tumors. Am J Surg Pathol 22:327, 1998.
317. Ordi J, de Alava E, Torné A, et al. Intra-abdominal desmoplastic small round cell tumor with EWS/ERG fusion transcript. Am J Surg Pathol 22:1026, 1998.
318. Ordóñez NG. Desmoplastic small round cell tumor. I. A histopathologic study of 39 cases with emphasis on unusual histological patterns. Am J Surg Pathol 22:1303, 1998.
319. Ordóñez NG. Desmoplastic small round cell tumor. II. An ultrastructural and immunohistochemical study with emphasis on new immunohistochemical markers. Am J Surg Pathol 22: 1314, 1998.
320. Ordóñez NG, el-Naggar AK, Ro JY, et al. Intraabdominal desmoplatic small cell tumor: a light microscopic, immunocytochemical, ultrastructural, and flow cytometric study. Hum Pathol 24:850, 1993.
321. Ordóñez NG, Sahin AA. CA125 production in desmoplastic small round cell minor: report of a case with elevated serum levels and prominent signet ring morphology. Hum Pathol 29: 294, 1998.
322. Ordóñez NG, Zirkin R, Bloom RE. Malignant small-cell epithelial tumor of the peritoneum coexpressing mesenchymal type intermediate filaments. Am J Surg Pathol 13:413, 1989.
323. Parkash V, Gerald WL, Parma A, et al. Desmoplastic small round cell tumor of the pleura. Am J Surg Pathol 19:659, 1995.
324. Roberts P, Burchill SA, Beddow RA, et al. A combined cytogenetic and molecular approach to diagnosis in a case of desmoplastic small round cell tumor with a complex translocation (11;22;21). Cancer Genet Cytogenet 108:19, 1999.
325. Rodriguez E, Sreekantaiah C, Gerald W, et al. A recurring translocation, t(11;22)(p13;q11.2), characterizes intra-abdominal desmoplastic small round-cell tumors. Cancer Genet Cytogenet 69:17, 1993.
326. Sawyer JR, Tryka AF, Lewis JM. A novel reciprocal chromosome translocation t(11;22) (p13;q12) in an intraabdominal desmoplastic small round-cell tumor. Am J Surg Pathol 16:411, 1992.
327. Schwarz RE, Gerald WL, Kushner BH, et al. Desmoplastic small round cell tumors: prognostic indicators and results of surgical management. Ann Surg Oncol 5:416, 1998.
328. Sesterhenn I, Davis CJ, Mostofi K. Undifferentiated malignant epithelial tumors involving serosal surfaces of scrotum and abdomen in young males [abstract]. J Urol 137:214, 1987.
329. Shimizu Y, Mitsui T, Kawakami T, et al. Novel breakpoints of the EWS gene and the WT1 gene in a desmoplastic small round cell tumor. Cancer Genet Cytogenet 106:156, 1998.

330. Tison V, Cerasoli S, Morigi F, et al. Intracranial desmoplastic small-cell tumor: report of a case. Am J Surg Pathol 20:112, 1996.
331. Trupiano JK, Machen SK, Barr FG, et al. Cytokeratin-negative desmoplastic small round cell tumor: a report of two cases emphasizing the utility of reverse transcriptase-polymerase chain reaction. Mod Pathol 12:849, 1999.
332. Van Muijen GNP, Ruiter DJ, Warnaar SO. Coexpression of intermediate filament polypeptides in human fetal and adult tissues. Lab Invest 57:359, 1987.
333. Variend S, Gerrard M, Norris PD, et al. Intraabdominal neuroectodermal tumour of childhood with divergent differentiation. Histopathology 18:45, 1991.
334. Wills EJ. Peritoneal desmoplastic small round cell tumors with divergent differentiation: a review. Ultrastruct Pathol 17:295, 1993.
335. Wolf AN, Ladanyi M, Paull G, et al. The expanding clinical spectrum of desmoplastic small round-cell tumor: a report of two cases with molecular confirmation. Hum Pathol 30:430, 1999.
336. Zaloudek C, Miller TR, Stern JL. Desmoplastic small cell tumor of the ovary: a unique polyphenotypic tumor with an unfavorable prognosis. Int J Gynecol Pathol 14:260, 1995.

### Malignant Extrarenal Rhabdoid Tumor

337. Besnard-Guerin C, Cavanee W, Newsham I. The t(11;22)(p15.5; q11.23) in a retroperitoneal rhabdoid tumor also includes a regional deletion distal to CRYBB2 on 22q. Genes Chromosomes Cancer 13:141, 1995.
338. Biegel JA, Rorke LB, Emanuel BS. Monosomy 22 in rhabdoid or atypical teratoid tumors of the brain. N Engl J Med 321:906, 1989.
339. Biegel JA, Zhou JY, Rorke LB, et al. Germ-line and acquired mutations of INI 1 in atypical teratoid and rhabdoid tumors. Cancer Res 59:74, 1999.
340. Bittesini L, Dei Tos AP, Fletcher CDM. Metastatic melanoma showing rhabdoid phenotype: further evidence of a non-histological pattern. Histopathology 20:167, 1992.
341. Borek BT, McKee PH, Freeman JA, et al. Primary malignant melanoma with rhabdoid features: a histologic and immunocytochemical study of three cases. Am J Dermatopathol 20:123, 1998.
342. Brooks JJ. The significance of double phenotypic patterns and markers in sarcomas: a new model of mesenchymal differentiation. Am J Pathol 125:113, 1986.
343. Buchino JJ. Atypical teratoid/rhabdoid tumor: a stereogram unveiled. Adv Anat Pathol 6:97, 1999.
344. Burger PC, Yu I-T, Tihan T, et al. Atypical teratoid/rhabdoid tumor of the central nervous system: a highly malignant tumor of infancy and childhood frequently mistaken for medulloblastoma: a Pediatric Oncology Group study. Am J Surg Pathol 22:1083, 1998.
345. Chang ES, Wick MR, Swanson PE, et al. Metastatic melanoma with "rhabdoid" features. Am J Clin Pathol 102:426, 1994.
346. Chetty R, Bhathal PS. Cecal adenocarcinoma with rhabdoid phenotype. Virchows Arch A Pathol Anat Histopathol 422:179, 1993.
347. Dabbs DJ, Park HK. Malignant rhabdoid skin tumor: an uncommon primary skin neoplasm: ultrastructural and immunohistochemical analysis. J Cutan Pathol 15:109, 1988.
348. Fanburg-Smith J, Hengge M, Hengge UR, et al. Extrarenal rhabdoid tumors of soft tissue: a clinicopathologic and immunohistochemical study of 18 cases and a review of the literature. Ann Diagn Pathol 2:1, 1998.
349. Ferreiro JA, Nascimento AG. Hyaline-cell rich chondroid syringoma: a tumor mimicking malignancy. Am J Surg Pathol 19:912, 1995.
350. Fletcher CDM. Pleomorphic malignant fibrous histiocytoma: fact of fiction? Am J Surg Pathol 16:213, 1992.
351. Foschini MP, Van Eyken P, Brock PR, et al. Malignant rhabdoid tumor of the liver: a case report. Histopathology 20:157, 1992.
352. Franquemont DW, Mills SE. Plasmacytoid monomorphic adenoma of salivary glands. Am J Surg Pathol 17:146, 1993.
352a. Gökden N, Nappi O, Swanson PE, et al. Renal cell carcinoma with rhabdoid features. Am J Surg Pathol 24:1329, 2000.
353. Haas JE, Palmer NE, Weinberg AG, et al. Ultrastructure of malignant rhabdoid tumor of the kidney. Hum Pathol 12:646, 1981.
354. Harris M, Eyden BP, Joglekar VM. Rhabdoid tumor of the bladder: a histological, ultrastructural, and immunohistochemical study. Histopathology 11:1083, 1987.
355. Hasserjian RP, Folkerth RD, Scott RM, et al. A clinicopathologic and cytogenetic analysis of malignant rhabdoid tumor of the central nervous system. J Neurooncol 25:193, 1995.
356. Hsueh S, Chang TC. Malignant rhabdoid tumor of the uterine corpus. Gynecol Oncol 61:142, 1996.
357. Kaiserling E, Ruck P, Handgretinger R, et al. Immunohistochemical and cytogenetic findings in malignant rhabdoid tumor. Gen Diagn Pathol 141:327, 1996.
358. Karnes PS, Tran TN, Cui MY, et al. Establishment of a rhabdoid tumor cell line with a specific chromosomal abnormality: 46 XY, t(11;22) (p15.5;q11.23). Cancer Genet Cytogenet 56:31, 1991.
359. Kodet R, Newton WA, Hamoudi AB, et al. Rhabdomyosarcomas with intermediate-filament inclusions and features of rhabdoid tumors: light microscopic and immunohistochemical study. Am J Surg Pathol 15:257, 1991.
360. Kudo E, Hirose T, Fuji Y, et al. Undifferentiated carcinoma of the vulva mimicking epithelioid sarcoma. Am J Surg Pathol 15:990, 1991.
361. Kumar S, Kumar D, Cowan DF. Transitional cell carcinoma with rhabdoid features. Am J Surg Pathol 16:515, 1992.
362. Laskin WB, Knittel DR, Frame JN. S100 protein and HMB-45 negative "rhaboid" malignant melanoma: a totally dedifferentiated malignant melanoma? Am J Clin Pathol 103:772, 1995.
363. Lemos LB, Hamoudi AB. Malignant thymic tumor in an infant (malignant histiocytoma). Arch Pathol Lab Med 102:84, 1978.
364. Leong FJW-M, Leong AS-Y. Malignant rhabdoid tumor in adults: heterogeneous tumors with a unique morphological phenotype. Pathol Res Pract 192:796, 1996.
365. Luppi G, Jin R, Clemente C. Malignant rhabdoid tumor of the vulva: a case report and a review of the literature. Tumori 82: 93, 1996.
366. Machen SK, Easley KA, Goldblum JR. Synovial sarcoma of the extremities: a clinicopathologic study of 34 cases, including semi-quantitative analysis of spindled, epithelial, and poorly differentiated areas. Am J Surg Pathol 23:268, 1999.
367. Marcus VA, Viloria J, Owen D, et al. Malignant rhabdoid tumor of the colon: report of a case with molecular analysis. Dis Colon Rectum 39:1322, 1996.
368. Matsukuma S, Aida S, Hata Y, et al. Localized malignant peritoneal mesothelioma containing rhabdoid cells. Pathol Int 46:389, 1996.
369. McCluggage WG, Date A, Bharucha H, et al. Endometrial stromal sarcoma with sex cord-like areas and focal rhabdoid differentiation. Histopathology 29:369, 1996.
370. Newsham I, Daub D, Besnard-Guerin C, et al. Molecular sublocalization and characterization of the 11;22 translocation breakpoint in a malignant rhabdoid tumor. Genomics 19:433, 1994.
371. Ogino S, Ro JY, Redline RW. Malignant rhabdoid tumor: a phenotype? An entity? A controversy revisited. Adv Anat Pathol 7:181, 2000.

372. Parham DM, Weeks, DA, Beckwith JB. The clinicopathologic spectrum of putative extrarenal rhabdoid tumors: an analysis of 42 cases studies with immunohistochemistry or electron microscopy. Am J Surg Pathol 18:1010, 1994.
373. Perlman E, Ali S, Robinson R, et al. Infantile extrarenal rhabdoid tumor. Pediatr Dev Pathol 1:149, 1998.
374. Perry A, Scheithauer BW, Stafford SL, et al. "Rhabdoid" meningioma: an aggressive variant. Am J Surg Pathol 22:1482, 1998.
375. Pinto JA, Gonazales-Alfonzo JE, Gonzalez L, et al. Well-differentiated gastric adenocarcinoma with rhabdoid areas: a case report with immunohistochemical analysis. Pathol Res Pract 193:801, 1997.
376. Rorke LB, Packer R, Biegel J. Central nervous system atypical teratoid/rhabdoid tumors of infancy and childhood. J Neurooncol 24:21, 1995.
377. Rorke LB, Packer RJ, Biegel JA. Central nervous system atypical teratoid/rhabdoid tumors of infancy and childhood: definition of an entity. J Neurosurg 85:56, 1996.
378. Rosson GB, Hazen-Martin DJ, Biegel JA, et al. Establishment and molecular characterization of five cell lines derived from renal and extrarenal malignant rhabdoid tumors. Mod Pathol 11:1228, 1998.
379. Rosty C, Peter M, Zucman J, et al. Cytogenetic and molecular analysis of a t(1;22) (p36;q11.2) in a rhabdoid tumor with a putative homozygous deletion of chromosome 22. Genes Chromosomes Cancer 21:82, 1998.
380. Schofield DE, Beckwith JB, Sklar J. Loss of heterozygosity at chromosome 22q11-12 and 11p15.5 in renal rhabdoid tumors. Genes Chromosomes Cancer 15:10, 1996.
381. Shashai V, Lovell MA, Von Kap-Herr C, et al. Malignant rhabdoid tumor of the kidney: involvement of chromosome 22. Genes Chromosomes Cancer 10:49, 1994.
382. Simons J, Teshima I, Zielenska M, et al. Analysis of chromosome 22q as an aid to the diagnosis of rhabdoid tumor: a case report. Am J Surg Pathol 23:982, 1999.
383. Sotelo-Avila C, Gonzalez-Crussi F, de Mello D, et al. Renal and extrarenal rhabdoid tumors in children: a clinicopathologic study of 14 patients. Semin Diagn Pathol 3:151, 1986.
384. Tsokos M, Kouraklis G, Chandra RS, et al. Malignant rhabdoid tumor of the kidney and soft tissues: evidence for a diverse morphological and immunocytochemical phenotype. Arch Pathol Lab Med 113:115, 1989.
385. Tsuneyoshi M, Daimaru Y, Hashimoto H, et al. The existence of rhabdoid cells in specified soft tissue sarcomas: histopathological, ultrastructural, and immunohistochemical evidence. Virchows Arch [Pathol Anat] 411:509, 1987.
386. Ueyama T, Nagai E, Yao T, et al. Vimentin-positive gastric carcinomas with rhabdoid features: a clinicopathologic and immunohistochemical study. Am J Surg Pathol 17:813, 1993.
387. Versteege I, Sevenet N, Lange J, et al. Truncating mutations of hSNF5/INI1 in an aggressive pediatric cancer. Nature 394:203, 1998.
388. Weeks DA, Beckwith JB, Mierau GW, et al. Renal neoplasms mimicking rhabdoid tumor of kidney: a report from the National Wilms' Tumor Study Pathology Center. Am J Surg Pathol 15:1042, 1991.
389. Weeks DA, Beckwith JB, Mierau GW, et al. Rhabdoid tumor of kidney: a report of 111 cases from the National Wilms' Tumor Study Pathology Center. Am J Surg Pathol 13:439, 1989.
390. Wick MR, Ritter JH. "Composite" malignant rhabdoid tumors of the viscera: models of clonal evolution. Pathol Res Pract 193:807, 1997.
391. Wick MR, Ritter JH, Dehner LP. Malignant rhabdoid tumors: a clinicopathologic review and conceptual discussion. Semin Diagn Pathol 12:233, 1995.
392. Yang AH, Chen WYK, Chiang H. Malignant rhabdoid tumour of colon. Histopathology 24:89, 1994.

### Malignant Mesenchymoma

393. Brady MS, Perino G, Tallini G, et al. Malignant mesenchymoma. Cancer 77:467, 1996.
394. Ewing MR, Harrison CV. Mesenchymoma. Br J Surg 44:408, 1956/1957.
395. Nash A, Stout AP. Malignant mesenchymomas in children. Cancer 14:524, 1961.
396. Newman PL, Fletcher CD. Malignant mesenchymoma: clinicopathologic analysis of a series with evidence of low-grade behavior. Am J Surg Pathol 15:607, 1991.
397. Stout AP. Mesenchymoma: the mixed tumor of mesenchymal derivatives. Ann Surg 127:278, 1948.
398. Symmers WSC, Nangle EJ. An unusual recurring tumor formed of connective tissues of embryonic type (so-called mesenchymoma). J Pathol Bacteriol 63:417, 1951.
399. Thomas A, Kothare SN. Malignant mesenchymomata of soft tissues. Indian J Cancer 11:227, 1974.

### Inflammatory Myxohyaline Tumors of the Distal Extremities

400. Meis-Kindblom JM, Kindblom L-G. Acral myxoinflammatory fibroblastic sarcoma: a low-grade tumor of the hands and feet. Am J Surg Pathol 22:911, 1998.
401. Michal M. Inflammatory myxoid tumor of the soft parts with bizarre giant cells. Pathol Res Pract 194:529, 1998.
402. Montgomery EA, Devaney KO, Giordano TJ, et al. Inflammatory myxohyaline tumor of distal extremities with virocyte or Reed-Sternberg-like cells: a distinctive lesion with features simulating inflammatory conditions, Hodgkins disease, and various sarcomas. Mod Pathol 11:384, 1998.
403. Montgomery EA, Devaney K, Weiss SW. Inflammatory myxohyaline tumor of distal extremities with Reed-Sternberg-like cells: a novel entity with features simulating myxoid malignant fibrous histiocytoma, inflammatory conditions and Hodgkin disease. Mod Pathol 10:47A, 1997.

# INDEX

Note: Page numbers in *italics* refer to illustrations; page numbers followed by t refer to tables.

ISBN 0-323-01200-0